DRUG INFORMATION HANDBOOK for NURSING

Including
Assessment, Administration, Monitoring Guidelines, and Patient Education

Beatrice B. Turkoski, RN, PhD
Brenda R. Lance, RN, MSN
Mark F. Bonfiglio, BS, PharmD, RPh

2007

8ᵗʰ Edition

LEXI-COMP

DRUG INFORMATION HANDBOOK for NURSING

Including
Assessment, Administration, Monitoring Guidelines, and Patient Education

Beatrice B. Turkoski, RN, PhD
Associate Professor, Graduate Faculty,
Advanced Pharmacology
College of Nursing
Kent State University
Kent, Ohio

Brenda R. Lance, RN, MSN
Program Development Director
Northcoast HealthCare Management Company
Northcoast Infusion Therapies
Oakwood Village, Ohio

Mark F. Bonfiglio, BS, PharmD, RPh
Chief Content Officer
Lexi-Comp, Inc
Hudson, Ohio

NOTICE

Drug information is constantly evolving because of ongoing research and clinical experience and is often subject to interpretation. While great care has been taken to ensure the accuracy of the information presented, the reader is advised that the authors, editors, reviewers, contributors, and publishers cannot be responsible for the continued currency of the information or for any errors, omissions, or the application of this information, or for any consequences arising therefrom. Therefore, the author(s) and/or the publisher shall have no liability to any person or entity with regard to claims, loss, or damage caused, or alleged to be caused, directly or indirectly, by the use of information contained herein. Because of the dynamic nature of drug information, readers are advised that decisions regarding drug therapy must be based on the independent judgment of the clinician, changing information about a drug (eg, as reflected in the literature and manufacturer's most current product information), and changing medical practices. The authors are not responsible for any inaccuracy of quotation or for any false or misleading implication that may arise due to the text or formulas as used or due to the quotation of revisions no longer official. Further, the *Drug Information Handbook for Nursing* is not offered as a guide to dosing. The reader, herewith, is advised that information shown under the heading **Dosing** is provided only as an indication of the amount of the drug typically given or taken during therapy. Actual dosing amount for any specific drug should be based on an in-depth evaluation of the individual patient's therapy requirement and strong consideration given to such issues as contraindications, warnings, precautions, adverse reactions, along with the interaction of other drugs. The manufacturers most current product information or other standard recognized references should always be consulted for such detailed information prior to drug use.

The authors and contributors have written this book in their private capacities. No official support or endorsement by any federal agency or pharmaceutical company is intended or inferred.

If you have any suggestions or questions regarding any information presented in this handbook, please contact our drug information pharmacists at **(330) 650-6506**.

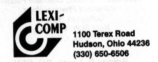

LEXI-COMP

1100 Terex Road
Hudson, Ohio 44236
(330) 650-6506

TABLE OF CONTENTS

PREFACE

The ever-expanding roles of nurses require them to be informed and knowledgeable about safe pharmacotherapy. Yet, at the same time, there is an expanding number and complexity of pharmacotherapeutic agents used in both outpatient and institutional settings. In addition, there is an increased availability of over-the-counter (OTC) agents and nonregulated biological and herbal products used by the public, whose information about use and safety may or may not be accurate.

The information about current drug therapy is voluminous and the quality of that information varies greatly. Compiling reliable information into a logical guide for nurses is difficult when facing the complexities of diverse disease states and the demands of today's changing healthcare environment. The authors of this book have extensively reviewed the available literature and have developed the *Drug Information Handbook for Nursing* with the intent to provide pertinent information related to pharmacotherapeutic agents.

The introductory section of the *Drug Information Handbook for Nursing* includes directions for using the book and a list of common abbreviations, General Nursing Issues (Assessment, Safe Administration, and Monitoring), Patient Factors That Influence Drug Therapy, and Therapeutic Nursing Management of Side Effects.

Each of the monographs presents information in a concise and consistent manner with appropriate referencing to an extensive appendix of helpful information. Each monograph includes pertinent therapeutic purpose, administration guidelines, possible adverse reactions, and medication safety issues. The section Nursing Actions, in each monograph, reflects both the therapeutic monitoring recommendations and specific information for patient education that addresses administration, possible adverse effects/interventions, and symptoms the patient should report to the prescriber.

The extensive appendix includes sections on common uses for herbs and natural products, administration guidelines, adverse reactions, pregnancy and breast-feeding information, OBRA recommendations for long-term care, and overdose/toxicology guidelines.

The introductory information, the format of the individual monographs, and the valuable appendix information in the *Drug Information Handbook for Nursing* was designed to provide Registered Professional Nurses and upper-division nursing students with information to facilitate safe clinical decision-making.

ABOUT THE AUTHORS

Beatrice B. Turkoski, RN, PhD

Dr Turkoski received her BSN from Alverno College in Wisconsin, an MS in Community Health Nursing from the University of Wisconsin-Milwaukee School of Nursing, and a PhD from the University of Wisconsin. Her extensive professional nursing experience includes several years as a clinician in critical care in Wisconsin and Israel, Director of Nursing, clinician, and researcher in gerontology and chronic adult illness in Wisconsin and Ohio, and clinical nurse specialist in family/community practice in Israel.

In her graduate faculty role at Kent State University College of Nursing, Dr Turkoski developed and teaches the Advanced Pharmacology course for graduate students in the Nurse Practitioner and Clinical Nurse Specialist programs. Her expertise in this area is highly regarded by both students and faculty. She also conducts continuing education programs and workshops in pharmacology and nursing practice, both in person and on the internet.

Dr Turkoski is an active member and past officer in several national and international professional organizations. She has made presentations at scientific conferences in the United States, Europe, China, Korea, Canada, and Israel. Dr Turkoski is also a frequent contributor to professional journals.

Brenda R. Lance, RN, MSN

Ms Lance received a diploma in nursing from Methodist Hospital School of Nursing in Lubbock, Texas. She also has earned bachelor's and master's degrees in nursing from Kent State University, Kent, Ohio.

Ms Lance's nursing experiences and expertise are numerous and varied. Her nursing career spans over 35 years, having worked in intensive care, emergency room, ambulatory care clinics, home health, and home infusion. She is currently the Program Development Director for Northcoast HealthCare Management Company and Northcoast Infusion Therapies located in Oakwood Village, Ohio.

In addition to many years of direct patient care experience, she is also certified in risk management, has extensive experience in Joint Commission on Accreditation of Healthcare Organizations standards and Medicare regulations for home health, and has been a military nurse for the past 30 years. She retired with the rank of Captain (0-6) from the U.S. Naval Reserve Nurse Corps.

Ms Lance is a member of the Sigma Theta Tau (National Honor Society of Nursing) and National Home Infusion Association.

Mark F. Bonfiglio, BS, PharmD, RPh

Dr Bonfiglio received his bachelor's degrees and undergraduate training from the University of Toledo (BA in Biology/BS in Pharmacy) and his PharmD from the Ohio State University. He completed a residency in Critical Care Pharmacy at University Hospitals in Columbus, Ohio. On completion of his training, he was employed by the College of Pharmacy at Ohio Northern University where he attained the rank of Associate Clinical Professor. During this time he maintained a clinical practice, initially as a Clinical Specialist in Critical Care in the SUMMA Health System, followed by a position as Pharmacotherapy Specialist in Internal Medicine at Akron General Medical Center. In addition to his current responsibilities at Lexi-Comp, he has continued to remain active in science and healthcare education. He currently coordinates the Advanced Pharmacology course for the College of Nursing at Malone College, and has served as Part-Time Faculty in the Department of Biological Sciences at Kent State University.

Dr Bonfiglio is currently the Chief Content Officer in the Medical Science Division of Lexi-Comp, Inc. He coordinates the development and maintenance of the core pharmacology database and serves as an author for several printed titles, including the *Drug Information Handbook for Advanced Practice Nursing* and *Drug Interactions Handbook*. He is also a contributing author to the *Pharmacogenomics Handbook*. Dr Bonfiglio maintains memberships in the Society for Critical Care Medicine (SCCM), the American Pharmacists Association (APhA), the American Society of Health-System Pharmacists (ASHP), the Ohio College of Clinical Pharmacy (OCCP), the American Society for Automation in Pharmacy (ASAP), and the American Association for the Advancement of Science (AAAS).

EDITORIAL ADVISORY PANEL

Barbara L. Gracious, MD
Assistant Professor of Psychiatry and Pediatrics
Case Western Reserve University
Director of Child Psychiatry and Training & Education
University Hospitals of Cleveland
Cleveland, Ohio

Larry D. Gray, PhD, ABMM
TriHealth Clinical Microbiology Laboratory
Bethesda and Good Samaritan Hospitals
Cincinnati, Ohio

James L. Gutmann, DDS
Professor and Director of Graduate Endodontics
The Texas A & M University System
Baylor College of Dentistry
Dallas, Texas

Tracey Hagemann, PharmD
Associate Professor
College of Pharmacy
The University of Oklahoma
Oklahoma City, Oklahoma

Charles E. Hawley, DDS, PhD
Professor Emeritus
Department of Periodontics
University of Maryland
Consultant on Periodontics
Commission on Dental Accreditation of the American Dental
Association

Martin D. Higbee, PharmD, CGP
Associate Professor
Department of Pharmacy Practice and Science
The University of Arizona
Tucson, Arizona

Jane Hurlburt Hodding, PharmD
Director, Pharmacy
Miller Children's Hospital
Long Beach, California

Collin A. Hovinga, PharmD
Neuropharmacologist
Miami Children's Hospital
Miami, Florida

Darrell T. Hulisz, PharmD
Department of Family Medicine
Case Western Reserve University
Cleveland, Ohio

David S. Jacobs, MD
President, Pathologists Chartered
Consultant in Pathology and Laboratory Medicine
Overland Park, Kansas

Polly E. Kintzel, PharmD, BCPS, BCOP
Clinical Pharmacy Specialist-Oncology
Spectrum Health
Grand Rapids, Michigan

Jill M. Kolesar, PharmD, FCCP, BCPS
Associate Professor of Pharmacy
University of Wisconsin
Madison, Wisconsin

Donna M. Kraus, PharmD, FAPhA
Associate Professor of Pharmacy Practice
Departments of Pharmacy Practice and Pediatrics
Pediatric Clinical Pharmacist
University of Illinois
Chicago, Illinois

Daniel L. Krinsky, RPh, MS
Director, Pharmacotherapy Sales and Marketing
Lexi-Comp, Inc
Hudson, Ohio

Kay Kyllonen, PharmD
Clinical Specialist
The Cleveland Clinic Children's Hospital
Cleveland, Ohio

Charles Lacy, RPh, PharmD, FCSHP
Vice President, Information Technologies
Professor, Pharmacy Practice
Professor, Business Leadership
University of Southern Nevada
Las Vegas, Nevada

Brenda R. Lance, RN, MSN
Program Development Director
Northcoast HealthCare Management Company
Northcoast Infusion Therapies
Oakwood Village, Ohio

Leonard L. Lance, RPh, BSPharm
Clinical Pharmacist
Lexi-Comp Inc
Hudson, Ohio

Jerrold B. Leikin, MD, FACP, FACEP, FACMT, FAACT
Director, Medical Toxicology
Evanston Northwestern Healthcare-OMEGA
Glenbrook Hospital
Glenview, Illinois
Associate Director
Toxikon Consortium at Cook County Hospital
Chicago, Illinois
Professor of Medicine
Pharmacology and Health Systems Management
Rush Medical College
Chicago, Ilinois
Professor of Medicine
Feinberg School of Medicine
Northwestern University
Chicago, Ilinois

Jeffrey D. Lewis, PharmD
Pharmacotherapy Specialist
Lexi-Comp, Inc
Hudson, Ohio

Jennifer K. Long, PharmD, BCPS
Infectious Diseases Clinical Specialist
The Cleveland Clinic Foundation
Cleveland, Ohio

Laurie S. Mauro, BS, PharmD
Associate Professor of Clinical Pharmacy
Department of Pharmacy Practice
College of Pharmacy
The University of Toledo
Toledo, Ohio

Vincent F. Mauro, BS, PharmD, FCCP
Professor of Clinical Pharmacy
College of Pharmacy
The University of Toledo
Adjunct Professor of Medicine
College of Medicine
Medical University of Ohio at Toledo
Toledo, Ohio

EDITORIAL ADVISORY PANEL *(Continued)*

ACKNOWLEDGMENTS

This handbook exists in its present form as the result of the concerted efforts of the following individuals: Robert D. Kerscher, publisher and chief executive officer of Lexi-Comp, Inc; Steven Kerscher, president and chief operating officer; Mark Bonfiglio, BS, PharmD, RPh, chief content officer; Stacy S. Robinson, editorial manager; Robin L. Farabee, project manager; David C. Marcus, chief information officer; Tracey J. Henterly, senior graphic designer; Alexandra Hart, composition specialist; Leslie Jo Hoppes, pharmacology database manager; Matthew C. Kerscher, business unit manager.

Much of the material contained in this book was a result of pharmacy contributors throughout the United States and Canada. Lexi-Comp has assisted many medical institutions to develop hospital-specific formulary manuals that contain clinical drug information as well as dosing. Working with clinical pharmacists, hospital pharmacy and therapeutics committees, and hospital drug information centers, Lexi-Comp has developed an evolutionary drug database that reflects the practice of pharmacy in these major institutions.

The authors also thank their families, friends, and colleagues, who supported them in their efforts to complete this handbook.

DESCRIPTION OF SECTIONS AND FIELDS

Introduction

This and other documents in this section provide guidelines for the use of the handbook including a brief overview of General Nursing Issues (Assessment, Administration, Monitoring, and Patient Education); Patient Factors That Influence Drug Therapy; and Therapeutic Nursing Management of Side Effects.

Individual Drug Monographs

Medications are arranged alphabetically by generic name. Abbreviated monographs contain unique information, commonly for combination formulations.

Monograph Fields

Generic Name	U.S. adopted name
Pronunciation	Phonetic pronunciation of generic name
U.S. Brand Names	Trade names (manufacturer-specific) found in the United States. The symbol [DSC] appears after trade names that have been recently discontinued.
Synonyms	Other name(s) or accepted abbreviation(s) of the generic drug
Restrictions	The controlled substance classification from the Drug Enforcement Agency (DEA); U.S. schedules are I-V; schedules vary by country and sometimes state (ie, Massachusetts uses I-VI)
Pharmacologic Category	Indicates one or more systematic classifications of the drug
Medication Safety Issues	In an effort to promote the safe use of medications, this field is intended to highlight possible sources of medication errors such as look-alike/sound-alike drugs or highly concentrated formulations which require vigilance on the part of healthcare professionals. In addition, medications which have been associated with severe consequences in the event of a medication error are also identified in this field.
Pregnancy Risk Factor	Indicates one or more of the five categories established by the FDA to indicate the potential of a systemically absorbed drug for causing birth defects
Lactation	Information describing characteristics of using the drug while breast-feeding (where recommendation of American Academy of Pediatrics differs, notation is made); the following distinctions are made:
	Does not enter breast milk
	Enters breast milk (may include: compatible, use caution, not recommended, contraindicated, or consult prescriber)
	Excretion in breast milk unknown (may include: compatible, use caution, not recommended, contraindicated, or consult prescriber)
	Not indicated for use in women
	No data available (may include: use caution)
Use	Description of FDA-approved indications of the drug
Unlabeled/Investigational Use	Information pertaining to non-FDA approved and investigational indications of the drug
Mechanism of Action/Effect	A brief description of how the drug works

Contraindications	Inappropriate use(s) of the drug or disease states and patient populations in which the drug should not be used, according to the FDA
Warnings/Precautions	Warnings include hazardous conditions related to use of the drug. Precautions include disease states or patient populations in which the drug should be used with caution.
Drug Interactions	Agents that, when combined with the drug, may affect therapy; may include the following:
Cytochrome P450 Effect	Drugs which are involved in possible interactions due to their activity with the hepatic cytochrome P450 system are identified, and their role for a specific isoenzyme is listed according to the degree of effect. Substrates are described as major or minor. Inhibitors are classified as weak, moderate, or strong. Inducers are defined as weak or strong.
Decreased Effect	Drug combinations that result in a decreased therapeutic effect between the drug listed in the monograph and other drugs or drug classes
Increased Effect/Toxicity	Drug combinations that result in a increased or toxic therapeutic effect between the drug listed in the monograph and other drugs or drug classes
Nutritional/Ethanol Interactions	Information regarding potential interactions with food, nutritional supplements (including herbal products and vitamins), ethanol, or cigarette smoking
Lab Interactions	A list of assay interferences when taking the drug
Adverse Reactions	Only side effects >1% are included and are grouped by percentage of incidence (if known) and/or body system
Overdose/Toxicology	Comment or considerations with signs or symptoms of excess drug ingestion
Pharmacodynamics/Kinetics	May include the following:
Onset of Action	The time after drug administration when therapeutic effect is observed; may also include time for peak therapeutic effect
Duration of Action	Length of therapeutic effect
Time to Peak	Describes the relative time after ingestion when concentration achieves the highest serum concentration
Protein Binding	The percent of drug listed in the monograph bound to circulating proteins (ie, albumin, etc)
Half-Life Elimination	The reported half-life of elimination for the parent or metabolites of the drug
Metabolism	Describes the site of metabolism and may include the percentage of active metabolites
Excretion	Route of drug elimination
Pharmacokinetic Note	Provides additional pharmacokinetic information when needed.
Available Dosage Forms	A description of the product form(s) including strength and formulation (ie, tablet, capsule, injection, syrup, etc)
Dosing	The amount of drug to be given during therapy; may include the following:
Adults	The recommended amount of drug to be given to adult patients
Adults and Elderly	This combined field is only used to indicate that no specific adjustments for elderly patients were identified. However, other issues should be considered (ie, renal or hepatic impairment). Also refer to Geriatric Considerations for additional information related to the elderly.

DESCRIPTION OF SECTIONS AND FIELDS *(Continued)*

Elderly — A suggested amount of drug to be given to elderly patients; may include adjustments from adult dosing (lack of information in the monograph may imply that the drug is not used in the elderly patient or no specific adjustments could be identified)

Pediatrics — Suggested amount of drug to be given to neonates, infants, and children

Renal Impairment — Suggested dosage adjustments based on compromised renal function; may include dosing instructions for patients on dialysis

Hepatic Impairment — Suggested dosage adjustments based on compromised liver function

Dosing Adjustment for Toxicity — Suggested dosage adjustments in the event specific toxicities related to therapy are noted, such as hematologic toxicities related to cancer chemotherapy

Administration

Oral
I.M.
I.V.
I.V. Detail
Inhalation
Topical
Other

The administration field contains subfields by route regarding issues relative to appropriately giving a medication; includes suggestions on final drug concentrations and/or rates of infusion for parenteral medications and comments regarding the timing of drug administration relative to meals.

Stability

Reconstitution — Includes comments on solution choice with time or conditions for the mixture to maintain full potency before administration

Compatibility — Provides information regarding stability of the drug in different solutions; known incompatibilities when admixed or coadministered with other drugs; and when it is administered through Y-site administration sets or syringe

Storage — Information relating to appropriate storage of the medication prior to opening the manufacturers original packaging; information is only given if recommendations are for storage at other than room temperature; includes storage requirements for reconstituted products

Laboratory Monitoring — Suggested laboratory tests to monitor for safety and efficacy of the drug

Nursing Actions

Physical Assessment — Monitoring guidelines

Patient Education — Suggested items to discuss with the patient or caregiver when taking the medication; may include issues regarding contraception, self-monitoring, precautions, and administration

Dietary Considerations — Includes information on how the medication should be taken relative to meals or food

Geriatric Considerations — Comments or suggestions of drug use in elderly patients; may include monitoring, dose adjustments, precautions, or comments on appropriateness of use

Breast-Feeding Issues — Provides further information relating to taking the drug while nursing

Pregnancy Issues — Comments related to safe drug administration during pregnancy, if appropriate

Other Issues — Additional pertinent information regarding nursing issues

Additional Information	Information about sodium content and/or pertinent information about specific brands
Related Information	Cross-reference to other pertinent drug information in this handbook

Appendix

The extensive appendix is filled with useful tables and text including conversions, laboratory information, adverse reaction information, comparison charts for selected classes of drugs, maternal and fetal guidelines, OBRA recommendations for long-term care, and overdose/toxicology information.

Controlled Substance Index

A list of drug names and their corresponding controlled substance classification

Alphabetical Index

This is an alphabetical index which provides a quick reference to the monograph section by using the generic names, synonyms, and U.S. brand names. From this index, the reader may also cross-reference to the appendix information.

FDA NAME DIFFERENTIATION PROJECT: THE USE OF TALL-MAN LETTERS

Confusion between similar drug names is an important cause of medication errors. For years, The Institute For Safe Medication Practices (ISMP), has urged generic manufacturers use a combination of large and small letters as well as bolding (ie, chlorproM-AZINE and chlorproPAMIDE) to help distinguish drugs with look-alike names, especially when they share similar strengths. Recently the FDA's Division of Generic Drugs began to issue recommendation letters to manufacturers suggesting this novel way to label their products to help reduce this drug name confusion. Although this project has had marginal success, the method has successfully eliminated problems with products such as diphenhydrAMINE and dimenhyDRINATE. Hospitals should also follow suit by making similar changes in their own labels, preprinted order forms, computer screens and printouts, and drug storage location labels.

Lexi-Comp Medical Publishing has adopted the use of these "Tall-Man" letters for the drugs suggested by the FDA.

The following is a list of product names and recommended FDA revisions.

DRUG PRODUCT	RECOMMENDED REVISION
acetazolamide	acetaZOLAMIDE
acetohexamide	acetoHEXAMIDE
bupropion	buPROPion
buspirone	busPIRone
chlorpromazine	chlorproMAZINE
chlorpropamide	chlorproPAMIDE
clomiphene	clomiPHENE
clomipramine	clomiPRAMINE
cycloserine	cycloSERINE
cyclosporine	cycloSPORINE
daunorubicin	DAUNOrubicin
dimenhydrinate	dimenhyDRINATE
diphenhydramine	diphenhydrAMINE
dobutamine	DOBUTamine
dopamine	DOPamine
doxorubicin	DOXOrubicin
glipizide	glipiZIDE
glyburide	glyBURIDE
hydralazine	hydrALAZINE
hydroxyzine	hydrOXYzine
medroxyprogesterone	medroxyPROGESTERone
methylprednisolone	methylPREDNISolone
methyltestosterone	methylTESTOSTERone
nicardipine	niCARdipine
nifedipine	NIFEdipine
prednisolone	prednisoLONE
prednisone	predniSONE
sulfadiazine	sulfaDIAZINE
sulfisoxazole	sulfiSOXAZOLE
tolazamide	TOLAZamide
tolbutamide	TOLBUTamide
vinblastine	vinBLAStine
vincristine	vinCRIStine

Institute for Safe Medication Practices. "New Tall-Man Lettering Will Reduce Mix-Ups Due to Generic Drug Name Confusion," *ISMP Medication Safety Alert*, September 19, 2001. Available at: http://www.ismp.org.
Institute for Safe Medication Practices. "Prescription Mapping, Can Improve Efficiency While Minimizing Errors With Look-Alike Products," *ISMP Medication Safety Alert*, October 6, 1999. Available at: http://www.ismp.org.
U.S. Pharmacopeia, "USP Quality Review: Use Caution-Avoid Confusion," March 2001, No. 76. Available at: http://www.usp.org.

ABBREVIATIONS AND SYMBOLS USED IN THIS HANDBOOK[1]

°C	degrees Celsius (Centigrade)
<	less than
>	greater than
≤	less than or equal to
≥	greater than or equal to
μg	microgram
μmol	micromole
AAPC	antibiotic associated pseudomembranous colitis
ABG	arterial blood gas
ABMT	autologous bone marrow transplant
ACE	angiotensin-converting enzyme
ACLS	advanced cardiac life support
ADH	antidiuretic hormone
AED	antiepileptic drug
AIDS	acquired immunodeficiency syndrome
ALL	acute lymphoblastic leukemia
ALT	alanine aminotransferase (formerly called SGPT)
AML	acute myeloblastic leukemia
ANA	antinuclear antibodies
ANC	absolute neutrophil count
ANLL	acute nonlymphoblastic leukemia
APTT	activated partial thromboplastin time
ASA (class I-IV)	American Society of Anesthesiology physical status classification of surgical patients according to their baseline health
	ASA I: Normal healthy patients
	ASA II: Patients having controlled disease states (eg, controlled hypertension)
	ASA III: Patients having a disease which compromises their organ function (eg, decompensated CHF, end stage renal failure)
	ASA IV: Patients who are extremely critically ill
AST	aspartate aminotransferase (formerly called SGOT)
AUC	area under the curve (area under the serum concentration-time curve)
A-V	atrial-ventricular
BMT	bone marrow transplant
BUN	blood urea nitrogen
cAMP	cyclic adenosine monophosphate
CBC	complete blood count
CHF	congestive heart failure
CI	cardiac index
Cl_{cr}	creatinine clearance
CMV	cytomegalovirus
CNS	central nervous system
COPD	chronic obstructive pulmonary disease
CSF	cerebrospinal fluid
CT	computed tomography
CVA	cerebral vascular accident
CVP	central venous pressure
d	day
D_5W	dextrose 5% in water
$D_5/1/2NS$	dextrose 5% in sodium chloride 0.45%
$D_{10}W$	dextrose 10% in water
DIC	disseminated intravascular coagulation
DL_{co}	pulmonary diffusion capacity for carbon monoxide
DNA	deoxyribonucleic acid
DVT	deep vein thrombosis
ECHO	echocardiogram
ECMO	extracorporeal membrane oxygenation
EEG	electroencephalogram
EKG	electrocardiogram
ESR	erythrocyte sedimentation rate
E.T.	endotracheal
FEV_1	forced expiratory volume exhaled after 1 second

ABBREVIATIONS AND SYMBOLS USED IN THIS HANDBOOK[1] *(Continued)*

FSH	follicle-stimulating hormone
FVC	forced vital capacity
g	gram
G-6-PD	glucose-6-phosphate dehydrogenase
GA	gestational age
GABA	gamma-aminobutyric acid
GE	gastroesophageal
GI	gastrointestinal
GU	genitourinary
h	hour
HIV	human immunodeficiency virus
HPLC	high performance liquid chromatography
IBW	ideal body weight
ICP	intracranial pressure
IgG	immune globulin G
I.M.	intramuscular
INR	international normalized ratio
int. unit	international units
I.O.	intraosseous
I & O	input and output
IOP	intraocular pressure
I.T.	intrathecal
I.V.	intravenous
IVH	intraventricular hemorrhage
IVP	intravenous push
JRA	juvenile rheumatoid arthritis
kg	kilogram
L	liter
LDH	lactate dehydrogenase
LE	lupus erythematosus
LH	luteinizing hormone
LP	lumbar puncture
LR	lactated Ringer's
MAC	*Mycobacterium avium* complex
MAO	monoamine oxidase
MAP	mean arterial pressure
mcg	microgram
mg	milligram
MI	myocardial infarction
min	minute
mL	milliliter
mo	month
mOsm	milliosmoles
MRI	magnetic resonance image
MRSA	methicillin-resistant *Staphylococcus aureus*
NCI	National Cancer Institute
ND	nasoduodenal
ng	nanogram
NG	nasogastric
NMDA	n-methyl-d-aspartate
nmol	nanomole
NPO	nothing per os (nothing by mouth)
NSAID	nonsteroidal anti-inflammatory drug
O.R.	operating room
OTC	over-the-counter (nonprescription)
PABA	para-aminobenzoic acid
PALS	pediatric advanced life support
PCA	postconceptional age
PCP	*Pneumocystis carinii* pneumonia
PCWP	pulmonary capillary wedge pressure

PDA	patent ductus arteriosus
PIP	peak inspiratory pressure
PNA	postnatal age
PSVT	paroxysmal supraventricular tachycardia
PT	prothrombin time
PTT	partial thromboplastin time
PUD	peptic ulcer disease
PVC	premature ventricular contraction
PVR	peripheral vascular resistance
qsad	add an amount sufficient to equal
RAP	right arterial pressure
RIA	radioimmunoassay
RNA	ribonucleic acid
S-A	sino-atrial
S_{cr}	serum creatinine
SIADH	syndrome of inappropriate antidiuretic hormone
S.L.	sublingual
SLE	systemic lupus erythematosus
SubQ	subcutaneous
SVR	systemic vascular resistance
SVT	supraventricular tachycardia
SWI	sterile water for injection
T_3	triiodothyronine
T_4	thyroxine
TIBC	total iron binding capacity
TPN	total parenteral nutrition
TSH	thyroid stimulating hormone
TT	thrombin time
UTI	urinary tract infection
V_d	volume of distribution
V_{dss}	volume of distribution at steady-state
VMA	vanillylmandelic acid
w/w	weight for weight
y	year

[1]Other than drug synonyms

FDA PREGNANCY CATEGORIES

Throughout this book there is a field labeled Pregnancy Risk Factor and the letter A, B, C, D, or X, immediately following, which signifies a category. The FDA has established these five categories to indicate the potential of a systemically-absorbed drug for causing birth defects. The key differentiation among the categories rests upon the reliability of documentation and the risk:benefit ratio. Category **X** is particularly notable, in that if any data exists that may implicate a drug as a teratogen, and the risk:benefit ratio is clearly negative, the drug is **contraindicated** during pregnancy.

These categories are summarized as follows:

A   Controlled studies in pregnant women fail to demonstrate a risk to the fetus in the first trimester with no evidence of risk in later trimesters. The possibility of fetal harm appears remote.

B   Either animal-reproduction studies have not demonstrated a fetal risk but there are no controlled studies in pregnant women, or animal-reproduction studies have shown an adverse effect (other than a decrease in fertility) that was not confirmed in controlled studies in women in the first trimester and there is no evidence of a risk in later trimesters.

C   Either studies in animals have revealed adverse effects on the fetus (teratogenic or embryocidal effects or other) and there are no controlled studies in women, or studies in women and animals are not available. Drugs should be given only if the potential benefits justify the potential risk to the fetus.

D   There is positive evidence of human fetal risk, but the benefits from use in pregnant women may be acceptable despite the risk (eg, if the drug is needed in a life-threatening situation or for a serious disease for which safer drugs cannot be used or are ineffective).

X   Studies in animals or human beings have demonstrated fetal abnormalities or there is evidence of fetal risk based on human experience, or both, and the risk of the use of the drug in pregnant women clearly outweighs any possible benefit. The drug is contraindicated in women who are or may become pregnant.

GENERAL NURSING ISSUES

ASSESSMENT

Assessment is the *primary* action in the nursing process and it is also a vital part of optimal drug therapy. Assessment activities must precede administering any medication. Appropriate assessment includes not just the particulars of the presenting complaint, but also must include what the patient understands or believes about the problem (eg, etiology and prognosis of complaint, impact of lifestyle habits, etc). Information gathered in primary assessment should serve as a guide to patient education and to identify specific areas that need close monitoring. Generally, assessment starts with a thorough patient history that can include:

- Current complaint: History, observation, laboratory results, other treatments, etc

- Other concurrent conditions: Chronic illnesses

- Past health problems and treatments: Resolved, chronic, treatments effective/noneffective

- Current drugs: Prescription, OTC, home remedies, herbs and herbal medicines

- Past drugs: Reason for taking, effectiveness, adverse effects

- Allergies or adverse effects: Drugs, household products, food products, environmental factors

- Health habits: Caffeine, alcohol, nicotine, street drugs, sleep, activity, nutrition, hydration, sexual activity, pregnant, lactating, use of contraceptives (barrier or oral)

- Physical: Vital signs, weight, height; may include particulars (as necessary) about any body system: pulmonary, cardiac, circulatory, hepatic, renal, gastrointestinal, genitourinary, integument, skeletal, or connective tissues systems

- Psychosocial support: Financial, religious, personal, community

SAFE ADMINISTRATION

Safe administration is grounded in the five "Right" principles: *Right Drug, Right Dose, Right Patient, Right Route, Right Time.*

Right drug – involves checking drug dispensed with the written prescription. Many drugs have similar names (terbutaline/tolbutamine, calciferol/calcitriol); caution must be used to determine the exact drug prescribed. In addition, a nurse must understand why any particular medication is being prescribed.

Right dose – requires checking the prescribed dosage, being aware of the "average" or "usual" dosage for that drug, or identifying any particular patient characteristics which may be rational for unusual dosing. Determining the right dose for some medications means titrating dose to monitored physiological parameters determined by hemodynamic or cardiac monitoring, according to kidney or liver function, or calculating dose according to body weight or body surface area.

Right patient – means identifying each individual patient. Patients in healthcare institutions most generally wear identifying namebands that can be checked prior to administration. When patients are not wearing namebands (eg, at home, in rehabilitation, in outpatient settings), asking patients to identify themselves will reduce medication misadventures.

Right route – includes consideration of traditional routes (P.O., I.V., I.M., or SubQ etc). Right route should also include knowledge about whether the dispensed oral drug form can be changed. Can the drug safely be crushed, chewed, dissolved, administered via a nasogastric or any other type of feeding tube. Extended-release formulations should never be crushed, chewed, or dissolved (see Oral Medications That Cannot Be Crushed *on page 1389*). Some intravenous drugs should be administered via a central line because the possibility of peripheral extravasation presents a serious risk for the patient. Some intravenous drugs (eg, ectoposide VP-16, idarubicin, hydroxyzine, ifosfamide, irinotecan, mannitol, mechlorethamine, mitomycin, nafcillin, norepinephrine, phenobarbital, phenylephrine, phenytoin, potassium chloride, vasopressin, etc) are extremely irritating to peripheral veins; this requires their administration via a central line or as dilute solutions at a slow rate given peripherally.

Right time – necessitates knowledge of a drug's bioavailability; knowing whether the drug should be given at around-the-clock intervals, or whether doses need to be timed in a specific manner. Are there specific dietary considerations? Food will slow the absorption time of many drugs, however, their overall effect will not be affected. Administering medications with food will often reduce the nausea or vomiting that occurs when medications are given on an empty stomach. The drug monographs clearly identify those drugs that must specifically be administered on an empty stomach or should definitely be administered with food. Some monographs include the recommendation for administering in the early part of the day, to reduce night-time sleep interruptions (diuretics).

GENERAL NURSING ISSUES *(Continued)*

MONITORING

Nursing Actions are found in each monograph and address a wide variety of assessment and monitoring activities. Advanced nurse practitioners may be responsible for both prescribing and monitoring. However, at all times, the nurse responsible for administering the medication or instructing the patient about administration is also responsible for monitoring effectiveness and adverse effects and communicating these details to the prescriber. Some common monitoring responsibilities are described in the following paragraphs.

Assessing patient knowledge/teaching. Specifics regarding the prescribed formulation of the drug and route of administration may require discussing that particular area of concern with a patient (or caregiver) and ensuring that their knowledge is correct and complete. If their knowledge is incomplete or incorrect, then it is vital to teach the patient (or caregiver) the necessary information (eg, correct procedure for using inhalators, instilling ophthalmic medications, inserting a suppository, administering injectable medications, or disposing of needles). Is the patient's knowledge about identifying signs and symptoms of opportunistic infections accurate? Is the patient aware of the precautions necessary with antihypertensives (eg, postural hypotension precautions)? Does the patient understand the rationale for contraception and the difference between oral and barrier forms of contraception? Sometime patients need to be referred to other professionals for advanced education pertaining to their disease and the prescribed drugs (eg, drug monographs for medications used to treat diabetics suggest referring the patient to a diabetic educator).

Monitoring vital signs means more than just identifying normal or abnormal patient responses. It also means communicating any adverse signs or symptoms to the prescriber. When the patient is in danger it may be necessary to discontinue a medication and notify the prescriber. In other instances, it will mean contacting the prescriber for further instructions. Some monitoring is constant, as with emergency drugs; and some is intermittent, as with patient administered medications. Awareness of the need for monitoring, the rationale behind monitoring instructions, and the type of monitoring required is a nursing responsibility.

Monitoring for adverse/toxic response. Known adverse reactions are categorized according to body systems in the Adverse Reactions field. Whenever possible, the frequency is either shown in parentheses next to the symptom or the symptoms are grouped in categories which are usually identified as >10%, 1% to 10%, and <1% (Limited to important or life-threatening). The Physical Assessment section of Nursing Actions also includes reminders about the necessity for monitoring the most threatening or severe of those possible side effects.

Monitoring laboratory test results includes knowing what tests are necessary to monitor drug response and ensuring that ordered tests are done at appropriate times. Communicating laboratory test results to the appropriate prescriber is frequently a nursing responsibility.

Some laboratory tests must be completed prior to administering the first dose of a drug (eg, culture and sensitivity tests, tests that indicate premedication status of liver, kidney, or other systems function). Standard peak and trough serum concentration recommendations are available from most laboratories. Since these may change somewhat among laboratories, it is always best to check with the laboratory that will be completing peak and trough assays to identify their exact timing regulations.

Patient Education sections in each drug monograph include the major points that patients need to know about administration safety, including appropriate timing, dietary considerations, drug interaction precautions, and possible actions the patient may take to reduce unpleasant inherent adverse effects (eg, postural hypotension precautions; caution against driving or engaging in hazardous activity because of confusion, dizziness, or impaired judgment; the need to prevent excessive exposure to sunlight because of photosensitivity; and strategies to reduce or prevent nausea and vomiting). Adverse effects that should be reported to the prescriber are also identified, including the necessity for informing the prescriber if the patient is pregnant or intends to be pregnant. In monographs for drugs classified as C, D, or X pregnancy risk factors, such information is included in both the Monitoring and Education sections.

Geriatric Considerations include information pertinent for that drug in relation to therapy for older patients. In addition to these precautions or information, it is necessary to remember the general effects of aging on drug response, especially the effects that impaired circulation or renal function may have on pharmacokinetics.

PATIENT FACTORS THAT INFLUENCE DRUG THERAPY

Many factors related to an individual patient, or a group of similar patients, can impact the pharmacokinetics of drugs and relate to adverse reactions.

PREGNANCY / LACTATION

The changes that occur during pregnancy may necessitate dosage changes for some drugs. Decreased gastric tract motility, increased blood volume, decreased protein binding sites, and increased glomerular filtration rates may alter the degree of anticipated pharmacotherapeutic response.

Primarily, the concern about drugs during pregnancy is the effect of drugs on the fetus, either teratogenic (causing birth defects) or systemic (causing addiction). Although many drugs cross the placenta, the type of drug, the concentration of that drug, and the gestational age at time of exposure of the fetus are primary determinants of fetal reaction. When prescribing or administering drugs to any childbearing age female, it is vital to ask when her last menstrual period was and, if necessary, to wait for the results of a pregnancy test before starting any drug therapy. Of course, it is best to avoid all drugs during pregnancy, however, in some cases, the physiological context (ie, cardiac output, renal blood flow, etc) may be altered enough to require the use of drugs that are not needed by the same woman when not pregnant.

Most systematically absorbed drugs have been assigned a pregnancy risk factor based on the drugs potential to cause birth defects. This permits an evaluation of the risk:benefit ratio when prescribing or administering drugs becomes necessary. Drugs in the risk factor class "A" are generally considered to be safe for use during pregnancy, class "X" drugs are never safe and are known to be positively teratogenic. See FDA Pregnancy Categories *on page 16.*

Contraception note: Many drugs will interact with and decrease the effect of oral contraceptives (eg, barbiturates, protease inhibitors, rifampin, and carbamazepine). When a second drug will decrease the effect of oral contraceptives, the patient needs to be educated about the necessity for using a "barrier" (nonhormonal) form of contraception. Barrier contraception (alone or in combination with some form of oral contraception) is often recommended for the patient who must take selected drugs with pregnancy risk factors "D" (idarubicin) or class "X" (isotretinoin).

Because many drugs and substances used by a mother appear in breast milk, care must be taken to evaluate the drug effects on the lactating woman and the infant. Some drugs are identified as being clearly contraindicated during lactation, others may cross into breast milk but adverse side effects on the fetus have not been identified, and for some drugs the administration times should be distanced from nursing time. Nurses should advise lactating women about the effects that drugs may have on the infant.

AGE

All pharmacokinetics (absorption, distribution, metabolism, and excretion) are different in infants, young adults, and elderly patients. Elderly patients may have mildly decreased or severely decreased blood flow to all organs, gastric motility may be slowed, kidney function may be reduced, decreased nutrition may result in decreased albumin, and sedentary lifestyles may have an impact on drug response. Slower gastric motility means that absorption is slowed, resulting in longer time periods to clinical response. Decreased blood flow means that distribution is altered, resulting in decreased response or longer response time. Excretion may be altered with decreased glomerular filtration rates or slower gastric emptying which can result in increased levels of drug remaining in the system.

The ratio between total body water and total body fat also changes with age; older persons have decreased amounts of total body water and higher body fat. This aspect of aging also influences the blood concentration of some drugs. In a person with increased body fat, fat-soluble drugs are distributed to tissues more than to plasma; resulting in a longer response time as the drug must then be redistributed from tissue to plasma. The idiosyncratic response incidence also increases with an aging population. Responses to drugs may be both more exaggerated or diminished with the "usual" doses of some drugs.

In addition, and of major concern with elderly patients, is the incidence of poly-pharmacy; the increased numbers of drugs the patient may be taking. Older patients may have 2, 3, 4, or 5 (or more) chronic conditions for which they are taking medication. In addition, they may be seeing a different prescriber for each of these conditions. Often, it is a nurse who identifies and coordinates the care of these elderly patients, and the nurse must be aware of the possibility for increased incidence of adverse effects.

BODY WEIGHT / BUILD

Most "recommended" dosages of drugs are based on the average size, young or middle aged adult (usually males). Extremely obese or extremely thin patients may be prone to adverse effects as a result of "nonindividualized" prescribing. Serum creatinine is a breakdown product of skeletal muscle and its levels in the serum are frequently used to estimate renal function. Decreased muscle mass can result in reduced creatinine from muscle breakdown, leading to a serum creatinine, which is artificially low or appears normal. When dosing is based on estimated creatinine clearance (which is calculated based on the serum creatinine) rather than "actual" creatinine clearance, normal doses may be administered to patients with a diminished capacity for excretion, potentially leading to accumulation and toxicity. This is a particular problem in elderly and/or debilitated patients.

SMOKING, ALCOHOL, NUTRITION, AND HYDRATION

Smoking has a direct impact on liver enzyme activity, blood flow, and the central nervous system. Excessive alcohol intake impacts liver enzymes, renal function, and has an additive effect with most antipsychotic, sedative, or anxiolytic medications, as well as altering responses to many other medications. Nutrition and hydration also play an important part in drug responses and possible adverse reactions. Poor hydration may result in reduced blood flow and excretion. Decreased or prolonged gastric motility can result in slowed excretion and/or prolonged absorption. Poor or inadequate nutrition may result in decreased protein available for binding.

It is vital that a patient's current habits are considered when prescribing, administering, or monitoring drug therapy, but in addition, patients must be aware of the need to inform their professional care provider that they have changed their smoking, alcohol, or dietary patterns. When dosage of theophylline is based on the fact that the patient is a smoker, the theophylline dosage must be

PATIENT FACTORS THAT INFLUENCE DRUG THERAPY *(Continued)*

adjusted to prevent overdose, if the patient quits smoking. When a patient is on warfarin, drastic increases in the amount of vitamin K intake through increased green leafy vegetables can dramatically alter the dose of warfarin.

OTHER PATIENT FACTORS THAT INFLUENCE DRUG RESPONSE

– Genetic variations

– Differences in circadian patterns

– Disease states

– Psychological temperament

Genetic differences in enzymes may influence the effectiveness of therapy or the incidence of adverse effects (fast acetylators or slow acetylators). The emerging science of pharmacogenomics is devoted to the investigation of these genetic differences in drug response, and offers the hope of truly individualized therapy. Circadian rhythms differ among individuals and have an impact on absorption patterns, hormone secretion, or urinary excretion patterns. Disease states can and do change all aspects of pharmacokinetics. Cirrhosis can impair liver enzyme metabolism rate. Kidney disease will reduce excretion rates for many drugs. Abnormal thyroid function can influence drug metabolism. Diseases which affect blood circulation (eg, hypertension, CHF, Raynaud's phenomena, malignancies, etc) can have an impact on absorption, distribution, and excretion. Diabetes impacts the response to many drugs. Malnutrition, commonly associated with disease, can drastically reduce albumin levels.

See Therapeutic Nursing Management of Side Effects *on page 21.*

THERAPEUTIC NURSING MANAGEMENT OF SIDE EFFECTS

MANAGEMENT OF DRUG-RELATED PROBLEMS

Patients may experience some type of side effect or adverse drug reaction as a result of their drug therapy. The type of effect, the severity, and the frequency of occurrence is dependent on the medication and dose being used, as well as the individual's response to therapy. The following information is presented as helpful tips to assist the patient through these drug-related problems. Pharmacological support may also be required for their management.

Alopecia

- Your hair loss is temporary. Hair usually will begin to grow within 3-6 months of completing drug therapy.
- Your hair may come back with a different texture, color, or thickness.
- Avoid excessive shampooing and hair combing, or harsh hair care products.
- Avoid excessive drying of hair.
- Avoid use of permanents, dyes, or hair sprays.
- Always cover head in cold weather or sunshine.

Anemia

- Observe all bleeding precautions (see Thrombocytopenia).
- Get adequate sleep and rest.
- Be alert for potential for dizziness, fainting, or extreme fatigue.
- Maintain adequate nutrition and hydration.
- Have laboratory tests done as recommended.
- If unusual bleeding occurs, notify prescriber.

Anorexia

- Small frequent meals containing favorite foods may tempt appetite.
- Eat simple foods such as toast, rice, bananas, mashed potatoes, scrambled eggs.
- Eat in a pleasant environment conducive to eating.
- When possible, eat with others.
- Avoid noxious odors when eating.
- Use nutritional supplements high in protein and calories.
- Freezing nutritional supplements sometimes makes them more palatable.
- A small glass of wine (if not contraindicated) may stimulate appetite.
- Mild exercise or short walks may stimulate appetite.
- Request antiemetic medication to reduce nausea or vomiting.

Diarrhea

- Include fiber, high protein foods, and fruits in dietary intake.
- Drink plenty of liquids.
- Buttermilk, yogurt, or boiled milk may be helpful.
- Antidiarrheal agents may be needed. Consult your prescriber.
- Include regular rest periods in your activities.
- Institute skin care regimen to prevent breakdown and promote comfort.

Fluid Retention/Edema

- Elevate legs when sitting.
- Wear support hose.
- Increase physical exercise.
- Maintain adequate hydration; avoiding fluids will not reduce edema.
- Weigh yourself regularly.
- If your prescriber has advised you to limit your salt intake, avoid foods such as ham, bacon, processed meats, and canned foods. Many foods are high in salt content. Read labels carefully.
- Report to prescriber if any of the following occur: sudden weight gain, decrease in urination, swelling of hands or feed, increase in waist size, wet cough, or difficulty breathing.

Headache

- Lie down.
- Use cool cloth on forehead.
- Avoid caffeine.
- Use mild analgesics. Consult prescriber.

Leukopenia/Neutropenia

- Monitor for signs of infections: persistent sore throat, fever, chills, fatigue, headache, flu-like symptoms, vaginal discharge, foul-smelling stools.
- Prevent infection. Maintain strict handwashing at all times. Avoid crowds when possible. Avoid exposure to infected persons.
- Avoid exposure to temperature changes.
- Maintain adequate nutrition and hydration.
- Maintain good personal hygiene.

THERAPEUTIC NURSING MANAGEMENT OF SIDE EFFECTS *(Continued)*

- Avoid injury or skin breaks.
- Avoid vaccinations (unless recommended by healthcare provider).
- Avoid sunburn.

Nausea and Vomiting

- Eat food served cold or at room temperature. Ice chips are sometimes helpful.
- Drink clear liquids in severe cases of nausea. Avoid carbonated beverages.
- Sip liquids slowly.
- Avoid spicy food. Bland foods are easier to digest.
- Rinse mouth with lemon water. Practice good oral hygiene.
- Avoid sweet, fatty, salty foods and foods with strong odors.
- Eat small frequent meals rather than heavy meals.
- Use relaxation techniques and guided imagery.
- Use distractions such as meals, television, reading, games, etc.
- Sleep during intense periods of nausea.
- Chew gum or suck on hard candy or lozenges.
- Eat in an upright (sitting position), rather than semirecumbant.
- Avoid tight constrictive clothing at meal time.
- Use some mild exercise following light meals rather than lying down.
- Request antiemetic medication to reduce nausea or vomiting.

Postural Hypotension

- Use care and rise slowly from sitting or lying position to standing.
- Use care when climbing stairs.
- Initiate ambulation slowly. Get your bearings before you start walking.
- Do not bend over; always squat slowly if you must pick up something from floor.
- Use caution when showering or bathing (use secure handrails).

Stomatitis

- Perform good oral hygiene frequently, especially before and after meals.
- Avoid use of strong or alcoholic commercial mouthwashes.
- Keep lips well lubricated.
- Avoid tobacco or other products that are irritating to the oral mucosa.
- Avoid hot, spicy, excessively salty foods.
- Eat soft foods and drink adequate fluids.
- Request topical or systemic analgesics for painful ulcerations.
- Be alert for and report signs of oral fungal infections.

Thrombocytopenia

- Avoid aspirin and aspirin-containing products.
- Use electric or safety razor and blunt scissors.
- Use soft toothbrush or cotton swabs for oral care. Avoid use of dental floss.
- Avoid use of enemas, cathartics, and suppositories unless approved by prescriber.
- Avoid valsalva maneuvers such as straining at stool.
- Use stool softeners if necessary to prevent constipation. Consult prescriber.
- Avoid blowing nose forcefully.
- Never go barefoot, wear protective foot covering.
- Use care when trimming nails (if necessary).
- Maintain safe environment; arrange furniture to provide safe passageway.
- Maintain adequate lighting in darkened areas to avoid bumping into objects.
- Avoid handling sharp tools or instruments.
- Avoid contact sports or activities that might result in injury.
- Promptly report signs of bleeding; abdominal pain; blood in stool, urine, or vomitus; unusual fatigue; easy bruising; bleeding around gums; or nosebleeds.
- If injection or bloodsticks are necessary, inform healthcare provider that you may have excess bleeding.

Vertigo

- Observe postural hypotension precautions.
- Use caution when driving or using any machinery.
- Avoid sudden position shifts; do not "rush".
- Utilize appropriate supports (eg, cane, walker) to prevent injury.

ALPHABETICAL LISTING OF DRUGS

Abacavir (a BAK a veer)

U.S. Brand Names Ziagen®

Synonyms Abacavir Sulfate; ABC

Restrictions An FDA-approved medication guide is available at http://www.fda.gov/cder/Offices/ODS/labeling.htm; distribute to each patient to whom this medication is dispensed.

Pharmacologic Category Antiretroviral Agent, Reverse Transcriptase Inhibitor (Nucleoside)

Pregnancy Risk Factor C

Lactation Excretion in breast milk unknown/contraindicated

Use Treatment of HIV infections in combination with other antiretroviral agents

Mechanism of Action/Effect Nucleoside reverse transcriptase inhibitor which interferes with HIV viral RNA-dependent DNA polymerase resulting in inhibition of viral replication

Contraindications Hypersensitivity to abacavir (or carbovir) or any component of the formulation (do not rechallenge patients who have experienced hypersensitivity to abacavir); moderate-to-severe hepatic impairment

Warnings/Precautions Abacavir should always be used as a component of a multidrug regimen. Serious and sometimes fatal hypersensitivity reactions have occurred. **Patients exhibiting symptoms from two or more of the following: Fever, skin rash, constitutional symptoms (malaise, fatigue, aches), respiratory symptoms (eg, pharyngitis, dyspnea, cough), and GI symptoms (eg, abdominal pain, diarrhea, nausea, vomiting) should discontinue therapy immediately and call for medical attention. Abacavir should be permanently discontinued if hypersensitivity cannot be ruled out, even when other diagnoses are possible. Abacavir SHOULD NOT be restarted because more severe symptoms may occur within hours, including LIFE-THREATENING HYPOTENSION AND DEATH.** Fatal hypersensitivity reactions have occurred following the reintroduction of abacavir in patients whose therapy was interrupted (ie, interruption in drug supply, temporary discontinuation while treating other conditions). Reactions occurred within hours. In some cases, signs of hypersensitivity may have been previously present, but attributed to other medical conditions (eg, acute onset respiratory diseases, gastroenteritis, reactions to other medications). If abacavir is restarted following an interruption in therapy, evaluate the patient for previously unsuspected symptoms of hypersensitivity. Do not restart if hypersensitivity is suspected or if hypersensitivity cannot be ruled out. To report these events on abacavir hypersensitivity, a registry has been established (1-800-270-0425). Use with caution in patients with mild hepatic dysfunction (contraindicated in moderate-to-severe dysfunction). Lactic acidosis and severe hepatomegaly with steatosis (sometimes fatal) have occurred with antiretroviral nucleoside analogues; female gender, obesity, and prolonged treatment may increase the risk of hepatotoxicity.

Drug Interactions

Increased Effect/Toxicity: Abacavir increases the blood levels of amprenavir. Abacavir may decrease the serum concentration of methadone in some patients. Concomitant use of ribavirin and nucleoside analogues may increase the risk of developing lactic acidosis (includes adefovir, didanosine, lamivudine, stavudine, zalcitabine, zidovudine).

Nutritional/Ethanol Interactions Ethanol: Ethanol may increase the risk of toxicity.

Adverse Reactions Hypersensitivity reactions (which may be fatal) occur in ~5% of patients (see Warnings/Precautions). Symptoms may include anaphylaxis, fever, rash (including erythema multiforme), fatigue, diarrhea, abdominal pain; respiratory symptoms (eg, pharyngitis, dyspnea, cough, adult respiratory distress syndrome, or respiratory failure); headache, malaise, lethargy, myalgia, myolysis, arthralgia, edema, paresthesia, nausea and vomiting, mouth ulcerations, conjunctivitis, lymphadenopathy, hepatic failure, and renal failure.

Note: Rates of adverse reactions were defined during combination therapy with other antiretrovirals (lamivudine and efavirenz **or** lamivudine and zidovudine). Only reactions which occurred at a higher frequency than in the comparator group are noted. Adverse reaction rates attributable to abacavir alone are not available.

>10%:

Central nervous system: Headache (7% to 13%), fatigue and malaise (7% to 12%)

Gastrointestinal: Nausea (7% to 19%, children 9%)

1% to 10%:

Central nervous system: Depression (6%), dizziness (6%), fever (6%, children 9%), anxiety (5%), abnormal dreams (10%)

Dermatologic: Rash (5% to 6%, children 7%)

Gastrointestinal: Diarrhea (7%), vomiting (2% to 10%, children 9%), abdominal pain (6%)

Hematologic: Thrombocytopenia (1%)

Hepatic: AST increased (6%)

Neuromuscular and skeletal: Musculoskeletal pain (5% to 6%)

Respiratory: Bronchitis (4%), respiratory viral infection (5%)

Miscellaneous: Hypersensitivity reactions (9%; may include reactions to other components of antiretroviral regimen), infection (EENT 5%)

Pharmacodynamics/Kinetics

Time to Peak: 0.7-1.7 hours

Protein Binding: 50%

Half-Life Elimination: 1.5 hours

Metabolism: Hepatic via alcohol dehydrogenase and glucuronyl transferase to inactive carboxylate and glucuronide metabolites

Excretion: Primarily urine (as metabolites, 1.2% as unchanged drug); feces (16% total dose)

Available Dosage Forms

Solution, oral: 20 mg/mL (240 mL) [strawberry-banana flavor]

Tablet: 300 mg

Dosing

Adults & Elderly: HIV treatment: Oral: 300 mg twice daily or 600 mg once daily in combination with other antiretroviral agents

Pediatrics: HIV treatment: Oral: 3 months to 16 years: 8 mg/kg body weight twice daily (maximum: 300 mg twice daily) in combination with other antiretroviral agents

Hepatic Impairment:

Mild dysfunction (Child-Pugh score 5-6): 200 mg twice daily (oral solution is recommended)

Moderate-to-severe dysfunction: Use is contraindicated by the manufacturer

Administration

Oral: May be administered with or without food.

Stability

Storage: Store oral solution and tablets at controlled room temperature of 20°C to 25°C (68°F to 77°F). Oral solution may be refrigerated; do not freeze.

Nursing Actions

Physical Assessment: Assess closely for any previous exposure/allergy to abacavir prior to beginning treatment. Assess other pharmacological or herbal products patient may be taking for potential interactions. A list of medications that should not be used is available in each bottle; patients should be provided with this information. **Note:** Monitor patient closely for any sign of hypersensitivity reaction; can occur within hours or at any time and may be fatal (See Warnings/Precautions). Monitor laboratory tests, effectiveness of therapy, and adverse reactions periodically during therapy. Teach patient proper use (eg, timing of multiple medications and drugs that should not be used concurrently), possible side effects/appropriate interventions, and importance of reporting any sign of hypersensitivity (eg, anaphylaxis, fever, rash, respiratory changes, abdominal pain, gastrointestinal distress, lethargy, myalgia, headache).

Patient Education: You will be provided with a list of specific medications that should not be used during therapy; do not take any new prescriptions, over-the-counter medications, or herbal products (even if they are not on the list) without consulting prescriber. This drug will not cure HIV, nor has it been found to reduce transmission of HIV; use appropriate precautions to prevent spread to other persons. This drug is prescribed as one part of a multidrug combination; take exactly as directed for full course of therapy. Maintain adequate hydration (2-3 L/day of fluids) unless advised by prescriber to restrict fluids. Avoid alcohol to decrease risk of hypersensitivity reaction. You may be susceptible to infection; avoid crowds and exposure to known infections and do not have any vaccinations without consulting prescriber. Frequent blood tests may be required with prolonged therapy. May cause dizziness or weakness (use caution when driving or engaging in tasks requiring alertness until response to drug is known); nausea and vomiting (small frequent meals, frequent mouth care, chewing gum, or sucking lozenges may help). **Note:** Stop drug and report immediately symptoms of hypersensitivity (eg, fever; rash; fatigue, malaise, lethargy; persistent nausea, vomiting, diarrhea, abdominal pain; mouth sores; sore throat, cough, difficulty breathing; headache; swelling of face, mouth or throat; numbness or loss of sensation; pain, tingling, or numbness in toes, feet, muscles or joints; swollen glands; alterations in urinary pattern; swelling of extremities or weight gain). Do not restart without specific instruction by your prescriber. If you are instructed to stop the medication, do not restart in the future. **Pregnancy/breast-feeding precautions:** Inform prescriber if you are or intend to become pregnant. Do not breast-feed.

Dietary Considerations May be taken with or without food.

Breast-Feeding Issues HIV-infected mothers are discouraged from breast-feeding to decrease potential transmission of HIV.

Pregnancy Issues It is not known if abacavir crosses the human placenta. Cases of lactic acidosis/hepatic steatosis syndrome have been reported in pregnant women receiving nucleoside analogues. It is not known if pregnancy itself potentiates this known side effect; however, pregnant women may be at increased risk of lactic acidosis and liver damage. Hepatic enzymes and electrolytes should be monitored frequently during the 3rd trimester of pregnancy in women receiving nucleoside analogues. The pharmacokinetics of abacavir during pregnancy are currently under study. The Perinatal HIV Guidelines Working Group considers abacavir to be an alternative NRTI in dual nucleoside combination regimens. Health professionals are encouraged to contact the antiretroviral pregnancy registry to monitor outcomes of pregnant women exposed to antiretroviral medications (1-800-258-4263 or www.APRegistry.com).

Additional Information A medication guide is available and should be dispensed with each prescription or refill for abacavir. A warning card is also available and patients should be instructed to carry this card with them.

A high rate of early virologic nonresponse was observed when abacavir, lamivudine, and tenofovir were used as the initial regimen in treatment-naive patients. Use of this combination is not recommended; patients currently on this regimen should be closely monitored for modification of therapy.

Abacavir and Lamivudine
(a BAK a veer & la MI vyoo deen)

U.S. Brand Names Epzicom™
Synonyms Abacavir Sulfate and Lamivudine; Lamivudine and Abacavir
Restrictions An FDA-approved medication guide is available at www.fda.gov/cder/Offices/ODS/labeling.htm; distribute to each patient to whom this medication is dispensed.
Pharmacologic Category Antiretroviral Agent, Reverse Transcriptase Inhibitor (Nucleoside)
Pregnancy Risk Factor C
Lactation Enters breast milk/contraindicated
Use Treatment of HIV infections in combination with other antiretroviral agents
Available Dosage Forms Tablet: Abacavir 600 mg and lamivudine 300 mg
Dosing
Adults: HIV: Oral: One tablet (abacavir 600 mg and lamivudine 300 mg) once daily
Renal Impairment: Cl_{cr} <50 mL/minute: Use not recommended
Hepatic Impairment: Use not recommended.
Nursing Actions
Physical Assessment: See individual agents.

Abacavir, Lamivudine, and Zidovudine
(a BAK a veer, la MI vyoo deen, & zye DOE vyoo deen)

U.S. Brand Names Trizivir®
Synonyms Azidothymidine, Abacavir, and Lamivudine; AZT, Abacavir, and Lamivudine; Compound S, Abacavir, and Lamivudine; Lamivudine, Abacavir, and Zidovudine; 3TC, Abacavir, and Zidovudine; ZDV, Abacavir, and Lamivudine; Zidovudine, Abacavir, and Lamivudine
Restrictions An FDA-approved medication guide is available at www.fda.gov/cder/Offices/ODS/labeling.htm; distribute to each patient to whom this medication is dispensed.
Pharmacologic Category Antiretroviral Agent, Reverse Transcriptase Inhibitor (Nucleoside)
Pregnancy Risk Factor C
Lactation See individual agents.
Use Treatment of HIV infection (either alone or in combination with other antiretroviral agents) in patients whose regimen would otherwise contain the components of Trizivir®
Available Dosage Forms Tablet: Abacavir 300 mg, lamivudine 150 mg, and zidovudine 300 mg
Dosing
Adults: HIV treatment: Oral: 1 tablet twice daily. **Note:** Not recommended for patients <40 kg.
Elderly: Use with caution.
Pediatrics: HIV treatment: Adolescents: Refer to adult dosing (not recommended for patients <40 kg).
Renal Impairment: Cl_{cr} ≤50 mL/minute: Avoid use.
Hepatic Impairment: Use not recommended.
Nursing Actions
Physical Assessment: See individual agents.
Patient Education: You will be provided with a list of specific medications that should not be used during therapy; do not take any new prescriptions, over-the-counter medications, or herbal products
(Continued)

Abacavir, Lamivudine, and Zidovudine
(Continued)

during therapy (even if they are not on the list) without consulting prescriber. This drug will not cure HIV, nor has it been found to reduce transmission of HIV; use appropriate precautions to prevent spread to other persons. This drug is prescribed as one part of a multidrug combination; take exactly as directed for full course of therapy. Maintain adequate hydration (2-3 L/day of fluids) unless advised by prescriber to restrict fluids. Avoid alcohol to decrease risk of hypersensitivity reaction. You may be susceptible to infection; avoid crowds and exposure to known infections and do not have any vaccinations without consulting prescriber. Frequent blood tests may be required with prolonged therapy. May cause dizziness or weakness (use caution when driving or engaging in tasks requiring alertness until response to drug is known); nausea and vomiting (small frequent meals, frequent mouth care, chewing gum, or sucking lozenges may help). **Note:** Stop drug and report immediately symptoms of hypersensitivity (eg, fever; rash; fatigue, malaise, or lethargy; persistent nausea, vomiting, diarrhea, or abdominal pain; mouth sores; sore throat, cough, difficulty breathing; headache; swelling of face, mouth, or throat; numbness or loss of sensation; pain, tingling, or numbness in toes, feet, muscles or joints; swollen glands; alterations in urinary pattern; swelling of extremities or weight gain). Do not restart without specific instruction by your prescriber. If you are instructed to stop the medication, do not restart in the future. **Pregnancy/breast-feeding precautions:** Inform prescriber if you are or intend to become pregnant. Do not breast-feed.

Related Information
Abacavir on page 24
Lamivudine on page 704
Zidovudine on page 1300

Abarelix (a ba REL iks)

U.S. Brand Names Plenaxis™ [DSC]

Synonyms PPI-149; R-3827

Restrictions Abarelix is not distributed through retail pharmacies. Prescribing and distribution of abarelix is limited to physicians and hospital pharmacies participating in the Plenaxis™ PLUS program. See Additional Information, or contact Praecis Pharmaceuticals at www.plenaxisplus.com or by calling 1-877-772-3247.

Pharmacologic Category Gonadotropin Releasing Hormone Antagonist

Pregnancy Risk Factor X

Lactation Excretion in breast milk unknown/not indicated in women

Use Palliative treatment of advanced symptomatic prostate cancer; treatment is limited to men who are not candidates for LHRH therapy, refuse surgical castration, and have one or more of the following complications due to metastases or local encroachment: 1) risk of neurological compromise, 2) ureteral or bladder outlet obstruction, or 3) severe bone pain (persisting despite narcotic analgesia)

Mechanism of Action/Effect Competes with naturally-occurring GnRH for binding on receptors of the pituitary. Suppresses LH and FSH, resulting in decreased testosterone.

Contraindications Hypersensitivity to abarelix or any component of the formulation

Warnings/Precautions Hazardous agent — use appropriate precautions for handling and disposal. Has been associated with immediate-onset allergic reactions; may occur with initial dose and risk increases with duration of treatment. Observe for signs/symptoms of allergic reactions (which may include hypotension and/or syncope) for at least 30 minutes following each injection. Abarelix may cause prolongation of the QT interval; consider risk:benefit in patients with baseline QT_c values >450 msec or patients receiving concurrent medications which prolong the QT_c interval (class Ia and class III antiarrhythmics). Efficacy may diminish during prolonged treatment, particularly in patients weighing >225 pounds; monitor serum testosterone levels to identify treatment failures. Monitor transaminase levels and hepatic function during therapy. Extended treatment may result in a decrease in bone mineral density. Not indicated for use in women or children.

Drug Interactions

Increased Effect/Toxicity: When used with other QT_c-prolonging agents, additive QT_c prolongation may occur; Life-threatening ventricular arrhythmias may result; example drugs include class Ia and class III antiarrhythmics, cisapride, selected quinolones, erythromycin, pimozide, mesoridazine, and thioridazine.

Adverse Reactions

>10%:
    Cardiovascular: Hot flushes (79%), peripheral edema (15%)
    Central nervous system: Sleep disturbance (44%), pain (31%), dizziness (12%), headache (12%)
    Endocrine & metabolic: Breast enlargement (30%), nipple discharge/tenderness (20%)
    Gastrointestinal: Constipation (15%), diarrhea (11%)
    Neuromuscular & skeletal: Back pain (17%)
    Respiratory: Upper respiratory infection (12%)
1% to 10%:
    Central nervous system: Fatigue (10%)
    Endocrine & metabolic: Serum triglycerides increased (10%)
    Gastrointestinal: Nausea (10%)
    Genitourinary: Dysuria (10%), micturition frequency (10%), urinary retention (10%), urinary tract infection (10%)
    Hepatic: Transaminases increased (2% to 8%)
    Miscellaneous: Allergic reactions (urticaria, pruritus, syncope, hypotension): risk increases with prolonged treatment

Overdosage/Toxicology No experience in overdose. Treatment is symptomatic and supportive.

Pharmacodynamics/Kinetics

Time to Peak: Serum: 3 days (following I.M. administration)

Half-Life Elimination: 13 days

Metabolism: Hepatic, via peptide hydrolysis

Excretion: Urine (13% as unchanged drug)

Available Dosage Forms [DSC] = Discontinued product
Injection, powder for reconstitution [preservative free]: 113 mg [provides 100 mg/2 mL depot suspension when reconstituted; packaged with diluent and syringe] [DSC]

Dosing

Adults & Elderly: Male prostate cancer: I.M.: 100 mg administered on days 1, 15, 29 (week 4), then every 4 weeks

Administration

I.M.: Administer intramuscularly (to the buttock).

Stability

Reconstitution: Reconstitute vial with 2.2 mL of NS; reconstituted solutions contain abarelix 50 mg/mL.

Storage: Store at room temperature: 25°C (77°F); excursions permitted to 15°C to 30°C (58°F to 86°F). Reconstituted solution is stable for at least 8 hours at 30°C.

Laboratory Monitoring Obtain transaminase levels at baseline and periodically during treatment. Serum testosterone (to identify treatment failure) just prior to abarelix administration, beginning on day 29 and every

8 weeks thereafter. PSA and bone mineral density may be monitored as needed.

Nursing Actions

Physical Assessment: Refer to Additional Information for **required Plenaxis™ PLUS program** prior to prescribing. Assess potential for interactions with other prescription, OTC medications, or herbal products patient may be using. Monitor laboratory tests and adverse reactions with each injection and frequently throughout therapy. **Note:** Monitor patient for adverse reactions for a minimum of 30 minutes following each injection. Teach patient possible side effects/appropriate interventions and adverse symptoms to report. **Pregnancy risk factor X:** Not indicated for use in women. May cause fetal harm if administered to a pregnant woman.

Patient Education: Do not take any new medications during therapy without consulting prescriber. This drug must be administered via injections. You will be monitored closely following the injections. Report immediately any feelings of flushing, dizziness, difficulty swallowing difficulty breathing, or chest tightness. You will be scheduled for injections and frequent laboratory tests. It is important to maintain adequate nutrition (frequent small meals) and hydration (2 L/day) unless advised to restrict fluids by prescriber. You may experience hot flashes (cool clothes and temperatures may help); swelling of extremities; sleep disturbances, dizziness, headache (use caution when driving or engaging in hazardous tasks until response to drug is known); breast enlargement, nipple tenderness/discharge; gastrointestinal disturbances (frequent small meals and frequent mouth care may help); constipation (increased dietary fiber and fluid and increased exercise may help); diarrhea (boiled milk or yogurt may help); or back pain (consult prescriber for analgesic). Report any palpitations or chest pain, respiratory difficulty, rash, or any other persistent adverse reaction.

Breast-Feeding Issues Not indicated for use in women

Pregnancy Issues Not indicated for use in women; may cause fetal harm if administered to a pregnant woman.

Additional Information Prior to distribution, Praecis Pharmaceuticals must enroll prescribing physicians and/or hospital pharmacies in the Plenaxis™ user safety program (Plenaxis™ PLUS). A Physician Attestation form must be used to document the physician's qualifications and acceptance of responsibilities concerning patient education and adverse effect reporting. Physicians must obtain the patient's signature and personally cosign the two-part Plenaxis™ Patient Information leaflet. The original signed copy should be retained in the patient's medical record while the other copy should be given to the patient. Hospital pharmacies must submit a hospital pharmacy agreement form to allow dispensing, which will be limited to physicians enrolled in the prescriber's registry. Confirmation of physician enrollment may be obtained by calling 1-866-753-6294. All doses must be dispensed with a Patient Information leaflet. Distributors must restrict shipment to physicians or hospital pharmacies enrolled in the Plenaxis™ prescribing program. Additional details and/or forms may be obtained through Praecis Pharmaceuticals at www.plenaxisplus.com or by calling 1-877-772-3247.

Abatacept (ab a TA sept)

U.S. Brand Names Orencia®
Synonyms CTLA-4Ig

Pharmacologic Category Antirheumatic, Disease Modifying

Pregnancy Risk Factor C

Lactation Excretion in breast milk unknown/not recommended

Use Treatment of rheumatoid arthritis not responsive to other disease-modifying antirheumatic drugs (DMARD); may be used as monotherapy or in combination with other DMARDs (**not** in combination with TNF-blocking agents)

Mechanism of Action/Effect Prevents activation of T cells

Contraindications Hypersensitivity to abatacept or any component of the formulation; concurrent use with tumor necrosis factor (TNF) blocking agents (eg, adalimumab, etanercept, infliximab)

Warnings/Precautions Caution should be exercised when considering the use of abatacept in patients with a history of recurrent infections, with conditions that predispose them to infections, or with chronic, latent, or localized infections. Patients who develop a new infection while undergoing treatment should be monitored closely. If a patient develops a serious infection, abatacept should be discontinued. Screen patients for latent tuberculosis infection prior to initiating abatacept; safety in tuberculosis-positive patients has not been established. Patients receiving abatacept in combination with TNF-blocking agents had higher rates of infections (including serious infections) than patients on TNF-blocking agents alone. The manufacturer does not recommend concurrent use with anakinra. Due to the affect of T-cell inhibition on host defenses, abatacept may affect immune responses against infections and malignancies; impact on the development and course of malignancies is not fully defined.

Use caution with chronic obstructive pulmonary disease (COPD), higher incidences of adverse effects (COPD exacerbation, cough, rhonchi, dyspnea) have been observed; monitor closely. May cause hypersensitivity, anaphylaxis, or anaphylactoid reactions; medications for the treatment of hypersensitivity reactions should be available for immediate use. Safety and efficacy in children have not been established.

Drug Interactions

Decreased Effect: Abatacept may decrease the efficacy of immune response to live vaccines.

Increased Effect/Toxicity: Abatacept may increase the risk of infections associated with vaccines (live organism). TNF-blocking agents used in combination with abatacept is contraindicated (may increase risk of infections).

Adverse Reactions Note: Percentages not always reported; COPD patients experienced a higher frequency of COPD-related adverse reactions (COPD exacerbation, cough, dyspnea, pneumonia, rhonchi)
>10%:
Central nervous system: Headache (18%)
Gastrointestinal: Nausea
Respiratory: Nasopharyngitis (12%), upper respiratory tract infection
Miscellaneous: Infection
1% to 10%:
Cardiovascular: Hypertension (7%)
Central nervous system: Dizziness (9%)
Dermatologic: Rash (4%), herpes simplex
Gastrointestinal: Dyspepsia (6%)
Genitourinary: Urinary tract infection (6%)
Neuromuscular & skeletal: Back pain (7%), limb pain (3%)
Respiratory: Cough (8%), bronchitis, pneumonia, rhinitis, sinusitis
(Continued)

Abatacept *(Continued)*

Miscellaneous: Infusion-related reactions (9%), influenza

Overdosage/Toxicology Doses up to 50 mg/kg have been tolerated. In the event of an overdose, monitor for signs and symptoms of adverse reactions; treatment should be symptom-directed and supportive.

Pharmacodynamics/Kinetics
Half-Life Elimination: 8-25 days

Available Dosage Forms Injection, powder for reconstitution [preservative free]: 250 mg

Dosing
Adults: Rheumatoid arthritis: I.V.: Dosing is according to body weight: Repeat dose at 2 weeks and 4 weeks after initial dose, and every 4 weeks thereafter:

<60 kg: 500 mg

60-100 kg: 750 mg

>100 kg: 1000 mg

Elderly: Refer to adult dosing. Due to potential for higher rates of infections and malignancies, use caution.

Dosing Adjustment for Toxicity: Withhold therapy for patients with serious infections.

Administration
I.V.: Infuse over 30 minutes. Administer through a 0.2-1.2 micron low protein-binding. filter

I.V. Detail: pH: 7-8

Stability
Reconstitution: Reconstitute each vial with 10 mL SWFI using a silicone-free disposable syringe (discard solutions accidentally reconstituted with siliconized syringe as they may develop translucent particles). Inject SWFI down the side of the vial to avoid foaming. Gently rotate or swirl vial to dissolve; do not shake. Upon dissolution, vent vial to dissipate foaming. After reconstitution, each mL will contain 25 mg abatacept. Further dilute (using a silicone-free syringe) to a final concentration of 5-10 mg/mL in 100 mL NS; gently mix.

Storage: Prior to reconstitution, store at 2°C to 8°C (36°F to 46°F); protect from light. After dilution, may be stored for up to 24 hours at room temperature or refrigerated at 2°C to 8°C (36°F to 46°F). Must be used within 24 hours of reconstitution.

Nursing Actions
Physical Assessment: Monitor therapeutic response and adverse reactions. Perform testing for tuberculosis prior to initiating therapy. Teach patient appropriate interventions to reduce side effects and adverse symptoms to report.

Patient Education: This drug can only be administered by infusion. You may be more susceptible to infections. Report signs of infection. Avoid immunizations unless approved by prescriber. You may experience headache, sore throat, and nausea. Report immediately respiratory difficulty, hives, dizziness, nausea, flushing, cough, or wheezing. **Pregnancy/breast-feeding precautions:** Inform prescriber if you are or intend to become pregnant. Breast-feeding is not recommended.

Breast-Feeding Issues Due to the potential for adverse reactions and possible effects on the developing immune system, breast-feeding is not recommended.

Pregnancy Issues Teratogenic effects were not observed in animal studies. There are no adequate and well-controlled studies in pregnant women. Due to the potential risk for development of autoimmune disease in the fetus, use during pregnancy only if clearly needed.

Acamprosate *(a kam PROE sate)*

U.S. Brand Names Campral®

Synonyms Acamprosate Calcium; Calcium Acetylhomotaurinate

Pharmacologic Category GABA Agonist/Glutamate Antagonist

Pregnancy Risk Factor C

Lactation Excretion in breast milk unknown/use caution

Use Maintenance of alcohol abstinence

Mechanism of Action/Effect Mechanism not fully defined. Structurally similar to GABA, acamprosate appears to restore balance to GABA and glutamate activities which are disrupted in alcohol dependence. During therapeutic use, alcohol intake is reduced, but does not cause a disulfiram-like reaction following alcohol ingestion.

Contraindications Hypersensitivity to acamprosate or any component of the formulation; severe renal impairment (Cl$_{cr}$ <30 mL/minute)

Warnings/Precautions Should be used as part of a comprehensive program to treat alcohol dependence. Treatment should be initiated as soon as possible following the period of alcohol withdrawal, when the patient has achieved abstinence. Acamprosate does not eliminate or diminish the symptoms of alcohol withdrawal. Use caution in moderate renal impairment (Cl$_{cr}$ 30-50 mL/minute). Suicidal ideation, attempted and completed suicides have occurred in acamprosate-treated patients; monitor for depression and/or suicidal thinking. Traces of sulfites may be present in the formulation. Safety and efficacy have not been established in pediatric patients.

Drug Interactions
Decreased Effect: No clinically-significant drug-to-drug interactions have been identified.

Nutritional/Ethanol Interactions
Ethanol: Abstinence is required during treatment. Ethanol does not affect the pharmacokinetics of acamprosate; however, the continued use of ethanol will decrease desired efficacy of acamprosate.

Food: Food decreases absorption of acamprosate (not clinically significant).

Adverse Reactions
Note: Many adverse effects associated with treatment may be related to alcohol abstinence; reported frequency range may overlap with placebo.

>10%: Gastrointestinal: Diarrhea (10% to 17%)

1% to 10%:

Cardiovascular: Syncope, palpitation, edema (peripheral)

Central nervous system: Insomnia (6% to 9%), anxiety (5% to 8%), depression (4% to 8%), dizziness (3% to 4%), pain (2% to 4%), paresthesia (2% to 3%), headache, somnolence, amnesia, tremor, chills

Dermatologic: Pruritus (3% to 4%), rash

Endocrine and metabolic: Weight gain, libido decreased

Gastrointestinal: Anorexia (2% to 5%), flatulence (1% to 3%), nausea (3% to 4%), abdominal pain, dry mouth (1% to 3%), vomiting, dyspepsia, constipation, appetite increased, taste perversion

Genitourinary: Impotence

Neuromuscular & skeletal: Weakness (5% to 7%), back pain, myalgia, arthralgia

Ocular: Abnormal vision

Respiratory: Rhinitis, dyspnea, pharyngitis, bronchitis

Miscellaneous: Diaphoresis (2% to 3%), suicide attempt

Overdosage/Toxicology Symptoms may include diarrhea and (in chronic overdose) hypercalcemia. Treatment is symptom-directed and supportive.

Pharmacodynamics/Kinetics

Protein Binding: Negligible

Half-Life Elimination: 20-33 hours

Metabolism: Not metabolized

Excretion: Urine (as unchanged drug)

Available Dosage Forms Tablet, enteric coated, delayed release, as calcium: 333 mg [contains calcium 33 mg and sulfites]

Dosing

Adults & Elderly: Alcohol abstinence: Oral: 666 mg 3 times/day (a lower dose may be effective in some patients).

Adjustment in patients with low body weight (unlabeled): A lower dose (4 tablets/day) may be considered in patients with low body weight (eg, <60 kg).

Note: Treatment should be initiated as soon as possible following the period of alcohol withdrawal, when the patient has achieved abstinence.

Renal Impairment:

Cl_{cr} 30-50 mL/minute: Initial dose should be reduced to 333 mg 3 times/day.

Cl_{cr} <30 mL/minute: Contraindicated in severe renal impairment.

Administration

Oral: May be administered without regard to meals. Tablet should be swallowed whole; do not crush or chew.

Stability

Storage: Store at 25°C (77°F); excursions permitted to 15°C to 30°C (59°F to 86°F)

Nursing Actions

Physical Assessment: Assess other medications patient may be taking for effectiveness and potential interactions. Can cause depression. Monitor for suicide ideation.

Patient Education: Taking this medication helps maintain abstinence only when used as part of a treatment program that includes counseling and support. Swallow tablet whole. Do not chew or crush. Maintain adequate hydration (2-3 L/day of fluids) unless instructed to restrict fluid intake by prescriber. Can cause drowsiness (use caution when driving or engaging in activities requiring alertness until response to drug is known). You may experience diarrhea (buttermilk, boiled milk, or yogurt may help), peripheral edema, insomnia, anxiety, depression, and generalized weakness. Report persistent diarrhea, excessive or sudden weight gain, swelling of extremities, respiratory difficulties, fainting, or thoughts of suicide. **Pregnancy/breast-feeding precautions:** Inform prescriber if you are or intend to become pregnant. Consult prescriber before breast-feeding.

Dietary Considerations May be taken without regard to meals. Each 333 mg tablet contains 33 mg of elemental calcium.

Geriatric Considerations Initial studies did not include sufficient geriatric patients to be able to derive sufficient data to compare elderly to younger adults. Only 41 out of 4234 patients in clinical trials ≥65 years of age with none ≥75 years. However, since this medication is cleared renally exclusively, caution should be used since many elderly have Cl_{cr} 30-50 mL/minute where dosage reduction is required (see Dosing).

Acarbose (AY car bose)

U.S. Brand Names Precose®

Pharmacologic Category Antidiabetic Agent, Alpha-Glucosidase Inhibitor

Medication Safety Issues

Sound-alike/look-alike issues:

Precose® may be confused with PreCare®

Pregnancy Risk Factor B

Lactation Excretion in breast milk unknown/use caution

Use

Monotherapy, as indicated as an adjunct to diet to lower blood glucose in patients with type 2 diabetes mellitus (noninsulin dependent, NIDDM) whose hyperglycemia cannot be managed on diet alone

Combination with a sulfonylurea, metformin, or insulin in patients with type 2 diabetes mellitus (noninsulin dependent, NIDDM) when diet plus acarbose do not result in adequate glycemic control. The effect of acarbose to enhance glycemic control is additive to that of other hypoglycemic agents when used in combination.

Mechanism of Action/Effect Delays glucose absorption and lowers postprandial hyperglycemia.

Contraindications Hypersensitivity to acarbose or any component of the formulation; patients with diabetic ketoacidosis or cirrhosis; patients with inflammatory bowel disease, colonic ulceration, partial intestinal obstruction, or in patients predisposed to intestinal obstruction; patients who have chronic intestinal diseases associated with marked disorders of digestion or absorption, and in patients who have conditions that may deteriorate as a result of increased gas formation in the intestine

Warnings/Precautions Acarbose given in combination with a sulfonylurea will cause a further lowering of blood glucose and may increase the hypoglycemic potential of the sulfonylurea. If hypoglycemia occurs, appropriate adjustments in the dosage of these agents should be made. Oral glucose (dextrose) should be used in the treatment of mild-to-moderate hypoglycemia.

Treatment-emergent elevations of serum transaminases (AST and/or ALT) occurred in 15% of acarbose-treated patients in long-term studies. These serum transaminase elevations appear to be dose related and were asymptomatic, reversible, more common in females, and, in general, were not associated with other evidence of liver dysfunction.

Drug Interactions

Decreased Effect: The effect of acarbose is antagonized/decreased by thiazide and related diuretics, corticosteroids, phenothiazines, thyroid products, estrogens, oral contraceptives, phenytoin, nicotinic acid, sympathomimetics, calcium channel-blocking drugs, isoniazid, intestinal adsorbents (eg, charcoal), and digestive enzyme preparations (eg, amylase, pancreatin). Acarbose decreases the absorption/serum concentration of digoxin.

Increased Effect/Toxicity: Acarbose may increase the risk of hypoglycemia when used with oral hypoglycemics. See Warnings/Precautions.

Nutritional/Ethanol Interactions Ethanol: Limit ethanol.

Adverse Reactions >10%:

Gastrointestinal: Abdominal pain (21%) and diarrhea (33%) tend to return to pretreatment levels over time, and the frequency and intensity of flatulence (77%) tend to abate with time

Hepatic: Transaminases increased

Overdosage/Toxicology An overdose of acarbose will not result in hypoglycemia. An overdose may result in transient increases in flatulence, diarrhea, and abdominal discomfort which shortly subside. However, acarbose may complicate the treatment of hypoglycemia (Continued)

Acarbose (Continued)

from other causes, since it will inhibit the absorption of oral disaccharides (sucrose). Oral glucose (dextrose) should be used in mild-to-moderate hypoglycemia; severe hypoglycemia should be treated with I.V. glucose. In cases of overdosage, the patient should not be given fluids or food containing carbohydrates (polysaccharides, oligosaccharides, or disaccharides) for 4-6 hours following overdose.

Pharmacodynamics/Kinetics

Metabolism: Exclusively via GI tract, principally by intestinal bacteria and digestive enzymes; 13 metabolites identified

Excretion: Urine (~34%)

Available Dosage Forms Tablet: 25 mg, 50 mg, 100 mg

Dosing

Adults & Elderly: Type 2 diabetes: Oral:

Initial: 25 mg 3 times/day

Maintenance dose: Should be adjusted at 4- to 8-week intervals based on 1-hour postprandial glucose levels and tolerance until maintenance dose is reached; maintenance dose: 50-100 mg 3 times/day. Dosage must be individualized on the basis of effectiveness and tolerance while not exceeding the maximum recommended dose.

Maximum:

≤60 kg: 50 mg 3 times/day

>60 kg: 100 mg 3 times/day

Patients receiving sulfonylureas: Acarbose given in combination with a sulfonylurea will cause a further lowering of blood glucose and may increase the hypoglycemic potential of the sulfonylurea. If hypoglycemia occurs, appropriate adjustments in the dosage of these agents should be made.

Renal Impairment: Cl_{cr} <25 mL/minute: Peak plasma concentrations were 5 times higher and AUCs were 6 times larger than in volunteers with normal renal function; however, long-term clinical trials in diabetic patients with significant renal dysfunction have not been conducted and treatment of these patients with acarbose is not recommended

Administration

Oral: Should be **administered with the first bite of each main meal.**

Stability

Storage: Store at <25°C (77°F) and protect from moisture.

Laboratory Monitoring Postprandial glucose, glycosylated hemoglobin levels, and serum transaminase levels should be checked every 3 months during the first year of treatment and periodically thereafter.

Nursing Actions

Physical Assessment: Assess potential for interactions with other prescriptions, OTC medications, or herbal products patient may be taking. Monitor laboratory tests, therapeutic effectiveness, and adverse response on a regular basis throughout therapy. Teach patient proper use (or refer patient to diabetic educator), possible side effects/appropriate interventions (eg, importance of adequate hydration), and adverse symptoms to report.

Patient Education: Do not take any new medication during therapy unless approved by prescriber. Take this medication exactly as directed, with the first bite of each main meal. Do not change dosage or discontinue this medicine without first consulting prescriber. Do not take other medications with or within 2 hours of this medication unless advised by prescriber. Avoid alcohol. It is important to follow dietary and lifestyle recommendations of prescriber. You will be instructed in signs of hypo- or hyperglycemia by prescriber or diabetic educator. If combining acarbose with other diabetic medication (eg, sulfonylureas, insulin), keep

source of glucose (sugar) on hand in case hypoglycemia occurs. May cause mild side effects during first weeks of acarbose therapy (eg, bloating, flatulence, diarrhea, abdominal discomfort); these should diminish over time. Report severe or persistent side effects, fever, extended vomiting or flu, or change in color of urine or stool. **Breast-feeding precaution:** Consult prescriber if breast-feeding.

Geriatric Considerations Monitor change in preprandial blood glucose concentrations to account for potential age-related changes in postprandial glucose.

Pregnancy Issues Abnormal blood glucose levels are associated with a higher incidence of congenital abnormalities. Insulin is the drug of choice for the control of diabetes mellitus during pregnancy.

Acetaminophen (a seet a MIN oh fen)

U.S. Brand Names Acephen® [OTC]; Aspirin Free Anacin® Maximum Strength [OTC]; Cetafen® [OTC]; Cetafen Extra® [OTC]; Comtrex® Sore Throat Maximum Strength [OTC]; ElixSure™ Fever/Pain [OTC]; FeverALL® [OTC]; Genapap® [OTC]; Genapap® Children [OTC]; Genapap® Extra Strength [OTC]; Genapap® Infant [OTC]; Genebs® [OTC]; Genebs® Extra Strength [OTC]; Mapap® [OTC]; Mapap® Arthritis [OTC]; Mapap® Children's [OTC]; Mapap® Extra Strength [OTC]; Mapap® Infants [OTC]; Redutemp® [OTC]; Silapap® Children's [OTC]; Silapap® Infants [OTC]; Tylenol® [OTC]; Tylenol® 8 Hour [OTC]; Tylenol® Arthritis Pain [OTC]; Tylenol® Children's [OTC]; Tylenol® Extra Strength [OTC]; Tylenol® Infants [OTC]; Tylenol® Junior [OTC]; Tylenol® Sore Throat [OTC]; Valorin [OTC]; Valorin Extra [OTC]

Synonyms APAP; N-Acetyl-P-Aminophenol; Paracetamol

Pharmacologic Category Analgesic, Miscellaneous

Medication Safety Issues

Sound-alike/look-alike issues:

Acephen® may be confused with AcipHex®

FeverALL® may be confused with Fiberall®

Tylenol® may be confused with atenolol, timolol, Tuinal®, Tylox®

Pregnancy Risk Factor B

Lactation Enters breast milk/compatible

Use Treatment of mild-to-moderate pain and fever (antipyretic/analgesic); does not have antirheumatic or anti-inflammatory effects

Mechanism of Action/Effect Reduces fever by acting on the hypothalamus to cause vasodilatation and sweating

Contraindications Hypersensitivity to acetaminophen or any component of the formulation

Warnings/Precautions Limit dose to <4 g/day. May cause severe hepatic toxicity on acute overdose; in addition, chronic daily dosing in adults has resulted in liver damage in some patients. Use with caution in patients with alcoholic liver disease; consuming ≥3 alcoholic drinks/day may increase the risk of liver damage. Use caution in patients with known G6PD deficiency.

OTC labeling: When used for self-medication, patients should be instructed to contact healthcare provider if used for fever lasting >3 days or for pain lasting >10 days in adults or >5 days in children.

Drug Interactions

Cytochrome P450 Effect: Substrate (minor) of CYP1A2, 2A6, 2C8/9, 2D6, 2E1, 3A4; **Inhibits** CYP3A4 (weak)

Decreased Effect: Barbiturates, carbamazepine, hydantoins, rifampin, and sulfinpyrazone may decrease the analgesic effect of acetaminophen. Cholestyramine may decrease acetaminophen absorption (separate dosing by at least 1 hour).

Increased Effect/Toxicity: Barbiturates, carbamazepine, hydantoins, isoniazid, rifampin, sulfinpyrazone may increase the hepatotoxic potential of acetaminophen. Chronic ethanol abuse increases risk for acetaminophen toxicity; effect of warfarin may be enhanced.

Nutritional/Ethanol Interactions

Ethanol: Excessive intake of ethanol may increase the risk of acetaminophen-induced hepatotoxicity. Avoid ethanol or limit to <3 drinks/day.

Food: Rate of absorption may be decreased when given with food.

Herb/Nutraceutical: St John's wort may decrease acetaminophen levels.

Lab Interactions Increased chloride, bilirubin, uric acid, glucose, ammonia (B), chloride (S), uric acid (S), alkaline phosphatase (S), chloride (S); decreased sodium, bicarbonate, calcium (S)

Adverse Reactions Frequency not defined.

Dermatologic: Rash

Endocrine & metabolic: May increase chloride, uric acid, glucose; may decrease sodium, bicarbonate, calcium

Hematologic: Anemia; blood dyscrasias (neutropenia, pancytopenia, leukopenia)

Hepatic: Bilirubin increased, alkaline phosphatase increased

Renal: Ammonia increased, nephrotoxicity with chronic overdose, analgesic nephropathy

Miscellaneous: Hypersensitivity reactions (rare)

Overdosage/Toxicology Symptoms of overdose include hepatic necrosis, transient azotemia, renal tubular necrosis with acute toxicity, anemia, and GI disturbances with chronic toxicity. Treatment consists of acetylcysteine 140 mg/kg orally (loading) followed by 70 mg/kg every 4 hours for 17 doses; therapy should be initiated based upon laboratory analysis suggesting a high probability of hepatotoxic potential. Activated charcoal is very effective at binding acetaminophen. Intravenous acetylcysteine should be reserved for patients unable to take oral forms.

Pharmacodynamics/Kinetics

Onset of Action: <1 hour

Duration of Action: 4-6 hours

Time to Peak: Serum: Oral: 10-60 minutes; may be delayed in acute overdoses

Protein Binding: 8% to 43% at toxic doses

Half-Life Elimination: Prolonged following toxic doses

Neonates: 2-5 hours; Adults: 1-3 hours (may be increased in elderly; however, this should not affect dosing)

Metabolism: At normal therapeutic dosages, hepatic to sulfate and glucuronide metabolites, while a small amount is metabolized by CYP to a highly reactive intermediate (acetylimidoquinone) which is conjugated with glutathione and inactivated; at toxic doses (as little as 4 g daily) glutathione conjugation becomes insufficient to meet the metabolic demand causing an increase in acetylimidoquinone concentration, thought to cause hepatic cell necrosis

Excretion: Urine (2% to 5% unchanged; 55% as glucuronide metabolites; 30% as sulphate metabolites)

Available Dosage Forms [DSC] = Discontinued product

Caplet (Cetafen Extra® Strength, Genapap® Extra Strength, Genebs® Extra Strength, Mapap® Extra Strength, Tylenol® Extra Strength): 500 mg

Caplet, extended release (Mapap® Arthritis, Tylenol® 8 Hour, Tylenol® Arthritis Pain): 650 mg

Capsule (Mapap® Extra Strength): 500 mg

Elixir: 160 mg/5 mL (120 mL, 480 mL, 3780 mL)

Mapap® Children's: 160 mg/5 mL (120 mL) [alcohol free; contains benzoic acid and sodium benzoate; cherry flavor]

Gelcap (Mapap® Extra Strength, Tylenol® Extra Strength): 500 mg

Geltab (Mapap® Extra Strength, Tylenol® Extra Strength): 500 mg

Geltab, extended release (Tylenol® 8 Hour): 650 mg

Liquid, oral: 500 mg/15 mL (240 mL)

Comtrex® Sore Throat Maximum Strength: 500 mg/15 mL (240 mL) [contains sodium benzoate; honey lemon flavor]

Genapap® Children: 160 mg/5 mL (120 mL) [contains sodium benzoate; cherry and grape flavors]

Silapap®: 160 mg/5 mL (120 mL, 240 mL, 480 mL) [sugar free; contains sodium benzoate; cherry flavor]

Tylenol® Extra Strength: 500 mg/15 mL (240 mL) [contains sodium benzoate; cherry flavor]

Tylenol® Sore Throat: 500 mg/15 mL (240 mL) [contains sodium benzoate; cherry and honey-lemon flavors]

Solution, oral drops: 80 mg/0.8 mL (15 mL) [droppers are marked at 0.4 mL (40 mg) and at 0.8 mL (80 mg)]

Genapap® Infant: 80 mg/0.8 mL (15 mL) [fruit flavor]

Silapap® Infant's: 80 mg/0.8 mL (15 mL, 30 mL) [contains sodium benzoate; cherry flavor]

Solution, oral: 160 mg/5 mL (120 mL, 480 mL)

Suppository, rectal: 120 mg, 325 mg, 650 mg

Acephen®: 120 mg, 325 mg, 650 mg

FeverALL®: 80 mg, 120 mg, 325 mg, 650 mg

Mapap®: 125 mg, 650 mg

Suspension, oral:

Mapap® Children's: 160 mg/5 mL (120 mL) [contains sodium benzoate; cherry flavor]

Tylenol® Children's: 160 mg/5 mL (120 mL, 240 mL) [contains sodium benzoate; bubble gum yum, cherry blast, dye free cherry, grape splash, and very berry strawberry flavors]

Suspension, oral drops:

Mapap® Infants: 80 mg/0.8 mL (15 mL, 30 mL) [contains sodium benzoate; cherry flavor]

Tylenol® Infants: 80 mg/0.8 mL (15 mL, 30 mL) [contains sodium benzoate; cherry, dye free cherry, and grape flavors]

Syrup, oral (ElixSure™ Fever/Pain): 160 mg/5 mL (120 mL) [bubble gum, cherry, and grape flavors]

Tablet: 325 mg, 500 mg

Aspirin Free Anacin® Extra Strength, Genapap® Extra Strength, Genebs® Extra Strength, Mapap® Extra Strength, Redutemp®, Tylenol® Extra Strength, Valorin Extra: 500 mg

Cetafen®, Genapap®, Genebs®, Mapap®, Tylenol®, Valorin®: 325 mg

Tablet, chewable: 80 mg

Genapap® Children: 80 mg [contains phenylalanine 6 mg/tablet; fruit and grape flavors]

Mapap® Children's: 80 mg [contains phenylalanine 3 mg/tablet; bubble gum, fruit, and grape flavors]

Mapap® Junior Strength: 160 mg [contains phenylalanine 12 mg/tablet; grape flavor]

Tylenol® Children's: 80 mg [fruit and grape flavors contain phenylalanine 3 mg/tablet; bubble gum flavor contains phenylalanine 6 mg/tablet] [DSC]

Tylenol® Junior: 160 mg [contains phenylalanine 6 mg/tablet; fruit and grape flavors] [DSC]

Tablet, orally disintegrating:

Tylenol® Children's Meltaways: 80 mg [bubble gum, grape, and watermelon flavors]

Tylenol® Junior Meltaways: 160 mg [bubble gum and grape flavors]

Dosing

Adults & Elderly: Pain or fever: Oral, rectal: 325-650 mg every 4-6 hours or 1000 mg 3-4 times/day; do **not** exceed 4 g/day.

Pediatrics: Pain or fever: Oral, rectal: Children <12 years: 10-15 mg/kg/dose every 4-6 hours as needed; do **not** exceed 5 doses (2.6 g) in 24 hours; alternatively, the the following doses may be used; see table on next page.

Note: Higher rectal doses have been studied for use in preoperative pain control in children. However, specific guidelines are not available

(Continued)

Acetaminophen *(Continued)*

and dosing may be product dependent. The safety and efficacy of alternating acetaminophen and ibuprofen dosing has not been established.

Acetaminophen Dosing

Age	Dosage (mg)	Age	Dosage (mg)
0-3 mo	40	4-5 y	240
4-11 mo	80	6-8 y	320
1-2 y	120	9-10 y	400
2-3 y	160	11 y	480

Renal Impairment:

Cl_{cr} 10-50 mL/minute: Administer every 6 hours.

Cl_{cr} <10 mL/minute: Administer every 8 hours (metabolites accumulate).

Moderately dialyzable (20% to 50%)

Hepatic Impairment: Use with caution. Limited, low-dose therapy is usually well tolerated in hepatic disease/cirrhosis. However, cases of hepatotoxicity at daily acetaminophen dosages <4 g/day have been reported. Avoid chronic use in hepatic impairment.

Administration

Oral: Shake suspension well before pouring dose.

Stability

Storage: Do not freeze suppositories.

Laboratory Monitoring Serum APAP levels with long-term use in patients with hepatic disease

Nursing Actions

Physical Assessment: Assess patient for history of liver disease or ethanol abuse (acetaminophen and excessive ethanol may have adverse liver effects). Assess other medications patient may be taking for additive or adverse interactions. Monitor therapeutic effectiveness and for signs of overdose. Monitor vital signs and signs of adverse reactions at beginning of therapy and at regular intervals with long-term use. Assess knowledge/teach patient appropriate use. Teach patient to monitor for adverse reactions and appropriate interventions to reduce side effects.

Patient Education: Take exactly as directed; do not increase dose or frequency. Most adverse effects are related to excessive use. Take with food or milk. While using this medication, avoid or limit alcohol to <3 drinks/day and avoid other prescription or OTC medications that contain acetaminophen. Maintain adequate hydration (2-3 L/day of fluids) unless instructed to restrict fluid intake. This medication will not reduce inflammation; consult prescriber for anti-inflammatory, if needed. Report unusual bleeding (stool, mouth, urine) or bruising; unusual fatigue and weakness; change in elimination patterns; or change in color of urine or stool.

Dietary Considerations Chewable tablets may contain phenylalanine (amount varies, ranges between 3-12 mg/tablet); consult individual product labeling.

Related Information

Overdose and Toxicology *on page 1423*

Acetaminophen and Codeine
(a seet a MIN oh fen & KOE deen)

U.S. Brand Names Capital® and Codeine; Tylenol® With Codeine

Synonyms Codeine and Acetaminophen

Restrictions C-III; C-V

Note: In countries outside of the U.S., some formulations of Tylenol® with Codeine (eg, Tylenol® No. 3) include caffeine.

Pharmacologic Category Analgesic, Narcotic

Pregnancy Risk Factor C

Lactation Enters breast milk/use caution

Use Relief of mild-to-moderate pain

Available Dosage Forms [DSC] = Discontinued product; [CAN] = Canadian brand name

Caplet:
ratio-Lenoltec No. 1 [CAN], Tylenol No. 1 [CAN]: Acetaminophen 300 mg, codeine phosphate 8 mg, and caffeine 15 mg [not available in the U.S.]

Tylenol No. 1 Forte [CAN]: Acetaminophen 500 mg, codeine phosphate 8 mg, and caffeine 15 mg [not available in the U.S.]

Elixir, oral [C-V]: Acetaminophen 120 mg and codeine phosphate 12 mg per 5 mL (5 mL, 10 mL, 12.5 mL, 15 mL, 120 mL, 480 mL) [contains alcohol 7%]

Tylenol® with Codeine [DSC]: Acetaminophen 120 mg and codeine phosphate 12 mg per 5 mL (480 mL) [contains alcohol 7%; cherry flavor]

Tylenol Elixir with Codeine [CAN]: Acetaminophen 160 mg and codeine phosphate 8 mg per 5 mL (500 mL) [contains alcohol 7%, sucrose 31%; cherry flavor; not available in the U.S.]

Suspension, oral [C-V] (Capital® and Codeine): Acetaminophen 120 mg and codeine phosphate 12 mg per 5 mL (480 mL) [alcohol free; fruit punch flavor]

Tablet [C-III]: Acetaminophen 300 mg and codeine phosphate 15 mg; acetaminophen 300 mg and codeine phosphate 30 mg; acetaminophen 300 mg and codeine phosphate 60 mg

ratio-Emtec [CAN], Triatec-30 [CAN]: Acetaminophen 300 mg and codeine phosphate 30 mg [not available in the U.S.]

ratio-Lenoltec No. 1 [CAN]: Acetaminophen 300 mg, codeine phosphate 8 mg, and caffeine 15 mg [not available in the U.S.]

ratio-Lenoltec No. 2 [CAN], Tylenol No. 2 with Codeine [CAN]: Acetaminophen 300 mg, codeine phosphate 15 mg, and caffeine 15 mg [not available in the U.S.]

ratio-Lenoltec No. 3 [CAN], Tylenol No. 3 with Codeine [CAN]: Acetaminophen 300 mg, codeine phosphate 30 mg, and caffeine 15 mg [not available in the U.S.]

ratio-Lenoltec No. 4 [CAN], Tylenol No. 4 with Codeine [CAN]: Acetaminophen 300 mg and codeine phosphate 60 mg [not available in the U.S.]

Triatec-8 [CAN]: Acetaminophen 325 mg, codeine phosphate 8 mg, and caffeine 30 mg [not available in the U.S.]

Triatec-8 Strong [CAN]: Acetaminophen 500 mg, codeine phosphate 8 mg, and caffeine 30 mg [not available in the U.S.]

Tylenol® with Codeine No. 3: Acetaminophen 300 mg and codeine phosphate 30 mg [contains sodium metabisulfite]

Tylenol® with Codeine No. 4: Acetaminophen 300 mg and codeine phosphate 60 mg [contains sodium metabisulfite]

Dosing

Adults: Doses should be adjusted according to severity of pain and response of the patient. Adult doses ≥60 mg codeine fail to give commensurate relief of pain but merely prolong analgesia and are associated with an appreciably increased incidence of side effects.

Cough (Antitussive): Oral: Based on codeine (15-30 mg/dose) every 4-6 hours (maximum: 360 mg/24 hours based on codeine component)

Pain (Analgesic): Oral: Based on codeine (30-60 mg/dose) every 4-6 hours (maximum: 4000 mg/24 hours based on acetaminophen component)

1-2 tablets every 4 hours to a maximum of 12 tablets/24 hours

Elderly: Doses should be titrated to appropriate analgesic effect.

1 Tylenol® [#3] or 2 Tylenol® [#2] tablets every 4 hours; do **not** exceed 4 g/day acetaminophen.

Pediatrics:

Analgesic: Oral:

Codeine: 0.5-1 mg codeine/kg/dose every 4-6 hours

Acetaminophen: 10-15 mg/kg/dose every 4 hours up to a maximum of 2.6 g/24 hours for children <12 years

3-6 years: 5 mL 3-4 times/day as needed of elixir

7-12 years: 10 mL 3-4 times/day as needed of elixir

Children >12 years: 15 mL every 4 hours as needed of elixir

Renal Impairment: See individual agents.

Hepatic Impairment: Use with caution. Limited, low-dose therapy is usually well tolerated in hepatic disease/cirrhosis; however, cases of hepatotoxicity at daily acetaminophen dosages <4 g/day have been reported. Avoid chronic use in hepatic impairment.

Nursing Actions

Physical Assessment: See individual agents.

Patient Education: See individual agents. **Pregnancy/breast-feeding precautions:** Inform prescriber if you are or intend to become pregnant. Consult prescriber if breast-feeding.

Related Information

Acetaminophen *on page 30*

Codeine *on page 296*

Acetaminophen, Isometheptene, and Dichloralphenazone

(a seet a MIN oh fen, eye soe me THEP teen, & dye KLOR al FEN a zone)

U.S. Brand Names Amidrine; Duradrin®; Midrin®; Migquin; Migratine; Migrazone®; Migrin-A

Synonyms Acetaminophen, Dichloralphenazone, and Isometheptene; Dichloralphenazone, Acetaminophen, and Isometheptene; Dichloralphenazone, Isometheptene, and Acetaminophen; Isometheptene, Acetaminophen, and Dichloralphenazone; Isometheptene, Dichloralphenazone, and Acetaminophen

Restrictions C-IV

Pharmacologic Category Analgesic, Miscellaneous

Medication Safety Issues

Sound-alike/look-alike issues:

Midrin® may be confused with Mydfrin®

Lactation Excretion in breast milk unknown/use caution

Use Relief of migraine and tension headache

Contraindications Hypersensitivity to acetaminophen, isometheptene, dichloralphenazone, or any component of the formulation; glaucoma; severe renal disease; hypertension; organic heart disease; hepatic disease; MAO inhibitor therapy

Drug Interactions

Cytochrome P450 Effect: Acetaminophen: **Substrate** (minor) of CYP1A2, 2A6, 2C8/9, 2D6, 2E1, 3A4; **Inhibits** CYP3A4 (weak)

Decreased Effect: See individual agents.

Increased Effect/Toxicity: See individual agents.

Nutritional/Ethanol Interactions Ethanol: Excessive intake of ethanol may increase the risk of acetaminophen-induced hepatotoxicity. Avoid ethanol or limit to <3 drinks/day.

Adverse Reactions Frequency not defined.

Central nervous system: Transient dizziness

Dermatological: Rash

Available Dosage Forms

Capsule: Acetaminophen 325 mg, isometheptene mucate 65 mg, dichloralphenazone 100 mg

Amidrine, Duradrin®, Midrin®, Migquin, Migrazone®, Migratine, Migrin-A: Acetaminophen 325 mg, isometheptene mucate 65 mg, and dichloralphenazone 100 mg

Dosing

Adults & Elderly:

Migraine headache: Oral: 2 capsules to start, followed by 1 capsule every hour until relief is obtained (maximum: 5 capsules/12 hours)

Tension headache: Oral: 1-2 capsules every 4 hours (maximum: 8 capsules/24 hours)

Hepatic Impairment: Use with caution. Limited, low-dose therapy usually well tolerated in hepatic disease/cirrhosis; however, cases of hepatotoxicity at daily acetaminophen dosages <4 g/day have been reported. Avoid chronic use in hepatic impairment.

Nursing Actions

Physical Assessment: Monitor therapeutic effectiveness. Instruct patient in appropriate use.

Patient Education: Can cause dizziness. Use caution when driving or engaging in hazardous tasks until response to drug is known. **Breast-feeding precaution:** Consult prescriber if breast-feeding.

Breast-Feeding Issues Acetaminophen and dichloralphenazone are excreted in breast milk; excretion of isometheptene is not known.

Related Information

Acetaminophen *on page 30*

AcetaZOLAMIDE (a set a ZOLE a mide)

U.S. Brand Names Diamox® Sequels®

Pharmacologic Category Anticonvulsant, Miscellaneous; Carbonic Anhydrase Inhibitor; Diuretic, Carbonic Anhydrase Inhibitor; Ophthalmic Agent, Antiglaucoma

Medication Safety Issues

Sound-alike/look-alike issues:

AcetaZOLAMIDE may be confused with acetoHEXAMIDE

Diamox® Sequels® may be confused with Dobutrex®, Trimox®

Pregnancy Risk Factor C

Lactation Enters breast milk/not recommended (AAP rates "compatible")

Use Treatment of glaucoma (chronic simple open-angle, secondary glaucoma, preoperatively in acute angle-closure); drug-induced edema or edema due to congestive heart failure (adjunctive therapy); centrencephalic epilepsies (immediate release dosage form); prevention or amelioration of symptoms associated with acute mountain sickness

Unlabeled/Investigational Use Urine alkalinization; respiratory stimulant in COPD; metabolic alkalosis

Mechanism of Action/Effect Reversible inhibition of the enzyme carbonic anhydrase resulting in reduction of hydrogen ion secretion at renal tubule and an increased renal excretion of sodium, potassium, bicarbonate, and water. Decreases production of aqueous humor; also inhibits carbonic anhydrase in central nervous system to retard abnormal and excessive discharge from CNS neurons.

(Continued)

AcetaZOLAMIDE *(Continued)*

Contraindications Hypersensitivity to acetazolamide, sulfonamides, or any component of the formulation; hepatic disease or insufficiency; decreased sodium and/ or potassium levels; adrenocortical insufficiency; cirrhosis; hyperchloremic acidosis, severe renal disease or dysfunction; severe pulmonary obstruction; long-term use in noncongestive angle-closure glaucoma

Warnings/Precautions Use in impaired hepatic function may result in coma. Use with caution in patients with respiratory acidosis and diabetes mellitus. Impairment of mental alertness and/or physical coordination may occur. I.M. administration is painful (use by this route is not recommended). Drug may cause substantial increase in blood glucose in some diabetic patients. Malaise and complaints of tiredness and myalgia are signs of excessive dosing and acidosis in the elderly. Cross-sensitivity between sulfonamide antibiotics and sulfonamide diuretics including various thiazide diuretics. Discontinue if signs of hypersensitivity are noted. **Sustained release is not recommended for anticonvulsant use.**

Drug Interactions

Cytochrome P450 Effect: Inhibits CYP3A4 (weak)

Decreased Effect: Methenamine's efficacy may be reduced. Primidone and/or lithium serum concentrations may be decreased.

Increased Effect/Toxicity: Amphetamines, carbamazepine, memantine, phenytoin, and quinidine may have increased effects with concurrent use. Cyclosporine concentrations may be increased by acetazolamide. Salicylate use may result in carbonic anhydrase inhibitor accumulation and toxicity.

Lab Interactions May cause false-positive results for urinary protein with Albustix®, Labstix®, Albutest®, Bumintest®. Interferes with HPLC theophylline assay and serum uric acid levels.

Adverse Reactions Frequency not defined.

Cardiovascular: Flushing

Central nervous system: Ataxia, confusion, convulsions, depression, dizziness, drowsiness, excitement, fatigue, fever, headache, malaise

Dermatologic: Allergic skin reactions, photosensitivity, Stevens-Johnson syndrome, toxic epidermal necrolysis, urticaria

Endocrine & metabolic: Electrolyte imbalance, growth retardation (children), hyperglycemia, hypoglycemia, hypokalemia, hyponatremia, metabolic acidosis

Gastrointestinal: Appetite decreased, diarrhea, melena, nausea, taste alteration, vomiting

Genitourinary: Crystalluria, glycosuria, hematuria, polyuria, renal failure

Hematologic: Agranulocytosis, aplastic anemia, leukopenia, thrombocytopenia, thrombocytopenic purpura

Hepatic: Cholestatic jaundice, fulminant hepatic necrosis, hepatic insufficiency, liver function tests abnormal

Local: Pain at injection site

Neuromuscular & skeletal: Flaccid paralysis, paresthesia

Ocular: Myopia

Otic: Hearing disturbance, tinnitus

Miscellaneous: Anaphylaxis

Overdosage/Toxicology Symptoms of overdose include low blood sugar, tingling of lips and tongue, nausea, yawning, confusion, agitation, tachycardia, sweating, convulsions, stupor, and coma. Hypoglycemia should be managed with 50 mL I.V. dextrose 50% followed immediately with a continuous infusion of 10% dextrose in water (administer at a rate sufficient enough to approach a serum glucose level of 100 mg/dL). The use of corticosteroids to treat hypoglycemia is controversial, however, adding 100 mg of hydrocortisone to the dextrose infusion may prove helpful. In certain instances, hemodialysis may be helpful.

Pharmacodynamics/Kinetics

Onset of Action: Capsule, extended release: 2 hours; I.V.: 2 minutes

Peak effect: Capsule, extended release: 8-12 hours; I.V.: 15 minutes; Tablet: 2-4 hours

Duration of Action: Inhibition of aqueous humor secretion: Capsule, extended release: 18-24 hours; I.V.: 4-5 hours; Tablet: 8-12 hours

Excretion: Urine (70% to 100% as unchanged drug)

Available Dosage Forms

Capsule, extended release:

Diamox® Sequels®: 500 mg

Injection, powder for reconstitution: 500 mg

Tablet: 125 mg, 250 mg

Dosing

Adults: Note: I.M. administration is not recommended.

Glaucoma:

Chronic simple (open-angle): Oral: 250 mg 1-4 times/day or 500 mg extended release capsule twice daily

Secondary, acute (closed-angle): I.V.: 250-500 mg, may repeat in 2-4 hours to a maximum of 1 g/day

Edema: Oral, I.V.: 250-375 mg once daily

Epilepsy: Oral: 8-30 mg/kg/day in 1-4 divided doses, not to exceed 1 g/day. **Note:** Extended release capsule is not recommended for treatment of epilepsy.

Metabolic alkalosis (unlabeled use): I.V. 250 mg every 6 hours for 4 doses or 500 mg single dose; reassess need based upon acid-base status

Mountain sickness: Oral: 250 mg every 8-12 hours (or 500 mg extended release capsules every 12-24 hours). Therapy should begin 24-48 hours before and continue during ascent and for at least 48 hours after arrival at the high altitude.

Note: In situations of rapid ascent (such as rescue or military operations), 1000 mg/day is recommended.

Urine alkalinization (unlabeled use): Oral: 5 mg/kg/ dose repeated 2-3 times over 24 hours

Respiratory stimulant in COPD (unlabeled use): Oral, I.V.: 250 mg twice daily

Elderly: Oral: Initial: 250 mg once or twice daily; use lowest effective dose possible.

Pediatrics: Note: I.M. administration is not recommended.

Glaucoma:

Oral: 8-30 mg/kg/day or 300-900 mg/m^2/day divided every 8 hours

I.V.: 20-40 mg/kg/24 hours divided every 6 hours, not to exceed 1 g/day

Edema: Oral, I.V.: 5 mg/kg or 150 mg/m^2 once every day

Epilepsy: Oral: Refer to adult dosing.

Renal Impairment:

Cl_{cr} 10-50 mL/minute: Administer every 12 hours.

Cl_{cr} <10 mL/minute: Avoid use (ineffective).

Moderately dialyzable (20% to 50%)

Administration

Oral: Oral: May cause an alteration in taste, especially carbonated beverages. Short-acting tablets may be crushed and suspended in cherry or chocolate syrup to disguise the bitter taste of the drug; do not use fruit juices. Alternatively, submerge tablet in 10 mL of hot water and add 10 mL honey or syrup.

I.M.:

I.M. administration is painful because of the alkaline pH of the drug; use by this route is not recommended.

I.V. Detail: pH: 9.2

Stability

Reconstitution: Injection: Reconstitute with at least 5 mL sterile water to provide a solution containing not more than 100 mg/mL. Further dilute in D_5W or NS for I.V. infusion.

Compatibility: Stable in dextran 6% in D_5W, dextran 6% in NS, D_5LR, D_5NS, $D_5\frac{1}{2}NS$, $D_5\frac{1}{4}NS$, D_5W, $D_{10}W$, LR, NS, $\frac{1}{2}NS$

Compatibility when admixed: Incompatible with multivitamins

Storage:

Capsules, tablets: Store at controlled room temperature.

Injection: Store vial for injection (prior to reconstitution) at controlled room temperature. Reconstituted solution may be refrigerated (2°C to 8°C) for 1 week, however, use within 12 hours is recommended. Stability of IVPB solution is 5 days at room temperature (25°C) and 44 days at refrigeration (5°C).

Laboratory Monitoring Intraocular pressure, serum electrolytes, periodic CBC with differential

Physical Assessment: Assess allergy history prior to beginning therapy. Assess effectiveness and interactions of other medications patient may be taking. Monitor for signs of excessive fatigue, malaise, and myalgia. Monitor therapeutic effectiveness, laboratory tests, and adverse response. Monitor growth in pediatric patients. Monitor blood glucose levels closely if diabetic. Assess knowledge/teach patient appropriate use, possible side effects/appropriate interventions, and adverse symptoms to report.

Patient Education: Take as directed; do not chew or crush long-acting capsule (contents may be sprinkled on soft food). May be administered with food to decrease GI upset. You will need periodic ophthalmic examinations while taking this medication. You may experience drowsiness, dizziness, or weakness (use caution when driving or engaging in tasks that require alertness until response to drug is known); or nausea, loss of appetite, or altered taste (small, frequent meals, frequent mouth care, sucking lozenges, or chewing gum may help). Monitor serum glucose closely (may cause altered blood glucose in some patients with diabetes, or unusual response to some forms of glucose testing). You may experience increased sensitivity to sunlight (use sunblock, protective clothing, and avoid exposure to direct sunlight). Report unusual and persistent tiredness; numbness, burning, or tingling of extremities or around mouth, lips, or anus; muscle weakness; black stool; or excessive depression. **Pregnancy/breast-feeding precautions:** Inform prescriber if you are or intend to become pregnant. Consult prescriber if breast-feeding.

Dietary Considerations May be taken with food to decrease GI upset. May have additive effects with other folic acid antagonists. Sodium content of 500 mg injection: 47.2 mg (2.05 mEq).

Geriatric Considerations Malaise and complaints of tiredness and myalgia are signs of excessive dosing and acidosis in the elderly. Assess blood pressure (orthostatic hypotension can occur).

Related Information

FDA Name Differentiation Project: The Use of Tall-Man Letters *on page 12*

Acetic Acid, Propylene Glycol Diacetate, and Hydrocortisone

(a SEE tik AS id, PRO pa leen GLY kole dye AS e tate, & hye droe KOR ti sone)

U.S. Brand Names Acetasol® HC; VoSol® HC

Synonyms Acetic Acid, Hydrocortisone, and Propylene Glycol Diacetate; Hydrocortisone, Acetic Acid, and Propylene Glycol Diacetate; Propylene Glycol Diacetate, Acetic Acid, and Hydrocortisone

Pharmacologic Category Otic Agent, Anti-infective

Use Treatment of superficial infections of the external auditory canal caused by organisms susceptible to the action of the antimicrobial, complicated by swelling

Available Dosage Forms Solution, otic drops: Acetic acid 2%, propylene glycol diacetate 3%, and hydrocortisone 1% (10 mL)

Dosing

Adults & Elderly: Otitis externa (superficial): Otic: Instill 4 drops in ear(s) 3-4 times/day

Pediatrics: Refer to adult dosing.

Physical Assessment: Refer to Hydrocortisone.

Related Information

Hydrocortisone *on page 617*

Acetylcysteine (a se teel SIS teen)

U.S. Brand Names Acetadote®

Synonyms Acetylcysteine Sodium; Mercapturic Acid; Mucomyst; NAC; N-Acetylcysteine; N-Acetyl-L-cysteine

Pharmacologic Category Antidote; Mucolytic Agent

Medication Safety Issues

Sound-alike/look-alike issues:

Acetylcysteine may be confused with acetylcholine

Mucomyst® may be confused with Mucinex®

Pregnancy Risk Factor B

Lactation Excretion in breast milk unknown/use caution

Use Adjunctive mucolytic therapy in patients with abnormal or viscid mucous secretions in acute and chronic bronchopulmonary diseases; pulmonary complications of surgery and cystic fibrosis; diagnostic bronchial studies; antidote for acute acetaminophen toxicity

Unlabeled/Investigational Use Prevention of radiocontrast-induced renal dysfunction (oral, I.V.); distal intestinal obstruction syndrome (DIOS, previously referred to as meconium ileus equivalent)

Mechanism of Action/Effect Exerts mucolytic action through its free sulfhydryl group which opens up the disulfide bonds in the mucoproteins thus lowering mucous viscosity. The exact mechanism of action in acetaminophen toxicity is unknown. It is thought to act by providing substrate for conjugation with the toxic metabolite.

Contraindications Hypersensitivity to acetylcysteine or any component of the formulation

Warnings/Precautions

Inhalation: Since increased bronchial secretions may develop after inhalation, percussion, postural drainage, and suctioning should follow. If bronchospasm occurs, administer a bronchodilator; discontinue acetylcysteine if bronchospasm progresses.

Intravenous: Acute flushing and erythema have been reported; usually occurs within 30-60 minutes and may resolve spontaneously. Serious anaphylactoid reactions have also been reported. Acetylcysteine infusion may be interrupted until treatment of allergic symptoms is initiated; the infusion can then be carefully restarted. Treatment for anaphylactic reactions should be immediately available. Use caution with asthma or history of bronchospasm.

Acetaminophen overdose: The modified Rumack-Matthew nomogram allows for stratification of patients into risk categories based on the relationship between the serum acetaminophen level and time after ingestion. There are several situations where the nomogram is of limited use. Serum acetaminophen levels obtained prior to 4-hour postingestion are not interpretable; patients presenting late may

(Continued)

Acetylcysteine *(Continued)*

have undetectable serum concentrations, but have received a lethal dose. The nomogram is less predictive in a chronic ingestion or in an overdose with an extended release product. Acetylcysteine should be administered for any signs of hepatotoxicity even if acetaminophen serum level is low or undetectable. The nomogram also does not take into account patients at higher risk of acetaminophen toxicity (eg, alcoholics, malnourished patients).

Drug Interactions

Decreased Effect: Adsorbed by activated charcoal; clinical significance is minimal, though, once a pure acetaminophen ingestion requiring N-acetylcysteine is established; further charcoal dosing is unnecessary once the appropriate initial charcoal dose is achieved (5-10 g:g acetaminophen)

Adverse Reactions

Inhalation: Frequency not defined.

Central nervous system: Drowsiness, chills, fever

Gastrointestinal: Vomiting, nausea, stomatitis

Local: Irritation, stickiness on face following nebulization

Respiratory: Bronchospasm, rhinorrhea, hemoptysis

Miscellaneous: Acquired sensitization (rare), clamminess, unpleasant odor during administration

Intravenous:

>10%: Miscellaneous: Anaphylactoid reaction (~17%; reported as severe in 1% or moderate in 10% of patients within 15 minutes of first infusion; severe in 1% or mild to moderate in 6% to 7% of patients after 60-minute infusion)

1% to 10%:

Cardiovascular: Angioedema (2% to 8%), vasodilation (1% to 6%), hypotension (1% to 4%), tachycardia (1% to 4%), syncope (1% to 3%), chest tightness (1%), flushing (1%)

Central nervous system: Dysphoria (<1% to 2%)

Dermatologic: Urticaria (2% to 7%), rash (1% to 5%), facial erythema (≤1%), palmar erythema (≤1%), pruritus (≤1% to 3%), pruritus with rash and vasodilation (2% to 9%)

Gastrointestinal: Vomiting (<1% to 10%), nausea (1% to 10%), dyspepsia (≤1%)

Neuromuscular & skeletal: Gait disturbance (<1% to 2%)

Ocular: Eye pain (<1% to 3%)

Otic: Ear pain (1%)

Respiratory: Bronchospasm (1% to 6%), cough (1% to 4%), dyspnea (<1% to 3%), pharyngitis (1%), rhinorrhea (1%), rhonchi (1%), throat tightness (1%)

Miscellaneous: Diaphoresis (≤1%)

Overdosage/Toxicology Treatment of acetylcysteine toxicity is usually aimed at reversing anaphylactoid symptoms or controlling nausea and vomiting. The use of epinephrine, antihistamines, and steroids may be beneficial.

Pharmacodynamics/Kinetics

Onset of Action: Inhalation: 5-10 minutes

Duration of Action: Inhalation: >1 hour

Time to Peak: Plasma: Oral: 1-2 hours

Protein Binding: Plasma: 83%

Half-Life Elimination: Reduced acetylcysteine: 2 hours; Total acetylcysteine: Adults: 5.5 hours; Newborns: 11 hours

Excretion: Urine

Available Dosage Forms

Injection, solution:

Acetadote®: 20% [200 mg/mL] (30 mL) [contains disodium edetate]

Solution, inhalation/oral: 10% [100 mg/mL] (4 mL, 10 mL, 30 mL); 20% [200 mg/mL] (4 mL, 10 mL, 30 mL)

Dosing

Adults & Elderly:

Acetaminophen poisoning:

Oral: 140 mg/kg; followed by 17 doses of 70 mg/kg every 4 hours; repeat dose if emesis occurs within 1 hour of administration; therapy should continue until acetaminophen levels are undetectable and there is no evidence of hepatotoxicity.

I.V. (Acetadote®): Loading dose: 150 mg/kg over 60 minutes. Loading dose is followed by 2 additional infusions: Initial maintenance dose of 50 mg/kg infused over 4 hours, followed by a second maintenance dose of 100 mg/kg infused over 16 hours. To avoid fluid overload in patients <40 kg and those requiring fluid restriction, decrease volume of D$_5$W proportionally. Total dosage: 300 mg/kg administered over 21 hours.

Note: If commercial I.V. form is unavailable, the following dose has been reported using solution for oral inhalation (unlabeled): Loading dose: 140 mg/kg, followed by 70 mg/kg every 4 hours, for a total of 13 doses (loading dose and 48 hours of treatment); infuse each dose over 1 hour through a 0.2 micron Millipore filter (in-line).

Experts suggest that the duration of acetylcysteine administration may vary depending upon serial acetaminophen levels and liver function tests obtained during treatment. In general, patients without measurable acetaminophen levels and without significant LFT elevations (>3 times the ULN) can safely stop acetylcysteine after ≤24 hours of treatment. The patients who still have detectable levels of acetaminophen, and/or LFT elevations (>1000 units/L) continue to benefit from addition acetylcysteine administration

Adjuvant therapy in respiratory conditions:

Note: Patients should receive bronchodilator 15 minutes prior to dose.

Inhalation, nebulization (face mask, mouth piece, tracheostomy): Acetylcysteine 10% and 20% solution (dilute 20% solution with sodium chloride or sterile water for inhalation); 10% solution may be used undiluted: 3-5 mL of 20% solution or 6-10 mL of 10% solution until nebulized given 3-4 times/day; dosing range: 1-10 mL of 20% solution or 2-20 mL of 10% solution every 2-6 hours

Inhalation, nebulization (tent, croupette): Dose must be individualized; may require up to 300 mL solution/treatment

Direct instillation:

Into tracheostomy: 1-2 mL of 10% to 20% solution every 1-4 hours

Through percutaneous intratracheal catheter: 1-2 mL of 20% or 2-4 mL of 10% solution every 1-4 hours via syringe attached to catheter

Diagnostic bronchogram: Nebulization or intratracheal: 1-2 mL of 20% solution or 2-4 mL of 10% solution administered 2-3 times prior to procedure

Prevention of radiocontrast-induced renal dysfunction (unlabeled use): Oral: 600 mg twice daily for 2 days (beginning the day before the procedure); may be given as powder in capsules, some centers use solution (diluted in cola beverage or juice). Hydrate patient with saline concurrently.

Pediatrics:

Acetaminophen poisoning: Refer to adult dosing.

Adjuvant therapy in respiratory conditions:

Note: Patients should receive an aerosolized bronchodilator 10-15 minutes prior to acetylcysteine

Inhalation, nebulization (face mask, mouth piece, tracheostomy): Acetylcysteine 10% and 20% solution (dilute 20% solution with sodium chloride or sterile water for inhalation); 10% solution may be used undiluted.

Infants: 1-2 mL of 20% solution or 2-4 mL 10% solution until nebulized given 3-4 times/day

Children: Refer to adult dosing.

Inhalation, nebulization (tent, croupette): Children: Refer to adult dosing.

Administration

Oral: For treatment of acetaminophen overdosage, administer orally as a 5% solution. Dilute the 20% solution 1:3 with a cola, orange juice, or other soft drink. Use within 1 hour of preparation. Unpleasant odor becomes less noticeable as treatment progresses. If patient vomits within 1 hour of dose, readminister.

I.V.: Intravenous formulation (Acetadote®): Administer loading dose of 150 mg/kg over 60 minutes, followed by two separate maintenance infusions: 50 mg/kg over 4 hours followed by 100 mg/kg over 16 hours.

If not using commercially available I.V. formulation, use a 0.2-μ millipore filter (in-line).

Inhalation: Acetylcysteine is incompatible with tetracyclines, erythromycin, amphotericin B, iodized oil, chymotrypsin, trypsin, and hydrogen peroxide. Administer separately. Intermittent aerosol treatments are commonly given when patient arises, before meals, and just before retiring at bedtime.

Stability
Reconstitution:

Solution for injection (Acetadote®): To avoid fluid overload in patients <40 kg and those requiring fluid restriction, decrease volume of D₅W proportionally. Discard unused portion.

Loading dose: Dilute 150 mg/kg in D₅W 200 mL

Initial maintenance dose: Dilute 50 mg/kg in D₅W 500 mL

Second maintenance dose: Dilute 100 mg/kg in D₅W 1000 mL

Solution for inhalation (Mucomyst®): The 20% solution may be diluted with sodium chloride or sterile water; the 10% solution may be used undiluted.

Intravenous administration of solution for inhalation (unlabeled route): Using D₅W, dilute acetylcysteine 20% oral solution to a 3% solution.

Compatibility:

Inhalation: **Incompatible** with rubber and metals (particularly iron, copper, and nickel); do not mix with ampicillin, tetracycline, oxytetracycline, erythromycin

Intravenous: **Incompatible** with rubber and metals (particularly iron, copper, and nickel)

Storage:

Solution for injection (Acetadote®): Store vials at room temperature, 20°C to 25°C (68°F to 77°F). Following reconstitution with D₅W, solution is stable for 24 hours at room temperature.

Solution for inhalation (Mucomyst®): Store unopened vials at room temperature; once opened, store under refrigeration and use within 96 hours. A color change may occur in opened vials (light purple) and does not affect the safety or efficacy.

Laboratory Monitoring Acetaminophen overdose: AST, ALT, bilirubin, PT, serum creatinine, BUN, serum glucose, and electrolytes. Acetaminophen levels at ~4 hours postingestion (every 4-6 hours if extended release acetaminophen; plot on the nomogram) and every 4-6 hours to assess serum levels, and LFTs for possible hepatotoxicity.

Nursing Actions

Physical Assessment: Monitor effectiveness of therapy and advent of adverse/allergic effects. Monitor pulmonary function and response to therapy.

If giving I.V., monitor for possible anaphylactoid reactions and be prepared to treat appropriately if needed. Instruct patient on appropriate use, adverse effects to report, and interventions to reduce side effects.

Patient Education: Pulmonary treatment: Prepare solution (may dilute with sterile water to reduce concentrate from impeding nebulizer) and use as directed. Clear airway by coughing deeply before using aerosol. Wash face and face mask after treatment to remove any residual. You may experience drowsiness (use caution when driving or engaging in tasks requiring alertness), nausea, or vomiting (small, frequent meals may help). Report persistent chills or fever, adverse change in respiratory status, palpitations, or extreme anxiety or nervousness. **Breast-feeding precaution:** Inform prescriber if you are breast-feeding.

Pregnancy Issues Based on limited reports using acetylcysteine to treat acetaminophen overdose in pregnant women, acetylcysteine has been shown to cross the placenta and may provide protective levels in the fetus.

Acrivastine and Pseudoephedrine
(AK ri vas teen & soo doe e FED rin)

U.S. Brand Names Semprex®-D

Synonyms Pseudoephedrine Hydrochloride and Acrivastine

Pharmacologic Category Antihistamine

Pregnancy Risk Factor B

Lactation Enters breast milk/contraindicated

Use Temporary relief of nasal congestion, decongest sinus openings, running nose, itching of nose or throat, and itchy, watery eyes due to hay fever or other upper respiratory allergies

Available Dosage Forms Capsule: Acrivastine 8 mg and pseudoephedrine hydrochloride 60 mg

Dosing

Adults & Elderly: Rhinitis, nasal congestion, allergic symptoms: Oral: 1 capsule 3-4 times/day

Renal Impairment: Do not use.

Nursing Actions

Physical Assessment: Assess effectiveness and interactions of other medications patient may be taking. Monitor effectiveness of therapy and adverse reactions at beginning of therapy and periodically with long-term use. Assess knowledge/teach patient appropriate use, interventions to reduce side effects, and adverse symptoms to report.

Patient Education: Take as directed; do not exceed recommended dose. Avoid use of other depressants, alcohol, or sleep-inducing medications unless approved by prescriber. You may experience drowsiness or dizziness (use caution when driving or engaging in hazardous activity until response to drug is known); or dry mouth, nausea, or vomiting (small frequent meals, frequent mouth care, chewing gum, or sucking lozenges may help). Report persistent dizziness, sedation, or agitation; chest pain, rapid heartbeat, or palpitations; respiratory difficulty or increased cough; changes in urinary pattern; muscle weakness; or lack of improvement or worsening of condition. **Breast-feeding precaution:** Do not breast-feed.

Related Information

Pseudoephedrine *on page 1047*

Acyclovir (ay SYE kloe veer)

U.S. Brand Names Zovirax®
Synonyms Aciclovir; ACV; Acycloguanosine
Pharmacologic Category Antiviral Agent
Medication Safety Issues
Sound-alike/look-alike issues:
Zovirax® may be confused with Zostrix®, Zyvox™
Pregnancy Risk Factor B
Lactation Enters breast milk/use with caution (AAP rates "compatible")
Use Treatment of genital herpes simplex virus (HSV), herpes labialis (cold sores), herpes zoster (shingles), HSV encephalitis, neonatal HSV, mucocutaneous HSV in immunocompromised patients, varicella-zoster (chickenpox)
Unlabeled/Investigational Use Prevention of HSV reactivation in HIV-positive patients; prevention of HSV reactivation in hematopoietic stem-cell transplant (HSCT); prevention of HSV reactivation during periods of neutropenia in patients with acute leukemia
Mechanism of Action/Effect Inhibits DNA synthesis and viral replication
Contraindications Hypersensitivity to acyclovir, valacyclovir, or any component of the formulation
Warnings/Precautions Use with caution in immunocompromised patients; thrombocytopenic purpura/hemolytic uremic syndrome (TTP/HUS) has been reported. Use caution in the elderly, pre-existing renal disease, or in those receiving other nephrotoxic drugs. Maintain adequate hydration during oral or intravenous therapy. Use I.V. preparation with caution in patients with underlying neurologic abnormalities, serious hepatic or electrolyte abnormalities, or substantial hypoxia.

Safety and efficacy of oral formulations have not been established in pediatric patients <2 years of age.

Chickenpox: Treatment should begin within 24 hours of appearance of rash; oral route not recommended for routine use in otherwise healthy children with varicella, but may be effective in patients at increased risk of moderate to severe infection (>12 years of age, chronic cutaneous or pulmonary disorders, long-term salicylate therapy, corticosteroid therapy).

Genital herpes: Physical contact should be avoided when lesions are present; transmission may also occur in the absence of symptoms. Treatment should begin with the first signs or symptoms.

Herpes labialis: For external use only to the lips and face; do not apply to eye or inside the mouth or nose. Treatment should begin with the first signs or symptoms.

Herpes zoster: Acyclovir should be started within 72 hours of appearance of rash to be effective.
Nutritional/Ethanol Interactions Food: Does not affect absorption of oral acyclovir.
Adverse Reactions
Systemic: Oral:
>10%: Central nervous system: Malaise (12%)
1% to 10%:
Central nervous system: Headache (2%)
Gastrointestinal: Nausea (2% to 5%), vomiting (3%), diarrhea (2% to 3%)
Systemic: Parenteral:
1% to 10%:
Dermatologic: Hives (2%), itching (2%), rash (2%)
Gastrointestinal: Nausea/vomiting (7%)
Hepatic: Liver function tests increased (1% to 2%)
Local: Inflammation at injection site or phlebitis (9%)
Renal: BUN increased (5% to 10%), creatinine increased (5% to 10%), acute renal failure

Topical:
>10%: Dermatologic: Mild pain, burning, or stinging (ointment 30%)
1% to 10%: Dermatologic: Pruritus (ointment 4%), itching
Overdosage/Toxicology Overdoses of up to 20 g have been reported. Symptoms of overdose include agitation, seizures, somnolence, confusion, elevated serum creatinine, and renal failure. In the event of overdose, sufficient urine flow must be maintained to avoid drug precipitation within renal tubules. Hemodialysis has resulted in up to 60% reduction in serum acyclovir levels.
Pharmacodynamics/Kinetics
Time to Peak: Serum: Oral: Within 1.5-2 hours
Protein Binding: 9% to 33%
Half-Life Elimination: Terminal: Neonates: 4 hours; Children 1-12 years: 2-3 hours; Adults: 3 hours
Metabolism: Converted by viral enzymes to acyclovir monophosphate, and further converted to diphosphate then triphosphate (active form) by cellular enzymes
Excretion: Urine (62% to 90% as unchanged drug and metabolite)
Available Dosage Forms
Capsule: 200 mg
Zovirax®: 200 mg
Cream, topical:
Zovirax®: 5% (2 g)
Injection, powder for reconstitution, as sodium: 500 mg, 1000 mg
Zovirax®: 500 mg
Injection, solution, as sodium [preservative free]: 25 mg/mL (20 mL, 40 mL); 50 mg/mL (10 mL, 20 mL)
Ointment, topical:
Zovirax®: 5% (15 g)
Suspension, oral: 200 mg/5 mL (480 mL)
Zovirax®: 200 mg/5 mL (480 mL) [banana flavor]
Tablet: 400 mg, 800 mg
Zovirax®: 400 mg, 800 mg
Dosing
Adults & Elderly: Note: Obese patients should be dosed using ideal body weight
Genital HSV:
I.V.: Immunocompetent: Initial episode, severe: 5 mg/kg every 8 hours for 5-7 days
Oral:
Initial episode: 200 mg every 4 hours while awake (5 times/day) for 10 days (per manufacturer's labeling); 400 mg 3 times/day for 5-10 days has also been reported
Recurrence: 200 mg every 4 hours while awake (5 times/day) for 5 days (per manufacturer's labeling; begin at earliest signs of disease); 400 mg 3 times/day for 5 days has also been reported
Chronic suppression: 400 mg twice daily or 200 mg 3-5 times/day, for up to 12 months followed by re-evaluation (per manufacturer's labeling); 400-1200 mg/day in 2-3 divided doses has also been reported
Topical: Immunocompromised: Ointment: Initial episode: ½" ribbon of ointment for a 4" square surface area every 3 hours (6 times/day) for 7 days
Herpes labialis (cold sores): Topical: Apply 5 times/day for 4 days

Herpes zoster (shingles):
Oral: Immunocompetent: 800 mg every 4 hours (5 times/day) for 7-10 days
I.V.: Immunocompromised: 10 mg/kg/dose or 500 mg/m² /dose every 8 hours for 7 days
HSV encephalitis: I.V.: 10 mg/kg/dose every 8 hours for 10 days (per manufacturer's labeling); 10-15 mg/kg/dose every 8 hours for 14-21 days also reported

Mucocutaneous HSV:
I.V.: Immunocompromised: 5 mg/kg/dose every 8 hours for 7 days (per manufacturer's labeling); dosing for up to 14 days also reported
Oral: Immunocompromised (unlabeled use): 400 mg 5 times a day for 7-14 days
Topical: Ointment: Nonlife-threatening, immunocompromised: $1/2$" ribbon of ointment for a 4" square surface area every 3 hours (6 times/day) for 7 days

Varicella-zoster (chickenpox): Begin treatment within the first 24 hours of rash onset:
Oral: >40 kg (immunocompetent): 800 mg/dose 4 times a day for 5 days
I.V.: Immunocompromised (unlabeled use): 1500 mg/m^2/day divided every 8 hours or 10 mg/kg/dose every 8 hours for 7-10 days

Prevention of HSV reactivation in HIV-positive patients, for use only when recurrences are frequent or severe (unlabeled use): Oral: 200 mg 3 times/day or 400 mg 2 times/day

Prevention of HSV reactivation in HSCT (unlabeled use): Note: Start at the beginning of conditioning therapy and continue until engraftment or until mucositis resolves (~30 days)
Oral: 200 mg 3 times/day
I.V.: 250 mg/m^2/dose every 12 hours

Bone marrow transplant recipients (unlabeled use): I.V.: Allogeneic patients who are HSV and CMV seropositive: 500 mg/m^2/dose (10 mg/kg) every 8 hours; for clinically-symptomatic CMV infection, consider replacing acyclovir with ganciclovir

Pediatrics: Note: Obese patients should be dosed using ideal body weight
Genital HSV:
I.V.: Children ≥12 years: Refer to adult dosing.
Oral:
Initial episode (unlabeled use): 40-80 mg/kg/day divided into 3-4 doses for 5-10 days (maximum: 1 g/day)
Chronic suppression (unlabeled use; limited data): 80 mg/kg/day in 3 divided doses (maximum: 1 g/day), re-evaluate after 12 months of treatment

Herpes labialis (cold sores): Topical: Children ≥12 years: Refer to adult dosing.
Herpes zoster (shingles): I.V.:
Children <12 years (immunocompromised): 20 mg/kg/dose every 8 hours for 7 days
Children ≥12 years: Refer to adult dosing.

HSV encephalitis: I.V.:
Children 3 months to 12 years: 20 mg/kg/dose every 8 hours for 10 days (per manufacturer's labeling); dosing for 14-21 days also reported
Children ≥12 years: Refer to adult dosing.

Mucocutaneous HSV: I.V.:
Children <12 years (immunocompromised): 10 mg/kg/dose every 8 hours for 7 days
Children ≥12 years: Refer to adult dosing.

Neonatal HSV: I.V.: Neonate: Birth to 3 months: 10 mg/kg/dose every 8 hours for 10 days (manufacturer's labeling); 15 mg/kg/dose or 20 mg/kg/dose every 8 hours for 14-21 days has also been reported

Varicella-zoster (chickenpox): Begin treatment within the first 24 hours of rash onset:
Oral:
Children ≥2 years and ≤40 kg (immunocompetent): 20 mg/kg/dose (up to 800 mg/dose) 4 times/day for 5 days
Children >40 kg: Refer to adult dosing.
I.V.:
Children <1 year (immunocompromised, unlabeled use): 10 mg/kg/dose every 8 hours for 7-10 days
Children ≥1 year: Refer to adult dosing.

Prevention of HSV reactivation in HIV-positive patients, for use only when recurrences are frequent or severe (unlabeled use): Oral: 80 mg/kg/day in 3-4 divided doses

Prevention of HSV reactivation in HSCT (unlabeled use): Note: Start at the beginning of conditioning therapy and continue until engraftment or until mucositis resolves (~30 days): I.V.: 250 mg/m^2/dose every 8 hours or 125 mg/m^2/dose every 6 hours

Bone marrow transplant recipients (unlabeled use): I.V.: Refer to adult dosing.

Renal Impairment:
Oral:
Cl$_{cr}$ 10-25 mL/minute/1.73 m^2: Normal dosing regimen 800 mg every 4 hours: Administer 800 mg every 8 hours
Cl$_{cr}$ <10 mL/minute/1.73 m^2:
Normal dosing regimen 200 mg every 4 hours, 200 mg every 8 hours, or 400 mg every 12 hours: Administer 200 mg every 12 hours
Normal dosing regimen 800 mg every 4 hours: Administer 800 mg every 12 hours
I.V.:
Cl$_{cr}$ 25-50 mL/minute/1.73 m^2: Administer recommended dose every 12 hours
Cl$_{cr}$ 10-25 mL/minute/1.73 m^2: Administer recommended dose every 24 hours
Cl$_{cr}$ <10 mL/minute/1.73 m^2: Administer 50% of recommended dose every 24 hours
Hemodialysis: Administer dose after dialysis
Peritoneal dialysis: No supplemental dose needed
CAVH: 3.5 mg/kg/day
CVVHD/CVVH: Adjust dose based upon Cl$_{cr}$ 30 mL/minute

Administration
Oral: May be administered with or without food.
I.V.: For I.V. infusion only. Avoid rapid infusion. Infuse over 1 hour to prevent renal damage. Maintain adequate hydration of patient. Check for phlebitis and rotate infusion sites.
I.V. Detail: pH: 10.5-11.6 (reconstituted solution)
Topical: Not for use in the eye. Apply using a finger cot or rubber glove to avoid transmission to other parts of the body or to other persons.

Stability
Reconstitution: Powder for injection: Reconstitute acyclovir 500 mg with SWFI 10 mL; do not use bacteriostatic water containing benzyl alcohol or parabens. For intravenous infusion, dilute to final concentration of ≤7 mg/mL. Concentrations >10 mg/mL increase the risk of phlebitis.
Compatibility: Stable in D$_5$W, D$_5$NS, D$_5$1/4NS, D$_5$1/2NS, LR, NS
Incompatible with blood products and protein-containing solutions
Y-site administration: Incompatible with amifostine, amsacrine, aztreonam, cefepime, dobutamine, dopamine, fludarabine, foscarnet, gemcitabine, idarubicin, levofloxacin, ondansetron, piperacillin/tazobactam, sargramostim, vinorelbine
Compatibility when admixed: Incompatible with dobutamine, dopamine

Storage:
Capsule, tablet: Store at controlled room temperature of 15°C to 25°C (59°F to 77°F); protect from moisture.
Cream, suspension: Store at controlled room temperature of 15°C to 25°C (59°F to 77°F).
Ointment: Store at controlled room temperature of 15°C to 25°C (59°F to 77°F) in a dry place.
Injection: Store powder at controlled room temperature of 15°C to 25°C (59°F to 77°F). Reconstituted solutions remain stable for 12 hours at room
(Continued)

Acyclovir (Continued)

temperature. Do not refrigerate reconstituted solutions as they may precipitate. Once diluted for infusion, use within 24 hours.

Laboratory Monitoring Urinalysis, BUN, serum creatinine, liver enzymes, CBC

Nursing Actions

Physical Assessment: Assess potential for interactions with other prescriptions, OTC, or herbal medications patient may be taking. Patient should be adequately hydrated during I.V. therapy and monitored closely during intravenous administration. Monitor laboratory tests, therapeutic effects, and adverse responses according to purpose for use and formulation. Teach patient proper use (if self-administered), possible side effects/appropriate interventions, and adverse symptoms to report.

Patient Education: Do not take any new medication during therapy (including creams, lotions, or ointments) unless approved by prescriber. This is not a cure for herpes (recurrences tend to continually reappear every 3-6 months after original infection), nor will this medication reduce the risk of transmission to others when lesions are present; avoid sexual intercourse when visible lesions are present. Use as directed for full course of therapy; do not discontinue even if feeling better. Oral doses may be taken with food. Maintain adequate hydration (2-3 L/day of fluids) unless instructed to restrict fluid intake. May cause nausea or vomiting (small, frequent meals, frequent mouth care, sucking lozenges, or chewing gum may help); lightheadedness or dizziness (use caution when driving or engaging in tasks that require alertness until response to drug is known); or headache, fever, muscle pain (consult prescriber for approved analgesic). Report any change in urination (difficulty urinating, dark colored or concentrated urine); persistent lethargy; acute headache; severe nausea or vomiting; confusion or hallucinations; rash; or respiratory difficulty.

Topical: Apply as directed. Use gloves or finger cot when applying.

Dietary Considerations May be taken with or without food. Acyclovir 500 mg injection contains sodium ~50 mg (~2 mEq).

Geriatric Considerations Calculate creatinine clearance. Dose adjustment may be necessary depending on renal function.

Breast-Feeding Issues Nursing mothers with herpetic lesions near or on the breast should avoid breast-feeding. Limited data suggest exposure to the nursing infant of ~0.3 mg/kg/day following oral administration of acyclovir to the mother.

Pregnancy Issues Teratogenic effects were not observed in animal studies. Acyclovir has been shown to cross the human placenta. There are no adequate and well-controlled studies in pregnant women. Results from a pregnancy registry, established in 1984 and closed in 1999, did not find an increase in the number of birth defects with exposure to acyclovir when compared to those expected in the general population. However, due to the small size of the registry and lack of long-term data, the manufacturer recommends using during pregnancy with caution and only when clearly needed. Data from the pregnancy registry may be obtained from Glaxo-SmithKline.

Adalimumab (a da LIM yoo mab)

U.S. Brand Names Humira®

Synonyms Antitumor Necrosis Factor Apha (Human); D2E7; Human Antitumor Necrosis Factor Alpha

Pharmacologic Category Antirheumatic, Disease Modifying; Monoclonal Antibody; Tumor Necrosis Factor (TNF) Blocking Agent

Medication Safety Issues
Sound-alike/look-alike issues:
Humira® may be confused with Humulin®

Pregnancy Risk Factor B

Lactation Excretion in breast milk unknown/not recommended

Use Treatment of active rheumatoid and active psoriatic arthritis (moderate to severe). **Note:** May be used alone or in combination with disease-modifying antirheumatic drugs (DMARDs).

Mechanism of Action/Effect Adalimumab decreases signs and symptoms of psoriatic and rheumatoid arthritis and inhibits progression of structural damage in rheumatoid arthritis.

Contraindications Hypersensitivity to adalimumab or any component of the formulation

Warnings/Precautions Use caution with chronic infection, history of recurrent infection, or predisposition to infection. Do not give to patients with a clinically-important, active infection. Tuberculosis (disseminated or extrapulmonary) has been reactivated while on adalimumab. Most cases have been reported within the first 8 months of treatment. Patients should be evaluated for latent tuberculosis infection with a tuberculin skin test prior to therapy. Treatment of latent tuberculosis should be initiated before adalimumab is used. Rare reactivation of hepatitis B has occurred in chronic virus carriers; evaluate prior to initiation and during treatment. Adalimumab may affect defenses against infections and malignancies; serious infections (including sepsis and fatal infections) have been reported in patients receiving TNF-blocking agents, including adalimumab. Many of the serious infections have occurred in patients on concomitant immunosuppressive therapy. Other opportunistic infections (*Histoplasma*, *Aspergillus*, and *Nocardia*) have occurred during therapy. Use caution in patients who have resided in regions where histoplasmosis is endemic. Patients who develop a new infection while undergoing treatment with adalimumab should be monitored closely. If a patient develops a serious infection or sepsis, adalimumab should be discontinued. Rare cases of lymphoma have also been reported in association with adalimumab. Impact on the development and course of malignancies is not fully defined.

May exacerbate pre-existing or recent-onset demyelinating CNS disorders. Worsening and new-onset CHF has been reported; use caution in patients with decreased left ventricular function. Use caution in patients with CHF. Patients should be brought up to date with all immunizations before initiating therapy. No data are available concerning the effects of adalimumab on vaccination. Live vaccines should not be given concurrently. No data are available concerning secondary transmission of live vaccines in patients receiving adalimumab. Rare cases of pancytopenia (including aplastic anemia) have been reported with TNF-blocking agents; with significant hematologic abnormalities, consider discontinuing therapy. Positive antinuclear antibody titers have been detected in patients (with negative baselines) treated with adalimumab. Rare cases of autoimmune disorder, including lupus-like syndrome, have been reported; monitor and discontinue adalimumab if symptoms develop. May cause hypersensitivity reactions, including anaphylaxis; monitor. Safety and efficacy have not been established in pediatric patients.

Drug Interactions

Decreased Effect: Concomitant use with vaccines (live) has not be studied; currently recommended not to administer live vaccines during adalimumab therapy.

Increased Effect/Toxicity: Concomitant use with anakinra may increase risk of infections; not recommended.

Adverse Reactions

>10%:

Central nervous system: Headache (12%)

Dermatologic: Rash (12%)

Local: Injection site reaction (20%; includes erythema, itching, hemorrhage, pain, swelling)

Respiratory: Upper respiratory tract infection (17%), sinusitis (11%)

5% to 10%:

Cardiovascular: Hypertension (5%)

Endocrine & metabolic: Hyperlipidemia (7%), hypercholesterolemia (6%)

Gastrointestinal: Nausea (9%), abdominal pain (7%)

Genitourinary: Urinary tract infection (8%)

Hepatic: Alkaline phosphatase increased (5%)

Local: Injection-site reaction (8%; other than erythema, itching, hemorrhage, pain, swelling)

Neuromuscular & skeletal: Back pain (6%)

Renal: Hematuria (5%)

Miscellaneous: Accidental injury (10%), flu-like syndrome (7%)

<5%:

Cardiovascular: Arrhythmia, atrial fibrillation, chest pain, CHF, coronary artery disorder, heart arrest, hypertensive encephalopathy, myocardial infarct, palpitation, pericardial effusion, pericarditis, peripheral edema, syncope, tachycardia, thrombosis (leg), vascular disorder

Central nervous system: Confusion, fever, multiple sclerosis, pain in extremity, paresthesia, subdural hematoma, tremor

Dermatologic: Cellulitis

Endocrine & metabolic: Dehydration, menstrual disorder, parathyroid disorder

Gastrointestinal: Diverticulitis, esophagitis, gastroenteritis, gastrointestinal hemorrhage, vomiting

Genitourinary: Cystitis, pelvic pain

Hematologic: Agranulocytosis, granulocytopenia, leukopenia, pancytopenia, polycythemia

Hepatic: Cholecystitis, cholelithiasis, hepatic necrosis

Neuromuscular & skeletal: Arthritis, bone fracture, bone necrosis, joint disorder, muscle cramps, myasthenia, pyogenic arthritis, synovitis, tendon disorder

Ocular: Cataract

Renal: Kidney calculus, paraproteinemia, pyelonephritis

Respiratory: Asthma, bronchospasm, dyspnea, lung function decreased, pleural effusion, pneumonia

Miscellaneous: Adenoma, allergic reactions (1%), carcinoma (including breast, gastrointestinal, skin, urogenital), erysipelas, healing abnormality, herpes zoster, ketosis, lupus erythematosus syndrome, lymphoma, melanoma, postsurgical infection, sepsis, tuberculosis (reactivation of latent infection)

Overdosage/Toxicology Doses of up to 10 mg/kg have been tolerated in clinical trials. In case of overdose, treatment should be symptomatic and supportive.

Pharmacodynamics/Kinetics

Time to Peak: Serum: SubQ: 131 ± 56 hours

Half-Life Elimination: Terminal: ~2 weeks (range 10-20 days)

Excretion: Clearance increased in the presence of antiadalimumab antibodies; decreased in patients 40 years and older

Available Dosage Forms Injection, solution [preservative free]: 40 mg/0.8 mL (1 mL) [prefilled glass syringe; packaged with alcohol preps; needle cover contains latex]

Dosing

Adults & Elderly:

Rheumatoid arthritis: SubQ: 40 mg every other week; may be administered with other DMARDs; patients not taking methotrexate may increase dose to 40 mg every week

Psoriatic arthritis: SubQ: 40 mg every other week

Administration

Other: For SubQ injection; rotate injection sites. Do not use if solution is discolored. Do not administer to skin which is red, tender, bruised, or hard.

Stability

Storage: Store under refrigeration at 2°C to 8°C (36°F to 46°F). Do not freeze. Protect from light.

Nursing Actions

Physical Assessment: Monitor for signs and symptoms of infection. Assess for liver dysfunction (unusual fatigue, easy bruising or bleeding, jaundice). Assess potential for interactions with other prescriptions, OTC medications, and herbal products patient may be taking. Monitor laboratory tests (PDD), therapeutic effectiveness (eg, pain, range of movement, mobility), and adverse response at regular intervals during treatment. Teach patient proper use if self-injected (appropriate injection technique and syringe/needle disposal), possible side effects/appropriate interventions, and adverse symptoms to report.

Patient Education: Inform prescriber of all prescriptions, OTC medications, or herbal products you are taking, allergies, history of tuberculosis, or any kind of infection you have. Do not take any new medication during therapy without consulting prescriber. If self-administered, follow directions for injection and needle/syringe disposal exactly. Do not have any vaccinations while using this medication without consulting prescriber first. May cause headache or dizziness (use caution when driving or engaged in potentially hazardous tasks); if persistent, consult prescriber for approved analgesic. Report persistent fever, respiratory tract infection, unhealed or infected wounds, urinary tract infection, or flu-like symptoms. Stop drug and report immediately persistent nausea, abdominal pain; numbness or tingling; problems with vision; weakness in legs; chest pains, respiratory difficulty; joint pain; skin rash; redness, swelling, or pain at injection site. **Breast-feeding precaution:** Breast-feeding is not recommended.

Pregnancy Issues Teratogenic effects were not observed in animal studies, however, there are no adequate and well-controlled studies in pregnant women. Use during pregnancy only if clearly needed. A pregnancy registry has been established to monitor outcomes of women exposed to adalimumab during pregnancy (877-311-8972).

Adapalene (a DAP a leen)

U.S. Brand Names Differin®

Pharmacologic Category Acne Products

Pregnancy Risk Factor C

Lactation Excretion in breast milk unknown/use caution

Use Treatment of acne vulgaris

Mechanism of Action/Effect Retinoid-like compound which is a modulator of cellular differentiation, keratinization, and inflammatory processes, all of which represent important features in the pathology of acne vulgaris

Contraindications Hypersensitivity to adapalene or any component in the vehicle gel

Warnings/Precautions Use with caution in patients with eczema. Avoid excessive exposure to sunlight and sunlamps. Avoid contact with abraded skin, mucous membranes, eyes, mouth, and angles of the nose. (Continued)

Adapalene (Continued)

Adverse Reactions >10%: Dermatologic: Erythema, scaling, dryness, pruritus, burning, pruritus or burning immediately after application

Overdosage/Toxicology Toxic signs of overdose commonly respond to drug discontinuation, with spontaneous resolution in a few days to weeks. When confronted with signs of increased intracranial pressure, treatment with mannitol (0.25 g/kg I.V. up to 1 g/kg/dose repeated every 5 minutes as needed), dexamethasone (1.5 mg/kg I.V. load followed with 0.375 mg/kg every 6 hours for 5 days), and/or hyperventilation should be employed.

Pharmacodynamics/Kinetics
Excretion: Bile

Available Dosage Forms [DSC] = Discontinued product

Cream, topical: 0.1% (15 g, 45 g)
Gel, topical: 0.1% (15 g, 45 g) [alcohol free]
Pledget, topical: 0.1% (60s) [DSC]
Solution, topical: 0.1% (30 mL) [DSC]

Dosing
Adults & Elderly: Acne: Topical: Apply once daily before bedtime; results appear after 8-12 weeks of therapy.
Pediatrics: Children >12 years: Refer to adult dosing.

Nursing Actions
Physical Assessment: Monitor effectiveness of therapy and adverse reactions at beginning and periodically during therapy. Assess knowledge/teach patient appropriate use and adverse symptoms to report.

Patient Education: Apply with gloves in thin film at night to thoroughly clean/dry skin; avoid area around eyes or mouth. Do not apply occlusive dressing. Results may take 8-12 weeks to appear. You may experience transient burning or stinging immediately after applying. Report worsening of condition or skin redness, dryness, peeling, or burning that persists between applications. Avoid excessive exposure to sunlight or sunlamps.

Adefovir (a DEF o veer)

U.S. Brand Names Hepsera™
Synonyms Adefovir Dipivoxil
Pharmacologic Category Antiretroviral Agent, Reverse Transcriptase Inhibitor (Nucleoside)
Pregnancy Risk Factor C
Lactation Excretion in breast milk unknown/not recommended
Use Treatment of chronic hepatitis B with evidence of active viral replication (based on persistent elevation of ALT/AST or histologic evidence), including patients with lamivudine-resistant hepatitis B
Mechanism of Action/Effect Acyclic nucleotide reverse transcriptase inhibitor (adenosine analog) which interferes with HBV viral DNA polymerase resulting in inhibition of viral replication
Contraindications Hypersensitivity to adefovir or any component of the formulation
Warnings/Precautions Use with caution in patients with renal dysfunction or in patients at risk of renal toxicity (including concurrent nephrotoxic agents or NSAIDs). Chronic administration may result in nephrotoxicity. Dosage adjustment is required in patients with renal dysfunction or in patients who develop renal dysfunction during therapy. May cause the development of resistance in patients with unrecognized or untreated HIV infection. Lactic acidosis and severe hepatomegaly with steatosis (sometimes fatal) have occurred with antiretroviral nucleoside analogues; female gender, obesity, and prolonged treatment may increase the risk

of hepatotoxicity. Treatment should be discontinued in patients with lactic acidosis or signs/symptoms of hepatotoxicity (which may occur without marked transaminase elevations). Acute exacerbations of hepatitis may occur (in up to 25% of patients) when antihepatitis therapy is discontinued. Exacerbations typically occur within 12 weeks; monitor patients following discontinuation of therapy. Safety and efficacy in pediatric patients have not been established.

Drug Interactions
Increased Effect/Toxicity: Ibuprofen increases the bioavailability of adefovir. Concurrent use of nephrotoxic agents (including aminoglycosides, cyclosporine, NSAIDs, tacrolimus, vancomycin) may increase the risk of nephrotoxicity.

Nutritional/Ethanol Interactions
Ethanol: Should be avoided in hepatitis B infection due to potential hepatic toxicity.
Food: Does not have a significant effect on adefovir absorption.

Adverse Reactions
>10%: Renal: Hematuria (11% vs 10% in placebo-treated)
1% to 10%:
Central nervous system: Fever, headache
Dermatologic: Rash, pruritus
Gastrointestinal: Dyspepsia (3%), nausea, vomiting, flatulence, diarrhea, abdominal pain
Hepatic: AST/ALT increased, abnormal liver function, hepatic failure
Neuromuscular & skeletal: Weakness
Renal: Serum creatinine increased (4%), renal failure, renal insufficiency
Note: In patients with baseline renal dysfunction, frequency of increased serum creatinine has been observed to be as high as 26% to 37%; the role of adefovir in these changes could not be established.
Respiratory: Cough increased, sinusitis, pharyngitis

Overdosage/Toxicology Limited experience in acute overdose. Chronic overdose may be associated with renal toxicity and gastrointestinal adverse effects. Hemodialysis may be effective in the removal of adefovir (35% of a 10 mg dose removed in 4 hours).

Pharmacodynamics/Kinetics
Time to Peak: 1.75 hours
Protein Binding: ≤4%
Half-Life Elimination: 7.5 hours; prolonged in renal impairment
Metabolism: Prodrug; rapidly converted to adefovir (active metabolite) in intestine
Excretion: Urine (45% as active metabolite within 24 hours)

Available Dosage Forms Tablet, as dipivoxil: 10 mg
Dosing
Adults & Elderly: Hepatitis B (chronic): Oral: 10 mg once daily
Renal Impairment:
Cl$_{cr}$ 20-49 mL/minute: 10 mg every 48 hours
Cl$_{cr}$ 10-19 mL/minute: 10 mg every 72 hours
Hemodialysis: 10 mg every 7 days (following dialysis)
Hepatic Impairment: No adjustment required.

Administration
Oral: May be administered without regard to food.
Stability
Storage: Store at 25°C (77 °F); excursions permitted to 15°C to 30°C (59°F to 86°F).
Laboratory Monitoring Serum creatinine (prior to initiation and during therapy); viral load
Nursing Actions
Physical Assessment: Assess potential for interactions with other prescriptions, OTC medications, or herbal products patient may be taking. Monitor laboratory tests, patient response, and adverse reactions (eg, altered hepatic status) on a regular basis

throughout therapy. Teach patient proper use, possible side effects/appropriate interventions, and adverse symptoms to report.

Patient Education: Do not take any new medication during therapy without consulting prescriber. Use appropriate precautions to prevent spread to other persons. Take as directed. Do not discontinue medication without consulting prescriber. You will require frequent blood tests; follow recommended schedule. Maintain adequate hydration (2-3 L/day of fluids) unless instructed to restrict fluid intake. You may be more susceptible to infection (avoid crowds and exposure to infection and do not have any vaccinations without consulting prescriber). May cause headache or abdominal pain (consult prescriber for approved analgesia); or nausea or vomiting (small, frequent meals, frequent mouth care, sucking lozenges, or chewing gum may help). Report unusual bleeding (blood in urine, tarry stools, or easy bruising); unresolved nausea or vomiting (eg, fever, chills, sore throat, burning urination, flu-like symptoms); persistent fatigue; muscle weakness; changes in urinary pattern; or other persistent adverse effects. **Pregnancy/breast-feeding precautions:** Inform prescriber if you are or intend to become pregnant. Breast-feeding is not recommended.

Dietary Considerations May be taken without regard to food.

Additional Information Adefovir dipivoxil is a prodrug, rapidly converted to the active component (adefovir). It was previously investigated as a treatment for HIV infections (at dosages substantially higher than the approved dose for hepatitis B). The NDA was withdrawn, and no further studies in the treatment of HIV are anticipated (per manufacturer).

Adenosine (a DEN oh seen)

U.S. Brand Names Adenocard®; Adenoscan®
Synonyms 9-Beta-D-ribofuranosyladenine
Pharmacologic Category Antiarrhythmic Agent, Class IV; Diagnostic Agent
Pregnancy Risk Factor C
Lactation Excretion in breast milk unknown
Use
Adenocard®: Treatment of paroxysmal supraventricular tachycardia (PSVT) including that associated with accessory bypass tracts (Wolff-Parkinson-White syndrome); when clinically advisable, appropriate vagal maneuvers should be attempted prior to adenosine administration; **not effective in atrial flutter, atrial fibrillation, or ventricular tachycardia**

Adenoscan®: Pharmacologic stress agent used in myocardial perfusion thallium-201 scintigraphy

Unlabeled/Investigational Use
Adenoscan®: Acute vasodilator testing in pulmonary artery hypertension

Mechanism of Action/Effect Slows conduction time through the AV node and restores normal sinus rhythm

Contraindications Hypersensitivity to adenosine or any component of the formulation; second- or third-degree AV block or sick sinus syndrome (except in patients with a functioning artificial pacemaker), atrial flutter, atrial fibrillation, and ventricular tachycardia (this drug is not effective in converting these arrhythmias to sinus rhythm). The manufacturer states that Adenoscan® should be avoided in patients with known or suspected bronchoconstrictive or bronchospastic lung disease.

Warnings/Precautions Adenosine decreases conduction through the AV node and may produce first-, second-, or third-degree heart block. Patients with pre-existing S-A nodal dysfunction may experience prolonged sinus pauses after adenosine; use caution in patients with first-degree AV block or bundle branch block; avoid use of adenosine for pharmacologic stress testing in patients with high-grade AV block or sinus node dysfunction (unless a functional pacemaker is in place). There have been reports of atrial fibrillation/flutter in patients with PSVT associated with accessory conduction pathways after adenosine. Rare, prolonged episodes of asystole have been reported, with fatal outcomes in some cases. Use caution in patients receiving other drugs which slow AV conduction (eg, digoxin, verapamil). Drugs which affect adenosine (theophylline, caffeine) should be withheld for five half-lives prior to adenosine use. Avoid dietary caffeine for 12-24 hours prior to pharmacologic stress testing.

Adenosine may also produce profound vasodilation with subsequent hypotension. When used as a bolus dose (PSVT), effects are generally self-limiting (due to the short half-life of adenosine). However, when used as a continuous infusion (pharmacologic stress testing), effects may be more pronounced and persistent, corresponding to continued exposure. Adenosine infusions should be used with caution in patients with autonomic dysfunction, stenotic valvular heart disease, pericarditis, pleural effusion, carotid stenosis (with cerebrovascular insufficiency), or uncorrected hypovolemia. Use caution in elderly patients; may be at increased risk of hemodynamic effects, bradycardia, and/or AV block.

A limited number of patients with asthma have received adenosine and have not experienced exacerbation of their asthma. Adenosine may cause bronchoconstriction in patients with asthma, and should be used cautiously in patients with obstructive lung disease not associated with bronchoconstriction (eg, emphysema, bronchitis).

Adenocard®: Transient AV block is expected. When used in PSVT, at the time of conversion to normal sinus rhythm, a variety of new rhythms may appear on the ECG. Administer as a rapid bolus, either directly into a vein or (if administered into an I.V. line), as close to the patient as possible (followed by saline flush).

Drug Interactions
Decreased Effect: Methylxanthines (eg, caffeine, theophylline) antagonize the effect of adenosine.

Increased Effect/Toxicity: Dipyridamole potentiates effects of adenosine. Use with carbamazepine may increase heart block.

Nutritional/Ethanol Interactions Food: Avoid food or drugs with caffeine. Adenosine's therapeutic effect may be decreased if used concurrently with caffeine. Avoid dietary caffeine for 12-24 hours prior to pharmacologic stress testing.

Adverse Reactions
Note: Frequency varies based on use; higher frequency of infusion-related effects, such as flushing and lightheadedness, were reported with continuous infusion (Adenoscan®).

>10%:
Cardiovascular: Facial flushing (18% to 44%)
Central nervous system: Headache (2% to 18%), lightheadedness (2% to 12%)
Neuromuscular & skeletal: Discomfort of neck, throat, jaw (<1% to 15%)
Respiratory: Dyspnea (12% to 28%), chest pressure/discomfort (7% to 40%)

1% to 10%:
Cardiovascular: Hypotension (<1% to 2%), AV block (infusion 6%; third degree <1%), ST segment depression (3%), palpitation, chest pain
Central nervous system: Dizziness, nervousness (2%), apprehension
Gastrointestinal: Nausea (3%)
Neuromuscular & skeletal: Upper extremity discomfort (up to 4%), numbness (up to 2%), paresthesia (up to 2%)
Respiratory: Hyperventilation
Miscellaneous: Diaphoresis
(Continued)

Adenosine (Continued)

Overdosage/Toxicology Since adenosine half-life is <10 seconds, adverse effects are rapidly self-limiting. Treatment of prolonged effects requires individualization. To reverse the effects of Adenoscan®, administer theophylline 50-125 mg slow I.V. push.

Pharmacodynamics/Kinetics
Onset of Action: Rapid

Duration of Action: Very brief

Half-Life Elimination: <10 seconds

Metabolism: Blood and tissue to inosine then to adenosine monophosphate (AMP) and hypoxanthine

Available Dosage Forms
Injection, solution [preservative free]: 3 mg/mL (2 mL)

Adenocard®: 3 mg/mL (2 mL, 4 mL)

Adenoscan®: 3 mg/mL (20 mL, 30 mL)

Dosing
Adults:

Paroxysmal supraventricular tachycardia (Adenocard®): I.V. (rapid - over 1-2 seconds, via peripheral line): 6 mg; if not effective within 1-2 minutes, 12 mg may be given; may repeat 12 mg bolus if needed; maximum single dose: 12 mg.

Follow each I.V. bolus of adenosine with normal saline flush.

Note: Preliminary results in adults suggest adenosine may be administered via a central line at lower doses (ie, initial adult dose: 3 mg).

Pharmacologic stress agent (Adenoscan®): I.V.: Continuous I.V. infusion via peripheral line: 140 mcg/kg/minute for 6 minutes using syringe or columetric infusion pump; total dose: 0.84 mg/kg. Thallium-201 is injected at midpoint (3 minutes) of infusion.

Acute vasodilator testing (unlabeled use) (Adenoscan®): I.V.: Initial: 50 mcg/kg/minute increased by 50 mcg/kg/minute every 2 minutes to a maximum dose of 500 mcg/kg/minute; acutely assess vasodilator response

Elderly: Refer to adult dosing. Elderly may be more sensitive to effects of adenosine.

Pediatrics:

Paroxysmal supraventricular tachycardia (Adenocard®): Rapid I.V. push (over 1-2 seconds) via peripheral line: Infants and Children (manufacturer's recommendation):

Children <50 kg: 0.05-0.1 mg/kg. If conversion of PSVT does not occur within 1-2 minutes, may increase dose by 0.05-0.1 mg/kg. May repeat until sinus rhythm is established or to a maximum single dose of 0.3 mg/kg or 12 mg. Follow each dose with normal saline flush.

Children ≥50 kg: Refer to adult dosing.

Pediatric advanced life support (PALS): Treatment of SVT: I.V., I.O.: 0.1 mg/kg; if not effective, administer 0.2 mg/kg; maximum single dose: 12 mg. Follow each dose with normal saline flush.

Renal Impairment:
Hemodialysis: Significant drug removal is unlikely based on physiochemical characteristics.

Peritoneal dialysis: Significant drug removal is unlikely based on physiochemical characteristics.

Note: Higher doses may be needed for administration via peripheral versus central vein.

Administration
I.V.: For rapid bolus I.V. use only. Administer I.V. push over 1-2 seconds at a peripheral I.V. site as proximal as possible to trunk (ie, not in lower arm, hand, lower leg, or foot). If administered into an I.V. line, administer as close to the patient's heart as possible (followed by saline flush).

I.V. Detail: Do not mix with any other drugs in syringe or solution.

Stability
Compatibility: Stable in D₅LR, D₅W, LR, NS

Storage: Store at controlled room temperature of 15°C to 30°C (59°F to 86°F). Do **not** refrigerate; precipitation may occur (may dissolve by warming to room temperature).

Nursing Actions
Physical Assessment: Assess other medications patient may be taking for effectiveness and interactions. Requires use of infusion pump and continuous cardiac and hemodynamic monitoring during infusion. Monitor for adverse reactions. Note that adenosine could produce bronchoconstriction in patients with asthma.

Patient Education: Adenosine is administered in emergencies; patient education should be appropriate to the situation. May cause facial flushing. Report chest pain or pressure, difficulty breathing immediately. **Pregnancy precautions:** Inform prescriber if you are pregnant.

Dietary Considerations Avoid dietary caffeine for 12-24 hours prior to pharmacologic stress testing.

Geriatric Considerations Geriatric patients may be more sensitive to the effects of this medication.

Other Issues Confirm labeling before administration. **Do not use adenosine phosphate (given I.M. for symptomatic relief of varicose veins complications). Have emergency resuscitation and equipment available when using this drug.**

Albendazole (al BEN da zole)

U.S. Brand Names Albenza®

Pharmacologic Category Anthelmintic

Pregnancy Risk Factor C

Lactation Excretion in breast milk unknown/not recommended

Use Treatment of parenchymal neurocysticercosis caused by *Taenia solium* and cystic hydatid disease of the liver, lung, and peritoneum caused by *Echinococcus granulosus*

Unlabeled/Investigational Use Albendazole has activity against *Ascaris lumbricoides* (roundworm); *Ancylostoma caninum*; *Ancylostoma duodenale* and *Necator americanus* (hookworms); cutaneous larva migrans; *Enterobius vermicularis* (pinworm); *Gnathostoma spinigerum*; *Gongylonema* sp; *Hymenolepis nana* sp (tapeworms); *Mansonella perstans* (filariasis); *Opisthorchis sinensis* and *Opisthorchis viverrini* (liver flukes); *Strongyloides stercoralis* and *Trichuris trichiura* (whipworm); visceral larva migrans (toxocariasis); activity has also been shown against the liver fluke *Clonorchis sinensis*, *Giardia lamblia*, *Cysticercus cellulosae*, and *Echinococcus multilocularis*. Albendazole has also been used for the treatment of intestinal microsporidiosis (*Encephalitozoon intestinalis*), disseminated microsporidiosis (*E. hellem*, *E. cuniculi*, *E. intestinalis*, *Pleistophora* sp, *Trachipleistophora* sp, *Brachiola vesicularum*), and ocular microsporidiosis (*E. hellem*, *E. cuniculi*, *Vittaforma corneae*).

Mechanism of Action/Effect Active metabolite, albendazole, causes selective degeneration of cytoplasmic microtubules in intestinal and tegmental cells of intestinal helminths and larvae; glycogen is depleted, glucose uptake and cholinesterase secretion are impaired, and desecratory substances accumulate intracellular. ATP production decreases causing energy depletion, immobilization, and worm death.

Contraindications Hypersensitivity to albendazole or any component of the formulation

Warnings/Precautions Discontinue therapy if LFT elevations are significant; may restart treatment when decreased to pretreatment values. Becoming pregnant within 1 month following therapy is not advised.

Neurocysticercosis: Corticosteroids should be administered 1-2 days before albendazole therapy to minimize inflammatory reactions. Steroid and anticonvulsant therapy should be used concurrently during the first week of therapy to prevent cerebral hypertension. If retinal lesions exist, weigh risk of further retinal damage due to albendazole-induced changes to the retinal lesion vs benefit of disease treatment.

Drug Interactions
Cytochrome P450 Effect: Substrate (minor) of CYP1A2, 3A4; **Inhibits** CYP1A2 (weak)

Nutritional/Ethanol Interactions Food: Albendazole serum levels may be increased if taken with a fatty meal (increases the oral bioavailability by 4-5 times).

Adverse Reactions
N = Neurocysticercosis; H = Hydatid disease

>10%:
Central nervous system: Headache (11% - N; 1% - H)
Hepatic: LFTs increased (~15% - H; <1% - N)

1% to 10%:
Central nervous system: Dizziness, vertigo, fever (≤1%), intracranial pressure increased (1% - N), meningeal signs (1% - N)
Dermatologic: Alopecia (2% - H; <1% - N)
Gastrointestinal: Abdominal pain (6% - H; 0% - N), nausea/vomiting (3% to 6%)
Hematologic: Leukopenia (reversible) (<1%)
Miscellaneous: Allergic reactions (<1%)

Pharmacodynamics/Kinetics
Time to Peak: Serum: 2-2.4 hours
Protein Binding: 70%
Half-Life Elimination: 8-12 hours
Metabolism: Hepatic; extensive first-pass effect; pathways include rapid sulfoxidation (major), hydrolysis, and oxidation
Excretion: Urine (<1% as active metabolite); feces

Available Dosage Forms Tablet: 200 mg

Dosing
Adults & Elderly:
Neurocysticercosis: Oral:
<60 kg: 15 mg/kg/day in 2 divided doses (maximum: 800 mg/day) for 8-30 days
≥60 kg: 400 mg twice daily for 8-30 days
Note: Give concurrent anticonvulsant and steroid therapy during first week.

Hydatid: Oral:
<60 kg: 15 mg/kg/day in 2 divided doses (maximum: 800 mg/day)
≥60 kg: 400 mg twice daily
Note: Administer dose for three 28-day cycles with a 14-day drug-free interval in between.

Ancylostoma caninum, Ascaris lumbricoides (roundworm), ***Ancylostoma duodenale*, and *Necator americanus* (hookworms) (unlabeled use):** Oral: 400 mg as a single dose

***Clonorchis sinensis* (Chinese liver fluke) (unlabeled use):** Oral: 10 mg/kg for 7 days

Cutaneous larva migrans (unlabeled use): Oral: 400 mg once daily for 3 days

***Enterobius vermicularis* (pinworm) (unlabeled use):** Oral: 400 mg as a single dose; may repeat in 2 weeks

***Gnathostoma spinigerum* (unlabeled use):** Oral: 400 mg twice daily for 21 days

Gongylonemiasis (unlabeled use): Oral: 10 mg/kg/day for 3 days

***Mansonella perstans* (unlabeled use):** Oral: 400 mg twice daily for 10 days

Visceral larva migrans (toxocariasis) (unlabeled use): Oral: 400 mg twice daily for 5 days

***Cysticercus cellulosae* (unlabeled use):** Oral: 400 mg twice daily for 8-30 days; may be repeated as necessary

Disseminated microsporidiosis (unlabeled use): Oral: 400 mg twice daily

***Echinococcus granulosus* (tapeworm) (unlabeled use):** Oral: 400 mg twice daily for 1-6 months

Intestinal microsporidiosis (unlabeled use): Oral: 400 mg twice daily for 21 days

Ocular microsporidiosis (unlabeled use): Oral: 400 mg twice daily, in combination with fumagillin

Pediatrics:

Neurocysticercosis: Oral: Refer to adult dosing.

Hydatid: Oral: Refer to adult dosing.

***Cysticercus cellulosae* (unlabeled use):** Oral: 15 mg/kg/day (maximum: 800 mg/day) in 2 divided doses for 8-30 days; may be repeated as necessary

***Echinococcus granulosus* (tapeworm) (unlabeled use):** Oral: 15 mg/kg/day (maximum: 800 mg) divided twice daily for 1-6 months

For the following unlabeled uses, refer to adult dosing:

Ancylostoma caninum, Ascaris lumbricoides (roundworm), *Ancylostoma duodenale, Clonorchis sinensis,* (Chinese liver fluke), cutaneous larva migrans, *Enterobius vermicularis* (pinworm), *Gnathostoma spinigerum,* gongylonemiasis, *Mansonella perstans, Necator americanus* (hookworms), visceral larva migrans (toxocariasis)

Administration
Oral: Administer with meals; administer anticonvulsant and steroid therapy during first week of neurocysticercosis therapy

Laboratory Monitoring Monitor fecal specimens for ova and parasites for 3 weeks after treatment; if positive, retreat; monitor LFTs and clinical signs of hepatotoxicity; CBC at start of each 28-day cycle and every 2 weeks during therapy

Nursing Actions
Physical Assessment: Pretreatment may be recommended. Monitor laboratory tests (reduction or elimination of ova and parasites) and adverse reactions (eg, elevated LFTs, leukopenia). Teach patient appropriate use, possible side effects/appropriate interventions, and adverse symptoms to report.

Patient Education: You may be prescribed other medications to take during first week of therapy. Do not take any other new medication during therapy unless approved by prescriber. Laboratory tests may be required; maintain recommended schedule. Take as directed, with a high-fat meal. Follow prescriber's suggestions to prevent reinfection. May cause loss of hair (reversible); nausea or vomiting (small, frequent meals, frequent mouth care, sucking lozenges, or chewing gum may help); or dizziness or headaches (use caution when driving or engaging in tasks that require alertness until response to drug is known). Report unusual fever, persistent or unresolved abdominal pain, vomiting, yellowing of skin or eyes, darkening of urine, or light colored stools. **Pregnancy/breast-feeding precautions:** Inform prescriber if you are or intend to become pregnant. Breast-feeding is not recommended. Becoming pregnant within 1 month following therapy is not advised.

Dietary Considerations Should be taken with a high-fat meal.

Pregnancy Issues Albendazole has been shown to be teratogenic in laboratory animals and should not be used during pregnancy, if at all possible. Women should be advised to avoid pregnancy for at least 1 month following therapy. Discontinue if pregnancy occurs during treatment.

Albumin (al BYOO min)

U.S. Brand Names Albumarc®; Albuminar®; Albutein®; Buminate®; Flexbumin; Plasbumin®

Synonyms Albumin (Human); Normal Human Serum Albumin; Normal Serum Albumin (Human); Salt Poor Albumin; SPA

Pharmacologic Category Blood Product Derivative; Plasma Volume Expander, Colloid

Medication Safety Issues
Sound-alike/look-alike issues:
Albutein® may be confused with albuterol
Buminate® may be confused with bumetanide

Pregnancy Risk Factor C

Lactation Excretion in breast milk unknown/compatible

Use Plasma volume expansion and maintenance of cardiac output in the treatment of certain types of shock or impending shock; may be useful for burn patients, ARDS, and cardiopulmonary bypass; other uses considered by some investigators (but not proven) are retroperitoneal surgery, peritonitis, and ascites; unless the condition responsible for hypoproteinemia can be corrected, albumin can provide only symptomatic relief or supportive treatment

Unlabeled/Investigational Use In cirrhotics, administered with diuretics to help facilitate diuresis; large volume paracentesis; volume expansion in dehydrated, mildly-hypotensive cirrhotics

Mechanism of Action/Effect Restores plasma volume

Contraindications Hypersensitivity to albumin or any component of the formulation; patients with severe anemia or cardiac failure

Warnings/Precautions Use with caution in patients with hepatic or renal failure because of added protein load; rapid infusion of albumin solutions may cause vascular overload. All patients should be observed for signs of hypervolemia such as pulmonary edema. Use with caution in those patients for whom sodium restriction is necessary. Avoid 25% concentration in preterm infants due to risk of intraventricular hemorrhage. Nutritional supplementation is not an appropriate indication for albumin.

Drug Interactions
Increased Effect/Toxicity: ACE inhibitors: May have increased risk of atypical reactions; withhold ACEIs for at least 24 hours prior to plasma exchanges using large volumes of albumin

Adverse Reactions Frequency not defined.
Cardiovascular: CHF precipitation, edema, hyper-/hypotension, hypervolemia, tachycardia
Central nervous system: Chills, fever, headache
Dermatologic: Pruritus, rash, urticaria
Gastrointestinal: Nausea, vomiting
Respiratory: Bronchospasm, pulmonary edema
Miscellaneous: Anaphylaxis

Overdosage/Toxicology Symptoms of overdose include hypervolemia, congestive heart failure, and pulmonary edema.

Available Dosage Forms
Injection, solution, human [preservative free]: 5% [50 mg/mL] (50 mL, 250 mL, 500 mL) [contains sodium 130-160 mEq/L]; 25% [250 mg/mL] (50 mL, 100 mL) [contains sodium 130-160 mEq/L]
Albumarc®: 5% [50 mg/mL] (250 mL, 500 mL) [contains sodium 130-160 mEq/L]; 25% [250 mg/mL] (50 mL, 100 mL) [contains sodium 130-160 mEq/L]
Albuminar®: 5% [50 mg/mL] (50 mL, 250 mL, 500 mL, 1000 mL) [contains sodium 130-160 mEq/L]; 25% [250 mg/mL] (20 mL, 50 mL, 100 mL) [contains sodium 130-160 mEq/L]
Albutein®, Buminate®: 5% [50 mg/mL] (250 mL, 500 mL) [contains sodium 130-160 mEq/L]; 25% [250 mg/mL] (20 mL, 50 mL, 100 mL) [contains sodium 130-160 mEq/L]

Flexbumin: 25% [250 mg/mL] (50 mL, 100 mL) [contains sodium 130-160 mEq/L]
Plasbumin®: 5% [50 mg/mL] (50 mL, 250 mL, 500 mL) [contains sodium ~145 mEq/L]; 25% [250 mg/mL] (20 mL, 50 mL, 100 mL) [contains sodium ~145 mEq/L]

Dosing
Adults & Elderly:
Note: Use 5% solution in hypovolemic patients or intravascularly-depleted patients. Use 25% solution in patients in whom fluid and sodium intake is restricted.
Usual dose: 25 g; initial dose may be repeated in 15-30 minutes if response is inadequate; no more than 250 g should be administered within 48 hours.
Hypoproteinemia: I.V.: 0.5-1 g/kg/dose; repeat every 1-2 days as calculated to replace ongoing losses.
Hypovolemia: I.V.: 0.5-1 g/kg/dose; repeat as needed; maximum: 6 g/kg/day

Pediatrics:
Note: 5% should be used in hypovolemic patients or intravascularly-depleted patients. 25% should be used in patients in whom fluid and sodium intake must be minimized.
Dose depends on condition of patient: Hypovolemia: I.V.: 0.5-1 g/kg/dose (10-20 mL/kg/dose of albumin 5%); maximum dose: 6 g/kg/day

Administration
I.V.: For I.V. administration only. Use within 4 hours after opening vial; discard unused portion. In emergencies, may administer as rapidly as necessary to improve clinical condition. After initial volume replacement:
5%: Do not exceed 2-4 mL/minute in patients with normal plasma volume; 5-10 mL/minute in patients with hypoproteinemia
25%: Do not exceed 1 mL/minute in patients with normal plasma volume; 2-3 mL/minute in patients with hypoproteinemia
I.V. Detail: Do not dilute 5% solution. Rapid infusion may cause vascular overload. Albumin 25% may be given undiluted or diluted in normal saline. May give in combination or through the same administration set as saline or carbohydrates. Do not use with ethanol or protein hydrolysates, precipitation may form.

pH: 6.4-7.4

Stability
Reconstitution: If 5% human albumin is unavailable, it may be prepared by diluting 25% human albumin with 0.9% sodium chloride or 5% dextrose in water. Do not use sterile water to dilute albumin solutions, as this has been associated with hypotonic-associated hemolysis.
Compatibility: Stable in dextran 6% in D_5W, dextran 6% in NS, D_5LR, D_5NS, D_5-1/2NS, $D_5$1/4NS, D_5W, $D_{10}W$, LR, NS, 1/2NS; incompatible with sterile water
Y-site administration: Incompatible with midazolam, vancomycin, verapamil
Compatibility when admixed: Incompatible with verapamil
Storage: Store at a temperature ≤30°C (86°F); do not freeze. Do not use solution if it is turbid or contains a deposit; use within 4 hours after opening vial; discard unused portion.

Laboratory Monitoring Hematocrit

Nursing Actions
Physical Assessment: Monitor patient closely for pulmonary edema and cardiac failure (vital signs, central venous pressure) during administration, with frequent assessment for hypovolemia or fluid overload. If adverse reactions (eg, fever, tachycardia, hypotension, or dyspnea) occur, stop infusion and notify prescriber. Teach patient adverse symptoms to report.

Patient Education: Education is provided as appropriate for patient condition. This medication can only be administered intravenously. You will be monitored closely during the infusion. Report immediately any pain or bruising at infusion site, acute headache, difficulty breathing, chills, chest pain or tightness, palpitations, or sudden pain. **Pregnancy precaution:** Inform prescriber if you are pregnant.

Dietary Considerations
Albumarc®, Albuminar®, Albutein®, Buminate®, Flexbumin: 5% [50 mg/mL] and 25% [250 mg/mL] contain sodium 130-160 mEq/L]
Plasbumin®: 5%[50 mg/mL] and 25% [250 mg/mL] contain sodium ~145 mEq/L

Additional Information Albumin 5% and 25% solutions contain 130-160 mEq/L sodium and are considered isotonic with plasma. Dilution of albumin 25% solution with sterile water produces a hypotonic solution; administration of such can cause hemolysis and/or renal failure. An albumin 5% solution is osmotically equivalent to an equal volume of plasma, whereas a 25% solution is osmotically equivalent to 5 times its volume of plasma. Albumin solutions are heated to 60°C for 10 hours, decreasing any possible risk of viral hepatitis transmission. To date, there have been no reports of viral transmission using these products.

Albuterol (al BYOO ter ole)

U.S. Brand Names AccuNeb™; Proventil®; Proventil® HFA; Ventolin® HFA; VoSpire ER®
Synonyms Albuterol Sulfate; Salbutamol
Pharmacologic Category Beta₂-Adrenergic Agonist
Medication Safety Issues
Sound-alike/look-alike issues:
Albuterol may be confused with Albutein®, atenolol
Proventil® may be confused with Bentyl®, Prilosec® Prinivil®
Salbutamol may be confused with salmeterol
Ventolin® may be confused with phentolamine, Benlysta®, Vantin®
Volmax® may be confused with Flomax®

Pregnancy Risk Factor C
Lactation Excretion in breast milk unknown/use caution
Use Bronchodilator in reversible airway obstruction due to asthma or COPD; prevention of exercise-induced bronchospasm
Mechanism of Action/Effect Relaxes bronchial smooth muscle by action on beta₂-receptors with little effect on heart rate
Contraindications Hypersensitivity to albuterol, adrenergic amines, or any component of the formulation
Warnings/Precautions Optimize anti-inflammatory treatment before initiating maintenance treatment with albuterol. Do not use as a component of chronic therapy without an anti-inflammatory agent. Only the mildest forms of asthma (Step 1 and/or exercise-induced) would not require concurrent use based upon asthma guidelines. Patient must be instructed to seek medical attention in cases where acute symptoms are not relieved or a previous level of response is diminished. The need to increase frequency of use may indicate deterioration of asthma, and treatment must not be delayed.

Use caution in patients with cardiovascular disease (arrhythmia or hypertension or CHF), convulsive disorders, diabetes, glaucoma, hyperthyroidism, or hypokalemia. Beta agonists may cause elevation in blood pressure, heart rate, and result in CNS stimulation/excitation. Beta₂ agonists may increase risk of arrhythmia, increase serum glucose, or decrease serum potassium.

Do not exceed recommended dose; serious adverse events, including fatalities, have been associated with excessive use of inhaled sympathomimetics. Rarely, paradoxical bronchospasm may occur with use of inhaled bronchodilating agents; this should be distinguished from inadequate response. All patients should utilize a spacer device when using a metered-dose inhaler; in addition, face masks should be used in children <4 years of age.

Because of its minimal effect on beta₁-receptors and its relatively long duration of action, albuterol is a rational choice in the elderly when an inhaled beta agonist is indicated. Oral use should be avoided in the elderly due to adverse effects. Patient response may vary between inhalers that contain chlorofluorocarbons and those which are chlorofluorocarbon-free.

Drug Interactions
Cytochrome P450 Effect: Substrate of CYP3A4 (major)
Decreased Effect: When used with nonselective beta-adrenergic blockers (eg, propranolol) the effect of albuterol is decreased. Levels/effects of albuterol may be decreased by aminoglutethimide, carbamazepine, nafcillin, nevirapine, phenobarbital, phenytoin, rifamycins, and other CYP3A4 inducers.
Increased Effect/Toxicity: When used with inhaled ipratropium, an increased duration of bronchodilation may occur. Cardiovascular effects are potentiated in patients also receiving MAO inhibitors, tricyclic antidepressants, and sympathomimetic agents (eg, amphetamine, dopamine, dobutamine). Albuterol may increase the risk of malignant arrhythmias with inhaled anesthetics (eg, enflurane, halothane).

Nutritional/Ethanol Interactions
Food: Avoid or limit caffeine (may cause CNS stimulation).
Herb/Nutraceutical: Avoid ephedra, yohimbe (may cause CNS stimulation).

Lab Interactions Increased renin (S), aldosterone (S)
Adverse Reactions Incidence of adverse effects is dependent upon age of patient, dose, and route of administration.
Cardiovascular: Angina, atrial fibrillation, chest discomfort, extrasystoles, flushing, hypertension, palpitation, tachycardia
Central nervous system: CNS stimulation, dizziness, drowsiness, headache, insomnia, irritability, lightheadedness, migraine, nervousness, nightmares, restlessness, sleeplessness, tremor
Dermatologic: Angioedema, erythema multiforme, rash, Stevens-Johnson syndrome, urticaria
Endocrine & metabolic: Hypokalemia, serum glucose increased, serum potassium decreased
Gastrointestinal: Diarrhea, dry mouth, gastroenteritis, nausea, unusual taste, vomiting, tooth discoloration
Genitourinary: Micturition difficulty
Neuromuscular & skeletal: Muscle cramps, weakness
Otic: Otitis media, vertigo
Respiratory: Asthma exacerbation, bronchospasm, cough, epistaxis, laryngitis, oropharyngeal drying/irritation, oropharyngeal edema
Miscellaneous: Allergic reaction, lymphadenopathy

Overdosage/Toxicology Symptoms of overdose include tachycardia, tremor, hypertension, angina, and seizures. Hypokalemia also may occur. Cardiac arrest and death may be associated with abuse of beta-agonist bronchodilators. Treatment includes immediate discontinuation and symptomatic and supportive therapies. Cautious use of beta-adrenergic blocking agents may be considered in severe cases.

Pharmacodynamics/Kinetics
Onset of Action: Peak effect:
Nebulization/oral inhalation: 0.5-2 hours
CFC-propelled albuterol: 10 minutes
Ventolin® HFA: 25 minutes
Oral: 2-3 hours
Duration of Action: Nebulization/oral inhalation: 3-4 hours; Oral: 4-6 hours
Half-Life Elimination: Inhalation: 3.8 hours; Oral: 3.7-5 hours
(Continued)

Albuterol *(Continued)*

Metabolism: Hepatic to an inactive sulfate

Excretion: Urine (30% as unchanged drug)

Available Dosage Forms

Aerosol, for oral inhalation: 90 mcg/dose (17 g) [200 doses; contains chlorofluorocarbons]

Proventil®: 90 mcg/dose (17 g) [200 doses; contains chlorofluorocarbons]

Aerosol, for oral inhalation: 90 mcg/dose (6.7 g) [200 doses; chlorofluorocarbon free]

Proventil® HFA: 90 mcg/dose (6.7 g) [200 doses; chlorofluorocarbon free]

Ventolin® HFA: 90 mcg/dose (18 g) [200 doses; chlorofluorocarbon free]

Solution for nebulization: 0.083% (3 mL); 0.5% (20 mL)

AccuNeb™: 0.63 mg/3 mL (3 mL); 1.25 mg/3 mL (3 mL)

Proventil®: 0.083% (3 mL); 0.5% (20 mL)

Syrup, as sulfate: 2 mg/5 mL (480 mL)

Tablet: 2 mg, 4 mg

Tablet, extended release:

VoSpire ER®: 4 mg, 8 mg

Dosing

Adults:

Acute treatment of bronchospasm:

Inhalation: MDI 90 mcg/puff: 4-8 puffs every 20 minutes for up to 4 hours, then every 1-4 hours as needed

Nebulization: 2.5 mg, diluted to a total of 3 mL, 3-4 times/day over 5-15 minutes

NIH guidelines: 1.25-5 mg every 4-8 hours

Bronchospasm in ICU patients (acute):

Nebulization: 2.5-5 mg every 20 minutes for 3 doses, then 2.5-10 mg every 1-4 hours as needed, **or** 10-15 mg/hour continuously

Chronic treatment of bronchospasm:

Inhalation: MDI 90 mcg/puff: 1-2 inhalations every 4-6 hours; maximum: 12 inhalations/day

NIH guidelines: 2 puffs 3-4 times a day as needed; may double dose for mild exacerbations

Oral:

Regular release: 2-4 mg/dose 3-4 times/day; maximum dose not to exceed 32 mg/day (divided doses)

Extended release: 8 mg every 12 hours; maximum dose not to exceed 32 mg/day (divided doses). A 4 mg dose every 12 hours may be sufficient in some patients, such as adults of low body weight.

Prophylaxis of exercise-induced bronchospasm:

Inhalation: MDI 90 mcg/puff: 2 puffs 5-30 minutes prior to exercise

Elderly:

Inhalation: Refer to adult dosing.

Bronchospasm (treatment): Oral: 2 mg 3-4 times/day; maximum: 8 mg 4 times/day

Pediatrics:

Bronchospasm (acute):

Inhalation: MDI 90 mcg/puff:

Children ≤12 years: 4-8 puffs every 20 minutes for 3 doses, then every 1-4 hours; spacer/holding-chamber device should be used

Children >12 years: Refer to adult dosing.

Nebulization:

Children ≤12 years: Solution 0.5%: 0.15 mg/kg (minimum dose: 2.5 mg) every 20 minutes for 3 doses, then 0.15-0.3 mg/kg (up to 10 mg) every 1-4 hours as needed; may also use 0.5 mg/kg/hour by continuous infusion. Continuous nebulized albuterol at 0.3 mg/kg/hour has been used safely in the treatment of severe status asthmaticus in children; continuous nebulized doses of 3 mg/kg/hour ± 2.2 mg/kg/hour in children whose mean age was 20.7 months resulted in no cardiac toxicity; the optimal dosage for continuous nebulization remains to be determined.

Children >12 years: Refer to adult dosing.

Prophylaxis of exercise-induced bronchospasm:

Inhalation: MDI 90 mcg/puff:

Children ≤12 years: 1-2 puffs 5 minutes prior to exercise

Children >12 years: Refer to adult dosing.

Chronic treatment of bronchospasm:

Inhalation: MDI 90 mcg/puff: Children ≥4 years: Refer to adult dosing.

Oral:

Children: 2-6 years: 0.1-0.2 mg/kg/dose 3 times/day; maximum dose not to exceed 12 mg/day (divided doses)

Children: 6-12 years: 2 mg/dose 3-4 times/day; maximum dose not to exceed 24 mg/day (divided doses)

Extended release: 4 mg every 12 hours; maximum dose not to exceed 24 mg/day (divided doses)

Children >12 years: Refer to adult dosing.

Nebulization:

Children ≤12 years: 0.05 mg/kg every 4-6 hours; minimum dose: 1.25 mg, maximum dose: 2.5 mg

2-12 years: AccuNeb™: 0.63 mg or 1.25 mg 3-4 times/day, as needed, delivered over 5-15 minutes

Note: Use of the 0.5% solution should be used for bronchospasm (acute or treatment) in children <15 kg.

Children >40 kg, patients with more severe asthma, or children 11-12 years: May respond better with a 1.25 mg dose

Children >12 years: Refer to adult dosing.

Renal Impairment: Not removed by hemodialysis

Administration

Oral: Do not crush or chew extended release tablets.

Inhalation: MDI: Shake well before use; prime prior to first use, and whenever inhaler has not been used for >2 weeks or when it has been dropped, by releasing 4 test sprays into the air (away from face)

Stability

Reconstitution: Nebulization 0.5% solution: To prepare a 2.5 mg dose, dilute 0.5 mL of solution to a total of 3 mL with normal saline; also compatible with cromolyn or ipratropium nebulizer solutions.

Storage:

Syrup, nebulization 0.5% solution: Store at 2°C to 30°C (36°F to 86°F)

HFA aerosols: Store at 15°C to 25°C (59°F to 77°F)

Ventolin® HFA: Discard after using 200 actuations or 3 months after removal from protective pouch, whichever comes first. Store with mouthpiece down.

Inhalation solution: AccuNeb™: Store at 2°C to 25°C (36°F to 77°F). Do not use if solution changes color or becomes cloudy. Use within 1 week of opening foil pouch.

Laboratory Monitoring Arterial or capillary blood gases (if patients condition warrants); FEV$_1$, peak flow, and/or other pulmonary function tests; serum potassium, serum glucose (in selected patients)

Nursing Actions

Physical Assessment: Assess effectiveness and interactions of other medications patient may be taking. Monitor effectiveness of therapy (relief of airway obstruction) and adverse reactions (eg, cardiac and CNS changes; see Adverse Reactions) at beginning of therapy and periodically with long-term use. For inpatient care, monitor vital signs and lung sounds prior to and periodically during therapy. Assess knowledge/teach patient appropriate use, interventions to reduce side effects, and adverse symptoms to report.

Patient Education: Use exactly as directed; do not use more often than recommended. Take oral medicine with water 1 hour before or 2 hours after meals. Maintain adequate hydration (2-3 L/day of fluids) unless instructed to restrict fluid intake. You may experience nervousness, dizziness, or fatigue (use caution when driving or engaging in hazardous activities until response to drug is known); dry mouth, unpleasant taste, stomach upset (frequent, small meals, frequent mouth care, chewing gum, or sucking lozenges may help); or difficulty urinating (always void before treatment). Report unresolved GI upset, dizziness or fatigue, vision changes, chest pain or palpitations, persistent inability to void, nervousness or insomnia, muscle cramping or tremor, or unusual cough.

Self-administered inhalation: Do not freeze. Shake canister before using. Sit when using medication. Close eyes when administering albuterol to avoid spray getting into eyes. Exhale slowly and completely through nose; inhale deeply through mouth while administering aerosol. Hold breath for 5-10 seconds after inhalation. Wait at least 1 full minute between inhalations. Wash mouthpiece between use. If more than one inhalation medication is used, use albuterol first and wait 5 minutes between medications. Prime inhaler prior to first use, and whenever the inhaler has not been used for more than 2 weeks, by releasing 4 test sprays into the air (away from face). Discard inhaler after labeled number of doses are used, even if the canister does not feel empty. **Ventolin® HFA:** Discard canister after 200 actuations or 3 months after removal from foil pouch, whichever comes first. Store with mouthpiece down. Do not allow metal canister to become wet.

Self-administered nebulizer: Wash hands before and after treatment. Wash and dry nebulizer after each treatment. Twist open the top of one unit-dose vial and squeeze contents into nebulizer reservoir. Connect nebulizer reservoir to the mouthpiece or face mask. Connect nebulizer to compressor. Sit in comfortable, upright position. Place mouthpiece in your mouth or put on face mask and turn on compressor. If face mask is used, avoid leakage around the mask to avoid mist getting into eyes which may cause vision problems. Breathe calmly and deeply until no more mist is formed in nebulizer (about 5 minutes). At this point, treatment is finished.

Volmax®: Tablets should be swallowed whole; do not crush or chew. Outer coating of tablet is not absorbed and may be found eliminated in stool.

Dietary Considerations Oral forms should be administered with water 1 hour before or 2 hours after meals.

Geriatric Considerations Because of its minimal effect on beta$_1$-receptors and its relatively long duration of action, albuterol is a rational choice in the elderly when a beta agonist is indicated. Elderly patients may find it beneficial to utilize a spacer device when using a metered dose inhaler. The Ventolin Rotahaler® is an alternative for patients who have difficulty using the metered dose inhaler. Oral use should be avoided due to adverse effects.

Pregnancy Issues Albuterol crosses the placenta; tocolytic effects, fetal tachycardia, fetal hypoglycemia secondary to maternal hyperglycemia with oral or intravenous routes reported. Available evidence suggests safe use during pregnancy.

Aldesleukin (al des LOO kin)

U.S. Brand Names Proleukin®

Synonyms Epidermal Thymocyte Activating Factor; ETAF; IL-2; Interleukin-2; Lymphocyte Mitogenic Factor; NSC-373364; T-Cell Growth Factor; TCGF; Thymocyte Stimulating Factor

Pharmacologic Category Biological Response Modulator

Medication Safety Issues
Sound-alike/look-alike issues:
Aldesleukin may be confused with oprelvekin
Proleukin® may be confused with oprelvekin

Pregnancy Risk Factor C

Lactation Enters breast milk/contraindicated

Use Treatment of metastatic renal cell cancer, melanoma

Unlabeled/Investigational Use Investigational: Multiple myeloma, HIV infection, and AIDS; may be used in conjunction with lymphokine-activated killer (LAK) cells, tumor-infiltrating lymphocyte (TIL) cells, interleukin-1, and interferons; colorectal cancer; non-Hodgkin's lymphoma

Mechanism of Action/Effect Aldesleukin promotes proliferation, differentiation, and recruitment of T and B cells, natural killer (NK) cells, and thymocytes; causes cytolytic activity in a subset of lymphocytes and subsequent interactions between the immune system and malignant cells; can stimulate lymphokine-activated killer (LAK) cells and tumor-infiltrating lymphocytes (TIL) cells.

Contraindications Hypersensitivity to aldesleukin or any component of the formulation; patients with abnormal thallium stress or pulmonary function tests; patients who have had an organ allograft; retreatment in patients who have experienced sustained ventricular tachycardia (≥5 beats), refractory cardiac rhythm disturbances, recurrent chest pain with ECG changes consistent with angina or myocardial infarction, intubation ≥72 hours, pericardial tamponade, renal dialysis for ≥72 hours, coma or toxic psychosis lasting ≥48 hours, repetitive or refractory seizures, bowel ischemia/perforation, GI bleeding requiring surgery

Warnings/Precautions Hazardous agent - use appropriate precautions for handling and disposal. Has been associated with capillary leak syndrome (CLS) resulting in hypotension and reduced organ perfusion which may be severe and can result in death. Therapy should be restricted to patients with normal cardiac and pulmonary functions as defined by thallium stress and formal pulmonary function testing. Extreme caution should be used in patients with a history of prior cardiac or pulmonary disease.

May exacerbate pre-existing or initial presentation of autoimmune diseases and inflammatory disorders. Patients should be evaluated and treated for CNS metastases and have a negative scan prior to treatment. Mental status changes (irritability, confusion, depression) can occur and may indicate bacteremia, hypoperfusion, CNS malignancy, or CNS toxicity.

Drug Interactions

Decreased Effect: Corticosteroids have been shown to decrease toxicity of aldesleukin, but may reduce the efficacy of the lymphokine.

Increased Effect/Toxicity: Aldesleukin may affect central nervous system; therefore, interactions could occur following concomitant administration of psychotropic drugs (eg, narcotics, analgesics, antiemetics, sedatives, tranquilizers).

Concomitant administration of drugs possessing nephrotoxic (eg, aminoglycosides, indomethacin), myelotoxic (eg, cytotoxic chemotherapy), cardiotoxic (eg, doxorubicin), or hepatotoxic effects with aldesleukin may increase toxicity in these organ systems.
(Continued)

Aldesleukin *(Continued)*

Beta-blockers and other antihypertensives may potentiate the hypotension seen with aldesleukin.

Nutritional/Ethanol Interactions Ethanol: May increase CNS adverse effects.

Adverse Reactions

>10%:

Cardiovascular: Hypotension (85%), dose-limiting, possibly fatal; sinus tachycardia (70%); arrhythmia (22%); edema (47%); angina

Central nervous system: Mental status changes (transient memory loss, confusion, drowsiness) (73%); dizziness (17%); cognitive changes, fatigue, malaise, somnolence, and disorientation (25%); headaches; insomnia; paranoid delusion

Dermatologic: Macular erythematous rash (100% of patients on high-dose therapy), pruritus (48%), erythema (41%), rash (26%), exfoliative dermatitis (14%), dry skin (15%)

Endocrine & metabolic: Fever and chills (89%), electrolyte levels decreased (magnesium, calcium, phosphate, potassium, sodium) (1% to 15%)

Gastrointestinal: Nausea and vomiting (87%), diarrhea (76%), stomatitis (32%), GI bleeding (13%), weight gain (23%), anorexia (27%)

Hematologic: Anemia (77%), thrombocytopenia (64%), leukopenia (34%) - may be dose-limiting, coagulation disorders (10%)

Hepatic: Transient elevations of bilirubin (64%) and enzymes (56%), jaundice (11%)

Neuromuscular & skeletal: Weakness; rigors - respond to acetaminophen, diphenhydramine, an NSAID, or meperidine

Renal: Oliguria/anuria (63%, severe in 5% to 6%); proteinuria (12%); renal failure (dose-limiting toxicity) manifested as oliguria noted within 24-48 hours of initiation of therapy; marked fluid retention, azotemia, and increased serum creatinine seen, which may return to baseline within 7 days of discontinuation of therapy; hypophosphatemia

Respiratory: Congestion (54%), dyspnea (27% to 52%)

Miscellaneous: Pain (54%), infection (including sepsis and endocarditis) due to neutrophil impairment (23%)

1% to 10%:

Cardiovascular: Capillary leak syndrome, including peripheral edema, ascites, pulmonary infiltration, and pleural effusion (2% to 4%), may be dose-limiting and potentially fatal; MI (2%)

Central nervous system: Seizures (1%)

Endocrine & metabolic: Hypo- and hyperglycemia (2%), electrolyte levels increased (magnesium, calcium, phosphate, potassium, sodium) (1%), hypothyroidism

Hepatic: Ascites (4%)

Neuromuscular & skeletal: Arthralgia (6%), myalgia (6%)

Renal: Hematuria (9%), creatinine increased (5%)

Respiratory: Pleural effusions, edema (10%)

Overdosage/Toxicology Side effects following the use of aldesleukin are dose related. Administration of more than the recommended dose has been associated with a more rapid onset of expected dose-limiting toxicities. Adverse reactions generally will reverse when the drug is stopped, particularly because of its short serum half-life. Provide supportive treatment of any continuing symptoms. Life-threatening toxicities have been ameliorated by the I.V. administration of dexamethasone, but may decrease the therapeutic effect of aldesleukin.

Pharmacodynamics/Kinetics

Half-Life Elimination: Initial: 6-13 minutes; Terminal: 80-120 minutes

Available Dosage Forms Injection, powder for reconstitution: 22 x 10^6 int. units [18 million int. units/mL = 1.1 mg/mL when reconstituted]

Dosing

Adults & Elderly: Refer to individual protocols.

Renal cell carcinoma: I.V.: 600,000 int. units/kg every 8 hours for a maximum of 14 doses; repeat after 9 days for a total of 28 doses per course. Retreat if needed 7 weeks after previous course.

Melanoma:

I.V.:

Single-agent use: 600,000 int. units/kg every 8 hours for a maximum of 14 doses; repeat after 9 days for a total of 28 doses per course. Retreat if needed 7 weeks after previous course.

In combination with cytotoxic agents: 24 million int. units/m^2 days 12-16 and 19-23

SubQ:

Single-agent doses: 3-18 million int. units/day for 5 days each week, up to 6 weeks

In combination with interferon:

5 million int. units/m^2 3 times/week

1.8 million int. units/m^2 twice daily 5 days/week for 6 weeks

Investigational regimen: SubQ: 11 million int. units (flat dose) daily for 4 days per week for 4 consecutive weeks; repeat every 6 weeks

Renal Impairment: No specific recommendations by manufacturer. Use with caution.

Administration

I.V.: Infuse over 15 minutes.

I.V. Detail: Management of symptoms related to vascular leak syndrome:

If actual body weight increases >10% above baseline, or rales or rhonchi are audible:

Administer furosemide at dosage determined by patient response.

Administer dopamine hydrochloride 2-4 mcg/kg/minute to maintain renal blood flow and urine output.

If patient has dyspnea at rest: Give supplemental oxygen by facemask.

If patient has severe respiratory distress: Intubate patient and provide mechanical ventilation. Administer ranitidine (as the hydrochloride salt) 50 mg I.V. every 8-12 hours as prophylaxis against stress ulcers.

Other: May be administered by SubQ injection.

Stability

Reconstitution: Reconstitute vials with 1.2 mL SWFI. Gently swirl; do not shake. Further dilute with 50 mL of D_5W. Smaller volumes of D_5W should be used for doses <1.5 mg; avoid concentrations <30 mcg/mL and >70 mcg/mL (an increased variability in drug delivery has been seen).

Final Dilution Concentration (mcg/mL)	Final Dilution Concentration (10^6 int. units/mL)	Stability
<30	<0.49	Albumin must be added to bag **prior to addition** of aldesleukin at a final concentration of 0.1% (1 mg/mL) albumin; stable at room temperature or at ≥32°C (89°F) for 6 days[1,2]
≥30 to ≤70	≥0.49 to ≤1.1	Stable at room temperature at 6 days without albumin added or at ≥32°C (89°F) for 6 days only if albumin is added (0.1%)[1,2]
70-100	1.2-1.6	Unstable; avoid use
>100-500	1.7-8.2	Stable at room temperature and at ≥32°C (89°F) for 6 days[1,2]

[1]These solutions do not contain a preservative; use for more than 24 hours may not be advisable.

[2]Continuous infusion via ambulatory infusion device raises aldesleukin to this temperature.

Note: Filtration will result in significant loss of bioactivity.

Compatibility: Stable in D_5W

Y-site administration: Incompatible with ganciclovir, lorazepam, pentamidine, prochlorperazine edisylate, promethazine

Compatibility when admixed: Incompatible with NS

Storage: Store vials of lyophilized injection in a refrigerator at 2°C to 8°C (36°F to 46°F). Reconstituted vials and solutions diluted for infusion are stable for 48 hours at room temperature or refrigerated, per the manufacturer. Solution diluted with D_5W to a concentration of 220 mg/mL and repackaged into tuberculin syringes was reported to be stable for 14 days refrigerated.

Laboratory Monitoring CBC, differential, and platelet counts; blood chemistries including electrolytes, renal and hepatic function; chest x-rays

Nursing Actions

Physical Assessment: Assess potential for interactions with other prescriptions, OTC medications, or herbal products patient may be taking. See Administration I.V. specifics. Monitor vital signs; cardiac, respiratory, and CNS status; fluid balance; signs of systemic sepsis; changes in mental status; and laboratory tests daily prior to beginning infusion and for 2 hours following infusion. Closely monitor infusion site for extravasation. Teach patient possible side effects/appropriate interventions and adverse symptoms to report.

Patient Education: Do not take any new medication during therapy unless approved by prescriber. Avoid alcohol. Maintain adequate hydration (2-3 L/day of fluids) unless instructed to restrict fluid intake. You will be susceptible to infection (avoid crowds and exposure to infection and do not have any vaccinations without consulting prescriber). May cause increased sensitivity to sunlight (use sunblock 15 SPF or greater, wear protective clothing, avoid direct sun exposure); or nausea, vomiting, stomatitis, anorexia (frequent mouth care, small frequent meals, chewing gum, or sucking lozenges may help). This drug may result in many side effects; you will be monitored and assessed closely during therapy, however, it is important that you report any changes or problems for evaluation. Report any changes in urination, unusual bruising or bleeding, chest pain or palpitations, acute dizziness, respiratory difficulty, fever or chills, changes in cognition, rash, feelings of pain or numbness in extremities, severe or persistent GI upset or diarrhea, vaginal discharge or mouth sores, yellowing of eyes or skin, or changes in color of urine or stool. **Pregnancy/breast-feeding precautions:** Inform prescriber if you are pregnant. Do not breast-feed.

Pregnancy Issues Use during pregnancy only if benefits to the mother outweigh potential risk to the fetus. Contraception is recommended for fertile males or females using this medication.

Additional Information

1 Cetus unit = 6 int. units

1.1 mg = 18×10^6 int. units (or 3×10^6 Cetus units)

1 Roche unit (Teceleukin) = 3 int. units

Alefacept (a LE fa sept)

U.S. Brand Names Amevive®

Synonyms B 9273; BG 9273; Human LFA-3/IgG(1) Fusion Protein; LFA-3/IgG(1) Fusion Protein, Human

Restrictions Alefacept will be distributed directly to physician offices or to a specialty pharmacy; injections are intended to be administered in the physician's office

Pharmacologic Category Monoclonal Antibody

Pregnancy Risk Factor B

Lactation Excretion in breast milk unknown/not recommended

Use Treatment of moderate to severe chronic plaque psoriasis in adults who are candidates for systemic therapy or phototherapy

Mechanism of Action/Effect Alefacept is a monoclonal antibody against a specific receptor on T lymphocytes, and reduces the number of both CD4+ and CD8+ T lymphocytes. It improves symptoms of psoriasis by decreasing the number of activated T lymphocytes, and their production of inflammatory mediators such as interferon gamma.

Contraindications Hypersensitivity to alefacept or any component of the formulation; history of severe malignancy; patients with HIV infection or other clinically-important infections

Warnings/Precautions Alefacept induces a decline in circulating T-lymphocytes (CD4+ and CD8+); CD4+ lymphocyte counts should be monitored every 2 weeks throughout therapy. Do not initiate in pre-existing depression of CD4+ lymphocytes and withhold treatment in any patient who develops a depressed CD4+ lymphocyte count (<250 cells/μL) during treatment; permanently discontinue if CD4+ lymphocyte counts remain <250 cells/μL for 1 month.

Alefacept may increase the risk of malignancies; use caution in patients at high risk for malignancy. Discontinue if malignancy develops during therapy. Alefacept may increase the risk of infection and may reactivate latent infection; monitor for new infections. Avoid use in patients receiving other immunosuppressant drugs or phototherapy. May cause serious liver damage; discontinue if signs and symptoms of hepatic injury occur. Safety and efficacy of live or attenuated vaccines have not been evaluated. Safety and efficacy have not been established in pediatric patients.

Drug Interactions

Decreased Effect: No formal drug interaction studies have been completed.

Increased Effect/Toxicity: No formal drug interaction studies have been completed.

Nutritional/Ethanol Interactions Ethanol: Avoid ethanol (may increase risk of liver toxicity).

Adverse Reactions

≥10%:

Hematologic: Lymphopenia (up to 10% of patients required temporary discontinuation, up to 17% during a second course of therapy)

Local: Injection site reactions (up to 16% of patients; includes pain, inflammation, bleeding, edema, or other reaction)

1% to 10%:

Central nervous system: Chills (6%; primarily during intravenous administration), dizziness (≥2%)

Dermatologic: Pruritus (≥2%)

Gastrointestinal: Nausea (≥2%)

Neuromuscular & skeletal: Myalgia (≥2%)

Respiratory: Pharyngitis (≥2%), cough increased (≥2%)

Miscellaneous: Malignancies (1% vs 0.5% in placebo), antibodies to alefacept (3%; significance unknown), infection (1% requiring hospitalization)

Overdosage/Toxicology No specific experience in overdose. Symptoms observed at 0.75 mg/kg I.V. included chills, headache, arthralgia, and sinusitis. Reductions in lymphocyte populations should be closely monitored. Treatment is supportive.

Pharmacodynamics/Kinetics

Half-Life Elimination: 270 hours (following I.V. administration)

Excretion: Clearance: 0.25 mL/hour/kg

Available Dosage Forms

Injection, powder for reconstitution:

Amevive®: 15 mg [for I.M. administration; contains sucrose 12.5 mg; supplied with SWFI]

(Continued)

Alefacept *(Continued)*

Dosing

Adults & Elderly: Psoriasis (moderate-to-severe chronic plaque psoriasis):

I.M.: 15 mg once weekly; usual duration of treatment: 12 weeks

Second course: A second course of treatment may be initiated at least 12 weeks after completion of the initial course of treatment, provided CD4+ T-lymphocyte counts are within the normal range.

Note: CD4+ T-lymphocyte counts should be monitored before initiation of treatment and every 2 weeks during therapy. Dosing should be withheld if CD4+ counts are <250 cells/μL, and dosing should be permanently discontinued if CD4+ lymphocyte counts remain at <250 cell/μL for longer than 1 month.

Renal Impairment: No dosage adjustment required.

Administration

I.M.: I.M. injections should be administered at least 1 inch from previous administration sites.

Stability

Reconstitution: Reconstitute 15 mg vial for I.M. solution with 0.6 mL of SWFI (supplied); 0.5 mL of reconstituted solution contains 15 mg of alefacept. Gently swirl to avoid foaming. Do not filter reconstituted solutions. Do not mix with other medications or solutions.

Compatibility: Do not mix with other medications or solutions.

Storage: Store under refrigeration at 2°C to 8°C (36°F to 46°F); protect from light. Following reconstitution, may be stored for up to 4 hours at 2°C to 8°C (36°F to 46°F). Discard any unused solution after 4 hours.

Laboratory Monitoring Baseline CD4+ T-lymphocyte counts prior to initiation and every 2 weeks during treatment course

Nursing Actions

Physical Assessment: Monitor closely for the development of malignancies or infections. Monitor laboratory tests, therapeutic effectiveness, and adverse reactions. Teach patient possible side effects/appropriate interventions and adverse symptoms to report.

Patient Education: This medication can only be administered by injection; report immediately any pain, redness, swelling at injection site, chills, rash, difficulty swallowing or breathing, or feelings of tightness in chest. Avoid alcohol. You will need weekly blood tests while receiving this medication. May cause nausea or muscle pain. Report unusual feelings of fatigue or weakness; signs of infection (eg, cough, runny nose, sore throat, unusual cough, swollen glands, mouth sores, vaginal itching or discharge, burning on urination, fever, chills, or unhealed sores); abdominal pain; jaundice; easy bruising; dark urine; or pale stools. Notify prescriber if pregnancy occurs during therapy or within 8 weeks of treatment. **Breast-feeding precaution:** Breast-feeding is not recommended.

Breast-Feeding Issues It is not known whether alefacept is excreted in breast milk. Since alefacept is an immunosuppressant, and transfer of proteins into breast milk may occur, breast-feeding women are cautioned to discontinue breast-feeding or to discontinue use of the drug while breast-feeding (recommendations per manufacturer).

Pregnancy Issues Patients who become pregnant during therapy or within 8 weeks of treatment are advised to enroll in pregnancy registry (866-263-8483).

Alendronate *(a LEN droe nate)*

U.S. Brand Names Fosamax®
Synonyms Alendronate Sodium
Pharmacologic Category Bisphosphonate Derivative
Medication Safety Issues
Sound-alike/look-alike issues:
Fosamax® may be confused with Flomax®
Pregnancy Risk Factor C
Lactation Excretion in breast milk unknown/use caution
Use Treatment and prevention of osteoporosis in postmenopausal females; treatment of osteoporosis in males; Paget's disease of the bone in patients who are symptomatic, at risk for future complications, or with alkaline phosphatase ≥2 times the upper limit of normal; treatment of glucocorticoid-induced osteoporosis in males and females with low bone mineral density who are receiving a daily dosage ≥7.5 mg of prednisone (or equivalent)
Mechanism of Action/Effect A bisphosphonate which inhibits bone resorption via actions on osteoclasts or on osteoclast precursors; decreases the rate of bone resorption, leading to an indirect increase in bone mineral density. In Paget's disease, characterized by disordered resorption and formation of bone, inhibition of resorption leads to an indirect decrease in bone formation; but the newly-formed bone has a more normal architecture.
Contraindications Hypersensitivity to alendronate, other bisphosphonates, or any component of the formulation; hypocalcemia; abnormalities of the esophagus which delay esophageal emptying such as stricture or achalasia; inability to stand or sit upright for at least 30 minutes; oral solution should not be used in patients at risk of aspiration
Warnings/Precautions Use caution in patients with renal impairment (not recommended for use in patients with Cl$_{cr}$ <35 mL/minute); hypocalcemia must be corrected before therapy initiation; ensure adequate calcium and vitamin D intake. May cause irritation to upper gastrointestinal mucosa. Esophagitis, esophageal ulcers, esophageal erosions, and esophageal stricture (rare) have been reported; risk increases in patients unable to comply with dosing instructions. Use with caution in patients with dysphagia, esophageal disease, gastritis, duodenitis, or ulcers (may worsen underlying condition).

Bisphosphonate therapy has been associated with osteonecrosis, primarily of the jaw; this has been observed mostly in cancer patients, but also in patients with postmenopausal osteoporosis and other diagnoses. Dental exams and preventative dentistry should be performed prior to placing patients with risk factors on chronic bisphosphonate therapy. Invasive dental procedures should be avoided during treatment.

Infrequent reports of severe and occasionally debilitating bone, joint, and/or muscle pain during bisphosphonate treatment; onset of pain ranged from a single day to several months, with relief in most cases upon discontinuation of the drug. Some patients experienced recurrence when rechallenged with same drug or another bisphosphonate.

Safety and efficacy in children have not been established.
Drug Interactions
Decreased Effect: The following agents may decrease the absorption of oral bisphosphonate derivatives: Antacids (aluminum, calcium, magnesium), oral calcium salts, oral iron salts, and oral magnesium salts.
Increased Effect/Toxicity: Aminoglycosides may lower serum calcium levels with prolonged administration; concomitant use may have an additive hypocalcemic effect. NSAIDs may enhance the

gastrointestinal adverse/toxic effects (increased incidence of GI ulcers) of bisphosphonate derivatives. Bisphosphonate derivatives may enhance the hypocalcemic effect of phosphate supplements.

Nutritional/Ethanol Interactions

Ethanol: Avoid ethanol (may increase risk of osteoporosis and gastric irritation).

Food: All food and beverages interfere with absorption. Coadministration with caffeine may reduce alendronate efficacy. Coadministration with dairy products may decrease alendronate absorption. Beverages (especially orange juice and coffee) and food may reduce the absorption of alendronate as much as 60%.

Lab Interactions Bisphosphonates may interfere with diagnostic imaging agents such as technetium-99m-diphosphonate in bone scans.

Adverse Reactions Note: Incidence of adverse effects (mostly GI) increases significantly in patients treated for Paget's disease at 40 mg/day.

>10%: Endocrine & metabolic: Hypocalcemia (transient, mild, 18%); hypophosphatemia (transient, mild, 10%)

1% to 10%:

Central nervous system: Headache (up to 3%)

Gastrointestinal: Abdominal pain (1% to 7%), acid reflux (1% to 4%), dyspepsia (1% to 4%), nausea (1% to 4%), flatulence (up to 4%), diarrhea (1% to 3%), gastroesophageal reflux disease (1% to 3%), constipation (up to 3%), esophageal ulcer (up to 2%), abdominal distension (up to 1%), gastritis (up to 1%), vomiting (up to 1%), dysphagia (up to 1%), gastric ulcer (1%), melena (1%)

Neuromuscular & skeletal: Musculoskeletal pain (up to 6%), muscle cramps (up to 1%)

Overdosage/Toxicology Symptoms of overdose include hypocalcemia, hypophosphatemia, and upper GI adverse affects (eg, upset stomach, heartburn, esophagitis, gastritis, or ulcer). Treat with milk or antacids to bind alendronate. Dialysis would not be beneficial. Do not induce vomiting (due to the risk of esophageal irritation); keep fully upright.

Pharmacodynamics/Kinetics

Protein Binding: ~78%

Half-Life Elimination: Exceeds 10 years

Metabolism: None

Excretion: Urine; feces (as unabsorbed drug)

Available Dosage Forms

Solution, oral, as monosodium trihydrate: 70 mg/75 mL [contains parabens; raspberry flavor]

Tablet, as sodium: 5 mg, 10 mg, 35 mg, 40 mg, 70 mg

Dosing

Adults & Elderly: Note: Patients treated with glucocorticoids and those with Paget's disease should receive adequate amounts of calcium and vitamin D.

Osteoporosis in postmenopausal females: Oral:
Prophylaxis: 5 mg once daily **or** 35 mg once weekly
Treatment: 10 mg once daily **or** 70 mg once weekly

Osteoporosis in males: Oral: 10 mg once daily **or** 70 mg once weekly

Osteoporosis secondary to glucocorticoids in males and females: Oral: Treatment: 5 mg once daily; a dose of 10 mg once daily should be used in postmenopausal females who are not receiving estrogen.

Paget's disease of bone in males and females:
Oral: 40 mg once daily for 6 months

Retreatment: Relapses during the 12 months following therapy occurred in 9% of patients who responded to treatment. Specific retreatment data are not available. Following a 6-month post-treatment evaluation period, treatment with alendronate may be considered in patients who have relapsed based on increases in serum alkaline phosphatase, which should be measured periodically. Retreatment may also be considered

in those who failed to normalize their serum alkaline phosphatase.

Renal Impairment:
Cl$_{cr}$ 35-60 mL/minute: None necessary.
Cl$_{cr}$ <35 mL/minute: Alendronate is not recommended due to lack of experience.

Hepatic Impairment: No adjustment necessary.

Administration

Oral: Alendronate must be taken with plain water (tablets 6-8 oz; oral solution follow with 2 oz) first thing in the morning and ≥30 minutes before the first food, beverage, or other medication of the day. Do not take with mineral water or with other beverages. Patients should be instructed to stay upright (not to lie down) for at least 30 minutes **and** until after first food of the day (to reduce esophageal irritation). Patients should receive supplemental calcium and vitamin D if dietary intake is inadequate.

Stability

Storage: Store tablets and oral solution at room temperature of 15°C to 30°C (59°F to 86°F). Keep in well-closed container.

Laboratory Monitoring Alkaline phosphatase should be periodically measured; serum calcium and phosphorus; hormonal status (male and female) prior to therapy; bone mineral density (should be done prior to initiation of therapy and after 6-12 months of combined glucocorticoid and alendronate treatment)

Nursing Actions

Physical Assessment: Monitor laboratory tests, effectiveness of treatment, and development of adverse reactions. Assess ability of patient to comply with administration directions. Teach appropriate use and administration of medication, lifestyle and dietary changes that will have a beneficial impact on Paget's disease or osteoporosis, possible side effects/appropriate interventions, and adverse reactions to report.

Patient Education: Do not take any new medication during therapy unless approved by prescriber. Take as directed, with a full glass of water first thing in the morning and at least 30 minutes before the first food or beverage of the day. Wait at least 30 minutes after taking alendronate before taking anything else. Stay in sitting or standing position for 30 minutes following administration and until after the first food of the day to reduce potential for esophageal irritation. Consult prescriber to determine necessity of lifestyle changes (eg, decreased smoking, decreased alcohol intake, dietary supplements of calcium or vitamin D). May cause flatulence, bloating, nausea, or acid regurgitation; small, frequent meals may help. Report acute headache or gastric pain, unresolved GI upset, or acid stomach. **Pregnancy/breast-feeding precautions:** Inform prescriber if you are or intend to become pregnant. Consult prescriber if breast-feeding.

Dietary Considerations Ensure adequate calcium and vitamin D intake; however, wait at least 30 minutes after taking alendronate before taking any supplement. Alendronate must be taken with plain water first thing in the morning and at least 30 minutes before the first food or beverage of the day.

Geriatric Considerations Since many elderly patients receive diuretics, evaluation of electrolyte status (calcium, phosphate, magnesium, potassium) may need to be done periodically due to the drug class (bisphosphonate). Should assure immobile patients are at least sitting up for 30 minutes after swallowing tablets. Drink a full glass of water with each dose.

Pregnancy Issues Safety and efficacy have not been established in pregnant women. Animal studies have shown delays in delivery and fetal/neonatal death (secondary to hypocalcemia). Bisphosphonates are incorporated into the bone matrix and gradually released over time. Theoretically, there may be a risk of fetal harm when pregnancy follows the completion of therapy. Based on limited case reports with (Continued)

Alendronate *(Continued)*

pamidronate, serum calcium levels in the newborn may be altered if administered during pregnancy.

Alfuzosin *(al FYOO zoe sin)*

U.S. Brand Names Uroxatral®

Synonyms Alfuzosin Hydrochloride

Pharmacologic Category Alpha$_1$ Blocker

Pregnancy Risk Factor B

Lactation Not indicated for use in women

Use Treatment of the functional symptoms of benign prostatic hyperplasia (BPH)

Mechanism of Action/Effect An antagonist of alpha$_1$ adrenoreceptors in the lower urinary tract. Blockade of these adrenoreceptors can cause smooth muscles in the bladder neck and prostate to relax, resulting in an improvement in urine flow rate and a reduction in symptoms of BPH.

Contraindications Hypersensitivity to alfuzosin or any component of the formulation; moderate or severe hepatic insufficiency (Child-Pugh class B and C); potent CYP3A4 inhibitors (eg, itraconazole, ketoconazole, ritonavir)

Warnings/Precautions Not intended for use as an antihypertensive drug. May cause orthostasis, syncope, or dizziness. Patients should avoid situations where injury may occur as a result of syncope. Discontinue if symptoms of angina occur or worsen. Use caution with history of QT prolongation or use with medications which may prolong the QT interval. Rule out prostatic carcinoma before beginning therapy. Use caution with renal or mild hepatic impairment. Intraoperative floppy iris syndrome has been observed in cataract surgery patients who were on or were previously treated with alpha$_1$ blockers. Causality has not been established and there appears to be no benefit in discontinuing alpha blocker therapy prior to surgery. Safety and efficacy in children have not been established.

Drug Interactions

Cytochrome P450 Effect: Substrate of CYP3A4 (major)

Decreased Effect: Levels/effects of alfuzosin may be decreased by aminoglutethimide, carbamazepine, nafcillin, nevirapine, phenobarbital, phenytoin, rifamycins, and other CYP3A4 inducers.

Increased Effect/Toxicity: Alfuzosin levels/effects may be increased by azole antifungals, clarithromycin, diclofenac, doxycycline, erythromycin, imatinib, isoniazid, nefazodone, nicardipine, propofol, protease inhibitors, quinidine, verapamil, telithromycin, and other CYP3A4 inhibitors. Concurrent use of itraconazole, ketoconazole, or ritonavir is contraindicated.

Nutritional/Ethanol Interactions Food: Food increases the extent of absorption.

Adverse Reactions 1% to 10%:

Central nervous system: Dizziness (6%), fatigue (3%), headache (3%), pain (1% to 2%)

Gastrointestinal: Abdominal pain (1% to 2%), constipation (1% to 2%), dyspepsia (1% to 2%), nausea (1% to 2%)

Genitourinary: Impotence (1% to 2%)

Respiratory: Upper respiratory tract infection (3%), bronchitis (1% to 2%), pharyngitis (1% to 2%), sinusitis (1% to 2%)

Overdosage/Toxicology Hypotension would be expected in case of overdose. Treatment is symptom-directed and supportive. Dialysis not likely to benefit.

Pharmacodynamics/Kinetics

Time to Peak: Plasma: 8 hours following a meal

Protein Binding: 82% to 90%

Half-Life Elimination: 10 hours

Metabolism: Hepatic, primarily via CYP3A4; metabolism includes oxidation, O-demethylation, and N-dealkylation; forms metabolites (inactive)

Excretion: Feces (69%); urine (24%)

Available Dosage Forms Tablet, extended release, as hydrochloride: 10 mg

Dosing

Adults & Elderly: Benign prostatic hyperplasia (BPH): Oral: 10 mg once daily

Renal Impairment: Bioavailability and maximum serum concentrations are increased by ~50% with mild, moderate, or severe renal impairment.

Note: Safety has not been evaluated in patients with creatinine clearances <30 mL/minute.

Hepatic Impairment:

Mild hepatic impairment: Use has not been studied.

Moderate or severe hepatic impairment (Child-Pugh class B and C): Clearance is decreased $\frac{1}{3}$ to $\frac{1}{4}$ and serum concentration is increased three- to fourfold; use is contraindicated.

Administration

Oral: Tablet should be swallowed whole; do not crush or chew. Administer once daily (with a meal); should be taken at the same time each day.

Stability

Storage: Store at controlled room temperature of 15°C to 30°C (59°F to 86°F). Protect from light and moisture.

Nursing Actions

Physical Assessment: Monitor for patient response (eg, improved urine flow) and adverse reactions (hypotension) at beginning of therapy and on a regular basis with long-term therapy. Teach patient proper use, possible side effects/appropriate interventions, and adverse symptoms to report.

Patient Education: Do not take any new medication during therapy without consulting prescriber. Take exactly as directed, with a meal at the same time each day. Swallow tablet whole; do not crush or chew. May cause drowsiness, dizziness, impaired judgment (use caution when driving or engaging in tasks that require alertness until response to drug is known), or postural hypotension (use caution when rising from sitting or lying position or when climbing stairs). Report unusual chest pain, respiratory difficulty, or any persistent adverse reactions.

Dietary Considerations Take following a meal at the same time each day.

Alglucerase *(al GLOO ser ase)*

U.S. Brand Names Ceredase®

Synonyms Glucocerebrosidase

Pharmacologic Category Enzyme

Medication Safety Issues

Sound-alike/look-alike issues:

Ceredase® may be confused with Cerezyme®

Pregnancy Risk Factor C

Lactation Excretion in breast milk unknown/use caution

Use Replacement therapy for Gaucher's disease (type 1)

Mechanism of Action/Effect Replaces the missing enzyme, glucocerebrosidase, associated with Gaucher's disease

Contraindications Hypersensitivity to any component of the formulation

Warnings/Precautions Prepared from pooled human placental tissue that may contain the causative agents of some viral diseases. Patients who develop IgG antibodies may be at a higher risk for developing hypersensitivity. Use caution with androgen-sensitive malignancies or prior allergies to hCG. May cause early virilization in males <10 years of age.

Lab Interactions False-positive pregnancy tests

Adverse Reactions Frequency not defined.

Cardiovascular: Peripheral edema

Central nervous system: Chills, fatigue, fever, headache, lightheadedness

Endocrine & metabolic: Hot flashes, menstrual abnormalities

Gastrointestinal: Abdominal discomfort, diarrhea, nausea, oral ulcerations, vomiting

Local: Injection site: Abscess, burning, discomfort, pruritus, swelling

Neuromuscular & skeletal: Backache, weakness

Miscellaneous: Dysosmia; hypersensitivity reactions (abdominal cramping, angioedema, chest discomfort, flushing, hypotension, nausea, pruritus, respiratory symptoms, urticaria); IgG antibody formation (~13%)

Overdosage/Toxicology No obvious toxicity has been detected after single doses up to 234 units/kg.

Pharmacodynamics/Kinetics

Half-Life Elimination: ~3-11 minutes

Available Dosage Forms [DSC] = Discontinued product

Injection, solution [preservative free]: 10 units/mL (5 mL) [DSC]; 80 units/mL (5 mL) [contains human albumin 1%]

Dosing

Adults & Elderly: Gaucher's disease: I.V.: Initial: 30-60 units/kg every 2 weeks; dosing is individualized based on disease severity; average dose: 60 units/kg every 2 weeks. Range: 2.5 units/kg 3 times/week to 60 units/kg 1-4 times/week. Once patient response is well established, dose may be reduced every 3-6 months to determine maintenance therapy.

Pediatrics: Refer to adult dosing.

Administration

I.V.: Infuse I.V. over 1-2 hours; use of an in-line filter is recommended.

I.V. Detail: Effective only via I.V. Filter during administration. Do not shake, shaking may render glycoprotein inactive. Dilute with NS only.

Stability

Reconstitution: Dilute with NS to a final volume ≤200 mL. Do not shake.

Compatibility:

Do not mix with any other additives.

Storage: Refrigerate (4°C), do not freeze. Contains no preservatives. Do not store opened vials for future use. Once diluted, 100 mL and 200 mL solutions for infusion are stable for 18 hours when stored at 2°C to 8°C.

Laboratory Monitoring CBC, platelets, acid phosphatase (AP), plasma glucocerebroside, IgG antibody formation

Nursing Actions

Physical Assessment: Must be infused via filter (see I.V. Detail). Monitor laboratory tests (see above) and therapeutic response (eg, vital signs, energy level, change in bleeding tendency, reduced joint swelling, or bone pain). Teach patient possible side effects/appropriate interventions and adverse symptoms to report.

Patient Education: Inform prescriber of all prescriptions, OTC medications, or herbal products you are taking, and any allergies you have. Do not take any new medication during therapy unless approved by prescriber. This medication will not cure Gaucher's disease, but rather, may help control it. Treatment is required for life. May cause abdominal discomfort, nausea, or vomiting (small, frequent meals, good mouth care, chewing gum, or sucking lozenges may help); these symptoms should go away with continued

use. Inform prescriber if pain, swelling, or redness occurs at injection site or if GI symptoms persist. **Pregnancy/breast-feeding precautions:** Inform prescriber if you are or intend to become pregnant. Consult prescriber if breast-feeding.

Alitretinoin (a li TRET i noyn)

U.S. Brand Names Panretin®

Pharmacologic Category Antineoplastic Agent, Miscellaneous

Medication Safety Issues

Sound-alike/look-alike issues:

Panretin® may be confused with pancreatin

Pregnancy Risk Factor D

Lactation Excretion in breast milk unknown/not recommended

Use Orphan drug: Topical treatment of cutaneous lesions in AIDS-related Kaposi's sarcoma

Unlabeled/Investigational Use Cutaneous T-cell lymphomas

Mechanism of Action/Effect Binds to retinoid receptors to inhibit growth of Kaposi's sarcoma

Contraindications Hypersensitivity to alitretinoin, other retinoids, or any component of the formulation; pregnancy

Warnings/Precautions May cause fetal harm if absorbed by a woman who is pregnant. Do not use concurrently with topical products containing DEET (a common component of insect repellent products). Safety in pediatric patients or geriatric patients has not been established.

Drug Interactions

Increased Effect/Toxicity: Increased toxicity of DEET may occur if products containing this compound are used concurrently with alitretinoin. Due to limited absorption after topical application, interaction with systemic medications is unlikely.

Adverse Reactions

>10%:

Central nervous system: Pain (0% to 34%)

Dermatologic: Rash (25% to 77%), pruritus (8% to 11%)

Neuromuscular & skeletal: Paresthesia (3% to 22%)

5% to 10%:

Cardiovascular: Edema (3% to 8%)

Dermatologic: Exfoliative dermatitis (3% to 9%), skin disorder (0% to 8%)

Overdosage/Toxicology There has been no experience with human overdosage of alitretinoin, and overdose is unlikely following topical application. Treatment is symptomatic and supportive.

Available Dosage Forms Gel: 0.1% (60 g tube)

Dosing

Adults & Elderly:

Kaposi's sarcoma: Topical: Apply gel twice daily to cutaneous lesions.

T-cell lymphomas (unlabeled use): Topical: Apply gel twice daily to cutaneous lesions.

Administration

Topical: Do not use occlusive dressings.

Stability

Storage: Store at room temperature.

Nursing Actions

Physical Assessment: Monitor effectiveness of therapy and adverse reactions at beginning and periodically during therapy. Teach patient appropriate use and adverse symptoms to report.

Patient Education: For external use only. Use exactly as directed; do not overuse. Avoid use of any product such as insect repellents which contain DEET (check with your pharmacist). Wear protective clothing and/or avoid exposure to direct sun or sunlamps. Wash

(Continued)

Alitretinoin (Continued)

hands thoroughly before applying. Avoid applying skin products that contain alcohol or harsh chemicals during treatment. Do not apply occlusive dressings. Stop treatment and inform prescriber if rash, skin irritation, redness, scaling, or excessive dryness appears. **Pregnancy/breast-feeding precautions:** Do not get pregnant while taking this medication. Consult prescriber for appropriate contraceptive measures. Breast-feeding is not recommended.

Breast-Feeding Issues Excretion in human breast milk is unknown; women are advised to discontinue breast-feeding prior to using this medication.

Pregnancy Issues Potentially teratogenic and/or embryotoxic; limb, craniofacial, or skeletal defects have been observed in animal models. If used during pregnancy or if the patient becomes pregnant while using alitretinoin, the woman should be advised of potential harm to the fetus. Women of childbearing potential should avoid becoming pregnant.

Allopurinol (al oh PURE i nole)

U.S. Brand Names Aloprim™; Zyloprim®

Synonyms Allopurinol Sodium

Pharmacologic Category Xanthine Oxidase Inhibitor

Medication Safety Issues
Sound-alike/look-alike issues:
Allopurinol may be confused with Apresoline
Zyloprim® may be confused with Xylo-Pfan®, ZORprin®

Pregnancy Risk Factor C

Lactation Enters breast milk/use caution (AAP rates "compatible")

Use
Oral: Prevention of attack of gouty arthritis and nephropathy; treatment of secondary hyperuricemia which may occur during treatment of tumors or leukemia; prevention of recurrent calcium oxalate calculi
I.V.: Treatment of elevated serum and urinary uric acid levels when oral therapy is not tolerated in patients with leukemia, lymphoma, and solid tumor malignancies who are receiving cancer chemotherapy

Mechanism of Action/Effect Allopurinol inhibits xanthine oxidase, the enzyme responsible for the conversion of hypoxanthine to xanthine to uric acid. Allopurinol is metabolized to oxypurinol which is also an inhibitor of xanthine oxidase; allopurinol acts on purine catabolism, reducing the production of uric acid without disrupting the biosynthesis of vital purines.

Contraindications Hypersensitivity to allopurinol or any component of the formulation

Warnings/Precautions Do not use to treat asymptomatic hyperuricemia. Discontinue at first signs of rash. Caution in renal impairment, dosage adjustments needed. Use with caution in patients taking diuretics concurrently. Risk of skin rash may be increased in patients receiving amoxicillin or ampicillin. The risk of hypersensitivity may be increased in patients receiving thiazides, and possibly ACE inhibitors. Use caution with mercaptopurine or azathioprine.

Drug Interactions
Decreased Effect: Ethanol decreases effectiveness.
Increased Effect/Toxicity: Allopurinol may increase the effects of azathioprine, chlorpropamide, mercaptopurine, theophylline, and oral anticoagulants. An increased risk of bone marrow suppression may occur when given with myelosuppressive agents (cyclophosphamide, possibly other alkylating agents). Amoxicillin/ampicillin, ACE inhibitors, and thiazide diuretics have been associated with hypersensitivity reactions when combined with allopurinol (rare), and

the incidence of rash may be increased with penicillins (ampicillin, amoxicillin). Urinary acidification with large amounts of vitamin C may increase kidney stone formation.

Nutritional/Ethanol Interactions
Ethanol: May decrease effectiveness.
Iron supplements: Hepatic iron uptake may be increased.
Vitamin C: Large amounts of vitamin C may acidify urine and increase kidney stone formation.

Adverse Reactions
>1%:
Dermatologic: Rash (increased with ampicillin or amoxicillin use, 1.5% per manufacturer, >10% in some reports)
Gastrointestinal: Nausea (1.3%), vomiting (1.2%)
Renal: Renal failure/impairment (1.2%)

Overdosage/Toxicology If significant amounts of allopurinol have been absorbed, it is theoretically possible that oxypurinol stones could form, but no record of such occurrence exists. Alkalinization of urine and forced diuresis can help prevent potential xanthine stone formation.

Pharmacodynamics/Kinetics
Onset of Action: Peak effect: 1-2 weeks
Time to Peak: Plasma: Oral: 30-120 minutes
Protein Binding: <1%
Half-Life Elimination:
Normal renal function: Parent drug: 1-3 hours; Oxypurinol: 18-30 hours
End-stage renal disease: Prolonged
Metabolism: ~75% to active metabolites, chiefly oxypurinol
Excretion: Urine (76% as oxypurinol, 12% as unchanged drug)
Allopurinol and oxypurinol are dialyzable

Available Dosage Forms
Injection, powder for reconstitution, as sodium (Aloprim™): 500 mg
Tablet (Zyloprim®): 100 mg, 300 mg

Dosing
Adults: Doses >300 mg should be given in divided doses.
Gout: Oral: Mild: 200-300 mg/day; Severe: 400-600 mg/day; to reduce the possibility of acute gouty attacks, initiate dose at 100 mg/day and increase weekly to recommended dosage. Maximum daily dose: 800 mg/day.
Secondary hyperuricemia associated with chemotherapy:
Oral: 600-800 mg/day in 2-3 divided doses for prevention of acute uric acid nephropathy for 2-3 days starting 1-2 days before chemotherapy
I.V.: 200-400 mg/m²/day (maximum: 600 mg/day)
Note: Intravenous daily dose can be given as a single infusion or in equally divided doses at 6-, 8-, or 12-hour intervals. A fluid intake sufficient to yield a daily urinary output of at least 2 L in adults and the maintenance of a neutral or, preferably, slightly alkaline urine are desirable.
Recurrent calcium oxalate stones: 200-300 mg/day in single or divided doses
Elderly: Oral: Initial: 100 mg/day; increase until desired uric acid level is obtained. Refer to adult dosing.
Pediatrics:
Gout: Children >10 years: Refer to adult dosing.
Recurrent calcium oxalate stones: Children >10 years: Refer to adult dosing.
Secondary hyperuricemia associated with chemotherapy:
Oral: Children ≤10 years: 10 mg/kg/day in 2-3 divided doses or 200-300 mg/m²/day in 2-4 divided doses, maximum: 800 mg/24 hours, for prevention of acute uric acid nephropathy (begin 1-2 days before chemotherapy)

Alternative (manufacturer labeling):
<6 years: 150 mg/day in 3 divided doses
6-10 years: 300 mg/day in 2-3 divided doses
>10 years: Refer to adult dosing.

I.V.:
Children ≤10 years: Starting dose: 200 mg/m²/day
Note: Intravenous daily dose can be given as a single infusion or in equally divided doses at 6-, 8-, or 12-hour intervals. Adequate fluid intake and the maintenance of a neutral or, preferably, slightly alkaline urine are desirable.
Children >10 years: Refer to adult dosing.

Renal Impairment:
Oral:
Must be adjusted due to accumulation of allopurinol and metabolites; see table.

Adult Maintenance Doses of Allopurinol[1]

Creatinine Clearance (mL/min)	Maintenance Dose of Allopurinol (mg)
140	400 daily
120	350 daily
100	300 daily
80	250 daily
60	200 daily
40	150 daily
20	100 daily
10	100 every 2 days
0	100 every 3 days

[1]This table is based on a standard maintenance dose of 300 mg of allopurinol per day for a patient with a creatinine clearance of 100 mL/min.

Hemodialysis: Administer dose after hemodialysis or administer 50% supplemental dose.
I.V.:
Cl$_{cr}$ 10-20 mL/minute: Administer 200 mg/day.
Cl$_{cr}$ 3-10 mL/minute: Administer 100 mg/day.
Cl$_{cr}$ <3 mL/minute: Administer 100 mg/day at extended intervals.

Administration
Oral: Should be administered after meals with plenty of fluid.
I.V.: Infuse over 15-60 minutes. The rate of infusion depends on the volume of the infusion. Whenever possible, therapy should be initiated at 24-48 hours before the start of chemotherapy known to cause tumor lysis (including adrenocorticosteroids). I.V. daily dose can be administered as a single infusion or in equally divided doses at 6-, 8-, or 12-hour intervals.

Stability
Reconstitution: Further dilution with NS or D$_5$W (50-100 mL) to ≤6 mg/mL is recommended.
Compatibility: Stable in D$_5$W, NS, SWFI
Y-site administration: Incompatible with amikacin, amphotericin B, carmustine, cefotaxime, chlorpromazine, cimetidine, clindamycin, cytarabine, dacarbazine, daunorubicin, diphenhydramine, doxorubicin, doxycycline, droperidol, floxuridine, gentamicin, haloperidol, hydroxyzine, idarubicin, imipenem/cilastatin, mechlorethamine, meperidine, methylprednisolone sodium succinate, metoclopramide, minocycline, nalbuphine, netilmicin, ondansetron, prochlorperazine edisylate, promethazine, sodium bicarbonate, streptozocin, tobramycin, vinorelbine

Storage:
Powder for injection: Store at controlled room temperature of 15°C to 30°C (59°F to 86°F). Following reconstitution, intravenous solutions should be stored at 20°C to 25°C. Do not refrigerate reconstituted and/or diluted product. Must be administered within 10 hours of solution preparation.

Tablet: Store at controlled room temperature of 15°C to 25°C (59°F to 77°F).
Laboratory Monitoring CBC, serum uric acid levels, hepatic and renal function, especially at start of therapy

Nursing Actions
Physical Assessment: Assess effectiveness and interactions of other medications patient may be taking. Monitor laboratory values, effectiveness of therapy, frequency and severity of gouty attacks, and adverse reactions at beginning of therapy and periodically with long-term use. Assess knowledge/teach patient appropriate use, interventions to reduce side effects, and adverse symptoms to report.
Patient Education: Take as directed. Maintain adequate hydration (2-3 L/day of fluids) unless instructed to restrict fluid intake. While using this medication, do not use alcohol, other prescriptions, OTC medications, or vitamins without consulting prescriber. You may experience drowsiness (use caution when driving or engaging in tasks requiring alertness until response to drug is known); nausea, vomiting, or heartburn (small frequent meals, frequent mouth care, chewing gum, or sucking lozenges may help); or hair loss (reversible). Report skin rash or lesions; painful urination or blood in urine or stool; unresolved nausea or vomiting; numbness of extremities; pain or irritation of the eyes; swelling of lips, mouth, or tongue; unusual fatigue; easy bruising or bleeding; yellowing of skin or eyes; or any change in color of urine or stool. **Pregnancy/breast-feeding precautions:** Inform prescriber if you are or intend to become pregnant. Consult prescriber if breast-feeding.
Dietary Considerations Should administer oral forms after meals with plenty of fluid. Fluid intake should be administered to yield neutral or slightly alkaline urine and an output of ~2 L (in adults).
Geriatric Considerations Adjust dose based on renal function.

Almotriptan (al moh TRIP tan)

U.S. Brand Names Axert™
Synonyms Almotriptan Malate
Pharmacologic Category Serotonin 5-HT$_{1D}$ Receptor Agonist
Medication Safety Issues
Sound-alike/look-alike issues:
Axert™ may be confused with Antivert®
Pregnancy Risk Factor C
Lactation Excretion in breast milk unknown/use caution
Use Acute treatment of migraine with or without aura
Mechanism of Action/Effect The therapeutic effect for migraine is due to serotonin agonist activity.
Contraindications Hypersensitivity to almotriptan or any component of the formulation; use as prophylactic therapy for migraine; hemiplegic or basilar migraine; cluster headache; known or suspected ischemic heart disease (angina pectoris, MI, documented silent ischemia, coronary artery vasospasm, Prinzmetal's variant angina); peripheral vascular syndromes (including ischemic bowel disease); uncontrolled hypertension; use within 24 hours of another 5-HT$_1$ agonist; use within 24 hours of ergotamine derivative; concurrent administration or within 2 weeks of discontinuing an MAO inhibitor (specifically MAO type A inhibitors)
Warnings/Precautions Indicated for migraine headaches only. Not for patients with risk factors for coronary artery disease; need cardiac evaluation first. If patient's cardiovascular evaluation is good, healthcare provider should administer the first dose and cardiovascular status should be periodically evaluated. Vasospastic events may occur in the heart, peripheral vascular, or (Continued)

Almotriptan *(Continued)*

gastrointestinal system. Cerebral/subarachnoid hemorrhage, stroke, and hypertensive crisis have occurred. Use with caution in liver or renal dysfunction. Safety and efficacy in pediatric patients have not been established.

Drug Interactions
Cytochrome P450 Effect: Substrate (minor) of CYP2D6, 3A4
Increased Effect/Toxicity: Ergot-containing drugs prolong vasospastic reactions; ketoconazole increases almotriptan serum concentration; select serotonin reuptake inhibitors may increase symptoms of hyper-reflexia, weakness, and incoordination; MAO inhibitors may increase toxicity

Adverse Reactions 1% to 10%:
Central nervous system: Headache (>1%), dizziness (>1%), somnolence (>1%)
Gastrointestinal: Nausea (1% to 2%), xerostomia (1%)
Neuromuscular & skeletal: Paresthesia (1%)

Overdosage/Toxicology Hypertension or more serious cardiovascular symptoms may occur. Clinical and electrocardiographic monitoring needed for at least 20 hours even if patient is asymptomatic. Treatment is symptom-directed and supportive.

Pharmacodynamics/Kinetics
Time to Peak: 1-3 hours
Protein Binding: ~35%
Half-Life Elimination: 3-4 hours
Metabolism: MAO type A oxidative deamination (~27% of dose); via CYP3A4 and 2D6 (~12% of dose) to inactive metabolites
Excretion: Urine: 40% (as unchanged drug); feces (13% unchanged and metabolized)

Available Dosage Forms Tablet, as malate: 6.25 mg, 12.5 mg

Dosing
Adults & Elderly: Migraine: Oral: Initial: 6.25-12.5 mg in a single dose; if the headache returns, repeat the dose after 2 hours; no more than 2 doses in 24-hour period
Note: If the first dose is ineffective, diagnosis needs to be re-evaluated. Safety of treating more than 4 migraines/month has not been established.
Renal Impairment: Initial: 6.25 mg in a single dose; maximum daily dose: ≤12.5 mg
Hepatic Impairment: Initial: 6.25 mg in a single dose; maximum daily dose: ≤12.5 mg

Stability
Storage: Store at 15°C to 30°C (59°F to 86°F).

Nursing Actions
Physical Assessment: Assess potential for interactions with other prescriptions, OTC medications, or herbal products patient may be taking (eg, ergot-containing drugs, SSRIs, MAO inhibitors). Monitor effectiveness of therapy (relief of migraines) and adverse response (eg, hypertension; see Adverse Reactions). Teach patient proper use, possible side effects/appropriate interventions, and adverse symptoms to report.
Patient Education: Inform prescriber of all prescriptions (including oral contraceptives), OTC medications, or herbal products you are taking, and any allergies you have. This drug is to be used to reduce your migraine, not to prevent or reduce the number of attacks. Follow exact instructions for use. Do not use more than two doses in 24 hours and do not take within 24 hours of any other migraine medication without consulting prescriber. May cause dizziness, fatigue, or drowsiness (use caution when driving or engaging in tasks requiring alertness until response to drug is known). Report immediately any chest pain, palpitations, or throbbing; feelings of tightness or pressure in jaw or throat; acute headache or dizziness; muscle cramping, pain, or tremors; skin rash; hallucinations, anxiety, panic; or other adverse reactions. **Pregnancy/breast-feeding precautions:** Inform prescriber if you are or intend to become pregnant. Consult prescriber if breast-feeding.

Dietary Considerations May be taken without regard to meals

Alprazolam *(al PRAY zoe lam)*

U.S. Brand Names Alprazolam Intensol®; Niravam™; Xanax®; Xanax XR®
Restrictions C-IV
Pharmacologic Category Benzodiazepine
Medication Safety Issues
Sound-alike/look-alike issues:
Alprazolam may be confused with alprostadil, lorazepam, triazolam
Xanax® may be confused with Lanoxin®, Tenex®, Tylox®, Xopenex®, Zantac®, Zyrtec®

Pregnancy Risk Factor D
Lactation Enters breast milk/not recommended (AAP rates "of concern")
Use Treatment of anxiety disorder (GAD); panic disorder, with or without agoraphobia; anxiety associated with depression
Unlabeled/Investigational Use Anxiety in children
Mechanism of Action/Effect Binds to stereospecific benzodiazepine receptors on the postsynaptic GABA neuron at several sites within the central nervous system, including the limbic system, reticular formation. Enhancement of the inhibitory effect of GABA on neuronal excitability results by increased neuronal membrane permeability to chloride ions. This shift in chloride ions results in hyperpolarization (a less excitable state) and stabilization.
Contraindications Hypersensitivity to alprazolam or any component of the formulation (cross-sensitivity with other benzodiazepines may exist); narrow-angle glaucoma; concurrent use with ketoconazole or itraconazole; pregnancy
Warnings/Precautions Rebound or withdrawal symptoms, including seizures, may occur 18 hours to 3 days following abrupt discontinuation or large decreases in dose (more common in patients receiving >4 mg/day or prolonged treatment). Breakthrough anxiety may occur at the end of dosing interval. Use with caution in patients receiving concurrent CYP3A4 inhibitors. Use with caution in renal impairment or predisposition to urate nephropathy. Use in elderly or debilitated patients, patients with hepatic disease (including alcoholics), renal impairment, or obese patients.

Causes CNS depression (dose related) which may impair physical and mental capabilities. Patients must be cautioned about performing tasks that require mental alertness (eg, operating machinery or driving). Effects with other sedative drugs or ethanol may be potentiated. Benzodiazepines have been associated with falls and traumatic injury and should be used with extreme caution in patients who are at risk of these events (especially the elderly). Use with caution in patients with respiratory disease or impaired gag reflex.

Use caution in patients with depression, particularly if suicidal risk may be present. Episodes of mania or hypomania have occurred in depressed patients treated with alprazolam. May cause physical or psychological dependence. Acute withdrawal may be precipitated in patients after administration of flumazenil.

Benzodiazepines have been associated with anterograde amnesia. Paradoxical reactions have been reported with benzodiazepines, particularly in adolescent/pediatric or psychiatric patients. Does not have analgesic, antidepressant, or antipsychotic properties.

Drug Interactions

Cytochrome P450 Effect: Substrate of CYP3A4 (major)

Decreased Effect: Aminoglutethimide, carbamazepine, nafcillin, nevirapine, phenobarbital, phenytoin, rifamycins, and other CYP3A4 inducers may decrease the levels/effects of alprazolam.

Increased Effect/Toxicity: Alprazolam serum levels/effects may be increased by azole antifungals, clarithromycin, diclofenac, doxycycline, erythromycin, fluoxetine, imatinib, isoniazid, nefazodone, nicardipine, oral contraceptives, propofol, protease inhibitors, quinidine, telithromycin, verapamil, and other inhibitors of CYP3A4. Contraindicated with itraconazole or ketoconazole. Alprazolam potentiates the CNS depressant effects of narcotic analgesics, barbiturates, phenothiazines, ethanol, antihistamines, MAO inhibitors, sedative-hypnotics, and cyclic antidepressants. Alprazolam increases plasma concentrations of imipramine and desipramine.

Nutritional/Ethanol Interactions

Cigarette smoking: May decrease alprazolam concentrations up to 50%.

Ethanol: Avoid ethanol (may increase CNS depression).

Food: Alprazolam serum concentration is unlikely to be increased by grapefruit juice because of alprazolam's high oral bioavailability. The C_{max} of the extended release formulation is increased by 25% when a high-fat meal is given 2 hours before dosing. T_{max} is decreased 30% when food is given immediately prior to dose. T_{max} is increased by 30% when food is given ≥1 hour after dose.

Herb/Nutraceutical: St John's wort may decrease alprazolam levels. Avoid valerian, St John's wort, kava kava, gotu kola (may increase CNS depression).

Lab Interactions Increased with alkaline phosphatase

Adverse Reactions

>10%:

Central nervous system: Abnormal coordination, cognitive disorder, depression, drowsiness, fatigue, irritability, lightheadedness, memory impairment, sedation, somnolence

Gastrointestinal: Appetite increased/decreased, constipation, salivation decreased, weight gain/loss, xerostomia

Genitourinary: Micturition difficulty

Neuromuscular & skeletal: Dysarthria

1% to 10%:

Cardiovascular: Hypotension

Central nervous system: Agitation, attention disturbance, confusion, depersonalization, derealization, disorientation, disinhibition, dizziness, dream abnormalities, fear, hallucinations, hypersomnia, nightmares, seizure, talkativeness

Dermatologic: Dermatitis, pruritus, rash

Endocrine & metabolic: Libido decreased/increased, menstrual disorders

Gastrointestinal: Salivation increased

Genitourinary: Incontinence

Hepatic: Bilirubin increased, jaundice, liver enzymes increased

Neuromuscular & skeletal: Arthralgia, ataxia, myalgia, paresthesia

Ocular: Diplopia

Respiratory: Allergic rhinitis, dyspnea

Overdosage/Toxicology

Symptoms of overdose include somnolence, confusion, coma, and diminished reflexes. Treatment for benzodiazepine overdose is supportive. Flumazenil has been shown to selectively block the binding of benzodiazepines to CNS receptors, resulting in a reversal of benzodiazepine-induced sedation; however, its use may not reverse respiratory depression.

Pharmacodynamics/Kinetics

Time to Peak: Serum: 1-2 hours

Protein Binding: 80%

Half-Life Elimination: Healthy adults: 11.2 hours (range: 6.3-26.9); Elderly: 16.3 hours (range: 9-26.9 hours); Alcoholic liver disease: 19.7 hours (range: 5.8-65.3 hours); Obesity: 21.8 hours (range: 9.9-40.4 hours)

Metabolism: Hepatic via CYP3A4; forms two active metabolites (4-hydroxyalprazolam and α-hydroxyalprazolam)

Excretion: Urine (as unchanged drug and metabolites)

Available Dosage Forms

Solution, oral [concentrate]:

Alprazolam Intensol®: 1 mg/mL (30 mL)

Tablet: 0.25 mg, 0.5 mg, 1 mg, 2 mg

Xanax®: 0.25 mg, 0.5 mg, 1 mg, 2 mg

Tablet, extended release: 0.5 mg, 1 mg, 2 mg, 3 mg

Xanax XR®: 0.5 mg, 1 mg, 2 mg, 3 mg

Tablet, orally disintegrating:

Niravam™: 0.25 mg, 0.5 mg, 1 mg, 2 mg [orange flavor]

Dosing

Adults: Note: Treatment >4 months should be re-evaluated to determine the patient's continued need for the drug

Anxiety: Oral: *Immediate release:* Effective doses are 0.5-4 mg/day in divided doses; the manufacturer recommends starting at 0.25-0.5 mg 3 times/day; titrate dose upward; usual maximum: 4 mg/day. Patients requiring doses >4 mg/day should be increased cautiously. Periodic reassessment and consideration of dosage reduction is recommended.

Anxiety associated with depression: Oral: *Immediate release:* Average dose required: 2.5-3 mg/day in divided doses

Ethanol withdrawal (unlabeled use): Oral: *Immediate release:* Usual dose: 2-2.5 mg/day in divided doses

Panic disorder: Oral:

Immediate release: Initial: 0.5 mg 3 times/day; dose may be increased every 3-4 days in increments ≤1 mg/day. Mean effective dosage: 5-6 mg/day; many patients obtain relief at 2 mg/day, as much as 10 mg/day may be required

Extended release: 0.5-1 mg once daily; may increase dose every 3-4 days in increments ≤1 mg/day (range: 3-6 mg/day)

Switching from immediate release to extended release: Patients may be switched to extended release tablets by taking the total daily dose of the immediate release tablets and giving it once daily using the extended release preparation.

Preoperative sedation: Oral: 0.5 mg in evening at bedtime and 0.5 mg 1 hour before procedure

Dose reduction: Abrupt discontinuation should be avoided. Daily dose may be decreased by 0.5 mg every 3 days; however, some patients may require a slower reduction. If withdrawal symptoms occur, resume previous dose and discontinue on a less rapid schedule.

Elderly: Initial: 0.125-0.25 mg twice daily; increase by 0.125 mg/day as needed. The smallest effective dose should be used.

Immediate release: Initial 0.25 mg 2-3 times/day

Extended release: Initial: 0.5 mg once daily

Pediatrics:

Anxiety (unlabeled use): Oral: Immediate release: Initial: 0.005 mg/kg/dose or 0.125 mg/dose 3 times/day; increase in increments of 0.125-0.25 mg, up to a maximum of 0.02 mg/kg/dose or 0.06 mg/kg/dose (0.375-3 mg/day). See "Dose Reduction" comment in adult dosing.

Note: Treatment >4 months should be re-evaluated to determine the patient's continued need for the drug.

(Continued)

Alprazolam *(Continued)*

Renal Impairment: No guidelines for adjustment; use caution.

Hepatic Impairment: Oral: Reduce dose by 50% to 60% or avoid in cirrhosis.

Administration

Oral:

Immediate release preparations: Can be administered sublingually with comparable onset and completeness of absorption.

Extended release tablet: Should be taken once daily in the morning; do not crush, break, or chew.

Orally-disintegrating tablets: Using dry hands, place tablet on top of tongue. If using one-half of tablet, immediately discard remaining half (may not remain stable). Administration with water is not necessary.

Stability

Storage:

Orally-disintegrating tablet: Store at room temperature of 20°C to 25°C (68°F to 77°F). Protect from moisture. Seal bottle tightly and discard any cotton packaged inside bottle.

Nursing Actions

Physical Assessment: Assess other medications patient may be taking for effectiveness and interactions. Assess for signs of CNS depression (sedation, dizziness, confusion, or ataxia). Assess for history of addiction; long-term use can result in dependence, abuse, or tolerance; periodically evaluate need for continued use. For inpatient use, institute safety measures and monitor effectiveness and adverse reactions. For outpatients, monitor therapeutic effectiveness and adverse reactions at beginning of therapy and periodically with long-term use. Taper dosage slowly when discontinuing. Assess knowledge/teach patient appropriate use, interventions to reduce side effects, and adverse symptoms to report.

Patient Education: Take exactly as directed; do not increase dose or frequency. Drug may cause physical and/or psychological dependence. Avoid alcohol and do not take other prescription or OTC medications (especially pain medications, sedatives, antihistamines, or hypnotics) without consulting prescriber. Do not stop medication or reduce dosage abruptly without consulting prescriber. Maintain adequate hydration (2-3 L/day of fluids) unless instructed to restrict fluid intake. You may experience drowsiness, lightheadedness, impaired coordination, dizziness, or blurred vision (use caution when driving or engaging in hazardous tasks until response to drug is known); nausea, vomiting, or dry mouth (small frequent meals, frequent mouth care, chewing gum, or sucking lozenges may help); constipation (increased exercise, fluids, fruit, and fiber may help); altered sexual drive or ability (reversible); or photosensitivity (use sunscreen, wear protective clothing and eyewear, and avoid direct sunlight). Report persistent CNS effects (eg, confusion, depression, increased sedation, excitation, headache, agitation, insomnia or nightmares, dizziness, fatigue, impaired coordination, changes in personality, or changes in cognition); changes in urinary pattern; muscle cramping, weakness, tremors, or rigidity; ringing in ears or visual disturbances; chest pain, palpitations, or rapid heartbeat; excessive perspiration; excessive GI symptoms (eg, cramping, constipation, vomiting, anorexia); or worsening of condition. **Pregnancy/breast-feeding precautions:** Do not get pregnant while taking this medication; use appropriate contraceptive measures as recommended by your prescriber. Breast-feeding is not recommended.

Geriatric Considerations Due to short duration of action, it is considered to be a benzodiazepine of choice in the elderly.

Breast-Feeding Issues Symptoms of withdrawal, lethargy, and loss of body weight have been reported in infants exposed to alprazolam and/or benzodiazepines while nursing. Breast-feeding is not recommended.

Pregnancy Issues Benzodiazepines cross the placenta. The association between benzodiazepine exposure and malformations remains controversial. A number of types of malformation have been reported (oral cleft, inguinal hernia, cardiac defects, spina bifida, dysmorphic facial features, skeletal defects); however, confounding factors make a clear association difficult. Overall, the risk to the fetus may be low. Nonteratogenic effects (including neonatal flaccidity, respiratory and feeding problems, and withdrawal symptoms) during the postnatal period have also been reported with benzodiazepine use.

Additional Information Not intended for management of anxieties and minor distresses associated with everyday life. Treatment longer than 4 months should be re-evaluated to determine the patient's need for the drug. Patients who become physically dependent on alprazolam tend to have a difficult time discontinuing it; withdrawal symptoms may be severe. To minimize withdrawal symptoms, taper dosage slowly; do not discontinue abruptly. Abrupt discontinuation after sustained use (generally >10 days) may cause withdrawal symptoms.

Related Information

Anxiolytic / Hypnotic Use in Long-Term Care Facilities *on page 1418*

Federal OBRA Regulations Recommended Maximum Doses *on page 1421*

Alprostadil *(al PROS ta dill)*

U.S. Brand Names Caverject®; Caverject Impulse®; Edex®; Muse®; Prostin VR Pediatric®

Synonyms PGE$_1$; Prostaglandin E$_1$

Pharmacologic Category Prostaglandin

Medication Safety Issues

Sound-alike/look-alike issues:

Alprostadil may be confused with alprazolam

Pregnancy Risk Factor X/C (Muse®)

Lactation Not indicated for use in women

Use

Prostin VR Pediatric®: Temporary maintenance of patency of ductus arteriosus in neonates with ductal-dependent congenital heart disease until surgery can be performed. These defects include cyanotic (eg, pulmonary atresia, pulmonary stenosis, tricuspid atresia, Fallot's tetralogy, transposition of the great vessels) and acyanotic (eg, interruption of aortic arch, coarctation of aorta, hypoplastic left ventricle) heart disease.

Caverject®: Treatment of erectile dysfunction of vasculogenic, psychogenic, or neurogenic etiology; adjunct in the diagnosis of erectile dysfunction

Edex®, Muse®: Treatment of erectile dysfunction of vasculogenic, psychogenic, or neurogenic etiology

Unlabeled/Investigational Use Investigational: Treatment of pulmonary hypertension in infants and children with congenital heart defects with left-to-right shunts

Mechanism of Action/Effect

Erectile dysfunction: Causes vasodilation by dilation of cavernosal arteries when injected along the penile shaft, allowing blood flow to, and entrapment in, the lacunar spaces of the penis (ie, corporeal veno-occlusive mechanism)

Neonate: Has direct effects on smooth muscle of ductus arteriosus.

Contraindications Hypersensitivity to alprostadil or any component of the formulation; hyaline membrane disease or persistent fetal circulation and when a dominant left-to-right shunt is present; respiratory distress syndrome; conditions predisposing patients to priapism (sickle cell anemia, multiple myeloma, leukemia);

patients with anatomical deformation of the penis, penile implants; use in men for whom sexual activity is inadvisable or contraindicated; pregnancy

Warnings/Precautions Use cautiously in neonates with bleeding tendencies. Apnea may occur in 10% to 12% of neonates with congenital heart defects, especially in those weighing <2 kg at birth. Apnea usually appears during the first hour of drug infusion.

When used in erectile dysfunction, priapism may occur. Patient must be instructed to report to physician or seek immediate medical assistance if an erection persists for longer than 4 hours. Treat immediately to avoid penile tissue damage and permanent loss of potency; discontinue therapy if signs of penile fibrosis develop (penile angulation, cavernosal fibrosis, or Peyronie's disease). Syncope occurring within 1 hour of administration has been reported. The potential for drug-drug interactions may occur when prescribed concomitantly with antihypertensives. Some lowering of blood pressure may occur without symptoms, and swelling of leg veins, leg pain, perineal pain, and rapid pulse have been reported in <2% of patients during in-clinic titration and home treatment.

Drug Interactions

Increased Effect/Toxicity: Risk of hypotension and syncope may be increased with antihypertensives.

Nutritional/Ethanol Interactions Ethanol: Avoid concurrent use (vasodilating effect).

Adverse Reactions

Intraurethral:

>10%: Genitourinary: Penile pain, urethral burning

2% to 10%:

Central nervous system: Headache, dizziness, pain

Genitourinary: Vaginal itching (female partner), testicular pain, urethral bleeding (minor)

Intracavernosal injection:

>10%: Genitourinary: Penile pain

1% to 10%:

Cardiovascular: Hypertension

Central nervous system: Headache, dizziness

Genitourinary: Prolonged erection (>4 hours, 4%), penile fibrosis, penis disorder, penile rash, penile edema

Local: Injection site hematoma and/or bruising

Intravenous:

>10%:

Cardiovascular: Flushing

Central nervous system: Fever

Respiratory: Apnea

1% to 10%:

Cardiovascular: Bradycardia, hyper-/hypotension, tachycardia, cardiac arrest, edema

Central nervous system: Seizures, headache, dizziness

Endocrine & metabolic: Hypokalemia

Gastrointestinal: Diarrhea

Hematologic: Disseminated intravascular coagulation

Neuromuscular & skeletal: Back pain

Respiratory: Upper respiratory infection, flu syndrome, sinusitis, nasal congestion, cough

Miscellaneous: Sepsis, localized pain in structures other than the injection site

Overdosage/Toxicology Symptoms of overdose when treating patent ductus arteriosus include apnea, bradycardia, hypotension, and flushing. If hypotension or pyrexia occurs, the infusion rate should be reduced until symptoms subside. Apnea or bradycardia requires drug discontinuation. If intracavernous overdose occurs, supervise until systemic effects have resolved or until penile detumescence has occurred.

Pharmacodynamics/Kinetics

Onset of Action: Rapid

Duration of Action: <1 hour

Protein Binding: Plasma: 81% to albumin

Half-Life Elimination: 5-10 minutes

Metabolism: ~75% by oxidation in one pass via lungs

Excretion: Urine (90% as metabolites) within 24 hours

Available Dosage Forms [DSC] = Discontinued product

Injection, powder for reconstitution:

Caverject®: 20 mcg, 40 mcg [contains lactose; diluent contains benzyl alcohol]

Caverject Impulse®: 10 mcg, 20 mcg [prefilled injection system; contains lactose; diluent contains benzyl alcohol]

Edex®: 10 mcg, 20 mcg, 40 mcg [contains lactose; packaged in kits containing diluent, syringe, and alcohol swab]

Injection, solution: 500 mcg/mL (1 mL)

Prostin VR Pediatric®: 500 mcg/mL (1 mL) [contains dehydrated alcohol]

Pellet, urethral (Muse®): 125 mcg (6s), 250 mcg (6s), 500 mcg (6s), 1000 mcg (6s)

Dosing

Adults & Elderly:

Erectile dysfunction:

Intracavernous (Caverject®, Edex®): Individualize dose by careful titration; doses >40 mcg (Edex®) or >60 mcg (Caverject®) are not recommended: Initial dose must be titrated in physician's office. Patient must stay in the physician's office until complete detumescence occurs; if there is no response, then the next higher dose may be given within 1 hour; if there is still no response, a 1-day interval before giving the next dose is recommended; increasing the dose or concentration in the treatment of impotence results in increasing pain and discomfort

Vasculogenic, psychogenic, or mixed etiology: Initiate dosage titration at 2.5 mcg, increasing by 2.5 mcg to a dose of 5 mcg and then in increments of 5-10 mcg depending on the erectile response until the dose produces an erection suitable for intercourse, not lasting >1 hour; if there is absolutely no response to initial 2.5 mcg dose, the second dose may be increased to 7.5 mcg, followed by increments of 5-10 mcg

Neurogenic etiology (eg, spinal cord injury): Initiate dosage titration at 1.25 mcg, increasing to a dose of 2.5 mcg and then 5 mcg; increase further in increments 5 mcg until the dose is reached that produces an erection suitable for intercourse, not lasting >1 hour

Maintenance: Once appropriate dose has been determined, patient may self-administer injections at a frequency of no more than 3 times/ week with at least 24 hours between doses

Intraurethral (Muse® Pellet):

Initial: 125-250 mcg

Maintenance: Administer as needed to achieve an erection; duration of action is about 30-60 minutes; use only two systems per 24-hour period

Pediatrics:

Patent ductus arteriosus I.V.:

Prostin VR Pediatric®: I.V. continuous infusion into a large vein, or alternatively through an umbilical artery catheter placed at the ductal opening: 0.05-0.1 mcg/kg/minute with therapeutic response, rate is reduced to lowest effective dosage. With unsatisfactory response, rate is increased gradually; maintenance: 0.01-0.4 mcg/kg/minute.

Note: PGE₁ is usually given at an infusion rate of 0.1 mcg/kg/minute, but it is often possible to reduce the dosage to ½ or even ¹⁄₁₀ without losing

(Continued)

Alprostadil *(Continued)*

the therapeutic effect. The mixing schedule is shown in the table.

Alprostadil

Add 1 Ampul (500 mcg) to:	Concentration (mcg/mL)	Infusion Rate	
		mL/min/kg Needed to Infuse 0.1 mcg/kg/min	mL/kg/24 h
250 mL	2	0.05	72
100 mL	5	0.02	28.8
50 mL	10	0.01	14.4
25 mL	20	0.005	7.2

Note: Therapeutic response is indicated by increased pH in those with acidosis or by an increase in oxygenation (PO_2) usually evident within 30 minutes.

Administration

Other: Erectile dysfunction: Use a $1/2$ inch, 27- to 30-gauge needle. Inject into the dorsolateral aspect of the proximal third of the penis, avoiding visible veins; alternate side of the penis for injections.

Stability

Reconstitution:

Caverject® Impulse™: Provided as a dual-chamber syringe with diluent in one chamber. To mix, hold syringe with needle pointing upward and turn plunger clockwise; turn upside down several times to mix. Device can be set to deliver specified dose, each device can be set at various increments.

Caverject® powder: Use only the supplied diluent for reconstitution (ie, bacteriostatic/sterile water with benzyl alcohol 0.945%).

Edex®: Reconstitute with NS.

Storage:

Caverject® Impulse™: Store at controlled room temperature of 15°C to 30°C (59°F to 86°F). Following reconstitution, use within 24 hours and discard any unused solution.

Caverject® powder: The 5 mcg, 10 mcg, and 20 mcg vials should be stored at or below 25°C (77°F); The 40 mcg vial should be stored at 2°C to 8°C until dispensed. After dispensing, stable for up to 3 months at or below 25°C. Following reconstitution, all strengths should be stored at or below 25°C (77°F); do not refrigerate or freeze; use within 24 hours.

Caverject® solution: Prior to dispensing, store frozen at -20°C to -10°C (-4°F to -14°F). Once dispensed, may be stored frozen for up to 3 months, or under refrigeration at 2°C to 8°C (36°F to 46°F) for up to 7 days. Do not refreeze. Once removed from foil wrap, solution may be allowed to warm to room temperature prior to use. If not used immediately, solution should be discarded. Shake well prior to use.

Edex®: Store at controlled room temperature of 15°C to 30°C (59°F to 86°F); following reconstitution, use immediately and discard any unused solution.

Muse®: Refrigerate at 2°C to 8°C (36°F to 46°F); may be stored at room temperature for up to 14 days

Prostin VR Pediatric®: Refrigerate at 2°C to 8°C (36°F to 46°F). Prior to infusion, dilute with D_5W or NS; use within 24 hours.

Nursing Actions

Physical Assessment: Neonate: Monitor closely; apnea has occurred during first hour after administration. **Erectile dysfunction:** After individual dose titration is determined by physician, the Caverject® injection (or Muse®) is generally self-administered.

Teach patient proper use if self-administered (appropriate injection technique and syringe/needle disposal), possible side effects/appropriate interventions, and adverse symptoms to report. **Pregnancy risk factor X:** See Pregnancy Issues.

Patient Education: Use only as directed, no more than 3 times/week, allowing 24 hours between injections. Avoid alcohol. Store in refrigerator and dilute with supplied diluent immediately before use. Use alternate sides of penis with each injection. Dispose of syringes and needle and single-dose vials in a safe manner (do not share medication, syringes, or needles). Note that the risk of transmitting blood-borne disease is increased with use of alprostadil injections since a small amount of bleeding at injection site is possible. Stop using and contact prescriber immediately if signs of priapism occur, erections last more than 4 hours, or you experience moderate to severe penile pain. Report penile problems (eg, nodules, new penile pain, rash, bruising, numbness, swelling, signs of infection, abnormal ejaculations); cardiac symptoms (hypo- or hypertension, chest pain, palpitations, irregular heartbeat); flushing, fever, flu-like symptoms; respiratory difficulty or wheezing; or other adverse reactions. Refer to prescriber every 3 months to ensure proper technique and for dosage evaluation. **Pregnancy precautions:** Consult prescriber about use of contraceptives. Do not give blood while taking this medication and for 1 month following discontinuance.

Geriatric Considerations Elderly may have concomitant diseases which would contraindicate the use of alprostadil. Other forms of attaining penile tumescence are recommended.

Pregnancy Issues Alprostadil is embryotoxic in animal studies. It is not indicated for use in women. The manufacturer of Muse® recommends a condom barrier when being used during sexual intercourse with a pregnant women.

Alteplase *(AL te plase)*

U.S. Brand Names Activase®; Cathflo® Activase®

Synonyms Alteplase, Recombinant; Alteplase, Tissue Plasminogen Activator, Recombinant; tPA

Pharmacologic Category Thrombolytic Agent

Medication Safety Issues

Sound-alike/look-alike issues:

Alteplase may be confused with Altace®

"tPA" abbreviation should not be used when writing orders for this medication; has been misread as TNKase (tenecteplase)

Pregnancy Risk Factor C

Lactation Excretion in breast milk unknown/use caution

Use Management of acute myocardial infarction for the lysis of thrombi in coronary arteries; management of acute massive pulmonary embolism (PE) in adults

Acute myocardial infarction (AMI): Chest pain ≥20 minutes, ≤12-24 hours; S-T elevation ≥0.1 mV in at least two ECG leads

Acute pulmonary embolism (APE): Age ≤75 years: Documented massive pulmonary embolism by pulmonary angiography or echocardiography or high probability lung scan with clinical shock

Cathflo® Activase®: Restoration of central venous catheter function

Unlabeled/Investigational Use Acute peripheral arterial occlusive disease

Mechanism of Action/Effect Dissolves thrombus (clot)

Contraindications Hypersensitivity to alteplase or any component of the formulation

Treatment of acute MI or PE: Active internal bleeding; history of CVA; recent intracranial or intraspinal surgery or trauma; intracranial neoplasm; arteriovenous malformation or aneurysm; known bleeding diathesis; severe uncontrolled hypertension

Treatment of acute ischemic stroke: Evidence of intracranial hemorrhage or suspicion of subarachnoid hemorrhage on pretreatment evaluation; recent (within 3 months) intracranial or intraspinal surgery; prolonged external cardiac massage; suspected aortic dissection; serious head trauma or previous stroke; history of intracranial hemorrhage; uncontrolled hypertension at time of treatment (eg, >185 mm Hg systolic or >110 mm Hg diastolic); seizure at the onset of stroke; active internal bleeding; intracranial neoplasm; arteriovenous malformation or aneurysm; known bleeding diathesis including but not limited to: current use of anticoagulants or an INR >1.7, administration of heparin within 48 hours preceding the onset of stroke and an elevated aPTT at presentation, platelet count <100,000/mm³.

Other exclusion criteria (NINDS recombinant tPA study): Stroke or serious head injury within 3 months, major surgery or serious trauma within 2 weeks, GI or urinary tract hemorrhage within 3 weeks, aggressive treatment required to lower blood pressure, glucose level <50 mg/dL or >400 mg/dL, arterial puncture at a noncompressible site or lumbar puncture within 1 week, clinical presentation suggesting post-MI pericarditis, pregnancy, breast-feeding

Warnings/Precautions Concurrent heparin anticoagulation may contribute to bleeding. Monitor all potential bleeding sites. Doses >150 mg are associated with increased risk of intracranial hemorrhage. Intramuscular injections and nonessential handling of the patient should be avoided. Venipunctures should be performed carefully and only when necessary. If arterial puncture is necessary, use an upper extremity vessel that can be manually compressed. If serious bleeding occurs, the infusion of alteplase and heparin should be stopped.

For the following conditions, the risk of bleeding is higher with use of alteplase and should be weighed against the benefits of therapy: Recent major surgery (eg, CABG, obstetrical delivery, organ biopsy, previous puncture of noncompressible vessels), cerebrovascular disease, recent gastrointestinal or genitourinary bleeding, recent trauma, hypertension (systolic BP >175 mm Hg and/or diastolic BP >110 mm Hg), high likelihood of left heart thrombus (eg, mitral stenosis with atrial fibrillation), acute pericarditis, subacute bacterial endocarditis, hemostatic defects including ones caused by severe renal or hepatic dysfunction, significant hepatic dysfunction, pregnancy, diabetic hemorrhagic retinopathy or other hemorrhagic ophthalmic conditions, septic thrombophlebitis or occluded AV cannula at seriously infected site, advanced age (eg, >75 years), patients receiving oral anticoagulants, any other condition in which bleeding constitutes a significant hazard or would be particularly difficult to manage because of location.

Coronary thrombolysis may result in reperfusion arrhythmias. Treatment of patients with acute ischemic stroke more than 3 hours after symptom onset is not recommended. Treatment of patients with minor neurological deficit or with rapidly improving symptoms is not recommended.

Cathflo® Activase®: When used to restore catheter function, use Cathflo® cautiously in those patients with known or suspected catheter infections. Evaluate catheter for other causes of dysfunction before use. Avoid excessive pressure when instilling into catheter.

Drug Interactions
Decreased Effect: Aminocaproic acid (an antifibrinolytic agent) may decrease the effectiveness of thrombolytic therapy. Nitroglycerin may increase the hepatic clearance of alteplase, potentially reducing lytic activity (limited clinical information).

Increased Effect/Toxicity: The potential for hemorrhage with alteplase is increased by oral anticoagulants (warfarin), heparin, low molecular weight heparins, and drugs which affect platelet function (eg, NSAIDs, dipyridamole, ticlopidine, clopidogrel, IIb/IIIa antagonists). Concurrent use with aspirin and heparin may increase the risk of bleeding. However, aspirin and heparin were used concomitantly with alteplase in the majority of patients in clinical studies.

Nutritional/Ethanol Interactions Herb/Nutraceutical: Avoid cat's claw, dong quai, evening primrose, feverfew, red clover, horse chestnut, garlic, green tea, ginseng, ginkgo (all have additional antiplatelet activity).

Lab Interactions Altered results of coagulation and fibrinolytic agents

Adverse Reactions As with all drugs which may affect hemostasis, bleeding is the major adverse effect associated with alteplase. Hemorrhage may occur at virtually any site. Risk is dependent on multiple variables, including the dosage administered, concurrent use of multiple agents which alter hemostasis, and patient predisposition. Rapid lysis of coronary artery thrombi by thrombolytic agents may be associated with reperfusion-related atrial and/or ventricular arrhythmia. **Note:** Lowest rate of bleeding complications expected with dose used to restore catheter function.

1% to 10%:
Cardiovascular: Hypotension
Central nervous system: Fever
Dermatologic: Bruising (1%)
Gastrointestinal: GI hemorrhage (5%), nausea, vomiting
Genitourinary: GU hemorrhage (4%)
Hematologic: Bleeding (0.5% major, 7% minor: GUSTO trial)
Local: Bleeding at catheter puncture site (15.3%, accelerated administration)
Additional cardiovascular events associated **with use in MI:** AV block, cardiogenic shock, heart failure, cardiac arrest, recurrent ischemia/infarction, myocardial rupture, electromechanical dissociation, pericardial effusion, pericarditis, mitral regurgitation, cardiac tamponade, thromboembolism, pulmonary edema, asystole, ventricular tachycardia, bradycardia, ruptured intracranial AV malformation, seizure, hemorrhagic bursitis, cholesterol crystal embolization
Additional events associated **with use in pulmonary embolism:** Pulmonary re-embolization, pulmonary edema, pleural effusion, thromboembolism
Additional events associated **with use in stroke:** Cerebral edema, cerebral herniation, seizure, new ischemic stroke

Overdosage/Toxicology Symptoms of overdose include increased incidence of intracranial bleeding.

Pharmacodynamics/Kinetics
Duration of Action: >50% present in plasma cleared ~5 minutes after infusion terminated, ~80% cleared within 10 minutes
Excretion: Clearance: Rapidly from circulating plasma (550-650 mL/minute), primarily hepatic; >50% present in plasma is cleared within 5 minutes after the infusion is terminated, ~80% cleared within 10 minutes

Available Dosage Forms
Injection, powder for reconstitution, recombinant:
Activase®: 50 mg [29 million int. units; contains polysorbate 80; packaged with diluent]; 100 mg [58 million int. units; contains polysorbate 80; packaged with diluent and transfer device]
Cathflo® Activase®: 2 mg [contains polysorbate 80]

Dosing
Adults & Elderly:
Coronary artery thrombi: I.V. Front loading dose (weight-based):
Patients >67 kg: Total dose: 100 mg over 1.5 hours; infuse 15 mg over 1-2 minutes. Infuse 50 mg over 30 minutes. See "Note" on next page.
(Continued)

Alteplase (Continued)

Patients ≤67 kg: Total dose: 1.25 mg/kg; infuse 15 mg I.V. bolus over 1-2 minutes, then infuse 0.75 mg/kg (not to exceed 50 mg) over next 30 minutes, followed by 0.5 mg/kg over next 60 minutes (not to exceed 35 mg). See "Note".

Note: Concurrently, begin heparin 60 units/kg bolus (maximum: 4000 units) followed by continuous infusion of 12 units/kg/hour (maximum: 1000 units/hour) and adjust to aPTT target of 1.5-2 times the upper limit of control. Infuse remaining 35 mg of alteplase over the next hour.

Acute pulmonary embolism: I.V.: 100 mg over 2 hours.

Acute ischemic stroke: I.V.: Doses should be given within the first 3 hours of the onset of symptoms; recommended total dose: 0.9 mg/kg (maximum dose should not exceed 90 mg) infused over 60 minutes.

Load with 0.09 mg/kg (10% of the 0.9 mg/kg dose) as an I.V. bolus over 1 minute, followed by 0.81 mg/kg (90% of the 0.9 mg/kg dose) as a continuous infusion over 60 minutes. Heparin should not be started for 24 hours or more after starting alteplase for stroke.

Central venous catheter clearance: Intracatheter (Cathflo® Activase® 1 mg/mL):

Patients <30 kg: 110% of the internal lumen volume of the catheter, not to exceed 2 mg/2 mL; retain in catheter for 0.5-2 hours; may instill a second dose if catheter remains occluded

Patients ≥30 kg: 2 mg (2 mL); retain in catheter for 0.5-2 hours; may instill a second dose if catheter remains occluded

Acute peripheral arterial occlusive disease (unlabeled use): Intra-arterial: 0.02-0.1 mg/kg/hour for up to 36 hours

Advisory Panel to the Society for Cardiovascular and Interventional Radiology on Thrombolytic Therapy recommendation: ≤2 mg/hour and subtherapeutic heparin (aPTT <1.5 times baseline)

Pediatrics: Central venous catheter clearance: Intracatheter: Patients <30 kg: 110% of the internal lumen volume of the catheter, not to exceed 2 mg/2 mL; retain in catheter for 0.5-2 hours; may instill a second dose if catheter remains occluded

Administration

I.V.: Activase®: Acute MI: Accelerated infusion:

Bolus dose may be prepared by one of three methods:

1) removal of 15 mL reconstituted (1 mg/mL) solution from vial

2) removal of 15 mL from a port on the infusion line after priming

3) programming an infusion pump to deliver a 15 mL bolus at the initiation of infusion

Remaining dose may be administered as follows:

50 mg vial: Either PVC bag or glass vial and infusion set

100 mg vial: Insert spike end of the infusion set through the same puncture site created by transfer device and infuse from vial

If further dilution is desired, may be diluted in equal volume of 0.9% sodium chloride or D₅W to yield a final concentration of 0.5 mg/mL AD

I.V. Detail: Reconstituted solution should be clear or pale yellow and transparent. Avoid agitation during dilution.

pH: 5-7.3

Other: Cathflo® Activase®: Intracatheter: Instill dose into occluded catheter. Do not force solution into catheter. After a 30-minute dwell time, assess catheter function by attempting to aspirate blood. If catheter is functional, aspirate 4-5 mL of blood in patients ≥10 kg or 3 mL in patients <10 kg to remove Cathflo® Activase® and residual clots. Gently irrigate the catheter with NS. If catheter remains nonfunctional, let Cathflo® Activase® dwell for another 90 minutes (total dwell time: 120 minutes) and reassess function. If catheter function is not restored, a second dose may be instilled.

Stability

Reconstitution:

Activase®:

50 mg vial: Use accompanying diluent (50 mL sterile water for injection); do not shake; final concentration: 1 mg/mL

100 mg vial: Use transfer set with accompanying diluent (100 mL vial of sterile water for injection); no vacuum is present in 100 mg vial; final concentration: 1 mg/mL

Cathflo® Activase®: Add 2.2 mL SWFI to vial; do not shake. Final concentration: 1 mg/mL.

Compatibility: Stable in NS, SWFI; **incompatible** with bacteriostatic water

Y-site administration: Incompatible with dobutamine, dopamine, heparin, nitroglycerin

Compatibility when admixed: Incompatible with dobutamine, dopamine, heparin

Storage:

Activase®: The lyophilized product may be stored at room temperature (not to exceed 30°C/86°F), or under refrigeration; once reconstituted it should be used within 8 hours

Cathflo® Activase®: Store lyophilized product in refrigerated. Once reconstituted, store at 2°C to 30°C (36°F to 86°F) and use within 8 hours.

Laboratory Monitoring CBC, PTT

Nursing Actions

Physical Assessment: Assess potential for interactions with other prescriptions, OTC medications, or herbal products patient may be taking (especially those medications that may affect coagulation or platelet function). See specific instructions for safe I.V. administration. Monitor vital signs, laboratory results, and ECG prior to, during, and after therapy. Report abnormalities to prescriber immediately. Arrhythmias may occur; have antiarrhythmic drugs available. Assess infusion site and monitor for hemorrhage every 10 minutes (or according to institutional policy) during therapy and for 1 hour following therapy. Maintain strict bedrest. Monitor for excess bleeding and use/teach bleeding precautions (avoid invasive procedures and activities that could cause trauma). Patient instruction is determined by patient condition.

Patient Education: This medication can only be administered by infusion; you will be monitored closely during and after treatment. You will have a tendency to bleed easily; use caution to prevent injury (use electric razor, soft toothbrush, and use caution with knives, needles, or anything sharp). Follow instructions for strict bedrest to reduce the risk of injury. If bleeding occurs, report immediately and apply pressure to bleeding spot until bleeding stops completely. Report unusual pain (acute headache, joint pain, chest pain); unusual bruising or bleeding; blood in urine, stool, or vomit; bleeding gums; vision changes; or respiratory difficulty. **Pregnancy/breast-feeding precautions:** Inform prescriber if you are or intend to become pregnant. Consult prescriber if breast-feeding. **Other issues:** Drug is frequently administered with heparin. Discontinue both if serious bleeding occurs. Avoid invasive procedures.

Other Issues Drug is frequently administered with heparin. Discontinue both if serious bleeding occurs. Avoid invasive procedures.

Altretamine (al TRET a meen)

U.S. Brand Names Hexalen®

Synonyms Hexamethylmelamine; HEXM; HMM; HXM; NSC-13875

Pharmacologic Category Antineoplastic Agent, Miscellaneous

Pregnancy Risk Factor D

Lactation Excretion in breast milk unknown

Use Palliative treatment of persistent or recurrent ovarian cancer

Mechanism of Action/Effect Exact mechanism of action that causes cell death is not known. Metabolism in the liver is required for cytotoxicity. Although altretamine's clinical antitumor spectrum resembles that of alkylating agents, the drug has demonstrated activity in alkylator-resistant patients. The drug selectively inhibits the incorporation of radioactive thymidine and uridine into DNA and RNA, inhibiting DNA and RNA synthesis. Reactive intermediates covalently bind to microsomal proteins and DNA; can spontaneously degrade to demethylated melamines and formaldehyde which are also cytotoxic.

Contraindications Hypersensitivity to altretamine or any component of the formulation; pre-existing severe bone marrow suppression or severe neurologic toxicity; pregnancy

Warnings/Precautions The U.S. Food and Drug Administration (FDA) currently recommends that procedures for proper handling and disposal of antineoplastic agents be considered. Use with caution in patients previously treated with other myelosuppressive drugs or with pre-existing neurotoxicity. Use with caution in patients with renal or hepatic dysfunction.

Drug Interactions

Decreased Effect: Phenobarbital may increase metabolism of altretamine which may decrease the effect.

Increased Effect/Toxicity: Altretamine may cause severe orthostatic hypotension when administered with MAO inhibitors. Cimetidine may decrease metabolism of altretamine.

Adverse Reactions

>10%:

Central nervous system: Peripheral sensory neuropathy, neurotoxicity (21%; may be progressive and dose-limiting)

Gastrointestinal: Nausea/vomiting (50% to 70%), anorexia (48%), diarrhea (48%)

Hematologic: Anemia, thrombocytopenia (31%), leukopenia (62%), neutropenia

1% to 10%:

Central nervous system: Seizures

Gastrointestinal: Stomach cramps

Hepatic: Alkaline phosphatase increased

Overdosage/Toxicology Symptoms of overdose include nausea, vomiting, peripheral neuropathy, severe bone marrow suppression. Treatment is supportive.

Pharmacodynamics/Kinetics

Time to Peak: Plasma: 0.5-3 hours

Half-Life Elimination: 13 hours

Metabolism: Hepatic; rapid and extensive demethylation; active metabolites

Excretion: Urine (<1% as unchanged drug)

Available Dosage Forms Gelcap: 50 mg [contains lactose]

Dosing

Adults & Elderly: Ovarian cancer (palliative): Oral: 4-12 mg/kg/day in 3-4 divided doses for 21-90 days

Alternatively: 240-320 mg/m²/day in 3-4 divided doses per day for 21 days, repeated every 6 weeks

Alternatively: 260 mg/m²/day in 4 divided doses per day for 14-21 days of a 28-day cycle

Alternatively: 150 mg/m²/day in 3-4 divided doses for 14 days of a 28-day cycle

Administration

Oral: Administer total daily dose as 3-4 divided doses after meals and at bedtime.

Laboratory Monitoring CBC with platelet count and differential should be done routinely before and after drug therapy.

Nursing Actions

Physical Assessment: Monitor results of laboratory tests and adverse response (eg, neuropathy, gastrointestinal upset, anemia). Teach patient appropriate use, possible side effects/appropriate interventions, and adverse symptoms to report.

Patient Education: Do not take any new medications (including aspirin or any aspirin-containing products) during treatment unless approved by prescriber. Take exactly as directed, preferably after meals. Avoid alcohol. May cause nausea or vomiting (small, frequent meals, good mouth care, chewing gum, or sucking lozenges may help). You will be more susceptible to infection (avoid crowds and exposure to infection). Report any numbness, tingling, or pain in extremities; unrelieved nausea or vomiting; tremors; yellowing of skin or eyes; fever; chills; easy bruising or unusual bleeding; extreme weakness; or increased fatigue. **Pregnancy/breast-feeding precautions:** Do not get pregnant while taking this medication. Consult prescriber for appropriate barrier contraceptive measures. Consult prescriber if breast-feeding.

Dietary Considerations Should be taken after meals at bedtime.

Aluminum Hydroxide (a LOO mi num hye DROKS ide)

U.S. Brand Names ALternaGel® [OTC]; Dermagran® [OTC]

Pharmacologic Category Antacid; Antidote; Protectant, Topical

Pregnancy Risk Factor C

Lactation Excretion in breast milk unknown

Use Treatment of hyperacidity; hyperphosphatemia; temporary protection of minor cuts, scrapes, and burns

Mechanism of Action/Effect Neutralizes or reduces gastric acidity, resulting in increased gastric pH and inhibition of pepsin activity

Contraindications Hypersensitivity to aluminum salts or any component of the formulation

Warnings/Precautions

Oral: Binds with phosphate ions. Hypophosphatemia may occur with prolonged administration or large doses. Use with caution in patients with CHF, renal failure, edema, cirrhosis, and low sodium diets, and patients who have recently suffered GI hemorrhage. Uremic patients not receiving dialysis may develop aluminum intoxication or osteomalacia and osteoporosis due to phosphate depletion.

Topical: Not for application over deep wounds, puncture wounds, infected areas, or lacerations. When used for self medication (OTC use), consult with healthcare provider if needed for >7 days or for use in children <6 months of age.

Drug Interactions

Decreased Effect: Aluminum hydroxide may decrease the absorption of allopurinol, antibiotics (tetracyclines, quinolones, some cephalosporins), bisphosphonate derivatives, corticosteroids, cyclosporine, delavirdine, iron salts, imidazole antifungals, isoniazid, mycophenolate, penicillamine, phosphate supplements, phenytoin, phenothiazines, trientine. Absorption of aluminum hydroxide may be decreased by citric acid derivatives.

(Continued)

Aluminum Hydroxide *(Continued)*

Lab Interactions Decreased phosphorus, inorganic (S); may interfere with some gastric imaging techniques or gastric acid secretion tests

Adverse Reactions Frequency not defined.

Gastrointestinal: Constipation, stomach cramps, fecal impaction, nausea, vomiting, discoloration of feces (white speckles)

Endocrine & metabolic: Hypophosphatemia, hypomagnesemia

Overdosage/Toxicology Aluminum antacids may cause constipation, phosphate depletion, and bezoar or fecalith formation. In patients with renal failure, aluminum may accumulate to toxic levels. Deferoxamine, traditionally used as an iron chelator, has been shown to increase urinary aluminum output. Deferoxamine chelation of aluminum has resulted in improvement of clinical symptoms and bone histology; however, this remains an experimental treatment for aluminum poisoning and has significant potential for adverse effects.

Available Dosage Forms

Ointment:

Dermagran®: 0.275% (120 g)

Suspension, oral: 320 mg/5 mL (473 mL)

ALternaGel®: 600 mg/5 mL (360 mL)

Dosing

Adults & Elderly:

Hyperphosphatemia: Oral: Initial: 300-600 mg 3 times/day with meals

Hyperacidity: Oral: 600-1200 mg between meals and at bedtime

Skin protectant: Topical: Apply to affected area as needed; reapply at least every 12 hours

Pediatrics:

Hyperphosphatemia: Oral: 50-150 mg/kg/24 hours in divided doses every 4-6 hours, titrate dosage to maintain serum phosphorus within normal range

Skin protectant: Topical: Refer to adult dosing.

Renal Impairment: Aluminum may accumulate in renal impairment.

Administration

Oral: Dose should be followed with water.

Topical: Apply as needed to affected area; reapply at least every 12 hours

Laboratory Monitoring Monitor calcium and phosphate levels periodically when patient is on chronic therapy

Nursing Actions

Physical Assessment: Monitor appropriate laboratory tests and effectiveness of treatment. Assess for constipation.

Patient Education: Take as directed, preferably 1-3 hours after meals (when used as an antacid) or with any other medications. When used to decrease phosphorus, take within 20 minutes of a meal. Do not increase sodium intake and maintain adequate hydration (2-3 L/day of fluids) unless instructed to restrict fluid intake. You may experience constipation (increased exercise, fluids, fruit, or fiber may help; if unresolved, contact prescriber). Report unresolved nausea, malaise, muscle weakness, blood in stool or black stool, or abdominal pain. **Pregnancy/breast-feeding precautions:** Inform prescriber if you are or intend to become pregnant. Consult prescriber if breast-feeding.

Dietary Considerations Should be taken 1-3 hours after meals when used as an antacid. When used to decrease phosphorus, should be taken within 20 minutes of a meal.

Geriatric Considerations Elderly, due to disease and/or drug therapy, may be predisposed to constipation and fecal impaction. This may be managed with a stool softener or laxatives. Careful evaluation of possible drug interactions must be done. Consider renal insufficiency (<30 mL/minute) as predisposition to aluminum toxicity.

Amantadine *(a MAN ta deen)*

U.S. Brand Names Symmetrel®

Synonyms Adamantanamine Hydrochloride; Amantadine Hydrochloride

Pharmacologic Category Anti-Parkinson's Agent, Dopamine Agonist; Antiviral Agent, Adamantane

Medication Safety Issues

Sound-alike/look-alike issues:

Amantadine may be confused with ranitidine, rimantadine

Symmetrel® may be confused with Synthroid®

Pregnancy Risk Factor C

Lactation Enters breast milk/not recommended

Use Prophylaxis and treatment of influenza A viral infection; treatment of parkinsonism; treatment of drug-induced extrapyramidal symptoms

Mechanism of Action/Effect As an antiviral, blocks the uncoating of influenza A virus preventing penetration of virus into host; antiparkinsonian activity may be due to its blocking the reuptake of dopamine into presynaptic neurons or by increasing dopamine release from presynaptic fibers

Contraindications Hypersensitivity to amantadine, rimantadine, or any component of the formulation

Warnings/Precautions Use with caution in patients with liver disease, history of recurrent and eczematoid dermatitis, uncontrolled psychosis or severe psychoneurosis, seizures, and in those receiving CNS stimulant drugs. Reduce dose in renal disease. When treating Parkinson's disease, do not discontinue abruptly. In many patients, the therapeutic benefits of amantadine are limited to a few months. Elderly patients may be more susceptible to CNS effects (using 2 divided daily doses may minimize this effect). Has been associated with neuroleptic malignant syndrome (associated with dose reduction or abrupt discontinuation). Has not been shown to prevent bacterial infection or complications when used as prophylaxis or treatment of influenza A. Use with caution in patients with CHF, peripheral edema, or orthostatic hypotension. Avoid in angle closure glaucoma.

Drug Interactions

Increased Effect/Toxicity: Anticholinergics (benztropine and trihexyphenidyl) may potentiate CNS side effects of amantadine. Hydrochlorothiazide, triamterene, and/or trimethoprim may increase toxicity of amantadine; monitor for altered response.

Nutritional/Ethanol Interactions Ethanol: Avoid ethanol (may increase CNS adverse effects).

Adverse Reactions 1% to 10%:

Cardiovascular: Orthostatic hypotension, peripheral edema

Central nervous system: Insomnia, depression, anxiety, irritability, dizziness, hallucinations, ataxia, headache, somnolence, nervousness, dream abnormality, agitation, fatigue, confusion

Dermatologic: Livedo reticularis

Gastrointestinal: Nausea, anorexia, constipation, diarrhea, xerostomia

Respiratory: Dry nose

Overdosage/Toxicology Symptoms of overdose include nausea, vomiting, slurred speech, blurred vision, lethargy, hallucinations, seizures, and myoclonic jerking. Acute toxicity may be primarily due to anticholinergic effects. The minimum lethal dose may be as low as 1 g. Treatment should be directed at reducing CNS stimulation, controlling seizures, and maintaining cardiovascular function.

Pharmacodynamics/Kinetics

Onset of Action: Antidyskinetic: Within 48 hours

Protein Binding: Normal renal function: ~67%; Hemodialysis: ~59%

Half-Life Elimination: Normal renal function: 16 ± 6 hours (9-31 hours); End-stage renal disease: 7-10 days

Metabolism: Not appreciable; small amounts of an acetyl metabolite identified

Excretion: Urine (80% to 90% unchanged) by glomerular filtration and tubular secretion; Total clearance: 2.5-10.5 L/hour

Available Dosage Forms [DSC] = Discontinued product

Capsule, as hydrochloride: 100 mg

Syrup, as hydrochloride: 50 mg/5 mL (480 mL)

Symmetrel®: 50 mg/5 mL (480 mL) [raspberry flavor] [DSC]

Tablet, as hydrochloride (Symmetrel®): 100 mg

Dosing

Adults:

Influenza A treatment: Oral: 100 mg twice daily; initiate within 24-48 hours after onset of symptoms; discontinue as soon as possible based on clinical response (generally within 3-5 days or within 24-48 hours after symptoms disappear).

Influenza A prophylaxis: Oral: 100 mg twice daily; continue treatment throughout the peak influenza activity in the community or throughout the entire influenza season in patients who cannot be vaccinated. Development of immunity following vaccination takes ~2 weeks; amantadine therapy should be considered for high-risk patients from the time of vaccination until immunity has developed.

Drug-induced extrapyramidal symptoms: Oral: 100 mg twice daily; may increase to 300-400 mg/day, if needed

Parkinson's disease or Creutzfeldt-Jakob disease (unlabeled use): Oral: 100 mg twice daily as sole therapy; may increase to 400 mg/day if needed with close monitoring; initial dose: 100 mg/day if with other serious illness or with high doses of other anti-Parkinson drugs

Elderly: Adjust dose based on renal function; some patients tolerate the drug better when it is given in 2 divided daily doses (to avoid adverse neurologic reactions).

Influenza A prophylaxis or treatment: ≤100 mg/day in patients ≥65 years

Pediatrics:

Influenza A treatment: Oral: **Note:** Initiate within 24-48 hours after onset of symptoms; discontinue as soon as possible based on clinical response (generally within 3-5 days or within 24-48 hours after symptoms disappear)

1-9 years: 5 mg/kg/day in 2 divided doses (manufacturers range: 4.4-8.8 mg/kg/day); maximum dose: 150 mg/day

≥10 years and <40 kg: 5 mg/kg/day; maximum dose: 150 mg/day

≥10 years and ≥40 kg: Refer to adult dosing.

Influenza A prophylaxis: Oral: Refer to "Influenza A treatment" dosing. Continue treatment throughout the peak influenza activity in the community or throughout the entire influenza season in patients who cannot be vaccinated. Development of immunity following vaccination takes ~2 weeks; amantadine therapy should be considered for high-risk patients from the time of vaccination until immunity has developed. For children <9 years receiving influenza vaccine for the first time, amantadine prophylaxis should continue for 6 weeks (4 weeks after the first dose and 2 weeks after the second dose)

Renal Impairment:

Cl$_{cr}$ 30-50 mL/minute: Administer 200 mg on day 1, then 100 mg/day

Cl$_{cr}$ 15-29 mL/minute: Administer 200 mg on day 1, then 100 mg on alternate days

Cl$_{cr}$ <15 mL/minute: Administer 200 mg every 7 days

Hemodialysis: Administer 200 mg every 7 days

Peritoneal dialysis: No supplemental dose is needed

Continuous arteriovenous or venous-venous hemofiltration: No supplemental dose is needed

Stability

Storage: Store at 15°C to 30°C (59°F to 86°F). Protect from freezing.

Laboratory Monitoring Renal function

Nursing Actions

Physical Assessment: Assess effectiveness and interactions of other medications patient may be taking. Monitor renal function, therapeutic response (eg, Parkinsonian symptoms), and adverse reactions (opportunistic infection: fever, mouth and vaginal sores or plaques, unhealed wounds, etc and CNS changes) at beginning of therapy and periodically throughout therapy. Assess blood pressure; monitor for signs of fluid retention. When treating Parkinson's disease, taper slowly when discontinuing. Assess knowledge/teach patient appropriate use, interventions to reduce side effects, and adverse symptoms to report.

Patient Education: Take as directed; do not increase dosage, take more often than prescribed, or discontinue medication without consulting prescriber. Maintain adequate hydration (2-3 L/day of fluids) unless instructed to restrict fluid intake and void before taking medication. Take last dose of day in the afternoon to reduce incidence of insomnia. Avoid alcohol, sedatives, or hypnotics unless consulting prescriber. You may experience decreased mental alertness or coordination (use caution when driving, climbing stairs, or engaging in tasks requiring alertness until response to drug is known); or nausea or dry mouth (small frequent meals, frequent mouth care, sucking lozenges, or chewing gum may help). Report unusual swelling of extremities, respiratory difficulty or shortness of breath, change in gait or increased tremors, or changes in mentation (eg, depression, anxiety, irritability, hallucination, slurred speech). **Pregnancy/breast-feeding precautions:** Inform prescriber if you are pregnant. Breast-feeding is not recommended.

Geriatric Considerations Elderly patients may be more susceptible to the CNS effects of amantadine; using 2 divided daily doses may minimize this effect. The syrup may be used to administer doses <100 mg.

Pregnancy Issues Impaired fertility has also been reported during animal studies and during human in vitro fertilization.

Additional Information Patients with intolerable CNS side effects often do better with rimantadine.

Ambenonium (am be NOE nee um)

U.S. Brand Names Mytelase®

Synonyms Ambenonium Chloride

Pharmacologic Category Cholinergic Agonist

Pregnancy Risk Factor C

Lactation Excretion in breast milk unknown/not recommended

Use Treatment of myasthenia gravis

Mechanism of Action/Effect Action increases acetylcholine concentration at transmission sites in parasympathetic neurons and skeletal muscles by inhibiting acetylcholinesterase

Contraindications Routine administration of atropine or other belladonna alkaloids with ambenonium is contraindicated because they may suppress the muscarinic symptoms of excessive gastrointestinal stimulation, leaving only the more serious symptoms of muscle fasciculations and paralysis as signs of overdosage; should not be administered to patients receiving mecamylamine

(Continued)

Ambenonium (Continued)

Warnings/Precautions Prolonged action after cholinergics; drug should be discontinued until the patient is stabilized. Use with caution in patients with asthma, epilepsy, bradycardia, hyperthyroidism, or peptic ulcer. Differentiation of cholinergic/myasthenia crisis is critical; use edrophonium and clinical judgment. Anticholinergic insensitivity may develop for brief or prolonged periods. Reduce or withhold dosages until the patient becomes sensitive again. May require respiratory support.

Drug Interactions

Decreased Effect: Corticosteroids antagonize effects of anticholinesterases in myasthenia gravis. Procainamide or quinidine may reverse ambenonium cholinergic effects on muscle.

Increased Effect/Toxicity: Succinylcholine neuromuscular blockade may be prolonged.

Lab Interactions Increased aminotransferase [ALT (SGPT)/AST (SGOT)] (S), amylase (S)

Adverse Reactions Frequency not defined.

Cardiovascular: Arrhythmias (especially bradycardia), hypotension, carbon monoxide decreased, tachycardia, AV block, nodal rhythm, ECG changes (nonspecific), cardiac arrest, syncope, flushing

Central nervous system: Convulsions, dysarthria, dysphonia, dizziness, loss of consciousness, drowsiness, headache

Dermatologic: Skin rash, thrombophlebitis (I.V.), urticaria

Gastrointestinal: Hyperperistalsis, nausea, vomiting, salivation, diarrhea, stomach cramps, dysphagia, flatulence

Genitourinary: Urinary urgency

Neuromuscular & skeletal: Weakness, fasciculations, muscle cramps, spasms, arthralgia

Ocular: Small pupils, lacrimation

Respiratory: Bronchial secretions increased, laryngospasm, bronchiolar constriction, respiratory muscle paralysis, dyspnea, respiratory depression, respiratory arrest, bronchospasm

Miscellaneous: Diaphoresis increased, anaphylaxis, allergic reactions

Overdosage/Toxicology Have atropine on hand to reverse cholinergic crisis or hypersensitivity reaction.

Available Dosage Forms Caplet, as chloride [scored]: 10 mg [contains lactose and sucrose]

Dosing

Adults & Elderly: Myasthenia gravis: Oral: 5-25 mg 3-4 times/day

Nursing Actions

Physical Assessment: Assess bladder and sphincter adequacy prior to administering medication. Assess other medications patient may be taking for effectiveness and interactions. Monitor therapeutic effectiveness and adverse reactions: cholinergic crisis (DUMBELS - diarrhea, urination, miosis, bronchospasm/bradycardia, excitability, lacrimation, and salivation/excessive sweating. Assess knowledge/teach patient appropriate use, interventions to reduce side effects, and adverse symptoms to report.

Patient Education: This drug will not cure myasthenia gravis, but it may reduce the symptoms. Use as directed; do not increase dose or discontinue medication without consulting prescriber. Maintain adequate hydration (2-3 L/day of fluids) unless instructed to restrict fluid intake. May cause dizziness, drowsiness, or postural hypotension (rise slowly from sitting or lying position and use caution when driving or climbing stairs); vomiting or loss of appetite (small frequent meals, frequent mouth care, sucking lozenges, or chewing gum may help); or diarrhea (boiled milk, yogurt, or buttermilk may help). Report persistent abdominal discomfort; significantly increased salivation, sweating, tearing, or urination; flushed skin; chest pain or palpitations; acute headache; unresolved diarrhea; excessive fatigue, insomnia, dizziness, or depression; increased muscle, joint, or body pain; vision changes or blurred vision; or shortness of breath or wheezing. **Pregnancy/breast-feeding precautions:** Inform prescriber if you are or intend to become pregnant. Breast-feeding is not recommended.

Amifostine (am i FOS teen)

U.S. Brand Names Ethyol®

Synonyms Ethiofos; Gammaphos; WR-2721; YM-08310

Pharmacologic Category Adjuvant, Chemoprotective Agent (Cytoprotective); Antidote

Medication Safety Issues

Sound-alike/look-alike issues:

Ethyol® may be confused with ethanol

Pregnancy Risk Factor C

Lactation Excretion in breast milk unknown/contraindicated

Use Reduce the incidence of moderate to severe xerostomia in patients undergoing postoperative radiation treatment for head and neck cancer, where the radiation port includes a substantial portion of the parotid glands; reduce the cumulative renal toxicity associated with repeated administration of cisplatin in patients with advanced ovarian cancer or nonsmall cell lung cancer

Mechanism of Action/Effect Reduces the toxic effects of cisplatin, cyclophosphamide, radiation therapy

Contraindications Hypersensitivity to aminothiol compounds, mannitol, or any component of the formulation

Warnings/Precautions Patients who are hypotensive or in a state of dehydration should not receive amifostine. Interrupt antihypertensive therapy for 24 hours before amifostine. Patients receiving antihypertensive therapy that cannot be stopped for 24 hours preceding amifostine treatment also should not receive amifostine.

It is recommended that antiemetic medication, including dexamethasone 20 mg I.V. and a serotonin 5-HT$_3$ receptor antagonist be administered prior to and in conjunction with amifostine. Rare hypersensitivity reactions, including anaphylaxis and severe cutaneous reactions, including anaphylaxis and severe cutaneous reaction, have been reported with a higher frequency in patients receiving amifostine as a radioprotectant. Discontinue if allergic reaction occurs; do not rechallenge.

Reports of clinically-relevant hypocalcemia are rare, but serum calcium levels should be monitored in patients at risk of hypocalcemia, such as those with nephrotic syndrome.

Drug Interactions

Increased Effect/Toxicity: Special consideration should be given to patients receiving antihypertensive medications or other drugs that could potentiate hypotension.

Adverse Reactions >10%:

Cardiovascular: Flushing; hypotension (62%)

Central nervous system: Chills, dizziness, somnolence

Gastrointestinal: Nausea/vomiting (may be severe)

Respiratory: Sneezing

Miscellaneous: Feeling of warmth/coldness, hiccups

Overdosage/Toxicology Symptoms of overdose include hypotension, nausea, and vomiting. Treatment includes supportive measures as clinically indicated.

Pharmacodynamics/Kinetics

Half-Life Elimination: 9 minutes

Metabolism: Hepatic dephosphorylation to two metabolites (active-free thiol and disulfide)

Excretion: Urine

Clearance, plasma: 2.17 L/minute

Available Dosage Forms Injection, powder for reconstitution: 500 mg

Dosing

Adults & Elderly: Note: It is recommended that antiemetic medication, including dexamethasone 20 mg I.V. and a serotonin 5-HT^3 receptor antagonist, be administered prior to and in conjunction with amifostine.

Cisplatin-induced renal toxicity, reduction: I.V.: 740-910 mg/m^2 once daily 30 minutes prior to cytotoxic therapy

Note: Doses >740 mg/m^2 are associated with a higher incidence of hypotension and may require interruption of therapy or dose modification for subsequent cycles. For 910 mg/m^2 doses, the manufacturer suggests the following blood pressure-based adjustment schedule:

The infusion of amifostine should be interrupted if the systolic blood pressure decreases significantly from baseline, as defined below:

Decrease of 20 mm Hg if baseline systolic blood pressure <100

Decrease of 25 mm Hg if baseline systolic blood pressure 100-119

Decrease of 30 mm Hg if baseline systolic blood pressure 120-139

Decrease of 40 mm Hg if baseline systolic blood pressure 140-179

Decrease of 50 mm Hg if baseline systolic blood pressure ≥180

If blood pressure returns to normal within 5 minutes (assisted by fluid administration and postural management) and the patient is asymptomatic, the infusion may be restarted so that the full dose of amifostine may be administered. If the full dose of amifostine cannot be administered, the dose of amifostine for subsequent cycles should be 740 mg/m^2.

Xerostomia from head and neck cancer, reduction:

I.V.: 200 mg/m^2/day during radiation therapy **or** SubQ: 500 mg/day during radiation therapy

Administration

I.V.: Administer over 3-15 minutes; administration as a longer infusion is associated with a higher incidence of side effects. **Note:** SubQ administration has been used.

I.V. Detail: pH: 7

Stability

Reconstitution: Reconstitute intact vials with 9.7 mL of sterile 0.9% sodium chloride injection. For I.V. infusion, dilute in 50-250 mL of 0.9% sodium chloride. Amifostine should be further diluted in 0.9% sodium chloride to a concentration of 5-40 mg/mL. For SubQ administration, reconstitute with 2.4 mL NS or SWFI.

Compatibility: Stable in NS

Y-site administration: Incompatible with acyclovir, amphotericin B, cefoperazone, chlorpromazine, cisplatin, ganciclovir, hydroxyzine, minocycline, prochlorperazine edisylate

Storage: Store intact vials of lyophilized powder at room temperature of 20°C to 25°C (68°F to 77°F). Reconstituted solutions (500 mg/10 mL) are chemically stable for up to 5 hours at room temperature (25°C) or up to 24 hours under refrigeration 2°C to 8°C.

Nursing Actions

Physical Assessment: Monitor blood pressure closely during infusion (continuously or every 5-7 minutes; see Dosing). Can cause hypotension. Monitor nausea and treat with antiemetic per prescriber's orders.

Patient Education: This I.V. medication is given to help reduce side effects of your chemotherapy and/or radiation therapy. Report immediately any nausea; you will be given medication. Report chills, severe dizziness, tremors or shaking, or sudden onset of hiccups. **Breast-feeding precaution:** Do not breast-feed.

Additional Information Mean onset of hypotension is 14 minutes into the 15-minute infusion and the mean duration 6 minutes.

Amikacin (am i KAY sin)

U.S. Brand Names Amikin®

Synonyms Amikacin Sulfate

Pharmacologic Category Antibiotic, Aminoglycoside

Medication Safety Issues

Sound-alike/look-alike issues:

Amikacin may be confused with Amicar®, anakinra

Amikin® may be confused with Amicar®

Pregnancy Risk Factor D

Lactation Enters breast milk/compatible

Use Treatment of serious infections due to organisms resistant to gentamicin and tobramycin, including *Pseudomonas*, *Proteus*, *Serratia*, and other gram-negative bacilli (bone infections, respiratory tract infections, endocarditis, and septicemia); documented infection of mycobacterial organisms susceptible to amikacin

Mechanism of Action/Effect Inhibits protein synthesis in susceptible bacteria by binding to ribosomal subunits

Contraindications Hypersensitivity to amikacin sulfate or any component of the formulation; cross-sensitivity may exist with other aminoglycosides

Warnings/Precautions Dose and/or frequency of administration must be monitored and modified in patients with renal impairment. Drug should be discontinued if signs of ototoxicity, nephrotoxicity, or hypersensitivity occur. Ototoxicity is proportional to the amount of drug given and the duration of treatment. Tinnitus or vertigo may be indications of vestibular injury and impending bilateral **irreversible** damage. Renal damage is usually reversible.

Drug Interactions

Increased Effect/Toxicity: Amikacin may increase or prolong the effect of neuromuscular blocking agents. Concurrent use of amphotericin (or other nephrotoxic drugs) may increase the risk of amikacin-induced nephrotoxicity. The risk of ototoxicity from amikacin may be increased with other ototoxic drugs.

Lab Interactions Some penicillin derivatives may accelerate the degradation of aminoglycosides *in vitro*, leading to a potential underestimation of aminoglycoside serum concentration.

Adverse Reactions 1% to 10%:

Central nervous system: Neurotoxicity

Otic: Ototoxicity (auditory), ototoxicity (vestibular)

Renal: Nephrotoxicity

Overdosage/Toxicology Symptoms of overdose include ototoxicity, nephrotoxicity, and neuromuscular toxicity. Treatment of choice, following a single acute overdose, appears to be maintenance of urine output of at least 3 mL/kg/hour during the acute treatment phase. Dialysis is of questionable value in enhancing aminoglycoside elimination. If required, hemodialysis is preferred over peritoneal dialysis in patients with normal renal function.

Pharmacodynamics/Kinetics

Time to Peak: Serum: I.M.: 45-120 minutes

Half-Life Elimination: Renal function and age dependent:

Infants: Low birth weight (1-3 days): 7-9 hours; Full-term >7 days: 4-5 hours

Children: 1.6-2.5 hours

Adults: Normal renal function: 1.4-2.3 hours; Anuria/end-stage renal disease: 28-86 hours

Excretion: Urine (94% to 98%)

Available Dosage Forms [DSC] = Discontinued product

(Continued)

Amikacin *(Continued)*

Injection, solution, as sulfate: 50 mg/mL (2 mL, 4 mL); 62.5 mg/mL (8 mL) [DSC]; 250 mg/mL (2 mL, 4 mL)

Amikin®: 50 mg/mL (2 mL, 4 mL); 250 mg/mL (2 mL, 4 mL) [contains metabisulfite]

Dosing

Adults & Elderly: Individualization is critical because of the low therapeutic index

Note: Use of ideal body weight (IBW) for determining the mg/kg/dose appears to be more accurate than dosing on the basis of total body weight (TBW)

In morbid obesity, dosage requirement may best be estimated using a dosing weight of IBW + 0.4 (TBW - IBW)

Susceptible infections: I.M., I.V.: 5-7.5 mg/kg/dose every 8 hours

Hospital-acquired pneumonia (HAP): 20 mg/kg/day with antipseudomonal beta-lactam or carbapenem (American Thoracic Society/ATS guidelines)

Meningitis *(Pseudomonas aeruginosa):* 5 mg/kg every 8 hours (administered with another bacteriocidal drug)

Adjustment: Initial and periodic peak and trough plasma drug levels should be determined, particularly in critically-ill patients with serious infections or in disease states known to significantly alter aminoglycoside pharmacokinetics (eg, cystic fibrosis, burns, or major surgery)

Note: Some clinicians suggest a daily dose of 15-20 mg/kg for all patients with normal renal function. This dose is at least as efficacious with similar, if not less, toxicity than conventional dosing.

Pediatrics: Infants and Children: Refer to adult dosing.

Renal Impairment: Individualization is critical because of the low therapeutic index. Some patients may require larger or more frequent doses if serum levels document the need (ie, cystic fibrosis or febrile granulocytopenic patients).

Cl_{cr} ≥60 mL/minute: Administer every 8 hours

Cl_{cr} 40-60 mL/minute: Administer every 12 hours

Cl_{cr} 20-40 mL/minute: Administer every 24 hours

Cl_{cr} <20 mL/minute: Loading dose, then monitor levels

Dialyzable (50% to 100%)

Administer dose postdialysis or administer ²/₃ normal dose as a supplemental dose postdialysis and follow levels.

Peritoneal dialysis effects: Dose as for Cl_{cr} <20 mL/minute: Follow levels.

Continuous arteriovenous or venovenous hemodiafiltration effects: Dose as for Cl_{cr} 10-40 mL/minute: Follow levels.

Administration

I.M.: Administer I.M. injection in large muscle mass. Administer around-the-clock to promote less variation in peak and trough serum levels. Do not mix with other drugs, administer separately.

I.V.: Infuse over 30-60 minutes.

Some penicillins (eg, carbenicillin, ticarcillin, and piperacillin) have been shown to inactivate *in vitro.* This has been observed to a greater extent with tobramycin and gentamicin, while amikacin has shown greater stability against inactivation. Concurrent use of these agents may pose a risk of reduced antibacterial efficacy *in vivo,* particularly in the setting of profound renal impairment. However, definitive clinical evidence is lacking. If combination penicillin/aminoglycoside therapy is desired in a patient with renal dysfunction, separation of doses (if feasible), and routine monitoring of aminoglycoside levels, CBC, and clinical response should be considered.

I.V. Detail: Administer around-the-clock to promote less variation in peak and trough serum levels. Do not mix with other drugs, administer separately.

pH: 3.5-5.5

Stability

Compatibility: Stable in dextran 75 6% in NS, D_5LR, $D_5^{1}/_4NS$, $D_5^{1}/_3NS$, $D_5^{1}/_2NS$, D_5NS, $D_{10}NS$, D_5W, $D_{10}W$, $D_{20}W$, mannitol 20%, ¹/₄NS, ¹/₂NS, NS

Y-site administration: Incompatible with allopurinol, amphotericin B cholesteryl sulfate complex, hetastarch, propofol

Compatibility in syringe: Incompatible with heparin

Compatibility when admixed: Incompatible with amphotericin B, ampicillin, cefazolin, chlorothiazide, heparin, phenytoin, thiopental, vitamin B complex with C

Storage: Stable for 24 hours at room temperature and 2 days at refrigeration when mixed in D_5W, $D_5^{1}/_4NS$, $D_5^{1}/_2NS$, NS, LR.

Laboratory Monitoring Perform culture and sensitivity testing prior to initiating therapy. Urinalysis, BUN, serum creatinine, appropriately timed peak and trough concentrations. Initial and periodic peak and trough plasma drug levels should be determined, particularly in critically-ill patients with serious infections or in disease states known to significantly alter aminoglycoside pharmacokinetics (eg, cystic fibrosis, burns, or major surgery). Aminoglycoside levels measured from blood taken from Silastic® central catheters can sometimes give falsely high readings (draw levels from alternate lumen or peripheral stick, if possible). Some penicillin derivatives may accelerate the degradation of aminoglycosides.

Nursing Actions

Physical Assessment: Assess allergy history prior to beginning therapy. Assess potential for interactions with other prescriptions, OTC medications, or herbal products patient may be taking. Assess results of laboratory tests, therapeutic effectiveness, and adverse response. Monitor for ototoxicity, nephrotoxicity, neurotoxicity. Hearing and renal status should be assessed before, during, and after therapy. Teach patient possible side effects/appropriate interventions and adverse symptoms to report.

Patient Education: Do not take any new medication during therapy unless approved by prescriber. This drug can only be administered by I.V. or I.M. injection. It is important to maintain adequate hydration (2-3 L/day of fluids) unless instructed to restrict fluid intake. Report immediately any change in hearing acuity, ringing or roaring in ears, alteration in balance, vertigo, feeling of fullness in head; pain, tingling, or numbness of any body part; or change in urinary pattern or decrease in urine. Report signs of opportunistic infection (eg, white plaques in mouth, vaginal discharge, unhealed sores, sore throat, unusual fever, chills); pain, redness, or swelling at injection site; or other adverse reactions. **Pregnancy precaution:** Inform prescriber if you are or intend to become pregnant.

Dietary Considerations Sodium content of 1 g: 29.9 mg (1.3 mEq)

Geriatric Considerations Adjust dose based on renal function.

Breast-Feeding Issues No specific recommendations. However, aminoglycosides are not systemically available when taken orally. Therefore, the risk to the infant is minimal if ingested with breast milk.

Additional Information Aminoglycoside levels measured from blood taken from Silastic® central catheters can sometimes give falsely high readings (draw levels from alternate lumen or peripheral stick, if possible).

Related Information

Peak and Trough Guidelines *on page 1387*

Amiloride (a MIL oh ride)

U.S. Brand Names Midamor® [DSC]

Synonyms Amiloride Hydrochloride

Pharmacologic Category Diuretic, Potassium-Sparing

Medication Safety Issues

Sound-alike/look-alike issues:

Amiloride may be confused with amiodarone, amlodipine, amrinone

Pregnancy Risk Factor B

Lactation Excretion in breast milk unknown/contraindicated

Use Counteracts potassium loss induced by other diuretics in the treatment of hypertension or edematous conditions including CHF, hepatic cirrhosis, and hypoaldosteronism; usually used in conjunction with more potent diuretics such as thiazides or loop diuretics

Unlabeled/Investigational Use Investigational: Cystic fibrosis; reduction of lithium-induced polyuria

Mechanism of Action/Effect Decreases potassium and calcium excretion in distal tubule, cortical collecting tubule, and collecting direct by inhibiting sodium, potassium, and ATPase; increases sodium, magnesium, and water excretion

Contraindications Hypersensitivity to amiloride or any component of the formulation; presence of elevated serum potassium levels (>5.5 mEq/L); if patient is receiving other potassium-conserving agents (eg, spironolactone, triamterene) or potassium supplementation (medicine, potassium-containing salt substitutes, potassium-rich diet); anuria; acute or chronic renal insufficiency; evidence of diabetic nephropathy. Patients with evidence of renal impairment or diabetes mellitus should not receive this medicine without close, frequent monitoring of serum electrolytes and renal function.

Warnings/Precautions May cause hyperkalemia (patients with renal impairment or diabetes and the elderly are at greatest risk). Should be stopped at least 3 days before glucose tolerance testing. Use caution in severely ill patients in whom respiratory or metabolic acidosis may occur.

Drug Interactions

Decreased Effect: Decreased effect of amiloride with use of NSAIDs. Amoxicillin's absorption may be reduced with concurrent use.

Increased Effect/Toxicity: Increased risk of amiloride-associated hyperkalemia with triamterene, spironolactone, ACE inhibitors or angiotensin receptor antagonists, potassium preparations, cyclosporine, tacrolimus, and indomethacin. Amiloride may increase the toxicity of amantadine and lithium by reduction of renal excretion. Quinidine and amiloride together may increase risk of malignant arrhythmias.

Nutritional/Ethanol Interactions Food: Hyperkalemia may result if amiloride is taken with potassium-containing foods.

Lab Interactions Increased potassium (S)

Adverse Reactions 1% to 10%:

Central nervous system: Headache, fatigue, dizziness

Endocrine & metabolic: Hyperkalemia (up to 10%; risk reduced in patients receiving kaliuretic diuretics), hyperchloremic metabolic acidosis, dehydration, hyponatremia, gynecomastia

Gastrointestinal: Nausea, diarrhea, vomiting, abdominal pain, gas pain, appetite changes, constipation

Genitourinary: Impotence

Neuromuscular & skeletal: Muscle cramps, weakness

Respiratory: Cough, dyspnea

Overdosage/Toxicology Clinical signs of toxicity are consistent with dehydration and electrolyte disturbance. Large amounts may result in life-threatening hyperkalemia (>6.5 mEq/L). This can be treated with I.V. glucose (dextrose 25% in water), rapid-acting insulin, concurrent I.V. sodium bicarbonate, and (if needed) Kayexalate® oral or rectal solution in sorbitol. Persistent hyperkalemia may require dialysis.

Pharmacodynamics/Kinetics

Onset of Action: 2 hours

Duration of Action: 24 hours

Time to Peak: Serum: 6-10 hours

Protein Binding: 23%

Half-Life Elimination: Normal renal function: 6-9 hours; End-stage renal disease: 8-144 hours

Metabolism: No active metabolites

Excretion: Urine and feces (equal amounts as unchanged drug)

Available Dosage Forms Tablet, as hydrochloride: 5 mg

Dosing

Adults: Hypertension, edema (to limit potassium loss): Oral: Initial: 5-10 mg/day (up to 20 mg)

Hypertension (JNC 7): 5-10 mg/day in 1-2 divided doses

Elderly: Oral: Initial: 5 mg once daily or every other day

Pediatrics: Edema, hypertension: Oral: Although safety and efficacy in children have not been established by the FDA, a dosage of 0.625 mg/kg/day has been used in children weighing 6-20 kg.

Renal Impairment: Oral:

Cl_{cr} 10-50 mL/minute: Administer 50% of normal dose.

Cl_{cr} <10 mL/minute: Avoid use.

Administration

Oral: Administer with food or meals to avoid GI upset.

Laboratory Monitoring Serum electrolytes, renal function

Nursing Actions

Physical Assessment: Assess potential for interactions with other prescriptions, OTC medications, or herbal products patient may be taking. Monitor laboratory tests (electrolytes), fluid status (I & O, weight, blood pressure), and adverse effects (eg, hyperkalemia, hyperchloremic metabolic acidosis, hyponatremia). Teach patient proper use, possible side effects/appropriate interventions, and adverse symptoms to report.

Patient Education: Do not take any new medication during therapy unless approved by prescriber. Take as directed, preferably early in day with food. Do not increase dietary intake of potassium unless instructed by prescriber (too much potassium can be as harmful as too little). May cause dizziness or fatigue (use caution when driving or engaging in tasks that require alertness until response to drug is known); constipation (increased exercise, fluids, fruit, and fiber may help); impotence (reversible); or loss of hair (rare). Report muscle cramping or weakness, unresolved nausea or vomiting, palpitations, or respiratory difficulty. **Breast-feeding precaution:** Do not breast-feed.

Dietary Considerations Take with food or meals to avoid GI upset. Do not use salt substitutes or low salt milk without checking with your healthcare provider; too much potassium can be as harmful as too little.

Geriatric Considerations Use lower initial dose, and adjust dose for renal impairment.

Additional Information Medication should be discontinued if potassium level exceeds 6.5 mEq/L. Combined with hydrochlorothiazide as Moduretic®. Amiloride is considered an alternative to triamterene or spironolactone.

Amiloride and Hydrochlorothiazide
(a MIL oh ride & hye droe klor oh THYE a zide)

Synonyms Hydrochlorothiazide and Amiloride
Pharmacologic Category Diuretic, Combination
Pregnancy Risk Factor B
Lactation Excretion in breast milk unknown/contraindicated
Use Potassium-sparing diuretic; antihypertensive
Available Dosage Forms Tablet: 5/50: Amiloride hydrochloride 5 mg and hydrochlorothiazide 50 mg
Dosing
Adults: Hypertension, edema: Oral: Initial: 1 tablet/day; may be increased to 2 tablets/day if needed; usually given in a single dose
Elderly: Oral: Initial: ½ to 1 tablet/day
Renal Impairment: See individual agents.
Nursing Actions
Physical Assessment: See individual agents.
Patient Education: See individual agents.
Breast-feeding precaution: Do not breast-feed.
Related Information
Amiloride *on page 71*
Hydrochlorothiazide *on page 610*

Aminoglutethimide
(a mee noe gloo TETH i mide)

U.S. Brand Names Cytadren®
Synonyms AG; AGT; BA-16038; Elipten
Pharmacologic Category Antineoplastic Agent, Aromatase Inhibitor; Aromatase Inhibitor; Enzyme Inhibitor; Hormone Antagonist, Anti-Adrenal; Nonsteroidal Aromatase Inhibitor
Medication Safety Issues
Sound-alike/look-alike issues:
Cytadren® may be confused with cytarabine
Pregnancy Risk Factor D
Lactation Excretion in breast milk unknown/contraindicated
Use Suppression of adrenal function in selected patients with Cushing's syndrome
Unlabeled/Investigational Use Treatment of breast and prostate cancer (androgen synthesis inhibitor)
Mechanism of Action/Effect Blocks the conversion of cholesterol to delta-5-pregnenolone, thereby reducing the synthesis of adrenal glucocorticoids, mineralocorticoids, estrogens, aldosterone, and androgens. This inhibits growth of tumors that need estrogen to thrive.
Contraindications Hypersensitivity to aminoglutethimide, glutethimide, or any component of the formulation; pregnancy
Warnings/Precautions Monitor blood pressure in all patients at appropriate intervals. Hypothyroidism may occur. **Mineralocorticoid replacement is necessary in up to 50% of patients.** Glucocorticoid replacement is necessary in most patients.
Drug Interactions
Cytochrome P450 Effect: Induces CYP1A2 (strong), 2C19 (strong), 3A4 (strong)
Decreased Effect: Aminoglutethimide may decrease therapeutic effect of dexamethasone, digitoxin (after 3-8 weeks), warfarin, medroxyprogesterone, megestrol, and tamoxifen. Aminoglutethimide may decrease the levels/effects of aminophylline, benzodiazepines, calcium channel blockers, citalopram, clarithromycin, cyclosporine, diazepam, erythromycin, estrogens, fluvoxamine, methsuximide, mirtazapine, nateglinide, nefazodone, nevirapine, phenytoin, proton pump inhibitors, protease inhibitors, ropinirole, sertraline, tacrolimus, theophylline, venlafaxine, voriconazole,

and other drugs metabolized by CYP1A2, 2C19, or 3A4.
Lab Interactions Increased alkaline phosphatase (S), AST (SGOT), TSH; decreased plasma cortisol, thyroxine (S), and urinary aldosterone
Adverse Reactions Most adverse effects will diminish in incidence and severity after the first 2-6 weeks
>10%:
Central nervous system: Headache, dizziness, drowsiness, lethargy, clumsiness
Dermatologic: Skin rash
Gastrointestinal: Nausea, anorexia
Hepatic: Cholestatic jaundice
Neuromuscular & skeletal: Myalgia
Renal: Nephrotoxicity
Respiratory: Pulmonary alveolar damage
1% to 10%:
Cardiovascular: Hypotension, tachycardia, orthostasis
Dermatologic: Hirsutism, pruritus
Endocrine & metabolic: Adrenocortical insufficiency
Gastrointestinal: Vomiting
Overdosage/Toxicology Symptoms of overdose include ataxia, somnolence, lethargy, dizziness, distress, fatigue, coma, hyperventilation, respiratory depression, hypovolemia, and shock. Treatment is supportive.
Pharmacodynamics/Kinetics
Onset of Action: Adrenal suppression: 3-5 days; following withdrawal of therapy, adrenal function returns within 72 hours
Protein Binding: Plasma: 20% to 25%
Half-Life Elimination: 7-15 hours; shorter following multiple doses
Metabolism: Major metabolite is N-acetylaminoglutethimide; induces its own metabolism
Excretion: Urine (34% to 50% as unchanged drug, 25% as metabolites)
Available Dosage Forms Tablet [scored]: 250 mg
Dosing
Adults & Elderly:
Cushing disease: Oral: 250 mg every 6 hours may be increased at 1- to 2-week intervals to a total of 2 g/day
Breast cancer, prostate cancer (unlabeled use): Oral: 250 mg 4 times/day
Renal Impairment: Dose reduction may be necessary.
Administration
Oral: Administer every 6 hours to reduce incidence of nausea and vomiting
Stability
Storage: Store at controlled room temperature not >30°C (86°F).
Laboratory Monitoring Thyroid function tests, CBC, liver function, electrolytes. Follow adrenal cortical response by careful monitoring of plasma cortisol until the desired level of suppression is achieved.
Nursing Actions
Physical Assessment: Assess potential for interactions with other medications patient may be taking. Monitor laboratory tests, therapeutic response, and adverse reactions (eg, hypotension, slow pulse, lethargy, dry skin, thick tongue, hirsutism, mood swings, increased susceptibility to infection). Teach patient possible side effects/appropriate interventions and adverse symptoms to report.
Patient Education: Do not take any new medication during therapy unless approved by prescriber. Take exactly as directed; may be taken with food to reduce incidence of nausea. May cause drowsiness or dizziness (avoid driving or engaging in tasks that require alertness until response to drug is known); nausea or vomiting (small, frequent meals, frequent mouth care,

chewing gum or sucking lozenges may reduce incidence of nausea or vomiting); or masculinization (reversible when treatment is discontinued). Report rash, unresolved nausea or vomiting, lethargy, yellowing of skin or eyes, easy bruising or bleeding, change in color of urine or stool, increased growth of facial hair, thick tongue, severe mood swings, palpitations, or respiratory difficulty. **Pregnancy/breast-feeding precautions:** Do not get pregnant while taking this medication. Consult prescriber for appropriate barrier contraceptive measures. Do not breast-feed.

Pregnancy Issues Suspected of causing virilization when given throughout pregnancy

---

Aminosalicylic Acid
(a mee noe sal i SIL ik AS id)

U.S. Brand Names Paser®

Synonyms Aminosalicylate Sodium; 4-Aminosalicylic Acid; Para-Aminosalicylate Sodium; PAS; Sodium PAS

Pharmacologic Category Salicylate

Pregnancy Risk Factor C

Lactation Enters breast milk/not recommended

Use Adjunctive treatment of tuberculosis used in combination with other antitubercular agents

Unlabeled/Investigational Use Crohn's disease

Mechanism of Action/Effect Aminosalicylic acid (PAS) is a highly-specific bacteriostatic agent active against *M. tuberculosis*. Most strains of *M. tuberculosis* are sensitive to a concentration of 1 mcg/mL. Structurally related to para-aminobenzoic acid (PABA) and its mechanism of action is thought to be similar to the sulfonamides, a competitive antagonism with PABA. Disrupts plate biosynthesis in sensitive organisms.

Contraindications Hypersensitivity to aminosalicylic acid or any component of the formulation

Warnings/Precautions Use with caution in patients with hepatic or renal dysfunction and patients with gastric ulcer.

Drug Interactions
Decreased Effect: Aminosalicylic acid may decrease serum levels of digoxin and vitamin B_{12}.

Adverse Reactions Frequency not defined.
Cardiovascular: Pericarditis, vasculitis
Central nervous system: Encephalopathy, fever
Dermatologic: Skin eruptions
Endocrine & metabolic: Goiter (with or without myxedema), hypoglycemia
Gastrointestinal: Abdominal pain, diarrhea, nausea, vomiting
Hematologic: Agranulocytosis, anemia (hemolytic), leukopenia, thrombocytopenia
Hepatic: Hepatitis, jaundice
Ocular: Optic neuritis
Respiratory: Eosinophilic pneumonia

Overdosage/Toxicology Acute overdose results in crystalluria and renal failure, nausea, and vomiting. Alkalinization of urine with sodium bicarbonate and forced diuresis can prevent crystalluria and nephrotoxicity.

Pharmacodynamics/Kinetics
Time to Peak: Serum: 6 hours
Protein Binding: 50% to 60%
Half-Life Elimination: Reduced with renal impairment
Metabolism: Hepatic (>50%) via acetylation
Excretion: Urine (>80% as unchanged drug and metabolites)

Available Dosage Forms
Granules, delayed release:
Paser®: 4 g/packet (30s)

Dosing
Adults & Elderly:
Tuberculosis: Oral: 150 mg/kg/day in 2-3 equally divided doses
Crohn's disease (unlabeled use): 1.5 g/day
Pediatrics: Tuberculosis: Oral: 200-300 mg/kg/day in 3-4 equally divided doses
Renal Impairment:
Cl_{cr} 10-50 mL/minute: Administer 50% to 75% of dose.
Cl_{cr} <10 mL/minute: Administer 50% of dose.
Administer after hemodialysis: Administer 50% of dose.
Continuous arteriovenous hemofiltration: Dose for Cl_{cr} <10 mL/minute
Hepatic Impairment: Use with caution.

Administration
Oral: Do not use granules if packet is swollen or if granules are discolored (ie, brown or purple). Granules may be sprinkled on applesauce or yogurt (do not chew) or suspended in tomato or orange juice.

Stability
Storage: Prior to dispensing, store granules below 15°C (59°F). Once dispensed, packets may be stored at room temperature for short periods of time. Do not use if packet is swollen or if granules are dark brown or purple.

Nursing Actions
Physical Assessment: Monitor for effectiveness of treatment and indications of adverse effects.
Patient Education: May be taken with food; may sprinkle on applesauce or yogurt, or suspend in tomato or orange juice. Do not use granules if discolored (brown or purple) or if packet is swollen; see pharmacist for new prescription. Do not stop taking without consulting prescriber. Report persistent sore throat, fever, unusual bleeding or bruising, persistent nausea or vomiting, or abdominal pain. **Pregnancy/breast-feeding precautions:** Inform prescriber if you are or intend to become pregnant. Breast-feeding is not recommended.

Dietary Considerations May be taken with food.

Geriatric Considerations See Warnings/Precautions; elderly may require lower recommended dose.

Amiodarone (a MEE oh da rone)

U.S. Brand Names Cordarone®; Pacerone®

Synonyms Amiodarone Hydrochloride

Restrictions An FDA-approved medication guide is available at www.fda.gov/cder/Offices/ODS/labeling.htm; distribute to each patient to whom this medication is dispensed.

Pharmacologic Category Antiarrhythmic Agent, Class III

Medication Safety Issues
Sound-alike/look-alike issues:
Amiodarone may be confused with amiloride, amrinone
Cordarone® may be confused with Cardura®, Cordran®

High alert medication: The Institute for Safe Medication Practices (ISMP) includes this medication among its list of drugs which have a heightened risk of causing significant patient harm when used in error.

Pregnancy Risk Factor D

Lactation Enters breast milk/not recommended (AAP rates "of concern")

Use Management of life-threatening recurrent ventricular fibrillation (VF) or hemodynamically-unstable ventricular tachycardia (VT) refractory to other antiarrhythmic agents or in patients intolerant of other agents used for these conditions
(Continued)

Amiodarone *(Continued)*

Unlabeled/Investigational Use

Conversion of atrial fibrillation to normal sinus rhythm; maintenance of normal sinus rhythm

Prevention of postoperative atrial fibrillation during cardiothoracic surgery

Paroxysmal supraventricular tachycardia (SVT)

Control of rapid ventricular rate due to accessory pathway conduction in pre-excited atrial arrhythmias [ACLS guidelines]

Cardiac arrest with persistent ventricular tachycardia (VT) or ventricular fibrillation (VF) if defibrillation, CPR, and vasopressor administration have failed [ACLS/PALS guidelines]

Control of hemodynamically-stable VT, polymorphic VT with a normal QT interval, or wide-complex tachycardia of uncertain origin [ACLS/PALS guidelines]

Mechanism of Action/Effect
Class III antiarrhythmic agent which inhibits adrenergic stimulation, prolongs the action potential and refractory period in myocardial tissue; decreases AV conduction and sinus node function. Amiodarone shows beta-blocker-like and calcium channel blocker-like effects on SA and AV nodes.

Contraindications
Hypersensitivity to amiodarone, iodine, or any component of the formulation; severe sinus-node dysfunction; second- and third-degree heart block (except in patients with a functioning artificial pacemaker); bradycardia causing syncope (except in patients with a functioning artificial pacemaker); pregnancy

Warnings/Precautions
Monitor for pulmonary toxicity, liver toxicity, or exacerbation of the arrhythmia (including torsade de pointes). Use very cautiously and with close monitoring in patients with thyroid or liver disease. May cause hyper- or hypothyroidism. Hyperthyroidism may aggravate or cause breakthrough arrhythmias. Significant heart block or sinus bradycardia can occur. Patients should be hospitalized when amiodarone is initiated. Amiodarone is a potent inhibitor of CYP enzymes and transport proteins (including p-glycoprotein), which may lead to increased serum concentrations/toxicity of a number of medications. Particular caution must be used when a drug with QT_c-prolonging potential relies on metabolism via these enzymes, since the effect of elevated concentrations may be additive with the effect of amiodarone. Carefully assess risk:benefit of coadministration of other drugs which may prolong QT_c interval. Correct electrolyte disturbances, especially hypokalemia or hypomagnesemia, prior to use and throughout therapy.

Pre-existing pulmonary disease does not increase risk of developing pulmonary toxicity, but if pulmonary toxicity develops then the prognosis is worse. Due to complex pharmacokinetics, it is difficult to predict when an arrhythmia or interaction with a subsequent treatment will occur following discontinuation of amiodarone. May cause optic neuropathy and/or optic neuritis, usually resulting in visual impairment. Corneal microdeposits occur in a majority of patients, and may cause visual disturbances in some patients (blurred vision, halos); these are not generally considered a reason to discontinue treatment.

May cause hypotension and bradycardia (infusion-rate related). Caution in surgical patients; may enhance hemodynamic effect of anesthetics; associated with increased risk of adult respiratory distress syndrome (ARDS) postoperatively. Injection contains benzyl alcohol, which has been associated with "gasping syndrome" in neonates. Safety and efficacy of amiodarone in children has not been fully established.

Drug Interactions

Cytochrome P450 Effect: Substrate of CYP1A2 (minor), 2C8/9 (major at low concentration), 2C19 (minor), 2D6 (minor), 3A4 (major); **Inhibits** CYP1A2 (strong), 2A6 (moderate), 2B6 (weak), 2C8/9 (moderate), 2C19 (weak), 2D6 (moderate), 3A4 (moderate)

Decreased Effect: Levels/effects of amiodarone may be decreased by aminoglutethimide, carbamazepine, nafcillin, nevirapine, phenobarbital, phenytoin, rifampin, rifapentine, secobarbital, and other CYP2C8/9 inducers and CYP3A4 inducers. Amiodarone may decrease the levels/effects of codeine, hydrocodone, oxycodone, tramadol, and other prodrug substrates of CYP2D6. Amiodarone may alter thyroid function and response to thyroid supplements; monitor closely.

Increased Effect/Toxicity: Note: Due to the long half-life of amiodarone, drug interactions may take 1 or more weeks to develop. The effect of drugs which prolong the QT interval, including amitriptyline, azole antifungals, bepridil, cisapride, clarithromycin, disopyramide, erythromycin, gatifloxacin, haloperidol, imipramine, moxifloxacin, quinidine, pimozide, procainamide, sotalol, sparfloxacin, theophylline, and thioridazine may be increased. Cisapride and sparfloxacin are contraindicated. Use of amiodarone with diltiazem, verapamil, digoxin, beta-blockers, and other drugs which delay AV conduction may cause excessive AV block (amiodarone may also decrease the metabolism of some of these agents - see below).

Amiodarone may increase the levels of digoxin (reduce dose by 50% on initiation), flecainide (decrease dose up to 33%), phenothiazines, procainamide (reduce dose), and quinidine. Amiodarone may increase the levels/effects of aminophylline, amphetamines, selected benzodiazepines, selected beta-blockers, calcium channel blockers, cyclosporine, dexmedetomidine, dextromethorphan, fluoxetine, fluvoxamine, glimepiride, glipizide, ifosfamide, imatinib, isoniazid, lidocaine, mexiletine, mirtazapine, nateglinide, nefazodone, paroxetine, phenytoin, pioglitazone, risperidone, ritonavir, ropinirole, rosiglitazone, sildenafil (and other PDE-5 inhibitors), sertraline, tacrolimus, telithromycin, theophylline, thioridazine, tricyclic antidepressants, trifluoperazine, venlafaxine, warfarin, and other CYP1A2, 2A6, 2C8/9, 2D6, and/or CYP3A4 substrates. Selected benzodiazepines (midazolam, triazolam), cisapride, ergot alkaloids, selected HMG-CoA reductase inhibitors (lovastatin and simvastatin), mesoridazine, pimozide, and thioridazine are generally contraindicated with strong CYP3A4 inhibitors; example CYP3A4 inhibitors include azole antifungals, clarithromycin, diclofenac, doxycycline, erythromycin, imatinib, isoniazid, nefazodone, nicardipine, propofol, protease inhibitors, quinidine, telithromycin, and verapamil. When used with strong CYP3A4 inhibitors, dosage adjustment/limits are recommended for sildenafil and other PDE-5 inhibitors; consult individual monographs.

The levels/effects of amiodarone may be increased by amprenavir, cimetidine, delavirdine, fluconazole, gemfibrozil, indinavir, ketoconazole, nelfinavir, nicardipine, NSAIDs, pioglitazone, ritonavir, sulfonamides, and other CYP2C8/9 inhibitors.

Concurrent use of fentanyl may lead to bradycardia, sinus arrest, and hypotension. Amiodarone may alter thyroid function and response to thyroid supplements. Amiodarone enhances the myocardial depressant and conduction effects of inhalation anesthetics (monitor).

Nutritional/Ethanol Interactions

Food: Increases the rate and extent of absorption of amiodarone. Grapefruit juice increases bioavailability of oral amiodarone by 50% and decreases the conversion of amiodarone to N-DEA (active metabolite); altered effects are possible; use should be avoided during therapy.

Herb/Nutraceutical: St John's wort may decrease amiodarone levels or enhance photosensitization. Avoid ephedra (may worsen arrhythmia). Avoid dong quai.

Adverse Reactions In a recent meta-analysis, patients taking lower doses of amiodarone (152-330 mg daily for at least 12 months) were more likely to develop thyroid, neurologic, skin, ocular, and bradycardic abnormalities than those taking placebo. Pulmonary toxicity was similar in both the low dose amiodarone group and in the placebo group but there was a trend towards increased toxicity in the amiodarone group. Gastrointestinal and hepatic events were seen to a similar extent in both the low dose amiodarone group and placebo group. As the frequency of adverse events varies considerably across studies as a function of route and dose, a consolidation of adverse event rates is provided by Goldschlager, *Arch Intern Med*, 2000, 160(12):1741-8.

>10%:

Cardiovascular: Hypotension (I.V. 16%, refractory in rare cases)

Central nervous system (3% to 40%): Abnormal gait/ataxia, dizziness, fatigue, headache, malaise, impaired memory, involuntary movement, insomnia, poor coordination, peripheral neuropathy, sleep disturbances, tremor

Dermatologic: Photosensitivity (10% to 75%)

Endocrine & Metabolic: Hypothyroidism (1% to 22%)

Gastrointestinal: Nausea, vomiting, anorexia, and constipation (10% to 33%); AST or ALT level >2x normal (15% to 50%)

Ocular: Corneal microdeposits (>90%; causes visual disturbance in <10%)

1% to 10%:

Cardiovascular: CHF (3%), bradycardia (3% to 5%), AV block (5%), conduction abnormalities, SA node dysfunction (1% to 3%), cardiac arrhythmia, flushing, edema. Additional effects associated with I.V. administration include asystole, cardiac arrest, electromechanical dissociation, ventricular tachycardia, and cardiogenic shock.

Dermatologic: Slate blue skin discoloration (<10%)

Endocrine & metabolic: Hyperthyroidism (<3%), libido decreased

Gastrointestinal: Abdominal pain, abnormal salivation, abnormal taste (oral)

Hematologic: Coagulation abnormalities

Hepatic: Hepatitis and cirrhosis (<3%)

Local: Phlebitis (I.V., with concentrations >3 mg/mL)

Ocular: Visual disturbances (2% to 9%), halo vision (<5% occurring especially at night), optic neuritis (1%)

Respiratory: Pulmonary toxicity has been estimated to occur at a frequency between 2% and 7% of patients (some reports indicate a frequency as high as 17%). Toxicity may present as hypersensitivity pneumonitis; pulmonary fibrosis (cough, fever, malaise); pulmonary inflammation; interstitial pneumonitis; or alveolar pneumonitis. ARDS has been reported in up to 2% of patients receiving amiodarone, and postoperatively in patients receiving oral amiodarone.

Miscellaneous: Abnormal smell (oral)

Overdosage/Toxicology Symptoms of overdose include extension of pharmacologic effects, sinus bradycardia and/or heart block, hypotension, and QT prolongation. Patients should be monitored for several days following ingestion. Intoxication with amiodarone necessitates ECG monitoring. Bradycardia may be atropine resistant. Injectable isoproterenol or a temporary pacemaker may be required. Dialysis is not beneficial.

Pharmacodynamics/Kinetics

Onset of Action: Oral: 2 days to 3 weeks; I.V.: May be more rapid; Peak effect: 1 week to 5 months

Duration of Action: After discontinuing therapy: 7-50 days

Note: Mean onset of effect and duration after discontinuation may be shorter in children than adults

Protein Binding: 96%

Half-Life Elimination: Terminal: 40-55 days (range: 26-107 days); shorter in children than adults

Metabolism: Hepatic via CYP2C8 and 3A4 to active N-desethylamiodarone metabolite; possible enterohepatic recirculation

Excretion: Feces; urine (<1% as unchanged drug)

Available Dosage Forms [DSC] = Discontinued product

Injection, solution, as hydrochloride: 50 mg/mL (3 mL, 9 mL, 18 mL) [contains benzyl alcohol and polysorbate (Tween®) 80]

Cordarone®: 50 mg/mL (3 mL) [contains benzyl alcohol and polysorbate (Tween®) 80]

Tablet, as hydrochloride [scored]: 200 mg, 400 mg

Cordarone®: 200 mg

Pacerone®: 100 mg [not scored], 200 mg, 300 mg [DSC], 400 mg

Dosing

Adults & Elderly: Note: Lower loading and maintenance doses are preferable in women and all patients with low body weight.

Ventricular arrhythmias: Oral: 800-1600 mg/day in 1-2 doses for 1-3 weeks, then 600-800 mg/day in 1-2 doses for 1 month; maintenance: 400 mg/day; lower doses are recommended for supraventricular arrhythmias.

Breakthrough VF or VT: I.V.: 150 mg supplemental doses in 100 mL D_5W over 10 minutes

Pulseless VF or VT: I.V. push: Initial: 300 mg in 20-30 mL NS or D_5W; if VF or VT recurs, supplemental dose of 150 mg followed by infusion of 1 mg/minute for 6 hours, then 0.5 mg/minute (maximum daily dose: 2.1 g)

Note: When switching from I.V. to oral therapy, use the following as a guide:

<1 week I.V. infusion: 800-1600 mg/day

1- to 3-week I.V. infusion: 600-800 mg/day

>3 week I.V. infusion: 400 mg

Recommendations for conversion to intravenous amiodarone after oral administration: During long-term amiodarone therapy (ie, ≥4 months), the mean plasma-elimination half-life of the active metabolite of amiodarone is 61 days. Replacement therapy may not be necessary in such patients if oral therapy is discontinued for a period <2 weeks, since any changes in serum amiodarone concentrations during this period may **not** be clinically significant.

Unlabeled uses:

Prophylaxis of atrial fibrillation following open heart surgery (unlabeled use): Note: A variety of regimens have been used in clinical trials, including oral and intravenous regimens:

Oral: 400 mg twice daily (starting in postop recovery) for up to 7 days. An alternative regimen of amiodarone 600 mg/day for 7 days prior to surgery, followed by 200 mg/day until hospital discharge has also been shown to decrease the risk of postoperative atrial fibrillation.

I.V.: 1000 mg infused over 24 hours (starting at postop recovery) for 2 days has been shown to reduce the risk of postoperative atrial fibrillation

Recurrent atrial fibrillation (unlabeled use): No standard regimen defined; examples of regimens include: Oral: Initial: 10 mg/kg/day for 14 days; followed by 300 mg/day for 4 weeks, followed by maintenance dosage of 100-200 mg/day (Roy D, 2000). Other regimens have been described and are used clinically (ie, 400 mg 3 times/day for 5-7 days, then 400 mg/day for 1 month, then 200 mg/day).

Stable VT or SVT (unlabeled use): I.V.: First 24 hours: 1050 mg according to following regimen

(Continued)

Amiodarone *(Continued)*

Step 1: 150 mg (100 mL) over first 10 minutes (mix 3 mL in 100 mL D₅W)

Step 2: 360 mg (200 mL) over next 6 hours (mix 18 mL in 500 mL D₅W): 1 mg/minute

Step 3: 540 mg (300 mL) over next 18 hours: 0.5 mg/minute

Note: After the first 24 hours: 0.5 mg/minute utilizing concentration of 1-6 mg/mL

Pediatrics:

Arrhythmias (unlabeled use):

Loading dose: Oral: 10-20 mg/kg/day in 1-2 doses for 4-14 days or until adequate control of arrhythmia or prominent adverse effects occur; alternative loading dose in children <1 year: 600-800 mg/1.73 m²/day in 1-2 divided doses/day.

Maintenance dose: Oral: Dose may be reduced to 5 mg/kg/day for several weeks (or 200-400 mg/1.73 m²/day given once daily); if no recurrence of arrhythmia, dose may be further reduced to 2.5 mg/kg/day; maintenance doses may be given 5-7 days/week.

Arrhythmias (unlabeled use, dosing based on limited data):

Loading dose: I.V.: 5 mg/kg over 30 minutes; may repeat up to 3 times if no response.

Maintenance dose: I.V.: 2-20 mg/kg/day (5-15 mcg/kg/minute) by continuous infusion.

Note: I.V. administration at low flow rates (potentially associated with use in pediatrics) may result in leaching of plasticizers (DEHP) from intravenous tubing. DEHP may adversely affect male reproductive tract development. Alternative means of dosing and administration (1 mg/kg aliquots) may need to be considered.

Pulseless VF or VT (PALS dosing): I.V.: 5 mg/kg rapid I.V. bolus or I.O.; repeat up to a maximum dose of 15 mg/kg (300 mg)

Perfusing tachycardias (PALS dosing): I.V.: Loading dose: 5 mg/kg I.V. over 20-60 minutes or I.O.; may repeat up to maximum dose of 15 mg/kg/day

Renal Impairment:

Hemodialysis effects: Not removed by hemodialysis or peritoneal dialysis (0% to 5%); no supplemental doses required.

Hepatic Impairment: Dosage adjustment is probably necessary in substantial hepatic impairment. No specific guidelines available.

Administration

Oral: Administer consistently with regard to meals. Take in divided doses with meals if high daily dose or if GI upset occurs. If GI intolerance occurs with single-dose therapy, use twice daily dosing.

I.V.: Adjust administration rate to urgency (give more slowly when perfusing arrhythmia present). Give I.V. therapy using an infusion pump at a concentration <2 mg/mL. Slow the infusion rate if hypotension or bradycardia develops. Infusions >2 hours must be administered in glass or polyolefin bottles. **Note:** I.V. administration at lower flow rates (potentially associated with use in pediatrics) and higher concentrations than recommended may result in leaching of plasticizers (DEHP) from intravenous tubing. DEHP may adversely affect male reproductive tract development. Alternative means of dosing and administration (1 mg/kg aliquots) may need to be considered. Use only volumetric infusion pump; use of drop counting may lead to under-dosing. Administer through I.V. line with in-line filter.

I.V. Detail: Incompatible with heparin. Flush with saline prior to and following infusion.

pH: 4.08

Stability

Compatibility:

Y-site administration: Incompatible with aminophylline, cefamandole, heparin, sodium bicarbonate

Compatibility in syringe: Incompatible with heparin

Compatibility when admixed: Incompatible with floxacillin

Storage: Store at room temperature; protect from light. When admixed in D₅W to a final concentration of 1-6 mg/mL, the solution is stable at room temperature for 24 hours in polyolefin or glass, or for 2 hours in PVC. Infusions >2 hours must be administered in glass or polyolefin bottles.

Laboratory Monitoring Thyroid function, pulmonary function, liver enzymes, serum electrolytes (potassium, magnesium)

Nursing Actions

Physical Assessment: Assess other medications patient may be taking for effectiveness and interactions. Eye examinations should be performed periodically. Monitor cardiac status closely and assess for CNS changes (ie, abnormal gait/ataxia, dizziness, impaired memory, involuntary movement, poor coordination, peripheral neuropathy, tremor). **I.V.:** Requires continuous cardiac/hemodynamic monitoring during infusion. Be alert for adverse reactions. **Oral:** Monitor laboratory tests, therapeutic response (cardiac status), and symptoms of adverse effects at beginning of therapy and regularly during long-term therapy.

Patient Education:

I.V.: Emergency use: Patient condition will determine amount of patient education.

Oral: May be taken with food to reduce GI disturbance, but be consistent. Always take with food or always take without food. Do not change dosage or discontinue drug without consulting prescriber. Regular blood work, ophthalmic exams, and cardiac assessment will be necessary while taking this medication on a long-term basis. You may experience dizziness, weakness, or insomnia (use caution when driving, climbing stairs, or engaging in tasks requiring alertness until response to drug is known); hypotension (use caution when rising from sitting or lying position); nausea, vomiting, loss of appetite, stomach discomfort, or abnormal taste (small frequent meals, frequent mouth care, chewing gum, or sucking lozenges may help); photosensitivity (use sunscreen, wear protective clothing and eyewear, and avoid direct sunlight); or decreased libido (reversible). Report persistent dry cough or shortness of breath; chest pain, palpitations, irregular or slow heartbeat; unusual bruising or bleeding; blood in urine, feces (black stool), vomitus; warmth, swelling, pain in calves; heat or cold intolerance; weight loss or gain; restlessness; hair thinning; changes in menses; sweating; swelling in neck; muscle tremor, weakness, numbness, or changes in gait; skin rash (bluish-gray color) or irritation; visual disturbances; or changes in urinary patterns. **Pregnancy/breast-feeding precautions:** Do not get pregnant while taking this medication; use appropriate contraceptive measures. Do not breast-feed.

Dietary Considerations Administer consistently with regard to meals. Amiodarone contains iodine 37.3% by weight. Grapefruit juice is not recommended.

Geriatric Considerations Information describing the clinical use and pharmacokinetics in older adults is lacking; however, the elderly may be predisposed to toxicity. See Drug Interactions. Half-life may be prolonged due to decreased clearance; monitor closely. It is recommended to start dosing at the lower end of dosing range.

Breast-Feeding Issues Hypothyroidism may occur in nursing infants. Both amiodarone and its active metabolite are excreted in human milk. Breast-feeding may lead to significant infant exposure and potential toxicity.

Pregnancy Issues May cause fetal harm when administered to a pregnant woman, leading to congenital goiter and hypo- or hyperthyroidism.

Amitriptyline (a mee TRIP ti leen)

U.S. Brand Names Elavil® [DSC]

Synonyms Amitriptyline Hydrochloride

Restrictions A medication guide concerning the use of antidepressants in children and teenagers can be found on the FDA website at www.fda.gov/cder/Offices/ODS/labeling.htm. It should be dispensed to parents or guardians of children and teenagers receiving this medication.

Pharmacologic Category Antidepressant, Tricyclic (Tertiary Amine)

Medication Safety Issues

Sound-alike/look-alike issues:

Amitriptyline may be confused with aminophylline, imipramine, nortriptyline

Elavil® may be confused with Aldoril®, Eldepryl®, enalapril, Equanil®, Mellaril®, Oruvail®, Plavix®

Pregnancy Risk Factor C

Lactation Enters breast milk/not recommended (AAP rates "of concern")

Use Relief of symptoms of depression

Unlabeled/Investigational Use Analgesic for certain chronic and neuropathic pain; prophylaxis against migraine headaches; treatment of depressive disorders in children

Mechanism of Action/Effect Increases the synaptic concentration of serotonin and/or norepinephrine in the central nervous system by inhibition of their reuptake by the presynaptic neuronal membrane

Contraindications Hypersensitivity to amitriptyline or any component of the formulation (cross-sensitivity with other tricyclics may occur); use of MAO inhibitors within past 14 days; acute recovery phase following myocardial infarction; concurrent use of cisapride

Warnings/Precautions Antidepressants increase the risk of suicidal thinking and behavior in children and adolescents with major depressive disorder (MDD) and other depressive disorders; consider risk prior to prescribing. All patients must be closely monitored for clinical worsening, suicidality, or unusual changes in behavior, especially during the initiation of therapy or following an increase or decrease in dosage. When used in children, the child's family or caregiver should be instructed to closely observe the patient and communicate condition with healthcare provider. A medication guide should be dispensed with each prescription. **Amitriptyline is not FDA approved for use in children <12 years of age.**

The possibility of a suicide attempt is inherent in major depression and may persist until remission occurs. Use caution in high-risk patients. Worsening depression and severe abrupt suicidality that are not part of the presenting symptoms may require discontinuation or modification of drug therapy. The patient's family or caregiver should be alerted to monitor patients for the emergence of suicidality and associated behaviors (such as agitation, irritability, hostility, impulsivity, and hypomania) and notify healthcare provider.

May worsen psychosis in some patients or precipitate a shift to mania or hypomania in patients with bipolar disorder. Patients presenting with depressive symptoms should be screened for bipolar disorder. Monotherapy in patients with bipolar disorder should be avoided. **Amitriptyline is not FDA approved for bipolar depression.**

The degree of sedation, anticholinergic effects, orthostasis, and conduction abnormalities are high relative to other antidepressants. Amitriptyline often causes drowsiness/sedation, resulting in impaired performance of tasks requiring alertness (eg, operating machinery or driving). Sedative effects may be additive with other CNS depressants and/or ethanol. Use with caution in patients with a history of cardiovascular disease (including previous MI, stroke, tachycardia, or conduction abnormalities). Use with caution in patients with urinary retention, benign prostatic hyperplasia, narrow-angle glaucoma, xerostomia, visual problems, constipation, or a history of bowel obstruction.

May alter glucose control - use with caution in patients with diabetes. May cause hyponatremia/SIADH. Consider discontinuing, when possible, prior to elective surgery. Therapy should not be abruptly discontinued in patients receiving high doses for prolonged periods. May lower seizure threshold - use caution in patients with a previous seizure disorder or condition predisposing to seizures such as brain damage, alcoholism, or concurrent therapy with other drugs which lower the seizure threshold. May increase the risks associated with electroconvulsive therapy. Use with caution in hyperthyroid patients or those receiving thyroid supplementation. Use with caution in patients with hepatic or renal dysfunction and in elderly patients.

Drug Interactions

Cytochrome P450 Effect: Substrate of CYP1A2 (minor), 2B6 (minor), 2C8/9 (minor), 2C19 (minor), 2D6 (major), 3A4 (minor); **Inhibits** CYP1A2 (weak), 2C8/9 (weak), 2C19 (weak), 2D6 (weak), 2E1 (weak)

Decreased Effect: Amitriptyline inhibits the antihypertensive response to bethanidine, clonidine, debrisoquin, guanadrel, guanethidine, guanabenz, or guanfacine. Cholestyramine and colestipol may bind TCAs and reduce their absorption.

Increased Effect/Toxicity: Amitriptyline increases the effects of amphetamines, anticholinergics, other CNS depressants (sedatives, hypnotics, or ethanol), carbamazepine, tolazamide, chlorpropamide, and warfarin. When used with MAO inhibitors, hyperpyrexia, hypertension, tachycardia, confusion, seizures, and **deaths have been reported** (serotonin syndrome). Serotonin syndrome has also been reported with ritonavir (rare). Levels/effects of amitriptyline may be increased by chlorpromazine, delavirdine, fluoxetine, miconazole, paroxetine, pergolide, quinidine, quinine, ritonavir, ropinirole, and other CYP2D6 inhibitors. Cimetidine, fenfluramine, grapefruit juice, indinavir, methylphenidate, diltiazem, valproate, and verapamil may increase the serum concentrations of tricyclic antidepressants (TCAs). Use of lithium with a TCA may increase the risk for neurotoxicity. Phenothiazines may increase concentration of some TCAs and TCAs may increase the concentration of phenothiazines. Pressor response to I.V. epinephrine, norepinephrine, and phenylephrine may be enhanced in patients receiving TCAs. (**Note:** Effect is unlikely with epinephrine or levonordefrin dosages typically administered as infiltration in combination with local anesthetics.) Combined use of beta-agonists or drugs which prolong QT$_c$ (including quinidine, procainamide, disopyramide, cisapride, sparfloxacin, gatifloxacin, moxifloxacin) with TCAs may predispose patients to cardiac arrhythmias.

Nutritional/Ethanol Interactions

Ethanol: Avoid ethanol (may increase CNS depression).

Food: Grapefruit juice may inhibit the metabolism of some TCAs and clinical toxicity may result.

Herb/Nutraceutical: St John's wort may decrease amitriptyline levels. Avoid valerian, St John's wort, kava kava, gotu kola (may increase CNS depression).

Lab Interactions Amitriptyline may increase or decrease serum glucose levels, may elevate liver function tests, and may prolong conduction time.
(Continued)

Amitriptyline *(Continued)*

Adverse Reactions Anticholinergic effects may be pronounced; moderate to marked sedation can occur (tolerance to these effects usually occurs).

Frequency not defined.

Cardiovascular: Orthostatic hypotension, tachycardia, ECG changes (nonspecific), AV conduction changes, cardiomyopathy (rare), MI, stroke, heart block, arrhythmia, syncope, hypertension, palpitation

Central nervous system: Restlessness, dizziness, insomnia, sedation, fatigue, anxiety, cognitive function (impaired), seizure, extrapyramidal symptoms, coma, hallucinations, confusion, disorientation, coordination impaired, ataxia, headache, nightmares, hyperpyrexia

Dermatologic: Allergic rash, urticaria, photosensitivity, alopecia

Endocrine & metabolic: Syndrome of inappropriate ADH secretion

Gastrointestinal: Weight gain, xerostomia, constipation, paralytic ileus, nausea, vomiting, anorexia, stomatitis, peculiar taste, diarrhea, black tongue

Genitourinary: Urinary retention

Hematologic: Bone marrow depression, purpura, eosinophilia

Neuromuscular & skeletal: Numbness, paresthesia, peripheral neuropathy, tremor, weakness

Ocular: Blurred vision, mydriasis, ocular pressure increased

Otic: Tinnitus

Miscellaneous: Diaphoresis, withdrawal reactions (nausea, headache, malaise)

Overdosage/Toxicology Symptoms of overdose include agitation, confusion, hallucinations, urinary retention, hypothermia, hypotension, ventricular tachycardia, and seizures. Treatment is symptomatic and supportive. Alkalinization by sodium bicarbonate and/or hyperventilation may limit cardiac toxicity.

Pharmacodynamics/Kinetics

Onset of Action: Migraine prophylaxis: 6 weeks, higher dosage may be required in heavy smokers because of increased metabolism; Depression: 4-6 weeks, reduce dosage to lowest effective level

Time to Peak: Serum: ~4 hours

Half-Life Elimination: Adults: 9-27 hours (average: 15 hours)

Metabolism: Hepatic to nortriptyline (active), hydroxy and conjugated derivatives; may be impaired in the elderly

Excretion: Urine (18% as unchanged drug); feces (small amounts)

Available Dosage Forms

Tablet, as hydrochloride: 10 mg, 25 mg, 50 mg, 75 mg, 100 mg, 150 mg

Dosing

Adults:

Depression:

Oral: 50-150 mg/day single dose at bedtime or in divided doses; dose may be gradually increased up to 300 mg/day.

Chronic pain management (unlabeled use): Oral: Initial: 25 mg at bedtime; may increase as tolerated to 100 mg/day.

Migraine prophylaxis (unlabeled use): Oral: Initial: 10-25 mg at bedtime; usual dose: 150 mg; reported dosing ranges: 10-400 mg/day

Elderly: Depression: Oral: Initial: 10-25 mg at bedtime; dose should be increased in 10-25 mg increments every week if tolerated; dose range: 25-150 mg/day. See Renal/Hepatic Impairment.

Pediatrics:

Chronic pain management (unlabeled use): Oral: Initial: 0.1 mg/kg at bedtime, may advance as tolerated over 2-3 weeks to 0.5-2 mg/kg at bedtime

Depressive disorders:

Children (unlabeled use): Oral: Initial doses of 1 mg/kg/day given in 3 divided doses with increases to 1.5 mg/kg/day have been reported in a small number of children (n=9) 9-12 years of age; clinically, doses up to 3 mg/kg/day (5 mg/kg/day if monitored closely) have been proposed

Adolescents: Initial: 25-50 mg/day; may administer in divided doses; increase gradually to 100 mg/day in divided doses.

Migraine prophylaxis (unlabeled use): Oral: Initial: 0.25 mg/kg/day, given at bedtime; increase dose by 0.25 mg/kg/day to maximum 1 mg/kg/day. Reported dosing ranges: 0.1-2 mg/kg/day; maximum suggested dose: 10 mg.

Renal Impairment: Nondialyzable

Hepatic Impairment: Use with caution and monitor plasma levels and patient response.

Stability

Storage: Protect injection and Elavil® 10 mg tablets from light

Nursing Actions

Physical Assessment: Assess other medications patient may be taking for effectiveness and interactions. Assess for suicidal tendencies or unusual changes in behavior before beginning therapy and periodically thereafter. May cause physiological or psychological dependence, tolerance, or abuse; evaluate need for continued use periodically. Caution patients with diabetes; may increase or decrease serum glucose levels. Monitor therapeutic response and adverse reactions at beginning of therapy and periodically with long-term use. Taper dosage slowly when discontinuing. Teach patient appropriate use, interventions to reduce side effects, and adverse symptoms to report.

Patient Education: Take exactly as directed; do not increase dose or frequency. It may take several weeks to achieve desired results. Restrict use of alcohol and caffeine; avoid grapefruit juice. Maintain adequate hydration (2-3 L/day of fluids) unless instructed to restrict fluid intake. If you have diabetes, monitor glucose levels closely; this medication may alter glucose levels. May turn urine blue-green (normal). May cause drowsiness, lightheadedness, impaired coordination, dizziness, or blurred vision (use caution when driving or engaging in tasks requiring alertness until response to drug is known); constipation (increased exercise, fluids, fruit, or fiber may help); urinary retention (void before taking medication); postural hypotension (use caution climbing stairs or when changing position from lying or sitting to standing); altered sexual drive or ability (reversible); or photosensitivity (use sunscreen, wear protective clothing and eyewear, and avoid direct sunlight). Report persistent CNS effects (eg, nervousness, restlessness, insomnia, headache, agitation, impaired coordination, changes in cognition); muscle cramping, weakness, tremors, or rigidity; ringing in ears or visual disturbances; chest pain, palpitations, or irregular heartbeat; blurred vision; or worsening of condition. **Pregnancy/breast-feeding precautions:** Do not get pregnant while taking this medication. Consult prescriber for appropriate contraceptive measures. Breast-feeding is not recommended.

Geriatric Considerations The most anticholinergic and sedating of the antidepressants. Due to pronounced effects on the cardiovascular system (hypotension), many psychiatrists agree it is best to avoid in the elderly.

Breast-Feeding Issues Generally, it is not recommended to breast-feed if taking antidepressants because of the long half-life, active metabolites, and the potential for side effects in the infant.

Pregnancy Issues Teratogenic effects have been observed in animal studies. Amitriptyline crosses the human placenta; CNS effects, limb deformities and developmental delay have been noted in case reports.

Related Information
Antidepressant Medication Guidelines *on page 1414*
Federal OBRA Regulations Recommended Maximum Doses *on page 1421*
Peak and Trough Guidelines *on page 1387*

Amlexanox (am LEKS an oks)

U.S. Brand Names Aphthasol®
Pharmacologic Category Anti-inflammatory, Locally Applied
Pregnancy Risk Factor B
Lactation Excretion in breast milk unknown/use caution
Use Treatment of aphthous ulcers (ie, canker sores)
Unlabeled/Investigational Use Allergic disorders
Mechanism of Action/Effect As a benzopyrano-bipyridine carboxylic acid derivative, amlexanox has anti-inflammatory and antiallergic properties; it inhibits chemical mediatory release of the slow-reacting substance of anaphylaxis (SRS-A) and may have antagonistic effects on interleukin-3
Contraindications Hypersensitivity to amlexanox or any component of the formulation
Warnings/Precautions Discontinue therapy if rash or contact mucositis develops.
Adverse Reactions 1% to 2%:
Dermatologic: Allergic contact dermatitis
Gastrointestinal: Oral irritation
Pharmacodynamics/Kinetics
Time to Peak: Serum: 2 hours
Half-Life Elimination: 3.5 hours
Metabolism: Hydroxylated and conjugated metabolites
Excretion: Urine (17% as unchanged drug)
Available Dosage Forms Paste: 5% (5 g) [contains benzyl alcohol]
Dosing
Adults & Elderly: Aphthous ulcers: Topical: Administer (0.5 cm - ¼") directly on ulcers 4 times/day following oral hygiene, after meals, and at bedtime.
Nursing Actions
Physical Assessment: Assess knowledge/teach patient appropriate application and use, adverse effects to report, and interventions for side effects.
Patient Education: This medication is only for treatment of mouth ulcers; do not apply to ulcers of the eye or any other part of the body. Use as directed. Apply after eating. Wash hands before and after use. Brush teeth and rinse mouth before applying directly to ulcers. Squeeze a small amount of paste on your clean finger tip and dab paste onto each ulcer in the mouth, using gentle pressure. Wash eyes immediately if any paste should come into contact with eyes. Notify prescriber or dentist if rash or irritation occurs, or if condition does not improve after 10 days use. **Breast-feeding precaution:** Consult prescriber if breast-feeding.

Amlodipine (am LOE di peen)

U.S. Brand Names Norvasc®
Synonyms Amlodipine Besylate
Pharmacologic Category Calcium Channel Blocker
Medication Safety Issues
Sound-alike/look-alike issues:
Amlodipine may be confused with amiloride
Norvasc® may be confused with Navane®, Norvir®, Vascor®
Pregnancy Risk Factor C

Lactation Excretion in breast milk unknown/not recommended
Use Treatment of hypertension; treatment of symptomatic chronic stable angina, vasospastic (Prinzmetal's) angina (confirmed or suspected); prevention of hospitalization due to angina with documented CAD (limited to patients without heart failure or ejection fraction <40%)
Mechanism of Action/Effect Inhibits calcium ion from entering the "slow channels" or select voltage-sensitive areas of vascular smooth muscle and myocardium during depolarization
Contraindications Hypersensitivity to amlodipine or any component of the formulation
Warnings/Precautions Increased angina and/or MI has occurred with initiation or dosage titration of calcium channel blockers. Use caution in severe aortic stenosis. Use caution in patients with severe hepatic impairment. Dosage titration should occur after 7-14 days on a given dose.
Drug Interactions
Cytochrome P450 Effect: Substrate of CYP3A4 (major); **Inhibits** CYP1A2 (moderate), 2A6 (weak), 2B6 (weak), 2C8/9 (weak), 2D6 (weak), 3A4 (weak)
Decreased Effect: Calcium may reduce the calcium channel blocker's hypotensive effects. Levels/effects of amlodipine may be decreased by aminoglutethimide, carbamazepine, nafcillin, nevirapine, phenobarbital, phenytoin, rifamycins, and other CYP3A4 inducers.
Increased Effect/Toxicity: Amlodipine may increase the levels/effects of aminophylline, fluvoxamine, mexiletine, mirtazapine, ropinirole, theophylline, trifluoperazine and other CYP1A2 substrates. Levels/effects of amlodipine may be increased by azole antifungals, clarithromycin, diclofenac, doxycycline, erythromycin, imatinib, isoniazid, nefazodone, nicardipine, propofol, protease inhibitors, quinidine, telithromycin, verapamil, and other CYP3A4 inhibitors. Cyclosporine levels may be increased by amlodipine. Blood pressure-lowering effects of sildenafil, tadalafil, and vardenafil are additive with amlodipine (use caution).
Nutritional/Ethanol Interactions
Food: Grapefruit juice may modestly increase amlodipine levels.
Herb/Nutraceutical: St John's wort may decrease amlodipine levels. Avoid dong quai if using for hypertension (has estrogenic activity). Avoid ephedra, yohimbe, ginseng (may worsen hypertension). Avoid garlic (may have increased antihypertensive effects).
Adverse Reactions
>10%: Cardiovascular: Peripheral edema (2% to 15% dose related)
1% to 10%:
Cardiovascular: Flushing (1% to 3%), palpitation (1% to 4%)
Central nervous system: Headache (7%; similar to placebo 8%), dizziness (1% to 3%), fatigue (4%), somnolence (1% to 2%)
Dermatologic: Rash (1% to 2%), pruritus (1% to 2%)
Endocrine & metabolic: Male sexual dysfunction (1% to 2%)
Gastrointestinal: Nausea (3%), abdominal pain (1% to 2%), dyspepsia (1% to 2%), gingival hyperplasia
Neuromuscular & skeletal: Muscle cramps (1% to 2%), weakness (1% to 2%)
Respiratory: Dyspnea (1% to 2%), pulmonary edema (15% from PRAISE trial, CHF population)
Overdosage/Toxicology Primary cardiac symptoms of calcium channel blocker overdose include hypotension and bradycardia. Noncardiac symptoms include confusion, stupor, nausea, vomiting, metabolic acidosis, and hyperglycemia. Treat other signs and symptoms symptomatically.
(Continued)

Amlodipine (Continued)

Pharmacodynamics/Kinetics

Onset of Action: Antihypertensive: 30-50 minutes

Duration of Action: Antihypertensive effect: 24 hours

Time to Peak: Plasma: 6-12 hours

Protein Binding: 93% to 98%

Half-Life Elimination: 30-50 hours; increased with hepatic dysfunction

Metabolism: Hepatic (>90%) to inactive metabolite

Excretion: Urine (10% as parent, 60% as metabolite)

Available Dosage Forms Tablet: 2.5 mg, 5 mg, 10 mg

Dosing

Adults:

Hypertension: Oral: Initial dose: 5 mg once daily; maximum dose: 10 mg once daily. In general, titrate in 2.5 mg increments over 7-14 days. Usual dosage range (JNC 7): 2.5-10 mg once daily.

Angina: Oral: Usual dose: 5-10 mg; lower dose suggested in elderly or hepatic impairment; most patients require 10 mg for adequate effect.

Elderly: Dosing should start at the lower end of dosing range due to possible increased incidence of hepatic, renal, or cardiac impairment. Elderly patients also show decreased clearance of amlodipine.

Hypertension: Oral: 2.5 mg once daily

Angina: Oral: 5 mg once daily

Pediatrics: Hypertension: Oral: Children 6-17 years: 2.5-5 mg once daily

Hepatic Impairment:

Hypertension: Administer 2.5 mg once daily

Angina: Administer 5 mg once daily

Administration

Oral: May be administered without regard to meals.

Stability

Storage: Store at room temperature of 15°C to 30°C (59°F to 86°F).

Nursing Actions

Physical Assessment: Assess potential for interactions with other prescriptions, OTC medications, or herbal products patient may be taking (eg, nitrates or drugs that effect blood pressure). Monitor blood pressure, cardiac rhythm, frequency and intensity of angina, I & O ratio, weight, edema, and signs or symptoms of adverse reactions at beginning of therapy, when changing dose, and periodically during long-term therapy. Teach patient proper use, possible side effects/appropriate interventions, and adverse symptoms to report.

Patient Education: Do not take any new medication during therapy unless approved by prescriber. Take exactly as directed; do not alter dose or discontinue medication without consulting prescriber. May cause headache (if unrelieved, consult prescriber); nausea or vomiting (small, frequent meals, frequent mouth care, chewing gum or sucking lozenges may help); constipation (increased dietary bulk and fluids may help); or drowsiness (use caution when driving or engaging in tasks that require alertness until response to drug is known). Report unrelieved headache; vomiting, constipation; palpitations; peripheral or facial swelling; weight gain >5 lb/week; or respiratory changes. **Pregnancy/breast-feeding precautions:** Inform prescriber if you are or intend to become pregnant. Consult prescriber if breast-feeding.

Dietary Considerations May be taken without regard to meals.

Geriatric Considerations Older adults may experience a greater hypotensive response. Constipation may be more of a problem in older adults. Calcium channel blockers are no more effective in older adults than other therapies, however, they do not cause significant CNS effects which is an advantage over some antihypertensive agents.

Amlodipine and Atorvastatin

(am LOW di peen & a TORE va sta tin)

U.S. Brand Names Caduet®

Synonyms Atorvastatin Calcium and Amlodipine Besylate

Pharmacologic Category Antilipemic Agent, HMG-CoA Reductase Inhibitor; Calcium Channel Blocker

Pregnancy Risk Factor X

Lactation Excretion in breast milk unknown/contraindicated

Use For use when treatment with both agents is appropriate:

Amlodipine is used for the treatment of hypertension and angina.

Atorvastatin is used with dietary therapy for the following:

Hyperlipidemias: To reduce elevations in total cholesterol, LDL-C, apolipoprotein B, and triglycerides in patients with primary hypercholesterolemia (elevations of 1 or more components are present in Fredrickson type IIa, IIb, III, and IV hyperlipidemias); treatment of homozygous familial hypercholesterolemia

Heterozygous familial hypercholesterolemia (HeFH): In adolescent patients (10-17 years of age, females >1 year postmenarche) with HeFH having LDL-C ≥190 mg/dL **or** LDL-C ≥160 mg/dL with positive family history of premature cardiovascular disease (CVD) or with two or more CVD risk factors in the adolescent patient

Primary prevention of CVD in high-risk patients

Available Dosage Forms Tablet:

2.5/10: Amlodipine 2.5 mg and atorvastatin 10 mg

2.5/20: Amlodipine 2.5 mg and atorvastatin 20 mg

2.5/40: Amlodipine 2.5 mg and atorvastatin 40 mg

5/10: Amlodipine 5 mg and atorvastatin 10 mg

5/20: Amlodipine 5 mg and atorvastatin 20 mg

5/40: Amlodipine 5 mg and atorvastatin 40 mg

5/80: Amlodipine 5 mg and atorvastatin 80 mg

10/10: Amlodipine 10 mg and atorvastatin 10 mg

10/20: Amlodipine 10 mg and atorvastatin 20 mg

10/40: Amlodipine 10 mg and atorvastatin 40 mg

10/80: Amlodipine 10 mg and atorvastatin 80 mg

Dosing

Adults: Treatment of hypertension/angina and hyperlipidemias: Oral: Dose is individualized, given once daily and substituted for each individual component. See individual agents. Maximum dose: Amlodipine 10 mg/day, atorvastatin 80 mg/day.

Pediatrics: Treatment of hypertension/angina and hyperlipidemias: Oral: Children 10-17 years (females >1 year postmenarche): Refer to adult dosing.

Renal Impairment: See individual agents.

Hepatic Impairment: Use of atorvastatin is contraindicated.

Nursing Actions

Physical Assessment: See individual agents. **Pregnancy risk factor X** - determine that patient is not pregnant before starting therapy. Do not give to child-bearing-age females unless capable of complying with effective contraceptive measures. Breast-feeding is contraindicated.

Patient Education: See individual agents. **Pregnancy/breast-feeding precautions:** Inform prescriber if you are pregnant. Do not get pregnant during therapy. Consult prescriber for instructions in appropriate contraceptive measures. This drug can cause severe fetal defects. Do not donate blood while taking this medication and for some period of time after discontinuing. Do not breast-feed.

Amlodipine and Benazepril
(am LOE di peen & ben AY ze pril)

U.S. Brand Names Lotrel®

Synonyms Benazepril Hydrochloride and Amlodipine Besylate

Pharmacologic Category Antihypertensive Agent, Combination

Pregnancy Risk Factor C/D (2nd and 3rd trimesters)

Lactation
Amlodipine: Excretion in breast milk unknown
Benazepril: Enters breast milk

Use Treatment of hypertension

Available Dosage Forms Capsule:
Lotrel® 2.5/10: Amlodipine 2.5 mg and benazepril hydrochloride 10 mg
Lotrel® 5/10: Amlodipine 5 mg and benazepril hydrochloride 10 mg
Lotrel® 5/20: Amlodipine 5 mg and benazepril hydrochloride 20 mg
Lotrel® 10/20: Amlodipine 10 mg and benazepril hydrochloride 20 mg

Dosing
Adults: Hypertension: Oral: 2.5-10 mg (amlodipine) and 10-20 mg (benazepril) once daily; maximum: Amlodipine: 10 mg/day; benazepril: 40 mg/day
Elderly: Initial dose: 2.5 mg (based on amlodipine component). Refer to adult dosing.
Renal Impairment: Cl$_{cr}$ ≤30 mL/minute: Use of combination product is not recommended.
Hepatic Impairment: Initial dose: 2.5 mg based on amlodipine component.

Nursing Actions
Physical Assessment: See individual agents.
Patient Education: See individual agents. **Pregnancy/breast-feeding precautions:** Inform prescriber if you are or intend to become pregnant. Consult prescriber if breast-feeding.

Related Information
Amlodipine *on page 79*
Benazepril *on page 142*

Amoxicillin (a moks i SIL in)

U.S. Brand Names Amoxil®; DisperMox™ [DSC]; Moxilin®; Trimox®

Synonyms Amoxicillin Trihydrate; Amoxycillin; *p*-Hydroxyampicillin

Pharmacologic Category Antibiotic, Penicillin

Medication Safety Issues
Sound-alike/look-alike issues:
Amoxicillin may be confused with amoxapine, Amoxil®, Atarax®
Amoxil® may be confused with amoxapine, amoxicillin
Trimox® may be confused with Diamox®, Tylox®

Pregnancy Risk Factor B

Lactation Enters breast milk/compatible

Use Treatment of otitis media, sinusitis, and infections caused by susceptible organisms involving the respiratory tract, skin, and urinary tract; prophylaxis of bacterial endocarditis in patients undergoing surgical or dental procedures; as part of a multidrug regimen for *H. pylori* eradication

Unlabeled/Investigational Use Postexposure prophylaxis for anthrax exposure with documented susceptible organisms

Mechanism of Action/Effect Interferes with bacterial cell wall synthesis during active multiplication, causing cell wall death and resultant bactericidal activity against susceptible bacteria

Contraindications Hypersensitivity to amoxicillin, penicillin, or any component of the formulation

Warnings/Precautions In patients with renal impairment, doses and/or frequency of administration should be modified in response to the degree of renal impairment. A high percentage of patients with infectious mononucleosis have developed rash during therapy with amoxicillin.

Drug Interactions
Decreased Effect: Decreased effectiveness with tetracyclines and chloramphenicol. Although anecdotal reports suggest oral contraceptive efficacy could be reduced by penicillins, this has been refuted by more rigorous scientific and clinical data.
Increased Effect/Toxicity: Disulfiram and probenecid may increase amoxicillin levels. Amoxicillin may increase the effects of oral anticoagulants (warfarin). Theoretically, allopurinol taken with amoxicillin has an additive potential for amoxicillin rash. Penicillins may increase the exposure to methotrexate during concurrent therapy; monitor.

Lab Interactions Altered response to Benedict's reagent in Clinitest®
Some penicillin derivatives may accelerate the degradation of aminoglycosides *in vitro*, leading to a potential underestimation of aminoglycoside serum concentration.

Adverse Reactions Frequency not defined.
Central nervous system: Hyperactivity, agitation, anxiety, insomnia, confusion, convulsions, behavioral changes, dizziness
Dermatologic: Acute exanthematous pustulosis, erythematous maculopapular rash, erythema multiforme, Stevens-Johnson syndrome, exfoliative dermatitis, toxic epidermal necrolysis, hypersensitivity vasculitis, urticaria
Gastrointestinal: Nausea, vomiting, diarrhea, hemorrhagic colitis, pseudomembranous colitis, tooth discoloration (brown, yellow, or gray; rare)
Hematologic: Anemia, hemolytic anemia, thrombocytopenia, thrombocytopenia purpura, eosinophilia, leukopenia, agranulocytosis
Hepatic: AST (SGOT) and ALT (SGPT) increased, cholestatic jaundice, hepatic cholestasis, acute cytolytic hepatitis
Renal: Crystalluria

Overdosage/Toxicology Symptoms of penicillin overdose include neuromuscular hypersensitivity (eg, agitation, hallucinations, asterixis, encephalopathy, confusion, and seizures). Interstitial nephritis and/or crystalluria, possibly resulting in renal failure, may occur; hydration and diuresis may be beneficial. Electrolyte imbalance may occur if the preparation contains potassium or sodium salts, especially in renal failure. A study of 51 pediatric overdose victims suggests that ingestion of doses ≤250 mg/kg does not manifest significant clinical symptoms, and thus does not require gastric lavage. Hemodialysis may be helpful to aid in removal of the drug from blood; otherwise, treatment is symptom-directed and supportive.

Pharmacodynamics/Kinetics
Time to Peak: Capsule: 2 hours; Suspension: 1 hour
Protein Binding: 17% to 20%
Half-Life Elimination:
Neonates, full-term: 3.7 hours
Infants and Children: 1-2 hours
Adults: Normal renal function: 0.7-1.4 hours
Cl$_{cr}$ <10 mL/minute: 7-21 hours
Metabolism: Partially hepatic
Excretion: Urine (80% as unchanged drug); lower in neonates

Available Dosage Forms [DSC] = Discontinued product
Capsule, as trihydrate: 250 mg, 500 mg
Amoxil®: 500 mg
Moxilin®, Trimox®: 250 mg, 500 mg
Powder for oral suspension, as trihydrate: 125 mg/5 mL (80 mL, 100 mL, 150 mL); 200 mg/5 mL (50 mL, 75
(Continued)

Amoxicillin *(Continued)*

mL, 100 mL); 250 mg/5 mL (80 mL, 100 mL, 150 mL); 400 mg/5 mL (50 mL, 75 mL, 100 mL)

Amoxil®: 200 mg/5 mL (5 mL, 50 mL, 75 mL, 100 mL) [contains sodium benzoate; bubble gum flavor]; 250 mg/5 mL (100 mL, 150 mL) [contains sodium benzoate; bubble gum flavor]; 400 mg/5 mL (5 mL, 50 mL, 75 mL, 100 mL) [contains sodium benzoate; bubble gum flavor]

Moxilin®: 250 mg/5 mL (100 mL, 150 mL)

Trimox®: 125 mg/5 mL (80 mL, 100 mL, 150 mL); 250 mg/5 mL (80 mL, 100 mL, 150 mL) [contains sodium benzoate; raspberry-strawberry flavor]

Powder for oral suspension, as trihydrate [drops] (Amoxil®): 50 mg/mL (30 mL) [bubble gum flavor]

Tablet, as trihydrate (Amoxil®): 500 mg, 875 mg

Tablet, chewable, as trihydrate: 125 mg, 200 mg, 250 mg, 400 mg

Amoxil®: 200 mg [contains phenylalanine 1.82 mg/tablet; cherry banana peppermint flavor]; 400 mg [contains phenylalanine 3.64 mg/tablet; cherry banana peppermint flavor]

Tablet, for oral suspension, as trihydrate (DisperMox™): 200 mg [contains phenylalanine 5.6 mg; strawberry flavor]; 400 mg [contains phenylalanine 5.6 mg; strawberry flavor]; 600 mg [contains phenylalanine 11.23 mg; strawberry flavor] [DSC]

Dosing

Adults & Elderly:

Usual dosage range: Oral: 250-500 mg every 8 hours or 500-875 mg twice daily

Anthrax exposure (CDC guidelines): Oral: **Note:** Postexposure prophylaxis in pregnant or nursing women only with documented susceptible organisms: 500 mg every 8 hours

Ear, nose, throat, genitourinary tract, or skin/skin structure infections:
Mild to moderate: Oral: 500 mg every 12 hours **or** 250 mg every 8 hours
Severe: Oral: 875 mg every 12 hours **or** 500 mg every 8 hours

Endocarditis prophylaxis: Oral: 2 g 1 hour before procedure

***Helicobacter pylori* eradication:** Oral: 1000 mg twice daily; requires combination therapy with at least one other antibiotic and an acid-suppressing agent (proton pump inhibitor or H₂ blocker)

Lower respiratory tract infections: Oral: 875 mg every 12 hours **or** 500 mg every 8 hours

Lyme disease: Oral: 500 mg every 6-8 hours (depending on size of patient) for 21-30 days

Pediatrics:

Usual dosage range:
Children ≤3 months: Oral: 20-30 mg/kg/day divided every 12 hours
Children >3 months and <40 kg: Oral: 20-50 mg/kg/day in divided doses every 8-12 hours

Acute otitis media: Children >3 months and <40 kg: Oral: 80-90 mg/kg/day divided every 12 hours

Anthrax exposure (CDC guidelines): Children >3 months and <40 kg: Oral: **Note:** Postexposure prophylaxis only with documented susceptible organisms: 80 mg/kg/day in divided doses every 8 hours (maximum: 500 mg/dose)

Ear, nose, throat, genitourinary tract, or skin/skin structure infections: Children >3 months and <40 kg: Oral:
Mild to moderate: 25 mg/kg/day in divided doses every 12 hours **or** 20 mg/kg/day in divided doses every 8 hours
Severe: 45 mg/kg/day in divided doses every 12 hours **or** 40 mg/kg/day in divided doses every 8 hours

Endocarditis (subacute bacterial) prophylaxis: Children >3 months and <40 kg: Oral: 50 mg/kg 1 hour before procedure

Lower respiratory tract infections: Children >3 months and <40 kg: Oral: 45 mg/kg/day in divided doses every 12 hours **or** 40 mg/kg/day in divided doses every 8 hours

Lyme disease: Children >3 months and <40 kg: Oral: 25-50 mg/kg/day divided every 8 hours (maximum: 500 mg)

Pneumonia:
4 months to 5 years: Oral: 100 mg/kg/day divided every 8 hours
5-15 years: Oral: 100 mg/kg/day divided every 8 hours with clarithromycin, azithromycin, or doxycycline

Renal Impairment:

The 875 mg tablet should not be used in patients with Cl$_{cr}$ <30 mL/minute.

Cl$_{cr}$ 10-30 mL/minute: 250-500 mg every 12 hours

Cl$_{cr}$ <10 mL/minute: 250-500 mg every 24 hours

Moderately dialyzable (20% to 50%) by hemodialysis or peritoneal dialysis; approximately 50 mg of amoxicillin per liter of filtrate is removed by continuous arteriovenous or venovenous hemofiltration. Dose as per Cl$_{cr}$ <10 mL/minute guidelines.

Administration

Oral: Administer around-the-clock to promote less variation in peak and trough serum levels. The appropriate amount of suspension may be mixed with formula, milk, fruit juice, water, ginger ale, or cold drinks; administer dose immediately after mixing.

DisperMox™: Dissolve 1 tablet in ~10 mL of water immediately before administration. Rinse container with additional water and drink entire contents to ensure that complete dose is taken. Do not chew or swallow tablet whole.

Some penicillins (eg, carbenicillin, ticarcillin, and piperacillin) have been shown to inactivate aminoglycosides *in vitro*. This has been observed to a greater extent with tobramycin and gentamicin, while amikacin has shown greater stability against inactivation. Concurrent use of these agents may pose a risk of reduced antibacterial efficacy *in vivo*, particularly in the setting of profound renal impairment. However, definitive clinical evidence is lacking. If combination penicillin/aminoglycoside therapy is desired in a patient with renal dysfunction, separation of doses (if feasible), and routine monitoring of aminoglycoside levels, CBC, and clinical response should be considered.

Stability

Reconstitution: DisperMox™: Dissolve 1 tablet in ~10 mL water immediately before use.

Storage: Amoxil®: Oral suspension remains stable for 14 days at room temperature or if refrigerated (refrigeration preferred); unit-dose antibiotic oral syringes are stable for 48 hours.

Laboratory Monitoring Perform culture and sensitivity testing prior to initiating therapy.

Nursing Actions

Physical Assessment: Assess for allergy history prior to starting therapy. Assess potential for interactions with other medications patient may be taking. Monitor for therapeutic effect and adverse reactions (eg, opportunistic infection [fever, chills, unhealed sores, white plaques in mouth or vagina, purulent vaginal discharge, fatigue]). Advise patients with diabetes about use of Clinitest®. Teach patient proper use, possible side effects/appropriate interventions, and adverse symptoms to report.

Patient Education: Do not take any new medication during therapy unless approved by prescriber. Take entire prescription, even if you are feeling better. Take at equal intervals around-the-clock. May be taken with milk, juice, or food. If you have diabetes, drug may cause false test results with Clinitest® urine glucose monitoring; use of another type of glucose monitoring is preferable. May cause nausea or vomiting (small, frequent meals, frequent mouth care, sucking lozenges, or chewing gum may help). Report rash; unusual diarrhea; vaginal itching, burning, or pain; unresolved vomiting or constipation; fever or chills; abdominal pain; jaundice; unusual bruising or bleeding; opportunistic infection [fever, chills, unhealed sores, white plaques in mouth or vagina, purulent vaginal discharge, fatigue]; or if condition being treated worsens or does not improve by the time prescription is completed.

Dietary Considerations May be taken with food. Amoxil® chewable contains phenylalanine 1.82 mg per 200 mg tablet, phenylalanine 3.64 mg per 400 mg tablet. DisperMox™ contains phenylalanine 5.6 mg in each 200 mg and 400 mg tablet.

Geriatric Considerations Resistance to amoxicillin has been a problem in patients on frequent antibiotics or in nursing homes. Alternative antibiotics may be necessary in these populations. Consider renal function.

Amoxicillin and Clavulanate Potassium
(a moks i SIL in & klav yoo LAN ate poe TASS ee um)

U.S. Brand Names Augmentin®; Augmentin ES-600®; Augmentin XR™

Synonyms Amoxicillin and Clavulanic Acid; Clavulanic Acid and Amoxicillin

Pharmacologic Category Antibiotic, Penicillin

Medication Safety Issues
Sound-alike/look-alike issues:
Augmentin® may be confused with Azulfidine®

Pregnancy Risk Factor B

Lactation Enters breast milk/use caution (AAP rates "compatible")

Use Treatment of otitis media, sinusitis, and infections caused by susceptible organisms involving the lower respiratory tract, skin and skin structure, and urinary tract; spectrum same as amoxicillin with additional coverage of beta-lactamase producing *B. catarrhalis, H. influenzae, N. gonorrhoeae,* and *S. aureus* (not MRSA). The expanded coverage of this combination makes it a useful alternative when amoxicillin resistance is present and patients cannot tolerate alternative treatments.

Mechanism of Action/Effect Interferes with bacterial cell wall synthesis during active multiplication, causing cell wall death and resultant bactericidal activity against susceptible bacteria. Clavulanic acid binds and inhibits beta-lactamases that inactivate amoxicillin resulting in amoxicillin having an expanded spectrum of activity.

Contraindications Hypersensitivity to amoxicillin, clavulanic acid, penicillin, or any component of the formulation; history of cholestatic jaundice or hepatic dysfunction with amoxicillin/clavulanate potassium therapy; Augmentin XR™: severe renal impairment (Cl_cr <30 mL/minute) and hemodialysis patients

Warnings/Precautions Hypersensitivity reactions, including anaphylaxis (some fatal), have been reported. Prolonged use may result in superinfection, including *Pseudomembranous colitis.* In patients with renal impairment, doses and/or frequency of administration should be modified in response to the degree of renal impairment. High percentage of patients with infectious mononucleosis have developed rash during therapy. Incidence of diarrhea is higher than with amoxicillin alone. Use caution in patients with hepatic dysfunction. Hepatic dysfunction, although rare, is more common in elderly and/or males, and occurs more frequently with prolonged treatment, and may occur after therapy is complete. Due to differing content of clavulanic acid, not all formulations are interchangeable. Low incidence of cross-allergy with cephalosporins exists. Some products contain phenylalanine.

Drug Interactions
Decreased Effect: Although anecdotal reports suggest oral contraceptive efficacy could be reduced by penicillins, this has been refuted by more rigorous scientific and clinical data.

Increased Effect/Toxicity: Probenecid may increase amoxicillin levels (concomitant use is not recommended). Increased effect of anticoagulants with amoxicillin. Allopurinol taken with Augmentin® has an additive potential for rash. Penicillins may increase the exposure to methotrexate during concurrent therapy; monitor.

Lab Interactions Urinary glucose (Benedict's solution, Clinitest®, Fehling's solution)
Some penicillin derivatives may accelerate the degradation of aminoglycosides *in vitro,* leading to a potential underestimation of aminoglycoside serum concentration.

Adverse Reactions
>10%: Gastrointestinal: Diarrhea (3% to 34%; incidence varies upon dose and regimen used)
1% to 10%:
Dermatologic: Diaper rash, skin rash, urticaria
Gastrointestinal: Abdominal discomfort, loose stools, nausea, vomiting
Genitourinary: Vaginitis, vaginal mycosis
Miscellaneous: Moniliasis

Additional adverse reactions seen with **ampicillin-class antibiotics:** Agitation, agranulocytosis, alkaline phosphatase increased, anaphylaxis, anemia, angioedema, anxiety, behavioral changes, bilirubin increased, black "hairy" tongue, confusion, convulsions, crystalluria, dizziness, enterocolitis, eosinophilia, erythema multiforme, exanthematous pustulosis, exfoliative dermatitis, gastritis, glossitis, hematuria, hemolytic anemia, hemorrhagic colitis, indigestion, insomnia, hyperactivity, interstitial nephritis, leukopenia, mucocutaneous candidiasis, pruritus, pseudomembranous colitis, serum sickness-like reaction, Stevens-Johnson syndrome, stomatitis, transaminases increased, thrombocytopenia, thrombocytopenic purpura, tooth discoloration, toxic epidermal necrolysis

Overdosage/Toxicology Symptoms of overdose may include abdominal pain, diarrhea, drowsiness, rash, hyperactivity, stomach pain, and vomiting. Interstitial nephritis and/or crystalluria, possibly resulting in renal failure, may occur; hydration and diuresis may be beneficial. Electrolyte imbalance may occur, especially in renal failure. A study of 51 pediatric overdose victims suggests that ingestion of amoxicillin at doses ≤250 mg/kg do not manifest significant clinical symptoms, and thus do not require gastric lavage. Hemodialysis may be helpful to aid in removal of the drug from blood; otherwise, treatment is supportive or symptom-directed.

Pharmacodynamics/Kinetics
Metabolism:
Clavulanic acid: Hepatic
Excretion:
Clavulanic acid: Urine (30% to 40% as unchanged drug)

Pharmacokinetic Note Amoxicillin pharmacokinetics are not affected by clavulanic acid. See Amoxicillin.

Available Dosage Forms
Powder for oral suspension: 200: Amoxicillin 200 mg and clavulanate potassium 28.5 mg per 5 mL (100 mL) [contains phenylalanine]; 400: Amoxicillin 400 mg and clavulanate potassium 57 mg per 5 mL (100 mL) [contains phenylalanine]; 600: Amoxicillin 600 mg and clavulanic potassium 42.9 mg per 5 mL (75 mL, 125 mL, 200 mL) [contains phenylalanine]
Augmentin®:
125: Amoxicillin 125 mg and clavulanate potassium 31.25 mg per 5 mL (75 mL, 100 mL, 150 mL) [banana flavor]
200: Amoxicillin 200 mg and clavulanate potassium 28.5 mg per 5 mL (50 mL, 75 mL, 100 mL)
(Continued)

Amoxicillin and Clavulanate Potassium
(Continued)

[contains phenylalanine 7 mg/5 mL; orange-raspberry flavor]

250: Amoxicillin 250 mg and clavulanate potassium 62.5 mg per 5 mL (75 mL, 100 mL, 150 mL) [orange flavor]

400: Amoxicillin 400 mg and clavulanate potassium 57 mg per 5 mL (50 mL, 75 mL, 100 mL) [contains phenylalanine 7 mg/5 mL; orange-raspberry flavor]

Augmentin ES-600®: Amoxicillin 600 mg and clavulanic potassium 42.9 mg per 5 mL (75 mL, 125 mL, 200 mL) [contains phenylalanine 7 mg/5 mL; strawberry cream flavor]

Tablet: 500: Amoxicillin trihydrate 500 mg and clavulanate potassium 125 mg; 875: Amoxicillin trihydrate 875 mg and clavulanate potassium 125 mg

Augmentin®:

250: Amoxicillin trihydrate 250 mg and clavulanate potassium 125 mg

500: Amoxicillin trihydrate 500 mg and clavulanate potassium 125 mg

875: Amoxicillin trihydrate 875 mg and clavulanate potassium 125 mg

Tablet, chewable: 200: Amoxicillin trihydrate 200 mg and clavulanate potassium 28.5 mg [contains phenylalanine]; 400: Amoxicillin trihydrate 400 mg and clavulanate potassium 57 mg [contains phenylalanine]

Augmentin®:

125: Amoxicillin trihydrate 125 mg and clavulanate potassium 31.25 mg [lemon-lime flavor]

200: Amoxicillin trihydrate 200 mg and clavulanate potassium 28.5 mg [contains phenylalanine 2.1 mg/tablet; cherry-banana flavor]

250: Amoxicillin trihydrate 250 mg and clavulanate potassium 62.5 mg [lemon-lime flavor]

400: Amoxicillin trihydrate 400 mg and clavulanate potassium 57 mg [contains phenylalanine 4.2 mg/tablet; cherry-banana flavor]

Tablet, extended release (Augmentin XR™): Amoxicillin 1000 mg and clavulanic acid 62.5 mg [contains potassium 29.3 mg (1.27 mEq) and sodium 12.6 mg (0.32 mEq)]

Dosing

Adults & Elderly: Note: Dose is based on the amoxicillin component; see "Augmentin® Product-Specific Considerations" table.

Susceptible infections: Children >40 kg and Adults: Oral: 250-500 mg every 8 hours or 875 mg every 12 hours

Acute bacterial sinusitis: Oral: Extended release tablet: Two 1000 mg tablets every 12 hours for 10 days

Bite wounds (animal/human): Oral: 875 mg every 12 hours or 500 mg every 8 hours

Chronic obstructive pulmonary disease: Oral: 875 mg every 12 hours or 500 mg every 8 hours

Diabetic foot: Oral: Extended release tablet: Two 1000 mg tablets every 12 hours for 7-14 days

Diverticulitis, perirectal abscess: Oral: Extended release tablet: Two 1000 mg tablets every 12 hours for 7-10 days

Erysipelas: Oral: 875 mg every 12 hours or 500 mg every 8 hours

Febrile neutropenia: Oral: 875 mg every 12 hours

Pneumonia:

Aspiration: Oral: 875 mg every 12 hours

Community-acquired: Oral: Extended release tablet: Two 1000 mg tablets every 12 hours for 7-10 days

Pyelonephritis (acute, uncomplicated): Oral: 875 mg every 12 hours or 500 mg every 8 hours

Skin abscess: Oral: 875 mg every 12 hours

Augmentin® Product-Specific Considerations

Strength	Form	Consideration
125 mg	CT, S	q8h dosing
	S	For adults having difficulty swallowing tablets, 125 mg/5 mL suspension may be substituted for 500 mg tablet.
200 mg	CT, S	q12h dosing
	CT	Contains phenylalanine
	S	For adults having difficulty swallowing tablets, 200 mg/5 mL suspension may be substituted for 875 mg tablet.
250 mg	CT, S, T	q8h dosing
	CT	Contains phenylalanine
	T	Not for use in patients <40 kg
	CT, T	Tablet and chewable tablet are not interchangeable due to differences in clavulanic acid.
	S	For adults having difficulty swallowing tablets, 250 mg/5 mL suspension may be substituted for 500 mg tablet.
400 mg	CT, S	q12h dosing
	CT	Contains phenylalanine
	S	For adults having difficulty swallowing tablets, 400 mg/5 mL suspension may be substituted for 875 mg tablet.
500 mg	T	q8h or q12h dosing
600 mg	S	q12h dosing
		Contains phenylalanine
		Not for use in adults or children ≥40 kg
		600 mg/5 mL suspension is not equivalent to or interchangeable with 200 mg/5 mL or 400 mg/5 mL due to differences in clavulanic acid.
875 mg	T	q12h dosing; not for use in Cl_{cr} <30 mL/minute
1000 mg	XR	q12h dosing
		Not for use in children <16 years of age
		Not interchangeable with two 500 mg tablets
		Not for use if Cl_{cr} <30 mL/minute or hemodialysis

Legend: CT = chewable tablet, S = suspension, T = tablet, XR = extended release.

Pediatrics: Note: Dose is based on the amoxicillin component; see "Augmentin® Product-Specific Considerations table".

Susceptible infections: Infants <3 months: Oral: 30 mg/kg/day divided every 12 hours using the 125 mg/5 mL suspension

Lower respiratory tract infections, severe infections, sinusitis: Children ≥3 months and <40 kg: Oral: 45 mg/kg/day divided every 12 hours or 40 mg/kg/day divided every 8 hours

Mild-to-moderate infections: Children ≥3 months and <40 kg: Oral: 25 mg/kg/day divided every 12 hours or 20 mg/kg/day divided every 8 hours

Otitis media (Augmentin® ES-600): Children ≥3 months and <40 kg: Oral: 90 mg/kg/day divided every 12 hours for 10 days in children with severe illness and when coverage for β-lactamase positive *H. influenzae* and *M. catarrhalis* is needed.

Children >40 kg: Refer to adult dosing.

Renal Impairment:

Cl_{cr} <30 mL/minute: Do not use 875 mg tablet or extended release tablets.

Cl_{cr} 10-30 mL/minute: 250-500 mg every 12 hours

Cl_{cr} <10 mL/minute: 250-500 mg every 24 hours

Hemodialysis: Moderately dialyzable (20% to 50%) 250-500 mg every 24 hours; administer dose during and after dialysis. Do not use extended release tablets.

Peritoneal dialysis: Moderately dialyzable (20% to 50%)

Amoxicillin: Administer 250 mg every 12 hours

Clavulanic acid: Dose for Cl$_{cr}$ <10 mL/minute

Continuous arteriovenous or venovenous hemofiltration effects:

Amoxicillin: ~50 mg of amoxicillin/L of filtrate is removed

Clavulanic acid: Dose for Cl$_{cr}$ <10 mL/minute

Administration

Oral: Administer around-the-clock to promote less variation in peak and trough serum levels. Administer with food to decrease stomach upset; shake suspension well before use. Extended release tablets should be administered with food.

Some penicillins (eg, carbenicillin, ticarcillin, and piperacillin) have been shown to inactivate aminoglycosides *in vitro*. This has been observed to a greater extent with tobramycin and gentamicin, while amikacin has shown greater stability against inactivation. Concurrent use of these agents may pose a risk of reduced antibacterial efficacy *in vivo*, particularly in the setting of profound renal impairment. However, definitive clinical evidence is lacking. If combination penicillin/aminoglycoside therapy is desired in a patient with renal dysfunction, separation of doses (if feasible), and routine monitoring of aminoglycoside levels, CBC, and clinical response should be considered.

Stability

Reconstitution: Reconstitute powder for oral suspension with appropriate amount of water as specified on the bottle. Shake vigorously until suspended. Reconstituted oral suspension should be kept in refrigerator. Discard unused suspension after 10 days. Unit-dose antibiotic oral syringes are stable for 48 hours.

Storage:

Powder for oral suspension: Store dry powder at room temperature of 25°C (77°F).

Tablet: Store at room temperature of 25°C (77°F).

Laboratory Monitoring Renal, hepatic, and hematologic function periodically with prolonged therapy. Perform culture and sensitivity testing prior to initiating therapy.

Nursing Actions

Physical Assessment: Assess for allergy history prior to starting therapy. Assess potential for interactions with other prescriptions, OTC medications, or herbal products patient may be taking. Advise patients with diabetes about use of Clinitest®. Monitor therapeutic effect and adverse reactions (eg, hypersensitivity reaction, hepatic dysfunction, opportunistic infection [fever, chills, unhealed sores, white plaques in mouth or vagina, purulent vaginal discharge, fatigue]). Teach patient proper use, possible side effects/appropriate interventions, and adverse symptoms to report.

Patient Education: Do not take any new medication during therapy unless approved by prescriber. Take as directed, for as long as directed, even if you are feeling better. (For small children, bottles may contain more suspension than needed, take for number of days prescribed.) Take at equal intervals around-the-clock; may be taken with milk, juice, or food. Extended release tablets should be taken with food. If you have diabetes, drug may cause false test results with Clinitest® urine glucose monitoring; use of another type of glucose monitoring is preferable. May cause nausea or vomiting (small, frequent meals, frequent mouth care, sucking lozenges, or chewing gum may help). Report rash; unusual diarrhea; vaginal itching, burning, or pain; unresolved vomiting or constipation; fever or chills; abdominal pain; jaundice; unusual bruising or bleeding; or if condition being treated worsens or does not improve by the time prescription is completed. Some products contain phenylalanine. If you have phenylketonuria or PKU, avoid use. **Breast-feeding precaution:** Consult prescriber if breast-feeding.

Dietary Considerations May be taken with meals or on an empty stomach; take with meals to increase absorption and decrease GI intolerance; may mix with milk, formula, or juice. Extended release tablets should be taken with food. Some products contain phenylalanine; avoid use in phenylketonurics. All dosage forms contain potassium.

Geriatric Considerations Resistance to amoxicillin has been a problem in patients on frequent antibiotics or in nursing homes. However, expanded coverage of this combination makes it a useful alternative when amoxicillin resistance is present and patients cannot tolerate alternative treatments. Consider renal function. Considered one of the drugs of choice in the outpatient treatment of community-acquired pneumonia in older adults.

Breast-Feeding Issues The AAP considers amoxicillin to be "compatible" with breast-feeding.

Pregnancy Issues Both amoxicillin and clavulanate potassium cross the human placenta. Teratogenic effects have not been reported. Use in women with premature rupture of fetal membranes may increase risk of necrotizing enterocolitis in neonates.

Additional Information Two 250 mg tablets are not equivalent to a 500 mg tablet (both tablet sizes contain equivalent clavulanate). Two 500 mg tablets are not equivalent to a single 1000 mg extended release tablet.

Related Information

Amoxicillin *on page 81*

Amphotericin B Cholesteryl Sulfate Complex

(am foe TER i sin bee kole LES te ril SUL fate KOM plecks)

U.S. Brand Names Amphotec®

Synonyms ABCD; Amphotericin B Colloidal Dispersion

Pharmacologic Category Antifungal Agent, Parenteral

Medication Safety Issues

Safety issues:

Lipid-based amphotericin formulations (Amphotec®) may be confused with conventional formulations (Amphocin®, Fungizone®)

Large overdoses have occurred when conventional formulations were dispensed inadvertently for lipid-based products. Single daily doses of conventional amphotericin formulation never exceed 1.5 mg/kg.

Pregnancy Risk Factor B

Lactation Excretion in breast milk unknown/contraindicated

Use Treatment of invasive aspergillosis in patients who have failed amphotericin B deoxycholate treatment, or who have renal impairment or experience unacceptable toxicity which precludes treatment with amphotericin B deoxycholate in effective doses.

Unlabeled/Investigational Use Effective in patients with serious *Candida* species infections

Mechanism of Action/Effect Binds to ergosterol altering cell membrane permeability in susceptible fungi and causing leakage of cell components with subsequent cell death

Contraindications Hypersensitivity to amphotericin B or any component of the formulation

Warnings/Precautions Anaphylaxis has been reported. Facilities for cardiopulmonary resuscitation should be available. Infusion reactions, sometimes severe, usually subside with continued therapy.

Drug Interactions

Decreased Effect: Pharmacologic antagonism may occur with azole antifungals (eg, ketoconazole, miconazole).

(Continued)

Amphotericin B Cholesteryl Sulfate Complex (Continued)

Increased Effect/Toxicity: Toxic effect with other nephrotoxic drugs (eg, cyclosporine and aminoglycosides) may be additive. Corticosteroids may increase potassium depletion caused by amphotericin. Amphotericin B may predispose patients receiving digitalis glycosides or neuromuscular blocking agents to toxicity secondary to hypokalemia.

Adverse Reactions

>10%: Central nervous system: Chills, fever

1% to 10%:

Cardiovascular: Hypotension, tachycardia

Central nervous system: Headache

Dermatologic: Rash

Endocrine & metabolic: Hypokalemia, hypomagnesemia

Gastrointestinal: Nausea, diarrhea, abdominal pain

Hematologic: Thrombocytopenia

Hepatic: LFT change

Neuromuscular & skeletal: Rigors

Renal: Creatinine increased

Respiratory: Dyspnea

Note: Amphotericin B colloidal dispersion has an improved therapeutic index compared to conventional amphotericin B, and has been used safely in patients with amphotericin B-related nephrotoxicity; however, continued decline of renal function has occurred in some patients.

Overdosage/Toxicology Symptoms of overdose include renal dysfunction, anemia, thrombocytopenia, granulocytopenia, fever, nausea, and vomiting. Treatment is supportive.

Pharmacodynamics/Kinetics

Half-Life Elimination: 28-29 hours; prolonged with higher doses

Available Dosage Forms Injection, powder for reconstitution: 50 mg, 100 mg

Dosing

Adults & Elderly:

Note: Premedication: For patients who experience chills, fever, hypotension, nausea, or other nonanaphylactic infusion-related immediate reactions, premedicate with the following drugs 30-60 minutes prior to drug administration: A nonsteroidal (eg, ibuprofen, choline magnesium trisalicylate) with or without diphenhydramine **or** acetaminophen with diphenhydramine **or** hydrocortisone 50-100 mg. If the patient experiences rigors during the infusion, meperidine may be administered.

Usual dosage: I.V.: 3-4 mg/kg/day (infusion of 1 mg/kg/hour); maximum: 7.5 mg/kg/day

A regimen of 6 mg/kg/day has been used for treatment of life-threatening invasive mold infections in immunocompromised patients; maximum: 7.5 mg/kg/day.

Initially infuse at 1 mg/kg/hour. Rate of infusion may be increased with subsequent doses to 3 mg/kg/hour as patient tolerance allows. Treatment should continue as patient tolerance allows, until complete resolution of microbiologic and clinical evidence of fungal disease.

Pediatrics: Refer to adult dosing.

Administration

I.V.: For a patient who experiences chills, fever, hypotension, nausea, or other nonanaphylactic infusion-related reactions, premedicate with the following drugs 30-60 minutes prior to drug administration: A nonsteroidal (eg, ibuprofen, choline magnesium trisalicylate) with or without diphenhydramine **or** acetaminophen with diphenhydramine **or** hydrocortisone 50-100 mg. If the patient experiences rigors during the infusion, meperidine may be administered. If severe

respiratory distress occurs, the infusion should be immediately discontinued.

I.V. Detail: Avoid injection faster than 1 mg/kg/hour

Stability

Reconstitution: Reconstitute 50 mg and 100 mg vials with 10 mL and 20 mL of SWI, respectively. The reconstituted vials contain 5 mg/mL of amphotericin B. Shake the vial gently by hand until all solid particles have dissolved. Further dilute amphotericin B colloidal dispersion with dextrose 5% in water.

Compatibility: Stable in D$_5$W; **incompatible** with NS

Y-site administration: Incompatible with alfentanil, amikacin, ampicillin, ampicillin/sulbactam, atenolol, aztreonam, bretylium, buprenorphine, butorphanol, calcium chloride, calcium gluconate, carboplatin, cefazolin, cefepime, cefoperazone, ceftazidime, ceftriaxone, chlorpromazine, cimetidine, cisatracurium, cisplatin, cyclophosphamide, cyclosporine, cytarabine, diazepam, digoxin, diphenhydramine, dobutamine, dopamine, doxorubicin, doxorubicin liposome, droperidol, enalaprilat, esmolol, famotidine, fluconazole, fluorouracil, gatifloxacin, gentamicin, haloperidol, heparin, hydromorphone, hydroxyzine, imipenem/cilastatin, labetalol, leucovorin, lidocaine, magnesium sulfate, meperidine, mesna, metoclopramide, metoprolol, metronidazole, midazolam, mitoxantrone, morphine, nalbuphine, naloxone, ofloxacin, ondansetron, paclitaxel, pentobarbital, phenobarbital, phenytoin, piperacillin, piperacillin/tazobactam, potassium chloride, prochlorperazine, promethazine, propranolol, ranitidine, remifentanil, sodium bicarbonate, ticarcillin, ticarcillin/clavulanate, tobramycin, vancomycin, vecuronium, verapamil, vinorelbine

Storage: Store intact vials under refrigeration. After reconstitution, the solution should be refrigerated at 2°C to 8°C (36°F to 46°F) and used within 24 hours. Concentrations of 0.1-2 mg/mL in dextrose 5% in water are stable for 14 days at 4°C and 23°C if protected from light, however, due to the occasional formation of subvisual particles, solutions should be used within 48 hours.

Laboratory Monitoring Monitor serum electrolytes (especially potassium and magnesium), liver function, and CBC. Perform culture and sensitivity testing prior to initiating therapy.

Nursing Actions

Physical Assessment: Culture and sensitivity and patient history of exposure to amphotericin B should be assessed prior to beginning treatment. Assess potential for interactions with other medications patient may be taking. Premedication may be ordered to reduce incidence/severity of infusion reaction. See Administration and Compatibility/Incompatibility prior to administering first dose. Monitor patient closely for infusion related reactions (eg, anaphylaxis, chills, fever, nausea, vomiting, rigors, hypotension, acute respiratory distress) and facilities for cardiopulmonary resuscitation should be available. Monitor laboratory tests, therapeutic effectiveness, and adverse response on a regular basis during therapy. Teach patient possible side effects/appropriate interventions and adverse symptoms to report.

Patient Education: Do not take any new medication during therapy unless approved by prescriber. This medication can only be administered by infusion and therapy may last several weeks. You will be monitored closely during and after infusion; report immediately any pain or swelling at infusion site, chills, nausea, chest pain, swelling of face or mouth, difficulty breathing, muscle cramping, acute anxiety, or other infusion reactions. Maintain adequate hydration (2-3 L/day of fluids) unless instructed to restrict fluid intake. May cause postural hypotension (use caution when changing from lying or sitting position to standing or when climbing stairs); or nausea or vomiting (small, frequent meals, frequent mouth care, sucking lozenges, or chewing gum may help). Report chest pain or palpitations; CNS disturbances; skin rash; unusual chills or fever; persistent nausea, vomiting, or abdominal pain; sore throat; excessive fatigue; swelling of extremities or unusual weight gain; difficulty breathing; pain at infusion site; muscle cramping or weakness; or other adverse reactions. **Breast-feeding precaution:** Do not breast-feed.

Geriatric Considerations The pharmacokinetics and dosing of amphotericin have not been studied in the elderly. It appears that use is similar to young adults. Caution should be exercised and renal function and desired effect monitored closely.

Breast-Feeding Issues Due to limited data, consider discontinuing nursing during therapy.

Additional Information Controlled trials which compare the original formulation of amphotericin B to the newer liposomal formulations (ie, Amphotec®) are lacking. Thus, comparative data discussing differences among the formulations should be interpreted cautiously. Although the risk of nephrotoxicity and infusion-related adverse effects may be less with Amphotec®, the efficacy profiles of Amphotec® and the original amphotericin formulation are comparable. Consequently, Amphotec® should be restricted to those patients who cannot tolerate or fail a standard amphotericin B formulation.

Related Information
Compatibility of Drugs *on page 1370*

Amphotericin B (Conventional)
(am foe TER i sin bee con VEN sha nal)

U.S. Brand Names Amphocin®
Synonyms Amphotericin B Desoxycholate
Pharmacologic Category Antifungal Agent, Parenteral
Medication Safety Issues
Safety issues:
Conventional amphotericin formulations (Amphocin®, Fungizone®) may be confused with lipid-based formulations (AmBisome®, Abelcet®, Amphotec®).
Large overdoses have occurred when conventional formulations were dispensed inadvertently for lipid-based products. Single daily doses of conventional amphotericin formulation never exceed 1.5 mg/kg.

Pregnancy Risk Factor B
Lactation Excretion in breast milk unknown/contraindicated

Use Treatment of severe systemic and central nervous system infections caused by susceptible fungi such as *Candida* species, *Histoplasma capsulatum*, *Cryptococcus neoformans*, *Aspergillus* species, *Blastomyces dermatitidis*, *Torulopsis glabrata*, and *Coccidioides immitis*; fungal peritonitis; irrigant for bladder fungal infections; used in fungal infection in patients with bone marrow transplantation, amebic meningoencephalitis, ocular aspergillosis (intraocular injection), candidal cystitis (bladder irrigation), chemoprophylaxis (low-dose I.V.), immunocompromised patients at risk of aspergillosis (intranasal/nebulized), refractory meningitis (intrathecal), coccidioidal arthritis (intra-articular/I.M.).

Low-dose amphotericin B has been administered after bone marrow transplantation to reduce the risk of invasive fungal disease.

Mechanism of Action/Effect Binds to ergosterol altering cell membrane permeability in susceptible fungi and causing leakage of cell components with subsequent cell death

Contraindications Hypersensitivity to amphotericin or any component of the formulation

Warnings/Precautions Avoid use with other nephrotoxic drugs. Monitor BUN and serum creatinine, potassium, and magnesium levels every 2-4 days, and daily in patients at risk for acute renal dysfunction. The standard dosage of lipid-based amphotericin B formulations, including amphotericin B cholesteryl sulfate (Amphotec®), amphotericin B lipid complex (Abelcet®), and liposomal amphotericin B (AmBisome®) is many fold greater than the dosage of conventional amphotericin B. To prevent inadvertent overdose, the product name and dosage must be verified for any amphotericin B dosage exceeding 1.5 mg/kg. Amphotericin B has been administered to pregnant women without obvious deleterious effects to the fetus, but the number of cases reported is small. Use during pregnancy only if absolutely necessary.

Drug Interactions
Decreased Effect: Pharmacologic antagonism may occur with azole antifungal agents (ketoconazole, miconazole).
Increased Effect/Toxicity: Use of amphotericin with other nephrotoxic drugs (eg, cyclosporine and aminoglycosides) may result in additive toxicity. Amphotericin may increase the toxicity of flucytosine. Antineoplastic agents may increase the risk of amphotericin-induced nephrotoxicity, bronchospasms, and hypotension. Corticosteroids may increase potassium depletion caused by amphotericin. Amphotericin B may predispose patients receiving digitalis glycosides or neuromuscular-blocking agents to toxicity secondary to hypokalemia.

Lab Interactions Increased BUN (S), serum creatinine, alkaline phosphate, bilirubin; decreased magnesium, potassium (S)

Adverse Reactions
>10%:
Central nervous system: Fever, chills, headache, malaise, generalized pain
Endocrine & metabolic: Hypokalemia, hypomagnesemia
Gastrointestinal: Anorexia
Hematologic: Anemia
Renal: Nephrotoxicity
1% to 10%:
Cardiovascular: Hypotension, hypertension, flushing
Central nervous system: Delirium, arachnoiditis, pain along lumbar nerves
Gastrointestinal: Nausea, vomiting
Genitourinary: Urinary retention
Hematologic: Leukocytosis
Local: Thrombophlebitis
Neuromuscular & skeletal: Paresthesia (especially with I.T. therapy)
Renal: Renal tubular acidosis, renal failure

Overdosage/Toxicology Symptoms of overdose include renal dysfunction, cardiac arrest, anemia, thrombocytopenia, granulocytopenia, fever, nausea, and vomiting. Treatment is supportive.

Pharmacodynamics/Kinetics
Time to Peak: Within 1 hour following a 4- to 6-hour dose
Protein Binding: Plasma: 90%
Half-Life Elimination: Biphasic: Initial: 15-48 hours; Terminal: 15 days
Excretion: Urine (2% to 5% as biologically active form); ~40% eliminated over a 7-day period and may be detected in urine for at least 7 weeks after discontinued use

Available Dosage Forms Injection, powder for reconstitution, as desoxycholate: 50 mg

Dosing
Adults & Elderly:
Note: **Premedication:** For patients who experience infusion-related immediate reactions, premedicate with the following drugs 30-60 minutes prior to drug
(Continued)

Amphotericin B (Conventional)
(Continued)

administration: NSAID (with or without diphenhydramine) **or** acetaminophen with diphenhydramine **or** hydrocortisone 50-100 mg. If the patient experiences rigors during the infusion, meperidine may be administered.

Test dose: I.V.: 1 mg infused over 20-30 minutes. Many clinicians believe a test dose is unnecessary.

Systemic fungal infections: I.V.: Maintenance dose: Usual: 0.25-1.5 mg/kg/day; 1-1.5 mg/kg over 4-6 hours every other day may be given once therapy is established. Aspergillosis, mucormycosis, rhinocerebral phycomycosis often require 1-1.5 mg/kg/day; do not exceed 1.5 mg/kg/day.

Duration of therapy varies with nature of infection: Usual duration is 4-12 weeks or cumulative dose of 1-4 g.

Meningitis, coccidioidal or cryptococcal: I.T.: Initial: 25-300 mcg every 48-72 hours; increase to 500 mcg to 1 mg as tolerated; maximum total dose: 15 mg has been suggested.

Cystitis (Candidal): Bladder irrigation: Irrigate with 50 mcg/mL solution instilled periodically or continuously for 5-10 days or until cultures are clear.

Bone marrow transplantation (prophylaxis): I.V.: Low-dose amphotericin B 0.1-0.25 mg/kg/day has been administered after bone marrow transplantation to reduce the risk of invasive fungal disease.

Note: Alternative routes of administration and extemporaneous preparations have been used when standard antifungal therapy is not available (eg, inhalation, intraocular injection, subconjunctival application, intracavitary administration into various joints and the pleural space).

Pediatrics:
Note: Premedication: For patients who experience infusion-related immediate reactions, premedicate with the following drugs 30-60 minutes prior to drug administration: NSAID (with or without diphenhydramine) **or** acetaminophen with diphenhydramine **or** hydrocortisone 50-100 mg. If the patient experiences rigors during the infusion, meperidine may be administered.

Test dose: I.V.: Infants and Children: 0.1 mg/kg/dose to a maximum of 1 mg; infuse over 30-60 minutes. Many clinicians believe a test dose is unnecessary.

Susceptible fungal infections: I.V.: Infants and Children: Maintenance dose: 0.25-1 mg/kg/day given once daily; infuse over 2-6 hours. Once therapy has been established, amphotericin B can be administered on an every-other-day basis at 1-1.5 mg/kg/dose; cumulative dose: 1.5-2 g over 6-10 weeks

Note: Duration of therapy varies with nature of infection: Usual duration is 4-12 weeks or cumulative dose of 1-4 g.

Meningitis, coccidioidal or cryptococcal: I.T.: Children: 25-100 mcg every 48-72 hours; increase to 500 mcg as tolerated

Renal Impairment:
If renal dysfunction is due to the drug, the daily total can be decreased by 50% or the dose can be given every other day. I.V. therapy may take several months.

Poorly dialyzed; no supplemental dose is necessary when using hemo- or peritoneal dialysis or CAVH/CAVHD.

Administration in dialysate: 1-2 mg/L of peritoneal dialysis fluid either with or without low-dose I.V. amphotericin B (a total dose of 2-10 mg/kg given over 7-14 days).

Administration
I.V.: May be infused over 4-6 hours. For a patient who experiences chills, fever, hypotension, nausea, or other nonanaphylactic infusion-related reactions,

premedicate with the following drugs 30-60 minutes prior to drug administration: A nonsteroidal (eg, ibuprofen, choline magnesium trisalicylate) with or without diphenhydramine **or** acetaminophen with diphenhydramine **or** hydrocortisone 50-100 mg. If the patient experiences rigors during the infusion, meperidine may be administered. Bolus infusion of normal saline immediately preceding, or immediately preceding and following amphotericin B may reduce drug-induced nephrotoxicity. Risk of nephrotoxicity increases with amphotericin B doses >1 mg/kg/day. Infusion of admixtures more concentrated than 0.25 mg/mL should be limited to patients absolutely requiring volume contraction.

I.V. Detail: Precipitate may form in ionic dialysate solutions.

pH: 5.7 (100 mg/L in D_5W)

Stability
Reconstitution: Add 10 mL of SWFI (without a bacteriostatic agent) to each vial of amphotericin B. Further dilute with 250-500 mL D_5W; final concentration should not exceed 0.1 mg/mL (peripheral infusion) or 0.25 mg/mL (central infusion).

Compatibility: Solution is **incompatible** with ampicillin, calcium gluconate, carbenicillin, cimetidine, dopamine, gentamicin, lidocaine, potassium chloride, sodium chloride, tetracycline, verapamil.

Storage: Store intact vials under refrigeration; protect from light. Reconstituted vials are stable, protected from light, for 24 hours at room temperature and 1 week when refrigerated. Parenteral admixtures are stable, protected from light, for 24 hours at room temperature and 2 days under refrigeration. Short-term exposure (<24 hours) to light during I.V. infusion does **not** appreciably affect potency.

Laboratory Monitoring BUN and serum creatinine levels should be determined every other day when therapy is increased and at least weekly thereafter. Monitor serum electrolytes (especially potassium and magnesium), liver function, and CBC. Perform culture and sensitivity testing prior to initiating therapy.

Nursing Actions
Physical Assessment: Culture and sensitivity and patient history of exposure to amphotericin B should be assessed prior to beginning treatment. Assess potential for interactions with other medications patient may be taking. Premedication may be ordered to reduce incidence/severity of infusion reaction. Monitor patient closely for infusion-related reactions (eg, anaphylaxis, chills, fever, nausea, vomiting, rigors, hypotension, acute respiratory distress) and facilities for cardiopulmonary resuscitation should be available. If acute respiratory distress occurs stop infusion and notify prescriber. Monitor results of laboratory tests, therapeutic effectiveness, and adverse response on a regular basis during therapy. Teach patient appropriate use, possible side effects/appropriate interventions, and adverse symptoms to report.

Patient Education: Do not take any new medication during therapy unless approved by prescriber. I.V.: You will be monitored closely during and after infusion; report immediately any pain or swelling at infusion site, chills, nausea, chest pain, swelling of face or mouth, difficulty breathing, muscle cramping, acute anxiety, or other infusion reactions. Take entire prescription, even if you are feeling better. Maintain adequate hydration (2-3 L/day of fluids) unless instructed to restrict fluid intake. May cause nausea, vomiting, or anorexia (small, frequent meals, frequent mouth care, sucking lozenges, or chewing gum may help); generalized muscle or joint pain (consult prescriber for approved analgesic); or hypotension (use caution when rising from sitting or lying position or when climbing stairs). Report severe muscle cramping or weakness; chest pain or palpitations; CNS disturbances; skin rash; change in urinary patterns or difficulty voiding; black stool; unusual bruising or bleeding; or pain, redness, or swelling at infusion site. **Breast-feeding precaution:** Do not breast-feed.

Geriatric Considerations Caution should be exercised and renal function and desired effect monitored closely in older adults.

Additional Information Premedication with diphenhydramine and acetaminophen may reduce the severity of acute infusion-related reactions. Meperidine reduces the duration of amphotericin B-induced rigors and chilling. Hydrocortisone may be used in patients with severe or refractory infusion-related reactions. Bolus infusion of normal saline immediately preceding, or immediately preceding and following amphotericin B may reduce drug-induced nephrotoxicity. Risk of nephrotoxicity increases with amphotericin B doses >1 mg/kg/day. Infusion of admixtures more concentrated than 0.25 mg/mL should be limited to patients absolutely requiring volume restriction. Amphotericin B does not have a bacteriostatic constituent, subsequently admixture expiration is determined by sterility more than chemical stability.

Related Information
Compatibility of Drugs *on page 1370*

Amphotericin B (Lipid Complex)
(am foe TER i sin bee LIP id KOM pleks)

U.S. Brand Names Abelcet®
Synonyms ABLC
Pharmacologic Category Antifungal Agent, Parenteral
Medication Safety Issues
Safety issues:
Lipid-based amphotericin formulations (Abelcet®) may be confused with conventional formulations (Amphocin®, Fungizone®)
Large overdoses have occurred when conventional formulations were dispensed inadvertently for lipid-based products. Single daily doses of conventional amphotericin formulation never exceed 1.5 mg/kg.

Pregnancy Risk Factor B
Lactation Enters breast milk/contraindicated
Use Treatment of aspergillosis or any type of progressive fungal infection in patients who are refractory to or intolerant of conventional amphotericin B therapy
Unlabeled/Investigational Use Effective in patients with serious *Candida* species infections
Mechanism of Action/Effect Mechanism is like amphotericin - includes binding to ergosterol altering cell membrane permeability in susceptible fungi and causing leakage of cell components with subsequent cell death.
Contraindications Hypersensitivity to amphotericin or any component of the formulation
Warnings/Precautions Anaphylaxis has been reported with amphotericin B-containing drugs. If severe respiratory distress occurs, the infusion should be immediately discontinued. During the initial dosing, the drug should be administered under close clinical observation. Acute reactions (including fever and chills) may occur 1-2 hours after starting an intravenous infusion. These reactions are usually more common with the first few doses and generally diminish with subsequent doses.

Drug Interactions
Decreased Effect: See Drug Interactions - Decreased Effect in Amphotericin B (Conventional).
Increased Effect/Toxicity: See Drug Interactions - Increased Effect/Toxicity in Amphotericin B (Conventional).
Lab Interactions Increased BUN (S), serum creatinine, alkaline phosphate, bilirubin; decreased magnesium, potassium (S)

Adverse Reactions Nephrotoxicity and infusion-related hyperpyrexia, rigor, and chilling are reduced relative to amphotericin deoxycholate.
>10%:
Central nervous system: Chills, fever
Renal: Serum creatinine increased
Miscellaneous: Multiple organ failure
1% to 10%:
Cardiovascular: Hypotension, cardiac arrest
Central nervous system: Headache, pain
Dermatologic: Rash
Endocrine & metabolic: Bilirubinemia, hypokalemia, acidosis
Gastrointestinal: Nausea, vomiting, diarrhea, gastrointestinal hemorrhage, abdominal pain
Renal: Renal failure
Respiratory: Respiratory failure, dyspnea, pneumonia

Pharmacodynamics/Kinetics
Half-Life Elimination: ~24 hours
Excretion: Clearance: Increases with higher doses (5 mg/kg/day): 400 mL/hour/kg

Available Dosage Forms Injection, suspension [preservative free]: 5 mg/mL (20 mL)

Dosing
Adults & Elderly:
Note: Premedication: For patients who experience infusion-related immediate reactions, premedicate with the following drugs 30-60 minutes prior to drug administration: A nonsteroidal anti-inflammatory agent ± diphenhydramine **or** acetaminophen with diphenhydramine **or** hydrocortisone 50-100 mg. If the patient experiences rigors during the infusion, meperidine may be administered.
Usual dosage: I.V.: 2.5-5 mg/kg/day as a single infusion
Pediatrics: Refer to adult dosing.
Renal Impairment: The effects of renal impairment on drug pharmacokinetics or pharmacodynamics are currently unknown. The dose of amphotericin B lipid complex may be adjusted or drug administration may have to be interrupted in patients with acute kidney dysfunction to reduce the magnitude of renal impairment.

Hemodialysis: Supplemental dose is not necessary.
Peritoneal dialysis: Supplemental dose is not necessary.
Continuous arteriovenous or venovenous hemofiltration: Supplemental dose is not necessary.

Administration
I.V.: For patients who experience nonanaphylactic infusion-related reactions, premedicate 30-60 minutes prior to drug administration with a nonsteroidal anti-inflammatory agent ± diphenhydramine **or** acetaminophen with diphenhydramine **or** hydrocortisone 50-100 mg. If the patient experiences rigors during the infusion, meperidine may be administered.
Invert infusion container several times prior to administration and every 2 hours during infusion.
I.V. Detail: Do not use an in-line filter. Flush line with dextrose; normal saline may cause precipitate.

Stability
Reconstitution: Shake vial gently to disperse yellow sediment at bottom of container. Dilute with D_5W to 1-2 mg/mL.
Compatibility: Do not admix or Y-site with any blood products, intravenous drugs, or intravenous fluids other than D_5W.
Storage: Intact vials should be stored at 2°C to 8°C (35°F to 46°F) and protected from exposure to light; do not freeze intact vials. Solutions for infusion are stable for 48 hours under refrigeration and 6 hours at room temperature.

Laboratory Monitoring BUN and serum creatinine levels should be determined every other day while therapy is increased and at least weekly thereafter. (Continued)

Amphotericin B (Lipid Complex)
(Continued)

Monitor serum electrolytes (especially potassium and magnesium), liver function, and CBC. Perform culture and sensitivity testing prior to initiating therapy.

Nursing Actions

Physical Assessment: Patient history of previous exposure to amphotericin B should be assessed before beginning treatment. Assess potential for interactions with other medications patient may be taking. Premedication may be ordered to reduce incidence/severity of infusion reaction. See Administration and Compatibility/Incompatibility prior to administering first dose. Monitor patient closely for infusion related reactions (eg, anaphylaxis, chills, fever, nausea, vomiting, rigors, hypotension, acute respiratory distress) and facilities for cardiopulmonary resuscitation should be available. If acute respiratory distress occurs, stop infusion and notify prescriber. Monitor laboratory tests, therapeutic effectiveness, and adverse response on a regular basis during therapy. Teach patient possible side effects/appropriate interventions and adverse symptoms to report.

Patient Education: Do not take any new medication during therapy unless approved by prescriber. This medication can only be administered by infusion and therapy may last several weeks. Maintain good personal hygiene to reduce spread and recurrence of lesions. Maintain adequate hydration (2-3 L/day of fluids) unless instructed to restrict fluid intake. May cause postural hypotension (use caution when changing from lying or sitting position to standing or when climbing stairs); or nausea or vomiting (small, frequent meals, frequent mouth care, sucking lozenges, or chewing gum may help). Report chest pain or palpitations; CNS disturbances; skin rash; chills or fever; persistent nausea, vomiting, or abdominal pain; sore throat; excessive fatigue; swelling of extremities or unusual weight gain; respiratory difficulty; pain at infusion site; muscle cramping or weakness; or other adverse reactions. **Breast-feeding precaution:** Do not breast-feed.

Geriatric Considerations Caution should be exercised and renal function and desired effect monitored closely in older adults.

Breast-Feeding Issues Due to limited data, consider discontinuing nursing during therapy.

Additional Information As a modification of dimyristoyl phosphatidylcholine:dimyristoyl phosphatidylglycerol 7:3 (DMPC:DMPG) liposome, amphotericin B lipid-complex has a higher drug to lipid ratio and the concentration of amphotericin B is 33 M. ABLC is a ribbon-like structure, not a liposome.

Controlled trials which compare the original formulation of amphotericin B to the newer liposomal formulations (ie, Abelcet®) are lacking. Thus, comparative data discussing differences among the formulations should be interpreted cautiously. Although the risk of nephrotoxicity and infusion-related adverse effects may be less with Abelcet®, the efficacy profiles of Abelcet® and the original amphotericin formulation are comparable. Consequently, Abelcet® should be restricted to those patients who cannot tolerate or fail a standard amphotericin B formulation.

Related Information

Compatibility of Drugs *on page 1370*

Amphotericin B (Liposomal)
(am foe TER i sin bee lye po SO mal)

U.S. Brand Names AmBisome®

Synonyms L-AmB

Pharmacologic Category Antifungal Agent, Parenteral

Medication Safety Issues

Safety issues:

Lipid-based amphotericin formulations (AmBisome®) may be confused with conventional formulations (Amphocin®, Fungizone®)

Large overdoses have occurred when conventional formulations were dispensed inadvertently for lipid-based products. Single daily doses of conventional amphotericin formulation never exceed 1.5 mg/kg.

Pregnancy Risk Factor B

Lactation Excretion in breast milk unknown/contraindicated

Use Empirical therapy for presumed fungal infection in febrile, neutropenic patients; treatment of patients with *Aspergillus* species, *Candida* species, and/or *Cryptococcus* species infections refractory to amphotericin B desoxycholate, or in patients where renal impairment or unacceptable toxicity precludes the use of amphotericin B desoxycholate; treatment of cryptococcal meningitis in HIV-infected patients; treatment of visceral leishmaniasis

Unlabeled/Investigational Use Effective in patients with serious *Candida* species infections

Mechanism of Action/Effect Amphotericin B, the active ingredient, acts by binding to the sterol component of a cell membrane leading to alterations in cell permeability and cell death. While amphotericin B has a higher affinity for the ergosterol component of the fungal cell membrane, it can also bind to the cholesterol component of the mammalian cell leading to cytotoxicity. AmBisome®, the liposomal preparation of amphotericin B, has been shown to penetrate the cell wall of both extracellular and intracellular forms of susceptible fungi.

Contraindications Hypersensitivity to amphotericin B or any component of the formulation unless, in the opinion of the treating physician, the benefit of therapy outweighs the risk

Warnings/Precautions Although amphotericin B (liposomal) has been shown to be significantly less toxic than amphotericin B desoxycholate, adverse events may still occur. Patients should be under close clinical observation during initial dosing. As with other amphotericin B-containing products, anaphylaxis has been reported. Facilities for cardiopulmonary resuscitation should be available during administration, and the drug should be administered by medically-trained personnel. Acute reactions (including fever and chills) may occur 1-2 hours after starting infusions; reactions are more common with the first few doses and generally diminish with subsequent doses. Immediately discontinue infusion if severe respiratory distress occurs; the patient should not receive further infusions. Safety and efficacy have not been established in patients <1 year of age.

Drug Interactions

Increased Effect/Toxicity: Drug interactions have not been studied in a controlled manner; however, drugs that interact with conventional amphotericin B may also interact with amphotericin B liposome for injection. See Drug Interactions - Increased Effect/Toxicity in Amphotericin B (Conventional) monograph.

Adverse Reactions Percentage of adverse reactions is dependent upon population studied and may vary with respect to premedications and underlying illness. Incidence of decreased renal function and infusion-related events are lower than rates observed with amphotericin B deoxycholate.

>10%:

Cardiovascular: Peripheral edema (15%), edema (12% to 14%), tachycardia (9% to 18%), hypotension (7% to 14%), hypertension (8% to 20%), chest pain (8% to 12%), hypervolemia (8% to 12%)

Central nervous system: Chills (29% to 48%), insomnia (17% to 22%), headache (9% to 20%), anxiety (7% to 14%), pain (14%), confusion (9% to 13%)

Dermatologic: Rash (5% to 25%), pruritus (11%)

Endocrine & metabolic: Hypokalemia (31% to 51%), hypomagnesemia (15% to 50%), hyperglycemia (8% to 23%), hypocalcemia (5% to 18%), hyponatremia (8% to 12%)

Gastrointestinal: Nausea (16% to 40%), vomiting (10% to 32%), diarrhea (11% to 30%), abdominal pain (7% to 20%), constipation (15%), anorexia (10% to 14%)

Hematologic: Anemia (27% to 48%), blood transfusion reaction (9% to 18%), leukopenia (15% to 17%), thrombocytopenia (6% to 13%)

Hepatic: Alkaline phosphatase increased (7% to 22%), BUN increased (7% to 21%), bilirubinemia (9% to 18%), ALT increased (15%), AST increased (13%), liver function tests abnormal (not specified) (4% to 13%)

Local: Phlebitis (9% to 11%)

Neuromuscular & skeletal: Weakness (6% to 13%), back pain (12%)

Renal: Creatinine increased (18% to 40%), hematuria (14%)

Respiratory: Dyspnea (18% to 23%), lung disorder (14% to 18%), cough increased (2% to 18%), epistaxis (8% to 15%), pleural effusion (12%), rhinitis (11%)

Miscellaneous: Sepsis (7% to 14%), infection (11% to 12%)

2% to 10%:

Cardiovascular: Arrhythmia, atrial fibrillation, bradycardia, cardiac arrest, cardiomegaly, facial swelling, flushing, postural hypotension, valvular heart disease, vascular disorder

Central nervous system: Agitation, abnormal thinking, coma, convulsion, depression, dysesthesia, dizziness (7% to 8%), hallucinations, malaise, nervousness, somnolence

Dermatologic: Alopecia, bruising, cellulitis, dry skin, maculopapular rash, petechia, purpura, skin discoloration, skin disorder, skin ulcer, urticaria, vesiculobullous rash

Endocrine & metabolic: Acidosis, fluid overload, hypernatremia (4%), hyperchloremia, hyperkalemia, hypermagnesemia, hyperphosphatemia, hypophosphatemia, hypoproteinemia, lactate dehydrogenase increased, nonprotein nitrogen increased

Gastrointestinal: Constipation, dry mouth, dyspepsia, abdomen enlarged, amylase increased, eructation, fecal incontinence, flatulence, gastrointestinal hemorrhage (10%), hematemesis, hemorrhoids, gum/oral hemorrhage, ileus, mucositis, rectal disorder, stomatitis, ulcerative stomatitis

Genitourinary: Vaginal hemorrhage

Hematologic: Coagulation disorder, hemorrhage, decreased prothrombin, thrombocytopenia

Hepatic: Hepatocellular damage, hepatomegaly, veno-occlusive liver disease

Local: Injection site inflammation

Neuromuscular & skeletal: Arthralgia, bone pain, dystonia, myalgia, neck pain, paresthesia, rigors, tremor

Ocular: Conjunctivitis, dry eyes, eye hemorrhage

Renal: Abnormal renal function, acute kidney failure, dysuria, kidney failure, toxic nephropathy, urinary incontinence

Respiratory: Asthma, atelectasis, cough, dry nose, hemoptysis, hyperventilation, lung edema, pharyngitis, pneumonia, respiratory alkalosis, respiratory insufficiency, respiratory failure, sinusitis, hypoxia (6% to 8%)

Miscellaneous: Allergic reaction, cell-mediated immunological reaction, flu-like syndrome, graft-versus-host disease, herpes simplex, hiccup, procedural complication (8% to 10%), diaphoresis (7%)

Overdosage/Toxicology The toxicity due to overdose has not been defined. Repeated daily doses up to 7.5 mg/kg have been administered in clinical trials with no reported dose-related toxicity. If overdosage should occur, cease administration immediately. Symptomatic supportive measures should be instituted. Particular attention should be given to monitoring renal function.

Pharmacodynamics/Kinetics

Half-Life Elimination: Terminal: 174 hours

Available Dosage Forms

Injection, powder for reconstitution:
AmBisome®: 50 mg [contains soy and sucrose]

Dosing

Adults & Elderly: Note: Premedication: For patients who experience chills, fever, hypotension, nausea, or other nonanaphylactic infusion-related immediate reactions, premedicate with the following drugs 30-60 minutes prior to drug administration: A nonsteroidal (eg, ibuprofen, choline magnesium trisalicylate) with or without diphenhydramine **or** acetaminophen with diphenhydramine **or** hydrocortisone 50-100 mg. If the patient experiences rigors during the infusion, meperidine may be administered.

Candidal infection:

Endocarditis: 3-6 mg/kg/day with flucytosine 25-37.5 mg/kg 4 times daily

Meningitis: 5 mg/kg/day with flucytosine 100 mg/kg/day

Cryptococcal meningitis (HIV-positive): 6 mg/kg/day

Note: IDSA guidelines (April, 2000) report doses of 3-6 mg/kg/day, noting that 4 mg/kg/day was effective in a small, open-label trial. The manufacturer's labeled dose of 6 mg/kg/day was approved in June, 2000.

Empiric therapy: 3 mg/kg/day

Fungal sinusitis: 5-7.5 mg/kg/day

Note: Use azole antifungal if causative organism is *Pseudallescheria boydii* (*Scedosporium* sp).

Systemic fungal infections (*Aspergillus, Candida, Cryptococcus*): 3-5 mg/kg/day

Visceral leishmaniasis:

Immunocompetent: 3 mg/kg/day on days 1-5, and 3 mg/kg/day on days 14 and 21; a repeat course may be given in patients who do not achieve parasitic clearance

Note: Alternate regimen of 2 mg/kg/day for 5 days has been reportedly effective.

Immunocompromised: 4 mg/kg/day on days 1-5, and 4 mg/kg/day on days 10, 17, 24, 31, and 38

Pediatrics: Note: Premedication: For patients who experience chills, fever, hypotension, nausea, or other nonanaphylactic infusion-related immediate reactions, premedicate with the following drugs 30-60 minutes prior to drug administration: A nonsteroidal (eg, ibuprofen, choline magnesium trisalicylate) with or without diphenhydramine **or** acetaminophen with diphenhydramine **or** hydrocortisone 50-100 mg. If the patient experiences rigors during the infusion, meperidine may be administered.

Candidal infection: I.V.: Refer to adult dosing.

Cryptococcal meningitis (HIV-positive): I.V.: Refer to adult dosing.

Empiric therapy: I.V.: Refer to adult dosing.

Systemic fungal infections (*Aspergillus, Candida, Cryptococcus*): I.V.: Refer to adult dosing.

(Continued)

Amphotericin B (Liposomal)

(Continued)

Visceral leishmaniasis: I.V.: Refer to adult dosing.

Renal Impairment:

Dosing adjustment in renal impairment: None necessary; effects of renal impairment are not currently known.

Hemodialysis: Supplemental dose is not necessary.

Peritoneal dialysis effects: Supplemental dose is not necessary.

Continuous arteriovenous or venovenous hemofiltration: Supplemental dose is not necessary.

Administration

I.V.: Should be administered by intravenous infusion, using a controlled infusion device, over a period of approximately 2 hours. Infusion time may be reduced to approximately 1 hour in patients in whom the treatment is well-tolerated. If the patient experiences discomfort during infusion, the duration of infusion may be increased. Administer at a rate of 2.5 mg/kg/hour. Discontinue if severe respiratory distress occurs.

For a patient who experiences chills, fever, hypotension, nausea, or other nonanaphylactic infusion-related reactions, premedicate with the following drugs, 30-60 minutes prior to drug administration: A nonsteroidal (eg, ibuprofen, choline magnesium trisalicylate) with or without diphenhydramine **or** acetaminophen with diphenhydramine **or** hydrocortisone 50-100 mg. If the patient experiences rigors during the infusion, meperidine may be administered.

I.V. Detail: Existing intravenous line should be flushed with D$_5$W prior to infusion (if not feasible, administer through a separate line). An in-line membrane filter (not less than 1 micron) may be used.

Stability

Reconstitution: Must be reconstituted using sterile water for injection, USP (without a bacteriostatic agent). Vials containing 50 mg of amphotericin B are prepared as follows:

1. Aseptically add 12 mL of sterile water for injection, USP to each vial to yield a preparation containing 4 mg amphotericin B/mL. **Caution:** Do not reconstitute with saline or add saline to the reconstituted concentration, or mix with other drugs. The use of any solution other than those recommended, or the presence of a bacteriostatic agent in the solution, may cause precipitation.

2. Immediately after the addition of water, **shake the vial vigorously** for 30 seconds to completely disperse the powder; it then forms a yellow, translucent suspension. Visually inspect the vial for particulate matter and continue shaking until completely dispersed.

Filtration and Dilution:

3. Calculate the amount of reconstituted (4 mg/mL) to be further diluted.

4. Withdraw this amount of reconstituted powder into a sterile syringe.

5. Attach the 5-micron filter, provided, to the syringe. Inject the syringe contents through the filter, into the appropriate amount of 5% dextrose injection. (Use only one filter per vial.)

6. Must be diluted with 5% dextrose injection to a final concentration of 1-2 mg/mL prior to administration. Lower concentrations (0.2-0.5 mg/mL) may be appropriate for infants and small children to provide sufficient volume for infusion. **Discard partially used vials.** Injection should commence within 6 hours of dilution with 5% dextrose injection. An in-line membrane filter may be used for the intravenous infusion, provided, **the mean pore diameter of the filter is not less than 1 micron.**

Storage: Unopened vials should be stored at temperatures ≤25°C (77°F).

Laboratory Monitoring BUN and serum creatinine levels should be determined every other day while therapy is increased and at least weekly thereafter. Serum potassium and magnesium should be monitored closely. Monitor electrolytes, liver function, hematocrit, and CBC regularly.

Nursing Actions

Physical Assessment: Patient history of previous exposure to amphotericin B should be assessed before beginning treatment. Assess potential for interactions with medications patient may be taking. Premedication may be ordered to reduce incidence/severity of infusion reaction. See Administration and Compatibility/Incompatibility prior to administering first dose. Monitor patient closely for infusion related reactions (eg, anaphylaxis, chills, fever, nausea, vomiting, rigors, hypotension, acute respiratory distress) and facilities for cardiopulmonary resuscitation should be available. If acute respiratory distress occurs, stop infusion and notify prescriber. Monitor laboratory tests, therapeutic effectiveness, and adverse response on a regular basis during therapy. Teach patient interventions to reduce side effects, and adverse symptoms to report.

Patient Education: Do not take any new medication during therapy unless approved by prescriber. This medication can only be administered by infusion and therapy may last several weeks. You will be monitored closely during and after infusion; report immediately any pain or swelling at infusion site, chills, nausea, chest pain, swelling of face or mouth, difficulty breathing, muscle cramping, acute anxiety, or other infusion reactions. Maintain adequate hydration (2-3 L/day of fluids) unless instructed to restrict fluid intake. May cause postural hypotension (use caution when changing from lying or sitting position to standing or when climbing stairs); or nausea or vomiting (small, frequent meals, frequent mouth care, sucking lozenges, or chewing gum may help). Report chest pain or palpitations, CNS disturbances, skin rash, unusual chills or fever, persistent nausea, vomiting, abdominal pain, sore throat, excessive fatigue, swelling of extremities, unusual weight gain, difficulty breathing, pain at infusion site, muscle cramping or weakness, or other adverse reactions. **Breast-feeding precaution:** Do not breast-feed.

Additional Information Amphotericin B (liposomal) is a true single bilayer liposomal drug delivery system. Liposomes are closed, spherical vesicles created by mixing specific proportions of amphiphilic substances such as phospholipids and cholesterol so that they arrange themselves into multiple concentric bilayer membranes when hydrated in aqueous solutions. Single bilayer liposomes are then formed by microemulsification of multilamellar vesicles using a homogenizer. Amphotericin B (liposomal) consists of these unilamellar bilayer liposomes with amphotericin B intercalated within the membrane. Due to the nature and quantity of amphiphilic substances used, and the lipophilic moiety in the amphotericin B molecule, the drug is an integral part of the overall structure of the amphotericin B liposomal liposomes. Amphotericin B (liposomal) contains true liposomes that are <100 nm in diameter.

Ampicillin (am pi SIL in)

U.S. Brand Names Principen®

Synonyms Aminobenzylpenicillin; Ampicillin Sodium; Ampicillin Trihydrate

Pharmacologic Category Antibiotic, Penicillin

Medication Safety Issues
Sound-alike/look-alike issues:
Ampicillin may be confused with aminophylline

Pregnancy Risk Factor B

Lactation Enters breast milk/use caution

Use Treatment of susceptible bacterial infections (nonbeta-lactamase-producing organisms); susceptible bacterial infections caused by streptococci, pneumococci, nonpenicillinase-producing staphylococci, *Listeria*, meningococci; some strains of *H. influenzae*, *Salmonella*, *Shigella*, *E. coli*, *Enterobacter*, and *Klebsiella*

Mechanism of Action/Effect Interferes with bacterial cell wall synthesis during active multiplication, causing cell wall death and resultant bactericidal activity against susceptible bacteria

Contraindications Hypersensitivity to ampicillin, any component of the formulation, or other penicillins

Warnings/Precautions Dosage adjustment may be necessary in patients with renal impairment. A low incidence of cross-allergy with other beta-lactams exists. High percentage of patients with infectious mononucleosis have developed rash during therapy with ampicillin. Appearance of a rash should be carefully evaluated to differentiate a nonallergic ampicillin rash from a hypersensitivity reaction. Ampicillin rash is a generalized dull red, maculopapular rash, generally appearing 3-14 days after the start of therapy. It normally begins on the trunk and spreads over most of the body. It may be most intense at pressure areas, elbows, and knees.

Drug Interactions

Decreased Effect: Although anecdotal reports suggest oral contraceptive efficacy could be reduced by penicillins, this has been refuted by more rigorous scientific and clinical data.

Increased Effect/Toxicity: Ampicillin increases the effect of disulfiram and anticoagulants. Probenecid may increase penicillin levels. Theoretically, allopurinol taken with ampicillin has an additive potential for rash. Penicillins may increase the exposure to methotrexate during concurrent therapy; monitor.

Nutritional/Ethanol Interactions Food: Food decreases ampicillin absorption rate; may decrease ampicillin serum concentration.

Lab Interactions Increased protein, positive Coombs' [direct]; alters result of urinary glucose (Benedict's solution, Clinitest®)
Some penicillin derivatives may accelerate the degradation of aminoglycosides *in vitro*, leading to a potential underestimation of aminoglycoside serum concentration.

Adverse Reactions Frequency not defined.
Central nervous system: Fever, penicillin encephalopathy, seizure
Dermatologic: Erythema multiforme, exfoliative dermatitis, rash, urticaria
Note: Appearance of a rash should be carefully evaluated to differentiate (if possible) nonallergic ampicillin rash from hypersensitivity reaction. Incidence is higher in patients with viral infection, *Salmonella* infection, lymphocytic leukemia, or patients that have hyperuricemia.
Gastrointestinal: Black hairy tongue, diarrhea, enterocolitis, glossitis, nausea, pseudomembranous colitis, sore mouth or tongue, stomatitis, vomiting
Hematologic: Agranulocytosis, anemia, hemolytic anemia, eosinophilia, leukopenia, thrombocytopenia purpura
Hepatic: AST increased

Renal: Interstitial nephritis (rare)
Respiratory: Laryngeal stridor
Miscellaneous: Anaphylaxis, serum sickness-like reaction

Overdosage/Toxicology Symptoms of penicillin overdose include neuromuscular hypersensitivity (eg, agitation, hallucinations, asterixis, encephalopathy, confusion, and seizures). Electrolyte imbalance may occur if the preparation contains potassium or sodium salts, especially in renal failure. Hemodialysis may be helpful to aid in removal of the drug from blood; otherwise, treatment is supportive or symptom-directed.

Pharmacodynamics/Kinetics
Time to Peak: Oral: Within 1-2 hours
Protein Binding: 15% to 25%
Half-Life Elimination:
Children and Adults: 1-1.8 hours
Anuria/end-stage renal disease: 7-20 hours
Excretion: Urine (~90% as unchanged drug) within 24 hours

Available Dosage Forms
Capsule (Principen®): 250 mg, 500 mg
Injection, powder for reconstitution, as sodium: 125 mg, 250 mg, 500 mg, 1 g, 2 g, 10 g
Powder for oral suspension (Principen®): 125 mg/5 mL (100 mL, 200 mL); 250 mg/5 mL (100 mL, 200 mL)

Dosing
Adults:
Usual dosage range:
Oral: 250-500 mg every 6 hours
I.M., I.V.: 250-500 mg every 6 hours
Actinomycosis: I.V.: 50 mg/kg/day for 4-6 weeks then oral amoxicillin
Cholangitis (acute): I.V.: 2 g every 4 hours with gentamicin
Diverticulitis: I.M., I.V.: 2 g every 6 hours with metronidazole
Endocarditis:
Infective: I.V.: 12 g/day via continuous infusion or divided every 4 hours
Prophylaxis: Dental, oral, respiratory tract, or esophageal procedures: I.M., I.V.: 2 g within 30 minutes prior to procedure in patients unable to take oral amoxicillin
Genitourinary and gastrointestinal tract (except esophageal) procedures: I.M., I.V.:
High-risk patients: 2 g within 30 minutes prior to procedure, followed by ampicillin 1 g (or amoxicillin 1g orally) 6 hours later; must be used in combination with gentamicin.
Moderate-risk patients: 2 g within 30 minutes prior to procedure
Group B strep prophylaxis (intrapartum): I.V.: 2 g initial dose, then 1 g every 4 hours until delivery
Listeria infections: I.V.: 200 mg/kg/day divided every 6 hours
Sepsis/meningitis: I.M., I.V.: 150-250 mg/kg/day divided every 3-4 hours (range: 6-12 g/day)
Urinary tract infections (enterococcus suspected): I.V.: 1-2 g every 6 hours with gentamicin
Elderly: Administer usual adult dose unless renal function is markedly reduced.
Pediatrics:
Endocarditis prophylaxis: Infants and Children: I.M., I.V.:
Dental, oral, respiratory tract, or esophageal procedures: 50 mg/kg within 30 minutes prior to procedure in patients unable to take oral amoxicillin
Genitourinary and gastrointestinal tract (except esophageal) procedures:
High-risk patients: 50 mg/kg (maximum: 2 g) within 30 minutes prior to procedure, followed by ampicillin 25 mg/kg (or amoxicillin 25 mg/kg orally) 6 hours later; must be used in combination with gentamicin.

(Continued)

Ampicillin *(Continued)*

Moderate-risk patients: 50 mg/kg within 30 minutes prior to procedure.

Mild-to-moderate infections: Infants and Children:
Oral: 50-100 mg/kg/day in doses divided every 6 hours (maximum: 2-4 g/day)

I.M., I.V.: 100-150 mg/kg/day in divided doses every 6 hours (maximum: 2-4 g/day)

Severe infections/meningitis: Infants and Children:
I.M., I.V.: 200-400 mg/kg/day in divided doses every 6 hours (maximum: 6-12 g/day)

Renal Impairment:

Cl_{cr} >50 mL/minute: Administer every 6 hours

Cl_{cr} 10-50 mL/minute: Administer every 6-12 hours

Cl_{cr} <10 mL/minute: Administer every 12-24 hours

Hemodialysis: Moderately dializable (20% to 50%); administer dose after dialysis

Peritoneal dialysis: Moderately dializable (20% to 50%)

Administer 250 mg every 12 hours

Continuous arteriovenous or venovenous hemofiltration effects: Dose as for Cl_{cr} 10-50 mL/minute; ~50 mg of ampicillin per liter of filtrate is removed

Administration

Oral: Administer around-the-clock to promote less variation in peak and trough serum levels. Administer on an empty stomach (ie, 1 hour prior to, or 2 hours after meals) to increase total absorption.

I.V.: Administer around-the-clock to promote less variation in peak and trough serum levels. Administer over 3-5 minutes (125-500 mg) or over 10-15 minutes (1-2 g). More rapid infusion may cause seizures. Ampicillin and gentamicin should not be mixed in the same I.V. tubing.

Some penicillins (eg, carbenicillin, ticarcillin, and piperacillin) have been shown to inactivate aminoglycosides *in vitro.* This has been observed to a greater extent with tobramycin and gentamicin, while amikacin has shown greater stability against inactivation. Concurrent use of these agents may pose a risk of reduced antibacterial efficacy *in vivo,* particularly in the setting of profound renal impairment. However, definitive clinical evidence is lacking. If combination penicillin/aminoglycoside therapy is desired in a patient with renal dysfunction, separation of doses (if feasible), and routine monitoring of aminoglycoside levels, CBC, and clinical response should be considered.

I.V. Detail: pH: 8-10 (reconstituted solution)

Stability

Reconstitution: I.V.: Minimum volume: Concentration should not exceed 30 mg/mL due to concentration-dependent stability restrictions. Standard diluent: 500 mg/50 mL NS; 1 g/50 mL NS; 2 g/100 mL NS

Compatibility: Incompatible with D_5W, D_5NS, $D_{10}W$, fat emulsion 10%, hetastarch 6%, LR

Y-site administration: Incompatible with amphotericin B cholesteryl sulfate complex, epinephrine, fluconazole, hydralazine, midazolam, ondansetron, sargramostim, verapamil, vinorelbine

Compatibility in syringe: Incompatible with erythromycin lactobionate, gentamicin, hydromorphone, kanamycin, lincomycin, metoclopramide

Compatibility when admixed: Incompatible with amikacin, chlorpromazine, dopamine, gentamicin, hydralazine, prochlorperazine

Storage:

Oral: Oral suspension is stable for 7 days at room temperature or for 14 days under refrigeration.

I.V.: Solutions for I.M. or direct I.V. should be used within 1 hour. Solutions for I.V. infusion will be inactivated by dextrose at room temperature. If dextrose-containing solutions are to be used, the resultant solution will only be stable for 2 hours versus 8 hours in the 0.9% sodium chloride injection. D_5W has limited stability.

Stability of parenteral admixture in NS at room temperature (25°C) is 8 hours.

Stability of parenteral admixture in NS at refrigeration temperature (4°C) is 2 days.

Laboratory Monitoring Perform culture and sensitivity testing prior to initiating therapy.

Nursing Actions

Physical Assessment: Allergy history should be assessed prior to starting therapy. Assess potential for interactions with other medications patient may be taking. Advise patients with diabetes about use of Clinitest®. Monitor therapeutic effectiveness and adverse reactions (eg, opportunistic infection [fever, chills, unhealed sores, white plaques in mouth or vagina, purulent vaginal discharge, fatigue]). Teach patient proper use, possible side effects/appropriate interventions, and adverse symptoms to report.

Patient Education: Do not take any new medication during therapy unless approved by prescriber. Take entire prescription, even if you are feeling better. Take at equal intervals around-the-clock; preferably on an empty stomach with a full glass of water (1 hour before or 2 hours after meals). Maintain adequate hydration (2-3 L/day of fluids) unless instructed to restrict fluid intake. If you have diabetes, drug may cause false test results with Clinitest® urine glucose monitoring; use of another type of glucose monitoring is preferable. May cause nausea or vomiting (small, frequent meals, frequent mouth care, sucking lozenges, or chewing gum may help); or diarrhea (buttermilk, boiled milk, or yogurt may help). Report immediately any rash; swelling of face, tongue, mouth, or throat; or chest tightness. Report if condition being treated worsens or does not improve by the time prescription is completed.

Dietary Considerations Take on an empty stomach 1 hour before or 2 hours after meals.

Sodium content of 5 mL suspension (250 mg/5 mL): 10 mg (0.4 mEq)

Sodium content of 1 g: 66.7 mg (3 mEq)

Geriatric Considerations See Drug Interactions and Renal Impairment. Adjust dose for renal impairment.

Related Information

Compatibility of Drugs *on page 1370*

Ampicillin and Sulbactam
(am pi SIL in & SUL bak tam)

U.S. Brand Names Unasyn®

Synonyms Sulbactam and Ampicillin

Pharmacologic Category Antibiotic, Penicillin

Pregnancy Risk Factor B

Lactation Enters breast milk/use caution

Use Treatment of susceptible bacterial infections involved with skin and skin structure, intra-abdominal infections, gynecological infections; spectrum is that of ampicillin plus organisms producing beta-lactamases such as *S. aureus, H. influenzae, E. coli, Klebsiella, Acinetobacter, Enterobacter,* and anaerobes

Mechanism of Action/Effect Interferes with bacterial cell wall synthesis during active multiplication, causing cell wall death and resultant bactericidal activity against susceptible bacteria. The addition of sulbactam, a beta-lactamase inhibitor, to ampicillin extends the spectrum of ampicillin to include beta-lactamase-producing organisms.

Contraindications Hypersensitivity to ampicillin, sulbactam, penicillins, or any component of the formulations

Warnings/Precautions Dosage adjustment may be necessary in patients with renal impairment. A low incidence of cross-allergy with other beta-lactams exists. A high percentage of patients with infectious mononucleosis have developed rash during therapy with ampicillin.

Appearance of a rash should be carefully evaluated to differentiate a nonallergic ampicillin rash from a hypersensitivity reaction.

Drug Interactions

Decreased Effect: Although anecdotal reports suggest oral contraceptive efficacy could be reduced by penicillins, this has been refuted by more rigorous scientific and clinical data.

Increased Effect/Toxicity: Disulfiram or probenecid can increase ampicillin levels. Theoretically, allopurinol taken with ampicillin has an additive potential for rash. Penicillins may increase the exposure to methotrexate during concurrent therapy; monitor.

Lab Interactions False-positive urinary glucose levels (Benedict's solution, Clinitest®); may cause temporary decreases in serum estrogens in pregnant women.

Some penicillin derivatives may accelerate the degradation of aminoglycosides in vitro, leading to a potential underestimation of aminoglycoside serum concentration.

Adverse Reactions Also see Ampicillin.

>10%: Local: Pain at injection site (I.M.)

1% to 10%:

Dermatologic: Rash

Gastrointestinal: Diarrhea

Local: Pain at injection site (I.V.), thrombophlebitis

Miscellaneous: Allergic reaction (may include serum sickness, urticaria, bronchospasm, hypotension, etc)

Overdosage/Toxicology Symptoms of penicillin overdose include neuromuscular hypersensitivity (eg, agitation, hallucinations, asterixis, encephalopathy, confusion, and seizures). Electrolyte imbalance may occur if the preparation contains potassium or sodium salts, especially in renal failure. Hemodialysis may be helpful to aid in removal of the drug from blood; otherwise, treatment is supportive or symptom-directed.

Pharmacodynamics/Kinetics

Protein Binding:

Sulbactam: 38%

Half-Life Elimination:

Sulbactam: Normal renal function: 1-1.3 hours

Excretion:

Sulbactam: Urine (~75% to 85% as unchanged drug) within 8 hours

Pharmacokinetic Note Also see Ampicillin.

Available Dosage Forms Injection, powder for reconstitution (Unasyn®): 1.5 g [ampicillin sodium 1 g and sulbactam sodium 0.5 g]; 3 g [ampicillin sodium 2 g and sulbactam sodium 1 g]; 15 g [ampicillin sodium 10 g and sulbactam sodium 5 g] [bulk package]

Dosing

Adults & Elderly: Doses expressed as ampicillin/ sulbactam combination.

Susceptible infections: I.M., I.V.: 1.5-3 g every 6 hours (maximum: Unasyn® 12 g)

Amnionitis, cholangitis, diverticulitis, endometritis, endophthalmitis, epididymitis/orchitis, liver abscess, osteomyelitis (diabetic foot), peritonitis: I.V.: 3 g every 6 hours

Endocarditis: I.V.: 3 g every 6 hours with gentamicin or vancomycin for 4-6 weeks

Orbital cellulitis: I.V.: 1.5 g every 6 hours

Parapharyngeal space infections: I.V.: 3 g every 6 hours

Pasteurella multocida (human, canine/feline bites): I.V.: 1.5-3 g every 6 hours

Pelvic inflammatory disease: I.V.: 3 g every 6 hours with doxycycline

Peritonitis (CAPD): Intraperitoneal:

Anuric, intermittent: 3 g every 12 hours

Anuric, continuous: Loading dose: 1.5 g; maintenance dose: 150 mg

Pneumonia:

Aspiration, community-acquired: I.V.: 1.5-3 g every 6 hours

Hospital-acquired: I.V.: 3 g every 6 hours

Urinary tract infections, pyelonephritis: I.V.: 3 g every 6 hours for 14 days

Pediatrics:

Epiglottitis: Children ≥1 year: I.V.: 100-200 mg ampicillin/kg/day divided in 4 doses

Mild-to-moderate infections: Children ≥1 year: I.V.: 100-200 mg ampicillin/kg/day (150-300 mg Unasyn®) divided every 6 hours (maximum: 8 g ampicillin/day, 12 g Unasyn®)

Peritonsillar and retropharyngeal abscess: Children ≥1 year: I.V.: 50 mg ampicillin/kg/dose every 6 hours

Severe infections: Children ≥1 year: I.M., I.V.: 200-400 mg ampicillin/kg/day divided every 6 hours (maximum: 8 g ampicillin/day, 12 g Unasyn®)

Note: The American Academy of Pediatrics recommends a dose of up to 300 mg/kg/day for severe infection in infants >1 month of age.

Renal Impairment:

Cl$_{cr}$ 15-29 mL/minute: Administer every 12 hours

Cl$_{cr}$ 5-14 mL/minute: Administer every 24 hours

Administration

I.V.: Administer around-the-clock to promote less variation in peak and trough serum levels. Administer by slow injection over 10-15 minutes or I.V. over 15-30 minutes. Ampicillin and gentamicin should not be mixed in the same I.V. tubing.

Some penicillins (eg, carbenicillin, ticarcillin, and piperacillin) have been shown to inactivate aminoglycosides in vitro. This has been observed to a greater extent with tobramycin and gentamicin, while amikacin has shown greater stability against inactivation. Concurrent use of these agents may pose a risk of reduced antibacterial efficacy in vivo, particularly in the setting of profound renal impairment. However, definitive clinical evidence is lacking. If combination penicillin/aminoglycoside therapy is desired in a patient with renal dysfunction, separation of doses (if feasible), and routine monitoring of aminoglycoside levels, CBC, and clinical response should be considered.

I.V. Detail: pH: 8-10

Stability

Reconstitution: I.M. and direct I.V. administration: Use within 1 hour after preparation. Reconstitute with sterile water for injection or 0.5% or 2% lidocaine hydrochloride injection (I.M.). Sodium chloride 0.9% (NS) is the diluent of choice for I.V. piggyback use.

Compatibility: Stable in NS

Y-site administration: Incompatible with aminoglycosides (eg, gentamicin, tobramycin), amphotericin B cholesteryl sulfate complex, ciprofloxacin, idarubicin, ondansetron, sargramostim

Compatibility when admixed: Incompatible with aminoglycosides

Storage: Prior to reconstitution, store at ≤30°C (86°F). Solutions made in NS are stable up to 72 hours when refrigerated whereas dextrose solutions (same concentration) are stable for only 4 hours.

Laboratory Monitoring Hematologic, renal, and hepatic function with prolonged therapy. Perform culture and sensitivity testing prior to initiating therapy.

Nursing Actions

Physical Assessment: Assess for allergy history prior to starting therapy. Assess potential for interactions with other prescriptions, OTC medications, or herbal products patient may be taking. Advise patients with diabetes about use of Clinitest®. Monitor laboratory tests and patient response (eg, opportunistic infection [fever, chills, unhealed sores, white plaques in mouth or vagina, purulent vaginal discharge, fatigue]). Teach possible side effects/ appropriate interventions and adverse symptoms to report.

(Continued)

Ampicillin and Sulbactam *(Continued)*

Patient Education: Do not take any new medication during therapy unless approved by prescriber. This medication is administered by infusion/injection. Report immediately pain, redness, swelling, or burning at injection/infusion site or feelings of acute anxiety, chest tightness, or difficulty swallowing. Maintain adequate hydration (2-3 L/day of fluids) unless instructed to restrict fluid intake. If you have diabetes, drug may cause false test results with Clinitest® urine glucose monitoring; use of another type of glucose monitoring is preferable. May cause diarrhea (if persistent, consult prescriber for approved medication). Report rash or opportunistic infection (eg, fever, chills, unhealed sores, white plaques in mouth or vagina, purulent vaginal discharge, fatigue). **Breast-feeding precaution:** Consult prescriber if breast-feeding.

Dietary Considerations Sodium content of 1.5 g injection: 115 mg (5 mEq)

Geriatric Considerations Adjust dose for renal function.

Related Information
Ampicillin *on page 93*

Amprenavir *(am PREN a veer)*

U.S. Brand Names Agenerase®

Pharmacologic Category Antiretroviral Agent, Protease Inhibitor

Pregnancy Risk Factor C

Lactation Excretion in breast milk unknown/contraindicated

Use Treatment of HIV infections in combination with at least two other antiretroviral agents; oral solution should only be used when capsules or other protease inhibitors are not therapeutic options

Mechanism of Action/Effect Binds to the protease activity site and inhibits the activity of the enzyme. HIV protease is required for the cleavage of viral polyprotein precursors into individual functional proteins found in infectious HIV. Inhibition prevents cleavage of these polyproteins, resulting in the formation of immature, noninfectious viral particles.

Contraindications Hypersensitivity to amprenavir or any component of the formulation; concurrent therapy with cisapride, ergot derivatives, midazolam, pimozide, and triazolam; severe previous allergic reaction to sulfonamides; oral solution is contraindicated in infants or children <4 years of age, pregnant women, patients with renal or hepatic failure, and patients receiving concurrent metronidazole or disulfiram

Warnings/Precautions Because of hepatic metabolism and effect on cytochrome P450 enzymes, amprenavir should be used with caution in combination with other agents metabolized by this system (see Contraindications and Drug Interactions). Avoid use of lovastatin and simvastatin (risk of rhabdomyolysis increases). Avoid concurrent use of hormonal contraceptives, rifampin, and/or St John's wort (may lead to loss of virologic response and/or resistance). New onset or worsening diabetes mellitus and hyperglycemia have been reported, including cases of diabetic ketoacidosis; use with caution in patients with impaired glucose control. Use with caution in patients with sulfonamide allergy, hepatic impairment, or hemophilia. Redistribution of fat may occur (eg, buffalo hump, peripheral wasting, cushingoid appearance). Immune reconstitution syndrome may develop resulting in the occurrence of an inflammatory response to an indolent or residual opportunistic infection; further evaluation and treatment may be required.

Amprenavir formulations contain vitamin E; additional vitamin E supplements should be avoided. Certain ethnic populations (Asians, Eskimos, Native Americans) may be at increased risk of propylene glycol-associated adverse effects; therefore, use of the oral solution of amprenavir should be avoided. Use oral solution only when capsules or other protease inhibitors are not options. Safety and efficacy in children <4 years of age have not been established.

Drug Interactions
Cytochrome P450 Effect: Substrate of CYP2C8/9 (minor), 3A4 (major); **Inhibits** CYP2C19 (weak), 3A4 (strong)

Decreased Effect: Serum concentrations of estrogen (oral contraceptives) may be decreased, use alternative (nonhormonal) forms of contraception. Serum concentrations of delavirdine may be decreased; may lead to loss of virologic response and possible resistance to delavirdine; concomitant use is not recommended. Efavirenz and nevirapine may decrease serum concentrations of amprenavir (dosing for combinations not established). Avoid St John's wort (may lead to subtherapeutic concentrations of amprenavir). Effect of amprenavir may be diminished when administered with methadone (consider alternative antiretroviral); in addition, effect of methadone may be reduced (dosage increase may be required). The levels/effects of amprenavir may be decreased by include aminoglutethimide, carbamazepine, nafcillin, nevirapine, phenobarbital, phenytoin, rifamycins, and other CYP3A4 inducers. The administration of antacids and didanosine (buffered formulation) should be separated from amprenavir by 1 hour to limit interaction between formulations.

Increased Effect/Toxicity: Concurrent use of cisapride, midazolam, pimozide, quinidine, or triazolam is contraindicated. Concurrent use of ergot alkaloids (dihydroergotamine, ergotamine, ergonovine, methylergonovine) with amprenavir is also contraindicated (may cause vasospasm and peripheral ischemia). Concurrent use of oral solution with disulfiram or metronidazole is contraindicated, due to the risk of propylene glycol toxicity.

Serum concentrations of amiodarone, bepridil, lidocaine, quinidine, and other antiarrhythmics may be increased, potentially leading to toxicity; when amprenavir is coadministered with ritonavir, flecainide and propafenone are contraindicated. HMG-CoA reductase inhibitors serum concentrations may be increased by amprenavir, increasing the risk of myopathy/rhabdomyolysis; lovastatin and simvastatin are not recommended; fluvastatin and pravastatin may be safer alternatives.

Amprenavir may increase the levels/effects of selected benzodiazepines (midazolam and triazolam are contraindicated), calcium channel blockers, cyclosporine, mirtazapine, nateglinide, nefazodone, quinidine, sildenafil (and other PDE-5 inhibitors), tacrolimus, venlafaxine, and other CYP3A4 substrates. Amprenavir may increase the levels/effects of trazodone (monitor for signs of hypotension/syncope); reduce dose of trazodone. When used with strong CYP3A4 inhibitors, dosage adjustment/limits are recommended for sildenafil and other PDE-5 inhibitors; refer to individual monographs. Amprenavir may increase the levels/effects of inhaled corticosteroids; monitor for adrenal suppression, Cushing's syndrome; concomitant use of fluticasone with amprenavir/ritonavir is not recommended.

Concurrent therapy with ritonavir may result in increased serum concentrations: dosage adjustment is recommended; avoid concurrent use of amprenavir and ritonavir oral solutions due to metabolic competition between formulation components. Clarithromycin, indinavir, nelfinavir may increase serum concentrations of amprenavir.

Nutritional/Ethanol Interactions
Ethanol: Avoid ethanol with amprenavir oral solution.
Food: Levels increased sixfold with high-fat meals.
Herb/Nutraceutical: Amprenavir serum concentration may be decreased by St John's wort; avoid concurrent use. Formulations contain vitamin E; avoid additional supplements.

Adverse Reactions
>10%:
Central nervous system: Depression/mood disorder (9% to 16%), paresthesia (peripheral 10% to 14%)
Dermatologic: Rash (20% to 27%)
Endocrine & metabolic: Hyperglycemia (>160 mg/dL: 37% to 41%), hypertriglyceridemia (>399 mg/dL: 36% to 47%; >750 mg/dL: 8% to 13%)
Gastrointestinal: Nausea (43% to 74%), vomiting (24% to 34%), diarrhea (39% to 60%), abdominal symptoms
Miscellaneous: Perioral tingling/numbness (26% to 31%)

1% to 10%:
Central nervous system: Headache, fatigue
Dermatologic: Stevens-Johnson syndrome (1% of total, 4% of patients who develop a rash)
Endocrine & metabolic: Hypercholesterolemia (>260 mg/dL: 4% to 9%), hyperglycemia (>251 mg/dL: 2% to 3%), fat redistribution
Gastrointestinal: Taste disorders (2% to 10%), amylase increased (3% to 4%)
Hepatic: AST increased (3% to 5%), ALT increased (4%)

Overdosage/Toxicology Monitor for signs and symptoms of propylene glycol toxicity if the oral solution is administered.

Pharmacodynamics/Kinetics
Time to Peak: 1-2 hours
Protein Binding: 90%
Half-Life Elimination: 7.1-10.6 hours
Metabolism: Hepatic via CYP (primarily CYP3A4)
Excretion: Feces (75%, ~68% as metabolites); urine (14% as metabolites)

Available Dosage Forms
Capsule: 50 mg [contains vitamin E 36.3 int. units (as TPGS)]
Solution, oral [use only when there are no other options]: 15 mg/mL (240 mL) [contains propylene glycol 550 mg/mL and vitamin E 46 int. units/mL; grape-bubble gum-peppermint flavor]

Dosing
Adults & Elderly: Note: Capsule and oral solution are not interchangeable on a mg-per-mg basis.
HIV infection: Oral:
Capsule:
<50 kg: 20 mg/kg twice daily (maximum: 2400 mg/day)
≥50 kg: 1200 mg twice daily
Dosage adjustments for amprenavir when administered in combination therapy:
Efavirenz: Adjustments necessary for both agents:
Amprenavir 1200 mg 3 times/day (single protease inhibitor) **or**
Amprenavir 1200 mg twice daily plus ritonavir 200 mg twice daily
Ritonavir: Adjustments necessary for both agents:
Amprenavir 1200 mg plus ritonavir 200 mg once daily **or**
Amprenavir 600 mg plus ritonavir 100 mg twice daily
Note: Oral solution of ritonavir and amprenavir should not be coadministered.
Solution:
<50 kg: 22.5 mg/kg (maximum: 2800 mg/day)

≥50 kg: 1400 mg twice daily
Pediatrics: Note: Capsule and oral solution are **not** interchangeable on a mg-per-mg basis.
HIV infection: Oral:
Capsule:
Children 4-12 years **or** 13-16 years (<50 kg): 20 mg/kg twice daily or 15 mg/kg 3 times daily; maximum: 2400 mg/day
Children >13 years (≥50 kg): 1200 mg twice daily
Solution:
Children 4-12 years **or** 13-16 years (<50 kg): 22.5 mg/kg twice daily or 17 mg/kg 3 times daily; maximum: 2800 mg/day
Children >13 years (≥50 kg): 1400 mg twice daily
Renal Impairment: Oral solution is contraindicated in renal failure.
Hepatic Impairment:
Child-Pugh score between 5-8:
Capsule: 450 mg twice daily
Solution: 513 mg twice daily; contraindicated in hepatic failure.
Child-Pugh score between 9-12:
Capsule: 300 mg twice daily
Solution: 342 mg twice daily; contraindicated in hepatic failure.

Laboratory Monitoring Viral load

Nursing Actions

Physical Assessment: Assess potential for interactions with other pharmacological agents and herbal products patient may be taking. A list of medications that should not be used is available in each bottle and patients should be provided with this information. Monitor laboratory tests, patient response, and adverse reactions (eg, gastrointestinal disturbance, nausea, vomiting, diarrhea that can lead to dehydration and weight loss; hyperlipidemia and redistribution of body fat; rash; CNS effects, malaise, insomnia, abnormal thinking; electrolyte imbalance) at regular intervals during therapy. Teach patient proper use (eg, timing of multiple medications and drugs that should not be used concurrently), possible side effects/appropriate interventions (eg, glucose testing; protease inhibitors may cause hyperglycemia, exacerbation, or new-onset diabetes; use of barrier contraceptives, protease inhibitors may decrease effectiveness of oral contraceptives), and adverse symptoms to report.

Patient Education: You will be provided with a list of specific medications that should not be used during therapy; do not take any new prescriptions, over-the-counter medications, or herbal products (even if they are not on the list) without consulting prescriber. This drug will not cure HIV, nor has it been found to reduce transmission of HIV; use appropriate precautions to prevent spread to other persons. This drug is prescribed as one part of a multidrug combination; take exactly as directed for full course of therapy. May take with light meal (eg, dry toast, skim milk, corn flakes) to reduce GI upset. Maintain adequate hydration (2-3 L/day of fluids) unless advised by prescriber to restrict fluids. Do not take antacids within one hour of this medication. You may be susceptible to infection; avoid crowds and exposure to known infections and do not have any vaccinations without consulting prescriber. Frequent blood tests may be required with prolonged therapy. You may be advised to check your glucose levels; medication can cause hyperglycemia. May cause body changes due to redistribution of body fat, facial atrophy, or breast enlargement (normal effects of drug); nausea or vomiting (small frequent meals, frequent mouth care, chewing gum, or sucking lozenges may help); muscle weakness or flank pain (consult prescriber for approved analgesic); headache or insomnia (consult prescriber for medication); or diarrhea (boiled milk, buttermilk, or yogurt may help). Inform prescriber if you experience muscle numbness (Continued)

Amprenavir *(Continued)*

or tingling; unresolved persistent vomiting, diarrhea, or abdominal pain; respiratory difficulty or chest pain; unusual skin rash; unusual depression; change in color of stool or urine; or any persistent adverse effects. **Pregnancy/breast-feeding precautions:**Inform prescriber if you are pregnant. This drug decreases the effect of oral contraceptives; use of alternative (nonhormonal) forms of contraception is recommended; consult prescriber for use of appropriate barrier contraceptives. Do not breast-feed.

Dietary Considerations May be taken with or without food; do not take with high-fat meal. The 50 mg capsules contain 36.3 int. units of vitamin E per capsule; oral solution contains 46 int. units of vitamin E per mL; avoid additional vitamin E-containing supplements.

Breast-Feeding Issues HIV-infected mothers are discouraged from breast-feeding to decrease potential transmission of HIV.

Pregnancy Issues It is not known if amprenavir crosses the human placenta and there are no clinical studies currently underway to evaluate its use in pregnant women. Pregnancy and protease inhibitors are both associated with an increased risk of hyperglycemia. Glucose levels should be closely monitored. Health professionals are encouraged to contact the antiretroviral pregnancy registry to monitor outcomes of pregnant women exposed to antiretroviral medications (1-800-258-4263 or www.APRegistry.com).

Additional Information Propylene glycol is included in the oral solution; a dose of 22.5 mg/kg twice daily corresponds to an intake of 1650 mg/kg of propylene glycol. Capsule and oral solution are not interchangeable on a mg-per-mg basis.

Anastrozole *(an AS troe zole)*

U.S. Brand Names Arimidex®
Synonyms ICI-D1033; ZD1033
Pharmacologic Category Aromatase Inhibitor
Pregnancy Risk Factor D
Lactation Excretion in breast milk unknown/use caution
Use Treatment of locally-advanced or metastatic breast cancer (ER-positive or hormone receptor unknown) in postmenopausal women; treatment of advanced breast cancer in postmenopausal women with disease progression following tamoxifen therapy; adjuvant treatment of early ER-positive breast cancer in postmenopausal women

Mechanism of Action/Effect Potent and selective nonsteroidal aromatase inhibitor. By inhibiting aromatase, the conversion of androstenedione to estrone, and testosterone to estradiol, is prevented. Anastrozole causes an 85% decrease in estrone sulfate levels.

Contraindications Hypersensitivity to anastrozole or any component of the formulation; pregnancy

Warnings/Precautions Use with caution in patients with hyperlipidemias; total cholesterol and LDL-cholesterol increase in patients receiving anastrozole. Exclude pregnancy before initiating therapy. Anastrozole may be associated with a reduction in bone mineral density. Safety and efficacy in premenopausal women or pediatric patients have not been established.

Drug Interactions
Cytochrome P450 Effect: Inhibits CYP1A2 (weak), 2C8/9 (weak), 3A4 (weak)

Nutritional/Ethanol Interactions Herb/Nutraceutical: Avoid black cohosh, hops, licorice, red clover, thyme, and dong quai.

Lab Interactions Lab test abnormalities: GGT, AST, ALT, alkaline phosphatase, total cholesterol, and LDL increased; threefold elevations of mean serum GGT levels have been observed among patients with liver metastases. These changes were likely related to the progression of liver metastases in these patients, although other contributing factors could not be ruled out. Mean serum total cholesterol levels increased by 0.5 mmol/L among patients.

Adverse Reactions
>10%:
Cardiovascular: Vasodilatation (25% to 36%), hypertension (5% to 13%)
Central nervous system: Mood disturbance (19%), pain (11% to 17%), headache (10% to 13%), depression (5% to 13%)
Dermatologic: Rash (6% to 11%)
Endocrine & metabolic: Hot flashes (12% to 36%)
Gastrointestinal: Nausea (11% to 19%), vomiting (8% to 13%)
Neuromuscular & skeletal: Weakness (16% to 19%), arthritis (17%), arthralgia (2% to 15%), back pain (10% to 12%), bone pain (6% to 11%), osteoporosis (11%)
Respiratory: Cough increased (8% to 11%), pharyngitis (6% to 14%)

1% to 10%:
Cardiovascular: Peripheral edema (5% to 10%), chest pain (5% to 7%), ischemic cardiovascular disease (4%), venous thromboembolic events (3% to 4%), ischemic cerebrovascular events (2%), angina (2%)
Central nervous system: Insomnia (6% to 10%), dizziness (8%), anxiety (6%), fever (2% to 5%), malaise (2% to 5%), confusion (2% to 5%), nervousness (2% to 5%), somnolence (2% to 5%), lethargy (1%)
Dermatologic: Alopecia (2% to 5%), pruritus (2% to 5%)
Endocrine & metabolic: Hypercholesterolemia (9%), breast pain (2% to 8%)
Gastrointestinal: Constipation (7% to 9%), abdominal pain (7% to 9%), diarrhea (7% to 9%), anorexia (5% to 7%), xerostomia (6%), dyspepsia (7%), weight gain (2% to 9%), weight loss (2% to 5%)
Genitourinary: Urinary tract infection (8%), vulvovaginitis (6%), pelvic pain (5%), vaginal bleeding (1% to 5%), vaginitis (4%), vaginal discharge (4%), vaginal hemorrhage (2% to 4%), leukorrhea (2% to 3%), vaginal dryness (2%)
Hematologic: Anemia (2% to 5%), leukopenia (2% to 5%)
Hepatic: Liver function tests increased (2% to 5%), alkaline phosphatase increased (2% to 5%), gamma GT increased (2% to 5%)
Local: Thrombophlebitis (2% to 5%)
Neuromuscular & skeletal: Fracture (10%), arthrosis (7%), paresthesia (5% to 7%), joint disorder (6%), myalgia (2% to 6%), neck pain (2% to 5%), hypertonia (3%)
Ocular: Cataracts (6%)
Respiratory: Dyspnea (8% to 10%), sinusitis (6%), bronchitis (5%), rhinitis (2% to 5%)
Miscellaneous: Lymph edema (10%), infection (2% to 9%), flu-like syndrome (2% to 7%), diaphoresis (2% to 5%), cyst (5%)

Overdosage/Toxicology Symptoms of overdose include severe irritation to the stomach (necrosis, gastritis, ulceration, and hemorrhage). There is no specific antidote; treatment must be symptomatic. Dialysis may be helpful because anastrozole is not highly protein bound.

Pharmacodynamics/Kinetics
Onset of Action: Onset of estradiol reduction: 24 hours (70% reduction; 80% after 2 weeks therapy)
Duration of Action: Duration of estradiol reduction: 6 days

Protein Binding: Plasma: 40%

Half-Life Elimination: 50 hours

Metabolism: Extensively hepatic (85%) via N-dealkylation, hydroxylation, and glucuronidation; primary metabolite inactive

Excretion: Feces (~75%); urine (10% as unchanged drug; 60% as metabolites)

Available Dosage Forms Tablet: 1 mg

Dosing

Adults & Elderly: Breast cancer: Oral (refer to individual protocols): 1 mg once daily

Renal Impairment: Dosage adjustment is not necessary.

Hepatic Impairment: Mild-to-moderate impairment: Plasma concentrations in subjects with stable hepatic cirrhosis were within the range concentrations in normal subjects across all clinical trials; therefore, no dosage adjustment required; however, patients should be monitored for side effects. Safety and efficacy in severe hepatic impairment have not been established.

Stability

Storage: Store at 20°C to 25°C (68°F to 77°F).

Laboratory Monitoring Bone mineral density; total cholesterol and LDL

Nursing Actions

Physical Assessment: Assess potential for interactions with other pharmacological agents and herbal products patient may be taking (tamoxifen and estrogens). Monitor laboratory tests (may decrease bone mineral density and elevate serum cholesterol). Therapeutic effectiveness and adverse reactions (eg, hyperlipidemia, hypotension, CNS changes, thrombophlebitis, bone pain or fracture) should be monitored periodically during therapy. Teach patient proper use, possible side effects/appropriate interventions, and adverse symptoms to report.

Patient Education: Do not take any new medication during therapy unless approved by prescriber. Take exactly as directed. Maintain adequate hydration (2-3 L/day of fluids) unless instructed to restrict fluid intake. May cause headache (consult prescriber for approved analgesic); drowsiness, dizziness, anxiety (use caution when driving or engaging in tasks that require alertness until response to drug is known); nausea or vomiting (small, frequent meals, frequent mouth care, chewing gum, or sucking lozenges may help); or increased pelvic, bone or tumor pain (may lessen with continued use; if not, consult prescriber for approved analgesic); or hot flashes (cool cloths may help). Report unresolved nausea or vomiting; pain or burning on urination; severe mood swings, confusion, anxiety; palpitations; swelling of extremities; unusual chest pain; flu-like symptoms; persistent bone or joint pain; respiratory difficulty; or other persistent adverse effects. **Pregnancy/breast-feeding precautions:** Do not get pregnant while taking this medication. Consult prescriber for appropriate contraceptive measures. Consult prescriber if breast-feeding.

Pregnancy Issues Anastrozole can cause fetal harm when administered to a pregnant woman.

Anthralin (AN thra lin)

U.S. Brand Names Dritho-Scalp®; Psoriatec™

Synonyms Dithranol

Pharmacologic Category Antipsoriatic Agent; Keratolytic Agent

Pregnancy Risk Factor C

Lactation Excretion in breast milk unknown/not recommended

Use Treatment of psoriasis (quiescent or chronic psoriasis)

Mechanism of Action/Effect Inhibits synthesis of nucleic protein from inhibition of DNA synthesis to affected areas

Contraindications Hypersensitivity to anthralin or any component of the formulation; acute psoriasis (acutely or actively inflamed psoriatic eruptions)

Warnings/Precautions If redness is observed, reduce frequency of dosage or discontinue application; avoid eye contact; should generally not be applied to opposing skin surfaces that may rub or touch (eg, skin folds of the groin, axilla, and breasts) and high strengths should not be used on these sites; do not apply to genitalia. Use caution in patients with renal disease and in those having extensive and prolonged applications. May stain skin, hair, fingernails (temporary); or fabrics (may be permanent).

Drug Interactions

Increased Effect/Toxicity: Long-term use of topical corticosteroids may destabilize psoriasis and withdrawal may also give rise to a "rebound" phenomenon. Allow an interval of at least 1 week between the discontinuance of topical corticosteroids and the commencement of therapy.

Adverse Reactions Frequency not defined: Dermatologic: Transient primary irritation of uninvolved skin; temporary discoloration of skin, hair, and fingernails; contact allergic reactions; erythema

Available Dosage Forms

Cream:

Dritho-Scalp®: 0.5% (50 g)

Psoriatec™: 1% (50 g)

Dosing

Adults & Elderly:

Psoriasis: Topical: Generally, apply once a day or as directed. The irritant potential of anthralin is directly related to the strength being used and each patient's individual tolerance. Always commence treatment using a short, daily contact time (5-10 minutes) for at least 1 week using the lowest strength possible. Contact time may be gradually increased (to 20-30 minutes) as tolerated.

Skin application: Apply sparingly only to psoriatic lesions and rub gently and carefully into the skin until absorbed. Avoid applying an excessive quantity which may cause unnecessary soiling and staining of the clothing or bed linen.

Scalp application: Comb hair to remove scalar debris, wet hair and, after suitably parting, rub cream well into the lesions, taking care to prevent the cream from spreading onto the forehead,

Note: Remove by washing or showering; optimal period of contact will vary according to the strength used and the patient's response to treatment. Continue treatment until the skin is entirely clear (ie, when there is nothing to feel with the fingers and the texture is normal).

Pediatrics: Unlabeled use: Refer to adult dosing.

Administration

Topical: May apply using latex gloves to prevent staining of fingers. Apply directly to plaques; rub in gently but thoroughly; avoid application to unaffected skin. When applying to scalp, part hair in one-inch segments to reach plaques. Remove by washing after conclusion of prescribed contact period. When rinsing, take care to avoid contact with eyes. Immediately clean tub or shower to prevent staining. Dry off using old towel (stains on fabric may be permanent). Petroleum jelly may be used around the edges of plaques, in body folds, or skin creases to prevent irritation of unaffected skin.

Stability

Storage: Store at controlled room temperature of 15°C to 30°C (59°F to 86°F). Avoid excessive heat.

Nursing Actions

Physical Assessment: When applied to large areas of skin or for extensive periods of time, monitor for

(Continued)

Anthralin *(Continued)*

adverse skin or systemic reactions. Assess knowledge/teach patient appropriate application and use and adverse symptoms to report.

Patient Education: For external use only. Use exactly as directed; do not overuse. Before using, wash and dry area gently. Wear gloves to apply a thin film to affected area and rub in gently. Remove by washing; may discolor fabric, skin, or hair. Use a porous dressing if necessary. For lesions on scalp, comb hair to remove scalar debris, part hair, and rub cream into lesions. Do not allow cream to spread to forehead or onto neck. Remove by washing hair. Avoid contact with eyes. Avoid exposing treated areas to direct sunlight; sunburn can occur. Optimal period of contact will vary according to strength used and response to treatment. Report increased swelling, redness, rash, itching, signs of infection, worsening of condition, or lack of healing. **Pregnancy/breast-feeding precautions:** Inform prescriber if you are or intend to become pregnant. Breast-feeding is not recommended.

Antihemophilic Factor (Human)
(an tee hee moe FIL ik FAK tor HYU man)

U.S. Brand Names Alphanate®; Hemofil® M; Humate-P®; Koāte®-DVI; Monarc® M; Monoclate-P®

Synonyms AHF (Human); Factor VIII (Human)

Pharmacologic Category Antihemophilic Agent; Blood Product Derivative

Pregnancy Risk Factor C

Lactation Excretion in breast milk unknown/use caution

Use Management of hemophilia A for patients in whom a deficiency in factor VIII has been demonstrated; can be of significant therapeutic value in patients with acquired factor VIII inhibitors not exceeding 10 Bethesda units/mL

Humate-P®: In addition, indicated as treatment of spontaneous bleeding in patients with severe von Willebrand disease and in mild and moderate von Willebrand disease where desmopressin is known or suspected to be inadequate

Orphan status: Alphanate®: Management of von Willebrand disease

Mechanism of Action/Effect Protein (factor VIII) in normal plasma which is necessary for clot formation and maintenance of hemostasis; activates factor X in conjunction with activated factor IX; activated factor X converts prothrombin to thrombin, which converts fibrinogen to fibrin, and with factor XIII forms a stable clot

Contraindications Hypersensitivity to any component of the formulation or to mouse protein (Monoclate-P®, Hemofil® M)

Warnings/Precautions Risk of viral transmission is not totally eradicated. Because antihemophilic factor is prepared from pooled plasma, it may contain the causative agent of viral hepatitis and other viral diseases. Hepatitis B vaccination is recommended for all patients. Hepatitis A vaccination is also recommended for seronegative patients. Antihemophilic factor contains trace amounts of blood groups A and B isohemagglutinins and when large or frequently repeated doses are given to individuals with blood groups A, B, and AB, the patient should be monitored for signs of progressive anemia and the possibility of intravascular hemolysis should be considered. Natural rubber latex is a component of Hemofil® M packaging. Products vary by preparation method; final formulations contain human albumin.

Overdosage/Toxicology Massive doses have been reported to cause acute hemolytic anemia, increased bleeding tendency, or hyperfibrinogenemia. Occurrence is rare.

Pharmacodynamics/Kinetics

Half-Life Elimination: Mean: 12-17 hours with hemophilia A; consult specific product labeling

Available Dosage Forms Injection, human [single-dose vial]: Labeling on cartons and vials indicates number of int. units

Dosing

Adults: Hemophilia: I.V.: Individualize dosage based on coagulation studies performed prior to treatment and at regular intervals during treatment. 1 AHF unit is the activity present in 1 mL of normal pooled human plasma. Dosage should be adjusted to actual vial size currently stocked in the pharmacy. (General guidelines presented; consult individual product labeling for specific dosing recommendations.)

Dosage based on desired factor VIII increase (%):

To calculate dosage needed based on desired factor VIII increase (%):

Body weight (kg) x 0.5 int. units/kg x desired factor VIII increase (%) = int. units factor VIII required

For example:

50 kg x 0.5 int. units/kg x 30 (% increase) = 750 int. units factor VIII

Dosage based on expected factor VIII increase (%):

It is also possible to calculate the **expected** % factor VIII increase:

(# int. units administered x 2%/int. units/kg) divided by body weight (kg) = expected % factor VIII increase

For example:

(1400 int. units x 2%/int. units/kg) divided by 70 kg = 40%

General guidelines:

Minor hemorrhage: Required peak postinfusion AHF level: 20% to 40% (10-20 int. units/kg): Repeat dose every 12-24 hours for 1-3 days until bleeding is resolved or healing achieved; mild superficial or early hemorrhages may respond to a single dose.

Moderate hemorrhage: Required peak postinfusion AHF level: 30% to 60% (15-30 int. units/kg): Infuse every 12-24 hours for ≥3 days until pain and disability are resolved.

Alternatively, a loading dose to achieve 50% (25 int. units/kg) may be given, followed by 10-15 int. units/kg dose given every 8-12 hours; may be needed for >7 days.

Severe/life-threatening hemorrhage: Required peak postinfusion AHF level: 60% to 100% (30-50 int. units/kg): Infuse every 8-24 hours until threat is resolved.

Alternatively, a loading dose to achieve 80% to 100% (40-50 int. units/kg) may be given, followed by 20-25 int. units/kg dose given every 8-12 hours for ≥14 days.

Minor surgery: Required peak postinfusion AHF level: 30% to 80% (15-40 int. units/kg): Highly dependent upon procedure and specific product recommendations; for some procedures, may be administered as a single infusion plus oral antifibrinolytic therapy within 1 hour. In other procedures, may repeat dose every 12-24 hours as needed.

Major surgery: Required peak pre- and postsurgery AHF level: 80% to 100% (40-50 int. units/kg): Administer every 6-24 hours until healing is complete (10-14 days).

Prophylaxis: May also be given on a regular schedule to prevent bleeding.

If bleeding is not controlled with adequate dose, test for presence of inhibitor. It may not be possible or practical to control bleeding if inhibitor titers are >10 Bethesda units/mL; antihemophilic factor (porcine) may be considered as an alternative.

von Willebrand disease: I.V.:

Treatment of hemorrhage in von Willebrand disease (Humate-P®): 1 int. units of factor VIII per kg of body weight would be expected to raise circulating vWF:RC of approximately 3.5-4 int. units/dL.

Type 1, mild (if desmopressin is not appropriate):
Major hemorrhage:
Loading dose: 40-60 int. units/kg
Maintenance dose: 40-50 int. units/kg every 8-12 hours for 3 days, keeping vWF:RC of nadir >50%; follow with 40-50 int. units/kg daily for up to 7 days

Type 1, moderate or severe:
Minor hemorrhage: 40-50 int. units/kg for 1-2 doses
Major hemorrhage:
Loading dose: 50-75 int. units/kg
Maintenance dose: 40-60 int. units/kg daily for up to 7 days

Types 2 and 3:
Minor hemorrhage: 40-50 int. units/kg for 1-2 doses
Major hemorrhage:
Loading dose: 60-80 int. units/kg
Maintenance dose: 40-60 int. units/kg every 8-12 hours for 3 days, keeping vWF:RC of nadir >50%; follow with 40-60 int. units/kg daily for up to 7 days

Elderly: Refer to adult dosing. Dosage should be individualized.

Pediatrics: Refer to adult dosing.

Administration

I.V.: Over 5-10 minutes (maximum: 10 mL/minute). Infuse Monoclate-P® at 2 mL/minute.

Stability

Reconstitution:
Gently agitate or rotate vial after adding diluent; do not shake vigorously.

Storage: Store under refrigeration, 2°C to 8°C (36°F to 46°F); avoid freezing. If refrigerated, the dried concentrate and diluent should be warmed to room temperature before reconstitution. Use within 3 hours of reconstitution. Do not refrigerate after reconstitution, precipitation may occur.

Alphanate®: May be stored at room temperature for ≤2 months.
Hemofil® M: May be stored at room temperature for ≤12 months.
Humate-P®, Koāte®-DVI; Monoclate-P®: May also be stored at room temperature for ≤6 months.

Laboratory Monitoring In patients with circulating inhibitors, the inhibitor level should be monitored; hematocrit

Nursing Actions

Physical Assessment: Assess potential for interactions with other pharmacological agents patient may be taking that may affect coagulation or platelet function. Monitor patient closely during and after infusion for any change in vital signs, cardiac and CNS status, or hypersensitivity reactions (chills, fever, chest pain, respiratory difficulty). Monitor therapeutic response (eg, results of laboratory tests, bleeding and coagulation status) and adverse reactions (eg, signs of intravascular hemolysis, increased bleeding or anemia). Provide patient education according to patient condition.

Patient Education: This medication can only be given intravenously. Report immediately any sudden-onset headache, rash, chest or back pain, wheezing or respiratory difficulties, hives, itching, low-grade fever, stomach pain, or nausea/vomiting to prescriber. Wear identification indicating that you have a hemophilic condition. **Pregnancy/breast-feeding precautions:** Inform prescriber if you are or intend to become pregnant. Consult prescriber if breast-feeding.

Pregnancy Issues Safety and efficacy in pregnant women have not been established. Use during pregnancy only if clearly needed. Parvovirus B19, which may be present in the solution, may seriously affect a pregnant woman.

Antihemophilic Factor (Recombinant)
(an tee hee moe FIL ik FAK tor ree KOM be nant)

U.S. Brand Names Advate; Helixate® FS; Kogenate® FS; Recombinate™; ReFacto®

Synonyms AHF (Recombinant); Factor VIII (Recombinant); rAHF

Pharmacologic Category Antihemophilic Agent

Pregnancy Risk Factor C

Lactation Excretion in breast milk unknown/use caution

Use Management of hemophilia A (classic hemophilia) for patients in whom a deficiency in factor VIII has been demonstrated; prevention and control of bleeding episodes; perioperative management of hemophilia A; can be of significant therapeutic value in patients with acquired factor VIII inhibitors ≤10 Bethesda units/mL

Mechanism of Action/Effect Factor VIII replacement, necessary for clot formation and maintenance of hemostasis. It activates factor X in conjunction with activated factor IX; activated factor X converts prothrombin to thrombin, which converts fibrinogen to fibrin, and with factor XIII forms a stable clot.

Contraindications Hypersensitivity to mouse or hamster protein (Advate, Helixate® FS, Kogenate® FS); hypersensitivity to mouse, hamster, or bovine protein (Recombinate™, ReFacto®); hypersensitivity to any component of the formulation

Warnings/Precautions Monitor for signs of formation of antibodies to factor VIII; may occur at anytime but more common in young children with severe hemophilia. The dosage requirement will vary in patients with inhibitors; optimal treatment should be determined by clinical response. Monitor for allergic hypersensitivity reactions. Products vary by preparation method. Recombinate™ is stabilized using human albumin. Helixate® FS and Kogenate® FS are stabilized with sucrose. Not indicated for the treatment of von Willebrand's disease.

Overdosage/Toxicology Massive doses of antihemophilic factor (human) have been reported to cause acute hemolytic anemia, increased bleeding tendency, or hyperfibrinogenemia. Occurrence is rare.

Pharmacodynamics/Kinetics
Half-Life Elimination: Mean: 13-16 hours

Available Dosage Forms

Injection, powder for reconstitution, recombinant [preservative free]:
Advate: 250 int. units, 500 int. units, 1000 int. units, 1500 int. units [plasma/albumin free]
Helixate® FS, Kogenate® FS: 250 int. units, 500 int. units, 1000 int. units [contains sucrose 28 mg/vial]
Recombinate™: 250 int. units, 500 units, 1000 int. units [contains human albumin 12.5 mg/mL; packaging contains natural rubber latex]
ReFacto®: 250 int. units, 500 units, 1000 int. units, 2000 int. units [contains sucrose]

Dosing
Adults: Hemophilia: I.V.: Individualize dosage based on coagulation studies. performed prior to treatment and at regular intervals during treatment; 1 AHF unit is the activity present in 1 mL of normal pooled human plasma; dosage should be adjusted to actual vial size
(Continued)

Antihemophilic Factor (Recombinant)
(Continued)

currently stocked in the pharmacy. (General guidelines presented; consult individual product labeling for specific dosing recommendations.)

Dosage based on desired factor VIII increase (%):
To calculate dosage needed based on desired factor VIII increase (%):
[Body weight (kg) x desired factor VIII increase (%)] divided by 2%/int. units/kg = int. units factor VIII required
For example:
50 kg x 30 (% increase) divided by 2%/int. units/kg = 750 int. units factor VIII

Dosage based on expected factor VIII increase (%):
It is also possible to calculate the **expected** % factor VIII increase:
(# int. units administered x 2%/int. units/kg) divided by body weight (kg) = expected % factor VIII increase
For example:
(1400 int. units x 2%/int. units/kg) divided by 70 kg = 40%

General guidelines:
Minor hemorrhage: Required peak postinfusion AHF level: 20% to 40% (10-20 int. units/kg); mild superficial or early hemorrhages may respond to a single dose; may repeat dose every 12-24 hours for 1-3 days until bleeding is resolved or healing achieved

Moderate hemorrhage/minor surgery: Required peak postinfusion AHF level: 30% to 60% (15-30 int. units/kg); repeat dose at 12-24 hours if needed; some products suggest continuing for ≥3 days until pain and disability are resolved

Severe/life-threatening hemorrhage: Required peak postinfusion AHF level: Initial dose: 80% to 100% (40-50 int. units/kg); maintenance dose: 40% to 50% (20-25 int. units/kg) every 8-12 hours until threat is resolved

Major surgery: Required peak pre- and postsurgery AHF level: ~100% (50 int. units/kg): Give first dose prior to surgery and repeat every 6-12 hours until healing complete (10-14 days)

Prophylaxis: May also be given on a regular schedule to prevent bleeding

If bleeding is not controlled with adequate dose, test for presence of inhibitor. It may not be possible or practical to control bleeding if inhibitor titers >10 Bethesda units/mL; antihemophilic factor (porcine) may be considered as an alternative.

Elderly: Refer to adult dosing. Dosage should be individualized.

Pediatrics: Refer to adult dosing.

Administration
I.V.: Infuse over 5-10 minutes (maximum: 10 mL/minute)
Advate: Infuse over ≤5 minutes (maximum: 10 mL/minute)

Stability
Reconstitution:
Gently agitate or rotate vial after adding diluent, do not shake vigorously.

Storage: Store under refrigeration, 2°C to 8°C (36°F to 46°F); avoid freezing. Use within 3 hours of reconstitution. Do not refrigerate after reconstitution, a precipitation may occur.
Advate: May also be stored at room temperature for up to 6 months.
Helixate® FS, Kogenate® FS, Recombinate™, ReFacto®: May also be stored at room temperature for up to 3 months; avoid prolonged exposure to light during storage.

If refrigerated, the dried concentrate and diluent should be warmed to room temperature before reconstitution.

Laboratory Monitoring Development of circulating inhibitors; bleeding

Nursing Actions
Physical Assessment: Assess potential for interactions with other pharmacological agents patient may be taking that may affect coagulation or platelet function. Monitor patient closely during and after infusion for any change in vital signs, cardiac and CNS status, or hypersensitivity reactions (chills, fever, chest pain, respiratory difficulty). Monitor therapeutic response (results of laboratory tests, bleeding and coagulation status) and adverse reactions (bleeding or anemia). Provide patient education according to patient condition.

Patient Education: This medication can only be given intravenously. Immediately report any sudden-onset headache, rash, chest or back pain, wheezing or respiratory difficulties, hives, itching, low grade fever, stomach pain, nausea, or vomiting to prescriber. Wear identification indicating that you have a hemophilic condition. **Pregnancy/breast-feeding precautions:** Inform prescriber if you are pregnant. Consult prescriber if breast-feeding.

Anti-inhibitor Coagulant Complex
(an tee-in HI bi tor coe AG yoo lant KOM pleks)

U.S. Brand Names Autoplex® T [DSC]; Feiba VH
Synonyms AICC; Coagulant Complex Inhibitor
Pharmacologic Category Activated Prothrombin Complex Concentrate (aPCC); Antihemophilic Agent; Blood Product Derivative
Pregnancy Risk Factor C
Lactation Excretion in breast milk unknown/use caution
Use Hemophilia A & B patients with factor VIII inhibitors who are to undergo surgery or those who are bleeding
Contraindications Hypersensitivity to any component of the formulation; disseminated intravascular coagulation (DIC); fibrinolysis; patients with normal coagulation mechanism
Warnings/Precautions Products are prepared from pooled human plasma; such plasma may contain the causative agents of viral diseases. Tests used to control improvement, such as aPTT, WBCT, and TEG, do not correlate with clinical efficacy. Dosing to normalize these values may result in DIC. Identification of the clotting deficiency as caused by factor VIII inhibitors is essential prior to starting therapy. Use with extreme caution in patients with impaired hepatic function. Thrombotic complications have been associated with high doses of Feiba VH; single doses should not exceed 100 units/kg and daily doses should not exceed 200 units/kg. Products may contain natural rubber latex. Products may contain minute amounts of factor VIII which may cause an anamnestic response.

Drug Interactions
Increased Effect/Toxicity: Coadministration of aminocaproic acid or tranexamic acid may increase risk of thrombosis.

Lab Interactions Increased/decreased PT, PTT; increased fibrin split products; decreased WBCT, fibrin, platelets

Adverse Reactions Frequency not defined.
Cardiovascular: Blood pressure changes, flushing, MI, pulse rate changes
Central nervous system: Headache, lethargy
Dermatologic: Rash, urticaria
Gastrointestinal: Nausea
Hematologic: DIC
Miscellaneous: Allergic reaction, anamnestic response, infusion-related reactions (fever, chills)

Overdosage/Toxicology Rapid infusion may cause hypotension. Excessive administration can cause DIC.

Available Dosage Forms Injection, powder for reconstitution:

Autoplex® T: Each bottle is labeled with correctional units of factor VIII [contains heparin 2 units/mL and sodium 162-192 mEg/L; packaging contains natural rubber latex] [DSC]

Feiba VH: Each bottle is labeled with Immuno units of factor VIII [heparin free; contains sodium 8 mg/mL; packaging contains natural rubber latex]

Dosing

Adults & Elderly: Control of bleeding: I.V.:

Autoplex® T: Dosage range: 25-100 factor VIII correctional units per kg depending on the severity of hemorrhage; may repeat in ~ 6 hours if needed. Adjust dose based on patient response.

Feiba VH: General dosing guidelines: 50-100 units/kg (maximum 200 units/kg)

Joint hemorrhage: 50 units/kg every 12 hours; may increase to 100 units/kg; continue until signs of clinical improvement occur

Mucous membrane bleeding: 50 units/kg every 6 hours; may increase to 100 units/kg (maximum: 2 administrations/day or 200 units/kg/day

Soft tissue hemorrhage: 100 units/kg every 12 hours (maximum: 200 units/kg/day)

Other severe hemorrhage: 100 units/kg every 12 hours; may be used every 6 hours if needed; continue until clinical improvement

Pediatrics: Refer to adult dosing.

Administration

I.V.:

Autoplex® T: Initial rate of infusion: 2 mL/minute; may gradually increase to 10 mL/minute as tolerated. Infusion should be completed within 1 hour of reconstitution.

Feiba VH: Maximum infusion rate: 2 units/kg/minute. Following reconstitution, complete infusion within 3 hours

Stability

Reconstitution: Prior to reconstitution, bring to room temperature. Reconstitute with provided SWI. Swirl to gently dissolve powder; do not shake vigorously. Do **not** refrigerate after reconstitution.

Storage: Store at 2°C to 8°C (36°F to 46°F); avoid freezing. Feiba VH may be stored at room temperature of 25°C (77°F) for up to 6 months prior to reconstitution; do not re-refrigerate.

Laboratory Monitoring Monitor for control of bleeding; signs and symptoms of DIC (blood pressure changes, pulse rate changes, chest pain/cough, fibrinogen decreased, platelet count decreased, fibrin-fibrinogen degradation products, significantly-prolonged thrombin time, PT, or partial thromboplastin time); hypotension; have epinephrine ready to treat hypersensitivity reactions. **Note:** Tests used to control efficacy such as aPTT, WBCT, and TEG do not correlate with clinical improvement. Dosing to normalize these values may result in DIC.

Nursing Actions

Physical Assessment: Assess potential for interactions with pharmacological agents patient may be taking that may affect coagulation or platelet function. Monitor patient closely during and after infusion for any change in vital signs, cardiac and CNS status, or hypersensitivity reactions (chills, fever, chest pain, respiratory difficulty). **Caution:** See Monitoring Laboratory Tests. If hypotension develops, the rate of infusion should be slowed and prescriber notified. Provide patient education according to patient condition.

Patient Education: This medication can only be administered by infusion; you will be monitored during and after infusion. Report immediately any sudden onset headache, rash, chest or back pain, wheezing

or respiratory difficulties, hives, itching, low-grade fever, stomach pain, or nausea/vomiting to prescriber. Wear identification indicating that you have a hemophilic condition. **Pregnancy/breast-feeding precautions:** Inform prescriber if you are pregnant. Consult prescriber if breast-feeding.

Dietary Considerations Autoplex® T contains sodium 162-192 mEg/L; Feiba VH contains sodium 8 mg/mL

Pregnancy Issues Reproduction studies have not been conducted.

Antithymocyte Globulin (Equine)
(an te THY moe site GLOB yu lin, E kwine)

U.S. Brand Names Atgam®

Synonyms Antithymocyte Immunoglobulin; ATG; Horse Antihuman Thymocyte Gamma Globulin; Lymphocyte Immune Globulin

Pharmacologic Category Immunosuppressant Agent

Medication Safety Issues

Sound-alike/look-alike issues:

Atgam® may be confused with Ativan®

Pregnancy Risk Factor C

Lactation Excretion in breast milk unknown/use caution

Use Prevention and treatment of acute renal allograft rejection; treatment of moderate to severe aplastic anemia in patients not considered suitable candidates for bone marrow transplantation

Unlabeled/Investigational Use Prevention and treatment of other solid organ allograft rejection; prevention of graft-versus-host disease following bone marrow transplantation

Mechanism of Action/Effect May involve elimination of antigen-reactive T lymphocytes (killer cells) in peripheral blood or alteration of T-cell function

Contraindications Hypersensitivity to lymphocytic immune globulin, any component of the formulation, or other equine gamma globulins

Warnings/Precautions For I.V. use only. Must be administered via central line due to chemical phlebitis. Should only be used by physicians experienced in immunosuppressive therapy or management of solid organ or bone marrow transplant patients. Adequate laboratory and supportive medical resources must be readily available in the facility for patient management. Rash, dyspnea, hypotension, or anaphylaxis precludes further administration of the drug. Discontinue if severe and unremitting thrombocytopenia and/or leukopenia occur. Dose must be administered over at least 4 hours. Patient may need to be pretreated with an antipyretic, antihistamine, and/or corticosteroid.

Adverse Reactions

>10%:

Central nervous system: Fever, chills

Dermatologic: Pruritus, rash, urticaria

Hematologic: Leukopenia, thrombocytopenia

1% to 10%:

Cardiovascular: Bradycardia, chest pain, CHF, edema, encephalitis, hyper-/hypotension, myocarditis, tachycardia

Central nervous system: Agitation, headache, lethargy, lightheadedness, listlessness, seizure

Gastrointestinal: Diarrhea, nausea, stomatitis, vomiting

Hepatic: Hepatosplenomegaly, liver function tests abnormal

Local: Pain at injection site, phlebitis, thrombophlebitis, burning soles/palms

Neuromuscular & skeletal: Myalgia, back pain, arthralgia

Ocular: Periorbital edema

Renal: Abnormal renal function tests

Respiratory: Dyspnea, respiratory distress

(Continued)

Antithymocyte Globulin (Equine)
(Continued)

Miscellaneous: Anaphylaxis, serum sickness, viral infection, night sweats, diaphoresis, lymphadenopathy

Pharmacodynamics/Kinetics

Half-Life Elimination: Plasma: 1.5-12 days

Excretion: Urine (~1%)

Available Dosage Forms Injection, solution: 50 mg/mL (5 mL)

Dosing

Adults & Elderly: Note: An intradermal skin test is recommended prior to administration of the initial dose of ATG; use 0.1 mL of a 1:1000 dilution of ATG in normal saline. A positive skin reaction consists of a wheal ≥10 mm in diameter. If a positive skin test occurs, the first infusion should be administered in a controlled environment with intensive life support immediately available. A systemic reaction precludes further administration of the drug. The absence of a reaction does **not** preclude the possibility of an immediate sensitivity reaction.

Note: Premedication with diphenhydramine, hydrocortisone, and is recommended prior to first dose.

Aplastic anemia protocol: I.V.: 10-20 mg/kg/day for 8-14 days, then give every other day for 7 more doses for a total of 21 doses in 28 days.

Renal allograft rejection, prevention: I.V.: 15 mg/kg/day for 14 days, then give every other day for 7 more doses for a total of 21 doses in 28 days; initial dose should be administered within 24 hours before or after transplantation.

Renal allograft rejection, treatment: I.V.: 10-15 mg/kg/day for 14 days, then give every other day for 7 more doses.

Pediatrics: Note: See adult dosing for notes on intradermal skin testing and premedication.

Aplastic anemia protocol: I.V.: 10-20 mg/kg/day for 8-14 days; then administer every other day for 7 more doses; addition doses may be given every other day for 21 total doses in 28 days.

Renal allograft: I.V.: 5-25 mg/kg/day

Administration

I.V.: Infuse dose over at least 4 hours. Any severe systemic reaction to the skin test, such as generalized rash, tachycardia, dyspnea, hypotension, or anaphylaxis, should preclude further therapy. Epinephrine and resuscitative equipment should be nearby. Patient may need to be pretreated with an antipyretic, antihistamine, and/or corticosteroid. Mild itching and erythema can be treated with antihistamines. Infuse into a vascular shunt, arterial venous fistula, or high-flow central vein through a 0.2-1 micron in-line filter.

First dose: Premedicate with diphenhydramine orally 30 minutes prior to and hydrocortisone I.V. 15 minutes prior to infusion and acetaminophen 2 hours after start of infusion.

Stability

Reconstitution: Dilute into inverted bottle of sterile vehicle to ensure that undiluted lymphocyte immune globulin does not contact air. Gently rotate or swirl to mix. Final concentration should be 4 mg/mL. May be diluted in NS, $D_5$1/4NS, $D_5$1/2NS.

Storage: Ampuls must be refrigerated; do not freeze. Diluted solution is stable for 24 hours (including infusion time) at refrigeration.

Laboratory Monitoring Lymphocyte profile, CBC with differential, platelet count

Nursing Actions

Physical Assessment: Assess for history of previous allergic reactions. Monitor vital signs during infusion and observe for adverse or allergic reactions. Teach patient adverse symptoms to report.

Patient Education: This medication can only be administered by infusion. You will be closely monitored during the infusion. Do not get up alone; ask for assistance if you must get up or change position. Do not have any vaccinations for the next 3 months without consulting prescriber. Immediately report chills; persistent dizziness or nausea; itching or stinging; acute back pain; chest pain, tightness, or rapid heartbeat; or respiratory difficulty. **Pregnancy/breast-feeding precautions:** Inform prescriber if you are pregnant. Consult prescriber if breast-feeding.

Pregnancy Issues Reproduction studies have not been conducted; use during pregnancy is not recommended. Women exposed to Atgam® during pregnancy may be enrolled in the National Transplantation Pregnancy Registry (877-955-6877).

Apomorphine (a poe MOR feen)

U.S. Brand Names Apokyn™

Synonyms Apomorphine Hydrochloride; Apomorphine Hydrochloride Hemihydrate

Pharmacologic Category Anti-Parkinson's Agent, Dopamine Agonist

Pregnancy Risk Factor C

Lactation Excretion in breast milk unknown/contraindicated

Use Treatment of hypomobility, "off" episodes with Parkinson's disease

Unlabeled/Investigational Use Treatment of erectile dysfunction

Mechanism of Action/Effect Improves motor function in Parkinson's disease

Contraindications Hypersensitivity to apomorphine or any component of the formulation; **concomitant use with 5HT$_3$ antagonists**; intravenous administration

Warnings/Precautions May cause orthostatic hypotension, especially during dosage escalation; use extreme caution, especially in patients on antihypertensives and/or vasodilators. Orthostasis peaks 20 minutes after dosing and lasts at least 90 minutes. If patient develops clinically-significant orthostatic hypotension with test dose, then apomorphine should not be used. **Pretreatment with antiemetic is necessary;** avoid pretreatment with antidopaminergic and antiserotonin antiemetic agents (antiemetic experience is greatest with trimethobenzamide). Monitor patients for drowsiness; patients may not be aware of drowsiness and may fall asleep without warning. Use caution in patients with risk factors for torsade de pointes (hypokalemia, hypomagnesemia, bradycardia, concurrent use of drugs that prolong QT$_c$, or genetic predisposition).

Use caution in cardiovascular and cerebrovascular disease; hypotension may cause coronary and/or cerebral ischemia. Use caution in patients with hepatic or renal dysfunction. Neuroleptic malignant syndrome has been reported with other dopamine agonists. Retinal degeneration has been observed in animal studies when using dopamine agonists for prolonged periods. Rare cases of abuse have been reported. Contains metabisulfite which may cause allergic reactions in some individuals. Safety and efficacy in pediatric patients have not been established.

Drug Interactions

Cytochrome P450 Effect: Substrate (minor) of CYP1A2, 3A4, 2C19; **Inhibits** CYP1A2 (weak), 3A (weak), 2C19 (weak)

Decreased Effect: Typical antipsychotics may decrease the efficacy of apomorphine.

Increased Effect/Toxicity: Antihypertensives, vasodilators, and 5HT$_3$ antagonists may increase risk of hypotension. QT$_c$ prolongation may rarely occur with concurrent use of QT$_c$-prolonging agents. Effects of concomitant levodopa may be increased.

Nutritional/Ethanol Interactions

Ethanol: Caution with ethanol consumption; may increase risk of hypotension.

Adverse Reactions

>10%:

Cardiovascular: Chest pain/pressure or angina (15%)

Central nervous system: Drowsiness or somnolence (35%), dizziness or orthostatic hypotension (20%)

Gastrointestinal: Nausea and/or vomiting (30%)

Neuromuscular & skeletal: Falls (30%), dyskinesias (24% to 35%)

Respiratory: Yawning (40%), rhinorrhea (20%)

1% to 10%:

Cardiovascular: Edema (10%), vasodilation (3%), hypotension (2%), syncope (2%), CHF

Central nervous system: Hallucinations or confusion (10%), anxiety, depression, fatigue, headache, insomnia, pain

Dermatologic: Bruising

Endocrine & metabolic: Dehydration

Gastrointestinal: Constipation, diarrhea

Local: Injection site reactions

Neuromuscular & skeletal: Arthralgias, weakness

Miscellaneous: Diaphoresis increased

Overdosage/Toxicology An accidental overdose of 25 mg SubQ was reported, resulting in nausea, loss of consciousness, bradycardia, and hypotension. Treatment should be supportive and symptomatic.

Pharmacodynamics/Kinetics

Onset of Action: SubQ: Rapid

Time to Peak: Plasma: Improved motor scores: 20 minutes

Half-Life Elimination: Terminal: 40 minutes

Metabolism: Not established; potential routes of metabolism include sulfation, N-demethylation, glucuronidation, and oxidation; catechol-O methyltransferase and nonenzymatic oxidation. CYP isoenzymes do not appear to play a significant role.

Excretion: Urine 93% (as metabolites); feces 16%

Available Dosage Forms Injection, solution, as hydrochloride: 10 mg/mL (2 mL) [contains sodium metabisulfite]; (3 mL) [multidose cartridge; contains sodium metabisulfite and benzyl alcohol]

Dosing

Adults & Elderly: Begin antiemetic therapy 3 days prior to initiation and continue for 2 months before reassessing need.

Parkinson's disease, "off" episode: SubQ: Initial test dose 2 mg, **medical supervision required; see "Note".** Subsequent dosing is based on both tolerance and response to initial test dose.

If patient tolerates test dose and responds: Starting dose: 2 mg as needed; may increase dose in 1 mg increments every few days; maximum dose: 6 mg

If patient tolerates but does not respond to 2 mg test dose: Second test dose: 4 mg

If patient tolerates and responds to 4 mg test dose: Starting dose: 3 mg, as needed for "off" episodes; may increase dose in 1 mg increments every few days; maximum dose 6 mg

If patient does not tolerate 4 mg test dose: Third test dose: 3 mg

If patient tolerates 3 mg test dose: Starting dose: 2 mg as needed for "off" episodes; may increase dose in 1 mg increments to a maximum of 3 mg

If therapy is interrupted for >1 week, restart at 2 mg and gradually titrate dose.

Note: Medical supervision is required for all test doses with standing and supine blood pressure

monitoring predose and 20-, 40-, and 60 minutes postdose. If subsequent test doses are required, wait >2 hours before another test dose is given; next test dose should be timed with another "off" episode. If a single dose is ineffective for a particular "off" episode, then a second dose should not be given. The average dosing frequency was 3 times/day in the development program with limited experience in dosing >5 times/day and with total daily doses >20 mg. Apomorphine is intended to treat the "off" episodes associated with levodopa therapy of Parkinson's disease and has not been studied in levodopa-naive Parkinson's patients.

Renal Impairment:

Mild-to-moderate impairment: Reduce test dose and starting dose: 1 mg

Severe impairment: Has not been studied

Hepatic Impairment:

Mild-to-moderate impairment: Use caution

Severe impairment: Has not been studied

Administration

I.V.: Not for I.V. administration.

Other: SubQ: Initiate antiemetic 3 days before test dose of apomorphine and continue for 2 months (if patient to be treated) before reassessment. Administer in abdomen, upper arm, or upper leg; change site with each injection. 3 mL cartridges are used with a manual, reusable, multidose injector pen. Injector pen can deliver doses up to 1 mL in 0.02 mL increments. Do not give intravenously; thrombus formation or pulmonary embolism may occur.

Stability

Storage: Store at 15°C to 30°C (59°F to 86°F).

Nursing Actions

Physical Assessment: Monitor patient closely for 90 minutes following each test dose (eg, orthostatic hypotension). Premedication with antiemetic is required prior to each dose. Monitor for therapeutic effectiveness and adverse response (eg, orthostatic hypotension, nausea, vomiting, dyskinesias, excessive sedation or somnolence) at beginning of therapy, with each change in dose, and at regular intervals during therapy. Teach patient (or caregiver) proper use (injection pen or syringe, needle disposal), possible side effects/appropriate interventions, and adverse symptoms to report.

Patient Education: Do not take any new medications during therapy without consulting prescriber. Follow specific directions for administration with injection pen or syringe and needle disposal. Avoid alcohol while taking Apokyn™. An antiemetic may be prescribed to reduce nausea or vomiting; take as directed. May cause headache, drowsiness, or dizziness (use caution when climbing stairs, driving, or engaged in potentially hazardous tasks until response to drug is known); postural hypotension (use caution climbing stairs or when changing position from lying or sitting to standing); or nausea or vomiting (if antiemetic medication does not relieve this, contact prescriber). Report immediately any irregular or rapid heartbeat, chest pain, palpitations, difficulty breathing, shortness of breath; unusual or sudden sleepiness; unusual muscle or skeletal movements or weakness, tremors, or altered gait; CNS changes (hallucinations, confusion, insomnia, anxiety, or depression); redness, swelling, or irritation at injection site; or other persistent side effects. **Pregnancy/breast-feeding precautions:** Inform prescriber if you are or intend to become pregnant. Breast-feeding is contraindicated.

Dietary Considerations Avoid ethanol consumption.

Apraclonidine (a pra KLOE ni deen)

U.S. Brand Names Iopidine®
Synonyms Aplonidine; Apraclonidine Hydrochloride; p-Aminoclonidine
Pharmacologic Category Alpha$_2$ Agonist, Ophthalmic
Medication Safety Issues
Sound-alike/look-alike issues:
Iopidine® may be confused with indapamide, iodine, Lodine®
Pregnancy Risk Factor C
Lactation Excretion in breast milk unknown/use caution
Use Prevention and treatment of postsurgical intraocular pressure (IOP) elevation; short-term, adjunctive therapy in patients who require additional reduction of IOP
Mechanism of Action/Effect Apraclonidine is a potent alpha-adrenergic agent similar to clonidine; relatively selective for alpha$_2$-receptors but does retain some binding to alpha$_1$-receptors; appears to result in reduction of aqueous humor formation; its penetration through the blood-brain barrier is more polar than clonidine which reduces its penetration through the blood-brain barrier and suggests that its pharmacological profile is characterized by peripheral rather than central effects.
Contraindications Hypersensitivity to apraclonidine, clonidine, or any component of the formulation; use with or within 14 days of MAO inhibitors
Warnings/Precautions IOP-lowering efficacy decreases over time in some patients. Most patients will experience decreased benefit from therapy lasting longer than 1 month. Closely monitor patients who develop exaggerated reductions in intraocular pressure. Use with caution in patients with cardiovascular disease, coronary insufficiency, recent myocardial infarction, cerebrovascular disease, history of vasovagal reactions, Raynaud's disease, thromboangiitis obliterans, depression, chronic renal failure, or severe renal or hepatic impairment.
Drug Interactions
Increased Effect/Toxicity: Topical beta-blockers, pilocarpine may have an additive effect on intraocular pressure. Apraclonidine may reduce pulse and blood pressure; use systemic agents with caution. Adverse effects may be additive with CNS-depressant agents. Use with MAO inhibitors is contraindicated.
Adverse Reactions
Ocular:
5% to 15%: Discomfort, hyperemia, pruritus
1% to 5%: Blanching, blurred vision, conjunctivitis, discharge, dry eye, foreign body sensation, lid edema, tearing
Other body systems:
1% to 10%: Gastrointestinal: Dry mouth (10%)
<3%:
Cardiovascular: Arrhythmia, chest pain, facial edema, peripheral edema
Central nervous system: Depression, dizziness, headache, insomnia, malaise, nervousness, somnolence
Dermatologic: Contact dermatitis, dermatitis
Gastrointestinal: Constipation, nausea, taste perversion
Neuromuscular & skeletal: Abnormal coordination, myalgia, paresthesia, weakness
Respiratory: Asthma, dry nose, dyspnea, parosmia, pharyngitis, rhinitis
Overdosage/Toxicology Bradycardia, drowsiness, and hypothermia have been reported following ingestion of the ophthalmic solution.
Pharmacodynamics/Kinetics
Onset of Action: 1 hour; Peak effect: Decreased intraocular pressure: 3-5 hours
Half-Life Elimination: Systemic: 8 hours
Available Dosage Forms Solution, ophthalmic, as hydrochloride: 0.5% (5 mL, 10 mL); 1% (0.1 mL) [contains benzalkonium chloride]

Dosing
Adults & Elderly: Postsurgical intraocular pressure elevation (prevention/treatment): Ophthalmic:
0.5%: Instill 1-2 drops in the affected eye(s) 3 times/day
1%: Instill 1 drop in operative eye 1 hour prior to anterior segment laser surgery, second drop in eye immediately upon completion of procedure
Renal Impairment: Although the topical use of apraclonidine has not been studied in renal failure patients, structurally-related clonidine undergoes a significant increase in half-life in patients with renal impairment. Close monitoring of cardiovascular parameters in patients with impaired renal function is advised.
Hepatic Impairment: Close monitoring of cardiovascular parameters in patients with impaired liver function is advised because the systemic dosage form of clonidine is partially metabolized in the liver.
Administration
Other: Wait 5 minutes between instillation of other ophthalmic agents to avoid washout of previous dose. After topical instillation, finger pressure should be applied to lacrimal sac to decrease drainage into the nose and throat and minimize possible systemic absorption.
Stability
Storage: Store between 2°C to 27°C (36°F to 80°F). Protect from freezing and light.
Nursing Actions
Physical Assessment: Assess potential for interactions with other pharmacological agents patient may be taking. Monitor patient response and adverse effects (ocular and other systems; see Adverse Reactions). Teach patient proper use, side effects/appropriate interventions, and adverse symptoms to report.
Patient Education: For use in eyes only. May sting on instillation, do not touch dropper to eye. Visual acuity may be decreased after administration. Night vision may be decreased. Distance vision may be altered. Read package instructions for insertion. **Pregnancy/breast-feeding precautions:** Inform prescriber if you are or intend to become pregnancy. Consult prescriber if breast-feeding.

Aprepitant (ap RE pi tant)

U.S. Brand Names Emend®
Synonyms L 754030; MK 869
Pharmacologic Category Antiemetic; Substance P/Neurokinin 1 Receptor Antagonist
Pregnancy Risk Factor B
Lactation Excretion in breast milk unknown/not recommended
Use Prevention of acute and delayed nausea and vomiting associated with moderately- and highly-emetogenic chemotherapy in combination with a corticosteroid and 5-HT$_3$ receptor antagonist
Mechanism of Action/Effect Prevents acute and delayed vomiting at the substance P/neurokinin 1 (NK$_1$) receptor.
Contraindications Hypersensitivity to aprepitant or any component of the formulation; use with cisapride or pimozide
Warnings/Precautions Use caution with agents primarily metabolized via CYP3A4. Use caution with hepatic impairment. Not intended for treatment of nausea and vomiting or for chronic continuous therapy. Safety and efficacy in pediatric patients have not been established.
Drug Interactions
Cytochrome P450 Effect: Substrate of CYP1A2 (minor), 2C19 (minor), 3A4 (major); **Inhibits** CYP2C8/

9 (weak), 2C19 (weak), 3A4 (moderate); **Induces** CYP2C9 (weak), 3A4 (weak)

Decreased Effect: CYP3A4 inducers may decrease the levels/effects of aprepitant; example inducers include aminoglutethimide, carbamazepine, nafcillin, nevirapine, phenobarbital, phenytoin, and rifamycins. Metabolism of warfarin may be induced; monitor INR following the start of each cycle. Efficacy of oral contraceptives may be decreased (plasma levels of ethinyl estradiol and norethindrone decreased with concomitant use).

Increased Effect/Toxicity: Use with cisapride or pimozide is contraindicated. CYP3A4 inhibitors may increase the levels/effects of aprepitant; example inhibitors include azole antifungals, clarithromycin, diclofenac, diltiazem, doxycycline, erythromycin, imatinib, isoniazid, nefazodone, nicardipine, propofol, protease inhibitors, quinidine, telithromycin, and verapamil. Aprepitant may increase the bioavailability of corticosteroids; dose adjustment of dexamethasone and methylprednisolone is needed. Aprepitant may increase the levels/effects of CYP3A4 substrates; example substrates include benzodiazepines, calcium channel blockers, ergot derivatives, mirtazapine, nateglinide, nefazodone, tacrolimus, and venlafaxine.

Nutritional/Ethanol Interactions

Food: Aprepitant serum concentration may be increased when taken with grapefruit juice; avoid concurrent use.

Herb/Nutraceutical: St John's wort may decrease aprepitant levels.

Adverse Reactions Note: Adverse reaction percentages reported as part of combination chemotherapy regimen.

>10%:

Central nervous system: Fatigue (18% to 22%)

Dermatologic: Alopecia (24%; placebo 22%)

Gastrointestinal: Nausea (7% to 13%), constipation (10% to 12%)

Neuromuscular & skeletal: Weakness (3% to 18%)

Miscellaneous: Hiccups (11%)

1% to 10%:

Central nervous system: Dizziness (3% to 7%)

Endocrine & metabolic: Dehydration (6%), hot flushing (3%)

Gastrointestinal: Diarrhea (6% to 10%), dyspepsia (8%), abdominal pain (5%), stomatitis (5%), epigastric discomfort (4%), gastritis (4%), mucous membrane disorder (3%), throat pain (3%)

Hematologic: Neutropenia (3% to 9%), leukopenia (9%), hemoglobin decreased (2% to 5%)

Hepatic: ALT increased (6%), AST increased (3%)

Renal: BUN increased (5%), proteinuria (7%), serum creatinine increased (4%)

Overdosage/Toxicology Limited data available; single doses to 600 mg and daily doses of 375 mg for up to 42 days were well-tolerated in healthy subjects; drowsiness and headache were noted at a dose of 1440 mg. In cancer patients, a single dose of 375 mg followed by 250 mg on days 2 to 5 was well tolerated. In case of overdose, treatment should be symptom-directed and supportive. Not removed by hemodialysis.

Pharmacodynamics/Kinetics

Time to Peak: Plasma: 4 hours

Protein Binding: >95%

Half-Life Elimination: Terminal: 9-13 hours

Metabolism: Extensively hepatic via CYP3A4 (major); CYP1A2 and CYP2C19 (minor); forms seven metabolites (weakly active)

Available Dosage Forms

Capsule: 80 mg, 125 mg

Combination package: Capsule 80 mg (2s), capsule 125 mg (1s)

Dosing

Adults & Elderly: Antiemetic: Oral: 125 mg on day 1, followed by 80 mg on days 2 and 3; should be used in combination with a corticosteroid and 5-HT$_3$ receptor antagonist

In clinical trials, the following regimens were used:

For highly-emetogenic chemotherapy:

Aprepitant: Oral: 125 mg on day 1, followed by 80 mg on days 2 and 3

Dexamethasone: Oral: 12 mg on day 1, followed 8 mg on days 2, 3, and 4

Ondansetron: I.V.: 32 mg on day 1

For moderately-emetogenic chemotherapy:

Aprepitant: Oral: 125 mg on day 1, followed by 80 mg on days 2 and 3

Dexamethasone: Oral: 12 mg on day 1 only

Ondansetron: Oral: Two 8 mg doses on day 1 only

Renal Impairment: No dose adjustment necessary in patients with renal disease or end-stage renal disease maintained on hemodialysis.

Hepatic Impairment:

Mild-to-moderate impairment (Child-Pugh score 5-9): No adjustment necessary.

Severe impairment (Child-Pugh score >9): No data available.

Administration

Oral: May be administered with or without food. First dose should be given 1 hour prior to chemotherapy; subsequent doses should be given in the morning.

Stability

Storage: Store at controlled room temperature of 20°C to 25°C (68°F to 77°F).

Nursing Actions

Physical Assessment: To be used in combination with other medications (corticosteroid and 5-HT$_3$ receptor antagonist). Assess potential for interactions with pharmacological agents or herbal products patient may be taking. Monitor therapeutic effectiveness (decreased nausea/vomiting) and adverse effects (fatigue, weakness, gastrointestinal upset, dehydration). Teach patient proper use, possible side effects/appropriate interventions, and adverse symptoms to report.

Patient Education: This medication will be prescribed in combination with other medications; follow directions and timing exactly. May take with or without food; avoid grapefruit juice and St John's wort while taking this medication. Report unusual fatigue, weakness, dizziness, disorientation, abdominal discomfort, chest pain, respiratory distress, or other persistent side effects to prescriber. **Breast-feeding precautions:** Breast-feeding is not recommended.

Dietary Considerations May be taken with or without food.

Geriatric Considerations In two studies by the manufacturer, with a total of 544 patients, 31% were >65 years of age, while 5% were >75 years. No differences in safety and efficacy were noted between elderly subjects and younger adults. No dosing adjustment is necessary.

Argatroban (ar GA troh ban)

Pharmacologic Category Anticoagulant, Thrombin Inhibitor

Medication Safety Issues

Sound-alike/look-alike issues:

Argatroban may be confused with Aggrastat®

Pregnancy Risk Factor B

Lactation Excretion in breast milk unknown/not recommended

(Continued)

Argatroban *(Continued)*

Use Prophylaxis or treatment of thrombosis in adults with heparin-induced thrombocytopenia; adjunct to percutaneous coronary intervention (PCI) in patients who have or are at risk of thrombosis associated with heparin-induced thrombocytopenia

Mechanism of Action/Effect A direct, highly-selective thrombin inhibitor. Reversibly binds to the active thrombin site of free and clot-associated thrombin. Inhibits fibrin formation; activation of coagulation factors V, VIII, and XIII; protein C; and platelet aggregation.

Contraindications Hypersensitivity to argatroban or any component of the formulation; overt major bleeding

Warnings/Precautions Hemorrhage can occur at any site in the body. Extreme caution should be used when there is an increased danger of hemorrhage, such as severe hypertension, immediately following lumbar puncture, spinal anesthesia, major surgery (including brain, spinal cord, or eye surgery), congenital or acquired bleeding disorders, and gastrointestinal ulcers. Use caution in critically-ill patients; reduced clearance may require dosage reduction. Use caution with hepatic dysfunction. Concomitant use with warfarin will cause increased prolongation of the PT and INR greater than that of warfarin alone; alternative guidelines for monitoring therapy should be followed. Safety and efficacy for use with other thrombolytic agents has not been established. Discontinue all parenteral anticoagulants prior to starting therapy. Allow reversal of heparin's effects before initiation. Patients with hepatic dysfunction may require >4 hours to achieve full reversal of argatroban's anticoagulant effect following treatment. Avoid use during PCI in patients with elevations of ALT/AST (>3 times ULN); the use of argatroban in these patients has not been evaluated. Safety and efficacy in children <18 years of age have not been established.

Drug Interactions

Cytochrome P450 Effect: Substrate of CYP3A4 (minor)

Increased Effect/Toxicity: Drugs which affect platelet function (eg, aspirin, NSAIDs, dipyridamole, ticlopidine, clopidogrel), anticoagulants, or thrombolytics may potentiate the risk of hemorrhage. Sufficient time must pass after heparin therapy is discontinued; allow heparin's effect on the aPTT to decrease.

Concomitant use of argatroban with warfarin increases PT and INR greater than that of warfarin alone. Argatroban is commonly continued during the initiation of warfarin therapy to assure anticoagulation and to protect against possible transient hypercoagulability.

Adverse Reactions As with all anticoagulants, bleeding is the major adverse effect of argatroban. Hemorrhage may occur at virtually any site. Risk is dependent on multiple variables, including the intensity of anticoagulation and patient susceptibility.

>10%:

Cardiovascular: Chest pain (<1% to 15%), hypotension (7% to 11%)

Gastrointestinal: Gastrointestinal bleed (minor, 3% to 14%)

Genitourinary: Genitourinary bleed and hematuria (minor, 2% to 12%)

1% to 10%:

Cardiovascular: Cardiac arrest (6%), ventricular tachycardia (5%), bradycardia (5%), myocardial infarction (PCI: 4%), atrial fibrillation (3%), angina (2%), CABG-related bleeding (minor, 2%), myocardial ischemia (2%), cerebrovascular disorder (<1% to 2%), thrombosis (<1% to 2%)

Central nervous system: Fever (<1% to 7%), headache (5%), pain (5%), intracranial bleeding (1% to 4%)

Gastrointestinal: Nausea (5% to 7%), diarrhea (6%), vomiting (4% to 6%), abdominal pain (3% to 4%), bleeding (major, <1% to 2%)

Genitourinary: Urinary tract infection (5%)

Hematologic: Hemoglobin (<2 g/dL) and hematocrit (minor, 2% to 10%) decreased

Local: Bleeding at injection or access site (minor, 2% to 5%)

Neuromuscular & skeletal: Back pain (8%)

Renal: Abnormal renal function (3%)

Respiratory: Dyspnea (8% to 10%), cough (3% to 10%), hemoptysis (minor, <1% to 3%), pneumonia (3%)

Miscellaneous: Sepsis (6%), infection (4%)

Overdosage/Toxicology No specific antidote is available. Treatment should be symptomatic and supportive. Discontinue or decrease infusion to control excessive anticoagulation with or without bleeding. Reversal of anticoagulant effects may be longer than 4 hours in patients with hepatic impairment. Hemodialysis may remove up to 20% of the drug; however, this is considered clinically insignificant.

Pharmacodynamics/Kinetics

Onset of Action: Immediate

Time to Peak: Steady-state: 1-3 hours

Protein Binding: Albumin: 20%; α_1-acid glycoprotein: 35%

Half-Life Elimination: 39-51 minutes; Hepatic impairment: ≤181 minutes

Metabolism: Hepatic via hydroxylation and aromatization. Metabolism via CYP3A4/5 to four known metabolites plays a minor role. Unchanged argatroban is the major plasma component. Plasma concentration of metabolite M1 is 0% to 20% of the parent drug and is three- to fivefold weaker.

Excretion: Feces (65%); urine (22%); low quantities of metabolites M2-4 in urine

Available Dosage Forms Injection, solution: 100 mg/mL (2.5 mL) [contains dehydrated alcohol 1000 mg/mL]

Dosing

Adults & Elderly:

Prophylaxis of thrombosis (heparin-induced thrombocytopenia): I.V.:

Initial dose: 2 mcg/kg/minute

Maintenance dose: Measure aPTT after 2 hours, adjust dose until the steady-state aPTT is 1.5-3.0 times the initial baseline value, not exceeding 100 seconds; dosage should not exceed 10 mcg/kg/minute

Conversion to oral anticoagulant: Because there may be a combined effect on the INR when argatroban is combined with warfarin, loading doses of warfarin should not be used. Warfarin therapy should be started at the expected daily dose.

Patients receiving ≤2 mcg/kg/minute of argatroban: Argatroban therapy can be stopped when the combined INR on warfarin and argatroban is >4; repeat INR measurement in 4-6 hours; if INR is below therapeutic level, argatroban therapy may be restarted. Repeat procedure daily until desired INR on warfarin alone is obtained.

Patients receiving >2 mcg/kg/minute of argatroban: Reduce dose of argatroban to 2 mcg/kg/minute; measure INR for argatroban and warfarin 4-6 hours after dose reduction; argatroban therapy can be stopped when the combined INR on warfarin and argatroban is >4. Repeat INR measurement in 4-6 hours; if INR is below therapeutic level, argatroban therapy may be restarted. Repeat procedure daily until desired INR on warfarin alone is obtained.

Note: Critically-ill patients with normal hepatic function became excessively anticoagulated with

FDA-approved or lower starting doses of argatroban (Reichert MG, 2003). Doses between 0.15-1.3 mcg/kg/minute were required to maintain aPTTs in the target range. Another report of a cardiac patient with anasarca secondary to acute renal failure had a reduction in argatroban clearance similar to patients with hepatic dysfunction (de Denus S, 2003). Reduced clearance may have been attributed to reduced perfusion to the liver. Consider reducing starting dose to 0.5-1 mcg/kg/minute in critically-ill patients who may have impaired hepatic perfusion (eg, patients requiring vasopressors, having decreased cardiac output, having fluid overload). In a retrospective review of critical care patients (Baghdasarian, 2004), patients with three organ system failure required 0.5 mcg/kg/minute. The mean argatroban dose of ICU patients was 0.9 mcg/kg/minute.

Percutaneous coronary intervention (PCI): I.V.:

Initial: Begin infusion of 25 mcg/minute and administer bolus dose of 350 mcg/kg (over 3-5 minutes). ACT should be checked 5-10 minutes after bolus infusion; proceed with procedure if ACT >300 seconds. Following initial bolus:

ACT <300 seconds: Give an additional 150 mcg/kg bolus, and increase infusion rate to 30 mcg/kg/minute (recheck ACT in 5-10 minutes)

ACT >450 seconds: Decrease infusion rate to 15 mcg/kg/minute (recheck ACT in 5-10 minutes)

Once a therapeutic ACT (300-450 seconds) is achieved, infusion should be continued at this dose for the duration of the procedure.

If dissection, impending abrupt closure, thrombus formation during PCI, or inability to achieve ACT >300 sec: An additional bolus of 150 mcg/kg, followed by an increase in infusion rate to 40 mcg/kg/minute may be administered.

Note: Post-PCI anticoagulation, if required, may be achieved by continuing infusion at a reduced dose of 2-10 mcg/kg/minute, with close monitoring of aPTT.

Renal Impairment: Removal during hemodialysis and continuous venovenous hemofiltration is clinically insignificant. No dosage adjustment required.

Hepatic Impairment: Decreased clearance and increased elimination half-life are seen with hepatic impairment; dose should be reduced. Initial dose for moderate hepatic impairment is 0.5 mcg/kg/minute.

Note: During PCI, avoid use in patients with elevations of ALT/AST (>3 times ULN); the use of argatroban in these patients has not been evaluated.

Administration

I.V.: Solution **must be diluted to 1 mg/mL** prior to administration.

Stability

Reconstitution: May be mixed with 0.9% sodium chloride injection, 5% dextrose injection, or lactated Ringer's injection. Do not mix with other medications. To prepare solution for I.V. administration, dilute each 250 mg vial with 250 mL of diluent. Mix by repeated inversion for one minute. Once mixed, final concentration should be 1 mg/mL. A slight but brief haziness may occur prior to mixing.

Compatibility: Stable in 0.9% NS, D₅W, LR

Y-site administration: Incompatible with other medications

Compatibility when admixed: Incompatible with other medications

Storage: Prior to use, store at 15°C to 30°C (59°F to 86°F). Protect from light. The prepared solution is stable for 24 hours at 15°C to 30°C (59°F to 86°F) in ambient indoor light. Do not expose to direct sunlight. Prepared solutions that are protected from light and kept at controlled room temperature of 20°C to 25°C (68°F to 77°F) or under refrigeration at 2°C to 8°C (36°F to 46°F) are stable for up to 96 hours.

Laboratory Monitoring Hemoglobin, hematocrit

Nursing Actions

Physical Assessment: Assess potential for interactions with other pharmacological agents patient may be taking (especially drugs that affect platelet function or coagulation). Monitor therapeutic effectiveness (eg, laboratory results) and adverse reactions (abnormal bleeding, GI pain, epistaxis, hematuria, irritation at infusion site) frequently during therapy. Observe bleeding precautions and teach patient interventions to reduce side effects and adverse reactions to report.

Patient Education: This medication can only be administered by intravenous infusion and you will be monitored with blood tests during therapy. You may have a tendency to bleed easily; use electric razor, brush teeth with soft brush, floss with waxed floss, avoid all scissors or sharp instruments (knives, needles, etc), and avoid injury or bruising. Report stomach cramping or pain; dark or bloody stools; blood in urine; acute headache or confusion; respiratory difficulty; nosebleed; or bleeding from gums. **Breast-feeding precaution:** Breast-feeding is not recommended.

Breast-Feeding Issues It is not known if argatroban is excreted in human milk. Because of the serious potential of adverse effects to the nursing infant, a decision to discontinue nursing or discontinue argatroban should be considered.

Additional Information Platelet counts recovered by day 3 in 53% of patients with heparin-induced thrombocytopenia and in 58% of patients with heparin-induced thrombocytopenia with thrombosis syndrome.

Aripiprazole (ay ri PIP ray zole)

U.S. Brand Names Abilify®

Synonyms BMS 337039; OPC-14597

Pharmacologic Category Antipsychotic Agent, Atypical

Medication Safety Issues

Sound-alike/look-alike issues:

Aripiprazole may be confused with proton pump inhibitors (eg, rabeprazole)

Pregnancy Risk Factor C

Lactation Excretion in breast milk unknown/not recommended

Use Treatment of schizophrenia; stabilization and maintenance therapy of bipolar disorder (with acute manic or mixed episodes)

Unlabeled/Investigational Use Depression with psychotic features

Mechanism of Action/Effect Aripiprazole (quinolinone antipsychotic) is a dopamine-serotonin system stabilizer with activity at dopamine and serotonin receptors. It improves symptoms of schizophrenia.

Contraindications Hypersensitivity to aripiprazole or any component of the formulation

Warnings/Precautions Patients with dementia-related behavioral disorders treated with atypical antipsychotics are at an increased risk of death compared to placebo. Aripiprazole is not approved for this indication.

May cause extrapyramidal symptoms, including pseudoparkinsonism, acute dystonic reactions, akathisia, and tardive dyskinesia (risk of these reactions is very low relative to typical/conventional antipsychotics, frequencies reported are similar to placebo). May be associated with neuroleptic malignant syndrome (NMS).

May be sedating, use with caution in disorders where CNS depression is a feature. May cause orthostatic hypotension (although reported rates are similar to (Continued)

Aripiprazole *(Continued)*

placebo); use caution in patients at risk of this effect or those who would not tolerate transient hypotensive episodes (cerebrovascular disease, cardiovascular disease, or other medications which may predispose). Clinical data have demonstrated an increased incidence of serious, including fatal, cerebrovascular events in elderly patients.

Use caution in patients with Parkinson's disease; hemodynamic instability; bone marrow suppression; predisposition to seizures; subcortical brain damage; and severe cardiac, hepatic, renal, or respiratory disease. Esophageal dysmotility and aspiration have been associated with antipsychotic use; use caution in patients at risk of pneumonia (ie, Alzheimer's disease). May alter temperature regulation or mask toxicity of other drugs due to antiemetic effects. Use caution in patients with a history of drug abuse.

Atypical antipsychotics have been associated with development of hyperglycemia; in some cases, may be extreme and associated with ketoacidosis, hyperosmolar coma, or death. Reports of hyperglycemia with aripiprazole therapy have been few and specific risk associated with this agent is not known. Use caution in patients with diabetes or other disorders of glucose regulation; monitor for worsening of glucose control.

The possibility of a suicide attempt is inherent in psychotic illness or bipolar disorder; use caution in high-risk patients during initiation of therapy. Prescriptions should be written for the smallest quantity consistent with good patient care. Safety and efficacy in pediatric patients have not been established.

Drug Interactions
Cytochrome P450 Effect: Substrate (major) of CYP2D6, 3A4
Decreased Effect: CYP3A4 inducers may decrease the levels/effects of aripiprazole; example inducers include aminoglutethimide, carbamazepine, nafcillin, nevirapine, phenobarbital, phenytoin, and rifamycins. Manufacturer recommends a doubling of the aripiprazole dose when carbamazepine is added. Similar increases may be required with other inducers.

Increased Effect/Toxicity: CYP2D6 inhibitors may increase the levels/effects of aripiprazole; example inhibitors include chlorpromazine, delavirdine, fluoxetine, miconazole, paroxetine, pergolide, quinidine, quinine, ritonavir, and ropinirole. CYP3A4 inhibitors may increase the levels/effects of aripiprazole; example inhibitors include azole antifungals, clarithromycin, diclofenac, doxycycline, erythromycin, imatinib, isoniazid, nefazodone, nicardipine, propofol, protease inhibitors, quinidine, telithromycin, and verapamil. Manufacturer recommends a 50% reduction in dose during concurrent ketoconazole therapy. Similar reductions in dose may be required with other potent inhibitors. Acetylcholinesterase inhibitors (central) may increase the risk of antipsychotic-related extrapyramidal symptoms.

Nutritional/Ethanol Interactions
Ethanol: Avoid ethanol (may increase CNS depression).
Food: Ingestion with a high-fat meal delays time to peak plasma level.
Herb/Nutraceutical: St John's wort may decrease aripiprazole levels. Avoid kava kava, gotu kola, valerian, St John's wort (may increase CNS depression).

Adverse Reactions
>10%:
Central nervous system: Headache (31%), agitation (25%), anxiety (20%), insomnia (20%), extrapyramidal symptoms (6% to 17%), somnolence (12% to 15%, dose related), akathisia (12%), lightheadedness (11%)
Gastrointestinal: Nausea (16%), dyspepsia (15%), constipation (11%), vomiting (11%), weight gain

(8% to 30%, highest frequency in patients with BMI <23):
1% to 10%:
Cardiovascular: Edema (peripheral 2%), hypertension (2%), tachycardia, hypotension, bradycardia, chest pain
Central nervous system: Fever, depression, nervousness, mania, confusion, hallucination, hostility, paranoid reaction, suicidal thought, delusion, abnormal dream
Dermatologic: Dry skin, skin ulcer
Endocrine & metabolic: Dehydration
Gastrointestinal: Salivation increased (3%), weight loss
Genitourinary: Urinary incontinence, pelvic pain
Hematologic: Anemia, bruising
Neuromuscular & skeletal: Tremor (4% to 9%), weakness (8%), myalgia (4%), neck pain, neck rigidity, muscle cramp, CPK increased, abnormal gait
Ocular: Blurred vision (3%), conjunctivitis
Respiratory: Rhinitis (4%), pharyngitis (4%), cough (3%), asthma, dyspnea, pneumonia, sinusitis
Miscellaneous: Accidental injury (5%), flu-like syndrome, diaphoresis

Overdosage/Toxicology Seventy-six cases of accidental or deliberate overdose have been reported world-wide, with no reported fatalities. Ingestion of 1080 mg has been reported, with full recovery. Common symptoms of overdose include somnolence, tremor, and vomiting. Treatment is supportive and symptom-directed. An ECG should be obtained and cardiac monitoring initiated if QT_c prolongation is present. Administration of 50 g activated charcoal 1 hour after a 15 mg dose reportedly decreased AUC and C_{max} values by 50%. Due to the high degree of protein binding, hemodialysis is unlikely to be effective in removing aripiprazole.

Pharmacodynamics/Kinetics
Onset of Action: Initial: 1-3 weeks
Time to Peak: Plasma: 3-5 hours; delayed with high-fat meal (aripiprazole: 3 hours; dehydro-aripiprazole: 12 hours)
Protein Binding: 99%, primarily to albumin
Half-Life Elimination:
Aripiprazole: 75 hours; dehydro-aripiprazole: 94 hours
CYP2D6 poor metabolizers: Aripiprazole: 146 hours
Metabolism: Hepatic, via CYP2D6, CYP3A4 (dehydro-aripiprazole metabolite has affinity for D_2 receptors similar to the parent drug and represents 40% of the parent drug exposure in plasma)
Excretion: Feces (55%), urine (25%); primarily as metabolites

Available Dosage Forms
Solution, oral: 1 mg/mL (150 mL) [contains sucrose 400 mg/mL and fructose 200 mg/mL; orange cream flavor]
Tablet: 2 mg, 5 mg, 10 mg, 15 mg, 20 mg, 30 mg

Dosing
Adults & Elderly: Note: Oral solution may be substituted for the oral tablet on a mg-per-mg basis, up to 25 mg. Patients receiving 30 mg tablets should be given 25 mg oral solution.

Schizophrenia: Oral: 10-15 mg once daily; may be increased to a maximum of 30 mg once daily (efficacy at dosages above 10-15 mg has not been shown to be increased). Dosage titration should not be more frequent than every 2 weeks.
Bipolar disorder (acute manic or mixed episodes):
Stabilization: Oral: 30 mg once daily; may require a decrease to 15 mg based on tolerability (15% of patients had dose decreased); safety of doses >30 mg/day has not been evaluated
Maintenance: Continue stabilization dose for up to 6 weeks; efficacy of continued treatment >6 weeks has not been established.

Dosage adjustment with concurrent CYP3A4 inducer therapy:

CYP3A4 inducers (eg, carbamazepine): Aripiprazole dose should be doubled (20-30 mg/day); dose should be subsequently reduced (10-15 mg/day) if concurrent inducer agent discontinued.

CYP3A4 inhibitors (eg, ketoconazole): Aripiprazole dose should be reduced to $^1/_2$ of the usual dose, and proportionally increased upon discontinuation of the inhibitor agent.

CYP2D6 inhibitors (eg, fluoxetine, paroxetine): Aripiprazole dose should be reduced to $^1/_2$ of the usual dose, and proportionally increased upon discontinuation of the inhibitor agent.

Renal Impairment: No dosage adjustment required.

Hepatic Impairment: No dosage adjustment required.

Administration

Oral: May be administered with or without food. Tablet and oral solution may be interchanged on a mg-per-mg basis, up to 25 mg. Doses using 30 mg tablets should be exchanged for 25 mg oral solution.

Stability

Storage:

Oral solution: Store at 25°C (77°F); excursions permitted to 15°C to 30°C (59°F to 86°F). Use within 6 months after opening.

Tablet: Store at 25°C (77°F); excursions permitted to 15°C to 30°C (59°F to 86°F).

Laboratory Monitoring Fasting lipid profile and fasting blood glucose/Hb A_{1c} (prior to treatment, at 3 months, then annually); BMI

Nursing Actions

Physical Assessment: Assess vital signs, blood pressure, mental status, thoughts of suicide ideation, abnormal involuntary movements, and extrapyramidal symptoms. Weight and waist circumference should be assessed prior to treatment, at 4 weeks, 8 weeks, 12 weeks, and then at quarterly intervals. This drug may alter glucose regulation and control. Monitor closely. Assess potential for interactions with other prescriptions, OTC medications, or herbal products patient may be taking. Monitor therapeutic effectiveness and adverse response (eg, extrapyramidal symptoms, neuroleptic malignant syndrome) at beginning of and at regular intervals during therapy. Teach patient proper use, possible side effects/appropriate interventions, and adverse symptoms to report.

Patient Education: Do not take any new medication during therapy without consulting prescriber. Take exactly as directed at the same time of day, without regard to meals. Do not alter dose; it may take some time to achieve desired results. Avoid alcohol. May cause headache, dizziness, lightheadedness, anxiety (use caution when driving or engaged in potentially hazardous tasks until response to drug is known), nausea or vomiting (small frequent meals and frequent mouth care may help), or orthostatic hypotension (use caution when changing position from lying or sitting to standing and when climbing stairs). Report chest pain or palpitations; persistent gastrointestinal effects; muscle or skeletal pain, weakness, cramping, or tremors; involuntary movements, altered gait; change in vision; change in mental status (especially suicide ideation); increased weight gain or loss; or respiratory changes or flu-like symptoms.

Dietary Considerations May be taken with or without food. Oral solution contains sucrose 400 mg/mL and fructose 200 mg/mL.

Geriatric Considerations Elderly patients have an increased risk of adverse response to side effects or adverse reactions to antipsychotics. Aripiprazole has been studied in elderly patients with psychosis associated with Alzheimer's disease. The package insert does not provide the outcomes of this study other than somnolence was more frequent with aripiprazole (8%) than placebo (1%). Clinical data have shown an increased incidence of serious cerebrovascular events in the elderly, some fatal. Aripiprazole's delayed onset of action and long half-life may limit its role in treating older persons with psychosis.

Pregnancy Issues Aripiprazole demonstrated developmental toxicity and teratogenic effects in animal models. There are no adequate and well-controlled trials in pregnant women. Should be used in pregnancy only when potential benefit to mother outweighs possible risk to the fetus.

Arsenic Trioxide (AR se nik tri OKS id)

U.S. Brand Names Trisenox™

Synonyms As_2O_3; NSC-706363

Pharmacologic Category Antineoplastic Agent, Miscellaneous

Pregnancy Risk Factor D

Lactation Excretion in breast milk unknown/contraindicated

Use Induction of remission and consolidation in patients with relapsed or refractory acute promyelocytic leukemia (APL) which is specifically characterized by t(15;17) translocation or PML/RAR-alpha gene expression.

Orphan drug: Treatment of myelodysplastic syndrome; multiple myeloma; chronic myeloid leukemia (CML); acute myelocytic leukemia (AML)

Mechanism of Action/Effect Not fully understood; causes *in vitro* morphological changes and DNA fragmentation to NB4 human promyelocytic leukemia cells; also damages or degrades the fusion protein PML-RAR alpha

Contraindications Hypersensitivity to arsenic or any component of the formulation; pregnancy

Warnings/Precautions Hazardous agent — use appropriate precautions for handling and disposal. May prolong the QT interval. A baseline 12-lead ECG, serum electrolytes (potassium, calcium, magnesium), and creatinine should be obtained. Correct electrolyte abnormalities prior to treatment and monitor potassium and magnesium levels during therapy (potassium should stay >4 mEq/dL and magnesium >1.8 mg/dL). Correct QT_c >500 msec prior to treatment. Discontinue therapy and hospitalize patient if QT_c >500 msec, syncope, or irregular heartbeats develop during therapy; do not reinitiate until QT_c<460 msec. May lead to torsade de pointes or complete AV block. Risk factors for torsade de pointes include CHF, a history of torsade de pointes, pre-existing QT interval prolongation, patients taking potassium-wasting diuretics, and conditions which cause hypokalemia or hypomagnesemia. If possible, discontinue all medications known to prolong the QT interval. May cause retinoic-acid-acute promyelocytic leukemia (RA-APL) syndrome or APL differentiation syndrome; high-dose steroids (eg, dexamethasone 10 mg I.V. twice daily for at least 3 days) have been used for treatment. May lead to the development of hyperleukocytosis. Use with caution in renal impairment. Safety and efficacy in children <5 years of age have not been established (limited experience with children 5-16 years of age).

Drug Interactions

Increased Effect/Toxicity: Use caution with medications causing hypokalemia or hypomagnesemia (ampho B, aminoglycosides, diuretics, cyclosporin). Use caution with medications that prolong the QT interval, avoid concurrent use if possible; includes type Ia and type III antiarrhythmic agents, selected quinolones (sparfloxacin, gatifloxacin, moxifloxacin, grepafloxacin), cisapride, dolasetron, palonosetron, thioridazine, and other agents.

(Continued)

Arsenic Trioxide *(Continued)*

Nutritional/Ethanol Interactions Herb/Nutraceutical: Avoid homeopathic products (arsenic is present in some homeopathic medications). Avoid hypoglycemic herbs, including alfalfa, bilberry, bitter melon, burdock, celery, damiana, fenugreek, garcinai, garlic, ginger, ginseng, gymnema, marshmallow, and stinging nettle (may enhance the hypoglycemic effect of arsenic trioxide).

Adverse Reactions

>10%:

Cardiovascular: Tachycardia (55%), edema (40%), QT interval >500 msec (40%), chest pain (25%), hypotension (25%)

Central nervous system: Fatigue (63%), fever (63%), headache (60%), insomnia (43%), anxiety (30%), dizziness (23%), depression (20%), pain (15%)

Dermatologic: Dermatitis (43%), pruritus (33%), bruising (20%), dry skin (13%)

Endocrine & metabolic: Hypokalemia (50%), hyperglycemia (45%), hypomagnesemia (45%), hyperkalemia (18%)

Gastrointestinal: Nausea (75%), abdominal pain (58%), vomiting (58%), diarrhea (53%), sore throat (35% to 40%), constipation (28%), anorexia (23%), appetite decreased (15%), weight gain (13%)

Genitourinary: Vaginal hemorrhage (13%)

Hematologic: Leukocytosis (50%), APL differentiation syndrome (23%), anemia (20%), thrombocytopenia (18%), febrile neutropenia (13%)

Hepatic: ALT increased (20%), AST increased (13%)

Local: Injection site: Pain (20%), erythema (13%)

Neuromuscular & skeletal: Neuropathy (43%), rigors (38%), arthralgia (33%), paresthesia (33%), myalgia (25%), bone pain (23%), back pain (18%), limb pain (13%), neck pain (13%), tremor (13%)

Respiratory: Cough (65%), dyspnea (38% to 53%), epistaxis (25%), hypoxia (23%), pleural effusion (20%), sinusitis (20%), postnasal drip (13%), upper respiratory tract infection (13%), wheezing (13%)

Miscellaneous: Herpes simplex (13%)

1% to 10%:

Cardiovascular: Hypertension (10%), flushing (10%), pallor (10%), palpitation (10%), facial edema (8%), abnormal ECG (not QT prolongation) (7%)

Central nervous system: Convulsion (8%), somnolence (8%), agitation (5%), coma (5%), confusion (5%)

Dermatologic: Erythema (10%), hyperpigmentation (8%), petechia (8%), skin lesions (8%), urticaria (8%), local exfoliation (5%)

Endocrine & metabolic: Hypocalcemia (10%), hypoglycemia (8%), acidosis (5%)

Gastrointestinal: Dyspepsia (10%), loose stools (10%), abdominal distension (8%), abdominal tenderness (8%), xerostomia (8%), fecal incontinence (8%), gastrointestinal hemorrhage (8%), hemorrhagic diarrhea (8%), oral blistering (8%), weight loss (8%), oral candidiasis (8%)

Genitourinary: Intermenstrual bleeding (8%), incontinence (5%)

Hematologic: Neutropenia (10%), DIC (8%), hemorrhage (8%), lymphadenopathy (8%)

Local: Injection site edema (8%)

Neuromuscular & skeletal: Weakness (10%)

Ocular: Blurred vision (10%), eye irritation (10%), dry eye (8%), eyelid edema (5%), painful eye (5%)

Otic: Earache (8%), tinnitus (5%)

Renal: Renal failure (8%), renal impairment (8%), oliguria (5%)

Respiratory: Crepitations (10%), breath sounds decreased (10%), rales (10%), hemoptysis (8%), rhonchi (8%), tachypnea (8%), nasopharyngitis (5%)

Miscellaneous: Diaphoresis increased (10%), bacterial infection (8%), herpes zoster (8%), night sweats (8%), hypersensitivity (5%), sepsis (5%)

Overdosage/Toxicology Symptoms of arsenic toxicity include convulsions, muscle weakness, and confusion. Discontinue treatment and consider chelation therapy. One suggested adult protocol: Dimercaprol 3 mg/kg I.M. every 4 hours; continue until life-threatening toxicity has subsided. Follow with penicillamine 250 mg orally up to 4 times/day (total daily dose ≤1 g).

Pharmacodynamics/Kinetics

Metabolism: Hepatic; pentavalent arsenic is reduced to trivalent arsenic (active) by arsenate reductase; trivalent arsenic is methylated to monomethylarsinic acid, which is then converted to dimethylarsinic acid via methyltransferases

Excretion: Urine (as methylated metabolite); disposition not yet studied

Available Dosage Forms Injection, solution [preservative free]: 1 mg/mL (10 mL)

Dosing

Adults:

Antineoplastic:

Induction: I.V.: 0.15 mg/kg/day; administer daily until bone marrow remission; maximum induction: 60 doses

Consolidation: I.V.: 0.15 mg/kg/day starting 3-6 weeks after completion of induction therapy; maximum consolidation: 25 doses over 5 weeks

Elderly: Safety and efficacy have not been established. Clinical trials included patients ≤72 years of age. Use with caution due to the increased risk of renal impairment in the elderly.

Pediatrics: Children >5 years: Refer to adult dosing.

Renal Impairment: Safety and efficacy have not been established; use with caution due to renal elimination.

Hepatic Impairment: Safety and efficacy have not been established.

Administration

I.V.: I.V. infusion over 1-2 hours. If acute vasomotor reactions occur, infuse over a maximum of 4 hours. Does not require administration via a central venous catheter.

I.V. Detail: pH: 7.5-8.5

Stability

Reconstitution: Dilute in 100-250 mL D₅W or 0.9% NaCl. Discard unused portion.

Storage: Store at room temperature, 25°C (77°F); do not freeze. Following dilution, stable for 24 hours at room temperature or 48 hours when refrigerated.

Laboratory Monitoring Baseline then weekly 12-lead ECG, baseline then twice weekly serum electrolytes, hematologic and coagulation profiles at least twice weekly; more frequent monitoring may be necessary in unstable patients.

Nursing Actions

Physical Assessment: To be used only by physicians experienced with the treatment of acute leukemia. Assess potential for interactions with other pharmacological agents or herbal products patient may be taking (especially anything that may cause hypokalemia or hypomagnesemia, or antiarrhythmic agents). Monitor laboratory tests and patient response at beginning and periodically during therapy (especially cardiac and electrolyte status). Teach patient possible side effects/appropriate interventions and adverse symptoms to report.

Patient Education: Do not take any new medication during therapy unless approved by prescriber. This medication can only be administered by intravenous infusion. Report immediately any redness, swelling, pain, or burning at infusion site. May cause dizziness, fatigue, blurred vision (use caution when driving or engaging in tasks requiring alertness until response to drug is known); or nausea, vomiting, diarrhea, or decreased appetite (small, frequent meals, frequent mouth care, sucking lozenges, or chewing gum may help). Report immediately unexplained fever; respiratory difficulty; chest pain or palpitations; confusion, lightheadedness, or fainting; or other persistent adverse effects. **Pregnancy/breast-feeding precautions:** Inform prescriber if you are pregnant. Do not get pregnant while take this medication. Consult prescriber for appropriate contraceptive methods. Do not breast-feed.

Pregnancy Issues Animal studies have demonstrated teratogenicity and fetal loss. There are no adequate and well-controlled studies in pregnant women. May cause harm to the fetus. Pregnancy should be avoided.

Additional Information Arsenic is stored in liver, kidney, heart, lung, hair, and nails. Arsenic trioxide is a human carcinogen.

Asparaginase (a SPEAR a ji nase)

U.S. Brand Names Elspar®

Synonyms *E. coli* Asparaginase; *Erwinia* Asparaginase; L-asparaginase; NSC-106977 (*Erwinia*); NSC-109229 (*E. coli*)

Pharmacologic Category Antineoplastic Agent, Miscellaneous

Medication Safety Issues
Sound-alike/look-alike issues:
Asparaginase may be confused with pegaspargase

Pregnancy Risk Factor C

Lactation Excretion in breast milk unknown/not recommended

Use Treatment of acute lymphocytic leukemia, lymphoma

Mechanism of Action/Effect Asparaginase inhibits protein synthesis by hydrolyzing asparagine to aspartic acid and ammonia. Leukemia cells, especially lymphoblasts, require exogenous asparagine; normal cells can synthesize asparagine. Asparaginase is cycle-specific for the G_1 phase.

Contraindications Hypersensitivity to asparaginase or any component of the formulation; history of anaphylaxis to asparaginase; pancreatitis (active or any history of); if a reaction occurs to Elspar®, pegaspargase may be used cautiously

Warnings/Precautions Hazardous agent - use appropriate precautions for handling and disposal. Monitor for severe allergic reactions. May alter hepatic function. Use cautiously in patients with an underlying coagulopathy. Up to 33% of patients who have an allergic reaction to *E. coli* asparaginase will also react to the *Erwinia* form or pegaspargase.

A test dose is often recommended prior to the first dose of asparaginase, or prior to restarting therapy after a hiatus of several days. **False-negative rates of up to 80% to test doses of 2-50 units are reported.** Desensitization may be performed in patients found to be hypersensitive by the intradermal test dose or who have received previous courses of therapy with the drug.

Drug Interactions
Decreased Effect: Asparaginase terminates methotrexate action.

Increased Effect/Toxicity: Increased toxicity has been noticed when asparaginase is administered with vincristine (neuropathy) and prednisone (hyperglycemia). Decreased metabolism when used with cyclophosphamide. Increased hepatotoxicity when used with mercaptopurine.

Lab Interactions Decreased thyroxine and thyroxine-binding globulin

Adverse Reactions Note: Immediate effects: Fever, chills, nausea, and vomiting occur in 50% to 60% of patients.

>10%:
Central nervous system: Fatigue, fever, chills, somnolence, depression, hallucinations, agitation, disorientation, or convulsions (10% to 60%), stupor, confusion, coma (25%)

Endocrine & metabolic: Hyperglycemia (10%)

Gastrointestinal: Nausea, vomiting (50% to 60%), anorexia, abdominal cramps (70%), acute pancreatitis (15%, may be severe in some patients)

Hematologic: Hypofibrinogenemia and depression of clotting factors V and VIII, variable decrease in factors VII and IX, severe protein C deficiency and decrease in antithrombin III (may be dose limiting or fatal)

Hepatic: Transaminases, bilirubin, and alkaline phosphatase increased (transient)

Hypersensitivity: Acute allergic reactions (fever, rash, urticaria, arthralgia, hypotension, angioedema, bronchospasm, anaphylaxis (15% to 35%); may be dose limiting in some patients, may be fatal)

Renal: Azotemia (66%)

1% to 10%:
Endocrine & metabolic: Hyperuricemia
Gastrointestinal: Stomatitis

Overdosage/Toxicology Symptoms of overdose include nausea and diarrhea.

Pharmacodynamics/Kinetics
Half-Life Elimination: 8-30 hours
Metabolism: Systemically degraded
Excretion: Urine (trace amounts)
Clearance: Unaffected by age, renal or hepatic function

Available Dosage Forms Injection, powder for reconstitution: 10,000 units

Dosing
Adults & Elderly: Refer to individual protocols.

Single agent induction:
I.V. infusion:
200 units/kg/day for 28 days **or**
5000-10,000 units/m²/day for 7 days every 3 weeks **or**
10,000-40,000 units every 2-3 weeks
I.M.: 6000-12,000 units/m²; reconstitution to 10,000 units/mL may be necessary

Notes: Some institutions recommended the following precautions for asparaginase administration: Have parenteral epinephrine, diphenhydramine, and hydrocortisone available at the bedside. Have a freely running I.V. in place. Have a physician readily accessible. Monitor the patient closely for 30-60 minutes. Avoid administering the drug at night.

Test dose: A test dose is often recommended prior to the first dose of asparaginase, or prior to restarting therapy after a hiatus of several days. Most commonly, 0.1-0.2 mL of a 20-250 units/mL (2-50 units) is injected intradermally, and the patient observed for 15-30 minutes. False-negative rates of up to 80% to test doses of 2-50 units are reported.

Some practitioners recommend a desensitization regimen for patients who react to a test dose, or are being retreated following a break in therapy. Doses are doubled and given every 10 minutes until the total daily dose for that day has been administered.

One schedule begins with a total of 1 unit given I.V. and doubles the dose every 10 minutes until the total amount given is the planned dose for that day. For example, if a patient was to receive a total dose of 4000 units, he/she would receive injections 1 through 12 during the desensitization. See table on next page.

Pediatrics: Refer to individual protocols.
Infusion for induction:
I.V.: 1000 units/kg/day for 10 days; consolidation: 6000-10,000 units/m²/day for 14 days
I.M.: 6000 units/m² on days 4, 7, 10, 13, 16, 19, 22, 25, 28
Note: Refer to information in adult dosing.

Administration
I.M.: Doses should be given as a deep intramuscular injection into a large muscle.
(Continued)

Asparaginase *(Continued)*

I.V.:

Note: I.V. administration greatly increases the risk of allergic reactions and should be avoided if possible.

The following precautions should be taken when administering. Administer in 50-250 mL of D_5W over at least 60 minutes. The manufacturer recommends a test dose (0.1 mL of a dilute 20 unit/mL solution) prior to initial administration and when given after an interval of 7 days or more. Institutional policies vary. The skin test site should be observed for at least 1 hour for a wheal or erythema. Note that a negative skin test does not preclude the possibility of an allergic reaction. Desensitization may be performed in patients who have been found to be hypersensitive by the intradermal skin test or who have received previous courses of therapy with the drug. Have epinephrine, diphenhydramine, and hydrocortisone at the bedside. Have a running I.V. in place. A physician should be readily accessible.

I.V. Detail: The intradermal skin test is commonly given prior to the initial injection, using a dose of 0.1 mL of 20 units/mL solution (~2 units). The skin test site should be observed for at least 1 hour for a wheal or erythema. Do not infuse through filter.

Gelatinous fiber-like particles may develop on standing. Filtration through a 5-micron filter during administration will remove the particles with no loss of potency.

pH: 7.4; 6.5-8 (active enzyme)

Asparaginase Desensitization

Injection No.	Elspar Dose (int. units)	Accumulated Total Dose
1	1	1
2	2	3
3	4	7
4	8	15
5	16	31
6	32	63
7	64	127
8	128	255
9	256	511
10	512	1023
11	1024	2047
12	2048	4095
13	4096	8191
14	8192	16,383
15	16,384	32,767
16	32,768	65,535
17	65,536	131,071
18	131,072	262,143

Stability

Reconstitution: Lyophilized powder should be reconstituted with 1-5 mL sterile water for injection or NS for I.V. administration; NS for I.M. use. Shake well, but not too vigorously. A 5 micron filter may be used to remove fiber-like particles in the solution (do not use a 0.2 micron filter; has been associated with loss of potency).

Standard I.M. dilution: 2000, 5000, or 10,000 int. units/mL.

Standard I.V. dilution: Dilute in 50-250 mL NS or D_5W

Compatibility: Stable in D_5W, NS

Storage: Intact vials of powder should be refrigerated (<8°C). Reconstituted solutions are stable 1 week at room temperature. Solutions for I.V. infusion are stable for 8 hours at room temperature or under refrigeration.

Laboratory Monitoring CBC, serum amylase, blood glucose, uric acid, liver function prior to and frequently during therapy

Nursing Actions

Physical Assessment: Assess potential for interactions with other pharmacological agents patient may be taking. Monitor skin tests and regular laboratory tests prior to and frequently during therapy. With each dose, monitor patient closely for adverse reactions; CNS changes, acute hypersensitivity reaction (may occur in 10% to 40% of patients and may be fatal), hyperglycemia, or nausea or vomiting. In the event of hypersensitivity or hyperglycemia, stop infusion and notify prescriber immediately. Teach patient possible side effects/appropriate interventions and adverse symptoms to report.

Patient Education: Do not take any new medication during therapy unless approved by prescriber. This medication can only be given I.M. or I.V. Report immediately any pain or burning at infusion/injection site, rash, chest pain, respiratory difficulty or chest tightness, difficulty swallowing, or sharp back pain. It is vital to maintain adequate hydration (2-3 L/day of fluids) unless instructed to restrict fluid intake, and good nutritional status (small, frequent meals may help). May cause acute nausea or vomiting (small, frequent meals, frequent mouth care, chewing gum, or sucking lozenges may help - or consult prescriber for approved antiemetic). Report unusual fever or chills; confusion, agitation, depression; yellowing of skin or eyes; unusual bleeding or bruising; unhealed sores; or vaginal discharge. **Pregnancy/breast-feeding precautions:** Inform prescriber if you are or intend to become pregnant. Consult prescriber if breast-feeding.

Breast-Feeding Issues Due to the potential for serious adverse reactions, breast-feeding is not recommended.

Pregnancy Issues Decreased weight gain, resorptions, gross abnormalities, and skeletal abnormalities were observed in animal studies.

Additional Information The *E. coli* and the *Erwinia* strains of asparaginase differ slightly in their gene sequencing, and have slight differences in their enzyme characteristics. Both are highly specific for asparagine and have <10% activity for the D-isomer. The *E. coli* form is more commonly used. The *Erwinia* variety is no longer available.

Aspirin *(AS pir in)*

U.S. Brand Names Ascriptin® [OTC]; Ascriptin® Extra Strength [OTC]; Aspercin [OTC]; Aspercin Extra [OTC]; Aspergum® [OTC]; Bayer® Aspirin [OTC]; Bayer® Aspirin Extra Strength [OTC]; Bayer® Aspirin Regimen Adult Low Strength [OTC]; Bayer® Aspirin Regimen Children's [OTC]; Bayer® Aspirin Regimen Regular Strength [OTC]; Bayer® Extra Strength Arthritis Pain Regimen [OTC]; Bayer® Plus Extra Strength [OTC]; Bayer® Women's Aspirin Plus Calcium [OTC]; Bufferin® [OTC]; Bufferin® Extra Strength [OTC]; Buffinol [OTC]; Buffinol Extra [OTC]; Easprin®; Ecotrin® [OTC]; Ecotrin® Low Strength [OTC]; Ecotrin® Maximum Strength [OTC]; Halfprin® [OTC]; St. Joseph® Adult Aspirin [OTC]; Sureprin 81™ [OTC]; ZORprin®

Synonyms Acetylsalicylic Acid; ASA

Pharmacologic Category Salicylate

Medication Safety Issues

Sound-alike/look-alike issues:

Aspirin may be confused with Afrin®, Asendin®

Ascriptin® may be confused with Aricept®

Ecotrin® may be confused with Akineton®, Edecrin®, Epogen®

Halfprin® may be confused with Halfan®, Haltran®
ZORprin® may be confused with Zyloprim®

Pregnancy Risk Factor C/D (full-dose aspirin in 3rd trimester - expert analysis)

Lactation Enters breast milk/use caution

Use Treatment of mild-to-moderate pain, inflammation, and fever; may be used as prophylaxis of myocardial infarction; prophylaxis of stroke and/or transient ischemic episodes; management of rheumatoid arthritis, rheumatic fever, osteoarthritis, and gout (high dose); adjunctive therapy in revascularization procedures (coronary artery bypass graft [CABG], percutaneous transluminal coronary angioplasty [PTCA], carotid endarterectomy), stent implantation

Unlabeled/Investigational Use Low doses have been used in the prevention of pre-eclampsia, complications associated with autoimmune disorders such as lupus or antiphospholipid syndrome

Mechanism of Action/Effect Inhibits prostaglandin synthesis, acts on the hypothalamus heat-regulating center to reduce fever, blocks prostaglandin synthetase action which prevents formation of the platelet-aggregating substance thromboxane A_2

Contraindications Hypersensitivity to salicylates, other NSAIDs, or any component of the formulation; asthma; rhinitis; nasal polyps; inherited or acquired bleeding disorders (including factor VII and factor IX deficiency); do not use in children (<16 years of age) for viral infections (chickenpox or flu symptoms), with or without fever, due to a potential association with Reye's syndrome; pregnancy (3rd trimester especially)

Warnings/Precautions Use with caution in patients with platelet and bleeding disorders, renal dysfunction, dehydration, erosive gastritis, or peptic ulcer disease. Heavy ethanol use (>3 drinks/day) can increase bleeding risks. Avoid use in severe renal failure or in severe hepatic failure. Discontinue use if tinnitus or impaired hearing occurs. Caution in mild-to-moderate renal failure (only at high dosages). Patients with sensitivity to tartrazine dyes, nasal polyps, and asthma may have an increased risk of salicylate sensitivity. Surgical patients should avoid ASA if possible, for 1-2 weeks prior to surgery, to reduce the risk of excessive bleeding.

When used for self-medication (OTC labeling): Children and teenagers who have or are recovering from chickenpox or flu-like symptoms should not use this product. Changes in behavior (along with nausea and vomiting) may be an early sign of Reye's syndrome; patients should be instructed to contact their healthcare provider if these occur.

Drug Interactions

Cytochrome P450 Effect: Substrate of CYP2C8/9 (minor)

Decreased Effect: The effects of ACE inhibitors may be blunted by aspirin administration (may be significant only at higher aspirin dosages). Aspirin may decrease the effects of beta-blockers, loop diuretics (furosemide), thiazide diuretics, and probenecid. Aspirin may cause a decrease in NSAIDs serum concentration and decrease the effects of probenecid. Increased serum salicylate levels when taken with with urine acidifiers (ammonium chloride, methionine). Ibuprofen, and possibly other COX-1 inhibitors, may reduce the cardioprotective effects of aspirin.

Increased Effect/Toxicity: Aspirin may increase methotrexate serum levels/toxicity and may displace valproic acid from binding sites which can result in toxicity. NSAIDs and aspirin increase GI adverse effects (ulceration). Aspirin with oral anticoagulants (warfarin), thrombolytic agents, heparin, low molecular weight heparins, and antiplatelet agents (ticlopidine, clopidogrel, dipyridamole, NSAIDs, and IIb/IIIa antagonists) may increase risk of bleeding. Bleeding times may be additionally prolonged with verapamil. The effects of older sulfonylurea agents

(tolazamide, tolbutamide) may be potentiated due to displacement from plasma proteins. This effect does not appear to be clinically significant for newer sulfonylurea agents (glyburide, glipizide, glimepiride).

Nutritional/Ethanol Interactions

Ethanol: Avoid ethanol (may enhance gastric mucosal damage).

Food: Food may decrease the rate but not the extent of oral absorption.

Folic acid: Hyperexcretion of folate; folic acid deficiency may result, leading to macrocytic anemia.

Iron: With chronic aspirin use and at doses of 3-4 g/day, iron-deficiency anemia may result.

Sodium: Hypernatremia resulting from buffered aspirin solutions or sodium salicylate containing high sodium content. Avoid or use with caution in CHF or any condition where hypernatremia would be detrimental.

Benedictine liqueur, prunes, raisins, tea, and gherkins: Potential salicylate accumulation.

Fresh fruits containing vitamin C: Displace drug from binding sites, resulting in increased urinary excretion of aspirin.

Herb/Nutraceutical: Avoid cat's claw, dong quai, evening primrose, feverfew, garlic, ginger, ginkgo, red clover, horse chestnut, green tea, ginseng (all have additional antiplatelet activity). Limit curry powder, paprika, licorice; may cause salicylate accumulation. These foods contain 6 mg salicylate/100 g. An ordinarily American diet contains 10-200 mg/day of salicylate.

Lab Interactions False-negative results for glucose oxidase urinary glucose tests (Clinistix®). Interferes with Gerhardt test, VMA determination; 5-HIAA, xylose tolerance test and T_3 and T_4.

Adverse Reactions As with all drugs which may affect hemostasis, bleeding is associated with aspirin. Hemorrhage may occur at virtually any site. Risk is dependent on multiple variables including dosage, concurrent use of multiple agents which alter hemostasis, and patient susceptibility. Many adverse effects of aspirin are dose related, and are rare at low dosages. Other serious reactions are idiosyncratic, related to allergy or individual sensitivity. Accurate estimation of frequencies is not possible. The reactions listed below have been reported for aspirin (frequency not defined).

Cardiovascular: Hypotension, tachycardia, dysrhythmias, edema

Central nervous system: Fatigue, insomnia, nervousness, agitation, confusion, dizziness, headache, lethargy, cerebral edema, hyperthermia, coma

Dermatologic: Rash, angioedema, urticaria

Endocrine & metabolic: Acidosis, hyperkalemia, dehydration, hypoglycemia (children), hyperglycemia, hypernatremia (buffered forms)

Gastrointestinal: Nausea, vomiting, dyspepsia, epigastric discomfort, heartburn, stomach pain, gastrointestinal ulceration (6% to 31%), gastric erosions, gastric erythema, duodenal ulcers

Hematologic: Anemia, disseminated intravascular coagulation, prothrombin times prolonged, coagulopathy, thrombocytopenia, hemolytic anemia, bleeding, iron deficiency anemia

Hepatic: Hepatotoxicity, transaminases increased, hepatitis (reversible)

Neuromuscular & skeletal: Rhabdomyolysis, weakness, acetabular bone destruction (OA)

Otic: Hearing loss, tinnitus

Renal: Interstitial nephritis, papillary necrosis, proteinuria, renal impairment, renal failure (including cases caused by rhabdomyolysis), BUN increased, serum creatinine increased

Respiratory: Asthma, bronchospasm, dyspnea, laryngeal edema, hyperpnea, tachypnea, respiratory alkalosis, noncardiogenic pulmonary edema

(Continued)

Aspirin *(Continued)*

Miscellaneous: Anaphylaxis, prolonged pregnancy and labor, stillbirths, low birth weight, peripartum bleeding, Reye's syndrome

Overdosage/Toxicology Symptoms of overdose include tinnitus, headache, dizziness, confusion, metabolic acidosis, hyperpyrexia, hypoglycemia, and coma. Treatment should be based upon symptomatology.

Pharmacodynamics/Kinetics

Duration of Action: 4-6 hours

Time to Peak: Serum: ~1-2 hours

Half-Life Elimination: Parent drug: 15-20 minutes; Salicylates (dose dependent): 3 hours at lower doses (300-600 mg), 5-6 hours (after 1 g), 10 hours with higher doses

Metabolism: Hydrolyzed to salicylate (active) by esterases in GI mucosa, red blood cells, synovial fluid, and blood; metabolism of salicylate occurs primarily by hepatic conjugation; metabolic pathways are saturable

Excretion: Urine (75% as salicyluric acid, 10% as salicylic acid)

Available Dosage Forms

Caplet:
  Bayer® Aspirin: 325 mg
  Bayer® Aspirin Extra Strength: 500 mg
  Bayer® Extra Strength Arthritis Pain Regimen: 500 mg [enteric coated]
  Bayer® Women's Aspirin Plus Calcium: 81 mg [contains elemental calcium 300 mg]
  Caplet, buffered (Ascriptin® Extra Strength): 500 mg [contains aluminum hydroxide, calcium carbonate, and magnesium hydroxide]
Gelcap (Bayer® Aspirin Extra Strength): 500 mg
Gum (Aspergum®): 227 mg [cherry or orange flavor]
Suppository, rectal: 300 mg, 600 mg
Tablet: 325 mg
  Aspercin: 325 mg
  Aspercin Extra: 500 mg
  Bayer® Aspirin: 325 mg [film coated]
Tablet, buffered: 325 mg
  Ascriptin®: 325 mg [contains aluminum hydroxide, calcium carbonate, and magnesium hydroxide]
  Bayer® Plus Extra Strength: 500 mg [contains calcium carbonate]
  Bufferin®: 325 mg [contains citric acid]
  Bufferin® Extra Strength: 500 mg [contains citric acid]
  Buffinol: 325 mg [contains magnesium oxide]
  Buffinol Extra: 500 mg [contains magnesium oxide]
Tablet, chewable: 81 mg
  Bayer® Aspirin Regimen Children's Chewable: 81 mg [cherry, mint or orange flavor]
  St. Joseph® Adult Aspirin: 81 mg [orange flavor]
Tablet, controlled release (ZORprin®): 800 mg
Tablet, enteric coated: 81 mg, 325 mg, 500 mg, 650 mg
  Bayer® Aspirin Regimen Adult Low Strength, Ecotrin® Low Strength, St. Joseph Adult Aspirin: 81 mg
  Bayer® Aspirin Regimen Regular Strength, Ecotrin®: 325 mg
  Easprin®: 975 mg
  Ecotrin® Maximum Strength: 500 mg
  Halfprin®: 81 mg, 162 mg
  Sureprin 81™: 81 mg

Dosing

Adults & Elderly:

Analgesic and antipyretic: Oral, rectal: 325-650 mg every 4-6 hours up to 4 g/day

Anti-inflammatory: Oral: Initial: 2.4-3.6 g/day in divided doses; usual maintenance: 3.6-5.4 g/day; monitor serum concentrations

Acute myocardial infarction: 160-325 mg/day (have patient chew tablet if not taking aspirin before presentation)

Myocardial infarction prophylaxis: 75-325 mg/day; use of a lower aspirin dosage has been recommended in patients receiving ACE inhibitors

CABG: 75-325 mg/day starting 6 hours following procedure; if bleeding prevents administration at 6 hours after CABG, initiate as soon as possible

PTCA: Initial: 80-325 mg/day starting 2 hours before procedure; longer pretreatment durations (up to 24 hours) should be considered if lower dosages (80-100 mg) are used

Stent implantation: Oral: 325 mg 2 hours prior to implantation and 160-325 mg daily thereafter

Carotid endarterectomy: 81-325 mg/day preoperatively and daily thereafter

Acute stroke: 160-325 mg/day, initiated within 48 hours (in patients who are not candidates for thrombolytics and are not receiving systemic anticoagulation)

Stroke prevention/TIA: 30-325 mg/day (dosages up to 1300 mg/day in 2-4 divided doses have been used in clinical trials)

Pre-eclampsia prevention (unlabeled use): 60-80 mg/day during gestational weeks 13-26 (patient selection criteria not established)

Pediatrics:

Analgesic and antipyretic: Oral, rectal: 10-15 mg/kg/dose every 4-6 hours, up to a total of 4 g/day

Anti-inflammatory: Oral: Initial: 60-90 mg/kg/day in divided doses; usual maintenance: 80-100 mg/kg/day divided every 6-8 hours; monitor serum concentrations

Antiplatelet effects: Oral: Adequate pediatric studies have not been performed; pediatric dosage is derived from adult studies and clinical experience and is not well established; suggested doses have ranged from 3-5 mg/kg/day to 5-10 mg/kg/day given as a single daily dose. Doses are rounded to a convenient amount (eg, ½ of 80 mg tablet).

Mechanical prosthetic heart valves: Oral: 6-20 mg/kg/day given as a single daily dose (used in combination with an oral anticoagulant in children who have systemic embolism despite adequate oral anticoagulation therapy (INR 2.5-3.5) and used in combination with low-dose anticoagulation (INR 2-3) and dipyridamole when full-dose oral anticoagulation is contraindicated)

Blalock-Taussig shunts: Oral: 3-5 mg/kg/day given as a single daily dose

Kawasaki disease: Oral: 80-100 mg/kg/day divided every 6 hours; monitor serum concentrations; after fever resolves: 3-5 mg/kg/day once daily; in patients without coronary artery abnormalities, use lower dose for at least 6-8 weeks or until ESR and platelet count are normal; in patients with coronary artery abnormalities, low-dose aspirin should be continued indefinitely

Antirheumatic: Oral: 60-100 mg/kg/day in divided doses every 4 hours

Renal Impairment:

Cl_{cr} Cl_{cr} <10 mL/minute: Avoid use.

Dialyzable (50% to 100%)

Hepatic Impairment: Avoid use in severe liver disease.

Administration

Oral: Do not crush sustained release or enteric coated tablet. Administer with food or a full glass of water to minimize GI distress. For acute myocardial infarction, have patient chew tablet.

Stability

Storage: Keep suppositories in refrigerator; do not freeze. Hydrolysis of aspirin occurs upon exposure to water or moist air, resulting in salicylate and acetate, which possess a vinegar-like odor. Do not use if a strong odor is present.

Nursing Actions

Physical Assessment: Do not use for persons with allergic reaction to salicylate or other NSAIDs. Assess other medications patient may be taking for additive or adverse interactions. Monitor therapeutic effectiveness and for signs of adverse reactions or overdose at beginning of therapy and periodically with long-term therapy. Assess knowledge/teach patient appropriate use. Teach patient to monitor for adverse reactions, adverse reactions to report, and appropriate interventions to reduce side effects.

Patient Education: If self-administered, use exactly as directed; do not increase dose or frequency. Adverse reactions can occur with overuse. Take with food or milk. Do not use aspirin with strong vinegar-like odor. Do not crush or chew extended release products. While using this medication, avoid alcohol, excessive amounts of vitamin C, or salicylate-containing foods (eg, curry powder, prunes, raisins, tea, or licorice), other prescription or OTC medications containing aspirin or salicylate, or other NSAIDs without consulting prescriber. Maintain adequate hydration (2-3 L/day of fluids) unless instructed to restrict fluid intake. You may experience nausea, vomiting, gastric discomfort (frequent mouth care, small frequent meals, sucking lozenges, or chewing gum may help); GI bleeding, ulceration, or perforation (can occur with or without pain); or discoloration of stool (pink/red). Stop taking aspirin and report ringing in ears; persistent stomach pain; unresolved nausea or vomiting; respiratory difficulty or shortness of breath; unusual bruising or bleeding (mouth, urine, stool); or skin rash. **Pregnancy/breast-feeding precautions:** Inform prescriber if you are or intend to become pregnant. Consult prescriber if breast-feeding.

Dietary Considerations Take with food or large volume of water or milk to minimize GI upset.

Geriatric Considerations Elderly are at high risk for adverse effects from NSAIDs. Elderly with GI complications can develop peptic ulceration and/or hemorrhage asymptomatically. The concomitant use of H_2 blockers and sucralfate is not effective as prophylaxis with the exception of NSAID-induced duodenal ulcers which may be prevented by the use of ranitidine. Misoprostol and proton pump inhibitors are the only prophylactic agents proven effective. Also, concomitant disease and drug use contribute to the risk for GI adverse effects. Use lowest effective dose for shortest period possible. Consider renal function decline with age. Use of NSAIDs can compromise existing renal function, especially when Cl_{cr} is ≤30 mL/minute. Tinnitus may be a difficult and unreliable indication of toxicity due to age-related hearing loss or eighth cranial nerve damage. CNS adverse effects such as confusion, agitation, and hallucination are generally seen in overdose or high-dose situations, but elderly may demonstrate these adverse effects at lower doses than younger adults.

Breast-Feeding Issues Low amounts of aspirin can be found in breast milk. Milk/plasma ratios ranging from 0.03-0.3 have been reported. Peak levels in breast milk are reported to be at ~9 hours after a dose. Metabolic acidosis was reported in one infant following an aspirin dose of 3.9 g/day in the mother. The AAP states that aspirin should be used with caution while breast-feeding. The WHO considers occasional doses of aspirin to be compatible with breast-feeding, but to avoid long-term therapy and consider monitoring the infant for adverse effects. Other sources suggest avoiding aspirin while breast-feeding due to the theoretical risk of Reye's syndrome.

Pregnancy Issues Salicylates have been noted to cross the placenta and enter fetal circulation. Adverse effects reported in the fetus include mortality, intrauterine growth retardation, salicylate intoxication, bleeding abnormalities, and neonatal acidosis. Use of aspirin close to delivery may cause premature closure of the ductus arteriosus. Adverse effects reported in the mother include anemia, hemorrhage, prolonged gestation, and prolonged labor. Aspirin has been used for the prevention of pre-eclampsia; however, the ACOG currently recommends that it not be used in low-risk women. Low-dose aspirin is used to treat complications resulting from antiphospholipid syndrome in pregnancy (either primary or secondary to SLE). In general, low doses during pregnancy needed for the treatment of certain medical conditions have not been shown to cause fetal harm, however, discontinuing therapy prior to delivery is recommended. Use of safer agents for routine management of pain or headache should be considered.

Aspirin and Codeine (AS pir in & KOE deen)

Synonyms Codeine Phosphate and Aspirin
Restrictions C-III
Pharmacologic Category Analgesic, Narcotic
Pregnancy Risk Factor D
Lactation Enters breast milk/use caution
Use Relief of mild-to-moderate pain
Available Dosage Forms Tablet:
#3: Aspirin 325 mg and codeine phosphate 30 mg
#4: Aspirin 325 mg and codeine phosphate 60 mg
Dosing
Adults: Management of pain: Oral: 1-2 tablets (#3 tablet) every 4-6 hours as needed for pain
Elderly: One ASA with codeine 30 mg (#3 tablet), or two ASA with codeine 15 mg (#2 tablet) every 4-6 hours as needed for pain
Pediatrics:
Aspirin: 10 mg/kg/dose every 4 hours
Codeine: 0.5-1 mg/kg/dose every 4 hours
Renal Impairment:
Cl_{cr} 10-50 mL/minute: Administer 75% of dose.
Cl_{cr} <10 mL/minute: Avoid use.
Hepatic Impairment: Avoid use in severe liver disease.

Nursing Actions

Physical Assessment: See individual agents.
Patient Education: See individual agents. **Pregnancy/breast-feeding precautions:** Inform prescriber if you are or intend to become pregnant. Consult prescriber if breast-feeding.
Related Information
Aspirin on page 114
Codeine on page 296

Aspirin and Dipyridamole
(AS pir in & dye peer ID a mole)

U.S. Brand Names Aggrenox®
Synonyms Aspirin and Extended-Release Dipyridamole; Dipyridamole and Aspirin
Pharmacologic Category Antiplatelet Agent
Pregnancy Risk Factor D
Lactation Enters breast milk/use caution
Use Reduction in the risk of stroke in patients who have had transient ischemia of the brain or completed ischemic stroke due to thrombosis
Available Dosage Forms Capsule: Dipyridamole (extended release) 200 mg and aspirin 25 mg [contains lactose]
Dosing
Adults & Elderly: Stroke prevention: Oral: 1 capsule (200 mg dipyridamole, 25 mg aspirin) twice daily
Renal Impairment: Avoid use in patients with severe renal dysfunction (Cl_{cr} <10 mL/minute).
Hepatic Impairment: Avoid use in patients with severe hepatic impairment.

Nursing Actions

Physical Assessment: Assess for previous drug allergies before administering first dose. Assess other medications patient may be taking for effectiveness
(Continued)

Aspirin and Dipyridamole *(Continued)*

and interactions. Monitor for signs of stroke or bleeding, laboratory results, adverse reactions, and overdose. Assess knowledge/teach patient appropriate use, interventions to reduce side effects, and adverse reactions to report.

Patient Education: See individual agents. **Pregnancy/breast-feeding precautions:** Notify prescriber if you are or intend to become pregnant. Do not breast-feed.

Related Information
Aspirin *on page 114*
Dipyridamole *on page 379*

Aspirin and Meprobamate
(AS pir in & me proe BA mate)

U.S. Brand Names Equagesic®

Synonyms Meprobamate and Aspirin

Restrictions C-IV

Pharmacologic Category Antianxiety Agent, Miscellaneous

Pregnancy Risk Factor D

Lactation Enters breast milk/use caution due to aspirin content

Use Adjunct to treatment of skeletal muscular disease in patients exhibiting tension and/or anxiety

Available Dosage Forms Tablet: Aspirin 325 mg and meprobamate 200 mg

Dosing
  Adults: Muscular disorders, anxiety (adjunct): Oral: 1 tablet 3-4 times/day

  Elderly: Refer to adult dosing and dosing in individual agents; use with caution.

Nursing Actions
  Physical Assessment: See individual components listed in Related Information. **Pregnancy risk factor D** - determine that patient is not pregnant before beginning treatment. Instruct patients of childbearing age about appropriate barrier contraceptive measures. Note breast-feeding caution.

  Patient Education: See individual agents. **Pregnancy/breast-feeding precautions:** Inform prescriber if you are or intend to become pregnant. Consult prescriber if breast-feeding.

Related Information
Aspirin *on page 114*
Meprobamate *on page 779*

Aspirin and Pravastatin
(AS pir in & PRA va stat in)

U.S. Brand Names Pravigard™ PAC [DSC]

Synonyms Buffered Aspirin and Pravastatin Sodium; Pravastatin and Aspirin

Pharmacologic Category Antilipemic Agent, HMG-CoA Reductase Inhibitor; Salicylate

Pregnancy Risk Factor X

Lactation Enters breast milk/contraindicated

Use Combination therapy in patients who need treatment with aspirin and pravastatin to reduce the incidence of cardiovascular events, including myocardial infarction, stroke, and death.

Available Dosage Forms [DSC] = Discontinued product

Combination package (Pravigard™ PAC) [each administration card contains] [DSC]:

81/20:
  Tablet: Aspirin, buffered 81 mg (5/card) [contains calcium carbonate, and magnesium oxide, and magnesium carbonate]
  Tablet (Pravachol®): Pravastatin sodium 20 mg (5/card) [contains lactose]

81/40:
  Tablet: Aspirin, buffered 81 mg (5/card) [contains calcium carbonate, and magnesium oxide, and magnesium carbonate]
  Tablet (Pravachol®): Pravastatin sodium 40 mg (5/card) [contains lactose]

81/80:
  Tablet: Aspirin, buffered 81 mg (5/card) [contains calcium carbonate, and magnesium oxide, and magnesium carbonate]
  Tablet (Pravachol®): Pravastatin sodium 80 mg (5/card) [contains lactose]

325/20:
  Tablet: Aspirin, buffered 325 mg (5/card) [contains calcium carbonate, and magnesium oxide, and magnesium carbonate]
  Tablet (Pravachol®): Pravastatin sodium 20 mg (5/card) [contains lactose]

325/40:
  Tablet: Aspirin, buffered 325 mg (5/card) [contains calcium carbonate, and magnesium oxide, and magnesium carbonate]
  Tablet (Pravachol®): Pravastatin sodium 40 mg (5/card) [contains lactose]

325/80:
  Tablet: Aspirin, buffered 325 mg (5/card) [contains calcium carbonate, and magnesium oxide, and magnesium carbonate]
  Tablet (Pravachol®): Pravastatin sodium 80 mg (5/card) [contains lactose]

Dosing
  Adults:

  Reduction in cardiac events: Initial: Oral: Pravastatin 40 mg with aspirin (either 81 mg or 325 mg); both medications taken once daily. If pravastatin 40 mg does not achieve the desired cholesterol result, dosage may be increased to 80 mg once daily with aspirin (either 81 mg or 325 mg) once daily. Some patients may achieve/maintain goal cholesterol levels at a pravastatin dosage of 20 mg.

  See Pravastatin for dosing in renal or hepatic impairment, as well as, dosing with concurrent immunosuppressant therapy.

Nursing Actions
  Physical Assessment: See individual agents. **Pregnancy risk factor X** - determine that patient is not pregnant before starting therapy. Do not give to females of childbearing age unless capable of complying with barrier contraceptive use. Breast-feeding is contraindicated.

  Patient Education: See individual agents. **Pregnancy/breast-feeding precautions:** Inform prescriber if you are pregnant. Consult prescriber for appropriate barrier contraceptive measures to use during and for 1 month following therapy. This drug may cause severe fetal defects. Do not donate blood during or for 1 month following therapy. Do not breast-feed during or for 1 month following therapy.

Related Information
Aspirin *on page 114*
Pravastatin *on page 1015*

Atenolol (a TEN oh lole)

U.S. Brand Names Tenormin®

Pharmacologic Category Beta Blocker, Beta₁ Selective

Medication Safety Issues

Sound-alike/look-alike issues:

Atenolol may be confused with albuterol, Altenol®, timolol, Tylenol®

Tenormin® may be confused with Imuran®, Norpramin®, thiamine, Trovan®

Pregnancy Risk Factor D

Lactation Enters breast milk/use caution

Use Treatment of hypertension, alone or in combination with other agents; management of angina pectoris, postmyocardial infarction patients

Unlabeled/Investigational Use Acute ethanol withdrawal, supraventricular and ventricular arrhythmias, and migraine headache prophylaxis

Mechanism of Action/Effect Competitively blocks response to beta-adrenergic stimulation, selectively blocks beta₁-receptors with little or no effect on beta₂-receptors except at high doses

Contraindications Hypersensitivity to atenolol or any component of the formulation; sinus bradycardia; sinus node dysfunction; heart block greater than first-degree (except in patients with a functioning artificial pacemaker); cardiogenic shock; uncompensated cardiac failure; pulmonary edema; pregnancy

Warnings/Precautions Safety and efficacy in children have not been established. Administer cautiously in compensated heart failure and monitor for a worsening of the condition (efficacy of atenolol in heart failure has not been established). Use caution with concurrent use of beta-blockers and either verapamil or diltiazem; bradycardia or heart block can occur. Avoid concurrent I.V. use of both agents. Beta-blockers should be avoided in patients with bronchospastic disease (asthma) and peripheral vascular disease (may aggravate arterial insufficiency). Atenolol, with B1 selectivity, has been used cautiously in bronchospastic disease with close monitoring. Use cautiously in patients with diabetes - may mask hypoglycemic symptoms. May mask signs of thyrotoxicosis. May cause fetal harm when administered in pregnancy. Use cautiously in the renally impaired (dosage adjustment required). Use care with anesthetic agents which decrease myocardial function. Caution in patients with myasthenia gravis. Beta-blocker therapy should not be withdrawn abruptly (particularly in patients with CAD), but gradually tapered to avoid acute tachycardia, hypertension, and/or ischemia.

Drug Interactions

Decreased Effect: Decreased effect of atenolol with aluminum salts, barbiturates, calcium salts, cholestyramine, colestipol, NSAIDs, penicillins (ampicillin), rifampin, salicylates, and sulfinpyrazone due to decreased bioavailability and plasma levels. Beta-blockers may decrease the effect of sulfonylureas.

Increased Effect/Toxicity: Atenolol may increase the effects of other drugs which slow AV conduction (digoxin, verapamil, diltiazem), alpha-blockers (prazosin, terazosin), and alpha-adrenergic stimulants (epinephrine, phenylephrine). Atenolol may mask the tachycardia from hypoglycemia caused by insulin and oral hypoglycemics. In patients receiving concurrent therapy, the risk of hypertensive crisis is increased when either clonidine or the beta-blocker is withdrawn. Reserpine has been shown to enhance the effect of atenolol. Beta-blockers may increase the action or levels of ethanol, disopyramide, nondepolarizing muscle relaxants, and theophylline although the effects are difficult to predict.

Nutritional/Ethanol Interactions

Food: Atenolol serum concentrations may be decreased if taken with food.

Herb/Nutraceutical: Avoid dong quai if using for hypertension (has estrogenic activity). Avoid ephedra, yohimbe, ginseng (may worsen hypertension). Avoid garlic (may have increased antihypertensive effect).

Lab Interactions Increased glucose; decreased HDL

Adverse Reactions 1% to 10%:

Cardiovascular: Persistent bradycardia, hypotension, chest pain, edema, heart failure, second- or third-degree AV block, Raynaud's phenomenon

Central nervous system: Dizziness, fatigue, insomnia, lethargy, confusion, mental impairment, depression, headache, nightmares

Gastrointestinal: Constipation, diarrhea, nausea

Genitourinary: Impotence

Miscellaneous: Cold extremities

Overdosage/Toxicology Symptoms of toxicity include lethargy, respiratory drive disorder, wheezing, sinus pause, and bradycardia. Additional effects associated with any beta-blocker are congestive heart failure, hypotension, bronchospasm, and hypoglycemia. Treatment includes removal of unabsorbed drug by induced emesis, gastric lavage, or administration of activated charcoal and symptomatic treatment of toxic responses. Atenolol can be removed by hemodialysis.

Pharmacodynamics/Kinetics

Onset of Action: Peak effect: Oral: 2-4 hours

Duration of Action: Normal renal function: 12-24 hours

Protein Binding: 3% to 15%

Half-Life Elimination: Beta:

Neonates: ≤35 hours; Mean: 16 hours

Children: 4.6 hours; children >10 years may have prolonged half-life (>5 hours) compared to children 5-10 years (<5 hours)

Adults: Normal renal function: 6-9 hours, prolonged with renal impairment; End-stage renal disease: 15-35 hours

Metabolism: Limited hepatic

Excretion: Feces (50%); urine (40% as unchanged drug)

Available Dosage Forms

Injection, solution: 0.5 mg/mL (10 mL)

Tablet: 25 mg, 50 mg, 100 mg

Dosing

Adults & Elderly:

Hypertension:

Oral: 25-50 mg once daily, may increase to 100 mg/day. Doses >100 mg are unlikely to produce any further benefit.

I.V.: Dosages of 1.25-5 mg every 6-12 hours have been used in short-term management of patients unable to take oral enteral beta-blockers

Angina pectoris: Oral: 50 mg once daily, may increase to 100 mg/day. Some patients may require 200 mg/day.

Postmyocardial infarction:

I.V.: Early treatment: 5 mg slow I.V. over 5 minutes; may repeat in 10 minutes. If both doses are tolerated, may start oral atenolol 50 mg every 12 hours or 100 mg/day for 6-9 days postmyocardial infarction.

Oral: Follow I.V. dose with 100 mg/day or 50 mg twice daily for 6-9 days postmyocardial infarction.

Pediatrics:

Hypertension: Oral: Children: 0.8-1 mg/kg/dose given daily; range of 0.8-1.5 mg/kg/day; maximum dose: 2 mg/kg/day

Renal Impairment:

Cl$_{cr}$ 15-35 mL/minute: Administer 50 mg/day maximum.

Cl$_{cr}$ <15 mL/minute: Administer 50 mg every other day maximum.

(Continued)

Atenolol *(Continued)*

Hemodialysis effects: Moderately dialyzable (20% to 50%) via hemodialysis. Administer dose postdialysis or administer 25-50 mg supplemental dose. Elimination is not enhanced with peritoneal dialysis. Supplemental dose is not necessary.

Administration
I.V.: When administered acutely for cardiac treatment, monitor ECG and blood pressure. The injection can be administered undiluted or diluted with a compatible I.V. solution. May administer by rapid infusion (I.V. push) at a rate of 1 mg/minute or by slow infusion over ~30 minutes. Necessary monitoring for surgical patients who are unable to take oral beta-blockers (prolonged ileus) has not been defined. Some institutions require monitoring of baseline and postinfusion heart rate and blood pressure when a patient's response to beta-blockade has not been characterized (ie, the patient's initial dose or following a change in dose). Consult individual institutional policies and procedures.

I.V. Detail: pH: 5.5-6.5

Stability
Compatibility: Stable in D$_5$W, NS

Y-site administration: Incompatible with amphotericin B cholesteryl sulfate complex

Storage: Protect from light.

Nursing Actions
Physical Assessment: Assess potential for interactions with other prescriptions, OTC medications, or herbal products patient may be taking. **I.V.:** Requires cardiac and hemodynamic monitoring and hypotensive precautions. **Oral:** Monitor blood pressure and heart rate prior to and following first dose and any change in dosage. Monitor for adverse effects (eg, CHF, edema, new cough, dyspnea, unresolved fatigue). Advise patients with diabetes to monitor glucose levels closely (beta-blockers may alter glucose tolerance). Drug should not be stopped abruptly; taper dose gradually when discontinuing. Teach patient appropriate use, possible side effects/appropriate interventions (hypotension precautions), and adverse symptoms to report.

Patient Education: Do not take any new medication during therapy unless approved by prescriber. Take exactly as directed; with or without regard to meals; do not take with antacids. Do not adjust dosage or discontinue medication without consulting prescriber. Take pulse daily (prior to medication) and follow prescriber's instruction about holding medication. If you have diabetes, monitor serum sugar closely (drug may alter glucose tolerance or mask signs of hypoglycemia). May cause fatigue, dizziness, or postural hypotension (use caution when changing position from lying or sitting to standing, when driving, or climbing stairs until response to medication is known). Alteration in sexual performance (reversible); or constipation (increased dietary bulk and fluids and exercise may help). Report unresolved swelling of extremities, respiratory difficulty or new cough, unresolved fatigue, unusual weight gain, unresolved constipation, or unusual muscle weakness. **Pregnancy/breast-feeding precautions:** Do not get pregnant or cause a pregnancy (males) while using this medication. Consult prescriber for appropriate contraceptive measures. Consult prescriber if breast-feeding.

Dietary Considerations May be taken without regard to meals.

Geriatric Considerations Due to alterations in the beta-adrenergic autonomic nervous system, beta-adrenergic blockade may result in less hemodynamic response than seen in younger adults.

Breast-Feeding Issues Symptoms of beta-blockade including cyanosis, hypothermia, and bradycardia have been reported in nursing infants.

Pregnancy Issues Atenolol crosses the placenta; beta-blockers have been associated with persistent bradycardia, hypotension, and IUGR; IUGR is probably related to maternal hypertension. Available evidence suggests beta-blockers are generally safe during pregnancy (JNC 7). Cases of neonatal hypoglycemia have been reported following maternal use of beta-blockers at parturition or during breast-feeding. Monitor breast-fed infant for symptoms of beta-blockade.

Atenolol and Chlorthalidone
(a TEN oh lole & klor THAL i done)

U.S. Brand Names Tenoretic®
Synonyms Chlorthalidone and Atenolol
Pharmacologic Category Antihypertensive Agent, Combination
Pregnancy Risk Factor D
Lactation Excretion in breast milk unknown/use caution
Use Treatment of hypertension with a cardioselective beta-blocker and a diuretic
Available Dosage Forms Tablet:
50: Atenolol 50 mg and chlorthalidone 25 mg
100: Atenolol 100 mg and chlorthalidone 25 mg

Dosing
Adults & Elderly: Hypertension: Oral: Initial: 1 (50) tablet once daily, then individualize dose until optimal dose is achieved
Renal Impairment:
Cl$_{cr}$ 15-35 mL/minute: Administer 50 mg/day.
Cl$_{cr}$ <15 mL/minute: Administer 50 mg every other day.

Nursing Actions
Physical Assessment: See individual agents.
Patient Education: See individual agents. **Pregnancy/breast-feeding precautions:** Inform prescriber if you are or intend to become pregnant. Consult prescriber if breast-feeding.

Related Information
Atenolol *on page 119*
Chlorthalidone *on page 255*

Atomoxetine (AT oh mox e teen)

U.S. Brand Names Strattera®
Synonyms Atomoxetine Hydrochloride; LY139603; Methylphenoxy-Benzene Propanamine; Tomoxetine
Restrictions A medication guide concerning the use of atomoxetine in children and teenagers can be found on the FDA website at http://www.fda.gov/cder/Offices/ODS/labeling.htm. It should be dispensed to parents or guardians of children and teenagers receiving this medication.
Pharmacologic Category Norepinephrine Reuptake Inhibitor, Selective
Pregnancy Risk Factor C
Lactation Excretion in breast milk unknown/use caution
Use Treatment of attention deficit/hyperactivity disorder (ADHD)
Mechanism of Action/Effect Selectively inhibits the reuptake of norepinephrine (Ki 4.5nM) with little to no activity at the other neuronal reuptake pumps or receptor sites.
Contraindications Hypersensitivity to atomoxetine or any component of the formulation; use with or within 14 days of MAO inhibitors; narrow-angle glaucoma
Warnings/Precautions Use caution with hepatic and renal impairment (dosage adjustments necessary in

hepatic impairment). Use may be associated with rare but severe hepatotoxicity; discontinue if signs or symptoms of hepatotoxic reaction (eg, jaundice, pruritus, flu-like symptoms) are noted. May cause increased heart rate or blood pressure; use caution with hypertension or other cardiovascular disease. Use caution in patients who are poor metabolizers of CYP2D6 metabolized drugs ("poor metabolizers"), bioavailability increases. May cause urinary retention/hesitancy; use caution in patients with history of urinary retention or bladder outlet obstruction. Allergic reactions (including angioneurotic edema, urticaria, and rash) may occur. Growth should be monitored during treatment. Height and weight gain may be reduced during the first 9-12 months of treatment, but should recover by 3 years of therapy. Use caution in pediatric patients; may be an increased risk of suicidal ideation. Additional family/caregiver and healthcare provider monitoring suggested during initial months of therapy or at times of dosage changes. Safety and efficacy have not been evaluated in pediatric patients <6 years of age.

Drug Interactions

Cytochrome P450 Effect: Substrate of CYP2C19 (minor), 2D6 (major)

Increased Effect/Toxicity: MAO inhibitors may increase risk of CNS toxicity (combined use is contraindicated). CYP2D6 inhibitors may increase the levels/effects of atomoxetine (dose adjustment may be needed in patients who are extensive metabolizers of CYP2D6); example inhibitors include chlorpromazine, delavirdine, fluoxetine, miconazole, paroxetine, pergolide, quinidine, quinine, ritonavir, and ropinirole. Albuterol may increase risk of cardiovascular toxicity.

Adverse Reactions Percentages as reported in children and adults; some adverse reactions may be increased in "poor metabolizers" (CYP2D6).

>10%:
Central nervous system: Headache (17% to 27%), insomnia (16%)
Gastrointestinal: Xerostomia (4% to 21%), abdominal pain (20%), vomiting (15%), appetite decreased (10% to 14%), nausea (12%)
Respiratory: Cough (11%)

1% to 10%:
Cardiovascular: Palpitations (4%), diastolic pressure increased (<1% to 5%), systolic blood pressure increased (2% to 9%), orthostatic hypotension (2%), tachycardia (2% to 3%)
Central nervous system: Fatigue/lethargy (7% to 9%), irritability (8%), somnolence (7%), dizziness (6%), mood swings (5%), abnormal dreams (4%), sleep disturbance (4%), pyrexia (3%), rigors (3%), crying (2%)
Dermatologic: Dermatitis (2% to 4%)
Endocrine & metabolic: Dysmenorrhea (7%), libido decreased (6%), menstruation disturbance (2% to 3%), hot flashes (3%), orgasm abnormal (2%)
Gastrointestinal: Dyspepsia (4% to 6%), diarrhea (4%), flatulence (2%), constipation (3% to 10%), weight loss (2%)
Genitourinary: Erectile disturbance (7%), ejaculatory disturbance (5%), prostatitis (3%), impotence (3%)
Neuromuscular & skeletal: Paresthesia (4%), myalgia (3%)
Otic: Ear infection (3%)
Renal: Urinary retention/hesitation (3% to 8%)
Respiratory: Rhinorrhea (4%), sinus headache (3%), sinusitis (6%)
Miscellaneous: Diaphoresis increased (4%), influenza (3%)

Overdosage/Toxicology Somnolence, agitation, hyperactivity, abnormal behavior, mydriasis, tachycardia, dry mouth and GI symptoms have been reported with acute and chronic overdose. Gastric emptying and use of activated charcoal may prevent drug absorption; monitor patient and provide supportive care. Dialysis is not likely to provide benefit.

Pharmacodynamics/Kinetics
Time to Peak: Plasma: 1-2 hours
Protein Binding: 98%, primarily albumin
Half-Life Elimination: Atomoxetine: 5 hours (up to 24 hours in poor metabolizers); Active metabolites: 4-hydroxyatomoxetine: 6-8 hours; N-desmethylatomoxetine: 6-8 hours (34-40 hours in poor metabolizers)
Metabolism: Hepatic, via CYP2D6 and CYP2C19; forms metabolites (4-hydroxyatomoxetine, active, equipotent to atomoxetine; N-desmethylatomoxetine in poor metabolizers, limited activity)
Excretion: Urine (80%, as conjugated 4-hydroxy metabolite); feces (17%)

Available Dosage Forms Capsule: 10 mg, 18 mg, 25 mg, 40 mg, 60 mg, 80 mg, 100 mg

Dosing
Adults:
Treatment of ADHD: Oral: Initial: 40 mg/day, increased after minimum of 3 days to ~80 mg/day; may administer as either a single daily dose or 2 evenly divided doses in morning and late afternoon/early evening. May increase to 100 mg in 2-4 additional weeks to achieve optimal response.
Dosage adjustment in patients receiving strong CYP2D6 inhibitors (eg, paroxetine, fluoxetine, quinidine): Do not exceed 80 mg/day; dose adjustments should occur only after 4 weeks.
Note: Atomoxetine may be discontinued without the need for tapering dose.
Elderly: Use has not been evaluated in the elderly.
Pediatrics: Treatment of ADHD:
Children and Adolescents ≤70 kg: Oral: Initial: 0.5 mg/kg/day, increase after minimum of 3 days to ~1.2 mg/kg/day; may administer as either a single daily dose or 2 evenly divided doses in morning and late afternoon/early evening. Maximum daily dose: 1.4 mg/kg or 100 mg, whichever is less.
Dosage adjustment in patients receiving strong CYP2D6 inhibitors (eg, paroxetine, fluoxetine, quinidine): Do not exceed 1.2 mg/kg/day; dose adjustments should occur only after 4 weeks.
Children and Adolescents >70 kg: Refer to adult dosing.
Note: Atomoxetine may be discontinued without the need for tapering dose.
Renal Impairment: No adjustment needed.
Hepatic Impairment:
Moderate hepatic insufficiency (Child-Pugh class B): All doses should be reduced to 50% of normal.
Severe hepatic insufficiency (Child-Pugh class C): All doses should be reduced to 25% of normal.

Administration
Oral: May be administered with or without food.

Stability
Storage: Store at room temperature of 25°C (77°F).

Nursing Actions
Physical Assessment: Assess other pharmacological agents patient may be taking for potential for interactions. Monitor therapeutic effectiveness and adverse response at regular intervals during therapy. Teach patient proper use, possible side effects/appropriate interventions, and adverse symptoms to report.
Patient Education: Do not take any new medication during therapy without consulting prescriber. Take exactly as directed at the same time of day, without regard for meals. Do not discontinue or alter dose without consulting prescriber. Avoid alcohol. May cause CNS changes; fatigue/lethargy, irritability, sleep disturbances (use caution when driving or engaged in potentially hazardous tasks until response to drug is known); diarrhea or constipation; menstrual disturbances, abnormal orgasm, erectile or ejaculatory disturbance, impotence; muscle, bone, or joint pain. Report chest pain, palpitations, rapid heartbeat, (Continued)

Atomoxetine *(Continued)*

persistent CNS changes (especially any increase in aggression or hostility), gastrointestinal effects, muscle or skeletal pain or weakness, dark urine, jaundice, right upper-quadrant pain, unexplained flu-like symptoms, or other persistent adverse effects. **Pregnancy/breast-feeding precautions:** Inform prescriber if you are or intend to become pregnant. Consult prescriber if breast-feeding.

Dietary Considerations May be taken with or without food.

Atorvastatin *(a TORE va sta tin)*

U.S. Brand Names Lipitor®

Pharmacologic Category Antilipemic Agent, HMG-CoA Reductase Inhibitor

Medication Safety Issues
Sound-alike/look-alike issues:
Lipitor® may be confused with Levatol®

Pregnancy Risk Factor X

Lactation Enters breast milk/contraindicated

Use Treatment of dyslipidemias or primary prevention of cardiovascular disease (atherosclerotic) as detailed below:
Primary prevention of cardiovascular disease (high-risk for CVD): To reduce the risk of MI or stroke in patients without evidence of heart disease who have multiple CVD risk factors or type 2 diabetes. Treatment reduces the risk for angina or revascularization procedures in patients with multiple risk factors.
Treatment of dyslipidemias: To reduce elevations in total cholesterol, LDL-C, apolipoprotein B, and triglycerides in patients with elevations of one or more components, and/or to increase HDL-C as present in Fredrickson type IIa, IIb, III, and IV hyperlipidemias; treatment of primary dysbetalipoproteinemia, homozygous familial hypercholesterolemia
Treatment of heterozygous familial hypercholesterolemia (HeFH) in adolescent patients (10-17 years of age, females >1 year postmenarche) having LDL-C ≥190 mg/dL or LDL-C ≥160 mg/dL with positive family history of premature cardiovascular disease (CVD) or with two or more CVD risk factors.

Mechanism of Action/Effect Inhibitor of 3-hydroxy-3-methylglutaryl coenzyme A (HMG-CoA) reductase, the rate-limiting enzyme in cholesterol synthesis (reduces the production of mevalonic acid from HMG-CoA); this then results in a compensatory increase in the expression of LDL receptors on hepatocyte membranes and a stimulation of LDL catabolism

Contraindications Hypersensitivity to atorvastatin or any component of the formulation; active liver disease; unexplained persistent elevations of serum transaminases; pregnancy

Warnings/Precautions Secondary causes of hyperlipidemia should be ruled out prior to therapy. May cause hepatic dysfunction. Use with caution in patients who consume large amounts of ethanol or have a history of liver disease. Monitoring is recommended. Rhabdomyolysis with acute renal failure has occurred. Risk is dose related and is increased with concurrent use of lipid-lowering agents which may cause rhabdomyolysis (gemfibrozil, fibric acid derivatives, or niacin at doses ≥1 g/day) or during concurrent use with potent CYP3A4 inhibitors (including amiodarone, clarithromycin, cyclosporine, erythromycin, itraconazole, ketoconazole, nefazodone, grapefruit juice in large quantities, verapamil, or protease inhibitors such as indinavir, nelfinavir, or ritonavir). Weigh the risk versus benefit when combining any of these drugs with atorvastatin. Discontinue in any patient experiencing an acute or serious condition predisposing to renal failure secondary to rhabdomyolysis. Safety and efficacy have not been established in patients <10 years of age or in premenarcheal girls.

Drug Interactions
Cytochrome P450 Effect: Substrate of CYP3A4 (major); **Inhibits** CYP3A4 (weak)
Decreased Effect: Colestipol, antacids decreased plasma concentrations but effect on LDL-cholesterol was not altered. Cholestyramine may decrease absorption of atorvastatin when administered concurrently.
Increased Effect/Toxicity: CYP3A4 inhibitors may increase the levels/effects of atorvastatin; example inhibitors include azole antifungals, clarithromycin, diclofenac, doxycycline, erythromycin, imatinib, isoniazid, nefazodone, nicardipine, propofol, protease inhibitors, quinidine, telithromycin, and verapamil. The risk of myopathy and rhabdomyolysis due to concurrent use of a CYP3A4 inhibitor with atorvastatin is probably less than lovastatin or simvastatin. Cyclosporine, clofibrate, fenofibrate, gemfibrozil, and niacin may also increase the risk of myopathy and rhabdomyolysis. The effect/toxicity of levothyroxine may be increased by atorvastatin. Levels of digoxin and ethinyl estradiol may be increased by atorvastatin.

Nutritional/Ethanol Interactions
Ethanol: Avoid excessive ethanol consumption (due to potential hepatic effects).
Food: Atorvastatin serum concentrations may be increased by grapefruit juice; avoid concurrent intake of large quantities (>1 quart/day). Red yeast rice contains an estimated 2.4 mg lovastatin per 600 mg rice.
Herb/Nutraceutical: St John's wort may decrease atorvastatin levels.

Adverse Reactions
>10%: Central nervous system: Headache (3% to 17%)
2% to 10%:
Cardiovascular: Chest pain, peripheral edema
Central nervous system: Insomnia, dizziness
Dermatologic: Rash (1% to 4%)
Gastrointestinal: Abdominal pain (up to 4%), constipation (up to 3%), diarrhea (up to 4%), dyspepsia (1% to 3%), flatulence (1% to 3%), nausea
Genitourinary: Urinary tract infection
Hepatic: Transaminases increased (2% to 3% with 80 mg/day dosing)
Neuromuscular & skeletal: Arthralgia (up to 5%), arthritis, back pain (up to 4%), myalgia (up to 6%), weakness (up to 4%)
Respiratory: Sinusitis (up to 6%), pharyngitis (up to 3%), bronchitis, rhinitis
Miscellaneous: Infection (3% to 10%), flu-like syndrome (up to 3%), allergic reaction (up to 3%)

Additional class-related events or case reports (not necessarily reported with atorvastatin therapy): Alkaline phosphatase increased, cataracts, cirrhosis, CPK increased (>10x normal), dermatomyositis, eosinophilia, erectile dysfunction, extraocular muscle movement impaired, fulminant hepatic necrosis, gynecomastia, hemolytic anemia, memory loss, ophthalmoplegia, peripheral nerve palsy, polymyalgia rheumatica, positive ANA, renal failure (secondary to rhabdomyolysis), systemic lupus erythematosus-like syndrome, thyroid dysfunction, tremor, vasculitis, vertigo

Overdosage/Toxicology Treatment is supportive.

Pharmacodynamics/Kinetics
Onset of Action: Initial changes: 3-5 days; Maximal reduction in plasma cholesterol and triglycerides: 2 weeks
Time to Peak: Serum: 1-2 hours
Protein Binding: ≥98%
Half-Life Elimination: Parent drug: 14 hours
Metabolism: Hepatic; forms active ortho- and parahydroxylated derivates and an inactive beta-oxidation product

Excretion: Bile; urine (2% as unchanged drug)
Available Dosage Forms Tablet: 10 mg, 20 mg, 40 mg, 80 mg

Dosing

Adults & Elderly:

Hyperlipidemias: Oral: Initial: 10-20 mg once daily; patients requiring >45% reduction in LDL-C may be started at 40 mg once daily; range: 10-80 mg once daily

Note: Doses should be individualized according to the baseline LDL-cholesterol levels, the recommended goal of therapy, and patient response; adjustments should be made at intervals of 2-4 weeks

Primary prevention of CVD: Oral: 10 mg once daily

Pediatrics:

HeFH: Children 10-17 years (females >1 year postmenarche): Oral: 10 mg once daily (maximum: 20 mg/day)

Note: Doses should be individualized according to the baseline LDL-cholesterol levels, the recommended goal of therapy, and patient response; adjustments should be made at intervals of 2-4 weeks

Renal Impairment: No adjustment is necessary.
Hepatic Impairment: Decrease dosage with severe disease (eg, chronic alcoholic liver disease).

Administration

Oral: May be administered with food if desired; may take without regard to time of day.

Laboratory Monitoring Monitor lipid levels after 2-4 weeks; LFTs prior to initiation and 12 weeks after initiation or first dose or dose elevation, and periodically (semiannually) thereafter; CPK

Nursing Actions

Physical Assessment: Assess risk potential for interactions with other prescriptions or herbal products patient may be taking (especially those that may increase risk of rhabdomyolysis). Schedule and monitor laboratory tests (eg, liver function tests, lipid levels, CPK) prior to initiation and at regular intervals during therapy. Monitor therapeutic response (decreased lipid levels) and adverse effects regularly during therapy. Teach patient proper use, possible side effects/appropriate interventions, and adverse symptoms to report. **Pregnancy risk factor X** - determine that patient is not pregnant before beginning treatment. Instruct patients of childbearing age about appropriate barrier contraceptive measures.

Patient Education: Do not take any new medication during therapy unless approved by prescriber. May take without regard to food. Maintain adequate hydration (2-3 L/day of fluids) unless instructed to restrict fluid intake. You will need laboratory evaluation during therapy. May cause headache (consult prescriber for approved analgesic); diarrhea (buttermilk, boiled milk, or yogurt may help); euphoria, giddiness, or confusion (use caution when driving or engaging in tasks that require alertness until response to medication is known). Report unresolved diarrhea, unusual muscle cramping or weakness, changes in mood or memory, yellowing of skin or eyes, easy bruising or bleeding, or unusual fatigue. **Pregnancy/breast-feeding precautions:** Inform prescriber if you are pregnant. Do not get pregnant during therapy. Consult prescriber for instructions on appropriate contraceptive measures. This drug can cause severe fetal defects. Do not donate blood while taking this medication and for same period of time after discontinuing. Do not breast-feed.

Dietary Considerations May take with food if desired; may take without regard to time of day. Before initiation of therapy, patients should be placed on a standard cholesterol-lowering diet for 3-6 months and the diet should be continued during drug therapy. Red yeast rice contains an estimated 2.4 mg lovastatin per 600 mg rice.

Geriatric Considerations Effective and well tolerated in elderly. The definition of and, therefore, when to treat hyperlipidemia in the elderly is a controversial issue. The National Cholesterol Education Program recommends that all adults maintain a plasma cholesterol <160 mg/dL. In elderly patients with one additional risk factor, goal LDL would decrease to <130 mg/dL. Pharmacologic treatment should be reserved for those who are unable to obtain a desirable plasma cholesterol concentration by diet alone and for whom the benefits of treatment are believed to outweigh the potential adverse effects, drug interactions, and cost of treatment.

Pregnancy Issues Cholesterol biosynthesis may be important in fetal development. Contraindicated in pregnancy. Administer to women of childbearing potential only when conception is highly unlikely and patients have been informed of potential hazards.

Atovaquone (a TOE va kwone)

U.S. Brand Names Mepron®
Pharmacologic Category Antiprotozoal
Pregnancy Risk Factor C
Lactation Excretion in breast milk unknown/use caution
Use Acute oral treatment of mild-to-moderate *Pneumocystis carinii* pneumonia (PCP) in patients who are intolerant to co-trimoxazole; prophylaxis of PCP in patients intolerant to co-trimoxazole; treatment/suppression of *Toxoplasma gondii* encephalitis; primary prophylaxis of *Toxoplasma gondii* encephalitis in HIV-infected persons at high risk for developing *Toxoplasma gondii* encephalitis

Mechanism of Action/Effect Has not been fully elucidated; may inhibit electron transport in mitochondria inhibiting metabolic enzymes

Contraindications Life-threatening allergic reaction to the drug or formulation

Warnings/Precautions Has only been used in mild-to-moderate PCP. Use with caution in elderly patients due to potentially impaired renal, hepatic, and cardiac function.

Drug Interactions

Decreased Effect: Rifamycins (rifampin) used concurrently decrease the steady-state plasma concentrations of atovaquone.

Increased Effect/Toxicity: Possible increased toxicity with other highly protein-bound drugs.

Nutritional/Ethanol Interactions Food: Ingestion with a fatty meal increases absorption.

Adverse Reactions Note: Adverse reaction statistics have been compiled from studies including patients with advanced HIV disease; consequently, it is difficult to distinguish reactions attributed to atovaquone from those caused by the underlying disease or a combination thereof.

>10%:

Central nervous system: Headache, fever, insomnia, anxiety

Dermatologic: Rash

Gastrointestinal: Nausea, diarrhea, vomiting

Respiratory: Cough

1% to 10%:

Central nervous system: Dizziness

Dermatologic: Pruritus

Endocrine & metabolic: Hypoglycemia, hyponatremia

Gastrointestinal: Abdominal pain, constipation, anorexia, dyspepsia, amylase increased

Hematologic: Anemia, neutropenia, leukopenia

Hepatic: Liver enzymes increased

Neuromuscular & skeletal: Weakness

Renal: BUN/creatinine increased

Miscellaneous: Oral moniliasis

(Continued)

Atovaquone (Continued)

Pharmacodynamics/Kinetics
Protein Binding: >99%
Half-Life Elimination: 2-3 days
Metabolism: Undergoes enterohepatic recirculation
Excretion: Feces (94% as unchanged drug)

Available Dosage Forms Suspension, oral: 750 mg/5 mL (5 mL, 210 mL) [contains benzyl alcohol; citrus flavor]

Dosing
Adults & Elderly:
Prevention of PCP: Oral: 1500 mg once daily with food
Treatment of mild-to-moderate PCP: Oral: 750 mg twice daily with food for 21 days
Pediatrics: Adolescents 13-16 years: Refer to adult dosing.

Stability
Storage: Do not freeze.

Nursing Actions
Physical Assessment: Monitor for CNS and respiratory changes and patient's knowledge of adverse reactions. Assess for interactions with other prescription or OTC medications.
Patient Education: Take as directed. Take with high-fat meals. You may experience dizziness or lightheadedness; use caution when driving or engaging in tasks that require alertness until response to drug is known. Small meals may help reduce nausea. Report unresolved diarrhea, fever, mouth sores (use good mouth care), unresolved headache, or vomiting. **Pregnancy/breast-feeding precautions:** Inform prescriber if you are or intend to become pregnant. Consult prescriber if breast-feeding.

Atovaquone and Proguanil
(a TOE va kwone & pro GWA nil)

U.S. Brand Names Malarone®
Synonyms Proguanil and Atovaquone
Pharmacologic Category Antimalarial Agent
Pregnancy Risk Factor C
Lactation
Atovaquone: Excretion in breast milk unknown/use caution
Proguanil: Enters breast milk (small amounts)/use caution

Use Prevention or treatment of acute, uncomplicated *P. falciparum* malaria

Mechanism of Action/Effect
Atovaquone: Selectively inhibits parasite mitochondrial electron transport.
Proguanil: The metabolite cycloguanil inhibits dihydrofolate reductase, disrupting deoxythymidylate synthesis. Together, atovaquone/cycloguanil affect the erythrocytic and exoerythrocytic stages of development.

Contraindications Hypersensitivity to atovaquone, proguanil, or any component of the formulation; prophylactic use in severe renal impairment

Warnings/Precautions Not indicated for severe or complicated malaria. Absorption of atovaquone may be decreased in patients who have diarrhea or vomiting; monitor closely and consider use of an antiemetic. If severe, consider use of an alternative antimalarial. Do not use with other medications containing proguanil. Administer with caution to patients with pre-existing renal disease. Not for use in patients <5 kg (treatment) or <11 kg (prophylaxis). Delayed cases of *P. falciparum* malaria may occur after stopping prophylaxis; travelers returning from endemic areas who develop febrile illnesses should be evaluated for malaria. Recrudescent infections or infections following prophylaxis with this agent should be treated with alternative agent(s).

Drug Interactions
Cytochrome P450 Effect: Proguanil: **Substrate** (minor) of 1A2, 2C19, 3A4
Decreased Effect: Metoclopramide decreases bioavailability of atovaquone. Rifabutin decreases atovaquone levels by 34%. Rifampin decreases atovaquone levels by 50%. Tetracycline decreases plasma concentrations of atovaquone by 40%.
Nutritional/Ethanol Interactions Food: Atovaquone taken with dietary fat increases the rate and extent of absorption.

Adverse Reactions The following adverse reactions were reported in patients being treated for malaria. When used for prophylaxis, reactions are similar to those seen with placebo.

>10%: Gastrointestinal: Abdominal pain (17%), nausea (12%), vomiting (children 10% to 13%, adults 12%)
1% to 10%:
Central nervous system: Headache (10%), dizziness (5%)
Dermatologic: Pruritus (children 6%)
Gastrointestinal: Diarrhea (children 6%, adults 8%), anorexia (5%)
Neuromuscular & skeletal: Weakness (8%)

Overdosage/Toxicology
Atovaquone: Overdoses of up to 31,500 mg have been reported. Rash has been reported as well as methemoglobinemia in one patient also taking dapsone. There is no known antidote and it is unknown if it is dialyzable.
Proguanil: Single doses of 1500 mg and 700 mg twice daily for 2 weeks have been reported without toxicity. Reversible hair loss, scaling of skin, reversible aphthous ulceration, and hematologic side effects have occurred. Epigastric discomfort and vomiting would also be expected.
There have been no reported overdoses with the atovaquone/proguanil combination.

Pharmacodynamics/Kinetics
Protein Binding: Proguanil: 75%
Half-Life Elimination: Proguanil: 12-21 hours
Metabolism: Proguanil: Hepatic to active metabolites, cycloguanil (via CYP2C19) and 4-chlorophenylbiguanide
Excretion: Proguanil: Urine (40% to 60%)
Pharmacokinetic Note See Atovaquone.

Available Dosage Forms
Tablet: Atovaquone 250 mg and proguanil hydrochloride 100 mg
Tablet, pediatric: Atovaquone 62.5 mg and proguanil hydrochloride 25 mg

Dosing
Adults: Doses given in mg of atovaquone and proguanil:
Prevention of malaria: Oral: Atovaquone/proguanil 250 mg/100 mg once daily; start 1-2 days prior to entering a malaria-endemic area, continue throughout the stay and for 7 days after returning.
Treatment of acute malaria: Oral: Atovaquone/proguanil 1 g/400 mg as a single dose, once daily for 3 consecutive days
Elderly: Refer to adult dosing. Use with caution due to possible decrease in renal and hepatic function, as well as possible decreases in cardiac function, concomitant diseases, or other drug therapy.
Pediatrics: Doses given in mg of atovaquone and proguanil (dosage based on body weight):
Prevention of malaria: Oral: Start 1-2 days prior to entering a malaria-endemic area, continue throughout the stay and for 7 days after returning. Take as a single dose, once daily.
11-20 kg: Atovaquone/proguanil 62.5 mg/25 mg
21-30 kg: Atovaquone/proguanil 125 mg/50 mg
31-40 kg: Atovaquone/proguanil 187.5 mg/75 mg
>40 kg: Atovaquone/proguanil 250 mg/100 mg

Treatment of acute malaria: Oral: Take as a single dose, once daily for 3 consecutive days.
5-8 kg: Atovaquone/proguanil 125 mg/50 mg
9-10 kg: Atovaquone/proguanil 187.5 mg/75 mg
11-20 kg: Atovaquone/proguanil 250 mg/100 mg
21-30 kg: Atovaquone/proguanil 500 mg/200 mg
31-40 kg: Atovaquone/proguanil 750 mg/300 mg
>40 kg: Atovaquone/proguanil 1 g/400 mg

Renal Impairment: Should not be used as prophylaxis in severe renal impairment (Cl_{cr} <30 mL/minute). Alternative treatment regimens should be used in patients with Cl_{cr} <30 mL/minute. No dosage adjustment required in mild-to-moderate renal impairment.

Hepatic Impairment: No dosage adjustment required in mild-to-moderate hepatic impairment. No data available for use in severe hepatic impairment.

Administration

Oral: Administer with food or milk at the same time each day. If patient vomits within 1 hour of administration, repeat the dose. For children who have difficulty swallowing tablets, tablets may be crushed and mixed with condensed milk just prior to administration.

Stability
Storage: Store tablets at 25°C (77°F).

Nursing Actions

Physical Assessment: Assess other medications patient may be taking for effectiveness and interactions. Monitor effectiveness (according to purpose for use), adverse reactions to report, and interventions to reduce side effects.

Patient Education: Do not take any new medication during therapy without consulting prescriber. Complete full course of therapy; do not discontinue or alter dosage without consulting prescriber. Take at the same time each day with full glass of milk or food. If vomiting occurs within 1 hour of taking dose, you may repeat the dose. You may experience nausea, vomiting, or loss of appetite (small frequent meals may help); or headache (if persistent, contact prescriber). Follow recommended precautions to avoid malaria exposure (use insect repellent, bednets, protective clothing). Notify prescriber if you develop fever after returning from or while visiting a malaria-endemic area. **Pregnancy/breast-feeding precautions:** Inform prescriber if you are or intend to become pregnant. Consult prescriber if breast-feeding.

Dietary Considerations Must be taken with food or a milky drink.

Pregnancy Issues Because falciparum malaria can cause maternal death and fetal loss, pregnant women traveling to malaria-endemic areas must use personal protection against mosquito bites.

Related Information
Atovaquone *on page 123*

Atracurium (a tra KYOO ree um)

U.S. Brand Names Tracrium®
Synonyms Atracurium Besylate
Pharmacologic Category Neuromuscular Blocker Agent, Nondepolarizing
Pregnancy Risk Factor C
Lactation Excretion in breast milk unknown/use caution
Use Adjunct to general anesthesia to facilitate endotracheal intubation and to relax skeletal muscles during surgery; to facilitate mechanical ventilation in ICU patients; does not relieve pain or produce sedation
Mechanism of Action/Effect Blocks neural transmission at the myoneural junction by binding with cholinergic receptor sites
Contraindications Hypersensitivity to atracurium besylate or any component of the formulation

Warnings/Precautions Reduce initial dosage and inject slowly (over 1-2 minutes) in patients in whom substantial histamine release would be potentially hazardous (eg, patients with clinically-important cardiovascular disease). Maintenance of an adequate airway and respiratory support is critical. Certain clinical conditions may result in potentiation or antagonism of neuromuscular blockade:

Potentiation: Electrolyte abnormalities, severe hyponatremia, severe hypocalcemia, severe hypokalemia, hypermagnesemia, neuromuscular diseases, acidosis, acute intermittent porphyria, renal failure, hepatic failure

Antagonism: Alkalosis, hypercalcemia, demyelinating lesions, peripheral neuropathies, diabetes mellitus

Increased sensitivity in patients with myasthenia gravis, Eaton-Lambert syndrome; resistance in burn patients (>30% of body) for period of 5-70 days postinjury; resistance in patients with muscle trauma, denervation, immobilization, infection, chronic treatment with atracurium. Cross-sensitivity with other neuromuscular-blocking agents may occur; use extreme caution in patients with previous anaphylactic reactions. Bradycardia may be more common with atracurium than with other neuromuscular-blocking agents since it has no clinically-significant effects on heart rate to counteract the bradycardia produced by anesthetics.

Drug Interactions

Decreased Effect: Effect of nondepolarizing neuromuscular blockers may be reduced by carbamazepine (chronic use), corticosteroids (also associated with myopathy - see increased effect), phenytoin (chronic use), sympathomimetics, and theophylline.

Increased Effect/Toxicity: Increased effects are possible with aminoglycosides, beta-blockers, clindamycin, calcium channel blockers, halogenated anesthetics, imipenem, ketamine, lidocaine, loop diuretics (furosemide), macrolides (case reports), magnesium sulfate, procainamide, quinidine, quinolones, tetracyclines, and vancomycin. May increase risk of myopathy when used with high-dose corticosteroids for extended periods.

Adverse Reactions Mild, rare, and generally suggestive of histamine release
1% to 10%: Cardiovascular: Flushing

Causes of prolonged neuromuscular blockade: Excessive drug administration; cumulative drug effect; metabolism/excretion decreased (hepatic and/or renal impairment); accumulation of active metabolites; electrolyte imbalance (hypokalemia, hypocalcemia, hypermagnesemia, hypernatremia); hypothermia

Overdosage/Toxicology
Symptoms of overdose include respiratory depression and cardiovascular collapse.
Neostigmine 1-3 mg slow I.V. push in adults (0.5 mg in children) antagonizes the neuromuscular blockade and should be administered with or immediately after atropine 1-1.5 mg I.V. push (adults). This may be especially useful in the presence of bradycardia.

Pharmacodynamics/Kinetics
Onset of Action: Dose dependent: 2-3 minutes
Duration of Action: Recovery begins in 20-35 minutes following initial dose of 0.4-0.5 mg/kg under balanced anesthesia; recovery to 95% of control takes 60-70 minutes
Half-Life Elimination: Biphasic: Adults: Initial (distribution): 2 minutes; Terminal: 20 minutes
Metabolism: Undergoes ester hydrolysis and Hofmann elimination (nonbiologic process independent of renal, hepatic, or enzymatic function); metabolites have no neuromuscular blocking properties; laudanosine, a product of Hofmann elimination, is a CNS stimulant and can accumulate with prolonged use. Laudanosine is hepatically metabolized.

(Continued)

Atracurium (Continued)

Excretion: Urine (<5%)

Available Dosage Forms

Injection, as besylate: 10 mg/mL (10 mL) [contains benzyl alcohol]

Injection, as besylate [preservative free]: 10 mg/mL (5 mL)

Dosing

Adults & Elderly: For I.V. administration only (not to be used I.M.): Dose to effect; doses must be individualized due to interpatient variability; use ideal body weight for obese patients.

Adjunct to surgical anesthesia (neuromuscular blockade):

I.V. (bolus): 0.4-0.5 mg/kg, then 0.08-0.1 mg/kg 20-45 minutes after initial dose to maintain neuromuscular block, followed by repeat doses of 0.08-0.1 mg/kg at 15- to 25-minute intervals

Initial dose after succinylcholine for intubation (balanced anesthesia): 0.2-0.4 mg/kg

Pretreatment/priming: I.V.: 10% of intubating dose given 3-5 minutes before initial dose

I.V. continuous infusion: Initial: 9-10 mcg/kg/minute at initial signs of recovery from bolus dose; block is usually maintained by a rate of 5-9 mcg/kg/minute under balanced anesthesia.

ICU neuromuscular blockade: I.V.: Initial (bolus) 0.4-0.5 mg/kg, followed by I.V. continuous infusion at an initial rate of 5-10 mcg/kg/minute; block is usually maintained by rate of 11-13 mcg/kg/minute (rates for pediatric patients may be higher).

Pediatrics:

Adjunct to surgical anesthesia: I.V. (not to be used I.M.): Dose to effect; doses must be individualized due to interpatient variability; use ideal body weight for obese patients

Children 1 month to 2 years: Initial: 0.3-0.4 mg/kg followed by maintenance doses as needed to maintain neuromuscular blockade

Children >2 years: Refer to adult dosing.

Renal Impairment: No adjustment is necessary.

Hepatic Impairment: No adjustment is necessary.

Administration

I.M.: Not for I.M. injection due to tissue irritation.

I.V.: May be given undiluted as a bolus injection. Administration via infusion requires the use of an infusion pump. Use infusion solutions within 24 hours of preparation.

I.V. Detail: pH: 3.25-2.65 (adjusted)

Stability

Compatibility: Stable in D$_5$W, NS, D$_5$NS; **incompatible** with LR

Y-site administration: Incompatible with diazepam, propofol, thiopental

Compatibility when admixed: Incompatible with aminophylline, cefazolin, heparin, quinidine gluconate, ranitidine, sodium nitroprusside

Storage: Refrigerate; unstable in alkaline solutions.

Laboratory Monitoring Renal function (serum creatinine, BUN) and liver function when in ICU

Nursing Actions

Physical Assessment: Only clinicians experienced in the use of neuromuscular-blocking drugs should administer and/or manage the use of atracurium. Ventilatory support must be instituted and maintained until adequate respiratory muscle function and/or airway protection are assured. Assess other medications for effectiveness and safety. Other drugs that affect neuromuscular activity may increase/decrease neuromuscular block induced by atracurium. This drug does not cause anesthesia or analgesia; pain must be treated with appropriate analgesic agents. Continuous monitoring of vital signs, cardiac status,

respiratory status, and degree of neuromuscular block (objective assessment with peripheral external nerve stimulator) is mandatory during infusion and until full muscle tone has returned. Muscle tone returns in a predictable pattern, starting with diaphragm, abdomen, chest, limbs, and finally muscles of the neck, face, and eyes. Safety precautions must be maintained until full muscle tone has returned. **Note:** It may take longer for return of muscle tone in obese or elderly patients or patients with renal or hepatic disease, myasthenia gravis, myopathy, other neuromuscular disease, dehydration, electrolyte imbalance, or severe acid/base imbalance. Provide appropriate patient teaching/support prior to and following administration.

Long-term use: Monitor fluid levels (intake and output) during and following infusion. Reposition patient and provide appropriate skin care, mouth care, and care of patient's eyes every 2-3 hours while sedated. Provide appropriate emotional and sensory support (auditory and environmental).

Patient Education: Patient will usually be unconscious prior to administration. Patient education should be appropriate to individual situation. Reassurance of constant monitoring and emotional support to reduce fear and anxiety should precede and follow administration. Following return of muscle tone, do not attempt to change position or rise from bed without assistance. Report immediately any skin rash or hives, pounding heartbeat, respiratory difficulty, or muscle tremors. **Pregnancy/breast-feeding precautions:** Inform prescriber if you are pregnant. Consult prescriber if breast-feeding.

Additional Information Atracurium is classified as an intermediate-duration neuromuscular-blocking agent. It does not appear to have a cumulative effect on the duration of blockade. It does not relieve pain or produce sedation.

Atropine (A troe peen)

U.S. Brand Names AtroPen®; Atropine-Care®; Isopto® Atropine; Sal-Tropine™

Synonyms Atropine Sulfate

Restrictions The AtroPen® formulation is available for use primarily by the Department of Defense.

Pharmacologic Category Anticholinergic Agent; Anticholinergic Agent, Ophthalmic; Antidote; Antispasmodic Agent, Gastrointestinal; Ophthalmic Agent, Mydriatic

Pregnancy Risk Factor C

Lactation Enters breast milk (trace amounts)/use caution (AAP rates "compatible")

Use

Injection: Preoperative medication to inhibit salivation and secretions; treatment of symptomatic sinus bradycardia; AV block (nodal level); ventricular asystole; antidote for organophosphate pesticide poisoning

Ophthalmic: Produce mydriasis and cycloplegia for examination of the retina and optic disc and accurate measurement of refractive errors; uveitis

Oral: Inhibit salivation and secretions

Unlabeled/Investigational Use Pulseless electric activity, asystole, neuromuscular blockade reversal; treatment of nerve agent toxicity (chemical warfare) in combination with pralidoxime

Mechanism of Action/Effect Blocks the action of acetylcholine at parasympathetic sites in smooth muscle, secretory glands, and the CNS; increases cardiac output, dries secretions, antagonizes histamine and serotonin

Contraindications Hypersensitivity to atropine or any component of the formulation; narrow-angle glaucoma; adhesions between the iris and lens; tachycardia;

obstructive GI disease; paralytic ileus; intestinal atony of the elderly or debilitated patient; severe ulcerative colitis; toxic megacolon complicating ulcerative colitis; hepatic disease; obstructive uropathy; renal disease; myasthenia gravis (unless used to treat side effects of acetylcholinesterase inhibitor); asthma; thyrotoxicosis; Mobitz type II block

Warnings/Precautions Heat prostration can occur in the presence of a high environmental temperature. Psychosis can occur in sensitive individuals. The elderly may be sensitive to side effects. Use caution in patients with myocardial ischemia. Use caution in hyperthyroidism, autonomic neuropathy, BPH, CHF, tachyarrhythmias, hypertension, and hiatal hernia associated with reflux esophagitis. Use with caution in children with spastic paralysis.

AtroPen®: There are no absolute contraindications for the use of atropine in organophosphate poisonings, however, use caution in those patients where the use of atropine would be otherwise contraindicated. Formulation for use by trained personnel only.

Drug Interactions

Decreased Effect: Effect of some phenothiazines may be antagonized. Levodopa effects may be decreased (limited clinical validation). Drugs with cholinergic mechanisms (metoclopramide, cisapride, bethanechol) decrease anticholinergic effects of atropine.

Increased Effect/Toxicity: Antihistamines, phenothiazines, TCAs, and other drugs with anticholinergic activity may increase anticholinergic effects of atropine when used concurrently. Sympathomimetic amines may cause tachyarrhythmias; avoid concurrent use.

Adverse Reactions Severity and frequency of adverse reactions are dose related and vary greatly; listed reactions are limited to significant and/or life-threatening.

Cardiovascular: Arrhythmia, flushing, hypotension, palpitation, tachycardia

Central nervous system: Ataxia, coma, delirium, disorientation, dizziness, drowsiness, excitement, fever, hallucinations, headache, insomnia, nervousness

Dermatologic: Anhidrosis, urticaria, rash, scarlatiniform rash

Gastrointestinal: Bloating, constipation, delayed gastric emptying, loss of taste, nausea, paralytic ileus, vomiting, xerostomia

Genitourinary: Urinary hesitancy, urinary retention

Neuromuscular & skeletal: Weakness

Ocular: Angle-closure glaucoma, blurred vision, cycloplegia, dry eyes, mydriasis, ocular tension increased

Respiratory: Dyspnea, laryngospasm, pulmonary edema

Miscellaneous: Anaphylaxis

Overdosage/Toxicology Symptoms of overdose include dilated, unreactive pupils; blurred vision; hot, dry flushed skin; dryness of mucous membranes; difficulty swallowing; foul breath; diminished or absent bowel sounds; urinary retention; tachycardia; hyperthermia; hypertension; and increased respiratory rate. For anticholinergic overdose with severe life-threatening symptoms, physostigmine 1-2 mg SubQ or I.V. slowly, may be given to reverse these effects.

Pharmacodynamics/Kinetics

Onset of Action: I.V.: Rapid

Half-Life Elimination: 2-3 hours

Metabolism: Hepatic

Excretion: Urine (30% to 50% as unchanged drug and metabolites)

Available Dosage Forms

Injection, solution, as sulfate: 0.05 mg/mL (5 mL); 0.1 mg/mL (5 mL, 10 mL); 0.4 mg/mL (0.5 mL, 1 mL, 20 mL); 0.5 mg/mL (1 mL); 1 mg/mL (1 mL)

AtroPen® [prefilled autoinjector]: 0.5 mg/0.7 mL (0.7 mL); 1 mg/0.7 mL (0.7 mL); 2 mg/0.7 mL (0.7 mL)

Ointment, ophthalmic, as sulfate: 1% (3.5 g)

Solution, ophthalmic, as sulfate: 1% (5 mL, 15 mL)

Atropine-Care®: 1% (2 mL)

Isopto® Atropine: 1% (5 mL, 15 mL)

Tablet, as sulfate (Sal-Tropine™): 0.4 mg

Dosing

Adults: Doses <0.5 mg have been associated with paradoxical bradycardia.

Asystole:

I.V.: 1 mg; repeat in 3-5 minutes if asystole persists; total dose of 0.04 mg/kg.

Intratracheal: Administer 2-2.5 times the recommended I.V. dose; dilute in 10 mL NS or distilled water. **Note:** Absorption is greater with distilled water, but causes more adverse effects on PaO_2.

Inhibit salivation and secretions (preanesthesia):

I.M., I.V., SubQ: 0.4-0.6 mg 30-60 minutes preop and repeat every 4-6 hours as needed.

Oral: 0.4 mg, may repeat every 4-6 hours

Bradycardia: I.V.: 0.5-1 mg every 5 minutes, not to exceed a total of 3 mg or 0.04 mg/kg; may give intratracheal in 1 mg/10 mL dilution only, intratracheal dose should be 2-2.5 times the I.V. dose.

Neuromuscular blockade reversal: I.V.: 25-30 mcg/kg 30-60 seconds before neostigmine or 7-10 mcg/kg 30-60 seconds before edrophonium

Organophosphate or carbamate poisoning:

I.V.: 2 mg, followed by 2 mg every 15 minutes until adequate atropinization has occurred; initial doses of up to 6 mg may be used in life-threatening cases

I.M.: AtroPen®: Mild symptoms: Administer 2 mg as soon as exposure is known or suspected. If severe symptoms develop after first dose, 2 additional doses should be repeated in 10 minutes; do not administer more than 3 doses. Severe symptoms: Immediately administer three 2 mg doses.

Nerve agent toxicity management (unlabeled use):

I.M.: See **Note**. Prehospital ("in the field") or hospital/emergency department: Mild-to-moderate symptoms: 2-4 mg; severe symptoms: 6 mg

Note: Pralidoxime is a component of the management of nerve agent toxicity; consult Pralidoxime for specific route and dose.

Prehospital ("in the field") management: Repeat atropine I.M. (2 mg) at 5-10 minute intervals until secretions have diminished and breathing is comfortable or airway resistance has returned to near normal.

Hospital management: Repeat atropine I.M. (2 mg) at 5-10 minute intervals until secretions have diminished and breathing is comfortable or airway resistance has returned to near normal.

Mydriasis, cycloplegia (preprocedure): Ophthalmic (1% solution): Instill 1-2 drops 1 hour before the procedure.

Uveitis: Ophthalmic:

1% solution: Instill 1-2 drops 4 times/day.

Ointment: Apply a small amount in the conjunctival sac up to 3 times/day. Compress the lacrimal sac by digital pressure for 1-3 minutes after instillation.

Elderly: Refer to adult dosing.

Nerve agent toxicity management (unlabeled use):

See **Note**. I.M.: Elderly and frail patients:

Prehospital ("in the field"): Mild-to-moderate symptoms: 1 mg; severe symptoms: 2-4 mg

Hospital/emergency department: Mild-to-moderate symptoms: 1 mg; severe symptoms: 2 mg

Note: Pralidoxime is a component of the management of nerve agent toxicity.

Prehospital ("in the field") management: Repeat atropine I.M. (2 mg) at 5-10 minute intervals until secretions have diminished and breathing is comfortable or airway resistance has returned to near normal.

(Continued)

Atropine (Continued)

Hospital management: Repeat atropine I.M. (2 mg) at 5-10 minute intervals until secretions have diminished and breathing is comfortable or airway resistance has returned to near normal.

Pediatrics: Note: Doses <0.1 mg have been associated with paradoxical bradycardia.

Inhibit salivation and secretions (preanesthesia): Oral, I.M., I.V., SubQ: Neonates, Infants, and Children:

Children <5 kg: 0.02 mg/kg/dose 30-60 minutes preop then every 4-6 hours as needed. Use of a minimum dosage of 0.1 mg in neonates <5 kg will result in dosages >0.02 mg/kg. There is no documented minimum dosage in this age group.

Children >5 kg: 0.01-0.02 mg/kg/dose to a maximum 0.4 mg/dose 30-60 minutes preop; minimum dose: 0.1 mg

Alternate dosing:

3-7 kg (7-16 lb): 0.1 mg
8-11 kg (17-24 lb): 0.15 mg
11-18 kg (24-40 lb): 0.2 mg
18-29 kg (40-65 lb): 0.3 mg
>30 kg (>65 lb): 0.4 mg

Bradycardia: I.V., intratracheal: Neonates, Infants, and Children: 0.02 mg/kg, minimum dose 0.1 mg, maximum single dose: 0.5 mg in children and 1 mg in adolescents; may repeat in 5-minute intervals to a maximum total dose of 1 mg in children or 2 mg in adolescents. (**Note:** For intratracheal administration, the dosage must be diluted with normal saline to a total volume of 1-5 mL). When treating bradycardia in neonates, reserve use for those patients unresponsive to improved oxygenation and epinephrine.

Organophosphate or carbamate poisoning:

I.V.: Children: 0.03-0.05 mg/kg every 10-20 minutes until atropine effect, then every 1-4 hours for at least 24 hours

I.M. (AtroPen®): Children: Mild symptoms: Administer dose listed below as soon as exposure is known or suspected. If severe symptoms develop after first dose, 2 additional doses should be repeated in 10 minutes; do not administer more than 3 doses. Severe symptoms: Immediately administer 3 doses as follows:

<6.8 kg (15 lb): Use of **AtroPen® formulation not recommended;** administer atropine 0.05 mg/kg
6.8-18 kg (15-40 lb): 0.5 mg/dose
18-41 kg (40-90 lb): 1 mg/dose
>41 kg (>90 lb): 2 mg/dose

Nerve agent toxicity management (unlabeled use):

I.M.: Infants and Children: See following **Note.**

Prehospital ("in the field"):

Birth to <2 years: Mild-to-moderate symptoms: 0.05 mg/kg; severe symptoms: 0.1 mg/kg
2-10 years: Mild-to-moderate symptoms: 1 mg; severe symptoms: 2 mg
>10 years: Mild-to-moderate symptoms: 2 mg; severe symptoms: 4 mg

Hospital/emergency department:

Birth to <2 years: Mild-to-moderate symptoms: 0.05 mg/kg I.M. **or** 0.02 mg/kg I.V.; severe symptoms: 0.1 mg/kg I.M. **or** 0.02 mg/kg I.V.
2-10 years: Mild-to-moderate symptoms: 1 mg; severe symptoms: 2 mg
>10 years: Mild-to-moderate symptoms: 2 mg; severe symptoms: 4 mg

Note: Pralidoxime is a component of the management of nerve agent toxicity; consult Pralidoxime for specific route and dose.

Prehospital ("in the field") management: Repeat atropine I.M. (0.05-0.1 mg/kg) at 5-10 minute intervals until secretions have diminished and breathing is comfortable or airway resistance has returned to near normal.

Hospital management: Repeat atropine I.M. (infants: 1 mg; all others: 2 mg) at 5-10 minute intervals until secretions have diminished and breathing is comfortable or airway resistance has returned to near normal.

Administration

I.M.: AtroPen®: Administer to outer thigh. May be given through clothing as long as pockets at the injection site are empty. Hold autoinjector in place for 10 seconds following injection; massage the injection site.

I.V.: Administer undiluted by rapid I.V. injection; slow injection may result in paradoxical bradycardia.

I.V. Detail: pH: 3-6.5; AtroPen®: pH: 4-5

Other: Intratracheal: Dilute in NS or distilled water. Absorption is greater with distilled water, but causes more adverse effects on PaO_2. Pass catheter beyond tip of tracheal tube, stop compressions, spray drug quickly down tube. Follow immediately with several quick insufflations and continue chest compressions.

Stability

Compatibility:

Y-site administration: Incompatible with thiopental

Compatibility in syringe: Incompatible with cimetidine/pentobarbital

Compatibility when admixed: Incompatible with floxacillin, metaraminol, methohexital, norepinephrine

Storage: Store injection at controlled room temperature of 15°C to 30°C (59°F to 86°F); avoid freezing. In addition, AtroPen® should be protected from light.

Nursing Actions

Physical Assessment: Assess other medications patient may be taking for effectiveness and interactions. Monitor for tachycardia, hypotension especially if cardiac problems are present. Ensure patient safety (side rails up, call light within reach), have patient void prior to administration, and ensure adequate hydration. Be alert to the potential of heat prostration in the presence of high temperatures. Assess knowledge/teach patient appropriate use, interventions to reduce side effects, and adverse symptoms to report.

Patient Education: Take oral forms exactly as directed, 30 minutes before meals. Maintain adequate hydration (2-3 L/day of fluids) unless instructed to restrict fluid intake. Void before taking medication. You may experience dizziness, blurred vision, sensitivity to light (use caution when driving or engaging in tasks requiring alertness until response to drug is known); dry mouth, nausea, or vomiting (small frequent meals, frequent mouth care, sucking lozenges, or chewing gum may help); orthostatic hypotension (use caution when climbing stairs and when rising from lying or sitting position); constipation (increased exercise, fluids, fruit, or fiber may help; if not effective, consult prescriber); increased sensitivity to heat and decreased perspiration (avoid extremes of heat, reduce exercise in hot weather); or decreased milk if breast-feeding. Report hot, dry, flushed skin; blurred vision or vision changes; difficulty swallowing; chest pain, palpitations, or rapid heartbeat; painful or difficult urination; increased confusion, depression, or loss of memory; rapid or difficult respirations; muscle weakness or tremors; or eye pain.

Ophthalmic: Instill as often as recommended. Wash hands before using. Sit or lie down, open eye, look at ceiling, and instill prescribed amount of solution. Do not blink for 30 seconds, close eye and roll eye in all directions, and apply gentle pressure to inner corner of eye for 1-2 minutes. Do not let tip of applicator touch eye; do not contaminate tip of applicator (may cause eye infection, eye damage, or vision loss). Temporary stinging or blurred vision may occur.

Pregnancy/breast-feeding precautions: Inform prescriber if you are or intend to become pregnant. Consult prescriber if breast-feeding.

Geriatric Considerations Anticholinergic agents are generally not well tolerated in the elderly and their use should be avoided when possible (see Warnings/Precautions, Adverse Reactions). In the elderly, anticholinergic agents should not be used as prophylaxis against extrapyramidal symptoms.

Breast-Feeding Issues Anticholinergic agents may suppress lactation.

Related Information
Compatibility of Drugs *on page 1370*
Compatibility of Drugs in Syringe *on page 1372*

Azacitidine (ay za SYE ti deen)

U.S. Brand Names Vidaza™

Synonyms AZA-CR; 5-Azacytidine; 5-AZC; Ladakamycin; NSC-102816

Pharmacologic Category Antineoplastic Agent, Antimetabolite (Pyrimidine)

Pregnancy Risk Factor D

Lactation Excretion in breast milk unknown/not recommended

Use Treatment of myelodysplastic syndrome (MDS)

Unlabeled/Investigational Use Investigational: Refractory acute lymphocytic and myelogenous leukemia

Mechanism of Action/Effect Antineoplastic effects may be a result of azacitidine's ability to promote hypomethylation of DNA leading to direct toxicity of abnormal hematopoietic cells in the bone marrow.

Contraindications Hypersensitivity to azacitidine, mannitol, or any component of the formulation; advanced malignant hepatic tumors; pregnancy

Warnings/Precautions The U.S. Food and Drug Administration (FDA) currently recommends that procedures for proper handling and disposal of antineoplastic agents be considered. Azacitidine may be hepatotoxic, use caution with hepatic impairment. Progressive hepatic coma leading to death has been reported (rare) in patients with extensive tumor burden, especially those with a baseline albumin <30 g/L. Use caution with renal impairment; dose adjustment may be required.

Adverse Reactions Note: Percentages reported are following SubQ administration unless otherwise noted.
>10%:
Cardiovascular: Hypotension (7%; I.V. 6% to 66% - incidence may be related to dose and rate of infusion), chest pain (16%), pallor (15%), peripheral edema (19%), pitting edema (14%)
Central nervous system: Pyrexia (52%), fatigue (13% to 36%), headache (22%), dizziness (19%), anxiety (13%), depression (12%), insomnia (11%), malaise (11%), pain (11%)
Dermatologic: Alopecia (I.V. 20%), bruising (30%), petechiae (24%), erythema (17%), skin lesion (14%), rash (14%)
Gastrointestinal: Nausea (70%; more common/more severe with I.V. administration), vomiting (54%; more common/more severe with I.V. administration), mucositis (I.V. 23% to 45%), diarrhea (36%), constipation (34%), anorexia (21%), weight loss (16%), abdominal pain (15%), appetite decreased (13%), abdominal tenderness (12%)
Hematologic: Anemia (70%), thrombocytopenia (66%), leukopenia (48%), neutropenia (32%), febrile neutropenia (16%)
Nadir: Day 10-17
Recovery: Day 28-31
Hepatic: Hepatic enzymes increased (I.V. 37%)
Local: Injection site:
I.V.: Redness, irritation, and induration (80%)

SubQ: Erythema (35%), pain (23%), bruising (14%)
Neuromuscular & skeletal: Weakness (30%), rigors (26%), arthralgia (22%), limb pain (20%), back pain (19%), myalgia (16%)
Respiratory: Cough (30%), dyspnea (5% to 30%), pharyngitis (20%), epistaxis (16%), nasopharyngitis (14%), upper respiratory tract infection (13%), productive cough (11%), pneumonia (11%)
Miscellaneous: Contusion (19%)
5% to 10%:
Cardiovascular: Cardiac murmur (10%), tachycardia (9%), peripheral swelling (7%), syncope (6%), chest wall pain (5%), hypoesthesia (5%), postprocedural pain (5%)
Central nervous system: Lethargy (8%)
Dermatologic: Cellulitis (8%), urticaria (6%), dry skin (5%), skin nodule (5%)
Gastrointestinal: Upper abdominal pain (10%), gingival bleeding (9%), oral mucosal petechiae (8%), stomatitis (8%), dyspepsia (7%), hemorrhoids (7%), abdominal distension (6%), loose stools (5%), dysphagia (5%), tongue ulceration (5%)
Genitourinary: Dysuria (8%), urinary tract infection (8%)
Hematologic: Hematoma (9%), postprocedural hemorrhage (6%)
Local: Injection site: Pruritus (7%), granuloma (5%), pigmentation change (5%), swelling (5%)
Neuromuscular & skeletal: Muscle cramps (6%)
Respiratory: Crackles (10%), rhinorrhea (10%), wheezing (9%), breath sounds decreased (8%), pleural effusion (6%), postnasal drip (6%), rhonchi (6%), nasal congestion (5%), atelectasis (5%), sinusitis (5%)
Miscellaneous: Diaphoresis (10%), lymphadenopathy (9%), herpes simplex (9%), night sweats (9%), transfusion reaction (7%), mouth hemorrhage (5%)

Overdosage/Toxicology Diarrhea, nausea, and vomiting were reported following a single I.V. dose of 290 mg/m^2. Treatment should be supportive.

Pharmacodynamics/Kinetics
Time to Peak: 30 minutes
Half-Life Elimination: ~4 hours
Metabolism: Hepatic; hydrolysis to several metabolites
Excretion: Urine (50% to 85%); feces (minor)

Available Dosage Forms Injection, powder for suspension: 100 mg [contains mannitol 100 mg]

Dosing
Adults & Elderly: Note: I.V. administration is an unlabeled use; doses reported in combination regimens.
Acute leukemia: I.V.:
50-150 mg/m^2 days 1 through 5 of induction
200 mg/m^2 CIVI days 7 through 9 of induction
AML induction: I.V.: 150 mg/m^2 days 3 through 5 and 8 through 10, **then**
150 mg/m^2 days 1 through 5 and 8 through 10 (cycle 2 consolidation)
AML consolidation: I.V.: 150 mg/m^2 CIVI days 1 through 7 for 3 cycles
AML maintenance: I.V.: 150 mg/m^2 days 1 through 3 every 6 weeks
CML (accelerated phase and blast crisis): I.V.: 50-150 mg/m^2 days 1 through 5 of induction
MDS:
I.V.: 75-150 mg/m^2 CIVI days 1 through 7 every 4 weeks
SubQ: 75 mg/m^2/day for 7 days repeated every 4 weeks. Dose may be increased to 100 mg/m^2/day if no benefit is observed after 2 cycles and no toxicity other than nausea and vomiting have occurred. Treatment is recommended for at least 4 cycles.
(Continued)

Azacitidine *(Continued)*

Dosage adjustment based on hematology: SubQ:
For baseline WBC ≥3.0 x 10⁹/L, ANC ≥1.5 x 10⁹/L, and platelets ≥75 x 10⁹/L:

Nadir count: ANC <0.5 x 10⁹/L and platelets <25 x 10⁹/L: Administer 50% of dose during next treatment course

Nadir count: ANC 0.5-1.5 x 10⁹/L and platelets 25-50 x 10⁹/L: Administer 67% of dose during next treatment course

Nadir count: ANC >1.5 x 10⁹/L and platelets >50 x 10⁹/L: Administer 100% of dose during next treatment course

For baseline WBC <3 x 10⁹/L, ANC 1.5 x 10⁹/L, or platelets <75 x 10⁹/L: Adjust dose as follows based on nadir counts and bone marrow biopsy cellularity at the time of nadir, unless clear improvement in differentiation at the time of the next cycle:

WBC or platelet nadir decreased 50% to 75% from baseline and bone marrow biopsy cellularity at time of nadir 30% to 60%: Administer 100% of dose during next treatment course

WBC or platelet nadir decreased 50% to 75% from baseline and bone marrow biopsy cellularity at time of nadir 15% to 30%: Administer 50% of dose during next treatment course

WBC or platelet nadir decreased 50% to 75% from baseline and bone marrow biopsy cellularity at time of nadir <15%: Administer 33% of dose during next treatment course

WBC or platelet nadir decreased >75% from baseline and bone marrow biopsy cellularity at time of nadir 30% to 60%: Administer 75% of dose during next treatment course

WBC or platelet nadir decreased >75% from baseline and bone marrow biopsy cellularity at time of nadir 15% to 30%: Administer 50% of dose during next treatment course

WBC or platelet nadir decreased >75% from baseline and bone marrow biopsy cellularity at time of nadir <15%: Administer 33% of dose during next treatment course

Note: If a nadir defined above occurs, administer the next treatment course 28 days after the start of the preceding course as long as WBC and platelet counts are >25% above the nadir and rising. If a >25% increase above the nadir is not seen by day 28, reassess counts every 7 days. If a 25% increase is not seen by day 42, administer 50% of the scheduled dose.

Dosage adjustment base on serum electrolytes: If serum bicarbonate falls to <20 mEq/L (unexplained decrease): Reduce dose by 50% for next treatment course

Pediatrics: Note: Unlabeled use; doses reported in combination regimens:
Pediatric AML and ANLL: I.V.: 250 mg/m² days 4 and 5 every 4 weeks
Pediatric AML induction: I.V.: 300 mg/m² days 5 and 6

Renal Impairment: Adults: If unexplained increases in BUN or serum creatinine occur, delay next cycle until values reach baseline or normal, then reduce dose by 50% for next treatment course.

Administration

I.V.: Premedication for nausea and vomiting is recommended. Administer as short (15 minutes to 2 hours) bolus or continuous (24 hours) infusion. Due to azacitidine's limited stability, for continuous infusions the daily dose should be divided by 12, and a freshly prepared bag, using a freshly reconstituted vial, started every 2 hours.

Other: SubQ: Premedication for nausea and vomiting is recommended. Doses >50 mg (2 mL) should be divided into two syringes and injected into two separate sites. Allow refrigerated suspensions to come to room temperature (up to 30 minutes) prior to administration. Resuspend by gently rolling the syringe between the palms for 30 seconds. If azacitidine suspension comes in contact with the skin, immediately wash with soap and water.

Stability
Reconstitution:

SubQ: Slowly add 4 mL SWFI to each vial. Invert vial 2-3 times and gently rotate until a suspension is formed.

I.V.: Reconstitute vial with 19.9 mL of lactated Ringer's injection, 0.9% sodium chloride, or 5% dextrose to form a 5 mg/mL solution. Mix in 50-250 mL (final concentration ≥2 mg/mL) lactated Ringer's injection for infusion.

Storage:

SubQ: Prior to reconstitution, store powder at room temperature of 15°C to 30°C (59°F to 86°F). Following reconstitution, suspension may be stored at room temperature for up to 1 hour, or immediately refrigerated at 2°C to 8°C (36°F to 46°F) and stored for up to 8 hours.

I.V.: Solutions for injection have very limited stability and must be prepared fresh immediately prior to each dose. Solutions (≥2 mg/mL) in lactated Ringer's injection are stable for 3 hours; solutions in 5% dextrose in water or 0.9% sodium chloride injection are only stable for ~1 hour.

Laboratory Monitoring Liver function tests, electrolytes, CBC, renal function tests (BUN and serum creatinine) should be obtained prior to initiation of therapy. Electrolytes, renal function (BUN and creatinine), CBC should be monitored periodically to monitor response and toxicity. At a minimum, CBC should be repeated prior to each cycle.

Nursing Actions

Physical Assessment: Pretreatment with antiemetic is recommended to reduce nausea and vomiting. Solutions have limited stability; note specific administration, reconstitution, and storage instructions. Monitor laboratory tests prior to beginning therapy and prior to each cycle. Monitor patient closely for adverse effects (eg, hypotension, CNS changes, gastrointestinal, hematologic, and hepatic effects). Teach patient (or caregiver) possible side effects/appropriate intervention and adverse symptoms to report.

Patient Education: Do not take anything new during treatment unless approved by prescriber. This medication can only be administered by injection (or I.V.); report immediately any pain, burning, or swelling at injection/infusion site. Limit oral intake for 4-6 hours before therapy to reduce potential for nausea/vomiting. It is important that you maintain adequate nutrition between treatments (small, frequent meals may help) and adequate hydration (2-3 L/day of fluids), unless advised by prescriber to restrict fluids. You may be susceptible to infection (avoid crowds and exposure to infection and do not have any vaccinations without consulting prescriber). May cause nausea, vomiting, or anorexia (small, frequent meals, frequent mouth care, chewing gum, or sucking lozenges may help - if nausea/vomiting are severe, request antiemetic); mouth sores (use soft toothbrush or cotton swabs for mouth care); or loss of hair (reversible). Report chest pain or palpitations; sore throat, fever, chills, unusual weakness or fatigue; unusual bruising/bleeding; change in color of urine or stool; difficulty breathing; change in visual acuity; pain, redness, or swelling at injection site; or any other adverse reactions. **Pregnancy/breast-feeding precautions:** Inform prescriber if you are pregnant. Do not get pregnant or cause a pregnancy (males) during therapy. Consult prescriber for instruction on appropriate contraceptive measures. This drug may cause severe fetal defects. Breast-feeding is not recommended.

Geriatric Considerations Monitor renal function

Pregnancy Issues Embryotoxicity, fetal death, and fetal abnormalities were observed in animal studies. Women of childbearing potential should be advised to avoid pregnancy during treatment. In addition, males should be advised to avoid fathering a child while on azacitidine therapy.

Azathioprine (ay za THYE oh preen)

U.S. Brand Names Azasan®; Imuran®

Synonyms Azathioprine Sodium

Pharmacologic Category Immunosuppressant Agent

Medication Safety Issues
Sound-alike/look-alike issues:
Azathioprine may be confused with azatadine, azidothymidine, Azulfidine®
Imuran® may be confused with Elmiron®, Enduron®, Imdur®, Inderal®, Tenormin®

Pregnancy Risk Factor D

Lactation Enters breast milk/not recommended

Use Adjunctive therapy in prevention of rejection of kidney transplants; active rheumatoid arthritis

Unlabeled/Investigational Use Adjunct in prevention of rejection of solid organ (nonrenal) transplants; maintenance of remission in Crohn's disease

Mechanism of Action/Effect Antagonizes purine metabolism and may inhibit synthesis of DNA, RNA, and proteins; may also interfere with cellular metabolism and inhibit mitosis; the 6-thioguanine nucleotides appear to mediate the majority of azathioprine's immunosuppressive and toxic effects

Contraindications Hypersensitivity to azathioprine or any component of the formulation; pregnancy

Warnings/Precautions Chronic immunosuppression increases the risk of neoplasia and serious infections. Azathioprine has mutagenic potential to both men and women and with possible hematologic toxicities; hematologic toxicities are dose related and may be more severe with renal transplants undergoing rejection. Gastrointestinal toxicity may occur within the first several weeks of therapy and is reversible. Symptoms may include severe nausea, vomiting, diarrhea, rash, fever, malaise, myalgia, hypotension, and liver enzyme abnormalities. Use with caution in patients with liver disease, renal impairment; monitor hematologic function closely. Patients with genetic deficiency of thiopurine methyltransferase (TPMT) or concurrent therapy with drugs which may inhibit TPMT may be sensitive to myelosuppressive effects.

Drug Interactions
Decreased Effect: Azathioprine may result in decreased action of warfarin.

Increased Effect/Toxicity: Allopurinol may increase serum levels of azathioprine's active metabolite (mercaptopurine). Decrease azathioprine dose to $1/3$ to $1/4$ of normal dose. Azathioprine and ACE inhibitors may induce anemia and severe leukopenia. Aminosalicylates (olsalazine, mesalamine, sulfasalazine) may inhibit TPMT, increasing toxicity/myelosuppression of azathioprine.

Nutritional/Ethanol Interactions Herb/Nutraceutical: Avoid cat's claw, echinacea (have immunostimulant properties).

Adverse Reactions Frequency not defined; dependent upon dose, duration, and concomitant therapy.
Central nervous system: Fever, malaise
Dermatologic: Alopecia, rash
Gastrointestinal: Diarrhea, nausea, pancreatitis, vomiting
Hematologic: Bleeding, leukopenia, macrocytic anemia, pancytopenia, thrombocytopenia

Hepatic: Hepatotoxicity, hepatic veno-occlusive disease, steatorrhea
Neuromuscular & skeletal: Arthralgia, myalgia
Respiratory: Interstitial pneumonitis
Miscellaneous: Hypersensitivity reactions (rare), infection secondary to immunosuppression, neoplasia

Overdosage/Toxicology Symptoms of overdose include nausea, vomiting, diarrhea, and hematologic toxicity. Following initiation of essential overdose management, symptomatic and supportive treatment should be instituted. Dialysis has been reported to remove significant amounts of the drug and its metabolites, and should be considered as a treatment option in those patients who deteriorate despite established forms of therapy.

Pharmacodynamics/Kinetics
Time to Peak: Plasma: 1-2 hours (including metabolites)

Protein Binding: ~30%

Half-Life Elimination: Parent drug: 12 minutes; mercaptopurine: 0.7-3 hours; End-stage renal disease: Slightly prolonged

Metabolism: Hepatic, to 6-mercaptopurine (6-MP), possibly by glutathione S-transferase (GST). Further metabolism of 6-MP (in the liver and GI tract), via three major pathways: Hypoxanthine guanine phosphoribosyltransferase (to 6-thioguanine-nucleotides, or 6-TGN), xanthine oxidase (to 6-thiouric acid), and thiopurine methyltransferase (TPMT), which forms 6-methylmercaptopurine (6-MMP).

Excretion: Urine (primarily as metabolites)

Available Dosage Forms
Injection, powder for reconstitution: 100 mg
Tablet [scored]: 50 mg
Azasan®: 75 mg, 100 mg
Imuran®: 50 mg

Dosing
Adults & Elderly: I.V. dose is equivalent to oral dose.
Renal transplantation: Oral, I.V.: Initial: 3-5 mg/kg/day usually given as a single daily dose, then 1-3 mg/kg/day maintenance
Rheumatoid arthritis: Oral:
Initial: 1 mg/kg/day given once daily or divided twice daily, for 6-8 weeks; increase by 0.5 mg/kg every 4 weeks until response or up to 2.5 mg/kg/day; an adequate trial should be a minimum of 12 weeks
Maintenance dose: Reduce dose by 0.5 mg/kg every 4 weeks until lowest effective dose is reached; optimum duration of therapy not specified; may be discontinued abruptly
Adjunctive management of severe recurrent aphthous stomatitis (unlabeled use): Oral: 50 mg once daily in conjunction with prednisone

Pediatrics: Renal transplantation, rheumatoid arthritis (unlabeled uses): Refer to adult dosing.

Renal Impairment:
Cl_{cr} 10-50 mL/minute: Administer 75% of normal dose.
Cl_{cr} <10 mL/minute: Administer 50% of normal dose.
Hemodialysis: Dialyzable (~45% removed in 8 hours)
Administer dose posthemodialysis: CAPD effects: Unknown; CAVH effects: Unknown

Administration
Oral: Administering tablets after meals or in divided doses may decrease adverse GI events.
I.V.: Can be administered IVP over 5 minutes at a concentration not to exceed 10 mg/mL **or** azathioprine can be further diluted with normal saline or D_5W and administered by intermittent infusion usually over 30-60 minutes; may be extended up to 8 hours.
I.V. Detail: pH: 9.6

Stability
Compatibility: Stable in neutral or acid solutions, but is hydrolyzed to mercaptopurine in alkaline solutions. Stable in D_5W, $1/2NS$, NS.
(Continued)

Azathioprine *(Continued)*

Storage:

Tablet: Store at room temperature of 15°C to 25°C (59°F to 77°F); protect from light.

Powder for injection: Store at room temperature of 15°C to 25°C (59°F to 77°F) and protect from light. Parenteral admixture is stable at room temperature (25°C) for 24 hours, and stable under refrigeration (4°C) for 16 days.

Laboratory Monitoring
CBC, platelet counts, total bilirubin, liver function tests, TPMT genotyping or phenotyping

Nursing Actions

Physical Assessment: Assess effectiveness and interactions of other medications patient may be taking. Monitor laboratory tests, therapeutic response (according to purpose for use) and adverse reactions at beginning of therapy and periodically throughout therapy, especially opportunistic infection (eg, fever, mouth and vaginal sores or plaques, unhealed wounds). Assess knowledge/teach patient appropriate use, interventions to reduce side effects, and adverse symptoms to report.

Patient Education: Take as prescribed (may take in divided doses or with food if GI upset occurs). You will be susceptible to infection (avoid crowds and exposure to infection and do not have any vaccinations unless approved by prescriber). You may experience nausea, vomiting, loss of appetite (small frequent meals, frequent mouth care, chewing gum, or sucking lozenges may help). Report abdominal pain and unresolved GI upset (eg, persistent vomiting or diarrhea); unusual fever or chills; bleeding or bruising; sore throat, unhealed sores, or signs of infection; yellowing of skin or eyes; or change in color of urine or stool.

Rheumatoid arthritis: Response may not occur for up to 3 months; do not discontinue medication without consulting prescriber.

Organ transplant: Azathioprine will usually be prescribed with other antirejection medications.

Pregnancy/breast-feeding precautions: Do not get pregnant while taking this medication; use appropriate contraceptive measures. Breast-feeding is not recommended.

Dietary Considerations
May be taken with food.

Geriatric Considerations
Immunosuppressive toxicity is increased in the elderly. Signs or symptoms of infection may differ in the elderly. Lethargy or confusion may be the first signs of infection.

Breast-Feeding Issues
Due to risk of immunosuppression, breast-feeding is not recommended.

Pregnancy Issues
Azathioprine crosses the placenta in humans; congenital anomalies, immunosuppression and intrauterine growth retardation have been reported. There are no adequate and well-controlled studies in pregnant women. Azathioprine should not be used to treat arthritis during pregnancy. The potential benefit to the mother versus possible risk to the fetus should be considered when treating other disease states.

Azithromycin *(az ith roe MYE sin)*

U.S. Brand Names
Zithromax®; Zmax™

Synonyms
Azithromycin Dihydrate; Zithromax® TRI-PAK™; Zithromax® Z-PAK®

Pharmacologic Category
Antibiotic, Macrolide

Medication Safety Issues

Sound-alike/look-alike issues:

Azithromycin may be confused with erythromycin

Zithromax® may be confused with Zinacef®

Pregnancy Risk Factor
B

Lactation
Enters breast milk/use caution

Use
Treatment of acute otitis media due to *H. influenzae, M. catarrhalis,* or *S. pneumoniae;* pharyngitis/tonsillitis due to *S. pyogenes;* treatment of mild-to-moderate upper and lower respiratory tract infections, infections of the skin and skin structure, community-acquired pneumonia, pelvic inflammatory disease (PID), sexually-transmitted diseases (urethritis/cervicitis), pharyngitis/tonsillitis (alternative to first-line therapy), and genital ulcer disease (chancroid) due to susceptible strains of *C. trachomatis, M. catarrhalis, H. influenzae, S. aureus, S. pneumoniae, Mycoplasma pneumoniae,* and *C. psittaci;* acute bacterial exacerbations of chronic obstructive pulmonary disease (COPD) due to *H. influenzae, M. catarrhalis,* or *S. pneumoniae;* acute bacterial sinusitis

Unlabeled/Investigational Use
Prevention of (or to delay onset of) or treatment of MAC in patients with advanced HIV infection; prophylaxis of bacterial endocarditis in patients who are allergic to penicillin and undergoing surgical or dental procedures; pertussis

Mechanism of Action/Effect
Inhibits RNA-dependent protein synthesis at the chain elongation step; binds to the 50S ribosomal subunit resulting in blockage of transpeptidation

Contraindications
Hypersensitivity to azithromycin, other macrolide antibiotics, or any component of the formulation

Warnings/Precautions
Use with caution in patients with hepatic dysfunction; hepatic impairment with or without jaundice has occurred chiefly in older children and adults. It may be accompanied by malaise, nausea, vomiting, abdominal colic, and fever; discontinue use if these occur. May mask or delay symptoms of incubating gonorrhea or syphilis, so appropriate culture and susceptibility tests should be performed prior to initiating azithromycin. Pseudomembranous colitis has been reported with use of macrolide antibiotics; use caution with renal dysfunction. Prolongation of the QT_c interval has been reported with macrolide antibiotics; use caution in patients at risk of prolonged cardiac repolarization. Safety and efficacy have not been established in children <6 months of age with acute otitis media, acute bacterial sinusitis, or community-acquired pneumonia, or in children <2 years of age with pharyngitis/tonsillitis. Suspensions (immediate release and extended release) are not interchangeable.

Drug Interactions

Cytochrome P450 Effect: Substrate of CYP3A4 (minor); **Inhibits** CYP3A4 (weak)

Decreased Effect: Decreased azithromycin peak serum concentrations with aluminum- and magnesium-containing antacids (by 24%), however, total absorption is unaffected.

Increased Effect/Toxicity: Concurrent use of pimozide is contraindicated due to potential cardiotoxicity. The manufacturer warns that azithromycin potentially may increase levels of tacrolimus, phenytoin, ergot alkaloids, alfentanil, bromocriptine, carbamazepine, cyclosporine, digoxin, disopyramide, and triazolam. However, azithromycin did not affect the response/ levels of carbamazepine, theophylline, or warfarin in specific interaction studies; caution is advised when administered together. Nelfinavir may increase azithromycin serum levels (monitor for adverse effects).

Nutritional/Ethanol Interactions
Food: Rate and extent of GI absorption may be altered depending upon the formulation. Azithromycin suspension, not tablet form, has significantly increased absorption (46%) with food.

Adverse Reactions

>10%: Gastrointestinal: Diarrhea (4% to 11%)

1% to 10%:

Central nervous system: Headache

Gastrointestinal: Nausea, abdominal pain, cramping, vomiting (especially with high single-dose regimens)

Overdosage/Toxicology Symptoms of overdose include nausea, vomiting, diarrhea, and prostration. Treatment is supportive and symptomatic.

Pharmacodynamics/Kinetics

Time to Peak: Serum: Immediate release: 2-3 hours; Extended release: 5 hours

Protein Binding: Concentration dependent: 7% to 51%

Half-Life Elimination: Terminal: Immediate release: 68-72 hours; Extended release: 59 hours

Metabolism: Hepatic

Excretion: Biliary (major route); urine (6%)

Available Dosage Forms Note: Strength expressed as base

Injection, powder for reconstitution, as dihydrate (Zithromax®): 500 mg [contains sodium 114 mg (4.96 mEq) per vial]

Microspheres for oral suspension, extended release, as dihydrate (Zmax™): 2 g [single-dose bottle; contains sodium 148 mg per bottle; cherry and banana flavor]

Powder for oral suspension, immediate release, as dihydrate (Zithromax®): 100 mg/5 mL (15 mL) [contains sodium 3.7 mg/ 5 mL; cherry creme de vanilla and banana flavor]; 200 mg/5 mL (15 mL, 22.5 mL, 30 mL) [contains sodium 7.4 mg/5 mL; cherry creme de vanilla and banana flavor]; 1 g [single-dose packet; contains sodium 37 mg per packet; cherry creme de vanilla and banana flavor]

Tablet, as dihydrate:

Zithromax®: 250 mg [contains sodium 0.9 mg per tablet]; 500 mg [contains sodium 1.8 mg per tablet]; 600 mg [contains sodium 2.1 mg per tablet]

Zithromax® TRI-PAK™ [unit-dose pack]: 500 mg (3s)

Zithromax® Z-PAK™ [unit-dose pack]: 250 mg (6s)

Tablet, as monohydrate: 250 mg, 500 mg, 600 mg

Dosing

Adults & Elderly: Note: Extended release suspension (Zmax™) is not interchangeable with immediate release formulations. Use should be limited to approved indications. All doses are expressed as immediate release azithromycin unless otherwise specified.

Mild to moderate respiratory tract, skin, and soft tissue infections: Oral: 500 mg in a single loading dose on day 1 followed by 250 mg/day as a single dose on days 2-5

Alternative regimen: Bacterial exacerbation of COPD: 500 mg/day for a total of 3 days

Bacterial sinusitis: Oral: 500 mg/day for a total of 3 days

Extended release suspension (Zmax™): 2 g as a single dose

Community-acquired pneumonia: I.V.: 500 mg as a single dose for at least 2 days, follow I.V. therapy by the oral route with a single daily dose of 500 mg to complete a 7- to 10-day course of therapy.

Urethritis/cervicitis:

Due to *C. trachomatis*: Oral: 1 g as a single dose

Due to *N. gonorrhoeae*: Oral: 2 g as a single dose

Chancroid due to *H. ducreyi*: Oral: 1 g as a single dose

Pelvic inflammatory disease (PID): I.V.: 500 mg as a single dose for 1-2 days, follow I.V. therapy by the oral route with a single daily dose of 250 mg to complete a 7-day course of therapy.

Pertussis (CDC guidelines): Oral: 500 mg on day 1 followed by 250 mg/day on days 2-5 (maximum: 500 mg/day)

Prophylaxis for bacterial endocarditis (unlabeled use): Oral: 500 mg 1 hour prior to the procedure

Disseminated *M. avium* complex disease in patient with advanced HIV infection (unlabeled use):

Prophylaxis: Oral: 1200 mg once weekly (may be combined with rifabutin)

Treatment: Oral: 600 mg daily in combination with ethambutol 15 mg/kg

Pediatrics: Note: Adolescents ≥16 years: Refer to adult dosing.

Community-acquired pneumonia: Oral: Children ≥6 months: 10 mg/kg on day 1 (maximum: 500 mg/day) followed by 5 mg/kg/day once daily on days 2-5 (maximum: 250 mg/day)

Bacterial sinusitis: Oral: Children ≥6 months: 10 mg/kg once daily for 3 days (maximum: 500 mg/day)

Otitis media: Oral: Children ≥6 months:

1-day regimen: 30 mg/kg as a single dose (maximum dose: 1500 mg)

3-day regimen: 10 mg/kg once daily for 3 days (maximum: 500 mg/day)

5-day regimen: 10 mg/kg on day 1 (maximum: 500 mg/day) followed by 5 mg/kg/day once daily on days 2-5 (maximum: 250 mg/day)

Pharyngitis, tonsillitis: Oral: Children ≥2 years: 12 mg/kg/day once daily for 5 days (maximum: 500 mg/day)

Pertussis (CDC guidelines):

Children <6 months: 10 mg/kg/day for 5 day

Children ≥6 months: 10 mg/kg on day 1 (maximum: 500 mg/day) followed by 5 mg/kg/day once daily on days 2-5 (maximum: 250 mg/day)

Disseminated *M. avium*-infected patients with acquired immunodeficiency syndrome (unlabeled use): Oral: 5 mg/kg/day once daily (maximum dose: 250 mg/day) or 20 mg/kg (maximum dose: 1200 mg) once weekly given alone or in combination with rifabutin

Treatment and secondary prevention of disseminated MAC (unlabeled use): Oral: 5 mg/kg/day once daily (maximum dose: 250 mg/day) in combination with ethambutol, with or without rifabutin

Prophylaxis for bacterial endocarditis (unlabeled use): Oral: 15 mg/kg 1 hour before procedure

Uncomplicated chlamydial urethritis or cervicitis (unlabeled use): Children ≥45 kg: 1 g as a single dose

Renal Impairment: Use caution in patients with Cl$_{cr}$ <10 mL/minute

Hepatic Impairment: Use with caution due to potential for hepatotoxicity (rare). Specific guidelines for dosing in hepatic impairment have not been established.

Administration

Oral: Immediate release suspension and tablet may be taken without regard to food; extended release suspension should be taken on an empty stomach (at least 1 hour before or 2 hours following a meal), within 12 hours of reconstitution.

I.V.: Other medications should not be infused simultaneously through the same I.V. line.

I.V. Detail: Infusate concentration and rate of infusion for azithromycin for injection should be either 1 mg/mL over 3 hours or 2 mg/mL over 1 hour.

Stability

Reconstitution: Injection: Prepare initiation solution by adding 4.8 mL of sterile water for injection to the 500 mg vial (resulting concentration: 100 mg/mL). Use of a standard syringe is recommended due to the vacuum in the vial (which may draw additional solution through an automated syringe).

The initial solution should be further diluted to a concentration of 1 mg/mL (500 mL) to 2 mg/mL (250 mL) in 0.9% sodium chloride, 5% dextrose in water, or lactated Ringer's. The diluted solution is stable for 24 hours at or below room temperature (30°C or 86°F) and for 7 days if stored under refrigeration (5°C or 41°F).

Compatibility: Other medications should not be infused simultaneously through the same I.V. line. (Continued)

Azithromycin (Continued)

Storage:
Injection: Store intact vials of injection at room temperature. Reconstituted solution is stable for 24 hours when stored below 30°C/86°F.

Suspension, immediate release: Store dry powder below 30°C (86°F). Following reconstitution, store at 5°C to 30°C (41°F to 86°F).

Suspension, extended release: Store dry powder below 30°C (86°F). Following reconstitution, store at 15°C to 30°C (59°F to 86°F); do not freeze. Should be consumed within 12 hours following reconstitution.

Tablets: Store between 15°C to 30°C (59°F to 86°F).

Laboratory Monitoring Liver function, CBC with differential. Perform culture and sensitivity testing prior to initiating therapy.

Nursing Actions
Physical Assessment: Assess allergy history prior to beginning therapy. Assess potential for interactions with other pharmacological agents patient may be taking. Monitor laboratory tests (LFTS, CBC with differential), therapeutic effectiveness, and adverse effects. Instruct patients being treated for STDs about preventing transmission. Teach patient appropriate use, possible side effects/appropriate interventions, and adverse symptoms to report.

Patient Education: Take as directed. Take all of prescribed medication and do not discontinue until prescription is completed. Take extended release suspension 1 hour before or 2 hours after meals; immediate release suspension and tablets may be taken with or without food; tablet form may be taken with meals to decrease GI effects. Do not take with antacids that contain aluminum or magnesium. Maintain adequate hydration (2-3 L/day of fluids) unless instructed to restrict fluid intake. If taken to treat a sexually-transmitted disease, follow advice of prescriber related to sexual intercourse and preventing transmission. May cause transient abdominal distress, diarrhea, and headache. Report signs of additional infections (eg, sores in mouth or vagina, vaginal discharge, unresolved fever, severe vomiting, or loose or foul-smelling stools). **Breast-feeding precaution:** Consult prescriber if breast-feeding.

Dietary Considerations
Oral suspension, immediate release, may be administered with or without food.

Oral suspension, extended release, should be taken on an empty stomach (at least 1 hour before or 2 hours following a meal).

Tablet may be administered with food to decrease GI effects.

Sodium content:
Injection: 114 mg (4.96 mEq) per vial

Oral suspension, immediate release: 3.7 mg per 100 mg/5 mL of constituted suspension; 7.4 mg per 200 mg/5 mL of constituted suspension; 37 mg per 1 g single-dose packet

Oral suspension, extended release: 148 mg per 2 g constituted suspension

Tablet: 0.9 mg/250 mg tablet; 1.8 mg/500 mg tablet; 2.1 mg/600 mg tablet

Geriatric Considerations Dosage adjustment does not appear to be necessary in the elderly. Considered one of the drugs of choice in the treatment of outpatient treatment of community-acquired pneumonia in older adults.

Breast-Feeding Issues Based on one case report, azithromycin has been shown to accumulate in breast milk.

Additional Information Capsules are no longer being produced in the United States.

Zithromax® tablets and immediate release suspension may be interchanged (eg, two 250 Zithromax® tablets may be substituted for a 500 mg Zithromax® tablet or the tablets may be substituted with the immediate release suspension); however, the extended release suspension (Zmax™) is not bioequivalent with Zithromax® and therefore should not be interchanged.

Aztreonam (AZ tree oh nam)

U.S. Brand Names Azactam®

Synonyms Azthreonam

Pharmacologic Category Antibiotic, Miscellaneous

Medication Safety Issues
Sound-alike/look-alike issues:
Aztreonam may be confused with azidothymidine

Pregnancy Risk Factor B

Lactation Enters breast milk/not recommended (AAP rates "compatible")

Use Treatment of patients with urinary tract infections, lower respiratory tract infections, septicemia, skin/skin structure infections, intra-abdominal infections, and gynecological infections caused by susceptible gram-negative bacilli

Mechanism of Action/Effect Monobactam which is active only against gram-negative bacilli; inhibits bacterial cell wall synthesis during active multiplication, causing cell wall destruction

Contraindications Hypersensitivity to aztreonam or any component of the formulation

Warnings/Precautions Rare cross-allergenicity to penicillins and cephalosporins has been reported. Use caution in renal impairment; dosing adjustment required.

Drug Interactions
Decreased Effect: Avoid antibiotics that induce beta-lactamase production (cefoxitin, imipenem).

Lab Interactions Urine glucose (Clinitest®), positive Coombs' test

Adverse Reactions As reported in adults:
1% to 10%:
Dermatologic: Rash
Gastrointestinal: Diarrhea, nausea, vomiting
Local: Thrombophlebitis, pain at injection site

Overdosage/Toxicology Symptoms of overdose include seizures. Treatment is supportive. If necessary, dialysis can reduce the drug concentration in the blood.

Pharmacodynamics/Kinetics
Time to Peak: I.M., I.V. push: Within 60 minutes; I.V. infusion: 1.5 hours

Protein Binding: 56%

Half-Life Elimination:
Children 2 months to 12 years: 1.7 hours
Adults: Normal renal function: 1.7-2.9 hours
End-stage renal disease: 6-8 hours

Metabolism: Hepatic (minor %)

Excretion: Urine (60% to 70% as unchanged drug); feces (~13% to 15%)

Available Dosage Forms
Infusion [premixed]: 1 g (50 mL); 2 g (50 mL)
Injection, powder for reconstitution: 500 mg, 1 g, 2 g

Dosing
Adults & Elderly:
Urinary tract infection: I.M., I.V.: 500 mg to 1 g every 8-12 hours

Moderately severe systemic infections:
I.M.: 1 g every 8-12 hours
I.V.: 1-2 g every 8-12 hours

Severe systemic or life-threatening infections (especially caused by Pseudomonas aeruginosa): I.V.: 2 g every 6-8 hours; maximum: 8 g/day

Meningitis (gram-negative): I.V.: 2 g every 6-8 hours

Pediatrics:
Susceptible infections: I.M., I.V.: Children >1 month:
Mild-to-moderate infections: 30 mg/kg every 8 hours

Moderate-to-severe infections: 30 mg/kg every 6-8 hours; maximum: 120 mg/kg/day (8 g/day)

Infection in children with cystic fibrosis: I.V.: Children >1 month: 50 mg/kg/dose every 6-8 hours (ie, up to 200 mg/kg/day); maximum: 8 g/day

Renal Impairment: Adults: Following initial dose, maintenance doses should be given as follows:

Cl_{cr} 10-30 mL/minute: 50% of usual dose at the usual interval

Cl_{cr} <10 mL/minute: 25% of usual dosage at the usual interval

Hemodialysis: Moderately dialyzable (20% to 50%); $^1/_8$ of initial dose after each hemodialysis session (given in addition to the maintenance doses)

Peritoneal dialysis: Administer as for Cl_{cr} <10 mL/minute

Continuous arteriovenous or venovenous hemofiltration: Dose as for Cl_{cr} 10-30 mL/minute

Administration

I.M.: Administer by deep injection into large muscle mass, such as upper outer quadrant of gluteus maximus or the lateral part of the thigh. Doses >1 g should be administered I.V.

I.V.: I.V. route is preferred for doses >1 g or in patients with severe life-threatening infections. Administer by IVP over 3-5 minutes or by intermittent infusion over 20-60 minutes at a final concentration not to exceed 20 mg/mL.

I.V. Detail: Monitor infusion/injection sites carefully. Administer around-the-clock to promote less variation in peak and trough serum levels.

pH: 4.5-7.5 (aqueous solution)

Stability

Reconstitution: Reconstituted solutions are colorless to light yellow straw and may turn pink upon standing without affecting potency. Use reconstituted solutions and I.V. solutions (in NS and D_5W) within 48 hours if kept at room temperature (25°C) or 7 days if kept in refrigerator (4°C).

I.M.: Reconstitute with at least 3 mL SWFI, sterile bacteriostatic water for injection, NS, or bacteriostatic sodium chloride.

I.V.:

Bolus injection: Reconstitute with 6-10 mL SWFI.

Infusion: Reconstitute to a final concentration ≤2%. Solution for infusion may be frozen at less than -2°C (less than -4°F) for up to 3 months. Thawed solution should be used within 24 hours if thawed at room temperature or within 72 hours if thawed under refrigeration. **Do not refreeze.**

Compatibility: Solution for infusion: Stable in D_5LR, $D_5^1/_4NS$, $D_5^1/_2NS$, D_5NS, D_5W, $D_{10}W$, mannitol 5%, mannitol 10%, LR, NS

Y-site administration: Incompatible with acyclovir, alatrofloxacin, amphotericin B, amphotericin B cholesteryl sulfate complex, amsacrine, chlorpromazine, daunorubicin, ganciclovir, lorazepam, metronidazole, mitomycin, mitoxantrone, prochlorperazine edisylate, streptozocin

Compatibility when admixed: Incompatible with metronidazole, nafcillin

Storage: Prior to reconstitution, store at room temperature. Avoid excessive heat.

Laboratory Monitoring Obtain specimens for culture and sensitivity before the first dose.

Nursing Actions

Physical Assessment: Allergy history should be assessed prior to beginning treatment. I.V.: Infusion site should be monitored closely. Assess therapeutic effectiveness and adverse response. Advise patients with diabetes about use of Clinitest®. Teach patient possible side effects and adverse symptoms to report.

Patient Education: Do not take any new medication during therapy unless approved by prescriber. This medication can only be administered by injection or infusion. Report immediately any burning, pain,

swelling, or redness at infusion/injection site. May cause nausea or GI distress (frequent mouth care, frequent small meals, sucking lozenges, or chewing gum may help relieve these symptoms). If you have diabetes, drug may cause false tests with Clinitest® urine glucose monitoring; use of another type of glucose monitoring is preferable. Report any persistent and unrelieved diarrhea or vomiting, pain at injection site, unresolved fever, unhealed or new sores in mouth or vagina, vaginal discharge, or acute onset of respiratory difficulty. **Breast-feeding precaution:** Consult prescriber if breast-feeding.

Geriatric Considerations Adjust dose relative to renal function.

Breast-Feeding Issues Aztreonam is excreted in breast milk at levels <1% of the maternal serum concentration. The manufacturer recommends temporary discontinuation of nursing during therapy.

Additional Information Although marketed as an agent similar to aminoglycosides, aztreonam is a monobactam antimicrobial with almost pure gram-negative aerobic activity. It cannot be used for gram-positive infections. Aminoglycosides are often used for synergy in gram-positive infections.

Bacitracin (bas i TRAY sin)

U.S. Brand Names AK-Tracin® [DSC]; Baciguent® [OTC]; BaciIM®

Pharmacologic Category Antibiotic, Miscellaneous; Antibiotic, Ophthalmic; Antibiotic, Topical

Medication Safety Issues

Sound-alike/look-alike issues:

Bacitracin may be confused with Bactrim®, Bactroban®

Pregnancy Risk Factor C

Lactation Excretion in breast milk unknown/use caution

Use Treatment of susceptible bacterial infections mainly; has activity against gram-positive bacilli; due to toxicity risks, systemic and irrigant uses of bacitracin should be limited to situations where less toxic alternatives would not be effective

Unlabeled/Investigational Use Oral administration: Successful in antibiotic-associated colitis; has been used for enteric eradication of vancomycin-resistant enterococci (VRE)

Mechanism of Action/Effect Inhibits bacterial cell wall synthesis by preventing transfer of mucopeptides into the growing cell wall

Contraindications Hypersensitivity to bacitracin or any component of the formulation; I.M. use is contraindicated in patients with renal impairment

Warnings/Precautions Prolonged use may result in overgrowth of nonsusceptible organisms. I.M. use may cause renal failure due to tubular and glomerular necrosis. **Do not administer intravenously** because severe thrombophlebitis occurs.

Drug Interactions

Increased Effect/Toxicity: Nephrotoxic drugs, neuromuscular blocking agents, and anesthetics (increased neuromuscular blockade).

Adverse Reactions 1% to 10%:

Cardiovascular: Hypotension, edema of the face/lips, chest tightness

Central nervous system: Pain

Dermatologic: Rash, itching

Gastrointestinal: Anorexia, nausea, vomiting, diarrhea, rectal itching

Hematologic: Blood dyscrasias

Miscellaneous: Diaphoresis

Overdosage/Toxicology Symptoms of overdose include nephrotoxicity (parenteral), nausea, and vomiting (oral). Treatment is symptomatic and supportive.

(Continued)

Bacitracin *(Continued)*

Pharmacodynamics/Kinetics

Duration of Action: 6-8 hours

Time to Peak: Serum: I.M.: 1-2 hours

Protein Binding: Plasma: Minimal

Excretion: Urine (10% to 40%) within 24 hours

Available Dosage Forms [DSC] = Discontinued product

Injection, powder for reconstitution (BaciiM®): 50,000 units

Ointment, ophthalmic (AK-Tracin® [DSC]): 500 units/g (3.5 g)

Ointment, topical: 500 units/g (0.9 g, 15 g, 30 g, 120 g, 454 g)

Baciguent®: 500 units/g (15 g, 30 g)

Dosing

Adults & Elderly: Do not administer I.V.:

Antibiotic-associated colitis: Oral: 25,000 units 4 times/day for 7-10 days

VRE eradication (unlabeled use): Oral: 25,000 units 4 times/day for 7-10 days

Superficial dermal infection: Topical: Apply 1-5 times/day.

Ophthalmic infection: Ophthalmic (ointment): Instill ¼" to ½" ribbon every 3-4 hours into conjunctival sac for acute infections, or 2-3 times/day for mild-to-moderate infections for 7-10 days.

Local irrigation: Solution: 50-100 units/mL in normal saline, lactated Ringer's, or sterile water for irrigation; soak sponges in solution for topical compresses 1-5 times/day or as needed during surgical procedures.

Pediatrics: Do not administer I.V.

Treatment of infection:

Infants: I.M.:

≤2.5 kg: 900 units/kg/day in 2-3 divided doses

>2.5 kg: 1000 units/kg/day in 2-3 divided doses

Children: I.M.: 800-1200 units/kg/day divided every 8 hours

Superficial dermal infection: Topical: Refer to adult dosing.

Ophthalmic infection: Ophthalmic (ointment): Refer to adult dosing.

Local irrigation: Solution: Refer to adult dosing.

Administration

Oral: The injection formulation is extemporaneously prepared and flavored to improve palatability.

I.M.: For I.M. administration only. pH of urine should be kept >6 by using sodium bicarbonate. Bacitracin sterile powder should be dissolved in 0.9% sodium chloride injection containing 2% procaine hydrochloride. Do not use diluents containing parabens.

I.V.: Not for I.V. administration.

Stability

Reconstitution: For I.M. use only. Bacitracin sterile powder should be dissolved in 0.9% sodium chloride injection containing 2% procaine hydrochloride. Once reconstituted, bacitracin is stable for 1 week under refrigeration (2°C to 8°C). Sterile powder should be stored in the refrigerator. Do not use diluents containing parabens.

Laboratory Monitoring I.M.: Urinalysis, renal function

Nursing Actions

Physical Assessment: Do not administer I.V. Assess potential for interactions with other pharmacological agents patient may be taking (eg, nephrotoxic drugs, neuromuscular blocking agents, and anesthetics). Monitor laboratory test (urinalysis and renal function with I.M.), effectiveness of therapy, and adverse reactions. Teach patient proper use, possible side effects/ appropriate interventions, and adverse symptoms to report.

Patient Education: Oral/I.M.: Maintain adequate hydration (2-3 L/day of fluids) unless instructed to restrict fluid intake. Report rash, redness, or itching; change in urinary pattern; acute dizziness; swelling of face or lips; chest pain or tightness; acute nausea or vomiting; or loss of appetite (small, frequent meals or frequent mouth care may help).

Ophthalmic: Instill as many times per day as directed. Wash hands before using. Gently pull lower eyelid forward, instill prescribed amount of ointment into lower eyelid. Close eye and roll eyeball in all directions. May cause blurred vision; use caution when driving or engaging in tasks that require clear vision. Report any adverse reactions such as rash or itching, swelling of face or lips, burning or pain in eye, worsening of condition, or if condition does not improve.

Topical: Apply a thin film as many times a day as prescribed to the affected area. May cover with porous sterile bandage (avoid occlusive dressings). Do not use longer than 1 week unless advised by prescriber. **Pregnancy/breast-feeding precautions:** Inform prescriber if you are or intend to become pregnant. Consult prescriber if breast-feeding.

Additional Information 1 unit is equivalent to 0.026 mg

Bacitracin and Polymyxin B

(bas i TRAY sin & pol i MIKS in bee)

U.S. Brand Names AK-Poly-Bac®; Betadine® First Aid Antibiotics + Moisturizer [OTC]; Polysporin® Ophthalmic; Polysporin® Topical [OTC]

Synonyms Polymyxin B and Bacitracin

Pharmacologic Category Antibiotic, Ophthalmic; Antibiotic, Topical

Pregnancy Risk Factor C

Lactation Excretion in breast milk unknown/use caution

Use Treatment of superficial infections caused by susceptible organisms

Available Dosage Forms

Ointment, ophthalmic (AK-Poly-Bac®, Polysporin®): Bacitracin 500 units and polymyxin B sulfate 10,000 units per g (3.5 g)

Ointment, topical [OTC]: Bacitracin 500 units and polymyxin B sulfate 10,000 units per g in white petrolatum (15 g, 30 g)

Betadine® First Aid Antibiotics + Moisturizer: Bacitracin 500 units and polymyxin B sulfate 10,000 units per g (14 g)

Polysporin®: Bacitracin 500 units and polymyxin B sulfate 10,000 units per g (15 g, 30 g)

Powder, topical (Polysporin®): Bacitracin 500 units and polymyxin B sulfate 10,000 units per g (10 g)

Dosing

Adults & Elderly:

Ophthalmic infection: Ophthalmic (ointment): Instill ½" ribbon in the affected eye(s) every 3-4 hours for acute infections or 2-3 times/day for mild-to-moderate infections for 7-10 days.

Superficial dermal infection: Topical ointment/ powder: Apply to affected area 1-4 times/day; may cover with sterile bandage if needed.

Pediatrics: Refer to adult dosing.

Nursing Actions

Physical Assessment: See individual agents.

Patient Education: See individual agents. **Pregnancy/breast-feeding precautions:** Inform prescriber if you are or intend to become pregnant. Consult prescriber if breast-feeding.

Related Information

Bacitracin *on page 135*

Polymyxin B *on page 1005*

Bacitracin, Neomycin, and Polymyxin B

(bas i TRAY sin, nee oh MYE sin, & pol i MIKS in bee)

U.S. Brand Names Neosporin® Neo To Go® [OTC]; Neosporin® Ophthalmic Ointment [DSC]; Neosporin® Topical [OTC]

Synonyms Neomycin, Bacitracin, and Polymyxin B; Polymyxin B, Bacitracin, and Neomycin; Triple Antibiotic

Pharmacologic Category Antibiotic, Ophthalmic; Antibiotic, Topical

Pregnancy Risk Factor C

Lactation Excretion in breast milk unknown/use caution

Use Helps prevent infection in minor cuts, scrapes, and burns; short-term treatment of superficial external ocular infections caused by susceptible organisms

Available Dosage Forms [DSC] = Discontinued product

Ointment, ophthalmic (Neosporin® [DSC]): Bacitracin 400 units, neomycin 3.5 mg, and polymyxin B 10,000 units per g (3.5 g)

Ointment, topical: Bacitracin 400 units, neomycin 3.5 mg, and polymyxin B 5000 units per g (0.9 g, 15 g, 30 g, 454 g)

Neosporin®: Bacitracin 400 units, neomycin 3.5 mg, and polymyxin B 5000 units per g (15 g, 30 g)

Neosporin® Neo To Go®: Bacitracin 400 units, neomycin 3.5 mg, and polymyxin B 5000 units per g (0.9 g)

Dosing

Adults & Elderly:

Ophthalmic infection: Ophthalmic ointment: Instill ½" into the conjunctival sac every 3-4 hours for 7-10 days for acute infections

Superficial dermal infection: Topical: Apply 1-3 times/day to infected area; may cover with sterile bandage if necessary.

Pediatrics: Refer to adult dosing.

Nursing Actions

Physical Assessment: See individual agents.

Patient Education: See individual agents. **Pregnancy/breast-feeding precautions:** Inform prescriber if you are or intend to become pregnant. Consult prescriber if breast-feeding.

Related Information

Bacitracin on page 135
Neomycin on page 872
Polymyxin B on page 1005

Bacitracin, Neomycin, Polymyxin B, and Hydrocortisone

(bas i TRAY sin, nee oh MYE sin, pol i MIKS in bee, & hye droe KOR ti sone)

U.S. Brand Names Cortisporin® Ointment

Synonyms Hydrocortisone, Bacitracin, Neomycin, and Polymyxin B; Neomycin, Bacitracin, Polymyxin B, and Hydrocortisone; Polymyxin B, Bacitracin, Neomycin, and Hydrocortisone

Pharmacologic Category Antibiotic, Ophthalmic; Antibiotic, Otic; Antibiotic, Topical; Corticosteroid, Ophthalmic; Corticosteroid, Otic; Corticosteroid, Topical

Pregnancy Risk Factor C

Lactation Excretion in breast milk unknown/use caution

Use Prevention and treatment of susceptible inflammatory conditions where bacterial infection (or risk of infection) is present

Available Dosage Forms [DSC] = Discontinued product

Ointment, ophthalmic (Cortisporin® [DSC]): Bacitracin 400 units, neomycin sulfate 3.5 mg, polymyxin B 10,000 units, and hydrocortisone 10 mg per g (3.5 g)

Ointment, topical (Cortisporin®): Bacitracin 400 units, neomycin 3.5 mg, polymyxin B 5000 units, and hydrocortisone 10 mg per g (15 g)

Dosing

Adults & Elderly:

Ophthalmic infection: Ophthalmic (ointment): Instill ½" ribbon to inside of lower lid every 3-4 hours until improvement occurs.

Superficial dermal infection: Topical: Apply sparingly 2-4 times/day.

Pediatrics: Refer to adult dosing.

Nursing Actions

Physical Assessment: See individual agents.

Patient Education: See individual agents. **Pregnancy/breast-feeding precautions:** Inform prescriber if you are or intend to become pregnant. Consult prescriber if breast-feeding.

Related Information

Bacitracin on page 135
Hydrocortisone on page 617
Neomycin on page 872
Polymyxin B on page 1005

Baclofen (BAK loe fen)

U.S. Brand Names Lioresal®

Pharmacologic Category Skeletal Muscle Relaxant

Medication Safety Issues

Sound-alike/look-alike issues:

Baclofen may be confused with Bactroban®

Lioresal® may be confused with lisinopril, Loniten®, Lotensin®

Pregnancy Risk Factor C

Lactation Enters breast milk (small amounts)/compatible

Use Treatment of reversible spasticity associated with multiple sclerosis or spinal cord lesions

Orphan drug: Intrathecal: Treatment of intractable spasticity caused by spinal cord injury, multiple sclerosis, and other spinal disease (spinal ischemia or tumor, transverse myelitis, cervical spondylosis, degenerative myelopathy)

Unlabeled/Investigational Use Intractable hiccups, intractable pain relief, bladder spasticity, trigeminal neuralgia, cerebral palsy, Huntington's chorea

Mechanism of Action/Effect Inhibits the transmission of both monosynaptic and polysynaptic reflexes at the spinal cord level, possibly by hyperpolarization of primary afferent fiber terminals, with resultant relief of muscle spasticity

Contraindications Hypersensitivity to baclofen or any component of the formulation

Warnings/Precautions Use with caution in patients with seizure disorder or impaired renal function. Avoid abrupt withdrawal of the drug; abrupt withdrawal of intrathecal baclofen has resulted in severe sequelae (hyperpyrexia, obtundation, rebound/exaggerated spasticity, muscle rigidity, and rhabdomyolysis), leading to organ failure and some fatalities. Risk may be higher in patients with injuries at T-6 or above, history of baclofen withdrawal, or limited ability to communicate. Elderly are more sensitive to the effects of baclofen and are more likely to experience adverse CNS effects at higher doses.

Drug Interactions

Increased Effect/Toxicity: Effects may be additive with CNS depressants.

Nutritional/Ethanol Interactions

Ethanol: Avoid ethanol (may increase CNS depression).

Herb/Nutraceutical: Avoid valerian, St John's wort, kava kava, gotu kola.

(Continued)

Baclofen (Continued)

Lab Interactions Increased alkaline phosphatase, AST, glucose, ammonia (B); decreased bilirubin (S)

Adverse Reactions

>10%:

Central nervous system: Drowsiness, vertigo, psychiatric disturbances, insomnia, slurred speech, ataxia, hypotonia

Neuromuscular & skeletal: Weakness

1% to 10%:

Cardiovascular: Hypotension

Central nervous system: Fatigue, confusion, headache

Dermatologic: Rash

Gastrointestinal: Nausea, constipation

Genitourinary: Polyuria

Overdosage/Toxicology Symptoms of overdose include vomiting, muscle hypotonia, salivation, drowsiness, coma, seizures, and respiratory depression. Atropine has been used to improve ventilation, heart rate, blood pressure, and core body temperature. Treatment is symptom-directed and supportive.

For toxicity following intrathecal administration: For adults, administer physostigmine 2 mg I.M. or I.V. (not to exceed 1 mg/minute). For pediatric patients, administer physostigmine 0.02 mg/kg I.M. or I.V. (not to exceed 0.5 mg/minute). Consider withdrawal of 30-40 mL of CSF to reduce baclofen concentration. Abrupt withdrawal of intrathecal baclofen has resulted in severe sequelae (hyperpyrexia, obtundation, muscle rigidity, and rhabdomyolysis).

Pharmacodynamics/Kinetics

Onset of Action: 3-4 days; Peak effect: 5-10 days

Time to Peak: Serum: Oral: Within 2-3 hours

Protein Binding: 30%

Half-Life Elimination: 3.5 hours

Metabolism: Hepatic (15% of dose)

Excretion: Urine and feces (85% as unchanged drug)

Available Dosage Forms

Injection, solution, intrathecal [preservative free] (Lioresal®): 50 mcg/mL (1 mL); 500 mcg/mL (20 mL); 2000 mcg/mL (5 mL)

Tablet: 10 mg, 20 mg

Dosing

Adults:

Spasticity:

Oral: 5 mg 3 times/day, may increase 5 mg/dose every 3 days to a maximum of 80 mg/day

Intrathecal:

Test dose: 50-100 mcg, doses >50 mcg should be given in 25 mcg increments, separated by 24 hours. A screening dose of 25 mcg may be considered in very small patients. Patients not responding to screening dose of 100 mcg should not be considered for chronic infusion/implanted pump.

Maintenance: After positive response to test dose, a maintenance intrathecal infusion can be administered via an implanted intrathecal pump. Initial dose via pump: Infusion at a 24-hourly rate dosed at twice the test dose. Avoid abrupt discontinuation.

Hiccups (unlabeled use): Oral: 10-20 mg 2-3 times/day

Elderly: Oral (the lowest effective dose is recommended): Initial: 5 mg 2-3 times/day, increasing gradually as needed; if benefits are not seen withdraw the drug slowly.

Pediatrics:

Spasticity:

Oral (avoid abrupt withdrawal of drug): Children:

2-7 years: Initial: 10-15 mg/24 hours divided every 8 hours; titrate dose every 3 days in increments of 5-15 mg/day to a maximum of 40 mg/day.

≥8 years: Maximum: 60 mg/day in 3 divided doses

Intrathecal: Refer to adult dosing.

Renal Impairment: May be necessary to reduce dosage; no specific guidelines have been established

Administration

I.V. Detail: pH: 5-7

Other: Intrathecal: For screening dosages, dilute with preservative-free sodium chloride to a final concentration of 50 mcg/mL for bolus injection into the subarachnoid space. For maintenance infusions, concentrations of 500-2000 mcg/mL may be used.

Stability

Compatibility: Stable in sterile, preservative free NS

Nursing Actions

Physical Assessment: Assess effectiveness and interactions of other medications patient may be taking. Monitor effectiveness of therapy (according to rational for therapy) and adverse reactions (eg, cardiovascular and CNS status) at beginning of therapy and periodically with long-term use. Assess knowledge/teach patient appropriate use, interventions to reduce side effects, and adverse symptoms to report.

Patient Education: Take this drug as prescribed. Do not discontinue this medicine without consulting prescriber (abrupt discontinuation may cause hallucinations). Do not take any prescription or OTC sleep-inducing drugs, sedatives, or antispasmodics without consulting prescriber. Avoid alcohol use. You may experience transient drowsiness, lethargy, or dizziness; use caution when driving or engaging in tasks requiring alertness until response to drug is known. Frequent small meals or lozenges may reduce GI upset.

Intrathecal use: Keep scheduled pump refill visits; abrupt interruption can cause serious withdrawal symptoms. Report increased spasticity, itching, numbness, unresolved insomnia, painful urination, change in urinary patterns, constipation, high fever, or persistent confusion.

Pregnancy precaution: Inform prescriber if you are or intend to become pregnant.

Geriatric Considerations The elderly are more sensitive to the effects of baclofen and are more likely to experience adverse CNS effects at higher doses. Two cases of encephalopathy were reported after inadvertent high doses (50 mg/day and 90 mg/day) were given to elderly patients.

Basiliximab (ba si LIK si mab)

U.S. Brand Names Simulect®

Pharmacologic Category Monoclonal Antibody

Pregnancy Risk Factor B (manufacturer)

Lactation Excretion in breast milk unknown/not recommended

Use Prophylaxis of acute organ rejection in renal transplantation

Mechanism of Action/Effect Mouse-derived monoclonal IgG antibody which blocks the alpha-chain of the interleukin-2 (IL-2) receptor complex; this receptor is expressed on activated T lymphocytes and is a critical pathway for activating cell-mediated allograft rejection

Contraindications Hypersensitivity to basiliximab, murine proteins, or any component of the formulation

Warnings/Precautions To be used as a component of immunosuppressive regimen which includes cyclosporine and corticosteroids. The incidence of lymphoproliferative disorders and/or opportunistic infections may be increased by immunosuppressive therapy. Severe hypersensitivity reactions, occurring within 24 hours, have been reported. Reactions, including anaphylaxis, have occurred both with the initial exposure and/or following re-exposure after several months. Use caution during re-exposure to a subsequent course of therapy in a patient who has previously received basiliximab. Discontinue the drug permanently if a reaction occurs. Medications for the treatment of hypersensitivity reactions should be available for immediate use. Treatment may result in the development of human antimurine antibodies (HAMA); however, limited evidence suggesting the use of muromonab-CD3 or other murine products is not precluded.

Drug Interactions
Decreased Effect: Basiliximab is an immunoglobulin; specific drug interactions have not been evaluated, but are not anticipated. It is not known if the immune response to vaccines will be impaired during or following basiliximab therapy.

Increased Effect/Toxicity: Basiliximab is an immunoglobulin; specific drug interactions have not been evaluated, but are not anticipated.

Adverse Reactions Administration of basiliximab did not appear to increase the incidence or severity of adverse effects in clinical trials. Adverse events were reported in 96% of both the placebo and basiliximab groups.

>10%:
Cardiovascular: Peripheral edema, hypertension, atrial fibrillation
Central nervous system: Fever, headache, insomnia, pain
Dermatologic: Wound complications, acne
Endocrine & metabolic: Hypokalemia, hyperkalemia, hyperglycemia, hyperuricemia, hypophosphatemia, hypercholesterolemia
Gastrointestinal: Constipation, nausea, diarrhea, abdominal pain, vomiting, dyspepsia
Genitourinary: Urinary tract infection
Hematologic: Anemia
Neuromuscular & skeletal: Tremor
Respiratory: Dyspnea, infection (upper respiratory)
Miscellaneous: Viral infection

3% to 10%:
Cardiovascular: Chest pain, cardiac failure, hypotension, arrhythmia, tachycardia, generalized edema, abnormal heart sounds, angina pectoris
Central nervous system: Hypoesthesia, neuropathy, agitation, anxiety, depression, malaise, fatigue, rigors, dizziness
Dermatologic: Cyst, hypertrichosis, pruritus, rash, skin disorder, skin ulceration
Endocrine & metabolic: Dehydration, diabetes mellitus, fluid overload, hypercalcemia, hyperlipidemia, hypoglycemia, hypomagnesemia, acidosis, hypertriglyceridemia, hypocalcemia, hyponatremia
Gastrointestinal: Flatulence, gastroenteritis, GI hemorrhage, gingival hyperplasia, melena, esophagitis, stomatitis, abdomen enlarged, moniliasis, ulcerative stomatitis, weight gain
Genitourinary: Impotence, genital edema, albuminuria, bladder disorder, hematuria, urinary frequency, oliguria, renal function abnormal, renal tubular necrosis, ureteral disorder, urinary retention, dysuria
Hematologic: Hematoma, hemorrhage, purpura, thrombocytopenia, thrombosis, polycythemia, leukopenia
Neuromuscular & skeletal: Arthralgia, arthropathy, cramps, fracture, hernia, myalgia, paresthesia, weakness, back pain, leg pain
Ocular: Cataract, conjunctivitis, abnormal vision
Respiratory: Bronchitis, bronchospasm, pneumonia, pulmonary edema, sinusitis, rhinitis, cough, pharyngitis
Miscellaneous: Accidental trauma, facial edema, sepsis, infection, glucocorticoids increased, herpes infection

Overdosage/Toxicology There have been no reports of overdose.

Pharmacodynamics/Kinetics
Duration of Action: Mean: 36 days (determined by IL-2R alpha saturation)
Half-Life Elimination: Children: 9.4 days; Adults: Mean: 7.2 days
Excretion: Clearance: Children: 20 mL/hour; Adults: Mean: 41 mL/hour
Available Dosage Forms Injection, powder for reconstitution: 10 mg, 20 mg

Dosing
Adults & Elderly: Note: Patients previously administered basiliximab should only be re-exposed to a subsequent course of therapy with extreme caution.
Renal transplantation: I.V.: 20 mg within 2 hours prior to transplant surgery, followed by a second 20 mg dose 4 days after transplantation. The second dose should be withheld if complications occur (including severe hypersensitivity reactions or graft loss).

Pediatrics: Note: Patients previously administered basiliximab should only be re-exposed to a subsequent course of therapy with extreme caution.
Renal transplantation: I.V.:
Children <35 kg: 10 mg within 2 hours prior to transplant surgery, followed by a second 10 mg dose 4 days after transplantation; the second dose should be withheld if complications occur (including severe hypersensitivity reactions or graft loss)
Children ≥35 kg: Refer to adult dosing
Renal Impairment: No specific dosing adjustment is recommended.
Hepatic Impairment: No specific dosing adjustment is recommended.

Administration
I.V.: For intravenous administration only. Infuse over 20-30 minutes.

Stability
Reconstitution: Reconstitute vials with sterile water for injection, USP. Shake the vial gently to dissolve. Further dilute reconstituted solution with 0.9% sodium chloride or dextrose 5% in water. When mixing the solution, gently invert the bag to avoid foaming. Do not shake.
Storage: Store intact vials under refrigeration 2°C to 8°C (36°F to 46°F). It is recommended that after reconstitution, the solution should be used immediately. If not used immediately, it can be stored at 2°C to 8°C for up to 24 hours or at room temperature for up to 4 hours. Discard the reconstituted solution within 24 hours.

Nursing Actions
Physical Assessment: Monitor infusion site, cardiovascular, respiratory, and renal function during infusion. Monitor for adverse reactions during infusion and periodically following infusion. Monitor closely for opportunistic infection (eg, chills, fever, sore throat, easy bruising or bleeding, mouth sores, unhealed sores). Assess knowledge/teach patient possible side effects/interventions and adverse symptoms to report as inpatient or following discharge.
Patient Education: This medication, which may help to reduce transplant rejection, can only be given by infusion. You will be monitored and assessed closely during infusion and thereafter. It is important that you report any changes or problems for evaluation. You will be susceptible to infection (avoid crowds and exposure to infection). Frequent mouth care and small frequent meals may help counteract any GI effects you may experience and will help maintain adequate nutrition and fluid intake. Report any changes in urination; unusual bruising or bleeding; chest pain or palpitations; acute dizziness; respiratory difficulty; fever or chills; changes in cognition; rash; feelings of pain or
(Continued)

Basiliximab *(Continued)*

numbness in extremities; severe GI upset or diarrhea; unusual back or leg pain or muscle tremors; vision changes; or any sign of infection (eg, chills, fever, sore throat, easy bruising or bleeding, mouth sores, unhealed sores, vaginal discharge). **Breast-feeding precaution:** Breast-feeding is not recommended.

Breast-Feeding Issues It is not known whether basiliximab is excreted in human milk. Because many immunoglobulins are secreted in milk and the potential for serious adverse reactions exists, a decision should be made whether to discontinue nursing or discontinue the drug, taking into account the importance of the drug to the mother.

Pregnancy Issues IL-2 receptors play an important role in the development of the immune system. Use in pregnant women only when benefit exceeds potential risk to the fetus. Women of childbearing potential should use effective contraceptive measures before beginning treatment and for 4 months after completion of therapy with this agent.

Beclomethasone *(be kloe METH a sone)*

U.S. Brand Names Beconase® AQ; QVAR®

Synonyms Beclomethasone Dipropionate

Pharmacologic Category Corticosteroid, Inhalant (Oral); Corticosteroid, Nasal

Medication Safety Issues
Sound-alike/look-alike issues:
Vanceril® may be confused with Vancenase®

Pregnancy Risk Factor C

Lactation Excretion in breast milk unknown/use caution

Use
Oral inhalation: Maintenance and prophylactic treatment of asthma; includes those who require corticosteroids and those who may benefit from a dose reduction/elimination of systemically-administered corticosteroids. Not for relief of acute bronchospasm.

Nasal aerosol: Symptomatic treatment of seasonal or perennial rhinitis; prevent recurrence of nasal polyps following surgery.

Mechanism of Action/Effect Acts at cellular level to prevent or control inflammation

Contraindications Hypersensitivity to beclomethasone or any component of the formulation; status asthmaticus

Warnings/Precautions Not to be used in status asthmaticus or for the relief of acute bronchospasm. Safety and efficacy in children <5 years of age have not been established. May cause suppression of hypothalamic-pituitary-adrenal (HPA) axis, particularly in younger children or in patients receiving high doses for prolonged periods. Fatalities have occurred due to adrenal insufficiency in asthmatic patients during and after transfer from systemic corticosteroids to aerosol steroids; aerosol steroids do **not** provide the systemic steroid needed to treat steroid-dependent patients having trauma, surgery, or infections. Withdrawal and discontinuation of the corticosteroid should be done slowly and carefully.

Controlled clinical studies have shown that orally-inhaled and intranasal corticosteroids may cause a reduction in growth velocity in pediatric patients, which appears to be related to dose and duration of exposure.

May suppress the immune system, patients may be more susceptible to infection. Use with caution in patients with systemic infections or ocular herpes simplex. Avoid exposure to chickenpox and measles. Corticosteroids should be used with caution in patients with diabetes, hypertension, osteoporosis, peptic ulcer, glaucoma, cataracts, or tuberculosis. Use caution in hepatic impairment.

Drug Interactions
Increased Effect/Toxicity: The addition of salmeterol has been demonstrated to improve response to inhaled corticosteroids (as compared to increasing steroid dosage).

Adverse Reactions Frequency not defined.

Central nervous system: Agitation, depression, dizziness, dysphonia, headache, lightheadedness, mental disturbances

Dermatologic: Acneiform lesions, angioedema, atrophy, bruising, pruritus, purpura, striae, rash, urticaria

Endocrine & metabolic: Cushingoid features, growth velocity reduction in children and adolescents, HPA function suppression, weight gain

Gastrointestinal: Dry/irritated nose, throat and mouth, hoarseness, localized *Candida* or *Aspergillus* infection, loss of smell, loss of taste, nausea, unpleasant smell, unpleasant taste, vomiting

Local: Nasal spray: Burning, epistaxis, localized *Candida* infection, nasal septum perforation (rare), nasal stuffiness, nosebleeds, rhinorrhea, sneezing, transient irritation, ulceration of nasal mucosa (rare)

Ocular: Cataracts, glaucoma, intraocular pressure increased

Respiratory: Cough, paradoxical bronchospasm, pharyngitis, sinusitis, wheezing

Miscellaneous: Anaphylactic/anaphylactoid reactions, death (due to adrenal insufficiency, reported during and after transfer from systemic corticosteroids to aerosol in asthmatic patients), immediate and delayed hypersensitivity reactions

Overdosage/Toxicology Symptoms of overdose include irritation and burning of the nasal mucosa, sneezing, intranasal and pharyngeal *Candida* infections, nasal ulceration, epistaxis, rhinorrhea, nasal stuffiness, and headache. When consumed in high doses over prolonged periods, systemic hypercorticism and adrenal suppression may occur. In those cases, discontinuation of the corticosteroid should be done judiciously.

Pharmacodynamics/Kinetics
Onset of Action: Therapeutic effect: 1-4 weeks

Protein Binding: 87%

Half-Life Elimination: Initial: 3 hours

Metabolism: Hepatic via CYP3A4 to active metabolites

Excretion: Feces (60%); urine (12%)

Available Dosage Forms
Aerosol for oral inhalation, as dipropionate (QVAR®): 40 mcg/inhalation [100 metered doses] (7.3 g); 80 mcg/inhalation [100 metered doses] (7.3 g)

Suspension, intranasal, aqueous, as dipropionate [spray] (Beconase® AQ): 42 mcg/inhalation [180 metered doses] (25 g)

Dosing
Adults & Elderly: Nasal inhalation and oral inhalation dosage forms are not to be used interchangeably.

Rhinitis, nasal polyps: Inhalation, nasal (Beconase® AQ): 1-2 inhalations each nostril twice daily; total dose 168-336 mcg/day

Asthma: Inhalation, oral (doses should be titrated to the lowest effective dose once asthma is controlled) (QVAR®):

Patients previously on bronchodilators only: Initial dose 40-80 mcg twice daily; maximum dose 320 mcg twice day

Patients previously on inhaled corticosteroids: Initial dose 40-160 mcg twice daily; maximum dose 320 mcg twice daily

NIH Asthma Guidelines (NAEPP, 2002; NIH, 1997): HFA formulation (eg, QVAR®): Administer in divided doses:
"Low" dose: 80-240 mcg/day
"Medium" dose: 240-480 mcg/day
"High" dose: >480 mcg/day

Oral inflammation (unlabeled dental use) (QVAR®): Initial: 40-160 mcg twice daily; maximum dose: 320 mcg twice daily. Apply spray to back of oral cavity.

Pediatrics: Nasal inhalation and oral inhalation dosage forms are not to be used interchangeably.

Rhinitis, nasal polyps: Inhalation, nasal (Beconase® AQ): Children ≥6 years: Refer to adult dosing

Asthma: Inhalation, oral (doses should be titrated to the lowest effective dose once asthma is controlled) (QVAR®):

Children 5-11 years: Initial: 40 mcg twice daily; maximum dose: 80 mcg twice daily

Children ≥12 years: Refer to adult dosing

NIH Asthma Guidelines (NAEPP, 2002; NIH, 1997): HFA formulation (eg, QVAR®): Administer in divided doses:

Children ≤12 years:

"Low" dose: 80-160 mcg/day

"Medium" dose: 160-320 mcg/day

"High" dose: >320 mcg/day

Children >12 years: Refer to adult dosing.

Administration

Inhalation:

Beconase AQ®: Shake well before use. Nasal applicator and dust cap may be washed in warm water and dry thoroughly.

QVAR®: Rinse mouth and throat after use to prevent *Candida* infection. Do not wash or put inhaler in water; mouth piece may be cleaned with a dry tissue or cloth. Prime canister before using.

Stability

Storage: Do not store near heat or open flame. Do not puncture canisters. Store at room temperature. Rest QVAR® on concave end of canister with actuator on top.

Nursing Actions

Physical Assessment: Not to be used to treat status asthmaticus or fungal infections of nasal passages. Monitor therapeutic effectiveness and adverse reactions. When changing from systemic steroids to inhalational steroids, taper reduction of systemic medication slowly. Assess knowledge/teach patient appropriate use, interventions to reduce side effects, and adverse symptoms to report.

Patient Education: Use as directed; do not increase dosage or discontinue abruptly without consulting prescriber. It may take 1-4 weeks for you to realize full effects of treatment. Review use of inhaler or spray with prescriber or follow package insert for directions. Keep oral inhaler clean and unobstructed. Always rinse mouth and throat after use of inhaler to prevent infection. If you are also using an inhaled bronchodilator, wait 10 minutes before using this steroid aerosol. Report adverse effects such as skin redness, rash, or irritation; pain or burning of nasal mucosa; white plaques in mouth or fuzzy tongue; unresolved headache; or worsening of condition or lack of improvement. Discard after date calculated by prescriber; the amount of medication in canister cannot be guaranteed after using the labeled number of actuations (sprays) even though it may not feel empty. **Pregnancy/breast-feeding precautions:** Inform prescriber if you are or intend to become pregnant. Consult prescriber if breast-feeding.

Inhalation: Sit when using. Take deep breaths for 3-5 minutes, and clear nasal passages before administration (use decongestant as needed). Hold breath for 5-10 seconds after use, and wait 1-3 minutes between inhalations. Follow package insert instructions for use. Do not exceed maximum dosage. If also using inhaled bronchodilator, use before beclomethasone. Rinse mouth and throat after use to reduce aftertaste and prevent candidiasis.

Geriatric Considerations Older patients may have difficulty with oral metered dose inhalers and may benefit from the use of a spacer or chamber device.

Breast-Feeding Issues Other corticosteroids have been found in breast milk; however, information for beclomethasone is not available. Inhaled corticosteroids are recommended for the treatment of asthma (most information available using budesonide) while breast-feeding.

Pregnancy Issues Teratogenic effects were observed in animal studies. No human data on beclomethasone crossing the placenta or effects on the fetus. A decrease in fetal growth has not been observed with inhaled corticosteroid use during pregnancy. Inhaled corticosteroids are recommended for the treatment of asthma (most information available using budesonide) and allergic rhinitis during pregnancy.

Additional Information Effects of inhaled/intranasal steroids on growth have been observed in the absence of laboratory evidence of HPA axis suppression, suggesting that growth velocity is a more sensitive indicator of systemic corticosteroid exposure in pediatric patients than some commonly used tests of HPA axis function. The long-term effects of this reduction in growth velocity associated with orally-inhaled and intranasal corticosteroids, including the impact on final adult height, are unknown. The potential for "catch up" growth following discontinuation of treatment with inhaled corticosteroids has not been adequately studied.

Belladonna and Opium

(bel a DON a & OH pee um)

U.S. Brand Names B&O Supprettes®

Synonyms Opium and Belladonna

Restrictions C-II

Pharmacologic Category Analgesic Combination (Narcotic); Antispasmodic Agent, Urinary

Pregnancy Risk Factor C

Lactation Excretion in breast milk unknown/use caution

Use Relief of moderate-to-severe pain associated with rectal or bladder tenesmus that may occur in postoperative states and neoplastic situations; pain associated with ureteral spasms not responsive to non-narcotic analgesics and to space intervals between injections of opiates

Mechanism of Action/Effect Anticholinergic alkaloids act primarily by competitive inhibition of the muscarinic actions of acetylcholine on structures innervated by postganglionic cholinergic neurons and on smooth muscle; resulting effects include antisecretory activity on exocrine glands and intestinal mucosa and smooth muscle relaxation. Contains many narcotic alkaloids including morphine; its mechanism for gastric motility inhibition is primarily due to this morphine content, resulting in a decrease in digestive secretions, an increase in GI muscle tone, and therefore a reduction in GI propulsion.

Contraindications Glaucoma; severe renal or hepatic disease; bronchial asthma; respiratory depression; convulsive disorders; acute alcoholism; premature labor

Warnings/Precautions Usual precautions of opiate agonist therapy should be observed. Use with caution and generally in reduced doses in the very young or geriatric patients.

Drug Interactions

Decreased Effect: May decrease effects of drugs with cholinergic mechanisms. Antipsychotic efficacy of phenothiazines may be decreased.

Increased Effect/Toxicity: Additive effects with CNS depressants. May increase effects of digoxin and atenolol. Coadministration with other anticholinergic agents (phenothiazines, tricyclic antidepressants, amantadine, and antihistamines) may increase effects (Continued)

Belladonna and Opium *(Continued)*

such as dry mouth, constipation, and urinary retention.

Nutritional/Ethanol Interactions Ethanol: Avoid ethanol (may increase sedation).

Lab Interactions Increased aminotransferase [ALT (SGPT)/AST (SGOT)] (S)

Adverse Reactions

>10%:
Dermatologic: Dry skin
Gastrointestinal: Constipation, dry throat, xerostomia
Respiratory: Dry nose
Miscellaneous: Diaphoresis decreased

1% to 10%:
Dermatologic: Light sensitivity increased
Endocrine & metabolic: Breast milk flow decreased
Gastrointestinal: Dysphagia

Overdosage/Toxicology Primary attention should be directed to ensuring adequate respiratory exchange. Opiate agonist-induced respiratory depression may be reversed with parenteral naloxone hydrochloride. Anticholinergic toxicity may be caused by strong binding of a belladonna alkaloid to cholinergic receptors. Physostigmine 1-2 mg given slowly SubQ or I.V. may be administered to reverse overdose with life-threatening effects.

Pharmacodynamics/Kinetics

Onset of Action:
Opium: Within 30 minutes

Metabolism:
Opium: Hepatic, with formation of glucuronide metabolites

Available Dosage Forms Suppository:
#15 A: Belladonna extract 16.2 mg and opium 30 mg
#16 A: Belladonna extract 16.2 mg and opium 60 mg

Dosing

Adults & Elderly: Rectal/bladder tenesmus or ureteral spasm: Rectal: 1 suppository 1-2 times/day, up to 4 doses/day

Administration

Other: Prior to rectal insertion, the finger and suppository should be moistened. Assist with ambulation.

Stability

Storage: Store at 15°C to 30°C; avoid freezing.

Nursing Actions

Physical Assessment: Assess other medications patient may be taking for additive or adverse interactions (additive effects with all CNS depressants, tricyclic antidepressants, and other anticholinergics). Monitor for effectiveness of pain relief and monitor for signs of overdose. Monitor blood pressure, CNS and respiratory status, and degree of sedation at beginning of therapy and at regular intervals with long-term use. May cause physical and/or psychological dependence. For inpatients, implement safety measures (eg, side rails up, call light within reach, instructions to call for assistance). Assess knowledge/teach patient appropriate use if self-administered. Teach patient to monitor for adverse reactions, adverse reactions to report, and appropriate interventions to reduce side effects.

Patient Education: If self-administered, use exactly as directed; do not increase dose or frequency. Drug may cause physical and/or psychological dependence. While using this medication, do not use alcohol and other prescription or OTC medications (especially sedatives, tranquilizers, antihistamines, or pain medications) without consulting prescriber. Maintain adequate hydration (2-3 L/day of fluids) unless instructed to restrict fluid intake. May cause hypotension, dizziness, or drowsiness; use caution when driving, climbing stairs, or changing position (rising from sitting or lying to standing) or when engaging in tasks requiring alertness (until response to drug is known); dry mouth or throat (frequent mouth care, frequent sips of fluids, chewing gum, or sucking lozenges may help); constipation (increased exercise, fluids, fruit, or fiber may help; if unresolved, consult prescriber about use of stool softeners); photosensitivity (use sunscreen, wear protective clothing and eyewear, and avoid direct sunlight); or decreased perspiration (avoid extremes in temperature or excessive activity in hot environments). Report chest pain or palpitations; persistent dizziness; changes in mentation; changes in gait; blurred vision; shortness of breath or respiratory difficulty. **Pregnancy/breast-feeding precautions:** Inform prescriber if you are or intend to become pregnant. Consult prescriber if breast-feeding.

Related Information
Opium Tincture *on page 915*

Benazepril *(ben AY ze pril)*

U.S. Brand Names Lotensin®

Synonyms Benazepril Hydrochloride

Pharmacologic Category Angiotensin-Converting Enzyme (ACE) Inhibitor

Medication Safety Issues
Sound-alike/look-alike issues:
Benazepril may be confused with Benadryl®
Lotensin® may be confused with Lioresal®, Loniten®, lovastatin

Pregnancy Risk Factor C (1st trimester)/D (2nd and 3rd trimesters)

Lactation Enters breast milk/compatible

Use Treatment of hypertension, either alone or in combination with other antihypertensive agents

Mechanism of Action/Effect Competitive inhibitor of angiotensin-converting enzyme (ACE); prevents conversion of angiotensin I to angiotensin II, a potent vasoconstrictor; results in lower levels of angiotensin II which causes an increase in plasma renin activity and a reduction in aldosterone secretion

Contraindications Hypersensitivity to benazepril or any component of the formulation; angioedema or serious hypersensitivity related to previous treatment with an ACE inhibitor; bilateral renal artery stenosis; patients with idiopathic or hereditary angioedema; pregnancy (2nd and 3rd trimesters)

Warnings/Precautions Anaphylactic reactions can occur. Angioedema can occur at any time during treatment (especially following first dose). Angioedema can occur at any time during treatment (especially following first dose). It may involve head and neck (potentially affecting the airway) or the intestine (presenting with abdominal pain). Prolonged monitoring may be required especially if tongue, glottis, or larynx are involved as they are associated with airway obstruction. Those with a history of airway surgery in this situation have a higher risk. Careful blood pressure monitoring with first dose (hypotension can occur especially in volume-depleted patients). Dosage adjustment needed in renal impairment. Use with caution in hypovolemia; collagen vascular diseases; valvular stenosis (particularly aortic stenosis); hyperkalemia; or before, during, or immediately after anesthesia. Avoid rapid dosage escalation which may lead to renal insufficiency. Rare toxicities associated with ACE inhibitors include cholestatic jaundice (which may progress to hepatic necrosis) and neutropenia/agranulocytosis with myeloid hyperplasia. Hypersensitivity reactions may be seen during hemodialysis with high-flux dialysis membranes (eg, AN69). Deterioration in renal function can occur with initiation. Use with caution in unilateral renal artery stenosis and pre-existing renal insufficiency.

Drug Interactions

Decreased Effect: Aspirin (high dose) may reduce the therapeutic effects of ACE inhibitors; at low dosages this does not appear to be significant. Rifampin may decrease the effect of ACE inhibitors. Antacids may decrease the bioavailability of ACE inhibitors (may be more likely to occur with captopril); separate administration times by 1-2 hours. NSAIDs, specifically indomethacin, may reduce the hypotensive effects of ACE inhibitors.

Increased Effect/Toxicity: Potassium supplements, co-trimoxazole (high dose), angiotensin II receptor antagonists (eg, candesartan, losartan, irbesartan), or potassium-sparing diuretics (amiloride, spironolactone, triamterene) may result in elevated serum potassium levels when combined with ACE inhibitors. ACE inhibitor effects may be increased by phenothiazines or probenecid (increases levels of captopril). ACE inhibitors may increase serum concentrations/effects of lithium. Diuretics have additive hypotensive effects with ACE inhibitors, and hypovolemia increases the potential for adverse renal effects of ACE inhibitors. In patients with compromised renal function, coadministration with NSAIDs may result in further deterioration of renal function. Allopurinol and ACE inhibitors may cause a higher risk of hypersensitivity reaction when taken concurrently.

Nutritional/Ethanol Interactions Herb/Nutraceutical: Avoid dong quai if using for hypertension (has estrogenic activity). Avoid ephedra, yohimbe, ginseng (may worsen hypertension). Avoid garlic (may have increased antihypertensive effect).

Adverse Reactions 1% to 10%:
Cardiovascular: Postural dizziness (2%)
Central nervous system: Headache (6%), dizziness (4%), fatigue (3%), somnolence (2%)
Endocrine & metabolic: Hyperkalemia (1%), uric acid increased
Gastrointestinal: Nausea (2%)
Renal: Serum creatinine increased (2%), worsening of renal function may occur in patients with bilateral renal artery stenosis or hypovolemia
Respiratory: Cough (1% to 10%)
Eosinophilic pneumonitis, neutropenia, anaphylaxis, renal insufficiency, and renal failure have been reported with other ACE inhibitors. In addition, a syndrome including fever, myalgia, arthralgia, interstitial nephritis, vasculitis, rash, eosinophilia, and elevated ESR has been reported to be associated with ACE inhibitors.

Overdosage/Toxicology Mild hypotension has been the primary toxic effect seen with acute overdose. Bradycardia may also occur. Hyperkalemia occurs even with therapeutic doses, especially in patients with renal insufficiency and those taking NSAIDs. Treatment is symptom-directed and supportive.

Pharmacodynamics/Kinetics
Onset of Action:
Reduction in plasma angiotensin-converting enzyme (ACE) activity: Peak effect: 1-2 hours after 2-20 mg dose
Reduction in blood pressure: Peak effect: Single dose: 2-4 hours; Continuous therapy: 2 weeks
Duration of Action: Reduction in plasma angiotensin-converting enzyme (ACE) activity: >90% inhibition for 24 hours after 5-20 mg dose
Time to Peak: Parent drug: 0.5-1 hour
Half-Life Elimination: Benazeprilat: Effective: 10-11 hours; Terminal: Children: 5 hours, Adults: 22 hours
Metabolism: Rapidly and extensively hepatic to its active metabolite, benazeprilat, via enzymatic hydrolysis; extensive first-pass effect
Excretion: Clearance: Nonrenal clearance (ie, biliary, metabolic) appears to contribute to the elimination of benazeprilat (11% to 12%), particularly patients with severe renal impairment; hepatic clearance is the main elimination route of unchanged benazepril

Dialysis: ~6% of metabolite removed within 4 hours of dialysis following 10 mg of benazepril administered

2 hours prior to procedure; parent compound not found in dialysate

Available Dosage Forms Tablet, as hydrochloride: 5 mg, 10 mg, 20 mg, 40 mg

Dosing
Adults: Hypertension: Oral: Initial: 10 mg/day in patients not receiving a diuretic; 20-40 mg/day as a single dose or 2 divided doses; the need for twice-daily dosing should be assessed by monitoring peak (2-6 hours after dosing) and trough responses.
Note: Patients taking diuretics should have them discontinued 2-3 days prior to starting benazepril. If they cannot be discontinued, then initial dose should be 5 mg; restart after blood pressure is stabilized if needed.
Elderly: Oral: Initial: 5-10 mg/day in single or divided doses; usual range: 20-40 mg/day; adjust for renal function. Also see "Note" in adult dosing.
Pediatrics: Hypertension: Children ≥6 years: Oral: Initial: 0.2 mg/kg/day as monotherapy; dosing range: 0.1-0.6 mg/kg/day (maximum dose: 40 mg/day)
Renal Impairment:
Cl_{cr} <30 mL/minute:
Children: Use is not recommended.
Adults: Administer 5 mg/day initially; maximum daily dose: 40 mg.
Hemodialysis: Moderately dialyzable (20% to 50%); administer dose postdialysis or administer 25% to 35% supplemental dose.
Peritoneal dialysis: Supplemental dose is not necessary.

Laboratory Monitoring CBC, renal function tests, electrolytes

Nursing Actions
Physical Assessment: Assess other pharmacological or herbal products patient may be taking for potential interactions. Assess results of laboratory tests, therapeutic effectiveness (blood pressure should be monitored after first doses and periodically during therapy), and adverse response on a regular basis during therapy. Teach patient proper use, possible side effects/appropriate interventions, and adverse symptoms to report.
Patient Education: Do not take any new medication during therapy without consulting prescriber. Take exactly as directed; do not alter dose or discontinue drug without consulting prescriber. Take first dose at bedtime. Do not take potassium supplements or salt substitutes containing potassium without consulting prescriber. This drug does not eliminate need for diet or exercise regimen as recommended by prescriber. May cause dizziness, fainting, or lightheadedness (use caution when driving or engaging in tasks that require alertness until response to drug is known); postural hypotension (use caution when rising from lying or sitting position or climbing stairs); nausea, vomiting, abdominal pain, dry mouth, or transient loss of appetite (small, frequent meals, frequent mouth care, sucking lozenges, or chewing gum may help); report if these side effects persist. Report mouth sores; fever or chills; swelling of extremities, face, mouth, or tongue; respiratory difficulty or unusual cough; or other persistent adverse reactions. **Pregnancy precaution:** Inform prescriber if you are or intend to become pregnant. This drug should not be used in the 2nd or 3rd trimester of pregnancy. Consult prescriber for appropriate contraceptive measures.

Geriatric Considerations Due to frequent decreases in glomerular filtration (also creatinine clearance) with aging, elderly patients may have exaggerated responses to ACE inhibitors. Differences in clinical response due to hepatic changes are not observed. ACE inhibitors may be preferred agents in elderly patients with congestive heart failure and diabetes mellitus. Diabetic proteinuria is reduced and insulin sensitivity is enhanced. In general, the side effect profile (Continued)

Benazepril *(Continued)*

is favorable in elderly and causes little or no CNS confusion. Use lowest dose recommendations initially.

Pregnancy Issues ACE inhibitors can cause fetal injury or death if taken during the 2nd or 3rd trimester. Discontinue ACE inhibitors as soon as pregnancy is detected.

Benazepril and Hydrochlorothiazide
(ben AY ze pril & hye droe klor oh THYE a zide)

U.S. Brand Names Lotensin® HCT

Synonyms Hydrochlorothiazide and Benazepril

Pharmacologic Category Antihypertensive Agent, Combination

Pregnancy Risk Factor C/D (2nd and 3rd trimesters)

Lactation Enters breast milk/compatible

Use Treatment of hypertension

Available Dosage Forms Tablet:

5/6.25: Benazepril 5 mg and hydrochlorothiazide 6.25 mg

10/12.5: Benazepril 10 mg and hydrochlorothiazide 12.5 mg

20/12.5: Benazepril 20 mg and hydrochlorothiazide 12.5 mg

20/25: Benazepril 20 mg and hydrochlorothiazide 25 mg

Dosing

Adults: Hypertension: Oral: Dose is individualized (range: benazepril: 5-20 mg; hydrochlorothiazide: 6.25-25 mg/day)

Elderly: Dose is individualized.

Renal Impairment: Cl$_{cr}$ <30 mL/minute: Not recommended; loop diuretics are preferred.

Nursing Actions

Physical Assessment: See individual agents.

Patient Education: See individual agents. **Pregnancy precaution:** Do not get pregnant while taking this medication; use appropriate contraceptive measures.

Related Information

Benazepril *on page 142*
Hydrochlorothiazide *on page 610*

Benzocaine (BEN zoe kane)

U.S. Brand Names Americaine® [OTC]; Americaine® Hemorrhoidal [OTC]; Anbesol® [OTC]; Anbesol® Baby [OTC]; Anbesol® Cold Sore Therapy [OTC]; Anbesol® Jr. [OTC]; Anbesol® Maximum Strength [OTC]; Benzodent® [OTC]; Cepacol® Sore Throat [OTC]; Chiggerex® [OTC]; Chiggertox® [OTC]; Cylex® [OTC]; Dentapaine [OTC]; Dent's Extra Strength Toothache [OTC]; Dent's Maxi-Strength Toothache [OTC]; Dermoplast® Antibacterial [OTC]; Dermoplast® Pain Relieving [OTC]; Detane® [OTC]; Foille® [OTC]; HDA® Toothache [OTC]; Hurricaine® [OTC]; Ivy-Rid® [OTC]; Kanka® Soft Brush™ [OTC]; Lanacane® [OTC]; Lanacane® Maximum Strength [OTC]; Mycinettes® [OTC]; Orabase® with Benzocaine [OTC]; Orajel® Baby Daytime and Nighttime [OTC]; Orajel® Baby Teething [OTC]; Orajel® Baby Teething Nighttime [OTC]; Orajel® Denture Plus [OTC]; Orajel® Maximum Strength [OTC]; Orajel® Medicated Toothache [OTC]; Orajel® Mouth Sore [OTC]; Orajel® Multi-Action Cold Sore [OTC]; Orajel PM® [OTC]; Orajel® Ultra Mouth Sore [OTC]; Oticaine™; Otocaine™; Outgro® [OTC]; Red Cross™ Canker Sore [OTC]; Rid-A-Pain Dental Drops [OTC]; Skeeter Stik [OTC]; Sting-Kill [OTC]; Tanac® [OTC]; Thorets [OTC]; Trocaine® [OTC]; Zilactin®-B [OTC]; Zilactin Toothache and Gum Pain® [OTC]

Synonyms Ethyl Aminobenzoate

Pharmacologic Category Local Anesthetic

Medication Safety Issues

Sound-alike/look-alike issues:

Orabase®-B may be confused with Orinase®

Pregnancy Risk Factor C

Lactation Excretion in breast milk unknown/use caution

Use Temporary relief of pain associated with pruritic dermatosis, pruritus, minor burns, acute congestive and serous otitis media, swimmer's ear, otitis externa, bee stings, insect bites; mouth and gum irritations (toothache, minor sore throat pain, canker sores, dentures, orthodontia, teething, mucositis, stomatitis); sunburn; hemorrhoids; anesthetic lubricant for passage of catheters and endoscopic tubes

Mechanism of Action/Effect Benzocaine blocks both the initiation and conduction of nerve impulses by decreasing the neuronal membrane's permeability to sodium ions, which results in inhibition of depolarization with resultant blockade of conduction. As a diet aide, the anesthetic effect appears to decrease the ability to detect degrees of sweetness by taste perception.

Contraindications Hypersensitivity to benzocaine, other ester-type local anesthetics, or any component of the formulation; secondary bacterial infection of area; ophthalmic use; otic preparations are also contraindicated in the presence of perforated tympanic membrane

Warnings/Precautions Methemoglobinemia has been reported following topical use (rare). When applied as a spray to the mouth or throat, multiple sprays (or sprays of longer than indicated duration) are not recommended. Use caution with breathing problems (asthma, bronchitis, emphysema, in smokers), heart disease, children <6 months of age, and hemoglobin or enzyme abnormalities (glucose-6-phosphodiesterase deficiency, hemoglobin-M disease, NADH-methemoglobin reductase deficiency, pyruvate-kinase deficiency).

When used for self-medication (OTC), notify healthcare provider if condition worsens or does not improve within 7 days, or if swelling, rash, or fever develops. Do not use on open wounds. Avoid contact with the eyes.

Drug Interactions

Decreased Effect: May antagonize actions of sulfonamides.

Adverse Reactions Frequency not defined.

Hematologic: Methemoglobinemia

Local: Burning, contact dermatitis, edema, erythema, pruritus, rash, stinging, tenderness, urticaria

Miscellaneous: Hypersensitivity

Overdosage/Toxicology Methemoglobinemia has been reported with benzocaine in oral overdose. Treatment is primarily symptomatic and supportive. Termination of anesthesia by pneumatic tourniquet inflation should be attempted when the agent is administered by infiltration or regional injection. Methemoglobinemia may be treated with methylene blue, 1-2 mg/kg I.V. infused over several minutes. Seizures commonly respond to diazepam, while hypotension responds to I.V. fluids and Trendelenburg positioning. Bradyarrhythmias (when the heart rate is <60) can be treated with I.V., I.M., or SubQ atropine 15 mcg/kg. With the development of metabolic acidosis, I.V. sodium bicarbonate 0.5-2 mEq/kg and ventilatory assistance should be instituted.

Pharmacodynamics/Kinetics

Metabolism: Hepatic (to a lesser extent) and plasma via hydrolysis by cholinesterase

Excretion: Urine (as metabolites)

Available Dosage Forms

Aerosol, oral spray (Hurricaine®): 20% (60 mL) [dye free; cherry flavor]

Aerosol, topical spray:

Americaine®: 20% (60 mL)

Dermoplast® Antibacterial: 20% (83 mL) [contains aloe vera, benzethonium chloride, menthol]

Dermoplast® Pain Relieving: 20% (60 mL, 83 mL) [contains menthol]

Foille®: 5% (92 g) [contains chloroxylenol 0.63% and corn oil]

Ivy-Rid®: 2% (83 mL)

Lanacane® Maximum Strength: 20% (120 mL) [contains alcohol]

Solarcaine®: 20% (120 mL) [contains triclosan 0.13%, alcohol 35%]

Combination package (Orajel® Baby Daytime and Nighttime):

Gel, oral [Daytime Regular Formula]: 7.5% (5.3 g)

Gel, oral [Nighttime Formula]: 10% (5.3 g)

Cream, oral:

Benzodent®: 20% (7.5 g, 30 g)

Orajel PM®: 20% (5.3 g, 7 g)

Cream, topical:

Lanacane®: 6% (30 g, 60 g)

Lanacane® Maximum Strength: 20% (30 g)

Gel, oral:

Anbesol®: 10% (7.5 g) [contains benzyl alcohol; cool mint flavor]

Anbesol® Baby: 7.5% (7.5 g) [contains benzoic acid; grape flavor]

Anbesol® Jr.: 10% (7 g) [contains benzyl alcohol; bubble gum flavor]

Anbesol® Maximum Strength: 20% (7.5 g, 10 g) [contains benzyl alcohol]

Dentapaine: 20% (11 g) [contains clove oil]

HDA® Toothache: 6.5% (15 mL) [contains benzyl alcohol]

Hurricaine®: 20% (5 g) [dye free; wild cherry flavor]; (30 g) [dye free; mint, pina colada, watermelon, and wild cherry flavors]

Kanka® Soft Brush™: 20% (2 mL) [packaged in applicator with brush tip]

Orabase® with Benzocaine®: 20% (7 g) [contains ethyl alcohol 48%; mild mint flavor]

Orajel®: 10% (5.3 g, 7 g, 9.4 g)

Orajel® Baby Teething: 7.5% (9.4 g, 11.9 g) [cherry flavor]

Orajel® Baby Teething Nighttime: 10% (5.3 g)

Orajel® Denture Plus: 15% (9 g) [contains menthol 2%, ethyl alcohol 66.7%]

Orajel® Maximum Strength: 20% (5.3 g, 7 g, 9.4 g, 11.9 g)

Orajel® Mouth Sore: 20% (5.3 g, 9.4 g, 11.9 g) [contains benzalkonium chloride 0.02%, zinc chloride 0.1%]

Orajel® Multi-Action Cold Sore: 20% (9.4 g) [contains allantoin 0.5%, camphor 3%, dimethicone 2%]

Orajel® Ultra Mouth Sore: 15% (9.4 g) [contains ethyl alcohol 66.7%, menthol 2%]

Zilactin®-B: 10% (7.5 g)

Gel, topical (Detane®): 7.5% (15 g)

Liquid, oral:

Anbesol®: 10% (9 mL) [cool mint flavor]

Anbesol® Maximum Strength: 20% (9 mL) [contains benzyl alcohol]

Hurricaine®: 20% (30 mL) [pina colada and wild cherry flavors]

Orajel® Baby Teething: 7.5% (13 mL) [very berry flavor]

Orajel® Maximum Strength: 20% (13 mL) [contains ethyl alcohol 44%, tartrazine]

Liquid, oral drop:

Dent's Maxi-Strength Toothache: 20% (3.7 mL) [contains alcohol 74%]

Rid-A-Pain Dental Drops: 6.3% (30 mL) [contains alcohol 70%]

Liquid, topical:

Chiggertox®: 2% (30 mL)

Outgro®: 20% (9 mL)

Skeeter Stik: 5% (14 mL) [contains menthol]

Tanac®: 10% (13 mL) [contains benzalkonium chloride]

Lozenge: 6 mg (18s) [contains menthol]; 15 mg (10s)

Cepacol® Sore Throat: 10 mg (18s) [contains cetylpyridinium, menthol; cherry, citrus, honey lemon, and menthol flavors]

Cepacol® Sore Throat: 10 mg (16s) [sugar free; contains cetylpyridinium, menthol; cherry and menthol flavors]

Cylex®: 15 mg [sugar free; contains cetylpyridinium chloride 5 mg; cherry flavor]

Mycinettes®: 15 mg (12s) [sugar free; contains sodium 9 mg; cherry or regular flavor]

Thorets: 18 mg (500s) [sugar free]

Trocaine®: 10 mg (40s, 400s)

Ointment, oral:

Anbesol® Cold Sore Therapy: 20% (7.1 g) [contains benzyl alcohol, allantoin, aloe, camphor, menthol, vitamin E]

Red Cross™ Canker Sore: 20% (7.5 g) [contains coconut oil]

Ointment, rectal (Americaine® Hemorrhoidal): 20% (30 g)

Ointment, topical:

Chiggerex®: 2% (50 g) [contains aloe vera]

Foille®: 5% (3.5 g, 14 g, 28 g) [contains chloroxylenol 0.1%, benzyl alcohol; corn oil base]

Pads, topical (Sting-Kill): 20% (8s) [contains menthol and tartrazine]

Paste, oral (Orabase® with Benzocaine): 20% (6 g)

Solution, otic drops (Oticaine, Otocaine™): 20% (15 mL)

Swabs, oral:

Hurricaine®: 20% (6s, 100s) [dye free; wild cherry flavor]

Orajel® Baby Teething: 7.5% (12s) [berry flavor]

Orajel® Medicated Mouth Sore, Orajel® Medicated Toothache: 20% (8s, 12s) [contains tartrazine]

Zilactin® Toothache and Gum Pain: 20% (8s) [grape flavor]

Swabs, topical (Sting-Kill): 20% (5s) [contains menthol and tartrazine]

Wax, oral (Dent's Extra Strength Toothache Gum): 20% (1 g)

Dosing

Adults & Elderly: Note: These are general dosing guidelines; Refer to specific product labeling for dosing instructions.

Bee stings, insect bites, minor burns, sunburn: Topical 5% to 20%: Apply to affected area 3-4 times a day as needed. In cases of bee stings, remove stinger before treatment.

Lubricant for passage of catheters and instruments: Topical 20%: Apply evenly to exterior of instrument prior to use.

Mouth and gum irritation: Topical (oral) 10% to 20%: Apply thin layer to affected area up to 4 times daily

Sore throat: Oral: Allow one lozenge (10-15 mg) to dissolve slowly in mouth; may repeat every 2 hours as needed

Hemorrhoids: Rectal 5% to 20%: Apply externally to affected area up to 6 times daily

Otitis: Otic 20%: Instill 4-5 drops into external auditory canal; may repeat in 1-2 hours if needed

Pediatrics: Note: These are general dosing guidelines; refer to specific product labeling for dosing instructions.

Teething pain: Children ≥4 months: Topical (oral): 7.5% to 10%: Apply to affected gum area up to 4 times daily

Bee stings, insect bites, minor burns, sunburn: Topical: Children ≥2 years: Refer to adult dosing.

Lubricant for passage of catheters and instruments: Topical: Children ≥2 years: Refer to adult dosing.

Mouth and gum irritation: Topical (oral) 10% to 20%: Children ≥2 years: Refer to adult dosing.

Sore throat: Oral: Children ≥5 years: Refer to adult dosing.

(Continued)

Benzocaine *(Continued)*

Hemorrhoids: Rectal 5% to 20%: Children ≥12 years: Refer to adult dosing.

Administration

Topical: Avoid application to large areas of broken skin, especially in children. When possible, apply to clean, dry area.

Nursing Actions

Physical Assessment: Monitor for effectiveness of application and adverse reactions. **Oral:** Use caution to prevent gagging or choking and avoid food or drink for 1 hour. Teach patient possible side effects/appropriate interventions and adverse symptoms to report.

Patient Education: Use as directed; do not overuse. Do not apply when infections are present and do not apply to large areas of broken skin. Do not eat or drink for 1 hour following oral application. Discontinue application and report if swelling of mouth, lips, tongue, or throat occurs; or if skin irritation occurs at application site. When using as a self-medication (OTC), notify prescriber if condition worsens or does not improve within 7 days or if swelling, rash, or fever develops. **Pregnancy/breast-feeding precautions:** Inform prescriber if you are pregnant. Consult prescriber if breast-feeding.

Benzonatate *(ben ZOE na tate)*

U.S. Brand Names Tessalon®
Pharmacologic Category Antitussive
Pregnancy Risk Factor C
Lactation Excretion in breast milk unknown/use caution
Use Symptomatic relief of nonproductive cough
Mechanism of Action/Effect Suppresses cough by topical anesthetic action on the respiratory stretch receptors
Contraindications Hypersensitivity to benzonatate, related compounds (such as tetracaine), or any component of the formulation
Adverse Reactions 1% to 10%:
Central nervous system: Sedation, headache, dizziness
Dermatologic: Rash
Gastrointestinal: GI upset
Neuromuscular & skeletal: Chest numbness
Ocular: Burning sensation in eyes
Respiratory: Nasal congestion
Overdosage/Toxicology Symptoms of overdose include restlessness, tremor, and CNS stimulation. Benzonatate's local anesthetic activity can reduce the patient's gag reflex and, therefore, may contradict the use of ipecac following ingestion. Treatment is supportive and symptomatic.
Pharmacodynamics/Kinetics
Onset of Action: Therapeutic: 15-20 minutes
Duration of Action: 3-8 hours
Available Dosage Forms
Capsule: 100 mg
Tessalon®: 100 mg, 200 mg
Dosing
Adults & Elderly: Cough: Oral: 100 mg 3 times/day or every 4 hours up to 600 mg/day
Pediatrics: Children >10 years: Refer to adult dosing.

Administration

Oral: Swallow capsule whole (do not break or chew).

Nursing Actions

Physical Assessment: Assess patient response, effectiveness of therapy (relief of cough, lung sounds, and respiratory pattern), and adverse reactions (eg, CNS changes) at beginning of therapy and periodically with long-term use. Teach patient appropriate use, possible side effects/interventions, and adverse symptoms to report.

Patient Education: Do not take any new medications (especially depressants or sleep-inducing agents) without consulting prescriber. Take only as prescribed; do not exceed prescribed dose or frequency. Do not break or chew capsule. Maintain adequate hydration (2-3 L/day of fluids) unless instructed to restrict fluid intake. You may experience drowsiness, impaired coordination, blurred vision, or increased anxiety (use caution when driving or engaging in tasks requiring alertness until response to drug is known); or upset stomach or nausea (small, frequent meals, frequent mouth care, chewing gum, or sucking hard candy may help). Report persistent CNS changes (dizziness, sedation, tremor, or agitation); numbness in chest or feeling of chill; visual changes or burning in eyes; numbness of mouth or difficulty swallowing; or lack of improvement or worsening or condition. **Pregnancy/breast-feeding precautions:** Inform prescriber if you are or intend to become pregnant. Consult prescriber if breast-feeding.

Geriatric Considerations No specific geriatric information is available about benzonatate. Avoid use in patients with impaired gag reflex or who cannot swallow the capsule whole.

Benzoyl Peroxide and Hydrocortisone *(BEN zoe il peer OKS ide & hye droe KOR ti sone)*

U.S. Brand Names Vanoxide-HC®
Synonyms Hydrocortisone and Benzoyl Peroxide
Pharmacologic Category Topical Skin Product; Topical Skin Product, Acne
Pregnancy Risk Factor C
Lactation For topical use
Use Treatment of acne vulgaris and oily skin
Available Dosage Forms Lotion: Benzoyl peroxide 5% and hydrocortisone acetate 0.5% (25 mL)
Dosing
Adults & Elderly: Acne vulgaris: Topical: Shake well; apply thin film 1-3 times/day; gently massage into skin
Pediatrics: Adolescents: Refer to adult dosing.

Nursing Actions

Physical Assessment: See individual agents.
Patient Education: See individual agents. **Pregnancy precaution:** Inform prescriber if you are or intend to become pregnant.
Related Information
Hydrocortisone *on page 617*

Benztropine *(BENZ troe peen)*

U.S. Brand Names Cogentin®
Synonyms Benztropine Mesylate
Pharmacologic Category Anti-Parkinson's Agent, Anticholinergic; Anticholinergic Agent
Medication Safety Issues
Sound-alike/look-alike issues:
Benztropine may be confused with bromocriptine
Pregnancy Risk Factor C
Lactation Excretion in breast milk unknown/use caution
Use Adjunctive treatment of Parkinson's disease; treatment of drug-induced extrapyramidal symptoms (except tardive dyskinesia)
Mechanism of Action/Effect Possesses both anticholinergic and antihistaminic effects. *In vitro* anticholinergic activity approximates that of atropine; *in vivo* it is only about half as active as atropine. Animal data suggest its antihistaminic activity and duration of action approach that of pyrilamine maleate. May also inhibit the reuptake and storage of dopamine and thereby, prolong the action of dopamine.

Contraindications Hypersensitivity to benztropine or any component of the formulation; pyloric or duodenal obstruction, stenosing peptic ulcers; bladder neck obstructions; achalasia; myasthenia gravis; children <3 years of age

Warnings/Precautions Use with caution in older children (dose has not been established). Use with caution in hot weather or during exercise. May cause anhydrosis and hyperthermia, which may be severe. The risk is increased in hot environments, particularly in the elderly, alcoholics, patients with CNS disease, and those with prolonged outdoor exposure.

Elderly patients frequently develop increased sensitivity and require strict dosage regulation - side effects may be more severe in elderly patients with atherosclerotic changes. Use with caution in patients with tachycardia, cardiac arrhythmias, hypertension, hypotension, prostatic hyperplasia (especially in the elderly), any tendency toward urinary retention, liver or kidney disorders, and obstructive disease of the GI or GU tract. When given in large doses or to susceptible patients, may cause weakness and inability to move particular muscle groups.

May be associated with confusion or hallucinations (generally at higher dosages). Intensification of symptoms or toxic psychosis may occur in patients with mental disorders. Benztropine does not relieve symptoms of tardive dyskinesia.

Drug Interactions

Cytochrome P450 Effect: Substrate of CYP2D6 (minor)

Decreased Effect: May increase gastric degradation of levodopa and decrease the amount of levodopa absorbed by delaying gastric emptying. Therapeutic effects of cholinergic agents (tacrine, donepezil) and neuroleptics may be antagonized.

Increased Effect/Toxicity: Central and/or peripheral anticholinergic syndrome can occur when benztropine is administered with amantadine, rimantadine, narcotic analgesics, phenothiazines and other antipsychotics (especially with high anticholinergic activity), tricyclic antidepressants, quinidine and some other antiarrhythmics, and antihistamines. Benztropine may increase the absorption of digoxin.

Nutritional/Ethanol Interactions Ethanol: Avoid ethanol (may increase CNS depression).

Adverse Reactions Frequency not defined.

Cardiovascular: Tachycardia

Central nervous system: Confusion, disorientation, memory impairment, toxic psychosis, visual hallucinations

Dermatologic: Rash

Endocrine & metabolic: Heat stroke, hyperthermia

Gastrointestinal: Xerostomia, nausea, vomiting, constipation, ileus

Genitourinary: Urinary retention, dysuria

Ocular: Blurred vision, mydriasis

Miscellaneous: Fever

Overdosage/Toxicology Symptoms of overdose include CNS depression, confusion, nervousness, hallucinations, dizziness, blurred vision, nausea, vomiting, and hyperthermia. For anticholinergic overdose with severe life-threatening symptoms, physostigmine 1-2 mg SubQ or I.V. slowly, may be given to reverse these effects.

Pharmacodynamics/Kinetics

Onset of Action: Oral: Within 1 hour; Parenteral: Within 15 minutes

Duration of Action: 6-48 hours

Metabolism: Hepatic (N-oxidation, N-dealkylation, and ring hydroxylation)

Available Dosage Forms

Injection, solution, as mesylate (Cogentin®): 1 mg/mL (2 mL)

Tablet, as mesylate: 0.5 mg, 1 mg, 2 mg

Dosing

Adults:

Drug-induced extrapyramidal symptom: Oral, I.M., I.V.: 1-4 mg/dose 1-2 times/day

Acute dystonia: I.M., I.V.: 1-2 mg

Parkinsonism: Oral: 0.5-6 mg/day in 1-2 divided doses; if one dose is greater, give at bedtime. Titrate dose in 0.5 mg increments at 5- to 6-day intervals.

Elderly: Oral: Initial: 0.5 mg once or twice daily; titrate dose in 0.5 mg increments at every 5-6 days; maximum: 4 mg/day.

Pediatrics: Note: Use in children ≤3 years of age should be reserved for life-threatening emergencies.

Drug-induced extrapyramidal symptoms: Oral, I.M., I.V.: Children >3 years: 0.02-0.05 mg/kg/dose 1-2 times/day

Administration

I.V. Detail: pH: 5-8

Nursing Actions

Physical Assessment: Assess effectiveness and interactions of other medications patient may be taking. Monitor renal function, therapeutic response (eg, Parkinsonian symptoms), and adverse reactions such as anticholinergic syndrome (dry mouth and mucous membranes, constipation, epigastric distress, CNS disturbances, paralytic ileus) at beginning of therapy and periodically throughout therapy. Assess knowledge/teach patient appropriate use, interventions to reduce side effects, and adverse symptoms to report.

Patient Education: Take exactly as directed; do not increase, decrease, or discontinue this medicine without consulting prescriber. Take at the same time each day. Do not use alcohol and any prescription or OTC sedatives or CNS depressants without consulting prescriber. You may experience drowsiness, dizziness, confusion, and blurred vision (use caution when driving, climbing stairs, or engaging in tasks requiring alertness until response to drug is known); increased susceptibility to heat stroke, decreased perspiration (use caution in hot weather, maintain adequate fluids and reduce exercise activity); or constipation (increased exercise, fluids, fruit, or fiber may help). Report unresolved nausea, vomiting, or gastric disturbances; rapid or pounding heartbeat, chest pain, or palpitation; respiratory difficulty; CNS changes (hallucination, loss of memory, nervousness, etc); eye pain; prolonged fever; painful or difficult urination; unresolved constipation; increased muscle spasticity or rigidity; skin rash; or significant worsening of condition. **Pregnancy/breast-feeding precautions:** Inform prescriber if you are or intend to become pregnant. Consult prescriber if breast-feeding.

Geriatric Considerations Anticholinergic agents are generally not well tolerated in the elderly and their use should be avoided when possible (see Warnings/Precautions and Adverse Reactions). In the elderly, anticholinergic agents should not be used as prophylaxis against extrapyramidal symptoms.

Additional Information No significant difference in onset of I.M. or I.V. injection, therefore, there is usually no need to use the I.V. route. Improvement is sometimes noticeable a few minutes after injection.

Betamethasone (bay ta METH a sone)

U.S. Brand Names Beta-Val®; Celestone®; Celestone® Soluspan®; Diprolene®; Diprolene® AF; Luxiq®; Maxivate®

Synonyms Betamethasone Dipropionate; Betamethasone Dipropionate, Augmented; Betamethasone Sodium Phosphate; Betamethasone Valerate; Flubenisolone

Pharmacologic Category Corticosteroid, Systemic; Corticosteroid, Topical

Medication Safety Issues
Sound-alike/look-alike issues:
Luxiq® may be confused with Lasix®

Pregnancy Risk Factor C

Lactation Excretion in breast milk unknown/use caution

Use Inflammatory dermatoses such as seborrheic or atopic dermatitis, neurodermatitis, anogenital pruritus, psoriasis, inflammatory phase of xerosis

Mechanism of Action/Effect Binds to corticosteroid receptors in cell and acts to prevent or control inflammation

Contraindications Hypersensitivity to betamethasone, other corticosteroids, or any component of the formulation; systemic fungal infections

Warnings/Precautions Topical use in patients ≤12 years of age is not recommended. May cause suppression of hypothalamic-pituitary-adrenal (HPA) axis, particularly in younger children or in patients receiving high doses for prolonged periods.

Very high potency topical products are not for treatment of rosacea, perioral dermatitis; not for use on face, groin, or axillae. Not for use in a diapered area. Avoid concurrent use of other corticosteroids.

May suppress the immune system; patients may be more susceptible to infection. Use with caution in patients with systemic infections or ocular herpes simplex. Avoid exposure to chickenpox and measles.

Use with caution in patients with hypothyroidism, cirrhosis, ulcerative colitis; do not use occlusive dressings on weeping or exudative lesions and general caution with occlusive dressings should be observed; adverse effects may be increased. Discontinue if skin irritation or contact dermatitis should occur; do not use in patients with decreased skin circulation.

Drug Interactions
Cytochrome P450 Effect: Inhibits CYP3A4 (weak)
Decreased Effect: May induce cytochrome P450 enzymes, which may lead to decreased effect of any drug metabolized by P450 (ie, barbiturates, phenytoin, rifampin). Decreased effectiveness of salicylates when taken with betamethasone.
Increased Effect/Toxicity: Inhibitors of CYP3A4 (including erythromycin, diltiazem, itraconazole, ketoconazole, quinidine, and verapamil) may decrease metabolism of betamethasone.

Nutritional/Ethanol Interactions
Ethanol: Avoid ethanol (may enhance gastric mucosal irritation).
Food: Betamethasone interferes with calcium absorption.
Herb/Nutraceutical: Avoid cat's claw, echinacea (have immunostimulant properties).

Adverse Reactions
Systemic:
Cardiovascular: Congestive heart failure, edema, hyper-/hypotension
Central nervous system: Dizziness, headache, insomnia, intracranial pressure increased, lightheadedness, nervousness, pseudotumor cerebri, seizure, vertigo
Dermatologic: Ecchymoses, facial erythema, fragile skin, hirsutism, hyper-/hypopigmentation, perioral dermatitis (oral), petechiae, striae, wound healing impaired
Endocrine & metabolic: Amenorrhea, Cushing's syndrome, diabetes mellitus, growth suppression, hyperglycemia, hypokalemia, menstrual irregularities, pituitary-adrenal axis suppression, protein catabolism, sodium retention, water retention
Local: Injection site reactions (intra-articular use), sterile abscess
Neuromuscular & skeletal: Arthralgia, muscle atrophy, fractures, muscle weakness, myopathy, osteoporosis, necrosis (femoral and humeral heads)
Ocular: Cataracts, glaucoma, intraocular pressure increased
Miscellaneous: Anaphylactoid reaction, diaphoresis, hypersensitivity, secondary infection

Topical:
Dermatologic: Acneiform eruptions, allergic dermatitis, burning, dry skin, erythema, folliculitis, hypertrichosis, irritation, miliaria, pruritus, skin atrophy, striae, vesiculation
Endocrine and metabolic effects have occasionally been reported with topical use.

Overdosage/Toxicology When consumed in high doses for prolonged periods, systemic hypercorticism and adrenal suppression may occur. In those cases, discontinuation of the corticosteroid should be done judiciously.

Pharmacodynamics/Kinetics
Time to Peak: Serum: I.V.: 10-36 minutes
Protein Binding: 64%
Half-Life Elimination: 6.5 hours
Metabolism: Hepatic
Excretion: Urine (<5% as unchanged drug)

Available Dosage Forms [DSC] = Discontinued product
Note: Potency expressed as betamethasone base.
Cream, topical, as dipropionate: 0.05% (15 g, 45 g)
Maxivate®: 0.05% (45 g)
Cream, topical, as dipropionate augmented (Diprolene® AF): 0.05% (15 g, 50 g)
Cream, topical, as valerate (Beta-Val®): 0.1% (15 g, 45 g)
Foam, topical, as valerate (Luxiq®): 0.12% (50 g, 100 g, 150 g) [contains alcohol 60.4%]
Gel, topical, as dipropionate augmented: 0.05% (15 g, 50 g)
Injection, suspension (Celestone® Soluspan®): Betamethasone sodium phosphate 3 mg/mL and betamethasone acetate 3 mg/mL [6 mg/mL] (5 mL)
Lotion, topical, as dipropionate (Maxivate®): 0.05% (60 mL)
Lotion, topical, as dipropionate augmented (Diprolene®): 0.05% (30 mL, 60 mL)
Lotion, topical, as valerate (Beta-Val®): 0.1% (60 mL)
Ointment, topical, as dipropionate: 0.05% (15 g, 45 g)
Maxivate®: 0.05% (45 g)
Ointment, topical, as dipropionate augmented (Diprolene®): 0.05% (15 g, 50 g)
Ointment, topical, as valerate: 0.1% (15 g, 45 g)
Syrup, as base (Celestone®): 0.6 mg/5 mL (118 mL)

Dosing
Adults: Base dosage on severity of disease and patient response
Inflammatory conditions:
Oral: 2.4-4.8 mg/day in 2-4 doses; range: 0.6-7.2 mg/day
I.M.: Betamethasone sodium phosphate and betamethasone acetate: 0.6-9 mg/day (generally, 1/3 to 1/2 of oral dose) divided every 12-24 hours
Psoriasis (scalp): Topical (foam): Apply to the scalp twice daily, once in the morning and once at night.
Rheumatoid arthritis/osteoarthritis:
Intrabursal, intra-articular, intradermal: 0.25-2 mL
Intralesional:
Very large joints: 1-2 mL

Large joints: 1 mL

Medium joints: 0.5-1 mL

Small joints: 0.25-0.5 mL

Steroid-responsive dermatoses: Therapy should be discontinued when control is achieved; if no improvement is seen, reassessment of diagnosis may be necessary.

Gel, augmented formulation: Apply once or twice daily; rub in gently. **Note:** Do not exceed 2 weeks of treatment or 50 g/week.

Lotion: Apply a few drops twice daily

Augmented formulation: Apply a few drops once or twice daily; rub in gently. **Note:** Do not exceed 2 weeks of treatment or 50 mL/week.

Cream/ointment: Apply once or twice daily

Augmented formulation: Apply once or twice daily. **Note:** Do not exceed 2 weeks of treatment or 45 g/week.

Elderly: Refer to adult dosing. Use the lowest effective dose.

Pediatrics: Base dosage on severity of disease and patient response.

Inflammatory conditions: Note: Use lowest dose listed as initial dose for adrenocortical insufficiency (physiologic replacement).

I.M.:

Children ≤12 years: 0.0175-0.125 mg base/kg/day divided every 6-12 hours **or** 0.5-7.5 mg base/m^2/day divided every 6-12 hours

Children >13 years: Refer to adult dosing.

Oral:

Children ≤12 years: 0.0175-0.25 mg/kg/day divided every 6-8 hours **or** 0.5-7.5 mg/m^2/day divided every 6-8 hours

Children >13 years: Refer to adult dosing.

Topical: Children ≥13 years (use in children ≤12 years is not recommended): Use minimal amount for shortest period of time to avoid HPA axis suppression

Steroid-responsive dermatoses: Topical: Refer to adult dosing

Hepatic Impairment: Adjustments may be necessary in patients with liver failure because betamethasone is extensively metabolized in the liver

Administration

Oral: Not for alternate day therapy; once daily doses should be given in the morning.

I.M.: Do **not** give injectable sodium phosphate/acetate suspension I.V.

Topical: Apply topical sparingly to areas. Not for use on broken skin or in areas of infection. Do not apply to wet skin unless directed; do not cover with occlusive dressing. Do not apply very high potency agents to face, groin, axillae, or diaper area.

Foam: Invert can and dispense a small amount onto a saucer or other cool surface. Do not dispense directly into hands. Pick up small amounts of foam and gently massage into affected areas until foam disappears. Repeat until entire affected scalp area is treated.

Nursing Actions

Physical Assessment: Assess potential for interactions with other prescriptions, OTC medications, or herbal products patient may be taking. Monitor therapeutic response and adverse effects according to indications for therapy, dose, route (systemic or topical), and duration of therapy. When used for long-term therapy (longer than 10-14 days), dosage should be decreased incrementally. Growth should be routinely monitored in pediatric patients. With systemic administration, caution patients with diabetes to monitor glucose levels closely (corticosteroids may alter glucose levels). Teach patient proper use (according to formulation), side effects/appropriate interventions, and symptoms to report.

Patient Education: Do not take any new medication during therapy unless approved by prescriber. Take exactly as directed; do not increase dose or discontinue this medicine abruptly without consulting prescriber. Take oral medication with or after meals. Avoid alcohol and limit intake of caffeine or stimulants. Prescriber may recommend increased dietary vitamins, minerals, or iron. If you have diabetes, monitor glucose levels closely (antidiabetic medication may need to be adjusted). Inform prescriber if you are experiencing greater-than-normal levels of stress (medication may need adjustment). You may be more susceptible to infection (avoid crowds and exposure to infection and do not have any vaccination without consulting prescriber). Some forms of this medication may cause GI upset (small frequent meals and frequent mouth care may help or oral medication may be taken with meals to reduce GI upset). Report promptly excessive nervousness or sleep disturbances; signs of infection (eg, sore throat, unhealed injuries); excessive growth of body hair or loss of skin color; vision changes; excessive or sudden weight gain (>5 lb/week); swelling of face or extremities; respiratory difficulty; muscle weakness; change in color of stools (tarry) or persistent abdominal pain; or worsening of condition or failure to improve.

Topical: For external use only. Do not use for eyes, mucous membranes, or open wounds. Use exactly as directed. Before using, wash and dry area gently. Apply in a thin layer (may rub in lightly). Apply light dressing (if necessary) to area being treated. Do not use occlusive dressing unless so advised by prescriber. Avoid prolonged or excessive use around sensitive tissues, genital, or rectal areas. Avoid exposing treated area to direct sunlight. Inform prescriber if condition worsens (redness, swelling, irritation, signs of infection, or open sores) or fails to improve.

Pregnancy/breast-feeding precautions: Inform prescriber if you are or intend to become pregnant. Consult prescriber if breast-feeding.

Dietary Considerations May be taken with food to decrease GI distress.

Geriatric Considerations Because of the risk of adverse effects, systemic corticosteroids should be used cautiously in the elderly, in the smallest possible dose, and for the shortest possible time.

Breast-Feeding Issues Systemic corticosteroids are excreted in human milk. The extent of topical absorption is variable. Use with caution while breast-feeding; do not apply to nipples.

Pregnancy Issues There are no reports linking the use of betamethasone with congenital defects in the literature. Betamethasone is often used in patients with premature labor [26-34 weeks gestation] to stimulate fetal lung maturation.

Additional Information

Very high potency: Augmented betamethasone dipropionate ointment, lotion

High potency: Augmented betamethasone dipropionate cream, betamethasone dipropionate cream and ointment

Intermediate potency: Betamethasone dipropionate lotion, betamethasone valerate cream

Betamethasone and Clotrimazole
(bay ta METH a sone & kloe TRIM a zole)

U.S. Brand Names Lotrisone®

Synonyms Clotrimazole and Betamethasone

Pharmacologic Category Antifungal Agent, Topical; Corticosteroid, Topical

Pregnancy Risk Factor C

Lactation Excretion in breast milk unknown/use caution

Use Topical treatment of various dermal fungal infections (including tinea pedis, cruris, and corpora in patients ≥17 years of age)

Available Dosage Forms

Cream: Betamethasone dipropionate 0.05% and clotrimazole 1% (15 g, 45 g) [contains benzyl alcohol]

Lotion: Betamethasone dipropionate 0.05% and clotrimazole 1% (30 mL) [contains benzyl alcohol]

Dosing

Adults:

Allergic or inflammatory diseases: Topical: Apply to affected area twice daily, morning and evening

Tinea corporis, tinea cruris: Topical: Massage into affected area twice daily, morning and evening. Do not use for longer than 2 weeks; re-evaluate after 1 week if no clinical improvement. Do not exceed 45 g cream/week or 45 mL lotion/week.

Tinea pedis: Topical: Massage into affected area twice daily, morning and evening. Do not use for longer than 4 weeks; re-evaluate after 2 weeks if no clinical improvement. Do not exceed 45 g cream/week or 45 mL lotion/week.

Elderly: Refer to adult dosing. Use with caution. Skin atrophy and skin ulceration (rare) have been reported in patients with thinning skin. Do not use for diaper dermatitis or under occlusive dressings.

Pediatrics:

Children <17 years: Do not use.

Children ≥17 years: Refer to adult dosing.

Nursing Actions

Physical Assessment: See individual agents.

Patient Education: This medication is for topical use only. Avoid contact with the eyes or mouth. Do not use intravaginally. Do not use longer than recommended. Do not use under dressings or diapers. Shake lotion well before use. Notify prescriber if the condition does not improve or if side effects occur.

Pregnancy/breast-feeding precautions: Inform prescriber if you are or intend to become pregnant. Consult prescriber if breast-feeding.

Related Information

Betamethasone *on page 148*

Clotrimazole *on page 291*

Betaxolol (be TAKS oh lol)

U.S. Brand Names Betoptic® S; Kerlone®

Synonyms Betaxolol Hydrochloride

Pharmacologic Category Beta Blocker, Beta₁ Selective

Medication Safety Issues

Sound-alike/look-alike issues:

Betaxolol may be confused with bethanechol, labetalol

Pregnancy Risk Factor C (manufacturer); D (2nd and 3rd trimesters - expert analysis)

Lactation Oral: Enters breast milk/use caution

Use Treatment of chronic open-angle glaucoma and ocular hypertension; management of hypertension

Mechanism of Action/Effect Competitively blocks beta₁-receptors, with little or no effect on beta₂-receptors; ophthalmic reduces intraocular pressure by reducing the production of aqueous humor

Contraindications Hypersensitivity to betaxolol or any component of the formulation; sinus bradycardia; heart block greater than first-degree (except in patients with a functioning artificial pacemaker); cardiogenic shock; uncompensated cardiac failure; pulmonary edema; pregnancy (2nd and 3rd trimester)

Warnings/Precautions Administer cautiously in compensated heart failure and monitor for a worsening of the condition. Beta-blocker therapy should not be withdrawn abruptly (particularly in patients with CAD), but gradually tapered to avoid acute tachycardia, hypertension, and/or ischemia. Use caution with concurrent use of beta-blockers and either verapamil or diltiazem; bradycardia or heart block can occur. Use caution in patients with PVD (can aggravate arterial insufficiency). In general, beta-blockers should be avoided in patients with bronchospastic disease. Betaxolol, with beta₁ selectivity, should be used cautiously in bronchospastic disease with close monitoring. Use cautiously in patients with diabetes because it can mask prominent hypoglycemic symptoms. Can mask signs of thyrotoxicosis. Dosage adjustment required in severe renal impairment and in patients on dialysis. Use care with anesthetic agents which decrease myocardial function. Safety and efficacy in pediatric patients have not been established.

Drug Interactions

Cytochrome P450 Effect: Substrate (major) of CYP1A2, 2D6; **Inhibits** CYP2D6 (weak)

Decreased Effect: Barbiturates, CYP1A2 inducers, NSAIDs, and rifamycin derivatives may decrease the effects of beta-blockers. Beta₂-agonists may decrease the bradycardic effect of beta-blockers. Beta-blockers may decrease the bronchodilatory effect of theophylline.

Increased Effect/Toxicity: Acetylcholinesterase inhibitors, amiodarone, cardiac glycosides, dipyridamole, disopyramide, and SSRIs may enhance the bradycardic effects of beta-blockers. Beta-blockers may enhance the vasopressor effects of alpha-/ beta-agonists, the orthostatic effects of alpha₁-agonists, and the rebound hypertensive effect of alpha₂-agonists after abrupt withdrawal. Aminoquinolones (amtimalarial), antipsychotic agents, calcium channel blockers, CYP1A2 inhibitors, 2D6 inhibitors, and propoxyphene may increase the effects of beta-blockers. Beta-blockers may enhance the effects of insulin(hypoglycemia), lidocaine, and sulfonylureas (hypoglycemia).

Nutritional/Ethanol Interactions Herb/Nutraceutical: Avoid bayberry; blue cohosh, cayenne, ephedra, ginger, ginseng (American), kola, and licorice (may worsen hypertension). Avoid black cohosh, California poppy, coleus, golden seal, hawthorn, mistletoe, periwinkle, quinine, shepherd's purse (may have increased antihypertensive effects).

Adverse Reactions

Ophthalmic:

>10%: Ocular: Short-term discomfort (25%)

Frequency not defined: Ocular: Anisocoria, blurred vision, corneal sensitivity decreased, corneal staining, crusty lashes, discharge, dry eyes, edema, erythema, foreign body sensation, inflammation, itching sensation, keratitis, photophobia, tearing, visual acuity decreased

Systemic:

>10%:

Central nervous system: Drowsiness, insomnia

Endocrine & metabolic: Sexual ability decreased

1% to 10%:

Cardiovascular: Bradycardia, palpitation, edema, CHF, peripheral circulation reduced

Central nervous system: Mental depression

Gastrointestinal: Diarrhea or constipation, nausea, vomiting, stomach discomfort

Respiratory: Bronchospasm

Miscellaneous: Cold extremities

Overdosage/Toxicology Symptoms of significant overdose include bradycardia, hypotension, AV block, CHF, bronchospasm, hypoglycemia. Treat initially with fluids. Sympathomimetics (eg, epinephrine or dopamine), glucagon, or a pacemaker can be used to treat toxic bradycardia, asystole, and/or hypotension.

Pharmacodynamics/Kinetics
Onset of Action: Ophthalmic: 30 minutes; Oral: 1-1.5 hours
Duration of Action: Ophthalmic: ≥12 hours
Time to Peak: Ophthalmic: ~2 hours; Oral: 1.5-6 hours
Protein Binding: Oral: 50%
Half-Life Elimination: Oral: 12-22 hours
Metabolism: Hepatic to multiple metabolites
Excretion: Urine

Available Dosage Forms
Solution, ophthalmic, as hydrochloride: 0.5% (5 mL, 10 mL, 15 mL) [contains benzalkonium chloride]
Suspension, ophthalmic, as hydrochloride (Betoptic® S): 0.25% (2.5 mL, 5 mL, 10 mL, 15 mL) [contains benzalkonium chloride]
Tablet, as hydrochloride (Kerlone®): 10 mg, 20 mg

Dosing
Adults:
Glaucoma: Ophthalmic: Instill 1-2 drops twice daily.
Hypertension, angina: Oral: 5-10 mg/day; may increase dose to 20 mg/day after 7-14 days if desired response is not achieved
Elderly:
Ophthalmic: Refer to adult dosing.
Hypertension: Oral: Initial: 5 mg/day
Renal Impairment: Oral: Administer 5 mg/day; can increase every 2 weeks up to a maximum of 20 mg/day.
Cl_{cr} <10 mL/minute: Administer 50% of usual dose.

Administration
Other: Ophthalmic: Shake suspension well before using. Tilt head back and instill in eye. Keep eye open and do not blink for 30 seconds. Apply gentle pressure to lacrimal sac for 1 minute. Wipe away excess from skin. Do not touch applicator to eye and do not contaminate tip of applicator.

Stability
Storage: Avoid freezing. Store ophthalmic drops at room temperature.

Laboratory Monitoring Ophthalmic: Intraocular pressure

Nursing Actions
Physical Assessment: Assess potential for interactions with other prescriptions, OTC medications, or herbal products patient may be taking (especially products that affect cardiac function or blood pressure). Monitor therapeutic response and adverse effects. Patients with diabetes should be cautioned that beta-blockers may mask prominent hypoglycemic symptoms. Teach patient proper use (according to formulation), side effects/appropriate interventions, and symptoms to report. Systemic absorption from ophthalmic instillation is minimal. Intraocular pressure should be measured periodically.

Patient Education: Do not take any new medication during therapy unless approved by prescriber.

Oral: Use as directed and do not discontinue this medicine without consulting prescriber. May cause dizziness or blurred vision (use caution when driving or engaging in tasks requiring alertness until response to drug is known); or nausea or vomiting (small frequent meals, frequent mouth care, sucking lozenges, or chewing gum may help). If diabetic, may mask prominent hypoglycemic symptoms. Monitor blood glucose levels closely. Report chest pain, palpitations or irregular heartbeat; persistent GI upset (eg, nausea, vomiting, diarrhea, or constipation); unusual cough; respiratory difficulty; swelling or coolness of extremities; or unusual mental depression. **Pregnancy/breast-feeding precautions:** Inform prescriber if you are or intend to become pregnant. Consult prescriber if breast-feeding.

Ophthalmic: Shake suspension well before using. Tilt head back and instill in eye. Keep eye open; do not blink for 30 seconds. Apply gentle pressure to corner of eye for 1 minute. Wipe away excess from skin. Do not let tip of applicator touch eye; do not contaminate tip of applicator (may cause eye infection, eye damage, or vision loss). Report if condition does not improve or if you experience eye pain, vision changes, or other adverse eye response.

Geriatric Considerations Oral: Due to alterations in the beta-adrenergic autonomic nervous system, beta-adrenergic blockade may result in less hemodynamic response than seen in younger adults.

Bethanechol (be THAN e kole)

U.S. Brand Names Urecholine®
Synonyms Bethanechol Chloride
Pharmacologic Category Cholinergic Agonist
Medication Safety Issues
Sound-alike/look-alike issues:
Bethanechol may be confused with betaxolol
Pregnancy Risk Factor C
Lactation Excretion in breast milk unknown/contraindicated
Use Nonobstructive urinary retention and retention due to neurogenic bladder
Unlabeled/Investigational Use Treatment and prevention of bladder dysfunction caused by phenothiazines; diagnosis of flaccid or atonic neurogenic bladder; gastroesophageal reflux
Mechanism of Action/Effect Stimulates cholinergic receptors in the smooth muscle of the urinary bladder and GI tract resulting in increased peristalsis, increased GI and pancreatic secretions, bladder muscle contraction, and increased ureteral peristaltic waves
Contraindications Hypersensitivity to bethanechol or any component of the formulation; mechanical obstruction of the GI or GU tract or when the strength or integrity of the GI or bladder wall is in question; hyperthyroidism, peptic ulcer disease, epilepsy, obstructive pulmonary disease, bradycardia, vasomotor instability, atrioventricular conduction defects, hypotension, or parkinsonism
Warnings/Precautions Potential for reflux infection if the sphincter fails to relax as bethanechol contracts the bladder. Safety and efficacy in children have not been established.

Drug Interactions
Decreased Effect: Procainamide, quinidine may decrease the effects of bethanechol. Anticholinergic agents (atropine, antihistamines, TCAs, phenothiazines) may decrease effects.
Increased Effect/Toxicity: Bethanechol and ganglionic blockers may cause a critical fall in blood pressure. Cholinergic drugs or anticholinesterase agents may have additive effects with bethanechol.

Lab Interactions Increased lipase, AST, amylase (S), bilirubin, aminotransferase [ALT (SGPT)/AST (SGOT)] (S)

Adverse Reactions Frequency not defined.
Cardiovascular: Hypotension, tachycardia, flushed skin
Central nervous system: Headache, malaise
Gastrointestinal: Abdominal cramps, diarrhea, nausea, vomiting, salivation, eructation
Genitourinary: Urinary urgency
Ocular: Lacrimation, miosis
Respiratory: Asthmatic attacks, bronchial constriction
Miscellaneous: Diaphoresis
(Continued)

Bethanechol *(Continued)*

Overdosage/Toxicology Symptoms of overdose include nausea, vomiting, abdominal cramps, diarrhea, involuntary defecation, flushed skin, hypotension, and bronchospasm. Treat symptomatically; atropine for severe muscarinic symptoms, epinephrine to reverse severe cardiovascular or pulmonary sequelae.

Pharmacodynamics/Kinetics
Onset of Action: 30-90 minutes
Duration of Action: Up to 6 hours
Available Dosage Forms Tablet, as chloride: 5 mg, 10 mg, 25 mg, 50 mg

Dosing
Adults:
Urinary retention, neurogenic bladder, and/or bladder atony:
Oral: Initial: 10-50 mg 2-4 times/day (some patients may require dosages of 50-100 mg 4 times/day). To determine effective dose, may initiate at a dose of 5-10 mg, with additional doses of 5-10 mg hourly until an effective cumulative dose is reached. Cholinergic effects at higher oral dosages may be cumulative.
SubQ: Initial: 2.575 mg, may repeat in 15-30 minutes (maximum cumulative initial dose: 10.3 mg); subsequent doses may be given 3-4 times daily as needed (some patients may require more frequent dosing at 2.5- to 3-hour intervals). Chronic neurogenic atony may require doses of 7.5-10 every 4 hours.
Gastroesophageal reflux (unlabeled): Oral: 25 mg 4 times/day
Elderly: Refer to adult dosing. Use the lowest effective dose.
Pediatrics:
Urinary retention (unlabeled use): Oral: 0.6 mg/kg/day divided 3-4 times/day
Gastroesophageal reflux (unlabeled use): Oral: 0.1-0.2 mg/kg/dose given 30 minutes to 1 hour before each meal to a maximum of 4 times/day

Stability
Storage: Store at room temperature of 15°C to 30°C (59°F to 86°F).

Nursing Actions
Physical Assessment: Assess bladder and sphincter adequacy prior to administering medication. Assess other medications patient may be taking for effectiveness and interactions. Monitor therapeutic effect and adverse reactions (eg, cholinergic crisis - DUMBELS - diarrhea, urination, miosis, bronchospasm/bradycardia, excitability, lacrimation, and salivation/excessive sweating). Assess knowledge/teach patient appropriate use, interventions to reduce side effects, and adverse symptoms to report.
Patient Education: Take as directed, on an empty stomach to avoid nausea or vomiting. Do not discontinue this medicine without consulting prescriber. Maintain adequate hydration (2-3 L/day of fluids) unless instructed to restrict fluid intake. May cause dizziness or hypotension (rise slowly from sitting or lying position and use caution when driving or climbing stairs); or vomiting or loss of appetite (small frequent meals, frequent mouth care, sucking lozenges, or chewing gum may help). Report persistent abdominal discomfort; significantly increased salivation, sweating, tearing, or urination; flushed skin; chest pain or palpitations; acute headache; unresolved diarrhea; excessive fatigue, insomnia, dizziness, or depression; increased muscle, joint, or body pain; vision changes or blurred vision; or respiratory difficulty or wheezing. **Pregnancy/breast-feeding precautions:** Inform prescriber if you are or intend to become pregnant. Do not breast-feed.
Dietary Considerations Should be taken 1 hour before meals or 2 hours after meals.

Geriatric Considerations Urinary incontinence in an elderly patient should be investigated. Bethanechol may be used for overflow incontinence (dribbling) caused by an atonic or hypotonic bladder, but clinical efficacy is variable (see Contraindications, Warnings/Precautions, and Adverse Reactions).

Bevacizumab *(be vuh SIZ uh mab)*

U.S. Brand Names Avastin™
Synonyms Anti-VEGF Monoclonal Antibody; NSC-704865; rhuMAb-VEGF
Pharmacologic Category Antineoplastic Agent, Monoclonal Antibody; Vascular Endothelial Growth Factor (VEGF) Inhibitor
Medication Safety Issues
Sound-alike/look-alike issues:
Bevacizumab may be confused with cetuximab
Pregnancy Risk Factor C
Lactation Excretion in breast milk unknown/not recommended
Use Treatment of metastatic colorectal cancer (in combination with I.V. fluorouracil-based regimen)
Unlabeled/Investigational Use Breast cancer, malignant mesothelioma, prostate cancer, lung cancer (nonsmall cell), renal cell cancer
Investigational: Ovarian cancer (earlier stage)
Mechanism of Action/Effect Bevacizumab is a monoclonal antibody which binds to (and neutralizes) vascular endothelial growth factor (VEGF), preventing its association with endothelial receptors. It blocks the formation of new blood vessels which in turn may slow the growth of all tissues (including metastatic tissue).
Contraindications Hypersensitivity to bevacizumab, murine products, or any component of the formulation
Warnings/Precautions Gastrointestinal perforation, intra-abdominal abscess, and wound dehiscence have been reported in patients receiving bevacizumab (not related to treatment duration); monitor patients for signs/symptoms of abdominal pain, constipation, or vomiting. Permanently discontinue in patients who develop these complications. The appropriate intervals between administration of bevacizumab and surgical procedures to avoid impairment in wound healing has not been established. Do not initiate therapy within 28 days of major surgery and only following complete healing of the incision. Bevacizumab should be discontinued prior to elective surgery and the estimated half-life (20 days) should be considered.

Use with caution in patients with cardiovascular disease; patients with significant recent cardiovascular disease were excluded from clinical trials. An increased risk for arterial thromboembolic events (eg, stroke, MI, TIA, angina) is associated with bevacizumab use in combination with chemotherapy. History of arterial thromboembolism or ≥65 years of age may present an even greater risk; permanently discontinue if serious arterial thromboembolic events occur.

May cause CHF and/or potentiate cardiotoxic effects of anthracyclines. Bevacizumab may cause and/or worsen hypertension significantly; use caution in patients with pre-existing hypertension and monitor BP closely in all patients. Permanent discontinuation is recommended in patients who experience a hypertensive crisis. Temporarily discontinue in patients who develop uncontrolled hypertension. Discontinue if reversible posterior leukoencephalopathy syndrome (RPLS) occurs.

Avoid use in patients with recent hemoptysis; significant pulmonary bleeding has been reported in patients receiving bevacizumab (primarily in patients with nonsmall cell lung cancer). Avoid use in patients with CNS metastases; patients with CNS metastases were excluded from clinical trials due to concerns for bleeding. Other serious bleeding events may occur, but with a lower frequency; discontinuation of treatment is recommended in all patients with serious hemorrhage.

Interrupt therapy in patients experiencing severe infusion reactions; there are no data to address reinstitution of therapy in patients who experience CHF and/or severe infusion reactions. Proteinuria and/or nephrotic syndrome has been associated with bevacizumab; discontinuation of therapy is recommended in patients with nephrotic syndrome. Safety and efficacy in children have not been established.

Drug Interactions
Increased Effect/Toxicity: Bevacizumab may potentiate the cardiotoxic effects of anthracyclines. Serum concentrations of irinotecan's active metabolite may be increased by bevacizumab; an approximate 33% increase has been observed.

Adverse Reactions Percentages reported as part of a combination chemotherapy regimen.

>10%:

Cardiovascular: Hypertension (23% to 34%; grades 3/4: 12%); thromboembolism (18%); hypotension (7% to 15%)

Central nervous system: Pain (61% to 62%); headache (26%); dizziness (19% to 26%)

Dermatologic: Alopecia (6% to 32%), dry skin (7% to 20%), exfoliative dermatitis (3% to 19%), skin discoloration (2% to 16%)

Endocrine & metabolic: Weight loss (15% to 16%), hypokalemia (12% to 16%)

Gastrointestinal: Abdominal pain (50% to 61%); diarrhea (grades 3/4: 34%); vomiting (47% to 52%); anorexia (35% to 43%); constipation (29% to 40%); stomatitis (30% to 32%); gastrointestinal hemorrhage (19% to 24%), dyspepsia (17% to 24%); taste disorder (14% to 21%), flatulence (11% to 19%)

Hematologic: Leukopenia (grades 3/4: 37%), neutropenia (grades 3/4: 21%)

Neuromuscular & skeletal: Weakness (73% to 74%); myalgia (8% to 15%)

Ocular: Tearing increased (6% to 18%)

Renal: Proteinuria (36%)

Respiratory: Upper respiratory infection (40% to 47%), epistaxis (32% to 35%), dyspnea (25% to 26%)

1% to 10%:

Cardiovascular: DVT (6% to 9%; grades 3/4: 9%); arterial thrombosis (4%); syncope (grades 3/4: 3%), intra-abdominal venous thrombosis (grades 3/4: 3%), cardio-/cerebrovascular arterial thrombotic event (2%), CHF (2%)

Central nervous system: Confusion (1% to 6%), abnormal gait (1% to 5%)

Dermatologic: Nail disorder (2% to 8%), skin ulcer (6%)

Gastrointestinal: Xerostomia (4% to 7%), colitis (1% to 6%), gingival bleeding (2%)

Genitourinary: Polyuria/urgency (3% to 6%), vaginal hemorrhage (4%)

Hematologic: Thrombocytopenia (5%)

Hepatic: Bilirubinemia (1% to 6%)

Respiratory: Voice alteration (6% to 9%)

Miscellaneous: Infusion reactions (<3%)

Overdosage/Toxicology Treatment is symptom-directed and supportive.

Pharmacodynamics/Kinetics
Half-Life Elimination: Half-life elimination: 20 days (range: 11-50 days)

Excretion: Clearance: 2.75-5 mL/kg/day

Available Dosage Forms Injection, solution [preservative free]: 25 mg/mL (4 mL, 16 mL)

Dosing
Adults & Elderly:

Colorectal cancer: I.V.: 5 mg/kg every 2 weeks; higher doses (unlabeled) up to 10 mg/kg every 2 weeks have been used.

Breast cancer (unlabeled use): I.V.: 3 mg/kg or 10 mg/kg or 20 mg/kg every 2 weeks

Head and neck cancer (unlabeled use): 5 mg/kg or 10 mg/kg, or 15 mg/kg every 3 weeks

Prostate cancer (unlabeled use): I.V.: 10 mg/kg every 2 weeks

Lung cancer, nonsmall cell (unlabeled use): 15 mg/kg every 3 weeks

Renal cell cancer (unlabeled use): 3 mg/kg or 10 mg/kg every 2 weeks

Dosing Adjustment for Toxicity: Temporary suspension is recommended in moderate-to-severe proteinuria or in patients with severe hypertension which is not controlled with medical management. Permanent discontinuation is recommended in patients who develop wound dehiscence requiring intervention, gastrointestinal perforation, hypertensive crisis, serious bleeding, or nephrotic syndrome.

Administration
I.V.: Infusion, usually after the other antineoplastic agents. Infuse the initial dose over 90 minutes. Infusion may be shortened to 60 minutes if the initial infusion is well tolerated. The third and subsequent infusions may be shortened to 30 minutes if the 60-minute infusion is well tolerated.

I.V. Detail: Monitor closely during the infusion for signs/symptoms of an infusion reaction.

Stability
Reconstitution: Prior to infusion, dilute prescribed dose of bevacizumab in 100 mL NS. Do not mix with dextrose-containing solutions.

Storage: Store vials at 2°C to 8°C (36°F to 46°F). Protect from light; do not freeze or shake. Diluted solutions are stable for up to 8 hours under refrigeration.

Laboratory Monitoring CBC with differential; urinalysis

Nursing Actions
Physical Assessment: Assess other pharmacological or herbal products patient may be taking for potential interactions. Monitor patient closely during and following infusion for infusion reaction. Monitor laboratory tests, therapeutic effectiveness, and adverse response (abdominal pain, constipation, vomiting, bleeding events, hypertension, nephritic syndrome) at each infusion and throughout therapy. Teach patient possible side effects/appropriate interventions, and adverse symptoms to report.

Patient Education: Do not take any new medication during therapy unless approved by prescriber. This medication can only be administered by infusion and you will be closely monitored during infusion; report immediately unusual back or abdominal pain; acute headache; difficulty breathing or chest tightness; difficulty swallowing; itching or rash; or redness, swelling, or pain at infusion site. Maintain adequate hydration (2-3 L/day of fluids) unless instructed to restrict fluid intake and nutrition (small frequent meals). You may experience dry mouth or taste changes (frequent oral care, sucking lozenges, or chewing gum may help); or loss of hair (will grow back when therapy is completed). Report any chest pain, palpitations, or change in heart rate; acute headache, dizziness; abdominal pain, vomiting, or constipation; changes in urinary pattern; pain, redness or swelling, or loss of sensation in extremities; any unusual bleeding; skin rash; or any other adverse reactions. **Pregnancy precautions:** Inform prescriber if you are or intend to become pregnant.

Geriatric Considerations Elderly patients ≥65 years of age had an increased incidence of arterial thromboembolic events; other serious adverse events occurring (Continued)

Bevacizumab *(Continued)*

often include weakness, sepsis, hyper-/hypotension, CHF, constipation, anorexia, anemia, hyper-/hypokalemia, and diarrhea.

Breast-Feeding Issues Immunoglobulins are excreted in breast milk, and it is assumed that bevacizumab may appear in breast milk. Due to concerns for effects on the infant, breast-feeding is not recommended. The half-life of bevacizumab is up to 50 days (average 20 days), and this should be considered when decisions are made concerning breast-feeding resumption.

Pregnancy Issues There are no adequate or well-controlled studies in pregnant women. Angiogenesis is of critical importance to fetal development, and bevacizumab is likely to have adverse consequences in terms of fetal development. Adequate contraception during therapy is recommended. The risk and benefit of treatment should be evaluated in pregnant women. Patients should also be counseled regarding prolonged exposure following discontinuation of therapy due to the long half-life of bevacizumab.

Bexarotene *(beks AIR oh teen)*

U.S. Brand Names Targretin®

Pharmacologic Category Antineoplastic Agent, Miscellaneous

Pregnancy Risk Factor X

Lactation Excretion in breast milk unknown/contraindicated

Use

Oral: Treatment of cutaneous manifestations of cutaneous T-cell lymphoma in patients who are refractory to at least one prior systemic therapy

Topical: Treatment of cutaneous lesions in patients with refractory cutaneous T-cell lymphoma (stage 1A and 1B) or who have not tolerated other therapies

Mechanism of Action/Effect Exact mechanism in is unknown. Acts to inhibit the growth of some tumor cell lines of hematopoietic and squamous cell origin.

Contraindications Hypersensitivity to bexarotene or any component of the formulation; pregnancy

Warnings/Precautions Pregnancy test needed 1 week before initiation and every month thereafter. Effective contraception must be in place 1 month before initiation, during therapy, and for at least 1 month after discontinuation. Male patients with sexual partners who are pregnant, possibly pregnant, or who could become pregnant, must use condoms during sexual intercourse during treatment and for 1 month after last dose. Induces significant lipid abnormalities in a majority of patients (triglyceride, total cholesterol, and HDL); reversible on discontinuation. Use extreme caution in patients with underlying hypertriglyceridemia. Pancreatitis secondary to hypertriglyceridemia has been reported. Monitor for liver function test abnormalities and discontinue drug if tests are three times the upper limit of normal values for AST (SGOT), ALT (SGPT), or bilirubin. Hypothyroidism occurs in about a third of patients. Monitor for signs and symptoms of infection about 4-8 weeks after initiation (leukopenia may occur). Any new visual abnormalities experienced by the patient should be evaluated by an ophthalmologist (cataracts can form, or worsen, especially in the geriatric population). May cause photosensitization. Safety and efficacy are not established in the pediatric population. Avoid use in hepatically-impaired patients. Limit additional vitamin A intake to <15,000 int. units/day. Use caution with diabetic patients.

Drug Interactions

Cytochrome P450 Effect: Substrate of CYP3A4 (minor); **Induces** CYP3A4 (weak)

Decreased Effect: Bexarotene may decrease the plasma levels of hormonal contraceptives and tamoxifen.

Increased Effect/Toxicity: Bexarotene plasma concentrations may be increased by gemfibrozil. Bexarotene may increase the toxicity of DEET.

Nutritional/Ethanol Interactions

Food: Take with a fat-containing meal. Bexarotene serum levels may be increased by grapefruit juice; avoid concurrent use.

Herb/Nutraceutical: Avoid dong quai, St John's wort (may also cause photosensitization). St John's wort may decrease bexarotene levels. Additional vitamin A supplements may lead to vitamin A toxicity (dry skin, irritation, arthralgias, myalgias, abdominal pain, hepatic changes).

Adverse Reactions First percentage is at a dose of 300 mg/m^2/day; the second percentage is at a dose >300 mg/m^2/day.

>10%:
Cardiovascular: Peripheral edema (13% to 11%)
Central nervous system: Headache (30% to 42%), chills (10% to 13%)
Dermatologic: Rash (17% to 23%), exfoliative dermatitis (10% to 28%)
Endocrine & metabolic: Hyperlipidemia (about 79% in both dosing ranges), hypercholesteremia (32% to 62%), hypothyroidism (29% to 53%)
Hematologic: Leukopenia (17% to 47%)
Neuromuscular & skeletal: Weakness (20% to 45%)
Miscellaneous: Infection (13% to 23%)

<10%:
Cardiovascular: Hemorrhage, hypertension, angina pectoris, right heart failure, tachycardia, cerebrovascular accident
Central nervous system: Fever (5% to 17%), insomnia (5% to 11%), subdural hematoma, syncope, depression, agitation, ataxia, confusion, dizziness, hyperesthesia
Dermatologic: Dry skin (about 10% for both dosing ranges), alopecia (4% to 11%), skin ulceration, acne, skin nodule, maculopapular rash, serous drainage, vesicular bullous rash, cheilitis
Endocrine & metabolic: Hypoproteinemia, hyperglycemia, weight loss/gain, breast pain
Gastrointestinal: Abdominal pain (11% to 4%), nausea (16% to 8%), diarrhea (7% to 42%), vomiting (4% to 13%), anorexia (2% to 23%), constipation, xerostomia, flatulence, colitis, dyspepsia, gastroenteritis, gingivitis, melena, pancreatitis, serum amylase increased
Genitourinary: Albuminuria, hematuria, urinary incontinence, urinary tract infection, urinary urgency, dysuria, kidney function abnormality
Hematologic: Hypochromic anemia (4% to 13%), anemia (6% to 25%), eosinophilia, thrombocythemia, coagulation time increased, lymphocytosis, thrombocytopenia
Hepatic: LDH increase (7% to 13%), hepatic failure
Neuromuscular & skeletal: Back pain (2% to 11%), arthralgia, myalgia, bone pain, myasthenia, arthrosis, neuropathy
Ocular: Dry eyes, conjunctivitis, blepharitis, corneal lesion, visual field defects, keratitis
Otic: Ear pain, otitis externa
Renal: Creatinine increased
Respiratory: Pharyngitis, rhinitis, dyspnea, pleural effusion, bronchitis, cough increased, lung edema, hemoptysis, hypoxia
Miscellaneous: Flu-like syndrome (4% to 13%), bacterial infection (1% to 13%)

Topical:
Cardiovascular: Edema (10%)
Central nervous system: Headache (14%), weakness (6%), pain (30%)

Dermatologic: Rash (14% to 72%), pruritus (6% to 40%), contact dermatitis (14%), exfoliative dermatitis (6%)

Hematologic: Leukopenia (6%), lymphadenopathy (6%)

Neuromuscular & skeletal: Paresthesia (6%)

Respiratory: Cough (6%), pharyngitis (6%)

Miscellaneous: Diaphoresis (6%), infection (18%)

Overdosage/Toxicology Doses up to 1000 mg/m^2/day have been used in humans without acute toxic effects. Any overdose should be treated with supportive care focused on the symptoms exhibited.

Pharmacodynamics/Kinetics
Time to Peak: 2 hours
Protein Binding: >99%
Half-Life Elimination: 7 hours
Metabolism: Hepatic via CYP3A4 isoenzyme; four metabolites identified; further metabolized by glucuronidation
Excretion: Primarily feces; urine (<1% as unchanged drug and metabolites)

Available Dosage Forms
Capsule: 75 mg
Gel: 1% (60 g)

Dosing
Adults & Elderly:
Cutaneous T-cell lymphoma: Oral: 300-400 mg/m^2/day taken as a single daily dose.
Cutaneous lesions of T-cell lymphoma: Topical: Apply to lesions once every other day for first week, then increase on a weekly basis to once daily, 2 times/day, 3 times/day, and finally 4 times/day, according to tolerance.
Renal Impairment: No studies have been conducted; however, renal insufficiency may result in significant protein binding changes and alter pharmacokinetics of bexarotene.
Hepatic Impairment: No studies have been conducted; however, hepatic impairment would be expected to result in decreased clearance of bexarotene due to the extensive hepatic contribution to elimination.

Administration
Oral: Administer capsule following a fat-containing meal.
Topical: Allow gel to dry before covering with clothing. Avoid application to normal skin. Use of occlusive dressings is not recommended.

Stability
Storage: Store at 2°C to 25°C (36°F to 77°F). Protect from light.

Laboratory Monitoring If female, pregnancy test 1 week before initiation then monthly while on bexarotene; lipid panel before initiation, then weekly until lipid response established and then at 8-week intervals thereafter; baseline LFTs, repeat at 1, 2, and 4 weeks after initiation then at 8-week intervals thereafter if stable; baseline and periodic thyroid function tests; baseline CBC with periodic monitoring

Nursing Actions
Physical Assessment: Assess other pharmacological or herbal products patient may be taking for potential interactions. Monitor laboratory tests (pregnancy, lipid panel, LFTs, thyroid function, CBC) prior to and during therapy. Monitor therapeutic response (reduction of cutaneous lesions), and adverse reactions (eg, CNS or cardiovascular effects, opportunistic infection, visual abnormalities, hypoglycemia). Teach patient proper use according to formulation, side effects/appropriate interventions, and symptoms to report. **Pregnancy risk factor X** - determine that patient is not pregnant before beginning treatment. Instruct female patients of childbearing age and males who may have intercourse with females of childbearing age about appropriate use of barrier contraceptives 1 month prior to, during, and 1 month following treatment.

Patient Education: Do not take any new medication during therapy unless approved by prescriber. Use exactly as directed; it is preferable to take capsules after a fat-containing meal. Maintain adequate hydration (2-3 L/day of fluids) unless instructed to restrict fluid intake. Avoid grapefruit juice, St John's wort, or additional vitamin A supplements while using this medication. You may be more susceptible to infection (avoid crowds and exposure to infection and do not have any vaccinations without consulting prescriber). May cause nausea, vomiting, anorexia, flatulence (frequent, small meals, good mouth care, chewing gum, or sucking lozenges may help); constipation (increased exercise, fluid, fruit, or fiber may help); diarrhea (buttermilk, boiled milk, or yogurt may help); headache, back or muscle pain (consult prescriber for mild analgesic); or photosensitivity (avoid direct sunlight, wear protective clothing and hat, use sunblock, and protective eyewear). Report chest pain, rapid heartbeat; unresolved GI effects; headache, back or muscle pain; skin dryness, skin rash or peeling; mucous membrane lesions; altered urinary patterns; flu syndrome or opportunistic infection (eg, weakness, fatigue, white plaques or sores in mouth, vaginal discharge, chills, fever); CNS disturbances (insomnia, dizziness, agitation, confusion, depression); vision or hearing changes; or any other adverse effects. **Pregnancy/breast-feeding precautions:** Pregnancy test is needed 1 week before initiation of therapy and every month during therapy. Consult prescriber for appropriate barrier contraceptives. Effective contraception must be in place 1 month before initiation, during therapy, and for at least 1 month after discontinuation. Male patients with sexual partners who are pregnant, possibly pregnant, or who could become pregnant, must use condoms when having sexual intercourse while using this medication and for 1 month after last dose. Do not breast-feed.

Oral: Take exactly as directed, at the same time each day with a fat-containing meal. If you miss a dose, take as soon as possible. If it is almost time for next dose, skip the missed dose and continue on regular schedule. Do not double doses.

Topical: Apply as directed. Allow gel to dry before covering. Avoid applying to normal skin or mucous membranes. Do not use occlusive dressings.

Dietary Considerations It is preferable to take the oral capsule following a fat-containing meal.

Pregnancy Issues Bexarotene caused birth defects when administered orally to pregnant rats. It must not be given to a pregnant woman or a woman who intends to become pregnant. If a woman becomes pregnant while taking the drug, it must be stopped immediately and appropriate counseling be given.

Bicalutamide (bye ka LOO ta mide)

U.S. Brand Names Casodex®
Synonyms CDX; ICI-176334; NC-722665
Pharmacologic Category Antineoplastic Agent, Antiandrogen
Pregnancy Risk Factor X
Lactation Excretion in breast milk unknown/contraindicated
Use In combination therapy with LHRH agonist analogues in treatment of metastatic prostate cancer
Unlabeled/Investigational Use Monotherapy for locally-advanced prostate cancer
(Continued)

Bicalutamide *(Continued)*

Mechanism of Action/Effect Nonsteroidal antiandrogen that inhibits androgen uptake or inhibits binding of androgen in target tissues

Contraindications Hypersensitivity to bicalutamide or any component of the formulation; female patients; pregnancy

Warnings/Precautions Hazardous agent — use appropriate precautions for handling and disposal. Rare cases of death or hospitalization due to hepatitis have been reported postmarketing. Use with caution in moderate-to-severe hepatic dysfunction. Hepatotoxicity generally occurs within the first 3-4 months of use; patients should be monitored for signs and symptoms of liver dysfunction. Bicalutamide should be discontinued if patients have jaundice or ALT is >2 times the upper limit of normal. May cause gynecomastia, breast pain, or lead to spermatogenesis inhibition.

Adverse Reactions Adverse reaction percentages reported as part of combination regimen with an LHRH analogue.

>10%:
  Cardiovascular: Peripheral edema (13%)
  Central nervous system: Pain (35%)
  Endocrine & metabolic: Hot flashes (53%)
  Gastrointestinal: Constipation (22%), nausea (15%), diarrhea (12%), abdominal pain (11%)
  Genitourinary: Pelvic pain (21%), nocturia (12%), hematuria (12%)
  Hematologic: Anemia (11%)
  Neuromuscular & skeletal: Back pain (25%), weakness (22%)
  Respiratory: Dyspnea (13%)
  Miscellaneous: Infection (18%)

≥2% to 10%:
  Cardiovascular: Chest pain (8%), hypertension (8%), angina pectoris (2% to <5%), CHF (2% to <5%), edema (2% to <5%), MI (2% to <5%), coronary artery disorder (2% to <5%), syncope (2% to <5%)
  Central nervous system: Dizziness (10%), headache (7%), insomnia (7%), anxiety (5%), depression (4%), chills (2% to <5%), confusion (2% to <5%), fever (2% to <5%), nervousness (2% to <5%), somnolence (2% to <5%)
  Dermatologic: Rash (9%), alopecia (2% to <5%), dry skin (2% to <5%), herpes zoster (2% to <5%), pruritus (2% to <5%), skin carcinoma (2% to <5%)
  Endocrine & metabolic: Gynecomastia (9%), breast pain (6%; up to 39% as monotherapy), hyperglycemia (6%), dehydration (2% to <5%), gout (2% to <5%), hypercholesterolemia (2% to <5%), libido decreased (2% to <5%)
  Gastrointestinal: Dyspepsia (7%), weight loss (7%), anorexia (6%), flatulence (6%), vomiting (6%), weight gain (5%), dysphagia (2% to <5%), gastrointestinal carcinoma (2% to <5%), melena (2% to <5%), periodontal abscess (2% to <5%), rectal hemorrhage (2% to <5%), xerostomia (2% to <5%)
  Genitourinary: Urinary tract infection (9%), impotence (7%), polyuria (6%), urinary retention (5%), urinary impairment (5%), urinary incontinence (4%), dysuria (2% to <5%), urinary urgency (2% to <5%)
  Hepatic: LFTs increased (7%), alkaline phosphatase increased (5%)
  Neuromuscular & skeletal: Bone pain (9%), paresthesia (8%), myasthenia (7%), arthritis (5%), pathological fracture (4%), hypertonia (2% to <5%), leg cramps (2% to <5%), myalgia (2% to <5%), neck pain (2% to <5%), neuropathy (2% to <5%)
  Ocular: Cataract (2% to <5%)
  Renal: BUN increased, creatinine increased, hydronephrosis
  Respiratory: Cough (8%), pharyngitis (8%), bronchitis (6%), pneumonia (4%), rhinitis (4%), asthma (2% to <5%), epistaxis (2% to <5%), sinusitis (2% to <5%)
  Miscellaneous: Flu syndrome (7%), diaphoresis (6%), cyst (2% to <5%), hernia (2% to <5%), sepsis (2% to <5%)

Overdosage/Toxicology Doses up to 200 mg daily have been well tolerated in long term clinical trials. Symptoms of overdose may include hypoactivity, ataxia, anorexia, vomiting, slow respiration, and lacrimation. Vomiting may be induced if the patient is alert. Vital signs should be monitored frequently. Treatment is symptom-directed and supportive. Dialysis is of no benefit.

Pharmacodynamics/Kinetics
Time to Peak: 31 hours
Protein Binding: 96%
Half-Life Elimination: Active enantiomer ~6 days, ~10 days in severe liver disease
Metabolism: Extensively hepatic; glucuronidation and oxidation of the R (active) enantiomer to inactive metabolites
Excretion: Urine (36%, as inactive metabolites); feces (42%, as unchanged drug and inactive metabolites)

Available Dosage Forms Tablet: 50 mg

Dosing
Adults & Elderly:
  Metastatic prostate cancer: Oral: 50 mg once daily (in combination with an LHRH analogue)
  Locally-advanced prostate cancer (unlabeled use): Oral: 150 mg once daily (as monotherapy)
Renal Impairment: No adjustment required
Hepatic Impairment: No adjustment required for mild, moderate, or severe hepatic impairment; use caution with moderate-to-severe impairment. Discontinue if ALT >2 times ULN or patient develops jaundice.

Administration
Oral: Dose should be taken at the same time each day with or without food. Treatment should be started concomitantly with an LHRH analogue.

Stability
Storage: Store at room temperature of 20°C to 25°C (68°F to 77°F).

Laboratory Monitoring Liver function tests should be obtained at baseline and repeated regularly during the first 4 months of treatment, and periodically thereafter (in addition to monitoring signs/symptoms of liver dysfunction). Discontinue if jaundice is noted or ALT is >2 times the upper limit of normal. Periodically monitor CBC, ECG, echocardiograms, serum testosterone, luteinizing hormone, and prostate specific antigen.

Nursing Actions
Physical Assessment: Monitor laboratory tests (eg, LFTs) at baseline and regularly during therapy. Monitor patient response (therapeutic effectiveness and adverse effects). Advise patients with diabetes to monitor glucose levels closely (may induce hyperglycemia). Teach patient appropriate use, possible side effects/appropriate interventions, and adverse symptoms to report. **Pregnancy risk factor X:** Instruct patient on absolute need for barrier contraceptives.

Patient Education: Do not take any new medication during therapy unless approved by prescriber. Take as directed, at the same time each day, with or without food. Do not alter dose or discontinue this medicine without consulting prescriber. If you have diabetes, monitor serum glucose closely and notify prescriber of changes (this medication may alter glucose levels). May cause dizziness, confusion, or drowsiness (use caution when driving or engaging in tasks that require alertness until response to drug is known); nausea or vomiting (small, frequent meals, frequent mouth care, sucking lozenges, or chewing gum may help); constipation (increased exercise, fluids, fruit, or fiber may help); hair loss; or impotence. Report easy bruising or bleeding; yellowing of skin or eyes; change in color of urine or stool; unresolved CNS changes (eg, nervousness, chills, insomnia, somnolence); skin rash, redness, or irritation; chest pain or palpitations; respiratory difficulty; urinary retention or inability to void; muscle weakness, tremors, or pain; persistent nausea, vomiting, diarrhea, constipation; or other unusual signs or adverse reactions. **Pregnancy/breast-feeding precautions:** This drug will cause fetal abnormalities - consult prescriber for effective contraceptives.

Dietary Considerations May be taken with or without food.

Geriatric Considerations Renal impairment has no clinically-significant changes in elimination of the parent compound or active metabolite; therefore, no dosage adjustment is needed in the elderly. In dosage studies, no difference was found between young adults and elderly with regard to steady-state serum concentrations for bicalutamide and its active R-enantiomer metabolite.

Breast-Feeding Issues Bicalutamide is not indicated for use in women.

Bimatoprost (bi MAT oh prost)

U.S. Brand Names Lumigan®

Pharmacologic Category Ophthalmic Agent, Antiglaucoma; Prostaglandin, Ophthalmic

Pregnancy Risk Factor C

Lactation Excretion in breast milk unknown/use caution

Use Reduction of intraocular pressure (IOP) in patients with open-angle glaucoma or ocular hypertension; should be used in patients who are intolerant of other IOP-lowering medications or failed treatment with another IOP-lowering medication

Mechanism of Action/Effect Decreases intraocular pressure by increasing outflow of aqueous humor

Contraindications Hypersensitivity to bimatoprost or any component of the formulation

Warnings/Precautions May cause permanent changes in eye color (increases the amount of brown pigment in the iris), the eyelid skin, and eyelashes. In addition, may increase the length and/or number of eyelashes (may vary between eyes). Use caution in patients with intraocular inflammation, aphakic patients, pseudophakic patients with a torn posterior lens capsule, or patients with risk factors for macular edema. Contains benzalkonium chloride (may be adsorbed by contact lenses). Safety and efficacy have not been determined for use in patients with renal impairment or angle-closure, inflammatory, or neovascular glaucoma. Safety and efficacy in pediatric patients have not been not established.

Drug Interactions
Increased Effect/Toxicity:

Combination therapy with latanoprost may result in higher IOP than either agent alone.

Adverse Reactions

>10%: Ocular (15% to 45%): Conjunctival hyperemia, growth of eyelashes, ocular pruritus

1% to 10%:

Central nervous system: Headache (1% to 5%)

Dermatologic: Hirsutism (1% to 5%)

Hepatic: Liver function tests abnormal (1% to 5%)

Neuromuscular & skeletal: Weakness (1% to 5%)

Ocular:

3% to 10%: Blepharitis, burning, cataract, dryness, eyelid redness, eyelash darkening, foreign body sensation, irritation, pain, pigmentation of periocular skin, superficial punctate keratitis, visual disturbance

1% to 3%: Allergic conjunctivitis, asthenopia, conjunctival edema, discharge, iris pigmentation increased, photophobia, tearing

Respiratory: Upper respiratory tract infection (10%)

Overdosage/Toxicology No information available; treatment is symptom-directed and supportive.

Pharmacodynamics/Kinetics

Onset of Action: Reduction of IOP: ~4 hours; Peak effect: Maximum reduction of IOP: ~8-12 hours

Time to Peak: 10 minutes

Protein Binding: ~88%

Half-Life Elimination: I.V.: 45 minutes

Metabolism: Undergoes oxidation, N-demethylation, and glucuronidation after reaching systemic circulation; forms metabolites

Excretion: Urine (67%); feces (25%)

Available Dosage Forms Solution, ophthalmic: 0.03% (2.5 mL, 5 mL, 7.5 mL) [contains benzalkonium chloride]

Dosing

Adults & Elderly: Open-angle glaucoma or ocular hypertension: Ophthalmic: Instill 1 drop into affected eye(s) once daily in the evening; do not exceed once-daily dosing (may decrease IOP-lowering effect). If used with other topical ophthalmic agents, separate administration by at least 5 minutes.

Administration

Other: May be used with other eye drops to lower intraocular pressure. If using more than one ophthalmic product, wait at least 5 minutes in between application of each medication. Remove contact lenses prior to administration and wait 15 minutes before reinserting.

Stability

Storage: Store between 2°C to 25°C (36°F to 77°F).

Nursing Actions

Physical Assessment: Assess potential for interactions with other prescriptions, OTC medications, or herbal products patient may be taking. Monitor patient response and adverse effects. Teach patient proper use, side effects/appropriate interventions, and symptoms to report.

Patient Education: For use in eyes only. Wash hands before instilling. Sit or lie down to instill. Open eye, look at ceiling, and instill prescribed amount of solution. Apply gentle pressure to inner corner of eye. Do not let tip of applicator touch eye; do not contaminate tip of applicator (may cause eye infection, eye damage, or vision loss). Contact prescriber concerning continued use of drops if eye infection develops, trauma occurs to the eye, and prior to eye surgery. This product contains benzalkonium chloride which may be adsorbed by contact lenses; remove contacts prior to administration and wait 15 minutes before reinserting. May cause permanent changes in eye color (increases the amount of brown pigment in the iris), eyelid, and eyelashes. May also increase the length and/or number of eyelashes. Changes may occur slowly (months to years). May be used with other eye drops to lower intraocular pressure. If using more than one eye drop medicine, wait at least 5 minutes in between application of each medication. Notify prescriber if conjunctivitis or eyelid reactions occur with use of this product. **Pregnancy/breast-feeding precautions:** Inform prescriber if you are pregnant or breast-feeding.

Additional Information The IOP-lowering effect was shown to be 7-8 mm Hg in clinical studies.

Bismuth (BIZ muth)

U.S. Brand Names Diotame® [OTC]; Kaopectate® [OTC]; Kaopectate® Extra Strength [OTC]; Kaopectolin *(new formulation)* [OTC]; Maalox® Total Stomach Relief® [OTC]; Pepto-Bismol® [OTC]; Pepto-Bismol® Maximum Strength [OTC]

Synonyms Bismatrol; Bismuth Subgallate; Bismuth Subsalicylate; Pink Bismuth

Pharmacologic Category Antidiarrheal

Medication Safety Issues
Sound-alike/look-alike issues:
Kaopectate® may be confused with Kayexalate®

Pregnancy Risk Factor C/D (3rd trimester)

Lactation Excretion in breast milk unknown (salicylates enter breast milk)/use caution

Use
Subsalicylate formulation: Symptomatic treatment of mild, nonspecific diarrhea; control of traveler's diarrhea (enterotoxigenic *Escherichia coli*); as part of a multidrug regimen for *H. pylori* eradication to reduce the risk of duodenal ulcer recurrence

Subgallate formulation: An aid to reduce fecal odors from a colostomy or ileostomy

Mechanism of Action/Effect Bismuth subsalicylate exhibits both antisecretory and antimicrobial action. This agent may provide some anti-inflammatory action as well. The salicylate moiety provides antisecretory effect and the bismuth exhibits antimicrobial directly against bacterial and viral gastrointestinal pathogens.

Contraindications Hypersensitivity to bismuth or any component of the formulation

Subsalicylate formulation: Do not use subsalicylate in patients with influenza or chickenpox because of risk of Reye's syndrome; hypersensitivity to salicylates or any component of the formulation; history of severe GI bleeding; history of coagulopathy; pregnancy (3rd trimester)

Warnings/Precautions Subsalicylate should be used with caution if patient is taking aspirin. Use with caution in children, especially those <3 years of age and those with viral illness. May be neurotoxic with very large doses.

When used for self-medication (OTC labeling): Children and teenagers who have or are recovering from chickenpox or flu-like symptoms should not use subsalicylate. Changes in behavior (along with nausea and vomiting) may be an early sign of Reye's syndrome; patients should be instructed to contact their healthcare provider if these occur. Patients should be instructed to contact healthcare provider for diarrhea lasting >2 days, hearing loss, or ringing in the ears. Not labeled for OTC use in children <12 years of age.

Drug Interactions
Decreased Effect: The effects of tetracyclines and uricosurics may be decreased.

Increased Effect/Toxicity: Toxicity of aspirin, warfarin, and/or hypoglycemics may be increased.

Lab Interactions Increased uric acid, AST; may interfere with radiologic tests since bismuth is radiopaque.

Adverse Reactions Frequency not defined; subsalicylate formulation:
Central nervous system: Anxiety, confusion, headache, mental depression, slurred speech
Gastrointestinal: Discoloration of the tongue (darkening), grayish black stools, impaction may occur in infants and debilitated patients
Neuromuscular & skeletal: Muscle spasms, weakness
Ocular: Hearing loss, tinnitus

Overdosage/Toxicology
Symptoms of toxicity:
Subsalicylate: Hyperpnea, nausea, vomiting, tinnitus, hyperpyrexia, metabolic acidoses/respiratory alkalosis, tachycardia, and confusion; seizures in severe overdose, pulmonary or cerebral edema, respiratory failure, cardiovascular collapse, coma, and death. **Note:** Each 262.4 mg tablet of bismuth subsalicylate contains an equivalent of 130 mg aspirin (150 mg/kg of aspirin is considered to be toxic; serious life-threatening toxicity occurs with >300 mg/kg)

Bismuth: Rare with short-term administrations of bismuth salts; encephalopathy, methemoglobinemia, seizures

Treatment: Gastrointestinal decontamination (activated charcoal for immediate release formulations (10x dose of ASA in g), whole bowel irrigation for enteric-coated tablets, or when serially increasing ASA plasma levels indicate the presence of an intestinal bezoar); supportive and symptomatic treatment with emphasis on correcting fluid, electrolyte, blood glucose, and acid-base disturbances. Elimination is enhanced with urinary alkalinization (sodium bicarbonate infusion with potassium), multiple dose activated charcoal, and hemodialysis. Chelation with dimercaprol in doses of 3 mg/kg or penicillamine 100 mg/kg/day for 5 days can hasten recovery from bismuth-induced encephalopathy; methylene blue 1-2 mg/kg in a 1% sterile aqueous solution I.V. push over 4-6 minutes for methemoglobinemia. This may be repeated within 60 minutes if necessary, up to a total dose of 7 mg/kg. Seizures usually respond to I.V. diazepam.

Pharmacodynamics/Kinetics
Half-Life Elimination: Terminal: Bismuth: Highly variable

Metabolism: Bismuth subsalicylate is converted to salicylic acid and insoluble bismuth salts in the GI tract.

Excretion: Bismuth: Urine and feces; Salicylate: Urine

Available Dosage Forms
Caplet, as subsalicylate (Pepto-Bismol®): 262 mg [sugar free; contains sodium 2 mg]
Liquid, as subsalicylate: 262 mg/15 mL (240 mL, 360 mL, 480 mL); 525 mg/15 mL (240 mL, 360 mL)
Diotame®: 262 mg/15 mL (30 mL)
Kaopectate®: 262 mg/15 mL (180 mL, 240 mL, 360 mL) [contains sodium 10 mg/15 mL; regular and peppermint flavor]
Kaopectate® Extra Strength: 525 mg/15 mL (240 mL) [contains sodium 11 mg/15 mL; peppermint flavor]
Maalox® Total Stomach Relief®: 525 mg/15 mL (360 mL) [contains sodium 3.3 mg/15mL; strawberry flavor]
Pepto-Bismol®: 262 mg/15 mL (120 mL, 240 mL, 360 mL, 480 mL) [sugar free; contains sodium 6 mg/15 mL and benzoic acid; wintergreen flavor]
Pepto-Bismol® Maximum Strength: 525 mg/15 mL (120 mL, 240 mL, 360 mL) [sugar free; contains sodium 6 mg/15 mL and benzoic acid; wintergreen flavor]
Suspension (Kaopectolin): 262 mg/15 mL (480 mL)
Tablet, as subgallate: 200 mg
Tablet, chewable, as subsalicylate: 262 mg
Diotame®: 262 mg
Pepto-Bismol®: 262 mg [sugar free; contains sodium <1 mg; cherry flavor]

Dosing
Adults & Elderly:
Treatment of nonspecific diarrhea, control/relieve traveler's diarrhea: Oral: Subsalicylate (doses based on 262 mg/15 mL liquid or 262 mg tablets): 2 tablets or 30 mL every 30 minutes to 1 hour as needed up to 8 doses/24 hours
Helicobacter pylori **eradication:** Oral: 524 mg 4 times/day with meals and at bedtime; requires combination therapy
Control of fecal odor in ileostomy or colostomy: Oral: Subgallate: 200-400 mg up to 4 times/day

Pediatrics:

Nonspecific diarrhea, control/relieve traveler's diarrhea: Subsalicylate (doses based on 262 mg/5 mL liquid or 262 mg tablet): Oral:

Children: Up to 8 doses/24 hours:

3-6 years: $^1/_3$ tablet or 5 mL every 30 minutes to 1 hour as needed

6-9 years: $^2/_3$ tablet or 10 mL every 30 minutes to 1 hour as needed

9-12 years: 1 tablet or 15 mL every 30 minutes to 1 hour as needed

>12 years: Refer to adult dosing

Control of fecal odor in ileostomy or colostomy: Children≥12 years: Oral: Refer to adult dosing

Renal Impairment: Should probably be avoided in patients with renal impairment.

Administration

Oral: Subsalicylate tablets should be taken at least 3 hours apart from other medications.

Nursing Actions

Physical Assessment: Patient's history with aspirin products should be assessed prior to beginning treatment (contains ASA). Assess other pharmacological or herbal products patient may be taking for potential iteractions (eg, aspirin products). Monitor therapeutic effectiveness (reduction in diarrhea) and adverse response (eg, CNS changes, impactions, tinnitus). Teach patient appropriate use, possible side effects/appropriate interventions, and adverse symptoms to report.

Patient Education: Do not take any new medication during therapy unless approved by prescriber. Chew tablet well or shake suspension well before using. Maintain adequate fluid intake to prevent dehydration: 2-3 L/day of fluids (unless instructed to restrict fluid intake). May darken stools and turn tongue black. If diarrhea persists for more than 2 days, consult healthcare provider. If tinnitus (ringing in the ears) occurs this may indicate toxicity; discontinue use and notify healthcare provider. **Pregnancy/breast-feeding precautions:** Inform prescriber if you are or intend to be pregnant or breast-feed.

Dietary Considerations Drink plenty of fluids to help prevent dehydration caused by diarrhea. Different dosage forms contain variable amounts of sodium; consult individual product labeling.

Bismuth Subsalicylate, Metronidazole, and Tetracycline

(BIZ muth sub sa LIS i late, me troe NI da zole, & tet ra SYE kleen)

U.S. Brand Names Helidac®

Synonyms Bismuth Subsalicylate, Tetracycline, and Metronidazole; Metronidazole, Bismuth Subsalicylate, and Tetracycline; Tetracycline, Metronidazole, and Bismuth Subsalicylate

Pharmacologic Category Antibiotic, Tetracycline Derivative; Antidiarrheal

Pregnancy Risk Factor D (tetracycline); B (metronidazole)

Lactation Enters breast milk/contraindicated

Use In combination with an H_2 antagonist, as part of a multidrug regimen for *H. pylori* eradication to reduce the risk of duodenal ulcer recurrence

Available Dosage Forms Combination package [each package contains 14 blister cards (2-week supply); each card contains the following]:

Capsule: Tetracycline hydrochloride: 500 mg (4)

Tablet: Bismuth subsalicylate [chewable]: 262.4 mg (8)

Tablet: Metronidazole: 250 mg (4)

Dosing

Adults & Elderly: Duodenal ulcer associated with *H. pylori* infection: Oral: Chew 2 bismuth subsalicylate 262.4 mg tablets, swallow 1 metronidazole 250 mg tablet, and swallow 1 tetracycline 500 mg capsule plus an H_2 antagonist 4 times/day at meals and bedtime for 14 days; follow with 8 oz of water.

Nursing Actions

Physical Assessment: See individual agents.

Patient Education: See individual agents. **Pregnancy/breast-feeding precautions:** Inform prescriber if you are or intend to become pregnant. Do not breast-feed.

Related Information

Bismuth *on page 158*
Metronidazole *on page 815*
Tetracycline *on page 1192*

Bisoprolol (bis OH proe lol)

U.S. Brand Names Zebeta®

Synonyms Bisoprolol Fumarate

Pharmacologic Category Beta Blocker, Beta$_1$ Selective

Medication Safety Issues

Sound-alike/look-alike issues:

Zebeta® may be confused with DiaBeta®

Pregnancy Risk Factor C (manufacturer); D (2nd and 3rd trimesters - expert analysis)

Lactation Enters breast milk/use caution

Use Treatment of hypertension, alone or in combination with other agents

Unlabeled/Investigational Use Angina pectoris, supraventricular arrhythmias, PVCs, CHF

Mechanism of Action/Effect Selective inhibitor of beta$_1$-adrenergic receptors; little or no effect on beta$_2$-receptors at doses <10 mg

Contraindications Hypersensitivity to bisoprolol or any component of the formulation; sinus bradycardia; heart block greater than first-degree (except in patients with a functioning artificial pacemaker); cardiogenic shock; uncompensated cardiac failure; pulmonary edema; pregnancy (2nd and 3rd trimesters)

Warnings/Precautions Administer cautiously in compensated heart failure and monitor for a worsening of the condition. Beta-blocker therapy should not be withdrawn abruptly (particularly in patients with CAD), but gradually tapered to avoid acute tachycardia, hypertension, and/or ischemia. Use caution in patients with PVD (can aggravate arterial insufficiency). Use caution with concurrent use of beta-blockers and either verapamil or diltiazem; bradycardia or heart block can occur. In general, beta-blockers should be avoided in patients with bronchospastic disease. Bisoprolol, with B1 selectivity, has been used cautiously in bronchospastic disease with close monitoring. Use cautiously in patients with diabetes because it can mask prominent hypoglycemic symptoms. Can mask signs of thyrotoxicosis. Can cause fetal harm when administered in pregnancy. Dosage adjustment is required in patients with significant hepatic or renal dysfunction. Use care with anesthetic agents which decrease myocardial function.

Drug Interactions

Cytochrome P450 Effect: Substrate of CYP2D6 (minor), 3A4 (major)

Decreased Effect: Decreased effect of bisoprolol with aluminum salts, calcium salts, cholestyramine, colestipol, NSAIDs, penicillins (ampicillin), and salicylates due to decreased bioavailability and plasma levels. The effect of sulfonylureas may be decreased by beta-blockers. CYP3A4 inducers may decrease the levels/effects of bisoprolol; example inducers include aminoglutethimide, carbamazepine, nafcillin, nevirapine, phenobarbital, phenytoin, and rifamycins. (Continued)

Bisoprolol *(Continued)*

Increased Effect/Toxicity: Bisoprolol may increase the effects of other drugs which slow AV conduction (digoxin, verapamil, diltiazem), alpha-blockers (prazosin, terazosin), and alpha-adrenergic stimulants (epinephrine, phenylephrine). Bisoprolol may mask the tachycardia from hypoglycemia caused by insulin and oral hypoglycemics. In patients receiving concurrent therapy, the risk of hypertensive crisis is increased when either clonidine or the beta-blocker is withdrawn. Reserpine has been shown to enhance the effect of beta-blockers. Beta-blockers may increase the action or levels of ethanol, disopyramide, nondepolarizing muscle relaxants, and theophylline although the effects are difficult to predict. CYP3A4 inhibitors may increase the levels/effects of bisoprolol; example inhibitors include azole antifungals, clarithromycin, diclofenac, doxycycline, erythromycin, imatinib, isoniazid, nefazodone, nicardipine, propofol, protease inhibitors, quinidine, telithromycin, and verapamil.

Nutritional/Ethanol Interactions Herb/Nutraceutical: Avoid dong quai if using for hypertension (has estrogenic activity). Avoid ephedra, yohimbe, ginseng (may worsen hypertension). Avoid garlic (may have increased antihypertensive effect).

Lab Interactions Increased thyroxine (S), cholesterol (S), glucose, triglycerides, uric acid; decreased HDL; possible false glucose tolerance tests

Adverse Reactions
>10%:
Central nervous system: Drowsiness, insomnia
Endocrine & metabolic: Sexual ability decreased
1% to 10%:
Cardiovascular: Bradycardia, palpitation, edema, CHF, peripheral circulation reduced
Central nervous system: Mental depression
Gastrointestinal: Diarrhea, constipation, nausea, vomiting, stomach discomfort
Ocular: Mild ocular stinging and discomfort, tearing, photophobia, corneal sensitivity decreased, keratitis
Respiratory: Bronchospasm
Miscellaneous: Cold extremities

Overdosage/Toxicology Symptoms of overdose include severe hypotension, bradycardia, heart failure, bronchospasm, and hypoglycemia. Treat initially with I.V. fluids. Sympathomimetics (eg, epinephrine or dopamine), glucagon, or a pacemaker can be used to treat toxic bradycardia, asystole, and/or hypotension. Bisoprolol may be removed by hemodialysis. Other treatment is symptomatic and supportive.

Pharmacodynamics/Kinetics
Onset of Action: 1-2 hours
Time to Peak: 1.7-3 hours
Protein Binding: 26% to 33%
Half-Life Elimination: 9-12 hours
Metabolism: Extensively hepatic; significant first-pass effect
Excretion: Urine (3% to 10% as unchanged drug); feces (<2%)
Available Dosage Forms Tablet, as fumarate: 5 mg, 10 mg
Dosing
Adults:
Hypertension: Oral: 2.5-5 mg once daily; may be increased to 10 mg and then up to 20 mg once daily, if necessary; usual dose range (JNC 7): 2.5-10 mg once daily
CHF (unlabeled use): Initial: 1.25 mg once daily; maximum recommended dose: 10 mg once daily
Elderly: Oral: Initial: 2.5 mg/day; may be increased by 2.5-5 mg/day; maximum recommended dose: 20 mg/day
Renal Impairment: Cl$_{cr}$ <40 mL/minute: Oral: Initial: 2.5 mg/day; increase cautiously.
Not dialyzable

Laboratory Monitoring Serum glucose regularly (if diabetic)

Nursing Actions
Physical Assessment: Assess potential for interactions with other prescriptions, OTC medications, or herbal products patient may be taking (see Drug Interactions). Monitor blood pressure and heart rate prior to and following first dose and with any change in dosage. Monitor therapeutic effectiveness and adverse effects (eg, CHF). Instruct patients with diabetes to monitor glucose levels closely (beta-blockers may alter glucose tolerance). Teach patient proper use, possible side effects/appropriate interventions (hypotension precautions), and adverse symptoms to report.

Patient Education: Do not take any new medication during therapy unless approved by prescriber. Take exactly as directed, with or without regard to meals. Do not take with antacids. Do not adjust dosage or discontinue medication without consulting prescriber. Take pulse daily (prior to medication) and follow prescriber's instruction about holding medication. If you have diabetes, monitor serum sugar closely (drug may alter glucose tolerance or mask signs of hypoglycemia). May cause fatigue, dizziness, or postural hypotension (use caution when changing position from lying or sitting to standing, when driving, or climbing stairs until response to medication is known); alteration in sexual performance (reversible); or constipation (increased dietary bulk and fluids and exercise may help). Report unresolved swelling of extremities, respiratory difficulty or new cough, unresolved fatigue, unusual weight gain, unresolved constipation, or unusual muscle weakness. **Pregnancy/breast-feeding precautions:** Inform prescriber if you are or intend to become pregnant. Consult prescriber if breast-feeding.

Dietary Considerations May be taken without regard to meals.

Geriatric Considerations Due to alterations in the beta-adrenergic autonomic nervous system, beta-adrenergic blockade may result in less hemodynamic response than seen in younger adults.

Pregnancy Issues No data available on whether bisoprolol crosses the placenta. Beta-blockers have been associated with persistent bradycardia, hypotension, and IUGR; IUGR is probably related to maternal hypertension. Available evidence suggests beta-blockers are generally safe during pregnancy (JNC 7). Cases of neonatal hypoglycemia have been reported following maternal use of beta-blockers at parturition or during breast-feeding. Monitor breast-fed infant for symptoms of beta-blockade.

Bisoprolol and Hydrochlorothiazide
(bis OH proe lol & hye droe klor oh THYE a zide)

U.S. Brand Names Ziac®
Synonyms Hydrochlorothiazide and Bisoprolol
Pharmacologic Category Antihypertensive Agent, Combination
Pregnancy Risk Factor C/D (2nd and 3rd trimesters)
Lactation Enters breast milk/use caution
Use Treatment of hypertension
Available Dosage Forms Tablet:
2.5/6.25: Bisoprolol fumarate 2.5 mg and hydrochlorothiazide 6.25 mg
5/6.25: Bisoprolol fumarate 5 mg and hydrochlorothiazide 6.25 mg
10/6.25: Bisoprolol fumarate 10 mg and hydrochlorothiazide 6.25 mg

Dosing

Adults & Elderly: Hypertension: Oral: Dose is individualized, given once daily.

Hepatic Impairment: Caution should be used in dosing/titrating patients.

Nursing Actions

Physical Assessment: See individual agents.

Patient Education: See individual agents. **Pregnancy/breast-feeding precautions:** Inform prescriber if you are or intend to become pregnant. Consult prescriber if breast-feeding.

Related Information

Bisoprolol *on page 159*
Hydrochlorothiazide *on page 610*

Bleomycin (blee oh MYE sin)

U.S. Brand Names Blenoxane®

Synonyms Bleo; Bleomycin Sulfate; BLM; NSC-125066

Pharmacologic Category Antineoplastic Agent, Antibiotic

Medication Safety Issues

Sound-alike/look-alike issues:
Bleomycin may be confused with Cleocin®

Pregnancy Risk Factor D

Lactation Excretion in breast milk unknown/not recommended

Use Treatment of squamous cell carcinomas, melanomas, sarcomas, testicular carcinoma, Hodgkin's lymphoma, and non-Hodgkin's lymphoma

Orphan drug: Sclerosing agent for malignant pleural effusion

Mechanism of Action/Effect Inhibits synthesis of DNA

Contraindications Hypersensitivity to bleomycin or any component of the formulation; severe pulmonary disease; pregnancy

Warnings/Precautions Hazardous agent — use appropriate precautions for handling and disposal. Occurrence of pulmonary fibrosis is higher in elderly patients, patients receiving >400 units total, smokers, and patients with prior radiation therapy. A severe idiosyncratic reaction consisting of hypotension, mental confusion, fever, chills, and wheezing is possible. Follow manufacturer recommendations for administering O_2 during surgery to patients who have received bleomycin.

Drug Interactions

Decreased Effect: Bleomycin may decrease plasma levels of digoxin. Concomitant therapy with phenytoin results in decreased phenytoin levels.

Increased Effect/Toxicity: Cisplatin may decrease bleomycin elimination.

Adverse Reactions

>10%:
Cardiovascular: Raynaud's phenomenon
Dermatologic: Pain at the tumor site, phlebitis. About 50% of patients develop erythema, induration, hyperkeratosis, and peeling of the skin, particularly on the palmar and plantar surfaces of the hands and feet. Hyperpigmentation (50%), alopecia, nailbed changes may also occur. These effects appear dose related and reversible with discontinuation of the drug.
Gastrointestinal: Stomatitis and mucositis (30%), anorexia, weight loss
Respiratory: Tachypnea, rales, acute or chronic interstitial pneumonitis, and pulmonary fibrosis (5% to 10%); hypoxia and death (1%). Symptoms include cough, dyspnea, and bilateral pulmonary infiltrates. The pathogenesis is not certain, but may be due to damage of pulmonary, vascular, or connective tissue. Response to steroid therapy is variable and somewhat controversial.

Miscellaneous: Acute febrile reactions (25% to 50%); anaphylactoid reactions characterized by hypotension, confusion, fever, chills, and wheezing. Onset may be immediate or delayed for several hours.
1% to 10%:
Dermatologic: Rash (8%), skin thickening, diffuse scleroderma, onycholysis
Miscellaneous: Acute anaphylactoid reactions

Overdosage/Toxicology Symptoms of overdose include chills, fever, pulmonary fibrosis, and hyperpigmentation. Treatment is supportive.

Pharmacodynamics/Kinetics

Time to Peak: Serum: I.M.: Within 30 minutes

Protein Binding: 1%

Half-Life Elimination: Biphasic: Renal function dependent:
Normal renal function: Initial: 1.3 hours; Terminal: 9 hours
End-stage renal disease: Initial: 2 hours; Terminal: 30 hours

Metabolism: Via several tissues including hepatic, GI tract, skin, pulmonary, renal, and serum

Excretion: Urine (50% to 70% as active drug)

Available Dosage Forms Injection, powder for reconstitution, as sulfate: 15 units, 30 units

Dosing

Adults: Maximum cumulative lifetime dose: 400 units; refer to individual protocols; 1 unit = 1 mg; may be administered I.M., I.V., SubQ, or intracavitary.

Test dose for lymphoma patient: I.M., I.V., SubQ: Because of the possibility of an anaphylactoid reaction, ≤2 units of bleomycin for the first 2 doses; monitor vital signs every 15 minutes; wait a minimum of 1 hour before administering remainder of dose; if no acute reaction occurs, then the regular dosage schedule may be followed. **Note:** Test doses may produce false-negative results.

Single agent therapy:
I.M./I.V./SubQ: Squamous cell carcinoma, lymphosarcoma, reticulum cell sarcoma, testicular carcinoma: 0.25-0.5 units/kg (10-20 units/m²) 1-2 times/week
Continuous intravenous infusion: 15 units/m² over 24 hours/day for 4 days

Pleural sclerosing: Intracavitary: 60 units as a single infusion. Dose may be repeated at intervals of several days if fluid continues to accumulate (mix in 50-100 mL of D_5W, NS, or SWFI); may add lidocaine 100-200 mg to reduce local discomfort.

Elderly: Refer to adult dosing. Some recommend limiting the dose in the elderly to 40 units/m², maximum: 60 units.

Pediatrics: Refer to adult dosing.

Renal Impairment:
Cl_{cr} 10-50 mL/minute: Administer 75% of normal dose.
Cl_{cr} <10 mL/minute: Administer 50% of normal dose.

Administration

I.M.: May cause pain at injection site.

I.V.: May be an irritant. I.V. doses should be administered slowly (manufacturer recommends giving over a period of 10 minutes).

I.V. Detail: pH: 4.5-6.0 (reconstituted solution, varies depending on diluent)

Other: SubQ: May cause pain at injection site.

Stability

Reconstitution: Reconstitute powder with 1-5 mL BWFI or BNS which is stable at room temperature or under refrigeration for 28 days.

Standard I.V. dilution: Dose/50-1000 mL NS or D_5W

Compatibility: Stable in NS

Compatibility when admixed: Incompatible with aminophylline, ascorbic acid injection, cefazolin, diazepam, hydrocortisone sodium succinate, methotrexate, mitomycin, nafcillin, penicillin G sodium, terbutaline

(Continued)

Bleomycin *(Continued)*

Storage: Refrigerate intact vials of powder; intact vials are stable for up to 1 month at 45°C.

Laboratory Monitoring Pulmonary function (total lung volume, forced vital capacity, carbon monoxide diffusion), renal function, chest x-ray, liver function

Nursing Actions

Physical Assessment: Pulmonary and pregnancy status should be evaluated prior to beginning therapy. Assess other pharmacological or herbal products patient may be taking for potential interactions. Monitor pulmonary status for fine rales prior to each treatment (may be the first symptom of pulmonary toxicity) and notify prescriber of any changes. Monitor patients with lymphoma closely for 1 hour following test dose before remainder of dose is administered. Infusion or injection site must be monitored closely to avoid extravasation. Monitor laboratory tests (pulmonary, renal, and hepatic function), therapeutic effectiveness, and adverse reactions regularly during therapy. Teach patient possible side effects/appropriate interventions and adverse symptoms to report.

Patient Education: Do not take any new medications during treatment unless approved by prescriber. This medication can only be administered by injection or infusion; report immediately any redness, burning, pain, or swelling at injection/infusion site. May cause loss of appetite, nausea, or vomiting (small, frequent meals, sucking lozenges, or chewing gum may help); mouth sores (frequent mouth care with soft swabs and mouth rinses may help); fever or chills (will usually resolve); redness, peeling, or increased color of skin; or loss of hair (reversible after cessation of therapy). Report any change in respiratory status; respiratory difficulty; wheezing; air hunger; increased secretions; difficulty expectorating secretions; confusion; unresolved fever or chills; sores in mouth; vaginal itching, burning, or discharge; sudden onset of dizziness; acute headache; or burning, stinging, redness, or swelling at injection site. **Pregnancy/breast-feeding precautions:** Inform prescriber if you are pregnant. Do not get pregnant during or for 1 month following therapy. Consult prescriber for instruction on appropriate contraceptives. This drug may cause severe fetal defects. Breast-feeding is not recommended

Geriatric Considerations Pulmonary toxicity has been reported more frequently in geriatric patients (>70 years of age).

Bortezomib *(bore TEZ oh mib)*

U.S. Brand Names Velcade®

Synonyms LDP-341; MLN341; PS-341

Pharmacologic Category Antineoplastic Agent; Proteasome Inhibitor

Pregnancy Risk Factor D

Lactation Excretion in breast milk unknown/not recommended

Use Treatment of multiple myeloma in patients who have had at least one prior therapy

Mechanism of Action/Effect Reversibly inhibits enzyme complexes (proteosomes) which control intracellular protein homeostasis. Inhibition leads to cell death (apoptosis).

Contraindications Hypersensitivity to bortezomib, boron, mannitol, or any component of the formulation; pregnancy

Warnings/Precautions Hazardous agent - use appropriate precautions for handling and disposal. May cause peripheral neuropathy (usually sensory but may be mixed sensorimotor); risk may be increased with previous use of neurotoxic agents or pre-existing peripheral neuropathy; adjustment of dose and schedule may be required. May cause orthostatic/postural hypotension; use caution with dehydration, history of syncope, or medications associated with hypotension. Has been associated with the development or exacerbation of congestive heart failure; use caution in patients with risk factors or existing heart disease. May cause tumor lysis syndrome; risk is increased in patients with large tumor burden prior to treatment. Hematologic toxicity with severe thrombocytopenia may occur; risk is increased in patients with pretreatment platelet counts <75,000 μL; frequent monitoring is required throughout treatment. Use caution with hepatic or renal impairment. Safety and efficacy have not been established in pediatric patients.

Drug Interactions

Cytochrome P450 Effect: Substrate of CYP1A2 (minor), 2C8/9 (minor), 2C19 (minor), 2D6 (minor), 3A4 (major); **Inhibits** CYP1A2 (weak), 2C8/9 (weak), 2C19 (moderate), 2D6 (weak), 3A4 (weak)

Decreased Effect: Levels/effects of bortezomib may be decreased by aminoglutethimide, carbamazepine, nafcillin, nevirapine, phenobarbital, phenytoin, rifamycins, and other CYP3A4 inducers.

Increased Effect/Toxicity: Bortezomib may increase the levels/effects citalopram, diazepam, methsuximide, phenytoin, propranolol, sertraline, and other CYP2C19 substrates. Levels/effects of bortezomib may be increased by azole antifungals, clarithromycin, diclofenac, doxycycline, erythromycin, imatinib, isoniazid, nefazodone, nicardipine, propofol, protease inhibitors, quinidine, telithromycin, verapamil, and other CYP3A4 inhibitors.

Adverse Reactions

>10%:

Cardiovascular: Edema (25%), hypotension (12%)

Central nervous system: Pyrexia (35% to 36%), psychiatric disturbance (35%), headache (26% to 28%), insomnia (27%), dizziness (14% to 21%, excludes vertigo), anxiety (14%)

Dermatologic: Rash (18% to 21%), pruritus (11%)

Endocrine & metabolic: Dehydration (18%)

Gastrointestinal: Nausea (57% to 64%), diarrhea (51% to 57%), appetite decreased (43%), constipation (42% to 43%), vomiting (35% to 36%), abdominal pain (13% to 16%), abnormal taste (13%), dyspepsia (13%)

Hematologic: Thrombocytopenia (35% to 43%, Grade 3: 26% to 27%, Grade 4: 3%; Nadir: Day 11), anemia (26% to 32%, Grade 3: 9%), neutropenia (19% to 24%, Grade 3: 13%, Grade 4: 3%)

Neuromuscular & skeletal: Asthenic conditions (61% to 65%, Grade 3: 12% to 18% - includes fatigue, malaise, weakness), peripheral neuropathy (36% to 37%, Grade 3: 7% to 14%), arthralgia (14% to 26%), limb pain (26%), paresthesia and dysesthesia (23%), bone pain (16%), back pain (14%), muscle cramps (12% to 14%), myalgia (12% to 14%), rigors (11% to 12%)

Ocular: Blurred vision (11%)

Respiratory: Dyspnea (20% to 22%), upper respiratory tract infection (18%), cough (17% to 21%), lower respiratory infection (15%), nasopharyngitis (14%)

Miscellaneous: Herpes zoster (11% to 13%)

1% to 10%: Respiratory: Pneumonia (10%)

Overdosage/Toxicology In case of overdose, treatment should be symptom directed and supportive.

Pharmacodynamics/Kinetics

Protein Binding: ~83%

Half-Life Elimination: 9-15 hours

Metabolism: Hepatic via CYP 1A2, 2C9, 2C19, 2D6, 3A4; forms metabolites (inactive)

Available Dosage Forms Injection, powder for reconstitution [preservative free]: 3.5 mg [contains mannitol 35 mg]

Dosing

Adults & Elderly: Multiple myeloma: I.V.: 1.3 mg/m² twice weekly for 2 weeks on days 1, 4, 8, 11, every 21 days. Consecutive doses should be separated by at least 72 hours.

Renal Impairment: Specific guidelines are not available; studies did not include patients with Cl_{cr} <13 mL/minute and patients on hemodialysis. Monitor closely for toxicity.

Hepatic Impairment: Specific guidelines are not available; clearance may be decreased; monitor closely for toxicity.

Dosing Adjustment for Toxicity:

Grade 3 nonhematological (excluding neuropathy) or Grade 4 hematological toxicity: Withhold until toxicity resolved; may reinitiate at a 25% reduced dose

Neuropathic pain and/or peripheral sensory neuropathy:

Grade 1 without pain or loss of function: No action needed

Grade 1 with pain or Grade 2 interfering with function but not activities of daily living: Reduce dose to 1 mg/m²

Grade 2 with pain or Grade 3 interfering with activities of daily living: Withhold until toxicity resolved, may reinitiate at 0.7 mg/m² once weekly

Grade 4: Discontinue therapy

Administration

I.V.: Administer via rapid I.V. push (3-5 seconds).

Stability

Reconstitution: Dilute each 3.5 mg vial with 3.5 mL NS.

Storage: Prior to reconstitution, store at controlled room temperature, 15°C to 30°C (59°F to 86°F). Protect from light. Once reconstituted, may be stored at room temperature for up to 3 days, or under refrigeration for up to 5 days, in vial or syringe; protect from light.

Laboratory Monitoring CBC

Nursing Actions

Physical Assessment: Assess potential for interactions with other prescriptions, OTC medications, or herbal products patient may be taking. See Administration specifics. Monitor laboratory results, therapeutic effectiveness, and adverse response on regular basis during therapy (eg, peripheral neuropathy, postural hypotension, dehydration, congestive heart failure, infections). Monitor for psychiatric disturbances. Teach patient possible side effects/appropriate interventions and adverse symptoms to report.

Patient Education: Do not take any new medication during therapy without consulting prescriber. This medication can only be administered intravenously; you will be monitored during and following infusion. Maintain adequate hydration (2-3 L/day of fluids) unless instructed to restrict fluid intake. May cause headache, dizziness (use caution when changing positions), anxiety, or fatigue (use caution when driving or engaging in hazardous tasks until response to drug is known); nausea, vomiting, or abnormal taste (small frequent meals, frequent mouth care, chewing gum, or sucking lozenges may help) or diarrhea (boiled milk, yogurt, or buttermilk may help). Report immediately any chest pain, respiratory difficulty, itching, rash, acute headache, throat tightness, pain, redness, or swelling at infusion site. Report chest pain or shortness of breath, swelling in extremities, recent weight gain (>3-5 pounds/week), persistent headache; muscle, bone, or back pain; cramping or loss of sensation; changes in vision; psychiatric disturbances; or other persistent adverse reactions.

Pregnancy/breast-feeding precautions: Inform prescriber if you are pregnant. Do not get pregnant or cause a pregnancy (males) during therapy or for 1 month following therapy. Consult prescriber for instructions on appropriate nonhormonal contraceptive measures. This drug may cause fetal defects. Breast-feeding is not recommended.

Breast-Feeding Issues Breast-feeding should be avoided.

Pregnancy Issues Adverse effects were observed in animal studies. Effective contraception is recommended for women of childbearing potential.

Additional Information Bortezomib was FDA approved under an accelerated approval program. Clinical trials have shown safety and efficacy as well as a decrease in tumor size. Studies addressing clinical benefit (including impact on survival) are ongoing.

Bretylium (bre TIL ee um)

Synonyms Bretylium Tosylate

Pharmacologic Category Antiarrhythmic Agent, Class III

Medication Safety Issues
Sound-alike/look-alike issues:
Bretylium may be confused with Brevibloc®

Pregnancy Risk Factor C

Lactation Excretion in breast milk unknown

Use Treatment of ventricular tachycardia and fibrillation; treatment of other serious ventricular arrhythmias resistant to lidocaine

Mechanism of Action/Effect Class III antiarrhythmic; after an initial release of norepinephrine at the peripheral adrenergic nerve terminals, bretylium inhibits further release by postganglionic nerve endings in response to sympathetic nerve stimulation

Contraindications Hypersensitivity to bretylium or any component of the formulation; severe aortic stenosis; severe pulmonary hypertension

Warnings/Precautions Use only in areas where there is equipment and staff familiar with management of life-threatening arrhythmias. Use continuous cardiac and blood pressure monitoring. Keep patients supine (postural hypotension common). Initially, may see transient hypertension and increased frequency of arrhythmias. Adjust dose in patients with impaired renal function. Give to a pregnant woman only if clearly needed. Rapid I.V. administration may cause nausea and vomiting, and a higher risk of orthostatic hypotension (particularly in elderly patients).

Drug Interactions

Increased Effect/Toxicity: Other antiarrhythmic agents may potentiate or antagonize cardiac effects of bretylium. Toxic effects may be additive. The vasopressor effects of catecholamines may be enhanced by bretylium. Toxicity of agents which may prolong QT interval (including cisapride, tricyclic antidepressants, antipsychotics, erythromycin, Class Ia and Class III antiarrhythmics) and specific quinolones (sparfloxacin, gatifloxacin, moxifloxacin) may be increased. Digoxin toxicity may be aggravated by bretylium.

Adverse Reactions
>10%: Cardiovascular: Hypotension (both postural and supine)

1% to 10%: Gastrointestinal: Nausea, vomiting

Overdosage/Toxicology Symptoms of overdose include significant hypertension followed by severe hypotension. Administration of a short-acting hypotensive agent should be used for the hypertensive response. Treatment is symptomatic and supportive. Dialysis is not useful.

Pharmacodynamics/Kinetics
Onset of Action: I.M.: May require 2 hours; I.V.: 6-20 minutes; Peak effect: 6-9 hours
(Continued)

Bretylium *(Continued)*

Duration of Action: 6-24 hours
Protein Binding: 1% to 6%
Half-Life Elimination: 7-11 hours; Mean: 4-17 hours; End-stage renal disease: 16-32 hours
Metabolism: None
Excretion: Urine (70% to 80% as unchanged drug) within 24 hours
Available Dosage Forms [DSC] = Discontinued product

Injection, solution, as tosylate: 50 mg/mL (10 mL) [DSC]
Injection, solution, as tosylate [premixed in D_5W]: 2 mg/mL (250 mL); 4 mg/mL (250 mL) [DSC]

Dosing

Adults & Elderly: (Note: Patients should undergo defibrillation/cardioversion before and after bretylium doses as necessary.)

Immediate life-threatening ventricular arrhythmias, ventricular fibrillation, unstable ventricular tachycardia: I.V.: Initial: 5 mg/kg (undiluted) over 1 minute; if arrhythmia persists, give 10 mg/kg (undiluted) over 1 minute and repeat as necessary (usually at 15- to 30-minute intervals) up to a total dose of 30-35 mg/kg

Other life-threatening ventricular arrhythmias: I.M., I.V.:

Initial: 5-10 mg/kg, may repeat every 1-2 hours if arrhythmia persist; give I.V. dose (diluted) over 8-10 minutes

Maintenance dose: I.M.: 5-10 mg/kg every 6-8 hours; I.V. (diluted): 5-10 mg/kg every 6 hours; I.V. infusion (diluted): 1-2 mg/minute (little experience with doses >40 mg/kg/day)

Pediatrics: Note: Patients should undergo defibrillation/cardioversion before and after bretylium doses as necessary.

Arrhythmias:

Note: Not well established, although the following dosing has been suggested:

I.M.: 2-5 mg/kg as a single dose
I.V.: Acute ventricular fibrillation: Initial: 5 mg/kg, then attempt electrical defibrillation; repeat with 10 mg/kg if ventricular fibrillation persists at 15- to 30-minute intervals to maximum total of 30 mg/kg
Maintenance dose: I.M., I.V.: 5 mg/kg every 6 hours

Renal Impairment:

Cl_{cr} 10-50 mL/minute: Administer 25% to 50% of dose.
Cl_{cr} <10 mL/minute: Administer 25% of dose.
Not dialyzable

Administration

I.M.: I.M. injection in adults should not exceed 5 mL volume in any one site.

I.V.: 2 g/250 mL D_5W (infusion pump should be used for I.V. infusion)

Bolus, emergency: Infuse rapidly (1 minute).
Bolus, nonemergency: May be given over 8-10 minutes.

Suggested rate of I.V. infusion: 1-4 mg/minute.

1 mg/minute = 7 mL/hour
2 mg/minute = 15 mL/hour
3 mg/minute = 22 mL/hour
4 mg/minute = 30 mL/hour

I.V. Detail: An initial worsening of arrhythmia, as well as nausea, may occur with bolus. During continuous infusions, hypotension may occur.

pH: 4.5-7 (injection); 4.5 (premixed infusion)

Stability

Reconstitution: Standard diluent: 2 g/250 mL D_5W
Compatibility: Stable in D_5LR, $D_5^{1}/_2NS$, D_5NS, D_5W, mannitol 20%, LR, sodium bicarbonate 5%, NS
Y-site administration: Incompatible with amphotericin B cholesteryl sulfate complex, propofol, warfarin

Compatibility when admixed: Incompatible with phenytoin

Storage: The premix infusion should be stored at room temperature and protected from freezing.

Nursing Actions

Physical Assessment: Assess other medications patient may be taking for effectiveness and interactions. **I.V.:** Requires use of infusion pump and continuous cardiac and hemodynamic monitoring during infusion. Be alert for cardiovascular adverse reactions. Patient education/instruction is according to patient condition.

Patient Education: Emergency use: Patient education is determined by patient condition. You may experience nausea or vomiting (call for assistance if this occurs, do not try to get out of bed or change position on your own). Report chest pain, acute dizziness, or respiratory difficulty immediately. **Breast-feeding precaution:** Consult prescriber if breast-feeding.

Geriatric Considerations Elderly are particularly at risk of orthostatic hypotension. See Warnings/Precautions and Adverse Reactions.

Brimonidine (bri MOE ni deen)

U.S. Brand Names Alphagan® P
Synonyms Brimonidine Tartrate
Pharmacologic Category Alpha$_2$ Agonist, Ophthalmic; Ophthalmic Agent, Antiglaucoma
Medication Safety Issues

Sound-alike/look-alike issues:
Brimonidine may be confused with bromocriptine

Pregnancy Risk Factor B
Lactation Excretion in breast milk unknown/not recommended
Use Lowering of intraocular pressure (IOP) in patients with open-angle glaucoma or ocular hypertension
Mechanism of Action/Effect Decreases IOP by reducing aqueous humor formation and increasing uveoscleral outflow
Contraindications Hypersensitivity to brimonidine tartrate or any component of the formulation; during or within 14 days of MAO inhibitor therapy
Warnings/Precautions Exercise caution in treating patients with severe cardiovascular disease. Use with caution in patients with depression, cerebral or coronary insufficiency, Raynaud's phenomenon, orthostatic hypotension, or thromboangiitis obliterans. Use with caution in patients with hepatic or renal impairment. May cause drowsiness or fatigue; use caution performing tasks which require alertness. Safety and efficacy in children <2 years of age have not been established.

Products may contain benzalkonium chloride which may be absorbed by contact lenses; remove contacts prior to administration and wait 15 minutes before reinserting. The IOP-lowering efficacy observed with brimonidine tartrate during the first of month of therapy may not always reflect the long-term level of IOP reduction. Routinely monitor IOP.

Drug Interactions

Decreased Effect: Tricyclic antidepressants can affect the metabolism and uptake of circulating amines.

Increased Effect/Toxicity: CNS depressants (eg, ethanol, barbiturates, opiates, sedatives, anesthetics) may have additive or potentiating effect; topical beta-blockers, pilocarpine may have additive decreased intraocular pressure; antihypertensives, cardiac glycosides may increase effects. Concomitant use of MAO inhibitors is contraindicated.

Adverse Reactions Actual frequency of adverse reactions may be formulation dependant; percentages reported with Alphagan® P:

>10%: Ocular: Allergic conjunctivitis, conjunctival hyperemia, eye pruritus

1% to 10% (unless otherwise noted 1% to 4%):

Cardiovascular: Hypertension (5% to 9%), hypotension

Central nervous system: Dizziness, fatigue, headache, insomnia, somnolence

Dermatologic: Rash

Endocrine & metabolic: Hypercholesterolemia

Gastrointestinal: Xerostomia (5% to 9%), dyspepsia

Ocular: Burning sensation (5% to 9%), conjunctival folliculosis (5% to 9%), ocular allergic reaction (5% to 9%), visual disturbance (5% to 9%), blepharitis, blepharoconjunctivitis, blurred vision, cataract, conjunctival edema, conjunctival hemorrhage, conjunctivitis, dry eye, eye discharge, irritation, epiphora, eyelid disorder, eyelid edema, eyelid erythema, follicular conjunctivitis, foreign body sensation, keratitis, pain, photophobia, stinging, superficial punctate keratopathy, visual acuity worsened, visual field defect, vitreous detachment, vitreous floaters, watery eyes

Respiratory: Bronchitis, cough, dyspnea, pharyngitis, rhinitis, sinus infection, sinusitis

Miscellaneous: Allergic reaction, flu-like syndrome, infection

Overdosage/Toxicology No information is available on overdosage in humans. Treatment is supportive and symptomatic.

Pharmacodynamics/Kinetics
Onset of Action: Peak effect: 2 hours
Time to Peak: Plasma: 0.5-2.5 hours
Half-Life Elimination: 2-3 hours
Metabolism: Hepatic
Excretion: Urine (74%)

Available Dosage Forms

Solution, ophthalmic, as tartrate: 0.2% (5 mL, 10 mL, 15 mL) [may contain benzalkonium chloride]

Alphagan® P: 0.1% (5 mL, 10 mL, 15 mL) [contains Purite® as preservative]; 0.15% (5 mL, 10 mL, 15 mL) [contains Purite® as preservative]

Dosing
Adults & Elderly: Glaucoma: Ophthalmic: Instill 1 drop in affected eye(s) 3 times/day (approximately every 8 hours)
Pediatrics: Children ≥2 years of age: Refer to adult dosing.

Administration
Other: Remove contact lenses prior to administration; wait 15 minutes before reinserting if using products containing benzalkonium chloride. Separate administration of other ophthalmic agents by 5 minutes.

Stability
Storage: Store between 15°C to 25°C (59°F to 77°F).

Nursing Actions
Physical Assessment: Assess potential for interactions with other prescriptions, OTC medications, or herbal products patient may be taking. Monitor patient response and adverse effects. Teach patient proper use, side effects/appropriate interventions, and symptoms to report.

Patient Education: For use in eyes only. Wash hands before instilling. Remove contacts prior to administration and wait 15 minutes before reinserting. Sit or lie down to instill. Open eye, look at ceiling, and instill prescribed amount of solution. Apply gentle pressure to inner corner of eye. Do not let tip of applicator touch eyes; do not contaminate tip of applicator (may cause eye infection, eye damage, or vision loss). Brimonidine tartrate may cause fatigue or drowsiness in some patients. Avoid engaging in hazardous activities due to potential for decreased mental alertness.

Wait at least 15 minutes after instilling brimonidine tartrate before reinserting soft contact lenses.
Breast-feeding precaution: Do not breast-feed.

Additional Information The use of Purite® as a preservative in Alphagan® P has lead to a reduced incidence of certain adverse effects associated with products using benzalkonium chloride as a preservative. The 0.1% and 0.15% solutions are comparable to the 0.2% solution in lowering intraocular pressure.

Brinzolamide (brin ZOH la mide)

U.S. Brand Names Azopt®
Pharmacologic Category Carbonic Anhydrase Inhibitor; Ophthalmic Agent, Antiglaucoma
Pregnancy Risk Factor C
Lactation Excretion in breast milk unknown/not recommended
Use Lowers intraocular pressure in patients with ocular hypertension or open-angle glaucoma
Mechanism of Action/Effect Brinzolamide inhibits carbonic anhydrase, leading to decreased aqueous humor secretion. This results in a reduction of intraocular pressure.
Contraindications Hypersensitivity to brinzolamide, sulfonamides, or any component of the formulation
Warnings/Precautions Effects of prolonged use on corneal epithelial cells have not been evaluated; has not been studied in acute angle-closure glaucoma. Use caution with renal impairment (parent and metabolite may accumulate). Systemic absorption may cause serious hypersensitivity reactions to recur. Chemical similarities are present among sulfonamides, sulfonylureas, carbonic anhydrase inhibitors, thiazides, and loop diuretics (except ethacrynic acid). In patients with allergy to one of these compounds, a risk of cross-reaction exists; avoid use when previous reaction has been severe. Safety and efficacy have not been established with hepatic impairment or in pediatric patients.

Drug Interactions
Cytochrome P450 Effect: Substrate of CYP3A4 (minor)
Increased Effect/Toxicity: Concurrent use of oral carbonic anhydrase inhibitors (CAIs) may lead to additive effects and toxicity (use is not recommended). High-dose salicylates may result in toxicity from CAIs.

Adverse Reactions
1% to 10%:
Dermatologic: Dermatitis (1% to 5%)
Gastrointestinal: Taste disturbances (5% to 10%)
Ocular: Blurred vision (5% to 10%), blepharitis (1% to 5%), dry eye (1% to 5%), foreign body sensation (1% to 5%), eye discharge (1% to 5%), eye pain (1% to 5%), itching of eye (1% to 5%)
Respiratory: Rhinitis (1% to 5%)

Overdosage/Toxicology Theoretically, overdose could lead to electrolyte imbalance, acidosis, and CNS effects; monitor serum electrolytes and blood pH. Treatment is supportive.

Pharmacodynamics/Kinetics
Onset of Action: Peak effect: 2 hours
Duration of Action: 8-12 hours
Metabolism: To N-desmethyl brinzolamide
Excretion: Urine (as unchanged drug and metabolites)

Available Dosage Forms Suspension, ophthalmic: 1% (5 mL, 10 mL, 15 mL) [contains benzalkonium chloride]

Dosing
Adults & Elderly: Glaucoma: Ophthalmic: Instill 1 drop in affected eye(s) 3 times/day
(Continued)

Brinzolamide *(Continued)*

Administration
Other: May be used concomitantly with other topical ophthalmic drug products to lower intraocular pressure. If more than one topical ophthalmic drug is being used, administer drugs at least 10 minutes apart.

Stability
Storage: Store at 4°C to 30°C (39°F to 86°F). Shake well before use.

Nursing Actions
Physical Assessment: Assess potential for interactions with other prescriptions, OTC medications, or herbal products patient may be taking. Monitor patient response and adverse effects. Teach patient proper use, side effects/appropriate interventions, and symptoms to report.

Patient Education: For use in eyes only. Tilt head back, place medication in conjunctival sac, and close eyes. Apply finger pressure at corner of eye for 1 minute following application. Do not let tip of applicator touch eye; do not contaminate tip of applicator (may cause eye infection, eye damage, or vision loss). If using other ophthalmic preparations, administer 10 minutes apart. Avoid excessive use of aspirin or aspirin-containing medications (may cause toxicity). May cause taste changes; runny nose; or vision changes (blurred vision, dry eye, foreign body sensation, eye discharge, temporary sensitivity to bright light, blurring or stinging, altered distance perception, reduced night vision acuity). Report persistent dizziness or headache, skin rash, loss of hair, unresolved GI disturbance, difficulty breathing, or persistent sore throat. **Pregnancy/breast-feeding precautions:** Inform prescriber if you are or intend to become pregnant. Breast-feeding is not recommended.

Bromfenac *(BROME fen ak)*

U.S. Brand Names Xibrom™
Synonyms Bromfenac Sodium
Pharmacologic Category Nonsteroidal Anti-inflammatory Drug (NSAID), Ophthalmic
Pregnancy Risk Factor C/D (3rd trimester)
Lactation
Excretion in breast milk unknown/use caution
Use Treatment of postoperative inflammation and reduction in ocular pain following cataract removal
Mechanism of Action/Effect Inhibits prostaglandin synthesis by decreasing the activity of the enzyme, cyclooxygenase, which results in decreased formation of prostaglandin precursors.
Warnings/Precautions Use caution in patients with previous sensitivity to aspirin or other NSAIDs, including patients who experience bronchospasm, asthma, rhinitis, or urticaria following NSAID or aspirin. May slow/delay healing or prolong bleeding time following surgery. Use caution in patients with a predisposition to bleeding (bleeding tendencies or medications which interfere with coagulation).

May cause keratitis; continued use of bromfenac in a patient with keratitis may cause severe corneal adverse reactions, potentially resulting in loss of vision. Immediately discontinue use in patients with evidence of corneal epithelial damage.

Use caution in patients with complicated ocular surgeries, corneal denervation, corneal epithelial defects, diabetes mellitus, ocular surface disease, rheumatoid arthritis, or repeat ocular surgeries (within a short timeframe); may be at risk of corneal adverse events, potentially resulting in loss of vision. Patients using ophthalmic drops should not wear soft contact lenses.

Contains sulfites, which may cause allergic reactions. Safety and efficacy not established in patients <18 years of age.
Drug Interactions
Decreased Effect: Bromfenac may decrease the reduction in IOP produced by latanoprost.
Increased Effect/Toxicity: Concurrent use of ophthalmic corticosteroids may increase the risk of healing problems.
Adverse Reactions 2% to 7%:
Central nervous system: Headache
Ocular: Abnormal vision, abnormal sensation, conjunctival hyperemia, eye pain, iritis, pruritus
Pharmacodynamics/Kinetics
Half-Life Elimination: 0.5-4 hours (following oral administration)
Metabolism: Hepatic
Available Dosage Forms Solution, ophthalmic: 0.09% (5 mL) [contains benzoic acid and sodium sulfite]
Dosing
Adults & Elderly: Ophthalmic: Instill 1 drop into affected eye(s) twice daily beginning 24 hours after surgery and continuing for 2 weeks postoperatively
Renal Impairment: No adjustment required.
Stability
Storage: Store at 15°C to 25°C (59°F to 77°F).
Nursing Actions
Physical Assessment: Assess for intraocular bleeding. Evaluate allergy history with aspirin or other NSAIDs. Assess knowledge/teach patient appropriate use, interventions to reduce side effects, and adverse symptoms to report
Patient Education: Do not wear contact lenses while using this medication. Report any abnormal sensation in eye, redness, severe headache, or pain.
Pregnancy Issues Safety and efficacy in pregnant women have not been established. Exposure to nonsteroidal anti-inflammatory drugs late in pregnancy may lead to premature closure of the ductus arteriosus and may inhibit uterine contractions.
Additional Information An oral formulation of bromfenac was previously available and was withdrawn from the market following reports of idiosyncratic hepatotoxicity.

Bromocriptine *(broe moe KRIP teen)*

U.S. Brand Names Parlodel®
Synonyms Bromocriptine Mesylate
Pharmacologic Category Anti-Parkinson's Agent, Dopamine Agonist; Ergot Derivative
Medication Safety Issues
Sound-alike/look-alike issues:
Bromocriptine may be confused with benztropine, brimonidine
Parlodel® may be confused with pindolol, Provera®
Pregnancy Risk Factor B
Lactation Enters breast milk/contraindicated
Use Treatment of hyperprolactinemia associated with amenorrhea with or without galactorrhea, infertility, or hypogonadism; treatment of prolactin-secreting adenomas; treatment of acromegaly; treatment of Parkinson's disease
Unlabeled/Investigational Use Neuroleptic malignant syndrome
Mechanism of Action/Effect Semisynthetic ergot alkaloid derivative and a dopamine receptor agonist which activates postsynaptic dopamine receptors to decrease prolactin secretion (tuberoinfundibular pathway) and enhance coordinated motor control (nigrostriatal pathways).
Contraindications Hypersensitivity to bromocriptine, ergot alkaloids, or any component of the formulation;

ergot alkaloids are contraindicated with potent inhibitors of CYP3A4 (includes protease inhibitors, azole antifungals, and some macrolide antibiotics); uncontrolled hypertension; severe ischemic heart disease or peripheral vascular disorders; pregnancy (risk to benefit evaluation must be performed in women who become pregnant during treatment for acromegaly, prolactinoma, or Parkinson's disease - hypertension during treatment should generally result in efforts to withdraw)

Warnings/Precautions Complete evaluation of pituitary function should be completed prior to initiation of treatment. Use caution in patients with impaired renal or hepatic function, a history of peptic ulcer disease, dementia, psychosis, or cardiovascular disease (myocardial infarction, arrhythmia). Symptomatic hypotension may occur in a significant number of patients. In addition, hypertension, seizures, MI, and stroke have been rarely associated with bromocriptine therapy. Severe headache or visual changes may precede events. The onset of reactions may be immediate or delayed (often may occur in the second week of therapy).

Concurrent antihypertensives or drugs which may alter blood pressure should be used with caution. Concurrent use with levodopa has been associated with an increased risk of hallucinations. Consider dosage reduction and/or discontinuation in patients with hallucinations. Hallucinations may require weeks to months before resolution.

In the treatment of acromegaly, discontinuation is recommended if tumor expansion occurs during therapy. Digital vasospasm (cold sensitive) may occur in some patients with acromegaly; may require dosage reduction. Patients who receive bromocriptine during and immediately following pregnancy as a continuation of previous therapy (eg, acromegaly) should be closely monitored for cardiovascular effects. Should not be used post-partum in women with coronary artery disease or other cardiovascular disease. Use of bromocriptine to control or prevent lactation or in patients with uncontrolled hypertension is not recommended.

Monitoring and careful evaluation of visual changes during the treatment of hyperprolactinemia is recommended to differentiate between tumor shrinkage and traction on the optic chiasm; rapidly progressing visual field loss requires neurosurgical consultation. Discontinuation of bromocriptine in patients with macroadenomas has been associated with rapid regrowth of tumor and increased prolactin serum levels. Pleural and retroperitoneal fibrosis have been reported with prolonged daily use. Cardiac valvular fibrosis has also been associated with ergot alkaloids. Safety and effectiveness in patients <15 years of age (for pituitary adenoma) have not been established.

Drug Interactions

Cytochrome P450 Effect: Substrate of CYP3A4 (major); **Inhibits** CYP1A2 (weak), 3A4 (weak)

Decreased Effect: Effects of bromocriptine may be diminished by antipsychotics, metoclopramide.

Increased Effect/Toxicity: Effect/toxicity of bromocriptine may be increased by alpha agonists/ sympathomimetics, antifungals (azole derivatives), macrolide antibiotics, protease inhibitors, and MAO inhibitors. Bromocriptine may increase the effects of sibutramine and other serotonin agonists (serotonin syndrome). CYP3A4 inhibitors may increase the levels/effects of bromocriptine; example inhibitors include azole antifungals, clarithromycin, diclofenac, doxycycline, erythromycin, imatinib, isoniazid, nefazodone, nicardipine, propofol, protease inhibitors, quinidine, telithromycin, and verapamil. Concurrent use of bromocriptine with antihypertensive agents may increase the risk of hypotension. Concurrent use of levodopa may increase the risk of hallucinations (dose-dependant).

Nutritional/Ethanol Interactions

Ethanol: Avoid ethanol (may increase GI side effects or ethanol intolerance).

Herb/Nutraceutical: St John's wort may decrease bromocriptine levels.

Adverse Reactions Note: Frequency of adverse effects may vary by dose and/or indication.

>10%:

Cardiovascular: Hypotension (up to 30%)

Central nervous system: Headache, dizziness

Gastrointestinal: Nausea, constipation

1% to 10%:

Cardiovascular: Orthostasis, vasospasm (cold-sensitive), Raynaud's syndrome, syncope

Central nervous system: Fatigue, lightheadedness, drowsiness

Gastrointestinal: Anorexia, vomiting, abdominal cramps, diarrhea, dyspepsia, GI bleeding, xerostomia

Respiratory: Nasal congestion

Withdrawal reactions: Abrupt discontinuation has resulted in rare cases of a withdrawal reaction with symptoms similar to neuroleptic malignant syndrome.

Overdosage/Toxicology Symptoms of overdose include nausea, vomiting, and hypotension. Treatment is symptomatic and supportive.

Pharmacodynamics/Kinetics

Time to Peak: Serum: 1-2 hours

Protein Binding: 90% to 96%

Half-Life Elimination: Biphasic: Initial: 6-8 hours; Terminal: 50 hours

Metabolism: Primarily hepatic

Excretion: Feces; urine (2% to 6% as unchanged drug)

Available Dosage Forms

Capsule, as mesylate: 5 mg

Parlodel®: 5 mg

Tablet, as mesylate: 2.5 mg

Parlodel®: 2.5 mg

Dosing

Adults & Elderly:

Parkinsonism: Oral: 1.25 mg twice daily, increased by 2.5 mg/day in 2- to 4-week intervals (usual dose range is 30-90 mg/day in 3 divided doses), though elderly patients can usually be managed on lower doses.

Neuroleptic malignant syndrome (unlabeled use): Oral: 2.5-5 mg 3 times/day

Acromegaly: Oral: Initial: 1.25-2.5 mg daily increasing by 1.25-2.5 mg as necessary every 3-7 days; usual dose: 20-30 mg/day (maximum: 100 mg/day)

Hyperprolactinemia: Oral: Initial: 1.25-2.5 mg/day; may be increased by 2.5 mg/day as tolerated every 2-7 days until optimal response (range: 2.5-15 mg/day)

Pediatrics:

Hyperprolactinemia: Oral:

Children 11-15 years (based on limited information): Initial: 1.25-2.5 mg daily. Dosage may be increased as tolerated to achieve a therapeutic response (range 2.5-10 mg daily).

Children ≥16 years: Refer to adult dosing.

Hepatic Impairment: No guidelines are available, however, adjustment may be necessary.

Laboratory Monitoring Pregnancy test during amenorrheic peroid; growth hormone and prolactin levels

Nursing Actions

Physical Assessment: Assess effectiveness and interactions of other medications patient may be taking. Monitor therapeutic response (eg, mental status, involuntary movements) and adverse reactions at beginning of therapy and periodically throughout therapy. Assess knowledge/teach patient appropriate (Continued)

Bromocriptine *(Continued)*

use, interventions to reduce side effects, and adverse symptoms to report.

Patient Education: Take exactly as directed (may be prescribed in conjunction with levodopa/carbidopa); do not change dosage or discontinue this medicine without consulting prescriber. Therapeutic effects may take several weeks or months to achieve and you may need frequent monitoring during first weeks of therapy. Take with meals if GI upset occurs, before meals if dry mouth occurs, or after eating if drooling or if nausea occurs. Take at the same time each day. Maintain adequate hydration (2-3 L/day of fluids) unless instructed to restrict fluid intake; void before taking medication. Do not use alcohol, prescription or OTC sedatives, or CNS depressants without consulting prescriber. Urine or perspiration may appear darker. You may experience drowsiness, dizziness, confusion, or vision changes (use caution when driving, climbing stairs, or engaging in tasks requiring alertness until response to drug is known); orthostatic hypotension (use caution when rising from sitting or lying position); constipation (increased exercise, fluids, fruit, or fiber may help); nasal congestion (consult prescriber for appropriate relief); or nausea, vomiting, loss of appetite, or stomach discomfort (small frequent meals, frequent mouth care, chewing gum, or sucking lozenges may help). Report unresolved constipation or vomiting; chest pain or irregular heartbeat; acute headache or dizziness; CNS changes (eg, hallucination, loss of memory, seizures, acute headache, nervousness); painful or difficult urination; increased muscle spasticity, rigidity, or involuntary movements; skin rash; or significant worsening of condition. **Breast-feeding precaution:** Do not breast-feed.

Dietary Considerations May be taken with food to decrease GI distress.

Geriatric Considerations See Adverse Reactions; elderly patients are usually managed on lower doses.

Breast-Feeding Issues A previous indication for prevention of postpartum lactation was withdrawn voluntarily by the manufacturer following reports of serious adverse reactions, including stroke, MI, seizures, and severe hypertension. Based on the risk/benefit assessment, other treatments should be considered for lactation suppression.

Pregnancy Issues Bromocriptine is used for ovulation induction in women with hyperprolactinemia. In general, therapy should be discontinued if pregnancy is confirmed unless needed for treatment of macroprolactinoma. Data collected from women taking bromocriptine during pregnancy suggest the incidence of birth defects is not increased with use. However, the majority of women discontinued use within 8 weeks of pregnancy. Women not seeking pregnancy should be advised to use appropriate contraception.

Additional Information Usually used with levodopa or levodopa/carbidopa to treat Parkinson's disease. When adding bromocriptine, the dose of levodopa/carbidopa can usually be decreased.

Budesonide *(byoo DES oh nide)*

U.S. Brand Names Entocort™ EC; Pulmicort Respules®; Pulmicort Turbuhaler®; Rhinocort® Aqua®

Pharmacologic Category Corticosteroid, Inhalant (Oral); Corticosteroid, Nasal; Corticosteroid, Systemic

Pregnancy Risk Factor C/B (Pulmicort Respules® and Turbuhaler®, Rhinocort® Aqua®)

Lactation Enters breast milk/use caution

Use

Intranasal: Children ≥6 years of age and Adults: Management of symptoms of seasonal or perennial rhinitis

Nebulization: Children 12 months to 8 years: Maintenance and prophylactic treatment of asthma

Oral capsule: Treatment of active Crohn's disease (mild to moderate) involving the ileum and/or ascending colon; maintenance of remission (for up to 3 months) of Crohn's disease (mild to moderate) involving the ileum and/or ascending colon

Oral inhalation: Maintenance and prophylactic treatment of asthma; includes patients who require corticosteroids and those who may benefit from systemic dose reduction/elimination

Mechanism of Action/Effect Anti-inflammatory effect on nasal tissues

Contraindications Hypersensitivity to budesonide or any component of the formulation

Inhalation: Contraindicated in primary treatment of status asthmaticus, acute episodes of asthma; not for relief of acute bronchospasm

Warnings/Precautions May cause hypercorticism and/or suppression of hypothalamic-pituitary-adrenal (HPA) axis, particularly in younger children or in patients receiving high doses for prolonged periods. Particular care is required when patients are transferred from systemic corticosteroids to products with lower systemic bioavailability (ie, inhalation). May lead to possible adrenal insufficiency or withdrawal from steroids, including an increase in allergic symptoms. Patients receiving prolonged therapy ≥20 mg per day of prednisone (or equivalent) may be most susceptible. Aerosol steroids do **not** provide the systemic steroid needed to treat patients having trauma, surgery, or infections.

Controlled clinical studies have shown that orally-inhaled and intranasal corticosteroids may cause a reduction in growth velocity in pediatric patients. (In studies of orally-inhaled corticosteroids, the mean reduction in growth velocity was approximately 1 centimeter per year [range 0.3-1.8 cm per year] and appears to be related to dose and duration of exposure.) To minimize the systemic effects of orally-inhaled and intranasal corticosteroids, each patient should be titrated to the lowest effective dose. Growth should be routinely monitored in pediatric patients.

May suppress the immune system; patients may be more susceptible to infection. Use with caution in patients with systemic infections or ocular herpes simplex. Avoid exposure to chickenpox and measles. Corticosteroids should be used with caution in patients with diabetes, hypertension, osteoporosis, peptic ulcer, glaucoma, cataracts, or tuberculosis. Use caution in hepatic impairment. Enteric-coated capsules should not be crushed or chewed.

Drug Interactions

Cytochrome P450 Effect: Substrate of CYP3A4 (major)

Decreased Effect: Theoretically, proton pump inhibitors (omeprazole, pantoprazole) alter gastric pH and may affect the rate of dissolution of enteric-coated capsules. Administration with omeprazole did not alter kinetics of budesonide capsules.

Increased Effect/Toxicity: Cimetidine may decrease the clearance and increase the bioavailability of budesonide, increasing its serum concentrations. In addition, CYP3A4 inhibitors may increase the serum level and/or toxicity of budesonide this effect was shown with ketoconazole, but not erythromycin. Other potential inhibitors include amiodarone, cimetidine, clarithromycin, delavirdine, diltiazem, dirithromycin, disulfiram, fluoxetine, fluvoxamine, grapefruit juice, indinavir, itraconazole, ketoconazole, nefazodone, nevirapine, propoxyphene, quinupristin-dalfopristin, ritonavir, saquinavir, telithromycin, verapamil, zafirlukast, and zileuton. The addition of salmeterol has been demonstrated to improve response to inhaled corticosteroids (as compared to increasing steroid dosage).

Nutritional/Ethanol Interactions

Food: Grapefruit juice may double systemic exposure of orally-administered budesonide. Administration of capsules with a high-fat meal delays peak concentration, but does not alter the extent of absorption.

Herb/Nutraceutical: St John's wort may decrease budesonide levels.

Adverse Reactions Reaction severity varies by dose and duration; not all adverse reactions have been reported with each dosage form.

>10%:

Central nervous system: Headache (up to 21%)
Gastrointestinal: Nausea (up to 11%)
Respiratory: Respiratory infection, rhinitis
Miscellaneous: Symptoms of HPA axis suppression and/or hypercorticism may occur in >10% of patients following administration of dosage forms which result in higher systemic exposure (ie, oral capsule), but may be less frequent than rates observed with comparator drugs (prednisolone). These symptoms may be rare (<1%) following administration via methods which result in lower exposures (topical).

1% to 10%:

Cardiovascular: Chest pain, edema, flushing, hypertension, palpitation, syncope, tachycardia
Central nervous system: Dizziness, dysphonia, emotional lability, fatigue, fever, insomnia, migraine, nervousness, pain, vertigo
Dermatologic: Acne, alopecia, bruising, contact dermatitis, eczema, hirsutism, pruritus, pustular rash, rash, striae
Endocrine & metabolic: Adrenal insufficiency, hypokalemia, menstrual disorder
Gastrointestinal: Abdominal pain, anorexia, diarrhea, dry mouth, dyspepsia, flatulence, gastroenteritis, oral candidiasis, taste perversion, vomiting, weight gain
Genitourinary: Dysuria, hematuria, nocturia, pyuria
Hematologic: Cervical lymphadenopathy, leukocytosis, purpura
Hepatic: Alkaline phosphatase increased
Neuromuscular & skeletal: Arthralgia, back pain, fracture, hyperkinesis, hypertonia, myalgia, neck pain, weakness, paresthesia
Ocular: Conjunctivitis, eye infection
Otic: Earache, ear infection, external ear infection
Respiratory: Bronchitis, bronchospasm, cough, epistaxis, nasal irritation, pharyngitis, sinusitis, stridor
Miscellaneous: Abscess, allergic reaction, C-reactive protein increased, erythrocyte sedimentation rate increased, fat distribution (moon face, buffalo hump), flu-like syndrome, herpes simplex, infection, moniliasis, viral infection, voice alteration

Overdosage/Toxicology

Inhaled formulations: Symptoms of overdose include irritation and burning of the nasal mucosa, sneezing, intranasal and pharyngeal *Candida* infections, nasal ulceration, epistaxis, rhinorrhea, nasal stuffiness, headache.

When consumed in excessive quantities, systemic hypercorticism and adrenal suppression may occur. In those cases discontinuation and withdrawal of the corticosteroid should be done judiciously. Treatment should be symptomatic and supportive.

Pharmacodynamics/Kinetics

Onset of Action: Respules®: 2-8 days; Rhinocort® Aqua®: ~10 hours; Turbuhaler®: 24 hours
Peak effect: Respules®: 4-6 weeks; Rhinocort® Aqua®: ~2 weeks; Turbuhaler®: 1-2 weeks

Time to Peak: Capsule: 0.5-10 hours (variable in Crohn's disease); Respules®: 10-30 minutes; Turbuhaler®: 1-2 hours; Nasal: 1 hour

Protein Binding: 85% to 90%

Half-Life Elimination: 2-3.6 hours

Metabolism: Hepatic via CYP3A4 to two metabolites: 16 alpha-hydroxyprednisolone and 6 beta-hydroxybudesonide; minor activity

Excretion: Urine (60%) and feces as metabolites

Available Dosage Forms [CAN] = Canadian brand name

Capsule, enteric coated (Entocort™ EC): 3 mg
Powder for oral inhalation:
  Pulmicort Turbuhaler®: 200 mcg/inhalation (104 g) [delivers ~160 mcg/inhalation; 200 metered doses]
  Pulmicort Turbuhaler® [CAN]: 100 mcg/inhalation [delivers 200 metered doses]; 200 mcg/inhalation [delivers 200 metered doses]; 400 mcg/inhalation [delivers 200 metered doses] [not available in the U.S.]

Suspension, intranasal [spray] (Rhinocort® Aqua®): 32 mcg/inhalation (8.6 g) [120 metered doses]
Suspension for nebulization (Pulmicort Respules®): 0.25 mg/2 mL (30s), 0.5 mg/2 mL (30s)

Dosing

Adults & Elderly:

Asthma: Inhalation: 1- to 4-inhalations twice daily using Pulmicort Turbuhaler® device; maintenance therapy may be gradually reduced to a single daily inhalation. See table.

Budesonide

Previous Therapy	Recommended Starting Dose	Highest Recommended Dose
Bronchodilators alone	200-400 mcg twice daily	400 mcg twice daily
Inhaled corticosteroids[1]	200-400 mcg twice daily	800 mcg twice daily
Oral corticosteroids	400-800 mcg twice daily	800 mcg twice daily

[1]In patients with mild-to-moderate asthma who are well controlled on inhaled corticosteroids, dosing with Pulmicort Turbuhaler® 200 mcg or 400 mcg once daily may be considered. Pulmicort Turbuhaler® can be administered once daily either in the morning or in the evening.

Crohn's disease (active): Oral: 9 mg once daily in the morning for up to 8 weeks; recurring episodes may be treated with a repeat 8-week course of treatment

Note: Patients receiving CYP3A4 inhibitors should be monitored closely for signs and symptoms of hypercorticism; dosage reduction may be required. If switching from oral prednisolone, prednisolone dosage should be tapered while budesonide (Entocort™ EC) treatment is initiated.

Crohn's disease, maintenance of remission: Following treatment of active disease (control of symptoms with CDAI <150), treatment may be continued at a dosage of 6 mg once daily for up to 3 months. If symptom control is maintained for 3 months, tapering of the dosage to complete cessation is recommended. Continued dosing beyond 3 months has not been demonstrated to result in substantial benefit.

(Continued)

Budesonide *(Continued)*

Rhinitis: Nasal inhalation (Rhinocort® Aqua®): 64 mcg/day as a single 32 mcg spray in each nostril. Some patients who do not achieve adequate control may benefit from increased dosage. A reduced dosage may be effective after initial control is achieved.

Maximum dose: Children <12 years: 129 mcg/day; Adults: 256 mcg/day

Pediatrics:

Asthma:

Nasal inhalation: ≥6 years: Refer to adult dosing.

Oral inhalation: ≥6 years:

Previous therapy of bronchodilators alone: 200 mcg twice initially which may be increased up to 400 mcg twice daily

Previous therapy of inhaled corticosteroids: 200 mcg twice initially which may be increased up to 400 mcg twice daily

Previous therapy of oral corticosteroids: The highest recommended dose in children is 400 mcg twice daily

NIH Guidelines (NIH, 1997) (give in divided doses twice daily):

"Low" dose: 100-200 mcg/day

"Medium" dose: 200-400 mcg/day (1-2 inhalations/day)

"High" dose: >400 mcg/day (>2 inhalation/day)

Nebulization: Children 12 months to 8 years: Pulmicort Respules®: Titrate to lowest effective dose once patient is stable; start at 0.25 mg/day or use as follows:

Previous therapy of bronchodilators alone: 0.5 mg/day administered as a single dose or divided twice daily (maximum daily dose: 0.5 mg)

Previous therapy of inhaled corticosteroids: 0.5 mg/day administered as a single dose or divided twice daily (maximum daily dose: 1 mg)

Previous therapy of oral corticosteroids: 1 mg/day administered as a single dose or divided twice daily (maximum daily dose: 1 mg)

Hepatic Impairment: Monitor closely for signs and symptoms of hypercorticism; dosage reduction may be required.

Administration

Oral: Oral capsule: Capsule should be swallowed whole; do not crush or chew.

Inhalation:

Inhalation: Inhaler should be shaken well immediately prior to use. While activating inhaler, deep breathe for 3-5 seconds, hold breath for ~10 seconds, and allow ≥1 minute between inhalations. Rinse mouth with water after use to reduce aftertaste and incidence of candidiasis.

Nebulization: Shake well before using. Use Pulmicort Respules® with jet nebulizer connected to an air compressor; administer with mouthpiece or facemask. Do not use ultrasonic nebulizer. Do not mix with other medications in nebulizer. Rinse mouth following treatments to decrease risk of oral candidiasis (wash face if using face mask).

Stability

Storage:

Nebulizer: Store upright at 20°C to 25°C (68°F to 77°F) and protect from light. Do not refrigerate or freeze. Once aluminum package is opened, solution should be used within 2 weeks. Continue to protect from light.

Nasal inhaler: Store with valve up at 15°C to 30°C (59°F to 86°F). Use within 6 months after opening aluminum pouch. Protect from high humidity.

Nasal spray: Store with valve up at 20°C to 25°C (68°F to 77°F) and protect from light. Do not freeze.

Nursing Actions

Physical Assessment: Monitor therapeutic effectiveness and adverse reactions. When changing from systemic steroids to inhalational steroids, taper reduction of systemic medication slowly (may take several months). Growth should be routinely monitored in pediatric patients. Assess knowledge/teach patient appropriate use, interventions to reduce side effects, and adverse symptoms to report.

Patient Education: Use as directed; do not increase dosage or discontinue abruptly without consulting prescriber. May be more susceptible to infection; avoid exposure to chickenpox and measles unless immunity has been established. If exposure to measles or chickenpox occurs, notify your prescriber immediately. Report acute nervousness or inability to sleep; severe sneezing or nosebleed; respiratory difficulty, sore throat, hoarseness, bronchitis, or bronchospasms; disturbed menstrual pattern; vision changes; loss of taste or smell perception; or worsening of condition or lack of improvement. **Pregnancy/breast-feeding precautions:** Inform prescriber if you are or intend to become pregnant. Consult prescriber if breast-feeding.

Oral capsule: Swallow whole; do not crush or chew capsule.

Inhalation/nebulization: This is not a bronchodilator and will not relieve acute asthma attacks. It may take several days for you to realize full effects of treatment. If you are also using an inhaled bronchodilator, wait 10 minutes before using this steroid aerosol. Take 5-10 deep breaths. Use inhaler on inspiration. Hold breath for 5-10 seconds after inhalation. Allow 1 full minute between inhalations. You may experience dizziness, anxiety, or blurred vision (rise slowly from sitting or lying position and use caution when driving or engaging in tasks requiring alertness until response to drug is known); or taste disturbance or aftertaste (frequent mouth care and mouth rinses may help). Rinse mouth with water following oral treatments to decrease risk of oral candidiasis (wash face if using a face mask).

Dietary Considerations Avoid grapefruit juice when using oral capsules.

Geriatric Considerations Ensure that patients can correctly use nasal inhaler.

Pregnancy Issues There are no adequate and well-controlled studies in pregnant women; use only if potential benefit to the mother outweighs the possible risk to the fetus. Hypoadrenalism has been reported in infants.

Additional Information Effects of inhaled/intranasal steroids on growth have been observed in the absence of laboratory evidence of HPA axis suppression, suggesting that growth velocity is a more sensitive indicator of systemic corticosteroid exposure in pediatric patients than some commonly used tests of HPA axis function. The long-term effects of this reduction in growth velocity associated with orally-inhaled and intranasal corticosteroids, including the impact on final adult height, are unknown. The potential for "catch up" growth following discontinuation of treatment with inhaled corticosteroids has not been adequately studied.

Bumetanide (byoo MET a nide)

U.S. Brand Names Bumex®

Pharmacologic Category Diuretic, Loop

Medication Safety Issues
Sound-alike/look-alike issues:
Bumetanide may be confused with Buminate®
Bumex® may be confused with Brevibloc®, Buprenex®, Permax®

Pregnancy Risk Factor C (manufacturer); D (expert analysis)

Lactation Excretion in breast milk unknown/use caution

Use Management of edema secondary to congestive heart failure or hepatic or renal disease including nephrotic syndrome; may be used alone or in combination with antihypertensives in the treatment of hypertension; can be used in furosemide-allergic patients

Mechanism of Action/Effect Inhibits reabsorption of sodium and chloride in the ascending loop of Henle and proximal renal tubule, causing increased excretion of water, sodium, chloride, magnesium, phosphate, and calcium

Contraindications Hypersensitivity to bumetanide, any component of the formulation, or sulfonylureas; anuria; patients with hepatic coma or in states of severe electrolyte depletion until the condition improves or is corrected; pregnancy (based on expert analysis)

Warnings/Precautions In cirrhosis, avoid electrolyte and acid/base imbalances that might lead to hepatic encephalopathy. Ototoxicity is associated with I.V. rapid administration, renal impairment, excessive doses, and concurrent use of other ototoxins. Hypersensitivity reactions can rarely occur. Monitor fluid status and renal function in an attempt to prevent oliguria, azotemia, and reversible increases in BUN and creatinine. May cause significant electrolyte disturbances or volume depletion. Coadministration of antihypertensives may increase the risk of hypotension.

Chemical similarities are present among sulfonamides, sulfonylureas, carbonic anhydrase inhibitors, thiazides, and loop diuretics (except ethacrynic acid). Use in patients with sulfonylurea allergy is specifically contraindicated in product labeling, however, a risk of cross-reaction exists in patients with allergy to any of these compounds; avoid use when previous reaction has been severe.

Drug Interactions
Decreased Effect: Glucose tolerance may be decreased by loop diuretics, requiring adjustment of hypoglycemic agents. Cholestyramine or colestipol may reduce bioavailability of bumetanide. Indomethacin (and other NSAIDs) may reduce natriuretic and hypotensive effects of diuretics. Hypokalemia may reduce the efficacy of some antiarrhythmics.

Increased Effect/Toxicity: Bumetanide-induced hypokalemia may predispose to digoxin toxicity and may increase the risk of arrhythmia with drugs which may prolong QT interval, including type Ia and type III antiarrhythmic agents, cisapride, and some quinolones (sparfloxacin, gatifloxacin, and moxifloxacin). The risk of toxicity from lithium and salicylates (high dose) may be increased by loop diuretics. Hypotensive effects and/or adverse renal effects of ACE inhibitors and NSAIDs are potentiated by bumetanide-induced hypovolemia. The effects of peripheral adrenergic-blocking drugs or ganglionic blockers may be increased by bumetanide.

Bumetanide may increase the risk of ototoxicity with other ototoxic agents (aminoglycosides, cis-platinum), especially in patients with renal dysfunction. Synergistic diuretic effects occur with thiazide-type diuretics. Diuretics tend to be synergistic with other antihypertensive agents, and hypotension may occur.

Nutritional/Ethanol Interactions Herb/Nutraceutical: Avoid ephedra, yohimbe, ginseng (may worsen hypertension). Avoid dong quai if using for hypertension (has estrogenic activity). Avoid garlic (may have increased antihypertensive effect).

Adverse Reactions
>10%:
Endocrine & metabolic: Hyperuricemia (18%), hypochloremia (15%), hypokalemia (15%)
Renal: Azotemia (11%)
1% to 10%:
Central nervous system: Dizziness (1%)
Endocrine & metabolic: Hyponatremia (9%); hyperglycemia (7%); variations in phosphorus (5%), CO_2 content (4%), bicarbonate (3%), and calcium (2%)
Neuromuscular & skeletal: Muscle cramps (1%)
Otic: Ototoxicity (1%)
Renal: Serum creatinine increased (7%)

Overdosage/Toxicology Symptoms of overdose include electrolyte and volume depletion. Treatment is symptomatic and supportive.

Pharmacodynamics/Kinetics
Onset of Action: Oral, I.M.: 0.5-1 hour; I.V.: 2-3 minutes
Duration of Action: 4-6 hours
Protein Binding: 95%
Half-Life Elimination: Neonates: ~6 hours; Infants (1 month): ~2.4 hours; Adults: 1-1.5 hours
Metabolism: Partially hepatic
Excretion: Primarily urine (as unchanged drug and metabolites)

Available Dosage Forms
Injection, solution: 0.25 mg/mL (2 mL, 4 mL, 10 mL) [contains benzyl alcohol]
Tablet (Bumex®): 0.5 mg, 1 mg, 2 mg

Dosing
Adults:
Edema:
Oral: 0.5-2 mg/dose (maximum dose: 10 mg/day) 1-2 times/day
I.M., I.V.: 0.5-1 mg/dose; may repeat in 2-3 hours for up to 2 doses if needed (maximum dose: 10 mg/day)
Continuous I.V. infusion: Initial: 1 mg load then 0.5-2 mg/hour (ACC/AHA 2005 practice guidelines for chronic heart failure)
Hypertension: Oral: 0.5 mg daily (maximum dose: 5 mg/day)
Usual dosage range (JNC 7): 0.5-2 mg/day in 2 divided doses
Elderly: Initial: Oral: 0.5 mg once daily, increase as necessary
Pediatrics: Edema (diuresis): Oral, I.M., I.V.:
Neonates (see Warnings/Precautions): 0.01-0.05 mg/kg/dose every 24-48 hours
Infants and Children: 0.015-0.1 mg/kg/dose every 6-24 hours (maximum dose: 10 mg/day)

Administration
I.V.: Administer I.V. slowly, over 1-2 minutes. An alternate-day schedule or a 3-4 daily dosing regimen with rest periods of 1-2 days in between may be the most tolerable and effective regimen for the continued control of edema. Reserve I.V. administration for those unable to take oral medications.
I.V. Detail: pH: 6.8-7.8 (adjusted)
Stability
Compatibility: Stable in D_5W, NS, LR
Y-site administration: Incompatible with midazolam
Compatibility when admixed: Incompatible with dobutamine, milrinone
Storage:
I.V.: Store vials at 15°C to 30°C (59°F to 86°F). Infusion solutions should be used within 24 hours after preparation. Light sensitive; discoloration may occur when exposed to light.
Tablet: Store at 15°C to 30°C (59°F to 86°F).
(Continued)

Bumetanide *(Continued)*

Laboratory Monitoring Serum electrolytes, renal function

Nursing Actions

Physical Assessment: Assess history of allergies, renal, electrolyte, hepatic, and pregnancy status prior to beginning treatment. Assess other pharmacological or herbal products patient may be taking for potential interactions (eg, increased risk of hyperglycemia, hypotension, arrhythmias, ototoxicity). Blood pressure, weight, and fluid status should be monitored at beginning of therapy and periodically during therapy. Glucose levels for patients with diabetes should be monitored closely (glucose tolerance may be decreased by loop diuretics, requiring adjustment of hypoglycemic agents). Assess results of laboratory tests (electrolytes and renal function), therapeutic effectiveness (reduced edema and cardiopulmonary symptoms), and adverse effects (hypotension, electrolyte imbalance, ototoxicity). Teach patient proper use, possible side effects/appropriate interventions, and adverse symptoms to report.

Patient Education: Do not take any new medication during therapy unless approved by prescriber. May be taken with food to reduce GI effects. If taking one dose daily, take single dose early in day; if taking twice daily, take last dose early in afternoon to prevent sleep interruptions. Include orange juice or bananas (or other sources of potassium-rich foods) in your daily diet, but do not take supplemental potassium without consulting prescriber. If you have diabetes, monitor glucose levels closely (glucose tolerance may be decreased by loop diuretics), and notify prescriber of noted changes (hypoglycemic agent may need to be adjusted). May cause dizziness, hypotension, lightheadedness, or weakness (use caution when changing position from sitting or lying position, when driving, exercising, climbing stairs, or performing hazardous tasks until response to drug is known). Report palpitations or chest pain; swelling of ankles or feet; weight increase or decrease (>3 lb in any one day); increased fatigue, muscle cramps, or trembling; and any changes in hearing. **Pregnancy/breast-feeding precautions:** Inform prescriber if you are or intend to become pregnant; contraceptives may be recommended. Consult prescriber if breast-feeding.

Dietary Considerations May require increased intake of potassium-rich foods.

Geriatric Considerations See Warnings/Precautions. Severe loss of sodium and/or increases in BUN can cause confusion. For any change in mental status in patients on bumetanide, monitor electrolytes and renal function.

Bupivacaine *(byoo PIV a kane)*

U.S. Brand Names Marcaine®; Marcaine® Spinal; Sensorcaine®; Sensorcaine®-MPF

Synonyms Bupivacaine Hydrochloride

Pharmacologic Category Local Anesthetic

Medication Safety Issues

Sound-alike/look-alike issues:

Bupivacaine may be confused with mepivacaine, ropivacaine

Marcaine® may be confused with Narcan®

Pregnancy Risk Factor C

Lactation Enters breast milk/not recommended

Use Local anesthetic (injectable) for peripheral nerve block, infiltration, sympathetic block, caudal or epidural block, retrobulbar block

Mechanism of Action/Effect Blocks both the initiation and conduction of nerve impulses by decreasing the neuronal membrane's permeability to sodium ions, which results in inhibition of depolarization with resultant blockade of conduction

Contraindications Hypersensitivity to bupivacaine hydrochloride, amide-type local anesthetics, or any component of the formulation; obstetrical paracervical block anesthesia

Warnings/Precautions Use with caution in patients with hepatic impairment. Not recommended for use in children <12 years of age. The solution for spinal anesthesia should not be used in children <18 years of age. **Do not use solutions containing preservatives for caudal or epidural block.** Local anesthetics have been associated with rare occurrences of sudden respiratory arrest; convulsions due to systemic toxicity leading to cardiac arrest have also been reported, presumably following unintentional intravascular injection. The 0.75% is **not** recommended for obstetrical anesthesia. A test dose is recommended prior to epidural administration (prior to initial dose) and all reinforcing doses with continuous catheter technique. Use caution with cardiovascular dysfunction. Use caution in debilitated, elderly, or acutely ill patients; dose reduction may be required.

Drug Interactions

Cytochrome P450 Effect: Substrate (minor) of CYP1A2, 2C19, 2D6, 3A4

Adverse Reactions Note: Incidence of adverse reactions is difficult to define. Most effects are dose related, and are often due to accelerated absorption from the injection site, unintentional intravascular injection, or slow metabolic degradation. The development of any central nervous system symptoms may be an early indication of more significant toxicity (seizure).

Cardiovascular: Hypotension, bradycardia, palpitation, heart block, ventricular arrhythmia, cardiac arrest

Central nervous system: Restlessness, anxiety, dizziness, seizure (0.1%); rare symptoms (usually associated with unintentional subarachnoid injection during high spinal anesthesia) include persistent anesthesia, paresthesia, paralysis, headache, septic meningitis, and cranial nerve palsies

Gastrointestinal: Nausea, vomiting; rare symptoms (usually associated with unintentional subarachnoid injection during high spinal anesthesia) include fecal incontinence and loss of sphincter control

Genitourinary: Rare symptoms (usually associated with unintentional subarachnoid injection during high spinal anesthesia) include urinary incontinence, loss of perineal sensation, and loss of sexual function

Neuromuscular & skeletal: Weakness

Ocular: Blurred vision, pupillary constriction

Otic: Tinnitus

Respiratory: Apnea, hypoventilation (usually associated with unintentional subarachnoid injection during high spinal anesthesia)

Miscellaneous: Allergic reactions (urticaria, pruritus, angioedema), anaphylactoid reactions

Overdosage/Toxicology Treatment is symptomatic and supportive. Termination of anesthesia by pneumatic tourniquet inflation should be attempted when bupivacaine is administered by infiltration or regional injection. Treatment is symptomatic and supportive. Methemoglobinemia should be treated with methylene blue 1-2 mg/kg in a 1% sterile aqueous solution by I.V. push over 4-6 minutes, repeated up to a total dose of 7 mg/kg.

Pharmacodynamics/Kinetics

Onset of Action: Anesthesia (route and dose dependent): 1-17 minutes

Duration of Action: Route and dose dependent: 2-9 hours

Protein Binding: ~95%

Half-Life Elimination: Age dependent: Neonates: 8.1 hours; Adults: 1.5-5.5 hours

Metabolism: Hepatic; forms metabolite (PPX)
Excretion: Urine (~6% unchanged)

Available Dosage Forms

Injection, solution, as hydrochloride [preservative free]: 0.25% [2.5 mg/mL] (10 mL, 20 mL, 30 mL, 50 mL); 0.5% [5 mg/mL] (10 mL, 20 mL, 30 mL); 0.75% [7.5 mg/mL] (10 mL, 20 mL, 30 mL)

Marcaine®: 0.25% [2.5 mg/mL] (10 mL, 30 mL); 0.5% [5 mg/mL] (10 mL, 30 mL); 0.75% [7.5 mg/mL] (10 mL, 30 mL)

Marcaine® Spinal: 0.75% [7.5 mg/mL] (2 mL) [in dextrose 8.25%]

Sensorcaine®-MPF: 0.25% [2.5 mg/mL] (10 mL, 30 mL); 0.5% [5 mg/mL] (10 mL, 30 mL); 0.75% [7.5 mg/mL] (10 mL, 30 mL)

Injection, solution, as hydrochloride (Marcaine®, Sensorcaine®): 0.25% [2.5 mg/mL] (50 mL); 0.5% [5 mg/mL] (50 mL) [contains methylparaben]

Dosing

Adults & Elderly: Note: Dose varies with procedure, depth of anesthesia, vascularity of tissues, duration of anesthesia, and condition of patient. Do not use solutions containing preservatives for caudal or epidural block.

Local anesthesia: Infiltration: 0.25% infiltrated locally; maximum: 175 mg

Caudal block) (preservative free: 15-30 mL of 0.25% or 0.5%

Epidural block (other than caudal block; preservative free): Administer in 3-5 mL increments, allowing sufficient time to detect toxic manifestations of inadvertent I.V. or I.T. administration: 10-20 mL of 0.25% or 0.5%

Surgical procedures requiring a high degree of muscle relaxation and prolonged effects **only:** 10-20 mL of 0.75% (**Note:** Not to be used in obstetrical cases)

Peripheral nerve block: 5 mL of 0.25 or 0.5%; maximum: 400 mg/day

Sympathetic nerve block: 20-50 mL of 0.25%

Retrobulbar anesthesia: 2-4 mL of 0.75%

Spinal anesthesia: Preservative free solution of 0.75% bupivacaine in 8.25% dextrose:

Lower extremity and perineal procedures: 1 mL

Lower abdominal procedures: 1.6 mL

Normal vaginal delivery: 0.8 mL (higher doses may be required in some patients)

Cesarean section: 1-1.4 mL

Pediatrics: Note: Dose varies with procedure, depth of anesthesia, vascularity of tissues, duration of anesthesia, and condition of patient. Do not use solutions containing preservatives for caudal or epidural block.

Caudal block, epidural block, local anesthesia: Children >12 years: Refer to adult dosing.

Peripheral or sympathetic nerve block: Children >12 years: Refer to adult dosing.

Retrobulbar anesthesia: Children >12 years: Refer to adult dosing.

Administration

I.V. Detail: pH: 4.0-6.5

Other: Solutions containing preservatives should not be used for epidural or caudal blocks.

Stability

Compatibility: Stable in NS

Storage: Store at controlled room temperature of 15°C to 30°C (59°F to 86°F).

Nursing Actions

Physical Assessment: Assess other medications patient may be taking for additive or adverse interactions. Monitor for effectiveness of anesthesia and adverse reactions. Monitor for return of sensation. Teach patient adverse reactions to report; use and teach appropriate interventions to promote safety.

Patient Education: This medication is given to reduce sensation in the injected area. You will experience decreased sensation to pain, heat, or cold in the area

and/or decreased muscle strength (depending on area of application) until the effects wear off; use necessary caution to reduce incidence of possible injury until full sensation returns. If used in mouth, do not eat or drink until full sensation returns. Immediately report chest pain or palpitations; increased restlessness, anxiety, or dizziness; skeletal or muscle weakness; respiratory difficulty; ringing in ears; or vision changes. **Pregnancy/breast-feeding precautions:** Inform prescriber if you are pregnant. Do not breast-feed.

Pregnancy Issues Bupivacaine is approved for use at term in obstetrical anesthesia or analgesia. Bupivacaine 0.75% solutions have been associated with cardiac arrest following epidural anesthesia in obstetrical patients and use of this concentration is not recommended for this purpose. Use in obstetrical paracervical block anesthesia is contraindicated.

Buprenorphine (byoo pre NOR feen)

U.S. Brand Names Buprenex®; Subutex®

Synonyms Buprenorphine Hydrochloride

Restrictions Injection: C-V; Tablet: C-III

Prescribing of tablets for opioid dependence is limited to physicians who have met the qualification criteria and have received a DEA number specific to prescribing this product. Tablets will be available through pharmacies and wholesalers which normally provide controlled substances.

Pharmacologic Category Analgesic, Narcotic

Medication Safety Issues

Sound-alike/look-alike issues:

Buprenex® may be confused with Brevibloc®, Bumex®

Pregnancy Risk Factor C

Lactation Enters breast milk/not recommended

Use

Injection: Management of moderate to severe pain

Tablet: Treatment of opioid dependence

Unlabeled/Investigational Use Injection: Heroin and opioid withdrawal

Mechanism of Action/Effect Buprenorphine exerts its analgesic effect via high affinity binding to μ opiate receptors in the CNS; displays both agonist and antagonist activity

Contraindications Hypersensitivity to buprenorphine or any component of the formulation

Warnings/Precautions An opioid-containing analgesic regimen should be tailored to each patient's needs and based upon the type of pain being treated (acute versus chronic), the route of administration, degree of tolerance for opioids (naive versus chronic user), age, weight, and medical condition. The optimal analgesic dose varies widely among patients. Doses should be titrated to pain relief/prevention.

May cause CNS depression, which may impair physical or mental abilities. Effects with other sedative drugs or ethanol may be potentiated. Elderly may be more sensitive to CNS depressant and constipating effects. May cause respiratory depression - use caution in patients with respiratory disease or pre-existing respiratory depression. Potential for drug dependency exists, abrupt cessation may precipitate withdrawal. Use caution in elderly, debilitated, pediatric patients, depression or suicidal tendencies, or in patients with a history of drug abuse. Tolerance, psychological and physical dependence may occur with prolonged use. Partial antagonist activity may precipitate acute narcotic withdrawal in opioid-dependent individuals.

Use with caution in patients with hepatic, pulmonary, or renal function impairment. Also use caution in patients with head injury or increased ICP, biliary tract dysfunction, pancreatitis, patients with history of ileus or bowel (Continued)

Buprenorphine *(Continued)*

obstruction, glaucoma, hyperthyroidism, adrenal insufficiency, prostatic hyperplasia, urinary stricture, CNS depression, toxic psychosis, alcoholism, delirium tremens, or kyphoscoliosis.

Tablets, which are used for induction treatment of opioid dependence, should not be started until effects of withdrawal are evident.

Drug Interactions

Cytochrome P450 Effect: Substrate of CYP3A4 (major); **Inhibits** CYP1A2 (weak), 2A6 (weak), 2C19 (weak), 2D6 (weak)

Decreased Effect: CYP3A4 inducers may decrease the levels/effects of buprenorphine; example inducers include aminoglutethimide, carbamazepine, nafcillin, nevirapine, phenobarbital, phenytoin, and rifamycins. Naltrexone may antagonize the effect of narcotic analgesics; concurrent use or use within 7-10 days of injection for pain relief is contraindicated.

Increased Effect/Toxicity: Barbiturate anesthetics and other CNS depressants may produce additive respiratory and CNS depression. Respiratory and CV collapse was reported in a patient who received diazepam and buprenorphine. Effects may be additive with other CNS depressants. CYP3A4 inhibitors may increase the levels/effects of buprenorphine; example inhibitors include azole antifungals, clarithromycin, diclofenac, doxycycline, erythromycin, imatinib, isoniazid, nefazodone, nicardipine, propofol, protease inhibitors, quinidine, and verapamil.

Nutritional/Ethanol Interactions

Ethanol: Avoid ethanol (may increase CNS depression).
Herb/Nutraceutical: Avoid valerian, St John's wort, kava kava, gotu kola (may increase CNS depression).

Adverse Reactions

Injection:
>10%: Central nervous system: Sedation
1% to 10%:
Cardiovascular: Hypotension
Central nervous system: Respiratory depression, dizziness, headache
Gastrointestinal: Vomiting, nausea
Ocular: Miosis
Otic: Vertigo
Miscellaneous: Diaphoresis

Tablet:
>10%:
Central nervous system: Headache (30%), pain (24%), insomnia (21% to 25%), Oralety (12%), depression (11%)
Gastrointestinal: Nausea (10% to 14%), abdominal pain (12%), constipation (8% to 11%)
Neuromuscular & skeletal: Back pain (14%), weakness (14%)
Respiratory: Rhinitis (11%)
Miscellaneous: Withdrawal syndrome (19%; placebo 37%), infection (12% to 20%), diaphoresis (12% to 13%)
1% to 10%:
Central nervous system: Chills (6%), nervousness (6%), somnolence (5%), dizziness (4%), fever (3%)
Gastrointestinal: Vomiting (5% to 8%), diarrhea (5%), dyspepsia (3%)
Ocular: Lacrimation (5%)
Respiratory: Cough (4%), pharyngitis (4%)
Miscellaneous: Flu-like syndrome (6%)

Overdosage/Toxicology Symptoms of overdose include CNS depression, pinpoint pupils, hypotension, and bradycardia. Treatment is supportive. Naloxone may have limited effects in reversing respiratory depression; doxapram has also been used to stimulate respirations.

Pharmacodynamics/Kinetics

Onset of Action: Analgesic: 10-30 minutes
Duration of Action: 6-8 hours
Protein Binding: High
Half-Life Elimination: 2.2-3 hours
Metabolism: Primarily hepatic; extensive first-pass effect
Excretion: Feces (70%); urine (20% as unchanged drug)

Available Dosage Forms

Injection, solution (Buprenex®): 0.3 mg/mL (1 mL)
Tablet, sublingual (Subutex®): 2 mg, 8 mg
Additional dosage strength available in Canada: 0.4 mg

Dosing

Adults: Long-term use is not recommended
Note: These are guidelines and do not represent the maximum doses that may be required in all patients. Doses should be titrated to pain relief/prevention. In high-risk patients (eg, elderly, debilitated, presence of respiratory disease) and/or concurrent CNS depressant use, reduce dose by one-half. Buprenorphine has an analgesic ceiling.
Acute pain (moderate to severe):
I.M.: Initial: Opiate-naive: 0.3 mg every 6-8 hours as needed; initial dose (up to 0.3 mg) may be repeated once in 30-60 minutes after the initial dose if needed; usual dosage range: 0.15-0.6 mg every 4-8 hours as needed
Slow I.V.: Initial: Opiate-naive: 0.3 mg every 6-8 hours as needed; initial dose (up to 0.3 mg) may be repeated once in 30-60 minutes after the initial dose if needed
Heroin or opiate withdrawal (unlabeled use): I.M., slow I.V.: Variable; 0.1-0.4 mg every 6 hours
Opioid dependence: Sublingual:
Induction: Range: 12-16 mg/day (doses during an induction study used 8 mg on day 1, followed by 16 mg on day 2; induction continued over 3-4 days). Treatment should begin at least 4 hours after last use of heroin or short-acting opioid, preferably when first signs of withdrawal appear. Titrating dose to clinical effectiveness should be done as rapidly as possible to prevent undue withdrawal symptoms and patient drop-out during the induction period.
Maintenance: Target dose: 16 mg/day; range: 4-24 mg/day; patients should be switched to the buprenorphine/naloxone combination product for maintenance and unsupervised therapy
Elderly: Moderate to severe pain: I.M., slow I.V.: 0.15 mg every 6 hours; elderly patients are more likely to suffer from confusion and drowsiness compared to younger patients. **Long-term use is not recommended.**
Pediatrics:
Acute pain (moderate to severe):
Children 2-12 years: I.M., slow I.V.: 2-6 mcg/kg every 4-6 hours
Children ≥13 years: Refer to adult dosing.
Opioid dependence: Children ≥13 years: Refer to adult dosing.

Administration

Oral: Sublingual: Tablet should be placed under the tongue until dissolved; should not be swallowed. If two or more tablets are needed per dose, all may be placed under the tongue at once, or two at a time. To ensure consistent bioavailability, subsequent doses should always be taken the same way.
I.V.: Administer slowly, over at least 2 minutes.
I.V. Detail: pH: 3.5-5.5

Stability

Compatibility: Injection:
Y-site administration: Incompatible with amphotericin B cholesteryl sulfate complex, doxorubicin liposome

Compatibility when admixed: Incompatible with diazepam, floxacillin, furosemide, lorazepam

Storage:

Injection: Protect from excessive heat >40°C (>104°F) and light.

Tablet: Store at room temperature at 25°C (77°F).

Laboratory Monitoring LFTs

Nursing Actions

Physical Assessment: Assess other medications patient may be taking for possible additive or adverse interactions. Monitor for effectiveness of pain relief and monitor for signs of overdose (can cause respiratory depression). Monitor blood pressure, CNS and respiratory status, and degree of sedation at beginning of therapy and at regular intervals with long-term use. For inpatients, implement safety measures (eg, side rails up, call light within reach, instructions to call for assistance). Assess knowledge/teach patient appropriate use (if self-administered). Teach patient to monitor and report adverse reactions and appropriate interventions to reduce side effects.

Patient Education: If self-administered, use exactly as directed; do not increase dose or frequency. While using this medication, do not use alcohol and other prescription or OTC medications (especially sedatives, tranquilizers, antihistamines, or pain medications) without consulting prescriber. May cause dizziness, drowsiness, confusion, or blurred vision (use caution when driving, climbing stairs, rising from sitting or lying position, or engaging in tasks requiring alertness until response to drug is known). You may experience nausea or vomiting (frequent mouth care, small frequent meals, sucking lozenges, or chewing gum may help); or constipation (increased exercise, fluids, or dietary fruit and fiber may help). If constipation is unresolved, consult prescriber about use of stool softeners and/or laxatives. Report unresolved nausea or vomiting; respiratory difficulty or shortness of breath; excessive sedation or unusual weakness; or rapid heartbeat or palpitations. **Pregnancy/breast-feeding precautions:** Inform prescriber if you are or intend to become pregnant. Breast-feeding is not recommended.

Pregnancy Issues Withdrawal has been reported in infants of women receiving buprenorphine during pregnancy. Onset of symptoms ranged from day 1 to day 8 of life, most occurring on day 1.

Additional Information

Buprenorphine injection: 0.3 mg = 10 mg morphine or 75 mg meperidine, has longer duration of action than either agent

Subutex® (buprenorphine) should be limited to supervised use whenever possible; patients should be switched to Suboxone® (buprenorphine/naloxone) for maintenance and unsupervised therapy

---

Buprenorphine and Naloxone
(byoo pre NOR feen & nal OKS one)

U.S. Brand Names Suboxone®

Synonyms Buprenorphine Hydrochloride and Naloxone Hydrochloride Dihydrate; Naloxone and Buprenorphine; Naloxone Hydrochloride Dihydrate and Buprenorphine Hydrochloride

Restrictions C-III; Prescribing of tablets for opioid dependence is limited to physicians who have met the qualification criteria and have received a DEA number specific to prescribing this product. Tablets will be available through pharmacies and wholesalers which normally provide controlled substances.

Pharmacologic Category Analgesic, Narcotic

Pregnancy Risk Factor C

Lactation Buprenorphine: Enters breast milk/not recommended

Use Treatment of opioid dependence

Available Dosage Forms Tablet, sublingual: Buprenorphine 2 mg and naloxone 0.5 mg; buprenorphine 8 mg and naloxone 2 mg [lemon-lime flavor]

Dosing

Adults: Opioid dependence: Sublingual: **Note:** This combination product is not recommended for use during the induction period; initial treatment should begin using buprenorphine oral tablets. Patients should be switched to the combination product for maintenance and unsupervised therapy.

Maintenance: Target dose (based on buprenorphine content): 16 mg/day; range: 4-24 mg/day

Pediatrics: Opioid dependence: Children ≥16 years: Refer to adult dosing.

Nursing Actions

Physical Assessment: See individual agents.

Patient Education: If self-administered, use exactly as directed; do not increase dose or frequency. While using this medication, do not use alcohol, other prescriptions, or OTC medications (especially sedatives, tranquilizers, antihistamines, or pain medications) without consulting prescriber. May cause dizziness, drowsiness, confusion, or blurred vision (use caution when driving, climbing stairs, or changing position - rising from sitting or lying to standing, or when engaging in tasks requiring alertness until response to drug is known). You may experience nausea or vomiting (frequent mouth care, small frequent meals, sucking lozenges, or chewing gum may help); or constipation (increased exercise, fluids, or dietary fruit and fiber may help). If constipation is unresolved, consult prescriber about use of stool softeners and/or laxatives. Report unresolved nausea or vomiting; respiratory difficulty or shortness of breath; excessive sedation or unusual weakness; or rapid heartbeat or palpitations. In case of an emergency, notify prescriber and emergency room staff you are taking this medication. **Pregnancy/breast-feeding precautions:** Inform prescriber if you are or intend to become pregnant. Breast-feeding is not recommended.

Related Information

Buprenorphine *on page 173*
Naloxone *on page 860*

BuPROPion (byoo PROE pee on)

U.S. Brand Names Budeprion™ SR; Buproban™; Wellbutrin®; Wellbutrin SR®; Wellbutrin XL™; Zyban®

Restrictions A medication guide concerning the use of antidepressants in children and teenagers can be found on the FDA website at http://www.fda.gov/cder/Offices/ODS/labeling.htm. It should be dispensed to parents or guardians of children and teenagers receiving this medication.

Pharmacologic Category Antidepressant, Dopamine-Reuptake Inhibitor; Smoking Cessation Aid

Medication Safety Issues

Sound-alike/look-alike issues:

BuPROPion may be confused with busPIRone
Wellbutrin SR® may be confused with Wellbutrin XL™
Wellbutrin XL™ may be confused with Wellbutrin SR®
Zyban® may be confused with Zagam®

Pregnancy Risk Factor B

Lactation Enters breast milk/not recommended (AAP rates "of concern")

Use Treatment of depression; adjunct in smoking cessation

Unlabeled/Investigational Use Attention-deficit/hyperactivity disorder (ADHD)

Mechanism of Action/Effect Antidepressant structurally different from all other marketed antidepressants; (Continued)

BuPROPion (Continued)

like other antidepressants the mechanism of bupropion's activity is not fully understood; relatively weak inhibitor of the neuronal uptake of serotonin, norepinephrine, and dopamine

Contraindications Hypersensitivity to bupropion or any component of the formulation; seizure disorder; anorexia/bulimia; use of MAO inhibitors within 14 days; patients undergoing abrupt discontinuation of ethanol or sedatives (including benzodiazepines); patients receiving other dosage forms of bupropion

Warnings/Precautions Antidepressants increase the risk of suicidal thinking and behavior in children and adolescents with major depressive disorder (MDD) and other depressive disorders; consider risk prior to prescribing. All patients must be closely monitored for clinical worsening, suicidality, or unusual changes in behavior, especially during the initiation of therapy or following an increase or decrease in dosage. When used in children, the child's family or caregiver should be instructed to closely observe the patient and communicate condition with healthcare provider. A medication guide should be dispensed with each prescription. **Bupropion is not FDA approved for use in children.**

The possibility of a suicide attempt is inherent in major depression and may persist until remission occurs. Use caution in high-risk patients. Worsening depression and severe abrupt suicidality that are not part of the presenting symptoms may require discontinuation or modification of drug therapy. The patient's family or caregiver should be alerted to monitor patients for the emergence of suicidality and associated behaviors (such as agitation, irritability, hostility, impulsivity, and hypomania) and notify the healthcare provider.

May worsen psychosis in some patients or precipitate a shift to mania or hypomania in patients with bipolar disorder. Patients presenting with depressive symptoms should be screened for bipolar disorder. Monotherapy in patients with bipolar disorder should be avoided. **Bupropion is not FDA approved for bipolar depression.**

When using immediate release tablets, seizure risk is increased at total daily dosage >450 mg, individual dosages >150 mg, or by sudden, large increments in dose. Data for the immediate-release formulation of bupropion revealed a seizure incidence of 0.4% in patients treated at doses in the 300-450 mg/day range. The estimated seizure incidence increases almost 10-fold between 450 mg and 600 mg per day. Data for the sustained release dosage form revealed a seizure incidence of 0.1% in patients treated at a dosage range of 100-300 mg/day, and increases to ~0.4% at the maximum recommended dose of 400 mg/day. The risk of seizures is increased in patients with a history of seizures, anorexia/bulimia, head trauma, CNS tumor, severe hepatic cirrhosis, abrupt discontinuation of sedative-hypnotics or ethanol, medications which lower seizure threshold (antipsychotics, antidepressants, theophyllines, systemic steroids), stimulants, or hypoglycemic agents. Discontinue and do not restart in patients experiencing a seizure. May cause CNS stimulation (restlessness, anxiety, insomnia) or anorexia. May increase the risks associated with electroconvulsive therapy. Consider discontinuing, when possible, prior to elective surgery. May cause weight loss; use caution in patients where weight loss is not desirable. The incidence of sexual dysfunction with bupropion is generally lower than with SSRIs.

Use caution in patients with cardiovascular disease, history of hypertension, or coronary artery disease; treatment-emergent hypertension (including some severe cases) has been reported, both with bupropion alone and in combination with nicotine transdermal systems. Use with caution in patients with hepatic or renal dysfunction and in elderly patients. Elderly patients may be at greater risk of accumulation during chronic dosing. May cause motor or cognitive impairment in some patients; use with caution if tasks requiring alertness such as operating machinery or driving are undertaken. Arthralgia, myalgia, and fever with rash and other symptoms suggestive of delayed hypersensitivity resembling serum sickness reported.

Drug Interactions

Cytochrome P450 Effect: Substrate of CYP1A2 (minor), 2A6 (minor), 2B6 (major), 2C8/9 (minor), 2D6 (minor), 2E1 (minor), 3A4 (minor); **Inhibits** CYP2D6 (weak)

Decreased Effect: CYP2B6 inducers may decrease the levels/effects of bupropion; example inducers include carbamazepine, nevirapine, phenobarbital, phenytoin, and rifampin. Effect of warfarin may be altered by bupropion.

Increased Effect/Toxicity: Treatment-emergent hypertension may occur in patients treated with bupropion and nicotine patch. Cimetidine may inhibit the metabolism (increase clinical/adverse effects) of bupropion. Toxicity of bupropion is enhanced by levodopa and phenelzine (MAO inhibitors). Risk of seizures may be increased with agents that may lower seizure threshold (antipsychotics, antidepressants, theophylline, abrupt discontinuation of benzodiazepines, systemic steroids). Effect of warfarin may be altered by bupropion. Concurrent use with amantadine appears to result in a higher incidence of adverse effects; use caution. CYP2B6 inhibitors may increase the levels/effects of bupropion; example inhibitors include desipramine, paroxetine, and sertraline. Combined use of CYP2B6 inhibitors (orphenadrine, thiotepa, cyclophosphamide) with bupropion may increase serum concentrations and may result in seizures.

Nutritional/Ethanol Interactions

Ethanol: Ethanol (may increase CNS depression).

Herb/Nutraceutical: Avoid valerian, St John's wort, SAMe, gotu kola, kava kava (may increase CNS depression).

Lab Interactions Decreased prolactin levels

Adverse Reactions Frequencies, when reported, reflect highest incidence reported with sustained release product.

>10%:

Central nervous system: Dizziness (11%), headache (25%), insomnia (16%)

Gastrointestinal: Nausea (18%), xerostomia (24%)

Respiratory: Pharyngitis (11%)

1% to 10%:

Cardiovascular: Arrhythmias, chest pain (4%), flushing, hypertension (may be severe), hypotension, palpitation (5%), syncope, tachycardia

Central nervous system: Agitation (9%), anxiety (6%), confusion, depression, euphoria, hostility, irritability (2%), memory decreased (3%), migraine, nervousness (3%), sleep disturbance, somnolence (3%)

Dermatologic: Pruritus (4%), rash (4%), sweating increased (5%), urticaria (1%)

Endocrine & metabolic: Hot flashes, libido decreased, menstrual complaints

Gastrointestinal: Abdominal pain, anorexia (3%), appetite increased, constipation (5%), diarrhea (7%), dyspepsia, dysphagia (2%), taste perversion (4%), vomiting (2%)

Genitourinary: Urinary frequency (5%)

Neuromuscular & skeletal: Arthralgia (4%), arthritis (2%), myalgia (6%), neck pain, paresthesia (2%), tremor (3%), twitching (2%)

Ocular: Amblyopia (2%), blurred vision

Otic: Auditory disturbance, tinnitus (6%)

Respiratory: Cough increased (2%), sinusitis (1%)

Miscellaneous: Allergic reaction (including anaphylaxis, pruritus, urticaria), infection

Overdosage/Toxicology

Symptoms of overdose include labored breathing, salivation, ataxia, and convulsions. Dialysis may be of limited value after drug absorption because of slow tissue-to-plasma diffusion. Treatment is symptomatic and supportive.

Pharmacodynamics/Kinetics

Time to Peak: Bupropion: Serum: ~3 hours; Bupropion extended release: Serum: ~5 hours
Metabolites (hydroxybupropion, erythrohydrobupropion, threohydrobupropion): 6 hours

Protein Binding: 82% to 88%

Half-Life Elimination: Half-life:
Distribution: 3-4 hours
Elimination: 21 ± 9 hours; Metabolites: Hydroxybupropion: 20 ± 5 hours; Erythrohydrobupropion: 33 ± 10 hours; Threohydrobupropion: 37 ± 13 hours

Metabolism: Extensively hepatic to 3 active metabolites: Hydroxybupropion, erythrohydrobupropion, threohydrobupropion (metabolite activity ranges from $\frac{1}{5}$ to $\frac{1}{2}$ potency of bupropion)

Excretion: Urine (87%); feces (10%)

Available Dosage Forms

Tablet, as hydrochloride (Wellbutrin®): 75 mg, 100 mg
Tablet, extended release, as hydrochloride:
Budeprion™ SR: 100 mg [contains tartrazine; equivalent to Wellbutrin® SR], 150 mg [equivalent to Wellbutrin® SR]
Buproban™: 150 mg [equivalent to Zyban®]
Wellbutrin XL™: 150 mg, 300 mg
Tablet, sustained release, as hydrochloride: 100 mg, 150 mg [equivalent to Wellbutrin® SR], 150 mg [equivalent to Zyban®]
Wellbutrin® SR: 100 mg, 150 mg, 200 mg
Zyban®: 150 mg

Dosing

Adults:

Depression: Oral:
Immediate release: 100 mg 3 times/day; begin at 100 mg twice daily; may increase to a maximum dose of 450 mg/day.
Sustained release: Initial: 150 mg/day in the morning; may increase to 150 mg twice daily by day 4 if tolerated; target dose: 300 mg/day given as 150 mg twice daily; maximum dose: 400 mg/day given as 200 mg twice daily.
Extended release: Initial: 150 mg/day in the morning; may increase as early as day 4 of dosing to 300 mg/day; maximum dose: 450 mg/day

Smoking cessation (Zyban®): Oral: Initiate with 150 mg once daily for 3 days; increase to 150 mg twice daily; treatment should continue for 7-12 weeks.

Elderly:

Depression: Oral: Initial: 37.5 mg of immediate release tablets twice daily or 100 mg/day of sustained release tablets; increase by 37.5-100 mg every 3-4 days as tolerated. **Note:** There is evidence that the elderly respond at 150 mg/day in divided doses, but some may require a higher dose.
Smoking cessation: Refer to adult dosing.

Pediatrics: ADHD (unlabeled use): Oral: Children and Adolescents: 1.4-6 mg/kg/day

Renal Impairment: Effect of renal disease on bupropion's pharmacokinetics has not been studied; elimination of the major metabolites of bupropion may be affected by reduced renal function. Patients with renal failure should receive a reduced dosage initially and be closely monitored.

Hepatic Impairment:

Mild-to-moderate hepatic impairment: Use with caution and/or reduced dose/frequency
Severe hepatic cirrhosis: Use with extreme caution; maximum dose:
Wellbutrin®: 75 mg/day;
Wellbutrin SR®: 100 mg/day or 150 mg every other day

Wellbutrin XL™: 150 mg every other day
Zyban®: 150 mg every other day
Note: The mean AUC increased by ~1.5-fold for hydroxybupropion and ~2.5-fold for erythro/threohydrobupropion; median T_{max} was observed 19 hours later for hydroxybupropion, 31 hours later for erythro/threohydrobupropion; mean half-life for hydroxybupropion increased fivefold, and increased twofold for erythro/threohydrobupropion in patients with severe hepatic cirrhosis compared to healthy volunteers.

Administration

Oral: May be taken without regard to meals. Zyban® and extended release tablets should be swallowed whole; do not crush, chew, or divide. The insoluble shell of the extended-release tablet may remain intact during GI transit and is eliminated in the feces. Wellbutrin® SR may be divided, but not crushed or chewed.

Stability

Storage: Store at controlled of 20°C to 25°C (68°F to 77°F).

Nursing Actions

Physical Assessment: Assess other medications patient may be taking for effectiveness and interactions. Monitor therapeutic response, and adverse reactions at beginning of therapy and periodically with long-term use. Monitor for clinical worsening and suicidality, especially at the beginning of therapy or when dose changes occur. Taper dosage slowly when discontinuing. Assess knowledge/teach patient appropriate use, interventions to reduce side effects, and adverse symptoms to report.

Patient Education: Be aware that bupropion is marketed under different names and should not be taken together; Zyban® is for smoking cessation and Wellbutrin® is for treatment of depression. **Note:** Excessive use or abrupt discontinuation of alcohol or sedatives may alter seizure threshold.

Depression: Take as directed, in equally divided doses; do not take in larger dose or more often than recommended. Do not discontinue this medicine without consulting prescriber. Do not use alcohol or OTC medications not approved by prescriber. May cause drowsiness, clouded sensorium, headache, restlessness, or agitation (use caution when driving or engaging in tasks requiring alertness until response to drug is known); nausea, vomiting, or dry mouth (small, frequent meals, frequent mouth care, chewing gum, or sucking lozenges may help); constipation (increased exercise, fluids, fruit, or fiber may help); or impotence (reversible). Report persistent CNS effects (eg, agitation, confusion, anxiety, restlessness, insomnia, psychosis, hallucinations, seizures); suicidal ideation; muscle weakness or tremor; skin rash or irritation; chest pain or palpitations, abdominal pain or blood in stools; yellowing of skin or eyes; or respiratory difficulty, bronchitis, or unusual cough.

Smoking cessation: Use as directed; do not take extra doses. Do not combine nicotine patches with use of Zyban® unless approved by prescriber. May cause dry mouth and insomnia (these may resolve with continued use). Report any respiratory difficulty, unusual cough, dizziness, or muscle tremors.

Breast-feeding precaution: Breast-feeding is not recommended.

Geriatric Considerations Limited data is available about the use of bupropion in the elderly. Two studies have found it equally effective when compared to imipramine. Its side effect profile (minimal anticholinergic and blood pressure effects) may make it useful in persons who do not tolerate traditional cyclic antidepressants.

Breast-Feeding Issues Generally, it is not recommended to breast-feed if taking antidepressants
(Continued)

BuPROPion *(Continued)*

because of the long half-life, active metabolites, and the potential for side effects in the infant.

Related Information
Antidepressant Medication Guidelines *on page 1414*
FDA Name Differentiation Project: The Use of Tall-Man Letters *on page 12*

BusPIRone *(byoo SPYE rone)*

U.S. Brand Names BuSpar®
Synonyms Buspirone Hydrochloride
Pharmacologic Category Antianxiety Agent, Miscellaneous
Medication Safety Issues
Sound-alike/look-alike issues:
BusPIRone may be confused with buPROPion
Pregnancy Risk Factor B
Lactation Excretion in breast milk unknown/not recommended
Use Management of generalized anxiety disorder (GAD)
Unlabeled/Investigational Use Management of aggression in mental retardation and secondary mental disorders; major depression; potential augmenting agent for antidepressants; premenstrual syndrome
Mechanism of Action/Effect The mechanism of action of buspirone is unknown. Buspirone has a high affinity for serotonin $5\text{-}HT_{1A}$ and $5\text{-}HT_2$ receptors, without affecting benzodiazepine-GABA receptors. Buspirone has moderate affinity for dopamine D_2 receptors.
Contraindications Hypersensitivity to buspirone or any component of the formulation
Warnings/Precautions Use in hepatic or renal impairment is not recommended; does not prevent or treat withdrawal from benzodiazepines. Low potential for cognitive or motor impairment. Use with MAO inhibitors may result in hypertensive reactions.

Drug Interactions
Cytochrome P450 Effect: Substrate of CYP2D6 (minor), 3A4 (major)
Decreased Effect: CYP3A4 inducers may decrease the levels/effects of buspirone; example inducers include aminoglutethimide, carbamazepine, nafcillin, nevirapine, phenobarbital, phenytoin, and rifamycins.
Increased Effect/Toxicity: Concurrent use of buspirone with SSRIs or trazodone may cause serotonin syndrome. Buspirone should not be used concurrently with an MAO inhibitor due to reports of increased blood pressure; theoretically, a selective MAO type B inhibitors (selegiline) has a lower risk of this reaction. Concurrent use of buspirone with nefazodone may increase risk of CNS adverse events; limit buspirone initial dose (eg, 2.5 mg/day). CYP3A4 inhibitors may increase the levels/effects of buspirone; example inhibitors include azole antifungals, clarithromycin, diclofenac, doxycycline, erythromycin, imatinib, isoniazid, nefazodone, nicardipine, propofol, protease inhibitors, quinidine, telithromycin, and verapamil.
Nutritional/Ethanol Interactions
Ethanol: Ethanol (may increase CNS depression).
Food: Food may decrease the absorption of buspirone, but it may also decrease the first-pass metabolism, thereby increasing the bioavailability of buspirone. Grapefruit juice may cause increased buspirone concentrations; avoid concurrent use.
Herb/Nutraceutical: St John's wort may decrease buspirone levels or increase CNS depression. Avoid valerian, gotu kola, kava kava (may increase CNS depression).
Lab Interactions Increased AST, ALT, growth hormone(s), prolactin (S)
Adverse Reactions
>10%: Central nervous system: Dizziness

1% to 10%:
Central nervous system: Drowsiness, EPS, serotonin syndrome, confusion, nervousness, lightheadedness, excitement, anger, hostility, headache
Dermatologic: Rash
Gastrointestinal: Diarrhea, nausea
Neuromuscular & skeletal: Muscle weakness, numbness, paresthesia, incoordination, tremor
Ocular: Blurred vision, tunnel vision
Miscellaneous: Diaphoresis, allergic reactions
Overdosage/Toxicology Symptoms of overdose include dizziness, drowsiness, pinpoint pupils, nausea, and vomiting. There is no known antidote for buspirone. Treatment is supportive.
Pharmacodynamics/Kinetics
Time to Peak: Serum: Within 0.7-1.5 hours
Protein Binding: 95%
Half-Life Elimination: Mean: 2.4 hours (range: 2-11 hours)
Metabolism: Hepatic via oxidation; extensive first-pass effect
Excretion: Urine: 65%; feces: 35%; ~1% dose excreted unchanged
Available Dosage Forms
Tablet, as hydrochloride: 5 mg, 7.5 mg, 10 mg, 15 mg, 30 mg
BuSpar®: 5 mg, 10 mg, 15 mg, 30 mg
Dosing
Adults: Anxiety disorders (GAD): Oral: 15 mg/day (7.5 mg twice daily); may increase in increments of 5 mg/day every 2-4 days to a maximum of 60 mg/day. Target dose for most people is 30 mg/day (15 mg twice daily).
Elderly: Oral: Initial: 5 mg twice daily, increase by 5 mg/day every 2-3 days as needed up to 20-30 mg/day; maximum daily dose: 60 mg/day (see Geriatric Considerations).
Pediatrics:
Generalized anxiety disorder (GAD): Children and Adolescents: Oral: Initial: 5 mg daily; increase in increments of 5 mg/day at weekly intervals as needed, to a maximum dose of 60 mg/day divided into 2-3 doses
Renal Impairment: Use in patients with severe renal impairment cannot be recommended.
Hepatic Impairment: Buspirone is metabolized by the liver and excreted by the kidneys. Patients with impaired hepatic or renal function demonstrated increased plasma levels and a prolonged half-life of buspirone. Therefore, use in patients with severe hepatic or renal impairment cannot be recommended.
Nursing Actions
Physical Assessment: Assess other medications patient may be taking for effectiveness and interactions. Monitor therapeutic response and adverse reactions at beginning of therapy and periodically with long-term use. Assess knowledge/teach patient appropriate use, interventions to reduce side effects, and adverse symptoms to report.
Patient Education: Take only as directed; do not increase dose or take more often than prescribed. May take 2-3 weeks to see full effect; do not discontinue this medicine without consulting prescriber. Do not use alcohol or other prescription or OTC medications (especially pain medications, sedatives, antihistamines, or hypnotics) without consulting prescriber. Maintain adequate hydration (2-3 L/day of fluids) unless instructed to restrict fluid intake. You may experience drowsiness, lightheadedness, impaired coordination, dizziness, or blurred vision (use caution when driving or engaging in tasks requiring alertness until response to drug is known); or upset stomach, nausea (small frequent meals, frequent mouth care, chewing gum, or sucking lozenges may help). Report persistent vomiting; chest pain or rapid heartbeat; persistent CNS effects (eg, confusion, restlessness,

anxiety, insomnia, excitation, headache, dizziness, fatigue, impaired coordination); or worsening of condition. **Breast-feeding precaution:** Breast-feeding is not recommended.

Geriatric Considerations Because buspirone is less sedating than other anxiolytics, it may be a useful agent in geriatric patients when an anxiolytic is indicated.

Additional Information Has shown little potential for abuse; needs continuous use. Because of slow onset, not appropriate for "as needed" (prn) use or for brief, situational anxiety. Ineffective for treatment of benzodiazepine or ethanol withdrawal.

Related Information
FDA Name Differentiation Project: The Use of Tall-Man Letters *on page 12*

Busulfan (byoo SUL fan)

U.S. Brand Names Busulfex®; Myleran®
Pharmacologic Category Antineoplastic Agent, Alkylating Agent
Medication Safety Issues
Sound-alike/look-alike issues:
Busulfan may be confused with Butalan®
Myleran® may be confused with melphalan, Mylicon®
Pregnancy Risk Factor D
Lactation Contraindicated
Use
Oral: Chronic myelogenous leukemia; conditioning regimens for bone marrow transplantation
I.V.: Combination therapy with cyclophosphamide as a conditioning regimen prior to allogeneic hematopoietic progenitor cell transplantation for chronic myelogenous leukemia
Unlabeled/Investigational Use Oral: Bone marrow disorders, such as polycythemia vera and myeloid metaplasia; thrombocytosis
Mechanism of Action/Effect Interferes with DNA function; cytotoxic
Contraindications Hypersensitivity to busulfan or any component of the formulation; failure to respond to previous courses; pregnancy
Warnings/Precautions Hazardous agent — use appropriate precautions for handling and disposal. May induce severe bone marrow hypoplasia. Use caution in patients predisposed to seizures. Discontinue if lung toxicity develops. Busulfan has been causally related to the development of secondary malignancies (tumors and acute leukemias). Busulfan has been associated with ovarian failure (including failure to achieve puberty) in females. High busulfan area under the concentration versus time curve (AUC) values (>1500 µM/minute) are associated with increased risk of hepatic veno-occlusive disease during conditioning for allogenic BMT.

Drug Interactions
Cytochrome P450 Effect: Substrate of CYP3A4 (major)
Decreased Effect: CYP3A4 inducers may decrease the levels/effects of busulfan; example inducers include aminoglutethimide, carbamazepine, nafcillin, nevirapine, phenobarbital, phenytoin, and rifamycins.
Increased Effect/Toxicity: CYP3A4 inhibitors may increase the levels/effects of busulfan; example inhibitors include azole antifungals, clarithromycin, diclofenac, doxycycline, erythromycin, imatinib, isoniazid, nefazodone, nicardipine, propofol, protease inhibitors, quinidine, telithromycin, and verapamil. Metronidazole may increase busulfan plasma levels. Pulmonary toxicity of other cytotoxic agents may be additive.
Nutritional/Ethanol Interactions
Ethanol: Avoid ethanol due to GI irritation.
Food: No clear or firm data on the effect of food on busulfan bioavailability.

Herb/Nutraceutical: St John's wort may decrease busulfan levels.
Adverse Reactions
>10%: Hematologic: Severe pancytopenia, leukopenia, thrombocytopenia, anemia, and bone marrow suppression
Myelosuppressive:
WBC: Moderate
Platelets: Moderate
Onset: 7-10 days
Nadir: 14-21 days
Recovery: 28 days
1% to 10%:
Dermatologic: Hyperpigmentation skin (busulfan tan), urticaria, erythema, alopecia
Endocrine & metabolic: Amenorrhea
Gastrointestinal: Nausea, vomiting, diarrhea; drug has little effect on the GI mucosal lining
Neuromuscular & skeletal: Weakness
Overdosage/Toxicology Symptoms of overdose include leukopenia and thrombocytopenia. Induction of vomiting or gastric lavage is indicated for recent ingestion; the effects of dialysis are unknown.
Pharmacodynamics/Kinetics
Duration of Action: 28 days
Time to Peak: Serum: Oral: Within 4 hours; I.V.: Within 5 minutes
Protein Binding: ~14%
Half-Life Elimination: After first dose: 3.4 hours; After last dose: 2.3 hours
Metabolism: Extensively hepatic (may increase with multiple dosing)
Excretion: Urine (10% to 50% as metabolites) within 24 hours (<2% as unchanged drug)
Available Dosage Forms
Injection, solution (Busulfex®): 6 mg/mL (10 mL)
Tablet (Myleran®): 2 mg
Dosing
Adults:
CML remission induction: Oral: 4-8 mg/day (may be as high as 12 mg/day); Maintenance doses: 1-4 mg/day to 2 mg/week to maintain WBC 10,000-20,000 cells/mm^3
BMT marrow-ablative conditioning regimen:
Oral: 1 mg/kg/dose (ideal body weight) every 6 hours for 16 doses
I.V.: 0.8 mg/kg (ideal body weight or actual body weight, whichever is lower) every 6 hours for 4 days (a total of 16 doses)
Polycythemia vera (unlabeled use): Oral: 2-6 mg/day
Thrombocytosis (unlabeled use): Oral: 4-6 mg/day
Elderly: Oral (refer to individual protocols): Start with lowest recommended doses for adults.
Pediatrics:
CML remission: Oral: Induction: 0.06-0.12 mg/kg/day or 1.8-4.6 mg/m^2/day; titrate dosage to maintain leukocyte count above 40,000/mm^3; reduce dosage by 50% if the leukocyte count reaches 30,000-40,000/mm^3; discontinue drug if counts fall to ≤20,000/mm^3.
BMT marrow-ablative conditioning regimen:
Oral: 1 mg/kg/dose (ideal body weight) every 6 hours for 16 doses
I.V.:
≤12 kg: 1.1 mg/kg/dose (ideal body weight) every 6 hours for 16 doses
>12 kg: 0.8 mg/kg/dose (ideal body weight) every 6 hours for 16 doses
Adjust dose to desired AUC [1125 µmol(min)] using the following formula:
Adjusted dose (mg) = Actual dose (mg) x [target AUC µmol(min) / actual AUC µmol(min)]
Administration
Oral: BMT only: To facilitate ingestion of high oral doses, insert multiple tablets into gelatin capsules.
(Continued)

Busulfan *(Continued)*

I.V.: Intravenous busulfan should be administered as a 2-hour infusion, every 6 hours for 4 consecutive days for a total of 16 doses.

Stability

Reconstitution: Dilute (using manufacturer provided filters) in 0.9% sodium chloride injection or dextrose 5% in water. The dilution volume of busulfan injection, ensuring that the final concentration of busulfan is 0.5 mg/mL.

Storage: Store unopened ampuls (injection) under refrigeration (2°C to 8°C). Final solution is stable for up to 8 hours at room temperature (25°C) but the infusion must also be completed within that 8-hour timeframe. Dilution of busulfan injection in 0.9% sodium chloride is stable for up to 12 hours at refrigeration (2°C to 8°C), but the infusion must also be completed within that 12-hour timeframe.

Laboratory Monitoring CBC with differential and platelet count, liver function

Nursing Actions

Physical Assessment: Assess other pharmacological or herbal products patient may be taking for potential interactions (eg, anything that may increase or decrease levels/effects of busulfan). Dosing should be based on adjusted ideal body weight (refer to individual protocols). BMT: Phenytoin or clonazepam should be administered prophylactically during and for at least 48 hours following completion of busulfan to reduce risk of seizures. Monitor laboratory tests (CBC with differential, platelet count, LFTs), adverse effects (eg, pulmonary fibrosis, fever, cough, difficulty breathing), or hematologic effects (bleeding or easy bruising, uricemia, black stools), anemia (fatigue, loss of appetite, pale skin), and leukopenia (infection) during therapy and for several months following therapy. Teach patient proper use (oral), possible side effects/appropriate interventions, and adverse symptoms to report.

Patient Education: Do not take any new medication during therapy unless approved by prescriber. Take oral medication as directed with chilled liquids. Maintain adequate hydration (2-3 L/day of fluids) unless instructed to restrict fluid intake. Avoid alcohol and acidic or spicy foods. You will be more susceptible to infection (avoid crowds and exposure to infection and do not have any vaccinations unless approved by prescriber). May cause mouth sores (brush teeth with soft toothbrush or cotton swab); loss of hair or darkening of skin color (reversible when medication is discontinued); nausea, vomiting, or anorexia (small, frequent meals, chewing gum, or sucking hard candy may help); constipation (increased exercise, fruit, fluids, or fiber may help); amenorrhea; sterility; or skin rash. Report palpitations or chest pain, excessive dizziness, confusion, respiratory difficulty, numbness or tingling of extremities, unusual bruising or bleeding, pain or changes in urination, or other adverse effects. **Pregnancy/breast-feeding precautions:** Inform prescriber if you are pregnant. Do not get pregnant during or for 1 month following therapy. Consult prescriber for instruction on appropriate barrier contraceptive measures. This drug may cause severe fetal defects. Do not breast-feed.

Geriatric Considerations Toxicity to immunosuppressives is increased in the elderly. Start with lowest recommended adult doses. Signs of infection, such as fever and rise in WBCs, may not occur. Lethargy and confusion may be more prominent signs of infection.

Butalbital, Acetaminophen, and Caffeine
(byoo TAL bi tal, a seet a MIN oh fen, & KAF een)

U.S. Brand Names Anolor 300; Dolgic® LQ; Dolgic® Plus; Esgic®; Esgic-Plus™; Fioricet®; Medigesic®; Repan®; Zebutal™

Synonyms Acetaminophen, Butalbital, and Caffeine

Pharmacologic Category Barbiturate

Pregnancy Risk Factor C

Lactation Enters breast milk/not recommended

Use Relief of the symptomatic complex of tension or muscle contraction headache

Available Dosage Forms

Capsule:

Anolor 300, Esgic®, Medigesic®: Butalbital 50 mg, caffeine 40 mg, and acetaminophen 325 mg

Dolgic® Plus: Butalbital 50 mg, caffeine 40 mg, and acetaminophen 750 mg

Esgic-Plus™, Zebutal™: Butalbital 50 mg, caffeine 40 mg, and acetaminophen 500 mg

Elixir (Dolgic® LQ): Butalbital 50 mg, caffeine 40 mg, and acetaminophen 325 mg per 15 mL (480 mL) [contains alcohol 7%; fruit flavor]

Tablet: Butalbital 50 mg, caffeine 40 mg, and acetaminophen 325 mg; butalbital 50 mg, caffeine 40 mg, and acetaminophen 500 mg

Esgic®, Fioricet®, Repan®: Butalbital 50 mg, caffeine 40 mg, and acetaminophen 325 mg

Dosing

Adults: Tension or muscle contraction headache: Oral: 1-2 tablets or capsules (or 15-30 mL elixir) every 4 hours; not to exceed 6 tablets or capsules (or 180 mL elixir) daily

Elderly: Not recommended for use in the elderly.

Renal Impairment: Dosage should be reduced.

Hepatic Impairment: Dosage should be reduced.

Nursing Actions

Physical Assessment: Assess patient for history of liver disease or ethanol abuse (acetaminophen and excessive ethanol may have adverse liver effects). Assess other medications patient may be taking for additive or adverse interactions. Monitor therapeutic effectiveness. Assess knowledge/teach patient appropriate use, adverse reactions to report, and appropriate interventions to reduce side effects.

Patient Education: If self-administered, use exactly as directed; do not increase dose or frequency. Drug may cause physical and/or psychological dependence. Take with food or milk. While using this medication, do not use alcohol and other prescription or OTC medications (especially sedatives, tranquilizers, antihistamines, or pain medications) without consulting prescriber. Maintain adequate hydration (2-3 L/day of fluids) unless instructed to restrict fluid intake. May cause dizziness, lightheadedness, confusion, or drowsiness (use caution when driving, climbing stairs, or changing position - rising from sitting or lying to standing, or when engaging in tasks requiring alertness until response to drug is known); heartburn or epigastric discomfort (frequent mouth care, frequent sips of fluids, chewing gum, or sucking lozenges may help); or constipation (increased exercise, fluids, fruit, or fiber may help). Report chest pain or palpitations; persistent dizziness; confusion; nightmares, excitation, or changes in mentation; shortness of breath or respiratory difficulty; skin rash; unusual bleeding or bruising; or unusual fatigue and weakness.

Related Information

Acetaminophen *on page 30*

Butalbital, Acetaminophen, Caffeine, and Codeine

(byoo TAL bi tal, a seet a MIN oh fen, KAF een, & KOE deen)

U.S. Brand Names Fioricet® with Codeine

Synonyms Acetaminophen, Caffeine, Codeine, and Butalbital; Caffeine, Acetaminophen, Butalbital, and Codeine; Codeine, Acetaminophen, Butalbital, and Caffeine

Restrictions C-III

Pharmacologic Category Analgesic Combination (Narcotic); Barbiturate

Pregnancy Risk Factor C (per manufacturer); D (prolonged use or high doses at term)

Lactation Enters breast milk/not recommended

Use Relief of symptoms of complex tension (muscle contraction) headache

Available Dosage Forms Capsule: Butalbital 50 mg, caffeine 40 mg, acetaminophen 325 mg, and codeine phosphate 30 mg

Dosing

Adults & Elderly: Oral: Adults: 1-2 capsules every 4 hours. Total daily dosage should not exceed 6 capsules.

Hepatic Impairment: Use with caution. Limited, low-dose therapy usually well tolerated in hepatic disease/cirrhosis. However, cases of hepatotoxicity at daily acetaminophen dosages <4 g/day have been reported. Avoid chronic use in hepatic impairment.

Nursing Actions

Physical Assessment: Assess effectiveness and interactions of other prescriptions, OTC medications, or herbal products patient may be taking. Assess history for allergies to butalbital, codeine, barbiturates, or acetaminophen. Monitor for effectiveness of therapy, signs of overdose, and adverse reactions. Dosage should be discontinued slowly after long-term use. For inpatient use, implement safety precautions. Teach patient proper use, appropriate interventions to reduce side effects, and adverse symptoms to report.

Patient Education: Do not take any new medication during therapy unless approved by prescriber. Take oral medication as directed with chilled liquids. Use exactly as directed; do not increase dose or frequency. Drug may cause physical and/or psychological dependence. Take with food or milk. Do not use alcohol, other prescriptions, OTC medications, or herbal products (especially sedatives, tranquilizers, antihistamines, or pain medications) without consulting prescriber. Maintain adequate hydration (2-3 L/day of fluids) unless instructed to restrict fluid intake. May cause dizziness, lightheadedness, confusion, or drowsiness (use caution when driving, climbing stairs, or changing position sitting or lying to standing, or when engaging in tasks requiring alertness until response to drug is known); heartburn, nausea (small, frequent meals, frequent mouth care, chewing gum, or sucking lozenges may help); or constipation (increased exercise, fluids, fruit, or fiber may help; if unresolved, contact prescriber). Report chest pain or palpitation; persistent dizziness; confusion; nightmares; excitation or changes in mentation; shortness of breath or respiratory difficulty; skin rash or irritation; unusual muscle weakness or leg pain; or ringing in ears. **Pregnancy/breast-feeding precautions:** Inform prescriber if you are or intend to become pregnant. Breast-feeding is not recommended.

Related Information

Acetaminophen on page 30
Codeine on page 296

Butalbital, Aspirin, and Caffeine

(byoo TAL bi tal, AS pir in, & KAF een)

U.S. Brand Names Fiorinal®

Synonyms Aspirin, Caffeine, and Butalbital; Butalbital Compound

Restrictions C-III

Pharmacologic Category Barbiturate

Pregnancy Risk Factor C/D (prolonged use or high doses at term)

Lactation Enters breast milk/use caution due to aspirin content

Use Relief of the symptomatic complex of tension or muscle contraction headache

Available Dosage Forms Capsule: Butalbital 50 mg, caffeine 40 mg, and aspirin 325 mg

Dosing

Adults: Tension or muscle contraction headache: Oral: 1-2 tablets or capsules every 4 hours; not to exceed 6 tablets or capsules/day

Elderly: Not recommended for use in the elderly.

Renal Impairment: Dosage should be reduced.

Hepatic Impairment: Dosage should be reduced.

Nursing Actions

Physical Assessment: Monitor for effectiveness of pain relief. Monitor CNS status, heart rate, blood pressure, fluid balance (I & O), and elimination regularly. Combination drug contains aspirin; assess for aspirin sensitivity.

Patient Education: Take as directed; do not exceed prescribed amount. Avoid alcohol, aspirin or aspirin-containing medications, or any OTC medications unless approved by prescriber. Maintain adequate hydration to prevent constipation (2-3 L/day) unless instructed to restrict fluid intake. You may experience drowsiness, impaired judgment or coordination; use caution when driving or engaging in tasks that require alertness until response to drug is known. Small frequent meals may help reduce GI upset. Report any ringing in ears; abdominal pain; easy bruising or bleeding; blood in urine; severe weakness; acute unresolved dizziness or confusion; nervousness, nightmares, insomnia; or skin rash. **Pregnancy/breast-feeding precautions:** Inform prescriber if you are or intend to become pregnant. Consult prescriber if breast-feeding.

Related Information

Aspirin on page 114

Butalbital, Aspirin, Caffeine, and Codeine

(byoo TAL bi tal, AS pir in, KAF een, & KOE deen)

U.S. Brand Names Fiorinal® With Codeine; Phrenilin® With Caffeine and Codeine

Synonyms Aspirin, Caffeine, Codeine, and Butalbital; Butalbital Compound and Codeine; Codeine and Butalbital Compound; Codeine, Butalbital, Aspirin, and Caffeine

Restrictions C-III

Pharmacologic Category Analgesic Combination (Narcotic); Barbiturate

Pregnancy Risk Factor C/D (prolonged use or high doses at term)

Lactation Excretion in breast milk unknown/use caution

Use Mild-to-moderate pain when sedation is needed

Available Dosage Forms

Capsule: Butalbital 50 mg, caffeine 40 mg, aspirin 325 mg, and codeine phosphate 30 mg

Fioricet® with Codeine: Butalbital 50 mg, caffeine 40 mg, acetaminophen 325 mg, and codeine phosphate 30 mg [may contain benzyl alcohol]

(Continued)

Butalbital, Aspirin, Caffeine, and Codeine *(Continued)*

Phrenilin® with Caffeine and Codeine: Butalbital 50 mg, caffeine 40 mg, acetaminophen 325 mg, and codeine phosphate 30 mg [contains benzyl alcohol and lactose]

Dosing

Adults: Mild-to-moderate pain (sedation desired): Oral: 1-2 capsules every 4 hours as needed; up to 6 capsules/day

Elderly: Not recommended for use in the elderly.

Nursing Actions

Physical Assessment: Do not use for persons with allergic reaction to aspirin, opium, or codeine. Assess other medications patient may be taking for additive or adverse interactions. Monitor vital signs, effectiveness of pain relief, signs of overdose, and adverse reactions especially gastrointestinal bleeding at beginning of therapy and at regular intervals with long-term use. May cause physical and/or psychological dependence. Discontinue slowly after long-term use. For inpatients, implement safety measures (eg, side rails up, call light within reach, instructions to call for assistance). Assess knowledge/teach patient appropriate use if self-administered. Teach patient to monitor for adverse reactions, adverse reactions to report, and appropriate interventions to reduce side effects.

Patient Education: If self-administered, use exactly as directed; do not increase dose or frequency. Drug may cause physical and/or psychological dependence. Take with food or milk. While using this medication, do not use alcohol and other prescription or OTC medications (especially sedatives, tranquilizers, antihistamines, or pain medications) without consulting prescriber. Maintain adequate hydration (2-3 L/day of fluids) unless instructed to restrict fluid intake. May cause dizziness, lightheadedness, confusion, or drowsiness (use caution when driving, climbing stairs, or changing position - rising from sitting or lying to standing, or when engaging in tasks requiring alertness until response to drug is known); heartburn or epigastric discomfort (frequent mouth care, frequent sips of fluids, chewing gum, or sucking lozenges may help); or constipation (increased exercise, fluids, fruit, or fiber may help; if unresolved, consult prescriber about use of stool softeners). Report chest pain or palpitations; persistent dizziness; confusion, nightmares, excitation, or changes in mentation; shortness of breath or respiratory difficulty; skin rash, unusual bleeding or bruising; or unusual fatigue and weakness. **Pregnancy/breast-feeding precautions:** Inform prescriber if you are or intend to become pregnant. Consult prescriber if breast-feeding.

Related Information

Aspirin *on page 114*
Codeine *on page 296*

Butorphanol *(byoo TOR fa nole)*

U.S. Brand Names Stadol®

Synonyms Butorphanol Tartrate

Restrictions C-IV

Pharmacologic Category Analgesic, Narcotic

Medication Safety Issues

Sound-alike/look-alike issues:
Stadol® may be confused with Haldol®, sotalol

Pregnancy Risk Factor C/D (prolonged use or high doses at term)

Lactation Enters breast milk/use caution (AAP rates "compatible")

Use

Parenteral: Management of moderate-to-severe pain; preoperative medication; supplement to balanced anesthesia; management of pain during labor

Nasal spray: Management of moderate-to-severe pain, including migraine headache pain

Mechanism of Action/Effect Mixed narcotic agonist-antagonist with central analgesic actions; binds to opiate receptors in the CNS, causing inhibition of ascending pain pathways, altering the perception of and response to pain; produces generalized CNS depression

Contraindications Hypersensitivity to butorphanol or any component of the formulation; avoid use in opiate-dependent patients who have not been detoxified, may precipitate opiate withdrawal; pregnancy (prolonged use or high doses at term)

Warnings/Precautions An opioid-containing analgesic regimen should be tailored to each patient's needs and based upon the type of pain being treated (acute versus chronic), the route of administration, degree of tolerance for opioids (naive versus chronic user), age, weight, and medical condition. The optimal analgesic dose varies widely among patients. Doses should be titrated to pain relief/prevention. May cause CNS depression, which may impair physical or mental abilities. Effects with other sedative drugs or ethanol may be potentiated. Use with caution in patients with hepatic/renal dysfunction. Tolerance or drug dependence may result from extended use. Concurrent use of sumatriptan nasal spray and butorphanol nasal spray may increase risk of transient high blood pressure.

Drug Interactions

Increased Effect/Toxicity: Increased toxicity with CNS depressants, phenothiazines, barbiturates, skeletal muscle relaxants, alfentanil, guanabenz, and MAO inhibitors.

Nutritional/Ethanol Interactions

Ethanol: Avoid or limit ethanol (may increase CNS depression). Watch for sedation.

Herb/Nutraceutical: Avoid valerian, St John's wort, kava kava, gotu kola (may increase CNS depression).

Adverse Reactions

>10%:
Central nervous system: Drowsiness (43%), dizziness (19%), insomnia (Stadol® NS)
Gastrointestinal: Nausea/vomiting (13%)
Respiratory: Nasal congestion (Stadol® NS)

1% to 10%:
Cardiovascular: Vasodilation, palpitation
Central nervous system: Lightheadedness, headache, lethargy, anxiety, confusion, euphoria, somnolence
Dermatologic: Pruritus
Gastrointestinal: Anorexia, constipation, xerostomia, stomach pain, unpleasant aftertaste
Neuromuscular & skeletal: Tremor, paresthesia, weakness
Ocular: Blurred vision
Otic: Ear pain, tinnitus
Respiratory: Bronchitis, cough, dyspnea, epistaxis, nasal irritation, pharyngitis, rhinitis, sinus congestion, sinusitis, upper respiratory infection
Miscellaneous: Diaphoresis increased

Overdosage/Toxicology Symptoms of overdose include respiratory depression, cardiac and CNS depression. Treatment is supportive. Naloxone, 2 mg I.V. with repeat administration as necessary up to a total of 10 mg, can also be used to reverse toxic effects of the opiate.

Pharmacodynamics/Kinetics

Onset of Action: I.M.: 5-10 minutes; I.V.: <10 minutes; Nasal: Within 15 minutes
Peak effect: I.M.: 0.5-1 hour; I.V.: 4-5 minutes

Duration of Action: I.M., I.V.: 3-4 hours; Nasal: 4-5 hours

Protein Binding: 80%
Half-Life Elimination: 2.5-4 hours
Metabolism: Hepatic
Excretion: Primarily urine

Available Dosage Forms

Injection, solution, as tartrate [preservative free] (Stadol®): 1 mg/mL (1 mL); 2 mg/mL (1 mL, 2 mL)

Injection, solution, as tartrate [with preservative] (Stadol®): 2 mg/mL (10 mL)

Solution, intranasal, as tartrate [spray]: 10 mg/mL (2.5 mL) [14-15 doses]

Dosing

Adults: Note: These are guidelines and do not represent the maximum doses that may be required in all patients. Doses should be titrated for pain relief/prevention. Butorphanol has an analgesic ceiling.

Acute pain (moderate to severe):

I.M.: Initial: 2 mg, may repeat every 3-4 hours as needed; usual range: 1-4 mg every 3-4 hours as needed

I.V.: Initial: 1 mg, may repeat every 3-4 hours as needed; usual range: 0.5-2 mg every 3-4 hours as needed

Intranasal (spray) (includes use for migraine headache pain): Initial: 1 spray (~1 mg per spray) in 1 nostril; if adequate pain relief is not achieved within 60-90 minutes, an additional 1 spray in 1 nostril may be given; may repeat initial dose sequence in 3-4 hours after the last dose as needed

Alternatively, an initial dose of 2 mg (1 spray in each nostril) may be used in patients who will be able to remain recumbent (in the event drowsiness or dizziness occurs); additional 2 mg doses should not be given for 3-4 hours

Note: In some clinical trials, an initial dose of 2 mg (as 2 doses 1 hour apart or 2 mg initially - 1 spray in each nostril) has been used, followed by 1 mg in 1 hour; side effects were greater at these dosages

Migraine: Nasal spray: Refer to "moderate to severe pain" indication

Preoperative medication: I.M.: 2 mg 60-90 minutes before surgery

Supplement to balanced anesthesia: I.V.: 2 mg shortly before induction and/or an incremental dose of 0.5-1 mg (up to 0.06 mg/kg), depending on previously administered sedative, analgesic, and hypnotic medications

Pain during labor (fetus >37 weeks gestation and no signs of fetal distress):

I.M., I.V.: 1-2 mg; may repeat in 4 hours

Note: Alternative analgesia should be used for pain associated with delivery or if delivery is anticipated within 4 hours

Elderly:

I.M., I.V.: Initial dosage should generally be ½ of the recommended dose; repeated dosing must be based on initial response rather than fixed intervals, but generally should be at least 6 hours apart

Nasal spray: Initial dose should not exceed 1 mg; a second dose may be given after 90-120 minutes

Renal Impairment:

I.M., I.V.: Initial dosage should generally be ½ of the recommended dose; repeated dosing must be based on initial response rather than fixed intervals, but generally should be at least 6 hours apart

Nasal spray: Initial dose should not exceed 1 mg; a second dose may be given after 90-120 minutes

Hepatic Impairment:

I.M., I.V.: Initial dosage should generally be ½ of the recommended dose; repeated dosing must be based on initial response rather than fixed intervals, but generally should be at least 6 hours apart

Nasal spray: Initial dose should not exceed 1 mg; a second dose may be given after 90-120 minutes

Administration

I.V. Detail: pH: 3.0-5.5

Inhalation: See Dosing.

Other: Intranasal: Consider avoiding simultaneous intranasal migraine sprays; may want to separate by at least 30 minutes

Stability

Compatibility:

Y-site administration: Incompatible with amphotericin B cholesteryl sulfate complex, midazolam

Compatibility in syringe: Incompatible with dimenhydrinate, pentobarbital

Storage: Store at room temperature; protect from freezing.

Nursing Actions

Physical Assessment: Assess other medications patient may be taking for possible additive or adverse interactions. Monitor for effectiveness of pain relief, signs of overdose, and adverse effects. Monitor blood pressure, CNS and respiratory status, and degree of sedation at beginning of therapy and at regular intervals with long-term use. For inpatients, implement safety measures (eg, side rails up, call light within reach, instructions to call for assistance). May cause physical and/or psychological dependence. Assess knowledge/teach patient appropriate use (if self-administered). Teach patient adverse reactions to report and appropriate interventions to reduce side effects.

Patient Education: If self-administered, use exactly as directed; do not increase dose or frequency. Drug may cause physical and/or psychological dependence. While using this medication, do not use alcohol and other prescription or OTC medications (especially sedatives, tranquilizers, antihistamines, or pain medications) without consulting prescriber. May cause dizziness, drowsiness, confusion, or blurred vision (use caution when driving, climbing stairs, or changing position - rising from sitting or lying to standing, or when engaging in tasks requiring alertness until response to drug is known); nausea or vomiting, or loss of appetite (frequent mouth care, small frequent meals, sucking lozenges, or chewing gum may help). Report unresolved nausea or vomiting; respiratory difficulty or shortness of breath; restlessness, insomnia, euphoria, or nightmares; excessive sedation or unusual weakness; facial flushing, rapid heartbeat, or palpitations; urinary difficulty; or vision changes. **Pregnancy/breast-feeding precautions:** Inform prescriber if you are or intend to become pregnant. If you are breast-feeding, take dose immediately after breast-feeding or 3-4 hours prior to next feeding.

Nasal administration: Do not use more frequently than prescribed. Blow nose prior to administering. Follow directions on package insert. Insert nozzle of applicator gently into one nostril and exhale. With next breath, squeeze applicator once firmly and quickly once as you breath in. If adequate relief from headache is not achieved within 60-90 minutes, an additional 1 spray may be given. May be repeated in 3-4 hours following last dose, as needed. **Alternatively:** Two sprays may be given - one spray in each nostril, if you are able to remain lying down (in the event of drowsiness or dizziness). Additional doses should not be taken for 3-4 hours. Avoid using simultaneously with intranasal migraine sprays. Separate by at least 30 minutes.

Geriatric Considerations Adjust dose for renal function in the elderly.

Related Information

Compatibility of Drugs in Syringe *on page 1372*

Caffeine (KAF een)

U.S. Brand Names Cafcit®; Caffedrine® [OTC]; Enerjets [OTC]; Lucidex [OTC]; No Doz® Maximum Strength [OTC]; Vivarin® [OTC]

Synonyms Caffeine and Sodium Benzoate; Caffeine Citrate; Sodium Benzoate and Caffeine

Pharmacologic Category Stimulant

Pregnancy Risk Factor C

Lactation Enters breast milk/use caution (AAP rates "compatible")

Use
Caffeine citrate: Treatment of idiopathic apnea of prematurity

Caffeine and sodium benzoate: Treatment of acute respiratory depression (not a preferred agent)

Caffeine [OTC labeling]: Restore mental alertness or wakefulness when experiencing fatigue

Unlabeled/Investigational Use Caffeine and sodium benzoate: Treatment of spinal puncture headache; CNS stimulant; diuretic

Mechanism of Action/Effect CNS stimulant which increases respiratory center sensitivity to carbon dioxide, stimulates central inspiratory drive, and improves skeletal muscle contraction (diaphragmatic contractility); prevention of apnea may occur by competitive inhibition of adenosine

Contraindications Hypersensitivity to caffeine or any component of the formulation; sodium benzoate is not for use in neonates

Warnings/Precautions Use with caution in patients with a history of peptic ulcer, gastroesophageal reflux, impaired renal or hepatic function, seizure disorders, or cardiovascular disease. Avoid use in patients with symptomatic cardiac arrhythmias, agitation, anxiety, or tremor. Over-the-counter [OTC] products contain an amount of caffeine similar to one cup of coffee; limit the use of other caffeine-containing beverages or foods.

Caffeine citrate should not be interchanged with caffeine and sodium benzoate. Avoid use of products containing sodium benzoate in neonates; has been associated with a potentially fatal toxicity ("gasping syndrome"). Neonates receiving caffeine citrate should be closely monitored for the development of necrotizing enterocolitis. Caffeine serum levels should be closely monitored to optimize therapy and prevent serious toxicity.

Drug Interactions
Cytochrome P450 Effect: Substrate of CYP1A2 (major), 2C8/9 (minor), 2D6 (minor), 2E1 (minor), 3A4 (minor); **Inhibits** CYP1A2 (weak), 3A4 (moderate)

Decreased Effect: Caffeine may diminish the sedative or anxiolytic effects of benzodiazepines. CYP1A2 inducers may decrease the levels/effects of caffeine; example inducers include aminoglutethimide, carbamazepine, phenobarbital, and rifampin.

Increased Effect/Toxicity: Quinolones (specifically ciprofloxacin, norfloxacin, ofloxacin) and CYP1A2 inhibitors may increase the levels/effects of caffeine; example inhibitors include amiodarone, fluvoxamine, ketoconazole, and rofecoxib

Adverse Reactions Frequency not specified; primarily serum-concentration related.
Cardiovascular: Angina, arrhythmia (ventricular), chest pain, flushing, palpitation, sinus tachycardia, tachycardia (supraventricular), vasodilation

Central nervous system: Agitation, delirium, dizziness, hallucinations, headache, insomnia, irritability, psychosis, restlessness

Dermatologic: Urticaria

Gastrointestinal: Esophageal sphincter tone decreased, gastritis

Neuromuscular & skeletal: Fasciculations

Ocular: Intraocular pressure increased (>180 mg caffeine), miosis

Renal: Diuresis

Overdosage/Toxicology Symptoms of overdose may include CNS stimulation, tachyarrhythmias, and tremor. Treatment is symptomatic and supportive.

Pharmacodynamics/Kinetics
Time to Peak: Serum: Oral: Within 30 minutes to 2 hours

Protein Binding: 17% (children) to 36% (adults)

Half-Life Elimination:
Neonates: 72-96 hours (range: 40-230 hours)
Children >9 months and Adults: 5 hours

Metabolism: Hepatic, via demethylation by CYP1A2.
Note: In neonates, interconversion between caffeine and theophylline has been reported (caffeine levels are ~25% of measured theophylline after theophylline administration and ~3% to 8% of caffeine would be expected to be converted to theophylline)

Excretion:
Neonates ≤1 month: 86% excreted unchanged in urine
Infants >1 month and Adults: In urine, as metabolites

Available Dosage Forms
Caplet (Caffedrine®, Vivarin®): 200 mg [OTC]

Injection, solution, as citrate [preservative free] (Cafcit®): 20 mg/mL (3 mL) [equivalent to 10 mg/mL caffeine base]

Injection, solution [with sodium benzoate]: Caffeine 125 mg/mL and sodium benzoate 125 mg/mL (2 mL); caffeine 121 mg/mL and sodium benzoate 129 mg/mL (2 mL)

Lozenge (Enerjets): 75 mg [OTC; Hazelnut coffee or mochamint flavor]

Solution, oral, as citrate (Cafcit®): 20 mg/mL (3 mL) [equivalent to 10 mg/mL caffeine base]

Tablet:
Lucidex: 100 mg [OTC]
NoDoz® Maximum Strength, Vivarin®: 200 mg [OTC]

Dosing
Adults & Elderly:
Note: Caffeine citrate should not be interchanged with the caffeine sodium benzoate formulation.

Caffeine and sodium benzoate:
Respiratory depression: I.M., I.V.: 250 mg as a single dose; may repeat as needed. Maximum single dose should be limited to 500 mg; maximum amount in any 24-hour period should generally be limited to 2500 mg.

Spinal puncture headache (unlabeled use):
I.V.: 500 mg in 1000 mL NS infused over 1 hour, followed by 1000 mL NS infused over 1 hour; a second course of caffeine can be given for unrelieved headache pain in 4 hours.

Oral: 300 mg as a single dose

Stimulant/diuretic (unlabeled use): I.M., I.V.: 500 mg, maximum single dose: 1 g

OTC labeling (stimulant): Oral: 100-200 mg every 3-4 hours as needed

Pediatrics:
Note: Caffeine citrate should not be interchanged with the caffeine sodium benzoate formulation.

Caffeine citrate: Apnea of prematurity: Neonates: Oral, I.V.:
Loading dose: 10-20 mg/kg as caffeine citrate (5-10 mg/kg as caffeine base). If theophylline has been administered to the patient within the previous 3 days, a full or modified loading dose (50% to 75% of a loading dose) may be given.

Maintenance dose: 5 mg/kg/day as caffeine citrate (2.5 mg/kg/day as caffeine base) once daily starting 24 hours after the loading dose. Maintenance dose is adjusted based on patient's response and serum caffeine concentrations.

Caffeine and sodium benzoate: Stimulant:

I.M., I.V., SubQ: 8 mg/kg every 4 hours as needed
Oral: OTC labeling: Children ≥12 years: Refer to adult dosing.

Renal Impairment: No dosage adjustment required.

Administration

Oral: May be administered without regard to feedings or meals. May administer injectable formulation (caffeine citrate) orally.

I.M.: Parenteral: **Caffeine and sodium benzoate:** May administer I.M. undiluted

I.V.: Parenteral:

Caffeine citrate: Infuse loading dose over at least 30 minutes; maintenance dose may be infused over at least 10 minutes. May administer without dilution or diluted with D_5W to 10 mg caffeine citrate/mL.

Caffeine and sodium benzoate: I.V. as slow direct injection. For spinal headaches, dilute in 1000 mL NS and infuse over 1 hour. Follow with 1000 mL NS; infuse over 1 hour. May administer I.M. undiluted.

Stability

Storage: Store at 20°C to 25°C (68°F to 77°F).

Nursing Actions

Physical Assessment: Assess other prescription and OTC medications the patient may be taking to avoid duplications and interactions. Assess knowledge/teach patient appropriate use, side effects, and symptoms to report.

Patient Education: Take as directed. Do not exceed recommended dosage. Maintain adequate hydration (2-3 L/day of fluids) unless instructed to restrict fluid intake by prescriber. You may experience CNS stimulation, excitability, sensorium changes, flushing, dizziness, insomnia, or agitation. Report excessive excitability or nervousness, rapid heartbeat or palpitations, chest pain, or respiratory difficulty. **Pregnancy/breast-feeding precaution:** Inform prescriber if you are or intend to become pregnant. Consult prescriber if breast-feeding.

Breast-Feeding Issues Irritability and poor sleeping patterns have been reported following maternal consumption of large amounts of caffeine. Moderate intake (2-3 cups/day) is considered to be compatible with breast-feeding.

Calcipotriene (kal si POE try een)

U.S. Brand Names Dovonex®

Pharmacologic Category Topical Skin Product; Vitamin D Analog

Pregnancy Risk Factor C

Lactation Excretion in breast milk unknown/use caution

Use Treatment of plaque psoriasis

Mechanism of Action/Effect Synthetic vitamin D_3 analog which regulates skin cell production and proliferation

Contraindications Hypersensitivity to calcipotriene or any component of the formulation; patients with demonstrated hypercalcemia or evidence of vitamin D toxicity; use on the face

Warnings/Precautions Use may cause irritations of lesions and surrounding uninvolved skin. If irritation develops, discontinue use. Transient, rapidly reversible elevation of serum calcium has occurred during use. If elevation in serum calcium occurs above the normal range, discontinue treatment until calcium levels are normal. For external use only; not for ophthalmic, oral, or intravaginal use. Avoid or limit excessive exposure to natural or artificial sunlight, or phototherapy. Safety and efficacy have not been established in children.

Drug Interactions
Decreased Effect: No data reported
Increased Effect/Toxicity: No data reported
Adverse Reactions Frequency may vary with site of application.

>10%: Dermatologic: Burning, itching, rash, skin irritation, stinging, tingling
1% to 10%: Dermatologic: Dermatitis, dry skin, erythema, peeling, worsening of psoriasis
Note: Skin atrophy, hyperpigmentation, folliculitis, and hypercalcemia are potential adverse effects of calcipotriene.

Pharmacodynamics/Kinetics
Onset of Action:
Improvement begins after 2 weeks; marked improvement seen after 8 weeks
Metabolism:
Converted in the skin to inactive metabolites
Available Dosage Forms
Cream: 0.005% (60 g, 120 g)
Ointment: 0.005% (60 g, 120 g)
Solution, topical: 0.005% (60 mL)

Dosing
Adults & Elderly: Psoriasis: Topical: Apply in a thin film to the affected skin twice daily and rub in gently and completely.

Administration
Topical: For external use only.
Cream: Apply to affected skin; rub in gently and completely
Solution: Prior to using scalp solution, comb hair to remove debris; apply only to lesions. Rub in gently and completely. Avoid solution spreading or dripping onto forehead.

Stability
Storage: Store at 15° to 25°C (59° to 77°F). Do not freeze. Solution should be kept away from open flame; avoid sunlight.

Laboratory Monitoring Serum calcium

Nursing Actions
Physical Assessment: When applied to large areas of skin or for extensive periods of time, monitor for adverse skin or systemic reactions. Assess knowledge/teach patient appropriate application and use and adverse symptoms to report.

Patient Education: For external use only. Use exactly as directed; do not overuse. Before using, wash and dry area gently. Wear gloves to apply a thin film to affected area and rub in gently. If dressing is necessary, use a porous dressing. Avoid contact with eyes. Avoid exposing treated area to direct sunlight; sunburn can occur. Report increased swelling, redness, rash, itching, signs of infection, worsening of condition, or lack of healing. **Pregnancy/breast-feeding precautions:** Inform prescriber if you are or intend to become pregnant. Consult prescriber if breast-feeding.

Calcipotriene and Betamethasone
(kal si POE try een & bay ta METH a sone)

U.S. Brand Names Taclonex®

Synonyms Betamethasone Dipropionate and Calcipotriene Hydrate; Calcipotriol and Betamethasone Dipropionate

Pharmacologic Category Corticosteroid, Topical; Vitamin D Analog

Pregnancy Risk Factor C

Lactation Excretion in breast milk unknown/not recommended

Use Treatment of psoriasis vulgaris

Unlabeled/Investigational Use Treatment of corticosteroid-responsive dermatoses
(Continued)

Calcipotriene and Betamethasone
(Continued)

Available Dosage Forms [CAN] = Canadian brand name

Cream, topical (Dovobet®) [CAN]: Calcipotriol 50 mcg and betamethasone 0.5 mg per gram (3 g, 30 g, 60 g, 100 g, 120 g) [not available in the U. S.]

Ointment, topical (Taclonex®): Calcipotriene 0.005% and betamethasone 0.064% (15 g, 30 g, 60 g)

Dosing

Adults & Elderly:

Psoriasis vulgaris: Topical: Apply to affected area once daily for up to 4 weeks (maximum recommended dose: 100 g/week). Application to >30% of body surface area is not recommended.

Renal Impairment: Safety and efficacy have not been established with severe renal impairment.

Hepatic Impairment: Safety and efficacy have not been established with severe hepatic impairment.

Nursing Actions

Physical Assessment: Monitor therapeutic response and adverse reactions at the beginning and periodically throughout therapy.

Patient Education: For external use only. Unless directed by prescriber to do so, avoid use of occlusive dressing, concomitant use of other corticosteroids, and excessive exposure of the affected skin to natural or artificial light. Do not use on face, axillae, or groin. Skin should be cleansed prior to use. Wash hands after applying. You may experience a scaly rash, burning sensation on skin, or itching. **Pregnancy/breast-feeding precautions:** Inform prescriber if you are or intend to become pregnant. Do not breast-feed.

Related Information

Betamethasone *on page 148*
Calcipotriene *on page 185*

Calcitonin (kal si TOE nin)

U.S. Brand Names Fortical®; Miacalcin®

Synonyms Calcitonin (Salmon)

Pharmacologic Category Antidote; Hormone

Medication Safety Issues

Sound-alike/look-alike issues:
Calcitonin may be confused with calcitriol
Miacalcin® may be confused with Micatin®

Pregnancy Risk Factor C

Lactation Excretion in breast milk unknown/not recommended

Use Calcitonin (salmon): Treatment of Paget's disease of bone (osteitis deformans); adjunctive therapy for hypercalcemia; postmenopausal osteoporosis

Mechanism of Action/Effect Peptide sequence similar to human calcitonin; functionally antagonizes the effects of parathyroid hormone. Directly inhibits osteoclastic bone resorption; promotes the renal excretion of calcium, phosphate, sodium, magnesium, and potassium by decreasing tubular reabsorption; increases the jejunal secretion of water, sodium, potassium, and chloride

Contraindications Hypersensitivity to calcitonin salmon or any component of the formulation

Warnings/Precautions A skin test should be performed prior to initiating therapy of calcitonin salmon in patients with suspected sensitivity. Have epinephrine immediately available for a possible hypersensitivity reaction. Use caution with renal insufficiency, pernicious anemia. A detailed skin testing protocol is available from the manufacturers. Temporarily withdraw use of nasal spray if ulceration of nasal mucosa occurs. Safety and efficacy have not been established in pediatric patients.

Nutritional/Ethanol Interactions Ethanol: Avoid ethanol (may increase risk of osteoporosis).

Adverse Reactions Unless otherwise noted, frequencies reported are with nasal spray.

>10%: Respiratory: Rhinitis (12%)

1% to 10%:
Cardiovascular: Flushing (nasal spray: <1%; injection: 2% to 5%), angina (1% to 3%), hypertension (1% to 3%)
Central nervous system: Depression (1% to 3%), dizziness (1% to 3%), fatigue (1% to 3%)
Dermatologic: Erythematous rash (1% to 3%)
Gastrointestinal: Abdominal pain (1% to 3%), constipation (1% to 3%), diarrhea (1% to 3%), dyspepsia (1% to 3%), nausea (injection: 10%; nasal spray: 1% to 3%)
Genitourinary: Cystitis (1% to 3%)
Hematologic: Lymphadenopathy (1% to 3%)
Local: Injection site reactions (injection: 10%)
Neuromuscular & skeletal: Back pain (5%), arthrosis (1% to 3%), myalgia (1% to 3%), paresthesia (1% to 3%)
Ocular: Conjunctivitis (1% to 3%), lacrimation abnormality (1% to 3%)
Respiratory: Bronchospasm (1% to 3%), sinusitis (1% to 3%), upper respiratory tract infection (1% to 3%)
Miscellaneous: Flu-like symptoms (1% to 3%), infection (1% to 3%)

Overdosage/Toxicology Symptoms of overdose include nausea, vomiting, hypocalcemia, and hypocalcemic tetany. Treatment should be symptom-directed and supportive.

Pharmacodynamics/Kinetics

Onset of Action: Hypercalcemia: I.M. or SubQ: ~2 hours

Duration of Action: Hypercalcemia: I.M. or SubQ: 6-8 hours

Time to Peak: Nasal: ~30-40 minutes

Half-Life Elimination: SubQ: 1.2 hours; Nasal: 43 minutes

Excretion: Urine (as inactive metabolites)

Available Dosage Forms

Injection, solution, calcitonin-salmon: (Miacalcin®): 200 int. units/mL (2 mL)

Solution, nasal spray, calcitonin-salmon:
Fortical®: 200 int. units/0.09 mL (3.7 mL) [rDNA origin; contains benzyl alcohol; delivers 30 doses, 200 units/actuation]
Miacalcin®: 200 int. units/0.09 mL (3.7 mL) [contains benzalkonium chloride; delivers 30 doses, 200 units/actuation]

Dosing

Adults & Elderly:

Paget's disease *(Miacalcin®)*: I.M., SubQ: Initial: 100 units/day; maintenance: 50 units/day or 50-100 units every 1-3 days

Hypercalcemia *(Miacalcin®)*: Initial: I.M., SubQ: 4 units/kg every 12 hours; may increase up to 8 units/kg every 12 hours to a maximum of every 6 hours

Postmenopausal osteoporosis:
Miacalcin®: I.M., SubQ: 100 units/every other day
Fortical®, Miacalcin®: Intranasal: 200 units (1 spray)/day

Administration

I.M.: Administer injection solution I.M. or SubQ; intramuscular route is recommended over the subcutaneous route when the volume of calcitonin to be injected exceeds 2 mL.

Inhalation: Nasal spray: Before first use, allow bottle to reach room temperature, then prime pump by releasing at least 5 sprays until full spray is produced. To administer, place nozzle into nostril with head in upright position. Alternate nostrils daily. Do not prime pump before each daily use. Discard after 30 doses.

Stability

Reconstitution: Injection: NS has been recommended for the dilution to prepare a skin test in patients with suspected sensitivity.

Storage:

Injection: Store under refrigeration at 2°C to 8°C (36°F to 46°F); protect from freezing.

Nasal: Store unopened bottle under refrigeration at 2°C to 8°C (36°F to 46°F).

Fortical®: After opening, store for up to 30 days at 20°C to 25°C (68°F to 77°F); excursions permitted to 15°C to 30°C (59°F to 86°F). Store in upright position.

Miacalcin®: After opening, store for up to 35 days at room temperature of 15°C to 30°C (59°F to 86°F). Store in upright position.

Laboratory Monitoring Serum electrolytes and calcium, alkaline phosphatase and 24-hour urine collection for hydroxyproline excretion (Paget's disease); bone mineral density

Nursing Actions

Physical Assessment: Skin test should be administered before initiating therapy (increased erythema or skin wheal indicates positive reaction and allergy). Assess potential for interactions with other prescriptions, OTC medications, or herbal products patient may be taking. Monitor laboratory tests and patient response (eg, hypocalcemic tetany, hypercalcemia) at regular intervals during therapy. Teach patient appropriate administration (eg, subcutaneous or I.M. injections or nasal spray), dietary requirements (low calcium diet if used for hypercalcemia), possible side effects/appropriate interventions, and adverse symptoms to report.

Patient Education: Do not take any new medication during therapy unless approved by prescriber. If administered by injection, you or a significant other will be instructed on how to give the injections and dispose of syringes/needles (follow directions exactly). Keep drug vials in refrigerator; do not freeze. May cause increased warmth and flushing (this should only last about 1 hour after administration; taking drug in evening may minimize these discomforts). Report significant nasal irritation if using nasal spray. Immediately report twitching, muscle spasm, dark-colored urine, hives, significant skin rash, palpitations, or respiratory difficulty. **Pregnancy/breast-feeding precautions:** Inform prescriber if you are or intend to become pregnant. Consult prescriber if breast-feeding.

Dietary Considerations Adequate vitamin D and calcium intake is essential for preventing/treating osteoporosis. Patients with Paget's disease and hypercalcemia should follow a low calcium diet as prescribed.

Geriatric Considerations Calcitonin may be the drug of choice for postmenopausal women unable to take estrogens to increase bone density and reduce fractures. Calcium and vitamin D supplements should also be given. Calcitonin may also be effective in steroid-induced osteoporosis and other states associated with high bone turnover.

Breast-Feeding Issues Has been shown to decrease milk production in animals.

Pregnancy Issues Decreased birth weight was observed in animal studies. Calcitonin does not cross the placental barrier. There are no adequate and well-controlled studies in pregnant women.

Calcitriol (kal si TRYE ole)

U.S. Brand Names Calcijex®; Rocaltrol®
Synonyms 1,25 Dihydroxycholecalciferol
Pharmacologic Category Vitamin D Analog
Medication Safety Issues
Sound-alike/look-alike issues:
Calcitriol may be confused with calcifediol, Calciferol®, calcitonin

Dosage is expressed in mcg (micrograms), **not** mg (milligrams); rare cases of acute overdose have been reported

Pregnancy Risk Factor C (manufacturer); A/D (dose exceeding RDA recommendation) (expert analysis)
Lactation Enters breast milk/not recommended
Use Management of hypocalcemia in patients on chronic renal dialysis; management of secondary hyperparathyroidism in moderate-to-severe chronic renal failure; management of hypocalcemia in hypoparathyroidism and pseudohypoparathyroidism
Unlabeled/Investigational Use Decrease severity of psoriatic lesions in psoriatic vulgaris; vitamin D-resistant rickets
Mechanism of Action/Effect Promotes absorption of calcium in the intestines and retention at the kidneys thereby increasing calcium levels in the serum; decreases excessive serum phosphatase levels, parathyroid hormone levels, and decreases bone resorption; increases renal tubule phosphate resorption
Contraindications Hypercalcemia; vitamin D toxicity; abnormal sensitivity to the effects of vitamin D; pregnancy (dose exceeding RDA)
Warnings/Precautions Adequate dietary (supplemental) calcium is necessary for clinical response to vitamin D. Monitor serum calcium and phosphate concentrations. Avoid hypercalcemia; calcium-phosphate product (serum calcium times phosphorus) must not exceed 70. Immobilization or excessive doage may increase risk of hypercalcemia and/or hypercalciuria. Maintain adequate hydration. Use caution in patients with malabsorption syndromes (efficacy may be limited and/or response may be unpredictable).
Drug Interactions
Cytochrome P450 Effect: Induces CYP3A4 (weak)
Decreased Effect: Cholestyramine and colestipol decrease absorption/effect of calcitriol. Thiazide diuretics and corticosteroids may reduce the effect of calcitriol.
Increased Effect/Toxicity: Risk of hypercalcemia with thiazide diuretics. Risk of hypermagnesemia with magnesium-containing antacids. Risk of digoxin toxicity may be increased (if hypercalcemia occurs).
Lab Interactions Increased calcium, cholesterol, magnesium, BUN, AST, ALT, calcium (S), cholesterol (S); decreased alkaline phosphatase
Adverse Reactions
>10%: Endocrine & metabolic: Hypercalcemia (33%)
Frequency not defined:
Cardiovascular: Cardiac arrhythmia, hyper-/hypotension
Central nervous system: Headache, irritability, seizure (rare), somnolence, psychosis
Dermatologic: Pruritus, erythema multiforme
Endocrine & metabolic: Hypermagnesemia, hyperphosphatemia, polydipsia
Gastrointestinal: Anorexia, constipation, metallic taste, nausea, pancreatitis, vomiting, xerostomia
Hepatic: LFTs increased
Neuromuscular & skeletal: Bone pain, myalgia, dystrophy, soft tissue calcification
Ocular: Conjunctivitis, photophobia
Renal: Polyuria
(Continued)

Calcitriol (Continued)

Overdosage/Toxicology Toxicity rarely occurs from acute overdose. Symptoms of chronic overdose include hypercalcemia, hypercalciuria with weakness, altered mental status, GI upset, renal tubular injury, and occasionally cardiac arrhythmias. Following withdrawal of the drug, treatment consists of bedrest, liberal fluid intake, reduced calcium intake, and cathartic administration. Severe hypercalcemia requires I.V. hydration and forced diuresis. I.V. saline may increase excretion of calcium. Calcitonin, cholestyramine, prednisone, sodium EDTA, bisphosphonates, and mithramycin have all been used successfully to treat the more resistant cases of vitamin D-induced hypercalcemia. Use of peritoneal dialysis against a calcium-free dialysate has been reported.

Pharmacodynamics/Kinetics
Onset of Action: ~2-6 hours
Duration of Action: 3-5 days
Protein Binding: 99.9%
Half-Life Elimination: 3-8 hours
Metabolism: Primarily to 1,24,25-trihydroxycholecalciferol and 1,24,25-trihydroxy ergocalciferol
Excretion: Primarily feces; urine (4% to 6%)

Available Dosage Forms
Capsule (Rocaltrol®): 0.25 mcg, 0.5 mcg [each strength contains coconut oil]
Injection, solution: 1 mcg/mL (1 mL); 2 mcg/mL (2 mL)
Calcijex®: 1 mcg/mL (1 mL)
Solution, oral (Rocaltrol®): 1 mcg/mL (15 mL) [contains palm seed oil]

Dosing
Adults & Elderly: Individualize dosage to maintain calcium levels of 9-10 mg/dL.
Renal failure:
Oral: 0.25 mcg/day or every other day (may require 0.5-1 mcg/day)
I.V.: 0.5 mcg (0.01 mcg/kg) 3 times/week; most doses in the range of 0.5-3 mcg (0.01-0.05 mcg/kg) 3 times/week
Hypoparathyroidism/pseudohypoparathyroidism: Oral: 0.5-2 mcg/day
Vitamin D-dependent rickets: Oral: 1 mcg once daily
Vitamin D-resistant rickets (familial hypophosphatemia): Oral: Initial: 0.015-0.02 mcg/kg once daily; maintenance: 0.03-0.06 mcg/kg once daily; maximum dose: 2 mcg once daily
Pediatrics: Individualize dosage to maintain calcium levels of 9-10 mg/dL.
Renal failure:
Oral: 0.25-2 mcg/day have been used (with hemodialysis); 0.014-0.041 mcg/kg/day (not receiving hemodialysis); increases should be made at 4- to 8-week intervals.
I.V.: 0.01-0.05 mcg/kg 3 times/week if undergoing hemodialysis
Hypoparathyroidism/pseudohypoparathyroidism: Oral (evaluate dosage at 2- to 4-week intervals):
<1 year: 0.04-0.08 mcg/kg once daily
1-5 years: 0.25-0.75 mcg once daily
≥6 years: 0.5-2 mcg once daily
Vitamin D-dependent rickets: Refer to adult dosing.
Vitamin D-resistant rickets (familial hypophosphatemia): Refer to adult dosing.
Dosing Adjustment for Toxicity: Hypercalcemia:
Adults:
Dialysis or hypoparathyroidism: Discontinue calcitriol and calcium supplements; initiate low-calcium diet. In dialysis patients with persistent hypercalcemia, may dialyze against calcium-free dialysate.
Predialysis:
Discontinue or reduce calcium supplements.
If taking calcitriol 0.5 mcg once daily, reduce to 0.25 mcg once daily.

If taking calcitriol 0.25 mcg once daily, discontinue until serum calcium normalizes. Restart at 0.25 mcg every other day.

Administration
Oral: May be administered without regard to food. Give with meals to reduce GI problems.
I.V.: May be administered as a bolus dose I.V. through the catheter at the end of hemodialysis.
I.V. Detail: pH: 7.2 (target); 6.5-8.0 (range)

Stability
Compatibility: Stable in D₅W, NS, SWFI
Storage: Store in tight, light-resistant container. Calcitriol degrades upon prolonged exposure to light.
Laboratory Monitoring Serum calcium and phosphorus, and renal function. The serum calcium times phosphate product should not be allowed to exceed 70.

Nursing Actions
Physical Assessment: Assess effectiveness and interactions of other medications patient may be taking. Monitor lab tests, effectiveness of therapy, and adverse effects at beginning of therapy and regularly with long-term use. Assess knowledge/teach patient appropriate use, appropriate nutritional counseling, possible side effects/interventions, and adverse symptoms to report.

Patient Education: Take exact dose as prescribed; do not increase dose. Maintain recommended diet and calcium supplementation. Avoid taking magnesium-containing antacids. You may experience nausea, vomiting, loss of appetite, or metallic taste (small frequent meals, frequent mouth care, chewing gum, or sucking lozenges may help); or hypotension (use caution when rising from sitting or lying position or when climbing stairs or bending over). Report chest pain or palpitations; acute headache; skin rash; change in vision or eye irritation; CNS changes; unusual weakness or fatigue; persistent nausea, vomiting, cramps, or diarrhea; or muscle or bone pain. **Pregnancy/breast-feeding precautions:** Inform prescriber if you are or intend to become pregnant. Breast-feeding is not recommended.

Dietary Considerations May be taken without regard to food. Give with meals to reduce GI problems.

Geriatric Considerations Appetite and caloric requirements may decrease with advanced age. Assess diet for adequate nutrient intake with regard to vitamins and minerals. (Daily vitamin supplements are sometimes recommended). Persons >65 years of age have decreased absorption and may have decreased intake of vitamin D. This may require supplement with daily vitamin D intake, especially for those with high risk for osteoporosis.

Calcium Acetate (KAL see um AS e tate)

U.S. Brand Names PhosLo®
Pharmacologic Category Antidote; Calcium Salt; Phosphate Binder
Pregnancy Risk Factor C
Use
Oral: Control of hyperphosphatemia in end-stage renal failure; does not promote aluminum absorption
I.V.: Calcium supplementation in parenteral nutrition therapy
Available Dosage Forms [DSC] = Discontinued product. **Note:** Elemental calcium listed in brackets:
Gelcap (PhosLo®): 667 mg [169 mg]
Injection, solution: 0.5 mEq/mL (10 mL, 50 mL, 100 mL)
Tablet (PhosLo®): 667 mg [169 mg] [DSC]
Dosing
Adults & Elderly:
Dietary Reference Intake:
Adults, Male/Female:
19-50 years: 1000 mg/day

≥51 years: 1200 mg/day
Female: Pregnancy: Same as for Adults, Male/Female
Female: Lactating: Same as for Adults, Male/Female

Control of hyperphosphatemia (ESRD, on dialysis): Oral: Initial: 1334 mg with each meal, can be increased gradually to bring the serum phosphate value <6 mg/dL as long as hypercalcemia does not develop (usual dose: 2001-2868 mg calcium acetate with each meal); do not give additional calcium supplements

Calcium supplementation (parenteral): I.V.: Dose is dependent on the requirements of the individual patient; in central venous total parental nutrition (TPN), calcium is administered at a concentration of 5 mEq (10 mL)/L of TPN solution

Pediatrics:

Dietary Reference Intake:
0-6 months: 210 mg/day
7-12 months: 270 mg/day
1-3 years: 500 mg/day
4-8 years: 800 mg/day
9-18 years: 1300 mg/day

Calcium supplementation (parenteral): I.V.: Dose is dependent on the requirements of the individual patient; in central venous total parental nutrition (TPN), calcium is administered at a concentration of 5 mEq (10 mL)/L of TPN solution; the additive maintenance dose in neonatal TPN is 0.5 mEq calcium/kg/day (1mL/kg/day)
Neonates: 70-200 mg/kg/day
Infants and Children: 70-150 mg/kg/day
Adolescents: 18-35 mg/kg/day

Renal Impairment: Refer to adult dosing.

Nursing Actions

Patient Education: Inform prescriber of any other medications or dietary supplements you are taking. Do not take any new medication during therapy without consulting prescriber. Follow exact instructions for dosing. Take with meals. Avoid alcohol, other antacids, caffeine, or other calcium supplements unless approved by prescriber. May cause constipation (increased exercise, fluids, fiber, or fruits may help) or dry mouth (frequent mouth care, chewing gum, or sucking lozenges may help). Report severe, unresolved GI disturbances and unusual emotional lability (mood swings). **Pregnancy precaution:** Inform prescriber if you are or intend to become pregnant.

Calcium Carbonate (KAL see um KAR bun ate)

U.S. Brand Names Alcalak [OTC]; Alka-Mints® [OTC]; Amitone® [OTC] [DSC]; Calcarb 600 [OTC]; Calci-Chew® [OTC]; Calci-Mix® [OTC]; Cal-Gest [OTC]; Cal-Mint [OTC]; Caltrate® 600 [OTC]; Children's Pepto [OTC]; Chooz® [OTC]; Florical® [OTC]; Maalox® Quick Dissolve [OTC]; Mylanta® Children's [OTC]; Nephro-Calci® [OTC]; Nutralox® [OTC]; Os-Cal® 500 [OTC]; Oysco 500 [OTC]; Oyst-Cal 500 [OTC]; Rolaids® Softchews [OTC]; Titralac™ [OTC]; Titralac™ Extra Strength [OTC]; Tums® [OTC]; Tums® E-X [OTC]; Tums® Extra Strength Sugar Free [OTC]; Tums® Smoothies™ [OTC]; Tums® Ultra [OTC]

Pharmacologic Category Antacid; Antidote; Calcium Salt; Electrolyte Supplement, Oral

Medication Safety Issues
Sound-alike/look-alike issues:
Florical® may be confused with Fiorinal®
Mylanta® may be confused with Mynatal®
Nephro-Calci® may be confused with Nephrocaps®
Os-Cal® may be confused with Asacol®

Use As an antacid; treatment and prevention of calcium deficiency or hyperphosphatemia (eg, osteoporosis, osteomalacia, mild/moderate renal insufficiency, hypoparathyroidism, postmenopausal osteoporosis, rickets); has been used to bind phosphate

Mechanism of Action/Effect As dietary supplement, used to prevent or treat negative calcium balance; in osteoporosis, it helps to prevent or decrease the rate of bone loss. The calcium in calcium salts moderates nerve and muscle performance and allows normal cardiac function. Also used to treat hyperphosphatemia in patients with advanced renal insufficiency by combining with dietary phosphate to form insoluble calcium phosphate, which is excreted in feces. Calcium salts as antacids neutralize gastric acidity resulting in increased gastric and duodenal bulb pH; they additionally inhibit proteolytic activity of peptic if the pH is increased >4 and increase lower esophageal sphincter tone.

Contraindications Hypercalcemia, renal calculi, hypophosphatemia; patients with suspected digoxin toxicity

Warnings/Precautions Calcium carbonate absorption is impaired in achlorhydria (common in elderly - use alternate salt, administer with food). Administration is followed by increased gastric acid secretion within 2 hours of administration. While hypercalcemia and hypercalciuria may result when therapeutic replacement amounts are given for prolonged periods, they are most likely to occur in hypoparathyroid patients receiving high doses of vitamin D.

Drug Interactions

Decreased Effect: Absorption of tetracycline, atenolol (and potentially other beta-blockers), iron, quinolone antibiotics, alendronate, sodium fluoride, and zinc absorption may be significantly decreased; space administration times. Effects of calcium channel blockers (eg, verapamil) effects may be diminished. Polystyrene sulfonate's potassium-binding ability may be reduced; avoid concurrent administration.

Increased Effect/Toxicity: High doses of calcium with thiazide diuretics may result in milk-alkali syndrome and hypercalcemia; monitor response. Calcium salts may decrease T_4 absorption; separate dose from levothyroxine by at least 4 hours. Calcium acetate may potentiate digoxin toxicity.

Nutritional/Ethanol Interactions
Ethanol: Avoid ethanol (may increase risk of osteoporosis).
Food: Food may increase calcium absorption. Calcium may decrease iron absorption. Bran, foods high in oxalates, or whole grain cereals may decrease calcium absorption.

Lab Interactions Increased calcium (S); decreased magnesium

Adverse Reactions Well tolerated
1% to 10%:
Central nervous system: Headache
Endocrine & metabolic: Hypophosphatemia, hypercalcemia
Gastrointestinal: Constipation, laxative effect, acid rebound, nausea, vomiting, anorexia, abdominal pain, xerostomia, flatulence
Miscellaneous: Milk-alkali syndrome with very high, chronic dosing and/or renal failure (headache, nausea, irritability, weakness, alkalosis, hypercalcemia, renal impairment)

Overdosage/Toxicology
Acute single ingestions of calcium salts may produce mild gastrointestinal distress, but hypercalcemia or other toxic manifestations are extremely unlikely. Treatment is supportive.

Pharmacodynamics/Kinetics
Excretion: Primarily feces (as unabsorbed calcium); urine (20%)

Available Dosage Forms
[DSC] = Discontinued product
(Continued)

Calcium Carbonate *(Continued)*

Capsule:

Calci-Mix®: 1250 mg [equivalent to elemental calcium 500 mg]

Florical®: 364 mg [equivalent to elemental calcium 145.6 mg; contains sodium fluoride 3.75 mg]

Gum, chewing: 250 mg (30s)

Chooz®: 500 mg [equivalent to elemental calcium 200 mg; mint flavor]

Powder: 4000 mg/teaspoonful (480 g) [equivalent to 1600 mg elemental calcium/teaspoonful]

Suspension, oral: 1250 mg/5 mL (5 mL, 500 mL) [equivalent to elemental calcium 500 mg/5 mL; mint flavor]

Tablet: 1250 mg [equivalent to elemental calcium 500 mg]; 1500 mg [equivalent to elemental calcium 600 mg]

Calcarb 600, Caltrate® 600, Nephro-Calci®: 1500 mg [equivalent to elemental calcium 600 mg]

Florical®: 364 mg [equivalent to elemental calcium 145.6 mg; contains sodium fluoride 8.3 mg]

Os-Cal® 500: 1250 mg [equivalent to elemental calcium 500 mg; contains tartrazine]

Oysco 500, Oyst-Cal 500: 1250 mg [equivalent to elemental calcium 500 mg]

Tablet, chewable: 500 mg [equivalent to elemental calcium 200 mg]; 650 mg [equivalent to elemental calcium 260 mg]; 750 mg [equivalent to elemental calcium 300 mg]

Alcalak: 420 mg [equivalent to elemental calcium 168 mg; mint flavor]

Alka-Mints®: 850 mg [equivalent to elemental calcium 340 mg; spearmint flavor]

Amitone®: 420 mg [equivalent to elemental calcium 168 mg; spearmint flavor] [DSC]

Cal-Gest: 500 mg [equivalent to elemental calcium 200 mg; assorted flavors]

Calci-Chew®: 1250 mg [equivalent to elemental calcium 500 mg; cherry, lemon, and orange flavors]

Cal-Mint: 650 mg [equivalent to elemental calcium 260 mg; mint flavor]

Children's Pepto: 400 mg [equivalent to elemental calcium 161 mg; bubble gum or watermelon flavors]

Maalox® Quick Dissolve: 600 mg [equivalent to elemental calcium 222 mg; contains phenylalanine 0.5 mg/tablet; lemon flavor]

Mylanta® Children's: 400 mg [equivalent to elemental calcium 160 mg; bubble gum flavor]

Nutralox®: 420 mg [equivalent to elemental calcium 168 mg; sugar free; mint flavor]

Os-Cal® 500: 1250 mg [equivalent to elemental calcium 500 mg; Bavarian cream flavor] [DSC]

Titralac™: 420 mg [equivalent to elemental calcium 168 mg; sugar free; contains sodium 1.1 mg/tablet; spearmint flavor]

Titralac™ Extra Strength: 750 mg [equivalent to elemental calcium 300 mg; sugar free; contains sodium 1.1 mg/tablet; spearmint flavor]

Tums®: 500 mg [equivalent to elemental calcium 200 mg; contains tartrazine; assorted fruit and peppermint flavors]

Tums® E-X: 750 mg [equivalent to elemental calcium 300 mg; contains tartrazine; assorted fruit, cool relief mint, fresh blend, tropical assorted fruit, wintergreen, and assorted berry flavors]

Tums® Extra Strength Sugar Free: 750 mg [equivalent to elemental calcium 300 mg; sugar free; contains phenylalanine <1 mg/tablet; orange cream flavor]

Tums® Smoothies™: 750 mg [equivalent to elemental calcium 300 mg; contains tartrazine; assorted fruit, assorted tropical fruit, peppermint flavors]

Tums® Ultra®: 1000 mg [equivalent to elemental calcium 400 mg; contains tartrazine; assorted berry, assorted fruit, assorted tropical fruit, peppermint, and spearmint flavors]

Tablet, softchew (Rolaids®): 1177 mg [equivalent to elemental calcium 471 mg; contains coconut oil and soy lecithin; vanilla creme and wild cherry flavors]

Dosing

Adults & Elderly: Dosage is in terms of elemental calcium:

Dietary Reference Intake: Oral:

Adults, Male/Female:

19-50 years: 1000 mg/day

≥51 years: 1200 mg/day

Female: Pregnancy: Same as for Adults, Male/Female

Female: Lactating: Same as for Adults, Male/Female

Hypocalcemia (dose depends on clinical condition and serum calcium level): Oral: Dose expressed in mg of **elemental calcium**: 1-2 g or more/day in 3-4 divided doses

Dietary supplementation: Oral: 500 mg to 2 g divided 2-4 times/day

Antacid: Oral: Dosage based on acid-neutralizing capacity of specific product; generally, 1-2 tablets or 5-10 mL every 2 hours; maximum: 7000 mg calcium carbonate per 24 hours; specific product labeling should be consulted

Osteoporosis: Oral: Adults >51 years: 1200 mg/day

Pediatrics: Dosage is in terms of elemental calcium:

Dietary Reference Intake: Oral:

0-6 months: 210 mg/day

7-12 months: 270 mg/day

1-3 years: 500 mg/day

4-8 years: 800 mg/day

9-19 years: 1300 mg/day

Hypocalcemia (dose depends on clinical condition and serum calcium level): Oral: Dose expressed in mg of **elemental calcium**

Neonates: 50-150 mg/kg/day in 4-6 divided doses; not to exceed 1 g/day

Children: 45-65 mg/kg/day in 4 divided doses

Antacid: Oral:

Children 2-5 years (24-47 lb): Elemental calcium 161 mg as needed; maximum 483 mg per 24 hours

Children 6-11 years (48-95 lb): Elemental calcium 322 mg as needed; maximum: 966 mg per 24 hours

Renal Impairment: Cl_{cr} <25 mL/minute: Dosage adjustments may be necessary depending on the serum calcium levels.

Stability

Compatibility: Admixture **incompatibilities** include carbonates, phosphates, sulfates, tartrates

Nursing Actions

Physical Assessment: Assess other medications patient may be taking for effectiveness and interactions. Monitor results of laboratory tests, therapeutic effectiveness, and adverse/toxic effects. Assess knowledge/teach patient proper use, appropriate interventions to reduce side effects, and adverse symptoms to report.

Patient Education: Follow instructions for dosing. Take with a full glass of water or juice 1-2 hours before any iron supplements and 1-3 hours after meals or other medications. Avoid alcohol, other antacids, caffeine, or other calcium supplements, unless approved by prescriber. You may experience constipation (increased exercise, fluids, fiber, or fruit may help) or dry mouth (sucking lozenges or hard candy may help). Report severe, unresolved GI disturbances and unusual emotional liability (mood swings).

Pregnancy precaution: Inform prescriber if you are or intend to become pregnant.

Dietary Considerations As a dietary supplement, should be given with meals to increase absorption. May decrease iron absorption, so should be administered 1-2

hours before or after iron supplementation. Limit intake of bran, foods high in oxalates, or whole grain cereals which may decrease calcium absorption.

Maalox® Quick Dissolve 600 mg tablet contains phenylalanine 0.5 mg/tablet.

Tums® Extra Strength Sugar Free 750 mg tablet contains phenylalanine <1 mg/tablet.

Titralac™ 420 mg tablet and Titralac™ Extra Strength 750 mg tablet each contain sodium 1.1 mg/tablet.

Additional Information 20 mEq calcium/g; 400 mg elemental calcium/g calcium carbonate (40% elemental calcium)

Calcium Chloride (KAL see um KLOR ide)

Pharmacologic Category Calcium Salt; Electrolyte Supplement, Parenteral

Pregnancy Risk Factor C

Use Cardiac resuscitation when epinephrine fails to improve myocardial contractions, cardiac disturbances of hyperkalemia, hypocalcemia; emergent treatment of hypocalcemic tetany; treatment of hypermagnesemia

Unlabeled/Investigational Use

Calcium channel blocker overdose

Available Dosage Forms Injection, solution [preservative free]: 10% [100 mg/mL] (10 mL) [equivalent to elemental calcium 27.2 mg/mL, calcium 1.36 mEq/mL]

Dosing

Adults & Elderly: Note: Calcium chloride has 3 times more elemental calcium than calcium gluconate. Calcium chloride is 27% elemental calcium; calcium gluconate is 9% elemental calcium. One gram of calcium chloride is equal to 270 mg of elemental calcium; one gram of calcium gluconate is equal to 90 mg of elemental calcium. Dosages are expressed in terms of the calcium chloride salt based on a solution concentration of 100 mg/mL (10%) containing 1.4 mEq (27.3 mg)/mL elemental calcium.

Cardiac arrest in the presence of hyperkalemia or hypocalcemia, magnesium toxicity: I.V.: 2-4 mg/kg, repeated every 10 minutes if necessary

Calcium channel blocker overdose (unlabeled use):

I.V.: 1 g every 15-20 minutes (total of 4 doses) **or** 1 g every 2-3 minutes until clinical effect is achieved

I.V. infusion: 0.2-0.4 mL/kg/hour

Hypocalcemia: I.V.: 500 mg to 1 g/dose repeated every 4-6 hours if needed

Hypocalcemic tetany: I.V.: 1 g over 10-30 minutes; may repeat after 6 hours

Hypocalcemia secondary to citrated blood transfusion: I.V.: 200-500 mg per 500 mL of citrated blood (infused into another vein)

Note: Routine administration of calcium, in the absence of signs/symptoms of hypocalcemia, is generally not recommended. A number of recommendations have been published seeking to address potential hypocalcemia during massive transfusion of citrated blood; however, many practitioners recommend replacement only as guided by clinical evidence of hypocalcemia and/or serial monitoring of ionized calcium.

Pediatrics: Note: Calcium chloride has 3 times more elemental calcium than calcium gluconate. Calcium chloride is 27% elemental calcium; calcium gluconate is 9% elemental calcium. One gram of calcium chloride is equal to 270 mg of elemental calcium; one gram of calcium gluconate is equal to 90 mg of elemental calcium. Dosages are expressed in terms of the calcium chloride salt based on a solution concentration of 100 mg/mL (10%) containing 1.4 mEq (27.3 mg)/mL elemental calcium.

Cardiac arrest in the presence of hyperkalemia or hypocalcemia, magnesium toxicity: I.V.:

Infants and Children: 20 mg/kg; may repeat in 10 minutes if necessary

Adolescents: Refer to adult dosing.

Hypocalcemia: I.V.:

Children (manufacturer's recommendation): 2.7-5 mg/kg/dose every 4-6 hours

Alternative pediatric dosing: Infants and Children: 10-20 mg/kg/dose; repeat every 4-6 hours if needed

Hypocalcemic tetany: I.V.:

Neonates: Divided doses totaling approximately 170 mg/kg/24 hours

Infants and Children: 10 mg/kg over 5-10 minutes; may repeat after 6-8 hours or follow with an infusion with a maximum dose of 200 mg/kg/day; alternatively, higher doses of 35-50 mg/kg/dose repeated every 6-8 hours have been used

Hypocalcemia secondary to citrated blood transfusion: I.V.: Neonates, Infants, and Children: Give 32 mg (0.45 mEq **elemental** calcium) for each 100 mL citrated blood infused.

Note: Routine administration of calcium, in the absence of signs/symptoms of hypocalcemia, is generally not recommended. A number of recommendations have been published seeking to address potential hypocalcemia during massive transfusion of citrated blood; however, many practitioners recommend replacement only as guided by clinical evidence of hypocalcemia and/or serial monitoring of ionized calcium.

Renal Impairment: Cl_{cr} <25 mL/minute: Dosage adjustments may be necessary depending on the serum calcium levels.

Nursing Actions

Physical Assessment:

Assess other medications or herbal/natural products the patient may be taking for effectiveness and interactions. Assess results of laboratory tests, therapeutic effect, and adverse/toxic effects. Infusion site should be monitored closely to prevent extravasation (see Administration).

Patient Education: This medication can only be given intravenously. Do not make rapid postural changes while calcium is infusing. Report any feelings of excitation, chest pain, irregular or pounding heartbeat, vomiting, acute headache, or dizziness.

Calcium Citrate (KAL see um SIT rate)

U.S. Brand Names Cal-Citrate® 250 [OTC]; Citracal® [OTC]

Pharmacologic Category Calcium Salt

Medication Safety Issues

Sound-alike/look-alike issues:

Citracal® may be confused with Citrucel®

Pregnancy Risk Factor C

Use Antacid; treatment and prevention of calcium deficiency or hyperphosphatemia (eg, osteoporosis, osteomalacia, mild/moderate renal insufficiency, hypoparathyroidism, postmenopausal osteoporosis, rickets)

Contraindications Hypersensitivity to any component of the formulation; hypercalcemia, renal calculi, ventricular fibrillation

Warnings/Precautions Calcium absorption is impaired in achlorhydria (citrate may be preferred due to limited impact on absorption). Hypercalcemia and hypercalciuria may result when therapeutic replacement amounts are given for prolonged periods. They are most likely to occur in hypoparathyroid patients receiving high doses of vitamin D. Use with caution in digitalized patients, respiratory failure, or acidosis. Hypercalcemia may
(Continued)

Calcium Citrate *(Continued)*

occur in patients with renal failure, and frequent determination of serum calcium is necessary.

Drug Interactions

Decreased Effect: Absorption of tetracycline, atenolol (and potentially other beta-blockers), iron, quinolone antibiotics, alendronate, sodium fluoride, and zinc absorption may be significantly decreased; space administration times. Effects of calcium channel blockers (eg, verapamil) effects may be diminished. Polystyrene sulfonate's potassium-binding ability may be reduced; avoid concurrent administration.

Increased Effect/Toxicity: High doses of calcium with thiazide diuretics may result in milk-alkali syndrome and hypercalcemia; monitor response. Calcium salts may decrease T_4 absorption; separate dose from levothyroxine by at least 4 hours. Calcium acetate may potentiate digoxin toxicity.

Nutritional/Ethanol Interactions Ethanol: Avoid ethanol (may increase risk of osteoporosis).

Adverse Reactions Frequency not defined:

Mild hypercalcemia (calcium: >10.5 mg/dL) may be asymptomatic or manifest itself as constipation, anorexia, nausea, and vomiting

More severe hypercalcemia (calcium: >12 mg/dL) is associated with confusion, delirium, stupor, and coma

Frequency not defined:

Central nervous system: Headache

Endocrine & metabolic: Hypophosphatemia, hypercalcemia

Gastrointestinal: Nausea, anorexia, vomiting, abdominal pain, constipation

Miscellaneous: Thirst

Available Dosage Forms

Granules: 760 mg/teaspoonful (480 g)

Tablet: Elemental calcium 200 mg, 250 mg

Cal-Citrate®: Elemental calcium 250 mg

Citracal®: 950 mg [equivalent to elemental calcium 200 mg]

Dosing

Adults & Elderly: Oral: Dosage is in terms of elemental calcium

Dietary Reference Intake:

Adults, Male/Female:

19-50 years: 1000 mg/day

≥51 years: 1200 mg/day

Female: Pregnancy: Same as for Adults, Male/Female

Female: Lactating: Same as for Adults, Male/Female

Dietary supplement: Oral: Usual dose: 500 mg to 2 g 2-4 times/day

Pediatrics: Oral: Dosage is in terms of elemental calcium

Dietary Reference Intake:

0-6 months: 210 mg/day

7-12 months: 270 mg/day

1-3 years: 500 mg/day

4-8 years: 800 mg/day

9-18 years: 1300 mg/day

Nursing Actions

Physical Assessment:

Assess other medications patient may be taking for effectiveness and interactions. Monitor therapeutic effect, and adverse/toxic effects. Assess knowledge/teach patient proper use, appropriate interventions to reduce side effects, and adverse symptoms to report.

Patient Education: Inform prescriber of any other medications or dietary supplements you are taking. Do not take any new medication during therapy without consulting prescriber. Follow exact instructions for dosing. Take with a full glass of water or juice, 1-3 hours after other medications, and 1-2 hours

before any approved iron supplements. Avoid alcohol, other antacids, caffeine, or other calcium supplements unless approved by prescriber. May cause constipation (increased exercise, fluids, fiber, or fruits may help) or dry mouth (frequent mouth care, chewing gum, or sucking lozenges may help). Report severe, unresolved GI disturbances and unusual emotional lability (mood swings). **Pregnancy precaution:** Inform prescriber if you are or intend to become pregnant.

Calcium Glubionate

(KAL see um gloo BYE oh nate)

Pharmacologic Category Calcium Salt

Pregnancy Risk Factor C

Use Adjunct in treatment and prevention of postmenopausal osteoporosis; treatment and prevention of calcium depletion or hyperphosphatemia (eg, osteoporosis, osteomalacia, mild-to-moderate renal insufficiency, hypoparathyroidism, rickets)

Available Dosage Forms Syrup: 1.8 g/5 mL (480 mL) [equivalent to elemental calcium 115 mg/5 mL]

Dosing

Adults & Elderly: Dosage is in terms of **elemental** calcium

Dietary Reference Intake:

Adults, Male/Female:

19-50 years: 1000 mg/day

≥51 years: 1200 mg/day

Female: Pregnancy: Same as for Adults, Male/Female

Female: Lactating: Same as for Adults, Male/Female

Syrup is a hyperosmolar solution; dosage is in terms of calcium glubionate, elemental calcium is in parentheses: 6-18 g (~0.5-1 g Ca++)/day in divided doses

Pediatrics: Dosage is in terms of **elemental** calcium

Dietary Reference Intake:

0-6 months: 210 mg/day

7-12 months: 270 mg/day

1-3 years: 500 mg/day

4-8 years: 800 mg/day

9-18 years: 1300 mg/day

Note: Syrup is a hyperosmolar solution; dosage is in terms of calcium glubionate, elemental calcium is in parentheses

Neonatal hypocalcemia: 1200 mg (77 mg Ca++)/kg/day in 4-6 divided doses

Maintenance: Infants and Children: 600-2000 mg (38-128 mg Ca++)/kg/day in 4 divided doses up to a maximum of 9 g (575 mg Ca++)/day

Renal Impairment: Cl_{cr} <25 mL/minute: Dosage adjustments may be necessary depending on the serum calcium levels.

Nursing Actions

Patient Education: Do not take any new medication during therapy without consulting prescriber. Follow exact instructions for dosing. Take with a full glass of water or juice, 1-3 hours after meals and other medications, and 1-2 hours before any approved iron supplements. Avoid alcohol, other antacids, caffeine, or other calcium supplements unless approved by prescriber. May cause constipation (increased exercise, fluids, fiber, or fruits may help) or dry mouth (frequent mouth care, chewing gum, or sucking lozenges may help). Report severe, unresolved GI disturbances and unusual emotional lability (mood swings). **Pregnancy precaution:** Inform prescriber if you are or intend to become pregnant.

Calcium Gluconate
(KAL see um GLOO koe nate)

Pharmacologic Category Calcium Salt; Electrolyte Supplement, Oral; Electrolyte Supplement, Parenteral

Medication Safety Issues
Sound-alike/look-alike issues:
Calcium gluconate may be confused with calcium glubionate

Pregnancy Risk Factor C

Lactation Enters breast milk

Use Treatment and prevention of hypocalcemia; treatment of tetany, cardiac disturbances of hyperkalemia, cardiac resuscitation when epinephrine fails to improve myocardial contractions, hypocalcemia; calcium supplementation

Unlabeled/Investigational Use Hydrofluoric acid (HF) burns; calcium channel blocker overdose

Mechanism of Action/Effect As dietary supplement, used to prevent or treat negative calcium balance; in osteoporosis, it helps to prevent or decrease the rate of bone loss. The calcium in calcium salts moderates nerve and muscle performance and allows normal cardiac function.

Contraindications Ventricular fibrillation during cardiac resuscitation; digitalis toxicity or suspected digoxin toxicity; hypercalcemia

Warnings/Precautions Injection solution is for I.V. use only; do not inject SubQ or I.M. Avoid too rapid I.V. administration and avoid extravasation. Use with caution in digitalized patients, severe hyperphosphatemia, respiratory failure or acidosis. May produce cardiac arrest. Hypercalcemia may occur in patients with renal failure; frequent determination of serum calcium is necessary. Use caution with renal disease. Solutions may contain aluminum; toxic levels may occur following prolonged administration in premature neonates or patients with renal dysfunction.

Drug Interactions
Decreased Effect: Bisphosphonate derivative absorption may be decreased by calcium salts. Calcium channel blockers (eg, verapamil) effects may be diminished; monitor response. Calcium salts may diminish the therapeutic effect of dobutamine. Calcium carbonate (and possibly other calcium salts) may decrease T_4 absorption; separate dose from levothyroxine by at least 4 hours. Calcium salts may decrease the absorption of phosphate supplements. Calcium salts may decrease the absorption of quinolone antibiotics with oral adminstration of both agents.

Increased Effect/Toxicity: Calcium salts may potentiate digoxin toxicity. Thiazide diuretics may decrease the excretion of calcium salts. Continued concomitant use can also result in metabolic alkalosis.

Lab Interactions Increased calcium (S); decreased magnesium

Adverse Reactions Frequency not defined.
I.V.:
Cardiovascular: Arrhythmia, bradycardia, cardiac arrest, hypotension, vasodilation, and syncope may occur following rapid I.V. injection
Central nervous system: Sense of oppression
Gastrointestinal: Chalky taste
Local: Abscess and necrosis following I.M. administration
Neuromuscular & skeletal: Tingling sensation
Miscellaneous: Heat waves

Oral: Gastrointestinal: Constipation

Overdosage/Toxicology
Acute single oral ingestions of calcium salts may produce mild gastrointestinal distress, but hypercalcemia or other toxic manifestations are extremely unlikely. Symptoms of hypercalcemia include lethargy, nausea, vomiting, and coma.
Treatment is supportive. Severe hypercalcemia following parenteral overdose requires I.V. hydration. Urine output should be monitored and maintained at >3 mL/kg/hour. I.V. saline and natriuretic agents (eg, furosemide) can quickly and significantly increase excretion of calcium into urine.

Pharmacodynamics/Kinetics
Protein Binding: Primarily albumin
Excretion: Primarily feces (as unabsorbed calcium); urine (20%)

Available Dosage Forms
Injection, solution [preservative free]: 10% [100 mg/mL] (10 mL, 50 mL, 100 mL, 200 mL) [equivalent to elemental calcium 9 mg/mL; calcium 0.46 mEq/mL]
Powder: 347 mg/tablespoonful (480 g)
Tablet: 500 mg [equivalent to elemental calcium 45 mg]; 650 mg [equivalent to elemental calcium 58.5 mg]; 975 mg [equivalent to elemental calcium 87.75 mg]

Dosing
Adults & Elderly:
Adequate Intake (as elemental calcium):
Adults, Male/Female:
19-50 years: 1000 mg/day
≥51 years: 1200 mg/day
Female: Pregnancy: Same as for Adults, Male/Female
Female: Lactating: Same as for Adults, Male/Female

Dosage note: Calcium chloride has 3 times more elemental calcium than calcium gluconate. Calcium chloride is 27% elemental calcium; calcium gluconate is 9% elemental calcium. One gram of calcium chloride is equal to 270 mg of elemental calcium; 1 gram of calcium gluconate is equal to 90 mg of elemental calcium. The following dosages are expressed in terms of the calcium gluconate salt based on a solution concentration of 100 mg/mL (10%) containing 0.465 mEq (9.3 mg)/mL elemental calcium:

Hypocalcemia:
I.V.: 2-15 g/24 hours as a continuous infusion or in divided doses
Oral: 500 mg to 2 g 2-4 times/day

Hypocalcemia secondary to citrated blood infusion: I.V.: 500 mg to 1 g per 500 mL of citrated blood (infused into another vein). Single doses up to 2 g have also been recommended.
Note: Routine administration of calcium, in the absence of signs/symptoms of hypocalcemia, is generally not recommended. A number of recommendations have been published seeking to address potential hypocalcemia during massive transfusion of citrated blood; however, many practitioners recommend replacement only as guided by clinical evidence of hypocalcemia and/or serial monitoring of ionized calcium.

Hypocalcemic tetany: I.V.: 1-3 g/dose may be administered until therapeutic response occurs

Magnesium intoxication or cardiac arrest in the presence of hyperkalemia or hypocalcemia: I.V.: 500-800 mg/dose (maximum: 3 g/dose)

Maintenance electrolyte requirements for TPN: I.V.: Daily requirements: 1.7-3.4 g/1000 kcal/24 hours

Calcium channel blocker overdose (unlabeled use): I.V. infusion: 10% solution: 0.6-1.2 mL/kg/hour or I.V. 0.2-0.5 ml/kg every 15-20 minutes for 4 doses (maximum: 2-3 g/dose). In life-threatening situations, 1 g has been given every 1-10 minutes until clinical effect is achieved (case reports of resistant hypotension reported use of 12-18 g total).

Pediatrics:
Adequate Intake (as elemental calcium):
0-6 months: 210 mg/day
(Continued)

Calcium Gluconate *(Continued)*

7-12 months: 270 mg/day
1-3 years: 500 mg/day
4-8 years: 800 mg/day
9-18 years: 1300 mg/day

Dosage note: Calcium chloride has 3 times more elemental calcium than calcium gluconate. Calcium chloride is 27% elemental calcium; calcium gluconate is (9% elemental calcium). One gram of calcium chloride is equal to 270 mg of elemental calcium; 1 gram of calcium gluconate is equal to 90 mg of elemental calcium. The following dosages are expressed in terms of the calcium gluconate salt based on a solution concentration of 100 mg/mL (10%) containing 0.465 mEq (9.3 mg)/mL elemental calcium:

Hypocalcemia:
I.V.:
Neonates: 200-800 mg/kg/day as a continuous infusion or in 4 divided doses (maximum: 1 g/ dose)
Infants and Children: 200-500 mg/kg/day as a continuous infusion or in 4 divided doses (maximum: 2-3 g/dose)
Oral: Children: 200-500 mg/kg/day divided every 6 hours

Hypocalcemia secondary to citrated blood infusion: I.V.: Neonates, Infants, and Children: Give 98 mg (0.45 mEq **elemental** calcium) for each 100 mL citrated blood infused.

Note: Routine administration of calcium, in the absence of signs/symptoms of hypocalcemia, is generally not recommended. A number of recommendations have been published seeking to address potential hypocalcemia during massive transfusion of citrated blood; however, many practitioners recommend replacement only as guided by clinical evidence of hypocalcemia and/ or serial monitoring of ionized calcium.

Hypocalcemic tetany: I.V.: Infants and Children: 100-200 mg/kg/dose over 5-10 minutes; may repeat every 6-8 hours **or** follow with an infusion of 500 mg/kg/day

Magnesium intoxication or cardiac arrest in the presence of hyperkalemia or hypocalcemia: I.V.: Infants and Children: 60-100 mg/kg/dose (maximum: 3 g/dose)

Renal Impairment: Cl_{cr} <25 mL/minute: Dosage adjustments may be necessary depending on the serum calcium levels.

Administration
I.M.: Not for I.M. or SubQ administration
I.V.: For I.V. administration only; administer slowly (~1.5 mL calcium gluconate 10% per minute) through a small needle into a large vein in order to avoid too rapid increased in serum calcium and extravasation
Other: Not for SubQ administration.

Stability
Compatibility: Stable in D_5LR, D_5NS, D_5W, $D_{10}W$, $D_{20}W$, LR, NS; **incompatible** in fat emulsion 10%
Y-site administration: Incompatible with amphotericin B cholesteryl sulfate complex, fluconazole, indomethacin
Compatibility in syringe: Incompatible with metoclopramide
Compatibility when admixed: Incompatible with amphotericin B, cefamandole, cefazolin, clindamycin, dobutamine, floxacillin, methylprednisolone sodium succinate

Storage:
Do not refrigerate solutions. IVPB solutions/I.V. infusion solutions are stable for 24 hours at room temperature.
Standard diluent: 1 g/100 mL D_5W or NS; 2 g/100 mL D_5W or NS

Maximum concentration in parenteral nutrition solutions is variable depending upon concentration and solubility (consult detailed reference).

Nursing Actions
Physical Assessment:
Assess other medications patient may be taking for effectiveness and interactions. Monitor results of laboratory tests, therapeutic effect, and adverse/toxic effects. Assess knowledge/teach patient proper use, appropriate interventions to reduce side effects, and adverse symptoms to report. If administered I.V., monitor ECG, vital signs, and CNS. Observe infusion site closely. Avoid extravasation.

Patient Education: Do not take any new medication during therapy without consulting prescriber. Follow exact instructions for dosing. Oral: Take with a full glass of water or juice, 1-3 hours after other medications, and 1-2 hours before any approved iron supplements. Avoid alcohol, other antacids, caffeine, or other calcium supplements unless approved by prescriber. May cause constipation (increased exercise, fluids, fiber, or fruits may help) or dry mouth (frequent mouth care, chewing gum, or sucking lozenges may help). Report severe, unresolved GI disturbances and unusual emotional lability (mood swings). **Pregnancy precaution:** Inform prescriber if you are or intend to become pregnant.

Breast-Feeding Issues Endogenous calcium is excreted in breast milk.

Additional Information A topical 2.5% to 5% calcium gel for the treatment of hydrofluoric acid (HF) burns can be prepared by adding calcium gluconate to a surgical lubricant (water soluble such as K-Y® Jelly). Calcium chloride should not be used for this purpose. Use of injectable calcium gluconate (I.V., SubQ) has also been reported in the literature for the treatment of HF burns not amenable to topical treatment.

Related Information
Compatibility of Drugs *on page 1370*

Calcium Lactate (KAL see um LAK tate)

Pharmacologic Category Calcium Salt
Pregnancy Risk Factor C
Use Adjunct in prevention of postmenopausal osteoporosis; treatment and prevention of calcium depletion
Available Dosage Forms Tablet: 650 mg [equivalent to elemental calcium 84.5 mg]
Dosing
Adults & Elderly: Dosage in terms of calcium lactate
Dietary Reference Intake (in terms of elemental calcium):
Adults, Male/Female:
19-50 years: 1000 mg/day
≥51 years: 1200 mg/day
Female: Pregnancy: Same as Adults, Male/Female
Female: Lactating: Same as Adults, Male/Female

Calcium supplement, osteoporosis prevention:
Oral: 1.5-3 g divided every 8 hours
Pediatrics: Oral (in terms of calcium lactate):
Dietary Reference Intake (in terms of elemental calcium):
0-6 months: 210 mg/day
7-12 months: 270 mg/day
1-3 years: 500 mg/day
4-8 years: 800 mg/day
9-18 years: 1300 mg/day

Calcium supplement: 500 mg/kg/day divided every 6-8 hours; maximum daily dose: 9 g
Renal Impairment: Cl_{cr} <25 mL/minute: Dosage adjustments may be necessary depending on the serum calcium levels.

Nursing Actions

Patient Education: Do not take any new medication during therapy without consulting prescriber. Follow exact instructions for dosing. Take with a full glass of water or juice, 1-3 hours after other medications, and 1-2 hours before any approved iron supplements. Avoid alcohol, other antacids, caffeine, or other calcium supplements unless approved by prescriber. May cause constipation (increased exercise, fluids, fiber, or fruits may help) or dry mouth (frequent mouth care, chewing gum, or sucking lozenges may help). Report severe, unresolved GI disturbances and unusual emotional lability (mood swings). **Pregnancy precaution:** Inform prescriber if you are or intend to become pregnant.

Calcium Phosphate (Tribasic)
(KAL see um FOS fate tri BAY sik)

U.S. Brand Names Posture® [OTC]
Synonyms Tricalcium Phosphate
Pharmacologic Category Calcium Salt
Use Dietary supplement
Available Dosage Forms Tablet: 1565.2 mg [equivalent to elemental calcium 600 mg; sugar free]
Dosing
Adults & Elderly:
Adequate Intake (as elemental calcium): Oral:
Male/Female:
19-50 years: 1000 mg/day
≥51 years: 1200 mg/day
Female: Pregnancy: Same as for nonpregnant females
Female: Lactating: Same as for nonlactating females
Dietary supplement: Oral: 2 tablets daily
Pediatrics: Adequate Intake (as elemental calcium): Oral:
0-6 months: 210 mg/day
7-12 months: 270 mg/day
1-3 years: 500 mg/day
4-8 years: 800 mg/day
9-18 years: 1300 mg/day
Renal Impairment: Cl_{cr} <25 mL/minute: Dosage adjustments may be necessary depending on the serum calcium levels.

Nursing Actions

Patient Education: Do not take any new medication during therapy without consulting prescriber. Follow exact instructions for dosing. Take with a full glass of water or juice, 1-3 hours after meals and other medications, and 1-2 hours before any approved iron supplements. Avoid alcohol, other antacids, caffeine, or other calcium supplements unless approved by prescriber. May cause constipation (increased exercise, fluids, fiber, or fruits may help) or dry mouth (frequent mouth care, chewing gum, or sucking lozenges may help). Report severe, unresolved GI disturbances and unusual emotional lability (mood swings). **Pregnancy precaution:** Inform prescriber if you are or intend to become pregnant.

Candesartan (kan de SAR tan)

U.S. Brand Names Atacand®
Synonyms Candesartan Cilexetil
Pharmacologic Category Angiotensin II Receptor Blocker

Pregnancy Risk Factor C/D (2nd and 3rd trimesters)
Lactation Enters breast milk/contraindicated
Use Alone or in combination with other antihypertensive agents in treating essential hypertension; treatment of heart failure (NYHA class II-IV)
Mechanism of Action/Effect Blocks the vasoconstrictor and aldosterone-secreting effects of angiotensin II by binding of angiotensin II at the AT1 receptor in many tissues, such as vascular smooth muscle and the adrenal gland. Independent of pathways for angiotensin II synthesis. Does not affect the response to bradykinin; does not bind to block other hormone receptors or ion channels known to be important in cardiovascular regulation.
Contraindications Hypersensitivity to candesartan or any component of the formulation; hypersensitivity to other A-II receptor antagonists; bilateral renal artery stenosis; pregnancy (2nd and 3rd trimesters)
Warnings/Precautions Avoid use or use a smaller dose in patients who are volume depleted; correct depletion first. May be associated with deterioration of renal function and/or increases in serum creatinine, particularly in patients dependent on renin-angiotensin-aldosterone system; deterioration may result in oliguria, acute renal failure and progressive azotemia. Small increases in serum creatinine may occur following initiation; consider discontinuation only in patients with progressive and/or significant deterioration in renal function. Use with caution in unilateral renal artery stenosis, hepatic dysfunction, pre-existing renal insufficiency, or significant aortic/mitral stenosis. Use caution when initiating in heart failure; may need to adjust dose, and/or concurrent diuretic therapy, because of candesartan-induced hypotension. Although some properties may be shared between these agents, concurrent therapy with ACE-inhibitor may be rational in selected patients.

Drug Interactions
Cytochrome P450 Effect: Substrate of CYP2C8/9 (minor); **Inhibits** CYP2C8/9 (weak)
Increased Effect/Toxicity: The risk of lithium toxicity may be increased by candesartan; monitor lithium levels. Concurrent use with potassium-sparing diuretics (amiloride, spironolactone, triamterene), potassium supplements, or trimethoprim (high-dose) may increase the risk of hyperkalemia.

Nutritional/Ethanol Interactions
Food: Food reduces the time to maximal concentration and increases the C_{max}
Herb/Nutraceutical: Avoid dong quai if using for hypertension (has estrogenic activity). Avoid ephedra, yohimbe, ginseng (may worsen hypertension). Avoid garlic (may have increased antihypertensive effect).

Adverse Reactions
Cardiovascular: Angina, hypotension (CHF 19%), MI, palpitation, tachycardia
Central nervous system: Dizziness, lightheadedness, drowsiness, headache, vertigo, anxiety, depression, somnolence, fever
Dermatologic: Angioedema, rash
Endocrine & metabolic: Hyperglycemia, hyperkalemia (CHF <1% to 6%), hypertriglyceridemia, hyperuricemia
Gastrointestinal: Dyspepsia, gastroenteritis
Genitourinary: Hematuria
Neuromuscular & skeletal: Back pain, CPK increased, myalgia, paresthesia, weakness
(Continued)

Candesartan *(Continued)*

Renal: Serum creatinine increased (up to 13% in patients with CHF with drug discontinuation required in 6%)

Respiratory: Dyspnea, epistaxis, pharyngitis, rhinitis, upper respiratory tract infection

Miscellaneous: Diaphoresis increased

Overdosage/Toxicology Symptoms of overdose include hypotension and tachycardia. Treatment is supportive.

Pharmacodynamics/Kinetics

Onset of Action: 2-3 hours; Peak effect: 6-8 hours

Duration of Action: >24 hours

Time to Peak: 3-4 hours

Protein Binding: 99%

Half-Life Elimination: Dose dependent: 5-9 hours

Metabolism: To candesartan by the intestinal wall cells

Excretion: Urine (26%)

Clearance: Total body: 0.37 mL/kg/minute; Renal: 0.19 mL/kg/minute

Available Dosage Forms Tablet, as cilexetil: 4 mg, 8 mg, 16 mg, 32 mg

Dosing

Adults:

Hypertension: Oral: 4-32 mg once daily. Dosage must be individualized. Blood pressure response is dose related over the range of 2-32 mg. The usual recommended starting dose is 16 mg once daily when it is used as monotherapy in patients who are not volume depleted. It can be administered once or twice daily with total daily doses ranging from 8-32 mg; larger doses do not appear to have a greater effect and there is relatively little experience with such doses.

Congestive heart failure: Oral: Initial: 4 mg once daily; double the dose at 2-week intervals, as tolerated; target dose: 32 mg

Note: In selected cases, concurrent therapy with an ACE inhibitor may provide additional benefit.

Elderly: Refer to adult dosing. No initial dosage adjustment is necessary for elderly patients (although higher concentrations (C_{max}) and AUC were observed in these populations), for patients with mildly impaired renal function, or for patients with mildly impaired hepatic function.

Hepatic Impairment: No initial dosage adjustment required in mild hepatic impairment. Consider initiation at lower dosages in moderate hepatic impairment (AUC increased by 145%). No data available concerning dosing in severe hepatic impairment.

Laboratory Monitoring Electrolytes, serum creatinine, BUN, urinalysis; in CHF, serum potassium during dose escalation and periodically thereafter

Nursing Actions

Physical Assessment: Assess other pharmacological or herbal products patient may be taking for potential interactions (eg, increased risk for hypotension, hyperkalemia). Monitor laboratory tests, effectiveness of therapy (reduced hypertension), and adverse response (eg, tachycardia, CNS changes, hyperglycemia, hypotension) at beginning of therapy, when changing dose, and on a regular basis during long-term therapy. Teach patient proper use, possible side effects/appropriate interventions, and adverse symptoms to report.

Patient Education: Do not take any new medication during therapy unless approved by prescriber. Take exactly as directed and do not discontinue medication without consulting prescriber. Preferable to take on an empty stomach, 1 hour before or 2 hours after meals. This drug does not eliminate need for diet or exercise regimen as recommended by prescriber. May cause dizziness, fainting, or lightheadedness (use caution when driving or engaging in tasks that require alert-ness until response to drug is known); postural hypotension (use caution when rising from lying or sitting position or climbing stairs); nausea or vomiting (small, frequent meals, frequent mouth care, chewing gum, or sucking lozenges may help); or diarrhea (boiled milk, buttermilk, or yogurt may help). Report chest pain or palpitations; unusual weight gain or swelling of ankles and hands; persistent fatigue; unusual flu or cold symptoms or dry cough; respiratory difficulty; swelling of eyes, face, or lips; skin rash; muscle pain or weakness; unusual bleeding (blood in urine or stool, or from gums); or excessive sweating. **Pregnancy/breast-feeding precautions:** Inform prescriber if you are or intend to become pregnant. This drug should not be used in the 2nd or 3rd trimester of pregnancy. Consult prescriber for appropriate contraceptive measures if necessary. Do not breast-feed.

Geriatric Considerations High concentrations occur in the elderly compared to younger subjects. AUC may be doubled in patients with renal impairment. No initial dose adjustment necessary since repeated dose did not demonstrate accumulation of drug or metabolites in elderly.

Pregnancy Issues The drug should be discontinued as soon as possible when pregnancy is detected. Drugs which act directly on renin-angiotensin can cause fetal and neonatal morbidity and death.

Additional Information May have an advantage over losartan due to minimal metabolism requirements and consequent use in mild-to-moderate hepatic impairment

Candesartan and Hydrochlorothiazide

(kan de SAR tan & hye droe klor oh THYE a zide)

U.S. Brand Names Atacand HCT™

Synonyms Candesartan Cilexetil and Hydrochlorothiazide

Pharmacologic Category Angiotensin II Receptor Blocker Combination; Antihypertensive Agent, Combination; Diuretic, Thiazide

Pregnancy Risk Factor C/D (2nd and 3rd trimesters)

Lactation Enters breast milk/contraindicated

Use Treatment of hypertension; combination product should not be used for initial therapy

Available Dosage Forms Tablet:

16-12.5: Candesartan 16 mg and hydrochlorothiazide 12.5 mg

32-12.5: Candesartan 32 mg and hydrochlorothiazide 12.5 mg

Dosing

Adults & Elderly: Hypertension, replacement therapy: Oral: Combination product can be substituted for individual agents; maximum therapeutic effect would be expected within 4 weeks

Usual dosage range:

Candesartan: 8-32 mg/day, given once daily or twice daily in divided doses

Hydrochlorothiazide: 12.5-50 mg once daily

Renal Impairment: Serum levels of candesartan are increased and the half-life of hydrochlorothiazide is prolonged in patients with renal impairment. Do not use if Cl_{cr} is <30 mL/minute.

Hepatic Impairment: Use with caution.

Nursing Actions

Physical Assessment: See individual agents.

Patient Education: See individual agents. **Pregnancy/breast-feeding precautions:** Inform prescriber if you are or intend to become pregnant; contraceptives may be recommended. Do not breast-feed.

Related Information

Candesartan *on page 195*
Hydrochlorothiazide *on page 610*

Capecitabine (ka pe SITE a been)

U.S. Brand Names Xeloda®

Synonyms NSC-712807

Pharmacologic Category Antineoplastic Agent, Antimetabolite

Medication Safety Issues

Sound-alike/look-alike issues:

Xeloda® may be confused with Xenical®

Pregnancy Risk Factor D

Lactation Excretion in breast milk unknown/not recommended

Use Treatment of metastatic colorectal cancer; adjuvant therapy of Dukes' C colon cancer; treatment of metastatic breast cancer

Mechanism of Action/Effect Capecitabine is a prodrug of fluorouracil. It undergoes hydrolysis in the liver and tissues to form fluorouracil. It interferes with DNA (and to a lesser degree RNA) synthesis. Appears to be specific for G$_1$ and S phases of the cell cycle.

Contraindications Hypersensitivity to capecitabine, fluorouracil, or any component of the formulation; known deficiency of dihydropyrimidine dehydrogenase (DPD); severe renal impairment (Cl$_{cr}$ <30 mL/minute); pregnancy

Warnings/Precautions Hazardous agent — use appropriate precautions for handling and disposal. Use with caution in patients with bone marrow suppression, poor nutritional status, ≥80 years of age, or renal or hepatic dysfunction. Patients with baseline moderate renal impairment require dose reduction. Patients with mild-to-moderate renal impairment require careful monitoring and subsequent dose reduction with any grade 2 or higher adverse event. Use with caution in patients who have received extensive pelvic radiation or alkylating therapy. Use cautiously with warfarin. Rare and unexpected severe toxicity may be attributed to dihydropyrimidine dehydrogenase (DPD) deficiency.

Capecitabine can cause severe diarrhea; median time to first occurrence is 34 days. Subsequent doses should be reduced after grade 3 or 4 diarrhea or recurrence of grade 2 diarrhea.

Hand-and-foot syndrome is characterized by numbness, dysesthesia/paresthesia, tingling, painless or painful swelling, erythema, desquamation, blistering, and severe pain. If grade 2 or 3 hand-and-foot syndrome occurs, interrupt administration of capecitabine until decreases to grade 1. Following grade 3 hand-and-foot syndrome, decrease subsequent doses of capecitabine.

There has been cardiotoxicity associated with fluorinated pyrimidine therapy. May be more common in patients with a history of coronary artery disease.

Safety and efficacy in children <18 years of age have not been established.

Drug Interactions

Increased Effect/Toxicity: Phenytoin and warfarin levels or effects may be increased.

Nutritional/Ethanol Interactions Food: Food reduced the rate and extent of absorption of capecitabine.

Adverse Reactions Frequency listed derived from monotherapy trials.

>10%:

Cardiovascular: Edema (9% to 15%)

Central nervous system: Fatigue (16% to 42%), fever (7% to 18%), pain (12%)

Dermatologic: Palmar-plantar erythrodysesthesia (hand-and-foot syndrome) (54% to 60%); grade 3: 11% to 17%; may be dose limiting), dermatitis (27% to 37%)

Gastrointestinal: Diarrhea (47% to 57%; may be dose limiting; grade 3: 12% to 13%; grade 4: 2% to 3%), nausea (34% to 53%), vomiting (15% to 37%), abdominal pain (7% to 35%), stomatitis (22% to 25%), appetite decreased (26%), anorexia (9% to 23%), constipation (9% to 15%)

Hematologic: Lymphopenia (94%; grade 4: 14%), anemia (72% to 80%; grade 4: <1% to 1%), neutropenia (2% to 26%; grade 4: 2%), thrombocytopenia (24%; grade 4: 1%)

Hepatic: Bilirubin increased (22% to 48%; grades 3/4: 11% to 23%)

Neuromuscular & skeletal: Paresthesia (21%)

Ocular: Eye irritation (13% to 15%)

Respiratory: Dyspnea (14%)

5% to 10%:

Cardiovascular: Venous thrombosis (8%), chest pain (6%)

Central nervous system: Headache (5% to 10%), lethargy (10%), dizziness (6% to 8%), insomnia (7% to 8%), mood alteration (5%), depression (5%)

Dermatologic: Nail disorder (7%), rash (7%), skin discoloration (7%), alopecia (6%), erythema (6%)

Endocrine & metabolic: Dehydration (7%)

Gastrointestinal: Motility disorder (10%), oral discomfort (10%), dyspepsia (6% to 8%), upper GI inflammatory disorders (colorectal cancer: 8%), hemorrhage (6%), ileus (6%), taste perversion (colorectal cancer: 6%)

Neuromuscular & skeletal: Back pain (10%), weakness (10%), neuropathy (10%), myalgia (9%), arthralgia (8%), limb pain (6%)

Ocular: Abnormal vision (colorectal cancer: 5%), conjunctivitis (5%)

Respiratory: Cough (7%)

Miscellaneous: Viral infection (colorectal cancer: 5%)

Overdosage/Toxicology Symptoms of overdose include myelosuppression, nausea, vomiting, diarrhea, and gastrointestinal irritation/bleeding. No specific antidote exists. Monitor hematologically for at least 4 weeks. Dialysis may be of benefit in reducing levels of the metabolite 5'-DFUR. Treatment is symptom-directed and supportive.

Pharmacodynamics/Kinetics

Time to Peak: 1.5 hours; Fluorouracil: 2 hours

Protein Binding: <60%; ~35% to albumin

Half-Life Elimination: 0.5-1 hour

Metabolism: Hepatic: Inactive metabolites: 5'-deoxy-5-fluorocytidine, 5'-deoxy-5-fluorouridine; Tissue: Active metabolite: Fluorouracil

Excretion: Urine (96%, 57% as α-fluoro-β-alanine); feces (<3%)

Available Dosage Forms Tablet: 150 mg, 500 mg

Dosing

Adults: Metastatic breast carcinoma, metastatic colorectal cancer: Oral: 1250 mg/m^2 twice daily (morning and evening) for 2 weeks, every 21-28 days

Adjuvant therapy of Dukes' C colon cancer: Recommended for a total of 24 weeks (8 cycles of 2 weeks of drug administration and 1 week rest period.

Elderly: The elderly may be more sensitive to the toxic effects of fluorouracil. Insufficient data are available to provide dosage modifications.

Renal Impairment:

Cl$_{cr}$ 51-80 mL/minute: No adjustment of initial dose.

Cl$_{cr}$ 30-50 mL/minute: Administer 75% of normal dose.

Cl$_{cr}$ <30 mL/minute: Use is contraindicated.

Hepatic Impairment:

Mild-to-moderate impairment: No starting dose adjustment is necessary; however, carefully monitor patients.

Severe hepatic impairment: Patients have not been studied.

Dosing Adjustment for Toxicity: Dosage modification guidelines: See table on next page.

(Continued)

Capecitabine *(Continued)*

Refer to package labeling for modifications when administered in combination with docetaxel.

Recommended Dose Modifications

Toxicity NCI Grades	During a Course of Therapy (Monotherapy)	Dose Adjustment for Next Cycle (% of starting dose)
Grade 1	Maintain dose level	Maintain dose level
Grade 2		
1st appearance	Interrupt until resolved to grade 0-1	100%
2nd appearance	Interrupt until resolved to grade 0-1	75%
3rd appearance	Interrupt until resolved to grade 0-1	50%
4th appearance	Discontinue treatment permanently	
Grade 3		
1st appearance	Interrupt until resolved to grade 0-1	75%
2nd appearance	Interrupt until resolved to grade 0-1	50%
3rd appearance	Discontinue treatment permanently	
Grade 4		
1st appearance	Discontinue permanently **or** If physician deems it to be in the patient's best interest to continue, interrupt until resolved to grade 0-1	50%

Administration

Oral: Usually administered in 2 divided doses taken 12 hours apart. Doses should be taken with water within 30 minutes after a meal.

Stability

Storage: Store at room temperature between 15°C and 30°C (59°F and 86°F).

Laboratory Monitoring Renal function should be estimated at baseline to determine initial dose. During therapy, CBC with differential, hepatic function, and renal function should be monitored.

Nursing Actions

Physical Assessment: Monitor laboratory tests at baseline and regularly during therapy (including INR for patients receiving oral coumarin-derivative anticoagulants). Assess for adverse reactions periodically during therapy (eg, gastrointestinal upset [nausea, vomiting, pain, dehydration, or severe diarrhea that can occur at any time during therapy]; hematologic [lymphopenia, anemia, thrombocytopenia], cardiovascular [edema, chest pain], or paresthesia regularly during therapy. Teach patient proper use, necessity for contraception with sexually-active female patients, possible side effects/appropriate interventions, and adverse symptoms to report.

Patient Education: Do not take any new medication during therapy unless approved by prescriber. Take with water within 30 minutes after meal. Avoid use of antacids within 2 hours of taking this medication. Do not crush, chew, or dissolve tablets. Maintain adequate hydration (2-3 L/day of fluids) unless instructed to restrict fluid intake. You may be more susceptible to infection (avoid crowds and exposure to infection and do not have any vaccinations without consulting prescriber). May cause lethargy, dizziness, visual changes, confusion, anxiety (avoid driving or engaging in tasks requiring alertness until response to drug is known); nausea, vomiting, loss of appetite, or dry mouth (small, frequent meals, frequent mouth care, chewing gum, or sucking lozenges may help); loss of hair (will grow back when treatment is discontinued); photosensitivity (use sunscreen, wear protective clothing and eyewear, and avoid direct sunlight); or dry, itchy, skin, and dry or irritated eyes (avoid contact lenses). Report persistent diarrhea or abdominal pain; skin rash, pain, tenderness, or peeling (especially hands and feet); chills or fever, confusion, persistent or violent vomiting; respiratory difficulty; chest pain or palpitations; unusual bleeding or bruising; bone pain; muscle spasms/tremors; or vision changes immediately. **Pregnancy/breast-feeding precautions:** Inform prescriber if you are pregnant. Do not get pregnant while taking this medication. Consult prescriber for appropriate contraceptive measures. Breast-feeding is not recommended.

Dietary Considerations Because current safety and efficacy data are based upon administration with food, it is recommended that capecitabine be administered with food. In all clinical trials, patients were instructed to take with water within 30 minutes after a meal.

Geriatric Considerations Patients ≥80 years of age may experience a greater incidence of grade 3 or 4 adverse events (diarrhea, hand-and-foot syndrome, nausea/vomiting).

Breast-Feeding Issues It is not known if the drug is excreted in breast milk. Because of the potential for serious adverse reactions in nursing infants, it is recommended that nursing be discontinued when receiving capecitabine therapy.

Pregnancy Issues Animal studies have demonstrated teratogenicity and fetal loss. There are no adequate and well-controlled studies in pregnant women; however, fetal harm may occur. Women of childbearing potential should avoid pregnancy.

Captopril *(KAP toe pril)*

U.S. Brand Names Capoten®

Synonyms ACE

Pharmacologic Category Angiotensin-Converting Enzyme (ACE) Inhibitor

Medication Safety Issues
Sound-alike/look-alike issues:
Captopril may be confused with Capitrol®, carvedilol

Pregnancy Risk Factor C (1st trimester)/D (2nd and 3rd trimesters)

Lactation Enters breast milk/not recommended (AAP rates "compatible")

Use Management of hypertension; treatment of congestive heart failure, left ventricular dysfunction after myocardial infarction, diabetic nephropathy

Unlabeled/Investigational Use Treatment of hypertensive crisis, rheumatoid arthritis; diagnosis of anatomic renal artery stenosis, hypertension secondary to scleroderma renal crisis; diagnosis of aldosteronism, idiopathic edema, Bartter's syndrome, postmyocardial infarction for prevention of ventricular failure; increase circulation in Raynaud's phenomenon, hypertension secondary to Takayasu's disease

Mechanism of Action/Effect Competitive inhibitor of angiotensin-converting enzyme (ACE); prevents conversion of angiotensin I to angiotensin II, a potent vasoconstrictor; results in lower levels of angiotensin II which causes an increase in plasma renin activity and a reduction in aldosterone secretion

Contraindications Hypersensitivity to captopril or any component of the formulation; angioedema related to previous treatment with an ACE inhibitor; idiopathic or hereditary angioedema; bilateral renal artery stenosis; pregnancy (2nd or 3rd trimester)

Warnings/Precautions Anaphylactic reactions can occur. Angioedema can occur at any time during treatment (especially following first dose). It may involve head and neck (potentially affecting the airway) or the intestine (presenting with abdominal pain). Prolonged monitoring may be required especially if tongue, glottis, or larynx are involved as they are associated with airway obstruction. Those with a history of airway surgery in this situation have a higher risk. Careful blood pressure monitoring with first dose (hypotension can occur especially in volume-depleted patients). Dosage adjustment needed in renal impairment. Use with caution in hypovolemia; collagen vascular diseases; valvular stenosis (particularly aortic stenosis); hyperkalemia; or before, during, or immediately after anesthesia. Avoid rapid dosage escalation which may lead to renal insufficiency. Rare toxicities associated with ACE inhibitors include cholestatic jaundice (which may progress to hepatic necrosis) and neutropenia/agranulocytosis with myeloid hyperplasia. Additional hematologic monitoring required in patients with baseline renal impairment. Deterioration in renal function can occur with initiation. Use with caution in unilateral renal artery stenosis and pre-existing renal insufficiency.

Drug Interactions

Cytochrome P450 Effect: Substrate of CYP2D6 (major)

Decreased Effect: Aspirin (high dose) may reduce the therapeutic effects of ACE inhibitors; at low dosages this does not appear to be significant. Rifampin may decrease the effect of ACE inhibitors. Antacids may decrease the bioavailability of ACE inhibitors (may be more likely to occur with captopril); separate administration times by 1-2 hours. NSAIDs, specifically indomethacin, may reduce the hypotensive effects of ACE inhibitors. More likely to occur in low renin or volume-dependent hypertensive patients.

Increased Effect/Toxicity: Potassium supplements, co-trimoxazole (high dose), angiotensin II receptor antagonists (candesartan, losartan, irbesartan, etc), or potassium-sparing diuretics (amiloride, spironolactone, triamterene) may result in elevated serum potassium levels when combined with captopril. CYP2D6 inhibitors may increase the levels/effects of captopril; example inhibitors include chlorpromazine, delavirdine, fluoxetine, miconazole, paroxetine, pergolide, quinidine, quinine, ritonavir, and ropinirole. ACE inhibitor effects may be increased by phenothiazines or probenecid (increases levels of captopril). ACE inhibitors may increase serum concentrations/effects of lithium.

Diuretics have additive hypotensive effects with ACE inhibitors, and hypovolemia increases the potential for adverse renal effects of ACE inhibitors. In patients with compromised renal function, coadministration with NSAIDs may result in further deterioration of renal function. Allopurinol and ACE inhibitors may cause a higher risk of hypersensitivity reaction when taken concurrently.

Nutritional/Ethanol Interactions

Food: Captopril serum concentrations may be decreased if taken with food. Long-term use of captopril may result in a zinc deficiency which can result in a decrease in taste perception.

Herb/Nutraceutical: Avoid dong quai if using for hypertension (has estrogenic activity). Avoid ephedra, yohimbe, ginseng (may worsen hypertension). Avoid garlic (may have increased antihypertensive effect).

Lab Interactions Increased BUN, creatinine, potassium, positive Coombs' [direct]; decreased cholesterol (S); may cause false-positive results in urine acetone determinations using sodium nitroprusside reagent

Adverse Reactions

1% to 10%:
Cardiovascular: Hypotension (1% to 3%), tachycardia (1%), chest pain (1%), palpitation (1%)

Dermatologic: Rash (maculopapular or urticarial) (4% to 7%), pruritus (2%); in patients with rash, a positive ANA and/or eosinophilia has been noted in 7% to 10%.

Endocrine & metabolic: Hyperkalemia (1% to 11%)

Hematologic: Neutropenia may occur in up to 4% of patients with renal insufficiency or collagen-vascular disease.

Renal: Proteinuria (1%), serum creatinine increased, worsening of renal function (may occur in patients with bilateral renal artery stenosis or hypovolemia)

Respiratory: Cough (<1% to 2%)

Miscellaneous: Hypersensitivity reactions (rash, pruritus, fever, arthralgia, and eosinophilia) have occurred in 4% to 7% of patients (depending on dose and renal function); dysgeusia - loss of taste or diminished perception (2% to 4%)

Frequency not defined:

Cardiovascular: Angioedema, cardiac arrest, cerebrovascular insufficiency, rhythm disturbances, orthostatic hypotension, syncope, flushing, pallor, angina, MI, Raynaud's syndrome, CHF

Central nervous system: Ataxia, confusion, depression, nervousness, somnolence

Dermatologic: Bullous pemphigus, erythema multiforme, Stevens-Johnson syndrome, exfoliative dermatitis

Endocrine & metabolic: Alkaline phosphatase increased, bilirubin increased, gynecomastia

Gastrointestinal: Pancreatitis, glossitis, dyspepsia

Genitourinary: Urinary frequency, impotence

Hematologic: Anemia, thrombocytopenia, pancytopenia, agranulocytosis, anemia

Hepatic: Jaundice, hepatitis, hepatic necrosis (rare), cholestasis, hyponatremia (symptomatic), transaminases increased

Neuromuscular & skeletal: Asthenia, myalgia, myasthenia

Ocular: Blurred vision

Renal: Renal insufficiency, renal failure, nephrotic syndrome, polyuria, oliguria

Respiratory: Bronchospasm, eosinophilic pneumonitis, rhinitis

Miscellaneous: Anaphylactoid reactions

Overdosage/Toxicology Mild hypotension has been the primary toxic effect seen with acute overdose. Bradycardia may also occur. Hyperkalemia occurs even with therapeutic doses, especially in patients with renal insufficiency and those taking NSAIDs. Treatment is symptom-directed and supportive.

Pharmacodynamics/Kinetics

Onset of Action: Peak effect: Blood pressure reduction: 1-1.5 hours after dose

Duration of Action: Dose related, may require several weeks of therapy before full hypotensive effect

Protein Binding: 25% to 30%

Half-Life Elimination: Renal and cardiac function dependent: Adults: Healthy volunteers: 1.9 hours; Congestive heart failure: 2.06 hours; Anuria: 20-40 hours

Metabolism: 50%

Excretion: Urine (95%) within 24 hours

Available Dosage Forms Tablet: 12.5 mg, 25 mg, 50 mg, 100 mg

Dosing

Adults & Elderly: Note: Dosage must be titrated according to patient's response

Acute hypertension (urgency/emergency): Oral: 12.5-25 mg, may repeat as needed (may be given sublingually, but no therapeutic advantage demonstrated)

Hypertension: Oral: Initial: 12.5-25 mg 2-3 times/day; may increase by 12.5-25 mg/dose at 1- to 2-week intervals up to 50 mg 3 times/day. Maximum: 150 mg

(Continued)

Captopril *(Continued)*

3 times/day. Add diuretic before further dosage increases.

Usual dose range (JNC 7): 25-100 mg/day in 2 divided doses

Congestive heart failure: Oral:

Initial: 6.25-12.5 mg 3 times/day in conjunction with cardiac glycoside and diuretic therapy. Initial dose depends upon patient's fluid/electrolyte status.

Target: 50 mg 3 times/day

Prevention of LV dysfunction following MI: Oral: Initial: 6.25 mg; followed by 12.5 mg 3 times/day; increase to 25 mg 3 times/day over the next few days; following gradual increase to a goal of 50 mg 3 times/day (Some dosage schedules increase the dosage more aggressively to achieve goal dosage within the first few days of initiation).

Diabetic nephropathy: Oral:

25 mg 3 times/day. May be taken with other antihypertensive therapy if required to further lower blood pressure.

Pediatrics: Note: Dosage must be titrated according to patient's response.

Hypertension: Oral:

Infants: Initial: 0.15-0.3 mg/kg/dose; titrate dose upward to maximum of 6 mg/kg/day in 1-4 divided doses; usual required dose: 2.5-6 mg/kg/day

Children: Initial: 0.5 mg/kg/dose; titrate upward to maximum of 6 mg/kg/day in 2-4 divided doses.

Older Children: Initial: 6.25-12.5 mg/dose every 12-24 hours; titrate upward to maximum of 6 mg/kg/day.

Adolescents: Initial: 12.5-25 mg/dose given every 8-12 hours; increase by 25 mg/dose to maximum of 450 mg/day.

Renal Impairment:

Cl_{cr} 10-50 mL/minute: Administer 75% of normal dose.

Cl_{cr} <10 mL/minute: Administer 50% of normal dose.

Note: Smaller dosages given every 8-12 hours are indicated in patients with renal dysfunction. Renal function and leukocyte count should be carefully monitored during therapy.

Hemodialysis effects: Moderately dialyzable (20% to 50%); administer dose postdialysis or administer 25% to 35% supplemental dose.

Peritoneal dialysis: Supplemental dose is not necessary.

Administration

Oral: Unstable in aqueous solutions; to prepare solution for oral administration, mix prior to administration and use within 10 minutes.

Laboratory Monitoring BUN, serum creatinine, urine dipstick for protein, CBC, electrolytes. If patient has renal impairment, a baseline WBC with differential and serum creatinine should be evaluated and monitored closely during the first 3 months of therapy.

Nursing Actions

Physical Assessment: Assess other pharmacological or herbal products patient may be taking for potential interactions (especially anything that may impact renal function). Monitor patient closely when beginning therapy (anaphylactic reaction or severe angioedema can occur). Monitor laboratory tests (renal function), therapeutic effectiveness (blood pressure), and adverse response (eg, hypovolemia, angioedema, postural hypotension) when beginning therapy, adjusting dosage, and on a regular basis during therapy. Teach patient proper use, possible side effects/appropriate interventions, and adverse symptoms to report.

Patient Education: Do not take any new medication during therapy unless approved by prescriber. Do not use potassium supplement or salt substitutes without consulting prescriber. Take exactly as directed; do not discontinue this medication without consulting prescriber. Take first dose at bedtime. Take all doses on an empty stomach, 1 hour before or 2 hours after meals. This drug does not eliminate need for diet or exercise regimen as recommended by prescriber. May cause dizziness, fainting, or lightheadedness (use caution when driving or engaging in tasks that require alertness until response to drug is known); postural hypotension (use caution when rising from lying or sitting position or climbing stairs); or nausea, vomiting, abdominal pain, dry mouth, or transient loss of appetite (small, frequent meals, frequent mouth care, sucking lozenges, or chewing gum may help). Report immediately swelling or numbness of face, mouth, or throat; unusual chest pain or palpitations; decreased urinary output; fever or chills; swelling of extremities; skin rash; numbness, tingling, or pain in muscles; respiratory difficulty or unusual cough; and other persistent adverse reactions. **Pregnancy precautions** Inform prescriber if you are or intend to become pregnant. This drug should not be used in the 2nd or 3rd trimester of pregnancy. Consult prescriber for appropriate contraceptive measures if necessary.

Dietary Considerations Should be taken at least 1 hour before or 2 hours after eating.

Geriatric Considerations Due to frequent decreases in glomerular filtration (also creatinine clearance) with aging, elderly patients may have exaggerated responses to ACE inhibitors. Differences in clinical response due to hepatic changes are not observed.

Pregnancy Issues ACE inhibitors can cause fetal injury or death if taken during the 2nd or 3rd trimester. Discontinue ACE inhibitors as soon as pregnancy is detected.

Captopril and Hydrochlorothiazide
(KAP toe pril & hye droe klor oh THYE a zide)

U.S. Brand Names Capozide®

Synonyms Hydrochlorothiazide and Captopril

Pharmacologic Category Antihypertensive Agent, Combination

Pregnancy Risk Factor C/D (2nd and 3rd trimesters)

Lactation Enters breast milk/compatible

Use Management of hypertension and treatment of congestive heart failure

Available Dosage Forms Tablet:

25/15: Captopril 25 mg and hydrochlorothiazide 15 mg

25/25: Captopril 25 mg and hydrochlorothiazide 25 mg

50/15: Captopril 50 mg and hydrochlorothiazide 15 mg

50/25: Captopril 50 mg and hydrochlorothiazide 25 mg

Dosing

Adults: Hypertension, CHF: May be substituted for previously titrated dosages of the individual components; alternatively, may initiate as follows: Oral:

Initial: Single tablet (captopril 25 mg/hydrochlorothiazide 15 mg) taken once daily; daily dose of captopril should not exceed 150 mg; daily dose of hydrochlorothiazide should not exceed 50 mg

Elderly: Refer to dosing in individual monographs.

Renal Impairment: May respond to smaller or less frequent doses.

Nursing Actions

Physical Assessment: See individual agents.

Patient Education: See individual agents. **Pregnancy precaution:** Inform prescriber if you are or intend to become pregnant.

Related Information

Captopril *on page 198*

Hydrochlorothiazide *on page 610*

Carbamazepine (kar ba MAZ e peen)

U.S. Brand Names Carbatrol®; Epitol®; Equetro™; Tegretol®; Tegretol®-XR

Synonyms CBZ; SPD417

Pharmacologic Category Anticonvulsant, Miscellaneous

Medication Safety Issues
Sound-alike/look-alike issues:
Carbatrol® may be confused with Cartrol®
Epitol® may be confused with Epinal®
Tegretol®, Tegretol®-XR may be confused with Mebaral®, Tegrin®, Toprol-XL®, Toradol®, Trental®

Pregnancy Risk Factor D

Lactation Enters breast milk/not recommended (AAP rates "compatible")

Use
Carbatrol®, Tegretol®, Tegretol®-XR: Partial seizures with complex symptomatology (psychomotor, temporal lobe), generalized tonic-clonic seizures (grand mal), mixed seizure patterns, trigeminal neuralgia
Equetro™: Acute manic and mixed episodes associated with bipolar 1 disorder

Unlabeled/Investigational Use Treatment of resistant schizophrenia, ethanol withdrawal, restless leg syndrome, psychotic behavior associated with dementia, post-traumatic stress disorders

Mechanism of Action/Effect In addition to anticonvulsant effects, carbamazepine has anticholinergic, antineuralgic, antidiuretic, muscle relaxant, antimanic, antidepressive, and and antiarrhythmic properties; may depress activity in the nucleus ventralis of the thalamus or decrease synaptic transmission or decrease summation of temporal stimulation leading to neural discharge by limiting influx of sodium ions across cell membrane or other unknown mechanisms; stimulates the release of ADH and potentiates its action in promoting reabsorption of water; chemically related to tricyclic antidepressants

Contraindications Hypersensitivity to carbamazepine, tricyclic antidepressants, or any component of the formulation; bone marrow depression; with or within 14 days of MAO inhibitor use; pregnancy

Warnings/Precautions Administer carbamazepine with caution to patients with history of cardiac damage, hepatic or renal disease; potentially fatal blood cell abnormalities have been reported. Patients with a previous history of adverse hematologic reaction to any drug may be at increased risk. Prescriptions should be written for the smallest quantity consistent with good patient care. The smallest effective dose is suggested for use in bipolar disorder to reduce the risk for overdose; high-risk patients should be monitored. Actuation of latent psychosis is possible.

Carbamazepine is not effective in absence, myoclonic, or akinetic seizures; exacerbation of certain seizure types have been seen after initiation of carbamazepine therapy in children with mixed seizure disorders. Abrupt discontinuation is not recommended in patients being treated for seizures. Dizziness or drowsiness may occur; caution should be used when performing tasks which require alertness until the effects are known. Coadministration of carbamazepine and delavirdine may lead to loss of virologic response and possible resistance. Elderly may have increased risk of SIADH-like syndrome. Carbamazepine has mild anticholinergic activity; use with caution in patients with increased intraocular pressure, or sensitivity to anticholinergic effects. Severe dermatologic reactions, including Lyell and Stevens-Johnson syndromes, although rarely reported, have resulted in fatalities. Discontinue if there are any signs of hypersensitivity.

Drug Interactions

Cytochrome P450 Effect: Substrate of CYP2C8/9 (minor), 3A4 (major); **Induces** CYP1A2 (strong), 2B6 (strong), 2C8/9 (strong), 2C19 (strong), 3A4 (strong)

Decreased Effect: The levels/effects of carbamazepine may be decreased by aminoglutethimide, nafcillin, nevirapine, phenobarbital, phenytoin, and rifamycins, and other CYP3A4 inducers. Carbamazepine may induce its own metabolism. Carbamazepine suspension is incompatible with chlorpromazine solution and thioridazine liquid. Schedule carbamazepine suspension at least 1-2 hours apart from other liquid medicinals. Concomitant use of antimalarial drugs (chloroquine, mefloquine) with carbamazepine may reduce seizure control by lowering plasma levels.

Carbamazepine may decrease the effect of clozapine, corticosteroids, cyclosporine, delavirdine, doxycycline, ethosuximide, felbamate, felodipine, haloperidol, mebendazole, methadone, oral contraceptives, thyroid hormones, tricyclic antidepressants, and valproic acid. Carbamazepine may decrease the levels/effects of aminophylline, amiodarone, benzodiazepines, bupropion, calcium channel blockers, citalopram, clarithromycin, cyclosporine, diazepam, efavirenz, erythromycin, estrogens, fluoxetine, fluvoxamine, glimepiride, glipizide, losartan, methsuximide, mirtazapine, nateglinide, nefazodone, nevirapine, pioglitazone, promethazine, propranolol, protease inhibitors, proton pump inhibitors, ropinirole, rosiglitazone, selegiline, sertraline, sulfonamides, tacrolimus, theophylline, venlafaxine. voriconazole, warfarin, zafirlukast, and other CYP1A2, 2B6, 2C8/9, 2C19, or 3A4 substrates.

Increased Effect/Toxicity: Carbamazepine may enhance the hepatotoxic potential of acetaminophen. Neurotoxicity may result in patients receiving lithium and carbamazepine concurrently. CYP3A4 inhibitors may increase the levels/effects of carbamazepine; example inhibitors include azole antifungals, clarithromycin, diclofenac, doxycycline, erythromycin, imatinib, isoniazid, nefazodone, nicardipine, propofol, protease inhibitors, quinidine, telithromycin, and verapamil. Carbamazepine may increase the levels/effects of phenytoin.

Nutritional/Ethanol Interactions

Ethanol: Avoid ethanol (may increase CNS depression).

Food: Carbamazepine serum levels may be increased if taken with food. Carbamazepine serum concentration may be increased if taken with grapefruit juice; avoid concurrent use.

Herb/Nutraceutical: Avoid evening primrose (seizure threshold decreased). Avoid valerian, St John's wort, kava kava, gotu kola (may increase CNS depression).

Lab Interactions May interact with some pregnancy tests; increased BUN, AST, ALT, bilirubin, alkaline phosphatase (S); decreased calcium, T_3, T_4, sodium (S)

Adverse Reactions Frequency not defined, unless otherwise specified.

Cardiovascular: Arrhythmias, AV block, bradycardia, chest pain (bipolar use), CHF, edema, hyper-/hypotension, lymphadenopathy, syncope, thromboembolism, thrombophlebitis

Central nervous system: Amnesia (bipolar use), anxiety (bipolar use), aseptic meningitis (case report), ataxia (bipolar use 15%), confusion, depression (bipolar use), dizziness (bipolar use 44%), fatigue, headache (bipolar use 22%), sedation, slurred speech, somnolence (bipolar use 32%)

Dermatologic: Alopecia, alterations in skin pigmentation, erythema multiforme, exfoliative dermatitis, photosensitivity reaction, pruritus (bipolar use 8%), purpura, rash, Stevens-Johnson syndrome, toxic epidermal necrolysis, urticaria

Endocrine & metabolic: Chills, fever, hyponatremia, syndrome of inappropriate ADH secretion (SIADH)
(Continued)

Carbamazepine *(Continued)*

Gastrointestinal: Abdominal pain, anorexia, constipation, diarrhea, dyspepsia (bipolar use), gastric distress, nausea (bipolar use 29%), pancreatitis, vomiting (bipolar use 18%), xerostomia (bipolar use)

Genitourinary: Azotemia, impotence, renal failure, urinary frequency, urinary retention

Hematologic: Acute intermittent porphyria, agranulocytosis, aplastic anemia, bone marrow suppression, eosinophilia, leukocytosis, leukopenia, pancytopenia, thrombocytopenia

Hepatic: Abnormal liver function tests, hepatic failure, hepatitis, jaundice

Neuromuscular & skeletal: Back pain, pain (bipolar use 12%), peripheral neuritis, weakness

Ocular: Blurred vision, conjunctivitis, lens opacities, nystagmus

Otic: Hyperacusis, tinnitus

Miscellaneous: Diaphoresis, hypersensitivity (including multiorgan reactions, may include disorders mimicking lymphoma, eosinophilia, hepatosplenomegaly, vasculitis); infection (bipolar use 12%)

Overdosage/Toxicology Symptoms of overdose include dizziness ataxia, drowsiness, nausea, vomiting, tremor, agitation, nystagmus, urinary retention, dysrhythmias, coma, seizures, twitches, respiratory depression, and neuromuscular disturbances. Severe cardiac complications occur with very high doses. Activated charcoal is effective at binding carbamazepine. Other treatment is supportive and symptomatic.

Pharmacodynamics/Kinetics

Time to Peak: Unpredictable:

Immediate release: Suspension: 1.5 hour; tablet: 4-5 hours

Extended release: Carbatrol®, Equetro™: 12-26 hours (single dose), 4-8 hours (multiple doses); Tegretol®-XR: 3-12 hours

Protein Binding: Carbamazepine: 75% to 90%, may be decreased in newborns; Epoxide metabolite: 50%

Half-Life Elimination:

Carbamazepine: Initial: 18-55 hours; Multiple doses: Children: 8-14 hours; Adults: 12-17 hours

Epoxide metabolite: Initial: 25-43 hours

Metabolism: Hepatic via CYP3A4 to active epoxide metabolite; induces hepatic enzymes to increase metabolism

Excretion: Urine 72% (1% to 3% as unchanged drug); feces (28%)

Available Dosage Forms

Capsule, extended release (Carbatrol®, Equetro™): 100 mg, 200 mg, 300 mg

Suspension, oral: 100 mg/5 mL (10 mL, 450 mL)

Tegretol®: 100 mg/5 mL (450 mL) [citrus vanilla flavor]

Tablet (Epitol®, Tegretol®): 200 mg

Tablet, chewable (Tegretol®): 100 mg

Tablet, extended release (Tegretol®-XR): 100 mg, 200 mg, 400 mg

Dosing

Adults: Dosage must be adjusted according to patient's response and serum concentrations. Administer tablets (chewable or conventional) in 2-3 divided doses daily and suspension in 4 divided doses daily. (See Additional Information for investigational oral loading dose and rectal maintenance dose information.) Oral:

Epilepsy: Initial: 200 mg twice daily (tablets, extended release tablets, or extended release capsules) or 100 mg of suspension 4 times/day (400 mg daily); increase by up to 200 mg/day at weekly intervals using a twice daily regimen of extended release tablets or capsules, or a 3-4 times/day regimen of other formulations until optimal response and therapeutic levels are achieved; usual dose: 800-1200 mg/day

Maximum recommended dose: 1600 mg/day; however, some patients have required up to 1.6-2.4 g/day

Trigeminal or glossopharyngeal neuralgia: Oral: Initial: 100 mg twice daily with food, gradually increasing in increments of 100 mg twice daily as needed

Maintenance: Usual: 400-800 mg daily in 2 divided doses; maximum dose: 1200 mg/day

Bipolar disorder (Equetro™): Oral: Initial: 400 mg/day in divided doses, twice daily; may adjust by 200 mg daily increments; maximum dose: 1600 mg/day

Elderly: 100 mg 1-2 times daily, increase in increments of 100 mg/day at weekly intervals until therapeutic level is achieved; usual dose: 400-1000 mg/day

Pediatrics: Dosage must be adjusted according to patient's response and serum concentrations. Administer tablets (chewable or conventional) in 2-3 divided doses daily and suspension in 4 divided doses daily. (See Additional Information for investigational oral loading dose and rectal maintenance dose information.)

Epilepsy: Oral:

Children <6 years: Initial: 10-20 mg/kg/day divided twice or 3 times daily as tablets or 4 times/day as suspension; increase dose every week until optimal response and therapeutic levels are achieved

Maintenance dose: Divide into 3-4 doses daily (tablets or suspension); maximum recommended dose: 35 mg/kg/day

Children 6-12 years: Initial: 100 mg twice daily (tablets or extended release tablets) or 50 mg of suspension 4 times/day (200 mg/day); increase by up to 100 mg/day at weekly intervals using a twice daily regimen of extended release tablets or 3-4 times daily regimen of other formulations until optimal response and therapeutic levels are achieved

Maintenance: Usual: 400-800 mg/day; maximum recommended dose: 1000 mg/day

Note: Children <12 years who receive ≥400 mg/day of carbamazepine may be converted to extended release capsules (Carbatrol®) using the same total daily dosage divided twice daily

Children >12 years: Refer to adult dosing.

Maximum recommended doses:

Children 12-15 years: 1000 mg/day

Children >15 years: 1200 mg/day

Administration

Oral:

Suspension: Must be given on a 3-4 times/day schedule versus tablets which can be given 2-4 times/day. When carbamazepine suspension has been combined with chlorpromazine or thioridazine solutions, a precipitate forms which may result in loss of effect. Therefore, it is recommended that the carbamazepine suspension dosage form not be administered at the same time with other liquid medicinal agents or diluents. Since a given dose of suspension will produce higher peak levels than the same dose given as the tablet form, patients given the suspension should be started on lower doses and increased slowly to avoid unwanted side effects. Should be administered with meals.

Extended release capsule (Carbatrol®, Equetro™): Consists of three different types of beads: Immediate release, extended-release, and enteric release. The bead types are combined in a ratio to allow twice daily dosing. May be opened and contents sprinkled over food such as a teaspoon of applesauce; may be administered with or without food; do not crush or chew.

Extended release tablet: Should be inspected for damage. Damaged extended release tablets (without release portal) should not be administered.

Should be administered with meals; swallow whole, do not crush or chew.

Laboratory Monitoring CBC with platelet count, reticulocytes, serum iron, liver function tests, urinalysis, BUN, serum carbamazepine levels, thyroid function tests, serum sodium

Nursing Actions

Physical Assessment: Assess effectiveness and interactions of other medications patient may be taking. Monitor therapeutic response (seizure activity, force, type, duration), laboratory values, and adverse reactions at beginning of therapy and periodically with long-term use. Taper dosage slowly when discontinuing. Observe and teach seizure/safety precautions. Monitor for mental and CNS changes, excessive sedation (especially when initiating or increasing therapy), suicide ideation. Assess knowledge/teach patient appropriate use, interventions to reduce side effects, and adverse symptoms to report.

Patient Education: Take exactly as directed; do not increase dose or frequency or discontinue this medication without consulting prescriber. Do not use extended release tablets which have been damaged or crushed. While using this medication, do not use alcohol and other prescription or OTC medications (especially when pain medications, sedatives, antihistamines, or hypnotics) without consulting prescriber. Maintain adequate hydration (2-3 L/day of fluids) unless instructed to restrict fluid intake. You may experience drowsiness, dizziness, or blurred vision (use caution when driving or engaging in tasks requiring alertness until response to drug is known); or nausea, vomiting, loss of appetite, or dry mouth (small frequent meals, frequent mouth care, chewing gum, or sucking lozenges may help). Wear identification of epileptic status and medications. Report CNS changes, mentation changes, or changes in cognition; muscle cramping, weakness, tremors, sore throat, mouth ulcers, swollen glands, jaundice, changes in gait; persistent GI symptoms (cramping, constipation, vomiting, anorexia); rash or skin irritations; unusual bruising or bleeding (mouth, urine, stool); or worsening of seizure activity, or loss of seizure control. **Pregnancy/breast-feeding precautions:** Inform prescriber if you are or intend to become pregnant. Breast-feeding is not recommended.

Dietary Considerations Drug may cause GI upset, take with large amount of water or food to decrease GI upset. May need to split doses to avoid GI upset.

Geriatric Considerations Elderly may have increased risk of SIADH-like syndrome.

Breast-Feeding Issues Carbamazepine and its metabolites are found in breast milk. The manufacturer does not recommend use while breast-feeding. However, AAP rates this medication "compatible" in breast-feeding.

Pregnancy Issues Crosses the placenta. Dysmorphic facial features, cranial defects, cardiac defects, spina bifida, IUGR, and multiple other malformations have been reported. Epilepsy itself, number of medications, genetic factors, or a combination of these probably influence the teratogenicity of anticonvulsant therapy. Benefit:risk ratio usually favors continued use during pregnancy.

Other Issues

Timing of serum samples: Absorption is slow, peak levels occur 6-8 hours after ingestion of the first dose. The half-life ranges from 8-60 hours; therefore, steady-state is achieved in 2-5 days.

Therapeutic levels: 6-12 mcg/mL (SI: 25-51 µmol/L)

Toxic concentration: >15 mcg/mL. Patients who require higher levels of 8-12 mcg/mL (SI: 34-51 µmol/L) should be watched closely. Side effects including CNS effects occur commonly at higher dosage levels. If other anticonvulsants are given therapeutic range is 4-8 mcg/mL.

Additional Information Investigationally, loading doses of the suspension (10 mg/kg for children <12 years of age and 8 mg/kg for children >12 years of age) were given (via NG or ND tubes followed by 5-10 mL of water to flush through tube) to PICU patients with frequent seizures/status. Five of 6 patients attained mean Cp of 4.3 mcg/mL and 7.3 mcg/mL at 1 and 2 hours postload. Concurrent enteral feeding or ileus may delay absorption.

Related Information

Overdose and Toxicology *on page 1423*
Peak and Trough Guidelines *on page 1387*

Carbenicillin (kar ben i SIL in)

U.S. Brand Names Geocillin®

Synonyms Carbenicillin Indanyl Sodium; Carindacillin

Pharmacologic Category Antibiotic, Penicillin

Pregnancy Risk Factor B

Lactation Enters breast milk/use caution

Use Treatment of serious urinary tract infections and prostatitis caused by susceptible gram-negative aerobic bacilli

Mechanism of Action/Effect Interferes with bacterial cell wall synthesis during active multiplication

Contraindications Hypersensitivity to carbenicillin, penicillins, or any component of the formulation

Warnings/Precautions Do not use in patients with severe renal impairment (Cl$_{cr}$ <10 mL/minute); dosage modification required in patients with impaired renal and/or hepatic function; oral carbenicillin should be limited to treatment of urinary tract infections. Use with caution in patients with history of hypersensitivity to cephalosporins.

Drug Interactions

Decreased Effect: Decreased effectiveness with tetracyclines. Although anecdotal reports suggest oral contraceptive efficacy could be reduced by penicillins, this has been refuted by more rigorous scientific and clinical data.

Increased Effect/Toxicity: Increased bleeding effects if taken with high doses of heparin or oral anticoagulants. Aminoglycosides may be synergistic against selected organisms. Penicillins may increase the exposure to methotrexate during concurrent therapy; monitor. Probenecid and disulfiram may increase levels of penicillins (carbenicillin).

Lab Interactions May interfere with urinary glucose tests using cupric sulfate (Benedict's solution, Clinitest®); false-positive urine or serum proteins

Some penicillin derivatives may accelerate the degradation of aminoglycosides *in vitro*, leading to a potential underestimation of aminoglycoside serum concentration.

Adverse Reactions

>10%: Gastrointestinal: Diarrhea

1% to 10%: Gastrointestinal: Nausea, bad taste, vomiting, flatulence, glossitis

Overdosage/Toxicology Symptoms of overdose include neuromuscular hypersensitivity and convulsions. Hemodialysis may be helpful to aid in removal of the drug from blood; otherwise, treatment is supportive or symptom-directed.

Pharmacodynamics/Kinetics

Time to Peak: Serum: Normal renal function: 0.5-2 hours; concentrations are inadequate for treatment of systemic infections

Protein Binding: ~50%

Half-Life Elimination: Children: 0.8-1.8 hours; Adults: 1-1.5 hours, prolonged to 10-20 hours with renal insufficiency

(Continued)

Carbenicillin *(Continued)*

Excretion: Urine (~80% to 99% as unchanged drug)

Available Dosage Forms Tablet: 382 mg [contains sodium 23 mg/tablet]

Dosing

Adults & Elderly:

Prostatitis: Oral: 2 tablets every 6 hours

Urinary tract infections: Oral: 1-2 tablets every 6 hours

Pediatrics: Susceptible infections: Oral: Children: 30-50 mg/kg/day divided every 6 hours (maximum dose: 2-3 g/day)

Renal Impairment:

Cl_{cr} 10-50 mL/minute: Administer every 12-24 hours.

Cl_{cr} <10 mL/minute: Administer every 24-48 hours.

Moderately dialyzable (20% to 50%)

Administration

Oral: Administer around-the-clock to promote less variation in peak and trough serum levels.

Some penicillins (eg, carbenicillin, ticarcillin and piperacillin) have been shown to inactivate aminoglycosides *in vitro*. This has been observed to a greater extent with tobramycin and gentamicin, while amikacin has shown greater stability against inactivation. Concurrent use of these agents may pose a risk of reduced antibacterial efficacy *in vivo*, particularly in the setting of profound renal impairment. However, definitive clinical evidence is lacking. If combination penicillin/aminoglycoside therapy is desired in a patient with renal dysfunction, separation of doses (if feasible), and routine monitoring of aminoglycoside levels, CBC, and clinical response should be considered.

Stability

Compatibility: Solution is **incompatible** with aminophylline, amphotericin B, epinephrine, erythromycin, gentamicin, levarterenol, tetracycline, vitamin B and C complex.

Laboratory Monitoring Renal and hepatic function, CBC, serum potassium, bleeding times. Perform culture and sensitivity testing prior to initiating therapy.

Nursing Actions

Physical Assessment: Results of culture/sensitivity tests and patient's allergy history should be assessed prior to beginning treatment. Assess other pharmacological or herbal products patient may be taking for potential interactions. Assess results of laboratory tests, therapeutic effectiveness, and adverse response. Advise patients with diabetes about use of Clinitest®. Teach patient proper use, possible side effects/appropriate interventions, and adverse symptoms to report.

Patient Education: Do not take any new medication during therapy unless approved by prescriber. Take as prescribed, at equal intervals around-the-clock, with a full glass of water, and preferably on an empty stomach, 1 hour before or 2 hours after meals. Do not skip doses and take full course of treatment even if feeling better. If you have diabetes, drug may cause false test results with Clinitest® urine glucose monitoring; use of another form of glucose monitoring is preferable. May cause diarrhea (boiled milk, buttermilk, or yogurt may help - if diarrhea persists for more than 2 days, contact prescriber for approved antidiarrhea medication); or dry mouth and bitter aftertaste (frequent mouth care may help). Report respiratory difficulty; easy bruising or bleeding; rash, itching, hives; or signs of opportunistic infection (eg, sore throat, fever, chills, fatigue, thrush, vaginal discharge, diarrhea). **Breast-feeding precaution:** Consult prescriber if breast-feeding.

Dietary Considerations Should be taken with water on empty stomach. Sodium content of 382 mg tablet: 23 mg (1 mEq).

Geriatric Considerations Has not been studied in the elderly.

Related Information

Compatibility of Drugs *on page 1370*

Carbetapentane and Chlorpheniramine

(kar bay ta PEN tane & klor fen IR a meen)

U.S. Brand Names Tannate 12 S; Tannic-12; Tannic-12 S; Tannihist-12 RF; Tussi-12®; Tussi-12 S™; Tussizone-12 RF™

Synonyms Carbetapentane Tannate and Chlorpheniramine Tannate; Chlorpheniramine and Carbetapentane

Pharmacologic Category Antihistamine/Antitussive

Pregnancy Risk Factor C

Lactation Excretion in breast milk unknown/contraindicated

Use Symptomatic relief of cough associated with upper respiratory tract conditions, such as the common cold, bronchitis, bronchial asthma

Available Dosage Forms

Suspension:

Tannate 12 S: Carbetapentane tannate 30 mg and chlorpheniramine tannate 4 mg per 5 mL (120 mL, 480 mL)

Tannic-12 S: Carbetapentane tannate 30 mg and chlorpheniramine tannate 4 mg per 5 mL (120 mL) [contains benzoic acid; strawberry flavor]

Tannihist-12 RF: Carbetapentane tannate 30 mg and chlorpheniramine tannate 4 mg per 5 mL (120 mL, 480 mL) [strawberry-black currant flavor]

Tussi-12 S™: Carbetapentane tannate 30 mg and chlorpheniramine tannate 4 mg per 5 mL (120 mL) [contains benzoic acid and tartrazine; strawberry-currant flavor]

Tussizone-12 RF™: Carbetapentane tannate 30 mg and chlorpheniramine tannate 4 mg per 5 mL (120 mL, 480 mL) [contains benzoic acid and tartrazine; strawberry-black currant flavor]

Tablet (Tannic-12, Tussi-12®, Tussizone-12 RF™): Carbetapentane tannate 60 mg and chlorpheniramine tannate 5 mg

Dosing

Adults: Cough and upper respiratory symptoms: Oral (based on carbetapentane 60 mg and chlorpheniramine 5 mg per tablet): 1-2 tablets every 12 hours

Pediatrics: Cough and upper respiratory symptoms: Oral (based on carbetapentane 30 mg and chlorpheniramine 4 mg per 5 mL suspension): Children:

2-6 years: 2.5-5 mL every 12 hours

>6 years: 5-10 mL every 12 hours

Carbetapentane, Phenylephrine, and Chlorpheniramine

(kar bay ta PEN tane, fen il EF rin, & klor fen IR a meen)

U.S. Brand Names Carbaphen 12®; Carbaphen 12 Ped®; XiraTuss™

Synonyms Chlorpheniramine, Carbetapentane, and Phenylephrine; Phenylephrine, Chlorpheniramine, and Carbetapentane

Pharmacologic Category Antihistamine/Decongestant/Antitussive; Antitussive; Histamine H₁ Antagonist; Sympathomimetic

Pregnancy Risk Factor C

Lactation Excretion in breast milk unknown/contraindicated

Use Symptomatic relief of cough, nasal congestion, and discharge associated with the common cold, bronchial asthma, acute and chronic bronchitis, and other respiratory tract conditions

Available Dosage Forms

Suspension:

Carbaphen 12®: Carbetapentane tannate 60 mg, phenylephrine tannate 20 mg, and chlorpheniramine tannate 8 mg per 5 mL (480 mL) [contains benzoic acid, phenylalanine 1 mg/5 mL; alcohol free, sugar free; blueberry-banana flavor]

Carbaphen 12 Ped®: Carbetapentane tannate 15 mg, phenylephrine tannate 2.5 mg, and chlorpheniramine tannate 2 mg per mL (60 mL) [contains benzoic acid, phenylalanine 1.6 mg/mL; alcohol free, sugar free; blueberry-banana flavor]

XiraTuss™: Carbetapentane tannate 30 mg, phenylephrine tannate 12.5 mg, and chlorpheniramine tannate 4 mg per 5 mL (120 mL) [strawberry flavor]

Tablet (XiraTuss™): Carbetapentane tannate 60 mg, phenylephrine tannate 10 mg, and chlorpheniramine tannate 5 mg

Dosing

Adults: Relief of cough, congestion: Oral:
Carbaphen 12®: 5-10 mL every 12 hours
XiraTuss tablet: 1-2 tablets every 12 hours

Pediatrics: Relief of cough, congestion: Oral:
Children 2-6 years:
Carbaphen 12 Ped®: 1-2 mL every 12 hours
XiraTuss suspension: 2.5-5 mL every 12 hours
Children 6-12 years:
Carbaphen 12 Ped®: 2-4 mL every 12 hours
XiraTuss suspension: 5-10 mL every 12 hours
Children >12 years: Refer to adult dosing.

Related Information

Phenylephrine *on page 980*

Carbinoxamine and Pseudoephedrine
(kar bi NOKS a meen & soo doe e FED rin)

U.S. Brand Names Andehist NR Drops; Carbaxefed RF; Carboxine-PSE; Cordron-D NR; Hydro-Tussin™-CBX; Palgic®-D; Palgic®-DS; Pediatex™-D; Rondec® Drops [DSC]; Rondec® Tablets; Rondec-TR®; Sildec

Synonyms Pseudoephedrine and Carbinoxamine

Pharmacologic Category Adrenergic Agonist Agent; Antihistamine, H_1 Blocker; Decongestant

Pregnancy Risk Factor C

Lactation Enters breast milk/contraindicated

Use Seasonal and perennial allergic rhinitis; vasomotor rhinitis

Mechanism of Action/Effect Carbinoxamine is an antihistamine; pseudoephedrine is a decongestant

Contraindications Hypersensitivity to carbinoxamine, pseudoephedrine, or any component of the formulation; severe hypertension or coronary artery disease; MAO inhibitor therapy; GI or GU obstruction; peptic ulcer disease; narrow-angle glaucoma; avoid use in premature or term infants due to a possible association with SIDS; acute asthma attack

Warnings/Precautions Use caution with hypertension, ischemic heart disease, hyperthyroidism, increased intraocular pressure, diabetes mellitus, BPH, and patients >60 years of age. May cause decreased mental alertness; excitation in younger children; paradoxical reactions (manifested by hyperexcitability) in older children. The elderly may be more sensitive to anticholinergic and antihistamine effects and experience increased adverse effects. Use caution in atopic children. Safety and efficacy in children <1 month of age have not been established.

Drug Interactions

Decreased Effect: May decrease effects of antihypertensive agents.

Increased Effect/Toxicity: Increased sedation/CNS depression with barbiturates and other CNS depressants; anticholinergic effects may be increased by MAO inhibitors, tricyclic antidepressants

Nutritional/Ethanol Interactions Ethanol: Avoid ethanol (may increase CNS depression).

Adverse Reactions Frequency not defined.

Cardiovascular: Arrhythmias, cardiovascular collapse, hypertension, pallor, tachycardia

Central nervous system: Anxiety, convulsions, CNS stimulation, dizziness, excitability (children; rare), fear, hallucinations, headache, insomnia, nervousness, restlessness, sedation

Gastrointestinal: Anorexia, diarrhea, dyspepsia, nausea, vomiting, xerostomia

Neuromuscular skeletal: Tremors, weakness

Ocular: Diplopia

Renal: Dysuria, polyuria, urinary retention (with BPH)

Respiratory: Respiratory difficulty

Overdosage/Toxicology Symptoms of overdose include dry mouth, flushed skin, dilated pupils, and CNS depression. There is no specific treatment for antihistamine overdose. Clinical toxicity is due to blockade of cholinergic receptors. For anticholinergic overdose with severe life-threatening symptoms, physostigmine 1-2 mg I.V. slowly, may be given to reverse these effects.

Available Dosage Forms [DSC] = Discontinued product

Liquid:

Cordron-D NR: Carbinoxamine maleate 2 mg and pseudoephedrine hydrochloride 12.5 mg per 5 mL (480 mL) [cotton candy flavor]

Pediatex™-D: Carbinoxamine maleate 2 mg and pseudoephedrine hydrochloride 20 mg per 5 mL (480 mL) [alcohol free, dye free, sugar free; cotton candy flavor]

Solution, oral drops:

Andehist NR: Carbinoxamine maleate 1 mg and pseudoephedrine hydrochloride 15 mg per mL (30 mL) [alcohol and sugar free; raspberry flavor]

Carbaxefed RF, Rondec® [DSC]: Carbinoxamine maleate 1 mg and pseudoephedrine hydrochloride 15 mg per mL (30 mL) [alcohol free; contains sodium benzoate; cherry flavor]

Sildec: Carbinoxamine maleate 1 mg and pseudoephedrine hydrochloride 15 mg per mL (30 mL) [raspberry flavor]

Solution: Carbinoxamine maleate 2 mg and pseudoephedrine hydrochloride 25 mg per 5 mL (480 mL)

Carboxine-PSE: Carbinoxamine maleate 2 mg and pseudoephedrine hydrochloride 20 mg per 5 mL (480 mL) [peach flavor]

Syrup: Carbinoxamine maleate 2 mg and pseudoephedrine hydrochloride 25 mg per 5 mL (480 mL)

Hydro-Tussin™-CBX, Palgic®-DS: Carbinoxamine maleate 2 mg and pseudoephedrine hydrochloride 25 mg per 5 mL (480 mL) [alcohol, dye, and sugar free; strawberry/pineapple flavor]

Tablet (Rondec®): Carbinoxamine maleate 4 mg and pseudoephedrine hydrochloride 60 mg

Tablet, timed release:

Palgic®-D: Carbinoxamine maleate 8 mg and pseudoephedrine hydrochloride 80 mg [dye free]

Rondec-TR®: Carbinoxamine maleate 8 mg and pseudoephedrine hydrochloride 120 mg

Dosing

Adults & Elderly: Nasal congestion, allergic symptoms: Oral:

Liquid (Pediatex™-D): 10 mL 4 times/day

Syrup (Hydro-Tussin™-CBX, Palgic®-DS): 10 mL 4 times/day

Tablet (Rondec®): 1 tablet 4 times a day

Tablet, timed release (Palgic®-D, Rondec-TR®): 1 tablet every 12 hours

Pediatrics: Nasal congestion, allergic symptoms: Oral:
Children:

Drops (Andehist NR, Carbaxefed RF, Rondec®, Sildec):
1-3 months: 0.25 mL 4 times/day
3-6 months: 0.5 mL 4 times/day

(Continued)

Carbinoxamine and Pseudoephedrine
(Continued)

6-12 months: 0.75 mL 4 times/day

12-24 months: 1 mL 4 times/day

Liquid (Pediatex™-D):

1-3 months: 1.25 mL up to 4 times/day

3-6 months: 2.5 mL up to 4 times/day

6-9 months: 3.75 mL up to 4 times/day

9-18 months: 3.75-5 mL up to 4 times/day

18 months to 6 years: 5 mL 3-4 times/day

>6 years: Refer to adult dosing.

Syrup (Hydro-Tussin™-CBX, Palgic®-DS):

1-3 months: 1.25 mL up to 4 times/day

3-6 months: 2.5 mL up to 4 times/day

6-9 months: 3.75 mL up to 4 times/day

9-18 months: 3.75-5 mL up to 4 times/day

18 months to 6 years: 5 mL 3-4 times/day

>6 years: Refer to adult dosing.

Tablet (Rondec®): ≥6 years: Refer to adult dosing.

Tablet, timed release:

6-12 years (Palgic®-D): One-half tablet every 12 hours

≥12 years (Palgic®-D, Rondec-TR®): Refer to adult dosing.

Administration

Oral:

Palgic®-D: Tablets may be broken in half; do not crush or chew

Rondec-TR®: Do not crush or chew

Stability

Storage: Store at room temperature of 15°C to 30°C (59°F to 86°F).

Nursing Actions

Physical Assessment: Assess potential for interactions with other medications patient may be taking. Monitor effectiveness of therapy and adverse reactions at beginning of therapy and periodically with long-term use. Teach patient proper use, possible side effects/appropriate interventions, and adverse symptoms to report.

Patient Education: Take as directed; do not exceed recommended dose. Maintain adequate hydration (2-3 L/day of fluids) unless instructed to restrict fluid intake. Avoid use of other depressants, alcohol, or sleep-inducing medications unless approved by prescriber. You may experience drowsiness, impaired coordination, blurred vision, or increased anxiety (use caution when driving or engaging in tasks requiring alertness until response to drug is known); or dry mouth or nausea (small frequent meals, frequent mouth care, chewing gum, or sucking hard candy may help). Report persistent dizziness, sedation, or agitation; respiratory difficulty or increased cough; changes in urinary pattern; muscle weakness; or lack of improvement or worsening of condition. **Pregnancy/breast-feeding precautions:** Inform prescriber if you are or intend to become pregnant or breast-feed.

Geriatric Considerations Elderly are more predisposed to adverse effects of sympathomimetics since they frequently have cardiovascular diseases and diabetes mellitus as well as multiple drug therapies. It may be advisable to treat with a short-acting/immediate-release formulation before initiating sustained-release/long-acting formulations.

Breast-Feeding Issues Small amounts of antihistamines and pseudoephedrine are excreted in breast milk. Premature infants and newborns have a higher risk of intolerance to antihistamines. Antihistamines may inhibit lactation.

Related Information

Pseudoephedrine *on page 1047*

Carboplatin (KAR boe pla tin)

U.S. Brand Names Paraplatin®

Synonyms CBDCA

Pharmacologic Category Antineoplastic Agent, Alkylating Agent

Medication Safety Issues

Sound-alike/look-alike issues:

Carboplatin may be confused with cisplatin

Paraplatin® may be confused with Platinol®

Pregnancy Risk Factor D

Lactation Excretion in breast milk unknown/contraindicated

Use Treatment of ovarian cancer

Unlabeled/Investigational Use Lung cancer, head and neck cancer, endometrial cancer, esophageal cancer, bladder cancer, breast cancer, cervical cancer, CNS tumors, germ cell tumors, osteogenic sarcoma, and high-dose therapy with stem cell/bone marrow support

Mechanism of Action/Effect Carboplatin is an alkylating agent which covalently binds to DNA; possible cross-linking and interference with the function of DNA

Contraindications History of severe allergic reaction to cisplatin, carboplatin, other platinum-containing formulations, mannitol, or any component of the formulation; pregnancy

Warnings/Precautions Hazardous agent — use appropriate precautions for handling and disposal. High doses have resulted in severe abnormalities of liver function tests. Bone marrow suppression, which may be severe, and vomiting are dose related; reduce dosage in patients with bone marrow suppression and impaired renal function. Increased risk of allergic reactions in patients previously exposed to platinum therapy. When administered as sequential infusions, taxane derivatives (docetaxel, paclitaxel) should be administered before the platinum derivatives (carboplatin, cisplatin) to limit myelosuppression and to enhance efficacy.

Drug Interactions

Increased Effect/Toxicity: Nephrotoxic drugs; aminoglycosides increase risk of ototoxicity. When administered as sequential infusions, observational studies indicate a potential for increased toxicity when platinum derivatives (carboplatin, cisplatin) are administered before taxane derivatives (docetaxel, paclitaxel).

Nutritional/Ethanol Interactions Herb/Nutraceutical: Avoid black cohosh, dong quai in estrogen-dependent tumors.

Adverse Reactions

>10%:

Dermatologic: Alopecia

Endocrine & metabolic: Hypomagnesemia, hypokalemia, hyponatremia, hypocalcemia; less severe than those seen after cisplatin (usually asymptomatic)

Gastrointestinal: Nausea, vomiting, stomatitis

Hematologic: Myelosuppression (dose related and dose limiting); thrombocytopenia (37% to 80%); leukopenia (27% to 38%)

Nadir: ~21 days following a single dose

Hepatic: Alkaline phosphatase increased, AST increased (usually mild and reversible)

Otic: Hearing loss at high tones (above speech ranges, up to 19%); clinically-important ototoxicity is not usually seen

Renal: BUN and/or creatinine increased

1% to 10%:

Gastrointestinal: Diarrhea, anorexia

Hematologic: Hemorrhagic complications

Local: Pain at injection site

Neuromuscular & skeletal: Peripheral neuropathy (4% to 6%; up to 10% in older and/or previously-treated patients)

Otic: Ototoxicity

Overdosage/Toxicology Symptoms of overdose include bone marrow suppression and hepatic toxicity. Treatment is symptomatic and supportive.

Pharmacodynamics/Kinetics

Protein Binding: 0%; platinum is 30% irreversibly bound

Half-Life Elimination: Terminal: 22-40 hours; Cl_{cr} >60 mL/minute: 2.5-5.9 hours

Metabolism: Minimally hepatic to aquated and hydroxylated compounds

Excretion: Urine (~60% to 90%) within 24 hours

Available Dosage Forms

Injection, powder for reconstitution: 50 mg, 150 mg, 450 mg

Injection, solution: 10 mg/mL (5 mL, 15 mL, 45 mL, 60 mL)

Dosing

Adults & Elderly: Refer to individual protocols: **Note:** Doses are usually determined by the AUC using the Calvert formula.

IVPB, I.V. infusion, intraperitoneal:

Autologous BMT: I.V.: 1600 mg/m^2 (total dose) divided over 4 days

Ovarian cancer: 300-360 mg/m^2 I.V. every 3-4 weeks

Pediatrics: Refer to individual protocols: **Note:** Doses are usually determined by the AUC using the Calvert formula.

IVPB, I.V. infusion, intraperitoneal:

Solid tumor: 300-600 mg/m^2 once every 4 weeks

Brain tumor: 175 mg/m^2 weekly for 4 weeks every 6 weeks, with a 2-week recovery period between courses

Renal Impairment:

No guidelines are available.

Hepatic Impairment: No guidelines are available.

Administration

I.V.: Administer over 15 minutes, up to 24 hours. May also be administered intraperitoneally. When administered as sequential infusions, taxane derivatives (docetaxel, paclitaxel) should be administered before platinum derivatives to limit myelosuppression and to enhance efficacy.

I.V. Detail: Observe serum creatinine. Carboplatin is nephrotoxic and drug accumulation occurs with decreased creatinine clearance.

pH: 5-7

Stability

Reconstitution: Reconstitute powder to yield a final concentration of 10 mg/mL; reconstituted carboplatin 10 mg/mL should be further diluted to a final concentration of 0.5-2 mg/mL with D_5W or NS for administration

Compatibility: Stable in $D_5\frac{1}{4}NS$, $D_5\frac{1}{2}NS$, D_5NS, D_5W, NS

Y-site administration: Incompatible with amphotericin B cholesteryl sulfate complex

Compatibility when admixed: Incompatible with fluorouracil, mesna

Storage: Store intact vials at room temperature of 15°C to 30°C (59°F to 86°F); protect from light. Further dilution to a concentration as low as 0.5 mg/mL is stable at room temperature (25°C) or under refrigeration for 8 days in D_5W.

Powder for reconstitution: Reconstituted to a final concentration of 10 mg/mL is stable for 5 days at room temperature (25°C).

Solution for injection: Multidose vials are stable for up to 14 days after opening when stored at room temperature.

Laboratory Monitoring CBC with differential and platelet count, serum electrolytes, creatinine clearance, liver function

Nursing Actions

Physical Assessment: Patient allergy history must be assessed prior to therapy. Assess other pharmacological or herbal products patient may be taking for potential interactions (especially products that may be ototoxic or nephrotoxic and need for sequencing with taxane derivatives). Monitor laboratory tests (hematology, electrolytes, renal and hepatic function), prior to treatment and on a regular basis during therapy. Monitor patient response (eg, nausea and vomiting; pretreatment with antiemetic may be required), ototoxicity (audiometry may be advisable), bone marrow depression, anemia, bleeding, peripheral neuropathy frequently throughout therapy. Teach patient (or caregiver) possible side effects/appropriate interventions and adverse symptoms to report.

Patient Education: Do not take any new medication during therapy unless approved by healthcare provider. This medicine can only be administered intravenously. Report immediately any redness, burning, pain, or swelling at infusion site. It is important that you maintain adequate nutrition (small, frequent meals may help) and adequate hydration (2-3 L/day of fluids) unless instructed to restrict fluid intake. You will be susceptible to infection (avoid crowds and exposure to infection and do not have any vaccinations without consulting prescriber). May cause nausea and vomiting (small, frequent meals, frequent mouth care, chewing gum, or sucking lozenges may help - if unresolved, consult prescriber for antiemetic); mouth sores (use soft toothbrush or cotton swabs for mouth care); or loss of hair (reversible). Report chest pain or palpitations; sore throat, fever, chills, unusual fatigue; unusual bruising/bleeding; respiratory difficulty; numbness, pain, or tingling in extremities; muscle cramps or twitching; change in hearing acuity; or other persistent adverse effects. **Pregnancy/breast-feeding precautions:** Inform prescriber if you are pregnant. Do not get pregnant during or for 1 month following therapy. Male: Do not cause a female to become pregnant. Male/female: Consult prescriber for instruction on appropriate contraceptive measures. This drug may cause severe fetal defects. Do not breast-feed.

Geriatric Considerations Peripheral neuropathy is more frequent in patients >65 years of age.

Other Issues Carboplatin is sometimes confused with cisplatin. Institute measures to prevent mix-ups.

Carboprost Tromethamine
(KAR boe prost tro METH a meen)

U.S. Brand Names Hemabate®

Synonyms Carboprost

Pharmacologic Category Abortifacient; Prostaglandin

Pregnancy Risk Factor X

Lactation Excretion in breast milk unknown/opportunity for use is minimal

Use Termination of pregnancy and refractory postpartum uterine bleeding

Unlabeled/Investigational Use Investigational: Hemorrhagic cystitis

Mechanism of Action/Effect Carboprost tromethamine is a prostaglandin similar to prostaglandin F_2. Carboprost tromethamine stimulates the gravid uterus to contract, which usually results in expulsion of the products of conception. Used to induce abortion between 13-20 weeks of pregnancy.

Contraindications Hypersensitivity to carboprost tromethamine or any component of the formulation; acute pelvic inflammatory disease; pregnancy

Warnings/Precautions Use with caution in patients with history of asthma, hypotension or hypertension, cardiovascular, adrenal, renal or hepatic disease, (Continued)

Carboprost Tromethamine (Continued)

anemia, jaundice, diabetes, epilepsy, or compromised uterus.

Drug Interactions
Increased Effect/Toxicity: Toxicity may be increased by oxytocic agents.

Adverse Reactions
>10%: Gastrointestinal: Nausea (33%)

1% to 10%: Cardiovascular: Flushing (7%)

Pharmacodynamics/Kinetics
Excretion: Urine

Available Dosage Forms Injection, solution: Carboprost 250 mcg and tromethamine 83 mcg per mL (1 mL) [contains benzyl alcohol]

Dosing
Adults & Elderly:

Abortion: I.M.: 250 mcg to start, 250 mcg at 1½-hour to 3½-hour intervals depending on uterine response; a 500 mcg dose may be given if uterine response is not adequate after several 250 mcg doses; do not exceed 12 mg total dose.

Refractory postpartum uterine bleeding: I.M.: Initial: 250 mcg; may repeat at 15- to 90-minute intervals to a total dose of 2 mg

Hemorrhagic cystitis: Bladder irrigation (refer to individual protocols): [0.4-1.0 mg/dL as solution] 50 mL instilled into bladder 4 times/day for 1 hour

Administration
I.M.: Give deep I.M.; rotate site if repeat injections are required.

I.V.: Do not inject I.V.; may result in bronchospasm, hypertension, vomiting, and anaphylaxis.

Stability
Reconstitution: Bladder irrigation: Dilute immediately prior to administration in NS; stability unknown.

Storage: Refrigerate ampuls.

Nursing Actions
Physical Assessment: Note that nausea or vomiting may be significant; premedication with an antiemetic may be considered. Assess for therapeutic effectiveness (eg, uterine contractions) and adverse reactions (eg, hypertension, hemorrhage, or respiratory effects, prolonged or excessively elevated temperature). Report contractions lasting longer than 1 minute or absence of contractions to prescriber. Assess for complete expulsion of uterine contents (fetal tissue). Assess knowledge/instruct patient on adverse symptoms to report. If used to treat hemorrhagic cystitis (bladder irrigation). **Pregnancy risk factor X.**

Patient Education: This medication is used to stimulate expulsion of uterine contents (fetal tissue) or stimulate uterine contractions to reduce uterine bleeding. Report increased blood loss, acute abdominal cramping, foul-smelling vaginal discharge, or persistent elevation of temperature. Increased temperature (elevated temperature) may occur 1-16 hours after therapy and last for several hours. **Pregnancy precaution:** If being treated for hemorrhagic cystitis, inform prescriber if you are pregnant.

Carisoprodol (kar eye soe PROE dole)

U.S. Brand Names Soma®

Synonyms Carisoprodate; Isobamate

Pharmacologic Category Skeletal Muscle Relaxant

Pregnancy Risk Factor C

Lactation Enters breast milk (high concentrations)/not recommended

Use Skeletal muscle relaxant

Mechanism of Action/Effect Precise mechanism is not yet clear, but many effects have been ascribed to its central depressant actions.

Contraindications Hypersensitivity to carisoprodol, meprobamate or any component of the formulation; acute intermittent porphyria

Warnings/Precautions May cause CNS depression, which may impair physical or mental abilities. Effects with other sedative drugs or ethanol may be potentiated. Use with caution in patients with hepatic/renal dysfunction. Tolerance or drug dependence may result from extended use.

Drug Interactions
Cytochrome P450 Effect: Substrate of CYP2C19 (major)

Increased Effect/Toxicity: CYP2C19 inhibitors may increase the levels/effects of carisoprodol; example inhibitors include delavirdine, fluconazole, fluvoxamine, gemfibrozil, isoniazid, omeprazole, and ticlopidine. Ethanol, CNS depressants, psychotropic drugs, and phenothiazines may increase toxicity.

Nutritional/Ethanol Interactions Ethanol: Avoid ethanol (may increase CNS depression).

Adverse Reactions
>10%: Central nervous system: Drowsiness

1% to 10%:

Cardiovascular: Tachycardia, tightness in chest, flushing of face, syncope

Central nervous system: Mental depression, allergic fever, dizziness, lightheadedness, headache, paradoxical CNS stimulation

Dermatologic: Angioedema

Gastrointestinal: Nausea, vomiting, stomach cramps

Neuromuscular & skeletal: Trembling

Ocular: Burning eyes

Respiratory: Dyspnea

Miscellaneous: Hiccups

Overdosage/Toxicology Symptoms of overdose include CNS depression, stupor, coma, shock, and respiratory depression. Treatment is supportive.

Pharmacodynamics/Kinetics
Onset of Action: ~30 minutes

Duration of Action: 4-6 hours

Half-Life Elimination: 8 hours

Metabolism: Hepatic

Excretion: Urine

Available Dosage Forms Tablet: 350 mg

Dosing
Adults: Muscle spasm (including spasm associated with acute temporomandibular joint pain): Oral: 350 mg 3-4 times/day; take last dose at bedtime; compound: 1-2 tablets 4 times/day

Elderly: Not recommended for use in the elderly (see Geriatric Considerations).

Administration
Oral: Give with food to decrease GI upset.

Nursing Actions
Physical Assessment: Assess effectiveness and interactions of other medications patient may be taking. Monitor effectiveness of therapy (according to rationale for therapy) and adverse reactions (eg, cardiovascular, CNS status, excessive drowsiness) at beginning of therapy and periodically with long-term use. Do not discontinue abruptly; taper dosage slowly (withdrawal symptoms such as abdominal cramping, headache, insomnia may occur). Assess knowledge/teach patient appropriate use, interventions to reduce side effects (postural hypotension precautions), and adverse symptoms to report.

Patient Education: Take exactly as directed with food. Do not increase dose or discontinue this medication without consulting prescriber. Do not use alcohol, prescriptive or OTC antidepressants, sedatives, and pain medications without consulting prescriber. You may experience drowsiness, dizziness, lightheadedness (avoid driving or engaging in tasks requiring alertness until response to drug is known); nausea, vomiting, or cramping (small frequent meals, frequent mouth care, or sucking hard candy may help); or postural hypotension (change position slowly when rising from sitting or lying or when climbing stairs). Report excessive drowsiness or mental agitation; palpitations, rapid heartbeat, chest pain; skin rash; muscle cramping or tremors; or respiratory difficulty. **Pregnancy/breast-feeding precautions:** Inform prescriber if you are or intend to become pregnant. Breast-feeding is not recommended.

Geriatric Considerations Because of the risk of orthostatic hypotension and CNS depression, avoid or use with caution in the elderly. Not considered a drug of choice in the elderly.

Carisoprodol and Aspirin
(kar eye soe PROE dole & AS pir in)

U.S. Brand Names Soma® Compound
Synonyms Aspirin and Carisoprodol
Pharmacologic Category Skeletal Muscle Relaxant
Pregnancy Risk Factor C/D (full-dose aspirin in 3rd trimester)
Lactation Enters breast milk/contraindicated
Use Skeletal muscle relaxant
Available Dosage Forms Tablet: Carisoprodol 200 mg and aspirin 325 mg
Dosing
Adults: Skeletal muscle relaxant (including TMJ pain/spasm): Oral: 1 or 2 tablets 4 times/day
Elderly: Avoid use in the elderly due to risk of orthostatic hypotension and CNS depression.
Nursing Actions
Physical Assessment: See individual agents.
Patient Education: See individual agents. **Pregnancy/breast-feeding precautions:** Inform prescriber if you are or intend to become pregnant. Do not breast-feed.
Related Information
Aspirin *on page 114*
Carisoprodol *on page 208*

Carisoprodol, Aspirin, and Codeine
(kar eye soe PROE dole, AS pir in, and KOE deen)

U.S. Brand Names Soma® Compound w/Codeine
Synonyms Aspirin, Carisoprodol, and Codeine; Codeine, Aspirin, and Carisoprodol
Restrictions C-III
Pharmacologic Category Skeletal Muscle Relaxant
Pregnancy Risk Factor C/D (full-dose aspirin in 3rd trimester)
Lactation Enters breast milk/contraindicated
Use Skeletal muscle relaxant
Available Dosage Forms Tablet: Carisoprodol 200 mg, aspirin 325 mg, and codeine phosphate 16 mg
Dosing
Adults: Skeletal muscle relaxant, analgesic: Oral: 1 or 2 tablets 4 times/day
Elderly: Avoid use in the elderly due to the risk of orthostatic hypotension and CNS depression.
Nursing Actions
Physical Assessment: See individual agents.
Patient Education: See individual agents. **Pregnancy/breast-feeding precautions:** Inform prescriber if you are or intend to become pregnant. Do not breast-feed.
Related Information
Aspirin *on page 114*
Carisoprodol *on page 208*
Codeine *on page 296*

Carmustine (kar MUS teen)

U.S. Brand Names BiCNu®; Gliadel®
Synonyms BCNU; bis-chloronitrosourea; Carmustinum; NSC-409962; WR-139021
Pharmacologic Category Antineoplastic Agent; Antineoplastic Agent, Alkylating Agent (Nitrosourea); Antineoplastic Agent, DNA Adduct-Forming Agent; Antineoplastic Agent, DNA Binding Agent
Medication Safety Issues
Sound-alike/look-alike issues:
Carmustine may be confused with lomustine
Pregnancy Risk Factor D
Lactation Excretion in breast milk unknown/contraindicated
Use
Injection: Treatment of brain tumors (glioblastoma, brainstem glioma, medulloblastoma, astrocytoma, ependymoma, and metastatic brain tumors), multiple myeloma, Hodgkin's disease, non-Hodgkin's lymphomas, melanoma, lung cancer, colon cancer
Wafer (implant): Adjunct to surgery in patients with recurrent glioblastoma multiforme; adjunct to surgery and radiation in patients with high-grade malignant glioma
Mechanism of Action/Effect Interferes with the normal function of DNA by alkylation and cross-linking the strands of DNA, and by possible protein modification
Contraindications Hypersensitivity to carmustine or any component of the formulation; myelosuppression; pregnancy
Warnings/Precautions Hazardous agent — use appropriate precautions for handling and disposal. Administer with caution to patients with depressed platelet, leukocyte or erythrocyte counts, renal or hepatic impairment. Diluent contains significant amounts of ethanol; use caution with aldehyde dehydrogenase-2 deficiency or history of "alcohol flushing syndrome."
Drug Interactions
Increased Effect/Toxicity: Carmustine given in combination with cimetidine is reported to cause bone marrow depression. Carmustine given in combination with etoposide is reported to cause severe hepatic dysfunction with hyperbilirubinemia, ascites, and thrombocytopenia. Diluent for infusion contains alcohol; avoid concurrent use of medications that inhibit aldehyde dehydrogenase-2 or cause disulfiram-like reactions.
Nutritional/Ethanol Interactions Ethanol: Avoid ethanol.
Adverse Reactions
>10%:
Cardiovascular: Hypotension (with high dose therapy, due to the alcohol content of the diluent)
Central nervous system: Dizziness, ataxia; Wafers: Seizures (54%) postoperatively
Dermatologic: Hyperpigmentation of skin (with skin contact)
Gastrointestinal: Severe nausea and vomiting, usually begins within 2-4 hours of drug administration and lasts for 4-6 hours; dose related. Patients should receive a prophylactic antiemetic regimen.
Hematologic: Myelosuppression - cumulative, dose related, delayed, thrombocytopenia is usually more common and more severe than leukopenia
Onset (days): 7-14
Nadir (days): 21-35
Recovery (days): 42-56
Hepatic: Reversible increases in bilirubin, alkaline phosphatase, and SGOT occur in 20% to 25% of patients
Local: Pain and burning at injection site; phlebitis
Ocular: Ocular toxicities (transient conjunctival flushing and blurred vision), retinal hemorrhages
(Continued)

Carmustine *(Continued)*

Respiratory: Interstitial fibrosis occurs in up to 50% of patients receiving a cumulative dose >1400 mg/m^2, or bone marrow transplantation doses; may be delayed up to 3 years; rare in patients receiving lower doses. A history of lung disease or concomitant bleomycin therapy may increase the risk of this reaction. Patients with forced vital capacity (FVC) or carbon monoxide diffusing capacity of the lungs (DLCO) <70% of predicted are at higher risk.

1% to 10%:

Central nervous system: Wafers: Amnesia, aphasia, ataxia, cerebral edema, confusion, convulsion, depression, diplopia, dizziness, headache, hemiplegia, hydrocephalus, insomnia, meningitis, somnolence, stupor

Dermatologic: Facial flushing, probably due to the alcohol diluent; alopecia

Gastrointestinal: Anorexia, constipation, diarrhea, stomatitis

Hematologic: Anemia

Overdosage/Toxicology Symptoms of overdose include nausea, vomiting, thrombocytopenia, and leukopenia. Treatment is symptomatic and supportive.

Pharmacodynamics/Kinetics

Half-Life Elimination: Biphasic: Initial: 1.4 minutes; Secondary: 20 minutes (active metabolites: plasma half-life of 67 hours)

Metabolism: Rapidly hepatic

Excretion: Urine (~60% to 70%) within 96 hours; lungs (6% to 10% as CO$_2$)

Available Dosage Forms

Injection, powder for reconstitution (BiCNu®): 100 mg [packaged with 3 mL of absolute alcohol as diluent]

Wafer (Gliadel®): 7.7 mg (8s)

Dosing

Adults & Elderly: Refer to individual protocols.

Usual dosage (per manufacturer labeling): I.V.: 150-200 mg/m^2 every 6 weeks as a single dose or divided into daily injections on 2 successive days

Alternative regimens:

75-120 mg/m^2 days 1 and 2 every 6-8 weeks **or** 50-80 mg/m^2 days 1,2,3 every 6-8 weeks

Primary brain cancer:

150-200 mg/m^2 every 6-8 weeks as a single dose **or**

75-120 mg/m^2 days 1 and 2 every 6-8 weeks **or**

20-65 mg/m^2 every 4-6 weeks **or**

0.5-1 mg/kg every 4-6 weeks **or**

40-80 mg/m^2/day for 3 days every 6-8 weeks

Autologous BMT: I.V.: ALL OF THE FOLLOWING DOSES ARE FATAL WITHOUT BMT

Combination therapy: Up to 300-900 mg/m^2

Single-agent therapy: Up to 1200 mg/m^2 (fatal necrosis is associated with doses >2 g/m^2)

Glioblastoma multiforme (recurrent), malignant glioma: Implantation (wafer): Up to 8 wafers may be placed in the resection cavity (total dose 62.6 mg); should the size and shape not accommodate 8 wafers, the maximum number of wafers allowed should be placed

Pediatrics: Refer to individual protocols: Children: I.V.: 200-250 mg/m^2 every 4-6 weeks as a single dose

Hepatic Impairment: Dosage adjustment may be necessary; however, no specific guidelines are available.

Administration

I.V.: Irritant (alcohol-based diluent). Injection: Significant absorption to PVC containers - should be administered in either glass or Excel® container. I.V. infusion over 1-2 hours is recommended; infusion through a free-flowing saline or dextrose infusion, or administration through a central catheter can alleviate venous pain/irritation

High-dose carmustine: Maximum rate of infusion of ≤3 mg/m^2/minute to avoid excessive flushing, agitation, and hypotension; infusions should run over at least 2 hours; some investigational protocols dictate shorter infusions.

Fatal doses if not followed by bone marrow or peripheral stem cell infusions.

I.V. Detail:

Extravasation management: Elevate extremity. Inject long-acting dexamethasone (Decadron® LA) or by hyaluronidase throughout tissue with a 25- to 37-gauge needle. Apply warm, moist compresses.

BMT only: Vital signs must be monitored frequently during the infusion of high-dose carmustine.

BMT only: Patients receiving high-dose carmustine must be supine and may require the Trendelenburg position, fluid support, and vasopressor support.

Infusion-related cardiovascular effects are primarily due to concomitant ethanol and acetaldehyde. Use with great caution in patients with aldehyde dehydrogenase-2 deficiency or history of "alcohol flushing syndrome". Acute lung injury tends to occur 1-3 months following carmustine infusion. Patients must be counseled to contact their BMT physician for dyspnea, cough, or fever following carmustine. Acute lung injury is managed with a course of corticosteroids.

pH: 5.6-6.0

Stability

Reconstitution: Injection: Initially, dilute with 3 mL of absolute alcohol. Further dilute with SWFI (27 mL) to a concentration of 3.3 mg/mL; protect from light; may further dilute with D$_5$W or NS.

Compatibility: Stable in NS

Y-site administration: Incompatible with allopurinol

Compatibility when admixed: Incompatible with sodium bicarbonate

Storage:

Injection: Store intact vials under refrigeration; vials are stable for 36 days at room temperature. Reconstituted solutions are stable for 8 hours at room temperature (25°C) and 24 hours under refrigeration (2°C to 8°C) and protected from light. Further dilution in D$_5$W or NS is stable for 8 hours at room temperature (25°C) and 48 hours under refrigeration (4°C) in glass or Excel® protected from light.

Wafer: Store at or below -20°C (-4°F). May be kept at room temperature for up to 6 hours.

Laboratory Monitoring CBC with differential, platelet count, pulmonary function, liver and renal function

Nursing Actions

Physical Assessment: Assess other pharmacological or herbal products patient may be taking for potential interactions. An antiemetic including a serotonin [5-HT$_3$] antagonist and dexamethasone) may be ordered prior to therapy. Monitor infusion site closely to prevent extravasation. Patients should be supine and vital signs closely monitored during high dose infusion (may require the Trendelenburg position, fluid support, and vasopressor support). Monitor laboratory tests (eg, hematology, pulmonary, hepatic and renal function) at baseline and periodically during therapy. Monitor therapeutic response and adverse effects regularly during and for some time following therapy. Pulmonary function should be assessed for extended periods following high dose or BMT doses; acute lung injury can occur 1-3 months after treatment and pulmonary fibrosis may be delayed up to 3 years. Teach patient (or caregiver) possible side effects/appropriate interventions and adverse symptoms to report.

Patient Education: Do not take any new medication during therapy unless approved by prescriber. This medication can only be administered intravenously.

Report immediately any pain, burning, swelling at infusion site; sudden onset chest pain; respiratory difficulty; difficulty swallowing. Limit oral intake for 4-6 hours before therapy to reduce potential for nausea/vomiting. It is important that you maintain adequate nutrition between treatments (small, frequent meals may help) and adequate hydration (2-3 L/day of fluids) unless instructed to restrict fluid intake. You will be susceptible to infection (avoid crowds and exposure to infection and do not have any vaccinations without consulting prescriber). May cause nausea, vomiting, or anorexia (small, frequent meals, frequent mouth care, chewing gum, or sucking lozenges may help - if nausea/vomiting are severe, request antiemetic); mouth sores (use soft toothbrush or cotton swabs for mouth care); hyperpigmentation of skin and loss of hair (reversible); or sensitivity to sunlight (use sunblock, wear protective clothing and dark glasses, and avoid direct exposure to sunlight). Report immediately any dyspnea, cough, or fever; chest pain or palpitations; sore throat, chills, persistent unusual fatigue; unusual bruising/bleeding; change in color of urine or stool, change in urinary pattern; change in visual acuity. **Pregnancy/breast-feeding precautions:** Inform prescriber if you are pregnant. Do not get pregnant or cause a pregnancy (males) during therapy or for 1 month following therapy. Consult prescriber for instruction on appropriate contraceptive measures. This drug may cause severe fetal defects. Do not breast-feed.

Breast-Feeding Issues It is not known if carmustine is excreted in human breast milk. Due to potential harm to infant, breast-feeding is not recommended.

Pregnancy Issues Carmustine can cause fetal harm if administered to a pregnant woman.

Additional Information Accidental skin contact may cause transient burning and brown discoloration of the skin. Delayed onset pulmonary fibrosis occurring up to 17 years after treatment has been reported in patients who received cumulative >1400 mg/m^2.

Carvedilol (KAR ve dil ole)

U.S. Brand Names Coreg®

Pharmacologic Category Beta Blocker With Alpha-Blocking Activity

Medication Safety Issues
Sound-alike/look-alike issues:
Carvedilol may be confused with captopril, carteolol

Pregnancy Risk Factor C (manufacturer); D (2nd and 3rd trimesters - expert analysis)

Lactation Excretion in breast milk unknown/contraindicated

Use Mild to severe heart failure of ischemic or cardiomyopathic origin (usually in addition to standardized therapy); left ventricular dysfunction following myocardial infarction (MI); management of hypertension

Unlabeled/Investigational Use Angina pectoris

Mechanism of Action/Effect Nonselective beta-adrenoreceptor and alpha-adrenergic blocking agent, lowers heart rate and blood pressure. Has been shown to lower risk of hospitalization and increase survival in patients with mild to severe heart failure.

Contraindications Hypersensitivity to carvedilol or any component of the formulation; patients with decompensated cardiac failure requiring intravenous inotropic therapy; bronchial asthma or related bronchospastic conditions; second- or third-degree AV block, sick sinus syndrome, and severe bradycardia (except in patients with a functioning artificial pacemaker); cardiogenic shock; severe hepatic impairment; pregnancy (2nd and 3rd trimesters)

Warnings/Precautions Initiate cautiously and monitor for possible deterioration in patient status (including

symptoms of CHF). Adjustment of other medications (ACE inhibitors and/or diuretics) may be required. In severe chronic heart failure, trial patients were excluded if they had cardiac-related rales, ascites, or a serum creatinine >2.8 mg/dL. Congestive heart failure patients may experience a worsening of renal function; risks include ischemic disease, diffuse vascular disease, underlying renal dysfunction; systolic BP <100 mm Hg. Patients should be advised to avoid driving or other hazardous tasks during initiation of therapy due to the risk of syncope. Avoid abrupt discontinuation (may exacerbate underlying condition), particularly in patients with coronary artery disease; dose should be tapered over 1-2 weeks with close monitoring.

Manufacturer recommends discontinuation of therapy if liver injury occurs (confirmed by laboratory testing). Use caution in patients with PVD (can aggravate arterial insufficiency). Use caution with concurrent use of verapamil or diltiazem; bradycardia or heart block can occur. Use caution in patients with bronchospastic disease. Use cautiously in patients with diabetes because it can mask prominent hypoglycemic symptoms. May mask signs of thyrotoxicosis. Use care with anesthetic agents that decrease myocardial contractility. Safety and efficacy in children <18 years of age have not been established.

Drug Interactions

Cytochrome P450 Effect: Substrate of CYP1A2 (minor), 2C8/9 (major), 2D6 (major), 2E1 (minor), 3A4 (minor)

Decreased Effect: CYP2C8/9 inducers may decrease the levels/effects of carvedilol; example inducers include carbamazepine, phenobarbital, phenytoin, rifampin, rifapentine, and secobarbital. Decreased antihypertensive effect of beta-blockers has occurred with concurrent NSAID or salicylate use. Beta-blockers may alter the effect of sulfonylureas. Disopyramide may exacerbate heart failure or enhance bradycardic effect of beta-blockers. Beta-blockers may counteract desired effects of beta-agonists.

Increased Effect/Toxicity: CYP2C8/9 inhibitors may increase the levels/effects of carvedilol; example inhibitors include delavirdine, fluconazole, gemfibrozil, ketoconazole, nicardipine, NSAIDs, pioglitazone, and sulfonamides. CYP2D6 inhibitors may increase the levels/effects of carvedilol; example inhibitors include chlorpromazine, delavirdine, fluoxetine, miconazole, paroxetine, pergolide, quinidine, quinine, ritonavir, and ropinirole. Cimetidine increase the serum levels and effects of carvedilol. Carvedilol may increase the effects of other drugs which slow AV conduction (digoxin, verapamil, diltiazem) and alpha-blockers (prazosin, terazosin). Carvedilol may mask the tachycardia from hypoglycemia caused by insulin and oral hypoglycemics. SSRIs may decrease the metabolism of carvedilol.

Nutritional/Ethanol Interactions Herb/Nutraceutical: Avoid dong quai if using for hypertension (has estrogenic activity). Avoid ephedra, yohimbe, ginseng (may worsen hypertension). Avoid garlic (may have increased antihypertensive effect).

Lab Interactions Increased hepatic enzymes, BUN, NPN, alkaline phosphatase; decreased HDL

Adverse Reactions Note: Frequency ranges include data from hypertension and heart failure trials. Higher rates of adverse reactions have generally been noted in patients with CHF. However, the frequency of adverse effects associated with placebo is also increased in this population. Events occurring at a frequency > placebo in clinical trials.

>10%:
Cardiovascular: Hypotension (9% to 20%)
Central nervous system: Dizziness (6% to 32%), fatigue (4% to 24%)
Endocrine & metabolic: Hyperglycemia (5% to 12%), weight gain (10% to 12%)
(Continued)

Carvedilol (Continued)

Gastrointestinal: Diarrhea (2% to 12%)
Neuromuscular & skeletal: Weakness (11%)
1% to 10%:
Cardiovascular: Bradycardia (2% to 10%), hypertension (3%), AV block (3%), angina (2% to 6%), postural hypotension (2%), syncope (3% to 8%), dependent edema (4%), palpitation, peripheral edema (1% to 7%), generalized edema (5% to 6%)
Central nervous system: Headache (5% to 8%), fever (3%), paresthesia (2%), somnolence (2%), insomnia (2%), malaise, hypoesthesia, vertigo
Endocrine & metabolic: Alkaline phosphatase increased, gout (6%), hypercholesterolemia (4%), dehydration (2%), hyperkalemia (3%), hypervolemia (2%), hypertriglyceridemia (1%), hyperuricemia, hypoglycemia, hyponatremia
Gastrointestinal: Nausea (4% to 9%), vomiting (6%), melena, periodontitis
Genitourinary: Hematuria (3%), impotence
Hematologic: Thrombocytopenia (1% to 2%), decreased prothrombin, purpura
Hepatic: Transaminases increased
Neuromuscular & skeletal: Back pain (2% to 7%), arthralgia (6%), myalgia (3%), muscle cramps
Ocular: Blurred vision (3% to 5%), lacrimation
Renal: BUN increased (6%), abnormal renal function, albuminuria, glycosuria, creatinine increased (3%), kidney failure
Respiratory: Rhinitis (2%), increased cough (5%)
Miscellaneous: Injury (3% to 6%), allergy, sudden death

Overdosage/Toxicology Symptoms of intoxication include cardiac disturbances, CNS toxicity, bronchospasm, hypoglycemia, and hyperkalemia. The most common cardiac symptoms include hypotension and bradycardia. Atrioventricular block, intraventricular conduction disturbances, cardiogenic shock, and asystole may occur with severe overdose, especially with membrane-depressant drugs (eg, propranolol). CNS effects include convulsions, coma, and respiratory arrest (commonly seen with propranolol and other membrane-depressant and lipid-soluble drugs). Treatment is symptom-directed and supportive. Carvedilol does not appear to be significantly cleared by hemodialysis.

Pharmacodynamics/Kinetics
Onset of Action: 1-2 hours; Peak antihypertensive effect: ~1-2 hours
Protein Binding: >98%, primarily to albumin
Half-Life Elimination: 7-10 hours
Metabolism: Extensively hepatic, via **CYP2D6, 2C9, 3A4**, and 2C19 (2% excreted unchanged); three active metabolites (4-hydroxyphenyl metabolite is 13 times more potent than parent drug for beta-blockade); first-pass effect; plasma concentrations in the elderly and those with cirrhotic liver disease are 50% and 4-7 times higher, respectively
Excretion: Primarily feces

Available Dosage Forms
Tablet: 3.125 mg, 6.25 mg, 12.5 mg, 25 mg

Dosing
Adults & Elderly: Reduce dosage if heart rate drops to <55 beats/minute.
Hypertension: Oral: 6.25 mg twice daily; if tolerated, dose should be maintained for 1-2 weeks, then increased to 12.5 mg twice daily. Dosage may be increased to a maximum of 25 mg twice daily after 1-2 weeks. Maximum dose: 50 mg/day
Congestive heart failure: Oral: 3.125 mg twice daily for 2 weeks; if this dose is tolerated, may increase to 6.25 mg twice daily. Double the dose every 2 weeks to the highest dose tolerated by patient. (Prior to initiating therapy, other heart failure medications should be stabilized and fluid retention minimized.)

Maximum recommended dose: Oral:
Mild-to-moderate heart failure:
<85 kg: 25 mg twice daily
>85 kg: 50 mg twice daily
Severe heart failure: Oral: 25 mg twice daily
Left ventricular dysfunction following MI: Initial 3.125-6.25 mg twice daily; increase dosage incrementally (ie, from 6.25 to 12.5 mg twice daily) at intervals of 3-10 days, based on tolerance, to a target dose of 25 mg twice daily. **Note:** Should be initiated only after patient is hemodynamically stable and fluid retention has been minimized.
Angina pectoris (unlabeled use): Oral: 25-50 mg twice daily
Renal Impairment: None necessary
Hepatic Impairment: Use is contraindicated in severe liver dysfunction.

Administration
Oral: Administer with food.

Stability
Storage: Store at 30°C (86°F).
Laboratory Monitoring Renal studies, BUN, liver function

Nursing Actions
Physical Assessment: Assess potential for interactions with other prescriptions, OTC medications, or herbal products patient may be taking (especially anything that will effect blood pressure). Take blood pressure and heart rate prior to and following first doses and with any change in dosage. Caution patients with diabetes to monitor glucose levels closely (beta-blockers may alter glucose tolerance). Monitor laboratory tests, therapeutic effectiveness (eg, hypertension, reduction of angina), and adverse response (eg, CHF). Teach patient proper use, possible side effects/appropriate interventions, and adverse symptoms to report.

Patient Education: Do not take any new medication during therapy unless approved by prescriber. Take exactly as directed. Do not alter dose or discontinue this medication without consulting prescriber. Take pulse daily, prior to taking medication; follow prescriber's instruction about holding medication. If you have diabetes, monitor serum glucose closely (drug may alter glucose tolerance or mask signs of hypoglycemia). You may experience fatigue, dizziness, or postural hypotension (use caution when changing position from lying or sitting to standing, driving, or climbing stairs until response to medication is known); alteration in sexual performance (reversible); or diarrhea (buttermilk, boiled milk, or yogurt may help). Report unresolved swelling of extremities; respiratory difficulty or new cough; unresolved fatigue; unusual weight gain (>5 lb/week); unresolved constipation or diarrhea; or unusual muscle weakness.

Pregnancy/breast-feeding precautions: Inform prescriber if you are pregnant. Do not get pregnant while taking this medications. Consult prescriber for appropriate contraceptive use. Do not breast-feed.

Dietary Considerations Should be taken with food to minimize the risk of orthostatic hypotension.

Geriatric Considerations Due to alterations in the beta-adrenergic autonomic nervous system, beta-adrenergic blockade may result in less hemodynamic response than seen in younger adults. In U.S. trials conducted by the manufacturer, hypertension patients who were elderly (>65%) had a higher incidence of dizziness (8.8% vs 6%) than seen in younger patients. No other differences noted between young and old in these trials.

Pregnancy Issues No data available on whether carvedilol crosses the placenta; beta-blockers have been associated with persistent bradycardia, hypotension, and IUGR; IUGR probably related to maternal hypertension. Cases of neonatal hypoglycemia have been reported following maternal use of beta-blockers at parturition or during breast-feeding. Use during pregnancy only if the potential benefit justifies the risk.

Additional Information Fluid retention during therapy should be treated with an increase in diuretic dosage.

Caspofungin (kas poe FUN jin)

U.S. Brand Names Cancidas®
Synonyms Caspofungin Acetate
Pharmacologic Category Antifungal Agent, Parenteral; Echinocandin
Pregnancy Risk Factor C
Lactation Excretion in breast milk unknown/use caution
Use Treatment of invasive *Aspergillus* infections in patients who are refractory or intolerant of other therapy; treatment of candidemia and other *Candida* infections (intra-abdominal abscesses, esophageal, peritonitis, pleural space); empirical treatment for presumed fungal infections in febrile neutropenic patient
Mechanism of Action/Effect Blocks synthesis of a vital component of fungal cell wall, limiting its growth. The cell wall component is unique to specific fungi, limiting any potential for toxicity in mammals.
Contraindications Hypersensitivity to caspofungin or any component of the formulation
Warnings/Precautions Concurrent use of cyclosporine should be limited to patients for whom benefit outweighs risk, due to a high frequency of hepatic transaminase elevations observed during concurrent use. Limited data are available concerning treatment durations longer than 4 weeks; however, treatment appears to be well tolerated. Use caution in hepatic impairment; dosage reduction required in moderate impairment. Safety and efficacy in pediatric patients have not been established.
Drug Interactions
Decreased Effect: Caspofungin may decrease blood concentrations of tacrolimus. Dosage adjustment of caspofungin to 70 mg is required for patients on rifampin.
Increased Effect/Toxicity: Concurrent administration of cyclosporine may increase caspofungin concentrations; hepatic serum transaminases may be observed.
Adverse Reactions
>10%:
Central nervous system: Headache (up to 11%), fever (3% to 26%), chills (up to 14%)
Endocrine & metabolic: Hypokalemia (4% to 11%)
Hematologic: Hemoglobin decreased (1% to 12%)
Hepatic: Serum alkaline phosphatase (3% to 11%) increased, transaminases increased (up to 13%)
Local: Infusion site reactions (2% to 12%), phlebitis/thrombophlebitis (up to 16%)
1% to 10%:
Cardiovascular: Flushing (2% to 3%), facial edema (up to 3%), hypertension (1% to 2%), tachycardia (1% to 2%), hypotension (1%)
Central nervous system: Dizziness (2%), pain (1% to 5%), insomnia (1%)
Dermatologic: Rash (<1% to 6%), pruritus (1% to 3%), erythema (1% to 2%)
Gastrointestinal: Nausea (2% to 6%), vomiting (1% to 4%), abdominal pain (1% to 4%), diarrhea (1% to 4%), anorexia (1%)
Hematologic: Eosinophils increased (3%), neutrophils decreased (2% to 3%), WBC decreased (5% to 6%), anemia (up to 4%), platelet count decreased (2% to 3%)
Hepatic: Bilirubin increased (3%)
Local: Induration (up to 3%)
Neuromuscular & skeletal: Myalgia (up to 3%), paresthesia (1% to 3%), tremor (≤2%)
Renal: Nephrotoxicity (8%)*, proteinuria (5%), hematuria (2%), serum creatinine increased (<1% to 4%), urinary WBCs increased (up to 8%), urinary RBCs

increased (1% to 4%), blood urea nitrogen increased (1%)
*Nephrotoxicity defined as serum creatinine ≥2X baseline value or ≥1 mg/dL in patients with serum creatinine above ULN range (patients with Cl$_{cr}$ <30 mL/minute were excluded)
Miscellaneous: Flu-like syndrome (3%), diaphoresis (up to 3%)
Overdosage/Toxicology No experience with overdosage has been reported. Caspofungin is not dialyzable. Treatment is symptomatic and supportive.
Pharmacodynamics/Kinetics
Protein Binding: 97% to albumin
Half-Life Elimination: Beta (distribution): 9-11 hours; Terminal: 40-50 hours
Metabolism: Slowly, via hydrolysis and N-acetylation as well as by spontaneous degradation, with subsequent metabolism to component amino acids. Overall metabolism is extensive.
Excretion: Urine (41% as metabolites, 1% to 9% unchanged) and feces (35% as metabolites)
Available Dosage Forms Injection, powder for reconstitution, as acetate: 50 mg [contains sucrose 39 mg], 70 mg [contains sucrose 54 mg]
Dosing
Adults & Elderly: Note: Duration of caspofungin treatment should be determined by patient status and clinical response. Empiric therapy should be given until neutropenia resolves. In patients with positive cultures, treatment should continue until 14 days after last positive culture. In neutropenic patients, treatment should be given at least 7 days after both signs and symptoms of infection **and** neutropenia resolve.
Empiric therapy: Initial dose: 70 mg on day 1; subsequent dosing: 50 mg/day; may increase up to 70 mg/day if tolerated, but clinical response is inadequate.
Invasive *Aspergillus*, candidiasis: I.V.: Initial dose: 70 mg on day 1; subsequent dosing: 50 mg/day
Esophageal candidiasis: I.V.: 50 mg/day; **Note:** The majority of patients studied for this indication also had oropharyngeal involvement.

Dosage adjustment with concomitant use of an enzyme inducer:
Patients receiving rifampin: 70 mg caspofungin daily
Patients receiving carbamazepine, dexamethasone, efavirenz, nevirapine, or phenytoin (and possibly other enzyme inducers) may require an increased daily dose of caspofungin (70 mg/day).
Pediatrics: Safety and efficacy in pediatric patients have not been established.
Renal Impairment: No specific dosage adjustment is required; supplemental dose is not required following dialysis.
Hepatic Impairment:
Mild hepatic insufficiency (Child-Pugh score 5-6): No adjustment necessary.
Moderate hepatic insufficiency (Child-Pugh score 7-9): 35 mg/day; initial 70 mg loading dose should still be administered in treatment of invasive infections.
Severe hepatic insufficiency (Child-Pugh score >9): No clinical experience.
Administration
I.V.: Infuse slowly, over 1 hour.
I.V. Detail: Monitor during infusion. Isolated cases of possible histamine-related reactions have occurred during clinical trials (rash, flushing, pruritus, facial edema).
Stability
Reconstitution: Bring refrigerated vial to room temperature. Reconstitute vials using 0.9% sodium chloride for injection, SWFI, or bacteriostatic water for injection. Mix gently until clear solution is formed; do
(Continued)

Caspofungin *(Continued)*

not use if cloudy or contains particles. Solution should be further diluted with 0.9%, 0.45%, or 0.225% sodium chloride or LR. Do not mix with dextrose-containing solutions. Do not coadminister with other medications.

Compatibility: Do not mix with dextrose-containing solutions.

Storage: Store vials at 2°C to 8°C (36°F to 46°F). Reconstituted solution may be stored at less than 25°C (77°F) for 1 hour prior to preparation of infusion solution. Infusion solutions may be stored at less than 25°C (77°F) and should be used within 24 hours; up to 48 hours if stored at 2°C to 8°C (36°F to 46°F).

Nursing Actions

Physical Assessment: Assess therapeutic response and adverse reactions (see Adverse Reactions). See Administration I.V. specifics. Teach patient possible side effects/appropriate interventions and adverse symptoms to report.

Patient Education: This medication can only be administered by infusion. Report immediately any pain, burning, or swelling at infusion site, or any signs of allergic reaction (eg, respiratory difficulty or swallowing, back pain, chest tightness, rash, hives, or swelling of lips or mouth). Report nausea, vomiting, abdominal pain, or diarrhea. **Pregnancy/breast-feeding precautions:** Inform prescriber if you are or intend to become pregnant. Consult prescriber if breast-feeding.

Cefaclor *(SEF a klor)*

U.S. Brand Names Raniclor™

Pharmacologic Category Antibiotic, Cephalosporin (Second Generation)

Medication Safety Issues

Sound-alike/look-alike issues:

Cefaclor may be confused with cephalexin

Pregnancy Risk Factor B

Lactation Enters breast milk/use caution

Use Treatment of susceptible bacterial infections including otitis media, lower respiratory tract infections, acute exacerbations of chronic bronchitis, pharyngitis and tonsillitis, urinary tract infections, skin and skin structure infections

Mechanism of Action/Effect Inhibits bacterial cell wall synthesis by binding to one or more of the penicillin-binding proteins (PBPs)

Contraindications Hypersensitivity to cefaclor, any component of the formulation, or other cephalosporins

Warnings/Precautions Modify dosage in patients with severe renal impairment. Prolonged use may result in superinfection. Use with caution in patients with a history of penicillin allergy especially IgE-mediated reactions (eg, anaphylaxis, urticaria). Beta-lactamase-negative, ampicillin-resistant (BLNAR) strains of *H. influenzae* should be considered resistant to cefaclor. Extended release tablets are not approved for use in children <16 years of age.

Drug Interactions

Increased Effect/Toxicity: Probenecid may decrease cephalosporin elimination. Furosemide, aminoglycosides when taken with cefaclor may result in additive nephrotoxicity.

Nutritional/Ethanol Interactions

Food: Cefaclor serum levels may be decreased slightly if taken with food. The bioavailability of cefaclor extended release tablets is decreased 23% and the maximum concentration is decreased 67% when taken on an empty stomach.

Lab Interactions Positive direct Coombs', false-positive urinary glucose test using cupric sulfate (Benedict's solution, Clinitest®, Fehling's solution), false-positive serum or urine creatinine with Jaffé reaction

Adverse Reactions

1% to 10%:

Dermatologic: Rash (maculopapular, erythematous, or morbilliform) (1% to 2%)

Gastrointestinal: Diarrhea (3%)

Genitourinary: Vaginitis (2%)

Hematologic: Eosinophilia (2%)

Hepatic: Transaminases increased (3%)

Miscellaneous: Moniliasis (2%)

Reactions reported with other cephalosporins include fever, abdominal pain, superinfection, renal dysfunction, toxic nephropathy, hemorrhage, cholestasis

Overdosage/Toxicology Symptoms of overdose include diarrhea, epigastric distress, nausea, and vomiting. Many beta-lactam containing antibiotics have the potential to cause neuromuscular hyperirritability or seizures. Hemodialysis may be helpful to aid in removal of the drug from blood; otherwise, treatment is supportive and symptom-directed.

Pharmacodynamics/Kinetics

Time to Peak: Capsule: 60 minutes; Suspension: 45 minutes

Protein Binding: 25%

Half-Life Elimination: 0.5-1 hour; prolonged with renal impairment

Metabolism: Partially hepatic

Excretion: Urine (80% as unchanged drug)

Available Dosage Forms

Capsule: 250 mg, 500 mg

Powder for oral suspension: 125 mg/5 mL (75 mL, 150 mL); 187 mg/5 mL (50 mL, 100 mL); 250 mg/5 mL (75 mL, 150 mL); 375 mg/5 mL (50 mL, 100 mL)

Tablet, chewable (Raniclor™): 125 mg [contains phenylalanine 2.8 mg; fruity flavor], 187 mg [contains phenylalanine 4.2 mg; fruity flavor]

Dosing

Adults & Elderly: Susceptible infections: Oral: Dosing range: 250-500 mg every 8 hours

Pediatrics: Susceptible infections: Oral: Children >1 month: Dosing range: 20-40 mg/kg/day divided every 8-12 hours; maximum dose: 1 g/day

Otitis media: Oral: 40 mg/kg/day divided every 12 hours

Pharyngitis: Oral: 20 mg/kg/day divided every 12 hours

Renal Impairment:

Cl_{cr} 10-50 mL/minute: Administer 50% to 100% of dose

Cl_{cr} <10 mL/minute: Administer 50% of dose

Hemodialysis: Moderately dialyzable (20% to 50%)

Administration

Oral: Administer around-the-clock to promote less variation in peak and trough serum levels.

Chewable tablet: Should be chewed before swallowing; should not be swallowed whole.

Oral suspension: Shake well before using.

Stability

Storage: Store at controlled room temperature. Refrigerate suspension after reconstitution. Discard after 14 days. Do not freeze.

Laboratory Monitoring Perform culture and sensitivity studies prior to initiating drug therapy; renal function

Nursing Actions

Physical Assessment: Results of culture/sensitivity tests and patient's allergy history should be assessed prior to therapy. Assess other pharmacological or herbal products patient may be taking for potential interactions (eg, nephrotoxicity). Monitor laboratory tests, therapeutic effectiveness, and adverse effects (hypersensitivity can occur days after therapy is started) regularly during therapy. Advise patients with diabetes about use of Clinitest®. Teach patient proper use, possible side effects/appropriate interventions, and adverse symptoms to report (eg, hypersensitivity, opportunistic infections).

Patient Education: Do not take any new medication during therapy unless approved by prescriber. Take as directed, at regular intervals around-the-clock (with or without food). Chilling oral suspension improves flavor (do not freeze). Do not chew or crush extended release tablets. Maintain adequate hydration (2-3 L/day of fluids) unless instructed to restrict fluid intake. Complete full course of medication, even if you feel better. May cause false test results with Clinitest®; use of another type of testing is preferable. May cause diarrhea (yogurt, boiled milk, or buttermilk may help). Report rash; breathing or swallowing difficulty; persistent diarrhea, nausea, vomiting, or abdominal pain; changes in urinary pattern or pain on urination; opportunistic infection (eg, vaginal itching or drainage; sores in mouth; blood in stool or urine, vaginal itching or drainage, unusual fever or chills); or CNS changes (eg, irritability, agitation, nervousness, insomnia, hallucinations); or other adverse reactions. **Breast-feeding precaution:** Consult prescriber if breast-feeding.

Dietary Considerations Capsule, chewable tablet, and suspension may be taken with or without food. Raniclor™ contains phenylalanine 2.8 mg/cefaclor 125 mg.

Breast-Feeding Issues Theoretically, drug absorbed by nursing infant may change bowel flora or affect fever work-up result. Small amounts can be detected in breast milk (trace amounts after 1 hour, increasing to 0.16 mcg/mL at 5 hours). **Note:** As a class, cephalosporins are used to treat bacterial infections in infants.

Cefadroxil (sef a DROKS il)

U.S. Brand Names Duricef®

Synonyms Cefadroxil Monohydrate

Pharmacologic Category Antibiotic, Cephalosporin (First Generation)

Pregnancy Risk Factor B

Lactation Enters breast milk (small amounts)/use caution (AAP rates "compatible")

Use Treatment of susceptible bacterial infections, including those caused by group A beta-hemolytic *Streptococcus*; prophylaxis against bacterial endocarditis in patients who are allergic to penicillin and undergoing surgical or dental procedures

Mechanism of Action/Effect Inhibits bacterial cell wall synthesis by binding to one or more of the penicillin-binding proteins (PBPs)

Contraindications Hypersensitivity to cefadroxil, other cephalosporins, or any component of the formulation

Warnings/Precautions Modify dosage in patients with severe renal impairment; prolonged use may result in superinfection; use with caution in patients with a history of penicillin allergy especially IgE-mediated reactions (eg, anaphylaxis, angioedema, urticaria). May cause antibiotic-associated colitis or colitis secondary to *C. difficile*.

Drug Interactions

Increased Effect/Toxicity: Bleeding may occur when administered with anticoagulants. Probenecid may decrease cephalosporin elimination.

Nutritional/Ethanol Interactions Food: Concomitant administration with food, infant formula, or cow's milk does **not** significantly affect absorption.

Lab Interactions Positive direct Coombs', false-positive urinary glucose test using cupric sulfate (Benedict's solution, Clinitest®, Fehling's solution), false-positive serum or urine creatinine with Jaffé reaction

Adverse Reactions

1% to 10%: Gastrointestinal: Diarrhea

Reactions reported with other cephalosporins include toxic epidermal necrolysis, abdominal pain, superinfection. renal dysfunction, toxic nephropathy, aplastic anemia, hemolytic anemia, hemorrhage, prolonged prothrombin time, increased BUN, increased creatinine, eosinophilia, pancytopenia, seizure

Overdosage/Toxicology Symptoms of overdose include neuromuscular hypersensitivity and convulsions. Many beta-lactam containing antibiotics have the potential to cause neuromuscular hyperirritability or convulsive seizures. Hemodialysis may be helpful to aid in removal of the drug from blood; otherwise, treatment is supportive or symptom-directed.

Pharmacodynamics/Kinetics

Time to Peak: Serum: 70-90 minutes

Protein Binding: 20%

Half-Life Elimination: 1-2 hours; Renal failure: 20-24 hours

Excretion: Urine (>90% as unchanged drug)

Available Dosage Forms

Capsule, as monohydrate: 500 mg
Duricef®: 500 mg
Powder for oral suspension, as monohydrate: 250 mg/5 mL (50 mL, 100 mL); 500 mg/5 mL (75 mL, 100 mL)
Duricef®: 250 mg/5 mL (50 mL, 100 mL); 500 mg/5 mL (75 mL, 100 mL) [contains sodium benzoate; orange-pineapple flavor]
Tablet, as monohydrate: 1 g
Duricef®: 1 g

Dosing

Adults & Elderly:

Susceptible infections: Oral: 1-2 g/day in 2 divided doses

Prophylaxis against bacterial endocarditis: Oral: 2 g 1 hour prior to the procedure

Pediatrics:

Susceptible infections: Oral: Children: 30 mg/kg/day divided twice daily up to a maximum of 2 g/day

Prophylaxis against bacterial endocarditis: Oral: Children: 50 mg/kg 1 hour prior to the procedure

Renal Impairment:

Cl_{cr} 10-25 mL/minute: Administer every 24 hours.

Cl_{cr} <10 mL/minute: Administer every 36 hours.

Administration

Oral: Administer around-the-clock to promote less variation in peak and trough serum levels.

Stability

Reconstitution: Refrigerate suspension after reconstitution. Discard after 14 days.

Laboratory Monitoring Perform culture and sensitivity studies prior to initiating drug therapy; renal function

Nursing Actions

Physical Assessment: Results of culture/sensitivity tests and patient's allergy history should be assessed prior to therapy. Assess other pharmacological or herbal products patient may be taking for potential interactions (eg, anticoagulants). Monitor laboratory tests, therapeutic response, and adverse effects (eg, hypersensitivity can occur several days after therapy is started) regularly during therapy. Advise patients with diabetes about use of Clinitest®. Teach patient proper use, possible side effects/appropriate interventions, and adverse symptoms to report (eg, hypersensitivity, opportunistic infection, renal dysfunction, anemia).

Patient Education: Do not take any new medication during therapy unless approved by prescriber. Take as directed, at regular intervals around-the-clock (with or without food). Chilling oral suspension improves flavor (do not freeze). Maintain adequate hydration (2-3 L/day of fluids) unless instructed to restrict fluid intake. Complete full course of medication, even if you feel better. May cause false test results with Clinitest®; use of another type of glucose testing is preferable. May cause diarrhea (yogurt, boiled milk, or buttermilk (Continued)

Cefadroxil (Continued)

may help). Report rash; breathing or swallowing difficulty; persistent diarrhea, nausea, vomiting, or abdominal pain; changes in urinary pattern or pain on urination; opportunistic infection (eg, vaginal itching or drainage; sores in mouth; blood in urine or stool; unusual fever or chills); or CNS changes (eg, irritability, agitation, nervousness, insomnia, hallucinations); or other adverse reactions. **Breast-feeding precaution:** Consult prescriber if breast-feeding.

Geriatric Considerations Adjust dose for renal function in the elderly.

Breast-Feeding Issues Theoretically, drug absorbed by nursing infant may change bowel flora or affect fever work-up result. **Note:** As a class, cephalosporins are used to treat infections in infants.

Cefazolin (sef A zoe lin)

U.S. Brand Names Ancef®

Synonyms Cefazolin Sodium

Pharmacologic Category Antibiotic, Cephalosporin (First Generation)

Medication Safety Issues
Sound-alike/look-alike issues:
Cefazolin may be confused with cefprozil, cephalexin, cephalothin
Kefzol® may be confused with Cefzil®

Pregnancy Risk Factor B

Lactation Enters breast milk (small amounts)/use caution (AAP rates "compatible")

Use Treatment of respiratory tract, skin and skin structure, genital, urinary tract, biliary tract, bone and joint infections, and septicemia due to susceptible gram-positive cocci (except enterococcus); some gram-negative bacilli including *E. coli, Proteus,* and *Klebsiella* may be susceptible; perioperative prophylaxis

Unlabeled/Investigational Use Prophylaxis against bacterial endocarditis

Mechanism of Action/Effect Inhibits bacterial cell wall synthesis by binding to one or more of the penicillin-binding proteins (PBPs)

Contraindications Hypersensitivity to cefazolin sodium, any component of the formulation, or other cephalosporins

Warnings/Precautions Modify dosage in patients with severe renal impairment; prolonged use may result in superinfection; use with caution in patients with a history of penicillin allergy especially IgE-mediated reactions (eg, anaphylaxis, angioedema, urticaria). May cause antibiotic-associated colitis or colitis secondary to *C. difficile.*

Drug Interactions
Increased Effect/Toxicity: High-dose probenecid decreases clearance and increases effect of cefazolin. Aminoglycosides increase nephrotoxic potential when taken with cefazolin. Cefazolin may increase the hypothrombinemic response to warfarin (due to alteration of GI microbial flora).

Lab Interactions Positive direct Coombs', false-positive urinary glucose test using cupric sulfate (Benedict's solution, Clinitest®, Fehling's solution), false-positive serum or urine creatinine using Jaffé reaction
Some penicillin derivatives may accelerate the degradation of aminoglycosides *in vitro,* leading to a potential underestimation of aminoglycoside serum concentration.

Adverse Reactions Frequency not defined.
Central nervous system: Fever, seizure
Dermatologic: Rash, pruritus, Stevens-Johnson syndrome
Gastrointestinal: Diarrhea, nausea, vomiting, abdominal cramps, anorexia, pseudomembranous colitis, oral candidiasis
Genitourinary: Vaginitis
Hepatic: Transaminases increased, hepatitis
Hematologic: Eosinophilia, neutropenia, leukopenia, thrombocytopenia, thrombocytosis
Local: Pain at injection site, phlebitis
Renal: BUN increased, serum creatinine increased, renal failure
Miscellaneous: Anaphylaxis

Reactions reported with other cephalosporins include toxic epidermal necrolysis, abdominal pain, cholestasis, superinfection, toxic nephropathy, aplastic anemia, hemolytic anemia, hemorrhage, prolonged prothrombin time, pancytopenia

Overdosage/Toxicology Symptoms of overdose include neuromuscular hypersensitivity and convulsions. Many beta-lactam containing antibiotics have the potential to cause neuromuscular hyperirritability or convulsive seizures. Hemodialysis may be helpful to aid in the removal of drug from blood; otherwise, treatment is supportive or symptom-directed.

Pharmacodynamics/Kinetics
Time to Peak: Serum: I.M.: 0.5-2 hours
Protein Binding: 74% to 86%
Half-Life Elimination: 90-150 minutes; prolonged with renal impairment
Metabolism: Minimally hepatic
Excretion: Urine (80% to 100% as unchanged drug)

Available Dosage Forms [DSC] = Discontinued product
Infusion [premixed in D_5W]: 500 mg (50 mL); 1 g (50 mL)
Injection, powder for reconstitution: 500 mg, 1 g, 10 g, 20 g
Ancef®: 1 g; 10 g [DSC]

Dosing
Adults & Elderly:
Usual dosage range: I.M., I.V.: 1-2 g every 8 hours, depending on severity of infection; maximum: 12 g/day
Mild-to-moderate infections: 500 mg to 1 g every 6-8 hours
Mild infection with gram-positive cocci: 250-500 mg every 8 hours
Perioperative prophylaxis: 1 g given 30 minutes prior to surgery (repeat with 500 mg to 1 g during prolonged surgery); followed by 500 mg to 1 g every 6-9 hours for 24 hours postop
Pneumococcal pneumonia: 500 mg every 12 hours
Severe infection: 1-2 g every 6 hours
Prophylaxis against bacterial endocarditis (unlabeled use): 1 g 30 minutes before procedure
UTI (uncomplicated): 1 g every 12 hours
Pediatrics:
Usual dosage range: I.M., I.V.: Children >1 month: 25-100 mg/kg/day divided every 6-8 hours; maximum: 6 g/day
Prophylaxis against bacterial endocarditis (unlabeled use): Infants and Children: 25 mg/kg 30 minutes before procedure; maximum dose: 1 g
Renal Impairment:
Cl_{cr} 10-30 mL/minute: Administer every 12 hours.
Cl_{cr} <10 mL/minute: Administer every 24 hours.
Moderately dialyzable (20% to 50%); administer dose postdialysis or administer supplemental dose of 0.5-1 g after dialysis.
Peritoneal dialysis: Administer 0.5 g every 12 hours.
Continuous arteriovenous or venovenous hemofiltration: Dose as for Cl_{cr} 10-30 mL/minute. Removes 30 mg of cefazolin per liter of filtrate per day.

Administration

I.M.: Inject deep I.M. into large muscle mass.

I.V.: Inject direct I.V. over 5 minutes. Infuse intermittent infusion over 30-60 minutes.

Some penicillins (eg, carbenicillin, ticarcillin and piperacillin) have been shown to inactivate aminoglycosides *in vitro*. This has been observed to a greater extent with tobramycin and gentamicin, while amikacin has shown greater stability against inactivation. Concurrent use of these agents may pose a risk of reduced antibacterial efficacy *in vivo*, particularly in the setting of profound renal impairment. However, definitive clinical evidence is lacking. If combination penicillin/aminoglycoside therapy is desired in a patient with renal dysfunction, separation of doses (if feasible), and routine monitoring of aminoglycoside levels, CBC, and clinical response should be considered.

I.V. Detail: pH: 4.5-6.0

Stability

Reconstitution: Dilute large vial with 2.5 mL SWFI; 10 g vial may be diluted with 45 mL to yield 1 g/5 mL or 96 mL to yield 1 g/10 mL. May be injected or further dilution for I.V. administration in 50-100 mL compatible solution. Standard diluent is 1 g/50 mL D$_5$W or 2 g/50 mL D$_5$W.

Compatibility: Stable in D$_5$W, D$_5$LR, D$_5$¼NS, D$_5$½NS, D$_5$NS, D$_{10}$W,LR, NS

Y-site administration: Incompatible with amphotericin B cholesteryl sulfate complex, idarubicin, pentamidine, vinorelbine

Compatibility in syringe: Incompatible with ascorbic acid injection, cimetidine, lidocaine

Compatibility when admixed: Incompatible with amikacin, amobarbital, atracurium, bleomycin, calcium gluconate, clindamycin with gentamicin, colistimethate, kanamycin, pentobarbital, polymyxin B sulfate, ranitidine

Storage: Store intact vials at room temperature and protect from temperatures exceeding 40°C. Reconstituted solutions of cefazolin are light yellow to yellow. Protection from light is recommended for the powder and for the reconstituted solutions. Reconstituted solutions are stable for 24 hours at room temperature and for 10 days under refrigeration. Stability of parenteral admixture at room temperature (25°C) is 48 hours. Stability of parenteral admixture at refrigeration temperature (4°C) is 14 days.

DUPLEX™: Store at 20°C to 25°C (68°F to 77°F); excursions permitted to 15°C to 30°C (59°F to 86°F) prior to activation. Following activation, stable for 24 hours at room temperature and for 7 days under refrigeration.

Laboratory Monitoring Perform culture and sensitivity studies prior to initiating drug therapy; renal function

Nursing Actions

Physical Assessment: Assess results of culture/sensitivity tests and patient's allergy history prior to therapy. Assess other pharmacological or herbal products patient may be taking for potential interactions (eg, anticoagulants). Monitor results of laboratory tests, therapeutic effectiveness, and adverse response (eg, hypersensitivity can occur several days after therapy is started) regularly during therapy. Advise patients with diabetes about use of Clinitest®. Teach patient proper use, possible side effects/appropriate interventions, and adverse symptoms to report (eg, hypersensitivity, opportunistic infection, renal dysfunction, anemia).

Patient Education: Do not take any new medication during therapy unless approved by prescriber. This medication is administered by injection or infusion. Report immediately any redness, swelling, burning, or pain at injection/infusion site; rash or hives; or respiratory difficulty, chest pain, or difficulty swallowing. Maintain adequate hydration (2-3 L/day of fluids)

unless instructed to restrict fluid intake. If you have diabetes, drug may cause false test results with Clinitest® urine glucose monitoring; use of another type of glucose monitoring is preferable. May cause diarrhea (yogurt, boiled milk, or buttermilk may help). Report rash; breathing or swallowing difficulty; persistent diarrhea, nausea, vomiting, or abdominal pain; changes in urinary pattern or pain on urination; opportunistic infection (eg, vaginal itching or drainage; sores in mouth; blood in stool or urine; unusual fever or chills); or CNS changes (eg, irritability, agitation, nervousness, insomnia, hallucinations); or other adverse reactions. **Breast-feeding precautions:** Consult prescriber if breast-feeding.

Dietary Considerations Sodium content of 1 g: 48 mg (2 mEq)

Geriatric Considerations Adjust dose for renal function.

Breast-Feeding Issues Theoretically, drug absorbed by nursing infant may change bowel flora or affect fever work-up result. **Note:** As a class, cephalosporins are used to treat infections in infants.

Related Information
Compatibility of Drugs *on page 1370*

Cefdinir (SEF di ner)

U.S. Brand Names Omnicef®

Synonyms CFDN

Pharmacologic Category Antibiotic, Cephalosporin (Third Generation)

Pregnancy Risk Factor B

Lactation Excretion in breast milk unknown/use caution

Use Treatment of community-acquired pneumonia, acute exacerbations of chronic bronchitis, acute bacterial otitis media, acute maxillary sinusitis, pharyngitis/tonsillitis, and uncomplicated skin and skin structure infections.

Mechanism of Action/Effect Inhibits bacterial cell wall synthesis by binding to one or more of the penicillin-binding proteins (PBPs) which in turn inhibits the final transpeptidation step of peptidoglycan synthesis in bacterial cell walls, thus inhibiting cell wall biosynthesis. Bacteria eventually lyse due to ongoing activity of cell wall autolytic enzymes (autolysins and murein hydrolases) while cell wall assembly is arrested.

Contraindications Hypersensitivity to cefdinir, other cephalosporins, related antibiotics, or any component of the formulation

Warnings/Precautions Administer cautiously to penicillin-sensitive patients, especially IgE-mediated reactions (eg, anaphylaxis, urticaria). There is evidence of partial cross-allergenicity and cephalosporins cannot be assumed to be an absolutely safe alternative to penicillin in the penicillin-allergic patient. Serum sickness-like reactions have been reported. Signs and symptoms occur after a few days of therapy and resolve a few days after drug discontinuation with no serious sequelae. Pseudomembranous colitis occurs; consider its diagnosis in patients who develop diarrhea with antibiotic use. Use caution with renal dysfunction; dose adjustment may be required.

Drug Interactions

Decreased Effect: Coadministration with iron or antacids reduces the rate and extent of cefdinir absorption.

Increased Effect/Toxicity: Probenecid may increase the effects of cefdinir by decreasing renal elimination (peak plasma levels of cefdinir are increased by 54% and half-life is prolonged by 50%).

Adverse Reactions

>10%: Gastrointestinal: Diarrhea (8% to 15%)

1% to 10%:
  Central nervous system: Headache (2%)
  Dermatologic: Rash (≤3%)

(Continued)

Cefdinir *(Continued)*

Gastrointestinal: Nausea (≤3%), abdominal pain (≤1%), vomiting (≤1%)

Genitourinary: Vaginal moniliasis (≤4%), urine leukocytes increased (2%), urine protein increased (1% to 2%), vaginitis (≤1%)

Hematologic: Eosinophils increased (1%)

Hepatic: Alkaline phosphatase increased (≤1%), platelets increased (1%)

Renal: Microhematuria (1%)

Miscellaneous: Lymphocytes increased (≤2%), GGT increased (1%), lactate dehydrogenase increased (≤1%), bicarbonate decreased (≤1%), lymphocytes decreased (≤1%), PMN changes (≤1%)

Reactions reported with other cephalosporins include dizziness, fever, encephalopathy, asterixis, neuromuscular excitability, seizure, aplastic anemia, interstitial nephritis, toxic nephropathy, angioedema, hemorrhage, prolonged PT, and superinfection.

Overdosage/Toxicology After acute overdose, most agents cause only nausea, vomiting, and diarrhea, although neuromuscular hypersensitivity and seizures are possible, especially in patients with renal insufficiency. Hemodialysis may be helpful to aid in the removal of the drug from the blood but not usually indicated, otherwise most treatment is supportive or symptom-directed following GI decontamination.

Pharmacodynamics/Kinetics

Protein Binding: 60% to 70%

Half-Life Elimination: 100 minutes

Metabolism: Minimally hepatic

Excretion: Primarily urine

Available Dosage Forms

Capsule: 300 mg

Powder for oral suspension: 125 mg/5 mL (60 mL, 100 mL) [contains sodium benzoate and sucrose 2.86 g/5 mL; strawberry flavor]; 250 mg/5 mL (60 mL, 100 mL) [contains sodium benzoate and sucrose 2.86 g/5 mL; strawberry flavor]

Dosing

Adults & Elderly:

Acute exacerbations of chronic bronchitis, pharyngitis/tonsillitis: Oral: 300 mg twice daily for 5-10 days or 600 mg once daily for 10 days

Acute maxillary sinusitis: Oral: 300 mg twice daily or 600 mg once daily for 10 days

Community-acquired pneumonia, uncomplicated skin and skin structure infections: Oral: 300 mg twice daily for 10 days

Pediatrics:

Children 6 months to 12 years:

Acute bacterial otitis media, pharyngitis/tonsillitis: Oral: 7 mg/kg/dose twice daily for 5-10 days or 14 mg/kg/dose once daily for 10 days (maximum: 600 mg/day)

Acute maxillary sinusitis: Oral: 7 mg/kg/dose twice daily or 14 mg/kg/dose once daily for 10 days (maximum: 600 mg/day)

Uncomplicated skin and skin structure infections: Oral: 7 mg/kg/dose twice daily for 10 days (maximum: 600 mg/day)

Children >12 years: Refer to adult dosing.

Renal Impairment:

Children: 7 mg/kg once daily (maximum: 300 mg/day)

Adults: 300 mg once daily

Administration

Oral: Twice daily doses should be given every 12 hours. May be taken with or without food. The suspension should be shaken well before each administration.

Stability

Reconstitution: Oral suspension should be mixed with 38 mL water for the 60 mL bottle and 63 mL of water for the 120 mL bottle.

Storage: Capsules and unmixed powder should be stored at room temperature of 25°C (77°F). After mixing, the suspension can be stored at room temperature of 25°C (77°F) for 10 days.

Laboratory Monitoring Perform culture and sensitivity studies prior to initiating drug therapy; renal function

Nursing Actions

Physical Assessment: Results of culture/sensitivity tests and patient's allergy history should be assessed prior to therapy. Assess other pharmacological or herbal products patient may be taking for potential interactions. Monitor therapeutic response and adverse effects during therapy. Teach patient proper use, possible side effects/appropriate interventions, and adverse symptoms to report (eg, opportunistic infection, hypersensitivity).

Patient Education: Take as directed, at regular intervals around-the-clock (with or without food). Chilling oral suspension improves flavor (do not freeze). Complete full course of medication, even if you feel better. Maintain adequate hydration (2-3 L/day of fluids) unless instructed to restrict fluid intake. May cause diarrhea (yogurt, boiled milk, or buttermilk may help); or nausea, vomiting, flatulence (small frequent meals, frequent mouth care, chewing gum, or sucking lozenges may help). Report rash; breathing or swallowing difficulty; persistent diarrhea, nausea, vomiting, or abdominal pain; changes in urinary pattern or pain on urination; opportunistic infection (eg, vaginal itching or drainage; sores in mouth; blood in stool or urine, unusual fever or chills); CNS changes (eg, irritability, agitation, nervousness, insomnia, hallucinations); or other adverse reactions. **Breast-feeding precaution:** Consult prescriber if breast-feeding.

Dietary Considerations Suspension contains sucrose 2.86 g/5 mL

Breast-Feeding Issues Following a single 600 mg dose, cefdinir was not detected in breast milk; information following multiple doses is not available.

Cefditoren (sef de TOR en)

U.S. Brand Names Spectracef™

Synonyms Cefditoren Pivoxil

Pharmacologic Category Antibiotic, Cephalosporin

Pregnancy Risk Factor B

Lactation Excretion in breast milk unknown/use caution

Use Treatment of acute bacterial exacerbation of chronic bronchitis or community-acquired pneumonia (due to susceptible organisms including *Haemophilus influenzae, Haemophilus parainfluenzae, Streptococcus pneumoniae*-penicillin susceptible only, *Moraxella catarrhalis*); pharyngitis or tonsillitis (*Streptococcus pyogenes*); and uncomplicated skin and skin-structure infections (*Staphylococcus aureus* - not MRSA, *Streptococcus pyogenes*)

Mechanism of Action/Effect Has bactericidal activity against susceptible gram-positive and gram-negative pathogens. Inhibits bacterial cell wall synthesis by binding to one or more of the penicillin-binding proteins (PBPs)

Contraindications Hypersensitivity to cefditoren, other cephalosporins, milk protein, or any component of the formulation; carnitine deficiency

Warnings/Precautions Use with caution in patients with a history of penicillin allergy, especially IgE-mediated reactions (eg, anaphylaxis, urticaria). May cause antibiotic-associated colitis or colitis secondary to *C. difficile*. Prolonged use may result in superinfection. Caution in individuals with seizure disorders. Use caution in patients with renal or hepatic impairment; modify dosage in patients with severe renal impairment; Cefditoren causes renal excretion of carnitine; do not use in patients with carnitine deficiency; not for long-term therapy due to the possible development of carnitine deficiency over time. May prolong prothrombin time; use with caution in patients with a history of bleeding disorder. Cefditoren tablets contain sodium caseinate, which may cause hypersensitivity reactions in patients with milk protein hypersensitivity; this does not affect patients with lactose intolerance. Safety and efficacy have not been established in children <12 years of age.

Drug Interactions

Increased Effect/Toxicity: Increased levels of cefditoren with probenecid. Prothrombin time may be prolonged with warfarin.

Nutritional/Ethanol Interactions Food: Moderate- to high-fat meals increase bioavailability and maximum plasma concentration.

Lab Interactions May induce a positive direct Coomb's test. May cause a false-negative ferricyanide test; Glucose oxidase or hexokinase methods recommended for blood/plasma glucose determinations. False-positive urine glucose test when using copper reduction based assays (eg, Clinitest®).

Adverse Reactions

>10%: Gastrointestinal: Diarrhea (11% to 15%)

1% to 10%:

Central nervous system: Headache (2% to 3%)

Endocrine & metabolic: Glucose increased (1% to 2%)

Gastrointestinal: Nausea (4% to 6%), abdominal pain (2%), dyspepsia (1% to 2%), vomiting (1%)

Genitourinary: Vaginal moniliasis (3% to 6%)

Hematologic: Hematocrit decreased (2%)

Renal: Hematuria (3%), urinary white blood cells increased (2%)

Additional adverse effects seen with cephalosporin antibiotics: Anaphylaxis, aplastic anemia, cholestasis, erythema multiforme, hemorrhage, hemolytic anemia, renal dysfunction, reversible hyperactivity, serum sickness-like reaction, Stevens-Johnson syndrome, toxic epidermal necrolysis, toxic nephropathy

Overdosage/Toxicology Specific information not available. General symptoms of cephalosporin overdose may include nausea, vomiting, epigastric distress, diarrhea, and seizures. Treatment should be symptom-directed and supportive. Hemodialysis may be helpful (removes ~30% from circulation).

Pharmacodynamics/Kinetics

Time to Peak: 1.5-3 hours

Protein Binding: 88% (*in vitro*), primarily to albumin

Half-Life Elimination: 1.6 ± 0.4 hours

Metabolism: Cefditoren pivoxil is hydrolyzed to cefditoren (active) and pivalate

Excretion: Urine (as cefditoren and pivaloylcarnitine)

Available Dosage Forms Tablet, as pivoxil: 200 mg [equivalent to cefditoren; contains sodium caseinate]

Dosing

Adults & Elderly:

Acute bacterial exacerbation of chronic bronchitis: Oral: 400 mg twice daily for 10 days

Community-acquired pneumonia: Oral: 400 mg twice daily for 14 days

Dental infections (unlabeled use): Oral: 400 mg twice daily for 10 days

Pharyngitis, tonsillitis, uncomplicated skin and skin structure infections: Oral: 200 mg twice daily for 10 days

Pediatrics: Children ≥12 years: Refer to adult dosing.

Renal Impairment:

Cl$_{cr}$ 30-49 mL/minute/1.73 m^2: Maximum dose: 200 mg twice daily

Cl$_{cr}$ <30 mL/minute/1.73 m^2: Maximum dose: 200 mg once daily

End-stage renal disease: Appropriate dosing not established

Hepatic Impairment:

Mild or moderate impairment: Adjustment not required

Severe impairment (Child-Pugh class C): Specific guidelines not available

Administration

Oral: Should be taken with meals.

Stability

Storage: Store at controlled room temperature of 15°C to 30°C (59°F to 86°F). Protect from light and moisture.

Laboratory Monitoring Perform culture and sensitivity studies prior to initiating drug therapy; renal function

Nursing Actions

Physical Assessment: Results of culture/sensitivity tests and patient's allergy history should be assessed prior to therapy. Assess therapeutic response and adverse effects during therapy. Advise patients with diabetes about use of Clinitest®. Teach patient proper use, possible side effects/appropriate interventions, and adverse symptoms to report (eg, hypersensitivity, opportunistic infection, gastrointestinal upset, diarrhea).

Patient Education: Do not take any new medication during therapy without consulting prescriber. Take as directed, at regular intervals around-the-clock, with food. Maintain adequate hydration (2-3 L/day of fluids unless instructed to restrict fluid intake). Complete full course of medication, even if you feel better. If you have diabetes, monitor glucose levels closely; may cause false test results with Clinitest® urine glucose monitoring; use of another type of glucose monitoring is preferable. May cause diarrhea (yogurt, buttermilk, or boiled milk may help); or nausea or vomiting (small, frequent meals, frequent mouth care, sucking lozenges, or chewing gum may help). Report rash; breathing or swallowing difficulty; persistent diarrhea, nausea, vomiting, or abdominal pain; opportunistic infection (eg, vaginal itching or drainage, sores in mouth, blood in stool or urine, or unusual fever or chills); or CNS changes (eg, irritability, agitation, nervousness, insomnia, hallucinations); or other adverse reactions. **Breast-feeding precaution:** Consult prescriber if breast-feeding.

Dietary Considerations Cefditoren should be taken with meals. Plasma carnitine levels are decreased during therapy (39% with 200 mg dosing, 63% with 400 mg dosing); normal concentrations return within 7-10 days after treatment is discontinued.

Cefepime (SEF e pim)

U.S. Brand Names Maxipime®

Synonyms Cefepime Hydrochloride

Pharmacologic Category Antibiotic, Cephalosporin (Fourth Generation)

Pregnancy Risk Factor B

Lactation Enters breast milk/use caution

Use Treatment of uncomplicated and complicated urinary tract infections, including pyelonephritis caused by typical urinary tract pathogens; monotherapy for febrile neutropenia; uncomplicated skin and skin structure infections caused by *Streptococcus pyogenes*; moderate to severe pneumonia caused by pneumococcus, *Pseudomonas aeruginosa*, and other gram-negative organisms; complicated intra-abdominal infections (in combination with metronidazole). Also active against methicillin-susceptible staphylococci, *Enterobacter* sp, and many other gram-negative bacilli.

Children 2 months to 16 years: Empiric therapy of febrile neutropenia, uncomplicated skin/soft tissue infections, pneumonia, and uncomplicated/complicated urinary tract infections.

Mechanism of Action/Effect Inhibits bacterial cell wall synthesis by binding to one or more of the penicillin-binding proteins (PBPs) (Continued)

Cefepime *(Continued)*

Contraindications Hypersensitivity to cefepime, any component of the formulation, or other cephalosporins

Warnings/Precautions Modify dosage in patients with severe renal impairment; prolonged use may result in superinfection; use with caution in patients with a history of penicillin or cephalosporin allergy, especially IgE-mediated reactions (eg, anaphylaxis, urticaria). May cause antibiotic-associated colitis or colitis secondary to *C. difficile*. Use in patients <2 months of age has not been established.

Drug Interactions

Increased Effect/Toxicity: High-dose probenecid decreases clearance and increases effect of cefepime. Aminoglycosides increase nephrotoxic potential when taken with cefepime.

Lab Interactions Positive direct Coombs', false-positive urinary glucose test using cupric sulfate (Benedict's solution, Clinitest®, Fehling's solution), false-positive serum or urine creatinine with Jaffé reaction

Adverse Reactions

>10%: Hematologic: Positive Coombs' test without hemolysis

1% to 10%:

Central nervous system: Fever (1%), headache (1%)

Dermatologic: Rash, pruritus

Gastrointestinal: Diarrhea, nausea, vomiting

Local: Pain, erythema at injection site

Reactions reported with other cephalosporins include aplastic anemia, erythema multiforme, hemolytic anemia, hemorrhage, pancytopenia, prolonged PT, renal dysfunction, Stevens-Johnson syndrome, superinfection, toxic epidermal necrolysis, toxic nephropathy, vaginitis

Overdosage/Toxicology Symptoms of overdose include neuromuscular hypersensitivity and CNS toxicity (including hallucinations, confusion, seizures, and coma). Many beta-lactam containing antibiotics have the potential to cause neuromuscular hyperirritability or convulsive seizures. Hemodialysis may be helpful to aid in removal of the drug from blood; otherwise, treatment is supportive and symptom-directed.

Pharmacodynamics/Kinetics

Time to Peak: 0.5-1.5 hours

Protein Binding: Plasma: 16% to 19%

Half-Life Elimination: 2 hours

Metabolism: Minimally hepatic

Excretion: Urine (85% as unchanged drug)

Available Dosage Forms Injection, powder for reconstitution, as hydrochloride: 500 mg, 1 g, 2 g

Dosing

Adults & Elderly:

Brain abscess (*Pseudomonas*) and meningitis (postsurgical): I.V.: 2 g every 8 hours; if treating *Pseudomonas*, the addition of an aminoglycoside should be considered

Hospital"acquired pneumonia (HAP): I.V.: 1-2 g every 8-12 hours (American Thoracic Society/ATS guidelines)

Monotherapy for febrile neutropenic patients: I.V.: 2 g every 8 hours for 7 days or until neutropenia resolves

Otitis externa (malignant) and pneumonia: I.V.: 2 g every 12 hours

Peritonitis (spontaneous): I.V.: 2 g every 12 hours with metronidazole

Septic lateral/cavernous sinus thrombosis: I.V.: 2 g every 6 hours; with metronidazole for lateral

Susceptible infections: I.V.: 1-2 g every 12 hours for 7-10 days; higher doses or more frequent administration may be required in pseudomonal infections

Urinary tract infections, mild to moderate: I.M., I.V.: 500-1000 mg every 12 hours

Pediatrics:

Febrile neutropenia: I.V.: Children >2 months of age: 50 mg/kg every 8 hours for 7-10 days

Uncomplicated skin/soft tissue infections, pneumonia, and complicated/uncomplicated UTI: I.V.: Children >2 months of age: 50 mg/kg twice daily

Renal Impairment:

Adjustment of recommended maintenance schedule is required:

Normal dosing schedule: 500 mg every 12 hours

Cl_{cr} 30-60 mL/minute: 500 mg every 24 hours

Cl_{cr} 11-29 mL/minute: 500 mg every 24 hours

Cl_{cr} <11 mL/minute: 250 mg every 24 hours

Normal dosing schedule: 1 g every 12 hours

Cl_{cr} 30-60 mL/minute: 1 g every 24 hours

Cl_{cr} 11-29 mL/minute: 500 mg every 24 hours

Cl_{cr} <11 mL/minute: 250 mg every 24 hours

Normal dosing schedule: 2 g every 12 hours

Cl_{cr} 30-60 mL/minute: 2 g every 24 hours

Cl_{cr} 11-29 mL/minute: 1 g every 24 hours

Cl_{cr} <11 mL/minute: 500 mg every 24 hours

Normal dosing schedule: 2 g every 8 hours

Cl_{cr} 30-60 mL/minute: 2 g every 12 hours

Cl_{cr} 11-29 mL/minute: 2 g every 24 hours

Cl_{cr} <11 mL/minute: 1 g every 24 hours

Hemodialysis effects: Initial: 1 g (single dose) on day 1. Maintenance: 500 mg once daily (1 g once daily in febrile neutropenic patients). Dosage should be administered after dialysis on dialysis days.

Peritoneal dialysis effects: Removed to a lesser extent than hemodialysis; administer 250 mg every 48 hours.

Continuous arteriovenous hemofiltration: Dose as for Cl_{cr} >30 mL/minute.

Administration

I.M.: Inject deep I.M. into large muscle mass.

I.V.: Inject direct I.V. over 5 minutes. Infuse intermittent infusion over 30-60 minutes.

I.V. Detail: pH: 4-6

Stability

Compatibility: Stable in D_5LR, D_5NS, D_5W, $D_{10}W$, NS, bacteriostatic water, SWFI

Y-site administration: Incompatible with acyclovir, amphotericin B, amphotericin B cholesteryl sulfate complex, chlordiazepoxide, chlorpromazine, cimetidine, ciprofloxacin, cisplatin, dacarbazine, daunorubicin, diazepam, diphenhydramine, dobutamine, dopamine, doxorubicin, droperidol, enalaprilat, etoposide, etoposide phosphate, famotidine, filgrastim, floxuridine, ganciclovir, haloperidol, hydroxyzine, idarubicin, ifosfamide, magnesium sulfate, mannitol, mechlorethamine, meperidine, metoclopramide, mitomycin, mitoxantrone, morphine, nalbuphine, ofloxacin, ondansetron, plicamycin, prochlorperazine edisylate, promethazine, streptozocin, vancomycin, vinblastine, vincristine

Compatibility when admixed: Incompatible with aminophylline, gentamicin, netilmicin, tobramycin, vancomycin

Storage: Cefepime is **compatible** and stable with normal saline, D_5W, and a variety of other solutions for 24 hours at room temperature and 7 days refrigerated

Laboratory Monitoring Perform culture and sensitivity studies prior to initiating drug therapy; renal function

Nursing Actions

Physical Assessment: Results of culture/sensitivity tests and patient's allergy history should be assessed prior to therapy. Assess other pharmacological or herbal products patient may be taking for potential interactions. Note I.V. or I.M. administration specifics prior to starting treatment. Monitor laboratory tests (prothrombin time), therapeutic response, and adverse effects during therapy. Advise patients with diabetes about use of Clinitest®. Teach patient proper use, possible side effects/appropriate interventions, and adverse symptoms to report (eg, hypersensitivity, nephrotoxicity, opportunistic infection).

Patient Education: Do not take any new medication during therapy unless approved by prescriber. This medication is administered by infusion or injection. Report immediately any redness, swelling, burning, or pain at injection/infusion site; itching or hives; chest pain; difficulty swallowing or breathing. Maintain adequate hydration (2-3 L/day of fluids unless instructed to restrict fluid intake). May cause false test results with Clinitest®; use of another type of glucose testing is preferable. May cause diarrhea (yogurt, boiled milk, or buttermilk may help); nausea and vomiting (small, frequent meals, frequent mouth care, chewing gum, or sucking lozenges may help). Report rash; breathing or swallowing difficulty; persistent diarrhea, nausea, vomiting, or abdominal pain; changes in urinary pattern or pain on urination; opportunistic infection (eg, vaginal itching or drainage, sores in mouth, blood in stool or urine, unusual fever or chills); CNS changes (eg, irritability, agitation, nervousness, insomnia, hallucinations); or other adverse reactions. **Breast-feeding precaution:** Consult prescriber if breast-feeding.

Geriatric Considerations Adjust dose for changes in renal function.

Breast-Feeding Issues Theoretically, drug absorbed by nursing infant may change bowel flora or affect fever work-up result. **Note:** As a class, cephalosporins are used to treat infections in infants.

Cefixime (sef IKS eem)

U.S. Brand Names Suprax®

Pharmacologic Category Antibiotic, Cephalosporin (Third Generation)

Medication Safety Issues
Sound-alike/look-alike issues:
Suprax® may be confused with Sporanox®, Surbex®

Pregnancy Risk Factor B

Lactation Excretion in breast milk unknown/use caution

Use Treatment of urinary tract infections, otitis media, respiratory infections due to susceptible organisms including *S. pneumoniae* and *S. pyogenes*, *H. influenzae* and many Enterobacteriaceae; uncomplicated cervical/urethral gonorrhea due to *N. gonorrhoeae*

Mechanism of Action/Effect Inhibits bacterial cell wall synthesis by binding to one or more of the penicillin-binding proteins (PBPs)

Contraindications Hypersensitivity to cefixime, any component of the formulation, or other cephalosporins

Warnings/Precautions Prolonged use may result in superinfection; modify dosage in patients with renal impairment; use with caution in patients with a history of penicillin allergy especially IgE-mediated reactions (eg, anaphylaxis, urticaria). May cause antibiotic-associated colitis or colitis secondary to *C. difficile*.

Drug Interactions
Increased Effect/Toxicity: Aminoglycosides and furosemide may be possible additives to nephrotoxicity. Probenecid increases cefixime concentration. Cefixime may increase carbamazepine. Cefixime may increase prothrombin time when administered with warfarin.

Nutritional/Ethanol Interactions Food: Delays cefixime absorption.

Lab Interactions Positive direct Coombs', false-positive urinary glucose test using cupric sulfate (Benedict's solution, Clinitest®, Fehling's solution), false-positive serum or urine creatinine with Jaffé reaction

Adverse Reactions
>10%: Gastrointestinal: Diarrhea (16%)

2% to 10%: Gastrointestinal: Abdominal pain, nausea, dyspepsia, flatulence, loose stools

Reactions reported with other cephalosporins include interstitial nephritis, aplastic anemia, hemolytic anemia, hemorrhage, pancytopenia, agranulocytosis, colitis, superinfection

Overdosage/Toxicology Symptoms of overdose include neuromuscular hypersensitivity and convulsions. Many beta-lactam containing antibiotics have the potential to cause neuromuscular hyperirritability or convulsive seizures. Hemodialysis may be helpful to aid in the removal of drug from blood; otherwise, treatment is supportive or symptom-directed.

Pharmacodynamics/Kinetics
Time to Peak: Serum: 2-6 hours; delayed with food
Protein Binding: 65%
Half-Life Elimination: Normal renal function: 3-4 hours; Renal failure: Up to 11.5 hours
Excretion: Urine (50% of absorbed dose as active drug); feces (10%)

Available Dosage Forms Powder for oral suspension: 100 mg/5 mL (50 mL, 75 mL, 100 mL) [contains sodium benzoate; strawberry flavor]

Dosing
Adults & Elderly:
Susceptible infections: Oral: 400 mg/day divided every 12-24 hours
S. pyogenes infections: Treat for 10 days
Typhoid fever: Oral: 20-30 mg/kg/day in 2 divided doses for 7-14 days after I.V. therapy
Uncomplicated cervical/urethral gonorrhea due to *N. gonorrhoeae*: Oral: 400 mg as a single dose
Pediatrics:
Susceptible infections: Oral:
Children ≥6 months: 8 mg/kg/day divided every 12-24 hours
Children >50 kg or >12 years: Refer to adult dosing.
S. pyogenes infections: Treat for 10 days
Typhoid fever: Oral: 20 mg/kg/day for 10-14 days; maximum 400 mg
Renal Impairment:
Cl_{cr} 21-60 mL/minute: Administer 75% of the standard dose.
Cl_{cr} <20 mL/minute: Administer 50% of the standard dose.
10% removed by hemodialysis

Administration
Oral: Shake oral suspension well before use. May be administered with or without food. Administer with food to decrease GI distress.

Stability
Storage: After reconstitution, suspension may be stored for 14 days at room temperature or under refrigeration.

Laboratory Monitoring Perform culture and sensitivity studies prior to initiating drug therapy; renal function

Nursing Actions
Physical Assessment: Results of culture/sensitivity tests and patient's allergy history should be assessed prior to therapy. Assess other pharmacological or herbal products patient may be taking for potential interactions. Monitor laboratory tests (prothrombin time), therapeutic response, and adverse effects (eg, anemia, hemorrhage, pancytopenia, agranulocytosis, colitis) during therapy. Advise patients with diabetes about use of Clinitest®. Teach patient proper use, possible side effects/appropriate interventions, and adverse symptoms to report (eg, hypersensitivity, opportunistic infection).

Patient Education: Do not take any new medication during therapy unless approved by prescriber. Take as directed, at regular intervals around-the-clock (with or without food). Chilling oral suspension improves flavor (do not freeze); shake suspension thoroughly before using. Maintain adequate hydration (2-3 L/day of fluids) unless instructed to restrict fluid intake. (Continued)

Cefixime *(Continued)*

Complete full course of medication, even if you feel better. May cause false test results with Clinitest®; use of another type of glucose testing is preferable. May cause nausea or vomiting (small, frequent meals, frequent mouth care, sucking lozenges, or chewing gum may help); or diarrhea (yogurt, boiled milk, or buttermilk may help). Report rash; breathing or swallowing difficulty; persistent diarrhea, nausea, vomiting, or abdominal pain; changes in urinary pattern or pain on urination; opportunistic infection (eg, vaginal itching or drainage; sores in mouth; blood in stool or urine; unusual fever or chills); CNS changes (eg, irritability, agitation, nervousness, insomnia, hallucinations); or other adverse reactions. **Breast-feeding precaution:** Consult prescriber if breast-feeding.

Dietary Considerations May be taken with food.

Geriatric Considerations Adjust dose for renal function.

Breast-Feeding Issues Theoretically, drug absorbed by nursing infant may change bowel flora or affect fever work-up result. **Note:** As a class, cephalosporins are used to treat infections in infants.

Cefotaxime *(sef oh TAKS eem)*

U.S. Brand Names Claforan®
Synonyms Cefotaxime Sodium
Pharmacologic Category Antibiotic, Cephalosporin (Third Generation)
Medication Safety Issues
Sound-alike/look-alike issues:
Cefotaxime may be confused with cefoxitin, ceftizoxime, cefuroxime

Pregnancy Risk Factor B
Lactation Enters breast milk/use caution (AAP rates "compatible")

Use Treatment of susceptible infection in respiratory tract, skin and skin structure, bone and joint, urinary tract, gynecologic as well as septicemia, and documented or suspected meningitis. Active against most gram-negative bacilli (not *Pseudomonas*) and gram-positive cocci (not enterococcus). Active against many penicillin-resistant pneumococci.

Mechanism of Action/Effect Inhibits bacterial cell wall synthesis by binding to one or more of the penicillin-binding proteins (PBPs)

Contraindications Hypersensitivity to cefotaxime, any component of the formulation, or other cephalosporins

Warnings/Precautions Modify dosage in patients with severe renal impairment; prolonged use may result in superinfection; a potentially life-threatening arrhythmia has been reported in patients who received a rapid bolus injection via central line. Use caution in patients with colitis; minimize tissue inflammation by changing infusion sites when needed. Use with caution in patients with a history of penicillin allergy especially IgE-mediated reactions (eg, anaphylaxis, urticaria). May cause antibiotic-associated colitis or colitis secondary to *C. difficile*.

Drug Interactions
Increased Effect/Toxicity: Probenecid may decrease cephalosporin elimination resulting in increased levels. Furosemide, aminoglycosides in combination with cefotaxime may result in additive nephrotoxicity.

Lab Interactions Positive direct Coombs', false-positive urinary glucose test using cupric sulfate (Benedict's solution, Clinitest®, Fehling's solution), false-positive serum or urine creatinine with Jaffé reaction

Adverse Reactions
1% to 10%:
Dermatologic: Rash, pruritus

Gastrointestinal: Diarrhea, nausea, vomiting, colitis
Local: Pain at injection site
Reactions reported with other cephalosporins include agranulocytosis, aplastic anemia, cholestasis, hemolytic anemia, hemorrhage, nephropathy, pancytopenia, renal dysfunction, seizure, superinfection.

Overdosage/Toxicology Symptoms of overdose include neuromuscular hypersensitivity and convulsions. Many beta-lactam containing antibiotics have the potential to cause neuromuscular hyperirritability or convulsive seizures. Hemodialysis may be helpful to aid in removal of the drug from blood; otherwise, treatment is supportive or symptom-directed.

Pharmacodynamics/Kinetics
Time to Peak: Serum: I.M.: Within 30 minutes
Half-Life Elimination:
Cefotaxime: Premature neonates <1 week: 5-6 hours; Full-term neonates <1 week: 2-3.4 hours; Adults: 1-1.5 hours, prolonged with renal and/or hepatic impairment
Desacetylcefotaxime: 1.5-1.9 hours; prolonged with renal impairment
Metabolism: Partially hepatic to active metabolite, desacetylcefotaxime
Excretion: Urine (as unchanged drug and metabolites)
Available Dosage Forms
Infusion, as sodium [premixed in D$_5$W]: 1 g (50 mL); 2 g (50 mL)
Injection, powder for reconstitution, as sodium: 500 mg, 1 g, 2 g, 10 g, 20 g
Claforan®: 500 mg, 1 g, 2 g, 10 g [contains sodium 50.5 mg (2.2 mEq) per cefotaxime 1 g]
Dosing
Adults & Elderly:
Arthritis (septic): I.V.: 1 g every 8 hours
Brain abscess and meningitis: I.V.: 2 g every 4-6 hours
C-section: 1 g as soon as the umbilical cord is clamped, then 1 g I.M., I.V. at 6- and 12-hours intervals.
Epiglottitis: I.V.: 2 g every 4-8 hours
Gonorrhea: I.M.: 1 g as a single dose; disseminated 1 g every 8 hours
Life-threatening infections: I.V.: 2 g every 4 hours
Liver abscess: I.V.: 1-2 g every 6 hours
Lyme disease:
Cardiac manifestations: I.V.: 2 g every 4 hours
CNS manifestations: I.V.: 2 g every 8 hours for 14-28 days
Moderate/severe infections: I.M., I.V.: 1-2 g every 8 hours
Orbital cellulitis: I.V.: 2 g every 4 hours
Peritonitis (spontaneous): I.V.: 2 g every 8 hours, unless life-threatening then 2 g every 4 hours
Septicemia: I.V.: 2 g every 6-8 hours
Skin and soft tissue:
Mixed, necrotizing: I.V.: 2 g every 6 hours, with metronidazole or clindamycin
Bite wounds (animal): I.V.: 2 g every 6 hours
Surgical prophylaxis: I.M., I.V.: 1 g 30-90 minutes before surgery
Uncomplicated infections: I.M., I.V.: 1 g every 12 hours
Pediatrics:
Susceptible infections: I.M., I.V.: Infants and Children 1 month to 12 years: <50 kg: 50-200 mg/kg/day in divided doses every 4-6 hours
Epiglottitis: I.M., I.V.: 150-200 mg/kg/day in 4 divided doses with clindamycin for 7-10 days
Meningitis: I.M., I.V.: 200 mg/kg/day in divided doses every 6 hours
Pneumonia: I.V.: 200 mg/kg/day divided every 8 hours
Sepsis: I.V.: 150 mg/kg/day divided every 8 hours
Typhoid fever: I.M., I.V.: 150-200 mg/kg/day in 3-4 divided doses (maximum 12 g/day); fluoroquinolone

resistant: 80 mg/kg/day in 3-4 divided doses (maximum 12 g/day)

Children >12 years: Refer to adult dosing.

Renal Impairment:

Cl_{cr} 10-50 mL/minute: Administer every 8-12 hours.

Cl_{cr} <10 mL/minute: Administer every 24 hours.

Moderately dialyzable (20% to 50%)

Continuous arteriovenous hemofiltration: 1 g every 12 hours.

Hepatic Impairment: Moderate dosage reduction is recommended in severe liver disease.

Administration

I.M.: Inject deep I.M. into large muscle mass.

I.V.: Inject direct I.V. over 3-5 minutes. Infuse intermittent infusion over 30 minutes.

I.V. Detail: pH: 5.0-7.5 (injectable solution)

Stability

Reconstitution: Reconstituted solution is stable for 12-24 hours at room temperature and 7-10 days when refrigerated and for 13 weeks when frozen; for I.V. infusion in NS or D_5W, solution is stable for 24 hours at room temperature, 5 days when refrigerated, or 13 weeks when frozen in Viaflex® plastic containers; thawed solutions previously of frozen premixed bags are stable for 24 hours at room temperature or 10 days when refrigerated.

Compatibility: Stable in $D_5^1/_4NS$, $D_5^1/_2NS$, D_5NS, D_5W, $D_{10}W$, LR, NS

Y-site administration: Incompatible with allopurinol, filgrastim, fluconazole, gemcitabine, hetastarch, pentamidine

Compatibility in syringe: Incompatible with doxapram

Compatibility when admixed: Incompatible with aminoglycosides, aminophylline, sodium bicarbonate

Laboratory Monitoring Perform culture and sensitivity studies prior to initiating drug therapy; CBC with differential (especially with long courses); renal function

Nursing Actions

Physical Assessment: Assess results of culture/sensitivity tests and patient's allergy history prior to therapy. Assess other pharmacological or herbal products patient may be taking for potential interactions (eg, nephrotoxicity). Evaluate results of laboratory tests (prothrombin time, CBC with differential), therapeutic response, and adverse effects (diarrhea, nausea/vomiting, nephrotoxicity) regularly during therapy. Advise patients with diabetes about use of Clinitest®. Teach patient proper use, possible side effects/appropriate interventions, and adverse symptoms to report (eg, hypersensitivity, opportunistic infection).

Patient Education: Do not take any new medication during therapy unless approved by prescriber. This medication is administered by injection or infusion. Report immediately any redness, swelling, burning, or pain at injection/infusion site; chest pain, palpitations, respiratory difficulty or swallowing; or itching or hives. Maintain adequate hydration (2-3 L/day of fluids) unless instructed to restrict fluid intake. May cause false test results with Clinitest®; use of another type of glucose testing is preferable. May cause diarrhea (yogurt, boiled milk, or buttermilk may help); GI distress or nausea (small, frequent meals, frequent oral care, chewing gum, or sucking lozenges may help). Report unresolved diarrhea; opportunistic infection (vaginal itching or drainage; sores in mouth; blood in stool or urine; easy bleeding or bruising, unusual fever or chills); or respiratory difficulty. **Breast-feeding precaution:** Consult prescriber if breast-feeding.

Dietary Considerations Sodium content of 1 g: 50.5 mg (2.2 mEq)

Geriatric Considerations Adjust dose for renal function.

Breast-Feeding Issues Theoretically, drug absorbed by nursing infant may change bowel flora or affect fever work-up result. **Note:** As a class, cephalosporins are used to treat infections in infants.

Cefotetan (SEF oh tee tan)

U.S. Brand Names Cefotan® [DSC]

Synonyms Cefotetan Disodium

Pharmacologic Category Antibiotic, Cephalosporin (Second Generation)

Medication Safety Issues

Sound-alike/look-alike issues:

Cefotetan may be confused with cefoxitin, Ceftin®

Cefotan® may be confused with Ceftin®

Pregnancy Risk Factor B

Lactation Enters breast milk (small amounts)/use caution

Use Surgical prophylaxis; intra-abdominal infections and other mixed infections; respiratory tract, skin and skin structure, bone and joint, urinary tract and gynecologic as well as septicemia; active against gram-negative enteric bacilli including *E. coli*, *Klebsiella*, and *Proteus*; less active against staphylococci and streptococci than first generation cephalosporins, but active against anaerobes including *Bacteroides fragilis*

Mechanism of Action/Effect Inhibits bacterial cell wall synthesis by binding to one or more of the penicillin-binding proteins (PBPs)

Contraindications Hypersensitivity to cefotetan, any component of the formulation, or other cephalosporins; previous cephalosporin-associated hemolytic anemia

Warnings/Precautions Modify dosage in patients with severe renal impairment; prolonged use may result in superinfection; although cefotetan contains the methyltetrazolethiol side chain, bleeding has not been a significant problem; use with caution in patients with a history of penicillin allergy especially IgE-mediated reactions (eg, anaphylaxis, urticaria). Cefotetan has been associated with a higher risk of hemolytic anemia relative to other cephalosporins (approximately threefold); monitor carefully during use and consider cephalosporin-associated immune anemia in patients who have received cefotetan within 2-3 weeks (either as treatment or prophylaxis). May cause antibiotic-associated colitis or colitis secondary to *C. difficile*.

Drug Interactions

Increased Effect/Toxicity: Disulfiram-like reaction may occur if ethanol is consumed by a patient taking cefotetan. Probenecid may increase cefotetan plasma levels. Cefotetan may increase risk of bleeding in patients receiving warfarin.

Nutritional/Ethanol Interactions Ethanol: Avoid ethanol (may cause a disulfiram-like reaction).

Lab Interactions Positive direct Coombs', false-positive urinary glucose test using cupric sulfate (Benedict's solution, Clinitest®, Fehling's solution), false-positive serum or urine creatinine with Jaffé reaction

Adverse Reactions

1% to 10%:

Gastrointestinal: Diarrhea (1%)

Hepatic: Transaminases increased (1%)

Miscellaneous: Hypersensitivity reactions (1%)

Reactions reported with other cephalosporins include seizure, Stevens-Johnson syndrome, toxic epidermal necrolysis, renal dysfunction, toxic nephropathy, cholestasis, aplastic anemia, hemolytic anemia, hemorrhage, pancytopenia, agranulocytosis, colitis, superinfection

Overdosage/Toxicology Symptoms of overdose include neuromuscular hypersensitivity and convulsions. Many beta-lactam containing antibiotics have the potential to cause neuromuscular hyperirritability or convulsive seizures. Hemodialysis may be helpful to aid *(Continued)*

Cefotetan (Continued)

in removal of the drug from blood; otherwise, treatment is supportive or symptom-directed.

Pharmacodynamics/Kinetics
Time to Peak: Serum: I.M.: 1.5-3 hours
Protein Binding: 76% to 90%
Half-Life Elimination: 3-5 hours
Excretion: Primarily urine (as unchanged drug); feces (20%)

Available Dosage Forms [DSC] = Discontinued product
Infusion [premixed iso-osmotic solution]: 1 g (50 mL); 2 g (50 mL) [contains sodium 80 mg/g (3.5 mEq/g)] [DSC]
Injection, powder for reconstitution: 1 g, 2 g [contains sodium 80 mg/g (3.5 mEq/g)] [DSC]

Dosing
Adults & Elderly:
Susceptible infections: I.M., I.V.: 1-6 g/day in divided doses every 12 hours; usual dose: 1-2 g every 12 hours for 5-10 days; 1-2 g may be given every 24 hours for urinary tract infection
Orbital cellulitis, odontogenic infections: I.V.: 2 g every 12 hours
Pelvic inflammatory disease: I.V.: 2 g every 12 hours; used in combination with doxycycline
Preoperative prophylaxis: I.M., I.V.: 1-2 g 30-60 minutes prior to surgery; when used for cesarean section, dose should be given as soon as umbilical cord is clamped
Urinary tract infection: I.M., I.V.: 1-2 g may be given every 24 hours

Pediatrics:
Severe infections (unlabeled use): I.M., I.V.: 20-40 mg/kg/dose every 12 hours (maximum: 6 g/day)
Preoperative prophylaxis (unlabeled use): I.M., I.V.: 40 mg/kg 30-60 minutes prior to surgery
Pelvic inflammatory disease: Adolescents: I.V.: Refer to adult dosing.

Renal Impairment: I.M., I.V.:
Cl_{cr} 10-30 mL/minute: Administer every 24 hours
Cl_{cr} <10 mL/minute: Administer every 48 hours
Hemodialysis: Dialyzable (5% to 20%); administer ¼ the usual dose every 24 hours on days between dialysis; administer ½ the usual dose on the day of dialysis.
Continuous arteriovenous or venovenous hemodiafiltration effects: Administer 750 mg every 12 hours

Administration
I.M.: Inject deep I.M. into large muscle mass.
I.V.: Inject direct I.V. over 3-5 minutes. Infuse intermittent infusion over 30 minutes.
I.V. Detail: pH: 4.5-6.5 (reconstituted solution)

Stability
Reconstitution: Reconstituted solution is stable for 24 hours at room temperature and 96 hours when refrigerated. For I.V. infusion in NS or D_5W solution and after freezing, thawed solution is stable for 24 hours at room temperature or 96 hours when refrigerated. Frozen solution is stable for 12 weeks.
Compatibility: Stable in D_5W, NS
Y-site administration: Incompatible with promethazine, vinorelbine
Compatibility in syringe: Incompatible with doxapram, promethazine
Compatibility when admixed: Incompatible with gentamicin, heparin, tetracyclines

Laboratory Monitoring Prothrombin time; perform culture and sensitivity studies prior to initiating drug therapy; renal function

Nursing Actions
Physical Assessment: Assess results of culture/sensitivity tests and patient's allergy history prior to therapy. Assess other pharmacological or herbal products patient may be taking for potential interactions. Assess results of laboratory tests (prothrombin time), therapeutic response, and adverse effects (eg, hemolytic anemia, hypoprothrombinemia, and bleeding) regularly during therapy. Advise patients with diabetes about use of Clinitest® (may cause false-positive test). Teach patient possible side effects/appropriate interventions and adverse symptoms to report (eg, nephrotoxicity, opportunistic infection, hypersensitivity reaction).

Patient Education: Do not take any new medication during therapy unless approved by prescriber. This medication is administered by injection or infusion. Report immediately any redness, swelling, burning, or pain at injection/infusion site, or immediately report any itching, hives, difficulty swallowing or respiratory difficulty. Maintain adequate hydration (2-3 L/day of fluids) unless instructed to restrict fluid intake. Avoid alcohol during therapy and for 72 hours after last dose (may cause severe disulfiram-like reactions). May cause false test results with Clinitest®; use of another type of glucose testing is preferable. May cause diarrhea (yogurt, boiled milk, or buttermilk may help). Report rash; breathing or swallowing difficulty; persistent diarrhea, nausea, vomiting, or abdominal pain; changes in urinary pattern or pain on urination; opportunistic infection (eg, vaginal itching or drainage; sores in mouth; blood in stool or urine; unusual fever or chills); CNS changes (eg, irritability, agitation, nervousness, insomnia, hallucinations); or other adverse reactions. **Breast-feeding precaution:** Consult prescriber if breast-feeding.

Dietary Considerations Contains sodium of 80 mg (3.5 mEq) per cefotetan 1 g
Geriatric Considerations Cefotetan has not been studied in the elderly. Adjust dose for renal function in the elderly.
Breast-Feeding Issues Theoretically, drug absorbed by nursing infant may change bowel flora or affect fever work-up result. **Note:** As a class, cephalosporins are used to treat infections in infants.

Cefoxitin (se FOKS i tin)

U.S. Brand Names Mefoxin®
Synonyms Cefoxitin Sodium
Pharmacologic Category Antibiotic, Cephalosporin (Second Generation)

Medication Safety Issues
Sound-alike/look-alike issues:
Cefoxitin may be confused with cefotaxime, cefotetan, Cytoxan®
Mefoxin® may be confused with Lanoxin®

Pregnancy Risk Factor B
Lactation Enters breast milk (small amounts)/use caution (AAP rates "compatible")
Use Less active against staphylococci and streptococci than first generation cephalosporins, but active against anaerobes including *Bacteroides fragilis*; active against gram-negative enteric bacilli including *E. coli, Klebsiella,* and *Proteus;* used predominantly for respiratory tract, skin and skin structure, bone and joint, urinary tract and gynecologic as well as septicemia; surgical prophylaxis; intra-abdominal infections and other mixed infections; indicated for bacterial *Eikenella corrodens* infections
Mechanism of Action/Effect Inhibits bacterial cell wall synthesis by binding to one or more of the penicillin-binding proteins (PBPs)
Contraindications Hypersensitivity to cefoxitin, any component of the formulation, or other cephalosporins
Warnings/Precautions Use with caution in patients with history of colitis; cefoxitin may increase resistance of organisms by inducing beta-lactamase; modify dosage in patients with severe renal impairment;

prolonged use may result in superinfection; use with caution in patients with a history of penicillin allergy especially IgE-mediated reactions (eg, anaphylaxis, urticaria). May cause antibiotic-associated colitis or colitis secondary to *C. difficile.*

Drug Interactions

Increased Effect/Toxicity: Probenecid may decrease cephalosporin elimination. Furosemide, aminoglycosides in combination with cefoxitin may result in additive nephrotoxicity.

Lab Interactions Positive direct Coombs', false-positive urinary glucose test using cupric sulfate (Benedict's solution, Clinitest®, Fehling's solution), false-positive serum or urine creatinine with Jaffé reaction

Adverse Reactions

1% to 10%: Gastrointestinal: Diarrhea

Reactions reported with other cephalosporins include Agranulocytosis, aplastic anemia, cholestasis, colitis, erythema multiforme, hemolytic anemia, hemorrhage, pancytopenia, renal dysfunction, serum-sickness reactions, seizure, Stevens-Johnson syndrome, superinfection, toxic nephropathy, vaginitis

Overdosage/Toxicology Symptoms of overdose include neuromuscular hypersensitivity and convulsions. Many beta-lactam containing antibiotics have the potential to cause neuromuscular hyperirritability or convulsive seizures. Hemodialysis may be helpful to aid in removal of the drug from blood; otherwise, treatment is supportive or symptom-directed.

Pharmacodynamics/Kinetics

Time to Peak: Serum: I.M.: 20-30 minutes

Protein Binding: 65% to 79%

Half-Life Elimination: 45-60 minutes; significantly prolonged with renal impairment

Excretion: Urine (85% as unchanged drug)

Available Dosage Forms

Infusion, as sodium [premixed iso-osmotic solution]: 1 g (50 mL); 2 g (50 mL) [contains sodium 53.8 mg/g (2.3 mEq/g)]

Injection, powder for reconstitution, as sodium: 1 g, 2 g, 10 g [contains sodium 53.8 mg/g (2.3 mEq/g)]

Dosing

Adults & Elderly: Susceptible infections: I.M., I.V.: 1-2 g every 6-8 hours (I.M. injection is painful); up to 12 g/day

Amnionitis and endomyometritis: I.M., I.V.: 2 g every 6-8 hours

Aspiration pneumonia, empyema, orbital cellulitis, parapharyngeal space, and human bites: I.M., I.V.: 2 g every 8 hours

Liver abscess: I.V.: 1 g every 4 hours

Mycobacterium species, not MTB or MAI: I.V.: 12 g/day with amikacin

Pelvic inflammatory disease:

Inpatients: I.V.: 2 g every 6 hours **plus** doxycycline 100 mg I.V. or 100 mg orally every 12 hours until improved, followed by doxycycline 100 mg orally twice daily to complete 14 days

Outpatients: I.M.: 2 g **plus** probenecid 1 g orally as a single dose, followed by doxycycline 100 mg orally twice daily for 14 days

Perioperative prophylaxis: I.M., I.V.: 1-2 g 30-60 minutes prior to surgery followed by 1-2 g every 6-8 hours for no more than 24 hours after surgery depending on the procedure

Pediatrics:

Perioperative prophylaxis: I.V.:

Infants >3 months and Children: 30-40 mg/kg 30-60 minutes prior to surgery followed by 30-40 mg/kg/dose every 6 hours for no more than 24 hours after surgery depending on the procedure

Adolescents: Refer to adult dosing.

Mild-to-moderate infection: I.M., I.V.: Infants >3 months and Children: 80-100 mg/kg/day in divided doses every 4-6 hours

Severe infection: I.M., I.V.: Infants >3 months and Children: 100-160 mg/kg/day in divided doses every 4-6 hours

Maximum dose: 12 g/day

Renal Impairment: I.M., I.V.:

Cl_{cr} 30-50 mL/minute: Administer 1-2 g every 8-12 hours

Cl_{cr} 10-29 mL/minute: Administer 1-2 g every 12-24 hours

Cl_{cr} 5-9 mL/minute: Administer 0.5-1 g every 12-24 hours

Cl_{cr} <5 mL/minute: Administer 0.5-1 g every 24-48 hours

Hemodialysis: Moderately dialyzable (20% to 50%); administer a loading dose of 1-2 g after each hemodialysis; maintenance dose as noted above based on Cl_{cr}

Continuous arteriovenous or venovenous hemodiafiltration effects: Dose as for Cl_{cr} 10-50 mL/minute

Administration

I.M.: Inject deep I.M. into large muscle mass.

I.V.: Can be administered IVP over 3-5 minutes at a maximum concentration of 100 mg/mL or I.V. intermittent infusion over 10-60 minutes at a final concentration for I.V. administration not to exceed 40 mg/mL

I.V. Detail: pH: 4.2-7.0 (reconstituted solution); 6.5 (frozen premixed solution)

Stability

Reconstitution: Reconstitute vials with SWFI, bacteriostatic water for injection, NS, or D_5W. For I.V. infusion, solutions may be further diluted in NS, $D_5^1/_4NS$, $D_5^1/_2NS$, D_5NS, D_5W, $D_{10}W$, LR, D_5LR, mannitol 10%, or sodium bicarbonate 5%.

Compatibility: Stable in D_5LR, $D_5^1/_4NS$, $D_5^1/_2NS$, D_5NS, D_5W, $D_{10}W$, LR, NS, mannitol 10%, sodium bicarbonate 5%

Y-site administration: Incompatible with filgrastim, gatifloxacin, hetastarch, pentamidine

Compatibility when admixed: Incompatible with ranitidine

Storage: Reconstituted solution is stable for 6 hours at room temperature or 7 days when refrigerated; I.V. infusion in NS or D_5W solution is stable for 18 hours at room temperature or 48 hours when refrigerated. Premixed frozen solution, when thawed, is stable for 24 hours at room temperature or 21 days when refrigerated.

Laboratory Monitoring Prothrombin times; perform culture and sensitivity studies prior to initiating drug therapy; renal function

Nursing Actions

Physical Assessment: Results of culture/sensitivity tests and patient's allergy history should be assessed prior to therapy. Assess other pharmacological or herbal products patient may be taking for potential interactions (eg, nephrotoxicity). Monitor laboratory tests (prothrombin time, CBC with differential, therapeutic response, and adverse effects (diarrhea, nausea/vomiting, nephrotoxicity) on a regular basis during therapy. Advise patients with diabetes about use of Clinitest®. Teach patient proper use, possible side effects/appropriate interventions, and adverse symptoms to report (eg, hypersensitivity, opportunistic infection).

Patient Education: Do not take any new medication during therapy unless approved by prescriber. This medication is administered by injection or infusion. Report immediately any redness, swelling, burning, or pain at injection/infusion site; chest pain, palpitations, respiratory difficulty or swallowing; itching or hives. Maintain adequate hydration (2-3 L/day of fluids) unless instructed to restrict fluid intake. May cause false test results with Clinitest®; use of another type of glucose testing is preferable. May cause diarrhea (yogurt, boiled milk, or buttermilk may help); GI distress or nausea (small, frequent meals, frequent (Continued)

Cefoxitin (Continued)

oral care, chewing gum, or sucking lozenges may help). Report rash; breathing or swallowing difficulty; persistent diarrhea, nausea, vomiting, or abdominal pain; changes in urinary pattern or pain on urination; opportunistic infection (eg, vaginal itching or drainage; sores in mouth; blood in stool or urine; unusual fever or chills); CNS changes (eg, irritability, agitation, nervousness, insomnia, hallucinations); or other adverse reactions. **Breast-feeding precaution:** Consult prescriber if breast-feeding.

Dietary Considerations Sodium content of 1 g: 53 mg (2.3 mEq)

Geriatric Considerations Adjust dose for renal function in the elderly.

Breast-Feeding Issues Theoretically, drug absorbed by nursing infant may change bowel flora or affect fever work-up result. **Note:** As a class, cephalosporins are used to treat infections in infants.

Cefpodoxime (sef pode OKS eem)

U.S. Brand Names Vantin®

Synonyms Cefpodoxime Proxetil

Pharmacologic Category Antibiotic, Cephalosporin (Third Generation)

Medication Safety Issues
Sound-alike/look-alike issues:
Vantin® may be confused with Ventolin®

Pregnancy Risk Factor B

Lactation Enters breast milk (small amounts)/use caution

Use Treatment of susceptible acute, community-acquired pneumonia caused by *S. pneumoniae* or nonbeta-lactamase producing *H. influenzae*; acute uncomplicated gonorrhea caused by *N. gonorrhoeae*; uncomplicated skin and skin structure infections caused by *S. aureus* or *S. pyogenes*; acute otitis media caused by *S. pneumoniae*, *H. influenzae*, or *M. catarrhalis*; pharyngitis or tonsillitis; and uncomplicated urinary tract infections caused by *E. coli*, *Klebsiella*, and *Proteus*

Mechanism of Action/Effect Inhibits bacterial cell wall synthesis by binding to one or more of the penicillin-binding proteins (PBPs)

Contraindications Hypersensitivity to cefpodoxime, any component of the formulation, or other cephalosporins

Warnings/Precautions Modify dosage in patients with severe renal impairment; prolonged use may result in superinfection. Use with caution in patients with a history of penicillin allergy especially IgE-mediated reactions (eg, anaphylaxis, urticaria).

Drug Interactions
Decreased Effect: Antacids and H_2-receptor antagonists reduce absorption and serum concentration of cefpodoxime.
Increased Effect/Toxicity: Probenecid may decrease cephalosporin elimination. Furosemide, aminoglycosides in combination with cefpodoxime may result in additive nephrotoxicity.

Nutritional/Ethanol Interactions Food: Food delays absorption; cefpodoxime serum levels may be increased if taken with food.

Lab Interactions Positive direct Coombs', false-positive urinary glucose test using cupric sulfate (Benedict's solution, Clinitest®, Fehling's solution), false-positive serum or urine creatinine with Jaffé reaction

Adverse Reactions
>10%:
Dermatologic: Diaper rash (12%)
Gastrointestinal: Diarrhea in infants and toddlers (15%)
1% to 10%:
Central nervous system: Headache (1%)
Dermatologic: Rash (1%)

Gastrointestinal: Diarrhea (7%), nausea (4%), abdominal pain (2%), vomiting (1% to 2%)
Genitourinary: Vaginal infection (3%)
Reactions reported with other cephalosporins include seizure, Stevens-Johnson syndrome, toxic epidermal necrolysis, erythema multiforme, urticaria, serum-sickness reactions, renal dysfunction, interstitial nephritis toxic nephropathy, cholestasis, aplastic anemia, hemolytic anemia, hemorrhage, pancytopenia, agranulocytosis, colitis, vaginitis, superinfection

Overdosage/Toxicology Symptoms of overdose include neuromuscular hypersensitivity and convulsions. Many beta-lactam containing antibiotics have the potential to cause neuromuscular hyperirritability or convulsive seizures. Hemodialysis may be helpful to aid in removal of the drug from blood; otherwise, treatment is supportive or symptom-directed.

Pharmacodynamics/Kinetics
Time to Peak: Within 1 hour
Protein Binding: 18% to 23%
Half-Life Elimination: 2.2 hours; prolonged with renal impairment
Metabolism: De-esterified in GI tract to active metabolite, cefpodoxime
Excretion: Urine (80% as unchanged drug) in 24 hours

Available Dosage Forms
Granules for oral suspension: 50 mg/5 mL (50 mL, 75 mL, 100 mL); 100 mg/5 mL (50 mL, 75 mL, 100 mL) [contains sodium benzoate; lemon creme flavor]
Tablet: 100 mg, 200 mg

Dosing
Adults & Elderly:
Acute community-acquired pneumonia and bacterial exacerbations of chronic bronchitis: Oral: 200 mg every 12 hours for 14 days and 10 days, respectively
Acute maxillary sinusitis: Oral: 200 mg every 12 hours for 10 days
Pharyngitis/tonsillitis: Oral: 100 mg every 12 hours for 5-10 days
Skin and skin structure: Oral: 400 mg every 12 hours for 7-14 days
Uncomplicated gonorrhea (male and female) and rectal gonococcal infections (female): Oral: 200 mg as a single dose
Uncomplicated urinary tract infection: Oral: 100 mg every 12 hours for 7 days
Pediatrics:
Acute maxillary sinusitis: Oral: Children:
2 months to 12 years: 10 mg/kg/day divided every 12 hours for 10 days (maximum: 200 mg/dose)
Acute otitis media: Oral: Children 2 months to 12 years: 10 mg/kg/day divided every 12 hours (400 mg/day) for 5 days (maximum: 200 mg/dose)
≥12 years: Refer to adult dosing.
Pharyngitis/tonsillitis: Oral: Children:
2 months to 12 years: 10 mg/kg/day in 2 divided doses for 5-10 days (maximum: 100 mg/dose)
≥12 years: Refer to adult dosing.
Renal Impairment:
Cl_{cr} <30 mL/minute: Administer every 24 hours.
Hemodialysis: Dose 3 times/week following dialysis.
Hepatic Impairment: Dose adjustment is not necessary in patients with cirrhosis.

Administration
Oral: Administer around-the-clock to promote less variation in peak and trough serum levels.

Stability
Reconstitution: After mixing, keep suspension in refrigerator, shake well before using. Discard unused portion after 14 days.

Laboratory Monitoring Perform culture and sensitivity studies prior to initiating drug therapy; renal function

Nursing Actions

Physical Assessment: Results of culture/sensitivity tests and patient's allergy history should be assessed prior to therapy. Assess other pharmacological or herbal products patient may be taking for potential interactions. Monitor laboratory tests (prothrombin time), therapeutic response, and adverse effects (eg, hemolytic anemia, hypoprothrombinemia, and bleeding) regularly during therapy. Advise patients with diabetes about use of Clinitest® (may cause false-positive test). Teach patient possible side effects/appropriate interventions and adverse symptoms to report (eg, nephrotoxicity, opportunistic infection, hypersensitivity reaction).

Patient Education: Do not take any new medication during therapy unless approved by prescriber. Take as directed, at regular intervals around-the-clock (with or without food). Chilling oral suspension improves flavor (do not freeze); shake well before using. Maintain adequate hydration (2-3 L/day of fluids) unless instructed to restrict fluid intake. Complete full course of medication, even if you feel better. May cause false test results with Clinitest®; use of another type of glucose testing is preferable. May cause nausea or vomiting (small, frequent meals, frequent mouth care, sucking lozenges, or chewing gum may help); or diarrhea (yogurt, boiled milk, or buttermilk may help). Report rash; breathing or swallowing difficulty; persistent diarrhea, nausea, vomiting, or abdominal pain; changes in urinary pattern or pain on urination; opportunistic infection (eg, vaginal itching or drainage; sores in mouth; blood in stool or urine; unusual fever or chills; CNS changes (eg, irritability, agitation, nervousness, insomnia, hallucinations); or other adverse reactions. **Breast-feeding precaution:** Consult prescriber if breast-feeding.

Dietary Considerations May be taken with food.

Geriatric Considerations Considered one of the drugs of choice for outpatient treatment of community-acquired pneumonia in older adults. Adjust dosage with renal impairment.

Breast-Feeding Issues Theoretically, drug absorbed by nursing infant may change bowel flora or affect fever work-up result. **Note:** As a class, cephalosporins are used to treat infections in infants.

Cefprozil (sef PROE zil)

U.S. Brand Names Cefzil®

Pharmacologic Category Antibiotic, Cephalosporin (Second Generation)

Medication Safety Issues
Sound-alike/look-alike issues:
Cefprozil may be confused with cefazolin, cefuroxime
Cefzil® may be confused with Cefol®, Ceftin®, Kefzol®

Pregnancy Risk Factor B

Lactation Enters breast milk/use caution (AAP rates "compatible")

Use Treatment of otitis media and infections involving the respiratory tract and skin and skin structure; active against methicillin-sensitive staphylococci, many streptococci, and various gram-negative bacilli including *E. coli*, some *Klebsiella*, *P. mirabilis*, *H. influenzae*, and *Moraxella*.

Mechanism of Action/Effect Inhibits bacterial cell wall synthesis by binding to one or more of the penicillin-binding proteins (PBPs)

Contraindications Hypersensitivity to cefprozil, any component of the formulation, or other cephalosporins

Warnings/Precautions Modify dosage in patients with severe renal impairment; prolonged use may result in superinfection; use with caution in patients with a history of penicillin allergy especially IgE-mediated reactions (eg, anaphylaxis, urticaria). May cause antibiotic-associated colitis or colitis secondary to *C. difficile*.

Drug Interactions

Increased Effect/Toxicity: Probenecid may decrease cephalosporin elimination. Furosemide, aminoglycosides in combination with cefprozil may result in additive nephrotoxicity.

Nutritional/Ethanol Interactions Food: Food delays cefprozil absorption.

Lab Interactions Positive direct Coombs', false-positive urinary glucose test using cupric sulfate (Benedict's solution, Clinitest®, Fehling's solution), false-positive serum or urine creatinine with Jaffé reaction

Adverse Reactions
1% to 10%:
Central nervous system: Dizziness (1%)
Dermatologic: Diaper rash (2%)
Gastrointestinal: Diarrhea (3%), nausea (4%), vomiting (1%), abdominal pain (1%)
Genitourinary: Vaginitis, genital pruritus (2%)
Hepatic: Transaminases increased (2%)
Miscellaneous: Superinfection
Reactions reported with other cephalosporins include seizure, toxic epidermal necrolysis, renal dysfunction, interstitial nephritis, toxic nephropathy, aplastic anemia, hemolytic anemia, hemorrhage, pancytopenia, agranulocytosis, colitis, vaginitis, superinfection

Overdosage/Toxicology Symptoms of overdose include neuromuscular hypersensitivity and convulsions. Many beta-lactam containing antibiotics have the potential to cause neuromuscular hyperirritability or convulsive seizures. Hemodialysis may be helpful to aid in removal of the drug from blood; otherwise, treatment is supportive or symptom-directed.

Pharmacodynamics/Kinetics

Time to Peak: Serum: Fasting: 1.5 hours

Protein Binding: 35% to 45%

Half-Life Elimination: Normal renal function: 1.3 hours

Excretion: Urine (61% as unchanged drug)

Available Dosage Forms
Powder for oral suspension, as anhydrous: 125 mg/5 mL (50 mL, 75 mL, 100 mL); 250 mg/5 mL (50 mL, 75 mL, 100 mL)
Cefzil®: 125 mg/5 mL (50 mL, 75 mL, 100 mL) [contains phenylalanine 28 mg/5 mL and sodium benzoate; bubble gum flavor]; 250 mg/5 mL (50 mL, 75 mL, 100 mL) [contains phenylalanine 28 mg/5 mL and sodium benzoate; bubble gum flavor]
Tablet, as anhydrous: 250 mg, 500 mg
Cefzil®: 250 mg, 500 mg

Dosing

Adults & Elderly:

Pharyngitis/tonsillitis: Oral: 500 mg every 24 hours for 10 days

Secondary bacterial infection of acute bronchitis or acute bacterial exacerbation of chronic bronchitis: Oral: 500 mg every 12 hours for 10 days

Uncomplicated skin and skin structure infections: Oral: 250 mg every 12 hours, or 500 mg every 12-24 hours for 10 days

Pediatrics:

Otitis media: Oral: Children >6 months to 12 years: 15 mg/kg every 12 hours for 10 days

Pharyngitis/tonsillitis: Oral: Children:
2-12 years: 7.5-15 mg/kg/day divided every 12 hours for 10 days (administer for >10 days if due to *S. pyogenes*); maximum: 1 g/day
>13 years: Refer to adult dosing.

Uncomplicated skin and skin structure infections: Oral:
2-12 years: 20 mg/kg every 24 hours for 10 days; maximum: 1 g/day
>13 years: Refer to adult dosing.

(Continued)

Cefprozil *(Continued)*

Renal Impairment:
Cl$_{cr}$ <30 mL/minute: Reduce dose by 50%.

Hemodialysis effects: 55% is removed by hemodialysis.

Administration
Oral: Administer around-the-clock to promote less variation in peak and trough serum levels. Chilling the reconstituted oral suspension improves flavor (do not freeze).

Laboratory Monitoring Perform culture and sensitivity studies prior to initiating drug therapy; renal function

Nursing Actions
Physical Assessment: Results of culture/sensitivity tests and patient's allergy history should be assessed prior to therapy. Assess other pharmacological or herbal products patient may be taking for potential interactions. Monitor laboratory tests (prothrombin time), therapeutic response, and adverse effects (eg, interstitial nephritis, hemolytic anemia, hemorrhage). Advise patients with diabetes about use of Clinitest® (may cause false-positive test). Teach patient possible side effects/appropriate interventions and adverse symptoms to report (eg, opportunistic infection, hypersensitivity reaction).

Patient Education: Do not take any new medication during therapy unless approved by prescriber. Take as directed, at regular intervals around-the-clock (with or without food). Chilling oral suspension improves flavor (do not freeze). Maintain adequate hydration (2-3 L/day of fluids) unless instructed to restrict fluid intake. Complete full course of medication, even if you feel better. May cause false test results with Clinitest®; use of another type of glucose testing is preferable. May cause dizziness (use caution when driving or engaging in potentially hazardous tasks until response to drug is known); nausea or vomiting (small, frequent meals, frequent mouth care, sucking lozenges, or chewing gum may help); or diarrhea (yogurt, boiled milk, or buttermilk may help). Report rash; breathing or swallowing difficulty; persistent diarrhea, nausea, vomiting, or abdominal pain; changes in urinary pattern or pain on urination; opportunistic infection (eg, vaginal itching or drainage; sores in mouth; blood in stool or urine; unusual fever or chills); CNS changes (eg, irritability, agitation, nervousness, insomnia, hallucinations); or other adverse reactions. **Breast-feeding precaution:** Consult prescriber if breast-feeding.

Dietary Considerations May be taken with food. Oral suspension contains phenylalanine 28 mg/5 mL.

Geriatric Considerations Has not been studied exclusively in the elderly. Adjust dose for estimated renal function.

Breast-Feeding Issues Theoretically, drug absorbed by nursing infant may change bowel flora or affect fever work-up result. **Note:** As a class, cephalosporins are used to treat infections in infants.

Ceftazidime (SEF tay zi deem)

U.S. Brand Names Ceptaz® [DSC]; Fortaz®; Tazicef®

Pharmacologic Category Antibiotic, Cephalosporin (Third Generation)

Medication Safety Issues
Sound-alike/look-alike issues:
Ceftazidime may be confused with ceftizoxime
Ceptaz® may be confused with Septra®
Tazicef® may be confused with Tazidime®
Tazidime® may be confused with Tazicef®

Pregnancy Risk Factor B

Lactation Enters breast milk (small amounts)/use caution (AAP rates "compatible")

Use Treatment of documented susceptible *Pseudomonas aeruginosa* infection and infections due to other susceptible aerobic gram-negative organisms; empiric therapy of a febrile, granulocytopenic patient

Mechanism of Action/Effect Inhibits bacterial cell wall synthesis by binding to one or more of the penicillin-binding proteins (PBPs)

Contraindications Hypersensitivity to ceftazidime, any component of the formulation, or other cephalosporins

Warnings/Precautions Modify dosage in patients with severe renal impairment; prolonged use may result in superinfection; use with caution in patients with a history of penicillin allergy especially IgE-mediated reactions (eg, anaphylaxis, urticaria). May cause antibiotic-associated colitis or colitis secondary to *C. difficile*.

Drug Interactions
Increased Effect/Toxicity: Probenecid may decrease cephalosporin elimination. Aminoglycosides: *in vitro* studies indicate additive or synergistic effect against some strains of Enterobacteriaceae and *Pseudomonas aeruginosa*. Furosemide, aminoglycosides in combination with ceftazidime may result in additive nephrotoxicity.

Lab Interactions Positive direct Coombs', false-positive urinary glucose test using cupric sulfate (Benedict's solution, Clinitest®, Fehling's solution), false-positive serum or urine creatinine with Jaffé reaction

Adverse Reactions
1% to 10%:
Gastrointestinal: Diarrhea (1%)
Local: Pain at injection site (1%)
Miscellaneous: Hypersensitivity reactions (2%)
Reactions reported with other cephalosporins include seizure, urticaria, serum-sickness reactions, renal dysfunction, interstitial nephritis, toxic nephropathy, elevated BUN, elevated creatinine, cholestasis, aplastic anemia, hemolytic anemia, pancytopenia, agranulocytosis, colitis, prolonged PT, hemorrhage, superinfection

Overdosage/Toxicology Symptoms of overdose include neuromuscular hypersensitivity and convulsions. Many beta-lactam containing antibiotics have the potential to cause neuromuscular hyperirritability or convulsive seizures. Hemodialysis may be helpful to aid in removal of the drug from blood; otherwise, treatment is supportive or symptom-directed.

Pharmacodynamics/Kinetics
Time to Peak: Serum: I.M.: ~1 hour
Protein Binding: 17%
Half-Life Elimination: 1-2 hours, prolonged with renal impairment; Neonates <23 days: 2.2-4.7 hours

Excretion: Urine (80% to 90% as unchanged drug)

Available Dosage Forms [DSC] = Discontinued product
Infusion, as sodium [premixed iso-osmotic solution] (Fortaz®): 1 g (50 mL); 2 g (50 mL)
Injection, powder for reconstitution:
Ceptaz® [DSC]: 10 g [L-arginine formulation]
Fortaz®: 500 mg, 1 g, 2 g, 6 g [contains sodium carbonate]
Tazicef®: 1 g, 2 g, 6 g [contains sodium carbonate]

Dosing
Adults:
Bacterial arthritis (gram negative bacilli): I.V.: 1-2 g every 8 hours
Bone and joint infections: I.V.: 2 g every 12 hours
Cystic fibrosis, lung infection caused by *Pseudomonas* spp: I.V.: 30-50 mg/kg every 8 hours (maximum 6 g/day)
Melioidosis: I.V.: 40 mg/kg every 8 hours for 10 days, followed by oral therapy with doxycycline or TMP/SMX
Otitis externa: I.V.: 2 g every 8 hours
Peritonitis (CAPD):
Anuric, intermittent: 1000-1500 mg/day

Anuric, continuous (per liter exchange): Loading dose: 250 mg; maintenance dose: 125 mg

Pneumonia: I.V.:
Uncomplicated: 500 mg to 1 g every 8 hours
Complicated or severe: 2 g every 8 hours

Skin and soft tissue infections: I.V., I.M.: 500 mg to 1 g every 8 hours

Severe infections, including meningitis, complicated pneumonia, endophthalmitis, CNS infection, osteomyelitis, intra-abdominal and gynecological, skin and soft tissue: I.V.: 2 g every 8 hours

Urinary tract infections: I.V., I.M.:
Uncomplicated: 250 mg every 12 hours
Complicated: 500 mg every 8-12 hours

Elderly: I.M., I.V.: Dosage should be based on renal function with a dosing interval not more frequent then every 12 hours.

Pediatrics: Susceptible infections: I.V.:
Children 1 month to 12 years: 30-50 mg/kg/dose every 8 hours; maximum dose: 6 g/day (higher doses reserved for immunocompromised patients, cystic fibrosis, or meningitis)
Children ≥12 years: Refer to adult dosing.

Renal Impairment:
Cl$_{cr}$ 30-50 mL/minute: Administer every 12 hours
Cl$_{cr}$ 10-30 mL/minute: Administer every 24 hours
Cl$_{cr}$ <10 mL/minute: Administer every 48-72 hours
Hemodialysis: Dialyzable (50% to 100%)
Continuous arteriovenous or venovenous hemodiafiltration effects: Dose as for Cl$_{cr}$ 30-50 mL/minute

Administration
I.M.: Inject deep I.M. into large mass muscle.
I.V.: Ceftazidime can be administered IVP over 3-5 minutes or I.V. intermittent infusion over 15-30 minutes.
I.V. Detail: Any carbon dioxide bubbles that may be present in the withdrawn solution should be expelled prior to injection. Administer around-the-clock to promote less variation in peak and trough serum levels.

pH: 5-8 (Fortaz®); 5.0-7.5 (Ceptaz®)

Stability
Reconstitution: Reconstituted solution and I.V. infusion in NS or D$_5$W solution are stable for 24 hours at room temperature, 10 days when refrigerated, or 12 weeks when frozen. After freezing, thawed solution is stable for 24 hours at room temperature or 4 days when refrigerated. After mixing for 96 hours refrigerated.

Compatibility: Stable in D$_5$NS, D$_5$W, NS, SWFI
Y-site administration: Incompatible with alatrofloxacin, amphotericin B cholesteryl sulfate complex, amsacrine, doxorubicin liposome, fluconazole, idarubicin, midazolam, pentamidine, warfarin
Compatibility when admixed: Incompatible with aminoglycosides in same bottle/bag, aminophylline, ranitidine

Laboratory Monitoring Perform culture and sensitivity studies prior to initiating drug therapy; renal function

Nursing Actions
Physical Assessment: Results of culture/sensitivity tests and patient's allergy history should be assessed prior to therapy. Assess other pharmacological or herbal products patient may be taking for potential interactions (eg, nephrotoxicity). Monitor laboratory tests (prothrombin time), therapeutic response, and adverse effects (eg, hemolytic anemia, hypoprothrombinemia, and bleeding) during therapy. Advise patients with diabetes about use of Clinitest® (may cause false-positive test). Teach patient possible side effects/appropriate interventions and adverse symptoms to report (eg, opportunistic infection, hypersensitivity reaction).

Patient Education: Do not take any new medication during therapy unless approved by prescriber. This medication is administered by infusion or injection. Report immediately any redness, swelling, burning, or pain at injection/infusion site. Maintain adequate hydration (2-3 L/day of fluids) unless instructed to restrict fluid intake. May cause false test results with Clinitest®; use of another type of glucose testing is preferable. May cause diarrhea (yogurt, boiled milk, or buttermilk may help). Report rash; breathing or swallowing difficulty; persistent diarrhea, nausea, vomiting, or abdominal pain; changes in urinary pattern or pain on urination; opportunistic infection (eg, vaginal itching or drainage; sores in mouth; blood in stool or urine; unusual fever or chills); CNS changes (eg, irritability, agitation, nervousness, insomnia, hallucinations); or other adverse reactions. **Breast-feeding precaution:** Consult prescriber if breast-feeding.

Dietary Considerations Sodium content of 1 g: 2.3 mEq

Geriatric Considerations Changes in renal function associated with aging and corresponding alterations in pharmacokinetics result in every 12-hour dosing being an adequate dosing interval. Adjust dose based on renal function.

Breast-Feeding Issues Theoretically, drug absorbed by nursing infant may change bowel flora or affect fever work-up result. **Note:** As a class, cephalosporins are used to treat infections in infants.

Additional Information With some organisms, resistance may develop during treatment (including *Enterobacter* spp and *Serratia* spp); consider combination therapy or periodic susceptibility testing for organisms with inducible resistance

---

Ceftibuten (sef TYE byoo ten)

U.S. Brand Names Cedax®
Pharmacologic Category Antibiotic, Cephalosporin (Third Generation)
Pregnancy Risk Factor B
Lactation Excretion in breast milk unknown/use caution
Use Oral cephalosporin for treatment of bronchitis, otitis media, and pharyngitis/tonsillitis due to *H. influenzae* and *M. catarrhalis*, both beta-lactamase-producing and nonproducing strains, as well as *S. pneumoniae* (weak) and *S. pyogenes*
Mechanism of Action/Effect Inhibits bacterial cell wall synthesis by binding to one or more of the penicillin-binding proteins (PBPs)
Contraindications Hypersensitivity to ceftibuten, any component of the formulation, or other cephalosporins
Warnings/Precautions Modify dosage in patients with severe renal impairment, prolonged use may result in superinfection; use with caution in patients with a history of penicillin allergy, especially IgE-mediated reactions (eg, anaphylaxis, urticaria). May cause antibiotic-associated colitis or colitis secondary to *C. difficile*.

Drug Interactions
Increased Effect/Toxicity: High-dose probenecid decreases clearance. Aminoglycosides in combination with ceftibuten may increase nephrotoxic potential.

Lab Interactions Positive direct Coombs', false-positive urinary glucose test using cupric sulfate (Benedict's solution, Clinitest®, Fehling's solution), false-positive serum or urine creatinine with Jaffé reaction

Adverse Reactions
1% to 10%:
Central nervous system: Headache (3%), dizziness (1%)
Gastrointestinal: Nausea (4%), diarrhea (3%), dyspepsia (2%), vomiting (1%), abdominal pain (1%)
Hematologic: Increased eosinophils (3%), decreased hemoglobin (2%), thrombocytosis
(Continued)

Ceftibuten *(Continued)*

Hepatic: Increased ALT (1%), increased bilirubin (1%)

Renal: Increased BUN (4%)

Reactions reported with other cephalosporins include anaphylaxis, fever, paresthesia, pruritus, Stevens-Johnson syndrome, toxic epidermal necrolysis, erythema multiforme, angioedema, pseudomembranous colitis, hemolytic anemia, candidiasis, vaginitis, encephalopathy, asterixis, neuromuscular excitability, seizure, serum-sickness reactions, renal dysfunction, interstitial nephritis, toxic nephropathy, cholestasis, aplastic anemia, hemolytic anemia, pancytopenia, agranulocytosis, colitis, prolonged PT, hemorrhage, superinfection

Overdosage/Toxicology Symptoms of overdose include neuromuscular hypersensitivity and convulsions. Many beta-lactam containing antibiotics have the potential to cause neuromuscular hyperirritability or convulsive seizures. Hemodialysis may be helpful to aid in the removal of drug from blood; otherwise, treatment is supportive or symptom-directed.

Pharmacodynamics/Kinetics

Time to Peak: 2-3 hours

Half-Life Elimination: 2 hours

Excretion: Urine

Available Dosage Forms

Capsule: 400 mg

Powder for oral suspension: 90 mg/5 mL (30 mL, 60 mL, 120 mL) [contains sodium benzoate; cherry flavor]

Dosing

Adults & Elderly: Susceptible infections: Oral: 400 mg once daily for 10 days; maximum: 400 mg

Pediatrics: Susceptible infections: Oral:

<12 years: 9 mg/kg/day for 10 days; maximum daily dose: 400 mg

≥12 years: Refer to adult dosing.

Renal Impairment:

Cl_{cr} 30-49 mL/minute: Administer 4.5 mg/kg or 200 mg every 24 hours.

Cl_{cr} 5-29 mL/minute: Administer 2.25 mg/kg or 100 mg every 24 hours.

Administration

Oral: Administer at the same time each day to maintain adequate blood levels. Shake suspension well before use.

Stability

Storage: Reconstituted suspension is stable for 14 days in the refrigerator.

Laboratory Monitoring Renal, hepatic, and hematologic function periodically with prolonged therapy; perform culture and sensitivity studies prior to initiating drug therapy

Nursing Actions

Physical Assessment: Results of culture/sensitivity tests and patient's allergy history should be assessed prior to therapy. Assess other pharmacological or herbal products patient may be taking for potential interactions (eg, nephrotoxicity). Assess results of laboratory tests, therapeutic response, and adverse effects (eg, hemolytic anemia, hypoprothrombinemia, and bleeding) regularly during therapy. Advise patients with diabetes about use of Clinitest® (may cause false-positive test). Teach patient possible side effects/appropriate interventions and adverse symptoms to report (eg, opportunistic infection, hypersensitivity reaction).

Patient Education: Do not take any new medication during therapy unless approved by prescriber. Take as directed, at regular intervals around-the-clock (take capsules with or without food; take suspension 2 hours before or 1 hour after meals). Chilling oral suspension improves flavor (do not freeze). Maintain adequate hydration (2-3 L/day of fluids) unless instructed to restrict fluid intake. Complete full course of medication, even if you feel better. May cause false

test results with Clinitest®; use of another type of testing is preferable. May cause headache or dizziness (use caution when driving or engaging in potentially hazardous tasks until response to drug is known); nausea or vomiting (small, frequent meals, frequent mouth care, sucking lozenges, or chewing gum may help); or diarrhea (yogurt, boiled milk, or buttermilk may help). Report rash; breathing or swallowing difficulty; persistent diarrhea, nausea, vomiting, or abdominal pain; changes in urinary pattern or pain on urination; opportunistic infection (eg, vaginal itching or drainage; sores in mouth; blood in stool or urine; unusual fever or chills); CNS changes (eg, irritability, agitation, nervousness, insomnia, hallucinations); or other adverse reactions. **Breast-feeding precaution:** Consult prescriber if breast-feeding.

Dietary Considerations

Capsule: Take without regard to food.

Suspension: Take 2 hours before or 1 hour after meals; contains 1 g of sucrose per 5 mL

Geriatric Considerations Has not been studied specifically in the elderly. Adjust dose for renal function.

Breast-Feeding Issues Theoretically, drug absorbed by nursing infant may change bowel flora or affect fever work-up result. **Note:** As a class, cephalosporins are used to treat infections in infants.

Ceftizoxime *(sef ti ZOKS eem)*

U.S. Brand Names Cefizox®

Synonyms Ceftizoxime Sodium

Pharmacologic Category Antibiotic, Cephalosporin (Third Generation)

Medication Safety Issues

Sound-alike/look-alike issues:

Ceftizoxime may be confused with cefotaxime, ceftazidime, cefuroxime

Pregnancy Risk Factor B

Lactation Enters breast milk (small amounts)/use caution

Use Treatment of susceptible bacterial infection, mainly respiratory tract, skin and skin structure, bone and joint, urinary tract and gynecologic, as well as septicemia; active against many gram-negative bacilli (not *Pseudomonas*), some gram-positive cocci (not *Enterococcus*), and some anaerobes

Mechanism of Action/Effect Inhibits bacterial cell wall synthesis by binding to one or more of the penicillin-binding proteins (PBPs)

Contraindications Hypersensitivity to ceftizoxime, any component of the formulation, or other cephalosporins

Warnings/Precautions Modify dosage in patients with severe renal impairment, prolonged use may result in superinfection; use with caution in patients with a history of penicillin allergy, especially IgE-mediated reactions (eg, anaphylaxis, urticaria). May cause antibiotic-associated colitis or colitis secondary to *C. difficile*.

Drug Interactions

Increased Effect/Toxicity: Probenecid may decrease cephalosporin elimination. Furosemide, aminoglycosides in combination with ceftizoxime may result in additive nephrotoxicity.

Lab Interactions Positive direct Coombs', false-positive urinary glucose test using cupric sulfate (Benedict's solution, Clinitest®, Fehling's solution), false-positive serum or urine creatinine with Jaffé reaction

Adverse Reactions

1% to 10%:

Central nervous system: Fever

Dermatologic: Rash, pruritus

Hematologic: Eosinophilia, thrombocytosis

Hepatic: Alkaline phosphatase increased, transaminases increased

Local: Pain, burning at injection site

Other reactions reported with cephalosporins include Stevens-Johnson syndrome, toxic epidermal necrolysis, erythema multiforme, pseudomembranous colitis, angioedema, hemolytic anemia, candidiasis, encephalopathy, asterixis, neuromuscular excitability, seizure, serum-sickness reactions, renal dysfunction, interstitial nephritis, toxic nephropathy, cholestasis, aplastic anemia, hemolytic anemia, pancytopenia, agranulocytosis, colitis, prolonged PT, hemorrhage, superinfection

Overdosage/Toxicology Symptoms of overdose include neuromuscular hypersensitivity and convulsions. Many beta-lactam containing antibiotics have the potential to cause neuromuscular hyperirritability or convulsive seizures. Hemodialysis may be helpful to aid in removal of the drug from blood; otherwise, treatment is supportive or symptom-directed.

Pharmacodynamics/Kinetics
Time to Peak: Serum: I.M.: 0.5-1 hour
Protein Binding: 30%
Half-Life Elimination: 1.6 hours; Cl_{cr} <10 mL/minute: 25 hours
Excretion: Urine (as unchanged drug)
Available Dosage Forms
Infusion [premixed iso-osmotic solution]: 1 g (50 mL); 2 g (50 mL)
Injection, powder for reconstitution: 1 g, 2 g, 10 g
Dosing
Adults & Elderly: Usual dosage: I.M., I.V.: 1-2 g every 8-12 hours, up to 2 g every 4 hours or 4 g every 8 hours for life-threatening infections
Gonococcal:
Disseminated infection: I.M., I.V.: 1 g every 8 hours
Uncomplicated: I.M.: 1 g as single dose
Life-threatening infections: I.V.: 2 g every 4 hours or 4 g every 8 hours
Pediatrics: Usual dosage: I.M., I.V.: Children ≥6 months: 150-200 mg/kg/day divided every 6-8 hours (maximum: 12 g/24 hours)
Renal Impairment:
Cl_{cr} 50-79 mL/minute: Administer 500-1500 mg every 8 hours.
Cl_{cr} 5-49 mL/minute: Administer 250-1000 mg every 12 hours.
Cl_{cr} 0-4 mL/minute: Administer 500-1000 mg every 48 hours or 250-500 mg every 24 hours.
Moderately dialyzable (20% to 50%)
Continuous arteriovenous hemofiltration: Dose as for Cl_{cr} 10-50 mL/minute.
Administration
I.M.: Inject deep I.M. into large muscle mass.
I.V.: Inject direct I.V. over 3-5 minutes. Infuse intermittent infusion over 30 minutes.
I.V. Detail: pH: 6-8 (reconstituted solution); 5.5-8.0 (frozen premixed infusion solution)
Stability
Reconstitution: Reconstituted solution is stable for 24 hours at room temperature and 96 hours when refrigerated. For I.V. infusion in NS or D_5W, solution is stable for 24 hours at room temperature, 96 hours when refrigerated or 12 weeks when frozen. After freezing, thawed solution is stable for 24 hours at room temperature or 10 days when refrigerated.
Compatibility: Stable in $D_5^{1/4}NS$, $D_5^{1/2}NS$, D_5NS, D_5W, $D_{10}W$, LR, NS, sodium bicarbonate 5%
Y-site administration: Incompatible with filgrastim
Laboratory Monitoring Perform culture and sensitivity studies prior to initiating drug therapy; renal function
Nursing Actions
Physical Assessment: Results of culture/sensitivity tests and patient's allergy history should be assessed prior to therapy. Assess other pharmacological or herbal products patient may be taking for potential interactions. Monitor laboratory tests (prothrombin times), therapeutic response, and adverse effects (eg,

hemolytic anemia, hypoprothrombinemia, and bleeding) regularly during therapy. Advise patients with diabetes about use of Clinitest® (may cause false-positive test). Teach patient possible side effects/appropriate interventions and adverse symptoms to report (eg, opportunistic infection, hypersensitivity reactions).
Patient Education: Do not take any new medication during therapy unless approved by prescriber. This medication is administered by infusion or injection. Report immediately any redness, swelling, burning, or pain at injection/infusion site; itching or hives; or difficulty swallowing or breathing. Maintain adequate hydration (2-3 L/day of fluids) unless instructed to restrict fluid intake. May cause false test results with Clinitest®; use of another type of glucose testing is preferable. Report rash; breathing or swallowing difficulty; persistent diarrhea, nausea, vomiting, or abdominal pain; changes in urinary pattern or pain on urination; opportunistic infection (eg, vaginal itching or drainage; sores in mouth; blood in stool or urine; unusual fever or chills); CNS changes (eg, irritability, agitation, nervousness, insomnia, hallucinations); or other adverse reactions. **Breast-feeding precaution:** Consult prescriber if breast-feeding.
Dietary Considerations Sodium content of 1 g: 60 mg (2.6 mEq)
Geriatric Considerations Adjust dose for renal function in the elderly.
Breast-Feeding Issues Theoretically, drug absorbed by nursing infant may change bowel flora or affect fever work-up result. **Note:** As a class, cephalosporins are used to treat infections in infants.

Ceftriaxone (sef trye AKS one)

U.S. Brand Names Rocephin®
Synonyms Ceftriaxone Sodium
Pharmacologic Category Antibiotic, Cephalosporin (Third Generation)
Medication Safety Issues
Sound-alike/look-alike issues:
Rocephin® may be confused with Roferon®
Pregnancy Risk Factor B
Lactation Enters breast milk/use caution (AAP rates "compatible")
Use Treatment of lower respiratory tract infections, acute bacterial otitis media, skin and skin structure infections, bone and joint infections, intra-abdominal and urinary tract infections, pelvic inflammatory disease (PID), uncomplicated gonorrhea, bacterial septicemia, and meningitis; used in surgical prophylaxis
Unlabeled/Investigational Use Treatment of chancroid, epididymitis, complicated gonococcal infections; sexually-transmitted diseases (STD); periorbital or buccal cellulitis; salmonellosis or shigellosis; atypical community-acquired pneumonia; Lyme disease; used in chemoprophylaxis for high-risk contacts and persons with invasive meningococcal disease; sexual assault
Mechanism of Action/Effect Inhibits bacterial cell wall synthesis by binding to one or more of the penicillin-binding proteins (PBPs)
Contraindications Hypersensitivity to ceftriaxone sodium, any component of the formulation, or other cephalosporins; **do not use in hyperbilirubinemic neonates**, particularly those who are premature since ceftriaxone is reported to displace bilirubin from albumin binding sites
Warnings/Precautions Modify dosage in patients with severe renal impairment, prolonged use may result in superinfection. Use with caution in patients with a history of penicillin allergy, especially IgE-mediated reactions (eg, anaphylaxis, urticaria). May cause antibiotic-associated colitis or colitis secondary to *C. difficile.*
(Continued)

Ceftriaxone *(Continued)*

Discontinue in patients with signs and symptoms of gall-bladder disease.

Drug Interactions

Decreased Effect: Uricosuric agents (eg, probenecid, sulfinpyrazone) may decrease the excretion of cephalosporin; monitor for toxic effects.

Increased Effect/Toxicity: Cephalosporins may increase the anticoagulant effect of coumarin derivatives (eg, dicumarol, warfarin).

Lab Interactions Positive direct Coombs', false-positive urinary glucose test using cupric sulfate (Benedict's solution, Clinitest®, Fehling's solution), false-positive serum or urine creatinine with Jaffé reaction

Adverse Reactions

1% to 10%:

Dermatologic: Rash (2%)

Gastrointestinal: Diarrhea (3%)

Hematologic: Eosinophilia (6%), thrombocytosis (5%), leukopenia (2%)

Hepatic: Transaminases increased (3.1% to 3.3%)

Local: Pain, induration at injection site (I.V. 1%); warmth, tightness, induration (5% to 17%) following I.M. injection

Renal: Increased BUN (1%)

Overdosage/Toxicology
Symptoms of overdose include neuromuscular hypersensitivity and convulsions. Many beta-lactam containing antibiotics have the potential to cause neuromuscular hyperirritability or convulsive seizures. Hemodialysis may be helpful to aid in removal of the drug from blood; otherwise, treatment is supportive or symptom-directed.

Pharmacodynamics/Kinetics

Time to Peak: Serum: I.M.: 1-2 hours

Protein Binding: 85% to 95%

Half-Life Elimination: Normal renal and hepatic function: 5-9 hours

Excretion: Urine (33% to 65% as unchanged drug); feces

Available Dosage Forms Note: Contains sodium 83 mg (3.6 mEq) per ceftriaxone 1 g

Infusion [premixed in dextrose]: 1 g (50 mL); 2 g (50 mL)

Injection, powder for reconstitution: 250 mg, 500 mg, 1 g, 2 g, 10 g

Dosing

Adults & Elderly:

Dosage range: Usual dose: 1-2 g every 12-24 hours, depending on the type and severity of infection

Arthritis (septic): I.V.: 1-2 g once daily

Brain abscess and necrotizing fasciitis: I.V.: 2 g every 12 hours

Cavernous sinus thrombosis: I.V.: 1 g every 12 hours with vancomycin or linezolid

Chancroid (unlabeled use): I.M.: 250 mg as single dose

Chemoprophylaxis for high-risk contacts and persons with invasive meningococcal disease (unlabeled use): I.M.: 250 mg in a single dose

Endocarditis, acute native valve: I.V.: 2 g once daily for 2-4 weeks

Epididymitis, acute (unlabeled use) and prostatitis: I.M.: 250 mg in a single dose with doxycycline

Gonococcal infections:

Conjunctivitis, complicated (unlabeled use): I.M., I.V.: 1 g in a single dose

Disseminated (unlabeled use): I.M., I.V.: 1 g once daily for 7 days

Endocarditis (unlabeled use): I.M., I.V.: 1-2 g every 12 hours for at least 28 days

Uncomplicated: I.M.: 125-250 mg in a single dose

Lyme disease: I.V.: 2 g once daily for 14-28 days

Mastoiditis (hospitalized): I.V.: 2 g once daily; >60 years old: 1 g once daily

Meningitis: I.V.: 2 g every 12 hours for 7-14 days (longer courses may be necessary for selected organisms

Orbital cellulitis (unlabeled use) and endophthalmitis: I.V.: 2 g once daily

PID: I.M.: 250 mg in a single dose

Pneumonia, community-acquired: I.V.: 2 g once daily; >65 years of age: 1 g once daily

Septic/toxic shock: I.V.: 2 g once daily; with clindamycin for toxic shock

Surgical prophylaxis: I.V.: 1 g 30 minutes to 2 hours before surgery

Syphilis: I.M., I.V.: 1 g once daily for 8-10 days

Typhoid fever: I.V.: 2-3 g once daily for 7-14 days

Pediatrics:

Dosage range: Infants and Children: Usual dose: I.M., I.V.:

Mild-to-moderate infections: 50-75 mg/kg/day in 1-2 divided doses every 12-24 hours (maximum: 2 g/day); continue until at least 2 days after signs and symptoms of infection have resolved

Serious infections: 80-100 mg/kg/day in 1-2 divided doses (maximum: 4 g/day)

Epiglottis: I.M., I.V.: 50-100 mg/kg once daily for 7-10 days with clindamycin

Gonococcal infections:

Conjunctivitis, complicated (unlabeled use): I.M.:

<45 kg: 50 mg/kg in a single dose (maximum: 1 g)

>45 kg: 1 g in a single dose

Disseminated (unlabeled use): I.M., I.V.:

<45 kg: 25-50 mg/kg once daily (maximum: 1 g)

>45 kg: 1 g once daily for 7 days

Endocarditis (unlabeled use):

<45 kg: I.M., I.V.: 50 mg/kg/day every 12 hours (maximum: 2 g/day) for at least 28 days

>45 kg: I.V.: 1-2 g every 12 hours, for at least 28 days

Uncomplicated: I.M.: 125 mg in a single dose

Meningitis: I.M., I.V.:

Uncomplicated: Loading dose of 100 mg/kg (maximum: 4 g), followed by 100 mg/kg/day divided every 12-24 hours (maximum: 4 g/day); usual duration of treatment is 7-14 days

Gonococcal, complicated:

<45 kg: 50 mg/kg/day given every 12 hours (maximum: 2 g/day); usual duration of treatment is 10-14 days

>45 kg: I.V.: 1-2 g every 12 hours; usual duration of treatment is 10-14 days

Otitis media: I.M., I.V.:

Acute: 50 mg/kg in a single dose (maximum: 1 g)

Persistent or relapsing (unlabeled use): 50 mg/kg once daily for 3 days

Pneumonia: I.V.: 50-75 mg/kg once daily

STD, sexual assault (unlabeled uses): 125 mg in a single dose

Typhoid fever: I.V.: 100 mg/kg once daily, maximum 4 g

Chemoprophylaxis for high-risk contacts and persons with invasive meningococcal disease (unlabeled use):

Children ≤15 years: I.M.: 125 mg in a single dose

Children >15 years: Refer to adult dosing.

Epididymitis, acute: Children >8 years (≥45 kg) and Adolescents (unlabeled use): I.M.: 125 mg in a single dose

Renal Impairment:

No adjustment is necessary.

Not dialyzable (0% to 5%)

Administer dose postdialysis.

Peritoneal dialysis effects: Administer 750 mg every 12 hours.

Continuous arteriovenous or venovenous hemofiltration: Removes 10 mg of ceftriaxone of liter of filtrate per day.

Hepatic Impairment: No adjustment necessary.

Administration

I.M.: Inject deep I.M. into large muscle mass; a concentration of 250 mg/mL or 350 mg/mL is recommended for all vial sizes except the 250 mg size (250 mg/mL is suggested); can be diluted with 1:1 water and 1% lidocaine for I.M. administration

I.V.: Do not admix with aminoglycosides in same bottle/bag. Infuse intermittent infusion over 30 minutes.

I.V. Detail: pH: 6.6 (premixed infusion solution); 6.7 (1% aqueous solution)

Stability

Reconstitution:

I.M. injection: Vials should be reconstituted with appropriate volume of diluent (including D₅W, NS, or 1% lidocaine) to make a final concentration of 250 mg/mL or 350 mg/mL.

Volume to add to create a **250 mg/mL** solution:
250 mg vial: 0.9 mL
500 mg vial: 1.8 mL
1 g vial: 3.6 mL
2 g vial: 7.2 mL

Volume to add to create a **350 mg/mL** solution:
500 mg vial: 1.0 mL
1 g vial: 2.1 mL
2 g vial: 4.2 mL

I.V. infusion: Infusion is prepared in two stages: Initial reconstitution of powder, followed by dilution to final infusion solution.

Vials: Reconstitute powder with appropriate I.V. diluent (including SWFI, D₅W, NS) to create an initial solution of ~100 mg/mL. Recommended volume to add:
250 mg vial: 2.4 mL
500 mg vial: 4.8 mL
1 g vial: 9.6 mL
2 g vial: 19.2 mL

Note: After reconstitution of powder, further dilution into a volume of compatible solution (eg, 50-100 mL of D₅W or NS) is recommended.

Piggyback bottle: Reconstitute powder with appropriate I.V. diluent (D₅W or NS) to create a resulting solution of ~100 mg/mL. Recommended initial volume to add:
1 g bottle:10 mL
2 g bottle: 20 mL

Note: After reconstitution, to prepare the final infusion solution, further dilution to 50 mL or 100 mL volumes with the appropriate I.V. diluent (including D₅W or NS) is recommended.

Compatibility: Stable in D₅W with KCl 10 mEq, D₅¼NS with KCl 20 mEq, D₅½ NS, D₅W, D₁₀W, NS, mannitol 5%, mannitol 10%, sodium bicarbonate 5%, bacteriostatic water, SWFI

Y-site administration: Incompatible with alatrofloxacin, amphotericin B cholesteryl sulfate complex, amsacrine, filgrastim, fluconazole, labetalol, pentamidine, vinorelbine

Compatibility when admixed: Incompatible with aminophylline, clindamycin, linezolid, theophylline

Storage:

Powder for injection: Prior to reconstitution, store at room temperature of 25°C (77°F); protect from light.

Premixed solution (manufacturer premixed): Store at -20°C; once thawed, solutions are stable for 3 days at room temperature of 25°C (77°F) or for 21 days refrigerated at 5°C (41°F). Do not refreeze.

Stability of reconstituted solutions:

10-40 mg/mL: Reconstituted in D₅W or NS: Stable for 2 days at room temperature of 25°C (77°F) or for 10 days when refrigerated at 5°C (41°F).

100 mg/mL:
Reconstituted in D₅W or NS: Stable for 2 days at room temperature of 25°C (77°F) or for 10 days when refrigerated at 5°C (41°F). Stable for 26 weeks when frozen at -20°C. Once thawed, solutions are stable for 2 days at room temperature of 25°C (77°F) or for 10 days when refrigerated at 5°C (41°F); does not apply to manufacturer's premixed bags. Do not refreeze.

Reconstituted in lidocaine 1% solution: Stable for 24 hours at room temperature of 25°C (77°F) or for 10 days when refrigerated at 5°C (41°F).

250-350 mg/mL: Reconstituted in D₅W, NS, lidocaine 1% solution, or SWFI: Stable for 24 hours at room temperature of 25°C (77°F) or for 3 days when refrigerated at 5°C (41°F).

Laboratory Monitoring Prothrombin times; perform culture and sensitivity studies prior to initiating drug therapy.

Nursing Actions

Physical Assessment: Results of culture/sensitivity tests and patient's allergy history should be assessed prior to therapy. Assess potential for interactions with other pharmacological agents patient may be taking (especially coumarin derivatives). Monitor laboratory tests (prothrombin times), therapeutic response, and adverse effects (eg, hemolytic anemia, hypoprothrombinemia, and bleeding). Advise patients with diabetes about use of Clinitest® (may cause false-positive test). Teach patient possible side effects/appropriate interventions and adverse symptoms to report (eg, opportunistic infection, hypersensitivity reaction).

Patient Education: Do not take any new medication during therapy unless approved by prescriber. This medication is administered by infusion or injection. Report immediately any redness, swelling, burning or pain at injection/infusion site; rash, itching, or hives. Maintain adequate hydration (2-3 L/day of fluids) unless instructed to restrict fluid intake. May cause false test results with Clinitest®; use of another type of glucose testing is preferable. May cause diarrhea (yogurt, boiled milk, or buttermilk may help). Report rash; breathing or swallowing difficulty; persistent diarrhea, nausea, vomiting, or abdominal pain; changes in urinary pattern or pain on urination; opportunistic infection (eg, vaginal itching or drainage, sores in mouth, blood in stool or urine, unusual fever or chills); CNS changes (eg, irritability, agitation, nervousness, insomnia, hallucinations); or other adverse reactions.**Breast-feeding precaution:** Consult prescriber if breast-feeding.

Dietary Considerations Sodium contents: 83 mg (3.6 mEq) per ceftriaxone 1 g

Geriatric Considerations No adjustment for changes in renal function necessary.

Breast-Feeding Issues Theoretically, drug absorbed by nursing infant may change bowel flora or affect fever work-up result. **Note:** As a class, cephalosporins are used to treat infections in infants.

Cefuroxime (se fyoor OKS eem)

U.S. Brand Names Ceftin®; Zinacef®

Synonyms Cefuroxime Axetil; Cefuroxime Sodium

Pharmacologic Category Antibiotic, Cephalosporin (Second Generation)

Medication Safety Issues

Sound-alike/look-alike issues:

Cefuroxime may be confused with cefotaxime, cefprozil, ceftizoxime, deferoxamine

Ceftin® may be confused with Cefotan®, cefotetan, Cefzil®, Cipro®

Zinacef® may be confused with Zithromax®

Pregnancy Risk Factor B

Lactation Enters breast milk/use caution

Use Treatment of infections caused by staphylococci, group B streptococci, *H. influenzae* (type A and B), *E. coli*, *Enterobacter*, *Salmonella*, and *Klebsiella*; treatment
(Continued)

Cefuroxime *(Continued)*

of susceptible infections of the lower respiratory tract, otitis media, urinary tract, skin and soft tissue, bone and joint, sepsis and gonorrhea

Mechanism of Action/Effect Inhibits bacterial cell wall synthesis by binding to one or more of the penicillin-binding proteins (PBPs)

Contraindications Hypersensitivity to cefuroxime, any component of the formulation, or other cephalosporins

Warnings/Precautions Modify dosage in patients with severe renal impairment, prolonged use may result in superinfection; use with caution in patients with a history of penicillin allergy, especially IgE-mediated reactions (eg, anaphylaxis, urticaria). May cause antibiotic-associated colitis or colitis secondary to *C. difficile*. May be associated with increased INR, especially in nutritionally-deficient patients, prolonged treatment, hepatic or renal disease. Tablets and oral suspension are not bioequivalent (do not substitute on a mg-per-mg basis).

Drug Interactions
Increased Effect/Toxicity: High-dose probenecid decreases clearance. Aminoglycosides in combination with cefuroxime may result in additive nephrotoxicity.

Nutritional/Ethanol Interactions Food: Bioavailability is increased with food; cefuroxime serum levels may be increased if taken with food or dairy products.

Lab Interactions Positive direct Coombs', false-positive urinary glucose test using cupric sulfate (Benedict's solution, Clinitest®, Fehling's solution), false-positive serum or urine creatinine with Jaffé reaction

Adverse Reactions
1% to 10%:
Endocrine & metabolic: Alkaline phosphatase increased (2%)

Hematologic: Eosinophilia (7%), decreased hemoglobin and hematocrit (10%)

Hepatic: Transaminases increased (4%)

Local: Thrombophlebitis (2%)

Reactions reported with other cephalosporins include agranulocytosis, aplastic anemia, asterixis, encephalopathy, hemorrhage, neuromuscular excitability, serum-sickness reactions, superinfection, toxic nephropathy

Overdosage/Toxicology Symptoms of overdose include neuromuscular hypersensitivity and convulsions. Many beta-lactam containing antibiotics have the potential to cause neuromuscular hyperirritability or convulsive seizures. Hemodialysis may be helpful to aid in removal of the drug from blood; otherwise, treatment is supportive or symptom-directed.

Pharmacodynamics/Kinetics
Time to Peak: Serum: I.M.: ~15-60 minutes; I.V.: 2-3 minutes

Protein Binding: 33% to 50%

Half-Life Elimination: Adults: 1-2 hours; prolonged with renal impairment

Excretion: Urine (66% to 100% as unchanged drug)

Available Dosage Forms
Infusion, as sodium [premixed] (Zinacef®): 750 mg (50 mL); 1.5 g (50 mL) [contains sodium 4.8 mEq (111 mg) per 750 mg]

Injection, powder for reconstitution, as sodium (Zinacef®): 750 mg, 1.5 g, 7.5 g [contains sodium 4.8 mEq (111 mg) per 750 mg]

Powder for oral suspension, as axetil (Ceftin®): 125 mg/5 mL (100 mL) [contains phenylalanine 11.8 mg/5 mL; tutti-frutti flavor]; 250 mg/5 mL (50 mL, 100 mL) [contains phenylalanine 25.2 mg/5 mL; tutti-frutti flavor]

Tablet, as axetil (Ceftin®): 250 mg, 500 mg

Dosing
Adults & Elderly: Note: Cefuroxime axetil film-coated tablets and oral suspension are not bioequivalent and are not substitutable on a mg/mg basis.

Acute bacterial maxillary sinusitis: Oral: 250 mg twice daily for 10 days

Bronchitis, acute (and exacerbations of chronic bronchitis):
Oral: 250-500 mg every 12 hours for 10 days
I.V.: 500-750 mg every 8 hours (complete therapy with oral dosing)

Cellulitis:
Oral: 500 mg every 12 hours
Orbital: I.V.: 1.5 g every 8 hours

Gonorrhea:
Disseminated: I.M., I.V.: 750 mg every 8 hours
Uncomplicated:
Oral: 1 g as a single dose
I.M.: 1.5 g as single dose (administer in 2 different sites with probenecid)

Lyme disease (early): Oral: 500 mg twice daily for 20 days

Pharyngitis/tonsillitis and sinusitis: Oral: 250 mg twice daily for 10 days

Skin/skin structure infection, uncomplicated:
Oral: 250-500 mg every 12 hours for 10 days
I.M., I.V.: 750 mg every 8 hours

Pneumonia, uncomplicated: I.M., I.V.: 750 mg every 8 hours

Severe or complicated infections: I.M., I.V.: 1.5 g every 8 hours (up to 1.5 g every 6 hours in life-threatening infections)

Surgical prophylaxis:
I.V.: 1.5 g 30 minutes to 1 hour prior to procedure (if procedure is prolonged can give 750 mg every 8 hours I.M.)
Open heart: I.V.: 1.5 g every 12 hours to a total of 6 g

Urinary tract infection, uncomplicated:
Oral: 125-250 mg twice daily for 7-10 days
I.V., I.M.: 750 mg every 8 hours

Pediatrics: Note: Cefuroxime axetil film-coated tablets and oral suspension are not bioequivalent and are not substitutable on a mg/mg basis.

Children ≥3 months to 12 years:
Epiglottitis: 150 mg/kg/day in 3 divided doses for 7-10 days

Acute otitis media, impetigo:
Oral:
Suspension: 30 mg/kg/day (maximum: 1 g/day) in 2 divided doses
Tablet: 250 mg every 12 hours
I.M., I.V.: 75-150 mg/kg/day divided every 8 hours (maximum dose: 6 g/day)

Acute bacterial maxillary sinusitis: Oral:
Suspension: 30 mg/kg/day in 2 divided doses for 10 days (maximum dose: 1 g/day)
Tablet: 250 mg twice daily for 10 days

Meningitis: NOT recommended (doses of 200-240 mg/kg/day divided every 6-8 hours have been used) (maximum dose: 9 g/day)

Pharyngitis, tonsillitis:
Oral:
Suspension: 20 mg/kg/day (maximum: 500 mg/day) in 2 divided doses for 10 days
Tablet: 125 mg every 12 hours for 10 days
I.M., I.V.: 75-150 mg/kg/day divided every 8 hours; maximum dose: 6 g/day

Children ≥13 years: Refer to adult dosing.

Renal Impairment:
Cl$_{cr}$ 10-20 mL/minute: Administer every 12 hours.
Cl$_{cr}$ <10 mL/minute: Administer every 24 hours.
Hemodialysis: Dialyzable (25%)
Note: Cefuroxime axetil film-coated tablets and oral suspension are not bioequivalent and are not substitutable on a mg/mg basis.

Continuous arteriovenous or venovenous hemodiafiltration effects: Dose as for Cl_{cr} 10-20 mL/minute.

Administration

Oral: Administer around-the-clock to promote less variation in peak and trough serum levels. Oral suspension: Administer with food. Shake well before use.

I.M.: Inject deep I.M. into large muscle mass.

I.V.: Inject direct I.V. over 3-5 minutes. Infuse intermittent infusion over 15-30 minutes.

I.V. Detail: pH: 6.0-8.5 (vials); 5.0-7.5 (frozen premixed solution)

Stability
Reconstitution:

Injectable: Reconstituted solution is stable for 24 hours at room temperature and 48 hours when refrigerated. I.V. infusion in NS or D_5W solution is stable for 24 hours at room temperature, 7 days when refrigerated, or 26 weeks when frozen. After freezing, thawed solution is stable for 24 hours at room temperature or 21 days when refrigerated.

Oral suspension: Store in refrigerator or at room temperature. Discard after 10 days.

Compatibility: Stable in $D_5{}^1/_4NS$, $D_5{}^1/_2NS$, D_5NS, D_5W, $D_{10}W$, LR, NS

Y-site administration: Incompatible with clarithromycin, filgrastim, fluconazole, midazolam, vinorelbine

Compatibility in syringe: Incompatible with doxapram

Compatibility when admixed: Incompatible with aminoglycosides, sodium bicarbonate

Laboratory Monitoring Perform culture and sensitivity studies prior to initiating therapy; renal function

Nursing Actions

Physical Assessment: Results of culture/sensitivity tests and patient's allergy history should be assessed prior to therapy. Assess other pharmacological or herbal products patient may be taking for potential interactions (eg, nephrotoxicity). Monitor laboratory tests (prothrombin times), therapeutic response, and adverse effects (eg, hemolytic anemia, hypoprothrombinemia, and bleeding) regularly during therapy. Advise patients with diabetes about use of Clinitest® (may cause false-positive test). Teach patient possible side effects/appropriate interventions and adverse symptoms to report (eg, opportunistic infection, hypersensitivity reaction).

Patient Education: Do not take any new medication during therapy unless approved by prescriber. If administered by injection or infusion, report immediately any swelling, redness, or pain at injection/infusion site; respiratory difficulty or swallowing; chest pain; or rash. Oral tablets or suspension should be taken as directed, at regular intervals around-the-clock (with or without food). Chilling oral suspension improves flavor (do not freeze); shake well before using. Complete full course of medication, even if you feel better. Maintain adequate hydration (2-3 L/day of fluids) unless instructed to restrict fluid intake. May cause false test results with Clinitest®; use of another type of glucose testing is preferable. Report rash; breathing or swallowing difficulty; persistent diarrhea, nausea, vomiting, or abdominal pain; changes in urinary pattern or pain on urination; opportunistic infection (eg, vaginal itching or drainage, sores in mouth, blood in stool or urine, unusual fever or chills); CNS changes (eg, irritability, agitation, nervousness, insomnia, hallucinations); or other adverse reactions. **Breast-feeding precaution:** Consult prescriber if breast-feeding.

Dietary Considerations May be taken with food.

Zinacef®: Sodium content: 4.8 mEq (111 mg) per 750 mg

Ceftin®: Powder for oral suspension 125 mg/5 mL contains phenylalanine 11.8 mg/5 mL; 250 mg/5 mL contains phenylalanine 25.2 mg/5 mL.

Geriatric Considerations Adjust dose for renal function in the elderly. Considered one of the drugs of choice for outpatient treatment of community-acquired pneumonia in the older adult.

Breast-Feeding Issues Theoretically, drug absorbed by nursing infant may change bowel flora or affect fever work-up result. **Note:** As a class, cephalosporins are used to treat infections in infants.

Celecoxib (se le KOKS ib)

U.S. Brand Names Celebrex®

Restrictions A medication guide should be dispensed with each prescription. A template for the required MedGuide can be found on the FDA website at http://www.fda.gov/medwatch/SAFETY/2005/safety05.htm#NSAID

Pharmacologic Category Nonsteroidal Anti-inflammatory Drug (NSAID), COX-2 Selective

Medication Safety Issues

Sound-alike/look-alike issues:

Celebrex® may be confused with Celexa™, cerebra, Cerebyx®

Pregnancy Risk Factor C/D (3rd trimester)

Lactation Enters breast milk/not recommended (contraindicated in Canadian labeling)

Use Relief of the signs and symptoms of osteoarthritis, ankylosing spondylitis, and rheumatoid arthritis; management of acute pain; treatment of primary dysmenorrhea; decreasing intestinal polyps in familial adenomatous polyposis (FAP). **Note:** The Notice of Compliance for the use of celecoxib in FAP has been suspended by Health Canada.

Mechanism of Action/Effect Inhibits prostaglandin synthesis by decreasing the activity of the enzyme, cyclooxygenase-2 (COX-2), which results in decreased formation of prostaglandin precursors. Celecoxib does not inhibit cyclooxygenase-1 (COX-1) at therapeutic concentrations.

Contraindications Hypersensitivity to celecoxib, sulfonamides, aspirin, other NSAIDs, or any component of the formulation; perioperative pain in the setting of coronary artery bypass surgery (CABG); pregnancy (3rd trimester)

Warnings/Precautions NSAIDs are associated with an increased risk of adverse cardiovascular events, including MI, and new onset or worsening of pre-existing hypertension. Risk may be increased with duration of use or pre-existing cardiovascular risk-factors or disease. Carefully evaluate individual cardiovascular risk profiles prior to prescribing. Use caution with fluid retention, CHF, cerebrovascular disease, ischemic heart disease, or hypertension.

NSAIDs may increase risk of gastrointestinal irritation, ulceration, bleeding, and perforation. These events may occur at any time during therapy and without warning. Use caution with a history of GI disease (bleeding or ulcers), concurrent therapy with aspirin, anticoagulants and/or corticosteroids, smoking, use of alcohol, the elderly or debilitated patients.

Use the lowest effective dose for the shortest duration of time, consistent with individual patient goals, to reduce risk of cardiovascular or GI adverse events. Alternate therapies should be considered for patients at high risk.

NSAIDs may cause serious skin adverse events including exfoliative dermatitis, Stevens-Johnson syndrome (SJS), and toxic epidermal necrolysis (TEN). Anaphylactoid reactions may occur, even without prior exposure; patients with "aspirin triad" (bronchial asthma, aspirin intolerance, rhinitis) may be at increased risk. Do not use in patients who experience bronchospasm, asthma, rhinitis, or urticaria with NSAID or aspirin therapy.

(Continued)

Celecoxib *(Continued)*

Use with caution in patients with dehydration, decreased renal or hepatic function. Use of NSAIDs can compromise existing renal function especially when Cl_{cr} <30 mL/minute. Not recommended for use in severe renal or hepatic impairment.

Use caution in patients with known or suspected deficiency of cytochrome P450 isoenzyme 2C9. Safety and efficacy have not been established in patients <18 years of age.

Drug Interactions

Cytochrome P450 Effect: Substrate (minor) of CYP2C8/9, 3A4; **Inhibits** CYP2D6 (weak)

Decreased Effect: Efficacy of thiazide diuretics, loop diuretics (furosemide), ACE inhibitors, beta-blockers, and hydralazine may be diminished by celecoxib. Celecoxib may decrease excretion of vancomycin and aminoglycosides; monitor levels. Bile acid sequestrants may decrease absorption of NSAIDs.

Increased Effect/Toxicity: Fluconazole increases celecoxib concentrations twofold. Lithium and methotrexate concentrations may be increased by celecoxib. Celecoxib may be used with low-dose aspirin, however, rates of gastrointestinal bleeding may be increased with coadministration. Bleeding events (including rare intracranial hemorrhage in association with increased prothrombin time) have been reported with concomitant warfarin use; monitor closely (especially in the elderly). NSAIDs may increase levels/nephrotoxicity of cyclosporine.

Nutritional/Ethanol Interactions

Ethanol: Avoid ethanol (increased GI irritation).

Food: Peak concentrations are delayed and AUC is increased by 10% to 20% when taken with a high-fat meal.

Adverse Reactions

>10%: Central nervous system: Headache (16%)

2% to 10%:

Cardiovascular: Peripheral edema (2%)

Central nervous system: Insomnia (2%), dizziness (2%)

Dermatologic: Skin rash (2%)

Gastrointestinal: Dyspepsia (9%), diarrhea (6%), abdominal pain (4%), nausea (4%), flatulence (2%)

Neuromuscular & skeletal: Back pain (3%)

Respiratory: Upper respiratory tract infection (8%), sinusitis (5%), pharyngitis (2%), rhinitis (2%)

Miscellaneous: Accidental injury (3%)

0.1% to 2%:

Cardiovascular: Hypertension (aggravated), chest pain, MI, palpitation, tachycardia, facial edema

Central nervous system: Migraine, vertigo, hypoesthesia, fatigue, fever, pain, hypotonia, anxiety, depression, nervousness, somnolence

Dermatologic: Alopecia, dermatitis, photosensitivity, pruritus, rash (maculopapular), rash (erythematous), dry skin, urticaria

Endocrine & metabolic: Hot flashes, diabetes mellitus, hyperglycemia, hypercholesterolemia, breast pain, dysmenorrhea, menstrual disturbances, hypokalemia .

Gastrointestinal: Constipation, tenesmus, diverticulitis, eructation, esophagitis, gastroenteritis, vomiting, gastroesophageal reflux, hemorrhoids, hiatal hernia, melena, stomatitis, anorexia, increased appetite, taste disturbance, dry mouth, tooth disorder, weight gain

Genitourinary: Prostate disorder, vaginal bleeding, vaginitis, monilial vaginitis, dysuria, cystitis, urinary frequency, incontinence, urinary tract infection.

Hematologic: Anemia, thrombocytopenia, ecchymosis

Hepatic: Alkaline phosphatase increased, transaminases increased

Neuromuscular & skeletal: Leg cramps, increased CPK, neck stiffness, arthralgia, myalgia, bone

disorder, fracture, synovitis, tendonitis, neuralgia, paresthesia, neuropathy, weakness

Ocular: Glaucoma, blurred vision, cataract, conjunctivitis, eye pain

Otic: Deafness, tinnitus, earache, otitis media

Renal: Increased BUN, increased creatinine, albuminuria, hematuria, renal calculi

Respiratory: Bronchitis, bronchospasm, cough, dyspnea, laryngitis, pneumonia, epistaxis

Miscellaneous: Allergic reactions, diaphoresis increased, flu-like syndrome, breast cancer, herpes infection, bacterial infection, moniliasis, viral infection

Overdosage/Toxicology Doses up to 2400 mg/day for up to 10 days have been reported without serious toxicity. Symptoms of overdose may include epigastric pain, drowsiness, lethargy, nausea, and vomiting; gastrointestinal bleeding may occur. Rare manifestations include hypertension, respiratory depression, coma, and acute renal failure. Treatment is symptomatic and supportive. Forced diuresis, hemodialysis and/or urinary alkalinization may not be useful.

Pharmacodynamics/Kinetics

Time to Peak: 3 hours

Protein Binding: 97% to albumin

Half-Life Elimination: 11 hours (fasted)

Metabolism: Hepatic via CYP2C9; forms inactive metabolites

Excretion: Urine (27% as metabolites, <3% as unchanged drug); feces (57%)

Available Dosage Forms Capsule: 100 mg, 200 mg, 400 mg

Dosing

Adults:

Osteoarthritis: Oral: 200 mg/day as a single dose or in divided dose twice daily

Ankylosing spondylitis: Oral: 200 mg/day as a single dose or in divided doses twice daily; if no effect after 6 weeks, may increase to 400 mg/day. If no response following 6 weeks of treatment with 400 mg/day, consider discontinuation and alternative treatment.

Rheumatoid arthritis: Oral: 100-200 mg twice daily

Familial adenomatous polyposis: Oral: 400 mg twice daily

Acute pain or primary dysmenorrhea: Oral: Initial dose: 400 mg, followed by an additional 200 mg if needed on day 1; maintenance dose: 200 mg twice daily as needed

Elderly: Refer to adult dosing. No specific adjustment is recommended. However, the AUC in elderly patients may be increased by 50% as compared to younger subjects. Use the lowest recommended dose in patients weighing <50 kg.

Renal Impairment: No specific dosage adjustment is recommended. Not recommended in patients with advanced renal disease.

Hepatic Impairment: Reduced dosage is recommended (AUC may be increased by 40% to 180%). Decrease dose by 50% in patients with moderate hepatic impairment (Child-Pugh class B).

Stability

Storage: Store at controlled room temperature of 25°C (77°F).

Nursing Actions

Physical Assessment: Assess effectiveness and interactions of other medications patient may be taking (ie, monitor patients taking lithium closely). Assess allergy history (aspirin, NSAIDs, salicylates). Monitor blood pressure at the beginning of therapy and periodically during use. Monitor effectiveness of therapy (pain, range of motion, mobility, ADL function, inflammation). Assess knowledge/teach patient appropriate use, possible side effects/interventions, and adverse symptoms to report.

Patient Education: Do not take more than recommended dose. May be taken with food to reduce GI upset. Do not take with antacids. Avoid alcohol, aspirin, and OTC medication unless approved by prescriber. You may experience dizziness, confusion, or blurred vision (avoid driving or engaging in tasks requiring alertness until response to drug is known); anorexia, nausea, vomiting, taste disturbance, gastric distress (small frequent meals, frequent mouth care, sucking lozenges, or chewing gum may help). GI bleeding, ulceration, or perforation can occur with or without pain. It is unclear whether celecoxib has rates of these events which are similar to nonselective NSAIDs. Stop taking medication and report immediately stomach pain or cramping; unusual bleeding or bruising (blood in vomitus, stool, or urine). Report persistent insomnia; skin rash; unusual fatigue, muscle pain, tremors, or weakness; sudden weight gain or edema; chest pain; shortness of breath; changes in hearing (ringing in ears) or vision; changes in urination pattern; or respiratory difficulty. **Pregnancy/breast-feeding precautions:** Inform your prescriber if you are or intend to become pregnant. This drug should not be used in the 3rd trimester of pregnancy. Breast-feeding is not recommended.

Dietary Considerations Lower doses (200 mg twice daily) may be taken without regard to meals. Larger doses should be taken with food to improve absorption.

Geriatric Considerations The elderly are at increased risk for adverse effects from NSAIDs. As many as 60% of elderly can develop peptic ulceration and/or hemorrhage asymptomatically. CNS adverse effects such as confusion, agitation, and hallucination are generally seen in overdose or high-dose situations; however, elderly patients may demonstrate these adverse effects at lower doses than younger adults. The elderly are also at increased risk of renal toxicity.

Breast-Feeding Issues Based on limited data, celecoxib has been found to be excreted in milk; a decision should be made whether to discontinue nursing or discontinue the drug, taking into account the importance of the drug to the mother.

Pregnancy Issues In late pregnancy, this drug may cause premature closure of the ductus arteriosus.

Cephalexin (sef a LEKS in)

U.S. Brand Names Biocef®; Keflex®; Panixine DisperDose™ [DSC]

Synonyms Cephalexin Monohydrate

Pharmacologic Category Antibiotic, Cephalosporin (First Generation)

Medication Safety Issues
Sound-alike/look-alike issues:
Cephalexin may be confused with cefaclor, cefazolin, cephalothin, ciprofloxacin

Pregnancy Risk Factor B

Lactation Enters breast milk (small amounts)/use caution

Use Treatment of susceptible bacterial infections including respiratory tract infections, otitis media, skin and skin structure infections, bone infections and genitourinary tract infections, including acute prostatitis; alternative therapy for acute bacterial endocarditis prophylaxis

Mechanism of Action/Effect Inhibits bacterial cell wall synthesis by binding to one or more of the penicillin-binding proteins (PBPs)

Contraindications Hypersensitivity to cephalexin, any component of the formulation, or other cephalosporins

Warnings/Precautions Modify dosage in patients with severe renal impairment, prolonged use may result in superinfection; use with caution in patients with a history of penicillin allergy, especially IgE-mediated reactions

(eg, anaphylaxis, urticaria). May cause antibiotic-associated colitis or colitis secondary to *C. difficile*.

Drug Interactions
Increased Effect/Toxicity: High-dose probenecid may decrease clearance of cephalexin. Aminoglycosides in combination with cephalexin may result in additive nephrotoxicity.

Nutritional/Ethanol Interactions Food: Peak antibiotic serum concentration is lowered and delayed, but total drug absorbed is not affected. Cephalexin serum levels may be decreased if taken with food.

Lab Interactions Positive direct Coombs', false-positive urinary glucose test using cupric sulfate (Benedict's solution, Clinitest®, Fehling's solution), false-positive serum or urine creatinine with Jaffé reaction

Adverse Reactions Frequency not defined.
Central nervous system: Agitation, confusion, dizziness, fatigue, hallucinations, headache
Dermatologic: Angioedema, erythema multiforme (rare), rash, Stevens-Johnson syndrome (rare), toxic epidermal necrolysis (rare), urticaria
Gastrointestinal: Abdominal pain, diarrhea, dyspepsia, gastritis, nausea (rare), pseudomembranous colitis, vomiting (rare)
Genitourinary: Genital pruritus, genital moniliasis, vaginitis, vaginal discharge
Hematologic: Eosinophilia, neutropenia, thrombocytopenia
Hepatic: AST/ALT increased, cholestatic jaundice (rare), transient hepatitis (rare)
Neuromuscular & skeletal: Arthralgia, arthritis, joint disorder
Renal: Interstitial nephritis (rare)
Miscellaneous: Allergic reactions

Overdosage/Toxicology Symptoms of overdose include epigastric distress, diarrhea, hematuria, nausea, and vomiting. Many beta-lactam containing antibiotics have the potential to cause neuromuscular hyperirritability or seizures. Hemodialysis may be helpful to aid in removal of the drug from blood; otherwise, treatment is supportive and symptom-directed.

Pharmacodynamics/Kinetics
Time to Peak: Serum: ~1 hour
Protein Binding: 6% to 15%
Half-Life Elimination: Adults: 0.5-1.2 hours; prolonged with renal impairment
Excretion: Urine (80% to 100% as unchanged drug) within 8 hours

Available Dosage Forms [DSC] = Discontinued product
Capsule: 250 mg, 500 mg
Biocef®: 500 mg
Keflex®: 250 mg, 500 mg
Powder for oral suspension: 125 mg/5 mL (100 mL, 200 mL); 250 mg/5 mL (100 mL, 200 mL)
Biocef®: 125 mg/5 mL (100 mL); 250 mg/5 mL (100 mL)
Keflex®: 125 mg/5 mL (100 mL, 200 mL); 250 mg/5 mL (100 mL, 200 mL)
Tablet, for oral suspension (Panixine DisperDose™): 125 mg [contains phenylalanine 2.8 mg; peppermint flavor], 250 mg [contains phenylalanine 5.6 mg; peppermint flavor] [DSC]

Dosing
Adults & Elderly:
Dosing range: Oral: 250-1000 mg every 6 hours (maximum: 4 g/day)
Cellulitis and mastitis: Oral 500 mg every 6 hours
Furunculosis/skin abscess: Oral: 250 mg 4 times/day
Prophylaxis of bacterial endocarditis (dental, oral, respiratory tract, or esophageal procedures): Oral: 2 g 1 hour prior to procedure
Streptococcal pharyngitis, skin and skin structure infections: Oral: 500 mg every 12 hours
(Continued)

Cephalexin *(Continued)*

Uncomplicated cystitis: Oral: 500 mg every 12 hours for 7-14 days

Pediatrics:

Usual dose: Oral: Children >1 year: Dosing range: 25-100 mg/kg/day in divided doses every 6-8 hours (maximum: 4 g/day)

Furunculosis: Oral: 25-50 mg/kg/day in 4 divided doses

Impetigo: Oral: 25 mg/kg/day in 4 divided doses

Otitis media: 75-100 mg/kg/day in 4 divided doses

Prophylaxis of bacterial endocarditis (dental, oral, respiratory tract, or esophageal procedures): 50 mg/kg 1 hour prior to procedure (maximum: 2 g)

Severe infections: Oral: 50-100 mg/kg/day in divided doses every 6-8 hours

Skin abscess: Oral: 50 mg/kg/day in 4 divided doses (maximum 4 g)

Streptococcal pharyngitis, skin and skin structure infections: 25-50 mg/kg/day divided every 12 hours

Uncomplicated cystitis: Children >15 years: Refer to adult dosing.

Renal Impairment:

Cl_{cr} <10 mL/minute: Adults: 250-500 mg every 12 hours

Hemodialysis: Moderately dialyzable (20% to 50%)

Administration

Oral: Take without regard to food. If GI distress, take with food. Give around-the-clock to promote less variation in peak and trough serum levels.

Panixine DisperDose™: Tablets should be mixed in ~10 mL of water immediately prior to administration. Drink entire solution, then rinse glass with additional water and drink contents to ensure entire dose has been taken. Tablets should not be chewed or swallowed whole.

Stability

Reconstitution: Tablets for oral suspension (Panixine DisperDose™): Tablets must be dissolved in ~10 mL water prior to administration.

Storage: Refrigerate suspension after reconstitution; discard after 14 days. Tablets for suspension should be used immediately after dissolving.

Laboratory Monitoring Renal, hepatic, and hematologic function periodically with prolonged therapy; perform culture and sensitivity studies prior to initiating drug therapy.

Nursing Actions

Physical Assessment: Assess results of culture/sensitivity tests and patient's allergy history prior to therapy. Assess other pharmacological or herbal products patient may be taking for potential interactions (eg, nephrotoxicity). Monitor laboratory tests, therapeutic response, and adverse reactions (see Adverse Reactions). Advise patients with diabetes about use of Clinitest® (may cause false-positive test). Teach patient possible side effects/appropriate interventions and adverse symptoms to report (eg, opportunistic infection, hypersensitivity reaction).

Patient Education: Do not take any new medication during therapy unless approved by prescriber. Take as directed, at regular intervals around-the-clock (with or without food). Take complete prescription even if feeling better. Maintain adequate hydration (2-3 L/day of fluids) unless instructed to restrict fluid intake. May cause false test results with Clinitest®; use of another type of glucose testing is preferable. May cause diarrhea (yogurt, boiled milk, or buttermilk may help). Report rash; breathing or swallowing difficulty; persistent diarrhea, nausea, vomiting, or abdominal pain; changes in urinary pattern or pain on urination; opportunistic infection (eg, vaginal itching or drainage, sores in mouth, blood in stool or urine, unusual fever

or chills); CNS changes (eg, irritability, agitation, nervousness, insomnia, hallucinations); or other adverse reactions. **Breast-feeding precaution:** Consult prescriber if breast-feeding.

Dietary Considerations Take without regard to food. If GI distress, take with food. Panixine DisperDose™ contains phenylalanine 2.8 mg/cephalexin 125 mg.

Geriatric Considerations Adjust dose for renal function.

Breast-Feeding Issues Theoretically, drug absorbed by nursing infant may change bowel flora or affect fever work-up result. Cephalexin levels can be detected in breast milk, reaching a maximum concentration 4 hours after a single oral dose and gradually decreasing by 8 hours after administration. **Note:** As a class, cephalosporins are used to treat bacterial infections in infants.

Cephradine *(SEF ra deen)*

U.S. Brand Names Velosef®

Pharmacologic Category Antibiotic, Cephalosporin (First Generation)

Medication Safety Issues

Sound-alike/look-alike issues:

Cephradine may be confused with cephapirin

Velosef® may be confused with Vasosulf®

Pregnancy Risk Factor B

Lactation Enters breast milk/use caution

Use Treatment of infections when caused by susceptible strains in respiratory, genitourinary, gastrointestinal, skin and soft tissue, bone and joint infections; treatment of susceptible gram-positive bacilli and cocci (never enterococcus); some gram-negative bacilli including *E. coli, Proteus,* and *Klebsiella* may be susceptible

Mechanism of Action/Effect Inhibits bacterial cell wall synthesis by binding to one or more of the penicillin-binding proteins (PBPs)

Contraindications Hypersensitivity to cephradine, any component of the formulation, or cephalosporins

Warnings/Precautions Use caution with renal impairment; dose adjustment required. Prolonged use may result in superinfection; use with caution in patients with a history of penicillin allergy, especially IgE-mediated reactions (eg, anaphylaxis, urticaria). May cause antibiotic-associated colitis or colitis secondary to *C. difficile.*

Drug Interactions

Increased Effect/Toxicity: High-dose probenecid decreases clearance of cephradine. Aminoglycosides in combination with cephradine may result in additive nephrotoxicity.

Nutritional/Ethanol Interactions Food: Food delays cephradine absorption but does not decrease extent.

Lab Interactions Positive direct Coombs', false-positive urinary glucose test using cupric sulfate (Benedict's solution, Clinitest®, Fehling's solution), false-positive serum or urine creatinine with Jaffé reaction

Adverse Reactions Frequency not defined.

Central nervous system: Dizziness

Dermatologic: Rash, pruritus

Gastrointestinal: Diarrhea, nausea, vomiting, pseudomembranous colitis

Hematologic: Leukopenia, neutropenia, eosinophilia

Neuromuscular & skeletal: Joint pain

Renal: BUN increased, creatinine increased

Reactions reported with other cephalosporins include anaphylaxis, erythema multiforme, toxic epidermal necrolysis, Stevens-Johnson syndrome, fever, headache, encephalopathy, asterixis, neuromuscular excitability, seizure, agranulocytosis, pancytopenia, aplastic anemia, hemolytic anemia, interstitial nephritis, toxic nephropathy, vaginitis, angioedema, cholestasis, hemorrhage, prolonged PT, serum-sickness reactions, superinfection

Overdosage/Toxicology Symptoms of overdose include neuromuscular hypersensitivity and convulsions. Many beta-lactam containing antibiotics have the potential to cause neuromuscular hyperirritability or convulsive seizures. Hemodialysis may be helpful to aid in removal of the drug from blood; otherwise, treatment is supportive or symptom-directed.

Pharmacodynamics/Kinetics

Time to Peak: Serum: 1-2 hours

Protein Binding: 18% to 20%

Half-Life Elimination: 1-2 hours; prolonged with renal impairment

Excretion: Urine (~80% to 90% as unchanged drug) within 6 hours

Available Dosage Forms [DSC] = Discontinued product

Capsule: 250 mg, 500 mg [DSC]

Powder for oral suspension: 250 mg/5 mL (100 mL) [fruit flavor]

Dosing

Adults & Elderly:

Susceptible infections, usual dose: Oral: 250-500 mg every 6-12 hours

Pediatrics:

Usual dose: Oral: Children ≥9 months: 25-100 mg/kg/day in divided doses every 6 or 12 hours (maximum: 4 g/day)

Otitis media: Oral: Children ≥9 months: 75-100 mg/kg/day in divided doses every 6 or 12 hours (maximum: 4 g/day)

Renal Impairment:

Cl_{cr} 10-50 mL/minute: Administer 50% of dose.

Cl_{cr} <10 mL/minute: Administer 25% of dose.

Administration

Oral: Administer around-the-clock to promote less variation in peak and trough serum levels. Shake oral suspension well.

Stability

Storage:

Capsule: Store at controlled room temperature.

Powder for oral suspension: Store at controlled room temperature. Following reconstitution, refrigerated storage of oral suspension maintains potency for 14 days. Room temperature storage maintains potency for 7 days.

Laboratory Monitoring Perform culture and sensitivity studies prior to initiating drug therapy; renal function

Nursing Actions

Physical Assessment: Assess results of culture/sensitivity tests and patient's allergy history prior to therapy. Assess other pharmacological or herbal products patient may be taking for potential interactions (eg, nephrotoxicity). Monitor laboratory tests, therapeutic response, and adverse effects (see Adverse Reactions). Advise patients with diabetes about use of Clinitest® (may cause false-positive test). Teach patient possible side effects/appropriate interventions and adverse symptoms to report (eg, opportunistic infection, hypersensitivity reaction).

Patient Education: Do not take any new medication during therapy unless approved by prescriber. Take as directed, at regular intervals around-the-clock (with or without food). Take complete prescription even if feeling better. Chilling oral suspension improves flavor (do not freeze). Maintain adequate hydration (2-3 L/day of fluids) unless instructed to restrict fluid intake. May cause false test results with Clinitest®; use of another type of glucose testing is preferable. May cause diarrhea (yogurt, boiled milk, or buttermilk may help). Report rash; breathing or swallowing difficulty;

persistent diarrhea, nausea, vomiting, or abdominal pain; changes in urinary pattern or pain on urination; opportunistic infection (eg, vaginal itching or drainage, sores in mouth, blood in stool or urine, unusual fever or chills); CNS changes (eg, irritability, agitation, nervousness, insomnia, hallucinations); or other adverse reactions. **Breast-feeding precaution:** Consult prescriber if breast-feeding.

Dietary Considerations May administer with food to decrease GI distress.

Geriatric Considerations Cephradine has not been studied in the elderly. Adjust dose for renal function in the elderly.

Breast-Feeding Issues Theoretically, drug absorbed by nursing infant may change bowel flora or affect fever work-up result. **Note:** As a class, cephalosporins are used to treat infections in infants.

Cetirizine (se TI ra zeen)

U.S. Brand Names Zyrtec®

Synonyms Cetirizine Hydrochloride; P-071; UCB-P071

Pharmacologic Category Antihistamine

Medication Safety Issues

Sound-alike/look-alike issues:

Zyrtec® may be confused with Serax®, Xanax®, Zantac®, Zyprexa®

Pregnancy Risk Factor B

Lactation Enters breast milk/not recommended

Use Perennial and seasonal allergic rhinitis and other allergic symptoms including urticaria; chronic idiopathic urticaria

Mechanism of Action/Effect Competes with histamine for H_1-receptor sites on effector cells in the GI tract, blood vessels, and respiratory tract

Contraindications Hypersensitivity to cetirizine, hydroxyzine, or any component of the formulation

Warnings/Precautions Cetirizine should be used cautiously in patients with hepatic or renal dysfunction, or the elderly. May cause drowsiness, use caution performing tasks which require alertness (eg, operating machinery or driving). Safety and efficacy in pediatric patients <6 months of age have not been established.

Drug Interactions

Cytochrome P450 Effect: Substrate of CYP3A4 (minor)

Increased Effect/Toxicity: Increased toxicity with CNS depressants and anticholinergics.

Nutritional/Ethanol Interactions Ethanol: Avoid ethanol (may increase CNS depression).

Adverse Reactions

>10%: Central nervous system: Headache (children 11% to 14%, placebo 12%), somnolence (adults 14%, children 2% to 4%)

2% to 10%:

Central nervous system: Insomnia (children 9%, adults <2%), fatigue (adults 6%), malaise (4%), dizziness (adults 2%)

Gastrointestinal: Abdominal pain (children 4% to 6%), dry mouth (adults 5%), diarrhea (children 2% to 3%), nausea (children 2% to 3%, placebo 2%), vomiting (children 2% to 3%)

Respiratory: Epistaxis (children 2% to 4%, placebo 3%), pharyngitis (children 3% to 6%, placebo 3%), bronchospasm (children 2% to 3%, placebo 2%)

Overdosage/Toxicology Symptoms of overdose may include somnolence, restlessness, or irritability. Treatment is symptomatic and supportive. Cetirizine is not removed by dialysis.

(Continued)

Cetirizine (Continued)

Pharmacodynamics/Kinetics
Onset of Action: 15-30 minutes
Time to Peak: Serum: 1 hour
Half-Life Elimination: 8 hours
Metabolism: Limited hepatic
Excretion: Urine (70%); feces (10%)

Available Dosage Forms
Syrup, as hydrochloride: 5 mg/5 mL (120 mL, 480 mL) [banana-grape flavor]
Tablet, as hydrochloride: 5 mg, 10 mg
Tablet, chewable, as hydrochloride: 5 mg, 10 mg [grape flavor]

Dosing
Adults: Perennial or seasonal allergic rhinitis, chronic urticaria: Oral: 5-10 mg once daily, depending upon symptom severity

Elderly: Oral: Initial: 5 mg once daily; may increase to 10 mg/day
  Note: Manufacturer recommends 5 mg/day in patients ≥77 years of age.

Pediatrics:
  Perennial allergic rhinitis, chronic urticaria: Oral: Children:
    6-12 months: 2.5 mg once daily
    12 months to <2 years: 2.5 mg once daily; may increase to 2.5 mg every 12 hours if needed
  Perennial or seasonal allergic rhinitis, chronic urticaria: Oral: Children:
    2-5 years: Initial: 2.5 mg once daily; may be increased to 2.5 mg every 12 hours or 5 mg once daily
    ≥6 years Refer to adult dosing.

Renal Impairment:
  Children <6 years: Cetirizine use not recommended.
  Children 6-11 years: <2.5 mg once daily
  Children ≥12 and Adults:
    Cl_{cr} 11-31 mL/minute or hemodialysis: Administer 5 mg once daily
    Cl_{cr} <11 mL/minute, not on dialysis: Cetirizine use not recommended.

Hepatic Impairment:
  Children <6 years: Cetirizine use not recommended.
  Children 6-11 years: <2.5 mg once daily
  Children ≥12 and Adults: Administer 5 mg once daily

Administration
Oral: May be administered with or without food.

Stability
Storage:
  Syrup: Store at room temperature of 15°C to 30°C (59°F to 86°F), or under refrigeration at 2°C to 8°C (36°F to 46°F).
  Tablet: Store at room temperature of 15°C to 30°C (59°F to 86°F).

Nursing Actions
Physical Assessment: Assess effectiveness and interactions of other medications patient may be taking. Monitor effectiveness of therapy and adverse reactions at beginning of therapy and periodically with long-term use. Assess knowledge/teach patient appropriate use, interventions to reduce side effects, and adverse symptoms to report. Breast-feeding is not recommended.

Patient Education: Take as directed; do not exceed recommended dose. Avoid use of other depressants, alcohol, or sleep-inducing medications unless approved by prescriber. You may experience drowsiness or dizziness (use caution when driving or engaging in tasks requiring alertness until response to drug is known); or dry mouth (frequent small meals, frequent mouth care, chewing gum, or sucking hard candy may help). Report persistent sedation, confusion, or agitation; persistent nausea or vomiting;

changes in urinary pattern; blurred vision; chest pain or palpitations; persistent headaches; or lack of improvement or worsening of condition.
Breast-feeding precaution: Breast-feeding is not recommended.

Dietary Considerations May be taken with or without food.

Geriatric Considerations Adjust dose for renal function.

Cetrorelix (set roe REL iks)

U.S. Brand Names Cetrotide®
Synonyms Cetrorelix Acetate
Pharmacologic Category Gonadotropin Releasing Hormone Antagonist
Pregnancy Risk Factor X
Lactation Excretion in breast milk unknown/not recommended
Use Inhibits premature luteinizing hormone (LH) surges in women undergoing controlled ovarian stimulation
Mechanism of Action/Effect Competes with naturally occurring GnRH for binding on receptors of the pituitary. This delays luteinizing hormone surge, preventing ovulation until the follicles are of adequate size.
Contraindications Hypersensitivity to cetrorelix or any component of the formulation; extrinsic peptide hormones, mannitol, gonadotropin releasing hormone (GnRH) or GnRH analogs; severe renal impairment; pregnancy
Warnings/Precautions Should only be prescribed by fertility specialists. Monitor carefully after first injection for possible hypersensitivity reactions. Use caution in women with active allergic conditions or a history of allergies; use in women with severe allergic conditions is not recommended. Pregnancy should be excluded before treatment is begun.

Drug Interactions
Decreased Effect: No formal studies have been performed.
Increased Effect/Toxicity: No formal studies have been performed.

Adverse Reactions
1% to 10%:
  Central nervous system: Headache (1%)
  Endocrine & metabolic: Ovarian hyperstimulation syndrome, WHO grade II or III (4%)
  Gastrointestinal: Nausea (1%)
  Hepatic: Increased ALT, AST, GGT, and alkaline phosphatase (1% to 2%)

Overdosage/Toxicology No cases of overdose have been reported. In nonfertility studies, single doses of up to 120 mg have been well tolerated.

Pharmacodynamics/Kinetics
Onset of Action: 0.25 mg dose: 2 hours; 3 mg dose: 1 hour
Duration of Action: 3 mg dose (single dose): 4 days
Time to Peak: 0.25 mg dose: 1 hour; 3 mg dose: 1.5 hours
Protein Binding: 86%
Half-Life Elimination: 0.25 mg dose: 5 hours; 0.25 mg multiple doses: 20.6 hours; 3 mg dose: 62.8 hours
Metabolism: Transformed by peptidases; cetrorelix and peptides (1-9), (1-7), (1-6), and (1-4) are found in the bile; peptide (1-4) is the predominant metabolite
Excretion: Feces (5% to 10% as unchanged drug and metabolites); urine (2% to 4% as unchanged drug); within 24 hours

Available Dosage Forms Injection, powder for reconstitution: 0.25 mg, 3 mg [supplied with SWFI in prefilled syringe]

Dosing

Adults:

Controlled ovarian stimulation in conjunction with gonadotropins (FSH, HMG): Female: SubQ:

Single-dose regimen: 3 mg given when serum estradiol levels show appropriate stimulation response, usually stimulation day 7 (range days 5-9). If hCG is not administered within 4 days, continue cetrorelix at 0.25 mg/day until hCG is administered

Multiple-dose regimen: 0.25 mg morning or evening of stimulation day 5, or morning of stimulation day 6; continue until hCG is administered.

Elderly: Not intended for use in women ≥65 years of age (Phase 2 and Phase 3 studies included women 19-40 years of age).

Renal Impairment:

Severe impairment: Use is contraindicated.

Mild-to-moderate impairment: No specific guidelines are available.

Administration

Other: Cetrorelix is administered by SubQ injection following proper aseptic technique procedures. Injections should be to the lower abdomen, preferably around the navel (but staying at least 1 inch from the navel). The injection site should be rotated daily. The needle should be inserted completely into the skin at a 45-degree angle.

Stability

Storage: Store in outer carton. Once mixed, solution should be used immediately.

0.25 mg vials: Store under refrigeration at 2°C to 8°C (36°F to 46°F).

3 mg vials: Store at controlled room temperature at 25°C (77°F).

Nursing Actions

Physical Assessment: This medication should only be prescribed by a fertility specialist. Teach patient proper use if self-administered (appropriate injection technique and syringe/needle disposal), possible side effects/appropriate interventions, and adverse symptoms to report. **Pregnancy risk factor X:** Pregnancy must be excluded before starting medication. Breast-feeding is not recommended.

Patient Education: This drug can only be given by injection as demonstrated. An instructional leaflet will be provided if you will be administering this medication to yourself. Instructions will be given on how to administer SubQ injections and proper disposal of syringes and needles. Give at a similar time each day as instructed by prescriber. Do not skip any doses. If you miss an injection, do not double next dose; contact your prescriber. You must keep all scheduled ultrasound appointments. Store in refrigerator in outer carton. Solution should be used immediately after mixing. You may experience headache (use of mild analgesic may help); or nausea (small frequent meals, good mouth care, chewing gum, or sucking hard candy may help). Report immediately any sudden or acute abdominal pain; shortness of breath; vaginal bleeding; or pain, itching, or signs of infection at injection site. **Pregnancy/breast-feeding precautions:** Do not get pregnant while taking this drug. Breast-feeding is not recommended.

Pregnancy Issues Animal studies have shown fetal resorption and implantation losses following administration. Resorption resulting in fetal loss would be expected if used in a pregnant woman.

Cetuximab (se TUK see mab)

U.S. Brand Names Erbitux®

Synonyms C225; IMC-C225; NSC-714692

Pharmacologic Category Antineoplastic Agent, Monoclonal Antibody; Epidermal Growth Factor Receptor (EGFR) Inhibitor

Medication Safety Issues

Sound-alike/look-alike issues:

Cetuximab may be confused with bevacizumab

Pregnancy Risk Factor C

Lactation Excretion in breast milk is unknown/not recommended

Use Treatment of metastatic colorectal cancer; treatment of squamous cell cancer of the head and neck

Unlabeled/Investigational Use Breast cancer, tumors overexpressing EGFR

Mechanism of Action/Effect Inhibits cell growth, induces apoptosis and decreases matrix metalloproteinase and vascular endothelial growth factor production.

Contraindications Hypersensitivity to cetuximab, murine proteins, or any component of the formulation

Warnings/Precautions Severe infusion reactions (bronchospasm, stridor, hoarseness, urticaria, hypotension, cardiac arrest) have been reported in ~3% of patients (~90% with the first infusion despite the use of prophylactic antihistamines). **Note:** Although a 20 mg test dose was used in some studies, it did not reliably predict the risk of an infusion reaction, and is not recommended. In case of severe reaction, treatment should be stopped and permanently discontinued. Immediate treatment for anaphylactic/anaphylactoid reactions should be available during administration. Patients should be monitored for at least 1 hour following completion of infusion, or longer if a reaction occurs. Mild-to-moderate infusion reactions (chills, fever, dyspnea) are managed by slowing the infusion rate and administering antihistamines.

Cardiopulmonary arrest has been reported in patients receiving radiation therapy in combination with cetuximab; use caution with history of coronary artery disease, CHF, and arrhythmias. Close monitoring of serum electrolytes (magnesium, potassium, calcium) during and after cetuximab therapy is recommended. Interstitial lung disease (ILD) has been reported; use caution with pre-existing lung disease. Dermatologic toxicities have been reported, including a 90% incidence of acneform rash (may require dose modification); sunlight may exacerbate skin reactions. Dermatologic toxicities should be treated with topical and/or oral antibiotics; topical corticosteroids are not recommended. Non-neutralizing anticetuximab antibodies were detected in 5% of evaluable patients. Relationship between the appearance of antibodies and the safety or antitumor activity of the molecule is unknown. Safety and efficacy in children have not been established.

Drug Interactions

Increased Effect/Toxicity: Interactions have not been evaluated in clinical trials.

Adverse Reactions Except where noted, percentages reported for cetuximab monotherapy.

>10%:

Central nervous system: Malaise (48%), pain (17% to 28%), fever (5% to 27%), headache (26%)

Dermatologic: Acneform rash (76% to 90%; grades 3/4: 1% to 8%), nail disorder (16%), pruritus (11%)

Endocrine & metabolic: Hypomagnesemia (50%; grades 3/4: 10% to 15%)

Gastrointestinal: Nausea (mild to moderate 29%), weight loss (7% to 27%), constipation (26%), abdominal pain (26%), diarrhea (25%), vomiting (25%), anorexia (23%)

Neuromuscular & skeletal: Weakness (45% to 48%)

(Continued)

Cetuximab *(Continued)*

Respiratory: Dyspnea (17%), cough (11%)

Miscellaneous: Infusion reaction (19% to 21%; grades 3/4: 2% to 4%; 90% with first infusion), infection (14%)

1% to 10%:

Cardiovascular: Peripheral edema (10%), cardiopulmonary arrest (2%; with radiation therapy)

Central nervous system: Insomnia (10%), depression (7%)

Dermatologic: Alopecia (4%), skin disorder (4%)

Endocrine & metabolic: Dehydration (2% to 10%)

Gastrointestinal: Stomatitis (10%), dyspepsia (6%)

Hematologic: Anemia (9%)

Hepatic: Alkaline phosphatase increased (5% to 10%), transaminases increased (5% to 10%)

Neuromuscular & skeletal: Back pain (10%)

Ocular: Conjunctivitis (7%)

Renal: Kidney failure (2%)

Respiratory: Pulmonary embolus (1%)

Miscellaneous: Sepsis (3%)

Overdosage/Toxicology Single doses >500 mg/m^2 have not been tested. Treatment is symptom-directed and supportive.

Pharmacodynamics/Kinetics

Half-Life Elimination: 112 hours (range: 63-230 hours)

Available Dosage Forms Injection, solution [preservative free]: 2 mg/mL (50 mL) [contains sodium chloride 8.48 mg/mL]

Dosing

Adults & Elderly:

Colorectal cancer: I.V.:

Initial loading dose: 400 mg/m^2 infused over 120 minutes

Maintenance dose: 250 mg/m^2 infused over 60 minutes weekly

Head and neck cancer:

Initial loading dose: 400 mg/m^2 infused over 120 minutes

Maintenance dose: 250 mg/m^2 infused over 60 minutes weekly

Note: If given in combination with radiation therapy, administer loading dose 1 week prior to initiation of radiation course. Administer weekly maintenance dose 1 hour prior to radiation for the duration of radiation therapy (6-7 weeks).

Breast cancer (unlabeled use): I.V.: 50-200 mg/m^2 weekly for 6 weeks

Tumors overexpressing EGFR (unlabeled use): I.V.:

5-100 mg/m^2 weekly

or

Loading dose: 100-500 mg/m^2

Maintenance dose: 5-400 mg/m^2 weekly

Renal Impairment: No adjustment required.

Hepatic Impairment: No adjustment required.

Dosing Adjustment for Toxicity:

Infusion reactions, mild to moderate (grade 1 or 2): Permanently reduce the infusion rate by 50% and continue to use prophylactic antihistamines

Infusion reactions, severe (grade 3 or 4): Immediately and permanently discontinue treatment

Skin toxicity, mild to moderate: No dosage modification required

Acneform rash, severe (grade 3 or 4):

First occurrence: Delay cetuximab infusion 1-2 weeks

If improvement, continue at 250 mg/m^2

If no improvement, discontinue therapy

Second occurrence: Delay cetuximab infusion 1-2 weeks

If improvement, continue at 200 mg/m^2

If no improvement, discontinue therapy

Third occurrence: Delay cetuximab infusion 1-2 weeks

If improvement, continue at 150 mg/m^2

If no improvement, discontinue therapy

Fourth occurrence: Discontinue therapy

Note: Dose adjustments are not recommended for severe **radiation** dermatitis.

Administration

I.V.: I.V. infusion; loading dose over 2 hours, weekly maintenance dose over 1 hour. Do not administer as I.V. push or bolus. Do not shake or dilute. Administer via infusion pump or syringe pump. Following the infusion, an observation period is recommended; longer observation time (following an infusion reaction) may be required. Premedication with antihistamines is recommended. The maximum infusion rate is 5 mL/minute. Administer through a low protein-binding 0.22 micrometer in-line filter. Use 0.9% NaCl to flush line at the end of infusion.

I.V. Detail: pH: 7-7.4; may contain a small amount of visible white, amorphous cetuximab particles

Stability

Reconstitution: Reconstitution is not required. Appropriate dose should be added to empty sterile container; do not shake or dilute.

Storage: Store unopened vials under refrigeration at 2°C to 8°C (36°F to 46°F). Do not freeze. Preparations in infusion containers are stable for up to 12 hours under refrigeration at 2°C to 8°C (36°F to 46°F) and up to 8 hours at controlled room temperature of 20°C to 25°C (68°F to 77°F).

Laboratory Monitoring EGF receptor expression testing should be completed prior to treatment (for colorectal cancer). Periodic monitoring of serum magnesium, calcium, and potassium are recommended to continue over an interval consistent with the half-life (8 weeks); monitor closely (during and after treatment) for cetuximab plus radiation therapy.

Nursing Actions

Physical Assessment: Premedication with antihistamines may be prescribed. Monitor patient closely for infusion reaction (eg, airway obstruction, hives, hypotension) during infusion and for 1 hour following infusion: treatment for anaphylactic reactions should be available. In case of severe infusion reaction, stop infusion and notify prescriber. Assess patient response. Teach patient possible side effects/interventions and adverse symptoms to report (eg, cough, dyspnea, gastrointestinal upset, opportunistic infection).

Patient Education: Do not take any new medication during therapy unless approved by prescriber. This medication can only be administered by infusion and you will be closely monitored during each infusion; report immediately unusual chest tightness; difficulty breathing or swallowing; itching or skin rash; back pain or acute headache; or redness, swelling, or pain at infusion site. Maintain adequate hydration (2-3 L/day of fluids) unless instructed to restrict fluid intake and nutrition (small frequent meals). You may experience feelings of weakness or fatigue (adequate rest is important); nausea, vomiting, loss of appetite (small frequent meals, sucking lozenges, chewing gum may help); diarrhea (boiled milk or yogurt may help); headache or back pain (consult prescriber for appropriate analgesic); skin rash or dryness (use only mild soap, apply nonmedicated lotion, and wear protective clothing); loss of hair or nail disorder (may grow back after therapy). Report persistent gastrointestinal disturbances (pain, constipation, diarrhea, vomiting); CNS changes (depression or insomnia); skin rash, dryness, or cracking; any signs of infection; or other persistent adverse reactions. **Pregnancy/breast-feeding precautions:** Inform prescriber if you are or intend to become pregnant. Do not breast-feed during therapy or for 60 days following completion.

Dietary Considerations

Injection solution 2 mg/mL (50 mL) contains sodium chloride 8.48 mg/mL.

Breast-Feeding Issues Breast-feeding should be discontinued during treatment and for 60 days following the last dose.

Pregnancy Issues Animal reproductive studies have not been conducted. There are no adequate and well-controlled studies in pregnant women. It is not known whether cetuximab can cause fetal harm or affect reproductive capacity. Because cetuximab inhibits epidermal growth factor (EGF), a component of fetal development, adverse effects on pregnancy would be expected. Cetuximab should only be given to a pregnant woman if the potential benefit justifies the potential risk to the fetus.

Additional Information Premedication with an H_1 antagonist (eg, diphenhydramine 50 mg I.V.) is recommended. EGFR expression is detected in nearly all patients with head and neck cancer; laboratory evidence of EGFR expression is not necessary for head and neck cancers.

Cevimeline (se vi ME leen)

U.S. Brand Names Evoxac®

Synonyms Cevimeline Hydrochloride

Pharmacologic Category Cholinergic Agonist

Medication Safety Issues

Sound-alike/look-alike issues:

Evoxac® may be confused with Eurax®

Pregnancy Risk Factor C

Lactation Excretion in breast milk unknown/not recommended

Use Treatment of symptoms of dry mouth in patients with Sjögren's syndrome

Mechanism of Action/Effect Binds to muscarinic (cholinergic) receptors, causing an increase in secretion of exocrine glands (including salivary glands)

Contraindications Hypersensitivity to cevimeline or any component of the formulation; uncontrolled asthma; narrow-angle glaucoma; acute iritis; other conditions where miosis is undesirable

Warnings/Precautions May alter cardiac conduction and/or heart rate; use caution in patients with significant cardiovascular disease, including angina, myocardial infarction, or conduction disturbances. Use with caution in patients with controlled asthma, COPD, or chronic bronchitis. May cause decreased visual acuity (particularly at night and in patients with central lens changes) and impaired depth perception. May cause a variety of parasympathomimetic effects, which may be particularly dangerous in elderly patients; excessive sweating may lead to dehydration in some patients.

Use with caution in patients with a history of biliary stones or nephrolithiasis; cevimeline may precipitate cholangitis, cholecystitis, biliary obstruction, renal colic, or ureteral reflux in susceptible patients. Patients with a known or suspected deficiency of CYP2D6 may be at higher risk of adverse effects. Safety and efficacy have not been established in pediatric patients.

Drug Interactions

Cytochrome P450 Effect: Substrate (minor) of CYP2D6, CYP3A4

Decreased Effect: Anticholinergic agents (atropine, TCAs, phenothiazines) may antagonize the effects of cevimeline.

Increased Effect/Toxicity: The effects of other cholinergic agents may be increased during concurrent administration with cevimeline. Concurrent use of cevimeline and beta-blockers may increase the potential for conduction disturbances.

Adverse Reactions

>10%:

Central nervous system: Headache (14%; placebo 20%)

Gastrointestinal: Nausea (14%), diarrhea (10%)

Respiratory: Rhinitis (11%), sinusitis (12%), upper respiratory infection (11%)

Miscellaneous: Diaphoresis increased (19%)

1% to 10%:

Cardiovascular: Peripheral edema, chest pain, edema, palpitation

Central nervous system: Dizziness (4%), fatigue (3%), pain (3%), insomnia (2%), anxiety (1%), fever, depression, migraine, hypoesthesia, vertigo

Dermatologic: Rash (4%; placebo 6%), pruritus, skin disorder, erythematous rash

Endocrine & metabolic: Hot flashes (2%)

Gastrointestinal: Dyspepsia (8%; placebo 9%), abdominal pain (8%), vomiting (5%), excessive salivation (2%), constipation, salivary gland pain, dry mouth, sialoadenitis, gastroesophageal reflux, flatulence, ulcerative stomatitis, eructation, increased amylase, anorexia, tooth disorder

Genitourinary: Urinary tract infection (6%), vaginitis, cystitis

Hematologic: Anemia

Local: Abscess

Neuromuscular & skeletal: Back pain (5%), arthralgia (4%), skeletal pain (3%), rigors (1%), hypertonia, tremor, myalgia, hyporeflexia, leg cramps

Ocular: Conjunctivitis (4%), abnormal vision, eye pain, eye abnormality, xerophthalmia

Otic: Ear ache, otitis media

Respiratory: Coughing (6%), bronchitis (4%), pneumonia, epistaxis

Miscellaneous: Flu-like syndrome, infection, fungal infection, allergy, hiccups

Overdosage/Toxicology Symptoms of toxicity may include headache, visual disturbances, lacrimation, sweating, gastrointestinal spasm, nausea, vomiting, diarrhea, AV block, mental confusion, tremor, cardiac depression, bradycardia, tachycardia, or bronchospasm. Atropine may be of value as an antidote, and epinephrine may be required for bronchoconstriction. Additional treatment is supportive. The effect of hemodialysis is unknown.

Pharmacodynamics/Kinetics

Time to Peak: 1.5-2 hours

Protein Binding: <20%

Half-Life Elimination: 5 hours

Metabolism: Hepatic via CYP2D6 and CYP3A4

Excretion: Urine (as metabolites and unchanged drug)

Available Dosage Forms Capsule, as hydrochloride: 30 mg

Dosing

Adults & Elderly: Xerostomia (in Sjögren's syndrome): Oral: 30 mg 3 times/day

Stability

Storage: Store at 25°C (77°F).

Nursing Actions

Physical Assessment: Assess other medications patient may be taking for effectiveness and interactions. Monitor for therapeutic effect and adverse reactions (especially with elderly persons). Assess knowledge/teach patient appropriate use, interventions to reduce side effects, and adverse reactions to report.

Patient Education: Take exactly as directed; do not alter dosage without consulting prescriber. Take with or without food. You may experience decreased visual acuity, especially at night (use caution when driving at night or when engaging in other activities in poorly lighted areas until response to medication is known); GI distress or nausea (small frequent meals, frequent mouth care, sucking lozenges, or chewing gum may help); headache (mild analgesic may help);

(Continued)

Cevimeline *(Continued)*

or diarrhea (boiled milk, yogurt, or buttermilk may help). Report unresolved diarrhea or constipation, abdominal pain, flatulence, anorexia, or excessive salivation; excessive sweating; unresolved respiratory distress, runny nose, cold or flu symptoms; joint, bone, or muscle weakness, pain, tremor, or cramping; chest pain or palpitations, swelling of extremities, weight gain; or other persistent adverse symptoms. **Pregnancy/breast-feeding precautions:** Inform prescriber if you are or intend to become pregnant. Breast-feeding is not recommended.

Dietary Considerations Take with or without food.

Charcoal *(CHAR kole)*

U.S. Brand Names Actidose-Aqua® [OTC]; Actidose® with Sorbitol [OTC]; Char-Caps [OTC]; CharcoAid G® [OTC] [DSC]; Charcoal Plus® DS [OTC]; Charcocaps® [OTC]; EZ-Char™ [OTC]; Kerr Insta-Char® [OTC]

Synonyms Activated Carbon; Activated Charcoal; Adsorbent Charcoal; Liquid Antidote; Medicinal Carbon; Medicinal Charcoal

Pharmacologic Category Antidote

Medication Safety Issues
Sound-alike/look-alike issues:
Actidose® may be confused with Actos®

Pregnancy Risk Factor C

Lactation Does not enter breast milk/compatible

Use Emergency treatment in poisoning by drugs and chemicals; aids the elimination of certain drugs and improves decontamination of excessive ingestions of sustained-release products or in the presence of bezoars; repetitive doses have proven useful to enhance the elimination of certain drugs (eg, theophylline, phenobarbital, and aspirin); repetitive doses for gastric dialysis in uremia to adsorb various waste products; dietary supplement (digestive aid)

Mechanism of Action/Effect Adsorbs toxic substances or irritants, thus inhibiting GI absorption; adsorbs intestinal gas; the addition of sorbitol results in hyperosmotic laxative action causing catharsis

Contraindications Intestinal obstruction; GI tract not anatomically intact; patients at risk of hemorrhage or GI perforation; if use would increase risk and severity of aspiration; not effective for cyanide, mineral acids, caustic alkalis, organic solvents, iron, ethanol, methanol poisoning, lithium; do not use charcoal with sorbitol in patients with fructose intolerance; charcoal with sorbitol not recommended in children <1 year of age

Warnings/Precautions When using ipecac with charcoal, induce vomiting with ipecac before administering activated charcoal since charcoal adsorbs ipecac syrup; charcoal may cause vomiting which is hazardous in petroleum distillate and caustic ingestions; if charcoal in sorbitol is administered, doses should be limited to prevent excessive fluid and electrolyte losses. Use caution with decreased peristalsis. Most effective when administered within 1 hour of ingestion for most ingestions.

Drug Interactions
Decreased Effect: Charcoal decreases the effect of ipecac syrup.

Nutritional/Ethanol Interactions Food: Do not mix with milk, ice cream, sherbet, or marmalade (may reduce charcoal's effectiveness).

Adverse Reactions Frequency not defined.
Endocrine & metabolic: Hypernatremia, hypokalemia, and hypermagnesemia may occur with coadministration of cathartics
Gastrointestinal: Vomiting (incidence may increase with sorbitol), diarrhea (with sorbitol), constipation, swelling of abdomen, bowel obstruction

Miscellaneous: Fecal discoloration (black)

Pharmacodynamics/Kinetics
Excretion: Feces (as charcoal)

Available Dosage Forms [DSC] = Discontinued product

Capsule, activated (Char-Caps, Charcocaps®): 260 mg
Granules, activated (CharcoAid G®): 15 g (120 mL) [DSC]
Liquid, activated:
Actidose-Aqua®: 15 g (72 mL); 25 g (120 mL); 50 g (240 mL)
Kerr Insta-Char®: 25 g (120 mL) [cherry flavor]; 50 g (240 mL) [unflavored or cherry flavor]
Liquid, activated [with sorbitol]:
Actidose® with Sorbitol: 25 g (120 mL); 50 g (240 mL)
Kerr Insta-Char®: 25 g (120 mL); 50 g (240 mL) [cherry flavor]
Pellets, activated (EZ-Char™): 25 g
Powder for suspension, activated: 30 g, 240 g
Tablets, activated (Charcoal Plus® DS): 250 mg

Dosing
Adults & Elderly:
Acute poisoning:
Oral: 25-100 g as a single dose; if multiple doses are needed, additional doses may be given as 12.5 g/hour or equivalent (ie, 25 g every 2 hours)
Note: ~10 g of activated charcoal for each 1 g of toxin is considered adequate; this may require multiple doses. If sorbitol is also used, sorbitol dose should not exceed 1.5 g/kg. When using multiple doses of charcoal, sorbitol should be given with every other dose (not to exceed 2 doses/day)
Dietary supplement: Oral: 500-520 mg after meals; may repeat in 2 hours if needed (maximum 10 g/day)

Pediatrics:
Acute poisoning: Oral:
Children: 1 g/kg as a single dose; if multiple doses are needed, additional doses can be given as 0.25 g/kg every hour or equivalent (ie, 0.5 g/kg every 2 hours) **or**
>1 year to 12 years: 25-50 g as a single dose; smaller doses (10-25 g) may be used in children 1-5 years due to smaller gut lumen capacity
>12 years: Refer to adult dosing.
Note: ~10 g of activated charcoal for each 1 g of toxin is considered adequate; this may require multiple doses. If sorbitol is also used, sorbitol dose should not exceed 1.5 g/kg. When using multiple doses of charcoal, sorbitol should be given with every other dose (not to exceed 2 doses/day).

Administration
Oral: Flavoring agents (eg, chocolate) and sorbitol can enhance charcoal's palatability. If treatment includes ipecac syrup, induce vomiting prior to administration of charcoal. Often given with a laxative or cathartic; check for presence of bowel sounds before administration.

Stability
Reconstitution: Powder: Dilute with at least 8 mL of water per 1 g of charcoal, or mix in a charcoal to water ratio of 1:4 to 1:8. Mix to form a slurry.
Storage: Adsorbs gases from air, store in closed container.

Nursing Actions
Physical Assessment: Monitor for active bowel sounds prior to administration. If antidote treatment includes ipecac syrup, induce vomiting before administering charcoal. May be administered with sorbitol or chocolate to improve palatability; do not administer with milk products.
Patient Education: Charcoal will cause your stools to turn black. Do not self-administer as an antidote

before calling the poison control center, hospital emergency room, or physician for instructions (charcoal is not the antidote for all poisons). **Pregnancy precaution:** Inform prescriber if you are pregnant.

Chloral Hydrate (KLOR al HYE drate)

U.S. Brand Names Aquachloral® Supprettes®; Somnote™

Synonyms Chloral; Hydrated Chloral; Trichloroacetaldehyde Monohydrate

Restrictions C-IV

Pharmacologic Category Hypnotic, Nonbenzodiazepine

Pregnancy Risk Factor C

Lactation Enters breast milk/compatible

Use Short-term sedative and hypnotic (<2 weeks), sedative/hypnotic for diagnostic procedures; sedative prior to EEG evaluations

Mechanism of Action/Effect Central nervous system depressant effects are due to its active metabolite trichloroethanol, mechanism unknown

Contraindications Hypersensitivity to chloral hydrate or any component of the formulation; hepatic or renal impairment; gastritis or ulcers; severe cardiac disease

Warnings/Precautions Use with caution in patients with porphyria. Use with caution in neonates, drug may accumulate with repeated use, prolonged use in neonates associated with hyperbilirubinemia. Tolerance to hypnotic effect develops, therefore, not recommended for use longer than 2 weeks. Taper dosage to avoid withdrawal with prolonged use. Trichloroethanol (TCE), a metabolite of chloral hydrate, is a carcinogen in mice; there is no data in humans. Chloral hydrate is considered a second line hypnotic agent in the elderly. Recent interpretive guidelines from the Centers for Medicare and Medicaid Services (CMS) discourage the use of chloral hydrate in residents of long-term care facilities.

Drug Interactions

Increased Effect/Toxicity: Chloral hydrate and ethanol (and other CNS depressants) have additive CNS depressant effects; monitor for CNS depression. Chloral hydrate's metabolite may displace warfarin from its protein binding sites resulting in an increase in the hypoprothrombinemic response to warfarin; warfarin dosages may need to be adjusted. Diaphoresis, flushing, and hypertension have occurred in patients who received I.V. furosemide within 24 hours after administration of chloral hydrate; consider using a benzodiazepine.

Nutritional/Ethanol Interactions

Ethanol: Avoid ethanol (may increase CNS depression). Herb/Nutraceutical: Avoid valerian, St John's wort, kava kava, gotu kola (may increase CNS depression).

Lab Interactions False-positive urine glucose using Clinitest® method; may interfere with fluorometric urine catecholamine and urinary 17-hydroxycorticosteroid tests

Adverse Reactions Frequency not defined.

Central nervous system: Ataxia, disorientation, sedation, excitement (paradoxical), dizziness, fever, headache, confusion, lightheadedness, nightmares, hallucinations, drowsiness, "hangover" effect

Dermatologic: Rash, urticaria

Gastrointestinal: Gastric irritation, nausea, vomiting, diarrhea, flatulence

Hematologic: Leukopenia, eosinophilia, acute intermittent porphyria

Miscellaneous: Physical and psychological dependence may occur with prolonged use of large doses

Overdosage/Toxicology Symptoms of overdose include hypotension, respiratory depression, coma,

hypothermia, and cardiac arrhythmias. Treatment is supportive and symptomatic.

Pharmacodynamics/Kinetics

Onset of Action: Peak effect: 0.5-1 hour

Duration of Action: 4-8 hours

Half-Life Elimination: Active metabolite: 8-11 hours

Metabolism: Rapidly hepatic to trichloroethanol (active metabolite); variable amounts hepatically and renally to trichloroacetic acid (inactive)

Excretion: Urine (as metabolites); feces (small amounts)

Available Dosage Forms

Capsule (Somnote™): 500 mg

Suppository, rectal (Aquachloral® Supprettes®): 325 mg [contains tartrazine], 650 mg

Syrup: 500 mg/5 mL (480 mL) [contains sodium benzoate]

Dosing

Adults:

Sedation, anxiety: Oral, rectal: 250 mg 3 times/day

Hypnotic: Oral, rectal: 500-1000 mg at bedtime or 30 minutes prior to procedure, not to exceed 2 g/24 hours

Discontinuation: Withdraw gradually over 2 weeks if patient has been maintained on high doses for prolonged period of time. Do not stop drug abruptly.

Elderly: Hypnotic: Initial: Oral: 250 mg at bedtime; adjust for renal impairment. See Geriatric Considerations.

Pediatrics:

Sedation, anxiety: Oral, rectal: 5-15 mg/kg/dose every 8 hours, maximum: 500 mg/dose

Prior to EEG: Oral, rectal: 20-25 mg/kg/dose, 30-60 minutes prior to EEG; may repeat in 30 minutes to maximum of 100 mg/kg or 2 g total

Hypnotic: Oral, rectal: 20-40 mg/kg/dose up to a maximum of 50 mg/kg/24 hours or 1 g/dose or 2 g/24 hours

Conscious sedation: Oral: 50-75 mg/kg/dose 30-60 minutes prior to procedure; may repeat 30 minutes after initial dose if needed, to a total maximum dose of 120 mg/kg or 1 g total

Discontinuation: Withdraw gradually over 2 weeks if patient has been maintained on high doses for prolonged period of time. Do not stop drug abruptly.

Renal Impairment:

Cl_{cr} <50 mL/minute: Avoid use.

Hemodialysis effects: Supplemental dose is not necessary; dializable (50% to 100%).

Hepatic Impairment: Avoid use in patients with severe hepatic impairment.

Administration

Oral: Chilling the syrup may help to mask unpleasant taste. Do not crush capsule (contains drug in liquid form). Gastric irritation may be minimized by diluting dose in water or other oral liquid.

Stability

Storage: Sensitive to light. Exposure to air causes volatilization. Store in light-resistant, airtight container.

Nursing Actions

Physical Assessment: For short-term use. Assess effectiveness and interactions of other medications patient may be taking. Assess for history of addiction; long-term use can result in dependence, abuse, or tolerance. Monitor for excessive sedation. Evaluate periodically for need for continued use (symptoms of dependence may resemble alcoholism, but usually there is more gastritis). After long-term use, taper dosage slowly when discontinuing. For inpatient use, institute safety measures (side rails, night light, call bell, assistance with ambulation) and monitor effectiveness and adverse reactions. For outpatients, monitor for effectiveness of therapy and adverse reactions at beginning of therapy and periodically with long-term use. Assess knowledge/teach patient (Continued)

Chloral Hydrate (Continued)

appropriate use, interventions to reduce side effects, and adverse symptoms to report.

Patient Education: Use exactly as directed; do not increase dose or frequency or discontinue this medication without consulting prescriber. Drug may cause physical and/or psychological dependence. While using this medication, do not use alcohol and other prescription or OTC medications (especially, pain medications, sedatives, antihistamines, or hypnotics) without consulting prescriber. Maintain adequate hydration (2-3 L/day of fluids) unless instructed to restrict fluid intake. You may experience drowsiness, dizziness, or blurred vision (use caution when driving or engaging in tasks requiring alertness until response to drug is known); nausea, vomiting, unpleasant taste (small frequent meals, frequent mouth care, chewing gum, or sucking lozenges may help); or diarrhea (buttermilk, boiled milk, yogurt may help). Report skin rash or irritation, CNS changes (confusion, depression, increased sedation, excitation, headache, insomnia, or nightmares), unresolved GI distress, chest pain or palpitations, or ineffectiveness of medication. **Pregnancy precaution:** Inform prescriber if you are or intend to become pregnant.

Geriatric Considerations Chloral hydrate is considered a second- or third-line hypnotic agent in the elderly. Interpretive guidelines from the Centers for Medicare and Medicaid Services (CMS) discourage the use of chloral hydrate in residents of long-term care facilities.

Additional Information Not an analgesic

Related Information

Anxiolytic / Hypnotic Use in Long-Term Care Facilities on page 1418
Federal OBRA Regulations Recommended Maximum Doses on page 1421

Chlorambucil (klor AM byoo sil)

U.S. Brand Names Leukeran®

Synonyms CB-1348; Chlorambucilum; Chloraminophene; Chlorbutinum; NSC-3088; WR-139013

Pharmacologic Category Antineoplastic Agent, Alkylating Agent

Medication Safety Issues
Sound-alike/look-alike issues:
Chlorambucil may be confused with Chloromycetin®
Leukeran® may be confused with Alkeran®, leucovorin, Leukine®

Pregnancy Risk Factor D

Lactation Excretion in breast milk unknown

Use Management of chronic lymphocytic leukemia, Hodgkin's and non-Hodgkin's lymphoma; breast and ovarian carcinoma; Waldenström's macroglobulinemia, testicular carcinoma, thrombocythemia, choriocarcinoma

Mechanism of Action/Effect Interferes with DNA replication and RNA transcription by alkylation and cross-linking the strands of DNA

Contraindications Hypersensitivity to chlorambucil or any component of the formulation; hypersensitivity to other alkylating agents (may have cross-hypersensitivity); pregnancy

Warnings/Precautions Hazardous agent — use appropriate precautions for handling and disposal. Use with caution in patients with seizure disorder and bone marrow suppression; reduce initial dosage if patient has received myelosuppressive therapy, or has a depressed baseline leukocyte or platelet count within the previous 4 weeks. Avoid administration of live vaccines to immunocompromised patients. Rare instances of severe skin reactions (eg, erythema multiforme, Stevens-Johnson syndrome) have been reported; discontinue if a reaction occurs.

Affects human fertility; carcinogenic in humans and probably mutagenic and teratogenic as well; chromosomal damage has been documented; secondary acute myelocytic leukemia may be associated with chronic therapy. Safety and efficacy in pediatric patients have not been established.

Drug Interactions

Decreased Effect: Patients may experience impaired immune response to vaccines; possible infection after administration of live vaccines in patients receiving immunosuppressants.

Nutritional/Ethanol Interactions Food: Avoid acidic foods and hot foods. Avoid spices.

Adverse Reactions Frequency not defined.

Central nervous system: Agitation, ataxia, confusion, focal/generalized seizures (rare), hallucinations

Dermatologic: Angioneurotic edema, erythema multiforme (rare), skin hypersensitivity, Stevens-Johnson syndrome (rare), toxic epidermal necrolysis (rare), urticaria

Endocrine & metabolic: Amenorrhea, azoospermia, chromosomal damage, infertility, sterility

Gastrointestinal: Hepatotoxicity, jaundice, diarrhea (infrequent), nausea (infrequent), stomatitis (infrequent), vomiting (infrequent)

Genitourinary: Sterile cystitis

Hematologic: Myelosuppression (common), leukemia, lymphopenia, neutropenia, secondary malignancies

Hepatic: Hepatotoxicity, jaundice

Neuromuscular & skeletal: Flaccid paresis, muscular twitching, myoclonia, neuropathy (peripheral), tremor

Respiratory: Interstitial pneumonia, pulmonary fibrosis, SIADH (rare)

Miscellaneous: Fever, secondary malignancies

Overdosage/Toxicology Symptoms of overdose include vomiting, ataxia, coma, seizures, and pancytopenia. There are no known antidotes for chlorambucil intoxication. Treatment is mainly supportive and symptomatic.

Pharmacodynamics/Kinetics

Time to Peak:
Within 1 hour; Phenylacetic acid mustard: 1.2-2.6 hours

Protein Binding: ~99%

Half-Life Elimination: ~1.5 hours; Phenylacetic acid mustard: 2.5 hours

Metabolism: Hepatic; active metabolite, phenylacetic acid mustard

Excretion: Urine (15% to 60% primarily as metabolites, <1% as unchanged drug or phenylacetic acid mustard: 2.5 hours)

Available Dosage Forms Tablet: 2 mg

Dosing

Adults: Refer to individual protocols.

Usual dose range: Oral: 0.1-0.2 mg/kg/day or
3-6 mg/m²/day for 3-6 weeks, then adjust dose on basis of blood counts or
0.4 mg/kg and increased by 0.1 mg/kg biweekly or monthly or
14 mg/m²/day for 5 days, repeated every 21-28 days

Elderly: Oral (refer to individual protocols): Use lowest recommended doses for adults; usual dose for elderly is 2-4 mg/day, particularly for use in treatment of rheumatoid arthritis.

Pediatrics: Refer to individual protocols.

General short courses: Oral: 0.1-0.2 mg/kg/day or 4.5 mg/m²/day for 3-6 weeks for remission induction (usual: 4-10 mg/day); maintenance therapy: 0.03-0.1 mg/kg/day (usual: 2-4 mg/day)

Nephrotic syndrome: Oral: 0.1-0.2 mg/kg/day every day for 5-15 weeks with low-dose prednisone

Chronic lymphocytic leukemia (CLL): Oral:

Biweekly regimen: Initial: 0.4 mg/kg/dose every 2 weeks; increase dose by 0.1 mg/kg every 2 weeks until a response occurs and/or myelosuppression occurs

Monthly regimen: Initial: 0.4 mg/kg, increase dose by 0.2 mg/kg every 4 weeks until a response occurs and/or myelosuppression occurs

Malignant lymphomas: Oral:

Non-Hodgkin's lymphoma: 0.1 mg/kg/day

Hodgkin's lymphoma: 0.2 mg/kg/day

Renal Impairment:

Hemodialysis: Supplemental dose is not necessary.

Peritoneal dialysis: Supplemental dose is not necessary.

Administration

Oral: Usually administered as a single dose; preferably on an empty stomach

Stability

Storage: Store in refrigerator at 2°C to 8°C (36°F to 46°F). Protect from light.

Laboratory Monitoring Liver function, CBC, platelet count, serum uric acid

Nursing Actions

Physical Assessment: Monitor laboratory tests and patient response (eg, hematologic myelosuppression, hypersensitivity rash, drug fever, seizures, gastrointestinal upset, hepatotoxicity) on a regular basis throughout therapy. Teach patient (or caregiver) proper use, necessity for contraception with sexually-active female patients, possible side effects/appropriate interventions, and adverse symptoms to report.

Patient Education: Do not take any new medication during therapy unless approved by prescriber. Take exactly as directed. Maintain adequate hydration (2-3 L/day of fluids) unless instructed to restrict fluid intake. Avoid alcohol, acidic, spicy, or hot foods. May cause menstrual irregularities and/or sterility. You will be more susceptible to infection (avoid crowds and exposure to infection and do not have any vaccinations without consulting prescriber). May cause nausea or vomiting (small, frequent meals, good mouth care, chewing gum or sucking lozenges may help); or mouth sores (use soft toothbrush or cotton swab for oral care). Report CNS changes (agitation, confusion, hallucinations, seizures); easy bruising or bleeding; unusual rash; persistent nausea, vomiting, or mouth sores; menstrual irregularities; yellowing of skin or dark urine; respiratory difficulty; or other adverse effects. **Pregnancy/breast-feeding precautions:** Inform prescriber if you are pregnant. Do not get pregnant during therapy. Consult prescriber for instruction on appropriate contraceptive measures. This drug may cause severe fetal defects. Consult prescriber if breast-feeding.

Geriatric Considerations Toxicity to immunosuppressives is increased in the elderly. Start with lowest recommended adult doses (see Dosing). Signs of infection, such as fever and rise in WBCs, may not occur. Lethargy and confusion may be more prominent signs of infection.

Pregnancy Issues Carcinogenic and mutagenic in humans.

Chloramphenicol (klor am FEN i kole)

U.S. Brand Names Chloromycetin® Sodium Succinate

Pharmacologic Category Antibiotic, Miscellaneous

Medication Safety Issues
Sound-alike/look-alike issues:
Chloromycetin® may be confused with chlorambucil, Chlor-Trimeton®

Pregnancy Risk Factor C

Lactation Enters breast milk/not recommended (AAP rates "of concern")

Use Treatment of serious infections due to organisms resistant to other less toxic antibiotics or when its penetrability into the site of infection is clinically superior to other antibiotics to which the organism is sensitive; useful in infections caused by *Bacteroides*, *H. influenzae*, *Neisseria meningitidis*, *Salmonella*, and *Rickettsia*; active against many vancomycin-resistant enterococci

Mechanism of Action/Effect Reversibly binds to 50S ribosomal subunits of susceptible organisms preventing amino acids from being transferred to growing peptide chains thus inhibiting protein synthesis

Contraindications Hypersensitivity to chloramphenicol or any component of the formulation

Warnings/Precautions Use with caution in patients with impaired renal or hepatic function and in neonates. Reduce dose with impaired liver function. Use with care in patients with glucose 6-phosphate dehydrogenase deficiency. Serious and fatal blood dyscrasias have occurred after both short-term and prolonged therapy. Should not be used when less potentially toxic agents are effective. Prolonged use may result in superinfection.

Drug Interactions

Cytochrome P450 Effect: Inhibits CYP2C8/9 (weak), 3A4 (weak)

Decreased Effect: Phenobarbital and rifampin may decrease serum concentrations of chloramphenicol.

Increased Effect/Toxicity: Chloramphenicol increases serum concentrations of chlorpropamide, phenytoin, and oral anticoagulants.

Nutritional/Ethanol Interactions Food: May decrease intestinal absorption of vitamin B_{12} may have increased dietary need for riboflavin, pyridoxine, and vitamin B_{12}.

Lab Interactions May cause false-positive results in urine glucose tests when using cupric sulfate (Benedict's solution, Clinitest®).

Adverse Reactions

Three (3) major toxicities associated with chloramphenicol include:

Aplastic anemia, an idiosyncratic reaction which can occur with any route of administration; usually occurs 3 weeks to 12 months after initial exposure to chloramphenicol

Bone marrow suppression is thought to be dose related with serum concentrations >25 mcg/mL and reversible once chloramphenicol is discontinued; anemia and neutropenia may occur during the first week of therapy

Gray syndrome is characterized by circulatory collapse, cyanosis, acidosis, abdominal distention, myocardial depression, coma, and death; reaction appears to be associated with serum levels ≥50 mcg/mL; may result from drug accumulation in patients with impaired hepatic or renal function

Additional adverse reactions, frequency not defined:

Central nervous system: Confusion, delirium, depression, fever, headache

Dermatologic: Angioedema, rash, urticaria

Gastrointestinal: Diarrhea, enterocolitis, glossitis, nausea, stomatitis, vomiting

Hematologic: Granulocytopenia, hypoplastic anemia, pancytopenia, thrombocytopenia

(Continued)

Chloramphenicol (Continued)

Ocular: Optic neuritis

Miscellaneous: Anaphylaxis, hypersensitivity reactions

Overdosage/Toxicology Symptoms of overdose include anemia, metabolic acidosis, hypotension, and hypothermia. Treatment is supportive.

Pharmacodynamics/Kinetics

Protein Binding: 60%

Half-Life Elimination:

Normal renal function: 1.6-3.3 hours

End-stage renal disease: 3-7 hours

Cirrhosis: 10-12 hours

Metabolism: Extensively hepatic (90%) to inactive metabolites, principally by glucuronidation; chloramphenicol sodium succinate is hydrolyzed by esterases to active base

Excretion: Urine (5% to 15%)

Available Dosage Forms Injection, powder for reconstitution: 1 g [contains sodium ~52 mg/g (2.25 mEq/g)]

Dosing

Adults & Elderly: Systemic infections: I.V.: 50-100 mg/kg/day in divided doses every 6 hours; maximum daily dose: 4 g/day.

Pediatrics:

Meningitis: I.V.: Infants >30 days and Children: 50-100 mg/kg/day divided every 6 hours

Other infections: I.V.: Infants >30 days and Children: 50-75 mg/kg/day divided every 6 hours; maximum daily dose: 4 g/day

Renal Impairment: Slightly dialyzable (5% to 20%) via hemo- and peritoneal dialysis; no supplemental doses are needed in dialysis or continuous arteriovenous or venovenous hemofiltration.

Hepatic Impairment: Avoid use in severe liver impairment as increased toxicity may occur.

Administration

I.V.: Do not administer I.M.; can be administered IVP over at least 1 minute at a concentration of 100 mg/mL, or I.V. intermittent infusion over 15-30 minutes at a final concentration for administration of ≤20 mg/mL.

I.V. Detail: pH: 6.4-7.0

Stability

Compatibility: Stable in dextran 6% in dextrose, dextran 6% in NS, D₅LR, D₅¼NS, D₅½NS, D₅NS, D₅W, D₁₀W, fat emulsion 10%, LR, ½NS, NS

Y-site administration: Incompatible with fluconazole

Compatibility in syringe: Incompatible with glycopyrrolate, metoclopramide

Compatibility when admixed: Incompatible with chlorpromazine, hydroxyzine, phenytoin, polymyxin B sulfate, prochlorperazine edisylate, prochlorperazine mesylate, promethazine, vancomycin

Storage: Store at room temperature prior to reconstitution; reconstituted solutions remain stable for 30 days; use only clear solutions; frozen solutions remain stable for 6 months

Laboratory Monitoring CBC with reticulocyte and platelet counts, periodic liver and renal function, serum drug concentration; culture and sensitivity prior to initiating therapy

Nursing Actions

Physical Assessment: Culture and sensitivity results and allergy history should be assessed prior to beginning therapy. See Administration for infusion specifics. Monitor laboratory tests, therapeutic response, and adverse reactions (eg, bone marrow depression or aplastic anemia [petechiae, sore throat, fatigue, unusual bleeding or bruising, abdominal or bone pain], circulatory collapse; CNS disturbances, opportunistic infection). Teach patient possible side

effects/appropriate interventions and adverse symptoms to report (eg, CNS changes, opportunistic infection, aplastic anemia) may occur 3 weeks to 12 months after initial exposure to chloramphenicol.

Patient Education: Do not take any new medication during therapy unless approved by prescriber. This medication can only be administered by infusion and you will be monitored during each infusion; report immediately unusual chest tightness, difficulty breathing or swallowing; itching or skin rash; back pain or acute headache, redness, swelling, or pain at infusion site. You may experience a bitter taste during infusion, this will pass. If you have diabetes, drug may cause false test results with Clinitest® glucose monitoring; use alternative glucose monitoring. May cause nausea, vomiting (small, frequent meals, frequent mouth care, sucking lozenges, or chewing gum may help). Report persistent rash, diarrhea; pain, burning, or numbness of extremities; petechiae; sore throat; fatigue; unusual bleeding or bruising; vaginal itching or discharge; mouth sores; yellowing of skin or eyes; dark urine or stool discoloration (blue); CNS disturbances (nightmares, acute headache); lack of improvement or worsening of condition. **Pregnancy/breast-feeding precautions:** Inform prescriber if you are or intend to become pregnant. Breast-feeding is not recommended.

Dietary Considerations May have increased dietary need for riboflavin, pyridoxine, and vitamin B₁₂. Sodium content of 1 g injection: ~52 mg (2.25 mEq).

Geriatric Considerations Chloramphenicol has not been studied in the elderly. It is not necessary to adjust the dose based upon the decrease in renal function associated with age. Chloramphenicol should be reserved for serious infections and the oral form avoided.

Breast-Feeding Issues Excreted in breast milk. Not recommended due to potential bone marrow suppression to the infant.

Pregnancy Issues Embryotoxic and teratogenic in animals, but there are no adequate and well-controlled trials in pregnant women. Has been shown to cross placental barrier.

Chlordiazepoxide (klor dye az e POKS ide)

U.S. Brand Names Librium®

Synonyms Methaminodiazepoxide Hydrochloride

Restrictions C-IV

Pharmacologic Category Benzodiazepine

Medication Safety Issues

Sound-alike/look-alike issues:

Librium® may be confused with Librax®

Pregnancy Risk Factor D

Lactation Enters breast milk/not recommended

Use Management of anxiety disorder or for the short-term relief of symptoms of anxiety; withdrawal symptoms of acute alcoholism; preoperative apprehension and anxiety

Mechanism of Action/Effect Binds to stereospecific benzodiazepine receptors on the postsynaptic GABA neuron at several sites within the central nervous system, including the limbic system, reticular formation. Enhancement of the inhibitory effect of GABA on neuronal excitability results by increased neuronal membrane permeability to chloride ions. This shift in chloride ions results in hyperpolarization (a less excitable state) and stabilization.

Contraindications Hypersensitivity to chlordiazepoxide or any component of the formulation (cross-sensitivity with other benzodiazepines may also exist); narrow-angle glaucoma; pregnancy

Warnings/Precautions Use with caution in renal impairment or predisposition to urate nephropathy, elderly or debilitated patients, patients with hepatic disease (including alcoholics), renal impairment, respiratory disease, impaired gag reflex, or obese patients. Use with caution in patients receiving concurrent CYP3A4 inhibitors, particularly when these agents are added to therapy. Use with caution in renal impairment or predisposition to urate nephropathy, elderly or debilitated patients with hepatic disease (including alcoholics), renal impairment, respiratory disease, impaired gag reflex, or obese patients.

Parenteral administration should be avoided in comatose patients or shock. Adequate resuscitative equipment/personnel should be available, and appropriate monitoring should be conducted at the time of injection and for several hours following administration. The parenteral formulation should be diluted for I.M. administration with the supplied diluent only. This diluent should not be used when preparing the drug for intravenous administration.

Causes CNS depression (dose related) which may impair physical and mental capabilities. Use with caution in patients receiving other CNS depressants or psychoactive agents. Benzodiazepines have been associated with falls and traumatic injury and should be used with extreme caution in patients who are at risk of these events (especially the elderly). Active metabolites with extended half-lives may lead to delayed accumulation and adverse effects.

Use caution in patients with depression, particularly if suicidal risk may be present. May cause physical or psychological dependence - use with caution in patients with a history of drug dependence.

Benzodiazepines have been associated with anterograde amnesia. Paradoxical reactions, including hyperactive or aggressive behavior, have been reported with benzodiazepines, particularly in adolescent/pediatric or psychiatric patients. Does not have analgesic, antidepressant, or antipsychotic properties.

Drug Interactions
Cytochrome P450 Effect: Substrate of CYP3A4 (major)

Decreased Effect: CYP3A4 inducers may decrease the levels/effects of chlordiazepoxide; example inducers include aminoglutethimide, carbamazepine, nafcillin, nevirapine, phenobarbital, phenytoin, and rifamycins.

Increased Effect/Toxicity: Chlordiazepoxide potentiates the CNS depressant effects of narcotic analgesics, barbiturates, phenothiazines, ethanol, antihistamines, MAO inhibitors, sedative-hypnotics, and cyclic antidepressants. CYP3A4 inhibitors may increase the levels/effects of chlordiazepoxide; example inhibitors include azole antifungals, clarithromycin, diclofenac, doxycycline, erythromycin, imatinib, isoniazid, nefazodone, nicardipine, propofol, protease inhibitors, quinidine, telithromycin, and verapamil.

Nutritional/Ethanol Interactions
Ethanol: Avoid ethanol (may increase CNS depression).
Food: Serum concentrations/effects may be increased with grapefruit juice, but unlikely because of high oral bioavailability of chlordiazepoxide.
Herb/Nutraceutical: Avoid valerian, St John's wort, kava kava, gotu kola (may increase CNS depression).

Lab Interactions Increased triglycerides (S); decreased HDL

Adverse Reactions
>10%:
Central nervous system: Drowsiness, fatigue, ataxia, lightheadedness, memory impairment, dysarthria, irritability
Dermatologic: Rash
Endocrine & metabolic: Decreased libido, menstrual disorders

Gastrointestinal: Xerostomia, decreased salivation, increased or decreased appetite, weight gain/loss
Genitourinary: Micturition difficulties
1% to 10%:
Cardiovascular: Hypotension
Central nervous system: Confusion, dizziness, disinhibition, akathisia, increased libido
Dermatologic: Dermatitis
Gastrointestinal: Increased salivation
Genitourinary: Sexual dysfunction, incontinence
Neuromuscular & skeletal: Rigidity, tremor, muscle cramps
Otic: Tinnitus
Respiratory: Nasal congestion

Overdosage/Toxicology Symptoms of overdose include hypotension, respiratory depression, coma, hypothermia, and cardiac arrhythmias. Treatment for benzodiazepine overdose is supportive. Flumazenil has been shown to selectively block the binding of benzodiazepines to CNS receptors, resulting in a reversal of benzodiazepine-induced CNS depression. Respiratory depression may not be reversed.

Pharmacodynamics/Kinetics
Time to Peak: Serum: Oral: Within 2 hours; I.M.: Results in lower peak plasma levels than oral
Protein Binding: 90% to 98%
Half-Life Elimination: 6.6-25 hours; End-stage renal disease: 5-30 hours; Cirrhosis: 30-63 hours
Metabolism: Extensively hepatic to desmethyldiazepam (active and long-acting)
Excretion: Urine (minimal as unchanged drug)

Available Dosage Forms
Capsule, as hydrochloride: 5 mg, 10 mg, 25 mg
Injection, powder for reconstitution, as hydrochloride: 100 mg [diluent contains benzyl alcohol, polysorbate 80, and propylene glycol]

Dosing
Adults:
Anxiety:
Oral: 15-100 mg divided 3-4 times/day
I.M., I.V.: Initial: 50-100 mg followed by 25-50 mg 3-4 times/day as needed
Preoperative anxiety: I.M.: 50-100 mg prior to surgery
Ethanol withdrawal symptoms: Oral, I.V.: 50-100 mg to start, dose may be repeated in 2-4 hours as necessary to a maximum of 300 mg/24 hours
Note: Up to 300 mg may be given I.M. or I.V. during a 6-hour period, but not more this in any 24-hour period.
Elderly: Anxiety: Oral: 5 mg 2-4 times/day; adjust for renal impairment. Avoid use if possible. See Geriatric Considerations.
Pediatrics: Anxiety: Oral, I.M.:
<6 years: Not recommended
>6 years: 0.5 mg/kg/24 hours divided every 6-8 hours
Renal Impairment:
Cl_cr <10 mL/minute: Administer 50% of dose.
Not dialyzable (0% to 5%)
Hepatic Impairment: Avoid use.

Administration
I.M.: Administer by deep I.M. injection slowly into the upper outer quadrant of the gluteus muscle; use only the diluent provided for I.M. use; solutions made with SWFI or NS cause pain with I.M. administration
I.V.: Administer slowly over at least 1 minute; do not use the diluent provided for I.M. use; air bubbles form during reconstitution
I.V. Detail: Rapid administration may cause symptoms of overdose.

pH: 2.5-3.5 (using I.M. diluent)
pH: 3 (using SWFI or NS as diluent)
(Continued)

Chlordiazepoxide *(Continued)*

Stability

Reconstitution:

I.M. use: Reconstitute by adding 2 mL of provided diluent; agitate gently until dissolved. Provided diluent is **not** for I.V. use.

I.V. use: Reconstitute by adding 5 mL NS or SWFI; agitate gently until dissolved; **do not administer this dilution I.M.**

Compatibility: Stable in D_5W; **incompatible** (consult detailed reference) in LR, NS

Y-site administration: Incompatible with cefepime

Storage: Injection: Prior to reconstitution, store under refrigeration and protect from light. Solution should be used immediately following reconstitution.

Nursing Actions

Physical Assessment: Assess other medications patient may be taking for effectiveness and interactions. Assess for signs of CNS depression (sedation, dizziness, confusion, or ataxia). Assess for history of addiction; long-term use can result in dependence, abuse, or tolerance; periodically evaluate need for continued use. For inpatient use, institute safety measures and monitor effectiveness and adverse reactions. For outpatients, monitor therapeutic effectiveness and adverse reactions at beginning of therapy and periodically with long-term use. Taper dosage slowly when discontinuing. Assess knowledge/teach patient appropriate use, interventions to reduce side effects, and adverse symptoms to report. **I.V.:** Monitor vital signs frequently during infusion, observe safety precautions (side rails up, etc), and maintain bedrest for 2-3 hours following infusion.

Patient Education: Oral: Take exactly as directed; do not increase dose or frequency. Drug may cause physical and/or psychological dependence. Do not use alcohol or other prescription or OTC medications (especially pain medications, sedatives, antihistamines, or hypnotics) without consulting prescriber. Maintain adequate hydration (2-3 L/day of fluids) unless instructed to restrict fluid intake. You may experience drowsiness, lightheadedness, impaired coordination, dizziness, or blurred vision (use caution when driving or engaging in tasks requiring alertness until response to drug is known); dry mouth (small frequent meals, frequent mouth care, chewing gum, or sucking lozenges may help); constipation (increased exercise, fluids, fruit, or fiber may help); or altered sexual drive or ability (reversible). Report persistent CNS effects (eg, euphoria, confusion, increased sedation, depression); chest pain, palpitations, or rapid heartbeat; muscle cramping, weakness, tremors, rigidity, or altered gait; or worsening of condition. **Pregnancy/breast-feeding precautions:** Do not get pregnant while taking this medication; use appropriate contraceptive measures. Breast-feeding is not recommended.

Geriatric Considerations Due to its long-acting metabolite, chlordiazepoxide is not considered a drug of choice in the elderly.

Breast-Feeding Issues There is no significant data for chlordiazepoxide, but a related compound diazepam has been shown to accumulate in nursing infants. It is recommended to discontinue nursing or the drug.

Pregnancy Issues Benzodiazepines cross the placenta. The association between benzodiazepine exposure and malformations remains controversial. A number of types of malformation have been reported (oral cleft, inguinal hernia, cardiac defects, spina bifida, dysmorphic facial features, skeletal defects); however, confounding factors make a clear association difficult. Overall, the risk to the fetus may be low. Nonteratogenic effects (including neonatal flaccidity, respiratory and feeding problems, and withdrawal symptoms) during the postnatal period have also been reported with benzodiazepine use.

Additional Information Abrupt discontinuation after sustained use (generally >10 days) may cause withdrawal symptoms.

Related Information

Anxiolytic / Hypnotic Use in Long-Term Care Facilities *on page 1418*

Federal OBRA Regulations Recommended Maximum Doses *on page 1421*

Chlordiazepoxide and Methscopolamine

U.S. Brand Names Librax® *[reformulation]* [DSC]

Synonyms Methscopolamine Nitrate and Chlordiazepoxide Hydrochloride

Restrictions C-IV

Pharmacologic Category Anticholinergic Agent; Benzodiazepine

Medication Safety Issues

Librax® formulation may be cause for confusion:

In November 2004, Valeant Pharmaceuticals licensed the Librax® trademark to Victory Pharmaceuticals. Subsequently, the product was reformulated to contain chlordiazepoxide and methscopolamine. In January 2006, Valeant Pharmaceuticals began redistributing the original formulation of Librax®, containing clidinium and chlordiazepoxide. Victory Pharmaceuticals has discontinued their product. **Note:** The formulation of Librax® distributed in Canada (Valeant Canada Ltd) always contained clidinium and clhordiazepoxide.

Pregnancy Risk Factor C

Lactation Excretion in breast milk unknown/not recommended

Use Adjunctive treatment of peptic ulcer; treatment of irritable bowel syndrome, acute enterocolitis

Mechanism of Action/Effect Chlordiazepoxide possesses sedative, hypnotic, anxiolytic, and muscle relaxant properties; methscopolamine reduces the volume and the total acid content of gastric secretions, inhibits salivation, and reduces gastrointestinal motility

Contraindications Hypersensitivity to chlordiazepoxide, methscopolamine, or any component of the formulation; glaucoma; prostatic hyperplasia; benign bladder neck obstruction

Warnings/Precautions Causes CNS depression; patients must be cautioned about performing tasks which require mental alertness (eg, operating machinery or driving). Use caution with hypersensitivity to other benzodiazepines (cross sensitivity may exist). Use caution in patients with depression, particularly if suicidal risk may be present. Use with caution in patients receiving other CNS depressants or psychoactive agents (lithium, phenothiazines). Effects with other sedative drugs or ethanol may be potentiated. Use with caution in elderly or debilitated patients, patients with hepatic disease or renal impairment. Benzodiazepines have been associated with dependence and acute withdrawal symptoms on discontinuation or reduction in dose. Do not abruptly discontinue this medication after prolonged use; taper dose gradually. Safety and efficacy have not been established in children.

Nutritional/Ethanol Interactions

Ethanol: Avoid ethanol (may increase CNS depression).

Herb/Nutraceutical: Avoid valerian, St John's wort, kava kava, gotu kola (may increase CNS depression).

Adverse Reactions See individual agents.

Overdosage/Toxicology See individual agents.

Pharmacokinetic Note See individual agents.

Available Dosage Forms Capsule: Chlordiazepoxide hydrochloride 5 mg and methscopolamine nitrate 2.5 mg [DSC]

Dosing

Adults: Peptic ulcer, irritable bowel syndrome, acute enterocolitis: Oral: 1-2 capsules 3-4 times/day; adjust dose based on individual response.

Elderly: Oral: Initial dose should not exceed 2 capsules/day; adjust dose as tolerated.

Administration

Oral: Administer before meals and at bedtime. Do not abruptly discontinue after prolonged use; taper dose gradually.

Stability

Storage: Store at room temperature of 15°C to 30°C (59°F to 86°F).

Nursing Actions

Physical Assessment: Monitor therapeutic response and adverse reactions at the beginning and periodically throughout therapy. Assess other prescription and OTC medications the patient may be taking to avoid duplications and interactions. Taper dosage slowly when discontinuing. Do not discontinue abruptly. Assess knowledge/teach patient appropriate use, side effects, and symptoms to report.

Patient Education:

Inform prescriber of all prescription medications, OTC medications, or herbal products you are taking. Avoid alcohol; may increase drowsiness. Take as directed. Do not increase dosage without consulting prescriber. May cause physical and psychological dependency. You may experience dizziness or lightheadedness. Use caution when driving or engaging in activities requiring alertness until response to drug is known. You may experience dry mouth (small, frequent meals, frequent mouth care, chewing gum, or sucking lozenges may help); blurring of vision, urinary hesitancy or constipation (increasing exercise, fluids, fruit/fiber may help). Maintain adequate hydration (2-3 L/day) unless instructed to restrict intake by prescriber. Report persistent CNS changes (euphoria, confusion, increased sedation, depression, suicide ideation). **Pregnancy/breast-feeding precautions:** Inform prescriber if you are or intend to become pregnant. Breast-feeding is not recommended.

Dietary Considerations Take before meals.

Geriatric Considerations Due to its long-acting metabolite, chlordiazepoxide is not considered a drug of choice in the elderly. The use of anticholinergic agents may cause problems with bladder emptying, constipation, or case confusion. This combination of benzodiazepine and anticholinergic agent may increase the risk of confusion.

Chlorophyllin, Papain, and Urea
(KLOR oh fil in, pa PAY in, & yoor EE a)

U.S. Brand Names Panafil®; Ziox™

Synonyms Chlorophyllin Copper Complex Sodium, Papain, and Urea; Papain, Urea, and Chlorophyllin; Urea, Chlorophyllin, and Papain

Pharmacologic Category Enzyme, Topical Debridement

Medication Safety Issues

Sound-alike/look-alike issues:

Ziox™ may be confused with Zyvox™

Use Treatment of acute and chronic lesions, such as varicose, diabetic decubitus ulcers, burns, postoperative wounds, pilonidal cyst wounds, carbuncles, and miscellaneous traumatic or infected wounds

Mechanism of Action/Effect

Papain: Promotes digestion of injured tissue; harmless to uninjured tissue

Urea: Promotes activation of papain and makes injured tissue ready for digestion

Chlorophyllin copper complex sodium: Contributes to wound healing by decreasing local inflammation, decreasing odors, and promoting healthy granulation

Contraindications Hypersensitivity to chlorophyllin, papain, urea, or any component of the formulation

Warnings/Precautions For topical use only; not for use in eyes.

Drug Interactions
Decreased Effect: Heavy metals, hydrogen peroxide

Adverse Reactions Local: Burning sensation, skin irritation

Available Dosage Forms

Ointment: Copper chlorophyllin complex sodium 0.5%, papain ≥521,700 units/g, and urea 10% (30 g)

Panafil®: Chlorophyllin copper complex sodium 0.5%, papain ≥409,500 units/g, and urea 10% (6 g, 30 g)

Ziox™: Chlorophyllin copper complex sodium 0.5%, papain ≥521,700 units/g, and urea 10% (3.5 g [single-dose packets], 30 g)

Spray:

Panafil®: Copper chlorophyllin complex sodium 0.5%, papain ≥521,700 units/g, and urea 10% (33 mL)

Dosing
Adults & Elderly:

Topical: Apply with each dressing change; daily or twice daily dressing changes are preferred, but may be every 2-3 days. Cover with dressing following application.

Ointment: Apply ¹/₈" thickness over the wound with clean applicator.

Spray: Completely cover the wound site so that the wound is not visible.

Administration

Topical: Cleanse wound prior to application. May apply under pressure dressings. Initially may require more frequent dressing changes to decrease irritation from enzymatic activity. Avoid cleansing with hydrogen peroxide solution. Avoid using heavy metal containing solutions (lead, mercury, silver). Do not use in or around the eyes.

Spray: Shake well before use. Prime pump (initial use only): Hold spray upright directly above the wound and prime the pump 6-8 times. Normal use: Allow a distance of 2-3 inches between the spray container and the wound; may hold spray at an angle or upright.

Stability
Storage:

Ointment: Store at room temperature of 15°C to 30°C (59°F to 86°F).

Spray: Store upright at controlled room temperature of 20°C to 25°C (68°F to 77°F).

Nursing Actions
Physical Assessment: Monitor therapeutic response and adverse reactions at the beginning and periodically throughout therapy.

Patient Education: For external use only. Skin should be cleansed prior to use. Hydrogen peroxide should not be used (may inactivate papain). Apply to entire wound area so that wound is not visible. Apply dressing (may use pressure dressings). Dressing changes are recommended once to twice daily. Do not use near eyes. **Pregnancy/breast-feeding precautions:** Inform prescriber if you are or intend to become pregnant. Consult prescriber if breast-feeding.

Chloroquine (KLOR oh kwin)

U.S. Brand Names Aralen®
Synonyms Chloroquine Phosphate
Pharmacologic Category Aminoquinoline (Antimalarial)
Pregnancy Risk Factor C
Lactation Enters breast milk/not recommended (AAP considers "compatible")
Use Suppression or chemoprophylaxis of malaria; treatment of uncomplicated or mild-to-moderate malaria; extraintestinal amebiasis
Unlabeled/Investigational Use Rheumatoid arthritis; discoid lupus erythematosus
Mechanism of Action/Effect Chloroquine concentrates within parasite acid vesicles and raises internal pH resulting in inhibition of parasite growth
Contraindications Hypersensitivity to chloroquine or any component of the formulation; retinal or visual field changes
Warnings/Precautions Use with caution in patients with liver disease, G6PD deficiency, alcoholism or in conjunction with hepatotoxic drugs. May exacerbate psoriasis or porphyria. Retinopathy (irreversible) has occurred with long or high-dose therapy; discontinue drug if any abnormality in the visual field or if muscular weakness develops during treatment. Use caution in patients with pre-existing auditory damage; discontinue immediately if hearing defects are noted. Use caution in patients with seizure disorders.

Drug Interactions
Cytochrome P450 Effect: Substrate (major) of CYP2D6, 3A4; **Inhibits** CYP2D6 (moderate)
Decreased Effect: Chloroquine levels may be decreased by antacids or kaolin. Chloroquine may decrease ampicillin and/or praziquantel levels. Chloroquine may decrease the levels/effects of CYP2D6 prodrug substrates; example prodrug substrates include codeine, hydrocodone, oxycodone, and tramadol. The levels/effects of chloroquine may be decreased by aminoglutethimide, carbamazepine, nafcillin, nevirapine, phenobarbital, phenytoin, rifamycins, and other CYP3A4 inducers.
Increased Effect/Toxicity: Chloroquine may increase the levels/effects of dextromethorphan, fluoxetine, lidocaine, mirtazapine, nefazodone, paroxetine, risperidone, ritonavir, thioridazine, tricyclic antidepressants, venlafaxine, and other CYP2D6 substrates. Chloroquine may increase the levels/effects of cyclosporine. The levels/effects of chloroquine may be increased by azole antifungals, chlorpromazine, cimetidine, clarithromycin, delavirdine, diclofenac, doxycycline, erythromycin, fluoxetine, imatinib, isoniazid, miconazole, nefazodone, nicardipine, paroxetine, pergolide, propofol, protease inhibitors, quinidine, quinine, ritonavir, ropinirole, telithromycin, verapamil, and other CYP2D6 or 3A4 inhibitors.
Nutritional/Ethanol Interactions Ethanol: Avoid ethanol (may increase GI irritation).
Adverse Reactions Frequency not defined.
Cardiovascular: Hypotension (rare), ECG changes (rare; including T-wave inversion), cardiomyopathy
Central nervous system: Fatigue, personality changes, headache, psychosis, seizure, delirium, depression
Dermatologic: Pruritus, hair bleaching, pleomorphic skin eruptions, alopecia, lichen planus eruptions, alopecia, mucosal pigmentary changes (blue-black), photosensitivity
Gastrointestinal: Nausea, diarrhea, vomiting, anorexia, stomatitis, abdominal cramps
Hematologic: Aplastic anemia, agranulocytosis (reversible), neutropenia, thrombocytopenia
Neuromuscular & skeletal: Rare cases of myopathy, neuromyopathy, proximal muscle atrophy, and depression of deep tendon reflexes have been reported
Ocular: Retinopathy (including irreversible changes in some patients long-term or high-dose therapy), blurred vision
Otic: Nerve deafness, tinnitus, reduced hearing (risk increased in patients with pre-existing auditory damage)
Overdosage/Toxicology Symptoms of overdose include headache, visual changes, cardiovascular collapse, shock, seizures, abdominal cramps, vomiting, cyanosis, methemoglobinemia, leukopenia, and respiratory and cardiac arrest. Following initial measures (immediate GI decontamination), treatment is supportive and symptomatic.

Pharmacodynamics/Kinetics
Duration of Action: Small amounts may be present in urine months following discontinuation of therapy
Time to Peak: Serum: 1-2 hours
Half-Life Elimination: 3-5 days
Metabolism: Partially hepatic
Excretion: Urine (~70% as unchanged drug); acidification of urine increases elimination
Available Dosage Forms
Tablet, as phosphate: 250 mg [equivalent to 150 mg base]; 500 mg [equivalent to 300 mg base]
Aralen®: 500 mg [equivalent to 300 mg base]
Dosing
Adults & Elderly:
Malaria, suppression or prophylaxis: Oral: 500 mg/week (300 mg base) on the same day each week; begin 1-2 weeks prior to exposure; continue for 4-6 weeks after leaving endemic area; if suppressive therapy is not begun prior to exposure, double the initial loading dose to 1 g (600 mg base) and administer in 2 divided doses 6 hours apart, followed by the usual dosage regimen.
Malaria, acute attack: Oral: 1 g (600 mg base) on day 1, followed by 500 mg (300 mg base) 6 hours later, followed by 500 mg (300 mg base) on days 2 and 3.
Extraintestinal amebiasis: Oral: 1 g/day (600 mg base) for 2 days followed by 500 mg/day (300 mg base) for at least 2-3 weeks.
Rheumatoid arthritis, lupus erythematosus (unlabeled uses): Oral: 250 mg (150 mg base) once daily; reduce dosage following maximal response (taper to discontinue after response in lupus); generally requires 3-6 weeks. **Note:** Not considered first-line agent.
Pediatrics:
Malaria, suppression or prophylaxis: Oral: Administer 5 mg base/kg/week on the same day each week (not to exceed 300 mg base/dose); begin 1-2 weeks prior to exposure; continue for 4-6 weeks after leaving endemic area; if suppressive therapy is not begun prior to exposure, double the initial loading dose to 10 mg base/kg and administer in 2 divided doses 6 hours apart, followed by the usual dosage regimen.
Malaria, acute attack: Oral: 10 mg/kg (base) on day 1, followed by 5 mg/kg (base) 6 hours later and 5 mg/kg (base) on days 2 and 3
Extraintestinal amebiasis: Oral: 10 mg/kg (base) once daily for 2-3 weeks (up to 300 mg base/day)
Renal Impairment:
Cl$_{cr}$ <10 mL/minute: Administer 50% of dose.
Hemodialysis effects: Minimally removed by hemodialysis
Administration
Oral: Chloroquine phosphate tablets have also been mixed with chocolate syrup or enclosed in gelatin capsules to mask the bitter taste.
Stability
Storage: Store tablets at 25°C (77°F). Excursions permitted at 15°C to 30°C (59°F to 86°F).

Laboratory Monitoring Periodic CBC

Nursing Actions

Physical Assessment: Assess other pharmacological or herbal products patient may be taking for potential interactions. Assess results of laboratory tests (CBC), therapeutic effectiveness (according to purpose for use), and adverse response (eg, retinopathy, hearing loss, myopathy) regularly during long-term therapy. Teach patient appropriate use, possible side effects/appropriate interventions, and adverse symptoms to report (eg, anemia, muscle weakness, visual or auditory changes).

Patient Education: Inform prescriber of all prescriptions, OTC medications, or herbal products you are taking, and any allergies you have. Do not take any new medication during therapy unless approved by prescriber. It is important to complete full course of therapy, which may take up to 6 months for full effect. May be taken with meals to decrease GI upset and bitter aftertaste. Avoid alcohol. You should have regular ophthalmic exams (every 4-6 months) if using this medication over extended periods. May cause skin discoloration (blue/black), hair bleaching, or skin rash. If you have psoriasis, may cause exacerbation. May turn urine black/brown (normal). May cause headache (if persistent, consult prescriber for analgesic); nausea, vomiting, or loss of appetite (small, frequent meals, frequent mouth care, sucking lozenges, or chewing gum may help); or increased sensitivity to sunlight (wear dark glasses and protective clothing, use sunblock, and avoid direct exposure to sunlight). Report vision changes; rash or itching; persistent diarrhea or GI disturbances; change in hearing acuity or ringing in the ears; chest pain or palpitation; CNS changes; unusual fatigue, easy bruising or bleeding; or any other persistent adverse reactions. **Pregnancy/breast-feeding precautions:** Inform prescriber if you are or intend to become pregnant. Consult prescriber if breast-feeding.

Dietary Considerations May be taken with meals to decrease GI upset.

Pregnancy Issues There are no adequate and well-controlled studies using chloroquine during pregnancy. However, based on clinical experience and because malaria infection in pregnant women may be more severe than in nonpregnant women, chloroquine prophylaxis may be considered in areas of chloroquine-sensitive *P. falciparum* malaria. Pregnant women should be advised not to travel to areas of *P. falciparum* resistance to chloroquine.

ChlorproMAZINE (klor PROE ma zeen)

Synonyms Chlorpromazine Hydrochloride; CPZ

Pharmacologic Category Antipsychotic Agent, Typical, Phenothiazine

Medication Safety Issues

Sound-alike/look-alike issues:

ChlorproMAZINE may be confused with chlorproPAMIDE, clomiPRAMINE, prochlorperazine, promethazine

Thorazine® may be confused with thiamine, thioridazine

Pregnancy Risk Factor C

Lactation Enters breast milk/not recommended (AAP rates "of concern")

Use Control of mania; treatment of schizophrenia; control of nausea and vomiting; relief of restlessness and apprehension before surgery; acute intermittent porphyria; adjunct in the treatment of tetanus; intractable hiccups; combativeness and/or explosive hyperexcitable behavior in children 1-12 years of age and in short-term treatment of hyperactive children

Unlabeled/Investigational Use Management of psychotic disorders

Mechanism of Action/Effect Chlorpromazine is an aliphatic phenothiazine antipsychotic which blocks postsynaptic mesolimbic dopaminergic receptors in the brain; exhibits a strong alpha-adrenergic blocking effect and depresses the release of hypothalamic and hypophyseal hormones; believed to depress the reticular activating system, thus affecting basal metabolism, body temperature, wakefulness, vasomotor tone, and emesis

Contraindications Hypersensitivity to chlorpromazine or any component of the formulation (cross-reactivity between phenothiazines may occur); severe CNS depression; coma

Warnings/Precautions Highly sedating, use with caution in disorders where CNS depression is a feature and in patients with Parkinson's disease. Use with caution in patients with hemodynamic instability, bone marrow suppression, predisposition to seizures, subcortical brain damage, severe cardiac, hepatic, renal, or respiratory disease. Esophageal dysmotility and aspiration have been associated with antipsychotic use - use with caution in patients at risk of aspiration pneumonia (ie, Alzheimer's disease). Caution in breast cancer or other prolactin-dependent tumors (may elevate prolactin levels). May alter temperature regulation or mask toxicity of other drugs due to antiemetic effects. May alter cardiac conduction - life-threatening arrhythmias have occurred with therapeutic doses of neuroleptics.

Use with caution in patients at risk of hypotension (orthostasis is common) or those who would tolerate transient hypotensive episodes (cerebrovascular disease, cardiovascular disease, or other medications which may predispose). Significant hypotension may occur, particularly with parenteral administration. Injection contains sulfites and benzyl alcohol.

Use with caution in patients with decreased gastrointestinal motility, urinary retention, BPH, xerostomia, or visual problems (ie, narrow-angle glaucoma - screening is recommended) and myasthenia gravis. Relative to other neuroleptics, chlorpromazine has a moderate potency of cholinergic blockade.

May cause extrapyramidal symptoms, neuroleptic malignant syndrome (NMS) or pigmentary retinopathy.

Drug Interactions

Cytochrome P450 Effect: Substrate of CYP1A2 (minor), 2D6 (major), 3A4 (minor); **Inhibits** CYP2D6 (strong), 2E1 (weak)

Decreased Effect: Chlorpromazine may decrease the levels/effects of CYP2D6 prodrug substrates; example prodrug substrates include codeine, hydrocodone, oxycodone, and tramadol. Phenothiazines inhibit the ability of bromocriptine to lower serum prolactin concentrations. Benztropine (and other anticholinergics) may inhibit the therapeutic response to chlorpromazine and excess anticholinergic effects may occur. Antihypertensive effects of guanethidine and guanadrel may be inhibited by chlorpromazine. Chlorpromazine may inhibit the antiparkinsonian effect of levodopa. Chlorpromazine and possibly other low potency antipsychotics may reverse the pressor effects of epinephrine.

Increased Effect/Toxicity: The levels/effects of chlorpromazine may be increased by delavirdine, fluoxetine, miconazole, paroxetine, pergolide, quinidine, quinine, ritonavir, ropinirole, and other CYP2D6 inhibitors. Effects on CNS depression may be additive when chlorpromazine is combined with CNS depressants (narcotic analgesics, ethanol, barbiturates, cyclic antidepressants, antihistamines, or sedative-hypnotics). Chlorpromazine may increase the levels/effects of amphetamines, selected (Continued)

ChlorproMAZINE *(Continued)*

beta-blockers, dextromethorphan, fluoxetine, lidocaine, mirtazapine, nefazodone, paroxetine, risperidone, ritonavir, thioridazine, tricyclic antidepressants, and venlafaxine and other CYP2D6 substrates. Chlorpromazine may increase the effects/toxicity of anticholinergics, antihypertensives, lithium (rare neurotoxicity), trazodone, or valproic acid. Concurrent use with TCA may produce increased toxicity or altered therapeutic response. Chloroquine and propranolol may increase chlorpromazine concentrations. Hypotension may occur when chlorpromazine is combined with epinephrine. May increase the risk of arrhythmia when combined with antiarrhythmics, cisapride, pimozide, sparfloxacin, or other drugs which prolong QT interval. Metoclopramide may increase risk of extrapyramidal symptoms (EPS). Acetylcholinesterase inhibitors (central) may increase the risk of antipsychotic-related EPS.

Nutritional/Ethanol Interactions

Ethanol: Avoid ethanol (may increase CNS depression).

Herb/Nutraceutical: Avoid St John's wort (may decrease chlorpromazine levels, increase photosensitization, or enhance sedative effect). Avoid dong quai (may enhance photosensitization). Avoid kava kava, gotu kola, valerian (may increase CNS depression).

Lab Interactions False-positives for phenylketonuria, amylase, uroporphyrins, urobilinogen. May cause false-positive pregnancy test.

Adverse Reactions Frequency not defined.

Cardiovascular: Postural hypotension, tachycardia, dizziness, nonspecific QT changes

Central nervous system: Drowsiness, dystonias, akathisia, pseudoparkinsonism, tardive dyskinesia, neuroleptic malignant syndrome, seizure

Dermatologic: Photosensitivity, dermatitis, skin pigmentation (slate gray)

Endocrine & metabolic: Lactation, breast engorgement, false-positive pregnancy test, amenorrhea, gynecomastia, hyper- or hypoglycemia

Gastrointestinal: Xerostomia, constipation, nausea

Genitourinary: Urinary retention, ejaculatory disorder, impotence

Hematologic: Agranulocytosis, eosinophilia, leukopenia, hemolytic anemia, aplastic anemia, thrombocytopenic purpura

Hepatic: Jaundice

Ocular: Blurred vision, corneal and lenticular changes, epithelial keratopathy, pigmentary retinopathy

Overdosage/Toxicology Symptoms of overdose include deep sleep, coma, extrapyramidal symptoms, abnormal involuntary muscle movements, and hypotension. Following initiation of essential overdose management, toxic symptom treatment and supportive treatment should be initiated. Neuroleptics often cause extrapyramidal symptoms (eg, dystonic reactions) requiring management with anticholinergic agents such as benztropine mesylate 1-2 mg for adult patients (oral, I.M., I.V.) or diphenhydramine 25-50 mg (oral, I.M., I.V.) may be effective.

Pharmacodynamics/Kinetics

Onset of Action: I.M.: 15 minutes; Oral: 30-60 minutes

Protein Binding: 92% to 97%

Half-Life Elimination: Biphasic: Initial: 2 hours; Terminal: 30 hours

Metabolism: Extensively hepatic to active and inactive metabolites

Excretion: Urine (<1% as unchanged drug) within 24 hours

Available Dosage Forms

Injection, solution, as hydrochloride: 25 mg/mL (1 mL, 2 mL)

Tablet, as hydrochloride: 10 mg, 25 mg, 50 mg, 100 mg, 200 mg

Dosing

Adults:

Schizophrenia/psychoses:

Oral: Range: 30-800 mg/day in 1-4 divided doses, initiate at lower doses and titrate as needed; usual dose: 200 mg/day; some patients may require 1-2 g/day

I.M., I.V.: Initial: 25 mg, may repeat (25-50 mg) in 1-4 hours, gradually increase to a maximum of 400 mg/dose every 4-6 hours until patient is controlled; usual dose: 300-800 mg/day

Intractable hiccups: Oral, I.M.: 25-50 mg 3-4 times/ day

Nausea and vomiting:

Oral: 10-25 mg every 4-6 hours

I.M., I.V.: 25-50 mg every 4-6 hours

Elderly:

Behavioral symptoms associated with dementia: Initial: 10-25 mg 1-2 times/day; increase at 4- to 7-day intervals by 10-25 mg/day. Increase dose intervals (eg, twice daily, 3 times/day) as necessary to control behavior response or side effects; maximum daily dose: 800 mg; gradual increases (titration) may prevent some side effects or decrease their severity.

Other indications: Refer to adult dosing.

Pediatrics:

Schizophrenia/psychoses: Children ≥6 months:

Oral: 0.5-1 mg/kg/dose every 4-6 hours; older children may require 200 mg/day or higher.

I.M., I.V.: 0.5-1 mg/kg/dose every 6-8 hours; maximum dose for <5 years (22.7 kg): 40 mg/day; maximum for 5-12 years (22.7-45.5 kg): 75 mg/ day

Nausea and vomiting: Children ≥6 months:

Oral: 0.5-1 mg/kg/dose every 4-6 hours as needed

I.M., I.V.: 0.5-1 mg/kg/dose every 6-8 hours; maximum dose for <5 years (22.7 kg): 40 mg/day; maximum for 5-12 years (22.7-45.5 kg): 75 mg/ day

Renal Impairment: Not dialyzable (0% to 5%)

Hepatic Impairment: Avoid use in severe hepatic dysfunction.

Administration

I.V.: Direct of intermittent infusion: Infuse 1 mg or portion thereof over 1 minute. **Note:** Avoid skin contact with solution; may cause contact dermatitis.

Stability

Reconstitution: Dilute injection (1 mg/mL) with NS for I.V. administration.

Compatibility: Stable in dextran 6% in dextrose, dextran 6% in NS, D_5LR, $D_5\frac{1}{4}NS$, $D_5\frac{1}{2}NS$, D_5NS, D_5W, $D_{10}W$, LR, $\frac{1}{2}NS$, NS

Y-site administration: Incompatible with allopurinol, amifostine, amphotericin B cholesteryl sulfate complex, aztreonam, cefepime, etoposide phosphate, fludarabine, furosemide, linezolid, melphalan, methotrexate, paclitaxel, piperacillin/ tazobactam, sargramostim

Compatibility in syringe: Incompatible with cimetidine, dimenhydrinate, heparin, pentobarbital, thiopental

Compatibility when admixed: Incompatible with aminophylline, amphotericin B, ampicillin, chloramphenicol, chlorothiazide, floxacillin, furosemide, methohexital, penicillin G potassium, penicillin G sodium, phenobarbital

Storage: Injection: Protect from light. A slightly yellowed solution does not indicate potency loss, but a markedly discolored solution should be discarded. Diluted injection (1 mg/mL) with NS and stored in 5 mL vials remains stable for 30 days.

Laboratory Monitoring Lipid profile, fasting blood glucose/Hgb A_{1c}; BMI

Nursing Actions

Physical Assessment: Assess other medications patient is taking for effectiveness and interactions. Review ophthalmic exam and monitor laboratory results, therapeutic response (eg, mental status, mood, affect, gait), and adverse reactions at beginning of therapy and periodically with long-term use (eg, excess sedation, extrapyramidal symptoms, CNS changes). **I.V./I.M.:** Significant hypotension may occur. Initiate at lower doses (see Dosing) and taper dosage slowly when discontinuing. Assess knowledge/teach patient appropriate use, interventions to reduce side effects, and adverse symptoms to report. **Note:** Chlorpromazine may cause false-positive pregnancy test.

Patient Education: Use exactly as directed; do not increase dose or frequency. Do not discontinue this medication without consulting prescriber. Tablets may be taken with food. Do not take within 2 hours of any antacid. Store away from light. Avoid alcohol or caffeine and other prescription or OTC medications not approved by prescriber. Maintain adequate hydration (2-3 L/day of fluids) unless instructed to restrict fluid intake. May turn urine red-brown (normal). You may experience excess drowsiness, lightheadedness, dizziness, or blurred vision (use caution driving or when engaging in tasks requiring alertness until response to drug is known); dry mouth, upset stomach, nausea, vomiting, anorexia (small frequent meals, frequent mouth care, sucking lozenges, or chewing gum may help); constipation (increased exercise, fluids, fruit, or fiber may help); postural hypotension (use caution climbing stairs or when changing position from lying or sitting to standing); urinary retention (void before taking medication); ejaculatory dysfunction (reversible); decreased perspiration (avoid strenuous exercise in hot environments); or photosensitivity (use sunscreen, wear protective clothing and eyewear, and avoid direct sunlight). Report persistent CNS effects (trembling fingers, altered gait or balance, excessive sedation, seizures, unusual movements, anxiety, abnormal thoughts, confusion, personality changes); chest pain, palpitations, rapid heartbeat, or severe dizziness; unresolved urinary retention or changes in urinary pattern; altered menstrual pattern, change in libido, swelling or pain in breasts (male or female); vision changes, skin rash, irritation, or changes in color of skin (gray-blue); or worsening of condition. **Pregnancy/breast-feeding precautions:** Inform prescriber if you are or intend to become pregnant. Breast-feeding is not recommended.

Geriatric Considerations See Warnings/Precautions, Adverse Reactions, and Overdose/Toxicology. Elderly patients have an increased risk of adverse response to side effects or adverse reactions to antipsychotics.

Breast-Feeding Issues Drowsiness and lethargy have been reported in nursing infants; galactorrhea has been reported in mother.

Related Information

Chlorthalidone (klor THAL i done)

U.S. Brand Names Thalitone®
Synonyms Hygroton
Pharmacologic Category Diuretic, Thiazide
Pregnancy Risk Factor B (manufacturer); D (expert analysis)
Lactation Enters breast milk/use caution (AAP rates "compatible")
Use Management of mild-to-moderate hypertension when used alone or in combination with other agents; treatment of edema associated with congestive heart failure or nephrotic syndrome. Recent studies have found chlorthalidone effective in the treatment of isolated systolic hypertension in the elderly.
Mechanism of Action/Effect Sulfonamide-derived diuretic that inhibits sodium and chloride reabsorption in the cortical-diluting segment of the ascending loop of Henle
Contraindications Hypersensitivity to chlorthalidone or any component of the formulation; cross-sensitivity with other thiazides or sulfonamides; anuria; renal decompensation; pregnancy
Warnings/Precautions Use with caution in patients with hypokalemia, renal disease, hepatic disease, gout, lupus erythematosus, or diabetes mellitus. Use with caution in severe renal diseases. Correct hypokalemia before initiating therapy. Chemical similarities are present among sulfonamides, sulfonylureas, carbonic anhydrase inhibitors, thiazides, and loop diuretics (except ethacrynic acid). Use in patients with thiazide or sulfonamide allergy is specifically contraindicated in product labeling, however, a risk of cross-reaction exists in patients with allergy to any of these compounds; avoid use when previous reaction has been severe.

Drug Interactions

Decreased Effect: Effects of oral hypoglycemics may be decreased. Decreased absorption of chlorthalidone with cholestyramine and colestipol. NSAIDs can decrease the efficacy of chlorthalidone, reducing the diuretic and antihypertensive effects.

Increased Effect/Toxicity: Increased effect of chlorthalidone with furosemide and other loop diuretics. Increased hypotension and/or renal adverse effects of ACE inhibitors may result in aggressively diuresed patients. Beta-blockers increase hyperglycemic effects of thiazides in Type 2 diabetes mellitus. Cyclosporine and thiazides can increase the risk of gout or renal toxicity. Digoxin toxicity can be exacerbated if a thiazide induces hypokalemia or hypomagnesemia. Lithium toxicity can occur with thiazides due to reduced renal excretion of lithium. Thiazides may prolong the duration of action with neuromuscular blocking agents.

Nutritional/Ethanol Interactions Herb/Nutraceutical: Avoid dong quai if using for hypertension (has estrogenic activity). Avoid dong quai, St John's Wort (may also cause photosensitization). Avoid ephedra, yohimbe, ginseng (may worsen hypertension).

Lab Interactions Increased creatine phosphokinase [CPK] (S), ammonia (B), amylase (S), calcium (S), chloride (S), cholesterol (S), glucose, acid (S); decreased chloride (S), magnesium, potassium (S), sodium (S)

Adverse Reactions 1% to 10%:
Dermatologic: Photosensitivity
Endocrine & metabolic: Hypokalemia
Gastrointestinal: Anorexia, epigastric distress

Overdosage/Toxicology Symptoms of overdose include hypermotility, diuresis, lethargy, confusion, muscle weakness, and coma. Treatment is supportive.

Pharmacodynamics/Kinetics

Onset of Action: Peak effect: 2-6 hours

Duration of Action:
24-72 hours
(Continued)

Chlorthalidone *(Continued)*

Half-Life Elimination: 35-55 hours; may be prolonged with renal impairment; Anuria: 81 hours

Metabolism: Hepatic

Excretion: Urine (~50% to 65% as unchanged drug)

Available Dosage Forms

Tablet: 25 mg, 50 mg, 100 mg

Thalitone®: 15 mg

Dosing

Adults:

Hypertension: Oral: 25-100 mg/day or 100 mg 3 times/week; usual dosage range (JNC 7): 12.5-25 mg/day

Edema: Initial: 50-100 mg/day or 100 mg on alternate days; maximum dose: 200 mg/day

Heart failure-associated edema: 12.5-25 mg once daily; maximum daily dose: 100 mg (ACC/AHA 2005 Heart Failure Guidelines)

Elderly: Oral: Initial: 12.5-25 mg/day or every other day; there is little advantage to using doses >25 mg/day.

Pediatrics: Oral: Children (nonapproved): 2 mg/kg/dose 3 times/week or 1-2 mg/kg/day

Renal Impairment: Cl_{cr} <10 mL/minute: Avoid use. Ineffective with low GFR (Aronoff G, 2002)

Note: ACC/AHA 2005 Heart Failure Guidelines suggest that thiazides lose their efficacy when Cl_{cr} <40 mL/minute

Laboratory Monitoring Serum electrolytes, renal function

Nursing Actions

Physical Assessment: Allergy history should be assessed prior to beginning therapy. Assess other pharmacological or herbal products patient may be taking for potential interactions. Monitor laboratory tests and patient response (eg, blood pressure, fluid status, and electrolyte balance) regularly during long-term therapy. Caution patients with diabetes to monitor glucose levels; may reduce effect of oral hypoglycemics. Teach patient appropriate use, possible side effects/appropriate interventions, and adverse symptoms to report (see Patient Education).

Patient Education: Do not take any new medication during therapy unless approved by prescriber. Take once-daily dose in morning or last of daily doses early in the day to avoid night-time disturbances. You may need to make dietary changes (eg, your prescriber may recommend a potassium supplement or foods high in potassium; do not increase your potassium intake unless recommended to do so). If using oral hypoglycemics, monitor glucose levels closely (this medication may reduce effect of oral hypoglycemics); contact prescriber with any major changes. May cause sensitivity to sunlight (use sunblock, wear protective clothing, and avoid direct sunlight); or anorexia or GI distress (small, frequent meals, frequent mouth care, chewing gum, or sucking lozenges may help). Report muscle twitching or cramps; nausea or vomiting; confusion; numbness of extremities; loss of appetite or GI distress; severe rash, redness, or itching of skin; chest pain or palpitations; respiratory difficulty; unusual weight loss; or other persistent adverse effects. **Pregnancy/breast-feeding precautions:** Do not get pregnant while taking this medication. Consult prescriber for appropriate contraceptive measures. Consult prescriber if breast-feeding.

Dietary Considerations This product may cause a potassium loss; your healthcare provider may prescribe a potassium supplement, another medication to help prevent the potassium loss, or recommend that you eat foods high in potassium, especially citrus fruits; do not change your diet on your own while taking this medication, especially if you are taking potassium supplements

or medications to reduce potassium loss; too much potassium can be as harmful as too little.

Geriatric Considerations Studies have found chlorthalidone effective in the treatment of isolated systolic hypertension in the elderly.

Chlorzoxazone *(klor ZOKS a zone)*

U.S. Brand Names Parafon Forte® DSC

Pharmacologic Category Skeletal Muscle Relaxant

Medication Safety Issues

Sound-alike/look-alike issues:

Parafon Forte® may be confused with Fam-Pren Forte

Pregnancy Risk Factor C

Lactation Excretion in breast milk unknown/not recommended

Use Symptomatic treatment of muscle spasm and pain associated with acute musculoskeletal conditions

Mechanism of Action/Effect Acts on the spinal cord and subcortical levels by depressing polysynaptic reflexes

Contraindications Hypersensitivity to chlorzoxazone or any component of the formulation; impaired liver function

Drug Interactions

Cytochrome P450 Effect: Substrate of CYP1A2 (minor), 2A6 (minor), 2D6 (minor), 2E1 (major), 3A4 (minor); **Inhibits** CYP2E1 (weak), 3A4 (weak)

Increased Effect/Toxicity: Effects of CNS depressants may be increased by chlorzoxazone. CYP2E1 inhibitors may increase the levels/effects of chlorzoxazone; example inhibitors include disulfiram, isoniazid, and miconazole. Disulfiram and isoniazid may increase chlorzoxazone concentration; monitor.

Nutritional/Ethanol Interactions Ethanol: Avoid ethanol (may increase CNS depression).

Adverse Reactions Frequency not defined.

Central nervous system: Dizziness, drowsiness lightheadedness, paradoxical stimulation, malaise

Dermatologic: Rash, petechiae, ecchymoses (rare), angioneurotic edema

Gastrointestinal: Nausea, vomiting, stomach cramps

Genitourinary: Urine discoloration

Hepatic: Liver dysfunction

Miscellaneous: Anaphylaxis (very rare)

Overdosage/Toxicology Symptoms of overdose include nausea, vomiting, diarrhea, drowsiness, dizziness, headache, absent tendon reflexes, and hypotension. Treatment is supportive following attempts to enhance drug elimination. Dialysis, hemoperfusion, and osmotic diuresis have all been useful in reducing serum drug concentrations. The patient should be observed for possible relapses due to incomplete gastric emptying.

Pharmacodynamics/Kinetics

Onset of Action: ~1 hour

Duration of Action: 6-12 hours

Metabolism: Extensively hepatic via glucuronidation

Excretion: Urine (as conjugates)

Available Dosage Forms

Caplet (Parafon Forte® DSC): 500 mg

Tablet: 250 mg, 500 mg

Dosing

Adults: Muscle spasm: Oral: 250-500 mg 3-4 times/day up to 750 mg 3-4 times/day

Elderly: Oral: Initial: 250 mg 2-4 times/day; increase as necessary to 750 mg 3-4 times/day.

Pediatrics: Muscle spasm: Oral: 20 mg/kg/day or 600 mg/m²/day in 3-4 divided doses

Laboratory Monitoring Periodic liver functions

Nursing Actions

Physical Assessment: Monitor results of laboratory tests, effectiveness of therapy (according to rationale for therapy), and adverse reactions at beginning of therapy and periodically with long-term use. Do not discontinue abruptly; taper dosage slowly. Assess knowledge/teach patient appropriate use, interventions to reduce side effects (postural hypotension precautions), and adverse symptoms to report.

Patient Education: Take exactly as directed with food. Do not increase dose or discontinue this medication without consulting prescriber. Do not use alcohol, prescriptive or OTC antidepressants, sedatives, or pain medications without consulting prescriber. May turn urine orange or red (normal). You may experience drowsiness, dizziness, lightheadedness (avoid driving or engaging in tasks that require alertness until response to drug is known); nausea, vomiting, or cramping (small frequent meals, frequent mouth care, or sucking hard candy may help); postural hypotension (change position slowly when rising from sitting or lying or when climbing stairs); or constipation (increased exercise, fluids, fruit, or fiber may help). Report excessive drowsiness or mental agitation; palpitations, rapid heartbeat, or chest pain; skin rash or swelling of mouth or face; persistent diarrhea or constipation; or unusual weakness or bleeding. **Pregnancy/breast-feeding precautions:** Inform prescriber if you are or intend to become pregnant. Breast-feeding is not recommended.

Geriatric Considerations Start dosing low and increase as necessary. The FDA recently approved a stronger warning about hepatotoxicity in the labeling of chlorzoxazone. Because it can cause unpredictable, fatal hepatic toxicity, the use of chlorzoxazone should be avoided.

Cholestyramine Resin
(koe LES teer a meen REZ in)

U.S. Brand Names Prevalite®; Questran®; Questran® Light

Pharmacologic Category Antilipemic Agent, Bile Acid Sequestrant

Pregnancy Risk Factor C

Lactation Does not enter breast milk/use caution

Use Adjunct in the management of primary hypercholesterolemia; pruritus associated with elevated levels of bile acids; diarrhea associated with excess fecal bile acids; binding toxicologic agents; pseudomembraneous colitis

Mechanism of Action/Effect Forms a nonabsorbable complex with bile acids in the intestine, releasing chloride ions in the process; inhibits enterohepatic reuptake of intestinal bile salts and thereby increases the fecal loss of bile salt-bound low density lipoprotein cholesterol

Contraindications Hypersensitivity to bile acid sequestering resins or any component of the formulation; complete biliary obstruction; bowel obstruction

Warnings/Precautions Not to be taken simultaneously with many other medicines (decreased absorption). Treat any diseases contributing to hypercholesterolemia first. May interfere with fat-soluble vitamins (A, D, E, K) and folic acid. Chronic use may be associated with bleeding problems (especially in high doses). May produce or exacerbate constipation problems. Fecal impaction may occur. Hemorrhoids may be worsened.

Drug Interactions
Decreased Effect:
Cholestyramine can reduce the absorption of numerous medications when used concurrently. Give other medications 1 hour before or 4-6 hours after giving cholestyramine. Medications which may be affected include HMG-CoA reductase inhibitors, thiazide diuretics, propranolol (and potentially other beta-blockers), corticosteroids, thyroid hormones, digoxin, valproic acid, NSAIDs, loop diuretics, sulfonylureas, troglitazone (and potentially other agents in this class).

Warfarin and other oral anticoagulants: Hypoprothrombinemic effects may be reduced by cholestyramine. Separate administration times (as detailed above) and monitor INR closely when initiating or discontinuing.

Nutritional/Ethanol Interactions
Food: Cholestyramine (especially high doses or long-term therapy) may decrease the absorption of folic acid, calcium, and iron.
Herb/Nutraceutical: Cholestyramine (especially high doses or long-term therapy) may decrease the absorption of fat-soluble vitamins (vitamins A, D, E, and K).

Lab Interactions Increased prothrombin time (S); decreased cholesterol (S), iron (B)

Adverse Reactions
>10%: Gastrointestinal: Constipation, heartburn, nausea, vomiting, stomach pain
1% to 10%:
Central nervous system: Headache
Gastrointestinal: Belching, bloating, diarrhea

Overdosage/Toxicology Symptoms of overdose include GI obstruction. Treatment is supportive.

Pharmacodynamics/Kinetics
Onset of Action: Peak effect: 21 days
Excretion: Feces (as insoluble complex with bile acids)

Available Dosage Forms
Powder for oral suspension: 4 g of resin/5.7 g of powder (5.7 g packets, 240 g can) [light formulation]; 4 g of resin/9 g of powder (9 g packets, 378 g can)
Prevalite®: 4 g of resin/5.5 g of powder (5.5 g packets, 231 g can) [contains phenylalanine 14.1 mg/5.5 g; orange flavor]
Questran®: 4 g of resin/9 g of powder (9 g packets, 378 g can)
Questran® Light: 4 g of resin/5 g of powder (5 g packets, 210 g can) [contains phenylalanine 16.8 g/5 g]

Dosing
Adults & Elderly: Dyslipidemia: Oral (dosages are expressed in terms of anhydrous resin): 4 g 1-2 times/day to a maximum of 16-24 g/day (and a maximum of 6 times/day)
Pediatrics: Dyslipidemia: Oral (dosages are expressed in terms of anhydrous resin): Children: 240 mg/kg/day in 3 divided doses; need to titrate dose depending on indication
Renal Impairment: Not removed by hemo- or peritoneal dialysis. Supplemental doses not necessary with dialysis or continuous arteriovenous or venovenous hemofiltration effects.

Administration
Oral: Mix powder with water or other fluid prior to administration; not to be taken in dry form. Suspension should not be sipped or held in mouth for prolonged periods (may cause tooth discoloration or enamel decay).

Stability
Storage: Store powder at controlled room temperature of 15°C to 30°C (59°F to 86°F). Mix contents of 1 packet or 1 level scoop of powder with 4-6 oz of beverage. Allow to stand 1-2 minutes prior to mixing. May also be mixed with highly-fluid soups, cereals, applesauce, etc. Suspension may be used for up to 48 hours after refrigeration.

Laboratory Monitoring Serum cholesterol and triglyceride levels before initiating treatment and periodically throughout treatment.

Nursing Actions
Physical Assessment: Assess other medications patient may be taking for effectiveness and interactions. Monitor laboratory results, therapeutic response, and adverse reactions (eg, GI effects and nutritional status) periodically throughout therapy. Assess knowledge/teach patient appropriate use, (Continued)

Cholestyramine Resin *(Continued)*

interventions to reduce side effects, and adverse symptoms to report.

Patient Education: Take once or twice a day as directed. Do not take the powder in its dry form; mix with fluid, applesauce, pudding, or jello. Take other medications 1 hour before or 4-6 hours after cholestyramine. Ongoing medical follow-up and laboratory tests may be required. You may experience GI effects (these should resolve after continued use); nausea and vomiting (small frequent meals, frequent mouth care, sucking lozenges, or chewing gum may help); or constipation (increased exercise, fluids, fruit, or fiber may help; consult prescriber about use of stool softener or laxative). Report unusual stomach cramping, pain or blood in stool; unresolved nausea, vomiting, or constipation. **Pregnancy/breast-feeding precautions:** Inform prescriber if you are or intend to become pregnant. Consult prescriber if breast-feeding.

Dietary Considerations Supplementation of vitamins A, D, E, and K, folic acid, and iron may be required with high-dose, long-term therapy.

Questran® Light contains phenylalanine 16.8 g/5 g powder.

Prevalite® contains phenylalanine 14.1 g/5.5 g powder.

Geriatric Considerations The definition of and, therefore, when to treat hyperlipidemia in the elderly is a controversial issue. Treatment is best reserved for those who are unable to obtain a desirable plasma cholesterol level by diet alone and for whom the benefits of treatment are believed to outweigh the potential adverse effects, drug interactions, and cost of treatment.

Choline Magnesium Trisalicylate
(KOE leen mag NEE zhum trye sa LIS i late)

U.S. Brand Names Trilisate® [DSC]

Synonyms Tricosal

Pharmacologic Category Salicylate

Pregnancy Risk Factor C/D (3rd trimester)

Lactation Enters breast milk/use caution

Use Management of osteoarthritis, rheumatoid arthritis, and other arthritis; acute painful shoulder

Mechanism of Action/Effect Inhibits prostaglandin synthesis; acts on the hypothalamus heat-regulating center to reduce fever; blocks the generation of pain impulses

Contraindications Hypersensitivity to salicylates, other nonacetylated salicylates, other NSAIDs, or any component of the formulation; bleeding disorders; pregnancy (3rd trimester)

Warnings/Precautions Salicylate salts may not inhibit platelet aggregation and, therefore, should not be substituted for aspirin in the prophylaxis of thrombosis. Use with caution in patients with impaired renal function, dehydration, erosive gastritis, asthma, or peptic ulcer. Discontinue use 1 week prior to surgical procedures. Children and teenagers who have or are recovering from chickenpox or flu-like symptoms should not use this product. Changes in behavior (along with nausea and vomiting) may be an early sign of Reye's syndrome; patients should be instructed to contact their healthcare provider if these occur.

Elderly are a high-risk population for adverse effects from NSAIDs. As many as 60% of elderly can develop peptic ulceration and/or hemorrhage asymptomatically. Use lowest effective dose for shortest period possible. CNS adverse effects may be observed in the elderly at lower doses than younger adults.

Drug Interactions

Decreased Effect: Antacids may decrease choline magnesium trisalicylate absorption/salicylate concentrations.

Increased Effect/Toxicity: Choline magnesium trisalicylate may increase the hypoprothrombinemic effect of warfarin.

Nutritional/Ethanol Interactions

Ethanol: Avoid ethanol (may enhance gastric mucosal irritation).

Food: May decrease the rate but not the extent of oral absorption.

Herb/Nutraceutical: Avoid cat's claw, dong quai, evening primrose, feverfew, garlic, ginger, ginkgo, red clover, horse chestnut, green tea, ginseng (all have additional antiplatelet activity). Limit curry powder, paprika, licorice, Benedictine liqueur, prunes, raisins, tea, and gherkins; may cause salicylate accumulation. These foods contain 6 mg salicylate/100 g.

Lab Interactions False-negative results for glucose oxidase urinary glucose tests (Clinistix®); false-positives using the cupric sulfate method (Clinitest®); also, interferes with Gerhardt test (urinary ketone analysis), VMA determination; 5-HIAA, xylose tolerance test, and T_3 and T_4; increased PBI; increased uric acid

Adverse Reactions

<20%:

Gastrointestinal: Nausea, vomiting, diarrhea, heartburn, dyspepsia, epigastric pain, constipation

Otic: Tinnitus

<2%:

Central nervous system: Headache, lightheadedness, dizziness, drowsiness, lethargy

Otic: Hearing impairment

Overdosage/Toxicology Symptoms of overdose include tinnitus, vomiting, acute renal failure, hyperthermia, irritability, seizures, coma, and metabolic acidosis. For acute ingestion, determine serum salicylate levels 6 hours after ingestion. Nomograms, such as the "Done" nomogram, may be helpful for estimating the severity of aspirin poisoning and directing treatment using serum salicylate levels. Treatment is based upon symptomatology.

Pharmacodynamics/Kinetics

Onset of Action: Peak effect: ~2 hours

Time to Peak: Serum: ~2 hours

Half-Life Elimination: Dose dependent: Low dose: 2-3 hours; High dose: 30 hours

Available Dosage Forms

Liquid: 500 mg/5 mL (240 mL) [choline salicylate 293 mg and magnesium salicylate 362 mg per 5 mL; cherry cordial flavor]

Tablet: 500 mg [choline salicylate 293 mg and magnesium salicylate 362 mg]; 750 mg [choline salicylate 440 mg and magnesium salicylate 544 mg]; 1000 mg [choline salicylate 587 mg and magnesium salicylate 725 mg]

Dosing

Adults & Elderly: Arthritis, pain: Oral (based on total salicylate content): 500 mg to 1.5 g 2-3 times/day **or** 3 g at bedtime; usual maintenance dose: 1-4.5 g/day

Pediatrics: Children: Oral (based on total salicylate content): <37 kg: 50 mg/kg/day given in 2 divided doses; 2250 mg/day for heavier children

Renal Impairment: Avoid use in severe renal impairment.

Administration

Oral: Liquid may be mixed with fruit juice just before drinking. Do not administer with antacids. Take with a full glass of water and remain in an upright position for 15-30 minutes after administration.

Stability

Storage: Store at controlled room temperature of 15°C to 30°C (59°F to 86°F).

Laboratory Monitoring Serum magnesium with high-dose therapy or in patients with impaired renal function, serum salicylate levels, renal function

Nursing Actions

Physical Assessment: Do not use for persons with allergic reaction to salicylates or other NSAIDs.

Assess other medications patient may be taking for additive or adverse interactions. Monitor for effectiveness of pain relief. Monitor for signs of adverse reactions or overdose at beginning of therapy and periodically during long-term therapy. Assess knowledge/teach patient appropriate use. Teach patient to monitor for adverse reactions, adverse reactions to report, and appropriate interventions to reduce side effects.

Patient Education: Use exactly as directed; do not increase dose or frequency. Adverse reactions can occur with overuse. Take with food or milk. While using this medication, do not use alcohol, excessive amounts of vitamin C, or salicylate-containing foods (curry powder, prunes, raisins, tea, or licorice), other prescription or OTC medications containing aspirin or salicylate, or other NSAIDs without consulting prescriber. Maintain adequate hydration (2-3 L/day of fluids) unless instructed to restrict fluid intake. You may experience nausea, vomiting, gastric discomfort (frequent mouth care, small frequent meals, sucking lozenges, or chewing gum may help). GI bleeding, ulceration, or perforation can occur with or without pain. Stop taking medication and report ringing in ears; persistent stomach pain; unresolved nausea or vomiting; respiratory difficulty or shortness of breath; or unusual bruising or bleeding (mouth, urine, stool); or skin rash. **Pregnancy/breast-feeding precautions:** Inform prescriber if you are or intend to become pregnant. Consult prescriber if breast-feeding.

Dietary Considerations Take with food or large volume of water or milk to minimize GI upset. Liquid may be mixed with fruit juice just before drinking. Hypermagnesemia resulting from magnesium salicylate; avoid or use with caution in renal insufficiency.

Geriatric Considerations Elderly are at high risk for adverse effects from nonsteroidal anti-inflammatory agents. As much as 60% of elderly can develop peptic ulceration and/or hemorrhage asymptomatically.

Breast-Feeding Issues Excreted in breast milk; peak levels occur 9-12 hours after dose. Use caution if used during breast-feeding.

Pregnancy Issues Animal reproduction studies have not been conducted. Due to the known effects of other salicylates (closure of ductus arteriosus), use during late pregnancy should be avoided.

Chorionic Gonadotropin (Human)
(kor ee ON ik goe NAD oh troe pin, HYU man)

U.S. Brand Names Novarel™; Pregnyl®

Synonyms CG; hCG

Pharmacologic Category Ovulation Stimulator

Pregnancy Risk Factor C

Lactation Excretion in breast milk unknown/unlikely to be used

Use Induces ovulation and pregnancy in anovulatory, infertile females; treatment of hypogonadotropic hypogonadism, prepubertal cryptorchidism; spermatogenesis induction with follitropin alfa or follitropin beta

Mechanism of Action/Effect Stimulates production of gonadal steroid hormones by causing production of androgen by the testis; as a substitute for luteinizing hormone (LH) to stimulate ovulation

Contraindications Hypersensitivity to chorionic gonadotropin or any component of the formulation; precocious puberty, prostatic carcinoma or similar neoplasms

Warnings/Precautions Use with caution in asthma, seizure disorders, migraine, cardiac or renal disease. **Not** effective in the treatment of obesity.

Adverse Reactions
1% to 10%:
Central nervous system: Mental depression, fatigue

Endocrine & metabolic: Pelvic pain, ovarian cysts, enlargement of breasts, precocious puberty

Local: Pain at the injection site

Neuromuscular & skeletal: Premature closure of epiphyses

Pharmacodynamics/Kinetics

Half-Life Elimination: Biphasic: Initial: 11 hours; Terminal: 23 hours

Excretion: Urine (as unchanged drug) within 3-4 days

Available Dosage Forms

Injection, powder for reconstitution: 10,000 units [packaged with diluent; diluent contains benzyl alcohol and mannitol]

Novarel™: 10,000 units [packaged with diluent; diluent contains benzyl alcohol and mannitol]

Pregnyl®: 10,000 units [packaged with diluent; diluent contains benzyl alcohol]

Dosing

Adults & Elderly:

Use with menotropins to stimulate spermatogenesis: I.M.: 5000 units 3 times/week for 4-6 months. With the beginning of menotropins therapy, hCG dose is continued at 2000 units 2 times/week.

Induction of ovulation and pregnancy: I.M.: 5000-10,000 units 1 day following last dose of menotropins

Spermatogenesis induction: Male: I.M.: Initial: 1500 int. units twice weekly to normalize serum testosterone levels. If no response in 8 weeks, increase dose to 3000 int. units twice weekly. After normalization of testosterone levels, combine with follitropin beta (Follistim®). Continue hCG at same dose used to normalize testosterone levels. Treatment response was noted at up to 12 months.

Pediatrics:

Prepubertal cryptorchidism: I.M.: Children: 1000-2000 units/m^2/dose 3 times/week for 3 weeks **or** 4000 units 3 times/week for 3 weeks **or** 5000 units every second day for 4 injections **or** 500 units 3 times/week for 4-6 weeks

Hypogonadotropic hypogonadism: I.M.: Children: 500-1000 units 3 times/week for 3 weeks, followed by the same dose twice weekly for 3 weeks **or** 1000-2000 units 3 times/week **or** 4000 units 3 times/week for 6-9 months; reduce dosage to 2000 units 3 times/week for additional 3 months.

Administration

I.M.: I.M. administration only

Stability

Reconstitution: Following reconstitution with the provided diluent, solutions are stable for 30-90 days, depending on the specific preparation, when stored at 2°C to 15°C.

Nursing Actions

Physical Assessment: Monitor therapeutic effectiveness (according to purpose for use) and adverse response regularly during long-term therapy. Teach patient proper use if self-administered (appropriate injection technique and syringe/needle disposal, possible side effects/appropriate interventions, and adverse symptoms to report.

Patient Education: This medication can only be administered by injection. If self-administered, follow instruction for reconstitution, injection, and needle disposal. Use exactly as directed; do not alter dosage or miss a dose. May cause headache, depression, irritability, or restlessness (use caution when driving or engaging in potentially hazardous tasks until response to drug is known). Contact prescriber if symptoms are severe or do not resolve with use. Contact prescriber if breasts swell; if you experience swelling of legs or feet; or if there is pain, redness, or swelling at injection site. **Pregnancy/breast-feeding precautions:** Inform prescriber if you are or intend to become pregnant. Consult prescriber if breast-feeding.

Chorionic Gonadotropin (Recombinant)

(kor ee ON ik goe NAD oh troe pin ree KOM be nant)

U.S. Brand Names Ovidrel®

Synonyms Choriogonadotropin Alfa; r-hCG

Pharmacologic Category Gonadotropin; Ovulation Stimulator

Pregnancy Risk Factor X

Lactation Excretion in breast milk unknown/use caution

Use As part of an assisted reproductive technology (ART) program, induces ovulation in infertile females who have been pretreated with follicle stimulating hormones (FSH); induces ovulation and pregnancy in infertile females when the cause of infertility is functional

Contraindications Hypersensitivity to hCG preparations or any component of the formulation; primary ovarian failure; uncontrolled thyroid or adrenal dysfunction; uncontrolled organic intracranial lesion (ie, pituitary tumor); abnormal uterine bleeding, ovarian cyst or enlargement of undetermined origin; sex hormone dependent tumors; pregnancy

Warnings/Precautions For use by infertility specialists; may cause ovarian hyperstimulation syndrome (OHSS); if severe, treatment should be discontinued and patient should be hospitalized. OHSS results in a rapid (<24 hours to 7 days) accumulation of fluid in the peritoneal cavity, thorax, and possibly the pericardium, which may become more severe if pregnancy occurs; monitor for ovarian enlargement; use may lead to multiple births; risk of arterial thromboembolism with hCG products; safety and efficacy in pediatric and geriatric patients have not been established.

Drug Interactions

Increased Effect/Toxicity: Specific drug interaction studies have not been conducted.

Lab Interactions May interfere with interpretation of pregnancy tests; may cross-react with radioimmunoassay of luteinizing hormone and other gonadotropins

Adverse Reactions

2% to 10%:

Endocrine & metabolic: Ovarian cyst (3%), ovarian hyperstimulation (<2% to 3%)

Gastrointestinal: Abdominal pain (3% to 4%), nausea (3%), vomiting (3%)

Local: Injection site: Pain (8%), bruising (3% to 5%), reaction (<2% to 3%), inflammation (<2% to 2%)

Miscellaneous: Postoperative pain (5%)

<2%:

Cardiovascular: Cardiac arrhythmia, heart murmur

Central nervous system: Dizziness, emotional lability, fever, headache, insomnia, malaise

Dermatologic: Pruritus, rash

Endocrine & metabolic: Breast pain, hot flashes, hyperglycemia, intermenstrual bleeding, vaginal hemorrhage

Gastrointestinal: Abdominal enlargement, diarrhea, flatulence

Genitourinary: Cervical carcinoma, cervical lesion, dysuria, genital herpes, genital moniliasis, leukorrhea, urinary incontinence, urinary tract infection, vaginitis

Hematologic: Leukocytosis

Neuromuscular & skeletal: Back pain, paresthesia

Renal: Albuminuria

Respiratory: Cough, pharyngitis, upper respiratory tract infection

Miscellaneous: Ectopic pregnancy, hiccups

In addition, the following have been reported with menotropin therapy: Adnexal torsion, hemoperitoneum, mild-to-moderate ovarian enlargement, pulmonary and vascular complications. Ovarian neoplasms have also been reported (rare) with multiple drug regimens used for ovarian induction (relationship not established).

Pharmacodynamics/Kinetics

Time to Peak: 12-24 hours

Half-Life Elimination: Initial: 4 hours; Terminal: 29 hours

Excretion: Urine (10% of dose)

Available Dosage Forms [DSC] = Discontinued product

Injection, powder for reconstitution: 285 mcg [packaged with 1 mL SWFI; delivers 250 mcg r-hCG following reconstitution] [DSC]

Injection, solution: 257.5 mcg/0.515 mL (0.515 mL) [prefilled syringe; delivers 250 mcg r-hCG/0.5 mL]

Dosing

Adults: Assisted reproductive technologies (ART) and ovulation induction in females: SubQ: 250 mcg given 1 day following the last dose of follicle stimulating agent. Use only after adequate follicular development has been determined. Hold treatment when there is an excessive ovarian response.

Elderly: Safety and efficacy have not been established.

Renal Impairment: Safety and efficacy have not been established.

Hepatic Impairment: Safety and efficacy have not been established.

Stability

Reconstitution: Powder for reconstitution: Mix vial with 1 mL sterile water for injection. Gently mix by rotating vial to dissolve powder; do not shake. Use immediately following reconstitution.

Storage:

Powder for reconstitution: Store in original package under refrigeration or at room temperature of 2°C to 25°C (36°F to 77°F). Protect from light.

Prefilled syringe: Prior to dispensing, store at 2°C to 8°C (36°F to 46°F). Patient may store at 25°C (77°F) for up to 30 days. Protect from light.

Nursing Actions

Physical Assessment: For use only under the supervision/direction of an infertility physician. Monitor for adverse reactions. Teach patient proper use if self-administered (storage, reconstitution, injection technique, needle/syringe disposal; recommend return demonstration), monitoring requirements, interventions to reduce side effects, and adverse reactions to report. **Pregnancy risk factor X:** Determine that patient is not pregnant before beginning treatment and monitor ovulation closely during treatment. Note breast-feeding caution.

Patient Education: Note that there is a risk of multiple births associated with treatment. This drug must be administered exactly as scheduled (1 day following last dose of follicle stimulating agent); maintain a calendar of treatment days. Follow administration directions exactly. Keep all ultrasound and laboratory appointments as instructed by prescriber. Avoid strenuous exercise, especially those with pelvic involvement. You may experience nausea, vomiting, or GI upset (small frequent meals, frequent mouth care, sucking lozenges, or chewing gum may help), hot flashes (cool clothes, cool room, adequate rest may help) if persistent consult prescriber. Report immediately any persistent abdominal pain, vomiting, or acute pelvic pain; chest pain or palpitations; shortness of breath; or urinary tract or vaginal infection or urinary incontinence. **Pregnancy/breast-feeding precautions:** Do not take this medicine if you are pregnant and report to prescriber immediately if you suspect you are pregnant. Consult prescriber if breast-feeding.

Pregnancy Issues Ectopic pregnancy, premature labor, postpartum fever, and spontaneous abortion have been reported in clinical trials. Congenital abnormalities have also been observed, however, the incidence is similar during natural conception.

Additional Information Clinical studies have shown r-hCG to be clinically and statistically equivalent to urinary-derived hCG products.

Cidofovir (si DOF o veer)

U.S. Brand Names Vistide®
Pharmacologic Category Antiviral Agent
Pregnancy Risk Factor C
Lactation Excretion in breast milk unknown/contraindicated
Use Treatment of cytomegalovirus (CMV) retinitis in patients with acquired immunodeficiency syndrome (AIDS). **Note:** Should be administered with probenecid.
Mechanism of Action/Effect Nucleotide analog that selectively inhibits viral DNA polymerase, suppressing viral DNA synthesis
Contraindications Hypersensitivity to cidofovir; history of clinically-severe hypersensitivity to probenecid or other sulfa-containing medications; serum creatinine >1.5 mg/dL; Cl$_{cr}$ <55 mL/minute; urine protein ≥100 mg/dL (≥2+ proteinuria); use with or within 7 days of nephrotoxic agents; direct intraocular injection
Warnings/Precautions Dose-dependent nephrotoxicity requires dose adjustment or discontinuation if changes in renal function occur during therapy (eg, proteinuria, glycosuria, decreased serum phosphate, uric acid or bicarbonate, and elevated creatinine); neutropenia and ocular hypotony have also occurred; safety and efficacy have not been established in children or the elderly; administration must be accompanied by oral probenecid and intravenous saline prehydration; prepare admixtures in a class two laminar flow hood, wearing protective gear; dispose of cidofovir as directed.

Drug Interactions
Increased Effect/Toxicity: Drugs with nephrotoxic potential (eg, amphotericin B, aminoglycosides, foscarnet, and I.V. pentamidine) should not be used with or within 7 days of cidofovir therapy. Due to concomitant probenecid administration, temporarily discontinue or decrease zidovudine dose by 50% on the day of cidofovir administration only.

Adverse Reactions
>10%:
   Central nervous system: Chills, fever, headache, pain
   Dermatologic: Alopecia, rash
   Gastrointestinal: Nausea, vomiting, diarrhea, anorexia
   Hematologic: Anemia, neutropenia
   Neuromuscular & skeletal: Weakness
   Ocular: Intraocular pressure decreased, iritis, ocular hypotony, uveitis
   Renal: Creatinine increased, proteinuria, renal toxicity
   Respiratory: Cough, dyspnea
   Miscellaneous: Infection, oral moniliasis, serum bicarbonate decreased
1% to 10%:
   Renal: Fanconi syndrome
   Respiratory: Pneumonia
   Frequency not defined (limited to important or life-threatening reactions):
   Cardiovascular: Cardiomyopathy, cardiovascular disorder, CHF, edema, postural hypotension, shock, syncope, tachycardia
   Central nervous system: Agitation, amnesia, anxiety, confusion, convulsion, dizziness, hallucinations, insomnia, malaise, vertigo
   Dermatologic: Photosensitivity reaction, skin discoloration, urticaria
   Endocrine & metabolic: Adrenal cortex insufficiency
   Gastrointestinal: Abdominal pain, aphthous stomatitis, colitis, constipation, dysphagia, fecal incontinence, gastritis, GI hemorrhage, gingivitis, melena, proctitis, splenomegaly, stomatitis, tongue discoloration
   Genitourinary: Urinary incontinence

Hematologic: Hypochromic anemia, leukocytosis, leukopenia, lymphadenopathy, lymphoma-like reaction, pancytopenia, thrombocytopenia, thrombocytopenic purpura
Hepatic: Hepatomegaly, hepatosplenomegaly, jaundice, liver function tests abnormal, liver damage, liver necrosis
Local: Injection site reaction
Neuromuscular & skeletal: Tremor
Ocular: Amblyopia, blindness, cataract, conjunctivitis, corneal lesion, diplopia, vision abnormal
Otic: Hearing loss
Miscellaneous: Allergic reaction, sepsis

Overdosage/Toxicology Hemodialysis and hydration may reduce drug plasma concentrations. Probenecid may assist in decreasing active tubular secretion.

Pharmacodynamics/Kinetics
Protein Binding: <6%
Half-Life Elimination: Plasma: ~2.6 hours
Metabolism: Minimal; phosphorylation occurs intracellularly
Excretion: Urine

Pharmacokinetic Note Data is based on a combination of cidofovir administered with probenecid.

Available Dosage Forms Injection, solution [preservative free]: 75 mg/mL (5 mL)

Dosing
Adults & Elderly: Treatment of cytomegalovirus (CMV) retinitis: I.V.:
   Induction treatment: 5 mg/kg once weekly for 2 consecutive weeks
   Maintenance treatment: 5 mg/kg administered once every 2 weeks
   Note: Probenecid must be administered orally with each dose of cidofovir.
   Probenecid dose: 2 g 3 hours prior to cidofovir dose, 1 g 2 hours and 8 hours after completion of the infusion; patients should also receive 1 L of normal saline intravenously prior to each infusion of cidofovir; saline should be infused over 1-2 hours.
Renal Impairment:
   Changes in renal function during therapy: If the creatinine increases by 0.3-0.4 mg/dL, reduce the cidofovir dose to 3 mg/kg; discontinue therapy for increases ≥0.5 mg/dL or development of ≥3+ proteinuria
   Pre-existing renal impairment: Use is contraindicated with serum creatinine >1.5 mg/dL, Cl$_{cr}$ <55 mL/minute, or urine protein ≥100 mg/dL (≥2+ proteinuria)

Administration
I.V.: For I.V. infusion only. Infuse over 1 hour. Hydrate with 1 L of 0.9% NS I.V. prior to cidofovir infusion; a second liter may be administered over a 1- to 3-hour period immediately following infusion, if tolerated
I.V. Detail: pH: 6.7-7.6

Stability
Reconstitution: Dilute dose in NS 100 mL prior to infusion.
Compatibility: Stable in D$_5$¼NS, D$_5$W, NS
Storage: Store at controlled room temperature 20°C to 25°C (68°F to 77°F). Store admixtures under refrigeration for ≤24 hours. Cidofovir infusion admixture should be administered within 24 hours of preparation at room temperature or refrigerated. Admixtures should be allowed to equilibrate to room temperature prior to use.

Laboratory Monitoring Serum creatinine, serum bicarbonate, acid-base status, urine protein, WBC should be monitored with each dose; monitor intraocular pressure frequently.

Nursing Actions
Physical Assessment: Administration must be accompanied by oral probenecid and intravenous saline prehydration. Assess other pharmacological or (Continued)

Cidofovir *(Continued)*

herbal products patient may be taking for potential interactions (especially anything that may be nephrotoxic). Pretreatment with probenecid and both pre- and post-treatment hydration may be ordered. Monitor infusion site closely to avoid extravasation. Monitor laboratory tests with each dose. Monitor patient response throughout therapy (eg, CNS changes, anemia, renal status, visual acuity). For patients with diabetes, serum glucose should be monitored closely (may cause hyperglycemia). Teach patient possible side effects/appropriate interventions and adverse symptoms to report (especially any changes in vision or eye pain).

Patient Education: Inform prescriber of all prescriptions, OTC medications, or herbal products you are taking, and any allergies you have. Do not take any new medication during therapy unless approved by prescriber. This drug can only be administered I.V. Report immediately any pain, stinging, swelling at infusion site. You may be more susceptible to infection (avoid crowds and exposure to infection and do not have any vaccinations without consulting prescriber). May cause hair loss (reversible); headache, anxiety, confusion (use caution when driving or engaging in tasks that require alertness until response to drug is known); diarrhea (buttermilk or yogurt may help); nausea, heartburn, or vomiting (small, frequent meals, frequent mouth care, sucking lozenges, or chewing gum may help); constipation (increased exercise, fluids, fruit, or fiber may help); or postural hypotension (use caution changing from lying to sitting or standing position and when climbing stairs). Report severe unresolved vomiting, constipation, or diarrhea; chills, fever, signs of infection; respiratory difficulty or unusual coughing; palpitations, chest pain, or syncope; CNS changes (eg, hallucinations, depression, excessive sedation, amnesia, seizures, insomnia); vision changes; or other serious side effects. **Pregnancy/breast-feeding precautions:** Inform prescriber if you are pregnant and do not get pregnant while taking this medicine. Consult prescriber for appropriate contraceptives. Do not breast-feed.

Geriatric Considerations Since elderly individuals frequently have reduced kidney function, particular attention should be paid to assessing renal function before and frequently during administration.

Breast-Feeding Issues The CDC recommends **not** to breast-feed if diagnosed with HIV to avoid postnatal transmission of the virus.

Pregnancy Issues Cidofovir was shown to be teratogenic and embryotoxic in animal studies, some at doses which also produced maternal toxicity. Reduced testes weight and hypospermia were also noted in animal studies. There are no adequate and well-controlled studies in pregnant women; use during pregnancy only if the potential benefit to the mother outweighs the possible risk to the fetus. Women of childbearing potential should use effective contraception during therapy and for 1 month following treatment. Males should use a barrier contraceptive during therapy and for 3 months following treatment.

Cilostazol *(sil OH sta zol)*

U.S. Brand Names Pletal®
Synonyms OPC-13013
Pharmacologic Category Antiplatelet Agent; Phosphodiesterase Enzyme Inhibitor
Medication Safety Issues
Sound-alike/look-alike issues:
Pletal® may be confused with Plendil®
Pregnancy Risk Factor C

Lactation Excretion in breast milk unknown/not recommended

Use Symptomatic management of peripheral vascular disease, primarily intermittent claudication

Unlabeled/Investigational Use Treatment of acute coronary syndromes and for graft patency improvement in percutaneous coronary interventions with or without stenting

Mechanism of Action/Effect Cilostazol and its metabolites are inhibitors of phosphodiesterase III. As a result, cyclic AMP is increased leading to reversible inhibition of platelet aggregation and vasodilation. Other effects of phosphodiesterase III inhibition include increased cardiac contractility, accelerated AV nodal conduction, increased ventricular automaticity, heart rate, and coronary blood flow.

Contraindications Hypersensitivity to cilostazol or any component of the formulation; heart failure (of any severity)

Warnings/Precautions Use with caution in patients receiving other platelet inhibitors or in patients with thrombocytopenia. Discontinue therapy if thrombocytopenia or leukopenia occur, progression to agranulocytosis (reversible) has been reported when cilostazol was not immediately stopped. When cilostazol and clopidogrel are used concurrently, manufacturer recommends checking bleeding times. Withhold prior to elective surgical procedures. Use with caution in patients receiving CYP3A4 inhibitors (eg, ketoconazole or erythromycin) or CYP2C19 inhibitors (eg, omeprazole); use with caution in severe underlying heart disease. Use caution in moderate to severe hepatic impairment. Use cautiously in severe renal impairment (Cl_{cr} <25 mL/minute). Safety and efficacy in pediatric patients have not been established.

Drug Interactions

Cytochrome P450 Effect: Substrate of CYP1A2 (minor), 2C19 (minor), 2D6 (minor), 3A4 (major)

Increased Effect/Toxicity: Cilostazol serum concentrations may be increased by antifungal agents (midazole), macrolide antibiotics, and omeprazole. Increased concentrations of cilostazol may be anticipated during concurrent therapy with other inhibitors of CYP3A4 (eg, clarithromycin, diclofenac, doxycycline, erythromycin, imatinib, isoniazid, nefazodone, nicardipine, propofol, protease inhibitors, quinidine, telithromycin, and verapamil) or inhibitors of CYP2C19 (eg, delavirdine, fluconazole, fluvoxamine, gemfibrozil, isoniazid, omeprazole, and ticlopidine). Aspirin-induced inhibition of platelet aggregation is potentiated by concurrent cilostazol. Concurrent use of drotrecogin alfa, NSAIDs, or treprostinil may cause increased bleeding.

Nutritional/Ethanol Interactions Food: Taking cilostazol with a high-fat meal may increase peak concentration by 90%. Avoid concurrent ingestion of grapefruit juice due to the potential to inhibit CYP3A4.

Adverse Reactions

>10%:
Central nervous system: Headache (27% to 34%)
Gastrointestinal: Abnormal stools (12% to 15%), diarrhea (12% to 19%)
Respiratory: Rhinitis (7% to 12%)
Miscellaneous: Infection (10% to 14%)

2% to 10%:
Cardiovascular: Peripheral edema (7% to 9%), palpitation (5% to 10%), tachycardia (4%)
Central nervous system: Dizziness (9% to 10%), vertigo (up to 3%)
Gastrointestinal: Dyspepsia (6%), nausea (6% to 7%), abdominal pain (4% to 5%), flatulence (2% to 3%)
Neuromuscular & skeletal: Back pain (6% to 7%), myalgia (2% to 3%)
Respiratory: Pharyngitis (7% to 10%), cough (3% to 4%)

Overdosage/Toxicology Experience with overdosage in humans is limited. Headache, diarrhea, hypotension, tachycardia, and/or cardiac arrhythmias may occur. Treatment is symptomatic and supportive. Hemodialysis is unlikely to be of value. In some animal models, high-dose or long-term administration was associated with a variety of cardiovascular lesions, including endocardial hemorrhage, hemosiderin deposition and left ventricular fibrosis, coronary arteritis, and periarteritis.

Pharmacodynamics/Kinetics

Onset of Action: 2-4 weeks; may require up to 12 weeks

Protein Binding: 97% to 98%

Half-Life Elimination: 11-13 hours

Metabolism: Hepatic via CYP3A4 (primarily), 1A2, 2C19, and 2D6; at least one metabolite has significant activity

Excretion: Urine (74%) and feces (20%) as metabolites

Available Dosage Forms Tablet: 50 mg, 100 mg

Dosing

Adults & Elderly: Peripheral vascular disease: Oral: 100 mg twice daily taken at least 30 minutes before or 2 hours after breakfast and dinner; dosage should be reduced to 50 mg twice daily during concurrent therapy with inhibitors of CYP3A4 or CYP2C19 (see Drug Interactions).

Nursing Actions

Physical Assessment: Assess effectiveness and interactions of other medications patient may be taking. Monitor effectiveness of therapy and adverse reactions at beginning of therapy and periodically with long-term use. Assess knowledge/teach patient appropriate use, interventions to reduce side effects, and adverse symptoms to report.

Patient Education: Use exactly as directed; do not discontinue this medication without consulting prescriber. Beneficial effect may take between 2-12 weeks. Take on empty stomach (30 minutes before or 2 hours after meals). Do not take with grapefruit juice. You may experience nervousness, dizziness, or fatigue (use caution when driving or engaging in tasks requiring alertness until response to treatment is known); nausea, vomiting, or flatulence (small frequent meals, frequent mouth care, chewing gum or sucking hard candy may help); or postural hypotension (change position slowly when rising from sitting or lying position or climbing stairs). Report chest pain, palpitations, unusual heartbeat, or swelling of extremities; unusual bleeding; unresolved GI upset or pain; dizziness, nervousness, sleeplessness, or fatigue; muscle cramping or tremor; unusual cough; or other adverse effects. **Pregnancy/breast-feeding precautions:** Inform prescriber if you are or intend to become pregnant. Breast-feeding is not recommended.

Dietary Considerations It is best to take cilostazol 30 minutes before or 2 hours after meals.

Breast-Feeding Issues It is not known whether cilostazol is excreted in human milk. Because of the potential risk to nursing infants, a decision to discontinue the drug or discontinue nursing should be made.

Pregnancy Issues In animal studies, abnormalities of the skeletal, renal and cardiovascular system were increased. In addition, the incidence of stillbirth and decreased birth weights were increased.

Cimetidine (sye MET i deen)

U.S. Brand Names Tagamet®; Tagamet® HB 200 [OTC]
Pharmacologic Category Histamine H_2 Antagonist
Medication Safety Issues
Sound-alike/look-alike issues:
Cimetidine may be confused with simethicone
Pregnancy Risk Factor B
Lactation Enters breast milk/not recommended
Use Short-term treatment of active duodenal ulcers and benign gastric ulcers; long-term prophylaxis of duodenal ulcer; gastric hypersecretory states; gastroesophageal reflux; prevention of upper GI bleeding in critically-ill patients; labeled for OTC use for prevention or relief of heartburn, acid indigestion, or sour stomach
Unlabeled/Investigational Use Part of a multidrug regimen for *H. pylori* eradication to reduce the risk of duodenal ulcer recurrence
Mechanism of Action/Effect Competitive inhibition of histamine at H_2 receptors of the gastric parietal cells resulting in reduced gastric acid secretion, gastric volume and hydrogen ion concentration reduced
Contraindications Hypersensitivity to cimetidine, any component of the formulation, or other H_2 antagonists
Warnings/Precautions Reversible confusional states, usually clearing within 3-4 days after discontinuation, have been linked to use. Increased age (>50 years) and renal or hepatic impairment are thought to be associated. Dosage should be adjusted in renal/hepatic impairment or in patients receiving drugs metabolized through the P450 system.

Over the counter (OTC) cimetidine should not be taken by individuals experiencing painful swallowing, vomiting with blood, or bloody or black stools; medical attention should be sought. A physician should be consulted prior to use when pain in the stomach, shoulder, arms or neck is present; if heartburn has occurred for >3 months; or if unexplained weight loss, or nausea and vomiting occur. Frequent wheezing, shortness of breath, lightheadedness, or sweating, especially with chest pain or heartburn, should also be reported. Consultation of a healthcare provider should occur by patients if also taking theophylline, phenytoin, or warfarin; if heartburn or stomach pain continues or worsens; or if use is required for >14 days. Pregnant or breast-feeding women should speak to a healthcare provider before use. OTC cimetidine is not approved for use in patients <12 years of age.

Drug Interactions

Cytochrome P450 Effect: Inhibits CYP1A2 (moderate), 2C8/9 (weak), 2C19 (moderate), 2D6 (moderate), 2E1 (weak), 3A4 (moderate)

Decreased Effect: Cimetidine may decrease the levels/effects of CYP2D6 prodrug substrates (eg, codeine, hydrocodone, oxycodone, and tramadol). Ketoconazole, fluconazole, itraconazole (especially capsule) decrease serum concentration; avoid concurrent use with H_2 antagonists. Absorption of delavirdine and atazanavir may be decreased; avoid concurrent use of delavirdine with H_2 antagonists.

Increased Effect/Toxicity: Cimetidine may increase the levels/effects of aminophylline, amphetamines, selected beta-blockers, selected benzodiazepines, calcium channel blockers, cyclosporine, dextromethorphan, dofetilide, ergot derivatives, lidocaine, meperidine, metformin, methsuximide, metronidazole, mexiletine, mirtazapine, moricizine, nateglinide, nefazodone, paroxetine (and other SSRIs), phenytoin, procainamide, propafenone, propranolol, quinidine, quinolone antibiotics, risperidone, ritonavir, ropinirole, sildenafil (and other PDE-5 inhibitors), sulfonylureas, tacrine, tacrolimus, theophylline, thioridazine, triamterene, tricyclic antidepressants, trifluoperazine, (Continued)

Cimetidine *(Continued)*

venlafaxine, and other CYP1A2, 2C19, or 2D6 substrates.

Cimetidine increases warfarin's effect in a dose-related manner. Cimetidine increases carmustine's myelotoxicity; avoid concurrent use.

Nutritional/Ethanol Interactions

Ethanol: Avoid ethanol (may enhance gastric mucosal irritation).

Food: Cimetidine may increase serum caffeine levels if taken with caffeine. Cimetidine peak serum levels may be decreased if taken with food.

Herb/Nutraceutical: St John's wort may decrease cimetidine levels.

Adverse Reactions 1% to 10%:

Central nervous system: Headache (2% to 4%), dizziness (1%), somnolence (1%), agitation

Endocrine & metabolic: Gynecomastia (<1% to 4%)

Gastrointestinal: Diarrhea (1%), nausea, vomiting

Adverse reactions reported with H_2 antagonists: Alopecia, AV heart block , bradycardia, erythema multiforme, exfoliative dermatitis, Stevens-Johnson syndrome, toxic epidermal necrolysis

Overdosage/Toxicology Reported ingestions of up to 20 g have resulted in transient side effects seen with recommended doses. Reports of ingestions up to 40 g have documented severe CNS depression, including unresponsiveness. Treatment is symptom-directed and supportive. Animal data suggests that ventilation assistance and beta-blocker treatment may be effective in managing the possible respiratory depression and tachycardia, respectively.

Pharmacodynamics/Kinetics

Onset of Action: 1 hour

Duration of Action: 4-8 hours

Time to Peak: Serum: Oral: 1-2 hours

Protein Binding: 20%

Half-Life Elimination: Neonates: 3.6 hours; Children: 1.4 hours; Adults: Normal renal function: 2 hours

Metabolism: Partially hepatic

Excretion: Primarily urine (48% as unchanged drug); feces (some)

Available Dosage Forms

Infusion, as hydrochloride [premixed in NS]: 300 mg (50 mL)

Injection, solution, as hydrochloride: 150 mg/mL (2 mL, 8 mL) [8 mL size contains benzyl alcohol]

Liquid, oral, as hydrochloride: 300 mg/5 mL (240 mL, 480 mL) [contains alcohol 2.8%; mint-peach flavor]

Tablet: 200 mg [OTC], 300 mg, 400 mg, 800 mg

Tagamet®: 300 mg, 400 mg

Tagamet® HB 200: 200 mg

Dosing

Adults & Elderly:

Short-term treatment of active ulcers:

Oral: 300 mg 4 times/day or 800 mg at bedtime or 400 mg twice daily for up to 8 weeks

Note: Higher doses of 1600 mg at bedtime for 4 weeks may be beneficial for a subpopulation of patients with larger duodenal ulcers (>1 cm defined endoscopically) who are also heavy smokers (≥1 pack/day).

I.M., I.V.: 300 mg every 6 hours or 37.5 mg/hour by continuous infusion; I.V. dosage should be adjusted to maintain an intragastric pH ≥5

Prevention of upper GI bleed in critically-ill patients: 50 mg/hour by continuous infusion; I.V. dosage should be adjusted to maintain an intragastric pH ≥5

Note: Reduce dose by 50% if Cl_{cr} <30 mL/minute; treatment >7 days has not been evaluated.

Duodenal ulcer prophylaxis: Oral: 400 mg at bedtime

Gastric hypersecretory conditions: Oral, I.M., I.V.: 300-600 mg every 6 hours; dosage not to exceed 2.4 g/day

Gastroesophageal reflux disease: Oral: 400 mg 4 times/day or 800 mg twice daily for 12 weeks

Peptic ulcer disease eradication of *Helicobacter pylori* (unlabeled use): Oral: 400 mg twice daily; requires combination therapy with antibiotics

Heartburn, acid indigestion, sour stomach (OTC labeling): Oral: 200 mg up to twice daily; may take 30 minutes prior to eating foods or beverages expected to cause heartburn or indigestion

Pediatrics:

Oral, I.M., I.V.: 20-40 mg/kg/day in divided doses every 6 hours

Heartburn, acid indigestion, sour stomach (OTC labeling): Children ≥12 years: Oral: Refer to adult dosing.

Renal Impairment:

Cl_{cr} 10-50 mL/minute: Administer 50% of normal dose

Cl_{cr} <10 mL/minute: Administer 25% of normal dose

Slightly dialyzable (5% to 20%); administer after dialysis

Hepatic Impairment: Usual dose is safe in mild liver disease but use with caution and in reduced dosage in severe liver disease. Increased risk of CNS toxicity in cirrhosis suggested by enhanced penetration of CNS.

Administration

Oral: Give with meals so that the drug's peak effect occurs at the proper time (peak inhibition of gastric acid secretion occurs at 1 and 3 hours after dosing in fasting subjects and approximately 2 hours in nonfasting subjects. This correlates well with the time food is no longer in the stomach offering a buffering effect). Stagger doses of antacids with cimetidine.

I.V.: May be administered as a slow I.V. push or preferably as an I.V. intermittent or I.V. continuous infusion. Administer each 300 mg (or fraction thereof) over a minimum of 5 minutes when giving I.V. push. Give intermittent infusion over 15-30 minutes for each 300 mg dose. Intermittent infusions are administered over 15-30 minutes at a final concentration not to exceed 6 mg/mL; for patients with an active bleed, preferred method of administration is continuous infusion.

I.V. Detail: Rapid infusion may cause cardiac arrhythmias and hypotension.

pH: 3.8-6.0 (injection); 5-7 (premixed infusion)

Stability

Compatibility: Stable in D_5LR, D_5¼NS, D_5½NS, D_5NS, D_5W, $D_{10}W$, $D_{10}NS$, LR, sodium bicarbonate 5%, NS

Y-site administration: Incompatible with allopurinol, amphotericin B cholesteryl sulfate complex, amsacrine, cefepime, indomethacin, warfarin

Compatibility in syringe: Incompatible with atropine/pentobarbital, cefamandole, cefazolin, chlorpromazine, ioxaglate meglumine and ioxaglate sodium, pentobarbital, secobarbital

Compatibility when admixed: Incompatible with amphotericin B, barbiturates

Storage:

Tablet: Store between 15°C and 30°C (59°F to 86°F); protect from light.

Solution for injection/infusion: Intact vials should be stored at room temperature, between 15°C and 30°C (59°F to 86°F); protect from light. May precipitate from solution upon exposure to cold, but can be redissolved by warming without degradation.

Stability at room temperature:

Prepared bags: 7 days

Premixed bags: Manufacturer expiration dating and out of overwrap stability: 15 days

Stable in parenteral nutrition solutions for up to 7 days when protected from light.

Physically Incompatible with barbiturates, amphotericin B, and cephalosporins

Laboratory Monitoring CBC, gastric pH, occult blood with GI bleeding; monitor renal function to correct dose.

Physical Assessment: Assess other pharmacological or herbal products patient may be taking for potential interactions. **I.V.:** Note administration specifics. Monitor laboratory tests, therapeutic effectiveness (according to purpose for use), and adverse response (eg, changes in CNS, agitation; gastric bleeding) regularly during therapy. Teach patient proper use, possible side effects/appropriate interventions, and adverse symptoms to report.

Patient Education: Do not take any new medication during therapy unless approved by prescriber. Take with meals. Do not increase dose or frequency without consulting prescriber. To be effective, continue to take for the prescribed time (possibly several weeks) even though symptoms may have improved. Smoking decreases the effectiveness of cimetidine (stop smoking if possible). Avoid excess alcohol and caffeine. May cause headache, dizziness, agitation (use caution when driving or engaging in any potentially hazardous tasks until response to drug is known); nausea or vomiting (small, frequent meals, frequent mouth care, chewing gum, or sucking lozenges may help); or diarrhea (buttermilk, boiled milk, or yogurt may help). Report chest pain or palpitations; CNS changes (confusion, agitation); persistent diarrhea, nausea, vomiting, or heartburn; black tarry stools or coffee ground-like emesis; rash; unusual bleeding or bruising; sore throat; or fever; unexplained weight lose or other adverse effects.

Geriatric Considerations Patients diagnosed with PUD should be evaluated for *Helicobacter pylori*. H₂ blockers are the preferred drugs for treating PUD in elderly due to cost and ease of administration. These agents are no less or more effective than any other therapy. The preferred agents, due to favorable pharmacokinetic, side effect and drug interaction profiles are ranitidine, famotidine, and nizatidine. Due to the potential for confusion and drug interactions, cimetidine has been identified by a panel of experts as a drug to avoid in the elderly.

Related Information
Compatibility of Drugs *on page 1370*
Compatibility of Drugs in Syringe *on page 1372*

Cinacalcet (sin a KAL cet)

U.S. Brand Names Sensipar™

Synonyms AMG 073; Cinacalcet Hydrochloride

Pharmacologic Category Calcimimetic

Pregnancy Risk Factor C

Lactation Excretion in breast milk unknown/not recommended

Use Treatment of secondary hyperparathyroidism in dialysis patients; treatment of hypercalcemia in patients with parathyroid carcinoma

Unlabeled/Investigational Use Primary hyperparathyroidism

Mechanism of Action/Effect Increases the sensitivity of the calcium-sensing receptor on the parathyroid gland

Contraindications Hypersensitivity to cinacalcet or any component of the formulation

Warnings/Precautions If hypocalcemia develops during treatment, consider initiating treatment or temporarily withholding cinacalcet. Use caution in patients with a seizure disorder; monitor calcium levels closely. Adynamic bone disease may develop if iPTH levels are suppressed (<100 pg/mL). Use caution in patients with

hepatic impairment. Safety and efficacy have not been established in pediatric patients.

Drug Interactions

Cytochrome P450 Effect: Substrate of CYP1A2, 2D6, 3A4; **Inhibits** CYP2D6

Increased Effect/Toxicity: Cinacalcet increases levels of amitriptyline and nortriptyline. Ketoconazole may increase cinacalcet levels.

Nutritional/Ethanol Interactions Food: Food increases bioavailability.

Adverse Reactions

>10%:
Endocrine & metabolic: Hypocalcemia
Gastrointestinal: Nausea (31%), vomiting (27%), diarrhea (21%)
Neuromuscular & skeletal: Myalgia (15%)

1% to 10%:
Cardiovascular: Hypertension (7%)
Central nervous system: Dizziness (10%), seizure (1%)
Endocrine & metabolic: Testosterone decreased
Gastrointestinal: Anorexia (6%)
Neuromuscular & skeletal: Weakness (7%), chest pain (6%)

Overdosage/Toxicology Overdose may cause hypocalcemia. Signs and symptoms may include paresthesias, myalgias, cramping, tetany, and seizures. Treatment is symptom-directed and supportive. Cinacalcet is not removed by dialysis.

Pharmacodynamics/Kinetics

Time to Peak: Nadir in iPTH levels: 2-6 hours postdose

Protein Binding: 93% to 97%

Half-Life Elimination: Terminal: 30-40 hours

Metabolism: Hepatic via CYP3A4, 2D6, 1A2; forms inactive metabolites

Excretion: Urine 80% (as metabolites); feces 15%

Available Dosage Forms Tablet: 30 mg, 60 mg, 90 mg

Dosing

Adults: Note: Do not titrate dose more frequently than every 2-4 weeks.

Secondary hyperparathyroidism: Oral: Initial: 30 mg once daily (maximum daily dose: 180 mg); increase dose incrementally (60 mg, 90 mg, 120 mg, 180 mg once daily) as necessary to maintain iPTH level between 150-300 pg/mL.

Parathyroid carcinoma: Oral: Initial: 30 mg twice daily (maximum daily dose: 360 mg daily as 90 mg 4 times/day); increase dose incrementally (60 mg twice daily, 90 mg twice daily, 90 mg 4 times/day) as necessary to normalize serum calcium levels.

Elderly: Refer to adult dosing. No adjustment required.

Renal Impairment: No adjustment required.

Hepatic Impairment: Patients with moderate to severe dysfunction have an increased exposure to cinacalcet and increased half-life.

Dosing Adjustment for Toxicity: Dosage adjustment for hypocalcemia:

If serum calcium >7.5 mg/dL but <8.4 mg/dL **or** if hypocalcemia symptoms occur: Use calcium-containing phosphate binders and/or vitamin D to raise calcium levels.

If serum calcium <7.5 mg/dL **or** if hypocalcemia symptoms occur and the dose of vitamin D cannot be increased: Discontinue cinacalcet until serum calcium ≥8 mg/dL or symptoms of hypocalcemia resolve. Reinitiate cinacalcet at the next lowest dose.

If iPTH <150-300 pg/mL: Reduce dose or discontinue cinacalcet and/or vitamin D.

Oral: Administer with food. Do not break tablet; should be taken whole.
(Continued)

Cinacalcet *(Continued)*

Stability

Storage: Store at 25°C (77°F).

Laboratory Monitoring

Hyperparathyroidism: Serum calcium levels prior to initiation and within a week of initiation or dosage adjustment; iPTH should be measured 1-4 weeks after initiation or dosage adjustment. After the maintenance dose is established, monthly calcium and phosphorus levels and iPTH every 1-3 months are required.

Parathyroid carcinoma: Serum calcium levels prior to initiation and within a week of initiation or dosage adjustment; once maintenance dose is established, obtain serum calcium level every 2 months.

Nursing Actions

Physical Assessment: Assess other pharmacological or herbal products patient may be taking for potential interactions. Monitor laboratory tests, therapeutic response (calcium levels), and adverse reactions (eg, hypocalcemia [paresthesias, myalgia, cramping, tetany, convulsions]) frequently at beginning of therapy and regularly thereafter. Teach patient possible aide effects, interventions to reduce side effects, and adverse symptoms to report.

Patient Education: Do not take any new medication during therapy unless approved by prescriber. Take exactly as directed with food; do not break, chew, or crush tablet (swallow whole). Do not take more than prescribed. You may experience dizziness (use caution when driving or engaged in potentially hazards tasks until response to drug is known); nausea, vomiting, or loss of appetite (good mouth care, small frequent meals, sucking lozenges, or chewing gum may help); diarrhea (yogurt or boiled milk may help). Report any muscle cramping, twitches, tremors, or spasms; chest pain or palpitations; unresolved gastrointestinal disturbance, or other persistent adverse effects. **Pregnancy/breast-feeding precautions:** Inform prescriber if you are or intend to become pregnant.

Dietary Considerations Take with food. May be taken with vitamin D and/or phosphate binders.

Breast-Feeding Issues The manufacturer recommends discontinuing nursing or discontinuing cinacalcet.

Ciprofloxacin *(sip roe FLOKS a sin)*

U.S. Brand Names Ciloxan®; Cipro®; Cipro® XR; Proquin® XR

Synonyms Ciprofloxacin Hydrochloride

Pharmacologic Category Antibiotic, Ophthalmic; Antibiotic, Quinolone

Medication Safety Issues

Sound-alike/look-alike issues:

Ciprofloxacin may be confused with cephalexin

Ciloxan® may be confused with cinoxacin, Cytoxan®

Cipro® may be confused with Ceftin®

Pregnancy Risk Factor C

Lactation Enters breast milk/not recommended (AAP rates "compatible")

Use

Children: Complicated urinary tract infections and pyelonephritis due to *E. coli*. **Note:** Although effective, ciprofloxacin is not the drug of first choice in children.

Children and adults: To reduce incidence or progression of disease following exposure to aerolized *Bacillus anthracis*. Ophthalmologically, for superficial ocular infections (corneal ulcers, conjunctivitis) due to susceptible strains

Adults: Treatment of the following infections when caused by susceptible bacteria: Urinary tract infections; acute uncomplicated cystitis in females; chronic bacterial prostatitis; lower respiratory tract infections

(including acute exacerbations of chronic bronchitis); acute sinusitis; skin and skin structure infections; bone and joint infections; complicated intra-abdominal infections (in combination with metronidazole); infectious diarrhea; typhoid fever due to *Salmonella typhi* (eradication of chronic typhoid carrier state has not been proven); uncomplicated cervical and urethra gonorrhea (due to *N. gonorrhoeae*); nosocomial pneumonia; empirical therapy for febrile neutropenic patients (in combination with piperacillin)

Unlabeled/Investigational Use Acute pulmonary exacerbations in cystic fibrosis (children); cutaneous/gastrointestinal/oropharyngeal anthrax (treatment, children and adults); disseminated gonococcal infection (adults); chancroid (adults); prophylaxis to *Neisseria meningitidis* following close contact with an infected person

Mechanism of Action/Effect Inhibits DNA-gyrase in susceptible organisms; inhibits relaxation of supercoiled DNA and promotes breakage of double-stranded DNA

Contraindications Hypersensitivity to ciprofloxacin, any component of the formulation, or other quinolones; concurrent administration of tizanidine

Warnings/Precautions CNS stimulation may occur (tremor, restlessness, confusion, and very rarely hallucinations or seizures). Use with caution in patients with known or suspected CNS disorder. Prolonged use may result in superinfection. Tendon inflammation and/or rupture have been reported with ciprofloxacin and other quinolone antibiotics. Risk may be increased with concurrent corticosteroids, particularly in the elderly. Discontinue at first sign of tendon inflammation or pain. Adverse effects, including those related to joints and/or surrounding tissues, are increased in pediatric patients and therefore, ciprofloxacin should not be considered as drug of choice in children (exception is anthrax treatment). Rare cases of peripheral neuropathy may occur.

Severe hypersensitivity reactions, including anaphylaxis, have occurred with quinolone therapy. Quinolones may exacerbate myasthenia gravis, use with caution (rare, potentially life-threatening weakness of respiratory muscles may occur). Use caution in renal impairment. Avoid excessive sunlight; may cause moderate-to-severe phototoxicity reactions.

Ciprofloxacin is a potent inhibitor of CYP1A2. Coadministration of drugs which depend on this pathway may lead to substantial increases in serum concentrations and adverse effects.

Drug Interactions

Cytochrome P450 Effect: Inhibits CYP1A2 (strong), 3A4 (weak)

Decreased Effect: Concurrent administration of metal cations, including most antacids, oral electrolyte supplements, quinapril, sucralfate, some didanosine formulations (chewable/buffered tablets and pediatric powder for oral suspension), other highly-buffered oral drugs, and sevelamer may decrease quinolone absorption; separate doses. Ciprofloxacin may decrease phenytoin levels.

Increased Effect/Toxicity: Ciprofloxacin may increase serum levels of tizanidine; concurrent administration is contraindicated. Ciprofloxacin may increase the effects/toxicity of caffeine, CYP1A2 substrates (eg, aminophylline, fluvoxamine, mexiletine, mirtazapine, ropinirole, tizanidine, and trifluoperazine), glyburide, methotrexate, ropivacaine, theophylline, and warfarin. Headache has been observed with concomitant pentoxifylline therapy. Concomitant use with corticosteroids may increase the risk of tendon rupture. Concomitant use with foscarnet may increase the risk of seizures. Probenecid may increase ciprofloxacin levels.

Nutritional/Ethanol Interactions

Food: Food decreases rate, but not extent, of absorption. Ciprofloxacin serum levels may be decreased if taken with dairy products or calcium-fortified juices.

Ciprofloxacin may increase serum caffeine levels if taken with caffeine.

Enteral feedings may decrease plasma concentrations of ciprofloxacin probably by >30% inhibition of absorption. Ciprofloxacin should not be administered with enteral feedings. The feeding would need to be discontinued for 1-2 hours prior to and after ciprofloxacin administration. Nasogastric administration produces a greater loss of ciprofloxacin bioavailability than does nasoduodenal administration.

Herb/Nutraceutical: Avoid dong quai, St John's wort (may also cause photosensitization).

Lab Interactions Some quinolones may produce a false-positive urine screening result for opiates using commercially-available immunoassay kits. This has been demonstrated most consistently for levofloxacin and ofloxacin, but other quinolones have shown cross-reactivity in certain assay kits. Confirmation of positive opiate screens by more specific methods should be considered.

Adverse Reactions
1% to 10%:

Central nervous system: Neurologic events (children 2%, includes dizziness, insomnia, nervousness, somnolence); fever (children 2%); headache (I.V. administration); restlessness (I.V. administration)

Dermatologic: Rash (children 2%, adults 1%)

Gastrointestinal: Nausea (children/adults 3%); diarrhea (children 5%, adults 2%); vomiting (children 5%, adults 1%); abdominal pain (children 3%, adults <1%); dyspepsia (children 3%)

Hepatic: ALT/AST increased (adults 1%)

Local: Injection site reactions (I.V. administration)

Respiratory: Rhinitis (children 3%)

Overdosage/Toxicology Symptoms of overdose include acute renal failure and seizures. Treatment is supportive and should include adequate hydration and renal function monitoring. Magnesium or calcium containing antacids may be given to decrease absorption of oral ciprofloxacin. Only a small amount of ciprofloxacin (<10%) is removed from the body after hemodialysis or peritoneal dialysis.

Pharmacodynamics/Kinetics
Time to Peak:

Oral:

Immediate release tablet: 0.5-2 hours

Extended release tablet: Cipro® XR: 1-2.5 hours, Proquin® XR: 3.5-8.7 hours

Protein Binding: 20% to 40%

Half-Life Elimination: Children: 2.5 hours; Adults: Normal renal function: 3-5 hours

Metabolism: Partially hepatic; forms 4 metabolites (limited activity)

Excretion: Urine (30% to 50% as unchanged drug); feces (15% to 43%)

Available Dosage Forms [DSC] = Discontinued product

Infusion [premixed in D₅W] (Cipro®): 200 mg (100 mL); 400 mg (200 mL) [latex free]

Injection, solution (Cipro®): 10 mg/mL (20 mL, 40 mL, 120 mL [DSC])

Microcapsules for oral suspension (Cipro®): 250 mg/5 mL (100 mL); 500 mg/5 mL (100 mL) [strawberry flavor]

Ointment, ophthalmic, as hydrochloride (Ciloxan®): 3.33 mg/g [0.3% base] (3.5 g)

Solution, ophthalmic, as hydrochloride (Ciloxan®): 3.5 mg/mL [0.3% base] (2.5 mL, 5 mL, 10 mL) [contains benzalkonium chloride]

Tablet: 250 mg, 500 mg, 750 mg

Cipro®: 100 mg, 250 mg, 500 mg, 750 mg

Tablet, extended release:

Cipro® XR: 500 mg [equivalent to ciprofloxacin hydrochloride 287.5 mg and ciprofloxacin base 212.6 mg]; 1000 mg [equivalent to ciprofloxacin hydrochloride 574.9 mg and ciprofloxacin base 425.2 mg]

Proquin® XR: 500 mg

Dosing
Adults: Note: Extended release tablets and immediate release formulations are not interchangeable. Unless otherwise specified, oral dosing reflects the use of immediate release formulations.

Anthrax:

Inhalational (postexposure prophylaxis):
Oral: 500 mg every 12 hours for 60 days
I.V.: 400 mg every 12 hours for 60 days

Cutaneous (treatment, CDC guidelines): Oral: Immediate release formulation: 500 mg every 12 hours for 60 days. **Note:** In the presence of systemic involvement, extensive edema, lesions on head/neck, refer to I.V. dosing for treatment of inhalational/gastrointestinal/oropharyngeal anthrax.

Inhalational/gastrointestinal/oropharyngeal (treatment, CDC guidelines): I.V.: 400 mg every 12 hours. **Note:** Initial treatment should include two or more agents predicted to be effective (per CDC recommendations). Agents suggested for use in conjunction with ciprofloxacin or doxycycline include rifampin, vancomycin, imipenem, penicillin, ampicillin, chloramphenicol, clindamycin, and clarithromycin. May switch to oral antimicrobial therapy when clinically appropriate. Continue combined therapy for 60 days.

Bacterial conjunctivitis:

Ophthalmic solution: Instill 1-2 drops in eye(s) every 2 hours while awake for 2 days and 1-2 drops every 4 hours while awake for the next 5 days

Ophthalmic ointment: Apply a ½" ribbon into the conjunctival sac 3 times/day for the first 2 days, followed by a ½" ribbon applied twice daily for the next 5 days

Bone/joint infections:
Oral: 500-750 mg twice daily for 4-6 weeks, depending on severity and susceptibility
I.V.:
Mild/moderate: 400 mg every 12 hours for 4-6 weeks
Severe/complicated: 400 mg every 8 hours for 4-6 weeks

Chancroid (CDC guidelines): Oral: 500 mg twice daily for 3 days

Corneal ulcer: Ophthalmic solution: Instill 2 drops into affected eye every 15 minutes for the first 6 hours, then 2 drops into the affected eye every 30 minutes for the remainder of the first day. On day 2, instill 2 drops into the affected eye hourly. On days 3-14, instill 2 drops into affected eye every 4 hours. Treatment may continue after day 14 if re-epithelialization has not occurred.

Febrile neutropenia (with piperacillin): I.V.: 400 mg every 8 hours for 7-14 days

Gonococcal infections:

Urethral/cervical gonococcal infections: Oral: 250-500 mg as a single dose (CDC recommends concomitant doxycycline or azithromycin due to developing resistance; avoid use in Asian or Western Pacific travelers)

Disseminated gonococcal infection (CDC guidelines): Oral: 500 mg twice daily to complete 7 days of therapy (initial treatment with ceftriaxone 1 g I.M./I.V. daily for 24-48 hours after improvement begins)

Infectious diarrhea: Oral:
Salmonella: 500 mg twice daily for 5-7 days
Shigella: 500 mg twice daily for 3 days
Traveler's diarrhea: Mild: 750 mg for one dose; Severe: 500 mg twice daily for 3 days
Vibrio cholerae: 1 g for one dose

Intra-abdominal (in combination with metronidazole):
Oral: 500 mg every 12 hours for 7-14 days

(Continued)

Ciprofloxacin (Continued)

I.V.: 400 mg every 12 hours for 7-14 days

Lower respiratory tract, skin/skin structure infections:

Oral: 500-750 mg twice daily for 7-14 days depending on severity and susceptibility

I.V.:

Mild/moderate: 400 mg every 12 hours for 7-14 days

Severe/complicated: 400 mg every 8 hours for 7-14 days

Nosocomial pneumonia: I.V.: 400 mg every 8 hours for 10-14 days

Prostatitis (chronic, bacterial):

Oral: 500 mg every 12 hours for 28 days

I.V.: 400 mg every 12 hours for 28 days

Sinusitis (acute):

Oral: 500 mg every 12 hours for 10 days

I.V.: 400 mg every 12 hours for 10 days

Typhoid fever: Oral: 500 mg every 12 hours for 10 days

Urinary tract infection:

Acute uncomplicated: Oral: Immediate release formulation: 250 mg every 12 hours for 3 days

Acute uncomplicated pyelonephritis: Oral: Extended release formulation (Cipro® XR): 1000 mg every 24 hours for 7-14 days

Uncomplicated/acute cystitis: Oral: Extended release formulation (Cipro® XR, Proquin® XR): 500 mg every 24 hours for 3 days

Mild/moderate:

Oral: Immediate release formulation: 250 mg every 12 hours for 7-14 days

I.V.: 200 mg every 12 hours for 7-14 days

Severe/complicated:

Oral:

Immediate release formulation: 500 mg every 12 hours for 7-14 days

Extended release formulation (Cipro® XR): 1000 mg every 24 hours for 7-14 days

I.V.: 400 mg every 12 hours for 7-14 days

Elderly: Refer to adult dosing. Adjust dose carefully based on renal function.

Pediatrics: See Warnings/Precautions. **Note:** Extended release tablets and immediate release formulations are not interchangeable. Unless otherwise specified, oral dosing reflects the use of immediate release formulations.

Anthrax:

Inhalational (postexposure prophylaxis):

Oral: 15 mg/kg/dose every 12 hours for 60 days; maximum: 500 mg/dose

I.V.: 10 mg/kg/dose every 12 hours for 60 days; do **not** exceed 400 mg/dose (800 mg/day)

Cutaneous (treatment, CDC guidelines): Oral: 10-15 mg/kg every 12 hours for 60 days (maximum: 1 g/day); amoxicillin 80 mg/kg/day divided every 8 hours is an option for completion of treatment after clinical improvement. **Note:** In the presence of systemic involvement, extensive edema, lesions on head/neck, refer to I.V. dosing for treatment of inhalational/gastrointestinal/ oropharyngeal anthrax.

Inhalational/gastrointestinal/oropharyngeal (treatment, CDC guidelines): I.V.: Initial: 10-15 mg/kg every 12 hours for 60 days (maximum: 500 mg/ dose); switch to oral therapy when clinically appropriate; refer to adult dosing for notes on combined therapy and duration

Bacterial conjunctivitis:

Ophthalmic solution: Children >1 year: Refer to adult dosing.

Ophthalmic ointment: Children >2 years: Refer to adult dosing.

Corneal ulcer: Children >1 year: Refer to adult dosing.

Cystic fibrosis (unlabeled use): Children 5-17 years:

Oral: 40 mg/kg/day divided every 12 hours administered following 1 week of I.V. therapy has been reported in a clinical trial; total duration of therapy: 10-21 days

I.V.: 30 mg/kg/day divided every 8 hours for 1 week, followed by oral therapy, has been reported in a clinical trial

Urinary tract infection (complicated) or pyelonephritis: Children 1-17 years:

Oral: 20-30 mg/kg/day in 2 divided doses (every 12 hours) for 10-21 days; maximum: 1.5 g/day

I.V.: 6-10 mg/kg every 8 hours for 10-21 days (maximum: 400 mg/dose)

Renal Impairment: Adults:

Cl$_{cr}$ 30-50 mL/minute: Oral: Administer 250-500 mg every 12 hours.

Cl$_{cr}$ <30 mL/minute: Acute uncomplicated pyelonephritis or complicated UTI: Oral: Extended release formulation: 500 mg every 24 hours

Cl$_{cr}$ 5-29 mL/minute:

Oral: Administer 250-500 mg every 18 hours.

I.V.: Administer 200-400 mg every 18-24 hours.

Dialysis: Only small amounts of ciprofloxacin are removed by hemo- or peritoneal dialysis (<10%); usual dose: Oral: 250-500 mg every 24 hours following dialysis.

Continuous arteriovenous or venovenous hemodiafiltration effects: Administer 200-400 mg I.V. every 12 hours.

Administration

Oral: May administer with food to minimize GI upset; avoid antacid use; maintain proper hydration and urine output. Administer immediate release ciprofloxacin and Cipro® XR at least 2 hours before or 6 hours after, and Proquin® XR at least 4 hours before or 6 hours after antacids or other products containing calcium, iron, or zinc (including dairy products or calcium-fortified juices). Separate oral administration from drugs which may impair absorption (see Drug Interactions).

Oral suspension: Should not be administered through feeding tubes (suspension is oil-based and adheres to the feeding tube). Patients should avoid chewing on the microcapsules.

Nasogastric/orogastric tube: Crush immediate-release tablet and mix with water. Flush feeding tube before and after administration. Hold tube feedings at least 1 hour before and 2 hours after administration.

Tablet, extended release: Do not crush, split, or chew. May be administered with meals containing dairy products (calcium content <800 mg), but not with dairy products alone. Proquin® XR should be administered with a main meal of the day; evening meal is preferred

I.V.: Administer by slow I.V. infusion over 60 minutes into a large vein.

I.V. Detail: Administer slowly to reduce the risk of venous irritation (burning, pain, erythema, and swelling).

pH: 3.3-3.9 (vials); 3.5-4.6 (PVC bags)

Stability

Reconstitution: Injection, vial: May be diluted with NS, D$_5$W, SWFI, D$_{10}$W, D$_5$¼NS, D$_5$½NS, LR.

Compatibility: Stable in D$_5$¼NS, D$_5$½NS, D$_5$W, D$_{10}$W, LR, NS

Y-site administration: Incompatible with aminophylline, ampicillin/sulbactam, cefepime, dexamethasone sodium phosphate, furosemide, heparin, hydrocortisone sodium succinate, methylprednisolone sodium succinate, phenytoin, propofol, sodium phosphates, warfarin

Compatibility when admixed: Incompatible with aminophylline, clindamycin, floxacillin, heparin

Storage:

Injection:

Premixed infusion: Store between 5°C to 25°C (41°F to 77°F). Protect from light. Avoid freezing.

Vial: Store between 5°C to 30°C (41°F to 86°F). Protect from light. Avoid freezing. Diluted solutions of 0.5-2 mg/mL are stable for up to 14 days refrigerated or at room temperature.

Ophthalmic solution/ointment: Store at 36°F to 77°F (2°C to 25°C). Protect from light.

Microcapsules for oral suspension: Prior to reconstitution, store below 25°C (77°F). Following reconstitution, store below 30°C (86°F) for up to 14 days. Protect from freezing.

Tablet:

Immediate release: Store below 30°C (86°F).

Extended release: Store at room temperature of 15°C to 30°C (59°F to 86°F).

Laboratory Monitoring CBC, renal and hepatic function during prolonged therapy; patients receiving concurrent ciprofloxacin, theophylline, or cyclosporine should have serum theophylline or cyclosporine levels monitored. Culture and sensitivity specimen should be taken prior to initiating therapy.

Nursing Actions

Physical Assessment: Results of culture and sensitivity tests should be assessed prior to beginning therapy. Assess other pharmacological or herbal products patient may be taking for potential interactions. **I.V.:** See Administration specifics. Monitor patient response (according to purpose for use) and adverse effects (eg, hypersensitivity reactions, severe reactions including anaphylaxis have occurred with quinolone therapy; changes in CNS, especially in elderly patients) regularly during therapy. Teach patient proper use (appropriate for formulation), possible side effects/appropriate interventions, and adverse symptoms to report.

Patient Education: Do not take any new medication during therapy unless approved by prescriber.

Infusion: Report immediately any redness, burning, or swelling at infusion site; tightness or swelling in mouth or throat, difficulty swallowing, difficulty breathing, skin rash, rapid heartbeat or palpitations, or onset of other adverse response.

Oral: Take exactly as directed, (at least 2 hours before or 6 hours after antacids or other drug products containing calcium, iron, or zinc). Extended release tablet may be taken with meals containing dairy products, but not with dairy products alone; do not crush, split, or chew extended release tablet. Swallow oral suspension; do not chew microcapsules. Shake bottle vigorously with each use. Take entire prescription, even if feeling better. Maintain adequate hydration to avoid concentrated urine and crystal formation (2-3 L/day) unless instructed to restrict fluid intake. You may experience nausea, vomiting, or anorexia (small frequent meals, frequent mouth care, sucking lozenges, or chewing gum may help); or increased sensitivity to sunlight (use sunscreen, wear protective clothing and dark glasses, and avoid direct exposure to sunlight). If signs of inflammation or tendon pain occur, discontinue use immediately and report to prescriber. If signs of allergic reaction (eg, itching, urticaria, respiratory difficulty, facial edema, difficulty swallowing, loss of consciousness, tingling, chest pain, palpitations) occur, discontinue use immediately and report to prescriber. Report unusual fever or chills, vaginal itching or foul-smelling vaginal discharge, easy bruising or bleeding, or tendon or muscle pain.

Ophthalmic: Use exactly as directed. Wash hands prior to instilling eye medication. Do not touch dropper to eye or any other surface. Do not wear contact lenses while using this medication (check with prescriber before using again). Tilt head back, look upward and pull lower eyelid down to make a pouch. Drop prescribed number of drops directly into eye. Close eye, place one finger at corner of eye near nose and apply gentle pressure. Do not blink or rub eye. If also using ointment, use drops before ointment. Use for exact time as prescribed, do not discontinue even if symptoms disappear. May cause temporary stinging or burning. Report persistent eye discomfort, itching, redness, unusual tearing, feeling as if something is in your eye, blurred vision, eye pain, worsening vision, a bad taste in your mouth, sensitivity to light, skin rash, difficulty breathing, or worsening of symptoms.

Pregnancy/breast-feeding precautions: Inform prescriber if you are or intend to become pregnant. Do not breast-feed.

Dietary Considerations

Food: Drug may cause GI upset; take without regard to meals (manufacturer prefers that immediate release tablet is taken 2 hours after meals). Extended release tablet may be taken with meals that contain dairy products (calcium content <800 mg), but not with dairy products alone.

Dairy products, calcium-fortified juices, oral multivitamins, and mineral supplements: Absorption of ciprofloxacin is decreased by divalent and trivalent cations. The manufacturer states that the usual dietary intake of calcium (including meals which include dairy products) has not been shown to interfere with ciprofloxacin absorption. Immediate release ciprofloxacin and Cipro® XR may be taken 2 hours before or 6 hours after, and Proquin® XR may be taken 4 hours before or 6 hours after, any of these products.

Caffeine: Patients consuming regular large quantities of caffeinated beverages may need to restrict caffeine intake if excessive cardiac or CNS stimulation occurs.

Geriatric Considerations Ciprofloxacin should not be used as first-line therapy unless the culture and sensitivity findings show resistance to usual therapy. The interactions with caffeine and theophylline can result in serious toxicity in the elderly. Adjust dose for renal function.

Breast-Feeding Issues Ciprofloxacin is excreted in breast milk; however, the exposure to the infant is considered small and one source suggests that the decision to breast-feed be independent of the need for the antibiotic in the mother. Another source recommends the mother wait 48 hours after the last dose of ciprofloxacin to continue nursing. The manufacturer recommends to discontinue nursing or to discontinue ciprofloxacin.

Pregnancy Issues Ciprofloxacin crosses the placenta and concentrates in amniotic fluid; maternal serum levels may be decreased during pregnancy. Reports of arthropathy (observed in immature animals and reported rarely in humans) have limited the use of fluoroquinolones in pregnancy. According to the FDA, the Teratogen Information System concluded that therapeutic doses during pregnancy are unlikely to produce substantial teratogenic risk, but data are insufficient to say that there is no risk. Since safer alternatives are usually available, quinolones should generally be avoided in pregnancy. When considering treatment for life-threatening infection and/or prolonged duration of therapy, the potential risk to the fetus must be balanced against the severity of the potential illness.

Ciprofloxacin and Dexamethasone
(sip roe FLOKS a sin & deks a METH a sone)

U.S. Brand Names Ciprodex®

Synonyms Ciprofloxacin Hydrochloride and Dexamethasone; Dexamethasone and Ciprofloxacin

Pharmacologic Category Antibiotic/Corticosteroid, Otic

Pregnancy Risk Factor C

Lactation Excretion in breast milk unknown/not recommended

Use Treatment of acute otitis media in pediatric patients with tympanostomy tubes or acute otitis externa in children and adults

Available Dosage Forms Suspension, otic: Ciprofloxacin 0.3% and dexamethasone 0.1% (7.5 mL) [contains benzalkonium chloride]

Dosing
Adults & Elderly: Acute otitis externa: Otic: Instill 4 drops into affected ear(s) twice daily for 7 days

Pediatrics: Acute otitis media in patients with tympanostomy tubes or acute otitis externa: Otic: Instill 4 drops into affected ear(s) twice daily for 7 days

Nursing Actions
Physical Assessment: See individual agents.

Patient Education: See individual agents. **Pregnancy/breast-feeding precautions:** Inform prescriber if you are or intend to become pregnant. Breast-feeding is not recommended.

Related Information
Ciprofloxacin *on page 266*
Dexamethasone *on page 343*

Ciprofloxacin and Hydrocortisone
(sip roe FLOKS a sin & hye droe KOR ti sone)

U.S. Brand Names Cipro® HC

Synonyms Hydrocortisone and Ciprofloxacin

Pharmacologic Category Antibiotic/Corticosteroid, Otic

Use Treatment of acute otitis externa, sometimes known as "swimmer's ear"

Available Dosage Forms Suspension, otic: Ciprofloxacin hydrochloride 0.2% and hydrocortisone 1% (10 mL) [contains benzyl alcohol]

Dosing
Adults & Elderly: Otitis externa: Otic: The recommended dosage for all patients is three drops of the suspension in the affected ear twice daily for seven day; twice-daily dosing schedule is more convenient for patients than that of existing treatments with hydrocortisone, which are typically administered three or four times a day; a twice-daily dosage schedule may be especially helpful for parents and caregivers of young children

Pediatrics: Children ≥1 year: Refer to adult dosing.

Nursing Actions
Physical Assessment: See individual agents.

Patient Education: Pregnancy/breast-feeding precautions: Inform prescriber if you are or intend to become pregnant. Consult prescriber if breast-feeding.

Related Information
Ciprofloxacin *on page 266*
Hydrocortisone *on page 617*

Cisapride (SIS a pride)

U.S. Brand Names Propulsid®

Restrictions In U.S., available via limited-access protocol only (1-800-JANSSEN).

Pharmacologic Category Gastrointestinal Agent, Prokinetic

Medication Safety Issues
Sound-alike/look-alike issues:
Propulsid® may be confused with propranolol

Pregnancy Risk Factor C

Lactation Enters breast milk/use caution (AAP rates "compatible")

Use Treatment of nocturnal symptoms of gastroesophageal reflux disease (GERD); has demonstrated effectiveness for gastroparesis, refractory constipation, and nonulcer dyspepsia

Mechanism of Action/Effect Enhances the release of acetylcholine at the myenteric plexus. *In vitro* studies have shown cisapride to have serotonin-4 receptor agonistic properties which may increase GI motility and cardiac rate; increases lower esophageal sphincter pressure and lower esophageal peristalsis; accelerates gastric emptying of both liquids and solids.

Contraindications
Hypersensitivity to cisapride or any component of the formulations; GI hemorrhage, mechanical obstruction, GI perforation, or other situations when GI motility stimulation is dangerous

Serious cardiac arrhythmias including ventricular tachycardia, ventricular fibrillation, torsade de pointes, and QT prolongation have been reported in patients taking cisapride with other drugs that inhibit CYP3A4. Some of these events have been fatal. Concomitant oral or intravenous administration of the following drugs with cisapride may lead to elevated cisapride blood levels and is contraindicated:
Antibiotics: Oral or I.V. erythromycin, clarithromycin, troleandomycin
Antidepressants: Nefazodone
Antifungals: Oral or I.V. fluconazole, itraconazole, miconazole, oral ketoconazole
Protease inhibitors: Indinavir, ritonavir, amprenavir, atazanavir

Cisapride is also contraindicated for patients with a prolonged electrocardiographic QT intervals (QT_c >450 msec), a history of QT_c prolongation, or known family history of congenital long QT syndrome; clinically significant bradycardia, renal failure, history of ventricular arrhythmias, ischemic heart disease, and congestive heart failure; uncorrected electrolyte disorders (hypokalemia, hypomagnesemia); respiratory failure; and concomitant medications known to prolong the QT interval and increase the risk of arrhythmia, such as certain antiarrhythmics, certain antipsychotics, certain antidepressants, bepridil, sparfloxacin, and terodiline. The preceding lists of drugs are not comprehensive. Cisapride should not be used in patients with uncorrected hypokalemia or hypomagnesemia or who might experience rapid reduction of plasma potassium such as those administered potassium-wasting diuretics and/or insulin in acute settings.

Warnings/Precautions Safety and effectiveness in children have not been established. Serious cardiac ventricular arrhythmias, including ventricular tachycardia, torsade de pointes, and QT prolongation have been reported in patients taking cisapride with other drugs that inhibit P450 3A4 (eg, clarithromycin, erythromycin, fluconazole, itraconazole, ketoconazole, miconazole injection, troleandomycin). Avoid other medications which may prolong QT. Avoid use when stimulation of GI motility may be dangerous (eg, obstruction, perforation, hemorrhage). Extreme caution with use in the elderly.

A 12-lead ECG should be performed prior to administration of cisapride. Treatment with cisapride should not be initiated if the QT_c value exceeds 450 milliseconds. Serum electrolytes (potassium, calcium, and magnesium) and creatinine should be assessed prior to administration of cisapride and whenever conditions develop that may affect electrolyte balance or renal function.

Drug Interactions

Cytochrome P450 Effect: Substrate of CYP1A2 (minor), 2A6 (minor), 2B6 (minor), 2C8/9 (minor), 2C19 (minor), 3A4 (major); **Inhibits** CYP2D6 (weak), 3A4 (weak)

Decreased Effect: Cisapride may decrease the effect of atropine and digoxin.

Increased Effect/Toxicity: Cisapride may increase blood levels of warfarin, diazepam, cimetidine, ranitidine, and CNS depressants. The risk of cisapride-induced malignant arrhythmias may be increased by azole antifungals (fluconazole, itraconazole, ketoconazole, miconazole), antiarrhythmics (Class Ia; quinidine, procainamide, and Class III; amiodarone, sotalol), bepridil, cimetidine, maprotiline, macrolide antibiotics (erythromycin, clarithromycin, troleandomycin), molindone, nefazodone, protease inhibitors (amprenavir, atazanavir, indinavir, nelfinavir, ritonavir), phenothiazines (eg, prochlorperazine, promethazine), sertindole, tricyclic antidepressants (eg amitriptyline), and some quinolone antibiotics (sparfloxacin, gatifloxacin, moxifloxacin). Other strong inhibitors of CYP3A4 (including diclofenac, doxycycline, imatinib, isoniazid, nefazodone, nicardipine, propofol, telithromycin, and verapamil) should be avoided. Cardiovascular disease or electrolyte imbalances (potentially due to diuretic therapy) increase the risk of malignant arrhythmias.

Nutritional/Ethanol Interactions

Ethanol: Avoid ethanol (may increase CNS depression).

Food: Coadministration of grapefruit juice with cisapride increases the bioavailability of cisapride and concomitant use should be avoided.

Herb/Nutraceutical: St John's wort may decrease cisapride levels.

Adverse Reactions

>5%:
Central nervous system: Headache
Dermatologic: Rash
Gastrointestinal: Diarrhea, GI cramping, dyspepsia, flatulence, nausea, xerostomia
Respiratory: Rhinitis

<5%:
Cardiovascular: Tachycardia
Central nervous system: Extrapyramidal effects, somnolence, fatigue, seizure, insomnia, anxiety
Hematologic: Thrombocytopenia, increased LFTs, pancytopenia, leukopenia, granulocytopenia, aplastic anemia
Respiratory: Sinusitis, cough, upper respiratory tract infection, increased incidence of viral infection

Pharmacodynamics/Kinetics

Onset of Action: 0.5-1 hour
Protein Binding: 97.5% to 98%
Half-Life Elimination: 6-12 hours
Metabolism: Extensively hepatic to norcisapride
Excretion: Urine and feces (<10%)

Dosing

Adults & Elderly: GERD or gastrointestinal dysmotility: Oral: Initial: 5-10 mg 4 times/day at least 15 minutes before meals and at bedtime; in some patients the dosage will need to be increased to 20 mg to obtain a satisfactory result.

Pediatrics: Gastrointestinal dysmotility: Oral: Children: 0.15-0.3 mg/kg/dose 3-4 times/day; maximum: 10 mg/dose

Hepatic Impairment: Initiate at 50% usual dose.

Laboratory Monitoring A 12-lead ECG should be performed prior to administration of cisapride. Treatment with cisapride should not be initiated if the QT_c value exceeds 450 milliseconds. Serum electrolytes (potassium, calcium, and magnesium) and creatinine should be assessed prior to administration of cisapride and whenever conditions develop that may affect electrolyte balance or renal function.

Nursing Actions

Physical Assessment: Cardiac status must be evaluated prior to therapy (12-lead ECG). Assess other pharmacological or herbal products patient may be taking for potential interactions (eg, anything that may increase risk of cardiac arrhythmias). Monitor laboratory tests (eg, ECG, electrolyte balance, and renal function), therapeutic effectiveness (relief of symptoms), and adverse response (eg, tachycardia, CNS changes, anemia, viral infection) regularly during therapy. Teach patient proper use, possible side effects/appropriate interventions, and adverse symptoms to report.

Patient Education: It is absolutely vital that you inform prescriber of all prescriptions, OTC medications, or herbal products you are taking, and any allergies you have. Do not take any new medication during therapy unless approved by prescriber. Take before meals. Avoid alcohol and grapefruit juice. May cause increased sedation, headache, anxiety (use caution when driving or engaging in hazardous tasks until response to drug is known). Immediately report rapid heartbeat, palpitations, chest pain, or tightness. Report severe abdominal pain, prolonged diarrhea, weight loss, extreme fatigue, or other persistent adverse effects. **Pregnancy/breast-feeding precautions:** Inform prescriber if you are or intend to become pregnant. Consult prescriber if breast-feeding.

Geriatric Considerations Steady-state serum concentrations are higher than those in younger adults; however, the therapeutic dose and pharmacologic effects are the same as those in younger adults and no adjustment in dose recommended for elderly.

Cisatracurium (sis a tra KYOO ree um)

U.S. Brand Names Nimbex®
Synonyms Cisatracurium Besylate
Pharmacologic Category Neuromuscular Blocker Agent, Nondepolarizing
Medication Safety Issues
Sound-alike/look-alike issues:
Nimbex® may be confused with Revex®
Pregnancy Risk Factor B
Lactation Excretion in breast milk unknown/use caution
Use Adjunct to general anesthesia to facilitate endotracheal intubation and to relax skeletal muscles during surgery; to facilitate mechanical ventilation in ICU patients; does not relieve pain or produce sedation
Mechanism of Action/Effect Blocks neural transmission at the myoneural junction by binding with cholinergic receptor sites
Contraindications Hypersensitivity to cisatracurium besylate or any component of the formulation
Warnings/Precautions Maintenance of an adequate airway and respiratory support is critical; certain clinical conditions may result in potentiation or antagonism of neuromuscular blockade:
Potentiation: Electrolyte abnormalities, severe hyponatremia, severe hypocalcemia, severe hypokalemia, hypermagnesemia, neuromuscular diseases, acidosis, acute intermittent porphyria, renal failure, hepatic failure
Antagonism: Alkalosis, hypercalcemia, demyelinating lesions, peripheral neuropathies, diabetes mellitus
(Continued)

Cisatracurium (Continued)

Increased sensitivity in patients with myasthenia gravis, Eaton-Lambert syndrome; resistance in burn patients (>30% of body) for period of 5-70 days postinjury; resistance in patients with muscle trauma, denervation, immobilization, infection. Cross-sensitivity with other neuromuscular-blocking agents may occur; use extreme caution in patients with previous anaphylactic reactions. Bradycardia may be more common with cisatracurium than with other neuromuscular blocking agents since it has no clinically significant effects on heart rate to counteract the bradycardia produced by anesthetics.

Drug Interactions

Decreased Effect: Effect of nondepolarizing neuromuscular blockers may be reduced by carbamazepine (chronic use), corticosteroids (also associated with myopathy - see increased effect), phenytoin (chronic use), sympathomimetics, and theophylline.

Increased Effect/Toxicity: Increased effects are possible with aminoglycosides, beta-blockers, clindamycin, calcium channel blockers, halogenated anesthetics, imipenem, ketamine, lidocaine, loop diuretics (furosemide), macrolides (case reports), magnesium sulfate, procainamide, quinidine, quinolones, tetracyclines, and vancomycin. May increase risk of myopathy when used with high-dose corticosteroids for extended periods.

Overdosage/Toxicology

Symptoms of overdose include respiratory depression and cardiovascular collapse.

Neostigmine 1-3 mg slow I.V. push in adults (0.5 mg in children) antagonizes the neuromuscular blockade, and should be administered with or immediately after atropine 1-1.5 mg I.V. push (adults). This may be especially useful in the presence of bradycardia.

Pharmacodynamics/Kinetics

Onset of Action: I.V.: 2-3 minutes; Peak effect: 3-5 minutes

Duration of Action: Recovery begins in 20-35 minutes when anesthesia is balanced; recovery is attained in 90% of patients in 25-93 minutes

Half-Life Elimination: 22-29 minutes

Metabolism: Undergoes rapid nonenzymatic degradation in the bloodstream (Hofmann elimination), additional metabolism occurs via ester hydrolysis; some active metabolites

Available Dosage Forms

Injection, solution: 2 mg/mL (5 mL); 10 mg/mL (20 mL)
Injection, solution: 2 mg/mL (10 mL) [contains benzyl alcohol]

Dosing

Adults & Elderly: Neuromuscular blockade: I.V. (not to be used I.M.):

Operating room administration:

Intubating doses: 0.15-0.2 mg/kg as components of propofol/nitrous oxide/oxygen induction-intubation technique. (**Note:** May produce generally good or excellent conditions for tracheal intubation in 1.5-2 minutes with clinically effective duration of action during propofol anesthesia of 55-61 minutes.) Initial dose after succinylcholine for intubation: 0.1 mg/kg; maintenance dose: 0.03 mg/kg 40-60 minutes after initial dose, then at ~20-minute intervals based on clinical criteria.

Continuous infusion: After an initial bolus, a diluted solution can be given by continuous infusion for maintenance of neuromuscular blockade during extended surgery; adjust the rate of administration according to the patient's response as determined by peripheral nerve stimulation. An initial infusion rate of 3 mcg/kg/minute may be required to rapidly counteract the spontaneous recovery of neuromuscular function; thereafter, a rate of 1-2 mcg/kg/minute should be adequate to maintain continuous neuromuscular block in the 89% to 99% range in most pediatric and adult patients. Consider reduction of the infusion rate by 30% to 40% when administering during stable isoflurane, enflurane, sevoflurane, or desflurane anesthesia. Spontaneous recovery from neuromuscular blockade following discontinuation of infusion of cisatracurium may be expected to proceed at a rate comparable to that following single bolus administration.

Intensive care unit administration: Follow the principles for infusion in the operating room. At initial signs of recovery from bolus dose, begin the infusion at a dose of 3 mcg/kg/minute and adjust rates accordingly; dosage ranges of 0.5-10 mcg/kg/minute have been reported. If patient is allowed to recover from neuromuscular blockade, readministration of a bolus dose may be necessary to quickly re-establish neuromuscular block prior to reinstituting the infusion. See table.

Cisatracurium Besylate Infusion Chart

Drug Delivery Rate (mcg/kg/min)	Infusion Rate (mL/kg/min) 0.1 mg/mL (10 mg/100 mL)	Infusion Rate (mL/kg/min) 0.4 mg/mL (40 mg/100 mL)
1	0.01	0.0025
1.5	0.015	0.00375
2	0.02	0.005
3	0.03	0.0075
5	0.05	0.0125

Pediatrics: Neuromuscular blockade:

Operating room administration:

Children 2-12 years: I.V. (Not to be used I.M.)

Intubating doses: 0.1 mg over 5-15 seconds during either halothane or opioid anesthesia. (**Note:** When given during stable opioid nitrous oxide/oxygen anesthesia, 0.1 mg/kg produces maximum neuromuscular block in an average of 2.8 minutes and clinically effective block for 28 minutes.)

Continuous infusion: Refer to adult dosing.

Intensive care unit administration: Refer to adult dosing.

Renal Impairment: Because slower times to onset of complete neuromuscular block were observed in renal dysfunction patients, extending the interval between the administration of cisatracurium and intubation attempt may be required to achieve adequate intubation conditions.

Administration

I.M.: Not for I.M. injection, too much tissue irritation.

I.V.: Administer I.V. only. The use of a peripheral nerve stimulator will permit the most advantageous use of cisatracurium, minimize the possibility of overdosage or underdosage and assist in the evaluation of recovery.

Give undiluted as a bolus injection. Continuous administration requires the use of an infusion pump.

Stability

Compatibility: Stable in D₅W, NS, D₅NS

Y-site administration: Incompatible with amphotericin B cholesteryl sulfate complex, cefoperazone

Compatibility when admixed: Incompatible with ketorolac, propofol

Storage: Refrigerate intact vials at 2°C to 8°C/36°F to 46°F. Use vials within 21 days upon removal from the refrigerator to room temperature (25°C to 77°F). Dilutions of 0.1-0.2 mg/mL in 0.9% sodium chloride or dextrose 5% in water are stable for up to 24 hours at room temperature.

Nursing Actions

Physical Assessment: Only clinicians experienced in the use of neuromuscular blocking drugs should administer and/or manage the use of cisatracurium. Ventilatory support must be instituted and maintained until adequate respiratory muscle function and/or airway protection are assured. Assess other medications for effectiveness and safety. Other drugs that affect neuromuscular activity may increase/decrease neuromuscular block induced by cisatracurium. This drug does not cause anesthesia or analgesia; pain must be treated with appropriate analgesic agents. Continuous monitoring of vital signs, cardiac status, respiratory status, and degree of neuromuscular block (objective assessment with peripheral external nerve stimulator) is mandatory during infusion and until full muscle tone has returned. Muscle tone returns in a predictable pattern, starting with diaphragm, abdomen, chest, limbs, and finally muscles of the neck, face, and eyes. Safety precautions must be maintained until full muscle tone has returned. **Note:** It may take longer for return of muscle tone in obese or elderly patients or patients with renal or hepatic disease, myasthenia gravis, myopathy, other neuromuscular disease, dehydration, electrolyte imbalance, or severe acid/base imbalance. Provide appropriate patient teaching/support prior to and following administration.

Long-term use: Monitor fluid levels (intake and output) during and following infusion. Reposition patient and provide appropriate skin care, mouth care, and care of patient's eyes every 2-3 hours while sedated. Provide appropriate emotional and sensory support (auditory and environmental).

Patient Education: Patient will usually be unconscious prior to administration. Patient education should be appropriate to individual situation. Reassurance of constant monitoring and emotional support to reduce fear and anxiety should precede and follow administration. Following return of muscle tone, do not attempt to change position or rise from bed without assistance. Report immediately any skin rash or hives, pounding heartbeat, respiratory difficulty, or muscle tremors. **Breast-feeding precaution:** Consult prescriber if breast-feeding.

Additional Information Cisatracurium is classified as an intermediate-duration neuromuscular-blocking agent. It does not appear to have a cumulative effect on the duration of blockade. Neuromuscular-blocking potency is 3 times that of atracurium; maximum block is up to 2 minutes longer than for equipotent doses of atracurium.

Cisplatin (SIS pla tin)

U.S. Brand Names Platinol®-AQ [DSC]

Synonyms CDDP

Pharmacologic Category Antineoplastic Agent, Alkylating Agent

Medication Safety Issues
Sound-alike/look-alike issues:
Cisplatin may be confused with carboplatin
Platinol®-AQ may be confused with Paraplatin®, Patanol®, Plaquenil®

Doses >100 mg/m^2 once every 3-4 weeks are rarely used and should be verified with the prescriber.

Pregnancy Risk Factor D

Lactation Enters breast milk/contraindicated

Use Treatment of bladder, testicular, and ovarian cancer

Unlabeled/Investigational Use Treatment of head and neck, breast, gastric, lung, esophageal, cervical, prostate and small cell lung cancer; Hodgkin's and non-Hodgkin's lymphoma; neuroblastoma; sarcomas, myeloma, melanoma, mesothelioma, and osteosarcoma

Mechanism of Action/Effect Inhibits DNA synthesis

Contraindications Hypersensitivity to cisplatin, other platinum-containing compounds, or any component of the formulation (anaphylactic-like reactions have been reported); pre-existing renal insufficiency; myelosuppression; hearing impairment; pregnancy

Warnings/Precautions Hazardous agent - use appropriate precautions for handling and disposal. Doses >100 mg/m^2 once every 3-4 weeks are rarely used and should be verified with the prescriber. All patients should receive adequate hydration, with or without diuretics, prior to and for 24 hours after cisplatin administration. Reduce dosage in renal impairment. Cumulative renal toxicity may be severe. Elderly patients may be more susceptible to nephrotoxicity; select dose cautiously and monitor closely. Dose-related toxicities include myelosuppression, nausea, and vomiting. Ototoxicity, especially pronounced in children, is manifested by tinnitus or loss of high frequency hearing and occasionally, deafness. **Serum magnesium, as well as other electrolytes, should be monitored both before and within 48 hours after cisplatin therapy.** When administered as sequential infusions, taxane derivatives (docetaxel, paclitaxel) should be administered before platinum derivatives (carboplatin, cisplatin).

Drug Interactions

Decreased Effect: Sodium thiosulfate and amifostine theoretically inactivate drug systemically; have been used clinically to reduce systemic toxicity with administration of cisplatin.

Increased Effect/Toxicity: Cisplatin and ethacrynic acid have resulted in severe ototoxicity in animals. Delayed bleomycin elimination with decreased glomerular filtration rate. When administered as sequential infusions, observational studies indicate a potential for increased toxicity when platinum derivatives (carboplatin, cisplatin) are administered before taxane derivatives (docetaxel, paclitaxel).

Nutritional/Ethanol Interactions Herb/Nutraceutical: Avoid black cohosh, dong quai in estrogen-dependent tumors.

Adverse Reactions
>10%:
Central nervous system: Neurotoxicity: Peripheral neuropathy is dose- and duration-dependent.
Dermatologic: Mild alopecia
Gastrointestinal: Nausea and vomiting (76% to 100%)
Hematologic: Myelosuppression (25% to 30%; mild with moderate doses, mild to moderate with high-dose therapy)
WBC: Mild
Platelets: Mild
Onset: 10 days
Nadir: 14-23 days
Recovery: 21-39 days
Hepatic: Liver enzymes increased
Renal: Nephrotoxicity (acute renal failure and chronic renal insufficiency)
Otic: Ototoxicity (10% to 30%; manifested as high frequency hearing loss; ototoxicity is especially pronounced in children)
1% to 10%:
Gastrointestinal: Diarrhea
Local: Tissue irritation

Overdosage/Toxicology Symptoms of overdose include severe myelosuppression, intractable nausea and vomiting, kidney and liver failure, deafness, ocular toxicity, and neuritis. Overdose may be fatal. There is no known antidote. Hemodialysis appears to have little effect. Treatment is symptom-directed and supportive.

Pharmacodynamics/Kinetics
Protein Binding: >90%
Half-Life Elimination: Initial: 20-30 minutes; Beta: 60 minutes; Terminal: ~24 hours; Secondary half-life: 44-73 hours
Metabolism: Nonenzymatic; inactivated (in both cell and bloodstream) by sulfhydryl groups; covalently binds to glutathione and thiosulfate
(Continued)

273

Cisplatin *(Continued)*

Excretion: Urine (>90%); feces (10%)

Available Dosage Forms [DSC] = Discontinued product

Injection, solution: 1 mg/mL (50 mL, 100 mL, 200 mL)

Platinol®-AQ: 1 mg/mL (50 mL, 100 mL) [contains sodium 9 mg/mL] [DSC]

Dosing

Adults & Elderly:

Advanced bladder cancer: 50-70 mg/m² every 3-4 weeks

Head and neck cancer (unlabeled use): 100-120 mg/m² every 3-4 weeks

Malignant pleural mesothelioma in combination with pemetrexed (unlabeled use): 75 mg/m² on day 1 of each 21-day cycle; see Pemetrexed monograph for additional details

Metastatic ovarian cancer: 75-100 mg/m² every 3-4 weeks

Intraperitoneal: Cisplatin has been administered intraperitoneal with systemic sodium thiosulfate for ovarian cancer; doses up to 90-270 mg/m² have been administered and retained for 4 hours before draining

Testicular cancer: 10-20 mg/m²/day for 5 days repeated every 3-4 weeks

High dose BMT: Continuous I.V.: 55 mg/m²/24 hours for 72 hours; total dose: 165 mg/m²

Pediatrics: Refer to individual protocols. VERIFY ANY CISPLATIN DOSE EXCEEDING 100 mg/m² PER COURSE.

Unlabeled pediatric uses:

Intermittent dosing schedule: 37-75 mg/m² once every 2-3 weeks or 50-100 mg/m² over 4-6 hours, once every 21-28 days

Daily dosing schedule: 15-20 mg/m²/day for 5 days every 3-4 weeks

Osteogenic sarcoma or neuroblastoma: 60-100 mg/m² on day 1 every 3-4 weeks

Recurrent brain tumors: 60 mg/m² once daily for 2 consecutive days every 3-4 weeks

Bone marrow/blood cell transfusion: Continuous Infusion: High dose: 55 mg/m²/day for 72 hours; total dose = 165 mg/m²

Renal Impairment: Note: The manufacturer(s) recommend that repeat courses of cisplatin should not be given until serum creatinine is <1.5 mg/100 mL and/or BUN is <25 mg/100 mL. There is no FDA-approved renal dosing adjustment guideline; the following guidelines have been used by some clinicians:

Kintzel, 1995:

Cl_{cr} 46-60 mL/minute: Reduce dose by 25%

Cl_{cr} 31-45 mL/minute: Reduce dose by 50%

Cl_{cr} <30 mL/minute: Consider use of alternative drug

Aronoff, 1999:

Cl_{cr} 10-50 mL/minute: Administer 75% of dose

Cl_{cr} <10 mL/minute: Administer 50% of dose

Hemodialysis: Partially cleared by hemodialysis. Administer dose posthemodialysis.

CAPD effects: Unknown

CAVH effects: Unknown

Administration

I.V.: Irritant. Perform pretreatment hydration (see Dosage).

I.V.: Rate of administration has varied from a 15- to 120-minute infusion, 1 mg/minute infusion, 6- to 8-hour infusion, 24-hour infusion, or per protocol. Maximum rate of infusion: 1 mg/minute in patients with CHF.

When administered as sequential infusions, taxane derivatives (docetaxel, paclitaxel) should be administered before platinum derivatives to limit myelosuppression and to enhance efficacy.

I.V. Detail:

Extravasation management: Large extravasations (>20 mL) of concentrated solutions (>0.5 mg/mL) produce tissue necrosis. **Treatment is not recommended unless a large amount of highly concentrated solution is extravasated.** Mix 4 mL of 10% sodium thiosulfate with 6 mL sterile water for injection: Inject 1-4 mL through existing I.V. line cannula. Administer 1 mL for each mL extravasated; inject SubQ if needle is removed.

pH: 3.5-5.5 (reconstituted solution); 3.7-6.0 (aqueous injection)

Stability

Reconstitution: Further dilutions in NS, D_5/0.45% NaCl or D_5/NS to a concentration of 0.05-2 mg/mL are stable for 72 hours at 4°C to 25°C. The infusion solution should have a final sodium chloride concentration of ≥0.2%.

Compatibility: Stable in $D_5^{1}/_4$NS, $D_5^{1}/_2$NS, D_5NS, $^{1}/_4$NS, $^{1}/_3$NS, $^{1}/_2$NS, NS; **incompatible** with sodium bicarbonate 5%

Y-site administration: Incompatible with amifostine, amphotericin B cholesteryl sulfate complex, cefepime, piperacillin/tazobactam, thiotepa

Compatibility when admixed: Incompatible with fluorouracil, mesna, thiotepa

Storage: Store intact vials at room temperature 15°C to 25°C (59°F to 77°F) and protect from light. Do not refrigerate solution as a precipitate may form. Further dilution **stability is dependent on the chloride ion concentration** and should be mixed in solutions of NS (at least 0.3% NaCl). After initial entry into the vial, solution is stable for 28 days protected from light or for at least 7 days under fluorescent room light at room temperature.

Laboratory Monitoring Renal function (serum creatinine, BUN, Cl_{cr}); electrolytes (particularly magnesium, calcium, potassium) before and within 48 hours after cisplatin therapy; liver function periodically, CBC with differential and platelet count, urinalysis

Nursing Actions

Physical Assessment: Assess potential for interactions with other pharmacological agents or herbal products patient may be taking (especially anything that is ototoxic or nephrotoxic). Patient should be vigorously hydrated prior to and for 24 hours following infusion. Cisplatin is highly emetogenic; antiemetic should be administered prior to each treatment and as needed between infusions. See Administration for detailed infusion specifics. Infusion site must be monitored closely to reduce potential for extravasation. Monitor laboratory tests and evaluate any changes in auditory status prior to each treatment and regularly during therapy. Patient response should be closely monitored during and following therapy (eg, acute or chronic renal failure; peripheral neuropathy and ototoxicity, may be irreversible). Teach patient (or caregiver) possible side effects/appropriate interventions (eg, importance of adequate hydration) and adverse symptoms to report. (see Warnings/Precautions for extensive use cautions).

Patient Education: Do not take any new medication during therapy unless approved by prescriber. This medication can only be administered by I.V. and numerous side-effects can occur. Report immediately any burning, pain, itching, or redness at infusion site. It is important that you maintain adequate hydration (2-3 L/day of fluids) unless instructed to restrict fluid intake, and adequate nutrition (small, frequent meals may help). May cause severe nausea or vomiting that can be delayed for up to 48 hours after infusion and last for 1 week (consult prescriber for appropriate antiemetic medication); mouth sores (use soft toothbrush or cotton swabs for mouth care); or loss of hair (reversible). You will be susceptible to infection (avoid crowds and exposure to infection and do not have any vaccinations without consulting prescriber). Report promptly any pain, tingling, loss of sensation or cramping in extremities; change in hearing; difficulty breathing or swallowing; fever or chills; unusual fatigue; unusual bruising/bleeding; or any other unusual symptoms. **Pregnancy/breast-feeding precautions:** Inform prescriber if you are pregnant. Do not get pregnant during therapy. Consult prescriber for instruction on appropriate contraceptive measures. This drug may cause severe fetal defects. Consult prescriber if breast-feeding.

Dietary Considerations Sodium content: 9 mg/mL (equivalent to 0.9% sodium chloride solution)

Pregnancy Issues Animal studies have demonstrated teratogenicity and embryotoxicity. There are no adequate and well-controlled studies in pregnant women. Women of childbearing potential should be advised to avoid pregnancy. If used in pregnancy, or if patient becomes pregnant during treatment, the patient should be apprised of potential hazard to the fetus.

Additional Information
Sodium content: 9 mg/mL (equivalent to 0.9% sodium chloride solution)

Osmolality of Platinol®-AQ = 285-286 mOsm

Recommendations for minimizing nephrotoxicity include:
Prepare cisplatin in saline-containing vehicles
Infuse dose over 24 hours
Vigorous hydration (125-150 mL/hour) before, during, and after cisplatin administration
Simultaneous administration of either mannitol or furosemide
Pretreatment with amifostine
Avoid other nephrotoxic agents (aminoglycosides, amphotericin, etc)

Citalopram (sye TAL oh pram)

U.S. Brand Names Celexa®

Synonyms Citalopram Hydrobromide; Nitalapram

Restrictions A medication guide concerning the use of antidepressants in children and teenagers can be found on the FDA website at http://www.fda.gov/cder/Offices/ODS/labeling.htm. It should be dispensed to parents or guardians of children and teenagers receiving this medication.

Pharmacologic Category Antidepressant, Selective Serotonin Reuptake Inhibitor

Medication Safety Issues
Sound-alike/look-alike issues:
Celexa™ may be confused with Celebrex®, Cerebra®, Cerebyx®, Zyprexa®

Pregnancy Risk Factor C

Lactation Enters breast milk/contraindicated

Use Treatment of depression

Unlabeled/Investigational Use Treatment of dementia, smoking cessation, ethanol abuse, obsessive-compulsive disorder (OCD) in children, diabetic neuropathy

Mechanism of Action/Effect A bicyclic phthalein derivative, citalopram selectively inhibits serotonin reuptake in the presynaptic neurons

Contraindications Hypersensitivity to citalopram or any component of the formulation; hypersensitivity or other adverse sequelae during therapy with other SSRIs; concomitant use with MAO inhibitors or within 2 weeks of discontinuing MAO inhibitors.

Warnings/Precautions Antidepressants increase the risk of suicidal thinking and behavior in children and adolescents with major depressive disorder (MDD) and other depressive disorders; consider risk prior to prescribing. All patients must be closely monitored for clinical worsening, suicidality, or unusual changes in behavior, especially during the initiation of therapy or following an increase or decrease in dosage. When used in children, the child's family or caregiver should be instructed to closely observe the patient and communicate condition with healthcare provider. A medication guide should be dispensed with each prescription. **Citalopram is not FDA approved for use in children.**

The possibility of a suicide attempt is inherent in major depression and may persist until remission occurs. Use caution in high-risk patients. Worsening depression and severe abrupt suicidality that are not part of the presenting symptoms may require discontinuation or modification of drug therapy. The patient's family or caregiver should be alerted to monitor patients for the emergence of suicidality and associated behaviors (such as agitation, irritability, hostility, impulsivity, and hypomania) and call healthcare provider.

May worsen psychosis in some patients or precipitate a shift to mania or hypomania in patients with bipolar disorder. Patients presenting with depressive symptoms should be screened for bipolar disorder. Monotherapy in patients with bipolar disorder should be avoided. **Citalopram is not FDA approved for the treatment of bipolar depression.**

The potential for severe reaction exists when used with MAO inhibitors; serotonin syndrome (hyperthermia, muscular rigidity, mental status changes/agitation, autonomic instability) may occur. May increase the risks associated with electroconvulsive therapy. Has a low potential to impair cognitive or motor performance; caution operating hazardous machinery or driving.

Use with caution in patients with hepatic or renal dysfunction, in elderly patients, concomitant CNS depressants, and pregnancy (high doses of citalopram have been associated with teratogenicity in animals). Use caution with concomitant use of NSAIDs, ASA, or other drugs that affect coagulation; the risk of bleeding is potentiated. May cause hyponatremia/SIADH. May cause or exacerbate sexual dysfunction. Upon discontinuation of citalopram therapy, gradually taper dose. If intolerable symptoms occur following a decrease in dosage or upon discontinuation of therapy, then resuming the previous dose with a more gradual taper should be considered.

Drug Interactions
Cytochrome P450 Effect: Substrate of CYP2C19 (major), 2D6 (minor), 3A4 (major); **Inhibits** CYP1A2 (weak), 2B6 (weak), 2C19 (weak), 2D6 (weak)

Decreased Effect: CYP2C19 inducers may decrease the levels/effects of citalopram; example inducers include aminoglutethimide, carbamazepine, phenytoin, and rifampin. Cyproheptadine may inhibit the effects of serotonin reuptake inhibitors. CYP3A4 inducers may decrease the levels/effects of citalopram; example inducers include aminoglutethimide, carbamazepine, nafcillin, nevirapine, phenobarbital, phenytoin, and rifamycins.

Increased Effect/Toxicity: Citalopram should not be used with nonselective MAO inhibitors (phenelzine, isocarboxazid) or other drugs with MAO inhibition (linezolid); fatal reactions have been reported. Wait 5 weeks after stopping citalopram before starting a nonselective MAO inhibitor and 2 weeks after stopping an MAO inhibitor before starting citalopram. Concurrent selegiline has been associated with mania, hypertension, or serotonin syndrome (risk may be reduced relative to nonselective MAO inhibitors).

CYP2C19 inhibitors may increase the levels/effects of citalopram; example inhibitors include delavirdine, fluconazole, fluvoxamine, gemfibrozil, isoniazid, omeprazole, and ticlopidine. CYP3A4 inhibitors may increase the levels/effects of citalopram; example inhibitors include azole antifungals, clarithromycin, diclofenac, doxycycline, erythromycin, imatinib, isoniazid, nefazodone, nicardipine, propofol, protease inhibitors, quinidine, telithromycin, and verapamil.

(Continued)

Citalopram (Continued)

Combined use of SSRIs and amphetamines, buspirone, meperidine, nefazodone, serotonin agonists (such as sumatriptan), sibutramine, other SSRIs, sympathomimetics, ritonavir, tramadol, and venlafaxine may increase the risk of serotonin syndrome. Risk of hyponatremia may increase with concurrent use of loop diuretics (bumetanide, furosemide, torsemide). Citalopram may increase the hypoprothrombinemic response to warfarin. Concomitant use of citalopram and NSAIDs, aspirin, or other drugs affecting coagulation has been associated with an increased risk of bleeding; monitor.

Combined use of sumatriptan (and other serotonin agonists) may result in toxicity; weakness, hyper-reflexia, and incoordination have been observed with sumatriptan and SSRIs. In addition, concurrent use may theoretically increase the risk of serotonin syndrome; includes sumatriptan, naratriptan, rizatriptan, and zolmitriptan.

Nutritional/Ethanol Interactions

Ethanol: Avoid ethanol (may increase CNS depression).
Herb/Nutraceutical: Avoid valerian, St John's wort, SAMe, kava kava, and gotu kola (may increase CNS depression).

Adverse Reactions

>10%:
Central nervous system: Somnolence, insomnia
Gastrointestinal: Nausea, xerostomia
Miscellaneous: Diaphoresis
<10%:
Central nervous system: Anxiety, anorexia, agitation, yawning
Dermatologic: Rash, pruritus
Endocrine & metabolic: Sexual dysfunction
Gastrointestinal: Diarrhea, dyspepsia, vomiting, abdominal pain, weight gain
Neuromuscular & skeletal: Tremor, arthralgia, myalgia
Respiratory: Cough, rhinitis, sinusitis

Overdosage/Toxicology

Symptoms of overdose include dizziness, nausea, vomiting, sweating, tremor, somnolence, and sinus tachycardia. Rare symptoms have included amnesia, confusion, coma, seizures, hyperventilation, and ECG changes (including QT_c prolongation, ventricular arrhythmia, and torsade de pointes). Management is supportive and symptomatic.

Pharmacodynamics/Kinetics

Time to Peak: Serum: 1-6 hours, average within 4 hours
Protein Binding: Plasma: ~80%
Half-Life Elimination: 24-48 hours (average: 35 hours); doubled with hepatic impairment
Metabolism: Extensively hepatic, including CYP, to N-demethylated, N-oxide, and deaminated metabolites
Excretion: Urine (10% as unchanged drug)
Note: Clearance was decreased, while AUC and half-life were significantly increased in elderly patients and in patients with hepatic impairment. Mild-to-moderate renal impairment may reduce clearance (17%) and prolong half-life of citalopram. No pharmacokinetic information is available concerning patients with severe renal impairment.

Available Dosage Forms

Solution, oral: 10 mg/5 mL (240 mL) [alcohol free, sugar free; peppermint flavor]
Tablet: 10 mg, 20 mg, 40 mg

Dosing

Adults: Depression: Oral: Initial: 20 mg/day, generally with an increase to 40 mg/day; doses of more than 40 mg are not usually necessary. Should a dose increase be necessary, it should occur in 20 mg increments at intervals of no less than 1 week. Maximum dose: 60 mg/day.

Elderly: Oral: Initial dose: 10-20 mg once daily. Increase dose to 40 mg/day only in nonresponders.
Pediatrics: Children and Adolescents: OCD (unlabeled use): Oral: 10-40 mg/day
Renal Impairment: None necessary in mild-moderate renal impairment; best avoided in severely impaired renal function (Cl_{cr} <20 mL/minute).
Hepatic Impairment: Reduce dosage in those with hepatic impairment.

Stability

Storage: Store below 25°C.

Laboratory Monitoring Liver function tests and CBC with continued therapy

Nursing Actions

Physical Assessment: Assess other medications patient may be taking for possible interaction (especially MAO inhibitors, P450 inhibitors, and other CNS active agents). Monitor for effectiveness of therapy and adverse reactions. Assess mental status for depression, suicidal ideation, anxiety, social functioning, mania, or panic attack. Assess knowledge/teach patient appropriate use, interventions to reduce side effects (eg, hypotensive precautions), and adverse symptoms to report.

Patient Education: It may take up to 3 weeks to see therapeutic effects from this medication. Take as directed; do not alter dose or frequency without consulting prescriber. May be taken with or without food. Avoid alcohol, caffeine, and CNS stimulants. Avoid use of aspirin or other NSAIDs unless approved by prescriber (may increase risk of bleeding). You may experience sexual dysfunction (reversible). May cause dizziness, anxiety, or blurred vision (rise slowly from sitting or lying position and use caution when driving or engaging in tasks requiring alertness until response to drug is known); or nausea or dry mouth (small frequent meals, frequent mouth care, chewing gum, or sucking lozenges may help). Report confusion or impaired concentration, thoughts of suicide, severe headache, palpitations, rash, insomnia or nightmares, changes in personality, muscle weakness or tremors, altered gait pattern, signs and symptoms of respiratory infection, or excessive perspiration. Pregnancy/breast-feeding precautions: Inform prescriber if you are or intend to become pregnant. Do not breast-feed.

Dietary Considerations May be taken without regard to food.

Geriatric Considerations Clearance was decreased, while AUC and half-life were significantly increased in elderly patients and in patients with hepatic impairment. Mild-to-moderate renal impairment may reduce clearance of citalopram (17% reduction noted in trials). No pharmacokinetic information is available concerning patients with severe renal impairment.

Breast-Feeding Issues Citalopram is excreted in human milk. Excessive somnolence, decreased feeding, and weight loss have been reported in breast-fed infants. A decision should be made whether to continue or discontinue nursing or discontinue the drug.

Pregnancy Issues Teratogenic effects have been observed in animal studies. Nonteratogenic effects including respiratory distress, cyanosis, apnea, seizures, temperature instability, feeding difficulty, vomiting, hypoglycemia, hypo- or hypertonia, hyper-reflexia, jitteriness, irritability, constant crying, and tremor have been reported in the neonate immediately following delivery after exposure late in the third trimester. Adverse effects may be due to toxic effects of SSRI or drug discontinuation. In some cases, may present clinically as serotonin syndrome. There are no adequate and well-controlled studies in pregnant women. Use during pregnancy only if the potential benefit to the mother outweighs the possible risk to the fetus. If treatment during pregnancy is required, consider tapering therapy during the third trimester.

Related Information
Antidepressant Medication Guidelines *on page 1414*

Cladribine (KLA dri been)

U.S. Brand Names Leustatin®
Synonyms 2-CdA; 2-Chlorodeoxyadenosine
Pharmacologic Category Adjuvant, Radiosensitizing Agent; Antineoplastic Agent; Antimetabolite; Antineoplastic Agent, Antimetabolite (Purine Antagonist)
Medication Safety Issues
Sound-alike/look-alike issues:
Leustatin® may be confused with lovastatin
Pregnancy Risk Factor D
Lactation Enters breast milk/contraindicated
Use Treatment of hairy cell leukemia, chronic lymphocytic leukemia (CLL), chronic myelogenous leukemia (CML)
Unlabeled/Investigational Use Non-Hodgkin's lymphomas, progressive multiple sclerosis
Mechanism of Action/Effect A prodrug which incorporates DNA causing breakage of DNA strands and shutdown of DNA synthesis. Cladribine is cell-cycle nonspecific.
Contraindications Hypersensitivity to cladribine or any component of the formulation; pregnancy
Warnings/Precautions Hazardous agent — use appropriate precautions for handling and disposal. Because of its myelosuppressive properties, cladribine should be used with caution in patients with pre-existing hematologic or immunologic abnormalities.
Nutritional/Ethanol Interactions Ethanol: Avoid ethanol (due to GI irritation).
Adverse Reactions
>10%:
Allergic: Fever (70%), chills (18%); skin reactions (erythema, itching) at the catheter site (18%)
Central nervous system: Fatigue (17%), headache (13%)
Dermatologic: Rash
Hematologic: Myelosuppression, common, dose-limiting; leukopenia (70%); anemia (37%); thrombocytopenia (12%)
Nadir: 5-10 days
Recovery: 4-8 weeks
1% to 10%:
Cardiovascular: Edema, tachycardia
Central nervous system: Dizziness; pains; chills; malaise; severe infection, possibly related to thrombocytopenia
Dermatologic: Pruritus, erythema
Gastrointestinal: Nausea, mild to moderate, usually not seen at doses <0.3 mg/kg/day; constipation; abdominal pain
Neuromuscular & skeletal: Myalgia, arthralgia, weakness
Renal: Renal failure at high (>0.3 mg/kg/day) doses
Miscellaneous: Diaphoresis, delayed herpes zoster infection, tumor lysis syndrome
Pharmacodynamics/Kinetics
Protein Binding: Plasma: 20%
Half-Life Elimination: Biphasic: Alpha: 25 minutes; Beta: 6.7 hours; Terminal, mean: Normal renal function: 5.4 hours
Metabolism: Hepatic; 5'-triphosphate moiety-active
Excretion: Urine (21% to 44%); Clearance: Estimated systemic: 640 mL/hour/kg
Available Dosage Forms Injection, solution [preservative free]: 1 mg/mL (10 mL)
Dosing
Adults & Elderly: Refer to individual protocols.
Hairy cell leukemia: I.V. Continuous infusion:
0.09-0.1 mg/kg/day days 1-7; may be repeated every 28-35 days **or**

3.4 mg/m²/day SubQ days 1-7
Chronic lymphocytic leukemia: I.V. Continuous infusion:
0.1 mg/kg/day days 1-7 **or**
0.028-0.14 mg/kg/day as a 2-hour infusion days 1-5
Chronic myelogenous leukemia: I.V. 15 mg/m²/day as a 1-hour infusion days 1-5; if no response increase dose to 20 mg/m²/day in the second course.
Pediatrics: Refer to individual protocols.
Acute leukemias: 6.2-7.5 mg/m²/day continuous infusion for days 1-5; maximum tolerated dose was 8.9 mg/m²/day.
Administration
I.V.: Administer as a 1- to 2-hour infusion or by continuous infusion
I.V. Detail: pH: 6.0-6.6
Stability
Reconstitution: Dilute in 250-1000 mL. Solutions for 7-day infusion should be prepared in bacteriostatic NS.
Compatibility: Stable in NS; **incompatible** with D₅W
Storage: Store intact vials under refrigeration 2°C to 8°C (36°F to 46°F). Dilutions in 500 mL NS are stable for 72 hours. Stable in PVC containers for 24 hours at room temperature of 15°C to 30°C (59°F to 86°F) and 7 days in Pharmacia Deltec® cassettes.
Laboratory Monitoring Liver and renal function tests, CBC with differential, platelets, uric acid
Nursing Actions
Physical Assessment: Monitor laboratory tests, therapeutic effectiveness, and adverse response (eg, myelosuppression, cardiac changes, renal failure) regularly during therapy and following therapy (patients should be considered immunosuppressed for up to 1 year after cladribine therapy). Teach patient (or caregiver) possible side effects/appropriate interventions and adverse symptoms to report.

Patient Education: Inform prescriber of all prescriptions, OTC medications, or herbal products you are taking, and any allergies you have. Do not take any new medication during therapy unless approved by prescriber. This drug can only be administered by infusion. It is important to maintain adequate hydration (2-3 L/day of fluids) unless instructed to restrict fluid intake, and nutrition during therapy (small, frequent meals may help). You will be more susceptible to infection during therapy and for up to 1 year following therapy (avoid crowds and exposure to infection and do not have any vaccinations without consulting prescriber). May cause nausea or vomiting (small, frequent meals, frequent mouth care, sucking lozenges, or chewing gum may help); muscle weakness or pain (consult prescriber for mild analgesics); or mouth sores (use frequent mouth care with soft toothbrush or cotton swabs and frequent mouth rinses). Report immediately rash, unusual excessive fatigue, and/or signs of infection. Report rapid heartbeat or palpitations; unusual bruising or bleeding; persistent GI disturbances; diarrhea or constipation; yellowing of eyes or skin; change in color of urine or stool; swelling, warmth, or pain in extremities; or difficult respirations. **Pregnancy/breast-feeding precautions:** Do not get pregnant while taking this medication. Consult prescriber for appropriate contraceptive measures. Do not breast-feed until prescriber advises it is safe.

Clarithromycin (kla RITH roe mye sin)

U.S. Brand Names Biaxin®; Biaxin® XL
Pharmacologic Category Antibiotic, Macrolide
Medication Safety Issues
Sound-alike/look-alike issues:
Clarithromycin may be confused with erythromycin
Pregnancy Risk Factor C
Lactation Excretion in breast milk unknown/use caution
Use
Children:
Pharyngitis/tonsillitis, acute maxillary sinusitis, uncomplicated skin/skin structure infections, and mycobacterial infections
Acute otitis media (*H. influenzae*, *M. catarrhalis*, or *S. pneumoniae*)
Prevention of disseminated mycobacterial infections due to MAC disease in patients with advanced HIV infection
Adults:
Pharyngitis/tonsillitis due to susceptible *S. pyogenes*
Acute maxillary sinusitis and acute exacerbation of chronic bronchitis due to susceptible *H. influenzae*, *M. catarrhalis*, or *S. pneumoniae*
Community-acquired pneumonia due to susceptible *H. influenzae*, *H. parainfluenzae*, *Mycoplasma pneumoniae*, *S. pneumoniae*, or *Chlamydia pneumoniae* (TWAR)
Uncomplicated skin/skin structure infections due to susceptible *S. aureus*, *S. pyogenes*
Disseminated mycobacterial infections due to *M. avium* or *M. intracellulare*
Prevention of disseminated mycobacterial infections due to *M. avium* complex (MAC) disease (eg, patients with advanced HIV infection)
Duodenal ulcer disease due to *H. pylori* in regimens with other drugs including amoxicillin and lansoprazole or omeprazole, ranitidine bismuth citrate, bismuth subsalicylate, tetracycline, and/or an H₂ antagonist
Alternate antibiotic for prophylaxis of bacterial endocarditis in patients who are allergic to penicillin and undergoing surgical or dental procedures
Unlabeled/Investigational Use Pertussis
Mechanism of Action/Effect Exerts its antibacterial action by binding to 50S ribosomal subunit resulting in inhibition of protein synthesis. The 14-OH metabolite of clarithromycin is twice as active as the parent compound against some organisms.
Contraindications Hypersensitivity to clarithromycin, erythromycin, or any macrolide antibiotic; use with ergot derivatives, pimozide, cisapride; combination with ranitidine bismuth citrate should not be used in patients with history of acute porphyria or Cl$_{cr}$ <25 mL/minute
Warnings/Precautions Dosage adjustment required with severe renal impairment, decreased dosage or prolonged dosing interval may be appropriate; antibiotic-associated colitis has been reported with use of clarithromycin. Macrolides (including clarithromycin) have been associated with rare QT prolongation and ventricular arrhythmias, including torsade de pointes. Avoid use of extended release tablets (Biaxin® XL) in patients with known stricture/narrowing of the GI tract. Safety and efficacy in children <6 months of age have not been established.
Drug Interactions
Cytochrome P450 Effect: Substrate of CYP3A4 (major); **Inhibits** CYP1A2 (weak), 3A4 (strong)
Decreased Effect: Therapeutic effect of clopidogrel may be decreased by clarithromycin. Peak levels (but not AUC) of zidovudine may be increased; other studies suggest levels may be decreased. The levels/effects of clarithromycin may be decreased by aminoglutethimide, carbamazepine, nafcillin, nevirapine, phenobarbital, phenytoin, rifamycins, and other CYP3A4 inducers.

Increased Effect/Toxicity: Avoid concomitant use of the following with clarithromycin due to increased risk of malignant arrhythmias: Cisapride, gatifloxacin, moxifloxacin, pimozide, sparfloxacin, thioridazine. Other agents that prolong the QT$_c$ interval, including type Ia (eg, quinidine) and type III antiarrhythmic agents, and selected antipsychotic agents (eg, thioridazine) should be used with extreme caution.

Clarithromycin is a strong CYP3A4 inhibitor, and may increase the levels/effects of selected benzodiazepines, calcium channel blockers, cyclosporine, mirtazapine, nateglinide, nefazodone, quinidine, sildenafil (and other PDE-5 inhibitors), tacrolimus, venlafaxine, and other CYP3A4 substrates. Selected benzodiazepines (midazolam, triazolam), cisapride, ergot alkaloids, selected HMG-CoA reductase inhibitors (lovastatin and simvastatin), and pimozide are generally contraindicated with strong CYP3A4 inhibitors. When used with strong CYP3A4 inhibitors, dosage adjustment/limits are recommended for sildenafil and other PDE-5 inhibitors; refer to individual monographs.

The effects of warfarin have been potentiated by clarithromycin. Clarithromycin serum concentrations may be increased by amprenavir (and possibly other protease inhibitors). Digoxin serum levels may be increased by clarithromycin; digoxin toxicity and potentially fatal arrhythmias have been reported; monitor digoxin levels. Fluconazole increases clarithromycin levels and AUC by ~25%. Peak levels (but not AUC) of zidovudine may be increased; other studies suggest levels may be decreased.

The levels/effects of clarithromycin may be increased by azole antifungals, diclofenac, doxycycline, erythromycin, imatinib, isoniazid, nefazodone, nicardipine, propofol, protease inhibitors, quinidine, telithromycin, verapamil, and other CYP3A4 inhibitors.
Nutritional/Ethanol Interactions
Food: Delays absorption; total absorption remains unchanged.
Herb/Nutraceutical: St John's wort may decrease clarithromycin levels.
Adverse Reactions 1% to 10%:
Central nervous system: Headache (adults and children 2%)
Dermatologic: Rash (children 3%)
Gastrointestinal: Abnormal taste (adults 3% to 7%), diarrhea (adults 3% to 6%; children 6%), vomiting (children 6%), nausea (adults 3%), heartburn (adults 2%), abdominal pain (adults 2%; children 3%), dyspepsia 2%
Hepatic: Prothrombin time increased (1%)
Renal: BUN increased (4%)
Overdosage/Toxicology Symptoms of overdose include nausea, vomiting, diarrhea, prostration, reversible pancreatitis, hearing loss with or without tinnitus, or vertigo. Treatment includes symptomatic and supportive care. Dialysis not likely to benefit.
Pharmacodynamics/Kinetics
Time to Peak: 2-4 hours
Half-Life Elimination: Clarithromycin: 3-7 hours; 14-OH-clarithromycin: 5-9 hours
Metabolism: Partially hepatic via CYP3A4; converted to 14-OH clarithromycin (active metabolite)
Excretion: Primarily urine
Clearance: Approximates normal GFR
Available Dosage Forms
Granules for oral suspension (Biaxin®): 125 mg/5 mL (50 mL, 100 mL); 250 mg/5 mL (50 mL, 100 mL) [fruit punch flavor]
Tablet (Biaxin®): 250 mg, 500 mg
Tablet, extended release (Biaxin® XL): 500 mg

Dosing

Adults & Elderly:

Usual dose: Oral: 250-500 mg every 12 hours **or** 1000 mg (two 500 mg extended release tablets) once daily for 7-14 days

Upper respiratory tract: Oral: 250-500 mg every 12 hours for 10-14 days

Pharyngitis/tonsillitis: 250 mg every 12 hours for 10 days

Acute maxillary sinusitis: 500 mg every 12 hours **or** 1000 mg (two 500 mg extended release tablets) once daily for 14 days

Lower respiratory tract: Oral: 250-500 mg every 12 hours for 7-14 days

Acute exacerbation of chronic bronchitis due to:

M. catarrhalis and *S. pneumoniae:* 250 mg every 12 hours for 7-14 days**or** 1000 mg (two 500 mg extended release tablets) once daily for 7 days

H. influenzae: 500 mg every 12 hours for 7-14 days or 1000 mg (two 500 mg extended release tablets) for 7 days

H. parainfluenzae: 500 mg every 12 hours for 7 days or 1000 mg (two 500 mg extended release tablets) for 7 days

Pneumonia due to:

C. pneumoniae, M. pneumoniae, and *S. pneumoniae:* 250 mg every 12 hours for 7-14 days **or** 1000 mg (two 500 mg extended release tablets) once daily for 7 days

H. influenzae: 250 mg every 12 hours for 7 days **or** 1000 mg (two 500 mg extended release tablets) once daily for 7 days

Mycobacterial infection (prevention and treatment): Oral: 500 mg twice daily (use with other antimycobacterial drugs, eg, ethambutol, clofazimine, or rifampin)

Pertussis (CDC guidelines): 500 mg twice daily for 7 days

Prophylaxis of bacterial endocarditis: Oral: 500 mg 1 hour prior to procedure

Uncomplicated skin and skin structure: Oral: 250 mg every 12 hours for 7-14 days

Peptic ulcer disease: Eradication of *Helicobacter pylori:* Oral: Dual or triple combination regimen with bismuth subsalicylate, tetracycline, clarithromycin, and an H₂-receptor; or combination of omeprazole and clarithromycin; 500 mg every 8-12 hours for 10-14 days

Pediatrics: Oral:

Children ≥1 months: **Pertussis (CDC guidelines):**15 mg/kg/day divided every 12 hours for 7 days; maximum: 1 g/day

Children ≥6 months: 15 mg/kg/day divided every 12 hours for 10 days

Community-acquired pneumonia, sinusitis, bronchitis, skin infections: 15 mg/kg/day divided every 12 hours for 10 days

Mycobacterial infection (prevention and treatment): 7.5 mg/kg twice daily, up to 500 mg twice daily. **Note:** Safety of clarithromycin for MAC not studied in children <20 months.

Prophylaxis of bacterial endocarditis: 15 mg/kg 1 hour before procedure (maximum dose: 500 mg)

Renal Impairment:

Cl$_{cr}$ <30 mL/minute: Half the normal dose or double the dosing interval.

In combination with ritonavir:

Cl$_{cr}$ 30-60 mL/minute: Reduce dose by 50%.

Cl$_{cr}$ <30 mL/minute: Reduce dose by 75%.

Hepatic Impairment: No dosing adjustment is needed as long as renal function is normal.

Administration

Oral: Clarithromycin may be given with or without meals. Give every 12 hours rather than twice daily to avoid peak and trough variation.

Biaxin® XL: Should be given with food. Do not crush or chew extended release tablet.

Stability

Reconstitution: Reconstituted oral suspension should not be refrigerated because it might gel. Microencapsulated particles of clarithromycin in suspension is stable for 14 days when stored at room temperature.

Storage: Store tablets and granules for oral suspension at controlled room temperature.

Laboratory Monitoring Perform culture and sensitivity studies prior to initiating drug therapy.

Nursing Actions

Physical Assessment: Results of culture/sensitivity tests and patient's allergy history should be assessed prior to therapy. Assess potential for interactions with other pharmacological agents or herbal products patient may be taking (eg, drugs that affect or are affected by CYP3A4 enzyme activity). Assess therapeutic effectiveness (according to purpose for use) and adverse reactions. Teach patient proper use, possible side effects/appropriate interventions, and adverse symptoms to report.

Patient Education: Do not take any new medication during therapy unless approved by prescriber. Take full course of therapy even if feeling better; do not discontinue this medication without consulting prescriber. Tablets or suspension may be taken with or without food or milk. Extended release tablets should be taken with food. Do not crush or chew extended release tablets. Do not refrigerate oral suspension (more palatable at room temperature). Maintain adequate hydration (2-3 L/day of fluids) unless instructed to restrict fluid intake. May cause nausea, heartburn, or abnormal taste (small frequent meals, frequent mouth care, chewing gum or sucking lozenges may help); diarrhea (buttermilk, boiled milk, or yogurt may help); or headache or abdominal cramps (consult prescriber for analgesic). Report rapid heartbeat or palpitations, persistent fever or chills, easy bruising or bleeding, joint pain, severe persistent diarrhea, skin rash, sores in mouth, foul-smelling urine, or respiratory difficulty. **Pregnancy/breast-feeding precautions:** Inform prescriber if you are or intend to become pregnant. Consult prescriber if breast-feeding.

Dietary Considerations May be taken with or without meals; may be taken with milk. Biaxin® XL should be taken with food.

Geriatric Considerations Considered one of the drugs of choice in the outpatient treatment of community-acquired pneumonia in older adults. After doses of 500 mg every 12 hours for 5 days, 12 healthy elderly had significantly increased C$_{max}$ and C$_{min}$, elimination half-lives of clarithromycin and 14-OH clarithromycin compared to 12 healthy young subjects. These changes were attributed to a significant decrease in renal clearance. At a dose of 1000 mg twice daily, 100% of 13 older adults experienced an adverse event compared to only 10% taking 500 mg twice daily.

Breast-Feeding Issues Erythromycins may be taken while breast-feeding. Use caution.

Pregnancy Issues There are no adequate and well-controlled studies in pregnant women. Due to adverse fetal effects reported in animal studies, the manufacturer recommends that clarithromycin not be used in a pregnant woman unless there are no alternatives to therapy.

Clindamycin (klin da MYE sin)

U.S. Brand Names Cleocin®; Cleocin HCl®; Cleocin Pediatric®; Cleocin Phosphate®; Cleocin T®; Clindagel®; ClindaMax™; Clindesse™; Clindets®; Evoclin™

Synonyms Clindamycin Hydrochloride; Clindamycin Palmitate; Clindamycin Phosphate

Pharmacologic Category Antibiotic, Lincosamide

Medication Safety Issues
Sound-alike/look-alike issues:
Cleocin® may be confused with bleomycin, Clinoril®, Lincocin®

Pregnancy Risk Factor B

Lactation Enters breast milk/compatible

Use Treatment against aerobic and anaerobic strepto-cocci (except enterococci), most staphylococci, *Bacteroides* sp and *Actinomyces*; bacterial vaginosis (vaginal cream, vaginal suppository); pelvic inflammatory disease (I.V.); topically in treatment of severe acne; vaginally for *Gardnerella vaginalis*

Unlabeled/Investigational Use May be useful in PCP; alternate treatment for toxoplasmosis

Mechanism of Action/Effect Reversibly binds to 50S ribosomal subunits preventing peptide bond formation thus inhibiting bacterial protein synthesis; bacteriostatic or bactericidal depending on drug concentration, infection site, and organism

Contraindications Hypersensitivity to clindamycin or any component of the formulation; previous pseudo-membranous colitis; regional enteritis, ulcerative colitis

Warnings/Precautions Dosage adjustment may be necessary in patients with severe hepatic dysfunction; can cause severe and possibly fatal colitis; discontinue drug if significant diarrhea, abdominal cramps, or passage of blood and mucus occurs. Vaginal products may weaken latex or rubber condoms, or contraceptive diaphragms. Barrier contraceptives are not recommended concurrently or for 3-5 days (depending on the product) following treatment. Some dosage forms contain benzyl alcohol or tartrazine. Use caution in atopic patients.

Drug Interactions
Increased Effect/Toxicity: Increased duration of neuromuscular blockade when given in conjunction with tubocurarine and pancuronium.

Nutritional/Ethanol Interactions
Food: Peak concentrations may be delayed with food.
Herb/Nutraceutical: St John's wort may decrease clinda-mycin levels.

Adverse Reactions
Systemic:
>10%: Gastrointestinal: Diarrhea, abdominal pain
1% to 10%:
Cardiovascular: Hypotension
Dermatologic: Urticaria, rash, Stevens-Johnson syndrome
Gastrointestinal: Pseudomembranous colitis, nausea, vomiting
Local: Thrombophlebitis, sterile abscess at I.M. injection site
Miscellaneous: Fungal overgrowth, hypersensitivity
Topical:
>10%: Dermatologic: Dryness, burning, itching, scaliness, erythema, or peeling of skin (lotion, solution); oiliness (gel, lotion)
1% to 10%: Central nervous system: Headache
Vaginal:
>10%: Genitourinary: Fungal vaginosis, vaginitis or vulvovaginal pruritus (from *Candida albicans*)
1% to 10%:
Central nervous system: Back pain, headache
Gastrointestinal: Constipation, diarrhea
Genitourinary: Urinary tract infection
Respiratory: Nasopharyngitis
Miscellaneous: Fungal infection

Overdosage/Toxicology Symptoms of overdose include diarrhea, nausea, and vomiting. Treatment is supportive.

Pharmacodynamics/Kinetics
Time to Peak: Serum: Oral: Within 60 minutes; I.M.: 1-3 hours
Half-Life Elimination: Neonates: Premature: 8.7 hours; Full-term: 3.6 hours; Adults: 1.6-5.3 hours (average: 2-3 hours)
Metabolism: Hepatic
Excretion: Urine (10%) and feces (~4%) as active drug and metabolites

Available Dosage Forms Note: Strength is expressed as base
Capsule, as hydrochloride: 150 mg, 300 mg
Cleocin HCl®: 75 mg [contains tartrazine], 150 mg [contains tartrazine], 300 mg
Cream, vaginal, as phosphate:
Cleocin®: 2% (40 g) [contains benzyl alcohol and mineral oil; packaged with 7 disposable applicators]
Clindesse™: 2% (5 g) [contains mineral oil; prefilled single disposable applicator]
Foam, topical, as phosphate (Evoclin™): 1% (50 g, 100 g) [contains ethanol 58%]
Gel, topical, as phosphate: 1% [10 mg/g] (30 g, 60 g)
Cleocin T®: 1% [10 mg/g] (30 g, 60 g)
Clindagel®: 1% [10 mg/g] (40 mL, 75 mL)
ClindaMax™: 1% (30 g, 60 g)
Granules for oral solution, as palmitate (Cleocin Pediatric®): 75 mg/5 mL (100 mL) [cherry flavor]
Infusion, as phosphate [premixed in D₅W] (Cleocin Phosphate®): 300 mg (50 mL); 600 mg (50 mL); 900 mg (50 mL)
Injection, solution, as phosphate (Cleocin Phosphate®): 150 mg/mL (2 mL, 4 mL, 6 mL, 60 mL) [contains benzyl alcohol and disodium edetate 0.5 mg]
Lotion, as phosphate (Cleocin T®, ClindaMax™): 1% [10 mg/mL] (60 mL)
Pledgets, topical: 1% (60s) [contains alcohol]
Cleocin T®: 1% (60s) [contains isopropyl alcohol 50%]
Clindets®: 1% (69s) [contains isopropyl alcohol 52%]
Solution, topical, as phosphate (Cleocin T®): 1% [10 mg/mL] (30 mL, 60 mL) [contains isopropyl alcohol 50%]
Suppository (ovule), vaginal, as phosphate (Cleocin®): 100 mg (3s) [contains oleaginous base; single reusable applicator]

Dosing
Adults & Elderly:
Usual dose:
Oral: 150-450 mg/dose every 6-8 hours; maximum dose: 1.8 g/day
I.M., I.V.: 1.2-1.8 g/day in 2-4 divided doses; maximum dose: 4.8 g/day
Acne: *Topical:*
Gel, pledget, lotion, solution: Apply a thin film twice daily
Foam (Evoclin™): Apply once daily
Amnionitis: *I.V.:* 450-900 mg every 8 hours
Anthrax: *I.V.:* 900 mg every 8 hours with ciprofloxacin or doxycycline
Babesiosis:
Oral: 600 mg 3 times/day for 7 days with quinine
I.V.: 1.2 g twice daily
Bacterial vaginosis: *Intravaginal:*
Suppositories: Insert one ovule (100 mg clinda-mycin) daily into vagina at bedtime for 3 days
Cream:
Cleocin®: One full applicator inserted intravaginally once daily before bedtime for 3 or 7 consecutive days in nonpregnant patients or for 7 consecutive days in pregnant patients
Clindesse™: One full applicator inserted intravaginally as a single dose at anytime during the day in nonpregnant patients
Bite wounds (canine): *Oral:* 300 mg 4 times/day with a fluoroquinolone

Gangrenous myositis: *I.V.:* 900 mg every 8 hours with penicillin G

Group B streptococcus (neonatal prophylaxis): *I.V.:* 900 mg every 8 hours until delivery

Orofacial/parapharyngeal space infections:
Oral: 150-450 mg every 6 hours for at least 7 days; maximum dose: 1.8 g/day
I.V.: 600-900 mg every 8 hours

Pelvic inflammatory disease: *I.V.:* 900 mg every 8 hours with gentamicin 2 mg/kg, then 1.5 mg/kg every 8 hours; continue after discharge with doxycycline 100 mg twice daily to complete 14 days of total therapy

Pneumonia due to *Pneumocystis jiroveci* (unlabeled use):
Oral: 300-450 mg 4 times/day with primaquine
I.M., I.V.: 1200-2400 mg/day with pyrimethamine
I.V.: 600 mg 4 times/day with primaquine

Prevention of bacterial endocarditis (unlabeled use):
Oral: 600 mg 1 hour before procedure with no follow-up dose needed
I.V.: 600 mg within 30 minutes before procedure

Toxic shock syndrome: *I.V.:* 900 mg every 8 hours with penicillin G or ceftriaxone

Toxoplasmosis (unlabeled use): *Oral, I.V.:* 600 mg every 6 hours with pyrimethamine and folinic acid

Pediatrics:

Usual dose:
Oral: Infants and Children: 8-20 mg/kg/day as hydrochloride; 8-25 mg/kg/day as palmitate in 3-4 divided doses; minimum dose of palmitate: 37.5 mg 3 times/day
I.M., I.V.:
<1 month: 15-20 mg/kg/day
>1 month: 20-40 mg/kg/day in 3-4 divided doses

Anthrax: *I.V.:* 7.5 mg/kg every 6 hours

Prevention of bacterial endocarditis (unlabeled use):
Oral: 20 mg/kg 1 hour before procedure with no follow-up dose needed
I.V.: 20 mg/kg within 30 minutes before procedure

Orofacial infections: 8-25 mg/kg in 3-4 equally divided doses

Acne: *Topical:* Children ≥12 years: Refer to adult dosing.

Babesiosis: *Oral:* 20-40 mg/kg divided every 8 hours for 7 days plus quinine

Hepatic Impairment: Systemic use: Adjustment is recommended in patients with severe hepatic disease.

Administration

Oral: Administer oral dosage form with a full glass of water to minimize esophageal ulceration. Give around-the-clock to promote less variation in peak and trough serum levels.

I.M.: Deep I.M. sites, rotate sites. Do not exceed 600 mg in a single injection.

I.V.: Never administer as bolus; administer by I.V. intermittent infusion over at least 10-60 minutes, at a rate **not** to exceed 30 mg/minute (not exceed 1200 mg/hour); final concentration for administration should not exceed 18 mg/mL

I.V. Detail: pH: 6.0-6.3 (usual); 5.5-7.0 (range)

Topical: Foam: Dispense directly into cap or onto a cool surface. Do not dispense directly into hands.

Other:
Intravaginal:
Cream: Insertion should be as far as possible into the vagina without causing discomfort
Ovule: The foil should be removed; if the applicator is used for insertion, it should be washed for additional use

Stability
Compatibility: Stable in D_5LR, $D_5^1/_2NS$, D_5NS, D_5W, $D_{10}W$, LR, NS

Y-site administration: Incompatible with allopurinol, filgrastim, fluconazole, idarubicin

Compatibility in syringe: Incompatible with tobramycin

Compatibility when admixed: Incompatible with aminophylline, barbiturates, calcium gluconate, ceftriaxone, ciprofloxacin, gentamicin with cefazolin, magnesium sulfate, phenytoin

Storage:
Capsule: Store at room temperature of 20°C to 25°C (68°F to 77°F).
Cream: Store at room temperature.
Foam: Store at room temperature of 20°C to 25°C (68°F to 77°F). Avoid fire, flame, or smoking during or following application.
Gel: Store at room temperature.
Clindagel®: Do not store in direct sunlight.
I.V.: Infusion solution in NS or D_5W solution is stable for 16 days at room temperature.
Lotion: Store at room temperature of 20°C to 25°C (68°F to 77°F).
Oral solution: Do not refrigerate reconstituted oral solution (it will thicken). Following reconstitution, oral solution is stable for 2 weeks at room temperature of 20°C to 25°C (68°F to 77°F).
Ovule: Store at room temperature of 15°C to 30°C (68°F to 77°F).
Pledget: Store at room temperature.
Topical solution: Store at room temperature of 20°C to 25°C (68°F to 77°F).

Laboratory Monitoring CBC, liver and renal function periodically with prolonged therapy

Nursing Actions

Physical Assessment: Previous allergy history should be assessed prior to beginning therapy. **I.V.:** Monitor cardiac status and blood pressure and keep patient recumbent after infusion until blood pressure is stabilized. Monitor laboratory tests and patient response according to dose, route of administration, and purpose of therapy. Teach patient proper use, possible side effects/appropriate interventions, and adverse symptoms to report (eg, severe diarrhea, opportunistic infection).

Patient Education:

I.M., I.V.: Report any burning, pain, swelling, or redness at infusion or injection site.

Oral: Take each dose with a full glass of water. Complete full prescription, even if feeling better. You may experience nausea or vomiting (small, frequent meals, frequent mouth care, chewing gum, or sucking lozenges may help). Report dizziness; persistent GI effects (pain, diarrhea, vomiting); skin redness, rash, or burning; fever; chills; unusual bruising or bleeding; signs of infection; excessive fatigue; yellowing of eyes or skin; change in color of urine or blackened stool; swelling, warmth, or pain in extremities; difficult respirations; bloody or fatty stool (do not take antidiarrheal without consulting prescriber); or lack of improvement or worsening of condition.

Topical, foam: Wash hands thoroughly or wear gloves. Do not dispense directly onto hands or face (foam will begin to melt on contact with warm skin). Dispense an amount the will cover the affected area directly into the cap or onto a cool surface. If can seems warm or foam seems runny, run can under cold water. Pick up small amounts of foam with fingertips and gently massage into affected areas until foam disappears. Wash hands thoroughly. Wait 30 minutes before shaving or applying make-up.

Topical gel, lotion, or solution: Wash hands thoroughly before applying or wear gloves. Apply thin film of gel, lotion, or solution to affected area. May apply porous dressing. Wash hands thoroughly. Wait 30 minutes before shaving or applying make-up. Report
(Continued)

Clindamycin *(Continued)*

persistent burning, swelling, itching, excessive dryness, or worsening of condition.

Vaginal: Wash hands before using. At bedtime: If using applicator, gently insert full applicator into vagina and expel cream. Wash applicator with soap and water following use. If using suppository, insert high into vagina. Remain lying down for 30 minutes following administration. Avoid intercourse during therapy. Report adverse reactions (dizziness, nausea, vomiting, stomach cramps, or headache) or lack of improvement or worsening of condition.

Dietary Considerations May be taken with food.

Geriatric Considerations Elderly patients are often at a higher risk for developing serious colitis and require close monitoring.

Related Information
Compatibility of Drugs *on page 1370*

ClomiPHENE (KLOE mi feen)

U.S. Brand Names Clomid®; Serophene®
Synonyms Clomiphene Citrate
Pharmacologic Category Ovulation Stimulator
Medication Safety Issues
Sound-alike/look-alike issues:
ClomiPHENE may be confused with clomiPRAMINE, clonidine
Clomid® may be confused with clonidine
Serophene® may be confused with Sarafem™

Pregnancy Risk Factor X
Lactation Excretion in breast milk unknown/contraindicated
Use Treatment of ovulatory failure in patients desiring pregnancy
Unlabeled/Investigational Use Male infertility
Mechanism of Action/Effect Induces ovulation by stimulating the release of pituitary gonadotropins
Contraindications Hypersensitivity to clomiphene citrate or any of its components; liver disease; abnormal uterine bleeding; enlargement or development of ovarian cyst; uncontrolled thyroid or adrenal dysfunction in the presence of an organic intracranial lesion such as pituitary tumor; pregnancy
Warnings/Precautions Use with caution in patients sensitive to pituitary gonadotropins (eg, polycystic ovary disease). Clomiphene may induce multiple pregnancies, ovarian enlargement, ovarian hyperstimulation syndrome, or abdominal pain, blurring or other visual symptoms.

Drug Interactions
Decreased Effect: Decreased response when used with danazol. Decreased estradiol response when used with clomiphene.
Lab Interactions Clomiphene may increase levels of serum thyroxine and thyroxine-binding globulin (TBG)
Adverse Reactions
>10%: Endocrine & metabolic: Hot flashes, ovarian enlargement
1% to 10%:
Cardiovascular: Thromboembolism
Central nervous system: Mental depression, headache
Endocrine & metabolic: Breast enlargement (males), breast discomfort (females), abnormal menstrual flow
Gastrointestinal: Distention, bloating, nausea, vomiting, hepatotoxicity
Ocular: Blurring of vision, diplopia, floaters, after-images, phosphenes, photophobia

Pharmacodynamics/Kinetics
Half-Life Elimination: 5-7 days

Metabolism: Undergoes enterohepatic recirculation

Excretion: Primarily feces; urine (small amounts)

Available Dosage Forms Tablet, as citrate: 50 mg

Dosing
Adults & Elderly:

Infertility (in males): Oral: 25 mg/day for 25 days with 5 days rest, or 100 mg every Monday, Wednesday, Friday

Ovulatory failure (females): Oral: 50 mg/day for 5 days (first course); start the regimen on or about the fifth day of cycle. The dose should be increased only in those patients who do not ovulate in response to cyclic 50 mg Clomid®. A low dosage or duration of treatment course is particularly recommended if unusual sensitivity to pituitary gonadotropin is suspected, such as in patients with polycystic ovary syndrome.

Repeat dosing; If ovulation does not appear to occur after the first course of therapy, a second course of 100 mg/day (two 50 mg tablets given as a single daily dose) for 5 days should be given. This course may be started as early as 30 days after the previous one after precautions are taken to exclude the presence of pregnancy. Increasing the dosage or duration of therapy beyond 100 mg/day for 5 days is not recommended. The majority of patients who are going to ovulate will do so after the first course of therapy. If ovulation does not occur after 3 courses of therapy, further treatment is not recommended and the patient should be re-evaluated. If 3 ovulatory responses occur, but pregnancy has not been achieved, further treatment is not recommended. If menses does not occur after an ovulatory response, the patient should be re-evaluated. Long-term cyclic therapy is not recommended beyond a total of about 6 cycles.

Stability
Storage: Protect from light.

Laboratory Monitoring Urine estrogens and estriol levels; normal levels indicate appropriateness for clomiphene therapy.

Nursing Actions
Physical Assessment: Monitor laboratory tests, therapeutic effectiveness (according to purpose for use), and adverse response regularly during therapy. Teach patient proper use (eg, measuring basal body temperature and timing intercourse), possible side effects/appropriate interventions, and adverse symptoms to report. **Pregnancy risk factor X**: Determine that patient is not pregnant before beginning treatment. Breast-feeding is contraindicated.

Patient Education: Inform prescriber of all prescriptions, OTC medications, or herbal products you are taking, and any allergies you have. Do not take any new medication during therapy unless approved by prescriber. Follow recommended schedule of dosing exactly. May cause hot flashes (cool clothes and cool environment may help). Report acute sudden headache; respiratory difficulty; warmth, swelling, pain, or redness in calves; breast enlargement (male) or breast discomfort (female); abnormal menstrual bleeding; vision changes (blurring, diplopia, photophobia, floaters); acute abdominal discomfort; or fever. **Breast-feeding precaution:** Do not breast-feed.

Related Information
FDA Name Differentiation Project: The Use of Tall-Man Letters *on page 12*

ClomiPRAMINE (kloe MI pra meen)

U.S. Brand Names Anafranil®

Synonyms Clomipramine Hydrochloride

Restrictions A medication guide concerning the use of antidepressants in children and teenagers can be found on the FDA website at http://www.fda.gov/cder/Offices/ODS/labeling.htm. It should be dispensed to parents or guardians of children and teenagers receiving this medication.

Pharmacologic Category Antidepressant, Tricyclic (Tertiary Amine)

Medication Safety Issues

Sound-alike/look-alike issues:

ClomiPRAMINE may be confused with chlorproMAZINE, clomiPHENE, desipramine, Norpramin®

Anafranil® may be confused with alfentanil, enalapril, nafarelin

Pregnancy Risk Factor C

Lactation Enters breast milk/contraindicated (AAP rates "of concern")

Use Treatment of obsessive-compulsive disorder (OCD)

Unlabeled/Investigational Use Depression, panic attacks, chronic pain

Mechanism of Action/Effect Clomipramine appears to affect serotonin uptake while its active metabolite, desmethylclomipramine, affects norepinephrine uptake

Contraindications Hypersensitivity to clomipramine, other tricyclic agents, or any component of the formulation; use of MAO inhibitors within 14 days; use in a patient during the acute recovery phase of MI

Warnings/Precautions Antidepressants increase the risk of suicidal thinking and behavior in children and adolescents with major depressive disorder (MDD) and other depressive disorders; consider risk prior to prescribing. All patients must be closely monitored for clinical worsening, suicidality, or unusual changes in behavior, especially during the initiation of therapy or following an increase or decrease in dosage. When used in children, the child's family or caregiver should be instructed to closely observe the patient and communicate condition with healthcare provider. A medication guide should be dispensed with each prescription. **Clomipramine is FDA approved for the treatment of OCD in children ≥10 years of age.**

The possibility of a suicide attempt is inherent in major depression and may persist until remission occurs. Use caution in high-risk patients. Worsening depression and severe abrupt suicidality that are not part of the presenting symptoms may require discontinuation or modification of drug therapy. The patient's family or caregiver should be alerted to monitor patients for the emergence of suicidality and associated behaviors (such as agitation, irritability, hostility, impulsivity, and hypomania) and notify the healthcare provider.

May worsen psychosis in some patients or precipitate a shift to mania or hypomania in patients with bipolar disorder. Patients presenting with depressive symptoms should be screened for bipolar disorder. Monotherapy in patients with bipolar disorder should be avoided. **Clomipramine is not FDA approved for bipolar depression.**

May cause seizures (relationship to dose and/or duration of therapy) - do not exceed maximum doses. Use caution in patients with a previous seizure disorder or condition predisposing to seizures such as brain damage, alcoholism, or concurrent therapy with other drugs which lower the seizure threshold. May increase the risks associated with electroconvulsive therapy. Has been associated with a high incidence of sexual dysfunction. Weight gain may occur.

The degree of sedation, anticholinergic effects, and conduction abnormalities are high relative to other antidepressants. Clomipramine often causes drowsiness/sedation, resulting in impaired performance of tasks requiring alertness (eg, operating machinery or driving). Sedative effects may be additive with other CNS depressants and/or ethanol. The risk of orthostasis is moderate-high relative to other antidepressants. Use with caution in patients with a history of cardiovascular disease (including previous MI, stroke, tachycardia, or conduction abnormalities). Use with caution in patients with urinary retention, benign prostatic hyperplasia, narrow-angle glaucoma, xerostomia, visual problems, constipation, or a history of bowel obstruction.

Consider discontinuing, when possible, prior to elective surgery. Therapy should not be abruptly discontinued in patients receiving high doses for prolonged periods. Use with caution in hyperthyroid patients or those receiving thyroid supplementation. Use with caution in patients with hepatic or renal dysfunction and in elderly patients.

Drug Interactions

Cytochrome P450 Effect: Substrate of CYP1A2 (major), 2C19 (major), 2D6 (major), 3A4 (minor); **Inhibits** CYP2D6 (moderate)

Decreased Effect: The levels/effects of clomipramine may be decreased by aminoglutethimide, carbamazepine, phenobarbital, phenytoin, rifampin, and other CYP1A2 or 2C19 inducers. Clomipramine may decrease the levels/effects of CYP2D6 prodrug substrates (eg, codeine, hydrocodone, oxycodone, tramadol). Clomipramine inhibits the antihypertensive response to bethanidine, clonidine, debrisoquin, guanadrel, guanethidine, guanabenz, and guanfacine. Cholestyramine and colestipol may decrease the absorption of clomipramine.

Increased Effect/Toxicity: The levels/effects of clomipramine may be increased by amiodarone, chlorpromazine, ciprofloxacin, delavirdine, fluconazole, fluoxetine, fluvoxamine, gemfibrozil, isoniazid, ketoconazole, miconazole, norfloxacin, ofloxacin, omeprazole, paroxetine, pergolide, quinidine, quinine, ritonavir, rofecoxib, ropinirole, ticlopidine, and other CYP1A2, 2C19, or 2D6 inhibitors. Clomipramine may increase the levels/effects of amphetamines, selected beta-blockers, dextromethorphan, fluoxetine, lidocaine, mirtazapine, nefazodone, paroxetine, risperidone, ritonavir, thioridazine, tricyclic antidepressants, venlafaxine, and other CYP2D6 substrates.

Clomipramine increases the effects of amphetamines, anticholinergics, lithium, other CNS depressants (sedatives, hypnotics, ethanol), chlorpropamide, tolazamide, phenothiazines, and warfarin. When used with MAO inhibitors or other serotonergic drugs, serotonin syndrome may occur. Serotonin syndrome has also been reported with ritonavir (rare). Pressor response to I.V. epinephrine, norepinephrine, and phenylephrine may be enhanced in patients receiving TCAs (**Note:** Effect is unlikely with epinephrine or levonordefrin dosages typically administered as infiltration in combination with local anesthetics). Combined use of beta-agonists or drugs which prolong QT$_c$ (including quinidine, procainamide, disopyramide, cisapride, sparfloxacin, gatifloxacin, moxifloxacin) with TCAs may predispose patients to cardiac arrhythmias.

Nutritional/Ethanol Interactions

Ethanol: Avoid ethanol (may increase CNS depression).

Food: Serum concentrations/toxicity may be increased by grapefruit juice.

Herb/Nutraceutical: Avoid valerian, St John's wort, SAMe, kava kava.

Lab Interactions Increased glucose
(Continued)

ClomiPRAMINE *(Continued)*

Adverse Reactions

>10%:

Central nervous system: Dizziness, drowsiness, headache, insomnia, nervousness

Endocrine & metabolic: Libido changes

Gastrointestinal: Xerostomia, constipation, increased appetite, nausea, weight gain, dyspepsia, anorexia, abdominal pain

Neuromuscular & skeletal: Fatigue, tremor, myoclonus

Miscellaneous: Diaphoresis increased

1% to 10%:

Cardiovascular: Hypotension, palpitation, tachycardia

Central nervous system: Confusion, hypertonia, sleep disorder, yawning, speech disorder, abnormal dreaming, paresthesia, memory impairment, anxiety, twitching, impaired coordination, agitation, migraine, depersonalization, emotional lability, flushing, fever

Dermatologic: Rash, pruritus, dermatitis

Gastrointestinal: Diarrhea, vomiting

Genitourinary: Difficult urination

Ocular: Blurred vision, eye pain

Overdosage/Toxicology
Symptoms of overdose include agitation, confusion, hallucinations, urinary retention, hypothermia, hypotension, tachycardia, ventricular tachycardia, seizures, and coma. Following initiation of essential overdose management, toxic symptoms should be treated.

Pharmacodynamics/Kinetics

Half-Life Elimination: 20-30 hours

Metabolism: Hepatic to desmethylclomipramine (active); extensive first-pass effect

Available Dosage Forms
Capsule, as hydrochloride: 25 mg, 50 mg, 75 mg

Dosing

Adults & Elderly: Treatment of OCD: Oral: Initial: 25 mg/day and gradually increase, as tolerated, to 100 mg/day the first 2 weeks, may then be increased to a total of 250 mg/day maximum

Pediatrics:

Treatment of OCD: Oral: Children >10 years: Initial: 25 mg/day and gradually increase, as tolerated, to a maximum of 3 mg/kg/day or 200 mg/day, whichever is smaller. **Note:** The safety and efficacy of clomipramine in pediatric patients <10 years of age have not been established and, therefore, dosing recommendations cannot be made.

Laboratory Monitoring
Monitor ECG/cardiac status in older adults and patients with cardiac disease

Nursing Actions

Physical Assessment: Assess other medications patient may be taking for effectiveness and interactions. Monitor therapeutic response and adverse reactions at beginning of therapy and periodically with long-term use. Assess mental status, affect, and suicidal tendencies. If history of cardiac problems, monitor cardiac status closely. Be alert to the potential of new or increased seizure activity. Observe for clinical worsening, suicidality, or unusual behavior changes, especially during the initial few months of therapy or during dosage changes. Taper dosage slowly when discontinuing. Assess knowledge/teach patient appropriate use, interventions to reduce side effects, and adverse symptoms to report.

Patient Education: Take multiple dose medication with meals to reduce side effects. Take single daily dose at bedtime to reduce daytime sedation. The effect of this drug may take several weeks to appear. Do not use alcohol, caffeine, and other prescriptive or OTC medications without consulting prescriber. May cause dizziness, drowsiness, headache, or seizures (use caution when driving or engaging in tasks that require alertness until response to drug is known); dry mouth or unpleasant aftertaste (sucking lozenges and frequent mouth care may help); constipation (increased exercise, fluids, fruit, or fiber may help); or orthostatic hypotension (use caution when rising from lying or sitting to standing position or when climbing stairs). Report unresolved constipation or GI upset, unusual muscle weakness, palpitations, or persistent CNS disturbances (hallucinations, suicidality, seizures, delirium, insomnia, or impaired gait). **Pregnancy/breast-feeding precautions:** Inform prescriber if you are or intend to become pregnant. Do not breast-feed.

Geriatric Considerations
Not approved as an antidepressant, clomipramine's anticholinergic and hypotensive effects limit its use versus other preferred antidepressants. Elderly patients were found to have higher dose-normalized plasma concentrations as a result of decreased demethylation (decreased 50%) and hydroxylation (25%).

Breast-Feeding Issues
Generally, it is not recommended to breast-feed if taking antidepressants because of the long half-life, active metabolites, and the potential for side effects in the infant.

Pregnancy Issues
There are no adequate and well-controlled studies in pregnant women. Withdrawal symptoms (including dizziness, nausea, vomiting, headache, malaise, sleep disturbance, hyperthermia, and/or irritability) have been observed in neonates whose mothers took clomipramine up to delivery. Use in pregnancy only if the benefits to the mother outweigh the potential risks to the fetus.

Related Information

Antidepressant Medication Guidelines *on page 1414*

FDA Name Differentiation Project: The Use of Tall-Man Letters *on page 12*

Clonazepam *(kloe NA ze pam)*

U.S. Brand Names
Klonopin®

Restrictions
C-IV

Pharmacologic Category
Benzodiazepine

Medication Safety Issues

Sound-alike/look-alike issues:

Clonazepam may be confused with clofazimine, clonidine, clorazepate, clozapine, lorazepam

Klonopin® may be confused with clofazimine, clonidine, clorazepate, clozapine, lorazepam

Pregnancy Risk Factor
D

Lactation
Enters breast milk/not recommended

Use
Alone or as an adjunct in the treatment of petit mal variant (Lennox-Gastaut), akinetic, and myoclonic seizures; petit mal (absence) seizures unresponsive to succimides; panic disorder with or without agoraphobia

Unlabeled/Investigational Use
Restless legs syndrome; neuralgia; multifocal tic disorder; parkinsonian dysarthria; bipolar disorder; adjunct therapy for schizophrenia

Mechanism of Action/Effect
The exact mechanism is unknown, but believed to be related to its ability to enhance the activity of GABA; suppresses the spike-and-wave discharge in absence seizures by depressing nerve transmission in the motor cortex

Contraindications
Hypersensitivity to clonazepam or any component of the formulation (cross-sensitivity with other benzodiazepines may exist); significant liver disease; narrow-angle glaucoma; pregnancy

Warnings/Precautions
Use with caution in elderly or debilitated patients, patients with hepatic disease (including alcoholics), or renal impairment. Use with caution in patients with respiratory disease or impaired gag reflex or ability to protect the airway from secretions (salivation may be increased). Worsening of seizures may occur when added to patients with multiple seizure types. Concurrent use with valproic acid may result in

absence status. Monitoring of CBC and liver function tests has been recommended during prolonged therapy.

Causes CNS depression (dose related) resulting in sedation, dizziness, confusion, or ataxia which may impair physical and mental capabilities. Use with caution in patients receiving other CNS depressants or ethanol. Benzodiazepines have been associated with falls and traumatic injury and should be used with extreme caution in patients who are at risk of these events (especially the elderly).

Use caution in patients with depression, particularly if suicidal risk may be present. Use with caution in patients with a history of drug dependence. Benzodiazepines have been associated with dependence and acute withdrawal symptoms, including seizures, on discontinuation or reduction in dose.

Benzodiazepines have been associated with anterograde amnesia. Paradoxical reactions, including hyperactive or aggressive behavior, have been reported with benzodiazepines, particularly in adolescent/pediatric or psychiatric patients. Does not have analgesic, antidepressant, or antipsychotic properties.

Drug Interactions
Cytochrome P450 Effect: Substrate of CYP3A4 (major)

Decreased Effect: The combined use of clonazepam and valproic acid has been associated with absence seizures. CYP3A4 inducers may decrease the levels/effects of clonazepam; example inducers include aminoglutethimide, carbamazepine, nafcillin, nevirapine, phenobarbital, phenytoin, and rifamycins.

Increased Effect/Toxicity: Combined use of clonazepam and valproic acid has been associated with absence seizures. Clonazepam potentiates the CNS depressant effects of narcotic analgesics, barbiturates, phenothiazines, ethanol, antihistamines, MAO inhibitors, sedative-hypnotics, and cyclic antidepressants. CYP3A4 inhibitors may increase the levels/effects of clonazepam; example inhibitors include azole antifungals, clarithromycin, diclofenac, doxycycline, erythromycin, imatinib, isoniazid, nefazodone, nicardipine, propofol, protease inhibitors, quinidine, telithromycin, and verapamil.

Nutritional/Ethanol Interactions
Ethanol: Avoid ethanol (may increase CNS depression).

Food: Clonazepam serum concentration is unlikely to be increased by grapefruit juice because of clonazepam's high oral bioavailability.

Herb/Nutraceutical: St John's wort may decrease clonazepam levels. Avoid valerian, St John's wort, kava kava, gotu kola (may increase CNS depression).

Adverse Reactions Reactions reported in patients with seizure and/or panic disorder. Frequency not defined.

Cardiovascular: Edema (ankle or facial), palpitation

Central nervous system: Amnesia, ataxia (seizure disorder ~30%; panic disorder 5%), behavior problems (seizure disorder ~25%), coma, confusion, depression, dizziness, drowsiness (seizure disorder ~50%), emotional lability, fatigue, fever, hallucinations, headache, hypotonia, hysteria, insomnia, intellectual ability reduced, memory disturbance, nervousness; paradoxical reactions (including aggressive behavior, agitation, anxiety, excitability, hostility, irritability, nervousness, nightmares, sleep disturbance, vivid dreams); psychosis, slurred speech, somnolence (panic disorder 37%), suicidal attempt, vertigo

Dermatologic: Hair loss, hirsutism, skin rash

Endocrine & metabolic: Dysmenorrhea, libido increased/decreased

Gastrointestinal: Abdominal pain, anorexia, appetite increased/decreased, coated tongue, constipation, dehydration, diarrhea, gastritis, gum soreness, nausea, weight changes (loss/gain), xerostomia

Genitourinary: Colpitis, dysuria, ejaculation delayed, enuresis, impotence, micturition frequency, nocturia, urinary retention, urinary tract infection

Hematologic: Anemia, eosinophilia, leukopenia, thrombocytopenia

Hepatic: Alkaline phosphatase increased (transient), hepatomegaly, serum transaminases increased (transient)

Neuromuscular & skeletal: Choreiform movements, coordination abnormal, dysarthria, muscle pain, muscle weakness, myalgia, tremor

Ocular: Blurred vision, eye movements abnormal, diplopia, nystagmus

Respiratory: Chest congestion, cough, bronchitis, hypersecretions, pharyngitis, respiratory depression, respiratory tract infection, rhinitis, rhinorrhea, shortness of breath, sinusitis

Miscellaneous: Allergic reaction, aphonia, dysdiadochokinesis, encopresis, "glassy-eyed" appearance, hemiparesis, lymphadenopathy

Overdosage/Toxicology May produce somnolence, confusion, ataxia, diminished reflexes, or coma. Treatment for benzodiazepine overdose is supportive. Flumazenil has been shown to selectively block the binding of benzodiazepines to CNS receptors, resulting in a reversal of benzodiazepine-induced CNS depression, but not respiratory depression.

Pharmacodynamics/Kinetics
Onset of Action: 20-60 minutes

Duration of Action: Infants and young children: 6-8 hours; Adults: ≤12 hours

Time to Peak: Serum: 1-3 hours; Steady-state: 5-7 days

Protein Binding: 85%

Half-Life Elimination: Children: 22-33 hours; Adults: 19-50 hours

Metabolism: Extensively hepatic via glucuronide and sulfate conjugation

Excretion: Urine (<2% as unchanged drug); metabolites excreted as glucuronide or sulfate conjugates

Available Dosage Forms
Tablet: 0.5 mg, 1 mg, 2 mg

Tablet, orally disintegrating [wafer]: 0.125 mg, 0.25 mg, 0.5 mg, 1 mg, 2 mg

Dosing
Adults:

Seizure disorders: Oral:
Initial daily dose not to exceed 1.5 mg given in 3 divided doses; may increase by 0.5-1 mg every third day until seizures are controlled or adverse effects seen (maximum: 20 mg/day)

Usual maintenance dose: 0.05-0.2 mg/kg; do not exceed 20 mg/day

Panic disorder: Oral: 0.25 mg twice daily; increase in increments of 0.125-0.25 mg twice daily every 3 days; target dose: 1 mg/day (maximum: 4 mg/day)

Discontinuation of treatment: To discontinue, treatment should be withdrawn gradually. Decrease dose by 0.125 mg twice daily every 3 days until medication is completely withdrawn.

Elderly: Refer to adult dosing. Initiate with low doses and observe closely.

Pediatrics:

Seizure disorders (see Use): Oral:
Children <10 years or 30 kg:
Initial daily dose: 0.01-0.03 mg/kg/day (maximum: 0.05 mg/kg/day) given in 2-3 divided doses; increase by no more than 0.5 mg every third day until seizures are controlled or adverse effects seen.

Usual maintenance dose: 0.1-0.2 mg/kg/day divided 3 times/day; not to exceed 0.2 mg/kg/day.

Children >10 years or 30 kg: Refer to adult dosing.

Renal Impairment: Hemodialysis: Supplemental dose is not necessary.
(Continued)

Clonazepam *(Continued)*

Administration

Oral: Orally-disintegrating tablet: Open pouch and peel back foil on the blister; do not push tablet through foil. Use dry hands to remove tablet and place in mouth. May be swallowed with or without water. Use immediately after removing from package.

Laboratory Monitoring Renal function

Nursing Actions

Physical Assessment: Assess effectiveness and interactions of other medications patient may be taking. Assess for signs of CNS depression (sedation, dizziness, confusion, or ataxia). Assess for history of addiction; long-term use can result in dependence, abuse, or tolerance; periodically evaluate need for continued use. For inpatient use, institute safety measures and monitor effectiveness and adverse reactions. For outpatients, monitor therapeutic effectiveness and adverse reactions at beginning of therapy and periodically with long-term use. Taper dosage slowly when discontinuing. Assess knowledge/teach patient seizure precautions (if administered for seizures), appropriate use, interventions to reduce side effects, and adverse symptoms to report.

Patient Education: Take exactly as directed; do not increase dose or frequency. Drug may cause physical and/or psychological dependence. While using this medication, do not use alcohol and other prescription or OTC medications (especially pain medications, sedatives, antihistamines, or hypnotics) without consulting prescriber. Maintain adequate hydration (2-3 L/day of fluids) unless instructed to restrict fluid intake. You may experience drowsiness, dizziness, or blurred vision (use caution when driving or engaging in tasks requiring alertness until response to drug is known); nausea, vomiting, loss of appetite, or dry mouth (small frequent meals, frequent mouth care, chewing gum, or sucking lozenges may help); or constipation (increased exercise, fluids, fruit, or fiber may help). If medication is used to control seizures, wear identification that you are taking an antiepileptic medication. Report excessive drowsiness, dizziness, fatigue, or impaired coordination; CNS changes (confusion, depression, increased sedation, excitation, headache, agitation, insomnia, or nightmares) or changes in cognition; respiratory difficulty or shortness of breath; changes in urinary pattern, changes in sexual activity; muscle cramping, weakness, tremors, or rigidity; ringing in ears or visual disturbances; excessive perspiration, or excessive GI symptoms (cramping, constipation, vomiting, anorexia); worsening of seizure activity, or loss of seizure control. **Pregnancy/breast-feeding precautions:** Inform prescriber if you are or intend to become pregnant. Breast-feeding is not recommended.

Geriatric Considerations Hepatic clearance may be decreased allowing accumulation of active drug. Also, metabolites of clonazepam are renally excreted and may accumulate in the elderly as renal function declines with age. Observe for signs of CNS and pulmonary toxicity.

Breast-Feeding Issues Clonazepam enters breast milk; clinical effects on the infant include CNS depression, respiratory depression reported (no recommendation from the AAP).

Pregnancy Issues Benzodiazepines cross the placenta. The association between benzodiazepine exposure and malformations remains controversial. A number of types of malformation have been reported (oral cleft, inguinal hernia, cardiac defects, spina bifida, dysmorphic facial features, skeletal defects); however, confounding factors make a clear association difficult. Overall, the risk to the fetus may be low. Nonteratogenic effects (including neonatal flaccidity, respiratory and feeding problems, and withdrawal symptoms) during the postnatal period have also been reported with benzodiazepine use.

Additional Information Ethosuximide or valproic acid may be preferred for treatment of absence (petit mal) seizures. Clonazepam-induced behavioral disturbances may be more frequent in mentally handicapped patients. Abrupt discontinuation after sustained use (generally >10 days) may cause withdrawal symptoms. Flumazenil, a competitive benzodiazepine antagonist at the CNS receptor site, reverses benzodiazepine-induced CNS depression.

Related Information
Anxiolytic / Hypnotic Use in Long-Term Care Facilities *on page 1418*

Clonidine (KLON i deen)

U.S. Brand Names Catapres®; Catapres-TTS®; Duraclon™

Synonyms Clonidine Hydrochloride

Pharmacologic Category Alpha$_2$-Adrenergic Agonist

Medication Safety Issues
Sound-alike/look-alike issues:
Clonidine may be confused with Clomid®, clomiPHENE, clonazepam, clozapine, Klonopin™, Loniten®, quinidine
Catapres® may be confused with Cataflam®, Cetapred®, Combipres®

Transdermal patch may contain conducting metal (eg, aluminum); remove patch prior to MRI.

Pregnancy Risk Factor C

Lactation Enters breast milk/not recommended

Use Management of mild-to-moderate hypertension; either used alone or in combination with other antihypertensives

Orphan drug: Duraclon™: For continuous epidural administration as adjunctive therapy with intraspinal opiates for treatment of cancer pain in patients tolerant to or unresponsive to intraspinal opiates

Unlabeled/Investigational Use Heroin or nicotine withdrawal; severe pain; dysmenorrhea; vasomotor symptoms associated with menopause; ethanol dependence; prophylaxis of migraines; glaucoma; diabetes-associated diarrhea; impulse control disorder, attention-deficit/hyperactivity disorder (ADHD), clozapine-induced sialorrhea

Mechanism of Action/Effect Stimulates alpha$_2$-adrenoceptors in the brain stem, thus activating an inhibitory neuron, resulting in reduced sympathetic outflow from the CNS, producing a decrease in peripheral resistance, renal vascular resistance, heart rate, and blood pressure; epidural clonidine may produce pain relief at spinal presynaptic and postjunctional alpha$_2$-adrenoceptors by preventing pain signal transmission; pain relief occurs only for the body regions innervated by the spinal segments where analgesic concentrations of clonidine exist

Contraindications Hypersensitivity to clonidine hydrochloride or any component of the formulation

Warnings/Precautions Gradual withdrawal is needed (over 1 week for oral, 2-4 days with epidural) if drug needs to be stopped. Patients should be instructed about abrupt discontinuation (causes rapid increase in BP and symptoms of sympathetic overactivity). In patients on both a beta-blocker and clonidine where withdrawal of clonidine is necessary, withdraw the beta-blocker first and several days before clonidine. Then slowly decrease clonidine.

Use with caution in patients with severe coronary insufficiency; conduction disturbances; recent MI, CVA, or chronic renal insufficiency. Caution in sinus node dysfunction. Discontinue within 4 hours of surgery then restart as soon as possible after. Clonidine injection should be administered via a continuous epidural infusion device. Epidural clonidine is not recommended for perioperative, obstetrical, or postpartum pain. It is not recommended for use in patients with severe cardiovascular disease or hemodynamic instability. In all cases, the epidural may lead to cardiovascular instability (hypotension, bradycardia). Transdermal patch may contain conducting metal (eg, aluminum); remove patch prior to MRI. Due to the potential for altered electrical conductivity, remove transdermal patch before cardioversion or defibrillation. Clonidine cause significant CNS depression and xerostomia. Caution in patients with pre-existing CNS disease or depression. Elderly may be at greater risk for CNS depressive effects, favoring other agents in this population.

Drug Interactions

Decreased Effect: Tricyclic antidepressants (TCAs) antagonize the hypotensive effects of clonidine.

Increased Effect/Toxicity: Concurrent use with antipsychotics (especially low potency), narcotic analgesics, or nitroprusside may produce additive hypotensive effects. Clonidine may decrease the symptoms of hypoglycemia with oral hypoglycemic agents or insulin. Alcohol, barbiturates, and other CNS depressants may have additive CNS effects when combined with clonidine. Epidural clonidine may prolong the sensory and motor blockade of local anesthetics. Clonidine may increase cyclosporine (and perhaps tacrolimus) serum concentrations. Beta-blockers may potentiate bradycardia in patients receiving clonidine and may increase the rebound hypertension of withdrawal. Tricyclic antidepressants may also enhance the hypertensive response associated with abrupt clonidine withdrawal.

Nutritional/Ethanol Interactions

Ethanol: Avoid ethanol (may increase CNS depression).

Herb/Nutraceutical: Avoid dong quai if using for hypertension (has estrogenic activity). Avoid ephedra, yohimbe, ginseng (may worsen hypertension). Avoid valerian, St John's wort, kava kava, gotu kola (may increase CNS depression).

Lab Interactions Increased sodium (S), transient serum glucose; decreased catecholamines (U); positive Coombs'

Adverse Reactions Incidence of adverse events is not always reported.

>10%:

Central nervous system: Drowsiness (35% oral, 12% transdermal), dizziness (16% oral, 2% transdermal)

Dermatologic: Transient localized skin reactions characterized by pruritus, and erythema (15% to 50% transdermal)

Gastrointestinal: Dry mouth (40% oral, 25% transdermal)

1% to 10%:

Cardiovascular: Orthostatic hypotension (3% oral)

Central nervous system: Headache (1% oral, 5% transdermal), sedation (3% transdermal), fatigue (6% transdermal), lethargy (3% transdermal), insomnia (2% transdermal), nervousness (3% oral, 1% transdermal), mental depression (1% oral)

Dermatologic: Rash (1% oral), allergic contact sensitivity (5% transdermal), localized vesiculation (7%), hyperpigmentation (5% at application site), edema (3%), excoriation (3%), burning (3%), throbbing, blanching (1%), papules (1%), and generalized macular rash (1%) has occurred in patients receiving transdermal clonidine.

Endocrine & metabolic: Sodium and water retention, sexual dysfunction (3% oral, 2% transdermal), impotence (3% oral, 2% transdermal), weakness (10% transdermal)

Gastrointestinal: Nausea (5% oral, 1% transdermal), vomiting (5% oral), anorexia and malaise (1% oral), constipation (10% oral, 1% transdermal), dry throat (2% transdermal), taste disturbance (1% transdermal), weight gain (1% oral)

Genitourinary: Nocturia (1% oral)

Hepatic: Liver function test (mild abnormalities, 1% oral)

Miscellaneous: Withdrawal syndrome (1% oral)

Overdosage/Toxicology Symptoms of overdose include bradycardia, CNS depression, hypothermia, diarrhea, respiratory depression, and apnea. Treatment is supportive and symptomatic. Naloxone may be utilized in treating CNS depression and/or apnea and should be given I.V., 0.4-2 mg, with repeated doses as needed up to a total of 10 mg, or as an infusion.

Pharmacodynamics/Kinetics

Onset of Action: Oral: 0.5-1 hour; Transdermal: Initial application: 2-3 days

Duration of Action: 6-10 hours

Time to Peak: 2-4 hours

Protein Binding: 20% to 40%

Half-Life Elimination: Adults: Normal renal function: 6-20 hours; Renal impairment: 18-41 hours

Metabolism: Extensively hepatic to inactive metabolites; undergoes enterohepatic recirculation

Excretion: Urine (65%, 32% as unchanged drug); feces (22%)

Available Dosage Forms

Injection, epidural solution, as hydrochloride [preservative free] (Duraclon™): 100 mcg/mL (10 mL); 500 mcg/mL (10 mL)

Patch, transdermal [once-weekly patch]:
Catapres-TTS®-1: 0.1 mg/24 hours (4s)
Catapres-TTS®-2: 0.2 mg/24 hours (4s)
Catapres-TTS®-3: 0.3 mg/24 hours (4s)

Tablet, as hydrochloride (Catapres®): 0.1 mg, 0.2 mg, 0.3 mg

Dosing

Adults:

Acute hypertension (urgency): Oral: Initial 0.1-0.2 mg; may be followed by additional doses of 0.1 mg every hour, if necessary, to a maximum total dose of 0.6 mg

Unlabeled route of administration: Sublingual clonidine 0.1-0.2 mg twice daily may be effective in patients unable to take oral medication

Hypertension:

Oral: Initial dose: 0.1 mg twice daily (maximum recommended dose: 2.4 mg/day); usual dose range (JNC 7): 0.1-0.8 mg/day in 2 divided doses

Transdermal: Apply once every 7 days; for initial therapy start with 0.1 mg and increase by 0.1 mg at 1- to 2-week intervals (dosages >0.6 mg do not improve efficacy); usual dose range (JNC 7): 0.1-0.3 mg once weekly

Note: If transitioning from oral to transdermal, overlap oral for 1-2 days. Transdermal route takes 2-3 days to achieve therapeutic effects.

Conversion from oral to transdermal:
Day 1: Place Catapres-TTS® 1; administer 100% of oral dose.
Day 2: Administer 50% of oral dose.
Day 3: Administer 25% of oral dose.
Day 4: Patch remains, no further oral supplement necessary.

Nicotine withdrawal symptoms: 0.1 mg twice daily to maximum of 0.4 mg/day for 3-4 weeks

Pain management: Epidural infusion: Starting dose: 30 mcg/hour; titrate as required for relief of pain or presence of side effects; minimal experience with doses >40 mcg/hour; should be considered an adjunct to intraspinal opiate therapy

Elderly: Oral: Initial: 0.1 mg once daily at bedtime, increase gradually as needed.

Pediatrics:

Hypertension: Oral: Initial: 5-10 mcg/kg/day in divided doses every 8-12 hours; increase gradually

(Continued)

Clonidine *(Continued)*

at 5- to 7-day intervals to 25 mcg/kg/day in divided doses every 6 hours; maximum: 0.9 mg/day.

Clonidine tolerance test (growth hormone release from pituitary): Oral: 0.15 mg/m^2 or 4 mcg/kg as single dose

ADHD (unlabeled use): Oral: Initial: 0.05 mg/day, increase every 3-7 days by 0.05 mg/day to 3-5 mcg/kg/day given in divided doses 3-4 times/day; maximum dose: 0.3-0.4 mg/day

Pain management: Epidural infusion: Reserved for patients with severe intractable pain, unresponsive to other analgesics or epidural or spinal opiates: Initial: 0.5 mcg/kg/hour; adjust with caution, based on clinical effect

Renal Impairment:
Cl$_{cr}$ <10 mL/minute: Administer 50% to 75% of normal dose initially.

Not dialyzable (0% to 5%) via hemo- or peritoneal dialysis; supplemental dose is not necessary.

Administration

Oral: Do not discontinue clonidine abruptly. if needed, gradually reduce dose over 2-4 days to avoid rebound hypertension.

I.V. Detail: pH: 5-7

Topical: Transdermal patches should be applied weekly at bedtime to a clean, hairless area of the upper outer arm or chest. Rotate patch sites weekly. Redness under patch may be reduced if a topical corticosteroid spray is applied to the area before placement of the patch.

Laboratory Monitoring Liver function tests

Nursing Actions

Physical Assessment: Assess potential for interactions with other pharmacological agents or herbal products patient may be taking (eg, potential for additive hypotension, bradycardia, CNS depression). Monitor results of laboratory tests, therapeutic effectiveness (according to purpose for use), and adverse response regularly during therapy. Advise patients using oral hypoglycemic agents or insulin to check glucose levels closely; clonidine may decrease the symptoms of hypoglycemia. When discontinuing, blood pressure should be monitored and dose tapered slowly over 1 week or more. Teach patient proper use (eg, do not discontinue abruptly), side effects/appropriate interventions, and adverse symptoms to report.

Patient Education: Do not take anything new (especially cough or cold remedies and sleep or stay-awake medications that might affect blood pressure) during treatment unless approved by prescriber. Take as directed, at bedtime. If using patch, check daily for correct placement. Do not skip doses or discontinue this medication without consulting prescriber (this drug must be discontinued on a specific schedule to prevent serious adverse effects). Follow dietary restrictions as recommended by prescriber. This medication may cause drowsiness, dizziness, or impaired judgment (use caution when driving or engaging in tasks that require alertness until response is known); decreased libido or sexual function (will resolve when drug is discontinued); postural hypotension (use caution when rising from sitting or lying position or when climbing stairs); constipation (increase roughage, bulk in diet); or dry mouth or nausea (frequent mouth care or sucking lozenges may help). Report difficulty, pain, or burning on urination; increased nervousness or depression; sudden weight gain (weigh yourself in the same clothes at the same time of day once a week); unusual or persistent swelling of ankles, feet, or extremities; wet cough or respiratory difficulty; chest pain or palpitations; muscle weakness, fatigue, or pain; or other persistent side effects. **Pregnancy/breast-feeding precautions:**

Inform prescriber if you are or intend to become pregnant. Breast-feeding is not recommended.

Dietary Considerations Hypertensive patients may need to decrease sodium and calories in diet.

Geriatric Considerations Because of its potential CNS adverse effects, clonidine may not be considered a drug of choice in the elderly. If the decision is to use clonidine, adjust dose based on response and adverse reactions.

Breast-Feeding Issues Enters breast milk; AAP has NO RECOMMENDATION.

Pregnancy Issues Clonidine crosses the placenta. Caution should be used with this drug due to the potential of rebound hypertension with abrupt discontinuation.

Additional Information Transdermal clonidine should only be used in patients unable to take oral medication. The transdermal product is much more expensive than oral clonidine and produces no better therapeutic effects.

Clonidine and Chlorthalidone
(KLON i deen & klor THAL i done)

U.S. Brand Names Clorpres®; Combipres® [DSC]
Synonyms Chlorthalidone and Clonidine
Pharmacologic Category Antihypertensive Agent, Combination
Pregnancy Risk Factor C
Lactation
Clonidine: Enters breast milk/not recommended
Chlorthalidone: Enters breast milk/compatible
Use Management of mild-to-moderate hypertension
Available Dosage Forms Tablet:
0.1: Clonidine hydrochloride 0.1 mg and chlorthalidone 15 mg
0.2: Clonidine hydrochloride 0.2 mg and chlorthalidone 15 mg
0.3: Clonidine hydrochloride 0.3 mg and chlorthalidone 15 mg

Dosing
Adults: Hypertension: Oral: 1 tablet 1-2 times/day
Elderly: May benefit from lower initial dose; see individual agents.

Nursing Actions
Physical Assessment: See individual agents.
Patient Education: See individual agents. **Pregnancy/breast-feeding precautions:** Inform prescriber if you are or intend to become pregnant. Breast-feeding is not recommended.

Related Information
Chlorthalidone *on page 255*
Clonidine *on page 286*

Clopidogrel (kloh PID oh grel)

U.S. Brand Names Plavix®
Synonyms Clopidogrel Bisulfate
Pharmacologic Category Antiplatelet Agent
Medication Safety Issues
Sound-alike/look-alike issues:
Plavix® may be confused with Elavil®, Paxil®
Pregnancy Risk Factor B
Lactation Excretion in breast milk unknown/not recommended
Use Reduce atherosclerotic events (myocardial infarction, stroke, vascular deaths) in patients with atherosclerosis documented by recent myocardial infarction (MI), recent stroke, or established peripheral arterial disease; acute coronary syndrome (unstable angina or non-Q-wave MI) managed medically or through PCI (with or without stent)

Unlabeled/Investigational Use In aspirin-allergic patients, prevention of coronary artery bypass graft closure (saphenous vein)

Mechanism of Action/Effect Blocks the ADP receptors, which prevent fibrinogen binding at that site and thereby reduce the possibility of platelet adhesion and aggregation.

Contraindications Hypersensitivity to clopidogrel or any component of the formulation; active pathological bleeding such as PUD or intracranial hemorrhage; coagulation disorders

Warnings/Precautions Use with caution in patients who may be at risk of increased bleeding, including patients with peptic ulcer disease, trauma, or surgery. Consider discontinuing 5 days before elective surgery. Use caution in concurrent treatment with other antiplatelet drugs; bleeding risk is increased. Use with caution in patients with severe liver disease (experience is limited). Cases of thrombotic thrombocytopenic purpura (usually occurring within the first 2 weeks of therapy) have been reported; urgent referral to a hematologist is required.

Drug Interactions

Cytochrome P450 Effect: Substrate (minor) of CYP1A2, 3A4; **Inhibits** CYP2C8/9 (weak)

Decreased Effect: Atorvastatin may attenuate the effects of clopidogrel; monitor. CYP3A4-inhibiting macrolide antibiotics may attenuate the effects of clopidogrel (including clarithromycin, erythromycin, and troleandomycin); monitor.

Increased Effect/Toxicity: At high concentrations, clopidogrel may interfere with the metabolism of amiodarone, cisapride, cyclosporine, diltiazem, fluvastatin, irbesartan, losartan, oral hypoglycemics, paclitaxel, phenytoin, quinidine, sildenafil, tamoxifen, torsemide, verapamil, and some NSAIDs which may result in toxicity. Clopidogrel and naproxen resulted in an increase of GI occult blood loss. Anticoagulants (warfarin, thrombolytics, drotrecogin alfa) or other antiplatelet agents may increase the risk of bleeding. Rifampin may increase the effects of clopidogrel (monitor).

Nutritional/Ethanol Interactions Herb/Nutraceutical: Avoid cat's claw, dong quai, evening primrose, feverfew, garlic, ginger, ginkgo, red clover, horse chestnut, green tea, ginseng (all have additional antiplatelet activity).

Adverse Reactions As with all drugs which may affect hemostasis, bleeding is associated with clopidogrel. Hemorrhage may occur at virtually any site. Risk is dependent on multiple variables, including the concurrent use of multiple agents which alter hemostasis and patient susceptibility.

>10%: Gastrointestinal: The overall incidence of gastrointestinal events (including abdominal pain, vomiting, dyspepsia, gastritis and constipation) has been documented to be 27% compared to 30% in patients receiving aspirin.

3% to 10%:
Cardiovascular: Chest pain (8%), edema (4%), hypertension (4%)
Central nervous system: Headache (3% to 8%), dizziness (2% to 6%), depression (4%), fatigue (3%), general pain (6%)
Dermatologic: Rash (4%), pruritus (3%)
Endocrine & metabolic: Hypercholesterolemia (4%)
Gastrointestinal: Abdominal pain (2% to 6%), dyspepsia (2% to 5%), diarrhea (2% to 5%), nausea (3%)
Genitourinary: Urinary tract infection (3%)
Hematologic: Bleeding (major 4%; minor 5%), purpura (5%), epistaxis (3%)
Hepatic: Liver function test abnormalities (<3%; discontinued in 0.11%)
Neuromuscular & skeletal: Arthralgia (6%), back pain (6%)

Respiratory: Dyspnea (5%), rhinitis (4%), bronchitis (4%), cough (3%), upper respiratory infection (9%)
Miscellaneous: Flu-like syndrome (8%)
1% to 3%:
Cardiovascular: Atrial fibrillation, cardiac failure, palpitation, syncope
Central nervous system: Fever, insomnia, vertigo, anxiety
Dermatologic: Eczema
Endocrine & metabolic: Gout, hyperuricemia
Gastrointestinal: Constipation, GI hemorrhage, vomiting
Genitourinary: Cystitis
Hematologic: Hematoma, anemia
Neuromuscular & skeletal: Arthritis, leg cramps, neuralgia, paresthesia, weakness
Ocular: Cataract, conjunctivitis

Overdosage/Toxicology

Symptoms of acute toxicity include vomiting, prostration, difficulty breathing, and gastrointestinal hemorrhage. Only one case of overdose with clopidogrel has been reported to date, no symptoms were reported with this case and no specific treatments were required.

Based on its pharmacology, platelet transfusions may be an appropriate treatment when attempting to reverse the effects of clopidogrel. After decontamination, treatment is symptomatic and supportive.

Pharmacodynamics/Kinetics

Onset of Action: Inhibition of platelet aggregation detected: 2 hours after 300 mg administered; after second day of treatment with 50-100 mg/day
Peak effect: 50-100 mg/day: Bleeding time: 5-6 days; Platelet function: 3-7 days

Time to Peak: Serum: ~1 hour

Half-Life Elimination: ~8 hours

Metabolism: Extensively hepatic via hydrolysis; biotransformation primarily to carboxyl acid derivative (inactive). The active metabolite that inhibits platelet aggregation has not been isolated.

Excretion: Urine

Available Dosage Forms Tablet: 75 mg

Dosing

Adults & Elderly:

Recent MI, recent stroke, or established arterial disease: Oral: 75 mg once daily

Acute coronary syndrome: Oral: Initial: 300 mg loading dose, followed by 75 mg once daily (in combination with aspirin 75-325 mg once daily).
Note: A loading dose of 600 mg has been used in some investigations; limited research exists comparing the two doses.

Prevention of coronary artery bypass graft closure (saphenous vein): Aspirin-allergic patients (unlabeled use): Oral: Loading dose: 300 mg 6 hours following procedure; maintenance: 50-100 mg/day

Renal Impairment: No adjustment is necessary.

Hepatic Impairment: Dose adjustment may be necessary for patients with moderate to severe hepatic disease.

Stability

Storage: Store at 25°C (77°F); excursions permitted to 15°C to 3°C (59°F to 86°F).

Laboratory Monitoring Hemoglobin and hematocrit periodically

Nursing Actions

Physical Assessment: Assess effectiveness or interactions of other medications patient may be taking. Monitor for unusual bleeding. Monitor therapeutic effectiveness and instruct patient what symptoms to report.

Patient Education: Take as directed. May cause headache or dizziness; use caution when driving or engaging in tasks that require alertness until response to drug is known. It may take longer than usual to stop bleeding. Small frequent meals, frequent mouth care, (Continued)

Clopidogrel (Continued)

sucking lozenges, or chewing gum may reduce nausea or vomiting. Mild analgesics may reduce arthralgia or back pain. Inform physicians and dentists that you are taking this medication prior to scheduling any surgery or dental procedure. Report immediately unusual or acute chest pain or respiratory difficulties; skin rash; unresolved bleeding, diarrhea, or GI distress; nosebleed; or acute headache. **Breast-feeding precaution:** Breast-feeding is not recommended.

Dietary Considerations May be taken without regard to meals.

Geriatric Considerations Plasma levels of the primary clopidogrel metabolite were significantly higher in the elderly (≥75 years). This was not associated with changes in bleeding time or platelet aggregation. No dosage adjustment is recommended.

Clorazepate (klor AZ e pate)

U.S. Brand Names Tranxene® SD™; Tranxene® SD™-Half Strength; Tranxene® T-Tab®

Synonyms Clorazepate Dipotassium; Tranxene T-Tab®

Restrictions C-IV

Pharmacologic Category Benzodiazepine

Medication Safety Issues

Sound-alike/look-alike issues:
Clorazepate may be confused with clofibrate, clonazepam

Pregnancy Risk Factor D

Lactation Excretion in breast milk unknown/not recommended

Use Treatment of generalized anxiety disorder; management of ethanol withdrawal; adjunct anticonvulsant in management of partial seizures

Mechanism of Action/Effect Binds to stereospecific benzodiazepine receptors on the postsynaptic GABA neuron at several sites within the central nervous system, including the limbic system, reticular formation. Enhancement of the inhibitory effect of GABA on neuronal excitability results by increased neuronal membrane permeability to chloride ions. This shift in chloride ions results in hyperpolarization (a less excitable state) and stabilization.

Contraindications Hypersensitivity to clorazepate or any component of the formulation (cross-sensitivity with other benzodiazepines may exist); narrow-angle glaucoma; pregnancy

Warnings/Precautions Causes CNS depression (dose related) which may impair physical and mental capabilities. Use with caution in patients receiving other CNS depressants or psychoactive agents. Benzodiazepines have been associated with falls and traumatic injury and should be used with extreme caution in patients who are at risk of these events (especially the elderly). May cause physical or psychological dependence - use with caution in patients with a history of drug dependence.

Active metabolites with extended half-lives may lead to delayed accumulation and adverse effects. Avoid use in patients with sleep apnea. Use with caution in patients receiving concurrent CYP3A4 inhibitors, particularly when these agents are added to therapy. Use with caution in elderly or debilitated patients, patients with hepatic disease (including alcoholics), renal impairment, respiratory disease, impaired gag reflex, or obese patients.

Benzodiazepines have been associated with anterograde amnesia. Paradoxical reactions, including hyperactive or aggressive behavior, have been reported with benzodiazepines, particularly in adolescent/pediatric or psychiatric patients. Does not have analgesic, antidepressant, or antipsychotic properties. Not recommended for use in patients <9 years of age.

Drug Interactions

Cytochrome P450 Effect: Substrate of CYP3A4 (major)

Decreased Effect: CYP3A4 inducers may decrease the levels/effects of clorazepate; example inducers include aminoglutethimide, carbamazepine, nafcillin, nevirapine, phenobarbital, phenytoin, and rifamycins.

Increased Effect/Toxicity: Clorazepate potentiates the CNS depressant effects of narcotic analgesics, barbiturates, phenothiazines, ethanol, antihistamines, MAO inhibitors, sedative-hypnotics, and cyclic antidepressants. CYP3A4 inhibitors may increase the levels/effects of clorazepate; example inhibitors include azole antifungals, clarithromycin, diclofenac, doxycycline, erythromycin, imatinib, isoniazid, nefazodone, nicardipine, propofol, protease inhibitors, quinidine, telithromycin, and verapamil.

Nutritional/Ethanol Interactions

Ethanol: Avoid ethanol (may increase CNS depression).

Food: Serum concentrations/toxicity may be increased by grapefruit juice.

Herb/Nutraceutical: Avoid valerian, St John's wort, kava kava, gotu kola (may increase CNS depression).

Lab Interactions Decreased hematocrit; abnormal liver and renal function tests

Adverse Reactions Frequency not defined.

Cardiovascular: Hypotension

Central nervous system: Drowsiness, fatigue, ataxia, lightheadedness, memory impairment, insomnia, anxiety, headache, depression, slurred speech, confusion, nervousness, dizziness, irritability

Dermatologic: Rash

Endocrine & metabolic: Decreased libido

Gastrointestinal: Xerostomia, constipation, diarrhea, decreased salivation, nausea, vomiting, increased or decreased appetite

Neuromuscular & skeletal: Dysarthria, tremor

Ocular: Blurred vision, diplopia

Overdosage/Toxicology May produce somnolence, confusion, ataxia, diminished reflexes, and coma. Treatment for benzodiazepine overdose is supportive. Rarely is mechanical ventilation required. Flumazenil has been shown to selectively block the binding of benzodiazepines to CNS receptors, resulting in a reversal of benzodiazepine-induced CNS depression, but not respiratory depression.

Pharmacodynamics/Kinetics

Onset of Action: 1-2 hours

Duration of Action: Variable, 8-24 hours

Time to Peak: Serum: ~1 hour

Half-Life Elimination: Adults: Desmethyldiazepam: 48-96 hours; Oxazepam: 6-8 hours

Metabolism: Rapidly decarboxylated to desmethyldiazepam (active) in acidic stomach prior to absorption; hepatically to oxazepam (active)

Excretion: Primarily urine

Available Dosage Forms

Tablet, as dipotassium: 3.75 mg, 7.5 mg, 15 mg

Tranxene® SD™: 22.5 mg [once daily]

Tranxene® SD™-Half Strength: 11.25 mg [once daily]

Tranxene® T-Tab®: 3.75 mg, 7.5 mg, 15 mg

Dosing

Adults:

Anxiety:
Regular release tablets (Tranxene® T-Tab®): 7.5-15 mg 2-4 times/day
Sustained release (Tranxene® SD): 11.25 or 22.5 mg once daily at bedtime

Ethanol withdrawal: Oral: Initial: 30 mg, then 15 mg 2-4 times/day on first day; maximum daily dose: 90 mg; gradually decrease dose over subsequent days.

Seizures (anticonvulsant): Oral: Initial: Up to 7.5 mg/dose 2-3 times/day; increase dose by 7.5 mg at weekly intervals; not to exceed 90 mg/day

Elderly: Oral: Anxiety: 7.5 mg 1-2 times/day; use is not recommended in the elderly.

Pediatrics:

Seizures (anticonvulsant): Oral:

Children 9-12 years: Initial: 3.75-7.5 mg/dose twice daily; increase dose by 3.75 mg at weekly intervals, not to exceed 60 mg/day in 2-3 divided doses.

Children >12 years: Refer to adult dosing.

Nursing Actions

Physical Assessment: Assess other medications patient may be taking for effectiveness and interactions. Assess for signs of CNS depression (sedation, dizziness, confusion, or ataxia). Assess for history of addiction; long-term use can result in dependence, abuse, or tolerance; periodically evaluate need for continued use. For inpatient use, institute safety measures and monitor effectiveness and adverse reactions. For outpatients, monitor therapeutic effectiveness and adverse reactions at beginning of therapy and periodically with long-term use. Taper dosage slowly when discontinuing. Assess knowledge/teach patient appropriate use, interventions to reduce side effects, and adverse symptoms to report.

Patient Education: Take exactly as directed; do not increase dose or frequency. Drug may cause physical and/or psychological dependence. Do not use alcohol and other prescription or OTC medications (especially pain medications, sedatives, antihistamines, or hypnotics) without consulting prescriber. Maintain adequate hydration (2-3 L/day of fluids) unless instructed to restrict fluid intake. You may experience drowsiness, lightheadedness, impaired coordination, dizziness, or blurred vision (use caution when driving or engaging in tasks requiring alertness until response to drug is known); nausea, vomiting, or dry mouth (small frequent meals, frequent mouth care, chewing gum, or sucking lozenges may help); constipation (increased exercise, fluids, fruit, or fiber may help); altered sexual drive or ability (reversible); or photosensitivity (use sunscreen, wear protective clothing and eyewear, and avoid direct sunlight). Report persistent CNS effects (eg, confusion, depression, increased sedation, excitation, headache, agitation, insomnia or nightmares, dizziness, fatigue, impaired coordination, changes in personality, or changes in cognition); changes in urinary pattern; muscle cramping, weakness, tremors, or rigidity; ringing in ears or visual disturbances; chest pain, palpitations, or rapid heartbeat; excessive perspiration; excessive GI symptoms (cramping, constipation, vomiting, anorexia); or worsening of condition. **Pregnancy/ breast-feeding precautions:** Do not get pregnant while using this medication; use appropriate contraceptive measures. Breast-feeding is not recommended.

Geriatric Considerations Clorazepate is not considered a drug of choice in the elderly. Long-acting benzodiazepines have been associated with falls in the elderly.

Breast-Feeding Issues No specific data for clorazepate; however, other benzodiazepines have been shown to be excreted in breast milk. Therefore, it is recommended not to nurse while taking clorazepate.

Pregnancy Issues Benzodiazepines cross the placenta. The association between benzodiazepine exposure and malformations remains controversial. A number of types of malformation have been reported (oral cleft, inguinal hernia, cardiac defects, spina bifida, dysmorphic facial features, skeletal defects); however, confounding factors make a clear association difficult. Overall, the risk to the fetus may be low. Nonteratogenic effects (including neonatal flaccidity, respiratory and feeding problems, and withdrawal symptoms) during the post-natal period have also been reported with benzodiazepine use.

Additional Information Abrupt discontinuation after sustained use (generally >10 days) may cause withdrawal symptoms.

Related Information

Anxiolytic / Hypnotic Use in Long-Term Care Facilities *on page 1418*

Federal OBRA Regulations Recommended Maximum Doses *on page 1421*

Clotrimazole (kloe TRIM a zole)

U.S. Brand Names Cruex® Cream [OTC]; Gyne-Lotrimin® 3 [OTC]; Lotrimin® AF Athlete's Foot Cream [OTC]; Lotrimin® AF Athlete's Foot Solution [OTC]; Lotrimin® AF Jock Itch Cream [OTC]; Mycelex®; Mycelex®-7 [OTC]; Mycelex® Twin Pack [OTC]

Pharmacologic Category Antifungal Agent, Oral Nonabsorbed; Antifungal Agent, Topical; Antifungal Agent, Vaginal

Medication Safety Issues

Sound-alike/look-alike issues:

Clotrimazole may be confused with co-trimoxazole

Lotrimin® may be confused with Lotrisone®, Otrivin®

Mycelex® may be confused with Myoflex®

Pregnancy Risk Factor B (topical); C (troches)

Lactation Excretion in breast milk unknown

Use Treatment of susceptible fungal infections, including oropharyngeal candidiasis, dermatophytoses, superficial mycoses, and cutaneous candidiasis, as well as vulvovaginal candidiasis; limited data suggest that clotrimazole troches may be effective for prophylaxis against oropharyngeal candidiasis in neutropenic patients

Mechanism of Action/Effect Binds to phospholipids in the fungal cell membrane altering cell wall permeability resulting in loss of essential intracellular elements

Contraindications Hypersensitivity to clotrimazole or any component of the formulation

Warnings/Precautions Clotrimazole should not be used for treatment of ocular or systemic fungal infection. Use with caution with hepatic impairment. Safety and effectiveness of clotrimazole lozenges (troches) in children <3 years of age have not been established. When using topical formulation, avoid contact with eyes.

Drug Interactions

Cytochrome P450 Effect: Inhibits CYP1A2 (weak), 2A6 (weak), 2B6 (weak), 2C8/9 (weak), 2C19 (weak), 2D6 (weak), 2E1 (weak), 3A4 (moderate)

Increased Effect/Toxicity: Clotrimazole may increase the levels/effects of selected benzodiazepines, calcium channel blockers, cisapride, cyclosporine, ergot derivatives, selected HMG-CoA reductase inhibitors, mesoridazine, mirtazapine, nateglinide, nefazodone, pimozide, quinidine, sildenafil (and other PDE-5 inhibitors), tacrolimus, thioridazine, venlafaxine, and other CYP3A4 substrates.

Adverse Reactions

Oral:

>10%: Hepatic: Abnormal liver function tests

1% to 10%:

Gastrointestinal: Nausea and vomiting may occur in patients on clotrimazole troches

Local: Mild burning, irritation, stinging to skin or vaginal area

Vaginal:

1% to 10%: Genitourinary: Vulvar/vaginal burning

Pharmacodynamics/Kinetics

Time to Peak: Serum:

Oral topical (troche): Salivary levels occur within 3 hours following 30 minutes of dissolution time

(Continued)

Clotrimazole *(Continued)*

Vaginal cream: High vaginal levels: 8-24 hours
Vaginal tablet: High vaginal levels: 1-2 days

Excretion: Feces (as metabolites)

Available Dosage Forms

Combination pack (Mycelex®-7): Vaginal tablet 100 mg (7s) and vaginal cream 1% (7 g)

Cream, topical: 1% (15 g, 30 g, 45 g)

Cruex®: 1% (15 g)

Lotrimin® AF Athlete's Foot: 1% (12 g, 24 g)

Lotrimin® AF Jock Itch: 1% (12 g)

Cream, vaginal: 2% (21 g)

Mycelex®-7: 1% (45 g)

Solution, topical: 1% (10 mL, 30 mL)

Lotrimin® AF Athlete's Foot: 1% (10 mL)

Tablet, vaginal (Gyne-Lotrimin® 3): 200 mg (3s)

Troche (Mycelex®): 10 mg

Dosing

Adults & Elderly:

Oropharyngeal candidiasis: Oral:

Prophylaxis: 10 mg troche dissolved 3 times/day for the duration of chemotherapy or until steroids are reduced to maintenance levels

Treatment: 10 mg troche dissolved slowly 5 times/ day for 14 consecutive days

Dermatophytosis, cutaneous candidiasis: Topical (cream, solution): Apply twice daily; if no improvement occurs after 4 weeks of therapy, re-evaluate diagnosis.

Vulvovaginal candidiasis: Intravaginal:

Cream (1%): Insert 1 applicatorful of 1% vaginal cream daily (preferably at bedtime) for 7 consecutive days.

Cream (2%): Insert 1 applicatorful of 2% vaginal cream daily (preferably at bedtime) for 3 consecutive days.

Tablet: Insert 100 mg/day for 7 days or 500 mg single dose.

Dermatologic infection (superficial): Topical (cream, solution): Apply to affected area twice daily (morning and evening) for 7 consecutive days.

Pediatrics:

Oropharyngeal candidiasis: Children >3 years: Refer to adult dosing.

Vaginal, Topical infections: Children >12 years: Refer to adult dosing.

Administration

Oral: Troche: Allow to dissolve slowly over 15-30 minutes.

Topical: For external use only. Apply sparingly. Protect hands with latex gloves. Do not use occlusive dressings.

Other: Avoid contact with eyes.

Laboratory Monitoring Periodic liver function during oral therapy with clotrimazole troche

Nursing Actions

Physical Assessment: Monitor laboratory values, effectiveness of treatment, and adverse reactions. Assess knowledge/teach patient appropriate use, interventions to reduce side effects, and adverse symptoms to report. Assess for opportunistic infection.

Patient Education:

Oral (troche): Do not swallow oral medication whole; allow to dissolve slowly in mouth. You may experience nausea or vomiting (small frequent meals, frequent mouth care, chewing gum, or sucking lozenges may help). Report signs of opportunistic infection (eg, white plaques in mouth, fever, chills, perianal itching, vaginal itching or discharge, fatigue, unhealed wounds or sores).

Topical: Avoid contact with eyes. Wash hands before applying or wear gloves. Apply thin film to affected area. May apply porous dressing. Report persistent burning, swelling, itching, worsening of condition, or lack of response to therapy.

Vaginal: Wash hands before using. Insert full applicator into vagina gently and expel cream, or insert tablet into vagina, at bedtime. Wash applicator with soap and water following use. Remain lying down for 30 minutes following administration. Avoid intercourse during therapy (sexual partner may experience penile burning or itching). Report adverse reactions (eg, vulvar itching, frequent urination), worsening of condition, or lack of response to therapy. Contact prescriber if symptoms do not improve within 3 days or you do not feel well within 7 days. Do not use tampons until therapy is complete. Contact prescriber immediately if you experience abdominal pain, fever, or foul-smelling discharge.

Pregnancy/breast-feeding precautions: Inform prescriber if you are pregnant. Consult prescriber if breast-feeding.

Geriatric Considerations Localized fungal infections frequently follow broad spectrum antimicrobial therapy. Specifically, oral and vaginal infections due to *Candida*.

Clozapine *(KLOE za peen)*

U.S. Brand Names Clozaril®; FazaClo®

Restrictions Patient-specific registration is required to dispense clozapine. Monitoring systems for individual clozapine manufacturers are independent. If a patient is switched from one brand/manufacturer of clozapine to another, the patient must be entered into a new registry (must be completed by the prescriber and delivered to the dispensing pharmacy). Healthcare providers, including pharmacists dispensing clozapine, should verify the patient's hematological status and qualification to receive clozapine with all existing registries. The manufacturer of Clozaril® requests that healthcare providers submit all WBC/ANC values following discontinuation of therapy to the Clozaril National Registry for all nonrechallengable patients until WBC ≥3500/mm^3 and ANC ≥2000/mm^3.

Pharmacologic Category Antipsychotic Agent, Atypical

Medication Safety Issues

Sound-alike/look-alike issues:

Clozapine may be confused with clofazimine, clonidine, Klonopin®

Clozaril® may be confused with Clinoril®, Colazal®

Pregnancy Risk Factor B

Lactation Enters breast milk/not recommended (AAP rates "of concern")

Use Treatment-refractory schizophrenia; to reduce risk of recurrent suicidal behavior in schizophrenia or schizoaffective disorder

Unlabeled/Investigational Use Schizoaffective disorder, bipolar disorder, childhood psychosis, severe obsessive-compulsive disorder

Mechanism of Action/Effect Clozapine (dibenzodiazepine antipsychotic) exhibits weak antagonism of D_1, D_2, D_3, and D_5 dopamine receptor subtypes, but shows high affinity for D_4; in addition, it blocks the serotonin (5HT$_2$), alpha-adrenergic, histamine H_1, and cholinergic receptors

Contraindications Hypersensitivity to clozapine or any component of the formulation; history of agranulocytosis or granulocytopenia with clozapine; uncontrolled epilepsy; severe central nervous system depression or comatose state; paralytic ileus; myeloproliferative disorders or use with other agents which have a well-known risk of agranulocytosis or bone marrow suppression

Warnings/Precautions Patients with dementia-related behavioral disorders treated with atypical antipsychotics are at an increased risk of death compared to placebo. Clozapine is not approved for this indication.

Significant risk of agranulocytosis, potentially life-threatening. Therapy should not be initiated in patients with WBC <3500 cells/mm³ or ANC <2000 cells/mm³ or history of myeloproliferative disorder. WBC testing should occur periodically on an on-going basis (see prescribing information for monitoring details) to ensure that acceptable WBC/ANC counts are maintained. Initial episodes of moderate leukopenia or granulopoietic suppression confer up to a 12-fold increased risk for subsequent episodes of agranulocytosis. WBCs must be monitored weekly for at least 4 weeks after therapy discontinuation or until WBC ≥3500/mm³ and ANC ≥2000/mm³. Use with caution in patients receiving other marrow suppressive agents. Eosinophilia has been reported to occur with clozapine and may require temporary or permanent interruption of therapy. Due to the significant risk of agranulocytosis, it is strongly recommended that a patient must fail at least two trials of other primary medications for the treatment of schizophrenia (of adequate dose and duration) before initiating therapy with clozapine.

Cognitive and/or motor impairment (sedation) is common with clozapine, resulting in impaired performance of tasks requiring alertness (eg, operating machinery or driving); use caution in patients receiving general anesthesia. Seizures have been associated with clozapine use in a dose-dependent manner; use with caution in patients at risk of seizures, including those with a history of seizures, head trauma, brain damage, alcoholism, or concurrent therapy with medications which may lower seizure threshold. Has been associated with benign, self-limiting fever (<100.4°F, usually within first 3 weeks). However, clozapine may also be associated with severe febrile reactions, including neuroleptic malignant syndrome (NMS). Clozapine's potential for extrapyramidal symptoms (including tardive dyskinesia) appears to be extremely low.

Deep vein thrombosis, myocarditis, pericarditis, pericardial effusion, cardiomyopathy, and CHF have also been associated with clozapine. Fatalities due to myocarditis have been reported; highest risk in the first month of therapy, however, later cases also reported. Clozapine should be discontinued in patients with confirmed cardiomyopathy unless benefit clearly outweighs risk. Rare cases of thromboembolism, including pulmonary embolism and stroke resulting in fatalities, have been associated with clozapine.

May cause anticholinergic effects; use with caution in patients with urinary retention, benign prostatic hyperplasia, narrow-angle glaucoma, xerostomia, visual problems, constipation, or history of bowel obstruction. May cause hyperglycemia; in some cases may be extreme and associated with ketoacidosis, hyperosmolar coma, or death. Use with caution in patients with diabetes or other disorders of glucose regulation; monitor for worsening of glucose control. Use with caution in patients with hepatic disease or impairment; hepatitis has been reported as a consequence of therapy.

Use caution with cardiovascular, renal, or pulmonary disease. May cause orthostatic hypotension (with or without syncope) and tachycardia; use with caution in patients at risk of hypotension or in patients where transient hypotensive episodes be poorly tolerated (cardiovascular disease or cerebrovascular disease). Concurrent use with benzodiazepines may increase the risk of severe cardiopulmonary reactions.

The possibility of a suicide attempt is inherent in psychotic illness or bipolar disorder; use caution in high-risk patients during initiation of therapy. Prescriptions should be written for the smallest quantity consistent with good patient care.

Medication should not be stopped abruptly; taper off over 1-2 weeks. If conditions warrant abrupt discontinuation (leukopenia, myocarditis, cardiomyopathy), monitor patient for psychosis and cholinergic rebound (headache, nausea, vomiting, diarrhea). Consider titrating to a different antipsychotic agent for a weight gain ≥5% of the initial weight). Elderly patients are more susceptible to adverse effects (including agranulocytosis, cardiovascular, anticholinergic, and tardive dyskinesia).

Drug Interactions

Cytochrome P450 Effect: Substrate of CYP1A2 (major), 2A6 (minor), 2C8/9 (minor), 2C19 (minor), 2D6 (minor), 3A4 (minor); **Inhibits** CYP1A2 (weak), 2C8/9 (weak), 2C19 (weak), 2D6 (moderate), 2E1 (weak), 3A4 (weak)

Decreased Effect: Clozapine may decrease the levels/effects of CYP2D6 prodrug substrates; example prodrug substrates include codeine, hydrocodone, oxycodone, and tramadol. The levels/effects of clozapine may be decreased by carbamazepine, phenobarbital, primidone, rifampin, and other CYP1A2 inducers. Cigarette smoking (nicotine) may enhance the metabolism of clozapine. Clozapine may reverse the pressor effect of epinephrine (avoid in treatment of drug-induced hypotension). Omeprazole may alter the concentrations/effects of clozapine.

Increased Effect/Toxicity: May potentiate anticholinergic and hypotensive effects of other drugs. Benzodiazepines in combination with clozapine may produce respiratory depression and hypotension, especially during the first few weeks of therapy. May potentiate effect/toxicity of risperidone. Clozapine serum concentrations may be increased by inhibitors of CYP1A2; example inhibitors include amiodarone, ciprofloxacin, fluvoxamine, ketoconazole, norfloxacin, ofloxacin, and rofecoxib. Clozapine may increase the levels/effects of amphetamines, selected beta-blockers, substrates; example substrates include dextromethorphan, fluoxetine, lidocaine, mirtazapine, nefazodone, paroxetine, risperidone, ritonavir, thioridazine, tricyclic antidepressants, venlafaxine, and other CYP2D6 substrates. Sedative effects may be additive with other CNS depressants (eg, ethanol, barbiturates, benzodiazepines, narcotic analgesics, and other sedatives). Metoclopramide may increase risk of extrapyramidal symptoms (EPS). Acetylcholinesterase inhibitors (central) may increase the risk of antipsychotic-related EPS. Citalopram may increase the levels/effects of clozapine. Omeprazole may alter the concentrations/effects of clozapine.

Nutritional/Ethanol Interactions

Ethanol: Avoid ethanol (may increase CNS depression).

Herb/Nutraceutical: St John's wort may decrease clozapine levels. Avoid kava kava, gotu kola, valerian, St John's wort (may increase CNS depression).

Adverse Reactions

>10%:

Cardiovascular: Tachycardia (25%)

Central nervous system: Drowsiness (39% to 46%), dizziness (19% to 27%), insomnia (2% to 20%)

Gastrointestinal: Constipation (14% to 25%), weight gain (4% to 31%), sialorrhea (31% to 48%), nausea/vomiting (3% to 17%)

1% to 10%:

Cardiovascular: Angina (1%), ECG changes (1%), hypertension (4%), hypotension (9%), syncope (6%)

Central nervous system: Akathisia (3%), seizure (3%), headache (7%), nightmares (4%), akinesia (4%), confusion (3%), myoclonic jerks (1%), restlessness (4%), agitation (4%), lethargy (1%), ataxia (1%), slurred speech (1%), depression (1%), anxiety (1%)

Dermatologic: Rash (2%)

(Continued)

Clozapine *(Continued)*

Gastrointestinal: Abdominal discomfort/heartburn (4% to 14%), anorexia (1%), diarrhea (2%), xerostomia (6%), throat discomfort (1%)

Genitourinary: Urinary abnormalities (eg, abnormal ejaculation, retention, urgency, incontinence; 1% to 2%)

Hematologic: Eosinophilia (1%), leukopenia, leukocytosis, agranulocytosis (1%)

Hepatic: Liver function tests abnormal (1%)

Neuromuscular & skeletal: Tremor (6%), hypokinesia (4%), rigidity (3%), hyperkinesia (1%), weakness (1%), pain (1%), spasm (1%)

Ocular: Visual disturbances (5%)

Respiratory: Dyspnea (1%), nasal congestion (1%)

Miscellaneous: Diaphoresis (increased), fever, tongue numbness (1%)

Overdosage/Toxicology Symptoms of overdose include altered states of consciousness (delirium, drowsiness, coma), tachycardia, hypotension, hypersalivation, and respiratory depression. Aspiration pneumonia and cardiac arrhythmias have also been reported. Fatal overdose generally at >2500 mg. Following initiation of essential overdose management, toxic symptom treatment and supportive treatment should be initiated.

Pharmacodynamics/Kinetics

Time to Peak: 2.5 hours (range: 1-6 hours)

Protein Binding: 97% to serum proteins

Half-Life Elimination: Steady state:12 hours (range: 4-66 hours)

Metabolism: Extensively hepatic; forms metabolites with limited or no activity

Excretion: Urine (~50%) and feces (30%) with trace amounts of unchanged drug

Available Dosage Forms

Tablet: 12.5 mg, 25 mg, 100 mg

Clozaril®: 25 mg, 100 mg

Tablet, orally disintegrating (FazaClo®): 25 mg [contains phenylalanine 1.75 mg; mint flavor], 100 mg [contains phenylalanine 6.96 mg; mint flavor]

Dosing

Adults:

Schizophrenia: Initial: 12.5 mg once or twice daily; increased, as tolerated, in increments of 25-50 mg/day to a target dose of 300-450 mg/day after 2-4 weeks, may require doses as high as 600-900 mg/day

Reduce risk of suicidal behavior: Initial: 12.5 mg once or twice daily; increased, as tolerated, in increments of 25-50 mg/day to a target dose of 300-450 mg/day after 2-4 weeks; median dose is ~300 mg/day (range: 12.5-900 mg)

Termination of therapy: If dosing is interrupted for ≥48 hours, therapy must be reinitiated at 12.5-25 mg/day; may be increased more rapidly than with initial titration, unless cardiopulmonary arrest occurred during initial titration.

In the event of planned termination of clozapine, gradual reduction in dose over a 1- to 2-week period is recommended. If conditions warrant abrupt discontinuation (leukopenia), monitor patient for psychosis and cholinergic rebound (headache, nausea, vomiting, diarrhea).

Patients discontinued on clozapine therapy due to WBC <2000/mm^3 or ANC <1000/mm^3 should not be restarted on clozapine.

Dosage adjustment for toxicity:

Moderate leukopenia or granulocytopenia (WBC <3000/mm^3 and ANC <1500/mm^3): Discontinue therapy; may rechallenge patient when WBC >3500/mm^3 and/or ANC >2000/mm^3. **Note:** Patient is at greater risk for developing agranulocytosis.

Severe leukopenia or granulocytopenia (WBC <2000/mm^3 and/or ANC <1000/mm^3): Discontinue therapy and do not rechallenge patient.

Elderly: Oral: Experience in the elderly is limited; initial dose should be 25 mg/day; increase as tolerated by 25 mg/day to desired response. Maximum daily dose in the elderly should probably be 450 mg. Dose titration to 300-450 mg/day may be attained in 2 weeks if tolerated; however, elderly may require slower titration and daily increases may not be tolerated.

Pediatrics: Children and Adolescents: Childhood psychosis (unlabeled use): Oral: Initial: 25 mg/day; increase to a target dose of 25-400 mg/day

Dosing Adjustment for Toxicity:

Moderate leukopenia or granulocytopenia (WBC <3000/mm^3 and/or ANC <1500/mm^3): Discontinue therapy; may rechallenge patient when WBC >3500/mm^3 and ANC >2000/mm^3. **Note:** Patient is at greater risk for developing agranulocytosis.

Severe leukopenia or granulocytopenia (WBC <2000/mm^3 and/or ANC <1000/mm^3): Discontinue therapy and do not rechallenge patient.

Administration

Oral: Orally-disintegrating tablet: Should be removed from foil blister by peeling apart (do not push tablet through the foil). Remove immediately prior to use. Place tablet in mouth and allow to dissolve; swallow with saliva. If dosing requires splitting tablet, throw unused portion away.

Stability

Storage: Dispensed in "clozapine patient system" packaging. Store at controlled room temperature. FazaClo™: Protect from moisture; do not remove from package until ready to use.

Laboratory Monitoring ECG; WBC (see below), fasting lipid profile and fasting blood glucose/Hgb A$_{1c}$ (prior to treatment, at 3 months, then annually; BMI, personal/family history of obesity; waist circumference (weight should be assessed prior to treatment, at 4 weeks, 8 weeks, 12 weeks, and then at quarterly intervals.

WBC and ANC should be obtained at baseline and at least weekly for the first 6 months of continuous treatment. If counts remain acceptable (WBC ≥3500/mm^3, ANC ≥2000/mm^3) during this time period, then they may be monitored every other week for the next 6 months. If WBC/ANC continue to remain within these acceptable limits after the second 6 months of therapy, monitoring can be decreased to every 4 weeks. (**Note:** The decease in monitoring to every 4 weeks is applicable in the United States. Blood monitoring requirements related to the use of clozapine have not changed in Canada). If clozapine is discontinued, a weekly WBC should be conducted for an additional 4 weeks or until WBC ≥3500/mm^3 and ANC ≥2000/mm^3. If clozapine therapy is interrupted due to moderate leukopenia, weekly WBC/ANC monitoring is required for 12 months in patients restarted on clozapine treatment. If therapy is interrupted for reasons other than leukopenia/granulocytopenia, the 6-month time period for initiation of biweekly WBCs may need to be reset. This determination depends upon the treatment duration, the length of the break in therapy, and whether or not an abnormal blood event occurred.

Consult full prescribing information for determination of appropriate WBC/ANC monitoring interval (http://www.clozaril.com/index.jsp).

Nursing Actions

Physical Assessment: Assess other medications patient is taking for effectiveness and interactions. Initiate at lower doses and taper dosage slowly when discontinuing. Instruct patients with diabetes to monitor blood glucose levels frequently; can cause hyperglycemia. Be alert to the potential of cardiac abnormalities. Monitor weight prior to initiating therapy and at least monthly. Review ophthalmic exam and monitor laboratory results, therapeutic response (mental status, mood, affect), and adverse reactions at beginning of therapy and periodically with long-term use (especially orthostatic hypotension, ECG changes, anticholinergic and extrapyramidal symptoms). Teach patient appropriate use, interventions to reduce side effects, and adverse symptoms to report.

Patient Education: Use exactly as directed; do not increase dose or frequency. Do not discontinue this medication without consulting prescriber. Avoid alcohol or caffeine and other prescription or OTC medications not approved by prescriber. Maintain adequate hydration (2-3 L/day of fluids) unless instructed to restrict fluid intake. If you have diabetes, monitor blood glucose levels frequently. You may experience headache, excess drowsiness, dizziness, or blurred vision (use caution driving or when engaging in tasks requiring alertness until response to drug is known); constipation, diarrhea; dry mouth, nausea, vomiting (small frequent meals, frequent mouth care, sucking lozenges, or chewing gum may help); or postural hypotension (use caution climbing stairs or when changing position from lying or sitting to standing). You may be prone to infections; report fever, sore throat or other possible signs of infection. Report persistent CNS effects (insomnia, depression, altered consciousness); palpitations, rapid heartbeat, severe dizziness; vision changes; hypersalivation, tearing, sweating; respiratory difficulty; or worsening of condition. Report seizures, flu-like symptoms, chest pain, shortness of breath, or excessive fatigue. **Breast-feeding precaution:** Breast-feeding is not recommended.

Dietary Considerations May be taken without regard to food. Fazaclo™ contains phenylalanine 1.75 mg per 25 mg tablet and phenylalanine 6.96 mg per 100 mg tablet.

Geriatric Considerations Not recommended for use in nonpsychotic patients. Studies in subjects >65 years of age have not been done. Orthostatic hypotension and sustained tachycardia have been noted in up to 25% of patients taking clozapine; therefore, elderly with cardiovascular disease may be at risk. The anticholinergic effects of clozapine may be prominent in elderly (eg, constipation, confusion, urinary retention).

Pregnancy Issues Teratogenic effects were not seen in animal studies; however, there are no adequate and well-controlled studies in pregnant women. Use during pregnancy only if clearly needed.

Related Information
Antipsychotic Medication Guidelines *on page 1415*
Federal OBRA Regulations Recommended Maximum Doses *on page 1421*

Cocaine (koe KANE)

Synonyms Cocaine Hydrochloride
Restrictions C-II
Pharmacologic Category Local Anesthetic
Pregnancy Risk Factor C/X (nonmedicinal use)
Lactation Enters breast milk/contraindicated
Use Topical anesthesia for mucous membranes
Mechanism of Action/Effect Blocks both the initiation and conduction of nerve impulses
Contraindications Hypersensitivity to cocaine or any component of the topical solution; ophthalmologic anesthesia (causing sloughing of the corneal epithelium); pregnancy (nonmedicinal use)
Warnings/Precautions For topical use only. Limit to office and surgical procedures only. Resuscitative equipment and drugs should be immediately available when any local anesthetic is used. Debilitated, elderly patients, acutely ill patients, and children should be given reduced doses consistent with their age and physical status. Use caution in patients with severely traumatized mucosa and sepsis in the region of the proposed application. Use with caution in patients with cardiovascular disease or a history of cocaine abuse. In patients being treated for cardiovascular complication of cocaine abuse, avoid beta-blockers for treatment.

Drug Interactions
Cytochrome P450 Effect: Substrate of CYP3A4 (major); **Inhibits** CYP2D6 (strong), 3A4 (weak)
Increased Effect/Toxicity: Cocaine may increase the levels/effects of CYP2D6 substrates (eg, amphetamines, selected beta-blockers, dextromethorphan, fluoxetine, lidocaine, mirtazapine, nefazodone, paroxetine, risperidone, ritonavir, thioridazine, tricyclic antidepressants, venlafaxine). Increased toxicity with MAO inhibitors. Use with epinephrine may cause extreme hypertension and/or cardiac arrhythmias. CYP3A4 inhibitors may increase the levels/effects of cocaine (eg, azole antifungals, clarithromycin, diclofenac, doxycycline, erythromycin, imatinib, isoniazid, nefazodone, nicardipine, propofol, protease inhibitors, quinidine, telithromycin, verapamil).

Adverse Reactions
>10%:
Central nervous system: CNS stimulation
Gastrointestinal: Loss of taste perception
Respiratory: Rhinitis, nasal congestion
Miscellaneous: Loss of smell
1% to 10%:
Cardiovascular: Heart rate (decreased) with low doses, tachycardia with moderate doses, hypertension, cardiomyopathy, cardiac arrhythmia, myocarditis, QRS prolongation, Raynaud's phenomenon, cerebral vasculitis, thrombosis, fibrillation (atrial), flutter (atrial), sinus bradycardia, CHF, pulmonary hypertension, sinus tachycardia, tachycardia (supraventricular), arrhythmia (ventricular), vasoconstriction
Central nervous system: Fever, nervousness, restlessness, euphoria, excitation, headache, psychosis, hallucinations, agitation, seizure, slurred speech, hyperthermia, dystonic reactions, cerebral vascular accident, vasculitis, clonic-tonic reactions, paranoia, sympathetic storm
Dermatologic: Skin infarction, pruritus, madarosis
Gastrointestinal: Nausea, anorexia, colonic ischemia, spontaneous bowel perforation
Genitourinary: Priapism, uterine rupture
Hematologic: Thrombocytopenia
Neuromuscular & skeletal: Chorea (extrapyramidal), paresthesia, tremor, fasciculations
Ocular: Mydriasis (peak effect at 45 minutes; may last up to 12 hours), sloughing of the corneal epithelium, ulceration of the cornea, iritis, mydriasis, chemosis
Renal: Myoglobinuria, necrotizing vasculitis
Respiratory: Tachypnea, nasal mucosa damage (when snorting), hyposmia, bronchiolitis obliterans organizing pneumonia
Miscellaneous: "Washed-out" syndrome

Overdosage/Toxicology Symptoms of overdose include anxiety, excitement, confusion, nausea, vomiting, headache, rapid pulse, irregular respiration, delirium, fever, seizures, respiratory arrest, hallucinations, dilated pupils, muscle spasms, sensory aberrations, and cardiac arrhythmias.
Fatal dose: Oral: 500 mg to 1.2 g; severe toxic effects have occurred with doses as low as 20 mg.

Since no specific antidote for cocaine exists, serious toxic effects are treated symptomatically.

Pharmacodynamics/Kinetics
Onset of Action: ~1 minute; Peak effect: ~5 minutes
Duration of Action: Dose dependent: ≥30 minutes; cocaine metabolites may appear in urine of neonates up to 5 days after birth due to maternal cocaine use shortly before birth
(Continued)

Cocaine *(Continued)*

Half-Life Elimination: 75 minutes

Metabolism: Hepatic; major metabolites are ecgonine methyl ester and benzoyl ecgonine

Excretion: Primarily urine (<10% as unchanged drug and metabolites)

Pharmacokinetic Note Data is based on topical administration to mucosa.

Available Dosage Forms

Powder, as hydrochloride: 1 g, 5 g, 25 g

Solution, topical, as hydrochloride: 4% [40 mg/mL] (4 mL, 10 mL); 10% [100 mg/mL] (4 mL, 10 mL)

Dosing

Adults: Topical application (ear, nose, throat, bronchoscopy): Dosage depends on the area to be anesthetized, tissue vascularity, technique of anesthesia, and individual patient tolerance; the lowest dose necessary to produce adequate anesthesia should be used; concentrations of 1% to 10% are used (not to exceed 1 mg/kg). Use reduced dosages for children, elderly, or debilitated patients.

Elderly: Refer to adult dosing; use with caution.

Administration

Topical: Use only on mucous membranes of the oral, laryngeal, and nasal cavities. Do not use on extensive areas of broken skin.

Stability

Storage: Store in well-closed, light-resistant containers.

Nursing Actions

Physical Assessment: Assess other medications patient may be taking for interactions. Monitor adverse effects (eg, cardiovascular, CNS, and respiratory effects) and teach patient adverse symptoms to report. **Pregnancy risk factor C/X (if nonmedicinal use).** Breast-feeding is contraindicated.

Patient Education: When used orally, do not take anything by mouth until full sensation returns. **Ocular:** Use caution when driving or engaging in tasks that require alert vision (mydriasis may last for several hours). At time of use or immediately thereafter, report any unusual cardiovascular, CNS, or respiratory symptoms. Following use, report skin irritation or eruption; alterations in vision, eye pain, or irritation; persistent GI effects; muscle or skeletal tremors, numbness, or rigidity; urinary or genital problems; or persistent fatigue. **Pregnancy/breast-feeding precautions:** Inform prescriber if you are pregnant. Do not breast-feed.

Breast-Feeding Issues Irritability, vomiting, diarrhea, tremors, and seizures have been reported in nursing infants.

Additional Information Cocaine intoxication of infants who are receiving breast milk from their mothers abusing cocaine has been reported.

Codeine (KOE deen)

Synonyms Codeine Phosphate; Codeine Sulfate; Methylmorphine

Restrictions C-II

Pharmacologic Category Analgesic, Narcotic; Antitussive

Medication Safety Issues

Sound-alike/look-alike issues:

Codeine may be confused with Cardene®, Cophene®, Cordran®, iodine, Lodine®

Pregnancy Risk Factor C/D (prolonged use or high doses at term)

Lactation Enters breast milk/use caution (AAP rates "compatible")

Use Treatment of mild-to-moderate pain; antitussive in lower doses; dextromethorphan has equivalent antitussive activity but has much lower toxicity in accidental overdose

Mechanism of Action/Effect Inhibits perception of and response to pain; causes cough supression; produces generalized CNS depression

Contraindications Hypersensitivity to codeine or any component of the formulation; pregnancy (prolonged use or high doses at term)

Warnings/Precautions An opioid-containing analgesic regimen should be tailored to each patient's needs and based upon the type of pain being treated (acute versus chronic), the route of administration, degree of tolerance for opioids (naive versus chronic user), age, weight, and medical condition. The optimal analgesic dose varies widely among patients. Doses should be titrated to pain relief/prevention.

Use with caution in patients with hypersensitivity reactions to other phenanthrene derivative opioid agonists (morphine, hydrocodone, hydromorphone, levorphanol, oxycodone, oxymorphone); respiratory diseases including asthma, emphysema, COPD, or severe liver or renal insufficiency; some preparations contain sulfites which may cause allergic reactions; tolerance or drug dependence may result from extended use

Not recommended for use for cough control in patients with a productive cough; not recommended as an antitussive for children <2 years of age; the elderly may be particularly susceptible to the CNS depressant and confusion as well as constipating effects of narcotics

Not approved for I.V. administration (although this route has been used clinically). If given intravenously, must be given slowly and the patient should be lying down. Rapid intravenous administration of narcotics may increase the incidence of serious adverse effects, in part due to limited opportunity to assess response prior to administration of the full dose. Access to respiratory support should be immediately available

Drug Interactions

Cytochrome P450 Effect: Substrate of CYP2D6 (major), 3A4 (minor); **Inhibits** CYP2D6 (weak)

Decreased Effect: CYP2D6 inhibitors may decrease the effects of codeine. Example inhibitors include chlorpromazine, delavirdine, fluoxetine, miconazole, paroxetine, pergolide, quinidine, quinine, ritonavir, and ropinirole. Decreased effect with cigarette smoking.

Increased Effect/Toxicity: May cause severely increased toxicity of codeine when taken with CNS depressants, phenothiazines, tricyclic antidepressants, other narcotic analgesics, guanabenz, MAO inhibitors, and neuromuscular blockers.

Nutritional/Ethanol Interactions

Ethanol: Avoid or limit ethanol (may increase CNS depression).

Herb/Nutraceutical: St John's wort may decrease codeine levels. Avoid valerian, St John's wort, kava kava, gotu kola (may increase CNS depression).

Lab Interactions Some quinolones may produce a false-positive urine screening result for opiates using commercially-available immunoassay kits. This has been demonstrated most consistently for levofloxacin and ofloxacin, but other quinolones have shown cross-reactivity in certain assay kits. Confirmation of positive opiate screens by more specific methods should be considered.

Adverse Reactions

Frequency not defined: Increased AST, ALT

>10%:

Central nervous system: Drowsiness

Gastrointestinal: Constipation

1% to 10%:

Cardiovascular: Tachycardia or bradycardia, hypotension

Central nervous system: Dizziness, lightheadedness, false feeling of well being, malaise, headache, restlessness, paradoxical CNS stimulation, confusion

Dermatologic: Rash, urticaria

Gastrointestinal: Xerostomia, anorexia, nausea, vomiting

Genitourinary: Decreased urination, ureteral spasm

Hepatic: Increased LFTs

Local: Burning at injection site

Neuromuscular & skeletal: Weakness

Ocular: Blurred vision

Respiratory: Dyspnea

Miscellaneous: Histamine release

Overdosage/Toxicology Symptoms of overdose include CNS and respiratory depression, GI cramping, and constipation. Naloxone, 2 mg I.V. with repeat administration as necessary up to a total of 10 mg, can also be used to reverse toxic effects of the opiate.

Pharmacodynamics/Kinetics

Onset of Action: Oral: 0.5-1 hour; I.M.: 10-30 minutes; Peak effect: Oral: 1-1.5 hours; I.M.: 0.5-1 hour

Duration of Action: 4-6 hours

Protein Binding: 7%

Half-Life Elimination: 2.5-3.5 hours

Metabolism: Hepatic to morphine (active)

Excretion: Urine (3% to 16% as unchanged drug, norcodeine, and free and conjugated morphine)

Available Dosage Forms [CAN] = Canadian brand name

Injection, as phosphate: 15 mg/mL (2 mL); 30 mg/mL (2 mL) [contains sodium metabisulfite]

Solution, oral, as phosphate: 15 mg/5 mL (5 mL, 500 mL) [strawberry flavor]

Tablet, as phosphate: 30 mg, 60 mg

Tablet, as sulfate: 15 mg, 30 mg, 60 mg

Tablet, controlled release (Codeine Contin®) [CAN]: 50 mg, 100 mg, 150 mg, 200 mg [not available in U.S.]

Dosing

Adults & Elderly: Note: These are guidelines and do not represent the maximum doses that may be required in all patients. Doses should be titrated to pain relief/prevention. Doses >1.5 mg/kg body weight are not recommended.

Pain management (analgesic):

Oral, regular release: 30 mg every 4-6 hours as needed; patients with prior opiate exposure may require higher initial doses. Usual range: 15-120 mg every 4-6 hours as needed

Oral, controlled release formulation (Codeine Contin®, not available in U.S.): 50-300 mg every 12 hours. **Note:** A patient's codeine requirement should be established using prompt release formulations; conversion to long acting products may be considered when chronic, continuous treatment is required. Higher dosages should be reserved for use only in opioid-tolerant patients.

I.M., SubQ: 30 mg every 4-6 hours as needed; patients with prior opiate exposure may require higher initial doses. Usual range: 15-120 mg every 4-6 hours as needed; more frequent dosing may be needed

Cough (antitussive): Oral (for nonproductive cough): 10-20 mg/dose every 4-6 hours as needed; maximum: 120 mg/day

Pediatrics: Note: These are guidelines and do not represent the maximum doses that may be required in all patients. Doses should be titrated to pain relief/prevention. Doses >1.5 mg/kg body weight are not recommended.

Analgesic: Oral, I.M., SubQ: Children: 0.5-1 mg/kg/dose every 4-6 hours as needed; maximum: 60 mg/dose

Antitussive: Oral (for nonproductive cough): Children: 1-1.5 mg/kg/day in divided doses every 4-6 hours as needed: Alternative dose according to age:

2-6 years: 2.5-5 mg every 4-6 hours as needed; maximum: 30 mg/day

6-12 years: 5-10 mg every 4-6 hours as needed; maximum: 60 mg/day

Renal Impairment:

Cl_{cr} 10-50 mL/minute: Administer 75% of dose.

Cl_{cr} <10 mL/minute: Administer 50% of dose.

Hepatic Impairment: Dosing adjustment is probably necessary in hepatic insufficiency.

Administration

I.V. Detail: pH: 3-6 (codeine phosphate)

Stability

Storage: Store injection between 15°C to 30°C, avoid freezing. Do not use if injection is discolored or contains a precipitate. Protect injection from light.

Nursing Actions

Physical Assessment: Assess other medications patient may be taking for possible additive or adverse interactions. Monitor for effectiveness of pain relief and monitor for signs of overdose. Monitor blood pressure, CNS and respiratory status, and degree of sedation at beginning of therapy and at regular intervals with long-term use. May cause physical and/or psychological dependence. For inpatients, implement safety measures (eg, side rails up, call light within reach, instructions to call for assistance). Assess knowledge/teach patient appropriate use (if self-administered). Teach patient to monitor for adverse reactions, adverse reactions to report, and appropriate interventions to reduce side effects.

Patient Education: If self-administered, use exactly as directed; do not increase dose or frequency. Drug may cause physical and/or psychological dependence. While using this medication, do not use alcohol and other prescription or OTC medications (especially sedatives, tranquilizers, antihistamines, or pain medications) without consulting prescriber. Maintain adequate hydration (2-3 L/day of fluids) unless instructed to restrict fluid intake. May cause dizziness, drowsiness, confusion, agitation, impaired coordination, or blurred vision (use caution when driving, climbing stairs, or changing position - rising from sitting or lying to standing, or when engaging in tasks requiring alertness until response to drug is known); nausea or vomiting, or loss of appetite (frequent mouth care, small frequent meals, sucking lozenges, or chewing gum may help); or constipation (increased exercise, fluids, fruit, or fiber may help; if unresolved, consult prescriber about use of stool softeners). Report confusion, insomnia, excessive nervousness, excessive sedation or drowsiness, or shakiness; acute GI upset; respiratory difficulty or shortness of breath; facial flushing, rapid heartbeat, or palpitations; urinary difficulty; unusual muscle weakness; or vision changes. **Pregnancy/breast-feeding precautions:** Inform prescriber if you are or intend to become pregnant. If you are breast-feeding, take medication immediately after breast-feeding or 3-4 hours prior to next feeding.

Geriatric Considerations The elderly may be particularly susceptible to CNS depression and confusion as well as the constipating effects of narcotics.

Colchicine (KOL chi seen)

Pharmacologic Category Colchicine

Medication Safety Issues

High alert medication: The Institute for Safe Medication Practices (ISMP) includes this medication among its list of drugs which have a heightened risk of causing significant patient harm when used in error.

Pregnancy Risk Factor C (oral); D (parenteral)

Lactation Enters breast milk/use caution (AAP rates "compatible")

Use Treatment of acute gouty arthritis attacks and prevention of recurrences of such attacks

Unlabeled/Investigational Use Primary biliary cirrhosis; management of familial Mediterranean fever; pericarditis

Mechanism of Action/Effect Reduces the deposition of urate crystals that perpetuates the inflammatory response

Contraindications Hypersensitivity to colchicine or any component of the formulation; severe renal, gastrointestinal, hepatic, or cardiac disorders; blood dyscrasias; pregnancy (parenteral)

Warnings/Precautions Use with caution in debilitated patients or elderly patients; use caution in patients with mild-to-moderate cardiac, GI, renal, or liver disease. Severe local irritation can occur following SubQ or I.M. administration. Dosage reduction is recommended in patients who develop weakness or gastrointestinal symptoms (anorexia, diarrhea, nausea, vomiting) related to drug therapy.

Intravenous: Use only with extreme caution; potential for serious, life-threatening complications. Should not be administered to patients with renal insufficiency, hepatobiliary obstruction, patients >70 years of age, or recent oral colchicine use. Should be reserved for hospitalized patients who are under the care of a physician experienced in the use of intravenous colchicine.

Drug Interactions

Cytochrome P450 Effect: Substrate of CYP3A4 (major); **Induces** CYP2C8/9 (weak), 2E1 (weak), 3A4 (weak)

Increased Effect/Toxicity: Concurrent use of cyclosporine with colchicine may increase toxicity of colchicine. CYP3A4 inhibitors may increase the levels/effects of colchicine (example inhibitors include azole antifungals, diclofenac, doxycycline, imatinib, isoniazid, nefazodone, nicardipine, propofol, protease inhibitors, quinidine, and verapamil. Macrolide antibiotics (clarithromycin, erythromycin, troleandomycin) and telithromycin may decrease the metabolism of colchicine resulting in severe colchicine toxicity; avoid, if possible. Verapamil may increase colchicine toxicity (especially nephrotoxicity).

Nutritional/Ethanol Interactions

Ethanol: Avoid ethanol.

Food: Cyanocobalamin (vitamin B_{12}): Malabsorption of the substrate. May result in macrocytic anemia or neurologic dysfunction.

Herb/Nutraceutical: Vitamin B_{12} absorption may be decreased by colchicine.

Lab Interactions May cause false-positive results in urine tests for erythrocytes or hemoglobin

Adverse Reactions

>10%: Gastrointestinal: Nausea, vomiting, diarrhea, abdominal pain

1% to 10%:

Dermatologic: Alopecia

Gastrointestinal: Anorexia

Overdosage/Toxicology Symptoms of overdose include acute nausea, vomiting, abdominal pain, shock, kidney damage, muscle weakness, burning in throat, watery to bloody diarrhea, hypotension, anuria, cardiovascular collapse, delirium, convulsions, and respiratory paralysis. Treatment includes gastric lavage and measures to prevent shock, hemodialysis or peritoneal dialysis. Atropine and morphine may relieve abdominal pain.

Pharmacodynamics/Kinetics

Onset of Action: Oral: Pain relief: ~12 hours if adequately dosed

Time to Peak: Serum: Oral: 0.5-2 hours, declining for the next 2 hours before increasing again due to enterohepatic recycling

Protein Binding: 10% to 31%

Half-Life Elimination: 12-30 minutes; End-stage renal disease: 45 minutes

Metabolism: Partially hepatic via deacetylation

Excretion: Primarily feces; urine (10% to 20%)

Available Dosage Forms

Injection, solution: 0.5 mg/mL (2 mL)

Tablet: 0.6 mg

Dosing

Adults:

Familial Mediterranean fever (unlabeled use): Prophylaxis: Oral: 1-2 mg daily in divided doses (occasionally reduced to 0.6 mg/day in patients with GI intolerance)

Gouty arthritis:

Prophylaxis of acute attacks: Oral: 0.6 mg twice daily; initial and/or subsequent dosage may be decreased (ie, 0.6 mg once daily) in patients at risk of toxicity or in those who are intolerant (including weakness, loose stools, or diarrhea); range: 0.6 mg every other day to 0.6 mg 3 times/day

Acute attacks:

Oral: Initial: 0.6-1.2 mg, followed by 0.6 every 1-2 hours; some clinicians recommend a maximum of 3 doses; more aggressive approaches have recommended a maximum dose of up to 6 mg. Wait at least 3 days before initiating another course of therapy

I.V.: Initial: 1-2 mg, then 0.5 mg every 6 hours until response, not to exceed total dose of 4 mg. If pain recurs, it may be necessary to administer additional daily doses. The amount of colchicine administered intravenously in an acute treatment period (generally ~1 week) should not exceed a total dose of 4 mg. Do not administer more colchicine by any route for at least 7 days after a full course of I.V. therapy.

Note: Many experts would avoid use because of potential for serious, life-threatening complications. Should not be administered to patients with renal insufficiency, hepatobiliary obstruction, patients >70 years of age, or recent oral colchicine use. Should be reserved for hospitalized patients who are under the care of a physician experienced in the use of intravenous colchicine.

Surgery: Gouty arthritis, prophylaxis of recurrent attacks: Oral: 0.6 mg/day or every other day; patients who are to undergo surgical procedures may receive 0.6 mg 3 times/day for 3 days before and 3 days after surgery

Primary biliary cirrhosis (unlabeled use): Oral: 0.6 mg twice daily

Pericarditis (unlabeled use): Oral: 0.6 mg twice daily

Elderly: Refer to adult dosing. Reduce maintenance/prophylactic dose by 50% in individuals >70 years.

Pediatrics: Prophylaxis of familial Mediterranean fever (unlabeled use): Oral:

Children ≤5 years: 0.5 mg/day

Children >5 years: 1-1.5 mg/day in 2-3 divided doses

Renal Impairment:

Gouty arthritis, acute attacks: Oral: Specific dosing recommendations not available from the manufacturer:

Prophylaxis:

Cl_{cr} 35-49 mL/minute: 0.6 mg once daily

Cl_{cr} 10-34 mL/minute: 0.6 mg every 2-3 days

Cl_{cr} <10 mL/minute: Avoid chronic use of colchicine. Use in serious renal impairment is contraindicated by the manufacturer.

Treatment: Cl_{cr} <10 mL/minute: Use in serious renal impairment is contraindicated by the manufacturer. If a decision is made to use colchicine, decrease dose by 75%.

Peritoneal dialysis: Supplemental dose is not necessary

Hepatic Impairment: Avoid in hepatobiliary dysfunction and in patients with hepatic disease.

Administration

Oral: Administer tablet orally with water and maintain adequate fluid intake.

I.V.: Injection should be made over 2-5 minutes into tubing of free-flowing I.V. with compatible fluid. Do not administer I.M. or SubQ; severe local irritation can occur following SubQ or I.M. administration. Extravasation can cause tissue irritation.

Stability

Compatibility: I.V. colchicine is **incompatible** with dextrose or I.V. solutions with preservatives.

Storage: Protect tablets from light.

Laboratory Monitoring CBC and renal function on a regular basis

Nursing Actions

Physical Assessment: Assess effectiveness and interactions of other medications patient may be taking. **I.V.:** Monitor therapeutic response (frequency and severity of gouty attacks), laboratory values, and adverse reactions at beginning of therapy and periodically with long-term use. Assess knowledge/teach patient appropriate use, interventions to reduce side effects, and adverse symptoms to report.

Patient Education: Take as directed; do not exceed recommended dosage. Consult prescriber about a low-purine diet. Maintain adequate hydration (2-3 L/day of fluids) unless instructed to restrict fluid intake. Do not use alcohol or aspirin-containing medication without consulting prescriber. You may experience nausea, vomiting, or anorexia (small frequent meals, frequent mouth care, chewing gum, or sucking lozenges may help); hair loss (reversible). Stop medication and report to prescriber if severe vomiting, watery or bloody diarrhea, or abdominal pain occurs. Report muscle tremors or weakness; fatigue; easy bruising or bleeding; yellowing of eyes or skin; or pale stool or dark urine. **Pregnancy/breast-feeding precautions:** Inform prescriber if you are or intend to become pregnant. Consult prescriber if breast-feeding.

Dietary Considerations May need to supplement with vitamin B_{12}.

Geriatric Considerations Colchicine appears to be more toxic in the elderly, particularly in the presence of renal, gastrointestinal, or cardiac disease. The most predictable oral side effects are (gastrointestinal) vomiting, abdominal pain, and nausea. If colchicine is stopped at this point, other more severe adverse effects may be avoided, such as bone marrow suppression, peripheral neuritis, etc.

Colchicine and Probenecid
(KOL chi seen & proe BEN e sid)

Synonyms ColBenemid; Probenecid and Colchicine

Pharmacologic Category Anti-inflammatory Agent; Antigout Agent; Uricosuric Agent

Pregnancy Risk Factor C

Lactation
Colchicine: Compatible
Probenecid: Excretion in breast milk unknown

Use Treatment of chronic gouty arthritis when complicated by frequent, recurrent acute attacks of gout

Available Dosage Forms Tablet: Colchicine 0.5 mg and probenecid 0.5 g

Dosing
Adults & Elderly: Gout: Oral: 1 tablet/day for 1 week, then 1 tablet twice daily thereafter

Renal Impairment: Probenecid may not be effective in patients with chronic renal insufficiency particularly when Cl_{cr} is ≤30 mL/minute.

Nursing Actions
Physical Assessment: See individual agents.

Patient Education: See individual agents. **Pregnancy/breast-feeding precautions:** Inform prescriber if you are or intend to become pregnant. Consult prescriber if breast-feeding.

Related Information
Colchicine on page 298
Probenecid on page 1025

Colesevelam (koh le SEV a lam)

U.S. Brand Names WelChol®

Pharmacologic Category Antilipemic Agent, Bile Acid Sequestrant

Pregnancy Risk Factor B

Lactation Excretion in breast milk unknown

Use Adjunctive therapy to diet and exercise in the management of elevated LDL in primary hypercholesterolemia (Fredrickson type IIa) when used alone or in combination with an HMG-CoA reductase inhibitor

Mechanism of Action/Effect Colesevelam binds bile acids including glycocholic acid in the intestine, impeding their reabsorption. Increases the fecal loss of bile salt-bound LDL-C.

Contraindications Hypersensitivity to colesevelam or any component of the formulation; bowel obstruction

Warnings/Precautions Use caution in treating patients with triglyceride levels >300 mg/dL (excluded from trials). Safety and efficacy not established in pediatric patients. Use caution in dysphagia, swallowing disorders, severe GI motility disorders, major GI tract surgery, or in patients susceptible to fat soluble vitamin deficiencies. Minimal effects are seen on HDL-C and triglyceride levels. Secondary causes of hypercholesterolemia should be excluded before initiation.

Drug Interactions
Decreased Effect: Sustained-release verapamil AUC and C_{max} were reduced. Clinical significance unknown.

Digoxin, lovastatin, metoprolol, quinidine, valproic acid, or warfarin absorption was not significantly affected with concurrent administration.

Clinical effects of atorvastatin, lovastatin, and simvastatin were not changed by concurrent administration.

Increased Effect/Toxicity: Refer to Decreased Effect.

Adverse Reactions
>10%: Gastrointestinal: Constipation (11%)
2% to 10%:
Gastrointestinal: Dyspepsia (8%)
(Continued)

Colesevelam (Continued)

Neuromuscular & skeletal: Weakness (4%), myalgia (2%)

Respiratory: Pharyngitis (3%)

Incidence less than or equal to placebo: Infection, headache, pain, back pain, abdominal pain, flu syndrome, flatulence, diarrhea, nausea, sinusitis, rhinitis, cough

Overdosage/Toxicology Systemic toxicity low since it is not absorbed.

Pharmacodynamics/Kinetics

Onset of Action: Peak effect: Therapeutic: ~2 weeks

Half-Life Elimination: 0.05% was excreted in the urine after 1 month of chronic dosing

Excretion: Urine (0.05%) after 1 month of chronic dosing

Available Dosage Forms Tablet, as hydrochloride: 625 mg

Dosing

Adults & Elderly:

Dyslipidemia: Oral:

Monotherapy: 3 tablets twice daily with meals or 6 tablets once daily with a meal; maximum dose: 7 tablets/day

Combination therapy with an HMG-CoA reductase inhibitor: 4-6 tablets daily; maximum dose: 6 tablets/day

Administration

Oral: Administer with meal(s). Make sure patient understands dietary guidelines.

Stability

Storage: Store at room temperature. Protect from moisture.

Laboratory Monitoring Serum cholesterol, LDL, and triglyceride levels should be obtained before initiating treatment and periodically thereafter (in accordance with NCEP guidelines).

Nursing Actions

Physical Assessment: Assess other medications patient may be taking for effectiveness and interactions. Administer other medication 1 hour before or 2 hours after colesevelam. Monitor laboratory results on a regular basis during therapy. Assess knowledge/teach patient appropriate use, possible adverse reactions and appropriate interventions, and symptoms to report.

Patient Education: Take medication exactly as directed; do not alter dosage without consulting prescriber. Other medications should be taken 1 hour before or 2 hours after colesevelam. You may experience constipation (increased exercise, increased exercise, fluids, fruit, fiber, or stool softener may help). Report persistent GI upset, skeletal or muscle pain or weakness, or respiratory difficulties. **Breast-feeding precaution:** Inform prescriber if breast-feeding.

Dietary Considerations Should be taken with meal(s). Follow dietary guidelines.

Colestipol (koe LES ti pole)

U.S. Brand Names Colestid®

Synonyms Colestipol Hydrochloride

Pharmacologic Category Antilipemic Agent, Bile Acid Sequestrant

Pregnancy Risk Factor C

Lactation Not recommended

Use Adjunct in management of primary hypercholesterolemia; regression of arteriolosclerosis; relief of pruritus associated with elevated levels of bile acids; possibly used to decrease plasma half-life of digoxin in toxicity

Mechanism of Action/Effect Increases fecal loss of low density lipoprotein cholesterol

Contraindications Hypersensitivity to bile acid sequestering resins or any component of the formulation; bowel obstruction

Warnings/Precautions Not to be taken simultaneously with many other medicines (decreased absorption). May interfere with fat soluble vitamins (A, D, E, K) and folic acid. Chronic use may be associated with bleeding problems. May produce or exacerbate constipation problems; fecal impaction may occur, hemorrhoids may be worsened.

Drug Interactions

Decreased Effect: Colestipol can reduce the absorption of numerous medications when used concurrently. Give other medications 1 hour before or 4 hours after giving colestipol. Medications which may be affected include HMG-CoA reductase inhibitors, thiazide diuretics, propranolol (and potentially other beta-blockers), corticosteroids, thyroid hormones, digoxin, valproic acid, NSAIDs, loop diuretics, sulfonylureas, troglitazone (and potentially other agents in this class - pioglitazone and rosiglitazone).

Warfarin and other oral anticoagulants: Absorption is reduced by cholestyramine and may also be reduced by colestipol. Separate administration times (as detailed above).

Lab Interactions Increased prothrombin time (S); decreased cholesterol (S)

Adverse Reactions

>10%: Gastrointestinal: Constipation

1% to 10%:

Central nervous system: Headache, dizziness, anxiety, vertigo, drowsiness, fatigue

Gastrointestinal: Abdominal pain and distention, belching, flatulence, nausea, vomiting, diarrhea

Overdosage/Toxicology Symptoms of overdose include GI obstruction, nausea, and GI distress. Treatment is supportive.

Pharmacodynamics/Kinetics

Excretion: Feces

Available Dosage Forms

Granules, as hydrochloride:

5 g/7.5 g packet (30s, 90s) [unflavored]

5 g/7.5 g (300 g, 500 g) [unflavored]

5 g/7.5 g packet (60s) [contains phenylalanine 18.2 mg/7.5 g; orange flavor]

5 g/7.5 g (450 g) [contains phenylalanine 18.2 mg/7.5 g; orange flavor]

Tablet, as hydrochloride: 1 g

Dosing

Adults & Elderly: Dyslipidemia: Oral: 5-30 g/day in divided doses 2-4 times/day

Administration

Oral: Dry powder should be added to at least 90 mL of liquid and stirred until completely mixed. Other drugs should be administered at least 1 hour before or 4 hours after colestipol.

Nursing Actions

Physical Assessment: Assess other medications the patient may be taking for effectiveness and interactions. Monitor knowledge/teach patient appropriate preparation and use, possible adverse reactions, and symptoms to report. Monitor bowel function. Be alert to potential of constipation or hemorrhoid problems.

Patient Education: Take granules with 3-4 oz of water or fruit juice. Rinse glass with small amount of water to ensure full dose is taken. Take tablets one at a time. Other medications should be taken 1 hour before or 4 hours after colestipol. You may experience constipation (increased exercise, fluids, fruit, fiber, or stool softener may help); or drowsiness or dizziness (use caution when driving or engaging in tasks that require alertness until response to drug is known). Report acute gastric pain, tarry stools, or respiratory difficulty. **Pregnancy/breast-feeding precautions:** Inform prescriber if you are or intend to become pregnant. Breast-feeding is not recommended.

Dietary Considerations Granules, orange flavor, contain phenylalanine 18.2 mg/7.5 g.

Geriatric Considerations Pharmacologic treatment should be reserved for those who are unable to obtain a desirable plasma cholesterol level by diet alone and for whom the benefits of treatment are believed to outweigh the potential adverse effects, drug interactions, and cost of treatment.

Collagenase (KOL la je nase)

U.S. Brand Names Santyl®

Pharmacologic Category Enzyme, Topical Debridement

Pregnancy Risk Factor C

Lactation Excretion in breast milk unknown

Use Promotes debridement of necrotic tissue in dermal ulcers and severe burns

Orphan drug: Injection: Treatment of Peyronie's disease; treatment of Dupytren's disease

Mechanism of Action/Effect Digests collagen in injured tissue. Collagenase will not attack collagen in healthy tissue or newly formed granulation tissue. In addition, it does not act on fat, fibrin, keratin, or muscle.

Contraindications Hypersensitivity to collagenase or any component of the formulation

Warnings/Precautions For external use only. Avoid contact with eyes. Monitor debilitated patients for systemic bacterial infections because debriding enzymes may increase the risk of bacteremia.

Drug Interactions

Decreased Effect: Enzymatic activity is inhibited by detergents, benzalkonium chloride, hexachlorophene, nitrofurazone, tincture of iodine, and heavy metal ions (silver and mercury).

Adverse Reactions Frequency not defined.

Local: Irritation, Pain and burning may occur at site of application

Overdosage/Toxicology Action of enzyme may be stopped by applying Burow's solution.

Available Dosage Forms Ointment: 250 units/g (15 g, 30 g)

Dosing

Adults & Elderly: Dermal ulcers, burns: Topical: Apply once daily.

Pediatrics: Refer to adult dosing.

Administration

Topical: For external use only. Clean target area of all interfering agents listed above. If infection is persistent, apply powdered antibiotic first. Do not introduce into major body cavities. Monitor debilitated patients for systemic bacterial infections.

Nursing Actions

Physical Assessment: For external use only. Clean target area of all interfering agents (eg, detergents, benzalkonium chloride, hexachlorophene, nitrofurazone, tincture of iodine, and heavy metal ions silver and mercury). If infection is persistent, apply powdered antibiotic first. Do not introduce into major body cavities. Monitor debilitated patients for systemic bacterial infections. When applied to large areas or for extensive periods of time, monitor for adverse reactions. Teach patient (or caregiver) appropriate application (if self administered) and adverse symptoms to report.

Patient Education: Use exactly as directed; do not overuse. Clean target area of all interfering agents (eg, detergents, benzalkonium chloride, hexachlorophene, nitrofurazone, tincture of iodine, and heavy metal ions silver and mercury). Wear gloves to apply a thin film to affected area. If dressing is necessary, use a porous dressing. Avoid contact with eyes. Report increased swelling, redness, rash, itching, signs of infection, worsening of condition, or lack of healing. **Pregnancy/breast-feeding precautions:** Inform prescriber if you are or intend to become pregnant. Consult prescriber if breast-feeding.

Geriatric Considerations Preventive skin care should be instituted in all older patients at high risk for pressure ulcers. Collagenase is indicated in stage 3 and 4 pressure ulcers.

Cromolyn (KROE moe lin)

U.S. Brand Names Crolom®; Gastrocrom®; Intal®; NasalCrom® [OTC]; Opticrom®

Synonyms Cromoglycic Acid; Cromolyn Sodium; Disodium Cromoglycate; DSCG

Pharmacologic Category Mast Cell Stabilizer

Medication Safety Issues

Sound-alike/look-alike issues:

Intal® may be confused with Endal®

NasalCrom® may be confused with Nasacort®, Nasalide®

Pregnancy Risk Factor B

Lactation Excretion in breast milk unknown/use caution

Use

Inhalation: May be used as an adjunct in the prophylaxis of allergic disorders, including asthma; prevention of exercise-induced bronchospasm

Nasal: Prevention and treatment of seasonal and perennial allergic rhinitis

Oral: Systemic mastocytosis

Ophthalmic: Treatment of vernal keratoconjunctivitis, vernal conjunctivitis, and vernal keratitis

Unlabeled/Investigational Use Oral: Food allergy, treatment of inflammatory bowel disease

Mechanism of Action/Effect Prevents the mast cell release of histamine, leukotrienes and slow-reacting substance of anaphylaxis

Contraindications Hypersensitivity to cromolyn or any component of the formulation; acute asthma attacks

Warnings/Precautions Severe anaphylactic reactions may occur rarely; cromolyn is a prophylactic drug with no benefit for acute situations; caution should be used when withdrawing the drug or tapering the dose as symptoms may reoccur; use with caution in patients with a history of cardiac arrhythmias. Transient burning and stinging may occur with ophthalmic use. Dosage of oral product should be decreased with hepatic or renal dysfunction.

Adverse Reactions

Inhalation: >10%: Gastrointestinal: Unpleasant taste in mouth

Nasal:

>10%: Respiratory: Increase in sneezing, burning, stinging, or irritation inside of nose

1% to 10%:

Central nervous system: Headache

Gastrointestinal: Unpleasant taste

Respiratory: Hoarseness, cough, postnasal drip

<1% (Limited to important or life-threatening): Anaphylactic reactions, epistaxis

Ophthalmic: Frequency not defined:

Ocular: Conjunctival injection, dryness around the eye, edema, eye irritation, immediate hypersensitivity reactions, itchy eyes, puffy eyes, styes, rash, watery eyes

Respiratory: Dyspnea

Systemic: Frequency not defined:

Cardiovascular: Angioedema, chest pain, edema, flushing, palpitation, premature ventricular contractions, tachycardia

(Continued)

Cromolyn *(Continued)*

Central nervous system: Anxiety, behavior changes, convulsions, depression, dizziness, fatigue, hallucinations, headache, irritability, insomnia, lethargy, migraine, nervousness, hypoesthesia, postprandial lightheadedness, psychosis

Dermatologic: Erythema, photosensitivity, pruritus, purpura, rash, urticaria

Gastrointestinal: Abdominal pain, constipation, diarrhea, dyspepsia, dysphagia, esophagospasm, flatulence, glossitis, nausea, stomatitis, unpleasant taste, vomiting

Genitourinary: Dysuria, urinary frequency

Hematologic: Neutropenia, pancytopenia, polycythemia

Hepatic: Liver function test abnormal

Local: Burning

Neuromuscular & skeletal: Arthralgia, leg stiffness, leg weakness, myalgia, paresthesia

Otic: Tinnitus

Respiratory: Dyspnea, pharyngitis

Miscellaneous: Lupus erythematosus

Overdosage/Toxicology Symptoms of overdose include bronchospasm, laryngeal edema, and dysuria. Treat symptomatically.

Pharmacodynamics/Kinetics

Onset of Action: Onset: Response to treatment:

Nasal spray: May occur at 1-2 weeks

Ophthalmic: May be seen within a few days; treatment for up to 6 weeks is often required

Oral: May occur within 2-6 weeks

Time to Peak: Serum: Inhalation: ~15 minutes

Half-Life Elimination: 80-90 minutes

Excretion: Urine and feces (equal amounts as unchanged drug); exhaled gases (small amounts)

Available Dosage Forms

Aerosol, for oral inhalation, as sodium (Intal®): 800 mcg/inhalation (8.1 g) [112 metered inhalations; 56 doses], (14.2 g) [200 metered inhalations; 100 doses]

Solution for nebulization, as sodium (Intal®): 20 mg/2 mL (60s, 120s)

Solution, intranasal, as sodium [spray] (NasalCrom®): 40 mg/mL (13 mL, 26 mL) [5.2 mg/inhalation; contains benzalkonium chloride]

Solution, ophthalmic, as sodium (Crolom®, Opticrom®): 4% (10 mL) [contains benzalkonium chloride]

Solution, oral, as sodium (Gastrocrom®): 100 mg/5 mL (96s)

Dosing

Adults & Elderly:

Allergic rhinitis (treatment and prophylaxis): Nasal: Instill 1 spray in each nostril 3-4 times/day

Asthma: For chronic control of asthma, taper frequency to the lowest effective dose (ie, 4 times/day to 3 times/day to twice daily). **Note:** Not effective for immediate relief of symptoms in acute asthmatic attacks; must be used at regular intervals for 2-4 weeks to be effective.

Nebulization solution: Initial: 20 mg 4 times/day; usual dose: 20 mg 3-4 times/day

Metered spray: Initial: 2 inhalations 4 times/day; usual dose: 2-4 inhalations 3-4 times/day

Prophylaxis of bronchospasm (allergen- or exercise-induced):

Note: Administer 10-15 minutes prior to exercise or allergen exposure but no longer than 1 hour before:

Nebulization solution: Single dose of 20 mg

Metered spray: Single dose of 2 inhalations

Conjunctivitis and keratitis: Ophthalmic: 1-2 drops in each eye 4-6 times/day

Mastocytosis: Oral: 200 mg 4 times/day; given $1/2$ hour prior to meals and at bedtime. If control of symptoms is not seen within 2-3 weeks, dose may be increased to a maximum 40 mg/kg/day

Food allergy and inflammatory bowel disease (unlabeled use): Oral: Initial dose: 200 mg 4 times/day; may double the dose if effect is not satisfactory within 2-3 weeks; up to 400 mg 4 times/day

Pediatrics:

Allergic rhinitis (treatment and prophylaxis): Nasal: Children ≥2 years: Refer to adult dosing.

Asthma: Inhalation:

Note: For chronic control of asthma, taper frequency to the lowest effective dose (ie, 4 times/day to 3 times/day to twice daily):

Nebulization solution: Children >2 years: Initial: 20 mg 4 times/day; usual dose: 20 mg 3-4 times/day

Metered spray:

Children 5-12 years: Initial: 2 inhalations 4 times/day; usual dose: 1-2 inhalations 3-4 times/day

Children ≥12 years: Refer to adult dosing.

Prevention of allergen- or exercise-induced bronchospasm:

Note: Administer 10-15 minutes prior to exercise or allergen exposure but no longer than 1 hour before:

Nebulization solution: Children >2 years: Refer to adult dosing.

Metered spray: Children >5 years: Single dose of 2 inhalations

Systemic mastocytosis: Oral:

Children 2-12 years: Initial: 100 mg 4 times/day; not to exceed 40 mg/kg/day; given $1/2$ hour prior to meals and at bedtime

Children >12 years: Refer to adult dosing.

Food allergy and inflammatory bowel disease (unlabeled use): Oral:

Children <2 years: Not recommended

Children 2-12 years: Initial dose: 100 mg 4 times/day; may double the dose if effect is not satisfactory within 2-3 weeks; not to exceed 40 mg/kg/day

Children >12 years: Refer to adult dosing.

Note: Once desired effect is achieved, dose may be tapered to lowest effective dose

Renal Impairment: Specific guidelines not available; consider lower dose of oral product.

Hepatic Impairment: Specific guidelines not available; consider lower dose of oral product.

Administration

Oral: Oral solution: Open ampul and squeeze contents into glass of water; stir well. Administer at least 30 minutes before meals and at bedtime.

Inhalation: Oral inhalation: Shake canister gently before use; do not immerse canister in water.

Other: Nasal inhalation: Clear nasal passages by blowing nose prior to use.

Stability

Compatibility: Nebulizer solution is **compatible** with metaproterenol sulfate, isoproterenol hydrochloride, 0.25% isoetharine hydrochloride, epinephrine hydrochloride, terbutaline sulfate, and 20% acetylcysteine solution for at least 1 hour after their admixture.

Storage: Store at room temperature of 15°C to 30°C (59°F to 86°F); protect from light. Do not use oral solution if solution becomes discolored or forms a precipitate.

Laboratory Monitoring Periodic pulmonary function

Nursing Actions

Physical Assessment: This is prophylactic therapy, not to be used for acute situations. Monitor laboratory tests (long-term use) and adverse reactions. Assess knowledge/teach patient appropriate use, interventions to reduce side effects, and adverse symptoms to report.

Patient Education: Oral: Use as directed; do not increase dosage or discontinue abruptly without consulting prescriber. Take at least 30 minutes before meals. You may experience dizziness or nervousness (use caution when driving or engaging in tasks requiring alertness until response to drug is known); diarrhea (boiled milk, yogurt, or buttermilk may help); or headache or muscle pain (mild analgesic may offer relief). Report persistent insomnia; skin rash or irritation; abdominal pain or difficulty swallowing; unusual cough, bronchospasm, or respiratory difficulty; decreased urination; or if condition worsens or fails to improve. **Breast-feeding precaution:** Consult prescriber if breast-feeding.

Nebulizer: Store nebulizer solution away from light. Prepare nebulizer according to package instructions. Clear as much mucus as possible before use. Rinse mouth following each use to prevent opportunistic infection and reduce unpleasant aftertaste. Report if symptoms worsen or condition fails to improve.

Nasal: Instill 1 spray into each nostril 3-4 times a day. You may experience unpleasant taste (rinsing mouth and frequent oral care may help); or headache (mild analgesic may help). Report increased sneezing, burning, stinging, or irritation inside of nose; sore throat, hoarseness, nosebleed; anaphylactic reaction (skin rash, fever, chills, backache, respiratory difficulty, chest pain); or worsening of condition or lack of improvement.

Ophthalmic: For ophthalmic use only. Wash hands before using. Tilt head back and look upward. Put drops of suspension inside lower eyelid. Close eye and roll eyeball in all directions. Do not blink for $\frac{1}{2}$ minute. Apply gentle pressure to inner corner of eye for 30 seconds. Do not let tip of applicator touch eye; do not contaminate tip of applicator (may cause eye infection, eye damage, or vision loss). Do not share medication with anyone else. Temporary stinging or blurred vision may occur. Inform prescriber if condition worsens or fails to improve or if you experience eye pain, redness, burning, watering, dryness, double vision, puffiness around eye, vision changes, or other adverse eye response; or worsening of condition or lack of improvement. Do not wear contact lenses during treatment.

Dietary Considerations Oral: Should be taken at least 30 minutes before meals.

Geriatric Considerations Assess the patient's ability to empty capsules via the Spinhaler®. Older persons often have difficulty with inhaled and ophthalmic dosage forms.

Breast-Feeding Issues No data available on whether cromolyn enters into breast milk or clinical effects on the infant.

Pregnancy Issues Available evidence suggests safe use during pregnancy.

Adverse Reactions Frequency not defined. Topical:
Dermatologic: Pruritus, contact dermatitis, rash
Local: Local irritation
Miscellaneous: Allergic sensitivity reactions, warm sensation

Overdosage/Toxicology Symptoms of ingestion include burning sensation in mouth, irritation of the buccal, esophageal and gastric mucosa, nausea, vomiting, and abdominal pain. There is no specific antidote. General measures to eliminate the drug and reduce its absorption, combined with symptomatic treatment, are recommended.

Available Dosage Forms
Cream: 10% (60 g)
Lotion: 10% (60 mL, 480 mL)

Dosing
Adults & Elderly:
Scabies: Topical: Wash thoroughly and scrub away loose scales, then towel dry; apply a thin layer and massage drug onto skin of the entire body from the neck to the toes (with special attention to skin folds, creases, and interdigital spaces). Repeat application in 24 hours. Take a cleansing bath 48 hours after the final application. Treatment may be repeated after 7-10 days if live mites are still present.
Pruritus: Topical: Massage into affected areas until medication is completely absorbed; repeat as necessary
Pediatrics: Refer to adult dosing.

Administration
Topical: For external use only. Shake lotion well before using. Avoid contact with face, eyes, mucous membranes, and urethral meatus.

Stability
Storage: Store at room temperature.

Nursing Actions
Physical Assessment: Assess knowledge/teach patient appropriate application and use and adverse symptoms to report.
Patient Education: For topical use only. Avoid eyes. **Pregnancy/breast-feeding precautions:** Inform prescriber if you are or intend to become pregnant. Consult prescriber if breast-feeding.

When used as scabicide, apply lotion and/or cream to whole body from the chin down being sure to cover all skin folds and creases; apply a second application 24 hours later. Take a bath 48 hours after application. All contaminated clothing and bed linen should be washed to avoid reinfestation. If cure is not achieved after 2 doses, use alternative therapy.

Crotamiton (kroe TAM i tonn)

U.S. Brand Names Eurax®
Pharmacologic Category Scabicidal Agent
Medication Safety Issues
Sound-alike/look-alike issues:
Eurax® may be confused with Efudex®, Eulexin®, Evoxac™, Serax®, Urex®

Pregnancy Risk Factor C
Lactation Excretion in breast milk unknown
Use Treatment of scabies (*Sarcoptes scabiei*) and symptomatic treatment of pruritus
Mechanism of Action/Effect Mechanism of action unknown
Contraindications Hypersensitivity to crotamiton or any component of the formulation; patients who manifest a primary irritation response to topical medications
Warnings/Precautions Avoid contact with face, eyes, mucous membranes, and urethral meatus. Do not apply to acutely inflamed or raw skin. For external use only.

Cyanocobalamin (sye an oh koe BAL a min)

U.S. Brand Names Nascobal®; Twelve Resin-K
Synonyms Vitamin B_{12}
Pharmacologic Category Vitamin, Water Soluble
Pregnancy Risk Factor A/C (dose exceeding RDA recommendation); C (intranasal)
Lactation Enters breast milk/compatible
Use Treatment of pernicious anemia; vitamin B_{12} deficiency due to malabsorption diseases, inadequaste secretion of intrinisic factor, and inadequate utilization of B_{12} (eg, during neoplastic treatment); increased B_{12} requirements due to pregnancy, thyrotoxicosis, hemorrhage, malignancy, liver or kidney disease
Mechanism of Action/Effect Coenzyme for various metabolic functions, including fat and carbohydrate metabolism and protein synthesis, used in cell replication and hematopoiesis
Contraindications Hypersensitivity to cyanocobalamin or any component of the formulation, cobalt; hereditary optic nerve atrophy (Leber's disease)
(Continued)

Cyanocobalamin (Continued)

Warnings/Precautions I.M. route used to treat pernicious anemia; vitamin B_{12} deficiency for >3 months results in irreversible degenerative CNS lesions; treatment of vitamin B_{12} megaloblastic anemia may result in severe hypokalemia, sometimes fatal, due to intracellular potassium shift upon anemia resolution. B_{12} deficiency masks signs of polycythemia vera; vegetarian diets may result in B_{12} deficiency; pernicious anemia occurs more often in gastric carcinoma than in general population. Patients with Leber's disease may suffer rapid optic atrophy when treated with vitamin B_{12}; an intradermal test dose of parenteral B_{12} is recommended prior to administration of intranasal product in patients suspected of cyanocobalamin sensitivity; do not use folic acid as substitute for vitamin B_{12} in preventing anemia, as progression of spinal cord degeneration may occur; some parenteral products contain aluminum: use caution in neonates and patients with renal impairment.

Drug Interactions

Decreased Effect: Ethanol and metformin may decrease B_{12} absorption. Chloramphenicol, cholestyramine, cimetidine, colchicine, neomycin, PAS, and potassium may reduce absorption and/or effect of cyanocobalamin.

Nutritional/Ethanol Interactions Ethanol: Heavy consumption may impair vitamin B_{12} absorption.

Lab Interactions Methotrexate, pyrimethamine, and most antibiotics invalidate folic acid and vitamin B_{12} diagnostic microbiological blood assays

Adverse Reactions

>10%:
  Cardiovascular: Peripheral vascular disease
  Central nervous system: Headache (2% to 11%)
1% to 10%:
  Central nervous system: Anxiety, dizziness, pain, nervousness, hypoesthesia
  Dermatologic: Itching
  Gastrointestinal: Sore throat, nausea and vomiting, dyspepsia, diarrhea
  Neuromuscular & skeletal: Weakness (1% to 4%), back pain, arthritis, myalgia, paresthesia, abnormal gait, incoordination
  Respiratory: Dyspnea, rhinitis
  Miscellaneous: Infection
Frequency not defined: Peripheral vascular thrombosis, urticaria, anaphylaxis, CHF, pulmonary edema, polycythemia vera, transient exanthema

Pharmacodynamics/Kinetics

Protein Binding: To transcobalamin II

Metabolism: Converted in tissues to active coenzymes, methylcobalamin and deoxyadenosylcobalamin

Available Dosage Forms [DSC] = Discontinued product

Gel, intranasal (Nascobal®): 500 mcg/0.1 mL (2.3 mL) [contains benzalkonium chloride; delivers 8 doses] [DSC]

Injection, solution: 1000 mcg/mL (1 mL, 10 mL, 30 mL) [may contain benzyl alcohol and/or aluminum]

Lozenge [OTC]: 100 mcg, 250 mcg, 500 mcg

Solution, intranasal spray (Nascobal®): 500 mcg/0.1 mL actuation (2.3 mL) [contains benzalkonium chloride; delivers 8 doses]

Tablet [OTC]: 50 mcg, 100 mcg, 250 mcg, 500 mcg, 1000 mcg, 5000 mcg

Twelve Resin-K: 1000 mcg [may be used as oral, sublingual, or buccal]

Tablet, extended release [OTC]: 1500 mcg

Tablet, sublingual [OTC]: 2500 mcg

Dosing

Adults & Elderly:

Recommended daily allowance (RDA): 2.4 mcg/day
  Pregnancy: 2.6 mcg/day
  Lactation: 2.8 mcg/day

Vitamin B_{12} deficiency:
  Intranasal: 500 mcg in one nostril once weekly
  Oral: 250 mcg/day
  I.M., deep SubQ: Initial: 30 mcg/day for 5-10 days; maintenance: 100-200 mcg/month

Pernicious anemia: I.M., deep SubQ (administer concomitantly with folic acid if needed, 1 mg/day for 1 month): 100 mcg/day for 6-7 days; if improvement, administer same dose on alternate days for 7 doses, then every 3-4 days for 2-3 weeks; once hematologic values have returned to normal, maintenance dosage: 100 mcg/month. **Note:** Alternative dosing of 1000 mcg/day for 5 days (followed by 500-1000 mcg/month) has been used.

Hematologic remission (without evidence of nervous system involvement):
  Intranasal gel: 500 mcg in one nostril once weekly
  Oral: 1000-2000 mcg/day
  I.M., SubQ: 100-1000 mcg/month

Schilling test: I.M.: 1000 mcg

Pediatrics:

Recommended daily allowance (RDA): 0.9-2.4 mcg/day

Vitamin B_{12} deficiency:
  Intranasal: 500 mcg in one nostril once weekly
  Oral: 250 mcg/day
  I.M., deep SubQ: Dosage in children not well established: 0.2 mcg/kg for 2 days, followed by 1000 mcg/day for 2-7 days, followed by 100 mcg/week for one month; for malabsorptive causes of B_{12} deficiency, monthly maintenance doses of 100 mcg have been recommended **or** as an alternative 100 mcg/day for 10-15 days, then once or twice weekly for several months

Pernicious anemia: I.M., deep SubQ (administer concomitantly with folic acid if needed, 1 mg/day for 1 month): 30-50 mcg/day for 2 or more weeks (to a total dose of 1000-5000 mcg), then follow with 100 mcg/month as maintenance dosage

Administration

Oral: Not recommended due to variable absorption; however, oral therapy of 1000-2000 mcg/day has been effective for anemia if I.M./SubQ routes refused or not tolerated.

I.M.: I.M. or deep SubQ are preferred routes of administration.

I.V.: Not recommended

I.V. Detail: pH: 4.5-7.0

Other: Intranasal: Nasal spray: Prior to initial dose, activate (prime) spray nozzle by pumping unit quickly and firmly until first appearance of spray, then prime twice more. The unit must be reprimed once immediately before each use.

Stability

Compatibility: Stable in dextran 6% in dextrose, dextran 6% in NS, D_5LR, $D_5\frac{1}{4}NS$, $D_5\frac{1}{2}NS$, D_5NS, D_5W, $D_{10}W$, $D_{10}NS$, LR, $\frac{1}{2}NS$, NS

Compatibility when admixed: Incompatible with chlorpromazine, phytonadione, prochlorperazine edisylate, warfarin

Storage: Injection: Clear pink to red solutions are stable at room temperature. Protect from light.

Laboratory Monitoring Erythrocyte and reticulocyte count, hemoglobin, hematocrit; monitor potassium concentrations during early therapy

Nursing Actions

Physical Assessment: Assess effectiveness and interactions of other medications patient may be taking. Monitor laboratory tests at beginning of therapy and periodically with long-term therapy. Teach patient proper use (injection technique and needle disposal), appropriate nutritional counseling, and adverse symptoms to report.

Patient Education: Use exactly as directed. Pernicious anemia may require monthly injections for life.

Report skin rash; swelling, pain, or redness of extremities; or acute persistent diarrhea. **Pregnancy precaution:** Inform prescriber if you are pregnant.

Dietary Considerations Vegetarian diets may result in vitamin B$_{12}$ deficiency; use intranasal product at least 1 hour before or after ingestion of hot foods or liquids due to increased nasal secretions

Geriatric Considerations There exists evidence that people, particularly elderly whose serum cobalamin concentrations <500 pg/mL, should receive replacement parenteral therapy.

Cyclobenzaprine (sye kloe BEN za preen)

U.S. Brand Names Flexeril®

Synonyms Cyclobenzaprine Hydrochloride

Pharmacologic Category Skeletal Muscle Relaxant

Medication Safety Issues
Sound-alike/look-alike issues:
Cyclobenzaprine may be confused with cycloSERINE, cyproheptadine
Flexeril® may be confused with Floxin®

Pregnancy Risk Factor B

Lactation Excretion in breast milk unknown/not recommended

Use Treatment of muscle spasm associated with acute painful musculoskeletal conditions

Mechanism of Action/Effect Centrally-acting skeletal muscle relaxant pharmacologically related to tricyclic antidepressants; reduces tonic somatic motor activity influencing both alpha and gamma motor neurons

Contraindications Hypersensitivity to cyclobenzaprine or any component of the formulation; do not use concomitantly or within 14 days of MAO inhibitors; hyperthyroidism; congestive heart failure; arrhythmias; acute recovery phase of MI

Warnings/Precautions Cyclobenzaprine shares the toxic potentials of the tricyclic antidepressants and the usual precautions of tricyclic antidepressant therapy should be observed; use with caution in patients with urinary hesitancy, angle-closure glaucoma, hepatic impairment, or in the elderly. Do not use concomitantly or within 14 days after MAO inhibitors; combination may cause hypertensive crisis, severe convulsions. Safety and efficacy have not been established in patients <15 years of age.

Drug Interactions

Cytochrome P450 Effect: Substrate of CYP1A2 (major), 2D6 (minor), 3A4 (minor)

Decreased Effect: Cyclobenzaprine may decrease effect of guanethidine; effect seen with tricyclic antidepressants and guanethidine

Increased Effect/Toxicity: CYP1A2 inhibitors may increase the levels/effects of cyclobenzaprine; example inhibitors include amiodarone, ciprofloxacin, fluvoxamine, ketoconazole, norfloxacin, ofloxacin, and rofecoxib. Because of cyclobenzaprine's similarities to the tricyclic antidepressants, there may be additive toxicities and side effects similar to tricyclic antidepressants. Cyclobenzaprine's toxicity may also be additive with other agents with anticholinergic properties. Cyclobenzaprine may enhance effects of CNS depressants. Do not use concomitantly or within 14 days of MAO inhibitors. Tramadol may increase risk of seizure; effect seen with tricyclic antidepressants and tramadol.

Nutritional/Ethanol Interactions
Ethanol: Avoid ethanol (may increase CNS depression).
Herb/Nutraceutical: Avoid valerian, kava kava, gotu kola (may increase CNS depression).

Adverse Reactions
>10%:
Central nervous system: Drowsiness (29% to 39%), dizziness (1% to 11%)

Gastrointestinal: Xerostomia (21% to 32%)
1% to 10%:
Central nervous system: Fatigue (1% to 6%), confusion (1% to 3%), headache (1% to 3%), irritability (1% to 3%), mental acuity decreased (1% to 3%), nervousness (1% to 3%)
Gastrointestinal: Abdominal pain (1% to 3%), constipation (1% to 3%), diarrhea (1% to 3%), dyspepsia (1% to 3%), nausea (1% to 3%)
Neuromuscular & skeletal: Muscle weakness (1% to 3%)
Ocular: Blurred vision (1% to 3%)
Respiratory: Pharyngitis (1% to 3%)

Overdosage/Toxicology Symptoms of overdose include troubled breathing, drowsiness, syncope, seizures, tachycardia, hallucinations, and vomiting. Following initiation of essential overdose management, treatment is supportive and symptomatic.

Pharmacodynamics/Kinetics

Onset of Action: ~1 hour

Duration of Action: 12-24 hours

Time to Peak: Serum: 3-8 hours

Half-Life Elimination: 18 hours (range: 8-37 hours)

Metabolism: Hepatic via CYP3A4, 1A2, and 2D6; may undergo enterohepatic recirculation

Excretion: Urine (as inactive metabolites); feces (as unchanged drug)

Available Dosage Forms
Tablet, as hydrochloride: 5 mg, 10 mg
Flexeril®: 5 mg, 10 mg

Dosing

Adults: Muscle spasm (including spasms associated with acute temporomandibular joint pain): Oral: Initial: 5 mg 3 times/day; may increase to 10 mg 3 times/day if needed. Do not use longer than 2-3 weeks.

Elderly: Plasma concentrations and adverse effects are increased in older patients. See Geriatric Considerations.

Hepatic Impairment:
Mild: 5 mg 3 times/day; use with caution and titrate slowly.
Moderate to severe: Use not recommended.

Stability
Storage: Store at room temperature 25°C (77°F); excursions permitted to 15°C to 30°C (59°F to 86°F).

Nursing Actions

Physical Assessment: Assess effectiveness and interactions of other medications patient may be taking. Monitor effectiveness of therapy (according to rationale for therapy) and adverse reactions at beginning and periodically during therapy. Assess knowledge/teach patient appropriate use, interventions to reduce side effects (postural hypotension precautions), and adverse symptoms to report.

Patient Education: Take exactly as directed. Do not increase dose or discontinue this medication without consulting prescriber. Do not use alcohol, prescriptive or OTC antidepressants, sedatives, or pain medications without consulting prescriber. You may experience drowsiness, dizziness, lightheadedness (avoid driving or engaging in tasks that require alertness until response to drug is known); or urinary retention (void before taking medication). Report excessive drowsiness or mental agitation, chest pain, skin rash, swelling of mouth/face, difficulty speaking, ringing in ears, or blurred vision. **Breast-feeding precaution:** Breast-feeding is not recommended.

Geriatric Considerations High doses in the elderly caused drowsiness and dizziness; therefore, use the lowest dose possible. Because cyclobenzaprine causes anticholinergic effects, it may not be the skeletal muscle relaxant of choice in the elderly.

Cyclophosphamide (sye kloe FOS fa mide)

U.S. Brand Names Cytoxan®

Synonyms CPM; CTX; CYT; NSC-26271

Pharmacologic Category Antineoplastic Agent, Alkylating Agent

Medication Safety Issues

Sound-alike/look-alike issues:

Cyclophosphamide may be confused with cyclo-SPORINE, ifosfamide

Cytoxan® may be confused with cefoxitin, Centoxin®, Ciloxan®, cytarabine, CytoGam®, Cytosar®, Cytosar-U®, Cytotec®

Pregnancy Risk Factor D

Lactation Enters breast milk/contraindicated

Use

Oncologic: Treatment of Hodgkin's and non-Hodgkin's lymphoma, Burkitt's lymphoma, chronic lymphocytic leukemia (CLL), chronic myelocytic leukemia (CML), acute myelocytic leukemia (AML), acute lymphocytic leukemia (ALL), mycosis fungoides, multiple myeloma, neuroblastoma, retinoblastoma, rhabdomyosarcoma, Ewing's sarcoma; breast, testicular, endometrial, ovarian, and lung cancers, and in conditioning regimens for bone marrow transplantation

Nononcologic: Prophylaxis of rejection for kidney, heart, liver, and bone marrow transplants, severe rheumatoid disorders, nephrotic syndrome, Wegener's granulomatosis, idiopathic pulmonary hemosideroses, myasthenia gravis, multiple sclerosis, systemic lupus erythematosus, lupus nephritis, autoimmune hemolytic anemia, idiopathic thrombocytic purpura (ITP), macroglobulinemia, and antibody-induced pure red cell aplasia

Mechanism of Action/Effect Interferes with the normal function of DNA by alkylation and cross-linking the strands of DNA, and by possible protein modification; cyclophosphamide also possesses potent immunosuppressive activity; note that cyclophosphamide must be metabolized to its active form in the liver

Contraindications Hypersensitivity to cyclophosphamide or any component of the formulation; pregnancy

Warnings/Precautions Hazardous agent - use appropriate precautions for handling and disposal. Dosage adjustment needed for renal or hepatic failure.

Drug Interactions

Cytochrome P450 Effect: Substrate of CYP2A6 (minor), 2B6 (major), 2C8/9 (minor), 2C19 (minor), 3A4 (major); **Inhibits** CYP3A4 (weak); **Induces** CYP2B6 (weak), 2C8/9 (weak)

Decreased Effect: Cyclophosphamide may decrease digoxin serum levels. CYP2B6 inhibitors may decrease the levels/effects of acrolein (the active metabolite of cyclophosphamide); example inhibitors include desipramine, paroxetine, and sertraline. CYP3A4 inhibitors may decrease the levels/effects of acrolein (the active metabolite of cyclophosphamide); example inhibitors include azole antifungals, ciprofloxacin, clarithromycin, diclofenac, doxycycline, erythromycin, imatinib, isoniazid, nefazodone, nicardipine, propofol, protease inhibitors, quinidine, and verapamil.

Increased Effect/Toxicity: Allopurinol may cause an increase in bone marrow depression and may result in significant elevations of cyclophosphamide cytotoxic metabolites.

Anesthetic agents: Cyclophosphamide reduces serum pseudocholinesterase concentrations and may prolong the neuromuscular blocking activity of succinylcholine. Use with caution with halothane, nitrous oxide, and succinylcholine.

Chloramphenicol causes prolonged cyclophosphamide half-life and increased toxicity.

CYP2B6 inducers: CYP2B6 inducers may increase the levels/effects of acrolein (the active metabolite of cyclophosphamide). Example inducers include carbamazepine, nevirapine, phenobarbital, phenytoin, and rifampin.

CYP3A4 inducers: CYP3A4 inducers may increase the levels/effects of acrolein (the active metabolite of cyclophosphamide). Example inducers include aminoglutethimide, carbamazepine, nafcillin, nevirapine, phenobarbital, phenytoin, and rifamycins.

Doxorubicin: Cyclophosphamide may enhance cardiac toxicity of anthracyclines.

Tetrahydrocannabinol results in enhanced immunosuppression in animal studies.

Thiazide diuretics: Leukopenia may be prolonged.

Nutritional/Ethanol Interactions Herb/Nutraceutical: Avoid black cohosh, dong quai in estrogen-dependent tumors.

Lab Interactions Increased uric acid in serum and urine; false-positive Pap test; suppression of some skin tests

Adverse Reactions

>10%:

Dermatologic: Alopecia (40% to 60%) but hair will usually regrow although it may be a different color and/or texture. Hair loss usually begins 3-6 weeks after the start of therapy.

Endocrine & metabolic: Fertility: May cause sterility; interferes with oogenesis and spermatogenesis; may be irreversible in some patients; gonadal suppression (amenorrhea)

Gastrointestinal: Nausea and vomiting, usually beginning 6-10 hours after administration; anorexia, diarrhea, mucositis, and stomatitis are also seen

Genitourinary: Severe, potentially fatal acute hemorrhagic cystitis (7% to 40%)

Hematologic: Thrombocytopenia and anemia are less common than leukopenia

Onset: 7 days

Nadir: 10-14 days

Recovery: 21 days

1% to 10%:

Cardiovascular: Facial flushing

Central nervous system: Headache

Dermatologic: Skin rash

Renal: SIADH may occur, usually with doses >50 mg/kg (or 1 g/m^2); renal tubular necrosis, which usually resolves with discontinuation of the drug, is also reported

Respiratory: Nasal congestion occurs when I.V. doses are administered too rapidly; patients experience runny eyes, rhinorrhea, sinus congestion, and sneezing during or immediately after the infusion.

Overdosage/Toxicology Symptoms of overdose include myelosuppression, alopecia, nausea, and vomiting. Treatment is supportive.

Pharmacodynamics/Kinetics

Time to Peak: Serum: Oral: ~1 hour

Protein Binding: 10% to 56%

Half-Life Elimination: 4-8 hours

Metabolism: Hepatic to active metabolites acrolein, 4-aldophosphamide, 4-hydroperoxycyclophosphamide, and nor-nitrogen mustard

Excretion: Urine (<30% as unchanged drug, 85% to 90% as metabolites)

Available Dosage Forms

Injection, powder for reconstitution (Cytoxan®): 500 mg, 1 g, 2 g [contains mannitol 75 mg per cyclophosphamide 100 mg]

Tablet (Cytoxan®): 25 mg, 50 mg

Dosing

Adults: Refer to individual protocols.

Usual dose:

Oral: 50-100 mg/m^2/day as continuous therapy or 400-1000 mg/m^2 in divided doses over 4-5 days as intermittent therapy

I.V.:

Single doses: 400-1800 mg/m² (30-50 mg/kg) per treatment course (1-5 days) which can be repeated at 2- to 4-week intervals

Continuous daily doses: 60-120 mg/m² (1-2.5 mg/kg) per day

JRA/vasculitis: I.V.: 10 mg/kg every 2 weeks

High dose BMT:

I.V.:

60 mg/kg/day for 2 days (total dose: 120 mg/kg)

50 mg/kg/day for 4 days (total dose: 200 mg/kg)

1.8 g/m²/day for 4 days (total dose: 7.2 g/m²)

Continuous I.V.:

1.5 g/m²/24 hours for 96 hours (total dose: 6 g/m²)

1875 mg/m²/24 hours for 72 hours (total dose: 5625 mg/m²)

Note: Duration of infusion is 1-24 hours; generally combined with other high-dose chemotherapeutic drugs, lymphocyte immune globulin, or total body irradiation (TBI).

Nephrotic syndrome: Oral: 2-3 mg/kg/day every day for up to 12 weeks when corticosteroids are unsuccessful

Elderly: Refer to individual protocols: Initial and maintenance for induction: 1-2 mg/kg/day; adjust for renal clearance.

Pediatrics: Refer to individual protocols. Children:

Chemotherapy: Refer to adult dosing.

SLE: I.V.: 500-750 mg/m² every month; maximum dose: 1 g/m²

JRA/vasculitis: I.V.: Refer to adult dosing.

Nephrotic syndrome: Refer to adult dosing.

Renal Impairment: A large fraction of cyclophosphamide is eliminated by hepatic metabolism; some authors recommend no dose adjustment unless severe renal insufficiency (Cl$_{cr}$ <20 mL/minute).

Cl$_{cr}$ >10 mL/minute: Administer 100% of normal dose.

Cl$_{cr}$ <10 mL/minute: Administer 75% of normal dose.

Hemodialysis effects: Moderately dialyzable (20% to 50%)

Administer dose posthemodialysis

CAPD effects: Unknown

CAVH effects: Unknown

Hepatic Impairment: The pharmacokinetics of cyclophosphamide are not significantly altered in the presence of hepatic insufficiency. No dosage adjustments are recommended.

Administration

Oral: Tablets are not scored and should not be cut or crushed; should be administered during or after meals.

I.V.: I.P., intrapleurally, IVPB, or continuous intravenous infusion; I.V. infusions may be administered over 1-24 hours. Doses >500 mg to approximately 2 g may be administered over 20-30 minutes.

To minimize bladder toxicity, increase normal fluid intake during and for 1-2 days after cyclophosphamide dose. Most adult patients will require a fluid intake of at least 2 L/day. High-dose regimens should be accompanied by vigorous hydration with or without mesna therapy.

I.V. Detail: Slow IVP in doses ≤1 g. High-dose regimens should be accompanied by vigorous hydration with or without mesna therapy.

BMT only: Approaches to reduction of hemorrhagic cystitis include infusion of 0.9% NaCl 3 L/m²/24 hours, infusion of 0.9% NaCl 3 L/m²/24 hours with continuous 0.9% NaCl bladder irrigation 300-1000 mL/hour, and infusion of 0.9% NaCl 1.5-3 L/m²/24 hours with intravenous mesna. Hydration should begin at least 4 hours before cyclophosphamide and continue at least 24 hours after completion of cyclophosphamide. The dose of daily mesna used should equal the daily dose of cyclophosphamide. Mesna can be administered as a continuous 24-hour intravenous infusion or be given in divided doses every 4 hours. Mesna should begin at the start of treatment, and continue at least 24 hours following the last dose of cyclophosphamide.

pH: 3-9 (reconstituted solution)

Stability

Reconstitution: Reconstitute vials with SWI, NS, or D₅W to a concentration of 20 mg/mL.

Compatibility: Stable in D₅LR, D₅NS, D₅W, LR, ½NS, NS

Y-site administration: Incompatible with amphotericin B cholesteryl sulfate complex

Storage: Store intact vials of powder at room temperature of (25°C to 35°C). Reconstituted solutions are stable for 24 hours at room temperature (25°C) and 6 days under refrigeration (5°C). Further dilutions in D₅W or NS are stable for 24 hours at room temperature (25°C) and 6 days at refrigeration (5°C).

Laboratory Monitoring CBC with differential, platelet count, ESR, BUN, UA, serum electrolytes, serum creatinine

Nursing Actions

Physical Assessment: Assess other pharmacological or herbal products patient may be taking for potential interactions (eg, potential for increased or prolonged nephrotoxicity, cardiotoxicity). Note infusion specifics in Administration; including recommendations for pre- and post-hydration. Monitor infusion site to prevent extravasation. Monitor laboratory tests, therapeutic effectiveness (according to purpose for use), and adverse response (hemorrhagic cystitis, leukopenia, renal tubular necrosis) prior to each infusion and regularly during therapy. Teach patient (or caregiver) proper use (oral), possible side effects/appropriate interventions (eg, importance of adequate hydration), and adverse symptoms to report.

Patient Education: Do not take any new medication during therapy unless approved by prescriber. Take exactly as directed, during or after meals; do not take at night. Maintain adequate hydration (2-3 L/day of fluids) unless instructed to restrict fluid intake and void frequently to reduce incidence of bladder irritation. You will be more susceptible to infection (avoid crowds and exposure to infection and do not have any vaccinations without consulting prescriber). May cause loss of hair (reversible, although regrowth hair may be different color or texture); fertility or amenorrhea; nausea or vomiting (small, frequent meals, good mouth care, chewing gum, or sucking lozenges may help - if persistent consult prescriber for antiemetic); headache (consult prescriber for analgesic); nasal congestion or cold symptoms (consult prescriber for decongestant); or mouth sores (use soft toothbrush or cotton swab for oral care). Report any difficulty or pain with urination; chest pain; rapid heartbeat, or palpitations; easy bruising or bleeding; unusual rash; persistent nausea or vomiting; menstrual irregularities; swelling of extremities; respiratory difficulty; or unusual fatigue. **Pregnancy/breast-feeding precautions:** Inform prescriber if you are pregnant. Do not get pregnant during therapy. Consult prescriber for instruction on appropriate contraceptive measures. This drug may cause severe fetal defects. Do not breast-feed.

Dietary Considerations Tablets should be administered during or after meals.

Geriatric Considerations Toxicity to immunosuppressives is increased in the elderly. Start with lowest recommended adult doses. Signs of infection, such as fever and WBC rise, may not occur. Lethargy and confusion may be more prominent signs of infection; adjust dose for renal function in the elderly.

CycloSERINE (sye kloe SER een)

U.S. Brand Names Seromycin®

Pharmacologic Category Antibiotic, Miscellaneous; Antitubercular Agent

Medication Safety Issues
Sound-alike/look-alike issues:
CycloSERINE may be confused with cyclobenzaprine, cycloSPORINE

Pregnancy Risk Factor C

Lactation Enters breast milk/compatible

Use Adjunctive treatment in pulmonary or extrapulmonary tuberculosis

Unlabeled/Investigational Use Treatment of Gaucher's disease

Mechanism of Action/Effect Inhibits bacterial cell wall synthesis by competing with amino acid (D-alanine) for incorporation into the bacterial cell wall; bacteriostatic or bactericidal

Contraindications Hypersensitivity to cycloserine or any component of the formulation

Warnings/Precautions Epilepsy, depression, severe anxiety, psychosis, severe renal insufficiency, chronic alcoholism.

Drug Interactions
Increased Effect/Toxicity: Alcohol, isoniazid, and ethionamide increase toxicity of cycloserine. Cycloserine inhibits the hepatic metabolism of phenytoin and may increase risk of epileptic seizures.

Nutritional/Ethanol Interactions
Ethanol: Avoid ethanol (may increase CNS depression).
Food: May increase vitamin B_{12} and folic acid dietary requirements.

Adverse Reactions Frequency not defined.
Cardiovascular: Cardiac arrhythmia
Central nervous system: Drowsiness, headache, dizziness, vertigo, seizure, confusion, psychosis, paresis, coma
Dermatologic: Rash
Endocrine & metabolic: Vitamin B_{12} deficiency
Hematologic: Folate deficiency
Hepatic: Liver enzymes increased
Neuromuscular & skeletal: Tremor

Overdosage/Toxicology Symptoms of overdose include confusion, CNS depression, psychosis, coma, and seizures. Decontaminate with activated charcoal. Can be hemodialyzed. Management is supportive. Administer 100-300 mg/day of pyridoxine to reduce neurotoxic effects. Acute toxicity can occur with ingestion >1 g.

Pharmacodynamics/Kinetics
Time to Peak: Serum: 3-4 hours
Half-Life Elimination: Normal renal function: 10 hours
Metabolism: Hepatic
Excretion: Urine (60% to 70% as unchanged drug) within 72 hours; feces (small amounts); remainder metabolized

Available Dosage Forms Capsule: 250 mg

Dosing
Adults & Elderly: Note: Some of the neurotoxic effects may be relieved or prevented by the concomitant administration of pyridoxine.

Tuberculosis: Oral: Initial: 250 mg every 12 hours for 14 days, then give 500 mg to 1 g/day in 2 divided doses for 18-24 months (maximum daily dose: 1 g)

Pediatrics: Note: Some of the neurotoxic effects may be relieved or prevented by the concomitant administration of pyridoxine.

Tuberculosis: Oral: Children: 10-20 mg/kg/day in 2 divided doses up to 1000 mg/day for 18-24 months

Renal Impairment:
Cl_{cr} 10-50 mL/minute: Administer every 12-24 hours.

Cl_{cr} <10 mL/minute: Administer every 24 hours.

Laboratory Monitoring Periodic renal, hepatic, hematological tests, plasma cycloserine concentrations

Nursing Actions
Physical Assessment: Assess other pharmacological or herbal products patient may be taking for potential interactions. Monitor laboratory tests, therapeutic effectiveness, and adverse response (eg, CNS changes, arrhythmias, vitamin B_{12} deficiency, folate deficiency) regularly during therapy. Teach patient proper use, possible side effects/appropriate interventions (eg, importance of adequate hydration), and adverse symptoms to report.

Patient Education: Take as prescribed; do not discontinue this medication without consulting prescriber. Avoid alcohol. Maintain recommended diet and adequate hydration (2-3 L/day of fluids) unless instructed to restrict fluid intake. May cause drowsiness or restlessness (use caution when driving or engaging in tasks that require alertness until response to drug is known). Report skin rash, acute headache, tremors or changes in mentation (confusion, nightmares, depression, or suicide ideation), or fluid retention (respiratory difficulty, swelling of extremities, unusual weight gain). **Pregnancy precaution:** Inform prescriber if you are or intend to become pregnant.

Dietary Considerations May be taken with food; may increase vitamin B_{12} and folic acid dietary requirements.

Geriatric Considerations Adjust dose for renal function.

Related Information
FDA Name Differentiation Project: The Use of Tall-Man Letters *on page 12*

CycloSPORINE (SYE kloe spor een)

U.S. Brand Names Gengraf®; Neoral®; Restasis™; Sandimmune®

Synonyms CsA; CyA; Cyclosporin A

Pharmacologic Category Immunosuppressant Agent

Medication Safety Issues
Sound-alike/look-alike issues:
CycloSPORINE may be confused with cyclophosphamide, Cyklokapron®, cycloSERINE
Gengraf® may be confused with Prograf®
Neoral® may be confused with Neurontin®, Nizoral®
Sandimmune® may be confused with Sandostatin®

Pregnancy Risk Factor C

Lactation Enters breast milk/contraindicated

Use Prophylaxis of organ rejection in kidney, liver, and heart transplants, has been used with azathioprine and/or corticosteroids; severe, active rheumatoid arthritis (RA) not responsive to methotrexate alone; severe, recalcitrant plaque psoriasis in nonimmunocompromised adults unresponsive to or unable to tolerate other systemic therapy

Ophthalmic emulsion (Restasis™): Increase tear production when suppressed tear production is presumed to be due to keratoconjunctivitis sicca-associated ocular inflammation (in patients not already using topical anti-inflammatory drugs or punctal plugs)

Unlabeled/Investigational Use Short-term, high-dose cyclosporine as a modulator of multidrug resistance in cancer treatment; allogenic bone marrow transplants for prevention and treatment of graft-versus-host disease; also used in some cases of severe autoimmune disease (ie, SLE, myasthenia gravis) that are resistant to corticosteroids and other therapy; focal segmental glomerulosclerosis

Mechanism of Action/Effect Inhibits T-lymphocytes and lymphokine production and release in a reversible manner.

Contraindications Hypersensitivity to cyclosporine or any component of the formulation. Rheumatoid arthritis and psoriasis: Abnormal renal function, uncontrolled hypertension, malignancies. Concomitant treatment with PUVA or UVB therapy, methotrexate, other immunosuppressive agents, coal tar, or radiation therapy are also contraindications for use in patients with psoriasis. Ophthalmic emulsion is contraindicated in patients with active ocular infections.

Warnings/Precautions Dose-related risk of nephrotoxicity and hepatotoxicity; monitor. Use caution with other potentially nephrotoxic drugs. Increased risk of lymphomas and other malignancies. Increased risk of infection. May cause hypertension. Use caution when changing dosage forms. Monitor cyclosporine concentrations closely following the addition, modification, or deletion of other medications; live, attenuated vaccines may be less effective; use should be avoided.

Transplant patients: May cause significant hyperkalemia and hyperuricemia, seizures (particularly if used with high dose corticosteroids), and encephalopathy. To avoid toxicity or possible organ rejection, make dose adjustments based on cyclosporine blood concentrations. Anaphylaxis has been reported with I.V. use; reserve for patients who cannot take oral form.

Psoriasis: Patients should avoid excessive sun exposure. Safety and efficacy in children <18 have not been established.

Rheumatoid arthritis: Safety and efficacy for use in juvenile rheumatoid arthritis have not been established. If receiving other immunosuppressive agents, radiation or UV therapy, concurrent use of cyclosporine is not recommended.

Ophthalmic emulsion: Has not been studied in patients with a history of herpes keratitis. Safety and efficacy have not been established in patients <16 years of age.

Products may contain corn oil, castor oil, ethanol, or propylene glycol; injection also contains Cremophor® EL (polyoxyethylated castor oil), which has been associated with rare anaphylactic reactions.

Drug Interactions

Cytochrome P450 Effect: Substrate of CYP3A4 (major); **Inhibits** CYP2C8/9 (weak), 3A4 (moderate)

Decreased Effect: Isoniazid and ticlopidine decrease cyclosporine concentrations. The levels/effects of cyclosporine may be decreased by aminoglutethimide, carbamazepine, nafcillin, nevirapine, phenobarbital, phenytoin, rifamycins, and other CYP3A4 inducers. Orlistat may decrease absorption of cyclosporine; avoid concomitant use. Vaccination may be less effective; avoid use of live vaccines during therapy. Sulfinpyrazone may decrease cyclosporine levels.

Increased Effect/Toxicity: The levels/effects of cyclosporine may be increased by allopurinol, azole antifungals, clarithromycin, diclofenac, doxycycline, erythromycin, imatinib, isoniazid, metoclopramide, nefazodone, nicardipine, octreotide, oral contraceptives (hormonal), propofol, protease inhibitors, quinidine, telithromycin, verapamil, and other CYP3A4 inhibitors. Cyclosporine (modified) may increase the levels/effects of sirolimus. Cyclosporine may increase the levels/effects of selected benzodiazepines, calcium channel blockers, cisapride, cyclosporine, ergot alkaloids, selected HMG-CoA reductase inhibitors, mesoridazine, mirtazapine, nateglinide, nefazodone, pimozide, prednisolone (dosage adjustment may be required), quinidine, sildenafil (and other PDE-5 inhibitors), tacrolimus, thioridazine, venlafaxine, and other CYP3A4 substrates. Drugs that enhance nephrotoxicity of cyclosporine include aminoglycosides, amphotericin B, acyclovir, cimetidine, ketoconazole, lovastatin, melphalan, NSAIDs, ranitidine, and trimethoprim and sulfamethoxazole.

Cyclosporine increases toxicity of digoxin, diuretics, methotrexate, nifedipine. Fibric acid derivatives may increase the risk of renal dysfunction and may alter CSA concentrations. Concurrent therapy with sirolimus may increase the risk of HUS/TTP/TMA.

Nutritional/Ethanol Interactions

Food: Grapefruit juice increases absorption; unsupervised use should be avoided.

Herb/Nutraceutical: Avoid St John's wort; as an enzyme inducer, it may increase the metabolism of and decrease plasma levels of cyclosporine; organ rejection and graft loss have been reported. Avoid cat's claw, echinacea (have immunostimulant properties).

Lab Interactions Specific whole blood, HPLC assay for cyclosporine may be falsely elevated if sample is drawn from the same line through which dose was administered (even if flush has been administered and/or dose was given hours before).

Adverse Reactions Adverse reactions reported with systemic use, including rheumatoid arthritis, psoriasis, and transplantation (kidney, liver, and heart). Percentages noted include the highest frequency regardless of indication/dosage. Frequencies may vary for specific conditions or formulation.

>10%:
Cardiovascular: Hypertension (8% to 53%), edema (5% to 14%)
Central nervous system: Headache (2% to 25%)
Dermatologic: Hirsutism (21% to 45%), hypertrichosis (5% to 19%)
Endocrine & metabolic: Triglycerides increased (15%), female reproductive disorder (9% to 11%)
Gastrointestinal: Nausea (23%), diarrhea (3% to 13%), gum hyperplasia (2% to 16%), abdominal discomfort (<1% to 15%), dyspepsia (2% to 12%)
Neuromuscular & skeletal: Tremor (7% to 55%), paresthesia (1% to 11%), leg cramps/muscle contractions (2% to 12%)
Renal: Renal dysfunction/nephropathy (10% to 38%), creatinine increased (16% to ≥50%)
Respiratory: Upper respiratory infection (1% to 14%)
Miscellaneous: Infection (3% to 25%)

Kidney, liver, and heart transplant only (≤2% unless otherwise noted):
Cardiovascular: Flushes (<1% to 4%), MI
Central nervous system: Convulsions (1% to 5%), anxiety, confusion, fever, lethargy
Dermatologic: Acne (1% to 6%), brittle fingernails, hair breaking, pruritus
Endocrine & metabolic: Gynecomastia (<1% to 4%), hyperglycemia
Gastrointestinal: Nausea (2% to 10%), vomiting (2% to 10%), diarrhea (3% to 8%), abdominal discomfort (<1% to 7%), cramps (0% to 4%), anorexia, constipation, gastritis, mouth sores, pancreatitis, swallowing difficulty, upper GI bleed, weight loss
Hematologic: Leukopenia (<1% to 6%), anemia, thrombocytopenia
Hepatic: Hepatotoxicity (<1% to 7%)
Neuromuscular & skeletal: Paresthesia (1% to 3%), joint pain, muscle pain, tingling, weakness
Ocular: Conjunctivitis, visual disturbance
Otic: Hearing loss, tinnitus
Renal: Hematuria
Respiratory: Sinusitis (<1% to 7%)
Miscellaneous: Lymphoma (<1% to 6%), allergic reactions, hiccups, night sweats

Rheumatoid arthritis only (1% to <3% unless otherwise noted):
Cardiovascular: Hypertension (8%), edema (5%), chest pain (4%), arrhythmia (2%), abnormal heart sounds, cardiac failure, MI, peripheral ischemia
Central nervous system: Dizziness (8%), pain (6%), insomnia (4%), depression (3%), migraine (2%), anxiety, hypoesthesia, emotional lability, impaired
(Continued)

CycloSPORINE *(Continued)*

concentration, malaise, nervousness, paranoia, somnolence, vertigo

Dermatologic: Purpura (3%), abnormal pigmentation, angioedema, cellulitis, dermatitis, dry skin, eczema, folliculitis, nail disorder, pruritus, skin disorder, urticaria

Endocrine & metabolic: Menstrual disorder (3%), breast fibroadenosis, breast pain, diabetes mellitus, goiter, hot flashes, hyperkalemia, hyperuricemia, hypoglycemia, libido increased/decreased

Gastrointestinal: Vomiting (9%), flatulence (5%), gingivitis (4%), gum hyperplasia (2%), constipation, dry mouth, dysphagia, enanthema, eructation, esophagitis, gastric ulcer, gastritis, gastroenteritis, gingival bleeding, glossitis, peptic ulcer, salivary gland enlargement, taste perversion, tongue disorder, tooth disorder, weight loss/gain

Genitourinary: Leukorrhea (1%), abnormal urine, micturition urgency, nocturia, polyuria, pyelonephritis, urinary incontinence, uterine hemorrhage

Hematologic: Anemia, leukopenia

Hepatic: Bilirubinemia

Neuromuscular & skeletal: Paresthesia (8%), tremor (8%), leg cramps/muscle contractions (2%), arthralgia, bone fracture, joint dislocation, myalgia, neuropathy, stiffness, synovial cyst, tendon disorder, weakness

Ocular: Abnormal vision, cataract, conjunctivitis, eye pain

Otic: Tinnitus, deafness, vestibular disorder

Renal: Increased BUN, hematuria, renal abscess

Respiratory: Cough (5%), dyspnea (5%), sinusitis (4%), abnormal chest sounds, bronchospasm, epistaxis

Miscellaneous: Infection (9%), abscess, allergy, bacterial infection, carcinoma, fungal infection, herpes simplex, herpes zoster, lymphadenopathy, moniliasis, diaphoresis increased, tonsillitis, viral infection

Psoriasis only (1% to <3% unless otherwise noted):

Cardiovascular: Chest pain, flushes

Central nervous system: Psychiatric events (4% to 5%), pain (3% to 4%), dizziness, fever, insomnia, nervousness, vertigo

Dermatologic: Hypertrichosis (5% to 7%), acne, dry skin, folliculitis, keratosis, pruritus, rash, skin malignancies

Endocrine & metabolic: Hot flashes

Gastrointestinal: Nausea (5% to 6%), diarrhea (5% to 6%), gum hyperplasia (4% to 6%), abdominal discomfort (3% to 6%), dyspepsia (2% to 3%), abdominal distention, appetite increased, constipation, gingival bleeding

Genitourinary: Micturition increased

Hematologic: Bleeding disorder, clotting disorder, platelet disorder, red blood cell disorder

Hepatic: Hyperbilirubinemia

Neuromuscular & skeletal: Paresthesia (5% to 7%), arthralgia (1% to 6%)

Ocular: Abnormal vision

Respiratory: Bronchospasm (5%), cough (5%), dyspnea (5%), rhinitis (5%), respiratory infection

Miscellaneous: Flu-like symptoms (8% to 10%)

Ophthalmic emulsion (Restasis™):

>10%: Ocular: Burning (17%)

1% to 10%: Ocular: Hyperemia (conjunctival 5%), eye pain, pruritus, stinging

Overdosage/Toxicology Symptoms of overdose include hepatotoxicity, nephrotoxicity, nausea, vomiting, tremor. CNS secondary to direct action of the drug may not be reflected in serum concentrations, may be more predictable by renal magnesium loss. Forced emesis may be beneficial if done within 2 hours of ingestion of cyclosporine capsules (modified). Treatment is symptomatic and supportive. Cyclosporine is not dialyzable.

Pharmacodynamics/Kinetics

Time to Peak: Serum: Oral:

Cyclosporine (non-modified): 2-6 hours; some patients have a second peak at 5-6 hours

Cyclosporine (modified): Renal transplant: 1.5-2 hours

Protein Binding: 90% to 98% to lipoproteins

Half-Life Elimination: Oral: May be prolonged with hepatic impairment and shorter in pediatric patients due to the higher metabolism rate

Cyclosporine (non-modified): Biphasic: Alpha: 1.4 hours; Terminal: 19 hours (range: 10-27 hours)

Cyclosporine (modified): Biphasic: Terminal: 8.4 hours (range: 5-18 hours)

Metabolism: Extensively hepatic via CYP; forms at least 25 metabolites; extensive first-pass effect following oral administration

Excretion: Primarily feces; urine (6%, 0.1% as unchanged drug and metabolites)

Available Dosage Forms

Capsule, soft gel, modified: 25 mg, 100 mg [contains castor oil, ethanol]

Gengraf®: 25 mg, 100 mg [contains ethanol, castor oil, propylene glycol]

Neoral®: 25 mg, 100 mg [contains dehydrated ethanol, corn oil, castor oil, propylene glycol]

Capsule, soft gel, non-modified (Sandimmune®): 25 mg, 100 mg [contains dehydrated ethanol, corn oil]

Emulsion, ophthalmic [preservative free, single-use vial] (Restasis™): 0.05% (0.4 mL) [contains glycerin, castor oil, polysorbate 80, carbomer 1342; 32 vials/box]

Injection, solution, non-modified (Sandimmune®): 50 mg/mL (5 mL) [contains Cremophor® EL (polyoxyethylated castor oil), ethanol]

Solution, oral, modified:

Gengraf®: 100 mg/mL (50 mL) [contains castor oil, propylene glycol]

Neoral®: 100 mg/mL (50 mL) [contains dehydrated ethanol, corn oil, castor oil, propylene glycol]

Solution, oral, non-modified (Sandimmune®): 100 mg/mL (50 mL) [contains olive oil, ethanol]

Dosing

Adults: Note: Neoral® and Sandimmune® are not bioequivalent and cannot be used interchangeably

Newly-transplanted patients: Adjunct therapy with corticosteroids is recommended. Initial dose should be given 4-12 hours prior to transplant or may be given postoperatively; adjust initial dose to achieve desired plasma concentration.

Oral: Dose is dependent upon type of transplant and formulation:

Cyclosporine (modified):

Renal: 9 ± 3 mg/kg/day, divided twice daily

Liver: 8 ± 4 mg/kg/day, divided twice daily

Heart: 7 ± 3 mg/kg/day, divided twice daily

Cyclosporine (non-modified): Initial dose: 15 mg/kg/day as a single dose (range 14-18 mg/kg); lower doses of 10-14 mg/kg/day have been used for renal transplants. Continue initial dose daily for 1-2 weeks; taper by 5% per week to a maintenance dose of 5-10 mg/kg/day; some renal transplant patients may be dosed as low as 3 mg/kg/day

Note: When using the non-modified formulation, cyclosporine levels may increase in liver transplant patients when the T-tube is closed; dose may need decreased

I.V.: Manufacturer's labeling: Cyclosporine (non-modified): Initial dose: 5-6 mg/kg/day as a single dose (¹/₃ the oral dose), infused over 2-6 hours; use should be limited to patients unable to take capsules or oral solution; patients should be switched to an oral dosage form as soon as possible

Note: Many transplant centers administer cyclosporine as "divided dose" infusions (in 2-3 doses/day) or as a continuous (24-hour) infusion; dosages range from 3-7.5 mg/kg/day. Specific institutional protocols should be consulted.

Note: Conversion to cyclosporine (modified) from cyclosporine (non-modified): Start with daily dose previously used and adjust to obtain preconversion cyclosporine trough concentration. Plasma concentrations should be monitored every 4-7 days and dose adjusted as necessary, until desired trough level is obtained. When transferring patients with previously poor absorption of cyclosporine (non-modified), monitor trough levels at least twice weekly (especially if initial dose exceeds 10 mg/kg/day); high plasma levels are likely to occur.

Rheumatoid arthritis: Oral: Cyclosporine (modified): Initial dose: 2.5 mg/kg/day, divided twice daily; salicylates, NSAIDs, and oral glucocorticoids may be continued (refer to Drug Interactions); dose may be increased by 0.5-0.75 mg/kg/day if insufficient response is seen after 8 weeks of treatment; additional dosage increases may be made again at 12 weeks (maximum dose: 4 mg/kg/day). Discontinue if no benefit is seen by 16 weeks of therapy.

Note: Increase the frequency of blood pressure monitoring after each alteration in dosage of cyclosporine. Cyclosporine dosage should be decreased by 25% to 50% in patients with no history of hypertension who develop sustained hypertension during therapy and, if hypertension persists, treatment with cyclosporine should be discontinued.

Psoriasis: Oral: Cyclosporine (modified): Initial dose: 2.5 mg/kg/day, divided twice daily; dose may be increased by 0.5 mg/kg/day if insufficient response is seen after 4 weeks of treatment; additional dosage increases may be made every 2 weeks if needed (maximum dose: 4 mg/kg/day). Discontinue if no benefit is seen by 6 weeks of therapy. Once patients are adequately controlled, the dose should be decreased to the lowest effective dose. Doses <2.5 mg/kg/day may be effective. Treatment longer than 1 year is not recommended.

Note: Increase the frequency of blood pressure monitoring after each alteration in dosage of cyclosporine. Cyclosporine dosage should be decreased by 25% to 50% in patients with no history of hypertension who develop sustained hypertension during therapy and, if hypertension persists, treatment with cyclosporine should be discontinued.

Focal segmental glomerulosclerosis: Initial: 3 mg/kg/day divided every 12 hours

Autoimmune diseases: 1-3 mg/kg/day

Keratoconjunctivitis sicca: Ophthalmic: Instill 1 drop in each eye every 12 hours

Elderly: Refer to adult dosing (**Note:** Sandimmune® and Neoral® are not bioequivalent and cannot be used interchangeably without physician supervision).

Pediatrics: Transplant: Refer to adult dosing; children may require, and are able to tolerate, larger doses than adults.

Renal Impairment: For severe psoriasis:

Serum creatinine levels ≥25% above pretreatment levels: Take another sample within 2 weeks; if the level remains ≥25% above pretreatment levels, decrease dosage of cyclosporine (modified) by 25% to 50%. If two dosage adjustments do not reverse the increase in serum creatinine, treatment should be discontinued.

Serum creatinine levels ≥50% above pretreatment levels: Decrease cyclosporine dosage by 25% to 50%. If two dosage adjustments do not

reverse the increase in serum creatinine levels, treatment should be discontinued.

Hemodialysis: Supplemental dose is not necessary.

Peritoneal dialysis: Supplemental dose is not necessary.

Hepatic Impairment: Dosage adjustment is probably necessary; monitor levels closely

Administration

Oral: Oral solution: Do not administer liquid from plastic or styrofoam cup. May dilute Neoral® oral solution with orange juice or apple juice. May dilute Sandimmune® oral solution with milk, chocolate milk, or orange juice. Avoid changing diluents frequently. Mix thoroughly and drink at once. Use syringe provided to measure dose. Mix in a glass container and rinse container with more diluent to ensure total dose is taken. Do not rinse syringe before or after use (may cause dose variation).

I.V.: The manufacturer recommends that following dilution, intravenous admixture be administered over 2-6 hours. However, many transplant centers administer as divided doses (2-3 doses/day) or as a 24-hour continuous infusion. Patients should be under continuous observation for at least the first 30 minutes of the infusion, and should be monitored frequently thereafter.

I.V. Detail: Anaphylaxis has been reported with I.V. use; reserve for patients who cannot take oral form. Patients should be under continuous observation for at least the first 30 minutes of the infusion, and should be monitored frequently thereafter. Maintain patent airway; other supportive measures and agents for treating anaphylaxis should be present when I.V. drug is given. Discard solution after 24 hours.

Other: Ophthalmic emulsion: Prior to use, invert vial several times to obtain a uniform emulsion. Remove contact lenses prior to instillation of drops; may be reinserted 15 minutes after administration. May be used with artificial tears; allow 15 minute interval between products.

Stability

Reconstitution:

Sandimmune® injection: Injection should be further diluted [1 mL (50 mg) of concentrate in 20-100 mL of D_5W or NS] for administration by intravenous infusion. Light protection is not required for intravenous admixtures of cyclosporine.

Stability of injection of parenteral admixture at room temperature (25°C) is 6 hours in PVC; 24 hours in Excel®, PAB® containers, or glass.

Polyoxyethylated castor oil (Cremophor® EL) surfactant in cyclosporine injection may leach phthalate from PVC containers such as bags and tubing. The actual amount of diethylhexyl phthalate (DEHP) plasticizer leached from PVC containers and administration sets may vary in clinical situations, depending on surfactant concentration, bag size, and contact time.

Compatibility: Stable in D_5W, fat emulsion 10%, fat emulsion 20%, NS

Y-site administration: Incompatible with amphotericin B cholesteryl sulfate complex

Compatibility when admixed: Incompatible with magnesium sulfate

Storage:

Capsule: Store at controlled room temperature

Injection: Store at controlled room temperature; do not refrigerate. Ampuls should be protected from light.

Ophthalmic emulsion: Store at 15°C to 25°C (59°F to 77°F). Vials are single-use; discard immediately following administration.

Oral solution: Store at controlled room temperature; do not refrigerate. Use within 2 months after opening; should be mixed in glass containers.

Laboratory Monitoring Cyclosporine levels, serum electrolytes, renal function, hepatic function

(Continued)

CycloSPORINE *(Continued)*

Nursing Actions

Physical Assessment: Assess effectiveness and interactions of other medications patient may be taking. Monitor kidney and hepatic function closely. Monitor blood pressure periodically while taking this medication. Monitor laboratory tests, therapeutic response, and adverse reactions at beginning of therapy and periodically throughout therapy, especially opportunistic infection (eg, fever, mouth and vaginal sores or plaques, unhealed wounds). **I.V.:** Monitor closely for first 30 minutes of infusion and frequently thereafter to assess for adverse reactions (CNS changes or hypertension). **Oral:** Teach patient appropriate administration, possible side effects, and symptoms to report.

Patient Education: Oral: Take dose at the same time each day. You will be susceptible to infection (avoid crowds and exposure to infection and do not have any vaccinations without consulting prescriber). Practice good oral hygiene to reduce gum inflammation; see a dentist regularly during treatment. Report severe headache; unusual hair growth or deepening of voice; mouth sores or swollen gums; persistent nausea, vomiting, or abdominal pain; muscle pain or cramping; tremors; unusual swelling of extremities, weight gain, or change in urination; or chest pain or rapid heartbeat. Increase in blood pressure or damage to the kidney is possible. Your prescriber will need to monitor you closely. Do not change one brand of cyclosporine for another; any changes must be done by your prescriber. If you are taking this medication for psoriasis, your risk of cancer may be increased when taking additional medications. **Oral solution:** Diluting oral solution improves flavor. Dilute Neoral® with orange juice or apple juice. Dilute Sandimmune® with milk, chocolate milk, or orange juice. Avoid changing what you mix with your cyclosporine. Mix thoroughly and drink at once. Use syringe provided to measure dose. Mix in a glass container (do not use plastic or styrofoam) and rinse container with more juice/milk to ensure total dose is taken. Do not rinse syringe before or after use (may cause dose variation). **Pregnancy/ breast-feeding precautions:** Inform prescriber if you are or intend to become pregnant. Do not breast-feed.

Dietary Considerations Administer this medication consistently with relation to time of day and meals.

Pregnancy Issues Cyclosporine crosses the placenta. Based on clinical use, premature births and low birth weight were consistently observed. Use only if the benefit to the mother outweighs the possible risks to the fetus.

Additional Information Cyclosporine (modified): Refers to the capsule dosage formulation of cyclosporine in an aqueous dispersion (previously referred to as "microemulsion"). Cyclosporine (modified) has increased bioavailability as compared to cyclosporine (non-modified) and cannot be used interchangeably without close monitoring.

Related Information

FDA Name Differentiation Project: The Use of Tall-Man Letters *on page 12*
Peak and Trough Guidelines *on page 1387*

Cyproheptadine *(si proe HEP ta deen)*

Synonyms Cyproheptadine Hydrochloride; Periactin
Pharmacologic Category Antihistamine
Medication Safety Issues
Sound-alike/look-alike issues:
Cyproheptadine may be confused with cyclobenzaprine
Periactin may be confused with Perative®, Percodan®, Persantine®

Pregnancy Risk Factor B
Lactation Excretion in breast milk unknown/contraindicated
Use Perennial and seasonal allergic rhinitis and other allergic symptoms including urticaria
Unlabeled/Investigational Use Appetite stimulation, blepharospasm, cluster headaches, migraine headaches, Nelson's syndrome, pruritus, schizophrenia, spinal cord damage associated spasticity, and tardive dyskinesia
Mechanism of Action/Effect A potent antihistamine and serotonin antagonist
Contraindications Hypersensitivity to cyproheptadine or any component of the formulation; narrow-angle glaucoma; bladder neck obstruction; acute asthmatic attack; stenosing peptic ulcer; GI tract obstruction; concurrent use of MAO inhibitors; avoid use in premature and term newborns due to potential association with SIDS
Warnings/Precautions Do not use in the presence of symptomatic prostate hypertrophy. Antihistamines are more likely to cause dizziness, excessive sedation, syncope, toxic confusion states, and hypotension in the elderly. In case reports, cyproheptadine has promoted weight gain in anorexic adults, though it has not been specifically studied in the elderly. All cases of weight loss or decreased appetite should be adequately assessed.

Drug Interactions

Increased Effect/Toxicity: Cyproheptadine may potentiate the effect of CNS depressants. MAO inhibitors may cause hallucinations when taken with cyproheptadine.
Nutritional/Ethanol Interactions Ethanol: Avoid ethanol (may increase CNS sedation).
Lab Interactions Diagnostic antigen skin tests; increased amylases (S); decreased fasting glucose (S)

Adverse Reactions

>10%:
Central nervous system: Slight to moderate drowsiness
Respiratory: Thickening of bronchial secretions
1% to 10%:
Central nervous system: Headache, fatigue, nervousness, dizziness
Gastrointestinal: Appetite stimulation, nausea, diarrhea, abdominal pain, xerostomia
Neuromuscular & skeletal: Arthralgia
Respiratory: Pharyngitis

Overdosage/Toxicology Symptoms of overdose include CNS depression or stimulation, dry mouth, flushed skin, fixed and dilated pupils, and apnea. There is no specific treatment for antihistamine overdose. Clinical toxicity is due to blockade of cholinergic receptors. For anticholinergic overdose with severe life-threatening symptoms, physostigmine 1-2 mg I.V. slowly, may be given to reverse these effects.

Pharmacodynamics/Kinetics

Metabolism: Almost completely hepatic
Excretion: Urine (>50% primarily as metabolites); feces (~25%)

Available Dosage Forms

Syrup, as hydrochloride: 2 mg/5 mL (473 mL) [contains alcohol 5%; mint flavor]
Tablet, as hydrochloride: 4 mg

Dosing

Adults:
Appetite stimulation (including anorexia nervosa): Oral: 2 mg 4 times/day; may be increased gradually over a 3-week period to 8 mg 4 times/day
Allergic conditions: Oral: 4-20 mg/day divided every 8 hours (not to exceed 0.5 mg/kg/day)
Cluster headaches: Oral: 4 mg 4 times/day
Migraine headaches: Oral: 4-8 mg 3 times/day
Spasticity associated with spinal cord damage: Oral: 4 mg at bedtime; increase by a 4 mg dose

every 3-4 days; average daily dose: 16 mg in divided doses; not to exceed 36 mg/day

Elderly: Oral: Initial: 4 mg twice daily

Pediatrics:

Allergic conditions: Oral: Children: 0.25 mg/kg/day or 8 mg/m²/day in 2-3 divided doses **or**

2-6 years: 2 mg every 8-12 hours (not to exceed 12 mg/day)

7-14 years: 4 mg every 8-12 hours (not to exceed 16 mg/day)

Migraine headaches: 4 mg 2-3 times/day

Spasticity associated with spinal cord damage: Oral: Children ≥12 years: Refer to adult dosing.

Appetite stimulation (Including anorexia nervosa): Children >13 years: Refer to adult dosing.

Hepatic Impairment: Dosage should be reduced in patients with significant hepatic dysfunction.

Nursing Actions

Physical Assessment: Assess effectiveness and interactions of other medications patient may be taking. Monitor weight periodically. Monitor effectiveness of therapy and adverse reactions (eg, excess anticholinergic effects) at beginning of therapy and periodically with long-term use. Assess knowledge/teach patient appropriate use, interventions to reduce side effects, and adverse symptoms to report.

Patient Education: Take as directed; do not exceed recommended dose. Avoid use of other depressants, alcohol, or sleep-inducing medications unless approved by prescriber. You may experience drowsiness or dizziness (use caution when driving or engaging in tasks requiring alertness until response to drug is known); or dry mouth, nausea, or abdominal pain (small frequent meals, frequent mouth care, chewing gum, or sucking hard candy may help). Report persistent sedation, confusion, or agitation; changes in urinary pattern; blurred vision; chest pain or palpitations; sore throat respiratory difficulty or expectorating (thick secretions); significant change in weight; or lack of improvement or worsening or condition. **Breast-feeding precaution:** Do not breast-feed.

Geriatric Considerations Elderly may not tolerate anticholinergic effects.

Additional Information May stimulate appetite; in case reports, cyproheptadine has promoted weight gain in anorexic adults.

Cytarabine (sye TARE a been)

U.S. Brand Names Cytosar-U®

Synonyms Arabinosylcytosine; Ara-C; Cytarabine Hydrochloride; Cytosine Arabinosine Hydrochloride; NSC-63878

Pharmacologic Category Antineoplastic Agent, Antimetabolite

Medication Safety Issues

Sound-alike/look-alike issues:

Cytarabine may be confused with Cytadren®, Cytosar®, Cytoxan®, vidarabine

Cytosar-U® may be confused with cytarabine, Cytovene®, Cytoxan®, Neosar®

Pregnancy Risk Factor D

Lactation Excretion in breast milk unknown/not recommended

Use Cytarabine is one of the most active agents in leukemia; also active against lymphoma, meningeal leukemia, and meningeal lymphoma; has little use in the treatment of solid tumors

Mechanism of Action/Effect Inhibition of DNA synthesis in S Phase of cell division; degree of its cytotoxicity correlates linearly with its incorporation into DNA, therefore, incorporation into the DNA is responsible for drug activity and toxicity

Contraindications Hypersensitivity to cytarabine or any component of the formulation

Warnings/Precautions The U.S. Food and Drug Administration (FDA) currently recommends that procedures for proper handling and disposal of antineoplastic agents be considered. Use with caution in patients with impaired renal and hepatic function.

Drug Interactions

Decreased Effect: Decreased effect of gentamicin, flucytosine. Decreased digoxin oral tablet absorption.

Increased Effect/Toxicity: Alkylating agents and radiation and purine analogs when coadministered with cytarabine may result in increased toxic effects. Methotrexate, when administered prior to cytarabine, may enhance the efficacy and toxicity of cytarabine; some combination treatment regimens (eg, hyper-CVAD) have been designed to take advantage of this interaction.

Adverse Reactions

>10%:

Central nervous system: Fever (>80%)

Dermatologic: Alopecia

Gastrointestinal: Nausea, vomiting, diarrhea, and mucositis which subside quickly after discontinuing the drug; GI effects may be more pronounced with divided I.V. bolus doses than with continuous infusion

Hematologic: Myelosuppression; neutropenia and thrombocytopenia are severe, anemia may also occur

Onset: 4-7 days

Nadir: 14-18 days

Recovery: 21-28 days

Hepatic: Hepatic dysfunction, mild jaundice, transaminases increased (acute)

Ocular: Tearing, ocular pain, foreign body sensation, photophobia, and blurred vision may occur with high-dose therapy; ophthalmic corticosteroids usually prevent or relieve the condition

1% to 10%:

Cardiovascular: Thrombophlebitis, cardiomegaly

Central nervous system: Dizziness, headache, somnolence, confusion, malaise; a severe cerebellar toxicity occurs in about 8% of patients receiving a high dose (>36-48 g/m²/cycle); it is irreversible or fatal in about 1%

Dermatologic: Skin freckling, itching, cellulitis at injection site; rash, pain, erythema, and skin sloughing of the palmar and plantar surfaces may occur with high-dose therapy. Prophylactic topical steroids and/or skin moisturizers may be useful.

Genitourinary: Urinary retention

Neuromuscular & skeletal: Myalgia, bone pain

Respiratory: Syndrome of sudden respiratory distress, including tachypnea, hypoxemia, interstitial and alveolar infiltrates progressing to pulmonary edema, pneumonia

Overdosage/Toxicology Symptoms of overdose include myelosuppression, megaloblastosis, nausea, vomiting, respiratory distress, and pulmonary edema. A syndrome of sudden respiratory distress progressing to pulmonary edema and cardiomegaly has been reported following high doses. Treatment is symptomatic and supportive.

Pharmacodynamics/Kinetics

Half-Life Elimination: Initial: 7-20 minutes; Terminal: 0.5-2.6 hours

Metabolism: Primarily hepatic; aracytidine triphosphate is the active moiety; about 86% to 96% of dose is metabolized to inactive uracil arabinoside

Excretion: Urine (~80% as metabolites) within 24-36 hours

Available Dosage Forms

Injection, powder for reconstitution: 100 mg, 500 mg, 1 g, 2 g

(Continued)

Cytarabine *(Continued)*

Injection, solution: 20 mg/mL (5 mL, 25 mL, 50 mL); 100 mg/mL (20 mL)

Dosing

Adults & Elderly: I.V. bolus, IVPB, and continuous intravenous infusion doses of cytarabine are very different. Bolus doses are relatively well tolerated since the drug is rapidly metabolized. Continuous infusion uniformly results in myelosuppression. Refer to individual protocols.

Induction remission:
I.V.: 200 mg/m^2/day for 5 days at 2-week intervals 100-200 mg/m^2/day for 5- to 10-day therapy course or every day until remission
I.T.: 5-75 mg/m^2 every 2-7 days until CNS findings normalize

Maintenance remission:
I.V.: 70-200 mg/m^2/day for 2-5 days at monthly intervals
I.M., SubQ: 1-1.5 mg/kg single dose for maintenance at 1- to 4-week intervals

High-dose therapies for leukemia/lymphoma:
Doses as high as 1-3 g/m^2 have been used for refractory or secondary leukemias or refractory non-Hodgkin's lymphoma.
Doses of 1-3 g/m^2 every 12 hours for up to 12 doses have been used

Bone marrow transplant: 1.5 g/m^2 continuous infusion over 48 hours

Pediatrics: I.V. bolus, IVPB, and CIV doses of cytarabine are very different. Bolus doses are relatively well tolerated since the drug is rapidly metabolized; bolus doses are associated with greater gastrointestinal and neurotoxicity; continuous infusion uniformly results in myelosuppression. Refer to individual protocols.

Induction remission:
I.V.: 200 mg/m^2/day for 5 days at 2-week intervals 100-200 mg/m^2/day for 5- to 10-day therapy course or every day until remission
I.T.: 5-75 mg/m^2 every 4 days until CNS findings normalize
or
<1 year: 20 mg
1-2 years: 30 mg
2-3 years: 50 mg
>3 years: 70 mg

Maintenance remission: Refer to adult dosing.

Renal Impairment: In one study, 76% of patients with a Cl$_{cr}$ <60 mL/minute experienced neurotoxicity. Dosage adjustment of high-dose therapy should be considered in patients with renal insufficiency.

Hepatic Impairment: Dose may need to be adjusted in patients with liver failure since cytarabine is partially detoxified in the liver.

Administration

I.V.: Can be administered I.M., I.V. infusion, I.T., or SubQ at a concentration not to exceed 100 mg/mL. I.V. may be administered either as a bolus, IVPB (high doses of >500 mg/m^2), or continuous intravenous infusion (doses of 100-200 mg/m^2). High-dose regimens are usually administered by I.V. infusion over 1-3 hours or as I.V. continuous infusion.

I.V. Detail: I.V. doses of ≥1.5 g/m^2 may produce conjunctivitis which can be ameliorated with prophylactic use of corticosteroid (0.1% dexamethasone) eye drops. Dexamethasone eye drops should be administered at 1-2 drops every 6 hours during and for 2-7 days after cytarabine is done.

BMT only: Risk of cerebellar toxicity increases with creatinine clearance <60 mL/minute, age older than 50 years, pre-existing CNS lesion, and alkaline phosphatase levels exceeding 3 times the upper limit of normal. Conjunctivitis is prevented and treated with saline or corticosteroid eye drops. As prophylaxis, eye drops should be started 6-12 hours before initiation of cytarabine and continued 24 hours following the last dose.

pH: 5

Other: Can be administered intrathecally.

Stability

Reconstitution: Reconstitute powder with bacteriostatic water for injection. High-dose regimens are usually administered by I.V. infusion over 1-3 hours or as I.V. continuous infusion; for I.T. use, reconstitute with preservative free saline or preservative free lactated Ringer's solution
Standard I.V. infusion dilution: Dose/250-1000 mL D$_5$W or NS.
Standard intrathecal dilutions: Dose/3-5 mL lactated Ringer's ± methotrexate (12 mg) ± hydrocortisone (15-50 mg)
Note: Solutions containing bacteriostatic agents should not be used for the preparation of either high doses or intrathecal doses of cytarabine; may be used for I.M., SubQ, and low-dose (100-200 mg/m^2) I.V. solution.

Compatibility: Stable in D$_5$LR, D$_5$¼NS, D$_5$NS, D$_{10}$NS, D$_5$W, LR, NS

Y-site administration: Incompatible with allopurinol, amphotericin B cholesteryl sulfate complex, ganciclovir

Compatibility when admixed: Incompatible with fluorouracil, gentamicin, heparin, insulin (regular), nafcillin, oxacillin, penicillin G sodium

Storage:
Powder for reconstitution: Store intact vials of powder at room temperature 15°C to 30°C (59°F to 86°F). Reconstituted solutions are for up to 8 days at room temperature.
Solution: Prior to dilution, store at room temperature, 15°C to 30°C (59°F to 86°F); protect from light.

Laboratory Monitoring Liver function, CBC with differential and platelet count, serum creatinine, BUN, serum uric acid

Nursing Actions

Physical Assessment: Assess other pharmacological or herbal products patient may be taking for potential interactions (eg, additive myelosuppression, increased risk of cardiomyopathy, pancreatitis). See Administration for I.V. specifics. Premedication with antiemetic and corticosteroid eye drops may be ordered to reduce adverse effects. Patient should be monitored closely for anaphylaxis, sudden onset respiratory distress (especially with high doses). Assess results of laboratory tests (BUN, urinalysis, and serum creatinine [hepatic function]; CBC and platelet count [myelosuppression]) prior to therapy and on a regular basis throughout therapy. Teach patient possible side effects/appropriate interventions (eg, importance of adequate hydration) and adverse symptoms to report.

Patient Education: Do not take any new medication during therapy unless approved by prescriber. This drug is administered by infusion. You will be monitored closely during infusion. Report immediately any redness, swelling, burning, or pain at injection/infusion site; sudden difficulty breathing or swallowing, chest pain, or chills. Maintain adequate hydration (2-3 L/day of fluids) unless instructed to restrict fluid intake. You will be more susceptible to infection (avoid crowds and exposure to infection and do not have any vaccinations without consulting prescriber). May cause nausea, vomiting or loss of appetite (small, frequent meals, frequent mouth care, sucking lozenges, or chewing gum may help - if ineffective, consult prescriber for antiemetic medication); diarrhea (buttermilk, boiled milk, or yogurt may help - if persistent, consult with prescriber); mouth sores (use soft toothbrush or cotton swabs for oral care); or dizziness, headache, or confusion (use caution when driving or engaging in potentially hazardous tasks until response to drug is known). Report immediately any signs of CNS changes, change in gait, respiratory distress or respiratory difficulty, easy bruising or bleeding, persistent GI upset, yellowing of eyes or skin, change in color of urine or blackened stool, or any other persistent adverse effects. **Pregnancy/ breast-feeding precautions:** Inform prescriber if you are pregnant. Consult prescriber for instruction on appropriate contraceptive measures. This drug may cause severe fetal defects. Breast-feeding is not recommended.

Pregnancy Issues Cytarabine is teratogenic in animal studies. Limb and ear defects have been noted in case reports when cytarabine has been used during pregnancy. The following have also been noted in the neonate: Pancytopenia, WBC depression, electrolyte abnormalities, prematurity, low birth weight, decreased hematocrit or platelets. Risk to the fetus is decreased if therapy is avoided during the 1st trimester; however, women of childbearing potential should be advised of the potential risks.

Additional Information Latex-free products: 100 mg, 500 mg, 1 g, 2 g vials (Cytosar-U®) by Pharmacia-Upjohn

Pyridoxine has been administered on days of high-dose Ara-C therapy for prophylaxis of CNS toxicity.

Cytarabine (Liposomal)
(sye TARE a been lip po SOE mal)

U.S. Brand Names DepoCyt™

Pharmacologic Category Antineoplastic Agent, Antimetabolite

Medication Safety Issues
Sound-alike/look-alike issues:
Cytarabine may be confused with Cytadren®, Cytosar®, Cytoxan®, vidarabine
DepoCyt™ may be confused with Depoject®

Pregnancy Risk Factor D

Lactation Excretion in breast milk unknown/not recommended

Use Treatment of neoplastic (lymphomatous) meningitis

Mechanism of Action/Effect This is a sustained-release formulation of the active ingredient cytarabine. Acts to inhibit DNA polymerase which decreases DNA synthesis and repair.

Contraindications Hypersensitivity to cytarabine or any component of the formulation; active meningeal infection; pregnancy

Warnings/Precautions Hazardous agent — use appropriate precautions for handling and disposal. The incidence and severity of chemical arachnoiditis is reduced by coadministration with dexamethasone. May cause neurotoxicity. Blockage to CSF flow may increase the risk of neurotoxicity.

Drug Interactions
Decreased Effect: No formal studies of interactions with other medications have been conducted. The limited systemic exposure minimizes the potential for interaction between liposomal cytarabine and other medications.

Increased Effect/Toxicity: No formal studies of interactions with other medications have been conducted. The limited systemic exposure minimizes the potential for interaction between liposomal cytarabine and other medications.

Lab Interactions Since cytarabine liposomes are similar in appearance to WBCs, care must be taken in interpreting CSF examinations in patients receiving liposomal cytarabine

Adverse Reactions
>10%:
Central nervous system: Headache (28%), confusion (14%), somnolence (12%), fever (11%), pain (11%); chemical arachnoiditis is commonly observed, and may include neck pain, neck rigidity, headache, fever, nausea, vomiting, and back pain; may occur in up to 100% of cycles without dexamethasone prophylaxis; incidence is reduced to 33% when dexamethasone is used concurrently
Gastrointestinal: Vomiting (12%), nausea (11%)
1% to 10%:
Cardiovascular: Peripheral edema (7%)
Gastrointestinal: Constipation (7%)
Genitourinary: Incontinence (3%)
Hematologic: Neutropenia (9%), thrombocytopenia (8%), anemia (1%)
Neuromuscular & skeletal: Back pain (7%), weakness (19%), abnormal gait (4%)

Overdosage/Toxicology No overdosage with liposomal cytarabine has been reported. See Cytarabine *on page 313* for toxicology related to systemic administration.

Pharmacodynamics/Kinetics
Time to Peak: CSF: Intrathecal: ~5 hours
Half-Life Elimination: CSF: 100-263 hours
Metabolism: In plasma to ara-U (inactive)
Excretion: Primarily urine (as metabolites - ara-U)

Available Dosage Forms Injection, suspension [preservative free]: 10 mg/mL (5 mL)

Dosing
Adults & Elderly: Note: Patients should be started on dexamethasone 4 mg twice daily (oral or I.V.) for 5 days, beginning on the day of liposomal cytarabine injection
Lymphomatous meningitis: I.T.:
Induction: 50 mg intrathecally every 14 days for a total of 2 doses (weeks 1 and 3)
Consolidation: 50 mg intrathecally every 14 days for 3 doses (weeks 5, 7, and 9), followed by an additional dose at week 13
Maintenance: 50 mg intrathecally every 28 days for 4 doses (weeks 17, 21, 25, and 29)
Dosage adjustment for toxicity: If drug-related neurotoxicity develops, dose should be reduced to 25 mg. If toxicity persists, treatment with liposomal cytarabine should be discontinued.

Administration
Other: For intrathecal use only. Dose should be removed from vial immediately before administration (must be administered within 4 hours of removal). An in-line filter should **not** be used. Administer directly into the CSF via an intraventricular reservoir or by direct injection into the lumbar sac. Injection should be made slowly (over 1-5 minutes). Patients should lie flat for 1 hour after lumbar puncture.

Stability
Storage: Store under refrigeration (2°C to 8°C); protect from freezing and avoid aggressive agitation. Solutions should be used within 4 hours of withdrawal from the vial. Particles may settle in diluent over time, and may be resuspended by gentle agitation or inversion of the vial.

Laboratory Monitoring Since cytarabine liposomes are similar in appearance to WBCs, care must be taken in interpreting CSF examinations in patients receiving liposomal cytarabine.

Nursing Actions
Physical Assessment: This medication is only for intrathecal administration. Monitor patient continuously for adverse reactions that can be immediate (eg, neurotoxicity [myelopathy, ataxia, confusion, coma] and chemical arachnoiditis [eg, neck pain, neck rigidity, headache, fever, nausea, vomiting, back
(Continued)

Cytarabine (Liposomal) *(Continued)*

pain]). Incidence and severity of chemical arachnoiditis may be reduced by coadministration with dexamethasone. Provide patient teaching according to patient condition.

Patient Education: Patient instruction will be according to mental status. This medication can only be given by infusion into the spinal cord. You will be monitored closely during and after each infusion. Report immediately any neck pain or rigidity, headache, fever, nausea, or vomiting. Report any swelling of extremities, acute weakness, unusual gait pattern, CNS changes (confusion, speech difficulty), or other adverse effects. **Pregnancy/breast-feeding precautions:** Inform prescriber if you are pregnant. Do not get pregnant during or for 1 month following therapy. Consult prescriber for instruction on appropriate barrier contraceptive measures. Breast-feeding is not recommended.

Pregnancy Issues Cytarabine may cause fetal harm if a pregnant woman is exposed systemically.

Cytomegalovirus Immune Globulin (Intravenous-Human)

(sye toe meg a low VYE rus i MYUN GLOB yoo lin in tra VEE nus HYU man)

U.S. Brand Names CytoGam®
Synonyms CMV-IGIV
Pharmacologic Category Immune Globulin
Medication Safety Issues

Sound-alike/look-alike issues:
CytoGam® may be confused with Cytoxan®, Gamimune® N

Pregnancy Risk Factor C
Lactation Excretion in breast milk unknown
Use Prophylaxis of cytomegalovirus (CMV) disease associated with kidney, lung, liver, pancreas, and heart transplants; concomitant use with ganciclovir should be considered in organ transplants (other than kidney) from CMV seropositive donors to CMV seronegative recipients
Unlabeled/Investigational Use Adjunct therapy in the treatment of CMV disease in immunocompromised patients
Mechanism of Action/Effect CMV-IGIV is a preparation of immunoglobulin G (as well as trace amounts of IgA and IgM) derived from pooled healthy blood donors with a high titer of CMV antibodies; administration provides a passive source of antibodies against cytomegalovirus
Contraindications Hypersensitivity to CMV-IGIV, other immunoglobulins, or any component of the formulation; immunoglobulin A deficiency
Warnings/Precautions Monitor for anaphylactic reactions during infusion. May theoretically transmit blood-borne viruses. Use with caution in patients with renal insufficiency, diabetes mellitus, patients >65 years of age, volume depletion, sepsis, paraproteinemia, or patients on concomitant nephrotoxic drugs. Stabilized with sucrose and albumin, contains no preservative.

Drug Interactions

Decreased Effect: Decreased effect of live vaccines may be seen if given within 3 months of IGIV administration. Defer vaccination or revaccinate.

Adverse Reactions <6%:
Cardiovascular: Flushing
Central nervous system: Fever, chills
Gastrointestinal: Nausea, vomiting
Neuromuscular & skeletal: Arthralgia, back pain, muscle cramps
Respiratory: Wheezing

Overdosage/Toxicology Symptoms related to volume overload would be expected to occur with overdose; treatment is symptom-directed and supportive.
Available Dosage Forms Injection, solution [preservative free]: 50 mg ± 10 mg/mL (50 mL) [contains human albumin and sucrose]
Dosing
Adults:
Kidney transplant: I.V.:
Initial dose (within 72 hours of transplant): 150 mg/kg/dose
2-, 4-, 6-, and 8 weeks after transplant: 100 mg/kg/dose
12 and 16 weeks after transplant: 50 mg/kg/dose
Liver, lung, pancreas, or heart transplant: I.V.:
Initial dose (within 72 hours of transplant): 150 mg/kg/dose
2-, 4-, 6-, and 8 weeks after transplant: 150 mg/kg/dose
12 and 16 weeks after transplant: 100 mg/kg/dose
Severe CMV pneumonia: I.V.: Various regimens have been used, including 400 mg/kg CMV-IGIV in combination with ganciclovir on days 1, 2, 7, or 8, followed by 200 mg/kg CMV-IGIV on days 14 and 21
Elderly: Use with caution in patients >65 years of age; elderly may be at increased risk of renal insufficiency.
Renal Impairment: Use with caution; specific dosing adjustments are not available. Infusion rate should be the minimum practical; do not exceed 180 mg/kg/hour.
Administration
I.V.: For I.V. use only. Administer as separate infusion. Infuse beginning at 15 mg/kg/hour, then increase to 30 mg/kg/hour after 30 minutes if no untoward reactions. May titrate up to 60 mg/kg/hour. Do not administer faster than 75 mL/hour. Begin infusion within 6 hours of entering vial, complete infusion within 12 hours.
I.V. Detail: Administer through an I.V. line containing an in-line filter (pore size 15 micron) using an infusion pump. Do not mix with other infusions; do not use if turbid. Begin infusion within 6 hours of entering vial, complete infusion within 12 hours.

Infuse at 15 mg/kg/hour. If no adverse reactions occur within 30 minutes, may increase rate to 30 mg/kg/hour. If no adverse reactions occur within the second 30 minutes, may increase rate to 60 mg/kg/hour; maximum rate of infusion: 75 mL/hour. When infusing subsequent doses, may decrease titration interval from 30 minutes to 15 minutes. If patient develops nausea, back pain, or flushing during infusion, slow the rate or temporarily stop the infusion. Discontinue if blood pressure drops or in case of anaphylactic reaction.
Stability
Reconstitution: Dilution is not recommended. Do not shake vials. Do not use if turbid.
Compatibility: Infusion with other products is not recommended. If unavoidable, may be piggybacked into an I.V. line of sodium chloride, 2.D₅W, D₅W, D₁₀W, or D₂₀W; do not dilute more than 1:2
Storage: Store between 2°C and 8°C (35.6°F and 46.4°F)
Nursing Actions
Physical Assessment: Assess for history of previous allergic reactions. Monitor vital signs during infusion and observe for adverse or allergic reactions. Teach patient adverse symptoms to report.
Patient Education: This medication can only be administered by infusion. You will be monitored closely during the infusion. If you experience nausea, ask for assistance; do not get up alone. Do not have any vaccinations for the next 3 months without consulting prescriber. Immediately report chills,

muscle cramping, low back pain, chest pain or tightness, or respiratory difficulty. **Pregnancy/breast-feeding precautions:** Inform prescriber if you are or intend to become pregnant. Consult prescriber if breast-feeding.

Dacarbazine (da KAR ba zeen)

U.S. Brand Names DTIC-Dome®

Synonyms DIC; Dimethyl Triazeno Imidazole Carboxamide; DTIC; Imidazole Carboxamide; Imidazole Carboxamide Dimethyltriazene; WR-139007

Pharmacologic Category Antineoplastic Agent, Alkylating Agent (Triazene)

Medication Safety Issues
Sound-alike/look-alike issues:
Dacarbazine may be confused with Dicarbosil®, procarbazine

Pregnancy Risk Factor C

Lactation Excretion in breast milk unknown/not recommended

Use Treatment of malignant melanoma, Hodgkin's disease, soft-tissue sarcomas, fibrosarcomas, rhabdomyosarcoma, islet cell carcinoma, medullary carcinoma of the thyroid, and neuroblastoma

Mechanism of Action/Effect Inhibits DNA/RNA and protein synthesis; alkylating agent

Contraindications Hypersensitivity to dacarbazine or any component of the formulation

Warnings/Precautions The U.S. Food and Drug Administration (FDA) currently recommends that procedures for proper handling and disposal of antineoplastic agents be considered. Use with caution in patients with bone marrow depression. In patients with renal and/or hepatic impairment, dosage reduction may be necessary.

Drug Interactions
Cytochrome P450 Effect: Substrate (major) of CYP1A2, 2E1
Decreased Effect: CYP1A2 inducers may decrease the levels/effects of dacarbazine; example inducers include aminoglutethimide, carbamazepine, phenobarbital, and rifampin. Patients may experience impaired immune response to vaccines; possible infection after administration of live vaccines in patients receiving immunosuppressants.
Increased Effect/Toxicity: CYP1A2 inhibitors may increase the levels/effects of dacarbazine; example inhibitors include amiodarone, ciprofloxacin, fluvoxamine, ketoconazole, norfloxacin, ofloxacin, and rofecoxib. CYP2E1 inhibitors may increase the levels/effects of dacarbazine; example inhibitors include disulfiram, isoniazid, and miconazole.

Nutritional/Ethanol Interactions
Ethanol: Avoid ethanol (due to GI irritation).
Herb/Nutraceutical: Avoid dong quai, St John's wort (may also cause photosensitization).

Adverse Reactions
>10%:
Gastrointestinal: Nausea and vomiting (>90%), can be severe and dose-limiting; nausea and vomiting decrease on successive days when dacarbazine is given daily for 5 days; diarrhea
Hematologic: Myelosuppression, leukopenia, thrombocytopenia - dose-limiting
Onset: 5-7 days
Nadir: 7-10 days
Recovery: 21-28 days
Local: Pain on infusion, may be minimized by administration through a central line, or by administration as a short infusion (eg, 1-2 hours as opposed to bolus injection)
1% to 10%:
Dermatologic: Alopecia, rash, photosensitivity

Gastrointestinal: Anorexia, metallic taste
Miscellaneous: Flu-like syndrome (fever, myalgia, malaise)

Overdosage/Toxicology Symptoms of overdose include myelosuppression and diarrhea. There are no known antidotes and treatment is symptomatic and supportive.

Pharmacodynamics/Kinetics
Onset of Action: I.V.: 18-24 days
Protein Binding: 5%
Half-Life Elimination: Biphasic: Initial: 20-40 minutes; Terminal: 5 hours
Metabolism: Extensively hepatic; hepatobiliary excretion is probably of some importance; metabolites may also have an antineoplastic effect
Excretion: Urine (~30% to 50% as unchanged drug)

Available Dosage Forms
Injection, powder for reconstitution: 100 mg, 200 mg, 500 mg
DTIC-Dome®: 200 mg

Dosing
Adults & Elderly: Refer to individual protocols. Some dosage regimens include:
Intra-arterial: 50-400 mg/m² for 5-10 days
Hodgkin's disease, ABVD: 375 mg/m² days 1 and 15 every 4 weeks **or** 100 mg/m²/day for 5 days
Metastatic melanoma (alone or in combination with other agents): I.V.: 150-250 mg/m² days 1-5 every 3-4 weeks
Metastatic melanoma: I.V.: 850 mg/m² every 3 weeks
High dose: Bone marrow/blood cell transplantation: I.V.: 1-3 g/m²; maximum dose as a single agent: 3.38 g/m²; generally combined with other high-dose chemotherapeutic drugs
Pediatrics: Refer to individual protocols.
Pediatric solid tumors: I.V.: 200-470 mg/m²/day over 5 days every 21-28 days
Pediatric neuroblastoma: I.V.: 800-900 mg/m² as a single dose on day 1 of therapy every 3-4 weeks in combination therapy
Hodgkin's disease, ABVD: I.V.: 375 mg/m² on days 1 and 15 of treatment course, repeat every 28 days
Renal Impairment: Adjustment is warranted.
Hepatic Impairment: Monitor closely for signs of toxicity.

Administration
I.V.: Irritant. Infuse over 30-60 minutes.
I.V. Detail: Rapid infusion may cause severe venous irritation.

Extravasation management: Local pain, burning sensation, and irritation at the injection site may be relieved by local application of hot packs. If extravasation occurs, apply cold packs. Protect exposed tissue from light following extravasation.

BMT only: Doses of 6591 mg/m² have been administered, although hypotension is considered the nonhematologic dose-limiting side effect for doses >3380 mg/m². Infusion-related hypotension may be secondary to calcium chelation by citric acid in formulation.

pH: 3-4
Stability
Reconstitution: Reconstitute with a minimum of 2 mL (100 mg vial) or 4 mL (200 mg vial) of SWI, D₅W, or NS. Dilute to a concentration of 10 mg/mL.
Standard I.V. dilution: 250-500 mL D₅W or NS
Compatibility: Stable in NS, SWFI
Y-site administration: Incompatible with allopurinol, cefepime, piperacillin/tazobactam
Compatibility when admixed: Incompatible with hydrocortisone sodium succinate
Storage: Store intact vials under refrigeration (2°C to 8°C) and protect from light. Vials are stable for 4 (Continued)

Dacarbazine *(Continued)*

weeks at room temperature. Reconstituted solution is stable for 24 hours at room temperature (20°C) and 96 hours under refrigeration (4°C). Solutions for infusion (in D₅W or NS) are stable for 24 hours at room temperature and protected from light. Decomposed drug turns pink.

Laboratory Monitoring CBC with differential, liver function

Nursing Actions

Physical Assessment: Assess other pharmacological or herbal products patient may be taking for potential interactions. Antiemetic premedication may be ordered (emetic potential is moderately high). Monitor infusion site closely; extravasation can cause severe cellulitis or tissue necrosis. Monitor laboratory tests, therapeutic effectiveness, and adverse response prior to each treatment and on a regular basis throughout therapy. Teach patient possible side effects/appropriate interventions and adverse symptoms to report.

Patient Education: Inform prescriber of all prescriptions, OTC medications, or herbal products you are taking, and any allergies you have. Do not take any new medication during therapy unless approved by prescriber. This drug can only be given by infusion. Report immediately any pain, burning, or swelling at infusion site. Limit oral intake for 4-6 hours before infusion. Maintain adequate hydration (2-3 L/day of fluids) unless instructed to restrict fluid intake, and nutrition (small, frequent meals). You will be more susceptible to infection (avoid crowds and exposure to infection and do not have any vaccinations without consulting prescriber). May cause nausea, vomiting, loss of appetite, or diarrhea (consult prescriber for medication); hair loss (reversible); or headache, fever, sinus congestion, or muscles aches (consult prescriber for analgesic). Report immediately any numbness in extremities or change in gait, respiratory distress or respiratory difficulty; rash; easy bruising or bleeding; yellowing of eyes or skin, change in color of urine or blackened stool; or any other persistent adverse effects. **Pregnancy/breast-feeding precautions:** Inform prescriber if you are pregnant. Breast-feeding is not recommended.

Daclizumab *(dac KLYE zue mab)*

U.S. Brand Names Zenapax®

Pharmacologic Category Immunosuppressant Agent

Pregnancy Risk Factor C

Lactation Excretion in breast milk unknown/use caution

Use Part of an immunosuppressive regimen (including cyclosporine and corticosteroids) for the prophylaxis of acute organ rejection in patients receiving renal transplant

Unlabeled/Investigational Use Graft-versus-host disease; prevention of organ rejection after heart transplant

Contraindications Hypersensitivity to daclizumab or any component of the formulation

Warnings/Precautions Patients on immunosuppressive therapy are at increased risk for infectious complications and secondary malignancies. Long-term effects of daclizumab on immune function are unknown. Severe hypersensitivity reactions have been rarely reported; anaphylaxis has been observed on initial exposure and following re-exposure; medications for the management of severe allergic reaction should be available for immediate use. Anti-idiotype antibodies have been measured in patients that have received daclizumab (adults 14%;

children 34%); detection of antibodies may be influenced by multiple factors and may therefore be misleading.

In cardiac transplant patients, the combined use of daclizumab, cyclosporine, mycophenolate mofetil, and corticosteroids has been associated with an increased mortality. Higher mortality may be associated with the use of antilymphocyte globulin and a higher incidence of severe infections.

Drug Interactions

Increased Effect/Toxicity: The combined use of daclizumab, cyclosporine, mycophenolate mofetil, and corticosteroids has been associated with an increased mortality in a population of cardiac transplant recipients, particularly in patients who received antilymphocyte globulin and in patients with severe infections.

Adverse Reactions Although reported adverse events are frequent, when daclizumab is compared with placebo the incidence of adverse effects is similar between the two groups. Many of the adverse effects reported during clinical trial use of daclizumab may be related to the patient population, transplant procedure, and concurrent transplant medications. Diarrhea, fever, postoperative pain, pruritus, respiratory tract infection, urinary tract infection, and vomiting occurred more often in children than adults.

≥5%:

Cardiovascular: Chest pain, edema, hyper-/hypotension, tachycardia, thrombosis

Central nervous system: Dizziness, fatigue, fever, headache, insomnia, pain, post-traumatic pain, tremor

Dermatologic: Acne, cellulitis, wound healing impaired

Gastrointestinal: Abdominal distention, abdominal pain, constipation, diarrhea, dyspepsia, epigastric pain, nausea, pyrosis, vomiting

Genitourinary: Dysuria

Hematologic: Bleeding

Neuromuscular & skeletal: Back pain, musculoskeletal pain

Renal: Oliguria, renal tubular necrosis

Respiratory: Cough, dyspnea, pulmonary edema,

Miscellaneous: Lymphocele, wound infection

≥2% to <5%:

Central nervous system: Anxiety, depression, shivering

Dermatologic: Hirsutism, pruritus, rash

Endocrine & metabolic: Dehydration, diabetes mellitus, fluid overload

Gastrointestinal: Flatulence, gastritis, hemorrhoids

Genitourinary: Urinary retention, urinary tract bleeding

Local: Application site reaction

Neuromuscular & skeletal: Arthralgia, leg cramps, myalgia, weakness

Ocular: Vision blurred

Renal: Hydronephrosis, renal damage, renal insufficiency

Respiratory: Atelectasis, congestion, hypoxia, pharyngitis, pleural effusion, rales, rhinitis

Miscellaneous: Night sweats, prickly sensation, diaphoresis

Overdosage/Toxicology Overdose has not been reported.

Pharmacodynamics/Kinetics

Half-Life Elimination: Estimated: Adults: Terminal: 20 days; Children: 13 days

Available Dosage Forms Injection, solution [preservative free]: 5 mg/mL (5 mL)

Dosing

Adults:

Note: Daclizumab is used adjunctively with other immunosuppressants (eg, cyclosporine, corticosteroids, mycophenolate mofetil, and azathioprine).

Immunoprophylaxis against acute renal allograft rejection: I.V.: 1 mg/kg infused over 15 minutes within 24 hours before transplantation (day 0), then every 14 days for 4 additional doses

Treatment of graft-versus-host disease (unlabeled use, limited data): I.V.: 0.5-1.5 mg/kg, repeat same dosage for transient response. Repeat doses have been administered 11-48 days following the initial dose.

Prevention of organ rejection after heart transplant (unlabeled use): 1 mg/kg up to a maximum of 100 mg; administer within 12 hours after heart transplant and on days 8, 22, 36, and 50 post-transplant

Elderly: Refer to adult dosing. Use with caution.

Pediatrics: Refer to adult dosing.

Renal Impairment: No dosage adjustment needed.

Hepatic Impairment: No data available for patients with severe impairment.

Administration

I.V.: For I.V. administration following dilution. Daclizumab solution should be administered within 4 hours of preparation if stored at room temperature; infuse over a 15-minute period via a peripheral or central vein.

Stability

Reconstitution: Dose should be further diluted in 50 mL 0.9% sodium chloride solution. When mixing, gently invert bag to avoid foaming; do not shake. Do not use if solution is discolored.

Compatibility: Do not mix with other medications or infuse other medications through same I.V. line.

Storage: Refrigerate vials at 2°C to 8°C (36°F to 46°F). Do not shake or freeze; protect undiluted solution against direct sunlight. Diluted solution is stable for 24 hours at 4°C or for 4 hours at room temperature.

Nursing Actions

Physical Assessment: Assess potential for interactions with other prescriptions, OTC medications, or herbal products patient may be taking. Monitor cardiorespiratory and renal function (eg, fluid overload) and adverse reactions during infusion and periodically between infusions. Be alert to the possibility of the development of infection or malignancies. **Note:** Hypersensitivity reactions can occur; medications for immediate treatment of severe allergic reactions should be available for immediate use. Teach patient possible side effects/appropriate interventions and adverse symptoms to report.

Patient Education: This medication, which may help transplant rejection, can only be administered by infusion. You will be monitored closely during infusion. Report immediately any respiratory or swallowing difficulty; tightness in jaw or throat; chest pain; or rash, pain, burning, redness, or swelling at infusion site. You will be more susceptible to infection (avoid crowds and exposure to infection and do not have any vaccinations without consulting prescriber). Maintain adequate hydration (2-3 L/day of fluids) unless instructed to restrict fluid intake and nutrition (small frequent meals may be advisable). May cause headache, dizziness, fatigue (use caution when driving or engaging in tasks that require alertness until response to drug is known): back pain, leg cramps, or musculoskeletal pain (consult prescriber for approved analgesic); or nausea, vomiting, dyspepsia, or abdominal discomfort (good mouth care, small frequent meals, chewing gum, or sucking lozenges may help). Report changes in urinary pattern; unusual bleeding or bruising; chest pain or palpitations; persistent dizziness, tremors, or headache; respiratory difficulty or unusual cough; rash; opportunistic infection (vaginal itching or drainage, sores in mouth, unusual fever or chills); or other persistent adverse effects. **Pregnancy/breast-feeding precautions:** Inform prescriber if you are or intend to become pregnant. Consult prescriber if breast-feeding.

Pregnancy Issues Animal reproduction studies have not been conducted. Generally, IgG molecules cross the placenta. Do not use during pregnancy unless the potential benefit to the mother outweighs the possible risk to the fetus. Women of childbearing potential should use effective contraception before, during, and for 4 months following treatment.

Dactinomycin (dak ti noe MYE sin)

U.S. Brand Names Cosmegen®

Synonyms ACT; Act-D; Actinomycin; Actinomycin Cl; Actinomycin D; DACT; NSC-3053

Pharmacologic Category Antineoplastic Agent, Antibiotic

Medication Safety Issues

Sound-alike/look-alike issues:

Dactinomycin may be confused with DAUNOrubicin

Actinomycin may be confused with Achromycin

Pregnancy Risk Factor D

Lactation Excretion in breast milk unknown/contraindicated

Use Treatment of testicular tumors, melanoma, choriocarcinoma, Wilms' tumor, neuroblastoma, retinoblastoma, rhabdomyosarcoma, uterine sarcomas, Ewing's sarcoma, Kaposi's sarcoma, sarcoma botryoides, and soft tissue sarcoma

Mechanism of Action/Effect Causes cell death by inhibiting messenger RNA

Contraindications Hypersensitivity to dactinomycin or any component of the formulation; patients with concurrent or recent chickenpox or herpes zoster; avoid in infants <6 months of age

Warnings/Precautions Hazardous agent - use appropriate precautions for handling and disposal. Dactinomycin is extremely irritating to tissues and must be administered I.V.; if extravasation occurs during I.V. use, severe damage to soft tissues will occur. Dosage is usually expressed in **MICRO**grams, **NOT** milligrams, and must be calculated on the basis of body surface area (BSA) in obese or edematous patients. Dactinomycin potentiates the effects of radiation therapy; use with caution in patients who have received radiation therapy; reduce dosages in patients who are receiving dactinomycin and radiation therapy simultaneously; combination with radiation therapy may result in increased GI toxicity and myelosuppression. Toxic effects may be delayed in onset (2-4 days following a course of treatment)and may require 1-2 weeks to reach maximum severity. Avoid administration of live vaccines. Use caution in hepatobiliary dysfunction; may cause potentially fatal veno-occlusive liver disease, increased risk in children <4 years of age. Long-term observation of cancer survivors is recommended due to the potential for secondary primary tumors following treatment with radiation and antineoplastic agents.

Drug Interactions

Increased Effect/Toxicity: Dactinomycin potentiates the effects of radiation therapy. Avoid administration of live vaccines in immunosuppressive therapy.

Lab Interactions May interfere with bioassays of antibacterial drug levels

Adverse Reactions Frequency not defined.

Central nervous system: Fatigue, fever, lethargy, malaise

Dermatologic: Acne, alopecia (reversible), cheilitis; increased pigmentation, sloughing, or erythema of previously irradiated skin; skin eruptions

Endocrine & metabolic: Growth retardation, hypocalcemia

(Continued)

Dactinomycin *(Continued)*

Gastrointestinal: Abdominal pain, anorexia, diarrhea, dysphagia, esophagitis, GI ulceration, mucositis, nausea, pharyngitis, proctitis, stomatitis, vomiting

Hematologic: Agranulocytosis, anemia, leukopenia, pancytopenia, reticulocytopenia, thrombocytopenia, myelosuppression (onset: 7 days, nadir: 14-21 days, recovery: 21-28 days)

Hepatic: Ascites, hepatic failure, hepatitis, hepatomegaly, hepatotoxicity, liver function test abnormality, veno-occlusive disease

Local: Tissue necrosis, pain, and ulceration (following extravasation)

Neuromuscular & skeletal: Myalgia

Renal: Renal function abnormality

Respiratory: Pneumonitis

Miscellaneous: Anaphylactoid reaction, infection

Overdosage/Toxicology Symptoms of overdose include nausea, vomiting, diarrhea, depression, GI ulceration, mucositis, severe myelosuppression, skin disorders (eg, exanthema, desquamation, epidermolysis), stomatitis, veno-occlusive disease, acute renal failure and fatality. Treatment is symptomatic and supportive. Toxic effects may not be apparent until 2-4 days after a treatment course (peak after 1-2 weeks).

Pharmacodynamics/Kinetics

Time to Peak: Serum: I.V.: 2-5 minutes

Half-Life Elimination: 36 hours

Metabolism: Hepatic, minimal

Excretion: Bile (50%); feces (14%); urine (~10% as unchanged drug)

Available Dosage Forms Injection, powder for reconstitution: 0.5 mg [contains mannitol 20 mg]

Dosing

Adults: Refer to individual protocols.

Note: Medication orders for dactinomycin are commonly written in MICROgrams (eg, 150 mcg) although many regimens list the dose in MILLIgrams (eg, mg/kg or mg/m²). One-time doses for >1000 mcg, or multiple-day doses for >500 mcg/ day are not common. The dose intensity per 2-week cycle for adults and children should not exceed 15 mcg/kg/day for 5 days or 400-600 mcg/m²/day for 5 days. Some practitioners recommend calculation of the dosage for obese or edematous patients on the basis of body surface area in an effort to relate dosage to lean body mass.

I.V.: 2.5 mg/m² in divided doses over 1 week, repeated every 2 weeks **or**

0.75-2 mg/m² every 1-4 weeks **or**

400-600 mcg/m²/day for 5 days, repeated every 3-6 weeks

Elderly: Refer to adult dosing. Elderly patients are at increased risk of myelosuppression; dosing should begin at the low end of the dosing range.

Pediatrics: Refer to individual protocols.

Note: Dactinomycin doses are almost ALWAYS expressed in MICROGRAMS rather than milligrams. The dose intensity per 2-week cycle for adults and children should not exceed 15 mcg/kg/ day for 5 days or 400-600 mcg/m²/day for 5 days. Some practitioners recommend calculation of the dosage for obese or edematous patients on the basis of body surface area in an effort to relate dosage to lean body mass.

Usual dose: I.V.: Children >6 months: 15 mcg/kg/day or 400-600 mcg/m²/day for 5 days every 3-6 weeks

Renal Impairment: No adjustment is necessary.

Administration

I.V.: Vesicant. Infuse over 10-15 minutes.

Accidental contact management: For eye contact, irrigate for 15 minutes with water, saline or eye irrigating solutions; ophthalmologic consult recommended. For skin contact, irrigate for 15 minutes with water, seek medical attention.

I.V. Detail: Avoid extravasation. Extremely damaging to soft tissue and will cause a severe local reaction if extravasation occurs. Administer slow I.V. push over 10-15 minutes. Do not give I.M. or SubQ

Extravasation management: Apply ice immediately for 30-60 minutes, then alternate off/on every 15 minutes for 3 days. Data is not currently available regarding potential antidotes for dactinomycin. Close observation is advised.

pH: 5.5-7.0 (reconstituted solution)

Stability

Reconstitution: Dilute with 1.1 mL of preservative-free SWI to yield a final concentration of 500 mcg/ mL; do not use preservative diluent as precipitation may occur.

Compatibility: Stable in D_5W, NS, SWFI

Y-site administration: Incompatible with filgrastim

Storage: Store at controlled room temperature of 15°C to 30°C (59°F to 86°F). Protect from light and humidity. Reconstituted solutions are chemically stable under refrigeration for up to 60 days. Solutions in 50 mL D_5W or NS are stable for 24 hours at room temperature.

Laboratory Monitoring CBC with differential and platelet count, liver and renal function

Nursing Actions

Physical Assessment: Monitor patient closely during infusion; extravasation is extremely damaging to soft tissue and will cause a severe local reaction (see Extravasation Management). Administer slow I.V. push over 10-15 minutes. Do not give I.M. or SubQ. Monitor results of laboratory tests (eg, hematological, renal, and hepatic function), therapeutic response, and adverse reactions (myelosuppression, nausea, vomiting, glossitis, and oral ulceration) prior to each treatment and on a regular basis throughout therapy. Teach patient possible side effects/appropriate interventions and adverse symptoms to report.

Patient Education: Do not take any new medication during therapy unless approved by prescriber. This drug can only be given by infusion; report immediately any pain, burning, or swelling at infusion site; sudden chest pain; difficulty breathing or swallowing; or chills. Limit oral intake for 4-6 hours immediately before infusion. Between infusions, maintain adequate hydration (2-3 L/day of fluids) unless instructed to restrict fluid intake and nutrition (small frequent meals). You will be more susceptible to infection (avoid crowds and exposure to infection and do not have any vaccinations without consulting prescriber). May cause fatigue or malaise (use caution when driving or engaging in potentially hazardous tasks until response to drug is known); nausea, vomiting, loss of appetite, or diarrhea (consult prescriber for appropriate medication); or hair loss (reversible). Report unresolved nausea, vomiting, diarrhea, or abdominal pain; difficulty swallowing; rash; or any other persistent adverse effects. **Pregnancy/breast-feeding precautions:** Inform prescriber if you are or intend to become pregnant. Do not breast-feed.

Breast-Feeding Issues It is not known if dactinomycin is excreted in human breast milk. Due to the potential for serious reactions in the infant, breast-feeding is not recommended.

Pregnancy Issues Animal studies have demonstrated teratogenic effects and fetal loss There are no adequate and well-controlled studies in pregnant women. Women of childbearing potential are advised not to become pregnant. Use only when potential benefit justifies potential risk to the fetus.

Dalteparin (dal TE pa rin)

U.S. Brand Names Fragmin®
Pharmacologic Category Low Molecular Weight Heparin
Pregnancy Risk Factor B
Lactation Excretion in breast milk unknown/use caution
Use Prevention of deep vein thrombosis which may lead to pulmonary embolism, in patients requiring abdominal surgery who are at risk for thromboembolism complications (eg, patients >40 years of age, obesity, patients with malignancy, history of deep vein thrombosis or pulmonary embolism, and surgical procedures requiring general anesthesia and lasting >30 minutes); prevention of DVT in patients undergoing hip-replacement surgery; patients immobile during an acute illness; acute treatment of unstable angina or non-Q-wave myocardial infarction; prevention of ischemic complications in patients on concurrent aspirin therapy
Unlabeled/Investigational Use Active treatment of deep vein thrombosis
Mechanism of Action/Effect Low molecular weight heparin analog; the commercial product contains 3% to 15% heparin; has been shown to inhibit both factor Xa and factor IIa (thrombin), however, the antithrombotic effect of dalteparin is characterized by a higher ratio of antifactor Xa to antifactor IIa activity (ratio = 4)
Contraindications Hypersensitivity to dalteparin or any component of the formulation; thrombocytopenia associated with a positive *in vitro* test for antiplatelet antibodies in the presence of dalteparin; hypersensitivity to heparin or pork products; patients with active major bleeding; patients with unstable angina or non-Q-wave MI undergoing regional anesthesia; not for I.M. or I.V. use
Warnings/Precautions Patients with recent or anticipated neuraxial anesthesia (epidural or spinal anesthesia) are at risk of spinal or epidural hematoma and subsequent paralysis. Consider risk versus benefit prior to neuraxial anesthesia. Risk is increased by concomitant agents which may alter hemostasis, as well as traumatic or repeated epidural or spinal puncture. Patient should be observed closely for bleeding if dalteparin is administered during or immediately following diagnostic lumbar puncture, epidural anesthesia, or spinal anesthesia.

Not to be used interchangeably (unit for unit) with heparin or any other low molecular weight heparins. Use caution in patients with known hypersensitivity to methylparaben or propylparaben, renal failure, or a history of heparin-induced thrombocytopenia. Monitor platelet count closely. Rare thrombocytopenia may occur. Consider discontinuation of dalteparin in any patient developing significant thrombocytopenia. Monitor patient closely for signs or symptoms of bleeding. Certain patients are at increased risk of bleeding. Risk factors include bacterial endocarditis; congenital or acquired bleeding disorders; active ulcerative or angiodysplastic GI diseases; severe uncontrolled hypertension; hemorrhagic stroke; or use shortly after brain, spinal, or ophthalmology surgery; in patient treated concomitantly with platelet inhibitors; recent GI bleeding; thrombocytopenia or platelet defects; severe liver disease; hypertensive or diabetic retinopathy; or in patients undergoing invasive procedures. Rare cases of thrombocytopenia with thrombosis have occurred. Multidose vials contain benzyl alcohol and should not be used in pregnant women. Heparin can cause hyperkalemia by affecting aldosterone. Similar reactions could occur with LMWHs. Monitor for hyperkalemia. Safety and efficacy in pediatric patients have not been established.

Drug Interactions
Increased Effect/Toxicity: The risk of bleeding with dalteparin may be increased by drugs which affect platelet function (eg, aspirin, NSAIDs, dipyridamole,

ticlopidine, clopidogrel), oral anticoagulants, and thrombolytic agents. Although the risk of bleeding may be increased during concurrent warfarin therapy, dalteparin is commonly continued during the initiation of warfarin therapy to assure anticoagulation and to protect against possible transient hypercoagulability.
Nutritional/Ethanol Interactions Herb/Nutraceutical: Avoid cat's claw, dong quai, evening primrose, garlic, ginseng (all have additional antiplatelet activity).
Lab Interactions Increased AST, ALT levels
Adverse Reactions 1% to 10%:
Hematologic: Bleeding (3% to 5%), wound hematoma (0.1% to 3%)
Local: Pain at injection site (up to 12%), injection site hematoma (0.2% to 7%)
Pharmacodynamics/Kinetics
Onset of Action: 1-2 hours
Duration of Action: >12 hours
Time to Peak: Serum: 4 hours
Half-Life Elimination: Route dependent: 2-5 hours
Available Dosage Forms
Injection, solution [multidose vial]: Antifactor Xa 10,000 int. units per 1 mL (9.5 mL) [contains benzyl alcohol]; antifactor Xa 25,000 units per 1 mL (3.8 mL) [contains benzyl alcohol]
Injection, solution [preservative free; prefilled syringe]: Antifactor Xa 2500 int. units per 0.2 mL (0.2 mL); antifactor Xa 5000 int. units per 0.2 mL (0.2 mL); antifactor Xa 7500 int. units per 0.3 mL (0.3 mL); antifactor Xa 10,000 int. units per 1 mL (1 mL)
Dosing
Adults & Elderly:
Abdominal surgery (DVT prophylaxis):
Low-to-moderate DVT risk: SubQ: 2500 int. units 1-2 hours prior to surgery, then once daily for 5-10 days postoperatively
High DVT risk: SubQ: 5000 int. units 1-2 hours prior to surgery and then once daily for 5-10 days postoperatively
Total hip surgery (DVT prophylaxis): SubQ: **Note:** Three treatment options are currently available. Dose is given for 5-10 days, although up to 14 days of treatment have been tolerated in clinical trials:
Postoperative start:
Initial: 2500 int. units 4-8 hours* after surgery
Maintenance: 5000 int. units once daily; start at least 6 hours after postsurgical dose
Preoperative (starting day of surgery):
Initial: 2500 int. units within 2 hours before surgery
Adjustment: 2500 int. units 4-8 hours* after surgery
Maintenance: 5000 int. units once daily; start at least 6 hours after postsurgical dose
Preoperative (starting evening prior to surgery):
Initial: 5000 int. units 10-14 hours before surgery
Adjustment: 5000 int. units 4-8 hours* after surgery
Maintenance: 5000 int. units once daily, allowing 24 hours between doses.
*Note: Dose may be delayed if hemostasis is not yet achieved.
Unstable angina or non-Q-wave myocardial infarction: SubQ: 120 int. units/kg body weight (maximum dose: 10,000 int. units) every 12 hours for 5-8 days with concurrent aspirin therapy. Discontinue dalteparin once patient is clinically stable.
Immobility/acute illness (DVT prophylaxis): 5000 int. units once daily
Administration
I.M.: Do not give I.M.
Other: For deep SubQ injection only. May be injected in a U-shape to the area surrounding the navel, the upper outer side of the thigh, or the upper outer quadrangle of the buttock. Apply pressure to injection (Continued)

Dalteparin *(Continued)*

site; do not massage. Use thumb and forefinger to lift a fold of skin when injecting dalteparin to the navel area or thigh. Insert needle at a 45- to 90-degree angle. The entire length of needle should be inserted. Do not expel air bubble from fixed-dose syringe prior to injection. Air bubble (and extra solution, if applicable) may be expelled from graduated syringes.

Administration once daily beginning prior to surgery and continuing 5-10 days after surgery prevents deep vein thrombosis in patients at risk for thromboembolic complications. For unstable angina or non-Q-wave myocardial infarction, dalteparin is administered every 12 hours until the patient is stable (5-8 days).

Stability

Storage: Store at temperatures 20°C to 25°C (68°F to 77°F).

Laboratory Monitoring Periodic CBC including platelet count, stool occult blood; monitoring of PT and PTT is not necessary.

Nursing Actions

Physical Assessment: Bleeding precautions should be observed for full period of therapy. Assess other pharmacological or herbal products patient may be taking for potential interactions (especially anything that will impact coagulation or platelet aggregation). Assess results of laboratory tests, therapeutic effectiveness (according to purpose for use), and adverse response (eg, thrombolytic reactions). Teach patient possible side effects/appropriate interventions (eg, bleeding precautions) and adverse symptoms to report.

Patient Education: Do not take any new medication during therapy unless approved by prescriber (especially anything containing aspirin). This drug can only be administered by injection. You may have a tendency to bleed easily while taking this drug (use caution to prevent falls or bruises or other accidents, brush teeth with soft brush, use waxed dental floss, use electric razor, avoid scissors or sharp knives, and potentially harmful activities). Report unusual fever; unusual bleeding or bruising (bleeding gums, nosebleed, blood in urine, dark stool); pain in joints or back; severe head pain; skin rash; or redness, swelling, or pain at injection site. **Breast-feeding precaution:** Consult prescriber if breast-feeding.

Pregnancy Issues Multiple-dose vials contain benzyl alcohol (avoid in pregnant women due to association with fetal syndrome in premature infants).

Additional Information Multidose vial contains 14 mg/mL benzyl alcohol.

Danazol *(DA na zole)*

U.S. Brand Names Danocrine® [DSC]

Pharmacologic Category Androgen

Medication Safety Issues

Sound-alike/look-alike issues:

Danazol may be confused with Dantrium®

Danocrine® may be confused with Dacriose®

Pregnancy Risk Factor X

Lactation Enters breast milk/contraindicated

Use Treatment of endometriosis, fibrocystic breast disease, and hereditary angioedema

Mechanism of Action/Effect Suppresses pituitary output of follicle-stimulating hormone and luteinizing hormone that causes regression and atrophy of normal and ectopic endometrial tissue; decreases rate of growth of abnormal breast tissue; reduces attacks associated with hereditary angioedema by increasing levels of C4 component of complement

Contraindications Hypersensitivity to danazol or any component of the formulation; undiagnosed genital bleeding; pregnancy; breast-feeding; porphyria; markedly impaired hepatic, renal, or cardiac function

Warnings/Precautions Use with caution in patients with seizure disorders, migraine, or conditions influenced by edema. Thromboembolism, thrombotic, and thrombophlebitic events have been reported (including life-threatening or fatal strokes). Peliosis hepatis and benign hepatic adenoma have been reported with long-term use. May cause benign intracranial hypertension. Breast cancer should be ruled out prior to treatment for fibrocystic breast disease. May increase risk of atherosclerosis and coronary artery disease. May cause nonreversible androgenic effects. Pregnancy must be ruled out prior to treatment. Safety and efficacy in pediatric patients have not been established.

Drug Interactions

Cytochrome P450 Effect: Inhibits CYP3A4 (weak)

Decreased Effect: Danazol may decrease effectiveness of hormonal contraceptives. Nonhormonal birth control methods are recommended.

Increased Effect/Toxicity: Danazol may increase serum levels of carbamazepine, cyclosporine, tacrolimus, and warfarin leading to toxicity; dosage adjustment may be needed; monitor. Concomitant use of danazol and HMG-CoA reductase inhibitors may lead to severe myopathy or rhabdomyolysis. Danazol may enhance the glucose-lowering effect of hypoglycemic agents.

Nutritional/Ethanol Interactions Food: Delays time to peak; high-fat meal increases plasma concentration

Lab Interactions Testosterone, androstenedione, dehydroepiandrosterone

Adverse Reactions Frequency not defined.

Cardiovascular: Benign intracranial hypertension (rare), edema, flushing, hypertension

Central nervous system: Anxiety (rare), chills (rare), convulsions (rare), depression, dizziness, emotional lability, fainting, fever (rare), Guillain-Barré syndrome, headache, nervousness, sleep disorders, tremor

Dermatologic: Acne, hair loss, mild hirsutism, maculopapular rash, papular rash, petechial rash, pruritus, purpuric rash, seborrhea, Stevens-Johnson syndrome (rare), photosensitivity (rare), urticaria, vesicular rash

Endocrine & metabolic: Amenorrhea (which may continue post therapy), breast size reduction, clitoris hypertrophy, glucose intolerance, HDL decreased, LDL increased, libido changes, nipple discharge, menstrual disturbances (spotting, altered timing of cycle), semen abnormalities (changes in volume, viscosity, sperm count/motility), spermatogenesis reduction

Gastrointestinal: Appetite changes (rare), bleeding gums (rare), constipation, gastroenteritis, nausea, pancreatitis (rare), vomiting, weight gain

Genitourinary: Vaginal dryness, vaginal irritation, pelvic pain

Hematologic: Eosinophilia, erythrocytosis (reversible), leukocytosis, leukopenia, platelet count increased, polycythemia, RBC increased, thrombocytopenia

Hepatic: Cholestatic jaundice, hepatic adenoma, jaundice, liver enzymes (elevated), malignant tumors (after prolonged use), peliosis hepatis

Neuromuscular & skeletal: Back pain, carpal tunnel syndrome (rare), extremity pain, joint lockup, joint pain, joint swelling, muscle cramps, neck pain, paresthesia, spasms, weakness

Ocular: Cataracts (rare), visual disturbances

Renal: Hematuria

Respiratory: Nasal congestion (rare)

Miscellaneous: Voice change (hoarseness, sore throat, instability, deepening of pitch), diaphoresis

Pharmacodynamics/Kinetics
Onset of Action: Therapeutic: ~4 weeks
Time to Peak: Serum: Within 2 hours
Half-Life Elimination: Variable: 4.5 hours
Metabolism: Extensively hepatic, primarily to 2-hydroxymethylethisterone
Excretion: Urine

Available Dosage Forms [DSC] = Discontinued product
Capsule: 50 mg, 100 mg, 200 mg
Danocrine®: 50 mg, 100 mg, 200 mg [DSC]

Dosing
Adults & Elderly:
Endometriosis: Oral: Initial: 200-400 mg/day in 2 divided doses for mild disease; individualize dosage. Usual maintenance dose: 800 mg/day in 2 divided doses to achieve amenorrhea and rapid response to painful symptoms. Continue therapy uninterrupted for 3-6 months (up to 9 months).
Fibrocystic breast disease (Female): Oral: Range: 100-400 mg/day in 2 divided doses
Hereditary angioedema (Male/Female): Oral: Initial: 200 mg 2-3 times/day; after favorable response, decrease the dosage by 50% or less at intervals of 1-3 months or longer if the frequency of attacks dictates. If an attack occurs, increase the dosage by up to 200 mg/day.

Stability
Storage: Store at controlled room temperature of 15°C to 30°C (59°F to 86°F).
Laboratory Monitoring Liver and renal function

Nursing Actions
Physical Assessment: Assess other pharmacological or herbal products patient may be taking for potential interactions (eg, anticoagulants and hypoglycemic agents). Monitor therapeutic effectiveness (according to purpose for use) and adverse response (eg, hypertension, increased LDL, CNS changes, jaundice, hematuria). Caution patients with diabetes to monitor glucose levels closely (may enhance the glucose-lowering effect of hypoglycemic agents). Teach patient proper use, possible side effects/appropriate interventions (eg, good self-breast exam technique), and adverse symptoms to report (refer to Patient Education). **Pregnancy risk factor X** - determine that patient is not pregnant before starting therapy. Do not give to women of childbearing age unless capable of complying with barrier contraceptive use. Instruct patient in appropriate contraceptive measures.

Patient Education: Inform prescriber of all prescriptions, OTC medications, or herbal products you are taking, and any allergies you have. Do not take any new medication during therapy unless approved by prescriber. Take as directed; do not discontinue without consulting prescriber. Therapy may take up to several months depending on purpose for therapy. If you have diabetes, monitor serum glucose closely and notify prescriber of changes; this medication can alter hypoglycemic requirements. Consult prescriber for appropriate self-breast-exam technique. May cause headache, sleeplessness, anxiety (use caution when driving or engaging in potentially hazardous tasks until response to drug is known); acne, growth of body hair, deepening of voice, loss of libido, impotence, or menstrual irregularity (usually reversible). Report changes in menstrual pattern; deepening of voice or unusual growth of body hair; persistent penile erections; fluid retention (eg, swelling of ankles, feet, or hands, respiratory difficulty, or sudden weight gain); change in color of urine or stool; yellowing of eyes or skin; unusual bruising or bleeding; or other adverse reactions. **Pregnancy/breast-feeding precautions:** Inform prescriber if you are pregnant. Consult prescriber for appropriate contraceptive measures. This drug may cause severe fetal defects.

Do not donate blood during or for 1 month following therapy. Do not breast-feed.
Pregnancy Issues Pregnancy should be ruled out prior to treatment using a sensitive test (beta subunit test, if available). Nonhormonal contraception should be used during therapy. May cause androgenic effects to the female fetus; clitoral hypertrophy, labial fusion, urogenital sinus defect, vaginal atresia, and ambiguous genitalia have been reported.

Dantrolene (DAN troe leen)

U.S. Brand Names Dantrium®
Synonyms Dantrolene Sodium
Pharmacologic Category Skeletal Muscle Relaxant
Medication Safety Issues
Sound-alike/look-alike issues:
Dantrium® may be confused with danazol, Daraprim®
Pregnancy Risk Factor C
Lactation Excretion in breast milk unknown/not recommended
Use Treatment of spasticity associated with spinal cord injury, stroke, cerebral palsy, or multiple sclerosis; treatment of malignant hyperthermia
Unlabeled/Investigational Use Neuroleptic malignant syndrome (NMS)
Mechanism of Action/Effect Acts directly on skeletal muscle by interfering with release of calcium ion from the sarcoplasmic reticulum; prevents or reduces the increase in myoplasmic calcium ion concentration that activates the acute catabolic processes associated with malignant hyperthermia
Contraindications Active hepatic disease; should not be used where spasticity is used to maintain posture or balance
Warnings/Precautions Use with caution in patients with impaired cardiac function or impaired pulmonary function. Has potential for hepatotoxicity. Overt hepatitis has been most frequently observed between the third and twelfth month of therapy. Hepatic injury appears to be greater in females and in patients >35 years of age.

Drug Interactions
Cytochrome P450 Effect: Substrate of CYP3A4 (major)
Decreased Effect: CYP3A4 inducers may decrease the levels/effects of dantrolene; example inducers include aminoglutethimide, carbamazepine, nafcillin, nevirapine, phenobarbital, phenytoin, and rifamycins.
Increased Effect/Toxicity: Increased toxicity with estrogens (hepatotoxicity), CNS depressants (sedation), MAO inhibitors, phenothiazines, clindamycin (increased neuromuscular blockade), verapamil (hyperkalemia and cardiac depression), warfarin, clofibrate, and tolbutamide. CYP3A4 inhibitors may increase the levels/effects of dantrolene; example inhibitors include azole antifungals, clarithromycin, diclofenac, doxycycline, erythromycin, imatinib, isoniazid, nefazodone, nicardipine, propofol, protease inhibitors, quinidine, telithromycin, and verapamil.
Nutritional/Ethanol Interactions
Ethanol: Avoid ethanol (may increase CNS depression).
Herb/Nutraceutical: Avoid valerian, St John's wort, kava kava, gotu kola (may increase CNS depression).
Lab Interactions Increased aminotransferase [ALT (SGPT)/AST (SGOT)] (S), alkaline phosphatase, LDH, BUN, and total serum bilirubin
Adverse Reactions
>10%:
Central nervous system: Drowsiness, dizziness, lightheadedness, fatigue
Dermatologic: Rash
Gastrointestinal: Diarrhea (mild), nausea, vomiting
Neuromuscular & skeletal: Muscle weakness
(Continued)

Dantrolene *(Continued)*

1% to 10%:
Cardiovascular: Pleural effusion with pericarditis
Central nervous system: Chills, fever, headache, insomnia, nervousness, mental depression
Gastrointestinal: Diarrhea (severe), constipation, anorexia, stomach cramps
Ocular: Blurred vision
Respiratory: Respiratory depression

Overdosage/Toxicology Symptoms of overdose include CNS depression, hypotension, nausea, and vomiting. For decontamination, lavage with activated charcoal and administer a cathartic. Do not use ipecac. Other treatment is supportive and symptomatic.

Pharmacodynamics/Kinetics
Half-Life Elimination: 8.7 hours
Metabolism: Hepatic
Excretion: Feces (45% to 50%); urine (25% as unchanged drug and metabolites)

Available Dosage Forms
Capsule, as sodium: 25 mg, 50 mg, 100 mg
Injection, powder for reconstitution, as sodium: 20 mg [contains mannitol 3 g]

Dosing
Adults & Elderly:
Spasticity: Oral: 25 mg/day to start, increase frequency to 2-4 times/day, then increase dose by 25 mg every 4-7 days to a maximum of 100 mg 2-4 times/day or 400 mg/day
Malignant hyperthermia:
Preoperative prophylaxis:
Oral: 4-8 mg/kg/day in 4 divided doses, begin 1-2 days prior to surgery with last dose 3-4 hours prior to surgery
I.V.: 2.5 mg/kg ~1¼ hours prior to anesthesia and infused over 1 hour with additional doses as needed and individualized
Crisis: I.V.: 2.5 mg/kg; may repeat dose up to cumulative dose of 10 mg/kg; if physiologic and metabolic abnormalities reappear, repeat regimen
Postcrisis follow-up: Oral: 4-8 mg/kg/day in 4 divided doses for 1-3 days; I.V. dantrolene may be used when oral therapy is not practical; individualize dosage beginning with 1 mg/kg or more as the clinical situation dictates
Neuroleptic malignant syndrome (unlabeled use): I.V.: 1 mg/kg; may repeat dose up to maximum cumulative dose of 10 mg/kg, then switch to oral dosage
Pediatrics:
Spasticity: Oral: Initial: 0.5 mg/kg/dose twice daily, increase frequency to 3-4 times/day at 4- to 7-day intervals, then increase dose by 0.5 mg/kg to a maximum of 3 mg/kg/dose 2-4 times/day up to 400 mg/day
Malignant hyperthermia: Refer to adult dosing.

Administration
I.V.: Therapeutic or emergency dose can be administered with rapid continuous I.V. push. Follow-up doses should be administered over 2-3 minutes.
I.V. Detail: Avoid extravasation; tissue irritant. 36 vials are needed for adequate hyperthermia therapy.

Stability
Reconstitution: Reconstitute vial by adding 60 mL of sterile water for injection USP (**not bacteriostatic water for injection**). Protect from light. Use within 6 hours. Avoid glass bottles for I.V. infusion.

Laboratory Monitoring Liver function for potential hepatotoxicity

Nursing Actions
Physical Assessment: Assess effectiveness and interactions of other medications patient may be taking. **I.V.:** Monitor vital signs, cardiac function, respiratory status, and I.V. site (extravasation very irritating to tissues) frequently during infusion. Monitor effectiveness of therapy (according to rationale for therapy) and adverse reactions at beginning and periodically during therapy. Assess knowledge/teach patient appropriate use, interventions to reduce side effects, and adverse symptoms to report.

Patient Education: Take exactly as directed. Do not increase dose or discontinue without consulting prescriber. Do not use alcohol, prescriptive or OTC antidepressants, sedatives, or pain medications without consulting prescriber. You may experience drowsiness, dizziness, lightheadedness (avoid driving or engaging in tasks that require alertness until response to drug is known); nausea or vomiting (small frequent meals, frequent mouth care, or sucking hard candy may help); or diarrhea (buttermilk, boiled milk, or yogurt may help). Report excessive confusion; drowsiness or mental agitation; chest pain, palpitations, or respiratory difficulty; skin rash; or vision changes. **Pregnancy/breast-feeding precautions:** Inform prescriber if you are or intend to become pregnant. Breast-feeding is not recommended.

Dapsone *(DAP sone)*

U.S. Brand Names Aczone™
Synonyms Diaminodiphenylsulfone
Pharmacologic Category Antibiotic, Miscellaneous
Medication Safety Issues
Sound-alike/look-alike issues:
Dapsone may be confused with Diprosone®

Pregnancy Risk Factor C
Lactation Enters breast milk/not recommended (AAP rates "compatible")
Use Treatment of leprosy and dermatitis herpetiformis (infections caused by *Mycobacterium leprae*); treatment of acne vulgaris

Unlabeled/Investigational Use Prophylaxis of toxoplasmosis in severely-immunocompromised patients; alternative agent for *Pneumocystis carinii* pneumonia prophylaxis (monotherapy) and treatment (in combination with trimethoprim)

Mechanism of Action/Effect Dapsone is a sulfone antimicrobial that prevents normal bacterial utilization of PABA for the synthesis of folic acid.

Contraindications Hypersensitivity to dapsone or any component of the formulation

Warnings/Precautions Use with caution in patients with severe anemia, G6PD deficiency, hypersensitivity to other sulfonamides, or restricted hepatic function. Safety and efficacy of topical dapsone has not been adequately evaluated in patient with G6PD deficiency or in patients <12 years of age.

Drug Interactions
Cytochrome P450 Effect: Substrate of CYP2C8/9 (minor), 2C19 (minor), 2E1 (minor), 3A4 (major)
Decreased Effect: CYP3A4 inducers may decrease the levels/effects of dapsone; example inducers include aminoglutethimide, carbamazepine, efavirenz, fosphenytoin, nafcillin, nevirapine, oxcarbazine, phenobarbital, phenytoin, primidone, and rifamycins. Didanosine (except enteric coated capsules) may decrease absorption of dapsone.

Increased Effect/Toxicity: Folic acid antagonists (methotrexate) may increase the risk of hematologic reactions of dapsone; probenecid decreases dapsone excretion; trimethoprim with dapsone may increase toxic effects of both drugs. CYP3A4 inhibitors may increase the levels/effects of dapsone; example inhibitors include azole antifungals, clarithromycin, diclofenac, doxycycline, erythromycin, imatinib, isoniazid, nefazodone, nicardipine, propofol, protease inhibitors, quinidine, telithromycin, and verapamil.

Nutritional/Ethanol Interactions Herb/Nutraceutical: St John's wort may decrease dapsone levels.

Adverse Reactions

>10%: Hematologic: Hemolysis (dose-related; seen in patients with and without G6PD deficiency), hemoglobin decrease (1-2 g/dL — almost all patients), reticulocyte increase (2% to 12%), methemoglobinemia, red cell life span shortened

Frequency not defined.

Cardiovascular: Tachycardia

Central nervous system: Fever, headache, insomnia, psychosis, tonic-clonic movement (topical), vertigo

Dermatologic: Bullous and exfoliative dermatitis, erythema nodosum, exfoliative dermatitis (oral), morbilliform and scarlatiniform reactions, phototoxicity (oral), Stevens-Johnson syndrome, toxic epidural necrolysis, urticaria

Endocrine & metabolic: Hypoalbuminemia (without proteinuria), male infertility

Gastrointestinal: Abdominal pain (oral, topical), nausea, pancreatitis (oral, topical), vomiting

Hematologic: Agranulocytosis, anemia, leukopenia, pure red cell aplasia (case report)

Hepatic: Cholestatic jaundice, hepatitis

Neuromuscular & skeletal: Drug-induced lupus erythematosus, lower motor neuron toxicity (prolonged therapy), peripheral neuropathy (rare, nonleprosy patients)

Ocular: Blurred vision

Otic: Tinnitus

Renal: Albuminuria, nephrotic syndrome, renal papillary necrosis

Respiratory: Interstitial pneumonitis, pharyngitis (topical), pulmonary eosinophilia

Miscellaneous: Infectious mononucleosis-like syndrome (rash, fever, lymphadenopathy, hepatic dysfunction)

Overdosage/Toxicology Symptoms of overdose include nausea, vomiting, hyperexcitability, methemoglobin-induced depression, seizures, cyanosis, and hemolysis. Following decontamination, methylene blue 1-2 mg/kg I.V. is the treatment of choice.

Pharmacodynamics/Kinetics

Half-Life Elimination: 30 hours (range: 10-50 hours)

Metabolism: Hepatic; forms metabolite

Excretion: Urine (~85%)

Available Dosage Forms

Gel, topical (Aczone™): 5% (30 g)

Tablet: 25 mg, 100 mg

Dosing

Adults & Elderly:

Leprosy: Oral: 50-100 mg/day for 3-10 years

Dermatitis herpetiformis: Oral: Initial: 50 mg/day, increase to 300. mg/day, or higher to achieve full control. Reduce dosage to minimum level as soon as possible.

Pneumonia caused by *Pneumocystis carinii* (unlabeled use): Oral:

Prophylaxis: 100 mg/day

Treatment: Adults: 100 mg/day in combination with trimethoprim (15-20 mg/kg/day) for 21 days

Acne vulgaris: Topical: Apply pea-sized amount twice daily.

Pediatrics:

Leprosy: Oral: Children: 1-2 mg/kg/24 hours, up to a maximum of 100 mg/day

Prophylaxis of *Pneumocystis carinii* pneumonia (unlabeled use): Oral: Children >1 month: 2 mg/kg/day once daily (maximum dose: 100 mg/day) or 4 mg/kg/dose once weekly (maximum dose: 200 mg)

Acne: Topical: Children ≥12 years: Refer to adult dosing.

Renal Impairment: No guidelines are available.

Oral: May give with meals if GI upset occurs.

Topical: Apply to clean, dry skin; rub in completely. Wash hands after application.

Stability

Storage:

Gel: Store at 20°C to 25°C (68°F to 76°F). Protect from freezing and from light. Keep tube in original box.

Tablet: Store at 20°C to 25°C (68°F to 76°F). Protect from light.

Laboratory Monitoring Liver function, CBC

Physical Assessment: Assess potential for interactions with other pharmacological agents or herbal products patient may be taking. Monitor laboratory tests (CBC and LFT), therapeutic effectiveness (according to purpose for use), and adverse response. Teach patient appropriate use, possible side effects/appropriate interventions, and adverse symptoms to report.

Patient Education: Do not take any new medication during therapy unless approved by prescriber. Take as directed; do not discontinue without consulting prescriber. Do not take with antacids, alkaline foods, or other medication. Therapy may take 3-10 years for leprosy. Frequent blood tests may be required. If rash develops, discontinue and notify prescriber. Report persistent sore throat, fever, chills; constant fatigue; yellowing of skin or eyes; or easy bruising or bleeding. **Pregnancy/breast-feeding precautions:** Inform prescriber if you are or intend to become pregnant. Consult prescriber if breast-feeding.

Dietary Considerations Do not administer with antacids, alkaline foods, or drugs.

Daptomycin (DAP toe mye sin)

U.S. Brand Names Cubicin®

Synonyms Cidecin; Dapcin; LY146032

Pharmacologic Category Antibiotic, Cyclic Lipopeptide

Pregnancy Risk Factor B

Lactation Excretion in breast milk unknown/use caution

Use Treatment of complicated skin and skin structure infections caused by susceptible aerobic Gram-positive organisms

Unlabeled/Investigational Use Treatment of bacteremia, endocarditis, and other severe infections caused by MRSA or VRE

Mechanism of Action/Effect Daptomycin binds to components of the cell membrane of susceptible organisms and causes rapid depolarization, inhibiting intracellular synthesis of DNA, RNA, and protein. Daptomycin is bactericidal in a concentration-dependent manner.

Contraindications Hypersensitivity to daptomycin or any component of the formulation

Warnings/Precautions May be associated with an increased incidence of myopathy; discontinue in patients with signs and symptoms of myopathy in conjunction with an increase in CPK (>5 times ULN or 1000 units/L) or in asymptomatic patients with a CPK ≥10 times ULN. Myopathy may occur more frequently at dose and/or frequency in excess of recommended dosages. Use caution in patients receiving other drugs associated with myopathy (eg, HMG-CoA reductase inhibitors). Not indicated for the treatment of pneumonia (poor lung penetration). Use caution in renal impairment (dosage adjustment required). Symptoms suggestive of peripheral neuropathy have been observed with treatment; monitor for new-onset or worsening neuropathy. Superinfection by resistant strains and/or pseudomembranous colitis may be associated with use. Safety and efficacy in patients <18 years of age have not been established.

(Continued)

Daptomycin *(Continued)*

Drug Interactions
Increased Effect/Toxicity: No clinically-significant interactions have been identified.

Adverse Reactions 1% to 10%:
Cardiovascular: Hypotension (2%), hypertension (1%)
Central nervous system: Headache (5%), insomnia (5%), dizziness (2%), fever (2%)
Dermatologic: Rash (4%), pruritus (3%)
Gastrointestinal: Constipation (6%), nausea (6%), diarrhea (5%), vomiting (3%), dyspepsia (1%)
Genitourinary: Urinary tract infection (2%)
Hematologic: Anemia (2%)
Hepatic: Transaminases increased (3%)
Local: Injection site reaction (6%)
Neuromuscular & skeletal: CPK increased (3%), limb pain (2%), arthralgia (1%)
Renal: Renal failure (2%)
Respiratory: Dyspnea (2%)
Miscellaneous: Infection (fungal, 3%)

Overdosage/Toxicology
Treatment is symptomatic and supportive; hemodialysis removes approximately 15% in 4 hours.

Pharmacodynamics/Kinetics
Protein Binding: 92%
Half-Life Elimination: 8-9 hours (up to 28 hours in renal impairment)
Excretion: Urine (78%; primarily as unchanged drug); feces (6%)
Available Dosage Forms Injection, powder for reconstitution: 250 mg, 500 mg

Dosing
Adults & Elderly:
Skin and/or skin structure infections (complicated): I.V.: 4 mg/kg once daily for 7-14 days
Bacteremia, endocarditis (unlabeled use): I.V.: 6 mg/kg once daily
Renal Impairment: Skin and soft tissue infections: Cl$_{cr}$ <30 mL/minute: 4 mg/kg every 48 hours
Hemodialysis (administer after hemodialysis) and/or CAPD: Dose as in Cl$_{cr}$ <30 mL/minute
Hepatic Impairment: No adjustment required for mild-to-moderate impairment (Child-Pugh Class A or B). Not evaluated in severe hepatic impairment.

Administration
I.V.: Infuse over 30 minutes.

Stability
Reconstitution: Reconstitute vial with NS (5 mL for 250 mg vial, 10 mL for 500 mg vial). Should be further diluted following reconstitution in an appropriate volume of NS.
Compatibility: Incompatible in dextrose-containing solutions
Storage: Store under refrigeration at 2°C to 8°C (36°F to 46°F). Reconstituted solution (either in vial or in infusion bag) is stable for a cumulative time of 12 hours at room temperature and 48 hours if refrigerated (2°C to 8°C).

Laboratory Monitoring
CPK should be monitored at least weekly during therapy.

Nursing Actions
Physical Assessment: Assess potential for interactions with other pharmacological agents (eg, HMG-CoA reductase inhibitors). Monitor laboratory tests (CPK), therapeutic effectiveness (eg, signs and symptoms of infection), and adverse reactions at beginning of therapy and on a regular basis during therapy. Should be infused over 30 minutes. Teach patient possible side effects and adverse symptoms to report (eg, rash, hypotension, CNS changes, limb pain, muscle pain or weakness, opportunistic infection).
Patient Education: This medication can only be administered via intravenous infusion. You will be monitored during and after each infusion. Report immediately any burning, pain, or redness at infusion site, any throat tightness, respiratory difficulty, or chest tightness. Use caution when driving or engaging in tasks that require mental alertness until response to drug is known. Report unusual headache, insomnia, nausea or vomiting, limb or joint pain, alteration in urination patterns, itching or pain on urination, or other possible adverse reactions. **Breast-feeding precaution:** Inform prescriber if you are or intend to breast-feed.
Geriatric Considerations The manufacturer reports that in studies of complicated skin and skin structure infections, elderly patients had a lower clinical success rate and a higher incidence of adverse effects (no quantitative data provided in product labeling). Refer to dosing in renal impairment.

Darbepoetin Alfa *(dar be POE e tin AL fa)*

U.S. Brand Names Aranesp®
Synonyms Erythropoiesis Stimulating Protein
Pharmacologic Category Colony Stimulating Factor; Growth Factor; Recombinant Human Erythropoietin
Medication Safety Issues
Sound-alike/look-alike issues:
Darbepoetin alfa may be confused with epoetin alfa
Pregnancy Risk Factor C
Lactation Excretion in breast milk unknown/use caution
Use Treatment of anemia associated with chronic renal failure (CRF), including patients on dialysis (ESRD) and patients not on dialysis; anemia associated with chemotherapy for nonmyeloid malignancies
Mechanism of Action/Effect Stimulates production of red blood cells within the bone marrow. There is a dose response relationship with this effect. This results in an increase in red blood cell counts followed by a rise in hematocrit and hemoglobin levels. When administered SubQ or I.V., darbepoetin's half-life is ~3 times that of epoetin alfa.
Contraindications Hypersensitivity to darbepoetin or any component of the formulation; uncontrolled hypertension
Warnings/Precautions Erythropoietic therapies may be associated with an increased risk of cardiovascular and/or neurologic events. Darbepoetin alfa should be managed carefully; avoid hemoglobin increases >1 g/dL in any 2-week period, and do not exceed a target level of 12 g/dL. Prior to and during therapy, iron stores must be evaluated. Supplemental iron is recommended if serum ferritin <100 mcg/mL or serum transferrin saturation <20%. In cancer patients, the risk of thrombotic events (eg, pulmonary emboli, thrombophlebitis, thrombosis) was increased by erythropoietic therapy.

Use with caution in patients with hypertension or with a history of seizures; hypertensive encephalopathy and seizures have been reported. If hypertension is difficult to control, reduce or hold darbepoetin alpha. **Not** recommended for acute correction of severe anemia or as a substitute for transfusion. Consider discontinuing in patients who receive a renal transplant.

Prior to treatment, correct or exclude deficiencies of vitamin B$_{12}$ and/or folate, as well as other factors which may impair erythropoiesis (aluminum toxicity, inflammatory conditions, infections). Poor response should prompt evaluation of these potential factors, as well as possible malignant processes, occult blood loss, hemolysis, and/or bone marrow fibrosis. Pure red cell aplasia (PRCA) with associated neutralizing antibodies to erythropoietin has been reported, predominantly in patients with CRF. Patients with loss of response to darbepoetin alfa should be evaluated. Discontinue treatment in patients with PRCA secondary to neutralizing antibodies to erythropoietin.

Due to the delayed onset of erythropoiesis, darbepoetin is of no value in the acute treatment of anemia. Safety and efficacy in patients with underlying hematologic diseases have not been established, including porphyria, thalassemia, hemolytic anemia, and sickle cell disease. Potentially serious allergic reactions have been reported. Do not shake solution; vigorous shaking may denature darbepoetin alfa, rendering it biologically inactive. Safety and efficacy (as initial treatment) in children have not been established; children >1 year of age with CRF have been converted from epoetin alfa to darbepoetin.

Nutritional/Ethanol Interactions Ethanol: Should be avoided due to adverse effects on erythropoiesis.

Adverse Reactions Note: Frequency of adverse events cited in patients with CRF or cancer and may be, in part, a reflection of population in which the drug is used and/or associated with dialysis procedures.

>10%:
Cardiovascular: Hypertension (4% to 23%), hypotension (22%), edema (21%), peripheral edema (11%)
Central nervous system: Fatigue (9% to 33%), fever (4% to 19%), headache (12% to 16%), dizziness (8% to 14%)
Gastrointestinal: Diarrhea (16% to 22%), constipation (5% to 18%), vomiting (2% to 15%), nausea (14%), abdominal pain (12%)
Neuromuscular & skeletal: Myalgia (8% to 21%), arthralgia (11% to 13%)
Respiratory: Upper respiratory infection (14%), dyspnea (2% to 12%)
Miscellaneous: Infection (27%)

1% to 10%:
Cardiovascular: Arrhythmia (10%), angina/chest pain (6% to 8%), fluid overload (6%), CHF (6%), thrombosis (6%), MI (2%)
Central nervous system: Seizure (≤1%), stroke (1%), TIA (1%)
Dermatologic: Pruritus (8%), rash (7%)
Endocrine & metabolic: Dehydration (3% to 5%)
Local: Vascular access thrombosis (8%), injection site pain (7%), vascular access hemorrhage (6%), vascular access infection (6%)
Neuromuscular & skeletal: Limb pain (10%), back pain (8%), weakness (5%)
Respiratory: Cough (10%), bronchitis (6%), pneumonia (3%), pulmonary embolism (1%)
Miscellaneous: Death (7%), flu-like symptoms (6%)

Postmarketing and/or case reports: Deep vein thrombosis, pure red cell aplasia, severe anemia (with or without other cytopenias), thromboembolism, thrombophlebitis

Overdosage/Toxicology The maximum amount of darbepoetin which may be safely administered has not been determined. However, cardiovascular and neurologic adverse events have been correlated to excessive and/or rapid rise in hemoglobin. Phlebotomy may be performed if clinically indicated.

Pharmacodynamics/Kinetics
Onset of Action: Increased hemoglobin levels not generally observed until 2-6 weeks after initiating treatment
Time to Peak: SubQ: CRF: 34 hours (range: 24-72 hours); Cancer: 90 hours (range: 71-123 hours)
Half-Life Elimination: CRF: Terminal: I.V.: 21 hours, SubQ: 49 hours; cancer: SubQ: 74 hours; **Note:** Half-life is ~3 times as long as epoetin alfa

Available Dosage Forms
Injection, solution, with human albumin 2.5 mg/mL [preservative free, single-dose vial]: 25 mcg/mL (1 mL); 40 mcg/mL (1 mL); 60 mcg/mL (1 mL); 100 mcg/mL (1 mL); 150 mcg/0.75 mL (0.75 mL); 200 mcg/mL (1 mL); 300 mcg/mL (1 mL)
Injection, solution, with human albumin 2.5 mg/mL [preservative free, prefilled syringe]: 25 mcg/0.42 mL (0.42 mL); 40 mcg/0.4 mL (0.4 mL); 60 mcg/0.3 mL (0.3 mL); 100 mcg/0.5 mL (0.5 mL); 200 mcg/0.4 mL (0.4 mL); 300 mcg/0.6 mL (0.6 mL); 500 mcg/mL (1 mL)

Dosing
Adults & Elderly:
Anemia associated with CRF: I.V., SubQ: Initial: 0.45 mcg/kg once weekly; titrate to response; some patients may respond to doses given once every 2 weeks
Unlabeled dosing:
Every 2-weeks: 0.75 mcg/kg every 2 weeks (Toto, 2004)
or
Every 4-weeks: 0.75 mcg/kg every 2 weeks; once titrated, multiply dose by 2 and give every 4 weeks (Jadoul, 2004).
Dosage adjustment:
Inadequate response: Increase dose by ~25% (not more frequently than once a month) for hemoglobin increase <1 g/dL after 4 weeks
Excessive response:
Decrease dose by ~25% when hemoglobin increases >1 g/dL in any 2-week period **or** hemoglobin increases and approaches 12 g/dL in any 2-week period
Hold dose, then decrease dose by ~25% when hemoglobin increases despite previous dose decrease (hold until hemoglobin decreases)
Anemia associated with chemotherapy: SubQ: Initial: 2.25 mcg/kg once weekly; with inadequate response after 6 weeks: 4.5 mcg/kg once weekly
or
500 mcg once every 3 weeks
Unlabeled dosing:
Every 2 weeks:
Initial: 200 mcg every 2 weeks; inadequate response: 300 mcg every 2 weeks (Thames, 2003)
or
Initial: 3 mcg/kg every 2 weeks; inadequate response: 5 mcg/kg every 2 weeks (Vadhan-Raj, 2003)
or
Every 3 weeks (front load): Initial:
4.5 mcg/kg every week until desired Hgb obtained; maintenance: 4.5 mcg/kg (or titrated dose) every 3 weeks (Hesketh, 2004)
or
Initial: 325 mcg every week until desired Hgb obtained; maintenance: 325 mcg every 3 weeks (Hesketh, 2004)
Dosage adjustment: Titration may be required to limit rises of Hgb to <1 g/dL over any 2-week interval and to reach a hemoglobin concentration not to exceed 12 g/dL.
Inadequate response: Increase dose up to 4.5 mcg/kg when hemoglobin increase <1 g/dL after 4-6 weeks
Excessive response:
Decrease dose by ~40% when hemoglobin increases >1 g/dL in any 2-week period **or** hemoglobin exceeds 11 g/dL in any 2-week period
Hold dose, then decrease dose by ~40% when hemoglobin increases despite previous dose decrease (hold until hemoglobin decreases) **or** when hemoglobin ≥13 g/dL (hold until hemoglobin ≤12 g/dL)
Conversion from epoetin alfa to darbepoetin alfa: See table on next page.
Renal Impairment: Dosage requirements for patients with chronic renal failure who do not require dialysis may be lower than in dialysis patients. Monitor patients closely during the time period in which a dialysis regimen is initiated, dosage requirement may increase.
(Continued)

Darbepoetin Alfa *(Continued)*

Conversion From Epoetin Alfa to Darbepoetin Alfa

Previous Dosage of Epoetin Alfa (units/week)	Children Darbepoetin Alfa Dosage (mcg/week)	Adults Darbepoetin Alfa Dosage (mcg/week)	Adults Darbepoetin Alfa Dosage (mcg/every 2 weeks)
<1500	Not established	6.25	12.5
1500-2499	6.25	6.25	12.5
2500-4999	10	12.5	25
5000-10,999	20	25	50
11,000-17,999	40	40	80
18,000-33,999	60	60	120
34,000-89,999	100	100	200
≥90,000	200	200	400

Note: In patients receiving epoetin alfa 2-3 times per week, darbepoetin alfa is administered once weekly. In patients receiving epoetin alfa once weekly, darbepoetin alfa is administered once every 2 weeks.

Administration

I.V.: May be administered by SubQ or I.V. injection. The I.V. route is recommended in hemodialysis patients. Do not shake; vigorous shaking may denature darbepoetin alfa, rendering it biologically inactive. Do not dilute or administer in conjunction with other drug solutions. Discard any unused portion of the vial; do not pool unused portions. Discontinue immediately if signs/symptoms of anaphylaxis occur.

Stability

Compatibility: Do not dilute or administer with other solutions.

Storage: Store at 2°C to 8°C (36°F to 46°F). Do not freeze or shake. Protect from light.

Laboratory Monitoring Hemoglobin (weekly); prior to and during therapy, iron stores must be evaluated (supplemental iron is recommended in any patient with a serum ferritin <100 mcg/mL or serum transferrin saturation <20%)

Nursing Actions

Physical Assessment: Assess potential for interactions with other prescriptions, OTC medications, or herbal products patient may be taking (eg, nutritional or supplemental iron). Monitor blood pressure and be alert for signs of fluid retention. Assess GI function. Monitor laboratory tests and patient response prior to and during therapy. Teach patient proper use if self-administered (appropriate injection technique and syringe/needle disposal, possible side effects/appropriate interventions, and adverse symptoms to report.

Patient Education: Do not take any new medication during therapy without consulting prescriber. This medication can only be administered by infusion or injection (if self-administered, follow exact directions for injection and needle disposal). You will need frequent blood tests to determine appropriate dosage. Avoid alcohol and do not make significant changes in your dietary iron without consulting prescriber. Check your blood pressure as frequently as recommended and report any significant changes. May cause nausea or vomiting (small frequent meals, frequent mouth care, sucking lozenges, or chewing gum may help); diarrhea (boiled milk, buttermilk, or yogurt may help); constipation (increased dietary fruit, fiber, fluids, and increased exercise may help); or dizziness, fatigue, or headache (use caution when driving or engaging in tasks that require alertness until response to drug is known). Report signs of edema (swollen extremities, respiratory difficulty); sudden onset of acute headache, back pain, or chest pain; muscle tremors or weakness; cough or signs of respiratory infection; or other adverse effects. **Pregnancy/breast-feeding precautions:** Inform prescriber if you are or intend to become pregnant. Consult prescriber if breast-feeding.

Dietary Considerations Supplemental iron intake may be required in patients with low iron stores.

Darifenacin *(dar i FEN a sin)*

U.S. Brand Names Enablex®

Synonyms Darifenacin Hydrobromide; UK-88,525

Pharmacologic Category Anticholinergic Agent

Pregnancy Risk Factor C

Lactation Excretion in breast milk unknown/use caution

Use Management of symptoms of bladder overactivity (urge incontinence, urgency, and frequency)

Mechanism of Action/Effect Blocks muscarinic/cholinergic receptors (M3 subtype) on the smooth muscle of the urinary bladder to limit bladder contractions, reducing the symptoms of bladder irritability/overactivity (urge incontinence, urgency and frequency).

Contraindications Hypersensitivity to darifenacin or any component of the formulation; uncontrolled narrow-angle glaucoma; urinary retention, paralytic ileus, GI or GU obstruction

Warnings/Precautions Use with caution with hepatic impairment; dosage limitation is required in moderate hepatic impairment (Child-Pugh Class B). Not recommended for use in severe hepatic impairment (Child-Pugh Class C). Use with caution in patients with clinically-significant bladder outlet obstruction or prostatic hyperplasia (nonobstructive).Use caution in patients with decreased GI motility, constipation, hiatal hernia, reflux esophagitis, and ulcerative colitis. Use caution in patients with myasthenia gravis. In patients with controlled narrow-angle glaucoma, darifenacin should be used with extreme caution and only when the potential benefit outweighs risks of treatment. Safety and efficacy have not been established in pediatric patients.

Drug Interactions

Cytochrome P450 Effect: Substrate of CYP2D6 (minor), CYP3A4 (major); **Inhibits** CYP2D6 (moderate), 3A4 (weak)

Decreased Effect: Darifenacin may decrease the levels/effects of CYP2D6 prodrug substrates; example prodrug substrates include codeine, hydrocodone, oxycodone, and tramadol. CYP3A4 inducers may decrease the levels/effects of darifenacin; example inducers include aminoglutethimide, carbamazepine, nafcillin, nevirapine, phenobarbital, phenytoin, and rifamycins. Concomitant use with acetylcholinesterase inhibitors may reduce the therapeutic efficacy of darifenacin.

Increased Effect/Toxicity: Adverse anticholinergic effects may be additive with other anticholinergic agents (includes tricyclic antidepressants, antihistamines, and phenothiazines). Coadministration with pramlintide may result an additive reduction in gut motility. Darifenacin may increase the levels/effects of CYP2D6 substrates; example substrates include amphetamines, selected beta-blockers, dextromethorphan, fluoxetine, lidocaine, mirtazapine, nefazodone, paroxetine, risperidone, ritonavir, thioridazine, tricyclic antidepressants, and venlafaxine. CYP3A4 inhibitors may increase the levels/effects of darifenacin; example inhibitors include azole antifungals, clarithromycin, diclofenac, doxycycline, erythromycin, imatinib, isoniazid, nefazodone, nicardipine, propofol, protease inhibitors, quinidine, telithromycin, and verapamil.

Adverse Reactions

>10%: Gastrointestinal: Xerostomia (19% to 35%), constipation (15% to 21%)

1% to 10%:
Cardiovascular: Hypertension, peripheral edema
Central nervous system: Headache (7%), dizziness (1% to 2%)
Dermatological: Dry skin, pruritis, rash
Gastrointestinal: Dyspepsia (3% to 8%), abdominal pain (2% to 4%), nausea (2% to 4%), diarrhea (1% to 2%), vomiting, weight gain
Genitourinary: Urinary tract infection (4% to 5%), urinary retention, urinary tract disorder, vaginitis
Neuromuscular & skeletal: Weakness (2% to 3%), arthralgia, back pain
Ocular: Dry eyes (2%), abnormal vision
Respiratory: Bronchitis, pharyngitis, rhinitis, sinusitis
Miscellaneous: Flu-like syndrome (<1% to 3%), accidental injury (<1% to 3%)

Overdosage/Toxicology Doses of up to 75 mg have been used in clinical trials, with abnormal vision as the primary adverse event. Overdose may result in severe antimuscarinic effects. Treatment should be symptom-directed and supportive. ECG monitoring is recommended.

Pharmacodynamics/Kinetics
Time to Peak: Plasma: 7 hours
Protein Binding: 98%
Half-Life Elimination: 13-19 hours
Metabolism: Hepatic, via CYP3A4 (major) and CYP2D6 (minor)
Excretion: Urine (60%), feces (40%); as metabolites (inactive)

Available Dosage Forms Tablet, extended release: 7.5 mg, 15 mg

Dosing
Adults & Elderly:
Symptoms of bladder overactivity: Oral: Initial: 7.5 mg once daily. If response is not adequate after a minimum of 2 weeks, dosage may be increased to 15 mg once daily.
Dosage adjustment with concomitant potent CYP3A4 inhibitors: Daily dosage should not exceed 7.5 mg/day
Renal Impairment: No adjustment required.
Hepatic Impairment:
Moderate impairment (Child-Pugh Class B): Daily dosage should not exceed 7.5 mg/day
Severe impairment (Child-Pugh Class C): Has not been evaluated; use is not recommended

Administration
Oral: Tablet should be taken with liquid and swallowed whole; do not chew, crush or split tablet. May be taken without regard to food.

Stability
Storage: Store at 25°C (77°F); excursions permitted to 15°C to 30°C (59°F to 86°F). Protect from light.

Nursing Actions
Physical Assessment: Assess potential for interactions with other prescriptions, OTC medications, or herbal products patient may be taking. Monitor therapeutic effectiveness and adverse reactions. Teach patient appropriate use, interventions to reduce side effects, and adverse symptoms to report.
Patient Education: Take as directed. Swallow tablet whole. May cause headache (consult prescriber for a mild analgesic); dizziness, nervousness, or sleepiness (use caution when driving, climbing stairs, or engaging in tasks requiring alertness until response to drug is known); or abdominal discomfort, diarrhea, constipation (increasing exercise, fluids, fruit/fiber may help); dry mouth, nausea, vomiting (small frequent meals, frequent mouth care, chewing gum, or sucking lozenges may help). Report back pain, muscle spasms, alteration in gait, or numbness of extremities; unresolved or persistent constipation, diarrhea, or vomiting; or symptoms of upper respiratory infection or flu. Report difficulty urinating, or pain on urination, or abdominal pain. **Pregnancy/**

breast-feeding precautions: Inform prescriber if you are or intend to become pregnant. Consult prescriber if considering breast-feeding.
Dietary Considerations May be taken without regard to meals, with or without food.
Geriatric Considerations There is a trend for decreased clearance with age, though no change in dose is recommended. The selectivity of darifenacin for the M3 receptor on the bladder may offer an advantage (less CNS and cardiovascular effects) over other anticholinergic agents used in the treatment of overactive bladder.
Breast-Feeding Issues Although human data are not available, darifenacin is excreted in the breast milk in animals.
Pregnancy Issues There are no adequate and well-controlled studies in pregnant women; should be used only if potential benefit outweighs possible risk to the fetus.

DAUNOrubicin Citrate (Liposomal)
(daw noe ROO bi sin SI trate lip po SOE mal)

U.S. Brand Names DaunoXome®
Pharmacologic Category Antineoplastic Agent, Anthracycline
Medication Safety Issues
Sound-alike/look-alike issues:
DAUNOrubicin may be confused with dactinomycin, DOXOrubicin, epirubicin, idarubicin
Liposomal formulations (DaunoXome®) may be confused with conventional formulations (Adriamycin PFS®, Adriamycin RDF®, Cerubidine®, Rubex®)
Pregnancy Risk Factor D
Lactation Excretion in breast milk unknown/not recommended
Use First-line cytotoxic therapy for advanced HIV-associated Kaposi's sarcoma
Mechanism of Action/Effect Binds to DNA and inhibits DNA synthesis causing cell death
Contraindications Hypersensitivity to daunorubicin or any component of the formulation; pregnancy
Warnings/Precautions Hazardous agent - use appropriate precautions for handling and disposal. Daunorubicin is associated with a dose-related cardiac toxicity. The risk of similar toxicity with liposome-encapsulated daunorubicin is not certain. Use caution in patients with previous therapy with high cumulative doses of anthracyclines, cyclophosphamide, or thoracic radiation, or who have pre-existing cardiac disease.
Drug Interactions
Decreased Effect: Patients may experience impaired immune response to vaccines; possible infection after administration of live vaccines in patients receiving immunosuppressants.
Adverse Reactions
>10%:
Central nervous system: Fatigue (51%), headache (28%), neuropathy (13%)
Hematologic: Myelosuppression, neutropenia (51%), thrombocytopenia, anemia
Onset: 7 days
Nadir: 14 days
Recovery: 21 days
Gastrointestinal: Abdominal pain, vomiting, anorexia (23%); diarrhea (38%); nausea (55%)
Respiratory: Cough (28%), dyspnea (26%), rhinitis
Miscellaneous: Allergic reactions (24%)
1% to 10%:
Cardiovascular: CHF (incidence unknown), hypertension, palpitation, syncope, tachycardia, chest pain, edema
Dermatologic: Alopecia (8%), pruritus (7%)
(Continued)

DAUNOrubicin Citrate (Liposomal)
(Continued)

Endocrine & metabolic: Hot flashes
Gastrointestinal: Constipation (7%), stomatitis (10%)
Neuromuscular & skeletal: Arthralgia (7%), myalgia (7%)
Ocular: Conjunctivitis, eye pain (5%)
Respiratory: Sinusitis

Overdosage/Toxicology Symptoms of acute overdose are increased severity of the observed dose-limiting toxicities of therapeutic doses, myelosuppression (especially granulocytopenia), fatigue, nausea, and vomiting. Treatment is symptomatic.

Pharmacodynamics/Kinetics
Half-Life Elimination: Distribution: 4.4 hours; Terminal: 3-5 hours
Metabolism: Similar to daunorubicin, but metabolite plasma levels are low
Excretion: Primarily feces; some urine
Clearance, plasma: 17.3 mL/minute

Available Dosage Forms Injection, solution [preservative free]: 2 mg/mL (25 mL) [contains sucrose 2125 mg/25 mL]

Dosing
Adults & Elderly: Refer to individual protocols.
Advanced HIV-associated Kaposi's sarcoma: I.V.: 20-40 mg/m^2 every 2 weeks
100 mg/m^2 every 3 weeks

Renal Impairment:
S_{cr} 1.2-3 mg/dL: Reduce dose to 75% of normal.
S_{cr} >3 mg/dL: Reduce dose to 50% of normal.

Hepatic Impairment:
Serum bilirubin 1.2-3 mg/dL: Reduce to 75% of normal dose.
Serum bilirubin >3 mg/dL: Reduce to 50% of normal dose.

Administration
I.V.: Vesicant. Infuse over 1 hour; do not mix with other drugs.
I.V. Detail: Extravasation management: Daunorubicin is a vesicant; infiltration can cause severe inflammation, tissue necrosis, and ulceration. If the drug is infiltrated, consult institutional policy, apply ice to the area, and elevate the limb.

Stability
Reconstitution: Only fluid which may be mixed with DaunoXome® is D$_5$W. Must not be mixed with saline, bacteriostatic agents such as benzyl alcohol, or any other solution.
Compatibility: Incompatible with sodium bicarbonate and fluorouracil, heparin, dexamethasone
Storage: Store in refrigerator 2°C to 8°C (37°F to 45°F); do not freeze. Protect from light.

Laboratory Monitoring Cardiac function, CBC with differential and platelet count, liver and renal function; repeat blood counts prior to each dose and withhold if the absolute granulocyte count is <750 cells/mm^3. Monitor serum uric acid levels.

Nursing Actions
Physical Assessment: Monitor infusion closely; extravasation can cause severe cellulitis or tissue necrosis. **Note:** Application of heat or sodium bicarbonate can be harmful and is contraindicated). Monitor laboratory tests and adverse reactions (eg, hypertension, tachycardia, cough, dyspnea, gastrointestinal upset) prior to each infusion and on a regular basis throughout therapy. Teach patient possible side effects/appropriate interventions and adverse symptoms to report.
Patient Education: Do not take any new medication during therapy unless approved by prescriber. This medication can only be administered by infusion. You will be monitored closely. Report immediately any swelling, pain, burning, or redness at infusion site;

chest pain or tightness; difficulty breathing or difficulty swallowing. It is important to maintain adequate hydration (2-3 L/day of fluids) unless instructed to restrict fluid intake, and nutrition (small, frequent meals may help). You will be more susceptible to infection (avoid crowds and exposure to infection and do not have any vaccinations without consulting prescriber). May cause nausea or vomiting (small, frequent meals, frequent mouth care, sucking lozenges, or chewing gum may help); diarrhea (buttermilk, boiled milk, or yogurt may help); loss of hair (reversible); or red-pink urine (normal). Report immediately chest pain, swelling of extremities, respiratory difficulty, palpitations, or rapid heartbeat. Report unresolved nausea, vomiting, or diarrhea; alterations in urinary pattern (increased or decreased); opportunistic infection (eg, fever, chills, unusual bruising or bleeding fatigue; purulent vaginal discharge; unhealed mouth sores); abdominal pain or blood in stools; excessive fatigue; or yellowing of eyes or skin. **Pregnancy/breast-feeding precautions:** Do not get pregnant or cause a pregnancy (males) while taking this medication. Consult prescriber for appropriate contraceptive measures. Breast-feeding is not recommended.

Related Information
FDA Name Differentiation Project: The Use of Tall-Man Letters *on page 12*

DAUNOrubicin Hydrochloride
(daw noe ROO bi sin hye droe KLOR ide)

U.S. Brand Names Cerubidine®
Synonyms Daunomycin; DNR; NSC-82151; Rubidomycin Hydrochloride
Pharmacologic Category Antineoplastic Agent, Anthracycline

Medication Safety Issues
Sound-alike/look-alike issues:
DAUNOrubicin may be confused with dactinomycin, DOXOrubicin, epirubicin, idarubicin
Conventional formulations (Cerubidine®) may be confused with liposomal formulations (DaunoXome®, Doxil®)

Pregnancy Risk Factor D
Lactation Excretion in breast milk unknown/not recommended
Use Treatment of acute lymphocytic (ALL) and nonlymphocytic (ANLL) leukemias
Mechanism of Action/Effect Inhibition of DNA and RNA synthesis by intercalation between DNA base pairs and by steric obstruction. Daunomycin intercalates at points of local uncoiling of the double helix. Although the exact mechanism is unclear, it appears that direct binding to DNA (intercalation) and inhibition of DNA repair (topoisomerase II inhibition) result in blockade of DNA and RNA synthesis and fragmentation of DNA.
Contraindications Hypersensitivity to daunorubicin or any component of the formulation; congestive heart failure or arrhythmias; previous therapy with high cumulative doses of daunorubicin and/or doxorubicin; pre-existing bone marrow suppression; pregnancy
Warnings/Precautions Hazardous agent — use appropriate precautions for handling and disposal. I.V. use only, severe local tissue necrosis will result if extravasation occurs. Reduce dose in patients with impaired hepatic, renal, or biliary function. Severe myelosuppression is possible when used in therapeutic doses. Total cumulative dose should take into account previous or concomitant treatment with cardiotoxic agents or irradiation of chest. Use caution in patients with previous therapy with anthracyclines, cyclophosphamide, thoracic radiation, or pre-existing cardiac disease.

Irreversible myocardial toxicity may occur as total dosage approaches:
550 mg/m^2 in adults
400 mg/m^2 in patients receiving chest radiation
300 mg/m^2 in children >2 years of age

Drug Interactions

Decreased Effect: Patients may experience impaired immune response to vaccines; possible infection after administration of live vaccines in patients receiving immunosuppressants.

Nutritional/Ethanol Interactions Ethanol: Avoid ethanol (due to GI irritation).

Lab Interactions Increased potassium (S)

Adverse Reactions

>10%:
Cardiovascular: Transient ECG abnormalities (supraventricular tachycardia, S-T wave changes, atrial or ventricular extrasystoles); generally asymptomatic and self-limiting. CHF, dose related, may be delayed for 7-8 years after treatment. Cumulative dose, radiation therapy, age, and use of cyclophosphamide all increase the risk. Recommended maximum cumulative doses:
No risk factors: 550-600 mg/m^2
Concurrent radiation: 450 mg/m^2
Regardless of cumulative dose, if the left ventricular ejection fraction is <30% to 40%, the drug is usually not given
Dermatologic: Alopecia, radiation recall
Gastrointestinal: Mild nausea or vomiting, stomatitis
Genitourinary: Discoloration of urine (red)
Hematologic: Myelosuppression, primarily leukopenia; thrombocytopenia and anemia
Onset: 7 days
Nadir: 10-14 days
Recovery: 21-28 days
1% to 10%:
Dermatologic: Skin "flare" at injection site; discoloration of saliva, sweat, or tears
Endocrine & metabolic: Hyperuricemia
Gastrointestinal: GI ulceration, diarrhea

Overdosage/Toxicology Symptoms of overdose include myelosuppression, nausea, vomiting, and stomatitis. There are no known antidotes. Treatment is symptomatic and supportive.

Pharmacodynamics/Kinetics

Half-Life Elimination: Distribution: 2 minutes; Elimination: 14-20 hours; Terminal: 18.5 hours; Daunorubicinol plasma half-life: 24-48 hours

Metabolism: Primarily hepatic to daunorubicinol (active), then to inactive aglycones, conjugated sulfates, and glucuronides

Excretion: Feces (40%); urine (~25% as unchanged drug and metabolites)

Available Dosage Forms

Injection, powder for reconstitution: 20 mg, 50 mg
Cerubidine®: 20 mg
Injection, solution: 5 mg/mL (4 mL, 10 mL)

Dosing

Adults & Elderly: Refer to individual protocols.
Range: I.V.: 30-60 mg/m^2/day for 3-5 days, repeat dose in 3-4 weeks
AML: I.V.:
Single agent induction: 60 mg/m^2/day for 3 days; repeat every 3-4 weeks
Combination therapy induction: 45 mg/m^2/day for 3 days of the first course of induction therapy; subsequent courses: Every day for 2 days
ALL combination therapy: I.V.: 45 mg/m^2/day for 3 days
Cumulative dose should not exceed 550 mg/m^2
Pediatrics: Refer to individual protocols.
ALL combination therapy: I.V.: Children: Remission induction: 25-45 mg/m^2 on day 1 every week for 4 cycles **or** 30-45 mg/m^2/day for 3 days

AML combination therapy: I.V.: Children: Induction (continuous infusion): 30-60 mg/m^2/day on days 1-3 of cycle
Note: In children <2 years or <0.5 m^2, daunorubicin should be based on weight - mg/kg: 1 mg/kg per protocol with frequency dependent on regimen employed
Cumulative dose should not exceed 300 mg/m^2 in children >2 years; maximum cumulative doses for younger children are unknown.

Renal Impairment:
Cl$_{cr}$ <10 mL/minute: Administer 75% of normal dose.
S$_{cr}$ >3 mg/dL: Administer 50% of normal dose.

Hepatic Impairment:
Serum bilirubin 1.2-3 mg/dL or AST 60-180 int. units: Reduce dose to 75%.
Serum bilirubin 3.1-5 mg/dL or AST >180 int. units: Reduce dose to 50%.
Serum bilirubin >5 mg/dL: Omit use.

Administration

I.V.: Vesicant. **Never** administer I.M. or SubQ. Administer IVP over 1-5 minutes.
I.V. Detail: Administer into the tubing of a rapidly infusing I.V. solution of D$_5$W or NS or dilute in 100 mL of D$_5$W or NS and infused over 15-30 minutes. Avoid extravasation, can cause severe tissue damage. Flush with 5-10 mL of I.V. solution before and after drug administration.

Extravasation management: Apply ice immediately for 30-60 minutes; then alternate off/on every 15 minutes for 1 day. Topical cooling may be achieved using ice packs or cooling pad with circulating ice water. Cooling of site for 24 hours as tolerated by the patient. Elevate and rest extremity 24-48 hours, then resume normal activity as tolerated. Application of cold inhibits vesicant's cytotoxicity. Application of heat or sodium bicarbonate can be harmful and is contraindicated. If pain, erythema, and/or swelling persist beyond 48 hours, refer patient immediately to plastic surgeon for consultation and possible debridement.

pH: 4.5-6.5

Stability

Reconstitution: Dilute vials with 4 mL SWFI for a final concentration of 5 mg/mL.
Compatibility: Stable in D$_5$W, LR, NS, SWFI
Incompatible with heparin, sodium bicarbonate, fluorouracil, and dexamethasone
Y-site administration: Incompatible with allopurinol, aztreonam, cefepime, fludarabine, piperacillin/tazobactam
Compatibility when admixed: Incompatible with dexamethasone sodium phosphate, heparin

Storage: Store intact vials at room temperature and protect from light. Reconstituted solution is stable for 4 days at 15°C to 25°C. Further dilution in D$_5$W, LR, or NS is stable at room temperature (25°C) for up to 4 weeks if protected from light.

Laboratory Monitoring CBC with differential, platelet count, liver function, ECG, ventricular ejection fraction, renal function

Nursing Actions

Physical Assessment: Monitor infusion site closely; extravasation can cause severe cellulitis or tissue necrosis (note application of heat or sodium bicarbonate can be harmful and is contraindicated). Monitor laboratory tests and patient response (eg, ECG abnormalities, CHF) prior to each infusion and on a regular basis throughout therapy. Teach patient possible side effects/appropriate interventions and adverse symptoms to report.

Patient Education: Do not take any new medication during therapy unless approved by prescriber. This medication can only be administered I.V. Report immediately any swelling, pain, burning, or redness at infusion site. Avoid alcohol. It is important to maintain
(Continued)

DAUNOrubicin Hydrochloride
(Continued)

adequate hydration (2-3 L/day of fluids) unless instructed to restrict fluid intake, and nutrition (small, frequent meals may help). You will be more susceptible to infection (avoid crowds and exposure to infection and do not have any vaccinations without consulting prescriber). May cause nausea or vomiting (small, frequent meals, frequent mouth care, sucking lozenges, or chewing gum may help); diarrhea (buttermilk, boiled milk, or yogurt may help); loss of hair (reversible); or red-pink urine (normal). Report immediately chest pain, swelling of extremities, respiratory difficulty, palpitations, or rapid heartbeat. Report unresolved nausea, vomiting, or diarrhea; alterations in urinary pattern (increased or decreased); opportunistic infection (eg, fever, chills, unusual bruising or bleeding fatigue, purulent vaginal discharge, unhealed mouth sores); abdominal pain or blood in stools; excessive fatigue; or yellowing of eyes or skin. **Pregnancy/breast-feeding precautions:** Do not get pregnant or cause a pregnancy (males) while taking this medication. Consult prescriber for appropriate contraceptive measures. Breast-feeding is not recommended.

Pregnancy Issues May cause fetal harm when administered to a pregnant woman. Animal studies have shown an increased incidence of fetal abnormalities.

Related Information
FDA Name Differentiation Project: The Use of Tall-Man Letters *on page 12*

Deferasirox (de FER a sir ox)

U.S. Brand Names Exjade®
Synonyms ICL670
Pharmacologic Category Antidote; Chelating Agent
Pregnancy Risk Factor B
Lactation Excretion in breast milk unknown/use caution
Use Treatment of chronic iron overload due to blood transfusions
Mechanism of Action/Effect Selectively binds iron, forming a complex which is excreted primarily through the feces.
Contraindications Hypersensitivity to deferasirox or any component of the formulation
Warnings/Precautions Dose-related elevations in serum creatinine have been reported; monitor and consider dose reduction, interruption, or discontinuation. May cause proteinuria; closely monitor. Hepatitis and elevated transaminases have been reported; monitor LFTs and consider dose modifications. May cause skin rash (dose-related); mild-to-moderate rashes may resolve without treatment interruption; for severe rash, interrupt and consider restarting at a lower dose with dose escalation and oral steroids. Auditory or ocular disturbances have been reported; monitor and consider dose reduction or treatment interruption. Use caution with hepatic impairment: limited experience. Do not combine with other iron chelation therapies; safety of combinations has not been established. May cause dizziness; use caution with driving or operating machinery. Safety and efficacy in children <2 years of age have not been established.

Drug Interactions
Decreased Effect: Aluminum-containing antacids may decrease absorption of deferasirox.

Adverse Reactions
>10%:
Central nervous system: Fever (19%), headache (16%)
Gastrointestinal: Abdominal pain (8% to 14%), diarrhea (12%), nausea (11%)

Renal: Serum creatinine increased (2% to 38%), proteinuria (19%)
Respiratory: Cough (14%), nasopharyngitis (13%), pharyngolaryngeal pain (11%)
Miscellaneous: Influenza (11%)
1% to 10%:
Central nervous system: Fatigue (6%)
Dermatologic: Rash (8%), urticaria (4%)
Gastrointestinal: Vomiting (10%)
Hepatic: ALT increased (6% to 8%), transaminitis (4%)
Neuromuscular & skeletal: Arthralgia (7%), back pain (6%)
Otic: Ear infection (5%)
Respiratory: Respiratory tract infection (10%), bronchitis (9%), pharyngitis (8%), acute tonsillitis (6%), rhinitis (6%)

Overdosage/Toxicology Single doses of up to 80 mg/kg have been tolerated with incidences of nausea and diarrhea. In case of overdose, induce vomiting and gastric lavage.

Pharmacodynamics/Kinetics
Time to Peak: 1-4 hours
Protein Binding: 99% to serum albumin
Half-Life Elimination: 8-16 hours
Metabolism: Hepatic via glucuronidation by UGT1A1 and UGT1A3; minor oxidation by CYP450; undergoes enterohepatic recirculation
Excretion: Feces (84%), urine (6% to 8%)
Available Dosage Forms Tablet, for oral suspension: 125 mg, 250 mg, 500 mg

Dosing
Adults & Elderly: Chronic iron overload due to blood transfusion: Oral: Initial: 20 mg/kg daily (calculate dose to nearest whole tablet)
Maintenance: Adjust dose every 3-6 months based on serum ferritin levels; increase by 5-10 mg/kg/day (calculate dose to nearest whole tablet); titrate. Maximum dose: 30 mg/kg/day; hold dose for serum ferritin <500 mcg/L. **Note:** Consider dose reduction or interruption for hearing loss or visual disturbances.

Pediatrics: Children ≥2 years: Refer to adult dosing.

Renal Impairment: Consider dose reduction, interruption, or discontinuation with serum creatinine elevation.

Hepatic Impairment: Consider dose adjustment or discontinuation for severe elevations in liver function tests.

Dosing Adjustment for Toxicity: Consider dose reduction or interruption for hearing loss or visual disturbances.

Administration
Oral: Do not chew or swallow whole tablets. Take at same time each day on an empty stomach, 30 minutes before food. Disperse tablets in water, orange juice, or apple juice (use 3.5 ounces for total doses <1 g; 7 ounces for doses >1 g); stir to form suspension and drink entire contents. Rinse remaining residue with more fluid; drink. Do not take simultaneously with aluminum-containing antacids.

Stability
Storage: Store at room temperature between 15°C and 30°C (59°F and 86°F). Protect from moisture.

Laboratory Monitoring
Serum creatinine, urine protein, liver function tests, and serum ferritin monthly

Nursing Actions
Physical Assessment: Assess hearing and vision prior to initiating therapy and periodically during treatment. Monitor lab results as indicated. Observe for skin rash. Mild-to-moderate rashes will usually resolve spontaneously. Assess for signs of liver dysfunction

(eg, unusual fatigue, easy bruising or bleeding, jaundice). Assess knowledge/teach patient appropriate use, side effects, and symptoms to report.

Patient Education: Take on an empty stomach at least 30 minutes prior to eating. Do not chew or swallow whole. Disperse in water, orange juice, or apple juice and drink immediately. Any residue remaining should be resuspended in a small volume of liquid and swallowed. Do not take with antacids. Maintain adequate hydration (2-3 L/day) unless instructed to restrict intake by prescriber. You may experience a fever, headache, abdominal pain, nausea, diarrhea, cough, sore throat, or dizziness (use caution when driving or engaging in activities requiring alertness until response to drug is known). Report severe rashes, changes in vision or hearing, unusual bleeding or bruising, change in color of urine or stool, yellowing of skin or eyes, or unusual fatigue. **Breast-feeding precaution:** Consult prescriber if breast-feeding.

Dietary Considerations Bioavailability increased variably when taken with food; take on empty stomach 30 minutes before a meal.

Geriatric Considerations Studies to date have not included sufficient numbers of subjects ≥65 years of age. Use caution in patients with liver dysfunction or low serum albumin. Monitor renal function.

Additional Information Deferasirox has a low affinity for binding with zinc and copper, may cause variable decreases in the serum concentration of these trace minerals.

Deferoxamine (de fer OKS a meen)

U.S. Brand Names Desferal®
Synonyms Deferoxamine Mesylate
Pharmacologic Category Antidote
Medication Safety Issues
Sound-alike/look-alike issues:
Deferoxamine may be confused with cefuroxime
Desferal® may be confused with desflurane, Dexferrum®, Disophrol®
Pregnancy Risk Factor C
Lactation Excretion in breast milk unknown/use caution
Use Acute iron intoxication or when clinical signs of significant iron toxicity exist; chronic iron overload secondary to multiple transfusions
Unlabeled/Investigational Use Removal of corneal rust rings following surgical removal of foreign bodies; diagnosis or treatment of aluminum induced toxicity associated with chronic kidney disease (CKD)
Mechanism of Action/Effect Complexes with trivalent ions (ferric ions) to form ferrioxamine, which are removed by the kidneys
Contraindications Hypersensitivity to deferoxamine or any component of the formulation; patients with severe renal disease and anuria; primary hemochromatosis
Warnings/Precautions Use with caution in patients with pyelonephritis; may increase susceptibility to *Yersinia enterocolitica.* Ocular and auditory disturbances and growth retardation (children only), have been reported following prolonged administration. Has been associated with adult respiratory distress syndrome (ARDS) following excessively high-dose treatment of acute intoxication. Caution must be used in performing tasks which require alertness (eg, operating machinery or driving). Patients should be informed that urine may have a reddish color.
Drug Interactions
Increased Effect/Toxicity: May cause loss of consciousness or coma when administered with prochlorperazine. Concomitant treatment with vitamin C (>500 mg/day) has been associated with cardiac impairment.

Lab Interactions TIBC may be falsely elevated with high serum iron concentrations or deferoxamine therapy.
Adverse Reactions Frequency not defined.
Cardiovascular: Flushing, hypotension, tachycardia, shock, edema
Central nervous system: Fever, dizziness, neuropathy, seizure, exacerbation of aluminum-related encephalopathy (dialysis), headache
Dermatologic: Angioedema, rash, urticaria
Endocrine & metabolic: Growth retardation (children), hypocalcemia
Gastrointestinal: Abdominal discomfort, abdominal pain, diarrhea, nausea, vomiting
Genitourinary: Dysuria
Hematologic: Thrombocytopenia, leukopenia
Local: Injection site: Burning, crust, edema, erythema, eschar, induration, infiltration, irritation, pain, pruritus, swelling, vesicles
Neuromuscular & skeletal: Arthralgia, leg cramps, myalgia, paresthesias
Ocular: Acuity decreased, blurred vision, dichromatopsia, visual loss, scotoma, visual field defects, optic neuritis, cataracts, retinal pigmentary abnormalities, night blindness
Otic: Hearing loss, tinnitus
Renal: Renal impairment, urine discoloration (vin-rose color)
Respiratory: Acute respiratory distress syndrome, asthma
Miscellaneous: Anaphylaxis, hypersensitivity reaction, infections (*Yersinia*, mucormycosis)
Overdosage/Toxicology Symptoms of overdose include aphasia, agitation, CNS depression, coma, bradycardia, acute renal failure, headache, hypotension, nausea, pallor, transient vision loss, and tachycardia. Treatment is symptomatic and supportive. Deferoxamine is dialyzable.
Pharmacodynamics/Kinetics
Half-Life Elimination: Parent drug: 6.1 hours; Ferrioxamine: 5.8 hours
Metabolism: Hepatic; binds with iron to form ferrioxamine
Excretion: Urine (as unchanged drug and ferrioxamine)
Available Dosage Forms Injection, powder for reconstitution, as mesylate: 500 mg, 2 g
Dosing
Adults & Elderly:
Acute iron toxicity:
I.M., I.V.: Initial: 1000 mg, may be followed by 500 mg every 4 hours for up to 2 doses; subsequent doses of 500 mg have been administered every 4-12 hours
Maximum recommended dose: 6 g/day (per manufacturer, however, higher doses have been administered)
Note: I.V. route is used when severe toxicity is evidenced by systemic symptoms (coma, shock, metabolic acidosis, or severe gastrointestinal bleeding) or potentially severe intoxications (serum iron level >500 mcg/dL). When severe symptoms are not present, the I.M. route may be preferred (per manufacturer); however, the use of deferoxamine in situations where the serum iron concentration is <500 mcg/dL or when severe toxicity is not evident is a subject of some clinical debate.
Chronic iron overload:
I.M., I.V.: 500-1000 mg/day I.M.; in addition, 2000 mg should be given I.V. with each unit of blood transfused (administer separately from blood); maximum: 6 g/day
SubQ: 1-2 g every day over 8-24 hours
Diagnosis of aluminum induced toxicity with CKD (unlabeled use): I.V.: Test dose: 5 mg/kg during the last hour of dialysis if serum aluminum levels
(Continued)

Deferoxamine *(Continued)*

are 60-200 mcg/L and there are clinical signs/symptoms of toxicity. Do not use if aluminum serum levels are >200 mcg/L

Treatment of aluminum toxicity with CKD (unlabeled use): I.V.: 5-10 mg/kg 4-6 hours before dialysis. Administer every 7-10 days with 3-4 dialysis procedures between doses. Do not use if aluminum serum levels are >200 mcg/L .

Pediatrics:

Acute iron toxicity: Refer to "Note" in adult dosing.

I.M.: 90 mg/kg/dose every 8 hours (maximum: 6 g/ 24 hours)

I.V.: 15 mg/kg/hour (maximum: 6 g/24 hours)

Chronic iron overload: SubQ: 20-40 mg/kg/day over 8-12 hours (maximum: 1000-2000 mg/day)

Diagnosis of aluminum induced toxicity with CKD (unlabeled use): Refer to adult dosing.

Treatment of aluminum toxicity with CKD (unlabeled use): Refer to adult dosing.

Renal Impairment: Cl_{cr} <10 mL/minute: Administer 50% of dose.

Administration

I.V.: Urticaria, hypotension, and shock have occurred following rapid I.V. administration; limiting infusion rate to 15mg/kg/hour may help avoid infusion-related adverse effects.

Acute iron toxicity: The manufacturer states that the I.M. route is preferred; however, the I.V. route is generally preferred in patients with severe toxicity (ie, patients in shock). For the first 1000 mg, infuse at 15 mg/kg/hour (although rates up to 40-50 mg/kg/ hour have been given in patients with massive iron intoxication). Subsequent doses may be given over 4-12 hours; maximum I.V. rate (per manufacturer): 15 mg/hour.

Diagnosis or treatment of aluminum induced toxicity with CKD: Administer dose over 1 hour

Other: SubQ: When administered for chronic iron overload, daily dose should be given over 8-24 hours using portable pump.

Stability

Reconstitution: Reconstitute using sterile water for injection to a final solution of 100 mg/mL (for I.V. administration).

Compatibility: Stable in D_5W, LR, NS, SWFI

Storage: Prior to reconstitution, do not store above 25°C (77°F). Following reconstitution, may be stored at room temperature for 7 days; protect from light. Do not refrigerate reconstituted solution.

Laboratory Monitoring Serum iron, total iron-binding capacity

Nursing Actions

Physical Assessment: Monitor laboratory tests. Infuse slowly and monitor infusion site. Monitor for acute reactions; urticaria, hypotension and shock can occur following rapid I.V. administration. With chronic therapy, perform ophthalmologic exam (fundoscopy, slit-lamp exam) and audiometry. Monitor for adverse reactions (eg, cardiac, respiratory, or CNS symptoms) and teach patient importance of reporting adverse symptoms.

Patient Education: Instructions depend on patient condition. You will be monitored closely for effects of this medication and frequent blood or urine tests may be necessary. Report chest pain, rapid heartbeat, headache, pain, swelling, or irritation at infusion site; skin rash; changes or loss of hearing or vision; or acute abdominal or leg cramps. **Pregnancy/ breast-feeding precautions:** Inform prescriber if you are or intend to become pregnant. Do not breast-feed.

Dietary Considerations Vitamin C supplements may need to be limited. The manufacturer recommends a maximum of 200 mg/day in adults (given in divided doses) and avoiding use in patients with heart failure.

Pregnancy Issues Skeletal anomalies and delayed ossification were observed in some but not all animal studies. Toxic amounts of iron or deferoxamine have not been noted to cross the placenta. In case of acute toxicity, treatment during pregnancy should not be withheld.

Delavirdine *(de la VIR deen)*

U.S. Brand Names Rescriptor®

Synonyms U-90152S

Pharmacologic Category Antiretroviral Agent, Reverse Transcriptase Inhibitor (Non-nucleoside)

Pregnancy Risk Factor C

Lactation Excretion in breast milk unknown/contraindicated

Use Treatment of HIV-1 infection in combination with at least two additional antiretroviral agents

Mechanism of Action/Effect Delavirdine binds directly to reverse transcriptase, blocking RNA-dependent and DNA-dependent DNA polymerase activities

Contraindications Hypersensitivity to delavirdine or any component of the formulation; concurrent use of alprazolam, cisapride, ergot alkaloids, midazolam, pimozide, or triazolam

Warnings/Precautions Avoid use with benzodiazepines, cisapride, clarithromycin, dapsone, enzyme-inducing anticonvulsants (carbamazepine, phenytoin, phenobarbital, rifampin, rifabutin, or St John's wort); may lead to loss of efficacy or development of resistance. Concurrent use of lovastatin or simvastatin should be avoided (use caution with other statins). Use caution with amphetamines, antacids, antiarrhythmics, benzodiazepines (alprazolam, midazolam, and triazolam are contraindicated), clarithromycin, dihydropyridine, calcium channel blockers, dapsone, immunosuppressants, methadone, oral contraceptives, or sildenafil.

Use with caution in patients with hepatic or renal dysfunction; due to rapid emergence of resistance, delavirdine should not be used as monotherapy; cross-resistance may be conferred to other non-nucleoside reverse transcriptase inhibitors, although potential for cross-resistance with protease inhibitors is low. Long-term effects of delavirdine are not known. Safety and efficacy have not been established in children. Rash, which occurs frequently, may require discontinuation of therapy; usually occurs within 1-3 weeks and lasts <2 weeks. Most patients may resume therapy following a treatment interruption.

Drug Interactions

Cytochrome P450 Effect: Substrate of CYP2D6 (minor), 3A4 (major); **Inhibits** CYP1A2 (weak), 2C8/9 (strong), 2C19 (strong), 2D6 (strong), 3A4 (strong)

Decreased Effect: Antacids, histamine-2 receptor antagonists, or proton pump inhibitors (omeprazole, lansoprazole) may reduce the absorption of delavirdine. Separate administration of didanosine buffered tablets or antacids and delavirdine by 1 hour. Concomitant use with histamine-2 receptor antagonists, omeprazole, or lansoprazole is not recommended.

Decreased delavirdine concentrations may occur when used with amprenavir and nelfinavir. Delavirdine decreases plasma concentrations of didanosine and didanosine may decrease plasma concentrations of delavirdine. Separate administration of didanosine buffered tablets and delavirdine by 1 hour.

Delavirdine may decrease the levels/effects of CYP2D6 prodrug substrates. Example prodrug substrates include codeine, hydrocodone, oxycodone, and tramadol. CYP3A4 inducers may decrease the levels/effects of delavirdine. Example inducers include aminoglutethimide, carbamazepine, nafcillin, nevirapine, phenobarbital, phenytoin, and rifamycins. Carbamazepine, phenobarbital, phenytoin and rifamycins should not be coadministered with delavirdine. Dexamethasone may decrease the plasma concentrations of delavirdine.

Increased Effect/Toxicity: Delavirdine has been reported to increase the serum concentrations of amprenavir, indinavir, nelfinavir, ritonavir, and saquinavir. Dose reduction of indinavir and saquinavir should be considered. Plasma concentrations of delavirdine may be increased by fluoxetine and ketoconazole. Clarithromycin and methadone serum concentrations may be increased by delavirdine.

Delavirdine may increase the levels/effects of CYP2C8/9, 2C19, or 2D6 substrates. Example substrates include amiodarone, amphetamines, selected beta-blockers, citalopram, dextromethorphan, diazepam, fluoxetine, glimepiride, glipizide, lidocaine, methsuximide, nateglinide, nefazodone, paroxetine, phenytoin, pioglitazone, propranolol, risperidone, ritonavir, rosiglitazone, sertraline, thioridazine, tricyclic antidepressants, venlafaxine, and warfarin.

Delavirdine may increase the levels/effects of CYP3A4 substrates. Example substrates include benzodiazepines, calcium channel blockers, cisapride, cyclosporine, mirtazapine, nateglinide, nefazodone, sildenafil (and other PDE-5 inhibitors), tacrolimus, and venlafaxine. Concomitant use with alprazolam, cisapride, ergot alkaloids, midazolam, pimozide, or triazolam is contraindicated. Use with lovastatin or simvastatin is not recommended.

Nutritional/Ethanol Interactions Herb/Nutraceutical: Delavirdine serum concentration may be decreased by St John's wort; avoid concurrent use.

Adverse Reactions

>10%: Dermatologic: Rash (3.2% required discontinuation)

1% to 10%:

Central nervous system: Headache, fatigue

Dermatologic: Pruritus

Gastrointestinal: Nausea, diarrhea, vomiting

Metabolic: Increased ALT (SGPT), increased AST (SGOT)

Overdosage/Toxicology Reports of human overdose with delavirdine are not available. GI decontamination and supportive measures are recommended. Dialysis is unlikely to be of benefit in removing this drug since it is extensively metabolized by the liver and is highly protein bound.

Pharmacodynamics/Kinetics
Time to Peak: Plasma: 1 hour

Protein Binding: ~98%, primarily to albumin

Half-Life Elimination: 2-11 hours

Metabolism: Hepatic via CYP3A4 and 2D6 (**Note:** May reduce CYP3A activity and inhibit its own metabolism.)

Excretion: Urine (51%, <5% as unchanged drug); feces (44%); nonlinear kinetics exhibited

Available Dosage Forms Tablet, as mesylate: 100 mg, 200 mg

Dosing
Adults & Elderly: HIV-1 infection (part of combination): Oral: 400 mg 3 times/day

Pediatrics:

HIV-1 infection (part of combination): Adolescents ≥16 years: Refer to adult dosing.

Administration
Oral: Patients with achlorhydria should take the drug with an acidic beverage. Antacids and delavirdine should be separated by 1 hour. A dispersion of delavirdine may be prepared by adding four 100 mg tablets to at least 3 oz of water. Allow to stand for a few minutes and stir until uniform dispersion. Drink immediately. Rinse glass and mouth, then swallow the rinse to ensure total dose administered. The 200 mg tablets should be taken intact.

Laboratory Monitoring Liver function tests if administered with saquinavir; viral load

Nursing Actions

Physical Assessment: Assess other pharmacological or herbal products patient may be taking for potential interactions. A list of medications that should not be used is available in each bottle and patients should be provided with this information. Monitor effectiveness of therapy (decrease in infections and progress of disease) and adverse reactions periodically during therapy. Teach patient proper use (eg, timing of multiple medications and drugs that should not be used concurrently), possible side effects/appropriate interventions, and adverse symptoms to report (eg, rash, gastrointestinal upset).

Patient Education: You will be provided with a list of specific medications that should not be used during therapy; do not take any new prescriptions, over-the-counter medications, or herbal products (even if they are not on the list) without consulting prescriber. This drug will not cure HIV, nor has it been found to reduce transmission of HIV; use appropriate precautions to prevent spread to other persons. This drug is prescribed as one part of a multidrug combination; take exactly as directed for full course of therapy. May be taken with or without food. Do not take antacids within 1 hour of delavirdine. Take 200 mg tablets intact (do not chew or dissolve). You may mix four 100 mg tablets in 3-5 oz of water, allow to stand a few minutes and stir; drink immediately; rinse glass and mouth (swallow rinse solution) following ingestion to ensure total dose administered. Maintain adequate hydration (2-3 L/day of fluids) unless advised by prescriber to restrict fluids. You may be susceptible to infection; avoid crowds and exposure to known infections and do not have any vaccinations without consulting prescriber. Frequent blood tests may be required with prolonged therapy. May cause nausea or vomiting (small frequent meals, frequent mouth care, sucking lozenges, or chewing gum may help). Consult prescriber if nausea or vomiting persists. Report skin rash or irritation, muscle weakness, persistent headache, fatigue or gastrointestinal upset. **Pregnancy/breast-feeding precautions:** Inform prescriber if you are or intend to become pregnant. Do not breast-feed.

Dietary Considerations May be taken without regard to food.

Breast-Feeding Issues HIV-infected mothers are discouraged from breast-feeding to decrease potential transmission of HIV.

Pregnancy Issues It is not known if delavirdine crosses the human placenta. Delavirdine was shown to be teratogenic in some animal studies. Health professionals are encouraged to contact the antiretroviral pregnancy registry to monitor outcomes of pregnant women exposed to antiretroviral medications (1-800-258-4263 or www.APRegistry.com).

Additional Information Potential compliance problems, frequency of administration, and adverse effects should be discussed with patients before initiating therapy to help prevent the emergence of resistance.

Demeclocycline (dem e kloe SYE kleen)

U.S. Brand Names Declomycin®

Synonyms Demeclocycline Hydrochloride; Demethyl-chlortetracycline

Pharmacologic Category Antibiotic, Tetracycline Derivative

Pregnancy Risk Factor D

Lactation Enters breast milk/not recommended (AAP rates tetracycline "compatible")

Use Treatment of susceptible bacterial infections (acne, gonorrhea, pertussis and urinary tract infections) caused by both gram-negative and gram-positive organisms

Unlabeled/Investigational Use Treatment of chronic syndrome of inappropriate secretion of antidiuretic hormone (SIADH)

Mechanism of Action/Effect Inhibits protein synthesis by binding with the 30S and possibly the 50S ribosomal subunit(s) of susceptible bacteria; may also cause alterations in the cytoplasmic membrane; inhibits actions of ADH in patients with SIADH

Contraindications Hypersensitivity to demeclocycline, tetracyclines, or any component of the formulation; children <8 years of age; concomitant use with methoxyflurane; pregnancy

Warnings/Precautions Photosensitivity reactions occur frequently with this drug, avoid prolonged exposure to sunlight, do not use tanning equipment. Use of tetracyclines during tooth development may cause permanent discoloration of the teeth and enamel, hypoplasia and retardation of skeletal development and bone growth with risk being the greatest for children <4 years and those receiving high doses; use caution in patients with renal or hepatic impairment (eg, elderly); dosage modification required in patients with renal impairment; may act as an antianabolic agent and increase BUN; pseudotumor cerebri has been reported with tetracycline use (usually resolves with discontinuation); outdated drug can cause nephropathy; superinfection possible

Drug Interactions

Decreased Effect: Antacid preparations containing calcium, magnesium, aluminum bismuth, or sodium bicarbonate may decrease tetracycline absorption; bile acid sequestrants, quinapril (magnesium-containing formulation), iron, or zinc may also decrease absorption; penicillin decrease therapeutic effect of tetracyclines. Although anecdotal reports suggest oral contraceptive efficacy could be reduced by tetracyclines, this has been refuted by more rigorous scientific and clinical data.

Increased Effect/Toxicity: Methoxyflurane anesthesia may cause fatal nephrotoxicity; retinoic acid derivatives may increase adverse and toxic effects; warfarin may result in increased anticoagulation; methotrexate levels may be increased

Nutritional/Ethanol Interactions

Food: Demeclocycline serum levels may be decreased if taken with food.

Herb/Nutraceutical: Avoid dong quai, St John's wort (may also cause photosensitization).

Lab Interactions May interfere with tests for urinary glucose (false-negative urine glucose using Clinistix®).

Adverse Reactions Frequency not defined.

Cardiovascular: Pericarditis

Central nervous system: Bulging fontanels (infants), dizziness, headache, pseudotumor cerebri (adults)

Dermatologic: Angioneurotic edema, erythema multiforme, erythematous rash, maculopapular rash, photosensitivity, pigmentation of skin, Stevens-Johnson syndrome (rare), urticaria

Endocrine & metabolic: Discoloration of thyroid gland (brown/black), nephrogenic diabetes insipidus

Gastrointestinal: Anorexia, diarrhea, dysphagia, enterocolitis, esophageal ulcerations, glossitis, nausea, pancreatitis, vomiting

Genitourinary: Balanitis

Hematologic: Eosinophilia, neutropenia, hemolytic anemia, thrombocytopenia

Hepatic: Hepatitis (rare), hepatotoxicity (rare), liver enzymes increased, liver failure (rare)

Neuromuscular & skeletal: Myasthenic syndrome, polyarthralgia, tooth discoloration (children <8 years, rarely in adults)

Ocular: Visual disturbances

Otic: Tinnitus

Renal: Acute renal failure

Respiratory: Pulmonary infiltrates

Miscellaneous: Anaphylaxis, anaphylactoid purpura, lupus-like syndrome, systemic lupus erythematosus exacerbation

Overdosage/Toxicology Treatment is supportive.

Pharmacodynamics/Kinetics

Onset of Action: SIADH: Several days

Time to Peak: Serum: 3-6 hours

Protein Binding: 41% to 50%

Half-Life Elimination: 10-17 hours

Metabolism: Hepatic (small amounts) to inactive metabolites; undergoes enterohepatic recirculation

Excretion: Urine (42% to 50% as unchanged drug)

Available Dosage Forms Tablet, as hydrochloride: 150 mg, 300 mg

Dosing

Adults & Elderly:

Susceptible infections: Oral: 150 mg 4 times/day or 300 mg twice daily

SIADH (unlabeled use): Oral: 900-1200 mg/day or 13-15 mg/kg/day divided every 6-8 hours initially, then decrease to 600-900 mg/day

Pediatrics: Susceptible infections: Oral: ≥8 years: 8-12 mg/kg/day divided every 6-12 hours

Renal Impairment: Should be avoided in patients with renal dysfunction.

Hepatic Impairment: Should be avoided in patients with hepatic dysfunction.

Administration

Oral: Administer 1 hour before or 2 hours after food or milk with plenty of fluid.

Laboratory Monitoring CBC, renal and hepatic function; perform culture and sensitivity studies prior to initiating therapy

Nursing Actions

Physical Assessment: Results of culture and sensitivity tests and patient's allergy history should be assessed prior to beginning therapy. Assess other pharmacological or herbal products patient may be taking for potential interactions (eg, increased risk of toxicity or decreased effectiveness). Monitor laboratory tests, therapeutic response, and adverse effects (eg, rash, anaphylactic reactions, anemia, CNS changes) on a regular basis throughout therapy. Advise patients with diabetes about use of Clinitest®. Teach patient proper use, possible side effects/appropriate interventions, and adverse symptoms to report.

Patient Education: Inform prescriber of all prescriptions, OTC medications, or herbal products you are taking, and any allergies you have. Do not take any new medication during therapy unless approved by prescriber. Take on an empty stomach (1 hour before or 2 hours after meals with plenty of fluid). Take at regularly scheduled intervals around-the-clock. Avoid antacids, iron, dairy products, and other medications within 2 hours of taking demeclocycline. May cause photosensitivity (use sunscreen, wear protective clothing and eyewear, and avoid direct sunlight); dizziness or lightheadedness (use caution when driving or engaging in tasks that require alertness until response to drug is known); nausea or vomiting (frequent, small meals, frequent mouth care, sucking lozenges, or chewing gum may help); or diarrhea (buttermilk, yogurt, or boiled milk may help). Report rash or intense itching, yellowing of skin or eyes, change in color of urine or stools, fever or chills, dark urine or pale stools, vaginal itching or discharge, foul-smelling stools, excessive thirst or urination, acute headache, unresolved diarrhea, or respiratory difficulty. **Pregnancy/breast-feeding precautions:** Inform prescriber if you are pregnant. Do not get pregnant while taking this medication. Consult prescriber for appropriate contraceptives. Breast-feeding is not recommended.

Dietary Considerations Should be taken 1 hour before or 2 hours after food or milk with plenty of fluid.

Geriatric Considerations Has not been studied exclusively in the elderly.

Pregnancy Issues Tetracyclines cross the placenta and enter fetal circulation; may cause permanent discoloration of teeth if used during the last half of pregnancy. Related antibiotics have been associated with mutagenesis, embryotoxicity, and oncogenic activity in animals.

Denileukin Diftitox (de ni LOO kin DIF ti toks)

U.S. Brand Names ONTAK®

Synonyms DAB$_{389}$IL-2; NSC-714744

Pharmacologic Category Antineoplastic Agent, Miscellaneous

Pregnancy Risk Factor C

Lactation Excretion in breast milk unknown/contraindicated

Use Treatment of persistent or recurrent cutaneous T-cell lymphoma whose malignant cells express the CD25 component of the IL-2 receptor

Mechanism of Action/Effect Interacts with receptors on surface of malignant cells to inhibit intracellular protein synthesis rapidly leading to cell death.

Contraindications Hypersensitivity to denileukin diftitox, diphtheria toxin, interleukin-2, or any component of the formulation

Warnings/Precautions Hazardous agent - use appropriate precautions for handling and disposal. Acute hypersensitivity reactions, including anaphylaxis, may occur; most events (eg, hypotension, back pain, dyspnea, vasodilation, rash, chest pain, tachycardia, dysphagia, syncope) occur during or within 24 hours of infusion; with ~50% occurring on the day one, regardless of treatment cycle. Denileukin diftitox has been associated with a delayed-onset vascular leak syndrome, which may be severe. The onset of symptoms (hypotension, edema, hypoalbuminemia) of vascular leak syndrome usually occurred within the first 2 weeks of infusion and may persist or worsen after cessation of denileukin diftitox. Use caution in patients with pre-existing cardiovascular disease. Pre-existing low serum albumin levels may predict or predispose to vascular leak syndrome; delay subsequent cycles until serum albumin ≥3 g/dL. Immunogenicity may develop; patients with antibodies have a two- to threefold increase in clearance. The presence of antibodies does not correlate with risk for hypersensitivity/infusion related reactions. Denileukin diftitox may impair immune function. Loss of visual acuity with loss of color vision (with or without retinal pigment mottling) has been reported. Use with caution in patients >65 years of age; adverse events (anemia, anorexia, confusion, hypotension, rash, nausea/vomiting) occur more frequently. Safety and efficacy in children have not been established.

Adverse Reactions
The following list of symptoms reported during treatment includes all levels of severity:

>10%:
Cardiovascular: Edema (47%; grade 3 and 4, 15%), hypotension (36%), chest pain (24%), vasodilation (22%), tachycardia (12%)
Central nervous system: Fever/chills (81%; grade 3 and 4, 22%), headache (26%), pain (48%; grade 3 and 4, 13%), dizziness (22%), nervousness (11%)
Dermatologic: Rash (34%; grade 3 and 4, 13%), pruritus (20%)
Endocrine & metabolic: Hypoalbuminemia (83%; grade 3 and 4, 14%), hypocalcemia (17%), weight loss (14%)
Gastrointestinal: Nausea/vomiting (64%; grade 3 and 4, 14%), anorexia (36%), diarrhea (29%)
Hematologic: Lymphocyte count decreased (34%), anemia (18%)
Hepatic: Transaminases increased (61%; grade 3 and 4, 15%)
Neuromuscular & skeletal: Weakness (66%; grade 3 and 4, 22%), myalgia (17%), paresthesia (13%)
Respiratory: Dyspnea (29%; grade 3 and 4, 14%), cough increased (26%), pharyngitis (17%), rhinitis (13%)
Miscellaneous: Flu-like syndrome (91%; beginning several hours to days following infusion), hypersensitivity (69%; reactions are variable, but may include hypotension, back pain, dyspnea, vasodilation, rash, chest pain, tachycardia, dysphagia, syncope, or anaphylaxis), infection (48%; grade 3 and 4, 24%), vascular leak syndrome (27%; characterized by hypotension, edema, or hypoalbuminemia; the syndrome usually developed within the first 2 weeks of infusion; 6% of patients who developed this syndrome required hospitalization; the symptoms may persist or even worsen despite cessation of denileukin diftitox)

1% to 10%:
Cardiovascular: Thrombotic events (7%), hypertension (6%), arrhythmia (6%), MI (1%)
Central nervous system: Insomnia (9%), confusion (8%)
Endocrine & metabolic: Dehydration (9%), hypokalemia (6%), hyperthyroidism (<5%), hypothyroidism (<5%)
Gastrointestinal: Constipation (9%), dyspepsia (7%), dysphagia (6%), oral ulcer (<5%), pancreatitis (<5%)
Hematologic: Thrombocytopenia (8%), leukopenia (6%)
Local: Injection site reaction (8%), anaphylaxis (1%)
Neuromuscular & skeletal: Arthralgia (8%)
Renal: Hematuria (10%), albuminuria (10%), pyuria (10%), creatinine increased (7%), acute renal insufficiency (<5%)
Respiratory: Lung disorder (8%)
Miscellaneous: Anaphylaxis (1%), diaphoresis decreased (10%)
Postmarketing and/or case reports: Toxic epidermal necrolysis, visual loss

Overdosage/Toxicology Although there is no human experience in overdose, dose-limiting toxicities include nausea, vomiting, fever, chills and persistent weakness. Treatment is supportive and symptom-directed. Fluid balance, as well as hepatic and renal function, should be closely monitored.

Pharmacodynamics/Kinetics
Half-Life Elimination: Distribution: 2-5 minutes; Terminal: 70-80 minutes
Metabolism: Hepatic via proteolytic degradation (animal studies)

Available Dosage Forms
Injection, solution [frozen]:
ONTAK®: 150 mcg/mL (2 mL) [contains EDTA]
(Continued)

Denileukin Diftitox *(Continued)*

Dosing

Adults & Elderly: Persistent or recurrent cutaneous T-cell lymphoma: I.V.: 9 or 18 mcg/kg/day days 1 through 5 every 21 days.

Administration

I.V.: For I.V. use only. Infuse over at least 15 minutes. Should not be given as an I.V. bolus. Discontinue or reduce infusion rate for infusion related reactions. There is no clinical experience with prolonged infusions (>80 minutes). Do not administer through an in-line filter. Consider premedication with antipyretics, antihistamines, and antiemetics.

I.V. Detail: pH: 6.9-7.2

Stability

Reconstitution: Must be brought to room temperature (25°C or 77°F) before preparing the dose. Do **not** heat vials. Thaw in refrigerator for not more than 24 hours or at room temperature for 1-2 hours. Avoid vigorous agitation. Solution may be mixed by gentle swirling. Dilute with NS to a concentration of ≥15 mcg/mL ; the concentration must be ≥15 mcg/mL during all steps of preparation. Add drug to the empty sterile I.V. bag first, then add NS.

Compatibility: Do **not** use glass syringes or containers.

Storage: Store frozen at or below -10°C (14°F); cannot be refrozen. Solutions ≥15 mcg/mL in NS should be used within 6 hours. DO NOT use glass syringes or containers.

Laboratory Monitoring Baseline CD25 expression (on malignant cells); CBC, blood chemistry panel, renal and hepatic function tests as well as a serum albumin level; these tests should be done prior to initiation of therapy and repeated at weekly intervals during therapy.

Nursing Actions

Physical Assessment: Monitor laboratory tests prior to therapy and weekly during therapy. Patient must be monitored closely for acute hypersensitivity reaction during and for 24 hours following first infusion. Following infusion, patient should be monitored or taught to monitor for delayed vascular leak syndrome (eg, hypotension, edema, or hypoalbuminemia) and other adverse reactions. Teach patient appropriate interventions to reduce side effects and adverse reactions to report.

Patient Education: This medication can only be administered via intravenous infusion. During infusion, report immediately any chills; chest pain, respiratory difficulty, or tightness in throat; or redness, swelling, pain, or burning at infusion site. Maintaining adequate nutrition and hydration is important (2-3 L/day) unless instructed to restrict fluid intake. You may be more susceptible to infection (avoid crowds and exposure to infection and do not have any vaccinations without consulting prescriber). May cause nausea, vomiting, anorexia, flatulence (small, frequent meals, good mouth care, chewing gum, or sucking lozenges may help); constipation (increased exercise, fluids, fruit, or fiber may help); diarrhea (buttermilk, boiled milk, or yogurt may help); headache, back or muscle pain (consult prescriber for mild analgesic); dizziness, weakness, or confusion (use caution when driving, engaging in hazardous activities, or climbing stairs until effect of medication is known). Report unresolved GI effects; headache, back or muscle pain; skin dryness, rash, or sores; altered urinary patterns; flu syndrome or infection (eg, weakness, fatigue, white plaques or sores in mouth, vaginal discharge, chills, fever); CNS disturbances (insomnia, dizziness, agitation, confusion, depression); unusual bleeding or bruising, blood in urine or stool; swelling of extremities; or any other adverse effects. **Pregnancy/breast-feeding precautions:** Inform prescriber if you are or intend to become pregnant. Do not breast-feed.

Breast-Feeding Issues The excretion of denileukin diftitox in breast milk is unknown, however, it is recommended that a breast-feeding woman who is treated with denileukin diftitox should discontinue nursing.

Additional Information Formulation includes polysorbate 20.

Desipramine *(des IP ra meen)*

U.S. Brand Names Norpramin®

Synonyms Desipramine Hydrochloride; Desmethylimipramine Hydrochloride

Restrictions A medication guide concerning the use of antidepressants in children and teenagers can be found on the FDA website at http://www.fda.gov/cder/Offices/ODS/labeling.htm. It should be dispensed to parents or guardians of children and teenagers receiving this medication.

Pharmacologic Category Antidepressant, Tricyclic (Secondary Amine)

Medication Safety Issues
Sound-alike/look-alike issues:
Desipramine may be confused with clomiPRAMINE, deserpidine, diphenhydrAMINE, disopyramide, imipramine, nortriptyline
Norpramin® may be confused with clomiPRAMINE, imipramine, Norpace®, nortriptyline, Tenormin®

Pregnancy Risk Factor C

Lactation Enters breast milk/not recommended (AAP rates "of concern")

Use Treatment of depression

Unlabeled/Investigational Use Analgesic adjunct in chronic pain; peripheral neuropathies; substance-related disorders; attention-deficit/hyperactivity disorder (ADHD)

Mechanism of Action/Effect Traditionally believed to increase the synaptic concentration of norepinephrine (and to a lesser extent, serotonin) in the central nervous system by inhibition of its reuptake by the presynaptic neuronal membrane. However, additional receptor effects have been found including desensitization of adenyl cyclase, down regulation of beta-adrenergic receptors, and down regulation of serotonin receptors.

Contraindications Hypersensitivity to desipramine, drugs of similar chemical class, or any component of the formulation; use of MAO inhibitors within 14 days; use in a patient during the acute recovery phase of MI

Warnings/Precautions Antidepressants increase the risk of suicidal thinking and behavior in children and adolescents with major depressive disorder (MDD) and other depressive disorders; consider risk prior to prescribing. All patients must be closely monitored for clinical worsening, suicidality, or unusual changes in behavior, especially during the initiation of therapy or following an increase or decrease in dosage. When used in children, the child's family or caregiver should be instructed to closely observe the patient and communicate condition with healthcare provider. A medication guide should be dispensed with each prescription. **Desipramine is FDA approved for the treatment of depression in adolescents.**

The possibility of a suicide attempt is inherent in major depression and may persist until remission occurs. Use caution in high-risk patients. Worsening depression and severe abrupt suicidality that are not part of the presenting symptoms may require discontinuation or modification of drug therapy. The patient's family or caregiver should be alerted to monitor patients for the emergence of suicidality and associated behaviors (such as agitation, irritability, hostility, impulsivity, and hypomania) and notify healthcare provider.

May worsen psychosis in some patients or precipitate a shift to mania or hypomania in patients with bipolar disorder. Patients presenting with depressive symptoms should be screened for bipolar disorder. Monotherapy in patients with bipolar disorder should be avoided. **Desipramine is not FDA approved for the treatment of bipolar depression.**

The degree of anticholinergic blockade produced by this agent is low relative to other cyclic antidepressants - however, caution should be used in patients with urinary retention, benign prostatic hyperplasia, narrow-angle glaucoma, xerostomia, visual problems, constipation, or a history of bowel obstruction. The degree of sedation and conduction disturbances with desipramine are low relative to other antidepressants. However, desipramine may cause drowsiness/sedation, resulting in impaired performance of tasks requiring alertness (eg, operating machinery or driving). Sedative effects may be additive with other CNS depressants and/or ethanol. The risk of orthostasis is moderate relative to other antidepressants. Use with caution in patients with a history of cardiovascular disease (including previous MI, stroke, tachycardia, or conduction abnormalities).

Consider discontinuing, when possible, prior to elective surgery. Therapy should not be abruptly discontinued in patients receiving high doses for prolonged periods. May lower seizure threshold - use caution in patients with a previous seizure disorder or condition predisposing to seizures such as brain damage, alcoholism, or concurrent therapy with other drugs which lower the seizure threshold. May increase the risks associated with electroconvulsive therapy. Use with caution in hyperthyroid patients or those receiving thyroid supplementation. Use with caution in patients with hepatic or renal dysfunction and in elderly patients.

Drug Interactions
Cytochrome P450 Effect: Substrate of CYP1A2 (minor), 2D6 (major); **Inhibits** CYP2A6 (moderate), 2B6 (moderate), 2D6 (moderate), 2E1 (weak), 3A4 (moderate)

Decreased Effect: Desipramine may decrease the levels/effects of CYP2D6 prodrug substrates (eg, codeine, hydrocodone, oxycodone, tramadol). Desipramine's serum levels/effect may be decreased by carbamazepine, cholestyramine, colestipol, phenobarbital, and rifampin. Desipramine inhibits the antihypertensive effect of to bethanidine, clonidine, debrisoquin, guanadrel, guanethidine, guanabenz, or guanfacine.

Increased Effect/Toxicity: Desipramine increases the effects of amphetamines, anticholinergics, other CNS depressants (sedatives, hypnotics, or ethanol), chlorpropamide, tolazamide, and warfarin. When used with MAO inhibitors, serotonin syndrome may occur. Serotonin syndrome has also been reported with ritonavir (rare). The levels/effects of desipramine may be increased by chlorpromazine, delavirdine, fluoxetine, miconazole, paroxetine, pergolide, quinidine, quinine, ritonavir, ropinirole, and other CYP2D6 inhibitors.

Cimetidine, grapefruit juice, indinavir, methylphenidate, diltiazem, and verapamil may increase the serum concentration of TCAs. Use of lithium with a TCA may increase the risk for neurotoxicity. Phenothiazines may increase concentration of some TCAs and TCAs may increase concentration of phenothiazines. Pressor response to I.V. epinephrine, norepinephrine, and phenylephrine may be enhanced in patients receiving TCAs (**Note:** Effect is unlikely with epinephrine or levonordefrin dosages typically administered as infiltration in combination with local anesthetics). Combined use of beta-agonists or drugs which prolong QT$_c$ (including quinidine, procainamide, disopyramide, cisapride, sparfloxacin, gatifloxacin, moxifloxacin) with TCAs may predispose patients to cardiac arrhythmias.

Desipramine may increase the levels/effects of selected benzodiazepines, bupropion, calcium channel blockers, cisapride, dexmedetomidine, dextromethorphan, ergot derivatives, ifosfamide, fluoxetine, selected HMG-CoA reductase inhibitors, lidocaine, mesoridazine, mirtazapine, nateglinide, nefazodone, paroxetine, pimozide, promethazine, propofol, quinidine, risperidone, ritonavir, selegiline, sertraline, sildenafil (and other PDE-5 inhibitors), tacrolimus, thioridazine, tricyclic antidepressants, venlafaxine, and other CYP2A6, 2B6, 2D6, or 3A4 substrates.

Nutritional/Ethanol Interactions
Ethanol: Avoid ethanol (may increase CNS depression).
Food: Grapefruit juice may inhibit the metabolism of some TCAs and clinical toxicity may result.
Herb/Nutraceutical: Avoid valerian, St John's wort, SAMe, kava kava (may increase risk of serotonin syndrome and/or excessive sedation).

Lab Interactions Increased glucose; decreased glucose has also been reported

Adverse Reactions Frequency not defined.
Cardiovascular: Arrhythmias, hyper-/hypotension, palpitation, heart block, tachycardia
Central nervous system: Dizziness, drowsiness, headache, confusion, delirium, hallucinations, nervousness, restlessness, parkinsonian syndrome, insomnia, disorientation, anxiety, agitation, hypomania, exacerbation of psychosis, incoordination, seizure, extrapyramidal symptoms
Dermatologic: Alopecia, photosensitivity, skin rash, urticaria
Endocrine & metabolic: Breast enlargement, galactorrhea, SIADH
Gastrointestinal: Xerostomia, decreased lower esophageal sphincter tone may cause GE reflux, constipation, nausea, unpleasant taste, weight gain/loss, anorexia, abdominal cramps, diarrhea, heartburn
Genitourinary: Difficult urination, sexual dysfunction, testicular edema
Hematologic: Agranulocytosis, eosinophilia, purpura, thrombocytopenia
Hepatic: Cholestatic jaundice, increased liver enzyme
Neuromuscular & skeletal: Fine muscle tremor, weakness, numbness, tingling, paresthesia of extremities, ataxia
Ocular: Blurred vision, disturbances of accommodation, mydriasis, increased intraocular pressure
Miscellaneous: Diaphoresis (excessive), allergic reactions

Overdosage/Toxicology Symptoms of overdose include agitation, confusion, hallucinations, hyperthermia, urinary retention, CNS depression, cyanosis, dry mucous membranes, cardiac arrhythmias, and seizures. Treatment is supportive. Ventricular arrhythmias and ECG changes (eg, QRS widening) often respond with concurrent systemic alkalinization (sodium bicarbonate 0.5-2 mEq/kg I.V. or hyperventilation). Arrhythmias unresponsive to phenytoin 15-20 mg/kg (adults) may respond to lidocaine. Physostigmine (1-2 mg I.V. slowly for adults) may be indicated for reversing life-threatening cardiac arrhythmias.

Pharmacodynamics/Kinetics
Onset of Action: 1-3 weeks; Maximum antidepressant effect: >2 weeks
Time to Peak: Plasma: 4-6 hours
Half-Life Elimination: Adults: 7-60 hours
Metabolism: Hepatic
Excretion: Urine (70%)
Available Dosage Forms Tablet, as hydrochloride: 10 mg, 25 mg, 50 mg, 75 mg, 100 mg, 150 mg

Dosing
Adults:
Depression: Oral: Initial: 75 mg/day in divided doses; increase gradually to 150-200 mg/day in divided or single dose; maximum: 300 mg/day
(Continued)

Desipramine *(Continued)*

Cocaine withdrawal (unlabeled use): 50-200 mg/day in divided or single dose

Elderly: Oral: Initial: 10-25 mg/day; increase by 10-25 mg every 3 days for inpatients and every week for outpatients if tolerated; usual maintenance dose: 75-100 mg/day, but doses up to 150 mg/day may be necessary.

Pediatrics: Depression: Oral:

Children 6-12 years (unlabeled use): 10-30 mg/day or 1-5 mg/kg/day in divided doses; do not exceed 5 mg/kg/day

Adolescents: Initial: 25-50 mg/day; gradually increase to 100 mg/day in single or divided doses; maximum: 150 mg/day

Renal Impairment: Hemodialysis/peritoneal dialysis effects: Supplemental dose is not necessary.

Nursing Actions

Physical Assessment: Assess potential for interactions with other prescriptions, OTC medications, or herbal products patient may be taking. Monitor CNS status. Assess for suicidal tendencies before beginning therapy. May cause physiological or psychological dependence, tolerance, or abuse; periodically evaluate need for continued use. Caution patients with diabetes to monitor glucose levels closely; may increase or decrease serum glucose levels. Monitor therapeutic response and adverse reactions at beginning of therapy and periodically with long-term use. Taper dose slowly when discontinuing. Teach patient proper use, appropriate interventions to reduce side effects, and adverse symptoms to report.

Patient Education: Do not take any new medication during therapy unless approved by prescriber. Take exactly as directed; do not increase dose or frequency. It may take 2-3 weeks to achieve desired results. This medicine may cause physical and/or psychological dependence. Avoid alcohol and grapefruit juice. Maintain adequate hydration (2-3 L/day of fluids) unless instructed to restrict fluid intake. May cause drowsiness, lightheadedness, impaired coordination, dizziness, or blurred vision (use caution when driving or engaging in tasks requiring alertness until response to drug is known); loss of appetite or disturbed taste (small frequent meals, good mouth care, chewing gum, or sucking lozenges may help); constipation (increased exercise, fluids, fruit, or fiber may help); urinary retention (void before taking medication); postural hypotension (use caution climbing stairs or when changing position from lying or sitting to standing); altered sexual drive or ability (reversible); or photosensitivity (use sunscreen, wear protective clothing and eyewear, and avoid direct sunlight). Report chest pain, palpitations, or rapid heartbeat; persistent adverse CNS effects (eg, suicidal ideation, nervousness, restlessness, insomnia, anxiety, excitation, headache, agitation, impaired coordination, changes in cognition); muscle cramping, weakness, tremors, or rigidity; blurred vision or eye pain; breast enlargement or swelling; yellowing of skin or eyes; or worsening of condition. **Pregnancy/breast-feeding precautions:** Inform prescriber if you are or intend to become pregnant. Breast-feeding is not recommended..

Geriatric Considerations Preferred agent because of its milder side effect profile; patients may experience excitation or stimulation, in such cases, give as a single morning dose or divided dose.

Breast-Feeding Issues Generally, it is not recommended to breast-feed if taking antidepressants because of the long half-life, active metabolites, and the potential for side effects in the infant.

Additional Information Less sedation and anticholinergic effects than with amitriptyline or imipramine

Related Information

Antidepressant Medication Guidelines *on page 1414*

Federal OBRA Regulations Recommended Maximum Doses *on page 1421*

Peak and Trough Guidelines *on page 1387*

Desloratadine *(des lor AT a deen)*

U.S. Brand Names Clarinex®

Pharmacologic Category Antihistamine, Nonsedating

Pregnancy Risk Factor C

Lactation Enters breast milk/not recommended

Use Relief of nasal and non-nasal symptoms of seasonal allergic rhinitis (SAR) and perennial allergic rhinitis (PAR); treatment of chronic idiopathic urticaria (CIU)

Mechanism of Action/Effect Desloratadine is a long-acting antihistamine with selective H_1 receptor antagonistic activity.

Contraindications Hypersensitivity to desloratadine, loratadine, or any component of the formulation

Warnings/Precautions Dose should be adjusted in patients with liver or renal impairment. Use with caution in patients known to be slow metabolizers of desloratadine (incidence of side effects may be increased). RediTabs® contain phenylalanine. Safety and efficacy have not been established for children <6 months of age.

Drug Interactions

Increased Effect/Toxicity: With concurrent use of desloratadine and erythromycin or ketoconazole, the C_{max} and AUC of desloratadine and its metabolite are increased; however, no clinically-significant changes in the safety profile of desloratadine were observed in clinical studies.

Nutritional/Ethanol Interactions Food: Does not affect bioavailability.

Adverse Reactions

>10%: Central nervous system: Headache (14%)

1% to 10%:

Central nervous system: Fatigue (2% to 5%), somnolence (2%), dizziness (4%)

Endocrine & metabolic: Dysmenorrhea (2%)

Gastrointestinal: Xerostomia (3%), nausea (5%), dyspepsia (3%)

Neuromuscular & skeletal: Myalgia (2% to 3%)

Respiratory: Pharyngitis (3% to 4%)

Overdosage/Toxicology Information is limited to doses studied during clinical trials (up to 45 mg/day). Symptoms included somnolence, and small increases in heart rate and QT_c interval (not clinically significant). In the event of an overdose, treatment should be symptom-directed and supportive. Desloratadine and its metabolite are not removed by hemodialysis.

Pharmacodynamics/Kinetics

Time to Peak: 3 hours

Protein Binding: Desloratadine: 82% to 87%; 3-hydroxydesloratadine: 85% to 89%

Half-Life Elimination: 27 hours

Metabolism: Hepatic to active metabolite, 3-hydroxydesloratadine (specific enzymes not identified); undergoes glucuronidation. Decreased in slow metabolizers of desloratadine. Not expected to affect or be affected by medications metabolized by CYP with normal doses.

Excretion: Urine and feces (as metabolites)

Available Dosage Forms

Syrup (Clarinex®): 0.5 mg/mL (120 mL, 480 mL) [bubble gum flavor]

Tablet (Clarinex®): 5 mg

Tablet, orally disintegrating (Clarinex® RediTabs®): 2.5 mg [contains phenylalanine 1.28 mg/tablet; tutti-frutti flavor]; 5 mg [contains phenylalanine 2.55 mg/tablet; tutti-frutti flavor]

Dosing

Adults & Elderly: Seasonal or perennial allergic rhinitis, chronic idiopathic urticaria: Oral: 5 mg once daily

Pediatrics: Seasonal or perennial allergic rhinitis, chronic idiopathic urticaria: Oral:

Children:

6-11 months: 1 mg once daily
12 months to 5 years: 1.25 mg once daily
6-11 years: 2.5 mg once daily
Children ≥12 years: Refer to adult dosing.

Renal Impairment:

Children: Not established
Adults: 5 mg every other day

Hepatic Impairment: 5 mg every other day

Administration

Oral: May be taken with or without food.

RediTabs® should be placed on the tongue; tablet will disintegrate immediately. May be taken with or without water.

Syrup: A commercially-available measuring dropper or syringe calibrated to deliver 2 mL or 2.5 mL should be used to administer age-appropriate doses in children.

Stability

Storage: Syrup, tablet, orally-disintegrating tablet: Store at 25°C (77°F); excursions permitted between 15°C to 30°C (59°F to 86°F). Protect from moisture and excessive heat (85°F). Use orally-disintegrating tablet immediately after opening blister package. Syrup should be protected from light.

Nursing Actions

Physical Assessment: Assess effectiveness and interactions of other medications patient may be taking. Monitor effectiveness of therapy and adverse reactions at beginning of therapy and periodically with long-term use. Assess knowledge/teach patient appropriate use, interventions to reduce side effects, and adverse symptoms to report.

Patient Education: Take as directed; do not exceed recommended dose. Avoid use of other depressants, alcohol, or sleep-inducing medications unless approved by prescriber. You may experience headache, drowsiness, or dizziness (use caution when driving or engaging in tasks that require alertness until response to drug is known); or dry mouth, dry throat, or nausea (small frequent meals, frequent mouth care, chewing gum, or sucking hard candy may help). Report rapid heartbeat, shortness of breath, skin rash, persistent flu-like symptoms, or muscle aches. **Pregnancy/breast-feeding precautions:** Inform prescriber if you are or intend to become pregnant. Breast-feeding is not recommended.

Dietary Considerations May be taken with or without food. Orally-disintegrating tablets contain phenylalanine.

Desmopressin (des moe PRES in)

U.S. Brand Names DDAVP®; Stimate™

Synonyms 1-Deamino-8-D-Arginine Vasopressin; Desmopressin Acetate

Pharmacologic Category Antihemophilic Agent; Hemostatic Agent; Vasopressin Analog, Synthetic

Pregnancy Risk Factor B

Lactation Excretion in breast milk unknown/use caution

Use

Injection: Treatment of diabetes insipidus; control of bleeding in hemophilia A, and mild-to-moderate classic von Willebrand disease (type I)

Tablet, nasal solution: Treatment of diabetes insipidus; primary nocturnal enuresis

Mechanism of Action/Effect Enhances reabsorption of water in the kidneys by increasing cellular permeability of the collecting ducts; possibly causes smooth muscle constriction with resultant vasoconstriction; raises plasma levels of von Willebrand factor and factor VIII

Contraindications Hypersensitivity to desmopressin or any component of the formulation; moderate to severe renal impairment (Cl_{cr}<50 mL/minute)

Warnings/Precautions Fluid intake should be adjusted downward in the elderly and very young patients to decrease the possibility of water intoxication and hyponatremia. Avoid overhydration especially when drug is used for its hemostatic effect. Use may rarely lead to extreme decreases in plasma osmolality, resulting in seizures and coma. Use caution with cystic fibrosis or other conditions associated with fluid and electrolyte imbalance due to potential hyponatremia. Use caution with coronary artery insufficiency or hypertensive cardiovascular disease; may increase or decrease blood pressure leading to changes in heart rate. Consider switching from nasal to intravenous solution if changes in the nasal mucosa (scarring, edema) occur leading to unreliable absorption. Use caution in patients predisposed to thrombus formation; thrombotic events (acute cerebrovascular thrombosis, acute myocardial infarction) have occurred (rare). Injection is not for use in hemophilia B, severe classic von Willebrand disease (type IIB), or in patients with factor VIII antibodies. In general, the injection is also not recommended for use in patients with ≤5% factor VIII activity level, although it may be considered in selected patients with activity levels between 2% and 5%. Some patients may demonstrate a change in response after long-term therapy (>6 months) characterized as decreased response or a shorter duration of response.

Drug Interactions

Decreased Effect: Demeclocycline and lithium may decrease ADH response.

Increased Effect/Toxicity: Chlorpropamide, fludrocortisone may increase ADH response.

Nutritional/Ethanol Interactions Ethanol: Avoid ethanol (may decrease antidiuretic effect).

Adverse Reactions Frequency not defined (may be dose or route related).

Cardiovascular: Acute cerebrovascular thrombosis, acute MI, blood pressure increased/decreased, chest pain, edema, facial flushing, palpitation

Central nervous system: Agitation, chills, coma, dizziness, headache, insomnia, somnolence

Dermatologic: Rash

Endocrine & metabolic: Hyponatremia, water intoxication

Gastrointestinal: Abdominal cramps, dyspepsia, nausea, sore throat, vomiting

Genitourinary: Balanitis, vulval pain

Local: Injection: Burning pain, erythema, and swelling at the injection site

Ocular: Conjunctivitis, eye edema, lacrimation disorder

Respiratory: Cough, epistaxis, nasal congestion, rhinitis

Miscellaneous: Allergic reactions (rare), anaphylaxis (rare)

Overdosage/Toxicology Symptoms of overdose include drowsiness, headache, confusion, anuria, and water intoxication. In case of overdose, decrease or discontinue desmopressin.

Pharmacodynamics/Kinetics

Onset of Action:

Intranasal administration: Onset of increased factor VIII activity: 30 minutes (dose related); peak effect 1.5 hours

I.V. infusion: Onset of increased factor VIII activity: 30 minutes (dose related); peak effect: 1.5-2 hours

Oral tablets: Onset of action: ADH: ~1 hour; peak effect: 4-7 hours

Half-Life Elimination:

I.V. infusion: Terminal: 3 hours (up to 9 hours in renal dysfunction)

Tablet: 1.5-2.5 hours

(Continued)

Desmopressin *(Continued)*

Metabolism: Unknown

Excretion: Urine

Available Dosage Forms

Injection, solution, as acetate (DDAVP®): 4 mcg/mL (1 mL, 10 mL)

Solution, intranasal, as acetate (DDAVP®): 100 mcg/mL (2.5 mL) [with rhinal tube]

Solution, intranasal, as acetate [spray]: 100 mcg/mL (5 mL) [delivers 10 mcg/spray]

DDAVP®: 100 mcg/mL (5 mL) [delivers 10 mcg/spray]

Stimate™: 1.5 mg/mL (2.5 mL) [delivers 150 mcg/spray]

Tablet, as acetate (DDAVP®): 0.1 mg, 0.2 mg

Dosing

Adults & Elderly:

Diabetes insipidus:

I.V., SubQ: 2-4 mcg/day (0.5-1 mL) in 2 divided doses or 1/10 of the maintenance intranasal dose

Intranasal (100 mcg/mL nasal solution): 10-40 mcg/day (0.1-0.4 mL) divided 1-3 times/day; adjust morning and evening doses separately for an adequate diurnal rhythm of water turnover. **Note:** The nasal spray pump can only deliver doses of 10 mcg (0.1 mL) or multiples of 10 mcg (0.1 mL); if doses other than this are needed, the rhinal tube delivery system is preferred.

Oral: Initial: 0.05 mg twice daily; total daily dose should be increased or decreased as needed to obtain adequate antidiuresis (range: 0.1-1.2 mg divided 2-3 times/day)

Nocturnal enuresis:

Intranasal (using 100 mcg/mL nasal solution): Initial: 20 mcg (0.2 mL) at bedtime; range: 10-40 mcg; it is recommended that ½ of the dose be given in each nostril. For 10 mcg dose, administer in one nostril. **Note:** The nasal spray pump can only deliver doses of 10 mcg (0.1 mL) or multiples of 10 mcg (0.1 mL); if doses other than this are needed, the rhinal tube delivery system is preferred.

Oral: 0.2 mg at bedtime; dose may be titrated up to 0.6 mg to achieve desired response. Patients previously on intranasal therapy can begin oral tablets 24 hours after the last intranasal dose.

Hemophilia A and mild-to-moderate von Willebrand disease (type I):

I.V.: 0.3 mcg/kg by slow infusion, begin 30 minutes before procedure

Nasal spray: Using high concentration spray (1.5 mg/mL): <50 kg: 150 mcg (1 spray); >50 kg: 300 mcg (1 spray each nostril); repeat use is determined by the patient's clinical condition and laboratory work. If using preoperatively, administer 2 hours before surgery.

Pediatrics:

Diabetes insipidus:

Intranasal (using 100 mcg/mL nasal solution):

Children 3 months to 12 years: Initial: 5 mcg/day (0.05 mL/day) divided 1-2 times/day; range: 5-30 mcg/day (0.05-0.3 mL/day) divided 1-2 times/day; adjust morning and evening doses separately for an adequate diurnal rhythm of water turnover; doses <10 mcg should be administered using the rhinal tube system

Children >12 years: Refer to adult dosing.

Oral: Children ≥4 years: Initial: 0.05 mg twice daily; total daily dose should be increased or decreased as needed to obtain adequate antidiuresis (range: 0.1-1.2 mg divided 2-3 times/day)

Hemophilia A and von Willebrand disease (type I):

I.V.: >3 months: 0.3 mcg/kg by slow infusion; may repeat dose if needed; begin 30 minutes before procedure

Intranasal: ≥11 months: Refer to adult dosing.

Nocturnal enuresis:

Children ≥6 years:

Intranasal (using 100 mcg/mL nasal solution): Initial: 20 mcg (0.2 mL) at bedtime; range: 10-40 mcg; it is recommended that ½ of the dose be given in each nostril. **Note:** The nasal spray pump can only deliver doses of 10 mcg (0.1 mL) or multiples of 10 mcg (0.1 mL); if doses other than this are needed, the rhinal tube delivery system is preferred. For 10 mcg dose, administer in one nostril.

Oral: 0.2 mg at bedtime. Dose may be titrated up to 0.6 mg to achieve desired response. Patients previously on intranasal therapy can begin oral tablets 24 hours after the last intranasal dose.

Children >12 years: Refer to adult dosing.

Renal Impairment: Cl_{cr} <50 mL/minute: Use is contraindicated.

Administration

I.V.: Infuse over 15-30 minutes

Other:

Intranasal:

DDAVP®: Nasal pump spray: Delivers 0.1 mL (10 mcg); for other doses which are not multiples, use rhinal tube. DDAVP® Nasal spray delivers fifty 10 mcg doses. For 10 mcg dose, administer in one nostril. Any solution remaining after 50 doses should be discarded. Pump must be primed prior to first use.

DDAVP® Rhinal tube: Insert top of dropper into tube (arrow marked end) in downward position. Squeeze dropper until solution reaches desired calibration mark. Disconnect dropper. Grasp the tube ¾inch from the end and insert tube into nostril until the fingertips reach the nostril. Place opposite end of tube into the mouth (holding breath). Tilt head back and blow with a strong, short puff into the nostril (for very young patients, an adult should blow solution into the child's nose). Reseal dropper after use.

Stability

Reconstitution: DDAVP®: Dilute solution for injection in 10-50 mL NS for I.V. infusion (10 mL for children ≤10 kg: 50 mL for adults and children >10 kg)

Storage:

DDAVP®:

Tablet, nasal spray: Store at controlled room temperature of 20°C to 25°C (68°F to 77°F). Keep nasal spray in upright position.

Rhinal tube: Store refrigerated at 2°C to 8°C (36°F to 46°F). May store at room temperature for up to 3 weeks.

Injection: Store refrigerated at 2°C to 8°C (36°F to 46°F).

Stimate™: Store refrigerated at 2°C to 8°C (36°F to 46°F). May store at room temperature for up to 3 weeks.

Laboratory Monitoring

Diabetes insipidus: Fluid intake, urine volume, specific gravity, plasma and urine osmolality, serum electrolytes

Hemophilia A: Factor VIII coagulant activity, Factor VIII ristocetin cofactor activity, and Factor VIII antigen levels, aPTT

Von Willebrand disease: Factor VIII coagulant activity, Factor VIII ristocetin cofactor activity, and Factor VIII von Willebrand antigen levels, bleeding time

Nocturnal enuresis: Serum electrolytes if used for >7 days

Nursing Actions

Physical Assessment: Monitor laboratory tests and therapeutic effectiveness (according to purpose for use) and adverse reactions (eg, thromboembolism, hyponatremia, water intoxication) regularly throughout therapy. Teach patient proper use (if self-administered), possible side effects/appropriate interventions, and adverse symptoms to report.

Patient Education: Do not take any new medication during therapy unless approved by prescriber. Use specific product as directed. Avoid alcohol; may decrease effect of medication. Diabetes insipidus: Avoid overhydration. Weigh yourself daily at the same time in the same clothes. Report increased weight or swelling of extremities. If using intranasal product, inspect nasal membranes regularly. Report swelling or increased nasal congestion.

All uses: Report unresolved headache; chest pain or palpitation; respiratory difficulty; acute heartburn, nausea, vomiting, or abdominal cramping; vulval pain; CNS changes (agitation, chills, coma, dizziness, insomnia, confusion); rash; or other adverse effects. **Breast-feeding precaution:** Consult prescriber if breast-feeding.

Geriatric Considerations Elderly patients should be cautioned not to increase their fluid intake beyond that sufficient to satisfy their thirst in order to avoid water intoxication and hyponatremia.

Additional Information 10 mcg of desmopressin acetate is equivalent to 40 int. units

---

Dexamethasone (deks a METH a sone)

U.S. Brand Names Decadron®; Decadron® Phosphate [DSC]; Dexamethasone Intensol®; DexPak® TaperPak®; Maxidex®

Synonyms Dexamethasone Sodium Phosphate

Pharmacologic Category Anti-inflammatory Agent; Anti-inflammatory Agent, Ophthalmic; Antiemetic; Corticosteroid, Ophthalmic; Corticosteroid, Systemic; Corticosteroid, Topical

Medication Safety Issues
Sound-alike/look-alike issues:
Dexamethasone may be confused with desoximetasone

Decadron® may be confused with Percodan®
Maxidex® may be confused with Maxzide®

Pregnancy Risk Factor C

Lactation Excretion in breast milk unknown

Use Systemically and locally for chronic swelling; allergic, hematologic, neoplastic, and autoimmune diseases; may be used in management of cerebral edema, septic shock, as a diagnostic agent, antiemetic

Unlabeled/Investigational Use General indicator consistent with depression; diagnosis of Cushing's syndrome

Mechanism of Action/Effect Decreases inflammation by suppression of neutrophil migration, decreased production of inflammatory mediators, and reversal of increased capillary permeability; suppresses normal immune response. Dexamethasone's mechanism of antiemetic activity is unknown.

Contraindications Hypersensitivity to dexamethasone or any component of the formulation; active untreated infections; ophthalmic use in viral, fungal, or tuberculosis diseases of the eye

Warnings/Precautions Use with caution in patients with hypothyroidism, cirrhosis, hypertension, CHF, ulcerative colitis, or thromboembolic disorders. Corticosteroids should be used with caution in patients with diabetes, osteoporosis, peptic ulcer, glaucoma, cataracts, or tuberculosis. Use caution following acute MI (corticosteroids have been associated with myocardial rupture). Use caution in hepatic impairment. Because of the risk of adverse effects, systemic corticosteroids should be used cautiously in the elderly in the smallest possible effective dose for the shortest duration.

May cause suppression of hypothalamic-pituitary-adrenal (HPA) axis, particularly in younger children or in patients receiving high doses for prolonged periods. Symptoms of adrenocortical insufficiency in suppressed patients may result from rapid discontinuation/withdrawal; deficits in HPA response may persist for months following discontinuation and require supplementation during metabolic stress. Patients receiving 20 mg/day of prednisone (or equivalent) may be most susceptible. Particular care is required when patients are transferred from systemic corticosteroids to inhaled products due to possible adrenal insufficiency or exacerbation of underlying disease, including an increase in allergic symptoms. Fatalities have occurred due to adrenal insufficiency in asthmatic patients during and after transfer from systemic corticosteroids to aerosol steroids; aerosol steroids do **not** provide the systemic steroid needed to treat patients having trauma, surgery, or infections. Dexamethasone does not provide adequate mineralocorticoid activity in adrenal insufficiency (may be employed as a single dose while cortisol assays are performed).

Controlled clinical studies have shown that orally-inhaled and intranasal corticosteroids may cause a reduction in growth velocity in pediatric patients. (In studies of orally-inhaled corticosteroids, the mean reduction in growth velocity was ~1 cm per year [range 0.3-1.8 cm per year] and appears to be related to dose and duration of exposure). The growth of pediatric patients receiving inhaled corticosteroids, should be monitored routinely (eg, via stadiometry). To minimize the systemic effects of orally-inhaled and intranasal corticosteroids, each patient should be titrated to the lowest effective dose.

May suppress the immune system; patients may be more susceptible to infection. Use with caution in patients with systemic infections or ocular herpes simplex. Avoid exposure to chickenpox and measles.

Drug Interactions

Cytochrome P450 Effect: Substrate of CYP3A4 (minor); **Induces** CYP2A6 (weak), 2B6 (weak), 2C8/9 (weak), 3A4 (weak)

Decreased Effect: Bile acid sequestrants may reduce the absorption of corticosteroids; separate administration by 2 hours. Aminoglutethimide may reduce the serum levels/effects of dexamethasone.

Serum concentrations of isoniazid and phenytoin may be decreased by corticosteroids. Corticosteroids may lead to a reduction in warfarin effect. Corticosteroids may suppress the response to vaccinations. The use of live vaccines is contraindicated in immunosuppressed patients. In patients receiving high doses of systemic corticosteroids for ≥14 days, wait at least 1 month between discontinuing steroid therapy and administering immunization.

Increased Effect/Toxicity: Aprepitant, azole antifungals, calcium channel blockers (nondihydropyridine), cyclosporine, and estrogens may increase the serum levels of corticosteroids. Antacids may increase the absorption of corticosteroids, separate administration by 2 hours. Corticosteroids may increase the serum levels of cyclosporine.

Concurrent use of nonsteroidal anti-inflammatory drugs (NSAIDs) and salicylates with corticosteroids may lead to an increased incidence of gastrointestinal adverse effects. Concurrent use with anticholinergic agents may lead to severe weakness in patients with myasthenia gravis. Concurrent use of fluoroquinolone antibiotics may increase the risk of tendon rupture, particularly in elderly patients (overall incidence rare). Concurrent use of neuromuscular-blocking agents with corticosteroids may increase the risk of myopathy. The concurrent use of thalidomide with corticosteroids may increase the risk of selected adverse effects (toxic epidermal necrolysis and DVT).
(Continued)

Dexamethasone *(Continued)*

Nutritional/Ethanol Interactions

Ethanol: Avoid ethanol (may enhance gastric mucosal irritation).

Food: Dexamethasone interferes with calcium absorption. Limit caffeine.

Herb/Nutraceutical: Avoid cat's claw, echinacea (have immunostimulant properties).

Adverse Reactions Frequency not defined.

Cardiovascular: Edema, hypertension, arrhythmia, cardiomyopathy, myocardial rupture (post-MI), syncope, thromboembolism, thrombophlebitis, vasculitis

Central nervous system: Insomnia, nervousness, vertigo, seizure, psychosis, pseudotumor cerebri (usually following discontinuation), headache, mood swings, delirium, hallucinations, euphoria

Dermatologic: Hirsutism, acne, skin atrophy, bruising, hyperpigmentation, pruritus (generalized), perianal pruritus (following I.V. injection), urticaria

Endocrine & metabolic: Diabetes mellitus, adrenal suppression, hyperlipidemia, Cushing's syndrome, pituitary-adrenal axis suppression, growth suppression, glucose intolerance, gynecomastia, hypokalemia, alkalosis, amenorrhea, sodium and water retention, hyperglycemia, hypercalciuria, weight gain

Gastrointestinal: Appetite increased, indigestion, peptic ulcer, nausea, vomiting, abdominal distention, ulcerative esophagitis, pancreatitis, intestinal perforation

Genitourinary: Altered (increased or decreased) spermatogenesis

Hematologic: Transient leukocytosis

Hepatic: Transaminases increased, hepatomegaly

Neuromuscular & skeletal: Arthralgia, muscle weakness, osteoporosis, fractures, myopathy (particularly in conjunction with neuromuscular disease or neuromuscular blocking agents), tendon rupture, vertebral compression fractures, neuropathy, neuritis, paresthesia

Ocular: Cataracts, glaucoma, exophthalmos, intraocular pressure increased

Miscellaneous: Infections, anaphylactoid reaction, anaphylaxis, angioedema, avascular necrosis, secondary malignancy, Kaposi's sarcoma, intractable hiccups, impaired wound healing, abnormal fat deposition, moon face

Overdosage/Toxicology When consumed in high doses over prolonged periods, systemic hypercorticism and adrenal suppression may occur. In these cases, discontinuation of the corticosteroid should be done judiciously.

Pharmacodynamics/Kinetics

Onset of Action: Acetate: Prompt

Duration of Action: Metabolic effect: 72 hours; acetate is a long-acting repository preparation

Time to Peak: Serum: Oral: 1-2 hours; I.M.: ~8 hours

Half-Life Elimination: Normal renal function: 1.8-3.5 hours; Biological half-life: 36-54 hours

Metabolism: Hepatic

Excretion: Urine and feces

Available Dosage Forms [DSC] = Discontinued product

Elixir, as base: 0.5 mg/5 mL (240 mL) [contains alcohol 5%; raspberry flavor]

Injection, solution, as sodium phosphate: 4 mg/mL (1 mL, 5 mL, 10 mL, 25 mL, 30 mL); 10 mg/mL (1 mL, 10 mL)

Decadron® Phosphate: 4 mg/mL (5 mL, 25 mL); 24 mg/mL (5 mL) [contains sodium bisulfite] [DSC]

Ointment, ophthalmic, as sodium phosphate: 0.05% (3.5 g)

Solution, ophthalmic, as sodium phosphate: 0.1% (5 mL)

Solution, oral: 0.5 mg/5 mL (500 mL) [cherry flavor]

Solution, oral concentrate (Dexamethasone Intensol®): 1 mg/mL (30 mL) [contains alcohol 30%]

Suspension, ophthalmic (Maxidex®): 0.1% (5 mL, 15 mL)

Tablet: 0.25 mg, 0.5 mg, 0.75 mg, 1 mg, 1.5 mg, 2 mg, 4 mg, 6 mg [some 0.5 mg tablets may contain tartrazine]

Decadron®: 0.5 mg, 0.75 mg, 4 mg

DexPak® TaperPak®: 1.5 mg [51 tablets on taper dose card]

Dosing

Adults:

Anti-inflammatory:

Oral, I.M., I.V. (injections should be given as sodium phosphate): 0.75-9 mg/day in divided doses every 6-12 hours

Intra-articular, intralesional, or soft tissue (as sodium phosphate): 0.4-6 mg/day

Extubation or airway edema: Oral, I.M., I.V. (injections should be given as sodium phosphate): 0.5-2 mg/kg/day in divided doses every 6 hours beginning 24 hours prior to extubation and continuing for 4-6 doses afterwards

Antiemetic:

Prophylaxis: Oral, I.V.: 10-20 mg 15-30 minutes before treatment on each treatment day

Continuous infusion regimen: Oral or I.V.: 10 mg every 12 hours on each treatment day

Mildly emetogenic therapy: Oral, I.M., I.V.: 4 mg every 4-6 hours

Delayed nausea/vomiting: Oral: 4-10 mg 1-2 times/day for 2-4 days **or**

8 mg every 12 hours for 2 days; then

4 mg every 12 hours for 2 days **or**

20 mg 1 hour before chemotherapy; then

10 mg 12 hours after chemotherapy; then

8 mg every 12 hours for 4 doses; then

4 mg every 12 hours for 4 doses

Ophthalmic anti-inflammatory:

Ophthalmic ointment: Apply thin coating into conjunctival sac 3-4 times/day; gradually taper dose to discontinue.

Ophthalmic suspension: Instill 2 drops into conjunctival sac every hour during the day and every other hour during the night; gradually reduce dose to every 3-4 hours, then to 3-4 times/day.

Steroid-responsive dermatoses: Topical: Apply 1-4 times/day. Therapy should be discontinued when control is achieved; if no improvement is seen, reassessment of diagnosis may be necessary.

Chemotherapy: Oral, I.V.: 40 mg every day for 4 days, repeated every 4 weeks (VAD regimen)

Cerebral edema: I.V. 10 mg stat, 4 mg I.M./I.V. (should be given as sodium phosphate) every 6 hours until response is maximized, then switch to oral regimen, then taper off if appropriate; dosage may be reduced after 24 days and gradually discontinued over 5-7 days

Dexamethasone suppression test (depression indicator) (unlabeled use): Oral: 1 mg at 11 PM, draw blood at 8 AM the following day for plasma cortisol determination

Cushing's syndrome, diagnostic: Oral: 1 mg at 11 PM, draw blood at 8 AM; greater accuracy for Cushing's syndrome may be achieved by the following:

Dexamethasone 0.5 mg by mouth every 6 hours for 48 hours (with 24-hour urine collection for 17-hydroxycorticosteroid excretion)

Differentiation of Cushing's syndrome due to ACTH excess from Cushing's due to other causes: Oral: Dexamethasone 2 mg every 6 hours for 48 hours (with 24-hour urine collection for 17-hydroxycorticosteroid excretion)

Multiple sclerosis (acute exacerbation): Oral: 30 mg/day for 1 week, followed by 4-12 mg/day for 1 month

Treatment of shock:

Addisonian crisis/shock (ie, adrenal insufficiency/ responsive to steroid therapy): I.V. (given as sodium phosphate): 4-10 mg as a single dose, which may be repeated if necessary

Unresponsive shock (ie, unresponsive to steroid therapy): I.V. (given as sodium phosphate): 1-6 mg/kg as a single I.V. dose or up to 40 mg initially followed by repeat doses every 2-6 hours while shock persists

Physiological replacement: Oral, I.M., I.V. (should be given as sodium phosphate): 0.03-0.15 mg/kg/ day **or** 0.6-0.75 mg/m²/day in divided doses every 6-12 hours

Elderly: Refer to adult dosing. Use cautiously in the elderly in the smallest possible dose.

Pediatrics:

Antiemetic (prior to chemotherapy): I.V. (should be given as sodium phosphate): 5-20 mg given 15-30 minutes before treatment

Anti-inflammatory and/or immunosuppressant: Oral, I.M., I.V. (injections should be given as sodium phosphate): 0.08-0.3 mg/kg/day **or** 2.5-10 mg/m²/ day in divided doses every 6-12 hours

Extubation or airway edema: Oral, I.M., I.V. (injections should be given as sodium phosphate): 0.5-2 mg/kg/day in divided doses every 6 hours beginning 24 hours prior to extubation and continuing for 4-6 doses afterwards

Cerebral edema: I.V. (should be given as sodium phosphate): Loading dose: 1-2 mg/kg/dose as a single dose; maintenance: 1-1.5 mg/kg/day (maximum: 16 mg/day) in divided doses every 4-6 hours for 5 days then taper for 5 days, then discontinue

Bacterial meningitis in infants and children >2 months: I.V. (should be given as sodium phosphate): 0.6 mg/kg/day in 4 divided doses every 6 hours for the first 4 days of antibiotic treatment; start dexamethasone at the time of the first dose of antibiotic

Physiologic replacement: Oral, I.M., I.V.: 0.03-0.15 mg/kg/day or 0.6-0.75 mg/m²/day in divided doses every 6-12 hours

Ophthalmic inflammation: Refer to adult dosing.

Renal Impairment: Hemodialysis or peritoneal dialysis: Supplemental dose is not necessary.

Administration

Oral: Administer oral formulation with meals to decrease GI upset.

I.M.: Acetate injection is **not** for I.V. use.

I.V.: Administer as a 5-10 minute bolus; rapid injection is associated with a high incidence of perianal discomfort.

I.V. Detail: pH: 7.0-8.5

Topical: Topical formation is for external use. Do not use on open wounds. Apply sparingly to occlusive dressings. Should not be used in the presence of open or weeping lesions.

Stability

Reconstitution: Injection should be diluted in 50-100 mL NS or D₅W.

Compatibility: Stable in D₅W, NS

Y-site administration: Incompatible with ciprofloxacin, idarubicin, midazolam, topotecan

Compatibility in syringe: Incompatible with doxapram, glycopyrrolate

Compatibility when admixed: Incompatible with daunorubicin, diphenhydramine with lorazepam and metoclopramide, metaraminol, vancomycin

Storage: Injection solution: Store at room temperature; protect from light and freezing.

Stability of injection of parenteral admixture at room temperature (25°C): 24 hours

Stability of injection of parenteral admixture at refrigeration temperature (4°C): 2 days; protect from light and freezing

Laboratory Monitoring Hemoglobin, occult blood loss, serum potassium, glucose

Dexamethasone suppression test, overnight: 8 AM cortisol <6 mg/100 mL (dexamethasone 1 mg). Plasma cortisol determination should be made on the day after giving dose.

Nursing Actions

Physical Assessment: Assess potential for interactions with other prescriptions, OTC medications, or herbal products patient may be taking. Monitor laboratory tests, patient response, and adverse effects according to indications for therapy, dose, route, and duration of therapy. When used for long-term therapy (>10-14 days) dosage should be reduced incrementally. With systemic administration, caution patients with diabetes to monitor glucose levels closely (corticosteroids may alter glucose levels). Teach patient proper use (according to formulation), side effects/appropriate interventions, and symptoms to report..

Patient Education: Do not take any new medication during therapy unless approved by prescriber. Take exactly as directed, do not increase dose or discontinue abruptly without consulting prescriber.

Oral: Take with or after meals. Avoid alcohol and limit intake of caffeine or stimulants. Prescriber may recommend increased dietary vitamins, minerals, or iron. If you have diabetes, monitor glucose levels closely (antidiabetic medication may need to be adjusted). Inform prescriber if you are experiencing greater-than-normal levels of stress (medication may need adjustment). You may be more susceptible to infection (avoid crowds and persons with contagious or infective conditions and do not have any vaccinations unless approved by prescriber). Some forms of this medication may cause GI upset (small frequent meals and frequent mouth care may help). Report promptly excessive nervousness or sleep disturbances; signs of infection (eg, sore throat, unhealed injuries); excessive growth of body hair or loss of skin color; vision changes; excessive or sudden weight gain (>3 lb/week); swelling of face or extremities; respiratory difficulty; muscle weakness; tarry stool; persistent abdominal pain; worsening of condition or failure to improve. **Pregnancy/breast-feeding precautions:** Inform prescriber if you are or intend to become pregnant. Consult prescriber if breast-feeding.

Ophthalmic: For use in eyes only. Wash hands before using. Lie down or tilt your head back and look upward. Put drops of suspension or apply thin ribbon of ointment inside lower eyelid. Close eye and roll eyeball in all directions. Do not blink for ½ minute. Apply gentle pressure to inner corner of eye for 30 seconds. Do not use any other eye preparation for at least 10 minutes. Do not let tip of applicator touch eye; do not contaminate tip of applicator (may cause eye infection, eye damage, or vision loss). Do not share medication with anyone else. Wear sunglasses when in sunlight; you may be more sensitive to bright light. Inform prescriber if condition worsens, fails to improve, or if you experience eye pain, disturbances of vision, or other adverse eye response.

Topical: For external use only. Do not use for eyes, mucous membranes, or open wounds. Use exactly as directed and for no longer than the period prescribed. Before using, wash and dry area gently. Apply in thin layer (may rub in lightly). Apply light dressing (if necessary) to area being treated. Do not use occlusive dressing unless so advised by prescriber. Avoid exposing treated area to sunlight (severe sunburn may occur). Inform prescriber if condition worsens (Continued)

Dexamethasone *(Continued)*

(swelling, redness, irritation, pain, open sores) or fails to improve.

Dietary Considerations May be taken with meals to decrease GI upset. May need diet with increased potassium, pyridoxine, vitamin C, vitamin D, folate, calcium, and phosphorus.

Geriatric Considerations Because of the risk of adverse effects, systemic corticosteroids should be used cautiously in the elderly in the smallest possible dose, and for the shortest possible time.

Pregnancy Issues Dexamethasone has been used in patients with premature labor (26-34 weeks gestation) to stimulate fetal lung maturation. Effects on the fetus: Crosses the placenta; transient leukocytosis has been reported. Available evidence suggests safe use during pregnancy.

Additional Information Effects of inhaled/intranasal steroids on growth have been observed in the absence of laboratory evidence of HPA axis suppression, suggesting that growth velocity is a more sensitive indicator of systemic corticosteroid exposure in pediatric patients than some commonly used tests of HPA axis function. The long-term effects of this reduction in growth velocity associated with orally-inhaled and intranasal corticosteroids, including the impact on final adult height, are unknown. The potential for "catch up" growth following discontinuation of treatment with inhaled corticosteroids has not been adequately studied.

Withdrawal/tapering of therapy: Corticosteroid tapering following short-term use is limited primarily by the need to control the underlying disease state; tapering may be accomplished over a period of days. Following longer-term use, tapering over weeks to months may be necessary to avoid signs and symptoms of adrenal insufficiency and to allow recovery of the HPA axis. Testing of HPA axis responsiveness may be of value in selected patients. Subtle deficits in HPA response may persist for months after discontinuation of therapy, and may require supplemental dosing during periods of acute illness or surgical stress.

Dexchlorpheniramine

(deks klor fen EER a meen)

Synonyms Dexchlorpheniramine Maleate

Pharmacologic Category Antihistamine

Pregnancy Risk Factor B

Lactation Excretion in breast milk unknown/not recommended

Use Perennial and seasonal allergic rhinitis and other allergic symptoms including urticaria

Mechanism of Action/Effect Competes with histamine for H_1-receptor sites on effector cells in the GI tract, blood vessels, and respiratory tract

Contraindications Hypersensitivity to dexchlorpheniramine or any component of the formulation; narrow-angle glaucoma

Warnings/Precautions Causes sedation, caution must be used in performing tasks which require alertness (eg, operating machinery or driving). Sedative effects of CNS depressants or ethanol are potentiated. Use with caution in patients with angle-closure glaucoma, pyloroduodenal obstruction (including stenotic peptic ulcer), urinary tract obstruction (including bladder neck obstruction and symptomatic prostatic hyperplasia), hyperthyroidism, increased intraocular pressure, and cardiovascular disease (including hypertension and tachycardia). High sedative and anticholinergic properties, therefore may not be considered the antihistamine of choice for prolonged use in the elderly. May cause paradoxical excitation in pediatric patients, and can result in hallucinations, coma, and death in overdose.

Drug Interactions

Decreased Effect: May increase gastric degradation of levodopa and decrease the amount of levodopa absorbed by delaying gastric emptying. Therapeutic effects of cholinergic agents (tacrine, donepezil) and neuroleptics may be antagonized.

Increased Effect/Toxicity: CNS depressants may increase the degree of sedation and respiratory depression with antihistamines. May increase the absorption of digoxin. Central and/or peripheral anticholinergic syndrome can occur when administered with amantadine, rimantadine, narcotic analgesics, phenothiazines and other antipsychotics (especially with high anticholinergic activity), tricyclic antidepressants, quinidine, disopyramide, procainamide, and antihistamines.

Nutritional/Ethanol Interactions Ethanol: Avoid ethanol (may increase CNS depression).

Lab Interactions May interfere with a methacholine bronchial challenge.

Adverse Reactions

>10%:

Central nervous system: Slight to moderate drowsiness

Respiratory: Thickening of bronchial secretions

1% to 10%:

Central nervous system: Headache, fatigue, nervousness, dizziness

Gastrointestinal: Appetite increase, weight gain, nausea, diarrhea, abdominal pain, xerostomia

Neuromuscular & skeletal: Arthralgia

Respiratory: Pharyngitis

Overdosage/Toxicology Symptoms of overdose include dry mouth, flushed skin, dilated pupils, CNS depression. There is no specific treatment for antihistamine overdose. Clinical toxicity is due to blockade of cholinergic receptors. For anticholinergic overdose with severe life-threatening symptoms, physostigmine 1-2 mg I.V. slowly, may be given to reverse these effects.

Pharmacodynamics/Kinetics

Onset of Action: ~1 hour

Duration of Action: 3-6 hours

Metabolism: Hepatic

Available Dosage Forms

Syrup, as maleate: 2 mg/5 mL (480 mL, 3840 mL) [contains alcohol 6%; orange flavor]

Tablet, sustained action, as maleate: 4 mg, 6 mg

Dosing

Adults & Elderly: Allergy symptoms: Oral: 2 mg every 4-6 hours or 4-6 mg timed release at bedtime or every 8-10 hours

Pediatrics: Allergy symptoms: Oral:

2-5 years: 0.5 mg every 4-6 hours (do not use timed release)

6-11 years: 1 mg every 4-6 hours or 4 mg timed release at bedtime

Nursing Actions

Physical Assessment: Assess effectiveness and interactions of other medications patient may be taking. Monitor effectiveness of therapy and adverse reactions (eg, excess anticholinergic effects) at beginning of therapy and periodically with long-term use. Assess knowledge/teach patient appropriate use, interventions to reduce side effects, and adverse symptoms to report.

Patient Education: Take as directed; do not exceed recommended dose. Do not chew or crush sustained release tablet. Take with food or water. Avoid use of other depressants, alcohol, or sleep-inducing medications unless approved by prescriber. You may experience drowsiness or dizziness (use caution when driving or engaging in tasks requiring alertness until response to drug is known); or dry mouth, nausea, or abdominal pain (small frequent meals, frequent mouth care, chewing gum, or sucking hard candy may help). Report persistent sedation, confusion, or agitation;

changes in urinary pattern; blurred vision; sore throat, respiratory difficulty or expectorating (thick secretions); or lack of improvement or worsening or condition. **Breast-feeding precaution:** Breast-feeding is not recommended.

Dietary Considerations May be taken with food or water.

Geriatric Considerations Anticholinergic action may cause significant confusional symptoms, constipation, or problems voiding urine.

Dexchlorpheniramine and Pseudoephedrine
(deks klor fen EER a meen & soo doe e FED rin)

U.S. Brand Names Duotan PD; Tanafed DP™

Synonyms Pseudoephedrine Tannate and Dexchlorpheniramine Tannate

Pharmacologic Category Alpha/Beta Agonist; Antihistamine

Pregnancy Risk Factor C

Lactation Excretion in breast milk unknown/not recommended

Use Relief of nasal congestion associated with the common cold, hay fever, and other allergies, sinusitis, and vasomotor and allergic rhinitis

Contraindications Hypersensitivity to dexchlorpheniramine, pseudoephedrine, or any component of the formulation; severe hypertension; severe cardiovascular disease; use with or within 2 weeks of discontinuing MAO inhibitor; narrow-angle glaucoma; urinary retention; peptic ulcer disease; breast-feeding

Warnings/Precautions Use caution with hypertension, diabetes, cardiovascular disease, hyperthyroidism, increased intraocular pressure, or prostatic hyperplasia. Causes sedation,:caution must be used in performing tasks which require alertness (eg, operating machinery or driving). Sedative effects of CNS depressants or ethanol are potentiated. Use caution in elderly patients (risk of CNS depression may be increased).

Drug Interactions
Cytochrome P450 Effect: See individual monographs for dexchlorpheniramine and pseudoephedrine.
Decreased Effect: See individual monographs for chlorpheniramine and pseudoephedrine.
Increased Effect/Toxicity: See individual monographs for dexchlorpheniramine and pseudoephedrine.

Nutritional/Ethanol Interactions Ethanol: Avoid ethanol (may increase CNS depression).

Adverse Reactions See individual monographs for dexchlorpheniramine and pseudoephedrine.

Available Dosage Forms Suspension: Dexchlorpheniramine tannate 2.5 mg and pseudoephedrine tannate 75 mg per 5 mL (120 mL, 480 mL) [contains sodium benzoate; strawberry-banana flavor]

Dosing
Adults: Rhinitis/decongestant: Oral: Dexchlorpheniramine tannate 2.5 mg and pseudoephedrine tannate 75 mg per 5 mL: 10-20 mL every 12 hours (maximum: 40 mL/24 hours)

Pediatrics: Rhinitis/decongestant: Oral: Dexchlorpheniramine tannate 2.5 mg and pseudoephedrine tannate 75 mg per 5 mL:
Children:
2-6 years: 2.5-5 mL every 12 hours (maximum: 10 mL/24 hours)
6-12 years: 5-10 mL every 12 hours (maximum: 20 mL/24 hours)
Children ≥12 years: Refer to adult dosing.

Administration
Oral: Shake suspension well prior to use.
Nursing Actions
Physical Assessment: Assess other prescription and OTC medications the patient may be taking to avoid duplications and interactions. Assess knowledge/teach patient appropriate use, side effects, and symptoms to report.

Patient Education: Do not exceed the recommended dosage. May cause drowsiness (use caution when driving or engaging in activities requiring alertness until response to drug is known). Avoid use of alcohol, sedatives, or tranquilizers without consulting prescriber. You may experience nervousness, excitability, restlessness, headache, and insomnia. Report persistent CNS changes (nervousness, dizziness, tremor, agitation, or convulsions); increased heart rate and palpitations; or sleeplessness to prescriber. **Pregnancy/Breast-feeding precaution:** Inform prescriber if you are or intend to become pregnant. Consult prescriber if breast-feeding.

Geriatric Considerations Elderly patients should be counseled about the proper use of over-the-counter cough and cold preparations. Elderly are more predisposed to adverse effects of sympathomimetics since they frequently have cardiovascular diseases and diabetes mellitus as well as multiple drug therapies. It may be advisable to treat with a short-acting/immediate-release formulation before initiating sustained-release/long-acting formulations. Anticholinergic action may cause significant confusional symptoms, constipation, or problems voiding urine.

Breast-Feeding Issues Pseudoephedrine is excreted in breast milk. The manufacturers do not recommend its use while breast-feeding; however, the AAP considers it to be "compatible" with breast-feeding. Information for dexchlorpheniramine is not available.

Dexmedetomidine (deks MED e toe mi deen)

U.S. Brand Names Precedex™

Synonyms Dexmedetomidine Hydrochloride

Pharmacologic Category Alpha$_2$-Adrenergic Agonist; Sedative

Medication Safety Issues
Sound-alike/look-alike issues:
Precedex™ may be confused with Peridex®

Pregnancy Risk Factor C

Lactation Excretion in breast milk unknown/use caution

Use Sedation of initially intubated and mechanically ventilated patients during treatment in an intensive care setting; duration of infusion should not exceed 24 hours

Unlabeled/Investigational Use Unlabeled uses include premedication prior to anesthesia induction with thiopental; relief of pain and reduction of opioid dose following laparoscopic tubal ligation; as an adjunct anesthetic in ophthalmic surgery; treatment of shivering; premedication to attenuate the cardiostimulatory and postanesthetic delirium of ketamine

Mechanism of Action/Effect Selective alpha$_2$-adrenoceptor agonist with sedative properties; alpha$_1$ activity was observed at high doses or after rapid infusions

Contraindications Hypersensitivity to dexmedetomidine or any component of the formulation; use outside of an intensive care setting

Warnings/Precautions Should be administered only by persons skilled in management of patients in intensive care setting. Patients should be continuously monitored. Episodes of bradycardia, hypotension, and sinus arrest have been associated with dexmedetomidine. Use caution in patients with heart block, severe ventricular dysfunction, hypovolemia, diabetes, chronic hypertension, and in the elderly. Use with caution in patients (Continued)

Dexmedetomidine *(Continued)*

receiving vasodilators or drugs which decrease heart rate. Transient hypertension has been primarily observed during the dose in association with the initial peripheral vasoconstrictive effects of dexmedetomidine. Treatment of this is not generally necessary; however, reduction of infusion rate may be desirable.

Drug Interactions
Cytochrome P450 Effect: Substrate of CYP2A6 (major); **Inhibits** CYP1A2 (weak), 2C8/9 (weak), 2D6 (strong), 3A4 (weak)
Decreased Effect: Dexmedetomidine may decrease the levels/effects of CYP2D6 prodrug substrates; example prodrug substrates include codeine, hydrocodone, oxycodone, and tramadol.
Increased Effect/Toxicity: The levels/effects of dexmedetomidine may be increased by isoniazid, methoxsalen, miconazole, and other CYP2A6 inhibitors. Dexmedetomidine may increase the levels/effects of amphetamines, selected beta-blockers, dextromethorphan, fluoxetine, lidocaine, mirtazapine, nefazodone, paroxetine, risperidone, ritonavir, thioridazine, tricyclic antidepressants, venlafaxine, and other CYP2D6 substrates. Hypotension and/or bradycardia may be increased by vasodilators and heart rate-lowering agents.

Adverse Reactions
>10%:
Cardiovascular: Hypotension (30%)
Gastrointestinal: Nausea (11%)
1% to 10%:
Cardiovascular: Bradycardia (8%), atrial fibrillation (7%)
Central nervous system: Pain (3%)
Hematologic: Anemia (3%), leukocytosis (2%)
Renal: Oliguria (2%)
Respiratory: Hypoxia (6%), pulmonary edema (2%), pleural effusion (3%)
Miscellaneous: Infection (2%), thirst (2%)

Overdosage/Toxicology In reports of overdosages where the blood concentration was 13 times the upper boundary of the therapeutic range, first-degree AV block and second degree heart block occurred. No hemodynamic compromise was noted with the AV block and the heart block resolved spontaneously within one minute. Two patients who received a 2 mcg/kg loading dose over 10 minutes experienced bradycardia and/or hypotension. One patient who received a loading dose of undiluted dexmedetomidine (19.4 mcg/kg) had cardiac arrest and was successfully resuscitated.

Pharmacodynamics/Kinetics
Onset of Action: Rapid
Protein Binding: 94%
Half-Life Elimination: 6 minutes; Terminal: 2 hours
Metabolism: Hepatic via glucuronidation and CYP2A6
Excretion: Urine (95%); feces (4%)
Available Dosage Forms Injection, solution [preservative free]: 100 mcg/mL (2 mL)

Dosing
Adults:
ICU sedation: I.V.: Initial: Loading infusion of 1 mcg/kg over 10 minutes, followed by a maintenance infusion of 0.2-0.7 mcg/kg/hour (individualized and titrated to desired clinical effect); not indicated for infusions lasting >24 hours
Note: Solution must be diluted prior to administration.
Elderly: Refer to adult dosing. Dosage reduction may need to be considered. No specific guidelines available. Dose selections should be cautious, at the low end of dosage range; titration should be slower, allowing adequate time to evaluate response.
Renal Impairment: Dosage reduction may need to be considered.
Hepatic Impairment: Dosage reduction may need to be considered. No specific guidelines available.

Administration
I.V.: Administer using a controlled infusion device. Must be diluted in 0.9% sodium chloride solution to achieve the required concentration prior to administration. Advisable to use administration components made with synthetic or coated natural rubber gaskets. Parenteral products should be inspected visually for particulate matter and discoloration prior to administration.

Stability
Compatibility: Stable in D_5W, LR, 0.9% NS, 20% mannitol, plasma substitute
May adsorb to certain types of natural rubber; use components made with synthetic or coated natural rubber gaskets whenever possible.

Nursing Actions
Physical Assessment: Administration should be managed by professionals experienced in anesthesia. Assess other medications for effectiveness and safety. Other drugs that cause CNS depression may increase CNS depression induced by dexmedetomidine. Continuous monitoring of vital signs, cardiac and respiratory status, and level of sedation is mandatory during infusion and until full consciousness is regained. Safety precautions must be maintained until patient is fully alert. Dexmedetomidine is an anesthetic; pain must be treated with appropriate analgesic agents. Do not discontinue abruptly (may result in agitation, anxiety, resistance to mechanical ventilation, headache, hypertension). Titrate infusion rate so patient awakes slowly. Monitor fluid levels (intake and output) during and following infusion. Reposition patient and provide appropriate skin, mouth, and eye care every 2-3 hours, while sedated. Provide appropriate emotional and sensory support (auditory and environmental).
Patient Education: This is an anesthetic. Patient education should be appropriate to individual situation. Following return of consciousness, do not attempt to change position or rise from bed without assistance. Report immediately any pounding or unusual heartbeat, respiratory difficulty, or acute dizziness. **Pregnancy/breast-feeding precautions:** Inform prescriber if you are pregnant. Consult prescriber if breast-feeding.

Dexmethylphenidate *(dex meth il FEN i date)*

U.S. Brand Names Focalin™; Focalin™ XR
Synonyms Dexmethylphenidate Hydrochloride
Restrictions C-II
Pharmacologic Category Central Nervous System Stimulant
Pregnancy Risk Factor C
Lactation Excretion in breast milk unknown/use caution
Use Treatment of attention-deficit/hyperactivity disorder (ADHD)
Mechanism of Action/Effect CNS stimulant
Contraindications Hypersensitivity to dexmethylphenidate, methylphenidate, or any component of the formulation; marked anxiety, tension, and agitation; glaucoma, motor tics, family history or diagnosis of Tourette's syndrome; use with or within 14 days following MAO inhibitor therapy
Warnings/Precautions Recommended to be used as part of a comprehensive treatment program for ADHD. Use with caution in patients with bipolar disorder, diabetes mellitus, cardiovascular disease, hyperthyroidism, seizure disorders, insomnia, porphyria, or hypertension. Use caution in patients with history of ethanol or drug abuse. May exacerbate symptoms of behavior and thought disorder in psychotic patients. Do not use to treat severe depression or fatigue states. Potential for drug dependency exists - avoid abrupt

discontinuation in patients who have received for prolonged periods. Visual disturbances have been reported with methylphenidate (rare). Stimulant use has been associated with growth suppression. Stimulants may unmask tics in individuals with coexisting Tourette's syndrome. Safety and efficacy in children <6 years of age not established.

Drug Interactions
Decreased Effect: Effectiveness of antihypertensive agents may be decreased. Carbamazepine may decrease the effect of methylphenidate.

Increased Effect/Toxicity: Methylphenidate may cause hypertensive effects when used in combination with MAO inhibitors or drugs with MAO-inhibiting activity (linezolid). Risk may be less with selegiline (MAO type B selective at low doses); it is best to avoid this combination. NMS has been reported in a patient receiving methylphenidate and venlafaxine. Methylphenidate may increase levels of phenytoin, phenobarbital, TCAs, and warfarin. Increased toxicity with clonidine and sibutramine.

Nutritional/Ethanol Interactions
Ethanol: Avoid ethanol (may cause CNS depression).
Food: High-fat meal may increase time to peak concentration.
Herb/Nutraceutical: Avoid ephedra (may cause hypertension or arrhythmias) and yohimbe (also has CNS stimulatory activity).

Adverse Reactions
>10%:
Central nervous system: Headache (25% to 26%), feeling jittery (12%)
Gastrointestinal: Appetite decreased (30%), abdominal pain (15%)
1% to 10%:
Central nervous system: Dizziness (6%), anxiety (5% to 6%), fever (5%)
Gastrointestinal: Nausea (9%), dyspepsia (5% to 8%), xerostomia (7%), anorexia (6%), pharyngolaryngeal pain (4%)

Also refer to Methylphenidate *on page 1140* for adverse effects seen with methylphenidate.

Overdosage/Toxicology Signs and symptoms of overdose may include agitation, cardiac arrhythmias, coma, confusion, convulsions, delirium, dry mucous membranes, euphoria, flushing, hallucinations, headache, hyper-reflexia, hyperpyrexia, hypertension, muscle twitching, mydriasis, palpitations, sweating, tachycardia, tremors and vomiting. Treatment is symptom-directed and supportive.

Pharmacodynamics/Kinetics
Time to Peak: Fasting:
Tablet: 1-1.5 hours
Capsule: First peak: 1.5 hours (range: 1-4 hours); Second peak: 6.5 hours (range: 4.5-7 hours)
Half-Life Elimination: 2-4.5 hours
Metabolism: Via de-esterification to inactive metabolite, *d*-α-phenyl-piperidine acetate (*d*-ritalinic acid)
Excretion: Urine (90%, primarily as inactive metabolite)

Available Dosage Forms
Capsule, extended release (Focalin™ XR): 5 mg, 10 mg, 20 mg [bimodal release]
Tablet, as hydrochloride (Focalin™): 2.5 mg, 5 mg, 10 mg

Dosing
Adults:
Treatment of ADHD: Patients not currently taking methylphenidate: Oral:
Tablet: Initial: 2.5 mg twice daily; dosage may be adjusted in increments of 2.5-5 mg at weekly intervals (maximum dose: 20 mg/day); doses should be taken at least 4 hours apart
Capsule: Initial: 10 mg/day; dosage may be adjusted in increments of 10 mg/day at weekly intervals (maximum dose: 20 mg/day)

Note:
Conversion to dexmethylphenidate from methylphenidate: Tablet, capsule: Initial: Half the total daily dose of racemic methylphenidate
Conversion from dexmethylphenidate immediate release to dexmethylphenidate extended release: When changing from Focalin™ tablets to Focalin™ XR capsules, patients may be switched to the same daily dose using Focalin™ XR (maximum dose: 20 mg/day)
Safety and efficacy for long-term use of dexmethylphenidate have not yet been established. Patients should be re-evaluated at appropriate intervals to assess continued need of the medication.
Dose reductions and discontinuation: Reduce dose or discontinue in patients with paradoxical aggravation. Discontinue if no improvement is seen after one month of treatment.

Pediatrics: Treatment of ADHD:
Children ≥6 years: Patients not currently taking methylphenidate: Oral:
Tablet: Initial: 2.5 mg twice daily; dosage may be adjusted in increments of 2.5-5 mg at weekly intervals (maximum dose: 20 mg/day); doses should be taken at least 4 hours apart
Capsule: Initial: 5 mg/day; dosage may be adjusted in increments of 5 mg/day at weekly intervals (maximum dose: 20 mg/day)
See "Note" in adult dosing.

Administration
Oral: Capsule: Should be taken once daily in the morning; do not crush or chew. Capsules may be opened and contents sprinkled over a spoonful of applesauce.
Tablet: Should be taken at least 4 hours apart; may be taken with or without food.

Stability
Storage: Store at 25°C (77°F). Protect from light and moisture.

Nursing Actions
Physical Assessment: Monitor for effectiveness and possible interactions of other medications patient may be taking. Monitor laboratory results for effectiveness of therapy, and adverse reactions at beginning of therapy and periodically with long-term use. Taper dosage when discontinuing from long-term therapy. Assess knowledge/teach patient appropriate use, interventions to reduce side effects, and importance of reporting adverse symptoms promptly.

Patient Education: Take exactly as directed; do not change dosage or discontinue without consulting prescriber. Response may take some time. Avoid alcohol, caffeine, or other stimulants. Maintain adequate hydration (2-3 L/day of fluids) unless instructed to restrict fluid intake. You may experience decreased appetite or weight loss (small frequent meals may help maintain adequate nutrition); or restlessness, impaired judgment, or dizziness (use caution when driving or engaging in tasks requiring alertness until response to drug is known). Report unresolved rapid heartbeat; excessive agitation, nervousness, insomnia, tremors, or dizziness; blackened stool; skin rash or irritation; or altered gait or movement. **Pregnancy/breast-feeding precautions:** Inform prescriber if you are or intend to become pregnant. Consult prescriber if breast-feeding.

Dietary Considerations May be taken with or without food. Food effects on Focalin™ XR have not been studied and may need to be individually adjusted.

Additional Information
Focalin™ XR capsules use a bimodal release where 1/2 the dose is provided in immediate release beads and 1/2 the dose is in delayed release beads. A single, once-daily dose of a capsule provides the same amount of dexmethylphenidate as two tablets given 4 hours apart.

Dexrazoxane (deks ray ZOKS ane)

U.S. Brand Names Zinecard®

Synonyms ICRF-187

Pharmacologic Category Cardioprotectant

Medication Safety Issues

Sound-alike/look-alike issues:

Zinecard® may be confused with Gemzar®

Pregnancy Risk Factor C

Lactation Excretion in breast milk unknown/not recommended

Use Reduction of the incidence and severity of cardiomyopathy associated with doxorubicin administration in women with metastatic breast cancer who have received a cumulative doxorubicin dose of 300 mg/m² and who would benefit from continuing therapy with doxorubicin. It is not recommended for use with the initiation of doxorubicin therapy.

Mechanism of Action/Effect Derivative of EDTA; potent intracellular chelating agent. The mechanism of cardioprotectant activity is not fully understood. Appears to be converted intracellularly to a ring-opened chelating agent that interferes with iron-mediated oxygen free radical generation thought to be responsible, in part, for anthracycline-induced cardiomyopathy.

Contraindications Hypersensitivity to dexrazoxane or any component of the formulation; use with chemotherapy regimens that do not contain an anthracycline

Warnings/Precautions Hazardous agent; use appropriate precautions for handling and disposal. Dexrazoxane may add to the myelosuppression caused by chemotherapeutic agents. Dexrazoxane does not eliminate the potential for anthracycline-induced cardiac toxicity. Carefully monitor cardiac function. Dosage adjustment required for moderate or severe renal insufficiency. Safety and efficacy in pediatric patients have not been established.

Adverse Reactions Adverse reactions listed are those which were greater in the dexrazoxane arm in a trial comparison of dexrazoxane plus fluorouracil, doxorubicin, and cyclophosphamide (FAC) to FAC alone. (Most adverse reactions are thought to be attributed to FAC except for myelosuppression (increased) and pain at injection site).

Central nervous system: Fatigue/malaise, fever

Dermatologic: Alopecia, extravasation, streaking/erythema

Endocrine & metabolic: Serum amylase increased, serum calcium decreased, serum triglycerides increased

Hematologic: Hemorrhage, granulocytopenia, leukopenia, myelosuppression, thrombocytopenia

Hepatic: AST/ALT increased, bilirubin increased

Local: Pain at injection site, phlebitis

Neuromuscular & skeletal: Neurotoxicity

Miscellaneous: Infection, sepsis

Overdosage/Toxicology Management includes supportive care until resolution of myelosuppression and related conditions is complete. Retention of a significant dose fraction of unchanged drug in the plasma pool, minimal tissue partitioning or binding, and availability of >90% of systemic drug levels in the unbound form suggest that dexrazoxane could be removed using conventional peritoneal or hemodialysis.

Pharmacodynamics/Kinetics

Protein Binding: None

Half-Life Elimination: 2.1-2.5 hours

Excretion: Urine (42%)

Clearance, renal: 3.35 L/hour/m²; Plasma: 6.25-7.88 L/hour/m²

Available Dosage Forms Injection, powder for reconstitution: 250 mg, 500 mg [10 mg/mL when reconstituted]

Dosing

Adults & Elderly: Prevention of doxorubicin cardiomyopathy: I.V.: A 10:1 ratio of dexrazoxane:doxorubicin (500 mg/m² dexrazoxane:50 mg/m² doxorubicin)

Renal Impairment: Moderate-to-severe (Cl_cr<40 mL/minute): A 5:1 ratio (250 mg/m² dexrazoxane:50 mg/m² doxorubicin).

Hepatic Impairment: Since doxorubicin dosage is reduced in hyperbilirubinemia, a proportional reduction in dexrazoxane dosage is recommended (maintain ratio of 10:1).

Administration

I.V.: Administer by slow I.V. push or rapid (5-15 minutes) I.V. infusion from a bag. Administer doxorubicin within 30 minutes after beginning the infusion with dexrazoxane.

Stability

Reconstitution: Must be reconstituted with 0.167 Molar (M/6) sodium lactate injection to a concentration of 10 mg dexrazoxane/mL sodium lactate. Reconstituted dexrazoxane solution may be diluted with either 0.9% sodium chloride injection or 5% dextrose injection to a concentration of 1.3-5 mg/mL in intravenous infusion bags.

Storage: Store intact vials at controlled room temperature (15°C to 30°C/59°F to 86°F). Reconstituted and diluted solutions are stable for 6 hours at controlled room temperature or under refrigeration (2°C to 8°C/36°F to 46°F).

Laboratory Monitoring Frequent complete blood counts are recommended; LFTs

Nursing Actions

Physical Assessment: Assess effectiveness and interactions of other medications patient may be taking. Monitor cardiac function closely. Assess infusion site frequently. Avoid extravasation. Monitor for effectiveness of therapy and adverse effects.

Patient Education: This I.V. medication is given to reduce incidence of cardiac complications with doxorubicin. Report promptly any pain at infusion site. You will be more susceptible to infections. Avoid crowds and exposure to infections whenever possible. Report shortness of breath, chest discomfort, or swelling of extremities. **Pregnancy/breast-feeding precautions:** Inform prescriber if you are pregnant. Breast-feeding is not recommended.

Breast-Feeding Issues Discontinue nursing during dexrazoxane therapy.

Other Issues Follow guidelines for handling cytotoxic agents. If drug comes in contact with skin or mucosa, wash immediately with soap and water.

Additional Information Reimbursement Guarantee Program: 1-800-808-9111

Dextran (DEKS tran)

U.S. Brand Names Gentran®; LMD®

Synonyms Dextran 40; Dextran 70; Dextran, High Molecular Weight; Dextran, Low Molecular Weight

Pharmacologic Category Plasma Volume Expander

Medication Safety Issues
Sound-alike/look-alike issues:
Dextran may be confused with Dexatrim®, Dexedrine®

Pregnancy Risk Factor C

Lactation Excretion in breast milk unknown

Use Blood volume expander used in treatment of shock or impending shock when blood or blood products are not available; dextran 40 is also used as a priming fluid in cardiopulmonary bypass and for prophylaxis of venous thrombosis and pulmonary embolism in surgical procedures associated with a high risk of thromboembolic complications

Mechanism of Action/Effect Produces plasma volume expansion by virtue of its highly colloidal starch structure, similar to albumin

Contraindications Hypersensitivity to dextran or any component of the formulation; marked hemostatic defects (thrombocytopenia, hypofibrinogenemia) of all types including those caused by drugs; marked cardiac decompensation; renal disease with severe oliguria or anuria

Warnings/Precautions Hypersensitivity reactions have been reported (dextran 40 rarely causes a reaction), usually early in the infusion. Monitor closely during infusion initiation for signs or symptoms of a hypersensitivity reaction. Dextran 1 is indicated for prophylaxis of serious anaphylactic reactions to dextran infusions. Administration can cause fluid or solute overload. Use caution in patients with fluid overload. Use with caution in patients with active hemorrhage. Use caution in patients receiving corticosteroids. Renal failure has been reported. Fluid status including urine output should be monitored closely. Exercise care to prevent a depression of hematocrit <30% (can cause hemodilution). Observe for signs of bleeding.

Drug Interactions
Increased Effect/Toxicity: Dextran may enhance the anticoagulant effect of abciximab; avoid concurrent use.

Overdosage/Toxicology Symptoms of overdose include fluid overload, pulmonary edema, increased bleeding time, and decreased platelet function. Treatment is supportive. Blood products containing clotting factors may be necessary.

Pharmacodynamics/Kinetics
Onset of Action: Minutes to 1 hour (depending upon the molecular weight polysaccharide administered)
Excretion: Urine (~75%) within 24 hours

Available Dosage Forms
Infusion [premixed in D_5W; high molecular weight]: 6% Dextran 70 (500 mL)
Infusion [premixed in D_5W; low molecular weight] (Gentran®, LMD®): 10% Dextran 40 (500 mL)
Infusion [premixed in $D_{10}W$; high molecular weight]: 32% Dextran 70 (500 mL)
Infusion [premixed in NS; high molecular weight] (Gentran®): 6% Dextran 70 (500 mL)
Infusion [premixed in NS; low molecular weight] (Gentran®, LMD®): 10% Dextran (500 mL)

Dosing
Adults:
Volume expansion/shock:
Children: Total dose should not exceed 20 mL/kg during first 24 hours
Adults: 500-1000 mL at a rate of 20-40 mL/minute; maximum daily dose: 20 mL/kg for first 24 hours; 10 mL/kg/day thereafter; therapy should not be continued beyond 5 days

Pump prime (Dextran 40): Varies with the volume of the pump oxygenator; generally, the 10% solution is added in a dose of 1-2 g/kg

Prophylaxis of venous thrombosis/pulmonary embolism (Dextran 40): Begin during surgical procedure and give 50-100 g on the day of surgery; an additional 50 g (500 mL) should be administered every 2-3 days during the period of risk (up to 2 weeks postoperatively); usual maximum infusion rate for nonemergency use: 4 mL/minute

Elderly: Use with extreme caution in patients with renal or hepatic impairment.

Pediatrics: Treatment of shock or impending shock (when blood or blood products are not available): I.V. (requires an infusion pump): Children: Total dose should not be >20 mL/kg during first 24 hours

Renal Impairment: Use with extreme caution.

Hepatic Impairment: Use with extreme caution.

Administration
I.V.: For I.V. infusion only (use an infusion pump). Infuse initial 500 mL at a rate of 20-40 mL/minute if hypervolemic. Reduce rate for additional infusion to 4 mL/minute. **Observe patients closely for anaphylactic reaction.**

I.V. Detail: Have other means of maintaining circulation with epinephrine and diphenhydramine available should dextran therapy result in an anaphylactoid reaction.

pH: 3-7 (dextran 40 10% in dextrose 5%); 3.5-7 (dextran 40 10% in sodium chloride)

Stability
Compatibility: Dextran 40 is stable in D_5W, NS
Solution **incompatible** with other drugs
To prevent coagulation of blood, flush tubing well or change I.V. tubing before infusing blood after dextran.
Compatibility when admixed: Incompatible with amoxicillin

Storage: Store at room temperature. Discard partially used containers.

Laboratory Monitoring Hemoglobin and hematocrit, electrolytes, serum protein

Nursing Actions
Physical Assessment: Patient should be monitored closely for fluid overload, anaphylactoid reaction, and bleeding (eg, fluid status [oliguria/anuria], vital signs, and CVP) during first 15 minutes of first hour and periodically thereafter. Other means of maintaining circulation (eg, with epinephrine and diphenhydramine) should be available in the event of an anaphylactoid reaction. Patient teaching should be appropriate to patient condition.

Patient Education: Since this medication is generally used in emergency situations, patient education should be appropriate to patient condition.

Additional Information Dextran 40 is known as low molecular weight dextran (LMD®) and has an average molecular weight of 40,000; dextran 75 has an average molecular weight of 75,000. Dextran 70 has an average molecular weight of 70,000; sodium content of 500 mL is 77 mEq, with pH ranging from 3.0-7.0.

Dextran 1 (DEKS tran won)

U.S. Brand Names Promit®

Pharmacologic Category Plasma Volume Expander

Medication Safety Issues
Sound-alike/look-alike issues:
Dextran may be confused with Dexatrim®, Dexedrine®

Pregnancy Risk Factor C

Lactation Excretion in breast milk unknown

Use Prophylaxis of serious anaphylactic reactions to I.V. infusion of dextran
(Continued)

Dextran 1 *(Continued)*

Mechanism of Action/Effect Binds to dextran-reactive immunoglobulin without bridge formation and no formation of large immune complexes

Contraindications Hypersensitivity to dextrans or any component of the formulation; **dextran** contraindicated

Warnings/Precautions Severe hypotension and bradycardia can occur. If any reaction occurs, do not administer dextran. Mild dextran-induced anaphylactic reactions are not prevented.

Available Dosage Forms Injection, solution: 150 mg/mL (20 mL)

Dosing

Adults & Elderly: Prophylaxis of severe reactions to dextran infusions: I.V.: 20 mL 1-2 minutes before infusion of dextran. Administer 1 dose only prior to dextran. Give 1-2 minutes before I.V. infusion of dextran. Time between dextran 1 and dextran solution should not exceed 15 minutes.

Pediatrics: Prophylaxis of severe adverse reactions to dextran: I.V. (time between dextran 1 and dextran solution should not exceed 15 minutes): Children: 0.3 mL/kg 1-2 minutes before I.V. infusion of dextran

Administration

I.V.: Infuse over 1 minute.

Stability

Compatibility: Do not dilute or admix with dextrans.

Storage: Protect from freezing.

Nursing Actions

Physical Assessment: Dextran 1 is to be infused not more than 15 minutes before dextran for prophylaxis of serious anaphylactic reactions to dextran infusions. Monitor patient during infusion; hypotension and bradycardia may occur. If reaction occurs, dextran should not be given. Patient teaching should be appropriate to patient condition.

Patient Education: Since this medication is generally administered in emergency situations, patient education should be supportive and appropriate to patient condition.

Dextroamphetamine

(deks troe am FET a meen)

U.S. Brand Names Dexedrine®; Dextrostat®

Synonyms Dextroamphetamine Sulfate

Restrictions C-II

Pharmacologic Category Stimulant

Medication Safety Issues

Sound-alike/look-alike issues:

Dexedrine® may be confused with dextran, Excedrin®

Pregnancy Risk Factor C

Lactation Enters breast milk/contraindicated

Use Narcolepsy; attention-deficit/hyperactivity disorder (ADHD)

Unlabeled/Investigational Use Exogenous obesity; depression; abnormal behavioral syndrome in children (minimal brain dysfunction)

Mechanism of Action/Effect Blocks reuptake of dopamine and norepinephrine from the synapse, thus increases the amount of circulating dopamine and norepinephrine in cerebral cortex to reticular activating system; inhibits the action of monoamine oxidase and causes catecholamines to be released. Peripheral actions include elevated blood pressure, weak bronchodilator, and respiratory stimulant action.

Contraindications Hypersensitivity or idiosyncrasy to dextroamphetamine or other sympathomimetic amines. Patients with advanced arteriosclerosis, symptomatic cardiovascular disease, moderate to severe hypertension (stage II or III), hyperthyroidism, glaucoma, diabetes mellitus, agitated states, patients with a history of drug abuse, and during or within 14 days following MAO inhibitor therapy. Stimulant medications are contraindicated for use in children with attention-deficit/hyperactivity disorders and concomitant Tourette's syndrome or tics.

Warnings/Precautions Use with caution in patients with bipolar disorder, cardiovascular disease, seizure disorders, insomnia, porphyria, mild hypertension (stage I), or history of substance abuse. May exacerbate symptoms of behavior and thought disorder in psychotic patients. Potential for drug dependency exists - avoid abrupt discontinuation in patients who have received for prolonged periods. Use in weight reduction programs only when alternative therapy has been ineffective. Products may contain tartrazine - use with caution in potentially sensitive individuals. Stimulant use in children has been associated with growth suppression.

Drug Interactions

Cytochrome P450 Effect: Substrate of CYP2D6 (major)

Decreased Effect: Amphetamines inhibit the antihypertensive response to guanethidine and guanadrel. Urinary acidifiers decrease the half-life and duration of action of amphetamines.

Increased Effect/Toxicity: CYP2D6 inhibitors may increase the levels/effects of dextroamphetamine; example inhibitors include chlorpromazine, delavirdine, fluoxetine, miconazole, paroxetine, pergolide, quinidine, quinine, ritonavir, and ropinirole. Dextroamphetamine may precipitate hypertensive crisis or serotonin syndrome in patients receiving MAO inhibitors (selegiline >10 mg/day, isocarboxazid, phenelzine, tranylcypromine, furazolidone). Serotonin syndrome has also been associated with combinations of amphetamines and SSRIs; these combinations should be avoided. TCAs may enhance the effects of amphetamines. Large doses of antacids or urinary alkalinizers increase the half-life and duration of action of amphetamines. May precipitate arrhythmias in patients receiving general anesthetics.

Nutritional/Ethanol Interactions

Ethanol: Avoid ethanol (may increase CNS depression).

Food: Dextroamphetamine serum levels may be altered if taken with acidic food, juices, or vitamin C.

Herb/Nutraceutical: Avoid ephedra (may cause hypertension or arrhythmias).

Adverse Reactions Frequency not defined.

Cardiovascular: Palpitations, tachycardia, hypertension, cardiomyopathy

Central nervous system: Overstimulation, euphoria, dyskinesia, dysphoria, exacerbation of motor and phonic tics, restlessness, insomnia, dizziness, headache, psychosis, Tourette's syndrome

Dermatologic: Rash, urticaria

Endocrine & metabolic: Changes in libido

Gastrointestinal: Diarrhea, constipation, anorexia, weight loss, xerostomia, unpleasant taste

Genitourinary: Impotence

Neuromuscular & skeletal: Tremor

Overdosage/Toxicology Symptoms of overdose include restlessness, tremor, confusion, hallucinations, panic, dysrhythmias, nausea, and vomiting. There is no specific antidote for dextroamphetamine intoxication and treatment is primarily supportive. Hyperactivity and agitation usually respond to reduced sensory input; however, with extreme agitation, haloperidol (2-5 mg I.M. for adults) may be required.

Pharmacodynamics/Kinetics

Onset of Action: 1-1.5 hours

Time to Peak: Serum: T_{max}: Immediate release: 3 hours; sustained release: 8 hours

Half-Life Elimination: Adults: 10-13 hours

Metabolism: Hepatic via CYP monooxygenase and glucuronidation

Excretion: Urine (as unchanged drug and inactive metabolites)

Available Dosage Forms

Capsule, sustained release, as sulfate: 5 mg, 10 mg, 15 mg

Dexedrine® Spansule®: 5 mg, 10 mg, 15 mg

Tablet, as sulfate: 5 mg, 10 mg

Dexedrine®: 5 mg [contains tartrazine]

Dextrostat®: 5 mg, 10 mg [contains tartrazine]

Dosing

Adults:

Narcolepsy: Oral: Initial: 10 mg/day, may increase at 10 mg increments in weekly intervals until side effects appear; maximum: 60 mg/day

Exogenous obesity (short-term adjunct): Oral: 5-30 mg/day in divided doses of 5-10 mg 30-60 minutes before meals

Elderly: Refer to adult dosing; start at lowest dose. Use with caution.

Pediatrics:

Narcolepsy: Oral: Children 6-12 years: Initial: 5 mg/day, may increase at 5 mg increments in weekly intervals until side effects appear; maximum dose: 60 mg/day

Attention-deficit/hyperactivity disorder (ADHD): Oral:

Children 3-5 years: Initial: 2.5 mg/day given every morning; increase by 2.5 mg/day in weekly intervals until optimal response is obtained, usual range: 0.1-0.5 mg/kg/dose every morning with maximum of 40 mg/day

Children ≥6 years: 5 mg once or twice daily; increase in increments of 5 mg/day at weekly intervals until optimal response is reached, usual range: 0.1-0.5 mg/kg/dose every morning (5-20 mg/day) with maximum of 40 mg/day

Administration

Oral: Do not crush sustained release drug product. Administer as single dose in morning or as divided doses with breakfast and lunch. Should be administered 30 minutes before meals and at least 6 hours before bedtime.

Stability

Storage: Protect from light.

Nursing Actions

Physical Assessment: Assess effectiveness and interactions of other medications patient may be taking. Assess for history of psychopathology, homicidal or suicidal tendencies, or addiction; long-term use can result in dependence, abuse, or tolerance. Periodically evaluate the need for continued use. Monitor therapeutic response, blood pressure, vital signs, and adverse reactions at start of therapy, when changing dosage, and at regular intervals during therapy Monitor serum glucose closely in patients with diabetes (amphetamines may alter antidiabetic requirements). Taper dosage slowly when discontinuing. Assess knowledge/teach patient appropriate use, possible side effects, and symptoms to report.

Patient Education: Take exactly as directed; do not increase dose or frequency without consulting prescriber. Drug may cause physical and/or psychological dependence. Take early in day to avoid sleep disturbance, 30 minutes before meals. Avoid alcohol, caffeine, or OTC medications that act as stimulants. You may experience restlessness, false sense of euphoria, or impaired judgment (use caution when driving or engaging in tasks requiring alertness until response to drug is known); dry mouth (frequent mouth care, sucking lozenges, or chewing gum may help); nausea or vomiting (small frequent meals, frequent mouth care may help); constipation (increased exercise, fluids, fruit, or fiber may help); diarrhea (buttermilk, boiled milk, or yogurt may help); or altered libido (reversible). Patients with diabetes need to monitor serum glucose closely (may alter antidiabetic medication requirements). Report chest pain, palpitations, or irregular heartbeat; extreme fatigue or depression; CNS changes (aggressiveness, restlessness, euphoria, sleep disturbances); severe unremitting abdominal distress or cramping; blackened stool; changes in sexual activity; or blurred vision. **Pregnancy/breast-feeding precautions:** Inform prescriber if you are or intend to become pregnant. Do not breast-feed.

Dietary Considerations Should be taken 30 minutes before meals and at least 6 hours before bedtime.

Dextroamphetamine and Amphetamine
(deks troe am FET a meen & am FET a meen)

U.S. Brand Names Adderall®; Adderall XR®

Synonyms Amphetamine and Dextroamphetamine

Restrictions C-II

Pharmacologic Category Stimulant

Medication Safety Issues

Sound-alike/look-alike issues:

Adderall® may be confused with Inderal®

Pregnancy Risk Factor C

Lactation Enters breast milk/contraindicated

Use Attention-deficit/hyperactivity disorder (ADHD); narcolepsy

Mechanism of Action/Effect Blocks reuptake of dopamine and norepinephrine from the synapse, thus increases the amount of circulating dopamine and norepinephrine in cerebral cortex to reticular activating system; inhibits the action of monoamine oxidase and causes catecholamines to be released. Peripheral actions include elevation of blood pressure, weak bronchodilation, and respiratory stimulation.

Contraindications Hypersensitivity to dextroamphetamine, amphetamine, or any component of the formulation; advanced arteriosclerosis; symptomatic cardiovascular disease; moderate to severe hypertension; hyperthyroidism; hypersensitivity or idiosyncrasy to the sympathomimetic amines; glaucoma; agitated states; patients with a history of drug abuse; with or within 14 days following MAO inhibitor (hypertensive crisis)

Warnings/Precautions Amphetamine has a high abuse potential; prolonged use may lead to dependency. Avoid use in patients with structural cardiac abnormalities; has been associated with sudden death. Use caution in patients with hypertension (including mildly hypertensive patients); sustained increases in blood pressure may require dosage reduction or antihypertensive therapy. Amphetamines may impair the ability to engage in potentially hazardous activities. In psychotic children, amphetamines may exacerbate symptoms of behavior disturbance and thought disorder. Stimulants may unmask tics in individuals with coexisting Tourette's syndrome. Appetite suppression may occur; monitor weight during therapy, particularly in children. Not recommended for children <3 years of age. Avoid abrupt discontinuation.

Drug Interactions

Cytochrome P450 Effect:

Dextroamphetamine: **Substrate** of CYP2D6 (major)

Amphetamine: **Substrate** of CYP2D6 (major); **Inhibits** CYP2D6 (weak)

Decreased Effect: Amphetamines inhibit the antihypertensive response to guanethidine and guanadrel. Urinary acidifiers decrease the half-life and duration of action of amphetamines. Efficacy of amphetamines may be decreased by antipsychotics.

Increased Effect/Toxicity: CYP2D6 inhibitors may increase the levels/effects of amphetamine and dextroamphetamine; example inhibitors include chlorpromazine, delavirdine, fluoxetine, miconazole, paroxetine, pergolide, quinidine, quinine, ritonavir, and ropinirole. Dextroamphetamine and amphetamine may precipitate hypertensive crisis or serotonin
(Continued)

Dextroamphetamine and Amphetamine
(Continued)

syndrome in patients receiving MAO inhibitors (selegiline >10 mg/day, isocarboxazid, phenelzine, tranylcypromine, furazolidone). Serotonin syndrome has also been associated with combinations of amphetamines and SSRIs; these combinations should be avoided. TCAs may enhance the effects of amphetamines, potentially leading to hypertensive crisis. Large doses of antacids or urinary alkalinizers increase the half-life and duration of action of amphetamines. May precipitate arrhythmias in patients receiving general anesthetics.

Nutritional/Ethanol Interactions
Ethanol: Avoid ethanol (may increase CNS depression).
Food: Dextroamphetamine serum levels may be altered if taken with acidic food, juices, or vitamin C. Avoid caffeine.
Herb/Nutraceutical: Avoid ephedra (may cause hypertension or arrhythmias).

Lab Interactions Increased corticosteroid levels (greatest in evening); may interfere with urinary steroid testing

Adverse Reactions
As reported with Adderall XR®:
>10%:
Central nervous system: Insomnia (12% to 27%), headache (up to 26% in adults)
Gastrointestinal: Appetite decreased (22% to 36%), abdominal pain (11% to 14%), dry mouth (2% to 35%), weight loss (4% to 11%)
1% to 10%:
Cardiovascular: Palpitation (2% to 4%), tachycardia (up to 6% in adults)
Central nervous system: Emotional lability (2% to 9%), agitation (up to 8% in adults), anxiety (8%), dizziness (2% to 7%), nervousness (6%), fever (5%), somnolence (2% to 4%)
Dermatologic: Photosensitization (2% to 4%)
Endocrine & metabolic: Dysmenorrhea (2% to 4%), impotence (2% to 4%), libido decreased (2% to 4%)
Gastrointestinal: Nausea (2% to 8%), vomiting (2% to 7%), diarrhea (2% to 6%), constipation (2% to 4%), dyspepsia (2% to 4%)
Neuromuscular & skeletal: Twitching (2% to 4%), weakness (2% to 6%)
Respiratory: Dyspnea (2% to 4%)
Miscellaneous: Diaphoresis (2% to 4%), infection (2% to 4%), speech disorder (2% to 4%)
<1% (Limited to important or life-threatening): MI, seizure, stroke, sudden death

Adverse reactions reported with other amphetamines include: Cardiomyopathy, dyskinesia, dysphoria, euphoria, exacerbation of motor and phonic tics, exacerbation of Tourette's syndrome, headache, hypertension, overstimulation, palpitation, psychosis, rash, restlessness, tachycardia, tremor, urticaria

Overdosage/Toxicology Manifestations of overdose vary widely. Symptoms of central stimulation are usually followed by fatigue and depression. Cardiovascular and gastrointestinal symptoms are also reported. Treatment is symptomatic and supportive. Chlorpromazine may be used to antagonize CNS effects.

Pharmacodynamics/Kinetics
Onset of Action: 30-60 minutes
Duration of Action: 4-6 hours
Time to Peak: T_{max}: Adderall®: 3 hours; Adderall XR®: 7 hours
Half-Life Elimination:
Children 6-12 years: d-amphetamine: 9 hours; l-amphetamine: 11 hours
Adolescents 13-17 years: d-amphetamine: 11 hours; l-amphetamine: 13-14 hours
Adults: d-amphetamine: 10 hours; l-amphetamine: 13 hours

Metabolism: Hepatic via cytochrome P450 monooxygenase and glucuronidation
Excretion: Urine (highly dependent on urinary pH); 70% of a single dose is eliminated within 24 hours; excreted as unchanged amphetamine (30%, may range from ~1% in alkaline urine to ~75% in acidic urine), benzoic acid, hydroxyamphetamine, hippuric acid, norephedrine, and p-hydroxynorephedrine
Pharmacokinetic Note See Dextroamphetamine monograph.

Available Dosage Forms
Capsule, extended release (Adderall XR®):
5 mg [dextroamphetamine sulfate 1.25 mg, dextroamphetamine saccharate 1.25 mg, amphetamine aspartate monohydrate 1.25 mg, amphetamine sulfate 1.25 mg (equivalent to amphetamine base 3.1 mg)]
10 mg [dextroamphetamine sulfate 2.5 mg, dextroamphetamine saccharate 2.5 mg, amphetamine aspartate monohydrate 2.5 mg, amphetamine sulfate 2.5 mg (equivalent to amphetamine base 6.3 mg)]
15 mg [dextroamphetamine sulfate 3.75 mg, dextroamphetamine saccharate 3.75 mg, amphetamine aspartate monohydrate 3.75 mg, amphetamine sulfate 3.75 mg (equivalent to amphetamine base 9.4 mg)]
20 mg [dextroamphetamine sulfate 5 mg, dextroamphetamine saccharate 5 mg, amphetamine aspartate monohydrate 5 mg, amphetamine sulfate 5 mg (equivalent to amphetamine base 12.5 mg)]
25 mg [dextroamphetamine sulfate 6.25 mg, dextroamphetamine saccharate 6.25 mg, amphetamine aspartate monohydrate 6.25 mg, amphetamine sulfate 6.25 mg (equivalent to amphetamine base 15.6 mg)]
30 mg [dextroamphetamine sulfate 7.5 mg, dextroamphetamine saccharate 7.5 mg, amphetamine aspartate monohydrate 7.5 mg, amphetamine sulfate 7.5 mg (equivalent to amphetamine base 18.8 mg)]
Tablet (Adderall®):
5 mg [dextroamphetamine sulfate 1.25 mg, dextroamphetamine saccharate 1.25 mg, amphetamine aspartate 1.25 mg, amphetamine sulfate 1.25 mg (equivalent to amphetamine base 3.13 mg)]
7.5 mg [dextroamphetamine 1.875 mg, dextroamphetamine saccharate 1.875 mg, amphetamine aspartate 1.875 mg, amphetamine sulfate 1.875 mg (equivalent to amphetamine base 4.7 mg)]
10 mg [dextroamphetamine sulfate 2.5 mg, dextroamphetamine saccharate 2.5 mg, amphetamine aspartate 2.5 mg, amphetamine sulfate 2.5 mg (equivalent to amphetamine base 6.3 mg)]
12.5 mg [dextroamphetamine sulfate 3.125 mg, dextroamphetamine saccharate 3.125 mg, amphetamine aspartate 3.125 mg, amphetamine sulfate 3.125 mg (equivalent to amphetamine base 7.8 mg)]
15 mg [dextroamphetamine sulfate 3.75 mg, dextroamphetamine saccharate 3.75 mg, amphetamine aspartate 3.75 mg, amphetamine sulfate 3.75 mg (equivalent to amphetamine base 9.4 mg)]
20 mg [dextroamphetamine sulfate 5 mg, dextroamphetamine saccharate 5 mg, amphetamine aspartate 5 mg, amphetamine sulfate 5 mg (equivalent to amphetamine base 12.6 mg)]
30 mg [dextroamphetamine sulfate 7.5 mg, dextroamphetamine saccharate 7.5 mg, amphetamine aspartate 7.5 mg, amphetamine sulfate 7.5 mg (equivalent to amphetamine base 18.8 mg)]

Dosing
Adults & Elderly: Note: Use lowest effective individualized dose; administer first dose as soon as awake; use intervals of 4-6 hours between additional doses.
ADHD: Oral:
Adderall®: Initial: 5 mg once or twice daily; increase daily dose in 5 mg increments at weekly intervals until optimal response is obtained; usual

maximum dose: 40 mg/day given in 1-3 divided doses per day.

Adderall XR®: Initial: 20 mg once daily in the morning; higher doses (up to 60 mg once daily) have been evaluated; however, there is not adequate evidence that higher doses afforded additional benefit

Narcolepsy: *Adderall®*: Oral: Initial: 10 mg/day; increase daily dose in 10 mg increments at weekly intervals until optimal response is obtained; maximum dose: 60 mg/day given in 1-3 divided doses per day.

Pediatrics:

Note: Use lowest effective individualized dose; administer first dose as soon as awake

ADHD: Oral:

Children: <3 years: Not recommended.

Children: 3-5 years (Adderall®): Initial 2.5 mg/day given every morning; increase daily dose in 2.5 mg increments at weekly intervals until optimal response is obtained; maximum dose: 40 mg/day given in 1-3 divided doses per day. Use intervals of 4-6 hours between additional doses.

Children: ≥6 years:

Adderall®: Initial: 5 mg once or twice daily; increase daily dose in 5 mg increments at weekly intervals until optimal response is obtained; usual maximum dose: 40 mg/day given in 1-3 divided doses per day. Use intervals of 4-6 hours between additional doses.

Adderall XR®: 5-10 mg once daily in the morning; if needed, may increase daily dose in 5-10 mg increments at weekly intervals (maximum dose: 30 mg/day)

Adolescents 13-17 years (Adderall XR®): 10 mg once daily in the morning ; maybe increased to 20 mg/day after 1 week if symptoms are not controlled; higher doses (up to 60 mg)/day have been evaluated; however, there is not adequate evidence that higher doses afforded additional benefit.

Narcolepsy: *Adderall®*: Oral:

Children: 6-12 years: Initial: 5 mg/day; increase daily dose in 5 mg increments at weekly intervals until optimal response is obtained; maximum dose: 60 mg/day given in 1-3 divided doses per day.

Children >12 years: Refer to adult dosing.

Administration

Oral:

Adderall®: To avoid insomnia, last daily dose should be administered no less than 6 hours before retiring.

Adderall XR®: Should be given by noon. Capsule may be swallowed whole or it may be opened and the contents sprinkled on applesauce. Applesauce should be consumed immediately without chewing. Do not divide the contents of the capsule.

Stability

Storage: Store at controlled room temperature of 15°C to 30°C (59°F to 86°F)

Nursing Actions

Physical Assessment: Assess effectiveness and interactions of other medications patient may be taking. Assess for history of psychopathology, homicidal or suicidal tendencies, or addiction; long-term use can result in dependence, abuse, or tolerance. Periodically evaluate the need for continued use. Monitor therapeutic response, vital signs, and adverse reactions at start of therapy, when changing dosage, and at regular intervals during therapy. Monitor serum glucose closely in patients with diabetes (amphetamines may alter antidiabetic requirements). May cause weight loss. Monitor weight periodically, especially in children. Taper dosage slowly when discontinuing. Assess knowledge/teach patient appropriate use, possible side effects, and symptoms to report.

Patient Education: Take exactly as directed; do not increase dose or frequency without consulting prescriber. Drug may cause physical and/or psychological dependence. Take early in the day to avoid sleep disturbance. If you miss a dose, take it as soon as you can. If it is almost time for your next dose, do not take double dose. Avoid alcohol, caffeine, or OTC medications that act as stimulants. You may experience restlessness, headaches, false sense of euphoria, or impaired judgment (use caution when driving or engaging in tasks requiring alertness until response to drug is known); dry mouth (frequent mouth care, sucking lozenges, or chewing gum may help); decreased appetite; nausea or vomiting (small frequent meals, frequent mouth care may help); constipation (increased exercise, fluids, fruit, or fiber may help); diarrhea (buttermilk, boiled milk, or yogurt may help); altered libido (reversible); or altered acuity of taste or smell. Patients with diabetes need to monitor serum glucose closely (may alter antidiabetic medication requirements). Report increased respirations, chest pain, palpitations, or irregular heartbeat; extreme fatigue or depression; CNS changes (aggressiveness, restlessness, euphoria, sleep disturbances); severe unremitting abdominal distress or cramping; blackened stool; changes in sexual activity; or blurred vision. **Pregnancy/breast-feeding precautions:** Inform prescriber if you are pregnant. Do not breast-feed.

Pregnancy Issues Use during pregnancy may lead to increased risk of premature delivery and low birth weight. Infants may experience symptoms of withdrawal. Teratogenic effects were reported when taken during the 1st trimester.

Additional Information Treatment of ADHD may include "drug holidays" or periodic discontinuation of medication in order to assess the patient's requirments, decrease tolerance, and limit suppression of linear growth and weight; the combination of equal parts of *d*, *l*-amphetamine aspartate, *d*, *l*-amphetamine sulfate, dextroamphetamine saccharate and dextroamphetamine sulfate results in a 75:25 ratio of the dextro and levo isomers of amphetamine.

The duration of action of Adderall® is longer than methylphenidate; behavioral effects of a single morning dose of Adderall® may last throughout the school day; a single morning dose of Adderall® has been shown in several studies to be as effective as twice daily dosing of methylphenidate for the treatment of ADHD (see Pelham et al, *Pediatrics*, 1999, 104(6):1300-11; Manos 1999; Pliszka 2000).

Related Information

Dextroamphetamine *on page 352*

Diazepam (dye AZ e pam)

U.S. Brand Names Diastat®; Diastat® AcuDial™; Diazepam Intensol®; Valium®

Restrictions C-IV

Pharmacologic Category Benzodiazepine

Medication Safety Issues

Sound-alike/look-alike issues:

Diazepam may be confused with diazoxide, Ditropan®, lorazepam

Valium® may be confused with Valcyte™

Pregnancy Risk Factor D

Lactation Enters breast milk/contraindicated (AAP rates "of concern")

(Continued)

Diazepam *(Continued)*

Use Management of anxiety disorders, ethanol withdrawal symptoms; skeletal muscle relaxant; treatment of convulsive disorders

Orphan drug: Viscous solution for rectal administration: Management of selected, refractory epilepsy patients on stable regimens of antiepileptic drugs (AEDs) requiring intermittent use of diazepam to control episodes of increased seizure activity

Unlabeled/Investigational Use Panic disorders; preoperative sedation, light anesthesia, amnesia

Mechanism of Action/Effect Binds to stereospecific benzodiazepine receptors on the postsynaptic GABA neuron at several sites within the central nervous system, including the limbic system, reticular formation. Enhancement of the inhibitory effect of GABA on neuronal excitability results by increased neuronal membrane permeability to chloride ions. This shift in chloride ions results in hyperpolarization (a less excitable state) and stabilization.

Contraindications Hypersensitivity to diazepam or any component of the formulation (cross-sensitivity with other benzodiazepines may exist); narrow-angle glaucoma; not for use in children <6 months of age (oral, rectal gel) or <30 days of age (parenteral); pregnancy

Warnings/Precautions Diazepam has been associated with increasing the frequency of grand mal seizures. Withdrawal has also been associated with an increase in the seizure frequency. Use with caution with drugs which may decrease diazepam metabolism. Use with caution in elderly or debilitated patients, patients with hepatic disease (including alcoholics), respiratory disease, impaired gag reflex, or renal impairment. Active metabolites with extended half-lives may lead to delayed accumulation and adverse effects.

Acute hypotension, muscle weakness, apnea, and cardiac arrest have occurred with parenteral administration. Acute effects may be more prevalent in patients receiving concurrent barbiturates, narcotics, or ethanol. Appropriate resuscitative equipment and qualified personnel should be available during administration and monitoring. Avoid use of the injection in patients with shock, coma, or acute ethanol intoxication. Intra-arterial injection or extravasation of the parenteral formulation should be avoided. Parenteral formulation contains propylene glycol, which has been associated with toxicity when administered in high dosages. Administration of rectal gel should only be performed by individuals trained to recognize characteristic seizure activity and monitor response.

Causes CNS depression (dose-related) resulting in sedation, dizziness, confusion, or ataxia which may impair physical and mental capabilities. Use with caution in patients receiving other CNS depressants or psychoactive agents. Effects with other sedative drugs or ethanol may be potentiated. The dosage of narcotics should be reduced by approximately 1/3 when diazepam is added. Benzodiazepines have been associated with falls and traumatic injury and should be used with extreme caution in patients who are at risk of these events (especially the elderly).

Use caution in patients with depression, particularly if suicidal risk may be present, or in patients with a history of drug dependence. Benzodiazepines have been associated with dependence and acute withdrawal symptoms on discontinuation or reduction in dose. Acute withdrawal, including seizures, may be precipitated in patients after administration of flumazenil to patients receiving long-term benzodiazepine therapy.

Diazepam has been associated with anterograde amnesia. Paradoxical reactions, including hyperactive or aggressive behavior, have been reported with benzodiazepines, particularly in adolescent/pediatric or psychiatric patients. Does not have analgesic, antidepressant, or antipsychotic properties.

Drug Interactions

Cytochrome P450 Effect: Substrate of CYP1A2 (minor), 2B6 (minor), 2C8/9 (minor), 2C19 (major), 3A4 (major); **Inhibits** CYP2C19 (weak), 3A4 (weak)

Decreased Effect: CYP2C19 inducers may decrease the levels/effects of diazepam; example inducers include aminoglutethimide, carbamazepine, phenytoin, and rifampin. CYP3A4 inducers may decrease the levels/effects of diazepam; example inducers include aminoglutethimide, carbamazepine, nafcillin, nevirapine, phenobarbital, phenytoin, and rifamycins.

Increased Effect/Toxicity: Diazepam potentiates the CNS depressant effects of narcotic analgesics, barbiturates, phenothiazines, ethanol, antihistamines, MAO inhibitors, sedative-hypnotics, and cyclic antidepressants. CYP2C19 inhibitors may increase the levels/effects of diazepam; example inhibitors include delavirdine, fluconazole, fluvoxamine, gemfibrozil, isoniazid, omeprazole, and ticlopidine. CYP3A4 inhibitors may increase the levels/effects of diazepam; example inhibitors include azole antifungals, clarithromycin, diclofenac, doxycycline, erythromycin, imatinib, isoniazid, nefazodone, nicardipine, propofol, protease inhibitors, quinidine, telithromycin, and verapamil.

Nutritional/Ethanol Interactions

Ethanol: Avoid ethanol (may increase CNS depression).

Food: Diazepam serum levels may be increased if taken with food. Diazepam effect/toxicity may be increased by grapefruit juice; avoid concurrent use.

Herb/Nutraceutical: St John's wort may decrease diazepam levels. Avoid valerian, St John's wort, kava kava, gotu kola (may increase CNS depression).

Lab Interactions False-negative urinary glucose determinations when using Clinistix® or Diastix®

Adverse Reactions Frequency not defined. Adverse reactions may vary by route of administration.

Cardiovascular: Hypotension, vasodilatation

Central nervous system: Agitation, amnesia, anxiety, ataxia, confusion, depression, dizziness, drowsiness, emotional lability, euphoria, fatigue, headache, incoordination, insomnia, memory impairment, paradoxical excitement or rage, seizure, slurred speech, somnolence, vertigo

Dermatologic: Rash

Endocrine & metabolic: Changes in libido

Gastrointestinal: Changes in salivation, constipation, diarrhea, nausea

Genitourinary: Incontinence, urinary retention

Hepatic: Jaundice

Local: Phlebitis, pain with injection

Neuromuscular & skeletal: Dysarthria, tremor, weakness

Ocular: Blurred vision, diplopia

Respiratory: Apnea, asthma, decrease in respiratory rate

Overdosage/Toxicology Symptoms of overdose include somnolence, confusion, coma, hypoactive reflexes, dyspnea, hypotension, slurred speech, or impaired coordination. Treatment for benzodiazepine overdose is supportive. Flumazenil has been shown to selectively block the binding of benzodiazepines to CNS receptors, resulting in a reversal of benzodiazepine-induced CNS depression, but not respiratory depression.

Pharmacodynamics/Kinetics

Onset of Action: I.V.: Status epilepticus: Almost immediate

Duration of Action: I.V.: Status epilepticus: 20-30 minutes

Protein Binding: 98%

Half-Life Elimination: Parent drug: Adults: 20-50 hours; increased half-life in neonates, elderly, and those with severe hepatic disorders; Active major metabolite (desmethyldiazepam): 50-100 hours; may be prolonged in neonates

Metabolism: Hepatic

Available Dosage Forms

Gel, rectal:

Diastat®: Pediatric rectal tip [4.4 cm]: 5 mg/mL (2.5 mg, 5 mg) [contains ethyl alcohol 10%, sodium benzoate, benzyl alcohol 1.5%; twin pack]

Diastat® AcuDial™ delivery system:

10 mg: Pediatric/adult rectal tip [4.4 cm]: 5 mg/mL (delivers set doses of 5 mg, 7.5 mg, and 10 mg) [contains ethyl alcohol 10%, sodium benzoate, benzyl alcohol 1.5%; twin pack]

20 mg: Adult rectal tip [6 cm]: 5 mg/mL (delivers set doses of 10 mg, 12.5 mg, 15 mg, 17.5 mg, and 20 mg) [contains ethyl alcohol 10%, sodium benzoate, benzyl alcohol 1.5%; twin pack]

Injection, solution: 5 mg/mL (2 mL, 10 mL) [may contain benzyl alcohol, sodium benzoate, benzoic acid]

Solution, oral: 5 mg/5 mL (5 mL, 500 mL) [winter-green-spice flavor]

Solution, oral concentrate (Diazepam Intensol®): 5 mg/mL (30 mL)

Tablet (Valium®): 2 mg, 5 mg, 10 mg

Dosing

Adults: Note: Oral absorption is more reliable than I.M.

Anticonvulsant (acute treatment): Rectal gel: 0.2 mg/kg. **Note:** Dosage should be rounded upward to the next available dose, 2.5, 5, 10, 12.5, 15, 17.5, and 20 mg/dose; dose may be repeated in 4-12 hours if needed; do not use for more than 5 episodes per month or more than one episode every 5 days.

Anxiety/sedation/skeletal muscle relaxation:

Oral: 2-10 mg 2-4 times/day

I.M., I.V.: 2-10 mg, may repeat in 3-4 hours if needed

Sedation in the ICU patient: I.V.: 0.03-0.1 mg/kg every 30 minutes to 6 hours

Status epilepticus: I.V.: 5-10 mg every 10-20 minutes, up to 30 mg in an 8-hour period; may repeat in 2-4 hours if necessary

Rapid tranquilization of agitated patient (administer every 30-60 minutes): Oral: 5-10 mg; average total dose for tranquilization: 20-60 mg

Elderly: Oral absorption is more reliable than I.M..

Oral: Initial:

Anxiety: 1-2 mg 1-2 times/day; increase gradually as needed, rarely need to use >10 mg/day.

Skeletal muscle relaxant: 2-5 mg 2-4 times/day

Rectal gel: Due to the increased half-life in elderly and debilitated patients, consider reducing dose.

Pediatrics:

Conscious sedation for procedures:

Oral:

Children: 0.2-0.3 mg/kg (maximum dose: 10 mg) 45-60 minutes prior to procedure

Adolescents: 10 mg

I.V.: Adolescents: 5 mg; may repeat with 2.5 mg if needed

Febrile seizure prophylaxis: Oral: Children: 1 mg/kg/day divided every 8 hours; initiate therapy at first sign of fever and continue for 24 hours after fever is gone

Sedation or muscle relaxation or anxiety:

Oral: Children: 0.12-0.8 mg/kg/day in divided doses every 6-8 hours

I.M., I.V.: Children: 0.04-0.3 mg/kg/dose every 2-4 hours to a maximum of 0.6 mg/kg within an 8-hour period if needed

Status epilepticus:

I.V.:

Infants >30 days and Children <5 years: 0.05-0.3 mg/kg/dose given over 3-5 minutes, every 15-30 minutes to a maximum total dose of 5 mg or 0.2-0.5 mg/dose every 2-5 minutes to a

maximum total dose of 5 mg; repeat in 2-4 hours as needed

Children ≥5 years: 0.05-0.3 mg/kg/dose given over 3-5 minutes, every 15-30 minutes to a maximum total dose of 10 mg **or** 1 mg/dose every 2-5 minutes to a maximum of 10 mg; repeat in 2-4 hours as needed

Rectal: 0.5 mg/kg/dose then 0.25 mg/kg/dose in 10 minutes if needed

Anticonvulsant (acute treatment): Rectal gel:

Infants <6 months: Not recommended

Children <2 years: Safety and efficacy have not been studied

Children 2-5 years: 0.5 mg/kg

Children 6-11 years: 0.3 mg/kg

Children ≥12 years: Refer to adult dosing.

Note: Dosage should be rounded upward to the next available dose, 2.5, 5, 10, 12.5, 15, 17.5, and 20 mg/dose; dose may be repeated in 4-12 hours if needed; do not use for more than 5 episodes per month or more than one episode every 5 days.

Muscle spasm associated with tetanus: I.V., I.M.:

Infants >30 days: 1-2 mg/dose every 3-4 hours as needed

Children ≥5 years: 5-10 mg/dose every 3-4 hours as needed

Renal Impairment: Hemodialysis effects: Not dialyzable (0% to 5%); supplemental dose is **not** necessary.

Hepatic Impairment: Reduce dose by 50% in cirrhosis and avoid in severe/acute liver disease.

Administration

Oral: Intensol® should be diluted before use.

I.V.: Continuous infusion is not recommended because of precipitation in I.V. fluids and absorption of drug into infusion bags and tubing. In children, do not exceed 1-2 mg/minute IVP; in adults 5 mg/minute.

I.V. Detail: pH: 6.2-6.9

Other: Rectal gel: Patient should be positioned on side (facing person responsible for monitoring), with top leg bent forward. Insert rectal tip (lubricated) into rectum and push in plunger gently over 3 seconds. Remove tip of rectal syringe after 3 additional seconds. Buttocks should be held together for 3 seconds after removal. Dispose of syringe appropriately.

Stability

Reconstitution: Most stable at pH 4-8, hydrolysis occurs at pH <3.

Compatibility: Do not mix I.V. product with other medications.

Y-site administration: Incompatible with amphotericin B cholesteryl sulfate complex, atracurium, cefepime, diltiazem, fluconazole, foscarnet, gatifloxacin, heparin, heparin with hydrocortisone sodium succinate, hydromorphone, linezolid, meropenem, pancuronium, potassium chloride, propofol, vecuronium, vitamin B complex with C

Compatibility in syringe: Incompatible with doxapram, glycopyrrolate, heparin, hydromorphone, nalbuphine, sufentanil

Compatibility when admixed: Incompatible with bleomycin, buprenorphine, dobutamine, doxorubicin, floxacillin, fluorouracil, furosemide

Storage:

Protect parenteral dosage form from light; potency is retained for up to 3 months when kept at room temperature.

Rectal gel: Store at 25°C (77°F); excursion permitted to 15°C to 30°C (59°F to 86°F).

Nursing Actions

Physical Assessment: Assess effectiveness and interactions of other medications patient may be taking. Assess for history of addiction; long-term use can result in dependence, abuse, or tolerance; periodically evaluate need for continued use. Monitor

(Continued)

Diazepam (Continued)

blood pressure, CNS status. For inpatient use, institute safety measures and monitor effectiveness and adverse reactions. For outpatients, monitor therapeutic effectiveness and adverse reactions at beginning of therapy and periodically with long-term use. Taper dosage slowly when discontinuing. Assess knowledge/teach patient seizure precautions (if administered for seizures), appropriate use, interventions to reduce side effects, and adverse symptoms to report..

Patient Education: Take exactly as directed; do not increase dose or frequency. Drug may cause physical and/or psychological dependence. While using this medication, do not use alcohol and other prescription or OTC medications (especially pain medications, sedatives, antihistamines, or hypnotics) without consulting prescriber. Maintain adequate hydration (2-3 L/day of fluids) unless instructed to restrict fluid intake. You may experience drowsiness, dizziness, or blurred vision (use caution when driving or engaging in tasks requiring alertness until response to drug is known); nausea, vomiting, loss of appetite, or dry mouth (small frequent meals, frequent mouth care, chewing gum, or sucking lozenges may help); constipation (increased exercise, fluids, fruit, or fiber may help). If medication is used to control seizures, wear identification that you are taking an antiepileptic medication. Report CNS changes (confusion, depression, increased sedation, excitation, headache, agitation, insomnia or nightmares, dizziness, fatigue, or impaired coordination) or changes in cognition; respiratory difficulty or shortness of breath; changes in urinary pattern; changes in sexual activity; muscle cramping, weakness, tremors, or rigidity; ringing in ears or visual disturbances; excessive perspiration; excessive GI symptoms (cramping, constipation, vomiting, anorexia); or worsening of seizure activity or loss of seizure control. **Pregnancy/breast-feeding precautions:** Do not get pregnant while taking this medication; use appropriate contraceptive measures. Do not breast-feed.

Geriatric Considerations Due to its long-acting metabolite, diazepam is not considered a drug of choice in the elderly. Long-acting benzodiazepines have been associated with falls in the elderly. Interpretive guidelines from the Centers for Medicare and Medicaid Services (CMS) strongly discourage the use of this agent in residents of long-term care facilities.

Breast-Feeding Issues Clinical effects on the infant include sedation; AAP reports that USE MAY BE OF CONCERN.

Pregnancy Issues Benzodiazepines cross the placenta. The association between benzodiazepine exposure and malformations remains controversial. A number of types of malformation have been reported (oral cleft, inguinal hernia, cardiac defects, spina bifida, dysmorphic facial features, skeletal defects); however, confounding factors make a clear association difficult. Overall, the risk to the fetus may be low. Nonteratogenic effects (including neonatal flaccidity, respiratory and feeding problems, and withdrawal symptoms) during the postnatal period have also been reported with benzodiazepine use.

Additional Information Diazepam does not have any analgesic effects.

Diastat®AcuDial™: When dispensing, consult package information for directions on setting patient's dose; confirm green "ready" band is visible prior to dispensing product.

Related Information

Anxiolytic / Hypnotic Use in Long-Term Care Facilities *on page 1418*
Compatibility of Drugs *on page 1370*
Federal OBRA Regulations Recommended Maximum Doses *on page 1421*

Diclofenac (dye KLOE fen ak)

U.S. Brand Names Cataflam®; Solaraze®; Voltaren®; Voltaren Ophthalmic®; Voltaren®-XR

Synonyms Diclofenac Potassium; Diclofenac Sodium

Restrictions A medication guide should be dispensed with each prescription. A template for the required MedGuide can be found on the FDA website at http://www.fda.gov/medwatch/SAFETY/2005/safety05.htm#NSAID

Pharmacologic Category Nonsteroidal Anti-inflammatory Drug (NSAID); Nonsteroidal Anti-inflammatory Drug (NSAID), Ophthalmic; Nonsteroidal Anti-inflammatory Drug (NSAID), Oral

Medication Safety Issues
Sound-alike/look-alike issues:
Diclofenac may be confused with Diflucan®, Duphalac®
Cataflam® may be confused with Catapres®
Voltaren® may be confused with tramadol, Ultram®, Verelan®

Pregnancy Risk Factor B (topical); C (oral)/D (3rd trimester)

Lactation Excretion in breast milk unknown/not recommended

Use
Immediate release: Ankylosing spondylitis; primary dysmenorrhea; acute and chronic treatment of rheumatoid arthritis, osteoarthritis
Delayed-release tablets: Acute and chronic treatment of rheumatoid arthritis, osteoarthritis, ankylosing spondylitis
Extended-release tablets: Chronic treatment of osteoarthritis, rheumatoid arthritis
Ophthalmic solution: Postoperative inflammation following cataract extraction; temporary relief of pain and photophobia in patients undergoing corneal refractive surgery
Topical gel: Actinic keratosis (AK) in conjunction with sun avoidance

Unlabeled/Investigational Use Juvenile rheumatoid arthritis

Mechanism of Action/Effect Inhibits prostaglandin synthesis by decreasing activity of the enzyme, cyclooxygenase, which results in decreased formation of prostaglandin precursors

Contraindications Hypersensitivity to diclofenac, aspirin, other NSAIDs, or any component of the formulation; perioperative pain in the setting of coronary artery bypass surgery (CABG); pregnancy (3rd trimester)

Warnings/Precautions NSAIDs are associated with an increased risk of adverse cardiovascular events, including MI, stroke, and new onset or worsening of pre-existing hypertension. Risk may be increased with duration of use or pre-existing cardiovascular risk factors or disease. Carefully evaluate individual cardiovascular risk profiles prior to prescribing. Use caution with fluid retention, CHF, or hypertension.

Use of NSAIDs can compromise existing renal function. Renal toxicity can occur in patient with impaired renal function, dehydration, heart failure, liver dysfunction, those taking diuretics and ACEI, and the elderly. Rehydrate patient before starting therapy. Monitor renal function closely. Not recommended for use in patients with advanced renal disease.

NSAIDs may increase risk of gastrointestinal irritation, ulceration, bleeding, and perforation. These events may occur at any time during therapy and without warning. Use caution with a history of GI disease (bleeding or ulcers), concurrent therapy with aspirin, anticoagulants and/or corticosteroids, smoking, use of alcohol, the elderly or debilitated patients.

Use the lowest effective dose for the shortest duration of time, consistent with individual patient goals, to reduce risk of cardiovascular or GI adverse events. Alternate therapies should be considered for patients at high risk.

NSAIDs may cause serious skin adverse events including exfoliative dermatitis, Stevens-Johnson syndrome (SJS), and toxic epidermal necrolysis (TEN). Anaphylactoid reactions may occur, even without prior exposure; patients with "aspirin triad" (bronchial asthma, aspirin intolerance, rhinitis) may be at increased risk. Do not use in patients who experience bronchospasm, asthma, rhinitis, or urticaria with NSAID or aspirin therapy.

Use with caution in patients with decreased hepatic function. Closely monitor patients with any abnormal LFT. Severe hepatic reactions (eg, fulminant hepatitis, liver failure) have occurred with NSAID use, rarely; discontinue if signs or symptoms of liver disease develop, or if systemic manifestations occur.

The elderly are at increased risk for adverse effects (especially peptic ulceration, CNS effects, renal toxicity) from NSAIDs even at low doses.

Withhold for at least 4-6 half-lives prior to surgical or dental procedures.

Topical gel should not be applied to the eyes, open wounds, infected areas, or to exfoliative dermatitis. Monitor patients for 1 year following application of ophthalmic drops for corneal refractive procedures. Patients using ophthalmic drops should not wear soft contact lenses. Ophthalmic drops may slow/delay healing or prolong bleeding time following surgery.

Drug Interactions

Cytochrome P450 Effect: Substrate (minor) of CYP1A2, 2B6, 2C8/9, 2C19, 2D6, 3A4; **Inhibits** CYP1A2 (moderate), 2C8/9 (weak), 2E1 (weak), 3A4 (strong)

Decreased Effect: Decreased effect of diclofenac with aspirin. Decreased effect of thiazides, furosemide.

Increased Effect/Toxicity: Increased toxicity of digoxin, methotrexate, cyclosporine, lithium, insulin, sulfonylureas, potassium-sparing diuretics, warfarin, and aspirin. Diclofenac may increase the levels/effects of aminophylline, selected benzodiazepines, calcium channel blockers, cyclosporine, fluvoxamine, mexiletine, mirtazapine, nateglinide, nefazodone, ropinirole, sildenafil (and other PDE-5 inhibitors), tacrolimus, theophylline, trifluoperazine, venlafaxine, and other CYP1A2 or 3A4 substrates. Selected benzodiazepines (midazolam and triazolam), cisapride, ergot alkaloids, selected HMG-CoA reductase inhibitors (lovastatin and simvastatin), mesoridazine, pimozide, and thioridazine are generally contraindicated with strong CYP3A4 inhibitors. When used with strong CYP3A4 inhibitors, dosage adjustment/limits are recommended for sildenafil and other PDE-5 inhibitors; refer to individual monographs.

Nutritional/Ethanol Interactions

Ethanol: Avoid ethanol (may enhance gastric mucosal irritation).

Herb/Nutraceutical: Avoid alfalfa, anise, bilberry, bladderwrack, bromelain, cat's claw, celery, coleus, cordyceps, dong quai, evening primrose, feverfew, fenugreek, garlic, ginger, ginkgo biloboa, red clover, horse chestnut, grapeseed, green tea, ginseng, guggul, horse chestnut seed, horseradish, licorice, prickly ash, red clover, reishi, SAMe, sweet clover, turmeric, white willow (all have additional antiplatelet activity).

Adverse Reactions

>10%:
Local: Application site reactions (gel): Pruritus (31% to 52%), rash (35% to 46%), contact dermatitis (19% to 33%), dry skin (25% to 27%), pain (15% to 26%), exfoliation (6% to 24%), paresthesia (8% to 20%)

Ocular: Ophthalmic drops (incidence may be dependent upon indication): Lacrimation (30%), keratitis (28%), elevated IOP (15%), transient burning/stinging (15%)

1% to 10%:
Central nervous system: Headache (7%), dizziness (3%)

Dermatologic: Pruritus (1% to 3%), rash (1% to 3%)

Endocrine & metabolic: Fluid retention (1% to 3%)

Gastrointestinal: Abdominal cramps (3% to 9%), abdominal pain (3% to 9%), constipation (3% to 9%), diarrhea (3% to 9%), flatulence (3% to 9%), indigestion (3% to 9%), nausea (3% to 9%), abdominal distention (1% to 3%), peptic ulcer/GI bleed (0.6% to 9%)

Hepatic: Increased ALT/AST (2%)

Local: Application site reactions (gel): Edema (4%)

Ocular: Ophthalmic drops: Abnormal vision, acute elevated IOP, blurred vision, conjunctivitis, corneal deposits, corneal edema, corneal opacity, corneal lesions, discharge, eyelid swelling, injection, iritis, irritation, itching, lacrimation disorder, ocular allergy

Otic: Tinnitus (1% to 3%)

Overdosage/Toxicology Symptoms of overdose include acute renal failure, vomiting, drowsiness, and leukocytosis. Management of NSAID intoxication is supportive and symptomatic.

Pharmacodynamics/Kinetics

Onset of Action: Cataflam® is more rapid than sodium salt (Voltaren®) because it dissolves in the stomach instead of the duodenum

Time to Peak: Serum: Cataflam®: ~1 hour; Voltaren®: ~2 hours

Protein Binding: 99% to albumin

Half-Life Elimination: 2 hours

Metabolism: Hepatic to several metabolites

Excretion: Urine (65%); feces (35%)

Available Dosage Forms [DSC] = Discontinued product

Gel, as sodium:
Solaraze®: 30 mg/g (50 g)

Solution, ophthalmic, as sodium:
Voltaren Ophthalmic®: 0.1% (2.5 mL, 5 mL)

Tablet, as potassium: 50 mg
Cataflam®: 50 mg

Tablet, delayed release, enteric coated, as sodium: 50 mg, 75 mg
Voltaren®: 25 mg [DSC], 50 mg [DSC], 75 mg

Tablet, extended release, as sodium: 100 mg
Voltaren®-XR: 100 mg

Dosing

Adults & Elderly:

Analgesia/primary dysmenorrhea: Oral: Starting dose: 50 mg 3 times/day; maximum dose: 150 mg/day

Rheumatoid arthritis: Oral: 150-200 mg/day in 2-4 divided doses (100 mg/day of sustained release product)

Osteoarthritis: Oral: 100-150 mg/day in 2-3 divided doses (100-200 mg/day of sustained release product)

Ankylosing spondylitis: Oral: 100-125 mg/day in 4-5 divided doses

Cataract surgery: Ophthalmic: Instill 1 drop into affected eye 4 times/day beginning 24 hours after cataract surgery and continuing for 2 weeks

Corneal refractive surgery: Ophthalmic: Instill 1-2 drops into affected eye within the hour prior to surgery, within 15 minutes following surgery, and then continue for 4 times/day, up to 3 days

Actinic keratosis (AK): Topical (gel): Apply gel to lesion area twice daily for 60-90 days

Renal Impairment: Not recommended in patients with advanced renal disease.
(Continued)

Diclofenac *(Continued)*

Hepatic Impairment: No adjustment necessary.

Administration

Oral: Do not crush tablets. Administer with food or milk to avoid gastric distress. Take with full glass of water to enhance absorption.

Topical: Topical gel: Cover lesion with gel and smooth into skin gently. Do not cover lesion with occlusive dressings or apply sunscreens, cosmetics, or other medications to affected area.

Other: Ophthalmic: Wait at least 5 minutes before administering other types of eye drops.

Stability

Storage: Store below 30°C (86°F); protect from moisture, store in tight container.

Laboratory Monitoring CBC, liver enzymes, urine output and BUN/serum creatinine in patients receiving diuretics, occult blood loss

Nursing Actions

Physical Assessment: Assess other medications patient may be taking for effectiveness and interactions. Monitor blood pressure at the beginning of therapy and periodically during use. Monitor laboratory tests, therapeutic response (eg, relief of pain and inflammation, increased activity tolerance), and adverse reactions (systemic or ophthalmic) at beginning of therapy and periodically throughout therapy. Schedule ophthalmic evaluations for patients who develop eye complaints during long-term NSAID therapy. Assess knowledge/teach patient appropriate use (oral, ophthalmic, gel), interventions to reduce side effects, and adverse symptoms to report.

Patient Education: Oral: Take this medication exactly as directed; do not increase dose without consulting prescriber. Do not crush or chew tablets. Take with 8 oz of water, along with food or milk products to reduce GI distress. Maintain adequate hydration (2-3 L/day of fluids) unless instructed to restrict fluid intake. Avoid alcohol, aspirin and aspirin-containing medication, or any other anti-inflammatory medications unless consulting prescriber. You may experience dizziness, nervousness, or headache (use caution when driving or engaging in tasks requiring alertness until response to drug is known); nausea, vomiting, dry mouth, or heartburn (small frequent meals, frequent mouth care, sucking lozenges, or chewing gum may help); or constipation (increased exercise, fluids, fruit, or fiber may help). GI bleeding, ulceration, or perforation can occur with or without pain; discontinue medication and contact prescriber if persistent abdominal pain or cramping, or blood in stool occurs. Report chest pain or palpitations; breathlessness or respiratory difficulty; unusual bruising/bleeding or blood in urine, stool, mouth, or vomitus; unusual fatigue; skin rash or itching; jaundice, unusual weight gain, or swelling of extremities; change in urinary pattern; change in vision or hearing (ringing in ears). **Pregnancy/breast-feeding precautions:** Consult prescriber if you are pregnant. This drug should not be used in the 3rd trimester of pregnancy. Consult prescriber if you are breast-feeding.

Ophthalmic: For ophthalmic use only. Apply prescribed amount as often as directed. Wash hands before using. Tilt head back and look upward. Gently pull down lower lid and put drop(s) in inner corner of eye. Do not let tip of applicator touch eye; do not contaminate tip of applicator (may cause eye infection, eye damage, or vision loss). Close eye and roll eyeball in all directions. Do not blink for ½minute. Apply gentle pressure to inner corner of eye for 30 seconds. Wipe away excess from skin around eye. Do not use any other eye preparation for at least 10 minutes. Do not share medication with anyone else. May cause sensitivity to bright light (dark glasses may help); temporary stinging or blurred vision may occur.

Inform prescriber if you experience eye pain, redness, burning, watering, dryness, double vision, puffiness around eye, vision changes, other adverse eye response, worsening of condition, or lack of improvement.

Gel: This preparation is for topical use only. Treatment may take up to 3 months. Do not use more often than recommended; use at regular intervals. Wash hands before and after use. Follow directions on prescription label. Gently apply enough of the gel to cover the lesion. Advise prescriber if you are using any other skin preparations. Avoid direct sunlight and sunlamps while using this medication. You may experience dry skin, itching, peeling, swelling, or tingling at site of application. If severe skin reaction develops, stop applications and notify your prescriber at once.

Dietary Considerations May be taken with food to decrease GI distress.
Diclofenac potassium = Cataflam®; potassium content: 5.8 mg (0.15 mEq) per 50 mg tablet

Geriatric Considerations The elderly are at increased risk for adverse effects from NSAIDs. As many as 60% of elderly can develop peptic ulceration and/or hemorrhage asymptomatically. CNS adverse effects such as confusion, agitation, and hallucination are generally seen in overdose or high-dose situations; however, elderly patients may demonstrate these adverse effects at lower doses than younger adults. The elderly are also at increased risk of renal toxicity.

Pregnancy Issues Safety and efficacy in pregnant women have not been established. Exposure late in pregnancy may lead to premature closure of the ductus arteriosus and may inhibit uterine contractions.

Diclofenac and Misoprostol
(dye KLOE fen ak & mye soe PROST ole)

U.S. Brand Names Arthrotec®

Synonyms Misoprostol and Diclofenac

Restrictions
A medication guide should be dispensed with each prescription. A template for the required MedGuide can be found on the FDA website at http://www.fda.gov/medwatch/SAFETY/2005/safety05.htm#NSAID

Pharmacologic Category Nonsteroidal Anti-inflammatory Drug (NSAID), Oral; Prostaglandin

Pregnancy Risk Factor X

Lactation Enters breast milk/contraindicated

Use The diclofenac component is indicated for the treatment of osteoarthritis and rheumatoid arthritis; the misoprostol component is indicated for the prophylaxis of NSAID-induced gastric and duodenal ulceration

Available Dosage Forms Tablet: Diclofenac sodium 50 mg and misoprostol 200 mcg; diclofenac sodium 75 mg and misoprostol 200 mcg

Dosing
Adults & Elderly:
Osteoarthritis: Oral: Arthrotec® 50: 1 tablet 2-3 times/day
Rheumatoid arthritis: Oral: Arthrotec® 50: 1 tablet 3-4 times/day
Note: For both regimens, if not tolerated by patient, the dose may be reduced to 1 tablet twice daily. Arthrotec® 75 may be used in patients who cannot tolerate full daily Arthrotec® 50 regimens. Dose: 1 tablet twice daily. However, the use of these tablets may not be as effective at preventing GI ulceration.

Renal Impairment: Not recommended for use in patients with advanced renal disease. In renal insufficiency, diclofenac should be used with caution due to potential detrimental effects on renal function, and misoprostol dosage reduction may be required if adverse effects occur (misoprostol is renally eliminated).

Nursing Actions

Physical Assessment: See individual agents. **Pregnancy risk factor X** - determine that patient is not pregnant before beginning treatment and do not give to women of childbearing age or to males who may have intercourse with women of childbearing age unless both male and female are capable of complying with barrier contraceptive measures during therapy and for 1 month following therapy. Breast-feeding is contraindicated.

Patient Education: See individual agents. Consult your prescriber before use if you have hypertension or heart failure. **Pregnancy/breast-feeding precautions:** Inform prescriber if you are pregnant. Do not get pregnant during or for 1 month following therapy. Male: Do not cause a female to become pregnant. Male/female: Consult prescriber for instruction on appropriate contraceptive measures. The misoprostol ingredient in this drug may cause severe fetal defects, miscarriage, or abortion; do not share medication with others. Do not breast-feed.

Related Information

Diclofenac *on page 358*
Misoprostol *on page 830*

Dicloxacillin (dye kloks a SIL in)

Synonyms Dicloxacillin Sodium

Pharmacologic Category Antibiotic, Penicillin

Pregnancy Risk Factor B

Lactation Excretion in breast milk unknown (probably similar to penicillin G)

Use Treatment of systemic infections such as pneumonia, skin and soft tissue infections, and osteomyelitis caused by penicillinase-producing staphylococci

Mechanism of Action/Effect Interferes with bacterial cell wall synthesis; causes cell wall death

Contraindications Hypersensitivity to dicloxacillin, penicillin, or any component of the formulation

Warnings/Precautions Monitor PT if patient concurrently on warfarin. Use with caution in patients allergic to cephalosporins.

Drug Interactions

Cytochrome P450 Effect: Induces CYP3A4 (weak)

Decreased Effect: Although anecdotal reports suggest oral contraceptive efficacy could be reduced by penicillins, this has been refuted by more rigorous scientific and clinical data. Decreased effect of (warfarin) anticoagulants.

Increased Effect/Toxicity: Disulfiram, probenecid may increase penicillin levels. Penicillins may increase the exposure to methotrexate during concurrent therapy; monitor.

Nutritional/Ethanol Interactions Food: Decreases drug absorption rate; decreases drug serum concentration.

Lab Interactions Positive Coombs' test [direct]

Adverse Reactions 1% to 10%: Gastrointestinal: Nausea, diarrhea, abdominal pain

Overdosage/Toxicology Symptoms of penicillin overdose include neuromuscular hypersensitivity (eg, agitation, hallucinations, asterixis, encephalopathy, confusion, and seizures). Electrolyte imbalance may occur if the preparation contains potassium or sodium salts, especially in renal failure. Hemodialysis may be helpful to aid in removal of the drug from blood; otherwise, treatment is supportive or symptom-directed.

Pharmacodynamics/Kinetics

Time to Peak: Serum: 0.5-2 hours

Protein Binding: 96%

Half-Life Elimination: 0.6-0.8 hour; slightly prolonged with renal impairment

Excretion: Feces; urine (56% to 70% as unchanged drug); prolonged in neonates

Available Dosage Forms Capsule: 250 mg, 500 mg

Dosing

Adults & Elderly:

Susceptible Infections: Oral: 125-500 mg every 6 hours

Erysipelas, furunculosis, impetigo, mastitis, otitis externa, septic bursitis, skin abscess: Oral: 500 mg every 6 hours

Prosthetic joint (long-term suppression therapy): Oral: 250 mg twice daily

***Staphylococcus aureus*, methicillin susceptible infection if no I.V. access:** Oral: 500-1000 mg every 6-8 hours

Pediatrics: Use in newborns is not recommended.

Susceptible infections: Oral:

Children <40 kg: 12.5-25 mg/kg/day divided every 6 hours; doses of 50-100 mg/kg/day in divided doses every 6 hours have been used for therapy of osteomyelitis

Children >40 kg: 125-250 mg every 6 hours

Furunculosis: Oral: 25-50 mg/kg/day divided every 6 hours

Osteomyelitis: Oral: 50-100 mg/kg/day in divided doses every 6 hours

Renal Impairment:

Dosage adjustment is not necessary.

Not dialyzable (0% to 5%); supplemental dose is not necessary.

Peritoneal dialysis effects: Supplemental dose is not necessary.

Continuous arteriovenous or venovenous hemofiltration: Supplemental dose is not necessary.

Administration

Oral: Administer 1 hour before or 2 hours after meals. Administer around-the-clock to promote less variation in peak and trough serum levels.

Laboratory Monitoring Perform culture and sensitivity studies prior to initiating therapy.

Nursing Actions

Physical Assessment: Assess allergy history prior to beginning therapy. Assess potential for interactions with other prescriptions, OTC medications, or herbal products patient may be taking. Monitor laboratory tests, therapeutic response, and adverse effects on a regular basis throughout therapy. Teach patient proper use, possible side effects/appropriate interventions, and adverse symptoms to report.

Patient Education: Do not take any new medication during therapy unless approved by prescriber. Take medication as directed, with a large glass of water 1 hour before or 2 hours after meals. Take at regular intervals around-the-clock and take for length of time prescribed. If you have diabetes, drug may cause false test results with Clinitest® urine glucose monitoring; use of another type of glucose monitoring is preferable. May cause some gastric distress (small, frequent meals may help) and diarrhea (if this persists, consult prescriber). Report fever, vaginal itching, sores in the mouth, loose foul-smelling stools, yellowing of skin or eyes, or change in color of urine or stool. **Breast-feeding precaution:** Consult prescriber if breast-feeding.

Dietary Considerations Administer on an empty stomach 1 hour before or 2 hours after meals. Sodium content of 250 mg capsule: 13 mg (0.6 mEq)

Breast-Feeding Issues No data reported; however, other penicillins may be taken while breast-feeding.

Didanosine (dye DAN oh seen)

U.S. Brand Names Videx®; Videx® EC
Synonyms ddl; Dideoxyinosine
Pharmacologic Category Antiretroviral Agent, Reverse Transcriptase Inhibitor (Nucleoside)
Medication Safety Issues
Sound-alike/look-alike issues:
Videx® may be confused with Lidex®
Pregnancy Risk Factor B
Lactation Excretion in breast milk unknown/contraindicated
Use Treatment of HIV infection; always to be used in combination with at least two other antiretroviral agents
Mechanism of Action/Effect Didanosine, a purine nucleoside (adenosine) analog and the deamination product of dideoxyadenosine (ddA), inhibits HIV replication in vitro in both T cells and monocytes. Didanosine is converted within the cell to the mono-, di-, and triphosphates of ddA. These ddA triphosphates act as substrate and inhibitor of HIV reverse transcriptase substrate and inhibitor of HIV reverse transcriptase thereby blocking viral DNA synthesis and suppressing HIV replication.
Contraindications Hypersensitivity to didanosine or any component of the formulation
Warnings/Precautions Pancreatitis (sometimes fatal) has been reported, incidence is dose related. Risk factors for developing pancreatitis include a previous history of the condition, concurrent cytomegalovirus or *Mycobacterium avium-intracellulare* infection, and concomitant use of stavudine, pentamidine, or co-trimoxazole. Discontinue didanosine if clinical signs of pancreatitis occur. Lactic acidosis, symptomatic hyperlactatemia, and severe hepatomegaly with steatosis (sometimes fatal) have occurred with antiretroviral nucleoside analogues, including didanosine. Hepatotoxicity may occur even in the absence of marked transaminase elevations; suspend therapy in any patient developing clinical/laboratory findings which suggest hepatotoxicity. Pregnant women may be at increased risk of lactic acidosis and liver damage.

Peripheral neuropathy occurs in ~20% of patients receiving the drug. Retinal changes (including retinal depigmentation) and optic neuritis have been reported in adults and children using didanosine. Patients should undergo retinal examination every 6-12 months. Use with caution in patients with decreased renal or hepatic function, phenylketonuria, sodium-restricted diets, or with edema, CHF, or hyperuricemia. Twice-daily dosing is the preferred dosing frequency for didanosine tablets. Didanosine delayed release capsules are indicated for once-daily use.
Drug Interactions
Decreased Effect: Didanosine buffered tablets and pediatric oral solution may decrease absorption of quinolones or tetracyclines (administer 2 hours prior to didanosine buffered formulations). Didanosine should be held during PCP treatment with pentamidine. Didanosine may decrease levels of indinavir. Drugs whose absorption depends on the level of acidity in the stomach such as ketoconazole, itraconazole, and dapsone should be administered at least 2 hours prior to the buffered formulations of didanosine (not affected by delayed release capsules). Methadone may decrease didanosine concentrations.
Increased Effect/Toxicity: Concomitant administration of other drugs which have the potential to cause peripheral neuropathy or pancreatitis may increase the risk of these toxicities Allopurinol may increase didanosine concentration; avoid concurrent use. Concomitant use of antacids with buffered tablet or pediatric didanosine solution may potentiate adverse effects of aluminum- or magnesium-containing antacids. Ganciclovir may increase didanosine

concentration; monitor. Hydroxyurea may precipitate didanosine-induced pancreatitis if added to therapy; concomitant use is not recommended. Coadministration with ribavirin or tenofovir may increase exposure to didanosine and/or its active metabolite increasing the risk or severity of didanosine toxicities, including pancreatitis, lactic acidosis, and peripheral neuropathy; monitor closely and suspend therapy if signs or symptoms of toxicity are noted. Additionally, concomitant tenofovir administration has been associated with hyperglycemia, decreased CD4 cell counts, and reduced virologic response.
Nutritional/Ethanol Interactions
Ethanol: Avoid ethanol (increases risk of pancreatitis).
Food: Decreases AUC and C_{max}. Didanosine serum levels may be decreased by 55% if taken with food.
Adverse Reactions As reported in monotherapy studies; risk of toxicity may increase when combined with other agents.

>10%:
Gastrointestinal: Increased amylase (15% to 17%), abdominal pain (7% to 13%), diarrhea (19% to 28%)
Neuromuscular & skeletal: Peripheral neuropathy (17% to 20%)
1% to 10%:
Dermatologic: Rash, pruritus
Endocrine & metabolic: Increased uric acid
Gastrointestinal: Pancreatitis; patients >65 years of age had a higher frequency of pancreatitis than younger patients
Hepatic: Increased SGOT, increased SGPT, increased alkaline phosphatase
Overdosage/Toxicology Chronic overdose may cause pancreatitis, peripheral neuropathy, diarrhea, hyperuricemia, and hepatic impairment. There is no known antidote for didanosine overdose. Treatment is symptomatic.
Pharmacodynamics/Kinetics
Time to Peak: Buffered tablets: 0.67 hours; Delayed release capsules: 2 hours
Protein Binding: <5%
Half-Life Elimination:
Children and Adolescents: 0.8 hour
Adults: Normal renal function: 1.5 hours; however, active metabolite, ddATP, has an intracellular half-life >12 hours in vitro; Renal impairment: 2.5-5 hours
Metabolism: Has not been evaluated in humans; studies conducted in dogs, show extensive metabolism with allantoin, hypoxanthine, xanthine, and uric acid being the major metabolites found in urine
Excretion: Urine (~55% as unchanged drug)
Clearance: Total body: Averages 800 mL/minute
Available Dosage Forms
Capsule, delayed release: 200 mg, 250 mg, 400 mg
Videx® EC: 125 mg, 200 mg, 250 mg, 400 mg
Powder for oral solution, pediatric (Videx®): 2 g, 4 g [makes 10 mg/mL solution after final mixing]
Tablet, buffered, chewable/dispersible (Videx®): 25 mg, 50 mg, 100 mg, 150 mg, 200 mg [all strengths contain phenylalanine 36.5 mg/tablet; orange flavor]
Dosing
Adults: Treatment of HIV infection: Oral (administer on an empty stomach): Oral:
Note: Preferred dosing frequency is twice daily for didanosine tablets
Chewable tablets, powder for oral solution:
<60 kg: 125 mg twice daily or 250 mg once daily
≥60 kg: 200 mg twice daily or 400 mg once daily
Note: Adults should receive 2-4 tablets per dose for adequate buffering and absorption; tablets should be chewed or dispersed (in 1 ounce of water).
Delayed release capsule (Videx® EC):
<60 kg: 250 mg once daily
≥60 kg; 400 mg once daily

Dosing adjustment with tenofovir (didanosine tablets or delayed release capsules; based on tenofovir product labeling):
<60 kg: 200 mg once daily
≥60 kg: 250 mg once daily

Elderly: Refer to adult dosing. Elderly patients have a higher frequency of pancreatitis (10% versus 5% in younger patients); monitor renal function and dose accordingly.

Pediatrics:

Treatment of HIV infection: Oral (administer on an empty stomach):

Children:

2 weeks to 8 months: 100 mg/m² twice daily is recommended by the manufacturer; 50 mg/m² may be considered in infants 2 weeks to 4 months

>8 months: 120 mg/m² twice daily; dosing range: 90-150 mg/m² twice daily; patients with CNS disease may require higher dose

Note: At least 2 tablets per dose should be administered for adequate buffering and absorption; tablets should be chewed or dispersed (in 1 ounce of water).

Adolescents: Refer to adult dosing.

Renal Impairment: See table.

Recommended Dose (mg) of Didanosine by Body Weight

Creatinine Clearance (mL/min)	≥60 kg		<60 kg	
	Tablet¹ (mg)	Delayed Release Capsule (mg)	Tablet¹ (mg)	Delayed Release Capsule (mg)
≥60	400 daily or 200 twice daily	400 daily	250 daily or 125 twice daily	250 daily
30-59	200 daily or 100 twice daily	200 daily	150 daily or 75 twice daily	125 daily
10-29	150 daily	125 daily	100 daily	125 daily
<10	100 daily	125 daily	75 daily	See footnote 2.

¹Chewable/dispersible buffered tablet; 2 tablets must be taken with each dose; different strengths of tablets may be combined to yield the recommended dose.

²Not suitable for use in patients <60 kg with Cl$_{cr}$ <10 mL/minute; use alternate formulation.

Patients requiring hemodialysis or CAPD: Dose per Cl$_{cr}$ 10 mL/minute

Hepatic Impairment: Should be considered; monitor for toxicity.

Administration

Oral:

Chewable/dispersible buffered tablets: The 200 mg tablet should only be used in once-daily dosing. At least 2 tablets, but no more than 4 tablets, should be taken together to allow adequate buffering. Tablets may be chewed or dispersed prior to consumption. To disperse, dissolve in 1 oz water, stir until uniform dispersion is formed, and drink immediately. May also add 1 oz of clear apple juice to initial dispersion if additional flavor is needed. The apple juice dilution is stable for 1 hour at room temperature.

Pediatric powder for oral solution: Prior to dispensing, the powder should be mixed with purified water USP to an initial concentration of 20 mg/mL and then further diluted with an appropriate antacid suspension to a final mixture of 10 mg/mL. Stable for 30 days under refrigeration. Shake well prior to use.

Stability

Reconstitution: Unbuffered powder for oral solution must be reconstituted and mixed with an equal volume of antacid at time of preparation.

Storage: Tablets and delayed release capsules should be stored in tightly closed bottles at 15°C to 30°C. Undergoes rapid degradation when exposed to an acidic environment. Tablets dispersed in water are stable for 1 hour at room temperature. Reconstituted pediatric solution is stable for 30 days if refrigerated.

Laboratory Monitoring Serum potassium, uric acid, creatinine, hemoglobin, CBC with neutrophil, platelet count, CD4 cells, liver function, amylase; viral load

Nursing Actions

Physical Assessment: Assess other pharmacological or herbal products patient may be taking for potential interactions. A list of medications that should not be used is available in each bottle and patients should be provided with this information. Monitor effectiveness of therapy (decrease in infections and progress of disease) and adverse reactions periodically during therapy. Teach patient proper use (eg, timing of multiple medications and drugs that should not be used concurrently), possible side effects/appropriate interventions (need for annual or semiannual retinal examinations), and adverse symptoms to report (eg, rash, gastrointestinal upset).

Patient Education: You will be provided with a list of specific medications that should not be used during therapy; do not take any new prescriptions, over-the-counter medications, or herbal products (even if they are not on the list) without consulting prescriber. This drug will not cure HIV, nor has it been found to reduce transmission of HIV; use appropriate precautions to prevent spread to other persons. This drug is prescribed as one part of a multidrug combination; take exactly as directed for full course of therapy. Take 30 minutes before or 2 hours after meals. Delayed release capsules should not be broken or chewed. Chewable/dispersible tablets can be chewed or mixed in water (water can be flavored with 1 ounce of apple juice; do not use other juices). Maintain adequate hydration (2-3 L/day of fluids) unless advised by prescriber to restrict fluids. You may be susceptible to infection; avoid crowds and exposure to known infections and do not have any vaccinations without consulting prescriber. Frequent blood tests may be required with prolonged therapy. May cause nausea or vomiting (small frequent meals, frequent mouth care, sucking lozenges, or chewing gum may help); consult prescriber if nausea or vomiting or diarrhea persists (boiled milk, yogurt, or buttermilk may help). Report immediately any loss of sensation, numbness, or tingling in fingers, toes, or feet; persistent unresolved abdominal distress (nausea, vomiting, diarrhea); or signs of infection (burning on urination, perineal itching, white plaques in mouth, unhealed sores, persistent sore throat or cough). **Pregnancy/breast-feeding precautions:** Inform prescriber if you are or intend to become pregnant. Do not breast-feed.

Dietary Considerations

Videx® EC: Take on an empty stomach; administer at least 1 hour before or 2 hours after eating

Chewable/dispersible tablet: Take on an empty stomach, 30 minutes before or 2 hours after eating. Chew well or mix in water; if mixed in water, may add 2 tablespoons (1 oz) apple juice for flavor. Do not use other juices. Each chewable tablet contains 36.5 mg phenylalanine and 8.6 mEq magnesium. Sodium content of buffered tablets: 264.5 mg (11.5 mEq).

Geriatric Considerations Since the elderly often have a creatinine clearance <60 mL/minute, monitor closely for adverse reactions and adjust dose accordingly to maintain efficacy (CD4 counts).

Breast-Feeding Issues HIV-infected mothers are discouraged from breast-feeding to decrease potential transmission of HIV.

Pregnancy Issues Cases of fatal and nonfatal lactic acidosis, with or without pancreatitis, have been

(Continued)

Didanosine *(Continued)*

reported in pregnant women. It is not known if pregnancy itself potentiates this known side effect; however, pregnant women may be at increased risk of lactic acidosis and liver damage. Hepatic enzymes and electrolytes should be monitored frequently during the 3rd trimester of pregnancy. Use during pregnancy only if the potential benefit to the mother outweighs the potential risk of this complication. Didanosine has been shown to cross the placenta. Pharmacokinetics are not significantly altered during pregnancy; dose adjustments are not needed. The Perinatal HIV Guidelines Working Group considers didanosine to be an alternative NRTI in dual nucleoside combination regimens; use with stavudine only if no other alternatives are available. Health professionals are encouraged to contact the antiretroviral pregnancy registry to monitor outcomes of pregnant women exposed to antiretroviral medications (1-800-258-4263 or www.APRegistry.com).

Additional Information A high rate of early virologic nonresponse was observed when didanosine, lamivudine, and tenofovir were used as the initial regimen in treatment-naive patients. Use of this combination is not recommended; patients currently on this regimen should be closely monitored for modification of therapy. Early virologic failure was also observed with tenofovir and didanosine delayed release capsules, plus either efavirenz or nevirapine; use caution in treatment-naive patients with high baseline viral loads.

Diethylpropion *(dye eth il PROE pee on)*

U.S. Brand Names Tenuate®; Tenuate® Dospan®
Synonyms Amfepramone; Diethylpropion Hydrochloride
Restrictions C-IV
Pharmacologic Category Anorexiant
Pregnancy Risk Factor B
Lactation Enters breast milk/not recommended
Use Short-term adjunct in a regimen of weight reduction based on exercise, behavioral modification, and caloric reduction in the management of exogenous obesity for patients with an initial body mass index $\geq$30 kg/m^2 or $\geq$27 kg/m^2 in the presence of other risk factors (diabetes, hypertension)

Unlabeled/Investigational Use Migraine

Mechanism of Action/Effect Diethylpropion is used as an anorexiant possessing pharmacological and chemical properties similar to those of amphetamines. The mechanism of action of diethylpropion in reducing appetite appears to be secondary to CNS effects, specifically stimulation of the hypothalamus to release catecholamines into the central nervous system. Anorexiant effects are mediated via norepinephrine and dopamine metabolism. An increase in physical activity and metabolic effects (inhibition of lipogenesis and enhancement of lipolysis) may also contribute to weight loss.

Contraindications Hypersensitivity or idiosyncrasy to sympathomimetic amines. Patients with advanced arteriosclerosis, symptomatic cardiovascular disease, moderate to severe hypertension (stage II or III), hyperthyroidism, glaucoma, agitated states, patients with a history of drug abuse, and during or within 14 days following MAO inhibitor therapy. Concurrent use with other anorectic agents; stimulant medications are contraindicated for use in children with attention-deficit/hyperactivity disorders and concomitant Tourette's syndrome or tics.

Warnings/Precautions Use with caution in patients with bipolar disorder, diabetes mellitus, cardiovascular disease, seizure disorders, insomnia, porphyria, or mild hypertension (stage I). May exacerbate symptoms of behavior and thought disorder in psychotic patients. Potential for drug dependency exists - avoid abrupt

discontinuation in patients who have received for prolonged periods. Stimulant use in children has been associated with growth suppression. Not recommended for use in patients <12 years of age.

Serious, potentially life-threatening toxicities may occur when thyroid hormones (at dosages above usual daily hormonal requirements) are used in combination with sympathomimetic amines to induce weight loss. Treatment of obesity is not an approved use for thyroid hormone.

Drug Interactions
Decreased Effect: Diethylpropion may displace guanethidine from the neuron and antagonize its antihypertensive effects; discontinue diethylpropion or use alternative antihypertensive.

Increased Effect/Toxicity: Concurrent use or use within 14 days following the administration of a MAO inhibitor is contraindicated (hypertensive crisis). Concurrent use of sibutramine and diethylpropion is contraindicated (severe hypertension, tachycardia). Concurrent use with TCAs may result in enhanced toxicity. Concurrent use with other anorectic agents may cause serious cardiac problems and is contraindicated.

Nutritional/Ethanol Interactions Ethanol: Avoid ethanol (may increase CNS depression).

Adverse Reactions Frequency not defined.
Cardiovascular: Hypertension, palpitation, tachycardia, chest pain, T-wave changes, arrhythmia, pulmonary hypertension, valvulopathy
Central nervous system: Euphoria, nervousness, insomnia, restlessness, dizziness, anxiety, headache, agitation, confusion, mental depression, psychosis, CVA, seizure
Dermatologic: Alopecia, urticaria, skin rash, ecchymosis, erythema
Endocrine & metabolic: Changes in libido, gynecomastia, menstrual irregularities, porphyria
Gastrointestinal: Nausea, vomiting, abdominal cramps, constipation, xerostomia, metallic taste
Genitourinary: Impotence
Hematologic: Bone marrow depression, agranulocytosis, leukopenia
Neuromuscular & skeletal: Tremor
Ocular: Blurred vision, mydriasis

Overdosage/Toxicology There is no specific antidote for amphetamine intoxication and treatment is primarily supportive. Hyperactivity and agitation usually respond to reduced sensory input; however, with extreme agitation, haloperidol (2-5 mg I.M. for adults) may be required.

Pharmacodynamics/Kinetics
Onset of Action: 1 hour
Duration of Action: 12-24 hours

Available Dosage Forms
Tablet, as hydrochloride (Tenuate®): 25 mg
Tablet, controlled release, as hydrochloride (Tenuate® Dospan®): 75 mg

Dosing
Adults & Elderly: Obesity (short-term adjunct): Oral:
Tablet: 25 mg 3 times/day before meals or food
Tablet, controlled release: 75 mg at midmorning

Administration
Oral: Do not crush 75 mg controlled release tablets. Dose should not be given in evening or at bedtime. Take tablets 1 hour before meals. Take controlled-release tablet at midmorning.

Nursing Actions
Physical Assessment: Assess effectiveness and interactions of other medications patient may be taking. Assess for history of psychopathology, homicidal or suicidal tendencies, or addiction; long-term use can result in dependence, abuse, or tolerance. Periodically evaluate the need for continued use. Monitor therapeutic response blood pressure, vital

signs, and adverse reactions at start of therapy, when changing dosage, and at regular intervals during therapy Monitor serum glucose closely in patients with diabetes (amphetamines may alter antidiabetic requirements). Taper dosage slowly when discontinuing. Assess knowledge/teach patient appropriate use, possible side effects, and symptoms to report.

Patient Education: Take exactly as directed; do not increase dose or frequency without consulting prescriber. Drug may cause physical and/or psychological dependence. Do not crush or chew extended release tablets. Take early in day to avoid sleep disturbance, 1 hour before meals. Avoid alcohol, caffeine, or OTC medications that act as stimulants. You may experience restlessness, false sense of euphoria, or impaired judgment (use caution when driving or engaging in tasks requiring alertness until response to drug is known); dry mouth (frequent mouth care, sucking lozenges, or chewing gum may help); nausea or vomiting (small frequent meals, frequent mouth care may help); constipation (increased exercise, fluids, fruit, or fiber may help); or diarrhea (buttermilk, boiled milk, or yogurt may help); or altered libido (reversible). Patients with diabetes need to monitor serum glucose closely (may alter antidiabetic medication requirements). Report chest pain, palpitations, or irregular heartbeat; muscle weakness or tremors; extreme fatigue or depression; CNS changes (aggressiveness, restlessness, euphoria, sleep disturbances); severe unremitting abdominal distress or cramping; changes in sexual activity; changes in urinary pattern; or blurred vision. **Breast-feeding precaution:** Breast-feeding is not recommended.

Difenoxin and Atropine
(dye fen OKS in & A troe peen)

U.S. Brand Names Motofen®
Synonyms Atropine and Difenoxin
Restrictions C-IV
Pharmacologic Category Antidiarrheal
Pregnancy Risk Factor C
Lactation Enters breast milk/contraindicated
Use Treatment of diarrhea
Available Dosage Forms Tablet: Difenoxin hydrochloride 1 mg and atropine sulfate 0.025 mg
Dosing
Adults: Diarrhea: Oral: Initial: 2 tablets, then 1 tablet after each loose stool; 1 tablet every 3-4 hours, up to 8 tablets in a 24-hour period; if no improvement after 48 hours, continued administration is not indicated
Elderly: Refer to adult dosing; use with caution.

Nursing Actions
Physical Assessment: Assess effects and interactions of other prescriptions, OTC medications, or herbal products patient may be taking. Monitor therapeutic effectiveness and adverse response. Teach patient proper use, possible side effects/appropriate interventions, and adverse effects to report.

Patient Education: Inform prescriber of all prescriptions, OTC medications, or herbal products you are taking, and any allergies you have. Do not take any new medication during therapy unless approved by prescriber. Take as directed; do not exceed recommended dose. If no relief in 48 hours, contact prescriber. Avoid alcohol. Keep out of reach of children; can cause severe and fatal respiratory depression if accidentally ingested. May cause lightheadedness, depression, dizziness, or weakness (use caution when driving or engaging in tasks that require alertness until response to drug is known). Report acute dizziness, headache, or GI symptoms. **Pregnancy/breast-feeding precautions:** Inform

prescriber if you are or intend to become pregnant. Do not breast-feed.
Related Information
Atropine on page 126

Diflunisal (dye FLOO ni sal)

U.S. Brand Names Dolobid® [DSC]
Restrictions A medication guide should be dispensed with each prescription. A template for the required MedGuide can be found on the FDA website at http://www.fda.gov/medwatch/SAFETY/2005/safety05.htm#NSAID
Pharmacologic Category Nonsteroidal Anti-inflammatory Drug (NSAID), Oral
Medication Safety Issues
Sound-alike/look-alike issues:
Dolobid® may be confused with Slo-Bid®
Pregnancy Risk Factor C (1st and 2nd trimesters)/D (3rd trimester)
Lactation Enters breast milk/not recommended
Use Management of inflammatory disorders usually including rheumatoid arthritis and osteoarthritis; can be used as an analgesic for treatment of mild to moderate pain
Mechanism of Action/Effect Inhibits prostaglandin synthesis by decreasing the activity of the enzyme, cyclooxygenase, which results in decreased formation of prostaglandin precursors
Contraindications Hypersensitivity to diflunisal, aspirin, other NSAIDs, or any component of the formulation; perioperative pain in the setting of coronary artery bypass surgery (CABG); pregnancy (3rd trimester)
Warnings/Precautions NSAIDs are associated with an increased risk of adverse cardiovascular events, including MI, stroke, and new onset or worsening of pre-existing hypertension. Risk may be increased with duration of use or pre-existing cardiovascular risk-factors or disease. Carefully evaluate individual cardiovascular risk profiles prior to prescribing. Use caution with fluid retention, CHF, or hypertension.

NSAIDs may increase risk of gastrointestinal irritation, ulceration, bleeding, and perforation. These events may occur at any time during therapy and without warning. Use caution with a history of GI disease (bleeding or ulcers), concurrent therapy with aspirin, anticoagulants and/or corticosteroids, smoking, use of alcohol, the elderly or debilitated patients.

Use of NSAIDs can compromise existing renal function. Renal toxicity can occur in patient with impaired renal function, dehydration, heart failure, liver dysfunction, those taking diuretics and ACEI and the elderly. Rehydrate patient before starting therapy. Monitor renal function closely. Diflunisal is not recommended for patients with advanced renal disease.

Use the lowest effective dose for the shortest duration of time, consistent with individual patient goals, to reduce risk of cardiovascular or GI adverse events. Alternate therapies should be considered for patients at high risk.

NSAIDs may cause serious skin adverse events including exfoliative dermatitis, Stevens-Johnson syndrome (SJS), and toxic epidermal necrolysis (TEN). Anaphylactoid reactions may occur, even without prior exposure; patients with "aspirin triad" (bronchial asthma, aspirin intolerance, rhinitis) may be at increased risk. Do not use in patients who experience bronchospasm, asthma, rhinitis, or urticaria with NSAID or aspirin therapy.

A hypersensitivity syndrome has been reported; monitor for constitutional symptoms and cutaneous findings; other organ dysfunction may be involved.
(Continued)

Diflunisal *(Continued)*

Use with caution in patients with decreased hepatic function. Closely monitor patients with any abnormal LFT. Severe hepatic reactions (eg, fulminant hepatitis, liver failure) have occurred with NSAID use, rarely; discontinue if signs or symptoms of liver disease develop, or if systemic manifestations occur.

Diflunisal is a derivative of acetylsalicylic acid and therefore may be associated with Reye's syndrome. Withhold for at least 4-6 half-lives prior to surgical or dental procedures. Safety and efficacy have not been established in children <12 years of age.

Drug Interactions
Decreased Effect: May reduce effect of some diuretics and antihypertensive effect of β-blockers, ACE inhibitors, angiotensin II inhibitors, hydralazine, verapamil. Cholestyramine and colestipol may reduce absorption of diflunisal.

Increased Effect/Toxicity: Diflunisal may increase effect/toxicity of anticoagulants (bleeding), antiplatelet agents (bleeding), aminoglycosides, biphosphonates (GI irritation), corticosteroids (GI irritation), cyclosporine (nephrotoxicity), lithium, methotrexate, pemetrexed, treprostinil (bleeding), vancomycin.

Nutritional/Ethanol Interactions
Ethanol: Avoid ethanol (may enhance gastric mucosal irritation).

Herb/Nutraceutical: Avoid alfalfa, anise, bilberry, bladderwrack, bromelain, cat's claw, celery, coleus, cordyceps, dong quai, evening primrose, feverfew, fenugreek, garlic, ginger, ginkgo biloboa, red clover, horse chestnut, grapeseed, green tea, ginseng, guggul, horse chestnut seed, horseradish, licorice, prickly ash, red clover, reishi, SAMe, sweet clover, turmeric, white willow (all have additional antiplatelet activity).

Lab Interactions
Falsely elevated increase in serum salicylate levels

Adverse Reactions
1% to 10%:
Central nervous system: Headache (3% to 9%), dizziness (1% to 3%), insomnia (1% to 3%), somnolence (1% to 3%), fatigue (1% to 3%)
Dermatologic: Rash (3% to 9%)
Gastrointestinal: Nausea (3% to 9%), dyspepsia (3% to 9%), GI pain (3% to 9%), diarrhea (3% to 9%), constipation (1% to 3%), flatulence (1% to 3%), vomiting (1% to 3%), GI ulceration
Otic: Tinnitus (1% to 3%)

Overdosage/Toxicology
Symptoms of overdose include drowsiness, nausea, vomiting, hyperventilation, tachycardia, tinnitus, stupor, coma, renal failure, and leukocytosis. Management of NSAID intoxication is supportive and symptomatic.

Pharmacodynamics/Kinetics
Onset of Action: Analgesic: ~1 hour; maximal effect: 2-3 hours
Duration of Action: 8-12 hours
Time to Peak: Serum: 2-3 hours
Protein Binding: >99%
Half-Life Elimination: 8-12 hours; prolonged with renal impairment
Metabolism: Extensively hepatic; metabolic pathways are saturable
Excretion: Urine (~3% as unchanged drug, 90% as glucuronide conjugates) within 72-96 hours

Available Dosage Forms
Tablet: 500 mg
Dolobid®: 250 mg, 500 mg [DSC]

Dosing
Adults & Elderly:
Mild-to-moderate pain: Oral: Initial: 500-1000 mg followed by 250-500 mg every 8-12 hours; maximum daily dose: 1.5 g
Arthritis: Oral: 500-1000 mg/day in 2 divided doses; maximum daily dose: 1.5 g

Renal Impairment:
Use with caution; Cl$_{cr}$ <50 mL/minute: Administer 50% of normal dose (Aronoff, 1998)
Hemodialysis: No supplement required
CAPD: No supplement require
CAVH: Dose for GFR 10-50

Administration
Oral: Tablet should be swallowed whole; do not crush or chew.

Nursing Actions
Physical Assessment: Assess patient for allergic reaction to salicylates or other NSAIDs. Assess other medications patient may be taking for additive or adverse interactions. Monitor blood pressure at the beginning of therapy and periodically during use. Monitor for effectiveness of pain relief. Monitor for signs of adverse reactions or overdose at beginning of therapy and periodically during long-term therapy. Schedule ophthalmic evaluations for patients who develop eye complaints during long-term NSAID therapy. Assess knowledge/teach patient appropriate use, adverse reactions, appropriate interventions to reduce side effects, and side effects to report.

Patient Education: If self-administered, use exactly as directed; do not increase dose or frequency. Adverse reactions can occur with overuse. Consult your prescriber before use if you have hypertension or heart failure. Do not take longer than 3 days for fever, or 10 days for pain without consulting medical advisor. Take with food or milk. While using this medication, do not use alcohol, excessive amounts of vitamin C, or salicylate-containing foods (curry powder, prunes, raisins, tea, or licorice), other prescription or OTC medications containing aspirin or salicylate, or other NSAIDs without consulting prescriber. Maintain adequate hydration (2-3 L/day of fluids) unless instructed to restrict fluid intake. You may experience nausea, vomiting, gastric discomfort (frequent mouth care, small frequent meals, chewing gum, or sucking lozenges may help). GI bleeding, ulceration, or perforation can occur with or without pain. Stop taking medication and report ringing in ears; persistent stomach pain; unresolved nausea or vomiting; respiratory difficulty or shortness of breath; unusual bruising or bleeding (mouth, urine, stool); skin rash; flu-like symptoms; unexplained weight gain; unusual swelling of extremities; chest pain; or palpitations.
Pregnancy/breast-feeding precautions: Inform prescriber if you are or intend to become pregnant. This drug should not be used in the 3rd trimester of pregnancy. Consult prescriber if breast-feeding.

Dietary Considerations
Should be taken with food to decrease GI distress.

Geriatric Considerations
The elderly are at increased risk for adverse effects from NSAIDs. As many as 60% of elderly can develop peptic ulceration and/or hemorrhage asymptomatically. CNS adverse effects such as confusion, agitation, and hallucination are generally seen in overdose or high-dose situations; however, elderly patients may demonstrate these adverse effects at lower doses than younger adults. The elderly are also at increased risk of renal toxicity.

Additional Information
Diflunisal is a salicylic acid derivative which is chemically different than aspirin and is not metabolized to salicylic acid. It is not considered a salicylate. Diflunisal 500 mg is equal in analgesic efficacy to aspirin 650 mg, acetaminophen 650 mg, and acetaminophen 650 mg/propoxyphene napsylate 100 mg, but has a longer duration of effect (8-12 hours). Not recommended as an antipyretic. Not found to be clinically useful to treat fever; at doses ≥2 g/day, platelets are reversibly inhibited in function. Diflunisal is uricosuric at 500-750 mg/day; causes less GI and renal toxicity than aspirin and other NSAIDs; fecal blood loss is 1/2 that of aspirin at 2.6 g/day.

Digoxin (di JOKS in)

U.S. Brand Names Digitek®; Lanoxicaps®; Lanoxin®
Pharmacologic Category Antiarrhythmic Agent, Class IV; Cardiac Glycoside
Medication Safety Issues
Sound-alike/look-alike issues:

Digoxin may be confused with Desoxyn®, doxepin

Lanoxin® may be confused with Lasix®, Levoxyl®, Levsinex®, Lomotil®, Lonox®, Mefoxin®, Xanax®
Pregnancy Risk Factor C
Lactation Enters breast milk (small amounts)/compatible
Use Treatment of congestive heart failure and to slow the ventricular rate in tachyarrhythmias such as atrial fibrillation, atrial flutter, and supraventricular tachycardia (paroxysmal atrial tachycardia); cardiogenic shock
Mechanism of Action/Effect
Congestive heart failure: Inhibition of the sodium/potassium ATPase pump which acts to increase the intracellular sodium-calcium exchange to increase intracellular calcium leading to increased contractility

Supraventricular arrhythmias: Direct suppression of the AV node conduction to increase effective refractory period and decrease conduction velocity - positive inotropic effect, enhanced vagal tone, and decreased ventricular rate to fast atrial arrhythmias. Atrial fibrillation may decrease sensitivity and increase tolerance to higher serum digoxin concentrations.

Contraindications Hypersensitivity to digoxin or any component of the formulation; hypersensitivity to cardiac glycosides (another may be tried); history of toxicity; ventricular tachycardia or fibrillation; idiopathic hypertrophic subaortic stenosis; constrictive pericarditis; amyloid disease; second- or third-degree heart block (except in patients with a functioning artificial pacemaker); Wolff-Parkinson-White syndrome and atrial fibrillation concurrently
Warnings/Precautions Withdrawal in CHF patients may lead to recurrence of CHF symptoms. Some arrhythmias that digoxin is used to treat may be exacerbated in digoxin toxicity. Sinus nodal disease may be worsened. Adjust doses in renal impairment and when verapamil, quinidine or amiodarone are added to a patient on digoxin. Correct hypokalemia and hypomagnesemia before initiating therapy. Calcium, especially when administered rapidly I.V., can produce serious arrhythmias. When used for rate control in atrial fibrillation, response may be better in a sedentary patients than in active/hypermetabolic patients. Use with caution in acute MI (within 6 months). Reduce or hold dose 1-2 days before elective electrical cardioversion.
Drug Interactions
Cytochrome P450 Effect: Substrate of CYP3A4 (minor)

Decreased Effect: Amiloride and spironolactone may reduce the inotropic response to digoxin. Cholestyramine, colestipol, kaolin-pectin, and metoclopramide may reduce digoxin absorption. Levothyroxine (and other thyroid supplements) may decrease digoxin blood levels. Penicillamine has been associated with reductions in digoxin blood levels The following reported interactions appear to be of limited clinical significance: Aminoglutethimide, aminosalicylic acid, aluminum-containing antacids, sucralfate, sulfasalazine, neomycin, ticlopidine.

Increased Effect/Toxicity: Beta-blocking agents (propranolol), verapamil, and diltiazem may have additive effects on heart rate. Carvedilol has additive effects on heart rate and inhibits the metabolism of digoxin. Digoxin levels may be increased by amiodarone (reduce digoxin dose 50%), bepridil, cyclosporine, diltiazem, indomethacin, itraconazole, some macrolides (erythromycin, clarithromycin), methimazole, nitrendipine, propafenone, propylthiouracil, quinidine (reduce digoxin dose 33% to 50% on initiation), tetracyclines, and verapamil. Moricizine may increase the toxicity of digoxin (mechanism undefined). Spironolactone may interfere with some digoxin assays, but may also increase blood levels directly. Succinylcholine administration to patients on digoxin has been associated with an increased risk of arrhythmias. Rare cases of acute digoxin toxicity have been associated with parenteral calcium (bolus) administration. The following medications have been associated with increased digoxin blood levels which appear to be of limited clinical significance: Famciclovir, flecainide, ibuprofen, fluoxetine, nefazodone, cimetidine, famotidine, ranitidine, omeprazole, trimethoprim.

Nutritional/Ethanol Interactions
Food: Digoxin peak serum levels may be decreased if taken with food. Meals containing increased fiber (bran) or foods high in pectin may decrease oral absorption of digoxin.

Herb/Nutraceutical: Avoid ephedra (risk of cardiac stimulation). Avoid natural licorice (causes sodium and water retention and increases potassium loss).

Adverse Reactions Incidence of reactions are not always reported.
Cardiovascular: Heart block; first-, second- (Wenckebach), or third-degree heart block; asystole; atrial tachycardia with block; AV dissociation; accelerated junctional rhythm; ventricular tachycardia or ventricular fibrillation; PR prolongation; ST segment depression

Central nervous system: Visual disturbances (blurred or yellow vision), headache (3%), dizziness (5%), apathy, confusion, mental disturbances (4%), anxiety, depression, delirium, hallucinations, fever

Dermatologic: Maculopapular rash (2%), erythematous, scarlatiniform, papular, vesicular or bullous rash, urticaria, pruritus, facial, angioneurotic or laryngeal edema, shedding of fingernails or toenails, alopecia

Gastrointestinal: Nausea (3%), vomiting (2%), diarrhea (3%), abdominal pain

Neuromuscular & skeletal: Weakness

Children are more likely to experience cardiac arrhythmia as a sign of excessive dosing. The most common are conduction disturbances or tachyarrhythmia (atrial tachycardia with or without block) and junctional tachycardia. Ventricular tachyarrhythmia are less common. In infants, sinus bradycardia may be a sign of digoxin toxicity. Any arrhythmia seen in a child on digoxin should be considered as digoxin toxicity. The gastrointestinal and central nervous system symptoms are not frequently seen in children.

Overdosage/Toxicology Manifested by a wide variety of signs and symptoms difficult to distinguish from effects associated with cardiac disease. Nausea and vomiting are common early signs of toxicity and may precede or follow evidence of cardiotoxicity. Other symptoms include anorexia, diarrhea, abdominal discomfort, headache, weakness, drowsiness, visual disturbances, mental depression, confusion, restlessness, disorientation, seizures, and hallucinations. Cardiac abnormalities include ventricular tachycardia, unifocal or multifocal PVCs (bigeminal, trigeminal), paroxysmal nodal rhythms, AV dissociation, excessive slowing of the pulse, AV block of varying degree, P-R prolongation, S-T depression, and occasional atrial fibrillation. Ventricular fibrillation is a common cause of death (alterations in cardiac rate and rhythm can result in any type of known arrhythmia).

Antidote: Life-threatening digoxin toxicity is treated with Digibind®. Administer potassium except in cases of complete heart block or renal failure. Digitalis-induced arrhythmias not responsive to potassium may be treated with phenytoin or lidocaine. Cholestyramine and colestipol may decrease absorption. Other agents to consider, based on ECG and clinical assessment, (Continued)

Digoxin *(Continued)*

include atropine, quinidine, procainamide, and propranolol. **Note:** Other antiarrhythmics appear more dangerous to use in toxicity.

Pharmacodynamics/Kinetics

Onset of Action: Oral: 1-2 hours; I.V.: 5-30 minutes; Peak effect: Oral: 2-8 hours; I.V.: 1-4 hours

Duration of Action: Adults: 3-4 days both forms

Time to Peak: Serum: Oral: ~1 hour

Protein Binding: 30%; in uremic patients, digoxin is displaced from plasma protein binding sites

Half-Life Elimination:

Age, renal and cardiac function dependent:

Neonates: Premature: 61-170 hours; Full-term: 35-45 hours

Infants: 18-25 hours

Children: 35 hours

Adults: 38-48 hours

Adults, anephric: 4-6 days

Parent drug: 38 hours; Metabolites: Digoxigenin: 4 hours; Monodigitoxoside: 3-12 hours

Metabolism: Via sequential sugar hydrolysis in the stomach or by reduction of lactone ring by intestinal bacteria (in ~10% of population, gut bacteria may metabolize up to 40% of digoxin dose); metabolites may contribute to therapeutic and toxic effects of digoxin; metabolism is reduced with CHF

Excretion: Urine (50% to 70% as unchanged drug)

Available Dosage Forms [DSC] = Discontinued product

Capsule (Lanoxicaps®): 50 mcg [DSC], 100 mcg, 200 mcg [contains ethyl alcohol]

Elixir: 50 mcg/mL (2.5 mL, 5 mL, 60 mL) [contains alcohol 10%; lime flavor]

Lanoxin® (pediatric): 50 mcg/mL (60 mL) [contains alcohol 10%; lime flavor] [DSC]

Injection: 250 mcg/mL (1 mL, 2 mL) [contains alcohol 10% and propylene glycol 40%]

Lanoxin®: 250 mcg/mL (2 mL) [contains alcohol 10% and propylene glycol 40%]

Injection, pediatric: 100 mcg/mL (1 mL) [contains alcohol 10% and propylene glycol 40%]

Tablet: 125 mcg, 250 mcg

Digitek®, Lanoxin®: 125 mcg, 250 mcg

Dosing

Adults:

Note: When changing from oral (tablets or liquid) or I.M. to I.V. therapy, dosage should be reduced by 20% to 25%.

Atrial dysrhythmias (rate control), CHF:

Initial: Total digitalizing dose: Give ½ of the total digitalizing dose (TDD) in the initial dose, then give ¼ of the TDD in each of two subsequent doses at 9- to 12-hour intervals. Obtain ECG 6 hours after each dose to assess potential toxicity.

Oral: 0.75-1.5 mg

I.V. or I.M.: 0.5-1 mg

Daily maintenance dose: Give once daily to children >10 years of age and adults.

Oral: 0.125-0.5 mg

I.V. or I.M.: 0.1-0.4 mg

Elderly: Dose is based on lean body weight and normal renal function for age. Decrease dose in patients with decreased renal function (see Dosing in Renal Impairment).

Pediatrics: Atrial dysrhythmias (rate control), CHF: When changing from oral (tablets or liquid) or I.M. to I.V. therapy, dosage should be reduced by 20% to 25%. See table.

Dosage Recommendations for Digoxin

Age	Total Digitalizing Dose[2] (mcg/kg[1])		Daily Maintenance Dose[3] (mcg/kg[1])	
	P.O.	I.V. or I.M.	P.O.	I.V. or I.M.
Preterm infant[1]	20-30	15-25	5-7.5	4-6
Full-term infant[1]	25-35	20-30	6-10	5-8
1 mo - 2 y[1]	35-60	30-50	10-15	7.5-12
2-5 y[1]	30-40	25-35	7.5-10	6-9
5-10 y[1]	20-35	15-30	5-10	4-8
>10 y[1]	10-15	8-12	2.5-5	2-3

[1]Based on lean body weight and normal renal function for age. Decrease dose in patients with ↓ renal function; digitalizing dose often not recommended in infants and children.

[2]Give one-half of the total digitalizing dose (TDD) in the initial dose, then give one-quarter of the TDD in each of two subsequent doses at 8- to 12-hour intervals. Obtain ECG 6 hours after each dose to assess potential toxicity.

[3]Divided every 12 hours in infants and children <10 years of age. Given once daily to children >10 years of age and adults.

Renal Impairment:

Cl_{cr} 10-50 mL/minute: Administer 25% to 75% of dose or every 36 hours.

Cl_{cr} <10 mL/minute: Administer 10% to 25% of dose or every 48 hours.

Reduce loading dose by 50% in ESRD.

Not dialyzable (0% to 5%)

Administration

I.M.: Inject no more than 2 mL per injection site. May cause intense pain.

I.V.: Inject slowly 1-5 minutes for undiluted form. May dilute up to fourfold with SWI, D_5W, or NS.

I.V. Detail: pH: 6.8-7.2

Stability

Compatibility: Stable in $D_5½NS$ with KCl 20 mEq, D_5W, $D_{10}W$, LR, ½NS, NS, and SWFI (when diluted fourfold or greater)

Y-site administration: Incompatible with amphotericin B cholesteryl sulfate complex, fluconazole, foscarnet, propofol

Compatibility in syringe: Incompatible with doxapram

Compatibility when admixed: Incompatible with dobutamine

Storage: Protect elixir and injection from light.

Laboratory Monitoring

When to draw serum digoxin concentrations: Digoxin serum levels should be drawn **at least 4 hours after an intravenous dose** and **at least 6 hours after an oral dose (optimally 12-24 hours after a dose).**

Initiation of therapy:

If a loading dose is given: Digoxin serum concentration may be drawn within 12-24 hours after the initial loading dose administration. Levels drawn this early may confirm the relationship of digoxin plasma levels and response but are of little value in determining maintenance doses.

If a loading dose is not given: Digoxin serum concentration should be obtained after 3-5 days of therapy.

Maintenance monitoring:

Trough concentrations should be followed just prior to the next dose or at a minimum of 4 hours after an I.V. dose and at least 6 hours after an oral dose.

Digoxin serum concentrations should be obtained within 5-7 days (approximate time to steady-state) after any dosage changes. Continue to obtain digoxin serum concentrations 7-14 days after any change in maintenance dose. **Note:** In patients with end-stage renal disease, it may take 15-20 days to reach steady-state.

Patients who are receiving potassium-depleting medications such as diuretics, should be monitored for potassium, magnesium, and calcium levels.

Digoxin serum concentrations should be obtained whenever any of the following conditions occur:

Questionable patient compliance or to evaluate clinical deterioration following an initial good response

Changing renal function

Suspected digoxin toxicity

Initiation or discontinuation of therapy with drugs (amiodarone, quinidine, verapamil) which potentially interact with digoxin; if quinidine therapy is started; digoxin levels should be drawn within the first 24 hours after starting quinidine therapy, then 7-14 days later or empirically skip one day's digoxin dose and decrease the daily dose by 50%.

Any disease changes (hypothyroidism)

Nursing Actions

Physical Assessment: Closely assess effects and interactions with other prescriptions, OTC medications, or herbal products patient may be taking. Monitor laboratory tests (when beginning or changing dosage, especially with I.V. administration and when patients are receiving diuretics or amphotericin). Monitor therapeutic response and adverse reactions at beginning of therapy, periodically throughout therapy, or when changing dosage. **I.V.:** Monitor ECG continuously. **Oral:** Monitor apical pulse before administering any dose. Assess knowledge/teach patient appropriate use, adverse reactions to report (especially noncardiac signs of toxicity — eg, anorexia, blurred vision, "yellow" vision, confusion) and appropriate interventions to reduce side effects.

Patient Education: Take as directed; do not discontinue without consulting prescriber. Maintain adequate dietary intake of potassium (do not increase without consulting prescriber). Adequate dietary potassium will reduce risk of digoxin toxicity. Take pulse at the same time each day; follow prescriber instructions for holding medication if pulse is <50. Notify prescriber of acute changes in pulse. Report loss of appetite, nausea, vomiting, persistent diarrhea, swelling of extremities, palpitations, "yellowing" or blurred vision, mental confusion or depression, or unusual fatigue. **Pregnancy precaution:** Inform prescriber if you are or intend to become pregnant.

Dietary Considerations Maintain adequate amounts of potassium in diet to decrease risk of hypokalemia (hypokalemia may increase risk of digoxin toxicity).

Geriatric Considerations Elderly may develop exaggerated serum/tissue concentrations due to age-related alterations in clearance and pharmacodynamic differences. Elderly are at risk for toxicity due to age-related changes.

Related Information
Peak and Trough Guidelines *on page 1387*

Digoxin Immune Fab (di JOKS in i MYUN fab)

U.S. Brand Names Digibind®; DigiFab™

Synonyms Antidigoxin Fab Fragments, Ovine

Pharmacologic Category Antidote

Pregnancy Risk Factor C

Lactation Excretion in breast milk unknown/use caution

Use Treatment of life-threatening or potentially life-threatening digoxin intoxication, including:

- acute digoxin ingestion (ie, >10 mg in adults or >4 mg in children)
- chronic ingestions leading to steady-state digoxin concentrations >6 ng/mL in adults or >4 ng/mL in children
- manifestations of digoxin toxicity due to overdose (life-threatening ventricular arrhythmias, progressive

bradycardia, second- or third-degree heart block not responsive to atropine, serum potassium >5 mEq/L in adults or >6 mEq/L in children)

Mechanism of Action/Effect Binds with molecules of digoxin or digitoxin and then is excreted by the kidneys and removed from the body

Contraindications Hypersensitivity to sheep products or any component of the formulation

Warnings/Precautions Suicidal attempts often involve multiple drugs. Consider other drug toxicities as well. Hypersensitivity reactions can occur. Epinephrine should be immediately available. Serum potassium levels should be monitored, especially during the first few hours after administration. Total serum digoxin concentrations will rise precipitously following administration of this drug (has no clinical meaning - avoid monitoring serum concentrations). If digoxin was being used to treat CHF then may see exacerbation of symptoms as digoxin level is reduced. Use with caution in renal failure (experience limited) - the complex will be removed from the body more slowly. Monitor for reoccurrence of digoxin toxicity. Has reversed thrombocytopenia induced by digoxin. Failure of response to adequate treatment may call diagnosis of digitalis toxicity into question. Digoxin immune Fab is processed with papain and may cause hypersensitivity reactions in patients allergic to papaya, other papaya extracts, papain, chymopapain, or the pineapple enzyme bromelain. There may also be cross allergy with dust mite and latex allergens.

Drug Interactions
Increased Effect/Toxicity: Digoxin: Following administration of digoxin immune Fab, serum digoxin levels are markedly increased due to bound complexes (may be clinically misleading, since bound complex cannot interact with receptors).

Lab Interactions Digibind® will interfere with digitalis immunoassay measurements - this will result in clinically misleading serum digoxin concentrations fragment is eliminated from the body (several days to >1 week after Digibind® administration).

Adverse Reactions Frequency not defined.

Cardiovascular: Effects (due to withdrawal of digitalis) include exacerbation of low cardiac output states and CHF, rapid ventricular response in patients with atrial fibrillation; postural hypotension

Endocrine & metabolic: Hypokalemia

Local: Phlebitis

Miscellaneous: Allergic reactions, serum sickness

Overdosage/Toxicology Symptoms of overdose include delayed serum sickness. Treatment of serum sickness includes acetaminophen, histamine$_1$ and possibly histamine$_2$ blockers, and corticosteroids.

Pharmacodynamics/Kinetics
Onset of Action: I.V.: Improvement in 2-30 minutes for toxicity

Half-Life Elimination: 15-20 hours; prolonged with renal impairment

Excretion: Urine; undetectable amounts within 5-7 days

Available Dosage Forms Injection, powder for reconstitution:

Digibind®: 38 mg

DigiFab™: 40 mg

Dosing
Adults & Elderly: Each vial of Digibind® 38 mg or DigiFab™ 40 mg will bind ~0.5 mg of digoxin or digitoxin.

Estimation of the dose is based on the body burden of digitalis. This may be calculated if the amount ingested is known or the postdistribution serum drug level is known (round dose to the nearest whole vial). See table on next page.

(Continued)

Digoxin Immune Fab (Continued)

Digoxin Immune Fab

Tablets Ingested (0.25 mg)	Fab Dose (vials)
5	2
10	4
25	10
50	20
75	30
100	40
150	60
200	80

Fab dose based on serum drug level postdistribution:

Digoxin: No. of vials = level (ng/mL) x body weight (kg) divided by 100

Digitoxin: No. of vials = digitoxin (ng/mL) x body weight (kg) divided by 1000

If neither amount ingested nor drug level are known, dose empirically as follows:

For acute toxicity: 20 vials, administered in 2 divided doses to decrease the possibility of a febrile reaction, and to avoid fluid overload in small children.

For chronic toxicity: 6 vials; for infants and small children (≤20 kg), a single vial may be sufficient.

Pediatrics:

Acute toxicity: I.V.: Refer to adult dosing.

Chronic toxicity: I.V.: If amount ingested and blood level are unknown:

Children ≤20 kg: 1 vial may be sufficient. If amount ingested or blood level is known, refer to adult dosing.

Children >20 kg: Refer to adult dosing.

Renal Impairment: Renal elimination of complexed digoxin may be decreased in renal failure. Potential "rebound" may occur when immune fragments are hepatically metabolized, leaving unbound digoxin.

Administration

I.V.: Continuous I.V. infusion over ≥30 minutes is preferred. Small doses (infants/small children) may be administered using tuberculin syringe.

I.V. Detail: Stopping the infusion and restarting at a slower rate may help if infusion-related reactions occur.

Stability

Reconstitution: Digoxin immune Fab is reconstituted by adding 4 mL sterile water, resulting in 10 mg/mL for I.V. infusion. The reconstituted solution may be further diluted with NS to a convenient volume (eg, 1 mg/mL). Reconstituted solutions should be used within 4 hours if refrigerated.

For very small doses, vial can be reconstituted by adding an additional 36 mL of sterile isotonic saline, to achieve a final concentration of 1 mg/mL.

Storage: Should be refrigerated at 2°C to 8°C.

Laboratory Monitoring Serum potassium, serum digoxin concentration prior to first dose of digoxin immune Fab, subsequent to start of Digibind® therapy; **digoxin levels will greatly increase and are not an accurate determination of body stores.**

Nursing Actions

Physical Assessment: Assess allergy history prior to administration. Monitor lab values, cardiac status, vital signs, blood pressure, and adverse reactions during and following infusion. Monitor for signs of reoccurrence of cardiac toxicity.

Patient Education: Patient education and instruction will be determined by patient condition and ability to understand. Immediately report dizziness, palpitations, cramping, respiratory difficulty, rash, or itching. **Pregnancy/breast-feeding precautions:** Inform prescriber if you are pregnant. Consult prescriber if breast-feeding.

Dihydrocodeine, Aspirin, and Caffeine
(dye hye droe KOE deen, AS pir in, & KAF een)

U.S. Brand Names Synalgos®-DC

Synonyms Dihydrocodeine Compound

Restrictions C-III

Pharmacologic Category Analgesic, Narcotic

Pregnancy Risk Factor B/D (prolonged use or high doses at term)

Lactation Excretion in breast milk unknown/use caution

Use Management of mild to moderate pain that requires relaxation

Available Dosage Forms Capsule: Dihydrocodeine bitartrate 16 mg, aspirin 356.4 mg, and caffeine 30 mg

Dosing

Adults: Pain: Oral: 1-2 capsules every 4-6 hours as needed

Elderly: Initial dosing should be cautious (low end of adult dosing range).

Nursing Actions

Physical Assessment: Assess for history of allergy (aspirin) and other medications patient may be taking for additive or adverse interactions. Monitor for effectiveness of pain relief and monitor for signs of overdose. Monitor blood pressure, CNS and respiratory status, and degree of sedation at beginning of therapy and at regular intervals with long-term use. May cause physical and/or psychological dependence. For inpatients, implement safety measures (eg, side rails up, call light within reach, instructions to call for assistance). Assess knowledge/teach patient appropriate use (if self-administered). Teach patient to monitor appropriate interventions to reduce side effects and adverse reactions to report.

Patient Education: If self-administered, use exactly as directed; do not increase dose or frequency. Drug may cause physical and/or psychological dependence. While using this medication, do not use alcohol and other prescription or OTC medications (especially sedatives, tranquilizers, antihistamines, or pain medications) without consulting prescriber. Maintain adequate hydration (2-3 L/day of fluids) unless instructed to restrict fluid intake. May cause dizziness, drowsiness, impaired coordination, or blurred vision (use caution when driving, climbing stairs, or changing position - rising from sitting or lying to standing or when engaging in tasks requiring alertness until response to drug is known); nausea or vomiting (frequent mouth care, small frequent meals, chewing gum, or sucking lozenges may help); or constipation (increased exercise, fluids, fruit, or fiber may help; if unresolved, consult prescriber about use of stool softeners). Report chest pain or rapid heartbeat; acute headache; swelling of extremities or unusual weight gain; changes in urinary elimination; acute headache; back or flank pain or spasms; or other adverse reactions. **Pregnancy/breast-feeding precautions:** Inform prescriber if you are or intend to become pregnant. Consult prescriber if breast-feeding.

Related Information
Aspirin *on page 114*

Dihydrocodeine, Pseudoephedrine, and Guaifenesin

(dye hye droe KOE, soo doe e FED rin, & gwye FEN e sin)

U.S. Brand Names DiHydro-GP; Hydro-Tussin™ EXP; Pancof®-EXP

Synonyms Guaifenesin, Dihydrocodeine, and Pseudoephedrine; Pseudoephedrine Hydrochloride, Guaifenesin, and Dihydrocodeine Bitartrate

Pharmacologic Category Antitussive/Decongestant/Expectorant

Pregnancy Risk Factor C

Use Temporary relief of cough and congestion associated with upper respiratory tract infections and allergies

Available Dosage Forms Syrup:

DiHydro-GP: Dihydrocodeine bitartrate 7.5 mg, pseudoephedrine hydrochloride 15 mg, and guaifenesin 100 mg per 5 mL (480 mL) [vanilla flavor]

Hydro-Tussin™ EXP, Pancof®-EXP: Dihydrocodeine bitartrate 7.5 mg, pseudoephedrine hydrochloride 15 mg, and guaifenesin 100 mg per 5 mL (480 mL) [alcohol free, dye free, sugar free]

Dosing

Adults:

Cough/congestion: Oral (Hydro-Tussin™ EXP, Pancof®-EXP): 5-10 mL every 4-6 hours as needed

Pediatrics:

Cough/congestion: Oral (Hydro-Tussin™ EXP, Pancof®-EXP): Children:

2-6 years: 1.25-2.5 mL every 4-6 hours as needed
6-12 years 2.5-5 mL every 4-6 hours as needed
≥12 years: Refer to adult dosing.

Nursing Actions

Physical Assessment: See individual agents.

Patient Education: See individual agents. **Pregnancy/breast-feeding precautions:** Inform prescriber if you are or intend to become pregnant. Consult prescriber if breast-feeding

---

Dihydroergotamine

(dye hye droe er GOT a meen)

U.S. Brand Names D.H.E. 45®; Migranal®

Synonyms DHE; Dihydroergotamine Mesylate

Pharmacologic Category Ergot Derivative

Pregnancy Risk Factor X

Lactation May be excreted in breast milk/contraindicated

Use Treatment of migraine headache with or without aura; injection also indicated for treatment of cluster headaches

Unlabeled/Investigational Use Adjunct for DVT prophylaxis for hip surgery, for orthostatic hypotension, xerostomia secondary to antidepressant use, and pelvic congestion with pain

Mechanism of Action/Effect Ergot alkaloid alpha-adrenergic blocker directly stimulates vascular smooth muscle to vasoconstrict peripheral and cerebral vessels; also has effects on serotonin receptors

Contraindications Hypersensitivity to dihydroergotamine or any component of the formulation; high-dose aspirin therapy; uncontrolled hypertension, ischemic heart disease, angina pectoris, history of MI, silent ischemia, or coronary artery vasospasm including Prinzmetal's angina; hemiplegic or basilar migraine; peripheral vascular disease; sepsis; severe hepatic or renal dysfunction; following vascular surgery; avoid use within 24 hours of sumatriptan, zolmitriptan, other serotonin agonists, or ergot-alkylating agents; avoid during or within 2 weeks of discontinuing MAO inhibitors; ergot alkaloids are contraindicated with potent inhibitors of CYP3A4 (includes protease inhibitors, azole antifungals, and some macrolide antibiotics); pregnancy

Warnings/Precautions Do not give to patients with risk factors for CAD until a cardiovascular evaluation has been performed; if evaluation is satisfactory, the healthcare provider should administer the first dose and cardiovascular status should be periodically evaluated. May cause vasospastic reactions; persistent vasospasm may lead to gangrene or death in patients with compromised circulation. Discontinue if signs of vasoconstriction develop. Rare reports of increased blood pressure in patients without history of hypertension. Rare reports of adverse cardiac events (acute MI, life-threatening arrhythmias, death) have been reported following use of the injection. Cerebral hemorrhage, subarachnoid hemorrhage, and stroke have also occurred following use of the injection. Not for prolonged use. Pleural and peritoneal fibrosis have been reported with prolonged daily use. Cardiac valvular fibrosis has also been associated with ergot alkaloids. Safety and efficacy in pediatric patients have not been established.

Drug Interactions

Cytochrome P450 Effect: Substrate of CYP3A4 (major); **Inhibits** CYP3A4 (weak)

Decreased Effect: Effects of dihydroergotamine may be diminished by antipsychotics, metoclopramide. Antianginal effects of nitrates may be reduced by ergot alkaloids.

Increased Effect/Toxicity: CYP3A4 inhibitors may increase the levels/effects of dihydroergotamine; example inhibitors include azole antifungals, clarithromycin, diclofenac, doxycycline, erythromycin, imatinib, isoniazid, nefazodone, nicardipine, propofol, protease inhibitors, quinidine, telithromycin, and verapamil. Ergot alkaloids are contraindicated with potent CYP3A4 inhibitors. Dihydroergotamine may increase the effects of 5-HT$_1$ agonists (eg, sumatriptan), MAO inhibitors, sibutramine, and other serotonin agonists (serotonin syndrome). Severe vasoconstriction may occur when peripheral vasoconstrictors or beta-blockers are used in patients receiving ergot alkaloids; concurrent use is contraindicated.

Adverse Reactions

>10%: Nasal spray: Respiratory: Rhinitis (26%)
1% to 10%: Nasal spray:

Central nervous system: Dizziness (4%), somnolence (3%)

Endocrine & metabolic: Hot flashes (1%)

Gastrointestinal: Nausea (10%), taste disturbance (8%), vomiting (4%), diarrhea (2%)

Local: Application site reaction (6%)

Neuromuscular & skeletal: Weakness (1%), stiffness (1%)

Respiratory: Pharyngitis (3%)

Overdosage/Toxicology Symptoms of overdose include peripheral ischemia, paresthesia, headache, nausea, and vomiting. Treatment is supportive. Activated charcoal is effective at binding ergot alkaloids.

Pharmacodynamics/Kinetics

Onset of Action: 15-30 minutes

Duration of Action: 3-4 hours

Time to Peak: Serum: I.M.: 15-30 minutes

Protein Binding: 93%

Half-Life Elimination: 1.3-3.9 hours

Metabolism: Extensively hepatic

Excretion: Primarily feces; urine (10% mostly as metabolites)

Available Dosage Forms

Injection, solution, as mesylate (D.H.E. 45®): 1 mg/mL (1 mL) [contains ethanol 94%]

Solution, intranasal spray, as mesylate (Migranal®): 4 mg/mL [0.5 mg/spray] (1 mL) [contains caffeine 10 mg/mL]

(Continued)

Dihydroergotamine *(Continued)*

Dosing

Adults:

Migraine, cluster headache:

I.M., SubQ: 1 mg at first sign of headache; repeat hourly to a maximum dose of 3 mg total; maximum dose: 6 mg/week

I.V.: 1 mg at first sign of headache; repeat hourly up to a maximum dose of 2 mg total; maximum dose: 6 mg/week

Intranasal: 1 spray (0.5 mg) of nasal spray should be administered into each nostril; if needed, repeat after 15 minutes, up to a total of 4 sprays. **Note:** Do not exceed 3 mg (6 sprays) in a 24-hour period and no more than 8 sprays in a week.

Elderly: Refer to adult dosing. Patients >65 years of age were not included in controlled clinical studies.

Renal Impairment: Contraindicated in severe renal impairment

Hepatic Impairment: Dosage reductions are probably necessary but specific guidelines are not available; contraindicated in severe hepatic dysfunction.

Administration

Other: Prior to administration of nasal spray, the nasal spray applicator must be primed (pumped 4 times); in order to let the drug be absorbed through the skin in the nose, patients should not inhale deeply through the nose while spraying or immediately after spraying; for best results, treatment should be initiated at the first symptom or sign of an attack; however, nasal spray can be used at any stage of a migraine attack

Stability

Storage:

Injection: Store below 25°C (77°F), do not refrigerate or freeze; protect from heat and light

Nasal spray: Prior to use, store below 25°C (77°F), do not refrigerate or freeze; once spray applicator has been prepared, use within 8 hours; discard any unused solution

Nursing Actions

Physical Assessment: Assess potential for interactions with other prescriptions, OTC medications, or herbal products patient may be taking. Monitor therapeutic response and adverse effects on a regular basis. Teach patient proper use for either nasal spray or injection (storage administration, injection technique, and syringe/needle disposal), possible side effects/appropriate interventions, and adverse symptoms to report. **Pregnancy risk factor X:** Determine that patient is not pregnant before starting therapy. Do not give to women of childbearing age, unless patient is capable of complying with contraceptive use. Breast-feeding is contraindicated.

Patient Education: Take this drug as rapidly as possible when first symptoms occur. May cause rare feelings of numbness or tingling of fingers, toes, or face (use caution and avoid injury) or drowsiness (use caution when driving or engaging in potentially hazardous tasks until response to drug is known). Report heart palpitations, severe nausea or vomiting, and severe numbness of fingers or toes.

Nasal spray: Follow directions for use on package insert. Wait 15 minutes between inhalations. Use no more than 4 inhalations (2 mg) for a single administration; do not use >3 mg (6 sprays) in a 24-hour period and no more than 8 sprays in a week.

I.M.: Follow directions for injections and needle disposal.

Pregnancy/breast-feeding precautions: Inform prescriber if you are pregnant. Consult prescriber for instruction on appropriate contraceptive measures. This drug may cause severe fetal defects. Do not breast-feed.

Geriatric Considerations Monitor cardiac and peripheral effects closely in the elderly since they often have cardiovascular disease and peripheral vascular impairment (ie, diabetes mellitus, PVD) that will complicate therapy and monitoring for adverse effects.

Breast-Feeding Issues Ergot derivatives inhibit prolactin and it is known that ergotamine is excreted in breast milk (vomiting, diarrhea, weak pulse, and unstable blood pressure have been reported in nursing infants). It is not known if dihydroergotamine would also cause these effects, however, it is likely that it is excreted in human breast milk. Do not use in nursing women.

Pregnancy Issues Dihydroergotamine is oxytocic and should not be used during pregnancy.

Diltiazem *(dil TYE a zem)*

U.S. Brand Names Cardizem®; Cardizem® CD; Cardizem® LA; Cardizem® SR [DSC]; Cartia XT™; Dilacor® XR; Diltia XT®; Taztia XT™; Tiazac®

Synonyms Diltiazem Hydrochloride

Pharmacologic Category Calcium Channel Blocker

Medication Safety Issues

Sound-alike/look-alike issues:

Diltiazem may be confused with Dilantin®

Cardizem® may be confused with Cardene®, Cardene SR®, Cardizem CD®, Cardizem SR®, cardiem

Cartia XT™ may be confused with Procardia XL®

Tiazac® may be confused with Tigan®, Ziac®

Pregnancy Risk Factor C

Lactation Enters breast milk/not recommended (AAP considers "compatible")

Use

Oral: Essential hypertension; chronic stable angina or angina from coronary artery spasm

Injection: Atrial fibrillation or atrial flutter; paroxysmal supraventricular tachycardia (PSVT)

Unlabeled/Investigational Use Investigational: Therapy of Duchenne muscular dystrophy

Mechanism of Action/Effect Inhibits calcium ion from entering the "slow channels" or select voltage-sensitive areas of vascular smooth muscle and myocardium during depolarization, producing a relaxation of coronary vascular smooth muscle and coronary vasodilation; increases myocardial oxygen delivery in patients with vasospastic angina

Contraindications Hypersensitivity to diltiazem or any component of the formulation; sick sinus syndrome; second- or third-degree AV block (except in patients with a functioning artificial pacemaker); hypotension (systolic <90 mm Hg); acute MI and pulmonary congestion

Warnings/Precautions Concomitant use with beta-blockers or digoxin can result in conduction disturbances. Avoid concurrent I.V. use of diltiazem and a beta-blocker. Use caution in left ventricular dysfunction (can exacerbate condition). Symptomatic hypotension can occur. Use with caution in hepatic or renal dysfunction.

Drug Interactions

Cytochrome P450 Effect: Substrate of CYP2C8/9 (minor), 2D6 (minor), 3A4 (major); **Inhibits** CYP2C8/9 (weak), 2D6 (weak), 3A4 (moderate)

Decreased Effect: Levels/effects of diltiazem may be decreased by aminoglutethimide, carbamazepine, nafcillin, nevirapine, phenobarbital, phenytoin, rifamycins, and other CYP3A4 inducers.

Increased Effect/Toxicity: Diltiazem effects may be additive with amiodarone, beta-blockers, or digoxin, which may lead to bradycardia, other conduction delays, and decreased cardiac output. The levels/effects of diltiazem may be increased by azole antifungals, clarithromycin, diclofenac, doxycycline, erythromycin, imatinib, isoniazid, nefazodone, nicardipine, propofol, protease inhibitors, quinidine, telithromycin, verapamil, and other CYP3A4 inhibitors.

Diltiazem may increase the levels/effects of selected benzodiazepines, calcium channel blockers, cisapride, cyclosporine, ergot alkaloids, selected HMG-CoA reductase inhibitors, mesoridazine, mirtazapine, nateglinide, nefazodone, pimozide, quinidine, sildenafil (and other PDE-5 inhibitors), tacrolimus, thioridazine, venlafaxine, and other CYP3A4 substrates. Blood pressure-lowering effects may be additive with sildenafil, tadalafil, and vardenafil (use caution).

Nutritional/Ethanol Interactions

Ethanol: Avoid ethanol (may increase risk of hypotension or vasodilation).

Food: Diltiazem serum levels may be elevated if taken with food. Serum concentrations were not altered by grapefruit juice in small clinical trials.

Herb/Nutraceutical: St John's wort may decrease diltiazem levels. Avoid dong quai if using for hypertension (has estrogenic activity). Avoid ephedra (may worsen arrhythmia or hypertension). Avoid yohimbe, ginseng (may worsen hypertension). Avoid garlic (may have increased antihypertensive effect).

Adverse Reactions Note: Frequencies represent ranges for various dosage forms. Patients with impaired ventricular function and/or conduction abnormalities may have higher incidence of adverse reactions.

>10%:

Cardiovascular: Edema (2% to 15%)

Central nervous system: Headache (5% to 12%)

2% to 10%:

Cardiovascular: AV block (first degree 2% to 8%), edema (lower limb 2% to 8%), pain (6%), bradycardia (2% to 6%), hypotension (<2% to 4%), vasodilation (2% to 3%), extrasystoles (2%), flushing (1% to 2%), palpitation (1% to 2%)

Central nervous system: Dizziness (3% to 10%), nervousness (2%)

Dermatologic: Rash (1% to 4%)

Endocrine & metabolic: Gout (1% to 2%)

Gastrointestinal: Dyspepsia (1% to 6%), constipation (<2% to 4%), vomiting (2%), diarrhea (1% to 2%)

Local: Injection site reactions: Burning, itching (4%)

Neuromuscular & skeletal: Weakness (1% to 4%), myalgia (2%)

Respiratory: Rhinitis (<2% to 10%), pharyngitis (2% to 6%), dyspnea (1% to 6%), bronchitis (1% to 4%), sinus congestion (1% to 2%)

Overdosage/Toxicology Primary cardiac symptoms of calcium blocker overdose include hypotension and bradycardia. Noncardiac symptoms include confusion, stupor, nausea, vomiting, metabolic acidosis, and hyperglycemia.

Following initial gastric decontamination, if possible, repeated calcium administration may promptly reverse depressed cardiac contractility (but not sinus node depression or peripheral vasodilation). Glucagon, epinephrine, and amrinone may treat refractory hypotension. Glucagon and epinephrine also increase heart rate (outside the U.S., 4-aminopyridine may be available as an antidote). Dialysis and hemoperfusion are not effective in enhancing elimination although repeat-dose activated charcoal may serve as an adjunct with sustained-release preparations.

Pharmacodynamics/Kinetics

Onset of Action: Oral: Immediate release tablet: 30-60 minutes

Time to Peak: Serum: Immediate release tablet: 2-4 hours

Protein Binding: 70% to 80%

Half-Life Elimination: Immediate release tablet: 3-4.5 hours, may be prolonged with renal impairment

Metabolism: Hepatic; extensive first-pass effect; following single I.V. injection, plasma concentrations of N-monodesmethyldiltiazem and desacetyldiltiazem are typically undetectable; however, these metabolites accumulate to detectable concentrations following 24-hour constant rate infusion. N-monodesmethyldiltiazem appears to have 20% of the potency of diltiazem; desacetyldiltiazem is about 25% to 50% as potent as the parent compound.

Excretion: Urine and feces (primarily as metabolites)

Available Dosage Forms [DSC] = Discontinued product

Capsule, extended release, as hydrochloride [once-daily dosing]: 120 mg, 180 mg, 240 mg, 300 mg

Cardizem® CD: 120 mg, 180 mg, 240 mg, 300 mg, 360 mg

Cartia XT™: 120 mg, 180 mg, 240 mg, 300 mg

Dilacor® XR, Diltia XT®: 120 mg, 180 mg, 240 mg

Taztia XT™: 120 mg, 180 mg, 240 mg, 300 mg, 360 mg

Tiazac®: 120 mg, 180 mg, 240 mg, 300 mg, 360 mg, 420 mg

Capsule, sustained release, as hydrochloride [twice-daily dosing] (Cardizem® SR [DSC]): 60 mg, 90 mg, 120 mg

Injection, solution, as hydrochloride: 5 mg/mL (5 mL, 10 mL, 25 mL)

Injection, powder for reconstitution, as hydrochloride (Cardizem®): 25 mg

Tablet, as hydrochloride (Cardizem®): 30 mg, 60 mg, 90 mg, 120 mg

Tablet, extended release, as hydrochloride (Cardizem® LA): 120 mg, 180 mg, 240 mg, 300 mg, 360 mg, 420 mg

Dosing

Adults:

Angina: Oral:

Capsule, extended release (Cardizem® CD, Cartia XT™, Dilacor® XR, Diltia XT®, Tiazac®): Initial: 120-180 mg once daily (maximum dose: 480 mg/day)

Tablet, extended release (Cardizem® LA): 180 mg once daily; may increase at 7- to 14-day intervals (maximum recommended dose: 360 mg/day)

Tablet, immediate release (Cardizem®): Usual starting dose: 30 mg 4 times/day; usual range: 180-360 mg/day

Hypertension: Oral:

Capsule, extended release (Cardizem® CD, Cartia XT™, Dilacor® XR, Diltia XT®, Tiazac®): Initial: 180-240 mg once daily; dose adjustment may be made after 14 days; usual dose range (JNC 7): 180-420 mg/day; Tiazac®: usual dose range: 120-540 mg/day

Capsule, sustained release (Cardizem® SR): Initial: 60-120 mg twice daily; dose adjustment may be made after 14 days; usual range: 240-360 mg/day

Tablet, extended release (Cardizem® LA): Initial: 180-240 mg once daily; dose adjustment may be made after 14 days; usual dose range (JNC 7): 120-540 mg/day

Atrial fibrillation, atrial flutter, PSVT: I.V.:

Initial bolus dose: 0.25 mg/kg actual body weight over 2 minutes (average adult dose: 20 mg)

Repeat bolus dose (may be administered after 15 minutes if the response is inadequate): 0.35 mg/kg actual body weight over 2 minutes (average adult dose: 25 mg)

Continuous infusion (requires an infusion pump; infusions >24 hours or infusion rates >15 mg/hour are not recommended): Initial infusion rate of 10 mg/hour; rate may be increased in 5 mg/hour increments up to 15 mg/hour as needed; some patients may respond to an initial rate of 5 mg/hour.

(Continued)

Diltiazem (Continued)

If diltiazem injection is administered by continuous infusion for >24 hours, the possibility of decreased diltiazem clearance, prolonged elimination half-life, and increased diltiazem and/or diltiazem metabolite plasma concentrations should be considered.

Conversion from I.V. diltiazem to oral diltiazem: Start oral approximately 3 hours after bolus dose.

Oral dose (mg/day) is approximately equal to [rate (mg/hour) x 3 + 3] x 10.

3 mg/hour = 120 mg/day
5 mg/hour = 180 mg/day
7 mg/hour = 240 mg/day
11 mg/hour = 360 mg/day

Elderly: Refer to adult dosing. **Note:** Patients ≥60 years may respond to a lower initial dose (eg, 120 mg once daily using extended release capsule)

Pediatrics:

Children: Minimal information available; some centers use the following:

Hypertension: Oral: Initial: 1.5-2 mg/kg/day in 3-4 divided doses; maximum dose: 3.5 mg/kg/day

Note: Doses up to 8 mg/kg/day given in 4 divided doses have been used for investigational therapy of Duchenne muscular dystrophy

Adolescents: Refer to adult dosing.

Renal Impairment: Use with caution as diltiazem is extensively metabolized by the liver and excreted in the kidneys and bile. Not removed by hemo- or peritoneal dialysis; supplemental dose is not necessary.

Hepatic Impairment: Use with caution as diltiazem is extensively metabolized by the liver and excreted in the kidneys and bile.

Administration

Oral: Do not crush long acting dosage forms.

Tiazac®: Capsules may be opened and sprinkled on a spoonful of applesauce. Applesauce should be swallowed without chewing, followed by drinking a glass of water.

I.V.: Bolus doses given over 2 minutes with continuous ECG and blood pressure monitoring. Continuous infusion should be via infusion pump.

I.V. Detail: Response to bolus may require several minutes to reach maximum. Response may persist for several hours after infusion is discontinued.

pH: 3.7-4.1

Stability

Compatibility: Stable in $D_5\frac{1}{2}NS$, D_5W, NS

Y-site administration: Incompatible with diazepam, furosemide, phenytoin, rifampin, thiopental

Storage:

Capsule, tablet: Store at controlled room temperature.

Solution for injection: Store in refrigerator at 2°C to 8°C (36°F to 46°F). May be stored at room temperature for up to one month; do not freeze. Following dilution with $D_5$1/2NS, D_5W, or NS, solution is stable for 24 hours at room temperature or under refrigeration.

Laboratory Monitoring Liver function tests

Nursing Actions

Physical Assessment: Assess other pharmacological or herbal products patient may be taking for potential interactions (eg, increased risk of bradycardia, conduction delays, decreased cardiac output). I.V. requires use of infusion pump and continuous cardiac and hemodynamic monitoring. Monitor therapeutic effectiveness according to purpose for use (hypertension, angina, atrial fib/flutter or PSVT) and adverse reactions (see Adverse Reactions) when beginning therapy, when changing dose, and periodically during long-term therapy. Teach patient appropriate use (oral), interventions to reduce side effects, and adverse symptoms to report.

Patient Education: Do not take any new medication during therapy unless approved by prescriber. Oral: Take as directed; do not alter dosage or discontinue therapy without consulting prescriber. Do not crush or chew extended release form. Avoid (or limit) alcohol and caffeine. May cause dizziness or lightheadedness (use caution when driving or engaging in tasks requiring alertness until response to drug is known); nausea or vomiting (small, frequent meals, frequent mouth care, chewing gum, or sucking lozenges may help); constipation (increased exercise, fluids, fruit, or fiber may help); or diarrhea (buttermilk, boiled milk, or yogurt may help). Report chest pain, palpitations, irregular heartbeat; unusual cough, respiratory difficulty; swelling of extremities; muscle tremors or weakness; confusion or acute lethargy; skin rash; or other adverse reactions. **Pregnancy/breast-feeding precautions:** Inform prescriber if you are or intend to become pregnant. Consult prescriber if breast-feeding.

Geriatric Considerations Elderly may experience a greater hypotensive response.

Breast-Feeding Issues Freely diffuses into breast milk; however, the AAP considers diltiazem to be **compatible** with breast-feeding. Available evidence suggest safe use during breast-feeding.

Pregnancy Issues Teratogenic and embryotoxic effects have been demonstrated in small animals.

Dimethyl Sulfoxide (dye meth il sul FOKS ide)

U.S. Brand Names Rimso®-50

Synonyms DMSO

Pharmacologic Category Urinary Tract Product

Pregnancy Risk Factor C

Lactation Excretion in breast milk unknown

Use Symptomatic relief of interstitial cystitis

Drug Interactions

Cytochrome P450 Effect: Inhibits CYP2C8/9 (weak), 2C19 (weak)

Adverse Reactions

>10%: Gastrointestinal: Garlic-like breath

1% to 10%:

Central nervous system: Headache, sedation

Gastrointestinal: Nausea, vomiting

Local: Local dermatitis

Ocular: Burning eyes

Available Dosage Forms Solution, intravesical: 50% [500 mg/mL] (50 mL)

Dosing

Adults & Elderly: Interstitial cystitis: Not for I.M. or I.V. administration; only for bladder instillation. Instill 50 mL of solution directly into bladder and allow to remain for 15 minutes. Repeat in 2 weeks or until symptoms are relieved, then increase intervals between treatments.

Nursing Actions

Physical Assessment: For bladder instillation only. Assess knowledge/teach patient interventions to reduce side effects and adverse symptoms to report.

Patient Education: This medication is only for use as a bladder instillation. Maintain adequate hydration (2-3 L/day of fluids) unless instructed to restrict fluid intake. Report persistent adverse reactions. **Pregnancy/breast-feeding precautions:** Inform prescriber if you are or intend to become pregnant. Note breast-feeding caution.

Dinoprostone (dye noe PROST one)

U.S. Brand Names Cervidil®; Prepidil®; Prostin E_2®

Synonyms PGE_2; Prostaglandin E_2

Pharmacologic Category Abortifacient; Prostaglandin

Medication Safety Issues

Sound-alike/look-alike issues:

Prepidil® may be confused with Bepridil®

Pregnancy Risk Factor C

Lactation Excretion in breast milk unknown/opportunity for use is minimal

Use

Gel: Promote cervical ripening prior to labor induction; usage for gel include any patient undergoing induction of labor with an unripe cervix, most commonly for pre-eclampsia, eclampsia, postdates, diabetes, intrauterine growth retardation, and chronic hypertension

Suppositories: Terminate pregnancy from 12th through 28th week of gestation; evacuate uterus in cases of missed abortion or intrauterine fetal death; manage benign hydatidiform mole

Vaginal insert: Initiation and/or cervical ripening in patients at or near term in whom there is a medical or obstetrical indication for the induction of labor

Mechanism of Action/Effect A synthetic prostaglandin E_2 abortifacient that stimulates uterine contractions similar to those seen during natural labor

Contraindications

Vaginal insert: Hypersensitivity to prostaglandins; fetal distress (suspicion or clinical evidence unless delivery is imminent); unexplained vaginal bleeding during this pregnancy; strong suspicion of marked cephalopelvic disproportion; patients in whom oxytoxic drugs are contraindicated or when prolonged contraction of the uterus may be detrimental to fetal safety or uterine integrity (including previous cesarean section or major uterine surgery); greater than 6 previous term pregnancies; patients already receiving oxytoxic drugs

Gel: Hypersensitivity to prostaglandins or any constituents of the cervical gel, history of asthma, contracted pelvis, malpresentation of the fetus. The following are "relative" contraindications and should only be considered by the physician under these circumstances: Patients in whom vaginal delivery is not indicated (ie, herpes genitalia with a lesion at the time of delivery), prior uterine surgery, breech presentation, multiple gestation, polyhydramnios, premature rupture of membranes

Suppository: Hypersensitivity to dinoprostone, acute pelvic inflammatory disease, uterine fibroids, cervical stenosis

Warnings/Precautions Dinoprostone should be used only by medically trained personnel in a hospital; caution in patients with cervicitis, infected endocervical lesions, acute vaginitis, compromised (scarred) uterus or history of asthma, hypertension or hypotension, epilepsy, diabetes mellitus, anemia, jaundice, or cardiovascular, renal, or hepatic disease. Oxytocin should not be used simultaneously with Prepidil® (>6 hours of the last dose of Prepidil®).

Drug Interactions

Increased Effect/Toxicity: Dinoprostone may increase the effect of oxytocin; wait 6-12 hours after dinoprostone administration before initiating oxytocin.

Adverse Reactions

>10%:

Central nervous system: Headache

Gastrointestinal: Vomiting, diarrhea, nausea

1% to 10%:

Cardiovascular: Bradycardia

Central nervous system: Fever

Neuromuscular & skeletal: Back pain

Overdosage/Toxicology Symptoms of overdose include vomiting, bronchospasm, hypotension, chest pain, abdominal cramps, and uterine contractions. Treatment is symptomatic.

Pharmacodynamics/Kinetics

Onset of Action: Uterine contractions: Within 10 minutes

Duration of Action: Up to 2-3 hours

Metabolism: In many tissues including the renal, pulmonary, and splenic systems

Excretion: Primarily urine; feces (small amounts)

Available Dosage Forms

Gel, endocervical (Prepidil®): 0.5 mg/3 g syringe [each package contains a 10 mm and 20 mm shielded catheter]

Insert, vaginal (Cervidil®): 10 mg [releases 0.3 mg/hour]

Suppository, vaginal (Prostin E_2®): 20 mg

Dosing

Adults & Elderly:

Abortifacient: Insert 1 suppository high in vagina, repeat at 3- to 5-hour intervals until abortion occurs up to 240 mg (maximum); continued administration for longer than 2 days is not advisable.

Cervical ripening:

Gel:

Intracervical: 0.25-1 mg

Intravaginal: 2.5 mg

Suppositories, intracervical: 2-3 mg

Vaginal insert (Cervidil®): Intracervical: 10 mg; remove upon onset of active labor or after 12 hours.

Administration

Other:

Endocervical gel: Intracervically: For cervical ripening, patient should be supine in the dorsal position

Vaginal insert: One vaginal insert is placed transversely in the posterior fornix of the vagina immediately after removal from its foil package. Patients should remain in the recumbent position for 2 hours after insertion, but thereafter may be ambulatory

Vaginal suppository: Bring to room temperature just prior to use. Patient should remain supine for 10 minutes following insertion.

Stability

Storage: Suppositories must be kept frozen, store in freezer not above -20°C (-4°F). Bring to room temperature just prior to use. Cervical gel should be stored under refrigeration 2°C to 8°C (36°F to 46°F).

Nursing Actions

Physical Assessment: Monitor temperature closely. Monitor uterine tone and vaginal discharge closely throughout procedure and postprocedure. Monitor abortion for completeness (other measures may be necessary if incomplete). Assess knowledge/teach patient interventions to reduce side effects and adverse symptoms to report.

Patient Education: Nausea and vomiting, cramping or uterine pain, or fever may occur. Report acute pain, respiratory difficulty, or skin rash. Closely monitor for vaginal discharge for several days. Report vaginal bleeding, itching, malodorous or bloody discharge, or severe cramping.

Additional Information Commercially available suppositories should not be used for extemporaneous preparation of any other dosage form of drug.

DiphenhydrAMINE (dye fen HYE dra meen)

U.S. Brand Names Aler-Cap [OTC]; Aler-Dryl [OTC]; Aler-Tab [OTC]; AllerMax® [OTC]; Altaryl [OTC]; Banophen® [OTC]; Banophen® Anti-Itch [OTC]; Benadryl® Allergy [OTC]; Benadryl® Children's Allergy [OTC]; Benadryl® Children's Allergy Fastmelt® [OTC]; Benadryl® Dye-Free Allergy [OTC]; Benadryl® Injection; Benadryl® Itch Stopping [OTC]; Benadryl® Itch Stopping Extra Strength [OTC]; Compoz® Nighttime Sleep Aid (Continued)

DiphenhydrAMINE *(Continued)*

[OTC]; Dermamycin® [OTC]; Dermarest® Insect Bite [OTC]; Dermarest® Plus [OTC]; Diphen® [OTC]; Diphen® AF [OTC]; Diphenhist [OTC]; Dytan™; Genahist® [OTC]; Hydramine® [OTC]; Nytol® Quick Caps [OTC]; Nytol® Quick Gels [OTC]; Q-Dryl [OTC]; Quenalin [OTC]; Siladryl® Allergy [OTC]; Siladryl® DAS [OTC]; Silphen® [OTC]; Simply Sleep® [OTC]; Sleep-ettes D [OTC]; Sleepinal® [OTC]; Sominex® [OTC]; Sominex® Maximum Strength [OTC]; Triaminic® Thin Strips™ Cough and Runny Nose [OTC]; Twilite® [OTC]; Unisom® Maximum Strength SleepGels® [OTC]

Synonyms Diphenhydramine Citrate; Diphenhydramine Hydrochloride; Diphenhydramine Tannate

Pharmacologic Category Antihistamine

Medication Safety Issues

Sound-alike/look-alike issues:

DiphenhydrAMINE may be confused with desipramine, dicyclomine, dimenhyDRINATE

Benadryl® may be confused with benazepril, Bentyl®, Benylin®, Caladryl®

Pregnancy Risk Factor B

Lactation Enters breast milk/contraindicated

Use Symptomatic relief of allergic symptoms caused by histamine release which include nasal allergies and allergic dermatosis; can be used for mild nighttime sedation; prevention of motion sickness and as an antitussive; has antinauseant and topical anesthetic properties; treatment of antipsychotic-induced extrapyramidal symptoms

Mechanism of Action/Effect Competes with histamine for H_1-receptor sites on effector cells in the gastrointestinal tract, blood vessels, and respiratory tract; anticholinergic and sedative effects are also seen

Contraindications Hypersensitivity to diphenhydramine or any component of the formulation; acute asthma; not for use in neonates

Warnings/Precautions Causes sedation, caution must be used in performing tasks which require alertness (eg, operating machinery or driving). Sedative effects of CNS depressants or ethanol are potentiated. Use with caution in patients with angle-closure glaucoma, pyloroduodenal obstruction (including stenotic peptic ulcer), urinary tract obstruction (including bladder neck obstruction and symptomatic prostatic hyperplasia), hyperthyroidism, increased intraocular pressure, and cardiovascular disease (including hypertension and tachycardia). Diphenhydramine has high sedative and anticholinergic properties, so it may not be considered the antihistamine of choice for prolonged use in the elderly. May cause paradoxical excitation in pediatric patients, and can result in hallucinations, coma, and death in overdose. Some preparations contain sodium bisulfite; syrup formulations may contain alcohol. Some preparations contain soy protein; patients with soy protein or peanut allergies should avoid.

Drug Interactions

Cytochrome P450 Effect: Inhibits CYP2D6 (moderate)

Decreased Effect: Diphenhydramine may decrease the levels/effects of CYP2D6 prodrug substrates; example prodrug substrates include codeine, hydrocodone, oxycodone, and tramadol. May increase gastric degradation of levodopa and decrease the amount of levodopa absorbed by delaying gastric emptying. Therapeutic effects of cholinergic agents (tacrine, donepezil) and neuroleptics may be antagonized.

Increased Effect/Toxicity: Diphenhydramine may increase the levels/effects of amphetamines, selected beta-blockers, dextromethorphan, fluoxetine, lidocaine, mirtazapine, nefazodone, paroxetine, risperidone, ritonavir, thioridazine, tricyclic antidepressants, venlafaxine and other CYP2D6 substrates. CNS depressants may increase the degree of sedation and

respiratory depression with diphenhydramine. May increase the absorption of digoxin. Central and/or peripheral anticholinergic syndrome can occur when administered with amantadine, rimantadine, narcotic analgesics, phenothiazines and other antipsychotics (especially with high anticholinergic activity), tricyclic antidepressants, quinidine, disopyramide, procainamide, and antihistamines. Syrup should not be given to patients taking drugs that can cause disulfiram reactions (ie, metronidazole, chlorpropamide) due to high alcohol content.

Nutritional/Ethanol Interactions

Ethanol: Avoid ethanol (may increase CNS depression).

Herb/Nutraceutical: Avoid valerian, St John's wort, kava kava, gotu kola (may increase CNS depression).

Lab Interactions May suppress the wheal and flare reactions to skin test antigens.

Adverse Reactions Frequency not defined.

Cardiovascular: Hypotension, palpitation, tachycardia

Central nervous system: Sedation, sleepiness, dizziness, disturbed coordination, headache, fatigue, nervousness, paradoxical excitement, insomnia, euphoria, confusion

Dermatologic: Photosensitivity, rash, angioedema, urticaria

Gastrointestinal: Nausea, vomiting, diarrhea, abdominal pain, xerostomia, appetite increase, weight gain, dry mucous membranes, anorexia

Genitourinary: Urinary retention, urinary frequency, difficult urination

Hematologic: Hemolytic anemia, thrombocytopenia, agranulocytosis

Neuromuscular & skeletal: Tremor, paresthesia

Ocular: blurred vision

Respiratory: Thickening of bronchial secretions

Overdosage/Toxicology Symptoms of overdose include CNS stimulation or depression; overdose may result in death in infants and children. There is no specific treatment for antihistamine overdose. Clinical toxicity is due to blockade of cholinergic receptors. For anticholinergic overdose with life-threatening symptoms, physostigmine 1-2 mg SubQ or I.V. slowly may be given to reverse these effects.

Pharmacodynamics/Kinetics

Onset of Action: Maximum sedative effect: 1-3 hours

Duration of Action: 4-7 hours

Time to Peak: Serum: 2-4 hours

Protein Binding: 78%

Half-Life Elimination: 2-8 hours; Elderly: 13.5 hours

Metabolism: Extensively hepatic; smaller degrees in pulmonary and renal systems; significant first-pass effect

Excretion: Urine (as unchanged drug)

Available Dosage Forms

Caplet, as hydrochloride: 25 mg, 50 mg

Aler-Dryl, AllerMax®, Compoz® Nighttime Sleep Aid, Sleep-ettes D, Sominex® Maximum Strength, Twilite®: 50 mg

Simply Sleep®, Nytol® Quick Caps: 25 mg

Capsule, as hydrochloride: 25 mg, 50 mg

Aler-Cap, Banophen®, Benadryl® Allergy, Diphen®, Diphenhist, Genahist®, Q-Dryl: 25 mg

Sleepinal®: 50 mg

Capsule, softgel, as hydrochloride: 50 mg

Benadryl® Dye-Free Allergy: 25 mg [dye-free]

Compoz® Nighttime Sleep Aid, Nytol® Quick Gels, Sleepinal®, Unisom® Maximum Strength Sleep-Gels®: 50 mg

Captab, as hydrochloride (Diphenhist®): 25 mg

Cream, as hydrochloride: 2% (30 g) [contains zinc acetate 0.1%]

Banophen® Anti-Itch: 2% (30 g) [contains zinc acetate 0.1%]

Benadryl® Itch Stopping: 1% (30 g) [contains zinc acetate 0.1%]

Benadryl® Itch Stopping Extra Strength: 2% (30 g) [contains zinc acetate 0.1%]

Diphenhist®: 2% (30 g) [contains zinc acetate 0.1%]

Elixir, as hydrochloride:

Altaryl: 12.5 mg/5 mL (120 mL, 480 mL, 3840 mL) [cherry flavor]

Banophen®: 12.5 mg/5 mL (120 mL)

Diphen AF: 12.5 mg/5 mL (120 mL, 240 mL, 480 mL) [alcohol free; cherry flavor]

Q-Dryl: 12.5 mg/5 mL (480 mL) [alcohol free]

Gel, topical, as hydrochloride:

Benadryl® Itch Stopping Extra Strength: 2% (120 mL)

Dermarest® Plus: 2% (28 g, 42 g) [contains menthol 1%]

Injection, solution, as hydrochloride: 50 mg/mL (1 mL)

Benadryl®: 50 mg/mL (1 mL, 10 mL)

Liquid, as hydrochloride:

AllerMax®: 12.5 mg/5 mL (120 mL)

Benadryl® Allergy: 12.5 mg/5 mL (120 mL, 240 mL) [alcohol free; contains sodium benzoate; cherry flavor]

Benadryl® Dye-Free Allergy: 12.5 mg/5 mL (120 mL) [alcohol free, dye free, sugar free; contains sodium benzoate; bubble gum flavor]

Genahist®: 12.5 mg/5 mL (120 mL) [alcohol free, sugar free; contains sodium benzoate; cherry flavor]

Hydramine®: 12.5 mg/5 mL (120 mL, 480 mL) [alcohol free]

Q-Dryl: 12.5 mg/5 mL (120 mL) [alcohol free; cherry flavor]

Quenalin: 12.5 mg/5 mL (120 mL) [fruit flavor]

Siladryl® Allergy: 12.5 mg/5 mL (120 mL, 240 mL, 480 mL) [alcohol free, sugar free; black cherry flavor]

Siladryl® DAS: 12.5 mg/5 mL (120 mL) [alcohol free, dye free, sugar free; black cherry flavor]

Liquid, topical, as hydrochloride [stick] (Benadryl® Itch Stopping Extra Strength): 2% (14 mL) [contains zinc acetate 0.1% and alcohol]

Solution, oral, as hydrochloride:

Banophen®: 12.5 mg/5mL (480 mL) [sugar free]

Diphenhist: 12.5 mg/5 mL (120 mL, 480 mL) [alcohol free; contains sodium benzoate]

Solution, topical, as hydrochloride [spray]:

Benadryl® Itch Stopping Extra Strength: 2% (60 mL) [contains zinc acetate 0.1% and alcohol]

Dermamycin®, Dermarest® Insect Bite: 2% (60 mL) [contains menthol 1%]

Strips, oral, as hydrochloride (Triaminic® Thin Strips™ Cough and Runny Nose): 12. 5 mg (16s) [grape flavor]

Suspension, as tannate (Dytan™): 25 mg/5 mL (120 mL) [strawberry flavor]

Syrup, as hydrochloride (Silphen® Cough): 12.5 mg/5 mL (120 mL, 240 mL, 480 mL) [contains alcohol; 5%; strawberry flavor]

Tablet, as hydrochloride: 25 mg, 50 mg

Aler-Tab, Benadryl® Allergy, Genahist®, Sleepinal®, Sominex®: 25 mg

Tablet, chewable, as hydrochloride (Benadryl® Children's Allergy): 12.5 mg [contains phenylalanine 4.2 mg/tablet; grape flavor]

Tablet, chewable, as tannate (Dytan™): 25 mg [contains phenylalanine; strawberry flavor]

Tablet, orally disintegrating, as citrate (Benadryl® Children's Allergy Fastmelt®): 19 mg [equivalent to diphenhydramine hydrochloride 12.5 mg; contains phenylalanine 4.5 mg/tablet and soy protein isolate; cherry flavor]

Dosing

Adults:

Minor allergic rhinitis or motion sickness: Oral: 25-50 mg every 4-6 hours; maximum: 300 mg/day

Moderate to severe allergic reactions:

Oral: 25-50 mg every 4 hours, not to exceed 400 mg/day

I.M., I.V.: 10-50 mg in a single dose every 2-4 hours, not to exceed 400 mg/day

Night-time sleep aid: Oral: 50 mg at bedtime

Dystonic reaction: I.M., I.V.: 50 mg in a single dose; may repeat in 20-30 minutes if necessary

Allergic dermatosis: Topical: For external application, not longer than 7 days

Elderly: Initial: 25 mg 2-3 times/day increasing as needed

Pediatrics:

Treatment of dystonic reactions and moderate to severe allergic reactions: Oral, I.M., I.V.: 5 mg/kg/day or 150 mg/m²/day in divided doses every 6-8 hours, not to exceed 300 mg/day

Minor allergic rhinitis or motion sickness: Oral, I.M., I.V.:

2 to <6 years: 6.25 mg every 4-6 hours; maximum: 37.5 mg/day

6 to <12 years: 12.5-25 mg every 4-6 hours; maximum: 150 mg/day

≥12 years: 25-50 mg every 4-6 hours; maximum: 300 mg/day

Night-time sleep aid: 30 minutes before bedtime: Oral, I.M., I.V.:

2 to <12 years: 1 mg/kg/dose; maximum: 50 mg/dose

≥12 years: 50 mg

Antitussive: Oral, I.M., I.V.:

2 to <6 years: 6.25 mg every 4 hours; maximum 37.5 mg/day

6 to <12 years: 12.5 mg every 4 hours; maximum 75 mg/day

≥12 years: 25 mg every 4 hours; maximum 150 mg/day

Administration

I.V. Detail: pH: 5-6

Stability

Compatibility: Stable in dextran 6% in dextrose, dextran 6% in NS, D₅LR, D₅¼NS, D₅½NS, D₅NS, D₅W, D₁₀W, fat emulsion 10%, LR, ½NS, NS

Y-site administration: Incompatible with allopurinol, amphotericin B cholesteryl sulfate complex, cefepime, foscarnet

Compatibility in syringe: Incompatible with diatrizoate meglumine 52% and diatrizoate sodium 8%, diatrizoate sodium 60%, haloperidol, iodipamide meglumine, iodipamide meglumine 52%, ioxaglate meglumine 39.3% and ioxaglate sodium 19.6%, pentobarbital, thiopental

Compatibility when admixed: Incompatible with amobarbital, amphotericin B, dexamethasone sodium phosphate with lorazepam and metoclopramide, iodipamide meglumine, phenytoin, phenobarbital, thiopental

Storage: Protect injection from light.

Nursing Actions

Physical Assessment: Assess effectiveness and interactions of other medications patient may be taking. Monitor effectiveness of therapy and adverse reactions (eg, excess anticholinergic effects) at beginning of therapy and periodically with long-term use. Assess knowledge/teach patient appropriate use, interventions to reduce side effects, and adverse symptoms to report.

Patient Education: Take as directed; do not exceed recommended dose. Avoid use of other depressants, alcohol, or sleep-inducing medications unless approved by prescriber. You may experience drowsiness or dizziness (use caution when driving or engaging in tasks requiring alertness until response to drug is known); or dry mouth, nausea, or vomiting (small frequent meals, frequent mouth care, chewing gum, or sucking hard candy may help). Report persistent sedation, confusion, or agitation; changes in urinary pattern; blurred vision; sore throat, respiratory difficulty, or expectorating (thick secretions); or lack of improvement or worsening or condition.

Breast-feeding precaution: Do not breast-feed.

(Continued)

DiphenhydrAMINE *(Continued)*

Dietary Considerations Tablet:

Chewable, as hydrochloride: Contains phenylalanine 4.2 mg per 12.5 mg tablet

Chewable, as tannate: Contains phenylalanine 1.5 mg per 25 mg tablet

Orally-disintegrating, as citrate: Contains phenylalanine 4.5 mg per 19 mg [equivalent to diphenhydramine hydrochloride 12.5 mg] tablet; contains soy protein isolate (contraindicated in patients with soy protein allergies; use caution in peanut allergic individuals, ~10% are estimated to also have soy protein allergies)

Geriatric Considerations Diphenhydramine has high sedative and anticholinergic properties, so it may not be considered the antihistamine of choice for prolonged use in the elderly. Its use as a sleep aid is discouraged due to its anticholinergic effects.

Breast-Feeding Issues Infants may be more sensitive to the effects of antihistamines.

Additional Information Its use as a sleep aid is discouraged due to its anticholinergic effects.

Related Information

Anxiolytic / Hypnotic Use in Long-Term Care Facilities *on page 1418*

Compatibility of Drugs in Syringe *on page 1372*

FDA Name Differentiation Project: The Use of Tall-Man Letters *on page 12*

Federal OBRA Regulations Recommended Maximum Doses *on page 1421*

Diphenoxylate and Atropine

(dye fen OKS i late & A troe peen)

U.S. Brand Names Lomotil®; Lonox®

Synonyms Atropine and Diphenoxylate

Restrictions C-V

Pharmacologic Category Antidiarrheal

Medication Safety Issues

Sound-alike/look-alike issues:

Lomotil® may be confused with Lamictal®, Lamisil®, lamotrigine, Lanoxin®, Lasix®, ludiomil

Lonox® may be confused with Lanoxin®, Loprox®

Pregnancy Risk Factor C

Lactation Use caution

Use Treatment of diarrhea

Mechanism of Action/Effect Diphenoxylate inhibits excessive GI motility and GI propulsion; commercial preparations contain a subtherapeutic amount of atropine to discourage abuse

Contraindications Hypersensitivity to diphenoxylate, atropine, or any component of the formulation; severe liver disease; jaundice; dehydration; narrow-angle glaucoma; not for use in children <2 years of age

Warnings/Precautions High doses may cause physical and psychological dependence with prolonged use. Use with caution in patients with ulcerative colitis, dehydration, and hepatic dysfunction. Reduction of intestinal motility may be deleterious in diarrhea resulting from *Shigella*, *Salmonella*, toxigenic strains of *E. coli*, and from pseudomembranous enterocolitis associated with broad spectrum antibiotics. If there is no response within 48 hours, the drug is unlikely to be effective and should be discontinued. If chronic diarrhea is not improved symptomatically within 10 days at maximum dosage of 20 mg/day, control is unlikely with further use.

Drug Interactions

Increased Effect/Toxicity: MAO inhibitors (hypertensive crisis), CNS depressants when taken with diphenoxylate may result in increased adverse effects, antimuscarinics (paralytic ileus). May prolong half-life of drugs metabolized in liver.

Nutritional/Ethanol Interactions Ethanol: Avoid ethanol (may increase CNS depression).

Adverse Reactions 1% to 10%:

Central nervous system: Nervousness, restlessness, dizziness, drowsiness, headache, mental depression

Gastrointestinal: Paralytic ileus, xerostomia

Genitourinary: Urinary retention and dysuria

Ocular: Blurred vision

Respiratory: Respiratory depression

Overdosage/Toxicology Symptoms of overdose include drowsiness, hypotension, blurred vision, flushing, dry mouth, and miosis. Administration of activated charcoal will reduce bioavailability of diphenoxylate. Naloxone, 2 mg I.V. with repeat administration as necessary up to a total of 10 mg, can also be used to reverse toxic effects of the opiate. For anticholinergic overdose with severe life-threatening symptoms, physostigmine 1-2 mg SubQ or I.V. slowly, may be given to reverse these effects.

Pharmacodynamics/Kinetics

Onset of Action:

Diphenoxylate: Antidiarrheal: 45-60 minutes; Peak antidiarrheal effect: ~2 hours

Duration of Action:

Diphenoxylate: Antidiarrheal: 3-4 hours

Time to Peak:

Diphenoxylate: Serum: 2 hours

Half-Life Elimination:

Diphenoxylate: 2.5 hours

Metabolism:

Diphenoxylate: Extensively hepatic to diphenoxylic acid (active)

Excretion:

Diphenoxylate: Primarily feces (as metabolites); urine (~14%, <1% as unchanged drug)

Pharmacokinetic Note See Atropine monograph.

Available Dosage Forms

Solution, oral: Diphenoxylate hydrochloride 2.5 mg and atropine sulfate 0.025 mg per 5 mL (5 mL, 10 mL, 60 mL)

Lomotil®: Diphenoxylate hydrochloride 2.5 mg and atropine sulfate 0.025 mg per 5 mL (60 mL) [contains alcohol 15%; cherry flavor]

Tablet (Lomotil®, Lonox®): Diphenoxylate hydrochloride 2.5 mg and atropine sulfate 0.025 mg

Dosing

Adults & Elderly: Diarrhea: Oral: 15-20 mg/day of diphenoxylate in 3-4 divided doses; maintenance: 5-15 mg/day in 2-3 divided doses

Pediatrics: Diarrhea: Oral: Use with caution in young children due to variable responses:

Liquid: 0.3-0.4 mg of diphenoxylate/kg/day in 2-4 divided doses **or**

<2 years: Not recommended

2-5 years: 2 mg of diphenoxylate 3 times/day

5-8 years: 2 mg of diphenoxylate 4 times/day

8-12 years: 2 mg of diphenoxylate 5 times/day

Stability

Storage: Protect from light.

Nursing Actions

Physical Assessment: Ascertain etiology of diarrhea before beginning treatment if possible. Assess effects and interactions of other prescriptions, OTC medications, or herbal products patient may be taking. Monitor therapeutic effectiveness and response. **Note:** There is potential for physical and psychological dependence with prolonged use. Teach patient proper use, possible side effects/appropriate interventions, and adverse effects to report.

Patient Education: Do not take any new medication during therapy unless approved by prescriber. Take as directed; do not exceed recommended dosage. If no response within 48 hours, notify prescriber. Avoid alcohol or other prescriptive or OTC sedatives or depressants. May cause drowsiness, blurred vision, impaired coordination (use caution when driving or engaging in tasks that require alertness until response to drug is known); dry mouth (sucking on lozenges or chewing gum may help). Report difficulty urinating, persistent unrelieved diarrhea, respiratory difficulties, fever, or palpitations. **Pregnancy/breast-feeding precautions:** Inform prescriber if you are or intend to become pregnant. Consult prescriber if breast-feeding.

Geriatric Considerations Elderly are particularly sensitive to fluid and electrolyte loss. Maintaining hydration and electrolyte balance is vital.

Related Information
Atropine *on page 126*

Dipyridamole (dye peer ID a mole)

U.S. Brand Names Persantine®

Pharmacologic Category Antiplatelet Agent; Vasodilator

Medication Safety Issues
Sound-alike/look-alike issues:
Dipyridamole may be confused with disopyramide
Persantine® may be confused with Periactin®, Permitil®

Pregnancy Risk Factor B

Lactation Enters breast milk/use caution

Use
Oral: Used with warfarin to decrease thrombosis in patients after artificial heart valve replacement
I.V.: Diagnostic agent in CAD

Unlabeled/Investigational Use Treatment of proteinuria in pediatric renal disease

Mechanism of Action/Effect Inhibits platelet aggregation and may cause vasodilation. May also stimulate release of prostacyclin or PGD_2 resulting in coronary vasodilation.

Contraindications Hypersensitivity to dipyridamole or any component of the formulation

Warnings/Precautions Use caution in patients with hypotension and severe cardiac disease. Use caution in patients on other antiplatelet agents or anticoagulation. Severe adverse reactions have occurred with I.V. administration (rarely); use the I.V. form with caution in patients with bronchospastic disease or unstable angina. Aminophylline should be available in case of urgency or emergency with I.V. use.

Drug Interactions
Decreased Effect: Decreased vasodilation from I.V. dipyridamole when given to patients taking theophylline. Theophylline may reduce the pharmacologic effects of dipyridamole (hold theophylline preparations for 36-48 hours before dipyridamole facilitated stress test). Dipyridamole may counteract effect of cholinesterase inhibitor and may aggravate myasthenia gravis.

Increased Effect/Toxicity: Adenosine blood levels and pharmacologic effects are increased with dipyridamole; consider reduced doses of adenosine.

Nutritional/Ethanol Interactions Herb/Nutraceutical: Avoid cat's claw, dong quai, evening primrose, feverfew, garlic, ginger, ginkgo, red clover, horse chestnut, green tea, ginseng (all have additional antiplatelet activity).

Adverse Reactions
Oral:
>10%: Dizziness (14%)
1% to 10%:
Central nervous system: Headache (2%)
Dermatologic: Rash (2%)
Gastrointestinal: Abdominal distress (6%)
Frequency not defined: Diarrhea, vomiting, flushing, pruritus, angina pectoris, liver dysfunction

I.V.:
>10%:
Cardiovascular: Exacerbation of angina pectoris (20%)
Central nervous system: Dizziness (12%), headache (12%)
1% to 10%:
Cardiovascular: Hypotension (5%), hypertension (2%), blood pressure lability (2%), ECG abnormalities (ST-T changes, extrasystoles; 5% to 8%), pain (3%), tachycardia (3%)
Central nervous system: Flushing (3%), fatigue (1%)
Gastrointestinal: Nausea (5%)
Neuromuscular & skeletal: Paresthesia (1%)
Respiratory: Dyspnea (3%)

Overdosage/Toxicology Symptoms of overdose include hypotension and peripheral vasodilation. Dialysis is not effective. Treatment is symptomatic and supportive.

Pharmacodynamics/Kinetics
Time to Peak: Serum: 2-2.5 hours
Protein Binding: 91% to 99%
Half-Life Elimination: Terminal: 10-12 hours
Metabolism: Hepatic
Excretion: Feces (as glucuronide conjugates and unchanged drug)

Available Dosage Forms
Injection, solution: 5 mg/mL (2 mL, 10 mL)
Tablet (Persantine®): 25 mg, 50 mg, 75 mg

Dosing
Adults & Elderly:
Adjunctive therapy for prophylaxis of thromboembolism with cardiac valve replacement: Oral: 75-100 mg 4 times/day
Evaluation of coronary artery disease: I.V.: 0.14 mg/kg/minute for 4 minutes; maximum dose: 60 mg

Pediatrics:
Proteinuria (unlabeled use): Oral: Doses of 4-10 mg/kg/day have been used investigationally to treat proteinuria in pediatric renal disease.
Mechanical prosthetic heart valves (unlabeled use): Oral: 2-5 mg/kg/day (used in combination with an oral anticoagulant in children who have systemic embolism despite adequate oral anticoagulant therapy, and used in combination with low-dose oral anticoagulation (INR 2-3) plus aspirin in children in whom full-dose oral anticoagulation is contraindicated).

Administration
Oral: Administer with water 1 hour before meals.
I.V.: I.V.: Infuse diluted solution over 4 minutes; following dipyridamole infusion, inject thallium-201 within 5 minutes. **Note:** Aminophylline should be available for urgent/emergent use; dosing of 50-100 mg (range: 50-250 mg) IVP over 30-60 seconds.

Stability
Reconstitution: Prior to administration, dilute solution for injection to a ≥1:2 ratio in NS, $\frac{1}{2}$NS, or D_5W. Total volume should be ~20-50 mL.
Storage: I.V.: Store between 15°C to 25°C (59°F to 77°F). Do not freeze, protect from light.

Nursing Actions
Physical Assessment: Assess effectiveness and interactions of other medications patient may be taking. Monitor therapeutic response (dependent on purpose for use) and adverse reactions. Observe bleeding precautions. **Oral:** Monitor blood pressure on a regular basis. **I.V.:** Continuous ECG and blood pressure monitoring during infusion. Assess knowledge/teach patient appropriate use, interventions to reduce side effects (eg, bleeding precautions), and adverse symptoms to report.

Patient Education: Take tablet exactly as directed, with water 1 hour before meals. You may experience mild headache, transient diarrhea, or temporary dizziness (sit or lie down when taking medication). You
(Continued)

Dipyridamole *(Continued)*

may have a tendency to bleed easily; use caution with sharps, needles, or razors. Report chest pain, redness around mouth, acute abdominal cramping or severe diarrhea, acute and persistent headache or dizziness, rash, respiratory difficulty, or swelling of extremities. **Breast-feeding precaution:** Consult prescriber if breast-feeding.

Dietary Considerations Should be taken with water 1 hour before meals.

Geriatric Considerations Since evidence suggests that clinically used doses are ineffective for prevention of platelet aggregation, consideration for low-dose aspirin (81-325 mg/day) alone may be necessary. This will decrease cost as well as inconvenience.

Breast-Feeding Issues Excretion in breast milk is reported to be minimal.

Disulfiram *(dye SUL fi ram)*

U.S. Brand Names Antabuse®

Pharmacologic Category Aldehyde Dehydrogenase Inhibitor

Medication Safety Issues
Sound-alike/look-alike issues:
Disulfiram may be confused with Diflucan®
Antabuse® may be confused with Anturane®

Pregnancy Risk Factor C

Lactation Excretion in breast milk unknown

Use Management of chronic alcoholism

Mechanism of Action/Effect Disulfiram is a thiuram derivative which interferes with aldehyde dehydrogenase. When taken concomitantly with alcohol, there is an increase in serum acetaldehyde levels. High acetaldehyde causes uncomfortable symptoms including flushing, nausea, thirst, palpitations, chest pain, vertigo, and hypotension. This reaction is the basis for disulfiram use in postwithdrawal long-term care of alcoholism.

Contraindications Hypersensitivity to disulfiram and related compounds or any component of the formulation; patients receiving or using ethanol, metronidazole, paraldehyde, or ethanol-containing preparations like cough syrup or tonics; psychosis; severe myocardial disease and coronary occlusion

Warnings/Precautions Use with caution in patients with diabetes, hypothyroidism, seizure disorders, nephritis (acute or chronic), hepatic cirrhosis or insufficiency. Should never be administered to a patient when he/she is in a state of ethanol intoxication, or without his/her knowledge. Patient must receive appropriate counseling, including information on "disguised" forms of alcohol (tonics, mouthwashes, etc) and the duration of the drug's activity (up to 14 days).

Drug Interactions

Cytochrome P450 Effect: Substrate (minor) of CYP1A2, 2A6, 2B6, 2D6, 2E1, 3A4; **Inhibits** CYP1A2 (weak), 2A6 (weak), 2B6 (weak), 2C8/9 (weak), 2D6 (weak), 2E1 (strong), 3A4 (weak)

Increased Effect/Toxicity: Disulfiram results in severe ethanol intolerance (disulfiram reaction) secondary to disulfiram's ability to inhibit aldehyde dehydrogenase; this combination should be avoided. Combined use with isoniazid, metronidazole, or MAO inhibitors may result in adverse CNS effects; this combination should be avoided. Some pharmaceutic dosage forms include ethanol, including elixirs and intravenous trimethoprim-sulfamethoxazole (contains 10% ethanol as a solubilizing agent); these may inadvertently provoke a disulfiram reaction. Disulfiram may increase the levels/effects of inhalational anesthetics, trimethadione, and other CYP2E1 substrates. Disulfiram may increase serum concentrations of benzodiazepines that undergo oxidative metabolism (all but oxazepam, lorazepam, temazepam). Disulfiram increases phenytoin and theophylline serum concentrations; toxicity may occur. Disulfiram inhibits the metabolism of warfarin resulting in an increased hypoprothrombinemic response.

Nutritional/Ethanol Interactions Ethanol: Disulfiram inhibits ethanol's usual metabolism. Avoid all ethanol. Patients can have a disulfiram reaction (headache, nausea, vomiting, chest, or abdominal pain) if they drink ethanol concurrently. Avoid cough syrups and elixirs containing ethanol. Avoid vinegars, cider, extracts, and foods containing ethanol.

Adverse Reactions Frequency not defined.

Central nervous system: Drowsiness, headache, fatigue, psychosis

Dermatologic: Rash, acneiform eruptions, allergic dermatitis

Gastrointestinal: Metallic or garlic-like aftertaste

Genitourinary: Impotence

Hepatic: Hepatitis (cholestatic and fulminant), hepatic failure (multiple case reports)

Neuromuscular & skeletal: Peripheral neuritis, polyneuritis, peripheral neuropathy

Ocular: Optic neuritis

Overdosage/Toxicology Management of disulfiram reaction: Institute support measures to restore blood pressure (vasopressors and fluids). Monitor for hypokalemia.

Pharmacodynamics/Kinetics

Onset of Action: Full effect: 12 hours

Duration of Action: ~1-2 weeks after last dose

Metabolism: To diethylthiocarbamate

Excretion: Feces and exhaled gases (as metabolites)

Available Dosage Forms Tablet: 250 mg

Dosing

Adults & Elderly: Note: Do not administer until the patient has abstained from ethanol for at least 12 hours.

Alcoholism: Oral: Initial: 500 mg/day as a single dose for 1-2 weeks; maximum daily dose is 500 mg. Average maintenance dose: 250 mg/day; range: 125-500 mg; duration of therapy is to continue until the patient is fully recovered socially and a basis for permanent self control has been established. Maintenance therapy may be required for months or even years.

Administration

Oral: Administration of any medications containing alcohol, including topicals, is contraindicated. Do not administer disulfiram if ethanol has been consumed within the prior 12 hours.

Laboratory Monitoring Monitor liver function before, 10-14 days after beginning therapy, and every 6 months during therapy.

Nursing Actions

Physical Assessment: Assess for adverse drug interactions with other prescription or OTC drugs. Do not administer until the patient has abstained from ethanol for 12 hours. Monitor laboratory tests and for CNS changes (eg, sedation, restlessness, peripheral neuropathy, and optic or retrobulbar neuritis) at beginning of therapy and periodically with long-term therapy. Advise patient about disulfiram reaction if alcohol is ingested. Assess knowledge/teach patient appropriate use, interventions to reduce side effects, and adverse symptoms to report.

Patient Education: Tablets can be crushed or mixed with water or juice. Metallic aftertaste may occur; this will go away. Do not drink any alcohol, including products containing alcohol (such as cough and cold syrups or some mouthwashes), or use alcohol-containing skin products while taking this medication and for at least 3 days (preferably 14 days) after stopping this medication. Drowsiness, tiredness, or visual changes may occur. Use care when driving or engaging in tasks requiring alertness until response to drug is known. Notify prescriber of any respiratory difficulty, weakness, nausea, vomiting, decreased appetite, yellowing of skin or eyes, or dark-colored urine. **Pregnancy/breast-feeding precautions:** Inform prescriber if you are or intend to become pregnant. Consult prescriber if breast-feeding.

DOBUTamine (doe BYOO ta meen)

Synonyms Dobutamine Hydrochloride
Pharmacologic Category Adrenergic Agonist Agent
Medication Safety Issues
Sound-alike/look-alike issues:
DOBUTamine may be confused with DOPamine
Pregnancy Risk Factor B
Lactation Excretion in breast milk unknown
Use Short-term management of patients with cardiac decompensation
Unlabeled/Investigational Use Positive inotropic agent for use in myocardial dysfunction of sepsis
Mechanism of Action/Effect Stimulates beta$_1$-adrenergic receptors, causing increased contractility and heart rate, with little effect on beta$_2$- or alpha-receptors
Contraindications Hypersensitivity to dobutamine or sulfites (some contain sodium metabisulfate), or any component of the formulation; idiopathic hypertrophic subaortic stenosis (IHSS)
Warnings/Precautions May increase heart rate. Patients with atrial fibrillation may experience an increase in ventricular response. An increase in blood pressure is more common, but occasionally a patient may become hypotensive. May exacerbate ventricular ectopy. If needed, correct hypovolemia first to optimize hemodynamics. Ineffective in the presence of mechanical obstruction such as severe aortic stenosis. Use caution post-MI (can increase myocardial oxygen demand). Use cautiously in the elderly starting at lower end of the dosage range.

Drug Interactions
Decreased Effect: Beta-adrenergic blockers may decrease effect of dobutamine and increase risk of severe hypotension.
Increased Effect/Toxicity: General anesthetics (eg, halothane or cyclopropane) and usual doses of dobutamine have resulted in ventricular arrhythmias in animals. Bretylium and may potentiate dobutamine's effects. Beta-blockers (nonselective ones) may increase hypertensive effect; avoid concurrent use. Cocaine may cause malignant arrhythmias. Guanethidine, MAO inhibitors, methyldopa, reserpine, and tricyclic antidepressants can increase the pressor response to sympathomimetics.
Lab Interactions May affect serum assay of chloramphenicol.
Adverse Reactions Incidence of adverse events is not always reported.
Cardiovascular: Increased heart rate, increased blood pressure, increased ventricular ectopic activity, hypotension, premature ventricular beats (5%, dose related), anginal pain (1% to 3%), nonspecific chest pain (1% to 3%), palpitation (1% to 3%)
Central nervous system: Fever (1% to 3%), headache (1% to 3%), paresthesia
Endocrine & metabolic: Slight decrease in serum potassium
Gastrointestinal: Nausea (1% to 3%)
Hematologic: Thrombocytopenia (isolated cases)
Local: Phlebitis, local inflammatory changes and pain from infiltration, cutaneous necrosis (isolated cases)
Neuromuscular & skeletal: Mild leg cramps
Respiratory: Dyspnea (1% to 3%)

Overdosage/Toxicology Symptoms of overdose include fatigue, nervousness, tachycardia, hypertension, and arrhythmias. Reduce rate of administration or discontinue infusion until condition stabilizes.
Pharmacodynamics/Kinetics
Onset of Action: I.V.: 1-10 minutes; Peak effect: 10-20 minutes
Half-Life Elimination: 2 minutes
Metabolism: In tissues and hepatically to inactive metabolites
Excretion: Urine (as metabolites)
Available Dosage Forms
Infusion, as hydrochloride [premixed in dextrose]: 1 mg/mL (250 mL, 500 mL); 2 mg/mL (250 mL); 4 mg/mL (250 mL)
Injection, solution, as hydrochloride: 12.5 mg/mL (20 mL, 40 mL, 100 mL) [contains sodium bisulfite]
Dosing
Adults & Elderly: Cardiac decompensation: I.V. infusion: 2.5-20 mcg/kg/minute; maximum: 40 mcg/kg/minute, titrate to desired response; see table.

Infusion Rates of Various Dilutions of Dobutamine

Desired Delivery Rate (mcg/kg/min)	Infusion Rate (mL/kg/min)	
	500 mcg/mL[1]	1000 mcg/mL[2]
2.5	0.005	0.0025
5.0	0.01	0.005
7.5	0.015	0.0075
10.0	0.02	0.01
12.5	0.025	0.0125
15.0	0.03	0.015

[1]500 mg per liter or 250 mg per 500 mL of diluent.

[2]1000 mg per liter or 250 mg per 250 mL of diluent.

Pediatrics: Cardiac decompensation: Refer to adult dosing.
Administration
I.V.: Always administer via infusion device; administer into large vein.
I.V. Detail: pH: 2.5-5.5
Stability
Reconstitution: Remix solution every 24 hours. Store reconstituted solution under refrigeration for 48 hours or 6 hours at room temperature. Pink discoloration of solution indicates slight oxidation but **no** significant loss of potency. Stability of parenteral admixture at room temperature (25°C) is 48 hours; at refrigeration (4°C) stability is 7 days.
Standard adult diluent: 250 mg/500 mL D$_5$W; 500 mg/500 mL D$_5$W
Compatibility: Do not give through same I.V. line as heparin, hydrocortisone sodium succinate, cefazolin, or penicillin. **Incompatible** with heparin, cefazolin, penicillin, and in alkaline solutions (sodium bicarbonate).
Stable in D$_5$LR, D$_5$^{1}/$_2$NS, D$_5$NS, D$_5$W, D$_{10}$W, LR, ^{1}/$_2$NS, NS, mannitol 20%; **incompatible** with sodium bicarbonate 5%
Y-site administration: Incompatible with acyclovir, alatrofloxacin, alteplase, aminophylline, amphotericin B cholesteryl sulfate complex, cefepime, foscarnet, indomethacin, phytonadione, piperacillin/tazobactam, thiopental, warfarin
Compatibility in syringe: Incompatible with doxapram
Compatibility when admixed: Incompatible with acyclovir, alteplase, aminophylline, bumetanide, calcium gluconate, diazepam, digoxin, floxacillin,
(Continued)

DOBUTamine *(Continued)*

furosemide, insulin (regular), magnesium sulfate, phenytoin, potassium phosphates, sodium bicarbonate

Laboratory Monitoring Serum glucose, renal function

Nursing Actions

Physical Assessment: Assess other medications patient may be taking for effectiveness and interactions. Infusion pump and continuous cardiac and hemodynamic monitoring are required. Monitor therapeutic response (cardiac status) and adverse reactions. Instruct patient on adverse symptoms to report.

Patient Education: When administered in emergencies, patient education should be appropriate to the situation. If patient is aware, instruct to promptly report chest pain, palpitations, rapid heartbeat, headache, nervousness, or restlessness, nausea or vomiting, or respiratory difficulty. **Breast-feeding precaution:** Consult prescriber if breast-feeding.

Geriatric Considerations Beneficial hemodynamic effects have been demonstrated in elderly patients; however, significant hypotension may occur more frequently in elderly patients; monitor closely.

Pregnancy Issues Since dobutamine has not been given to pregnant women, benefits of use should outweigh the risks.

Additional Information Dobutamine lowers central venous pressure and wedge pressure but has little effect on pulmonary vascular resistance.

Dobutamine therapy should be avoided in patients with stable heart failure due to an increase in mortality. In patients with intractable heart failure, dobutamine may be used as a short-term infusion to provide symptomatic benefit. It is not known whether short-term dobutamine therapy in end-stage heart failure has any outcome benefit.

Dobutamine infusion during echocardiography is used as a cardiovascular stress. Wall motion abnormalities developing with increasing doses of dobutamine may help to identify ischemic and/or hibernating myocardium.

Related Information

FDA Name Differentiation Project: The Use of Tall-Man Letters *on page 12*

Docetaxel *(doe se TAKS el)*

U.S. Brand Names Taxotere®

Synonyms NSC-628503; RP-6976

Pharmacologic Category Antineoplastic Agent, Natural Source (Plant) Derivative

Medication Safety Issues
Sound-alike/look-alike issues:
Taxotere® may be confused with Taxol®

Pregnancy Risk Factor D

Lactation Excretion in breast milk unknown/contraindicated

Use Treatment of locally-advanced or metastatic breast cancer; adjuvant treatment of operable node-positive breast cancer (in combination with doxorubicin and cyclophosphamide); treatment of locally-advanced or metastatic nonsmall cell lung cancer (NSCLC) in combination with cisplatin in treatment of patients who have not previously received chemotherapy for unresected NSCLC; treatment of prostate cancer (hormone refractory, metastatic)

Unlabeled/Investigational Use Investigational: Treatment of gastric, pancreatic, head and neck, and ovarian cancers, soft tissue sarcoma, and melanoma

Mechanism of Action/Effect Inhibits cancer cell division by acting on the microtubules

Contraindications Hypersensitivity to docetaxel or any component of the formulation; pre-existing bone marrow suppression (neutrophils <1500 cells/mm^3); pregnancy

Warnings/Precautions Hypersensitivity, including severe reactions, may occur; incidence up to 25% in patients who did not receive premedication; incidence reduced to 2.2% in patients who receive premedication. Patients should be premedicated with a steroid to prevent hypersensitivity reactions and fluid retention. A common regimen is dexamethasone 4-8 mg orally twice daily for 3-5 days, starting the day before docetaxel administration.

Fluid retention syndrome (pleural effusions, ascites, edema, and 2-15 kg weight gain) may occur. It has not been associated with cardiac, pulmonary, renal, hepatic, or endocrine dysfunction. The incidence and severity of the syndrome increase sharply at cumulative doses ≥400 mg/m^2.

Neutropenia was the dose-limiting toxicity. Patients with an absolute neutrophil count <1500 cells/mm^3 should not receive docetaxel. Hepatic dysfunction increases risk of neutropenia and severe infections. Should generally not be given to patients with bilirubin greater than the upper limit of normal or to patients with AST (SGOT) and/or ALT (SGPT) greater than 1.5x the upper limit of normal concomitantly with alkaline phosphatase greater than 2.5x the upper limit of normal. Obtain baseline levels prior to administration. If docetaxel contacts the skin, wash and flush thoroughly with water. Contains Polysorbate 80®; diluent contains ethanol.

When administered as sequential infusions, taxane derivatives (docetaxel, paclitaxel) should be administered before platinum derivatives (carboplatin, cisplatin) to limit myelosuppression and to enhance efficacy.

Drug Interactions

Cytochrome P450 Effect: Substrate of CYP3A4 (major); **Inhibits** CYP3A4 (weak)

Decreased Effect: CYP3A4 inducers may decrease the levels/effects of docetaxel; example inducers include aminoglutethimide, carbamazepine, nafcillin, nevirapine, phenobarbital, phenytoin, and rifamycins.

Increased Effect/Toxicity: CYP3A4 inhibitors may increase the levels/effects of docetaxel; example inhibitors include azole antifungals, clarithromycin, diclofenac, doxycycline, erythromycin, imatinib, isoniazid, nefazodone, nicardipine, propofol, protease inhibitors, quinidine, telithromycin, and verapamil. When administered as sequential infusions, observational studies indicate a potential for increased toxicity when platinum derivatives (carboplatin, cisplatin) are administered before taxane derivatives (docetaxel, paclitaxel).

Nutritional/Ethanol Interactions
Ethanol: Avoid ethanol (due to GI irritation).
Herb/Nutraceutical: St John's wort may decrease docetaxel levels.

Adverse Reactions Note: Frequencies cited for nonsmall cell lung cancer and breast cancer treatment. Exact frequency may vary based on tumor type, prior and/or current treatment, premedication, and dosage of docetaxel.

>10%:

Cardiovascular: Fluid retention, including peripheral edema, pleural effusion, and ascites (33% to 47%); may be more common at cumulative doses ≥400 mg/m^2. Up to 64% in breast cancer patients with dexamethasone premedication.

Dermatologic: Alopecia (56% to 76%); nail disorder (11% to 31%, banding, onycholysis, hypo- or hyperpigmentation)

Gastrointestinal: Mucositis/stomatitis (26% to 42%, severe in 6% to 7%), may be dose-limiting (premedication may reduce frequency and severity); nausea and vomiting (40% to 80%, severe in 1% to 5%); diarrhea (33% to 43%)

Hematologic: Myelosuppression, neutropenia (75% to 85%), thrombocytopenia, anemia
Onset: 4-7 days
Nadir: 5-9 days
Recovery: 21 days
Hepatic: Transaminases increased (18%)
Neuromuscular & skeletal: Myalgia (3% to 21%); neurosensory changes (paresthesia, dysesthesia, pain) noted in 23% to 49% (severe in up to 6%). Motor neuropathy (including weakness) noted in as many as 16% of lung cancer patients (severe in up to 5%). Neuropathy may be more common at higher cumulative docetaxel dosages or with prior cisplatin therapy.
Ocular: Epiphora associated with canalicular stenosis (up to 77% with weekly administration; up to 1% with every-3-week administration)
Miscellaneous: Hypersensitivity reactions (6% to 13%; angioedema, rash, flushing, fever, hypotension); frequency substantially reduced by premedication with dexamethasone starting one day prior to docetaxel administration.
1% to 10%:
Cardiovascular: Hypotension (3%)
Dermatologic: Rash and skin eruptions (6%)
Gastrointestinal: Taste perversion (6%)
Hepatic: Bilirubin increased (9%)
Neuromuscular & skeletal: Arthralgia (3% to 9%)
Miscellaneous: Infusion site reactions (up to 4%)

Pharmacodynamics/Kinetics

Protein Binding: 94%, primarily to alpha$_1$-acid glycoprotein, albumin, and lipoproteins

Half-Life Elimination: Alpha, beta, gamma: 4 minutes, 36 minutes, and 10-18 hours, respectively

Metabolism: Hepatic; oxidation via CYP3A4 to metabolites

Excretion: Feces (75%); urine (6%); ~80% within 48 hours
Clearance: Total body: Mean: 21 L/hour/m^2

Pharmacokinetic Note Exhibits linear pharmacokinetics at the recommended dosage range.

Available Dosage Forms Injection, solution [concentrate]: 20 mg/0.5 mL (0.5 mL, 2 mL) [contains Polysorbate 80®; diluent contains ethanol 13%]

Dosing

Adults & Elderly: Refer to individual protocols:
Breast cancer:
Locally-advanced or metastatic: I.V.: 60-100 mg/m^2 every 3 weeks; patients initially started at 60 mg/m^2 who do not develop toxicity may tolerate higher doses
Operable, node-positive (adjuvant treatment): 75 mg/m^2 every 3 weeks for 6 courses
Nonsmall-cell lung cancer: I.V.: 75 mg/m^2 every 3 weeks
Prostate cancer:: I.V.: 75 mg/m^2 every 3 weeks; prednisone (5 mg twice daily) is administered continuously

Pediatrics: Children ≥16 years: Refer to adult dosing.

Hepatic Impairment: Total bilirubin ≥ the upper limit of normal (ULN), or AST (SGOT)/ALT (SGPT) >1.5 times ULN concomitant with alkaline phosphatase >2.5 times ULN: Docetaxel **should not be administered.**

Dosing Adjustment for Toxicity: Note: Toxicity includes febrile neutropenia, neutrophils ≤500/mm^3 for >1 week, severe or cumulative cutaneous reactions; in nonsmall cell lung cancer, this may also include other grade 3/4 nonhematologic toxicities.
Breast cancer: Patients dosed initially at 100 mg/m^2; reduce dose to 75 mg/m^2; **Note:** If the patient continues to experience these adverse reactions, the dosage should be reduced to 55 mg/m^2 or therapy should be discontinued

Nonsmall cell lung cancer:
Monotherapy: Patients dosed initially at 75 mg/m^2 should have dose held until toxicity is resolved, then resume at 55 mg/m^2; discontinue patients who develop ≥ grade 3 peripheral neuropathy.
Combination therapy: Patients dosed initially at 75 mg/m^2, in combination with cisplatin, should have the docetaxel dosage reduced to 65 mg/m^2 in subsequent cycles; if further adjustment is required, dosage may be reduced to 50 mg/m^2
Prostate cancer: Reduce dose to 60 mg/m^2; discontinue therapy if adverse reactions persist at lower dose.

Administration

I.V.: Irritant.
Premedication with corticosteroids is recommended to prevent hypersensitivity reactions and pulmonary/peripheral edema (see Additional Information).
Administer I.V. infusion over 1-hour through nonsorbing (nonpolyvinylchloride) tubing; in-line filter is not necessary. When administered as sequential infusions, taxane derivatives should be administered before platinum derivatives (cisplatin, carboplatin) to limit myelosuppression and to enhance efficacy.

I.V. Detail: Follow guidelines for handling cytotoxic agents.

Stability

Reconstitution: Intact vials of solution should be diluted with 13% (w/w) ethanol/water to a final concentration of 10 mg/mL. Mix by repeated inversions; do not shake. Docetaxel dose should then be further diluted with NS or D$_5$W to a final concentration of 0.3-0.74 mg/mL and must be prepared in a glass bottle, polypropylene, or polyolefin plastic bag to prevent leaching of plasticizers.

Compatibility: Stable in D$_5$W, NS
Y-site administration: **Incompatible** with amphotericin B, doxorubicin liposome, methylprednisolone sodium succinate, nalbuphine

Storage: Intact vials should be stored at 2°C to 25°C (36°F to 77°F) and protected from light. Freezing does not adversely affect the product. Vials should be stored at room temperature for approximately 5 minutes before using. Following initial dilution, solution is stable for 8 hours at room temperature or under refrigeration. Following second dilution, the manufacturer recommends using within 4 hours. According to other references, the final diluted solutions are stable for up to 4 weeks at room temperature 15°C to 25°C (59°F to 77°F) in polyolefin containers. (Thiesen J, 1999).

Laboratory Monitoring CBC with differential and platelet count; liver function especially bilirubin, AST, ALT, and alkaline phosphatase

Nursing Actions

Physical Assessment: Assess potential for interactions with other pharmacological agents or herbal products patient may be taking (eg, drugs that may increase or decrease levels/effects of docetaxel). **Caution:** Severe hypersensitivity reactions have been reported; premedication with dexamethasone may be advisable. Assess vital signs and weight prior to administration and monitor patient continuously during infusion (dosing adjustment may be necessary). Monitor laboratory tests and adverse effects (eg, neutropenia, severe fluid retention, pleural effusion, opportunistic infections) prior to each infusion and on a regular basis throughout therapy. Teach patient possible side effects/appropriate interventions and adverse symptoms to report.

Patient Education: Do not take any new medication during therapy unless approved by prescriber. This medication can only be administered by infusion; report immediately any pain, burning, swelling, or (Continued)

Docetaxel (Continued)

redness at infusion site, difficulty breathing or swallowing, chest pain, or sudden chills. It is important to maintain adequate hydration (2-3 L/day of fluids) unless instructed to restrict fluid intake and adequate nutrition (small frequent meals may help). You will be more susceptible to infection (avoid crowds and exposure to infection and do not have any vaccinations without consulting prescriber). May cause nausea or vomiting (small frequent meals, frequent mouth care, sucking lozenges, or chewing gum may help); loss of hair (reversible); or diarrhea (buttermilk, boiled milk, or yogurt may help; if unresolved, contact prescriber for medication relief). Report immediately swelling of extremities, respiratory difficulty, unusual weight gain, abdominal distention, chest pain, palpitations, fever, chills, unusual bruising or bleeding, signs of infection, excessive fatigue, or rash. **Pregnancy/ breast-feeding precautions:** Inform prescriber if you are pregnant. Do not get pregnant while taking this drug. Consult prescriber for appropriate contraceptives. Do not breast-feed.

Breast-Feeding Issues The manufacturer recommends discontinuing nursing prior to treatment.

Pregnancy Issues Docetaxel was found to be embryotoxic and fetotoxic in animal studies. A pregnancy registry is available for all cancers diagnosed during pregnancy at Cooper Health (856-757-7876).

Additional Information Premedication with oral corticosteroids is recommended for all patients to decrease the incidence and severity of fluid retention and severity of hypersensitivity reactions. Suggested regimens include: Breast cancer, NSCLC: Dexamethasone 8-10 mg twice daily for 3-5 days. Start 1 day prior to docetaxel.

Prostate cancer: Dexamethasone 8 mg at 12 hours, 3 hours, and 1 hour before docetaxel infusion. Prednisone is also administered as a part of combination treatment.

Docusate (DOK yoo sate)

U.S. Brand Names Colace® [OTC]; Diocto® [OTC]; Docusoft-S™ [OTC]; DOK™ [OTC]; DOS® [OTC]; D-S-S® [OTC]; Dulcolax® Stool Softener [OTC]; Enemeez® [OTC]; Fleet® Sof-Lax® [OTC]; Genasoft® [OTC]; Phillips'® Stool Softener Laxative [OTC]; Silace [OTC]; Surfak® [OTC]

Synonyms Dioctyl Calcium Sulfosuccinate; Dioctyl Sodium Sulfosuccinate; Docusate Calcium; Docusate Potassium; Docusate Sodium; DOSS; DSS

Pharmacologic Category Stool Softener

Medication Safety Issues
Sound-alike/look-alike issues:
Docusate may be confused with Doxinate®
Colace® may be confused with Calan®
Surfak® may be confused with Surbex®

Pregnancy Risk Factor C

Lactation Excretion in breast milk unknown/compatible

Use Stool softener in patients who should avoid straining during defecation and constipation associated with hard, dry stools; prophylaxis for straining (Valsalva) following myocardial infarction. A safe agent to be used in elderly; some evidence that doses <200 mg are ineffective; stool softeners are unnecessary if stool is well hydrated or "mushy" and soft; shown to be ineffective used long-term.

Unlabeled/Investigational Use Ceruminolytic

Mechanism of Action/Effect Reduces surface tension of the oil-water interface of the stool resulting in enhanced incorporation of water and fat allowing for stool softening

Contraindications Hypersensitivity to docusate or any component of the formulation; concomitant use of mineral oil; intestinal obstruction, acute abdominal pain, nausea, or vomiting

Warnings/Precautions Prolonged, frequent, or excessive use may result in dependence or electrolyte imbalance.

Lab Interactions Decreased potassium (S), chloride (S)

Adverse Reactions 1% to 10%:
Gastrointestinal: Intestinal obstruction, diarrhea, abdominal cramping
Miscellaneous: Throat irritation

Overdosage/Toxicology Symptoms of overdose include abdominal cramps, diarrhea, fluid loss, and hypokalemia. Treatment is symptomatic.

Pharmacodynamics/Kinetics
Onset of Action: 12-72 hours
Excretion: Feces

Available Dosage Forms
Capsule, as calcium (Surfak®): 240 mg
Capsule, as sodium: 100 mg, 250 mg
Colace®: 50 mg [contains sodium 3 mg], 100 mg [contains sodium 5 mg]
Docusoft-S™: 100 mg [contains sodium 5 mg]
DOK™, Genasoft®: 100 mg
DOS®, D-S-S®: 100 mg, 250 mg
Dulcolax® Stool Softener: 100 mg [contains sodium 5 mg]
Phillips'® Stool Softener Laxative: 100 mg [contains sodium 5.2 mg]
Enema, rectal, as sodium (Enemeez®): 283 mg/5 mL 5 mL
Gelcap, as sodium (Fleet® Sof-Lax®): 100 mg
Liquid, as sodium: 150 mg/15 mL (480 mL)
Colace®: 150 mg/15 mL (30 mL) [contains sodium 1 mg/mL]
Diocto®: 150 mg/15 mL (480 mL) [vanilla flavor]
Silace: 150 mg/15 mL (480 mL) [lemon-vanilla flavor]
Syrup, as sodium: 60 mg/15 mL (480 mL)
Colace®, Diocto®: 60 mg/15 mL (480 mL) [alcohol free, sugar free; contains sodium 36 mg/5 mL]
Silace: 20 mg/5 mL (480 mL) [peppermint flavor]

Dosing
Adults & Elderly: Note: Docusate salts are interchangeable; the amount of sodium, calcium, or potassium per dosage unit is clinically insignificant.

Stool softener:
Oral: 50-500 mg/day in 1-4 divided doses
Rectal: Add 50-100 mg of docusate liquid to enema fluid (saline or water); give as retention or flushing enema

Pediatrics: Note: Docusate salts are interchangeable; the amount of sodium, calcium, or potassium per dosage unit is clinically insignificant.

Stool softener:
Oral:
Infants and Children <3 years: 10-40 mg/day in 1-4 divided doses
Children:
3-6 years: 20-60 mg/day in 1-4 divided doses
6-12 years: 40-150 mg/day in 1-4 divided doses
Adolescents: Refer to adult dosing.
Rectal: Older Children: Refer to adult dosing.

Administration
Oral: Docusate liquid should be given with milk, or fruit juice, to mask the bitter taste. Capsules should be administered with a full glass of water, milk, or fruit juice.

Nursing Actions
Physical Assessment: Monitor for effectiveness and instruct patient in proper use (avoid excessive or prolonged use) and adverse effects to report.
Patient Education: Docusate should be taken with a full glass of water, milk, or fruit juice. Do not use if abdominal pain, nausea, or vomiting are present. Laxative use should be used for a short period of time (<1 week). Prolonged use may result in abuse,

dependence, as well as fluid and electrolyte loss. Report bleeding or constipation. **Pregnancy precaution:** Inform prescriber if you are or intend to become pregnant.

Dietary Considerations Should be taken with a full glass of water, milk, or fruit juice.

Geriatric Considerations A safe agent to be used in the elderly. Some evidence that doses <200 mg are ineffective.

Docusate and Senna (DOK yoo sate & SEN na)

U.S. Brand Names Peri-Colace® *(reformulation)* [OTC]; Senokot-S® [OTC]

Synonyms Senna and Docusate; Senna-S

Pharmacologic Category Laxative, Stimulant; Stool Softener

Medication Safety Issues
Sound-alike/look-alike issues:
Senokot® may be confused with Depakote®

Use Short-term treatment of constipation

Unlabeled/Investigational Use Evacuate the colon for bowel or rectal examinations; management/prevention of opiate-induced constipation

Mechanism of Action/Effect Docusate is a stool softener; sennosides are laxatives

Contraindications Hypersensitivity to any component; intestinal obstruction; acute intestinal inflammation (eg, Crohn's disease); ulcerative colitis; appendicitis; abdominal pain of unknown origin; concurrent use of mineral oil; pregnancy (per Commission E for senna)

Warnings/Precautions Not recommended for over-the-counter (OTC) use in patients experiencing stomach pain, nausea, vomiting, or a sudden change in bowel movements which lasts >2 weeks. OTC labeling does not recommend for use longer than 1 week. Not recommended for OTC use in children <2 years of age.

Adverse Reactions Frequency not defined.
Gastrointestinal: Nausea, vomiting, diarrhea, abdominal cramps
Genitourinary: Urine discoloration (red/brown)

Available Dosage Forms
Tablet: Docusate sodium 50 mg and sennosides 8.6 mg
Peri-Colace® (reformulation): Docusate sodium 50 mg and sennosides 8.6 mg
Senokot-S®: Docusate sodium 50 mg and sennosides 8.6 mg [sugar free; contains sodium 3 mg/tablet]

Dosing
Adults: Constipation: OTC ranges: Oral: Initial: 2 tablets (17.2 mg sennosides plus 100 mg docusate) once daily (maximum: 4 tablets twice daily)
Elderly: Constipation: OTC ranges: Oral: Consider half the initial dose in older, debilitated patients
Pediatrics: Constipation: OTC ranges: Oral: Children:
2-6 years: Initial: 4.3 mg sennosides plus 25 mg docusate (½ tablet) once daily (maximum: 1 tablet twice daily)
6-12 years: Initial: 8.6 mg sennosides plus 50 mg docusate (1 tablet) once daily (maximum: 2 tablets twice daily)
≥12 years: Refer to adult dosing.

Administration
Oral: Once-daily doses should be taken at bedtime.

Nursing Actions
Physical Assessment: Determine cause of constipation before treating. Teach patient proper use, side effects/interventions, and symptoms to report.

Patient Education: Take exactly as directed. DO NOT exceed recommended dosage; prolonged use or excessive dosing may lead to dependence. Your urine may be discolored (red-brown) this is normal. Stop use and contact prescriber if you develop nausea, vomiting, persistent diarrhea, or abdominal

cramps. If constipation worsens or you experience no relief contact prescriber. **Note:** Increased fluids, fruits, fiber, and exercise may help relieve constipation.

Dietary Considerations Senokot-S®: Sodium content: 3 mg per tablet

Additional Information Individual product labeling should be consulted prior to dosing.

Related Information
Docusate *on page 384*

Dofetilide (doe FET il ide)

U.S. Brand Names Tikosyn™

Pharmacologic Category Antiarrhythmic Agent, Class III

Pregnancy Risk Factor C

Lactation Excretion in breast milk unknown/not recommended

Use Maintenance of normal sinus rhythm in patients with chronic atrial fibrillation/atrial flutter of longer than 1-week duration who have been converted to normal sinus rhythm; conversion of atrial fibrillation and atrial flutter to normal sinus rhythm

Mechanism of Action/Effect Blocks cardiac potassium ion channels and increases action potential duration due to delayed repolarization

Contraindications Hypersensitivity to dofetilide or any component of the formulation; patients with congenital or acquired long QT syndromes, do not use if a baseline QT interval or QT_c is >440 msec (500 msec in patients with ventricular conduction abnormalities); severe renal impairment (estimated Cl_{cr} <20 mL/minute); concurrent use with verapamil, cimetidine, hydrochlorothiazide (alone or in combinations), trimethoprim (alone or in combination with sulfamethoxazole), itraconazole, ketoconazole, prochlorperazine, or megestrol; baseline heart rate <50 beats/minute; other drugs that prolong QT intervals (phenothiazines, cisapride, bepridil, tricyclic antidepressants, sparfloxacin, gatifloxacin, moxifloxacin); hypokalemia or hypomagnesemia; concurrent amiodarone, clarithromycin, or erythromycin

Warnings/Precautions Note: Must be initiated (or reinitiated) by a cardiologist in a setting with continuous monitoring and staff familiar with the recognition and treatment of life-threatening arrhythmias. Patients must be monitored with continuous ECG for a minimum of 3 days, or for a minimum of 12 hours after electrical or pharmacological cardioversion to normal sinus rhythm, whichever is greater. Patients should be readmitted for continuous monitoring if dosage is later increased.

Reserve for patients who are highly symptomatic with atrial fibrillation/atrial flutter. Torsade de pointes significantly increases with doses >500 mcg twice daily. Hold class I or class III antiarrhythmics for at least three half-lives prior to starting dofetilide. Use in patients on amiodarone therapy only if serum amiodarone level is <0.3 mg/L or if amiodarone was stopped for >3 months previously. Correct hypokalemia or hypomagnesemia before starting dofetilide and maintained within normal limits during treatment. Risk of hypokalemia and/or hypomagnesemia may be increased by potassium-depleting diuretics, increasing the risk of torsade de pointes. Concurrent use with other drugs known to prolong QT_c interval is not recommended.

Patients with sick sinus syndrome or with second or third degree heart block should not receive dofetilide unless a functional pacemaker is in place. Defibrillation threshold is reduced in patients with ventricular tachycardia or ventricular fibrillation undergoing implantation of a cardioverter-defibrillator device. Safety/efficacy in children (<18 years of age) have not been established. Use with caution in renal impairment; not recommended
(Continued)

Dofetilide *(Continued)*

in patients receiving drugs which may compete for renal secretion via cationic transport. Use with caution in patients with severe hepatic impairment.

Drug Interactions

Cytochrome P450 Effect: Substrate of CYP3A4 (minor)

Increased Effect/Toxicity: Dofetilide concentrations are increased by cimetidine, verapamil, hydrochlorothiazide, ketoconazole, and trimethoprim (concurrent use of these agents is contraindicated). Dofetilide levels may also be increased by renal cationic transport inhibitors (including triamterene, metformin, amiloride, and megestrol). Diuretics and other drugs which may deplete potassium and/or magnesium (aminoglycoside antibiotics, amphotericin, cyclosporine) may increase dofetilide's toxicity (torsade de pointes); concurrent use of hydrochlorothiazide is contraindicated. Use of QT_c-prolonging agents (including bepridil, cisapride, clarithromycin, erythromycin, tricyclic antidepressants, phenothiazines, sparfloxacin, gatifloxacin, moxifloxacin) is contraindicated. Itraconazole may decrease the metabolism of dofetilide (concurrent use is contraindicated).

Nutritional/Ethanol Interactions Herb/Nutraceutical: St John's wort may decrease dofetilide levels. Avoid ephedra (may worsen arrhythmia).

Adverse Reactions

Supraventricular arrhythmia patients (incidence > placebo)

>10%: Central nervous system: Headache (11%)

2% to 10%:

Central nervous system: Dizziness (8%), insomnia (4%)

Cardiovascular: Ventricular tachycardia (2.6% to 3.7%), chest pain (10%), torsade de pointes (3.3% in CHF patients and 0.9% in patients with a recent MI; up to 10.5% in patients receiving doses in excess of those recommended). Torsade de pointes occurs most frequently within the first 3 days of therapy.

Dermatologic: Rash (3%)

Gastrointestinal: Nausea (5%), diarrhea (3%), abdominal pain (3%)

Neuromuscular & skeletal: Back pain (3%)

Respiratory: Dyspnea (6%), respiratory tract infection (7%)

Miscellaneous: Flu syndrome (4%)

<2%:

Central nervous system: CVA, facial paralysis, flaccid paralysis, migraine, paralysis

Cardiovascular: AV block (0.4% to 1.5%), ventricular fibrillation (0% to 0.4%), bundle branch block, heart block, edema, heart arrest, myocardial infarct, sudden death, syncope

Dermatologic: Angioedema

Gastrointestinal: Liver damage

Neuromuscular & skeletal: Paresthesia

Respiratory: Cough

>2% (incidence ≤ placebo): Anxiety, pain, angina, atrial fibrillation, hypertension, palpitation, supraventricular tachycardia, peripheral edema, urinary tract infection, weakness, arthralgia, diaphoresis

Overdosage/Toxicology The major dose-related toxicity is torsade de pointes. Treatment should be symptomatic and supportive. Watch for excessive prolongation of the QT interval in overdose situations. Continuous cardiac monitoring is necessary. A charcoal slurry is helpful when given early (15 minutes) after the overdose.

Pharmacodynamics/Kinetics

Time to Peak: Fasting: 2-3 hours

Protein Binding: 60% to 70%

Half-Life Elimination: 10 hours

Metabolism: Hepatic via CYP3A4, but low affinity for it; metabolites formed by N-dealkylation and N-oxidation

Excretion: Urine (80%, 80% as unchanged drug, 20% as inactive or minimally active metabolites); renal elimination consists of glomerular filtration and active tubular secretion via cationic transport system

Available Dosage Forms Capsule: 125 mcg, 250 mcg, 500 mcg

Dosing

Adults: Note: QT_c must be determined prior to first dose

Antiarrhythmic: Oral:

Initial: 500 mcg orally twice daily. Initial dosage must be adjusted in patients with estimated Cl_{cr} <60 mL/minute. Dofetilide may be initiated at lower doses than recommended based on physician discretion.

Modification of dosage in response to initial dose: QT_c interval should be measured 2-3 hours after the initial dose. If the QT_c >15% of baseline, or if the QT_c is >500 msec (550 msec in patients with ventricular conduction abnormalities), dofetilide should be adjusted. If the starting dose is 500 mcg twice daily, then adjust to 250 mcg twice daily. If the starting dose was 250 mcg twice daily, then adjust to 125 mcg twice daily. If the starting dose was 125 mcg twice daily, then adjust to 125 mcg every day.

Continued monitoring for doses 2-5: QT_c interval must be determined 2-3 hours after each subsequent dose of dofetilide for in-hospital doses 2-5. If the measured QT_c is >500 msec (550 msec in patients with ventricular conduction abnormalities) dofetilide should be stopped.

Elderly: Refer to adult dosing. No specific dosage adjustments are recommended based on age; however, careful assessment of renal function is particularly important in this population. See Special Geriatric Considerations.

Renal Impairment:

Cl_{cr} >60 mL/minute: Administer 500 mcg twice daily.

Cl_{cr} 40-60 mL/minute: Administer 250 mcg twice daily.

Cl_{cr} 20-39 mL/minute: Administer 125 mcg twice daily.

Cl_{cr} <20 mL/minute: Contraindicated in this group

Hepatic Impairment: No dosage adjustments required in Child-Pugh class A and B; patients with severe hepatic impairment were not studied.

Administration

Oral: Do not open capsules.

Laboratory Monitoring Serum creatinine; check serum potassium and magnesium levels if on medications where these electrolyte disturbances can occur, or if patient has a history of hypokalemia or hypomagnesemia.

Nursing Actions

Physical Assessment: Assess other medications patient may be taking for effectiveness and interactions. Must be initiated or reinitiated by a cardiologist in a setting with continuous ECG monitoring for a period of time at beginning or adjustment of therapy. Monitor for signs of electrolyte imbalance (muscle weakness, spasms, twitching, numbness, lethargy, irregular heartbeat, and seizures). Monitor laboratory results, therapeutic response, and adverse reactions at beginning of therapy and on a regular basis with long-term therapy. Assess knowledge/teach patient appropriate use, interventions to reduce side effects, and adverse reactions to report.

Patient Education: Take exactly as directed; do not take additional doses or discontinue without consulting prescriber. Do not open capsules. If you miss a dose, take your normal amount at the next scheduled time. You will need regular cardiac checkups and blood tests when taking this medication. You may experience headache, dizziness, or difficulty sleeping (use caution when driving or engaging in tasks requiring alertness until response to drug is known); or abdominal pain, diarrhea, or nausea (small frequent meals and increased dietary bulk may help). Inform prescriber immediately if you experience fainting; severe GI discomfort or diarrhea; chest palpitations, irregular heartbeat, or chest pain; increased thirst; respiratory difficulty; skin rash; back pain; or alteration in muscle strength or gait. **Pregnancy/breast-feeding precautions:** Inform your prescriber if you are or intend to become pregnant. Breast-feeding is not recommended.

Pregnancy Issues Dofetilide has been shown to adversely affect *in utero* growth, organogenesis, and survival of rats and mice. There are no adequate and well-controlled studies in pregnant women. Dofetilide should be used with extreme caution in pregnant women and in women of childbearing age only when the benefit to the patient unequivocally justifies the potential risk to the fetus.

Dolasetron (dol A se tron)

U.S. Brand Names Anzemet®

Synonyms Dolasetron Mesylate; MDL 73,147EF

Pharmacologic Category Antiemetic; Selective 5-HT$_3$ Receptor Antagonist

Medication Safety Issues
Sound-alike/look-alike issues:
Anzemet® may be confused with Aldomet®
Dolasetron may be confused with granisetron, ondansetron, palonosetron

Pregnancy Risk Factor B

Lactation Excretion in breast milk unknown/use caution

Use Prevention of nausea and vomiting associated with emetogenic cancer chemotherapy; prevention of postoperative nausea and vomiting; treatment of postoperative nausea and vomiting (injectable form only)

Not recommended for treatment of existing chemotherapy-induced emesis (CIE).

Mechanism of Action/Effect Selective 5-HT$_3$ receptor antagonist, blocking serotonin, both peripherally on vagal nerve terminals and centrally in the chemoreceptor trigger zone

Contraindications Hypersensitivity to dolasetron or any component of the formulation

Warnings/Precautions Administer with caution in patients who have or may develop prolongation of cardiac conduction intervals, particularly QT$_c$ intervals. These include patients with hypokalemia, hypomagnesemia, patients taking diuretics which may cause electrolyte disturbances, patients with congenital QT syndrome, patients taking antiarrhythmic drugs or drug which prolong QT interval, and cumulative high-dose anthracycline therapy. Safety and efficacy in children <2 years of age have not been established.

Drug Interactions
Cytochrome P450 Effect: Substrate (minor) of CYP2C8/9, 3A4; **Inhibits** CYP2D6 (weak)
Decreased Effect: Blood levels of active metabolite are decreased during coadministration of rifampin.
Increased Effect/Toxicity: Due to reports of profound hypotension during concomitant therapy with ondansetron, the manufacturer of apomorphine contraindicates its use with all 5-HT$_3$ antagonists. Use caution with QT$_c$-prolonging agents (includes but may not be limited to amitriptyline, bepridil, disopyramide, erythromycin, haloperidol, imipramine, quinidine, pimozide, procainamide, sotalol, and thioridazine);

effect/toxicity of dolasetron and other QT$_c$-prolonging agents may be increased

Nutritional/Ethanol Interactions Herb/Nutraceutical: St John's wort may decrease dolasetron levels.

Adverse Reactions Adverse events may vary according to indication
>10%:
Central nervous system: Headache (7% to 24%)
Gastrointestinal: Diarrhea (2% to 12%)
1% to 10%:
Cardiovascular: Bradycardia (5%), hypotension (5%), hypertension (2% to 3%), tachycardia (2% to 3%)
Central nervous system: Dizziness (1% to 6%), fatigue (3% to 6%), fever (3% to 5%), chills/shivering (1% to 2%), sedation (2%)
Dermatological: Pruritus (3% to 4%)
Gastrointestinal: Dyspepsia (2% to 3%), abdominal pain (3%)
Hepatic: Abnormal hepatic function (4%)
Neuromuscular & skeletal: Pain (3%)
Renal: Oliguria (1% to 3%), urinary retention (2%)

Overdosage/Toxicology Prolongation of QT, AV block, severe hypotension, and dizziness have been reported. Treatment is supportive, and continuous ECG monitoring (telemetry) is recommended.

Pharmacodynamics/Kinetics
Time to Peak:
1 hour
Protein Binding: Hydrodolasetron: 69% to 77% (50 bound to alpha$_1$-acid glycoprotein)
Half-Life Elimination: Dolasetron: 10 minutes; hydrodolasetron: 6-8 hours
Metabolism: Hepatic; reduction by carbonyl reductase to hydrodolasetron (active metabolite); further metabolized by CYP3A and flavin monooxygenase
Excretion: Urine ~67% (61% active metabolite); feces ~33%

Available Dosage Forms
Injection, solution, as mesylate: 20 mg/mL (0.625 mL) [single-use ampul, Carpuject®, or vial]; 20 mg/mL (5 mL) [single-use vial]; 20 mg/mL (25 mL) [multidose vial]
Tablet, as mesylate: 50 mg, 100 mg

Dosing
Adults & Elderly:
Nausea and vomiting associated with cancer chemotherapy:
Oral:100 mg single dose 1 hour prior to chemotherapy
I.V.: 1.8 mg/kg or 100 mg 30 minutes prior to chemotherapy
Postoperative nausea and vomiting:
Prevention:
Oral: 100 mg within 2 hours before surgery (doses of 25-200 mg have been used)
I.V.: 12.5 mg ~15 minutes before stopping anesthesia
Treatment: I.V. (only): 12.5 mg as soon as needed
Pediatrics:
Nausea and vomiting prophylaxis, chemotherapy-induced (including initial and repeat courses): Children 2-16 years:
Oral: 1.8 mg/kg within 1 hour before chemotherapy; maximum: 100 mg/dose
I.V.: 1.8 mg/kg ~30 minutes before chemotherapy; maximum: 100 mg/dose
Postoperative nausea and vomiting: Children 2-16 years:
Prevention:
Oral: 1.2 mg/kg within 2 hours before surgery; maximum: 100 mg/dose
I.V.: 0.35 mg/kg (maximum: 12.5 mg) ~15 minutes before stopping anesthesia
Treatment: I.V. (only): 0.35 mg/kg as soon as needed
(Continued)

Dolasetron *(Continued)*

Administration

Oral: Dolasetron injection may be diluted in apple or apple-grape juice and taken orally; this dilution is stable for 2 hours at room temperature.

I.V.: I.V. injection may be given either undiluted IVP over 30 seconds or diluted in 50 mL of compatible fluid and infused over 15 minutes. Line should be flushed, prior to and after, dolasetron administration.

Stability

Reconstitution: Dilute in 50-100 mL of a compatible solution.

Compatibility: Stable in 0.9% NS, D_5W, D_5W and 0.45% NS, D_5W and LR, LR, and 10% mannitol injection

Storage: Store intact vials and tablets at room temperature. Protect from light. Stock solution (20 mg/mL) drawn into syringes is stable for 8 months at room temperature. After dilution, I.V. dolasetron is stable under normal lighting conditions at room temperature for 24 hours or under refrigeration for 48 hours with the following **compatible** intravenous fluids: 0.9% sodium chloride injection, 5% dextrose injection, 5% dextrose and 0.45% sodium chloride injection, 5% dextrose and lactated Ringer's injection, lactated Ringer's injection, and 10% mannitol injection

Nursing Actions

Physical Assessment: Assess potential for interactions with other pharmacological agents or herbal products patient may be taking (eg, antiarrhythmics, diuretics). Monitor therapeutic effectiveness and adverse reactions (eg, cardiac abnormalities) on a regular basis. Teach patient possible side effects/appropriate interventions and adverse symptoms to report.

Patient Education: This drug is given to reduce the incidence of nausea and vomiting. May cause headache, drowsiness, or dizziness (request assistance when getting up or changing position and do not perform activities requiring alertness). Report immediately any chest pain, rapid heartbeat, or palpitations; unusual pain, chills, or fever; severe headache or diarrhea; chest pain, palpitations, or tightness; swelling of throat or feeling of tightness in throat; or difficulty urinating. **Breast-feeding precaution:** Consult prescriber if breast-feeding.

Additional Information Efficacy of dolasetron, for chemotherapy treatment, is enhanced with concomitant administration of dexamethasone 20 mg (increases complete response by 10% to 20%). Oral administration of the intravenous solution is equivalent to tablets. A single I.V. dose of dolasetron mesylate (1.8 or 2.4 mg/kg) has comparable safety and efficacy to a single 32 mg I.V. dose of ondansetron in patients receiving cisplatin chemotherapy.

Donepezil *(doh NEP e zil)*

U.S. Brand Names Aricept®; Aricept® ODT

Synonyms E2020

Pharmacologic Category Acetylcholinesterase Inhibitor (Central)

Medication Safety Issues
Sound-alike/look-alike issues:
Aricept® may be confused with AcipHex®, Ascriptin®

Pregnancy Risk Factor C

Lactation Excretion in breast milk unknown/not recommended

Use Treatment of mild to moderate dementia of the Alzheimer's type

Unlabeled/Investigational Use Attention-deficit/hyperactivity disorder (ADHD), behavioral syndromes in dementia

Mechanism of Action/Effect Alzheimer's disease is characterized by cholinergic deficiency in the cortex and basal forebrain, which contributes to cognitive deficits. Donepezil reversibly and noncompetitively inhibits centrally-active acetylcholinesterase, the enzyme responsible for hydrolysis of acetylcholine. This appears to result in increased concentrations of acetylcholine available for synaptic transmission in the central nervous system.

Contraindications Hypersensitivity to donepezil, piperidine derivatives, or any component of the formulation

Warnings/Precautions Cholinesterase inhibitors may have vagotonic effects which may cause bradycardia and/or heart block with or without a history of cardiac disease; syncopal episodes have been associated with donepezil. Use with caution with sick sinus syndrome or other supraventricular cardiac conduction abnormalities, with seizures, COPD, or asthma. Use with caution in patients at risk of ulcer disease (ie, previous history or NSAID use), or in patients with bladder outlet obstruction. May cause diarrhea, nausea, and/or vomiting, which may be dose-related.

Drug Interactions

Cytochrome P450 Effect: Substrate (minor) of CYP2D6, 3A4

Decreased Effect: Anticholinergic agents (benztropine) may inhibit the effects of donepezil. Acetylcholinesterase inhibitors (central) may increase the risk of antipsychotic-related extrapyramidal symptoms.

Increased Effect/Toxicity: A synergistic effect may be seen with concurrent administration of succinylcholine or cholinergic agonists (bethanechol).

Nutritional/Ethanol Interactions Herb/Nutraceutical: St John's wort may decrease donepezil levels.

Adverse Reactions
>10%:
Central nervous system: Insomnia (6% to 14%)
Gastrointestinal: Nausea (5% to 19%), diarrhea (8% to 15%)
1% to 10%:
Cardiovascular: Syncope (2%), chest pain, hyper-/hypotension, atrial fibrillation, hot flashes
Central nervous system: Abnormal dreams (3%), depression (3%), dizziness (8%), fatigue (3% to 8%), headache (10%), somnolence
Dermatologic: Bruising (4%), pruritus, urticaria
Endocrine & metabolic: Dehydration
Gastrointestinal: Anorexia (3% to 7%), vomiting (3% to 8%), weight loss (3%), fecal incontinence, GI bleeding, bloating, epigastric pain, toothache
Genitourinary: Frequent urination (2%), urinary incontinence, nocturia
Neuromuscular & skeletal: Muscle cramps (3% to 8%), arthritis (2%), body pain, bone fracture
Ocular: Blurred vision, cataract, eye irritation
Respiratory: Influenza, dyspnea, bronchitis
Miscellaneous: Diaphoresis

Overdosage/Toxicology Implement general supportive measures. Donepezil can cause a cholinergic crisis characterized by severe nausea, vomiting, salivation, sweating, bradycardia, hypotension, collapse, and convulsions. Increased muscle weakness is a possibility and may result in death if respiratory muscles are involved. The effectiveness of dialysis is unknown.

Tertiary anticholinergics, such as atropine, may be used as an antidote for overdose. I.V. atropine sulfate titrated to effect is recommended with an initial dose of 1-2 mg I.V., with subsequent doses based upon clinical response. Atypical increases in blood pressure and heart rate have been reported with other cholinomimetics when coadministered with quaternary anticholinergics such as glycopyrrolate.

Pharmacodynamics/Kinetics

Time to Peak: Plasma: 3-4 hours

Protein Binding: 96%, primarily to albumin (75%) and α_1-acid glycoprotein (21%)

Half-Life Elimination: 70 hours; time to steady-state: 15 days

Metabolism: Extensively to four major metabolites (two are active) via CYP2D6 and 3A4; undergoes glucuronidation

Excretion: Urine 57% (17% as unchanged drug); feces 15%

Available Dosage Forms

Tablet, as hydrochloride (Aricept®): 5 mg, 10 mg

Tablet, orally disintegrating, as hydrochloride (Aricept® ODT): 5 mg, 10 mg

Dosing

Adults & Elderly: Alzheimer's disease: Oral: Initial: 5 mg/day at bedtime; may increase to 10 mg/day at bedtime after 4-6 weeks.

Pediatrics: ADHD (unlabeled use): Oral: 5 mg/day

Administration

Oral:

Aricept® ODT: Allow tablet to dissolve completely on tongue and follow with water.

Nursing Actions

Physical Assessment: Assess bladder adequacy prior to administering medication. Assess other medications patient may be taking for effectiveness and interactions. Monitor laboratory tests, therapeutic effect, and adverse reactions: cholinergic crisis (DUMBELS - diarrhea, urination, miosis, bronchospasm/bradycardia, excitability, lacrimation, and salivation/excessive sweating). Monitor pulse. Assess knowledge/teach patient appropriate use, interventions to reduce side effects, and adverse symptoms to report.

Patient Education: This medication will not cure the disease, but may help reduce symptoms. Use as directed; do not increase dose or discontinue without consulting prescriber. Maintain adequate hydration (2-3 L/day of fluids) unless instructed to restrict fluid intake. May cause dizziness, sedation, or hypotension (rise slowly from sitting or lying position and use caution when driving or climbing stairs); vomiting or loss of appetite (small frequent meals, frequent mouth care, chewing gum, or sucking lozenges may help); or diarrhea (boiled milk, yogurt, or buttermilk may help). Report persistent abdominal discomfort; significantly increased salivation, sweating, tearing, or urination; flushed skin; chest pain or palpitations; acute headache; unresolved diarrhea; excessive fatigue, insomnia, dizziness, or depression; increased muscle, joint, or body pain; vision changes or blurred vision; or shortness of breath or wheezing. **Pregnancy/breast-feeding precautions:** Inform prescriber if you are or intend to become pregnant. Breast-feeding is not recommended.

Dietary Considerations

May take with or without food.

Geriatric Considerations Donepezil is an anticholinesterase for the treatment of Alzheimer's disease. It has been shown to cause an improvement in the ADAS-cog scores. As compared to tacrine, donepezil does **not** cause elevations in liver function tests and does not require routine laboratory monitoring. In addition, it is dosed once a day versus tacrine's four doses per day. For these reasons, donepezil may be preferred over tacrine in the treatment of mild to moderate dementia of the Alzheimer's type.

DOPamine (DOE pa meen)

Synonyms Dopamine Hydrochloride; Intropin

Pharmacologic Category Adrenergic Agonist Agent

Medication Safety Issues

Sound-alike/look-alike issues:

DOPamine may be confused with DOBUTamine, Dopram®

Pregnancy Risk Factor C

Lactation Excretion in breast milk unknown

Use Adjunct in the treatment of shock (eg, MI, open heart surgery, renal failure, cardiac decompensation) which persists after adequate fluid volume replacement

Unlabeled/Investigational Use Symptomatic bradycardia or heart block unresponsive to atropine or pacing

Mechanism of Action/Effect Stimulates both adrenergic and dopaminergic receptors, lower doses are mainly dopaminergic stimulating and produce renal and mesenteric vasodilation, higher doses also are both dopaminergic and beta$_1$-adrenergic stimulating and produce cardiac stimulation and renal vasodilation; large doses stimulate alpha-adrenergic receptors

Contraindications Hypersensitivity to sulfites (commercial preparation contains sodium bisulfite); pheochromocytoma; ventricular fibrillation

Warnings/Precautions Use with caution in patients with cardiovascular disease or cardiac arrhythmias or patients with occlusive vascular disease. Correct hypovolemia and electrolytes when used in hemodynamic support. May cause increases in HR and arrhythmia. Avoid infiltration - may cause severe tissue necrosis. Use with caution in post-MI patients. Avoid sudden discontinuation.

Drug Interactions

Decreased Effect: Tricyclic antidepressants may have a decreased effect when coadministered with dopamine. Guanethidine's hypotensive effects may only be partially reversed; may need to use a direct-acting sympathomimetic.

Increased Effect/Toxicity: Dopamine's effects are prolonged and intensified by MAO inhibitors, alpha- and beta-adrenergic blockers, cocaine, general anesthetics, methyldopa, phenytoin, reserpine, and TCAs.

Adverse Reactions Frequency not defined.

Cardiovascular: Ectopic beats, tachycardia, anginal pain, palpitation, hypotension, vasoconstriction

Central nervous system: Headache

Gastrointestinal: Nausea and vomiting

Respiratory: Dyspnea

Overdosage/Toxicology Symptoms of overdose include severe hypertension, cardiac arrhythmias, acute renal failure. Treat symptomatically.

Important: Antidote for peripheral ischemia: To prevent sloughing and necrosis in ischemic areas, the area should be infiltrated as soon as possible with 10-15 mL of saline solution containing 5-10 mg of Regitine (brand of phentolamine), an adrenergic blocking agent. A syringe with a fine hypodermic needle should be used, and the solution liberally infiltrated throughout the ischemic area. Sympathetic blockade with phentolamine causes immediate and conspicuous local hyperemic changes if the area is infiltrated within 12 hours. Therefore, phentolamine should be given as soon as possible after extravasation is noted.

Pharmacodynamics/Kinetics

Onset of Action: Adults: 5 minutes

Duration of Action: Adults: <10 minutes

Half-Life Elimination: 2 minutes

Metabolism: Renal, hepatic, plasma; 75% to inactive metabolites by monoamine oxidase and 25% to norepinephrine

(Continued)

DOPamine *(Continued)*

Excretion: Urine (as metabolites)

Clearance: Neonates: Varies and appears to be age related; prolonged clearance with combined hepatic and renal impairment

Pharmacokinetic Note Dopamine has exhibited nonlinear kinetics in children; with medication changes, may not achieve steady-state for ~1 hour rather than 20 minutes.

Available Dosage Forms

Infusion, as hydrochloride [premixed in D_5W]: 0.8 mg/mL (250 mL, 500 mL); 1.6 mg/mL (250 mL, 500 mL); 3.2 mg/mL (250 mL)

Injection, solution, as hydrochloride: 40 mg/mL (5 mL, 10 mL); 80 mg/mL (5 mL); 160 mg/mL (5 mL) [contains sodium metabisulfite]

Dosing

Adults & Elderly:

Hemodynamic support: I.V. infusion: 1-5 mcg/kg/minute up to 50 mcg/kg/minute, titrate to desired response; infusion may be increased by 1-4 mcg/kg/minute at 10- to 30-minute intervals until optimal response is obtained

Note: If dosages >20-30 mcg/kg/minute are needed, a more direct-acting vasopressor may be more beneficial (ie, epinephrine, norepinephrine).

Hemodynamic effects of dopamine are dose dependent:

Low-dose: 1-5 mcg/kg/minute, increased renal blood flow and urine output

Intermediate-dose: 5-15 mcg/kg/minute, increased renal blood flow, heart rate, cardiac contractility, and cardiac output

High-dose: >15 mcg/kg/minute, alpha-adrenergic effects begin to predominate, vasoconstriction, increased blood pressure

Pediatrics: Hemodynamic support: I.V. infusion:

Children: 1-20 mcg/kg/minute, maximum: 50 mcg/kg/minute continuous infusion, titrate to desired response.

Administration

I.V.: Vesicant. **Must be diluted prior to use.** Do not discontinue suddenly - sudden discontinuation may lead to marked hypotension.

I.V. Detail: Monitor continuously for free flow. Administration into an umbilical arterial catheter is not recommended; central line administration.

Extravasation management: Due to short half-life, withdrawal of drug is often only necessary treatment. Use phentolamine as antidote. Mix 5 mg with 9 mL of NS; inject a small amount of this dilution into extravasated area. Blanching should reverse immediately. Monitor site. If blanching should recur, additional injections of phentolamine may be needed.

pH: 3.3-3.6

Stability

Compatibility: Stable in D_5LR, $D_5\frac{1}{2}NS$, D_5NS, D_5W, $D_{10}W$, LR, mannitol 20%, NS; **incompatible** with sodium bicarbonate 5%, and alkaline solutions or iron salts.

Y-site administration: Incompatible with acyclovir, alteplase, amphotericin B cholesteryl sulfate complex, cefepime, indomethacin, insulin (regular), thiopental

Compatibility when admixed: Incompatible with acyclovir, alteplase, amphotericin B, ampicillin, metronidazole with sodium bicarbonate, penicillin G potassium

Storage: Protect from light. Solutions that are darker than slightly yellow should not be used.

Laboratory Monitoring Serum glucose, renal function

Physical Assessment: Assess other medications patient may be taking for effectiveness and interactions. Infusion pump and continuous cardiac and hemodynamic monitoring are required for inpatient therapy. Assess I.V. site frequently. Monitor therapeutic response (cardiac status, renal function) and adverse reactions including peripheral ischemia. Low-dose home infusion therapy requires frequent monitoring of cardiac and renal status and adverse reactions.

Patient Education: When administered in emergencies, patient education should be appropriate to the situation. If patient is aware, instruct to promptly report chest pain, palpitations, rapid heartbeat, headache, nervousness or restlessness, nausea or vomiting, or respiratory difficulty.

Geriatric Considerations Has not been specifically studied in the elderly.

Additional Information Dopamine is most frequently used for treatment of hypotension because of its peripheral vasoconstrictor action. In this regard, dopamine is often used together with dobutamine and minimizes hypotension secondary to dobutamine-induced vasodilation. Thus, pressure is maintained by increased cardiac output (from dobutamine) and vasoconstriction (by dopamine). It is critical neither dopamine nor dobutamine be used in patients in the absence of correcting any hypovolemia as a cause of hypotension.

Low-dose dopamine is often used in the intensive care setting for presumed beneficial effects on renal function. However, there is no clear evidence that low-dose dopamine confers any renal or other benefit. Indeed, dopamine may act on dopamine receptors in the carotid bodies causing chemoreflex suppression. In patients with heart failure, dopamine may inhibit breathing and cause pulmonary shunting. Both these mechanisms would act to decrease minute ventilation and oxygen saturation. This could potentially be deleterious in patients with respiratory compromise and patients being weaned from ventilators.

Related Information

Compatibility of Drugs *on page 1370*

FDA Name Differentiation Project: The Use of Tall-Man Letters *on page 12*

Dornase Alfa *(DOOR nase AL fa)*

U.S. Brand Names Pulmozyme®

Synonyms DNase; Recombinant Human Deoxyribonuclease

Pharmacologic Category Enzyme

Pregnancy Risk Factor B

Lactation Excretion in breast milk unknown

Use Management of cystic fibrosis patients to reduce the frequency of respiratory infections that require parenteral antibiotics, and to improve pulmonary function

Unlabeled/Investigational Use Treatment of chronic bronchitis

Mechanism of Action/Effect The hallmark of cystic fibrosis lung disease is the presence of abundant, purulent airway secretions composed primarily of highly polymerized DNA. Dornase selectively cleaves DNA, thus reducing mucous viscosity and as a result, airflow in the lung is improved and the risk of bacterial infection may be decreased.

Contraindications Hypersensitivity to dornase alfa, Chinese hamster ovary cell products (eg, epoetin alfa), or any component of the formulation

Warnings/Precautions No clinical trials have been conducted to demonstrate safety and effectiveness of dornase in children <5 years of age, in patients with pulmonary function <40% of normal, or in patients for longer treatment periods >12 months.

Adverse Reactions

>10%:

Respiratory: Pharyngitis

Miscellaneous: Voice alteration

1% to 10%:

Cardiovascular: Chest pain

Dermatologic: Rash

Ocular: Conjunctivitis

Respiratory: Laryngitis, cough, dyspnea, hemoptysis, rhinitis, hoarse throat, wheezing

Pharmacodynamics/Kinetics

Onset of Action: Nebulization: Enzyme levels are measured in sputum in ~15 minutes

Duration of Action: Rapidly declines

Available Dosage Forms Solution for nebulization: 1 mg/mL (2.5 mL)

Dosing

Adults & Elderly: Mucolytic: Inhalation: 2.5 mg once daily through selected nebulizers

Pediatrics:

Mucolytic (cystic fibrosis): Inhalation:

Children >3 months to Adults: 2.5 mg once daily through selected nebulizers; experience in children <5 years is limited

Note: Patients unable to inhale or exhale orally throughout the entire treatment period may use Pari-Baby™ nebulizer. Some patients may benefit from twice daily administration.

Stability

Compatibility: Should not be diluted or mixed with any other drugs in the nebulizer, this may inactivate the dornase alfa.

Storage: Must be stored in the refrigerator at 2°C to 8°C (36°F to 46°F) and protected from strong light. Should not be exposed to room temperature for a total of 24 hours.

Nursing Actions

Physical Assessment: Assess effectiveness of therapy and adverse reactions at beginning of therapy and periodically with long-term use. Teach patient or caregiver appropriate use of nebulizer, interventions to reduce side effects, and adverse symptoms to report.

Patient Education: Inform prescriber of any allergies you have. Use exactly as directed by prescriber (see following administration information). Report any signs of adverse response, skin rash, sore throat, respiratory difficulty, wheezing, or cough. **Breast-feeding precaution:** Consult prescriber if breast-feeding.

Self-administered nebulizer: Store in refrigerator, away from light. Do not combine with any other medications in the nebulizer. Wash hands before and after treatment. Wash and dry nebulizer after each treatment. Twist open the top of one unit dose vial and squeeze contents into nebulizer reservoir. Connect nebulizer reservoir to the mouthpiece or face mask. Connect nebulizer to compressor. Sit in comfortable, upright position. Put on face mask and turn on compressor. Avoid leakage around the mask to avoid mist getting into eyes. Breathe calmly and deeply until no more mist is formed in nebulizer (about 5 minutes). At this point treatment is finished.

Dorzolamide (dor ZOLE a mide)

U.S. Brand Names Trusopt®

Synonyms Dorzolamide Hydrochloride

Pharmacologic Category Carbonic Anhydrase Inhibitor; Ophthalmic Agent, Antiglaucoma

Pregnancy Risk Factor C

Lactation Excretion in breast milk unknown/not recommended

Use Lowers intraocular pressure in patients with ocular hypertension or open-angle glaucoma

Contraindications Hypersensitivity to dorzolamide or any component of the formulation

Warnings/Precautions Although administered topically, systemic absorption occurs. Similar adverse reactions attributed to sulfonamides may occur with topical administration. Chemical similarities are present among sulfonamides, sulfonylureas, carbonic anhydrase inhibitors, thiazides, and loop diuretics (except ethacrynic acid). In patients with allergy to one of these compounds, a risk of cross-reaction exists; avoid use when previous reaction has been severe. Not recommended for use in patients with severe renal impairment (Cl_{cr} <30 mL/minute); use with caution in patients with hepatic impairment. detachment has been reported after filtration procedures.

Contains benzalkonium chloride which may be absorbed by soft contact lenses. Dorzolamide should not be administered while wearing soft contact lenses. Safety and efficacy have not been established in children <2 years of age.

Drug Interactions

Cytochrome P450 Effect: Substrate (minor) of CYP2C8/9, 3A4

Increased Effect/Toxicity: High-dose salicylate therapy may result in carbonic anhydrase inhibitor accumulation and toxicity including CNS depression and metabolic acidosis; avoid use if possible.

Adverse Reactions

>10%:

Gastrointestinal: Bitter taste following administration (25%)

Ocular: Burning, stinging or discomfort immediately following administration (33%); superficial punctate keratitis (10% to 15%); signs and symptoms of ocular allergic reaction (10%)

1% to 5%: Ocular: Blurred vision, conjunctivitis, dryness, lid reactions, photophobia, tearing

Overdosage/Toxicology

Symptoms of overdose include electrolyte imbalance, development of an acidotic state and possible CNS effects. Treatment should be symptom-directed and supportive.

Pharmacodynamics/Kinetics

Onset of Action: Peak effect: 2 hours

Duration of Action: 8-12 hours

Protein Binding: 33%

Half-Life Elimination: Terminal RBC: 147 days; washes out of RBCs nonlinearly, resulting in a rapid decline of drug concentration initially, followed by a slower elimination phase with a half-life of about 4 months

Metabolism: To N-desethyl metabolite (less potent than parent drug)

Excretion: Urine (as unchanged drug and metabolite, N-desethyl)

Available Dosage Forms Solution, ophthalmic, as hydrochloride: 2% (5 mL, 10 mL) [contains benzalkonium chloride]

Dosing

Adults & Elderly: Reduction of intraocular pressure: Ophthalmic: Instill 1 drop in the affected eye(s) 3 times/day

(Continued)

Dorzolamide *(Continued)*

Pediatrics: Refer to adult dosing.

Administration

Other: If more than one topical ophthalmic drug is being used, administer the drugs at least 10 minutes apart. Instruct patients to avoid allowing the tip of the dispensing container to contact the eye or surrounding structures. Ocular solutions can become contaminated by common bacteria known to cause ocular infections. Serious damage to the eye and subsequent loss of vision may occur from using contaminated solutions.

Stability

Storage: Store at room temperature (25°C).

Nursing Actions

Physical Assessment: Assess potential for interactions with other prescriptions, OTC medications, or herbal products patient may be taking. Monitor patient response and adverse effects. Teach patient proper use, side effects/appropriate interventions, and symptoms to report.

Patient Education: For use in eyes only. If serious or unusual reactions or signs of hypersensitivity occur, discontinue use of the product. If any ocular reactions, particularly conjunctivitis and lid reactions, discontinue use and notify prescriber. If an intercurrent ocular condition (eg, trauma, ocular surgery, infection) occur, immediately seek your prescriber's advice concerning the continued use of the present multidose container. Avoid allowing the tip of the dispensing container to contact the eye or surrounding structures. Take out contact lenses before using medicine. Lenses can be replaced 15 minutes after medicine is given. **Pregnancy precaution:** Inform prescriber if you are pregnant.

Doxacurium *(doks a KYOO ri um)*

U.S. Brand Names Nuromax®

Synonyms Doxacurium Chloride

Pharmacologic Category Neuromuscular Blocker Agent, Nondepolarizing

Medication Safety Issues

Sound-alike/look-alike issues:

Doxacurium may be confused with doxapram, DOXOrubicin

Pregnancy Risk Factor C

Use Adjunct to general anesthesia to facilitate endotracheal intubation and to relax skeletal muscles during surgery; to facilitate mechanical ventilation in ICU patients; does not relieve pain or produce sedation; the characteristics of this agent make it especially useful in procedures requiring careful maintenance of hemodynamic stability for prolonged periods

Mechanism of Action/Effect Prevents depolarization of muscle membrane and subsequent muscle contraction by acting as a competitive antagonist to acetylcholine at the alpha subunits of the nicotinic cholinergic receptors on the motor endplates in skeletal muscle, also interferes with the mobilization of acetylcholine presynaptically; the neuromuscular blockade can be pharmacologically reversed with an anticholinesterase agent (neostigmine, edrophonium, pyridostigmine)

Contraindications Hypersensitivity to doxacurium or any component of the formulation

Warnings/Precautions Use with caution in the elderly, effects and duration are more variable; product contains benzyl alcohol, use with caution in newborns; use with caution in patients with renal or hepatic impairment; certain clinical conditions may result in potentiation or antagonism of neuromuscular blockade

Increased sensitivity in patients with myasthenia gravis, Eaton-Lambert syndrome; resistance in burn patients (>30% of body) for period of 5-70 days postinjury; resistance in patients with muscle trauma, denervation, immobilization, infection; does not counteract bradycardia produced by anesthetics/vagal stimulation. Cross-sensitivity with other neuromuscular-blocking agents may occur; use extreme caution in patients with previous anaphylactic reactions.

Drug Interactions

Decreased Effect: Effect of nondepolarizing neuromuscular blockers may be reduced by carbamazepine (chronic use), corticosteroids (also associated with myopathy - see increased effect), phenytoin (chronic use), sympathomimetics, and theophylline.

Increased Effect/Toxicity: Increased effects are possible with aminoglycosides, beta-blockers, clindamycin, calcium channel blockers, halogenated anesthetics, imipenem, ketamine, lidocaine, loop diuretics (furosemide), macrolides (case reports), magnesium sulfate, procainamide, quinidine, quinolones, tetracyclines, and vancomycin. May increase risk of myopathy when used with high- dose corticosteroids for extended periods.

Overdosage/Toxicology

Overdosage is manifested by prolonged neuromuscular blockage.

Treatment is supportive; reverse blockade with neostigmine, pyridostigmine, or edrophonium.

Pharmacodynamics/Kinetics

Onset of Action: 5-11 minutes

Duration of Action: 30 minutes (range: 12-54 minutes)

Protein Binding: 30%

Excretion: Primarily urine and feces (as unchanged drug); recovery time prolonged in elderly

Available Dosage Forms Injection, solution, as chloride: 1 mg/mL (5 mL) [contains benzyl alcohol]

Dosing

Adults & Elderly: Administer I.V.; dose to effect; doses will vary due to interpatient variability; use ideal body weight for obese patients.

Surgery (adjunct to anesthesia): I.V.: 0.05-0.08 mg/kg with thiopental/narcotic or 0.025 mg/kg after initial dose of succinylcholine for intubation; initial maintenance dose of 0.005-0.01 mg/kg after 100-160 minutes followed by repeat doses every 30-45 minutes

Pretreatment/priming: I.V.: 10% of intubating dose given 3-5 minutes before initial dose

Neuromuscular blockade in the ICU : I.V.: 0.05 mg/kg bolus followed by 0.025 mg/kg every 2-3 hours or 0.25-0.75 mcg/kg/minute once initial recovery from bolus dose observed

Pediatrics: *Note:* Administer I.V.; dose to effect; doses will vary due to interpatient variability; use ideal body weight for obese patients

Surgery (adjunct to anesthesia): Children >2 years: I.V.: Initial: 0.03-0.05 mg/kg followed by maintenance doses of 0.005-0.01 mg/kg after 30-45 minutes

Renal Impairment: Reduce initial dose and titrate carefully as duration may be prolonged.

Administration

I.V.: May be given rapid I.V. injection undiluted or via a continuous infusion using an infusion pump. Use infusion solutions within 24 hours of preparation.

Stability

Compatibility: Stable in D$_5$LR, D$_5$NS, D$_5$W, LR, NS

Storage: Stable for 24 hours at room temperature when diluted, up to 0.1 mg/mL in dextrose 5% or normal saline.

Nursing Actions

Physical Assessment: Only clinicians experienced in the use of neuromuscular-blocking drugs should administer and/or manage the use of doxacurium. Ventilatory support must be instituted and maintained until adequate respiratory muscle function and/or airway protection are assured. Assess other medications for effectiveness and safety. Other drugs that affect neuromuscular activity may increase/decrease neuromuscular block induced by doxacurium. This drug does not cause anesthesia or analgesia; pain must be treated with appropriate analgesic agents. Continuous monitoring of vital signs, cardiac status, respiratory status, and degree of neuromuscular block (objective assessment with peripheral external nerve stimulator) is mandatory during infusion and until full muscle tone has returned. Muscle tone returns in a predictable pattern, starting with diaphragm, abdomen, chest, limbs, and finally muscles of the neck, face, and eyes. Safety precautions must be maintained until full muscle tone has returned. **Note:** It may take longer for return of muscle tone in obese or elderly patients or patients with renal or hepatic disease, myasthenia gravis, myopathy, other neuromuscular disease, dehydration, electrolyte imbalance, or severe acid/base imbalance. Provide appropriate patient teaching/support prior to and following administration.

Long-term use: Monitor fluid levels (intake and output) during and following infusion. Reposition patient and provide appropriate skin care, mouth care, and care of patient's eyes every 2-3 hours while sedated. Provide appropriate emotional and sensory support (auditory and environmental).

Patient Education: Patient will usually be unconscious prior to administration. Patient education should be appropriate to individual situation. Reassurance of constant monitoring and emotional support to reduce fear and anxiety should precede and follow administration. Following return of muscle tone, do not attempt to change position or rise from bed without assistance. Report immediately any skin rash or hives, pounding heartbeat, respiratory difficulty, or muscle tremors. **Pregnancy precaution:** Inform prescriber if you are pregnant.

Additional Information Doxacurium is a long-acting nondepolarizing neuromuscular blocker with virtually no cardiovascular side effects. Characteristics of this agent make it especially useful in procedures requiring careful maintenance of hemodynamic stability for prolonged periods; reduce dosage in renal or hepatic impairment. It does not relieve pain or produce sedation. It does not appear to have a cumulative effect on duration of blockade.

Doxazosin (doks AY zoe sin)

U.S. Brand Names Cardura®
Synonyms Doxazosin Mesylate
Pharmacologic Category Alpha$_1$ Blocker
Medication Safety Issues
Sound-alike/look-alike issues:
Doxazosin may be confused with doxapram, doxepin, DOXOrubicin
Cardura® may be confused with Cardene®, Cordarone®, Cordran®, Coumadin®, K-Dur®, Ridaura®

Pregnancy Risk Factor C
Lactation Excretion in breast milk unknown
Use Treatment of hypertension alone or in conjunction with diuretics, cardiac glycosides, ACE inhibitors, or calcium antagonists (particularly appropriate for those with hypertension and other cardiovascular risk factors such as hypercholesterolemia and diabetes mellitus); treatment of urinary outflow obstruction and/or obstructive and irritative symptoms associated with benign prostatic hyperplasia (BPH), particularly useful in patients with troublesome symptoms who are unable or

unwilling to undergo invasive procedures, but who require rapid symptomatic relief; can be used in combination with finasteride

Mechanism of Action/Effect Competitively inhibits postsynaptic alpha-adrenergic receptors which results in vasodilation of veins and arterioles and a decrease in total peripheral resistance and blood pressure; approximately 50% as potent on a weight by weight basis as prazosin

Contraindications Hypersensitivity to quinazolines (prazosin, terazosin), doxazosin, or any component of the formulation; concurrent use with phosphodiesterase-5 (PDE-5) inhibitors including sildenafil (>25 mg), tadalafil, or vardenafil

Warnings/Precautions Can cause significant orthostatic hypotension and syncope, especially with first dose. Prostate cancer should be ruled out before starting for BPH. May need dosage adjustment in severe hepatic dysfunction. Anticipate a similar effect if therapy is interrupted for a few days, if dosage is rapidly increased, or if another antihypertensive drug is introduced.

Drug Interactions
Decreased Effect: Decreased hypotensive effect with NSAIDs.

Increased Effect/Toxicity: Increased hypotensive effect with beta-blockers, diuretics, ACE inhibitors, calcium channel blockers, other antihypertensive medications, sildenafil (use with extreme caution at a dose ≤25 mg), tadalafil (contraindicated by the manufacturer), and vardenafil (contraindicated by the manufacturer).

Nutritional/Ethanol Interactions Herb/Nutraceutical: Avoid dong quai if using for hypertension (has estrogenic activity). Avoid ephedra, yohimbe, ginseng (may worsen hypertension). Avoid saw palmetto when used for BPH (due to limited experience with this combination). Avoid garlic (may have increased antihypertensive effect).

Lab Interactions Increased urinary VMA 17%, norepinephrine metabolite 42%

Adverse Reactions Note: "Combination therapy" refers to doxazosin and finasteride.
>10%:
Cardiovascular: Postural hypotension (combination therapy 18%)
Central nervous system: Dizziness (16% to 19%; combination therapy 23%), headache (10% to 14%)
Endocrine & metabolic: Impotence (combination therapy 23%), libido decreased (combination therapy 12%)
Genitourinary: Ejaculation disturbances (combination therapy 14%)
Neuromuscular & skeletal: Weakness (combination therapy 17%)
1% to 10%:
Cardiovascular: Orthostatic hypotension (dose related; 0.3% up to 10%), edema (3% to 4%), hypotension (2%), palpitation (1% to 2%), chest pain (1% to 2%), arrhythmia (1%), syncope (2%), flushing (1%)
Central nervous system: Fatigue (8% to 12%), somnolence (3% to 5%), nervousness (2%), pain (2%), vertigo (2%), insomnia (1%), anxiety (1%), paresthesia (1%), movement disorder (1%), ataxia (1%), hypertonia (1%), depression (1%), weakness (1%)
Dermatologic: Rash (1%), pruritus (1%)
Endocrine & metabolic: Sexual dysfunction (2%)
Gastrointestinal: Abdominal pain (2%), diarrhea (2%), dyspepsia (1% to 2%), nausea (2% to 3%), xerostomia (1% to 2%), constipation (1%), flatulence (1%)
Genitourinary: Urinary tract infection (1%), impotence (1%), polyuria (2%), incontinence (1%)
(Continued)

Doxazosin *(Continued)*

Neuromuscular & skeletal: Back pain (2%), arthritis (1%), muscle weakness (1%), myalgia (1%), muscle cramps (1%)

Ocular: Abnormal vision (1% to 2%), conjunctivitis (1%)

Otic: Tinnitus (1%)

Respiratory: Rhinitis (3%), dyspnea (1% to 3%), respiratory disorder (1%), epistaxis (1%)

Miscellaneous: Diaphoresis increased (1%), flu-like syndrome (1%)

Overdosage/Toxicology Symptoms of overdose include severe hypotension, drowsiness, and tachycardia. Treatment is supportive and symptomatic.

Pharmacodynamics/Kinetics

Duration of Action: >24 hours

Time to Peak: Serum: 2-3 hours

Half-Life Elimination: 22 hours

Metabolism: Extensively hepatic

Excretion: Feces (63%); urine (9%)

Pharmacokinetic Note Not significantly affected by increased age.

Available Dosage Forms Tablet: 1 mg, 2 mg, 4 mg, 8 mg

Dosing

Adults: Hypertension or urinary outflow obstruction: Oral: 1 mg once daily in morning or evening; may be increased to 2 mg once daily; thereafter titrate upwards, if needed, over several weeks, balancing therapeutic benefit with doxazosin-induced postural hypotension; maximum dose for **hypertension:** 16 mg/day, for **BPH:** 8 mg/day (goal: 4-8 mg/day)

Elderly: Oral: Initial: 0.5 mg once daily

Administration

Oral: Syncope may occur usually within 90 minutes of the initial dose.

Laboratory Monitoring White blood count

Nursing Actions

Physical Assessment: Assess potential for interactions with other pharmacological agents or herbal products patient may be taking. Monitor therapeutic effectiveness (blood pressure) and adverse effects (eg, hypotension, CNS changes, urinary retention) at beginning of therapy and on a regular basis with long-term therapy. When discontinuing, monitor blood pressure and taper dose slowly over 1 week or more. Teach patient proper use, possible side effects/appropriate interventions, and adverse symptoms to report.

Patient Education: Do not take any new medication during therapy unless approved by prescriber. Take as directed, at bedtime. Do not skip dose or discontinue without consulting prescriber. Follow recommended diet and exercise program. May cause drowsiness, dizziness, or impaired judgment (use caution when driving or engaging in tasks that require alertness until response to drug is known); postural hypotension (use caution when rising from sitting or lying position or when climbing stairs); or dry mouth or nausea (frequent mouth care or sucking lozenges may help). Report increased nervousness or depression; sudden weight gain (weigh yourself in the same clothes at the same time of day once a week); unusual or persistent swelling of ankles, feet, or extremities; palpitations or rapid heartbeat; muscle weakness, fatigue, or pain; or other persistent side effects. **Pregnancy/breast-feeding precautions:** Inform prescriber if you are or intend to become pregnant. Consult prescriber if breast-feeding.

Geriatric Considerations Adverse reactions such as dry mouth and urinary problems can be particularly bothersome in the elderly.

Additional Information First-dose hypotension occurs less frequently with doxazosin as compared to prazosin; this may be due to its slower onset of action.

Doxepin (DOKS e pin)

U.S. Brand Names Prudoxin™; Sinequan® [DSC]; Zonalon®

Synonyms Doxepin Hydrochloride

Restrictions A medication guide concerning the use of antidepressants in children and teenagers can be found on the FDA website at http://www.fda.gov/cder/Offices/ODS/labeling.htm. It should be dispensed to parents or guardians of children and teenagers receiving this medication.

Pharmacologic Category Antidepressant, Tricyclic (Tertiary Amine); Topical Skin Product

Medication Safety Issues

Sound-alike/look-alike issues:

Doxepin may be confused with digoxin, doxapram, doxazosin, Doxidan®, doxycycline

Sinequan® may be confused with saquinavir, Serentil®, Seroquel®, Singulair®

Zonalon® may be confused with Zone-A Forte®

Pregnancy Risk Factor B (cream); C (all other forms)

Lactation Enters breast milk/not recommended (AAP rates "of concern")

Use

Oral: Depression

Topical: Short-term (<8 days) management of moderate pruritus in adults with atopic dermatitis or lichen simplex chronicus

Unlabeled/Investigational Use Analgesic for certain chronic and neuropathic pain; anxiety

Mechanism of Action/Effect Increases the synaptic concentration of serotonin and norepinephrine in the central nervous system by inhibition of their reuptake by the presynaptic neuronal membrane

Contraindications Hypersensitivity to doxepin, drugs from similar chemical class, or any component of the formulation; narrow-angle glaucoma; urinary retention; use of MAO inhibitors within 14 days; use in a patient during acute recovery phase of MI

Warnings/Precautions Antidepressants increase the risk of suicidal thinking and behavior in children and adolescents with major depressive disorder (MDD) and other depressive disorders; consider risk prior to prescribing. All patients must be closely monitored for clinical worsening, suicidality, or unusual changes in behavior, especially during the initiation of therapy or following an increase or decrease in dosage. When used in children, the child's family or caregiver should be instructed to closely observe the patient and communicate condition with healthcare provider. A medication guide should be dispensed with each prescription. **Doxepin is approved for treatment of depression in adolescents.**

The possibility of a suicide attempt is inherent in major depression and may persist until remission occurs. Use caution in high-risk patients. Worsening depression and severe abrupt suicidality that are not part of the presenting symptoms may require discontinuation or modification of drug therapy. The patient's family or caregiver should be alerted to monitor patients for the emergence of suicidality and associated behaviors (such as agitation, irritability, hostility, impulsivity, and hypomania) and call healthcare provider.

May worsen psychosis in some patients or precipitate a shift to mania or hypomania in patients with bipolar disorder. Patients presenting with depressive symptoms should be screened for bipolar disorder. Monotherapy in patients with bipolar disorder should be avoided. **Doxepin is not FDA approved for the treatment of bipolar depression.**

The risks of sedative and anticholinergic effects are high relative to other antidepressant agents. Doxepin frequently causes sedation, which may result in impaired performance of tasks requiring alertness (eg, operating machinery or driving). Sedative effects may be additive with other CNS depressants and/or ethanol. Also use caution in patients with benign prostatic hyperplasia, xerostomia, visual problems, constipation, or history of bowel obstruction.

May cause orthostatic hypotension or conduction disturbances (risks are moderate relative to other antidepressants). Use with caution in patients with a history of cardiovascular disease (including previous MI, stroke, tachycardia, or conduction abnormalities). Consider discontinuation, when possible, prior to elective surgery. Therapy should not be abruptly discontinued in patients receiving high doses for prolonged periods.

Use caution in patients with a previous seizure disorder or condition predisposing to seizures such as brain damage, alcoholism, or concurrent therapy with other drugs which lower the seizure threshold. Use with caution in hyperthyroid patients or those receiving thyroid supplementation. Use with caution in patients with hepatic or renal dysfunction and in elderly patients.

Cream formulation is for external use only (not for ophthalmic, vaginal, or oral use). Do not use occlusive dressings. Use for >8 days may increase risk of contact sensitization. Doxepin is significantly absorbed following topical administration; plasma levels may be similar to those achieved with oral administration.

Drug Interactions
Cytochrome P450 Effect: Substrate (major) of CYP1A2, 2D6, 3A4

Decreased Effect: CYP1A2 inducers may decrease the levels/effects of doxepin; example inducers include aminoglutethimide, carbamazepine, phenobarbital, and rifampin. Doxepin inhibits the antihypertensive response to bethanidine, clonidine, debrisoquin, guanadrel, guanethidine, guanabenz, and guanfacine. Cholestyramine and colestipol may bind TCAs and reduce their absorption. CYP3A4 inducers may decrease the levels/effects of doxepin; example inducers include aminoglutethimide, carbamazepine, nafcillin, nevirapine, phenobarbital, phenytoin, and rifamycins.

Increased Effect/Toxicity: Doxepin increases the effects of amphetamines, anticholinergics, other CNS depressants (sedatives, hypnotics, or ethanol), chlorpropamide, tolazamide, and warfarin. When used with MAO inhibitors, hyperpyrexia, hypertension, tachycardia, confusion, seizures, and **deaths have been reported** (serotonin syndrome). Serotonin syndrome has also been reported with ritonavir (rare).

CYP1A2 inhibitors may increase the levels/effects of doxepin; example inhibitors include amiodarone, ciprofloxacin, fluvoxamine, ketoconazole, norfloxacin, ofloxacin, and rofecoxib. CYP2D6 inhibitors may increase the levels/effects of doxepin; example inhibitors include chlorpromazine, delavirdine, fluoxetine, miconazole, paroxetine, pergolide, quinidine, quinine, ritonavir, and ropinirole. CYP3A4 inhibitors may increase the levels/effects of doxepin. Example inhibitors include azole antifungals, clarithromycin, diclofenac, doxycycline, erythromycin, imatinib, isoniazid, nefazodone, nicardipine, propofol, protease inhibitors, quinidine, telithromycin, and verapamil. Cimetidine, grapefruit juice, indinavir, methylphenidate, diltiazem, and verapamil may increase the serum concentrations of TCAs. Use of lithium with a TCA may increase the risk for neurotoxicity. Phenothiazines may increase concentration of some TCAs and TCAs may increase concentration of phenothiazines.

Pressor response to I.V. epinephrine, norepinephrine, and phenylephrine may be enhanced in patients receiving TCAs (**Note:** Effect is unlikely with epinephrine or levonordefrin dosages typically administered as infiltration in combination with local anesthetics).

Combined use of beta-agonists or drugs which prolong QT_c (including quinidine, procainamide, disopyramide, cisapride, sparfloxacin, gatifloxacin, moxifloxacin) with TCAs may predispose patients to cardiac arrhythmias.

Nutritional/Ethanol Interactions
Ethanol: Avoid ethanol (may increase CNS depression).
Food: Grapefruit juice may inhibit the metabolism of some TCAs and clinical toxicity may result.
Herb/Nutraceutical: Avoid valerian, St John's wort, SAMe, kava kava (may increase risk of serotonin syndrome and/or excessive sedation).

Lab Interactions
Increased glucose

Adverse Reactions
Oral: Frequency not defined.
Cardiovascular: Hyper-/hypotension, tachycardia
Central nervous system: Drowsiness, dizziness, headache, disorientation, ataxia, confusion, seizure
Dermatologic: Alopecia, photosensitivity, rash, pruritus
Endocrine & metabolic: Breast enlargement, galactorrhea, SIADH, increase or decrease in blood sugar, increased or decreased libido
Gastrointestinal: Xerostomia, constipation, vomiting, indigestion, anorexia, aphthous stomatitis, nausea, unpleasant taste, weight gain, diarrhea, trouble with gums, decreased lower esophageal sphincter tone may cause GE reflux
Genitourinary: Urinary retention, testicular edema
Hematologic: Agranulocytosis, leukopenia, eosinophilia, thrombocytopenia, purpura
Neuromuscular & skeletal: Weakness, tremor, numbness, paresthesia, extrapyramidal symptoms, tardive dyskinesia
Ocular: Blurred vision
Otic: Tinnitus
Miscellaneous: Diaphoresis (excessive), allergic reactions

Topical:
>10%:
Central nervous system: Drowsiness (22%)
Dermatologic: Stinging/burning (23%)
1% to 10%:
Cardiovascular: Edema: (1%)
Central nervous system: Dizziness (2%), emotional changes (2%)
Gastrointestinal: Xerostomia (10%), taste alteration (2%)

Overdosage/Toxicology Symptoms of overdose include confusion, hallucinations, seizures, urinary retention, hypothermia, hypotension, tachycardia, and cyanosis. Following initiation of essential overdose management, toxic symptoms should be treated symptomatically.

Pharmacodynamics/Kinetics
Onset of Action: Peak effect: Antidepressant: Usually >2 weeks; Anxiolytic: May occur sooner
Protein Binding: 80% to 85%
Half-Life Elimination: Adults: 6-8 hours
Metabolism: Hepatic; metabolites include desmethyldoxepin (active)
Excretion: Urine

Available Dosage Forms [DSC] = Discontinued product
Capsule, as hydrochloride: 10 mg, 25 mg, 50 mg, 75 mg, 100 mg, 150 mg
Sinequan®: 10 mg, 25 mg, 50 mg, 75 mg, 100 mg, 150 mg [DSC]
Cream, as hydrochloride:
Prudoxin™: 5% (45 g) [contains benzyl alcohol]
Zonalon®: 5% (30 g, 45 g) [contains benzyl alcohol]
Solution, oral concentrate, as hydrochloride (Sinequan®): 10 mg/mL (120 mL)
Sinequan®: 10 mg/mL (120 mL) [DSC]
(Continued)

Doxepin (Continued)

Dosing

Adults:

Depression and/or anxiety (unlabeled use): Oral: Initial: 25-150 mg/day at bedtime or in 2-3 divided doses; may gradually increase up to 300 mg/day; single dose should not exceed 150 mg; select patients may respond to 25-50 mg/day.

Chronic urticaria, angioedema, nocturnal pruritus: Oral: 10-30 mg/day

Pruritus: Topical: Apply a thin film 4 times/day with at least 3- to 4-hour interval between applications; not recommended for use >8 days. (Oral administration of doxepin 25-50 mg has also been used, but systemic adverse effects are increased.)

Elderly:

Depression and/or anxiety (unlabeled use): Oral: Initial: 10-25 mg at bedtime; increase by 10-25 mg every 3 days for inpatients and weekly for outpatients if tolerated. Rarely does the maximum dose required exceed 75 mg/day; a single bedtime dose is recommended.

Pruritus: Topical: Refer to adult dosing.

Pediatrics:

Depression and/or anxiety: Oral:

Children (unlabeled use): 1-3 mg/kg/day in single or divided doses

Adolescents: Initial: 25-50 mg/day in single or divided doses; gradually increase to 100 mg/day

Hepatic Impairment: Use a lower dose and adjust gradually.

Administration

Oral: Do not mix oral concentrate with carbonated beverages (physically incompatible).

Topical: Apply thin film to affected area; use of occlusive dressings is not recommended.

Stability

Storage: Protect from light.

Nursing Actions

Physical Assessment: Assess other medications patient may be taking for effectiveness and interactions. Monitor CNS status. Be alert for signs of clinical worsening, suicidal ideation, or other changes in behavior. Monitor laboratory tests, therapeutic response, and adverse reactions at beginning of therapy and periodically with long-term use. Taper dosage slowly when discontinuing. Assess knowledge/teach patient appropriate use (oral, topical), interventions to reduce side effects, and adverse symptoms to report.

Patient Education: Oral: Take exactly as directed; do not increase dose or frequency. It may take several weeks to achieve desired results. Avoid alcohol, caffeine, and other prescription or OTC medications not approved by prescriber. Maintain adequate hydration (2-3 L/day of fluids) unless instructed to restrict fluid intake. You may experience drowsiness, lightheadedness, impaired coordination, dizziness, or blurred vision (use caution when driving or engaging in tasks requiring alertness until response to drug is known); constipation (increased exercise, fluids, fruit, or fiber may help); urinary retention (void before taking medication); postural hypotension (use caution climbing stairs or when changing position from lying or sitting to standing); altered sexual drive or ability (reversible); or photosensitivity (use sunscreen, wear protective clothing and eyewear, and avoid direct sunlight). Report persistent CNS effects (eg, nervousness, restlessness, insomnia, anxiety, excitation, suicide ideation, headache, agitation, impaired coordination, changes in cognition); muscle cramping, weakness, tremors, or rigidity; chest pain, palpitations, or irregular heartbeat; blurred vision or eye pain; yellowing of skin or eyes; or worsening of condition. **Pregnancy/breast-feeding precautions:** Inform prescriber if you are or intend to become pregnant. Breast-feeding is not recommended.

Topical: Use as directed. Apply in thin layer; do not overuse. Report increased skin irritation, worsening of condition or lack of improvement.

Geriatric Considerations The oral form is the preferred agent when sedation is a desired property. Less potential for anticholinergic effects than amitriptyline and less orthostatic hypotension than imipramine. However, dosing should be approached cautiously, initiated at the low end of the dosage range.

Breast-Feeding Issues Generally, it is not recommended to breast-feed if taking antidepressants because of the long half-life, active metabolites, and the potential for side effects in the infant.

Related Information

Antidepressant Medication Guidelines on page 1414
Federal OBRA Regulations Recommended Maximum Doses on page 1421

Doxercalciferol (doks er kal si fe FEER ole)

U.S. Brand Names Hectorol®

Synonyms 1α-Hydroxyergocalciferol

Pharmacologic Category Vitamin D Analog

Pregnancy Risk Factor B

Lactation Excretion in breast milk unknown/not recommended

Use Treatment of secondary hyperparathyroidism in patients with chronic kidney disease

Mechanism of Action/Effect Doxercalciferol is metabolized to the active form of vitamin D.

Contraindications Hypersensitivity to any component of the formulation; history of hypercalcemia or evidence of vitamin D toxicity

Warnings/Precautions Other forms of vitamin D should be discontinued when doxercalciferol is started. Hyperphosphatemia should be corrected before initiating therapy. Use with caution in patients with hepatic impairment. Safety and efficacy have not been established in pediatric patients.

Drug Interactions

Decreased Effect: Absorption of doxercalciferol is reduced with mineral oil and cholestyramine.

Increased Effect/Toxicity: Doxercalciferol toxicity may be increased by concurrent use of other vitamin D supplements or magnesium-containing antacids and supplements.

Adverse Reactions

Note: As reported in dialysis patients.

>10%:
Cardiovascular: Edema (34%)
Central nervous system: Headache (28%), malaise (28%), dizziness (12%)
Gastrointestinal: Nausea/vomiting (24%)
Respiratory: Dyspnea (12%)

1% to 10%:
Cardiovascular: Bradycardia (7%)
Central nervous system: Sleep disorder (3%)
Dermatologic: Pruritus (8%)
Gastrointestinal: Anorexia (5%), constipation (3%), dyspepsia (5%), weight gain (5%)
Neuromuscular & skeletal: Arthralgia (5%)
Miscellaneous: Abscess (3%)

Overdosage/Toxicology Doxercalciferol, in excess, can cause hypercalcemia, hypercalciuria, hyperphosphatemia, and oversuppression of PTH secretion. Following withdrawal of the drug and calcium supplements, hypercalcemia treatment consists of a low calcium diet and monitoring. Adjustments of calcium in the dialysis bath can also be made if necessary. When calcium levels normalize, doxercalciferol can be restarted. Reduce each dose by at least 2.5 mcg. Monitor serum calcium levels closely.

Signs and symptoms of early hypercalcemia include: Anorexia, bone pain, constipation, headache, metallic taste, muscle pain, nausea, somnolence, vomiting, weakness, xerostomia

Signs and symptoms of late hypercalcemia include: Albuminuria, anorexia, apathy, AST/ALT increased, BUN increased, cardiac arrhythmias, conjunctivitis (calcific), dehydration, ectopic calcification, growth arrested, hypercholesterolemia, hypertension, hyperthermia, libido decreased, nocturia, pancreatitis, photophobia, polydipsia, polyuria, pruritus, psychosis (rare), rhinorrhea, sensory disturbances, urinary tract infections, weight loss

Pharmacodynamics/Kinetics
Half-Life Elimination: Active metabolite: 32-37 hours; up to 96 hours

Metabolism: Hepatic via CYP27

Available Dosage Forms
Capsule: 0.5 mcg, 2.5 mcg [contains coconut oil]

Injection, solution: 2 mcg/mL (2 mL) [contains disodium edetate]

Dosing
Adults & Elderly: Secondary hyperparathyroidism:
Oral:
Dialysis patients: Dose should be titrated to lower iPTH to 150-300 pg/mL; dose is adjusted at 8-week intervals (maximum dose: 20 mcg 3 times/week)
Initial dose: iPTH >400 pg/mL: 10 mcg 3 times/week at dialysis
Dose titration:
iPTH level decreased by 50% and >300 pg/mL: Dose can be increased to 12.5 mcg 3 times/week for 8 more weeks; this titration process can continue at 8-week intervals; each increase should be by 2.5 mcg/dose
iPTH level 150-300 pg/mL: Maintain current dose
iPTH level <100 pg/mL: Suspend doxercalciferol for 1 week; resume at a reduced dose; decrease each dose (not weekly dose) by at least 2.5 mcg
Predialysis patients: Dose should be titrated to lower iPTH to 35-70 pg/mL with stage 3 disease or to 70-110 pg/mL with stage 4 disease: Dose may be adjusted at 2-week intervals (maximum dose: 3.5 mcg/day)
Initial dose: 1 mcg/day
Dose titration:
iPTH level >70 pg/mL with stage 3 disease or >110 pg/mL with stage 4 disease: Increase dose by 0.5 mcg every 2 weeks as necessary
iPTH level 35-70 pg/mL with stage 3 disease or 70-110 pg/mL with stage 4 disease: Maintain current dose
iPTH level is <35 pg/mL with stage 3 disease or <70 pg/mL with stage 4 disease: Suspend doxercalciferol for 1 week, then resume at a reduced dose (at least 0.5 mcg lower)
I.V.:
Dialysis patients: Dose should be titrated to lower iPTH to 150-300 pg/mL; dose is adjusted at 8-week intervals (maximum dose: 18 mcg/week)
Initial dose: iPTH level >400 pg/mL: 4 mcg 3 times/week after dialysis, administered as a bolus dose
Dose titration:
iPTH level decreased by 50% and >300 pg/mL: Dose can be increased by 1-2 mcg at 8-week intervals, as necessary
iPTH level 150-300 pg/mL: Maintain the current dose
iPTH level <100 pg/mL: Suspend doxercalciferol for 1 week; resume at a reduced dose (at least 1 mcg lower)

Renal Impairment: No adjustment is required.

Hepatic Impairment: Use caution in these patients; no guidelines for dosage adjustment.

Stability
Storage: Store at controlled room temperature of 15°C to 30°C (59°F to 86°F). The injection should be protected from light.

Laboratory Monitoring
Dialysis patients: Before initiating, check iPTH, serum calcium and phosphorus. Check weekly thereafter until stable. Serum iPTH, calcium, phosphorus, and alkaline phosphatase should be monitored.

Predialysis patients: iPTH, serum calcium and phosphorus every 2 weeks for 3 months following initiation and dose adjustments, then monthly for 3 months, then every 3 months.

Nursing Actions
Physical Assessment: Monitor therapeutic response (laboratory results), adverse reactions. Monitor for fluid retention (swelling of extremities, sudden weight gain). Assess knowledge/teach patient appropriate use, interventions to reduce side effects, and adverse reactions to report.

Patient Education: Be clear on dose and directions for taking. Stop other vitamin D products. Do not miss doses. Avoid magnesium-containing antacids and supplements. Report headache, dizziness, weakness, sleepiness, severe nausea, vomiting, dry mouth, loss of appetite, constipation, metallic taste, muscle and/or bone pain, significant fluid retention, malaise, shortness of breath, and difficulty thinking or concentrating to your prescriber. Do not take over-the-counter medicines or supplements without first consulting your prescriber. Follow diet and calcium supplements as directed by your prescriber.

Dietary Considerations Based on serum levels, dietary phosphorus may be restricted and/or controlled with calcium-based phosphorus binders. The daily combined calcium intake (dietary and calcium based phosphate binder) should be 1.5-2 g. Additional vitamin D supplements and magnesium-containing antacids should be avoided. Capsules contain coconut oil.

Breast-Feeding Issues Excretion in breast milk is unknown. Other vitamin D derivatives are excreted in breast milk; there is a potential for adverse effects. Therefore, the manufacturer recommends that breast-feeding be discontinued or doxercalciferol discontinued, depending upon importance of the drug to the mother.

DOXOrubicin (doks oh ROO bi sin)

U.S. Brand Names Adriamycin PFS®; Adriamycin RDF®; Rubex®

Synonyms ADR (error-prone abbreviation); Adria; Doxorubicin Hydrochloride; Hydroxydaunomycin Hydrochloride; Hydroxyldaunorubicin Hydrochloride; NSC-123127

Pharmacologic Category Antineoplastic Agent, Anthracycline

Medication Safety Issues
Sound-alike/look-alike issues:
DOXOrubicin may be confused with dactinomycin, DAUNOrubicin, doxacurium, doxapram, doxazosin, epirubicin, idarubicin
Adriamycin PFS® may be confused with achromycin, Aredia®, Idamycin®
Rubex® may be confused with Robaxin®
Conventional formulations (Adriamycin PFS®, Adriamycin RDF®, Rubex®) may be confused with liposomal formulations (DaunoXome®, Doxil®)

ADR is an error-prone abbreviation

Pregnancy Risk Factor D

Lactation Enters breast milk/contraindicated
(Continued)

DOXOrubicin *(Continued)*

Use Treatment of leukemias, lymphomas, multiple myeloma, osseous and nonosseous sarcomas, mesotheliomas, germ cell tumors of the ovary or testis, and carcinomas of the head and neck, thyroid, lung, breast, stomach, pancreas, liver, ovary, bladder, prostate, uterus, and neuroblastoma

Mechanism of Action/Effect Inhibits DNA and RNA synthesis, active throughout cell cycle, results in cell death.

Contraindications Hypersensitivity to doxorubicin or any component of the formulation; congestive heart failure or arrhythmias; previous therapy with high cumulative doses of doxorubicin and/or daunorubicin; pre-existing bone marrow suppression; pregnancy

Warnings/Precautions Hazardous agent - use appropriate precautions for handling and disposal. Total dose should not exceed 550 mg/m^2 or 450 mg/m^2 in patients with previous or concomitant treatment with daunorubicin, cyclophosphamide, or irradiation of the cardiac region. Irreversible myocardial toxicity may occur as total dosage approaches 550 mg/m^2. I.V. use only, severe local tissue necrosis will result if extravasation occurs. Elderly and pediatric patients are at higher risk of cardiotoxicity (delayed). Reduce dose in patients with impaired hepatic function. Severe myelosuppression is also possible. Administration of live vaccines to immunosuppressed patients may be hazardous. Heart failure may occur during therapy or months to years after therapy. Treatment may increase the risk of other neoplasms. Secondary acute myelogenous leukemia may occur following treatment.

Drug Interactions
Cytochrome P450 Effect: Substrate (major) of CYP2D6, 3A4; **Inhibits** CYP2B6 (moderate), 2D6 (weak), 3A4 (weak)

Decreased Effect: The levels/effects of doxorubicin may be decreased by aminoglutethimide, carbamazepine, nafcillin, nevirapine, phenobarbital, phenytoin, rifamycins, and other CYP3A4 inducers. Doxorubicin may decrease plasma levels and effectiveness of digoxin. Doxorubicin may decrease the antiviral activity of zidovudine.

Increased Effect/Toxicity: Allopurinol may enhance the antitumor activity of doxorubicin (animal data only). Cyclosporine may increase doxorubicin levels, enhancing hematologic toxicity or may induce coma or seizures. Cyclophosphamide enhances the cardiac toxicity of doxorubicin by producing additional myocardial cell damage. Mercaptopurine increases doxorubicin toxicities. Streptozocin greatly enhances leukopenia and thrombocytopenia. Verapamil alters the cellular distribution of doxorubicin and may result in increased cell toxicity by inhibition of the P-glycoprotein pump. Paclitaxel reduces doxorubicin clearance and increases toxicity if administered prior to doxorubicin. High doses of progesterone enhance toxicity (neutropenia and thrombocytopenia).

Doxorubicin may increase the levels/effects of bupropion, promethazine, propofol, selegiline, sertraline, and other CYP2B6 substrates. The levels/effects of doxorubicin may be increased by azole antifungals, chlorpromazine, clarithromycin, delavirdine, diclofenac, doxycycline, erythromycin, fluoxetine, imatinib, isoniazid, miconazole, nefazodone, nicardipine, paroxetine, pergolide, propofol, protease inhibitors, quinidine, quinine, ritonavir, ropinirole, telithromycin, verapamil and other inhibitors of CYP2D6 or 3A4. Based on mouse studies, cardiotoxicity may be enhanced by verapamil. Concurrent therapy with actinomycin-D may result in recall pneumonitis following radiation.

Nutritional/Ethanol Interactions Herb/Nutraceutical: St John's wort may decrease doxorubicin levels. Avoid black cohosh, dong quai in estrogen-dependent tumors.

Adverse Reactions
>10%:
Dermatologic: Alopecia, radiation recall
Gastrointestinal: Nausea, vomiting, stomatitis, GI ulceration, anorexia, diarrhea
Genitourinary: Discoloration of urine, mild dysuria, urinary frequency, hematuria, bladder spasms, cystitis following bladder instillation
Hematologic: Myelosuppression, primarily leukopenia (75%); thrombocytopenia and anemia
Onset: 7 days
Nadir: 10-14 days
Recovery: 21-28 days
1% to 10%:
Cardiovascular: Transient ECG abnormalities (supraventricular tachycardia, S-T wave changes, atrial or ventricular extrasystoles); generally asymptomatic and self-limiting. CHF, dose related, may be delayed for 7-8 years after treatment. Cumulative dose, mediastinal/pericardial radiation therapy, cardiovascular disease, age, and use of cyclophosphamide (or other cardiotoxic agents) all increase the risk.
Recommended maximum cumulative doses:
No risk factors: 550 mg/m^2
Concurrent radiation: 450 mg/m^2
Note: Regardless of cumulative dose, if the left ventricular ejection fraction is <30% to 40%, the drug is usually not given.
Dermatologic: Skin "flare" at injection site; discoloration of saliva, sweat, or tears
Endocrine & metabolic: Hyperuricemia

Overdosage/Toxicology Symptoms of overdose include myelosuppression, nausea, vomiting, and myocardial toxicity. Treatment of acute overdose consists of treatment of the severely myelosuppressed patient with hospitalization, antibiotics, platelet and granulocyte transfusions, and symptomatic treatment of mucositis.

Pharmacodynamics/Kinetics
Protein Binding: Plasma: 70%
Half-Life Elimination:
Distribution: 10 minutes
Elimination: Doxorubicin: 1-3 hours; Metabolites: 3-3.5 hours
Terminal: 17-30 hours
Male: 54 hours; Female: 35 hours
Metabolism: Primarily hepatic to doxorubicinol (active), then to inactive aglycones, conjugated sulfates, and glucuronides
Excretion: Feces (~40% to 50% as unchanged drug); urine (~3% to 10% as metabolites, 1% doxorubicinol, <1% Adriamycin aglycones, and unchanged drug)
Clearance: Male: 113 L/hour; Female: 44 L/hour

Available Dosage Forms
Injection, powder for reconstitution, as hydrochloride: 10 mg, 20 mg, 50 mg [contains lactose]
Adriamycin RDF®: 10 mg, 20 mg, 50 mg, 150 mg [contains lactose; rapid dissolution formula]
Rubex®: 50 mg, 100 mg [contains lactose]
Injection, solution, as hydrochloride [preservative free]: 2 mg/mL (5 mL, 10 mL, 25 mL, 100 mL)
Adriamycin PFS® [preservative free]: 2 mg/mL (5 mL, 10 mL, 25 mL, 37.5 mL, 100 mL)

Dosing
Adults & Elderly: Refer to individual protocols.
Usual or typical dose: I.V.: 60-75 mg/m^2 as a single dose, repeat every 21 days or other dosage regimens like 20-30 mg/m^2/day for 2-3 days, repeat in 4 weeks or 20 mg/m^2 once weekly.
Pediatrics: Refer to individual protocols. Usual/typical dosages: I.V.:
Children:
35-75 mg/m^2 as a single dose, repeat every 21 days
or
20-30 mg/m^2 once weekly or

60-90 mg/m² given as a continuous infusion over 96 hours every 3-4 weeks

Renal Impairment:
Adjustments are not required.
Hemodialysis effects: Supplemental dose is not necessary.

Hepatic Impairment:
ALT/AST 2-3 times ULN: Administer 75% of dose
ALT/AST >3 times ULN **or** bilirubin 1.2-3 mg/dL (20-51 µmol/L): Administer 50% of dose
Bilirubin 3.1-5 mg/dL (51-85 µmol/L): Administer 25% of dose
Bilirubin >5 mg/dL (85 µmol/L): Do not administer

Administration

I.V.: Vesicant. I.V. push over 1-2 minutes or IVPB over 15-60 minutes. Infusion via central venous line recommended.

I.V. Detail: May be further diluted in either NS or D₅W for I.V. administration. Avoid extravasation associated with severe ulceration and soft tissue necrosis. Flush with 5-10 mL of I.V. solution before and after drug administration. Incompatible with heparin. Monitor for local erythematous streaking along vein and/or facial flushing (may indicate rapid infusion rate).

Extravasation management: Apply ice immediately for 30-60 minutes; then alternate off/on every 15 minutes for 1 day. Topical cooling may be achieved using ice packs or cooling pad with circulating ice water. Cooling of site for 24 hours as tolerated by the patient. Elevate and rest extremity 24-48 hours, then resume normal activity as tolerated. Application of cold inhibits vesicant's cytotoxicity. **Application of heat or sodium bicarbonate can be harmful and is contraindicated.** If pain, erythema, and/or swelling persist beyond 48 hours, refer patient immediately to plastic surgeon for consultation and possible debridement.

pH: 3.8-6.5 (lyophilized doxorubicin HCl reconstituted with sodium chloride 0.9%); 2.5-4.5 (adjusted solution)

Stability

Reconstitution: Reconstitute lyophilized powder with NS to a final concentration of 2 mg/mL (further dilution in 50-1000 mL D₅W or NS). Unstable in solutions with a pH <3 or >7.

Compatibility: Stable in D₅W, LR, NS

Y-site administration: Incompatible with allopurinol, amphotericin B cholesteryl sulfate complex, cefepime, ganciclovir, piperacillin/tazobactam, propofol

Compatibility in syringe: Incompatible with furosemide, heparin

Compatibility when admixed: Incompatible with aminophylline, diazepam, fluorouracil

Storage: Store intact vials of solution under refrigeration at 2°C to 8°C and protected from light. Store intact vials of lyophilized powder at room temperature (15°C to 30°C). Further dilution in 50-1000 mL D₅W or NS is stable for 48 hours at room temperature (25°C) when protected from light.

Laboratory Monitoring CBC with differential, platelet count, cardiac and liver function

Nursing Actions

Physical Assessment: Assess potential for interactions with other pharmacological agents or herbal products patient may be taking (eg, potential to reduce or increase levels/effects of doxorubicin). See Administration infusion specifics. Premedication with antiemetic may be ordered (especially with larger doses). Monitor infusion site closely; extravasation can cause sloughing or tissue necrosis (do not apply heat or sodium bicarbonate). Monitor laboratory tests and patient response prior to each treatment and on a regular basis throughout therapy. Teach patient possible side effects/appropriate interventions (eg,

importance of adequate hydration) and adverse symptoms to report.

Patient Education: Do not take any new medication during therapy unless approved by prescriber. This medication can only be administered intravenously. Report immediately any swelling, pain, burning, or redness at infusion site. Maintain adequate nutrition (small, frequent meals may help). You will be more susceptible to infection (avoid crowds and exposure to infection and do not have any vaccinations without consulting prescriber). May cause nausea or vomiting (small, frequent meals, frequent mouth care, sucking lozenges, or chewing gum may help); diarrhea (buttermilk, boiled milk, or yogurt may help); loss of hair (reversible); or darker yellow urine (normal). Report immediately chest pain, swelling of extremities, respiratory difficulty, palpitations, or rapid heartbeat. Report unresolved nausea, vomiting, or diarrhea; alterations in urinary pattern (increased or decreased); opportunistic infection (fever, chills, unusual bruising or bleeding fatigue, purulent vaginal discharge, unhealed mouth sores); abdominal pain or blood in stools; excessive fatigue; or yellowing of eyes or skin. **Pregnancy/breast-feeding precautions:** Inform prescriber if you are pregnant. Do not get pregnant while taking this medication or for 1 month following therapy. Consult prescriber for appropriate barrier contraceptives. Do not breast-feed.

Pregnancy Issues Advise patients to avoid becoming pregnant (females) and to avoid causing pregnancy (males).

Related Information
FDA Name Differentiation Project: The Use of Tall-Man Letters *on page 12*

DOXOrubicin (Liposomal)
(doks oh ROO bi sin lip pah SOW mal)

U.S. Brand Names Doxil®
Synonyms Doxorubicin Hydrochloride (Liposomal)
Pharmacologic Category Antineoplastic Agent, Anthracycline

Medication Safety Issues
Sound-alike/look-alike issues:
DOXOrubicin may be confused with dactinomycin, DAUNOrubicin, doxacurium, doxapram, doxazosin, epirubicin, idarubicin
Doxil® may be confused with Doxy®, Paxil®
Liposomal formulations (Doxil®) may be confused with conventional formulations (Adriamycin PFS®, Adriamycin RDF®, Cerubidine®, Rubex®).

Pregnancy Risk Factor D
Lactation Excretion in breast milk unknown/contraindicated

Use Treatment of AIDS-related Kaposi's sarcoma, breast cancer, ovarian cancer, solid tumors

Mechanism of Action/Effect Inhibits DNA and RNA synthesis of susceptible bacteria, active throughout cell cycle, results in cell death

Contraindications Hypersensitivity to doxorubicin, other anthracyclines, or any component of the formulation; breast-feeding, pregnancy

Warnings/Precautions The U.S. Food and Drug Administration (FDA) currently recommends that procedures for proper handling and disposal of antineoplastic agents be considered.

Doxorubicin is associated with dose-related myocardial damage leading to congestive heart failure. Doxorubicin and liposomal doxorubicin should be used cautiously in patients with high cumulative doses of anthracyclines, anthracenediones, and cyclophosphamide. Caution should also be used in patients with previous thoracic radiation or who have pre-existing cardiac disease. Total cumulative doses of anthracyclines, including (Continued)

DOXOrubicin (Liposomal) *(Continued)*

liposomal doxorubicin and anthracenediones should not exceed 550 mg/m^2 or 400 mg/m^2 in patients with previous or concomitant treatment (with daunorubicin, cyclophosphamide, or irradiation of the cardiac region); irreversible myocardial toxicity may occur at these doses. Symptoms of anthracycline-induced CHF and/or cardiomyopathy may be delayed in onset (up to 7-8 years in some cases). For I.V. use only; local tissue irritation will result if extravasation occurs; reduce dose in patients with impaired hepatic function; severe myelosuppression is also possible. Acute infusion reactions may occur, some may be serious/life-threatening. Liposomal formulations of doxorubicin should not be substituted for doxorubicin hydrochloride on a mg-per-mg basis.

Hand-foot syndrome (palmar-plantar erythrodysesthesia) has been reported in up to 51% of patients with ovarian cancer (and significantly lower frequency in patients with Kaposi's sarcoma). May occur early in treatment, but is usually seen after 2-3 treatment cycles. Dosage modification may be required. In severe cases, treatment discontinuation may be required.

Drug Interactions

Cytochrome P450 Effect: Substrate (major) of CYP2D6, 3A4; **Inhibits** CYP2B6 (moderate), 2D6 (weak), 3A4 (weak)

Decreased Effect: The levels/effects of doxorubicin may be decreased by aminoglutethimide, carbamazepine, nafcillin, nevirapine, phenobarbital, phenytoin, rifamycins, and other CYP3A4 inducers. Doxorubicin may decrease plasma levels and effectiveness of digoxin. Doxorubicin may decrease the antiviral activity of zidovudine.

Increased Effect/Toxicity: Allopurinol may enhance the antitumor activity of doxorubicin (animal data only). Cyclosporine may increase doxorubicin levels, enhancing hematologic toxicity or may induce coma or seizures. Cyclophosphamide enhances the cardiac toxicity of doxorubicin by producing additional myocardial cell damage. Mercaptopurine increases doxorubicin toxicities. Streptozocin greatly enhances leukopenia and thrombocytopenia. Verapamil alters the cellular distribution of doxorubicin and may result in increased cell toxicity by inhibition of the P-glycoprotein pump. Paclitaxel reduces doxorubicin clearance and increases toxicity if administered prior to doxorubicin. High doses of progesterone enhance toxicity (neutropenia and thrombocytopenia).

Doxorubicin may increase the levels/effects of bupropion, promethazine, propofol, selegiline, sertraline, and other CYP2B6 substrates. The levels/effects of doxorubicin may be increased by azole antifungals, chlorpromazine, clarithromycin, delavirdine, diclofenac, doxycycline, erythromycin, fluoxetine, imatinib, isoniazid, miconazole, nefazodone, nicardipine, paroxetine, pergolide, propofol, protease inhibitors, quinidine, quinine, ritonavir, ropinirole, telithromycin, verapamil and other inhibitors of CYP2D6 or 3A4. Based on mouse studies, cardiotoxicity may be enhanced by verapamil. Concurrent therapy with actinomycin-D may result in recall pneumonitis following radiation.

Nutritional/Ethanol Interactions

Ethanol: Avoid ethanol (due to GI irritation).

Herb/Nutraceutical: St John's wort may decrease doxorubicin levels. Avoid black cohosh, dong quai in estrogen-dependent tumors.

Adverse Reactions

>10%:

Cardiovascular: Peripheral edema (up to 11%)

Central nervous system: Fever (8% to 12%), headache (up to 11%), pain (up to 21%)

Dermatologic: Alopecia (9% to 19%); palmar-plantar erythrodysesthesia/hand-foot syndrome (up to 51% in ovarian cancer, 4% in Kaposi's sarcoma), rash (up to 29% in ovarian cancer, up to 5% in Kaposi's sarcoma)

Gastrointestinal: Stomatitis (5% to 41%), vomiting (8% to 33%), nausea (18% to 46%), mucositis (up to 14%), constipation (up to 30%), anorexia (up to 20%), diarrhea (5% to 21%), dyspepsia (up to 12%), intestinal obstruction (up to 11%)

Hematologic: Myelosuppression, neutropenia (12% to 62%), leukopenia (36%), thrombocytopenia (13% to 65%), anemia (6% to 74%)

Onset: 7 days

Nadir: 10-14 days

Recovery: 21-28 days

Neuromuscular & skeletal: Weakness (7% to 40%), back pain (up to 12%)

Respiratory: Pharyngitis (up to 16%), dyspnea (up to 15%)

1% to 10%:

Cardiovascular: Cardiac arrest, chest pain, edema, hypotension, pallor, tachycardia, vasodilation

Central nervous system: Agitation, anxiety, chills, confusion, depression, dizziness, emotional lability, insomnia, somnolence, vertigo

Dermatologic: Acne, dry skin (6%), dermatitis, furunculosis, herpes simplex/zoster, maculopapular rash, pruritus, rash, skin discoloration, vesiculobullous rash

Endocrine & metabolic: Dehydration, hyperbilirubinemia, hyperglycemia, hypocalcemia, hypokalemia, hyponatremia

Gastrointestinal: Abdomen enlarged, ascites, cachexia, dyspepsia, dysphagia, esophagitis, flatulence, gingivitis, glossitis, ileus, mouth ulceration, rectal bleeding, taste perversion, weight loss, xerostomia

Genitourinary: Cystitis, dysuria, leukorrhea, pelvic pain, polyuria, urinary incontinence, urinary tract infection, urinary urgency, vaginal bleeding

Hematologic: Ecchymosis, hemolysis, prothrombin time increased

Hepatic: ALT increased

Local: Thrombophlebitis

Neuromuscular & skeletal: Arthralgia, hypertonia, myalgia, neuralgia, neuritis (peripheral), neuropathy, paresthesia (up to 10%), pathological fracture,

Ocular: Conjunctivitis, dry eyes, retinitis

Otic: Ear pain

Renal: Albuminuria, hematuria

Respiratory: Apnea, cough increased (up to 10%), epistaxis, pleural effusion, pneumonia, rhinitis, sinusitis

Miscellaneous: Allergic reaction; infusion-related reactions (bronchospasm, chest tightness, chills, dyspnea, facial edema, flushing, headache, hypotension, pruritus); moniliasis, diaphoresis

Overdosage/Toxicology Symptoms of overdose include increases in mucositis, leukopenia, and thrombocytopenia. For acute overdose, treatment of the severely myelosuppressed patient consists of hospitalization, antibiotics, hematopoietic growth factors, platelet and granulocyte transfusion, and symptomatic treatment of mucositis.

Pharmacodynamics/Kinetics

Protein Binding: Unknown; nonliposomal doxorubicin 70%

Half-Life Elimination: Terminal: Distribution: 4.7-5.2 hours, Elimination: 44-55 hours

Metabolism: Hepatic and in plasma to doxorubicinol and the sulfate and glucuronide conjugates of 4-demethyl,7-deoxyaglycones

Excretion: Urine (5% as doxorubicin or doxorubicinol) Clearance: Mean: 0.041 L/hour/m^2

Available Dosage Forms Injection, solution, as hydrochloride: 2 mg/mL (10 mL, 25 mL)

Dosing

Adults & Elderly: Refer to individual protocols.

AIDS-KS: I.V.: 20 mg/m^2 every 3 weeks

Breast cancer: I.V.: 20-80 mg/m^2/dose every 8 weeks

Ovarian cancer: I.V.: 50 mg/m^2/dose every 4 weeks

Solid tumors: I.V.: 50-60 mg/m^2/dose every 3-4 weeks

Hepatic Impairment:

ALT/AST 2-3 times ULN: Administer 75% of dose

ALT/AST >3 times ULN **or** bilirubin 1.2-3 mg/dL (20-51 μmol/L): Administer 50% of dose

Bilirubin 3.1-5 mg/dL (51-85 μmol/L): Administer 25% of dose

Bilirubin >5 mg/dL (85 μmol/L): Do not administer

Dosing Adjustment for Toxicity:

Toxicity Grade 1

ANC 1500-1900; platelets 75,000-150,000: Resume treatment with no dose reduction

Toxicity Grade 2

ANC 1000-<1500; platelets 50,000-<75,000: Wait until ANC ≥1500 and platelets ≥75,000; redose with no dose reduction

Toxicity Grade 3

ANC 500-999; platelets 25,000-<50,000: Wait until ANC ≥1500 and platelets ≥75,000; redose with no dose reduction

Toxicity Grade 4

ANC <500; platelets <25,000: Wait until ANC ≥1500 and platelets ≥75,000; redose at 25% dose reduction or continue full dose with cytokine support

Administration

I.V.: Irritant. May be administered IVPB over 30 minutes; manufacturer recommends administering at initial rate of 1 mg/minute to minimize risk of infusion reactions until the absence of a reaction has been established, then increase the infusion rate for completion over 1 hour. Do not administer as a bolus injection or undiluted solution. **Do not administer intramuscular or subcutaneous. Do not use with in-line filters.**

I.V. Detail: Flush with 5-10 mL of D$_5$W solution before and after drug administration. Incompatible with heparin. Monitor for local erythematous streaking along vein and/or facial flushing (may indicate rapid infusion rate).

Stability

Reconstitution: Doses Doxil® ≤90 mg must be diluted in 250 mL of D$_5$W prior to administration. Doses >90 mg should be diluted in 500 mL D$_5$W.

Compatibility: Stable in D$_5$W

Y-site administration: Incompatible with amphotericin B, amphotericin B cholesteryl sulfate complex, buprenorphine, cefoperazone, ceftazidime, docetaxel, fluorouracil, furosemide, heparin, hydroxyzine, mannitol, meperidine, metoclopramide, mitoxantrone, morphine, ofloxacin, paclitaxel, piperacillin/tazobactam, promethazine, sodium bicarbonate

Storage: Store intact vials of solution under refrigeration (2°C to 8°C); avoid freezing. Prolonged freezing may adversely affect liposomal drug products, however, short-term freezing (<1 month) does not appear to have a deleterious effect. Diluted doxorubicin hydrochloride liposome injection may be refrigerated at 2°C to 8°C or at room temperature; administer within 24 hours. **Do not use with in-line filters.**

Laboratory Monitoring CBC with differential, platelet count, echocardiogram, liver function

Nursing Actions

Physical Assessment: Assess potential for interactions with other pharmacological agents or herbal products patient may be taking (eg, potential to reduce or increase levels/effects of doxorubicin). See Administration infusion specifics. Premedication with

antiemetic may be ordered (especially with larger doses). Monitor infusion site closely; extravasation can cause sloughing or tissue necrosis (do not apply heat or sodium bicarbonate). Monitor laboratory tests and patient response prior to each treatment and on a regular basis throughout therapy. Teach patient possible side effects/appropriate interventions (eg, importance of adequate hydration) and adverse symptoms to report.

Patient Education: Inform prescriber of all prescriptions, OTC medications, or herbal products you are taking, and any allergies you have. Do not take any new medication during therapy unless approved by prescriber. This medication can only be administered by infusion. Report immediately any swelling, pain, burning, or redness at infusion site. Avoid alcohol. It is important to maintain adequate hydration (2-3 L/day of fluids) unless instructed to restrict fluid intake, and adequate nutrition (small, frequent meals may help). You will be more susceptible to infection (avoid crowds and exposure to infection and do not have any vaccinations without consulting prescriber). May cause nausea or vomiting (small, frequent meals, frequent mouth care, sucking lozenges, or chewing gum may help); diarrhea (buttermilk, boiled milk, or yogurt may help); loss of hair (reversible); or red-pink urine (normal). Report immediately chest pain, swelling of extremities, respiratory difficulty, palpitations, or rapid heartbeat. Report unresolved nausea, vomiting, or diarrhea; alterations in urinary pattern (increased or decreased); opportunistic infection (fever, chills, unusual bruising or bleeding fatigue, purulent vaginal discharge, unhealed mouth sores); abdominal pain or blood in stools; excessive fatigue; or yellowing of eyes or skin. **Pregnancy/breast-feeding precautions:** Do not get pregnant while taking this medication or for 1 month following therapy. Consult prescriber for appropriate contraceptives. Do not breast-feed.

Pregnancy Issues Advise patients to avoid becoming pregnant (females) and to avoid causing pregnancy (males).

Doxycycline (doks i SYE kleen)

U.S. Brand Names Adoxa™; Doryx®; Doxy-100®; Monodox®; Periostat®; Vibramycin®; Vibra-Tabs®

Synonyms Doxycycline Calcium; Doxycycline Hyclate; Doxycycline Monohydrate

Pharmacologic Category Antibiotic, Tetracycline Derivative

Medication Safety Issues

Sound-alike/look-alike issues:

Doxycycline may be confused with dicyclomine, doxepin, doxylamine

Doxy-100® may be confused with Doxil®

Monodox® may be confused with Maalox®

Pregnancy Risk Factor D

Lactation Enters breast milk/not recommended

Use Principally in the treatment of infections caused by susceptible *Rickettsia*, *Chlamydia*, and *Mycoplasma*; alternative to mefloquine for malaria prophylaxis; treatment for syphilis, uncomplicated *Neisseria gonorrhoeae*, *Listeria*, *Actinomyces israelii*, and *Clostridium* infections in penicillin-allergic patients; used for community-acquired pneumonia and other common infections due to susceptible organisms; anthrax due to *Bacillus anthracis*, including inhalational anthrax (postexposure); treatment of infections caused by uncommon susceptible gram-negative and gram-positive organisms including *Borrelia recurrentis*, *Ureaplasma urealyticum*, *Haemophilus ducreyi*, *Yersinia pestis*, *Francisella tularensis*, *Vibrio cholerae*, *Campylobacter fetus*, *Brucella* (Continued)

Doxycycline *(Continued)*

spp, *Bartonella bacilliformis*, and *Calymmatobacterium granulomatis*

Unlabeled/Investigational Use Sclerosing agent for pleural effusion injection; vancomycin-resistant enterococci (VRE)

Mechanism of Action/Effect Inhibits protein synthesis by binding with the 30S and possibly the 50S ribosomal subunit(s) of susceptible bacteria; may also cause alterations in the cytoplasmic membrane

Doxycycline inhibits collagenase *in vitro* and has been shown to inhibit collagenase in the gingival crevicular fluid in adults with periodontitis

Contraindications Hypersensitivity to doxycycline, tetracycline or any component of the formulation; children <8 years of age, except in treatment of anthrax (including inhalational anthrax postexposure prophylaxis); severe hepatic dysfunction; pregnancy

Warnings/Precautions Do not use during pregnancy - use of tetracyclines during tooth development may cause permanent discoloration of the teeth and enamel hypoplasia. Prolonged use may result in superinfection, including oral or vaginal candidiasis. Photosensitivity reaction may occur with this drug; avoid prolonged exposure to sunlight or tanning equipment.

Drug Interactions

Cytochrome P450 Effect: Substrate of CYP3A4 (major); **Inhibits** CYP3A4 (moderate)

Decreased Effect: Decreased levels of doxycycline may occur when taken with antacids containing aluminum, calcium, or magnesium. Decreased levels when taken with iron, bismuth subsalicylate, barbiturates, sucralfate, didanosine, and quinapril. Concurrent use of tetracycline and Penthrane® has been reported to result in fatal renal toxicity. Although anecdotal reports suggest oral contraceptive efficacy could be reduced by tetracyclines, this has been refuted by more rigorous scientific and clinical data. The levels/effects of doxycycline may be decreased by include aminoglutethimide, carbamazepine, nafcillin, nevirapine, phenobarbital, phenytoin, rifamycins, and other CYP3A4 inducers.

Increased Effect/Toxicity: Increased digoxin toxicity when taken with digoxin. Increased prothrombin time with warfarin. Doxycycline may increase the levels/effects of selected benzodiazepines, calcium channel blockers, cyclosporine, mirtazapine, nateglinide, nefazodone, quinidine, sildenafil (and other PDE-5 inhibitors), tacrolimus, venlafaxine, and other CYP3A4 substrates. Selected benzodiazepines (midazolam, triazolam), cisapride, ergot alkaloids, selected HMG-CoA reductase inhibitors (lovastatin and simvastatin), mesoridazine, pimozide, and thioridazine are generally contraindicated with strong CYP3A4 inhibitors. When used with strong CYP3A4 inhibitors, dosage adjustment/limits are recommended

Nutritional/Ethanol Interactions

Ethanol: Chronic ethanol ingestion may reduce the serum concentration of doxycycline.

Food: Doxycycline serum levels may be slightly decreased if taken with food or milk. Administration with iron or calcium may decrease doxycycline absorption. May decrease absorption of calcium, iron, magnesium, zinc, and amino acids.

Herb/Nutraceutical: St John's wort may decrease doxycycline levels. Avoid dong quai, St John's wort (may also cause photosensitization).

Lab Interactions False-negative urine glucose using Clinistix®

Adverse Reactions Frequency not defined.

Cardiovascular: Intracranial hypertension, pericarditis

Dermatologic: Angioneurotic edema, exfoliative dermatitis (rare), photosensitivity, rash, urticaria

Endocrine & metabolic: Brown/black discoloration of thyroid gland (no dysfunction reported)

Gastrointestinal: Anorexia, diarrhea, dysphagia, enterocolitis, esophagitis (rare), esophageal ulcerations (rare), glossitis, inflammatory lesions in anogenital region, tooth discoloration (children)

Hematologic: Eosinophilia, hemolytic anemia, neutropenia, thrombocytopenia

Renal: Increased BUN

Miscellaneous: Anaphylactoid purpura, anaphylaxis, bulging fontanels (infants), SLE exacerbation

Note: Adverse effects in clinical trials with Periostat® occurring at a frequency more than 1% greater than placebo included nausea, dyspepsia, joint pain, diarrhea, menstrual cramp, and pain.

Overdosage/Toxicology Symptoms of overdose include nausea, anorexia, and diarrhea. Treatment is supportive.

Pharmacodynamics/Kinetics

Time to Peak: Serum: 1.5-4 hours

Protein Binding: 90%

Half-Life Elimination: 12-15 hours (usually increases to 22-24 hours with multiple doses); End-stage renal disease: 18-25 hours

Metabolism: Not hepatic; partially inactivated in GI tract by chelate formation

Excretion: Feces (30%); urine (23%)

Available Dosage Forms [DSC] = Discontinued product

Capsule, as hyclate: 50 mg, 100 mg

Vibramycin®: 100 mg

Capsule, as monohydrate (Monodox®): 50 mg, 100 mg

Capsule, coated pellets, as hyclate (Doryx®): 75 mg, 100 mg [DSC]

Injection, powder for reconstitution, as hyclate (Doxy-100®): 100 mg

Powder for oral suspension, as monohydrate (Vibramycin®): 25 mg/5 mL (60 mL) [raspberry flavor]

Syrup, as calcium (Vibramycin®): 50 mg/5 mL (480 mL) [contains sodium metabisulfite; raspberry-apple flavor]

Tablet, as hyclate: 100 mg

Periostat®: 20 mg

Vibra-Tabs®: 100 mg

Tablet, as monohydrate:

Adoxa™: 50 mg, 75 mg, 100 mg

Adoxa® Pak™ 1/75 [unit-dose pack]: 75 mg (31s)

Adoxa® Pak™ 1/100 [unit-dose pack]: 100 mg (31s)

Adoxa® Pak™ 1/150 [unit-dose pack]: 150 mg (30s)

Adoxa® Pak™ 2/100 [unit-dose pack]: 100 mg (60s)

Tablet, delayed-release coated pellets, as hyclate (Doryx®): 75 mg [contains sodium 4.5 mg (0.196 mEq)], 100 mg [contains sodium 6 mg (0.261 mEq)]

Dosing

Adults & Elderly:

Usual dosage range: Oral, I.V.: 100-200 mg/day in 1-2 divided doses

Acute gonococcal infection (PID) in combination with another antibiotic: 100 mg every 12 hours until improved, followed by 100 mg orally twice daily to complete 14 days

Community-acquired pneumonia, bronchitis: Oral, I.V.: 100 mg twice daily

Uncomplicated chlamydial infections: Oral: 100 mg twice daily for ≥7 days

Endometritis, salpingitis, parametritis, or peritonitis: 100 mg I.V. twice daily with cefoxitin 2 g every 6 hours for 4 days and for ≥48 hours after patient improves; then continue with oral therapy 100 mg twice daily to complete a 10- to 14-day course of therapy

Sclerosing agent for pleural effusion injection (unlabeled use): 500 mg as a single dose in 30-50 mL of NS or SWI

Lyme disease: Oral: 100 mg twice daily for 14-21 days

Syphilis:
Early syphilis: Oral, I.V.: 200 mg/day in divided doses for 14 days

Late syphilis: Oral, I.V.: 200 mg/day in divided doses for 28 days

Periodontitis: Oral (Periostat®): 20 mg twice daily as an adjunct following scaling and root planing; may be administered for up to 9 months. Safety beyond 12 months of treatment and efficacy beyond 9 months of treatment have not been established.

Anthrax:
Inhalational (postexposure prophylaxis): Oral, I.V. (use oral route when possible): 100 mg every 12 hours for 60 days (*MMWR*, 2001, 50:889-93); **Note:** Preliminary recommendation, FDA review and update is anticipated.

Cutaneous (treatment): Oral: 100 mg every 12 hours for 60 days. **Note:** In the presence of systemic involvement, extensive edema, lesions on head/neck, refer to I.V. dosing for treatment of inhalational/gastrointestinal/oropharyngeal anthrax

Inhalational/gastrointestinal/oropharyngeal (treatment): I.V.: Initial: 100 mg every 12 hours; switch to oral therapy when clinically appropriate; some recommend initial loading dose of 200 mg, followed by 100 mg every 8-12 hours (*JAMA*, 1997, 278:399-411).

Note: Initial treatment should include two or more agents predicted to be effective (per CDC recommendations). Agents suggested for use in conjunction with doxycycline or ciprofloxacin include rifampin, vancomycin, imipenem, penicillin, ampicillin, chloramphenicol, clindamycin, and clarithromycin. May switch to oral antimicrobial therapy when clinically appropriate. Continue combined therapy for 60 days.

Pediatrics:
Usual dosage range:
Children ≥8 years (<45 kg): Oral, I.V.: 2-5 mg/kg/day in 1-2 divided doses, not to exceed 200 mg/day

Children >8 years (>45 kg): Oral, I.V.: Refer to adult dosing.

Anthrax:
Inhalational (postexposure prophylaxis) (MMWR, 2001, 50:889-93): Oral, I.V. (use oral route when possible):
≤8 years: 2.2 mg/kg every 12 hours for 60 days
>8 years and ≤45 kg: 2.2 mg/kg every 12 hours for 60 days
>8 years and >45 kg: 100 mg every 12 hours for 60 days

Cutaneous (treatment): Oral: See dosing for "Inhalational (postexposure prophylaxis)"

Note: In the presence of systemic involvement, extensive edema, and/or lesions on head/neck, doxycycline should initially be administered I.V.

Inhalational/gastrointestinal/oropharyngeal (treatment): I.V.: Refer to dosing for inhalational anthrax (postexposure prophylaxis); switch to oral therapy when clinically appropriate.

Note: Initial treatment should include two or more agents predicted to be effective (per CDC recommendations). Agents suggested for use in conjunction with doxycycline or ciprofloxacin include rifampin, vancomycin, imipenem, penicillin, ampicillin, chloramphenicol, clindamycin, and clarithromycin. May switch to oral antimicrobial therapy when clinically appropriate. Continue combined therapy for 60 days

Renal Impairment: No adjustment necessary.
Not dialyzable; 0% to 5% by hemo- and peritoneal methods or by continuous arteriovenous or venovenous hemofiltration; supplemental dose is not necessary.

Administration
Oral: May give with meals to decrease GI upset. Capsule and tablet: Administer with at least 8 ounces of water and have patient sit up for at least 30 minutes after taking to reduce the risk of esophageal irritation and ulceration.

Doryx® capsules and tablets are bioequivalent. Doryx® capsules may be opened and contents sprinkled on applesauce. Applesauce should be swallowed immediately; do not chew. Follow with 8 ounces of water. Applesauce should not be hot and should be soft enough to swallow without chewing.

I.V.: Infuse slowly, usually over 1-4 hours. Avoid extravasation.

I.V. Detail: Avoid extravasation. Very irritating to vein; use central line if possible.

pH: 1.8-3.3 (reconstituted solution)

Stability
Reconstitution: I.V. infusion: Following reconstitution with sterile water for injection, dilute to a final concentration of 0.1-1 mg/mL using a compatible solution. Protect from light. Stability varies based on solution.

Compatibility: Stable in NS, D₅W, LR, D₅LR
Y-site administration: Incompatible with allopurinol, heparin, piperacillin/tazobactam

Storage: Capsule, tablet: Store at controlled room temperature 15°C to 30°C (59°F to 86°F). Protect from light.

Laboratory Monitoring Perform culture and sensitivity testing prior to initiating therapy.

Nursing Actions
Physical Assessment: Results of culture and sensitivity test and patient's allergy history should be assessed prior to beginning therapy. Assess potential for interactions with other pharmacological agents or herbal products patient may be taking. Monitor infusion site closely; extravasation can be very irritating to veins (use of central line is preferable). Monitor therapeutic effectiveness (resolution of infections) and adverse response (see Adverse Reactions) on a regular basis throughout therapy. Advise patients with diabetes about use of Clinistix®. Teach patient appropriate use/administration (oral), possible side effects, interventions to reduce side effects (eg, importance of adequate hydration), and adverse symptoms to report.

Patient Education: If administered by infusion, report immediately any acute back pain, difficulty breathing or swallowing, chest tightness, pain, redness, or swelling at infusion site. Oral: Do not take any new medication during therapy unless approved by prescriber. Take entire prescription as directed, even if you are feeling better. Take each regular dose with food or a full glass of water to reduce stomach upset. Do not chew, crush, or break extended release tablets. Avoid alcohol and maintain adequate hydration (2-3 L/day of fluids) unless instructed to restrict fluid intake. If you have diabetes, drug may cause false test results with Clinistix® urine glucose monitoring; use of another form of glucose monitoring is preferable. You may be very sensitive to sunlight (use sunblock, wear protective clothing and eyewear, or avoid exposure to direct sunlight). May cause lightheadedness, dizziness, or drowsiness (use caution when driving or engaging in tasks that require alertness until response to drug is known); nausea or vomiting (small, frequent meals, frequent mouth care, sucking lozenges, or chewing gum may help); or diarrhea (buttermilk, boiled milk, or yogurt may help). Report skin rash or itching; easy bruising or bleeding; yellowing of skin or eyes; pale stool or dark urine; unhealed mouth sores; vaginal itching or discharge; fever, chills, or unusual cough. **Pregnancy/breast-feeding precautions:** Inform prescriber if you are pregnant. Do not get pregnant while taking this (Continued)

Doxycycline (Continued)

medication. Consult prescriber for appropriate barrier contraceptive measures. Breast-feeding is not recommended.

Dietary Considerations

Take with food if gastric irritation occurs. While administration with food may decrease GI absorption of doxycycline by up to 20%, administration on an empty stomach is not recommended due to GI intolerance. Of currently available tetracyclines, doxycycline has the least affinity for calcium.

Doryx® 75 mg and 100 mg tablets contain sodium 4.5 mg and 6 mg, respectively.

Pregnancy Issues Exposure during the last half or pregnancy causes permanent yellow-gray-brown discoloration of the teeth. Tetracyclines also form a complex in bone-forming tissue, leading to a decreased fibula growth rate when given to premature infants. According to the FDA, the Teratogen Information System concluded that therapeutic doses during pregnancy are unlikely to produce substantial teratogenic risk, but data are insufficient to say that there is no risk. In general, reports of exposure have been limited to short durations of therapy in the first trimester. When considering treatment for life-threatening infection and/or prolonged duration of therapy (such as in anthrax), the potential risk to the fetus must be balanced against the severity of the potential illness.

Dronabinol (droe NAB i nol)

U.S. Brand Names Marinol®

Synonyms Delta-9-tetrahydro-cannabinol; Delta-9 THC; Tetrahydrocannabinol; THC

Restrictions C-III

Pharmacologic Category Antiemetic; Appetite Stimulant

Medication Safety Issues

Sound-alike/look-alike issues:

Dronabinol may be confused with droperidol

Pregnancy Risk Factor C

Lactation Enters breast milk/contraindicated

Use Chemotherapy-associated nausea and vomiting refractory to other antiemetic; AIDS-related anorexia

Unlabeled/Investigational Use

Cancer-related anorexia

Mechanism of Action/Effect Unknown, may inhibit endorphins in the emetic center, suppress prostaglandin synthesis, and/or inhibit medullary activity through an unspecified cortical action

Contraindications Hypersensitivity to dronabinol, cannabinoids, or any component of the formulation, or marijuana; should be avoided in patients with a history of schizophrenia

Warnings/Precautions Use with caution in patients with heart disease, hepatic disease, or seizure disorders. Reduce dosage in patients with severe hepatic impairment. May cause additive CNS effects with sedatives, hypnotics or other psychoactive agents; patients must be cautioned about performing tasks which require mental alertness (eg, operating machinery or driving). May have potential for abuse; drug is psychoactive substance in marijuana; use caution in patients with a history of substance abuse. May cause withdrawal symptoms upon abrupt discontinuation. Use with caution in patients with mania, depression, or schizophrenia; careful psychiatric monitoring is recommended.

Drug Interactions

Increased Effect/Toxicity: Sedative effects may be additive with CNS depressants (includes barbiturates, narcotic analgesics, and other sedative agents).

Nutritional/Ethanol Interactions

Ethanol: Avoid ethanol (may increase CNS depression).

Food: Administration with high-lipid meals may increase absorption.

Herb/Nutraceutical: St John's wort may decrease dronabinol levels.

Lab Interactions Decreased FSH, LH, growth hormone, testosterone

Adverse Reactions

>10%:

Central nervous system: Drowsiness (48%), sedation (53%), confusion (30%), dizziness (21%), detachment, anxiety, difficulty concentrating, mood change

Gastrointestinal: Appetite increased (when used as an antiemetic), xerostomia (38% to 50%)

1% to 10%:

Cardiovascular: Orthostatic hypotension, tachycardia

Central nervous system: Ataxia (4%), depression (7%), headache, vertigo, hallucinations (5%), memory lapse (4%)

Neuromuscular & skeletal: Paresthesia, weakness

Overdosage/Toxicology Symptoms of overdose may include tachycardia, hyper- or hypotension, behavioral disturbances, lethargy, panic reactions, seizures or motor incoordination. Benzodiazepines may be helpful for agitative behavior; Trendelenburg position and hydration may be helpful for hypotensive effects. For other manifestations, treatment should be symptom-directed and supportive.

Pharmacodynamics/Kinetics

Onset of Action: Within 1 hour; Peak effect: 2-4 hours

Duration of Action: 24 hours (appetite stimulation)

Time to Peak: Serum: 0.5-4 hours

Protein Binding: 97% to 99%

Half-Life Elimination: Dronabinol: 25-36 hours (terminal); Dronabinol metabolites: 44-59 hours

Metabolism: Hepatic to at least 50 metabolites, some of which are active; 11-hydroxy-delta-9-tetrahydrocannabinol (11-OH-THC) is the major metabolite; extensive first-pass effect

Excretion: Feces (35% as unconjugated metabolites, 5% as unchanged drug); urine (10% to 15% as acid metabolites and conjugates)

Available Dosage Forms Capsule, gelatin: 2.5 mg, 5 mg, 10 mg [contains sesame oil]

Dosing

Adults & Elderly:

Antiemetic: Oral: 5 mg/m^2 1-3 hours before chemotherapy, then give 5 mg/m^2/dose every 2-4 hours after chemotherapy for a total of 4-6 doses/day; dose may be increased up to a maximum of 15 mg/m^2/dose if needed (dosage may be increased by 2.5 mg/m^2 increments).

Appetite stimulant (AIDS-related): Oral: Initial: 2.5 mg twice daily (before lunch and dinner); titrate up to a maximum of 20 mg/day.

Pediatrics: Antiemetic: Oral: Refer to adult dosing.

Hepatic Impairment: Usual dose should be reduced in patients with severe liver failure.

Stability

Storage: Store under refrigeration (or in a cool environment) between 8°C and 15°C (46°F and 59°F). Protect from freezing.

Nursing Actions

Physical Assessment: Assess potential for interactions with other pharmacological agents or herbal products patient may be taking. Monitor effectiveness of therapy and adverse response (eg, CNS changes, psychotic reactions; this drug is the psychoactive substance in marijuana). Teach patient appropriate use, possible side effects/appropriate interventions, and adverse symptoms to report.

Patient Education: Do not take any new medication during therapy unless approved by prescriber (especially barbiturates, and benzodiazepines). Take exactly as directed; do not increase dose or take more often than prescribed. Avoid alcohol. May cause psychotic reaction, impaired coordination or judgment, faintness, dizziness, or drowsiness (do not drive or engage in activities that require alertness and coordination until response to drug is known); or clumsiness, unsteadiness, or muscular weakness (change position slowly and use caution when climbing stairs). Report excessive or persistent CNS changes (euphoria, anxiety, depression, memory lapse, bizarre thought patterns, excitability, inability to control thoughts or behavior, fainting); respiratory difficulties; rapid heartbeat; or other adverse reactions. **Pregnancy/breast-feeding precautions:** Inform prescriber if you are or intend to become pregnant. Do not breast-feed.

Dietary Considerations Capsules contain sesame oil.

Droperidol (droe PER i dole)

U.S. Brand Names Inapsine®
Synonyms Dehydrobenzperidol
Pharmacologic Category Antiemetic; Antipsychotic Agent, Typical
Medication Safety Issues
Sound-alike/look-alike issues:
Droperidol may be confused with dronabinol
Inapsine® may be confused with Nebcin®
Pregnancy Risk Factor C
Lactation Excretion in breast milk unknown
Use Antiemetic in surgical and diagnostic procedures; preoperative medication in patients when other treatments are ineffective or inappropriate
Mechanism of Action/Effect Droperidol is a butyrophenone antipsychotic; antiemetic effect is a result of blockade of dopamine stimulation of the chemoreceptor trigger zone. Other effects include alpha-adrenergic blockade, peripheral vascular dilation, and reduction of the pressor effect of epinephrine resulting in hypotension and decreased peripheral vascular resistance; may also reduce pulmonary artery pressure
Contraindications Hypersensitivity to droperidol or any component of the formulation; known or suspected QT prolongation, including congenital long QT syndrome (prolonged QT$_c$ is defined as >440 msec in males or >450 msec in females)
Warnings/Precautions May alter cardiac conduction. Cases of QT prolongation and torsade de pointes, including some fatal cases, have been reported. Use extreme caution in patients with bradycardia (<50 bpm), cardiac disease, concurrent MAOI therapy, Class I and Class III antiarrhythmics or other drugs known to prolong QT interval, and electrolyte disturbances (hypokalemia or hypomagnesemia), including concomitant drugs which may alter electrolytes (diuretics).

Use with caution in patients with seizures, bone marrow suppression, or severe liver disease. May be sedating, use with caution in disorders where CNS depression is a feature. Caution in patients with hemodynamic instability, predisposition to seizures, subcortical brain damage, renal or respiratory disease. Esophageal dysmotility and aspiration have been associated with antipsychotic use. Caution in breast cancer or other prolactin-dependent tumors. May cause orthostatic hypotension - use with caution in patients at risk of this effect. Significant hypotension may occur; injection contains benzyl alcohol; injection also contains sulfites which may cause allergic reaction.

Relative to other neuroleptics, droperidol has a low potency of cholinergic blockade. Use with caution in patients with decreased gastrointestinal motility, urinary retention, BPH, xerostomia, or visual problems. May worsen myasthenia gravis.

May cause extrapyramidal symptoms, including tardive dyskinesia. May be associated with neuroleptic malignant syndrome (NMS) or pigmentary retinopathy. Safety in children <6 months of age has not been established.

Drug Interactions
Increased Effect/Toxicity: Droperidol in combination with certain forms of conduction anesthesia may produce peripheral vasodilitation and hypotension. Droperidol and CNS depressants will likely have additive CNS effects. Droperidol and cyclobenzaprine may have an additive effect on prolonging the QT interval. Use caution with other agents known to prolong QT interval (Class I or Class III antiarrhythmics, some quinolone antibiotics, cisapride, some phenothiazines, pimozide, tricyclic antidepressants). Potassium- or magnesium-depleting agents (diuretics, aminoglycosides, amphotericin B, cyclosporine) may increase risk of arrhythmias. Metoclopramide may increase risk of extrapyramidal symptoms (EPS). Acetylcholinesterase inhibitors (central) may increase the risk of antipsychotic-related EPS.

Adverse Reactions
>10%:
Cardiovascular: QT$_c$ prolongation (dose dependent)
Central nervous system: Restlessness, anxiety, extrapyramidal symptoms, dystonic reactions, pseudoparkinsonian signs and symptoms, tardive dyskinesia, seizure, altered central temperature regulation, sedation, drowsiness
Endocrine & metabolic: Swelling of breasts
Gastrointestinal: Weight gain, constipation
1% to 10%:
Cardiovascular: Hypotension (especially orthostatic), tachycardia, abnormal T waves with prolonged ventricular repolarization, hypertension
Central nervous system: Hallucinations, persistent tardive dyskinesia, akathisia
Gastrointestinal: Nausea, vomiting
Genitourinary: Dysuria

Overdosage/Toxicology Symptoms of overdose include hypotension, tachycardia, hallucinations, and extrapyramidal symptoms. Following initiation of essential overdose management, toxic symptom treatment and supportive treatment should be initiated. Prolonged QT interval, seizures, and arrhythmias have been reported.

Pharmacodynamics/Kinetics
Onset of Action: Peak effect: Parenteral: Within 30 minutes
Duration of Action: Parenteral: 2-4 hours, may extend to 12 hours
Protein Binding: Extensive
Half-Life Elimination: Adults: 2.3 hours
Metabolism: Hepatic, to p-fluorophenylacetic acid, benzimidazolone, p-hydroxypiperidine
Excretion: Urine (75%, <1% as unchanged drug); feces (22%, 11% to 50% as unchanged drug)
Available Dosage Forms Injection, solution: 2.5 mg/mL (1 mL, 2 mL)

Dosing
Adults & Elderly: Titrate carefully to desired effect: Nausea and vomiting: I.M., I.V.: Initial: 2.5 mg; additional doses of 1.25 mg may be administered to achieve desired effect; administer additional doses with caution
Pediatrics: Titrate carefully to desired effect: Children 2-12 years: Nausea and vomiting: I.M., I.V.: 0.05-0.06 mg/kg (maximum initial dose: 0.1 mg/kg); additional doses may be repeated to achieve effect; administer additional doses with caution
(Continued)

Droperidol *(Continued)*

Administration

I.V.: Administer I.M. or I.V.; I.V. should be administered as a rapid IVP (over 30-60 seconds); for I.V. infusion, dilute in 50-100 mL NS or D_5W. ECG monitoring for 2-3 hours after administration is recommended.

I.V. Detail: pH: 3.0-3.8

Stability

Compatibility: Stable in D_5W, LR, NS

Y-site administration: Incompatible with allopurinol, amphotericin B cholesteryl sulfate complex, cefepime, fluorouracil, foscarnet, furosemide, leucovorin, nafcillin, piperacillin/tazobactam

Compatibility in syringe: Incompatible with fluorouracil, furosemide, heparin, leucovorin, methotrexate, ondansetron, pentobarbital

Storage: Droperidol ampuls/vials should be stored at room temperature and protected from light. Solutions diluted in NS or D_5W are stable at room temperature for up to 7 days.

Laboratory Monitoring To identify QT prolongation, a 12-lead ECG prior to use is recommended; ECG monitoring for 2-3 hours following administration is recommended. Lipid profile, fasting blood glucose/Hgb A_{1c}, serum magnesium and potassium; BMI

Nursing Actions

Physical Assessment: Assess other medications the patient may be taking for effectiveness and interactions. Monitor vital signs; cardiac and respiratory status on a frequent basis and especially immediately following administration and for several hours afterward. Monitor for extrapyramidal symptoms for 24-48 hours after therapy. Teach and use orthostatic hypotension precautions until the patient is stable. Teach adverse reactions to report.

Patient Education: This drug may cause you to feel very sleepy; do not attempt to get up without assistance. May cause orthostatic hypotension (use caution when changing position from lying or sitting to standing). You may experience constipation, (increasing exercise, fluids, fruit/fiber may help). Immediately report any respiratory difficulty, confusion, loss of thought processes, or palpitations. **Pregnancy/breast-feeding precautions:** Inform prescriber if you are pregnant. Consult prescriber if breast-feeding.

Geriatric Considerations Use of droperidol in the elderly may result in severe and often irreversible undesirable effects. Before initiating antipsychotic therapy, the clinician should investigate possible reversible causes.

Additional Information Does not possess analgesic effects; has little or no amnesic properties.

Drospirenone and Estradiol

(droh SPYE re none & es tra DYE ole)

U.S. Brand Names Angeliq®

Synonyms E2 and DRSP; Estradiol and Drospirenone

Pharmacologic Category Estrogen and Progestin Combination

Lactation Enters breast milk/not recommended

Use Treatment of moderate-to-severe vasomotor symptoms associated with menopause; treatment of vulvar and vaginal atrophy associated with menopause

Mechanism of Action/Effect

Drospirenone is a synthetic progestin and spironolactone analog with antimineralocorticoid and antiandrogenic activity. Counteracts estrogen effects causing endometrial thinning.

Estrogens are responsible for the development and maintenance of the female reproductive system and secondary sexual characteristics. Estradiol is the principal intracellular human estrogen and is more potent than estrone and estriol at the receptor level; it is the primary estrogen secreted prior to menopause. Following menopause, estrone and estrone sulfate are more highly produced. Estrogens modulate the pituitary secretion of gonadotropins, luteinizing hormone, and follicle-stimulating hormone through a negative feedback system; estrogen replacement reduces elevated levels of these hormones in postmenopausal women.

Contraindications Hypersensitivity to drospirenone, estradiol, or any component of the formulation; undiagnosed abnormal vaginal bleeding; history of current thrombophlebitis or venous thromboembolic disorders (including DVT, PE); active or recent (within 1 year) arterial thromboembolic disease (eg, stroke, MI); carcinoma of the breast; estrogen-dependent tumor; hepatic or renal dysfunction or disease; adrenal insufficiency; pregnancy

Warnings/Precautions Drospirenone has antimineralocorticoid activity that may lead to hyperkalemia in patients with renal insufficiency, hepatic dysfunction, or adrenal insufficiency. Use caution with medications that may increase serum potassium.

Cardiovascular-related considerations: Estrogens with or without progestin should not be used to prevent coronary heart disease. Use caution with cardiovascular disease or dysfunction. May increase the risks of hypertension, myocardial infarction (MI), stroke, pulmonary emboli (PE), and deep vein thrombosis; incidence of these effects was shown to be significantly increased in postmenopausal women using conjugated equine estrogens (CEE) in combination with medroxyprogesterone acetate (MPA). Nonfatal MI, PE, and thrombophlebitis have also been reported in males taking high doses of CEE (eg, for prostate cancer). Estrogen compounds are generally associated with lipid effects such as increased HDL-cholesterol and decreased LDL-cholesterol. Triglycerides may also be increased; use with caution in patients with familial defects of lipoprotein metabolism. Whenever possible, estrogens should be discontinued at least 4 weeks prior to and for 2 weeks following elective surgery associated with an increased risk of thromboembolism or during periods of prolonged immobilization.

Neurological considerations: The risk of dementia may be increased in postmenopausal women; increased incidence was observed in women ≥65 years of age taking CEE alone or in combination with MPA.

Cancer-related considerations: Unopposed estrogens may increase the risk of endometrial carcinoma in postmenopausal women. Estrogens may exacerbate endometriosis. Malignant transformation of residual endometrial implants has been reported posthysterectomy with estrogen only therapy. Estrogens may increase the risk of breast cancer. An increased risk of invasive breast cancer was observed in postmenopausal women using CEE in combination with MPA; a smaller increase in risk was seen with estrogen therapy alone in observational studies. An increase in abnormal mammograms has also been reported with estrogen and progestin therapy. Estrogen use may lead to severe hypercalcemia in patients with breast cancer and bone metastases; discontinue estrogen if hypercalcemia occurs.

Estrogens may cause retinal vascular thrombosis; discontinue permanently if papilledema or retinal vascular lesions are observed on examination. Use with caution in patients with diseases which may be exacerbated by fluid retention, including asthma, epilepsy, migraine, diabetes, or renal dysfunction. Use with caution in patients with a history of severe hypocalcemia, SLE, hepatic hemangiomas, porphyria, endometriosis, and gallbladder disease. Use caution with history of cholestatic jaundice associated with past estrogen use or pregnancy.

Before prescribing estrogen therapy to postmenopausal women, the risks and benefits must be weighed for each patient. Women should be informed of these risks and benefits, as well as possible effects of progestin when added to estrogen therapy. Estrogens with or without progestin should be used for shortest duration possible consistent with treatment goals. Conduct periodic risk:benefit assessments. When used solely for the treatment of vulvar and vaginal atrophy, topical vaginal products should be considered.

Drug Interactions
Cytochrome P450 Effect:
Drospirenone: **Substrate** of CYP3A4 (minor); **Inhibits** CYP1A2 (weak), 2C8/9 (weak), 2C19 (weak), 3A4 (weak)
Estradiol: **Substrate** of CYP1A2 (major), 2A6 (minor), 2B6 (minor), 2C8/9 (minor), 2C19 (minor), 2D6 (minor), 2E1 (minor), 3A4 (major); **Inhibits** CYP1A2 (weak); **Induces** CYP3A4 (weak)

Decreased Effect: Pregnancy has been reported following concomitant use of antibiotics (ampicillin, griseofulvin, tetracycline), however, pharmacokinetic studies have not shown consistent effects with these antibiotics on plasma concentrations of synthetic steroids. Oral contraceptives may increase or decrease the effects of coumarin derivatives. Anticonvulsants (carbamazepine, felbamate, phenobarbital, phenytoin, topiramate) increase the metabolism of ethinyl estradiol and/or some progestins, leading to possible decrease in contraceptive effectiveness. Phenylbutazones may decrease contraceptive effectiveness and increase menstrual irregularities.

Increased Effect/Toxicity: Potential for hyperkalemia with concomitant use of ACE inhibitors, aldosterone, angiotensin II receptor antagonists, heparin, NSAIDs (when taken daily, long term), and potassium-sparing diuretics; monitor serum potassium during first cycle. Potential for hyperkalemia with concomitant use of aldosterone antagonists; monitor serum potassium during first cycle. Aminoglutethimide may increase CYP metabolism of progestins. Oral contraceptives may increase or decrease the effects of coumarin derivatives.

Nutritional/Ethanol Interactions Ethanol: Avoid ethanol (routine use increases estrogen level and risk of breast cancer). Ethanol may also increase the risk of osteoporosis.

Lab Interactions Pathologist should be advised of estrogen/progesterone therapy when specimens are submitted. Reduced response to metyrapone test.

Adverse Reactions
>10%:
Endocrine & metabolic: Breast pain (19%)
Gastrointestinal: Abdominal pain (11%)
Respiratory: Upper respiratory tract infection (19%)
1% to 10%:
Cardiovascular: Peripheral edema (2%)
Central nervous system: Headache (10%), pain (8%)
Gastrointestinal: Abdomen enlarged (7%)
Genitourinary: Vaginal hemorrhage (9%), endometrial disorder (2%), leukorrhea (1%)
Neuromuscular & skeletal: Back pain (7%)
Respiratory: Flu-like syndrome (7%), sinusitis (5%)
Additional adverse effects reported with estrogens and/ or progestins: Abdominal cramps, acne, abnormal uterine bleeding, aggravation of porphyria, amenorrhea, anaphylactoid reactions, anaphylaxis, antifactor Xa decreased, antithrombin III decreased, appetite changes, bloating, breast enlargement, breast tenderness, cerebral embolism, cerebral thrombosis, chloasma, cholestatic jaundice, cholecystitis, cholelithiasis, chorea, contact lens intolerance,

cystitis-like syndrome, decreased carbohydrate tolerance, depression, dementia, dizziness, dysmenorrhea; factors VII, VIII, IX, X, XII, VII-X complex, and II-VII-X complex increased; endometrial hyperplasia, erythema multiforme, erythema nodosum, galactorrhea, hemorrhagic eruption, fatigue, fibrinogen increased, impaired glucose tolerance, HDL-cholesterol increased, hirsutism, hypertension, increase in size of uterine leiomyomata, gallbladder disease, insomnia, LDL-cholesterol decreased, libido changes, loss of scalp hair, melasma, migraine, mood disturbances, nausea, nervousness, optic neuritis, pancreatitis, platelet aggregability and platelet count increased, premenstrual-like syndrome, PT and PTT accelerated, pulmonary embolism, pyrexia, retinal thrombosis, somnolence, steepening of corneal curvature, stroke, thrombophlebitis, thyroid-binding globulin increased, total thyroid hormone (T_4) increased, triglycerides increased, urticaria, vaginal candidiasis, vomiting, weight gain/loss

Overdosage/Toxicology Overdose may cause nausea; withdrawal bleeding may occur in females. Monitor potassium and sodium serum concentrations. Treatment should be symptom directed and supportive.

Pharmacodynamics/Kinetics
Time to Peak:
Drospirenone: 1 hour; Estradiol: 6-8 hours
Protein Binding:
Drospirenone: 97%; does not bind to sex hormone binding globulin or corticosteroid binding globulin
Estradiol: 37% bound to sex hormone binding globulin; 61% bound to albumin
Metabolism: Hepatic
Drospirenone forms two metabolites (inactive)
Estradiol: Converted to estrone and estriol; also undergoes enterohepatic recirculation; estrone sulfite is the main metabolite in postmenopausal women

Available Dosage Forms Tablet: Drospirenone 0.5 mg and estradiol 1 mg

Dosing
Adults & Elderly:
Moderate-to-severe vasomotor symptoms associated with menopause: Oral: One tablet daily; re-evaluate patients at 3- and 6-month intervals to determine if treatment is still necessary.
Atrophic vaginitis in females with an intact uterus: Oral: One tablet daily; re-evaluate patients at 3- and 6-month intervals to determine if treatment is still necessary.
Note: The lowest dose of estrogen/progestin that will control symptoms should be used; medication should be discontinued as soon as possible.
Renal Impairment: Use in contraindicated.
Hepatic Impairment: Use in contraindicated.

Stability
Storage: Store at controlled room temperature of 15°C to 30°C (59°F to 86°F).

Laboratory Monitoring Glycemic control in diabetics; lipid profiles in patients being treated for hyperlipidemias; thyroid function in patients on thyroid hormone replacement therapy

Nursing Actions
Physical Assessment: Assess other prescription and OTC medications the patient may be taking to avoid duplications and interactions. Stress need for annual gynecological exam and performing self-breast examination. Monitor blood pressure at beginning of therapy and periodically while taking this medication. Assess knowledge/teach patient appropriate use, side effects, and symptoms to report.

Patient Education: Avoid alcohol. Maintain adequate hydration (2-3 L/day) unless instructed to restrict intake by prescriber. If diabetic, monitor blood glucose levels closely. May impair glucose tolerance. You may experience headache, pain in your breast, irregular
(Continued)

Drospirenone and Estradiol *(Continued)*

vaginal bleeding or spotting, abdominal cramps, bloated sensation, nausea and vomiting, or hair loss. Report lumps in the breast, unusual vaginal bleeding, dizziness or faintness (use caution when driving or engaging in activities requiring alertness until response to drug is known), changes in speech, severe headaches, chest pain, shortness of breath, pain or swelling in legs, changes in vision, upper respiratory infection, or severe vomiting. **Breast-feeding precaution:** Breast-feeding is not recommended.

Geriatric Considerations Before prescribing estrogen therapy to postmenopausal women, the risks and benefits must be weighed for each patient. Women should be informed of these risks and benefits, as well as possible side effects and the return of menstrual bleeding (when cycled with a progestin), and be involved in the decision to prescribe. A higher incidence of stroke and invasive breast cancer was observed in women >75 years in a WHI substudy. Oral therapy may be more convenient for vaginal atrophy and urinary incontinence.

Breast-Feeding Issues Following administration of an oral contraceptive agent containing drospirenone, ~0.02% of the dose was detected in breast milk, resulting in a maximum of ~3 mcg/day drospirenone to the infant. Estrogens may decrease the quality and quantity of breast milk.

Drotrecogin Alfa *(dro TRE coe jin AL fa)*

U.S. Brand Names Xigris®

Synonyms Activated Protein C, Human, Recombinant; Drotrecogin Alfa, Activated; Protein C (Activated), Human, Recombinant

Pharmacologic Category Protein C (Activated)

Pregnancy Risk Factor C

Lactation Excretion in breast milk unknown/not recommended

Use Reduction of mortality from severe sepsis (associated with organ dysfunction) in adults at high risk of death (eg, APACHE II score ≥25)

Unlabeled/Investigational Use Purpura fulminans

Mechanism of Action/Effect Decreases mortality from severe sepsis by blocking thrombotic activity. Blocks factor Va and VIIIa. In addition, may have other anti-inflammatory effects.

Contraindications Hypersensitivity to drotrecogin alfa or any component of the formulation; active internal bleeding; recent hemorrhagic stroke (within 3 months); severe head trauma (within 2 months); recent intracranial or intraspinal surgery (within 2 months); intracranial neoplasm or mass lesion; evidence of cerebral herniation; presence of an epidural catheter; trauma with an increased risk of life-threatening bleeding

Warnings/Precautions Increases risk of bleeding; careful evaluation of risks and benefit is required prior to initiation (see Contraindications). Bleeding risk is increased in patients receiving concurrent therapeutic heparin, oral anticoagulants, glycoprotein IIb/IIIa antagonists, platelet aggregation inhibitors, or aspirin at a dosage of >650 mg/day (within 7 days). In addition, an increased bleeding risk is associated with prolonged INR (>3.0), gastrointestinal bleeding (within 6 weeks), decreased platelet count (<30,000/mm³), thrombolytic therapy (within 3 days), recent ischemic stroke (within 3 months), intracranial AV malformation or aneurysm, known bleeding diathesis, severe hepatic disease (chronic), or other condition where bleeding is a significant hazard or difficult to manage due to its location. Discontinue if significant bleeding occurs (may consider continued use after stabilization). Treatment interruption required for invasive procedures. During treatment, aPTT cannot be used to assess coagulopathy (PT/INR not affected).

Efficacy not established in adult patients at a low risk of death. Patients with pre-existing nonsepsis-related medical conditions with a poor prognosis (anticipated survival <28 days), patients with acute pancreatitis (no established source of infection), HIV-infected patients with a CD4 count ≤50 cells/mm³, chronic dialysis patients, pre-existing hypercoagulable conditions, and patients who had received bone marrow, liver, lung, pancreas, or small bowel transplants were excluded from the clinical trial which established benefit. In addition, patients with a high body weight (>135 kg) were not evaluated. Safety and efficacy have not been established in pediatric patients.

Drug Interactions

Increased Effect/Toxicity: Concurrent use of antiplatelet agents, including aspirin (>650 mg/day, recent use within 7 days), cilostazol, clopidogrel, dipyridamole, ticlopidine, NSAIDs, or glycoprotein IIb/IIIa antagonists (recent use within 7 days) may increase risk of bleeding. Concurrent use of low molecular weight heparins or heparin at therapeutic rates of infusion may increase the risk of bleeding. However, the use of low-dose prophylactic heparin does not appear to affect safety. Recent use of thrombolytic agents (within 3 days) may increase the risk of bleeding. Recent use of warfarin (within 7 days or elevation of INR ≥3) may increase the risk of bleeding. Other drugs which interfere with coagulation may increase risk of bleeding (including antithrombin III, danaproid, direct thrombin inhibitors)

Nutritional/Ethanol Interactions Herb/Nutraceutical: Recent use/intake of herbs with anticoagulant or antiplatelet activity (including cat's claw, feverfew, garlic, ginkgo, ginseng, and horse chestnut seed) may increase the risk of bleeding.

Lab Interactions May interfere with one-stage coagulation assays based on the aPTT (such as factor VIII, IX, and XI assays).

Adverse Reactions As with all drugs which may affect hemostasis, bleeding is the major adverse effect associated with drotrecogin alfa. Hemorrhage may occur at virtually any site. Risk is dependent on multiple variables, including the dosage administered, concurrent use of multiple agents which alter hemostasis, and patient predisposition.

>10%:
Dermatologic: Bruising
Gastrointestinal: Gastrointestinal bleeding

1% to 10%: Hematologic: Bleeding (serious 2.4% during infusion vs 3.5% during 28-day study period; individual events listed as <1%)

Overdosage/Toxicology No reported experience with overdose. Hemorrhagic complications are likely consequence of overdose. Treatment is supportive, including immediate interruption of the infusion and monitoring for hemorrhagic complications. No known antidote.

Pharmacodynamics/Kinetics

Duration of Action: Plasma nondetectable within 2 hours of discontinuation

Half-Life Elimination: 1.6 hours

Metabolism: Inactivated by endogenous plasma protease inhibitors; mean clearance: 40 L/hour; increased with severe sepsis (~50%)

Available Dosage Forms Injection, powder for reconstitution [preservative free]: 5 mg [contains sucrose 31.8 mg], 20 mg [contains sucrose 124.9 mg]

Dosing

Adults:
Purpura fulminans (unlabeled use): 24 mcg/kg/hour
Severe sepsis: I.V.: 24 mcg/kg/hour for a total of 96 hours; stop infusion **immediately** if clinically-important bleeding is identified.

Pediatrics: Purpura fulminans (unlabeled use): Refer to adult dosing.

Renal Impairment: No specific adjustment recommended.

Administration

I.V.: Administer via infusion pump. Administration must be completed within 12 hours of solution preparation. Suspend administration for 2 hours prior to invasive procedures or other procedure with significant bleeding risk; may continue treatment immediately following uncomplicated, minimally-invasive procedures, but delay for 12 hours after major invasive procedures/surgery.

I.V. Detail: Compatible with 0.9% sodium chloride; normal saline, dextrose, lactated Ringer's or dextrose/saline mixtures may be infused through the same infusion line. Compatible with ceftriaxone, cisatracurium, fluconazole, nitroglycerin, potassium chloride, and vasopressin.

Stability

Reconstitution: Reconstitute 5 mg vials with 2.5 mL and 20 mg vials with 10 mL sterile water for injection (resultant solution ~2 mg/mL). Must be further diluted (within 3 hours of reconstitution) in 0.9% sodium chloride, typically to a concentration between 100 mcg/mL and 200 mcg/mL when using infusion pump and between 100 mcg/mL and 1000 mcg/mL when infused via syringe pump. Although product information states administration must be completed within 12 hours of preparation, additional studies (data on file, Lilly Research Laboratories) show that the final solution is stable for 14 hours at 15°C to 30°C (59°F to 86°F). If not used immediately, a prepared solution may be stored in the refrigerator for up to 12 hours. The total expiration time (refrigeration and administration) should be ≤24 hours from time of preparation.

Compatibility: Stable in NS; only NS, dextrose, LR, or dextrose/saline mixtures may be infused through the same line.

Y-site administration: Incompatible: Amiodarone, ampicillin/sulbactam sodium, ceftazidime, ciprofloxacin, clindamycin, cyclosporine, dobutamine hydrochloride, dopamine hydrochloride, epinephrine hydrochloride, fosphenytoin, furosemide, gentamicin sulfate, heparin sodium, human serum albumin, imipenem/cilastatin sodium, insulin human (regular), levofloxacin, magnesium sulfate, metronidazole, midazolam hydrochloride, nitroprusside sodium, norepinephrine bitartrate, piperacillin/tazobactam sodium, potassium phosphate, ranitidine hydrochloride, ticarcillin/clavulanate, tobramycin sulfate, vancomycin hydrochloride

Storage: Store vials under refrigeration at 2°C to 8°C (36°F to 46°F). Protect from light. Do not freeze.

Laboratory Monitoring Hemoglobin/hematocrit, PT/INR, platelet count

Nursing Actions

Physical Assessment: Assess interactions with other prescription, OTC medications, or herbal products patient may be taking (especially drugs affecting coagulation or platelet activity). Monitor laboratory tests prior to, during, and following therapy. Monitor patient very closely for bleeding during and following infusion (hemorrhage may occur at virtually any site). If significant bleeding occurs, stop infusion and notify prescriber immediately. Observe bleeding precautions. Patient instruction should be according to patient condition.

Patient Education: Inform prescriber of all prescriptions, OTC medications, or herbal products you are taking, and any allergies you have. This medication can only be administered by infusion. You will be monitored closely. Report immediately any unusual or acute abdominal pain or headache, or respiratory difficulty. You will be more susceptible to bleeding and bruising; remain in bed and ring for assistance to avoid falling or injuring yourself. Avoid sharps of any kind (knives, scissors, needles, nail clippers, etc;

shave with a safety razor). **Pregnancy/breast-feeding precautions:** Inform prescriber if you are pregnant. Breast-feeding is not recommended.

Additional Information Prepared by recombinant DNA technology in human cell line

---

Duloxetine (doo LOX e teen)

U.S. Brand Names Cymbalta®

Synonyms Duloxetine Hydrochloride; LY248686; (+)-(S)-N-Methyl-γ-(1-naphthyloxy)-2-thiophenepropylamine Hydrochloride

Restrictions A medication guide concerning the use of antidepressants in children and teenagers can be found on the FDA website at http://www.fda.gov/cder/Offices/ODS/labeling.htm. It should be dispensed to parents or guardians of children and teenagers receiving this medication.

Pharmacologic Category Antidepressant, Serotonin/Norepinephrine Reuptake Inhibitor

Medication Safety Issues
Sound-alike/look-alike issues:
Duloxetine may be confused with fluoxetine.

Pregnancy Risk Factor C

Lactation Enters breast milk/not recommended

Use Treatment of major depressive disorder; management of pain associated with diabetic neuropathy

Unlabeled/Investigational Use Treatment of stress incontinence; management of chronic pain syndromes; management of fibromyalgia

Mechanism of Action/Effect Inhibits reuptake of both norepinephrine and serotonin (SNRI); improves symptoms of depression.

Contraindications Hypersensitivity to duloxetine or any component of the formulation; concomitant use or within 2 weeks of MAO inhibitors; uncontrolled narrow angle glaucoma

Warnings/Precautions Antidepressants increase the risk of suicidal thinking and behavior in children and adolescents with major depressive disorder (MDD) and other depressive disorders; consider risk prior to prescribing. All patients must be closely monitored for clinical worsening, suicidality, or unusual changes in behavior, especially during the initiation of therapy or following an increase or decrease in dosage. When used in children, the child's family or caregiver should be instructed to closely observe the patient and communicate condition with healthcare provider. A medication guide should be dispensed with each prescription. **Duloxetine is not FDA approved for use in children.**

The possibility of a suicide attempt is inherent in major depression and may persist until remission occurs. Use caution in high-risk patients. Worsening depression and severe abrupt suicidality that are not part of the presenting symptoms may require discontinuation or modification of drug therapy. The patient's family or caregiver should be alerted to monitor patients for the emergence of suicidality and associated behaviors (such as agitation, irritability, hostility, impulsivity, and hypomania) and call healthcare provider.

May worsen psychosis in some patients or precipitate a shift to mania or hypomania in patients with bipolar disorder. Patients presenting with depressive symptoms should be screened for bipolar disorder. Monotherapy in patients with bipolar disorder should be avoided. **Duloxetine is not FDA approved for the treatment of bipolar depression.**

Duloxetine may cause increased urinary resistance; advise patient to report symptoms of urinary hesitation/difficulty. Has a low potential to impair cognitive or motor performance. Use caution with a previous seizure disorder or condition predisposing to seizures such as brain damage or alcoholism. May cause hepatotoxicity; (Continued)

Duloxetine (Continued)

avoid use in patients with substantial alcohol intake, evidence of chronic liver disease, or hepatic impairment. Use with caution in patients with controlled narrow angle glaucoma. May cause or exacerbate sexual dysfunction. Use caution with renal impairment or with concomitant CNS depressants.

A potential exists for severe reactions when used with MAO inhibitors; serotonin syndrome (hyperthermia, muscular rigidity, mental status changes/agitation, autonomic instability) may occur. Use caution during concurrent therapy with other drugs which lower the seizure threshold.

Upon discontinuation of duloxetine therapy, gradually taper dose. If intolerable symptoms occur following a decrease in dosage or upon discontinuation of therapy, then resuming the previous dose with a more gradual taper should be considered. May increase the risks associated with electroconvulsive therapy. Consider discontinuing, when possible, prior to elective surgery.

Drug Interactions

Cytochrome P450 Effect: Substrate (major) of CYP1A2, 2D6; **inhibits** CYP2D6 (moderate)

Decreased Effect: CYP1A2 inducers may decrease the levels/effects of duloxetine. Example inducers include aminoglutethimide, carbamazepine, phenobarbital, and rifampin.

Increased Effect/Toxicity: Hyperpyrexia, hypertension, tachycardia, confusion, seizures, and deaths have been reported with MAO inhibitors (serotonin syndrome); this combination is contraindicated. Avoid use of linezolid (due to MAO activity). Duloxetine may increase serum concentrations of thioridazine, which has been associated with the development of malignant ventricular arrhythmias. Serum levels/effects of tricyclic antidepressants may be increased by duloxetine.

Concurrent use of duloxetine with buspirone, meperidine, moclobemide, nefazodone, SSRIs, sibutramine, tramadol and trazodone and venlafaxine may cause serotonin syndrome; avoid concurrent use. Concurrent use of selegiline with SSRIs has been reported to cause serotonin syndrome (less than with nonselective MAO inhibitors). Concurrent use of sumatriptan and similar drugs (serotonin agonists) may result in weakness, hyper-reflexia, and incoordination.

CYP1A2 and CYP2D6 inhibitors may increase the levels/effects of duloxetine. Example inhibitors include amiodarone, chlorpromazine, ciprofloxacin, delavirdine, fluvoxamine, fluoxetine, ketoconazole, miconazole, norfloxacin, ofloxacin, paroxetine, pergolide, quinidine, quinine, rofecoxib, ritonavir, and ropinirole.

Nutritional/Ethanol Interactions

Ethanol: Avoid ethanol (may increase CNS depression and/or hepatotoxic potential of duloxetine).

Herb/Nutraceutical: Avoid valerian, St John's wort, SAMe, kava kava, and gotu kola (may increase CNS depression).

Adverse Reactions

>10%:
Central nervous system: Somnolence (7% to 15%), dizziness (6% to 14%), headache (13%), insomnia (8% to 11%)
Gastrointestinal: Nausea (14% to 22%), xerostomia (5% to 15%), diarrhea (8% to 13%), constipation (5% to 11%)

1% to 10%:
Cardiovascular: Palpitations (1%)
Central nervous system: Fatigue (2% to 10%), anxiety (3%), fever (1% to 2%), hypoesthesia (1%), irritability (1%), lethargy (1%), nervousness (1%), nightmares (1%), restlessness (1%), sleep disorder (1%), vertigo (1%), yawning (1%)

Dermatologic: Hyperhydrosis (6%), pruritus (1%), rash (1%)
Endocrine & metabolic: Libido decreased (3% to 6%), orgasm abnormality (3% to 4%), hot flushes (2%), anorgasmia (1%), hypoglycemia (1%)
Gastrointestinal: Appetite decreased (3% to 8%), vomiting (5% to 6%), dyspepsia (4%), loose stools (2% to 3%), weight loss (1% to 2%), gastritis (1%)
Genitourinary: Erectile dysfunction (1% to 4%), ejaculation delayed (3%), ejaculatory dysfunction (3%), pollakiuria (1% to 3%), dysuria (1%), urinary symptoms (hesitancy, obstructive symptoms; 1%)
Hepatic: Transaminases increased: Occasionally associated with hyperbilirubinemia and/or increased alkaline phosphatase (1%)
Neuromuscular & skeletal: Muscle cramp (4% to 5%), weakness (2% to 4%), myalgia (1% to 3%), tremor (1% to 3%), muscle tightness (1%), muscle twitching (1%), rigors (1%)
Ocular: Blurred vision (4%)
Respiratory: Nasopharyngitis (7% to 9%), cough (3% to 6%), pharyngolaryngeal pain (1% to 3%)
Miscellaneous: Diaphoresis increased (6%), night sweats (1%)

Overdosage/Toxicology Treatment is symptomatic and supportive.

Pharmacodynamics/Kinetics

Time to Peak: 6 hours
Protein Binding: >90%
Half-Life Elimination: 12 hours (range 8-17 hours)
Metabolism: Hepatic, via CYP1A2 and CYP2D6; forms multiple metabolites (inactive)
Excretion: As metabolites; urine (70%), feces (20%)
Available Dosage Forms Capsule: 20 mg, 30 mg, 60 mg [contains enteric coated pellets]

Dosing

Adults:
Treatment of depression: Oral: Initial: 40-60 mg/day; dose may be divided (ie, 20 or 30 mg twice daily) or given as a single daily dose of 60 mg; maximum dose: 60 mg/day
Management of diabetic neuropathy: Oral: 60 mg once daily. Lower initial doses may be considered in patients where tolerability is a concern and/or renal impairment is present.
Management of chronic pain syndromes (unlabeled use): Oral: 60 mg once daily
Management of fibromyalgia (unlabeled use): 60 mg twice daily
Management of stress incontinence (unlabeled use): Oral: 40 mg twice daily

Elderly:
Treatment of major depressive disorder: Oral: Initial dose: 20 mg 1-2 times/day; increase to 40-60 mg/day as a single daily dose or in divided doses
Other indications: Refer to adult dosing.

Renal Impairment: Not recommended for use in Cl$_{cr}$ <30 mL/minute or ESRD. In mild-moderate impairment, lower initial doses may be considered with titration guided by response and tolerability.

Hepatic Impairment: Not recommended for use in hepatic impairment.

Administration

Oral: Capsule should be swallowed whole; do not break open or crush.

Stability

Storage: Store at 25°C (77°F), excursions permitted to 15°C to 30°C (59°F to 86°F)

Nursing Actions

Physical Assessment: Assess other medications patient may be taking for effectiveness and potential interactions. Monitor blood pressure (can cause elevation) at the beginning of treatment and periodically throughout treatment. Monitor for worsening of depression and suicide ideation. Taper dosage slowly when discontinuing. Do not discontinue abruptly.

Assess knowledge/teach appropriate use of this medication, interventions to reduce side effects and adverse reactions.

Patient Education: Take exactly as directed. Swallow capsule whole; do not open or crush. It may take 2-3 weeks to achieve desired results. Inform prescriber of all prescription medications, OTC medications, or herbal products you are taking. Maintain adequate hydration (2-3 L/day of fluid) unless instructed to restrict fluid intake by prescriber. Avoid alcohol use. Can cause drowsiness, dizziness, fatigue, insomnia (use caution when driving or engaging in activities requiring alertness until response to drug is known). You may experience headache, nausea, diarrhea (buttermilk, yogurt, or boiled milk may help), constipation (increased exercise, fluids, fruit, or fiber may help), appetite decrease, or xerostomia. Report persistent insomnia, dizziness, headache, thoughts of suicide, worsening of anxiety, panic attacks, agitation, irritability, akathisia, hostility, hypomania, mania. **Pregnancy/breast-feeding precautions:** Inform prescriber if you are or intend to become pregnant. Consult prescriber before breast-feeding.

Dietary Considerations May be taken without regard to meals.

Geriatric Considerations Has not been studied exclusively in the elderly, however, its low anticholinergic activity, minimal sedation, and hypotension makes this a potentially valuable antidepressant in treating elderly with depression. No dose adjustment is necessary for age alone, additional studies are necessary; adjust dose for renal function in the elderly. Higher doses required for the treatment of the urinary stress incontinence and neuropathic pain.

Breast-Feeding Issues SSRIs have been associated with excessive somnolence, decreased feeding, and weight loss in nursing infants (relevance to SNRIs is not clearly established).

Pregnancy Issues Nonteratogenic effects including respiratory distress, cyanosis, apnea, seizures, temperature instability, feeding difficulty, vomiting, hypoglycemia, hypo- or hypertonia, hyper-reflexia, jitteriness, irritability, constant crying, and tremor have been reported in the neonate immediately following delivery after exposure late in the third trimester. Adverse effects may be due to toxic effects of SNRI or drug discontinuation. There are no adequate and well-controlled studies in pregnant women. Use during pregnancy only if the potential benefit to the mother outweighs the possible risk to the fetus. If treatment during pregnancy is required, consider tapering therapy during the third trimester.

Dyclonine (DYE kloe neen)

U.S. Brand Names Cēpacol® Dual Action Maximum Strength [OTC]; Sucrets® [OTC]

Synonyms Dyclonine Hydrochloride

Pharmacologic Category Local Anesthetic, Oral

Medication Safety Issues

Sound-alike/look-alike issues:

Dyclonine may be confused with dicyclomine

Use Temporary relief of pain associated with oral mucosa

Contraindications Hypersensitivity to dyclonine or any component of the formulation

Warnings/Precautions Topical anesthetics should be used with caution in patients with sepsis or traumatized mucosa in the area of application to avoid rapid systemic absorption. Topical anesthetics may impair swallowing, eating, and may enhance the danger of

aspiration. Topical anesthetics should be used with caution in debilitated, elderly, acute ill or pediatric patients.

When used for self-medication (OTC) patients should contact healthcare provider if symptoms worsen or last for >7 days. When treating a severe sore throat, patients should contact healthcare provider if symptoms lasts >2 days, occur with fever, headache, rash, nausea, or vomiting. Not for OTC use in children <2 years of age.

Adverse Reactions The following were reported with the previously available 0.5% and 1% topical solutions; effects are similar to other local anesthetic agents and are generally dose related; frequency not defined:

Cardiovascular: Bradycardia, hypotension

Central nervous system: Apprehension, confusion, convulsion, dizziness, drowsiness, euphoria, light-headedness, nervousness

Gastrointestinal: Vomiting

Neuromuscular & skeletal: Numbness, tremor, twitching

Ocular: Blurred vision, double vision

Otic: Tinnitus

Respiratory: Respiratory depression

Miscellaneous: Allergic reactions, cold/heat sensation

Pharmacodynamics/Kinetics

Onset of Action: Local anesthetic: 2-10 minutes

Duration of Action: ~30 minutes

Available Dosage Forms

Lozenge, as hydrochloride (Sucrets®): 1.2 mg [children's cherry flavor]; 2 mg [wild cherry and assorted flavors]; 3 mg [vapor black cherry and wintergreen flavors]

Spray, oral, as hydrochloride (Cēpacol® Dual Action Maximum Strength): 0.1% (120 mL) [contains glycerin 33%; cherry, honey lemon and cool menthol flavors]

Dosing

Adults & Elderly: Temporary relief of pain: Oral topical:

Lozenge: One lozenge every 2 hours as needed (maximum: 10 lozenges/day)

Spray: 1-4 sprays, up to 4 times a day

Pediatrics: Temporary relief of pain: Oral topical:

Lozenge: Children ≥2 years: Refer to adult dosing.

Spray:

Children ≥3-12 years: 1-3 sprays, up to 4 times a day

Children ≥12 years: Refer to adult dosing.

Administration

Oral: Allow lozenge to slowly dissolve in mouth.

Nursing Actions

Physical Assessment: Observe condition of mucous membranes in area to be treated; avoid use in traumatized areas. Monitor for effectiveness of anesthesia and for adverse or toxic reactions (seizures, hypotension, cardiac depression). Monitor for return of sensation (swallowing). Teach patient adverse reactions to report; use and teach appropriate interventions to promote safety.

Patient Education: This medication is given to reduce sensation in the injected area. When used in mouth or throat; do not eat or drink anything for at least 1 hour following treatment. Take small sips of water at first to ensure that you can swallow without difficulty. Your tongue and mouth may be numb, use caution to avoid biting yourself. Immediately report swelling of face, lips, tongue; chest pain or palpitations; increased restlessness, confusion, anxiety, or dizziness. **Pregnancy/breast-feeding precautions:** Inform prescriber if you are or intend to become pregnant. Consult prescriber if breast-feeding.

Dietary Considerations Topical anesthetics may impair swallowing or eating.

Edrophonium (ed roe FOE nee um)

U.S. Brand Names Enlon®; Reversol®

Synonyms Edrophonium Chloride

Pharmacologic Category Antidote; Cholinergic Agonist; Diagnostic Agent

Pregnancy Risk Factor C

Lactation Excretion in breast milk unknown

Use Diagnosis of myasthenia gravis; differentiation of cholinergic crises from myasthenia crises; reversal of nondepolarizing neuromuscular blockers; adjunct treatment of respiratory depression caused by curare overdose

Mechanism of Action/Effect Inhibits destruction of acetylcholine by acetylcholinesterase. This facilitates transmission of impulses across myoneural junction and results in increased cholinergic responses such as miosis, increased tonus of intestinal and skeletal muscles, bronchial and ureteral constriction, bradycardia, and increased salivary and sweat gland secretions.

Contraindications Hypersensitivity to edrophonium, sulfites, or any component of the formulation; GI or GU obstruction

Warnings/Precautions Use with caution in patients with bronchial asthma and those receiving a cardiac glycoside. Atropine sulfate should always be readily available as an antagonist. Overdosage can cause cholinergic crisis which may be fatal (DUMBELS - diarrhea, urination, miosis, bronchospasm/bradycardia, excitability, lacrimation, salivation/excessive sweating), and acute muscle weakness. I.V. atropine should be readily available for treatment of cholinergic reactions.

Drug Interactions

Decreased Effect: Atropine, nondepolarizing muscle relaxants, procainamide, and quinidine may antagonize the effects of edrophonium.

Increased Effect/Toxicity: Digoxin may enhance bradycardia potential of edrophonium. Effects of succinylcholine, decamethonium, nondepolarizing muscle relaxants (eg, pancuronium, vecuronium) are prolonged by edrophonium. I.V. acetazolamide, neostigmine, physostigmine, and acute muscle weakness may increase the effects of edrophonium.

Lab Interactions Increased aminotransferase [ALT (SGPT)/AST (SGOT)] (S), amylase (S)

Adverse Reactions Frequency not defined.

Cardiovascular: Arrhythmias (especially bradycardia), hypotension, decreased carbon monoxide, tachycardia, AV block, nodal rhythm, nonspecific ECG changes, cardiac arrest, syncope, flushing

Central nervous system: Convulsions, dysarthria, dysphonia, dizziness, loss of consciousness, drowsiness, headache

Dermatologic: Skin rash, thrombophlebitis (I.V.), urticaria

Gastrointestinal: Hyperperistalsis, nausea, vomiting, salivation, diarrhea, stomach cramps, dysphagia, flatulence

Genitourinary: Urinary urgency

Neuromuscular & skeletal: Weakness, fasciculations, muscle cramps, spasms, arthralgia

Ocular: Small pupils, lacrimation

Respiratory: Increased bronchial secretions, laryngospasm, bronchiolar constriction, respiratory muscle paralysis, dyspnea, respiratory depression, respiratory arrest, bronchospasm

Miscellaneous: Diaphoresis (increased), anaphylaxis, allergic reactions

Overdosage/Toxicology Symptoms of overdose include muscle weakness, nausea, vomiting, miosis, bronchospasm, and respiratory paralysis. Maintain an adequate airway. For muscarinic symptoms, the antidote is atropine 0.4-0.5 mg I.V. repeated every 3-10 minutes (initial doses as high as 1.2 mg have been administered). Skeletal muscle effects of edrophonium are not alleviated by atropine.

Pharmacodynamics/Kinetics

Onset of Action: I.M.: 2-10 minutes; I.V.: 30-60 seconds

Duration of Action: I.M.: 5-30 minutes; I.V.: 10 minutes

Half-Life Elimination: Adults:1.2-2.4 hours; Anephric patients: 2.4-4.4 hours

Excretion: Adults: Primarily urine (67%)

Available Dosage Forms Injection, solution, as chloride:

Enlon®: 10 mg/mL (15 mL) [contains sodium sulfite]

Reversol®: 10 mg/mL (10 mL) [contains sodium sulfite]

Dosing

Adults & Elderly: Usually administered I.V., however, if not possible, I.M. or SubQ may be used.

Diagnosis of Myasthenia gravis:

I.V.: 2 mg test dose administered over 15-30 seconds; 8 mg given 45 seconds later if no response is seen. Test dose may be repeated after 30 minutes.

I.M.: Initial: 10 mg; if no cholinergic reaction occurs, give 2 mg 30 minutes later to rule out false-negative reaction.

Titration of oral anticholinesterase therapy: 1-2 mg given 1 hour after oral dose of anticholinesterase; if strength improves, an increase in neostigmine or pyridostigmine dose is indicated.

Differentiation of cholinergic from myasthenic crisis: I.V.: 1 mg; may repeat after 1 minute. **Note:** Intubation and controlled ventilation may be required if patient has cholinergic crisis.

Reversal of nondepolarizing neuromuscular blocking agents (neostigmine with atropine usually preferred): I.V.: 10 mg over 30-45 seconds; may repeat every 5-10 minutes up to 40 mg.

Termination of paroxysmal atrial tachycardia: I.V. rapid injection: 5-10 mg

Pediatrics: Usually administered I.V., however, if not possible, I.M. or SubQ may be used:

Infants:

I.M.: 0.5-1 mg

I.V.: Initial: 0.1 mg, followed by 0.4 mg if no response; total dose = 0.5 mg

Children:

Diagnosis: Initial: 0.04 mg/kg over 1 minute followed by 0.16 mg/kg if no response, to a maximum total dose of 5 mg for children <34 kg, or 10 mg for children >34 kg **or**

Alternative dosing (manufacturer's recommendation):

≤34 kg: 1 mg; if no response after 45 seconds, repeat dosage in 1 mg increments every 30-45 seconds, up to a total of 5 mg

>34 kg: 2 mg; if no response after 45 seconds, repeat dosage in 1 mg increments every 30-45 seconds, up to a total of 10 mg

I.M.:

<34 kg: 1 mg

>34 kg: 5 mg

Titration of oral anticholinesterase therapy: 0.04 mg/kg once given 1 hour after oral intake of the drug being used in treatment. If strength improves, an increase in neostigmine or pyridostigmine dose is indicated.

Renal Impairment: Dose may need to be reduced in patients with chronic renal failure.

Administration

I.V. Detail: pH: 5.4

Nursing Actions

Physical Assessment: Administration of edrophonium for MG diagnosis is supervised by a neurologist and use as a neuromuscular blocking agent is supervised by an anesthesiologist. Nursing responsibilities include careful monitoring of the patient during and following procedure, including careful monitoring for cholinergic crisis; keep atropine at hand for antidote. Ascertain that patients receiving the medication for MG testing will have been advised by their neurologist about drug effects. Those patients receiving medication for neuromuscular block will be unaware of drug effects. Patient should never be left alone until all drug effects and the possibility of cholinergic crisis have passed.

Patient Education: Pregnancy/breast-feeding precautions: Inform prescriber if you are or intend to become pregnant. Consult prescriber if breast-feeding.

Geriatric Considerations Many elderly will have diseases which may influence the use of edrophonium. Also, many elderly will need doses reduced 50% due to creatinine clearances in the 10-50 mL/minute range (common in the aged). Side effects or concomitant disease may warrant use of pyridostigmine.

Additional Information Atropine should be administered along with edrophonium when reversing the effects of nondepolarizing agents to antagonize the cholinergic effects at the muscarinic receptors, especially bradycardia. It is important to recognize the difference in dose for diagnosis of myasthenia gravis versus reversal of muscle relaxant, a much larger dose is needed for desired effect of reversal of muscle paralysis.

Edrophonium and Atropine
(ed roe FOE nee um & A troe peen)

U.S. Brand Names Enlon-Plus™

Synonyms Atropine Sulfate and Edrophonium Chloride; Edrophonium Chloride and Atropine Sulfate

Pharmacologic Category Anticholinergic Agent; Antidote; Cholinergic Agonist

Pregnancy Risk Factor C

Use Reversal of nondepolarizing neuromuscular blockers; adjunct treatment of respiratory depression caused by curare overdose

Available Dosage Forms Injection, solution, as chloride: Edrophonium 10 mg/mL and atropine 0.14 mg/mL (5 mL, 15 mL) [contains sodium sulfite]

Dosing
Adults & Elderly: Reversal of neuromuscular blockade: I.V.: 0.05 mL/kg given over 45-60 seconds. The dose delivered is 0.5-1 mg/kg of edrophonium and 0.007-0.015 mg/kg of atropine. An edrophonium dose of 1 mg/kg should rarely be exceeded. **Note:** Monitor closely for bradyarrhythmias. Have atropine on hand in case needed.

Renal Impairment: Adjustment not required.

Hepatic Impairment: Adjustment not required.

Nursing Actions
Physical Assessment: Only clinicians experienced in the use of neuromuscular-blocking drugs should administer and/or manage the use of this drug. Ventilatory support must be instituted and maintained until adequate respiratory muscle function and/or airway protection are assured. Assess other medications for effectiveness and safety; other drugs that affect neuromuscular activity may increase/decrease neuromuscular-blocking activity. Continuous monitoring of vital signs, cardiac and respiratory status, and degree of neuromuscular block is mandatory during infusion and until full muscles tone returns (typically starting with limbs, abdomen, chest diaphragm, intercostals, and finally muscles of the neck, face, and eyes). Safety precautions must be maintained until full muscle tone has returned.

Patient Education: Patient will usually be unconscious prior to administration. Education should be appropriate to individual situation. Reassurance of constant monitoring and emotional support to reduce fear and anxiety should precede and follow administration. Following return of muscle tone, do not attempt to change position or rise from bed without assistance. **Pregnancy/breast-feeding precautions:** Inform prescriber if you are or intend to become pregnant. Consult prescriber if breast-feeding.

Related Information
Atropine *on page 126*
Edrophonium *on page 412*

Efalizumab (e fa li ZOO mab)

U.S. Brand Names Raptiva®
Synonyms Anti-CD11a; hu1124
Pharmacologic Category Immunosuppressant Agent; Monoclonal Antibody
Pregnancy Risk Factor C
Lactation Excretion in breast milk unknown/not recommended
Use Treatment of chronic moderate-to-severe plaque psoriasis in patients who are candidates for systemic therapy or phototherapy
Mechanism of Action/Effect Efalizumab is a recombinant monoclonal antibody; efalizumab blocks multiple T-cell mediated responses involved in the pathogenesis of psoriatic plaques.
Contraindications Hypersensitivity to efalizumab or any component of the formulation
Warnings/Precautions May result in increased susceptibility to infections or reactivation of latent infection; use caution with chronic infections, history of recurrent infection, or the elderly. Avoid administration to patients with clinically important infection. Discontinue therapy if serious infection develops. Thrombocytopenia has been reported (rare) and may require treatment; discontinue if thrombocytopenia develops. Hemolytic anemia, which may occur after 4-6 months of treatment, has been reported; discontinue if signs and symptoms of hemolytic anemia occur. Use caution in patients at high risk for malignancy or history of malignancy; effects of efalizumab on the development of malignancies is unknown. Psoriasis and/or arthritis may worsen with efalizumab treatment or following discontinuation (rare). First-dose reactions have been reported; a lower, conditioning dose is recommended to reduce the incidence and severity of reactions. Concomitant use with other immunosuppressant agents is not recommended. Produced in a Chinese hamster cell medium. Safety and efficacy in pediatric patients or patients with renal or hepatic impairment have not been established.

Drug Interactions
Decreased Effect: Note: Formal drug interaction studies have not been conducted. Acellular, live, and live-attenuated vaccines should not be administered during therapy.

Increased Effect/Toxicity: Concurrent use of immunosuppressants may increase risk of infection.

Lab Interactions Increased lymphocytes (related to mechanism of action)

Adverse Reactions
>10%:
Central nervous system: Headache (32%), chills (13%)
Gastrointestinal: Nausea (11%)
Hematologic: Lymphocytosis (40%), leukocytosis (26%)
Miscellaneous: First-dose reaction (29%, described as chills, fever, headache, myalgia, and nausea occurring within 2 days of the first injection; percent reported in patients receiving a 1 mg/kg dose; severity decreased with 0.7 mg/kg dose); infection (29%, serious infection <1%)
(Continued)

Efalizumab (Continued)

1% to 10%:
Cardiovascular: Peripheral edema (1% to 2%)
Central nervous system: Pain (10%), fever (7%)
Dermatologic: Acne (4%), psoriasis (1% to 2%), urticaria (1%)
Hepatic: Alkaline phosphatase elevated (4%)
Neuromuscular & skeletal: Myalgia (8%), back pain (4%), arthralgia (1% to 2%), weakness (1% to 2%)
Miscellaneous: Antibodies to efalizumab (6%); hypersensitivity reaction, including asthma, dyspnea, angioedema, urticaria, or maculopapular rash (8%); flu-like syndrome (7%)

Overdosage/Toxicology Limited data. Severe vomiting reported in one patient receiving 10 mg/kg intravenously. In case of overdose, monitor for 24-48 hours.

Pharmacodynamics/Kinetics
Onset of Action: Reduction of CD11a expression and free CD11a-binding sites seen 1-2 days after the first dose; time to steady state serum concentration: 4 weeks

Response to therapy (75% reduction from baseline of PASI score): Observed after 12 weeks

Duration of Action: CD11a expression was ~74% of baseline at 5-13 weeks after discontinuing dose; free CD11a binding sites were at ~86% of baseline at 8-13 weeks following discontinuation; response to therapy (75% reduction from baseline PASI score) continued 1-2 months after discontinuation

Excretion: Time to eliminate (at steady state): 25 days (range: 13-35 days)

Available Dosage Forms Injection, powder for reconstitution: 150 mg [contains sucrose 123.2 mg/vial; delivers 125 mg/1.25 mL; packaged with prefilled syringe containing sterile water for injection]

Dosing
Adults: Psoriasis: SubQ: Initial: 0.7 mg/kg, followed by weekly dose of 1 mg/kg (maximum: 200 mg/dose)

Administration
Other: For SubQ injection in the abdomen, buttocks, thigh, or upper arm

Stability
Reconstitution: Slowly inject 1.3 mL of the provided diluent into vial; gently swirl to mix, do not shake.
Storage: Powder should be stored under refrigeration at 2°C to 8°C (36°F to 46°F) and protected from light. Following reconstitution, solution should be stored at room temperature and used within 8 hours. Discard unused solution.

Laboratory Monitoring Platelet counts (at least monthly at the start of treatment, every 3 months as therapy continues)

Nursing Actions
Physical Assessment: Monitor laboratory tests. Be alert to the possibility of the development of infection or malignancy. Assess therapeutic effectiveness and adverse reactions on a regular basis throughout therapy. Do not administer any immunizations with acellular, live, or live-attenuated vaccines during therapy with efalizumab. Teach patient possible side effects/appropriate interventions and adverse symptoms to report.

Patient Education: This medication can only be given by injection. Do not take any new medications during therapy without consulting prescriber. You may be more susceptible to infection while on this therapy; avoid crowds and exposure to infections, and do not have any immunizations while on this therapy. Notify prescriber of any allergic response (headache, chills, muscle pain, rash, difficulty breathing, or swelling around mouth within 3 days of first dose). May cause mild edema in extremities; back or muscle pain or flu-like syndrome (consult prescriber for appropriate analgesic). Report unusual infection or bleeding; weight gain >5 pounds in 1 week; persistent muscle or joint pain or weakness; other persistent reactions or worsening of psoriasis. **Pregnancy/breast-feeding precautions:** Inform prescriber if you are or intend to be pregnant. Do not breast-feed.

Breast-Feeding Issues A decrease in the ability to mount an antibody response was observed in the offspring of lactating mice. It is not known if efalizumab is excreted in human milk. However, since maternal immunoglobulins are present, and animal data suggest possible adverse effects in the nursing infant, it is recommended to discontinue nursing or discontinue efalizumab.

Pregnancy Issues
There are no adequate and well-controlled studies in pregnant women. Healthcare providers are encouraged to enroll patients who may become pregnant during therapy or within 6 weeks of discontinuing treatment in the Raptiva® registry (877-727-8482).

Efavirenz (e FAV e renz)

U.S. Brand Names Sustiva®
Pharmacologic Category Antiretroviral Agent, Reverse Transcriptase Inhibitor (Non-nucleoside)
Pregnancy Risk Factor D
Lactation Excretion is breast milk unknown/contraindicated
Use Treatment of HIV-1 infections in combination with at least two other antiretroviral agents
Mechanism of Action/Effect As a non-nucleoside reverse transcriptase inhibitor, efavirenz has activity against HIV-1 by binding to reverse transcriptase. It consequently blocks the RNA-dependent and DNA-dependent DNA polymerase activities including HIV-1 replication. It does not require intracellular phosphorylation for antiviral activity.
Contraindications Clinically-significant hypersensitivity to efavirenz or any component of the formulation; concurrent use of cisapride, midazolam, triazolam, voriconazole, or ergot alkaloids (includes dihydroergotamine, ergotamine, ergonovine, methylergonovine); pregnancy
Warnings/Precautions Do not use as single-agent therapy; avoid pregnancy; women of childbearing potential should undergo pregnancy testing prior to initiation of therapy; use caution with other agents metabolized by cytochrome P450 isoenzyme 3A4 (see Contraindications); use caution with history of mental illness/drug abuse (predisposition to psychological reactions); may cause CNS and psychiatric symptoms, which include impaired concentration, dizziness or drowsiness (avoid potentially hazardous tasks such as driving or operating machinery if these effects are noted); serious psychiatric side effects have been associated with efavirenz, including severe depression, suicide, paranoia, and mania; discontinue if severe rash (involving blistering, desquamation, mucosal involvement or fever) develops. Children are more susceptible to development of rash; prophylactic antihistamines may be used. Caution in patients with known or suspected hepatitis B or C infection (monitoring of liver function is recommended); hepatic impairment. Persistent elevations of serum transaminases >5 times the upper limit of normal should prompt evaluation - benefit of continued therapy should be weighed against possible risk of hepatotoxicity. Concomitant use with St John's wort is not recommended.
Drug Interactions
Cytochrome P450 Effect: Substrate (major) of CYP2B6, 3A4; **Inhibits** CYP2C8/9 (moderate), 2C19 (moderate), 3A4 (moderate); **Induces** CYP2B6 (weak), 3A4 (strong)
Decreased Effect: CYP2B6 inducers may decrease the levels/effects of efavirenz; example inducers

include carbamazepine, nevirapine, phenobarbital, phenytoin, and rifampin. St John's wort may decrease serum concentrations of efavirenz. Concentrations of atazanavir, indinavir, and/or lopinavir may be reduced; dosage adjustments required. Concentrations of saquinavir may be decreased (use as sole protease inhibitor is not recommended). Serum concentrations of methadone may be decreased; monitor for withdrawal. May decrease (or increase) effect of warfarin. Serum concentrations of sertraline may be decreased by efavirenz. CYP3A4 inducers may decrease the levels/effects of efavirenz; example inducers include aminoglutethimide, carbamazepine, nafcillin, nevirapine, phenobarbital, phenytoin, and rifamycins. Voriconazole serum levels may be reduced by efavirenz (concurrent use is contraindicated).

Efavirenz may increase the levels/effects of CYP2C8/9 substrates; example substrates include fluoxetine, glimepiride, glipizide, nateglinide, phenytoin, pioglitazone, rosiglitazone, sertraline, and warfarin. Efavirenz may increase the levels/effects of CYP2C19 substrates; example substrates include citalopram, diazepam, methsuximide, phenytoin, propranolol, and sertraline. Efavirenz may alter the levels/effects of CYP3A4 substrates; example substrates include benzodiazepines, calcium channel blockers, ergot derivatives, mirtazapine, nateglinide, nefazodone, tacrolimus, and venlafaxine.

Increased Effect/Toxicity: Coadministration with medications metabolized by these enzymes may lead to increased concentration-related effects. Cisapride, midazolam, triazolam, and ergot alkaloids may result in life-threatening toxicities; concurrent use is contraindicated. May increase (or decrease) effect of warfarin.

Nutritional/Ethanol Interactions
Ethanol: Avoid ethanol (hepatic and CNS adverse effects).

Food: Avoid high-fat meals (increase the absorption of efavirenz).

Herb/Nutraceutical: St John's wort may decrease efavirenz serum levels. Avoid concurrent use.

Lab Interactions False-positive test for cannabinoids have been reported when the CEDIA DAU Multilevel THC assay is used. False-positive results with other assays for cannabinoids have not been observed.

Adverse Reactions
>10%:
Central nervous system: Dizziness* (2% to 28%), depression (1% to 16%), insomnia (6% to 16%), anxiety (1% to 11%), pain* (1% to 13%)

Dermatologic: Rash* (NCI grade 1: 9% to 11%, NCI grade 2: 15% to 32%, NCI grade 3 or 4: <1%); 26% experienced new rash vs 17% in control groups; up to 46% of pediatric patients experience rash (median onset: 8 days)

Endocrine & metabolic: HDL increased (25% to 35%), total cholesterol increased (20% to 40%)

Gastrointestinal: Diarrhea* (3% to 14%), nausea* (2% to 12%)

1% to 10%:
Central nervous system: Impaired concentration (2% to 8%), headache* (2% to 7%), somnolence (2% to 7%), fatigue (2% to 7%), abnormal dreams (1% to 6%), nervousness (2% to 6%), severe depression (2%), hallucinations (1%)

Dermatologic: Pruritus (1% to 9%)

Gastrointestinal: Vomiting* (6% to 7%), dyspepsia (3%), abdominal pain (1% to 3%), anorexia (1% to 2%)

Miscellaneous: Diaphoresis increased (1% to 2%)

*Adverse effect reported in ≥10% of patients 3-16 years of age

Overdosage/Toxicology Increased central nervous system symptoms and involuntary muscle contractions

have been reported in accidental overdose. Treatment is supportive. Activated charcoal may enhance elimination; dialysis is unlikely to remove the drug.

Pharmacodynamics/Kinetics
Time to Peak: 3-8 hours

Protein Binding: >99%, primarily to albumin

Half-Life Elimination: Single dose: 52-76 hours; Multiple doses: 40-55 hours

Metabolism: Hepatic via CYP3A4 and 2B6; may induce its own metabolism

Excretion: Feces (16% to 41% primarily as unchanged drug); urine (14% to 34% as metabolites)

Available Dosage Forms
Capsule: 50 mg, 100 mg, 200 mg

Tablet: 600 mg

Dosing
Adults & Elderly: Dosing at bedtime is recommended to limit central nervous system effects; should not be used as single-agent therapy.

HIV infection (as part of combination): Oral: 600 mg once daily

Pediatrics: Dosing at bedtime is recommended to limit central nervous system effects; should not be used as single-agent therapy. Dosage is based on body weight.

HIV infection (as part of combination): Oral: Children ≥3 years:
10 kg to <15 kg: 200 mg once daily
15 kg to <20 kg: 250 mg once daily
20 kg to <25 kg: 300 mg once daily
25 kg to <32.5 kg: 350 mg once daily
32.5 kg to <40 kg: 400 mg once daily
≥40 kg: 600 mg once daily

Renal Impairment: No adjustment is necessary.

Hepatic Impairment: Limited clinical experience - use with caution.

Administration
Oral: Administer on an empty stomach. Capsules may be opened and added to liquids or small amounts of food.

Stability
Storage: Store below 25°C (77°F).

Laboratory Monitoring Monitor serum transaminases (discontinuation of treatment should be considered for persistent elevations greater than five times the upper limit of normal), cholesterol, and triglycerides.

Nursing Actions
Physical Assessment: Assess other pharmacological or herbal products patient may be taking for potential interactions or toxicity. Monitor laboratory tests, effectiveness of therapy (decrease in infections and progress of disease), and adverse reactions periodically during therapy. Teach patient proper use (eg, timing of multiple medications and drugs that should not be used concurrently), possible side effects/appropriate interventions, and adverse symptoms to report (eg, CNS changes, rash, gastrointestinal upset).

Patient Education: You will be provided with a list of specific medications that should not be used during therapy; do not take any new prescriptions, over-the-counter medications, or herbal products (even if they are not on the list) without consulting prescriber. This drug will not cure HIV, nor has it been found to reduce transmission of HIV; use appropriate precautions to prevent spread to other persons. This drug is prescribed as one part of a multidrug combination; take exactly as directed for full course of therapy. Take 30 minutes before or 2 hours after meals. Capsules may be opened and added to liquids or small amount of food. Maintain adequate hydration (2-3 L/day of fluids) unless advised by prescriber to restrict fluids. You may be susceptible to infection; avoid crowds and exposure to known infections and do not have any vaccinations without consulting

(Continued)

Efavirenz (Continued)

prescriber. Frequent blood tests may be required with prolonged therapy. May cause nausea or vomiting (small frequent meals, frequent mouth care, sucking lozenges, or chewing gum may help) or diarrhea (boiled milk, yogurt or buttermilk may help). Report immediately any CNS changes (depression, anxiety, insomnia, dizziness, hallucinations, impaired concentration, abnormal dreams), rash, or other persistent adverse effects. **Pregnancy/breast-feeding precautions:** Inform prescriber if you are pregnant. Do not get pregnant while taking this medication. Consult prescriber for appropriate contraceptives; some contraceptives are contraindicated with this medication. Do not breast-feed.

Dietary Considerations Should be taken on an empty stomach.

Breast-Feeding Issues HIV-infected mothers are discouraged from breast-feeding to decrease potential transmission of HIV.

Pregnancy Issues Teratogenic effects have been observed in Primates receiving efavirenz. Severe CNS defects have been reported in infants following efavirenz exposure in the first trimester. Pregnancy should be avoided and alternate therapy should be considered in women of childbearing potential. Women of childbearing potential should undergo pregnancy testing prior to initiation of efavirenz. Barrier contraception should be used in combination with other (hormonal) methods of contraception. If therapy with efavirenz is administered during pregnancy, avoid use during the first trimester. Health professionals are encouraged to contact the antiretroviral pregnancy registry to monitor outcomes of pregnant women exposed to antiretroviral medications (1-800-258-4263 or www.APRegistry.com).

Additional Information Efavirenz oral solution is available only through an expanded access (compassionate use) program. Enrollment information may be obtained by calling 1-877-372-7097.

Early virologic failure was observed with tenofovir and didanosine delayed release capsules, plus either efavirenz or nevirapine; use caution in treatment-naive patients with high baseline viral loads.

Eflornithine (ee FLOR ni theen)

U.S. Brand Names Vaniqa™
Synonyms DFMO; Eflornithine Hydrochloride
Pharmacologic Category Antiprotozoal; Topical Skin Product
Medication Safety Issues
Sound-alike/look-alike issues:
Vaniqa™ may be confused with Viagra®
Pregnancy Risk Factor C
Lactation Excretion in breast milk unknown/use caution
Use Cream: Females ≥12 years: Reduce unwanted hair from face and adjacent areas under the chin
  Orphan status: Injection: Treatment of meningoencephalitic stage of *Trypanosoma brucei gambiense* infection (sleeping sickness)
Mechanism of Action/Effect Eflornithine exerts antitumor and antiprotozoal effects through specific, irreversible ("suicide") inhibition of the enzyme ornithine decarboxylase (ODC). ODC is the rate-limiting enzyme in the biosynthesis of putrescine, spermine, and spermidine, the major polyamines in nucleated cells. Polyamines are necessary for the synthesis of DNA, RNA, and proteins and are, therefore, necessary for cell growth and differentiation. Although many microorganisms and higher plants are able to produce polyamines from alternate biochemical pathways, all mammalian cells depend on ornithine decarboxylase to produce polyamines. Eflornithine inhibits ODC and rapidly

depletes animal cells of putrescine and spermidine; the concentration of spermine remains the same or may even increase. Rapidly dividing cells appear to be most susceptible to the effects of eflornithine. Topically, the inhibition of ODC in the skin leads to a decreased rate of hair growth.

Contraindications Hypersensitivity to eflornithine or any component of the formulation

Warnings/Precautions
Injection: For I.V. use only; not for I.M. administration. Must be diluted before use. Frequent monitoring for myelosuppression should be done. Use with caution in patients with a history of seizures and in patients with renal impairment. Serial audiograms should be obtained. Due to the potential for relapse, patients should be followed up for at least 24 months.
Cream: For topical use by females only. Discontinue if hypersensitivity occurs. Safety and efficacy in children <12 years has not been studied.

Drug Interactions
  Decreased Effect: Cream: Possible interactions with other topical products have not been studied.
  Increased Effect/Toxicity: Cream: Possible interactions with other topical products have not been studied.

Adverse Reactions
Injection:
  >10%: Hematologic (reversible): Anemia (55%), leukopenia (37%), thrombocytopenia (14%)
  1% to 10%:
    Central nervous system: Seizures (may be due to the disease) (8%), dizziness
    Dermatologic: Alopecia
    Gastrointestinal: Vomiting, diarrhea
    Hematologic: Eosinophilia
    Otic: Hearing impairment
Topical:
  >10%: Dermatologic: Acne (11% to 21%), pseudofolliculitis barbae (5% to 15%)
  1% to 10%:
    Central nervous system: Headache (4% to 5%), dizziness (1%), vertigo (0.3% to 1%)
    Dermatologic: Pruritus (3% to 4%), burning skin (2% to 4%), tingling skin (1% to 4%), dry skin (2% to 3%), rash (1% to 3%), facial edema (0.3% to 3%), alopecia (1% to 2%), skin irritation (1% to 2%), erythema (0% to 2%), ingrown hair (0.3% to 2%), folliculitis (0% to 1%)
    Gastrointestinal: Dyspepsia (2%), anorexia (0.7% to 2%)

Overdosage/Toxicology No known antidote; treatment is supportive. In mice and rats, CNS depression, seizures, death have occurred. Overdose with topical product is not expected due to low percutaneous penetration.

Pharmacodynamics/Kinetics
  Half-Life Elimination: I.V.: 3-3.5 hours; Topical: 8 hours
  Excretion: Primarily urine (as unchanged drug)
Available Dosage Forms
Cream, topical, as hydrochloride: 13.9% (30 g)
Injection, solution, as hydrochloride: 200 mg/mL (100 mL) [orphan drug status]
Dosing
  Adults & Elderly:
    Unwanted facial hair (Females): Topical: Apply thin layer of cream to affected areas of face and adjacent chin twice daily, at least 8 hours apart.
    Treatment of infections caused by *Trypanosoma*: I.V. infusion (orphan drug): 100 mg/kg/dose given every 6 hours (over at least 45 minutes) for 14 days.
  Pediatrics: Unwanted facial hair (females): Children ≥12 years: Refer to adult dosing.
  Renal Impairment: Injection: Dose should be adjusted although no specific guidelines are available.

Administration

I.M.: Not for I.M. use.

I.V.: Can only be administered I.V.; infuse over 45 minutes.

Other: Apply thin layer of eflornithine cream to affected areas of face and adjacent chin area twice daily, at least 8 hours apart. Rub in thoroughly. Hair removal techniques must still be continued; wait at least 5 minutes after removing hair to apply cream. Do not wash affected area for at least 8 hours following application.

Stability
Storage:
Injection: Must be diluted before use and used within 24 hours of preparation.

Cream: Store at controlled room temperature 25°C (77°F); do not freeze.

Laboratory Monitoring CBC with platelet counts

Nursing Actions

Physical Assessment: Laboratory tests and results should be monitored on regular basis during therapy. Monitor effectiveness according to purpose for use. Patient should be monitored for adverse reactions, especially with infusion administration. Assess knowledge/teach patient appropriate use, adverse reactions and possible interventions, and adverse reactions to report.

Patient Education: I.V.: This medication can only be administered I.V.; you will be closely monitored during therapy. Report immediately any signs of acute GI upset, seizures, altered hearing. You may lose your hair, however, it will grow back when therapy is discontinued.

Cream: This medication is for external use only. It will not prevent hair growth, but may decrease rate of growth. You will still need to use hair removal techniques while using eflornithine cream. Use only as directed; do not use more often or discontinue without consulting prescriber. Wait at least 5 minutes after removing hair to apply cream. Wash hands thoroughly prior to using cream. Apply thin lay of cream to affected areas of face and chin twice daily (at least 8 hours apart). Rub in thoroughly. Wash hands thoroughly after rubbing cream in. Do not wash area for 8 hours following application. Once cream has dried you may apply make-up over the affected area. Improvement may be seen in 4-8 weeks. Following discontinuation of therapy you may see hair growth return in about 8 weeks. You may be required to have blood tests if used for extended period of time. Report any skin irritation, rash, tingling, or skin eruptions; persistent headache, dizziness; or GI disturbances.

Pregnancy/breast-feeding precautions: Inform prescriber if you are or intend to become pregnant. Consult prescriber if breast-feeding.

Eletriptan (el e TRIP tan)

U.S. Brand Names Relpax®

Synonyms Eletriptan Hydrobromide

Pharmacologic Category Serotonin 5-HT$_{1B, 1D}$ Receptor Agonist

Pregnancy Risk Factor C

Lactation Enters breast milk/use caution

Use Acute treatment of migraine, with or without aura

Mechanism of Action/Effect The therapeutic effect for migraine is due to serotonin agonist activity causing vasoconstriction in cranial arteries.

Contraindications Hypersensitivity to eletriptan or any component of the formulation; ischemic heart disease or signs or symptoms of ischemic heart disease (including Prinzmetal's angina, angina pectoris, MI, silent myocardial ischemia); cerebrovascular syndromes (including strokes, transient ischemic attacks); peripheral vascular syndromes (including ischemic bowel disease); uncontrolled hypertension; use within 24 hours of ergotamine derivatives; use within 24 hours of another 5-HT$_1$ agonist; use within 72 hours of potent CYP3A4 inhibitors; management of hemiplegic or basilar migraine; prophylactic treatment of migraine; severe hepatic impairment

Warnings/Precautions Eletriptan is indicated only in patients ≥18 years of age with a clear diagnosis of migraine headache. If a patient does not respond to the first dose, the diagnosis of migraine should be reconsidered. Do not give to patients with risk factors for CAD until a cardiovascular evaluation has been performed; if evaluation is satisfactory, the healthcare provider should administer the first dose and cardiovascular status should be periodically evaluated. Cardiac events (coronary artery vasospasm, transient ischemia, MI, ventricular tachycardia/fibrillation, cardiac arrest, and death), cerebral/subarachnoid hemorrhage, stroke, peripheral vascular ischemia, and colonic ischemia have been reported with 5-HT$_1$ agonist administration. Significant elevation in blood pressure, including hypertensive crisis, has also been reported on rare occasions in patients with and without a history of hypertension. Use with caution in renal or mild to moderate hepatic impairment. Safety and efficacy in pediatric patients have not been established.

Drug Interactions

Cytochrome P450 Effect: Substrate of CYP3A4 (major)

Increased Effect/Toxicity: CYP3A4 inhibitors increase serum concentration and half-life of eletriptan; do not use eletriptan within 72 hours of potent CYP3A4 inhibitors (eg, azole antifungals, clarithromycin, diclofenac, doxycycline, erythromycin, imatinib, isoniazid, nefazodone, nicardipine, propofol, protease inhibitors, quinidine, telithromycin, verapamil). Ergot-containing drugs prolong vasospastic reactions; do not use within 24 hours of eletriptan.

Nutritional/Ethanol Interactions Food: High-fat meal increases bioavailability.

Adverse Reactions 1% to 10%:

Cardiovascular: Chest pain/tightness (1% to 4%; placebo 1%), palpitation

Central nervous system: Dizziness (3% to 7%; placebo 3%), somnolence (3% to 7%; placebo 4%), headache (3% to 4%; placebo 3%), chills, pain, vertigo

Gastrointestinal: Nausea (4% to 8%; placebo 5%), xerostomia (2% to 4%, placebo 2%), dysphagia (1% to 2%), abdominal pain/discomfort (1% to 2%; placebo 1%), dyspepsia (1% to 2%; placebo 1%)

Neuromuscular & skeletal: Weakness (4% to 10%), paresthesia (3% to 4%), back pain, hypertonia, hypoesthesia

Respiratory: Pharyngitis

Miscellaneous: Diaphoresis

Overdosage/Toxicology Hypertension or more serious cardiovascular symptoms may occur. Clinical and electrocardiographic monitoring needed for at least 20 hours even if patient is asymptomatic. Treatment is symptom-directed and supportive.

Pharmacodynamics/Kinetics

Time to Peak: Plasma: 1.5-2 hours

Protein Binding: ~85%

Half-Life Elimination: 4 hours (Elderly: 4.4-5.7 hours); Metabolite: ~13 hours

Metabolism: Hepatic via CYP3A4; forms one metabolite (active)

Available Dosage Forms Tablet, as hydrobromide: 20 mg, 40 mg [as base]

Dosing

Adults: Acute migraine: Oral: 20-40 mg; if the headache improves but returns, dose may be repeated after 2 hours have elapsed since first dose; maximum 80 mg/day

(Continued)

Eletriptan *(Continued)*

Note: If the first dose is ineffective, diagnosis needs to be re-evaluated. Safety of treating >3 headaches/month has not been established.

Renal Impairment: No dosing adjustment needed; monitor for increased blood pressure.

Hepatic Impairment:

Mild to moderate impairment: No adjustment necessary.

Severe impairment: Use is contraindicated.

Stability

Storage: Store at 25°C (77°F). Excursions permitted to 15°C to 30°C (59°F to 86°F).

Nursing Actions

Physical Assessment: Assess for potential for interactions with other pharmacological agents or herbal products patient may be taking (eg, ergot-containing drugs, other 5-HT$_1$ agonists). Monitor therapeutic effectiveness (relief of migraine) and adverse response (hypertension, cardiac events). Teach patient proper use, possible side effects/appropriate interventions, and adverse symptoms to report.

Patient Education: This drug is to be used to reduce your migraine, not to prevent the number of attacks. Follow exact instructions for use. Do not crush, break, or chew tablet. Do not take within 24 hours of any other medication without first consulting prescriber. If headache improves but returns, dose may be repeated after 2 hours. Do not exceed two doses in 24 hours (may take either 20 mg or 40 mg twice daily). If you have no relief with the first dose, do not take a second dose without consulting prescriber. May cause dizziness or drowsiness (use caution when driving or engaging in tasks requiring alertness until response to drug is known); nausea, vomiting, or abdominal pain. Report immediately any chest pain, tightness, or palpitations; muscle weakness or tremors; back pain; respiratory difficulty; changes in CNS (abnormal thought processes, depression, insomnia, confusion, agitation); swelling of eyelids, face, lips, throat; rash, hives, or any other adverse reactions. **Pregnancy/breast-feeding precautions:** Inform prescriber if you are or intend to become pregnant. Consult prescriber if breast-feeding.

Emtricitabine *(em trye SYE ta been)*

U.S. Brand Names Emtriva®

Synonyms BW524W91; Coviracil; FTC

Pharmacologic Category Antiretroviral Agent, Reverse Transcriptase Inhibitor (Nucleoside)

Pregnancy Risk Factor B

Lactation Excretion in breast milk unknown/not recommended

Use Treatment of HIV infection in combination with at least two other antiretroviral agents

Unlabeled/Investigational Use Hepatitis B (with HIV coinfection)

Mechanism of Action/Effect Nucleoside reverse transcriptase inhibitor which interferes with viral RNA-dependent DNA synthesis, resulting in inhibition of viral replication.

Contraindications Hypersensitivity to emtricitabine or any component of the formulation

Warnings/Precautions Lactic acidosis, severe hepatomegaly, and hepatic failure have occurred rarely with emtricitabine (similar to other nucleoside analogues). Some cases have been fatal; stop treatment if lactic acidosis or hepatotoxicity occur. Prior liver disease, obesity, extended duration of therapy, and female gender may represent risk factors for severe hepatic reactions. Testing for hepatitis B is recommended prior to the initiation of therapy; hepatitis B may be exacerbated following discontinuation of emtricitabine. Immune reconstitution syndrome may develop resulting in the occurrence of an inflammatory response to an indolent or residual opportunistic infection; further evaluation and treatment may be required. Use caution in patients with renal impairment (dosage adjustment required). Safety and efficacy in children ≤3 years of age have not been established.

Drug Interactions

Increased Effect/Toxicity: Concomitant use of ribavirin and nucleoside analogues may increase the risk of developing lactic acidosis.

Nutritional/Ethanol Interactions Food: Food decreases peak plasma concentrations, but does not alter the extent of absorption or overall systemic exposure.

Adverse Reactions Clinical trials were conducted in patients receiving other antiretroviral agents, and it is not possible to correlate frequency of adverse events with emtricitabine alone. The range of frequencies of adverse events is generally comparable to comparator groups, with the exception of hyperpigmentation, which occurred more frequently in patients receiving emtricitabine. Unless otherwise noted, percentages are as reported in adults.

>10%:

Central nervous system: Dizziness (4% to 25%), headache (13% to 22%), fever (children 18%), insomnia (7% to 16%), abnormal dreams (2% to 11%)

Dermatologic: Hyperpigmentation (adults 2% to 4%; children 32%; primarily of palms and/or soles but may include tongue, arms, lip and nails; generally mild and nonprogressive without associated local reactions such as pruritus or rash); rash (17% to 30%; includes pruritus, maculopapular rash, vesiculobullous rash, pustular rash, and allergic reaction)

Gastrointestinal: Diarrhea (adults 23%; children 20%), vomiting (adults 9%; children 23%), nausea (13% to 18%), abdominal pain (8% to 14%), gastroenteritis (children 11%)

Neuromuscular & skeletal: Weakness (12% to 16%), CPK increased (11% to 12%)

Otic: Otitis media (children 23%)

Respiratory: Cough (adults 14%; children 28%), rhinitis (adults 12% to 18%; children 20%), pneumonia (children 15%)

Miscellaneous: Infection (children 44%)

1% to 10%:

Central nervous system: Depression (6% to 9%), neuropathy/neuritis (4%)

Endocrine & metabolic: Serum triglycerides increased (9% to 10%), disordered glucose homeostasis (2% to 3%), serum amylase increased (adults 2% to 5%; children 9%), serum lipase increased (≤1%)

Gastrointestinal: Dyspepsia (4% to 8%)

Hematologic: Anemia (children: 7%)

Hepatic: Transaminases increased (2% to 6%), bilirubin increased (1%)

Neuromuscular & skeletal: Myalgia (4% to 6%), paresthesia (5% to 6%), arthralgia (3% to 5%)

Overdosage/Toxicology Treatment is supportive and symptom-directed. Approximately 30% of a dose is removed by hemodialysis.

Pharmacodynamics/Kinetics

Protein Binding: <4%

Half-Life Elimination: Normal renal function: Adults: 10 hours; children: 5-18 hours

Metabolism: Limited, via oxidation and conjugation (not via CYP isoenzymes)

Excretion: Urine (86% primarily as unchanged drug, 13% as metabolites); feces (14%)

Available Dosage Forms

Capsule: 200 mg

Solution: 10 mg/mL (170 mL) [cotton candy flavor]
Dosing
Adults & Elderly: HIV infection: Oral:
Capsule: 200 mg once daily
Solution: 240 mg once daily
Pediatrics: HIV infection: Children 3 months to 17 years:
Capsule: Children >33 kg: 200 mg once daily
Solution: 6 mg/kg once daily; maximum: 240 mg/day
Renal Impairment: Adults (consider similar adjustments in children):
Cl_{cr} 30-49 mL/minute: Capsule: 200 mg every 48 hours; solution: 120 mg every 24 hours
Cl_{cr} 15-29 mL/minute: Capsule: 200 mg every 72 hours; solution: 80 mg every 24 hours
Cl_{cr} <15 mL/minute (including hemodialysis patients): Capsule: 200 mg every 96 hours; solution: 60 mg every 24 hours; administer after dialysis on dialysis days
Hepatic Impairment: No adjustment required.
Administration
Oral: May be administered with or without food.
Stability
Storage: Store capsules at 15°C to 30°C (59°F to 86°F). Solution should be stored under refrigeration at 2°C to 8°C (36°F to 46°F); once dispensed, may be stored at 15°C to 30°C (59°F to 86°F) if used within 3 months.
Laboratory Monitoring Viral load, CD4, liver function tests; hepatitis B testing is recommended prior to initiation of therapy
Nursing Actions
Physical Assessment: Assess other pharmacological or herbal products patient may be taking for potential interactions. Monitor effectiveness of therapy (decrease in infections and progress of disease) and adverse reactions periodically during therapy. Teach patient proper use (eg, timing of multiple medications), possible side effects/appropriate interventions, and adverse symptoms to report.

Patient Education: Do not take any new medications during treatment without consulting prescriber. This drug will not cure HIV, nor has it been found to reduce transmission of HIV; use appropriate precautions to prevent spread to other persons. This drug is prescribed as one part of a multidrug combination; take exactly as directed for full course of therapy. Maintain adequate hydration (2-3 L/day of fluids) unless advised by prescriber to restrict fluids. You may be susceptible to infection; avoid crowds and exposure to known infections and do not have any vaccinations without consulting prescriber. Frequent blood tests may be required with prolonged therapy. May cause hyperpigmentation of hands, soles or lips (normal). May cause headache, dizziness, or insomnia (use care when driving or engaging in potentially hazardous tasks until response to drug is known); nausea, vomiting, or abdominal pain (small frequent meals, chewing gum, good mouth care, sucking lozenges may help); or diarrhea (boiled milk, yogurt, or buttermilk may help). Report respiratory difficulty; rash; persistent or unresolved diarrhea; signs of infection (burning on urination, perineal itching, white plaques in mouth, unhealed sores, persistent sore throat or cough), or other persistent side effects. **Pregnancy/breast-feeding precautions:** Inform prescriber if you are or intend to become pregnant. Do not breast-feed.

Dietary Considerations May be taken with or without food.

Breast-Feeding Issues HIV-infected women are discouraged from breast-feeding to decrease the potential transmission of HIV.

Pregnancy Issues Cases of fatal and nonfatal lactic acidosis, with or without pancreatitis, have been reported in pregnant women receiving reverse transcriptase inhibitors. It is not known if pregnancy itself potentiates this known side effect; however, pregnant women may be at increased risk of lactic acidosis and liver damage. Hepatic enzymes and electrolytes should be monitored frequently during the 3rd trimester of pregnancy. There are no studies of emtricitabine during pregnancy. The Perinatal HIV Guidelines Working Group considers emtricitabine to be an alternative NRTI in dual nucleoside combination regimens. Health professionals are encouraged to contact the antiretroviral pregnancy registry to monitor outcomes of pregnant women exposed to antiretroviral medications (1-800-258-4263 or www.APRegistry.com).

Emtricitabine and Tenofovir
(em trye SYE ta been & te NOE fo veer)

U.S. Brand Names Truvada®
Synonyms Tenofovir and Emtricitabine
Pharmacologic Category Antiretroviral Agent, Reverse Transcriptase Inhibitor (Nucleoside); Antiretroviral Agent, Reverse Transcriptase Inhibitor (Nucleotide)
Pregnancy Risk Factor B
Lactation Excretion in breast milk unknown/not recommended
Use Treatment of HIV infection in combination with other antiretroviral agents
Available Dosage Forms Tablet: Emtricitabine 200 mg and tenofovir disoproxil fumarate 300 mg
Dosing
Adults: HIV: Oral: One tablet (emtricitabine 200 mg and tenofovir 300 mg) once daily
Elderly: See adult dosing.
Renal Impairment:
Cl_{cr} 30-49 mL/minute: Increase interval to every 48 hours.
Cl_{cr} <30 mL/minute or hemodialysis: Not recommended.
Nursing Actions
Physical Assessment: See individual agents.

Enalapril (e NAL a pril)

U.S. Brand Names Vasotec®
Synonyms Enalaprilat; Enalapril Maleate
Pharmacologic Category Angiotensin-Converting Enzyme (ACE) Inhibitor
Medication Safety Issues
Sound-alike/look-alike issues:
Enalapril may be confused with Anafranil®, Elavil®, Eldepryl®, nafarelin, ramipril
Pregnancy Risk Factor C (1st trimester)/D (2nd and 3rd trimesters)
Lactation Enters breast milk/not recommended (AAP rates "compatible")
Use Management of mild to severe hypertension; treatment of congestive heart failure, left ventricular dysfunction after myocardial infarction
Unlabeled/Investigational Use
Unlabeled: Hypertensive crisis, diabetic nephropathy, rheumatoid arthritis, diagnosis of anatomic renal artery stenosis, hypertension secondary to scleroderma renal crisis, diagnosis of aldosteronism, idiopathic edema, Bartter's syndrome, postmyocardial infarction for prevention of ventricular failure
Investigational: Severe congestive heart failure in infants, neonatal hypertension, acute pulmonary edema
(Continued)

Enalapril (Continued)

Mechanism of Action/Effect Competitive inhibitor of angiotensin-converting enzyme (ACE); prevents conversion of angiotensin I to angiotensin II, a potent vasoconstrictor; results in lower levels of angiotensin II which causes an increase in plasma renin activity and a reduction in aldosterone secretion

Contraindications Hypersensitivity to enalapril or enalaprilat; angioedema related to previous treatment with an ACE inhibitor; patients with idiopathic or hereditary angioedema; bilateral renal artery stenosis; pregnancy (2nd and 3rd trimesters)

Warnings/Precautions Anaphylactic reactions can occur. Angioedema can occur at any time during treatment (especially following first dose). It may involve head and neck (potentially affecting the airway) or the intestine (presenting with abdominal pain). Prolonged monitoring may be required especially if tongue, glottis, or larynx are involved as they are associated with airway obstruction. Those with a history of airway surgery in this situation have a higher risk. Careful blood pressure monitoring with first dose (hypotension can occur especially in volume-depleted patients). Dosage adjustment needed in renal impairment. Use with caution in hypovolemia; collagen vascular diseases; valvular stenosis (particularly aortic stenosis); hyperkalemia; or before, during, or immediately after anesthesia. Avoid rapid dosage escalation which may lead to renal insufficiency.

Rare toxicities associated with ACE inhibitors include cholestatic jaundice (which may progress to hepatic necrosis) and neutropenia/agranulocytosis with myeloid hyperplasia. Hypersensitivity reactions may be seen during hemodialysis with high-flux dialysis membranes (eg, AN69). Hyperkalemia may rarely occur. Use with caution in unilateral renal artery stenosis and pre-existing renal insufficiency.

Drug Interactions

Cytochrome P450 Effect: Substrate of CYP3A4 (major)

Decreased Effect: Aspirin (high dose) may reduce the therapeutic effects of ACE inhibitors; at low dosages this does not appear to be significant. Antacids may decrease the bioavailability of ACE inhibitors (may be more likely to occur with captopril); separate administration times by 1-2 hours. NSAIDs may reduce the hypotensive effects of ACE inhibitors. More likely to occur in low renin or volume-dependent hypertensive patients. CYP3A4 inducers may decrease the levels/effects of enalapril; example inducers include aminoglutethimide, carbamazepine, nafcillin, nevirapine, phenobarbital, phenytoin, and rifamycins.

Increased Effect/Toxicity: Potassium supplements, co-trimoxazole (high dose), angiotensin II receptor antagonists (eg, candesartan, losartan, irbesartan), or potassium-sparing diuretics (amiloride, spironolactone, triamterene) may result in elevated serum potassium levels when combined with enalapril. ACE inhibitor effects may be increased by phenothiazines or probenecid (increases levels of captopril). ACE inhibitors may increase serum concentrations/effects of lithium.

Diuretics have additive hypotensive effects with ACE inhibitors, and hypovolemia increases the potential for adverse renal effects of ACE inhibitors. In patients with compromised renal function, coadministration with NSAIDs may result in further deterioration of renal function. Allopurinol and ACE inhibitors may cause a higher risk of hypersensitivity reaction when taken concurrently.

Nutritional/Ethanol Interactions Herb/Nutraceutical: St John's wort may decrease enalapril levels. Avoid dong quai if using for hypertension (has estrogenic activity). Avoid ephedra, yohimbe, ginseng (may worsen hypertension). Avoid natural licorice (causes sodium and water retention and increases potassium loss).

Avoid garlic (may have increased antihypertensive effect).

Lab Interactions Positive Coombs' [direct]; may cause false-positive results in urine acetone determinations using sodium nitroprusside reagent

Adverse Reactions Note: Frequency ranges include data from hypertension and heart failure trials. Higher rates of adverse reactions have generally been noted in patients with CHF. However, the frequency of adverse effects associated with placebo is also increased in this population.

1% to 10%:
Cardiovascular: Hypotension (0.9% to 7%), chest pain (2%), syncope (0.5% to 2%), orthostasis (2%), orthostatic hypotension (2%)
Central nervous system: Headache (2% to 5%), dizziness (4% to 8%), fatigue (2% to 3%)
Dermatologic: Rash (2%)
Gastrointestinal: Abnormal taste, abdominal pain, vomiting, nausea, diarrhea, anorexia, constipation
Neuromuscular & skeletal: Weakness
Renal: Increased serum creatinine (0.2% to 20%), worsening of renal function (in patients with bilateral renal artery stenosis or hypovolemia)
Respiratory (1% to 2%): Bronchitis, cough, dyspnea

Overdosage/Toxicology Mild hypotension has been the primary toxic effect seen with acute overdose. Bradycardia may also occur. Hyperkalemia occurs even with therapeutic doses, especially in patients with renal insufficiency and those taking NSAIDs. Following initiation of essential overdose management, toxic symptom treatment and supportive treatment should be initiated.

Pharmacodynamics/Kinetics

Onset of Action: Oral: ~1 hour
Duration of Action: Oral: 12-24 hours
Time to Peak: Serum: Oral: Enalapril: 0.5-1.5 hours; Enalaprilat (active): 3-4.5 hours
Protein Binding: 50% to 60%
Half-Life Elimination:
Enalapril: Adults: Healthy: 2 hours; Congestive heart failure: 3.4-5.8 hours
Enalaprilat: Infants 6 weeks to 8 months old: 6-10 hours; Adults: 35-38 hours
Metabolism: Prodrug, undergoes hepatic biotransformation to enalaprilat
Excretion: Urine (60% to 80%); some feces

Available Dosage Forms

Injection, solution, as enalaprilat: 1.25 mg/mL (1 mL, 2 mL) [contains benzyl alcohol]
Tablet, as maleate (Vasotec®): 2.5 mg, 5 mg, 10 mg, 20 mg

Dosing

Adults & Elderly: Use lower listed initial dose in patients with hyponatremia, hypovolemia, severe congestive heart failure, decreased renal function, or in those receiving diuretics.

Asymptomatic left ventricular dysfunction: Oral: 2.5 mg twice daily, titrated as tolerated to 20 mg/day

Hypertension:
Oral: 2.5-5 mg/day then increase as required, usually at 1- to 2-week intervals; usual dose range (JNC 7): 2.5-40 mg/day in 1-2 divided doses. **Note:** Initiate with 2.5 mg if patient is taking a diuretic which cannot be discontinued. May add a diuretic if blood pressure cannot be controlled with enalapril alone.

I.V. (Enalaprilat): 1.25 mg/dose, given over 5 minutes every 6 hours; doses as high as 5 mg/dose every 6 hours have been tolerated for up to 36 hours. **Note:** If patients are concomitantly receiving diuretic therapy, begin with 0.625 mg I.V. over 5 minutes; if the effect is not adequate after 1 hour, repeat the dose and administer 1.25 mg at 6-hour intervals thereafter; if adequate, administer 0.625 mg I.V. every 6 hours.

Heart failure:
Oral: Initial: 2.5 mg once or twice daily (usual range: 5-40 mg/day in 2 divided doses). Titrate slowly at 1- to 2-week intervals. Target dose: 10-20 mg twice daily (ACC/AHA 2005 Heart Failure Guidelines)

I.V.: Avoid I.V. administration in patients with unstable heart failure or those suffering acute myocardial infarction.

Conversion from I.V. to oral therapy if not concurrently on diuretics: 5 mg once daily; subsequent titration as needed; if concurrently receiving diuretics and responding to 0.625 mg I.V. every 6 hours, initiate with 2.5 mg/day.

Pediatrics:

Hypertension: Oral: Children 1 month to 16 years: Initial: 0.08 mg/kg (up to 5 mg) once daily; adjust dosage based on patient response; doses >0.58 mg/kg (40 mg) have not been evaluated in pediatric patients

Heart failure (non-FDA approved):
Infants and Children:
Oral (Enalapril): Initial: 0.1 mg/kg/day in 1-2 divided doses; increase as required over 2 weeks to maximum of 0.5 mg/kg/day; mean dose required for CHF improvement in 39 children (9 days to 17 years) was 0.36 mg/kg/day; investigationally, select individuals have been treated with doses up to 0.94 mg/kg/day

I.V. (Enalaprilat): 5-10 mcg/kg/dose administered every 8-24 hours (as determined by blood pressure readings); monitor patients carefully; select patients may require higher doses

Adolescents: Refer to adult dosing.

Renal Impairment:
Oral: Enalapril: Hypertension:
Cl$_{cr}$ 30-80 mL/minute: Administer 5 mg/day titrated upwards to maximum of 40 mg.
Cl$_{cr}$ <30 mL/minute: Administer 2.5 mg day titrated upward until blood pressure is controlled up to a maximum of 40 mg.
For heart failure patients with sodium <130 mEq/L or serum creatinine >1.6 mg/dL, initiate dosage with 2.5 mg/day, increasing to twice daily as needed; increase further in increments of 2.5 mg/dose at >4-day intervals to a maximum daily dose of 40 mg.

I.V.: Enalaprilat:
Cl$_{cr}$ >30 mL/minute: Initiate with 1.25 mg every 6 hours and increase dose based on response.
Cl$_{cr}$ <30 mL/minute: Initiate with 0.625 mg every 6 hours and increase dose based on response.

Moderately dialyzable (20% to 50%)
Administer dose postdialysis (eg, 0.625 mg I.V. every 6 hours) or administer 20% to 25% supplemental dose following dialysis; Clearance: 62 mL/minute

Peritoneal dialysis effects: Supplemental dose is not necessary, although some removal of drug occurs.

Hepatic Impairment: Hydrolysis of enalapril to enalaprilat may be delayed and/or impaired in patients with severe hepatic impairment, but the pharmacodynamic effects of the drug do not appear to be significantly altered. No dosage adjustment is necessary.

Administration
I.V.: Give direct IVP over at least 5 minutes or dilute up to 50 mL and infuse.

Stability
Reconstitution: Enalaprilat: I.V. is stable for 24 hours at room temperature in D₅W or NS.
Compatibility: Stable in dextran 40 10% in dextrose, D₅LR, D₅NS, D₅W, hetastarch 6%, NS
Y-site administration: Incompatible with amphotericin B, amphotericin B cholesteryl sulfate complex, cefepime, phenytoin

Storage: Enalaprilat: Clear, colorless solution which should be stored at <30°C.

Laboratory Monitoring CBC, renal function tests, electrolytes. If patient has renal impairment then a baseline WBC with differential and serum creatinine should be evaluated and monitored closely during the first 3 months of therapy.

Nursing Actions

Physical Assessment: Assess potential for interactions with other pharmacological agents or herbal products patient may be taking (especially anything that may impact fluid balance or cardiac status). **Infusion.:** See Administration details. Monitor blood pressure closely with first dose or change in dose. Monitor laboratory tests closely during first 3 months and regularly thereafter. Monitor therapeutic effectiveness according to purpose for use and adverse response on a regular basis during therapy (eg, anaphylactic reaction, hypovolemia, angioedema, postural hypotension). Teach patient appropriate use, possible side effects/appropriate interventions, and adverse symptoms to report.

Patient Education: Do not take any new medication during therapy unless approved by prescriber. Do not use potassium supplement or salt substitutes without consulting prescriber. Take exactly as directed; do not discontinue without consulting prescriber. Take first dose at bedtime. Take all doses on an empty stomach, 1 hour before or 2 hours after meals. This drug does not eliminate need for diet or exercise regimen as recommended by prescriber. May cause dizziness, fainting, or lightheadedness (use caution when driving or engaging in tasks that require alertness until response to drug is known); postural hypotension (use caution when rising from lying or sitting position or climbing stairs); or nausea, vomiting, abdominal pain, dry mouth, or transient loss of appetite (small, frequent meals, frequent mouth care, sucking lozenges, or chewing gum may help). Report persistent nausea and vomiting; chest pain or palpitations; mouth sores; fever or chills; swelling of extremities, face, mouth, or tongue; skin rash; numbness, tingling, or pain in muscles; respiratory difficulty or unusual cough; or other persistent adverse reactions.
Pregnancy precaution: Inform prescriber if you are or intend to become pregnant. This drug should not be used in the 2nd or 3rd trimester of pregnancy. Consult prescriber for appropriate contraceptive measures if necessary.

Dietary Considerations Limit salt substitutes or potassium-rich diet.

Geriatric Considerations Due to frequent decreases in glomerular filtration (also creatinine clearance) with aging, elderly patients may have exaggerated responses to ACE inhibitors.

Pregnancy Issues ACE inhibitors can cause fetal injury or death if taken during the 2nd or 3rd trimester. Discontinue ACE inhibitors as soon as pregnancy is detected.

Enalapril and Felodipine
(e NAL a pril & fe LOE di peen)

U.S. Brand Names Lexxel®
Synonyms Felodipine and Enalapril
Pharmacologic Category Antihypertensive Agent, Combination
Pregnancy Risk Factor C/D (2nd and 3rd trimesters)
Lactation Enters breast milk/use caution
Use Treatment of hypertension, however, not indicated for initial treatment of hypertension; replacement therapy in patients receiving separate dosage forms for patient convenience); when monotherapy with one component fails to achieve desired antihypertensive *(Continued)*

Enalapril and Felodipine *(Continued)*

effect, or when dose-limiting adverse effects limit upward titration of monotherapy

Available Dosage Forms Tablet, extended release:

Enalapril maleate 5 mg and felodipine 2.5 mg

Enalapril maleate 5 mg and felodipine 5 mg

Dosing

Adults: Hypertension: Oral: 1 tablet/day, individualize dose to achieve optimal effect. In some patients, the effect of enalapril may diminish toward the end of the dosing interval. Twice daily dosing may be considered.

Elderly: Recommended initial dose of felodipine is 2.5 mg daily. Titration of individual components is preferred.

Renal Impairment: Cl_{cr} <30 mL/minute: Recommended initial dose of enalapril is 2.5 mg/day. Titration of individual components is preferred.

Hepatic Impairment: Recommended initial dose of felodipine is 2.5 mg daily. Titration of individual components is preferred.

Nursing Actions

Physical Assessment: See individual agents.

Patient Education: See individual agents. **Pregnancy/breast-feeding precautions:** Inform prescriber if you are or intend to become pregnant. Consult prescriber if breast-feeding.

Related Information

Enalapril *on page 419*
Felodipine *on page 502*

Enalapril and Hydrochlorothiazide

(e NAL a pril & hye droe klor oh THYE a zide)

U.S. Brand Names Vaseretic®

Synonyms Hydrochlorothiazide and Enalapril

Pharmacologic Category Antihypertensive Agent, Combination

Pregnancy Risk Factor C/D (2nd and 3rd trimesters)

Lactation Enters breast milk (both ingredients)/compatible

Use Treatment of hypertension

Available Dosage Forms Tablet:

5-12.5: Enalapril maleate 5 mg and hydrochlorothiazide 12.5 mg

10-25: Enalapril maleate 10 mg and hydrochlorothiazide 25 mg

Dosing

Adults: Hypertension: Dose is individualized based on components

Elderly: Refer to dosing in individual monographs; adjust for renal impairment.

Renal Impairment:

Cl_{cr} >30 mL/minute: Administer usual dose.

Severe renal failure: Avoid; loop diuretics are recommended.

Nursing Actions

Physical Assessment: See individual agents.

Patient Education: See individual agents. **Pregnancy precaution:** Inform prescriber if you are or intend to become pregnant.

Related Information

Enalapril *on page 419*
Hydrochlorothiazide *on page 610*

Enfuvirtide (en FYOO vir tide)

U.S. Brand Names Fuzeon™

Synonyms T-20

Pharmacologic Category Antiretroviral Agent, Fusion Protein Inhibitor

Pregnancy Risk Factor B

Lactation Excretion in breast milk unknown/contraindicated

Use Treatment of HIV-1 infection in combination with other antiretroviral agents in treatment-experienced patients with evidence of HIV-1 replication despite ongoing antiretroviral therapy

Mechanism of Action/Effect Inhibits the fusion of HIV-1 virus with CD4 cells

Contraindications Hypersensitivity to enfuvirtide or any component of the formulation

Warnings/Precautions Monitor closely for signs/symptoms of pneumonia; associated with an increased incidence during clinical trials, particularly in patients with a low CD4 cell count, high initial viral load, I.V. drug use, smoking, or a history of lung disease. May cause hypersensitivity reactions (symptoms may include rash, fever, nausea, vomiting, hypotension, and elevated transaminases). In addition, local injection site reactions may occur. An inflammatory response to indolent or residual opportunistic infections (immune reconstitution syndrome) has occurred with antiretroviral therapy; further investigation is warranted. Safety and efficacy have not been established in children <6 years of age.

Drug Interactions

Decreased Effect: No significant interactions identified.

Increased Effect/Toxicity: No significant interactions identified.

Adverse Reactions

>10%:

Central nervous system: Insomnia (11%)

Local: Injection site reactions (98%; may include pain, erythema, induration, pruritus, ecchymosis, nodule or cyst formation)

1% to 10%:

Central nervous system: Depression (9%), anxiety (6%)

Dermatologic: Pruritus (5%)

Endocrine & metabolic: Weight loss (7%), anorexia (3%)

Gastrointestinal: Triglycerides increased (9%), appetite decreased (6%), constipation (4%), abdominal pain (3%), pancreatitis (2%), taste disturbance (2%), serum amylase increased (6%)

Hematologic: Eosinophilia (8%), anemia (2%)

Hepatic: Transaminases increased (4%)

Local: Injection site infection (1%)

Neuromuscular & skeletal: Neuropathy (9%), weakness (6%), myalgia (5%)

Ocular: Conjunctivitis (2%)

Respiratory: Cough (7%), pneumonia (4.7 events per 100 patient years vs 0.61 events per 100 patient years in control group), sinusitis (6%)

Miscellaneous: Infections (4% to 6%), flu-like symptoms (2%), lymphadenopathy (2%)

Overdosage/Toxicology No clinical experience in overdosage. Treatment is supportive.

Pharmacodynamics/Kinetics

Time to Peak: 8 hours

Protein Binding: 92%

Half-Life Elimination: 3.8 hours

Metabolism: Proteolytic hydrolysis (CYP isoenzymes do not appear to contribute to metabolism); clearance: 24.8 mL/hour/kg

Available Dosage Forms Injection, powder for reconstitution [single-use vial]: 108 mg [90 mg/mL following reconstitution; available in convenience kit of 60 vials, SWFI, syringes, alcohol wipes, patient instructions]

Dosing

Adults: HIV Treatment: SubQ: 90 mg twice daily

Elderly: See adults dosing.

Pediatrics: HIV treatment: SubQ: Children ≥6 years: 2 mg/kg twice daily (maximum dose: 90 mg twice daily)

Renal Impairment: No dosage adjustment required.

Administration

Other: Inject subcutaneously into upper arm, abdomen, or anterior thigh. Do not inject into moles, scar tissue, bruises, or the navel. Rotate injection site, give injections at a site different from the preceding injection site; do not inject into any site where an injection site reaction is evident.

Stability

Reconstitution: Reconstitute with 1.1 mL SWFI; tap vial for 10 seconds and roll gently to ensure contact with diluent; then allow to stand until solution is completed; may require up to 45 minutes to form solution. Reconstituted solutions should be refrigerated and must be used within 24 hours.

Storage: Store powder at 25 °C (77°F). Excursions permitted to 15°C to 30°C (59 to 86°F).

Nursing Actions

Physical Assessment: Monitor therapeutic response and adverse reactions (eg, pneumonia, neuropathy, CNS changes) on a regular basis throughout therapy. Teach patient or caregiver proper use (eg, reconstitution, injection procedure, needle/syringe disposal and proper timing of mediations). Teach patient possible side effects/appropriate interventions and adverse symptoms to report (eg, hypersensitivity reaction, injection site infection).

Patient Education: Do not take any new medication during therapy unless approved by prescriber. This drug will not cure HIV, nor has it been found to reduce transmission of HIV; use appropriate precautions to prevent spread to other persons. This drug is prescribed as one part of a multidrug combination; take exactly as directed for full course of therapy. This drug can only be administered by injection, follow exact injection instructions that come with your medication. Do not mix any other medications in the same syringe. Inject into the upper arm, abdomen, or anterior thigh; do not inject in the same area you did the time before and do not inject around the naval, into scar tissues, a bruise, a mole, or where there is an injection site reaction. Make sure you have an adequate supply of medications on hand; do not allow supply to run out. Do not miss or skip a dose; if you miss a dose, take the missed dose as soon as you can and take the next dose as scheduled. If it is close to the time for the next dose, wait and take the next dose as regularly scheduled. Do not take two doses at the same time. Frequent blood tests may be required with prolonged therapy. May cause injection site reactions such as itching, swelling, redness, pain, hardened skin, or bumps (usually last for <7 days). May cause insomnia, anorexia (small, frequent meals may help), or constipation (increased dietary fiber, fruit, fluids, or exercise may help). Notify prescriber immediately if you experience a hypersensitivity reaction (rash, fever, nausea, vomiting, hypotension, blood in urine) or injection site becomes infected (red, painful, swollen, drainage). Report CNS disturbances (depression, anxiety); weakness, loss of feeling, or muscle pain; respiratory infections, difficulty breathing, flu-like symptoms, unusual cough, fever, alteration in urinary pattern; swelling of legs or feet; or any other persistent adverse reactions. **Pregnancy/breast-feeding precautions:** Notify prescriber if you are or intend to become pregnant. Do not breast feed.

Breast-Feeding Issues HIV-infected mothers are discouraged from breast-feeding to decrease potential transmission of HIV.

Pregnancy Issues Teratogenic effects were not observed in animal studies, however there are no studies in pregnant women. An antiretroviral registry has been established to monitor maternal and fetal outcomes in women receiving antiretroviral drugs. Physicians are encouraged to register patients at 1-800-258-4263 or www.APRegistry.com.

Enoxaparin (ee noks a PA rin)

U.S. Brand Names Lovenox®

Synonyms Enoxaparin Sodium

Pharmacologic Category Low Molecular Weight Heparin

Medication Safety Issues

Sound-alike/look-alike issues:

Lovenox® may be confused with Lotronex®, Protonix®

High alert medication: The Institute for Safe Medication Practices (ISMP) includes this medication among its list of drugs which have a heightened risk of causing significant patient harm when used in error.

Pregnancy Risk Factor B

Lactation Excretion in breast milk unknown/use caution

Use

DVT Treatment (acute): Inpatient treatment (patients with and without pulmonary embolism) and outpatient treatment (patients without pulmonary embolism)

DVT prophylaxis: Following hip or knee replacement surgery, abdominal surgery, or in medical patients with severely-restricted mobility during acute illness in patients at risk of thromboembolic complications

Note: High-risk patients include those with one or more of the following risk factors: >40 years of age, obesity, general anesthesia lasting >30 minutes, malignancy, history of deep vein thrombosis or pulmonary embolism

Unstable angina and non-Q-wave myocardial infarction (to prevent ischemic complications)

Unlabeled/Investigational Use Prophylaxis and treatment of thromboembolism in children

Mechanism of Action/Effect Low molecular weight heparin that blocks factor Xa and IIa to prevent thrombus and clot formation

Contraindications Hypersensitivity to enoxaparin, heparin, or any component of the formulation; thrombocytopenia associated with a positive *in vitro* test for antiplatelet antibodies in the presence of enoxaparin; hypersensitivity to pork products; active major bleeding; not for I.M. or I.V. use

Warnings/Precautions Patients with recent or anticipated neuraxial anesthesia (epidural or spinal anesthesia) are at risk of spinal or epidural hematoma and subsequent paralysis. Consider risk versus benefit prior to neuraxial anesthesia; risk is increased by concomitant agents which may alter hemostasis, as well as traumatic or repeated epidural or spinal puncture. Patient should be observed closely for bleeding if enoxaparin is administered during or immediately following diagnostic lumbar puncture, epidural anesthesia, or spinal anesthesia.

Not recommended for thromboprophylaxis in patients with prosthetic heart valves (especially pregnant women). Not to be used interchangeably (unit for unit) with heparin or any other low molecular weight heparins. Use caution in patients with history of heparin-induced thrombocytopenia. Monitor patient closely for signs or symptoms of bleeding. Certain patients are at increased risk of bleeding. Risk factors include bacterial endocarditis; congenital or acquired bleeding disorders; active ulcerative or angiodysplastic GI diseases; severe uncontrolled hypertension; hemorrhagic stroke; use shortly after brain, spinal, or ophthalmology surgery; patients treated concomitantly with platelet inhibitors; (Continued)

Enoxaparin (Continued)

recent GI bleeding; thrombocytopenia or platelet defects; severe liver disease; hypertensive or diabetic retinopathy; or in patients undergoing invasive procedures. Monitor platelet count closely. Rare cases of thrombocytopenia have occurred. Manufacturer recommends discontinuation of therapy if platelets are <100,000/mm³. Risk of bleeding may be increased in women <45 kg and in men <57 kg. Use caution in patients with renal failure; dosage adjustment needed if Cl$_{cr}$ <30 mL/minute. Safety and efficacy in pediatric patients have not been established. Use with caution in the elderly (delayed elimination may occur). Heparin can cause hyperkalemia by affecting aldosterone. Similar reactions could occur with LMWHs. Monitor for hyperkalemia. Multiple-dose vials contain benzyl alcohol (use caution in pregnant women).

Drug Interactions

Increased Effect/Toxicity: Risk of bleeding with enoxaparin may be increased with thrombolytic agents, oral anticoagulants (warfarin), drugs which affect platelet function (eg, aspirin, NSAIDs, dipyridamole, ticlopidine, clopidogrel, and IIb/IIIa antagonists). Although the risk of bleeding may be increased during concurrent therapy with warfarin, enoxaparin is commonly continued during the initiation of warfarin therapy to assure anticoagulation and to protect against possible transient hypercoagulability. Some cephalosporins and penicillins may block platelet aggregation, theoretically increasing the risk of bleeding.

Nutritional/Ethanol Interactions Herb/Nutraceutical: Avoid cat's claw, dong quai, evening primrose, feverfew, garlic, ginger, ginkgo, red clover, horse chestnut, green tea, ginseng (all have additional antiplatelet activity).

Lab Interactions Increased AST, ALT levels

Adverse Reactions As with all anticoagulants, bleeding is the major adverse effect of enoxaparin. Hemorrhage may occur at virtually any site. Risk is dependent on multiple variables. At the recommended doses, single injections of enoxaparin do not significantly influence platelet aggregation or affect global clotting time (ie, PT or aPTT).

1% to 10%:

Central nervous system: Fever (5% to 8%), confusion, pain

Dermatologic: Erythema, bruising

Gastrointestinal: Nausea (3%), diarrhea

Hematologic: Hemorrhage (5% to 13%), thrombocytopenia (2%), hypochromic anemia (2%)

Hepatic: Increased ALT/AST

Local: Injection site hematoma (9%), local reactions (irritation, pain, ecchymosis, erythema)

Thrombocytopenia with thrombosis: Cases of heparin-induced thrombocytopenia (some complicated by organ infarction, limb ischemia, or death) have been reported.

Overdosage/Toxicology Symptoms of overdose include hemorrhage. Protamine sulfate has been used to reverse effects (protamine 1 mg neutralizes enoxaparin 1 mg). Monitor aPTT 2-4 hours after first infusion; consider readministration of protamine (50% of original dose). Note: anti-Xa activity is never completely neutralized (maximum of 60% to 75%). Avoid overdose of protamine.

Pharmacodynamics/Kinetics

Onset of Action: Peak effect: SubQ: Antifactor Xa and antithrombin (antifactor IIa): 3-5 hours

Duration of Action: 40 mg dose: Antifactor Xa activity: ~12 hours

Protein Binding: Does not bind to heparin binding proteins

Half-Life Elimination: Plasma: 2-4 times longer than standard heparin, independent of dose; based on anti-Xa activity: 4.5-7 hours

Metabolism: Hepatic, to lower molecular weight fragments (little activity)

Excretion: Urine (40% of dose; 10% as active fragments)

Available Dosage Forms

Injection, solution, as sodium [graduated prefilled syringe; preservative free]: 60 mg/0.6 mL (0.6 mL); 80 mg/0.8 mL (0.8 mL); 100 mg/mL (1 mL); 120 mg/0.8 mL (0.8 mL); 150 mg/mL (1 mL)

Injection, solution, as sodium [multidose vial]: 100 mg/mL (3 mL) [contains benzyl alcohol]

Injection, solution, as sodium [prefilled syringe; preservative free]: 30 mg/0.3 mL (0.3 mL); 40 mg/0.4 mL (0.4 mL)

Dosing

Adults:

DVT prophylaxis: SubQ:

Hip replacement surgery:

Twice-daily dosing: 30 mg twice daily, with initial dose within 12-24 hours after surgery, and every 12 hours until risk of DVT has diminished or the patient is adequately anticoagulated on warfarin.

Once-daily dosing: 40 mg once daily, with initial dose within 9-15 hours before surgery, and daily until risk of DVT has diminished or the patient is adequately anticoagulated on warfarin.

Knee replacement surgery: 30 mg twice daily, with initial dose within 12-24 hours after surgery, and every 12 hours until risk of DVT has diminished (usually 7-10 days).

Abdominal surgery: 40 mg once daily, with initial dose given 2 hours prior to surgery; continue until risk of DVT has diminished (usual 7-10 days).

Medical patients with severely-restricted mobility during acute illness: 40 mg once daily; continue until risk of DVT has diminished

DVT treatment (acute): SubQ: **Note:** Start warfarin within 72 hours and continue enoxaparin until INR is between 2.0 and 3.0 (usually 7 days).

Inpatient treatment (with or without pulmonary embolism): 1 mg/kg/dose every 12 hours or 1.5 mg/kg once daily.

Outpatient treatment (without pulmonary embolism): 1 mg/kg/dose every 12 hours.

Unstable angina or non-Q-wave MI: SubQ: 1 mg/kg twice daily in conjunction with oral aspirin therapy (100-325 mg once daily); continue until clinical stabilization (a minimum of at least 2 days)

Elderly: SubQ: Increased incidence of bleeding with doses of 1.5 mg/kg/day or 1 mg/kg every 12 hours. Injection-associated bleeding and serious adverse reactions are also increased in the elderly. Careful attention should be paid to elderly patients <45 kg.

Pediatrics: Thromboembolism (unlabeled use): SubQ:

Infants <2 months: Initial:

Prophylaxis: 0.75 mg/kg every 12 hours

Treatment: 1.5 mg/kg every 12 hours

Infants >2 months and Children ≤18 years: Initial:

Prophylaxis: 0.5 mg/kg every 12 hours

Treatment: 1 mg/kg every 12 hours

Maintenance: See **Dosage Titration** table.

Renal Impairment:

Cl$_{cr}$ ≥30 mL/minute: No specific adjustment recommended (per manufacturer); monitor closely for bleeding.

Cl$_{cr}$ <30 mL/minute:

DVT prophylaxis in abdominal surgery, hip replacement, knee replacement, or in medical patients during acute illness: SubQ: 30 mg once daily

DVT treatment (inpatient or outpatient treatment in conjunction with warfarin): SubQ: 1 mg/kg once daily

Unstable angina, non-Q-wave MI (with ASA): SubQ: 1 mg/kg once daily

Dialysis: Enoxaparin has not been FDA approved for use in dialysis patients. It's elimination is primarily via the renal route. Serious bleeding complications have been reported with use in patients who are dialysis dependent or have severe renal failure. LMWH administration at fixed doses without monitoring has greater unpredictable anticoagulant effects in patients with chronic kidney disease. If used, dosages should be reduced and anti-Xa activity frequently monitored, as accumulation may occur with repeated doses. Many clinicians would not use enoxaparin in this population especially without timely anti-Xa activity assay results.

Hemodialysis: Supplemental dose is not necessary.

Peritoneal dialysis: Significant drug removal is unlikely based on physiochemical characteristics.

Enoxaparin Pediatric Dosage Titration

Antifactor Xa	Dose Titration	Time to Repeat Antifactor Xa Level
<0.35 units/mL	Increase dose by 25%	4 h after next dose
0.35-0.49 units/mL	Increase dose by 10%	4 h after next dose
0.5-1 unit/mL	Keep same dosage	Next day, then 1 wk later, then monthly (4 h after dose)
1.1-1.5 units/mL	Decrease dose by 20%	Before next dose
1.6-2 units/mL	Hold dose for 3 h and decrease dose by 30%	Before next dose, then 4 h after next dose
>2 units/mL	Hold all doses until antifactor Xa is 0.5 units/mL, then decrease dose by 40%	Before next dose and every 12 h until antifactor Xa <0.5 units/mL

Modified from Monagle P, Michelson AD, Bovill E, et al, "Antithrombotic Therapy in Children," *Chest*, 2001, 119:344S-70S.

Administration
I.V. Detail: pH: 5.5-7.5

Other: Should be administered by deep SubQ injection to the left or right anterolateral and left or right posterolateral abdominal wall. To avoid loss of drug from the 30 mg and 40 mg syringes, do not expel the air bubble from the syringe prior to injection. In order to minimize bruising, do not rub injection site. An automatic injector (Lovenox EasyInjector™) is available with the 30 mg and 40 mg syringes to aid the patient with self-injections. **Note:** Enoxaparin is available in 100 mg/mL and 150 mg/mL concentrations.

Stability
Compatibility: Stable in NS

Storage: Store at 15°C to 25°C (59°F to 77°F). Do not freeze. Do not mix with other injections or infusions.

Laboratory Monitoring Platelets, occult blood, anti-Xa activity, if available; the monitoring of PT and/or aPTT is not necessary.

Nursing Actions
Physical Assessment: Use caution in presence or history of conditions that increase risk of bleeding. Assess potential for interactions with other pharmacological agents or herbal products patient may be taking (especially anything that will impact coagulation or platelet aggregation). Note specific injection directions (See Administration). Monitor therapeutic effectiveness according to purpose for use and adverse response (eg, bleeding, thrombosis). Teach patient possible side effects/appropriate interventions, and adverse symptoms to report.

Patient Education: Do not take any new medication during therapy without consulting prescriber. This drug can only be administered by injection. If self-administered, follow exact directions for injection and needle disposal. You may have a tendency to bleed easily while taking this drug (brush teeth with soft brush, use waxed dental floss, use electric razor, avoid scissors or sharp knives, and potentially harmful activities). Report chest pain; persistent constipation; persistent erection; unusual bleeding or bruising (bleeding gums, nosebleed, blood in urine, dark stool); pain in joints or back; or redness, swelling, burning, or pain at injection site. **Pregnancy/breast-feeding precautions:** Inform prescriber if you are pregnant. Consult prescriber if breast-feeding.

Geriatric Considerations No specific recommendations.

Breast-Feeding Issues This drug has a high molecular weight that would minimize excretion in breast milk and is inactivated by the GI tract which further reduces the risk to the infant.

Pregnancy Issues There are no adequate and well-controlled studies using enoxaparin in pregnant women. Postmarketing reports include congenital abnormalities (cause and effect not established) and also fetal death when used in pregnant women. In addition, prosthetic valve thrombosis, including fatal cases, has been reported in pregnant women receiving enoxaparin as thromboprophylaxis. Multiple-dose vials contain benzyl alcohol; use caution in pregnant women.

Entacapone (en TA ka pone)

U.S. Brand Names Comtan®

Pharmacologic Category Anti-Parkinson's Agent, COMT Inhibitor

Pregnancy Risk Factor C

Lactation Excretion in breast milk unknown/use caution

Use Adjunct to levodopa/carbidopa therapy in patients with idiopathic Parkinson's disease who experience "wearing-off" symptoms at the end of a dosing interval

Mechanism of Action/Effect Entacapone inhibits COMT peripherally and alters the pharmacokinetics of levodopa so serum levels of levodopa become more sustained when used with levodopa/carbidopa combinations.

Contraindications Hypersensitivity to entacapone or any of component of the formulation

Warnings/Precautions May increase risk of orthostatic hypotension and syncope. May cause diarrhea, hallucinations; may cause or exacerbate dyskinesia. This drug should be slowly withdrawn if discontinuation is needed. Use caution in patients with hepatic impairment and renal impairment. Other drugs metabolized by COMT (see drug interactions) may cause increases in heart rate, arrhythmias, and changes in blood pressure when used concurrently.

Drug Interactions

Cytochrome P450 Effect: Inhibits CYP1A2 (weak), 2A6 (weak), 2C8/9 (weak), 2C19 (weak), 2D6 (weak), 2E1 (weak), 3A4 (weak)

Increased Effect/Toxicity: Entacapone may decrease the metabolism and increase the side effects of COMT substrates (eg, apomorphine, bitolterol, dobutamine, dopamine, epinephrine, norepinephrine, isoproterenol, isoetharine, and methyldopa). Effects on mental status may be additive with other CNS depressants; includes barbiturates, benzodiazepines, TCAs, antipsychotics, ethanol, narcotic analgesics, and other sedative-hypnotics. Concurrent use of nonselective MAO inhibitors with entacapone may increase the risk of cardiovascular side effects; selective MAO inhibitors (eg, selegiline) appear to pose limited risk.

Nutritional/Ethanol Interactions Ethanol: Avoid ethanol (may increase CNS adverse effects).

Adverse Reactions
>10%:
Gastrointestinal: Nausea (14%)
(Continued)

Entacapone (Continued)

Neuromuscular & skeletal: Dyskinesia (25%), placebo (15%)

1% to 10%:

Cardiovascular: Orthostatic hypotension (4%), syncope (1%)

Central nervous system: Dizziness (8%), fatigue (6%), hallucinations (4%), anxiety (2%), somnolence (2%), agitation (1%)

Dermatologic: Purpura (2%)

Gastrointestinal: Diarrhea (10%), abdominal pain (8%), constipation (6%), vomiting (4%), dry mouth (3%), dyspepsia (2%), flatulence (2%), gastritis (1%), taste perversion (1%)

Genitourinary: Brown-orange urine discoloration (10%)

Neuromuscular & skeletal: Hyperkinesia (10%), hypokinesia (9%), back pain (4%), weakness (2%)

Respiratory: Dyspnea (3%)

Miscellaneous: Diaphoresis increased (2%), bacterial infection (1%)

Overdosage/Toxicology There have been no reported cases of overdose with this drug.

Pharmacodynamics/Kinetics

Onset of Action: Rapid; Peak effect: 1 hour

Time to Peak: Serum: 1 hour

Protein Binding: 98%, primarily to albumin

Half-Life Elimination: B phase: 0.4-0.7 hours; Y phase: 2.4 hours

Metabolism: Isomerization to the *cis*-isomer, followed by direct glucuronidation of the parent and *cis*-isomer

Excretion: Feces (90%); urine (10%)

Available Dosage Forms Tablet: 200 mg

Dosing

Adults & Elderly: Parkinson's disease: Oral: 200 mg with each dose of levodopa/carbidopa, up to a maximum of 8 times/day (maximum daily dose: 1600 mg/day). To optimize therapy, the dosage of levodopa may need reduced or the dosing interval may need extended. Patients taking levodopa ≥800mg/day or who had moderate-to-severe dyskinesias prior to therapy required an average decrease of 25% in the daily levodopa dose.

Renal Impairment: No adjustment is required; dialysis patients were not studied.

Hepatic Impairment: Dosage adjustment in chronic therapy with standard treatment has not been studied.

Nursing Actions

Physical Assessment: Assess other medications patient may be taking for effectiveness and interactions. Monitor therapeutic response (improved parkinsonian status), adverse reactions (eg, neuromuscular, CNS, GI reactions). Monitor blood pressure. Taper dosage when discontinuing. Assess knowledge/teach patient appropriate use, interventions to reduce side effects, and adverse reactions to report.

Patient Education: Take exactly as directed; do not alter dosage or discontinue without consulting prescriber. May be taken with food. Notify prescriber if any other prescription medications you are taking. Avoid all alcohol or OTC medications unless approved by your prescriber. Orange-brown urine is normal with this medication. You may experience dizziness, fatigue, or sleepiness (use caution when driving or engaging in tasks requiring alertness until response to drug is known); postural hypotension (rise slowly when getting up from chair or bed, when climbing stairs); or unusual taste, nausea, vomiting, flatulence, or upset stomach (small frequent meals, good mouth care, chewing gum, or sucking hard candy may help). Report any increased or abnormal skeletal movements or pain; unresolved sedation, nausea, diarrhea, constipation, or GI distress; signs of infection; persistent dizziness or sleepiness; or other unusual responses. **Pregnancy/breast-feeding precautions:**

Inform prescriber if you are or intend to become pregnant. Consult prescriber if breast-feeding.

Dietary Considerations May be taken with or without food.

Epinastine (ep i NAS teen)

U.S. Brand Names Elestat™

Synonyms Epinastine Hydrochloride

Pharmacologic Category Antihistamine, H₁ Blocker, Ophthalmic

Pregnancy Risk Factor C

Lactation Excretion in breast milk unknown/use caution

Use Treatment of allergic conjunctivitis

Mechanism of Action/Effect Selective H_1-receptor antagonist; inhibits release of histamine from the mast cell

Contraindications Hypersensitivity to epinastine or any component of the formulation

Warnings/Precautions Contains benzalkonium chloride; contact lenses should be removed prior to use. Not for the treatment of contact lens irritation. Safety and efficacy in children <3 years of age have not been established.

Adverse Reactions 1% to 10%:

Central nervous system: Headache (1% to 3%)

Ocular: Burning sensation, folliculosis, hyperemia, pruritus

Respiratory: Cough (1% to 3%), pharyngitis (1% to 3%), rhinitis (1% to 3%), sinusitis (1% to 3%)

Miscellaneous: Infection (10%; defined as cold symptoms and upper respiratory infection)

Pharmacodynamics/Kinetics

Onset of Action: 3-5 minutes

Duration of Action: 8 hours

Protein Binding: 64%

Half-Life Elimination: 12 hours

Metabolism: <10% metabolized

Excretion: I.V.: Urine (55%); feces (30%)

Available Dosage Forms Solution, ophthalmic, as hydrochloride: 0.05% (5 mL) [contains benzalkonium chloride]

Dosing

Adults & Elderly: Allergic conjunctivitis: Ophthalmic: Instill 1 drop into each eye twice daily. Continue throughout period of exposure, even in the absence of symptoms.

Pediatrics: Allergic conjunctivitis: Ophthalmic: Children ≥3 years: Refer to adult dosing.

Administration

Other: For ophthalmic use only; avoid touching tip of applicator to eye or other surfaces. Contact lenses should be removed prior to application, may be reinserted after 10 minutes. Do not wear contact lenses if eyes are red.

Stability

Storage: Store at controlled room temperature of 15°C to 25°C (59°F to 77°F). Keep tightly closed.

Nursing Actions

Physical Assessment: For ophthalmic use only. Assess therapeutic effectiveness and adverse reactions on a regular basis throughout therapy. Teach patient possible side effects/appropriate interventions and adverse symptoms to report.

Patient Education: For ophthalmic use only. Use exactly as directed. Do not wear contact lenses if eyes are red. May cause headache (consult prescriber for analgesic if persistent). Report unusual or persistent cough of cold symptoms related to use, or if condition does not improve. Wash hands before using. Remove contact lenses before application (may be reinserted after 10 minutes). Gently pull lower eyelid forward and instill prescribed amount in lower eyelid. Avoid touching tip of dropper to eye. Close eye and roll eyeball in all directions. May cause blurred vision, temporary stinging or burning sensation.

Geriatric Considerations No difference in safety and efficacy was observed between elderly and younger patients.

Epinephrine (ep i NEF rin)

U.S. Brand Names Adrenalin®; EpiPen®; EpiPen® Jr; Primatene® Mist [OTC]; Raphon [OTC]; S2® [OTC]; Twinject™

Synonyms Adrenaline; Epinephrine Bitartrate; Epinephrine Hydrochloride; Racepinephrine

Pharmacologic Category Alpha/Beta Agonist; Antidote

Medication Safety Issues
Sound-alike/look-alike issues:
Epinephrine may be confused with ephedrine
Epifrin® may be confused with ephedrine, EpiPen®
EpiPen® may be confused with Epifrin®

Medication errors have occurred due to confusion with epinephrine products expressed as ratio strengths (eg, 1:1000 vs 1:10,000).
Epinephrine 1:1000 = 1 mg/mL and is most commonly used SubQ.
Epinephrine 1:10,000 = 0.1 mg/mL and is used I.V.

Pregnancy Risk Factor C

Lactation Excretion in breast milk unknown

Use Treatment of bronchospasms, bronchial asthma, nasal congestion, viral croup, anaphylactic reactions, cardiac arrest; added to local anesthetics to decrease systemic absorption of local anesthetics and increase duration of action; decrease superficial hemorrhage

Unlabeled/Investigational Use ACLS guidelines: Ventricular fibrillation (VF) or pulseless ventricular tachycardia (VT) unresponsive to initial defibrillatory shocks; pulseless electrical activity, asystole, hypotension unresponsive to volume resuscitation; symptomatic bradycardia or hypotension unresponsive to atropine or pacing; inotropic support

Mechanism of Action/Effect Stimulates alpha-, beta$_1$-, and beta$_2$-adrenergic receptors resulting in relaxation of smooth muscle of the bronchial tree, cardiac stimulation, and dilation of skeletal muscle vasculature; small doses can cause vasodilation via beta$_2$-vascular receptors; large doses may produce constriction of skeletal and vascular smooth muscle

Contraindications Hypersensitivity to epinephrine or any component of the formulation; cardiac arrhythmias; angle-closure glaucoma

Warnings/Precautions Use with caution in elderly patients, patients with diabetes mellitus, cardiovascular diseases (angina, tachycardia, prostatic hyperplasia, history of seizures, renal dysfunction, myocardial infarction), thyroid disease, cerebral arteriosclerosis, or Parkinson's. Some products contain sulfites as preservatives. Rapid I.V. infusion may cause death from cerebrovascular hemorrhage or cardiac arrhythmias. Oral inhalation of epinephrine is **not** the preferred route of administration. Avoid topical application where reduced perfusion could lead to ischemic tissue damage (eg, penis, ears, digits).

Drug Interactions
Decreased Effect: Decreased bronchodilation with β-blockers. Decreases antihypertensive effects of methyldopa or guanethidine.

Increased Effect/Toxicity: Increased cardiac irritability if administered concurrently with halogenated inhalation anesthetics, beta-blocking agents, or alpha-blocking agents.

Nutritional/Ethanol Interactions Herb/Nutraceutical: Avoid ephedra, yohimbe (may cause CNS stimulation).

Lab Interactions Increased bilirubin (S), catecholamines (U), glucose, uric acid (S)

Adverse Reactions Frequency not defined.
Cardiovascular: Angina, cardiac arrhythmia, chest pain, flushing, hypertension, increased myocardial oxygen consumption, pallor, palpitation, sudden death, tachycardia (parenteral), vasoconstriction, ventricular ectopy
Central nervous system: Anxiety, dizziness, headache, insomnia, lightheadedness, nervousness, restlessness
Gastrointestinal: Dry throat, nausea, vomiting, xerostomia
Genitourinary: Acute urinary retention in patients with bladder outflow obstruction
Neuromuscular & skeletal: Trembling, weakness
Ocular: Allergic lid reaction, burning, eye pain, ocular irritation, precipitation of or exacerbation of narrow-angle glaucoma, transient stinging
Renal: Decreased renal and splanchnic blood flow
Respiratory: Dyspnea, wheezing
Miscellaneous: Diaphoresis (increased)

Overdosage/Toxicology Symptoms of overdose include arrhythmias, unusually large pupils, pulmonary edema, renal failure, metabolic acidosis; and hypertension, which may result in subarachnoid hemorrhage and hemiplegia. There is no specific antidote for epinephrine intoxication and treatment is primarily supportive.

Pharmacodynamics/Kinetics
Onset of Action: Bronchodilation: SubQ: ~5-10 minutes; Inhalation: ~1 minute

Metabolism: Taken up into the adrenergic neuron and metabolized by monoamine oxidase and catechol-o-methyltransferase; circulating drug hepatically metabolized

Excretion: Urine (as inactive metabolites, metanephrine, and sulfate and hydroxy derivatives of mandelic acid; small amounts as unchanged drug)

Available Dosage Forms
Aerosol for oral inhalation:
Primatene® Mist: 0.22 mg/inhalation (15 mL, 22.5 mL) [contains CFCs]
Injection, solution [prefilled auto injector]:
EpiPen®: 0.3 mg/0.3 mL [1:1000] (2 mL) [contains sodium metabisulfite; available as single unit or in double-unit pack with training unit]
EpiPen® Jr: 0.15 mg/0.3 mL [1:2000] (2 mL) [contains sodium metabisulfite; available as single unit or in double-unit pack with training unit]
Twinject™: 0.15 mg/0.15 mL [1:1000] (1.1 mL) [contains sodium bisulfite; two 0.15 mg doses per injector]; 0.3 mg/0.3 mL [1:1000] (1.1 mL) [contains sodium bisulfite; two 0.3 mg doses per injector]
Injection, solution, as hydrochloride: 0.1 mg/mL [1:10,000] (10 mL); 1 mg/mL [1:1000] (1 mL) [products may contain sodium metabisulfite]
Adrenalin®: 1 mg/mL [1:1000] (1 mL, 30 mL) [contains sodium bisulfite]
Solution for oral inhalation, as hydrochloride:
Adrenalin®: 1% [10 mg/mL, 1:100] (7.5 mL) [contains sodium bisulfite]
Solution for oral inhalation [racepinephrine]:
S2®: 2.25% (0.5 mL, 15 mL) [as d-epinephrine 1.125% and l-epinephrine 1.125%; contains metabisulfites]
Solution, topical [racepinephrine]:
Raphon: 2.25% (15 mL) [as d-epinephrine 1.125% and l-epinephrine 1.125%; contains metabisulfites]

Dosing
Adults & Elderly:
Asystole/pulseless arrest, bradycardia, VT/VF:
I.V., I.O.: 1 mg every 3-5 minutes; if this approach fails, higher doses of epinephrine (up to 0.2 mg/kg) may be indicated for treatment of specific problems (eg, beta-blocker or calcium channel blocker overdose)

(Continued)

Epinephrine *(Continued)*

Intratracheal: Administer 2-2.5 mg for VF or pulseless VT if I.V./I.O. access is delayed or cannot be established; dilute in 5-10 mL NS or distilled water. **Note:** Absorption is greater with distilled water, but causes more adverse effects on PaO$_2$.

Bradycardia (symptomatic) or hypotension (not responsive to atropine or pacing): *I.V. infusion:* 2-10 mcg/minute; titrate to desired effect

Bronchodilator:

SubQ: 0.3-0.5 mg **(1:1000)** every 20 minutes for 3 doses

Nebulization: 1-3 inhalations up to every 3 hours using solution prepared with 10 drops of the **1:100** product

S2® (racepinephrine, OTC labeling): 0.5 mL (~10 drops). Dose may be repeated not more frequently than very 3-4 hours if needed. Solution should be diluted if using jet nebulizer.

Inhalation: Primatene® Mist (OTC labeling): One inhalation, wait at least 1 minute; if relieved, may use once more. Do not use again for at least 3 hours.

Decongestant: *Intranasal:* Apply 1:1000 locally as drops or spray or with sterile swab

Hypersensitivity reaction:

I.M., SubQ: 0.3-0.5 mg (1:1000) every 15-20 minutes if condition requires (I.M route is preferred)

>30 kg: Twinject™: 0.3 mg (for self-administration following severe allergic reactions to insect stings, food, etc)

I.M.: >30 kg: Epipen®: 0.3 mg (for self-administration following severe allergic reactions to insect stings, food, etc)

I.V.: 0.1 mg (1:10,000) over 5 minutes. May infuse at 1-4 mcg/minute to prevent the need to repeat injections frequently.

Pediatrics:

Cardiac arrest: I.V.: Neonates: 0.01-0.03 mg/kg (0.1-0.3 mL/kg of **1:10,000** solution) every 3-5 minutes as needed. Although I.V. route is preferred, may consider administration of doses up to 0.1 mg/kg through the endotracheal tube until I.V. access established; dilute intratracheal doses to 1-2 mL with normal saline.

Asystole/pulseless arrest, bradycardia, VT/VF (after failed defibrillations):

I.V., I.O.: Infants and Children: 0.01 mg/kg (0.1 mL/kg of **1:10,000** solution) every 3-5 minutes as needed (maximum: 1 mg)

Intratracheal: Infants and Children: 0.1 mg/kg (0.1 mL/kg of **1:1000** solution) every 3-5 minutes (maximum: 10 mg)

Continuous I.V. infusion: Infants and Children: 0.1-1 mcg/kg/; doses <0.3 mcg/kg/minute generally produce β-adrenergic effects and higher doses generally produce α-adrenergic vasoconstriction; titrate dosage to desired effect

Bronchodilator: *SubQ:* Infants and Children:0.01 mg/kg (0.01 mL/kg of **1:1000**) (single doses not to exceed 0.5 mg) every 20 minutes for 3 doses

Nebulization: Infants and Children: 1-3 inhalations up to every 3 hours using solution prepared with 10 drops of **1:100**

Children <4 years: S2® (racepinephrine, OTC labeling): Croup: 0.05 mL/kg (max 0.5 mL/dose); dilute in NS 3 mL. Administer over ~15 minutes; do not administer more frequently than every 2 hours.

Inhalation: Children ≥4 years: Primatene® Mist: Refer to adult dosing.

Decongestant: Children ≥6 years: Refer to adult dosing.

Hypersensitivity reaction:

SubQ, I.V.: 0.01 mg/kg every 20 minutes; larger doses or continuous infusion may be needed for some anaphylactic reactions

SubQ, I.M.:

15-30 kg (Twinject™): 0.15 mg (for self-administration following severe allergic reactions to insect stings, food, etc)

>30 kg: Refer to adult dosing.

I.M.:

<30 kg (Epipen® Jr): 0.15 mg (for self-administration following severe allergic reactions to insect stings, food, etc)

>30 kg: Refer to adult dosing.

Administration

I.M.: I.M. administration into the buttocks should be avoided.

I.V.: Central line administration only. I.V. infusions require an infusion pump. Epinephrine solutions for injection can be administered SubQ, I.M., I.V., I.O.

I.V. Detail: Extravasation management: Use phentolamine as antidote. Mix 5 mg with 9 mL of NS. Inject a small amount of this dilution into extravasated area. Blanching should reverse immediately. Monitor site. If blanching should recur, additional injections of phentolamine may be needed.

pH: 2.5-5.0

Inhalation: S2®: Administer over ~15 minutes; must be diluted if using jet nebulizer

Other: Intratracheal: Dilute in NS or distilled water. Absorption is greater with distilled water, but causes more adverse effects on PaO$_2$. Pass catheter beyond tip of tracheal tube, stop compressions, spray drug quickly down tube. Follow immediately with several quick insufflations and continue chest compressions.

Stability

Reconstitution:

Standard I.V. diluent: 1 mg/250 mL NS

Preparation of adult I.V. infusion: Dilute 1 mg in 250 mL of D$_5$W or NS (4 mcg/mL). Administer at an initial rate of 1 mcg/minute and increase to desired effects. At 20 mcg/minute pure alpha effects occur.

S2®: Dilution not required when administered via hand-nebulizer; dilute with NS 3-5 mL if using jet nebulizer

Compatibility: Stable in dextran 6% in dextrose, dextran 6% in NS, D$_5$LR, D$_5$¼NS, D$_5$½NS, D$_5$NS, D$_5$W, D$_{10}$W, D$_{10}$NS, LR, NS; **incompatible** with sodium bicarbonate 5%

Y-site administration: Incompatible with ampicillin, thiopental

Compatibility when admixed: Incompatible with aminophylline, hyaluronidase, mephentermine, sodium bicarbonate

Storage: Epinephrine is sensitive to light and air. Protection from light is recommended. Oxidation turns drug pink, then a brown color. **Solutions should not be used if they are discolored or contain a precipitate.**

Adrenalin®: Store between 15°C to 25°C (59°F to 77°F); protect from light and freezing. The 1:1000 solution should be discarded 30 days after initial use.

Raphon: Store between 2°C to 25°C (36°F to 77°F). Refrigerate after opening.

Twinject™: Store between 20°C to 25°C (68°F to 77°F); protect from light and freezing. Do not refrigerate.

Stability of injection of parenteral admixture at room temperature (25°C) or refrigeration (4°C) is 24 hours.

Nursing Actions

Physical Assessment: Assess other medications patient may be taking for effectiveness and interactions. Monitor therapeutic response (according to purpose for use) and adverse reactions (eg, hypertension, CNS excitability, urinary retention, dysrhythmias, respiratory depression). Assess knowledge/teach patient appropriate use, interventions to reduce side effects, and adverse symptoms to report. **I.V.** (cardiovascular therapy): Central line with infusion pump and continuous cardiac/hemodynamic monitoring is necessary.

Patient Education: Use this medication exactly as directed; do not take more than recommended dosage. Avoid other stimulant prescriptive or OTC medications to avoid serious overdose reactions. You may experience dizziness, blurred vision, restlessness (use caution when driving or engaging in tasks requiring alertness until response to drug is known); or difficulty urinating (empty bladder immediately before taking this medication). Report excessive nervousness or excitation, inability to sleep, facial flushing, pounding heartbeat, muscle tremors or weakness, chest pain or palpitations, bronchial irritation or coughing, or increased sweating.

Aerosol: Use aerosol or nebulizer as per instructions. Clear as much mucus as possible before use. Rinse mouth following each use. If more than one inhalation is necessary, wait 1 minute between inhalations. May cause restlessness or nervousness; use caution when driving or engaging in hazardous activities until response to medication is known. Report persistent nervousness, restlessness, sleeplessness, palpitations, tachycardia, chest pain, muscle tremors, dizziness, flushing, or if breathing difficulty persists.

Pregnancy/breast-feeding precautions: Inform prescriber if you are or intend to become pregnant. Consult prescriber if breast-feeding.

Geriatric Considerations The use of epinephrine in the treatment of acute exacerbations of asthma was studied in older adults. A dose of 0.3 mg SubQ every 20 minutes for three doses was well tolerated in older patients with no history of angina or recent myocardial infarction. There was no significant difference in the incidence of ventricular arrhythmias in older adults versus younger adults.

Pregnancy Issues Crosses the placenta. Reported association with malformations in 1 study; may be secondary to severe maternal disease.

Related Information
Compatibility of Drugs *on page 1370*

Epirubicin (ep i ROO bi sin)

U.S. Brand Names Ellence®

Synonyms Pidorubicin; Pidorubicin Hydrochloride

Pharmacologic Category Antineoplastic Agent, Anthracycline

Medication Safety Issues
Sound-alike/look-alike issues:
Epirubicin may be confused with DOXOrubicin, DAUNOrubicin, idarubicin
Ellence® may be confused with Elase®

Pregnancy Risk Factor D

Lactation Excretion in breast milk unknown/contraindicated

Use Adjuvant therapy for primary breast cancer

Mechanism of Action/Effect Epirubicin inhibits DNA and RNA synthesis throughout the cell cycle.

Contraindications Hypersensitivity to epirubicin, other anthracyclines, or anthracenediones; severe myocardial insufficiency; severe arrhythmias; recent myocardial infarction; severe hepatic dysfunction; baseline neutrophil count 1500 cells/mm³; previous anthracycline treatment up to maximum cumulative dose; pregnancy

Warnings/Precautions Hazardous agent — use appropriate precautions for handling and disposal. The primary toxicity is myelosuppression; severe thrombocytopenia or anemia may occur. Thrombophlebitis and thromboembolic phenomena (including pulmonary embolism) have occurred.

Potential cardiotoxicity, particularly in patients who have received prior anthracyclines, prior radiotherapy to the mediastinal/pericardial area, or who have pre-existing cardiac disease, may occur. Acute toxicity (primarily arrhythmias) and delayed toxicity (CHF) have been described. Delayed toxicity usually develops late in the course of therapy or within 2-3 months after completion, however, events with an onset of several months to years after termination of treatment have been described. The risk of delayed cardiotoxicity increases more steeply at dosages above 900 mg/m², and this dose should be exceeded only with extreme caution. Toxicity may be additive with other anthracyclines or anthracenediones, and may be increased in pediatric patients. Regular monitoring of LVEF and discontinuation at the first sign of impairment is recommended especially in patients with risk factors or impaired cardiac function.

Reduce dosage and use with caution in mild to moderate hepatic impairment or in severe renal dysfunction (serum creatinine >5 mg/dL). May cause tumor lysis syndrome or radiation recall. Treatment with anthracyclines may increase the risk of secondary leukemias. For I.V. administration only, severe local tissue necrosis will result if extravasation occurs. Epirubicin is emetogenic. Women ≥70 years of age should be especially monitored for toxicity; women of childbearing age should be advised to avoid becoming pregnant.

Drug Interactions
Increased Effect/Toxicity: Cimetidine increased the blood levels of epirubicin (AUC increased by 50%).

Nutritional/Ethanol Interactions
Ethanol: Avoid ethanol (due to GI irritation).
Herb/Nutraceutical: St John's wort may decrease doxorubicin levels. Avoid black cohosh, dong quai in estrogen-dependent tumors.

Adverse Reactions
>10%:
Central nervous system: Lethargy (1% to 46%)
Dermatologic: Alopecia (69% to 95%)
Endocrine & metabolic: Amenorrhea (69% to 72%), hot flashes (5% to 39%)
Gastrointestinal: Nausea, vomiting (83% to 92%), mucositis (9% to 59%), diarrhea (7% to 25%)
Hematologic: Leukopenia (49% to 80%; Grade 3 and 4: 1.5% to 58.6%), neutropenia (54% to 80%), anemia (13% to 72%), thrombocytopenia (5% to 49%)
Local: Injection site reactions (3% to 20%)
Ocular: Conjunctivitis (1% to 15%)
Miscellaneous: Infection (15% to 21%)
1% to 10%:
Cardiovascular: CHF (0.4% to 1.5%), decreased LVEF (asymptomatic) (1.4% to 2.1%); recommended maximum cumulative dose: 900 mg/m²
Central nervous system: Fever (1% to 5%)
Dermatologic: Rash (1% to 9%), skin changes (0.7% to 5%)
Gastrointestinal: Anorexia (2% to 3%)
Other reactions (percentage not specified): Acute lymphoid leukemia, acute myelogenous leukemia (0.3% at 3 years, 0.5% at 5 years, 0.6% at 8 years), anaphylaxis, hypersensitivity, photosensitivity reaction, premature menopause in women, pulmonary embolism, radiation recall, skin and nail hyperpigmentation, thromboembolic phenomena, thrombophlebitis, transaminases increased, urticaria

Overdosage/Toxicology Symptoms of overdose are generally extensions of known cytotoxic effects, including myelosuppression, mucositis, gastrointestinal (Continued)

Epirubicin (Continued)

bleeding, lactic acidosis, multiple organ failure, and death. Treatment is supportive.

Pharmacodynamics/Kinetics

Protein Binding: 77% to albumin

Half-Life Elimination: Triphasic; Mean terminal: 33 hours

Metabolism: Extensive via hepatic and extrahepatic (including RBCs) routes

Excretion: Feces; urine (lesser extent)

Available Dosage Forms Injection, solution [preservative free]: 2 mg/mL (25 mL, 100 mL)

Dosing

Adults: I.V.: 100-120 mg/m^2 once weekly every 3-4 weeks **or** 50-60 mg/m^2 days 1 and 8 every 3-4 weeks

Breast cancer:

CEF-120: 60 mg/m^2 on days 1 and 8 every 28 days for 6 cycles

FEC-100: 100 mg/m^2 on day 1 every 21 days for 6 cycles

Note: Note: Patients receiving 120 mg/m^2/cycle as part of combination therapy should also receive prophylactic therapy with sulfamethoxazole/trimethoprim or a fluoroquinolone.

Dosage modifications:

Delay day 1 dose until platelets are ≥100,000/mm^3, ANC ≥1500/mm^3, and nonhematologic toxicities have recovered to ≤grade 1

Reduce day 1 dose in subsequent cycles to 75% of previous day 1 dose if patient experiences nadir platelet counts <50,000/mm^3, ANC <250/mm^3, neutropenic fever, or grade 3/4 nonhematologic toxicity during the previous cycle

For divided doses (day 1 and day 8), reduce day 8 dose to 75% of day 1 dose if platelet counts are 75,000-100,000/mm^3 and ANC is 1000-1499/mm^3; omit day 8 dose if platelets are <75,000/mm^3, ANC <1000/mm^3, or grade 3/4 nonhematologic toxicity

Dosage adjustment in bone marrow dysfunction: Heavily-treated patients, patients with pre-existing bone marrow depression or neoplastic bone marrow infiltration: Lower starting doses (75-90 mg/mm^2) should be considered.

Elderly: Plasma clearance of epirubicin in elderly female patients was noted to be reduced by 35%. Although no initial dosage reduction is specifically recommended, particular care should be exercised in monitoring toxicity and adjusting subsequent dosage in elderly patients (particularly females >70 years of age).

Renal Impairment: Severe renal impairment (serum creatinine >5 mg/dL): Lower doses should be considered.

Hepatic Impairment:

Bilirubin 1.2-3 mg/dL or AST 2-4 times the upper limit of normal: 50% of recommended starting dose.

Bilirubin >3 mg/dL or AST >4 times the upper limit of normal: 25% of recommended starting dose.

Administration

I.V.: The manufacturer recommends that starting doses of 100-120 mg/m^2 should be infused over 15-20 minutes; lower doses may be pushed into the tubing of a free-flowing intravenous infusion (NS or D$_5$W) over 3-10 minutes.

Stability

Reconstitution: May administer undiluted for IVP or dilute in 50-250 mL NS or D$_5$W for infusion.

Compatibility: Stable in D$_5$W, LR, NS; **incompatible** with any solution of alkaline pH

Incompatible with heparin, fluorouracil

Compatibility in syringe: Incompatible with fluorouracil, ifosfamide with mesna, any solution of alkaline pH

Storage: Store refrigerated at 2°C to 8°C (36°F to 46°F). Protect from light. Solution should be used within 24 hours.

Laboratory Monitoring CBC with differential and platelet count, liver function tests, renal function, ECG, and left ventricular ejection fraction (baseline and repeated measurement). The method used for assessment of LVEF (echocardiogram or MUGA) should be consistent during routine monitoring.

Nursing Actions

Physical Assessment: Note infusion specifics in Administration. Premedication with an antiemetic may be ordered (emetogenic). Monitor infusion site closely to prevent extravasation; severe local tissue necrosis will result if extravasation occurs. Monitor laboratory tests and patient response (eg, acute nausea and vomiting, anemia, cardiotoxicity, infection, bleeding) prior to each treatment and on a regular basis throughout therapy. Teach patient possible side effects/appropriate interventions (eg, importance of adequate hydration) and adverse symptoms to report.

Patient Education: Do not take any new medication during therapy unless approved by prescriber. This medication can only be administered by infusion. Report immediately any swelling, pain, burning, or redness at infusion site, sudden difficulty breathing or swallowing, chest pain, or chills. Maintain adequate hydration (2-3 L/day of fluids) unless instructed to restrict fluid intake, and adequate nutrition (small, frequent meals may help). You will be more susceptible to infection (avoid crowds and exposure to infection and do not have any vaccinations without consulting prescriber). May cause nausea or vomiting (small, frequent meals, frequent mouth care, sucking lozenges, or chewing gum may help); diarrhea (buttermilk, boiled milk, or yogurt may help); loss of hair (reversible); hyperpigmentation of skin or nails; mouth sores (frequent mouth care, soft toothbrush may help); or changes in menstrual cycle (consult prescriber). Report chest pain, swelling of extremities, palpitations, or rapid heartbeat; respiratory difficulty or unusual cough; pain, redness, unusual warmth in extremities; unresolved nausea, vomiting, or diarrhea; alterations in urinary pattern (increased or decreased); opportunistic infection (fever, chills, unusual bruising or bleeding, fatigue, purulent vaginal discharge, unhealed mouth sores); skin rash; abdominal pain; blood in urine or stool; or other unresolved reactions. **Pregnancy/breast-feeding precautions:** Do not get pregnant while taking this medication and for 1 month following therapy. Consult prescriber for appropriate barrier contraceptives. Do not breast-feed.

Breast-Feeding Issues Excretion in human breast milk is unknown, however, other anthracyclines are excreted. Breast-feeding is contraindicated.

Pregnancy Issues Epirubicin is mutagenic and carcinogenic. If a pregnant woman is treated with epirubicin, or if a woman becomes pregnant while receiving this drug, she should be informed of the potential hazard to the fetus. Women of childbearing potential should be advised to avoid becoming pregnant.

Eplerenone (e PLER en one)

U.S. Brand Names Inspra™

Pharmacologic Category Diuretic, Potassium-Sparing; Selective Aldosterone Blocker

Medication Safety Issues

Sound-alike/look-alike issues:

Inspra™ may be confused with Spiriva®

Pregnancy Risk Factor B

Lactation Excretion in breast milk unknown/not recommended

Use Treatment of hypertension (may be used alone or in combination with other antihypertensive agents); treatment of CHF following acute MI

Mechanism of Action/Effect Aldosterone increases blood pressure primarily by inducing sodium reabsorption. Eplerenone reduces blood pressure by blocking aldosterone binding at mineralocorticoid receptors found in the kidney, heart, blood vessels and brain.

Contraindications Hypersensitivity to eplerenone or any component of the formulation; serum potassium >5.5 mEq/L; Cl$_{cr}$ ≤30 mL/minute; concomitant use of strong CYP3A4 inhibitors (see Drug Interactions for details)

The following additional contraindications apply to patients with hypertension: Type 2 diabetes mellitus (noninsulin dependent, NIDDM) with microalbuminuria; serum creatinine >2.0 mg/dL in males or >1.8 mg/dL in females; Cl$_{cr}$ <50 mL/minute; concomitant use with potassium supplements or potassium-sparing diuretics

Warnings/Precautions Dosage adjustment needed for patients on moderate CYP3A4 inhibitors (see drug interactions for details). Monitor closely for hyperkalemia; increases in serum potassium were dose related during clinical trials and rates of hyperkalemia also increased with declining renal function. Safety and efficacy have not been established in pediatric patients or in patients with severe hepatic impairment. Use with caution in CHF patients post-MI with diabetes.

Drug Interactions

Cytochrome P450 Effect: Substrate of CYP3A4 (major)

Decreased Effect: NSAIDs may decrease the antihypertensive effects of eplerenone. CYP3A4 inducers may decrease the levels/effects of eplerenone; example inducers include aminoglutethimide, carbamazepine, nafcillin, nevirapine, phenobarbital, phenytoin, and rifamycins.

Increased Effect/Toxicity: ACE inhibitors, angiotensin II receptor antagonists, NSAIDs, potassium supplements, and potassium-sparing diuretics increase the risk of hyperkalemia; concomitant use with potassium supplements and potassium-sparing diuretics is contraindicated; monitor potassium levels with ACE inhibitors and angiotensin II receptor antagonists. Potent CYP3A4 inhibitors (eg, itraconazole, ketoconazole) lead to fivefold increase in eplerenone; concurrent use is contraindicated. Less potent CYP3A4 inhibitors (eg, erythromycin, fluconazole, saquinavir, verapamil) lead to approximately twofold increase in eplerenone; starting dose should be decreased to 25 mg/day. Although interaction studies have not been conducted, monitoring of lithium levels is recommended.

Nutritional/Ethanol Interactions

Food: Grapefruit juice increases eplerenone AUC ~25%.

Herb/Nutraceutical: St John's wort decreases eplerenone AUC ~30%.

Adverse Reactions

>10%: Endocrine & metabolic: Hypertriglyceridemia (1% to 15%, dose related)

1% to 10%:
Central nervous system: Dizziness (3%), fatigue (2%)
Endocrine & metabolic: Breast pain (males <1% to 1%), serum creatinine increased (6% in CHF), gynecomastia (males <1% to 1%), hyponatremia (2%, dose related), hypercholesterolemia (<1% to 1%); hyperkalemia (mild-to-moderate hypertension <1%; left ventricular dysfunction ~6% had serum potassium ≥6 mEq/L)
Gastrointestinal: Diarrhea (2%), abdominal pain (1%)
Genitourinary: Abnormal vaginal bleeding (<1% to 2%)
Renal: Albuminuria (1%)
Respiratory: Cough (2%)
Miscellaneous: Flu-like syndrome (2%)

Overdosage/Toxicology Cases of human overdose have not been reported; hypotension or hyperkalemia would be expected. Treatment should be symptom-directed and supportive. Eplerenone is not removed by hemodialysis; binds extensively to charcoal.

Pharmacodynamics/Kinetics

Time to Peak: Plasma: 1.5 hours; may take up to 4 weeks for full therapeutic effect

Protein Binding: ~50%; primarily to alpha$_1$-acid glycoproteins

Half-Life Elimination: 4-6 hours

Metabolism: Primarily hepatic via CYP3A4; metabolites inactive

Excretion: Urine (67%; <5% as unchanged drug), feces (32%)

Available Dosage Forms Tablet: 25 mg, 50 mg

Dosing

Adults:

Hypertension: Oral: Initial: 50 mg once daily; may increase to 50 mg twice daily if response is not adequate; may take up to 4 weeks for full therapeutic response. Doses >100 mg/day are associated with increased risk of hyperkalemia and no greater therapeutic effect.

Dose modification during concurrent use with moderate CYP3A4 inhibitors: Initial: 25 mg once daily

Congestive heart failure (post-MI): Oral: Initial: 25 mg once daily; dosage goal: titrate to 50 mg once daily within 4 weeks, as tolerated

Dosage adjustment per serum potassium concentrations for CHF:

Serum level <5.0 mEq/L:
Increase dose from 25 mg every other day to 25 mg daily **or**
Increase dose from 25 mg daily to 50 mg daily

5.0-5.4 mEq/L: No adjustment needed

5.5-5.9 mEq/L:
Decrease dose from 50 mg daily to 25 mg daily **or**
Decrease dose from 25 mg daily to 25 mg every other day **or**
Decrease does from 25 mg every other day to withhold medication

Potassium level ≥6.0 mEq/L: Withhold medication until potassium <5.5 mEq/L, then restart at 25 mg every other day

Elderly: See Geriatric Considerations.

Renal Impairment:

Patients with hypertension with Cl$_{cr}$ <50 mL/minute or serum creatinine >2.0 mg/dL in males or >1.8 mg/dL in females: Use is contraindicated; risk of hyperkalemia increases with declining renal function.

Patients with CHF post-MI: Use with caution.

Hepatic Impairment: No dosage adjustment needed for mild-to-moderate impairment. Safety and efficacy not established for severe impairment.

Administration

Oral: May be administered with or without food.

Stability

Storage: Store at controlled room temperature of 25°C (77°F).

Laboratory Monitoring Serum potassium (levels monitored every 2 weeks for the first 1-2 months, then monthly in clinical trials); renal function

Nursing Actions

Physical Assessment: Assess potential for interactions with other pharmacological agents or herbal products patient may be taking (eg, increased risk of toxicity). Monitor laboratory tests (eg, potassium levels, renal function) prior to and periodically during therapy, therapeutic effectiveness (blood pressure), and adverse response (eg, hypotension, hyperkalemia) at beginning of and at regular intervals during therapy. Teach patient proper use, possible side
(Continued)

Eplerenone *(Continued)*

effects/appropriate interventions, and adverse reactions to report.

Patient Education: Do not take any new medication during therapy without consulting prescriber. Take exactly as directed at the same time of day, without regard for meals. Do not alter dose or discontinue without consulting prescriber; it may take up to 4 weeks to achieve desired results. Do not use potassium supplement or salt substitutes without consulting prescriber. This drug does not eliminate need for diet or exercise regimen as recommended by prescriber. May cause dizziness, fainting, lightheadedness (use caution when driving or engaging in tasks that require alertness until response to drug is known); postural hypotension (use caution when rising from lying or sitting position or climbing stairs); diarrhea (boiled milk, buttermilk, or yogurt may help); breast pain (males); abnormal vaginal bleeding. Report chest pain, palpitations; unusual cough or flu-like symptoms; or other persistent or severe adverse effects.

Breast-feeding precaution: Breast-feeding is not recommended.

Dietary Considerations May be taken with or without food. Do not use salt substitutes containing potassium.

Geriatric Considerations Since this medication is contraindicated in patients with a Cl$_{cr}$ <50 mL/minute, it will have limited use in older adults. Due to physiologic changes older adults may be at increased risk of hyperkalemia when using this medication.

Epoetin Alfa *(e POE e tin AL fa)*

U.S. Brand Names Epogen®; Procrit®

Synonyms EPO; Erythropoietin; rHuEPO-α

Pharmacologic Category Colony Stimulating Factor

Medication Safety Issues
Sound-alike/look-alike issues:
Epoetin alfa may be confused with darbepoetin alfa

Pregnancy Risk Factor C

Lactation Excretion in breast milk unknown/use caution

Use Treatment of anemia related to HIV therapy, chronic renal failure, antineoplastic therapy; reduction of allogeneic blood transfusion for elective, noncardiac, nonvascular surgery

Unlabeled/Investigational Use Anemia associated with rheumatic disease; hypogenerative anemia of Rh hemolytic disease; sickle cell anemia; acute renal failure; Gaucher's disease; Castleman's disease; paroxysmal nocturnal hemoglobinuria; anemia of critical illness (limited documentation); anemia of prematurity

Mechanism of Action/Effect Induces red blood cell production in the bone marrow to be released into the blood stream where they mature to erythrocytes; results in rise in hematocrit and hemoglobin levels

Contraindications Hypersensitivity to albumin (human) or mammalian cell-derived products; uncontrolled hypertension

Warnings/Precautions Use caution with history of seizures or hypertension; blood pressure should be controlled prior to start of therapy and monitored closely throughout treatment. Excessive rate of rise of hematocrit may be possibly associated with the exacerbation of hypertension or seizures; decrease the epoetin dose if the hemoglobin increase exceeds 1 g/dL in any 2-week period. Use caution in patients at risk for thrombosis or with history of cardiovascular disease. Increased mortality has occurred when aggressive dosing is used in CHF or anginal patients undergoing hemodialysis.

Pure red cell aplasia (PRCA) with neutralizing antibodies to erythropoietin has been reported in limited patients treated with recombinant products; may occur more in patients with CRF.

Prior to and during therapy iron stores must be evaluated. Iron supplementation should be given during therapy. Use caution with porphyria. Not recommended for acute correction of severe anemia or as a substitute for transfusion.

Adverse Reactions Note: Adverse drug reaction incidences vary based on condition being treated and dose administered.

>10%:
Cardiovascular: Edema, hypertension
Central nervous system: Fever, headache, insomnia
Dermatologic: Pruritus, rash
Gastrointestinal: Dyspepsia, nausea, vomiting
Local: Injection site reaction
Neuromuscular & skeletal: Arthralgia, paresthesia, weakness
Respiratory: Congestion, cough, dyspnea, upper respiratory infection

1% to 10%:
Cardiovascular: Chest pain
Central nervous system: Fatigue, seizure
Gastrointestinal: Diarrhea
Hematologic: Clotted access, deep vein thrombosis

Overdosage/Toxicology Symptoms of overdose include erythrocytosis. Maintain adequate airway and provide other supportive measures and agents for treating anaphylaxis when the I.V. drug is given.

Pharmacodynamics/Kinetics
Onset of Action: Several days; Peak effect: 2-3 weeks
Time to Peak: Serum: SubQ: Chronic renal failure: 5-24 hours
Half-Life Elimination: Circulating: Chronic renal failure: 4-13 hours; Healthy volunteers: 20% shorter
Metabolism: Some degradation does occur
Excretion: Feces (majority); urine (small amounts, 10% unchanged in normal volunteers)

Available Dosage Forms
Injection, solution [preservative free]: 2000 units/mL (1 mL); 3000 units/mL (1 mL); 4000 units/mL (1 mL); 10,000 units/mL (1 mL); 40,000 units/mL (1 mL) [contains human albumin]
Injection, solution [with preservative]: 10,000 units/mL (2 mL); 20,000 units/mL (1 mL) [contains human albumin and benzyl alcohol]

Dosing
Adults & Elderly: Individuals with anemia due to iron deficiency, sickle cell disease, autoimmune hemolytic anemia, and bleeding, generally have appropriate endogenous EPO levels to drive erythropoiesis and would not ordinarily be candidates for EPO therapy.

Chronic renal failure patients: I.V., SubQ: Initial dose: 50-100 units/kg 3 times/week
Titration: Reduce dose by 25% when hemoglobin approaches 12 g/dL **or** when hemoglobin increases 1 g/dL in any 2-week period. Increase dose by 25% if hemoglobin does not increase by 2 g/dL after 8 weeks of therapy and hemoglobin is below suggested target range; suggested target hemoglobin range: 10-12 g/dL.
Maintenance dose: Individualize to target range; limit additional dosage increases to every 4 weeks (or longer)
Dialysis patients: Median dose: 75 units/kg 3 times/week
Nondialysis patients: Median dose: 75-150 units/kg

Zidovudine-treated, HIV-infected patients (patient with erythropoietin levels >500 mU/mL is unlikely to respond): I.V., SubQ: 100 units/kg 3 times/week for 8 weeks
Increase dose by 50-100 units/kg 3 times/week if response is not satisfactory in terms of reducing transfusion requirements or increasing hemoglobin after 8 weeks of therapy. Evaluate response every 4-8 weeks thereafter and adjust

the dose accordingly by 50-100 units/kg increments 3 times/week. If patient has not responded satisfactorily to a 300 unit/kg dose 3 times/week, a response to higher doses is unlikely. Stop dose if hemoglobin exceeds 13 g/dL and resume treatment at a 25% dose reduction when hemoglobin drops to 12 g/dL.

Cancer patients on chemotherapy: Treatment of patients with erythropoietin levels >200 mU/mL is **not recommended.** SubQ:

150 units/kg 3 times/week or 40,000 units once weekly; commonly used doses range from 10,000 units 3 times/week to 40,000-60,000 units once weekly.

Dose adjustment: If response is not satisfactory after a sufficient period of evaluation (8 weeks of 3 times/week and 4 weeks of once-weekly therapy), the dose may be increased every 4 weeks (or longer) up to 300 units/kg 3 times/week, **or** when dosed weekly, increased all at once to 60,000 units weekly. If patient does not respond, a response to higher doses is unlikely. Stop dose when hemoglobin drops to 12 g/dL; reduce dose by 25% if hemoglobin increases by 1 g/dL in any 2-week period.

Alternative dose (unlabeled dosing): Initial dose: 60,000 units once weekly for 8 weeks. **Dose adjustment:** If patient does not respond, a response to higher doses is unlikely. If response is adequate (hemoglobin increases >2 g/dL after 8 weeks), begin maintenance dose of 120,000 units, to be given once every 3 weeks. During any point of initial or maintenance therapy, if the hemoglobin increases 1.3 g/dL in a 2-week period, decrease dose to 40,000 units once weekly. Stop dose if hemoglobin exceeds 15 g/dL and resume treatment at 20,000 units once-weekly when hemoglobin drops to 13 g/dL (Patton, 2003).

Surgery patients: Prior to initiating treatment, obtain a hemoglobin to establish that is >10 mg/dL or ≤13 mg/dL: SubQ: Initial dose: 300 units/kg/day for 10 days before surgery, on the day of surgery, and for 4 days after surgery

Alternative dose: 600 units/kg in once weekly doses (21, 14, and 7 days before surgery) plus a fourth dose on the day of surgery

Anemia of critical illness (unlabeled use): SubQ: 40,000 units once weekly

Pediatrics:

Anemia of prematurity (unlabeled use): Infants: I.V., SubQ: Dosing range: 500-1250 units/kg/week; commonly used dose: 250 units/kg 3 times/week; supplement with oral iron therapy 3-8 mg/kg/day

Chronic renal failure patients: I.V., SubQ: Initial dose: 50 units/kg 3 times/week

Dosage adjustment: Reduce dose by 25% when hemoglobin approaches 12 g/dL **or** when hemoglobin increases 1 g/dL in any 2-week period. Increase dose by 25% if hemoglobin does not increase by 2 g/dL after 8 weeks of therapy and hemoglobin is below suggested target range; suggested target hemoglobin range: 10-12 g/dL

Maintenance dose: Individualize to target range; limit additional dosage increases to every 4 weeks (or longer)

Dialysis patients: Median dose: 167 units/kg/week **or** 76 units/kg 2-3 times/week

Nondialysis patients: Dosing range: 50-250 units/kg 1-3 times/week

Zidovudine-treated, HIV-infected patients (patient with erythropoietin levels >500 mU/mL is unlikely to respond): I.V., SubQ: Initial dose: Reported dosing range: 50-400 units/kg 2-3 times/week

Cancer patients on chemotherapy: Treatment of patients with erythropoietin levels >200 mU/mL is

not recommended: I.V., SubQ: Dosing range: 25-300 units/kg 3-7 times/week; commonly reported initial dose: 150 units/kg

Dosage adjustment: If response is not satisfactory after a sufficient period of evaluation (8 weeks), the dose may be increased every 4 weeks (or longer) up to 300 units/kg 3 times/week. If patient does not respond, a response to higher doses is unlikely. Stop dose if hemoglobin exceeds 13 g/dL and resume treatment at a 25% dose reduction when hemoglobin drops to 12 g/dL; reduce dose by 25% if hemoglobin increases by 1 g/dL in any 2-week period, or if hemoglobin approaches 12 g/dL.

Renal Impairment:

Dialysis patient: Usually administered as I.V. bolus 3 times/week. While administration is independent of the dialysis procedure, it may be administered into the venous line at the end of the dialysis procedure to obviate the need for additional venous access.

Chronic renal failure patients not on dialysis: May be given either as an I.V. or SubQ injection.

Hemodialysis: Supplemental dose is not necessary.

Peritoneal dialysis: Supplemental dose is not necessary.

Administration

I.V.: I.V. (not recommended; I.V. administration may require up to 40% more drug as SubQ/I.M. administration to achieve the same therapeutic result)

Patients with CRF on dialysis: May be administered I.V. bolus into the venous line after dialysis.

Patients with CRF not on dialysis: May be administered I.V. or SubQ

I.V. Detail: pH: 6.6-7.2 (single dose vial); 5.8-6.4 (multidose vial)

Stability

Reconstitution: Prior to SubQ administration, preservative free solutions may be mixed with bacteriostatic NS containing benzyl alcohol 0.9% in a 1:1 ratio. Dilutions of 1:10 in $D_{10}W$ with human albumin 0.05% or 0.1% are stable for 24 hours.

Compatibility: Stable in $D_{10}W$ with albumin 0.05%, $D_{10}W$ with albumin 0.1%; **incompatible** with $D_{10}W$ with albumin 0.01%, $D_{10}W$, NS

Storage: Vials should be stored at 2°C to 8°C (36°F to 46°F); **do not freeze or shake.**

Single-dose 1 mL vial contains no preservative: Use one dose per vial; do not re-enter vial; discard unused portions.

Single-dose vials (except 40,000 units/mL vial) are stable for 2 weeks at room temperature; single-dose 40,000 units/mL vial is stable for 1 week at room temperature.

Multidose 1 mL or 2 mL vial contains preservative; store at 2°C to 8°C after initial entry and between doses; discard 21 days after initial entry.

Multidose vials (with preservative) are stable for 1 week at room temperature.

Prefilled syringes containing the 20,000 units/mL formulation with preservative are stable for 6 weeks refrigerated (2°C to 8°C).

Laboratory Monitoring Hematocrit should be determined twice weekly until stabilization within the target range (30% to 36%), and twice weekly for at least 2-6 weeks after a dose increase. See table on next page.

Nursing Actions

Physical Assessment: Note administration specifics. I.V. lines should be monitored closely for possible clotting. Monitor frequent laboratory tests (eg, hematocrit determination twice weekly), therapeutic effectiveness (correction of anemia), and adverse response (eg, hypovolemia, angioedema, postural hypotension, anemia) on a regular basis during therapy. Teach patient proper use if self-administered (appropriate SubQ injection technique and syringe/needle disposal), possible side effects/appropriate

(Continued)

Epoetin Alfa (Continued)

interventions (importance of maintaining laboratory schedule), and adverse symptoms to report.

Test	Initial Phase Frequency	Maintenance Phase Frequency
Hematocrit/hemoglobin	2 x/week	2-4 x/month
Blood pressure	3 x/week	3 x/week
Serum ferritin	Monthly	Quarterly
Transferrin saturation	Monthly	Quarterly
Serum chemistries including CBC with differential, creatinine, blood urea nitrogen, potassium, phosphorous	Regularly per routine	Regularly per routine

Patient Education: Do not take any new medication during therapy without consulting prescriber. If self-administered, follow exact directions for injection and needle disposal. You will require frequent blood tests to determine appropriate dosage and reduce potential for severe adverse effects; maintaining laboratory testing schedule is vital. Do not make significant changes in your dietary iron without consulting prescriber. Report signs or symptoms of edema (eg, swollen extremities, respiratory difficulty, rapid weight gain); onset of severe headache; acute back pain; chest pain; or muscular tremors or seizure activity. **Pregnancy/breast-feeding precautions:** Inform prescriber if you are or intend to become pregnant. Consult prescriber if breast-feeding.

Geriatric Considerations There is limited information about the use of epoetin alfa in the elderly. Endogenous erythropoietin secretion has been reported to be decreased in older adults with normocytic or iron-deficiency anemias or those with a serum hemoglobin concentration <12 g/dL; one study did not find such a relationship in the elderly with chronic anemia. A blunted erythropoietin response to anemia has been reported in patients with cancer, rheumatoid arthritis, and AIDS.

Breast-Feeding Issues When administered enterally to neonates (mixed with human milk or infant formula), rHuEPO-α did not significantly increase serum EPO concentrations. If passage via breast milk does occur, risk to a nursing infant appears low.

Factors Limiting Response to Epoetin Alfa

Factor	Mechanism
Iron deficiency	Limits hemoglobin synthesis
Blood loss/hemolysis	Counteracts epoetin alfa-stimulated erythropoiesis
Infection/inflammation	Inhibits iron transfer from storage to bone marrow
	Suppresses erythropoiesis through activated macrophages
Aluminum overload	Inhibits iron incorporation into heme protein
Bone marrow replacement Hyperparathyroidism Metastatic, neoplastic	Limits bone marrow volume
Folic acid/vitamin B_{12} deficiency	Limits hemoglobin synthesis
Patient compliance	Self-administered epoetin alfa or iron therapy

Pregnancy Issues Epoetin alpha has been shown to have adverse effects in rats when given in doses 5 times the human dose. Use only if potential benefit justifies the potential risk to the fetus.

Additional Information Due to the delayed onset of erythropoiesis (7-10 days to increase reticulocyte count; 2-6 weeks to increase hemoglobin), erythropoietin is of no value in the acute treatment of anemia. See table "Factors Limiting Response to Epoetin Alfa". Emergency/stat orders for erythropoietin are inappropriate.

Professional Services:

Amgen (Epogen®): 1-800-772-6436

Ortho Biotech (Procrit®): 1-800-325-7504

Reimbursement Assistance:

Amgen: 1-800-272-9376

Ortho Biotech: 1-800-553-3851

Epoprostenol (e poe PROST en ole)

U.S. Brand Names Flolan®

Synonyms Epoprostenol Sodium; PGI_2; PGX; Prostacyclin

Restrictions Orders for epoprostenol are distributed by two sources in the United States. Information on orders or reimbursement assistance may be obtained from either Accredo Health, Inc (1-800-935-6526) or TheraCom, Inc (1-877-356-5264).

Pharmacologic Category Prostaglandin

Pregnancy Risk Factor B

Lactation Excretion in breast milk unknown/use caution

Use Treatment of idiopathic pulmonary arterial hypertension [IPAH]; pulmonary hypertension associated with the scleroderma spectrum of disease [SSD] in NYHA Class III and Class IV patients who do not respond adequately to conventional therapy

Mechanism of Action/Effect Naturally occurring prostacyclin (PGI_2) which acts as a strong vasodilator in all vascular beds; inhibits platelet aggregation

Contraindications Hypersensitivity to epoprostenol or to structurally-related compounds; chronic use in patients with CHF due to severe left ventricular systolic dysfunction; patients who develop pulmonary edema during dose initiation

Warnings/Precautions Abrupt interruptions or large sudden reductions in dosage may result in rebound pulmonary hypertension. Some patients with primary pulmonary hypertension have developed pulmonary edema during dose ranging, which may be associated with pulmonary veno-occlusive disease. During chronic use, unless contraindicated, anticoagulants should be coadministered to reduce the risk of thromboembolism. Use cautiously with patients who have bleeding tendencies (inhibits platelet aggregation).

Drug Interactions

Increased Effect/Toxicity: The hypotensive effects of epoprostenol may be exacerbated by other vasodilators, diuretics, or by using acetate in dialysis fluids. Patients treated with anticoagulants (heparins, warfarin, thrombin inhibitors) or antiplatelet agents (ticlopidine, clopidogrel, IIb/IIIa antagonists, aspirin) and epoprostenol should be monitored for increased bleeding risk.

Adverse Reactions

Note: Adverse events reported during dose initiation and escalation include flushing (58%), headache (49%), nausea/vomiting (32%), hypotension (16%), anxiety/nervousness/agitation (11%), chest pain (11%); abdominal pain, back pain, bradycardia, diaphoresis, dizziness, dyspepsia, dyspnea, hypoesthesia/paresthesia, musculoskeletal pain, and tachycardia are also reported. The following adverse events have been reported during chronic administration for IPAH. Although some may be related to the underlying disease state, anxiety, diarrhea, flu-like symptoms, flushing, headache, jaw pain, nausea, nervousness, and vomiting are clearly contributed to epoprostenol.

>10%:

Cardiovascular: Chest pain (67%), palpitation (63%), flushing (42%), tachycardia (35%), arrhythmia (27%), hemorrhage (19%), bradycardia (15%)

Central nervous system: Dizziness (83%), headache (83%), chills/fever/sepsis/flu-like symptoms (25%), anxiety/nervousness/tremor (21%)

Gastrointestinal: Nausea/vomiting (67%), diarrhea (37%)

Genitourinary: Weight loss (27%)

Local: Injection-site reactions: Infection (21%), pain (13%)

Neuromuscular & skeletal: Weakness (87%), jaw pain (54%), myalgia (44%), musculoskeletal pain (35%; predominantly involving legs and feet), hypoesthesia/hyperparesthesia/paresthesia (12%)

Respiratory: Dyspnea (90%)

1% to 10%:

Cardiovascular: Supraventricular tachycardia (8%), cerebrovascular accident (4%)

Central nervous system: Convulsion (4%)

Dermatologic: Rash (10%; conventional therapy 13%), pruritus (4%)

Endocrine & metabolic: Hypokalemia (6%)

Gastrointestinal: Constipation (6%), weight gain (6%)

Neuromuscular & skeletal: Arthralgia (6%)

Ocular: Amblyopia (8%), vision abnormality (4%)

Respiratory: Epistaxis (4%), pleural effusion (4%)

Overdosage/Toxicology Symptoms of overdose include headache, hypotension, tachycardia, nausea, vomiting, diarrhea, and flushing. If any of these symptoms occur, reduce the infusion rate until symptoms subside. If symptoms do not subside, consider drug discontinuation. Fatal cases of hypoxemia, hypotension, and respiratory arrest have been reported. Long-term overdose may lead to high output cardiac failure.

Pharmacodynamics/Kinetics

Half-Life Elimination: 6 minutes

Metabolism: Rapidly hydrolyzed; subject to some enzymatic degradation; forms one active metabolite and 13 inactive metabolites

Excretion: Urine (84%); feces (4%)

Available Dosage Forms Injection, powder for reconstitution, as sodium: 0.5 mg, 1.5 mg [provided with 50 mL sterile diluent]

Dosing

Adults & Elderly: IPAH or SSD: I.V.: Initial: 1-2 ng/kg/minute, increase dose in increments of 1-2 ng/kg/minute every 15 minutes or longer until dose-limiting side effects are noted or tolerance limit to epoprostenol is observed

Dose adjustment:

Increase dose in 1-2 ng/kg/minute increments at intervals of at least 15 minutes if symptoms persist or recur following improvement. In clinical trials, dosing increases occurred at intervals of 24-48 hours.

Decrease dose in 2 ng/kg/minute decrements at intervals of at least 15 minutes in case of dose-limiting pharmacologic events. Avoid abrupt withdrawal or sudden large dose reductions.

Lung transplant: In patients receiving lung transplants, epoprostenol was tapered after the initiation of cardiopulmonary bypass.

Pediatrics: Unlabeled use; refer to adult dosing.

Administration

I.V.:

The ambulatory infusion pump should be small and lightweight, be able to adjust infusion rates in 2 ng/kg/minute increments, have occlusion, end of infusion, and low battery alarms, have ± 6% accuracy of the programmed rate, and have positive continuous or pulsatile pressure with intervals ≤3 minutes between pulses. The reservoir should be made of

polyvinyl chloride, polypropylene, or glass. The infusion pump used in the most recent clinical trial was CADD-1 HFX 5100 (Pharmacia Deltec).

I.V. Detail: When given on an ongoing basis, must be infused through a central venous catheter. Peripheral infusion may be used temporarily until central line is established. Infuse using an infusion pump. Avoid abrupt withdrawal (including interruptions in delivery) or sudden large reductions in dosing. Patients should have access to a backup infusion pump and infusion sets.

pH: 10.2-10.8

Stability

Reconstitution: Reconstitute only with provided sterile diluent. See table.

Preparation of Epoprostenol Infusion

To make 100 mL of solution with concentration:	Directions
3000 ng/mL	Dissolve one 0.5 mg vial with 5 mL supplied diluent, withdraw 3 mL, and add to sufficient diluent to make a total of 100 mL.
5000 ng/mL	Dissolve one 0.5 mg vial with 5 mL supplied diluent, withdraw entire vial contents, and add a sufficient volume of diluent to make a total of 100 mL.
10,000 ng/mL	Dissolve two 0.5 mg vials each with 5 mL supplied diluent, withdraw entire vial contents, and add a sufficient volume of diluent to make a total of 100 mL.
15,000 ng/mL	Dissolve one 1.5 mg vial with 5 mL supplied diluent, withdraw entire vial contents, and add a sufficient volume of diluent to make a total of 100 mL.

Compatibility: Do not mix or administer with any other drugs prior to or during administration.

Storage: Prior to use, store vials at 15°C to 25°C (59°F to 77°F); protect from light, do not freeze. Following reconstitution, solution must be stored under refrigeration at 2°C to 8°C (36°F to 46°F) if not used immediately; protect from light, do not freeze; discard if refrigerated for >48 hours. During use, a single reservoir of solution may be used at room temperature for a total duration of 8 hours, or used with a cold pouch for administration up to 24 hours. Cold packs should be changed every 12 hours.

Nursing Actions

Physical Assessment: Institutional: Continuous pulmonary and hemodynamic arterial monitoring, protimes. **Noninstitutional:** Avoid sudden rate reduction or abrupt withdrawal or interruption of therapy. When adjustment in rate is made, monitor blood pressure (standing and supine) and pulse for several hours to ensure tolerance to new rate. Monitor for bleeding. Monitor (or teach appropriate caregiver or patient to monitor) vital signs on 3 times/day basis. Monitor for improved pulmonary function (decreased exertional dyspnea, fatigue, syncope, chest pain) and improved quality of life. Be alert for any infusion pump malfunction. Assess for signs of overdose (eg, hypoxia, flushing, tachycardia, fever, chills, anxiety, acute headache, tremor, vomiting, diarrhea).

Patient Education: Therapy on this drug will probably be prolonged, possibly for years. You may experience mild headache, nausea or vomiting, diarrhea, weight loss, nervousness, dizziness (use caution when driving or engaging in activities requiring alertness) and some muscular pains (use of a mild analgesia may be recommended by your prescriber). Report (Continued)

Epoprostenol (Continued)

immediately any signs or symptoms of acute or severe headache; back pain; increased difficult breathing; flushing; fever or chills; any unusual bleeding or bruising; chest pain; palpitations; irregular, slow or fast pulse; flushing; loss of sensation; or any onset of unresolved diarrhea. **Breast-feeding precaution:** Consult prescriber if breast-feeding.

Pregnancy Issues Teratogenic effects were not reported in animal studies. There are no adequate and well-controlled studies in pregnant women. Pregnant women with IPAH are encouraged to avoid pregnancy.

Eprosartan (ep roe SAR tan)

U.S. Brand Names Teveten®

Pharmacologic Category Angiotensin II Receptor Blocker

Pregnancy Risk Factor C (1st trimester); D (2nd and 3rd trimesters)

Lactation Not recommended

Use Treatment of hypertension; may be used alone or in combination with other antihypertensives

Mechanism of Action/Effect Eprosartan is an angiotensin receptor antagonist which blocks the vasoconstriction and aldosterone-secreting effects of angiotensin II.

Contraindications Hypersensitivity to eprosartan or any component of the formulation; sensitivity to other A-II receptor antagonists; bilateral renal artery stenosis; pregnancy (2nd and 3rd trimesters)

Warnings/Precautions Avoid use or use a smaller dose in patients who are volume depleted; correct depletion first. Deterioration in renal function can occur with initiation. Use with caution in unilateral renal artery stenosis and pre-existing renal insufficiency; significant aortic/mitral stenosis. Safety and efficacy in pediatric patients has not established.

Drug Interactions

Cytochrome P450 Effect: Inhibits CYP2C8/9 (weak)

Increased Effect/Toxicity: Eprosartan may increase risk of lithium toxicity. May increase risk of hyperkalemia with potassium-sparing diuretics (eg, amiloride, potassium, spironolactone, triamterene), potassium supplements, or high doses of trimethoprim.

Nutritional/Ethanol Interactions Herb/Nutraceutical: Avoid dong quai if using for hypertension (has estrogenic activity). Avoid ephedra, yohimbe, ginseng (may worsen hypertension). Avoid garlic (may have increased antihypertensive effect).

Adverse Reactions 1% to 10%:

Central nervous system: Fatigue (2%), depression (1%)

Endocrine & metabolic: Hypertriglyceridemia (1%)

Gastrointestinal: Abdominal pain (2%)

Genitourinary: Urinary tract infection (1%)

Respiratory: Upper respiratory tract infection (8%), rhinitis (4%), pharyngitis (4%), cough (4%)

Miscellaneous: Viral infection (2%), injury (2%)

Overdosage/Toxicology The most likely manifestations of overdose would be hypotension and tachycardia. Initiate supportive care for symptomatic hypotension.

Pharmacodynamics/Kinetics

Time to Peak: Serum: Fasting: 1-2 hours

Protein Binding: 98%

Half-Life Elimination: Terminal: 5-9 hours

Metabolism: Minimally hepatic

Excretion: Feces (90%); urine (7% primarily as unchanged drug)

Clearance: 7.9 L/hour

Available Dosage Forms Tablet: 400 mg, 600 mg

Dosing

Adults & Elderly: Hypertension: Oral: Dosage must be individualized. Can administer once or twice daily with total daily doses of 400-800 mg. Usual starting dose is 600 mg once daily as monotherapy in patients who are euvolemic. Limited clinical experience with doses >800 mg.

Renal Impairment: No starting dosage adjustment is necessary; however, carefully monitor the patient.

Hepatic Impairment: No starting dosage adjustment is necessary; however, carefully monitor the patient.

Laboratory Monitoring Electrolytes, serum creatinine, BUN, urinalysis

Nursing Actions

Physical Assessment: Assess potential for interactions with other pharmacological agents or herbal products patient may be taking. Monitor laboratory tests, therapeutic effectiveness, and adverse response (eg, hypotension) on a regular basis during therapy. Teach patient appropriate use, possible side effects/appropriate interventions, and adverse symptoms to report.

Patient Education: Do not take any new medication during therapy unless approved by prescriber. Take exactly as directed and do not discontinue without consulting prescriber. This drug does not eliminate need for diet or exercise regimen as recommended by prescriber. May cause dizziness, fainting, or light-headedness (use caution when driving or engaging in tasks that require alertness until response to drug is known); or postural hypotension (use caution when rising from lying or sitting position or climbing stairs). Report chest pain or palpitations; respiratory infection or cold symptoms; unusual cough; swelling of face, tongue, lips, or extremities; changes in urinary pattern; extreme fatigue; or other adverse response. **Pregnancy/breast-feeding precautions:** Inform prescriber if you are or intend to become pregnant. This drug should not be used in the 2nd or 3rd trimester of pregnancy. Consult prescriber for appropriate contraceptive measures if necessary. Breast-feeding is not recommended.

Pregnancy Issues Discontinue as soon as possible when pregnancy is detected. Drugs that act directly on renin-angiotensin can cause fetal and neonatal morbidity and death. Adverse effects to the fetus appear to be limited to the 2nd and 3rd trimesters.

Eprosartan and Hydrochlorothiazide
(ep roe SAR tan & hye droe klor oh THYE a zide)

U.S. Brand Names Teveten® HCT

Synonyms Eprosartan Mesylate and Hydrochlorothiazide; Hydrochlorothiazide and Eprosartan

Pharmacologic Category Angiotensin II Receptor Blocker Combination; Antihypertensive Agent, Combination; Diuretic, Thiazide

Pregnancy Risk Factor C/D (2nd and 3rd trimesters)

Lactation Excretion in breast milk unknown/not recommended

Use Treatment of hypertension (not indicated for initial treatment)

Available Dosage Forms Tablet:

600 mg/12.5 mg: Eprosartan 600 mg and hydrochlorothiazide 12.5 mg

600 mg/25 mg: Eprosartan 600 mg and hydrochlorothiazide 25 mg

Dosing

Adults & Elderly: Hypertension: Oral: Dose is individualized (combination substituted for individual components)

Usual recommended dose: Eprosartan 600 mg/hydrochlorothiazide 12.5 mg once daily (maximum dose: Eprosartan 600 mg/hydrochlorothiazide 25 mg once daily)

Renal Impairment: Initial dose adjustments not recommended by manufacturer; carefully monitor patient. Hydrochlorothiazide is ineffective in patients with Cl$_{cr}$ <30 mL/minute.

Hepatic Impairment: Initial dose adjustments not recommended by manufacturer; carefully monitor patient.

Nursing Actions
Physical Assessment: See individual components.

Patient Education: See individual agents. **Pregnancy/breast-feeding precautions:** Inform prescriber if you are or intend to become pregnant. Breast-feeding is not recommended.

Related Information
Eprosartan *on page 436*
Hydrochlorothiazide *on page 610*

Eptifibatide (ep TIF i ba tide)

U.S. Brand Names Integrilin®
Synonyms Intrifiban
Pharmacologic Category Antiplatelet Agent, Glycoprotein IIb/IIIa Inhibitor
Pregnancy Risk Factor B
Lactation Excretion in breast milk unknown/use caution
Use Treatment of patients with acute coronary syndrome (unstable angina/non-Q wave myocardial infarction [UA/NQMI]), including patients who are to be managed medically and those undergoing percutaneous coronary intervention (PCI including angioplasty, intracoronary stenting)

Mechanism of Action/Effect Eptifibatide is a IIb/IIa antagonist that reversibly blocks platelet aggregation and prevents thrombosis.

Contraindications Hypersensitivity to eptifibatide or any component of the product; active abnormal bleeding or a history of bleeding diathesis within the previous 30 days; history of CVA within 30 days or a history of hemorrhagic stroke; severe hypertension (systolic blood pressure >200 mm Hg or diastolic blood pressure >110 mm Hg) not adequately controlled on antihypertensive therapy; major surgery within the preceding 6 weeks; current or planned administration of another parenteral GP IIb/IIIa inhibitor; thrombocytopenia; dependency on renal dialysis

Warnings/Precautions Bleeding is the most common complication. Most major bleeding occurs at the arterial access site where the cardiac catheterization was done. When bleeding can not be controlled with pressure, discontinue infusion and heparin. Use caution in patients with hemorrhagic retinopathy or with other drugs that affect hemostasis. Concurrent use with thrombolytics has not been established as safe. Minimize other procedures including arterial and venous punctures, I.M. injections, nasogastric tubes, etc. Prior to sheath removal, the aPTT or ACT should be checked (do not remove unless aPTT is <45 seconds or the ACT <150 seconds). Use caution in renal dysfunction (estimated Cl$_{cr}$ <50 mL/minute); dosage adjustment required. Safety and efficacy in pediatric patients have not been determined.

Drug Interactions
Increased Effect/Toxicity: Eptifibatide effect may be increased by other drugs which affect hemostasis include thrombolytics, oral anticoagulants, NSAIDs, dipyridamole, heparin, low molecular weight heparins, ticlopidine, and clopidogrel. Avoid concomitant use of other IIb/IIIa inhibitors. Cephalosporins which contain the MTT side chain may theoretically increase the risk of hemorrhage. Use with aspirin and heparin may increase bleeding over aspirin and heparin alone. However, aspirin and heparin were used concurrently

in the majority of patients in the major clinical studies of eptifibatide. Antiplatelet agents (eg, eptifibatide) may enhance the adverse/toxic effect of drotrecogin alfa; bleeding may occur.

Nutritional/Ethanol Interactions Herb/Nutraceutical: Avoid alfalfa, anise, bilberry, bladderwrack, bromelain, cat's claw, celery, coleus, cordyceps, dong quai, evening primrose oil, fenugreek, feverfew, garlic, ginger, ginkgo biloba, ginseng (American), ginseng (Panax), ginseng (Siberian), grape seed, green tea, guggul, horse chestnut seed, horseradish, licorice, prickly ash, red clover, reishi, same (s-adenosylmethionine), sweet clover, turmeric, and white willow (all have additional antiplatelet activity).

Adverse Reactions Bleeding is the major drug-related adverse effect. Access site is often primary source of bleeding complications. Incidence of bleeding is also related to heparin intensity. Patients weighing <70 kg may have an increased risk of major bleeding.

>10%: Hematologic: Bleeding (major: 1% to 11%; minor: 3% to 14%; transfusion required: 2% to 13%)

1% to 10%:
Cardiovascular: Hypotension (up to 7%)
Hematologic: Thrombocytopenia (1% to 3%)
Local: Injection site reaction

Overdosage/Toxicology Two cases of human overdose have been reported; neither case was eventful or associated with major bleeding. Symptoms of overdose in animal studies include loss of righting reflex, dyspnea, ptosis, decreased muscle tone, and petechial hemorrhage. Treatment is supportive. Dialysis may be beneficial.

Pharmacodynamics/Kinetics
Onset of Action: Within 1 hour
Duration of Action: Platelet function restored ~4 hours following discontinuation
Protein Binding: ~25%
Half-Life Elimination: 2.5 hours
Excretion: Primarily urine (as eptifibatide and metabolites); significant renal impairment may alter disposition of this compound

Clearance: Total body: 55-58 mL/kg/hour; Renal: ~50% of total in healthy subjects

Available Dosage Forms Injection, solution: 0.75 mg/mL (100 mL); 2 mg/mL (10 mL, 100 mL)

Dosing
Adults:

Acute coronary syndrome: I.V.: Bolus of 180 mcg/kg (maximum: 22.6 mg) over 1-2 minutes, begun as soon as possible following diagnosis, followed by a continuous infusion of 2 mcg/kg/minute (maximum: 15 mg/hour) until hospital discharge or initiation of CABG surgery, up to 72 hours. Concurrent aspirin and heparin therapy (target aPTT 50-70 seconds) are recommended.

Percutaneous coronary intervention (PCI) with or without stenting: I.V.: Bolus of 180 mcg/kg (maximum: 22.6 mg) administered immediately before the initiation of PCI, followed by a continuous infusion of 2 mcg/kg/minute (maximum: 15 mg/hour). A second 180 mcg/kg bolus (maximum: 22.6 mg) should be administered 10 minutes after the first bolus. Infusion should be continued until hospital discharge or for up to 18-24 hours, whichever comes first. Concurrent aspirin (160-325 mg 1-24 hours before PCI and daily thereafter) and heparin therapy (ACT 200-300 seconds during PCI) are recommended. Heparin infusion after PCI is discouraged. In patients who undergo coronary artery bypass graft surgery, discontinue infusion prior to surgery.

Elderly: Refer to adult dosing. No dosing adjustment for the elderly appears to be necessary; adjust carefully to renal function.

Renal Impairment: Dialysis is a contraindication to use.

(Continued)

Eptifibatide *(Continued)*

Acute coronary syndrome: Cl$_{cr}$ <50 mL/minute: Use 180 mcg/kg bolus (maximum: 22.6 mg) and 1 mcg/kg/minute infusion (maximum: 7.5 mg/hour)

Percutaneous coronary intervention (PCI) with or without stenting: Cl$_{cr}$ <50 mL/minute: Use 180 mcg/kg bolus (maximum: 22.6 mg) administered immediately before the initiation of PCI and followed by a continuous infusion of 1 mcg/kg/minute (maximum: 7.5 mg/hour). A second 180 mcg/kg (maximum: 22.6 mg) bolus should be administered 10 minutes after the first bolus.

Administration

I.V.: Do not shake vial. Administer bolus doses by I.V. push over 1-2 minutes. Begin continuous infusion immediately following bolus administration; administer directly from the 100 mL vial.

I.V. Detail: Visually inspect for discoloration or particulate matter prior to administration. The bolus dose should be withdrawn from the 10 mL vial into a syringe. The 100 mL vial should be spiked with a vented infusion set.

Stability

Compatibility: Stable in NS (infusion may contain up to 60 mEq/L KCl), NS/D$_5$W (infusion may contain up to 60 mEq/L KCl)

Storage: Vials should be stored refrigerated at 2°C to 8°C (36°F to 46°F). Vials can be kept at room temperature for 2 months. Protect from light until administration. Do not use beyond the expiration date. Discard any unused portion left in the vial.

Laboratory Monitoring Laboratory tests at baseline and monitoring during therapy: Hematocrit and hemoglobin, platelet count, serum creatinine, PT/aPTT (maintain aPTT between 50-70 seconds unless PCI is to be performed), and ACT with PCI (maintain ACT between 200-300 seconds during PCI). Prior to sheath removal, the aPTT or ACT should be checked (do not remove unless aPTT is <45 seconds or the ACT <150 seconds).

Nursing Actions

Physical Assessment: Assess other medications for possible interactions or additive effects. Monitor vital signs and laboratory results prior to, during, and after therapy. Assess infusion insertion site during and after therapy (every 15 minutes or as institutional policy). Observe and teach patient bleeding precautions (avoid invasive procedures and activities that could result in injury). Monitor closely for signs of excessive bleeding (CNS changes; blood in urine, stool, or vomitus; unusual bruising or bleeding). Instruct patient about adverse reactions to report.

Patient Education: Emergency use may dictate depth of patient education. This medication can only be administered intravenously. You will have a tendency to bleed easily following this medication. Use caution to prevent injury (use electric razor, use soft toothbrush, use caution with sharps). If bleeding occurs, apply pressure to bleeding spot until bleeding stops completely. Report unusual bruising or bleeding (eg, blood in urine, stool, or vomitus, bleeding gums), dizziness or vision changes, or back pain. **Breast-feeding precaution:** Breast-feeding is not recommended.

Ergocalciferol *(er goe kal SIF e role)*

U.S. Brand Names Calciferol™; Drisdol®

Synonyms Activated Ergosterol; Viosterol; Vitamin D$_2$

Pharmacologic Category Vitamin D Analog

Medication Safety Issues
Sound-alike/look-alike issues:
Calciferol™ may be confused with calcitriol
Drisdol® may be confused with Drysol™

Pregnancy Risk Factor A/C (dose exceeding RDA recommendation)

Lactation Enters breast milk/compatible

Use Treatment of refractory rickets, hypophosphatemia, hypoparathyroidism; dietary supplement

Mechanism of Action/Effect Stimulates calcium and phosphate absorption from the small intestine, promotes secretion of calcium from bone to blood; promotes renal tubule phosphate resorption

Contraindications Hypersensitivity to ergocalciferol or any component of the formulation; hypercalcemia; malabsorption syndrome; evidence of vitamin D toxicity

Warnings/Precautions Administer with extreme caution in patients with impaired renal function, heart disease, renal stones, or arteriosclerosis. Must give concomitant calcium supplementation. Maintain adequate fluid intake. Avoid hypercalcemia. Renal function impairment with secondary hyperparathyroidism. Use as a dietary supplement is recommended for all breast-fed or nonbreast-fed infants receiving <500 mL/day of vitamin D-fortified formula, and in adults and children receiving <500 mL/day of vitamin D-fortified milk and who do not get regular sun exposure.

Drug Interactions

Decreased Effect: Cholestyramine, colestipol, mineral oil may decrease oral absorption.

Increased Effect/Toxicity: Thiazide diuretics may increase vitamin D effects. Cardiac glycosides may increase toxicity.

Adverse Reactions Generally well tolerated
Frequency not defined: Cardiac arrhythmia, hypertension (late), irritability, headache, psychosis (rare), somnolence, hyperthermia (late), pruritus, decreased libido (late), hypercholesterolemia, mild acidosis (late), polydipsia (late), nausea, vomiting, anorexia, pancreatitis, metallic taste, weight loss (rare), xerostomia, constipation, polyuria (late), increased BUN (late), increased LFTs (late), bone pain, myalgia, weakness, conjunctivitis, photophobia (late), vascular/nephrocalcinosis (rare)

Overdosage/Toxicology Symptoms of chronic overdose include hypercalcemia, weakness, fatigue, lethargy, and anorexia. Following withdrawal of the drug and oral decontamination, treatment consists of bedrest, liberal intake of fluids, reduced calcium intake, and cathartic administration. Severe hypercalcemia requires I.V. hydration and forced diuresis with I.V. furosemide. Urine output should be monitored and maintained at >2 mL/kg/hour during the acute treatment phase. I.V. saline can quickly and significantly increase excretion of calcium into urine. Calcitonin, mithramycin, and bisphosphonates have all been used successfully to treat the more resistant cases of vitamin D-induced hypercalcemia.

Pharmacodynamics/Kinetics

Onset of Action: Peak effect: ~1 month following daily doses

Metabolism: Inactive until hydroxylated hepatically and renally to calcifediol and then to calcitriol (most active form)

Available Dosage Forms [DSC] = Discontinued product
Capsule (Drisdol®): 50,000 int. units [1.25 mg; contains tartrazine and soybean oil]
Injection, solution (Calciferol™): 500,000 int. units/mL [12.5 mg/mL] (1 mL) [contains sesame oil] [DSC]

Liquid, drops (Calciferol™, Drisdol®): 8000 int. units/mL [200 mcg/mL] (60 mL) [OTC]

Dosing

Adults: Oral dosing is preferred; I.M. therapy is required with GI, liver, or biliary disease associated with malabsorption.

Dietary supplementation (each 1 mcg = 40 int. units): Oral:
18-50 years: 5 mcg/day (200 int. units/day)
51-70 years: 10 mcg/day (400 int. units/day)

Familial phosphatemia: 10,000-80,000 int. units/day and phosphorus 1-2 g/day

Renal failure: Oral: 500 mcg/day (20,000 int. units)

Hypoparathyroidism: Oral: 625 mcg to 5 mg/day (25,000-200,000 int. units) and calcium supplements

Vitamin D-dependent rickets: Oral: 250 mcg to 1.5 mg/day (10,000-60,000 int. units)

Nutritional rickets and osteomalacia: Oral:
With normal absorption: 25-125 mcg/day (1000-5000 int. units)
With malabsorption: 250-7500 mcg/day (10,000-300,000 int. units)

Vitamin D-resistant rickets: Oral: 250-1500 mcg/day (10,000-60,000 int. units) with phosphate supplements

Elderly: Refer to adult dosing (see Geriatric Considerations and Additional Information).
Dietary supplementation (each 1 mcg = 40 int. units):
>70 years: Oral: 15 mcg/day (600 int. units/day)

Pediatrics: Oral dosing is preferred; I.M. therapy is required with GI, liver, or biliary disease associated with malabsorption.

Dietary supplementation (each mcg = 40 int. units): Infants and Children: 5 mcg/day (200 int. units/day)

Renal failure: Children: 100-1000 mcg/day (4000-40,000 int. units)

Hypoparathyroidism: Children: 1.25-5 mg/day (50,000-200,000 int. units) and calcium supplements

Vitamin D-dependent rickets: Children: 75-125 mcg/day (3000-5000 int. units); maximum: 1500 mcg/day

Nutritional rickets and osteomalacia:
Children with normal absorption: 25-125 mcg/day (1000-5000 int. units)
Children with malabsorption: 250-625 mcg/day (10,000-25,000 int. units)

Vitamin D-resistant rickets: Children: Initial: 1000-2000 mcg/day (40,000-80,000 int. units) with phosphate supplements; daily dosage is increased at 3- to 4-month intervals in 250-500 mcg (10,000-20,000 int. units) increments

Familial hypophosphatemia: 10,000-80,000 units daily plus 1-2 g/day elemental phosphorus

Administration

I.M.: Parenteral injection is for I.M. use only.

Stability

Storage: Protect from light.

Laboratory Monitoring Serum calcium, BUN, phosphorus every 1-2 weeks

Nursing Actions

Physical Assessment: Assess effectiveness and interactions of other medications patient may be taking. Monitor lab tests, effectiveness of therapy, and adverse effects at beginning of therapy and regularly with long-term use. Teach patient proper use if self-administered (appropriate injection technique and syringe/needle disposal), appropriate nutritional counseling, possible side effects/interventions, and adverse symptoms to report.

Patient Education: Take exact dose prescribed; do not take more than recommended. Your prescriber may recommend a special diet; do not increase calcium intake without consulting prescriber. Avoid

magnesium supplements or magnesium-containing antacids. You may experience nausea, vomiting, or metallic taste (small frequent meals, frequent mouth care, or sucking hard candy may help). Report chest pain or palpitations; acute headache, dizziness, or feeling of weakness; unresolved nausea or vomiting; persistent metallic taste; unrelieved muscle or bone pain; or CNS irritability. **Pregnancy precaution:** Inform prescriber if you are pregnant.

Geriatric Considerations Recommended daily allowances (RDA) have not been developed for persons >65 years of age. Vitamin D, folate, and B_{12} (cyanocobalamin) have decreased absorption with age, but the clinical significance is yet unknown. Calorie requirements decrease with age and therefore, nutrient density must be increased to ensure adequate nutrient intake, including vitamins and minerals. Therefore, the use of a daily supplement with a multiple vitamin with minerals is recommended. Elderly consume less vitamin D, absorption may be decreased and many elderly have decreased sun exposure; therefore, elderly >70 years of age should receive supplementation with 600 units (15 mcg)/day. This is a recommendation of particular need to those with high risk for osteoporosis.

Additional Information Ergocalciferol 1.25 mg provides 50,000 int. units of vitamin D activity.

Erlotinib (er LOE tye nib)

U.S. Brand Names Tarceva™

Synonyms CP358774; Erlotinib Hydrochloride; NSC-718781; OSI-774; R 14-15

Pharmacologic Category Antineoplastic Agent, Tyrosine Kinase Inhibitor; Epidermal Growth Factor Receptor (EGFR) Inhibitor

Medication Safety Issues
Sound-alike/look-alike issues:
Erlotinib may be confused with gefitinib

Pregnancy Risk Factor D

Lactation Excretion in breast milk unknown/not recommended

Use Treatment of refractory advanced or metastatic nonsmall-cell lung cancer (NSCLC); pancreatic cancer (first-line therapy in combination with gemcitabine)

Unlabeled/Investigational Use Treatment of advanced or metastatic breast cancer, colorectal cancer, head and neck tumors, ovarian cancer, and renal cell cancer

Mechanism of Action/Effect Inhibits the intracellular phosphorylation of tyrosine kinase associated with epidermal growth factor receptor (EGFR) which is located on both normal and cancer cells causing cell death.

Contraindications Hypersensitivity to erlotinib or any component of the formulation; pregnancy

Warnings/Precautions Hazardous agent — use appropriate precautions for handling and disposal. Rare, sometimes fatal, pulmonary toxicity (interstitial pneumonia, interstitial lung disease, obliterative bronchiolitis, pulmonary fibrosis) has occurred; an interruption of therapy should occur with unexplained pulmonary symptoms (dyspnea, cough, and fever); use caution in hepatic or severe renal impairment. Use caution with cardiovascular disease; MI, CVA, and microangiopathic hemolytic anemia with thrombocytopenia have been noted in patients receiving concomitant erlotinib and gemcitabine. Elevated INR and bleeding events have been reported; use caution with concomitant anticoagulant therapy. Safety and efficacy in pediatric patients have not been established.

Drug Interactions

Cytochrome P450 Effect: Substrate of CYP1A2 (minor), 3A4 (major)
(Continued)

Erlotinib (Continued)

Decreased Effect: Rifamycins and CYP3A4 inducers may decrease erlotinib levels/effects; example inducers include aminoglutethimide, carbamazepine, nafcillin, nevirapine, phenobarbital, and phenytoin.

Increased Effect/Toxicity: Ketoconazole and CYP3A4 inhibitors may increase erlotinib levels/effects; example inhibitors include azole antifungals, clarithromycin, diclofenac, doxycycline, erythromycin, imatinib, isoniazid, nefazodone, nicardipine, propofol, protease inhibitors, quinidine, telithromycin, and verapamil.

Nutritional/Ethanol Interactions

Food: Erlotinib bioavailability is increased with food.

Herb/Nutraceutical: Avoid St John's wort (may increase metabolism and decrease erlotinib concentrations).

Adverse Reactions Percentages as reported with monotherapy; frequency of adverse event with combination chemotherapy (gemcitabine) noted where applicable

>10%:

Cardiovascular: Edema (37% combination)

Central nervous system: Fatigue (14% to 55%; 73% combination), pyrexia (36% combination), anxiety (21%), headache (17%), depression (16%; 19% combination), dizziness (15% combination), insomnia (12%; 15% combination)

Dermatologic: Acneiform rash (50% to 88%; grade 3/4: 9%), pruritus (13% to 55%), dry skin (12% to 35%), erythema (18%), alopecia (14% combination)

Gastrointestinal: Diarrhea (30% to 56%; grade 3/4: 6%), anorexia (23% to 52%), nausea (11% to 33%; 60% combination), vomiting (23%; 42% combination), mucositis (17% to 18%), glossodynia (18%), stomatitis (17%; 22% combination), xerostomia (17%), pain (14%), flatulence (13% combination); constipation (12%; 31% combination), dyspepsia (12%; 17% combination), dysphagia (12%), weight loss (12%; 39% combination), abnormal taste (11%), abdominal pain (11%; 46% combination)

Hepatic: ALT increased (4%; combination grade 2: 31%, grade 3: 13%, grade 4: <1%), AST increased (combination grade 2: 24%, grade 3: 10%, grade 4: <1%), hyperbilirubinemia (20%; combination grade 2: 17%, grade 3: 10%, grade 4: <1%)

Neuromuscular & skeletal: Bone pain (25% combination), myalgia (21% combination), arthralgia (14%), neuropathy (13% combination), rigors (12% combination), paresthesia (11%)

Ocular: Conjunctivitis (12%; <1% combination), keratoconjunctivitis sicca (12%)

Respiratory: Dyspnea (21% to 41%), cough (16% to 33%)

Miscellaneous: Infection (24%; 39% combination)

1% to 10%:

Cardiovascular (reported with combination chemotherapy): Deep venous thrombosis (4%), arrhythmia, cerebrovascular accidents (including cerebral hemorrhage), MI, myocardial ischemia, syncope

Gastrointestinal (reported with combination chemotherapy): Ileus, pancreatitis

Hematologic (reported with combination chemotherapy): Hemolytic anemia, microangiopathic hemolytic anemia with thrombocytopenia

Ocular: Keratitis (6%; <1% combination)

Renal (reported with combination chemotherapy): Renal insufficiency

Respiratory: Pneumonitis (6%)

Overdosage/Toxicology Single doses of up to 1000 mg in healthy patients and 1600 mg in cancer patients have been tolerated. Repeated doses of 200 mg twice daily in healthy subjects were poorly tolerated after a few days. Specific overdose-related toxicities include diarrhea, rash, and liver transaminase elevation. Overdose management should include withdrawal of erlotinib, and symptom-directed and supportive treatment.

Pharmacodynamics/Kinetics

Time to Peak: Plasma: 1-7 hours

Protein Binding: 92% to 95%, albumin and α_1-acid glycoprotein

Half-Life Elimination: 24-36 hours

Metabolism: Hepatic, CYP3A4 (major), CYP1A1 (minor), CYP1A2 (minor), and CYP1C (minor)

Excretion: Primarily as metabolites: Feces (83%); urine (8%)

Available Dosage Forms Tablet: 25 mg, 100 mg, 150 mg

Dosing

Adults & Elderly: Note: Treatment should continue until disease progression or unacceptable toxicity occurs.

NSCLC: Oral: 150 mg/day

Pancreatic cancer: Oral: 100 mg/day in combination with gemcitabine

Note: Dose reductions are more likely to be needed when erlotinib is administered concomitantly with strong CYP3A4 inhibitors. Dose reduction (if required) should be done in increments of 50 mg. Likewise, the CYP3A4 inducers may require increased doses; doses of >150 mg/day should be considered with rifampin. (See Drug Interactions for examples of CYP3A4 inhibitors and inducers).

Renal Impairment: No adjustment required.

Hepatic Impairment: Dose reduction or interruption should be considered if liver function changes are severe.

Dosing Adjustment for Toxicity: Patients experiencing poorly-tolerated diarrhea or a severe skin reaction may benefit from a brief therapy interruption. Patients experiencing acute onset (or worsening) of pulmonary symptoms should have therapy interrupted and be evaluated for drug-induced interstitial lung disease.

Administration

Oral: The manufacturer recommends administration on an empty stomach (at least 1 hour before or 2 hours after the ingestion of food) even though this reduces drug absorption by approximately 40%. Administration after a meal results in nearly 100% absorption.

Stability

Storage: Store at room temperature between 15°C and 30°C (59°F and 86°F).

Laboratory Monitoring Periodic liver function tests (asymptomatic increases in liver enzymes have occurred)

Nursing Actions

Physical Assessment: Assess potential for interactions with other pharmacological agents patient is taking, especially CYP3A4 inhibitors or inducers (dose reductions may be necessary). Monitor laboratory tests (LFTs), therapeutic response, and adverse reactions (eg, pulmonary toxicity, poorly-tolerated diarrhea, severe skin reactions). Teach patient/caregiver possible side effects, appropriate interventions, and adverse symptoms to report.

Patient Education: Do not take any new medication during therapy unless approved by prescriber. Take exactly as directed; 1 hour before or 2 hours after food. Maintain adequate hydration (2-3 L/day of fluids) unless instructed to restrict fluid intake, and adequate nutrition (small frequent meals may help). May cause fatigue (regular, adequate rest periods may help reduce fatigue); rash or dry skin (use nonirritating skin lotion that does not contain alcohol or other irritants); loss of hair (may grow back when treatment is completed); nausea or anorexia (small frequent meals, good mouth care, or sucking lozenges may help); diarrhea (boiled milk, yogurt). Report any persistent gastrointestinal changes (including diarrhea, abdominal pain, nausea, or vomiting); conjunctivitis or visual changes; any difficulty breathing, unusual cough or fever; signs of infection; or other persistent adverse effects. **Pregnancy/breast-feeding precautions:** Inform prescriber if you are pregnant. Do not get pregnant while taking this medication or for two weeks after discontinuing. This drug may cause fetal deformities or loss of pregnancy; see prescriber for appropriate contraceptives. Consult prescriber if breast-feeding.

Geriatric Considerations In clinical trials, there was no significant difference between older and younger adults in survival benefit, safety, or pharmacokinetics. No dosage adjustment necessary in elderly patients.

Ertapenem (er ta PEN em)

U.S. Brand Names Invanz®
Synonyms Ertapenem Sodium; L-749,345; MK0826
Pharmacologic Category Antibiotic, Carbapenem
Medication Safety Issues
Sound-alike/look-alike issues:
Invanz® may be confused with Avinza™

Pregnancy Risk Factor B
Lactation Enters breast milk/use caution
Use Treatment of the following moderate-severe infections: Complicated intra-abdominal infections, complicated skin and skin structure infections (including diabetic foot infections without osteomyelitis), complicated UTI (including pyelonephritis), acute pelvic infections, and community-acquired pneumonia. Antibacterial coverage includes aerobic gram-positive organisms, aerobic gram-negative organisms, anaerobic organisms.

Note: Methicillin-resistant *Staphylococcus*, *Enterococcus* spp, penicillin-resistant strains of *Streptococcus pneumoniae*, beta-lactamase-positive strains of *Haemophilus influenzae* are **resistant** to ertapenem, as are most *Pseudomonas aeruginosa*.

Mechanism of Action/Effect Inhibits cell wall biosynthesis; cell wall assembly is arrested and the bacteria eventually lyse.

Contraindications Hypersensitivity to ertapenem, other carbapenems, or any component of the formulation; anaphylactic reactions to beta-lactam antibiotics. If using intramuscularly, known hypersensitivity to local anesthetics of the amide type (lidocaine is the diluent).

Warnings/Precautions Use caution with renal impairment. Dosage adjustment required in patients with moderate-to-severe renal dysfunction; elderly patients often require lower doses (based upon renal function). Prolonged use may result in superinfection. Has been associated with CNS adverse effects, including confusional states and seizures; use caution with CNS disorders (eg, brain lesions, history of seizures). Serious hypersensitivity reactions, including anaphylaxis, have been reported (some without a history of previous allergic reactions to beta-lactams). Doses for I.M. administration are mixed with lidocaine; consult *Lidocaine on page 735* information for associated Warnings/Precautions. Safety and efficacy in patients <3 months of age have not been established.

Drug Interactions
Decreased Effect: Ertapenem may decrease valproic acid serum concentrations to subtherapeutic levels; monitor.

Increased Effect/Toxicity: Probenecid may increase serum concentrations of ertapenem; use caution.

Adverse Reactions Note: Percentages reported in adults.

1% to 10%:
Cardiovascular: Swelling/edema (3%), chest pain (1%), hypertension (0.7% to ≤2%), hypotension (1% to 2%), tachycardia (1% to 2%)

Central nervous system: Headache (6% to 7%), altered mental status (ie, agitation, confusion, disorientation, decreased mental acuity, changed mental status, somnolence, stupor) (3% to 5%), fever (2% to 5%), insomnia (3%), dizziness (2%), fatigue (1%), anxiety (0.8% to ≤1%)

Dermatologic: Rash (2% to 3%), pruritus (1% to 2%), erythema (1% to 2%)

Gastrointestinal: Diarrhea (9% to 10%), nausea (6% to 9%), abdominal pain (4%), vomiting (4%), constipation (3% to 4%), acid regurgitation (1% to 2%), dyspepsia (1%), oral candidiasis (0.1% to ≤1%)

Genitourinary: Vaginitis (1% to 3%)

Hematologic: Platelet count increased (4% to 7%), eosinophils increased (1% to 2%)

Hepatic: Hepatic enzyme elevations (7% to 9%), alkaline phosphatase increase (4% to 7%)

Local: Infused vein complications (5% to 7%), phlebitis/thrombophlebitis (2%), extravasation (0.7% to ≤2%)

Neuromuscular & skeletal: Leg pain (0.4% to 1%)

Respiratory: Dyspnea (1% to 3%), cough (1% to 2%), pharyngitis (0.7% to ≤1%), rales/rhonchi (0.5% to ≤1%), respiratory distress (0.2% to ≤1%)

Overdosage/Toxicology Treatment is symptom-directed and supportive. Ertapenem is removed by hemodialysis (plasma clearance increased by 30% following 4-hour session).

Pharmacodynamics/Kinetics
Time to Peak: I.M.: 2.3 hours
Protein Binding: Concentration dependent: 85% at 300 mcg/mL, 95% at <100 mcg/mL
Half-Life Elimination:
Children 3 months to 12 years: 2.5 hours
Children ≥13 years and Adults: 4 hours
Metabolism: Hydrolysis to inactive metabolite
Excretion: Urine (80% as unchanged drug and metabolite); feces (10%)

Available Dosage Forms Injection, powder for reconstitution: 1 g [contains sodium 137 mg/g (~6 mEq/g)]

Dosing
Adults & Elderly: Note: I.V. therapy may be administered for up to 14 days; I.M. for up to 7 days
Community-acquired pneumonia and urinary tract infections/pyelonephritis: I.M., I.V.: 1 g/day; duration of total antibiotic treatment: 10-14 days (**Note:** Duration includes possible switch to appropriate oral therapy after at least 3 days of parenteral treatment, once clinical improvement demonstrated.)

Intra-abdominal infection: I.M., I.V.: 1 g/day for 5-14 days

Pelvic infections (acute): I.M., I.V.: 1 g/day for 3-10 days

Skin and skin structure infections (including diabetic foot infections): I.M., I.V.: 1 g/day for 7-14 days

Pediatrics: Note: I.V. therapy may be administered for up to 14 days; I.M. therapy for up to 7 days

Children 3 months to 12 years:
Community-acquired pneumonia and urinary tract infections/pyelonephritis: I.M., I.V.: 15 mg/kg twice daily (maximum: 1 g/day); duration of total antibiotic treatment: 10-14 days (**Note:** Duration includes possible switch to appropriate oral therapy after at least 3 days of parenteral treatment, once clinical improvement demonstrated.)

Intra-abdominal infection: I.M., I.V.: 15 mg/kg twice daily (maximum: 1 g/day) for 5-14 days

Pelvic infections (acute): I.M., I.V.: 15 mg/kg twice daily (maximum: 1 g/day) for 3-10 days

(Continued)

Ertapenem (Continued)

Skin and skin structure infections: I.M., I.V.: 15 mg/kg twice daily (maximum: 1 g/day) for 7-14 days

Children ≥13 years: Refer to adult dosing.

Renal Impairment:

Children: No data available for pediatric patients with renal insufficiency.

Adults: Cl_{cr} <30 mL/minute and ESRD: 500 mg/day

Hemodialysis: When the daily dose is given within 6 hours prior to hemodialysis, a supplementary dose of 150 mg is required following hemodialysis.

Hepatic Impairment: Adjustments cannot be recommended (lack of experience and research in this patient population).

Administration

I.M.: Avoid injection into a blood vessel. Make sure patient does not have an allergy to lidocaine or another anesthetic of the amide type. Administer by deep I.M. injection into a large muscle mass (eg, gluteal muscle or lateral part of the thigh). Do not administer I.M. preparation or drug reconstituted for I.M. administration intravenously.

I.V.: Infuse over 30 minutes

I.V. Detail: pH 7.5

Stability

Reconstitution:

I.M.: Reconstitute 1 g vial with 3.2 mL of 1% lidocaine HCl injection (without epinephrine). Shake well.

I.V.: Reconstitute 1 g vial with 10 mL of water for injection, 0.9% sodium chloride injection, or bacteriostatic water for injection. Shake well. For adults, transfer dose to 50 mL of 0.9% sodium chloride injection; for children, dilute dose with NS to a final concentration of ≤20 mg/mL.

Compatibility: Do not mix with other medications or use diluents containing dextrose.

Storage: Before reconstitution store at ≤25°C (77°F).

I.M.: Use within 1 hour after preparation.

I.V.: Reconstituted I.V. solution may be stored at room temperature and used within 6 hours or refrigerated, stored for up to 24 hours and used within 4 hours after removal from refrigerator. Do not freeze.

Nursing Actions

Physical Assessment: Results of culture and sensitivity tests and patient history of previous allergies should be assessed prior to beginning treatment. See Administration for specific infusion/injection directions. Monitor closely for adverse reactions, especially CNS adverse effects (history of seizures, head injuries, or other CNS events increases risk). Teach patient interventions to reduce side effects and adverse symptoms to report.

Patient Education: This medication can only be administered intravenously or by intramuscular injections; report warmth, swelling, irritation at infusion or injection site. Maintain adequate hydration (2-3 L/day of fluids) unless instructed to restrict fluid intake, and nutrition. Report unresolved nausea or vomiting (small, frequent meals, frequent mouth care, and sucking hard candy may help). Report immediately any CNS changes (eg, dizziness, disorientation, visual disturbances, headaches, confusion, or seizures). Report prolonged GI effects, diarrhea, vomiting, abdominal pain; change in respirations or respiratory difficulty; chest pain or palpitations; skin rash; foul-smelling vaginal discharge; or white plaques in mouth. **Breast-feeding precaution:** Consult prescriber if breast-feeding.

Dietary Considerations Sodium content: 137 mg (~6 mEq) per gram of ertapenem

Breast-Feeding Issues The concentration in human breast milk within 24 hours of last dose (1 g I.V. for 3-10 days) ranged from <0.13 mcg/mL (lower limit of quantitation) to 0.38 mcg/mL. Five days after discontinuation

of therapy, the ertapenem level was undetectable in 80% (4 of 5 women) and below the lower limit of quantitation in 20% (1 of 5 women).

Erythromycin (er ith roe MYE sin)

U.S. Brand Names Akne-Mycin®; A/T/S®; E.E.S.®; Eryc®; Eryderm®; Erygel®; EryPed®; Ery-Tab®; Erythrocin®; PCE®; Romycin®; Staticin® [DSC]; Theramycin Z®; T-Stat® [DSC]

Synonyms Erythromycin Base; Erythromycin Estolate; Erythromycin Ethylsuccinate; Erythromycin Gluceptate; Erythromycin Lactobionate; Erythromycin Stearate

Pharmacologic Category Antibiotic, Macrolide; Antibiotic, Ophthalmic; Antibiotic, Topical; Topical Skin Product; Topical Skin Product, Acne

Medication Safety Issues

Sound-alike/look-alike issues:

Erythromycin may be confused with azithromycin, clarithromycin, Ethmozine®

Akne-Mycin® may be confused with AK-Mycin®

E.E.S.® may be confused with DES®

Eryc® may be confused with Emcyt®, Ery-Tab®

Ery-Tab® may be confused with Eryc®

Erythrocin® may be confused with Ethmozine®

Pregnancy Risk Factor B

Lactation Enters breast milk/use caution (AAP considers "compatible")

Use

Systemic: Treatment of susceptible bacterial infections including *S. pyogenes*, some *S. pneumoniae*, some *S. aureus*, *M. pneumoniae*, *Legionella pneumophila*, diphtheria, pertussis, chancroid, *Chlamydia*, erythrasma, *N. gonorrhoeae*, *E. histolytica*, syphilis and nongonococcal urethritis, and *Campylobacter* gastroenteritis; used in conjunction with neomycin for decontaminating the bowel

Ophthalmic: Treatment of superficial eye infections involving the conjunctiva or cornea; neonatal ophthalmia

Topical: Treatment of acne vulgaris

Unlabeled/Investigational Use Systemic: Treatment of gastroparesis

Mechanism of Action/Effect Inhibits RNA-dependent protein synthesis

Contraindications Hypersensitivity to erythromycin or any component of the formulation

Systemic: Pre-existing liver disease (erythromycin estolate); concomitant use with ergot derivatives, pimozide, or cisapride

Warnings/Precautions Systemic: Use caution with hepatic impairment with or without jaundice has occurred, it may be accompanied by malaise, nausea, vomiting, abdominal colic, and fever; discontinue use if these occur; avoid using erythromycin lactobionate in neonates since formulations may contain benzyl alcohol which is associated with toxicity in neonates; observe for superinfections. Use in infants has been associated with infantile hypertrophic pyloric stenosis (IHPS). Macrolides have been associated with rare QT prolongation and ventricular arrhythmias, including torsade de pointes.

Drug Interactions

Cytochrome P450 Effect: Substrate of CYP2B6 (minor), 3A4 (major); **Inhibits** CYP1A2 (weak), 3A4 (moderate)

Decreased Effect: Erythromycin may decrease the serum concentrations of zafirlukast. Erythromycin may antagonize the therapeutic effects of clindamycin and lincomycin. The levels/effects of erythromycin may be decreased by aminoglutethimide, carbamazepine, nafcillin, nevirapine, phenobarbital, phenytoin, rifamycins, and other CYP3A4 inducers.

Increased Effect/Toxicity: Avoid concomitant use of the following with erythromycin due to increased risk of malignant arrhythmias: Cisapride, gatifloxacin, moxifloxacin, pimozide, sparfloxacin, thioridazine. Other agents that prolong the QT_c interval, including type Ia (eg, quinidine) and type III antiarrhythmic agents, and selected antipsychotic agents (eg, mesoridazine, thioridazine) should be used with extreme caution. Concurrent use of ergot alkaloids with erythromycin is also contraindicated.

Erythromycin is a moderate CYP3A4 inhibitor, and may increase the levels/effects of selected benzodiazepines, calcium channel blockers, cyclosporine, mirtazapine, nateglinide, nefazodone, quinidine, sildenafil (and other PDE-5 inhibitors), tacrolimus, venlafaxine, and other CYP3A4 substrates. Selected benzodiazepines (midazolam, triazolam), cisapride, ergot alkaloids, selected HMG-CoA reductase inhibitors (lovastatin and simvastatin), and pimozide are generally contraindicated with strong CYP3A4 inhibitors. When used with strong CYP3A4 inhibitors, dosage adjustment/limits are recommended for sildenafil and other PDE-5 inhibitors; refer to individual monographs. The effects of neuromuscular-blocking agents and warfarin have been potentiated by erythromycin.

The levels/effects of erythromycin may be increased by azole antifungals, clarithromycin, diclofenac, doxycycline, imatinib, isoniazid, nefazodone, nicardipine, propofol, protease inhibitors, quinidine, telithromycin, verapamil, and other CYP3A4 inhibitors.

Nutritional/Ethanol Interactions
Ethanol: Avoid ethanol (may decrease absorption of erythromycin or enhance ethanol effects).

Food: Increased drug absorption with meals; erythromycin serum levels may be altered if taken with food.

Herb/Nutraceutical: St John's wort may decrease erythromycin levels.

Lab Interactions
False-positive urinary catecholamines

Adverse Reactions
Systemic:
Cardiovascular: Ventricular arrhythmia, QT_c prolongation, torsade de pointes (rare), ventricular tachycardia (rare)

Central nervous system: Headache (8%), pain (2%), fever, seizure

Dermatitis: Rash (3%), pruritus (1%)

Gastrointestinal: Abdominal pain (8%), cramping, nausea (8%), oral candidiasis, vomiting (3%), diarrhea (7%), dyspepsia (2%), flatulence (2%), anorexia, pseudomembranous colitis, hypertrophic pyloric stenosis (including cases in infants or IHPS), pancreatitis

Hematologic: Eosinophilia (1%)

Hepatic: Cholestatic jaundice (most common with estolate), increased liver function tests (2%)

Local: Phlebitis at the injection site, thrombophlebitis

Neuromuscular & skeletal: Weakness (2%)

Respiratory: Dyspnea (1%), cough (3%)

Miscellaneous: Hypersensitivity reactions, allergic reactions

Topical: 1% to 10%: Dermatologic: Erythema, desquamation, dryness, pruritus

Overdosage/Toxicology
Symptoms of overdose include nausea, vomiting, diarrhea, prostration, reversible pancreatitis, hearing loss with or without tinnitus or vertigo. Care is general and supportive only.

Pharmacodynamics/Kinetics
Time to Peak: Serum: Base: 4 hours; Ethylsuccinate: 0.5-2.5 hours; delayed with food due to differences in absorption

Protein Binding: 75% to 90%

Half-Life Elimination: Peak: 1.5-2 hours; End-stage renal disease: 5-6 hours

Metabolism: Hepatic via demethylation

Excretion: Primarily feces; urine (2% to 15% as unchanged drug)

Available Dosage Forms [DSC] = Discontinued product; [CAN] = Canadian brand name

Capsule, delayed release, enteric-coated pellets, as base (Eryc®): 250 mg

Gel, topical: 2% (30 g, 60 g)
A/T/S®: 2% (30 g) [contains alcohol 92%]
Erygel®: 2% (30 g, 60 g) [contains alcohol 92%]

Granules for oral suspension, as ethylsuccinate (E.E.S.®): 200 mg/5 mL (100 mL, 200 mL) [cherry flavor]

Injection, powder for reconstitution, as lactobionate (Erythrocin®): 500 mg, 1 g

Ointment, ophthalmic: 0.5% [5 mg/g] (1 g, 3.5 g)
Romycin®: 0.5% [5 mg/g] (3.5 g)

Ointment, topical (Akne-Mycin®): 2% (25 g)

Powder for oral suspension, as ethylsuccinate (EryPed®): 200 mg/5 mL (100 mL, 200 mL) [fruit flavor]; 400 mg/5 mL (100 mL, 200 mL) [banana flavor]

Powder for oral suspension, as ethylsuccinate [drops] (EryPed®): 100 mg/2.5 mL (50 mL) [fruit flavor]

Solution, topical: 2% (60 mL)
A/T/S®: 2% (60 mL) [contains alcohol 66%]
Eryderm®, T-Stat® [DSC], Theramycin Z®: 2% (60 mL) [contain alcohol]
Sans Acne® [CAN]: 2% (60 mL) [contains ethyl alcohol 44%; not available in U.S.]
Staticin®: 1.5% (60 mL) [DSC]

Suspension, oral, as estolate: 125 mg/5 mL (480 mL); 250 mg/5 mL (480 mL)

Suspension, oral, as ethylsuccinate: 200 mg/5 mL (480 mL); 400 mg/5 mL (480 mL)
E.E.S.®: 200 mg/5 mL (100 mL, 480 mL) [fruit flavor]; 400 mg/5 mL (100 mL, 480 mL) [orange flavor]

Swab (T-Stat® [DSC]): 2% (60s)

Tablet, chewable, as ethylsuccinate (EryPed®): 200 mg [fruit flavor] [DSC]

Tablet, delayed release, enteric coated, as base (Ery-Tab®): 250 mg, 333 mg, 500 mg

Tablet, as base: 250 mg, 500 mg

Tablet, as ethylsuccinate (E.E.S.®): 400 mg

Tablet, as stearate: 250 mg
Erythrocin®: 250 mg, 500 mg

Tablet [polymer-coated particles], as base (PCE®): 333 mg, 500 mg

Dosing
Adults & Elderly:
Usual dosage range:
Oral: (**Note:** Due to differences in absorption, 400 mg erythromycin ethylsuccinate produces the same serum levels as 250 mg erythromycin base, sterate or estolate)
Base: 30-50 mg/kg/day in 2-4 divided doses; do not exceed 2 g/day
Estolate: 30-50 mg/kg/day in 2-4 divided doses; do not exceed 2 g/day
Ethylsuccinate: 30-50 mg/kg/day in 2-4 divided doses; do not exceed 3.2 g/day
Stearate: 30-50 mg/kg/day in 2-4 divided doses; do not exceed 2 g/day
I.V.: Lactobionate: 15-20 mg/kg/day divided every 6 hours or 500 mg to 1 g every 6 hours, or given as a continuous infusion over 24 hours (maximum: 4 g/24 hours)

Ophthalmic infection: Ophthalmic: Instill ½" (1.25 cm) 2-6 times/day depending on the severity of the infection

Dermatologic infection: Topical: Apply over the affected area twice daily after the skin has been thoroughly washed and patted dry

Indication-specific dosing:
Cervicitis: Oral: 500 mg 4 times/day for 7 days
Chancroid (unlabeled use; not a preferred agent):
Oral: 500 mg 4 times/day for 7 days

(Continued)

Erythromycin (Continued)

Community-acquired pneumonia, bronchitis: Oral, I.V.: 500-1000 mg 4 times/day for 10-14 days. If *Legionella* is suspected/confirmed, 750-1000 mg 4 times/day for 21 days or more may be recommended. **Note:** Other macrolides and/or fluoroquinolones may be preferred and better tolerated.

Lymphogranuloma venereum: Oral: 500 mg 4 times/day for 21 days

Nongonococcal urethritis (recurrent): Oral: CDC Guidelines for the Treatment of Sexually Transmitted Diseases recommendation: Metronidazole (2 g as a single dose) plus 7 days of erythromycin base (500 mg 4 times/day) or erythromycin ethylsuccinate (800 mg 4 times/day)

Pertussis (CDC guidelines): Oral: 500 mg every 6 hours for 14 days

Preop bowel preparation (unlabeled use): Oral: 1 g erythromycin base at 1, 2, and 11 PM on the day before surgery combined with mechanical cleansing of the large intestine and oral neomycin

Gastrointestinal prokinetic (unlabeled use): Oral: Erythromycin has been used as a prokinetic agent to improve gastric emptying time and intestinal motility. In adults, 200 mg was infused I.V. initially followed by 250 mg orally 3 times/day 30 minutes before meals. Lower dosages have been used in some trials.

Pediatrics:

Prophylaxis of neonatal gonococcal or chlamydial conjunctivitis: Neonates: Ophthalmic: 0.5-1 cm ribbon of ointment should be instilled into each conjunctival sac

Usual dosage range: Infants and Children:

Oral: **Note:** Due to differences in absorption, 400 mg erythromycin ethylsuccinate produces the same serum levels as 250 mg erythromycin base, stearate or estolate).

Base: 30-50 mg/kg/day in 2-4 divided doses; do not exceed 2 g/day

Estolate: 30-50 mg/kg/day in 2-4 divided doses; do not exceed 2 g/day

Ethylsuccinate: 30-50 mg/kg/day in 2-4 divided doses; do not exceed 3.2 g/day

Stearate: 30-50 mg/kg/day in 2-4 divided doses; do not exceed 2 g/day

I.V. (as lactobionate): 15-50 mg/kg/day divided every 6 hours, not to exceed 4 g/day

Indication-specific dosing:

Acne vulgaris (unlabeled use): Adolescents: Oral: 250-1500 mg/day in 2 divided doses; therapy may be continued for 4-6 weeks at lowest possible dose

Pharyngitis: Oral: 40 mg/kg/day in 2 doses; maximum: 1600 mg/day; short-course therapy for 5 days may be considered

Pertussis (CDC guidelines): Oral: 40-50 mg/kg/day in 4 divided doses for 14 days; maximum 2 g/day (not preferred agent for infants <1 month

Preop bowel preparation: Oral: 20 mg/kg erythromycin base at 1, 2, and 11 PM on the day before surgery combined with mechanical cleansing of the large intestine and oral neomycin

Ophthalmic infection: Ophthalmic: Refer to adult dosing.

Topical: Refer to adult dosing.

Renal Impairment: Slightly dialyzable (5% to 20%); supplemental dose is not necessary in hemo- or peritoneal dialysis or in continuous arteriovenous or venovenous hemofiltration.

Administration

Oral: Do not crush enteric coated drug product. GI upset, including diarrhea, is common. May be administered with food to decrease GI upset. Do not give with milk or acidic beverages.

I.V.: Infuse 1 g over 20-60 minutes.

I.V. Detail: Some formulations may contain benzyl alcohol as a preservative. I.V. infusion may be very irritating to the vein. If phlebitis/pain occurs with used dilution, consider diluting further (eg, 1:5) if fluid status of the patient will tolerate, or consider administering in larger available vein. The addition of lidocaine or bicarbonate does not decrease the irritation of erythromycin infusions.

pH:

Erythromycin gluceptate: 7.7 (reconstituted solutions concentrated at 50 mg/mL)

Erythromycin lactobionate: 6.5-7.5 (reconstituted with sterile water for injection or D₅W to a 50 mg/mL concentration)

Other: Avoid contact of tip of ophthalmic ointment tube with affected eye.

Stability

Reconstitution: Erythromycin lactobionate should be reconstituted with sterile water for injection without preservatives to avoid gel formation. I.V. form has the longest stability in NS and should be prepared in this base solution whenever possible. Do not use D₅W as a diluent unless sodium bicarbonate is added to solution. If I.V. must be prepared in D₅W, 0.5 mL of the 8.4% sodium bicarbonate solution should be added per each 100 mL of D₅W.

Stability of parenteral admixture at room temperature (25°C) and at refrigeration temperature (4°C) is 24 hours.

Standard diluent: 500 mg/250 mL D₅W/NS; 750 mg/250 mL D₅W/NS; 1 g/250 mL D₅W/NS.

Compatibility: Erythromycin lactobionate: Stable in NS; incompatible with D₅LR, D₁₀W

Y-site administration: Incompatible with fluconazole

Compatibility in syringe: Incompatible with ampicillin, heparin

Compatibility when admixed: Incompatible with colistimethate, floxacillin, furosemide, heparin, metaraminol, metoclopramide, riboflavin, vitamin B complex with C

Storage:

Injection: Reconstituted solution is stable for 2 weeks when refrigerated or for 24 hours at room temperature. Erythromycin I.V. infusion solution is stable at pH 6-8; stability of lactobionate is pH dependent; I.V. form has longest stability in NS. Stability of parenteral admixture at room temperature (25°C) and at refrigeration temperature (4°C) is 24 hours.

Granules for oral suspension: After mixing, store under refrigeration and use within 10 days.

Powder for oral suspension: Refrigerate to preserve taste. Erythromycin ethylsuccinate may be stored at room temperature if used within 14 days. EryPed® drops should be used within 35 days following reconstitution; may store at room temperature or under refrigeration.

Topical and ophthalmic formulations: Store at room temperature.

Laboratory Monitoring Perform culture and sensitivity studies prior to initiating drug therapy.

Nursing Actions

Physical Assessment: Results of culture and sensitivity tests and patient's previous allergy history should be assessed prior to therapy. Assess potential for interactions with other pharmacological agents or herbal products patient may be taking (see Drug Interactions). Note Administration specifics. Assess therapeutic effectiveness and adverse reactions (see Adverse Reactions). Teach patient proper use (according to formulation and purpose for use), possible side effects/appropriate interventions, and adverse symptoms to report.

Patient Education: Do not take any new medication during therapy. Take as directed, around-the-clock, with a full glass of water (not juice or milk); may take with food to reduce GI upset. Do not chew or crush extended release capsules or tablets. Take complete prescription even if you are feeling better. Avoid alcohol (may cause adverse response). May cause nausea, vomiting, or mouth sores (small, frequent meals, frequent mouth care may help). Report immediately any unusual malaise, nausea, vomiting, abdominal colic, or fever; skin rash or itching; easy bruising or bleeding; vaginal itching or discharge; watery or bloody diarrhea; yellowing of skin or eyes, pale stool or dark urine; white plaques, sores, or fuzziness in mouth; or any change in hearing.

Dietary Considerations Systemic: Drug may cause GI upset; may take with food.

Geriatric Considerations Dose of erythromycin does not need to be adjusted in the elderly unless there is severe renal impairment or hepatic dysfunction. Elderly patients may be at an increased risk for torsade de pointes. Risk of ototoxicity may be increased in elderly, particularly when dose is ≥4 g/day in conjunction with renal or hepatic impairment.

Additional Information Due to differences in absorption, 400 mg erythromycin ethylsuccinate produces the same serum levels as 250 mg erythromycin base, stearate, or estolate. Do not use D_5W as a diluent unless sodium bicarbonate is added to solution; infuse over 20-60 minutes.

Related Information

Compatibility of Drugs *on page 1370*

Erythromycin and Benzoyl Peroxide

(er ith roe MYE sin & BEN zoe il per OKS ide)

U.S. Brand Names Benzamycin®; Benzamycin® Pak

Synonyms Benzoyl Peroxide and Erythromycin

Pharmacologic Category Topical Skin Product; Topical Skin Product, Acne

Pregnancy Risk Factor C

Lactation Excretion in breast milk unknown/use caution

Use Topical control of acne vulgaris

Available Dosage Forms Gel, topical:

Benzamycin®: Erythromycin 30 mg and benzoyl peroxide 50 mg per g (47 g)

Benzamycin® Pak: Erythromycin 30 mg and benzoyl peroxide 50 mg per 0.8 g packet (60s) [supplied with diluent containing alcohol]

Dosing

Adults & Elderly: Acne: Topical: Apply twice daily, morning and evening.

Pediatrics: Adolescents: Refer to adult dosing.

Nursing Actions

Physical Assessment: See individual agents.

Patient Education: See individual agents. This product contains benzoyl peroxide which may bleach or stain clothing. **Pregnancy/breast-feeding precautions:** Inform prescriber if you are or intend to become pregnant. Consult prescriber if breast-feeding.

Related Information

Erythromycin *on page 442*

Erythromycin and Sulfisoxazole

(er ith roe MYE sin & sul fi SOKS a zole)

U.S. Brand Names Pediazole®

Synonyms Sulfisoxazole and Erythromycin

Pharmacologic Category Antibiotic, Macrolide; Antibiotic, Macrolide Combination; Antibiotic, Sulfonamide Derivative

Pregnancy Risk Factor C

Lactation Enters breast milk/compatible

Use Treatment of susceptible bacterial infections of the upper and lower respiratory tract, otitis media in children caused by susceptible strains of *Haemophilus influenzae*, and many other infections in patients allergic to penicillin

Available Dosage Forms Powder for oral suspension: Erythromycin ethylsuccinate 200 mg and sulfisoxazole acetyl 600 mg per 5 mL (100 mL, 150 mL, 200 mL) [strawberry-banana flavor]

Dosing

Adults: Susceptible infections: Oral (dosage recommendation is based on the product's erythromycin content): 400 mg erythromycin and 1200 mg sulfisoxazole every 6 hours

Elderly: Not recommended for use in the elderly.

Pediatrics: Susceptible infections: Oral (dosage recommendation is based on the product's erythromycin content): ≥2 months: 50 mg/kg/day erythromycin and 150 mg/kg/day sulfisoxazole in divided doses every 6 hours; not to exceed 2 g erythromycin/day or 6 g sulfisoxazole/day for 10 days

Renal Impairment: Sulfisoxazole must be adjusted in renal impairment.

Cl_{cr} 10-50 mL/minute: Administer every 8-12 hours.

Cl_{cr} <10 mL/minute: Administer every 12-24 hours.

Nursing Actions

Physical Assessment: See individual agents.

Patient Education: See individual agents. **Pregnancy precaution:** Inform prescriber if you are or intend to become pregnant.

Related Information

Erythromycin *on page 442*

SulfiSOXAZOLE *on page 1158*

Escitalopram (es sye TAL oh pram)

U.S. Brand Names Lexapro®

Synonyms Escitalopram Oxalate; Lu-26-054; S-Citalopram

Restrictions A medication guide concerning the use of antidepressants in children and teenagers can be found on the FDA website at http://www.fda.gov/cder/Offices/ODS/labeling.htm. It should be dispensed to parents or guardians of children and teenagers receiving this medication.

Pharmacologic Category Antidepressant, Selective Serotonin Reuptake Inhibitor

Pregnancy Risk Factor C

Lactation Enters breast milk/not recommended

Use Treatment of major depressive disorder; generalized anxiety disorders (GAD)

Mechanism of Action/Effect Escitalopram is the S-enantiomer of the racemic derivative citalopram, which selectively inhibits the reuptake of serotonin with little to no effect on norepinephrine or dopamine reuptake. It has no or very low affinity for $5-HT_{1-7}$, alpha- and beta-adrenergic, D_{1-5}, H_{1-3}, M_{1-5}, and benzodiazepine receptors. Escitalopram does not bind or has low affinity for Na^+, K^+, Cl^-, and Ca^{++} ion channels.

Contraindications Hypersensitivity to escitalopram, citalopram, or any component of the formulation; concomitant use or within 2 weeks of MAO inhibitors (Continued)

445

Escitalopram *(Continued)*

Warnings/Precautions Antidepressants increase the risk of suicidal thinking and behavior in children and adolescents with major depressive disorder (MDD) and other depressive disorders; consider risk prior to prescribing. All patients must be closely monitored for clinical worsening, suicidality, or unusual changes in behavior, especially during the initiation of therapy or following an increase or decrease in dosage. When used in children, the child's family or caregiver should be instructed to closely observe the patient and communicate condition with healthcare provider. A medication guide should be dispensed with each prescription. **Escitalopram is not FDA approved for use in children.**

The possibility of a suicide attempt is inherent in major depression and may persist until remission occurs. Use caution in high-risk patients. Worsening depression and severe abrupt suicidality that are not part of the presenting symptoms may require discontinuation or modification of drug therapy. The patient's family or caregiver should be alerted to monitor patients for the emergence of suicidality and associated behaviors (such as agitation, irritability, hostility, impulsivity, and hypomania) and call healthcare provider.

May worsen psychosis in some patients or precipitate a shift to mania or hypomania in patients with bipolar disorder. Patients presenting with depressive symptoms should be screened for bipolar disorder. Monotherapy in patients with bipolar disorder should be avoided. **Escitalopram is not FDA approved for the treatment of bipolar depression.**

The potential for a severe reaction exists when used with MAO inhibitors; serotonin syndrome (hyperthermia, muscular rigidity, mental status changes/agitation, autonomic instability) may occur. May increase the risks associated with electroconvulsive therapy. Has a low potential to impair cognitive or motor performance; caution operating hazardous machinery or driving.

Use caution with a previous seizure disorder or condition predisposing to seizures such as brain damage, alcoholism, or concurrent therapy with other drugs which lower the seizure threshold. May cause hyponatremia/SIADH. May cause or exacerbate sexual dysfunction. Use caution with renal or liver impairment; concomitant CNS depressants; pregnancy (high doses of citalopram has been associated with teratogenicity in animals). Use caution with concomitant use of NSAIDs, ASA, or other drugs that affect coagulation; the risk of bleeding is potentiated.

Upon discontinuation of escitalopram therapy, gradually taper dose. If intolerable symptoms occur following a decrease in dosage or upon discontinuation of therapy, then resuming the previous dose with a more gradual taper should be considered.

Drug Interactions

Cytochrome P450 Effect: Substrate (major) of CYP2C19, 3A4; **Inhibits** CYP2D6 (weak)

Decreased Effect: CYP2C19 inducers may decrease the levels/effects of imipramine; example inducers include aminoglutethimide, carbamazepine, phenytoin, and rifampin. CYP3A4 inducers may decrease the levels/effects of escitalopram; example inducers include aminoglutethimide, carbamazepine, nafcillin, nevirapine, phenobarbital, phenytoin, and rifamycins.

Increased Effect/Toxicity: Escitalopram should not be used with nonselective MAO inhibitors (phenelzine, isocarboxazid) or other drugs with MAO inhibition (linezolid); fatal reactions have been reported. Wait 5 weeks after stopping escitalopram before starting a nonselective MAO inhibitor and 2 weeks after stopping an MAO inhibitor before starting escitalopram. Concurrent selegiline has been associated with mania, hypertension, or serotonin syndrome (risk may be reduced relative to nonselective MAO inhibitors).

CYP2C19 inhibitors may increase the levels/effects of imipramine; example inhibitors include delavirdine, fluconazole, fluvoxamine, gemfibrozil, isoniazid, omeprazole, and ticlopidine. CYP3A4 inhibitors may increase the levels/effects of escitalopram; example inhibitors include azole antifungals, clarithromycin, diclofenac, doxycycline, erythromycin, imatinib, isoniazid, nefazodone, nicardipine, propofol, protease inhibitors, quinidine, telithromycin, and verapamil.

Combined use of SSRIs and buspirone, meperidine, moclobemide, nefazodone, other SSRIs, tramadol, trazodone, and venlafaxine may increase the risk of serotonin syndrome. Escitalopram increases serum levels/effects of CYP2D6 substrates (tricyclic antidepressants). Escitalopram may increase desipramine levels.

Combined use of sumatriptan (and other serotonin agonists) may result in toxicity; weakness, hyper-reflexia, and incoordination have been observed with sumatriptan and SSRIs. In addition, concurrent use may theoretically increase the risk of serotonin syndrome; includes sumatriptan, naratriptan, rizatriptan, and zolmitriptan.

Concomitant use of escitalopram and NSAIDs, aspirin, or other drugs affecting coagulation has been associated with an increased risk of bleeding; monitor.

Nutritional/Ethanol Interactions

Ethanol: Avoid ethanol (may increase CNS depression).
Herb/Nutraceutical: Avoid valerian, St John's wort, SAMe, kava kava, and gotu kola (may increase CNS depression).

Adverse Reactions

>10%:
Central nervous system: Headache (24%), somnolence (6% to 13%), insomnia (9% to 12%)
Gastrointestinal: Nausea (15%)
Genitourinary: Ejaculation disorder (9% to 14%)

1% to 10%:
Cardiovascular: Chest pain, hypertension, palpitation
Central nervous system: Dizziness (5%), fatigue (5% to 8%), dreaming abnormal, concentration impaired, fever, irritability, lethargy, lightheadedness, migraine, vertigo, yawning
Dermatologic: Rash
Endocrine & metabolic: Libido decreased (3% to 7%), anorgasmia (2% to 6%), hot flashes, menstrual cramps, menstrual disorder
Gastrointestinal: Diarrhea (8%), xerostomia (6% to 9%), appetite decreased (3%), constipation (3% to 5%), indigestion (3%), abdominal pain (2%), abdominal cramps, appetite increased, flatulence, gastroenteritis, gastroesophageal reflux, heartburn, toothache, vomiting, weight gain/loss
Genitourinary: Impotence (3%), urinary tract infection, urinary frequency
Neuromuscular & skeletal: Arthralgia, limb pain, muscle cramp, myalgia, neck/shoulder pain, paresthesia, tremor
Ocular: Blurred vision
Otic: Earache, tinnitus
Respiratory: Rhinitis (5%), sinusitis (3%), bronchitis, cough, nasal or sinus congestion, sinus headache
Miscellaneous: Diaphoresis (4% to 5%), flu-like syndrome (5%), allergy

Overdosage/Toxicology
Treatment should be symptom-directed and supportive.

Pharmacodynamics/Kinetics

Time to Peak: Escitalopram: 5 ± 1.5 hours; S-desmethylcitalopram: 14 hours

Protein Binding: 56% to plasma proteins

Half-Life Elimination: Escitalopram: 27-32 hours; S-desmethylcitalopram: 59 hours

Metabolism: Hepatic via CYP2C19 and 3A4 to an active metabolite, S-desmethylcitalopram (S-DCT; 1/7 the activity); S-DCT is metabolized to S-didesmethylcitalopram (S-DDCT; active; 1/27 the activity) via CYP2D6

Excretion: Urine (Escitalopram: 8%; S-DCT: 10%)
Clearance: Total body: 37-40 L/hour; Renal: Escitalopram: 2.7 L/hour; S-desmethylcitalopram: 6.9 L/hour

Available Dosage Forms
Solution, oral: 1 mg/mL (240 mL) [peppermint flavor]
Tablet: 5 mg, 10 mg, 20 mg
Note: Cipralex® [CAN] is available only in 10 mg and 20 mg strengths.

Dosing
Adults: Depression, GAD: Oral: Initial: 10 mg/day; dose may be increased to 20 mg/day after at least 1 week
Elderly: Depression: Oral: 5-10 mg/day; doses may be increased by 5-10 mg/day after at least 1 week.
Renal Impairment:
Mild to moderate impairment: No dosage adjustment needed.
Severe impairment: Cl$_{cr}$ <20 mL/minute: Use caution.
Hepatic Impairment: 10 mg/day
Administration
Oral: Administer once daily (morning or evening), with or without food.
Stability
Storage: Store at 25°C (77°F).
Nursing Actions
Physical Assessment: Assess potential for interactions with other prescriptions, OTC medications, or herbal products patient may be taking (eg, MAO inhibitors and other SSRIs). Assess therapeutic effectiveness (mental status for depression, suicidal ideation, social functioning, mania, or panic attacks) and adverse reactions on a regular basis throughout therapy (eg, suicidal ideation, mania, or hypomania). Teach patient proper use, possible side effects/appropriate interventions, and adverse symptoms to report.
Patient Education: Do not take any new medication during therapy without consulting prescriber. Take exactly as directed; do not alter dose or discontinue without consulting prescriber (effects of medication may take up to 3 weeks to occur). Avoid other stimulants: caffeine or alcohol. May cause dizziness, light-headedness, insomnia, impaired concentration, headache (use caution when driving or engaging in tasks requiring alertness until response to drug is known); nausea, vomiting, loss or increase of appetite, indigestion, or heartburn (small frequent meals, frequent mouth care, sucking lozenges, or chewing gum may help); constipation (increased dietary fluid, fruit, fiber, and increased exercise may help); sexual dysfunction (reversible when drug is discontinued); hot flashes or menstrual cramps; or muscle pain, cramps, or tremor (consult prescriber for approved analgesia). Report immediately any CNS changes such as increased depression, confusion, impaired concentration, severe headache, insomnia, nightmares, irritability, acute anxiety, panic attacks, or thoughts of suicide; persistent GI changes; chest pain or palpitations; blurred vision or vision changes; ringing in ears; unusual cough; or other persistent adverse effects. **Pregnancy/breast-feeding precautions:** Inform prescriber if you are or intend to become pregnant. Breast-feeding is not recommended.
Dietary Considerations May be taken with or without food.
Breast-Feeding Issues Escitalopram is excreted in human milk. Excessive somnolence, decreased feeding and weight loss have been reported in breast-fed infants. A decision should be made whether to continue or discontinue nursing or discontinue the drug.

Pregnancy Issues Teratogenic effects have been reported in animal studies. Nonteratogenic effects including respiratory distress, cyanosis, apnea, seizures, temperature instability, feeding difficulty, vomiting, hypoglycemia, hypo- or hypertonia, hyper-reflexia, jitteriness, irritability, constant crying, and tremor have been reported in the neonate immediately following delivery after exposure late in the third trimester. Adverse effects may be due to toxic effects of SSRI or drug discontinuation. In some cases, may present clinically as serotonin syndrome. There are no adequate and well-controlled studies in pregnant women. Use during pregnancy only if the potential benefit to the mother outweighs the possible risk to the fetus. If treatment during pregnancy is required, consider tapering therapy during the third trimester.
Additional Information The tablet and oral solution dosage forms are bioequivalent. Clinically, escitalopram 20 mg is equipotent to citalopram 40 mg. Do not coadminister with citalopram.

Esmolol (ES moe lol)

U.S. Brand Names Brevibloc®
Synonyms Esmolol Hydrochloride
Pharmacologic Category Antiarrhythmic Agent, Class II; Beta Blocker, Beta$_1$ Selective
Medication Safety Issues
Sound-alike/look-alike issues:
Esmolol may be confused with Osmitrol®
Brevibloc® may be confused with bretylium, Brevital®, Bumex®, Buprenex®
Pregnancy Risk Factor C (manufacturer); D (2nd and 3rd trimesters - expert analysis)
Lactation Excretion in breast milk unknown/use with caution
Use Treatment of supraventricular tachycardia (SVT) and atrial fibrillation/flutter (control ventricular rate); treatment of tachycardia and/or hypertension (especially intraoperative or postoperative); treatment of noncompensatory sinus tachycardia
Unlabeled/Investigational Use In children, for SVT and postoperative hypertension
Mechanism of Action/Effect Class II antiarrhythmic: Beta$_1$ adrenergic receptor blocking agent that competes with beta$_1$ adrenergic agonists for available beta receptor sites; it is a selective beta$_1$ antagonist with a very short duration of action; has little if any intrinsic sympathomimetic activity; and lacks membrane stabilizing action; it is administered intravenously and is used when beta blockade of short duration is desired or in critically-ill patients in whom adverse effects of bradycardia, heart failure or hypotension may necessitate rapid withdrawal of the drug
Contraindications Hypersensitivity to esmolol or any component of the formulation; sinus bradycardia; heart block greater than first degree (except in patients with a functioning artificial pacemaker); cardiogenic shock; bronchial asthma (relative); uncompensated cardiac failure; hypotension; pregnancy (2nd and 3rd trimesters)
Warnings/Precautions Hypotension is common; patients need close blood pressure monitoring. Administer cautiously in compensated heart failure and monitor for a worsening of the condition. Use caution in patients with PVD (can aggravate arterial insufficiency). Use caution with concurrent use of beta-blockers and either verapamil or diltiazem; bradycardia or heart block can occur. Avoid concurrent I.V. use of both agents. Use beta-blockers cautiously in patients with bronchospastic disease; monitor pulmonary status closely. Use with caution in patients with diabetes - may mask prominent hypoglycemic symptoms. May mask signs of thyrotoxicosis. May cause fetal bradycardia when administered in the 3rd trimester of pregnancy or at delivery. Use (Continued)

Esmolol *(Continued)*

caution in patients with renal dysfunction (active metabolite retained). Do not use in the treatment of hypertension associated with vasoconstriction related to hypothermia. Extravasation can lead to skin necrosis and sloughing.

Drug Interactions

Decreased Effect: Alpha$_2$ agonists decrease the effectiveness of beta blockers (beta$_1$ selective). NSAIDs may diminish the antihypertensive effects of beta blockers.

Increased Effect/Toxicity: Anticholinesterase inhibitors, amiodarone, cardia glycosides dipyridamole (I.V.) increase bradycardia; beta blockers increase alpha$_1$ blockers orthostasis, alpha/beta agonists (direct acting) vasopressor effects, alpha$_2$ agonists rebound hypertension when withdrawn. Beta-blockers may enhance the hypoglycemia and mask most symptoms of hypoglycemia in patients on insulin or sulfonylureas. Calcium channel blockers increase hypotension

Lab Interactions Increased cholesterol (S), glucose

Adverse Reactions

>10%:
Cardiovascular: Asymptomatic hypotension (dose-related: 25% to 38%), symptomatic hypotension (dose-related: 12%)
Miscellaneous: Diaphoresis (10%)

1% to 10%:
Cardiovascular: Peripheral ischemia (1%)
Central nervous system: Dizziness (3%), somnolence (3%), confusion (2%), headache (2%), agitation (2%), fatigue (1%)
Gastrointestinal: Nausea (7%), vomiting (1%)
Local: Pain on injection (8%), infusion site reaction

Overdosage/Toxicology Symptoms of overdose include hypotension, bradycardia, bronchospasm, congestive heart failure, and heart block. Initially, a decrease/discontinuation of the esmolol infusion and administration of fluids may be the best treatment for hypotension. Sympathomimetics (eg, epinephrine or dopamine), glucagon, or an anticholinergic or a pacemaker can be used to treat the toxic bradycardia, asystole, and/or hypotension.

Pharmacodynamics/Kinetics

Onset of Action: Beta-blockade: I.V.: 2-10 minutes (quickest when loading doses are administered)

Duration of Action: Hemodynamic effects: 10-30 minutes; prolonged following higher cumulative doses, extended duration of use

Protein Binding: 55%

Half-Life Elimination: Adults: 9 minutes; elimination of metabolite decreases with end stage renal disease

Metabolism: In blood by red blood cell esterases

Excretion: Urine (~69% as metabolites, 2% unchanged drug)

Available Dosage Forms

Infusion [premixed in sodium chloride; preservative free] (Brevibloc®): 2000 mg (100 mL) [20 mg/mL; double strength]; 2500 mg (250 mL) [10 mg/mL]
Injection, solution, as hydrochloride: 10 mg/mL (10 mL) [premixed in sodium chloride]
Brevibloc®: 10 mg/mL (10 mL) [alcohol free; premixed in sodium chloride]; 20 mg/mL (5 mL, 100 mL) [alcohol free; double strength; premixed in sodium chloride]; 250 mg/mL (10 mL) [contains alcohol 25%, propylene glycol 25%; concentrate]

Dosing

Adults & Elderly: Infusion requires an infusion pump (must be adjusted to individual response and tolerance):

Intraoperative tachycardia and/or hypertension (immediate control): I.V.: Initial bolus: 80 mg (~1 mg/kg) over 30 seconds, followed by a 150 mcg/kg/minute infusion, if necessary. Adjust infusion rate as needed to maintain desired heart rate and/or blood pressure, up to 300 mcg/kg/minute.

For control of postoperative hypertension, as many as one-third of patients may require higher doses (250-300 mcg/kg/minute) to control blood pressure; the safety of doses >300 mcg/kg/minute has not been studied.

Supraventricular tachycardia or gradual control of postoperative tachycardia/hypertension: I.V.: Loading dose: 500 mcg/kg over 1 minute; follow with a 50 mcg/kg/minute infusion for 4 minutes; response to this initial infusion rate may be a rough indication of the responsiveness of the ventricular rate.

Infusion may be continued at 50 mcg/kg/minute or, if the response is inadequate, titrated upward in 50 mcg/kg/minute increments (increased no more frequently than every 4 minutes) to a maximum of 200 mcg/kg/minute.

Note: To achieve more rapid response, following the initial loading dose and 50 mcg/kg/minute infusion, rebolus with a second 500 mcg/kg loading dose over 1 minute, and increase the maintenance infusion to 100 mcg/kg/minute for 4 minutes. If necessary, a third (and final) 500 mcg/kg loading dose may be administered, prior to increasing to an infusion rate of 150 mcg/minute. After 4 minutes of the 150 mcg/kg/minute infusion, the infusion rate may be increased to a maximum rate of 200 mcg/kg/minute (without a bolus dose).

Supraventricular tachycardias (SVT); usual dose range: Usual dosage range: 50-200 mcg/kg/minute with average dose of 100 mcg/kg/minute.

Guidelines for transfer to oral therapy (beta blocker, calcium channel blocker):
Infusion should be reduced by 50% 30 minutes following the first dose of the alternative agent
Manufacturer suggests following the second dose of the alternative drug, patient's response should be monitored and if control is adequate for the first hours, esmolol may be discontinued.

Pediatrics:

Supraventricular tachycardias (unlabeled use): I.V.: A limited amount of information regarding esmolol use in pediatric patients is currently available. Some centers have utilized doses of 100-500 mcg/kg given over 1 minute for control of supraventricular tachycardias.

Postoperative hypertension (unlabeled use): I.V.: Loading doses of 500 mcg/kg/minute over 1 minute with maximal doses of 50-250 mcg/kg/minute (mean = 173) have been used in addition to nitroprusside to treat postoperative hypertension after coarctation of aorta repair.

Renal Impairment: Not removed by hemo- or peritoneal dialysis. Supplemental dose is not necessary.

Administration

I.V.: The 250 mg/mL ampul is **not** for direct I.V. injection, but rather must first be diluted to a final concentration of 10 mg/mL (ie, 2.5 g in 250 mL or 5 g in 500 mL). Concentrations >10 mg/mL or infusion into small veins or through a butterfly catheter should be avoided (can cause thrombophlebitis).

I.V. Detail: Infusions must be administered with an infusion pump. Decrease or discontinue infusion if hypotension, congestive heart failure occur.

pH: 3.5-5.5 (concentrate); 4.5-5.5 (ready to use)

Stability

Compatibility: Stable in D$_5$LR, D$_5$½NS, D$_5$NS, D$_5$W, D$_5$W with KCl 40 mEq/L, LR, ½NS, NS, sodium bicarbonate 5%

Y-site administration: Incompatible with amphotericin B cholesteryl sulfate complex, furosemide, warfarin

Compatibility when admixed: Incompatible with diazepam, procainamide, sodium bicarbonate, thiopental

Storage: Clear, colorless to light yellow solution which should be stored at 15°C to 30°C (59°F to 85°F); protect from freezing and excessive heat.

Nursing Actions

Physical Assessment: Assess other medications patient may be taking for effectiveness and interactions. Requires continuous cardiac, hemodynamic, and infusion site monitoring (extravasation). If diabetic, may mask signs of hypoglycemia. Monitor blood sugars closely. Monitor therapeutic response (cardiac status) and adverse reactions.

Patient Education: Esmolol is administered in emergencies, patient education should be appropriate to the situation. **Pregnancy/breast-feeding precautions:** Inform prescriber if you are pregnant. Consult prescriber if breast-feeding.

Geriatric Considerations Due to alterations in the beta-adrenergic autonomic nervous system, beta-adrenergic blockade may result in less hemodynamic response than seen in younger adults.

Esomeprazole (es oh ME pray zol)

U.S. Brand Names Nexium®

Synonyms Esomeprazole Magnesium

Pharmacologic Category Proton Pump Inhibitor; Substituted Benzimidazole

Pregnancy Risk Factor B

Lactation Excretion in breast milk unknown/not recommended

Use

Oral: Short-term (4-8 weeks) treatment of erosive esophagitis; maintaining symptom resolution and healing of erosive esophagitis; treatment of symptomatic gastroesophageal reflux disease (GERD); as part of a multidrug regimen for *Helicobacter pylori* eradication in patients with duodenal ulcer disease (active or history of within the past 5 years); prevention of gastric ulcers (in high-risk patients age >60 years and/or history of gastric ulcer) associated with continuous NSAID therapy

I.V.: Short-term (≤10 weeks) treatment of gastroesophageal reflux disease (GERD) when oral therapy is not possible or appropriate

Mechanism of Action/Effect Prevents gastric acid secretion

Contraindications Hypersensitivity to esomeprazole, substituted benzimidazoles (ie, lansoprazole, omeprazole, pantoprazole, rabeprazole), or any component of the formulation

Warnings/Precautions Relief of symptoms does not preclude the presence of a gastric malignancy. Atrophic gastritis (by biopsy) has been noted with long-term omeprazole therapy; this may also occur with esomeprazole. No reports of enterochromaffin-like (ECL) cell carcinoids, dysplasia, or neoplasia has occurred. Safety and efficacy in pediatric patients have not been established.

Drug Interactions

Cytochrome P450 Effect: Substrate of CYP2C19 (major), 3A4 (minor); **Inhibits** CYP2C19 (moderate)

Decreased Effect: CYP2C19 inducers may decrease the levels/effects of esomeprazole; example inducers include aminoglutethimide, carbamazepine, phenytoin, and rifampin. Proton pump inhibitors may decrease the absorption of atazanavir, indinavir, iron salts, itraconazole, and ketoconazole.

Increased Effect/Toxicity: Esomeprazole and omeprazole may increase the levels of carbamazepine, HMG CoA reductase inhibitors, and CYP2C19

substrates, including benzodiazepines metabolized by oxidation (eg, diazepam, midazolam, triazolam).

Nutritional/Ethanol Interactions Food: Absorption is decreased by 43% to 53% when taken with food.

Adverse Reactions Unless otherwise specified, percentages represent adverse reactions identified in clinical trials evaluating the intravenous formulation.

>10%: Central nervous system: Headache (I.V. 11%; oral 4% to 6%)

1% to 10%:

Central nervous system: Dizziness (3%)

Dermatologic: Pruritus (≤1%)

Gastrointestinal: Flatulence (10%), nausea (6%), aabdominal pain (6%; oral 4%), diarrhea (4%), xerostomia (4%), dyspepsia (<1% to 6%), constipation (3%)

Local: Injection site reaction (2%)

Respiratory: Sinusitis (≤2%), respiratory infection (1%)

Overdosage/Toxicology Doses up to 2400 mg have been reported. Symptoms of overdose may include confusion, drowsiness, blurred vision, tachycardia, nausea, sweating, headache or dry mouth. Treatment is symptom-directed and supportive; not dialyzable.

Pharmacodynamics/Kinetics

Time to Peak: 1.5 hours

Protein Binding: 97%

Half-Life Elimination: 1-1.5 hours

Metabolism: Hepatic via CYP2C19 and 3A4 enzymes to hydroxy, desmethyl, and sulfone metabolites (all inactive)

Excretion: Urine (80%); feces (20%)

Available Dosage Forms

Capsule, delayed release:

Nexium®: 20 mg, 40 mg

Injection, powder for reconstitution:

Nexium®: 20 mg, 40 mg [contains edetate sodium]

Dosing

Adults & Elderly:

Healing of erosive esophagitis: Oral: 20-40 mg once daily for 4-8 weeks; may consider an additional 4-8 weeks of treatment if patient is not healed

Maintenance of healing of erosive esophagitis: Oral: 20 mg once daily; clinical trials evaluated therapy for ≤6 months

Symptomatic gastroesophageal reflux: Oral: 20 mg once daily for 4 weeks; may consider an additional 4 weeks of treatment if symptoms do not resolve

Treatment of GERD (short-term): I.V.: 20 mg or 40 mg once daily for ≤10 days; change to oral therapy as soon as appropriate

Peptic ulcer disease: Eradication of *Helicobacter pylori*: Oral: 40 mg once daily for 10 days; requires combination therapy

Prevention of NSAID-induced gastric ulcers: 20-40 mg once daily for up to 6 months

Renal Impairment: No adjustment is necessary.

Hepatic Impairment:

Mild-to-moderate hepatic impairment (Child-Pugh Class A or B): No dosage adjustment needed.

Severe hepatic impairment (Child-Pugh Class C): Dose should not exceed 20 mg/day.

Administration

Oral: Capsule should be swallowed whole and taken at least 1 hour before eating (best if taken before breakfast). For patients with difficulty swallowing, open capsule and mix contents with 1 tablespoon of applesauce. Swallow immediately; mixture should not be chewed or warmed. The mixture should not be stored for future use.

I.V.:

May be administered by injection (≥3 minutes) or infusion (10-30 minutes). Flush line prior to and after administration with NS, LR, or D₅W.

Other: Nasogastric tube: Open capsule and place intact granules into a 60 mL syringe; mix with 50 mL of

(Continued)

Esomeprazole *(Continued)*

water. Replace plunger and shake vigorously for 15 seconds. Ensure that no granules remain in syringe tip. Do not administer if pellets dissolve or disintegrate. After administration, flush nasogastric tube with additional water. Use suspension immediately after preparation.

Stability

Reconstitution: Powder for injection:

For I.V. injection: Reconstitute powder with 5 mL NS.

For I.V. infusion: Initially reconstitute powder with 5 mL of NS, LR, or D₅W, then further dilute to a final volume of 50 mL.

Storage: Capsule: Store at 15°C to 30°C (59°F to 86°F). Keep container tightly closed.

Powder for injection: Store at 15°C to 30°C (59°F to 86°F). Protect from light. Following reconstitution, solution for injection prepared in NS, and solution for infusion prepared in NS or LR should be used within 12 hours. Following reconstitution, solution for infusion prepared in D₅W should be used within 6 hours. Refrigeration is not required following reconstitution.

Laboratory Monitoring Susceptibility testing is recommended in patients who fail *H. pylori* eradication regimen (esomeprazole, clarithromycin, and amoxicillin).

Nursing Actions

Physical Assessment: Assess other medications patient may be taking for effectiveness and interactions (especially those dependent on cytochrome P450 metabolism or those dependent on an acid environment for absorption). Monitor effectiveness of therapeutic response and adverse reactions at beginning of therapy and periodically throughout therapy. Assess knowledge/teach appropriate use of this medication, interventions to reduce side effects, and adverse symptoms to report.

Patient Education: Take as directed, 1 hour before eating at same time each day. Swallow capsule whole; do not crush or chew. If you cannot swallow capsule whole, open capsule, mix contents with 1 tablespoon of applesauce, and swallow immediately; do not store for future use. You may experience headache; constipation (increased exercise, fluids, fruit, or fiber may help); diarrhea (boiled milk, yogurt, or buttermilk may help); or abdominal pain (should diminish with use). Report persistent headache, diarrhea, constipation, abdominal pain, changes in urination or pain on urination, chest pain or palpitations, changes in respiratory status, CNS changes, persistent muscular aches or pain, ringing in ears or visual changes, or other adverse reactions. **Breast-feeding precaution:** Breast-feeding is not recommended.

Dietary Considerations Take at least 1 hour before meals; best if taken before breakfast. The contents of the capsule may be mixed in applesauce or water; pellets also remain intact when exposed to orange juice, apple juice, and yogurt.

Breast-Feeding Issues Esomeprazole excretion into breast milk has not been studied. However, omeprazole is excreted in breast milk, and therefore considered likely that esomeprazole is similarly excreted; breast-feeding is not recommended..

Additional Information Esomeprazole is the S-isomer of omeprazole.

Estradiol (es tra DYE ole)

U.S. Brand Names Alora®; Climara®; Delestrogen®; Depo®-Estradiol; Esclim®; Estrace®; Estraderm®; Estrasorb™; Estring®; EstroGel®; Femring™; Femtrace®; Gynodiol®; Menostar™; Vagifem®; Vivelle®; Vivelle-Dot®

Synonyms Estradiol Acetate; Estradiol Cypionate; Estradiol Hemihydrate; Estradiol Transdermal; Estradiol Valerate

Pharmacologic Category Estrogen Derivative

Medication Safety Issues

Sound-alike/look-alike issues:

Alora® may be confused with Aldara™

Estraderm® may be confused with Testoderm®

Transdermal patch may contain conducting metal (eg, aluminum); remove patch prior to MRI.

Pregnancy Risk Factor X

Lactation Enters breast milk/use caution

Use Treatment of moderate-to-severe vasomotor symptoms associated with menopause; treatment of vulvar and vaginal atrophy; hypoestrogenism (due to hypogonadism, castration, or primary ovarian failure); prostatic cancer (palliation); breast cancer (palliation); osteoporosis (prophylaxis); abnormal uterine bleeding due to hormonal imbalance; postmenopausal urogenital symptoms of the lower urinary tract (urinary urgency, dysuria)

Mechanism of Action/Effect Estrogens modulate the pituitary secretion of gonadotropins, luteinizing hormone, and follicle-stimulating hormone through a negative feedback system; estrogen replacement reduces elevated levels of these hormones in postmenopausal women.

Contraindications Hypersensitivity to estradiol or any component of the formulation; undiagnosed abnormal vaginal bleeding; history of or current thrombophlebitis or venous thromboembolic disorders (including DVT, PE); active or recent (within 1 year) arterial thromboembolic disease (eg, stroke, MI); carcinoma of the breast, except in appropriately selected patients being treated for metastatic disease; estrogen-dependent tumor; hepatic dysfunction or disease; porphyria; pregnancy

Warnings/Precautions

Cardiovascular-related considerations: Estrogens with or without progestin should not be used to prevent coronary heart disease. Use caution with cardiovascular disease or dysfunction. May increase the risks of hypertension, myocardial infarction (MI), stroke, pulmonary emboli (PE), and deep vein thrombosis; incidence of these effects was shown to be significantly increased in postmenopausal women using conjugated equine estrogens (CEE) in combination with medroxyprogesterone acetate (MPA). Nonfatal MI, PE, and thrombophlebitis have also been reported in males taking high doses of CEE (eg, for prostate cancer). Estrogen compounds are generally associated with lipid effects such as increased HDL-cholesterol and decreased LDL-cholesterol. Triglycerides may also be increased; use with caution in patients with familial defects of lipoprotein metabolism. Whenever possible, estrogens should be discontinued at least 4 weeks prior to and for 2 weeks following elective surgery associated with an increased risk of thromboembolism or during periods of prolonged immobilization.

Neurological considerations: The risk of dementia may be increased in postmenopausal women; increased incidence was observed in women ≥65 years of age taking CEE alone or in combination with MPA.

Cancer-related considerations: Unopposed estrogens may increase the risk of endometrial carcinoma in postmenopausal women. Estrogens may exacerbate endometriosis. Malignant transformation of residual endometrial implants has been reported post-hysterectomy with estrogen only therapy. Consider adding a progestin in women with residual endometriosis post-hysterectomy. Estrogens may increase the risk of breast cancer. An increased risk of invasive breast cancer was observed in postmenopausal women using CEE in combination with MPA; a smaller increase in risk was seen with estrogen therapy alone in observational studies. An increase in abnormal mammograms has also been reported with estrogen and progestin therapy. Estrogen use may lead to severe hypercalcemia in patients with breast cancer and bone metastases; discontinue estrogen if hypercalcemia occurs.

Estrogens may cause retinal vascular thrombosis; discontinue permanently if papilledema or retinal vascular lesions are observed on examination. Use with caution in patients with diseases which may be exacerbated by fluid retention, including asthma, epilepsy, migraine, diabetes or renal dysfunction. Use with caution in patients with a history of severe hypocalcemia, SLE, hepatic hemangiomas, endometriosis, and gallbladder disease. Use caution with history of cholestatic jaundice associated with past estrogen use or pregnancy. Safety and efficacy in pediatric patients have not been established. Prior to puberty, estrogens may cause premature closure of the epiphyses, premature breast development in girls or gynecomastia in boys. Vaginal bleeding and vaginal cornification may also be induced in girls.

Before prescribing estrogen therapy to postmenopausal women, the risks and benefits must be weighed for each patient. Women should be informed of these risks and benefits, as well as possible effects of progestin when added to estrogen therapy. Estrogens with or without progestin should be used for shortest duration possible consistent with treatment goals. Conduct periodic risk:benefit assessments.

When used solely for prevention of osteoporosis in women at significant risk, nonestrogen treatment options should be considered. When used solely for the treatment of vulvar and vaginal atrophy, topical vaginal products should be considered. Use caution when applying topical products to severely atrophic vaginal mucosa. Absorption of topical emulsion is increased by application of sunscreen; do not apply both products within close proximity of each other. Application of gel formulation with sunscreen has not been evaluated. Transdermal patch may contain conducting metal (eg, aluminum); remove patch prior to MRI.

Drug Interactions

Cytochrome P450 Effect: Substrate of CYP1A2 (major), 2A6 (minor), 2B6 (minor), 2C8/9 (minor), 2C19 (minor), 2D6 (minor), 2E1 (minor), 3A4 (major); **Inhibits** CYP1A2 (weak); **Induces** CYP3A4 (weak)

Decreased Effect: CYP1A2 inducers may decrease the levels/effects of estradiol; example inducers include aminoglutethimide, carbamazepine, phenobarbital, and rifampin. CYP3A4 inducers may decrease the levels/effects of estradiol; example inducers include aminoglutethimide, carbamazepine, nafcillin, nevirapine, phenobarbital, phenytoin, and rifamycins.

Increased Effect/Toxicity: Estradiol with hydrocortisone increases corticosteroid toxic potential. Anticoagulants and estradiol increase the potential for thromboembolic events.

Nutritional/Ethanol Interactions

Ethanol: Avoid ethanol (routine use increases estrogen level and risk of breast cancer). Ethanol may also increase the risk of osteoporosis.

Food: Folic acid absorption may be decreased

Herb/Nutraceutical: St John's wort may decrease estradiol levels. Avoid black cohosh, dong quai (has estrogenic activity). Avoid red clover, saw palmetto, ginseng.

Lab Interactions Increased Prothrombin and factors VII, VIII, IX, X; increased platelet aggregability, thyroid-binding globulin, total thyroid hormone (T_4), serum triglycerides/phospholipids; decreased antithrombin III, serum folate concentration

Adverse Reactions Frequency not defined.

Cardiovascular: Edema, hypertension, MI, venous thromboembolism

Central nervous system: Anxiety, dizziness, epilepsy exacerbation, headache, irritability, mental depression, migraine, mood disturbances, nervousness

Dermatologic: Chloasma, erythema multiforme, erythema nodosum, hemorrhagic eruption, hirsutism, loss of scalp hair, melasma, rash, pruritus

Endocrine & metabolic: Breast enlargement, breast tenderness, libido (changes in), increased thyroid-binding globulin, increased total thyroid hormone (T_4), increased serum triglycerides/phospholipids, increased HDL-cholesterol, decreased LDL-cholesterol, impaired glucose tolerance, hypercalcemia

Gastrointestinal: Abdominal cramps, abdominal pain, bloating, cholecystitis, cholelithiasis, diarrhea, flatulence, gallbladder disease, nausea, pancreatitis, vomiting, weight gain/loss

Genitourinary: Alterations in frequency and flow of menses, changes in cervical secretions, endometrial cancer, increased size of uterine leiomyomata, Pap smear suspicious, vaginal candidiasis

Vaginal: Trauma from applicator insertion may occur in women with severely atrophic vaginal mucosa

Hematologic: Aggravation of porphyria, antithrombin III and antifactor Xa decreased, levels of fibrinogen increased, platelet aggregability increased and platelet count; increased prothrombin and factors VII, VIII, IX, X

Hepatic: Cholestatic jaundice

Local: Transdermal patches: Burning, erythema, irritation, thrombophlebitis

Neuromuscular & skeletal: Chorea, back pain

Ocular: Intolerance to contact lenses, steeping of corneal curvature

Respiratory: Pulmonary thromboembolism

Miscellaneous: Anaphylactoid/anaphylactic reactions, carbohydrate intolerance

Overdosage/Toxicology Symptoms of overdose include fluid retention, jaundice, thrombophlebitis, nausea, and vomiting. Toxicity is unlikely following single exposure of excessive doses. Treatment following emesis and charcoal administration should be supportive and symptomatic.

Pharmacodynamics/Kinetics

Protein Binding: 37% to sex hormone-binding globulin; 61% to albumin

Metabolism: Hepatic via oxidation and conjugation in GI tract; hydroxylated via CYP3A4 to metabolites; first-pass effect; enterohepatic recirculation; reversibly converted to estrone and estriol

Excretion: Primarily urine (as metabolites estrone and estriol); feces (small amounts)

Available Dosage Forms

Cream, vaginal (Estrace®): 0.1 mg/g (12 g) [refill tube]; 0.1 mg/g (42.5 g) [tube with applicator]

Emulsion, topical, as hemihydrate (Estrasorb™): 2.5 mg/g (56s) [each pouch contains 4.35 mg estradiol hemihydrate; contents of two pouches delivers estradiol 0.05 mg/day]

Gel, topical (EstroGel®): 0.06% (93 g) [pump; delivers estradiol 0.75 mg/1.25 g; 64 doses]

Injection, oil, as cypionate (Depo®-Estradiol): 5 mg/mL (5 mL) [contains chlorobutanol; in cottonseed oil]

Injection, oil, as valerate (Delestrogen®):

10 mg/mL (5 mL) [contains chlorobutanol; in sesame oil]

20 mg/mL (5 mL) [contains benzyl alcohol; in castor oil]

40 mg/mL (5 mL) [contains benzyl alcohol; in castor oil]

(Continued)

Estradiol *(Continued)*

Ring, vaginal, as base (Estring®): 2 mg [total estradiol 2 mg; releases 7.5 mcg/day over 90 days] (1s)

Ring, vaginal, as acetate (Femring™): 0.05 mg [total estradiol 12.4 mg; releases 0.05 mg/day over 3 months] (1s); 0.1 mg [total estradiol 24.8 mg; releases 0.1 mg/day over 3 months] (1s)

Tablet, oral, as acetate (Femtrace®): 0.45 mg, 0.9 mg, 1.8 mg

Tablet, oral, micronized: 0.5 mg, 1 mg, 2 mg

Estrace®: 0.5 mg, 1 mg, 2 mg [2 mg tablets contain tartrazine]

Gynodiol®: 0.5 mg, 1 mg, 1.5 mg, 2 mg

Tablet, vaginal, as base (Vagifem®): 25 mcg [contains lactose]

Transdermal system: 0.025 mg/24 hours [once-weekly patch]; 0.05 mg/24 hours (4s) [once-weekly patch]; 0.075 mg/24 hours [once-weekly patch]; 0.1 mg/24 hours (4s) [once-weekly patch]

Alora® [twice-weekly patch]:
0.025 mg/24 hours [9 cm², total estradiol 0.77 mg] (8s)
0.05 mg/24 hours [18 cm², total estradiol 1.5 mg] (8s, 24s)
0.075 mg/24 hours [27 cm², total estradiol 2.3 mg] (8s)
0.1 mg/24 hours [36 cm², total estradiol 3.1 mg] (8s)

Climara® [once-weekly patch]:
0.025 mg/24 hours [6.5 cm², total estradiol 2.04 mg] (4s)
0.0375 mg/24 hours [9.375 cm², total estradiol 2.85 mg] (4s)
0.05 mg/24 hours [12.5 cm², total estradiol 3.8 mg] (4s)
0.06 mg/24 hours [15 cm², total estradiol 4.55 mg] (4s)
0.075 mg/24 hours [18.75 cm², total estradiol 5.7 mg] (4s)
0.1 mg/24 hours [25 cm², total estradiol 7.6 mg] (4s)

Esclim® [twice-weekly patch]:
0.025 mg/day [11 cm², total estradiol 5 mg] (8s)
0.0375 mg/day [16.5 cm², total estradiol 7.5 mg] (8s)
0.05 mg/day [22 cm², total estradiol 10 mg] (8s)
0.075 mg/day [33 cm², total estradiol 15 mg] (8s)
0.1 mg/day [44 cm², total estradiol 20 mg] (8s)

Estraderm® [twice-weekly patch]:
0.05 mg/24 hours [10 cm², total estradiol 4 mg] (8s)
0.1 mg/24 hours [20 cm², total estradiol 8 mg] (8s)

Menostar™ [once-weekly patch]: 0.014 mg/24 hours [3.25 cm², total estradiol 1 mg] (4s)

Vivelle® [twice-weekly patch]:
0.05 mg/24 hours [14.5 cm², total estradiol 4.33 mg] (8s)
0.1 mg/24 hours [29 cm², total estradiol 8.66 mg] (8s)

Vivelle-Dot® [twice-weekly patch]:
0.025 mg/day [2.5 cm², total estradiol 0.39 mg] (8s)
0.0375 mg/day [3.75 cm², total estradiol 0.585 mg] (8s)
0.05 mg/day [5 cm², total estradiol 0.78 mg] (8s)
0.075 mg/day [7.5 cm², total estradiol 1.17 mg] (8s)
0.1 mg/day [10 cm², total estradiol 1.56 mg] (8s)

Dosing

Adults & Elderly: All dosage needs to be adjusted based upon the patient's response:

Atrophic vaginitis, vulvar/vaginal atrophy:

Intravaginal:
Vaginal cream: Atrophic vaginitis, kraurosis vulvae: Insert 2-4 g/day for 2 weeks then gradually reduce to ½ the initial dose for 2 weeks followed by a maintenance dose of 1 g 1-3 times/week
Vaginal ring:
Postmenopausal vaginal atrophy, urogenital symptoms (Estring®): 2 mg intravaginally;

following insertion, ring should remain in place for 90 days
Vulvar/vaginal atrophy (Femring™): 0.05 mg intravaginally; following insertion, ring should remain in place for 3 months; dose may be increased to 0.1 mg if needed
Vaginal tablets (Vagifem®); Atrophic vaginitis: Initial: Insert 1 tablet once daily for 2 weeks; maintenance: Insert 1 tablet twice weekly. Attempts to discontinue or taper medication should be made at 3- to 6-month intervals
Topical gel: Vulvar/vaginal atrophy: 1.25 g/day applied at the same time each day
Transdermal: Refer to product-specific dosing (below)

Breast cancer (females; inoperable, progressing):
Oral: 10 mg 3 times/day for at least 3 months

Hypogonadism:
Oral: 1-2 mg/day in a cyclic regimen for 3 weeks on drug, then 1 week off drug
I.M.: Cypionate: 1.5-2 mg monthly; Valerate: 10-20 mg every 4 weeks
Transdermal: Refer to product-specific dosing (below)

Osteoporosis prevention (females):
Oral: 0.5 mg/day in a cyclic regimen (3 weeks on and 1 week off of drug)
Transdermal: Refer to product-specific dosing (below)

Prostate cancer:
I.M. (valerate): ≥30 mg or more every 1-2 weeks
Oral (androgen-dependent, inoperable, progressing): 10 mg 3 times/day for at least 3 months

Vasomotor symptoms (moderate-severe) associated with menopause:
Oral (in addition to I.M. dosing): 1-2 mg daily, adjusted as necessary to limit symptoms. Administrations should be cyclic (3 weeks on, 1 week off). Patients should be re-evaluated at 3-6 month intervals to determine if treatment is still necessary
I.M.: Cypionate: 1-5 mg every 3-4 weeks; Valerate: 10-20 mg every 4 weeks
Topical emulsion: 3.84 g applied once daily in the morning
Topical gel: 1.25 g/day applied at the same time each day
Vaginal ring (Femring™): 0.05 mg intravaginally; following insertion, ring should remain in place for 3 months; dose may be increased to 0.1 mg if needed
Transdermal: See product-specific dosing (below)

Transdermal product-specific dosing:
Note: Indicated dose may be used continuously in patients without an intact uterus. May be given continuously or cyclically (3 weeks on, 1 week off) in patients with an intact uterus **(exception - Menostar™, see specific dosing instructions).** When changing patients from oral to transdermal therapy, start transdermal patch 1 week after discontinuing oral hormone (may begin sooner if symptoms reappear within 1 week):

Transdermal once-weekly patch:
Moderate to severe vasomotor symptoms associated with menopause (Climara®): Apply 0.025 mg/day patch once weekly. Adjust dose as necessary to control symptoms. Patients should be re-evaluated at 3- to 6-month intervals to determine if treatment is still necessary.
Prevention of osteoporosis in postmenopausal women:
Climara®: Apply patch once weekly; minimum effective dose 0.025 mg/day; adjust dosage based on response to therapy as indicated by biological markers and bone mineral density.

Menostar™: Apply patch once weekly. In women with a uterus, also administer a progestin for 14 days every 6-12 months.

Transdermal twice-weekly patch (Alora®, Esclim®, Estraderm®, Vivelle®):

Moderate to severe vasomotor symptoms associated with menopause, vulvar/vaginal atrophy, female hypogonadism: Titrate to lowest dose possible to control symptoms, adjusting initial dose after the first month of therapy; re-evaluate therapy at 3- to 6-month intervals to taper or discontinue medication:

Alora®, Esclim®, Estraderm®, Vivelle-Dot®: Apply 0.05 mg patch twice weekly

Vivelle®: Apply 0.0375 mg patch twice weekly

Prevention of osteoporosis in postmenopausal women:

Alora®, Vivelle®, Vivelle-Dot®: Apply 0.025 mg patch twice weekly, increase dose as necessary

Estraderm®: Apply 0.05 mg patch twice weekly

Administration

I.M.: Injection for intramuscular administration only.

Topical:

Emulsion: Apply to clean dry skin while in a sitting position. Contents of two pouches (total 3.48 g) are to be applied individually, once daily in the morning. Apply contents of first pouch to left thigh, massage into skin of left thigh and calf until thoroughly absorbed (~3 minutes). Apply excess from both hands to the buttocks. Apply contents of second pouch to the right thigh, massage into skin of right thigh and calf until thoroughly absorbed (~3 minutes). Apply excess from both hands to buttocks. Wash hands with soap and water. Allow skin to dry before covering legs with clothing. Do not apply to other areas of body. Do not apply to red or irritated skin.

Gel: Apply to clean, dry, unbroken skin at the same time each day. Apply gel to the arm, from the wrist to the shoulder. Spread gel as thinly as possible over one arm. Allow to dry for 5 minutes prior to dressing. Gel is flammable; avoid fire or flame until dry. After application, wash hands with soap and water. Prior to the first use, pump must be primed. Do not apply gel to breast.

Transdermal patch: Aerosol topical corticosteroids applied under the patch may reduce allergic reactions. Do not apply transdermal system to breasts, but place on trunk of body (preferably abdomen). Rotate application sites allowing a 1-week interval between applications at a particular site. Do not apply to oily, damaged or irritated skin; avoid waistline or other areas where tight clothing may rub the patch off. Apply patch immediately after removing from protective pouch. In general, if patch falls off, the same patch may be reapplied or a new system may be used for the remainder of the dosing interval. Swimming, bathing, or showering are not expected to affect use of the patch. Note the following exceptions:

Estraderm®: Do not apply to an area exposed to direct sunlight.

Menostar™: Swimming, bathing, or wearing patch while in a sauna have not been studied; adhesion of patch may be decreased or delivery of estradiol may be affected. Remove patch slowly after use to avoid skin irritation. If any adhesive remains on the skin after removal, first allow skin to dry for 15 minutes, then gently rub area with an oil-based cream or lotion. If patch falls off, a new patch should be applied for the remainder of the dosing interval.

Other: Vaginal ring: Exact positioning is not critical for efficacy, however, patient should not feel anything once inserted. In case of discomfort, ring should be pushed further into vagina. If ring is expelled prior to 90 days, it may be rinsed off and reinserted.

Laboratory Monitoring Yearly Papanicolaou smear, mammogram. Adequate diagnostic measures, including endometrial sampling, if indicated, should be performed to rule out malignancy in all cases of undiagnosed abnormal vaginal bleeding.

Nursing Actions

Physical Assessment: Assess potential for interactions with other pharmacological agents or herbal products patient may be taking (eg, increased or decreased levels/effects of estradiol or increased potential for toxicity or thrombolic events). Monitor therapeutic effectiveness (dependent on rationale for use), and adverse effects (eg, CNS changes, hypertension, thromboembolism, fluid retention, edema, CHF, respiratory changes) on a regular basis during therapy. Caution patients with diabetes to monitor glucose levels closely (may impair glucose tolerance). Teach patient proper use and application (according to formulation), possible side effects/appropriate interventions, and adverse symptoms to report. Remind patient about the importance of frequent self-breast exams and the need for annual gynecological exam. **Pregnancy risk factor X:** Determine that patient is not pregnant before starting therapy. Do not give to females of childbearing age unless patient is capable of complying with contraceptive use. Advise patient about contraceptive measures as appropriate.

Patient Education: Do not take any new medication during therapy without consulting prescriber. Use/apply exactly as directed and maintain prescribed cycles or term as prescribed. Routine use of alcohol may increase estrogen level and risk of breast cancer. Annual gynecologic and regular self-breast exams are important. If you have diabetes, monitor glucose levels closely (may impair glucose tolerance). You may experience nausea, vomiting or abdominal pain (small, frequent meals may help); dizziness or mental depression (use caution when driving); rash; hair loss; headache; or breast pain, increased/decreased libido, or enlargement/tenderness of breasts. difficult/painful menstrual cycles. Report unusual swelling of extremities; sudden acute pain in legs or calves, chest, or abdomen; shortness of breath; severe headache or vomiting; sudden blindness; weakness or numbness of arm or leg; unusual vaginal bleeding; yellowing of skin or eyes; unusual bruising or bleeding, or other persistent adverse reactions. You may become intolerant to wearing contact lenses, notify prescriber if this occurs. **Pregnancy/breast-feeding precautions:** Inform prescriber if you are pregnant. Do not get pregnant while taking this medication. Consult prescriber for appropriate contraceptive measures. This medication may cause fetal defects and should not be used during pregnancy. Consult prescriber if breast-feeding.

Transdermal patch: Apply to clean dry skin. Do not apply transdermal patch to breasts. Apply to trunk of body (preferably abdomen). Rotate application sites. Aerosol topical corticosteroids may reduce allergic skin reaction; report persistent skin reaction.

Intravaginal cream: Insert high in vagina. Wash hands and applicator before and after use.

Topical emulsion: Contents of 2 pouches are applied one at time to each thigh and rubbed into thigh and calf. Excess on hands should be applied to buttocks. Wash hands with soap and water after application. Allow skin to dry before covering legs with clothes. Do not apply sunscreen soon after or before applying emulsion. Do not apply to red or irritated skin.

Topical gel: Apply dose to one arm (alternate arms daily) at the same time each day. Spread thinly from waist to shoulder. Allow to dry for 5 minutes prior to dressing. Wash hands with soap and water after
(Continued)

Estradiol (Continued)

application. Do not apply to red or irritated skin. Do not apply to breast.

Vaginal ring: Wash hands thoroughly before removing ring from pouch. In position that is comfortable for insertion (may be lying on your back with knees bent and resting apart), hold ring between thumb and forefinger and press sides together. Insert compressed ring gently into your vagina and push ring toward lower back. If the ring feels uncomfortable you may need to push ring further into vagina. If ring falls out, it may be washed with warm water and reinserted. Ring should be removed and replaced every 3 months.

Dietary Considerations Ensure adequate calcium and vitamin D intake when used for the prevention of osteoporosis.

Geriatric Considerations Before prescribing estrogen therapy to postmenopausal women, the risks and benefits must be weighed for each patient. Data in women 80 years and older is minimal and it is unclear if reduced risk is applicable to women in this age group. Women should be informed of risks and benefits, as well as possible side effects and the return of menstrual bleeding (when cycled with a progestin), and should be involved in the prescribing options. Oral therapy may be more convenient for vaginal atrophy and urinary incontinence.

Breast-Feeding Issues The AAP considers ethinyl estradiol, an estrogen derivative, to be "usually compatible" with breast-feeding. Estrogen has been shown to decrease the quantity and quality of human milk; use only if clearly needed; monitor the growth of the infant closely.

Pregnancy Issues Estrogens are not indicated for use during pregnancy or immediately postpartum. Increased risk of fetal reproductive tract disorders and other birth defects have been observed with diethylstilbestrol (DES); do not use during pregnancy.

Estradiol and Norethindrone
(es tra DYE ole & nor eth IN drone)

U.S. Brand Names Activella®; CombiPatch®

Synonyms Norethindrone and Estradiol

Pharmacologic Category Estrogen and Progestin Combination

Medication Safety Issues
Transdermal patch may contain conducting metal (eg, aluminum); remove patch prior to MRI.

Pregnancy Risk Factor X

Lactation Enters breast milk/use caution

Use Women with an intact uterus:
Tablet: Treatment of moderate-to-severe vasomotor symptoms associated with menopause; treatment of vulvar and vaginal atrophy; prophylaxis for postmenopausal osteoporosis

Transdermal patch: Treatment of moderate-to-severe vasomotor symptoms associated with menopause; treatment of vulvar and vaginal atrophy; treatment of hypoestrogenism due to hypogonadism, castration, or primary ovarian failure

Contraindications Hypersensitivity to estrogens, progestins, or any components; carcinoma of the breast; estrogen-dependent tumor; undiagnosed abnormal vaginal bleeding; history of or current thrombophlebitis or venous thromboembolic disorders (including DVT, PE); active or recent (within 1 year) arterial thromboembolic disease (eg, stroke, MI); hysterectomy; hepatic dysfunction or disease; pregnancy

Warnings/Precautions
Cardiovascular-related considerations: Estrogens with or without progestin should not be used to prevent coronary heart disease. Use caution with cardiovascular disease or dysfunction. May increase the risks of hypertension, myocardial infarction (MI), stroke, pulmonary emboli (PE), and deep vein thrombosis; incidence of these effects was shown to be significantly increased in postmenopausal women using conjugated equine estrogens (CEE) in combination with medroxyprogesterone acetate (MPA). Nonfatal MI, PE, and thrombophlebitis have also been reported in males taking high doses of CEE (eg, for prostate cancer). Estrogen compounds are generally associated with lipid effects such as increased HDL-cholesterol and decreased LDL-cholesterol. Triglycerides may also be increased; use with caution in patients with familial defects of lipoprotein metabolism. Whenever possible, combination hormonal contraceptives should be discontinued at least 4 weeks prior to and for 2 weeks following elective surgery associated with an increased risk of thromboembolism or during periods of prolonged immobilization.

Neurological considerations: The risk of dementia may be increased in postmenopausal women; increased incidence was observed in women ≥65 years of age taking CEE alone or in combination with MPA.

Cancer-related considerations: Unopposed estrogens may increase the risk of endometrial carcinoma in postmenopausal women. Estrogens may exacerbate endometriosis. Malignant transformation of residual endometrial implants has been reported post-hysterectomy with estrogen only therapy. Estrogens may increase the risk of breast cancer. An increased risk of invasive breast cancer was observed in postmenopausal women using CEE in combination with MPA; a smaller increase in risk was seen with estrogen therapy alone in observational studies. An increase in abnormal mammograms has also been reported with estrogen and progestin therapy. Estrogen use may lead to severe hypercalcemia in patients with breast cancer and bone metastases; discontinue estrogen if hypercalcemia occurs.

Estrogens may cause retinal vascular thrombosis; discontinue permanently if papilledema or retinal vascular lesions are observed on examination. Use with caution in patients with diseases which may be exacerbated by fluid retention, including asthma, epilepsy, migraine, diabetes or renal dysfunction. Use with caution in patients with a history of severe hypocalcemia, SLE, hepatic hemangiomas, porphyria, endometriosis, and gallbladder disease. Use caution with history of cholestatic jaundice associated with past estrogen use or pregnancy. Safety and efficacy in pediatric patients have not been established.

Before prescribing estrogen therapy to postmenopausal women, the risks and benefits must be weighed for each patient. Women should be informed of these risks and benefits, as well as possible effects of progestin when added to estrogen therapy. Estrogens with or without progestin should be used for shortest duration possible consistent with treatment goals. Conduct periodic risk:benefit assessments.

When used solely for prevention of osteoporosis in women at significant risk, nonestrogen treatment options should be considered. When used solely for the treatment of vulvar and vaginal atrophy, topical vaginal products should be considered.

Transdermal patch may contain conducting metal (eg, aluminum); remove patch prior to MRI.

Drug Interactions
Cytochrome P450 Effect:
Estradiol: **Substrate** of CYP1A2 (major), 2A6 (minor), 2B6 (minor), 2C8/9 (minor), 2C19 (minor), 2D6 (minor), 2E1 (minor), 3A4 (major); **Inhibits** CYP1A2 (weak); **Induces** CYP3A4 (weak)

Norethindrone: **Substrate** of CYP3A4 (major); **Induces** CYP2C19 (weak)

Nutritional/Ethanol Interactions

Ethanol: Avoid ethanol (routine use increases estrogen level and risk of breast cancer). Ethanol may also increase the risk of osteoporosis.

Food: Folic acid absorption may be decreased

Herb/Nutraceutical: St John's wort may decrease estradiol levels. Avoid black cohosh, dong quai (has estrogenic activity). Avoid red clover, saw palmetto, ginseng.

Adverse Reactions Frequency not defined.

Cardiovascular: Altered blood pressure, cardiovascular accident, edema, venous thromboembolism

Central nervous system: Dizziness, fatigue, headache, insomnia, mental depression, migraine, nervousness

Dermatologic: Chloasma, erythema multiforme, erythema nodosum, hemorrhagic eruption, hirsutism, itching, loss of scalp hair, melasma, pruritus, skin rash

Endocrine & metabolic: Breast enlargement, breast tenderness, breast pain, libido (changes in)

Gastrointestinal: Abdominal pain, bloating, changes in appetite, flatulence, gallbladder disease, nausea, pancreatitis, vomiting, weight gain/loss

Genitourinary: Alterations in frequency and flow of menses, changes in cervical secretions, cystitis-like syndrome, increased size of uterine leiomyomata, premenstrual-like syndrome, vaginal candidiasis, vaginitis

Hematologic: Aggravation of porphyria

Hepatic: Cholestatic jaundice

Local: Application site reaction (transdermal patch)

Neuromuscular & skeletal: Arthralgia, back pain, chorea, myalgia, weakness

Ocular: Intolerance to contact lenses, steeping of corneal curvature

Respiratory: Pharyngitis, pulmonary thromboembolism, rhinitis

Miscellaneous: Allergic reactions, carbohydrate intolerance, flu-like syndrome

Pharmacodynamics/Kinetics

Time to Peak: Activella®: Estradiol: 5-8 hours

Half-Life Elimination:

Activella®: Estradiol: 12-14 hours; Norethindrone: 8-11 hours

Pharmacokinetic Note See individual agents.

Available Dosage Forms [CAN] = Canadian brand name

Combination pack (Estalis-Sequi® [CAN; not available in U.S.]):

140/50:

Transdermal system (Vivelle®): Estradiol 50 mcg per day (4s) [14.5 sq cm; total estradiol 4.33 mg]

Transdermal system (Estalis®): Norethindrone acetate 140 mcg and estradiol 50 mcg per day (4s) [9 sq cm; total norethindrone acetate 2.7 mg, total estradiol 0.62 mg; not available in U.S.]

250/50:

Transdermal system (Vivelle®): Estradiol 50 mcg per day (4s) [14.5 sq cm; total estradiol 4.33 mg]

Transdermal system (Estalis®): Norethindrone acetate 250 mcg and estradiol 50 mcg per day (4s) [16 sq cm; total norethindrone acetate 4.8 mg, total estradiol 0.51 mg; not available in U.S.]

Tablet (Activella®): Estradiol 1 mg and norethindrone acetate 0.5 mg (28s)

Transdermal system:

CombiPatch®:

0.05/0.14: Estradiol 0.05 mg and norethindrone acetate 0.14 mg per day (8s) [9 sq cm]

0.05/0.25: Estradiol 0.05 mg and norethindrone acetate 0.25 mg per day (8s) [16 sq cm]

Estalis® [CAN]:

140/50: Norethindrone acetate 140 mcg and estradiol 50 mcg per day (8s) [9 sq cm; total norethindrone acetate 2.7 mg, total estradiol 0.62 mg; not available in U.S.]

250/50 Norethindrone acetate 250 mcg and estradiol 50 mcg per day (8s) [16 sq cm; total norethindrone acetate 4.8 mg, total estradiol 0.51 mg; not available in U.S.]

Dosing

Adults & Elderly:

Hypoestrogenism: Transdermal (patch):

Continuous combined regimen: Apply one patch twice weekly

Continuous sequential regimen: Apply estradiol-only patch for first 14 days of cycle, followed by one CombiPatch® applied twice weekly for the remaining 14 days of a 28-day cycle.

Osteoporosis, prevention in postmenopausal females (Activella®): Oral: 1 tablet daily

Menopause (moderate to severe vasomotor symptoms); vulvar and vaginal atrophy:

Oral (Activella®): 1 tablet daily

Transdermal (patch):

Continuous combined regimen: Apply one patch twice weekly

Continuous sequential regimen: Apply estradiol-only patch for first 14 days of cycle, followed by one CombiPatch® applied twice weekly for the remaining 14 days of a 28-day cycle.

Transdermal patch, combination pack (product-specific dosing for Canadian formulation):

Estalis®: Continuous combined regimen: Apply a new patch twice weekly during a 28-day cycle

Estalis-Sequi®: Continuous sequential regimen: Apply estradiol-only patch (Vivelle®) for first 14 days, followed by one Estalis® patch applied twice weekly during the last 14 days of a 28-day cycle

Note: In women previously receiving oral estrogens, initiate upon reappearance of menopausal symptoms following discontinuation of oral therapy.

Administration

Other: Transdermal patch: Apply to clean dry skin. Do not apply transdermal patch to breasts; apply to lower abdomen, avoiding waistline. Rotate application sites.

Nursing Actions

Physical Assessment: Assess potential for interactions with other prescriptions, OTC medications, or herbal products patient may be taking. Monitor therapeutic effectiveness (according to purpose for use) and adverse response (eg, CNS changes, hypertension, thromboembolism, fluid retention, edema, CHF, respiratory changes) on a regular basis during therapy. Caution patients with diabetes to monitor glucose levels closely (may impair glucose tolerance). Teach patient appropriate use (according to formulation), possible side effects/appropriate interventions, and adverse symptoms to report. **Pregnancy risk factor X:** Determine that patient is not pregnant before starting therapy

Patient Education: Do not take any new medication during therapy without consulting prescriber. Use/apply exactly as directed and maintain prescribed cycles or term as prescribed. Avoid routine use of alcohol (ethanol may increase the risk of breast cancer or osteoporosis). Annual gynecologic and regular self-breast exams are important. If you have diabetes, monitor glucose levels closely (may impair glucose tolerance). You may experience nausea, vomiting or abdominal pain (small frequent meals may help); dizziness or mental depression (use caution when driving); rash; hair loss; headache; or breast pain, increased/decreased libido, or enlargement/tenderness of breasts, difficult/painful menstrual cycles. Report significant swelling of extremities; sudden acute pain in legs or calves, chest, or abdomen; shortness of breath; severe headache or

(Continued)

Estradiol and Norethindrone
(Continued)

vomiting; sudden blindness; weakness or numbness of arm or leg; unusual vaginal bleeding; yellowing of skin or eyes; unusual bruising or bleeding, or other persistent adverse reactions. You may become intolerant to wearing contact lenses, notify prescriber if this occurs. **Pregnancy/breast-feeding precautions:** Inform prescriber if you are pregnant. Do not get pregnant while taking this medication. This medication may cause fetal defects and should not be used during pregnancy. Consult prescriber if breast-feeding.

Pregnancy Issues Estrogens/progestins should not be used during pregnancy.

Estrogens: Increased risk of fetal reproductive tract disorders and other birth defects; do not use during pregnancy.

Progestins: Associated with fetal genital abnormalities when used during the 1st trimester; not recommended for use during pregnancy.

Related Information
Estradiol *on page 450*
Norethindrone *on page 896*

Estramustine (es tra MUS teen)

U.S. Brand Names Emcyt®

Synonyms Estramustine Phosphate Sodium; NSC-89199

Pharmacologic Category Antineoplastic Agent, Alkylating Agent; Antineoplastic Agent, Hormone; Antineoplastic Agent, Hormone (Estrogen/Nitrogen Mustard)

Medication Safety Issues
Sound-alike/look-alike issues:
Emcyt® may be confused with Eryc®

Pregnancy Risk Factor C

Lactation Excretion in breast milk unknown/contraindicated

Use Palliative treatment of prostatic carcinoma (progressive or metastatic)

Mechanism of Action/Effect Mechanism is not completely clear. It appears to bind to microtubule proteins, preventing normal tubulin function. The antitumor effect may be due solely to an estrogenic effect. Estramustine causes a marked decrease in plasma testosterone and an increase in estrogen levels.

Contraindications Hypersensitivity to estramustine or any component, estradiol or nitrogen mustard; active thrombophlebitis or thromboembolic disorders

Warnings/Precautions Hazardous agent — use appropriate precautions for handling and disposal. Glucose tolerance may be decreased; elevated blood pressure may occur; exacerbation of peripheral edema or congestive heart disease may occur; use with caution in patients with impaired liver function, renal insufficiency, metabolic bone diseases, or history of cardiovascular disease (eg, thrombophlebitis, thrombosis, or thromboembolic disease). Patients with prostate cancer and osteoblastic metastases should have their calcium monitored regularly.

Drug Interactions
Decreased Effect: Milk products and calcium-rich foods/drugs may impair the oral absorption of estramustine phosphate sodium.

Nutritional/Ethanol Interactions Food: Estramustine serum levels may be decreased if taken with dairy products.

Adverse Reactions
>10%:
Cardiovascular: Impaired arterial circulation; ischemic heart disease; venous thromboembolism; cardiac

decompensation (58%), about 50% of complications occur within the first 2 months of therapy, 85% occur within the first year; edema

Endocrine & metabolic: Sodium and water retention, gynecomastia, breast tenderness, libido decreased

Gastrointestinal: Nausea, vomiting, may be dose-limiting

Hematologic: Thrombocytopenia

Local: Thrombophlebitis (nearly 100% with I.V. administration)

Respiratory: Dyspnea

1% to 10%:
Cardiovascular: Myocardial infarction
Central nervous system: Insomnia, lethargy
Gastrointestinal: Diarrhea, anorexia, flatulence
Hematologic: Leukopenia
Hepatic: Serum transaminases increased, jaundice
Neuromuscular & skeletal: Leg cramps
Respiratory: Pulmonary embolism

Overdosage/Toxicology Symptoms of overdose include nausea, vomiting, and myelosuppression. There are no known antidotes; treatment is symptomatic and supportive.

Pharmacodynamics/Kinetics
Time to Peak: Serum: 2-3 hours
Half-Life Elimination: Terminal: 20-24 hours
Metabolism: GI tract: Initial dephosphorylation; Hepatic: Oxidation and hydrolysis; metabolites include estramustine, estrone, estradiol, nitrogen mustard
Excretion: Feces (2.9% to 4.8% as unchanged drug)

Available Dosage Forms Capsule, as phosphate sodium: 140 mg

Dosing
Adults & Elderly: Refer to individual protocols.
Prostate carcinoma: Oral: 10-16 mg/kg/day (14 mg/kg/day is most common) or 140 mg 4 times/day (some patients have been maintained for >3 years on therapy) Refer to individual protocols.

Administration
Oral: Administer on an empty stomach, at least 1 hour before or 2 hours after eating.

Stability
Storage: Refrigerate at 2°C to 8°C (36°F to 46°F). Capsules may be stored outside of refrigerator for up to 24-48 hours without affecting potency.

Laboratory Monitoring Serum calcium, liver function tests

Nursing Actions
Physical Assessment: Assess potential for interactions with other pharmacological agents patient may be taking (see Drug Interactions). Assess results of laboratory tests, therapeutic effectiveness, and adverse response (eg, CNS changes, hypertension, thromboembolism) on a regular basis during therapy. Caution patients with diabetes to monitor glucose carefully; glucose intolerance may be decreased. Teach patient appropriate use, possible side effects/appropriate interventions, and adverse symptoms to report.

Patient Education: Do not take any new medication during therapy without consulting prescriber. It may take several weeks to manifest effects of this medication. Store capsules in refrigerator. Do not take with milk or milk products. Preferable to take on empty stomach, 1 hour before or 2 hours after meals. Diabetic patients should use caution and monitor glucose carefully; glucose intolerance may be decreased. May cause nausea or vomiting (small, frequent meals, frequent mouth care, chewing gum, or sucking lozenges may help); flatulence; diarrhea (buttermilk, boiled milk, or yogurt); decreased libido (reversible); or breast tenderness or enlargement. Report sudden acute pain or cramping in legs or calves, chest pain, shortness of breath, weakness or numbness of arms or legs, respiratory difficulty, or edema (increased weight, swelling of legs or feet).

Pregnancy/breast-feeding precautions: Male: Do not cause a female to become pregnant. Male/female: Consult prescriber for instruction on appropriate barrier contraceptive measures. This drug may cause severe fetal defects. Do not breast-feed.

Dietary Considerations Should be taken at least 1 hour before or 2 hours after eating.

Estrogens (Conjugated A/Synthetic)
(ES troe jenz, KON joo gate ed, aye, sin THET ik)

U.S. Brand Names Cenestin®

Pharmacologic Category Estrogen Derivative

Medication Safety Issues
Sound-alike/look-alike issues:
Cenestin® may be confused with Senexon®

Pregnancy Risk Factor X

Lactation Enters breast milk/use caution

Use Treatment of moderate to severe vasomotor symptoms of menopause; treatment of vulvar and vaginal atrophy

Mechanism of Action/Effect Estrogens modulate the pituitary secretion of gonadotropins, luteinizing hormone, and follicle-stimulating hormone through a negative feedback system; estrogen replacement reduces elevated levels of these hormones in postmenopausal women

Contraindications Hypersensitivity to estrogens or any component of the formulation; undiagnosed abnormal vaginal bleeding; history of or current thrombophlebitis or venous thromboembolic disorders (including DVT, PE); active or recent (within 1 year) arterial thromboembolic disease (eg, stroke, MI); carcinoma of the breast; estrogen-dependent tumor; hepatic dysfunction or disease; pregnancy

Warnings/Precautions

Cardiovascular-related considerations: Estrogens with or without progestin should not be used to prevent coronary heart disease. Use caution with cardiovascular disease or dysfunction. May increase the risks of hypertension, myocardial infarction (MI), stroke, pulmonary emboli (PE), and deep vein thrombosis; incidence of these effects was shown to be significantly increased in postmenopausal women using conjugated equine estrogens (CEE) in combination with medroxyprogesterone acetate (MPA). Nonfatal MI, PE, and thrombophlebitis have also been reported in males taking high doses of CEE (eg, for prostate cancer). Estrogen compounds are generally associated with lipid effects such as increased HDL-cholesterol and decreased LDL-cholesterol. Triglycerides may also be increased; use with caution in patients with familial defects of lipoprotein metabolism. Whenever possible, estrogens should be discontinued at least 4 weeks prior to and for 2 weeks following elective surgery associated with an increased risk of thromboembolism or during periods of prolonged immobilization.

Neurological considerations: The risk of dementia may be increased in postmenopausal women; increased incidence was observed in women ≥65 years of age taking CEE alone or in combination with MPA.

Cancer-related considerations: Unopposed estrogens may increase the risk of endometrial carcinoma in postmenopausal women. Estrogens may exacerbate endometriosis. Malignant transformation of residual endometrial implants has been reported post-hysterectomy with estrogen only therapy. Consider adding a progestin in women with residual endometriosis post-hysterectomy. Estrogens may increase the risk of breast cancer. An increased risk of invasive breast cancer was observed in postmenopausal women using CEE in combination with MPA; a smaller increase in risk was seen with estrogen therapy alone in observational studies. An increase in abnormal mammograms has also been reported with estrogen and progestin therapy. Estrogen use may lead to severe hypercalcemia in patients with breast cancer and bone metastases; discontinue estrogen if hypercalcemia occurs.

Estrogens may cause retinal vascular thrombosis; discontinue permanently if papilledema or retinal vascular lesions are observed on examination. Use with caution in patients with diseases which may be exacerbated by fluid retention, including asthma, epilepsy, migraine, diabetes or renal dysfunction. Use with caution in patients with a history of severe hypocalcemia, SLE, hepatic hemangiomas, porphyria, endometriosis, and gallbladder disease. Use caution with history of cholestatic jaundice associated with past estrogen use or pregnancy. Safety and efficacy in pediatric patients have not been established. Prior to puberty, estrogens may cause premature closure of the epiphyses, premature breast development in girls or gynecomastia in boys. Vaginal bleeding and vaginal cornification may also be induced in girls.

Before prescribing estrogen therapy to postmenopausal women, the risks and benefits must be weighed for each patient. Women should be informed of these risks and benefits, as well as possible effects of progestin when added to estrogen therapy. Estrogens with or without progestin should be used for shortest duration possible consistent with treatment goals. Conduct periodic risk:benefit assessments.

When used solely for prevention of osteoporosis in women at significant risk, nonestrogen treatment options should be considered. When used solely for the treatment of vulvar and vaginal atrophy, topical vaginal products should be considered.

Drug Interactions

Cytochrome P450 Effect:
Based on estradiol and estrone: **Substrate** of CYP1A2 (major), 2A6 (minor), 2B6 (minor), 2C8/9 (minor), 2C19 (minor), 2D6 (minor), 2E1 (minor), 3A4 (major); **Inhibits** CYP1A2 (weak); **Induces** CYP3A4 (weak)

Decreased Effect: CYP1A2 inducers may decrease the levels/effects of estrogens; example inducers include aminoglutethimide, carbamazepine, phenobarbital, and rifampin. CYP3A4 inducers may decrease the levels/effects of estrogen; example inducers include aminoglutethimide, carbamazepine, nafcillin, nevirapine, phenobarbital, phenytoin, and rifamycins.

Increased Effect/Toxicity: CYP3A4 enzyme inhibitors may increase estrogen plasma concentrations leading to increased incidence of adverse effects; examples of CYP3A4 enzyme inhibitors include clarithromycin, erythromycin, itraconazole, ketoconazole, and ritonavir. Anticoagulants increase the potential for thromboembolic events Estrogens may enhance the effects of hydrocortisone and prednisone

Nutritional/Ethanol Interactions
Ethanol: Avoid ethanol (routine use increases estrogen level and risk of breast cancer).
Food: Grapefruit juice may increase estrogen levels, leading to increased adverse effects.
Herb/Nutraceutical: St John's wort may decrease levels. Avoid black cohosh, dong quai (has estrogenic activity). Avoid red clover, saw palmetto, ginseng (due to potential hormonal effects).

Lab Interactions Pathologist should be advised of estrogen/progesterone therapy when specimens are submitted. Reduced response to metyrapone test observed with conjugated estrogens (equine).

Adverse Reactions Adverse effects associated with estrogen therapy; frequency not defined
Cardiovascular: Edema, hypertension, venous thromboembolism
(Continued)

457

Estrogens (Conjugated A/Synthetic)
(Continued)

Central nervous system: Dizziness, headache, mental depression, migraine

Dermatologic: Chloasma, erythema multiforme, erythema nodosum, hemorrhagic eruption, hirsutism, loss of scalp hair, melasma

Endocrine & metabolic: Breast enlargement, breast tenderness, libido (changes in), thyroid-binding globulin increased, total thyroid hormone (T_4) increased, serum triglycerides/phospholipids increased, HDL-cholesterol increased, LDL-cholesterol decreased, impaired glucose tolerance, hypercalcemia

Gastrointestinal: Abdominal cramps, bloating, cholecystitis, cholelithiasis, gallbladder disease, nausea, pancreatitis, vomiting, weight gain/loss

Genitourinary: Alterations in frequency and flow of menses, changes in cervical secretions, endometrial cancer, increased size of uterine leiomyomata, vaginal candidiasis

Hematologic: Aggravation of porphyria, antithrombin III and antifactor Xa decreased, levels of fibrinogen decreased, platelet aggregability and platelet count increased; prothrombin and factors VII, VIII, IX, X increased

Hepatic: Cholestatic jaundice

Neuromuscular & skeletal: Chorea

Ocular: Intolerance to contact lenses, steeping of corneal curvature

Respiratory: Pulmonary thromboembolism

Miscellaneous: Carbohydrate intolerance

Overdosage/Toxicology Symptoms of overdose include nausea and vomiting; withdrawal bleeding may occur in females. Toxicity is unlikely following single exposures of excessive doses, any treatment following emesis and charcoal administration should be supportive and symptomatic.

Pharmacodynamics/Kinetics

Time to Peak: 4-16 hours

Protein Binding: Sex hormone-binding globulin (SHBG) and albumin

Metabolism: Hepatic to metabolites

Excretion: Urine

Available Dosage Forms Tablet: 0.3 mg, 0.45 mg, 0.625 mg, 0.9 mg, 1.25 mg

Dosing

Adults: The lowest dose that will control symptoms should be used. Medication should be discontinued as soon as possible.

Menopause, moderate to severe vasomotor symptoms: Oral: 0.45 mg/day; may be titrated up to 1.25 mg/day; attempts to discontinue medication should be made at 3- to 6-month intervals

Vulvar and vaginal atrophy: Oral: 0.3 mg/day

Elderly: Refer to adult dosing. A higher incidence of stroke and invasive breast cancer were observed in women >75 years in a WHI substudy using conjugated equine estrogen.

Stability

Storage: Store at room temperature of 25°C (77°F).

Laboratory Monitoring Yearly Papanicolaou smear, mammogram. Adequate diagnostic measures, including endometrial sampling, if indicated, should be performed to rule out malignancy in all cases of undiagnosed abnormal vaginal bleeding.

Nursing Actions

Physical Assessment: Assess potential for interactions with other pharmacological agents or herbal products patient may be taking (eg, increased potential for decreased levels/effects or increased potential for toxicity or thrombolic events). Assess results of annual gynecological exam, therapeutic effectiveness (dependent on rationale for use), and adverse effects (eg, thromboembolism, hypertension, edema, CNS changes) on a regular basis during therapy. Caution patients with diabetes to monitor glucose levels closely (may impair glucose tolerance). Teach patient proper use, possible side effects/appropriate interventions, and adverse symptoms to report. Remind patient about the importance of frequent self-breast exams and the need for annual gynecological exam.

Pregnancy risk factor X: Determine that patient is not pregnant before starting therapy. Do not give to females of childbearing age unless patient is capable of complying with contraceptive use. Advise patient about contraceptive measures as appropriate.

Patient Education: Do not take any new medication during therapy without consulting prescriber. Take exactly as directed and maintain prescribed cycles or term as prescribed. Routine use of alcohol may increase estrogen level and risk of breast cancer. Annual gynecologic and regular self-breast exams are important. If you have diabetes, monitor glucose levels closely (may impair glucose tolerance). You may experience nausea, vomiting or abdominal pain (small, frequent meals may help); dizziness or mental depression (use caution when driving); rash; hair loss; headache; or breast pain, increased/decreased libido, or enlargement/tenderness of breasts. difficult/painful menstrual cycles. Report significant swelling of extremities; sudden acute pain in legs or calves, chest, or abdomen; shortness of breath; severe headache or vomiting; sudden blindness; weakness or numbness of arm or leg; unusual vaginal bleeding; yellowing of skin or eyes; unusual bruising or bleeding, or other persistent adverse reactions. You may become intolerant to wearing contact lenses, notify prescriber if this occurs. **Pregnancy/breast-feeding precautions:** Inform prescriber if you are pregnant. Do not get pregnant while taking this medication. Consult prescriber for appropriate contraceptive measures. This medication may cause fetal defects and should not be used during pregnancy. Consult prescriber if breast-feeding.

Additional Information Not biologically equivalent to conjugated estrogens from equine source. Contains 9 unique estrogenic compounds (equine source contains at least 10 active estrogenic compounds).

Estrogens (Conjugated/Equine)
(ES troe jenz KON joo gate ed, EE kwine)

U.S. Brand Names Premarin®

Synonyms CEE; C.E.S.; Estrogenic Substances, Conjugated

Pharmacologic Category Estrogen Derivative

Medication Safety Issues

Sound-alike/look-alike issues:

Premarin® may be confused with Primaxin®, Provera®, Remeron®

Pregnancy Risk Factor X

Lactation Enters breast milk/use caution

Use Treatment of moderate to severe vasomotor symptoms associated with menopause; treatment of vulvar and vaginal atrophy; hypoestrogenism (due to hypogonadism, castration, or primary ovarian failure); prostatic cancer (palliation); breast cancer (palliation); osteoporosis (prophylaxis, postmenopausal women at significant risk only); abnormal uterine bleeding

Unlabeled/Investigational Use Uremic bleeding

Mechanism of Action/Effect Estrogens modulate the pituitary secretion of gonadotropins, luteinizing hormone, and follicle-stimulating hormone through a negative feedback system; estrogen replacement reduces elevated levels of these hormones in postmenopausal women

Contraindications Hypersensitivity to estrogens or any component of the formulation; undiagnosed abnormal vaginal bleeding; history of or current thrombophlebitis or venous thromboembolic disorders (including DVT, PE); active or recent (within 1 year) arterial thromboembolic disease (eg, stroke, MI); carcinoma of the breast (except in appropriately selected patients being treated for metastatic disease); estrogen-dependent tumor; hepatic dysfunction or disease; pregnancy

Warnings/Precautions

Cardiovascular-related considerations: Estrogens with or without progestin should not be used to prevent coronary heart disease. Use caution with cardiovascular disease or dysfunction. May increase the risks of hypertension, myocardial infarction (MI), stroke, pulmonary emboli (PE), and deep vein thrombosis; incidence of these effects was shown to be significantly increased in postmenopausal women using conjugated equine estrogens (CEE) in combination with medroxyprogesterone acetate (MPA). Nonfatal MI, PE, and thrombophlebitis have also been reported in males taking high doses of CEE (eg, for prostate cancer). Estrogen compounds are generally associated with lipid effects such as increased HDL-cholesterol and decreased LDL-cholesterol. Triglycerides may also be increased; use with caution in patients with familial defects of lipoprotein metabolism. Whenever possible, estrogens should be discontinued at least 4 weeks prior to and for 2 weeks following elective surgery associated with an increased risk of thromboembolism or during periods of prolonged immobilization.

Neurological considerations: The risk of dementia may be increased in postmenopausal women; increased incidence was observed in women ≥65 years of age taking CEE alone or in combination with MPA.

Cancer-related considerations: Unopposed estrogens may increase the risk of endometrial carcinoma in postmenopausal women. Estrogens may exacerbate endometriosis. Malignant transformation of residual endometrial implants has been reported post-hysterectomy with estrogen only therapy. Consider adding a progestin in women with residual endometriosis post-hysterectomy. Estrogens may increase the risk of breast cancer. An increased risk of invasive breast cancer was observed in postmenopausal women using CEE in combination with MPA; a smaller increase in risk was seen with estrogen therapy alone in observational studies. An increase in abnormal mammograms has also been reported with estrogen and progestin therapy. Estrogen use may lead to severe hypercalcemia in patients with breast cancer and bone metastases; discontinue estrogen if hypercalcemia occurs.

Estrogens may cause retinal vascular thrombosis; discontinue permanently if papilledema or retinal vascular lesions are observed on examination. Use with caution in patients with diseases which may be exacerbated by fluid retention, including asthma, epilepsy, migraine, diabetes or renal dysfunction. Use with caution in patients with a history of severe hypocalcemia, SLE, hepatic hemangiomas, porphyria, endometriosis, and gallbladder disease. Use caution with history of cholestatic jaundice associated with past estrogen use or pregnancy. Safety and efficacy in pediatric patients have not been established. Prior to puberty, estrogens may cause premature closure of the epiphyses, premature breast development in girls or gynecomastia in boys. Vaginal bleeding and vaginal cornification may also be induced in girls.

Before prescribing estrogen therapy to postmenopausal women, the risks and benefits must be weighed for each patient. Women should be informed of these risks and benefits, as well as possible effects of progestin when added to estrogen therapy. Estrogens with or without progestin should be used for shortest duration possible consistent with treatment goals. Conduct periodic risk:benefit assessments.

When used solely for prevention of osteoporosis in women at significant risk, nonestrogen treatment options should be considered. When used solely for the treatment of vulvar and vaginal atrophy, topical vaginal products should be considered. Use caution applying topical products to severely atrophic vaginal mucosa.

Drug Interactions

Cytochrome P450 Effect:

Based on estradiol and estrone: **Substrate** of CYP1A2 (major), 2A6 (minor), 2B6 (minor), 2C8/9 (minor), 2C19 (minor), 2D6 (minor), 2E1 (minor), 3A4 (major); Inhibits CYP1A2 (weak); Induces CYP3A4 (weak)

Decreased Effect: CYP1A2 inducers may decrease the levels/effects of estrogens; example inducers include aminoglutethimide, carbamazepine, phenobarbital, and rifampin. CYP3A4 inducers may decrease the levels/effects of estrogens; example inducers include aminoglutethimide, carbamazepine, nafcillin, nevirapine, phenobarbital, phenytoin, and rifamycins.

Increased Effect/Toxicity: Hydrocortisone taken with estrogen may cause corticosteroid-induced toxicity. Increased potential for thromboembolic events with anticoagulants.

Nutritional/Ethanol Interactions

Ethanol: Avoid ethanol (routine use increases estrogen level and risk of breast cancer). Ethanol may also increase the risk of osteoporosis.

Food: Folic acid absorption may be decreased.

Herb/Nutraceutical: St John's wort may decrease levels. Avoid black cohosh, dong quai (has estrogenic activity). Avoid red clover, saw palmetto, ginseng (due to potential hormonal effects).

Lab Interactions Increased Prothrombin and factors VII, VIII, IX, X; increased platelet aggregability, thyroid-binding globulin, total thyroid hormone (T_4), serum triglycerides/phospholipids; decreased antithrombin III, serum folate concentration

Adverse Reactions

Note: Percentages reported in postmenopausal women.

>10%:

Central nervous system: Headache (26% to 32%; placebo 28%)

Endocrine & metabolic: Breast pain (7% to 12%; placebo 9%)

Gastrointestinal: Abdominal pain (15% to 17%)

Genitourinary: Vaginal hemorrhage (2% to 14%)

Neuromuscular & skeletal: Back pain (13% to 14%)

1% to 10%:

Central nervous system: Nervousness (2% to 5%)

Endocrine & metabolic: Leukorrhea (4% to 7%)

Gastrointestinal: Flatulence (6% to 7%)

Genitourinary: Vaginitis (5% to 7%), vaginal moniliasis (5% to 6%)

Neuromuscular & skeletal: Weakness (7% to 8%), leg cramps (3% to 7%)

In addition, the following have been reported with estrogen and/or progestin therapy:

Cardiovascular: Edema, hypertension, MI, stroke, venous thromboembolism

Central nervous system: Dizziness, epilepsy exacerbation, headache, irritability, mental depression, migraine, mood disturbances, nervousness

Dermatologic: Angioedema, chloasma, erythema multiforme, erythema nodosum, hemorrhagic eruption, hirsutism, loss of scalp hair, melasma, pruritus, rash, urticaria

Endocrine & metabolic: Breast cancer, breast enlargement, breast tenderness, libido (changes in), increased thyroid-binding globulin, increased total thyroid hormone (T_4), increased serum triglycerides/phospholipids, increased HDL-cholesterol, decreased LDL-cholesterol, impaired glucose tolerance, hypercalcemia, hypocalcemia

(Continued)

Estrogens (Conjugated/Equine)
(Continued)

Gastrointestinal: Abdominal cramps, bloating, cholecystitis, cholelithiasis, gallbladder disease, nausea, pancreatitis, vomiting, weight gain/loss

Genitourinary: Alterations in frequency and flow of menses, changes in cervical secretions, endometrial cancer, endometrial hyperplasia, increased size of uterine leiomyomata, vaginal candidiasis

Hematologic: Aggravation of porphyria, decreased antithrombin III and antifactor Xa, increased levels of fibrinogen, increased platelet aggregability and platelet count; increased prothrombin and factors VII, VIII, IX, X

Hepatic: Cholestatic jaundice, hepatic hemangiomas enlarged

Neuromuscular & skeletal: Arthralgias, chorea, leg cramps

Local: Thrombophlebitis

Ocular: Intolerance to contact lenses, retinal vascular thrombosis, steeping of corneal curvature

Respiratory: Asthma exacerbation, pulmonary thromboembolism

Miscellaneous: Anaphylactoid/anaphylactic reactions, carbohydrate intolerance

Overdosage/Toxicology Toxicity is unlikely following single exposures of excessive doses, any treatment following emesis and charcoal administration should be supportive and symptomatic. Effects noted after large doses include headache, nausea, and vomiting. Bleeding may occur in females.

Pharmacodynamics/Kinetics
Metabolism: Hepatic via CYP3A4; estradiol is converted to estrone and estriol; also undergoes enterohepatic recirculation; estrone sulfite is the main metabolite in postmenopausal women

Excretion: Urine (primarily estriol, also as estradiol, estrone, and conjugates)

Available Dosage Forms
Cream, vaginal: 0.625 mg/g (42.5 g)

Injection, powder for reconstitution: 25 mg [contains lactose 200 mg; diluent contains benzyl alcohol]

Tablet: 0.3 mg, 0.45 mg, 0.625 mg, 0.9 mg, 1.25 mg

Dosing
Adults:
Breast cancer palliation, metastatic disease in selected patients (male and female): Oral: 10 mg 3 times/day for at least 3 months

Uremic bleeding (unlabeled use): I.V.: 0.6 mg/kg/day for 5 days

Androgen-dependent prostate cancer palliation (males): Oral: 1.25-2.5 mg 3 times/day

Prevention of postmenopausal osteoporosis: Oral: Initial: 0.3 mg/day, cyclically* or daily, depending on medical assessment of patient. Dose may be adjusted based on bone mineral density and clinical response. The lowest effective dose should be used.

Menopause (moderate to severe vasomotor symptoms): Oral: Initial: 0.3 mg/day. May be given cyclically* or daily, depending on medical assessment of patient. The lowest dose that will control symptoms should be used. Medication should be discontinued as soon as possible.

Vulvar and vaginal atrophy: Oral: Initial: 0.3 mg/day. The lowest dose that will control symptoms should be used. May be given cyclically* or daily, depending on medical assessment of patient. Medication should be discontinued as soon as possible.

Vaginal cream: Intravaginal: ½ to 2 g/day given cyclically*

Female hypogonadism: Oral: 0.3-0.625 mg/day given cyclically*; dose may be titrated in 6- to 12-month intervals; progestin treatment should be added to maintain bone mineral density once skeletal maturity is achieved.

Female castration, primary ovarian failure: Oral: 1.25 mg/day given cyclically*; adjust according to severity of symptoms and patient response. For maintenance, adjust to the lowest effective dose.

Abnormal uterine bleeding:
Acute/heavy bleeding:
Oral (unlabeled route): 1.25 mg, may repeat every 4 hours for 24 hours, followed by 1.25 mg once daily for 7-10 days

I.M., I.V.: 25 mg, may repeat in 6-12 hours if needed

Note: Treatment should be followed by a low-dose oral contraceptive; medroxyprogesterone acetate along with or following estrogen therapy can also be given

Nonacute/lesser bleeding: Oral (unlabeled route): 1.25 mg once daily for 7-10 days

***Cyclic administration:** Either 3 weeks on, 1 week off **or** 25 days on, 5 days off

Elderly: Refer to adult dosing. A higher incidence of stroke and breast cancer was observed in women >75 years in a WHI substudy.

Pediatrics: Adolescents: Refer to adult dosing.

Hepatic Impairment:
Mild to moderate liver impairment: Dosage reduction of estrogens is recommended.

Severe liver impairment: **Not recommended.**

Administration
Oral: Give at bedtime to minimize adverse effects.

I.M.: May be administered intramuscularly.

I.V.: Administer I.V. doses slowly to avoid a flushing reaction.

Other: Vaginal cream: Administer at bedtime to minimize adverse effects.

Stability
Reconstitution: Injection: Reconstitute using provided diluent; do not shake violently.

Compatibility: Stable in D_5W and NS

Compatibility when admixed: Incompatible with ascorbic acid

Storage:
Injection: Refrigerate at 2°C to 8°C (36°F to 46°F) prior to reconstitution. Following reconstitution, solution may be stored under refrigeration for up to 60 days. Do not use if darkening or precipitation occurs.

Tablets, vaginal cream: Store at room temperature (25°C).

Laboratory Monitoring Yearly physical examination that includes blood pressure and Papanicolaou smear. Adequate diagnostic measures, including endometrial sampling, if indicated, should be performed to rule out malignancy in all cases of undiagnosed abnormal vaginal bleeding.

Nursing Actions
Physical Assessment: Assess potential for interactions with other pharmacological agents or herbal products patient may be taking (eg, increased potential for decreased levels/effects or increased potential for toxicity or thrombolic events). Monitor results of annual gynecological exam, therapeutic effectiveness (dependent on rationale for use), and adverse effects (eg, thromboembolism, hypertension, edema, CNS changes) on a regular basis during therapy. Caution patients with diabetes to monitor glucose levels closely (may impair glucose tolerance). Teach patient proper use, possible side effects/appropriate interventions, and adverse symptoms to report. Remind patient about the importance of frequent self-breast exams and the need for annual gynecological exam.

Pregnancy risk factor X: Determine that patient is not pregnant before starting therapy. Do not give to females of childbearing age unless patient is capable of complying with contraceptive use. Advise patient about appropriate contraceptive measures as appropriate.

Patient Education: Do not take any new medication during therapy without consulting prescriber. Use/apply exactly as directed and maintain prescribed cycles or term as prescribed. Routine use of alcohol may increase estrogen level and risk of breast cancer. Annual gynecologic exams and regular self-breast exams are important. If you have diabetes, monitor glucose levels closely (may impair glucose tolerance). You may experience nausea, vomiting or abdominal pain (small, frequent meals may help); dizziness or mental depression (use caution when driving); rash; hair loss; headache; or breast pain, increased/decreased libido, enlargement/tenderness of breasts; difficult/painful menstrual cycles. Report significant swelling of extremities; sudden acute pain in legs or calves, chest, or abdomen; shortness of breath; severe headache or vomiting; sudden blindness; weakness or numbness of arm or leg; unusual vaginal bleeding; yellowing of skin or eyes; unusual bruising or bleeding; or other persistent adverse reactions. You may become intolerant to wearing contact lenses, notify prescriber if this occurs. **Pregnancy/breast-feeding precautions:** Inform prescriber if you are pregnant. Do not get pregnant while taking this medication. Consult prescriber for appropriate contraceptive measures. This medication may cause fetal defects and should not be used during pregnancy. Consult prescriber if breast-feeding.

Dietary Considerations Ensure adequate calcium and vitamin D intake when used for the prevention of osteoporosis. Powder for reconstitution for injection (25 mg) contains lactose 200 mg.

Geriatric Considerations Before prescribing estrogen therapy to postmenopausal women, the risks and benefits must be weighed for each patient. Data in women 80 years and older is minimal and it is unclear if reduced risk is applicable to women in this age group. Women should be informed of risks and benefits, as well as possible side effects and the return of menstrual bleeding (when cycled with a progestin), and should be involved in prescribing options. Oral therapy may be more convenient for vaginal atrophy and urinary incontinence.

Breast-Feeding Issues The AAP considers ethinyl estradiol, an estrogen derivative, to be "usually compatible" with breast-feeding. Estrogen has been shown to decrease the quantity and quality of human milk. Use only if clearly needed. Monitor the growth of the infant closely.

Pregnancy Issues Increased risk of fetal reproductive tract disorders and other birth defects; do not use during pregnancy.

Estrogens (Conjugated/Equine) and Medroxyprogesterone
(ES troe jenz KON joo gate ed/EE kwine & me DROKS ee proe JES te rone)

U.S. Brand Names Premphase®; Prempro™

Synonyms Medroxyprogesterone and Estrogens (Conjugated); MPA and Estrogens (Conjugated)

Pharmacologic Category Estrogen and Progestin Combination

Medication Safety Issues
Sound-alike/look-alike issues:
Premphase® may be confused with Prempro™
Prempro™ may be confused with Premphase®

Pregnancy Risk Factor X

Lactation
Estrogens: Enters breast milk/use caution
Progestins: Enters breast milk/use caution

Use Women with an intact uterus: Treatment of moderate to severe vasomotor symptoms associated with menopause; treatment of atrophic vaginitis; osteoporosis (prophylaxis)

Mechanism of Action/Effect
Estrogens modulate the pituitary secretion of gonadotropins, luteinizing hormone, and follicle-stimulating hormone through a negative feedback system; estrogen replacement reduces elevated levels of these hormones in postmenopausal women.

In women with adequate estrogen, MPA transforms a proliferative endometrium into a secretory endometrium; when administered with conjugated estrogens, reduces the incidence of endometrial hyperplasia and risk of adenocarcinoma.

Contraindications Hypersensitivity to conjugated estrogens, medroxyprogesterone (MPA), or any component of the formulation; undiagnosed abnormal vaginal bleeding; history of or current thrombophlebitis or venous thromboembolic disorders (including DVT, PE); active or recent (within 1 year) arterial thromboembolic disease (eg, stroke, MI); carcinoma of the breast; estrogen-dependent tumor; hepatic dysfunction or disease; pregnancy

Warnings/Precautions

Cardiovascular-related considerations: Estrogens with or without progestin should not be used to prevent coronary heart disease. Use caution with cardiovascular disease or dysfunction. May increase the risks of hypertension, myocardial infarction (MI), stroke, pulmonary emboli (PE), and deep vein thrombosis; incidence of these effects was shown to be significantly increased in postmenopausal women using conjugated equine estrogens (CEE) in combination with medroxyprogesterone acetate (MPA). Nonfatal MI, PE, and thrombophlebitis have also been reported in males taking high doses of CEE (eg, for prostate cancer). Estrogen compounds are generally associated with lipid effects such as increased HDL-cholesterol and decreased LDL-cholesterol. Triglycerides may also be increased; use with caution in patients with familial defects of lipoprotein metabolism. Whenever possible, combination hormonal contraceptives should be discontinued at least 4 weeks prior to and for 2 weeks following elective surgery associated with an increased risk of thromboembolism or during periods of prolonged immobilization.

Neurological considerations: The risk of dementia may be increased in postmenopausal women; increased incidence was observed in women ≥65 years of age taking CEE alone or in combination with MPA.

Cancer-related considerations: Unopposed estrogens may increase the risk of endometrial carcinoma in postmenopausal women. Estrogens may exacerbate endometriosis. Malignant transformation of residual endometrial implants has been reported post-hysterectomy with estrogen only therapy. Estrogens may increase the risk of breast cancer. An increased risk of invasive breast cancer was observed in postmenopausal women using CEE in combination with MPA; a smaller increase in risk was seen with estrogen therapy alone in observational studies. An increase in abnormal mammograms has also been reported with estrogen and progestin therapy. Estrogen use may lead to severe hypercalcemia in patients with breast cancer and bone metastases; discontinue estrogen if hypercalcemia occurs.

Estrogens may cause retinal vascular thrombosis; discontinue permanently if papilledema or retinal vascular lesions are observed on examination. Use with caution in patients with diseases which may be exacerbated by fluid retention, including asthma, epilepsy, migraine, diabetes or renal dysfunction. Use with caution in patients with a history of severe hypocalcemia, SLE, hepatic hemangiomas, porphyria, endometriosis, and gallbladder disease. Use caution with history (Continued)

Estrogens (Conjugated/Equine) and Medroxyprogesterone *(Continued)*

of cholestatic jaundice associated with past estrogen use or pregnancy. Safety and efficacy in pediatric patients have not been established. Prior to puberty, estrogens may cause premature closure of the epiphyses, premature breast development in girls or gynecomastia in boys. Vaginal bleeding and vaginal cornification may also be induced in girls.

Before prescribing estrogen therapy to postmenopausal women, the risks and benefits must be weighed for each patient. Women should be informed of these risks and benefits, as well as possible effects of progestin when added to estrogen therapy. Estrogens with or without progestin should be used for shortest duration possible consistent with treatment goals. Conduct periodic risk:benefit assessments.

When used solely for prevention of osteoporosis in women at significant risk, nonstrogen treatment options should be considered. When used solely for the treatment of vulvar and vaginal atrophy, topical vaginal products should be considered.

Drug Interactions

Cytochrome P450 Effect:

Based on estradiol and estrone: **Substrate** of CYP1A2 (major), 2A6 (minor), 2B6 (minor), 2C8/9 (minor), 2C19 (minor), 2D6 (minor), 2E1 (minor), 3A4 (major); **Inhibits** CYP1A2 (weak); **Induces** CYP3A4 (weak)

Medroxyprogesterone: **Substrate** of CYP3A4 (major); **Induces** CYP3A4 (weak)

Decreased Effect:

Conjugated estrogens:

Anticonvulsants which are enzyme inducers (barbiturates, carbamazepine, phenobarbital, phenytoin, primidone) may potentially decrease estrogen levels.

Rifampin, nelfinavir, and ritonavir decrease estradiol serum concentrations

MPA: Aminoglutethimide: May decrease effects by increasing hepatic metabolism

Increased Effect/Toxicity: Hydrocortisone taken with estrogen may cause corticosteroid-induced toxicity. Increased potential for thromboembolic events with anticoagulants.

Nutritional/Ethanol Interactions

Ethanol: Avoid ethanol (routine use increases estrogen level and risk of breast cancer). Ethanol may also increase the risk of osteoporosis.

Food: Folic acid absorption may be decreased.

Herb/Nutraceutical: St John's wort may decrease levels. Avoid black cohosh, dong quai (has estrogenic activity). Avoid red clover, saw palmetto, ginseng (due to potential hormonal effects).

Lab Interactions Accelerated PT, partial thromboplastin time, and platelet aggregation time; increased platelet count; increased HDL; increased factors II, VII antigen, VIII coagulant activity, IX, X, XII, XII-X complex, II-VII-X complex, and beta-thromboglobulin; increased levels of fibrinogen and fibrinogen activity; increased plasminogen antigen and activity; increased thyroid-binding globulin; increased triglycerides; impaired glucose tolerance; reduced response to metyrapone test; reduced serum folate concentration; other binding proteins may be elevated; decreased LDL; decreased levels of antifactor Xa and antithrombin III; decreased antithrombin III activity

Adverse Reactions

>10%:

Central nervous system: Headache (28% to 37%), pain (11% to 13%), depression (6% to 11%)

Endocrine & metabolic: Breast pain (32% to 38%), dysmenorrhea (8% to 13%)

Gastrointestinal: Abdominal pain (16% to 23%), nausea (9% to 11%)

Neuromuscular & skeletal: Back pain (13% to 16%)

Respiratory: Pharyngitis (11% to 13%)

Miscellaneous: Infection (16% to 18%), flu-like syndrome (10% to 13%)

1% to 10%:

Cardiovascular: Peripheral edema (3% to 4%)

Central nervous system: Dizziness (3% to 5%)

Dermatologic: Pruritus (5% to 10%), rash (4% to 6%)

Endocrine & metabolic: Leukorrhea (5% to 9%)

Gastrointestinal: Flatulence (8% to 9%), diarrhea (5% to 6%), dyspepsia (5% to 6%)

Genitourinary: Vaginitis (5% to 7%), cervical changes (4% to 5%), vaginal hemorrhage (1% to 3%)

Neuromuscular & skeletal: Weakness (6% to 10%), arthralgia (7% to 9%), leg cramps (3% to 5%), hypertonia (3% to 4%)

Respiratory: Sinusitis (7% to 8%), rhinitis (6% to 8%)

Additional adverse effects reported with conjugated estrogens and/or progestins: Abdominal cramps, acne, abnormal uterine bleeding, aggravation of porphyria, amenorrhea, anaphylactoid reactions, anaphylaxis, antifactor Xa decreased, antithrombin III decreased, appetite changes, bloating, breast enlargement, breast tenderness, cerebral embolism, cerebral thrombosis, chloasma, cholestatic jaundice, cholecystitis, cholelithiasis, chorea, contact lens intolerance, cystitis-like syndrome, decreased carbohydrate tolerance, dizziness, factors VII, VIII, IX, X, XII, VII-X complex, and II-VII-X complex increased; endometrial hyperplasia, erythema multiforme, erythema nodosum, galactorrhea, hemorrhagic eruption, fatigue, fibrinogen increased, impaired glucose tolerance, HDL-cholesterol increased, hirsutism, hypertension, increase in size of uterine leiomyomata, gallbladder disease, insomnia, LDL-cholesterol decreased, libido changes, loss of scalp hair, melasma, migraine, nervousness, optic neuritis, pancreatitis, platelet aggregability and platelet count increased, premenstrual like syndrome, PT and PTT accelerated, pulmonary embolism, pyrexia, retinal thrombosis, somnolence, steepening of corneal curvature, thrombophlebitis, thyroid-binding globulin increased, total thyroid hormone (T$_4$) increased, triglycerides increased, urticaria, vaginal candidiasis, vomiting, weight gain/loss

Overdosage/Toxicology Effects noted after large doses include nausea, vomiting; withdrawal bleeding may occur in females. Treatment should be supportive and symptomatic.

Pharmacokinetic Note See individual agents.

Available Dosage Forms Tablet:

Premphase® [therapy pack contains 2 separate tablet formulations]: Conjugated estrogens 0.625 mg [14 maroon tablets] and conjugated estrogen 0.625 mg/ medroxyprogesterone acetate 5 mg [14 light blue tablets] (28s)

Prempro™:

0.3/1.5: Conjugated estrogens 0.3 mg and medroxyprogesterone acetate 1.5 mg (28s)

0.45/1.5: Conjugated estrogens 0.45 mg and medroxyprogesterone acetate 1.5 mg (28s)

0.625/2.5: Conjugated estrogens 0.625 mg and medroxyprogesterone acetate 2.5 mg (28s)

0.625/5: Conjugated estrogens 0.625 mg and medroxyprogesterone acetate 5 mg (28s)

Dosing

Adults:

Treatment of moderate to severe vasomotor symptoms associated with menopause or treatment of atrophic vaginitis in females with an intact uterus: (Note: The lowest dose that will control symptoms should be used; medication should be discontinued as soon as possible): Oral: *Premphase®:* One maroon conjugated estrogen 0.625 mg tablet daily on days 1 through 14 and one light blue conjugated estrogen 0.625 mg/ MPA 5 mg tablet daily on days 15 through 28; re-evaluate patients at 3- and 6-month intervals to determine if treatment is still necessary; monitor patients for signs of endometrial cancer; rule out malignancy if unexplained vaginal bleeding occurs

Prempro™: One conjugated estrogen 0.3 mg/MPA 1.5 mg tablet daily; re-evaluate at 3-and 6-month intervals to determine if therapy is still needed; dose may be increased to a maximum of one conjugated estrogen 0.625 mg/MPA 5 mg tablet daily in patients with bleeding or spotting, once malignancy has been ruled out

Osteoporosis prophylaxis in females with an intact uterus: Oral:

Premphase®: One maroon conjugated estrogen 0.625 tablet daily on days 1 through 14 and one light blue conjugated estrogen 0.625 mg/MPA 5 mg tablet daily on days 15 through 28; monitor patients for signs of endometrial cancer; rule out malignancy if unexplained vaginal bleeding occurs

Prempro™: One conjugated estrogen 0.3 mg/MPA 1.5 mg tablet daily; dose may be increased to one conjugated estrogen 0.625 mg/MPA 5 mg tablet daily; in patients with bleeding or spotting, once malignancy has been ruled out

Elderly: Refer to adult dosing. A higher incidence of stroke and breast cancer was observed in women >75 years in a WHI substudy.

Stability

Storage: Store at room temperature 20°C to 25°C (68°F to 77°F).

Laboratory Monitoring Serum cholesterol, HDL, LDL triglycerides

Nursing Actions

Physical Assessment: Assess potential for interactions with other prescriptions, OTC medications, or herbal products patient may be taking. Monitor laboratory tests, therapeutic effectiveness (according to purpose for use), and adverse response (eg, CNS changes, hypertension, thromboembolism, fluid retention, edema, CHF, respiratory changes) on a regular basis during therapy. Caution patients with diabetes to monitor glucose levels closely (may impair glucose tolerance). Teach patient appropriate use, possible side effects/appropriate interventions, and adverse symptoms to report. **Pregnancy risk factor X:** Determine that patient is not pregnant before beginning treatment.

Patient Education: Do not take any new medication during therapy without consulting prescriber. Take exactly as directed and maintain prescribed cycles or term as prescribed. Avoid routine use of alcohol (ethanol may increase the risk of breast cancer or osteoporosis). Annual gynecologic and regular self-breast exams are important. If you have diabetes, monitor glucose levels closely (may impair glucose tolerance). You may experience nausea, vomiting or abdominal pain (small frequent meals may help); dizziness or mental depression (use caution when driving); rash; hair loss; headache; or breast pain, increased/decreased libido, or enlargement/tenderness of breasts, difficult/painful menstrual cycles. Report significant swelling of extremities; sudden acute pain in legs or calves, chest, or abdomen; shortness of breath; severe headache or vomiting; sudden blindness; weakness or numbness of arm or leg; unusual vaginal bleeding; yellowing of skin or eyes; unusual bruising or bleeding, or other persistent adverse reactions. You may become intolerant to wearing contact lenses, notify prescriber if this occurs.

Pregnancy/breast-feeding precautions: Inform prescriber if you are pregnant. Do not get pregnant while taking this medication. This medication may cause fetal defects and should not be used during pregnancy.

Dietary Considerations Administration with food decreases nausea, administer with food. Ensure adequate calcium and vitamin D intake when used for the prevention of osteoporosis.

Breast-Feeding Issues The AAP considers ethinyl estradiol, an estrogen derivative, to be "usually compatible" with breast-feeding. Estrogen has been shown to decrease the quantity and quality of human milk. Monitor the growth of the infant closely. The AAP considers medroxyprogesterone to be "usually compatible" with breast-feeding.

Pregnancy Issues

Estrogens: Increased risk of fetal reproductive tract disorders and other birth defects; do not use during pregnancy.

Progestins: Associated with fetal genital abnormalities when used during the 1st trimester; not recommended for use during pregnancy.

Additional Information The use of estrogens for the prevention of other chronic diseases, as well as their potential negative effects on women's health, has been debated. Data published from the Women's Health Initiative (WHI) has provided some additional insight on this controversial topic. In the WHI, one arm of the study compared postmenopausal women with an intact uterus using CEE 0.625 mg in combination with MPA 2.5 mg daily, versus placebo. This arm of the study was stopped in 2002. In March, 2004, it was announced that the arm of the study comparing placebo to CEE alone in postmenopausal women without a uterus was ended.

Based on preliminary findings, the FDA has requested labeling changes be made to estrogen products used in postmenopausal women. The updates include information from the Women's Health Initiative Memory Study (WHIMS) as well as information collected from the completed CEE/MPA arm of the WHI study. Complete analysis of the WHI data is forthcoming, and will include all information collected through February, 2004.

Related Information

Estrogens (Conjugated/Equine) *on page 458*
MedroxyPROGESTERone *on page 767*

Estrogens (Esterified)
(ES troe jenz, es TER i fied)

U.S. Brand Names Menest®

Synonyms Esterified Estrogens

Pharmacologic Category Estrogen Derivative

Medication Safety Issues

Sound-alike/look-alike issues:

Estratab® may be confused with Estratest®, Estratest® H.S.

Pregnancy Risk Factor X

Lactation Enters breast milk/use caution

Use Treatment of moderate to severe vasomotor symptoms associated with menopause; treatment of vulvar and vaginal atrophy; hypoestrogenism (due to hypogonadism, castration, or primary ovarian failure); prostatic cancer (palliation); breast cancer (palliation); osteoporosis (prophylaxis, in women at significant risk only)

Mechanism of Action/Effect Esterified estrogens contain a mixture of estrogenic substances; the principle component is estrone. Estrogens modulate the pituitary secretion of gonadotropins, luteinizing hormone, and follicle-stimulating hormone through a negative feedback system; estrogen replacement reduces elevated levels of these hormones.

Contraindications Hypersensitivity to estrogens or any component of the formulation; undiagnosed abnormal vaginal bleeding; history of or current thrombophlebitis or venous thromboembolic disorders (including DVT, (Continued)

Estrogens (Esterified) (Continued)

PE); active or recent (within 1 year) arterial thromboembolic disease (eg, stroke, MI); carcinoma of the breast, except in appropriately selected patients being treated for metastatic disease; estrogen-dependent tumor; hepatic dysfunction or disease; pregnancy

Warnings/Precautions

Cardiovascular-related considerations: Estrogens with or without progestin should not be used to prevent coronary heart disease. Use caution with cardiovascular disease or dysfunction. May increase the risks of hypertension, myocardial infarction (MI), stroke, pulmonary emboli (PE), and deep vein thrombosis; incidence of these effects was shown to be significantly increased in postmenopausal women using conjugated equine estrogens (CEE) in combination with medroxyprogesterone acetate (MPA). Nonfatal MI, PE, and thrombophlebitis have also been reported in males taking high doses of CEE (eg, for prostate cancer). Estrogen compounds are generally associated with lipid effects such as increased HDL-cholesterol and decreased LDL-cholesterol. Triglycerides may also be increased; use with caution in patients with familial defects of lipoprotein metabolism. Whenever possible, estrogens should be discontinued at least 4 weeks prior to and for 2 weeks following elective surgery associated with an increased risk of thromboembolism or during periods of prolonged immobilization.

Neurological considerations: The risk of dementia may be increased in postmenopausal women; increased incidence was observed in women ≥65 years of age taking CEE alone or in combination with MPA.

Cancer-related considerations: Unopposed estrogens may increase the risk of endometrial carcinoma in postmenopausal women. Estrogens may exacerbate endometriosis. Malignant transformation of residual endometrial implants has been reported post-hysterectomy with estrogen only therapy. Consider adding a progestin in women with residual endometriosis post-hysterectomy. Estrogens may increase the risk of breast cancer. An increased risk of invasive breast cancer was observed in postmenopausal women using CEE in combination with MPA; a smaller increase in risk was seen with estrogen therapy alone in observational studies. An increase in abnormal mammograms has also been reported with estrogen and progestin therapy. Estrogen use may lead to severe hypercalcemia in patients with breast cancer and bone metastases; discontinue estrogen if hypercalcemia occurs.

Estrogens may cause retinal vascular thrombosis; discontinue permanently if papilledema or retinal vascular lesions are observed on examination. Use with caution in patients with diseases which may be exacerbated by fluid retention, including asthma, epilepsy, migraine, diabetes or renal dysfunction. Use with caution in patients with a history of severe hypocalcemia, SLE, hepatic hemangiomas, porphyria, endometriosis, and gallbladder disease. Use caution with history of cholestatic jaundice associated with past estrogen use or pregnancy. Safety and efficacy in pediatric patients have not been established. Prior to puberty, estrogens may cause premature closure of the epiphyses, premature breast development in girls or gynecomastia in boys. Vaginal bleeding and vaginal cornification may also be induced in girls.

Before prescribing estrogen therapy to postmenopausal women, the risks and benefits must be weighed for each patient. Women should be informed of these risks and benefits, as well as possible effects of progestin when added to estrogen therapy. Estrogens with or without progestin should be used for shortest duration possible consistent with treatment goals. Conduct periodic risk:benefit assessments.

When used solely for prevention of osteoporosis in women at significant risk, nonestrogen treatment options should be considered. When used solely for the treatment of vulvar and vaginal atrophy, topical vaginal products should be considered.

Drug Interactions

Cytochrome P450 Effect: Based on estrone: Substrate of CYP1A2 (major), 2B6 (minor), 2C8/9 (minor), 2E1 (minor), 3A4 (major)

Decreased Effect: CYP1A2 inducers may decrease the levels/effects of estrogens; example inducers include aminoglutethimide, carbamazepine, phenobarbital, and rifampin. CYP3A4 inducers may decrease the levels/effects of estrogens; example inducers include aminoglutethimide, carbamazepine, nafcillin, nevirapine, phenobarbital, phenytoin, and rifamycins.

Increased Effect/Toxicity: Hydrocortisone taken with estrogen may cause corticosteroid-induced toxicity. Increased potential for thromboembolic events with anticoagulants.

Nutritional/Ethanol Interactions

Ethanol: Avoid ethanol (routine use increases estrogen level and risk of breast cancer). Ethanol may also increase the risk of osteoporosis.

Food: Folic acid absorption may be decreased.

Herb/Nutraceutical: St John's wort may decrease levels. Avoid black cohosh, dong quai (has estrogenic activity). Avoid red clover, saw palmetto, ginseng (due to potential hormonal effects).

Lab Interactions Endocrine function test may be altered; increased prothrombin and factors VII, VIII, IX, X; increased platelet aggregability, thyroid-binding globulin, total thyroid hormone (T_4), serum triglycerides/phospholipids; decreased antithrombin III, serum folate concentration

Adverse Reactions Frequency not defined.

Cardiovascular: Edema, hypertension, venous thromboembolism

Central nervous system: Dizziness, headache, mental depression, migraine

Dermatologic: Chloasma, erythema multiforme, erythema nodosum, hemorrhagic eruption, hirsutism, loss of scalp hair, melasma

Endocrine & metabolic: Breast enlargement, breast tenderness, libido (changes in), increased thyroid-binding globulin, increased total thyroid hormone (T_4), increased serum triglycerides/phospholipids, increased HDL-cholesterol, decreased LDL-cholesterol, impaired glucose tolerance, hypercalcemia

Gastrointestinal: Abdominal cramps, bloating, cholecystitis, cholelithiasis, gallbladder disease, nausea, pancreatitis, vomiting, weight gain/loss

Genitourinary: Alterations in frequency and flow of menses, changes in cervical secretions, endometrial cancer, increased size of uterine leiomyomata, vaginal candidiasis

Hematologic: Aggravation of porphyria, decreased antithrombin III and antifactor Xa, increased levels of fibrinogen, increased platelet aggregability and platelet count; increased prothrombin and factors VII, VIII, IX, X

Hepatic: Cholestatic jaundice

Neuromuscular & skeletal: Chorea

Ocular: Intolerance to contact lenses, steeping of corneal curvature

Respiratory: Pulmonary thromboembolism

Miscellaneous: Carbohydrate intolerance

Overdosage/Toxicology Toxicity is unlikely following single exposures of excessive doses, any treatment following emesis and charcoal administration should be supportive and symptomatic. Effects noted after large doses include headache, nausea, and vomiting. Bleeding may occur in females.

Pharmacodynamics/Kinetics

Metabolism: Rapidly hepatic to estrone sulfate, conjugated and unconjugated metabolites; first-pass effect

Excretion: Urine (as unchanged drug and as glucuronide and sulfate conjugates)

Available Dosage Forms Tablet: 0.3 mg, 0.625 mg, 1.25 mg, 2.5 mg

Dosing

Adults:

Prostate cancer (palliation): Oral: 1.25-2.5 mg 3 times/day

Female hypogonadism: Oral: 2.5-7.5 mg of estrogen daily for 20 days followed by a 10-day rest period. Administer cyclically (3 weeks on and 1 week off). If bleeding does not occur by the end of the 10-day period, repeat the same dosing schedule; the number of courses dependent upon the responsiveness of the endometrium. If bleeding occurs before the end of the 10-day period, begin an estrogen-progestin cyclic regimen of 2.5-7.5 mg esterified estrogens daily for 20 days. During the last 5 days of estrogen therapy, give an oral progestin. If bleeding occurs before regimen is concluded, discontinue therapy and resume on the fifth day of bleeding.

Menopause, moderate to severe vasomotor symptoms: Oral: 1.25 mg/day administered cyclically (3 weeks on and 1 week off). If patient has not menstruated within the last 2 months or more, cyclic administration is started arbitrary. If the patient is menstruating, cyclical administration is started on day 5 of the bleeding. For short-term use only and should be discontinued as soon as possible. Re-evaluate at 3- to 6-month intervals for tapering or discontinuation of therapy.

Atopic vaginitis and kraurosis vulvae: Oral: 0.3 to ≥1.25 mg/day, depending on the tissue response of the individual patient. Administer cyclically. For short-term use only and should be discontinued as soon as possible. Re-evaluate at 3- to 6-month intervals for tapering or discontinuation of therapy.

Breast cancer (palliation): Oral: 10 mg 3 times/day for at least 3 months

Osteoporosis in postmenopausal women: Oral: Initial: 0.3 mg/day and increase to a maximum daily dose of 1.25 mg/day; initiate therapy as soon as possible after menopause; cyclically or daily, depending on medical assessment of patient. Monitor patients with an intact uterus for signs of endometrial cancer; rule out malignancy if unexplained vaginal bleeding occurs

Female castration and primary ovarian failure: Oral: 1.25 mg/day, cyclically. Adjust dosage upward or downward, according to the severity of symptoms and patient response. For maintenance, adjust dosage to lowest level that will provide effective control.

Elderly: Refer to adult dosing. A higher incidence of stroke and invasive breast cancer were observed in women >75 years in a WHI substudy using conjugated equine estrogen.

Hepatic Impairment:

Mild to moderate liver impairment: Dosage reduction of estrogens is recommended.

Severe liver impairment: **Not recommended.**

Stability

Storage: Store below 30°C (86°F); protect from moisture

Laboratory Monitoring Yearly Papanicolaou smear, mammogram. Adequate diagnostic measures, including endometrial sampling, if indicated, should be performed to rule out malignancy in all cases of undiagnosed abnormal vaginal bleeding.

Nursing Actions

Physical Assessment: Assess potential for interactions with other pharmacological agents or herbal products patient may be taking (eg, increased potential for decreased levels/effects or increased potential for toxicity or thrombolic events). Assess results of annual gynecological exam, therapeutic effectiveness (dependent on rationale for use), and adverse effects (eg, thromboembolism, hypertension, edema, CNS changes) on a regular basis during therapy. Caution patients with diabetes to monitor glucose levels closely (may impair glucose tolerance). Teach patient proper use, possible side effects/appropriate interventions, and adverse symptoms to report. Remind patient about the importance of frequent self-breast exams and the need for annual gynecological exam. **Pregnancy risk factor X:** Determine that patient is not pregnant before starting therapy. Do not give to females of childbearing age unless patient is capable of complying with barrier contraceptive use. Advise patient about contraceptive measures as appropriate.

Patient Education: Do not take any new medication during therapy without consulting prescriber. Take exactly as directed and maintain prescribed cycles or term as prescribed. Routine use of alcohol may increase estrogen level and risk of breast cancer. Annual gynecologic and regular self-breast exams are important. If you have diabetes, monitor glucose levels closely (may impair glucose tolerance). You may experience nausea, vomiting or abdominal pain (small, frequent meals may help); dizziness or mental depression (use caution when driving); rash; hair loss; headache; or breast pain, increased/decreased libido, or enlargement/tenderness of breasts. difficult/painful menstrual cycles. Report significant swelling of extremities; sudden acute pain in legs or calves, chest, or abdomen; shortness of breath; severe headache or vomiting; sudden blindness; weakness or numbness of arm or leg; unusual vaginal bleeding; yellowing of skin or eyes; unusual bruising or bleeding, or other persistent adverse reactions. You may become intolerant to wearing contact lenses, notify prescriber if this occurs. **Pregnancy/breast-feeding precautions:** Inform prescriber if you are pregnant. Do not get pregnant while taking this medication. Consult prescriber for appropriate contraceptive measures. This medication may cause fetal defects and should not be used during pregnancy. Consult prescriber if breast-feeding.

Dietary Considerations Should be taken with food at same time each day. Ensure adequate calcium and vitamin D intake when used for the prevention of osteoporosis.

Breast-Feeding Issues The AAP considers ethinyl estradiol, an estrogen derivative, to be "usually compatible" with breast-feeding. Estrogen has been shown to decrease the quantity and quality of human milk; use only if clearly needed; monitor the growth of the infant closely.

Pregnancy Issues Increased risk of fetal reproductive tract disorders and other birth defects; do not use during pregnancy.

Eszopiclone (es zoe PIK Ione)

U.S. Brand Names Lunesta™

Restrictions C-IV

Pharmacologic Category Hypnotic, Nonbenzodiazepine

Pregnancy Risk Factor C

Lactation Excretion in breast milk unknown/use caution

Use Treatment of insomnia

Mechanism of Action/Effect Interact with the GABA-receptor complex to promote sleep.

Contraindications Hypersensitivity to eszopiclone or any component of the formulation

(Continued)

Eszopiclone *(Continued)*

Warnings/Precautions Symptomatic treatment of insomnia should be initiated only after careful evaluation of potential causes of sleep disturbance. Tolerance did not develop over 6 months of use. Use with caution in patients with depression or a history of drug dependence. Abrupt discontinuance may lead to withdrawal symptoms. Use with caution in patients receiving other CNS depressants or psychoactive medications. May impair physical and mental capabilities. Use caution in patients with respiratory compromise or liver dysfunction. Safety and efficacy in children have not been established.

Drug Interactions

Cytochrome P450 Effect: Substrate of CYP2E1 (minor), 3A4 (major)

Decreased Effect: CYP3A4 inducers may decrease the levels/effects of eszopiclone; example inducers include aminoglutethimide, carbamazepine, nafcillin, nevirapine, phenobarbital, phenytoin, and rifamycins.

Increased Effect/Toxicity: CYP3A4 inhibitors may increase the levels/effects of eszopiclone; example inhibitors include azole antifungals, clarithromycin, diclofenac, doxycycline, erythromycin, imatinib, isoniazid, nefazodone, nicardipine, propofol, protease inhibitors, quinidine, telithromycin, and verapamil. Concurrent use with olanzapine may lead to decreased psychomotor function.

Nutritional/Ethanol Interactions

Ethanol: Use caution with concurrent use. Effects are additive and may decrease psychomotor function.

Food: Onset of action may be reduced if taken with or immediately after a heavy meal.

Herb/Nutraceutical: Avoid valerian, St John's wort, kava kava, gotu kola (may increase CNS depression).

Adverse Reactions

>10%:

Central nervous system: Headache (15% to 21%)

Gastrointestinal: Unpleasant taste (8% to 34%)

1% to 10%:

Cardiovascular: Chest pain, peripheral edema

Central nervous system: Somnolence (8% to 10%), dizziness (5% to 7%), hallucinations (1% to 3%), anxiety (1% to 3%), nervousness (up to 5%), confusion (up to 3%), depression (1% to 4%), abnormal dreams (1% to 3%), migraine

Dermatologic: Rash (3% to 4%), pruritus (1% to 4%)

Endocrine & metabolic: Libido decreased (up to 3%), dysmenorrhea (up to 3%), gynecomastia (males up to 3%)

Gastrointestinal: Xerostomia (3% to 7%), dyspepsia (5% to 6%), nausea (5%), diarrhea (2% to 4%), vomiting (up to 3%)

Genitourinary: Urinary tract infection (up to 3%)

Neuromuscular & skeletal: Neuralgia (up to 3%)

Miscellaneous: Infection (5% to 10%), viral infection (3%)

Overdosage/Toxicology Overdose symptoms range from somnolence to coma. Treatment is symptom-directed and supportive. Flumazenil may be useful.

Pharmacodynamics/Kinetics

Time to Peak: 1 hour

Protein Binding: 52% to 59%

Half-Life Elimination: 6 hours; Elderly (≥65 years): ~9 hours

Metabolism: Hepatic via oxidation and demethylation (CYP2E1, 3A4); 2 primary metabolites; one with activity less than parent

Excretion: Urine (75%, primarily as metabolites; <10% as parent drug)

Available Dosage Forms Tablet: 1 mg, 2 mg, 3 mg

Dosing

Adults:

Insomnia: Oral: Initial: 2 mg before bedtime (maximum dose: 3 mg)

Concurrent use with strong CYP3A4 inhibitor: 1 mg before bedtime; if needed, dose may be increased to 2 mg

Elderly:

Difficulty **falling** asleep: Initial: 1 mg before bedtime; maximum dose: 2 mg.

Difficulty **staying** asleep: 2 mg before bedtime.

Renal Impairment: No adjustment required.

Hepatic Impairment:

Mild-to-moderate: Use with caution; dosage adjustment unnecessary

Severe: Maximum dose: 2 mg

Administration

Oral: Because of the rapid onset of action, eszopiclone should be administered immediately prior to bedtime or after the patient has gone to bed and is having difficulty falling asleep. Do not take with, or immediately following, a high-fat meal. Do not crush or break tablet.

Stability

Storage: Store at 15°C to 30°C (59°F to 86°F).

Nursing Actions

Physical Assessment:

Evaluate potential causes of insomnia prior to initiating medication. Assess effectiveness and interactions of other medications patient may be taking Assess for history of addiction; long-term use can result in dependence, abuse, or tolerance. After long-term use, taper dosage slowly when discontinuing. Monitor for CNS depression. For inpatient use, institute safety measures (side rails, night light, call bell, assistance with ambulation) and monitor effectiveness and adverse reactions. For outpatients, monitor for effectiveness of therapy and adverse reactions at beginning of therapy and periodically with long-term use. Assess knowledge/teach patient appropriate use, interventions to reduce side effects, and adverse symptoms to report.

Patient Education:

Use exactly as directed; do not increase dose or frequency or discontinue without consulting prescriber. Drug may cause physical and/or psychological dependence. While using this medication, do not use alcohol or other prescription or OTC medications (especially, pain medications, sedatives, antihistamines, or hypnotics) without consulting prescriber. Take immediately prior to bedtime (quick onset) or when having difficulty falling asleep. Do not use unless you are able to get 8 or more hours of sleep before you must be active again. Swallow whole, do not crush or break tablet. Maintain adequate hydration (2-3 L/day of fluids) unless instructed to restrict fluid intake. You may experience drowsiness, dizziness, lightheadedness, or difficulty with coordination (use caution when driving or engaging in tasks requiring alertness until response to drug is known); headache, or unpleasant taste. Report CNS changes (confusion, depression, increased sedation, excitation, severe headache, abnormal thinking, insomnia, or nightmares). **Pregnancy/breast-feeding precautions:** Inform prescriber if you are or intend to become pregnant. Consult prescriber if breast-feeding.

Dietary Considerations Avoid taking after a heavy meal; may delay onset.

Geriatric Considerations In subjects >65 years of age, the AUC was increased by 41%. The manufacturer reports that in studies, the pattern of adverse reactions in elderly subjects was not different from that seen in younger adults. See Pharmacodynamics/Kinetics, Dosing, and Adverse Reactions.

Etanercept (et a NER sept)

U.S. Brand Names Enbrel®

Pharmacologic Category Antirheumatic, Disease Modifying; Tumor Necrosis Factor (TNF) Blocking Agent

Pregnancy Risk Factor B

Lactation Excretion in breast milk unknown/not recommended

Use Treatment of moderately- to severely-active rheumatoid arthritis, moderately- to severely-active polyarticular juvenile arthritis (in patients with inadequate response to at least one disease-modifying antirheumatic drug), psoriatic arthritis, active ankylosing spondylitis (AS); moderate-to-severe chronic plaque psoriasis

Mechanism of Action/Effect Etanercept is a recombinant DNA-derived protein composed of tumor necrosis factor receptor (TNFR) linked to the Fc portion of human IgG1. Etanercept binds tumor necrosis factor (TNF) and blocks its interaction with cell surface receptors. TNF plays an important role in the inflammatory processes and the resulting joint pathology of rheumatoid arthritis (RA), polyarticular-course juvenile arthritis (JRA), ankylosing spondylitis (AS), and plaque psoriasis.

Contraindications Hypersensitivity to etanercept or any component of the formulation; patients with sepsis (mortality may be increased); active infections (including chronic or local infection)

Warnings/Precautions Etanercept may affect defenses against infections and malignancies. Safety and efficacy in patients with immunosuppression or chronic infections have not been evaluated. Rare cases of tuberculosis have been reported. Rare reactivation of hepatitis B has occurred in chronic virus carriers; evaluate prior to initiation and during treatment. Discontinue administration if patient develops a serious infection. Do not start drug in patients with an active infection. Use caution in patients predisposed to infection, such as poorly-controlled diabetes.

Impact on the development and course of malignancies is not fully defined. As compared to the general population, an increased risk of lymphoma has been noted in clinical trials; however, rheumatoid arthritis has been previously associated with an increased rate of lymphoma. Etanercept is not recommended for use in patients with Wegener's granulomatosis who are receiving immunosuppressive therapy. Treatment may result in the formation of autoimmune antibodies; cases of autoimmune disease have not been described. Non-neutralizing antibodies to etanercept may also be formed. Rarely, a reversible lupus-like syndrome has occurred. The safety of etanercept has not been studied in children <4 years of age.

Use caution in patients with pre-existing or recent-onset demyelinating CNS disorders, CHF (has been associated with worsening and new-onset CHF), or a history of significant hematologic abnormalities. Discontinue if significant hematologic abnormalities are confirmed.

Allergic reactions may occur (<2%), but anaphylaxis has not been observed. If an anaphylactic reaction or other serious allergic reaction occurs, administration of etanercept should be discontinued immediately.

Patients should be brought up to date with all immunizations before initiating therapy. Live vaccines should not be given concurrently. Patients with a significant exposure to varicella virus should temporarily discontinue etanercept. Treatment with varicella zoster immune globulin should be considered.

Drug Interactions

Decreased Effect: Specific drug interaction studies have not been conducted with etanercept. Live vaccines should not be given during therapy.

Increased Effect/Toxicity: Specific drug interaction studies have not been conducted with etanercept. An increased rate of serious infections has been noted with concurrent anakinra therapy, without additional improvement in American College of Rheumatology (ACR) response criteria. Cyclophosphamide may increase the risk of noncutaneous solid malignancy when used with etanercept (concurrent therapy is not recommended).

Adverse Reactions

>10%:

Central nervous system: Headache (17%)

Local: Injection site reaction (14% to 37%)

Respiratory: Respiratory tract infection (upper, 29%; other than upper, 38%), rhinitis (12%)

Miscellaneous: Infection (35%), positive ANA (11%), positive antidouble-stranded DNA antibodies (15% by RIA, 3% by *Crithidia luciliae* assay)

≥3% to 10%:

Central nervous system: Dizziness (7%)

Dermatologic: Rash (5%)

Gastrointestinal: Abdominal pain (5%), dyspepsia (4%), nausea (9%), vomiting (3%)

Neuromuscular & skeletal: Weakness (5%)

Respiratory: Pharyngitis (7%), respiratory disorder (5%), sinusitis (3%), cough (6%)

Pediatric patients (JRA): The percentages of patients reporting abdominal pain (17%) and vomiting (13%) were higher than in adult RA. Two patients developed varicella infection associated with aseptic meningitis which resolved without complications (see Warnings/ Precautions).

Overdosage/Toxicology No dose-limiting toxicities have been observed during clinical trials. Single I.V. doses up to 60 mg/m^2 have been administered to healthy volunteers in an endotoxemia study without evidence of dose-limiting toxicities.

Pharmacodynamics/Kinetics

Onset of Action: ~2-3 weeks

Time to Peak: 72 hours (range: 48-96 hours)

Half-Life Elimination: 115 hours (range: 98-300 hours)

Excretion: Clearance: Children: 45.9 mL/hour/m^2; Adults: 89 mL/hour (52 mL/hour/m^2)

Available Dosage Forms

Injection, powder for reconstitution: 25 mg [diluent contains benzyl alcohol; packaging may contain dry natural rubber (latex)]

Injection, solution: 50 mg/mL (0.98 mL) [prefilled syringe with 27-gauge ½ inch needle]

Dosing

Adults:

Rheumatoid arthritis, psoriatic arthritis, ankylosing spondylitis: SubQ:

Once-weekly dosing: 50 mg once weekly

Twice-weekly dosing: 25 mg given twice weekly (individual doses should be separated by 72-96 hours)

Note: If the physician determines that it is appropriate, patients may self-inject after proper training in injection technique.

Elderly: SubQ: Although greater sensitivity of some elderly patients cannot be ruled out, no overall differences in safety or effectiveness were observed.

Pediatrics:

Juvenile rheumatoid arthritis: Children 4-17 years: SubQ:

Once-weekly dosing: 0.8 mg/kg (maximum: 50 mg/ dose) once weekly

Twice-weekly dosing: 0.4 mg/kg (maximum: 25 mg/ dose) twice weekly (individual doses should be separated by 72-96 hours)

Administration

Other: Administer subcutaneously. Rotate injection sites. New injections should be given at least one inch (Continued)

Etanercept *(Continued)*

from an old site and never into areas where the skin is tender, bruised, red, or hard.

Powder for reconstitution: Follow package instructions carefully for reconstitution. **Note:** The needle cover of the diluent syringe (multidose vial) may contain dry natural rubber (latex) which should not be handled by persons sensitive to this substance. The maximum amount injected at any single site should not exceed 25 mg.

Prefilled syringe: May be allowed to reach room temperature prior to injection.

Stability

Reconstitution: Reconstitute aseptically with 1 mL sterile bacteriostatic water for injection, USP (supplied). Do not filter reconstituted solution during preparation or administration. **Note:** The needle cover of the diluent syringe may contain dry natural rubber (latex), which should not be handled by persons sensitive to this substance. Swirl to mix; do not shake or vigorously agitate.

Storage: The prefilled syringe or dose tray containing etanercept (sterile powder) must be refrigerated at 2°C to 8°C (36°F to 46°F). Do not freeze. Reconstituted solutions of etanercept should be administered as soon as possible after reconstitution. If not administered immediately after reconstitution, etanercept may be stored in the vial at 2°C to 8°C (36°F to 46°F) for up to 14 days.

Nursing Actions

Physical Assessment: Monitor for signs and symptoms of infection. Assess for liver dysfunction (unusual fatigue, easy bruising or bleeding, jaundice). Monitor effectiveness of therapy (eg, pain, range of motion, mobility, ADL function, inflammation). Assess knowledge/teach patient appropriate administration (injection technique and needle disposal if self-administered), possible side effects/interventions, and adverse symptoms to report.

Patient Education: If self-injecting, follow instructions for injection and disposal of needles exactly. If redness, swelling, or irritation appears at the injection site, contact prescriber. Do not have any vaccinations while using this medication without consulting prescriber first. You may experience headache or dizziness (use caution when driving or engaging in tasks requiring alertness until response to drug is known). If stomach pain or cramping; unusual bleeding or bruising; persistent fever; paleness; blood in vomitus, stool, or urine occurs, stop medication and contact prescriber **immediately**. Also immediately report skin rash, unusual muscle or bone weakness, or signs of respiratory flu or other infection (eg, chills, fever, sore throat, easy bruising or bleeding, mouth sores, unhealed sores). **Breast-feeding precaution:** Breast-feeding is not recommended.

Breast-Feeding Issues It is not known whether etanercept is excreted in human milk or absorbed systemically after ingestion. Because many immunoglobulins are excreted in human milk, and because of the potential for serious adverse reactions in nursing infants from Enbrel®, a decision should be made whether to discontinue nursing or to discontinue the drug.

Ethacrynic Acid (eth a KRIN ik AS id)

U.S. Brand Names Edecrin®
Synonyms Ethacrynate Sodium
Pharmacologic Category Diuretic, Loop
Medication Safety Issues
Sound-alike/look-alike issues:
Edecrin® may be confused with Eulexin®, Ecotrin®

Pregnancy Risk Factor B
Lactation Contraindicated
Use Management of edema associated with congestive heart failure; hepatic cirrhosis or renal disease; short-term management of ascites due to malignancy, idiopathic edema, and lymphedema

Mechanism of Action/Effect Inhibits reabsorption of sodium and chloride in the ascending loop of Henle and distal renal tubule, interfering with the chloride-binding cotransport system, thus causing increased excretion of water, sodium, chloride, magnesium, and calcium

Contraindications Hypersensitivity to ethacrynic acid or any component of the formulation; anuria; history of severe watery diarrhea caused by this product; infants

Warnings/Precautions Adjust dose to avoid dehydration. In cirrhosis, avoid electrolyte and acid/base imbalances that might lead to hepatic encephalopathy. Ototoxicity is associated with rapid I.V. administration, renal impairment, excessive doses, and concurrent use of other ototoxins. Has been associated with a higher incidence of ototoxicity than other loop diuretics. Hypersensitivity reactions can rarely occur, however, ethacrynic acid has no cross-reactivity to sulfonamides or sulfonylureas. Monitor fluid status and renal function in an attempt to prevent oliguria, azotemia, and reversible increases in BUN and creatinine. Close medical supervision of aggressive diuresis required. Watch for and correct electrolyte disturbances. Coadministration of antihypertensives may increase the risk of hypotension.

Drug Interactions
Decreased Effect: Probenecid decreases diuretic effects of ethacrynic acid. Glucose tolerance may be decreased by loop diuretics, requiring adjustment of hypoglycemic agents. Cholestyramine or colestipol may reduce bioavailability of ethacrynic acid. Indomethacin (and other NSAIDs) may reduce natriuretic and hypotensive effects of diuretics.

Increased Effect/Toxicity: Ethacrynic acid-induced hypokalemia may predispose to digoxin toxicity and may increase the risk of arrhythmia with drugs which may prolong QT interval, including type Ia and type III antiarrhythmic agents, cisapride, and some quinolones (sparfloxacin, gatifloxacin, and moxifloxacin). The risk of toxicity from lithium and salicylates (high dose) may be increased by loop diuretics. Hypotensive effects and/or adverse renal effects of ACE inhibitors and NSAIDs are potentiated by ethacrynic acid-induced hypovolemia. The effects of peripheral adrenergic-blocking drugs or ganglionic blockers may be increased by ethacrynic acid.

Ethacrynic acid may increase the risk of ototoxicity with other ototoxic agents (aminoglycosides, cis-platinum), especially in patients with renal dysfunction. Synergistic diuretic effects occur with thiazide-type diuretics. Diuretics tend to be synergistic with other antihypertensive agents, and hypotension may occur. Nephrotoxicity has been associated with concomitant use of cephaloridine or cephalexin.

Adverse Reactions Frequency not defined.
Central nervous system: Headache, fatigue, apprehension, confusion, fever, chills, encephalopathy (patients with pre-existing liver disease); vertigo
Dermatologic: Skin rash, Henoch-Schönlein purpura (in patient with rheumatic heart disease)
Endocrine & metabolic: Hyponatremia, hyperglycemia, variations in phosphorus, CO_2 content, bicarbonate,

and calcium; reversible hyperuricemia, gout, hyperglycemia, hypoglycemia (occurred in two uremic patients who received doses above those recommended)

Gastrointestinal: Anorexia, malaise, abdominal discomfort or pain, dysphagia, nausea, vomiting, diarrhea, gastrointestinal bleeding, acute pancreatitis (rare)

Genitourinary: Hematuria

Hepatic: Jaundice, abnormal liver function tests

Hematology: Agranulocytosis, severe neutropenia, thrombocytopenia

Local: Thrombophlebitis (with intravenous use), local irritation and pain,

Ocular: Blurred vision

Otic: Tinnitus, temporary or permanent deafness

Renal: Serum creatinine increased

Overdosage/Toxicology Symptoms of overdose include electrolyte depletion, volume depletion, dehydration, and circulatory collapse. Treatment is supportive.

Pharmacodynamics/Kinetics

Onset of Action: Diuresis: Oral: ~30 minutes; I.V.: 5 minutes; Peak effect: Oral: 2 hours; I.V.: 30 minutes

Duration of Action: Oral: 12 hours; I.V.: 2 hours

Protein Binding: >90%

Half-Life Elimination: Normal renal function: 2-4 hours

Metabolism: Hepatic (35% to 40%) to active cysteine conjugate

Excretion: Feces and urine (30% to 60% as unchanged drug)

Available Dosage Forms

Injection, powder for reconstitution, as ethacrynate sodium: 50 mg

Tablet: 25 mg

Dosing

Adults: I.V. formulation should be diluted in D_5W or NS (1 mg/mL) and infused over several minutes.

Edema:

Oral: 50-100 mg/day in 1-2 divided doses; may increase in increments of 25-50 mg at intervals of several days to a maximum of 400 mg/24 hours.

I.V.: 0.5-1 mg/kg/dose (maximum: 100 mg/dose); repeat doses not routinely recommended; however, if indicated, repeat doses every 8-12 hours.

Elderly: Oral: Initial: 25-50 mg/day

Pediatrics:

Edema: Oral: Children: 1 mg/kg/dose once daily; increase at intervals of 2-3 days as needed, to a maximum of 3 mg/kg/day.

Renal Impairment:

Cl_{cr} <10 mL/minute: Avoid use.

Not removed by hemo- or peritoneal dialysis; supplemental dose is not necessary.

Administration

I.V.: Injection should **not** be given SubQ or I.M. due to local pain and irritation. Single I.V. doses should not exceed 100 mg. Administer each 10 mg over a minute.

I.V. Detail: If a second dose is needed, it is recommended to use a new injection site to avoid possible thrombophlebitis.

pH: 6.3-7.7

Stability

Compatibility: Stable in D_5NS, D_5W, LR, NS

Incompatible whole blood or its derivatives

Compatibility when admixed: Incompatible with hydralazine, procainamide, ranitidine, tolazoline, triflupromazine

Laboratory Monitoring Renal function, serum electrolytes

Nursing Actions

Physical Assessment: Assess potential for interactions with other pharmacological agents or herbal products patient may be taking (especially anything

that would impact blood pressure or add to risk of ototoxicity). **Infusion:** See Administration. Assess results of laboratory tests, therapeutic effectiveness (according to purpose for use), and adverse response (eg, dehydration, electrolyte imbalance, CNS changes) on a regular basis during therapy. Caution patients with diabetes to monitor glucose levels closely (may cause hyper/hypoglycemia). Teach patient appropriate use, possible side effects/appropriate interventions, and adverse symptoms to report.

Patient Education: Inform prescriber of all prescriptions, OTC medications, or herbal products you are taking, and any allergies you have. Do not take any new medication during therapy without consulting prescriber. Take prescribed dose with food early in day. Include orange juice or bananas (or other potassium-rich foods) in your diet, but do not take potassium supplements without consulting prescriber. If you have diabetes, monitor serum glucose closely (this medication may alter glucose levels). May cause postural hypotension (use caution when rising from lying or sitting position, when climbing stairs, or when driving); lightheadedness, dizziness, or drowsiness (use caution driving or when engaging in hazardous activities); diarrhea (buttermilk, boiled milk, or yogurt may help); or decreased accommodation to heat (avoid excessive exercise in hot weather). Report hearing changes (ringing in ears); persistent headache; unusual confusion or nervousness; abdominal pain or blood stool (black stool); palpitations, chest pain, rapid heartbeat; flu-like symptoms; skin rash or itching; blurred vision; swelling of ankles or feet; weight changes of more than 3 lb/day; increased fatigue; or joint/muscle swelling, pain, cramping, or trembling. **Breast-feeding precaution:** Do not breast-feed.

Dietary Considerations This product may cause a potassium loss. Your healthcare provider may prescribe a potassium supplement, another medication to help prevent the potassium loss, or recommend that you eat foods high in potassium, especially citrus fruits. Do not change your diet on your own while taking this medication, especially if you are taking potassium supplements or medications to reduce potassium loss. Too much potassium can be as harmful as too little.

Geriatric Considerations Ethacrynic acid is rarely used because of its increased incidence of ototoxicity as compared to the other loop diuretics.

Ethambutol (e THAM byoo tole)

U.S. Brand Names Myambutol®

Synonyms Ethambutol Hydrochloride

Pharmacologic Category Antitubercular Agent

Medication Safety Issues

Sound-alike/look-alike issues:

Myambutol® may be confused with Nembutal®

Pregnancy Risk Factor C

Lactation Enters breast milk/use caution (AAP considers "compatible")

Use Treatment of tuberculosis and other mycobacterial diseases in conjunction with other antituberculosis agents

Mechanism of Action/Effect Suppresses mycobacteria multiplication by interfering with RNA synthesis

Contraindications Hypersensitivity to ethambutol or any component of the formulation; optic neuritis; use in children, unconscious patients, or any other patient who may be unable to discern and report visual changes

Warnings/Precautions May cause optic neuritis, resulting in decreased visual acuity or other vision changes. Discontinue promptly in patients with changes in vision, color blindness, or visual defects (effects normally reversible, but reversal may require up to a (Continued)

Ethambutol *(Continued)*

year). Use only in children whose visual acuity can accurately be determined and monitored (not recommended for use in children <13 years of age). Dosage modification is required in patients with renal insufficiency. Hepatic toxicity has been reported, possibly due to concurrent therapy.

Drug Interactions

Decreased Effect: Decreased absorption with aluminum hydroxide. Avoid concurrent administration of aluminum-containing antacids for at least 4 hours following ethambutol.

Lab Interactions Increased uric acid (S)

Adverse Reactions Frequency not defined.

Cardiovascular: Myocarditis, pericarditis

Central nervous system: Headache, confusion, disorientation, malaise, mental confusion, fever, dizziness, hallucinations

Dermatologic: Rash, pruritus, dermatitis, exfoliative dermatitis

Endocrine & metabolic: Acute gout or hyperuricemia

Gastrointestinal: Abdominal pain, anorexia, nausea, vomiting

Hematologic: Leukopenia, thrombocytopenia, eosinophilia, neutropenia, lymphadenopathy

Hepatic: Abnormal LFTs, hepatotoxicity (possibly related to concurrent therapy), hepatitis

Neuromuscular & skeletal: Peripheral neuritis, arthralgia

Ocular: Optic neuritis; symptoms may include decreased acuity, scotoma, color blindness, or visual defects (usually reversible with discontinuation, irreversible blindness has been described)

Renal: Nephritis

Respiratory: Infiltrates (with or without eosinophilia), pneumonitis

Miscellaneous: Anaphylaxis, anaphylactoid reaction; hypersensitivity syndrome (rash, eosinophilia, and organ-specific inflammation)

Overdosage/Toxicology Symptoms of overdose include decrease in visual acuity, anorexia, joint pain, and numbness of extremities. Treatment is supportive.

Pharmacodynamics/Kinetics

Time to Peak: Serum: 2-4 hours

Protein Binding: 20% to 30%

Half-Life Elimination: 2.5-3.6 hours; End-stage renal disease: 7-15 hours

Metabolism: Hepatic (20%) to inactive metabolite

Excretion: Urine (~50%) and feces (20%) as unchanged drug

Available Dosage Forms Tablet, as hydrochloride: 100 mg, 400 mg

Dosing

Adults & Elderly:

Treatment of tuberculosis (suggested doses by lean body weight):

Daily therapy: 15-25 mg/kg

40-55 kg: 800 mg

56-75 kg: 1200 mg

76-90 kg: 1600 mg (maximum dose regardless of weight)

Twice weekly directly observed therapy (DOT): 50 mg/kg

40-55 kg: 2000 mg

56-75 kg: 2800 mg

76-90 kg: 4000 mg (maximum dose regardless of weight)

Three times/week DOT: 25-30 mg/kg (maximum: 2.5 g)

40-55 kg: 1200 mg

56-75 kg: 2000 mg

76-90 kg: 2400 mg (maximum dose regardless of weight)

Note: Used as part of a multidrug regimen. Treatment regimens consist of an initial 2 month phase, followed by a continuation phase of 4 or 7 additional months; frequency of dosing may differ depending on phase of therapy.

Disseminated *Mycobacterium avium* complex (MAC) in patients with advanced HIV infection: 15 mg/kg ethambutol in combination with azithromycin 600 mg daily

Pediatrics:

Treatment of tuberculosis Oral:

Daily therapy: 15-20 mg/kg/day (maximum: 1 g/day)

Twice weekly directly observed therapy (DOT): 50 mg/kg (maximum: 4 g/dose)

See "Note" in adult dosing.

Renal Impairment:

Cl_{cr} 10-50 mL/minute: Administer every 24-36 hours.

Cl_{cr} <10 mL/minute: Administer every 48 hours.

Slightly dialyzable (5% to 20%); administer dose postdialysis.

Peritoneal dialysis: Dose as for Cl_{cr} <10 mL/minute.

Continuous arteriovenous or venovenous hemofiltration: Administer every 24-36 hours.

Stability

Storage: Store at controlled room temperature of 20°C to 25°C (68°F to 77°F).

Laboratory Monitoring Baseline and periodic (monthly) visual testing (each eye individually, as well as both eyes tested together) in patients receiving >15 mg/kg/day; baseline and periodic renal, hepatic, and hematopoietic tests

Nursing Actions

Physical Assessment: Monitor baseline and periodic laboratory tests, therapeutic effectiveness, and adverse response (eg, CNS changes, neuritis, and ocular changes) on a regular basis during therapy. Teach patient appropriate use (need to adhere to dosing program), possible side effects/appropriate interventions (regular ophthalmic evaluations), and adverse symptoms to report.

Patient Education: Take as scheduled, with meals. Avoid missing doses and do not discontinue without consulting prescriber. Avoid aluminum-containing antacids for at least 4 hours following ethambutol. May cause GI distress (small, frequent meals and good oral care may help), dizziness, disorientation, drowsiness (avoid driving or engaging in tasks that require alertness until response to drug is known). You will need to have frequent ophthalmic exams and periodic medical check-ups to evaluate drug effects. Report vision changes, numbness or tingling of extremities, or persistent loss of appetite. **Pregnancy precaution:** Inform prescriber if you are or intend to become pregnant.

Dietary Considerations May be taken with food as absorption is not affected, may cause gastric irritation.

Geriatric Considerations Since most elderly patients acquired their tuberculosis before current antituberculin regimens were available, ethambutol is only indicated when patients are from areas where drug resistant *M. tuberculosis* is endemic, in HIV-infected elderly patients, and when drug resistant *M. tuberculosis* is suspected (see dose adjustments for renal impairment).

Breast-Feeding Issues The manufacturer suggests use during breast-feeding only if benefits to the mother outweigh the possible risk to the infant. Some references suggest that exposure to the infant is low and does not produce toxicity, and breast-feeding should not be discouraged. Other references recommend if breast-feeding, monitor the infant for rash, malaise, nausea, or vomiting.

Pregnancy Issues There are no adequate and well-controlled studies in pregnant women; teratogenic effects have been seen in animals. Ethambutol has been used safely during pregnancy.

Ethinyl Estradiol and Desogestrel

(ETH in il es tra DYE ole & des oh JES trel)

U.S. Brand Names Apri®; Cesia™; Cyclessa®; Desogen®; Kariva™; Mircette®; Ortho-Cept®; Reclipsen™; Solia™; Velivet™

Synonyms Desogestrel and Ethinyl Estradiol; Ortho Cept

Pharmacologic Category Contraceptive; Estrogen and Progestin Combination

Medication Safety Issues

Sound-alike/look-alike issues:

Ortho-Cept® may be confused with Ortho-Cyclen®

Pregnancy Risk Factor X

Lactation Enters breast milk/not recommended (AAP rates "compatible")

Use Prevention of pregnancy

Unlabeled/Investigational Use Treatment of hyper-menorrhea (menorrhagia); pain associated with endo-metriosis; dysmenorrhea; dysfunctional uterine bleeding

Mechanism of Action/Effect Combination hormonal contraceptives inhibit ovulation and also produce changes in the cervical mucus and endometrium creating an unfavorable environment for sperm penetration and nidation.

Contraindications Hypersensitivity to ethinyl estradiol, etonogestrel, desogestrel, or any component of the formulation; history of or current thrombophlebitis or venous thromboembolic disorders (including DVT, PE); active or recent (within 1 year) arterial thromboembolic disease (eg, stroke, MI); cerebral vascular disease, coronary artery disease, valvular heart disease with complications, severe hypertension; diabetes mellitus with vascular involvement; severe headache with focal neurological symptoms; known or suspected breast carcinoma, endometrial cancer, estrogen-dependent neoplasms, undiagnosed abnormal genital bleeding; hepatic dysfunction or tumor, cholestatic jaundice of pregnancy, jaundice with prior combination hormonal contraceptive use; major surgery with prolonged immobilization; heavy smoking (≥15 cigarettes/day) in patients >35 years of age; pregnancy

Warnings/Precautions Combination hormonal contraceptives do not protect against HIV infection or other sexually-transmitted diseases. The risk of cardiovascular side effects increases in women who smoke cigarettes, especially those who are >35 years of age; women who use combination hormonal contraceptives should be strongly advised not to smoke. Combination hormonal contraceptives may lead to increased risk of myocardial infarction, use with caution in patients with risk factors for coronary artery disease. May increase the risk of thromboembolism. Whenever possible, combination hormonal contraceptives should be discontinued at least 4 weeks prior to and for 2 weeks following elective surgery associated with an increased risk of thromboembolism or during periods of prolonged immobilization. Combination hormonal contraceptives may have a dose-related risk of vascular disease, hypertension, and gallbladder disease. Women with hypertension or renal disease should be encouraged to use another form of contraception. The use of combination hormonal contraceptives has been associated with a slight increase in frequency of breast cancer, however, studies are not consistent. Combination hormonal contraceptives may cause glucose intolerance. Retinal thrombosis has been reported (rarely). Use caution in conditions that may be aggravated by fluid retention, depression, or history of migraine. Not for use prior to menarche.

The minimum dosage combination of estrogen/progestin that will effectively treat the individual patient should be used. New patients should be started on products containing ≤0.035 mg of estrogen per tablet.

Drug Interactions

Cytochrome P450 Effect:

Ethinyl estradiol: **Substrate** of CYP2C8/9 (minor), 3A4 (major), 3A5-7 (minor); **Inhibits** CYP1A2 (weak), 2B6 (weak), 2C19 (weak), 3A4 (weak)

Desogestrel: **Substrate** of CYP2C19 (major)

Decreased Effect: CYP2C19 inducers may decrease the levels/effects of desogestrel; example inducers include aminoglutethimide, carbamazepine, phenytoin, and rifampin. CYP3A4 inducers may decrease the levels/effects of ethinyl estradiol; example inducers include aminoglutethimide, carbamazepine, nafcillin, phenobarbital, phenytoin, and rifamycins. Combination hormonal contraceptives may decrease plasma levels of acetaminophen, clofibric acid, lorazepam, morphine, oxazepam, salicylic acid, temazepam. Contraceptive effect decreased by acitretin, amprenavir, griseofulvin, lopinavir, nelfinavir, nevirapine, penicillins (effect not consistent), ritonavir, tetracyclines (effect not consistent), troglitazone. Combination hormonal contraceptives may decrease (or increase) the effects of coumarin derivatives.

Increased Effect/Toxicity: Acetaminophen, ascorbic acid, and repaglinide may increase plasma levels of estrogen component. Atorvastatin and indinavir increase plasma levels of combination hormonal contraceptives. Combination hormonal contraceptives increase the plasma levels of alprazolam, chlordiazepoxide, cyclosporine, diazepam, prednisolone, selegiline, theophylline, tricyclic antidepressants. Combination hormonal contraceptives may increase (or decrease) the effects of coumarin derivatives.

Nutritional/Ethanol Interactions

Food: CNS effects of caffeine may be enhanced if combination hormonal contraceptives are used concurrently with caffeine. Grapefruit juice increases ethinyl estradiol concentrations and would be expected to increase progesterone serum levels as well; clinical implications are unclear.

Herb/Nutraceutical: St John's wort may decrease the effectiveness of combination hormonal contraceptives by inducing hepatic enzymes. Avoid dong quai and black cohosh (have estrogen activity). Avoid saw palmetto, red clover, ginseng.

Lab Interactions Increased platelet aggregation, thyroid-binding globulin, total thyroid hormone (T_4), serum triglycerides/phospholipids; decreased antithrombin III, serum folate concentration

Adverse Reactions Frequency not defined.

Cardiovascular: Arterial thromboembolism, cerebral hemorrhage, cerebral thrombosis, edema, hypertension, mesenteric thrombosis, MI

Central nervous system: Depression, dizziness, headache, migraine, nervousness, premenstrual syndrome, stroke

Dermatologic: Acne, erythema multiforme, erythema nodosum, hirsutism, loss of scalp hair, melasma (may persist), rash (allergic)

Endocrine & metabolic: Amenorrhea, breakthrough bleeding, breast enlargement, breast secretion, breast tenderness, carbohydrate intolerance, lactation decreased (postpartum), glucose tolerance decreased, libido changes, menstrual flow changes, sex hormone-binding globulins (SHBG) increased, spotting, temporary infertility (following discontinuation), thyroid-binding globulin increased, triglycerides increased

Gastrointestinal: Abdominal cramps, appetite changes, bloating, cholestasis, colitis, gallbladder disease, jaundice, nausea, vomiting, weight gain/loss

Genitourinary: Cervical erosion changes, cervical secretion changes, cystitis-like syndrome, vaginal candidiasis, vaginitis

Hematologic: Antithrombin III decreased, folate levels decreased, hemolytic uremic syndrome, norepinephrine induced platelet aggregability increased, (Continued)

Ethinyl Estradiol and Desogestrel

(Continued)

porphyria, prothrombin increased; factors VII, VIII, IX, and X

Hepatic: Benign liver tumors, Budd-Chiari syndrome, cholestatic jaundice, hepatic adenomas

Local: Thrombophlebitis

Ocular: Cataracts, change in corneal curvature (steepening), contact lens intolerance, optic neuritis, retinal thrombosis

Renal: Impaired renal function

Respiratory: Pulmonary thromboembolism

Miscellaneous: Hemorrhagic eruption

Overdosage/Toxicology Toxicity is unlikely following single exposures of excessive doses. May cause withdrawal bleeding in females. Any treatment following emesis and charcoal administration should be supportive and symptomatic.

Pharmacodynamics/Kinetics

Protein Binding:

Desogestrel: Etonogestrel (active metabolite): 98%, primarily to sex hormone-binding globulin

Half-Life Elimination:

Desogestrel: 37.1 hours

Metabolism:

Desogestrel: Hepatic via CYP2C9 to active metabolite etonogestrel (3-keto-desogestrel); etonogestrel metabolized via CYP3A4

Excretion:

Desogestrel: Urine and feces (as metabolites)

Available Dosage Forms

Tablet, low-dose formulations:

Kariva™:

Day 1-21: Ethinyl estradiol 0.02 mg and desogestrel 0.15 mg [21 white tablets]

Day 22-23: 2 inactive light green tablets

Day 24-28: Ethinyl estradiol 0.01 mg [5 light blue tablets] (28s)

Mircette®:

Day 1-21: Ethinyl estradiol 0.02 mg and desogestrel 0.15 mg [21 white tablets]

Day 22-23: 2 inactive green tablets

Day 24-28: Ethinyl estradiol 0.01 mg [5 yellow tablets] (28s)

Tablet, monophasic formulations:

Apri® 28: Ethinyl estradiol 0.03 mg and desogestrel 0.15 mg [21 rose tablets and 7 white inactive tablets] (28s)

Desogen®, Reclipsen™, Solia™: Ethinyl estradiol 0.03 mg and desogestrel 0.15 mg [21 white tablets and 7 green inactive tablets] (28s)

Ortho-Cept® 28: Ethinyl estradiol 0.03 mg and desogestrel 0.15 mg [21 orange tablets and 7 green inactive tablets] (28s)

Tablet, triphasic formulations:

Cesia™, Cyclessa®:

Day 1-7:Ethinyl estradiol 0.025 mg and desogestrel 0.1 mg [7 light yellow tablets]

Day 8-14: Ethinyl estradiol 0.025 mg and desogestrel 0.125 mg [7 orange tablets]

Day 14-21: Ethinyl estradiol 0.025 mg and desogestrel 0.15 mg [7 red tablets]

Day 21-28: 7 green inactive tablets (28s)

Velivet™:

Day 1-7: Ethinyl estradiol 0.025 mg and desogestrel 0.1 mg [7 beige tablets]

Day 8-14: Ethinyl estradiol 0.025 mg and desogestrel 0.125 mg [7 orange tablets]

Day 14-21: Ethinyl estradiol 0.025 mg and desogestrel 0.15 mg [7 pink tablets]

Day 21-28: 7 white inactive tablets (28s)

Dosing

Adults: Female: Contraception: Oral:

Schedule 1 (Sunday starter): Dose begins on first Sunday after onset of menstruation; if the menstrual period starts on Sunday, take first tablet that very same day. **With a Sunday start, an additional method of contraception should be used until after the first 7 days of consecutive administration.**

For 21-tablet package: Dosage is 1 tablet daily for 21 consecutive days, followed by 7 days off of the medication; a new course begins on the 8th day after the last tablet is taken.

For 28-tablet package: Dosage is 1 tablet daily without interruption.

Schedule 2 (Day 1 starter): Dose starts on first day of menstrual cycle taking 1 tablet daily.

For 21-tablet package: Dosage is 1 tablet daily for 21 consecutive days, followed by 7 days off of the medication; a new course begins on the 8th day after the last tablet is taken.

For 28-tablet package: Dosage is 1 tablet daily without interruption.

If all doses have been taken on schedule and one menstrual period is missed, continue dosing cycle. If two consecutive menstrual periods are missed, pregnancy test is required before new dosing cycle is started.

Missed doses **monophasic formulations** (refer to package insert for complete information):

One dose missed: Take as soon as remembered or take 2 tablets next day

Two consecutive doses missed in the first 2 weeks: Take 2 tablets as soon as remembered or 2 tablets next 2 days. **An additional method of contraception should be used for 7 days after missed dose.**

Two consecutive doses missed in week 3 or three consecutive doses missed at any time: Schedule 1 (Sunday starter): Continue to take 1 tablet daily until Sunday, then discard the rest of the pack, and a new pack is started that same day. Schedule 2 (Day 1 starter): Current pack should be discarded, and a new pack started that same day. **An additional method of contraception should be used for 7 days after missed dose.**

Missed doses **biphasic/triphasic formulations** (refer to package insert for complete information):

One dose missed: Take as soon as remembered or take 2 tablets next day.

Two consecutive doses missed in week 1 or week 2 of the pack: Take 2 tablets as soon as remembered and 2 tablets the next day. Resume taking 1 tablet daily until the pack is empty. **An additional method of contraception should be used for 7 days after a missed dose.**

Two consecutive doses missed in week 3 of the pack; **an additional method of contraception must be used for 7 days after a missed dose:**

Schedule 1 (Sunday starter): Take 1 tablet every day until Sunday. Discard the remaining pack and start a new pack of pills on the same day.

Schedule 2 (Day 1 starter): Discard the remaining pack and start a new pack the same day.

Three or more consecutive doses missed; **an additional method of contraception must be used for 7 days after a missed dose:**

Schedule 1 (Sunday starter): Take 1 tablet every day until Sunday; on Sunday, discard the pack and start a new pack.

Schedule 2 (Day 1 starter): Discard the remaining pack and begin new pack of tablets starting on the same day.

Pediatrics: Female: Contraception: Oral: See adult dosing; not to be used prior to menarche.

Renal Impairment: Specific guidelines not available; use with caution and monitor blood pressure closely. Consider other forms of contraception.

Hepatic Impairment: Contraindicated in patients with hepatic impairment.

Administration

Oral: Administer at the same time each day.

Stability

Storage: Store at controlled room temperature of 25°C (77°F).

Nursing Actions

Physical Assessment: Monitor blood pressure on a regular basis. Assess for adverse reactions and potential drug interactions. Assess knowledge/teach importance of regular (monthly) blood pressure checks and annual physical assessment, Pap smear, and vision assessment. Teach importance of maintaining prescribed schedule of dosing. **Pregnancy risk factor X:** Do not use if patient is pregnant.

Patient Education: Oral contraceptives do not protect against HIV infection or other sexually-transmitted diseases. Take exactly as directed by prescriber (see package insert). You are at risk of becoming pregnant if doses are missed. Detailed and complete information on dosing and missed doses can be found in the package insert. Be aware that some medications may reduce the effectiveness of oral contraceptives; an alternate form of contraception may be needed. Check all medicines (prescription and over-the-counter), herbal and alternative products with prescriber. It is important that you check your blood pressure monthly (same day each month) and that you have an annual physical assessment, Pap smear, and vision exam while taking this medication. Avoid smoking while taking this medication; smoking increases risk of adverse effects, including thromboembolic events and heart attacks. You may experience loss of appetite (small frequent meals will help); or constipation (increased exercise, fluids, fruit, fiber, or stool softeners may help). If you have diabetes, use accurate serum glucose testing to identify any changes in glucose tolerance; notify prescriber of significant changes so antidiabetic medication can be adjusted if necessary. Report immediately pain or muscle soreness; warmth, swelling, pain, or redness in calves; shortness of breath; sudden loss of vision; unresolved leg/foot swelling; change in menstrual pattern (unusual bleeding, amenorrhea, breakthrough spotting); breast tenderness that does not go away; acute abdominal cramping; signs of vaginal infection (drainage, pain, itching); CNS changes (blurred vision, confusion, acute anxiety, or unresolved depression); chest pain; severe headache or vomiting; weakness in arm or leg; severe abdominal pain or tenderness; jaundice; or significant weight gain (>5 lb/week). Notify prescriber of changes in contact lens tolerance. **Pregnancy/breast-feeding precautions:** This medication should not be used during pregnancy. If you suspect you may become pregnant, contact prescriber immediately.

Dietary Considerations Should be taken at same time each day.

Breast-Feeding Issues Jaundice and breast enlargement in the nursing infant have been reported following the use of combination hormonal contraceptives. May decrease the quality and quantity of breast milk; a nonhormonal form of contraception is recommended.

Pregnancy Issues Pregnancy should be ruled out prior to treatment and discontinued if pregnancy occurs. In general, the use of combination hormonal contraceptives when inadvertently taken early in pregnancy have not been associated with teratogenic effects. Due to increased risk of thromboembolism postpartum, combination hormonal contraceptives should not be started earlier than 4-6 weeks following delivery.

Additional Information The World Health Organization (WHO) has issued revised management recommendations for missed combined oral contraceptive pills. Refer to the following reference for a complete presentation and discussion of the guidelines:

Faculty of Family Planning and Reproductive Health Care Clinical Effectiveness Unit, "Faculty Statement from the CEU on a New Publication: WHO Selected Practice Recommendations for Contraceptive Use Update. Missed Pills: New Recommendations," *J Fam Plann Reprod Health Care*, 2005, 31(2):153-5.

Ethinyl Estradiol and Drospirenone
(ETH in il es tra DYE ole & droh SPYE re none)

U.S. Brand Names Yasmin®; Yaz

Synonyms Drospirenone and Ethinyl Estradiol

Pharmacologic Category Contraceptive; Estrogen and Progestin Combination

Pregnancy Risk Factor X

Lactation Enters breast milk/not recommended

Use Prevention of pregnancy

Unlabeled/Investigational Use Treatment of hypermenorrhea (menorrhagia); pain associated with endometriosis; dysmenorrhea; dysfunctional uterine bleeding

Mechanism of Action/Effect Combination oral contraceptives inhibit ovulation and also produce changes in the cervical mucus and endometrium creating an unfavorable environment for sperm penetration and nidation.

Contraindications Hypersensitivity to ethinyl estradiol, drospirenone, or to any component of the formulation; history of or current thrombophlebitis or venous thromboembolic disorders (including DVT, PE); active or recent (within 1 year) arterial thromboembolic disease (eg, stroke, MI); cerebral vascular disease, coronary artery disease, severe hypertension; diabetes with vascular involvement; headache with focal neurological symptoms; known or suspected breast carcinoma; endometrial cancer, estrogen-dependent neoplasms, undiagnosed abnormal genital bleeding; renal insufficiency, hepatic dysfunction or tumor, adrenal insufficiency, cholestatic jaundice of pregnancy, jaundice with prior oral contraceptive use; heavy smoking (≥15 cigarettes/day) in patients >35 years of age; pregnancy

Warnings/Precautions Oral contraceptives do not protect against HIV infection or other sexually-transmitted diseases. The risk of cardiovascular side effects increases in women who smoke cigarettes, especially those who are >35 years of age; women who use oral contraceptives should be strongly advised not to smoke. Oral contraceptives may lead to increased risk of myocardial infarction, use with caution in patients with risk factors for coronary artery disease. May increase the risk of thromboembolism. Whenever possible, combination hormonal contraceptives should be discontinued at least 4 weeks prior to and for 2 weeks following elective surgery associated with an increased risk of thromboembolism or during periods of prolonged immobilization. Oral contraceptives may cause glucose intolerance. Retinal thrombosis has been reported (rarely) with oral contraceptive use. Use with caution in patients with conditions that may be aggravated by fluid retention, depression, or patients with history of migraine. Not for use prior to menarche.

Drospirenone has antimineralocorticoid activity that may lead to hyperkalemia in patients with renal insufficiency, hepatic dysfunction, or adrenal insufficiency. Use caution with medications that may increase serum potassium.

Drug Interactions

Cytochrome P450 Effect:

Ethinyl estradiol: **Substrate** of CYP2C9 (minor), 3A4 (major), 3A5-7 (minor); **Inhibits** CYP1A2 (weak), 2B6 (weak), 2C8 (weak), 2C19 (weak), 3A4 (weak)

(Continued)

Ethinyl Estradiol and Drospirenone
(Continued)

Drospirenone: **Substrate** of CYP3A4 (minor); **Inhibits** CYP1A2 (weak), 2C9 (weak), 2C19 (weak), 3A4 (weak)

Decreased Effect: Acitretin may diminish the therapeutic effect of progestins; contraceptive failure is possible. Oral contraceptives may decrease the plasma concentration of acetaminophen, clofibric acid, lamotrigine, morphine, salicylic acid, and temazepam. Aminoglutethimide, anticonvulsants (carbamazepine, felbamate, oxcarbazepine, phenobarbital, phenytoin, topiramate), aprepitant, phenylbutazone, rifampin, and ritonavir may increase metabolism leading to decreased effect of oral contraceptives. Griseofulvin may diminish the therapeutic effect of contraceptive (progestins). Oral contraceptives may decrease (or increase) the effects of coumarin derivatives. Modafinil and topiramate may decrease the serum concentration of oral contraceptive (estrogens).

Increased Effect/Toxicity: ACE inhibitors, aldosterone antagonists, angiotensin II receptor antagonists, heparin, NSAIDs (when taken daily, long term), and potassium-sparing diuretics increase risk of hyperkalemia with concomitant use. Acetaminophen, ascorbic acid, and atorvastatin may increase plasma concentrations of oral contraceptives. Ethinyl estradiol may increase plasma concentrations of cyclosporine, prednisolone, selegiline, and theophylline. Oral contraceptives may increase (or decrease) the effects of coumarin derivatives.

Nutritional/Ethanol Interactions

Food: CNS effects of caffeine may be enhanced if oral contraceptives are used concurrently with caffeine. Grapefruit juice increases ethinyl estradiol concentrations; clinical implications are unclear.

Herb/Nutraceutical: St John's wort may decrease the effectiveness of oral contraceptives by inducing hepatic enzymes; may also result in breakthrough bleeding.

Adverse Reactions

>1%:

Central nervous system: Depression, dizziness, emotional lability, fever, headache, migraine, nervousness

Dermatologic: Acne, pruritus, rash

Endocrine & metabolic: Amenorrhea, breast pain, dysmenorrhea, intermenstrual bleeding, menstrual irregularities

Gastrointestinal: Abdominal pain, diarrhea, dyspepsia, gastroenteritis, nausea, vomiting, weight gain

Genitourinary: Cystitis, leukorrhea, papanicolaou smear suspicious, pelvic pain, UTI, vaginal moniliasis, vaginitis

Neuromuscular & skeletal: Back pain, extremity pain, weakness

Respiratory: Bronchitis, cough, pharyngitis, rhinitis, sinusitis, upper respiratory infection

Miscellaneous: Allergic reaction, flu-like syndrome, infection

Adverse reactions reported with other oral contraceptives: Appetite changes, antithrombin III decreased, arterial thromboembolism, benign liver tumors, breast changes, Budd-Chiari syndrome, carbohydrate intolerance, cataracts, cerebral hemorrhage, cerebral thrombosis, cervical changes, change in corneal curvature (steepening), cholestatic jaundice, colitis, contact lens intolerance, decreased lactation (postpartum), deep vein thrombosis, diplopia, edema, erythema multiforme, erythema nodosum; factors VII, VIII, IX, X increased; folate serum concentrations decreased, gallbladder disease, glucose intolerance, hemorrhagic eruption, hemolytic uremic syndrome, hepatic adenomas, hirsutism, hypercalcemia, hypertension, hyperglycemia,

libido changes, melasma, mesenteric thrombosis, MI, papilledema, platelet aggregability increased, porphyria, premenstrual syndrome, proptosis, prothrombin increased, pulmonary thromboembolism, renal function impairment, retinal thrombosis, sex hormone-binding globulin increased, thrombophlebitis, thyroid-binding globulin increased, total thyroid hormone (T_4) increased, triglycerides/phospholipids increased, vaginal candidiasis, weight changes

Overdosage/Toxicology May cause nausea; withdrawal bleeding may occur in females. Due to antimineralocorticoid properties of drospirenone, monitor potassium and sodium serum concentrations and evidence of metabolic acidosis.

Pharmacodynamics/Kinetics

Time to Peak:
Drospirenone: 1-3 hours

Protein Binding:
Drospirenone: Serum proteins (excluding sex hormone-binding globulin and corticosteroid-binding globulin): 97%
Ethinyl estradiol: ~98%

Half-Life Elimination:
Drospirenone: 30 hours; Ethinyl estradiol: ~ 24 hours

Metabolism:
Drospirenone: To inactive metabolites, minor metabolism hepatically via CYP3A4
Ethinyl estradiol: Hepatic via CYP3A4; forms metabolites

Excretion:
Drospirenone, ethinyl estradiol: Urine and feces

Available Dosage Forms

Tablet:
Yasmin®: Ethinyl estradiol 0.03 mg and drospirenone 3 mg [21 yellow active tablets and 7 white inactive tablets] (28s)
Yaz: Ethinyl estradiol 0.02 mg and drospirenone 3 mg [24 light pink tablets and 4 white inactive tablets] (28s)

Dosing

Adults: Female: Contraception: Oral: Dosage is 1 tablet daily for 28 consecutive days. Dose should be taken at the same time each day, either after the evening meal or at bedtime. Dosing may be started on the first day of menstrual period (Day 1 starter) or on the first Sunday after the onset of the menstrual period (Sunday starter).

Day 1 starter: Dose starts on first day of menstrual cycle taking 1 tablet daily.

Sunday starter: Dose begins on first Sunday after onset of menstruation; if the menstrual period starts on Sunday, take first tablet that very same day. **With a Sunday start, an additional method of contraception should be used until after the first 7 days of consecutive administration.**

If all doses have been taken on schedule and one menstrual period is missed, continue dosing cycle. If two consecutive menstrual periods are missed, pregnancy test is required before new dosing cycle is started.

If doses have been missed during the first 3 weeks and the menstrual period is missed, pregnancy should be ruled out prior to continuing treatment.

Missed doses (monophasic formulations) (refer to package insert for complete information):

One dose missed: Take as soon as remembered or take 2 tablets next day

Two consecutive doses missed in the first 2 weeks: Take 2 tablets as soon as remembered or 2 tablets next 2 days. **An additional method of contraception should be used for 7 days after missed dose.**

Two consecutive doses missed in week 3 or three consecutive doses missed at any time: **An**

additional method of contraception must be used for 7 days after a missed dose.

Day 1 starter: Current pack should be discarded, and a new pack should be started that same day.

Sunday starter: Continue dose of 1 tablet daily until Sunday, then discard the rest of the pack, and a new pack should be started that same day.

Any number of doses missed in week 4: Continue taking one pill each day until pack is empty; no back-up method of contraception is needed

Pediatrics: Female: Contraception: Oral: Refer to adult dosing; not to be used prior to menarche.

Renal Impairment: Contraindicated in patients with renal dysfunction (Cl$_{cr}$ ≤50 mL/minute).

Hepatic Impairment: Contraindicated in patients with hepatic dysfunction.

Administration
Oral: To be taken at the same time each day, either after the evening meal or at bedtime

Stability
Storage: Store at 25°C (77°F).

Nursing Actions
Physical Assessment: Monitor or teach patient to monitor blood pressure on a regular (monthly) basis, and the importance of annual physical examinations (including Pap smear and vision exam). Assess knowledge/teach patient the importance of maintaining prescribed schedule of dosing, possible side effects, appropriate interventions, and adverse reactions to report. **Pregnancy risk factor X:** Determine patient is not pregnant prior to prescribing.

Patient Education: Take exactly as directed by prescriber (see package insert). An additional form of contraception should be used until after the first 7 consecutive days of administration. You are at risk of becoming pregnant if doses are missed. If you miss a dose, take as soon as possible or double the dose the next day. If two or more consecutive doses are missed, contact prescriber for restarting directions. Detailed and complete information on dosing and missed doses can be found in the package insert. If any number of doses are missed in week 4, continue taking one pill each day until pack is empty; no back-up method of contraception is needed. Be aware that some medications may reduce the effectiveness of oral contraceptives; an alternate form of contraception may be needed (see Drug Interactions). It is important that you check your blood pressure monthly (on same day each month) and report any increased blood pressure to prescriber. Have an annual physical assessment, Pap smear, and vision exam while taking this medication. Avoid smoking while taking this medication; smoking increases risk of adverse effects, including thromboembolic events and heart attacks. You may experience loss of appetite (small frequent meals may help); or constipation (increased exercise, fluids, fruit, fiber, or stool softeners may help). If you have diabetes, you should use accurate serum glucose testing to identify any changes in glucose tolerance; notify prescriber of significant changes so antidiabetic medication can be adjusted if necessary. Report immediately pain or muscle soreness; warmth, swelling, pain, or redness in calves; shortness of breath; sudden loss of vision; unresolved leg/foot swelling or weight gain (>5 lb); change in menstrual pattern (unusual bleeding, amenorrhea, breakthrough spotting); breast tenderness that does not go away; acute abdominal cramping; signs of vaginal infection (drainage, pain, itching); CNS changes (blurred vision, confusion, acute anxiety, or unresolved depression); chest pain; severe headache or vomiting; severe abdominal pain or tenderness; weakness in arm or leg; jaundice; or other persistent adverse effects. **Pregnancy/breast-feeding precautions:** Inform prescriber if you are pregnant. Breast-feeding is not recommended.

Breast-Feeding Issues The amount of drospirenone excreted in breast milk is ~0.02%, resulting in a maximum of ~3 mcg/day drospirenone to the infant. Jaundice and breast enlargement in the nursing infant have been reported following the use of other oral contraceptives. In addition, may decrease the quality and quantity of breast milk. Other forms of contraception are recommended while breast-feeding.

Pregnancy Issues In general, the use of oral contraceptives when inadvertently taken early in pregnancy have not been associated with teratogenic effects. Esophageal atresia was reported in one infant with a single-cycle exposure to ethinyl estradiol and drospirenone *in utero* (association not known). Pregnancy should be ruled out prior to treatment and discontinued if pregnancy occurs. Due to increased risk of thromboembolism postpartum, do not start oral contraceptives earlier than 4-6 weeks following delivery.

Additional Information The World Health Organization (WHO) has issued revised management recommendations for missed combined oral contraceptive pills. Refer to the following reference for a complete presentation and discussion of the guidelines:

Faculty of Family Planning and Reproductive Health Care Clinical Effectiveness Unit, "Faculty Statement from the CEU on a New Publication: WHO Selected Practice Recommendations for Contraceptive Use Update. Missed Pills: New Recommendations," *J Fam Plann Reprod Health Care*, 2005, 31(2):153-5.

Ethinyl Estradiol and Ethynodiol Diacetate
(ETH in il es tra DYE ole & e thye noe DYE ole dye AS e tate)

U.S. Brand Names Demulen®; Kelnor™; Zovia™

Synonyms Ethynodiol Diacetate and Ethinyl Estradiol

Pharmacologic Category Contraceptive; Estrogen and Progestin Combination

Medication Safety Issues
Sound-alike/look-alike issues:
Demulen® may be confused with Dalmane®, Demerol®

Pregnancy Risk Factor X

Lactation Enters breast milk/not recommended (AAP rates "compatible")

Use Prevention of pregnancy

Unlabeled/Investigational Use Treatment of hypermenorrhea (menorrhagia); pain associated with endometriosis; dysmenorrhea; dysfunctional uterine bleeding

Mechanism of Action/Effect Combination hormonal contraceptives inhibit ovulation and also produce changes in the cervical mucus and endometrium creating an unfavorable environment for sperm penetration and nidation.

Contraindications Hypersensitivity to ethinyl estradiol, ethynodiol diacetate, or any component of the formulation; history of or current thrombophlebitis or venous thromboembolic disorders (including DVT, PE); active or recent (within 1 year) arterial thromboembolic disease (eg, stroke, MI); cerebral vascular disease, coronary artery disease, valvular heart disease with complications, severe hypertension; diabetes mellitus with vascular involvement; severe headache with focal neurological symptoms; known or suspected breast carcinoma, endometrial cancer, estrogen-dependent neoplasms, undiagnosed abnormal genital bleeding; hepatic dysfunction or tumor, cholestatic jaundice of pregnancy, jaundice with prior combination hormonal (Continued)

Ethinyl Estradiol and Ethynodiol Diacetate *(Continued)*

contraceptive use; major surgery with prolonged immobilization; heavy smoking (≥15 cigarettes/day) in patients >35 years of age; pregnancy

Warnings/Precautions Combination hormonal contraceptives do not protect against HIV infection or other sexually-transmitted diseases. The risk of cardiovascular side effects increases in women who smoke cigarettes, especially those who are >35 years of age; women who use combination hormonal contraceptives should be strongly advised not to smoke. Combination hormonal contraceptives may lead to increased risk of myocardial infarction, use with caution in patients with risk factors for coronary artery disease. May increase the risk of thromboembolism. Whenever possible, combination hormonal contraceptives should be discontinued at least 4 weeks prior to and for 2 weeks following elective surgery associated with an increased risk of thromboembolism or during periods of prolonged immobilization. Combination hormonal contraceptives may have a dose-related risk of vascular disease, hypertension, and gallbladder disease. Women with hypertension or renal disease should be encouraged to use a nonhormonal form of contraception. The use of combination hormonal contraceptives has been associated with a slight increase in frequency of breast cancer, however, studies are not consistent. Combination hormonal contraceptives may cause glucose intolerance. Retinal thrombosis has been reported (rarely). Use caution with conditions that may be aggravated by fluid retention, depression, or history of migraine. Not for use prior to menarche.

The minimum dosage combination of estrogen/progestin that will effectively treat the individual patient should be used. New patients should be started on products containing ≤0.035 mg of estrogen per tablet.

Drug Interactions
Cytochrome P450 Effect: Ethinyl estradiol: **Substrate** of CYP2C8/9 (minor), 3A4 (major), 3A5-7 (minor); **Inhibits** CYP1A2 (weak), 2B6 (weak), 2C19 (weak), 3A4 (weak)

Decreased Effect: CYP3A4 inducers may decrease the levels/effects of ethinyl estradiol; example inducers include aminoglutethimide, carbamazepine, nafcillin, nevirapine, phenobarbital, phenytoin, and rifamycins. Combination hormonal contraceptives may decrease plasma levels of acetaminophen, clofibric acid, lorazepam, morphine, oxazepam, salicylic acid, temazepam. Contraceptive effect decreased by acitretin, aminoglutethimide, amprenavir, anticonvulsants, griseofulvin, lopinavir, nelfinavir, penicillins (effect not consistent), rifampin, ritonavir, tetracyclines (effect not consistent). Combination hormonal contraceptives may decrease (or increase) the effects of coumarin derivatives.

Increased Effect/Toxicity: Acetaminophen and ascorbic acid may increase plasma levels of estrogen component. Atorvastatin and indinavir increase plasma levels of combination hormonal contraceptives. Combination hormonal contraceptives increase the plasma levels of alprazolam, chlordiazepoxide, cyclosporine, diazepam, prednisolone, selegiline, theophylline, tricyclic antidepressants. Combination hormonal contraceptives may increase (or decrease) the effects of coumarin derivatives.

Nutritional/Ethanol Interactions
Food: CNS effects of caffeine may be enhanced if combination hormonal contraceptives are used concurrently with caffeine. Grapefruit juice increases ethinyl estradiol concentrations and would be expected to increase progesterone serum levels as well; clinical implications are unclear.

Herb/Nutraceutical: St John's wort may decrease the effectiveness of combination hormonal contraceptives by inducing hepatic enzymes. Avoid dong quai and black cohosh (have estrogen activity). Avoid saw palmetto, red clover, ginseng.

Lab Interactions Increased platelet aggregation, thyroid-binding globulin, total thyroid hormone (T_4), serum triglycerides/phospholipids; decreased antithrombin III, serum folate concentration

Adverse Reactions Frequency not defined.
Cardiovascular: Arterial thromboembolism, cerebral hemorrhage, cerebral thrombosis, edema, hypertension, mesenteric thrombosis, MI

Central nervous system: Depression, dizziness, headache, migraine, nervousness, premenstrual syndrome, stroke

Dermatologic: Acne, erythema multiforme, erythema nodosum, hirsutism, loss of scalp hair, melasma (may persist), rash (allergic)

Endocrine & metabolic: Amenorrhea, breakthrough bleeding, breast enlargement, breast secretion, breast tenderness, carbohydrate intolerance, lactation decreased (postpartum), glucose tolerance decreased, libido changes, menstrual flow changes, sex hormone-binding globulins (SHBG) increased, spotting, temporary infertility (following discontinuation), thyroid-binding globulin increased, triglycerides increased

Gastrointestinal: Abdominal cramps, appetite changes, bloating, cholestasis, colitis, gallbladder disease, jaundice, nausea, vomiting, weight gain/loss

Genitourinary: Cervical erosion changes, cervical secretion changes, cystitis-like syndrome, vaginal candidiasis, vaginitis

Hematologic: Antithrombin III decreased, folate levels decreased, hemolytic uremic syndrome, norepinephrine induced platelet aggregability increased, porphyria, prothrombin increased; factors VII, VIII, IX, and X increased

Hepatic: Benign liver tumors, Budd-Chiari syndrome, cholestatic jaundice, hepatic adenomas

Local: Thrombophlebitis

Ocular: Cataracts, change in corneal curvature (steepening), contact lens intolerance, optic neuritis, retinal thrombosis

Renal: Impaired renal function

Respiratory: Pulmonary thromboembolism

Miscellaneous: Hemorrhagic eruption

Overdosage/Toxicology Toxicity is unlikely following single exposures of excessive doses. May cause withdrawal bleeding in females. Any treatment following emesis and charcoal administration should be supportive and symptomatic.

Pharmacodynamics/Kinetics
Half-Life Elimination:
Ethynodiol diacetate (converted to norethindrone) Terminal: 5-14 hours

Metabolism:
Ethynodiol diacetate (converted to norethindrone): Hepatic conjugation

Available Dosage Forms
Tablet, monophasic formulations:
Demulen® 1/35-28: Ethinyl estradiol 0.035 mg and ethynodiol diacetate 1 mg [21 white tablets and 7 blue inactive tablets] (28s)

Kelnor™ 1/35: Ethinyl estradiol 0.035 mg and ethynodiol diacetate 1 mg [21 light yellow tablets and 7 white inactive tablets] (28s)

Zovia™ 1/35-28: Ethinyl estradiol 0.035 mg and ethynodiol diacetate 1 mg [21 light pink tablets and 7 white inactive tablets] (28s)

Zovia™ 1/50-28: Ethinyl estradiol 0.05 mg and ethynodiol diacetate 1 mg [21 pink tablets and 7 white inactive tablets] (28s)

Dosing

Adults:

Female: Contraception: Oral:

Schedule 1 (Sunday starter): Dose begins on first Sunday after onset of menstruation; if the menstrual period starts on Sunday, take first tablet that very same day. **With a Sunday start, an additional method of contraception should be used until after the first 7 days of consecutive administration:**

For 21-tablet package: 1 tablet/day for 21 consecutive days, followed by 7 days off of the medication; a new course begins on the 8th day after the last tablet is taken

For 28-tablet package: 1 tablet/day without interruption

Schedule 2 (Day-1 starter): Dose starts on first day of menstrual cycle taking 1 tablet/day:

For 21-tablet package: 1 tablet/day for 21 consecutive days, followed by 7 days off of the medication; a new course begins on the 8th day after the last tablet is taken

For 28-tablet package: 1 tablet/day without interruption

If all doses have been taken on schedule and one menstrual period is missed, continue dosing cycle. If two consecutive menstrual periods are missed, pregnancy test is required before new dosing cycle is started.

Missed doses **monophasic formulations** (refer to package insert for complete information):

One dose missed: Take as soon as remembered or take 2 tablets next day

Two consecutive doses missed in the first 2 weeks: Take 2 tablets as soon as remembered or 2 tablets next 2 days. **An additional method of contraception should be used for 7 days after missed dose.**

Two consecutive doses missed in week 3 or three consecutive doses missed at any time: **An additional method of contraception must be used for 7 days after a missed dose:**

Schedule 1 (Sunday starter): Continue dose of 1 tablet daily until Sunday, then discard the rest of the pack, and a new pack should be started that same day.

Schedule 2 (Day-1 starter): Current pack should be discarded, and a new pack should be started that same day.

Pediatrics: Female: Contraception: Oral: Refer to adult dosing; not to be used prior to menarche.

Renal Impairment: Specific guidelines not available; use with caution and monitor blood pressure closely. Consider other forms of contraception.

Hepatic Impairment: Contraindicated in patients with hepatic impairment.

Administration

Oral: Administer at the same time each day.

Stability

Storage: Store at controlled room temperature of 25°C (77°F).

Nursing Actions

Physical Assessment: Monitor or teach patient to monitor blood pressure on a regular basis. Monitor or teach patient to monitor for occurrence of adverse effects and symptoms to report (eg, thromboembolic disease, visual changes, neuromuscular weakness). Assess knowledge/teach importance of regular (monthly) blood pressure checks and annual physical assessment, Pap smear, and vision assessment. Teach importance of maintaining prescribed schedule

of dosing. **Pregnancy risk factor X:** Do not use if patient is pregnant.

Patient Education: Oral contraceptives do not protect against HIV or other sexually-transmitted diseases. Take exactly as directed by prescriber (also see package insert). You are at risk of becoming pregnant if doses are missed. Detailed and complete information on dosing and missed doses can be found in the package insert. Be aware that some medications may reduce the effectiveness of oral contraceptives; an alternate form of contraception may be needed. Check all medicines (prescription and OTC), herbal, and alternative products with prescriber. It is important that you check your blood pressure monthly (on same day each month) and that you have an annual physical assessment, Pap smear, and vision assessment while taking this medication. Avoid smoking while taking this medication; smoking increases risk of adverse effects, including thromboembolic events and heart attacks. You may experience loss of appetite (small frequent meals will help); or constipation (increased exercise, fluids, fruit, fiber, or stool softeners may help). If you have diabetes, use accurate serum glucose testing to identify any changes in glucose tolerance; notify prescriber of significant changes so antidiabetic medication can be adjusted if necessary. Report immediately pain or muscle soreness; warmth, swelling, pain, or redness in calves; shortness of breath; sudden loss of vision; unresolved leg/foot swelling; change in menstrual pattern (unusual bleeding, amenorrhea, breakthrough spotting); breast tenderness that does not go away; acute abdominal cramping; signs of vaginal infection (drainage, pain, itching); CNS changes (blurred vision, confusion, acute anxiety, or unresolved depression); chest pain; severe headache or vomiting; weakness in arm or leg; severe abdominal pain or tenderness; jaundice; or significant weight gain (>5 lb/week). Notify prescriber of changes in contact lens tolerance. **Pregnancy/breast-feeding precautions:** This medication should not be used during pregnancy. If you suspect you may become pregnant, contact prescriber immediately. Consult prescriber if breast-feeding.

Dietary Considerations Should be taken with food at same time each day.

Breast-Feeding Issues Jaundice and breast enlargement in the nursing infant have been reported following the use of combination hormonal contraceptives. May decrease the quality and quantity of breast milk; a nonhormonal form of contraception is recommended.

Pregnancy Issues Pregnancy should be ruled out prior to treatment and discontinued if pregnancy occurs. In general, the use of combination hormonal contraceptives when inadvertently taken early in pregnancy have not been associated with teratogenic effects. Due to increased risk of thromboembolism postpartum, combination hormonal contraceptives should not be started earlier than 4-6 weeks following delivery.

Additional Information The World Health Organization (WHO) has issued revised management recommendations for missed combined oral contraceptive pills. Refer to the following reference for a complete presentation and discussion of the guidelines:

Faculty of Family Planning and Reproductive Health Care Clinical Effectiveness Unit, "Faculty Statement from the CEU on a New Publication: WHO Selected Practice Recommendations for Contraceptive Use Update. Missed Pills: New Recommendations," *J Fam Plann Reprod Health Care*, 2005, 31(2):153-5.

Ethinyl Estradiol and Levonorgestrel
(ETH in il es tra DYE ole & LEE voe nor jes trel)

U.S. Brand Names Alesse®; Aviane™; Enpresse™; Lessina™; Levlen®; Levlite™; Levora®; Lutera™; Nordette®; Portia™; PREVEN®; Seasonale®; Tri-Levlen®; Triphasil®; Trivora®

Synonyms Levonorgestrel and Ethinyl Estradiol

Pharmacologic Category Contraceptive; Estrogen and Progestin Combination

Medication Safety Issues

Sound-alike/look-alike issues:

Alesse® may be confused with Aleve®

Nordette® may be confused with Nicorette®

PREVEN® may be confused with Prevnar®

Tri-Levlen® may be confused with Trilafon®

Triphasil® may be confused with Tri-Norinyl®

Pregnancy Risk Factor X

Lactation Enters breast milk/not recommended

Use Prevention of pregnancy; postcoital contraception

Unlabeled/Investigational Use Treatment of hypermenorrhea (menorrhagia); pain associated with endometriosis; dysmenorrhea; dysfunctional uterine bleeding

Mechanism of Action/Effect Combination oral contraceptives inhibit ovulation and also produce changes in the cervical mucus and endometrium creating an unfavorable environment for sperm penetration and nidation

Contraindications Hypersensitivity to ethinyl estradiol, levonorgestrel, or any component of the formulation; history of or current thrombophlebitis or venous thromboembolic disorders (including DVT, PE); active or recent (within 1 year) arterial thromboembolic disease (eg, stroke, MI); cerebral vascular disease, coronary artery disease, valvular heart disease with complications, severe hypertension; diabetes mellitus with vascular involvement; severe headache with focal neurological symptoms; known or suspected breast carcinoma, endometrial cancer, estrogen-dependent neoplasms, undiagnosed abnormal genital bleeding; hepatic dysfunction or tumor, cholestatic jaundice of pregnancy, jaundice with prior combination hormonal contraceptive use; major surgery with prolonged immobilization; heavy smoking (≥15 cigarettes/day) in patients >35 years of age; pregnancy

Warnings/Precautions Combination hormonal contraceptives do not protect against HIV infection or other sexually-transmitted diseases. The risk of cardiovascular side effects increases in women who smoke cigarettes, especially those who are >35 years of age; women who use combination hormonal contraceptives should be strongly advised not to smoke. Combination hormonal contraceptives may lead to increased risk of myocardial infarction, use with caution in patients with risk factors for coronary artery disease. May increase the risk of thromboembolism. Whenever possible, combination hormonal contraceptives should be discontinued at least 4 weeks prior to and for 2 weeks following elective surgery associated with an increased risk of thromboembolism or during periods of prolonged immobilization. Combination hormonal contraceptives may have a dose-related risk of vascular disease, hypertension, and gallbladder disease. Women with hypertension or renal disease should be encouraged to use another form of contraception. The use of combination hormonal contraceptives has been associated with a slight increase in frequency of breast cancer, however, studies are not consistent. Combination hormonal contraceptives may cause glucose intolerance. Retinal thrombosis has been reported (rarely). Use caution with conditions that may be aggravated by fluid retention, depression, or history of migraine. Not for use prior to menarche.

The minimum dosage combination of estrogen/progestin that will effectively treat the individual patient should be used. New patients should be started on products containing ≤0.035 mg of estrogen per tablet.

Drug Interactions

Cytochrome P450 Effect:

Ethinyl estradiol: **Substrate** of CYP2C8/9 (minor), 3A4 (major), 3A5-7 (minor); **Inhibits** CYP1A2 (weak), 2B6 (weak), 2C19 (weak), 3A4 (weak)

Levonorgestrel: **Substrate** of CYP3A4 (major)

Decreased Effect: CYP3A4 inducers may decrease the levels/effects of ethinyl estradiol and/or levonorgestrel; example inducers include aminoglutethimide, carbamazepine, nafcillin, nevirapine, phenobarbital, phenytoin, and rifamycins. Combination hormonal contraceptives may decrease plasma levels of acetaminophen, clofibric acid, lorazepam, morphine, oxazepam, salicylic acid, temazepam. Contraceptive effect decreased by acitretin, aminoglutethimide, amprenavir, anticonvulsants, griseofulvin, lopinavir, nelfinavir, penicillins (effect not consistent), rifampin, ritonavir, tetracyclines (effect not consistent). Combination hormonal contraceptives may decrease (or increase) the effects of coumarin derivatives.

Increased Effect/Toxicity: Acetaminophen and ascorbic acid may increase plasma levels of estrogen component. Atorvastatin and indinavir increase plasma levels of combination hormonal contraceptives. Combination hormonal contraceptives increase the plasma levels of alprazolam, chlordiazepoxide, cyclosporine, diazepam, prednisolone, selegiline, theophylline, tricyclic antidepressants. Combination hormonal contraceptives may increase (or decrease) the effects of coumarin derivatives.

Nutritional/Ethanol Interactions

Food: CNS effects of caffeine may be enhanced if combination hormonal contraceptives are used concurrently with caffeine. Grapefruit juice increases ethinyl estradiol concentrations and would be expected to increase progesterone serum levels as well; clinical implications are unclear.

Herb/Nutraceutical: St John's wort may decrease the effectiveness of combination hormonal contraceptives by inducing hepatic enzymes. Avoid dong quai and black cohosh (have estrogen activity). Avoid saw palmetto, red clover, ginseng.

Lab Interactions Increased prothrombin and factors VII, VIII, IX, X; increased platelet aggregability, thyroid-binding globulin, total thyroid hormone (T_4), serum triglycerides/phospholipids; decreased antithrombin III, serum folate concentration

Adverse Reactions Frequency not defined.

Cardiovascular: Arterial thromboembolism, cerebral hemorrhage, cerebral thrombosis, edema, hypertension, mesenteric thrombosis, MI

Central nervous system: Depression, dizziness, headache, migraine, nervousness, premenstrual syndrome, stroke

Dermatologic: Acne, erythema multiforme, erythema nodosum, hirsutism, loss of scalp hair, melasma (may persist), rash (allergic)

Endocrine & metabolic: Amenorrhea, breakthrough bleeding, breast enlargement, breast secretion, breast tenderness, carbohydrate intolerance, lactation decreased (postpartum), glucose tolerance decreased, libido changes, menstrual flow changes, sex hormone-binding globulins (SHBG) increased, spotting, temporary infertility (following discontinuation), thyroid-binding globulin increased, triglycerides increased

Gastrointestinal: Abdominal cramps, appetite changes, bloating, cholestasis, colitis, gallbladder disease, jaundice, nausea, vomiting, weight gain/loss

Genitourinary: Cervical erosion changes, cervical secretion changes, cystitis-like syndrome, vaginal candidiasis, vaginitis

Hematologic: Antithrombin III decreased, folate levels decreased, hemolytic uremic syndrome, norepinephrine induced platelet aggregability increased, porphyria, prothrombin increased; factors VII, VIII, IX, and X increased

Hepatic: Benign liver tumors, Budd-Chiari syndrome, cholestatic jaundice, hepatic adenomas

Local: Thrombophlebitis

Ocular: Cataracts, change in corneal curvature (steepening), contact lens intolerance, optic neuritis, retinal thrombosis

Renal: Impaired renal function

Respiratory: Pulmonary thromboembolism

Miscellaneous: Hemorrhagic eruption

Overdosage/Toxicology Toxicity is unlikely following single exposures of excessive doses. May cause withdrawal bleeding in females. Any treatment following emesis and charcoal administration should be supportive and symptomatic.

Pharmacokinetic Note See individual agents.

Available Dosage Forms

Tablet (PREVEN®): Ethinyl estradiol 0.05 mg and levonorgestrel 0.25 mg (4s) [also available as a kit containing 4 tablets and a pregnancy test]

Tablet, low-dose formulations:

Alesse® 28: Ethinyl estradiol 0.02 mg and levonorgestrel 0.1 mg [21 pink tablets and 7 light green inactive tablets] (28s)

Aviane™ 28: Ethinyl estradiol 0.02 mg and levonorgestrel 0.1 mg [21 orange tablets and 7 light green inactive tablets] (28s)

Lessina™ 28, Levlite™ 28: Ethinyl estradiol 0.02 mg and levonorgestrel 0.1 mg [21 pink tablets and 7 white inactive tablets] (28s)

Lutera™: Ethinyl estradiol 0.02 mg and levonorgestrel 0.1 mg [21 white tablets and 7 peach inactive tablets] (28s)

Tablet, monophasic formulations:

Levlen® 28: Ethinyl estradiol 0.03 mg and levonorgestrel 0.15 mg [21 light orange tablets and 7 pink inactive tablets] (28s)

Levora® 28: Ethinyl estradiol 0.03 mg and levonorgestrel 0.15 mg [21 white tablets and 7 peach inactive tablets] (28s)

Nordette® 21: Ethinyl estradiol 0.03 mg and levonorgestrel 0.15 mg [light orange tablets] (21s)

Nordette® 28: Ethinyl estradiol 0.03 mg and levonorgestrel 0.15 mg [21 light orange tablets and 7 pink inactive tablets] (28s)

Portia™ 28: Ethinyl estradiol 0.03 mg and levonorgestrel 0.15 mg [21 pink tablets and 7 white inactive tablets] (28s)

Seasonale®: Ethinyl estradiol 0.03 mg and levonorgestrel 0.15 mg [84 pink tablets and 7 white inactive tablets; extended cycle regimen]

Tablet, triphasic formulations:

Enpresse™:
Day 1-6: Ethinyl estradiol 0.03 mg and levonorgestrel 0.05 mg [6 pink tablets]
Day 7-11: Ethinyl estradiol 0.04 mg and levonorgestrel 0.075 mg [5 white tablets]
Day 12-21: Ethinyl estradiol 0.03 mg and levonorgestrel 0.125 mg [10 orange tablets]
Day 22-28: 7 light green inactive tablets (28s)

Tri-Levlen® 28, Triphasil® 28:
Day 1-6: Ethinyl estradiol 0.03 mg and levonorgestrel 0.05 mg [6 brown tablets]
Day 7-11: Ethinyl estradiol 0.04 mg and levonorgestrel 0.075 mg [5 white tablets]
Day 12-21: Ethinyl estradiol 0.03 mg and levonorgestrel 0.125 mg [10 light yellow tablets]
Day 22-28: 7 light green inactive tablets (28s)

Trivora®:
Day 1-6: Ethinyl estradiol 0.03 mg and levonorgestrel 0.05 mg [6 blue tablets]

Day 7-11: Ethinyl estradiol 0.04 mg and levonorgestrel 0.075 mg [5 white tablets]
Day 12-21: Ethinyl estradiol 0.03 mg and levonorgestrel 0.125 mg [10 pink tablets]
Day 22-28: 7 peach inactive tablets (28s)

Dosing

Adults: Female:

Contraception, 28-day cycle: Oral:

Schedule 1 (Sunday starter): Dose begins on first Sunday after onset of menstruation; if the menstrual period starts on Sunday, take first tablet that very same day. With a Sunday start, an additional method of contraception should be used until after the first 7 days of consecutive administration:

For 21-tablet package: 1 tablet/day for 21 consecutive days, followed by 7 days off of the medication; a new course begins on the 8th day after the last tablet is taken

For 28-tablet package: 1 tablet/day without interruption

Schedule 2 (Day-1 starter): Dose starts on first day of menstrual cycle taking 1 tablet/day:

For 21-tablet package: 1 tablet/day for 21 consecutive days, followed by 7 days off of the medication; a new course begins on the 8th day after the last tablet is taken

For 28-tablet package: 1 tablet/day without interruption

If all doses have been taken on schedule and one menstrual period is missed, continue dosing cycle. If two consecutive menstrual periods are missed, pregnancy test is required before new dosing cycle is started.

Missed doses **monophasic formulations** (refer to package insert for complete information):

One dose missed: Take as soon as remembered or take 2 tablets next day

Two consecutive doses missed in the first 2 weeks: Take 2 tablets as soon as remembered or 2 tablets next 2 days. An additional method of contraception should be used for 7 days after missed dose.

Two consecutive doses missed in week 3 or three consecutive doses missed at any time: An additional method of contraception must be used for 7 days after a missed dose:

Schedule 1 (Sunday starter): Continue dose of 1 tablet daily until Sunday, then discard the rest of the pack, and a new pack should be started that same day.

Schedule 2 (Day-1 starter): Current pack should be discarded, and a new pack should be started that same day.

Missed doses **biphasic/triphasic formulations** (refer to package insert for complete information):

One dose missed: Take as soon as remembered or take 2 tablets next day.

Two consecutive doses missed in week 1 or week 2 of the pack: Take 2 tablets as soon as remembered and 2 tablets the next day. Resume taking 1 tablet daily until the pack is empty. An additional method of contraception should be used for 7 days after a missed dose.

Two consecutive doses missed in week 3 of the pack: An additional method of contraception must be used for 7 days after a missed dose.

Schedule 1 (Sunday starter): Take 1 tablet every day until Sunday. Discard the remaining pack and start a new pack of pills on the same day.

Schedule 2 (Day-1 starter): Discard the remaining pack and start a new pack the same day.

Three or more consecutive doses missed: An additional method of contraception must be used for 7 days after a missed dose.

(Continued)

Ethinyl Estradiol and Levonorgestrel
(Continued)

Schedule 1 (Sunday starter): Take 1 tablet every day until Sunday; on Sunday, discard the pack and start a new pack.

Schedule 2 (Day-1 starter): Discard the remaining pack and begin new pack of tablets starting on the same day.

Contraception, 91-day cycle (Seasonale®): Oral: One active tablet/day for 84 consecutive days, followed by 1 inactive tablet/day for 7 days; if all doses have been taken on schedule and one menstrual period is missed, pregnancy should be ruled out prior to continuing therapy.

Missed doses:

One dose missed: Take as soon as remembered or take 2 tablets the next day

Two consecutive doses missed: Take 2 tablets as soon as remembered or 2 tablets the next 2 days. An additional nonhormonal method of contraception should be used for 7 consecutive days after the missed dose.

Three or more consecutive doses missed: Do not take the missed doses; continue taking 1 tablet/day until pack is complete. Bleeding may occur during the following week. An additional nonhormonal method of contraception should be used for 7 consecutive days after the missed dose.

Emergency contraception (PREVEN®): Oral: Initial: 2 tablets as soon as possible (but within 72 hours of unprotected intercourse), followed by a second dose of 2 tablets 12 hours later. Repeat dose or use antiemetic if vomiting occurs within 1 hour of dose.

Pediatrics: Female: Contraception or emergency contraception: Oral: Refer to adult dosing; not to be used prior to menarche.

Renal Impairment: Specific guidelines not available; use with caution and monitor blood pressure closely. Consider other forms of contraception.

Hepatic Impairment: Contraindicated in patients with hepatic impairment.

Administration

Oral: Administer at the same time each day.

Stability

Storage: Store at controlled room temperature of 25°C (77°F).

Nursing Actions

Physical Assessment: Monitor blood pressure on a regular basis. Assess for adverse reactions and potential drug interactions. Assess knowledge/teach importance of regular (monthly) blood pressure checks and annual physical assessment, Pap smear, and vision assessment. Teach importance of maintaining prescribed schedule of dosing (see Dosing for dosing and missed dose information). **Pregnancy risk factor X:** Do not use if patient is pregnant. Breast-feeding is not recommended.

Patient Education: Oral contraceptives do not protect against HIV or other sexually-transmitted diseases. Take exactly as directed by prescriber (also see package insert). You are at risk of becoming pregnant if doses are missed. Detailed and complete information on dosing and missed doses can be found in the package insert. Be aware that some medications may reduce the effectiveness of oral contraceptives; an alternate form of contraception may be needed. It is important that you check your blood pressure monthly (on same day each month) and that you have an annual physical assessment, Pap smear, and vision assessment while taking this medication. Avoid smoking while taking this medication; smoking increases risk of adverse effects, including thromboembolic events and heart attacks. You may experience loss of appetite (small frequent meals will help); or constipation (increased exercise, fluids, fruit, fiber, or stool softeners may help). If you have diabetes, use accurate serum glucose testing to identify any changes in glucose tolerance; notify prescriber of significant changes so antidiabetic medication can be adjusted if necessary. Report immediately pain or muscle soreness; warmth, swelling, pain, or redness in calves; shortness of breath; sudden loss of vision; unresolved leg/foot swelling; change in menstrual pattern (unusual bleeding, amenorrhea, breakthrough spotting); breast tenderness that does not go away; acute abdominal cramping; signs of vaginal infection (drainage, pain, itching); CNS changes (blurred vision, confusion, acute anxiety, or unresolved depression); chest pain; severe headache or vomiting; weakness in arm or leg; severe abdominal pain or tenderness; jaundice; or significant weight gain (>5 lb/week). Notify prescriber of changes in contact lens tolerance. **Pregnancy/breast-feeding precautions:** This medication should not be used during pregnancy. If you suspect you may become pregnant, contact prescriber immediately. Breast-feeding is not recommended.

Emergency contraceptive kit (PREVEN®) is **not** recommended for ongoing pregnancy protection or as a routine form of contraception. PREVEN® emergency contraceptive kit contains a pregnancy test. This test can be used to verify an existing pregnancy resulting from intercourse that occurred earlier in the concurrent menstrual cycle or the previous cycle. If a positive pregnancy result is obtained, the patient should **not** take the pills in the PREVEN® kit. The patient should be instructed that if she vomits within 1 hour of taking either dose of the medication, she should contact her healthcare professional to discuss whether to repeat that dose or to take an antiemetic.

Dietary Considerations Should be taken at the same time each day.

Breast-Feeding Issues Jaundice and breast enlargement in the nursing infant have been reported following the use of combination hormonal contraceptives. May decrease the quality and quantity of breast milk; alternative form of contraception is recommended.

Pregnancy Issues Pregnancy should be ruled out prior to treatment and discontinued if pregnancy occurs. In general, the use of combination hormonal contraceptives when inadvertently taken early in pregnancy have not been associated with teratogenic effects. Due to increased risk of thromboembolism postpartum, combination hormonal contraceptives should not be started earlier than 4-6 weeks following delivery.

Additional Information The World Health Organization (WHO) has issued revised management recommendations for missed combined oral contraceptive pills. Refer to the following reference for a complete presentation and discussion of the guidelines:

Faculty of Family Planning and Reproductive Health Care Clinical Effectiveness Unit, "Faculty Statement from the CEU on a New Publication: WHO Selected Practice Recommendations for Contraceptive Use Update. Missed Pills: New Recommendations," *J Fam Plann Reprod Health Care*, 2005, 31(2):153-5.

Related Information

Levonorgestrel *on page 730*

Ethinyl Estradiol and Norethindrone
(ETH in il es tra DYE ole & nor eth IN drone)

U.S. Brand Names Aranelle™; Brevicon®; Estrostep® Fe; femhrt®; Junel™; Junel™ Fe; Leena™; Loestrin®; Loestrin® 24 Fe; Loestrin® Fe; Microgestin™; Microgestin™ Fe; Modicon®; Necon® 0.5/35; Necon® 1/35; Necon® 7/7/7; Necon® 10/11; Norinyl® 1+35; Nortrel™; Nortrel™ 7/7/7; Ortho-Novum®; Ovcon®; Tri-Norinyl®

Synonyms Norethindrone Acetate and Ethinyl Estradiol; Ortho Novum

Pharmacologic Category Contraceptive; Estrogen and Progestin Combination

Medication Safety Issues
Sound-alike/look-alike issues:
femhrt® may be confused with Femara®
Modicon® may be confused with Mylicon®
Norinyl® may be confused with Nardil®
Tri-Norinyl® may be confused with Triphasil®

Pregnancy Risk Factor X

Lactation Enters breast milk/not recommended

Use Prevention of pregnancy; treatment of acne; moderate to severe vasomotor symptoms associated with menopause; prevention of osteoporosis (in women at significant risk only)

Unlabeled/Investigational Use Treatment of hypermenorrhea (menorrhagia); pain associated with endometriosis, dysmenorrhea; dysfunctional uterine bleeding

Mechanism of Action/Effect Combination oral contraceptives inhibit ovulation, and also produce changes in the cervical mucus and the endometrium, creating an unfavorable environment for sperm penetration and nidation. In postmenopausal women, exogenous estrogen is used to replace decreased endogenous production. The addition of progestin reduces the incidence of endometrial hyperplasia and risk of endometrial cancer in women with an intact uterus.

Contraindications Hypersensitivity to ethinyl estradiol, norethindrone, norethindrone acetate, or any component of the formulation; history of or current thrombophlebitis or venous thromboembolic disorders (including DVT, PE); active or recent (within 1 year) arterial thromboembolic disease (eg, stroke, MI); cerebral vascular disease, coronary artery disease, severe hypertension; diabetes mellitus with vascular involvement; severe headache with focal neurological symptoms; known or suspected breast carcinoma, endometrial cancer, estrogen-dependent neoplasms, undiagnosed abnormal genital bleeding; hepatic dysfunction or tumor, cholestatic jaundice of pregnancy, jaundice with prior combination hormonal contraceptive use; major surgery with prolonged immobilization; heavy smoking (≥15 cigarettes/day) in patients >35 years of age; pregnancy

Warnings/Precautions

Cardiovascular-related considerations: Use caution with cardiovascular disease or dysfunction. Combination estrogen/progestin therapy has been associated with an increased risk of cardiovascular disease, which may be dose related. May increase the risks of hypertension, myocardial infarction (MI), stroke, pulmonary emboli (PE), and deep vein thrombosis; incidence of these effects was shown to be significantly increased in postmenopausal women using conjugated equine estrogens (CEE) in combination with medroxyprogesterone acetate (MPA). Nonfatal MI, PE, and thrombophlebitis have also been reported in males taking high doses of CEE (eg, for prostate cancer). An increased risk of MI has been noted with use of combination hormonal contraceptives, primarily in women with underlying risk factors. The risk of cardiovascular events increases in women who smoke cigarettes, especially those who are >35 years of age; women who use combination hormonal contraceptives should be strongly advised not to smoke. Women with hypertension or renal disease should be encouraged to use another form of contraception. Estrogen compounds are generally associated with lipid effects such as increased HDL-cholesterol and decreased LDL-cholesterol. Triglycerides may also be increased; use with caution in patients with familial defects of lipoprotein metabolism. Estrogens with or without progestin should not be used to prevent coronary heart disease in postmenopausal women. Whenever possible, combination hormonal contraceptives should be discontinued at least 4 weeks prior to and for 2 weeks following elective surgery associated with an increased risk of thromboembolism or during periods of prolonged immobilization.

Cancer-related considerations: Estrogens may increase the risk of breast cancer. The use of combination hormonal contraceptives has been associated with a slight increase in frequency of breast cancer, however studies are not consistent. An increased risk of invasive breast cancer was observed in postmenopausal women using CEE in combination with MPA; a smaller increase in risk was seen with estrogen therapy alone in observational studies. An increase in abnormal mammograms has also been reported with estrogen and progestin therapy in postmenopausal women. Unopposed estrogens may increase the risk of endometrial carcinoma in postmenopausal women. Estrogens may exacerbate endometriosis. Malignant transformation of residual endometrial implants has been reported post-hysterectomy with estrogen only therapy. Consider adding a progestin in women with residual endometriosis post-hysterectomy. Estrogen use may lead to severe hypercalcemia in postmenopausal patients with breast cancer and bone metastases; discontinue estrogen if hypercalcemia occurs.

Use with caution in patients with diseases which may be exacerbated by fluid retention, including asthma, epilepsy, migraine, or diabetes. Use with caution in patients with a history of severe hypocalcemia, SLE, hepatic hemangiomas, porphyria, endometriosis, and gallbladder disease. Use caution with history of cholestatic jaundice associated with past estrogen use or pregnancy.

Estrogens may cause retinal vascular thrombosis. Discontinue pending examination in cases of sudden partial or complete vision loss, sudden onset of proptosis, diplopia, or migraine; discontinue permanently if papilledema or retinal vascular lesions are observed on examination.

Combination hormonal contraceptives do not protect against HIV infection or other sexually-transmitted diseases. The minimum dosage combination of estrogen/progestin that will effectively treat the individual patient should be used. New patients should be started on products containing ≤0.035 mg of estrogen per tablet. When used for acne, use only in females ≥15 years, who also desire combination hormonal contraceptive therapy, are unresponsive to topical treatments, and have no contraindications to combination hormonal contraceptive use. Not for use prior to menarche.

The risk of dementia may be increased in postmenopausal women; increased incidence was observed in women ≥65 years of age taking CEE alone or in combination with MPA. Before prescribing estrogen therapy to postmenopausal women, the risks and benefits must be weighed for each patient. Women should be informed of these risks and benefits, as well as possible effects of progestin when added to estrogen therapy. Estrogens with or without progestin should be used for shortest duration possible consistent with treatment goals. Conduct periodic risk:benefit assessments. When used solely for prevention of osteoporosis in women at significant risk, nonestrogen treatment options should be considered.
(Continued)

Ethinyl Estradiol and Norethindrone
(Continued)

Drug Interactions
Cytochrome P450 Effect:
Ethinyl estradiol: **Substrate** of CYP2C8/9 (minor), 3A4 (major), 3A5-7 (minor); **Inhibits** CYP1A2 (weak), 2B6 (weak), 2C19 (weak), 3A4 (weak)

Norethindrone: **Substrate** of CYP3A4 (major); Induces CYP2C19 (weak)

Decreased Effect: CYP3A4 inducers may decrease the levels/effects of ethinyl estradiol and norethindrone; example inducers include aminoglutethimide, carbamazepine, nafcillin, nevirapine, phenobarbital, phenytoin, and rifamycins. Combination hormonal contraceptives may decrease plasma levels of acetaminophen, clofibric acid, lorazepam, morphine, oxazepam, salicylic acid, temazepam. Contraceptive effect decreased by acitretin, aminoglutethimide, amprenavir, anticonvulsants, griseofulvin, lopinavir, nelfinavir, penicillins (effect not consistent), rifampin, ritonavir, tetracyclines (effect not consistent), troglitazone. Oral contraceptives may decrease (or increase) the effects of coumarin derivatives.

Increased Effect/Toxicity: Acetaminophen and ascorbic acid may increase plasma levels of estrogen component. Atorvastatin and indinavir increase plasma levels of combination hormonal contraceptives. Combination hormonal contraceptives increase the plasma levels of alprazolam, chlordiazepoxide, cyclosporine, diazepam, prednisolone, selegiline, theophylline, tricyclic antidepressants. Combination hormonal contraceptives may increase (or decrease) the effects of coumarin derivatives.

Nutritional/Ethanol Interactions
Ethanol: Routine use increases estrogen level and risk of breast cancer; avoid ethanol. Ethanol may also increase the risk of osteoporosis.

Food: CNS effects of caffeine may be enhanced if combination hormonal contraceptives are used concurrently with caffeine. Grapefruit juice increases ethinyl estradiol concentrations and would be expected to increase progesterone serum levels as well; clinical implications are unclear. Norethindrone absorption is increased by 27% following administration with food.

Herb/Nutraceutical: St John's wort may decrease the effectiveness of combination hormonal contraceptives by inducing hepatic enzymes. Avoid dong quai and black cohosh (have estrogen activity). Avoid saw palmetto, red clover, ginseng.

Lab Interactions
Increased prothrombin and factors VII, VIII, IX, X; increased platelet aggregability, thyroid-binding globulin, total thyroid hormone (T_4), serum triglycerides/phospholipids; decreased antithrombin III, serum folate concentration; pathologist should be advised of estrogen/progesterone therapy when specimens are submitted

Adverse Reactions
As reported with oral contraceptive agents. Frequency not defined.
Cardiovascular: Arterial thromboembolism, cerebral hemorrhage, cerebral thrombosis, edema, hypertension, mesenteric thrombosis, MI

Central nervous system: Depression, dizziness, headache, migraine, nervousness, premenstrual syndrome, stroke

Dermatologic: Acne, erythema multiforme, erythema nodosum, hirsutism, loss of scalp hair, melasma (may persist), rash (allergic)

Endocrine & metabolic: Amenorrhea, breakthrough bleeding, breast enlargement, breast secretion, breast tenderness, carbohydrate intolerance, lactation decreased (postpartum), glucose tolerance decreased, libido changes, menstrual flow changes, sex hormone-binding globulins (SHBG) increased, spotting, temporary infertility (following discontinuation), thyroid-binding globulin increased, triglycerides increased

Gastrointestinal: Abdominal cramps, appetite changes, bloating, cholestasis, colitis, gallbladder disease, jaundice, nausea, vomiting, weight gain/loss

Genitourinary: Cervical erosion changes, cervical secretion changes, cystitis-like syndrome, vaginal candidiasis, vaginitis

Hematologic: Antithrombin III decreased, folate levels decreased, hemolytic uremic syndrome, norepinephrine induced platelet aggregability increased, porphyria, prothrombin increased; factors VII, VIII, IX, and X

Hepatic: Benign liver tumors, Budd-Chiari syndrome, cholestatic jaundice, hepatic adenomas

Local: Thrombophlebitis

Ocular: Cataracts, change in corneal curvature (steepening), contact lens intolerance, optic neuritis, retinal thrombosis

Renal: Impaired renal function

Respiratory: Pulmonary thromboembolism

Miscellaneous: Hemorrhagic eruption

Overdosage/Toxicology Toxicity is unlikely following single exposures of excessive doses. May cause withdrawal bleeding in females. Any treatment following emesis and charcoal administration should be supportive and symptomatic.

Pharmacodynamics/Kinetics
Protein Binding: Ethinyl estradiol: >95% to albumin

Half-Life Elimination: Ethinyl estradiol: 19-24 hours

Metabolism: Ethinyl estradiol: Hepatic via oxidation and conjugation in GI tract; hydroxylated via CYP3A4 to metabolites; first-pass effect; enterohepatic recirculation; reversibly converted to estrone and estriol

Excretion: Ethinyl estradiol: Urine (as estradiol, estrone, and estriol); feces

Pharmacokinetic Note Norethindrone: See individual monograph.

Available Dosage Forms
Tablet (femhrt®):
1/5: Ethinyl estradiol 5 mcg and norethindrone acetate 1 mg [white tablets]
0.5/2.5: Ethinyl estradiol 2.5 mcg and norethindrone acetate 0.5 mg [white tablets]

Tablet, monophasic formulations:
Brevicon®: Ethinyl estradiol 0.035 mg and norethindrone 0.5 mg [21 blue tablets and 7 orange inactive tablets] (28s)
Junel™ 21 1/20: Ethinyl estradiol 0.02 mg and norethindrone acetate 1 mg [yellow tablets] (21s)
Junel™ 21 1.5/30: Ethinyl estradiol 0.03 mg and norethindrone acetate 1.5 mg [pink tablets] (21s)
Junel™ Fe 1/20: Ethinyl estradiol 0.02 mg and norethindrone acetate 1 mg [21 yellow tablets] and ferrous fumarate 75 mg [7 brown tablets] (28s)
Junel™ Fe 1.5/30: Ethinyl estradiol 0.03 mg and norethindrone acetate 1.5 mg [21 pink tablets] and ferrous fumarate 75 mg [7 brown tablets] (28s)
Loestrin® 21 1/20, Microgestin™ 1/20: Ethinyl estradiol 0.02 mg and norethindrone acetate 1 mg [white tablets] (21s)
Loestrin® 21 1.5/30, Microgestin™ 1.5/30: Ethinyl estradiol 0.03 mg and norethindrone acetate 1.5 mg [green tablets] (21s)
Loestrin® 24 Fe: 1/20: Ethinyl estradiol 0.02 mg and norethindrone acetate 1 mg [24 white tablets] and ferrous fumarate 75 mg [4 brown tablets] (28s)
Loestrin® Fe 1/20, Microgestin™ Fe 1/20: Ethinyl estradiol 0.02 mg and norethindrone acetate 1 mg [21 white tablets] and ferrous fumarate 75 mg [7 brown tablets] (28s)
Loestrin® Fe 1.5/30, Microgestin™ Fe 1.5/30: Ethinyl estradiol 0.03 mg and norethindrone acetate 1.5 mg [21 green tablets] and ferrous fumarate 75 mg [7 brown tablets] (28s)

Modicon® 28: Ethinyl estradiol 0.035 mg and norethindrone 0.5 mg [21 white tablets and 7 green inactive tablets] (28s)

Necon® 0.5/35-28: Ethinyl estradiol 0.035 mg and norethindrone 0.5 mg [21 light yellow tablets and 7 white inactive tablets] (28s)

Necon® 1/35-28: Ethinyl estradiol 0.035 mg and norethindrone 1 mg [21 dark yellow tablets and 7 white inactive tablets] (28s)

Norinyl® 1+35: Ethinyl estradiol 0.035 mg and norethindrone 1 mg [21 yellow-green tablets and 7 orange inactive tablets] (28s)

Nortrel™ 0.5/35 mg:
Ethinyl estradiol 0.035 mg and norethindrone 0.5 mg [light yellow tablets] (21s)
Ethinyl estradiol 0.035 mg and norethindrone 0.5 mg [21 light yellow tablets and 7 white inactive tablets] (28s)

Nortrel™ 1/35 mg:
Ethinyl estradiol 0.035 mg and norethindrone 1 mg [yellow tablets] (21s)
Ethinyl estradiol 0.035 mg and norethindrone 1 mg [21 yellow tablets and 7 white inactive tablets] (28s)

Ortho-Novum® 1/35 28: Ethinyl estradiol 0.035 mg and norethindrone 1 mg [21 peach tablets and 7 green inactive tablets] (28s)

Ovcon® 35 21-day: Ethinyl estradiol 0.035 mg and norethindrone 0.4 mg [peach tablets] (21s)

Ovcon® 35 28-day: Ethinyl estradiol 0.035 mg and norethindrone 0.4 mg [21 peach tablets and 7 green inactive tablets] (28s)

Ovcon® 50: Ethinyl estradiol 0.05 mg and norethindrone 1 mg [21 yellow tablets and 7 green inactive tablets] (28s)

Tablet, biphasic formulations:
Necon® 10/11-28:
Day 1-10: Ethinyl estradiol 0.035 mg and norethindrone 0.5 mg [10 light yellow tablets]
Day 11-21: Ethinyl estradiol 0.035 mg and norethindrone 1 mg [11 dark yellow tablets]
Day 22-28: 7 white inactive tablets (28s)

Ortho-Novum® 10/11-28:
Day 1-10: Ethinyl estradiol 0.035 mg and norethindrone 0.5 mg [10 white tablets]
Day 11-21: Ethinyl estradiol 0.035 mg and norethindrone 1 mg [11 peach tablets]
Day 22-28: 7 green inactive tablets (28s)

Tablet, triphasic formulations:
Aranelle™:
Day 1-7: Ethinyl estradiol 0.035 mg and norethindrone 0.5 mg [7 light yellow tablets]
Day 8-16: Ethinyl estradiol 0.035 mg and norethindrone 1 mg [9 white tablets]
Day 17-21: Ethinyl estradiol 0.035 mg and norethindrone 0.5 mg [5 light yellow tablets]
Day 22-28: 7 peach inactive tablets (28s)

Estrostep® Fe:
Day 1-5: Ethinyl estradiol 0.02 mg and norethindrone acetate 1 mg [5 white triangular tablets]
Day 6-12: Ethinyl estradiol 0.03 mg and norethindrone acetate 1 mg [7 white square tablets]
Day 13-21: Ethinyl estradiol 0.035 mg and norethindrone acetate 1 mg [9 white round tablets]
Day 22-28: Ferrous fumarate 75 mg [7 brown tablets] (28s)

Leena™:
Day 1-7: Ethinyl estradiol 0.035 mg and norethindrone 0.5 mg [7 light blue tablets]
Day 8-16: Ethinyl estradiol 0.035 mg and norethindrone 1 mg [9 light yellow-green tablets]
Day 17-21: Ethinyl estradiol 0.035 mg and norethindrone 0.5 mg [5 light blue tablets]
Day 22-28: 7 orange inactive tablets (28s)

Necon® 7/7/7, Ortho-Novum® 7/7/7 28:
Day 1-7: Ethinyl estradiol 0.035 mg and norethindrone 0.5 mg [7 white tablets]
Day 8-14: Ethinyl estradiol 0.035 mg and norethindrone 0.75 mg [7 light peach tablets]
Day 15-21: Ethinyl estradiol 0.035 mg and norethindrone 1 mg [7 peach tablets]
Day 22-28: 7 green inactive tablets (28s)

Nortrel™ 7/7/7 28:
Day 1-7: Ethinyl estradiol 0.035 mg and norethindrone 0.5 mg [7 light yellow tablets]
Day 8-14: Ethinyl estradiol 0.035 mg and norethindrone 0.75 mg [7 blue tablets]
Day 15-21: Ethinyl estradiol 0.035 mg and norethindrone 1 mg [7 peach tablets]
Day 22-28: 7 white inactive tablets (28s)

Ortho-Novum® 7/7/7 28:
Day 1-7: Ethinyl estradiol 0.035 mg and norethindrone 0.5 mg [7 white tablets]
Day 8-14: Ethinyl estradiol 0.035 mg and norethindrone 0.75 mg [7 light peach tablets]
Day 15-21: Ethinyl estradiol 0.035 mg and norethindrone 1 mg [7 peach tablets]
Day 22-28: 7 green inactive tablets (28s)

Tri-Norinyl® 28:
Day 1-7: Ethinyl estradiol 0.035 mg and norethindrone 0.5 mg [7 blue tablets]
Day 8-16: Ethinyl estradiol 0.035 mg and norethindrone 1 mg [9 yellow-green tablets]
Day 17-21: Ethinyl estradiol 0.035 mg and norethindrone 0.5 mg [5 blue tablets]
Day 22-28: 7 orange inactive tablets (28s)

Dosing
Adults:
Adolescents ≥15 years and Adults: Female: Acne: Estrostep®: Oral: Refer to dosing for contraception

Moderate-to-severe vasomotor symptoms associated with menopause: Initial: femhrt® 0.5/2.5: Oral: 1 tablet daily; patient should be re-evaluated at 3- to 6-month intervals to determine if treatment is still necessary; patient should be maintained on lowest effective dose

Prevention of osteoporosis: Initial: femhrt® 0.5/2.5: Oral: 1 tablet daily; patient should be maintained on lowest effective dose

Contraception: Oral:
Schedule 1 (Sunday starter): Dose begins on first Sunday after onset of menstruation; if the menstrual period starts on Sunday, take first tablet that very same day. With a Sunday start, an additional method of contraception should be used until after the first 7 days of consecutive administration.
For 21-tablet package: Dosage is 1 tablet daily for 21 consecutive days, followed by 7 days off of the medication; a new course begins on the 8th day after the last tablet is taken.
For 28-tablet package: Dosage is 1 tablet daily without interruption.
Schedule 2 (Day 1 starter): Dose starts on first day of menstrual cycle taking 1 tablet daily.
For 21-tablet package: Dosage is 1 tablet daily for 21 consecutive days, followed by 7 days off of the medication; a new course begins on the 8th day after the last tablet is taken.
For 28-tablet package: Dosage is 1 tablet daily without interruption.
If all doses have been taken on schedule and one menstrual period is missed, continue dosing cycle. If two consecutive menstrual periods are missed, pregnancy test is required before new dosing cycle is started.
Missed doses **monophasic formulations** (refer to package insert for complete information):
One dose missed: Take as soon as remembered or take 2 tablets next day Two consecutive doses missed in the first 2 weeks: Take 2

(Continued)

Ethinyl Estradiol and Norethindrone
(Continued)

tablets as soon as remembered or 2 tablets next 2 days. An additional method of contraception should be used for 7 days after missed dose.

Two consecutive doses missed in week 3 or three consecutive doses missed at any time: An additional method of contraception must be used for 7 days after a missed dose.

Schedule 1 (Sunday starter): Continue dose of 1 tablet daily until Sunday, then discard the rest of the pack, and a new pack should be started that same day.

Schedule 2 (Day 1 starter): Current pack should be discarded, and a new pack should be started that same day.

Missed doses **biphasic/triphasic formulations** (refer to package insert for complete information):

One dose missed: Take as soon as remembered or take 2 tablets next day.

Two consecutive doses missed in week 1 or week 2 of the pack: Take 2 tablets as soon as remembered and 2 tablets the next day. Resume taking 1 tablet daily until the pack is empty. An additional method of contraception should be used for 7 days after a missed dose.

Two consecutive doses missed in week 3 of the pack: An additional method of contraception must be used for 7 days after a missed dose.

Schedule 1 (Sunday Starter): Take 1 tablet every day until Sunday. Discard the remaining pack and start a new pack of pills on the same day.

Schedule 2 (Day 1 starter): Discard the remaining pack and start a new pack the same day.

Three or more consecutive doses missed: An additional method of contraception must be used for 7 days after a missed dose.

Schedule 1 (Sunday Starter): Take 1 tablet every day until Sunday; on Sunday, discard the pack and start a new pack.

Schedule 2 (Day 1 Starter): Discard the remaining pack and begin new pack of tablets starting on the same day.

Pediatrics: Female:

Acne: Oral (Estrostep®): For use in females ≥15 years; refer to adult dosing for contraception

Contraception: Oral: Refer to adult dosing; not to be used prior to menarche.

Renal Impairment: Specific guidelines not available; use with caution and monitor blood pressure closely. Consider other forms of contraception.

Hepatic Impairment: Contraindicated in patients with hepatic impairment.

Administration

Oral: Administer at the same time each day.

Stability

Storage: Store at controlled room temperature of 25°C (77°F).

Estrostep®: Protect from light.

Nursing Actions

Physical Assessment: Assess other medications patient may be taking for effectiveness and interactions. Teach patient importance of monthly blood pressure checks, annual physical assessment, Pap smear, vision assessment; and appropriate use (eg, maintaining prescribed schedule of dosing; see Dosing for dosing and missed dose information), and adverse symptoms to report. **Pregnancy risk factor X:** Do not use if patient is pregnant. Breast-feeding is not recommended.

Patient Education: Oral contraceptives do not protect against HIV infection or other sexually-transmitted diseases. Take exactly as directed by prescriber (detailed and complete information on dosing and missed doses can also be found in the package insert). You are at risk of becoming pregnant if doses are missed. Do not take any new medication during therapy without consulting prescriber. Avoid ethanol (routine use increases estrogen level and risk of breast cancer; may also increase risk of osteoporosis). Avoid smoking while taking this medication; smoking increases risk of adverse effects, including thromboembolic events and heart attacks. If you have diabetes, use accurate serum glucose testing to identify any changes in glucose tolerance (notify prescriber of significant changes). It is important that you check your blood pressure on the same day of each month (notify prescriber of significant changes) and that you have an annual physical assessment, Pap smear, and vision assessment while taking this medication. May cause loss of appetite (small frequent meals will help); or constipation (increased exercise, fluids, fruit, fiber, or stool softeners may help). Report immediately pain or muscle soreness; warmth, swelling, pain, or redness in calves; shortness of breath; sudden loss of vision; unresolved leg/foot swelling; change in menstrual pattern (unusual bleeding, amenorrhea, breakthrough spotting); breast tenderness that does not go away; acute abdominal cramping; signs of vaginal infection (drainage, pain, itching); CNS changes (blurred vision, confusion, acute anxiety, or unresolved depression); chest pain; severe headache or vomiting; weakness in arm or leg; severe abdominal pain or tenderness; jaundice; or significant weight gain (>5 lb/week). Notify prescriber of changes in contact lens tolerance. **Pregnancy/breast-feeding precautions:** This medication should not be used during pregnancy. Consult prescriber for appropriate form of contraception. If you suspect you may become pregnant, contact prescriber immediately. Breast-feeding is not recommended.

Dietary Considerations Should be taken at same time each day. May be taken with or without food. Ensure adequate calcium and vitamin D intake when used for the prevention of osteoporosis.

Breast-Feeding Issues Jaundice and breast enlargement in the nursing infant have been reported following the use of combination hormonal contraceptives. May decrease the quality and quantity of breast milk; alternative form of contraception is recommended.

Pregnancy Issues Pregnancy should be ruled out prior to treatment and discontinued if pregnancy occurs. In general, the use of combination hormonal contraceptives when inadvertently taken early in pregnancy have not been associated with teratogenic effects. Due to increased risk of thromboembolism postpartum, combination hormonal contraceptives should not be started earlier than 4-6 weeks following delivery.

Additional Information Norethindrone acetate 1 mg is equivalent to ethinyl estradiol 2.8 mcg.

The World Health Organization (WHO) has issued revised management recommendations for missed combined oral contraceptive pills. Refer to the following reference for a complete presentation and discussion of the guidelines:

Faculty of Family Planning and Reproductive Health Care Clinical Effectiveness Unit, "Faculty Statement from the CEU on a New Publication: WHO Selected Practice Recommendations for Contraceptive Use Update. Missed Pills: New Recommendations," *J Fam Plann Reprod Health Care*, 2005, 31(2):153-5.

Related Information

Norethindrone *on page 896*

Ethinyl Estradiol and Norgestimate
(ETH in il es tra DYE ole & nor JES ti mate)

U.S. Brand Names MonoNessa™; Ortho-Cyclen®; Ortho Tri-Cyclen®; Ortho Tri-Cyclen® Lo; Previfem™; Sprintec™; TriNessa™; Tri-Previfem™; Tri-Sprintec™

Synonyms Ethinyl Estradiol and NGM; Norgestimate and Ethinyl Estradiol; Ortho Cyclen; Ortho Tri Cyclen

Pharmacologic Category Contraceptive; Estrogen and Progestin Combination

Medication Safety Issues
Sound-alike/look-alike issues:
Ortho-Cyclen® may be confused with Ortho-Cept®

Pregnancy Risk Factor X

Lactation Enters breast milk/not recommended (AAP rates "compatible")

Use Prevention of pregnancy; treatment of acne

Unlabeled/Investigational Use Treatment of hypermenorrhea (menorrhagia); pain associated with endometriosis; dysmenorrhea; dysfunctional uterine bleeding

Mechanism of Action/Effect Combination hormonal contraceptives inhibit ovulation and also produce changes in the cervical mucus and endometrium creating an unfavorable environment for sperm penetration and nidation.

Contraindications Hypersensitivity to ethinyl estradiol, norgestimate, or any component of the formulation; history of or current thrombophlebitis or venous thromboembolic disorders (including DVT, PE); active or recent (within 1 year) arterial thromboembolic disease (eg, stroke, MI); cerebral vascular disease, coronary artery disease, valvular heart disease with complications, severe hypertension; severe headache with focal neurological symptoms; known or suspected breast carcinoma, endometrial cancer, estrogen-dependent neoplasms, undiagnosed abnormal genital bleeding; hepatic dysfunction or tumor, cholestatic jaundice of pregnancy, jaundice with prior combination hormonal contraceptive use; heavy smoking (≥15 cigarettes/day) in patients >35 years of age; pregnancy

Warnings/Precautions Combination hormonal contraceptives do not protect against HIV infection or other sexually-transmitted diseases. The risk of cardiovascular side effects increases in women who smoke cigarettes, especially those who are >35 years of age; women who use combination hormonal contraceptives should be strongly advised not to smoke. Combination hormonal contraceptives may lead to increased risk of myocardial infarction, use with caution in patients with risk factors for coronary artery disease. May increase the risk of thromboembolism. Whenever possible, combination hormonal contraceptives should be discontinued at least 4 weeks prior to and for 2 weeks following elective surgery associated with an increased risk of thromboembolism or during periods of prolonged immobilization. Combination hormonal contraceptives may have a dose-related risk of vascular disease, hypertension, and gallbladder disease. Women with hypertension or renal disease should be encouraged to use a nonhormonal form of contraception. The use of combination hormonal contraceptives has been associated with a slight increase in frequency of breast cancer, however, studies are not consistent. Combination hormonal contraceptives may cause glucose intolerance. Retinal thrombosis has been reported (rarely). Use caution with conditions that may be aggravated by fluid retention, depression, or history of migraine. Not for use prior to menarche.

The minimum dosage combination of estrogen/progestin that will effectively treat the individual patient should be used. New patients should be started on products containing ≤0.035 mg of estrogen per tablet.

Acne: For use only in females ≥15 years, who also desire combination hormonal contraceptive therapy, are unresponsive to topical treatments, and have no contraindications to combination hormonal contraceptive use.

Drug Interactions

Cytochrome P450 Effect: Ethinyl estradiol: **Substrate** of CYP2C8/9 (minor), 3A4 (major), 3A5-7 (minor); **Inhibits** CYP1A2 (weak), 2B6 (weak), 2C19 (weak), 3A4 (weak)

Decreased Effect: CYP3A4 inducers may decrease the levels/effects of ethinyl estradiol; example inducers include aminoglutethimide, carbamazepine, nafcillin, nevirapine, phenobarbital, phenytoin, and rifamycins. Combination hormonal contraceptives may decrease plasma levels of acetaminophen, clofibric acid, lorazepam, morphine, oxazepam, salicylic acid, temazepam. Contraceptive effect decreased by acitretin, aminoglutethimide, amprenavir, anticonvulsants, griseofulvin, lopinavir, nelfinavir, nevirapine, penicillins (effect not consistent), rifampin, ritonavir, tetracyclines (effect not consistent). Combination hormonal contraceptives may decrease (or increase) the effects of coumarin derivatives.

Increased Effect/Toxicity: Acetaminophen and ascorbic acid may increase plasma levels of estrogen component. Atorvastatin and indinavir increase plasma levels of combination hormonal contraceptives. Combination hormonal contraceptives increase the plasma levels of alprazolam, chlordiazepoxide, cyclosporine, diazepam, prednisolone, selegiline, theophylline, tricyclic antidepressants. Combination hormonal contraceptives may increase (or decrease) the effects of coumarin derivatives.

Nutritional/Ethanol Interactions

Food: CNS effects of caffeine may be enhanced if combination hormonal contraceptives are used concurrently with caffeine. Grapefruit juice increases ethinyl estradiol concentrations and would be expected to increase progesterone serum levels as well; clinical implications are unclear.

Herb/Nutraceutical: St John's wort may decrease the effectiveness of combination hormonal contraceptives by inducing hepatic enzymes. Avoid dong quai and black cohosh (have estrogen activity). Avoid saw palmetto, red clover, ginseng.

Lab Interactions Increased amylase (S), cholesterol (S), iron (B), sodium (S), thyroxine (S); decreased calcium (S), protein, prothrombin time

Adverse Reactions Frequency not defined.

Cardiovascular: Arterial thromboembolism, cerebral hemorrhage, cerebral thrombosis, edema, hypertension, mesenteric thrombosis, MI

Central nervous system: Depression, dizziness, headache, migraine, nervousness, premenstrual syndrome, stroke

Dermatologic: Acne, erythema multiforme, erythema nodosum, hirsutism, loss of scalp hair, melasma (may persist), rash (allergic)

Endocrine & metabolic: Amenorrhea, breakthrough bleeding, breast enlargement, breast secretion, breast tenderness, carbohydrate intolerance, lactation decreased (postpartum), glucose tolerance decreased, libido changes, menstrual flow changes, sex hormone-binding globulins (SHBG) increased, spotting, temporary infertility (following discontinuation), thyroid-binding globulin increased, triglycerides increased

Gastrointestinal: Abdominal cramps, appetite changes, bloating, cholestasis, colitis, gallbladder disease, jaundice, nausea, vomiting, weight gain/loss

Genitourinary: Cervical erosion changes, cervical secretion changes, cystitis-like syndrome, vaginal candidiasis, vaginitis

Hematologic: Antithrombin III decreased, folate levels decreased, hemolytic uremic syndrome, norepinephrine induced platelet aggregability increased, (Continued)

Ethinyl Estradiol and Norgestimate
(Continued)

porphyria, prothrombin increased; factors VII, VIII, IX, and X increased

Hepatic: Benign liver tumors, Budd-Chiari syndrome, cholestatic jaundice, hepatic adenomas

Local: Thrombophlebitis

Ocular: Cataracts, change in corneal curvature (steepening), contact lens intolerance, optic neuritis, retinal thrombosis

Renal: Impaired renal function

Respiratory: Pulmonary thromboembolism

Miscellaneous: Hemorrhagic eruption

Overdosage/Toxicology Toxicity is unlikely following single exposures of excessive doses. May cause withdrawal bleeding in females. Any treatment following emesis and charcoal administration should be supportive and symptomatic.

Pharmacodynamics/Kinetics

Protein Binding:
Norgestimate: To albumin and sex hormone-binding globulin (SHBG); SHBG capacity is affected by plasma ethinyl estradiol levels

Half-Life Elimination:
Norgestimate: 17-deacetylnorgestimate: 12-30 hours

Metabolism:
Norgestimate: Hepatic; forms 17-deacetylnorgestimate (major active metabolite) and other metabolites

Excretion:
Norgestimate: Urine and feces

Available Dosage Forms

Tablet, monophasic formulations:

MonoNessa™, Ortho-Cyclen®: Ethinyl estradiol 0.035 mg and norgestimate 0.25 mg [21 blue tablets and 7 green inactive tablets] (28s)

Previfem™: Ethinyl estradiol 0.035 mg and norgestimate 0.25 mg [21 blue tablets and 7 teal inactive tablets] (28s)

Sprintec™: Ethinyl estradiol 0.035 mg and norgestimate 0.25 mg [21 blue tablets and 7 white inactive tablets] (28s)

Tablet, triphasic formulations:

Ortho Tri-Cyclen®, TriNessa™:
Day 1-7: Ethinyl estradiol 0.035 mg and norgestimate 0.18 mg [7 white tablets]
Day 8-14: Ethinyl estradiol 0.035 mg and norgestimate 0.215 mg [7 light blue tablets]
Day 15-21: Ethinyl estradiol 0.035 mg and norgestimate 0.25 mg [7 blue tablets]
Day 22-28: 7 green inactive tablets (28s)

Tri-Previfem™:
Day 1-7: Ethinyl estradiol 0.035 mg and norgestimate 0.18 mg [7 white tablets]
Day 8-14: Ethinyl estradiol 0.035 mg and norgestimate 0.215 mg [7 light blue tablets]
Day 15-21: Ethinyl estradiol 0.035 mg and norgestimate 0.25 mg [7 blue tablets]
Day 22-28: 7 teal inactive tablets (28s)

Tri-Sprintec™:
Day 1-7: Ethinyl estradiol 0.035 mg and norgestimate 0.18 mg [7 gray tablets]
Day 8-14: Ethinyl estradiol 0.035 mg and norgestimate 0.215 mg [7 light blue tablets]
Day 15-21: Ethinyl estradiol 0.035 mg and norgestimate 0.25 mg [7 blue tablets]
Day 22-28: 7 white inactive tablets (28s)

Ortho Tri-Cyclen® Lo:
Day 1-7: Ethinyl estradiol 0.025 mg and norgestimate 0.18 mg [7 white tablets]
Day 8-14: Ethinyl estradiol 0.025 mg and norgestimate 0.215 mg [7 light blue tablets]
Day 15-21: Ethinyl estradiol 0.025 mg and norgestimate 0.25 mg [7 dark blue tablets]
Day 22-28: 7 green inactive tablets (28s)

Dosing

Adults: Female:

Acne (Ortho Tri-Cyclen®): Oral: Refer to dosing for contraception

Contraception: Oral:

Schedule 1 (Sunday starter): Dose begins on first Sunday after onset of menstruation; if the menstrual period starts on Sunday, take first tablet that very same day. **With a Sunday start, an additional method of contraception should be used until after the first 7 days of consecutive administration.**

For 21-tablet package: Dosage is 1 tablet daily for 21 consecutive days, followed by 7 days off of the medication; a new course begins on the 8th day after the last tablet is taken.

For 28-tablet package: Dosage is 1 tablet daily without interruption.

Schedule 2 (Day 1 starter): Dose starts on first day of menstrual cycle taking 1 tablet daily.

For 21-tablet package: Dosage is 1 tablet daily for 21 consecutive days, followed by 7 days off of the medication; a new course begins on the 8th day after the last tablet is taken.

For 28-tablet package: Dosage is 1 tablet daily without interruption.

If all doses have been taken on schedule and one menstrual period is missed, continue dosing cycle. If two consecutive menstrual periods are missed, pregnancy test is required before new dosing cycle is started.

Missed doses **monophasic formulations** (refer to package insert for complete information):

One dose missed: Take as soon as remembered or take 2 tablets next day

Two consecutive doses missed in the first 2 weeks: Take 2 tablets as soon as remembered or 2 tablets next 2 days. **An additional method of contraception should be used for 7 days after missed dose.**

Two consecutive doses missed in week 3 or three consecutive doses missed at any time: **An additional method of contraception must be used for 7 days after a missed dose:**

Schedule 1 (Sunday starter): Continue dose of 1 tablet daily until Sunday, then discard the rest of the pack, and a new pack should be started that same day.

Schedule 2 (Day 1 starter): Current pack should be discarded, and a new pack should be started that same day.

Missed doses **biphasic/triphasic formulations** (refer to package insert for complete information):

One dose missed: Take as soon as remembered or take 2 tablets next day.

Two consecutive doses missed in week 1 or week 2 of the pack: Take 2 tablets as soon as remembered and 2 tablets the next day. Resume taking 1 tablet daily until the pack is empty. **An additional method of contraception must be used for 7 days after a missed dose.**

Two consecutive doses missed in week 3 of the pack. **An additional method of contraception must be used for 7 days after a missed dose.**

Schedule 1 (Sunday starter): Take 1 tablet every day until Sunday. Discard the remaining pack and start a new pack of pills on the same day.

Schedule 2 (Day 1 starter): Discard the remaining pack and start a new pack the same day.

Three or more consecutive doses missed. **An additional method of contraception must be used for 7 days after a missed dose.**

Schedule 1 (Sunday starter): Take 1 tablet every day until Sunday; on Sunday, discard the pack and start a new pack.

Schedule 2 (Day 1 starter): Discard the remaining pack and begin new pack of tablets starting on the same day.

Pediatrics: Female:

Acne: Oral: Children ≥15 years; refer to adult dosing for contraception

Contraception: Oral: Refer to adult dosing; not to be used prior to menarche.

Renal Impairment: Specific guidelines not available; use with caution and monitor blood pressure closely. Consider other forms of contraception.

Hepatic Impairment: Contraindicated in patients with hepatic impairment.

Administration

Oral: Administer at the same time each day.

Stability

Storage: Store at controlled room temperature of 25°C (77°F).

Nursing Actions

Physical Assessment: Emphasize importance of monitoring blood pressure on a regular basis. Assess for adverse reactions and potential drug interactions. Assess knowledge/teach importance of regular (monthly) blood pressure checks and annual physical assessment, Pap smear, and vision assessment. Teach importance of maintaining prescribed schedule of dosing. **Pregnancy risk factor X:** Do not use if patient is pregnant.

Patient Education: Oral contraceptives do not protect against HIV or other sexually-transmitted diseases. Take exactly as directed by prescriber (also see package insert). You are at risk of becoming pregnant if doses are missed. Detailed and complete information on dosing and missed doses can be found in the package insert. Be aware that some medications may reduce the effectiveness of oral contraceptives; an alternate form of contraception may be needed. Check all medicines (prescription and OTC), herbal, and alternative products with prescriber. It is important that you check your blood pressure monthly (on same day each month) and that you have an annual physical assessment, Pap smear, and vision assessment while taking this medication. Avoid smoking while taking this medication; smoking increases risk of adverse effects, including thromboembolic events and heart attacks. You may experience loss of appetite (small frequent meals will help); or constipation (increased exercise, fluids, fruit, fiber, or stool softeners may help). If you have diabetes, use accurate serum glucose testing to identify any changes in glucose tolerance; notify prescriber of significant changes so antidiabetic medication can be adjusted if necessary. Report immediately pain or muscle soreness; warmth, swelling, pain, or redness in calves; shortness of breath; sudden loss of vision; unresolved leg/ foot swelling; change in menstrual pattern (unusual bleeding, amenorrhea, breakthrough spotting); breast tenderness that does not go away; acute abdominal cramping; signs of vaginal infection (drainage, pain, itching); CNS changes (blurred vision, confusion, acute anxiety, or unresolved depression); chest pain; severe headache or vomiting; weakness in arm or leg; severe abdominal pain or tenderness; jaundice; or significant weight gain (>5 lb/week). Notify prescriber of changes in contact lens tolerance. **Pregnancy/breast-feeding precautions:** This medication should not be used during pregnancy. If you suspect you may become pregnant, contact prescriber immediately. Consult prescriber if breast-feeding.

Dietary Considerations Should be taken at same time each day.

Breast-Feeding Issues Jaundice and breast enlargement in the nursing infant have been reported following the use of combination hormonal contraceptives. May decrease the quality and quantity of breast milk; a nonhormonal form of contraception is recommended.

Pregnancy Issues Pregnancy should be ruled out prior to treatment and discontinued if pregnancy occurs. In general, the use of combination hormonal contraceptives when inadvertently taken early in pregnancy have not been associated with teratogenic effects. Due to increased risk of thromboembolism postpartum, combination hormonal contraceptives should not be started earlier than 4-6 weeks following delivery.

Additional Information The World Health Organization (WHO) has issued revised management recommendations for missed combined oral contraceptive pills. Refer to the following reference for a complete presentation and discussion of the guidelines:

Faculty of Family Planning and Reproductive Health Care Clinical Effectiveness Unit, "Faculty Statement from the CEU on a New Publication: WHO Selected Practice Recommendations for Contraceptive Use Update. Missed Pills: New Recommendations," *J Fam Plann Reprod Health Care*, 2005, 31(2):153-5.

Ethosuximide (eth oh SUKS i mide)

U.S. Brand Names Zarontin®

Pharmacologic Category Anticonvulsant, Succinimide

Medication Safety Issues

Sound-alike/look-alike issues:

Ethosuximide may be confused with methsuximide

Zarontin® may be confused with Xalatan®, Zantac®, Zaroxolyn®

Pregnancy Risk Factor C

Lactation Enters breast milk/compatible

Use Management of absence (petit mal) seizures

Mechanism of Action/Effect Increases the seizure threshold and suppresses paroxysmal spike-and-wave pattern in absence seizures; depresses nerve transmission in the motor cortex

Contraindications Hypersensitivity to succinimides or any component of the formulation

Warnings/Precautions Use with caution in patients with hepatic or renal disease; abrupt withdrawal of the drug may precipitate absence status; ethosuximide may increase tonic-clonic seizures in patients with mixed seizure disorders; ethosuximide must be used in combination with other anticonvulsants in patients with both absence and tonic-clonic seizures. Succinimides have been associated with severe blood dyscrasias and cases of systemic lupus erythematosus. Consider evaluation of blood counts in patients with signs/symptoms of infection. Safety and efficacy in patients <3 years of age have not been established.

Drug Interactions

Cytochrome P450 Effect: Substrate of CYP3A4 (major)

Decreased Effect: CYP3A4 inducers may decrease the levels/effects of ethosuximide; example inducers include aminoglutethimide, carbamazepine, nafcillin, nevirapine, phenobarbital, phenytoin, and rifamycins.

Increased Effect/Toxicity: Ethosuximide may elevate phenytoin levels. Valproic acid has been reported to both increase and decrease ethosuximide levels. CYP3A4 inhibitors may increase the levels/effects of ethosuximide; example inhibitors include azole antifungals, clarithromycin, diclofenac, doxycycline, erythromycin, imatinib, isoniazid, nefazodone, nicardipine, propofol, protease inhibitors, quinidine, telithromycin, and verapamil.

Nutritional/Ethanol Interactions

Ethanol: Avoid ethanol (may increase CNS depression). (Continued)

Ethosuximide *(Continued)*

Herb/Nutraceutical: St John's wort may decrease ethosuximide levels.

Lab Interactions Increased alkaline phosphatase (S); positive Coombs' [direct]; decreased calcium (S)

Adverse Reactions Frequency not defined.

Central nervous system: Ataxia, drowsiness, sedation, dizziness, lethargy, euphoria, headache, irritability, hyperactivity, fatigue, night terrors, disturbance in sleep, inability to concentrate, aggressiveness, mental depression (with cases of overt suicidal intentions), paranoid psychosis

Dermatologic: Stevens-Johnson syndrome, SLE, rash, hirsutism

Endocrine & metabolic: Increased libido

Gastrointestinal: Weight loss, gastric upset, cramps, epigastric pain, diarrhea, nausea, vomiting, anorexia, abdominal pain, gum hypertrophy, tongue swelling

Genitourinary: Vaginal bleeding, microscopic hematuria

Hematologic: Leukopenia, agranulocytosis, pancytopenia, eosinophilia

Ocular: Myopia

Miscellaneous: Hiccups

Overdosage/Toxicology Acute overdose can cause CNS depression, ataxia, stupor, coma, hypotension. Chronic overdose can cause skin rash, confusion, ataxia, proteinuria, hepatic dysfunction, and hematuria. Treatment is supportive. Hemoperfusion and hemodialysis may be useful.

Pharmacodynamics/Kinetics

Time to Peak: Serum: Capsule: ~2-4 hours; Syrup: <2-4 hours

Half-Life Elimination: Serum: Children: 30 hours; Adults: 50-60 hours

Metabolism: Hepatic (~80% to 3 inactive metabolites)

Excretion: Urine, slowly (50% as metabolites, 10% to 20% as unchanged drug); feces (small amounts)

Available Dosage Forms

Capsule: 250 mg

Syrup: 250 mg/5 mL (473 mL) [contains sodium benzoate; raspberry flavor]

Dosing

Adults & Elderly: Management of absence (petit mal) seizures: Oral: Initial: 250 mg twice daily; increase by 250 mg as needed every 4-7 days up to 1.5 g/day in 2 divided doses; usual maintenance dose: 20-40 mg/kg/day in 2 divided doses

Pediatrics:

Absence (petit mal) seizures: Oral:

Children 3-6 years: Initial: 250 mg/day (or 15 mg/kg/day) in 2 divided doses; increase every 4-7 days; usual maintenance dose: 15-40 mg/kg/day in 2 divided doses.

Children >6 years: Refer to adult dosing.

Renal Impairment: Use with caution.

Hepatic Impairment: Use with caution.

Administration

Oral: Administer with food or milk to avoid GI upset.

Laboratory Monitoring Trough serum concentrations, CBC, platelets, liver enzymes, urinalysis

Nursing Actions

Physical Assessment: Assess effectiveness and interactions of other medications patient may be taking. Monitor therapeutic response (seizure activity, force, type, duration), laboratory values, and adverse reactions at beginning of therapy and periodically with long-term use. Observe and teach seizure/safety precautions. Taper dosage slowly when discontinuing. Assess knowledge/teach patient appropriate use, interventions to reduce side effects, and adverse symptoms to report.

Patient Education: Take exactly as directed; do not increase dose or frequency or discontinue without consulting prescriber. While using this medication, do not use alcohol and other prescription or OTC medications (especially pain medications, sedatives, antihistamines, or hypnotics) without consulting prescriber. Maintain adequate hydration (2-3 L/day of fluids) unless instructed to restrict fluid intake. You may experience drowsiness, dizziness, or blurred vision (use caution when driving or engaging in tasks requiring alertness until response to drug is known); nausea, vomiting, loss of appetite, or dry mouth (small frequent meals, frequent mouth care, chewing gum, or sucking lozenges may help); or constipation (increased exercise, fluids, fruit, or fiber may help). Wear identification of epileptic status and medications. Report CNS changes, mentation changes, or changes in cognition; muscle cramping, weakness, tremors, or changes in gait; persistent GI symptoms (cramping, constipation, vomiting, anorexia); rash or skin irritations; unusual bruising or bleeding (mouth, urine, stool); or worsening of seizure activity or loss of seizure control. **Pregnancy precaution:** Inform prescriber if you are or intend to become pregnant.

Dietary Considerations Increase dietary intake of folate; may be administered with food or milk.

Geriatric Considerations No specific studies with the use of this medication in the elderly. Consider renal function and proceed slowly with dosing increases; monitor closely.

Related Information

Peak and Trough Guidelines *on page 1387*

Etodolac *(ee.toe DOE lak)*

U.S. Brand Names Lodine® [DSC]; Lodine® XL [DSC]

Synonyms Etodolic Acid

Restrictions A medication guide should be dispensed with each prescription. A template for the required MedGuide can be found on the FDA website at http://www.fda.gov/medwatch/SAFETY/2005/safety05.htm#NSAID

Pharmacologic Category Nonsteroidal Anti-inflammatory Drug (NSAID), Oral

Medication Safety Issues

Sound-alike/look-alike issues:

Lodine® may be confused with codeine, iodine, Iopidine®, Lopid®

Pregnancy Risk Factor C/D (3rd trimester)

Lactation Excretion in breast milk unknown/not recommended

Use Acute and long-term use in the management of signs and symptoms of osteoarthritis; rheumatoid arthritis and juvenile rheumatoid arthritis; management of acute pain

Mechanism of Action/Effect Inhibits prostaglandin synthesis which results in decreased formation of prostaglandin precursors

Contraindications Hypersensitivity to etodolac, aspirin, other NSAIDs, or any component of the formulation; perioperative pain in the setting of coronary artery bypass surgery (CABG); pregnancy

Warnings/Precautions NSAIDs are associated with an increased risk of adverse cardiovascular events, including MI, stroke, and new onset or worsening of pre-existing hypertension. Risk may be increased with duration of use or pre-existing cardiovascular risk-factors or disease. Carefully evaluate individual cardiovascular risk profiles prior to prescribing. Use caution with fluid retention, CHF, or hypertension.

NSAIDs may increase risk of gastrointestinal irritation, ulceration, bleeding, and perforation. These events may occur at any time during therapy and without warning. Use caution with a history of GI disease (bleeding or ulcers), concurrent therapy with aspirin, anticoagulants and/or corticosteroids, smoking, use of alcohol, the elderly or debilitated patients.

Use of NSAIDs can compromise existing renal function. Renal toxicity can occur in patient with impaired renal function, dehydration, heart failure, liver dysfunction, those taking diuretics and ACE inhibitors and the elderly. Rehydrate patient before starting therapy. Monitor renal function closely. Etodolac is not recommended for patients with advanced renal disease.

Use the lowest effective dose for the shortest duration of time, consistent with individual patient goals, to reduce risk of cardiovascular or GI adverse events. Alternate therapies should be considered for patients at high risk.

NSAIDs may cause serious skin adverse events including exfoliative dermatitis, Stevens-Johnson syndrome (SJS), and toxic epidermal necrolysis (TEN). Anaphylactoid reactions may occur, even without prior exposure; patients with "aspirin triad" (bronchial asthma, aspirin intolerance, rhinitis) may be at increased risk. Do not use in patients who experience bronchospasm, asthma, rhinitis, or urticaria with NSAID or aspirin therapy.

Use with caution in patients with decreased hepatic function. Closely monitor patients with any abnormal LFT. Severe hepatic reactions (eg, fulminant hepatitis, liver failure) have occurred with NSAID use, rarely; discontinue if signs or symptoms of liver disease develop, or if systemic manifestations occur. The elderly are at increased risk for adverse effects (especially peptic ulceration, CNS effects, renal toxicity) from NSAIDs even at low doses.

Withhold for at least 4-6 half-lives prior to surgical or dental procedures.

Use of extended release product consisting of a nondeformable matrix should be avoided in patients with stricture/narrowing of the GI tract; symptoms of obstruction have been associated with nondeformable products.

Drug Interactions
Decreased Effect: May reduce effect of some diuretics and antihypertensive effect of beta-blockers, ACE inhibitors, angiotensin II inhibitors, hydralazine, verapamil. Cholestyramine and colestipol may reduce absorption of etodolac.

Increased Effect/Toxicity: Etodolac may increase effect/toxicity of anticoagulants (bleeding), antiplatelet agents (bleeding), aminoglycosides, biphosphonates (GI irritation), corticosteroids (GI irritation), cyclosporine (nephrotoxicity), lithium, methotrexate, pemetrexed, treprostinil (bleeding), vancomycin.

Nutritional/Ethanol Interactions
Ethanol: Avoid ethanol (may enhance gastric mucosal irritation).

Food: Etodolac peak serum levels may be decreased if taken with food.

Herb/Nutraceutical: Avoid alfalfa, anise, bilberry, bladderwrack, bromelain, cat's claw, celery, coleus, cordyceps, dong quai, evening primrose, feverfew, fenugreek, garlic, ginger, ginkgo biloba, red clover, horse chestnut, grapeseed, green tea, ginseng, guggul, horse chestnut seed, horseradish, licorice, prickly ash, red clover, reishi, SAMe, sweet clover, turmeric, white willow (all have additional antiplatelet activity)

Lab Interactions False-positive for urinary bilirubin and ketone

Adverse Reactions
1% to 10%:
Central nervous system: Dizziness (3% to 9 %), chills/fever (1% to 3%), depression (1% to 3%), nervousness (1% to 3%)
Dermatologic: Rash (1% to 3%), pruritus (1% to 3%)
Gastrointestinal: Abdominal cramps (3% to 9%), nausea (3% to 9%), vomiting (1% to 3%), dyspepsia (10%), diarrhea (3% to 9%), constipation (1% to

3%), flatulence (3% to 9%), melena (1% to 3%), gastritis (1% to 3%)
Genitourinary: Dysuria (1% to 3%)
Neuromuscular & skeletal: Weakness (3% to 9%)
Ocular: Blurred vision (1% to 3%)
Otic: Tinnitus (1% to 3%)
Renal: Polyuria (1% to 3%)

Overdosage/Toxicology Symptoms of overdose include acute renal failure, vomiting, drowsiness, leukocytosis. Management of NSAID intoxication is supportive and symptomatic. Emesis and/or activated charcoal and/or osmotic cathartic may be considered when overdoses are large (5-10 times usual dose) or recent (within 4 hours). Diuresis, urine alkalinization, hemodialysis, and hemoperfusion are not likely to be useful.

Pharmacodynamics/Kinetics
Onset of Action: Analgesic: 2-4 hours; Maximum anti-inflammatory effect: A few days
Time to Peak: Immediate release: Adults: 1-2 hours; Extended release: 5-7 hours, increased 1.4-3.8 hours with food
Protein Binding: ≥99%, primarily albumin
Half-Life Elimination: Terminal: Adults: 5-8 hours; Extended release: Children (6-16 years): 12 hours
Metabolism: Hepatic
Excretion: Urine 73% (1% unchanged); feces 16%

Available Dosage Forms [DSC] = Discontinued product
Capsule: 200 mg, 300 mg
Lodine®: 200 mg, 300 mg [DSC]
Tablet: 400 mg, 500 mg
Tablet, extended release (Lodine® XL): 400 mg, 500 mg [DSC]

Dosing
Adults & Elderly: Note: For chronic conditions, response is usually observed within 2 weeks.
Acute pain: Oral: 200-400 mg every 6-8 hours, as needed, not to exceed total daily doses of 1000 mg
Rheumatoid arthritis, osteoarthritis: Oral: 400 mg 2 times/day or 300 mg 2-3 times/day or 500 mg 2 times/day (doses >1000 mg/day have not been evaluated)
Lodine® XL: 400-1000 mg once daily
Pediatrics: Note: For chronic conditions, response is usually observed within 2 weeks.
Juvenile rheumatoid arthritis (Lodine® XL): Oral: Children 6-16 years:
20-30 kg: 400 mg once daily
31-45 kg: 600 mg once daily
46-60 kg: 800 mg once daily
Children >60 kg: 1000 mg once daily
Renal Impairment:
Mild to moderate: No adjustment required
Severe: Use not recommended; use with caution
Hemodialysis: Not removed
Hepatic Impairment:
No adjustment required.

Stability
Storage: Store at 20°C to 25°C (68°F to 77°F). Protect from moisture.

Laboratory Monitoring CBC, liver enzymes; in patients receiving diuretics, monitor BUN/serum creatinine.

Nursing Actions
Physical Assessment: Assess effectiveness and interactions of other medications patient may be taking. Monitor blood pressure at the beginning of therapy and periodically during use. Monitor laboratory tests and therapeutic response (eg, relief of pain and inflammation, activity tolerance) and adverse reactions (eg, gastrointestinal effects, cardiovascular complaints, or ototoxicity) at beginning of therapy and periodically throughout therapy. Assess knowledge/teach patient appropriate use, interventions to reduce side effects, and adverse symptoms to report.
(Continued)

Etodolac *(Continued)*

Patient Education: Take this medication exactly as directed; do not increase dose without consulting prescriber. Do not crush tablets or break capsules. Take with food or milk to reduce GI distress. Maintain adequate hydration (2-3 L/day of fluids) unless instructed to restrict fluid intake. Do not use alcohol, aspirin or aspirin-containing medication, or any other anti-inflammatory medications without consulting prescriber. You may experience anorexia, nausea, vomiting, or heartburn (small frequent meals, frequent mouth care, sucking lozenges, or chewing gum may help); drowsiness, dizziness, nervousness, or headache (use caution when driving or engaging in tasks requiring alertness until response to drug is known); or fluid retention (weigh yourself weekly and report unusual [3-5 lb/week] weight gain). GI bleeding, ulceration, or perforation can occur with or without pain; discontinue medication and contact prescriber if persistent abdominal pain or cramping, or blood in stool occurs. Report breathlessness, respiratory difficulty, or unusual cough; chest pain, rapid heartbeat; palpitations; unusual bruising/bleeding; blood in urine, stool, mouth, or vomitus; swollen extremities; skin rash, blisters, or itching; acute fatigue; fever; jaundice; abdominal tenderness; flu-like symptoms; or hearing changes (ringing in ears). **Pregnancy/breast-feeding precautions:** Inform prescriber if you are or intend to become pregnant. This drug should not be used in the 3rd trimester of pregnancy. Do not breast-feed.

Dietary Considerations May be taken with food to decrease GI distress.

Geriatric Considerations The elderly are at increased risk for adverse effects from NSAIDs. As many as 60% of elderly can develop peptic ulceration and/or hemorrhage asymptomatically. CNS adverse effects such as confusion, agitation, and hallucination are generally seen in overdose or high-dose situations; however, elderly patients may demonstrate these adverse effects at lower doses than younger adults. The elderly are also at increased risk of renal toxicity.

Etoposide *(e toe POE side)*

U.S. Brand Names Toposar®; VePesid®

Synonyms Epipodophyllotoxin; VP-16; VP-16-213

Pharmacologic Category Antineoplastic Agent, Podophyllotoxin Derivative

Medication Safety Issues
Sound-alike/look-alike issues:
Etoposide may be confused with teniposide
VePesid® may be confused with Versed

Pregnancy Risk Factor D

Lactation Enters breast milk/contraindicated

Use Treatment of refractory testicular tumors; treatment of small cell lung cancer

Unlabeled/Investigational Use Treatment of lymphomas, acute nonlymphocytic leukemia (ANLL); lung, bladder, and prostate carcinoma; hepatoma, rhabdomyosarcoma, uterine carcinoma, neuroblastoma, mycosis fungoides, Kaposi's sarcoma, histiocytosis, gestational trophoblastic disease, Ewing's sarcoma, Wilms' tumor, brain tumors

Mechanism of Action/Effect Inhibits DNA synthesis leading to cell death.

Contraindications Hypersensitivity to etoposide or any component of the formulation; pregnancy

Warnings/Precautions Hazardous agent — use appropriate precautions for handling and disposal. Severe myelosuppression with resulting infection or bleeding may occur. Treatment should be withheld for platelets <50,000/mm^3 or absolute neutrophil count (ANC) <500/mm^3. May cause anaphylactic reaction manifested by chills, fever, tachycardia, bronchospasm, dyspnea, and hypotension. In children, the use of concentrations higher than recommended were associated with higher rates of anaphylactic-like reactions. Infusion should be interrupted and medications for the treatment of anaphylaxis should be available for immediate use. Must be diluted; do not give I.V. push, infuse over at least 30-60 minutes; hypotension is associated with rapid infusion. Dosage should be adjusted in patients with hepatic or renal impairment. Injectable formula contains polysorbate 80; do not use in premature infants. May contain benzyl alcohol; do not use in newborn infants. Safety and efficacy in children have not been established.

Drug Interactions
Cytochrome P450 Effect: Substrate of CYP1A2 (minor), 2E1 (minor), 3A4 (major); **Inhibits** CYP2C8/9 (weak), 3A4 (weak)

Decreased Effect: Barbiturates and phenytoin may decrease the levels/effects of etoposide; monitor. CYP3A4 inducers may decrease the levels/effects of etoposide; example inducers include aminoglutethimide, carbamazepine, nafcillin, nevirapine, phenobarbital, phenytoin, and rifamycins.

Increased Effect/Toxicity: Cyclosporine may increase the levels of etoposide; consider reducing the dose of etoposide by 50%. Etoposide may increase the effects/toxicity of warfarin. CYP3A4 inhibitors may increase the levels/effects of etoposide; example inhibitors include azole antifungals, clarithromycin, diclofenac, doxycycline, erythromycin, imatinib, isoniazid, nefazodone, nicardipine, propofol, protease inhibitors, quinidine, telithromycin, and verapamil.

Nutritional/Ethanol Interactions
Ethanol: Avoid ethanol (may increase GI irritation).
Herb/Nutraceutical: Avoid concurrent St John's wort; may decrease etoposide levels.

Adverse Reactions
>10%:
Dermatologic: Alopecia (8% to 66%)
Endocrine & metabolic: Ovarian failure (38%), amenorrhea
Gastrointestinal: Nausea/vomiting (31% to 43%), anorexia (10% to 13%), diarrhea (1% to 13%), mucositis/esophagitis (with high doses)
Hematologic: Leukopenia (60% to 91%; grade 4: 3% to 17%; onset: 5-7 days; nadir: 7-14 days; recovery: 21-28 days), thrombocytopenia (22% to 41%; grades 3/4: 1% to 20%; nadir 9-16 days), anemia (up to 33%)
1% to 10%:
Cardiovascular: Hypotension (1% to 2%; due to rapid infusion)
Gastrointestinal: Stomatitis (1% to 6%), abdominal pain (up to 2%)
Hepatic: Hepatic toxicity (up to 3%)
Neuromuscular & skeletal: Peripheral neuropathy (1% to 2%)
Miscellaneous: Anaphylactic-like reaction (I.V. infusion: 1% to 2%; including chills, fever, tachycardia, bronchospasm, dyspnea)

Overdosage/Toxicology Symptoms of overdose include bone marrow suppression, leukopenia, thrombocytopenia, nausea, and vomiting. Treatment is symptom-directed and supportive.

Pharmacodynamics/Kinetics
Time to Peak: Serum: Oral: 1-1.5 hours
Protein Binding: 94% to 97%
Half-Life Elimination: Terminal: 4-11 hours; Children: Normal renal/hepatic function: 6-8 hours
Metabolism: Hepatic to hydroxy acid and cislactone metabolites
Excretion:
Children: Urine (≤55% as unchanged drug)

Adults: Urine (42% to 67%; 8% to 35% as unchanged drug) within 24 hours; feces (up to 44%)

Available Dosage Forms [DSC] = Discontinued product

Capsule, softgel (VePesid®): 50 mg

Injection, solution: 20 mg/mL (5 mL, 25 mL, 50 mL) [may contain benzyl alcohol or alcohol]

Toposar®: 20 mg/mL (5 mL, 10 mL, 25 mL) [contains benzyl alcohol]

VePesid®: 20 mg/mL (5 mL, 7.5 mL, 25 mL, 50 mL) [contains benzyl alcohol and alcohol 30%] [DSC]

Dosing

Adults & Elderly: Refer to individual protocols.

Small cell lung cancer (in combination with other approved chemotherapeutic drugs):

Oral: Due to poor bioavailability, oral doses should be twice the I.V. dose, rounded to the nearest 50 mg given once daily

I.V.: 35 mg/m^2/day for 4 days or 50 mg/m^2/day for 5 days every 3-4 weeks

IVPB: 60-100 mg/m^2/day for 3 days (with cisplatin)

CIV: 500 mg/m^2 over 24 hours every 3 weeks

Testicular cancer (in combination with other approved chemotherapeutic drugs):

IVPB: 50-100 mg/m^2/day for 5 days repeated every 3-4 weeks

I.V.: 100 mg/m^2 every other day for 3 doses repeated every 3-4 weeks

BMT/relapsed leukemia (unlabeled uses): I.V.: 2.4-3.5 g/m^2 or 25-70 mg/kg administered over 4-36 hours

Pediatrics: Refer to individual protocols.

Children (unlabeled uses): I.V.: 60-120 mg/m^2/day for 3-5 days every 3-6 weeks

AML: I.V.:

Remission induction: 150 mg/m^2/day for 2-3 days for 2-3 cycles

Intensification or consolidation: 250 mg/m^2/day for 3 days, courses 2-5

Brain tumor: I.V.: 150 mg/m^2/day on days 2 and 3 of treatment course

Neuroblastoma: I.V.: 100 mg/m^2/day over 1 hour on days 1-5 of cycle; repeat cycle every 4 weeks

BMT conditioning regimen used in patients with rhabdomyosarcoma or neuroblastoma: I.V.: continuous infusion: 160 mg/m^2/day for 4 days

Conditioning regimen for allogenic BMT: I.V.: 60 mg/kg/dose as a single dose

Renal Impairment:

Manufacturer recommended guidelines:

Cl$_{cr}$ 15-50 mL/minute: Administer 75% of normal dose

Cl$_{cr}$ <15 mL minute: Data not available, consider further dose reductions

Aronoff, 1999:

Cl$_{cr}$ 10-50 mL/minute: Administer 75% of normal dose

Cl$_{cr}$ <10 mL minute: Administer 50% of normal dose

Hemodialysis: Supplemental dose is not necessary

Peritoneal dialysis: Supplemental dose is not necessary

CAPD effects: Unknown

CAVH effects: Dose for Cl$_{cr}$ 10-50 mL/minute (Aronoff, 1999)

Hepatic Impairment:

Bilirubin 1.5-3 mg/dL or AST 60-180 units: Reduce dose by 50%.

Bilirubin >3 mg/dL or AST >180 units: Reduce by 75%.

Administration

Oral: Doses ≤400 mg/day as a single once daily dose; doses >400 mg should be divided. If necessary, the injection may be used for oral administration; etoposide injection diluted for oral use to 10 mg/mL in NS may be stored for 22 days in plastic oral syringes at room temperature. Mix with orange juice, apple juice, or lemonade to a concentration of ≤0.4 mg/mL, and use within a 3-hour period.

I.M.: Do not administer I.M. or SubQ (severe tissue necrosis).

I.V.: Irritant. Administer lower doses IVPB over at least 30 minutes to minimize the risk of hypotensive reactions.

I.V. Detail: Concentrations >0.4 mg/mL are very unstable and may precipitate within a few minutes. For large doses, where dilution to ≤0.4 mg/mL is not feasible, consideration should be given to slow infusion of the undiluted drug through a running normal saline, dextrose or saline/dextrose infusion; or use of etoposide phosphate. Etoposide solutions of 0.1-0.4 mg/mL may be filtered through a 0.22 micron filter without damage to the filter or significant loss of drug.

pH: 3-4

BMT only: The etoposide formulation contains ethanol 30.3% (v/v). Etoposide 2.4 mg/m^2 delivers ethanol 45 g/m^2 I.V. Adverse effects may be increased with administration of etoposide to patients with decreased creatinine clearance.

Stability

Reconstitution: Etoposide should be diluted to a concentration of 0.2-0.4 mg/mL in D$_5$W or NS for administration. Diluted solutions have concentration-dependent stability: More concentrated solutions have shorter stability times. Precipitation may occur with concentrations >0.4 mg/mL.

Compatibility: Variable stability (consult detailed reference) in D$_5$W, LR, NS

Y-site administration: Incompatible with cefepime, filgrastim, idarubicin

Storage: Store intact vials of injection at 15°C to 30°C (59°F to 86°F); protect from light. Store oral capsules at 2°C to 8°C (36°F to 46°F).

At room temperature in D$_5$W or NS in polyvinyl chloride, the concentration is stable as follows:

0.2 mg/mL: 96 hours

0.4 mg/mL: 24 hours

Laboratory Monitoring CBC with differential, platelet count, bilirubin, renal function

Nursing Actions

Physical Assessment: Assess potential for interactions with other pharmacological agents or herbal products patient may be taking (eg, potential for increasing/decreasing levels or effects of etoposide). Patient should be monitored closely for anaphylactic reaction (chills, fever, tachycardia, bronchospasm, dyspnea, hypotension). Emergency equipment should be available. See Reconstitution for specific directions. Assess results of laboratory tests and renal function, therapeutic effectiveness, and adverse response prior to each treatment and on a regular basis throughout therapy. Teach patient possible side effects/appropriate interventions and adverse symptoms to report.

Patient Education: Do not take any new medication during therapy unless approved by prescriber. This medication may be administered by infusion. Report immediately any swelling, pain, burning, or redness at infusion site; swelling of extremities; palpitations; rapid heartbeat; sudden difficulty breathing or swallowing; chest pain or chills. It is important to maintain adequate hydration (2-3 L/day of fluids) unless instructed to restrict fluid intake, and adequate nutrition (small, frequent meals may help). You will be more susceptible to infection (avoid crowds and exposure to infection and do not have any vaccinations without consulting prescriber). May cause nausea or vomiting (small, frequent meals, frequent mouth care, sucking lozenges, or chewing gum may help); diarrhea (buttermilk, boiled milk, or yogurt may help); loss

(Continued)

Etoposide (Continued)

of hair (reversible); or mouth sores (use soft toothbrush or cotton swabs for oral care and rinse mouth frequently). Report extreme fatigue, pain or numbness in extremities, severe GI upset or diarrhea, bleeding or bruising, fever, sore throat, vaginal discharge, yellowing of eyes or skin, or any changes in color of urine or stool. **Pregnancy/breast-feeding precautions:** Do not get pregnant while taking this medication. Consult prescriber for appropriate contraceptive measures to use during and for 1 month following therapy. Do not breast-feed.

Pregnancy Issues Animal studies have demonstrated teratogenicity and fetal loss. There are no adequate and well-controlled studies in pregnant women. Women of childbearing potential should be advised to avoid pregnancy.

Etoposide Phosphate
(e toe POE side FOS fate)

U.S. Brand Names Etopophos®

Pharmacologic Category Antineoplastic Agent, Podophyllotoxin Derivative

Medication Safety Issues
Sound-alike/look-alike issues:
Etoposide may be confused with teniposide
Etoposide phosphate is a prodrug of etoposide and is rapidly converted in the plasma to etoposide. To avoid confusion or dosing errors, **dosage should be expressed as the desired etoposide dose**, not as the etoposide phosphate dose (eg, etoposide phosphate equivalent to ____ mg etoposide).

Pregnancy Risk Factor D

Lactation Enters breast milk/contraindicated

Use Treatment of refractory testicular tumors; treatment of small cell lung cancer

Mechanism of Action/Effect Etoposide phosphate is converted *in vivo* to the active moiety, etoposide, by dephosphorylation. Etoposide inhibits mitotic activity; inhibits cells from entering prophase; inhibits DNA synthesis. Initially thought to be mitotic inhibitors similar to podophyllotoxin, but actually have no effect on microtubule assembly. However, later shown to induce DNA strand breakage and inhibition of topoisomerase II (an enzyme which breaks and repairs DNA); etoposide acts in late S or early G2 phases.

Contraindications Hypersensitivity to etoposide, etoposide phosphate, or any component of the formulation; pregnancy

Warnings/Precautions Hazardous agent - use appropriate precautions for handling and disposal. Severe myelosuppression with resulting infection or bleeding may occur. Treatment should be withheld for platelets <50,000/mm^3 or absolute neutrophil count (ANC) <500/mm^3. May cause anaphylactic reaction manifested by chills, fever, tachycardia, bronchospasm, dyspnea, and hypotension (higher concentrations were associated with higher rates of reactions in children). Infusion should be interrupted and medications for the treatment of anaphylaxis should be available for immediate use. Hypotension is associated with rapid infusion; infuse over at least 30-60 minutes. Dosage should be adjusted in patients with hepatic or renal impairment. Doses of etoposide phosphate >175mg/m^2 have not been evaluated. Use caution in elderly patients (may be more likely to develop severe myelosuppression and/or GI effects. Safety and efficacy in children have not been established.

Drug Interactions
Cytochrome P450 Effect: Substrate of CYP1A2 (minor), 2E1 (minor), 3A4 (major); **Inhibits** CYP2C8/9 (weak), 3A4 (weak)

Decreased Effect: Barbiturates and phenytoin may decrease the levels/effects of etoposide; monitor. CYP3A4 inducers may decrease the levels/effects of etoposide; example inducers include aminoglutethimide, carbamazepine, nafcillin, nevirapine, phenobarbital, phenytoin, and rifamycins.

Increased Effect/Toxicity: Cyclosporine may increase the levels of etoposide; consider reducing the dose of etoposide by 50%. Etoposide may increase the effects/toxicity of warfarin. CYP3A4 inhibitors may increase the levels/effects of etoposide; example inhibitors include azole antifungals, clarithromycin, diclofenac, doxycycline, erythromycin, imatinib, isoniazid, nefazodone, nicardipine, propofol, protease inhibitors, quinidine, telithromycin, and verapamil.

Nutritional/Ethanol Interactions
Ethanol: Avoid ethanol (may increase GI irritation).
Herb/Nutraceutical: St John's wort may decrease etoposide levels.

Adverse Reactions Note: Also see adverse reactions for **etoposide**. Since etoposide phosphate is converted to etoposide, adverse reactions experienced with etoposide would also be expected with etoposide phosphate.
>10%:
Central nervous system: Chills/fever (24%)
Dermatologic: Alopecia (33% to 44%)
Gastrointestinal: Nausea/vomiting (37%), anorexia (16%), mucositis (11%)
Hematologic: Leukopenia (91%; grade 4: 17%), neutropenia (88%; grade 4: 37%), anemia (72%; grades 3/4: 19%), thrombocytopenia (23%; grade 4: 9%)
Neuromuscular and skeletal: Weakness/malaise (39%)
1% to 10%:
Cardiovascular: Hypotension (5%), hypertension (3%), facial flushing (2%)
Central nervous system: Dizziness (5%)
Dermatologic: Skin rash (3%)
Gastrointestinal: Constipation (8%), abdominal pain (7%), diarrhea (6%), taste perversion (6%)
Local: Extravasation/phlebitis (5%)
Miscellaneous: Anaphylactic-type reactions (3%; including chills, diaphoresis, fever, rigor, tachycardia, bronchospasm, dyspnea, pruritus)

Overdosage/Toxicology Symptoms of overdose include bone marrow suppression, leukopenia, thrombocytopenia, nausea, and vomiting. Treatment is symptom-directed and supportive.

Pharmacodynamics/Kinetics
Protein Binding: 94% to 97%
Half-Life Elimination: Terminal: 4-11 hours; Children: Normal renal/hepatic function: 6-8 hours
Metabolism:
Etoposide phosphate: Rapidly and completely converted to etoposide in plasma
Etoposide: Hepatic to hydroxy acid and cislactone metabolites
Excretion: Urine (as unchanged drug and metabolites); feces (2% to 16%)
Children: I.V.: Urine (≤55% as unchanged drug)

Available Dosage Forms Injection, powder for reconstitution, as base: 100 mg

Dosing
Adults & Elderly: Refer to individual protocols. **Note:** Etoposide phosphate is a prodrug of etoposide, doses should be expressed as the desired **ETOPOSIDE** dose; **not** as the etoposide phosphate dose. (eg, etoposide phosphate equivalent to ____ mg etoposide).
Small cell lung cancer: I.V. (in combination with other approved chemotherapeutic drugs): Etoposide 35 mg/m^2/day for 4 days to 50 mg/m^2/day for 5 days. Courses are repeated at 3- to 4-week intervals after adequate recovery from any toxicity.

Testicular cancer: I.V. (in combination with other approved chemotherapeutic agents): Etoposide 50-100 mg/m²/day on days 1-5 to 100 mg/m²/day on days 1, 3, and 5. Courses are repeated at 3- to 4-week intervals after adequate recovery from any toxicity.

Renal Impairment:
Manufacturer recommended guidelines:
Cl$_{cr}$ 15-50 mL/minute: Administer 75% of normal dose
Cl$_{cr}$ <15 mL minute: Data are available; consider further dose reductions
Aronoff, 1999:
Cl$_{cr}$ 10-50 mL/minute: Administer 75% of normal dose
Cl$_{cr}$ <10 mL minute: Administer 50% of normal dose
Hemodialysis: Supplemental dose is not necessary
Peritoneal dialysis: Supplemental dose is not necessary
CAPD effects: Unknown
CAVH effects: Dose for Cl$_{cr}$ 10-50 mL/minute (Aronoff, 1999)

Hepatic Impairment:
Bilirubin 1.5-3 mg/dL or AST 60-180 units: Reduce dose by 50%.
Bilirubin 3-5 mg/dL or AST >180 units: Reduce dose by 75%.
Bilirubin >5 mg/dL: Do not administer.

Administration
I.V.: Infuse over 5-210 minutes.
I.V. Detail:
BMT only: In contrast to etoposide, metabolic acidosis is not a frequent adverse effect of high-dose etoposide phosphate.

pH: 2.9 (reconstituted with sterile water for injection)

Stability
Reconstitution: Reconstituted etoposide phosphate is stable refrigerated at 2°C to 8°C (36°F to 47°F) for 7 days. Undiluted solutions are stable for 24 hours at room temperature of 20°C to 25°C (68°F to 77°F) when reconstituted with SWI, D₅W or NS; and stable for 48 hours at room temperature when reconstituted with bacteriostatic SWI or NS. Further diluted solutions are stable at room temperature 20°C to 25°C (68°F to 77°F) or under refrigeration 2°C to 8°C (36°F to 47°F) for up to 24 hours.
Compatibility: Stable in D₅W, NS, SWFI
Y-site administration: Incompatible with amphotericin B, cefepime, chlorpromazine, imipenem/cilastatin, methylprednisolone sodium succinate, mitomycin, prochlorperazine edisylate
Storage: Store intact vials of injection under refrigeration 2°C to 8°C (36°F to 46°F). Protect from light. Reconstitute vials with 5 mL or 10 mL SWI, D₅W, NS, bacteriostatic SWI, or bacteriostatic NS to a concentration of 20 mg/mL or 10 mg/mL etoposide equivalent. These solutions may be administered without further dilution or may be diluted in 50-500 mL of D₅W or NS to a concentration as low as 0.1 mg/mL.

Laboratory Monitoring CBC with differential, platelet count, bilirubin, renal function

Nursing Actions
Physical Assessment: Use caution in presence of hepatic or renal impairment. Assess potential for interactions with other pharmacological agents or herbal products patient may be taking (potential for increasing/decreasing levels or effects of etoposide). See Reconstitution for specific directions. Assess results of laboratory tests and renal function, therapeutic effectiveness, and adverse response prior to each treatment and on a regular basis throughout therapy. Teach patient possible side effects/appropriate interventions and adverse symptoms to report (refer to Patient Education).

Patient Education: Do not take any new medication during therapy unless approved by prescriber. This medication is administered by infusion. Report immediately any swelling, pain, burning, or redness at infusion site. Avoid alcohol. It is important to maintain adequate hydration (2-3 L/day of fluids) unless instructed to restrict fluid intake, and adequate nutrition (small, frequent meals may help). You will be more susceptible to infection (avoid crowds and exposure to infection and do not have any vaccinations without consulting prescriber). May cause nausea or vomiting (small, frequent meals, frequent mouth care, sucking lozenges, or chewing gum may help); diarrhea (buttermilk, boiled milk, or yogurt may help); loss of hair (reversible); or mouth sores (use soft toothbrush or cotton swabs for oral care and rinse mouth frequently). Report immediately chest pain, swelling of extremities, respiratory difficulty, palpitations, or rapid heartbeat. Report extreme fatigue, pain or numbness in extremities, severe GI upset or diarrhea, bleeding or bruising, fever, chills, sore throat, vaginal discharge, respiratory difficulty, yellowing of eyes or skin, or changes in color of urine or stool. **Pregnancy/breast-feeding precautions:** Do not get pregnant while taking this medication. Consult prescriber for appropriate barrier contraceptive measures to use during and for 1 month following therapy. Do not breast-feed.

Geriatric Considerations Elderly patients may be more susceptible to severe myelosuppression. Other adverse effects including GI toxicity, infectious complications, weakness, and alopecia may occur more frequently in elderly.

Pregnancy Issues Animal studies have demonstrated teratogenicity and fetal loss. There are no adequate and well-controlled studies in pregnant women. Women of childbearing potential should be advised to avoid pregnancy.

Additional Information Etoposide phosphate 113.5 mg is equivalent to etoposide 100 mg. Dosages should always be expressed, and calculated, as the desired **etoposide** dose.

Exemestane (ex e MES tane)

U.S. Brand Names Aromasin®
Pharmacologic Category Antineoplastic Agent, Aromatase Inactivator
Pregnancy Risk Factor D
Lactation Excretion in breast milk unknown/use caution
Use Treatment of advanced breast cancer in postmenopausal women whose disease has progressed following tamoxifen therapy; adjuvant treatment of postmenopausal estrogen receptor-positive early breast cancer following 2-3 years of tamoxifen (for a total of 5 years of adjuvant therapy)
Mechanism of Action/Effect Exemestane prevents conversion of androgens to estrogens (Aromatase inhibitor) and lowers circulating estrogen levels.
Contraindications Hypersensitivity to exemestane or any component of the formulation; pregnancy
Warnings/Precautions Not indicated for premenopausal women; not to be given with estrogen-containing agents.
Drug Interactions
Cytochrome P450 Effect: Substrate of CYP3A4 (major)
Decreased Effect: CYP3A4 inducers may decrease the levels/effects of exemestane; example inducers include aminoglutethimide, carbamazepine, efavirenz, fosphenytoin, nafcillin, nevirapine, oxcarbazepine, pentobarbital, phenobarbital, phenytoin, primidone, rifabutin, rifampin, and rifapentine; adjustment required with potent inducers.
(Continued)

Exemestane (Continued)

Nutritional/Ethanol Interactions

Food: Plasma levels increased by 40% when exemestane was taken with a fatty meal.

Herb/Nutraceutical: St John's wort may decrease exemestane levels. Avoid black cohosh, dong quai in estrogen-dependent tumors.

Adverse Reactions

>10%:

Cardiovasuclar: Hypertension (5% to 15%)

Central nervous system: Fatigue (8% to 22%), insomnia (11% to 14%), pain (13%), headache (7% to 13%), depression (6% to 13%)

Dermatological: Hyperhidrosis (4% to 18%), alopecia (15%)

Endocrine & metabolic: Hot flashes (13% to 21%)

Gastrointestinal: Nausea (9% to 18%), abdominal pain (6% to 11%)

Hepatic: Alkaline phosphatase increased (14% to 15%)

Neuromuscular & skeletal: Arthralgia (15% to 29%)

1% to 10%:

Cardiovascular: Edema (6% to 7%); cardiac ischemic events (2%: MI, angina, myocardial ischemia); chest pain

Central nervous system: Dizziness (8% to 10%), anxiety (4% to 10%), fever (5%), confusion, hypoesthesia

Dermatologic: Dermatitis (8%), itching, rash

Endocrine & metabolic: Weight gain (8%)

Gastrointestinal: Diarrhea (4% to 10%), vomiting (7%), anorexia (6%), constipation (5%), appetite increased (3%), dyspepsia

Genitourinary: Urinary tract infection

Hepatic: Bilirubin increased (5% to 7%)

Neuromuscular & skeletal: Back pain (9%), limb pain (9%), osteoarthritis (6%), weakness (6%), osteoporosis (5%), pathological fracture (4%), paresthesia (3%), carpal tunnel syndrome (2%), cramps (2%)

Ocular: Visual disturbances (5%)

Renal: Creatinine increased (6%)

Respiratory: Dyspnea (10%), cough (6%), bronchitis, pharyngitis, rhinitis, sinusitis, upper respiratory infection

Miscellaneous: Influenza-like symptoms (6%), diaphoresis (6%), lymphedema, infection

A dose-dependent decrease in sex hormone-binding globulin has been observed with daily doses of 25 mg or more. Serum luteinizing hormone and follicle-stimulating hormone levels have increased with this medicine.

Overdosage/Toxicology In case of overdose, treatment should be symptom-directed and supportive.

Pharmacodynamics/Kinetics

Time to Peak: Women with breast cancer: 1.2 hours

Protein Binding: 90%, primarily to albumin and α_1-acid glycoprotein

Half-Life Elimination: 24 hours

Metabolism: Extensively hepatic; oxidation (CYP3A4) of methylene group, reduction of 17-keto group with formation of many secondary metabolites; metabolites are inactive

Excretion: Urine (<1% as unchanged drug, 39% to 45% as metabolites); feces (36% to 48%)

Available Dosage Forms Tablet: 25 mg

Dosing

Adults & Elderly: Breast cancer: Oral: 25 mg once daily

Dosage adjustment with CYP3A4 inducers: 50 mg once daily when used with potent inducers (eg, rifampin, phenytoin)

Renal Impairment: Safety of chronic dosing in renal impairment has not been established.

Hepatic Impairment: Safety of chronic dosing in hepatic impairment has not been established.

Administration

Oral: Administer after a meal.

Stability

Storage: Store at 25°C (77°F)

Nursing Actions

Physical Assessment: Not indicated for women who are premenopausal or those taking any estrogen containing products. Assess patient response prior to each treatment and on a regular basis throughout therapy. Teach patient proper use, possible side effects/appropriate interventions (eg, importance of adequate hydration), and adverse symptoms to report.

Patient Education: Do not take any new medication during therapy unless approved by prescriber. Take after meals at approximately the same time each day; may cause indigestion (small, frequent meals, and frequent mouth care may reduce GI upset). You may be more susceptible to infection (avoid crowds or exposure to infection and do not have any vaccinations unless approved by prescriber). May cause headache, dizziness, confusion, fatigue, anxiety, insomnia (use caution when driving or engaging in tasks requiring alertness until response to medication is known); nausea, vomiting, loss of appetite (small, frequent meals, good mouth care, chewing gum, or sucking hard candy may help); or hot flashes (cool dark room or cold compresses may help). Report chest pain, palpitations; acute headache, visual disturbances; unresolved GI problems; itching or burning on urination, vaginal discharge; acute joint, back, bone, or muscle pain; respiratory difficulty, unusual cough, respiratory infection; or other adverse response. **For use in postmenopausal women only.**

Dietary Considerations Take after a meal; patients on aromatase inhibitor therapy should receive vitamin D and calcium supplements.

Pregnancy Issues Exemestane has been associated with prolonged gestation, abnormal or difficult labor, increased resorption, reduced number of live fetuses, decreased fetal weight, and retarded ossification in rats. It is not indicated for premenopausal women, but if exposure occurred during pregnancy, risk to the fetus and potential risk for loss of the pregnancy should be discussed.

Exenatide (ex EN a tide)

U.S. Brand Names Byetta™

Synonyms AC002993; Exendin-4; LY2148568

Pharmacologic Category Antidiabetic Agent, Incretin Mimetic

Pregnancy Risk Factor C

Lactation Excretion in breast milk unknown/use caution

Use Management (adjunctive) of type 2 diabetes mellitus (noninsulin dependent, NIDDM)

Mechanism of Action/Effect Exenatide is an analog of the hormone incretin (glucagon-like peptide 1 or GLP-1) which increases insulin secretion, increases B-cell growth/replication, slows gastric emptying, and may decrease food intake. When added to sulfonylureas and/or metformin, it results in additional lowering of hemoglobin A_{1c} by approximately 0.5% to 1%.

Contraindications Hypersensitivity to exenatide or any component of the formulation; type 1 diabetes; diabetic ketoacidosis

Warnings/Precautions Should be used as an adjunct to diet and exercise in patients previously treated with a sulfonylurea, metformin, or a combination of these agents. Concurrent use with other hypoglycemic agents and/or insulin therapy has not been evaluated. May increase the risk of hypoglycemia in patients receiving sulfonylurea therapy (risk of hypoglycemia was not increased when added to metformin monotherapy). Risk of hypoglycemia is related to the dosage of both exenatide and the sulfonylurea.

Exenatide is frequently associated with gastrointestinal adverse effects and is not recommended for use in patients with gastroparesis or severe gastrointestinal disease. Gastrointestinal effects may be dose-related and may decrease in frequency/severity with gradual titration and continued use. Use may be associated with the development of anti-exenatide antibodies; low titers are not associated with a loss of efficacy, however high titers (observed in 6% of patients in clinical studies) may result in an attenuation of response. May be associated with weight loss (due to reduced intake) independent of the change in hemoglobin A_{1c}. Not recommended in severe renal impairment (Cl $_{cr}$<30 mL/minute). Safety and efficacy have not been established in children (<18 years of age).

Drug Interactions
Decreased Effect: Note: Due to its effects on gastric emptying, exenatide may reduce the rate and extent of absorption of orally-administered drugs. Should be used with caution in patients receiving medications which require rapid absorption from the gastrointestinal tract. Administration of medications 1 hour prior to the use of exenatide has been recommended by the manufacturer when optimal drug absorption and peak levels are important to the overall therapeutic effect (such as with antibiotics and/or oral contraceptives).

Nutritional/Ethanol Interactions Ethanol: Caution with ethanol (may cause hypoglycemia)
Adverse Reactions
>10%:
Endocrine & metabolic: Hypoglycemia (with concurrent sulfonylurea therapy 14% to 36%; frequency similar to placebo with metformin therapy)
Gastrointestinal: Nausea (44%), vomiting (13%), diarrhea (13%)
Miscellaneous: Anti-exenatide antibodies (low titers 38%, high titers 6%)
1% to 10%:
Central nervous system: Dizziness (9%), headache (9%)
Endocrine & metabolic: Appetite decreased
Gastrointestinal: Dyspepsia (6%), GERD
Neuromuscular & skeletal: Weakness
Miscellaneous: Feeling jittery (9%), diaphoresis increased

Pharmacodynamics/Kinetics
Time to Peak: SubQ: 2.1 hours
Half-Life Elimination: 2.4 hours
Metabolism: Minimal systemic metabolism; proteolytic degradation may occur following glomerular filtration
Excretion: Urine (majority of dose)
Available Dosage Forms Injection, solution [prefilled pen]: 250 mcg/mL (1.2 mL [provides 5 mcg/dose]; 2.4 mL [provides 10 mcg/dose])
Dosing
Adults & Elderly: Adjunctive therapy of type 2 diabetes: SubQ: Initial: 5 mcg twice daily within 60 minutes prior to a meal (morning and evening); after 1 month, may be increased to 10 mcg twice daily (based on response)
Renal Impairment:
Cl$_{cr}$ ≥30 mL/minute: No adjustment necessary.
Cl$_{cr}$ <30 mL/minute: Not recommended
Other: SubQ: Should be administered in the upper arm, thigh, or abdomen. Administer within 60 minutes prior to a meal (morning and evening).
Stability
Storage: Store under refrigeration at 2°C to 8°C (36°F to 46°F). Protect from light. Do not freeze (discard if

freezing occurs). Pen should be discarded 30 days after initial use
Laboratory Monitoring Serum glucose, hemoglobin A_{1c}, and renal function
Physical Assessment: Assess other prescription and OTC medications the patient may be taking to avoid duplications and interactions. Teach appropriate injection technique and disposal of needles. Assess knowledge/teach patient appropriate use, side effects, and symptoms to report.
Patient Education: Take as directed. Administer injection 30 minutes before meals. Do not administer after meal. Consume alcohol with caution; may cause hypoglycemia. It is important to follow dietary and lifestyle recommendations of prescriber. You may experience nausea (small, frequent meals, frequent oral care, sucking lozenges, or chewing gum may help), feeling jittery, dizziness, or lightheadedness (use caution when driving or engaging in activities requiring alertness until response to drug is known). Maintain adequate hydration (2-3 L/day) unless instructed to restrict intake by prescriber. Report persistent nausea, diarrhea, or dizziness. **Pregnancy/breast-feeding precautions:** Inform prescriber if you are or intend to become pregnant. Breast-feeding is not recommended
Additional Information A dosing strategy which employs progressive dose escalation of exenatide (initiating at 0.02 mcg/kg 3 times daily and increasing in increments of 0.02 mcg/kg every 3 days) has been described, limiting the frequency and severity of gastrointestinal adverse effects. The complexity of this regimen may limit its clinical application.

In animal models, exenatide has been a useful adjunctive therapy when added to immunotherapy protocols, resulting in recovery of beta cell function and sustained remission.

Ezetimibe (ez ET i mibe)

U.S. Brand Names Zetia™
Pharmacologic Category Antilipemic Agent, 2-Azetidinone
Medication Safety Issues
Sound-alike/look-alike issues:
Zetia™ may be confused with Zestril®
Pregnancy Risk Factor C
Lactation Excretion in breast milk unknown/not recommended
Use Use in combination with dietary therapy for the treatment of primary hypercholesterolemia (as monotherapy or in combination with HMG-CoA reductase inhibitors); homozygous sitosterolemia; homozygous familial hypercholesterolemia (in combination with atorvastatin or simvastatin)
Mechanism of Action/Effect Inhibits absorption of cholesterol at the brush border of the small intestine, leading to a decreased delivery of cholesterol to the liver, reduction of hepatic cholesterol stores and an increased clearance of cholesterol from the blood; decreases total C, LDL-C, ApoB, and triglycerides while increasing HDL-C
Contraindications Hypersensitivity to ezetimibe or any component of the formulation
Warnings/Precautions Secondary causes of hyperlipidemia should be ruled out prior to therapy. Use caution with renal or mild hepatic impairment; not recommended for use with moderate or severe hepatic impairment. Safety and efficacy have not been established in patients <10 years of age.
(Continued)

Ezetimibe *(Continued)*

Drug Interactions

Decreased Effect: Bile acid sequestrants may decrease ezetimibe bioavailability; administer ezetimibe ≥2 hours before or ≥4 hours after bile acid sequestrants.

Increased Effect/Toxicity: Cyclosporine may increase plasma levels of ezetimibe. Fibric acid derivatives may increase bioavailability of ezetimibe (safety and efficacy of concomitant use not established). Ezetimibe may increase serum levels of cyclosporine.

Adverse Reactions 1% to 10%:

Cardiovascular: Chest pain (3%), dizziness (3%), fatigue (2%)

Central nervous system: Headache (8%)

Gastrointestinal: Diarrhea (3% to 4%), abdominal pain (3%)

Neuromuscular & skeletal: Arthralgia (4%)

Respiratory: Sinusitis (4% to 5%), pharyngitis (2% to 3%, placebo 2%)

Overdosage/Toxicology Doses of up to 50 mg/day were well-tolerated. Treatment should be symptom-directed and supportive.

Pharmacodynamics/Kinetics

Time to Peak: Plasma: 4-12 hours

Protein Binding: >90% to plasma proteins

Half-Life Elimination: 22 hours (ezetimibe and metabolite)

Metabolism: Undergoes conjugation in the small intestine and liver; forms metabolite (active); may undergo enterohepatic recycling

Excretion: Feces (78%, 69% as ezetimibe); urine (11%, 9% as metabolite)

Available Dosage Forms Tablet: 10 mg [capsule shaped]

Dosing

Adults & Elderly:

Hyperlipidemias: Oral: 10 mg/day

Sitosterolemia: Oral: 10 mg/day

Pediatrics: Hyperlipidemias: Children ≥10 years: Refer to adult dosing.

Renal Impairment: Bioavailability increased with severe impairment; no dosing adjustment recommended.

Hepatic Impairment: Bioavailability increased with hepatic impairment

Mild impairment (Child-Pugh score 5-6): No dosing adjustment necessary.

Moderate to severe impairment (Child-Pugh score 7-15): Use of ezetimibe not recommended.

Administration

Oral: May be administered without regard to meals. May be taken at the same time as HMG-CoA reductase inhibitors. Administer ≥2 hours before or ≥4 hours after bile acid sequestrants.

Stability

Storage: Store at controlled room temperature of 15°C to 30°C (59°F to 86°F). Protect from moisture.

Laboratory Monitoring Total cholesterol profile prior to therapy, and when clinically indicated and/or periodically thereafter

Nursing Actions

Physical Assessment: Assess potential for interactions with other pharmacological agents or herbal products patient may be taking (eg, timing of concurrent medication). Monitor laboratory tests (lipid profile), therapeutic effectiveness, and adverse response at beginning of and at regular intervals during therapy. Teach patient proper use, possible side effects/appropriate interventions, and adverse reactions to report (eg, signs of hepatic, muscle, or pancreatic adverse reactions).

Patient Education: Do not take any new medication during therapy without consulting prescriber. Take at the same time of day, without regard for meals. Take 2 hours before or 4 hours after bile acid binding agents (ie, Questran®). This medication does not replace the need for dietary and exercise recommendations of prescriber. May cause headache, dizziness, or fatigue (use caution when driving or engaged in potentially hazardous tasks until response to drug is known); diarrhea (boiled milk, buttermilk, or yogurt may help); abdominal pain. Report any yellowing of skin or sclera; dark urine or pale stools; excessive tiredness; chest pain or palpitations; muscle, skeletal, or joint pain; twitching or numbness; increased perspiration; changes in urinary pattern; or other persistent side effects. **Pregnancy/breast-feeding precautions:** Inform prescriber if you are or intend to become pregnant. Breast-feeding is not recommended.

Dietary Considerations May be taken without regard to meals. Before initiation of therapy, patients should be placed on a standard cholesterol-lowering diet for 6 weeks and the diet should be continued during drug therapy.

Ezetimibe and Simvastatin

(ez ET i mibe & SIM va stat in)

U.S. Brand Names Vytorin™

Pharmacologic Category Antilipemic Agent, 2-Azetidinone; Antilipemic Agent, HMG-CoA Reductase Inhibitor

Pregnancy Risk Factor X

Lactation Excretion in breast milk unknown/contraindicated

Use Used in combination with dietary modification for the treatment of primary hypercholesterolemia and homozygous familial hypercholesterolemia

Available Dosage Forms Tablet:

10/10: Ezetimibe 10 mg and simvastatin 10 mg

10/20: Ezetimibe 10 mg and simvastatin 20 mg

10/40: Ezetimibe 10 mg and simvastatin 40 mg

10/80: Ezetimibe 10 mg and simvastatin 80 mg

Dosing

Adults & Elderly:

Homozygous familial hypercholesterolemia: Ezetimibe 10 mg and simvastatin 40 mg once daily or ezetimibe 10 mg and simvastatin 80 mg once daily in the evening

Hyperlipidemias: Oral: Initial: Ezetimibe 10 mg and simvastatin 20 mg once daily in the evening

Patients who require >55% reduction in LDL-C: Initial: Ezetimibe 10 mg and simvastatin 40 mg once daily

Dosage adjustment with concomitant medications: Oral:

Danazol or cyclosporine: Patient must first demonstrate tolerance to simvastatin ≥5 mg once daily. Dose should not exceed ezetimibe 10 mg and simvastatin 10 mg once daily.

Fibrates or niacin: Simvastatin dose should **not** exceed 10 mg/day.

Amiodarone or verapamil: Simvastatin dose should **not** exceed 20 mg/day.

Renal Impairment: Dosage adjustment unnecessary in mild to moderate renal dysfunction. In severe dysfunction, start only if patient tolerates 5 mg daily of simvastatin; monitor closely.

Hepatic Impairment: Dosage adjustment unnecessary in mild hepatic dysfunction.

Nursing Actions

Physical Assessment: See individual agents. **Pregnancy risk factor X** - determine that patient is not pregnant before starting therapy. Do not give to females of childbearing age unless patient is capable of complying with barrier contraceptive use. Breast-feeding is contraindicated.

Factor VIIa (Recombinant)
(FAK ter SEV en ree KOM be nant)

U.S. Brand Names NovoSeven®

Synonyms Coagulation Factor VIIa; Eptacog Alfa (Activated); rFVIIa

Pharmacologic Category Antihemophilic Agent; Blood Product Derivative

Medication Safety Issues
Sound-alike/look-alike issues:
NovoSeven® may be confused with Novacet®

Pregnancy Risk Factor C

Lactation Excretion in breast milk unknown/compatible

Use Treatment of bleeding episodes and prevention of bleeding in surgical interventions in patients with hemophilia A or B with inhibitors to factor VIII or factor IX and in patients with congenital factor VII deficiency

Mechanism of Action/Effect Promotes hemostasis by activating the extrinsic pathway of the coagulation cascade to promote formation of a fibrin-platelet hemostatic plug.

Contraindications Hypersensitivity to factor VII or any component of the formulation; hypersensitivity to mouse, hamster, or bovine proteins

Warnings/Precautions Patients should be monitored for signs and symptoms of activation of the coagulation system or thrombosis. Thrombotic events may be increased in patients with disseminated intravascular coagulation (DIC), advanced atherosclerotic disease, sepsis, crush injury, or concomitant treatment with prothrombin complex concentrates. Decreased dosage or discontinuation is warranted in confirmed DIC. Efficacy with prolonged infusions and data evaluating this agent's long-term adverse effects are limited.

Adverse Reactions 1% to 10%:
Cardiovascular: Hypertension
Central nervous system: Fever
Hematologic: Hemorrhage, decreased plasma fibrinogen
Neuromuscular & skeletal: Hemarthrosis

Overdosage/Toxicology Experience with overdose in humans is limited; an increased risk of thrombotic events may occur in overdosage. Treatment is symptomatic and supportive.

Pharmacodynamics/Kinetics
Half-Life Elimination: 2.3 hours (1.7-2.7)
Excretion: Clearance: 33 mL/kg/hour (27-49)

Available Dosage Forms Injection, powder for reconstitution [preservative free]: 1.2 mg, 2.4 mg, 4.8 mg [latex free; contains sodium 0.44 mEq/mg rFVIIa, polysorbate 80]

Dosing
Adults & Elderly: Hemophilia A or B with inhibitors: For I.V. administration only:
Bleeding episodes: 90 mcg/kg every 2 hours until hemostasis is achieved or until the treatment is judged ineffective. The dose and interval may be adjusted based upon the severity of bleeding and the degree of hemostasis achieved. For patients experiencing severe bleeds, dosing should be continued at 3- to 6-hour intervals after hemostasis has been achieved and the duration of dosing should be minimized.
Surgical interventions: 90 mcg/kg immediately before surgery, repeat at 2-hour intervals for the duration of surgery. Continue every 2 hours for 48 hours, then every 2-6 hours until healed for minor surgery; continue every 2 hours for 5 days, then every 4 hours until healed for major surgery.
Congenital factor VII deficiency: Bleeding episodes and surgical interventions: 15-30 mcg/kg every 4-6 hours until hemostasis. Doses as low as 10 mcg/kg have been effective.

Pediatrics: Refer to adult dosing.

Administration
I.V.: I.V. administration only; bolus over 2-5 minutes; administer within 3 hours after reconstitution
I.V. Detail: pH: 5.5

Stability
Reconstitution:
Prior to reconstitution, bring vials to room temperature. Reconstitute each vial to a final concentration of 0.6 mg/mL as follows:
1.2 mg vial: 2.2 mL sterile water
2.4 mg vial: 4.3 mL sterile water
4.8 mg vial: 8.5 mL sterile water
Add diluent along wall of vial, do not inject directly into powder. Gently swirl until dissolved.
Storage: Store under refrigeration (2°C to 8°C/36°F to 46°F). Protect from light. Reconstituted solutions may be stored at room temperature or under refrigeration, but must be infused within 3 hours of reconstitution.

Laboratory Monitoring Although the prothrombin time, aPTT, and factor VII clotting activity have no correlation with achieving hemostasis, these parameters may be useful as adjunct tests to evaluate efficacy and guide dose or interval adjustments

Nursing Actions
Physical Assessment: Assess potential for interactions with other pharmacological agents or herbal products patient may be taking that may affect coagulation or platelet function. Monitor patient closely (eg, vital signs, cardiac and CNS status, hemolytic status, hypersensitivity) during and after infusion. Provide patient education according to patient condition.
Patient Education: This medication can only be administered by infusion. Report immediately any swelling, pain, burning, or itching at infusion site. Report acute headache, visual changes, pain in joints or muscles, respiratory difficulty, chills, back pain, dizziness, nausea, or other unusual effects. **Pregnancy precaution:** Inform prescriber if you are or intend to become pregnant.

Dietary Considerations Contains sodium 0.44 mEq/mg rFVIIa

Famciclovir (fam SYE kloe veer)

U.S. Brand Names Famvir®

Pharmacologic Category Antiviral Agent

Pregnancy Risk Factor B

Lactation Excretion in breast milk unknown/use caution

Use Management of acute herpes zoster (shingles); treatment and suppression of recurrent episodes of genital herpes in immunocompetent patients; treatment of recurrent mucocutaneous/genital herpes simplex in HIV-infected patients

Mechanism of Action/Effect The prodrug famciclovir undergoes rapid biotransformation to the active compound, penciclovir, then intracellular conversion to triphosphate which is active against HSV-1, HSV-2, VZV, and EBV infected cells.

Contraindications Hypersensitivity to famciclovir, penciclovir, or any component of the formulation

Warnings/Precautions Has not been studied in immunocompromised patients or patients with ophthalmic or disseminated zoster. Dosage adjustment is required in patients with renal insufficiency and in patients with noncompensated hepatic disease. Tablets contain lactose; do not use with galactose intolerance, severe lactase deficiency, or glucose-galactose malabsorption syndromes. Safety and efficacy have not been established in children <18 years of age

Nutritional/Ethanol Interactions Food: Rate of absorption and/or conversion to penciclovir and peak concentration are reduced with food, but bioavailability is not affected.
(Continued)

Famciclovir *(Continued)*

Adverse Reactions
>10%:
Central nervous system: Headache (17% to 39%)
Gastrointestinal: Nausea (7% to 13%)
1% to 10%:
Central nervous system: Fatigue (4% to 6%), migraine (1% to 3%)
Dermatologic: Pruritus (1% to 4%), rash (<1% to 3%)
Endocrine and metabolic: Dysmenorrhea (up to 8%)
Gastrointestinal: Diarrhea (5% to 9%), flatulence (2% to 5%), vomiting (1% to 5%), abdominal pain (1% to 8%)
Hematologic: Neutropenia (3%), leukopenia (1%)
Hepatic: Transaminases increased (2% to 3%), bilirubin increased (2%)
Neuromuscular & skeletal: Paresthesia (1% to 3%)

Overdosage/Toxicology Supportive and symptomatic care is recommended. Hemodialysis may enhance elimination.

Pharmacodynamics/Kinetics
Time to Peak: 0.9 hours; C_{max} and T_{max} are decreased and prolonged with noncompensated hepatic impairment

Protein Binding: ≤20%

Half-Life Elimination: Penciclovir: 2-3 hours (10, 20, and 7 hours in HSV-1, HSV-2, and VZV-infected cells respectively); prolonged with renal impairment

Metabolism: Rapidly deacetylated and oxidized to penciclovir; not via CYP

Excretion: Urine (94% mostly as penciclovir)

Available Dosage Forms Tablet: 125 mg, 250 mg, 500 mg [contains lactose]

Dosing
Adults & Elderly:
Acute herpes zoster: Oral: 500 mg every 8 hours for 7 days (**Note:** Initiate therapy within 72 hours of rash onset.)

Recurrent genital herpes simplex in immunocompetent patients: Oral:
Initial: 125 mg twice daily for 5 days (**Note:** initiate therapy within 6 hours of symptoms/lesions.)
Suppressive therapy: 250 mg twice daily for up to 1 year

Recurrent mucocutaneous/genital herpes simplex in HIV patients: Oral: 500 mg twice daily for 7 days

Renal Impairment:
Herpes zoster:
Cl_{cr} 40-59 mL/minute: Administer 500 mg every 12 hours
Cl_{cr} 20-39 mL/minute: Administer 500 mg every 24 hours
Cl_{cr} <20 mL/minute: Administer 250 mg every 24 hours
Hemodialysis: Administer 250 mg after each dialysis session.
Recurrent genital herpes:
Cl_{cr} 20-39 mL/minute: Administer 125 mg every 24 hours
Cl_{cr} <20 mL/minute: Administer 125 mg every 24 hours
Hemodialysis: Administer 125 mg after each dialysis session.
Suppression of recurrent genital herpes:
Cl_{cr} 20-39 mL/minute: Administer 125 mg every 12 hours
Cl_{cr} <20 mL/minute: Administer 125 mg every 24 hours
Hemodialysis: Administer 125 mg after each dialysis session.
Recurrent orolabial or genital herpes in HIV-infected patients:
Cl_{cr} 20-39 mL/minute: Administer 500 mg every 24 hours
Cl_{cr} <20 mL/minute: Administer 250 mg every 24 hours
Hemodialysis: Administer 250 mg after each dialysis session.

Laboratory Monitoring Periodic CBC during long-term therapy

Nursing Actions
Physical Assessment: Assess potential for interactions with other pharmacological agents the patient may be taking. Monitor therapeutic effectiveness according to purpose for use and adverse response (eg, persistent fatigue, gastrointestinal upset). Teach patient proper use, possible side effects/appropriate interventions, and adverse symptoms to report.

Patient Education: Take for prescribed length of time, even if condition improves. Do not discontinue without consulting prescriber. This is not a cure for genital herpes. May cause mild GI disturbances (eg, nausea, vomiting, constipation, diarrhea), fatigue, headache, or muscle aches and pains. If these are severe, contact prescriber. **Breast-feeding precaution:** Do not breast-feed.

Dietary Considerations May be taken with food or on an empty stomach.

Geriatric Considerations For herpes zoster (shingles) infections, famciclovir should be started within 72 hours of the appearance of the rash to be effective. Famciclovir has been shown to accelerate healing, reduce the duration of viral shedding, and resolve posthepatic neuralgia faster than placebo. Comparison trials to acyclovir or valacyclovir are not available. Adjust dose for estimated renal function.

Breast-Feeding Issues There is no specific data describing the excretion of famciclovir in breast milk. Breast feeding should be avoided if herpes lesions are on breast in order to avoid transmission to infant.

Pregnancy Issues There are no adequate and well-controlled studies in pregnant women. Use only if benefit outweighs risk. A registry has been established for women exposed to famciclovir during pregnancy (888-669-6682).

Additional Information Most effective for herpes zoster if therapy is initiated within 48 hours of initial lesion. Resistance may occur by alteration of thymidine kinase, resulting in loss of or reduced penciclovir phosphorylation (cross-resistance occurs between acyclovir and famciclovir).

Famotidine *(fa MOE ti deen)*

U.S. Brand Names Fluxid™; Pepcid®; Pepcid® AC [OTC]

Pharmacologic Category Histamine H_2 Antagonist

Pregnancy Risk Factor B

Lactation Enters breast milk/not recommended

Use Therapy and treatment of duodenal ulcer, gastric ulcer, control gastric pH in critically-ill patients, symptomatic relief in gastritis, gastroesophageal reflux, active benign ulcer, and pathological hypersecretory conditions
OTC labeling: Relief of heartburn, acid indigestion, and sour stomach

Unlabeled/Investigational Use Part of a multidrug regimen for *H. pylori* eradication to reduce the risk of duodenal ulcer recurrence

Mechanism of Action/Effect Competitive inhibition of histamine at H_2 receptors of the gastric parietal cells, which inhibits gastric acid secretion

Contraindications Hypersensitivity to famotidine, other H_2 antagonists, or any component of the formulation

Warnings/Precautions Modify dose in patients with renal impairment; chewable tablets contain phenylalanine; multidose vials contain benzyl alcohol

OTC labeling: When used for self-medication, patients should be instructed not to use if they have difficulty swallowing, have vomiting with blood, or bloody or black stools. Not for use with other acid reducers.

Drug Interactions

Decreased Effect: Decreased serum levels of ketoconazole and itraconazole (reduced absorption).

Nutritional/Ethanol Interactions

Ethanol: Avoid ethanol (may cause gastric mucosal irritation).

Food: Famotidine bioavailability may be increased if taken with food.

Adverse Reactions

Note: Agitation and vomiting have been reported in up to 14% of pediatric patients <1 year of age.

1% to 10%:

Central nervous system: Dizziness (1%), headache (5%)

Gastrointestinal: Constipation (1%), diarrhea (2%)

Overdosage/Toxicology Symptoms of overdose include hypotension, tachycardia, vomiting, and drowsiness. Treatment is symptomatic and supportive.

Pharmacodynamics/Kinetics

Onset of Action: GI: Oral: Within 1-3 hour

Duration of Action: 10-12 hours

Time to Peak: Serum: Oral: ~1-3 hours

Protein Binding: 15% to 20%

Half-Life Elimination:

Injection, oral suspension, tablet: 2.5-3.5 hours; prolonged with renal impairment; Oliguria: 20 hours

Orally-disintegrating tablet: 2.5-5 hours

Excretion: Urine (as unchanged drug)

Available Dosage Forms [DSC] = Discontinued product

Gelcap (Pepcid® AC): 10 mg

Infusion [premixed in NS] (Pepcid®): 20 mg (50 mL)

Injection, solution: 10 mg/mL (4 mL, 20 mL, 50 mL) [contains benzyl alcohol]

Pepcid®: 10 mg/mL (4 mL [DSC], 20 mL)

Injection, solution [preservative free] (Pepcid®): 10 mg/mL (2 mL)

Powder for oral suspension (Pepcid®): 40 mg/5 mL (50 mL) [contains sodium benzoate; cherry-banana-mint flavor]

Tablet: 10 mg [OTC], 20 mg, 40 mg

Pepcid®: 20 mg, 40 mg

Pepcid® AC: 10 mg, 20 mg

Tablet, chewable (Pepcid® AC): 10 mg [contains phenylalanine 1.4 mg/tablet; mint flavor]

Tablet, orally disintegrating (Fluxid™): 20 mg, 40 mg [cherry flavor]

Dosing

Adults & Elderly:

Duodenal ulcer: Oral: Acute therapy: 40 mg/day at bedtime for 4-8 weeks; maintenance therapy: 20 mg/day at bedtime

Gastric ulcer: Oral: Acute therapy: 40 mg/day at bedtime

Hypersecretory conditions: Oral: Initial: 20 mg every 6 hours, may increase in increments up to 160 mg every 6 hours

GERD: Oral: 20 mg twice daily for 6 weeks

Esophagitis and accompanying symptoms due to GERD: Oral: 20 mg or 40 mg twice daily for up to 12 weeks

Peptic ulcer disease: Eradication of *Helicobacter pylori* (unlabeled use): Oral: 40 mg once daily; requires combination therapy with antibiotics

Patients unable to take oral medication: I.V.: 20 mg every 12 hours

Heartburn, indigestion, sour stomach: OTC labeling: Oral: 10-20 mg every 12 hours; dose may be taken 15-60 minutes before eating foods known to cause heartburn

Pediatrics: Treatment duration and dose should be individualized

Peptic ulcer: 1-16 years:

Oral: 0.5 mg/kg/day at bedtime or divided twice daily (maximum dose: 40 mg/day); doses of up to 1 mg/kg/day have been used in clinical studies

I.V.: 0.25 mg/kg every 12 hours (maximum dose: 40 mg/day); doses of up to 0.5 mg/kg have been used in clinical studies

GERD: Oral:

<3 months: 0.5 mg/kg once daily

3-12 months: 0.5 mg/kg twice daily

1-16 years: 1 mg/kg/day divided twice daily (maximum dose: 40 mg twice daily); doses of up to 2 mg/kg/day have been used in clinical studies

Heartburn, indigestion, sour stomach: OTC labeling: Oral: Children ≥12 years: Refer to adult dosing.

Renal Impairment: Cl$_{cr}$ <50 mL/minute: Manufacturer recommendation: Administer 50% of dose **or** increase the dosing interval to every 36-48 hours (to limit potential CNS adverse effects).

Administration

Oral:

Suspension: Shake vigorously before use. May be taken with or without food.

Tablet: May be taken with or without food.

Orally-disintegrating tablet: Place tablet on tongue with dry hands; tablet dissolves rapidly in saliva. May be taken with or without liquid or food. Do not break tablet.

I.V.:

I.V. push: Inject over at least 2 minutes

Solution for infusion: Administer over 15-30 minutes

I.V. Detail: pH: 5.7-6.4 (premixed solution); 5.0-5.6 (injection)

Stability

Reconstitution: Solution for injection:

I.V. push: Dilute famotidine with NS (or another compatible solution) to a total of 5-10 mL (some centers also administer undiluted).

Infusion: Dilute with D$_5$W 100 mL or another compatible solution.

Compatibility: Stable in D$_5$W, D$_{10}$W, LR, fat emulsion 10%, NS, sodium bicarbonate 5%

Y-site administration: Incompatible with alatrofloxacin, amphotericin B cholesteryl sulfate complex, cefepime, piperacillin/tazobactam

Storage:

Oral:

Powder for oral suspension: Prior to mixing, dry powder should be stored at room temperature of 25°C (77°F). Reconstituted oral suspension is stable for 30-days at room temperature. Do not freeze.

Tablet: Store at 20°C (77°F); excursions permitted between 15°C to 30°C (59°F to 86°F). Protect from moisture.

Orally-disintegrating tablet: Store at 20°C to 25°C (68°F to 77°F); excursions permitted between 15°C to 30°C (59°F to 86°F). Protect from moisture.

I.V.:

Solution for injection: Prior to use, store at 2°C to 8°C (36°F to 46°F). If solution freezes, allow to solubilize at room temperature.

I.V. push: Following reconstitution, solutions for I.V. push should be used immediately, or may be stored in refrigerator and used within 48 hours.

Infusion: Following reconstitution, solutions for infusion are stable for 7 days at room temperature.

Solution for injection, premixed bags: Store at room temperature of 25°C (77°F). Avoid excessive heat.

Nursing Actions

Physical Assessment: Monitor patient response on a regular basis throughout therapy. See Administration for I.V. specifics. Teach patient proper use, possible (Continued)

Famotidine *(Continued)*

side effects/appropriate interventions and adverse symptoms to report.

Patient Education: Do not take any new medication during therapy without consulting prescriber. Take as directed; do not alter dose or frequency or discontinue without consulting prescriber. May cause some drowsiness or dizziness (use caution when driving or engaging in tasks that require alertness until response to drug is known); constipation (increased exercise, fluids, fruit, or fiber may help); or diarrhea (buttermilk, boiled milk, or yogurt may help). Report acute headache, unresolved constipation or diarrhea, palpitations, vomiting with blood, black tarry stools, abdominal pain, rash, worsening of condition being treated, or recurrence of symptoms after therapy is completed.

Orally-disintegrating tablet: Do not break tablet.

Oral suspension: Shake well before use.

OTC: Do not use for more than 14 days unless recommended by prescriber.

Breast-feeding precaution: Breast-feeding is not recommended.

Dietary Considerations Phenylalanine content: Pepcid® AC chewable: Each 10 mg tablet contains phenylalanine 1.4 mg

Geriatric Considerations H₂ blockers are the preferred drugs for treating PUD in the elderly due to cost and ease of administration. They are no less or more effective than any other therapy. Famotidine is one of the preferred agents (due to side effects, drug interaction profile, and pharmacokinetics). Treatment for PUD in the elderly is recommended for 12 weeks since their lesions are typically larger; therefore, take longer to heal. Always adjust dose based upon creatinine clearance, since slight accumulation may result in CNS side effects, mainly confusion.

Breast-Feeding Issues Famotidine is concentrated in breast milk, but to a lesser degree than cimetidine or ranitidine; some sources prefer its use if one of these agents is needed.

Fat Emulsion *(fat e MUL shun)*

U.S. Brand Names Intralipid®; Liposyn® III
Synonyms Intravenous Fat Emulsion
Pharmacologic Category Caloric Agent
Pregnancy Risk Factor C
Lactation Excretion in breast milk unknown/compatible
Use Source of calories and essential fatty acids for patients requiring parenteral nutrition of extended duration
Mechanism of Action/Effect Essential for normal structure and function of cell membranes
Contraindications Hypersensitivity to fat emulsion or any component of the formulation; severe egg or legume (soybean) allergies; pathologic hyperlipidemia, lipoid nephrosis pancreatis with hyperlipemia
Warnings/Precautions Use caution in patients with severe liver damage, pulmonary disease, anemia, or blood coagulation disorder; use with caution in jaundiced, premature, and low birth weight children. Some formulations may contain aluminum which may accumulate following prolonged administration in renally-impaired patients. Premature neonates are particularly at risk of accumulation/toxicity from aluminum. To avoid hyperlipidemia and/or fat deposition, do not exceed recommended daily doses.
Adverse Reactions Frequency not defined.
Cardiovascular: Cyanosis, flushing, chest pain
Central nervous system: Headache, dizziness

Endocrine & metabolic: Hyperlipemia, hypertriglyceridemia
Gastrointestinal: Nausea, vomiting, diarrhea
Hematologic: Hypercoagulability, thrombocytopenia in neonates (rare)
Hepatic: Hepatomegaly, pancreatitis
Local: Thrombophlebitis
Respiratory: Dyspnea
Miscellaneous: Sepsis, diaphoresis, brown pigment deposition in the reticuloendothelial system (significance unknown)

Overdosage/Toxicology Rapid administration results in fluid or fat overload causing dilution of serum electrolytes, overhydration, pulmonary edema, impaired pulmonary diffusion capacity, and metabolic acidosis. Treatment is supportive.

Pharmacodynamics/Kinetics
Half-Life Elimination: 0.5-1 hour
Metabolism: Undergoes lipolysis to free fatty acids which are utilized by reticuloendothelial cells
Available Dosage Forms Injection, emulsion [soybean oil]:
Intralipid®: 10% [100 mg/mL] (100 mL, 250 mL, 500 mL); 20% [200 mg/mL] (50 mL, 100 mL, 250 mL, 500 mL, 1000 mL); 30% [300 mg/mL] (500 mL)
Liposyn® III: 10% [100 mg/mL] (200 mL, 500 mL); 20% [200 mg/mL] (200 mL, 500 mL); 30% [300 mg/mL] (500 mL)

Dosing
Adults & Elderly:
Caloric source: I.V. (fat emulsion should not exceed 60% of the total daily calories): Initial: 1 g/kg/day, increase by 0.5-1 g/kg/day to a maximum of 2.5 g/kg/day of 10% and 3 g/kg/day of 20%; maximum rate of infusion: 0.25 g/kg/hour (1.25 mL/kg/hour of 20% solution); do not exceed 50 mL/hour (20%) or 100 mL/hour (10%)
Prevention of fatty acid deficiency (8% to 10% of total caloric intake): I.V.: 0.5-1 g/kg/24 hours
500 mL twice weekly at rate of 1 mL/minute for 30 minutes, then increase to 500 mL over 4-6 hours
Note: May be used on a daily basis as a caloric source in TPN
Pediatrics:
Caloric source: I.V. (fat emulsion should not exceed 60% of the total daily calories):
Premature Infants: Initial dose: 0.25-0.5 g/kg/day, increase by 0.25-0.5 g/kg/day to a maximum of 3 g/kg/day depending on needs/nutritional goals; limit to 1 g/kg/day if on phototherapy; maximum rate of infusion: 0.15 g/kg/hour (0.75 mL/kg/hour of 20% solution)
Infants and Children: Initial dose: 0.5-1 g/kg/day, increase by 0.5 g/kg/day to a maximum of 3 g/kg/day depending on needs/nutritional goals; maximum rate of infusion: 0.25 g/kg/hour (1.25 mL/kg/hour of 20% solution)
Adolescents: Refer to adult dosing.
Prevention of essential fatty acid deficiency (8% to 10% of total caloric intake): I.V.: 0.5-1 g/kg/24 hours
Children: 5-10 mL/kg/day at 0.1 mL/minute then up to 100 mL/hour

Administration
I.V.: At the onset of therapy, the patient should be observed for any immediate allergic reactions such as dyspnea, cyanosis, and fever. Infuse for 10-15 minutes at a slower rate. Infuse 10% at 1 mL/minute. If no untoward effects, may increase rate to 500 mL over 4-6 hours. Infuse 20% at 0.5 mL/minute initially; increase to rate of 250 mL over 4-6 hours.
I.V. Detail: Change tubing after each infusion. May be simultaneously infused with amino acid dextrose mixtures by means of Y-connector located near infusion site. Hang fat emulsion higher than other fluids (has low specific gravity and could run up into other

lines). Infuse via pump using either peripheral or central venous line. Do not use filter in line.

Stability

Storage: May be stored at room temperature. Do not store partly used bottles for later use. Do not use if emulsion appears to be oiling out.

Laboratory Monitoring Serum triglycerides before initiation of therapy and at least weekly during therapy. Frequent (some advise daily) platelet counts should be performed in neonatal patients receiving parenteral lipids.

Nursing Actions

Physical Assessment: Assess for allergy to eggs prior to initiating therapy (pruritic urticaria can occur in patients allergic to eggs). Inspect emulsion before administering. Do not administer if oil separation or oiliness is noted. Monitor closely for allergic reactions, fluid overload, thrombosis or sepsis.

Patient Education: Report pain at infusion site, respiratory difficulty, chest pain, calf pain, or excessive sweating. **Pregnancy precaution:** Inform prescriber if you are pregnant

---

Felbamate (FEL ba mate)

U.S. Brand Names Felbatol®

Restrictions A patient "informed consent" form should be completed and signed by the patient and physician. Copies are available from Wallace Pharmaceuticals by calling 609-655-6147.

Pharmacologic Category Anticonvulsant, Miscellaneous

Pregnancy Risk Factor C

Lactation Enters breast milk/not recommended

Use Not as a first-line antiepileptic treatment; only in those patients who respond inadequately to alternative treatments and whose epilepsy is so severe that a substantial risk of aplastic anemia and/or liver failure is deemed acceptable in light of the benefits conferred by its use. Patient must be fully advised of risk and provide signed written informed consent. Felbamate can be used as either monotherapy or adjunctive therapy in the treatment of partial seizures (with and without generalization) and in adults with epilepsy.

Orphan drug: Adjunctive therapy in the treatment of partial and generalized seizures associated with Lennox-Gastaut syndrome in children

Mechanism of Action/Effect Mechanism of action is unknown but has properties in common with other marketed anticonvulsants. Has weak inhibitory effects on GABA-receptor binding, benzodiazepine receptor binding, and is devoid of activity at the MK-801 receptor binding site of the NMDA receptor-ionophore complex.

Contraindications Hypersensitivity to felbamate or any component of the formulation; use with caution in those patients who have demonstrated hypersensitivity reactions to other carbamates

Warnings/Precautions Use with caution in patients allergic to other carbamates (eg, meprobamate). Antiepileptic drugs should not be suddenly discontinued because of the possibility of increasing seizure frequency. **Reported 10 cases of aplastic anemia in the U.S. after 2 1/2 to 6 months of therapy.** Carter Wallace and the FDA recommended the use of this agent be suspended unless withdrawal of the product would place a patient at greater risk as compared to the frequently fatal form of anemia. Felbamate has also been associated with rare cases of hepatic failure (estimated >6 cases per 75,000 patients per year). Use caution in renal impairment (dose adjustment recommended). "Informed consent" (concerning hematological/hepatic risks) should be documented prior to initiation of therapy.

Drug Interactions

Cytochrome P450 Effect: Substrate of CYP2E1 (minor), 3A4 (major); **Inhibits** CYP2C19 (weak); **Induces** CYP3A4 (weak)

Decreased Effect: Felbamate may decrease carbamazepine levels and increase levels of the active metabolite of carbamazepine (10,11-epoxide) resulting in carbamazepine toxicity; monitor for signs of carbamazepine toxicity (dizziness, ataxia, nystagmus, drowsiness). CYP3A4 inducers may decrease the levels/effects of felbamate; example inducers include aminoglutethimide, carbamazepine, nafcillin, nevirapine, phenobarbital, phenytoin, and rifamycins.

Increased Effect/Toxicity: Felbamate increases serum phenytoin, phenobarbital, and valproic acid concentrations which may result in toxicity; consider decreasing phenytoin or phenobarbital dosage by 25%. A decrease in valproic acid dosage may also be necessary. CYP3A4 inhibitors may increase the levels/effects of felbamate; example inhibitors include azole antifungals, clarithromycin, diclofenac, doxycycline, erythromycin, imatinib, isoniazid, nefazodone, nicardipine, propofol, protease inhibitors, quinidine, telithromycin, and verapamil.

Nutritional/Ethanol Interactions

Ethanol: Avoid ethanol (may increase CNS depression).

Food: Food does not affect absorption.

Herb/Nutraceutical: Avoid evening primrose (seizure threshold decreased).

Lab Interactions Blood urea nitrogen is slightly lower (1.25 mg/dL). May cause slightly elevated serum cholesterol level (about 7 mg/dL) in patients receiving about 2.6 g/day.

Adverse Reactions

>10%:

 Central nervous system: Somnolence, headache, fatigue, dizziness

 Gastrointestinal: Nausea, anorexia, vomiting, constipation

1% to 10%:

 Cardiovascular: Chest pain, palpitation, tachycardia

 Central nervous system: Depression or behavior changes, nervousness, anxiety, ataxia, stupor, malaise, agitation, psychological disturbances, aggressive reaction

 Dermatologic: Skin rash, acne, pruritus

 Gastrointestinal: Xerostomia, diarrhea, abdominal pain, weight gain, taste perversion

 Neuromuscular & skeletal: Tremor, abnormal gait, paresthesia, myalgia

 Ocular: Diplopia, abnormal vision

 Respiratory: Sinusitis, pharyngitis

 Miscellaneous: ALT increase

Overdosage/Toxicology Symptoms of overdose include sedation, gastrointestinal upset, and tachycardia. Provide general supportive care.

Pharmacodynamics/Kinetics

Time to Peak: Serum: ~3 hours

Protein Binding: 22% to 25%, primarily to albumin

Half-Life Elimination: 20-23 hours (average); prolonged in renal dysfunction

Excretion: Urine (40% to 50% as unchanged drug, 40% as inactive metabolites)

Available Dosage Forms

Suspension, oral: 600 mg/5 mL (240 mL, 960 mL)

Tablet: 400 mg, 600 mg

Dosing

Adults & Elderly:

Anticonvulsant, monotherapy: Oral:

Initial: 1200 mg/day in divided doses 3 or 4 times/ day; titrate previously untreated patients under close clinical supervision, increasing the dosage in 600 mg increments every 2 weeks to 2400 mg/ day based on clinical response and thereafter to 3600 mg/day as clinically indicated

(Continued)

Felbamate (Continued)

Conversion to monotherapy: Initiate at 1200 mg/day in divided doses 3 or 4 times/day, reduce the dosage of the concomitant anticonvulsant(s) by 20% to 33% at the initiation of felbamate therapy; at week 2, increase the felbamate dosage to 2400 mg/day while reducing the dosage of the other anticonvulsant(s) up to an additional 33% of their original dosage; at week 3, increase the felbamate dosage up to 3600 mg/day and continue to reduce the dosage of the other anticonvulsant(s) as clinically indicated

Pediatrics:

Anticonvulsant, monotherapy: Oral: Children >14 years: Refer to adult dosing.

Adjunctive therapy, Lennox-Gastaut (ages 2-14 years): Oral:

Week 1: Felbamate: 15 mg/kg/day divided 3-4 times/day

Concomitant anticonvulsant(s): Reduce original dosage by 20% to 30%.

Week 2: Felbamate: 30 mg/kg/day divided 3-4 times/day

Concomitant anticonvulsant(s): Reduce original dosage up to an additional 33%.

Week 3: Felbamate: 45 mg/kg/day divided 3-4 times/day

Concomitant anticonvulsant(s): Reduce dosage as clinically indicated.

Adjunctive therapy: Children >14 years and Adults:

Week 1: Felbamate: 1200 mg/day initial dose

Concomitant anticonvulsant(s): Reduce original dosage by 20% to 33%.

Week 2: Felbamate: 2400 mg/day (therapeutic range)

Concomitant anticonvulsant(s): Reduce original dosage by up to an additional 33%.

Week 3: Felbamate: 3600 mg/day (therapeutic range)

Concomitant anticonvulsant(s): Reduce original dosage as clinically indicated.

Renal Impairment: Use caution; reduce initial and maintenance doses by 50% (half-life prolonged by 9-15 hours)

Administration

Oral: Administer on an empty stomach for best absorption.

Stability

Storage: Store medication in tightly closed container at room temperature away from excessive heat.

Laboratory Monitoring Monitor serum levels of concomitant anticonvulsant therapy; monitor AST, ALT, and bilirubin on a weekly basis. Hematologic evaluations before therapy begins, frequently during therapy, and for a significant period after discontinuation.

Nursing Actions

Physical Assessment: Assess effectiveness and interactions of other medications patient may be taking. Monitor therapeutic response (seizure activity, force, type, duration), laboratory values, and adverse reactions at beginning of therapy and periodically with long-term use. Taper dosage slowly when discontinuing. Use and teach seizure/safety precautions. Assess knowledge/teach patient appropriate use, interventions to reduce side effects, and adverse symptoms to report.

Patient Education: Take exactly as directed; do not increase dose or frequency or discontinue without consulting prescriber. While using this medication, do not use alcohol and other prescription or OTC medications (especially pain medications, sedatives, antihistamines, or hypnotics) without consulting prescriber. Maintain adequate hydration (2-3 L/day of fluids) unless instructed to restrict fluid intake. You may experience drowsiness, dizziness, or blurred vision (use caution when driving or engaging in tasks requiring alertness until response to drug is known); or nausea, vomiting, loss of appetite, or dry mouth (small frequent meals, frequent mouth care, chewing gum, or sucking lozenges may help). Wear identification of epileptic status and medications. Report CNS changes, mentation changes, or changes in cognition; muscle cramping, weakness, tremors, changes in gait; persistent GI symptoms (cramping, constipation, vomiting, anorexia); rash or skin irritations; unusual bruising or bleeding (mouth, urine, stool); cough, runny nose, sore throat, or respiratory difficulty; or worsening of seizure activity or loss of seizure control. **Pregnancy/breast-feeding precautions:** Inform prescriber if you are or intend to become pregnant. Breast-feeding is not recommended.

Dietary Considerations May be taken without regard to meals.

Geriatric Considerations Clinical studies have not included large numbers of patients >65 years of age. Due to decreased hepatic and renal function, dosing should start at the lower end of the dosage range.

Additional Information Monotherapy has not been associated with gingival hyperplasia, impaired concentration, weight gain, or abnormal thinking. Because felbamate is the only drug shown effective in Lennox-Gastaut syndrome, it is considered an orphan drug for this indication.

Felodipine (fe LOE di peen)

U.S. Brand Names Plendil®

Pharmacologic Category Calcium Channel Blocker

Medication Safety Issues

Sound-alike/look-alike issues:

Plendil® may be confused with Isordil®, pindolol, Pletal®, Prilosec®, Prinivil®

Pregnancy Risk Factor C

Lactation Excretion in breast milk unknown/not recommended

Use Treatment of hypertension

Mechanism of Action/Effect Inhibits calcium ions from entering the "slow channels" or select voltage-sensitive areas of vascular smooth muscle and myocardium during depolarization

Contraindications Hypersensitivity to felodipine, any component of the formulation, or other calcium channel blocker

Warnings/Precautions Use caution in patients with heart failure particularly with concurrent beta-blocker use. Elderly patients and patients with hepatic impairment should start off with a lower dose. Peripheral edema is the most common side effect (occurs within 2-3 weeks of starting therapy). May cause reflex tachycardia, hypotension, or syncope (rare). Use caution in hepatic impairment. Safety and efficacy in children have not been established. Dosage titration should occur after 14 days on a given dose.

Drug Interactions

Cytochrome P450 Effect: Substrate of CYP3A4 (major); **Inhibits** CYP2C8/9 (weak), 2D6 (weak), 3A4 (weak)

Decreased Effect: Felodipine may decrease pharmacologic actions of theophylline. Calcium may reduce the calcium channel blocker's effects, particularly hypotension. Felodipine may decrease pharmacologic actions of theophylline. CYP3A4 inducers may decrease the levels/effects of felodipine; example inducers include aminoglutethimide, carbamazepine, nafcillin, nevirapine, phenobarbital, phenytoin, and rifamycins.

Increased Effect/Toxicity: CYP3A4 inhibitors may increase the levels/effects of felodipine; example inhibitors include azole antifungals, clarithromycin, diclofenac, doxycycline, erythromycin, imatinib, isoniazid, nefazodone, nicardipine, propofol, protease inhibitors, quinidine, telithromycin, and verapamil. Beta-blockers may have increased pharmacokinetic or pharmacodynamic interactions with felodipine. Cyclosporine increases felodipine's serum concentration. Blood pressure-lowering effects may be additive with sildenafil, tadalafil, and vardenafil (use caution). Felodipine may increase tacrolimus serum levels (monitor).

Nutritional/Ethanol Interactions
Ethanol: Increases felodipine's absorption; watch for a greater hypotensive effect.
Food: Increased therapeutic and vasodilator side effects, including severe hypotension and myocardial ischemia, may occur if felodipine is taken with grapefruit juice; avoid concurrent use. High-fat/carbohydrate meals will increase C_{max} by 60%; grapefruit juice will increase C_{max} by twofold.
Herb/Nutraceutical: St John's wort may decrease felodipine levels. Avoid dong quai if using for hypertension (has estrogenic activity). Avoid ephedra, yohimbe, ginseng (may worsen hypertension). Avoid garlic (may have increased antihypertensive effect).

Adverse Reactions
>10%: Central nervous system: Headache (11% to 15%)
2% to 10%: Cardiovascular: Peripheral edema (2% to 17%), tachycardia (0.4% to 2.5%), flushing (4% to 7%)

Overdosage/Toxicology Primary cardiac symptoms of calcium blocker overdose include hypotension and bradycardia. Noncardiac symptoms include confusion, stupor, nausea, vomiting, metabolic acidosis, and hyperglycemia. Treat symptomatically.

Pharmacodynamics/Kinetics
Onset of Action: Antihypertensive: 2-5 hours
Duration of Action: Antihypertensive effect: 24 hours
Protein Binding: >99%
Half-Life Elimination: Immediate release: 11-16 hours
Metabolism: Hepatic; CYP3A4 substrate (major); extensive first-pass effect
Excretion: Urine (70% as metabolites); feces 10%
Available Dosage Forms Tablet, extended release: 2.5 mg, 5 mg, 10 mg

Dosing
Adults: Hypertension: Oral: 5-10 mg once daily; increase by 5 mg at 2-week intervals, as needed, to a maximum of 20 mg/day; usual dose range (JNC 7): 2.5-20 mg once daily.
Elderly: Oral: Initial 2.5 mg/day
Hepatic Impairment: Initial: 2.5 mg/day; monitor blood pressure

Administration
Oral: Do not crush or chew extended release tablets; swallow whole.

Nursing Actions
Physical Assessment: Assess potential for interactions with pharmacological agents or herbal products patient may be taking (eg, beta blockers or other drugs that effect blood pressure). Assess for therapeutic effectiveness and signs/symptoms of adverse reactions at beginning of therapy, when changing dosage, and periodically throughout long-term therapy. When discontinuing, taper gradually (over 2 weeks). Teach patient proper use, possible side effects/interventions, and adverse symptoms to report.
Patient Education: Do not take any new medication during therapy unless approved by prescriber. Take exactly as directed, without food. Avoid concurrent grapefruit juice and alcohol (may cause dangerous hypotension). Swallow whole, do not crush or chew. Do not alter dose or stop taking without consulting prescriber. May cause headache (consult prescriber

for analgesic); nausea or vomiting (small, frequent meals, frequent mouth care, chewing gum, or sucking lozenges may help); constipation (increased dietary bulk and fluids may help); or drowsiness (use caution when driving or engaging in tasks that require alertness until response to drug is known). Report irregular heartbeat, chest pain or palpitations; persistent headache; vomiting; constipation; peripheral or facial swelling; weight gain >5 lb/week; dyspnea or respiratory changes. **Pregnancy/breast-feeding precautions:** Inform prescriber if you are or intend to become pregnant. Consult prescriber if breast-feeding.

Dietary Considerations Should be taken without food.
Geriatric Considerations Elderly may experience a greater hypotensive response. Theoretically, constipation may be more of a problem in the elderly.
Pregnancy Issues Potentially, calcium channel blockers may prolong labor. There are no adequate or well-controlled studies in pregnant women.
Additional Information Felodipine maintains renal and mesenteric blood flow during hemorrhagic shock in animals.

Fenofibrate (fen oh FYE brate)

U.S. Brand Names Antara™; Lipofen™; Lofibra™; TriCor®; Triglide™
Synonyms Procetofene; Proctofene
Pharmacologic Category Antilipemic Agent, Fibric Acid
Pregnancy Risk Factor C
Lactation Excretion in breast milk unknown/not recommended
Use Adjunct to dietary therapy for the treatment of adults with elevations of serum triglyceride levels (types IV and V hyperlipidemia); adjunct to dietary therapy for the reduction of low density lipoprotein cholesterol (LDL-C), total cholesterol (total-C), triglycerides, and apolipoprotein B (apo B) in adult patients with primary hypercholesterolemia or mixed dyslipidemia (Fredrickson types IIa and IIb)
Mechanism of Action/Effect Fenofibric acid is believed to increase VLDL catabolism by enhancing the synthesis of lipoprotein lipase; as a result of a decrease in VLDL levels, total plasma triglycerides are reduced by 30% to 60%. Modest increase in HDL occurs in some hypertriglyceridemic patients.
Contraindications Hypersensitivity to fenofibrate or any component of the formulation; hepatic or severe renal dysfunction including primary biliary cirrhosis and unexplained persistent liver function abnormalities; pre-existing gallbladder disease
Warnings/Precautions Hepatic transaminases can become significantly elevated (dose-related); hepatocellular, chronic active, and cholestatic hepatitis have been reported. Regular monitoring of liver function tests is required. May cause cholelithiasis. Use caution with warfarin; adjustments in warfarin therapy may be required. Use caution with HMG-CoA reductase inhibitors (may lead to myopathy, rhabdomyolysis). Therapy should be withdrawn if an adequate response is not obtained after 2 months of therapy at the maximal daily dose. May cause mild to moderate decreases in hemoglobin, hematocrit and WBC upon initiation of therapy which usually stabilizes with long-term therapy. Rare hypersensitivity reactions may occur. Dose adjustment is required for renal impairment and elderly patients. Safety and efficacy in children have not been established.

Drug Interactions
Cytochrome P450 Effect: Substrate of CYP3A4 (minor); **Inhibits** CYP2A6 (weak), 2C8 (moderate), 2C9 (moderate), 2C19 weak
(Continued)

Fenofibrate *(Continued)*

Decreased Effect: Bile acid sequestrants may decrease absorption of fenofibrate (separate administration).

Increased Effect/Toxicity: Fenofibrate may increase the effects of sulfonylureas and warfarin. Concurrent use of fenofibrate with HMG-CoA reductase inhibitors may increase the risk of myopathy and rhabdomyolysis. Ezetimibe's serum concentration may be increased with concurrent use. Fenofibrate may increase the levels/effects of CYP2C8 substrates (example substrates include amiodarone, paclitaxel, pioglitazone, repaglinide, and rosiglitazone). Fenofibrate may increase the levels/effects of CYP2C9 substrates (example substrates include bosentan, dapsone, fluoxetine, glimepiride, glipizide, losartan, montelukast, nateglinide, paclitaxel, phenytoin, warfarin, and zafirlukast).

Adverse Reactions

>10%: Hepatic: ALT/AST increased (3% to 13%)

1% to 10%:

Gastrointestinal: Abdominal pain (5%), constipation (2%)

Neuromuscular & skeletal: Back pain (3%)

Respiratory: Respiratory disorder (6%), rhinitis (2%)

Frequency not defined:

Cardiovascular: Angina pectoris, arrhythmia, atrial fibrillation, cardiovascular disorder, chest pain, coronary artery disorder, edema, electrocardiogram abnormality, extrasystoles, hyper-/hypotension, MI, palpitation, peripheral edema, peripheral vascular disorder, phlebitis, tachycardia, varicose veins, vasodilatation

Central nervous system: Anxiety, depression, dizziness, fever, headache, insomnia, malaise, nervousness, neuralgia, pain, somnolence, vertigo

Dermatologic: Acne, alopecia, bruising, contact dermatitis, eczema, fungal dermatitis, maculopapular rash, nail disorder, photosensitivity reaction, pruritus, skin ulcer, Stevens-Johnson syndrome, toxic epidermal necrolysis, urticaria

Endocrine & metabolic: Diabetes mellitus, gout, gynecomastia, hypoglycemia, hyperuricemia, libido decreased

Gastrointestinal: Anorexia, appetite increased, colitis, diarrhea, dry mouth, duodenal ulcer, dyspepsia, eructation, esophagitis, flatulence, gastroenteritis, gastritis, gastrointestinal disorder, nausea, peptic ulcer, rectal disorder, rectal hemorrhage, tooth disorder, vomiting, weight gain/loss

Genitourinary: Cystitis, dysuria, prostatic disorder, libido decreased, pregnancy (unintended), urinary frequency, urolithiasis, vaginal moniliasis

Hematologic: Agranulocytosis, anemia, eosinophilia, leukopenia, lymphadenopathy, thrombocytopenia

Hepatic: Cholelithiasis, cholecystitis, creatine phosphokinase increased, fatty liver deposits, liver function tests abnormal

Neuromuscular & skeletal: Arthralgia, arthritis, arthrosis, bursitis, hypertonia, joint disorder, leg cramps, muscle pain, myalgia, myasthenia, myopathy, myositis, paresthesia, rhabdomyolysis, tenderness, tenosynovitis, weakness

Ocular: Abnormal vision, amblyopia, cataract, conjunctivitis, eye disorder, refraction disorder

Otic: Ear pain, otitis media

Renal: Creatinine increased, kidney function abnormality

Respiratory: Asthma, bronchitis, cough increased, dyspnea, laryngitis, pharyngitis, pneumonia, sinusitis

Miscellaneous: Allergic reaction, cyst, diaphoresis, hernia, herpes simplex, herpes zoster, hypersensitivity reaction, infection

Overdosage/Toxicology Symptoms of overdose include nausea, vomiting, diarrhea, and GI distress.

Treatment is supportive. Hemodialysis has no effect on removal of fenofibric acid from the plasma.

Pharmacodynamics/Kinetics

Time to Peak: 3-8 hours

Protein Binding: >99%

Half-Life Elimination: Half-life elimination: Fenofibric acid: Mean: 20 hours (range: 10-35 hours)

Metabolism: Tissue and plasma via esterases to active form, fenofibric acid; undergoes inactivation by glucuronidation hepatically or renally

Excretion: Urine (60% as metabolites); feces (25%); hemodialysis has no effect on removal of fenofibric acid from plasma

Available Dosage Forms [DSC] = Discontinued product

Capsule:

Lipofen™: 50 mg, 100 mg, 150 mg

Capsule [micronized]:

Antara™: 43 mg, 87 mg, 130 mg

Lofibra™: 67 mg, 134 mg, 200 mg

Tablet :

TriCor®: 48 mg, 54 mg [DSC], 145 mg, 160 mg [DSC]

Triglide™: 50 mg, 160 mg

Dosing

Adults:

Hypertriglyceridemia: Oral: Initial:

Antara™: 43-130 mg/day

Lipofen™: 50-150 mg/day; maximum dose: 150 mg/day

Lofibra™: 67 mg/day with meals, up to 200 mg/day

TriCor™: 48 mg/day, up to 145 mg/day

Triglide™: 50-160 mg/day

Hypercholesterolemia or mixed hyperlipidemia: Oral:

Antara™: 130 mg/day

Lipofen™: 150 mg/day

Lofibra™: 200 mg/day with meals

TriCor®: 145 mg/day

Triglide™: 160 mg/day

Elderly: Oral: Initial:

Antara™: 43 mg/day

Lipofen™: 50 mg/day

Lofibra™: 67 mg/day

TriCor™: 48 mg/day

Triglide™: 50 mg/day

Renal Impairment: Monitor renal function and lipid panel before adjusting. Decrease dose or increase dosing interval for patients with renal failure: Initial:

Antara™: 43 mg/day

Lipofen™: 50 mg/day

Lofibra™: 67 mg/day

TriCor®: 48 mg/day

Triglide™: 50 mg/day

Administration

Oral: 6-8 weeks of therapy is required to determine efficacy.

Lofibra™: Administer with meals.

Antara™, Lipofen™, TriCor®, Triglide™: May be administered with or without food.

Stability

Storage: Store at 15°C to 30°C (59°F to 86°F). Protect from moisture.

Laboratory Monitoring Total serum cholesterol and triglyceride concentration and CLDL, LDL, and HDL levels should be measured periodically; if only marginal changes are noted in 6-8 weeks, the drug should be discontinued. Serum transaminases should be measured every 3 months; if ALT values increase >100 units/L, therapy should be discontinued. Monitor LFTs prior to initiation, at 6 and 12 weeks after initiation or first dose, then periodically thereafter.

Nursing Actions

Physical Assessment: Assess potential for interactions with other pharmacological agents the patient may be taking (eg, increased risk of myopathy and rhabdomyolysis). Monitor laboratory tests and patient response (eg, arrhythmias, gastrointestinal upset, CNS changes, hypoglycemia, myalgia) on a regular basis during therapy. Teach patient possible side effects/appropriate interventions and adverse symptoms to report.

Patient Education: Do not take any new medication during therapy without consulting prescriber. Take as directed with food. Do not change dosage, dosage form, or frequency without consulting prescriber. Maintain diet and exercise program as prescribed. If you are a diabetic taking a sulfonylurea, monitor blood sugars closely; this medication may alter the effects of your antidiabetic medication. May cause mild GI disturbances (eg, gas, diarrhea, constipation, nausea); inform prescriber if these are severe. Report immediately unusual muscle pain or weakness; skin rash or irritation; insomnia; persistent dizziness; chest pain or palpitations; difficult respirations; or any other persistent adverse effects. **Pregnancy/breast-feeding precautions:** Inform prescriber if you are or intend to become pregnant. Breast-feeding is not recommended.

Dietary Considerations
Lofibra™: Take with meals.
Antara™, Lipofen™, TriCor®, Triglide™: May be taken with or without food.

Breast-Feeding Issues Tumor formation was observed in animal studies; nursing is not recommended if the medication cannot be discontinued.

Pregnancy Issues Although teratogenicity and mutagenicity tests in animals have been negative, significant risk has been identified with clofibrate. Use should be avoided, if possible, in pregnant women since the neonatal glucuronide conjugation pathways are immature.

Fenoprofen (fen oh PROE fen)

U.S. Brand Names Nalfon®

Synonyms Fenoprofen Calcium

Restrictions A medication guide should be dispensed with each prescription. A template for the required MedGuide can be found on the FDA website at http://www.fda.gov/medwatch/SAFETY/2005/safety05.htm#NSAID

Pharmacologic Category Nonsteroidal Anti-inflammatory Drug (NSAID), Oral

Medication Safety Issues
Sound-alike/look-alike issues:
Fenoprofen may be confused with flurbiprofen
Nalfon® may be confused with Naldecon®

Pregnancy Risk Factor C/D (3rd trimester)

Lactation Enters breast milk/not recommended

Use Symptomatic treatment of acute and chronic rheumatoid arthritis and osteoarthritis; relief of mild to moderate pain

Mechanism of Action/Effect Inhibits prostaglandin synthesis by decreasing the activity of the enzyme, cyclooxygenase, which results in decreased formation of prostaglandin precursors

Contraindications Hypersensitivity to fenoprofen, aspirin, or other NSAIDs, or any component of the formulation; perioperative pain in the setting of coronary artery bypass surgery (CABG); significant renal dysfunction; pregnancy (3rd trimester)

Warnings/Precautions NSAIDs are associated with an increased risk of adverse cardiovascular events, including MI, stroke, and new onset or worsening of pre-existing hypertension. Risk may be increased with duration of use or pre-existing cardiovascular risk-factors or disease. Carefully evaluate individual cardiovascular risk profiles prior to prescribing. Use caution with fluid retention, CHF, or hypertension.

Use of NSAIDs can compromise existing renal function. Renal toxicity can occur in patient with impaired renal function, dehydration, heart failure, liver dysfunction, those taking diuretics and ACEI, and the elderly. Rehydrate patient before starting therapy. Monitor renal function closely. Not recommended for use in patients with advanced renal disease.

NSAIDs may increase risk of gastrointestinal irritation, ulceration, bleeding, and perforation. These events may occur at any time during therapy and without warning. Use caution with a history of GI disease (bleeding or ulcers), concurrent therapy with aspirin, anticoagulants and/or corticosteroids, smoking, use of alcohol, the elderly or debilitated patients.

Use the lowest effective dose for the shortest duration of time, consistent with individual patient goals, to reduce risk of cardiovascular or GI adverse events. Alternate therapies should be considered for patients at high risk.

NSAIDs may cause serious skin adverse events including exfoliative dermatitis, Stevens-Johnson syndrome (SJS), and toxic epidermal necrolysis (TEN). Anaphylactoid reactions may occur, even without prior exposure; patients with "aspirin triad" (bronchial asthma, aspirin intolerance, rhinitis) may be at increased risk. Do not use in patients who experience bronchospasm, asthma, rhinitis, or urticaria with NSAID or aspirin therapy.

Use with caution in patients with decreased hepatic function. Closely monitor patients with any abnormal LFT. Severe hepatic reactions (eg, fulminant hepatitis, liver failure) have occurred with NSAID use, rarely; discontinue if signs or symptoms of liver disease develop, or if systemic manifestations occur.

Withhold for at least 4-6 half-lives prior to surgical or dental procedures. Safety and efficacy have not been established in children <18 years of age.

Drug Interactions
Decreased Effect: Decreased effect with phenobarbital. Thiazide efficacy (diuretic and antihypertensive effect) may be reduced (indomethacin may reduce this efficacy and it may be anticipated with any NSAID).

Increased Effect/Toxicity: Increased effect/toxicity of phenytoin, sulfonamides, sulfonylureas, salicylates, and oral anticoagulants. Serum concentration/toxicity of methotrexate may be increased.

Nutritional/Ethanol Interactions
Ethanol: Avoid ethanol (may enhance gastric mucosal irritation).
Food: Fenoprofen peak serum levels may be decreased if taken with food.
Herb/Nutraceutical: Avoid alfalfa, anise, bilberry, bladderwrack, bromelain, cat's claw, celery, coleus, cordyceps, dong quai, evening primrose, feverfew, fenugreek, garlic, ginger, ginkgo biloboa, red clover, horse chestnut, grapeseed, green tea, ginseng, guggul, horse chestnut seed, horseradish, licorice, prickly ash, red clover, reishi, SAMe, sweet clover, turmeric, white willow (all have additional antiplatelet activity).

Lab Interactions Increased chloride (S), sodium (S)

Adverse Reactions
>10%:
Central nervous system: Dizziness (7% to 15%), somnolence (9% to 15%)
Gastrointestinal: Abdominal cramps (2% to 4%), heartburn, indigestion, nausea (8% to 14%), dyspepsia (10% to 14%), flatulence (14%), anorexia (14%), constipation (7% to 14%), occult blood in stool (14%), vomiting (3% to 14%), diarrhea (2% to 14%)
1% to 10%:
Central nervous system: Headache (9%)
Dermatologic: Itching
(Continued)

Fenoprofen (Continued)

Endocrine & metabolic: Fluid retention

Overdosage/Toxicology Symptoms of overdose include acute renal failure, vomiting, drowsiness, and leukocytosis. Management of NSAID intoxication is supportive and symptomatic.

Pharmacodynamics/Kinetics

Onset of Action: A few days

Time to Peak: Serum: ~2 hours

Protein Binding: 99%

Half-Life Elimination: 2.5-3 hours

Metabolism: Extensively hepatic

Excretion: Urine (2% to 5% as unchanged drug); feces (small amounts)

Available Dosage Forms

Capsule, as calcium (Nalfon®): 200 mg, 300 mg

Tablet, as calcium: 600 mg

Dosing

Adults & Elderly:

Rheumatoid arthritis and osteoarthritis: Oral: 300-600 mg 3-4 times/day up to 3.2 g/day

Mild to moderate pain: Oral: 200 mg every 4-6 hours as needed

Renal Impairment: Not recommended in patients with advanced renal disease.

Administration

Oral: Do not crush tablets. Swallow whole with a full glass of water. Take with food to minimize stomach upset.

Laboratory Monitoring CBC, liver enzymes; urine output and BUN/serum creatinine in patients receiving diuretics

Nursing Actions

Physical Assessment: Assess effectiveness and interactions of other medications patient may be taking. Monitor blood pressure at the beginning of therapy and periodically during use. Monitor laboratory tests, therapeutic response (eg, relief of pain and inflammation, activity tolerance), and adverse reactions (eg, gastrointestinal effects or ototoxicity) at beginning of therapy and periodically throughout therapy. Assess knowledge/teach patient appropriate use, interventions to reduce side effects, and adverse symptoms to report.

Patient Education: Take this medication exactly as directed; do not increase dose without consulting prescriber. Do not crush tablets or break capsules. Take with food or milk to reduce GI distress. Maintain adequate hydration (2-3 L/day of fluids) unless instructed to restrict fluid intake. Do not use alcohol, aspirin or aspirin-containing medication, or any other anti-inflammatory medications without consulting prescriber. You may experience drowsiness, dizziness, nervousness, or headache (use caution when driving or engaging in tasks requiring alertness until response to drug is known); anorexia, nausea, vomiting, or heartburn (small frequent meals, frequent mouth care, sucking lozenges, or chewing gum may help); or fluid retention (weigh yourself weekly and report unusual (3-5 lb/week) weight gain). GI bleeding, ulceration, or perforation can occur with or without pain; discontinue medication and contact prescriber if persistent abdominal pain or cramping, or blood in stool occurs. Report breathlessness, respiratory difficulty, or unusual cough; chest pain, rapid heartbeat, palpitations; unusual bruising/bleeding; blood in urine, stool, mouth, or vomitus; swollen extremities; skin rash or itching; acute fatigue; or hearing changes (ringing in ears). **Pregnancy/breast-feeding precautions:** Inform prescriber if you are or intend to become pregnant. This drug should not be used in the 3rd trimester of pregnancy. Breast-feeding is not recommended.

Dietary Considerations May be taken with food to decrease GI distress.

Geriatric Considerations Elderly are at high risk for adverse effects from NSAIDs. As much as 60% of elderly can develop peptic ulceration and/or hemorrhage asymptomatically. The concomitant use of H_2 blockers, omeprazole, and sucralfate is not effective as prophylaxis with the exception of NSAID-induced duodenal ulcers which may be prevented by the use of ranitidine. Misoprostol is the only prophylactic agent proven effective. Also, concomitant disease and drug use contribute to the risk for GI adverse effects. Use lowest effective dose for shortest period possible. Consider renal function decline with age. Use of NSAIDs can compromise existing renal function especially when Cl_{cr} is ≤30 mL/minute. Tinnitus may be a difficult and unreliable indication of toxicity due to age-related hearing loss or eighth cranial nerve damage. CNS adverse effects such as confusion, agitation, and hallucination are generally seen in overdose or high-dose situations, but elderly may demonstrate these adverse effects at lower doses than younger adults.

Fentanyl (FEN ta nil)

U.S. Brand Names Actiq®; Duragesic®; Sublimaze®

Synonyms Fentanyl Citrate

Restrictions C-II

Pharmacologic Category Analgesic, Narcotic; General Anesthetic

Medication Safety Issues

Sound-alike/look-alike issues:

Fentanyl may be confused with alfentanil, sufentanil

New patch dosage form of Duragesic®-12 actually delivers 12.5 mcg/hour of fentanyl. Use caution, as orders may be written as "Duragesic 12.5" which can be erroneously interpreted as a 125 mcg dose.

Transdermal patch may contain conducting metal (eg, aluminum); remove patch prior to MRI.

Pregnancy Risk Factor C/D (prolonged use or high doses at term)

Lactation Enters breast milk/not recommended (AAP rates "compatible")

Use

Injection: Sedation, relief of pain, preoperative medication, adjunct to general or regional anesthesia

Transdermal: Management of moderate-to-severe chronic pain

Transmucosal (Actiq®): Management of breakthrough cancer pain

Mechanism of Action/Effect Binds with stereospecific receptors at many sites within the CNS, increases pain threshold, alters pain reception, inhibits ascending pain pathways

Contraindications Hypersensitivity to fentanyl or any component of the formulation; increased intracranial pressure; severe respiratory disease or depression including acute asthma (unless patient is mechanically ventilated); paralytic ileus; severe liver or renal insufficiency; pregnancy (prolonged use or high doses near term)

Transmucosal lozenges (Actiq®) or transdermal patches must not be used in patients who are not opioid tolerant. Patients are considered opioid-tolerant if they are taking at least 60 mg morphine/day, 30 mg oral oxycodone/day, 8 mg oral hydromorphone/day, 25 mcg transdermal fentanyl/hour, or an equivalent dose of another opioid for ≥1 week. Transdermal patches are not for use in acute pain, mild pain, intermittent pain, or postoperative pain management.

Warnings/Precautions An opioid-containing analgesic regimen should be tailored to each patient's needs and based upon the type of pain being treated (acute versus chronic), the route of administration, degree of tolerance for opioids (naive versus chronic user), age, weight, and medical condition. The optimal analgesic dose varies widely among patients. Doses should be titrated to pain relief/prevention. When using with other CNS depressants, reduce dose of one or both agents. Fentanyl shares the toxic potentials of opiate agonists, and precautions of opiate agonist therapy should be observed; use with caution in patients with bradycardia; rapid I.V. infusion may result in skeletal muscle and chest wall rigidity leading to respiratory distress and/or apnea, bronchoconstriction, laryngospasm; inject slowly over 3-5 minutes. Tolerance or drug dependence may result from extended use. Use caution in patients with a history of drug dependence or abuse. The elderly may be particularly susceptible to the CNS depressant and constipating effects of narcotics. Use extreme caution in patients with COPD or other chronic respiratory conditions.

Actiq® should be used only for the care of cancer patients and is intended for use by specialists who are knowledgeable in treating cancer pain. For patients who have received transmucosal product within 6-12 hours, it is recommended that if other narcotics are required, they should be used at starting doses ¼ to ⅓ those usually recommended. Actiq® preparations contain an amount of medication that can be fatal to children. Keep all units out of the reach of children and discard any open units properly. Patients and caregivers should be counseled on the dangers to children including the risk of exposure to partially-consumed units.

Topical patches: Serious or life-threatening hypoventilation may occur, even in opioid-tolerant patients. Serum fentanyl concentrations may increase approximately one-third for patients with a body temperature of 40°C secondary to a temperature-dependent increase in fentanyl release from the system and increased skin permeability. Avoid exposure of application site to direct external heat sources. Patients who experience adverse reactions should be monitored for at least 24 hours after removal of the patch. Transdermal patch may contain conducting metal (eg, aluminum); remove patch prior to MRI. Safety and efficacy of transdermal system have been limited to children ≥2 years of age who are opioid tolerant.

Drug Interactions

Cytochrome P450 Effect: Substrate of CYP3A4 (major); **Inhibits** CYP3A4 (weak)

Decreased Effect: CYP3A4 inducers (including carbamazepine, phenytoin, phenobarbital, rifampin) may decrease serum levels of fentanyl by increasing metabolism.

Increased Effect/Toxicity: Increased sedation with CNS depressants, phenothiazines. Tricyclic antidepressants may potentiate fentanyl's adverse effects. Potential for serotonin syndrome if combined with other serotonergic drugs. CYP3A4 inhibitors may increase the levels/effects of fentanyl; potentially fatal respiratory depression may occur when a potent inhibitor is used in a patient receiving chronic fentanyl (eg, transdermal); example inhibitors include azole antifungals, clarithromycin, diclofenac, doxycycline, erythromycin, imatinib, isoniazid, nefazodone, nicardipine, propofol, protease inhibitors, quinidine, telithromycin, and verapamil.

Nutritional/Ethanol Interactions

Ethanol: Avoid ethanol (may increase CNS depression).

Food: Glucose may cause hyperglycemia.

Herb/Nutraceutical: St John's wort may decrease fentanyl levels. Avoid valerian, St John's wort, kava kava, gotu kola (may increase CNS depression).

Adverse Reactions

>10%:

Cardiovascular: Hypotension, bradycardia

Central nervous system: CNS depression, confusion, drowsiness, sedation

Gastrointestinal: Nausea, vomiting, constipation, xerostomia

Neuromuscular & skeletal: Chest wall rigidity (high dose I.V.), weakness

Ocular: Miosis

Respiratory: Respiratory depression

Miscellaneous: Diaphoresis

1% to 10%:

Cardiovascular: Cardiac arrhythmia, edema, orthostatic hypotension, hypertension, syncope

Central nervous system: Abnormal dreams, abnormal thinking, agitation, amnesia, dizziness, euphoria, fatigue, fever, hallucinations, headache, insomnia, nervousness, paranoid reaction

Dermatologic: Erythema, papules, pruritus, rash

Gastrointestinal: Abdominal pain, anorexia, biliary tract spasm, diarrhea, dyspepsia, flatulence

Local: Application site reaction

Neuromuscular & skeletal: Abnormal coordination, abnormal gait, back pain, paresthesia, rigors, tremor

Respiratory: Apnea, bronchitis, dyspnea, hemoptysis, pharyngitis, rhinitis, sinusitis, upper respiratory infection

Miscellaneous: Hiccups, flu-like syndrome, speech disorder

Overdosage/Toxicology Symptoms of overdose include CNS depression, respiratory depression, and miosis; muscle and chest wall rigidity (may require nondepolarizing skeletal muscle relaxant). Treatment is supportive. Naloxone, 2 mg I.V. with repeat administration as necessary up to a total of 10 mg, can also be used to reverse toxic effects of the opiate. Patients who experience adverse reactions during use of transdermal fentanyl should be monitored for at least 24 hours after removal of the patch.

Pharmacodynamics/Kinetics

Onset of Action: Analgesic: I.M.: 7-15 minutes; I.V.: Almost immediate; Transmucosal: 5-15 minutes

Peak effect: Transmucosal: Analgesic: 20-30 minutes

Duration of Action: I.M.: 1-2 hours; I.V.: 0.5-1 hour; Transmucosal: Related to blood level; respiratory depressant effect may last longer than analgesic effect

Time to Peak: Transdermal: 24-72 hours

Half-Life Elimination: 2-4 hours; Transmucosal: 6.6 hours (range: 5-15 hours); Transdermal: 17 hours (half-life is influenced by absorption rate)

Metabolism: Hepatic, primarily via CYP3A4

Excretion: Urine (primarily as metabolites, 10% as unchanged drug)

Available Dosage Forms

Infusion [premixed in NS]: 0.05 mg (10 mL); 1 mg (100 mL); 1.25 mg (250 mL); 2 mg (100 mL); 2.5 mg (250 mL)

Injection, solution, as citrate [preservative free]: 0.05 mg/mL (2 mL, 5 mL, 10 mL, 20 mL, 30 mL, 50 mL)

Sublimaze®: 0.05 mg/mL (2 mL, 5 mL, 10 mL, 20 mL)

Lozenge, oral transmucosal, as citrate:

Actiq®: 200 mcg, 400 mcg, 600 mcg, 800 mcg, 1200 mcg, 1600 mcg [mounted on a plastic radiopaque handle; raspberry flavor]

Transdermal system: 25 mcg/hour [6.25 cm²] (5s); 50 mcg/hour [12.5 cm²] (5s); 75 mcg/hour [18.75 cm²]; 100 mcg/hour [25 cm²] (5s)

Duragesic®: 12 [delivers 12.5 mcg/hour; 5 cm²; contains alcohol 0.1 mL/10 cm²] (5s); 25 [delivers 25 mcg/hour; 10 cm²; contains alcohol 0.1 mL/10 cm²] (5s); 50 [delivers 50 mcg/hour; 20 cm²; contains alcohol 0.1 mL/10 cm²] (5s); 75 [delivers 75 mcg/hour; 30 cm²; contains alcohol 0.1 mL/10 cm²]; 100 [delivers 100 mcg/hour; 40 cm²; contains alcohol 0.1 mL/10 cm²] (5s)

Dosing

Adults: Note: These are guidelines and do not represent the maximum doses that may be required in all patients. Doses should be titrated to pain relief/
(Continued)

Fentanyl *(Continued)*

prevention. Monitor vital signs routinely. Single I.M. doses have a duration of 1-2 hours, single I.V. doses last 0.5-1 hour.

Sedation for minor procedures/analgesia: I.V.: 25-50 mcg; may repeat every 3-5 minutes to desired effect or adverse event; maximum dose of 500 mcg/4 hours; higher doses are used for major procedures

Surgery:

Premedication: I.M., slow I.V.: 25-100 mcg/dose 30-60 minutes prior to surgery

Adjunct to regional anesthesia: Slow I.V.: 25-100 mcg/dose over 1-2 minutes. **Note:** An I.V. should be in place with regional anesthesia so the I.M. route is rarely used but still maintained as an option in the package labeling.

Adjunct to general anesthesia: Slow I.V.:

Low dose: 0.5-2 mcg/kg/dose depending on the indication. For example, 0.5 mcg/kg will provide analgesia or reduce the amount of propofol needed for laryngeal mask airway insertion with minimal respiratory depression. However, to blunt the hemodynamic response to intubation 2 mcg/kg is often necessary.

Moderate dose: Initial: 2-15 mcg/kg/dose; maintenance (bolus or infusion): 1-2 mcg/kg/hour. Discontinuing fentanyl infusion 30-60 minutes prior to the end of surgery will usually allow adequate ventilation upon emergence from anesthesia. For "fast-tracking" and early extubation following major surgery, total fentanyl doses are limited to 10-15 mcg/kg.

High dose: **Note:** High-dose (20-50 mcg/kg/dose) fentanyl is rarely used, but is still maintained in the package labeling.

Acute pain management:

Severe: I.M, I.V.: 50-100 mcg/dose every 1-2 hours as needed; patients with prior opiate exposure may tolerate higher initial doses

Patient-controlled analgesia (PCA): I.V.: Usual concentration: 10 mcg/mL
Demand dose: Usual: 10 mcg; range: 10-50 mcg
Lockout interval: 5-8 minutes

Mechanically-ventilated patients (based on 70 kg patient): Slow I.V.: 0.35-1.5 mcg/kg every 30-60 minutes as needed; infusion: 0.7-10 mcg/kg/hour

Breakthrough cancer pain: Transmucosal: Actiq® dosing should be individually titrated to provide adequate analgesia with minimal side effects. For patients who are tolerant to and currently receiving opioid therapy for persistent cancer pain. Initial starting dose: 200 mcg; the second dose may be started 15 minutes after completion of the first dose. Consumption should be limited to 4 units/day or less. Patients needing more than 4 units/day should have the dose of their long-term opioid re-evaluated.

Chronic pain management: Opioid-tolerant patients: Transdermal:

Initial: To convert patients from oral or parenteral opioids to transdermal formulation, a 24-hour analgesic requirement should be calculated (based on prior opiate use). Using the tables, the appropriate initial dose can be determined. The initial fentanyl dosage may be approximated from the 24-hour morphine dosage and titrated to minimize adverse effects and provide analgesia. With the initial application, the absorption of transdermal fentanyl requires several hours to reach plateau; therefore transdermal fentanyl is inappropriate for management of acute pain. Change patch every 72 hours.

Conversion from continuous infusion of fentanyl: In patients who have adequate pain relief with a fentanyl infusion, fentanyl may be converted to transdermal dosing at a rate equivalent to the intravenous rate. A two-step taper of the infusion to be completed over 12 hours has been recommended (Kornick, 2001) after the patch is applied. The infusion is decreased to 50% of the original rate six hours after the application of the first patch, and subsequently discontinued twelve hours after application.

Titration: Short-acting agents may be required until analgesic efficacy is established and/or as supplements for "breakthrough" pain. The amount of supplemental doses should be closely monitored. Appropriate dosage increases may be based on daily supplemental dosage using the ratio of 45 mg/24 hours of oral morphine to a 12.5 mcg/hour increase in fentanyl dosage.

Frequency of adjustment: The dosage should not be titrated more frequently than every 3 days after the initial dose or every 6 days thereafter. Patients should wear a consistent fentanyl dosage through two applications (6 days) before dosage increase based on supplemental opiate dosages can be estimated.

Frequency of application: The majority of patients may be controlled on every 72-hour administration; however, a small number of patients require every 48-hour administration.

Dose conversion guidelines for transdermal fentanyl [1] (see tables).

Recommended Initial Duragesic® Dose Based Upon Daily Oral Morphine Dose[1]

Oral 24-Hour Morphine (mg/d)	Duragesic® Dose (mcg/h)
60-134[2]	25
135-224	50
225-314	75
315-404	100
405-494	125
495-584	150
585-674	175
675-764	200
765-854	225
855-944	250
945-1034	275
1035-1124	300

[1] The table should NOT be used to convert from transdermal fentanyl to other opioid analgesics. Rather, following removal of the patch, titrate the dose of the new opioid until adequate analgesia is achieved.

[2] Pediatric patients initiating therapy on a 25 mcg/hour Duragesic® system should be opioid-tolerant and receiving at least 60 mg oral morphine equivalents per day.

Elderly: Elderly have been found to be twice as sensitive as younger patients to the effects of fentanyl. A wide range of doses may be used. When choosing a dose, take into consideration the following patient factors: age, weight, physical status, underlying disease states, other drugs used, type of anesthesia used, and the surgical procedure to be performed.

Transmucosal: Dose should be reduced to 2.5-5 mcg/kg. Suck on lozenge vigorously approximately 20-40 minutes before the start of procedure.

Pediatrics: Note: These are guidelines and do not represent the maximum doses that may be required in all patients. Doses should be titrated to pain relief/prevention. Monitor vital signs routinely. Single I.M. doses have a duration of 1-2 hours, single I.V. doses last 0.5-1 hour.

Sedation for minor procedures/analgesia:

Children 1-12 years: I.M., I.V.: 1-2 mcg/kg/dose; may repeat at 30- to 60-minute intervals. **Note:** Children 18-36 months of age may require 2-3 mcg/kg/dose

Children >12 years: Refer to adult dosing.

Continuous sedation/analgesia: Children 1-12 years: Initial I.V. bolus: 1-2 mcg/kg; then 1-3 mcg/kg/hour to a maximum dose of 5 mcg/kg/hour

Chronic pain management: Children ≥2 years (opioid-tolerant patients): Transdermal: Refer to adult dosing.

Hepatic Impairment: Fentanyl kinetics may be altered in hepatic disease.

Administration

I.V.: Muscular rigidity may occur with rapid I.V. administration.

I.V. Detail: pH: 4.0-7.5

Topical: Transdermal: Apply to nonirritated and nonirradiated skin, such as chest, back, flank, or upper arm. Do not shave skin; hair at application site should be clipped. Prior to application, clean site with clear water and allow to dry completely. Do not use damaged or cut patches; a rapid release of fentanyl and increased systemic absorption may occur. Firmly press in place and hold for 30 seconds. Change patch every 72 hours. Do **not** use soap, alcohol, or other solvents to remove transdermal gel if it accidentally touches skin; use copious amounts of water. Avoid exposing application site to external heat sources (eg, heating pad, electric blanket, heat lamp, hot tub).

Other: Transmucosal: Foil overwrap should be removed just prior to administration. Place the unit in mouth and allow it to dissolve. Do **not** chew. Actiq® units may be moved from one side of the mouth to the other. The unit should be consumed over a period of 15 minutes. Unit should be removed after it is consumed or if patient has achieved an adequate response and/or shows signs of respiratory depression. For patients who have received transmucosal product within 6-12 hours, it is recommended that if other narcotics are required, they should be used at starting doses ¼ to ⅓ those usually recommended.

Opioid Analgesics Initial Oral Dosing Commonly Used for Severe Pain

Drug	Equianalgesic Dose (mg)		Initial Oral Dose	
	Oral[1]	Parenteral[2]	Children (mg/kg)	Adults (mg)
Buprenorphine	—	0.4	—	—
Butorphanol	—	2	—	—
Hydromorphone	7.5	1.5	0.06	4-8
Levorphanol	4 (acute) 1 (chronic)	2 (acute) 1 (chronic)	0.04	2-4
Meperidine	300	75	Not Recommended	
Methadone	10	5	0.2	0.2
Morphine	30	10	0.3	15-30
Nalbuphine	—	10	—	—
Pentazocine	50	30	—	—
Oxycodone	20	—	0.3	10-20
Oxymorphone	1	—	—	—

From "Principles of Analgesic Use in the Treatment of Acute Pain and Cancer Pain," *Am Pain Soc*, Fifth Ed.

[1]Elderly: Starting dose should be lower for this population group

[2]Standard parenteral doses for acute pain in adults; can be used to doses for I.V. infusions and repeated small I.V. boluses. Single I.V. boluses, use half the I.M. dose. Children >6 months: I.V. dose = parenteral equianalgesic dose x weight (kg)/100

Dosing Conversion Guidelines[1,2]

Current Analgesic	Daily Dosage (mg/day)			
Morphine (I.M./ I.V.)	10-22	23-37	38-52	53-67
Oxycodone (oral)	30-67	67.5-112	112.5-157	157.5-202
Oxycodone (I.M./ I.V.)	15-33	33.1-56	56.1-78	78.1-101
Codeine (oral)	150-447	448-747	748-1047	1048-1347
Hydro-morphone (oral)	8-17	17.1-28	28.1-39	39.1-51
Hydro-morphone (I.V.)	1.5-3.4	3.5-5.6	5.7-7.9	8-10
Meperidine (I.M.)	75-165	166-278	279-390	391-503
Methadone (oral)	20-44	45-74	75-104	105-134
Methadone (I.M.)	10-22	23-37	38-52	53-67
Fentanyl transdermal recommended dose (mcg/h)	25 mcg/h	50 mcg/h	75 mcg/h	100 mcg/h

[1] The table should NOT be used to convert from transdermal fentanyl to other opioid analgesics. Rather, following removal of the patch, titrate the dose of the new opioid until adequate analgesia is achieved.

[2] Duragesic® product insert, Janssen Pharmaceutica, Feb 2005.

Stability

Compatibility: Stable in D₅W, NS

Compatibility in syringe: Incompatible with pentobarbital

Compatibility when admixed: Incompatible with fluorouracil, methohexital, pentobarbital, thiopental

Storage:

Injection formulation: Store at controlled room temperature of 15°C to 25°C (59°F to 86°F). Protect from light.

Transdermal: Do not store above 25°C (77°F).

Transmucosal: Store at controlled room temperature of 15°C to 30°C (59°F to 86°F).

Nursing Actions

Physical Assessment: Assess other medications patient may be taking for additive or adverse interactions. Monitor therapeutic effectiveness and signs of adverse or overdose reactions. Monitor blood pressure, CNS and respiratory status, and degree of sedation at beginning of therapy and at regular intervals with long-term use. Monitor closely for 24 hours after transdermal product is removed. For inpatients, implement safety measures (eg, side rails up, call light within reach, instructions to call for assistance). May cause physical and/or psychological dependence. Assess knowledge/teach patient appropriate use (if self-administered), adverse reactions to report, and appropriate interventions to reduce side effects.

Patient Education: While using this medication, do not use alcohol and other prescription or OTC medications (especially sedatives, tranquilizers, antihistamines, or pain medications) without consulting prescriber. If using Actiq® oral transmucosal, you may be at risk for dental carries due to the sugar content. Maintain good oral hygiene. If using patch, avoid exposing application site to external heat sources (eg, heating pad, electric blanket, hot tub, heat lamp). Maintain adequate hydration (2-3 L/day of fluids) unless instructed to restrict fluid intake. May cause (Continued)

Fentanyl *(Continued)*

hypotension, dizziness, drowsiness, impaired coordination, or blurred vision (use caution when driving, climbing stairs, or changing position - rising from sitting or lying to standing, or when engaging in tasks requiring alertness until response to drug is known); nausea or vomiting (frequent mouth care, small frequent meals, chewing gum, or sucking lozenges may help); or constipation (increased exercise, fluids, fruit, or fiber may help; if unresolved, consult prescriber about use of stool softeners). Report acute dizziness, chest pain, slow or rapid heartbeat, acute headache; confusion or changes in mentation; changes in voiding frequency or amount; swelling of extremities or unusual weight gain; shortness of breath or respiratory difficulty; or vision changes. **Pregnancy/breast-feeding precautions:** Inform prescriber if you are or intend to become pregnant. Consult prescriber if breast-feeding.

Transdermal: Apply to clean, dry skin, immediately after removing from package. Firmly press in place and hold for 30 seconds.

Transmucosal (Actiq®): Contains an amount of medication that can be fatal to children. Keep all units out of the reach of children and discard any open units properly. Actiq® Welcome Kits are available which contain educational materials, safe storage, and disposal instructions.

Dietary Considerations Actiq® contains 2 g sugar per unit.

Geriatric Considerations The elderly may be particularly susceptible to the CNS depressant and constipating effects of narcotics; therefore, use with caution.

Breast-Feeding Issues Fentanyl is excreted in low concentrations into breast milk. Breast-feeding is considered acceptable following single doses to the mother; however, no information is available when used long-term.

Pregnancy Issues Fentanyl crosses the placenta and has been used safely during labor. Chronic use during pregnancy has shown detectable serum levels in the newborn with mild opioid withdrawal (case report).

Additional Information Fentanyl is 50-100 times as potent as morphine; morphine 10 mg I.M. is equivalent to fentanyl 0.1-0.2 mg I.M.; fentanyl has less hypotensive effects than morphine due to lack of histamine release. However, fentanyl may cause rigidity with high doses. If the patient has required high-dose analgesia or has used for a prolonged period (~7 days), taper dose to prevent withdrawal; monitor for signs and symptoms of withdrawal.

Transmucosal (oral lozenge): Disposal of Actiq® units: After consumption of a complete unit, the handle may be disposed of in a trash container that is out of the reach of children. For a partially-consumed unit, or a unit that still has any drug matrix remaining on the handle, the handle should be placed under hot running tap water until the drug matrix has dissolved. Special child-resistant containers are available to temporarily store partially consumed units that cannot be disposed of immediately.

Transdermal system (Duragesic®): Upon removal of the patch, ~17 hours are required before serum concentrations fall to 50% of their original values. Opioid withdrawal symptoms are possible. Gradual downward titration (potentially by the sequential use of lower-dose patches) is recommended. Keep transdermal product (both used and unused) out of the reach of children. Do **not** use soap, alcohol, or other solvents to remove transdermal gel if it accidentally touches skin as they may increase transdermal absorption, use copious amounts of water. Avoid exposure of direct external heat sources (eg, heating pads, electric blankets, heat lamps, saunas, hot tubs, heated water beds) to application site.

Related Information

Compatibility of Drugs *on page 1370*
Compatibility of Drugs in Syringe *on page 1372*

Ferric Gluconate (FER ik GLOO koe nate)

U.S. Brand Names Ferrlecit®

Synonyms Sodium Ferric Gluconate

Pharmacologic Category Iron Salt

Medication Safety Issues

Sound-alike/look-alike issues:

Ferrlecit® may be confused with Ferralet®

Pregnancy Risk Factor B

Lactation Excretion in breast milk unknown/use caution

Use Repletion of total body iron content in patients with iron-deficiency anemia who are undergoing hemodialysis in conjunction with erythropoietin therapy

Mechanism of Action/Effect Supplies a source to elemental iron necessary to the function of hemoglobin, myoglobin and specific enzyme systems; allows transport of oxygen via hemoglobin

Contraindications Hypersensitivity to ferric gluconate or any component of the formulation; use in any anemia not caused by iron deficiency; iron overload

Warnings/Precautions Potentially serious hypersensitivity reactions may occur. Fatal immediate hypersensitivity reactions have occurred with other iron carbohydrate complexes. Avoid rapid administration. Flushing and transient hypotension may occur. May augment hemodialysis-induced hypotension. Use with caution in elderly patients. Safety and efficacy in children <6 years of age have not been established. Contains benzyl alcohol; do not use in neonates.

Drug Interactions

Decreased Effect: Chloramphenicol may decrease effect of ferric gluconate injection; ferric gluconate injection may decrease the absorption of oral iron

Adverse Reactions Major adverse reactions include hypotension and hypersensitivity reactions. Hypersensitivity reactions have included pruritus, chest pain, hypotension, nausea, abdominal pain, flank pain, fatigue and rash.

Cardiovascular: Hypotension (serious hypotension in 1%), chest pain, hypertension, syncope, tachycardia, angina, MI, pulmonary edema, hypovolemia, peripheral edema

Central nervous system: Headache, fatigue, fever, malaise, dizziness, paresthesia, insomnia, agitation, somnolence, pain

Dermatologic: Pruritus, rash

Endocrine & metabolic: Hyperkalemia, hypoglycemia, hypokalemia

Gastrointestinal: Abdominal pain, nausea, vomiting, diarrhea, rectal disorder, dyspepsia, flatulence, melena, epigastric pain

Genitourinary: Urinary tract infection

Hematologic: Anemia, abnormal erythrocytes, lymphadenopathy

Local: Injection site reactions, pain

Neuromuscular & skeletal: Weakness, back pain, leg cramps, myalgia, arthralgia, paresthesia, groin pain

Ocular: Blurred vision, conjunctivitis

Respiratory: Dyspnea, cough, rhinitis, upper respiratory infection, pneumonia

Miscellaneous: Hypersensitivity reactions, infection, rigors, chills, flu-like syndrome, sepsis, carcinoma, diaphoresis increased

Overdosage/Toxicology Symptoms of iron overdose include CNS toxicity, acidosis, hepatic and renal impairment, hematemesis, and lethargy. A serum iron level ≥300 mcg/mL requires treatment due to severe toxicity. Treatment is generally symptomatic and supportive, but severe overdoses may be treated with deferoxamine. Deferoxamine may be administered I.V. (80 mg/kg over

24 hours) or I.M. (40-90 mg/kg every 8 hours). Usual toxic dose of elemental iron: ≥35 mg/kg.

Pharmacodynamics/Kinetics
Half-Life Elimination: Bound: 1 hour

Available Dosage Forms Injection, solution: Elemental iron 12.5 mg/mL (5 mL) [contains benzyl alcohol and sucrose 20%]

Dosing
Adults & Elderly: Note: A test dose of 2 mL diluted in 50 mL 0.9% sodium chloride over 60 minutes was previously recommended (not in current manufacturer labeling).

Repletion of iron in hemodialysis patients: I.V.: 125 mg elemental iron per 10 mL (either by I.V. infusion or slow I.V. injection). Most patients will require a cumulative dose of 1 g elemental iron over approximately 8 sequential dialysis treatments to achieve a favorable response.

Pediatrics: Repletion of iron in hemodialysis patients: I.V.: Children ≥6 years: 1.5 mg/kg (maximum: 125 mg/dose) diluted in NS 25 mL, administered over 60 minutes at 8 sequential dialysis sessions

Administration
I.V.:
Adults: May be diluted prior to administration; avoid rapid administration. Infusion rate should not exceed 2.1 mg/minute. If administered undiluted, infuse slowly at a rate of up to 12.5 mg/minute.

Stability
Reconstitution: For I.V. infusion, dilute 10 mL ferric gluconate in 0.9% sodium chloride (children: 25 mL NS, adults: 100 mL NS); use immediately after dilution. Do **not** mix with parenteral nutrition solutions or other medications.

Compatibility: Stable in NS
Do not mix with parenteral nutrition solutions or other medications.

Storage: Store at 20°C to 25°C (68°F to 77°F).

Laboratory Monitoring Hemoglobin and hematocrit, serum ferritin, iron saturation

Nursing Actions
Physical Assessment: Monitor results of test dose, infusion rate, effectiveness of therapy (laboratory results), and adverse reactions at beginning of therapy and periodically during therapy. Monitor blood pressure during infusion. Hypotension can occur. Be alert to the potential for hypersensitivity reactions. Assess knowledge/teach patient adverse symptoms to report.

Patient Education: This medication will be administered by I.V. in conjunction with your dialysis treatment. Report chest pain, rapid heartbeat, or palpitations; respiratory difficulty; headache, dizziness, agitation, or inability to sleep; nausea, vomiting, abdominal or flank pain; or skin rash, itching, or redness. **Breast-feeding precaution:** Consult prescriber if breast-feeding.

Ferrous Fumarate (FER us FYOO ma rate)

U.S. Brand Names Femiron® [OTC]; Feostat® [OTC] [DSC]; Ferretts [OTC]; Ferro-Sequels® [OTC]; Hemocyte® [OTC]; Ircon® [OTC]; Nephro-Fer® [OTC]

Synonyms Iron Fumarate

Pharmacologic Category Iron Salt

Pregnancy Risk Factor A

Use Prevention and treatment of iron-deficiency anemias

Available Dosage Forms [DSC] = Discontinued product
Tablet: 324 mg [elemental iron 106 mg]
Femiron®: 63 mg [elemental iron 20 mg]
Ferretts: 325 mg [elemental iron 106 mg]

Hemocyte®: 324 mg [elemental iron 106 mg]
Ircon®: 200 mg [elemental iron 66 mg]
Nephro-Fer®: 350 mg [elemental iron 115 mg; contains tartrazine]
Tablet, chewable (Feostat®): 100 mg [elemental iron 33 mg; chocolate flavor] [DSC]
Tablet, timed release (Ferro-Sequels®): 150 mg [elemental iron 50 mg; contains docusate sodium and sodium benzoate]

Dosing
Adults & Elderly: (Dose expressed in terms of elemental iron):
Treatment of iron deficiency: Oral: 60-100 mg twice daily up to 60 mg 2 times/day
Prophylaxis of iron deficiency: Oral: 60-100 mg/day
Note: To avoid GI upset, start with a single daily dose and increase by 1 tablet/day each week or as tolerated until desired daily dose is achieved

Pediatrics: (Dose expressed in terms of elemental iron):
Treatment of severe iron-deficiency anemia: Oral: 4-6 mg Fe/kg/day in 3 divided doses
Treatment of mild-to-moderate iron-deficiency anemia: Oral: 3 mg Fe/kg/day in 1-2 divided doses
Prophylaxis of iron deficiency: Oral: 1-2 mg Fe/kg/day

Nursing Actions
Patient Education: May color stool black. Take between meals for maximum absorption; take with food if GI upset occurs. Do not take with milk or antacids. Keep out of reach of children.

Ferrous Gluconate (FER us GLOO koe nate)

U.S. Brand Names Fergon® [OTC]

Synonyms Iron Gluconate

Pharmacologic Category Iron Salt

Pregnancy Risk Factor A

Use Prevention and treatment of iron-deficiency anemias

Available Dosage Forms
Tablet: 246 mg [elemental iron 28 mg]; 300 mg [elemental iron 34 mg]; 325 mg [elemental iron 36 mg]
Fergon®: 240 mg [elemental iron 27 mg]

Dosing
Adults & Elderly: (Dose expressed in terms of elemental iron):
Treatment of iron deficiency anemia: Oral: 60 mg twice daily up to 60 mg 4 times/day
Prophylaxis of iron deficiency: Oral: 60 mg/day

Pediatrics: (Dose expressed in terms of elemental iron):
Treatment of severe iron-deficiency anemia: Oral: 4-6 mg Fe/kg/day in 3 divided doses
Treatment of mild-to-moderate iron-deficiency anemia: Oral: 3 mg Fe/kg/day in 1-2 divided doses
Prophylaxis: Oral: 1-2 mg Fe/kg/day

Nursing Actions
Patient Education: May color stool black. Take between meals for maximum absorption; take with food if GI upset occurs. Do not take with milk or antacids. Keep out of reach of children.

Ferrous Sulfate (FER us SUL fate)

U.S. Brand Names Feosol® [OTC]; Feratab® [OTC]; Fer-Gen-Sol [OTC]; Fer-In-Sol® [OTC]; Fer-Iron® [OTC]; Slow FE® [OTC]

Synonyms FeSO$_4$; Iron Sulfate

Pharmacologic Category Iron Salt

Medication Safety Issues
Sound-alike/look-alike issues:
Feosol® may be confused with Feostat®, Fer-In-Sol® (Continued)

Ferrous Sulfate *(Continued)*

Fer-In-Sol® may be confused with Feosol®
Slow FE® may be confused with Slow-K®

Pregnancy Risk Factor A

Use Prevention and treatment of iron-deficiency anemias

Contraindications Hypersensitivity to iron salts or any component of the formulation; hemochromatosis, hemolytic anemia

Warnings/Precautions Administration of iron for >6 months should be avoided except in patients with continued bleeding, menorrhagia, or repeated pregnancies; avoid in patients with peptic ulcer, enteritis, or ulcerative colitis. Anemia in the elderly is often caused by "anemia of chronic disease" or associated with inflammation rather than blood loss. Iron stores are usually normal or increased, with a serum ferritin >50 ng/mL and a decreased total iron binding capacity. Hence, the "anemia of chronic disease" is not secondary to iron deficiency but the inability of the reticuloendothelial system to reclaim available iron stores.

Drug Interactions

Decreased Effect: Absorption of oral preparation of iron and tetracyclines are decreased when both of these drugs are given together. Absorption of fluoroquinolones, levodopa, methyldopa, and penicillamine may be decreased due to formation of a ferric ion-quinolone complex. Concurrent administration of antacids, H_2 blockers (cimetidine), or proton pump inhibitors may decrease iron absorption. Response to iron therapy may be delayed by chloramphenicol.

Increased Effect/Toxicity: Concurrent administration of ≥200 mg vitamin C per 30 mg elemental iron increases absorption of oral iron.

Nutritional/Ethanol Interactions Food: Cereals, dietary fiber, tea, coffee, eggs, and milk may decrease absorption.

Lab Interactions False-positive for blood in stool by the guaiac test

Adverse Reactions

>10%: Gastrointestinal: GI irritation, epigastric pain, nausea, dark stools, vomiting, stomach cramping, constipation

1% to 10%:

Gastrointestinal: Heartburn, diarrhea

Genitourinary: Discoloration of urine

Miscellaneous: Liquid preparations may temporarily stain the teeth

Overdosage/Toxicology

Symptoms of overdose include acute GI irritation; erosion of GI mucosa, hepatic and renal impairment, coma, hematemesis, lethargy, acidosis

Following treatment for fluid losses, metabolic acidosis, and shock, a severe iron overdose may be treated with deferoxamine. Deferoxamine may be administered I.V. (80 mg/kg over 24 hours) or I.M. (40-90 mg/kg every 8 hours). Usual toxic dose of elemental iron: ≥35 mg/kg.

Pharmacodynamics/Kinetics

Onset of Action: Hematologic response: Oral: ~3-10 days

Peak effect: Reticulocytosis: 5-10 days; hemoglobin increases within 2-4 weeks

Protein Binding: To transferrin

Excretion: Urine, sweat, sloughing of the intestinal mucosa, and menses

Available Dosage Forms

Elixir: 220 mg/5 mL (480 mL) [elemental iron 44 mg/5 mL; contains alcohol]

Liquid, oral drops: 75 mg/0.6 mL (50 mL) [elemental iron 15 mg/0.6 mL]

Fer-Gen-Sol: 75 mg/0.6 mL (50 mL) [elemental iron 15 mg/0.6 mL]

Fer-In-Sol®: 75 mg/0.6 mL (50 mL) [elemental iron 15 mg/0.6 mL; contains alcohol 0.2% and sodium bisulfite]

Fer-Iron®: 75 mg/0.6 mL (50 mL) [elemental iron 15 mg/0.6 mL]

Tablet: 324 mg [elemental iron 65 mg]; 325 mg [elemental iron 65 mg]

Feratab®: 300 mg [elemental iron 60 mg]

Tablet, exsiccated (Feosol®): 200 mg [elemental iron 65 mg]

Tablet, exsiccated, timed release (Slow FE®): 160 mg [elemental iron 50 mg]

Dosing

Adults & Elderly: Dose expressed in terms of ferrous sulfate:

Treatment of iron deficiency anemia: Oral: 300 mg twice daily up to 300 mg 4 times/day or 250 mg (extended release) 1-2 times/day

Prophylaxis of iron deficiency: Oral: 300 mg/day

Pediatrics: Dosage expressed in terms of elemental iron:

Treatment of severe iron-deficiency anemia: Oral: 4-6 mg Fe/kg/day in 3 divided doses

Treatment of mild-to-moderate iron-deficiency anemia: Oral: 3 mg Fe/kg/day in 1-2 divided doses

Prophylaxis: Oral: 1-2 mg Fe/kg/day up to a maximum of 15 mg/day

Laboratory Monitoring Serum iron, total iron binding capacity, reticulocyte count, hemoglobin

Nursing Actions

Physical Assessment: Monitor patient response and adverse effects. May cause GI irritation. Monitor GI function (observe for epigastric pain, nausea, dark stools, vomiting, stomach cramping, constipation).

Patient Education: May color stool black. Take between meals for maximum absorption; take with food if GI upset occurs. Do not take with milk or antacids. You may experience constipation; increasing exercise, fluids, fruit/fiber may help. Keep out of reach of children.

Dietary Considerations Should be taken with water or juice on an empty stomach; may be administered with food to prevent irritation; however, not with cereals, dietary fiber, tea, coffee, eggs, or milk.

Elemental iron content of iron salts in ferrous sulfate is 20% (ie, 300 mg ferrous sulfate is equivalent to 60 mg ferrous iron)

Fexofenadine *(feks oh FEN a deen)*

U.S. Brand Names Allegra®

Synonyms Fexofenadine Hydrochloride

Pharmacologic Category Antihistamine, Nonsedating

Medication Safety Issues

Sound-alike/look-alike issues:

Allegra® may be confused with Viagra®

Pregnancy Risk Factor C

Lactation Excretion in breast milk unknown/use caution (AAP rates "compatible")

Use Relief of symptoms associated with seasonal allergic rhinitis; treatment of chronic idiopathic urticaria

Mechanism of Action/Effect Fexofenadine is an active metabolite of terfenadine and like terfenadine it competes with histamine for H_1-receptor sites on effector cells in the GI tract, blood vessels, and respiratory tract; binds to lung receptors significantly greater than it binds to cerebellar receptors, resulting in a greatly reduced sedative potential

Contraindications Hypersensitivity to fexofenadine or any component of the formulation

Warnings/Precautions Safety and efficacy in children <6 years of age have not been established.

Drug Interactions

Cytochrome P450 Effect: Substrate of CYP3A4 (minor); **Inhibits** CYP2D6 (weak)

Decreased Effect: Aluminum- and magnesium-containing antacids decrease plasma levels of fexofenadine; separate administration is recommended.

Increased Effect/Toxicity: Erythromycin and ketoconazole increased the levels of fexofenadine; however, no increase in adverse events or QT_c intervals was noted. The effect of other macrolide agents or azoles has not been investigated.

Nutritional/Ethanol Interactions

Ethanol: Avoid ethanol (although limited with fexofenadine, may increase risk of sedation).

Food: Fruit juice (apple, grapefruit, orange, pineapple) may decrease bioavailability of fexofenadine by ~36%.

Herb/Nutraceutical: St John's wort may decrease fexofenadine levels.

Adverse Reactions

>10%: Central nervous system: Headache (5% to 11%)

1% to 10%:

Central nervous system: Fever (2%), dizziness (2%), pain (2%), drowsiness (1%), fatigue (1%)

Endocrine & metabolic: Dysmenorrhea (2%)

Gastrointestinal: Nausea (2%), dyspepsia (1% to 5%)

Neuromuscular & skeletal: Back pain (2% to 3%), myalgia (3%)

Otic: Otitis media (2%)

Respiratory: Cough (4%), upper respiratory tract infection (2% to 4%), nasopharyngitis (2%)

Miscellaneous: Viral infection (3%)

Overdosage/Toxicology Limited information from overdose describes dizziness, drowsiness, and dry mouth. Not effectively removed by hemodialysis. Doses up to 690 mg twice daily were administered for 1 month without significant adverse effects. Treatment is supportive.

Pharmacodynamics/Kinetics

Onset of Action: 60 minutes

Duration of Action: Antihistaminic effect: ≥12 hours

Time to Peak: Serum: ~2.6 hours

Protein Binding: 60% to 70%, primarily albumin and alpha$_1$-acid glycoprotein

Half-Life Elimination: 14.4 hours

Metabolism: Minimal (~5%)

Excretion: Feces (~80%) and urine (~11%) as unchanged drug

Available Dosage Forms Tablet, as hydrochloride: 30 mg, 60 mg, 180 mg

Dosing

Adults:

Allergic rhinitis, idiopathic urticaria: Oral: 60 mg twice daily **or** 180 mg once daily

Elderly: Starting dose: 60 mg once daily; adjust for renal impairment.

Pediatrics: Allergic rhinitis, idiopathic urticaria:

Children 6-11 years: Oral: 30 mg twice daily

Children ≥12 years: Refer to adult dosing.

Renal Impairment: Cl_{cr} <80 mL/minute:

Children 6-11 years: Initial: 30 mg once daily

Children ≥12 years and Adults: Initial: 60 mg once daily

Not effectively removed by hemodialysis

Administration

Oral: Administer with water.

Stability

Storage: Store at controlled room temperature of 20°C to 25°C (68°F to 77°F). Protect from excessive moisture.

Nursing Actions

Physical Assessment: Assess effectiveness and interactions of other medications patient may be taking. Monitor effectiveness of therapy and adverse reactions at beginning of therapy and periodically with long-term use. Assess knowledge/teach patient appropriate use, interventions to reduce side effects, and adverse symptoms to report.

Patient Education: Take as directed; do not exceed recommended dose. Store at room temperature in a dry place. If taking antacids, separate administration of antacid and this medication. Avoid use of other depressants, alcohol, or sleep-inducing medications unless approved by prescriber. You may experience mild drowsiness or dizziness (use caution when driving or engaging in tasks requiring alertness until response to drug is known); or nausea (small frequent meals, frequent mouth care, chewing gum, or sucking hard candy may help). Report persistent sedation or drowsiness, menstrual irregularities, or lack of improvement or worsening or condition. **Pregnancy/breast-feeding precautions:** Inform prescriber if you are or intend to become pregnant. Consult prescriber if breast-feeding.

Geriatric Considerations Plasma levels in the elderly are generally higher than those observed in other age groups. Once daily dosing is recommended when starting therapy in elderly patients or patients with decreased renal function.

Fexofenadine and Pseudoephedrine

(feks oh FEN a deen & soo doe e FED rin)

U.S. Brand Names Allegra-D® 12 Hour; Allegra-D® 24 Hour

Synonyms Pseudoephedrine and Fexofenadine

Pharmacologic Category Antihistamine/Decongestant Combination

Pregnancy Risk Factor C

Lactation Enters breast milk/use caution (AAP rates "compatible")

Use Relief of symptoms associated with seasonal allergic rhinitis in adults and children ≥12 years of age

Available Dosage Forms Tablet, extended release:

Allegra-D® 12 Hour: Fexofenadine hydrochloride 60 mg [immediate release] and pseudoephedrine hydrochloride 120 mg [extended release]

Allegra-D® 24 Hour: Fexofenadine hydrochloride 180 mg [immediate release] and pseudoephedrine hydrochloride 240 mg [extended release]

Dosing

Adults & Elderly: Allergic symptoms and nasal congestion: Oral:

Allegra-D® 12 Hour: One tablet twice daily

Allegra-D® 24 Hour: One tablet once daily

Pediatrics: Children ≥12 years: Refer to adult dosing.

Renal Impairment:

Allegra-D® 12 Hour: Cl_{cr} <80 mL/minute (based on fexofenadine component): One tablet once daily.

Allegra-D® 24 Hour: Avoid use.

Nursing Actions

Physical Assessment: See individual agents.

Patient Education: Patients should be instructed to take tablets only as prescribed. Do not exceed the recommended dose. If nervousness, dizziness, or sleeplessness occur, discontinue use and consult the physician. Patients should also be advised against the concurrent use of the tablets with over-the-counter antihistamines and decongestants. The product should not be used by patients who are hypersensitive to it or to any of its ingredients. Due to its pseudoephedrine component, this product should not be used by patients with narrow-angle glaucoma, urinary retention, or by patients receiving a monoamine oxidase (MAO) inhibitor or within 14 days of stopping use of MAO inhibitor. It also should not be used by patients with severe hypertension or severe coronary artery disease. Patients should be told that this product should be used in pregnancy or lactation only if the potential benefit justifies the potential risk to the fetus or nursing infant. Patients should be cautioned not to break or chew the tablet. Patients should be

(Continued)

Fexofenadine and Pseudoephedrine
(Continued)

directed to swallow the tablet whole. Patients should be instructed not to take the tablet with food. Patients should also be instructed to store the medication in a tightly closed container in a cool, dry place, away from children. **Pregnancy/breast-feeding precautions:** Inform prescriber if you are pregnant. Consult prescriber if breast-feeding.

Related Information
Fexofenadine *on page 512*
Pseudoephedrine *on page 1047*

Filgrastim (fil GRA stim)

U.S. Brand Names Neupogen®

Synonyms G-CSF; Granulocyte Colony Stimulating Factor

Pharmacologic Category Colony Stimulating Factor

Medication Safety Issues
Sound-alike/look-alike issues:
Neupogen® may be confused with Epogen®, Neumega®, Nutramigen®

Pregnancy Risk Factor C

Lactation Excretion in breast milk unknown/use caution

Use Stimulation of granulocyte production in chemotherapy-induced neutropenia (nonmyeloid malignancies, acute myeloid leukemia, and bone marrow transplantation); severe chronic neutropenia (SCN); patients undergoing peripheral blood progenitor cell (PBPC) collection

Mechanism of Action/Effect Stimulates the production, maturation, and activation of neutrophils, filgrastim activates neutrophils to increase both their migration and cytotoxicity. Natural proteins which stimulate hematopoietic stem cells to proliferate, prolong cell survival, stimulate cell differentiation, and stimulate functional activity of mature cells. CSFs are produced by a wide variety of cell types. Specific mechanisms of action are not yet fully understood, but possibly work by a second-messenger pathway with resultant protein production. See table.

Comparative Effects — Filgrastim vs Sargramostim

Proliferation/Differentiation	Filgrastim	Sargramostim
Neutrophils	Yes	Yes
Eosinophils	No	Yes
Macrophages	No	Yes
Neutrophil migration	Enhanced	Inhibited

Contraindications Hypersensitivity to filgrastim, *E. coli*-derived proteins, or any component of the formulation

Warnings/Precautions Do not use filgrastim in the period 24 hours before to 24 hours after administration of cytotoxic chemotherapy because of the potential sensitivity of rapidly dividing myeloid cells to cytotoxic chemotherapy. Precaution should be exercised in the usage of filgrastim in any malignancy with myeloid characteristics. Filgrastim can potentially act as a growth factor for any tumor type, particularly myeloid malignancies. Tumors of nonhematopoietic origin may have surface receptors for filgrastim. Safety and efficacy have not been established with patients receiving radiation therapy, or with chemotherapy associated with delayed myelosuppression (eg, nitrosoureas, mitomycin C).

Allergic-type reactions have occurred with first or later doses. Reactions tended to occur more frequently with intravenous administration and within 30 minutes of infusion. Rare cases of splenic rupture or adult respiratory distress syndrome have been reported in association with filgrastim; patients must be instructed to report left upper quadrant pain or shoulder tip pain or respiratory distress. Use caution in patients with sickle cell diseases; sickle cell crises have been reported following filgrastim therapy.

Adverse Reactions
>10%:
Central nervous system: Fever (12%)
Dermatologic: Petechiae (17%), rash (12%)
Gastrointestinal: Splenomegaly (≤33% of patients with cyclic neutropenia/congenital agranulocytosis receiving filgrastim for ≥14 days; rare in other patients)
Hepatic: Alkaline phosphatase increased (21%)
Neuromuscular & skeletal: Bone pain (22% to 33%), commonly in the lower back, posterior iliac crest, and sternum
Respiratory: Epistaxis (9% to 15%)
1% to 10%:
Cardiovascular: Hyper-/hypotension (4%), S-T segment depression (3%), myocardial infarction/arrhythmias (3%)
Central nervous system: Headache (7%)
Gastrointestinal: Nausea (10%), vomiting (7%), peritonitis (2%)
Hematologic: Leukocytosis (2%)

Overdosage/Toxicology No clinical adverse effects have been seen with high doses producing ANC >10,000/mm³. Filgrastim discontinuation should result in a 50% decrease in circulating neutrophils within 1-2 days and a return to pretreatment levels in 1-7 days.

Pharmacodynamics/Kinetics
Onset of Action: ~24 hours; plateaus in 3-5 days
Duration of Action: ANC decreases by 50% within 2 days after discontinuing filgrastim; white counts return to the normal range in 4-7 days; peak plasma levels can be maintained for up to 12 hours
Time to Peak: Serum: SubQ: 2-6 hours
Half-Life Elimination: 1.8-3.5 hours
Metabolism: Systemically degraded

Available Dosage Forms
Injection, solution [preservative free]: 300 mcg/mL (1 mL, 1.6 mL) [vial; contains sodium 0.035 mg/mL and sorbitol]
Injection, solution [preservative free]: 600 mcg/mL (0.5 mL, 0.8 mL) [prefilled Singleject® syringe; contains sodium 0.035 mg/mL and sorbitol]

Dosing
Adults & Elderly: Refer to individual protocols.
Note: Dosing should be based on actual body weight (even in morbidly obese patients). Rounding doses to the nearest vial size often enhances patient convenience and reduces costs without compromising clinical response.

Myelosuppressive therapy: I.V., SubQ: 5 mcg/kg/day; doses may be increased by 5 mcg/kg according to the duration and severity of the neutropenia; continue for up to 14 days or until the ANC reaches 10,000/mm³

Bone marrow transplantation: I.V., SubQ: 10 mcg/kg/day; doses may be increased by 5 mcg/kg according to the duration and severity of neutropenia; recommended steps based on neutrophil response:
When ANC >1000/mm³ for 3 consecutive days: Reduce filgrastim dose to 5 mcg/kg/day.
If ANC remains >1000/mm³ for 3 more consecutive days: Discontinue filgrastim.
If ANC decreases to <1000/mm³: Resume at 5 mcg/kg/day.
If ANC decreases <1000/mm³ during the 5 mcg/kg/day dose: Increase filgrastim to 10 mcg/kg/day and follow the above steps.

Peripheral blood progenitor cell (PBPC) collection: SubQ: 10 mcg/kg/day **or** 5-8 mcg/kg twice daily in donors. Begin at least 4 days before the first leukopheresis and continue until the last leukopheresis; the optimal timing and duration of growth factor stimulation has not been determined.

Severe chronic neutropenia: SubQ:
Congenital: 6 mcg/kg twice daily
Idiopathic/cyclic: 5 mcg/kg/day

Pediatrics: Children: Refer to adult dosing.

Administration

I.V.: May be administered undiluted by SubQ injection. May also be administered by I.V. bolus over 15-30 minutes in D_5W, or by continuous SubQ or I.V. infusion. Do not administer earlier than 24 hours after or in the 24 hours prior to cytotoxic chemotherapy.

I.V. Detail: pH: 4

Stability

Reconstitution:

Do not dilute with saline at any time; product may precipitate. Filgrastim may be diluted in dextrose 5% in water to a concentration 5-15 mcg/mL for I.V. infusion administration (minimum concentration: 5 mcg/mL). Dilution to <5 mcg/mL is not recommended. Concentrations 5-15 mcg/mL require addition of albumin (final concentration of 2 mg/mL) to the bag to prevent absorption to plastics.

Compatibility: Standard diluent: ≥375 mcg/25 mL D_5W. Stable in D_5W; **incompatible** with NS

Y-site administration: Incompatible with amphotericin B, cefepime, cefoperazone, cefotaxime, cefoxitin, ceftizoxime, ceftriaxone, cefuroxime, clindamycin, dactinomycin, etoposide, fluorouracil, furosemide, heparin, mannitol, methylprednisolone sodium succinate, metronidazole, mitomycin, piperacillin, prochlorperazine edisylate, thiotepa

Storage: Intact vials and prefilled syringes should be stored under refrigeration at 2°C to 8°C (36°F to 46°F) and protected from direct sunlight. Filgrastim should be protected from freezing and temperatures >30°C to avoid aggregation. If inadvertently frozen, thaw in a refrigerator and use within 24 hours; do not use if frozen >24 hours or frozen more than once. The solution should not be shaken since bubbles and/or foam may form. If foaming occurs, the solution should be left undisturbed for a few minutes until bubbles dissipate.

Filgrastim vials and prefilled syringes are stable for 7 days at 9°C to 30°C (47°F to 86°F), however, the manufacturer recommends discarding after 24 hours because of microbiological concerns. The product is packaged without a preservative.

Undiluted filgrastim is stable for 24 hours at 15°C to 30°C and for 2 weeks at 2°C to 8°C (36°F to 46°F) in tuberculin syringes. However, the manufacturer recommends to use immediately because of concern for bacterial contamination.

Filgrastim diluted for I.V. infusion (5-15 mcg/mL) is stable for 7 days at 2°C to 8°C (36°F to 46°F). Compatible with glass bottles, PVC and polyolefin I.V. bags, and polypropylene syringes when diluted in 5% dextrose or 5% dextrose with albumin.

Laboratory Monitoring CBC with differential prior to treatment and twice weekly during filgrastim treatment for chemotherapy-induced neutropenia (3 times a week following marrow transplantation). For severe chronic neutropenia, monitor CBC twice weekly during the first month of therapy and for 2 weeks following dose adjustments; monthly thereafter. Leukocytosis (white blood cell counts ≥100,000/mm³ has been observed in ~2% of patients receiving filgrastim at doses >5 mcg/kg/day.

Nursing Actions

Physical Assessment: Hypersensitivity to *E. coli* products should be assessed prior to beginning therapy. Monitor results of CBC and platelet counts twice weekly during therapy. Monitor therapeutic

effectiveness and signs/symptoms of adverse reactions at beginning of therapy and periodically throughout therapy (eg, allergic-type reactions have occurred in patients receiving G-CSF with first or later doses). If self-administered, teach patient (or caregiver) proper storage, administration, and syringe/needle disposal. Teach patient (or caregiver) possible side effects/appropriate interventions and adverse symptoms to report.

Patient Education: Do not take any new medication during therapy unless approved by prescriber. If self-administered, follow directions for proper storage and administration of SubQ medication. Never reuse syringes or needles. May cause bone pain (request analgesic); nausea or vomiting (small, frequent meals may help); hair loss (reversible); or sore mouth (frequent mouth care with soft toothbrush or cotton swab may help). Report immediately any respiratory difficulty or pain in left shoulder, chest or back. Report unusual fever or chills; unhealed sores; severe bone pain; pain, redness, or swelling at injection site; unusual swelling of extremities; or chest pain and palpitations. **Pregnancy/breast-feeding precautions:** Inform prescriber if you are or intend to become pregnant. Consult prescriber if breast-feeding.

Dietary Considerations Injection solution contains sodium 0.035 mg/mL and sorbitol.

Pregnancy Issues Animal studies have demonstrated adverse effects and fetal loss. Filgrastim has been shown to cross the placenta in humans. There are no adequate and well-controlled studies in pregnant women. Use only if potential benefit to mother justifies risk to the fetus.

Additional Information

Reimbursement Hotline: 1-800-272-9376
Professional Services [Amgen]: 1-800-77-AMGEN

Finasteride (fi NAS teer ide)

U.S. Brand Names Propecia®; Proscar®

Pharmacologic Category 5 Alpha-Reductase Inhibitor

Medication Safety Issues

Sound-alike/look-alike issues:
Proscar® may be confused with ProSom®, Prozac®, Psorcon®

Pregnancy Risk Factor X

Lactation Excretion in breast milk unknown/contraindicated

Use

Propecia®: Treatment of male pattern hair loss in **men only**. Safety and efficacy were demonstrated in men between 18-41 years of age.

Proscar®: Treatment of symptomatic benign prostatic hyperplasia (BPH); can be used in combination with an alpha blocker, doxazosin

Unlabeled/Investigational Use Adjuvant monotherapy after radical prostatectomy in the treatment of prostatic cancer; female hirsutism

Mechanism of Action/Effect Finasteride inhibits conversion of testosterone to dihydrotestosterone and markedly suppresses serum dihydrotestosterone levels

Contraindications Hypersensitivity to finasteride or any component of the formulation; pregnancy; not for use in children

Warnings/Precautions Hazardous agent - use appropriate precautions for handling and disposal. A minimum of 6 months of treatment may be necessary to determine whether an individual will respond to finasteride. Use with caution in those patients with hepatic dysfunction. Carefully monitor patients with a large residual urinary volume or severely diminished urinary flow for obstructive uropathy. These patients may not be candidates for finasteride therapy.
(Continued)

Finasteride (Continued)

Drug Interactions
Cytochrome P450 Effect: Substrate of CYP3A4 (minor)

Nutritional/Ethanol Interactions
Herb/Nutraceutical: St John's wort may decrease finasteride levels. Avoid saw palmetto (concurrent use has not been adequately studied).

Adverse Reactions Note: "Combination therapy" refers to finasteride and doxazosin.

>10%:
  Endocrine & metabolic: Impotence (19%; combination therapy 23%), libido decreased (10%; combination therapy 12%)
  Genitourinary: Neuromuscular & skeletal: Weakness (5%; combination therapy 17%)

1% to 10%:
  Cardiovascular: Postural hypotension (9%; combination therapy 18%), edema (1%, combination therapy 3%)
  Central nervous system: Dizziness (7%; combination therapy 23%), somnolence (2%; combination therapy 3%)
  Genitourinary: Ejaculation disturbances (7%; combination therapy 14%), decreased volume of ejaculate
  Endocrine & metabolic: Gynecomastia (2%)
  Respiratory: Dyspnea (1%; combination therapy 2%), rhinitis (1%; combination therapy 2%)

Pharmacodynamics/Kinetics
Onset of Action: 3-6 months of ongoing therapy
Duration of Action:
  After a single oral dose as small as 0.5 mg: 65% depression of plasma dihydrotestosterone levels persists 5-7 days
  After 6 months of treatment with 5 mg/day: Circulating dihydrotestosterone levels are reduced to castrate levels without significant effects on circulating testosterone; levels return to normal within 14 days of discontinuation of treatment
Time to Peak: Serum: 2-6 hours
Protein Binding: 90%
Half-Life Elimination: Elderly: 8 hours; Adults: 6 hours (3-16)
Metabolism: Hepatic via CYP3A4; two active metabolites (<20% activity of finasteride)
Excretion: Feces (57%) and urine (39%) as metabolites

Available Dosage Forms
Tablet:
  Propecia®: 1 mg
  Proscar®: 5 mg

Dosing
Adults & Elderly:
  Benign prostatic hyperplasia (Proscar®): Oral: 5 mg/day as a single dose; clinical responses occur within 12 weeks to 6 months of initiation of therapy; long-term administration is recommended for maximal response
  Male pattern baldness (Propecia®): Oral: 1 mg daily
  Female hirsutism (unlabeled use): Oral: 5 mg/day
Renal Impairment: No adjustment is necessary.
Hepatic Impairment: Use with caution in patients with liver function abnormalities because finasteride is metabolized extensively in the liver

Administration
Oral: Administration with food may delay the rate and reduce the extent of oral absorption. Women of childbearing age should not touch or handle broken tablets.

Stability
Storage: Store below 30°C (86°F). Protect from light.
Laboratory Monitoring Finasteride does not interfere with free PSA levels.

Nursing Actions
Physical Assessment: Assess potential for interactions with pharmacological agents or herbal products patient may be taking. Assess urinary pattern prior to therapy and periodically during therapy (obstructive uropathy). Assess therapeutic effectiveness and signs/symptoms of adverse reactions. Teach patient proper use (eg, a minimum of 6 months of treatment may be necessary to evaluate response), possible side effects/appropriate interventions, and adverse symptoms to report. **Pregnancy risk factor X** - instruct patient on absolute need for barrier contraceptives. Women of childbearing age should not touch or handle broken tablets.

Patient Education: Do not take any new medication during therapy unless approved by prescriber. Results of therapy may take several months. Take with or without meals. May cause decreased libido or impotence during therapy. Report any changes in urinary pattern (significant increase or decrease in volume or voiding patterns). Report changes in breast condition (pain, lumps, or nipple discharge) in male and female patients. **Pregnancy precautions:** This drug will cause fetal abnormalities - use barrier contraceptives and do not allow women of childbearing age to touch or handle broken or crushed tablets.

Geriatric Considerations Clearance of finasteride is decreased in the elderly, but no dosage reductions are necessary.

Breast-Feeding Issues Not indicated for use in women.

Flecainide (fle KAY nide)

U.S. Brand Names Tambocor™
Synonyms Flecainide Acetate
Pharmacologic Category Antiarrhythmic Agent, Class Ic

Medication Safety Issues
Sound-alike/look-alike issues:
  Flecainide may be confused with fluconazole
  Tambocor™ may be confused with tamoxifen

Pregnancy Risk Factor C
Lactation Enters breast milk/compatible

Use Prevention and suppression of documented life-threatening ventricular arrhythmias (eg, sustained ventricular tachycardia); controlling symptomatic, disabling supraventricular tachycardias in patients without structural heart disease in whom other agents fail

Mechanism of Action/Effect Class Ic antiarrhythmic; slows conduction in cardiac tissue by altering transport of ions across cell membranes; causes slight prolongation of refractory periods; decreases the rate of rise of the action potential without affecting its duration; increases electrical stimulation threshold of ventricle, His-Purkinje system; possesses local anesthetic and moderate negative inotropic effects

Contraindications Hypersensitivity to flecainide or any component of the formulation; pre-existing second- or third-degree AV block or with right bundle branch block when associated with a left hemiblock (bifascicular block) (except in patients with a functioning artificial pacemaker); cardiogenic shock; coronary artery disease (based on CAST study results); concurrent use of ritonavir or amprenavir

Warnings/Precautions Not recommend for patients with chronic atrial fibrillation. A worsening or new arrhythmia may occur (proarrhythmic effect). Use caution in heart failure (may precipitate or exacerbate CHF). Dose-related increases in PR, QRS, and QT intervals occur. Use with caution in sick sinus syndrome or with permanent pacemakers or temporary pacing wires (can increase endocardial pacing thresholds). Due to potential to exacerbate toxicity, pre-existing hypokalemia or hyperkalemia should be corrected before initiation of flecainide. Use caution in patients with significant hepatic impairment.

Drug Interactions

Cytochrome P450 Effect: Substrate of CYP1A2 (minor), 2D6 (major); **Inhibits** CYP2D6 (weak)

Decreased Effect: Smoking and acid urine increase flecainide clearance.

Increased Effect/Toxicity: CYP2D6 inhibitors may increase the levels/effects of flecainide; example inhibitors include chlorpromazine, delavirdine, fluoxetine, miconazole, paroxetine, pergolide, quinidine, quinine, ritonavir, and ropinirole. Flecainide concentrations may be increased by amiodarone (reduce flecainide 25% to 33%), and propranolol. Beta-adrenergic blockers, disopyramide, verapamil may enhance flecainide's negative inotropic effects. Alkalinizing agents (ie, high-dose antacids, cimetidine, carbonic anhydrase inhibitors, sodium bicarbonate) may decrease flecainide clearance, potentially increasing toxicity. Propranolol blood levels are increased by flecainide.

Nutritional/Ethanol Interactions Food: Clearance may be decreased in patients following strict vegetarian diets due to urinary pH ≥8. Dairy products (milk, infant formula, yogurt) may interfere with the absorption of flecainide in infants; there is one case report of a neonate (GA 34 weeks PNA >6 days) who required extremely large doses of oral flecainide when administered every 8 hours with feedings ("milk feeds"); changing the feedings from "milk feeds" to 5% glucose feeds alone resulted in a doubling of the flecainide serum concentration and toxicity.

Adverse Reactions

>10%:
Central nervous system: Dizziness (19% to 30%)
Ocular: Visual disturbances (16%)
Respiratory: Dyspnea (~10%)

1% to 10%:
Cardiovascular: Palpitations (6%), chest pain (5%), edema (3.5%), tachycardia (1% to 3%), proarrhythmic (4% to 12%), sinus node dysfunction (1.2%)
Central nervous system: Headache (4% to 10%), fatigue (8%), nervousness (5%) additional symptoms occurring at a frequency between 1% and 3%: fever, malaise, hypoesthesia, paresis, ataxia, vertigo, syncope, somnolence, tinnitus, anxiety, insomnia, depression
Dermatologic: Rash (1% to 3%)
Gastrointestinal: Nausea (9%), constipation (1%), abdominal pain (3%), anorexia (1% to 3%), diarrhea (0.7% to 3%)
Neuromuscular & skeletal: Tremor (5%), weakness (5%), paresthesia (1%)
Ocular: Diplopia (1% to 3%), blurred vision

Overdosage/Toxicology Flecainide has a narrow therapeutic index and severe toxicity may occur slightly above the therapeutic range, especially if combined with other antiarrhythmic drugs. (Acute single ingestion of twice the daily therapeutic dose is life-threatening). Symptoms of overdose include increase in P-R, QRS, or QT intervals and amplitude of the T wave, AV block, bradycardia, hypotension, ventricular arrhythmias (monomorphic or polymorphic ventricular tachycardia), and asystole. Other symptoms include dizziness, blurred vision, headache, and GI upset. Treatment is supportive.

Pharmacodynamics/Kinetics

Time to Peak: Serum: ~1.5-3 hours

Protein Binding: Alpha$_1$ glycoprotein: 40% to 50%

Half-Life Elimination: Infants: 11-12 hours; Children: 8 hours; Adults: 7-22 hours, increased with congestive heart failure or renal dysfunction; End-stage renal disease: 19-26 hours

Metabolism: Hepatic

Excretion: Urine (80% to 90%, 10% to 50% as unchanged drug and metabolites)

Available Dosage Forms Tablet, as acetate: 50 mg, 100 mg, 150 mg

Dosing

Adults & Elderly:

Life-threatening ventricular arrhythmias: Oral:
Initial: 100 mg every 12 hours; increase by 50-100 mg/day (given in 2 doses/day) every 4 days; maximum: 400 mg/day
For patients receiving 400 mg/day who are not controlled and have trough concentrations <0.6 mcg/mL, dosage may be increased to 600 mg/day.

Prevention of paroxysmal supraventricular arrhythmias: Oral:
Note: In patients with disabling symptoms but no structural heart disease
Initial: 50 mg every 12 hours; increase by 50 mg twice daily at 4-day intervals; maximum: 300 mg/day

Pediatrics:

Life-threatening ventricular arrhythmias: Oral: Children:
Initial: 3 mg/kg/day or 50-100 mg/m^2/day in 3 divided doses
Usual maintenance: 3-6 mg/kg/day or 100-150 mg/m^2/day in 3 divided doses; up to 11 mg/kg/day or 200 mg/m^2/day for uncontrolled patients with subtherapeutic levels

Renal Impairment:
Cl$_{cr}$ <10 mL/minute: Decrease usual dose by 25% to 50% in severe renal impairment.
Not dialyzable (0% to 5%) via hemo- or peritoneal dialysis; no supplemental dose is necessary.

Hepatic Impairment: Monitoring of plasma levels is recommended because half-life is significantly increased. When transferring from another antiarrhythmic agent, allow for 2-4 half-lives of the agent to pass before initiating flecainide therapy.

Administration

Oral: Administer around-the-clock to promote less variation in peak and trough serum levels.

Laboratory Monitoring Periodic serum concentrations, especially in patients with renal or hepatic impairment

Nursing Actions

Physical Assessment: Assess other medications patient may be taking for effectiveness and interactions. Monitor laboratory tests, therapeutic response (cardiac status), and adverse reactions when beginning therapy, when titrating dosage, and periodically during long-term therapy. **Note:** Flecainide has a low toxic:therapeutic ratio and overdose may easily produce severe and life-threatening reactions. Assess knowledge/teach patient appropriate use, interventions to reduce side effects, and adverse symptoms to report.

Patient Education: Take exactly as directed, around-the-clock. Do not discontinue without consulting prescriber. You will require frequent monitoring while taking this medication. You may experience lightheadedness, nervousness, dizziness, visual disturbances (use caution when driving or engaging in tasks requiring alertness until response to drug is known); or nausea, vomiting, or loss of appetite (small frequent meals may help). Report palpitations, chest pain, excessively slow or rapid heartbeat; acute nervousness, headache, or fatigue; unusual weight gain; unusual cough; respiratory difficulty; swelling of hands or ankles; or muscle tremor, numbness, or weakness. **Pregnancy precaution:** Inform prescriber if you are or intend to become pregnant.

Floxuridine (floks YOOR i deen)

U.S. Brand Names FUDR®

Synonyms Fluorodeoxyuridine; FUDR; 5-FUDR; NSC-27640

Pharmacologic Category Antineoplastic Agent, Antimetabolite (Pyrimidine Antagonist)

Medication Safety Issues
Sound-alike/look-alike issues:
Floxuridine may be confused with Fludara®, fludarabine
FUDR® may be confused with Fludara®

Pregnancy Risk Factor D

Lactation Excretion in breast milk unknown/contraindicated

Use Management of hepatic metastases of colorectal and gastric cancers

Mechanism of Action/Effect Mechanism of action and pharmacokinetics are very similar to fluorouracil; floxuridine is the deoxyribonucleotide of fluorouracil. Floxuridine is a fluorinated pyrimidine antagonist which inhibits DNA and RNA synthesis and methylation of deoxyuridylic acid to thymidylic acid.

Contraindications Hypersensitivity to floxuridine, fluorouracil, or any component of the formulation; pregnancy

Warnings/Precautions The U.S. Food and Drug Administration (FDA) currently recommends that procedures for proper handling and disposal of antineoplastic agents be considered.

Use caution in impaired kidney or liver function. Discontinue if intractable vomiting or diarrhea, precipitous fall in leukocyte or platelet counts, or myocardial ischemia occur. Use with caution in patients who have had high-dose pelvic radiation or previous use of alkylating agents. Use of floxuridine with pentostatin has been associated with a high incidence of fatal pulmonary toxicity; this combination is not recommended.

If floxuridine contacts the skin, wash and flush thoroughly with water.

Drug Interactions
Decreased Effect: Patients may experience impaired immune response to vaccines; possible infection after administration of live vaccines in patients receiving immunosuppressants.

Increased Effect/Toxicity: Any form of therapy which adds to the stress of the patient, interferes with nutrition, or depresses bone marrow function will increase the toxicity of floxuridine. Pentostatin and floxuridine administered together has resulted in fatal pulmonary toxicity.

Nutritional/Ethanol Interactions Ethanol: Avoid ethanol (due to GI irritation).

Lab Interactions Increased potassium (S)

Adverse Reactions
>10%:
Gastrointestinal: Stomatitis, diarrhea; may be dose-limiting
Hematologic: Myelosuppression, may be dose-limiting; leukopenia, thrombocytopenia, anemia
Onset: 4-7 days
Nadir: 5-9 days
Recovery: 21 days
1% to 10%:
Dermatologic: Alopecia, photosensitivity, hyperpigmentation of the skin, localized erythema, dermatitis
Gastrointestinal: Anorexia
Hepatic: Biliary sclerosis, cholecystitis, jaundice

Pharmacodynamics/Kinetics
Metabolism: Hepatic; Active metabolites: Floxuridine monophosphate (FUDR-MP) and fluorouracil; Inactive metabolites: Urea, CO_2, α-fluoro-β-alanine, α-fluoro-β-guanidopropionic acid, α-fluoro-β-ureidopropionic acid, and dihydrofluorouracil

Excretion: Urine: Fluorouracil, urea, α-fluoro-β-alanine, α-fluoro-β-guanidopropionic acid, α-fluoro-β-ureidopropionic acid and dihydrofluorouracil; exhaled gases (CO_2)

Available Dosage Forms Injection, powder for reconstitution: 500 mg

Dosing
Adults: Refer to individual protocols.
Colorectal or gastric metastases:
Intra-arterial: Primarily by an implantable pump: 0.1-0.6 mg/kg/day continuous intra-arterial administration for 14 days then heparinized saline is given for 14 days; toxicity requires dose reduction.
I.V.: Many regimens in use, examples:
0.15 mg/kg/day for 7-14 days
0.5-1 mg/kg/day for 6-15 days
30 mg/kg/day for 5 days, then 15 mg/kg/day every other day, up to 11 days

Elderly: Adjust dose since elderly patients are prone to toxicity.

Renal Impairment: Adjust dose relative to toxicity; patients with renal insufficiency are prone to toxicity.

Administration
I.V.: For intra-arterial use, use infusion pump, either external or implanted.

I.V. Detail: pH: 4.0-5.5

Stability
Reconstitution: Reconstitute with 5 mL SWI for a final concentration of 100 mg/mL; further dilute in 500-1000 mL D_5W or NS for I.V. infusion.

Compatibility: Stable in D_5W, NS, SWFI
Y-site administration: Incompatible with allopurinol, cefepime

Storage: Store intact vials at room temperature of 15°C to 30°C (59°F to 86°F). Reconstituted vials are stable for up to 2 weeks under refrigeration at 2°C to 8°C (36°C to 46°C). Further dilution in 500-1000 mL D_5W or NS is stable for 2 weeks at room temperature. Solutions in 0.9% sodium chloride are stable in some ambulatory infusion pumps for up to 21 days.

Laboratory Monitoring CBC, platelet count, liver function

Nursing Actions
Physical Assessment: Use caution with impaired liver or kidney function. Assess potential for interactions with other pharmacological agents or herbal products patient may be taking. See Administration for infusion specifics. Assess results of laboratory tests, therapeutic effectiveness, and adverse response (eg, CNS changes, acute gastrointestinal reactions [intractable vomiting or diarrhea may be dose limiting]) on a regular basis throughout therapy. Teach patient (caregiver) use and care of implantable pump, possible side effects/appropriate interventions, and adverse symptoms to report.

Patient Education: Do not take any new medication during therapy unless approved by prescriber. This drug can only be administered by infusion. Follow instructions of prescriber for care of implantable pump. Avoid alcohol. It is important to maintain adequate hydration (2-3 L/day of fluids) unless instructed to restrict fluid intake, and nutrition (small, frequent meals may help). You will be more susceptible to infection (avoid crowds and exposure to infection and do not have any vaccinations without consulting prescriber). May cause nausea or vomiting (small, frequent meals, frequent mouth care, sucking lozenges, or chewing gum may help); loss of hair (reversible); diarrhea (buttermilk, boiled milk, or yogurt may help reduce diarrhea); mouth sores (use a soft toothbrush or cotton swabs for oral care); or sterility. Increased emotional or physical stress will adversely affect the response to this medication. Notify prescriber if you are experiencing unusual or elevated levels of stress. Report extreme fatigue; pain or numbness in extremities; severe GI upset or diarrhea; bleeding or bruising; fever, chills, or sore throat; vaginal discharge; or signs of fluid retention (eg, swelling extremities, respiratory difficulty, unusual weight gain). **Pregnancy/breast-feeding precautions:** Do not get pregnant while taking this medication and for 1 month following therapy. Consult prescriber for appropriate barrier contraceptives. Do not breast-feed.

Fluconazole (floo KOE na zole)

U.S. Brand Names Diflucan®

Pharmacologic Category Antifungal Agent, Oral; Antifungal Agent, Parenteral

Medication Safety Issues

Sound-alike/look-alike issues:

Fluconazole may be confused with flecainide

Diflucan® may be confused with diclofenac, Diprivan®, disulfiram

Pregnancy Risk Factor C

Lactation Enters breast/not recommended (AAP rates "compatible")

Use Treatment of candidiasis (vaginal, oropharyngeal, esophageal, urinary tract infections, peritonitis, pneumonia, and systemic infections); cryptococcal meningitis; antifungal prophylaxis in allogeneic bone marrow transplant recipients

Mechanism of Action/Effect Interferes with cytochrome P450 activity, decreasing ergosterol synthesis (principal sterol in fungal cell membrane) and inhibiting cell membrane formation

Contraindications Hypersensitivity to fluconazole, other azoles, or any component of the formulation; concomitant administration with cisapride

Warnings/Precautions Should be used with caution in patients with renal and hepatic dysfunction or previous hepatotoxicity from other azole derivatives. Patients who develop abnormal liver function tests during fluconazole therapy should be monitored closely and discontinued if symptoms consistent with liver disease develop. Use caution in patients at risk of proarrhythmias.

Drug Interactions

Cytochrome P450 Effect: Inhibits CYP1A2 (weak), 2C8/9 (strong), 2C19 (strong), 3A4 (moderate)

Decreased Effect: Rifampin decreases concentrations of fluconazole.

Increased Effect/Toxicity: Concurrent use of fluconazole with cisapride is contraindicated due to the potential for malignant arrhythmias. Fluconazole may increase the levels/effects of amiodarone, selected benzodiazepines, calcium channel blockers, cisapride, citalopram, cyclosporine, diazepam, ergot derivatives, fluoxetine, glimepiride, glipizide, HMG-CoA reductase inhibitors, methsuximide, mirtazapine, nateglinide, nefazodone, phenytoin, pioglitazone, propranolol, rosiglitazone, sertraline, sildenafil (and other PDE-5 inhibitors), tacrolimus, venlafaxine, warfarin, and other substrates of CYP2C8/9, 2C19, and 3A4.

Adverse Reactions Frequency not always defined.

Cardiovascular: Angioedema, pallor, QT prolongation, torsade de pointes

Central nervous system: Headache (2% to 13%), seizure, dizziness

Dermatologic: Rash (2%), alopecia, toxic epidermal necrolysis, Stevens-Johnson syndrome

Endocrine & metabolic: Hypercholesterolemia, hypertriglyceridemia, hypokalemia

Gastrointestinal: Nausea (4% to 7%), vomiting (2%), abdominal pain (2% to 6%), diarrhea (2% to 3%), taste perversion, dyspepsia

Hematologic: Agranulocytosis, leukopenia, neutropenia, thrombocytopenia

Hepatic: Hepatic failure (rare), hepatitis, cholestasis, jaundice, increased ALT/AST, increased alkaline phosphatase

Respiratory: Dyspnea

Miscellaneous: Anaphylactic reactions (rare)

Overdosage/Toxicology Symptoms of overdose include decreased lacrimation, salivation, respiration and motility, urinary incontinence, and cyanosis. Treatment includes supportive measures. A 3-hour hemodialysis will remove 50%.

Pharmacodynamics/Kinetics

Time to Peak: Oral: 1-2 hours

Protein Binding: Plasma: 11% to 12%

Half-Life Elimination: Normal renal function: ~30 hours

Excretion: Urine (80% as unchanged drug)

Available Dosage Forms

Infusion [premixed in sodium chloride]: 2 mg/mL (100 mL, 200 mL)

Diflucan® [premixed in sodium chloride or dextrose] 2 mg/mL (100 mL, 200 mL)

Powder for oral suspension (Diflucan®): 10 mg/mL (35 mL); 40 mg/mL (35 mL) [contains sodium benzoate; orange flavor]

Tablet (Diflucan®): 50 mg, 100 mg, 150 mg, 200 mg

Dosing

Adults & Elderly: The daily dose of fluconazole is the same for both oral and I.V. administration

Usual dosage range: 200-400 mg daily; duration and dosage depends on severity of infection

Indication-specific dosing:

Candidiasis:

Candidemia, primary therapy, non-neutropenic: 400-800 mg/day for 14 days after last positive blood culture and resolution of signs/symptoms Alternate therapy: 800 mg/day with amphotericin B for 4-7 days followed by 800 mg/day for 14 days after last positive blood culture and resolution of signs/symptoms

Candidemia, secondary, neutropenic: 6-12 mg/kg/day for 14 days after last positive blood culture and resolution of signs/symptoms

Chronic, disseminated: 6 mg/kg/day for 3-6 months

Oropharyngeal (long-term suppression): 200 mg/day; chronic therapy is recommended in immunocompromised patients with history of oropharyngeal candidiasis (OPC)

Osteomyelitis: 6 mg/kg/day for 6-12 months

Esophageal: 200 mg on day 1, then 100-200 mg/day for 2-3 days after clinical improvement

Prophylaxis in bone marrow transplant: 400 mg/day; begin 3 days before onset of neutropenia and continue for 7 days after neutrophils >1000 cells/mm³

Urinary: 200 mg/day for 1-2 weeks

Vaginal: 150 mg as a single dose

Coccidiomycosis: 400 mg/day; doses of 800-1000 mg/day have been used for meningeal disease; usual duration of therapy ranges from 3-6 months for primary uncomplicated infections and up to 1 year for pulmonary (chronic and diffuse) infection

Endocarditis, prosthetic valve, early: 6-12 mg/kg/day for 6 weeks after valve replacement

Endophthalmitis: 6-12 mg/kg/day or 400-800 mg/day for 6-12 weeks after surgical intervention. **Note:** *C. krusei* and *C. galbrata* infection acquired exogenously should be treated with voriconazole.

Meningitis, cryptococcal: 400-800 mg/day for 10-12 weeks or with flucytosine 100-150 mg/day for 6 weeks; maintenance: 200-400 mg/day

(Continued)

Fluconazole (Continued)

Pneumonia, cryptococcal (mild-to-moderate): 200-400 mg/day for 6-12 months (life-long in HIV-positive patients)

Pediatrics: The daily dose of fluconazole is the same for oral and I.V. administration

Usual dosage ranges:

Neonates: First 2 weeks of life, especially premature neonates: Same dose as older children every 72 hours

Children: Loading dose: 6-12 mg/kg; maintenance: 3-12 mg/kg/day; duration and dosage depends on severity of infection

Indication-specific dosing:

Candidiasis:

Oropharyngeal: Loading dose: 6 mg/kg; maintenance: 3 mg/kg/day for 2 weeks

Esophageal: Loading dose: 6 mg/kg; maintenance: 3-12 mg/kg/day for 21 days and at least 2 weeks following resolution of symptoms

Systemic infection: 6 mg/kg every 12 hours for 28 days

Meningitis, cryptococcal: Loading dose: 12 mg/kg; maintenance: 6-12 mg/kg/day for 10-12 weeks following negative CSF culture; relapse suppression: 6 mg/kg/day

Renal Impairment:

No adjustment for vaginal candidiasis single-dose therapy

For multiple dosing, administer usual load then adjust daily doses

Cl$_{cr}$ ≤50 mL/minute (no dialysis): Administer 50% of recommended dose or administer every 48 hours.

Hemodialysis: 50% is removed by hemodialysis; administer 100% of daily dose (according to indication) after each dialysis treatment.

Continuous arteriovenous or venovenous hemofiltration: Dose as for Cl$_{cr}$ 10-50 mL/minute.

Administration

Oral: May be administered with or without food.

I.M.: For I.V. only; do not administer I.M. or SubQ

I.V.: Infuse over approximately 1-2 hours.

I.V. Detail: Do not use if cloudy or precipitated. Do not exceed 200 mg/hour when administering by I.V. infusion.

pH: 4-8 (sodium chloride diluent); 3.5-6.5 (dextrose)

Stability

Compatibility: Stable in D$_5$W, LR, NS

Y-site administration: Incompatible with amphotericin B, amphotericin B cholesteryl sulfate complex, ampicillin, calcium gluconate, cefotaxime, ceftazidime, ceftriaxone, cefuroxime, chloramphenicol, clindamycin, co-trimoxazole, diazepam, digoxin, erythromycin lactobionate, furosemide, haloperidol, hydroxyzine, imipenem/cilastatin, pentamidine, piperacillin, ticarcillin

Compatibility when admixed: Incompatible with co-trimoxazole

Storage:

Powder for oral suspension: Store dry powder at ≤30°C (86°F). Following reconstitution, store at 5°C to 30°C (41°F to 86°F). Discard unused portion after 2 weeks. Do not freeze.

Injection: Store injection in glass at 5°C to 30°C (41°F to 86°F). Store injection in Viaflex® at 5°C to 25°C (41°F to 77°F). Protect from freezing. Do not unwrap unit until ready for use.

Laboratory Monitoring Culture prior to beginning therapy, periodic liver function (AST, ALT, alkaline phosphatase) and renal function, potassium

Nursing Actions

Physical Assessment: Cultures should be obtained and allergy history assessed prior to beginning therapy. Assess potential for interactions with other pharmacological agents patient may be taking (eg, potential for toxicities). See Administration specifics for I.V. use. Assess results of laboratory tests (renal and hepatic function), therapeutic effectiveness (resolution of fungal infection), and adverse response (eg, hepatotoxicity [jaundice], skin disorders, abdominal pain) on a regular basis throughout therapy. Teach patient use (full course of therapy may require weeks or months after symptoms resolve), possible side effects/appropriate interventions, and adverse symptoms to report.

Patient Education: Do not take any new medication during therapy unless approved by prescriber. Take as directed, around-the-clock. Take full course of medication as ordered. Take with or without food. Follow good hygiene measures to prevent reinfection. Frequent blood tests may be required. Maintain adequate hydration (2-3 L/day of fluids) unless instructed to restrict fluid intake. May cause headache, dizziness, drowsiness (use caution when driving or engaging in tasks that require alertness until response to drug is known); or nausea, vomiting, or diarrhea (small, frequent meals, frequent mouth care, sucking lozenges, or chewing gum may help). Report skin rash, redness, or irritation; persistent GI upset; urinary pattern changes; excessively dry eyes or mouth; or changes in color of stool or urine. **Pregnancy/breast-feeding precautions:** Inform prescriber if you are or intend to become pregnant. Consult prescriber if breast-feeding.

Dietary Considerations Take with or without regard to food.

Geriatric Considerations Dose may need adjustment based on changes of renal function.

Breast-Feeding Issues Fluconazole is found in breast milk at concentration similar to plasma.

Pregnancy Issues When used in high doses, fluconazole is teratogenic in animal studies. Following exposure during the first trimester, case reports have noted similar malformations in humans when used in higher doses (400 mg/day) over extended periods of time. Use of lower doses (150 mg as a single dose or 200 mg/day) may have less risk; however, additional data is needed. Use during pregnancy only if the potential benefit to the mother outweighs any potential risk to the fetus.

Flucytosine (floo SYE toe seen)

U.S. Brand Names Ancobon®

Synonyms 5-FC; 5-Fluorocytosine; 5-Flurocytosine

Pharmacologic Category Antifungal Agent, Oral

Medication Safety Issues

Sound-alike/look-alike issues:

Flucytosine may be confused with fluorouracil

Ancobon® may be confused with Oncovin®

Pregnancy Risk Factor C

Lactation Excretion in breast milk unknown/not recommended

Use Adjunctive treatment of susceptible fungal infections (usually Candida or Cryptococcus); synergy with amphotericin B for certain fungal infections (Cryptococcus spp., Candida spp.)

Mechanism of Action/Effect Penetrates fungal cells and interferes with fungal RNA and protein synthesis

Contraindications Hypersensitivity to flucytosine or any component of the formulation

Warnings/Precautions Use with extreme caution in patients with renal dysfunction; dosage adjustment required. Avoid use as monotherapy; resistance rapidly develops. Use with caution in patients with bone marrow depression; patients with hematologic disease or who have been treated with radiation or drugs that suppress the bone marrow may be at greatest risk. Bone marrow toxicity can be irreversible.

Drug Interactions
Decreased Effect: Cytarabine may inactivate flucytosine activity.
Increased Effect/Toxicity: Increased effect with amphotericin B. Amphotericin B-induced renal dysfunction may predispose patient to flucytosine accumulation and myelosuppression.
Nutritional/Ethanol Interactions Food: Food decreases the rate, but not the extent of absorption.
Lab Interactions Flucytosine causes markedly false elevations in serum creatinine values when the Ektachem® analyzer is used.

Adverse Reactions Frequency not defined.
Cardiovascular: Cardiac arrest, myocardial toxicity, ventricular dysfunction, chest pain
Central nervous system: Confusion, headache, hallucinations, dizziness, drowsiness, psychosis, parkinsonism, ataxia, sedation, pyrexia, seizure, fatigue
Dermatologic: Rash, photosensitivity, pruritus, urticaria, Lyell's syndrome
Endocrine & metabolic: Temporary growth failure, hypoglycemia, hypokalemia
Gastrointestinal: Nausea, vomiting, diarrhea, abdominal pain, loss of appetite, dry mouth, hemorrhage, ulcerative colitis
Hematologic: Bone marrow suppression, anemia, leukopenia, thrombocytopenia, agranulocytosis, aplastic anemia, eosinophilia, pancytopenia
Hepatic: Liver enzymes increased, hepatitis, jaundice, azotemia, bilirubin increased
Neuromuscular & skeletal: Peripheral neuropathy, paresthesia, weakness
Otic: Hearing loss
Renal: BUN and serum creatinine increased, renal failure, azotemia, crystalluria
Respiratory: Respiratory arrest, dyspnea
Miscellaneous: Anaphylaxis, allergic reaction

Overdosage/Toxicology Symptoms of overdose include nausea, vomiting, diarrhea, hepatitis, and bone marrow suppression. Treatment is supportive. Removed by hemodialysis.

Pharmacodynamics/Kinetics
Time to Peak: Serum: ~2-6 hours
Protein Binding: 2% to 4%
Half-Life Elimination: Normal renal function: 2-5 hours; Anuria: 85 hours (range: 30-250); End stage renal disease: 75-200 hours
Metabolism: Minimally hepatic; deaminated, possibly via gut bacteria, to 5-fluorouracil
Excretion: Urine (>90% as unchanged drug)

Available Dosage Forms Capsule: 250 mg, 500 mg

Dosing
Adults & Elderly:
Endocarditis: Oral: 25-37.5 mg/kg 4 times/day (with amphotericin B) for at least 6 weeks after valve replacement
Fungal infections (adjunct): Oral: 50-150 mg/kg/day in divided doses every 6 hours
Meningoencephalitis, cryptococcal: Induction: Oral: 100 mg/kg/day (with amphotericin B) divided every 6 hours for 2 weeks; if clinical improvement, may discontinue both amphotericin and flucytosine and follow with an extended course of fluconazole; alternatively, may continue flucytosine for 6-10 weeks (with ampho B) without conversion to fluconazole treatment
Pneumonia, cryptococcal: HIV positive: Oral: 100-150 mg/kg/day for 10 weeks (with fluconazole 400 mg/day)
Pediatrics: Refer to adult dosing.
Renal Impairment: Use lower initial dose:
Cl_{cr} 20-40 mL/minute: Dose every 12 hours
Cl_{cr} 10-20 mL/minute: Dose every 24 hours
Cl_{cr} <10 mL/minute: Dose every 24-48 hours

Hemodialysis: Dialyzable (50% to 100%); administer dose posthemodialysis
Peritoneal dialysis: Adults: Administer 0.5-1 g every 24 hours
Continuous arteriovenous or venovenous hemodiafiltration effects: Dose as for Cl_{cr} 10-50 mL/minute

Administration
Oral: Administer around-the-clock to promote less variation in peak and trough serum levels. To avoid nausea and vomiting, administer a few capsules at a time over 15 minutes until full dose is taken.

Stability
Storage: Store at 25°C (77°F). Protect from light.

Laboratory Monitoring
Pretreatment: Electrolytes, CBC, BUN, renal function, blood culture
During treatment: CBC and LFTs frequently, serum flucytosine concentration, renal function

Nursing Actions
Physical Assessment: Assess potential for interactions with pharmacological agents patient may be taking. Monitor laboratory tests prior to and during treatment. Monitor therapeutic effectiveness (resolution of fungal infection) and adverse response (eg, cardiac incidents, CNS changes, bone marrow suppression, jaundice, skin reactions, hearing loss) on a regular basis throughout therapy. Teach patient use (full course of therapy may require some time after symptoms resolve), possible side effects/appropriate interventions, and adverse symptoms to report.

Patient Education: Do not take any new medication during therapy unless approved by prescriber. Take capsules one at a time over a few minutes with food to reduce GI upset. Take full course of medication as ordered. Do not discontinue without consulting prescriber. Practice good hygiene measures to prevent reinfection. Frequent blood tests may be required. May cause nausea and vomiting (small, frequent meals may help). Report rash; respiratory difficulty; CNS changes (eg, confusion, hallucinations, ataxia, acute headache); yellowing of skin or eyes; changes in color of stool or urine; unresolved diarrhea or anorexia; or unusual bleeding, fatigue, or weakness. **Pregnancy/breast-feeding precautions:** Inform prescriber if you are or intend to become pregnant. Breast-feeding is not recommended.

Geriatric Considerations Adjust for renal function.

Fludarabine (floo DARE a been)

U.S. Brand Names Fludara®
Synonyms Fludarabine Phosphate
Pharmacologic Category Antineoplastic Agent, Antimetabolite (Purine Antagonist)
Medication Safety Issues
Sound-alike/look-alike issues:
Fludarabine may be confused with floxuridine, Flumadine®
Fludara® may be confused with FUDR®
Pregnancy Risk Factor D
Lactation Excretion in breast milk unknown/contraindicated
Use
I.V.: Treatment of chronic lymphocytic leukemia (CLL) (including refractory CLL); non-Hodgkin's lymphoma in adults
Oral (formulation not available in U.S.): Approved in Canada for treatment of CLL
Unlabeled/Investigational Use Treatment of non-Hodgkin's lymphoma and acute leukemias in pediatric patients; reduced-intensity conditioning regimens prior to allogeneic hematopoietic stem cell transplantation (generally administered in combination with busulfan and antithymocyte globulin or lymphocyte (Continued)

Fludarabine *(Continued)*

immune globulin, or in combination with melphalan and alemtuzumab)

Mechanism of Action/Effect Inhibits DNA synthesis by inhibition of DNA polymerase and ribonucleotide reductase.

Contraindications Hypersensitivity of fludarabine or any component of the formulation; decompensated hemolytic anemia; breast-feeding, pregnancy

Warnings/Precautions Hazardous agent — use appropriate precautions for handling and disposal. Use with caution with renal insufficiency, patients with a fever, documented infection, or pre-existing hematological disorders (particularly granulocytopenia) or in patients with pre-existing central nervous system disorder (epilepsy), spasticity, or peripheral neuropathy. Life-threatening and sometimes fatal autoimmune hemolytic anemia have occurred. Severe myelosuppression (trilineage bone marrow hypoplasia/aplasia) has been reported (rare); the duration of significant cytopenias in these cases may be prolonged (up to 1 year).

Drug Interactions

Increased Effect/Toxicity: Combined use with pentostatin may lead to severe, even fatal, pulmonary toxicity.

Nutritional/Ethanol Interactions Ethanol: Avoid ethanol (due to GI irritation).

Adverse Reactions

>10%:

Cardiovascular: Edema

Central nervous system: Fatigue, somnolence (30%), chills, fever, pain

Dermatologic: Rash

Hematologic: Myelosuppression, common, dose-limiting toxicity, primarily leukopenia and thrombocytopenia

Nadir: 10-14 days

Recovery: 5-7 weeks

Neuromuscular & skeletal: Paresthesia, myalgia, weakness

Respiratory: Pneumonia

1% to 10%:

Cardiovascular: CHF

Central nervous system: Malaise, headache

Dermatologic: Alopecia

Endocrine & metabolic: Hyperglycemia, tumor lysis syndrome

Gastrointestinal: Anorexia, stomatitis (1.5%), diarrhea (1.8%), mild nausea/vomiting (3% to 10%)

Hematologic: Eosinophilia, hemolytic anemia, may be dose-limiting, possibly fatal in some patients

Overdosage/Toxicology High doses of fludarabine are associated with bone marrow depression including severe neutropenia and thrombocytopenia; irreversible central nervous system toxicity with delayed blindness, coma, and death has occurred. Discontinuation of drug and supportive therapy are recommended.

Pharmacodynamics/Kinetics

Half-Life Elimination: 2-fluoro-vidarabine: 9 hours

Metabolism: I.V.: Fludarabine phosphate is rapidly dephosphorylated to 2-fluoro-vidarabine, which subsequently enters tumor cells and is phosphorylated to the active triphosphate derivative; rapidly dephosphorylated in the serum

Excretion: Urine (60%, 23% as 2-fluoro-vidarabine) within 24 hours

Available Dosage Forms [CAN] = Canadian brand name

Injection, powder for reconstitution, as phosphate: 50 mg

Tablet, as phosphate [CAN]: 10 mg [not available in U.S.]

Dosing

Adults & Elderly:

Chronic lymphocytic leukemia (CLL):

I.V.: 25 mg/m^2/day for 5 days every 28 days

Oral: **Note:** Formulation available in Canada; not available in U.S.: 40 mg/m^2 once daily for 5 days every 28 days

Non-Hodgkin's lymphoma: Loading dose: 20 mg/m^2 followed by 30 mg/m^2/day for 48 hours

Reduced-intensity conditioning regimens prior to allogeneic hematopoietic stem cell transplantation (unlabeled use): 120-150 mg/m^2 administered in divided doses over 4-5 days

Pediatrics:

Acute leukemia (unlabeled use): 10 mg/m^2 bolus over 15 minutes followed by continuous infusion of 30.5 mg/m^2/day for 5 days **or**

10.5 mg/m^2 bolus over 15 minutes followed by 30.5 mg/m^2/day for 48 hours

Solid tumors (unlabeled use): 9 mg/m^2 bolus followed by 27 mg/m^2/day continuous infusion for 5 days

Renal Impairment:

Cl$_{cr}$ 30-70 mL/minute:

U.S. product labeling: Reduce dose by 20%

Canadian product labeling: Reduce dose by 50%

Cl$_{cr}$ <30 mL/minute: Not recommended

Administration

Oral: Tablet (formulation not available in U.S.) may be administered with or without food; should be swallowed whole; do not chew, break, or crush.

I.V.: Administer I.V. over 15-30 minutes or continuous infusion.

I.V. Detail: pH: 7.2-8.2

Stability

Reconstitution: Reconstitute vials with SWI, NS, or D$_5$W to a concentration of 10-25 mg/mL. Standard I.V. dilution: 50-100 mL D$_5$W or NS.

Compatibility: Stable in D$_5$W, NS, SWFI

Y-site administration: Incompatible Acyclovir, amphotericin B, chlorpromazine, daunorubicin, ganciclovir, hydroxyzine, prochlorperazine edisylate

Storage:

I.V.: Store intact vials under refrigeration at 2°C to 8°C (36°F to 46°F). Reconstituted vials are stable for 16 days at room temperature of 15°C to 30°C (59°F to 86°F) or refrigerated. Solutions diluted in saline or dextrose are stable for 48 hours at room temperature or under refrigeration.

Tablet (formulation not available in U.S.): Store between 15°C to 30°C (59°F to 86°F); should be kept within packaging until use.

Laboratory Monitoring CBC with differential, platelet count, AST, ALT, creatinine, serum albumin, uric acid

Nursing Actions

Physical Assessment: See Administration for infusion specifics. Monitor results of laboratory tests prior to each treatment and on a regular basis throughout therapy. Monitor patient response closely (especially CNS, hematological, and neuromuscular effects). Teach patient possible side effects/appropriate interventions and adverse symptoms to report.

Patient Education: Do not take any new medication during therapy unless approved by prescriber. This drug is administered by infusion; report any burning, pain, redness, or swelling at infusion site. It is important to maintain adequate hydration (2-3 L/day of fluids) unless instructed to restrict fluid intake and nutrition (small frequent meals may help). You will be more susceptible to infection (avoid crowds and exposure to infection and do not have any vaccinations without consulting prescriber). May cause mild nausea or vomiting (small frequent meals, frequent mouth care, sucking lozenges, or chewing gum may help); loss of hair (reversible); diarrhea (buttermilk, boiled milk, or yogurt may help); or mouth sores (use soft toothbrush or cotton swabs for oral care). Report extreme fatigue; pain or numbness in extremities; severe GI upset or diarrhea; bleeding or bruising; fever, chills, or sore throat; vaginal discharge; difficulty or pain on urination; muscle pain or weakness; unusual cough or respiratory difficulty; or other unusual side effects. **Pregnancy/breast-feeding precautions:** Inform prescriber if you are pregnant. Do not get pregnant while taking this medication and for 1 month following therapy. Consult prescriber for appropriate contraceptives. Do not breast-feed.

Fludrocortisone (floo droe KOR ti sone)

U.S. Brand Names Florinef®

Synonyms 9α-Fluorohydrocortisone Acetate; Fludrocortisone Acetate; Fluohydrisone Acetate; Fluohydrocortisone Acetate

Pharmacologic Category Corticosteroid, Systemic

Medication Safety Issues
Sound-alike/look-alike issues:
Florinef® may be confused with Fiorinal®

Pregnancy Risk Factor C

Lactation Excretion in breast milk unknown

Use Partial replacement therapy for primary and secondary adrenocortical insufficiency in Addison's disease; treatment of salt-losing adrenogenital syndrome

Mechanism of Action/Effect Promotes increased reabsorption of sodium and loss of potassium from renal distal tubules

Contraindications Hypersensitivity to fludrocortisone or any component of the formulation; systemic fungal infections

Warnings/Precautions Taper dose gradually when therapy is discontinued. Patients with Addison's disease are more sensitive to the action of the hormone and may exhibit side effects in an exaggerated degree.

Drug Interactions
Decreased Effect: Anticholinesterases effects are antagonized. Decreased corticosteroid effects by rifampin, barbiturates, and hydantoins. May decrease salicylate levels.

Adverse Reactions Frequency not defined.
Cardiovascular: Hypertension, edema, CHF
Central nervous system: Convulsions, headache, dizziness
Dermatologic: Acne, rash, bruising
Endocrine & metabolic: Hypokalemic alkalosis, suppression of growth, hyperglycemia, HPA suppression
Gastrointestinal: Peptic ulcer
Neuromuscular & skeletal: Muscle weakness
Ocular: Cataracts
Miscellaneous: Diaphoresis, anaphylaxis (generalized)

Overdosage/Toxicology Symptoms of overdose include hypertension, edema, hypokalemia, excessive weight gain. When consumed in excessive quantities, systemic hypercorticism and adrenal suppression may occur. In those cases, discontinuation of the corticosteroid should be done judiciously.

Pharmacodynamics/Kinetics
Time to Peak: Serum: ~1.7 hours
Protein Binding: 42%
Half-Life Elimination: Plasma: 30-35 minutes; Biological: 18-36 hours
Metabolism: Hepatic

Available Dosage Forms Tablet, as acetate: 0.1 mg

Dosing
Adults & Elderly: Mineralocorticoid deficiency: Oral: 0.05-0.2 mg/day with ranges of 0.1 mg 3 times/week to 0.2 mg/day
Pediatrics: Mineralocorticoid deficiency: Oral: Infants and Children: 0.05-0.1 mg/day

Administration
Oral: Administration in conjunction with a glucocorticoid is preferable.

Laboratory Monitoring Serum electrolytes, serum renin activity

Nursing Actions
Physical Assessment: Assess effectiveness and interactions of other medications patient may be taking. Monitor for effectiveness of therapy and adverse reactions according to dose and length of therapy. Assess knowledge/teach patient appropriate use, possible side effects/interventions, and adverse symptoms to report (eg, opportunistic infection, adrenal suppression). Instruct patients with diabetes to monitor serum glucose levels closely; corticosteroids can alter glycemic response. Dose may need to be increased if patient is experiencing higher than normal levels of stress. When discontinuing, taper dose and frequency slowly.

Patient Education: Take exactly as directed. Do not take more than prescribed dose and do not discontinue abruptly; consult prescriber. Take with or after meals. Take once-a-day dose with food in the morning. Limit intake of caffeine or stimulants. Maintain adequate nutrition; consult prescriber for possibility of special dietary recommendations. If you have diabetes, monitor serum glucose closely and notify prescriber of changes; this medication can alter glycemic response. Notify prescriber if you are experiencing higher than normal levels of stress; medication may need adjustment. Periodic ophthalmic examinations will be necessary with long-term use. You will be susceptible to infection (avoid crowds and exposure to infection). You may experience insomnia or nervousness; use caution when driving or engaging in tasks requiring alertness until response to drug is known. Report weakness, change in menstrual pattern, vision changes, signs of hyperglycemia, signs of infection (eg, fever, chills, mouth sores, perianal itching, vaginal discharge), other persistent side effects, or worsening of condition. **Pregnancy/breast-feeding precautions:** Inform prescriber if you are or intend to become pregnant. Consult prescriber if breast-feeding.

Dietary Considerations Systemic use of mineralocorticoids/corticosteroids may require a diet with increased potassium, vitamins A, B₆, C, D, folate, calcium, zinc, and phosphorus, and decreased sodium. With fludrocortisone, a decrease in dietary sodium is often not required as the increased retention of sodium is usually the desired therapeutic effect.

Geriatric Considerations The most common use of fludrocortisone in the elderly is orthostatic hypotension that is unresponsive to more conservative measures. Attempt nonpharmacologic measures (hydration, support stockings etc) before starting drug therapy.

Additional Information In patients with salt-losing forms of congenital adrenogenital syndrome, use along with cortisone or hydrocortisone. Fludrocortisone 0.1 mg has sodium retention activity equal to DOCA® 1 mg.

Flumazenil (FLOO may ze nil)

U.S. Brand Names Romazicon®

Pharmacologic Category Antidote

Pregnancy Risk Factor C

Lactation Excretion in breast milk unknown/use caution

Use Benzodiazepine antagonist; reverses sedative effects of benzodiazepines used in conscious sedation and general anesthesia; treatment of benzodiazepine overdose

Mechanism of Action/Effect Competitively inhibits the activity at the benzodiazepine recognition site on the GABA/benzodiazepine receptor complex. Flumazenil
(Continued)

Flumazenil *(Continued)*

does not antagonize the CNS effect of drugs affecting GABA-ergic neurons by means other than the benzodiazepine receptor (ethanol, barbiturates, general anesthetics) and does not reverse the effects of opioids.

Contraindications Hypersensitivity to flumazenil, benzodiazepines, or any component of the formulation; patients given benzodiazepines for control of potentially life-threatening conditions (eg, control of intracranial pressure or status epilepticus); patients who are showing signs of serious cyclic-antidepressant overdosage

Warnings/Precautions Benzodiazepine reversal may result in seizures in some patients. Patients who may develop seizures include patients on benzodiazepines for long-term sedation, tricyclic antidepressant overdose patients, concurrent major sedative-hypnotic drug withdrawal, recent therapy with repeated doses of parenteral benzodiazepines, myoclonic jerking or seizure activity prior to flumazenil administration. Flumazenil does not reverse respiratory depression/hypoventilation or cardiac depression. Resedation occurs more frequently in patients where a large single dose or cumulative dose of a benzodiazepine is administered along with a neuromuscular blocking agent and multiple anesthetic agents. Flumazenil should be used with caution in the intensive care unit because of increased risk of unrecognized benzodiazepine dependence in such settings. Should not be used to diagnose benzodiazepine-induced sedation. Reverse neuromuscular blockade before considering use. Flumazenil does not antagonize the CNS effects of other GABA agonists (such as ethanol, barbiturates, or general anesthetics); nor does it reverse narcotics. Use with caution in patients with a history of panic disorder; may provoke panic attacks. Use caution in drug and ethanol-dependent patients; these patients may also be dependent on benzodiazepines. Not recommended for treatment of benzodiazepine dependence. Use with caution in head injury patients. Use caution in patients with mixed drug overdoses; toxic effects of other drugs taken may emerge once benzodiazepine effects are reversed. Flumazenil does not consistently reverse amnesia; patient may not recall verbal instructions after procedure. Use caution in severe hepatic dysfunction and in patients relying on a benzodiazepine for seizure control. Safety and efficacy have not been established in children >1 year of age.

Drug Interactions
Increased Effect/Toxicity: Flumazenil reverses the effects of these nonbenzodiazepine hypnotics (zaleplon, zolpidem, zopiclone).

Adverse Reactions
>10%: Gastrointestinal: Vomiting, nausea
1% to 10%:
Cardiovascular: Palpitations
Central nervous system: Headache, anxiety, nervousness, insomnia, abnormal crying, euphoria, depression, agitation, dizziness, emotional lability, ataxia, depersonalization, increased tears, dysphoria, paranoia, fatigue, vertigo
Endocrine & metabolic: Hot flashes
Gastrointestinal: Xerostomia
Local: Pain at injection site
Neuromuscular & skeletal: Tremor, weakness, paresthesia
Ocular: Abnormal vision, blurred vision
Respiratory: Dyspnea, hyperventilation
Miscellaneous: Diaphoresis

Overdosage/Toxicology Excessively high doses may cause anxiety, agitation, increased muscle tone, hyperesthesia and seizures.

Pharmacodynamics/Kinetics
Onset of Action: 1-3 minutes; 80% response within 3 minutes; Peak effect: 6-10 minutes

Duration of Action: Resedation: ~1 hour; duration related to dose given and benzodiazepine plasma concentrations; reversal effects of flumazenil may wear off before effects of benzodiazepine

Protein Binding: 40% to 50%

Half-Life Elimination: Adults: Alpha: 7-15 minutes; Terminal: 41-79 minutes

Metabolism: Hepatic; dependent upon hepatic blood flow

Excretion: Feces; urine (0.2% as unchanged drug)

Available Dosage Forms Injection, solution: 0.1 mg/mL (5 mL, 10 mL) [contains edetate sodium]

Dosing
Adults: See table.

Flumazenil

Adult dosage for **reversal of conscious sedation and general anesthesia:**	
Initial dose	0.2 mg intravenously over 15 seconds
Repeat doses	If desired level of consciousness is not obtained, 0.2 mg may be repeated at 1-minute intervals.
Maximum total cumulative dose	1 mg (usual dose: 0.6-1 mg) **In the event of resedation:** Repeat doses may be given at 20-minute intervals with maximum of 1 mg/dose and 3 mg/hour.

Adult dosage for **suspected benzodiazepine overdose:**	
Initial dose	0.2 mg intravenously over 30 seconds; if the desired level of consciousness is not obtained, 0.3 mg can be given over 30 seconds
Repeat doses	0.5 mg over 30 seconds repeated at 1-minute intervals
Maximum total cumulative dose	3 mg (usual dose: 1-3 mg) Patients with a partial response at 3 mg may require additional titration up to a total dose of 5 mg. If a patient has not responded 5 minutes after cumulative dose of 5 mg, the major cause of sedation is not likely due to benzodiazepines. **In the event of resedation:** May repeat doses at 20-minute intervals with maximum of 1 mg/dose and 3 mg/hour.

Resedation: Repeated doses may be given at 20-minute intervals as needed; repeat treatment doses of 1 mg (at a rate of 0.5 mg/minute) should be given at any time and no more than 3 mg should be given in any hour. After intoxication with high doses of benzodiazepines, the duration of a single dose of flumazenil is not expected to exceed 1 hour; if desired, the period of wakefulness may be prolonged with repeated low intravenous doses of flumazenil, or by an infusion of 0.1-0.4 mg/hour. Most patients with benzodiazepine overdose will respond to a cumulative dose of 1-3 mg and doses >3 mg do not reliably produce additional effects. Rarely, patients with a partial response at 3 mg may require additional titration to a total dose of 5 mg. **If a patient has not responded 5 minutes after receiving a cumulative dose of 5 mg, the major cause of sedation is not likely to be due to benzodiazepines.**

Elderly: Refer to adult dosing. No differences in safety or efficacy have been reported; however, increased sensitivity may occur in some elderly patients.

Pediatrics:
Reversal of benzodiazepine when used in conscious sedation or general anesthesia: I.V.: Initial dose: 0.01 mg/kg (maximum dose: 0.2 mg) given over 15 seconds; may repeat 0.01 mg/kg (maximum dose: 0.2 mg) after 45 seconds, and then every minute (maximum: 4 doses) to a maximum of total cumulative dose of 0.05 mg/kg or

1 mg, whichever is lower; usual total dose: 0.08-1 mg (mean: 0.65 mg).

Renal Impairment: Not significantly affected by renal failure (Cl$_{cr}$ <10 mL/minute) or hemodialysis beginning 1 hour after drug administration.

Hepatic Impairment: Initial dose of flumazenil used for initial reversal of benzodiazepine effects is not changed; however, subsequent doses in liver disease patients should be reduced in amount or frequency.

Administration

I.V.: Administer in freely-running I.V. into large vein. Inject over 15 seconds for conscious sedation and general anesthesia and over 30 seconds for overdose.

I.V. Detail: pH: 4 (injection)

Stability

Reconstitution: For I.V. use only. Once drawn up in the syringe or mixed with solution use within 24 hours. Discard any unused solution after 24 hours.

Compatibility: Stable in D$_5$W, LR, NS

Storage: Store at 15°C to 30°C (59°F to 86°F).

Nursing Actions

Physical Assessment: Assess level of consciousness frequently. Monitor vital signs and airway closely. ECG monitoring and oxygenation via pulse oximetry is highly recommended. Observe continually for resedation, respiratory depression, preseizure activity, or other residual benzodiazepine effects. May require pain medication sooner after reversal. Assess for nausea and vomiting.

Patient Education: Flumazenil does not consistently reverse amnesia. Do not engage in activities requiring alertness for 18-24 hours after discharge. Avoid alcohol or OTC medications for 24 hours after receiving this medication, unless approved by prescriber. Resedation may occur in patients on long-acting benzodiazepines (such as diazepam).

Pregnancy/breast-feeding precautions: Inform prescriber if you are or intend to become pregnant. Consult prescriber if breast-feeding.

Flunisolide (floo NISS oh lide)

U.S. Brand Names AeroBid®; AeroBid®-M; Nasarel®

Pharmacologic Category Corticosteroid, Inhalant (Oral); Corticosteroid, Nasal

Medication Safety Issues

Sound-alike/look-alike issues:

Flunisolide may be confused with Flumadine®, fluocinonide

Nasarel® may be confused with Nizoral®

Pregnancy Risk Factor C

Lactation Excretion in breast milk unknown/use caution

Use Steroid-dependent asthma; nasal solution is used for seasonal or perennial rhinitis

Mechanism of Action/Effect Decreases inflammation by suppression of migration of polymorphonuclear leukocytes and reversal of increased capillary permeability; does not depress hypothalamus

Contraindications Hypersensitivity to flunisolide or any component of the formulation; acute status asthmaticus; viral, tuberculosis, fungal, or bacterial respiratory infections; infections of the nasal mucosa

Warnings/Precautions Not to be used in status asthmaticus or for the relief of acute bronchospasm. May cause suppression of hypothalamic-pituitary-adrenal (HPA) axis, particularly in younger children or in patients receiving high doses for prolonged periods. Fatalities have occurred due to adrenal insufficiency in asthmatic patients during and after transfer from systemic corticosteroids to aerosol steroids; aerosol steroids do **not** provide the systemic steroid needed to treat patients having trauma, surgery, or infections. Withdrawal and

discontinuation of the corticosteroid should be done slowly and carefully.

Controlled clinical studies have shown that orally-inhaled and intranasal corticosteroids may cause a reduction in growth velocity in pediatric patients, which appears to be related to dose and duration of exposure.

May suppress the immune system, patients may be more susceptible to infection. Use with caution in patients with systemic infections or ocular herpes simplex. Avoid exposure to chickenpox and measles.

Drug Interactions

Increased Effect/Toxicity: Expected interactions similar to other corticosteroids

Salmeterol: The addition of salmeterol has been demonstrated to improve response to inhaled corticosteroids (as compared to increasing steroid dosage).

Adverse Reactions

>10%:

Cardiovascular: Pounding heartbeat

Central nervous system: Dizziness, headache, nervousness

Dermatologic: Itching, rash

Endocrine & metabolic: Adrenal suppression, menstrual problems

Gastrointestinal: GI irritation, anorexia, sore throat, bitter taste

Local: Nasal burning, *Candida* infection of the nose or pharynx, atrophic rhinitis

Respiratory: Sneezing, cough, upper respiratory tract infection, bronchitis, nasal congestion, nasal dryness

Miscellaneous: Increased susceptibility to infection

1% to 10%:

Central nervous system: Insomnia, psychic changes

Dermatologic: Acne, urticaria

Gastrointestinal: Increase in appetite, xerostomia, dry throat, loss of taste perception

Ocular: Cataracts

Respiratory: Epistaxis

Miscellaneous: Diaphoresis, loss of smell

Overdosage/Toxicology When consumed in high doses over prolonged periods, systemic hypercorticism and adrenal suppression may occur. In those cases, discontinuation of the corticosteroid should be done judiciously.

Pharmacodynamics/Kinetics

Half-Life Elimination: 1.8 hours

Metabolism: Rapidly hepatic to active metabolites

Excretion: Urine and feces (equal amounts)

Available Dosage Forms

Aerosol for oral inhalation:

AeroBid®: 250 mcg/actuation (7 g) [100 metered inhalations; contains CFCs]

AeroBid®-M: 250 mcg/actuation (7 g) [100 metered inhalations; contains CFCs; menthol flavor]

Solution, intranasal [spray]: 29 mcg/actuation (25 mL) [200 sprays]

Nasarel®: 29 mcg/actuation (25 mL) [200 sprays; contains benzalkonium chloride]

Dosing

Adults & Elderly:

Asthma: Oral inhalation: 2 inhalations twice daily (morning and evening) up to 8 inhalations/day maximum

Seasonal allergic rhinitis: Nasal: 2 sprays in each nostril twice daily (morning and evening); maximum: 8 sprays/day in each nostril

Pediatrics:

Asthma (Children >6 years): Oral inhalation: 2 inhalations twice daily (morning and evening) up to 4 inhalations/day

Seasonal allergic rhinitis (Children >6 years): Intranasal: 1 spray each nostril twice daily (morning

(Continued)

Flunisolide (Continued)

and evening), not to exceed 4 sprays/day each nostril

Administration

Inhalation: Shake well before using. Do not use Nasalide® or Nasarel® orally. Throw out product after it has been opened for 3 months.

Nursing Actions

Physical Assessment: Not to be used to treat status asthmaticus or fungal infections of nasal passages. Monitor therapeutic effectiveness and adverse reactions. When changing from systemic steroids to inhalational steroid, taper reduction of systemic medication slowly. Assess knowledge/teach patient appropriate use, interventions to reduce side effects, and adverse symptoms to report.

Patient Education: Use as directed; do not use nasal preparations for oral inhalation. Do not increase dosage or discontinue abruptly without consulting prescriber. Review use of inhaler or spray with prescriber or follow package insert for directions. Keep oral inhaler clean and unobstructed. Always rinse mouth and throat after use of inhaler to prevent opportunistic infection. If you are also using an inhaled bronchodilator, wait 10 minutes before using this steroid aerosol. You may experience dizziness, anxiety, or blurred vision (rise slowly from sitting or lying position and use caution when driving or engaging in tasks requiring alertness until response to drug is known); or taste disturbance or aftertaste (frequent mouth care and mouth rinses may help). Report pounding heartbeat or chest pain; acute nervousness or inability to sleep; severe sneezing or nosebleed; respiratory difficulty, sore throat, hoarseness, or bronchitis; respiratory difficulty or bronchospasms; disturbed menstrual pattern; vision changes; loss of taste or smell perception; or worsening of condition or lack of improvement. **Pregnancy/breast-feeding precautions:** Inform prescriber if you are or intend to become pregnant. Consult prescriber if breast-feeding.

Inhaler: Sit when using. Take deep breaths for 3-5 minutes, and clear nasal passages before administration (use decongestant as needed). Hold breath for 5-10 seconds after use, and wait 1-3 minutes between inhalations. Follow package insert instructions for use. Do not exceed maximum dosage. If also using inhaled bronchodilator, use before flunisolide. Rinse mouth and throat after use to reduce aftertaste and prevent candidiasis.

Geriatric Considerations Many elderly patients have difficulty using metered dose inhalers, which can limit their effectiveness. Assess technique in all older patients. A spacer device may be beneficial for the oral inhaler.

Additional Information Does not contain fluorocarbons; contains polyethylene glycol vehicle.

Effects of inhaled/intranasal steroids on growth have been observed in the absence of laboratory evidence of HPA axis suppression, suggesting that growth velocity is a more sensitive indicator of systemic corticosteroid exposure in pediatric patients than some commonly used tests of HPA axis function. The long-term effects of this reduction in growth velocity associated with orally-inhaled and intranasal corticosteroids, including the impact on final adult height, are unknown. The potential for "catch up" growth following discontinuation of treatment with inhaled corticosteroids has not been adequately studied.

Fluocinolone (floo oh SIN oh lone)

U.S. Brand Names Capex™; Derma-Smoothe/FS®; Retisert™; Synalar®

Synonyms Fluocinolone Acetonide

Pharmacologic Category Corticosteroid, Ophthalmic; Corticosteroid, Topical

Medication Safety Issues
Sound-alike/look-alike issues:
Fluocinolone may be confused with fluocinonide

Pregnancy Risk Factor C

Lactation Excretion in breast milk unknown/use caution

Use Relief of susceptible inflammatory dermatosis [low, medium, high potency topical corticosteroid]; psoriasis of the scalp; atopic dermatitis in children ≥2 years of age
Ocular implant (Retisert™): Treatment of chronic, noninfectious uveitis affecting the posterior segment of the eye.

Mechanism of Action/Effect Topical corticosteroid with anti-inflammatory, antipruritic, and vasoconstrictive properties.

Contraindications Hypersensitivity to fluocinolone or any component of the formulation; TB of skin, herpes (including varicella)
Ocular implant: Additional contraindications include ocular infections of viral or fungal origin

Warnings/Precautions Adverse systemic effects may occur when used on large areas of the body, denuded areas, for prolonged periods of time, with an occlusive dressing, and/or in infants or small children. Infants and small children may be more susceptible to adrenal axis suppression from topical corticosteroid therapy. Derma-Smoothe/FS® contains peanut oil; use caution in peanut-sensitive children.
Ocular implant: May cause transient decrease in visual acuity of 1-4 weeks duration; caution with use in glaucoma patients; routine monitoring of IOP recommended. May require IOP-lowering treatments within 2 years postimplantation. Prolonged use of ocular corticosteroids may increase risk of secondary infection, cataract formation, optic nerve damage, and/or glaucoma. Recommend unilateral implantation only to minimize risk of postoperative infections developing in both eyes. Safety and efficacy have not been established in children <12 years of age.

Adverse Reactions Topical: Frequency not defined.
Dermatologic: Acneiform eruptions, allergic contact dermatitis, burning, dryness, folliculitis, irritation, itching, hypertrichosis, hypopigmentation, miliaria, perioral dermatitis, skin atrophy, striae
Endocrine & metabolic: Cushing's syndrome, HPA axis suppression
Miscellaneous: Secondary infection

Ocular implant:
>50%: Ocular: Cataract, intraocular pressure increased, eye pain; procedural complications (eg, cataract fragments, implant migration, wound complications)
10% to 35%:
Central nervous system: Dizziness (5% to 15%), headache (31%), pain (5% to 15%), pyrexia (5% to 15%)
Dermatologic: Rash (5% to 15%)
Gastrointestinal (5% to 15%): Nausea, vomiting
Neuromuscular & skeletal (5% to 15%): Arthralgia, back pain, limb pain
Ocular: Blurred vision, conjunctival hemorrhage, conjunctival hyperemia, dry eye, eye irritation/inflammation, eyelid edema, glaucoma, hypotony, maculopathy, pruritus, ptosis, tearing, visual acuity decrease, vitreous floaters, vitreous hemorrhage
Respiratory (5% to 15%): Cough, influenza, nasopharyngitis, sinusitis, upper respiratory infection

5% to 9%: Ocular: Blepharitis, choroidal detachment, conjunctival edema/chemosis, corneal edema, eye discharge, eye swelling, macular edema, photophobia, photopsia, retinal hemorrhage, visual disturbance, vitreous opacitites

Frequency not specified: Miscellaneous: Secondary infection (bacterial, viral, or fungal)

Overdosage/Toxicology Topically-applied products may be absorbed in sufficient amounts to produce systemic effects, particularly if applied to large surface area or to inflamed/damaged skin. Systemic hypercorticism and adrenal suppression may occur; in those cases, discontinuation and withdrawal of the corticosteroid should be done judiciously.

Pharmacodynamics/Kinetics
Duration of Action:
Ocular implant: Releases fluocinolone acetonide at a rate of 0.6 mcg/day, decreasing over 30 days to a steady-state release rate of 0.3-0.4 mcg/day for 30 months

Metabolism: Primarily in skin; small amount absorbed into systemic circulation is primarily hepatic to inactive compounds

Excretion: Urine (primarily as glucuronide and sulfate, also as unconjugated products); feces (small amounts)

Available Dosage Forms
Cream, as acetonide: 0.01% (15 g, 60 g); 0.025% (15 g, 60 g)
Synalar®: 0.025% (15 g, 60 g)
Oil, as acetonide:
Derma-Smoothe/FS® [eczema oil]: 0.01% (120 mL) [contains peanut oil]
Derma-Smoothe/FS® [scalp oil]: 0.01% (120 mL) [contains peanut oil; packaged with shower caps]
Ointment, as acetonide (Synalar®): 0.025% (15 g, 60 g)
Shampoo, as acetonide (Capex™): 0.01% (120 mL)
Solution, as acetonide: 0.01% (60 mL)
Synalar®: 0.01% (20 mL, 60 mL)
Tablet, ocular implant, as acetonide (Retisert™): 0.59 mg [enclosed in silicone elastomer]

Dosing
Adults & Elderly:
Corticosteroid-responsive dermatoses: Topical: Cream, ointment, solution: Apply a thin layer to affected area 2-4 times/day; may use occlusive dressings to manage psoriasis or recalcitrant conditions

Atopic dermatitis (Derma-Smoothe/FS®): Topical: Apply thin film to affected area 3 times/day

Scalp psoriasis (Derma-Smoothe/FS®): Topical: Massage thoroughly into wet or dampened hair/scalp; cover with shower cap. Leave on overnight (or for at least 4 hours). Remove by washing hair with shampoo and rinsing thoroughly.

Seborrheic dermatitis of the scalp (Capex™): Topical: Apply no more than 1 ounce to scalp once daily; work into lather and allow to remain on scalp for ~5 minutes. Remove from hair and scalp by rinsing thoroughly with water.

Chronic uveitis: Ocular implant: One silicone-encased tablet (0.59 mg) surgically implanted into the posterior segment of the eye is designed to release 0.6 mcg/day, decreasing over 30 days to a steady-state release rate of 0.3-0.4 mcg/day for 30 months. Recurrence of uveitis denotes depletion of tablet, requiring reimplantation.

Pediatrics: Children ≥2 years:
Atopic dermatitis (Derma-Smoothe/FS®): Topical: Moisten skin; apply to affected area twice daily; do not use for longer than 4 weeks

Corticosteroid-responsive dermatoses: Refer to adult dosing.

Administration
Topical: Apply thin film to affected area; avoid eyes.
Other:
Ocular implant: Handle only by suture tab to avoid damaging the tablet integrity and adversely affecting release characteristics. Maintain strict adherence to aseptic handling of product; do not resterilize.

Stability
Reconstitution: Capex™: Prior to dispensing, the contents of the capsule should be emptied into the liquid shampoo; shake well. Discard after 3 months.
Storage: Topical: Store at controlled room temperature in tightly-closed container.
Ocular implant (Retisert™): Store in original container at 15°C to 25°C (59°F to 77°F); protect from freezing

Nursing Actions
Physical Assessment: Assess potential for interactions with other prescriptions, OTC medications, or herbal products patient may be taking. Monitor patient response. Teach patient proper use (according to formulation), side effects/appropriate interventions, and symptoms to report.
Patient Education:
For external use only. Do not use for eyes, mucous membranes, or open wounds. Use exactly as directed and for no longer than the period prescribed. Before using, wash and dry area gently. Apply in a thin layer (may rub in lightly). Apply light dressing (if necessary) to area being treated. Do not use occlusive dressing unless so advised by prescriber. Avoid prolonged or excessive use around sensitive tissues, genital, or rectal areas. Avoid exposing treated area to direct sunlight. Inform prescriber if condition worsens (redness, swelling, irritation, signs of infection, or open sores) or fails to improve.
Pregnancy/breast-feeding precautions: Inform prescriber if you are or intend to become pregnant. Consult prescriber if breast-feeding.
Breast-Feeding Issues Systemic corticosteroids are excreted in human milk. It is not known if sufficient quantities of fluocinolone are absorbed following topical or ocular administration to produce detectable amounts in breast milk. Hypertension in the nursing infant has been reported following corticosteroid ointment applied to the nipples. Use with caution.
Pregnancy Issues In general, the use of topical corticosteroids during pregnancy is not considered to have significant risk, however, intrauterine growth retardation in the infant has been reported (rare). The use of large amounts or for prolonged periods of time should be avoided.

Fluocinolone, Hydroquinone, and Tretinoin
(floo oh SIN oh lone, HYE droe kwin one, & TRET i noyn)

U.S. Brand Names Tri-Luma™
Synonyms Hydroquinone, Fluocinolone Acetonide, and Tretinoin; Tretinoin, Fluocinolone Acetonide, and Hydroquinone
Pharmacologic Category Corticosteroid, Topical; Depigmenting Agent; Retinoic Acid Derivative
Pregnancy Risk Factor C
Lactation Excretion in breast milk unknown/use caution
Use Short-term treatment of moderate to severe melasma of the face
Available Dosage Forms Cream, topical: Hydroquinone 4%, tretinoin 0.05%, fluocinolone acetonide 0.01% (30 g) [contains sodium metabisulfite]
Dosing
Adults & Elderly: Melasma: Topical: Apply a thin film once daily to hyperpigmented areas of melasma
(Continued)

Fluocinolone, Hydroquinone, and Tretinoin *(Continued)*

(including ½ inch of normal-appearing surrounding skin). Apply 30 minutes prior to bedtime; not indicated for use beyond 8 weeks. Do not use occlusive dressings.

Renal Impairment: No dosage adjustment required.

Nursing Actions

Physical Assessment: Assess potential for interactions with other prescriptions, OTC medications, or herbal products patient may be taking (eg, anything with photosensitizing effect). Assess therapeutic effectiveness and adverse response. Teach patient use, possible side effects/interventions, and adverse symptoms to report.

Patient Education: This medication is for topical (skin) use only. Use exactly as directed (see below). Do not overuse or use for a longer period of time than prescribed. You will be sensitive to sunlight (avoid sunlight, wear sunscreen with SPF 30, and wear protective clothing); and sensitive to irritating skin products or cosmetics (avoid medicated preparations or agents with irritating or drying effects, you may use moisturizers and/or nonirritating cosmetics during the day). You may experience irritation and sensitivity to temperature changes, or excess bleaching effects. Report persistent burning, irritation, or eruptions on the skin; or if the condition being treated worsens or does not improve.

Application: Wash hands before beginning. Wash face with mild cleanser, rinse, and pat dry. Apply medication sparingly, in a very light film, rub in lightly. Avoid any contact with open or abraded skin, mucous membranes, eyes, mouth, or nose.

Pregnancy/breast-feeding precautions: Inform prescriber if you are or intend to become pregnant. Consult prescriber if breast-feeding.

Related Information

Fluocinolone *on page 526*
Hydroquinone *on page 623*
Tretinoin (Oral) *on page 1245*
Tretinoin (Topical) *on page 1247*

Fluocinonide *(floo oh SIN oh nide)*

U.S. Brand Names Lidex®; Lidex-E®; Vanos™
Pharmacologic Category Corticosteroid, Topical
Medication Safety Issues
Sound-alike/look-alike issues:
Fluocinonide may be confused with flunisolide, fluocinolone
Lidex® may be confused with Lasix®, Videx®, Wydase®

Pregnancy Risk Factor C
Use Anti-inflammatory, antipruritic; treatment of plaque-type psoriasis (up to 10% of body surface area) [high-potency topical corticosteroid]

Contraindications Hypersensitivity to fluocinonide or any component of the formulation; viral, fungal, or tubercular skin lesions; herpes simplex

Warnings/Precautions Adverse systemic effects may occur when used on large areas of the body, denuded areas, for prolonged periods of time, with an occlusive dressing, and/or in infants or small children. Pediatric patients may be more susceptible to HPA axis suppression. Lower-strength cream (0.05%) may be used cautiously on face or opposing skin surfaces that may rub or touch (eg, skin folds of the groin, axilla, and breasts); higher-strength (0.1%) should not be used on the face, groin, or axillae. Use of the 0.1% cream for >2

weeks or in patients <12 years of age is not recommended.

Drug Interactions

Increased Effect/Toxicity: No data reported. Concomitant use with other corticosteroids (by any route) may increase the risk of HPA axis suppression.

Adverse Reactions Frequency not defined.

Cardiovascular: Intracranial hypertension
Dermatologic: Acne, allergic dermatitis, contact dermatitis, dry skin, folliculitis, hypertrichosis, hypopigmentation, maceration of the skin, miliaria, perioral dermatitis, pruritus, skin atrophy, striae, telangiectasia
Endocrine & metabolic: Cushing's syndrome, growth retardation, HPA suppression, hyperglycemia
Local: Burning, irritation
Renal: Glycosuria
Miscellaneous: Secondary infection

Pharmacodynamics/Kinetics

Metabolism: Primarily in skin; small amount absorbed into systemic circulation is primarily hepatic to inactive compounds

Excretion: Urine (primarily as glucuronide and sulfate, also as unconjugated products); feces (small amounts as metabolites)

Available Dosage Forms

Cream, anhydrous, emollient (Lidex®): 0.05% (15 g, 30 g, 60 g)
Cream, aqueous, emollient (Lidex-E®): 0.05% (15 g, 30 g, 60 g)
Cream (Vanos™): 0.1% (30 g, 60 g)
Gel (Lidex®): 0.05% (15 g, 30 g, 60 g)
Ointment (Lidex®): 0.05% (15 g, 30 g, 60 g)
Solution (Lidex®): 0.05% (60 mL) [contains alcohol 35%]

Dosing

Adults & Elderly:

Pruritus and inflammation: Topical (0.5% cream): Apply thin layer to affected area 2-4 times/day depending on the severity of the condition. Therapy should be discontinued when control is achieved; if no improvement is seen, reassessment of diagnosis may be necessary.

Plaque-type psoriasis (Vanos™): Topical (0.1% cream): Apply a thin layer once or twice daily to affected areas (limited to <10% of body surface area). **Note:** Not recommended for use >2 consecutive weeks or >60 g/week total exposure. Discontinue when control is achieved.

Pediatrics:

Pruritus and inflammation: Refer to adult dosing.
Plaque-type psoriasis: Children ≥12 years: Refer to adult dosing.

Nursing Actions

Physical Assessment: Assess potential for interactions with other prescriptions, OTC medications, or herbal products patient may be taking. Monitor patient response. Teach patient proper use (according to formulation), side effects/appropriate interventions, and symptoms to report.

Patient Education: For external use only. Do not use for eyes, mucous membranes, or open wounds. Use exactly as directed and for no longer than the period prescribed. Before using, wash and dry area gently. Apply in a thin layer (may rub in lightly). Apply light dressing (if necessary) to area being treated. Do not use occlusive dressing unless so advised by prescriber. Avoid prolonged or excessive use around sensitive tissues, genital, or rectal areas. Avoid exposing treated area to direct sunlight. Inform prescriber if condition worsens (redness, swelling, irritation, signs of infection, or open sores) or fails to improve. **Pregnancy precaution:** Inform prescriber if you are or intend to become pregnant

Fluorometholone (flure oh METH oh lone)

U.S. Brand Names Eflone® [DSC]; Flarex®; Fluor-Op® [DSC]; FML®; FML® Forte

Pharmacologic Category Corticosteroid, Ophthalmic

Pregnancy Risk Factor C

Lactation Excretion in breast milk unknown/use caution

Use Treatment of steroid-responsive inflammatory conditions of the eye

Mechanism of Action/Effect Decreases inflammation by suppression of migration of polymorphonuclear leukocytes and reversal of increased capillary permeability

Contraindications Hypersensitivity to fluorometholone or any component of the formulation; viral diseases of the cornea and conjunctiva (including epithelial herpes simplex keratitis, vaccinia and varicella); mycobacterial or fungal infections of the eye; untreated eye infections which may be masked/enhanced by a steroid

Warnings/Precautions Not recommended in children <2 years of age. Prolonged use may result in glaucoma, elevated intraocular pressure, or other ocular damage. May exacerbate severity of viral infections, use caution in patients with history of herpes simplex. Re-evaluate after 2 days if symptoms have not improved. May delay healing following cataract surgery. Some products contain sulfites.

Adverse Reactions Frequency not defined.

Ocular: Anterior uveitis, burning upon application, cataract formation, conjunctival hyperemia, conjunctivitis, corneal ulcers, glaucoma with optic nerve damage, perforation of the globe, secondary ocular infection (bacterial, fungal, viral), intraocular pressure elevation, visual acuity and field defects, keratitis, mydriasis, stinging upon application, delayed wound healing

Miscellaneous: Systemic hypercorticoidism (rare) and taste perversion have also been reported

Overdosage/Toxicology When consumed in high doses over prolonged periods, systemic hypercorticism and adrenal suppression may occur. In those cases, discontinuation of the corticosteroid should be done judiciously.

Available Dosage Forms [DSC] = Discontinued product

Ointment, ophthalmic, as base (FML®): 0.1% (3.5 g)

Suspension, ophthalmic, as base: 0.1% (5 mL, 10 mL, 15 mL)

Fluor-Op®: 0.1% (5 mL, 10 mL, 15 mL) [contains benzalkonium chloride and polyvinyl alcohol] [DSC]

FML®: 0.1% (5 mL, 10 mL, 15 mL) [contains benzalkonium chloride]

FML® Forte: 0.25% (2 mL, 5 mL, 10 mL, 15 mL) [contains benzalkonium chloride]

Suspension, ophthalmic, as acetate:

Eflone®: 0.1% (5 mL, 10 mL) [DSC]

Flarex®: 0.1% (5 mL, 10 mL) [contains benzalkonium chloride]

Dosing

Adults & Elderly:

Occular inflammation: Ophthalmic:

Ointment: Apply small amount (~½ inch ribbon) to conjunctival sac every 4 hours in severe cases; 1-3 times/day in mild to moderate cases.

Solution: Instill 1-2 drops into conjunctival sac every hour during day, every 2 hours at night until favorable response is obtained, then use 1 drop every 4 hours; for mild to moderate inflammation, instill 1-2 drops into conjunctival sac 2-4 times/day.

Note: Re-evaluate therapy if improvement is not seen within 2 days; use care not to discontinue prematurely; in chronic conditions, gradually decrease dosing frequency prior to discontinuing treatment.

Pediatrics: Children >2 years: Refer to adult dosing.

Stability

Storage: Store at room temperature.

Nursing Actions

Physical Assessment: Monitor intraocular pressure in patients with glaucoma or when used for ≥10 days; monitor for presence of secondary infections (including the development of fungal infections and exacerbation of viral infections). Assess knowledge/teach patient appropriate use, interventions to reduce side effects, and adverse symptoms to report.

Patient Education: For ophthalmic use only. Apply prescribed amount as often as directed. Wash hands before using. Wipe away excess from skin around eye. Do not use any other eye preparation for at least 10 minutes. Do not touch tip of applicator to eye or any other surface. Do not share medication with anyone else. May cause sensitivity to bright light (dark glasses may help); temporary stinging or blurred vision may occur. Do not wear contacts during administration and for 15 minutes after. Inform prescriber if you experience eye pain, redness, burning, watering, dryness, double vision, puffiness around eye, vision changes, or other adverse eye response; worsening of condition or lack of improvement. **Pregnancy/breast-feeding precautions:** Inform prescriber if you are pregnant. Consult prescriber if breast-feeding.

Ointment: Gently squeeze the tube to apply to inside of lower lid. Close eye for 1-2 minutes and roll eyeball in all directions.

Suspension: Shake well before using. Tilt head back and look upward. Gently pull down lower lid and put drop(s) in inner corner of eye. Close eye and roll eyeball in all directions. Do not blink for 30 seconds. Apply gentle pressure to inner corner of eye for 30 seconds.

Fluorouracil (flure oh YOOR a sil)

U.S. Brand Names Adrucil®; Carac™; Efudex®; Fluoroplex®

Synonyms 5-Fluorouracil; FU; 5-FU

Pharmacologic Category Antineoplastic Agent, Antimetabolite (Pyrimidine Antagonist)

Medication Safety Issues

Sound-alike/look-alike issues:

Fluorouracil may be confused with flucytosine

Efudex® may be confused with Efidac (Efidac 24®), Eurax®

Pregnancy Risk Factor D (injection); X (topical)

Lactation Excretion in breast milk unknown/not recommended

Use Treatment of carcinomas of the breast, colon, head and neck, pancreas, rectum, or stomach; topically for the management of actinic or solar keratoses and superficial basal cell carcinomas

Mechanism of Action/Effect Interferes with DNA synthesis by blocking the methylation of deoxyuricytic acid.

Contraindications Hypersensitivity to fluorouracil or any component of the formulation; dihydropyrimidine dehydrogenase (DPD) enzyme deficiency; pregnancy

Warnings/Precautions Hazardous agent — use appropriate precautions for handling and disposal. Use with caution in patients with impaired kidney or liver function. The drug should be discontinued if intractable vomiting or diarrhea, precipitous falls in leukocyte or platelet counts, stomatitis, hemorrhage, or myocardial ischemia occurs. Use with caution in patients who have had high-dose pelvic radiation or previous use of alkylating agents. Palmar-plantar erythrodysesthesia (hand-foot) syndrome has been associated with use. Safety and efficacy have not been established in pediatric patients. (Continued)

Fluorouracil *(Continued)*

Administration to patients with a genetic deficiency of dihydropyrimidine dehydrogenase (DPD) has been associated with diarrhea, neutropenia, and neurotoxicity. Systemic toxicity normally associated with parenteral administration has also been associated with topical use, particularly in patients with DPD. Discontinue if symptoms of DPD occur. Avoid topical application to mucous membranes due to potential for local inflammation and ulceration. The use of occlusive dressings with topical preparations may increase the severity of inflammation in nearby skin areas. Avoid exposure to ultraviolet rays during and immediately following therapy.

Drug Interactions

Increased Effect/Toxicity: Fluorouracil may increase effects of warfarin.

Nutritional/Ethanol Interactions

Ethanol: Avoid ethanol (due to GI irritation).

Herb/Nutraceutical: Avoid black cohosh, dong quai in estrogen-dependent tumors.

Adverse Reactions Toxicity depends on route and duration of treatment

I.V.:

Cardiovascular: Angina, myocardial ischemia, nail changes

Central nervous system: Acute cerebellar syndrome, confusion, disorientation, euphoria, headache, nystagmus

Dermatologic: Alopecia, dermatitis, dry skin, fissuring, palmar-plantar erythrodysesthesia syndrome, pruritic maculopapular rash, photosensitivity, vein pigmentations

Gastrointestinal: Anorexia, bleeding, diarrhea, esophagopharyngitis, nausea, sloughing, stomatitis, ulceration, vomiting

Hematologic: Agranulocytosis, anemia, leukopenia, pancytopenia, thrombocytopenia

Myelosuppression:

Onset: 7-10 days

Nadir: 9-14 days

Recovery: 21-28 days

Local: Thrombophlebitis

Ocular: Lacrimation, lacrimal duct stenosis, photophobia, visual changes

Respiratory: Epistaxis

Miscellaneous: Anaphylaxis, generalized allergic reactions, loss of nails

Topical: Note: Systemic toxicity normally associated with parenteral administration (including neutropenia, neurotoxicity, and gastrointestinal toxicity) has been associated with topical use particularly in patients with a genetic deficiency of dihydropyrimidine dehydrogenase (DPD).

Central nervous system: Headache, insomnia, irritability

Dermatologic: Alopecia, photosensitivity, pruritus, rash, scarring, telangiectasia

Gastrointestinal: Medicinal taste, stomatitis

Hematologic: Leukocytosis, thrombocytopenia

Local: Application site reactions: Allergic contact dermatitis, burning, crusting, dryness, edema, erosion, erythema, hyperpigmentation, irritation, pain, soreness, ulceration

Ocular: Eye irritation (burning, watering, sensitivity, stinging, itching)

Miscellaneous: Birth defects, herpes simplex, miscarriage

Overdosage/Toxicology Symptoms of overdose include myelosuppression, nausea, vomiting, diarrhea, and alopecia. No specific antidote exists. Monitor hematologically for at least 4 weeks. Treatment is supportive.

Pharmacodynamics/Kinetics

Duration of Action: ~3 weeks

Half-Life Elimination: Biphasic: Initial: 6-20 minutes; two metabolites, FdUMP and FUTP, have prolonged half-lives depending on the type of tissue

Metabolism: Hepatic (90%) via dehydrogenase enzyme; FU must be metabolized to be active

Excretion: Lung (large amounts as CO_2); urine (5% as unchanged drug) in 6 hours

Available Dosage Forms

Cream, topical:

Carac™: 0.5% (30 g)

Efudex®: 5% (25 g, 40 g)

Fluoroplex®: 1% (30 g) [contains benzyl alcohol]

Injection, solution: 50 mg/mL (10 mL, 20 mL, 50 mL, 100 mL)

Adrucil®: 50 mg/mL (10 mL, 50 mL, 100 mL)

Solution, topical (Efudex®): 2% (10 mL); 5% (10 mL)

Dosing

Adults & Elderly:

Refer to individual protocols.

I.V. bolus: 500-600 mg/m² every 3-4 weeks **or** 425 mg/m² on days 1-5 every 4 weeks

Continuous I.V. infusion: 1000 mg/m²/day for 4-5 days every 3-4 weeks **or**

2300-2600 mg/m² on day 1 every week **or** 300-400 mg/m²/day **or**

225 mg/m²/day for 5-8 weeks (with radiation therapy)

Actinic keratoses: Topical:

Carac™: Apply thin film to lesions once daily for up to 4 weeks, as tolerated

Efudex®: Apply to lesions twice daily for 2-4 weeks; complete healing may not be evident for 1-2 months following treatment

Fluoroplex®: Apply to lesions twice daily for 2-6 weeks

Superficial basal cell carcinoma: Topical: Efudex® 5%: Apply to affected lesions twice daily for 3-6 weeks; treatment may be continued for up to 10-12 weeks

Pediatrics: Refer to adult dosing.

Renal Impairment: Hemodialysis: Administer dose following hemodialysis.

Hepatic Impairment: Bilirubin >5 mg/dL: Omit use.

Administration

Oral: I.V. formulation may be given orally mixed in water, grape juice, or carbonated beverage. It is generally best to drink undiluted solution, then rinse the mouth. CocaCola® has been recommended as the "best chaser" for oral fluorouracil.

I.V.: Irritant. Direct I.V. push injection (50 mg/mL solution needs no further dilution) or by I.V. infusion. Toxicity may be reduced by giving the drug as a constant infusion. Bolus doses may be administered by slow IVP or IVPB.

I.V. Detail: Warm to body temperature before using. After vial has been entered, any unused portion should be discarded within 1 hour. Continuous infusions may be administered in D_5W or NS. Solution should be protected from direct sunlight. Fluorouracil may also be administered intra-arterially or intrahepatically (refer to specific protocols).

pH: 9.2 (adjusted)

Topical: Topical: Apply 10 minutes after washing, rinsing, and drying the affected area. Apply using fingertip (wash hands immediately after application) or nonmetal applicator. Do not cover area with an occlusive dressing. Wash hands immediately after topical application of the 5% cream. Topical preparations are for external use only; not for ophthalmic, oral, or intravaginal use

Stability

Reconstitution: Dilute in 50-1000 mL NS, D_5W, or bacteriostatic NS for infusion.

Compatibility: Stable in D$_5$LR, D$_5$W, NS, bacteriostatic NS

Incompatible with concentrations >25 mg/mL of fluorouracil and >2 mg/mL of leucovorin (precipitation occurs)

Y-site administration: Incompatible with amphotericin B cholesteryl sulfate complex, droperidol, filgrastim, ondansetron, topotecan, vinorelbine

Compatibility in syringe: Incompatible with droperidol, epirubicin

Compatibility when admixed: Incompatible with carboplatin, cisplatin, cytarabine, diazepam, doxorubicin, fentanyl, leucovorin, metoclopramide, morphine

Storage:

Injection: Store intact vials at room temperature and protect from light; slight discoloration does not usually denote decomposition. If exposed to cold, a precipitate may form; **gentle** heating to 60°C will dissolve the precipitate without impairing the potency; solutions in 50-1000 mL NS or D$_5$W, or undiluted solutions in syringes are stable for 72 hours at room temperature.

Topical: Store at controlled room temperature of 15°C to 30°C (59°F to 86°F).

Laboratory Monitoring CBC with differential, platelet count, renal and liver function

Nursing Actions

Physical Assessment: Assess potential for interactions with other pharmacological agents or herbal products patient may be taking. Assess results of laboratory tests prior to each infusion and regularly with all formulations, including topical use. Assess patient response (eg, cardiovascular, respiratory, and renal function) prior to each infusion and on a regular basis throughout therapy. **Note:** Inform prescriber if intractable vomiting or diarrhea, precipitous fall in leukocyte or platelet counts, or myocardial ischemia occurs (drug may be discontinued). Teach patient proper use (topical application [avoid application to mucous membranes]; oral solution [rinse mouth thoroughly]), possible side effects/appropriate interventions (eg, importance of adequate hydration), and adverse symptoms to report. **Pregnancy risk factor D/X:** Determine that patient is not pregnant before starting therapy. Do not give to females of childbearing age unless patient is capable of complying with contraceptive use. Male/female: Advise patient about contraceptive measures as appropriate.

Patient Education: Do not take any new medication during therapy without consulting prescriber. Follow exact directions for use (oral solution or topical application). Avoid excessive alcohol (may increase gastrointestinal irritation). Maintain adequate nutrition and hydration (2-3 L/day of fluids) unless instructed to restrict fluid intake. May cause sensitivity to sunlight (use sunblock, wear protective clothing, and avoid direct sunlight); susceptibility to infection (avoid crowds and exposure to infection); nausea, vomiting, diarrhea, or loss of appetite (small frequent meals may help; request medication); weakness, lethargy, dizziness, decreased vision (use caution when driving or engaging in tasks requiring alertness until response to drug is known); or headache (request medication). Report signs and symptoms of infection (eg, fever, chills, sore throat, burning urination, vaginal itching or discharge, fatigue, mouth sores); bleeding (eg, black or tarry stools, easy bruising, unusual bleeding); vision changes; unremitting nausea, vomiting, or abdominal pain; CNS changes; respiratory difficulty; chest pain or palpitations; severe skin reactions to topical application; or any other adverse reactions.

Topical: Use as directed; do not overuse. Wash hands thoroughly before and after applying medication. Avoid contact with eyes, nostrils, and mouth. Avoid occlusive dressings; use a porous dressing. May cause local reaction (pain, burning, or swelling); if severe, contact prescriber.

Oral solution: May be mixed in water, grape juice, or carbonated beverage. It is generally best to drink undiluted solution, then rinse mouth thoroughly. CocaCola® has been recommended as the best rinse following oral fluorouracil.

Pregnancy/breast-feeding precautions: Inform prescriber if you are pregnant. Do not get pregnant during or for 1 month following therapy. Male: Do not cause a pregnancy. Male/female: Consult prescriber for instruction on appropriate contraceptive measures. This drug may cause severe fetal defects. Breast-feeding is not recommended.

Dietary Considerations Increase dietary intake of thiamine.

Pregnancy Issues There are no adequate and well-controlled studies in pregnant women, however, fetal defects and miscarriages have been reported following use of topical and intravenous products. Use is contraindicated during pregnancy.

Fluoxetine (floo OKS e teen)

U.S. Brand Names Prozac®; Prozac® Weekly™; Sarafem®

Synonyms Fluoxetine Hydrochloride

Restrictions A medication guide concerning the use of antidepressants in children and teenagers can be found on the FDA website at http://www.fda.gov/cder/Offices/ODS/labeling.htm. It should be dispensed to parents or guardians of children and teenagers receiving this medication.

Pharmacologic Category Antidepressant, Selective Serotonin Reuptake Inhibitor

Medication Safety Issues

Sound-alike/look-alike issues:

Fluoxetine may be confused with duloxetine, fluvastatin

Prozac® may be confused with Prilosec®, Proscar®, ProSom®, ProStep®

Sarafem® may be confused with Serophene®

Pregnancy Risk Factor C

Lactation Enters breast milk/not recommended (AAP rates "of concern")

Use Treatment of major depressive disorder (MDD); treatment of binge-eating and vomiting in patients with moderate-to-severe bulimia nervosa; obsessive-compulsive disorder (OCD); premenstrual dysphoric disorder (PMDD); panic disorder with or without agoraphobia

Unlabeled/Investigational Use Selective mutism

Mechanism of Action/Effect Inhibits CNS neuron serotonin reuptake; minimal or no effect on reuptake of norepinephrine or dopamine; does not significantly bind to alpha-adrenergic, histamine or cholinergic receptors

Contraindications Hypersensitivity to fluoxetine or any component of the formulation; patients currently receiving MAO inhibitors, pimozide, or thioridazine

Note: MAO inhibitor therapy must be stopped for 14 days before fluoxetine is initiated. Treatment with MAO inhibitors, thioridazine, or mesoridazine should not be initiated until 5 weeks after the discontinuation of fluoxetine.

Warnings/Precautions Antidepressants increase the risk of suicidal thinking and behavior in children and adolescents with major depressive disorder (MDD) and other depressive disorders; consider risk prior to prescribing. All patients must be closely monitored for clinical worsening, suicidality, or unusual changes in behavior, especially during the initiation of therapy or following an increase or decrease in dosage. When used in children, the child's family or caregiver should *(Continued)*

Fluoxetine (Continued)

be instructed to closely observe the patient and communicate condition with healthcare provider. A medication guide should be dispensed with each prescription. **Fluoxetine is FDA approved for the treatment of OCD in children ≥7 years of age and MDD in children ≥8 years of age.**

The possibility of a suicide attempt is inherent in major depression and may persist until remission occurs. Use caution in high-risk patients. Worsening depression and severe abrupt suicidality that are not part of the presenting symptoms may require discontinuation or modification of drug therapy. The patient's family or caregiver should be alerted to monitor patients for the emergence of suicidality and associated behaviors (such as agitation, irritability, hostility, impulsivity, and hypomania) and call healthcare provider.

May worsen psychosis in some patients or precipitate a shift to mania or hypomania in patients with bipolar disorder. Patients presenting with depressive symptoms should be screened for bipolar disorder. Monotherapy in patients with bipolar disorder should be avoided. **Fluoxetine is not FDA approved for the treatment of bipolar depression.** May cause insomnia, anxiety, nervousness or anorexia. Use with caution in patients where weight loss is undesirable. May impair cognitive or motor performance; caution operating hazardous machinery or driving.

The potential for severe reactions exists when used with MAO inhibitors; serotonin syndrome (hyperthermia, muscular rigidity, mental status changes/agitation, autonomic instability) may occur. Fluoxetine may elevate plasma levels of thioridazine and increase the risk of QT$_c$ interval prolongation. This may lead to serious ventricular arrhythmias such as torsade de pointes-type arrhythmias and sudden death. Fluoxetine use has been associated with occurrences of significant rash and allergic events, including vasculitis, lupus-like syndrome, laryngospasm, anaphylactoid reactions, and pulmonary inflammatory disease. Discontinue if underlying cause of rash cannot be identified.

Use caution in patients with a previous seizure disorder or condition predisposing to seizures such as brain damage, alcoholism, or concurrent therapy with other drugs which lower the seizure threshold. Use with caution in patients with hepatic or renal dysfunction and in elderly patients. May cause hyponatremia/SIADH. May increase the risks associated with electroconvulsive treatment. Use with caution in patients at risk of bleeding or receiving concurrent anticoagulant therapy - may cause impairment in platelet function. Use caution with history of MI or unstable hearst disease; use in these patients is limited. May alter glycemic control in patients with diabetes. Due to the long half-life of fluoxetine and its metabolites, the effects and interactions noted may persist for prolonged periods following discontinuation. May cause or exacerbate sexual dysfunction. Discontinuation symptoms (eg, dysphoric mood, irritability, agitation, confusion, anxiety, insomnia, hypomania) may occur upon abrupt discontinuation. Taper dose when discontinuing therapy.

Drug Interactions

Cytochrome P450 Effect: Substrate of CYP1A2 (minor), 2B6 (minor), 2C8/9 (major), 2C19 (minor), 2D6 (major), 2E1 (minor), 3A4 (minor); **Inhibits** CYP1A2 (moderate), 2B6 (weak), 2C8/9 (weak), 2C19 (moderate), 2D6 (strong), 3A4 (weak)

Decreased Effect: The levels/effects of fluoxetine may be decreased by carbamazepine, phenobarbital, phenytoin, rifampin, rifapentine, secobarbital and other CYP2C8/9 inducers. Fluoxetine may decrease the levels/effects of CYP2D6 prodrug substrates (eg, codeine, hydrocodone, oxycodone, tramadol). Cyproheptadine may inhibit the effects of serotonin

reuptake inhibitors. Lithium levels may be decreased by fluoxetine (in addition to reports of increased lithium levels).

Increased Effect/Toxicity: Fluoxetine should not be used with nonselective MAO inhibitors (phenelzine, isocarboxazid) or other drugs with MAO inhibition (linezolid); fatal reactions have been reported. Wait 5 weeks after stopping fluoxetine before starting a nonselective MAO inhibitor and 2 weeks after stopping an MAO inhibitor before starting fluoxetine. Concurrent selegiline has been associated with mania, hypertension, or serotonin syndrome (risk may be reduced relative to nonselective MAO inhibitors).

Due to potential QT$_c$ interval prolongation, concomitant use of pimozide is contraindicated. Fluoxetine may inhibit the metabolism of thioridazine, resulting in increased plasma levels and increasing the risk of QT$_c$ interval prolongation. This may lead to serious ventricular arrhythmias, such as torsade de pointes-type arrhythmias and sudden death. Do not use together. Wait at least 5 weeks after discontinuing fluoxetine prior to starting thioridazine.

Fluoxetine may increase the levels/effects of aminophylline, amphetamines, selected beta-blockers, citalopram, dextromethorphan, diazepam, fluvoxamine, lidocaine, mexiletine, methsuximide, mirtazapine, nefazodone, paroxetine, phenytoin, propranolol, risperidone, ritonavir, ropinirole, sertraline, theophylline, thioridazine, tricyclic antidepressants, trifluoperazine, venlafaxine, and other substrates of CYP1A2, 2C19, or 2D6.

Combined use of SSRIs and amphetamines, buspirone, meperidine, nefazodone, serotonin agonists (such as sumatriptan), sibutramine, other SSRIs, sympathomimetics, ritonavir, tramadol, and venlafaxine may increase the risk of serotonin syndrome. Combined use of sumatriptan (and other serotonin agonists) may result in toxicity; weakness, hyper-reflexia, and incoordination have been observed with sumatriptan and SSRIs. In addition, concurrent use may theoretically increase the risk of serotonin syndrome.

Concurrent lithium may increase risk of neurotoxicity, and lithium levels may be increased. Risk of hyponatremia may increase with concurrent use of loop diuretics (bumetanide, furosemide, torsemide). Fluoxetine may increase the hypoprothrombinemic response to warfarin. Concomitant use of fluoxetine and NSAIDs, aspirin, or other drugs affecting coagulation has been associated with an increased risk of bleeding; monitor.

The levels/effects of fluoxetine may be increased by chlorpromazine, delavirdine, fluconazole, gemfibrozil, ketoconazole, miconazole, nicardipine, NSAIDs, paroxetine, pergolide, pioglitazone, quinidine, quinine, ritonavir, ropinirole, sulfonamides, and other CYP2C8/9 or 2D6 inhibitors.

Nutritional/Ethanol Interactions

Ethanol: Avoid ethanol (may increase CNS depression). Depressed patients should avoid/limit intake.

Herb/Nutraceutical: Avoid valerian, St John's wort, kava kava, gotu kola (may increase CNS depression).

Lab Interactions Increased albumin in urine

Adverse Reactions Percentages listed for adverse effects as reported in placebo-controlled trials and were generally similar in adults and children; actual frequency may be dependent upon diagnosis and in some cases the range presented may be lower than or equal to placebo for a particular disorder.

>10%:

Central nervous system: Insomnia (10% to 33%), headache (21%), anxiety (6% to 15%), nervousness (8% to 14%), somnolence (5% to 17%)

Endocrine & metabolic: Libido decreased (1% to 11%)

Gastrointestinal: Nausea (12% to 29%), diarrhea (8% to 18%), anorexia (4% to 11%), xerostomia (4% to 12%)

Neuromuscular & skeletal: Weakness (7% to 21%), tremor (3% to 13%)

Respiratory: Pharyngitis (3% to 11%), yawn (<1% to 11%)

1% to 10%:

Cardiovascular: Vasodilation (1% to 5%), fever (2%), chest pain, hemorrhage, hypertension, palpitation

Central nervous system: Dizziness (9%), dream abnormality (1% to 5%), thinking abnormality (2%), agitation, amnesia, chills, confusion, emotional lability, sleep disorder

Dermatologic: Rash (2% to 6%), pruritus (4%)

Endocrine & metabolic: Ejaculation abnormal (<1% to 7%), impotence (<1% to 7%)

Gastrointestinal: Dyspepsia (6% to 10%), constipation (5%), flatulence (3%), vomiting (3%), weight loss (2%), appetite increased, taste perversion, weight gain

Genitourinary: Urinary frequency

Ocular: Vision abnormal (2%)

Otic: Ear pain, tinnitus

Respiratory: Sinusitis (1% to 6%)

Miscellaneous: Flu-like syndrome (3% to 10%), diaphoresis (2% to 8%)

Overdosage/Toxicology Among 633 adult patients who overdosed on fluoxetine alone, 34 resulted in a fatal outcome. Symptoms of overdose include ataxia, sedation, coma, and ECG abnormalities (QT prolongation, torsade de pointes). Respiratory depression may occur, especially with coingestion of ethanol or other drugs. Seizures rarely occur. Treatment is symptom-directed and supportive. Forced diuresis and dialysis are not likely to benefit.

Pharmacodynamics/Kinetics

Time to Peak: 6-8 hours

Protein Binding: 95%

Half-Life Elimination: Adults: Parent drug: 1-3 days (acute), 4-6 days (chronic), 7.6 days (cirrhosis); Metabolite (norfluoxetine): 9.3 days (range: 4-16 days), 12 days (cirrhosis)

Metabolism: Hepatic to norfluoxetine (activity equal to fluoxetine)

Excretion: Urine (10% as norfluoxetine, 2.5% to 5% as fluoxetine)

Pharmacokinetic Note Weekly formulation results in greater fluctuations between peak and trough concentrations of fluoxetine and norfluoxetine compared to once-daily dosing (24% daily/164% weekly; 17% daily/43% weekly, respectively). Trough concentrations are 76% lower for fluoxetine and 47% lower for norfluoxetine than the concentrations maintained by 20 mg once-daily dosing. Steady-state fluoxetine concentrations are ~50% lower following the once-weekly regimen compared to 20 mg once daily. Average steady-state concentrations of once-daily dosing were highest in children ages 6 to <13 (fluoxetine 171 ng/mL; norfluoxetine 195 ng/mL), followed by adolescents ages 13 to <18 (fluoxetine 86 ng/mL; norfluoxetine 113 ng/mL); concentrations were considered to be within the ranges reported in adults (fluoxetine 91-302 ng/mL; norfluoxetine 72-258 ng/mL).

Available Dosage Forms [DSC] = Discontinued product

Capsule, as hydrochloride: 10 mg, 20 mg, 40 mg

Prozac®: 10 mg, 20 mg, 40 mg

Sarafem®: 10 mg, 20 mg

Capsule, delayed release, as hydrochloride (Prozac® Weekly™): 90 mg

Solution, oral, as hydrochloride (Prozac®): 20 mg/5 mL (120 mL) [contains alcohol 0.23% and benzoic acid; mint flavor]

Tablet, as hydrochloride: 10 mg, 20 mg

Prozac® [scored]: 10 mg [DSC]

Dosing

Adults:

Depression, OCD, PMDD, bulimia: 20 mg/day in the morning; may increase after several weeks by 20 mg/day increments; maximum: 80 mg/day; doses >20 mg may be given once daily or divided twice daily. **Note:** Lower doses of 5-10 mg/day have been used for initial treatment.

Usual dosage range:

Depression: 20-40 mg/day; patients maintained on Prozac® 20 mg/day may be changed to Prozac® Weekly™ 90 mg/week, starting dose 7 days after the last 20 mg/day dose

Obsessive compulsive disorder (OCD): 40-80 mg/day

Premenstrual dysphoric disorder (Sarafem™): 20 mg/day continuously, **or** 20 mg/day starting 14 days prior to menstruation and through first full day of menses (repeat with each cycle)

Bulimia nervosa: 60-80 mg/day

Panic disorder: Initial: 10 mg/day; after 1 week, increase to 20 mg/day; may increase after several weeks; doses >60 mg/day have not been evaluated

Note: Upon discontinuation of fluoxetine therapy, gradually taper dose. If intolerable symptoms occur following a dose reduction, consider resuming the previously prescribed dose and/or decrease dose at a more gradual rate.

Elderly: Oral: Some patients may require an initial dose of 10 mg/day with dosage increases of 10 mg and 20 mg every several weeks as tolerated; should not be taken at night unless patient experiences sedation.

Pediatrics:

Depression: Oral: 8-18 years: 10-20 mg/day; lower-weight children can be started at 10 mg/day, may increase to 20 mg/day after 1 week if needed

OCD: Oral: 7-18 years: Initial: 10 mg/day; in adolescents and higher-weight children, dose may be increased to 20 mg/day after 2 weeks. Range: 10-60 mg/day

Selective mutism (unlabeled use): Oral:

<5 years: No dosing information available

5-18 years: Initial: 5-10 mg/day; titrate upwards as needed (usual maximum dose: 60 mg/day)

Note: Upon discontinuation of fluoxetine therapy, gradually taper dose. If intolerable symptoms occur following a dose reduction, consider resuming the previously prescribed dose and/or decrease dose at a more gradual rate.

Renal Impairment:

Single dose studies: Pharmacokinetics of fluoxetine and norfluoxetine were similar among subjects with all levels of impaired renal function, including anephric patients on chronic hemodialysis.

Chronic administration: Additional accumulation of fluoxetine or norfluoxetine may occur in patients with severely impaired renal function.

Not removed by hemodialysis; use of lower dose or less frequent dosing is not usually necessary.

Hepatic Impairment: Elimination half-life of fluoxetine is prolonged in patients with hepatic impairment. A lower dose or less frequent dosing of fluoxetine should be used in these patients.

Cirrhosis patient: Administer a lower dose or less frequent dosing interval.

Compensated cirrhosis without ascites: Administer 50% of normal dose.

Stability

Storage: All dosage forms should be stored at controlled room temperature of 15°C to 30°C (50°F to 86°F); oral liquid should be dispensed in a light-resistant container

Laboratory Monitoring Baseline liver and renal function before beginning drug therapy

(Continued)

Fluoxetine *(Continued)*

Nursing Actions

Physical Assessment: Assess other medications patient may be taking for effectiveness and interactions. Monitor laboratory tests, therapeutic response (eg, mental status, mode, affect, suicidal ideation), and adverse reactions at beginning of therapy and periodically with long-term use (eg, CNS and gastrointestinal). Taper dosage slowly when discontinuing. Assess mental status for depression, suicidal ideation, anxiety, social functioning, mania, or panic attack. Assess knowledge/teach patient appropriate use, interventions to reduce side effects and adverse symptoms to report.

Patient Education: Take exactly as directed; do not increase dose or frequency. It may take 2-3 weeks to achieve desired results. Take once-a-day dose in the morning to reduce incidence of insomnia. Avoid alcohol, caffeine, and other prescription or OTC medications not approved by prescriber. Maintain adequate hydration (2-3 L/day of fluids) unless instructed to restrict fluid intake. You may experience drowsiness, lightheadedness, impaired coordination, dizziness, or blurred vision (use caution when driving or engaging in tasks requiring alertness until response to drug is known); constipation (increased exercise, fluids, fruit, or fiber may help); anorexia (maintain regular dietary intake to avoid excessive weight loss); or postural hypotension (use caution when climbing stairs or changing position from lying or sitting to standing). If you have diabetes, monitor serum glucose closely (may cause hypoglycemia). Report persistent CNS effects (nervousness, restlessness, insomnia, anxiety, excitation, suicide ideation, headache, sedation); thoughts of suicide; rash or skin irritation; muscle cramping, tremors, or change in gait; respiratory depression or respiratory difficulty; or worsening of condition. **Pregnancy/breast-feeding precautions:** Inform prescriber if you are pregnant. Breast-feeding is not recommended.

Dietary Considerations May be taken with or without food.

Geriatric Considerations Fluoxetine's favorable side effect profile makes it a useful alternative to the traditional tricyclic antidepressants. Its potential stimulating and anorexic effects may be bothersome to some patients. Has not been shown to be superior in efficacy to the traditional tricyclic antidepressants or other SSRIs. The long half-life in the elderly makes it less attractive compared to other SSRIs. Data from a clinical trial comparing fluoxetine to tricyclics suggests that fluoxetine is significantly less effective than nortriptyline in hospitalized elderly patients with unipolar major affective disorder, especially those with melancholia and concurrent cardiovascular diseases. As with other SSRIs, fluoxetine has been associated with hyponatremia in elderly patients.

Breast-Feeding Issues Colic, irritability, slow weight gain, feeding and sleep disorders have been reported in nursing infants.

Pregnancy Issues Fluoxetine crosses the placenta. Nonteratogenic effects including respiratory distress, cyanosis, apnea, seizures, temperature instability, feeding difficulty, vomiting, hypoglycemia, hypo- or hypertonia, hyper-reflexia, jitteriness, irritability, constant crying, and tremor have been reported in the neonate immediately following delivery after exposure to other SSRIs late in the third trimester. Adverse effects may be due to toxic effects of SSRI or drug discontinuation. In some cases, may present clinically as serotonin syndrome. There are no adequate and well-controlled studies in pregnant women. Use during pregnancy only if the potential benefit to the mother outweighs the possible risk to the fetus. If treatment during pregnancy is required, consider tapering SSRI therapy during the third trimester.

Additional Information ECG may reveal S-T segment depression; not shown to be teratogenic in rodents; 15-60 mg/day, buspirone and cyproheptadine, may be useful in treatment of sexual dysfunction during treatment with a selective serotonin reuptake inhibitor.

Weekly capsules are a delayed release formulation containing enteric-coated pellets of fluoxetine hydrochloride, equivalent to 90 mg fluoxetine. Therapeutic equivalence of weekly formulation with daily formulation for delaying time to relapse has not been established.

Related Information

Antidepressant Medication Guidelines *on page 1414*

Fluphenazine *(floo FEN a zeen)*

U.S. Brand Names Prolixin® [DSC]; Prolixin Decanoate®

Synonyms Fluphenazine Decanoate

Pharmacologic Category Antipsychotic Agent, Typical, Phenothiazine

Medication Safety Issues

Sound-alike/look-alike issues:
Prolixin® may be confused with Proloprim®

Pregnancy Risk Factor C

Lactation Enters breast milk/not recommended

Use Management of manifestations of psychotic disorders and schizophrenia; depot formulation may offer improved outcome in individuals with psychosis who are nonadherent with oral antipsychotics

Unlabeled/Investigational Use Pervasive developmental disorder

Mechanism of Action/Effect Fluphenazine is a piperazine phenothiazine antipsychotic which blocks postsynaptic mesolimbic dopaminergic D_1 and D_2 receptors in the brain; depresses the release of hypothalamic and hypophyseal hormones; believed to depress the reticular activating system thus affecting basal metabolism, body temperature, wakefulness, vasomotor tone, and emesis

Contraindications Hypersensitivity to fluphenazine or any component of the formulation (cross-reactivity between phenothiazines may occur); severe CNS depression; coma; subcortical brain damage; blood dyscrasias; hepatic disease

Warnings/Precautions May be sedating, use with caution in disorders where CNS depression is a feature. Use with caution in Parkinson's disease. Caution in patients with hemodynamic instability; bone marrow suppression; predisposition to seizures; severe cardiac, renal, or respiratory disease. Esophageal dysmotility and aspiration have been associated with antipsychotic use - use with caution in patients at risk of pneumonia (ie, Alzheimer's disease). Caution in breast cancer or other prolactin-dependent tumors (may elevate prolactin levels). May alter temperature regulation or mask toxicity of other drugs due to antiemetic effects. May alter cardiac conduction; life-threatening arrhythmias have occurred with therapeutic doses of phenothiazines. Hypotension may occur, particularly with I.M. administration. May cause orthostatic hypotension - use with caution in patients at risk of this effect or those who would tolerate transient hypotensive episodes (cerebrovascular disease, cardiovascular disease, or other medications which may predispose). Adverse effects of depot injections may be prolonged.

Due to anticholinergic effects, use caution in patients with decreased gastrointestinal motility, urinary retention, BPH, xerostomia, visual problems, narrow-angle glaucoma (screening is recommended), and myasthenia gravis. Relative to other antipsychotics, fluphenazine has a low potency of cholinergic blockade.

May cause extrapyramidal symptoms, including pseudoparkinsonism, acute dystonic reactions, akathisia and tardive dyskinesia (risk of these reactions is high relative to other antipsychotics). May be associated with neuroleptic malignant syndrome (NMS) or pigmentary retinopathy.

Drug Interactions

Cytochrome P450 Effect: Substrate of CYP2D6 (major); **Inhibits** CYP1A2 (weak), 2C8/9 (weak), 2D6 (weak), 2E1 (weak)

Decreased Effect: Phenothiazines inhibit the activity of guanethidine, guanadrel, levodopa, and bromocriptine. Barbiturates and cigarette smoking may enhance the hepatic metabolism of fluphenazine. Fluphenazine and possibly other low potency antipsychotics may reverse the pressor effects of epinephrine.

Increased Effect/Toxicity: CYP2D6 inhibitors may increase the levels/effects of fluphenazine; example inhibitors include chlorpromazine, delavirdine, fluoxetine, miconazole, paroxetine, pergolide, quinidine, quinine, ritonavir, and ropinirole. Effects on CNS depression may be additive when fluphenazine is combined with CNS depressants (narcotic analgesics, ethanol, barbiturates, cyclic antidepressants, antihistamines, sedative-hypnotics). Fluphenazine may increase the effects/toxicity of anticholinergics, antihypertensives, lithium (rare neurotoxicity), trazodone, or valproic acid. Concurrent use with TCA may produce increased toxicity or altered therapeutic response. Chloroquine and propranolol may increase chlorpromazine concentrations. Hypotension may occur when fluphenazine is combined with epinephrine. May increase the risk of arrhythmia when combined with antiarrhythmics, cisapride, pimozide, sparfloxacin, or other drugs which prolong QT interval. Metoclopramide may increase risk of extrapyramidal symptoms (EPS). Acetylcholinesterase inhibitors (central) may increase the risk of antipsychotic-related EPS.

Nutritional/Ethanol Interactions

Ethanol: Avoid ethanol (may increase CNS depression). Herb/Nutraceutical: Avoid dong quai, St John's wort (may also cause photosensitization). Avoid kava kava, gotu kola, valerian, St John's wort (may increase CNS depression).

Lab Interactions Increased cholesterol (S), glucose; decreased uric acid (S)

Adverse Reactions Frequency not defined.

Cardiovascular: Hyper-/hypotension, tachycardia, fluctuations in blood pressure, arrhythmia, edema

Central nervous system: Parkinsonian symptoms, akathisia, dystonias, tardive dyskinesia, dizziness, hyper-reflexia, headache, cerebral edema, drowsiness, lethargy, restlessness, excitement, bizarre dreams, EEG changes, depression, seizure, NMS, altered central temperature regulation

Dermatologic: Dermatitis, eczema, erythema, itching, photosensitivity, rash, seborrhea, skin pigmentation, urticaria

Endocrine & metabolic: Changes in menstrual cycle, breast pain, amenorrhea, galactorrhea, gynecomastia, libido (changes in), elevated prolactin, SIADH

Gastrointestinal: Weight gain, loss of appetite, salivation, xerostomia, constipation, paralytic ileus, laryngeal edema

Genitourinary: Ejaculatory disturbances, impotence, polyuria, bladder paralysis, enuresis

Hematologic: Agranulocytosis, leukopenia, thrombocytopenia, nonthrombocytopenic purpura, eosinophilia, pancytopenia

Hepatic: Cholestatic jaundice, hepatotoxicity

Neuromuscular & skeletal: Trembling of fingers, SLE, facial hemispasm

Ocular: Pigmentary retinopathy, cornea and lens changes, blurred vision, glaucoma

Respiratory: Nasal congestion, asthma

Overdosage/Toxicology Symptoms of overdose include deep sleep, hypo- or hypertension, dystonia, seizures, extrapyramidal symptoms, and respiratory failure. Following initiation of essential overdose management, toxic symptom treatment and supportive treatment should be initiated.

Pharmacodynamics/Kinetics

Onset of Action: I.M., SubQ (derivative dependent): Hydrochloride salt: ~1 hour

Peak effect: Neuroleptic: Decanoate: 48-96 hours

Duration of Action: Hydrochloride salt: 6-8 hours; Decanoate: 24-72 hours

Protein Binding: 91% and 99%

Half-Life Elimination: Derivative dependent: Hydrochloride: 33 hours; Decanoate: 163-232 hours

Metabolism: Hepatic

Excretion: Urine (as metabolites)

Available Dosage Forms [DSC] = Discontinued product

Elixir, as hydrochloride (Prolixin®): 2.5 mg/5 mL (60 mL) [contains alcohol 14% and sodium benzoate] [DSC]

Injection, oil, as decanoate: 25 mg/mL (5 mL) [may contain benzyl alcohol, sesame oil]

Prolixin Decanoate®: 25 mg/mL (5 mL) [contains benzyl alcohol, sesame oil]

Injection, solution, as hydrochloride (Prolixin® [DSC]): 2.5 mg/mL (10 mL)

Solution, oral concentrate, as hydrochloride (Prolixin®): 5 mg/mL (120 mL) [contains alcohol 14%] [DSC]

Tablet, as hydrochloride: 1 mg, 2.5 mg, 5 mg, 10 mg

Prolixin®: 1 mg, 2.5 mg, 5 mg [contains tartrazine], 10 mg [DSC]

Dosing

Adults:

Psychosis:

Oral: 0.5-10 mg/day in divided doses at 6- to 8-hour intervals; some patients may require up to 40 mg/day

I.M.: 2.5-10 mg/day in divided doses at 6- to 8-hour intervals (parenteral dose is $^1/_3$ to $^1/_2$ the oral dose for the hydrochloride salts)

Long-acting maintenance injections (Depot):

I.M., SubQ (decanoate): 12.5 mg every 3 weeks

Conversion from hydrochloride to decanoate I.M.: 0.5 mL (12.5 mg) decanoate every 3 weeks is approximately equivalent to 10 mg hydrochloride/day

Elderly: Initial (nonpsychotic patient, dementia behavior): 1-2.5 mg/day; increase dose at 4- to 7-day intervals by 1-2.5 mg/day. Increase dosing intervals (bid, tid) as necessary to control response or side effects. Maximum daily dose: 20 mg; gradual increases (titration) may prevent some side effects or decrease their severity.

Pediatrics: Childhood-onset pervasive developmental disorder (unlabeled use): Oral: 0.04 mg/kg/day

Renal Impairment: Use with caution; not dialyzable (0% to 5%).

Hepatic Impairment: Use with caution.

Administration

Oral: Avoid contact of oral solution or injection with skin (contact dermatitis). Oral liquid should be diluted in the following **only:** Water, saline, homogenized milk, carbonated orange beverages, pineapple, apricot, prune, orange, tomato, and grapefruit juices. Do **not** dilute in beverages containing caffeine, tannics, or pectinate.

I.M.: Watch for hypotension when administering I.M.

I.V. Detail: pH: 4.8-5.2

Laboratory Monitoring CBC prior to and regularly during therapy, lipid profile, liver and kidney function, fasting blood glucose/Hgb A_{1c}; BMI

Nursing Actions

Physical Assessment: Assess other medications patient is taking for effectiveness and interactions. Review ophthalmic screening and monitor laboratory tests, therapeutic response (mental status, mood, affect), and adverse reactions at beginning of therapy *(Continued)*

Fluphenazine *(Continued)*

and periodically with long-term use (especially anticholinergic and extrapyramidal symptoms). With I.M. or SubQ use, monitor closely for hypotension. **Note:** Avoid skin contact with oral or injection medication; may cause contact dermatitis (wash immediately with warm, soapy water). Initiate at lower doses and taper dosage slowly when discontinuing. Assess knowledge/teach patient appropriate use, interventions to reduce side effects, and adverse symptoms to report.

Patient Education: Use exactly as directed; do not increase dose or frequency. Do not discontinue without consulting prescriber. Dilute with water, milk, orange or grapefruit juice; do not dilute with beverages containing caffeine, tannin, or pectinate (eg, coffee, colas, tea, or apple juice). Do not take within 2 hours of any antacid. Avoid alcohol or caffeine and other prescription or OTC medications not approved by prescriber. Avoid skin contact with medication; may cause contact dermatitis (wash immediately with warm, soapy water). Maintain adequate hydration (2-3 L/day of fluids) unless instructed to restrict fluid intake. You may experience excess drowsiness, lightheadedness, dizziness, or blurred vision (use caution driving or when engaging in tasks requiring alertness until response to drug is known); dry mouth, upset stomach, nausea, vomiting (small frequent meals, frequent mouth care, chewing gum, or sucking lozenges may help); constipation (increased exercise, fluids, fruits, or fiber may help); postural hypotension (use caution climbing stairs or when changing position from lying or sitting to standing); urinary retention (void before taking medication); ejaculatory dysfunction (reversible); decreased perspiration (avoid strenuous exercise in hot environments); or photosensitivity (use sunscreen, wear protective clothing and eyewear, and avoid direct sunlight). Report persistent CNS effects (eg, trembling fingers, altered gait or balance, excessive sedation, seizures, unusual movements, anxiety, abnormal thoughts, confusion, personality changes); chest pain, palpitations, rapid heartbeat, severe dizziness; unresolved urinary retention or changes in urinary pattern; altered menstrual pattern, change in libido, swelling or pain in breasts (male or female); vision changes; skin rash or irritation or yellowing of skin; or worsening of condition. **Pregnancy/breast-feeding precautions:** Inform prescriber if you are or intend to become pregnant. Breast-feeding is not recommended.

Geriatric Considerations (See Warnings/Precautions, Adverse Reactions, and Overdose/Toxicology.) Elderly patients have an increased risk of adverse response to side effects or adverse reactions to antipsychotics.

Additional Information Less sedative and hypotensive effects than chlorpromazine.

Related Information

Antipsychotic Medication Guidelines *on page 1415*
Federal OBRA Regulations Recommended Maximum Doses *on page 1421*

Flurazepam *(flure AZ e pam)*

U.S. Brand Names Dalmane®
Synonyms Flurazepam Hydrochloride
Restrictions C-IV
Pharmacologic Category Hypnotic, Benzodiazepine
Medication Safety Issues
Sound-alike/look-alike issues:
Flurazepam may be confused with temazepam
Dalmane® may be confused with Demulen®, Dialume®
Pregnancy Risk Factor X
Lactation Excretion in breast milk unknown/not recommended

Use Short-term treatment of insomnia

Mechanism of Action/Effect Binds to stereospecific benzodiazepine receptors on the postsynaptic GABA neuron at several sites within the central nervous system, including the limbic system, reticular formation. Enhancement of the inhibitory effect of GABA on neuronal excitability results by increased neuronal membrane permeability to chloride ions. This shift in chloride ions results in hyperpolarization (a less excitable state) and stabilization.

Contraindications Hypersensitivity to flurazepam or any component of the formulation (cross-sensitivity with other benzodiazepines may exist); narrow-angle glaucoma; pregnancy

Warnings/Precautions As a hypnotic, should be used only after evaluation of potential causes of sleep disturbance. Failure of sleep disturbance to resolve after 7-10 days may indicate psychiatric or medical illness. Use is not recommended in patients with depressive disorders or psychoses. Avoid use in patients with sleep apnea. Use with caution in patients receiving concurrent CYP3A4 inhibitors, particularly when these agents are added to therapy. Use with caution in elderly or debilitated patients, patients with hepatic disease (including alcoholics), renal impairment, respiratory disease, impaired gag reflex, or obese patients.

Causes CNS depression (dose-related) which may impair physical and mental capabilities. Use with caution in patients receiving other CNS depressants or psychoactive agents. Benzodiazepines have been associated with falls and traumatic injury and should be used with extreme caution in patients who are at risk of these events (especially the elderly). May cause physical or psychological dependence - use with caution in patients with a history of drug dependence.

Benzodiazepines have been associated with anterograde amnesia. Paradoxical reactions, including hyperactive or aggressive behavior, have been reported with benzodiazepines, particularly in adolescent/pediatric or psychiatric patients. Does not have analgesic, antidepressant, or antipsychotic properties.

Drug Interactions

Cytochrome P450 Effect: Substrate of CYP3A4 (major); **Inhibits** CYP2E1 (weak)

Decreased Effect: CYP3A4 inducers may decrease the levels/effects of flurazepam; example inducers include aminoglutethimide, carbamazepine, nafcillin, nevirapine, phenobarbital, phenytoin, and rifamycins.

Increased Effect/Toxicity: CYP3A4 inhibitors may increase the levels/effects of flurazepam; example inhibitors include azole antifungals, clarithromycin, diclofenac, doxycycline, erythromycin, imatinib, isoniazid, nefazodone, nicardipine, propofol, protease inhibitors, quinidine, telithromycin, and verapamil. Serum levels and response to flurazepam may be increased by cimetidine, clozapine, CNS depressants, diltiazem, disulfiram, digoxin, ethanol, fluconazole, fluoxetine, fluvoxamine, grapefruit juice, labetalol, levodopa, loxapine, metoprolol, metronidazole, nelfinavir, omeprazole, and valproic acid.

Nutritional/Ethanol Interactions
Ethanol: Avoid ethanol (may increase CNS depression).
Food: Serum levels and response to flurazepam may be increased by grapefruit juice, but unlikely because of flurazepam's high oral bioavailability.
Herb/Nutraceutical: Avoid valerian, St John's wort, kava kava, gotu kola (may increase CNS depression).

Lab Interactions Elevated alkaline phosphatase, AST, ALT, and bilirubin (total and direct)

Adverse Reactions Frequency not defined.
Cardiovascular: Palpitations, chest pain
Central nervous system: Drowsiness, ataxia, lightheadedness, memory impairment, depression, headache, hangover effect, confusion, nervousness, dizziness, falling, apprehension, irritability, euphoria, slurred

speech, restlessness, hallucinations, paradoxical reactions, talkativeness

Dermatologic: Rash, pruritus

Gastrointestinal: Xerostomia, constipation, increased/ excessive salivation, heartburn, upset stomach, nausea, vomiting, diarrhea, increased or decreased appetite, bitter taste, weight gain/loss

Hematologic: Granulocytopenia

Hepatic: Elevated AST/ALT, total bilirubin, alkaline phosphatase, cholestatic jaundice

Neuromuscular & skeletal: Dysarthria, body/joint pain, reflex slowing, weakness

Ocular: Blurred vision, burning eyes, difficulty focusing

Otic: Tinnitus

Respiratory: Apnea, dyspnea

Miscellaneous: Diaphoresis, drug dependence

Overdosage/Toxicology Symptoms of overdose include respiratory depression, hypoactive reflexes, unsteady gait, and hypotension. Treatment for benzodiazepine overdose is supportive. Flumazenil has been shown to selectively block the binding of benzodiazepines to CNS receptors, resulting in a reversal of benzodiazepine-induced CNS depression. Respiratory depression may not be reversed.

Pharmacodynamics/Kinetics

Onset of Action: Hypnotic: 15-20 minutes; Peak effect: 3-6 hours

Duration of Action: 7-8 hours

Half-Life Elimination: Desalkylflurazepam:

Adults: Single dose: 74-90 hours; Multiple doses: 111-113 hours

Elderly (61-85 years): Single dose: 120-160 hours; Multiple doses: 126-158 hours

Metabolism: Hepatic to N-desalkylflurazepam (active)

Available Dosage Forms Capsule, as hydrochloride: 15 mg, 30 mg

Dosing

Adults: Insomnia (short-term treatment): Oral: 15-30 mg at bedtime

Elderly: Oral: 15 mg at bedtime. Avoid use if possible.

Pediatrics: Hypnotic: Oral:

≤15 years: Dose not established

>15 years: 15 mg at bedtime

Administration

Oral: Give 30 minutes to 1 hour before bedtime on an empty stomach with full glass of water. May be taken with food if GI distress occurs.

Stability

Storage: Store in light-resistant containers.

Nursing Actions

Physical Assessment: For short-term use. Assess effectiveness and interactions of other medications patient may be taking. Assess for history of addiction; long-term use can result in dependence, abuse, or tolerance. Evaluate periodically for need for continued use. Monitor for CNS changes. After long-term use, taper dosage slowly when discontinuing. For inpatient use, institute safety measures and monitor effectiveness and adverse reactions. For outpatients, monitor therapeutic effectiveness and adverse reactions at beginning of therapy and periodically with long-term use. Assess knowledge/teach patient appropriate use, interventions to reduce side effects, and adverse symptoms to report. **Pregnancy risk factor X:** Determine that patient is not pregnant before starting therapy. Do not give to sexually-active female patients unless capable of complying with contraceptive use.

Patient Education: Use exactly as directed; do not increase dose or frequency or discontinue without consulting prescriber. Drug may cause physical and/ or psychological dependence. May take with food to decrease GI upset. While using this medication, do not use alcohol or other prescription or OTC medications (especially, pain medications, sedatives, antihistamines, or hypnotics) without consulting prescriber. Maintain adequate hydration (2-3 L/day of fluids)

unless instructed to restrict fluid intake. You may experience drowsiness, dizziness, lightheadedness, or blurred vision (use caution when driving or engaging in tasks requiring alertness until response to drug is known); dry mouth, nausea, or vomiting (small frequent meals, frequent mouth care, chewing gum, or sucking lozenges may help); difficulty urinating (void before taking medication); or altered libido (resolves when medication is discontinued). Report CNS changes (confusion, depression, increased sedation, excitation, headache, abnormal thinking, insomnia, or nightmares, memory impairment, impaired coordination); muscle pain or weakness; respiratory difficulty; persistent dizziness, chest pain, or palpitations; alterations in normal gait; vision changes; ringing in ears; or ineffectiveness of medication. **Pregnancy/breast-feeding precautions:** Inform prescriber if you are pregnant. Do not get pregnant during or for 1 month following therapy. Consult prescriber for instruction on appropriate contraceptive measures. This drug may cause severe fetal defects. Breast-feeding is not recommended.

Geriatric Considerations Due to its long-acting metabolite, flurazepam is not considered a drug of choice in the elderly. Long-acting benzodiazepines have been associated with falls in the elderly. Interpretive guidelines from the Centers for Medicare and Medicaid Services (CMS) discourage the use of this agent in residents of long-term care facilities.

Pregnancy Issues Benzodiazepines cross the placenta. The association between benzodiazepine exposure and malformations remains controversial. A number of types of malformation have been reported (oral cleft, inguinal hernia, cardiac defects, spina bifida, dysmorphic facial features, skeletal defects); however, confounding factors make a clear association difficult. Overall, the risk to the fetus may be low. Nonteratogenic effects (including neonatal flaccidity, respiratory and feeding problems, and withdrawal symptoms) during the postnatal period have also been reported with benzodiazepine use.

Related Information

Anxiolytic / Hypnotic Use in Long-Term Care Facilities on page 1418
Federal OBRA Regulations Recommended Maximum Doses on page 1421

Flurbiprofen (flure BI proe fen)

U.S. Brand Names Ansaid® [DSC]; Ocufen®

Synonyms Flurbiprofen Sodium

Restrictions A medication guide should be dispensed with each prescription. A template for the required MedGuide can be found on the FDA website at: http://www.fda.gov/medwatch/SAFETY/2005/safety05.htm#NSAID

Pharmacologic Category Nonsteroidal Anti-inflammatory Drug (NSAID), Ophthalmic; Nonsteroidal Anti-inflammatory Drug (NSAID), Oral

Medication Safety Issues

Sound-alike/look-alike issues:

Flurbiprofen may be confused with fenoprofen

Ansaid® may be confused with Asacol®, Axid®

Ocufen® may be confused with Ocuflox®, Ocupress®

Pregnancy Risk Factor C/D (3rd trimester)

Lactation Enters breast milk/not recommended

Use

Oral: Treatment of rheumatoid arthritis and osteoarthritis

Ophthalmic: Inhibition of intraoperative miosis

Mechanism of Action/Effect Inhibits prostaglandin synthesis by decreasing the activity of the enzyme, cyclooxygenase, which results in decreased formation of prostaglandin precursors

(Continued)

Flurbiprofen *(Continued)*

Contraindications Hypersensitivity to flurbiprofen, aspirin, other NSAIDs, or any component of the formulation; perioperative pain in the setting of coronary artery bypass surgery (CABG); dendritic keratitis; pregnancy (3rd trimester)

Warnings/Precautions NSAIDs are associated with an increased risk of adverse cardiovascular events, including MI, stroke, and new onset or worsening of pre-existing hypertension. Risk may be increased with duration of use or pre-existing cardiovascular risk-factors or disease. Carefully evaluate individual cardiovascular risk profiles prior to prescribing. Use caution with fluid retention, CHF, or hypertension.

Use of NSAIDs can compromise existing renal function. Renal toxicity can occur in patient with impaired renal function, dehydration, heart failure, liver dysfunction, those taking diuretics and ACEI, and the elderly. Rehydrate patient before starting therapy. Monitor renal function closely. Not recommended for use in patients with advanced renal disease.

NSAIDs may increase risk of gastrointestinal irritation, ulceration, bleeding, and perforation. These events may occur at any time during therapy and without warning. Use caution with a history of GI disease (bleeding or ulcers), concurrent therapy with aspirin, anticoagulants and/or corticosteroids, smoking, use of alcohol, the elderly or debilitated patients.

Use the lowest effective dose for the shortest duration of time, consistent with individual patient goals, to reduce risk of cardiovascular or GI adverse events. Alternate therapies should be considered for patients at high risk.

NSAIDs may cause serious skin adverse events including exfoliative dermatitis, Stevens-Johnson syndrome (SJS), and toxic epidermal necrolysis (TEN). Anaphylactoid reactions may occur, even without prior exposure; patients with "aspirin triad" (bronchial asthma, aspirin intolerance, rhinitis) may be at increased risk. Do not use in patients who experience bronchospasm, asthma, rhinitis, or urticaria with NSAID or aspirin therapy.

Use with caution in patients with decreased hepatic function. Closely monitor patients with any abnormal LFT. Severe hepatic reactions (eg, fulminant hepatitis, liver failure) have occurred with NSAID use, rarely; discontinue if signs or symptoms of liver disease develop, or if systemic manifestations occur.

The elderly are at increased risk for adverse effects (especially peptic ulceration, CNS effects, renal toxicity) from NSAIDs even at low doses.

Withhold for at least 4-6 half-lives prior to surgical or dental procedures. Safety and efficacy have not been established in children <18 years of age.

Drug Interactions

Cytochrome P450 Effect: Substrate of CYP2C8/9 (minor); **Inhibits** CYP2C8/9 (strong)

Decreased Effect: Ophthalmic: When used with concurrent administration of flurbiprofen, acetylcholine chloride and carbachol have been shown to be ineffective. Reports of acetylcholine chloride and carbachol being ineffective when used with flurbiprofen.

Increased Effect/Toxicity: Flurbiprofen may increase cyclosporine, digoxin, lithium, and methotrexate serum concentrations. The renal adverse effects of ACE inhibitors may be potentiated by NSAIDs. Corticosteroids may increase the risk of GI ulceration. Flurbiprofen may increase the levels/effects amiodarone, fluoxetine, glimepiride, glipizide, nateglinide, phenytoin, pioglitazone, rosiglitazone, sertraline, warfarin, and other CYP2C8/9 substrates.

Nutritional/Ethanol Interactions

Ethanol: Avoid ethanol (may enhance gastric mucosal irritation).

Food: Food may decrease the rate but not the extent of absorption.

Herb/Nutraceutical: Avoid alfalfa, anise, bilberry, bladderwrack, bromelain, cat's claw, celery, coleus, cordyceps, dong quai, evening primrose, feverfew, fenugreek, garlic, ginger, ginkgo biloboa, red clover, horse chestnut, grapeseed, green tea, ginseng, guggul, horse chestnut seed, horseradish, licorice, prickly ash, red clover, reishi, SAMe, sweet clover, turmeric, white willow (all have additional antiplatelet activity).

Adverse Reactions

Ophthalmic: Frequency not defined: Ocular: Slowing of corneal wound healing, mild ocular stinging, itching and burning, ocular irritation, fibrosis, miosis, mydriasis, bleeding tendency increased

Oral:

>1%:

Cardiovascular: Edema

Central nervous system: Amnesia, anxiety, depression, dizziness, headache, insomnia, malaise, nervousness, somnolence

Dermatologic: Rash

Gastrointestinal: Abdominal pain, constipation, diarrhea, dyspepsia, flatulence, GI bleeding, nausea, vomiting, weight changes

Hepatic: Liver enzymes elevated

Neuromuscular & skeletal: Reflexes increased, tremor, vertigo, weakness

Ocular: Vision changes

Otic: Tinnitus

Respiratory: Rhinitis

Overdosage/Toxicology Symptoms of overdose include apnea, metabolic acidosis, coma, nystagmus, leukocytosis, and renal failure. Management of NSAID intoxication is supportive and symptomatic. Since many NSAIDs undergo enterohepatic cycling, multiple doses of charcoal may be needed to reduce the potential for delayed toxicities.

Pharmacodynamics/Kinetics

Onset of Action: ~1-2 hours

Time to Peak: 1.5 hours

Protein Binding: 99%, primarily albumin

Half-Life Elimination: 5.7 hours

Metabolism: Hepatic via CYP2C9; forms metabolites such as 4-hydroxy-flurbiprofen (inactive)

Excretion: Urine (primarily as metabolites)

Available Dosage Forms [DSC] = Discontinued product

Solution, ophthalmic, as sodium (Ocufen®): 0.03% (2.5 mL) [contains thimerosal]

Tablet: 50 mg, 100 mg

Ansaid®: 50 mg, 100 mg [DSC]

Dosing

Adults & Elderly:

Rheumatoid arthritis and osteoarthritis: Oral: 200-300 mg/day in 2-, 3-, or 4 divided doses; do not administer more than 100 mg for any single dose; maximum: 300 mg/day

Management of postoperative dental pain: 100 mg every 12 hours

Ophthalmic anti-inflammatory/surgical aid: Ophthalmic: Instill 1 drop every 30 minutes, beginning 2 hours prior to surgery (total of 4 drops in each affected eye)

Renal Impairment: Not recommended in patients with advanced renal disease.

Administration

Oral: Take with a full glass of water.

Nursing Actions

Physical Assessment: Assess for allergic reaction to salicylate or other NSAIDs. Assess effectiveness and interactions of other medications patient may be taking. Monitor blood pressure at the beginning of therapy and periodically during use. Monitor therapeutic response (eg, relief of pain and inflammation, activity tolerance) and adverse reactions (eg, GI effects, hepatotoxicity, or ototoxicity) at beginning of therapy and periodically throughout therapy. Assess knowledge/teach patient proper use, appropriate interventions to reduce side effects, and adverse symptoms to report.

Patient Education: Oral: Take this medication exactly as directed; do not increase dose without consulting prescriber. Do not crush tablets. Take with food or milk to reduce GI distress. Maintain adequate hydration (2-3 L/day of fluids) unless instructed to restrict fluid intake. Do not use alcohol, aspirin or aspirin-containing medication, or any other anti-inflammatory medications without consulting prescriber. You may experience drowsiness, dizziness, nervousness, or headache (use caution when driving or engaging in tasks requiring alertness until response to drug is known); anorexia, nausea, vomiting, or heartburn (small frequent meals, frequent mouth care, sucking lozenges, or chewing gum may help); fluid retention (weigh yourself weekly and report unusual (3-5 lb/week) weight gain). GI bleeding, ulceration, or perforation can occur with or without pain; discontinue medication and contact prescriber if persistent abdominal pain or cramping, or blood in stool occurs. Report breathlessness, respiratory difficulty, or unusual cough; chest pain, rapid heartbeat, palpitations; unusual bruising/bleeding; blood in urine, stool, mouth, or vomitus; swollen extremities; skin rash or itching; acute fatigue; or hearing changes (ringing in ears). **Pregnancy/breast-feeding precautions:** Inform prescriber if you are or intend to become pregnant. This drug should not be used in the 3rd trimester of pregnancy. Breast-feeding is not recommended.

Ophthalmic: Wash hands before instilling. Sit or lie down to instill. Open eye, look at ceiling, and instill prescribed amount of medication. Close eye and roll eye in all directions, and apply gentle pressure to inner corner of eye. Do not let tip of applicator touch eye; do not contaminate tip of applicator (may cause eye infection, eye damage, or vision loss). Use protective dark eyewear until healed; avoid direct sunlight. Temporary stinging or burning may occur. Report persistent pain, burning, redness, vision changes, swelling, itching, or worsening of condition.

Dietary Considerations Tablet may be taken with food, milk, or antacid to decrease GI effects.

Geriatric Considerations Elderly are at high risk for adverse effects from NSAIDs. As much as 60% of elderly can develop peptic ulceration and/or hemorrhage asymptomatically. The concomitant use of H_2 blockers, omeprazole, and sucralfate is not effective as prophylaxis with the exception of NSAID-induced duodenal ulcers which may be prevented by the use of ranitidine. Misoprostol is the only prophylactic agent proven effective. Also, concomitant disease and drug use contribute to the risk for GI adverse effects. Use lowest effective dose for shortest period possible. Consider renal function decline with age. Use of NSAIDs can compromise existing renal function especially when Cl_{cr} is ≤30 mL/minute. Tinnitus may be a difficult and unreliable indication of toxicity due to age-related hearing loss or eighth cranial nerve damage. CNS adverse effects such as confusion, agitation, and hallucination are generally seen in overdose or high-dose situations, but elderly may demonstrate these adverse effects at lower doses than younger adults.

Flutamide (FLOO ta mide)

U.S. Brand Names Eulexin®

Synonyms Niftolid; NSC-147834; 4'-Nitro-3'-Trifluoro-methylisobutyrantide; SCH 13521

Pharmacologic Category Antineoplastic Agent, Antiandrogen

Medication Safety Issues
Sound-alike/look-alike issues:
Flutamide may be confused with Flumadine®, thalidomide
Eulexin® may be confused with Edecrin®, Eurax®

Pregnancy Risk Factor D

Lactation Excretion in breast milk unknown/not recommended

Use Treatment of metastatic prostatic carcinoma in combination therapy with LHRH agonist analogues

Unlabeled/Investigational Use Female hirsutism

Mechanism of Action/Effect Nonsteroidal antiandrogen that inhibits androgen uptake or inhibits binding of androgen in target tissues

Contraindications Hypersensitivity to flutamide or any component of the formulation; severe hepatic impairment; pregnancy

Warnings/Precautions Product labeling states flutamide is not for use in women, particularly for nonlife-threatening conditions. Patients with glucose-6 phosphate dehydrogenase deficiency or hemoglobin M disease or smokers are at risk of toxicities associated with aniline exposure, including methemoglobinemia, hemolytic anemia, and cholestatic jaundice. Monitor methemoglobin levels. Severe and potentially fatal hepatic injury may occur (50% of cases within first 3 months of therapy). Serum transaminases should be monitored at baseline and monthly for the first four months of therapy, and periodically thereafter. These should also be repeated at the first sign and symptom of liver dysfunction. Use of flutamide is not recommended in patients with baseline elevation of transaminase levels (>2 times the upper limit of normal). Flutamide should be discontinued immediately at any time if the patient develops jaundice or elevation in serum transaminase levels (>2 times upper limit of normal).

Drug Interactions

Cytochrome P450 Effect: Substrate (major) of CYP1A2, 3A4; **Inhibits** CYP1A2 (weak)

Decreased Effect: CYP1A2 inducers may decrease the levels/effects of flutamide; example inducers include aminoglutethimide, carbamazepine, phenobarbital, and rifampin. CYP3A4 inducers may decrease the levels/effects of flutamide; example inducers include aminoglutethimide, carbamazepine, nafcillin, nevirapine, phenobarbital, phenytoin, and rifamycins.

Increased Effect/Toxicity: CYP1A2 inhibitors may increase the levels/effects of flutamide; example inhibitors include amiodarone, ciprofloxacin, fluvoxamine, ketoconazole, lomefloxacin, ofloxacin, and rofecoxib. CYP3A4 inhibitors may increase the levels/effects of flutamide; example inhibitors include azole antifungals, clarithromycin, diclofenac, doxycycline, erythromycin, imatinib, isoniazid, nefazodone, nicardipine, propofol, protease inhibitors, quinidine, telithromycin, and verapamil. Warfarin effects may be increased.

Nutritional/Ethanol Interactions
Food: No effect on bioavailability of flutamide.
Herb/Nutraceutical: St John's wort may decrease flutamide levels.

Adverse Reactions
>10%:
Endocrine & metabolic: Gynecomastia, hot flashes, breast tenderness, galactorrhea (9% to 42%); impotence; decreased libido; tumor flare
Gastrointestinal: Nausea, vomiting (11% to 12%)
(Continued)

Flutamide *(Continued)*

Hepatic: Increased AST (SGOT) and LDH levels, transient, mild

1% to 10%:

Cardiovascular: Hypertension (1%), edema

Central nervous system: Drowsiness, confusion, depression, anxiety, nervousness, headache, dizziness, insomnia

Dermatologic: Pruritus, ecchymosis, photosensitivity, herpes zoster

Gastrointestinal: Anorexia, increased appetite, constipation, indigestion, upset stomach (4% to 6%); diarrhea

Hematologic: Anemia (6%), leukopenia (3%), thrombocytopenia (1%)

Neuromuscular & skeletal: Weakness (1%)

Overdosage/Toxicology Symptoms of overdose include hypoactivity, ataxia, anorexia, vomiting, slow respiration, and lacrimation. Induce vomiting. Management is supportive. Dialysis is of no benefit.

Pharmacodynamics/Kinetics

Protein Binding: Parent drug: 94% to 96%; 2-hydroxyflutamide: 92% to 94%

Half-Life Elimination: 5-6 hours (2-hydroxyflutamide)

Metabolism: Extensively hepatic to more than 10 metabolites, primarily 2-hydroxyflutamide (active)

Excretion: Primarily urine (as metabolites)

Available Dosage Forms Capsule: 125 mg

Dosing

Adults & Elderly: Refer to individual protocols.

Prostate carcinoma: Oral: 250 mg 3 times/day; alternatively, once-daily doses of 0.5-1.5 g have been used (unlabeled dosing)

Female hirsutism (unlabeled use): Oral: 250 mg daily

Administration

Oral: Usually administered orally in 3 divided doses; contents of capsule may be opened and mixed with applesauce, pudding, or other soft foods. Mixing with a beverage is not recommended.

Stability

Storage: Store at room temperature.

Laboratory Monitoring Serum transaminase levels should be obtained at baseline and repeated monthly for the first 4 months of therapy, and periodically thereafter. LFTs should be checked at the first sign or symptom of liver dysfunction. Other parameters include tumor reduction, testosterone/estrogen, prostate specific antigen, and phosphatase serum levels.

Nursing Actions

Physical Assessment: Assess potential for interactions with other pharmacological agents or herbal products patient may be taking (risk for increased or decreased levels/effects of flutamide). Assess results of laboratory tests prior to and periodically during therapy (eg, serum transaminase levels). Therapeutic effectiveness (eg, reduction of tumor) and adverse response should be assessed on a regular basis throughout therapy (eg, galactorrhea, CNS changes, ataxia, anorexia, vomiting, lacrimation, anemia, liver function). Teach patient proper use, possible side effects/appropriate interventions, and adverse symptoms to report (eg, chest pain, respiratory difficulty, abdominal pain, signs of liver dysfunction).

Patient Education: Do not take any new medication during therapy unless approved by prescriber. This medication will be prescribed in conjunction with another medication; take both exactly as directed; do not discontinue without consulting prescriber. May cause decreased libido, impotence, swelling of breasts, hot flashes, decreased appetite (small, frequent meals may help), or diarrhea (boiled milk, yogurt, or buttermilk may help). Report chest pain or palpitation; acute abdominal pain; pain, tingling, or numbness of extremities; swelling of extremities or

unusual weight gain; respiratory difficulty; yellowing of skin or sclera, dark urine, pale stool, unusual fatigue; or other persistent adverse effects. **Pregnancy/breast-feeding precautions:** Inform prescriber if you are pregnant and do not get pregnant during or for 1 month following therapy. Consult prescriber for instruction on appropriate barrier contraceptive measures. This drug may cause severe fetal defects. Breast-feeding is not recommended.

Geriatric Considerations A study has shown that the addition of flutamide to leuprolide therapy in patients with advanced prostatic cancer increased median actuarial survival time to 34.9 months versus 27.9 months with leuprolide alone. No specific dose alterations are necessary in the elderly.

Fluticasone *(floo TIK a sone)*

U.S. Brand Names Cutivate®; Flonase®; Flovent® HFA

Synonyms Fluticasone Propionate

Pharmacologic Category Corticosteroid, Inhalant (Oral); Corticosteroid, Nasal; Corticosteroid, Topical; Corticosteroid, Topical (Medium Potency)

Medication Safety Issues

Sound-alike/look-alike issues:

Cutivate® may be confused with Ultravate®

Pregnancy Risk Factor C

Lactation Excretion in breast milk unknown/use caution

Use

Inhalation: Maintenance treatment of asthma as prophylactic therapy. It is also indicated for patients requiring oral corticosteroid therapy for asthma to assist in total discontinuation or reduction of total oral dose

Intranasal: Management of seasonal and perennial allergic rhinitis and nonallergic rhinitis

Topical: Relief of inflammation and pruritus associated with corticosteroid-responsive dermatoses; atopic dermatitis

Mechanism of Action/Effect Fluticasone belongs to a new group of corticosteroids which utilizes a fluorocarbothioate ester linkage at the 17 carbon position; extremely potent vasoconstrictive and anti-inflammatory activity; has a weak HPA inhibitory potency when applied topically, which gives the drug a high therapeutic index. The effectiveness of inhaled fluticasone is due to its direct local effect. The mechanism of action for all topical corticosteroids is believed to be a combination of three important properties: anti-inflammatory activity, immunosuppressive properties, and antiproliferative actions.

Contraindications Hypersensitivity to fluticasone or any component of the formulation; primary treatment of status asthmaticus or acute bronchospasm

Topical: Do not use if infection is present at treatment site, in the presence of skin atrophy, or for the treatment of rosacea or perioral dermatitis

Warnings/Precautions May cause hypercorticism or suppression of hypothalamic-pituitary-adrenal (HPA) axis, particularly in younger children or in patients receiving high doses for prolonged periods. HPA axis suppression may lead to adrenal crisis. Fluticasone may cause less HPA axis suppression than therapeutically equivalent oral doses of prednisone. Particular care is required when patients are transferred from systemic corticosteroids to inhaled products due to possible adrenal insufficiency or withdrawal from steroids, including an increase in allergic symptoms. Patients receiving 20 mg per day of prednisone (or equivalent) may be most susceptible. Concurrent use of ritonavir (and potentially other strong inhibitors of CYP3A4) may increase fluticasone levels and effects on HPA suppression.

Controlled clinical studies have shown that orally-inhaled and intranasal corticosteroids may cause a reduction in growth velocity in pediatric patients. (In studies of orally-inhaled corticosteroids, the mean reduction in growth velocity was approximately 1 centimeter per year [range 0.3-1.8 cm per year] and appears to be related to dose and duration of exposure.) To minimize the systemic effects of orally-inhaled and intranasal corticosteroids, each patient should be titrated to the lowest effective dose. The risk of growth velocity reduction with intranasal administration of fluticasone may be very low.

May suppress the immune system, patients may be more susceptible to infection. Use with caution, if at all, in patients with systemic infections, active or quiescent tuberculosis infection, or ocular herpes simplex. Avoid exposure to chickenpox and measles.

Supplemental steroids (oral or parenteral) may be needed during stress or severe asthma attacks. Rare cases of vasculitis (Churg-Strauss syndrome) or other eosinophilic conditions can occur.

Inhalation: Not to be used in status asthmaticus or for the relief of acute bronchospasm. Flovent® Diskus® [CAN] contain lactose; very rare anaphylactic reactions have been reported in patients with severe milk protein allergy.

Topical: May also cause suppression of HPA axis, especially when used on large areas of the body, denuded areas, for prolonged periods of time or with an occlusive dressing. Pediatric patients may be more susceptible to systemic toxicity.

Drug Interactions
Cytochrome P450 Effect: Substrate of CYP3A4 (major)

Increased Effect/Toxicity: CYP3A4 inhibitors: May increase the levels/effects of fluticasone; example inhibitors include azole antifungals, clarithromycin, diclofenac, doxycycline, erythromycin, imatinib, isoniazid, nefazodone, nicardipine, propofol, protease inhibitors, quinidine, telithromycin, and verapamil. Ritonavir may increase serum levels (due to CYP3A4 inhibition) and the potential for steroid-related adverse effects (eg, Cushing syndrome, adrenal suppression). The addition of salmeterol has been demonstrated to improve response to inhaled corticosteroids (as compared to increasing steroid dosage).

Nutritional/Ethanol Interactions Herb/Nutraceutical: In theory, St John's wort may decrease serum levels of fluticasone by inducing CYP3A4 isoenzymes.

Adverse Reactions
Oral inhalation:
>10%:
Central nervous system: Headache (5% to 11%)
Respiratory: Upper respiratory tract infection (16% to 18%)
3% to 10%:
Respiratory: Throat irritation (8% to 10%), sinusitis/sinus infection (4% to 7%), cough (4% to 6%), bronchitis (2% to 6%), hoarseness/dysphonia (2% to 6%), upper respiratory tract inflammation (2% to 5%)
Miscellaneous: Candidiasis (2% to 5%)
1% to 3%:
Cardiovascular: Chest symptoms
Central nervous system: Dizziness, fever, migraine, pain
Gastrointestinal: Diarrhea, dyspepsia, gastrointestinal infection (viral), gastrointestinal discomfort/pain, hyposalivation
Genitourinary: Urinary tract infection
Neuromuscular & skeletal: Musculoskeletal pain, muscle pain, muscle stiffness/tightness/rigidity
Respiratory: Rhinitis, pharyngitis/throat infection, rhinorrhea/postnasal drip, nasal sinus disorder, laryngitis
Miscellaneous: Viral infection, injuries (including muscle, soft tissue)

Postmarketing and/or case reports: Aggression, agitation, anaphylactic reaction, angioedema, aphonia, asthma exacerbation, bronchospasm (immediate and delayed), cataracts, chest tightness, Churg-Strauss syndrome, contusion, Cushingoid features, cutaneous hypersensitivity, depression, dyspnea, ecchymoses, facial edema, growth velocity reduction in children/adolescents, HPA axis suppression, hyperglycemia, hypersensitivity reactions (immediate and delayed), oropharyngeal edema, osteoporosis, paradoxical bronchospasm, pneumonia, pruritus, rash, restlessness, throat soreness, urticaria, vasculitis, weight gain, wheeze

Nasal inhalation:
>10%: Central nervous system: Headache (7% to 16%)
1% to 10%:
Central nervous system: Dizziness (1% to 3%), fever (1% to 3%)
Gastrointestinal: Nausea/vomiting (3% to 5%), abdominal pain (1% to 3%), diarrhea (1% to 3%)
Respiratory: Pharyngitis (6% to 8%), epistaxis (6% to 7%), asthma symptoms (3% to 7%), cough (4%), blood in nasal mucous (1% to 3%), runny nose (1% to 3%), bronchitis (1% to 3%)
Miscellaneous: Aches and pains (1% to 3%), flu-like symptoms (1% to 3%)
<1% and postmarketing reports: Alteration or loss of sense of taste and/or smell, anaphylaxis/anaphylactoid reactions, angioedema, blurred vision, bronchospasm, cataracts, conjunctivitis, dry/irritated eyes, dry throat, dyspnea, edema (face and tongue), glaucoma, hoarseness, hypersensitivity reactions, increased intraocular pressure, nasal septal perforation (rare), nasal ulcer, pruritus, skin rash, sore throat, throat irritation, urticaria, voice changes, wheezing

Topical: 1% to 10%:
Dermatologic: Dry skin (7%), skin burning/stinging (2% to 5%), pruritus (3%), skin irritation (3%), viral skin infection (1% to 3%), exacerbation of eczema (2%)
Neuromuscular & skeletal: Numbness of fingers (1%)

Reported with other topical corticosteroids (in decreasing order of occurrence): Irritation, folliculitis, acneiform eruptions, hypopigmentation, perioral dermatitis, allergic contact dermatitis, secondary infection, skin atrophy, striae, miliaria, pustular psoriasis from chronic plaque psoriasis

Overdosage/Toxicology When consumed in high doses over prolonged periods, systemic hypercorticism and adrenal suppression may occur. In those cases, discontinuation of the corticosteroid should be done judiciously.

Pharmacodynamics/Kinetics
Onset of Action: Flovent® HFA: Maximal benefit may take 1-2 weeks or longer
Protein Binding: 91%
Metabolism: Hepatic via CYP3A4 to 17β-carboxylic acid (negligible activity)
Excretion: Feces (as parent drug and metabolites); urine (<5% as metabolites)

Available Dosage Forms [CAN] = Canadian brand name
Aerosol for oral inhalation, as propionate [CFC free]:
Flovent® HFA: 44 mcg/inhalation (10.6 g) [120 metered doses]
Flovent® HFA: 110 mcg/inhalation (12 g) [120 metered doses]
Flovent® HFA: 220 mcg/inhalation (12 g) [120 metered doses]
Cream, as propionate: 0.05% (15 g, 30 g, 60 g)
Cutivate®: 0.05% (15 g, 30 g, 60 g)
Lotion, as propionate:
Cutivate®: 0.05% (60 mL)
Ointment, as propionate: 0.005% (15 g, 30 g, 60 g)
Cutivate®: 0.005% (15 g, 30 g, 60 g)
(Continued)

Fluticasone *(Continued)*

Powder for oral inhalation, as propionate [prefilled blister pack]:

Flovent® Diskus®) [CAN]: 50 mcg (28s, 60s) [contains lactose] [not available in the U.S.]

Flovent® Diskus®) [CAN]: 100 mcg (28s, 60s) [contains lactose] [not available in the U.S.]

Flovent® Diskus®) [CAN]: 250 mcg (28s, 60s) [contains lactose] [not available in the U.S.]

Flovent® Diskus®) [CAN]: 500 mcg (28s, 60s) [contains lactose] [not available in the U.S.]

Suspension, intranasal spray, as propionate: 50 mcg/inhalation (16 g) [120 metered doses]

Flonase®: 50 mcg/inhalation (16 g) [120 metered doses]

Dosing

Adults & Elderly:

Asthma: Inhalation, oral: **Note:** Titrate to the lowest effective dose once asthma stability is achieved

Flovent® HFA: Manufacturers labeling: Dosing based on previous therapy

Bronchodilator alone: Recommended starting dose: 88 mcg twice daily; highest recommended dose: 440 mcg twice daily

Inhaled corticosteroids: Recommended starting dose: 88-220 mcg twice daily; highest recommended dose: 440 mcg twice daily; a higher starting dose may be considered in patients previously requiring higher doses of inhaled corticosteroids

Oral corticosteroids:

Recommended starting dose:

Flovent® HFA: 440 mcg twice daily

Highest recommended dose: 880 mcg twice daily; starting dose is patient dependent. In patients on chronic oral corticosteroids therapy, reduce prednisone dose no faster than 2.5-5 mg/day on a weekly basis; begin taper after 1 week of fluticasone therapy

NIH Asthma Guidelines (administer in divided doses twice daily).

"Low" dose: 88-264 mcg/day

"Medium" dose: 264-660 mcg/day

"High" dose: >660 mcg/day

Flovent® Diskus® [CAN]:

Mild asthma: 100-250 mcg twice daily

Moderate asthma: 250-500 mcg twice daily

Severe asthma: 500 mcg twice daily; may increase to 1000 mcg twice daily in very severe patients requiring high doses of corticosteroids

Corticosteroid-responsive dermatoses: Topical: Cream, lotion, ointment: Apply sparingly to affected area twice daily. If no improvement is seen within 2 weeks, reassessment of diagnosis may be necessary.

Atopic dermatitis: Topical: Cream, lotion: Apply sparingly to affected area once or twice daily. If no improvement is seen within 2 weeks, reassessment of diagnosis may be necessary.

Rhinitis: Intranasal: Initial: 2 sprays (50 mcg/spray) per nostril once daily; may also be divided into 100 mcg twice a day. After the first few days, dosage may be reduced to 1 spray per nostril once daily for maintenance therapy. Dosing should be at regular intervals.

Pediatrics:

Asthma: Inhalation, oral:

Flovent® HFA:

Children 4-11 years: 88 mcg twice daily

Children ≥12 years: Refer to adult dosing.

Note: NIH Asthma Guidelines (administer in divided doses twice daily):

"Low" dose: 88-176 mcg/day

"Medium" dose: 176-440 mcg/day

"High" dose: >440 mcg/day

Flovent® Diskus® [CAN]:

Children 4-16 years: Usual starting dose: 50-100 mcg twice daily; may increase to 200 mcg twice daily in patients not adequately controlled; titrate to the lowest effective dose once asthma stability is achieved

Children ≥16 years: Refer to adult dosing.

Corticosteroid-responsive dermatoses: Topical:

Children ≥3 months: Cream: Apply sparingly to affected area twice daily. If no improvement is seen within 2 weeks, reassessment of diagnosis may be necessary. **Note:** Safety and efficacy of treatment >4 weeks duration have not been established.

Atopic dermatitis: Topical:

Children ≥3 months: Cream: Apply sparingly to affected area 1-2 times/day. If no improvement is seen within 2 weeks, reassessment of diagnosis may be necessary.

Children ≥1 year: Lotion: Apply sparingly to affected area once daily.

Note: Safety and efficacy of treatment >4 weeks duration have not been established.

Rhinitis: Intranasal: Children ≥4 years and Adolescents: Initial: 1 spray (50 mcg/spray) per nostril once daily; patients not adequately responding or patients with more severe symptoms may use 2 sprays (100 mcg) per nostril. Depending on response, dosage may be reduced to 100 mcg daily. Total daily dosage should not exceed 2 sprays in each nostril (200 mcg)/day. Dosing should be at regular intervals.

Hepatic Impairment: Fluticasone is primarily cleared in the liver. Fluticasone plasma levels may be increased in patients with hepatic impairment, use with caution; monitor.

Administration

Inhalation:

Aerosol inhalation: Flovent® HFA: Shake container thoroughly before using. Take 3-5 deep breaths. Use inhaler on inspiration. Allow 1 full minute between inhalations. Rinse mouth with water after use to reduce aftertaste and incidence of candidiasis. Flovent® HFA inhaler must be primed before first use, when not used for 7 days, or if dropped. To prime the first time, release 4 sprays into air; shake well before each spray and spray away from face. If dropped or not used for 7 days, prime by releasing a single test spray. Discard after 120 actuations; do not use "float" test to determine contents

Nasal spray: Shake bottle gently before using. Prime pump prior to first use (press 6 times until fine spray appears). Blow nose to clear nostrils. Insert applicator into nostril, keeping bottle upright, and close off the other nostril. Breathe in through nose. While inhaling, press pump to release spray. Nasal applicator may be removed and rinsed with warm water to clean. Discard after labeled number of doses has been used, even if bottle is not completely empty.

Powder for oral inhalation: Flovent® Diskus® [CAN]: Do not use with a spacer device. Do not exhale into Diskus®. Do not wash or take apart. Use in horizontal position.

Topical: Cream, lotion, ointment: Apply sparingly in a thin film. Rub in lightly. Unless otherwise directed by healthcare professional, do not use with occlusive dressing; do not use on children's skin covered by diapers or plastic pants.

Stability

Storage:

Nasal spray: Store between 4°C to 30°C (39°F to 86°F).

Oral inhalation: Flovent®, Flovent® HFA: Store at 15°C to 30°C (59°F to 86°F). Store with mouthpiece down.

Powder for oral inhalation: Flovent® Diskus® [CAN]: Store between 2°C to 30°C in a dry place away from direct frost, heat, or sunlight. Do not store in a damp environment (eg, bathroom).

Topical, cream: Store at 15°C to 30°C (59°F to 86°F).

Cutivate® lotion: Store at 15°C to 30°C (59°F to 86°F). Do not refrigerate.

Cutivate® cream, ointment: Store at 2°C to 30°C (36°F to 86°F).

Nursing Actions

Physical Assessment: Monitor effectiveness of therapy and adverse reactions at beginning of therapy and periodically with long-term use. May take as long as 2 weeks before full benefit of medication is known. Assess knowledge/teach patient appropriate use, interventions to reduce side effects, and adverse symptoms to report. Monitor for possible eosinophilic conditions (including Churg-Strauss syndrome); growth (adolescents and children); and signs/symptoms of HPA axis suppression/adrenal insufficiency.

Patient Education: Use as directed; do not overuse and use only for length of time prescribed. Although you may see improvement within a few hours of use, the full benefit of the medication may not be achieved for several days. Do not change the prescribed dosage without consulting prescriber. Avoid exposure to chickenpox or measles. If exposed, inform your prescriber as soon as possible. **Pregnancy/breast-feeding precautions:** Inform prescriber if you are or intend to become pregnant. Consult prescriber if breast-feeding.

Metered-dose inhalation: Sit when using. Take deep breaths for 3-5 minutes, and clear nasal passages before administration (use decongestant as needed). Hold breath for 5-10 seconds after use, and wait 1-3 minutes between inhalations. Follow package insert instructions for use. Do not exceed maximum dosage. If also using inhaled bronchodilator, use before fluticasone. Rinse mouth and throat after use to reduce aftertaste and prevent candidiasis.

Nasal spray: Shake gently before use. Use at regular intervals, no more frequently than directed. Report unusual cough or spasm; persistent nasal bleeding, burning, or irritation; or worsening of condition.

Powder for oral inhalation: Flovent® Diskus® [CAN]: Do not attempt to take device apart. Do not use with a spacer device. Do not exhale into the Diskus®, use in a level horizontal position. Do not wash the mouthpiece.

Topical: For external use only. Apply thin film to affected area only; rub in lightly. Do not apply occlusive covering unless advised by prescriber. Wash hand thoroughly after use; avoid contact with eyes. Notify prescriber if skin condition persists or worsens. Do not use for treatment of diaper dermatitis or under diapers or plastic pants.

Dietary Considerations Flovent® Diskus® [CAN] contains lactose; very rare anaphylactic reactions have been reported with Flovent® Rotadisk® in patients with severe milk protein allergy.

Geriatric Considerations No specific information for the elderly patient is available.

Breast-Feeding Issues Systemic corticosteroids are excreted in human milk. The extent of topical absorption is variable. Use with caution while breast-feeding; do not apply to nipples.

Pregnancy Issues There are no adequate and well-controlled studies using inhaled fluticasone in pregnant women. Oral corticosteroid use has shown animals to be more prone to teratogenic effects than humans. Due to the natural increase in corticosteroid production during pregnancy, most women may require a lower steroid dose; use with caution.

Additional Information Effects of inhaled/intranasal steroids on growth have been observed in the absence of laboratory evidence of HPA axis suppression, suggesting that growth velocity is a more sensitive indicator of systemic corticosteroid exposure in pediatric patients than some commonly used tests of HPA axis function. The long-term effects of this reduction in growth velocity associated with orally-inhaled and intranasal corticosteroids, including the impact on final adult height, are unknown. The potential for "catch up" growth following discontinuation of treatment with inhaled corticosteroids has not been adequately studied. The product labeling notes that intranasal administration was not associated with a statistically-significant reduction in growth velocity (based on a small study conducted over 1 year).

In the United States, dosage for the metered dose inhaler (Flovent® HFA) is expressed as the amount of drug which leaves the actuater and is delivered to the patient. This differs from other countries, which express the dosage as the amount of drug which leaves the valve.

Fluticasone and Salmeterol
(floo TIK a sone & sal ME te role)

U.S. Brand Names Advair Diskus®

Synonyms Salmeterol and Fluticasone

Restrictions An FDA-approved medication guide is available at http://www.fda.gov/cder/Offices/ODS/labeling.htm; distribute to each patient to whom this medication is dispensed.

Pharmacologic Category Beta$_2$-Adrenergic Agonist; Corticosteroid, Inhalant (Oral)

Pregnancy Risk Factor C

Lactation

Fluticasone: Excretion in breast milk unknown/use caution

Salmeterol: Enters breast milk/use caution

Use Maintenance treatment of asthma in children ≥4 years and adults; maintenance treatment of COPD associated with chronic bronchitis

Available Dosage Forms Powder for oral inhalation:

100/50: Fluticasone propionate 100 mcg and salmeterol xinafoate 50 mcg (28s, 60s) [contains lactose]

250/50: Fluticasone propionate 250 mcg and salmeterol xinafoate 50 mcg (28s, 60s) [contains lactose]

500/50: Fluticasone propionate 500 mcg and salmeterol xinafoate 50 mcg (28s, 60s) [contains lactose]

Dosing

Adults & Elderly: Do not use to transfer patients from systemic corticosteroid therapy.

COPD: Oral inhalation: Fluticasone 250 mcg/salmeterol 50 mcg twice daily, 12 hours apart. **Note:** This is the maximum dose.

Asthma (maintenance): Oral inhalation: One inhalation twice daily, morning and evening, 12 hours apart

Note: Advair Diskus® is available in 3 strengths, initial dose prescribed should be based upon previous asthma therapy. Dose should be increased after 2 weeks if adequate response is not achieved. Patients should be titrated to lowest effective dose once stable. (Because each strength contains salmeterol 50 mcg/inhalation, dose adjustments should be made by changing inhaler strength. No more than 1 inhalation of any strength should be taken more than twice a day). Maximum dose: Fluticasone 500 mcg/salmeterol 50 mcg, one inhalation twice daily.

Patients not currently on inhaled corticosteroids: Fluticasone 100 mcg/salmeterol 50 mcg **or** fluticasone 250 mcg/salmeterol 50 mcg

Patients currently using inhaled beclomethasone dipropionate:

≤160 mcg/day: Fluticasone 100 mcg/salmeterol 50 mcg

(Continued)

Fluticasone and Salmeterol *(Continued)*

320 mcg/day: Fluticasone 250 mcg/salmeterol 50 mcg

650 mcg/day: Fluticasone 500 mcg/salmeterol 50 mcg

Patients currently using inhaled budesonide:

≤400 mcg/day: Fluticasone 100 mcg/salmeterol 50 mcg

800-1200 mcg/day: Fluticasone 250 mcg/salmeterol 50 mcg

1600 mcg/day: Fluticasone 500 mcg/salmeterol 50 mcg

Patients currently using inhaled flunisolide:

≤1000 mcg/day: Fluticasone 100 mcg/salmeterol 50 mcg

1250-2000 mcg/day: Fluticasone 250 mcg/salmeterol 50 mcg

Patients currently using inhaled fluticasone propionate aerosol:

≤176 mcg/day: Fluticasone 100 mcg/salmeterol 50 mcg

440 mcg/day: Fluticasone 250 mcg/salmeterol 50 mcg

660-880 mcg/day: Fluticasone 500 mcg/salmeterol 50 mcg

Patients currently using inhaled fluticasone propionate powder:

≤200 mcg/day: Fluticasone 100 mcg/salmeterol 50 mcg

500 mcg/day: Fluticasone 250 mcg/salmeterol 50 mcg

1000 mcg/day: Fluticasone 500 mcg/salmeterol 50 mcg

Patients currently using inhaled mometasone furoate powder:

220 mcg/day: Fluticasone 100 mcg/salmeterol 50 mcg

440 mcg/day: Fluticasone 250 mcg/salmeterol 50 mcg

880 mcg/day: Fluticasone 500 mcg/salmeterol 50 mcg

Patients currently using inhaled triamcinolone acetonide:

≤1000 mcg/day: Fluticasone 100 mcg/salmeterol 50 mcg

1100-1600 mcg/day: Fluticasone 250 mcg/salmeterol 50 mcg

Pediatrics: Asthma: Oral inhalation:

Children 4-11 years: Fluticasone 100 mcg/salmeterol 50 mcg twice daily, 12 hours apart. **Note:** This is the maximum dose.

Children ≥12 years: Refer to adult dosing.

Hepatic Impairment: Fluticasone is cleared by hepatic metabolism. No dosing adjustment suggested. Use with caution in patients with impaired liver function.

Nursing Actions

Physical Assessment: See individual agents.

Patient Education: See individual agents. **Pregnancy/breast-feeding precautions:** Inform prescriber if you are or intend to become pregnant. Consult prescriber if breast-feeding.

Related Information

Fluticasone *on page 540*
Salmeterol *on page 1106*

Fluvastatin (FLOO va sta tin)

U.S. Brand Names Lescol®; Lescol® XL

Pharmacologic Category Antilipemic Agent, HMG-CoA Reductase Inhibitor

Medication Safety Issues

Sound-alike/look-alike issues:

Fluvastatin may be confused with fluoxetine

Pregnancy Risk Factor X

Lactation Enters breast milk/contraindicated

Use To be used as a component of multiple risk factor intervention in patients at risk for atherosclerosis vascular disease due to hypercholesterolemia

Adjunct to dietary therapy to reduce elevated total cholesterol (total-C), LDL-C, triglyceride, and apolipoprotein B (apo-B) levels and to increase HDL-C in primary hypercholesterolemia and mixed dyslipidemia (Fredrickson types IIa and IIb); to slow the progression of coronary atherosclerosis in patients with coronary heart disease; reduce risk of coronary revascularization procedures in patients with coronary heart disease

Mechanism of Action/Effect Acts by competitively inhibiting 3-hydroxyl-3-methylglutaryl-coenzyme A (HMG-CoA) reductase, the enzyme that catalyzes the reduction of HMG-CoA to mevalonate; this is an early rate-limiting step in cholesterol biosynthesis. HDL is increased while total, LDL and VLDL cholesterols, apolipoprotein B, and plasma triglycerides are decreased.

Contraindications Hypersensitivity to fluvastatin or any component of the formulation; active liver disease; unexplained persistent elevations of serum transaminases; pregnancy; breast-feeding

Warnings/Precautions Secondary causes of hyperlipidemia should be ruled out prior to therapy. Liver function must be monitored by periodic laboratory assessment. Rhabdomyolysis with acute renal failure has occurred with fluvastatin and other HMG-CoA reductase inhibitors. Risk may be increased with concurrent use of other drugs which may cause rhabdomyolysis (including gemfibrozil, fibric acid derivatives, or niacin at doses ≥1 g/day). Temporarily discontinue in any patient experiencing an acute or serious condition predisposing to renal failure secondary to rhabdomyolysis. Use caution in patients with previous liver disease or heavy ethanol use. Treatment in patients <18 years of age is not recommended.

Drug Interactions

Cytochrome P450 Effect: Substrate (minor) of CYP2C8/9, 2D6, 3A4; **Inhibits** CYP1A2 (weak), 2C8/9 (moderate), 2D6 (weak), 3A4 (weak)

Decreased Effect: Administration of cholestyramine at the same time with fluvastatin reduces absorption and clinical effect of fluvastatin. Separate administration times by at least 4 hours. Rifampin and rifabutin may decrease fluvastatin blood levels.

Increased Effect/Toxicity: Cimetidine, omeprazole, ranitidine, and ritonavir may increase fluvastatin blood levels. Clofibrate, erythromycin, gemfibrozil, fenofibrate, and niacin may increase the risk of myopathy and rhabdomyolysis. Anticoagulant effect of warfarin may be increased by fluvastatin. Cholestyramine effect will be additive with fluvastatin if administration times are separated. Fluvastatin may increase C_{max} and decrease clearance of digoxin. Fluvastatin may increase the levels/effects of amiodarone, fluoxetine, glimepiride, glipizide, nateglinide, phenytoin, pioglitazone, rosiglitazone, sertraline, warfarin, and other CYP2C8/9 substrates.

Nutritional/Ethanol Interactions

Ethanol: Avoid excessive ethanol consumption (due to potential hepatic effects).

Food: Reduces rate but not the extent of absorption. Red yeast rice contains an estimated 2.4 mg lovastatin per 600 mg rice.

Lab Interactions Increased serum transaminases, CPK, alkaline phosphatase, and bilirubin and thyroid function tests

Adverse Reactions As reported with fluvastatin capsules; in general, adverse reactions reported with fluvastatin extended release tablet were similar, but the incidence was less.

1% to 10%:
Central nervous system: Headache (9%), fatigue (3%), insomnia (3%)
Gastrointestinal: Dyspepsia (8%), diarrhea (5%), abdominal pain (5%), nausea (3%)
Genitourinary: Urinary tract infection (2%)
Neuromuscular & skeletal: Myalgia (5%)
Respiratory: Sinusitis (3%), bronchitis (2%)

Overdosage/Toxicology GI complaints and elevated SGOT and SGPT have been reported following large doses of the extended release tablets. In case of overdose, supportive measure should be instituted, as required; dialyzability is not known.

Pharmacodynamics/Kinetics
Protein Binding: >98%
Half-Life Elimination: Capsule: <3 hours; Extended release tablet: 9 hours
Metabolism: To inactive and active metabolites [oxidative metabolism via CYP2C9 (75%), 2C8 (~5%), and 3A4 (~20%) isoenzymes]; active forms do not circulate systemically; extensive first-pass hepatic extraction
Excretion: Feces (90%): urine (5%)
Available Dosage Forms
Capsule (Lescol®): 20 mg, 40 mg
Tablet, extended release (Lescol® XL): 80 mg
Dosing
Adults & Elderly:
Dyslipidemia (also delay in progression of CAD): Oral:
Patients requiring ≥25% decrease in LDL-C: 40 mg capsule or 80 mg extended release tablet once daily in the evening; may also use 40 mg capsule twice daily
Patients requiring <25% decrease in LDL-C: 20 mg capsule once daily in the evening
Dosing range: 20-80 mg/day; adjust dose based on response to therapy; maximum response occurs within 4-6 weeks
Renal Impairment: Less than 6% is excreted renally. No dosage adjustment needed with mild to moderate renal impairment; use with caution in severe impairment.
Hepatic Impairment: Levels may accumulate in patients with liver disease (increased AUC and C_{max}). Use caution with severe hepatic impairment or heavy ethanol ingestion. Contraindicated in active liver disease or unexplained transaminase elevations. Decrease dose and monitor effects carefully in patients with hepatic insufficiency.

Administration
Oral: Patient should be placed on a standard cholesterol-lowering diet before and during treatment; fluvastatin may be taken without regard to meals; adjust dosage as needed in response to periodic lipid determinations during the first 4 weeks after a dosage change; lipid-lowering effects are additive when fluvastatin is combined with a bile-acid binding resin or niacin, however, it must be administered at least 2 hours following these drugs.

Stability
Storage: Store at 25°C (77°F); protect from light.
Laboratory Monitoring Obtain baseline LFTs and total cholesterol profile. Repeat tests at 12 weeks after initiation of therapy or elevation in dose, and periodically thereafter. Monitor LDL-C at intervals no less than 4 weeks.

Nursing Actions
Physical Assessment: Secondary causes of hyperlipidemia should be ruled out prior to beginning therapy. Assess potential for interactions with other pharmacological agents or herbal products patient may be taking (eg, increased risk of rhabdomyolysis, acute renal failure). Assess results of laboratory tests (eg, LFTs and cholesterol profile) at baseline and periodically thereafter. Monitor therapeutic effectiveness (reduced hyperlipemia) and adverse response (eg, myalgia, gastrointestinal disturbances; see Adverse Reactions) on a regular basis throughout therapy. Teach patient proper use, possible side effects/appropriate interventions, and adverse symptoms to report.
Pregnancy risk factor X - determine that patient is not pregnant before starting therapy. Do not give to sexually active female patients unless capable of complying with effective contraceptive use. Instruct patient in appropriate contraceptive measures. Breast-feeding is contraindicated.

Patient Education: Do not take any new medication during therapy unless approved by prescriber. Take as directed, with or without food. Follow diet and exercise regimen as prescribed. You will need periodic laboratory tests to evaluate response. You may experience nausea or dyspepsia (small, frequent meals, frequent mouth care, chewing gum, or sucking lozenges may help); diarrhea (buttermilk, boiled milk, or yogurt may help); or headache (consult prescriber for approved analgesic). Report muscle pain or cramping; tremor; or CNS changes (eg, memory loss, depression, personality changes; numbness, weakness, tingling or pain in extremities). **Pregnancy/breast-feeding precautions:** Inform prescriber if you are pregnant. Consult prescriber for instruction on appropriate contraceptive measures. This drug may cause severe fetal defects. Do not donate blood during or for 1 month following therapy (same reason). Do not breast-feed.

Dietary Considerations Before initiation of therapy, patients should be placed on a standard cholesterol-lowering diet for 3-6 months and the diet should be continued during drug therapy. May be taken without regard to meals. Red yeast rice contains an estimated 2.4 mg lovastatin per 600 mg rice.

Geriatric Considerations The definition of and, therefore, when to treat hyperlipidemia in the elderly is a controversial issue. The National Cholesterol Education Program recommends that all adults maintain a plasma cholesterol <160 mg/dL. In elderly patients with one additional risk factor, goal LDL would decrease to <130 mg/dL. Pharmacologic treatment should be reserved for those who are unable to obtain a desirable plasma cholesterol concentration by diet alone and for whom the benefits of treatment are believed to outweigh the potential adverse effects, drug interactions, and cost of treatment.

Breast-Feeding Issues Fluvastatin is excreted in human breast milk (milk plasma ratio 2:1); do not use in breast-feeding women.

Pregnancy Issues Cholesterol biosynthesis may be important in fetal development. Contraindicated in pregnancy. Administer to women of childbearing potential only when conception is highly unlikely and patients have been informed of potential hazards.

Fluvoxamine (floo VOKS a meen)

Synonyms Luvox

Restrictions A medication guide concerning the use of antidepressants in children and teenagers can be found on the FDA website at http://www.fda.gov/cder/Offices/ODS/labeling.htm. It should be dispensed to parents or guardians of children and teenagers receiving this medication.

Pharmacologic Category Antidepressant, Selective Serotonin Reuptake Inhibitor

Medication Safety Issues
Sound-alike/look-alike issues:
Fluvoxamine may be confused with flavoxate
Luvox may be confused with Lasix®, Levoxyl®

Pregnancy Risk Factor C

Lactation Enters breast milk/not recommended (AAP rates "of concern")

Use Treatment of obsessive-compulsive disorder (OCD) in children ≥8 years of age and adults

Unlabeled/Investigational Use Treatment of major depression; panic disorder; anxiety disorders in children

Mechanism of Action/Effect Inhibits CNS neuron serotonin uptake; minimal or no effect on reuptake of norepinephrine or dopamine; does not significantly bind to alpha-adrenergic, histamine or cholinergic receptors

Contraindications Hypersensitivity to fluvoxamine or any component of the formulation; concurrent use with alosetron, pimozide, thioridazine, tizanidine, mesoridazine, or cisapride; use of MAO inhibitors within 14 days

Warnings/Precautions Antidepressants increase the risk of suicidal thinking and behavior in children and adolescents with major depressive disorder (MDD) and other depressive disorders; consider risk prior to prescribing. All patients must be closely monitored for clinical worsening, suicidality, or unusual changes in behavior, especially during the initiation of therapy or following an increase or decrease in dosage. When used in children, the child's family or caregiver should be instructed to closely observe the patient and communicate condition with healthcare provider. A medication guide should be dispensed with each prescription. **Fluvoxamine is FDA approved for the treatment of OCD in children ≥8 years of age.**

The possibility of a suicide attempt is inherent in major depression and may persist until remission occurs. Use caution in high-risk patients. Worsening depression and severe abrupt suicidality that are not part of the presenting symptoms may require discontinuation or modification of drug therapy. The patient's family or caregiver should be alerted to monitor patients for the emergence of suicidality and associated behaviors (such as agitation, irritability, hostility, impulsivity, and hypomania) and call healthcare provider.

May worsen psychosis in some patients or precipitate a shift to mania or hypomania in patients with bipolar disorder. Patients presenting with depressive symptoms should be screened for bipolar disorder. Monotherapy in patients with bipolar disorder should be avoided. **Fluvoxamine is not FDA approved for the treatment of bipolar depression.**

The potential for severe reaction exits when used with MAO inhibitors - serotonin syndrome (hyperthermia, muscular rigidity, mental status changes/agitation, autonomic instability) may occur. Fluvoxamine has a low potential to impair cognitive or motor performance; caution operating hazardous machinery or driving. Use caution in patients with a previous seizure disorder or condition predisposing to seizures such as brain damage, alcoholism, or concurrent therapy with other drugs which lower the seizure threshold.

May increase the risks associated with electroconvulsive therapy. Use with caution in patients with hepatic or renal dysfunction and in elderly patients. May cause hyponatremia/SIADH. Use with caution in patients with renal insufficiency or other concurrent illness (cardiovascular disease). Use with caution in patients at risk of bleeding or receiving concurrent anticoagulant therapy, although not consistently noted, fluvoxamine may cause impairment in platelet function. May cause or exacerbate sexual dysfunction.

Drug Interactions
Cytochrome P450 Effect: Substrate (major) of CYP1A2, 2D6; **Inhibits** CYP1A2 (strong), 2B6 (weak), 2C8/9 (weak), 2C19 (strong), 2D6 (weak), 3A4 (weak)

Decreased Effect: The levels/effects of fluvoxamine may be decreased by aminoglutethimide, carbamazepine, phenobarbital, rifampin, and other CYP1A2 inducers. Cyproheptadine, a serotonin antagonist, may inhibit the effects of serotonin reuptake inhibitors (fluvoxamine); monitor for altered antidepressant response.

Increased Effect/Toxicity: Fluvoxamine should not be used with nonselective MAO inhibitors (phenelzine, isocarboxazid) and drugs with MAO inhibitor properties (linezolid); fatal reactions have been reported. Wait 5 weeks after stopping fluvoxamine before starting a nonselective MAO inhibitor and 2 weeks after stopping an MAO inhibitor before starting fluvoxamine. Concurrent selegiline has been associated with mania, hypertension, or serotonin syndrome (risk may be reduced relative to nonselective MAO inhibitors).

Fluvoxamine may inhibit the metabolism of thioridazine or mesoridazine, resulting in increased plasma levels and increasing the risk of QT_c interval prolongation. This may lead to serious ventricular arrhythmias, such as torsade de pointes-type arrhythmias and sudden death. Do not use together. Wait at least 5 weeks after discontinuing fluvoxamine prior to starting thioridazine. Fluvoxamine may increase the levels/effects of aminophylline, citalopram, diazepam, mexiletine, mirtazapine, methsuximide, phenytoin, propranolol, ropinirole, sertraline, theophylline, trifluoperazine and other substrates of CYP1A2 or 2C19. Fluvoxamine may increase the concentrations of alosetron and tizanidine; concurrent use is not recommended.

The levels/effects of fluvoxamine may be increased by amiodarone, amphetamines, selected beta-blockers, chlorpromazine, ciprofloxacin, delavirdine, fluoxetine, ketoconazole, miconazole, norfloxacin, ofloxacin, paroxetine, pergolide, quinidine, quinine, ritonavir, rofecoxib, ropinirole, and other CYP1A2 or 2D6 inhibitors.

Combined use of SSRIs and amphetamines, buspirone, meperidine, nefazodone, serotonin agonists (such as sumatriptan), sibutramine, other SSRIs, sympathomimetics, ritonavir, tramadol, and venlafaxine may increase the risk of serotonin syndrome. Combined use of sumatriptan (and other serotonin agonists) may result in toxicity; weakness, hyper-reflexia, and incoordination have been observed with sumatriptan and SSRIs. In addition, concurrent use may theoretically increase the risk of serotonin syndrome; includes sumatriptan, naratriptan, rizatriptan, and zolmitriptan.

Concurrent lithium may increase risk of nephrotoxicity. Risk of hyponatremia may increase with concurrent use of loop diuretics (bumetanide, furosemide, torsemide). Fluvoxamine may increase the hypoprothrombinemic response to warfarin. Concomitant use of fluvoxamine and NSAIDs, aspirin, or other drugs affecting coagulation has been associated with an increased risk of bleeding; monitor.

Nutritional/Ethanol Interactions

Ethanol: Avoid ethanol. Depressed patients should avoid/limit intake.

Food: The bioavailability of melatonin has been reported to be increased by fluvoxamine.

Herb/Nutraceutical: Avoid valerian, St John's wort, SAMe, kava kava (may increase risk of serotonin syndrome and/or excessive sedation).

Adverse Reactions

>10%:

Central nervous system: Headache (22%), somnolence (22%), insomnia (21%), nervousness (12%), dizziness (11%)

Gastrointestinal: Nausea (40%), diarrhea (11%), xerostomia (14%)

Neuromuscular & skeletal: Weakness (14%)

1% to 10%:

Cardiovascular: Palpitations

Central nervous system: Somnolence, mania, hypomania, vertigo, abnormal thinking, agitation, anxiety, malaise, amnesia, yawning, hypertonia, CNS stimulation, depression

Endocrine & metabolic: Decreased libido

Gastrointestinal: Abdominal pain, vomiting, dyspepsia, constipation, abnormal taste, anorexia, flatulence, weight gain

Genitourinary: Delayed ejaculation, impotence, anorgasmia, urinary frequency, urinary retention

Neuromuscular & skeletal: Tremors

Ocular: Blurred vision

Respiratory: Dyspnea

Miscellaneous: Diaphoresis

Overdosage/Toxicology

Symptoms of overdose include drowsiness, nausea, vomiting, abdominal pain, tremor, sinus bradycardia, and seizures. A specific antidote does not exist. Treatment is supportive.

Pharmacodynamics/Kinetics

Time to Peak: Plasma: 3-8 hours

Protein Binding: ~80%, primarily to albumin

Half-Life Elimination: ~15 hours

Metabolism: Hepatic

Excretion: Urine

Available Dosage Forms Tablet: 25 mg, 50 mg, 100 mg

Dosing

Adults: Obsessive-compulsive disorder: Oral: Initial: 50 mg at bedtime; adjust in 50 mg increments at 4- to 7-day intervals; usual dose range: 100-300 mg/day; divide total daily dose into 2 doses. Administer larger portion at bedtime.

Note: When total daily dose exceeds 50 mg, the dose should be given in 2 divided doses.

Elderly: Reduce dose, titrate slowly. See Geriatric Considerations.

Pediatrics: Obsessive-compulsive disorder: Oral: Children 8-17 years: Initial: 25 mg at bedtime; adjust in 25 mg increments at 4- to 7-day intervals, as tolerated, to maximum therapeutic benefit: Range: 50-200 mg/day

Maximum dose: Children: 8-11 years: 200 mg/day; Adolescents: 300 mg/day; lower doses may be effective in female versus male patients

Note: When total daily dose exceeds 50 mg, the dose should be given in 2 divided doses.

Hepatic Impairment: Reduce dose, titrate slowly.

Stability

Storage: Protect from high humidity and store at controlled room temperature 15°C to 30°C (59°F to 86°F); dispense in tight containers

Laboratory Monitoring Liver and kidney function assessment prior to beginning drug therapy

Physical Assessment: Assess other medications patient may be taking for effectiveness and interactions. Monitor laboratory tests, therapeutic response, and adverse reactions at beginning of therapy and periodically with long-term use (eg, CNS, and gastrointestinal). Taper dosage slowly when discontinuing. Assess mental status for depression, suicidal ideation, anxiety, social functioning, mania, or panic attack. Assess knowledge/teach patient appropriate use, interventions to reduce side effects, and adverse symptoms to report.

Patient Education: Take exactly as directed; do not increase dose or frequency. It may take 2-3 weeks to achieve desired results. Avoid alcohol, caffeine, and other prescription or OTC medications unless approved by prescriber. Maintain adequate hydration (2-3 L/day of fluids) unless instructed to restrict fluid intake. You may experience drowsiness, lightheadedness, impaired coordination, dizziness, or blurred vision (use caution when driving or engaging in tasks requiring alertness until response to drug is known); nausea, vomiting, or anorexia (small frequent meals, frequent mouth care, chewing gum, or sucking lozenges may help); constipation (increased exercise, fluids, fruits, or fiber may help); diarrhea (buttermilk, yogurt, or boiled milk may help); postural hypotension (use caution when climbing stairs or changing position from lying or sitting to standing); or decreased sexual function or libido (reversible). Report persistent CNS effects (nervousness, restlessness, insomnia, anxiety, excitation, suicide ideation, headache, sedation, seizures, mania, abnormal thinking); rash or skin irritation; muscle cramping, tremors, or change in gait; chest pain or palpitations; change in urinary pattern; or worsening of condition. **Pregnancy/breast-feeding precautions:** Inform prescriber if you are or intend to become pregnant. Breast-feeding is not recommended.

Geriatric Considerations Modify the initial dose and the subsequent dose titration in the elderly. It may be best to select a different agent when treating depression in the elderly.

Pregnancy Issues Nonteratogenic effects including respiratory distress, cyanosis, apnea, seizures, temperature instability, feeding difficulty, vomiting, hypoglycemia, hypo- or hypertonia, hyper-reflexia, jitteriness, irritability, constant crying, and tremor have been reported in the neonate immediately following delivery after exposure to other SSRIs late in the third trimester. Adverse effects may be due to toxic effects of SSRI or drug discontinuation. In some cases, may present clinically as serotonin syndrome. There are no adequate and well-controlled studies in pregnant women. Use during pregnancy only if the potential benefit to the mother outweighs the possible risk to the fetus. If treatment during pregnancy is required, consider tapering therapy during the third trimester.

Related Information

Antidepressant Medication Guidelines *on page 1414*

Folic Acid (FOE lik AS id)

Synonyms Folacin; Folate; Pteroylglutamic Acid

Pharmacologic Category Vitamin, Water Soluble

Medication Safety Issues

Sound-alike/look-alike issues:

Folic acid may be confused with folinic acid

Pregnancy Risk Factor A

Lactation Enters breast milk/compatible

Use Treatment of megaloblastic and macrocytic anemias due to folate deficiency; dietary supplement to prevent neural tube defects

Mechanism of Action/Effect Folic acid is necessary for formation of a number of coenzymes in many metabolic systems, particularly for purine and pyrimidine synthesis; required for nucleoprotein synthesis and maintenance in erythropoiesis; stimulates WBC and platelet production in folate deficiency anemia (Continued)

Folic Acid *(Continued)*

Contraindications Hypersensitivity to folic acid or any component of the formulation

Warnings/Precautions Not appropriate for monotherapy with pernicious, aplastic, or normocytic anemias when anemia is present with vitamin D deficiency. Doses >0.1 mg/day may obscure pernicious anemia with continuing irreversible nerve damage progression. Resistance to treatment may occur with depressed hematopoiesis, alcoholism, deficiencies of other vitamins. Injection contains benzyl alcohol (1.5%) as preservative (use care in administration to neonates).

Drug Interactions

Decreased Effect: Folic acid may decrease phenytoin concentrations. Folic acid may diminish the therapeutic effect of raltitrexed.

Lab Interactions Falsely low serum concentrations may occur with the *Lactobacillus casei* assay method in patients on anti-infectives (eg, tetracycline).

Adverse Reactions Frequency not defined.
Allergic reaction, bronchospasm, flushing (slight), malaise (general), pruritus, rash

Pharmacodynamics/Kinetics
Onset of Action: Peak effect: Oral: 0.5-1 hour

Available Dosage Forms
Injection, solution, as sodium folate: 5 mg/mL (10 mL) [contains benzyl alcohol]
Tablet: 0.4 mg, 0.8 mg, 1 mg

Dosing
Adults:
Anemia: Oral, I.M., I.V., SubQ: 0.4 mg/day
Pregnant and lactating women: 0.8 mg/day
RDA: Expressed as dietary folate equivalents: 400 mcg/day
Prevention of neural tube defects: Oral:
Females of childbearing potential: 400 mcg/day
Females at high risk or with family history of neural tube defects: 4 mg/day
Elderly: Refer to adults dosing. Vitamin B_{12} deficiency must be ruled out before initiating folate therapy due to frequency of combined nutritional deficiencies: RDA requirements (1999): 400 mcg/day (0.4 mg) minimum.
Pediatrics:
Anemia: Oral, I.M., I.V., SubQ:
Infants: 0.1 mg/day
Children <4 years: Up to 0.3 mg/day
Children >4 years and Adults: Refer to adult dosing.
RDA: Expressed as dietary folate equivalents: Oral:
Children:
1-3 years: 150 mcg/day
4-8 years: 200 mcg/day
9-13 years: 300 mcg/day
≥14 years: Refer to adult dosing.

Administration
I.M.: May also be administered by deep I.M. injection.
I.V. Detail: pH: 8-11

Stability
Compatibility: Stable in D_5W, $D_{20}W$, NS, fat emulsion 10%; **incompatible** with $D_{40}W$, $D_{50}W$
Compatibility in syringe: Incompatible with doxapram
Compatibility when admixed: Incompatible with calcium gluconate

Nursing Actions
Physical Assessment: Assess potential for interactions with other prescriptions, OTC medications, or herbal products patient may be taking. Monitor therapeutic effectiveness and adverse response on a regular basis throughout therapy. Teach patient proper use, possible side effects/appropriate interventions, and adverse symptoms to report.
Patient Education: Do not take any new medication during therapy unless approved by prescriber. Take exactly as prescribed. Toxicity can occur from

elevated doses. Increased intake of foods high in folic acid (eg, dried beans, nuts, bran, vegetables, fruits) may be recommended by prescriber. Excessive use of alcohol increases requirement for folic acid. May turn urine more intensely yellow. Report skin rash. **Pregnancy precaution:** Inform prescriber if you are pregnant.

Dietary Considerations As of January 1998, the FDA has required manufacturers of enriched flour, bread, corn meal, pasta, rice and other grain products to add folic acid to their products. The intent is to help decrease the risk of neural tube defects by increasing folic acid intake. Other foods which contain folic acid include dark green leafy vegetables, citrus fruits and juices, and lentils.

Geriatric Considerations Elderly frequently have combined nutritional deficiencies. Must rule out vitamin B_{12} deficiency before initiating folate therapy. Elderly RDA requirements from 1999 RDA are 400 mcg minimum (0.4 mg). Elderly, due to decreased nutrient intake, may benefit from daily intake of a multiple vitamin with minerals.

Additional Information The RDA for folic acid is presented as dietary folate equivalents (DFE). DFE adjusts for the difference in bioavailability of folic acid from food as compared to dietary supplements.

Follitropins *(foe li TRO pins)*

U.S. Brand Names Bravelle®; Follistim® AQ; Gonal-f®; Gonal-f® RFF

Synonyms Follitropin Alfa; Follitropin Alpha; Follitropin Beta; Recombinant Human Follicle Stimulating Hormone; rFSH-alpha; rFSH-beta; rhFSH-alpha; rhFSH-beta; Urofollitropin

Pharmacologic Category Gonadotropin; Ovulation Stimulator

Pregnancy Risk Factor X

Lactation Excretion in breast milk unknown/not recommended

Use
Urofollitropin (Bravelle®): Ovulation induction in patients who previously received pituitary suppression; Assisted Reproductive Technologies (ART)
Follitropin alfa:
Gonal-f®: Ovulation induction in patients in whom the cause of infertility is functional and not caused by primary ovarian failure; ART; spermatogenesis induction
Gonal-f® RFF: Ovulation induction in patients in whom the cause of infertility is functional and not caused by primary ovarian failure; ART
Follitropin beta (Follistim® AQ): Ovulation induction in patients in whom the cause of infertility is functional and not caused by primary ovarian failure; ART

Mechanism of Action/Effect Urofollitropin is a preparation of highly purified follicle-stimulating hormone (FSH) extracted from the urine of postmenopausal women. Follitropin alfa and follitropin beta are human FSH preparations of recombinant DNA origin. Follitropins stimulate ovarian follicular growth in women who do not have primary ovarian failure. FSH is required for normal follicular growth, maturation, and gonadal steroid production.

Contraindications Hypersensitivity to follitropins or any component of the formulation; high levels of FSH indicating primary gonadal failure (ovarian or testicular); uncontrolled thyroid or adrenal dysfunction; the presence of any cause of infertility other than anovulation; tumor of the ovary, breast, uterus, hypothalamus, testis, or pituitary gland; abnormal vaginal bleeding of undetermined origin; ovarian cysts or enlargement not due to polycystic ovary syndrome; pregnancy

Warnings/Precautions These medications should only be used by physicians who are thoroughly familiar with infertility problems and their management. To minimize risks, use only at the lowest effective dose. Monitor ovarian response with serum estradiol and vaginal ultrasound on a regular basis.

Ovarian enlargement which may be accompanied by abdominal distention or abdominal pain, occurs in ~20% of those treated with urofollitropin and hCG, and generally regresses without treatment in 2-3 weeks. If ovaries are abnormally enlarged on the last day of treatment, withhold hCG to reduce the risk of ovarian hyperstimulation syndrome (OHSS). OHSS is reported in about 6% of patients; it is characterized by severe ovarian enlargement, abdominal pain/distention, nausea, vomiting, diarrhea, dyspnea, and oliguria, and may be accompanied by ascites, pleural effusion, hypovolemia, electrolyte imbalance, hemoperitoneum, and thromboembolic events. If hyperstimulation occurs, stop treatment and hospitalize patient. This syndrome develops rapidly within 24 hours to several days and generally occurs during the 7-10 days immediately following treatment. Hemoconcentration associated with fluid loss into the abdominal cavity has occurred and should be assessed by fluid intake & output, weight, hematocrit, serum & urinary electrolytes, urine specific gravity, BUN and creatinine, and abdominal girth. Determinations should be performed daily or more often if the need arises. Treatment is primarily symptomatic and consists of bed rest, fluid and electrolyte replacement and analgesics. The ascitic, pleural and pericardial fluids should not be removed unless needed to relieve symptoms of cardiopulmonary distress.

Serious pulmonary conditions (atelectasis, acute respiratory distress syndrome and exacerbation of asthma) have been reported. Thromboembolic events, both in association with and separate from ovarian hyperstimulation syndrome, have been reported.

Multiple births may result from the use of these medications, including triplet and quintuplet gestations. Advise patient of the potential risk of multiple births before starting the treatment.

Follistim® AQ: Contains trace amounts of neomycin and streptomycin. Must be administered using the Follistim Pen™; dose adjustment required when switching from powder for injection to solution for injection due to accuracy of pen device.

Adverse Reactions Actual frequency varies by specific product, route of administration and indication.

Adverse reactions reported in females:

Cardiovascular: Hypertension, hypotension, palpitation, tachycardia

Central nervous system: Depression, dizziness, emotional lability, fatigue, febrile reaction, fever, headache, nervousness, pain, somnolence

Dermatologic: Acne, dry skin, erythema, exfoliative dermatitis, hair loss, hives, rash

Endocrine & metabolic: Adnexal torsion, breast pain, breast tenderness, hot flashes, OHSS, ovarian cyst, ovarian pain

Gastrointestinal: Abdomen enlarged, abdominal cramps, abdominal pain, constipation, diarrhea, dehydration, flatulence, nausea, weight gain

Genitourinary: Leukorrhea, ovarian enlargement, pelvic pain, uterine spasms, vaginal hemorrhage, vaginal spotting

Local: Injection site reaction

Neuromuscular & skeletal: Back pain, neck pain

Respiratory: Acute respiratory distress syndrome, anaphylactic reaction, atelectasis, dyspnea, hypersensitivity, sinusitis, tachypnea, upper respiratory tract infection

Miscellaneous: Flu-like syndrome, hemoperitoneum

Adverse reactions reported in males: Acne, breast pain, fatigue, gynecomastia, hemoptysis, injection site reaction, lymphadenopathy, pain, pilonidal cyst infection, varicocele

Overdosage/Toxicology Aside from possible ovarian hyperstimulation and multiple gestations, little is known concerning the consequences of an acute overdose. Treatment is symptomatic.

Pharmacodynamics/Kinetics

Onset of Action: Peak effect:

Spermatogenesis, median: 6.8-12.4 months (range 2.7-15.7 months)

Follicle development: Within cycle

Time to Peak:

Follitropin alfa: SubQ: 16 hours; I.M.: 25 hours

Follitropin beta: SubQ: 13 hours

Urofollitropin: Single dose: SubQ: 20 hours, I.M.: 17 hours; Multiple doses: I.M., SubQ: 10 hours

Half-Life Elimination:

Follitropin alfa:

I.M.:50 hours, 24 hours following multiple doses

SubQ: 24 hours

Follitropin beta: SubQ: 33.4 hours

Urofollitropin:

I.M.: 37 hours, 15 hours following multiple doses

SubQ: 32 hours, 21 hours following multiple doses

Excretion: Clearance: Follitropin alfa: I.V.: 0.6 L/hour

Available Dosage Forms

Injection, powder for reconstitution [packaged with diluent]:

Follitropin alfa [rDNA origin, multidose vial] (Gonal-f®): 450 int. units [contains sucrose 30 mg; packaged with calibrated syringes]

Follitropin alfa [rDNA origin, single-dose vial] (Gonal-f® RFF): 75 int. units [packaged with diluent in prefilled syringe]

Urofollitropin [urine derived] (Bravelle®): 75 int. units

Injection, solution:

Follitropin alfa [rDNA origin, prefilled multidose pen] (Gonal-f® RFF Pen): 300 int. units/0.5 mL (0.5 mL) [contains sucrose 60 mg/mL]; 450 int. units/0.7 mL (0.7 mL) [contains sucrose 60 mg/mL]; 900 int. units/1.5 mL (1.5 mL) [contains sucrose 60 mg/mL]

Follitropin beta [rDNA origin, prefilled cartridge] (Follistim® AQ):

175 int. units/0.21mL (0.21 mL) [equivalent to 833 int. units/mL; delivers 150 units; contains benzyl alcohol, sucrose 50 mg/mL; may contain trace amounts of neomycin and streptomycin]

350 int. units/0.42 mL (0.42 mL) [equivalent to 833 int. units/mL; delivers 300 units; contains benzyl alcohol, sucrose 50 mg/mL; may contain trace amounts of neomycin and streptomycin]

650 int. units/0.78 mL (0.78 mL) [equivalent to 833 int. units/mL; delivers 600 units; contains benzyl alcohol, sucrose 50 mg/mL; may contain trace amounts of neomycin and streptomycin]

977 int. units/1.17 mL (1.17 mL) [equivalent to 833 int. units/mL; delivers 900 units; contains benzyl alcohol, sucrose 50 mg/mL; may contain trace amounts of neomycin and streptomycin]

Follitropin beta [rDNA origin, single-use vial] (Follistim® AQ):

75 int. units/0.5 mL [contains sucrose 50 mg/mL; may contain trace amounts of neomycin and streptomycin]

150 int. units/0.5 mL [contains sucrose 50 mg/mL; may contain trace amounts of neomycin and streptomycin]

Dosing

Adults: Note: Use the lowest dose consistent with the expectation of good results. Over the course of treatment, doses may vary depending on individual patient response. When used for ovulation induction, if response to follitropin is appropriate, hCG is given 1 day following the last dose. Withhold hCG if serum estradiol is >2000 pg/mL, if the ovaries are abnormally enlarged, or if abdominal pain occurs.

(Continued)

Follitropins *(Continued)*

Urofollitropin: Bravelle®: Female:

Ovulation induction: I.M., SubQ: Initial: 150 int. units daily for the first 5 days of treatment. Dose adjustments of ≤75-150 int. units can be made every ≥2 days; maximum daily dose: 450 int. units; treatment >12 days is not recommended

ART: SubQ: 225 int. units for the first 5 days; dose may be adjusted based on patient response, but adjustments should not be made more frequently than once every 2 days; maximum adjustment: 75-150 int. units; maximum daily dose: 450 int. units; maximum duration of treatment: 12 days

Follitropin alfa: Gonal-f®, Gonal-f® RFF: Female:

Ovulation induction: SubQ: Initial: 75 int. units/day; consider dose adjustment after 5-7 days; additional dose adjustments of up to 37.5 int. units may be considered after 14 days; further dose increases of the same magnitude can be made, if necessary, every 7 days (maximum dose: 300 int. units)

ART: SubQ: Initiate therapy with follitropin alfa in the early follicular phase (cycle day 2 or day 3) at a dose of 150 int. units/day, until sufficient follicular development is attained. In most cases, therapy should not exceed 10 days. In patients whose endogenous gonadotropin levels are suppressed, initiate follitropin alfa at a dose of 225 int. units/day. Continue treatment until adequate follicular development is indicated as determined by ultrasound in combination with measurement of serum estradiol levels. Consider adjustments to dose after 5 days based on the patient's response; adjust subsequent dosage every 3-5 days by ≤75-150 int. units additionally at each adjustment. Doses >450 int. units/day are not recommended. Once adequate follicular development is evident, administer hCG (5000-10,000 units) to induce final follicular maturation in preparation for oocyte.

Follitropin alfa: Gonal-f®: Male:

Spermatogenesis induction: SubQ: Therapy should begin with hCG pretreatment until serum testosterone is in normal range, then 150 int. units 3 times/week with hCG 3 times/week; continue with lowest dose needed to induce spermatogenesis (maximum dose: 300 int. units 3 times/week); may be given for up to 18 months

Follitropin beta: Follistim® AQ: Female:

Ovulation induction: SubQ: Stepwise approach: Initiate therapy with 75 int. units/day for up to 7 days. A lower dose should be given if previous doses were administered using the powder for injection (see dosing conversion). Increase by 25 or 50 int. units at weekly intervals until follicular growth or serum estradiol levels indicate an adequate response. The maximum (individualized) daily dose that has been safely used for ovulation induction in patients during clinical trials is 175 int. units.

ART: SubQ: A starting dose of 150-225 int. units of follitropin beta is recommended for at least the first 5 days of treatment. The dose may be adjusted for the individual patient based upon their ovarian response. A lower dose should be given if previous doses were administered using the powder for injection (see dosing conversion). The maximum daily dose used in clinical studies is 450 int. units. When a sufficient number of follicles of adequate size are present, the final maturation of the follicles is induced by administering hCG at a dose of 5000-10,000 int. units. Oocyte retrieval is performed 34-36 hours later. Withhold hCG in cases where the ovaries are abnormally enlarged on the last day of follitropin beta therapy.

Follistim® AQ Dosing Conversion Guidelines: See table.

Follistim® AQ Dosing Conversion

Dose Administered Using Powder for Solution/ Conventional Syringe	Follistim® AQ Dose Administered Using Follistim Pen™
75 int. units	50 int. units
150 int. units	125 int. units
225 int. units	175 int. units
300 int. units	250 int. units
375 int. units	300 int. units
450 int. units	375 int. units

Elderly: Refer to adult dosing. Clinical studies did not include patients >65 years of age.

Administration

I.M.: Urofollitropin: Bravelle®: Administer I.M. or SubQ; gently massage site after administration. For I.M. injection, administer in upper quadrant of buttock near hip.

Other:

Urofollitropin: Bravelle®: Administer SubQ or I.M.; gently massage site after administration. For SubQ injection, administer on lower abdomen; thigh is not recommended unless abdomen cannot be used.

Follitropin alpha: Gonal-f®, Gonal-f® RFF: Administer SubQ. Contents of multidose vials should be administered using the calibrated syringes provided by the manufacturer. Do not shake solution; allow any bubbles to settle prior to administration.

Follitropin beta: Follistim® AQ: Administer SubQ only. Prefilled cartridges must be administered using the Follistim Pen™ which can be set to deliver the appropriate dose.

Stability

Reconstitution:

Urofollitropin: Bravelle®: Dissolve contents of vial in 1 mL **sterile saline**; gently swirl (do not shake); do not use if solution is not clear or contains particles. If more than 1 vial is required for a single dose, up to 6 vials can be reconstituted with 1 mL sterile saline and administered as a single injection. This is done by first reconstituting 1 vial with sterile saline as previously described, withdrawing the entire contents of the reconstituted vial and (using this as the diluent for the second vial) injecting into the second vial, etc. Use immediately after reconstitution.

Follitropin alfa:

Gonal-f®: Dissolve the contents of vial by slowly injecting bacteriostatic water for injection; do not shake. If bubbles appear, allow to settle prior to use. Final concentration: 600 int. units/mL.

Gonal-f® RFF vial: Dissolve contents of vial using diluent provided in prefilled syringe. Slowly inject diluent into vial and gently rotate vial until powder is dissolved; do not shake vial; if bubbles appear, allow to settle prior to use.

Storage:

Urofollitropin: Bravelle®: Lyophilized powder may be stored in the refrigerator or at room temperature of 3°C to 25°C (37°F to 77°F). Protect from light; use immediately after reconstitution.

Follitropin alfa:

Gonal-f®: Store powder refrigerated or at room temperature of 2°C to 25°C (36°F to 77°F). Protect from light. Following reconstitution, multidose vials may be stored under refrigeration or at room temperature for up to 28 days; protect from light.

Gonal-f® RFF:

Pen: Prior to dispensing, store under refrigeration at 2°C to 8°C (36°F to 46°F). Upon dispensing, patient may store under refrigeration until product expiration date or at room temperature of 20°C to 25°C (68°F to 77°F) for up to 1 month. Protect from light; do not freeze. After first use, use within 28 days.

Vial: Store at room temperature or under refrigeration; use immediately after reconstitution.

Follitropin beta: Follistim® AQ: Prior to dispensing, store refrigerated at 2°C to 8°C (36°F to 46°F). After dispensed, may be stored under refrigeration or at room temperature for up to 3 months. Once cartridge is pierced, must be stored in refrigerator and used within 28 days. Protect from light. Do not freeze.

Laboratory Monitoring Monitor sufficient follicular maturation. This may be directly estimated by sonographic visualization of the ovaries and endometrial lining or measuring serum estradiol levels. The combination of both ultrasonography and measurement of estradiol levels is useful for monitoring for the growth and development of follicles and timing hCG administration.

Spermatogenesis: Monitor serum testosterone levels, sperm count

Nursing Actions

Physical Assessment: This medication should only be prescribed by a fertility specialist. Laboratory tests and therapeutic response will need to be monitored by prescriber on a regular basis. Assess knowledge/teach patient appropriate use (injection technique and syringe disposal), interventions to reduce side effects, and adverse symptoms to report. **Pregnancy risk factor X:** Pregnancy must be excluded before starting medication.

Patient Education: This medication can only be administered by injection. If you are using this medication at home, follow exact instruction for administering injections and disposal of syringes. Administer exact amount as instructed; do not alter dosage or miss a dose. If dose is missed, notify prescriber. Frequent laboratory tests will be required while you are on this therapy; do not miss appointments for laboratory tests or ultrasound. You may experience headache, dizziness, or fever (use caution when driving or engaging in tasks requiring alertness until response to drug is known); or nausea or vomiting (small frequent meals, frequent oral care, sucking lozenges, or chewing gum may help). Report immediately abdominal pain/distension, bloating, persistent nausea, vomiting, diarrhea; dyspnea, respiratory difficulty, exacerbation of asthma; swelling, pain, or redness of extremities; itching or burning on urination; menstrual irregularity; acute backache; rash, pain, or inflammation at injection site; or other adverse response. **Pregnancy/breast-feeding precautions:** Inform your prescriber if you are pregnant. Breast-feeding is not recommended.

Pregnancy Issues Ectopic pregnancy, congenital abnormalities, and multiple births have been reported. The incidence of congenital abnormality may be slightly higher after ART than with spontaneous conception; higher incidence may be related to parenteral characteristics (maternal age, sperm characteristics)

Fondaparinux (fon da PARE i nuks)

U.S. Brand Names Arixtra®
Synonyms Fondaparinux Sodium
Pharmacologic Category Factor Xa Inhibitor
Pregnancy Risk Factor B
Lactation Excretion in breast milk unknown/use caution
Use Prophylaxis of deep vein thrombosis (DVT) in patients undergoing surgery for hip replacement, knee replacement, hip fracture (including extended prophylaxis following hip fracture surgery), or abdominal surgery (in patients at risk for thromboembolic complications); treatment of acute pulmonary embolism (PE); treatment of acute DVT without PE
Mechanism of Action/Effect Fondaparinux prevents factor Xa from binding with antithrombin III and inhibits thrombin formation and thrombus development.
Contraindications Hypersensitivity to fondaparinux or any component of the formulation; severe renal impairment (Cl$_{cr}$ <30 mL/minute); body weight <50 kg (prophylaxis); active major bleeding; bacterial endocarditis; thrombocytopenia associated with a positive *in vitro* test for antiplatelet antibody in the presence of fondaparinux
Warnings/Precautions Patients with recent or anticipated neuraxial anesthesia (epidural or spinal anesthesia) are at risk of spinal or epidural hematoma and subsequent paralysis. Not to be used interchangeably (unit-for-unit) with heparin, low molecular weight heparins (LMWHs), or heparinoids. Use caution in patients with moderate renal dysfunction (Cl$_{cr}$ 30-50 mL/minute). Discontinue if severe dysfunction or labile function develops.

Use caution in congenital or acquired bleeding disorders; active ulcerative or angiodysplastic gastrointestinal disease; hemorrhagic stroke; shortly after brain, spinal, or ophthalmologic surgery; or in patients taking platelet inhibitors. Risk of major bleeding may be increased if initial dose is administered earlier then recommended (initiation recommended at 6-8 hours following surgery). Discontinue agents that may enhance the risk of hemorrhage if possible. If thrombocytopenia occurs discontinue fondaparinux. Use caution in the elderly, patients with a history of heparin-induced thrombocytopenia, patients with a bleeding diathesis, uncontrolled hypertension, recent gastrointestinal ulceration, diabetic retinopathy, and hemorrhage. Use caution in patients <50 kg who are being treated for DVT/PE; fondaparinux clearance may be decreased. Safety and efficacy in pediatric patients have not been established.

Drug Interactions
Increased Effect/Toxicity: Anticoagulants, antiplatelet agents, drotrecogin alfa, NSAIDs, salicylates, and thrombolytic agents may enhance the anticoagulant effect and/or increase the risk of bleeding.
Nutritional/Ethanol Interactions Herb/Nutraceutical: Avoid alfalfa, anise, bilberry, bladderwrack, bromelain, cat's claw, celery, coleus, cordyceps, dong quai, evening primrose oil, fenugreek, feverfew, garlic, ginger, ginkgo biloba, ginseng (American/Panax/Siberian), grape seed, green tea, guggul, horse chestnut seed, horseradish, licorice, prickly ash, red clover, reishi, sweet clover, turmeric, white willow (all possess anticoagulant or antiplatelet activity and as such, may enhance the anticoagulant effects of fondaparinux).
Lab Interactions International standards of heparin or LMWH are not the appropriate calibrators for antifactor Xa activity of fondaparinux.
Adverse Reactions As with all anticoagulants, bleeding is the major adverse effect. Hemorrhage may occur at any site. Risk appears increased by a number of factors including renal dysfunction, age (>75 years), and weight (<50 kg).
(Continued)

Fondaparinux (Continued)

>10%:
Central nervous system: Fever (4% to 14%)
Gastrointestinal: Nausea (11%)
Hematologic: Anemia (20%)
1% to 10%:
Cardiovascular: Edema (9%), hypotension (4%), confusion (3%)
Central nervous system: Insomnia (5%), dizziness (4%), headache (2% to 5%), pain (2%)
Dermatologic: Rash (8%), purpura (4%), bullous eruption (3%)
Endocrine & metabolic: Hypokalemia (1% to 4%)
Gastrointestinal: Constipation (5% to 9%), nausea (3%), vomiting (6%), diarrhea (3%), dyspepsia (2%)
Genitourinary: Urinary tract infection (4%), urinary retention (3%)
Hematologic: Moderate thrombocytopenia (50,000-100,000/mm^3: 3%), major bleeding (1% to 3%), minor bleeding (2% to 4%), hematoma (3%); risk of major bleeding increased as high as 5% in patients receiving initial dose <6 hours following surgery
Hepatic: SGOT increased (2%), SGPT increased (3%)
Local: Injection site reaction (bleeding, rash, pruritus)
Miscellaneous: Wound drainage increased (5%)
Overdosage/Toxicology Treatment is symptom-directed and supportive. Hemodialysis may increase clearance by 20%.
Pharmacodynamics/Kinetics
Time to Peak: 2-3 hours
Protein Binding: ≥94% to antithrombin III
Half-Life Elimination: 17-21 hours; prolonged with worsening renal impairment
Excretion:
Urine (as unchanged drug); decreased clearance in patients <50 kg
Available Dosage Forms Injection, solution, as sodium [preservative free]: 2.5 mg/0.5 mL (0.5 mL); 5 mg/0.4 mL (0.4 mL); 7.5 mg/0.6 mL (0.6 mL); 10 mg/0.8 mL (0.8 mL) [prefilled syringe]
Dosing
Adults & Elderly:
DVT prophylaxis: SubQ: Adults ≥50 kg: 2.5 mg once daily. **Note:** Initiate dose after hemostasis has been established, 6-8 hours postoperatively.
Usual duration: 5-9 days (up to 10 days following abdominal surgery or up to 11 days following hip replacement or knee replacement).
Extended prophylaxis is recommended following hip fracture surgery (has been tolerated for up to 32 days).
Acute DVT/PE treatment: SubQ: **Note:** Concomitant treatment with warfarin sodium should be initiated as soon as possible, usually within 72 hours:
<50 kg: 5 mg once daily
50-100 kg: 7.5 mg once daily
>100 kg: 10 mg once daily
Usual duration: 5-9 days (has been administered up to 26 days)
Renal Impairment:
Cl$_{cr}$ 30-50 mL/minute: Use caution
Cl$_{cr}$ <30 mL/minute: Contraindicated
Administration
I.M.: Do not administer I.M.
Other: For SubQ administration only. Do not mix with other injections or infusions. Do not expel air bubble from syringe before injection. Administer according to recommended regimen; early initiation (before 6 hours after surgery) has been associated with increased bleeding.
Stability
Compatibility: Do not mix with other injections or infusions.

Storage: Store at 15°C to 30°C (59°F to 86°F).
Laboratory Monitoring CBC, platelet count, serum creatinine; stool occult blood tests
Nursing Actions
Physical Assessment: Assess potential for interactions with other prescription, OTC medications, or herbal products patient may be taking (especially anything that will affect coagulation or platelet function). Assess closely for bleeding; bleeding precautions should be observed. Monitor laboratory tests, therapeutic effectiveness, and adverse response regularly during therapy. Teach patient possible side effects/appropriate interventions (eg, bleeding precautions) and adverse symptoms to report.
Patient Education: Do not take any new medication during therapy without consulting prescriber. This drug can only be administered by injection. Report pain, burning, redness, or swelling at injection site. You may have a tendency to bleed easily while taking this drug (brush teeth with soft brush, floss with waxed floss, use electric razor, avoid scissors or sharp knives, and avoid potentially harmful activities). May cause nausea or vomiting (small frequent meals, frequent mouth care, chewing gum, or sucking lozenges may help); or dizziness, headache, insomnia (use caution when driving or engaging in tasks that require alertness until response to drug is known). Report unusual bleeding or bruising (bleeding gums, nosebleed, blood in urine, dark stool); pain in joints or back; CNS changes (fever, severe headache, confusion); unusual fever; persistent nausea or GI upset; changes in urinary pattern; or other persistent adverse response. **Breast-feeding precaution:** Consult prescriber if breast-feeding.
Geriatric Considerations Patients studied for DVT prophylaxis following elective knee or hip fracture surgery averaged 67.5 and 77 years of age, respectively. Use with caution in patients with estimated or actual creatinine clearance between 30-50 mL/minute. Contraindicated in patients whose Cl$_{cr}$ <30 mL/minute.
Pregnancy Issues Reproductive animal studies have not shown fetal harm. Based on case reports, small amounts of fondaparinux have been detected in the umbilical cord following multiple doses during pregnancy. There are no adequate and well-controlled studies in pregnant women; use only if clearly needed.

Formoterol (for MOH te rol)

U.S. Brand Names Foradil® Aerolizer™
Synonyms Formoterol Fumarate
Pharmacologic Category Beta$_2$-Adrenergic Agonist
Medication Safety Issues
Sound-alike/look-alike issues:
Foradil® may be confused with Toradol®
Foradil® capsules for inhalation are for administration via Aerolizer™ inhaler and are not for oral use.
Pregnancy Risk Factor C
Lactation Excretion in breast milk unknown/use caution
Use Maintenance treatment of asthma and prevention of bronchospasm in patients ≥5 years of age with reversible obstructive airway disease, including patients with symptoms of nocturnal asthma, who require regular treatment with inhaled, short-acting beta$_2$ agonists; maintenance treatment of bronchoconstriction in patients with COPD; prevention of exercise-induced bronchospasm in patients ≥5 years of age

Note: Oxeze® is also approved in Canada for acute relief of symptoms ("on demand" treatment) in patients ≥6 years of age.
Mechanism of Action/Effect Relaxes bronchial smooth muscle
Contraindications Hypersensitivity to adrenergic amines, formoterol, or any component of the formulation

Note: The approved U.S. labeling lists the need for acute bronchodilation as a contraindication; however, a formulation (Oxeze®) is approved for acute treatment in other countries (ie, Canada).

Warnings/Precautions Optimize anti-inflammatory treatment before initiating maintenance treatment with formoterol. Do not use as a component of chronic therapy without an anti-inflammatory agent. Patient must be instructed to seek medical attention in cases where acute symptoms are not relieved by rapid-onset beta-agonist or when a previous level of response is diminished. Treatment must not be delayed. Rarely, paradoxical bronchospasm may occur with use of inhaled bronchodilating agents; this should be distinguished from inadequate response.

Acute episodes should be treated with rapid-onset beta$_2$ agonist. The approved U.S. labeling states that formoterol is not meant to relieve acute asthmatic symptoms. Although, a formulation of formoterol (Oxeze®) is approved for acute treatment outside the U.S. (ie, Canada).

Do not exceed recommended dose; serious adverse events (including fatalities) have been associated with excessive use of inhaled sympathomimetics. Beta$_2$ agonists may increase risk of arrhythmias, decrease serum potassium, prolong QT$_c$ interval, or increase serum glucose. These effects may be exacerbated in hypoxemia. Use caution in patients with cardiovascular disease (arrhythmia or hypertension or CHF), convulsive disorders, diabetes, glaucoma, hyperthyroidism, or hypokalemia. Beta agonists may cause elevation in blood pressure, heart rate, and result in CNS stimulation/excitation. Safety and efficacy have not been established in children <5 years of age.

Drug Interactions
Cytochrome P450 Effect: Substrate (minor) of CYP2A6, 2C8/9, 2C19, 2D6

Increased Effect/Toxicity: Adrenergic agonists, antidepressants (tricyclic), beta-blockers, corticosteroids, diuretics, drugs that prolong QT$_c$ interval, MAO inhibitors, theophylline derivatives

Adverse Reactions Children are more likely to have infection, inflammation, abdominal pain, nausea, and dyspepsia.

>10%:
Endocrine & metabolic: Serum glucose increased, serum potassium decreased
Miscellaneous: Viral infection (17%)
1% to 10%:
Cardiovascular: Chest pain (2%)
Central nervous system: Tremor (2%), dizziness (2%), insomnia (2%), dysphonia (1%)
Dermatologic: Rash (1%)
Respiratory: Bronchitis (5%), infection (3%), dyspnea (2%), tonsillitis (1%)

Overdosage/Toxicology Symptoms of overdose include tachycardia, tremor, hypertension, angina, and seizures. Hypokalemia also may occur. Cardiac arrest and death may be associated with abuse of beta-agonist bronchodilators. Treatment includes immediate discontinuation and symptomatic and supportive therapies. Cautious use of beta-adrenergic blocking agents may be considered in severe cases.

Pharmacodynamics/Kinetics
Onset of Action: Within 3 minutes; 80% of peak effect within 15 minutes

Duration of Action: Improvement in FEV$_1$ observed for 12 hours in most patients

Time to Peak: Maximum improvement in FEV$_1$ in 1-3 hours

Protein Binding: 61% to 64% *in vitro* at higher concentrations than achieved with usual dosing

Half-Life Elimination: ~10-14 hours
Metabolism: Hepatic via direct glucuronidation and O-demethylation; CYP2D6, CYP2C19, CYP2C8/9, CYP2A6 involved in O-demethylation
Excretion:
Children 5-12 years: Urine (6% as unchanged drug, 7% to 9% as direct glucuronide metabolites)
Adults: Urine (15% to 18% as direct glucuronide metabolites, 10% as unchanged drug)
Available Dosage Forms [CAN] = Canadian brand name
Powder for oral inhalation, as fumarate:
Foradil® Aerolizer™ [capsule]: 12 mcg (12s, 60s) [contains lactose 25 mg]
Oxeze® Turbuhaler® [CAN]: 6 mcg/inhalation [delivers 60 metered doses; contains lactose 600 mcg/dose]; 12 mcg/inhalation [delivers 60 metered doses; contains lactose 600 mcg/dose] [not available in the U.S.]

Dosing
Adults & Elderly:
Asthma (maintenance): Inhalation: 12 mcg capsule every 12 hours
Oxeze® (CAN): **Note:** Not labeled for use in the U.S.: Inhalation: 6 mcg or 12 mcg every 12 hours. Maximum dose: Children: 24 mcg/day; Adults: 48 mcg/day
Exercise-induced bronchospasm: Inhalation: 12 mcg capsule at least 15 minutes before exercise on an "as needed" basis; additional doses should not be used for another 12 hours. **Note:** If already using for asthma maintenance then should not use additional doses for exercise-induced bronchospasm.
Oxeze® (CAN): **Note:** Not labeled for use in the U.S.: Children ≥6 years and Adults: Inhalation: 6 mcg or 12 mcg at least 15 minutes before exercise.
COPD (maintenance): Inhalation: 12 mcg capsule every 12 hours

Acute ("on demand") relief of bronchoconstriction: *Indication for Oxeze® approved in Canada:* 6 mcg or 12 mcg as a single dose (maximum dose: 72 mcg in any 24-hour period). The prolonged use of high dosages (48 mcg/day for ≥3 consecutive days) may be a sign of suboptimal control, and should prompt the re-evaluation of therapy.
Pediatrics:
Asthma maintenance: Inhalation: Children ≥5 years: Refer to adult dosing.
Exercise-induced bronchospasm: Inhalation: Children ≥5 years: Refer to adult dosing.
Acute "on demand" treatment of bronchospasm (Oxeze® [CAN]): Inhalation: Refer to adult dosing.
Renal Impairment: Not studied
Administration
Inhalation: Remove capsule from foil blister **immediately** before use. Place capsule in the capsule-chamber in the base of the Aerolizer™ Inhaler. Must only use the Aerolizer™ Inhaler. Press both buttons **once only** and then release. Keep inhaler in a level, horizontal position. Exhale fully. Do not exhale into inhaler. Tilt head slightly back and inhale (rapidly, steadily and deeply). Hold breath as long as possible. If any powder remains in capsule, exhale and inhale again. Repeat until capsule is empty. Throw away empty capsule; do not leave in inhaler. Do not use a spacer with the Aerolizer™ Inhaler. Always keep capsules and inhaler dry.
Stability
Storage: Prior to dispensing, store in refrigerator at 2°C to 8°C (36°F to 46°F); after dispensing, store at room temperature at 20°C to 25°C (68°F to 77°F). Protect from heat and moisture. Capsules should always be stored in the blister and only removed immediately before use. Always check expiration (Continued)

Formoterol *(Continued)*

date. Use within 4 months of purchase date or product expiration date, whichever comes first.

Laboratory Monitoring FEV$_1$, peak flow, and/or other pulmonary function tests; serum potassium, serum glucose (in selected patients)

Nursing Actions

Physical Assessment: Assess other medications patient may be taking for effectiveness and interactions. Monitor therapeutic response and adverse reactions at beginning of therapy and periodically throughout period of therapy. Assess knowledge/ teach appropriate use of medication, interventions to reduce side effects, and adverse symptoms to report.

Patient Education: Do not swallow capsules; this medication can only be used in the Aerolizer™ Inhaler. Use exactly as directed and do not use more often than recommended. Store capsules in blister and do not remove from blister until ready for treatment. Maintain adequate hydration (2-3 L/day of fluids) unless instructed to restrict fluid intake. It is recommended that you wear identification (Med-Alert bracelet) if you have an asthmatic condition. You may experience nervousness, dizziness, or insomnia (use caution when driving or engaging in hazardous activities until response to medication is known); dry mouth, nausea, or GI discomfort (small frequent meals, good mouth care, sucking lozenges, or chewing gum may help); or difficulty voiding (always void before treatment). Report any unresolved GI upset, nervousness or dizziness, muscle cramping, chest pain or palpitations, skin rash, signs of infection, unusual cough, or worsening of condition. **Pregnancy/breast-feeding precautions:** Inform prescriber if you are or intend to become pregnant. Consult prescriber if breast-feeding.

Administration: Follow directions for use and storage of inhaler exactly. Wash hands prior to treatment and sit in comfortable position for treatment. Remove capsule from foil blister immediately before treatment and place capsule in the capsule-chamber in the base of the Aerolizer™ Inhaler. Press both buttons once only and then release. Hold inhaler in a level, horizontal position, exhale fully (do not exhale into inhaler). Tilt head slightly back and inhale from inhaler rapidly, steadily, and deeply. Hold breath as long as possible. If any powder remains in capsule, exhale and inhale again. Repeat until capsule is empty. Throw away empty capsule. Do not use a spacer with Aerolizer™. Do not wash inhaler; store in dry place.

Pregnancy Issues There are no adequate and well-controlled studies in pregnant women. Use only if benefit outweighs risk to the fetus. Beta agonists interfere with uterine contractility so use during labor only if benefit outweighs risk to the fetus.

Fosamprenavir *(FOS am pren a veer)*

U.S. Brand Names Lexiva™

Synonyms Fosamprenavir Calcium; GW433908G

Pharmacologic Category Antiretroviral Agent, Protease Inhibitor

Medication Safety Issues

Sound-alike/look-alike issues:

Lexiva™ may be confused with Levitra®

Pregnancy Risk Factor C

Lactation Excretion in breast milk unknown/contraindicated

Use Treatment of HIV infections in combination with at least two other antiretroviral agents

Mechanism of Action/Effect Fosamprenavir is rapidly and almost completely converted to amprenavir *in vivo*.

Amprenavir binds to the protease activity site and inhibits the activity of the enzyme. HIV protease is required for the cleavage of viral polyprotein precursors into individual functional proteins found in infectious HIV. Inhibition prevents cleavage of these polyproteins, resulting in the formation of immature, noninfectious viral particles.

Contraindications Hypersensitivity to amprenavir or any component of the formulation; concurrent therapy with cisapride, ergot derivatives, midazolam, pimozide, and triazolam; severe previous allergic reaction to sulfonamides

Warnings/Precautions Because of hepatic metabolism and effect on cytochrome P450 enzymes, amprenavir should be used with caution in combination with other agents metabolized by this system (see Contraindications and Drug Interactions). Avoid concurrent administration of lovastatin or simvastatin (may increase the risk of rhabdomyolysis). Avoid use of hormonal contraceptives, rifampin, and/or St John's wort (may lead to loss of virologic response and/or resistance). Use with caution in patients with diabetes mellitus, sulfonamide allergy, hepatic impairment, or hemophilia. Redistribution of fat may occur (eg, buffalo hump, peripheral wasting, cushingoid appearance). Dosage adjustment is required for combination therapies (ritonavir and/or efavirenz); in addition, the risk of hyperlipidemia may be increased during concurrent therapy. Discontinue therapy in severe or dermatologic reactions or when a moderate rash is accompanied by systemic symptoms.

Drug Interactions

Cytochrome P450 Effect: As amprenavir: **Substrate** of CYP2C8/9 (minor), 3A4 (major); **Inhibits** CYP2C19 (weak), 3A4 (strong)

Decreased Effect: CYP3A4 inducers may decrease the levels/effects of amprenavir; example inducers include aminoglutethimide, carbamazepine, nafcillin, nevirapine, phenobarbital, phenytoin, and rifamycins. The administration of didanosine (buffered formulation) should be separated from amprenavir by 1 hour to limit interaction between formulations. Serum concentrations of estrogen (oral contraceptives) may be decreased, use alternative (nonhormonal) forms of contraception. Dexamethasone may decrease the therapeutic effect of amprenavir. Serum concentrations of delavirdine may be decreased; may lead to loss of virologic response and possible resistance to delavirdine; concomitant use is not recommended. Efavirenz and nevirapine may decrease serum concentrations of amprenavir (dosing for combinations not established). Avoid St John's wort (may lead to subtherapeutic concentrations of amprenavir). Effect of amprenavir may be diminished when administered with methadone (consider alternative antiretroviral); in addition, effect of methadone may be reduced (dosage increase may be required). Ranitidine may impair absorption of fosamprenavir, leading to reduced serum levels of amprenavir; separate doses.

Increased Effect/Toxicity: Concurrent use of cisapride, midazolam, pimozide, quinidine, or triazolam is contraindicated. Concurrent use of ergot alkaloids (dihydroergotamine, ergotamine, ergonovine, methylergonovine) with amprenavir is also contraindicated (may cause vasospasm and peripheral ischemia). Concurrent use of oral solution with disulfiram or metronidazole is contraindicated, due to the risk of propylene glycol toxicity.

Serum concentrations of amiodarone, bepridil, lidocaine, quinidine and other antiarrhythmics may be increased, potentially leading to toxicity; when amprenavir is coadministered with ritonavir, flecainide and propafenone are contraindicated. HMG-CoA reductase inhibitors serum concentrations may be increased by amprenavir, increasing the risk of myopathy/rhabdomyolysis; lovastatin and simvastatin are not recommended; fluvastatin and pravastatin may be safer alternatives.

Amprenavir may increase the levels/effects of selected benzodiazepines (midazolam and triazolam are contraindicated), calcium channel blockers, cyclosporine, mirtazapine, nateglinide, nefazodone, quinidine, sildenafil (and other PDE-5 inhibitors), tacrolimus, venlafaxine, and other CYP3A4 substrates. When used with strong CYP3A4 inhibitors, dosage adjustment/limits are recommended for sildenafil and other PDE-5 inhibitors; refer to individual monographs.

Concurrent therapy with ritonavir may result in increased serum concentrations: dosage adjustment is recommended. Clarithromycin, indinavir, nelfinavir may increase serum concentrations of amprenavir.

Nutritional/Ethanol Interactions Herb/Nutraceutical: Amprenavir serum concentration may be decreased by St John's wort; avoid concurrent use.

Adverse Reactions
>10%:
Central nervous system: Headache (19% to 21%), fatigue (10% to 18%)
Dermatologic: Rash (17% to 35%; moderate to severe reactions 3% to 8%)
Gastrointestinal: Nausea (37% to 39%), diarrhea (34% to 52%), vomiting (16% to 20%), abdominal pain (5% to 11%)
1% to 10%:
Central nervous system: Depression (8%), fatigue, headache, paresthesia
Dermatologic: Pruritus (3% to 8%)
Endocrine & metabolic: Hypertriglyceridemia (0% to 11%), serum lipase increased (6% to 8%), hyperglycemia (<1% to 2%)
Hematologic: Neutropenia (3%)
Hepatic: Transaminases increased (4% to 8%)
Miscellaneous: Perioral tingling/numbness (2% to 10%)

Overdosage/Toxicology Treatment is symptomatic and supportive.

Pharmacodynamics/Kinetics
Time to Peak: 1.5-4 hours
Protein Binding: 90%
Half-Life Elimination: 7.7 hours
Metabolism: Fosamprenavir is rapidly and almost completely converted to amprenavir by cellular phosphatases; amprenavir is hepatically metabolized via CYP isoenzymes (primarily CYP3A4)
Excretion: Feces (75%); urine (14% as metabolites; <1% as unchanged drug)

Available Dosage Forms Tablet, as calcium: 700 mg
Dosage formulation available in Canada [not available in U.S.]:
Suspension, oral, as calcium (Telzir®): 50 mg/mL (225 mL)

Dosing
Adults:
HIV infection: Oral:
Antiretroviral therapy-naive patients:
Unboosted regimen: 1400 mg twice daily (without ritonavir)
Ritonavir-boosted regimens:
Once-daily regimen: Fosamprenavir 1400 mg plus ritonavir 200 mg once daily
Twice-daily regimen: Fosamprenavir 700 mg plus ritonavir 100 mg twice daily. **Note:** Also used in protease inhibitor-experienced patients
Protease inhibitor-experienced patients: Fosamprenavir 700 mg plus ritonavir 100 mg twice daily. **Note:** Once-daily administration is not recommended in protease inhibitor-experienced patients.

Combination therapy with efavirenz (ritonavir-boosted regimen):
Once-daily regimen: Fosamprenavir 1400 mg daily plus ritonavir 300 mg once daily
Twice-daily regimen: No dosage adjustment recommended for twice-daily regimen
Combination therapy with nevirapine (ritonavir-boosted regimen): Fosampranavir 700 mg plus ritonavir 100 mg twice daily
Renal Impairment: No dosage adjustment required.
Hepatic Impairment:
Note: No recommendations are available for dosage adjustment in patients receiving ritonavir and fosamprenavir.
Mild-moderate impairment (Child-Pugh score 5-8): Reduce dosage of fosamprenavir to 700 mg twice daily (without concurrent ritonavir)
Severe impairment: Use is not recommended.

Stability
Storage: Store at 25°C (77°F); excursions permitted to 15°C to 30°C (59°F to 86°F).

Laboratory Monitoring Viral load

Nursing Actions
Physical Assessment: Assess potential for interactions with other pharmacological agents and herbal products patient may be taking. A list of medications that should not be used is available in each bottle and patients should be provided with this information. Monitor laboratory tests, patient response, and adverse reactions (eg, gastrointestinal disturbance [nausea, vomiting, diarrhea] that can lead to dehydration and weight loss; hyperlipidemia and redistribution of body fat; rash; CNS effects, malaise, insomnia, abnormal thinking; electrolyte imbalance) at regular intervals during therapy. Teach patient proper use (eg, timing of multiple medications and drugs that should not be used concurrently), possible side effects/appropriate interventions (eg, glucose testing; protease inhibitors may cause hyperglycemia, exacerbation or new-onset diabetes; use of barrier contraceptives; protease inhibitors may decrease effectiveness of oral contraceptives), and adverse symptoms to report.

Patient Education: You will be provided with a list of specific medications that should not be used during therapy; do not take any new prescriptions, over-the-counter medications, or herbal products (even if they are not on the list) without consulting prescriber. This is not a cure for HIV, nor has it been found to reduce transmission of HIV; use appropriate precautions to prevent spread to other persons. Take as directed with meals. Maintain adequate hydration (2-3 L/day of fluids) unless instructed to restrict fluid intake. This medication will be prescribed with a combination of other medications; time these medications as directed by prescriber. You may be advised to check your glucose levels; this class of drugs can cause hyperglycemia. Frequent blood tests may be required with prolonged therapy. You may be susceptible to infection; avoid crowds and exposure to known infections and do not have any vaccinations without consulting prescriber. May cause body changes due to redistribution of body fat, facial atrophy, or breast enlargement (normal effects of drug); headache, dizziness, or fatigue (use caution when driving or engaging in potentially hazardous tasks until response to drug is known); nausea or vomiting (small frequent meals, frequent mouth care, chewing gum, or sucking lozenges may help); diarrhea (buttermilk, boiled milk, or yogurt may help); back pain, or arthralgia (consult prescriber for approved analgesic). Inform prescriber if you experience muscle numbness or tingling; unresolved persistent vomiting, diarrhea, or abdominal pain; respiratory difficulty or chest pain; unusual skin rash; change in color of stool or urine; or any persistent adverse effects. **Pregnancy/**
(Continued)

Fosamprenavir (Continued)

breast-feeding precautions: Inform prescriber if you are or intend to become pregnant. Effectiveness of oral contraceptives may be decreased, use of alternative (nonhormonal) forms of contraception is recommended; consult prescriber for appropriate contraceptives. Do not breast-feed.

Dietary Considerations May be taken with or without food.

Breast-Feeding Issues HIV-infected mothers are discouraged from breast-feeding to decrease potential transmission of HIV.

Pregnancy Issues It is not known if amprenavir crosses the human placenta and there are no clinical studies currently underway to evaluate its use in pregnant women. Pregnancy and protease inhibitors are both associated with an increased risk of hyperglycemia. Glucose levels should be closely monitored. Health professionals are encouraged to contact the antiretroviral pregnancy registry to monitor outcomes of pregnant women exposed to antiretroviral medications (1-800-258-4263 or www.APRegistry.com).

Foscarnet (fos KAR net)

U.S. Brand Names Foscavir®

Synonyms PFA; Phosphonoformate; Phosphonoformic Acid

Pharmacologic Category Antiviral Agent

Pregnancy Risk Factor C

Lactation Excretion in breast milk unknown/contraindicated

Use

Treatment of herpes virus infections suspected to be caused by acyclovir-resistant (HSV, VZV) or ganciclovir-resistant (CMV) strains; this occurs almost exclusively in immunocompromised persons (eg, with advanced AIDS) who have received prolonged treatment for a herpes virus infection

Treatment of CMV retinitis in persons with AIDS

Unlabeled/Investigational Use Other CMV infections in persons unable to tolerate ganciclovir; may be given in combination with ganciclovir in patients who relapse after monotherapy with either drug

Mechanism of Action/Effect Pyrophosphate analogue which acts as a noncompetitive inhibitor of many viral RNA and DNA polymerases as well as HIV reverse transcriptase. Inhibitory effects occur at concentrations which do not affect host cellular DNA polymerases; however, some human cell growth suppression has been observed with high in vitro concentrations. Similar to ganciclovir, foscarnet is a virostatic agent. Foscarnet does not require activation by thymidine kinase.

Contraindications Hypersensitivity to foscarnet or any component of the formulation; Cl$_{cr}$ <0.4 mL/minute/kg during therapy

Warnings/Precautions Hazardous agent — use appropriate precautions for handling and disposal. Renal impairment occurs to some degree in the majority of patients treated with foscarnet. Renal impairment may occur at any time (usually reversible within 1 week following dose adjustment or discontinuation, but some severe cases). Renal function should be closely monitored. Foscarnet may cause tooth disorders. Safety and effectiveness in children have not been studied. Monitor electrolytes carefully, particularly calcium, magnesium, phosphate, and potassium. Seizures have been experienced by up to 10% of AIDS patients. Risk factors for seizures include a low baseline absolute neutrophil count (ANC), impaired baseline renal function and low total serum calcium. Some patients who have experienced seizures have died, while others have been able to continue or resume foscarnet treatment after their

mineral or electrolyte abnormality has been corrected, their underlying disease state treated, or their dose decreased. Foscarnet has been shown to be mutagenic in vitro and in mice at very high doses.

Drug Interactions

Increased Effect/Toxicity: Concurrent use with ciprofloxacin (or other fluoroquinolone) increases seizure potential. Acute renal failure (reversible) has been reported with cyclosporine due most likely to a synergistic toxic effect. Nephrotoxic drugs (amphotericin B, I.V. pentamidine, aminoglycosides, etc) should be avoided, if possible, to minimize additive renal risk with foscarnet. Concurrent use of pentamidine also increases the potential for hypocalcemia. Protease inhibitors (ritonavir, saquinavir) have been associated with an increased risk of renal impairment during concurrent use of foscarnet

Adverse Reactions

>10%:

Central nervous system: Fever (65%), headache (26%), seizure (10%)

Gastrointestinal: Nausea (47%), diarrhea (30%), vomiting

Hematologic: Anemia (33%)

Renal: Abnormal renal function/decreased creatinine clearance (27%)

1% to 10%:

Central nervous system: Fatigue, malaise, dizziness, hypoesthesia, depression/confusion/anxiety (≥5%)

Dermatologic: Rash

Endocrine & metabolic: Electrolyte imbalance (especially potassium, calcium, magnesium, and phosphorus)

Gastrointestinal: Anorexia

Hematologic: Granulocytopenia, leukopenia (≥5%), thrombocytopenia, thrombosis

Local: Injection site pain

Neuromuscular & skeletal: Paresthesia, involuntary muscle contractions, rigors, neuropathy (peripheral), weakness

Ocular: Vision abnormalities

Respiratory: Coughing, dyspnea (≥5%)

Miscellaneous: Sepsis, diaphoresis (increased)

Overdosage/Toxicology Symptoms of overdose include seizures, renal dysfunction, perioral or limb paresthesia, and hypocalcemia. Treatment is supportive.

Pharmacodynamics/Kinetics

Half-Life Elimination: ~3 hours

Metabolism: Biotransformation does not occur

Excretion: Urine (≤28% as unchanged drug)

Available Dosage Forms [DSC] = Discontinued product

Injection, solution: 24 mg/mL (250 mL [DSC], 500 mL)

Dosing

Adults & Elderly:

CMV retinitis: I.V.:

Induction treatment: 60 mg/kg/dose every 8 hours for 14-21 days

Maintenance therapy: 90-120 mg/kg/day as a single infusion

Acyclovir-resistant HSV induction treatment: I.V.: 40 mg/kg/dose every 8-12 hours for 14-21 days

Pediatrics: Adolescents: Refer to adult dosing.

Renal Impairment: See tables on next page.

Administration

I.V.: Use an infusion pump, at a rate not exceeding 1 mg/kg/minute. Adult induction doses of 60 mg/kg are administered over 1 hour. Adult maintenance doses of 90-120 mg/kg are infused over 2 hours.

I.V. Detail: Undiluted (24 mg/mL) solution can be administered without further dilution when using a central venous catheter for infusion. For peripheral vein administration, the solution **must** be diluted to a final concentration **not to exceed** 12 mg/mL.

The recommended dosage, frequency, and rate of infusion should not be exceeded.

pH: 7.4 (adjusted)

Induction Dosing of Foscarnet in Patients With Abnormal Renal Function

Cl_cr (mL/min/kg)	HSV Equivalent to 40 mg/kg q12h	HSV Equivalent to 40 mg/kg q8h	CMV Equivalent to 60 mg/kg q8h	CMV Equivalent to 90 mg/kg q12h
<0.4	Not recommended	Not recommended	Not recommended	Not recommended
≥0.4-0.5	20 mg/kg every 24 hours	35 mg/kg every 24 hours	50 mg/kg every 24 hours	50 mg/kg every 24 hours
>0.5-0.6	25 mg/kg every 24 hours	40 mg/kg every 24 hours	60 mg/kg every 24 hours	60 mg/kg every 24 hours
>0.6-0.8	35 mg/kg every 24 hours	25 mg/kg every 12 hours	40 mg/kg every 12 hours	80 mg/kg every 24 hours
>0.8-1.0	20 mg/kg every 12 hours	35 mg/kg every 12 hours	50 mg/kg every 12 hours	50 mg/kg every 12 hours
>1.0-1.4	30 mg/kg every 12 hours	30 mg/kg every 8 hours	45 mg/kg every 8 hours	70 mg/kg every 12 hours
>1.4	40 mg/kg every 12 hours	40 mg/kg every 8 hours	60 mg/kg every 8 hours	90 mg/kg every 12 hours

Maintenance Dosing of Foscarnet in Patients With Abnormal Renal Function

Cl_cr (mL/min/kg)	CMV Equivalent to 90 mg/kg q24h	CMV Equivalent to 120 mg/kg q24h
<0.4	Not recommended	Not recommended
≥0.4-0.5	50 mg/kg every 48 hours	65 mg/kg every 48 hours
>0.5-0.6	60 mg/kg every 48 hours	80 mg/kg every 48 hours
>0.6-0.8	80 mg/kg every 48 hours	105 mg/kg every 48 hours
>0.8-1.0	50 mg/kg every 24 hours	65 mg/kg every 24 hours
>1.0-1.4	70 mg/kg every 24 hours	90 mg/kg every 24 hours
>1.4	90 mg/kg every 24 hours	120 mg/kg every 24 hours

Stability
Reconstitution: Foscarnet should be diluted in D_5W or NS. For peripheral line administration, foscarnet **must** be diluted to ≤12 mg/mL with D_5W or NS. For central line administration, foscarnet may be administered undiluted.

Compatibility: Stable in D_5W, NS; **incompatible** with LR, dextrose 30%, TPN, I.V. solutions containing calcium, magnesium, or vancomycin

Y-site administration: Incompatible with acyclovir, amphotericin B, diazepam, digoxin, diphenhydramine, dobutamine, droperidol, ganciclovir, haloperidol, leucovorin, midazolam, pentamidine, prochlorperazine edisylate, promethazine, trimetrexate

Storage: Foscarnet injection is a clear, colorless solution. It should be stored at room temperature and protected from temperatures >40°C and from freezing. Diluted solution is stable for 24 hours at room temperature or under refrigeration.

Laboratory Monitoring: Renal function, CBC, electrolytes, calcium, magnesium

Nursing Actions
Physical Assessment: Evaluate electrolytes, renal status, and dental status prior to beginning therapy.

Assess potential for interactions with other pharmacological agents patient may be taking (eg, increased risk of seizures, renal failure, electrolyte imbalance). See Administration for infusion specifics. Assess results of laboratory tests (electrolytes) and renal function, therapeutic effectiveness (resolution of viral infection), and adverse response (eg, nephrotoxicity, electrolyte imbalance, seizures). Teach patient possible side effects/appropriate interventions (eg, need for regular dental evaluations) and adverse symptoms to report.

Patient Education: Do not take any new medication during therapy unless approved by prescriber. Foscarnet is not a cure for the disease; progression may occur during or following therapy. While on therapy, it is important to maintain adequate hydration (2-3 L/day of fluids) unless instructed to restrict fluid intake, and nutrition (small, frequent meals may help). Regular dental check-ups are recommended. May cause dizziness or confusion (use caution when driving or engaging in tasks that require alertness until response to drug is known); nausea and vomiting (small, frequent meals, frequent mouth care, chewing gum or sucking lozenges may help); or diarrhea (buttermilk, boiled milk, or yogurt may help). Report any change in sensorium or seizures; unresolved diarrhea or vomiting; unusual fever, chills, sore throat, unhealed sores, swollen lymph glands; or malaise. **Pregnancy/breast-feeding precautions:** Inform prescriber if you are pregnant. Barrier contraceptives are recommended to reduce transmission of disease. Do not breast-feed.

Geriatric Considerations Information on the use of foscarnet is lacking in the elderly. Dose adjustments and proper monitoring must be performed because of the decreased renal function common in older patients.

Breast-Feeding Issues The CDC recommends **not** to breast-feed if diagnosed with HIV to avoid postnatal transmission of the virus.

Additional Information Sodium loading with 500 mL of 0.9% sodium chloride solution before and after foscarnet infusion helps to minimize the risk of nephrotoxicity.

Fosinopril (foe SIN oh pril)

U.S. Brand Names Monopril®

Synonyms Fosinopril Sodium

Pharmacologic Category Angiotensin-Converting Enzyme (ACE) Inhibitor

Medication Safety Issues
Sound-alike/look-alike issues:
Fosinopril may be confused with lisinopril
Monopril® may be confused with Accupril®, minoxidil, moexipril, Monoket®, Monurol™, ramipril

Pregnancy Risk Factor C (1st trimester)/D (2nd and 3rd trimesters)

Lactation Enters breast milk/not recommended

Use Treatment of hypertension, either alone or in combination with other antihypertensive agents; treatment of congestive heart failure, left ventricular dysfunction after myocardial infarction

Mechanism of Action/Effect Competitive inhibitor of angiotensin-converting enzyme (ACE); prevents conversion of angiotensin I to angiotensin II, a potent vasoconstrictor; results in lower levels of angiotensin II which causes an increase in plasma renin activity and a reduction in aldosterone secretion; a CNS mechanism may also be involved in hypotensive effect as angiotensin II increases adrenergic outflow from CNS; vasoactive kallikreins may be decreased in conversion to active hormones by ACE inhibitors, thus reducing blood pressure

(Continued)

Fosinopril *(Continued)*

Contraindications Hypersensitivity to fosinopril or any component of the formulation; angioedema related to previous treatment with an ACE inhibitor; idiopathic or hereditary angioedema; bilateral renal artery stenosis; pregnancy (2nd and 3rd trimesters)

Warnings/Precautions Anaphylactic reactions can occur. Angioedema can occur at any time during treatment (especially following first dose). It may involve head and neck (potentially affecting the airway) or the intestine (presenting with abdominal pain). Prolonged monitoring may be required especially if tongue, glottis, or larynx are involved as they are associated with airway obstruction. Those with a history of airway surgery in this situation have a higher risk. Careful blood pressure monitoring (hypotension can occur especially in volume-depleted patients). Dosage adjustment needed in severe renal impairment (Cl_{cr} <10 mL/minute). Use with caution in hypovolemia; collagen vascular diseases; valvular stenosis (particularly aortic stenosis); hyperkalemia; or before, during, or immediately after anesthesia. Avoid rapid dosage escalation which may lead to renal insufficiency. Rare toxicities associated with ACE inhibitors include cholestatic jaundice (which may progress to hepatic necrosis) and neutropenia/agranulocytosis with myeloid hyperplasia. Hypersensitivity reactions may be seen during hemodialysis with high-flux dialysis membranes (eg, AN69). Hyperkalemia may rarely occur. Use with caution in unilateral renal artery stenosis and pre-existing renal insufficiency.

Drug Interactions

Decreased Effect: Aspirin (high dose) may reduce the therapeutic effects of ACE inhibitors; at low dosages this does not appear to be significant. Rifampin may decrease the effect of ACE inhibitors. Antacids may decrease the bioavailability of ACE inhibitors (may be more likely to occur with captopril); separate administration times by 1-2 hours. NSAIDs, specifically indomethacin, may reduce the hypotensive effects of ACE inhibitors. More likely to occur in low renin or volume dependent hypertensive patients.

Increased Effect/Toxicity: Potassium supplements, co-trimoxazole (high dose), angiotensin II receptor antagonists (eg, candesartan, losartan, irbesartan), or potassium-sparing diuretics (amiloride, spironolactone, triamterene) may result in elevated serum potassium levels when combined with fosinopril. ACE inhibitor effects may be increased by phenothiazines or probenecid (increases levels of captopril). ACE inhibitors may increase serum concentrations/effects of lithium.

Diuretics have additive hypotensive effects with ACE inhibitors, and hypovolemia increases the potential for adverse renal effects of ACE inhibitors. In patients with compromised renal function, coadministration with NSAIDs may result in further deterioration of renal function. Allopurinol and ACE inhibitors may cause a higher risk of hypersensitivity reaction when taken concurrently.

Nutritional/Ethanol Interactions Herb/Nutraceutical: Avoid dong quai if used for hypertension (has estrogenic activity). Avoid ephedra, garlic, yohimbe, ginseng (may worsen hypertension).

Lab Interactions Positive Coombs' (direct); may cause false-positive results in urine acetone determinations using sodium nitroprusside reagent; may cause false low serum digoxin levels with the Digi-Tab RIA kit for digoxin.

Adverse Reactions Note: Frequency ranges include data from hypertension and heart failure trials. Higher rates of adverse reactions have generally been noted in patients with CHF. However, the frequency of adverse effects associated with placebo is also increased in this population.

>10%: Central nervous system: Dizziness (2% to 12%)

1% to 10%:
Cardiovascular: Orthostatic hypotension (1% to 2%), palpitation (1%)
Central nervous system: Dizziness (1% to 2%; up to 12% in CHF patients), headache (3%), fatigue (1% to 2%)
Endocrine & metabolic: Hyperkalemia (2.6%)
Gastrointestinal: Diarrhea (2%), nausea/vomiting (1.2% to 2.2%)
Hepatic: Transaminases increased
Neuromuscular & skeletal: Musculoskeletal pain (<1% to 3%), noncardiac chest pain (<1% to 2%), weakness (1%)
Renal: Increased serum creatinine, worsening of renal function (in patients with bilateral renal artery stenosis or hypovolemia)
Respiratory: Cough (2% to 10%)
Miscellaneous: Upper respiratory infection (2%)

>1% but ≤ frequency in patients receiving placebo: Sexual dysfunction, fever, flu-like syndrome, dyspnea, rash, headache, insomnia

Other events reported with ACE inhibitors: Neutropenia, agranulocytosis, eosinophilic pneumonitis, cardiac arrest, pancytopenia, hemolytic anemia, anemia, aplastic anemia, thrombocytopenia, acute renal failure, hepatic failure, jaundice, symptomatic hyponatremia, bullous pemphigus, exfoliative dermatitis, Stevens-Johnson syndrome. In addition, a syndrome which may include fever, myalgia, arthralgia, interstitial nephritis, vasculitis, rash, eosinophilia and positive ANA, and elevated ESR has been reported for other ACE inhibitors.

Overdosage/Toxicology Mild hypotension has been the primary toxic effect seen with acute overdose. Bradycardia may also occur; hyperkalemia occurs even with therapeutic doses, especially in patients with renal insufficiency and those taking NSAIDs. Treatment is symptom-directed and supportive.

Pharmacodynamics/Kinetics

Onset of Action: 1 hour
Duration of Action: 24 hours
Time to Peak: Serum: ~3 hours
Protein Binding: 95%
Half-Life Elimination: Serum (fosinoprilat): 12 hours
Metabolism: Prodrug, hydrolyzed to its active metabolite fosinoprilat by intestinal wall and hepatic esterases
Excretion: Urine and feces (as fosinoprilat and other metabolites in roughly equal proportions, 45% to 50%)

Available Dosage Forms Tablet, as sodium: 10 mg, 20 mg, 40 mg

Dosing

Adults & Elderly:

Hypertension: Oral: Initial: 10 mg/day; increase to a maximum dose of 80 mg/day. Most patients are maintained on 20-40 mg/day. May need to divide the dose into two if trough effect is inadequate. Discontinue the diuretic, if possible 2-3 days before initiation of therapy. Resume diuretic therapy carefully, if needed.

Heart failure: Oral: Initial: 10 mg/day (5 mg if renal dysfunction present) and increase, as needed, to a maximum of 40 mg once daily over several weeks. Usual dose: 20-40 mg/day. If hypotension, orthostasis, or azotemia occurs during titration, consider decreasing concomitant diuretic dose, if any.

Pediatrics: Hypertension: Children >50 kg: Oral: Initial: 5-10 mg once daily

Renal Impairment: None needed since hepatobiliary elimination compensates adequately diminished renal elimination.
Hemodialysis: Moderately dialyzable (20% to 50%)

Hepatic Impairment: Decrease dose and monitor effects

Stability

Storage: Store at 25°C (77°F); excursions permitted to 15°C to 30°C (59°F to 86°F). Protect from moisture by keeping bottle tightly closed.

Laboratory Monitoring CBC, renal function tests, electrolytes. If patient has renal impairment, a baseline WBC with differential and serum creatinine should be evaluated and monitored closely during initial therapy.

Nursing Actions

Physical Assessment: Assess potential for interactions with other pharmacological agents or herbal products patient may be taking (especially anything that may impact fluid balance or cardiac status). Assess results of laboratory tests, therapeutic effectiveness according to purpose for use, and adverse response on a regular basis during therapy (eg, anaphylactic reactions, hypovolemia, angioedema, postural hypotension). Teach patient appropriate use, possible side effects/appropriate interventions, and adverse symptoms to report.

Patient Education: Inform prescriber of all prescriptions, OTC medications, or herbal products you are taking, and any allergies you have. Do not take any new medication during therapy unless approved by prescriber. Do not use potassium supplement or salt substitutes without consulting prescriber. Take exactly as directed; do not discontinue without consulting prescriber. This drug does not eliminate need for diet or exercise regimen as recommended by prescriber. May cause dizziness, fainting, or lightheadedness (use caution when driving or engaging in tasks that require alertness until response to drug is known); postural hypotension (use caution when rising from lying or sitting position or climbing stairs); or nausea, vomiting, abdominal pain, dry mouth, or loss of appetite (small, frequent meals, frequent mouth care, sucking lozenges, or chewing gum may help) - report if these persist. Report chest pain or palpitations; mouth sores; fever or chills; swelling of extremities, face, mouth, or tongue; skin rash; numbness, tingling, or pain in muscles; respiratory difficulty; unusual cough; or other persistent adverse reactions. **Pregnancy/breast-feeding precautions:** Inform prescriber if you are or intend to become pregnant. This drug should not be used in the 2nd or 3rd trimester of pregnancy. Consult prescriber for appropriate contraceptive measures if necessary. Breast-feeding is not recommended.

Dietary Considerations Should not take a potassium salt supplement without the advice of healthcare provider.

Geriatric Considerations Due to frequent decreases in glomerular filtration (also creatinine clearance) with aging, elderly patients may have exaggerated responses to ACE inhibitors. Differences in clinical response due to hepatic changes are not observed. ACE inhibitors may be preferred agents in elderly patients with congestive heart failure and diabetes mellitus. Diabetic proteinuria is reduced and insulin sensitivity is enhanced. In general, the side effect profile is favorable in the elderly and causes little or no CNS confusion; use lowest dose recommendations initially.

Pregnancy Issues ACE inhibitors can cause fetal injury or death if taken during the 2nd or 3rd trimester. Discontinue ACE inhibitors as soon as pregnancy is detected.

Fosphenytoin (FOS fen i toyn)

U.S. Brand Names Cerebyx®
Synonyms Fosphenytoin Sodium
Pharmacologic Category Anticonvulsant, Hydantoin
Medication Safety Issues
Sound-alike/look-alike issues:
Cerebyx® may be confused with Celebrex®, Celexa™, Cerezyme®

Pregnancy Risk Factor D
Lactation Excretion in breast milk unknown/not recommended
Use Used for the control of generalized convulsive status epilepticus and prevention and treatment of seizures occurring during neurosurgery; indicated for short-term parenteral administration when other means of phenytoin administration are unavailable, inappropriate or deemed less advantageous (the safety and effectiveness of fosphenytoin in this use has not been systematically evaluated for more than 5 days)
Mechanism of Action/Effect Diphosphate ester salt of phenytoin which acts as a water soluble prodrug of phenytoin; after administration, plasma esterases convert fosphenytoin to phosphate, formaldehyde and phenytoin as the active moiety; phenytoin works by stabilizing neuronal membranes and decreasing seizure activity by increasing efflux or decreasing influx of sodium ions across cell membranes in the motor cortex during generation of nerve impulses
Contraindications Hypersensitivity to phenytoin, other hydantoins, or any component of the formulation; patients with sinus bradycardia, sinoatrial block, second- and third-degree AV block, or Adams-Stokes syndrome; occurrence of rash during treatment (should not be resumed if rash is exfoliative, purpuric, or bullous); treatment of absence seizures
Warnings/Precautions Doses of fosphenytoin are expressed as their phenytoin sodium equivalent (PE). Antiepileptic drugs should not be abruptly discontinued. Hypotension may occur, especially after I.V. administration at high doses and high rates of administration. Administration of phenytoin has been associated with atrial and ventricular conduction depression and ventricular fibrillation. Careful cardiac monitoring is needed when administering I.V. loading doses of fosphenytoin. Acute hepatotoxicity associated with a hypersensitivity syndrome characterized by fever, skin eruptions, and lymphadenopathy has been reported to occur within the first 2 months of treatment. Discontinue if skin rash or lymphadenopathy occurs. Use with caution in patients with hypotension, severe myocardial insufficiency, diabetes mellitus, porphyria, hypoalbuminemia, hypothyroidism, fever, or hepatic or renal dysfunction.
Drug Interactions
Cytochrome P450 Effect: As phenytoin: **Substrate** of CYP2C8/9 (major), 2C19 (major), 3A4 (minor); **Induces** CYP2B6 (strong), 2C8/9 (strong), 2C19 (strong), 3A4 (strong)
Decreased Effect: Phenytoin may enhance the metabolism of estrogen and/or oral contraceptives, decreasing their clinical effect; an alternative method of contraception should be considered. Phenytoin may increase the metabolism of anticonvulsants including barbiturates, carbamazepine, ethosuximide, felbamate, lamotrigine, tiagabine, topiramate, and zonisamide. Valproic acid may increase, decrease, or have no effect on phenytoin serum concentrations. Phenytoin may also decrease the serum concentrations/effects of some antiarrhythmics (disopyramide, propafenone, quinidine, quetiapine) and tricyclic antidepressants may be reduced by phenytoin. Phenytoin may enhance the metabolism of doxycycline, decreasing its clinical effect; higher dosages may be required. Phenytoin may increase the metabolism of chloramphenicol or itraconazole.
(Continued)

Fosphenytoin *(Continued)*

Phenytoin may decrease the levels/effects of amiodarone, benzodiazepines, bupropion, calcium channel blockers, carbamazepine, citalopram, clarithromycin, cyclosporine, efavirenz, erythromycin, estrogens, fluoxetine, glimepiride, glipizide, losartan, methsuximide, mirtazapine, nateglinide, nefazodone, nevirapine, phenytoin, pioglitazone, promethazine, propranolol, protease inhibitors, proton pump inhibitors, rosiglitazone, selegiline, sertraline, sulfonamides, tacrolimus, venlafaxine, voriconazole, warfarin, zafirlukast, and other CYP2B6, 2C8/9, 2C19, or 3A4 substrates.

The levels/effects of phenytoin may be decreased by aminoglutethimide, carbamazepine, phenobarbital, rifampin, rifapentine, secobarbital, and other CYP2C8/9 or 2C19 inducers. Clozapine and vigabatrin may reduce phenytoin serum concentrations. Case reports indicate ciprofloxacin may increase or decrease serum phenytoin concentrations. Dexamethasone may decrease serum phenytoin concentrations. Replacement of folic acid has been reported to increase the metabolism of phenytoin, decreasing its serum concentrations and/or increasing seizures.

Initially, phenytoin increases the response to warfarin; this is followed by a decrease in response to warfarin. Phenytoin may inhibit the anti-Parkinson effect of levodopa. The duration of neuromuscular blockade from neuromuscular-blocking agents may be decreased by phenytoin. Phenytoin may enhance the metabolism of methadone resulting in methadone withdrawal. Phenytoin may decrease serum levels/effects of digitalis glycosides, theophylline, and thyroid hormones.

Several chemotherapeutic agents have been associated with a decrease in serum phenytoin levels; includes cisplatin, bleomycin, carmustine, methotrexate, and vinblastine. Enzyme-inducing anticonvulsant therapy may reduce the effectiveness of some chemotherapy regimens (specifically in ALL). Teniposide and methotrexate may be cleared more rapidly in these patients.

Increased Effect/Toxicity: The sedative effects of phenytoin may be additive with other CNS depressants including ethanol, barbiturates, sedatives, antidepressants, narcotic analgesics, and benzodiazepines. Selected anticonvulsants (felbamate, gabapentin, and topiramate) have been reported to increase phenytoin levels/effects. In addition, serum phenytoin concentrations may be increased by allopurinol, amiodarone, calcium channel blockers (including diltiazem and nifedipine), cimetidine, disulfiram, methylphenidate, metronidazole, omeprazole, selective serotonin reuptake inhibitors (SSRIs), ticlopidine, tricyclic antidepressants, trazodone, and trimethoprim. Case reports indicate ciprofloxacin may increase or decrease serum phenytoin concentrations.

The levels/effects of phenytoin may be increased by delavirdine, fluconazole, fluvoxamine, gemfibrozil, isoniazid, ketoconazole, nicardipine, NSAIDs, omeprazole, pioglitazone, sulfonamides, ticlopidine, and other CYP2C8/9 or 2C19 inhibitors.

Phenytoin enhances the conversion of primidone to phenobarbital resulting in elevated phenobarbital serum concentrations. Concurrent use of acetazolamide with phenytoin may result in an increased risk of osteomalacia. Concurrent use of phenytoin and lithium has resulted in lithium intoxication. Valproic acid (and sulfisoxazole) may displace phenytoin from binding sites; valproic acid may increase, decrease, or have no effect on phenytoin serum concentrations. Phenytoin transiently increased the response to warfarin initially; this is followed by an inhibition of the hypoprothrombinemic response. Phenytoin may enhance the hepatotoxic potential of acetaminophen overdoses. Concurrent use of dopamine and intravenous phenytoin may lead to an increased risk of hypotension.

Nutritional/Ethanol Interactions
Ethanol:
Acute use: Avoid or limit ethanol (inhibits metabolism of phenytoin); watch for sedation.
Chronic use: Avoid or limit ethanol (stimulates metabolism of phenytoin).

Lab Interactions May decrease serum concentrations of thyroxine; may produce artifactually low results in dexamethasone or metyrapone tests; may cause increase serum concentrations of glucose, alkaline phosphatase, and gamma glutamyl transpeptidase (GGT)

Adverse Reactions The more important adverse clinical events caused by the I.V. use of fosphenytoin or phenytoin are cardiovascular collapse and/or central nervous system depression. Hypotension can occur when either drug is administered rapidly by the I.V. route. Do not exceed a rate of 150 mg phenytoin equivalent/minute when administering fosphenytoin.

The adverse clinical events most commonly observed with the use of fosphenytoin in clinical trials were nystagmus, dizziness, pruritus, paresthesia, headache, somnolence, and ataxia. Paresthesia and pruritus were seen more often following fosphenytoin (versus phenytoin) administration and occurred more often with I.V. fosphenytoin than with I.M. administration. These events were dose- and rate-related (doses ≥15 mg/kg at a rate of 150 mg/minute). These sensations, generally described as itching, burning, or tingling are usually not at the infusion site. The location of the discomfort varied with the groin mentioned most frequently. The paresthesia and pruritus were transient events that occurred within several minutes of the start of infusion and generally resolved within 10 minutes after completion of infusion.

Transient pruritus, tinnitus, nystagmus, somnolence, and ataxia occurred 2-3 times more often at doses ≥15 mg/kg and rates ≥150 mg/minute.

I.V. administration (maximum dose/rate):
>10%:
Central nervous system: Nystagmus, dizziness, somnolence, ataxia
Dermatologic: Pruritus
1% to 10%:
Cardiovascular: Hypotension, vasodilation, tachycardia
Central nervous system: Stupor, incoordination, paresthesia, extrapyramidal syndrome, tremor, agitation, hypoesthesia, dysarthria, vertigo, brain edema, headache
Gastrointestinal: Nausea, tongue disorder, dry mouth, vomiting
Neuromuscular & skeletal: Pelvic pain, muscle weakness, back pain
Ocular: Diplopia, amblyopia
Otic: Tinnitus, deafness
Miscellaneous: Taste perversion
I.M. administration (substitute for oral phenytoin):
1% to 10%:
Central nervous system: Nystagmus, tremor, ataxia, headache, incoordination, somnolence, dizziness, paresthesia, reflexes decreased
Dermatologic: Pruritus
Gastrointestinal: Nausea, vomiting
Hematologic/lymphatic: Ecchymosis
Neuromuscular & skeletal: Muscle weakness

Overdosage/Toxicology Symptoms of fosphenytoin overdose include bradycardia, asystole, cardiac arrest, hypotension, vomiting, metabolic acidosis, and lethargy. Treatment is supportive for hypotension.

Pharmacodynamics/Kinetics

Time to Peak: Conversion to phenytoin: Following I.V. administration (maximum rate of administration): 15 minutes; following I.M. administration, peak phenytoin levels are reached in 3 hours

Protein Binding: Fosphenytoin: 95% to 99% to albumin; can displace phenytoin and increase free fraction (up to 30% unbound) during the period required for conversion of fosphenytoin to phenytoin

Half-Life Elimination: Fosphenytoin: 15 minutes; Phenytoin: Variable (mean: 12-29 hours); kinetics of phenytoin are saturable

Metabolism: Fosphenytoin is rapidly converted via hydrolysis to phenytoin; phenytoin is metabolized in the liver and forms metabolites

Excretion: Phenytoin: Urine (as inactive metabolites)

Pharmacokinetic Note Refer to Phenytoin monograph for additional information.

Available Dosage Forms Injection, solution, as sodium: 75 mg/mL [equivalent to phenytoin sodium 50 mg/mL] (2 mL, 10 mL)

Dosing

Adults:

The dose, concentration in solutions, and infusion rates for fosphenytoin are expressed as phenytoin sodium equivalents (PE); fosphenytoin should always be prescribed and dispensed in phenytoin sodium equivalents (PE)

Status epilepticus: I.V.: Loading dose: 15-20 mg PE/kg I.V. administered at 100-150 mg PE/minute

Nonemergent loading and maintenance dosing: I.V. or I.M.:

Loading dose: 10-20 mg PE/kg I.V. or I.M. (maximum I.V. rate: 150 mg PE/minute)

Initial daily maintenance dose: 4-6 mg PE/kg/day I.V. or I.M.

Substitution for oral phenytoin therapy: I.M. or I.V.: May be substituted for oral phenytoin sodium at the same total daily dose; however, Dilantin® capsules are ~90% bioavailable by the oral route; phenytoin, supplied as fosphenytoin, is 100% bioavailable by both the I.M. and I.V. routes; for this reason, plasma phenytoin concentrations may increase when I.M. or I.V. fosphenytoin is substituted for oral phenytoin sodium therapy; in clinical trials I.M. fosphenytoin was administered as a single daily dose utilizing either 1 or 2 injection sites; some patients may require more frequent dosing

Elderly: Phenytoin clearance is decreased in geriatric patients; lower doses may be required. In addition, older adults may have lower serum albumin which may increase the free fraction and, therefore, pharmacologic response. Refer to adult dosing.

Pediatrics:

Note: The dose, concentration in solutions, and infusion rates for fosphenytoin are expressed as phenytoin sodium equivalents (PE); fosphenytoin should always be prescribed and dispensed in phenytoin sodium equivalents (PE).

Infants and Children (unlabeled use): I.V.:

Loading dose: 10-20 mg PE/kg for the treatment of generalized convulsive status epilepticus.

Maintenance dosing: Phenytoin dosing guidelines in pediatric patients are used when dosing fosphenytoin using doses in PE equal to the phenytoin doses (ie, phenytoin 1 mg = fosphenytoin 1 PE); maintenance doses may be started 8-12 hours after a loading dose

Renal Impairment: Free phenytoin levels should be monitored closely in patients with renal disease or in those with hypoalbuminemia; furthermore, fosphenytoin clearance to phenytoin may be increased without a similar increase in phenytoin clearance in these patients leading to increase frequency and severity of adverse events.

Hepatic Impairment: Phenytoin clearance may be substantially reduced in cirrhosis and plasma level monitoring with dose adjustment advisable. Free phenytoin levels should be monitored closely in patients with hepatic disease or in those with hypoalbuminemia; furthermore, fosphenytoin clearance to phenytoin may be increased without a similar increase in phenytoin clearance in these patients leading to increase frequency and severity of adverse events.

Administration

I.M.: I.M. may be administered as a single daily dose using either 1 or 2 injection sites.

I.V.: Rates of infusion:

Children: 1-3 mg PE/kg/minute

Adults: Should not exceed 150 mg PE/minute

Stability

Reconstitution: Must be diluted to concentrations 1.5-25 mg PE/mL, in normal saline or D_5W, for I.V. infusion

Compatibility: Stable in D_5LR, $D_5\frac{1}{2}NS$, D_5W, $D_{10}W$, hetastarch 6% in NS, mannitol 20%, LR, NS

Y-site administration: Incompatible with midazolam

Storage: Refrigerate at 2°C to 8°C (36°F to 46°F). Do not store at room temperature for more than 48 hours. Do not use vials that develop particulate matter.

Laboratory Monitoring Serum phenytoin, renal function, albumin

Nursing Actions

Physical Assessment: Assess all other medications (prescription and OTC) or herbal products patient may be taking. Continuous hemodynamic monitoring and respiratory status are essential during infusion and for 30 minutes following infusion. Do not draw phenytoin levels until 2 hours following I.V. or 4 hours following I.M. administration. Monitor closely for adverse or overdose reactions during and following infusion.

Patient Education: Patients may not be in a position to evaluate their response. If conscious or alert, advise patient to report signs or symptoms of palpitations, racing or falling heartbeat, respiratory difficulty, acute faintness, or CNS disturbances (eg, somnolence, ataxia), and visual disturbances. **Pregnancy precaution:** Inform prescriber if you are pregnant.

Dietary Considerations Provides phosphate 0.0037 mmol/mg PE fosphenytoin

Geriatric Considerations No significant changes in fosphenytoin pharmacokinetics with age have been noted. Phenytoin clearance is decreased in the elderly and lower doses may be needed. Elderly may have reduced hepatic clearance due to age decline in Phase I metabolism. Elderly may have low albumin which will increase free fraction and, therefore, pharmacologic response. Monitor closely in those who are hypoalbuminemic. Free fraction measurements advised, also elderly may display a higher incidence of adverse effects (cardiovascular) when using the I.V. loading regimen; therefore, recommended to decrease loading I.V. dose to 25 mg/minute.

Breast-Feeding Issues Fosphenytoin is the prodrug of phenytoin. It is not known if fosphenytoin is excreted in breast milk prior to conversion to phenytoin. Refer to Phenytoin monograph for additional information.

Pregnancy Issues Fosphenytoin is the prodrug of phenytoin. Refer to Phenytoin monograph for additional information.

Additional Information 1.5 mg fosphenytoin is approximately equivalent to 1 mg phenytoin. Equimolar fosphenytoin dose is 375 mg (75 mg/mL solution) to phenytoin 250 mg (50 mg/mL).

Frovatriptan (froe va TRIP tan)

U.S. Brand Names Frova®

Synonyms Frovatriptan Succinate

Pharmacologic Category Antimigraine Agent; Serotonin 5-HT$_{1B, 1D}$ Receptor Agonist

Pregnancy Risk Factor C

Lactation Excretion in breast milk unknown/use caution

Use Acute treatment of migraine with or without aura in adults

Mechanism of Action/Effect Blocks 5-HT$_{1B}$ and 5-HT$_{1D}$ receptors. Relieves symptoms of migraine by blocking vasoconstrictive and other effects of serotonin.

Contraindications Hypersensitivity to frovatriptan or any component of the formulation; patients with ischemic heart disease or signs or symptoms of ischemic heart disease (including Prinzmetal's angina, angina pectoris, myocardial infarction, silent myocardial ischemia); cerebrovascular syndromes (including strokes, transient ischemic attacks); peripheral vascular syndromes (including ischemic bowel disease); uncontrolled hypertension; use within 24 hours of ergotamine derivatives; use within 24 hours of another 5-HT$_1$ agonist; management of hemiplegic or basilar migraine; prophylactic treatment of migraine; severe hepatic impairment

Warnings/Precautions Not intended for migraine prophylaxis, or treatment of cluster headaches, hemiplegic or basilar migraines. Cardiac events, cerebral/subarachnoid hemorrhage, and stroke have been reported with 5-HT$_1$ agonist administration. May cause vasospastic reactions resulting in colonic, peripheral, or coronary ischemia. Do not give to patients with risk factors for CAD until a cardiovascular evaluation has been performed. If the evaluation is satisfactory, the healthcare provider should administer the first dose and cardiovascular status should be periodically evaluated. Significant elevation in blood pressure has been reported on rare occasions in patients using other 5-HT$_{1D}$ agonists with and without a history of hypertension. Peripheral vascular ischemia and colonic ischemia with abdominal pain and bloody diarrhea have occurred. Use with caution in patients with a history of seizure disorder. Safety and efficacy in pediatric patients have not been established.

Drug Interactions
Cytochrome P450 Effect: Substrate of CYP1A2 (minor)

Increased Effect/Toxicity: The effects of frovatriptan may be increased by estrogen derivatives and propranolol. Ergot derivatives may increase the effects of frovatriptan (do not use within 24 hours of each other). SSRIs may exhibit additive toxicity with frovatriptan or other serotonin agonists (eg, antidepressants, dextromethorphan, tramadol) leading to serotonin syndrome.

Nutritional/Ethanol Interactions Food: Food does not affect frovatriptan bioavailability.

Adverse Reactions 1% to 10%:

Cardiovascular: Chest pain (2%), flushing (4%), palpitation (1%)

Central nervous system: Dizziness (8%), fatigue (5%), headache (4%), hot or cold sensation (3%), anxiety (1%), dysesthesia (1%), hypoesthesia (1%), insomnia (1%), pain (1%)

Gastrointestinal: Hyposalivation (3%), dyspepsia (2%), abdominal pain (1%), diarrhea (1%), vomiting (1%)

Neuromuscular & skeletal: Paresthesia (4%), skeletal pain (3%)

Ocular: Visual abnormalities (1%)

Otic: Tinnitus (1%)

Respiratory: Rhinitis (1%), sinusitis (1%)

Miscellaneous: Diaphoresis (1%)

Overdosage/Toxicology Single oral doses of up to 100 mg have been reported without adverse effects. Treatment of overdose should be supportive and symptomatic. Monitor for at least 48 hours or until signs and symptoms subside. It is not known if hemodialysis or peritoneal dialysis is effective.

Pharmacodynamics/Kinetics
Time to Peak: 2-4 hours

Protein Binding: 15%

Half-Life Elimination: 26 hours

Metabolism: Primarily hepatic via CYP1A2

Excretion: Feces (62%); urine (32%)

Available Dosage Forms Tablet, as base: 2.5 mg

Dosing
Adults & Elderly: Migraine: Oral: 2.5 mg; if headache recurs, a second dose may be given if first dose provided some relief and at least 2 hours have elapsed since the first dose (maximum daily dose: 7.5 mg)

Renal Impairment: No adjustment necessary.

Hepatic Impairment: No adjustment necessary in mild to moderate hepatic impairment; use with caution in severe impairment

Administration
Oral: Administer with fluids.

Stability
Storage: Store at room temperature of 25°C (77°F); protect from moisture and light.

Nursing Actions
Physical Assessment: Assess potential for interactions with other prescriptions, OTC medications, and herbal products patient may be taking (eg, ergot-containing drugs). Monitor laboratory tests and cardiovascular status periodically. Monitor effectiveness and adverse response. Teach patient proper use, possible side effects/appropriate interventions, and adverse symptoms to report.

Patient Education: This drug is to be used to reduce your migraine, not to prevent or reduce the number of attacks. Follow exact instructions for use. Do not take within 24 hours of any other migraine medication without first consulting prescriber. If first dose brings relief, a second dose may be taken anytime after 2 hours if migraine returns. Do not take more than three tablets (7.5 mg) in 24 hours without consulting prescriber. May cause dizziness, fatigue, insomnia, or drowsiness (use caution when driving or engaging in tasks requiring alertness until response to drug is known); dry mouth (frequent mouth care and sucking on lozenges may help); skin flushing or hot flashes (cool clothes or a cool environment may help); or mild abdominal discomfort or vomiting (small frequent meals, good mouth care, chewing gum, or sucking lozenges may help). Report immediately any chest pain, palpitations, or irregular heartbeat; severe dizziness, acute headache, stiff or painful neck, facial swelling, muscle weakness or pain, changes in mental acuity, blurred vision, eye pain, or ringing in ears; changes in urinary pattern; respiratory difficulty; or other persistent adverse effects. **Pregnancy/breast-feeding precautions:** Inform prescriber if you are or intend to become pregnant. Consult prescriber if breast-feeding.

Fulvestrant (fool VES trant)

U.S. Brand Names Faslodex®
Synonyms ICI-182,780; Zeneca 182,780; ZM-182,780
Pharmacologic Category Antineoplastic Agent, Estrogen Receptor Antagonist
Pregnancy Risk Factor D
Lactation Excretion in breast milk unknown/contraindicated

Use Treatment of hormone receptor positive metastatic breast cancer in postmenopausal women with disease progression following antiestrogen therapy.

Unlabeled/Investigational Use Endometriosis; uterine bleeding

Mechanism of Action/Effect Steroidal compound which competitively binds to estrogen receptors on tumors and other tissue targets; inhibits estrogen effects. Fulvestrant has no estrogen-receptor agonist activity. Causes down-regulation of estrogen receptors and inhibits tumor growth.

Contraindications Hypersensitivity to fulvestrant or any component of the formulation; contraindications to I.M. injections (bleeding diatheses, thrombocytopenia, or therapeutic anticoagulation); pregnancy

Warnings/Precautions Use caution in hepatic impairment.

Drug Interactions
Cytochrome P450 Effect: Substrate of CYP3A4 (minor)

Adverse Reactions
>10%:
Cardiovascular: Vasodilation (18%)
Central nervous system: Pain (19%), headache (15%)
Endocrine & metabolic: Hot flushes (19% to 24%)
Gastrointestinal: Nausea (26%), vomiting (13%), constipation (13%), diarrhea (12%), abdominal pain (12%)
Local: Injection site reaction (11%)
Neuromuscular & skeletal: Weakness (23%), bone pain (16%), back pain (14%)
Respiratory: Pharyngitis (16%), dyspnea (15%)
1% to 10%:
Cardiovascular: Edema (9%), chest pain (7%)
Central nervous system: Dizziness (7%), insomnia (7%), paresthesia (6%), fever (6%), depression (6%), anxiety (5%)
Dermatologic: Rash (7%)
Gastrointestinal: Anorexia (9%), weight gain (1% to 2%)
Genitourinary: Pelvic pain (10%), urinary tract infection (6%), vaginitis (2% to 3%)
Hematologic: Anemia (5%)
Neuromuscular and skeletal: Arthritis (3%)
Respiratory: Cough (10%)
Miscellaneous: Diaphoresis increased (5%)

Overdosage/Toxicology No specific experience in overdose. Treatment is supportive.

Pharmacodynamics/Kinetics
Duration of Action: I.M.: Plasma levels maintained for at least 1 month
Time to Peak: Plasma: I.M.: 7-9 days
Protein Binding: 99%
Half-Life Elimination: ~40 days
Metabolism: Hepatic via multiple pathways (CYP3A4 substrate, relative contribution to metabolism unknown)
Excretion: Feces (>90%); urine (<1%)

Available Dosage Forms Injection, solution: 50 mg/mL (2.5 mL, 5 mL) [prefilled syringe; contains alcohol, benzyl alcohol, benzyl stearate, castor oil]

Dosing
Adults: Metastatic breast cancer (postmenopausal women): I.M.: 250 mg at 1-month intervals

Renal Impairment: No dosage adjustment required.
Hepatic Impairment: Use in moderate to severe hepatic impairment has not been evaluated; use caution

Administration
I.M.: I.M. injection into a relatively large muscle (ie, buttock); do not administer I.V., SubQ, or intra-arterially. May be administered as a single 5 mL injection or two concurrent 2.5 mL injections.

Stability
Storage: Store under refrigeration at 2°C to 8°C (36°F to 46°F).

Nursing Actions
Physical Assessment: See Administration for injection specifics. Assess therapeutic effectiveness and adverse response (eg, vasodilation, edema, gastrointestinal disturbances, dyspnea, pain) on a regular basis throughout therapy. Teach patient use (if self-administered - injection technique and syringe/needle disposal), possible side effects/appropriate interventions, and adverse symptoms to report.

Patient Education: Do not take any new medication during therapy unless approved by prescriber. If self-administered, follow directions for injection and syringe/needle disposal. You may experience bone pain, back pain, or headache (consult prescriber for approved analgesic); nausea, vomiting, or loss of appetite (small, frequent meals, frequent mouth care, sucking lozenges, or chewing gum may help); dizziness (use caution when driving or engaging in tasks requiring alertness until response to drug is known); or increased perspiration. Report persistent pain; chest pain or palpitations; swelling of extremities or unusual weight gain (>5 lb/week); cough of respiratory difficulty; burning on urination or changes in urinary pattern; or other persistent, unrelieved adverse effects. **Pregnancy/breast-feeding precautions:** Approved only for postmenopausal women. Severe fetal damage can occur with this drug. Do not breast-feed.

Breast-Feeding Issues Approved for use only in postmenopausal women

Pregnancy Issues Antiestrogenic compounds have been associated with embryotoxicity, abnormalities in fetal development, and failure to maintain pregnancy in animal models. Approved for use only in postmenopausal women.

Furosemide (fyoor OH se mide)

U.S. Brand Names Lasix®
Synonyms Frusemide
Pharmacologic Category Diuretic, Loop
Medication Safety Issues
Sound-alike/look-alike issues:
Furosemide may be confused with torsemide
Lasix® may be confused with Esidrix®, Lanoxin®, Lidex®, Lomotil®, Luvox®, Luxiq®
Pregnancy Risk Factor C
Lactation Enters breast milk/use caution

Use Management of edema associated with congestive heart failure and hepatic or renal disease; alone or in combination with antihypertensives in treatment of hypertension

Mechanism of Action/Effect Inhibits reabsorption of sodium and chloride in the ascending loop of Henle and distal renal tubule, interfering with the chloride-binding cotransport system, thus causing increased excretion of water, sodium, chloride, magnesium, and calcium

Contraindications Hypersensitivity to furosemide, any component, or sulfonylureas; anuria; patients with hepatic coma or in states of severe electrolyte depletion until the condition improves or is corrected
(Continued)

Furosemide *(Continued)*

Warnings/Precautions In cirrhosis, avoid electrolyte and acid/base imbalances that might lead to hepatic encephalopathy. Ototoxicity is associated with rapid I.V. administration, renal impairment, excessive doses, and concurrent use of other ototoxins. Hypersensitivity reactions can rarely occur. Monitor fluid status and renal function in an attempt to prevent oliguria, azotemia, electrolyte disturbances, dehydration, and reversible increases in BUN and creatinine. Coadministration of antihypertensives may increase the risk of hypotension. Avoid use of medications in which the toxicity is enhanced by hypokalemia (including quinolones with QT prolongation).

Chemical similarities are present among sulfonamides, sulfonylureas, carbonic anhydrase inhibitors, thiazides, and loop diuretics (except ethacrynic acid). Use in patients with sulfonylurea allergy is specifically contraindicated in product labeling, however, a risk of cross-reaction exists in patients with allergy to any of these compounds; avoid use when previous reaction has been severe.

Drug Interactions

Decreased Effect: Indomethacin, aspirin, phenobarbital, phenytoin, and NSAIDs may reduce natriuretic and hypotensive effects of furosemide. Colestipol, cholestyramine, and sucralfate may reduce the effect of furosemide; separate administration by 2 hours. Furosemide may antagonize the effect of skeletal muscle relaxants (tubocurarine). Glucose tolerance may be decreased by furosemide, requiring an adjustment in the dose of hypoglycemic agents. Metformin may decrease furosemide concentrations.

Increased Effect/Toxicity: Furosemide-induced hypokalemia may predispose to digoxin toxicity and may increase the risk of arrhythmia with drugs which may prolong QT interval, including type Ia and type III antiarrhythmic agents, cisapride, and some quinolones (sparfloxacin, gatifloxacin, and moxifloxacin). The risk of toxicity from lithium and salicylates (high dose) may be increased by loop diuretics. Hypotensive effects and/or adverse renal effects of ACE inhibitors and NSAIDs are potentiated by furosemide-induced hypovolemia. The effects of peripheral adrenergic-blocking drugs or ganglionic blockers may be increased by furosemide.

Furosemide may increase the risk of ototoxicity with other ototoxic agents (aminoglycosides, cis-platinum), especially in patients with renal dysfunction. Synergistic diuretic effects occur with thiazide-type diuretics. Diuretics tend to be synergistic with other antihypertensive agents, and hypotension may occur.

Nutritional/Ethanol Interactions

Food: Furosemide serum levels may be decreased if taken with food.

Herb/Nutraceutical: Avoid dong quai if using for hypertension (has estrogenic activity). Avoid ephedra, yohimbe, ginseng (may worsen hypertension). Limit intake of natural licorice. Avoid garlic (may have increased antihypertensive effect).

Adverse Reactions Frequency not defined.

Cardiovascular: Orthostatic hypotension, necrotizing angiitis, thrombophlebitis, chronic aortitis, acute hypotension, sudden death from cardiac arrest (with I.V. or I.M. administration)

Central nervous system: Paresthesias, vertigo, dizziness, lightheadedness, headache, blurred vision, xanthopsia , fever, restlessness

Dermatologic: Exfoliative dermatitis, erythema multiforme, purpura, photosensitivity, urticaria, rash, pruritus, cutaneous vasculitis

Endocrine & metabolic: Hyperglycemia, hyperuricemia, hypokalemia, hypochloremia, metabolic alkalosis, hypocalcemia, hypomagnesemia, gout, hyponatremia

Gastrointestinal: Nausea, vomiting, anorexia, oral and gastric irritation, cramping, diarrhea, constipation, pancreatitis, intrahepatic cholestatic jaundice, ischemia hepatitis

Genitourinary: Urinary bladder spasm, urinary frequency

Hematological: Aplastic anemia (rare), thrombocytopenia, agranulocytosis (rare), hemolytic anemia, leukopenia, anemia, purpura

Neuromuscular & skeletal: Muscle spasm, weakness

Otic: Hearing impairment (reversible or permanent with rapid I.V. or I.M. administration), tinnitus, reversible deafness (with rapid I.V. or I.M. administration)

Renal: Vasculitis, allergic interstitial nephritis, glycosuria, fall in glomerular filtration rate and renal blood flow (due to overdiuresis), transient rise in BUN

Miscellaneous: Anaphylaxis (rare), exacerbate or activate systemic lupus erythematosus

Overdosage/Toxicology Symptoms of overdose include electrolyte depletion, volume depletion, hypotension, dehydration, and circulatory collapse. Treatment is supportive.

Pharmacodynamics/Kinetics

Onset of Action: Diuresis: Oral: 30-60 minutes; I.M.: 30 minutes; I.V.: ~5 minutes; Peak effect: Oral: 1-2 hours

Duration of Action: Oral: 6-8 hours; I.V.: 2 hours

Protein Binding: >98%

Half-Life Elimination: Normal renal function: 0.5-1.1 hours; End-stage renal disease: 9 hours

Metabolism: Minimally hepatic

Excretion: Urine (Oral: 50%, I.V.: 80%) within 24 hours; feces (as unchanged drug); nonrenal clearance prolonged with renal impairment

Available Dosage Forms

Injection, solution: 10 mg/mL (2 mL, 4 mL, 8 mL, 10 mL)

Solution, oral: 10 mg/mL (60 mL, 120 mL) [orange flavor]; 40 mg/5 mL (5 mL, 500 mL) [pineapple-peach flavor]

Tablet (Lasix®): 20 mg, 40 mg, 80 mg

Dosing

Adults:

Edema, CHF, or hypertension (diuresis):

Oral: 20-80 mg/dose initially increased in increments of 20-40 mg/dose at intervals of 6-8 hours; usual maintenance dose interval is twice daily or every day

Usual dosage range for hypertension (JNC 7): 20-80 mg/day in 2 divided doses

I.M., I.V.: 20-40 mg/dose, may be repeated in 1-2 hours as needed and increased by 20 mg/dose with each succeeding dose up to 1000 mg/day; usual dosing interval: 6-12 hours. **Note:** ACC/AHA 2005 guidelines for chronic congestive heart failure recommend a maximum single dose of 160-200 mg.

Continuous I.V. infusion: Initial I.V. bolus dose of 0.1 mg/kg followed by continuous I.V. infusion doses of 0.1 mg/kg/hour doubled every 2 hours to a maximum of 0.4 mg/kg/hour if urine output is <1 mL/kg/hour have been found to be effective and result in a lower daily requirement of furosemide than with intermittent dosing. Other studies have used 20-160 mg/hour continuous I.V. infusion. **Note:** ACC/AHA 2005 guidelines for chronic congestive heart failure recommend 40 mg I.V. load then 10-40 mg/hour infusion.

Refractory heart failure: Oral, I.V.: Doses up to 8 g/day have been used.

Elderly: Oral, I.M., I.V.: Initial: 20 mg/day; increase slowly to desired response.

Pediatrics:

Edema, CHF, or hypertension (diuresis): Infants and Children:

Oral: 1-2 mg/kg/dose increased in increments of 1 mg/kg/dose with each succeeding dose until a satisfactory effect is achieved to a maximum of 6 mg/kg/dose no more frequently than 6 hours

I.M., I.V.: 1 mg/kg/dose, increasing by each succeeding dose at 1 mg/kg/dose at intervals of 6-12 hours until a satisfactory response up to 6 mg/kg/dose

Renal Impairment:

Acute renal failure: Doses up to 1-3 g/day may be necessary to initiate desired response; avoid use in oliguric states.

Not removed by hemo- or peritoneal dialysis; supplemental dose is not necessary.

Hepatic Impairment: Diminished natriuretic effect with increased sensitivity to hypokalemia and volume depletion in cirrhosis. Monitor effects, particularly with high doses.

Administration

Oral: May be taken with or without food.

I.V.: I.V. injections should be given slowly. In adults, undiluted direct I.V. injections may be administered at a rate of 40 mg over 1-2 minutes; maximum rate of administration for IVPB or continuous infusion: 4 mg/minute. In children, a maximum rate of 0.5 mg/kg/minute has been recommended.

I.V. Detail: As a general guideline, I.V. bolus doses may be infused at a rate <20 mg/minute.

pH: 8-9.3

Stability

Reconstitution: I.V. infusion solution mixed in NS or D₅W solution is stable for 24 hours at room temperature. May also be diluted for infusion 1-2 mg/mL (maximum: 10 mg/mL) over 10-15 minutes (following infusion rate parameters).

Compatibility: Stable in D₅LR, D₅NS, D₅W, D₁₀W, D₂₀W, mannitol 20%, LR, NS

Y-site administration: Incompatible with alatrofloxacin, amiodarone, amsacrine, chlorpromazine, ciprofloxacin, clarithromycin, diltiazem, droperidol, esmolol, filgrastim, fluconazole, gatifloxacin, gemcitabine, gentamicin, hydralazine, idarubicin, levofloxacin, metoclopramide, midazolam, milrinone, netilmicin, nicardipine, ondansetron, quinidine gluconate, thiopental, vecuronium, vinblastine, vincristine, vinorelbine

Compatibility in syringe: Incompatible with doxapram, doxorubicin, droperidol, metoclopramide, milrinone, vinblastine, vincristine

Compatibility when admixed: Incompatible with buprenorphine, chlorpromazine, diazepam, dobutamine, erythromycin lactobionate, isoproterenol, meperidine, metoclopramide, netilmicin, prochlorperazine edisylate, promethazine

Storage: Furosemide injection should be stored at controlled room temperature and protected from light. Exposure to light may cause discoloration. Do not use furosemide solutions if they have a yellow color. Refrigeration may result in precipitation or crystallization, however, resolubilization at room temperature or warming may be performed without affecting the drugs stability.

Laboratory Monitoring Serum electrolytes, renal function

Nursing Actions

Physical Assessment: Allergy history should be assessed before beginning therapy. Assess potential for interactions with other pharmacological agents or herbal products patient may be taking (especially anything that may impact fluid balance, electrolyte balance, or increase potential for ototoxicity or hypotension). For intravenous use, see Administration specifics. Assess results of laboratory tests (electrolytes), therapeutic effectiveness, and adverse response on a regular basis during therapy (eg, dehydration, electrolyte imbalance, postural hypotension). Caution patients with diabetes about closely monitoring glucose levels (glucose tolerance may be decreased). Teach patient appropriate use, possible side effects/appropriate interventions, and adverse symptoms to report.

Patient Education: Do not take any new medication during therapy unless approved by prescriber. Take as directed with food or milk (to reduce GI distress) early in the day (daily), or if twice daily, take last dose in late afternoon in order to avoid sleep disturbance and achieve maximum therapeutic effect. Keep medication in original container, away from light; do not use discolored medication. Follow dietary advice of prescriber; include bananas or orange juice or other potassium-rich foods in daily diet. Do not take potassium supplements without advice of prescriber. If you are diabetic, monitor glucose levels closely (this medication may alter glucose tolerance requiring an adjustment in the dose of hypoglycemic agent). Weigh yourself each day, at the same time, in the same clothes when beginning therapy and weekly on long-term therapy. Report unusual or unanticipated weight gain or loss. May cause dizziness, blurred vision, or drowsiness (use caution when driving or engaging in tasks that require alertness until response to drug is known); postural hypotension (use caution when rising from lying or sitting position or when climbing stairs); or sensitivity to sunlight (use sunblock or wear protective clothing and sunglasses). Report signs of edema (eg, weight gains, swollen ankles, feet or hands), trembling, numbness or fatigue, cramping or muscle weakness, palpitations, unresolved nausea or vomiting, or change in hearing. **Pregnancy/breast-feeding precautions:** Inform prescriber if you are or intend to become pregnant. Consult prescriber if breast-feeding.

Dietary Considerations May cause a potassium loss; potassium supplement or dietary changes may be required. Administer on an empty stomach. May be administered with food or milk if GI distress occurs. Do not mix with acidic solutions.

Geriatric Considerations Severe loss of sodium and/or increase in BUN can cause confusion. For any change in mental status in patients on furosemide, monitor electrolytes and renal function.

Breast-Feeding Issues Crosses into breast milk; may suppress lactation. AAP has NO RECOMMENDATION.

Pregnancy Issues Crosses the placenta. Increased fetal urine production, electrolyte disturbances reported. Generally, use of diuretics during pregnancy is avoided due to risk of decreased placental perfusion.

Related Information

Compatibility of Drugs *on page 1370*

Gabapentin (GA ba pen tin)

U.S. Brand Names Neurontin®

Pharmacologic Category Anticonvulsant, Miscellaneous

Medication Safety Issues

Sound-alike/look-alike issues:

Neurontin® may be confused with Neoral®, Noroxin®

Pregnancy Risk Factor C

Lactation Enters breast milk/use caution

Use Adjunct for treatment of partial seizures with and without secondary generalized seizures in patients >12 years of age with epilepsy; adjunct for treatment of partial seizures in pediatric patients 3-12 years of age; management of postherpetic neuralgia (PHN) in adults

Unlabeled/Investigational Use Social phobia; chronic pain

Mechanism of Action/Effect Exact mechanism of action is not known, but does have properties in common with other anticonvulsants; although structurally related to GABA, it does not interact with GABA receptors

(Continued)

Gabapentin *(Continued)*

Contraindications Hypersensitivity to gabapentin or any component of the formulation

Warnings/Precautions Avoid abrupt withdrawal, may precipitate seizures; use cautiously in patients with severe renal dysfunction; male rat studies demonstrated an association with pancreatic adenocarcinoma (clinical implication unknown). May cause CNS depression, which may impair physical or mental abilities. Patients must be cautioned about performing tasks which require mental alertness (eg, operating machinery or driving). Effects with other sedative drugs or ethanol may be potentiated. Pediatric patients (3-12 years of age) have shown increased incidence of CNS-related adverse effects, including emotional lability, hostility, thought disorder, and hyperkinesia. Safety and efficacy in children <3 years of age have not been established.

Drug Interactions

Increased Effect/Toxicity: Sedative effects may be additive with CNS depressants; includes ethanol, barbiturates, narcotic analgesics, and other sedative agents; monitor for increased effect

Nutritional/Ethanol Interactions

Ethanol: Avoid ethanol (may increase CNS depression). Food: Does not change rate or extent of absorption. Herb/Nutraceutical: Avoid evening primrose (seizure threshold decreased). Avoid valerian, St John's wort, kava kava, gotu kola (may increase CNS depression).

Lab Interactions False positives have been reported with the Ames N-Multistix SG® dipstick test for urine protein

Adverse Reactions As reported in patients >12 years of age, unless otherwise noted in children (3-12 years)

>10%:

Central nervous system: Somnolence (20%; children 8%), dizziness (17% to 28%; children 3%), ataxia (13%), fatigue (11%)

Miscellaneous: Viral infection (children 11%)

1% to 10%:

Cardiovascular: Peripheral edema (2% to 8%), vasodilatation (1%)

Central nervous system: Fever (children 10%), hostility (children 8%), emotional lability (children 4%), fatigue (children 3%), headache (3%), ataxia (3%), abnormal thinking (2% to 3%; children 2%), amnesia (2%), depression (2%), dysarthria (2%), nervousness (2%), abnormal coordination (1% to 2%), twitching (1%), hyperesthesia (1%)

Dermatologic: Pruritus (1%), rash (1%)

Endocrine & metabolic: Hyperglycemia (1%)

Gastrointestinal: Diarrhea (6%), Nausea/vomiting (3% to 4%; children 8%), abdominal pain (3%), weight gain (adults and children 2% to 3%), dyspepsia (2%), flatulence (2%), dry throat (2%), xerostomia (2% to 5%), constipation (2% to 4%), dental abnormalities (2%), appetite stimulation (1%)

Genitourinary: Impotence (1%)

Hematologic: Leukopenia (1%), decreased WBC (1%)

Neuromuscular & skeletal: Tremor (7%), weakness (6%), hyperkinesia (children 3%), abnormal gait (2%), back pain (2%), myalgia (2%), fracture (1%)

Ocular: Nystagmus (8%), diplopia (1% to 6%), blurred vision (3% to 4%), conjunctivitis (1%)

Otic: Otitis media (1%)

Respiratory: Rhinitis (4%), bronchitis (children 3%), respiratory infection (children 3%), pharyngitis (1% to 3%), cough (2%)

Miscellaneous: Infection (5%)

Overdosage/Toxicology Acute oral overdoses of up to 49 g have been reported; double vision, slurred speech, drowsiness, lethargy, and diarrhea were observed. Patients recovered with supportive care. Decontaminate using lavage/activated charcoal with cathartic. Multiple dosing of activated charcoal may be useful; hemodialysis may be useful.

Pharmacodynamics/Kinetics

Protein Binding: 0%

Half-Life Elimination: 5-7 hours; anuria 132 hours; during dialysis 3.8 hours

Excretion: Proportional to renal function; urine (as unchanged drug)

Available Dosage Forms

Capsule (Neurontin®): 100 mg, 300 mg, 400 mg

Solution, oral (Neurontin®): 250 mg/5 mL (480 mL) [cool strawberry anise flavor]

Tablet: 100 mg, 300 mg, 400 mg

Neurontin®: 600 mg, 800 mg

Dosing

Adults:

Anticonvulsant: Oral:

Initial: 300 mg 3 times/day, if necessary the dose may be increased up to 1800 mg/day

Maintenance: 900-1800 mg/day administered in 3 divided doses; doses of up to 2400 mg/day have been tolerated in long-term clinical studies; up to 3600 mg/day has been tolerated in short-term studies

Note: If gabapentin is discontinued or if another anticonvulsant is added to therapy, it should be done slowly over a minimum of 1 week.

Chronic pain (unlabeled use): Oral: 300-1800 mg/day given in 3 divided doses has been the most common dosage range

Postoperative pain (unlabeled use): 300-1200 mg 1-2 hours before surgery

Postherpetic neuralgia: Day 1: 300 mg, Day 2: 300 mg twice daily, Day 3: 300 mg 3 times/day; dose may be titrated as needed for pain relief (range: 1800-3600 mg/day, daily doses >1800 mg do not generally show greater benefit)

Elderly: Studies in elderly patients have shown a decrease in clearance as age increases. This is most likely due to age-related decreases in renal function; dose reductions may be needed.

Pediatrics:

Anticonvulsant: Oral

Children 3-12 years: Initial: 10-15 mg/kg/day in 3 divided doses; titrate to effective dose over ~3 days; dosages of up to 50 mg/kg/day have been tolerated in clinical studies

Children 3-4 years: Effective dose: 40 mg/kg/day in 3 divided doses

Children ≥5-12 years: Effective dose: 25-35 mg/kg/day in 3 divided doses

Children >12 years: Refer to adult dosing.

Note: If gabapentin is discontinued or if another anticonvulsant is added to therapy, it should be done slowly over a minimum of 1 week

Renal Impairment: Children ≥12 years and Adults: See table.

Hemodialysis: Dialyzable

Gabapentin Dosing Adjustments in Renal Impairment

Creatinine Clearance (mL/min)	Daily Dose Range
≥60	300-1200 mg tid
>30-59	200-700 mg bid
>15-29	200-700 mg daily
15[1]	100-300 mg daily
Hemodialysis[2]	125-350 mg

[1]Cl$_{cr}$<15 mL/minute: Reduce daily dose in proportion to creatinine clearance.

[2]Single supplemental dose administered after each 4 hours of hemodialysis

Administration

Oral: Administer first dose on first day at bedtime to avoid somnolence and dizziness. Dosage must be adjusted for renal function; when given 3 times daily, the maximum time between doses should not exceed 12 hours.

Stability

Storage: Store at 25°C (77°F); excursions permitted to 15°C to 30°C (59°F to 86°F).

Laboratory Monitoring Monitor serum levels of concomitant anticonvulsant therapy. Routine monitoring of gabapentin levels is not mandatory.

Nursing Actions

Physical Assessment: Assess effectiveness and interactions of other medications patient may be taking. Monitor therapeutic response (seizure activity, force, type, duration), laboratory values, and adverse reactions at beginning of therapy and periodically with long-term use. Assess for CNS depression. Taper dosage slowly when discontinuing. Observe and teach seizure/safety precautions. Assess knowledge/teach patient appropriate use, interventions to reduce side effects, and adverse symptoms to report.

Patient Education: Take exactly as directed; do not increase dose or frequency. It may take 2-3 weeks to achieve desired results; may cause physical and/or psychological dependence. If prescribed once-a-day, take dose at bedtime. If taking antacids, take at least 2 hours after antacids. Do not stop medication abruptly, may lead to increased seizure activity. Avoid alcohol, caffeine, and other prescription or OTC medications not approved by prescriber. Maintain adequate hydration (2-3 L/day of fluids) unless instructed to restrict fluid intake. You may experience drowsiness, lightheadedness, impaired coordination, dizziness, or blurred vision (use caution when driving or engaging in tasks requiring alertness until response to drug is known); nausea, vomiting, or anorexia (small frequent meals, frequent mouth care, chewing gum, or sucking lozenges may help); constipation (increased exercise, fluids, fruit, or fiber may help); diarrhea (buttermilk, yogurt, or boiled milk may help); postural hypotension (use caution when climbing stairs or changing position from lying or sitting to standing); or decreased sexual function or libido (reversible). Report persistent CNS effects (nervousness, restlessness, insomnia, anxiety, excitation, headache, sedation, seizures, mania, abnormal thinking); rash or skin irritation; muscle cramping, tremors, or change in gait; chest pain or palpitations; change in urinary pattern; or worsening of condition.

Pregnancy/breast-feeding precautions: Inform prescriber if you are or intend to become pregnant. Breast-feeding is not recommended.

Dietary Considerations May be taken without regard to meals.

Geriatric Considerations No clinical studies to specifically evaluate this drug in the elderly have been performed; however, in premarketing studies, patients >65 years of age did not demonstrate any difference in side effect profiles from younger adults. Since gabapentin is eliminated renally, dose **must** be adjusted for creatinine clearance in the elderly patient.

Breast-Feeding Issues Gabapentin is excreted in human breast milk. A nursed infant could be exposed to ~1 mg/kg/day of gabapentin; the effect on the child is not known. Use in breast-feeding women only if the benefits to the mother outweigh the potential risk to the infant.

Pregnancy Issues No data on crossing the placenta; there have been reports of normal pregnancy outcomes, as well as respiratory distress, pyloric stenosis, and inguinal hernia following 1st trimester exposure to gabapentin plus carbamazepine; epilepsy itself, number of medications, genetic factors, or a combination of these probably influence the teratogenicity of anticonvulsant therapy. Use during pregnancy only if the potential benefit to the mother outweighs the potential risk to the fetus.

Galantamine (ga LAN ta meen)

U.S. Brand Names Razadyne™; Razadyne™ ER; Reminyl® [DSC]

Synonyms Galantamine Hydrobromide

Pharmacologic Category Acetylcholinesterase Inhibitor (Central)

Medication Safety Issues

Sound-alike/look-alike issues:

Reminyl® may be confused with Amaryl®

Due to patient safety concerns regarding prescribing and dispensing errors between Reminyl® and Amaryl®, Reminyl® (galantamine) is being renamed to Razadyne™ (immediate-release) and Razadyne™ ER (extended-release). The brand name Reminyl® will be discontinued with the July, 2005 distribution of Razadyne™.

Pregnancy Risk Factor B

Lactation Excretion in breast milk unknown/not recommended

Use Treatment of mild-to-moderate dementia of Alzheimer's disease

Mechanism of Action/Effect Increases the concentration of acetylcholine in the brain by slowing its metabolism.

Contraindications Hypersensitivity to galantamine or any component of the formulation; severe liver dysfunction (Child-Pugh score 10-15); severe renal dysfunction (Cl_{cr} <9 mL/minute)

Warnings/Precautions May exaggerate neuromuscular blockade effects of depolarizing neuromuscular-blocking agents like succinylcholine. Vagotonic effects on the SA and AV nodes may lead to bradycardia or AV block. Use caution in patients with supraventricular cardiac conduction delays (without a functional pacemaker in place) or patients taking concurrent medications that slow conduction through the SA or AV node. Use caution in peptic ulcer disease (or in patients at risk); seizure disorder; asthma; COPD; mild to moderate liver dysfunction; moderate renal dysfunction. May cause bladder outflow obstruction. Safety and efficacy in children have not been established.

Drug Interactions

Cytochrome P450 Effect: Substrate (minor) of CYP2D6, 3A4

Decreased Effect: Anticholinergic agents are antagonized by galantamine. CYP inducers may decrease galantamine levels.

Increased Effect/Toxicity: Succinylcholine: increased neuromuscular blockade. Amiodarone, beta-blockers without ISA activity, diltiazem, verapamil may increase bradycardia. NSAIDs increase risk of peptic ulcer. Other CYP3A4 inhibitors and other CYP2D6 inhibitors increase levels of galantamine. Concurrent cholinergic agents may have synergistic effects. Digoxin may lead to AV block. Acetylcholinesterase inhibitors (central) may increase the risk of antipsychotic-related extrapyramidal symptoms.

Nutritional/Ethanol Interactions

Ethanol: Avoid ethanol (may increase CNS adverse events).

Herb/Nutraceutical: St John's wort may decrease galantamine serum levels; avoid concurrent use.

Adverse Reactions

>10%: Gastrointestinal: Nausea (6% to 24%), vomiting (4% to 13%), diarrhea (6% to 12%)

1% to 10%:

Cardiovascular: Bradycardia (2% to 3%), syncope (0.4% to 2.2%: dose related), chest pain (≥1%)

Central nervous system: Dizziness (9%), headache (8%), depression (7%), fatigue (5%), insomnia (5%), somnolence (4%)

(Continued)

Galantamine *(Continued)*

Gastrointestinal: Anorexia (7% to 9%), weight loss (5% to 7%), abdominal pain (5%), dyspepsia (5%), flatulence (≥1%)

Genitourinary: Urinary tract infection (8%), hematuria (<1% to 3%), incontinence (≥1%)

Hematologic: Anemia (3%)

Neuromuscular & skeletal: Tremor (3%)

Respiratory: Rhinitis (4%)

Overdosage/Toxicology Symptoms of overdose may include bradycardia, collapse, convulsions, defecation, gastrointestinal cramping, hypotension, lacrimation, muscle fasciculations, muscle weakness, QT prolongation, respiratory depression, salivation, severe nausea, sweating, torsade de pointes, urination, ventricular tachycardia, vomiting. Treatment is symptom-directed and supportive. Atropine may be used as an antidote; initial dose 0.5-1 mg I.V. and titrate to effect. An atypical response in blood pressure and heart rate has been reported. Effects of hemodialysis are unknown.

Pharmacodynamics/Kinetics

Duration of Action: 3 hours; maximum inhibition of erythrocyte acetylcholinesterase ~40% at 1 hour post 8 mg oral dose; levels return to baseline at 30 hours

Time to Peak: Immediate release: 1 hour (2.5 hours with food); extended release: 4.5-5 hours

Protein Binding: 18%

Half-Life Elimination: 7 hours

Metabolism: Hepatic; linear, CYP2D6 and 3A4; metabolized to epigalanthaminone and galanthaminone both of which have acetylcholinesterase inhibitory activity 130 times less than galantamine

Excretion: Urine (25%)

Available Dosage Forms

Capsule, extended release, as hydrobromide (Razadyne™ ER): 8 mg, 16 mg, 24 mg [contains gelatin]

Solution, oral, as hydrobromide (Razadyne™): 4 mg/mL (100 mL) [with calibrated pipette]

Tablet, as hydrobromide (Razadyne™): 4 mg, 8 mg, 12 mg

Dosing

Adults & Elderly:

Alzheimer's dementia (mild-to-moderate): Oral:

Immediate release tablet or solution: Mild-to-moderate dementia of Alzheimer's: Initial: 4 mg twice a day for 4 weeks; if tolerated, increase to 8 mg twice daily for ≥4 weeks; if tolerated, increase to 12 mg twice daily

Range: 16-24 mg/day in 2 divided doses

Extended-release capsule: Initial: 8 mg once daily for 4 weeks; if tolerated, increase to 16 mg once daily for ≥4 weeks; if tolerated, increase to 24 mg once daily

Range: 16-24 mg once daily

Note: Oral solution and tablet should be taken with breakfast and dinner; capsule should be taken with breakfast. If therapy is interrupted for ≥3 days, restart at the lowest dose and increase to current dose.

Conversion to galantamine from other cholinesterase inhibitors: Patients experiencing poor tolerability with donepezil or rivastigmine should wait until side effects subside or allow a 7-day washout period prior to beginning galantamine. Patients not experiencing side effects with donepezil or rivastigmine may begin galantamine therapy the day immediately following discontinuation of previous therapy (Morris, 2001).

Renal Impairment:

Moderate renal impairment: Maximum dose: 16 mg/day.

Severe renal dysfunction (Cl$_{cr}$ <9 mL/minute): Use is not recommended

Hepatic Impairment:

Moderate liver dysfunction (Child-Pugh score 7-9): Maximum dose: 16 mg/day

Severe liver dysfunction (Child-Pugh score 10-15): Use is not recommended

Administration

Oral: Administer oral solution or tablet with breakfast and dinner; administer extended release capsule with breakfast. If therapy is interrupted for ≥3 days, restart at the lowest dose and increase to current dose. If using oral solution, mix dose with 3-4 ounces of any nonalcoholic beverage; mix well and drink immediately.

Stability

Storage: Store at 15°C to 30°C (59°F to 86°F). Do not freeze oral solution; protect from light.

Nursing Actions

Physical Assessment: Assess bladder and sphincter adequacy prior to administering. Note other medications patient may be taking for effectiveness and interactions. Monitor effectiveness of therapeutic response and adverse reactions at beginning of therapy and periodically throughout period of therapy (eg, cholinergic crisis). Assess knowledge/teach appropriate use, interventions to reduce side effects, and adverse symptoms to report.

Patient Education: This medication will not cure Alzheimer's disease, but may help reduce symptoms. Use exactly as directed; do not increase dose or discontinue without consulting prescriber. Maintain adequate hydration (2-3 L/day of fluids) unless instructed to restrict fluid intake. May cause dizziness, sedation, hypotension, or tremor (use caution when driving or engaging in hazardous tasks, rise slowly from sitting or lying position, and use caution when climbing stairs until response to drug is known); diarrhea (boiled milk, yogurt, or buttermilk may help); or nausea or vomiting (small frequent meals, good mouth care, sucking lozenges, or chewing gum may help). Report persistent GI disturbances; significantly increased salivation, sweating, or tearing; excessive fatigue, insomnia, dizziness, or depression; increased muscle, joint, or body pain or spasms; vision changes; respiratory changes, wheezing, or signs of dyspnea; chest pain or palpitations; or other adverse reactions. **Breast-feeding precaution:** Breast-feeding is not recommended.

Dietary Considerations

Administration with food is preferred, but not required; should be taken with breakfast and dinner (tablet or solution) or with breakfast (capsule).

Gallium Nitrate (GAL ee um NYE trate)

U.S. Brand Names Ganite™

Synonyms NSC-15200

Pharmacologic Category Calcium-Lowering Agent

Pregnancy Risk Factor C

Lactation Excretion in breast milk unknown/not recommended

Use Treatment of hypercalcemia

Mechanism of Action/Effect Inhibits bone resorption by inhibiting osteoclast function

Contraindications Hypersensitivity to gallium nitrate or any component of the formulation; severe renal dysfunction (creatinine >2.5 mg/dL)

Warnings/Precautions Hazardous agent - use appropriate precautions for handling and disposal. Use caution with renal impairment or when administering other nephrotoxic drugs (eg, aminoglycosides, amphotericin B); consider discontinuing gallium nitrate during treatment with nephrotoxic drugs. Maintain adequate hydration. Safety and efficacy in pediatric patients have not been established.

Drug Interactions

Increased Effect/Toxicity: Concurrent use of low-dose gallium nitrate with cyclophosphamide has been associated with dyspnea, stomatitis, asthenia, and rarely interstitial pneumonitis. Concurrent use nephrotoxic drugs (eg, aminoglycosides, amphotericin B) with gallium nitrate may increase nephrotoxic effects.

Adverse Reactions Not all frequencies defined.

Cardiovascular: Hypotension, tachycardia, edema of lower extremities

Central nervous system: Lethargy, confusion, dreams, hallucinations, hypothermia, fever

Dermatologic: Rash

Endocrine & metabolic: Hypophosphatemia (>50%, usually asymptomatic); hypocalcemia; mild respiratory alkalosis with hyperchloremia

Hematologic: Anemia, leukopenia

Gastrointestinal: Nausea (14%, generally mild), vomiting, diarrhea, constipation

Neuromuscular & skeletal: Paresthesia

Renal: Nephrotoxicity (>10%, generally reversible and reported to be minimized with adequate hydration and urine output)

Respiratory: Dyspnea, rales, rhonchi, pleural effusion, pulmonary infiltrates

Note: Toxicities reported with doses higher than those used to treat hypercalcemia (ie, in trials evaluating anticancer effect): Optic neuritis, tinnitus, hearing acuity decreased, metallic taste, hypomagnesemia, encephalopathy

Overdosage/Toxicology Symptoms of overdose include nausea, vomiting, and increased risk of nephrotoxicity.

Pharmacodynamics/Kinetics

Onset of Action: Onset of calcium lowering: Seen within 24-48 hours of beginning therapy, with normocalcemia achieved within 4-7 days of beginning therapy

Half-Life Elimination: Alpha: 1.25 hours; Beta: ~24 hours

Elimination half-life varies with method of administration (72-115 hours with prolonged intravenous infusion versus 24 hours with bolus administration); long elimination half-life may be related to slow release from tissue such as bone

Excretion: Primarily renal with no prior metabolism in the liver or kidney; long elimination half-life may be related to slow release from tissue such as bone; elimination half-life varies with method of administration (72-115 hours with prolonged intravenous infusion versus 24 hours with bolus administration)

Available Dosage Forms Injection, solution [preservative free]: 25 mg/mL (20 mL)

Dosing

Adults: Hypercalcemia: I.V.: 200 mg/m²/day for 5 days; duration may be shortened during a course if normocalcemia is achieved. If hypercalcemia is mild and with very few symptoms, 100 mg/m²/day may be used.

Renal Impairment:

Serum creatinine >2.5 mg/dL: Contraindicated

Serum creatinine 2 to <2.5 mg/dL: No guidelines exist; frequent monitoring is recommended.

Administration

I.V.: I.V. infusion over 30 minutes to 24 hours

Stability

Reconstitution: Dilute in 250-1000 mL NS or D₅W for infusion

Storage: Store unopened vials (25 mg/mL) at room temperature of 15°C to 30°C (59°F to 86°F); not light sensitive. Solutions in 0.9% NaCl or D₅W are stable for 48 hours at room temperature or for 7 days under refrigeration at 2°C to 8°C (36°F to 46°F).

Laboratory Monitoring Renal function, serum calcium (daily), serum phosphorus (twice weekly)

Nursing Actions

Physical Assessment: Assess potential for interactions with other pharmacological agents patient may be taking (eg, risk of nephrotoxicity). Assess results of laboratory tests, therapeutic effectiveness (calcium levels), and adverse response (eg, hypotension, tachycardia, gastrointestinal upset, hypocalcemia) on a regular basis throughout therapy. Teach patient possible side effects/appropriate interventions, and adverse symptoms to report.

Patient Education: This medication is given by intravenous infusion; report immediately any redness, swelling, or pain at infusion site. Report chest pain or palpitations, difficulty breathing, rash, CNS changes (confusion, dreams, hallucinations); numbness, pain, or tingling in extremities; unusual and persistent fatigue or lethargy; changes in urinary pattern or output; or other adverse reactions. **Pregnancy/breast-feeding precautions:** Inform prescriber if you are or intend to become pregnant. Inform prescriber if you intend to breast-feed.

Breast-Feeding Issues Due to the potential for adverse reactions in the nursing infant, it is recommended to discontinue nursing during treatment or discontinue gallium nitrate.

Ganciclovir (gan SYE kloe veer)

U.S. Brand Names Cytovene®; Vitrasert®

Synonyms DHPG Sodium; GCV Sodium; Nordeoxyguanosine

Pharmacologic Category Antiviral Agent

Medication Safety Issues

Sound-alike/look-alike issues:

Cytovene® may be confused with Cytosar®, Cytosar-U®

Pregnancy Risk Factor C

Lactation Excretion in breast milk unknown/contraindicated

Use

Parenteral: Treatment of CMV retinitis in immunocompromised individuals, including patients with acquired immunodeficiency syndrome; prophylaxis of CMV infection in transplant patients

Oral: Alternative to the I.V. formulation for maintenance treatment of CMV retinitis in immunocompromised patients, including patients with AIDS, in whom retinitis is stable following appropriate induction therapy and for whom the risk of more rapid progression is balanced by the benefit associated with avoiding daily I.V. infusions.

Implant: Treatment of CMV retinitis

Unlabeled/Investigational Use May be given in combination with foscarnet in patients who relapse after monotherapy with either drug

Mechanism of Action/Effect Ganciclovir is phosphorylated to a substrate which competitively inhibits the binding of deoxyguanosine triphosphate to DNA polymerase resulting in inhibition of viral DNA synthesis.

Contraindications Hypersensitivity to ganciclovir, acyclovir, or any component of the formulation; absolute neutrophil count <500/mm³; platelet count <25,000/mm³

Warnings/Precautions Hazardous agent - use appropriate precautions for handling and disposal. Dosage adjustment or interruption of ganciclovir therapy may be necessary in patients with neutropenia and/or thrombocytopenia and patients with impaired renal function. Use with extreme caution in children since long-term safety has not been determined and due to ganciclovir's potential for long-term carcinogenic and adverse reproductive effects. Ganciclovir may adversely affect spermatogenesis and fertility. Due to its mutagenic potential, contraceptive precautions for female and male patients need to be followed during and for at least 90 days after (Continued)

Ganciclovir *(Continued)*

therapy with the drug. Take care to administer only into veins with good blood flow.

Drug Interactions

Decreased Effect: A decrease in blood levels of ganciclovir AUC may occur when used with didanosine.

Increased Effect/Toxicity: Immunosuppressive agents may increase hematologic toxicity of ganciclovir. Imipenem/cilastatin may increase seizure potential. Oral ganciclovir increases blood levels of zidovudine, although zidovudine decreases steady-state levels of ganciclovir. Since both drugs have the potential to cause neutropenia and anemia, some patients may not tolerate concomitant therapy with these drugs at full dosage. Didanosine levels are increased with concurrent ganciclovir. Other nephrotoxic drugs (eg, amphotericin and cyclosporine) may have additive nephrotoxicity with ganciclovir.

Adverse Reactions

>10%:

Central nervous system: Fever (38% to 48%)

Dermatologic: Rash (15% and, 10% I.V.)

Gastrointestinal: Abdominal pain (17% to 19%), diarrhea (40%), nausea (25%), anorexia (15%), vomiting (13%)

Hematologic: Anemia (20% to 25%), leukopenia (30% to 40%)

1% to 10%:

Central nervous system: Confusion, neuropathy (8% to 9%), headache (4%)

Dermatologic: Pruritus (5%)

Hematologic: Thrombocytopenia (6%), neutropenia with ANC <500/mm^3 (5% oral, 14% I.V.)

Neuromuscular & skeletal: Paresthesia (6% to 10%), weakness (6%)

Ocular: Retinal detachment (8% oral, 11% I.V.; relationship to ganciclovir not established)

Miscellaneous: Sepsis (4% oral, 15% I.V.)

Overdosage/Toxicology Symptoms of overdose include neutropenia, vomiting, hypersalivation, bloody diarrhea, cytopenia, and testicular atrophy. Treatment is supportive. Hemodialysis removes 50% of the drug. Hydration may be of some benefit.

Pharmacodynamics/Kinetics

Protein Binding: 1% to 2%

Half-Life Elimination: 1.7-5.8 hours; prolonged with renal impairment; End-stage renal disease: 5-28 hours

Excretion: Urine (80% to 99% as unchanged drug)

Available Dosage Forms

Capsule: 250 mg, 500 mg

Cytovene®: 250 mg, 500 mg [DSC]

Implant, intravitreal (Vitrasert®): 4.5 mg [released gradually over 5-8 months]

Injection, powder for reconstitution, as sodium (Cytovene®): 500 mg

Dosing

Adults & Elderly: Dosing is based on total body weight.

CMV retinitis:

I.V. (slow infusion):

Induction therapy: 5 mg/kg/dose every 12 hours for 14-21 days followed by maintenance therapy

Maintenance therapy: 5 mg/kg/day as a single daily dose for 7 days/week or 6 mg/kg/day for 5 days/week

Oral: 1000 mg 3 times/day with food **or** 500 mg 6 times/day with food

Ocular implant: Intravitreally: One implant for 5- to 8-month period; following expected depletion of ganciclovir, as evidenced by progression of retinitis, implant may be removed and replaced

Prevention of CMV disease in patients with advanced HIV infection and normal renal function: Oral: 1000 mg 3 times/day with food

Prevention of CMV disease in transplant patients: Same initial and maintenance dose as CMV retinitis except duration of initial course is 7-14 days, duration of maintenance therapy is dependent on clinical condition and degree of immunosuppression

Pediatrics: CMV retinitis: Children >3 months: Refer to adult dosing.

Renal Impairment:

I.V. (Induction):

Cl_{cr} 50-69 mL/minute: Administer 2.5 mg/kg/dose every 12 hours.

Cl_{cr} 25-49 mL/minute: Administer 2.5 mg/kg/dose every 24 hours.

Cl_{cr} 10-24 mL/minute: Administer 1.25 mg/kg/dose every 24 hours.

Cl_{cr} <10 mL/minute: Administer 1.25 mg/kg/dose 3 times/week following hemodialysis.

I.V. (Maintenance):

Cl_{cr} 50-69 mL/minute: Administer 2.5 mg/kg/dose every 24 hours.

Cl_{cr} 25-49 mL/minute: Administer 1.25 mg/kg/dose every 24 hours.

Cl_{cr} 10-24 mL/minute: Administer 0.625 mg/kg/dose every 24 hours

Cl_{cr} <10 mL/minute: Administer 0.625 mg/kg/dose 3 times/week following hemodialysis.

Oral:

Cl_{cr} 50-69 mL/minute: Administer 1500 mg/day or 500 mg 3 times/day.

Cl_{cr} 25-49 mL/minute: Administer 1000 mg/day or 500 mg twice daily.

Cl_{cr} 10-24 mL/minute: Administer 500 mg/day.

Cl_{cr} <10 mL/minute: Administer 500 mg 3 times/week following hemodialysis.

Hemodialysis effects: Dialyzable (50%) following hemodialysis; administer dose postdialysis. During peritoneal dialysis, dose as for Cl_{cr} <10 mL/minute. During continuous arteriovenous or venovenous hemofiltration, administer 2.5 mg/kg/dose every 24 hours.

Administration

Oral: Should be administered with food.

I.V.: Should not be administered by I.M., SubQ, or rapid IVP. Administer by slow I.V. infusion over at least 1 hour. Too rapid infusion can cause increased toxicity and excessive plasma levels.

I.V. Detail: Flush line well with NS before and after administration.

pH: 11

Stability

Reconstitution: Reconstitute powder with unpreserved sterile water not bacteriostatic water because parabens may cause precipitation. Dilute in 250-1000 mL D_5W or NS to a concentration ≤10 mg/mL for infusion. Reconstituted solution is stable for 12 hours at room temperature, however, conflicting data indicates that reconstituted solution is stable for 60 days under refrigeration (4°C). Stability of parenteral admixture at room temperature (25°C) and at refrigeration temperature (4°C) is 5 days.

Compatibility: Stable in D_5W, LR, NS; **incompatible** with paraben preserved bacteriostatic water for injection (may cause precipitation)

Y-site administration: Incompatible with aldesleukin, amifostine, amsacrine, aztreonam, cefepime, cytarabine, doxorubicin, fludarabine, foscarnet, gemcitabine, ondansetron, piperacillin/tazobactam, sargramostim, vinorelbine

Storage: Intact vials should be stored at room temperature and protected from temperatures >40°C.

Laboratory Monitoring CBC with differential and platelet count, serum creatinine before beginning therapy and on a regular basis thereafter; liver function tests

Nursing Actions

Physical Assessment: Assess potential for interactions with other pharmacological agents patient may be taking that may result in increased risk for neutropenia, hematologic toxicity, or nephrotoxicity. **I.V.:** See Administration for infusion specifics. Assess results of laboratory tests prior to therapy and on a regular basis during therapy. Evaluate therapeutic effectiveness and adverse response (eg, paresthesia, neutropenia, anemia, nephrotoxicity, retinal detachment) throughout therapy. Teach proper use (according to formulation), possible side effects/appropriate interventions (importance of contraceptive precautions during and for 90 days following therapy), and adverse symptoms to report.

Patient Education: Do not take any new medication during therapy unless approved by prescriber. Ganciclovir is not a cure for CMV retinitis. For oral administration, take as directed and maintain adequate hydration (2-3 L/day of fluids) unless instructed to restrict fluid intake. You will need frequent blood tests and regular ophthalmic exams while taking this drug. You may experience increased susceptibility to infection (avoid crowds and exposure to infection and do not have any vaccinations without consulting prescriber). You may experience confusion or headache (use cautions when driving or engaging in potentially hazardous tasks until response to drug is known); nausea, vomiting, or anorexia (small, frequent meals, frequent mouth care, chewing gum, or sucking lozenges may help); diarrhea (buttermilk, boiled milk, or yogurt may help); or photosensitivity (use sunscreen, wear protective clothing and eyewear, and avoid direct sunlight). Report rash, infection (fever, chills, unusual bleeding or bruising, or unhealed sores or white plaques in mouth); abdominal pain; tingling, weakness, or pain in extremities; any vision changes; or pain, redness, swelling at injection site. **Pregnancy/breast-feeding precautions:** Inform prescriber if you are pregnant. Males and females should use appropriate barrier contraceptive measures during and for 60-90 days following end of therapy. Consult prescriber for appropriate barrier contraceptive measures. Do not breast-feed.

Dietary Considerations Sodium content of 500 mg vial: 46 mg

Geriatric Considerations Adjust dose based upon renal function.

Breast-Feeding Issues The CDC recommends **not** to breast-feed if diagnosed with HIV to avoid postnatal transmission of the virus.

Ganirelix (ga ni REL ix)

U.S. Brand Names Antagon®
Synonyms Ganirelix Acetate
Pharmacologic Category Gonadotropin Releasing Hormone Antagonist
Pregnancy Risk Factor X
Lactation Excretion in breast milk unknown/not recommended
Use Inhibits premature luteinizing hormone (LH) surges in women undergoing controlled ovarian hyperstimulation in fertility clinics.
Mechanism of Action/Effect Suppresses gonadotropin secretion and luteinizing hormone secretion to prevent ovulation until the follicles are of adequate size.
Contraindications Hypersensitivity to ganirelix or any component of the formulation; hypersensitivity to gonadotropin-releasing hormone or any other analog; known or suspected pregnancy

Warnings/Precautions Should only be prescribed by fertility specialists. The packaging contains natural rubber latex (may cause allergic reactions). Pregnancy must be excluded before starting medication.

Drug Interactions
Decreased Effect: No formal studies have been performed.
Increased Effect/Toxicity: No formal studies have been performed.

Adverse Reactions 1% to 10%:
Central nervous system: Headache (3%)
Endocrine & metabolic: Ovarian hyperstimulation syndrome (2%)
Gastrointestinal: Abdominal pain (5%), nausea (1%), and abdominal pain (1%)
Genitourinary: Vaginal bleeding (2%)
Local: Injection site reaction (1%)

Pharmacodynamics/Kinetics
Time to Peak: 1.1 hours
Protein Binding: 81.9%
Half-Life Elimination: 16.2 hours
Metabolism: Hepatic to two primary metabolites (1-4 and 1-6 peptide)
Excretion: Feces (75%) within 288 hours; urine (22%) within 24 hours

Available Dosage Forms Injection, solution, as acetate: 250 mcg/0.5 mL [prefilled glass syringe with 27-gauge x ½ inch needle]

Dosing
Adults & Elderly: Adjunct to controlled ovarian hyperstimulation: SubQ: 250 mcg/day during the mid-to-late phase after initiating follicle-stimulating hormone on day 2 or 3 of cycle. Treatment should be continued daily until the day of chorionic gonadotropin administration.

Stability
Storage: Store at controlled room temperature of 15°C to 30°C (59°F to 86°F).

Laboratory Monitoring Ultrasound to assess the follicle's size

Nursing Actions
Physical Assessment: This medication should only be prescribed by a fertility specialist. Assess/teach patient use (demonstrate injection procedures, syringe disposal), interventions to reduce side-effects, and adverse reactions to report. **Pregnancy risk factor X:** Pregnancy must be excluded before starting medication.

Patient Education: This drug can only be given by injection as demonstrated. Use this and any other medications as directed by prescriber; do not skip any doses. You must keep all scheduled ultrasound appointments. You may experience headache (use of mild analgesic may help); or nausea (small frequent meals, good mouth care, chewing gum, or sucking hard candy may help). Report immediately any sudden or acute abdominal pain; vaginal bleeding; or pain, itching, or signs of infection at injection site. **Note:** Packaging contains natural rubber latex; if you have a known latex allergy, advise prescriber. **Pregnancy/breast-feeding precautions:** Do not get pregnant while taking this drug. Breast-feeding is not recommended.

Pregnancy Issues Fetal resorption occurred in pregnant rats and rabbits. These effects are results of hormonal alterations and could result in fetal loss in humans. The drug should not be used in pregnant women.

Gatifloxacin (gat i FLOKS a sin)

U.S. Brand Names Tequin®; Zymar™

Pharmacologic Category Antibiotic, Ophthalmic; Antibiotic, Quinolone

Pregnancy Risk Factor C

Lactation Excretion in breast milk unknown/use caution

Use

Oral, I.V.: Treatment of the following infections when caused by susceptible bacteria: Acute bacterial exacerbation of chronic bronchitis; acute sinusitis; community-acquired pneumonia including pneumonia caused by multidrug-resistant *S. pneumoniae* (MDRSP); uncomplicated skin and skin structure infection; uncomplicated urinary tract infections (cystitis); complicated urinary tract infections; pyelonephritis; uncomplicated urethral and cervical gonorrhea; acute, uncomplicated rectal infections in women

Ophthalmic: Bacterial conjunctivitis

Unlabeled/Investigational Use *Legionella*

Mechanism of Action/Effect Inhibits bacterial DNA

Contraindications Hypersensitivity to gatifloxacin, other quinolone antibiotics, or any component of the formulation; diabetes mellitus

Warnings/Precautions Use with caution in patients with significant bradycardia (or receiving drugs which may cause bradycardia), acute myocardial ischemia, cardiovascular disease (especially with conduction disturbances), or individuals at risk of seizures (CNS disorders or concurrent therapy with medications which may lower seizure threshold). May cause increased CNS stimulation, increased intracranial pressure, convulsions, or psychosis. Discontinue in patients who experience significant CNS adverse effects (dizziness, hallucinations, suicidal ideation or actions), cardiovascular adverse effects (QT prolongation [concentration dependent], arrhythmia) or hypersensitivity reactions. Use caution in patients with known prolongation of QT interval, uncorrected hypokalemia, or concurrent administration of other medications known to prolong the QT interval (including Class Ia and Class III antiarrhythmics, cisapride, erythromycin, antipsychotics, and tricyclic antidepressants). Use caution in renal dysfunction and severe hepatic insufficiency. Serious disruptions in glucose regulation (including hyperglycemia and severe hypoglycemia) may occur, usually (but not always) in patients with diabetes. Other risk factors for glucose dysregulation include advanced age, renal insufficiency, and use of concurrent medications which alter glucose utilization. Hypoglycemia may be more prevalent in the initial 3 days of therapy while a greater risk of hyperglycemia may be present after the initial 3 days (particularly days 4-10). Monitor closely and discontinue if hyper- or hypoglycemia occur. Quinolones may exacerbate myasthenia gravis. May cause peripheral neuropathy (rare); discontinue if symptoms of sensory or sensorimotor neuropathy occur. Do not inject ophthalmic solution subconjunctivally or introduce directly into the anterior chamber of the eye.

Pseudomembranous colitis should be considered in all patients with diarrhea. Tendon inflammation and/or rupture has been reported with this and other quinolone antibiotics. Risk may be increased with concurrent corticosteroids, particularly in the elderly. Discontinue at first sign of tendon inflammation or pain. Safety and efficacy for ophthalmic use have not been established in children <1 year of age. Safety and efficacy for systemic use have not been established in patients <18 years of age.

Drug Interactions

Decreased Effect: Concurrent administration of metal cations, including most antacids (not calcium carbonate), oral electrolyte supplements, quinapril, sucralfate, some didanosine formulations (chewable/

buffered tablets and pediatric powder for oral suspension), and other highly-buffered oral drugs, may decrease quinolone levels; separate doses.

Increased Effect/Toxicity: Gatifloxacin may increase the effects/toxicity of hypoglycemic agents and warfarin. Concomitant use with corticosteroids may increase the risk of tendon rupture. Concomitant use with other QT_c-prolonging agents (eg, Class Ia and Class III antiarrhythmics, erythromycin, cisapride, antipsychotics, and cyclic antidepressants) may result in arrhythmias, such as torsade de pointes. Probenecid may increase gatifloxacin levels. Atypical antipsychotics and protease inhibitors may cause hyperglycemia; use with caution and monitor.

Nutritional/Ethanol Interactions

Ethanol: Caution with ethanol (may cause hypoglycemia).

Herb/Nutraceutical: Avoid dong quai, St John's wort (may also cause photosensitization); caution with chromium, garlic, gymnema (may cause hypoglycemia).

Lab Interactions Some quinolones may produce a false-positive urine screening result for opiates using commercially-available immunoassay kits. This has been demonstrated most consistently for levofloxacin and ofloxacin, but other quinolones have shown cross-reactivity in certain assay kits. Confirmation of positive opiate screens by more specific methods should be considered.

Adverse Reactions

Systemic therapy:

3% to 10%:

Central nervous system: Headache (3%), dizziness (3%)

Gastrointestinal: Nausea (8%), diarrhea (4%)

Genitourinary: Vaginitis (6%)

Local: Injection site reactions (5%)

0.1% to 3%: Abdominal pain, abnormal dreams, abnormal vision, agitation, alkaline phosphatase increased, allergic reaction, anorexia, anxiety, arthralgia, back pain, chest pain, chills, confusion, constipation, diaphoresis, dry skin, dyspepsia, dyspnea, dysuria, facial edema, fever, flatulence, gastritis, glossitis, hematuria, hyperglycemia, hypertension, insomnia, leg cramps, mouth ulceration, nervousness, oral candidiasis, palpitation, paresthesia, peripheral edema, pharyngitis, pruritus, rash, serum amylase increased, serum bilirubin increased, serum transaminases increased, somnolence, stomatitis, taste perversion, thirst, tinnitus, tremor, weakness, vasodilation, vertigo, vomiting

Ophthalmic therapy:

5% to 10%: Ocular: Conjunctival irritation, keratitis, lacrimation increased, papillary conjunctivitis

1% to 4%:

Central nervous system: Headache

Gastrointestinal: Taste disturbance

Ocular: Chemosis, conjunctival hemorrhage, discharge, dry eye, edema, irritation, pain, visual acuity decreased

Overdosage/Toxicology Potential symptoms of overdose may include CNS excitation, seizures, QT prolongation, and arrhythmias (including torsade de pointes). Patients should be monitored by continuous ECG in the event of an overdose. Management is supportive and symptomatic. Not removed by dialysis.

Pharmacodynamics/Kinetics

Time to Peak: Oral: 1 hour

Protein Binding: 20%

Half-Life Elimination: 7.1-13.9 hours; ESRD/CAPD: 30-40 hours

Metabolism: Only 1%; no interaction with CYP

Excretion: Excretion: Urine (70% as unchanged drug, <1% as metabolites); feces (5%)

Available Dosage Forms

Injection, infusion [premixed in D_5W] (Tequin®): 200 mg (100 mL); 400 mg (200 mL)

Injection, solution [preservative free] (Tequin®): 10 mg/mL (40 mL)

Solution, ophthalmic (Zymar™): 0.3% (2.5 mL, 5 mL) [contains benzalkonium chloride]

Tablet (Tequin®): 200 mg, 400 mg

Tequin® Teq-paq™ [unit-dose pack]: 400 mg (5s)

Dosing

Adults & Elderly:

Acute bacterial exacerbation of chronic bronchitis: Oral, I.V.: 400 mg every 24 hours for 5 days

Acute sinusitis: Oral, I.V.: 400 mg every 24 hours for 10 days

Bacterial conjunctivitis: Ophthalmic:

Days 1 and 2: Instill 1 drop into affected eye(s) every 2 hours while awake (maximum: 8 times/day)

Days 3-7: Instill 1 drop into affected eye(s) up to 4 times/day while awake

Community-acquired pneumonia: Oral, I.V.: 400 mg every 24 hours for 7-14 days

Legionella (unlabeled use): Oral, I.V.: 400 mg once daily for 10-21 days

Pyelonephritis (acute): Oral, I.V.: 400 mg every 24 hours for 7-10 days

Skin/skin structure infections (uncomplicated): Oral, I.V.: 400 mg every 24 hours for 7-10 days

Traveler's diarrhea (unlabeled use): Oral, I.V.: 400 mg once daily for 3 days

Urinary tract infections: Oral, I.V.:

Complicated: 400 mg every 24 hours for 7-10 days

Uncomplicated, cystitis: 400 mg single dose or 200 mg every 24 hours for 3 days

Urethral gonorrhea in men (uncomplicated), cervical or rectal gonorrhea in women and pharyngitis (gonococcal): Oral, I.V.: 400 mg single dose

Pediatrics: Bacterial conjunctivitis: Children ≥1 year: Ophthalmic: Refer to adult dosing.

Renal Impairment: Creatinine clearance <40 mL/minute (or patients on hemodialysis/CAPD) should receive an initial dose of 400 mg, followed by a subsequent dose of 200 mg every 24 hours. Patients receiving single-dose or 3-day therapy for appropriate indications do not require dosage adjustment. Administer after hemodialysis.

Hepatic Impairment: No dosage adjustment is required in mild-moderate hepatic disease. No data are available in severe hepatic impairment (Child-Pugh Class C).

Administration

Oral: May be administered with or without food, milk, or calcium supplements. Gatifloxacin should be taken 4 hours before supplements (including multivitamins) containing iron, zinc, or magnesium.

I.V.: For I.V. infusion only. Concentrated injection (10 mg/mL) must be diluted to 2 mg/mL prior to administration. No further dilution is required for premixed 100 mL and 200 mL solutions. Infuse over 60 minutes. Avoid rapid or bolus infusions.

Stability

Reconstitution:

Solution for injection: Single-use vials must be diluted to a concentration of 2 mg/mL prior to administration; may be diluted with D_5W, NS, D_5NS, D_5LR, 5% sodium bicarbonate, or Plasma-Lyte® 56 and D_5W. Do not dilute with SWFI (a hypertonic solution results).

Compatibility: Stable in D_5LR, D_5W, D_5NS, 5% dextrose or 0.45% sodium chloride containing up to 20 mEq/L potassium chloride, M/6 sodium lactate, NS, Plasma-Lyte® 56/5% dextrose injection, 5% sodium bicarbonate injection; **incompatible** with SWFI (results in a hypertonic solution)

Y-site administration: Incompatible with amphotericin B, amphotericin B cholesteryl sulfate complex, cefoperazone, cefoxitin, diazepam, furosemide, heparin, phenytoin, piperacillin, piperacillin/tazobactam, potassium phosphates, vancomycin

Storage:

Ophthalmic solution: Store between 15°C to 25°C (59°F to 77°F). Do not freeze.

Solution for injection: Store at 25°C (77°F). Do not freeze. Following dilution, stable for 14 days when stored between 20°C to 25°C or 2° to 8°C. Diluted solutions (except those prepared in 5% sodium bicarbonate) may also be frozen for up to 6 months when stored at -25°C to -10°C (-13°F to 14°F). Solutions may then be thawed at room temperature and should be used within 14 days (store between 20°C to 25°C or 2°C to 8°C). Do not refreeze.

Tablet: Store at 25°C (77°F).

Laboratory Monitoring WBC

Nursing Actions

Physical Assessment: Assess allergy history before initiating therapy. Assess potential for interactions with other pharmacological agents or herbal products patient may be taking (eg, increased risk of bradycardia, arrhythmias, tendon rupture, electrolyte imbalance). Assess WBC results, therapeutic effectiveness (resolution of infection), and adverse effects (eg, hyper/hypoglycemia, hypersensitivity, opportunistic infection, pseudomembraneous colitis, tendon inflammation) regularly during therapy. Caution patient with diabetes to monitor glucose levels closely; may cause serious disruptions in glucose regulation (hyperglycemia or severe hypoglycemia). Teach patient appropriate use (according to formulation), possible side effects/appropriate interventions, and adverse symptoms to report.

Patient Education: Do not take any new medication during therapy without consulting prescriber. **Pregnancy/breast-feeding precautions:** Inform prescriber if you are or intend to be pregnant. Breast-feeding is not recommended.

I.V.: Report any redness, pain, burning at infusion site, swelling of mouth or lips, difficulty breathing, or other adverse effects.

Ophthalmic: Tilt head back and instill drops in affected eye as often as directed for length of time prescribed. Do not allow dropper to touch any surface, including the eyes or hands. Apply light pressure to the inside corner of the eye (near the nose) after each drop. Do not wear contact lenses if being treated for a bacterial eye infection. May cause some temporary stinging, burning, itching, redness or tearing; eyelid swelling or itching, or a bad taste in mouth after instillation. Report persistent pain, burning, swelling, or visual disturbances.

Oral: Take exactly as directed with or without food. Should be taken at least 3 hours before or 2 hours after antacids or other drug products containing calcium, iron, magnesium, or zinc (including multivitamins). Take entire prescription even if feeling better. Maintain adequate hydration (2-3 L/day of fluids, unless instructed to restrict fluids). May cause headache or dizziness (use caution when driving or engaging in tasks requiring alertness until response is known); nausea, vomiting, or abdominal discomfort (small, frequent meals, good mouth care, chewing gum, or sucking hard candy may help); diarrhea (consult prescriber if persistent). If signs of inflammation or tendon pain occur, discontinue use immediately and report to prescriber. Discontinue use immediately and report to prescriber if you experience signs of allergic reaction (eg, itching, rash, respiratory difficulty, facial edema, or difficulty swallowing), chest (Continued)

Gatifloxacin (Continued)

pain or palpitations. Report CNS changes (hallucinations, suicidal ideation, seizures) or signs of opportunistic infection (unusual fever or chills; vaginal itching, foul smelling vaginal discharge; easy bruising or bleeding; tendon or muscle pain).

Dietary Considerations May take tablets with or without food, milk, or calcium supplements. Gatifloxacin should be taken 4 hours before supplements (including multivitamins) containing iron, zinc, or magnesium.

Breast-Feeding Issues Other quinolones are known to be excreted in breast milk. The manufacturer recommends using caution if gatifloxacin is administered while nursing.

Pregnancy Issues Reports of arthropathy (observed in immature animals and reported rarely in humans) have limited the use of fluoroquinolones during pregnancy. Gatifloxacin has been show to be fetotoxic in animal studies. There are no adequate and well-controlled studies in pregnant women. Based on limited data, quinolones are not expected to be a major human teratogen. Although quinolone antibiotics should not be used as first-line agents during pregnancy, when considering treatment for life-threatening infection and/or prolonged duration of therapy, the potential risk to the fetus must be balanced against the severity of the potential illness.

Gefitinib (ge Fl tye nib)

U.S. Brand Names IRESSA®

Synonyms NSC-715055; ZD1839

Restrictions As of September 15, 2005, distribution will be limited to patients enrolled in the Iressa Access Program. This has been developed as part of a risk-management plan by AstraZeneca and the FDA. Under this program, access to gefitinib will be limited to the following groups:

Patients who are currently receiving and benefitting from gefitinib (IRESSA®)

Patients who have previously received and benefited from gefitinib (IRESSA®)

Previously-enrolled patients or new patients in non-Investigational New Drug (IND) clinical trials involving gefitinib (IRESSA®) if these protocols were approved by an IRB prior to June 17, 2005

New patients may also receive Iressa if the manufacturer (AstraZeneca) decides to make it available under IND, and the patients meet the criteria for enrollment under the IND

Additional information on the IRESSA® Access Program, including enrollment forms, may be obtained by calling AstraZeneca at 1-800-601-8933 or via the web at www.Iressa-access.com

Pharmacologic Category Antineoplastic Agent, Tyrosine Kinase Inhibitor

Medication Safety Issues

Sound-alike/look-alike issues:

Gefitinib may be confused with erlotinib

Pregnancy Risk Factor D

Lactation Excretion in breast milk unknown/not recommended

Use

U.S. Labeling: Monotherapy for continued treatment of locally advanced or metastatic nonsmall cell lung cancer after failure of platinum-based and docetaxel therapies. Treatment is limited to patients who are benefiting or have benefited from treatment with gefitinib.

Note: Due to the lack of improved survival data from clinical trials of gefitinib, and in response to positive survival data with another EGFR inhibitor, physicians are advised to use other treatment options in advanced nonsmall cell lung cancer patients following one or two prior chemotherapy regimens

when they are refractory/intolerant to their most recent regimen.

Canada labeling: Approved indication is limited to NSCLC patients with epidermal growth factor receptor (EGFR) expression status positive or unknown.

Mechanism of Action/Effect The mechanism of gefitinib is not fully understood. Gefitinib inhibits tyrosine kinase activity, particularly in the epidermal growth factor receptor (EGFR), resulting in inhibition of cell growth and reproduction. It might also inhibit angiogenesis in the tumor.

Contraindications Hypersensitivity to gefitinib or any component of the formulation; pregnancy

Warnings/Precautions Rare, sometimes fatal, pulmonary toxicity (eg, alveolitis, interstitial pneumonia, pneumonitis) has occurred. Therapy should be interrupted in patients with acute onset or worsening pulmonary symptoms; discontinue gefitinib if interstitial pneumonitis is confirmed. Use caution in hepatic or severe renal impairment. May cause hepatic injury and elevation of transaminases; discontinue if elevations/changes are severe. Interruption of therapy may be required in patients with poorly tolerated diarrhea or adverse skin reactions. Eye pain should be promptly evaluated and therapy may be interrupted based on appropriate medical evaluation; may be re-initiated following resolution of symptoms and eye changes. Safety and efficacy in pediatric patients have not been established.

Drug Interactions

Cytochrome P450 Effect: Substrate of CYP3A4 (major); **Inhibits** CYP2C19 (weak), 2D6 (weak)

Decreased Effect: Gefitinib effects may be decreased by H_2-receptor blockers and sodium bicarbonate. CYP3A4 inducers may decrease the levels/effects of gefitinib; example inducers include aminoglutethimide, carbamazepine, nafcillin, nevirapine, phenobarbital, phenytoin, and rifamycins.

Increased Effect/Toxicity: Gefitinib may increase the effects of warfarin. CYP3A4 inhibitors may increase the levels/effects of gefitinib; example inhibitors include azole antifungals, clarithromycin, diclofenac, doxycycline, erythromycin, imatinib, isoniazid, nefazodone, nicardipine, propofol, protease inhibitors, quinidine, telithromycin, and verapamil.

Nutritional/Ethanol Interactions Food: Grapefruit juice may increase serum gefitinib concentrations; St John's wort may decrease serum gefitinib concentrations.

Adverse Reactions

>10%:

Dermatologic: Rash (43% to 54%), acne (25% to 33%), dry skin (13% to 26%)

Gastrointestinal: Diarrhea (48% to 76%), nausea (13% to 18%), vomiting (9% to 12%)

1% to 10%:

Cardiovascular: Peripheral edema (2%)

Dermatologic: Pruritus (8% to 9%)

Gastrointestinal: Anorexia (7% to 10%), weight loss (3% to 5%), mouth ulceration (1%)

Neuromuscular & skeletal: Weakness (4% to 6%)

Ocular: Amblyopia (2%), conjunctivitis (1%)

Respiratory: Dyspnea (2%), interstitial lung disease (1% to 2%)

Overdosage/Toxicology No specific overdose-related toxicities reported; Overdose management should be symptom-based and supportive.

Pharmacodynamics/Kinetics

Time to Peak: Plasma: Oral: 3-7 hours

Protein Binding: 90%, albumin and alpha$_1$-acid glycoprotein

Half-Life Elimination: I.V.: 48 hours

Metabolism: Hepatic, primarily via CYP3A4; forms metabolites

Excretion: Feces (86%); urine (<4%)

Available Dosage Forms Tablet: 250 mg

Dosing

Adults: Note: In response to the lack of improved survival data from the ISEL trial, AstraZeneca has temporarily suspended promotion of this drug.

Nonsmall cell lung cancer: Oral: 250 mg/day; consider 500 mg/day in patients receiving effective CYP3A4 inducers (eg, rifampin, phenytoin)

Elderly: No adjustment necessary. Refer to adult dosing.

Renal Impairment: No adjustment necessary.

Hepatic Impairment: No adjustment necessary.

Dosing Adjustment for Toxicity:

Consider interruption of therapy in any patient with evidence of pulmonary decompensation or severe hepatic injury; discontinuation may be required if toxicity is confirmed. Poorly tolerated diarrhea or adverse skin reactions may be managed by a brief interruption of therapy (up to 14 days), followed by reinitiation of therapy at 250 mg/day. Eye pain should be promptly evaluated and therapy may be interrupted based on appropriate medical evaluation; may be reinitiated following resolution of symptoms and eye changes.

Administration

Oral: May administer with or without food.

For patients unable to swallow tablets or for administration via NG tube: Tablets may be dispersed in noncarbonated drinking water. Drop whole tablet (do not crush) into ½ glass of water; stir until tablet is dispersed (~10 minutes). Drink immediately. Rinse with ½ glass of water and drink.

Stability

Storage: Store tablets at controlled room temperature of 20°C to 25°C (68°F to 77°F).

Laboratory Monitoring Periodic liver function tests (asymptomatic increases in liver enzymes have occurred)

Nursing Actions

Physical Assessment: Assess potential for interactions with other pharmacological agents or herbal products patient may be taking (eg, increased or decreased levels/effects of gefitinib). Assess results of liver function tests on a regular basis. Teach patient proper use, possible side effects/appropriate interventions, and adverse symptoms to report.

Patient Education: Do not take any new medication during therapy without consulting prescriber. Take exactly as directed with or without food. Do not take with grapefruit juice and do not take antacids 2 hours before or 2 hours after taking this mediation. You will need periodic laboratory tests while taking this medication. Maintain adequate hydration (2-3 L/day of fluids) unless instructed to restrict fluid intake. You may experience loss of appetite, nausea and vomiting (small, frequent meals and frequent mouth care may help), or diarrhea (buttermilk, boiled milk, or yogurt may help). Report immediately persistent diarrhea; skin rash; unusual or persistent respiratory difficulty or wheezing; chest pain or cough; any change in vision, eye pain, or signs of eye infection; unusual weakness or joint pain; or other persistent adverse reactions. **Pregnancy/breast-feeding precautions:** Inform prescriber if you are pregnant. Do not get pregnant. Consult prescriber for appropriate contraceptive measures while on this medication. Breast-feeding is not recommended.

Dietary Considerations Food does not affect gefitinib absorption.

Pregnancy Issues Animal studies have demonstrated fetal harm; there are no well-controlled studies in pregnant women. The risk of fetal harm should be carefully weighed. Women of childbearing potential should be advised to avoid pregnancy.

Gemcitabine (jem SITE a been)

U.S. Brand Names Gemzar®

Synonyms Gemcitabine Hydrochloride

Pharmacologic Category Antineoplastic Agent, Antimetabolite (Pyrimidine Antagonist)

Medication Safety Issues

Sound-alike/look-alike issues:

Gemzar® may be confused with Zinecard®

Pregnancy Risk Factor D

Lactation Excretion in breast milk unknown/contraindicated

Use

Adenocarcinoma of the pancreas: First-line therapy in locally-advanced (nonresectable stage II or stage III) or metastatic (stage IV) adenocarcinoma of the pancreas

Breast cancer: First-line therapy in metastatic breast cancer

Nonsmall-cell lung cancer: First-line therapy in locally-advanced (stage IIIA or IIIB) or metastatic (stage IV) nonsmall-cell lung cancer

Unlabeled/Investigational Use Bladder cancer, ovarian cancer

Mechanism of Action/Effect A pyrimidine antimetabolite that inhibits DNA synthesis by inhibition of DNA polymerase and ribonucleotide reductase, specific for the S-phase of the cycle.

Contraindications Hypersensitivity to gemcitabine or any component of the formulation; pregnancy

Warnings/Precautions Hazardous agent — use appropriate precautions for handling and disposal. Prolongation of the infusion time >60 minutes and more frequent than weekly dosing have been shown to increase toxicity. Gemcitabine can suppress bone marrow function manifested by leukopenia, thrombocytopenia and anemia, and myelosuppression is usually the dose-limiting toxicity. Gemcitabine may cause fever in the absence of clinical infection. Pulmonary toxicity has occurred; discontinue if severe. Use with caution in patients with pre-existing renal or hepatic impairment. Safety and efficacy have not been established with radiation therapy or in pediatric patients.

Drug Interactions

Decreased Effect: No confirmed interactions have been reported. No specific drug interaction studies have been conducted.

Nutritional/Ethanol Interactions Ethanol: Avoid ethanol (due to GI irritation).

Adverse Reactions Percentages reported with single-agent therapy for pancreatic cancer and other malignancies.

>10%:

Central nervous system: Pain (42% to 48%; grades 3 and 4: <1% to 9%), fever (38% to 41%; grades 3 and 4: ≤2%), somnolence (11%; grades 3 and 4: <1%). Fever was reported to occur in the absence of infection in pancreatic cancer treatment.

Dermatologic: Rash (28% to 30%; grades 3 and 4: <1%), alopecia (15% to 16%; grades 3 and 4: <1%). Rash in pancreatic cancer treatment was typically a macular or finely-granular maculopapular pruritic eruption of mild-to-moderate severity involving the trunk and extremities.

Gastrointestinal: Nausea and vomiting (69% to 71%; grades 3 and 4: 1% to 13%), constipation (23% to 31%; grades 3 and 4: <1% to 3%), diarrhea (19% to 30%; grades 3 and 4: ≤3%), stomatitis (10% to 11%; grades 3 and 4: <1%)

Hematologic: Anemia (73% to 68%; grades 3 and 4: 1% to 8%), leukopenia (62% to 64%; grades 3 and 4: <1% to 9%), neutropenia (61% to 63%; grades 3 and 4: 6% to 19%), thrombocytopenia (24% to 36%; grades 3 and 4: <1% to 7%), hemorrhage (4% to (Continued)

Gemcitabine *(Continued)*

17%; grades 3 or 4: <1%). Myelosuppression may be the dose-limiting toxicity with pancreatic cancer

Hepatic: Transaminases increased (68% to 78%; grades 3 and 4: 1% to 12%), alkaline phosphatase increased (55% to 77%; grades 3 and 4: 2% to 16%), bilirubin increased (13% to 26%; grades 3 or 4: <1% to 6%). Serious hepatotoxicity was reported rarely in pancreatic cancer treatment.

Renal: Proteinuria (32% to 45%; grades 3 and 4: <1%), hematuria (23% to 35%; grades 3 and 4: <1%), BUN increased (15% to 16%; grades 3 and 4: 0%)

Respiratory: Dyspnea (10% to 23%; grades 3 and 4: <1% to 3%)

Miscellaneous: Infection (10% to 16%; grades 3 or 4: <1% to 2%)

1% to 10%:

Local: Injection site reactions (4%)

Neuromuscular & skeletal: Paresthesias (10%)

Renal: Creatinine increased (6% to 8%)

Respiratory: Bronchospasm (<2%)

Overdosage/Toxicology Symptoms of overdose include myelosuppression, paresthesia, and severe rash. The principle toxicities were seen when a single dose as high as 5700 mg/m^2 was administered by I.V. infusion over 30 minutes every 2 weeks. Monitor blood counts and administer supportive therapy as needed.

Pharmacodynamics/Kinetics

Time to Peak: 30 minutes

Protein Binding: Low

Half-Life Elimination:

Gemcitabine: Infusion time ≤1 hour: 32-94 minutes; infusion time 3-4 hours: 4-10.5 hours

Metabolite (gemcitabine triphosphate), terminal phase: 1.7-19.4 hours

Metabolism: Hepatic, metabolites: di- and triphosphates (active); uridine derivative (inactive)

Excretion: Urine (99%, 92% to 98% as intact drug or inactive uridine metabolite); feces (<1%)

Available Dosage Forms Injection, powder for reconstitution, as hydrochloride: 200 mg, 1 g

Dosing

Adults & Elderly: Refer to individual protocols. **Note:** Prolongation of the infusion time >60 minutes and administration more frequently than once weekly have been shown to increase toxicity. I.V.:

Pancreatic cancer: Initial: 1000 mg/m^2 over 30 minutes once weekly for up to 7 weeks followed by 1 week rest; subsequent cycles once weekly for 3 consecutive weeks out of every 4 weeks.

Dose adjustment: Patients who complete an entire cycle of therapy may have the dose in subsequent cycles increased by 25% as long as the absolute granulocyte count (AGC) nadir is >1500 x 10^6/L, platelet nadir is >100,000 x 10^6/L, and nonhematologic toxicity is less than WHO Grade 1. If the increased dose is tolerated (with the same parameters) the dose in subsequent cycles may again be increased by 20%.

Nonsmall cell lung cancer:

28-day cycle: 1000 mg/m^2 over 30 minutes on days 1, 8, 15; repeat every 28 days

or

21-day cycle: 1250 mg/m^2 over 30 minutes on days 1, 8; repeat every 21 days

Breast cancer: 1250 mg/m^2 over 30 minutes on days 1 and 8 of each 21-day cycle

Bladder cancer (unlabeled use): 1000 mg/m^2 once weekly for 3 weeks; repeat cycle every 4 weeks

Ovarian cancer (unlabeled use): 1000 mg/m^2 once weekly for 3 weeks; repeat cycle every 4 weeks

Renal Impairment: Use with caution; has not been studied in patients with significant renal dysfunction.

Hepatic Impairment: Use with caution; gemcitabine has not been studied in patients with significant hepatic dysfunction.

Dosing Adjustment for Toxicity:

Pancreatic cancer: Hematologic toxicity:

AGC ≥1000 x 10^6/L and platelet count ≥100,000 x 10^6/L: Administer 100% of full dose

AGC 500-999 x 10^6/L or platelet count 50,000-90,000 x 10^6/L: Administer 75% of full dose

AGC <500 x 10^6/L or platelet count <50,000 x 10^6/L: Hold dose

Nonsmall-cell lung cancer:

Hematologic toxicity: Refer to guidelines for pancreatic cancer. Cisplatin dosage may also need adjusted.

Severe (grades 3 or 4) nonhematologic toxicity (except alopecia, nausea, and vomiting): Hold or decrease dose by 50%.

Breast cancer:

Hematologic toxicity: Adjustments based on granulocyte and platelet counts on day 8:

AGC ≥1200 x 10^6/L and platelet count ≥75,000 x 10^6/L: Administer 100% of full dose

AGC 1000-1199 x 10^6/L or platelet count ≥50,000-75,000 x 10^6/L: Administer 75% of full dose

AGC 700-999 x 10^6/L and platelet count ≥ 50,000 x 10^6/L: Administer 50% of full dose

AGC <700 x 10^6/L or platelet count <50,000 x 10^6/L: Hold dose

Severe (grades 3 or 4) nonhematologic toxicity (except alopecia, nausea, and vomiting): Hold or decrease dose by 50%. Paclitaxel dose may also need adjusted.

Administration

I.V.: Administer over 30 minutes. **Note:** Prolongation of the infusion time >60 minutes has been shown to increase toxicity.

Stability

Reconstitution: Reconstitute the 200 mg vial with preservative free 0.9% NaCl 5 mL or the 1000 mg vial with preservative free 0.9% NaCl 25 mL. Resulting solution is ~38 mg/mL, but is variable. Dilute with 50-500 mL 0.9% sodium chloride injection or D$_5$W to concentrations as low as 0.1 mg/mL.

Compatibility: Stable in D$_5$W, NS

Y-site administration: Incompatible with acyclovir, amphotericin B, cefoperazone, cefotaxime, furosemide, ganciclovir, imipenem/cilastatin, irinotecan, methotrexate, methylprednisolone sodium succinate, mitomycin, piperacillin, piperacillin/tazobactam, prochlorperazine edisylate

Storage: Store intact vials at room temperature (20°C to 25°C/68°F to 77°F). Reconstituted vials and infusion solutions diluted in 0.9% sodium chloride are stable up to 24 hours. Do not refrigerate.

Laboratory Monitoring Monitor CBC, including differential and platelet count, prior to each dose. Renal and hepatic function should be performed prior to initiation of therapy and periodically thereafter.

Nursing Actions

Physical Assessment: See specific Administration directions (adverse reactions increase when infused over >60 minutes). Assess results of laboratory tests (eg, CBC with differential and platelet count), prior to each dose. Monitor patient response (symptom relief) and adverse reactions (eg, CNS changes, rash, gastrointestinal upset, anemia, myelosuppression, dyspnea) prior to each treatment and on a regular basis throughout therapy. Teach patient possible side effects/appropriate interventions and adverse symptoms to report.

Patient Education: Do not take any new medication during therapy unless approved by prescriber. This drug can only be administered by infusion; report any redness, pain, or swelling at infusion site. During therapy, do not use alcohol. Maintain adequate hydration (2-3 L/day of fluids) unless instructed to restrict fluid intake, and nutrition (small, frequent meals may help). You will be more susceptible to infection (avoid crowds and exposure to infection and do not have any vaccinations without consulting prescriber). You may experience fatigue, lethargy, somnolence (use caution when driving or engaging in potentially hazardous tasks until response to drug is known); nausea or vomiting (small, frequent meals, frequent mouth care, sucking lozenges, or chewing gum may help); loss of hair (reversible); mouth sores (frequent mouth care and use of a soft toothbrush or cotton swabs may help); or diarrhea (buttermilk, boiled milk, or yogurt may help reduce diarrhea). This drug may cause sterility. Report extreme fatigue; severe GI upset or diarrhea; bleeding or bruising; fever, chills, sore throat; vaginal discharge; signs of fluid retention (swelling extremities, respiratory difficulty, unusual weight gain); yellowing of skin or eyes; change in color of urine or stool; muscle or skeletal pain or weakness; or other persistent adverse effects. **Pregnancy/breast-feeding precautions**: Inform prescriber if you are pregnant. Do not get pregnant while taking this medication. Consult prescriber for appropriate barrier contraceptive measures. This drug may cause severe fetal birth defects. Do not breast-feed.

Geriatric Considerations Clearance is affected by age. There is no evidence; however, that unusual dose adjustment is necessary in patients older than 65 years of age. In general, adverse reaction rates were similar to patients older and younger than 65 years. Grade 3/4 thrombocytopenia was more common in the elderly.

Pregnancy Issues It is embryotoxic causing fetal malformations (cleft palate, incomplete ossification, fused pulmonary artery, absence of gallbladder) in animals. There are no studies in pregnant women. If patient becomes pregnant she should be informed of risks.

Gemfibrozil (jem FI broe zil)

U.S. Brand Names Lopid®

Synonyms CI-719

Pharmacologic Category Antilipemic Agent, Fibric Acid

Medication Safety Issues
Sound-alike/look-alike issues:
Lopid® may be confused with Levbid®, Lodine®, Lorabid®, Slo-bid™

Pregnancy Risk Factor C

Lactation Excretion in breast milk unknown/contraindicated

Use Treatment of hypertriglyceridemia in types IV and V hyperlipidemia for patients who are at greater risk for pancreatitis and who have not responded to dietary intervention

Mechanism of Action/Effect Inhibits lipolysis and decreases subsequent hepatic fatty acid uptake and hepatic secretion of VLDL; decreases serum levels of VLDL and increases HDL levels

Contraindications Hypersensitivity to gemfibrozil or any component of the formulation; significant hepatic or renal dysfunction; primary biliary cirrhosis; pre-existing gallbladder disease

Warnings/Precautions Possible increased risk of malignancy and cholelithiasis. No evidence of cardiovascular mortality benefit. Anemia and leukopenia have been reported. Elevations in serum transaminases can be seen. Discontinue if lipid response not seen. Be careful in patient selection; this is not a first- or second-line choice. Other agents may be more suitable.

Adjustments in warfarin therapy may be required with concurrent use. Use caution when combining gemfibrozil with HMG-CoA reductase inhibitors (may lead to myopathy, rhabdomyolysis). Renal function deterioration has been seen in patients with a serum creatinine >2.0 mg/dL. Safety and efficacy in pediatric patients have not been established.

Drug Interactions

Cytochrome P450 Effect: Substrate of CYP3A4 (minor); **Inhibits** CYP1A2 (moderate), 2C8/9 (strong), 2C19 (strong)

Decreased Effect: Cyclosporine's blood levels may be reduced during concurrent therapy. Rifampin may decrease gemfibrozil blood levels.

Increased Effect/Toxicity: Gemfibrozil may potentiate the effects of bexarotene (avoid concurrent use), sulfonylureas (including glyburide, chlorpropamide), and warfarin. HMG-CoA reductase inhibitors (atorvastatin, fluvastatin, lovastatin, pravastatin, simvastatin) may increase the risk of myopathy and rhabdomyolysis. The manufacturer warns against the concurrent use of lovastatin (if unavoidable, limit lovastatin to <20 mg/day). Combination therapy with statins has been used in some patients with resistant hyperlipidemias (with great caution). Gemfibrozil may increase the serum concentration of repaglinide (resulting in severe, prolonged hypoglycemia); the addition of itraconazole may augment the effects of gemfibrozil on repaglinide (consider alternative therapy). Gemfibrozil may increase the levels/effects of aminophylline, amiodarone, citalopram, diazepam, fluoxetine, fluvoxamine, glimepiride, glipizide, methsuximide, mexiletine, mirtazapine, nateglinide, phenytoin, pioglitazone, propranolol, ropinirole, rosiglitazone, sertraline, theophylline, trifluoperazine, warfarin, and other substrates of CYP1A2, 2C8/9, or 2C19.

Nutritional/Ethanol Interactions Ethanol: Avoid ethanol to decrease triglycerides.

Adverse Reactions
>10%: Gastrointestinal: Dyspepsia (20%)
1% to 10%:
Central nervous system: Fatigue (4%), vertigo (2%), headache (1%)
Dermatologic: Eczema (2%), rash (2%)
Gastrointestinal: Abdominal pain (10%), diarrhea (7%), nausea/vomiting (3%), constipation (1%)

Reports where causal relationship has not been established: Weight loss, extrasystoles, pancreatitis, hepatoma, colitis, confusion, seizure, syncope, retinal edema, decreased fertility (male), renal dysfunction, positive ANA, drug-induced lupus-like syndrome, thrombocytopenia, anaphylaxis, vasculitis, alopecia, photosensitivity

Overdosage/Toxicology Symptoms of overdose include abdominal pain, diarrhea, nausea, and vomiting. Treatment is supportive.

Pharmacodynamics/Kinetics
Onset of Action: May require several days
Time to Peak: Serum: 1-2 hours
Protein Binding: 99%
Half-Life Elimination: 1.4 hours
Metabolism: Hepatic via oxidation to two inactive metabolites; undergoes enterohepatic recycling
Excretion: Urine (70% primarily as conjugated drug); feces (6%)

Available Dosage Forms Tablet: 600 mg

Dosing
Adults & Elderly: Hyperlipidemia/hypertriglyceridemia: Oral: 1200 mg/day in 2 divided doses, 30 minutes before breakfast and dinner

Renal Impairment: Hemodialysis effects: Not removed by hemodialysis; supplemental dose is not necessary.

Laboratory Monitoring Serum cholesterol, LFTs
(Continued)

577

Gemfibrozil *(Continued)*

Nursing Actions

Physical Assessment: Assess potential for interactions with other pharmacological agents patient may be taking (eg, increased risk of myopathy, rhabdomyolysis, hypoglycemia, and toxicity). Assess results of laboratory tests (serum cholesterol and LFTs), therapeutic effectiveness (decreased lipid levels), and adverse reactions periodically during therapy. Teach proper use, possible side effects/appropriate interventions, and adverse symptoms to report.

Patient Education: Do not take any new medication during therapy unless approved by prescriber. Should be taken 30 minutes before meals. Take with milk or meals if GI upset occurs. Avoid alcohol. Follow dietary recommendations of prescriber. You will need check-ups and blood work to assess effectiveness of therapy. You may experience loss of appetite and flatulence (small, frequent meals may help); or diarrhea (buttermilk, boiled milk, or yogurt may help). Report severe stomach pain, nausea, vomiting; headache; persistent diarrhea; or vision changes. **Pregnancy/breast-feeding precautions:** Inform prescriber if you are or intend to become pregnant. Do not breast-feed.

Dietary Considerations Before initiation of therapy, patients should be placed on a standard cholesterol-lowering diet for 3-6 months and the diet should be continued during drug therapy.

Geriatric Considerations Gemfibrozil is the drug of choice for the treatment of hypertriglyceridemia and hypoalphaproteinemia in the elderly; it is usually well tolerated; myositis may be more common in patients with poor renal function.

Gemifloxacin *(je mi FLOKS a sin)*

U.S. Brand Names Factive®

Synonyms DW286; Gemifloxacin Mesylate; LA 20304a; SB-265805

Pharmacologic Category Antibiotic, Quinolone

Pregnancy Risk Factor C

Lactation Excretion in breast milk unknown/not recommended

Use Treatment of acute exacerbation of chronic bronchitis; treatment of community-acquired pneumonia, including pneumonia caused by multidrug-resistant strains of *S. pneumoniae* (MDRSP)

Unlabeled/Investigational Use Acute sinusitis, uncomplicated urinary tract infection

Mechanism of Action/Effect Gemifloxacin is a DNA gyrase inhibitor and also inhibits topoisomerase IV. These enzymes are required for DNA replication and transcription, DNA repair, recombination, and transposition; quinolones are bactericidal

Contraindications Hypersensitivity to gemifloxacin, other fluoroquinolones, or any component of the formulation

Warnings/Precautions Fluoroquinolones may prolong QT_c interval; avoid use of gemifloxacin in patients with uncorrected hypokalemia, hypomagnesemia, or concurrent administration of other medications known to prolong the QT interval (including class Ia and class III antiarrhythmics, cisapride, erythromycin, antipsychotics, and tricyclic antidepressants). Use with caution in patients with significant bradycardia or acute myocardial ischemia. Use with caution in individuals at risk of seizures (CNS disorders or concurrent therapy with medications which may lower seizure threshold). Discontinue in patients who experience significant CNS adverse effects (dizziness, hallucinations, suicidal ideation or actions). Use caution in renal dysfunction (dosage adjustment required).

Severe hypersensitivity reactions, including anaphylaxis, have occurred with quinolone therapy. If an allergic reaction occurs (itching, urticaria, dyspnea or facial edema, loss of consciousness, tingling, cardiovascular collapse), discontinue drug immediately. Prolonged use may result in superinfection; pseudomembranous colitis may occur and should be considered in all patients who present with diarrhea. Tendon inflammation and/or rupture has been reported with other quinolone antibiotics; risk may increase with concurrent corticosteroids, particularly in the elderly. Discontinue at first sign of tendon inflammation or pain. Peripheral neuropathy has been linked to the use of quinolones; these cases were rare. Experience with quinolones in immature animals has resulted in permanent arthropathy. Safety and effectiveness in pediatric patients (<18 years of age) have not been established.

Drug Interactions

Decreased Effect: Concurrent administration of metal cations, including most antacids, oral electrolyte supplements, quinapril, sucralfate, some didanosine formulations (chewable/buffered tablets and pediatric powder for oral suspension), and other highly-buffered oral drugs, may decrease quinolone levels; separate doses.

Increased Effect/Toxicity: Gemifloxacin may increase the effects/toxicity of glyburide and warfarin. Concomitant use with corticosteroids may increase the risk of tendon rupture. Concomitant use with other QT_c-prolonging agents (eg, Class Ia and Class III antiarrhythmics, erythromycin, cisapride, antipsychotics, and cyclic antidepressants) may result in arrhythmias, such as torsade de pointes. Probenecid may increase gemifloxacin levels.

Nutritional/Ethanol Interactions Herb/Nutraceutical: Avoid dong quai, St John's wort (may also cause photosensitization).

Adverse Reactions

1% to 10%:

Central nervous system: Headache (1%), dizziness (1%)

Dermatologic: Rash (3%)

Gastrointestinal: Diarrhea (4%), nausea (3%), abdominal pain (1%), vomiting (1%)

Hepatic: Transaminases increased (1% to 2%)

Important adverse effects reported with other agents in this drug class include (not reported for gemifloxacin): Allergic reactions, CNS stimulation, hepatitis, jaundice, peripheral neuropathy, pneumonitis (eosinophilic); seizure; sensorimotor-axonal neuropathy (paresthesia, hypoesthesias, dysesthesias, weakness); severe dermatologic reactions (toxic epidermal necrolysis, Stevens-Johnson syndrome); tendon rupture, torsade de pointes, vasculitis

Overdosage/Toxicology Treatment should be symptom-directed and supportive; 20% to 30% removed by hemodialysis.

Pharmacodynamics/Kinetics

Time to Peak: Plasma: 1-2 hours

Protein Binding: 60% to 70%

Half-Life Elimination: 7 hours (range 4-12 hours)

Metabolism: Hepatic (minor); forms metabolites (CYP isoenzymes are not involved)

Excretion: Urine (30% to 40%); feces (60%)

Available Dosage Forms Tablet, as mesylate: 320 mg

Dosing

Adults & Elderly:

Susceptible infections: Oral: 320 mg once daily

Acute exacerbations of chronic bronchitis: Oral: 320 mg once daily for 5 days

Community-acquired pneumonia (mild to moderate): Oral: 320 mg once daily for 7 days

Sinusitis (unlabeled use): Oral: 320 mg once daily for 10 days

Renal Impairment: Cl_{cr} ≤40 mL/minute (or patients on hemodialysis/CAPD): 160 mg once daily (administer dose following hemodialysis)

Hepatic Impairment: No adjustment required.

Administration

Oral: May be administered with or without food, milk, or calcium supplements. Gemifloxacin should be taken 3 hours before or 2 hours after supplements (including multivitamins) containing iron, zinc, or magnesium.

Stability

Storage: Store at 25°C (77°F); excursions permitted to 15°C to 30°C (59°F to 86°F). Protect from light.

Laboratory Monitoring WBC

Nursing Actions

Physical Assessment: Allergy history should be ascertained prior to initiating therapy. Assess potential for interactions with other pharmacological agents or herbal products patient may be taking (eg, increased risk of tendon rupture or arrhythmias). Monitor therapeutic effectiveness (resolution of infection) and adverse effects regularly during therapy (eg, hypersensitivity, opportunistic infection, pseudomembraneous colitis, tendon inflammation). Teach patient proper use, possible side effects/appropriate interventions, and adverse symptoms to report.

Patient Education: Do not take any new medication during therapy without consulting prescriber. Take exactly as directed (with or without food). Should be taken at least 3 hours before or 2 hours after antacids or other drug products containing calcium, iron, magnesium, or zinc (including multivitamins). Take entire prescription, even if feeling better. Unless instructed to restrict fluid intake, maintain adequate hydration (2-3 L/day of fluids) to avoid concentrated urine and crystal formation. May cause headache or dizziness (use caution when driving or engaging in hazardous tasks until response to drug is known); nausea, vomiting, or abdominal discomfort (small, frequent meals, frequent mouth care, chewing gum, or sucking lozenges may help); diarrhea (consult prescriber if persistent). If signs of inflammation or tendon pain occur, discontinue use immediately and report to prescriber. Discontinue use immediately and report to prescriber if you experience signs of allergic reaction (eg, itching, rash, respiratory difficulty, facial edema, or difficulty swallowing); chest pain, or palpitations. Report CNS changes (eg, hallucinations, suicidal ideation, seizures) or signs of opportunistic infection (unusual fever or chills; vaginal itching or foul-smelling vaginal discharge; easy bruising or bleeding; tendon or muscle pain). **Pregnancy/breast-feeding precautions:** Inform prescriber if you are or intend to become pregnant. Breast-feeding is not recommended.

Dietary Considerations May take tablets with or without food, milk, or calcium supplements. Gemifloxacin should be taken 3 hours before or 2 hours after supplements (including multivitamins) containing iron, zinc, or magnesium.

Geriatric Considerations The risk of torsade de pointes and tendon inflammation and/or rupture associated with the concomitant use of corticosteroids and quinolones is increased in the elderly population. Adjust dose for renal function.

Breast-Feeding Issues Other quinolones are known to be excreted in breast milk. The manufacturer recommends using gemifloxacin while breast-feeding only if the possible benefit to the mother outweighs the possible risk to the infant.

Pregnancy Issues There are no adequate and well-controlled studies in pregnant women. Reports of arthropathy (observed in immature animals and reported rarely in humans) have limited the use of fluoroquinolones in pregnancy. Reversible fetal growth retardation was observed with gemifloxacin in some animal studies. Based on limited data, quinolones are not expected to be a major human teratogen. Although quinolone antibiotics should not be used as first-line agents during pregnancy, when considering treatment for life-threatening infection and/or prolonged duration of therapy, the potential risk to the fetus must be balanced against the severity of the potential illness.

Gemtuzumab Ozogamicin
(gem TOO zoo mab oh zog a MY sin)

U.S. Brand Names Mylotarg®

Synonyms CMA-676; NSC-720568

Pharmacologic Category Antineoplastic Agent, Monoclonal Antibody

Pregnancy Risk Factor D

Lactation Excretion in breast milk unknown/not recommended

Use Treatment of relapsed CD33 positive acute myeloid leukemia (AML) in patients ≥60 years of age who are not candidates for cytotoxic chemotherapy

Unlabeled/Investigational Use Salvage therapy for acute promyelocytic leukemia (APL), relapsed/ refractory CD33 positive acute myeloid leukemia in children and adults <60 years

Mechanism of Action/Effect Antibody to CD33 antigen, which is expressed on leukemic blasts in 80% of patients with acute myeloid leukemia (AML), as well as normal myeloid cells. Binding results in internalization of the antibody-antigen complex. Following internalization, the calicheamicin derivative is released inside the myeloid cell. The calicheamicin derivative binds to DNA resulting in double strand breaks and cell death. Pluripotent stem cells and nonhematopoietic cells are not affected.

Contraindications Hypersensitivity to gemtuzumab ozogamicin, calicheamicin derivatives, or any component of the formulation; patients with anti-CD33 antibody; pregnancy

Warnings/Precautions Hazardous agent - use appropriate precautions for handling and disposal. Gemtuzumab has been associated with severe veno-occlusive disease or hepatotoxicity. Risk may be increased by combination chemotherapy, previous hepatic disease, or hematopoietic stem cell transplant.

Infusion-related events are common, generally reported to occur with the first dose after the end of the 2-hour intravenous infusion. These symptoms usually resolved after 2-4 hours with a supportive therapy of acetaminophen, diphenhydramine, and intravenous fluids. Fewer infusion-related events were observed after the second dose. **Infusion-related reactions may be severe (including anaphylaxis, pulmonary edema, or ARDS).** Other severe and potentially fatal infusion related pulmonary events (including dyspnea, pulmonary infiltrates, pleural effusions, pulmonary edema, pulmonary insufficiency and hypoxia) have been reported infrequently. Symptomatic intrinsic lung disease or high peripheral blast counts may increase the risk of severe reactions. Consider discontinuation in patients who develop severe infusion-related reactions.

Severe myelosuppression occurs in all patients at recommended dosages. Use caution in patients with renal impairment (no clinical experience) and hepatic impairment (no clinical experience in patients with bilirubin >2 mg/dL). Tumor lysis syndrome may occur as a consequence of leukemia treatment, adequate hydration and prophylactic allopurinol must be instituted prior to use. Other methods to lower WBC <30,000 cells/mm^3 may be considered (hydroxyurea or leukapheresis) to minimize the risk of tumor lysis syndrome, and/or severe infusion reactions. Postinfusion reactions, which may include fever, chills, hypotension, or dyspnea, may occur during the first 24 hours after administration. (Continued)

Gemtuzumab Ozogamicin (Continued)

Safety and efficacy have not been established in pediatric patients, patients with poor performance status, or in patients with organ dysfunction.

Drug Interactions

Increased Effect/Toxicity: Monoclonal antibodies may increase the risk for allergic reactions to gemtuzumab due to the presence of HACA antibodies

Nutritional/Ethanol Interactions Ethanol: Avoid ethanol (due to GI irritation).

Lab Interactions None known

Adverse Reactions Percentages established in adults ≥60 years of age. **Note:** A postinfusion symptom complex (fever, chills, less commonly hypertension, and/or dyspnea) may occur within 24 hours of administration; the incidence of infusion-related events decreases with repeat administration.

>10%:
Cardiovascular: Peripheral edema (19%), hypotension (18%), hypertension (17%), tachycardia (11%)

Central nervous system: Fever (78%), chills (64%), headache (27%), pain (18%), insomnia (11%)

Dermatologic: Petechiae (19%), cutaneous herpes simplex (18%), rash (18%), bruising (11%)

Endocrine & metabolic: Hypokalemia (24%), hyperglycemia (11%)

Gastrointestinal: Nausea (63%), vomiting (53%), diarrhea (30%), anorexia (27%), abdominal pain (26%), constipation (23%), stomatitis/mucositis (22%)

Hematologic: Neutropenia (grades 3/4: 98%; median recovery 40.5 days), lymphopenia (grades 3/4: 93%), thrombocytopenia (49%; grades 3/4: 48%; median recovery 39 days), hemoglobin decreased (grades 3/4: 50%), leukopenia (grades 3/4: 43%), anemia (22%, grades 3/4: 12%)

Hepatic: Abnormal liver function tests (20%; grade 3/4: 7%), LDH increased (18%), hyperbilirubinemia (11%)

Local: Local reaction (17%)

Neuromuscular & skeletal: Weakness (36%), back pain (12%)

Respiratory: Dyspnea (26%), epistaxis (24%; grade 3/4: 3%), cough (18%), pneumonia (13%)

Miscellaneous: Sepsis (25%), neutropenic fever (19%)

1% to 10%:
Central nervous system: Anxiety (10%), depression (10%), dizziness (10%), cerebral hemorrhage (2%), intracranial hemorrhage (1%)

Dermatologic: Pruritus (4%)

Endocrine & metabolic: Hypocalcemia (10%), hypophosphatemia (6%) hypomagnesemia (3%)

Gastrointestinal: Dyspepsia (8%), gingival hemorrhage (5%)

Genitourinary: Vaginal hemorrhage (5%), vaginal bleeding 2%, hematuria (grade 3/4: 1%)

Hematologic: Hemorrhage (9%), disseminated intravascular coagulation (DIC) (1%)

Hepatic: Alkaline phosphatase increased (10%), PT/PTT increased, veno-occlusive disease (5% to 10%; up to 20% in relapsed patients; higher frequency in patients with prior history of subsequent hematopoietic stem cell transplant)

Neuromuscular & skeletal: Arthralgia (10%), myalgia (3%)

Respiratory: Pharyngitis (10%), rhinitis (7%), hypoxia (5%)

Miscellaneous: Infection (10%)

Overdosage/Toxicology Symptoms are unknown. Closely monitor vital signs and blood counts. Treatment is symptom-directed and supportive. Gemtuzumab ozogamicin is not dialyzable.

Pharmacodynamics/Kinetics

Time to Peak: Immediate; higher concentrations observed after repeat dose

Half-Life Elimination: Total calicheamicin: Initial: 41-45 hours, Repeat dose: 60-64 hours; Unconjugated: 100-143 hours (no change noted in repeat dosing)

Available Dosage Forms Injection, powder for reconstitution: 5 mg

Dosing

Adults & Elderly: Refer to individual protocols. **Note:** Patients should receive diphenhydramine 50 mg orally and acetaminophen 650-1000 mg orally 1 hour prior to administration of each dose. Acetaminophen dosage should be repeated as needed every 4 hours for 2 additional doses. Pretreatment with methylprednisolone may ameliorate infusion-related symptoms.

AML: I.V.:
≥60 years: 9 mg/m^2 infused over 2 hours. A full treatment course is a total of 2 doses administered with 14 days between doses. Full hematologic recovery is not necessary for administration of the second dose. There has been only limited experience with repeat courses of gemtuzumab ozogamicin.

<60 years (unlabeled use): 9 mg/m^2 infused over 2 hours. A full treatment course is a total of 2 doses administered with 14 days between doses.

APL (unlabeled use): I.V.: 6 mg/m^2 infused over 2 hours. A full treatment course is a total of 2 doses administered with 15 days between doses.

Pediatrics: AML (unlabeled use): 4-9 mg/m^2 infused over 2 hours every 2 weeks for a total of 1-3 doses per treatment course. Patients received the second and third doses and/or dose escalation if no dose limiting toxicities were observed. Patients should receive diphenhydramine (1 mg/kg) 1 hour prior to infusion and acetaminophen 15 mg/kg 1 hour prior to infusion and every 4 hours for 2 additional doses. (**Note:** Higher incidences of liver toxicities were observed in children at the 9 mg/m^2 dose level.)

Renal Impairment: No recommendation (not studied).

Hepatic Impairment: No recommendation (not studied).

Administration

I.V.: Do not administer as I.V. push or bolus. Administer via I.V. infusion, over at least 2 hours. Use of a low protein-binding (0.2-1.2 micron) in-line filter is recommended. Protect from light during infusion. Premedication with acetaminophen and diphenhydramine should be administered prior to each infusion.

Stability

Reconstitution: Prepare in biologic safety hood with the fluorescent light turned **off**. Allow to warm to room temperature prior to reconstitution. Reconstitute vial with 5 mL sterile water for injection, USP. Final concentration in vial is 1 mg/mL. Dilute desired dose in 100 mL of 0.9% sodium chloride injection. The resulting I.V. bag should be placed in a UV protectant bag and infused immediately.

Compatibility: No information; infuse via separate line

Storage: Light sensitive; protect from light. Store vials under refrigeration 2°C to 8°C (36°F to 46°F). Reconstituted solutions may be stored for up to 2 hours at room temperature or under refrigeration. Following dilution, solutions are stable for up to 16 hours at room temperature. Administration requires 2 hours; therefore, the maximum elapsed time from initial reconstitution to completion of infusion should be 20 hours.

Laboratory Monitoring Monitor electrolytes, LFTs, CBC with differential, and platelet counts frequently.

Nursing Actions

Physical Assessment: Premedication with acetaminophen and diphenhydramine should be administered one hour prior to infusion, and acetaminophen as needed postinfusion. Monitor patient closely during and for 4 hours following treatment for infusion-related reactions, which can be severe (eg, anaphylaxis, pulmonary edema, or ARDS). Assess results of laboratory tests, patient response, and adverse reactions for immediate 24 hours following infusion (eg, postinfusion symptom complex) and regularly between infusions (eg, tachycardia, hyper- or hypotension, CNS changes, gastrointestinal disturbance, hepatic reaction). Teach patient purpose for use, possible side effects/appropriate interventions, and adverse symptoms to report.

Patient Education: This medication can only be administered intravenously. During and immediately following infusion, you will be closely monitored; report immediately any burning, pain, or swelling at infusion site; difficulty breathing or swallowing; chest pain, chills, or sudden headache. You will need frequent laboratory tests during course of therapy. Do not use alcohol, aspirin-containing medications, any prescription or OTC medications between treatments without consulting your prescriber. It is important to maintain adequate hydration (2-3 L/day of fluids) unless instructed to restrict fluid intake and nutrition (small frequent meals will help). You will be susceptible to infection (avoid crowds and exposure to infection). You may experience nausea or vomiting (small frequent meals, good mouth care, sucking lozenges or chewing gum may help); contact prescriber if nausea and vomiting persists. Frequent mouth care with a soft toothbrush or soft swabs and avoidance of spicy or salty foods may reduce mouth sores. Report immediately any difficulty breathing, unusual cough, nose bleed, fever, or chills; unusual bleeding or bruising; signs of infection (eg, sore throat, cough, white plaques in mouth or perianal area, burning on urination); chest pain or palpitations; yellowing of the eyes or skin; swelling of extremities; rapid weight gain; right upper quadrant pain; rash; or other persistent adverse effects. **Pregnancy/breast-feeding precautions:** Inform prescriber if you are pregnant. Do not get pregnant while taking this medication; may cause fetal damage. Consult prescriber for appropriate contraceptives. Do not breast-feed

Breast-Feeding Issues Due to the potential for serious adverse reactions, breast-feeding is not recommended.

Pregnancy Issues Animal studies have demonstrated teratogenic effects, fetal loss, and maternal toxicity. There are no adequate and well-controlled studies in pregnant women. May cause fetal harm when administered to a pregnant woman. Women of childbearing potential should avoid becoming pregnant while receiving treatment.

Gentamicin (jen ta MYE sin)

U.S. Brand Names Genoptic® [DSC]; Gentak®

Synonyms Gentamicin Sulfate

Pharmacologic Category Antibiotic, Aminoglycoside; Antibiotic, Ophthalmic; Antibiotic, Topical

Medication Safety Issues
Sound-alike/look-alike issues:
Gentamicin may be confused with kanamycin
Garamycin® may be confused with kanamycin, Terramycin®

Pregnancy Risk Factor C

Lactation Enters breast milk (small amounts)/use caution (AAP rates "compatible")

Use Treatment of susceptible bacterial infections, normally gram-negative organisms including *Pseudomonas*, *Proteus*, *Serratia*, and gram-positive *Staphylococcus*; treatment of bone infections, respiratory tract infections, skin and soft tissue infections, as well as abdominal and urinary tract infections, endocarditis, and septicemia; used topically to treat superficial infections

of the skin or ophthalmic infections caused by susceptible bacteria; prevention of bacterial endocarditis prior to dental or surgical procedures

Mechanism of Action/Effect Bactericidal; interferes with bacterial protein synthesis resulting in cell death

Contraindications Hypersensitivity to gentamicin or other aminoglycosides

Warnings/Precautions Not intended for long-term therapy due to toxic hazards associated with extended administration. Pre-existing renal insufficiency, vestibular or cochlear impairment, myasthenia gravis, hypocalcemia, conditions which depress neuromuscular transmission.

Parenteral aminoglycosides have been associated with significant nephrotoxicity or ototoxicity. Ototoxicity may be directly proportional to the amount of drug given and the duration of treatment and may not be reversible. Tinnitus or vertigo are indications of vestibular injury and impending hearing loss. Renal damage is usually reversible.

Drug Interactions
Increased Effect/Toxicity: Penicillins, cephalosporins, amphotericin B, loop diuretics may increase nephrotoxic potential. Aminoglycosides may potentiate the effects of neuromuscular blocking agents.

Lab Interactions
Some penicillin derivatives may accelerate the degradation of aminoglycosides *in vitro*, leading to a potential underestimation of aminoglycoside serum concentration.

Adverse Reactions
>10%:
Central nervous system: Neurotoxicity (vertigo, ataxia)
Neuromuscular & skeletal: Gait instability
Otic: Ototoxicity (auditory), ototoxicity (vestibular)
Renal: Nephrotoxicity, decreased creatinine clearance
1% to 10%:
Cardiovascular: Edema
Dermatologic: Skin itching, reddening of skin, rash

Overdosage/Toxicology Symptoms of overdose include ototoxicity, nephrotoxicity, and neuromuscular toxicity. Serum level monitoring is recommended. The treatment of choice, following a single acute overdose, appears to be maintenance of urine output of at least 3 mL/kg/hour during the acute treatment phase. Dialysis is of questionable value in enhancing aminoglycoside elimination.

Pharmacodynamics/Kinetics
Time to Peak: Serum: I.M.: 30-90 minutes; I.V.: 30 minutes after 30-minute infusion
Protein Binding: <30%
Half-Life Elimination:
Infants: <1 week old: 3-11.5 hours; 1 week to 6 months old: 3-3.5 hours
Adults: 1.5-3 hours; End-stage renal disease: 36-70 hours
Excretion: Urine (as unchanged drug)
Clearance: Directly related to renal function

Available Dosage Forms [DSC] = Discontinued product
Cream, topical, as sulfate: 0.1% (15 g, 30 g)
Infusion, as sulfate [premixed in NS]: 40 mg (50 mL); 60 mg (50 mL, 100 mL); 70 mg (50 mL); 80 mg (50 mL, 100 mL); 90 mg (100 mL); 100 mg (50 mL, 100 mL); 120 mg (100 mL)
Injection, solution, as sulfate [ADD-Vantage® vial]: 10 mg/mL (6 mL, 8 mL, 10 mL)
Injection, solution, as sulfate: 40 mg/mL (2 mL, 20 mL) [may contain sodium metabisulfite]
Injection, solution, pediatric, as sulfate: 10 mg/mL (2 mL) [may contain sodium metabisulfite]
Injection, solution, pediatric, as sulfate [preservative free]: 10 mg/mL (2 mL)
(Continued)

Gentamicin *(Continued)*

Ointment, ophthalmic, as sulfate (Gentak®): 0.3% [3 mg/g] (3.5 g)

Ointment, topical, as sulfate: 0.1% (15 g, 30 g)

Solution, ophthalmic, as sulfate: 0.3% (5 mL, 15 mL) [contains benzalkonium chloride]

Genoptic®: 0.3% (1 mL) [contains benzalkonium chloride] [DSC]

Gentak®: 0.3% (5 mL; 15 mL [DSC]) [contains benzalkonium chloride]

Dosing

Adults & Elderly: Individualization is **critical** because of the low therapeutic index.

Use of ideal body weight (IBW) for determining the mg/kg/dose appears to be more accurate than dosing on the basis of total body weight (TBW). In morbid obesity, dosage requirement may best be estimated using a dosing weight of IBW + 0.4 (TBW - IBW).

Initial and periodic plasma drug levels (eg, peak and trough with conventional dosing) should be determined, particularly in critically-ill patients with serious infections or in disease states known to significantly alter aminoglycoside pharmacokinetics (eg, cystic fibrosis, burns, or major surgery).

Usual dosage ranges:

I.M., I.V.:

Conventional: 1-2.5 mg/kg/dose every 8-12 hours; to ensure adequate peak concentrations early in therapy, higher initial dosage may be considered in selected patients when extracellular water is increased (edema, septic shock, postsurgical, or trauma)

Once daily: 4-7 mg/kg/dose once daily; some clinicians recommend this approach for all patients with normal renal function; this dose is at least as efficacious with similar, if not less, toxicity than conventional dosing

Intrathecal: 4-8 mg/day

Ophthalmic:

Ointment: Instill 1/2" (1.25 cm) 2-3 times/day to every 3-4 hours

Solution: Instill 1-2 drops every 2-4 hours, up to 2 drops every hour for severe infections

Topical: Apply 3-4 times/day to affected area

Indication-specific dosing: I.M., I.V.:

Brucellosis: 240 mg (I.M.) daily or 5 mg/kg (I.V.) daily for 7 days; either regimen recommended in combination with doxycycline

Cholangitis: 4-6 mg/kg once daily with ampicillin

Diverticulitis (complicated): 1.5-2 mg/kg every 8 hours (with ampicillin and metronidazole)

Endocarditis prophylaxis: Dental, oral, upper respiratory procedures, GI/GU procedures: 1.5 mg/kg with ampicillin (50 mg/kg) 30 minutes prior to procedure

Endocarditis or synergy (for Gram-positive infections): 1 mg/kg every 8 hours (with ampicillin)

Meningitis, Listeria species: 5-7 mg/kg/day (with penicillin) for 1 week

Meningitis, neonatal:

0-7 days of age: <2000 g: 2.5 mg/kg every 18-24 hours; >2000 g: 2.5 mg/kg every 12 hours

8-28 days of age: <2000 g: 2.5 mg/kg every 8-12 hours; >2000 g: 2.5 mg/kg every 8 hours

Pelvic inflammatory disease: Loading dose: 2 mg/kg, then 1.5 mg/kg every 8 hours

Alternate therapy: 4.5 mg/kg once daily

Plague (Yersinia pestis): Treatment: 5 mg/kg/day, followed by postexposure prophylaxis with doxycycline

Pneumonia, hospital- or ventilator-associated: 7 mg/kg/day (with antipseudomonal beta-lactam or carbapenem)

Tularemia: 5 mg/kg/day divided every 8 hours for 1-2 weeks

Urinary tract infection: 1.5 mg/kg/dose every 8 hours

Pediatrics: Individualization is **critical** because of the low therapeutic index.

Use of ideal body weight (IBW) for determining the mg/kg/dose appears to be more accurate than dosing on the basis of total body weight (TBW). In morbid obesity, dosage requirement may best be estimated using a dosing weight of IBW + 0.4 (TBW - IBW).

Initial and periodic plasma drug levels (eg, peak and trough with conventional dosing) should be determined, particularly in critically-ill patients with serious infections or in disease states known to significantly alter aminoglycoside pharmacokinetics (eg, cystic fibrosis, burns, or major surgery).

Usual dosage ranges: I.M., I.V.:

Infants and Children <5 years: 2.5 mg/kg/dose every 8 hours*

Children ≥5 years: 2-2.5 mg/kg/dose every 8 hours*

*Note: Higher individual doses and/or more frequent intervals (eg, every 6 hours) may be required in selected clinical situations (cystic fibrosis) or serum levels document the need

CNS infections: Intrathecal: See adult dosing.

Ophthalmic, Dermatologic infections: See adult dosing.

Indication-specific dosing: See adult dosing.

Renal Impairment:

Conventional dosing:

Cl$_{cr}$ ≥60 mL/minute: Administer every 8 hours

Cl$_{cr}$ 40-60 mL/minute: Administer every 12 hours

Cl$_{cr}$ 20-40 mL/minute: Administer every 24 hours

Cl$_{cr}$ <20 mL/minute: Loading dose, then monitor levels

High-dose therapy: Interval may be extended (eg, every 48 hours) in patients with moderate renal impairment (Cl$_{cr}$ 30-59 mL/minute) and/or adjusted based on serum level determinations.

Hemodialysis: Dialyzable; removal by hemodialysis: 30% removal of aminoglycosides occurs during 4 hours of HD; administer dose after dialysis and follow levels

Removal by continuous ambulatory peritoneal dialysis (CAPD):

Administration via CAPD fluid:

Gram-negative infection: 4-8 mg/L (4-8 mcg/mL) of CAPD fluid

Gram-positive infection (eg, synergy): 3-4 mg/L (3-4 mcg/mL) of CAPD fluid

Administration via I.V., I.M. route during CAPD: Dose as for Cl$_{cr}$ <10 mL/minute and follow levels

Removal via continuous arteriovenous or venovenous hemofiltration: Dose as for Cl$_{cr}$ 10-40 mL/minute and follow levels

Hepatic Impairment: Monitor plasma concentrations.

Administration

I.M.: Administer by deep I.M. route if possible. Slower absorption and lower peak concentrations, probably due to poor circulation in the atrophic muscle, may occur following I.M. injection; in paralyzed patients, suggest I.V. route.

I.V.: Some penicillins (eg, carbenicillin, ticarcillin and piperacillin) have been shown to inactivate aminoglycosides *in vitro*. This has been observed to a greater extent with tobramycin and gentamicin, while amikacin has shown greater stability against inactivation. Concurrent use of these agents may pose a risk of reduced antibacterial efficacy *in vivo*, particularly in the setting of profound renal impairment. However, definitive clinical evidence is lacking. If combination penicillin/aminoglycoside therapy is desired in a patient with renal dysfunction, separation of doses (if feasible), and routine monitoring of aminoglycoside levels, CBC, and clinical response should be considered.

I.V. Detail: pH: 3.0-5.5 (I.V./I.M. injection); ph: 4 (premixed infusion in sodium chloride)

Other: Administer any other ophthalmics 10 minutes before or after gentamicin preparations.

Stability

Reconstitution: I.V. infusion solutions mixed in NS or D_5W solution are stable for 24 hours at room temperature and refrigeration.

Premixed bag: Manufacturer expiration date; remove from overwrap stability: 30 days

Compatibility: Stable in dextran 40, D_5W, $D_{10}W$, mannitol 20%, LR, NS; **incompatible** with fat emulsion 10%

Y-site administration: Incompatible with allopurinol, amphotericin B cholesteryl sulfate complex, cefamandole, furosemide, heparin, hetastarch, idarubicin, indomethacin, iodipamide meglumine, phenytoin, propofol, warfarin

Compatibility in syringe: Incompatible with ampicillin, cefamandole, heparin

Compatibility when admixed: Incompatible with amphotericin B, ampicillin, cefamandole, cefazolin with clindamycin, cefepime, heparin, nafcillin, ticarcillin

Storage: Gentamicin is a colorless to slightly yellow solution which should be stored between 2°C to 30°C, but refrigeration is not recommended.

Laboratory Monitoring Urinalysis, BUN, serum creatinine, plasma gentamicin levels (as appropriate to dosing method). Peak levels are drawn 30 minutes after the end of a 30-minute infusion or 1 hour after initiation of infusion or I.M. injection. The trough is drawn just before the next dose. Levels are typically obtained after the third dose in conventional dosing. Perform culture and sensitivity studies prior to initiating therapy to determine the causative organism and its susceptibility to gentamicin. Some penicillin derivatives may accelerate the degradation of aminoglycosides.

Nursing Actions

Physical Assessment: Assess effectiveness and interactions of other medications patient may be taking. Assess patient's hearing level before, during, and following therapy; report changes to prescriber immediately. Monitor therapeutic response, laboratory values, and adverse reactions (neurotoxicity [vertigo, ataxia], ototoxicity, decreased renal function, opportunistic infection [eg, fever, mouth and vaginal sores or plaques], unhealed wounds) at beginning of therapy and periodically throughout therapy. Assess knowledge/teach patient appropriate use, interventions to reduce side effects, and adverse symptoms to report.

Patient Education: Take exactly as directed and when prescribed. Drink adequate amounts of water (2-3 L/day) unless instructed to restrict fluid intake. You may experience headaches, ringing in ears, dizziness, blurred vision (use caution when driving or engaging in tasks requiring alertness until response to drug is known); GI upset, loss of appetite (small frequent meals and frequent mouth care may help); or photosensitivity (use sunscreen wear protective clothing and eyewear, and avoid direct sunlight). Report severe headache, changes in hearing acuity, ringing in ears, change in balance, changes in urine pattern, respiratory difficulty, rash, fever, unhealed sores, sores in mouth, vaginal drainage, muscle or bone pain, change in gait, or worsening of condition. **Pregnancy/breast-feeding precautions:** Inform prescriber if you are or intend to become pregnant. Consult prescriber if breast-feeding.

Ophthalmic: Wash hands before instilling. Sit or lie down to instill. Open eye, look at ceiling, and instill prescribed amount of solution; for ointment, pull lower lid down gently, instill thin ribbon of ointment inside lid. Close eye and roll eye in all directions, and apply gentle pressure to inner corner of eye. Do not let tip of applicator touch eye; do not contaminate tip of applicator (may cause eye infection, eye damage, or vision loss). Temporary stinging or blurred vision may occur. Report persistent pain, burning, vision changes, swelling, itching, or worsening of condition.

Topical: Apply thin film of ointment to affected area as often as recommended. May apply porous dressing. Report persistent burning, swelling, itching, worsening of condition, or lack of response to therapy.

Dietary Considerations Calcium, magnesium, potassium: Renal wasting may cause hypocalcemia, hypomagnesemia, and/or hypokalemia.

Geriatric Considerations Aminoglycosides are important therapeutic interventions for susceptible organisms and as empiric therapy in seriously ill patients. Their use is not without risk of toxicity, however. Additional studies comparing high-dose, once-daily aminoglycosides to traditional dosing regimens in the elderly are needed before once-daily aminoglycoside dosing can be routinely adopted to this patient population.

Breast-Feeding Issues No data reported; however, gentamicin is not absorbed orally and other aminoglycosides may be taken while breast-feeding.

Related Information
Compatibility of Drugs *on page 1370*
Peak and Trough Guidelines *on page 1387*

Glatiramer Acetate (gla TIR a mer AS e tate)

U.S. Brand Names Copaxone®

Synonyms Copolymer-1

Pharmacologic Category Biological, Miscellaneous

Medication Safety Issues
Sound-alike/look-alike issues:
Copaxone® may be confused with Compazine®

Pregnancy Risk Factor B

Lactation Excretion in breast milk unknown/use caution

Use Treatment of relapsing-remitting type multiple sclerosis; studies indicate that it reduces the frequency of attacks and the severity of disability; appears to be most effective for patients with minimal disability

Contraindications Previous hypersensitivity to any component of the copolymer formulation, glatiramer acetate, or mannitol

Warnings/Precautions For SubQ use only, **not for I.V. administration**. Glatiramer acetate is antigenic, and may possibly lead to the induction of untoward host responses. Systemic postinjection reactions occur in a substantial percentage of patients (~10% in premarketing studies). Safety and efficacy have not been established in patients <18 years of age.

Adverse Reactions Reported in >2% of patients in placebo-controlled trials:

>10%:
Cardiovascular: Chest pain (21%), vasodilation (27%), palpitation (17%)
Central nervous system: Pain (28%), anxiety (23%)
Dermatologic: Pruritus (18%), rash (18%), diaphoresis (15%)
Gastrointestinal: Nausea (22%), diarrhea (12%)
Local: Injection site reactions: Pain (73%), erythema (66%), inflammation (49%), pruritus (40%), mass (27%), induration (13%), welt (11%)
Neuromuscular & skeletal: Weakness (41%), arthralgia (24%), hypertonia (22%), back pain (16%)
Respiratory: Dyspnea (19%), rhinitis (14%)
Miscellaneous: Infection (50%), flu-like syndrome (19%), lymphadenopathy (12%)
(Continued)

Glatiramer Acetate (Continued)

1% to 10%:

Cardiovascular: Peripheral edema (7%), facial edema (6%), edema (3%), tachycardia (5%)

Central nervous system: Fever (8%), vertigo (6%), migraine (5%), syncope (5%), agitation (4%), chills (4%), confusion (2%), nervousness (2%), speech disorder (2%)

Dermatologic: Bruising (8%), erythema (4%), urticaria (4%), skin nodule (2%)

Endocrine & metabolic: Dysmenorrhea (6%)

Gastrointestinal: Anorexia (8%), vomiting (6%), gastrointestinal disorder (5%), gastroenteritis (3%), weight gain (3%)

Genitourinary: Urinary urgency (10%), vaginal moniliasis (8%)

Local: Injection site reactions: Hemorrhage (5%), urticaria (5%)

Neuromuscular & skeletal: Tremor (7%), foot drop (3%)

Ocular: Eye disorder (4%), nystagmus (2%)

Otic: Ear pain (7%)

Respiratory: Bronchitis (9%), laryngismus (5%)

Miscellaneous: Neck pain (8%), bacterial infection (5%), herpes simplex (4%), cyst (2%)

Overdosage/Toxicology Well tolerated; no serious toxicities can be anticipated

Pharmacodynamics/Kinetics

Metabolism: SubQ: Large percentage hydrolyzed locally

Available Dosage Forms Injection, solution [preservative free]: 20 mg/mL (1 mL) [prefilled syringe; contains mannitol; packaged with alcohol pads]

Dosing

Adults & Elderly: Multiple sclerosis (relapsing-remitting): SubQ: 20 mg daily

Administration

Other: For SubQ administration in the arms, abdomen, hips or thighs. Bring to room temperature prior to use.

Stability

Storage: Store in refrigerator at 2°C to 8°C (36°F to 46°F); excursions to room temperature for up to 1 week do not have a negative impact on potency.

Nursing Actions

Physical Assessment: Assess potential for interactions with other prescriptions, OTC medications, or herbal products patient may be taking. Assess effectiveness and adverse response (eg, postinjection reactions — self-resolving flushing, chest tightness, dyspnea, palpitations). Teach patient proper use (reconstitution, injection technique, and syringe/needle disposal, possible side effects/appropriate interventions, and adverse symptoms to report.

Patient Education: This drug will not cure MS, but may help relieve the severity and frequency of attacks. This drug can only be given by subcutaneous injection; your prescriber will instruct you in how to prepare the medication, proper injection technique, and syringe/needle disposal. If using prefilled glass syringe, use **only** the autoject® 2 *for glass syringe* device (not the original Copaxone® autoject). Do not stop or change doses without consulting your prescriber. May cause a transient reaction after injection, including flushing, chest tightness, dyspnea, or palpitations (usually last 30 minutes or less). May cause weakness, dizziness, confusion, nervousness, or anxiety (use caution when driving or engaging in tasks requiring alertness until response to drug is known); or nausea or vomiting (frequent mouth care and sucking on lozenges may help). Report chest pain or pounding heartbeat; persistent diarrhea or GI upset; infection (vaginal itching or drainage, sores in mouth, unusual fever or chills) or flu-like symptoms (swollen glands, chills, excessive sweating); bruising, rash, or skin irritation; joint pain or neck pain; swelling of puffiness of face; vision changes or ear pain; unusual cough or respiratory difficulty; alterations in menstrual pattern; skin depression, hard lump, redness, pain, or swelling at injection site; or any other persistent adverse reactions. **Breast-feeding precaution:** Consult prescriber if breast-feeding.

Glimepiride (GLYE me pye ride)

U.S. Brand Names Amaryl®

Pharmacologic Category Antidiabetic Agent, Sulfonylurea

Medication Safety Issues

Sound-alike/look-alike issues:

Glimepiride may be confused with glipiZIDE

Amaryl® may be confused with Altace®, Amerge®, Reminyl®

Pregnancy Risk Factor C

Lactation Excretion in breast milk unknown/contraindicated

Use Management of type 2 diabetes mellitus (noninsulin dependent, NIDDM) as an adjunct to diet and exercise to lower blood glucose; may be used in combination with metformin or insulin in patients whose hyperglycemia cannot be controlled by diet and exercise in conjunction with a single oral hypoglycemic agent

Mechanism of Action/Effect Stimulates insulin release from the pancreatic beta cells; reduces glucose output from the liver; insulin sensitivity is increased at peripheral target sites

Contraindications Hypersensitivity to glimepiride, any component of the formulation, or sulfonamides; diabetic ketoacidosis (with or without coma)

Warnings/Precautions The administration of oral hypoglycemic drugs (eg, tolbutamide) has been reported to be associated with increased cardiovascular mortality as compared to treatment with diet alone or diet plus insulin. All sulfonylurea drugs are capable of producing severe hypoglycemia. Hypoglycemia is more likely to occur when caloric intake is deficient, after severe or prolonged exercise, when ethanol is ingested, or when more than one glucose-lowering drug is used.

Chemical similarities are present among sulfonamides, sulfonylureas, carbonic anhydrase inhibitors, thiazides, and loop diuretics (except ethacrynic acid). Use in patients with sulfonamide allergy is specifically contraindicated in product labeling, however, a risk of cross-reaction exists in patients with allergy to any of these compounds; avoid use when previous reaction has been severe.

Product labeling states oral hypoglycemic drugs may be associated with an increased cardiovascular mortality. Data to support this association are limited, and several studies (UKPDS) have not supported an association. Safety and efficacy in pediatric patients have not been established.

Drug Interactions

Cytochrome P450 Effect: Substrate of CYP2C8/9 (major)

Decreased Effect: CYP2C8/9 inducers may decrease the levels/effects of glimepiride; example inducers include carbamazepine, phenobarbital, phenytoin, rifampin, rifapentine, and secobarbital. There may be a decreased effect of glimepiride with corticosteroids, estrogens, oral contraceptives, thiazide and other diuretics, phenothiazines, NSAIDs, thyroid products, nicotinic acid, isoniazid, sympathomimetics, urinary alkalinizers, and charcoal. **Note:** However, pooled data did **not** demonstrate drug interactions with calcium channel blockers, estrogens, NSAIDs, HMG-CoA reductase inhibitors, sulfonamides, or thyroid hormone.

Increased Effect/Toxicity: CYP2C8/9 inhibitors may increase the levels/effects of glimepiride; example inhibitors include delavirdine, ketoconazole, nicardipine, NSAIDs, and pioglitazone. Beta-blockers, chloramphenicol, cimetidine, fibric acid derivatives, fluconazole, pegvisomant, salicylates, sulfonamides, and tricyclic antidepressants may increase the hypoglycemic effects of glimepiride. Glimepiride may increase effects of cyclosporine. Sulfonylureas may induce a disulfiram-like reaction with ethanol.

Nutritional/Ethanol Interactions

Ethanol: Caution with ethanol (may cause hypoglycemia).

Herb/Nutraceutical: Caution with chromium, garlic, gymnema (may cause hypoglycemia).

Adverse Reactions

1% to 10%:

Central nervous system: Dizziness (2%), headache (2%)

Endocrine & metabolic: Hypoglycemia (1% to 2%)

Gastrointestinal: Nausea (1%)

Neuromuscular & skeletal: Weakness (2%)

Overdosage/Toxicology Symptoms of overdose include low blood sugar, tingling of lips and tongue, nausea, yawning, confusion, agitation, tachycardia, sweating, convulsions, stupor, and coma. Intoxication with sulfonylureas can cause hypoglycemia and are best managed with glucose administration (oral for milder hypoglycemia or by injection in more severe forms). Patients should be monitored for a minimum of 24-48 hours after ingestion.

Pharmacodynamics/Kinetics

Onset of Action: Peak effect: Blood glucose reductions: 2-3 hours

Duration of Action: 24 hours

Time to Peak: 2-3 hours

Protein Binding: >99.5%

Half-Life Elimination: 5-9 hours

Metabolism: Hepatic oxidation via CYP2C9 to M1 metabolite (~33% activity of parent compound); further oxidative metabolism to inactive M2 metabolite

Excretion: Urine (60%, 80% to 90% M1 and M2); feces (40%, 70% M1 and M2)

Available Dosage Forms Tablet: 1 mg, 2 mg, 4 mg

Dosing

Adults:

Type 2 diabetes: Oral:

Initial: 1-2 mg once daily, administered with breakfast or the first main meal

Adjustment: Allow several days between dose titrations: usual maintenance dose: 1-4 mg once daily; after a dose of 2 mg once daily, increase in increments of 2 mg at 1- to 2-week intervals based upon the patient's blood glucose response to a maximum of 8 mg once daily. If inadequate response to maximal dose, combination therapy with metformin may be considered.

Combination with insulin therapy:

Note: Fasting glucose level for instituting combination therapy is in the range of >150 mg/dL in plasma or serum depending on the patient)

Initial: 8 mg once daily with the first main meal

Adjustment: After starting with low-dose insulin, upward adjustments of insulin can be done approximately weekly as guided by frequent measurements of fasting blood glucose. Once stable, combination-therapy patients should monitor their capillary blood glucose on an ongoing basis, preferably daily.

Conversion from therapy with long half-life agents: Observe patient carefully for 1-2 weeks when converting from a longer half-life agent (eg, chlorpropamide) to glimepiride due to overlapping hypoglycemic effects.

Elderly: Initial: 1 mg/day; dose titration and maintenance dosing should be conservative to avoid hypoglycemia

Pediatrics: Type 2 diabetes: Oral: Children 10-18 years (unlabeled use): Initial: 1 mg once daily; maintenance: 1-4 mg once daily

Renal Impairment: Cl_{cr} <22 mL/minute: Initial starting dose should be 1 mg and dosage increments should be based on fasting blood glucose levels.

Administration

Oral: Administer once daily with breakfast or first main meal of the day. Patients who are NPO may need to have their dose held to avoid hypoglycemia.

Laboratory Monitoring Urine for glucose and ketones, fasting blood glucose, hemoglobin A_{1c}, fructosamine

Nursing Actions

Physical Assessment: Allergy history should be assessed prior to beginning therapy. Assess potential for interactions with other prescriptions, OTC medications, or herbal products patient may be taking. Monitor laboratory tests, therapeutic effectiveness, and adverse response at regular intervals during therapy. Teach patient proper use (or refer patient to diabetic educator for instruction), possible side effects/appropriate interventions, and adverse symptoms to report.

Patient Education: Do not take any new medication during therapy unless approved by prescriber. This medication is used to control diabetes; it is not a cure. Monitor glucose as recommended by prescriber. Other important components of treatment plan may include prescribed diet and exercise regimen (consult prescriber or diabetic educator). Always carry quick source of sugar with you. Take exactly as directed with breakfast or the first main meal of the day. Do not change dose or discontinue without consulting prescriber. Avoid alcohol while taking this medication; could cause severe reaction. Do not take other medication within 2 hours of this medication unless advised by prescriber. If you experience hypoglycemic reaction, contact prescriber immediately. You may experience side effects during first weeks of therapy (eg, headache, nausea); consult prescriber if these persist. Report severe or persistent side effects (eg, hypoglycemia: palpitations, sweaty palms, lightheadedness; extended vomiting or bleeding; or change in color of urine or stool). **Pregnancy/breast-feeding precautions:** Inform prescriber if you are or intend to become pregnant. Do not breast-feed.

Dietary Considerations Administer with breakfast or the first main meal of the day. Dietary modification based on ADA recommendations is a part of therapy. Decreases blood glucose concentration. Hypoglycemia may occur. Must be able to recognize symptoms of hypoglycemia (palpitations, sweaty palms, lightheadedness).

Geriatric Considerations Rapid and prolonged hypoglycemia (>12 hours) despite hypertonic glucose injections have been reported; age, hepatic, and renal impairment are independent risk factors for hypoglycemia; dosage titration should be made at weekly intervals. How "tightly" a geriatric patient's blood glucose should be controlled is controversial; however, a fasting blood sugar <150 mg/dL is now an acceptable end point. Such a decision should be based on the patient's functional and cognitive status, how well they recognize hypoglycemic or hyperglycemic symptoms, and how to respond to them and their other disease states.

Pregnancy Issues Abnormal blood glucose levels are associated with a higher incidence of congenital abnormalities. Insulin is the drug of choice for the control of diabetes mellitus during pregnancy.

GlipiZIDE (GLIP i zide)

U.S. Brand Names Glucotrol®; Glucotrol® XL

Synonyms Glydiazinamide

Pharmacologic Category Antidiabetic Agent, Sulfonylurea

Medication Safety Issues
Sound-alike/look-alike issues:
GlipiZIDE may be confused with glimepiride, glyBURIDE
Glucotrol® may be confused with Glucophage®, Glucotrol® XL, glyBURIDE
Glucotrol® XL may be confused with Glucotrol®

Pregnancy Risk Factor C

Lactation Excretion in breast milk unknown/not recommended

Use Management of type 2 diabetes mellitus (noninsulin dependent, NIDDM)

Mechanism of Action/Effect Stimulates insulin release from the pancreatic beta cells; reduces glucose output from the liver; insulin sensitivity is increased at peripheral target sites

Contraindications Hypersensitivity to glipizide or any component of the formulation, other sulfonamides; type 1 diabetes mellitus (insulin dependent, IDDM)

Warnings/Precautions Use with caution in patients with severe hepatic disease.

Chemical similarities are present among sulfonamides, sulfonylureas, carbonic anhydrase inhibitors, thiazides, and loop diuretics (except ethacrynic acid). Use in patients with sulfonamide allergy is specifically contraindicated in product labeling, however, a risk of cross-reaction exists in patients with allergy to any of these compounds; avoid use when previous reaction has been severe.

Avoid use of extended release tablets (Glucotrol® XL) in patients with known stricture/narrowing of the GI tract.

Product labeling states oral hypoglycemic drugs may be associated with an increased cardiovascular mortality as compared to treatment with diet alone or diet plus insulin. Data to support this association are limited, and several studies, including a large prospective trial (UKPDS) have not been supported an association.

Drug Interactions
Cytochrome P450 Effect: Substrate of 2C8/9 (major)
Decreased Effect: CYP2C8/9 inducers may decrease the levels/effects of glipizide; example inducers include carbamazepine, phenobarbital, phenytoin, rifampin, rifapentine, and secobarbital. Decreased effect of glipizide with beta-blockers, cholestyramine, hydantoins, thiazide diuretics, urinary alkalinizers, and charcoal.
Increased Effect/Toxicity: CYP2C8/9 inhibitors may increase the levels/effects of glipizide; example inhibitors include delavirdine, fluconazole, gemfibrozil, ketoconazole, nicardipine, NSAIDs, pioglitazone, and sulfonamides. Increased effects/hypoglycemic effects of glipizide with H_2 antagonists, anticoagulants, androgens, cimetidine, salicylates, tricyclic antidepressants, probenecid, MAO inhibitors, methyldopa, digitalis glycosides, and urinary acidifiers.

Nutritional/Ethanol Interactions
Ethanol: Caution with ethanol (may cause hypoglycemia or rare disulfiram reaction).
Food: A delayed release of insulin may occur if glipizide is taken with food. Immediate release tablets should be administered 30 minutes before meals to avoid erratic absorption.
Herb/Nutraceutical: Caution with chromium, garlic, gymnema (may cause hypoglycemia).

Adverse Reactions Frequency not defined.
Cardiovascular: Edema, syncope

Central nervous system: Anxiety, depression, dizziness, headache, insomnia, nervousness
Dermatologic: Rash, urticaria, photosensitivity, pruritus
Endocrine & metabolic: Hypoglycemia, hyponatremia, SIADH (rare)
Gastrointestinal: Anorexia, nausea, vomiting, diarrhea, epigastric fullness, constipation, heartburn, flatulence
Hematologic: Blood dyscrasias, aplastic anemia, hemolytic anemia, bone marrow suppression, thrombocytopenia, agranulocytosis
Hepatic: Cholestatic jaundice, hepatic porphyria
Neuromuscular & skeletal: Arthralgia, leg cramps, myalgia, tremor
Ocular: Blurred vision
Renal: Diuretic effect (minor)
Miscellaneous: Diaphoresis, disulfiram-like reaction

Overdosage/Toxicology Symptoms of overdose include low blood sugar, tingling of lips and tongue, nausea, yawning, confusion, agitation, tachycardia, sweating, convulsions, stupor, and coma. Intoxication with sulfonylureas can cause hypoglycemia and are best managed with glucose administration (oral for milder hypoglycemia or by injection in more severe forms).

Pharmacodynamics/Kinetics
Onset of Action: Peak effect: Blood glucose reductions: 1.5-2 hours
Duration of Action: 12-24 hours
Protein Binding: 92% to 99%
Half-Life Elimination: 2-4 hours
Metabolism: Hepatic with metabolites
Excretion: Urine (60% to 80%, 91% to 97% as metabolites); feces (11%)

Available Dosage Forms
Tablet (Glucotrol®): 5 mg, 10 mg
Tablet, extended release: 5 mg, 10 mg
Glucotrol® XL: 2.5 mg, 5 mg, 10 mg

Dosing
Adults:
Type 2 diabetes: Oral (allow several days between dose titrations): Initial: 5 mg/day; adjust dosage at 2.5-5 mg daily increments as determined by blood glucose response at intervals of several days.
Immediate release tablet: Maximum recommended once-daily dose: 15 mg; maximum recommended total daily dose: 40 mg
Extended release tablet (Glucotrol® XL): Maximum recommended dose: 20 mg
When transferring from insulin to glipizide:
Current insulin requirement ≤20 units: Discontinue insulin and initiate glipizide at usual dose
Current insulin requirement >20 units: Decrease insulin by 50% and initiate glipizide at usual dose; gradually decrease insulin dose based on patient response. Several days should elapse between dosage changes.
Elderly: Initial: 2.5 mg/day; increase by 2.5-5 mg/day at 1- to 2-week intervals.
Renal Impairment: Cl_{cr} <10 mL/minute: Some investigators recommend not using.
Hepatic Impairment: Initial dosage should be 2.5 mg/day.

Administration
Oral: Administer immediate release tablets 30 minutes before a meal to achieve greatest reduction in postprandial hyperglycemia. Extended release tablets should be given with breakfast. Patients who are NPO may need to have their dose held to avoid hypoglycemia.

Laboratory Monitoring Urine for glucose and ketones, fasting blood glucose, hemoglobin A_{1c}, fructosamine

Nursing Actions
Physical Assessment: Assess potential for interactions with other prescriptions, OTC medications, or herbal products patient may be taking, and any allergies they may have. Monitor laboratory tests and

patient response (eg, hypoglycemia) at regular intervals during therapy. Teach patient proper use (or refer patient to diabetic educator for instruction), possible side effects/appropriate interventions, and adverse symptoms to report.

Patient Education: Do not take any new medication during therapy unless approved by prescriber. This medication is used to control diabetes; it is not a cure. Monitor glucose as recommended by prescriber. Other important components of treatment plan may include prescribed diet and exercise regimen (consult prescriber or diabetic educator). Always carry quick source of sugar with you. Take exactly as directed. Immediate release tablets should be taken 30 minutes before meals, at the same time each day. Extended release tablets should be taken with breakfast. Do not chew or crush extended release tablets. Do not change dose or discontinue without consulting prescriber. Avoid alcohol while taking this medication; could cause severe reaction. Do not take other medication within 2 hours of this medication unless advised by prescriber. If you experience hypoglycemic reaction, contact prescriber immediately. You may experience more sensitivity to sunlight (use sunscreen, wear protective clothing and eyewear, and avoid direct sunlight); or headache or nausea (consult prescriber if these persist). Report severe or persistent side effects (eg, hypoglycemia: palpitations, sweaty palms, lightheadedness; extended vomiting; diarrhea or constipation; flu-like symptoms; skin rash; easy bruising or bleeding; or change in color of urine or stool). **Pregnancy/breast-feeding precautions:** Inform prescriber if you are or intend to become pregnant. Breast-feeding is not recommended

Dietary Considerations Take immediate release tablets 30 minutes before meals; extended release tablets should be taken with breakfast. Dietary modification based on ADA recommendations is a part of therapy. Decreases blood glucose concentration. Hypoglycemia may occur. Must be able to recognize symptoms of hypoglycemia (palpitations, sweaty palms, lightheadedness).

Geriatric Considerations Glipizide is a useful agent since there are few drug to drug interactions and elimination of the active drug is not dependent upon renal function. How "tightly" a geriatric patient's blood glucose should be controlled is controversial; however, a fasting blood sugar <150 mg/dL is now an acceptable end point. Such a decision should be based on the patient's functional and cognitive status, how well they recognize hypoglycemic or hyperglycemic symptoms, and how to respond to them and their other disease states.

Breast-Feeding Issues Due to risk of neonatal hypoglycemia, breast-feeding is not recommended. Discontinue nursing or consider switching to insulin if diet alone does not control blood glucose.

Pregnancy Issues Crosses the placenta. Abnormal blood glucose levels are associated with a higher incidence of congenital abnormalities. Insulin is the drug of choice for the control of diabetes mellitus during pregnancy. If glipizide is used during pregnancy, discontinue and change to insulin at least 1 month prior to delivery to decrease prolonged hypoglycemia in the neonate.

Related Information

FDA Name Differentiation Project: The Use of Tall-Man Letters *on page 12*

Glipizide and Metformin
(GLIP i zide & met FOR min)

U.S. Brand Names Metaglip™
Synonyms Glipizide and Metformin Hydrochloride; Metformin and Glipizide
Pharmacologic Category Antidiabetic Agent, Biguanide; Antidiabetic Agent, Sulfonylurea
Pregnancy Risk Factor C
Lactation Excretion in breast milk unknown/not recommended
Use Initial therapy for management of type 2 diabetes mellitus (noninsulin dependent, NIDDM) when hyperglycemia cannot be managed with diet and exercise alone. Second-line therapy for management of type 2 diabetes (NIDDM) when hyperglycemia cannot be managed with a sulfonylurea or metformin along with diet and exercise.

Available Dosage Forms Tablet:
2.5/250: Glipizide 2.5 mg and metformin 250 mg
2.5/500: Glipizide 2.5 mg and metformin 500 mg
5/500: Glipizide 5 mg and metformin 500 mg
Dosing
Adults:
Type 2 diabetes, first-line therapy: Oral: Initial: Glipizide 2.5 mg/metformin 250 mg once daily with a meal. Dose adjustment: Increase dose by 1 tablet/day every 2 weeks, up to a maximum of glipizide 10 mg/metformin 1000 mg daily
Patients with fasting plasma glucose (FPG) 280-320 mg/dL: Oral: Consider glipizide 2.5 mg/metformin 500 mg twice daily. Dose adjustment: Increase dose by 1 tablet/day every 2 weeks, up to a maximum of glipizide 10 mg/metformin 2000 mg daily in divided doses
Type 2 diabetes, second-line therapy: Oral: Glipizide 2.5 mg/metformin 500 mg **or** glipizide 5 mg/metformin 500 mg twice daily with morning and evening meals; starting dose should not exceed current daily dose of glipizide (or sulfonylurea equivalent) or metformin. Dose adjustment: Titrate dose in increments of no more than glipizide 5 mg/metformin 500 mg, up to a maximum dose of glipizide 20 mg/metformin 2000 mg daily.
Elderly: Conservative doses are recommended in the elderly due to potentially decreased renal function; **do not titrate to maximum dose**; should not be used in patients ≥80 years unless renal function is verified as normal
Renal Impairment: Risk of lactic acidosis increases with degree of renal impairment; contraindicated in renal disease or renal dysfunction (see Contraindications).
Hepatic Impairment: Use should be avoided; liver disease is a risk factor for the development of lactic acidosis during metformin therapy.
Nursing Actions
Physical Assessment: See individual agents.
Patient Education: Inform prescriber of all prescriptions, OTC medications, or herbal products you are taking, and any allergies you have. Do not take any new medication during therapy unless approved by prescriber. This medication is used to control diabetes; it is not a cure. Monitor glucose as recommended by prescriber. Other important components of treatment plan may include prescribed diet and exercise regimen (consult prescriber or diabetic educator). Always carry quick source of sugar with you. Take exactly as directed. All doses should be administered with a meal. Twice-daily dosing should be taken with the morning and evening meals. Do not change dose or discontinue without consulting prescriber. Avoid overuse of alcohol while taking this medication (could cause severe reaction). Do not take other medication within 2 hours of this medication
(Continued)

Glipizide and Metformin *(Continued)*

unless advised by prescriber. If you experience hypo-glycemic reaction, contact prescriber immediately. You may experience more sensitivity to sunlight (use sunscreen, wear protective clothing and eyewear, and avoid direct sunlight); drowsiness, dizziness, or head-ache (use caution driving or engaging in potentially hazardous tasks until response to drug is known); nausea or vomiting (taking with meals, eating small, frequent meals, frequent mouth care, or sucking lozenges may help). Report severe or persistent side effects (eg, hypoglycemia; palpitations, sweaty palms, lightheadedness; extended vomiting; diarrhea or constipation; flu-like symptoms; skin rash; easy bruising or bleeding; or change in color of urine or stool, sudden chest discomfort, slow or irregular heartbeat, or other adverse reactions). **Pregnancy/breast-feeding precautions:** Inform prescriber if you are or intend to become pregnant. Breast-feeding is not recommended.

Related Information
GlipiZIDE *on page 586*
Metformin *on page 789*

Glucagon *(GLOO ka gon)*

U.S. Brand Names GlucaGen®; GlucaGen® Diagnostic Kit; GlucaGen® HypoKit™; Glucagon Diagnostic Kit [DSC]; Glucagon Emergency Kit
Synonyms Glucagon Hydrochloride
Pharmacologic Category Antidote; Diagnostic Agent
Medication Safety Issues
Sound-alike/look-alike issues:
Glucagon may be confused with Glaucon®
Pregnancy Risk Factor B
Lactation Excretion in breast milk unknown/compatible
Use Management of hypoglycemia; diagnostic aid in radi-ologic examinations to temporarily inhibit GI tract move-ment
Unlabeled/Investigational Use Used with some success as a cardiac stimulant in management of severe cases of beta-adrenergic blocking agent over-dosage; treatment of myocardial depression due to calcium channel blocker overdose
Mechanism of Action/Effect Stimulates adenylate cyclase to produce increased cyclic AMP, which promotes hepatic glycogenolysis and gluconeogenesis, causing a raise in blood glucose levels
Contraindications Hypersensitivity to glucagon or any component of the formulation; insulinoma; pheochromo-cytoma
Warnings/Precautions Use caution with prolonged fasting, starvation, adrenal insufficiency or chronic hypo-glycemia; levels of glucose stores in liver may be decreased. Following response to therapy, oral carbo-hydrates should be administered to prevent hypogly-cemia.
Drug Interactions
Increased Effect/Toxicity: Oral anticoagulant: Hypo-prothrombinemic effects may be increased possibly with bleeding; effect seen with glucagon doses of 50 mg administered over 1-2 days
Nutritional/Ethanol Interactions Glucagon depletes glycogen stores.
Adverse Reactions Frequency not defined.
Cardiovascular: Hypotension (up to 2 hours after GI procedures), hypertension, tachycardia
Gastrointestinal: Nausea, vomiting (high incidence with rapid administration of high doses)
Miscellaneous: Hypersensitivity reactions, anaphylaxis
Overdosage/Toxicology Symptoms include hypoka-lemia, nausea and vomiting, inhibition of GI tract motility, decreased blood pressure, tachycardia

Pharmacodynamics/Kinetics
Onset of Action: Peak effect: Blood glucose levels:
Parenteral: I.V.: 5-20 minutes; I.M.: 30 minutes;
SubQ: 30-45 minutes
Duration of Action: Hyperglycemia: 60-90 minutes
Half-Life Elimination: Plasma: 3-10 minutes
Metabolism: Primarily hepatic; some inactivation occurring renally and in plasma
Available Dosage Forms Injection, powder for recon-stitution, as hydrochloride:
GlucaGen®: 1 mg [equivalent to 1 unit; contains lactose 107 mg]
GlucaGen® Diagnostic Kit: 1 mg [equivalent to 1 unit; contains lactose 107 mg; packaged with sterile water]
GlucaGen® HypoKit™: 1 mg [equivalent to 1 unit; contains lactose 107 mg; packaged with prefilled syringe containing sterile water]
Glucagon®: 1 mg [equivalent to 1 unit; contains lactose 49 mg]
Glucagon Diagnostic Kit, Glucagon Emergency Kit: 1 mg [equivalent to 1 unit; contains lactose 49 mg; packaged with diluent syringe containing glycerin 12 mg/mL and water for injection]

Dosing
Adults & Elderly:
Hypoglycemia or insulin shock therapy: I.M., I.V., SubQ: 1 mg; may repeat in 20 minutes as needed
Note: If patient fails to respond to glucagon, I.V. dextrose must be given.
Beta-blocker overdose, calcium channel blocker overdose (unlabeled use): I.V.: 5-10 mg over 1 minutes followed by an infusion of 1-10 mg/hour. The following has also been reported for beta-blocker overdose: 3-10 mg or initially 0.5-5 mg bolus followed by continuous infusion 1-5 mg/hour
Diagnostic aid: I.M., I.V.: 0.25-2 mg 10 minutes prior to procedure
Pediatrics:
Hypoglycemia or insulin shock therapy: I.M., I.V., SubQ:
Children <20 kg: 0.5 mg or 20-30 mcg/kg/dose; repeated in 20 minutes as needed
Children ≥20 kg: Refer to adult dosing.
Note: If patient fails to respond to glucagon, I.V. dextrose must be given.

Administration
I.V.: Bolus may be associated with nausea and vomiting. Continuous infusions may be used in beta-blocker overdose/toxicity.
Stability
Reconstitution: Reconstitute powder for injection by adding 1 mL of sterile diluent to a vial containing 1 unit of the drug, to provide solutions containing 1 mg of glucagon/mL. Gently roll vial to dissolve. If dose to be administered is <2 mg of the drug, then use only the diluent provided by the manufacturer. If >2 mg, use sterile water for injection. Use immediately after reconstitution. May be kept at 5°C for up to 48 hours if necessary.
Storage: Prior to reconstitution, store at controlled room temperature of 20°C to 25° (69°F to 77°F). Do not freeze.
Laboratory Monitoring Blood glucose

Nursing Actions
Physical Assessment: Arouse patient from hypogly-cemic or insulin shock as soon as possible and administer carbohydrates. Evaluate insulin dosage and patient's ability to administer appropriate dose. Instruct patient (or significant other) in appropriate administration procedures for emergency use of glucagon. If home glucose monitoring device is avail-able, check blood sugar as soon as possible.
Patient Education: Identify appropriate support person to administer glucagon if necessary. Follow prescribers instructions for administering glucagon.

Review diet, insulin administration, and testing procedures with prescriber or diabetic educator.

Dietary Considerations Administer carbohydrates to patient as soon as possible after response to treatment.

Additional Information 1 unit = 1 mg

Glutamine (GLOO ta meen)

U.S. Brand Names Enterex® Glutapak-10® [OTC]; NutreStore™; Resource® GlutaSolve® [OTC]; Sympt-X [OTC]; Sympt-X G.I. [OTC]

Synonyms Gln; L-Glutamine

Pharmacologic Category Amino Acid

Pregnancy Risk Factor C

Lactation Excretion in breast milk unknown/use caution

Use Treatment of short bowel syndrome when used in combination with nutritional support and growth hormone therapy; a medical food used to promote GI tract healing and nutritional supplementation with GI disorders, HIV/AIDS, cancer, and other critical illnesses

Mechanism of Action/Effect Glutamine regulates gastrointestinal cell growth, function, and regeneration. Considered a "conditionally essential" amino acid during metabolic stress and injury.

Warnings/Precautions Use caution with hepatic or renal impairment. NutreStore™ should be used with nutritional support based on individual patient requirements. Medical foods are intended to be used under the direction of a healthcare provider.

Adverse Reactions Frequency not defined.
Cardiovascular: Facial edema, peripheral edema
Central nervous system: Dizziness, fever, headache, pain
Dermatologic: Pruritus, rash
Gastrointestinal: Abdominal pain, flatulence, nausea, pancreatitis, tenesmus, vomiting
Neuromuscular & skeletal: Arthralgia, back pain, hypoesthesia
Otic: Ear or hearing symptoms
Respiratory: Rhinitis
Miscellaneous: Flu-like syndrome, infection, sepsis

Pharmacodynamics/Kinetics
Half-Life Elimination: I.V.: 1 hour
Metabolism: Via splanchnic tissue, lymphocytes, kidney, and liver to glutamate and ammonia

Pharmacokinetic Note As reported in healthy adults; parameters may vary following oral administration in patients with short bowel syndrome.

Available Dosage Forms Powder for oral solution:
Enterex® Glutapak-10®: 10 g/packet (50s)
NutreStore™: 5 g/packet
Resource® GlutaSolve®: 15 g/packet (56s)
Sympt-X, Sympt-X G.I.: 10 g/packet (60s)

Dosing
Adults:
Nutritional supplement (Enterex® Glutapak-10®, Resource® GlutaSolve®, Sympt-X, Sympt-X G.I.): Oral: Average dose: 10 g 3 times/day; dosing range: 5-30 g/day
Short bowel syndrome (NutreStore™): Oral: 30 g/day administered as 5 g 6 times/day (every 2-3 hours while awake) for up to 16 weeks; to be used in combination with growth hormone and nutritional support

Administration
Oral:
Enterex® Glutapak-10®: Prior to use, mix with clear liquids or semisolid food. If administering via feeding tube, mix each 10 g packet with ≥60 mL water. Use immediately after preparation. May also be added directly to enteral formula if used within 24 hours.
Resource® GlutaSolve®: Mix each 15 g packet with 120-240 mL of water. May also be mixed in hot or cold beverages, applesauce, or pudding. If administering via feeding tube, mix with 60-120 mL water. Use immediately after preparation.
NutreStore™: Mix each packet (5 g) with ~240 mL of water prior to administration. May be given with meals or snacks
Sympt-X, Sympt-X G.I.: Mix dose with 6-8 ounces of juice or another beverage, may also be mixed with applesauce or pudding. Administer with meals. If administering via feeding tube, mix with ≥60 mL water; do not add directly to feeding bag. Use immediately after preparation.

Stability
Storage: Store at controlled room temperature.

Laboratory Monitoring BUN

Nursing Actions
Physical Assessment: Assess therapeutic effectiveness according to purpose for use and adverse response (see Adverse Reactions). Teach patient proper use (reconstitution and storage), possible side effects/appropriate interventions, and adverse symptoms to report.

Patient Education: Prepare, store, and use exactly as directed. Do not exceed recommended dosage. May cause increased flatulence, nausea or vomiting, or abdominal pain; if persistent or severe contact prescriber. Report facial or peripheral swelling, rash; unusual back pain; or other persistent adverse reactions. **Pregnancy/breast-feeding precautions:** Inform prescriber if you are or intend to become pregnant or breast-feed.

Dietary Considerations NutreStore™: To be used in combination with a specialized diet. May be taken with food or a snack.

Breast-Feeding Issues The amount of total protein and free amino acids found in breast milk varies during lactation. Effects of the suggested oral dose of glutamine are unknown.

GlyBURIDE (GLYE byoor ide)

U.S. Brand Names Diaβeta®; Glynase® PresTab®; Micronase®

Synonyms Diabeta; Glibenclamide; Glybenclamide; Glybenzcyclamide

Pharmacologic Category Antidiabetic Agent, Sulfonylurea

Medication Safety Issues
Sound-alike/look-alike issues:
GlyBURIDE may be confused with glipiZIDE, Glucotrol®
Diaβeta® may be confused with Diabinese®, Zebeta®
Micronase® may be confused with microK®, miconazole, Micronor®

Pregnancy Risk Factor C

Lactation Does not enter breast milk/ use caution

Use Management of type 2 diabetes mellitus (noninsulin dependent, NIDDM)

Unlabeled/Investigational Use Alternative to insulin in women for the treatment of gestational diabetes (11-33 weeks gestation)

Mechanism of Action/Effect Stimulates insulin release from the pancreatic beta cells; reduces glucose output from the liver; insulin sensitivity is increased at peripheral target sites

Contraindications Hypersensitivity to glyburide, any component of the formulation, or other sulfonamides; type 1 diabetes mellitus (insulin dependent, IDDM), diabetic ketoacidosis with or without coma

Warnings/Precautions Elderly: Rapid and prolonged hypoglycemia (>12 hours) despite hypertonic glucose injections have been reported; age and hepatic and renal impairment are independent risk factors for hypoglycemia; dosage titration should be made at weekly (Continued)

GlyBURIDE (Continued)

intervals. Use with caution in patients with renal and hepatic impairment, malnourished or debilitated conditions, or adrenal or pituitary insufficiency.

Chemical similarities are present among sulfonamides, sulfonylureas, carbonic anhydrase inhibitors, thiazides, and loop diuretics (except ethacrynic acid). Use in patients with sulfonamide allergy is specifically contraindicated in product labeling, however, a risk of cross-reaction exists in patients with allergy to any of these compounds; avoid use when previous reaction has been severe.

Product labeling states oral hypoglycemic drugs may be associated with an increased cardiovascular mortality as compared to treatment with diet alone or diet plus insulin. Data to support this association are limited, and several studies, including a large prospective trial (UKPDS) have not supported an association.

Drug Interactions

Cytochrome P450 Effect: Inhibits CYP3A4 (weak)

Decreased Effect: Thiazides and other diuretics, corticosteroids may decrease effectiveness of glyburide.

Increased Effect/Toxicity: Increased hypoglycemic effects of glyburide may occur with oral anticoagulants (warfarin), phenytoin, other hydantoins, salicylates, NSAIDs, sulfonamides, and beta-blockers. Ethanol ingestion may cause disulfiram reactions.

Nutritional/Ethanol Interactions

Ethanol: Caution with ethanol (may cause hypoglycemia).

Herb/Nutraceutical: Caution with chromium, garlic, gymnema (may cause hypoglycemia).

Adverse Reactions Frequency not defined.

Central nervous system: Headache, dizziness

Dermatologic: Pruritus, rash, urticaria, photosensitivity reaction

Endocrine & metabolic: Hypoglycemia, hyponatremia (SIADH reported with other sulfonylureas)

Gastrointestinal: Nausea, epigastric fullness, heartburn, constipation, diarrhea, anorexia

Genitourinary: Nocturia

Hematologic: Leukopenia, thrombocytopenia, hemolytic anemia, aplastic anemia, bone marrow suppression, agranulocytosis

Hepatic: Cholestatic jaundice, hepatitis

Neuromuscular & skeletal: Arthralgia, paresthesia

Ocular: Blurred vision

Renal: Diuretic effect (minor)

Overdosage/Toxicology Symptoms of overdose include severe hypoglycemia, seizures, cerebral damage, tingling of lips and tongue, nausea, yawning, confusion, agitation, tachycardia, sweating, convulsions, stupor, and coma. Intoxication with sulfonylureas can cause hypoglycemia and is best managed with glucose administration (oral for milder hypoglycemia or by injection in more severe forms).

Pharmacodynamics/Kinetics

Onset of Action: Serum insulin levels begin to increase 15-60 minutes after a single dose

Duration of Action: ≤24 hours

Time to Peak: Serum: Adults: 2-4 hours

Protein Binding: Plasma: >99%

Half-Life Elimination: 5-16 hours; may be prolonged with renal or hepatic impairment

Metabolism: To one moderately active and several inactive metabolites

Excretion: Feces (50%) and urine (50%) as metabolites

Available Dosage Forms [DSC] = Discontinued product

Tablet (Diaβeta®, Micronase®): 1.25 mg, 2.5 mg, 5 mg

Tablet, micronized: 1.5 mg, 3 mg, 6 mg

Glynase® PresTab®: 1.5 mg [DSC], 3 mg, 6 mg

Dosing

Adults:

Type 2 diabetes: Oral:

Note: Regular tablets cannot be used interchangeably with micronized tablet formulations

Regular tablets (Diaβeta®, Micronase®):

Initial: 2.5-5 mg/day, administered with breakfast or the first main meal of the day. In patients who are more sensitive to hypoglycemic drugs, start at 1.25 mg/day.

Adjustment: Increase in increments of no more than 2.5 mg/day at weekly intervals based on the patient's blood glucose response

Maintenance: 1.25-20 mg/day given as single or divided doses; maximum: 20 mg/day

Micronized tablets (Glynase® PresTab®):

Initial: 1.5-3 mg/day, administered with breakfast or the first main meal of the day in patients who are more sensitive to hypoglycemic drugs, start at 0.75 mg/day. Increase in increments of no more than 1.5 mg/day in weekly intervals based on patient's blood glucose response.

Maintenance: 0.75-12 mg/day given as a single dose or in divided doses. Some patients (especially those receiving >6 mg/day) may have a more satisfactory response with twice-daily dosing.

Elderly: Regular tablets (Diaβeta®, Micronase®): Oral: Initial: 1.25-2.5 mg/day, increase by 1.25-2.5 mg/day every 1-3 weeks. Refer to adult dosing.

Renal Impairment: Cl$_{cr}$ <50 mL/minute: Not recommended

Hepatic Impairment: Use conservative initial and maintenance doses and avoid use in severe disease.

Administration

Oral: Administer with meals at the same time each day. Patients who are anorexic or NPO may need to have their dose held to avoid hypoglycemia.

Laboratory Monitoring Fasting blood glucose, hemoglobin A$_{1c}$, fructosamine

Nursing Actions

Physical Assessment: Allergy history should be evaluated prior to beginning therapy. Assess potential for interactions with other prescriptions, OTC medications, or herbal products patient may be taking. Monitor laboratory tests and patient response (eg, hypoglycemia) at regular intervals during therapy. Teach patient proper use (or refer patient to diabetic educator for instruction), possible side effects/appropriate interventions, and adverse symptoms to report.

Patient Education: Do not take any new medication during therapy unless approved by prescriber. This medication is used to control diabetes; it is not a cure. Monitor glucose as recommended by prescriber. Other important components of treatment plan may include prescribed diet and exercise regimen (consult prescriber or diabetic educator). If you experience hypoglycemic reaction, contact prescriber immediately. Always carry quick source of sugar with you. Take exactly as directed, 30 minutes before meal(s) at the same time each day. Do not change dose or discontinue without consulting prescriber. Avoid alcohol while taking this medication; could cause severe reaction. Do not take other medication within 2 hours of this medication unless advised by prescriber. You may experience more sensitivity to sunlight (use sunscreen, wear protective clothing and eyewear, and avoid direct sunlight); headache; or nausea (consult prescriber if these persist). Report severe or persistent side effects; hypoglycemia (palpitations, sweaty palms, lightheadedness); extended vomiting, diarrhea, or constipation; flu-like symptoms; skin rash; easy bruising or bleeding; or change in color of urine or stool. **Pregnancy/breast-feeding precautions:** Inform prescriber if you are or intend to become pregnant. Do not breast-feed.

Dietary Considerations Should be taken with meals at the same time each day. Dietary modification based on ADA recommendations is a part of therapy. Decreases blood glucose concentration. Hypoglycemia may occur. Must be able to recognize symptoms of hypoglycemia (palpitations, sweaty palms, lightheadedness).

Geriatric Considerations Rapid and prolonged hypoglycemia (>12 hours) despite hypertonic glucose injections have been reported; age, hepatic, and renal impairment are independent risk factors for hypoglycemia; conservative initial dosing and slow titration are required to avoid hypoglycemic reactions; dosage titration should be made at weekly intervals.

Breast-Feeding Issues Based on data from 11 women, glyburide was not detected in breast milk following a single-dose study (5 mg or 10 mg/dose), or a daily-dose study (5 mg/day). Hypoglycemia was not observed in the 3 nursing infants who were wholly breast fed.

Pregnancy Issues Glyburide was not found to significantly cross the placenta *in vitro*. Studies have shown glyburide to be an acceptable alternative to insulin when treatment is needed for gestational diabetes. However, one retrospective study comparing glyburide to insulin noted an increased risk of preeclampsia in women taking glyburide and a higher rate of phototherapy in neonates. Insulin is the drug of choice for the control of diabetes mellitus during pregnancy.

Related Information
FDA Name Differentiation Project: The Use of Tall-Man Letters *on page 12*

Glyburide and Metformin (GLYE byoor ide & met FOR min)

U.S. Brand Names Glucovance®

Synonyms Glyburide and Metformin Hydrochloride; Metformin and Glyburide

Pharmacologic Category Antidiabetic Agent, Biguanide; Antidiabetic Agent, Sulfonylurea

Pregnancy Risk Factor B (manufacturer); C (expert analysis)

Lactation No data available/use caution

Use Initial therapy for management of type 2 diabetes mellitus (noninsulin dependent, NIDDM). Second-line therapy for management of type 2 diabetes (NIDDM) when hyperglycemia cannot be managed with a sulfonylurea or metformin; combination therapy with a thiazolidinedione may be required to achieve additional control.

Available Dosage Forms Tablet:
1.25 mg/250 mg: Glyburide 1.25 mg and metformin hydrochloride 250 mg
2.5 mg/500 mg: Glyburide 2.5 mg and metformin hydrochloride 500 mg
5 mg/500 mg: Glyburide 5 mg and metformin hydrochloride 500 mg

Dosing
Adults: *Note:* Dose must be individualized. All doses should be taken with a meal. Twice daily dosage should be taken with the morning and evening meals. Dosages expressed as glyburide/metformin components.

Type 2 diabetes: Oral:
No prior treatment with sulfonylurea or metformin: Initial: 1.25 mg/250 mg once daily with a meal; patients with Hb A_{1c} >9% or fasting plasma glucose (FPG) >200 mg/dL may start with 1.25 mg/250 mg twice daily. Adjustment: Dosage may be increased in increments of 1.25 mg/250 mg, at intervals of not less than 2 weeks; maximum daily dose: 10 mg/2000 mg (limited experience with higher doses)
Previously treated with a sulfonylurea or metformin alone: Initial: 2.5 mg/500 mg or 5 mg/500 mg

twice daily; increase in increments no greater than 5 mg/500 mg; maximum daily dose: 20 mg/2000 mg
Note: When switching patients previously on a sulfonylurea and metformin together, do not exceed the daily dose of glyburide (or glyburide equivalent) or metformin.
Combination with thiazolidinedione: May be combined with a thiazolidinedione in patients with an inadequate response to glyburide/metformin therapy, however the risk of hypoglycemia may be increased.
Elderly: Refer to adult dosing. Adjust carefully to renal function. Should not be used in patients ≥80 years of age unless renal function is verified as normal.

Nursing Actions
Physical Assessment: See individual agents.
Patient Education: See individual agents. **Pregnancy/breast-feeding precautions:** Inform prescriber if you are or intend to become pregnant. Consult prescriber if breast-feeding.

Related Information
GlyBURIDE *on page 589*
Metformin *on page 789*

Glycopyrrolate (glye koe PYE roe late)

U.S. Brand Names Robinul®; Robinul® Forte

Synonyms Glycopyrronium Bromide

Pharmacologic Category Anticholinergic Agent

Pregnancy Risk Factor B

Lactation Excretion in breast milk unknown/use caution

Use Inhibit salivation and excessive secretions of the respiratory tract preoperatively; reversal of neuromuscular blockade; control of upper airway secretions; adjunct in treatment of peptic ulcer

Mechanism of Action/Effect Blocks the action of acetylcholine at parasympathetic sites in smooth muscle, secretory glands, and the CNS

Contraindications Hypersensitivity to glycopyrrolate or any component of the formulation; severe ulcerative colitis, toxic megacolon complicating ulcerative colitis, paralytic ileus, obstructive disease of GI tract, intestinal atony in the elderly or debilitated patient; unstable cardiovascular status in acute hemorrhage; narrow-angle glaucoma; acute hemorrhage; tachycardia; obstructive uropathy; myasthenia gravis

Warnings/Precautions Use caution in elderly, patients with autonomic neuropathy, hepatic or renal disease, ulcerative colitis may precipitate/aggravate toxic megacolon, hyperthyroidism, CAD, CHF, arrhythmias, tachycardia, BPH, or hiatal hernia with reflux. Use of anticholinergics in gastric ulcer treatment may cause a delay in gastric emptying due to antral statis. Caution should be used in individuals demonstrating decreased pigmentation (skin and iris coloration, dark versus light) since there has been some evidence that these individuals have an enhanced sensitivity to the anticholinergic response. May cause drowsiness, eye sensitivity to light, or blurred vision; caution should be used when performing tasks which require mental alertness, such as driving. Thr risk of heat stroke with this medication may be increased during exercise or hot weather. Infants, patients with Down syndrome, and children with spastic paralysis or brain damage may be hypersensitive to antimuscarine effects. Product packaging may contain latex. Injection contains benzyl alcohol (associated with gasping syndrome in neonates). Not recommended for use in children <12 years of age for the management of peptic ulcer or <16 years for preanesthetic use.

Drug Interactions
Increased Effect/Toxicity: Effects of other anticholinergic agents or medications with anticholinergic (Continued)

Glycopyrrolate *(Continued)*

activity may be increased by glycopyrrolate. Severity of potassium chloride-induced gastrointestinal lesions (when potassium is given in a wax matrix formulation, eg, Klor-Con®) may be increased by glycopyrrolate. Pramlinitide may enhance the anticholinergic effects of anticholinergics (effects are specific to the GI tract).

Adverse Reactions Frequency not defined. **Note:** Includes adverse effects which may occur as an extension of the pharmacologic action of anticholinergics (including glycopyrrolate) and adverse effects reported postmarketing with glycopyrrolate.

Cardiovascular: Arrhythmias, cardiac arrest, heart block, hyper-/hypotension, malignant hyperthermia, palpitation, QT_c interval prolongation, tachycardia

Central nervous system: Confusion, dizziness, drowsiness, excitement, headache, insomnia, nervousness, seizures

Dermatologic: Dry skin, pruritus, sensitivity to light increased

Endocrine & metabolic: Lactation suppression

Gastrointestinal: Bloated feeling, constipation, loss of taste, nausea, vomiting, xerostomia

Genitourinary: Impotence, urinary hesitancy, urinary retention

Local: Irritation at injection site

Neuromuscular & skeletal: Weakness

Ocular: Blurred vision, cycloplegia, mydriasis, ocular tension increased, photophobia, sensitivity to light increased

Respiratory: Respiratory depression

Miscellaneous: Anaphylactoid reactions, diaphoresis decreased, hypersensitivity reactions

Overdosage/Toxicology

Symptoms of overdose include blurred vision, urinary retention, tachycardia, and absent bowel sounds. For peripheral adverse effects, a quaternary ammonium anticholinesterase, such as neostigmine methylsulfate, may be given I.V. in increments of 0.25 mg in adults; may repeat every 5-10 minutes (up to a maximum of 2.5 mg) based upon decrease in heart rate and return of bowel sounds. For overdose exhibiting CNS symptoms (eg, excitement, restlessness, convulsions, psychotic behavior), physostigmine 0.5-2 mg I.V. slowly, may be given and repeated as necessary, up to 5 mg. Proportionally smaller doses should be used for pediatric patients. Artificial respiration should be given to individuals experiencing a neuromuscular or curare-like effect which could lead to muscular weakness or possible paralysis. Additional care should be symptomatic and supportive.

Pharmacodynamics/Kinetics

Onset of Action: Oral: 50 minutes; I.M.: 15-30 minutes; I.V.: ~1 minute

Peak effect: Oral: ~1 hour; I.M.: 30-45 minutes

Duration of Action: Vagal effect: 2-3 hours; Inhibition of salivation: Up to 7 hours; Anticholinergic: Oral 8-12 hours

Half-Life Elimination:

Infants: 22-130 minutes; Children 19-99 minutes; Adults: ~30-75 minutes

Metabolism: Hepatic (minimal)

Excretion: Urine (as unchanged drug, I.M.: 80%, I.V.: 85%); bile (as unchanged drug)

Available Dosage Forms

Injection, solution (Robinul®): 0.2 mg/mL (1 mL, 2 mL, 5 mL, 20 mL) [contains benzyl alcohol]

Tablet:

Robinul®: 1 mg

Robinul® Forte: 2 mg

Dosing

Adults & Elderly:

Reduction of secretions: I.M.:

Preoperative: I.M.: 4 mcg/kg 30-60 minutes before procedure

Intraoperative: I.V.: 0.1 mg repeated as needed at 2- to 3-minute intervals

Reversal of neuromuscular blockade: I.V.: 0.2 mg for each 1 mg of neostigmine or 5 mg of pyridostigmine administered or 5-15 mcg/kg glycopyrrolate with 25-70 mcg/kg of neostigmine or 0.1-0.3 mg/kg of pyridostigmine (agents usually administered simultaneously, but glycopyrrolate may be administered first if bradycardia is present)

Peptic ulcer:

Oral: 1-2 mg 2-3 times/day

I.M., I.V.: 0.1-0.2 mg 3-4 times/day

Pediatrics:

Reduction of secretions:

Preoperative: I.M.:

<2 years: 4-9 mcg/kg 30-60 minutes before procedure

>2 years: 4 mcg/kg 30-60 minutes before procedure

Intraoperative: I.V.: 4 mcg/kg not to exceed 0.1 mg; repeat at 2- to 3-minute intervals as needed.

Chronic:

Oral: 40-100 mcg/kg/dose 3-4 times/day

I.M., I.V.: 4-10 mcg/kg/dose every 3-4 hours; maximum: 0.2 mg/dose or 0.8 mg/24 hours

Reversal of neuromuscular blockade: Refer to adult dosing.

Administration

I.V.: Administer at a rate of 0.2 mg over 1-2 minutes.

I.V. Detail: For I.V. administration, glycopyrrolate may be administered by I.M. or I.V. without dilution. May also be administered via the tubing of a running I.V. infusion of a compatible solution. May be administered in the same syringe with neostigmine or pyridostigmine.

pH: 2-3

Stability

Compatibility: Stable in $D_5\frac{1}{2}NS$, D_5W, $D_{10}W$, LR, NS

Compatibility in syringe: Incompatible with chloramphenicol, dexamethasone sodium phosphate, diazepam, dimenhydrinate, methohexital, pentazocine, pentobarbital, secobarbital, sodium bicarbonate, thiopental

Compatibility when admixed: Incompatible with methylprednisolone sodium succinate

Storage: Store at 20°C to 25°C (68°F to 77°F).

Nursing Actions

Physical Assessment: Assess potential for interactions with other prescriptions, OTC medications, or herbal products patient may be taking (eg, anything that may add to anticholinergic effects). Monitor therapeutic effectiveness and adverse response. Teach patient proper use (self-administered), possible side effects/appropriate interventions, and adverse symptoms to report.

Patient Education: Do not take any new medication during therapy unless approved by prescriber. Take as directed before meals; do not increase dose and do not discontinue without consulting prescriber. Void before taking medication. You may experience dizziness or blurred vision (use caution when driving or engaging in tasks that require alertness until response to drug is known); dry mouth (sucking on lozenges may help); photosensitivity (wear dark glasses in bright sunlight); decreased ability to sweat (use caution in hot weather or hot rooms or engaging in strenuous activity); or impotence (temporary). Report excessive and persistent anticholinergic effects (blurred vision, headache, flushing, tachycardia, nervousness, constipation, dizziness, insomnia, mental confusion or excitement, dry mouth, altered taste perception, dysphagia, palpitations, bradycardia, urinary hesitancy or retention, impotence, decreased sweating). **Breast-feeding precaution:** Consult prescriber if breast-feeding.

Geriatric Considerations Anticholinergic agents are generally not well tolerated in the elderly and their use should be avoided when possible.

Breast-Feeding Issues May suppress lactation

Related Information
Compatibility of Drugs *on page 1370*
Compatibility of Drugs in Syringe *on page 1372*

Gonadorelin (goe nad oh RELL in)

U.S. Brand Names Factrel®

Synonyms GnRH; Gonadorelin Acetate; Gonadorelin Hydrochloride; Gonadotropin Releasing Hormone; LHRH; LRH; Luteinizing Hormone Releasing Hormone

Pharmacologic Category Diagnostic Agent; Gonadotropin

Medication Safety Issues
Sound-alike/look-alike issues:
Gonadorelin may be confused with gonadotropin, guanadrel
Factrel® may be confused with Sectral®
Gonadotropin may be confused with gonadorelin

Pregnancy Risk Factor B

Lactation Excretion in breast milk unknown

Use Evaluation of functional capacity and response of gonadotrophic hormones; evaluate abnormal gonadotropin regulation as in precocious puberty and delayed puberty.

Orphan drug: Lutrepulse®: Induction of ovulation in females with hypothalamic amenorrhea

Mechanism of Action/Effect Stimulates the release of luteinizing hormone (LH) from the anterior pituitary gland

Contraindications Hypersensitivity to gonadorelin or any component of the formulation; women with any condition that could be exacerbated by pregnancy; patients who have ovarian cysts or causes of anovulation other than those of hypothalamic origin; any condition that may worsened by reproductive hormones

Warnings/Precautions Hypersensitivity and anaphylactic reactions have occurred following multiple-dose administration. Use with caution in women in whom pregnancy could worsen pre-existing conditions (eg, pituitary prolactinemia). Multiple pregnancy is a possibility with gonadorelin.

Drug Interactions
Decreased Effect: Decreased levels/effect with oral contraceptives, digoxin, phenothiazines, and dopamine antagonists.
Increased Effect/Toxicity: Increased levels/effect with androgens, estrogens, progestins, glucocorticoids, spironolactone, and levodopa.

Adverse Reactions 1% to 10%: Local: Pain at injection site

Overdosage/Toxicology Symptoms of overdose include abdominal discomfort, nausea, headache, and flushing. Treatment is symptomatic.

Pharmacodynamics/Kinetics
Onset of Action: Peak effect: Maximal LH release: ~20 minutes
Duration of Action: 3-5 hours
Half-Life Elimination: 4 minutes

Available Dosage Forms Injection, powder for reconstitution, as hydrochloride: 100 mcg [diluent contains benzyl alcohol]

Dosing
Adults:
Diagnostic test: I.V., SubQ (hydrochloride salt): 100 mcg administered in women during early phase of menstrual cycle (day 1-7)
Primary hypothalamic amenorrhea: I.V. (acetate): 5 mcg every 90 minutes via Lutrepulse® pump kit at

treatment intervals of 21 days (pump will pulsate every 90 minutes for 7 days)
Pediatrics: Diagnostic test: Children >12 years: Refer to adult dosing.

Administration
I.V.:
Factrel®: Give I.V. push over 30 seconds.
Lutrepulse®: A presterilized reservoir bag with the infusion catheter set supplied with the kit should be filled with the reconstituted solution and administered I.V. using the Lutrepulse® pump. Set the pump to deliver 25-50 mL of solution, based upon the dose, over a pulse period of 1 minute and at a pulse frequency of 90 minutes.
I.V. Detail: Factrel®: Dilute in 3 mL of normal saline.

Stability
Reconstitution:
Factrel®: Prepare immediately prior to use. After reconstitution, store at room temperature and use within 1 day. Discard unused portion.
Lutrepulse®: Reconstitute with diluent immediately prior to use and transfer to plastic reservoir. The solution will supply 90-minute pulsatile doses for 7 consecutive days (Lutrepulse® pump).

Laboratory Monitoring LH, FSH

Nursing Actions
Physical Assessment: Assess other medications patient may be taking for effectiveness and interactions. When used for induction of ovulation, monitor laboratory tests and therapeutic response. Assess knowledge/teach patient appropriate use (use of pulsating pump if applicable), interventions to reduce side effects, and adverse symptoms to report.
Patient Education: If receiving this drug via pulsating pump, check all procedures with prescriber, and use exactly as prescribed. Report any rash, pain, or inflammation at injection site, and any change in respiratory status. **Breast-feeding precaution:** Consult prescriber if breast-feeding.

Goserelin (GOE se rel in)

U.S. Brand Names Zoladex®

Synonyms D-Ser(Bu^t)^6,Azgly^{10}-LHRH; Goserelin Acetate; ICI-118630; NSC-606864

Pharmacologic Category Gonadotropin Releasing Hormone Agonist

Pregnancy Risk Factor X (endometriosis, endometrial thinning); D (advanced breast cancer)

Lactation Enters breast milk/contraindicated

Use Palliative treatment of advanced breast cancer and carcinoma of the prostate; treatment of endometriosis, including pain relief and reduction of endometriotic lesions; endometrial thinning agent as part of treatment for dysfunctional uterine bleeding

Mechanism of Action/Effect LHRH synthetic analog of luteinizing hormone-releasing hormone also known as gonadotropin-releasing hormone (GnRH)

Contraindications Hypersensitivity to goserelin or any component of the formulation; pregnancy (or potential to become pregnant); breast-feeding

Warnings/Precautions Transient worsening of signs and symptoms (tumor flare) may develop during the first few weeks of treatment. Urinary tract obstruction or spinal cord compression have been reported when used for prostate cancer; closely observe patients for weakness, paresthesias, and urinary tract obstruction in first few weeks of therapy. Decreased bone density has been reported in women and may be irreversible; use caution if other risk factors are present; evaluate and institute preventative treatment if necessary. Rare cases of pituitary apoplexy (frequently secondary to pituitary adenoma) have been observed with leuprolide administration (onset from 1 hour to usually <2 weeks); may (Continued)

Goserelin (Continued)

present as sudden headache, vomiting, visual or mental status changes, and infrequently cardiovascular collapse; immediate medical attention required. Safety and efficacy have not been established in pediatric patients.

Lab Interactions Serum alkaline phosphatase, serum acid phosphatase, serum testosterone, serum LH and FSH, serum estradiol

Adverse Reactions Percentages reported in males with prostatic carcinoma and females with endometriosis using the 1-month implant:

>10%:

Central nervous system: Headache (female 75%, male 1% to 5%), emotional lability (female 60%), depression (female 54%, male 1% to 5%), pain (female 17%, male 8%), insomnia (female 11%, male 5%)

Endocrine & metabolic: Hot flashes (female 96%, male 62%), sexual dysfunction (21%), erections decreased (18%), libido decreased (female 61%), breast enlargement (female 18%)

Genitourinary: Lower urinary symptoms (male 13%), vaginitis (75%), dyspareunia (female 14%)

Miscellaneous: Diaphoresis (female 45%, male 6%); infection (female 13%)

1% to 10%:

Cardiovascular: CHF (male 5%), arrhythmia, cerebrovascular accident, hypertension, MI, peripheral vascular disorder, chest pain, palpitation, tachycardia, edema

Central nervous system: Lethargy (male 8%), dizziness (female 6%, male 5%), abnormal thinking, anxiety, chills, fever, malaise, migraine, somnolence

Dermatologic: Rash (female >1%, male 6%), alopecia, bruising, dry skin, skin discoloration

Endocrine & metabolic: Breast pain (female 7%), breast swelling/tenderness (male 1% to 5%), dysmenorrhea, gout, hyperglycemia

Gastrointestinal: Anorexia (female >1%, male 5%), nausea (male 5%), constipation, diarrhea, flatulence, dyspepsia, ulcer, vomiting, weight increased, xerostomia

Genitourinary: Renal insufficiency, urinary frequency, urinary obstruction, urinary tract infection, vaginal hemorrhage

Hematologic: Anemia, hemorrhage

Neuromuscular & skeletal: Arthralgia, bone mineral density decreased (female; ~4% decrease in 6 months), joint disorder, paresthesia

Ocular: Amblyopia, dry eyes

Respiratory: Upper respiratory tract infection (male 7%), COPD (male 5%), pharyngitis (female 5%), bronchitis, cough, epistaxis, rhinitis, sinusitis

Miscellaneous: Allergic reaction

Overdosage/Toxicology Symptomatic management

Pharmacodynamics/Kinetics

Time to Peak: SubQ: Male: 12-15 days, Female: 8-22 days

Half-Life Elimination: SubQ: Male: ~4 hours, Female: ~2 hours; Renal impairment: Male: 12 hours

Excretion: Urine (90%)

Pharmacokinetic Note Data reported using the 1-month implant.

Available Dosage Forms

Injection, solution, 1-month implant [disposable syringe; single-dose]: 3.6 mg [with 16-gauge hypodermic needle]

Injection, solution, 3-month implant [disposable syringe; single-dose]: 10.8 mg [with 14-gauge hypodermic needle]

Dosing

Adults & Elderly:

Prostate cancer: SubQ:

Monthly implant: 3.6 mg injected into upper abdomen every 28 days

3-month implant: 10.8 mg injected into the upper abdominal wall every 12 weeks

Breast cancer, endometriosis, endometrial thinning: SubQ: Monthly implant: 3.6 mg injected into upper abdomen every 28 days

Note: For breast cancer, treatment may continue indefinitely; for endometriosis, it is recommended that duration of treatment not exceed 6 months. Only 1-2 doses are recommended for endometrial thinning.

Administration

Other: Subcutaneous implant: Insert the hypodermic needle into the subcutaneous fat. Do not try to aspirate with the goserelin syringe. If the needle is in a large vessel, blood will immediately appear in the syringe chamber. Change the direction of the needle so it parallels the abdominal wall. Push the needle in until the barrel hub touches the patient's skin. Fully depress the plunger to discharge. Withdraw needle and bandage the site. Confirm discharge by ensuring tip of the plunger is visible within the tip of the needle.

Stability

Storage: Zoladex® should be stored at room temperature not to exceed 25°C (77°F). Protect from light. Should be dispensed in a lightproof bag.

Nursing Actions

Physical Assessment: Assess potential for interactions with other prescriptions, OTC medications, or herbal products patient may be taking. Monitor patient response periodically during therapy. Teach patient proper use, possible side effects/appropriate interventions, and adverse symptoms to report. **Pregnancy risk factor X:** Determine that patient is not pregnant before beginning treatment. Do not give to women of childbearing age unless female is capable of complying with contraceptive measures 1 month prior to therapy, during therapy, and at least 12 weeks following therapy. Instruct patient in appropriate contraceptive measures.

Patient Education: Do not take any new medication during therapy unless approved by prescriber. This drug must be implanted under the skin of your abdomen every 28 days; it is important to maintain appointment schedule. Males or females, you may experience systemic hot flashes (layered, cool clothes may help); headache (consult prescriber for approved analgesic); constipation (increased bulk and water in diet or stool softener may help); sexual dysfunction (decreased libido, males: decreased erection, females: vaginal dryness); or bone pain (consult prescriber for approved analgesic). Symptoms may worsen temporarily during first weeks of therapy. Report chest pain, palpitations, or respiratory difficulty; swelling of extremities; unusual persistent nausea, vomiting, or constipation; chest pain or respiratory difficulty; unresolved dizziness; or skin rash. **Pregnancy/breast-feeding precautions:** Inform prescriber if you are pregnant; do not get pregnant 1 month before, during, or for 1 month following therapy. Consult prescriber for instruction on appropriate contraceptive measures. This drug may cause severe fetal defects. Do not donate blood during or for 1 month following therapy (same reason). Do not breast-feed.

Pregnancy Issues Goserelin has been found to be teratogenic and increases pregnancy loss in animal studies. Women of childbearing potential should avoid pregnancy. Pregnancy must be ruled out prior to treatment. Use of nonhormonal contraception should be used during therapy and following discontinuation until the return of menses (or for at least 12 weeks).

Granisetron (gra NI se tron)

U.S. Brand Names Kytril®
Synonyms BRL 43694
Pharmacologic Category Antiemetic; Selective 5-HT$_3$ Receptor Antagonist
Medication Safety Issues
Sound-alike/look-alike issues:
Granisetron may be confused with dolasetron, ondansetron, palonosetron
Pregnancy Risk Factor B
Lactation Excretion in breast milk unknown/use caution
Use Prophylaxis of nausea and vomiting associated with emetogenic chemotherapy and radiation therapy, (including total body irradiation and fractionated abdominal radiation); prophylaxis and treatment of postoperative nausea and vomiting (PONV)

Generally **not** recommended for treatment of existing chemotherapy-induced emesis (CIE) or for prophylaxis of nausea from agents with a low emetogenic potential.
Mechanism of Action/Effect Selective 5-HT$_3$ receptor antagonist, blocking serotonin, both peripherally on vagal nerve terminals and centrally in the chemoreceptor trigger zone.
Contraindications Previous hypersensitivity to granisetron, other 5-HT$_3$ receptor antagonists, or any component of the formulation
Warnings/Precautions Chemotherapy-related emesis: **Granisetron should be used on a scheduled basis, not on an "as needed" (PRN) basis,** since data support the use of this drug in the prevention of nausea and vomiting and not in the rescue of nausea and vomiting. Granisetron should be used only in the first 24-48 hours of receiving chemotherapy or radiation. Data do not support any increased efficacy of granisetron in delayed nausea and vomiting. May be prescribed for patients who are refractory to or have severe adverse reactions to standard antiemetic therapy or young patients (ie, <45 years of age who are more likely to develop extrapyramidal symptoms to high-dose metoclopramide) who are to receive highly emetogenic chemotherapeutic agents. Should not be prescribed for chemotherapeutic agents with a low emetogenic potential (eg, bleomycin, busulfan, etoposide, 5-fluorouracil, vinblastine, vincristine).

Routine prophylaxis for PONV is not recommended. In patients where nausea and vomiting must be avoided postoperatively, administer to all patients even when expected incidence of nausea and vomiting is low. Use caution following abdominal surgery or in chemotherapy-induced nausea and vomiting; may mask progressive ileus or gastric distention. Use caution in patients with liver disease or in pregnancy. Safety and efficacy in children <2 years of age have not been established. Injection contains benzyl alcohol (1 mg/mL) and should not be used in neonates.

Drug Interactions
Cytochrome P450 Effect: Substrate of CYP3A4 (minor)
Increased Effect/Toxicity: Granisetron may enhance the hypotensive effect of apomorphine.
Nutritional/Ethanol Interactions Herb/Nutraceutical: St John's wort may decrease granisetron levels.
Adverse Reactions
>10%:
Central nervous system: Headache (9% to 21%)
Gastrointestinal: Constipation (3% to 18%)
Neuromuscular & skeletal: Weakness (5% to 18%)
1% to 10%:
Cardiovascular: Hypertension (1% to 2%)
Central nervous system: Pain (10%), fever (3% to 9%), dizziness (4% to 5%), insomnia (<2% to 5%), somnolence (1% to 4%), anxiety (2%), agitation (<2%), CNS stimulation (<2%)

Dermatologic: Rash (1%)
Gastrointestinal: Diarrhea (3% to 9%), abdominal pain (4% to 6%), dyspepsia (3% to 6%), taste perversion (2%)
Hepatic: Liver enzymes increased (5% to 6%)
Renal: Oliguria (2%)
Respiratory: Cough (2%)
Miscellaneous: Infection (3%)
Overdosage/Toxicology Overdoses of up to 38.5 mg have been reported without symptoms or with only slight headache. In the event of an overdose, treatment should be symptomatic and supportive.
Pharmacodynamics/Kinetics
Duration of Action: Generally up to 24 hours
Protein Binding: 65%
Half-Life Elimination: Terminal: 5-9 hours
Metabolism: Hepatic via N-demethylation, oxidation, and conjugation; some metabolites may have 5-HT$_3$ antagonist activity
Excretion: Urine (12% as unchanged drug, 48% to 49% as metabolites); feces (34% to 38% as metabolites)
Available Dosage Forms
Injection, solution: 1 mg/mL (1 mL, 4 mL) [contains benzyl alcohol]
Injection, solution [preservative free]: 0.1 mg/mL (1 mL)
Solution, oral: 2 mg/10 mL (30 mL) [contains sodium benzoate; orange flavor]
Tablet: 1 mg
Dosing
Adults & Elderly:
Prophylaxis of chemotherapy-related emesis:
Oral: 2 mg once daily up to 1 hour before chemotherapy or 1 mg twice daily; the first 1 mg dose should be given up to 1 hour before chemotherapy.
I.V.:
Within U.S.: 10 mcg/kg/dose (maximum: 1 mg/dose) given 30 minutes prior to chemotherapy; for some drugs (eg, carboplatin, cyclophosphamide) with a later onset of emetic action, 10 mcg/kg every 12 hours may be necessary.
Outside U.S.: 40 mcg/kg/dose (or 3 mg/dose); maximum: 9 mg/24 hours
Breakthrough: Granisetron has not been shown to be effective in terminating nausea or vomiting once it occurs and should not be used for this purpose.
Prophylaxis of radiation therapy-associated emesis: Oral: 2 mg once daily given 1 hour before radiation therapy.
Postoperative nausea and vomiting (PONV): I.V.:
Prevention: 1 mg given undiluted over 30 seconds; administer before induction of anesthesia or immediately before reversal of anesthesia
Treatment: 1 mg given undiluted over 30 seconds
Pediatrics: Prophylaxis associated with cancer chemotherapy: Children >2 years: Refer to adult dosing.
Renal Impairment: No dosage adjustment required.
Hepatic Impairment: Kinetic studies in patients with hepatic impairment showed that total clearance was approximately halved; however, standard doses were very well tolerated, and dose adjustments are not necessary.

Administration
Oral: Doses should be given up to 1 hour prior to initiation of chemotherapy/radiation
I.V.: Administer I.V. push over 30 seconds or as a 5-10 minute-infusion
Prevention of PONV: Administer before induction of anesthesia or immediately before reversal of anesthesia.
Treatment of PONV: Administer undiluted over 30 seconds.
(Continued)

Granisetron (Continued)

I.V. Detail: pH: 4.7-7.3

Stability

Compatibility: Stable in D₅½NS, D₅NS, D₅W, NS, bacteriostatic water

Y-site administration: Incompatible with amphotericin B

Storage:

I.V.: Store at 15°C to 30°C (59°F to 86°F). Protect from light. Do not freeze vials. Stable when mixed in NS or D₅W for 7 days under refrigeration and for 3 days at room temperature.

Oral: Store tablet or oral solution at 15°C to 30°C (59°F to 86°F). Protect from light.

Nursing Actions

Physical Assessment: Note: Oral and I.V. doses have different administration schedules and should not be administered on "as-needed" basis. Assess therapeutic effectiveness (prophylactic relief of nausea and vomiting associated with chemotherapy or radiation) and adverse response (eg, acute headache, CNS changes) periodically during therapy. Teach patient proper use (if self-administered oral), possible side effects/appropriate interventions and adverse symptoms to report.

Patient Education: This drug will be administered on days when you receive chemotherapy to reduce nausea and vomiting. If outpatient chemotherapy, you may be given oral medication to take after return home; take as directed. May also be given to prevent or treat nausea and vomiting after surgery; take as directed. You may experience drowsiness (use caution if driving); persistent or acute headache (request analgesic from prescriber); or nausea (frequent mouth care, chewing gum, or sucking on lozenges may help). Report unrelieved headache, fever, diarrhea, or constipation. **Breast-feeding precaution:** Consult prescriber if breast-feeding.

Geriatric Considerations Clinical trials with patients older than 65 years of age are limited; however, the data indicates that safety and efficacy are similar to that observed in younger adults. No adjustment in dose necessary for elderly.

Pregnancy Issues There are no adequate or well-controlled studies in pregnant women. Teratogenic effects were not observed in animal studies. Injection (1 mg/mL strength) contains benzyl alcohol which may cross the placenta. Use only if benefit exceeds the risk.

Griseofulvin (gri see oh FUL vin)

U.S. Brand Names Grifulvin® V; Gris-PEG®

Synonyms Griseofulvin Microsize; Griseofulvin Ultramicrosize

Pharmacologic Category Antifungal Agent, Oral

Medication Safety Issues

Sound-alike/look-alike issues:

Fulvicin® may be confused with Furacin®

Pregnancy Risk Factor C

Lactation Excretion in breast milk unknown

Use Treatment of susceptible tinea infections of the skin, hair, and nails

Mechanism of Action/Effect Inhibits fungal cell mitosis at metaphase; binds to human keratin making it resistant to fungal invasion

Contraindications Hypersensitivity to griseofulvin or any component of the formulation; severe liver disease; porphyria (interferes with porphyrin metabolism)

Warnings/Precautions Safe use in children ≤2 years of age has not been established; during long-term therapy, periodic assessment of hepatic, renal, and hematopoietic functions should be performed; may cause fetal harm when administered to pregnant women; avoid

exposure to intense sunlight to prevent photosensitivity reactions; hypersensitivity cross reaction between penicillins and griseofulvin is possible.

Drug Interactions

Cytochrome P450 Effect: Induces CYP1A2 (weak), 2C8/9 (weak), 3A4 (weak)

Decreased Effect: Barbiturates may decrease levels. Decreased warfarin activity. Decreased oral contraceptive effectiveness.

Increased Effect/Toxicity: Increased toxicity with ethanol, may cause tachycardia and flushing.

Nutritional/Ethanol Interactions

Ethanol: Avoid ethanol (may increase CNS depression). Ethanol will cause "disulfiram"-type reaction consisting of flushing, headache, nausea, and in some patients, vomiting and chest and/or abdominal pain.

Food: Griseofulvin concentrations may be increased if taken with food, especially with high-fat meals.

Lab Interactions False-positive urinary VMA levels

Adverse Reactions Frequency not defined.

Central nervous system: Headache, fatigue, dizziness, insomnia, mental confusion

Dermatologic: Rash (most common), urticaria (most common), photosensitivity, erythema multiforme, angioneurotic edema (rare)

Gastrointestinal: Nausea, vomiting, epigastric distress, diarrhea, GI bleeding

Genitourinary: Menstrual irregularities (rare)

Hematologic: Leukopenia, granulocytopenia

Neuromuscular & skeletal: Paresthesia (rare)

Renal: Hepatotoxicity, proteinuria, nephrosis

Miscellaneous: Oral thrush, drug-induced lupus-like syndrome (rare)

Overdosage/Toxicology Symptoms of overdose include lethargy, vertigo, blurred vision, nausea, vomiting, and diarrhea. Treatment is supportive.

Pharmacodynamics/Kinetics

Half-Life Elimination: 9-22 hours

Metabolism: Extensively hepatic

Excretion: Urine (<1% as unchanged drug); feces; perspiration

Available Dosage Forms

Suspension, oral, microsize (Grifulvin® V): 125 mg/5 mL (120 mL) [contains alcohol 0.2%]

Tablet, microsize (Grifulvin® V): 500 mg

Tablet, ultramicrosize: 125 mg, 250 mg, 330 mg

Gris-PEG®: 125 mg, 250 mg

Dosing

Adults & Elderly:

Tinea infections: Oral:

Microsize: 500-1000 mg/day in single or divided doses

Ultramicrosize: 330-375 mg/day in single or divided doses; doses up to 750 mg/day have been used for infections more difficult to eradicate such as tinea unguium and tinea pedis.

Note: Duration of therapy depends on the site of infection:

Tinea corporis: 2-4 weeks

Tinea capitis: 4-6 weeks or longer (up to 8-12 weeks)

Tinea pedis: 4-8 weeks

Tinea unguium: 4-6 months

Pediatrics:

Tinea infections: Oral: Children >2 years:

Microsize: 10-15 mg/kg/day in single or divided doses. In the treatment of tinea capitis, higher dosages (20-25 mg/kg/day for 8-12 weeks) have been recommended by some authors (unlabeled).

Ultramicrosize: 5.5-7.3 mg/kg/day in single or divided doses. In the treatment of tinea capitis, higher dosages (15 mg/kg/day for 8-12 weeks) have been recommended by some authors (unlabeled).

Administration

Oral: Oral: Administer with a fatty meal (peanuts or ice cream) to increase absorption, or with food or milk to avoid GI upset

Laboratory Monitoring Periodic renal, hepatic, and hematopoietic function especially with long-term use

Nursing Actions

Physical Assessment: Assess allergic history prior to beginning treatment (cross reaction with penicillin is possible). Assess potential for interactions with other pharmacological agents or herbal products patient may be taking (eg, decreased effectiveness of oral contraceptives). Assess results of laboratory tests, renal function, and hepatic function with long-term use, therapeutic effectiveness (resolution of viral infection), and adverse response (eg, CNS changes, gastrointestinal upset, rash, opportunistic infection) periodically during therapy. Teach patient proper use, possible side effects/appropriate interventions and adverse symptoms to report.

Patient Education: Do not take any new medication during therapy unless approved by prescriber. Take as directed, around-the-clock with food. Take full course of medication; do not discontinue without consulting prescriber. Avoid alcohol while taking this drug (disulfiram reactions). Practice good hygiene measures to prevent reinfection. Frequent blood tests may be required with prolonged therapy. You may experience confusion, dizziness, drowsiness (use caution when driving or engaging in tasks that require alertness until response to drug is known); nausea, vomiting, or diarrhea (small, frequent meals, frequent mouth care, sucking lozenges, or chewing gum may help); or increased sensitivity to sun (use sunscreen, wear protective clothing and eyewear, and avoid excessive exposure to direct sunlight). Report skin rash; respiratory difficulty; CNS changes (confusion, dizziness, acute headache); changes in color of stool or urine; white plaques in mouth; or worsening of condition. **Pregnancy/breast-feeding precautions:** Inform prescriber if you are or intend to become pregnant. Consult prescriber if breast-feeding.

Guaifenesin (gwye FEN e sin)

U.S. Brand Names Allfen Jr; Diabetic Tussin® EX [OTC]; Ganidin NR; Guiatuss™ [OTC]; Humibid® *e* [OTC]; Iophen NR; Mucinex® [OTC]; Naldecon Senior EX® [OTC] [DSC]; Organ-1 NR; Organidin® NR; Phanasin® [OTC]; Phanasin® Diabetic Choice [OTC]; Q-Tussin [OTC]; Robitussin® [OTC]; Scot-Tussin® Expectorant [OTC]; Siltussin DAS [OTC]; Siltussin SA [OTC]; Tussin [OTC]; Vicks® Casero™ [OTC]

Synonyms GG; Glycerol Guaiacolate

Pharmacologic Category Expectorant

Medication Safety Issues

Sound-alike/look-alike issues:

Guaifenesin may be confused with guanfacine

Mucinex® may be confused with Mucomyst®

Naldecon® may be confused with Nalfon®

Pregnancy Risk Factor C

Lactation Excretion in breast milk unknown/use caution

Use Help loosen phlegm and thin bronchial secretions to make coughs more productive

Mechanism of Action/Effect Thought to act as an expectorant by irritating the gastric mucosa and stimulating respiratory tract secretions, thereby increasing respiratory fluid volumes and decreasing mucus viscosity

Contraindications Hypersensitivity to guaifenesin or any component of the formulation

Warnings/Precautions Not for persistent cough such as occurs with smoking, asthma, chronic bronchitis, or emphysema or cough accompanied by excessive secretions. When used for self-medication (OTC), contact healthcare provider if needed for >7 days or for a cough with a fever, rash, or persistent headache.

Lab Interactions Possible color interference with determination of 5-HIAA and VMA; discontinue 48 hours prior to test

Adverse Reactions Frequency not defined.

Central nervous system: Dizziness, drowsiness, headache

Dermatologic: Rash

Endocrine & metabolic: Uric acid levels decreased

Gastrointestinal: Nausea, vomiting, stomach pain

Postmarketing and/or case reports: Kidney stone formation (with consumption of large quantities)

Overdosage/Toxicology Symptoms of overdose include vomiting, lethargy, coma, and respiratory depression. Treatment is supportive.

Pharmacodynamics/Kinetics

Half-Life Elimination: ~1 hour

Excretion: Urine (as unchanged drug and metabolites)

Available Dosage Forms [DSC] = Discontinued product

Liquid: 100 mg/5 mL (120 mL, 480 mL)

Diabetic Tussin EX®: 100 mg/5 mL (120 mL) [alcohol free, sugar free, dye free; contains phenylalanine 8.4 mg/5 mL]

Ganidin NR: 100 mg/5 mL (480 mL) [raspberry flavor]

Iophen NR: 100 mg/5 mL (480 mL)

Naldecon Senior EX®: 200 mg/5 mL (120 mL) [alcohol free, sugar free; contains sodium benzoate] [DSC]

Organidin® NR: 100 mg/5 mL (480 mL) [contains sodium benzoate; raspberry flavor]

Q-Tussin: 100 mg/5 mL (120 mL, 240 mL, 480 mL, 3840 mL) [alcohol free; cherry flavor]

Siltussin DAS: 100 mg/5 mL (120 mL) [alcohol free, dye free, sugar free; strawberry flavor]

Syrup: 100 mg/5 mL (120 mL, 480 mL)

Guiatuss™: 100 mg/5 mL (120 mL, 480 mL) [alcohol free; fruit-mint flavor]

Phanasin®: 100 mg/5 mL (120 mL, 240 mL) [alcohol free, sugar free; mint flavor]

Phanasin® Diabetic Choice: 100 mg/5 mL (120 mL) [alcohol free, sugar free; mint flavor]

Robitussin®: 100 mg/5 mL (5 mL, 10 mL, 15 mL, 30 mL, 120 mL, 240 mL, 480 mL) [alcohol free; contains sodium benzoate]

Scot-Tussin® Expectorant: 100 mg/5 mL (120 mL) [alcohol free, dye free, sugar free; contains benzoic acid; grape flavor]

Siltussin SA: 100 mg/5 mL (120 mL, 240 mL, 480 mL) [alcohol free, sugar free; strawberry flavor]

Tussin: 100 mg/5 mL (120 mL, 240 mL)

Vicks® Casero™: 100 mg/6.25 mL (120 mL, 480 mL) [contains phenylalanine 5.5 mg/12.5 mL, sodium 32 mg/12.5 mL, and sodium benzoate; honey menthol flavor]

Syrup, oral drops (Phanasin®): 50 mg/mL (50 mL) [alcohol free, sugar free; fruit flavor]

Tablet: 200 mg

Allfen Jr: 400 mg [dye free]

Humibid® *e*: 400 mg

Organ-1 NR, Organidin® NR: 200 mg

Tablet, extended release (Mucinex®): 600 mg

Dosing

Adults & Elderly:

Cough (expectorant): Oral: 200-400 mg every 4 hours to a maximum of 2.4 g/day

Extended release tablet: 600-1200 mg every 12 hours, not to exceed 2.4 g/day

Pediatrics:

Cough (expectorant): Oral: Children:

6 months to 2 years: 25-50 mg every 4 hours, not to exceed 300 mg/day

2-5 years: 50-100 mg every 4 hours, not to exceed 600 mg/day

(Continued)

Guaifenesin *(Continued)*

6-11 years: 100-200 mg every 4 hours, not to exceed 1.2 g/day

>12 years: Refer to adult dosing.

Administration

Oral: Do not crush, chew, or break extended release tablets. Administer with a full glass of water.

Nursing Actions

Physical Assessment: Monitor effectiveness of therapy and adverse reactions at beginning of therapy and periodically with long-term use. Teach patient appropriate use, interventions to reduce side effects, and adverse symptoms to report.

Patient Education: Do not take any new medication during therapy without consulting prescriber. Take as prescribed; do not exceed prescribed dose or frequency. Do not chew or crush extended release tablet; take with a full glass of water. Maintain adequate hydration (2-3 L/day of fluids) unless instructed to restrict fluid intake. You may experience some drowsiness (use caution when driving or engaging in tasks requiring alertness until response to drug is known). Report excessive drowsiness, respiratory difficulty, lack of improvement, or worsening of condition. **Pregnancy/breast-feeding precautions:** Inform prescriber if you are or intend to become pregnant. Consult prescriber if breast-feeding.

Dietary Considerations

Diabetic Tussin® EX contains phenylalanine 8.4 mg/5 mL.

Vicks® Casero™ contains phenylalanine 5.5 mg/12.5 mL and sodium 32 mg/12.5 mL.

Guaifenesin and Codeine

(gwye FEN e sin & KOE deen)

U.S. Brand Names Brontex®; Cheracol®; Cheratussin AC; Diabetic Tussin C®; Gani-Tuss® NR; Guaifen-C; Guaifenesin AC; Guaituss AC; Iophen-C NR; Kolephrin® #1; Mytussin® AC; Robafen® AC; Romilar® AC; Tussi-Organidin® NR; Tussi-Organidin® S-NR

Synonyms Codeine and Guaifenesin

Restrictions C-V

Pharmacologic Category Antitussive; Cough Preparation; Expectorant

Pregnancy Risk Factor C

Lactation Excretion in breast milk unknown/use caution

Use Temporary control of cough due to minor throat and bronchial irritation

Available Dosage Forms

Liquid:

Brontex®: Guaifenesin 75 mg and codeine phosphate 2.5 mg per 5 mL (480 mL) [alcohol free; strawberry mint flavor]

Diabetic Tussin C®: Guaifenesin 200 mg and codeine phosphate 10 mg per 5 mL (480 mL) [contains phenylalanine 0.03 mcg/5 mL; cherry vanilla flavor]

Gani-Tuss® NR: Guaifenesin 100 mg and codeine phosphate 10 mg per 5 mL (480 mL) [raspberry flavor]

Guaifen-C: Guaifenesin 75 mg and codeine phosphate 2.5 mg per 5 mL (480 mL) [cherry flavor]

Guaifenesin AC: Guaifenesin 100 mg and codeine phosphate 10 mg per 5 mL (120 mL, 480 mL) [alcohol free, sugar free; raspberry flavor]

Iophen-C NR: Guaifenesin 100 mg and codeine phosphate 10 mg per 5 mL (480 mL) [raspberry flavor]

Kolephrin® #1: Guaifenesin 100 mg and codeine phosphate 10 mg per 5 mL (120 mL) [contains sodium 1.1 mg/5 mL and sodium benzoate]

Tussi-Organidin® NR: Guaifenesin 100 mg and codeine phosphate 10 mg per 5 mL (480 mL) [contains sodium benzoate; raspberry flavor]

Tussi-Organidin® S-NR: Guaifenesin 100 mg and codeine phosphate 10 mg per 5 mL (120 mL) [contains sodium benzoate; raspberry flavor]

Syrup:

Cheracol®: Guaifenesin 100 mg and codeine phosphate 10 mg per 5 mL (120 mL) [contains alcohol 4.75% and benzoic acid]

Cheratussin AC: Guaifenesin 100 mg and codeine phosphate 10 mg per 5 mL (120 mL, 240 mL, 480 mL)

Guaituss AC: Guaifenesin 100 mg and codeine phosphate 10 mg per 5 mL (120 mL, 480 mL) [contains alcohol; sugar free; fruit-mint flavor]

Mytussin® AC: Guaifenesin 100 mg and codeine phosphate 10 mg per 5 mL (120 mL, 480 mL) [contains alcohol; sugar free; fruit flavor]

Robafen® AC: Guaifenesin 100 mg and codeine phosphate 10 mg per 5 mL (120 mL, 480 mL)

Romilar® AC: Guaifenesin 100 mg and codeine phosphate 10 mg per 5 mL (480 mL) [contains benzoic acid and phenylalanine; alcohol free, sugar free, dye free; grape flavor]

Tablet (Brontex®): Guaifenesin 300 mg and codeine phosphate 10 mg

Dosing

Adults & Elderly: Cough (antitussive/expectorant): Oral: 5-10 mL every 4-8 hours not to exceed 60 mL/24 hours

Pediatrics: Cough (antitussive/expectorant): Oral:

2-6 years: 1-1.5 mg/kg codeine/day divided into 4 doses administered every 4-6 hours (maximum: 30 mg/24 hours)

6-12 years: 5 mL every 4 hours, not to exceed 30 mL/24 hours

>12 years: 10 mL every 4 hours, up to 60 mL/24 hours

Nursing Actions

Physical Assessment: See individual agents.

Patient Education: See individual agents. **Pregnancy/breast-feeding precautions:** Inform prescriber if you are or intend to become pregnant. Consult prescriber if breast-feeding.

Related Information

Codeine *on page 296*

Guaifenesin *on page 597*

Guaifenesin and Dextromethorphan

(gwye FEN e sin & deks troe meth OR fan)

U.S. Brand Names Allfen-DM; Altarussin DM [OTC]; Amibid DM; Benylin® Expectorant [OTC] [DSC]; Cheracol® D [OTC]; Cheracol® Plus [OTC]; Coricidin HBP® Chest Congestion and Cough [OTC]; Diabetic Tussin® DM [OTC]; Diabetic Tussin® DM Maximum Strength [OTC]; Drituss DM; Duratuss® DM; Gani-Tuss DM NR; Genatuss DM® [OTC]; Guaicon DM [OTC]; Guaicon DMS [OTC]; Guaifenex® DM; Guia-D; Guiatuss-DM® [OTC]; Humibid® CS [OTC] [DSC]; Hydro-Tussin™ DM; Iophen DM NR; Kolephrin® GG/DM [OTC]; Mindal DM [DSC]; Mintab DM; Mucinex® DM [OTC]; Phanatuss® DM [OTC]; Q-Bid DM; Q-Tussin DM [OTC]; Respa-DM®; Robafen DM [OTC]; Robitussin® Cough and Congestion [OTC]; Robitussin® DM [OTC]; Robitussin® DM Infant [OTC]; Robitussin® Sugar Free Cough [OTC]; Safe Tussin® [OTC]; Scot-Tussin® Senior [OTC]; Silexin [OTC]; Siltussin DM [OTC]; Siltussin DM DAS [OTC]; Su-Tuss DM; Touro® DM; Vicks® 44E [OTC]; Vicks® Pediatric Formula 44E [OTC]; Z-Cof LA™

Synonyms Dextromethorphan and Guaifenesin

Pharmacologic Category Antitussive; Cough Preparation; Expectorant

Pregnancy Risk Factor C

Lactation Excretion in breast milk unknown/use caution

Use Temporary control of cough due to minor throat and bronchial irritation

Available Dosage Forms [DSC] = Discontinued product

Caplet, sustained release (Mindal DM [DSC]): Guaifenesin 500 mg and dextromethorphan hydrobromide 30 mg

Capsule, softgel (Coricidin HBP® Chest Congestion and Cough): Guaifenesin 200 mg and dextromethorphan hydrobromide 10 mg

Elixir:

Duratuss DM®: Guaifenesin 225 mg and dextromethorphan hydrobromide 25 mg per 5 mL (480 mL) [contains sodium benzoate; grape flavor]

Drituss DM: Guaifenesin 200 mg and dextromethorphan hydrobromide 20 mg per 5 mL (480 mL) [grape flavor]

Su-Tuss DM: Guaifenesin 200 mg and dextromethorphan hydrobromide 20 mg per 5 mL (480 mL) [fruit flavor]

Liquid: Guaifenesin 100 mg and dextromethorphan hydrobromide 10 mg per 5 mL (480 mL)

Diabetic Tussin® DM: Guaifenesin 100 mg and dextromethorphan hydrobromide 10 mg per 5 mL (120 mL) [alcohol free, sugar free, dye free; contains phenylalanine 8.4 mg/5 mL]

Diabetic Tussin® DM Maximum Strength: Guaifenesin 200 mg and dextromethorphan hydrobromide 10 mg per 5 mL (120 mL) [alcohol free, sugar free, dye free; contains phenylalanine 8.4 mg/5 mL]

Gani-Tuss® DM NR: Guaifenesin 100 mg and dextromethorphan hydrobromide 10 mg per 5 mL (480 mL) [raspberry flavor]

Hydro-Tussin™ DM: Guaifenesin 200 mg and dextromethorphan hydrobromide 20 mg per 5 mL (480 mL) [alcohol free, sugar free; contains sodium benzoate]

Iophen DM NR: Guaifenesin 100 mg and dextromethorphan hydrobromide 10 mg per 5 mL (480 mL) [raspberry flavor]

Kolephrin® GG/DM: Guaifenesin 150 mg and dextromethorphan hydrobromide 10 mg per 5 mL (120 mL) [alcohol free; cherry flavor]

Q-Tussin DM: Guaifenesin 100 mg and dextromethorphan hydrobromide 10 mg per 5 mL (120 mL, 240 mL, 480 mL, 3840 mL) [cherry flavor]

Safe Tussin®: Guaifenesin 100 mg and dextromethorphan hydrobromide 15 mg per 5 mL (120 mL) [alcohol free, sodium free, sugar free, dye free; mint flavor]

Scot-Tussin® Senior: Guaifenesin 200 mg and dextromethorphan hydrobromide 15 mg per 5 mL (120 mL) [alcohol free, sodium free, sugar free]

Vicks® 44E: Guaifenesin 200 mg and dextromethorphan hydrobromide 20 mg per 15 mL (120 mL, 235 mL) [contains sodium 31 mg/15 mL, alcohol, sodium benzoate]

Vicks® Pediatric Formula 44E: Guaifenesin 100 mg and dextromethorphan hydrobromide 10 mg per 15 mL (120 mL) [alcohol free; contains sodium 30 mg/15 mL, sodium benzoate; cherry flavor]

Liquid, oral drops (Robitussin® DM Infant): Guaifenesin 100 mg and dextromethorphan hydrobromide 5 mg per 2.5 mL (30 mL) [alcohol free; contains sodium benzoate; fruit punch flavor]

Syrup: Guaifenesin 100 mg and dextromethorphan hydrobromide 10 mg per 5 mL (120 mL, 480 mL)

Altarussin DM: Guaifenesin 100 mg and dextromethorphan hydrobromide 10 mg per 5 mL (120 mL, 240 mL, 480 mL, 3840 mL)

Benylin® Expectorant: Guaifenesin 100 mg and dextromethorphan hydrobromide 5 mg per 5 mL (120 mL) [alcohol free, sugar free; contains sodium benzoate; raspberry flavor] [DSC]

Cheracol® D: Guaifenesin 100 mg and dextromethorphan hydrobromide 10 mg per 5 mL (120 mL, 180 mL) [contains alcohol 4.75%, benzoic acid]

Cheracol® Plus: Guaifenesin 100 mg and dextromethorphan hydrobromide 10 mg per 5 mL (120 mL) [contains alcohol 4.75%, benzoic acid]

Genatuss DM®: Guaifenesin 100 mg and dextromethorphan hydrobromide 10 mg per 5 mL (120 mL)

Guiatuss® DM: Guaifenesin 100 mg and dextromethorphan hydrobromide 10 mg per 5 mL (120 mL, 480 mL, 3840 mL) [alcohol free; contains sodium benzoate]

Guaicon DM®: Guaifenesin 100 mg and dextromethorphan hydrobromide 10 mg per 5 mL (10 mL) [alcohol free]

Guaicon DMS®: Guaifenesin 100 mg and dextromethorphan hydrobromide 10 mg per 5 mL (10 mL) [alcohol free, sugar free]

Mintab DM: Guaifenesin 200 mg and dextromethorphan hydrobromide 10 mg per 5 mL (480 mL) [alcohol free, dye free; cherry vanilla flavor]

Phanatuss® DM: Guaifenesin 100 mg and dextromethorphan hydrobromide 10 mg per 5 mL (120 mL) [alcohol free, sugar free]

Robafen® DM: Guaifenesin 100 mg and dextromethorphan hydrobromide 10 mg per 5 mL (120 mL, 240 mL, 480 mL) [cherry flavor]

Robitussin® Cough and Congestion: Guaifenesin 100 mg and dextromethorphan hydrobromide 10 mg per 5 mL (120 mL) [alcohol free; contains sodium benzoate]

Robitussin®-DM: Guaifenesin 100 mg and dextromethorphan hydrobromide 10 mg per 5 mL (5 mL, 120 mL, 340 mL, 360 mL) [alcohol free; contains sodium benzoate]

Robitussin® Sugar Free Cough: Guaifenesin 100 mg and dextromethorphan hydrobromide 10 mg per 5 mL (120 mL) [alcohol free, sugar free; contains sodium benzoate]

Silexin: Guaifenesin 100 mg and dextromethorphan hydrobromide 10 mg per 5 mL (45 mL) [alcohol free, sugar free)]

Siltussin DM: Guaifenesin 100 mg and dextromethorphan hydrobromide 10 mg per 5 mL (120 mL, 240 mL, 480 mL) [strawberry flavor]

Siltussin DM DAS: Guaifenesin 100 mg and dextromethorphan hydrobromide 10 mg per 5 mL (120 mL) [alcohol free, dye free, sugar free; strawberry flavor]

Tablet:

Humibid® CS: Guaifenesin 400 mg and dextromethorphan hydrobromide 20 mg [DSC]

Silexin: Guaifenesin 100 mg and dextromethorphan hydrobromide 10 mg

Tablet, extended release: Guaifenesin 500 mg and dextromethorphan hydrobromide 30 mg

Amibid DM, Guaifenex® DM, Mucinex® DM, Q-Bid DM, Respa-DM®: Guaifenesin 600 mg and dextromethorphan hydrobromide 30 mg

Mucophen® DM: Guaifenesin 1000 mg and dextromethorphan hydrobromide 60 mg

Touro® DM: Guaifenesin 575 mg and dextromethorphan hydrobromide 30 mg

Tablet, long-acting: Guaifenesin 500 mg and dextromethorphan hydrobromide 30 mg; guaifenesin 1000 mg and dextromethorphan hydrobromide 50 mg; guaifenesin 1000 mg and dextromethorphan hydrobromide 60 mg

Z-Cof LA [scored]: Guaifenesin 650 mg and dextromethorphan hydrobromide 30 mg

Tablet, sustained release: Guaifenesin 800 mg and dextromethorphan hydrobromide 30 mg; guaifenesin 1000 mg and dextromethorphan hydrobromide 60 mg; guaifenesin 1200 mg and dextromethorphan hydrobromide 60 mg

Allfen-DM: Guaifenesin 1000 mg and dextromethorphan hydrobromide 55 mg

Tussi-Bid®: Guaifenesin 1200 mg and dextromethorphan hydrobromide 60 mg

(Continued)

Guaifenesin and Dextromethorphan
(Continued)

Tablet, timed release [scored] (Guia-D): Guaifenesin 1000 mg and dextromethorphan hydrobromide 60 mg [dye free]

Dosing

Adults & Elderly: Cough (antitussive/expectorant): Oral:

General dosing guidelines: Guaifenesin 200-400 mg and dextromethorphan 10-20 mg every 4 hours (maximum dose: Guaifenesin 2400 mg and dextromethorphan 120 mg per day)

Product-specific labeling:

Benylin®: 20 mL every 4 hours (maximum: 6 doses/24 hours)

Guaifenex® DM, Mucinex® DM, Touro® DM: 1-2 tablets every 12 hours (maximum: 4 tablets/24 hours)

Humibid® CD: 1 tablet every 4 hours (maximum: 6 tablets/24 hours)

Robitussin® DM, Robitussin® Sugar Free Cough: 10 mL every 4 hours (maximum: 6 doses/24 hours)

Vicks® 44E: 15 mL every 4 hours (maximum: 6 doses/24 hours)

Vicks® Pediatric Formula 44E: 30 mL every 4 hours (maximum: 6 doses/24 hours)

Z-Cof LA™: 1 tablet every 12 hours

Pediatrics: Cough (antitussive/expectorant): Oral:

Children:

2-6 years:

General dosing guidelines: Guaifenesin 50-100 mg and dextromethorphan 2.5-5 mg every 4 hours (maximum dose: Guaifenesin 600 mg and dextromethorphan 30 mg per day)

Product-specific labeling:

Benylin®: 5 mL every 4 hour (maximum: 6 doses/24 hours)

Guaifenex® DM, Touro® DM: ½ tablet every 12 hours (maximum: 1 tablet every 12 hour)

Robitussin® DM, Robitussin® DM Infant, Robitussin® Sugar Free Cough: 2.5 mL every 4 hours (maximum: 6 doses/24 hours)

Vicks® Pediatric Formula 44E: 7.5 mL every 4 hours (maximum: 6 doses/24 hours)

6-12 years:

General dosing guidelines: Guaifenesin 100-200 mg and dextromethorphan 5-10 mg every 4 hours (maximum dose: Guaifenesin 1200 mg and dextromethorphan 60 mg per day)

Product-specific labeling:

Benylin®: 10 mL every 4 hours (maximum: 6 doses/24 hours)

Guaifenex® DM, Touro® DM: 1 tablet every 12 hours (maximum: 2 tablets/24 hours)

Humibid® CS: ½ tablet every 4 hours (maximum: 6 doses/24 hours)

Robitussin® DM, Robitussin® Sugar Free Cough: 5 mL every 4 hours (maximum: 6 doses/24 hours)

Vicks® 44E: 7.5 mL every 4 hours (maximum: 6 doses/24 hours)

Vicks® Pediatric Formula 44E: 15 mL every 4 hours (maximum: 6 doses/24 hours)

Z-Cof LA™: ½ tablet very 12 hours

≥12 years: Refer to adult dosing.

Nursing Actions

Physical Assessment: See individual agents.

Patient Education: Also see Guaifenesin.

Based on Dextromethorphan component: Do not exceed recommended dosage; take with a large glass of water; if cough lasts more than 1 week or is accompanied by a rash, fever, or headache, notify physician.

Pregnancy/breast-feeding precautions: Inform prescriber if you are or intend to become pregnant. Consult prescriber if breast-feeding.

Related Information

Guaifenesin *on page 597*

Guaifenesin and Pseudoephedrine
(gwye FEN e sin & soo doe e FED rin)

U.S. Brand Names Ambifed-G; Ami-Tex PSE; Congestac® [OTC]; Dynex; Entex® PSE; Eudal®-SR; G-Phed; Guaifenex® GP; Guaifenex® PSE; Guaimax-D®; Levall G; Maxifed®; Maxifed-G®; Miraphen PSE; Mucinex®-D [OTC]; Nasatab® LA; PanMist®-JR; PanMist®-LA; PanMist®-S; Profen Forte®; Profen II®; Pseudo GG TR; Pseudovent™; Pseudovent™ 400; Pseudovent™-Ped; Refenesen Plus [OTC]; Respaire®-60 SR; Respaire®-120 SR; Robitussin-PE® [OTC]; Robitussin® Severe Congestion [OTC]; Sudafed® Non-Drying Sinus [OTC]; Touro LA®; Zephrex®; Zephrex LA®

Synonyms Pseudoephedrine and Guaifenesin

Pharmacologic Category Alpha/Beta Agonist; Expectorant

Pregnancy Risk Factor C

Lactation Enters breast milk/contraindicated (by some manufacturers)

Use Temporary relief of nasal congestion and to help loosen phlegm and thin bronchial secretions in the treatment of cough

Available Dosage Forms [DSC] = Discontinued product

Caplet (Congestac®, Refenesen Plus): Guaifenesin 400 mg and pseudoephedrine hydrochloride 60 mg

Caplet, long-acting (Touro LA®): Guaifenesin 500 mg and pseudoephedrine hydrochloride 120 mg

Caplet, prolonged release (Ambifed-G): Guaifenesin 1000 mg and pseudoephedrine hydrochloride 60 mg

Capsule, extended release:

Respaire®-60 SR: Guaifenesin 200 mg and pseudoephedrine hydrochloride 60 mg

Respaire®-120 SR: Guaifenesin 250 mg and pseudoephedrine hydrochloride 120 mg

Capsule, liquicap (Sudafed® Non-Drying Sinus): Guaifenesin 200 mg and pseudoephedrine hydrochloride 30 mg

Capsule, softgel (Robitussin® Severe Congestion): Guaifenesin 200 mg and pseudoephedrine hydrochloride 30 mg

Capsule, variable release:

Entex® PSE: Guaifenesin 400 mg [immediate release] and pseudoephedrine hydrochloride 120 mg [extended release]

G-Phed: Guaifenesin 250 mg [immediate release] and pseudoephedrine hydrochloride 120 mg [prolonged release]

Levall G: Guaifenesin 400 mg [immediate release] and pseudoephedrine hydrochloride 90 mg [extended release]

Pseudovent™: Guaifenesin 250 mg [immediate release] and pseudoephedrine hydrochloride 120 mg [prolonged release]

Pseudovent™-Ped: Guaifenesin 300 mg [immediate release] and pseudoephedrine hydrochloride 60 mg [prolonged release]

Pseudovent™ 400: Guaifenesin 400 mg [immediate release] and pseudoephedrine hydrochloride 120 mg [extended release]

Syrup: Guaifenesin 200 mg and pseudoephedrine hydrochloride 40 mg per 5 mL (480 mL)

PanMist®-S: Guaifenesin 200 mg and pseudoephedrine hydrochloride 40 mg per 5 mL (480 mL) [alcohol free; grape flavor]

Robitussin-PE®: Guaifenesin 100 mg and pseudoephedrine hydrochloride 30 mg per 5 mL (120 mL, 240 mL) [alcohol free; contains sodium benzoate]

Tablet (Zephrex®): Guaifenesin 400 mg and pseudoephedrine hydrochloride 60 mg

Tablet, extended release: Guaifenesin 550 mg and pseudoephedrine hydrochloride 60 mg; guaifenesin 595 mg and pseudoephedrine hydrochloride 48 mg; guaifenesin 600 mg and pseudoephedrine hydrochloride 60 mg; guaifenesin 600 mg and pseudoephedrine hydrochloride 120 mg; guaifenesin 795 mg and pseudoephedrine hydrochloride 85 mg; guaifenesin 800 mg and pseudoephedrine hydrochloride 45 mg; guaifenesin 800 mg and pseudoephedrine hydrochloride 60 mg; guaifenesin 800 mg and pseudoephedrine hydrochloride 90 mg; guaifenesin 1200 mg and pseudoephedrine hydrochloride 50 mg; guaifenesin 1200 mg and pseudoephedrine hydrochloride 60 mg; guaifenesin 1200 mg and pseudoephedrine hydrochloride 75 mg; guaifenesin 1200 mg and pseudoephedrine hydrochloride 90 mg; guaifenesin 1200 mg and pseudoephedrine hydrochloride 120 mg

Ami-Tex PSE, Guaimax-D®, Zephrex LA®: Guaifenesin 600 mg and pseudoephedrine hydrochloride 120 mg

Guaifenex® GP: Guaifenesin 1200 mg and pseudoephedrine hydrochloride 120 mg [dye free]

Guaifenex® PSE 60: Guaifenesin 600 mg and pseudoephedrine hydrochloride 60 mg

Guaifenex® PSE 80: Guaifenesin 800 mg and pseudoephedrine hydrochloride 80 mg

Maxifed®: Guaifenesin 700 mg and pseudoephedrine hydrochloride 80 mg

Maxifed-G®: Guaifenesin 550 mg and pseudoephedrine hydrochloride 60 mg

Mucinex®-D 600/60: Guaifenesin 600 mg and pseudoephedrine hydrochloride 60 mg

Mucinex®-D 1200/120: Guaifenesin 1200 mg and pseudoephedrine hydrochloride 120 mg

PanMist®-JR, Pseudo GG TR: Guaifenesin 595 mg and pseudoephedrine hydrochloride 48 mg

PanMist®-LA: Guaifenesin 795 mg and pseudoephedrine hydrochloride 85 mg

Profen II®: Guaifenesin 800 mg and pseudoephedrine hydrochloride 45 mg

Profen Forte®: Guaifenesin 800 mg and pseudoephedrine hydrochloride 90 mg

Tablet, long acting:
Dynex: Guaifenesin 1200 mg and pseudoephedrine hydrochloride 90 mg

Guaifenex® PSE 120: Guaifenesin 600 mg and pseudoephedrine hydrochloride 120 mg [dye free]

Miraphen PSE: Guaifenesin 600 mg and pseudoephedrine hydrochloride 120 mg

Tablet, sustained release (Nasatab® LA): Guaifenesin 500 mg and pseudoephedrine hydrochloride 120 mg

Dosing
Adults: Expectorant/decongestant: Oral:
Ambifed-G, Aquatab® D, Dynex, Entex® PSE, Eudal®-SR, G-Phed, Guaifenex® GP, Guaifenex® PSE 120, Guaimax-D®, Levall G, Miraphen PSE, Mucinex®-D 1200/120, Nasatab® LA, PanMist®-LA, Profen Forte®, Pseudovent™, Respaire®-120 SR, Touro LA, Zephrex® LA: One tablet or capsule every 12 hours (maximum: 2 tablets or capsules in 24 hours)

Congestac®: One caplet every 4-6 hours (maximum: 4 caplets in 24 hours)

Guaifenex® PSE 60, Maxifed-G®, Mucinex®-D 600/60, PanMist®-JR, Pseudovent™-Ped, Respaire®-60 SR: 1-2 tablets or capsules every 12 hours (maximum: 4 tablets or capsules/24 hours)

Guaifenex® PSE 80, PanMist®-LA: One tablet every twelve hours (maximum: 3 tablets/24 hours)

Guaifenex™ RX: 1-2 of the AM tablets every morning and 1-2 of the PM tablets 12 hours following morning dose

Maxifed®, Profen II®: One to 1½ tablets every 12 hours (maximum: 3 tablets/24 hours)

PanMist®-S: Up to 10 mL 4 times/day

Robitussin® PE: 10 mL every 4-6 hours (maximum: 4 doses/24 hours)

Robitussin® Severe Congestion, Sudafed® Non-Drying Sinus: Two capsules every 4 hours (maximum: 4 doses/24 hours)

Zephrex®: One tablet every 6 hours

Elderly: Refer to adult dosing; use with caution.
Pediatrics: Expectorant/decongestant: Oral:
Children 2-6 years:
Guaifenex® PSE 60: One-half tablet every 12 hours (maximum: 1 tablet/12 hours)

Maxifed-G®: One-third to ½ tablet every 12 hours (maximum: 1 tablet/12 hours)

PanMist® S: 2.5 mL 4 times/day (maximum: Pseudoephedrine 4 mg/kg/day)

Robitussin® PE: 2.5 mL every 4-6 hours (maximum: 4 doses/24 hours)

Children 6-12 years:
Ambifed-G, Dynex, Eudal-SR®, Guaimax-D®, Guaifenex® PSE 80, Guaifenex® PSE 120, Maxifed®, Miraphen PSE, Nasatab® LA, PanMist® LA, Profen II®, Profen Forte®, Zephrex® LA: One-half caplet or tablet every 12 hours (maximum: 1 tablet/24 hours)

Congestac®: One-half caplet every 4-6 hours (maximum: 2 caplets/24 hours)

Guaifenex® PSE 60, PanMist®-JR, Pseudovent™-Ped, Respaire®-60 SR: One tablet or capsule every 12 hours (maximum: 2 tablets or capsules every 24 hours)

Levall G: One capsule every 24 hours

Maxifed-G®: One-half to 1 tablet every 12 hours (maximum: 2 tablets/24 hours)

PanMist® S: 5 mL 4 times/day (maximum: Pseudoephedrine 4 mg/kg/day)

Robitussin® PE: 5 mL every 4-6 hours (maximum: 4 doses/24 hours)

Robitussin® Severe Congestion: One capsule every 4 hours (maximum: 4 doses/24 hours)

Zephrex®: One-half tablet every 6 hours
>12 years: Refer to adult dosing.

Nursing Actions
Physical Assessment: See individual agents.
Patient Education: See individual agents. **Pregnancy/breast-feeding precautions:** Inform prescriber if you are or intend to become pregnant. Consult prescriber if breast-feeding.

Related Information
Guaifenesin *on page 597*
Pseudoephedrine *on page 1047*

Guaifenesin, Pseudoephedrine, and Codeine
(gwye FEN e sin, soo doe e FED rin, & KOE deen)

U.S. Brand Names Guiatuss™ DAC®; Mytussin® DAC; Nucofed® Expectorant; Nucofed® Pediatric Expectorant
Synonyms Codeine, Guaifenesin, and Pseudoephedrine; Pseudoephedrine, Guaifenesin, and Codeine
Restrictions C-III; C-V
Pharmacologic Category Antitussive/Decongestant/ Expectorant
Pregnancy Risk Factor C
Lactation Excretion in breast milk unknown/use caution
Use Temporarily relieves nasal congestion and controls cough due to minor throat and bronchial irritation; helps loosen phlegm and thin bronchial secretions to make coughs more productive

Available Dosage Forms [DSC] = Discontinued product
Syrup:
Guiatuss™ DAC: Guaifenesin 100 mg, pseudoephedrine hydrochloride 30 mg, and codeine phosphate 10 mg per 5 mL (480 mL)

Mytussin® DAC: Guaifenesin 100 mg, pseudoephedrine hydrochloride 30 mg, and codeine phosphate
(Continued)

Guaifenesin, Pseudoephedrine, and Codeine (Continued)

10 mg per 5 mL (120 mL, 480 mL) [sugar free; contains alcohol 1.7%; strawberry-raspberry flavor]

Nucofed® Expectorant: Guaifenesin 200 mg, pseudoephedrine hydrochloride 60 mg, and codeine phosphate 20 mg per 5 mL (480 mL) [contains alcohol 12.5%; cherry flavor]

Nucofed® Pediatric Expectorant: Guaifenesin 100 mg, pseudoephedrine hydrochloride 30 mg, and codeine phosphate 10 mg per 5 mL (480 mL) [contains alcohol 6%; strawberry flavor]

Dosing

Adults: Expectorant/decongestant/cough suppressant: Oral: 10 mL syrup every 4 hours

Elderly: Refer to adult dosing; use with caution.

Pediatrics: Expectorant/decongestant/cough suppressant: Oral:

Children 6-12 years: 5 mL every 4 hours, not to exceed 40 mL/24 hours

Children >12 years: Refer to adult dosing.

Nursing Actions

Physical Assessment: See individual agents.

Patient Education: See individual agents. **Pregnancy/breast-feeding precautions:** Inform prescriber if you are or intend to become pregnant. Consult prescriber if breast-feeding.

Related Information

Codeine *on page 296*
Guaifenesin *on page 597*
Pseudoephedrine *on page 1047*

Halcinonide (hal SIN oh nide)

U.S. Brand Names Halog®

Pharmacologic Category Corticosteroid, Topical

Medication Safety Issues

Sound-alike/look-alike issues:

Halcinonide may be confused with Halcion®

Halog® may be confused with Haldol®, Mycolog®

Pregnancy Risk Factor C

Use Inflammation of corticosteroid-responsive dermatoses [high potency topical corticosteroid]

Contraindications Hypersensitivity to halcinonide or any component of the formulation; viral, fungal, or tubercular skin lesions

Warnings/Precautions Adverse systemic effects may occur when used on large areas of the body, denuded areas, for prolonged periods of time, with an occlusive dressing, and/or in infants or small children.

Adverse Reactions Frequency not defined: Itching; dry skin; folliculitis; hypertrichosis; acneiform eruptions; hypopigmentation; perioral dermatitis; allergic contact dermatitis; skin maceration; skin atrophy; striae; local burning, irritation, miliaria; secondary infection

Overdosage/Toxicology When consumed in excessive quantities, systemic hypercorticism and adrenal suppression may occur; in those cases, discontinuation and withdrawal of the corticosteroid should be done judiciously

Pharmacodynamics/Kinetics

Metabolism: Primarily hepatic

Excretion: Urine

Available Dosage Forms [DSC] = Discontinued product

Cream (Halog®): 0.1% (15 g, 30 g, 60 g, 240 g) [DSC]

Ointment (Halog®): 0.1% (15 g, 30 g, 60 g, 240 g) [DSC]

Solution, topical (Halog®): 0.1% (20 mL, 60 mL)

Dosing

Adults & Elderly: Steroid-responsive dermatoses: Topical: Apply sparingly 1-3 times/day, occlusive

dressing may be used for severe or resistant dermatoses; a thin film is effective; do not overuse. Therapy should be discontinued when control is achieved; if no improvement is seen, reassessment of diagnosis may be necessary.

Pediatrics: Refer to adult dosing.

Nursing Actions

Physical Assessment: Assess potential for interactions with other prescriptions, OTC medications, or herbal products patient may be taking. Monitor patient response. Teach patient proper use (according to formulation), side effects/appropriate interventions, and symptoms to report.

Patient Education: For external use only. Do not use for eyes, mucous membranes, or open wounds. Use exactly as directed and for no longer than the period prescribed. Before using, wash and dry area gently. Apply in a thin layer (may rub in lightly). Apply light dressing (if necessary) to area being treated. Do not use occlusive dressing unless so advised by prescriber. Avoid prolonged or excessive use around sensitive tissues, genital, or rectal areas. Avoid exposing treated area to direct sunlight. Inform prescriber if condition worsens (redness, swelling, irritation, signs of infection, or open sores) or fails to improve. **Pregnancy precaution:** Inform prescriber if you are or intend to become pregnant.

Haloperidol (ha loe PER i dole)

U.S. Brand Names Haldol®; Haldol® Decanoate

Synonyms Haloperidol Decanoate; Haloperidol Lactate

Pharmacologic Category Antipsychotic Agent, Typical

Medication Safety Issues

Sound-alike/look-alike issues:

Haloperidol may be confused Halotestin®

Haldol® may be confused with Halcion®, Halenol®, Halog®, Halotestin®, Stadol®

Pregnancy Risk Factor C

Lactation Enters breast milk/not recommended (AAP rates "of concern")

Use Management of schizophrenia; control of tics and vocal utterances of Tourette's disorder in children and adults; severe behavioral problems in children

Unlabeled/Investigational Use Treatment of psychosis; may be used for the emergency sedation of severely-agitated or delirious patients; adjunctive treatment of ethanol dependence; antiemetic

Mechanism of Action/Effect Haloperidol is a butyrophenone antipsychotic which blocks postsynaptic mesolimbic dopaminergic D_1 and D_2 receptors in the brain; depresses the release of hypothalamic and hypophyseal hormones; believed to depress the reticular activating system thus affecting basal metabolism, body temperature, wakefulness, vasomotor tone, and emesis

Contraindications Hypersensitivity to haloperidol or any component of the formulation; Parkinson's disease; severe CNS depression; bone marrow suppression; severe cardiac or hepatic disease; coma

Warnings/Precautions May be sedating, use with caution in disorders where CNS depression is a feature. Caution in patients with hemodynamic instability, predisposition to seizures, subcortical brain damage, renal or respiratory disease. Esophageal dysmotility and aspiration have been associated with antipsychotic use - use with caution in patients at risk of pneumonia (ie, Alzheimer's disease). Caution in breast cancer or other prolactin-dependent tumors (may elevate prolactin levels). May alter temperature regulation or mask toxicity of other drugs due to antiemetic effects. Hypotension may occur, particularly with parenteral administration. Decanoate form should never be administered I.V. Adverse effects of decanoate may be prolonged. Avoid in thyrotoxicosis.

May alter cardiac conduction - life-threatening arrhythmias have occurred with therapeutic doses of antipsychotics. Use with caution in patients at risk of hypotension (orthostasis) or those who would tolerate transient hypotensive episodes (cerebrovascular disease, cardiovascular disease, or other medications which may predispose).

Use with caution in patients with decreased gastrointestinal motility, urinary retention, BPH, xerostomia, or visual problems. May exacerbate narrow-angle glaucoma (screening is recommended) or worsen myasthenia gravis. Relative to other neuroleptics, haloperidol has a low potency of cholinergic blockade.

May cause extrapyramidal symptoms, including pseudoparkinsonism, acute dystonic reactions, akathisia, and tardive dyskinesia (risk of these reactions is high relative to other neuroleptics). May be associated with neuroleptic malignant syndrome (NMS) or pigmentary retinopathy. Some tablets contain tartrazine.

Drug Interactions

Cytochrome P450 Effect: Substrate of CYP1A2 (minor), 2D6 (major), 3A4 (major); **Inhibits** CYP2D6 (moderate), 3A4 (moderate)

Decreased Effect: Haloperidol may inhibit the ability of bromocriptine to lower serum prolactin concentrations. Benztropine (and other anticholinergics) may inhibit the therapeutic response to haloperidol and excess anticholinergic effects may occur. Barbiturates, carbamazepine, and cigarette smoking may enhance the hepatic metabolism of haloperidol. Haloperidol may inhibit the antiparkinsonian effect of levodopa; avoid this combination. The levels/effects of haloperidol may be decreased by aminoglutethimide, carbamazepine, nafcillin, nevirapine, phenobarbital, phenytoin, rifamycins, and other CYP3A4 inducers. Haloperidol may decrease the levels/effects of CYP2D6 prodrug substrates (eg, codeine, hydrocodone, oxycodone, tramadol).

Increased Effect/Toxicity: Haloperidol concentrations/effects may be increased by chloroquine, propranolol, and sulfadoxine-pyridoxine. The levels/effects of haloperidol may be increased by azole antifungals, chlorpromazine, clarithromycin, delavirdine, diclofenac, doxycycline, erythromycin, fluoxetine, imatinib, isoniazid, miconazole, nefazodone, nicardipine, paroxetine, pergolide, propofol, protease inhibitors, quinidine, quinine, ritonavir, ropinirole, telithromycin, verapamil, and other CYP2D6 or 3A4 inhibitors.

Haloperidol may increase the levels/effects of amphetamines, selected beta-blockers, selected benzodiazepines, calcium channel blockers, cisapride, cyclosporine, dextromethorphan, ergot alkaloids, fluoxetine, selected HMG-CoA reductase inhibitors, lidocaine, mesoridazine, mirtazapine, nateglinide, nefazodone, paroxetine, risperidone, ritonavir, sildenafil (and other PDE-5 inhibitors), tacrolimus, thioridazine, tricyclic antidepressants, venlafaxine, and other substrates of CYP2D6 or 3A4.

Haloperidol may increase the effects of antihypertensives, CNS depressants (ethanol, narcotics, sedative-hypnotics), lithium, trazodone, and TCAs. Haloperidol in combination with indomethacin may result in drowsiness, tiredness, and confusion. Metoclopramide may increase risk of extrapyramidal symptoms (EPS). Acetylcholinesterase inhibitors (central) may increase the risk of antipsychotic-related EPS.

Nutritional/Ethanol Interactions

Ethanol: Avoid ethanol (may increase CNS depression).

Herb/Nutraceutical: Avoid valerian, St John's wort, kava kava, gotu kola (may increase CNS depression).

Lab Interactions decreased cholesterol (S)

Adverse Reactions Frequency not defined.

Cardiovascular: Hyper-/hypotension, tachycardia, arrhythmia, abnormal T waves with prolonged ventricular repolarization, torsade de pointes (case-control study ~4%)

Central nervous system: Restlessness, anxiety, extrapyramidal symptoms, dystonic reactions, pseudoparkinsonian signs and symptoms, tardive dyskinesia, neuroleptic malignant syndrome (NMS), altered central temperature regulation, akathisia, tardive dystonia, insomnia, euphoria, agitation, drowsiness, depression, lethargy, headache, confusion, vertigo, seizure

Dermatologic: Hyperpigmentation, pruritus, rash, contact dermatitis, alopecia, photosensitivity (rare)

Endocrine & metabolic: Amenorrhea, galactorrhea, gynecomastia, sexual dysfunction, lactation, breast engorgement, mastalgia, menstrual irregularities, hyperglycemia, hypoglycemia, hyponatremia

Gastrointestinal: Nausea, vomiting, anorexia, constipation, diarrhea, hypersalivation, dyspepsia, xerostomia

Genitourinary: Urinary retention, priapism

Hematologic: Cholestatic jaundice, obstructive jaundice

Ocular: Blurred vision

Respiratory: Laryngospasm, bronchospasm

Miscellaneous: Heat stroke, diaphoresis

Overdosage/Toxicology Symptoms of overdose include deep sleep, dystonia, agitation, dysrhythmias, and extrapyramidal symptoms. Treatment is supportive and symptomatic.

Pharmacodynamics/Kinetics

Onset of Action: Sedation: I.V.: ~1 hour

Duration of Action: Decanoate: ~3 weeks

Time to Peak: Serum: 20 minutes

Protein Binding: 90%

Half-Life Elimination: 20 hours

Metabolism: Hepatic to inactive compounds

Excretion: Urine (33% to 40% as metabolites) within 5 days; feces (15%)

Available Dosage Forms [DSC] = Discontinued product. **Note:** Strength expressed as base.

Injection, oil, as decanoate (Haldol® Decanoate): 50 mg/mL (1 mL, 5 mL); 100 mg/mL (1 mL, 5 mL) [contains benzyl alcohol, sesame oil]

Injection, solution, as lactate: 5 mg/mL (1 mL, 10 mL)
Haldol®: 5 mg/mL (1 mL; 10 mL [DSC])

Solution, oral concentrate, as lactate: 2 mg/mL (15 mL, 120 mL)

Tablet: 0.5 mg, 1 mg, 2 mg, 5 mg, 10 mg, 20 mg

Dosing

Adults:

Psychosis:

Oral: 0.5-5 mg 2-3 times/day; usual maximum: 30 mg/day

I.M. (as lactate): 2-5 mg every 4-8 hours as needed

I.M. (as decanoate): Initial: 10-20 times the daily oral dose administered at 4-week intervals. Maintenance dose: 10-15 times initial oral dose; used to stabilize psychiatric symptoms

Delirium in the intensive care unit (unlabeled use, unlabeled route):

I.V.: 2-10 mg; may repeat bolus doses every 20-30 minutes until calm achieved then administer 25% of the maximum dose every 6 hours; monitor ECG and QT$_c$ interval

Intermittent I.V.: 0.03-0.15 mg/kg every 30 minutes to 6 hours

Oral: Agitation: 5-10 mg

Continuous I.V. infusion (100 mg/100 mL D$_5$W): Rates of 3-25 mg/hour have been used

Rapid tranquilization of severely-agitated patient (unlabeled use; administer every 30-60 minutes):

Oral: 5-10 mg

I.M.: 5 mg

Average total dose (oral or I.M.) for tranquilization: 10-20 mg

(Continued)

Haloperidol *(Continued)*

Elderly: Nonpsychotic patients, dementia behavior: Initial: Oral: 0.25-0.5 mg 1-2 times/day; increase dose at 4- to 7-day intervals by 0.25-0.5 mg/day. Increase dosing intervals (twice daily, 3 times/day, etc) as necessary to control response or side effects.

Pediatrics:

Sedation/psychotic disorders: Oral:

Children: 3-12 years (15-40 kg): Initial: 0.05 mg/kg/day or 0.25-0.5 mg/day given in 2-3 divided doses; increase by 0.25-0.5 mg every 5-7 days; maximum: 0.15 mg/kg/day

Usual maintenance:

Agitation or hyperkinesia: 0.01-0.03 mg/kg/day once daily

Nonpsychotic disorders: 0.05-0.075 mg/kg/day in 2-3 divided doses

Psychotic disorders: 0.05-0.15 mg/kg/day in 2-3 divided doses

Children 6-12 years: Sedation/psychotic disorders: I.M. (as lactate): 1-3 mg/dose every 4-8 hours to a maximum of 0.15 mg/kg/day; change over to oral therapy as soon as able.

Renal Impairment: Hemodialysis/peritoneal dialysis: Supplemental dose is not necessary.

Administration

Oral: Dilute the oral concentrate with water or juice before administration. **Note:** Avoid skin contact with oral medication; may cause contact dermatitis.

I.M.: The decanoate injectable formulation should be administered I.M. only; **do not give decanoate I.V.**

I.V.:

Decanoate: Do **not** administer I.V.

Lactate: Although not an FDA-approved route of administration, Haldol® has been administered by this route in many acute care settings.

I.V. Detail: The response to I.V. Haldol® may be delayed by several minutes.

pH: 3.0-3.6

Stability

Reconstitution: Haloperidol lactate may be administered IVPB or I.V. infusion in D_5W solutions. NS solutions should not be used due to reports of decreased stability and incompatibility.

Standardized dose: 0.5-100 mg/50-100 mL D_5W
Stability of standardized solutions is 38 days at room temperature (24°C).

Compatibility: Stable in D_5W

Y-site administration: Incompatible with allopurinol, amphotericin B cholesteryl sulfate complex, cefepime, fluconazole, foscarnet, heparin, piperacillin/tazobactam, sargramostim

Compatibility in syringe: Incompatible with diphenhydramine, heparin, hydroxyzine, ketorolac

Storage: Protect oral dosage forms from light. Haloperidol lactate injection should be stored at controlled room temperature and protected from light, freezing, and temperatures >40°C. Exposure to light may cause discoloration and the development of a grayish-red precipitate over several weeks.

Laboratory Monitoring Lipid profile, fasting blood glucose/Hgb A_{1c}; BMI

Nursing Actions

Physical Assessment: Assess other medications patient is taking for effectiveness and interactions (especially drugs metabolized by P450 enzymes). Review ophthalmic screening. Monitor therapeutic response (mental status, mood, affect) and adverse reactions at beginning of therapy and periodically with long-term use (sedation, anticholinergic, and extrapyramidal symptoms). With I.M. or I.V. use, monitor closely for hypotension. Initiate at lower doses and taper dosage slowly when discontinuing. **Note:** Avoid skin contact with oral medication; may cause contact dermatitis (wash immediately with warm, soapy water). Assess knowledge/teach patient appropriate use, interventions to reduce side effects, and adverse symptoms to report.

Patient Education: Use exactly as directed; do not increase dose or frequency. It may take 2-3 weeks to achieve desired results; do not discontinue without consulting prescriber. Dilute oral concentration with water or juice. Do not take within 2 hours of any antacid. Store away from light. Avoid alcohol or caffeine and other prescription or OTC medications not approved by prescriber. Maintain adequate hydration (2-3 L/day of fluids) unless instructed to restrict fluid intake. Avoid skin contact with medication; may cause contact dermatitis (wash immediately with warm, soapy water). You may experience excess drowsiness, restlessness, dizziness, or blurred vision (use caution driving or when engaging in tasks requiring alertness until response to drug is known); nausea or vomiting (small frequent meals, frequent mouth care, chewing gum, or sucking lozenges may help); constipation (increased exercise, fluids, fruit, or fiber may help); postural hypotension (use caution climbing stairs or when changing position from lying or sitting to standing); urinary retention (void before taking medication); or decreased perspiration (avoid strenuous exercise in hot environments). Report persistent CNS effects (eg, trembling fingers, altered gait or balance, excessive sedation, seizures, unusual movements, anxiety, abnormal thoughts, confusion, personality changes); chest pain, palpitations, rapid heartbeat, severe dizziness; unresolved urinary retention or changes in urinary pattern; vision changes; skin rash or yellowing of skin; respiratory difficulty; or worsening of condition. **Pregnancy/breast-feeding precautions:** Inform prescriber if you are or intend to become pregnant. Breast-feeding is not recommended.

Geriatric Considerations (See Warnings/Precautions, Adverse Reactions, and Overdose/Toxicology.) Elderly patients have an increased risk of adverse response to side effects or adverse reactions to antipsychotics.

Breast-Feeding Issues Decline in developmental scores may be seen in nursing infants.

Related Information

Antipsychotic Medication Guidelines *on page 1415*
Federal OBRA Regulations Recommended Maximum Doses *on page 1421*

Heparin *(HEP a rin)*

U.S. Brand Names HepFlush®-10; Hep-Lock®

Synonyms Heparin Calcium; Heparin Lock Flush; Heparin Sodium

Pharmacologic Category Anticoagulant

Medication Safety Issues

Sound-alike/look-alike issues:

Heparin may be confused with Hespan®

High alert medication: The Institute for Safe Medication Practices (ISMP) includes this medication among its list of drugs which have a heightened risk of causing significant patient harm when used in error.

Heparin lock flush solution is intended only to maintain patency of I.V. devices and is **not** to be used for anticoagulant therapy.

Note: The 100 unit/mL concentration should not be used in neonates or infants <10 kg, The 10 unit/mL concentration may cause systemic anticoagulation in infants <1 kg who receive frequent flushes.

Pregnancy Risk Factor C

Lactation Does not enter breast milk/compatible

Use Prophylaxis and treatment of thromboembolic disorders

Note: Heparin lock flush solution is intended only to maintain patency of I.V. devices and is **not** to be used for anticoagulant therapy.

Unlabeled/Investigational Use Acute MI — combination regimen of heparin (unlabeled dose), tenecteplase (half dose), and abciximab (full dose)

Mechanism of Action/Effect Potentiates the action of antithrombin III and thereby inactivates thrombin (as well as activated coagulation factors IX, X, XI, XII, and plasmin) and prevents the conversion of fibrinogen to fibrin; heparin also stimulates release of lipoprotein lipase (lipoprotein lipase hydrolyzes triglycerides to glycerol and free fatty acids)

Contraindications Hypersensitivity to heparin or any component of the formulation; severe thrombocytopenia; uncontrolled active bleeding except when due to DIC; suspected intracranial hemorrhage; not for I.M. use; not for use when appropriate monitoring parameters cannot be obtained

Warnings/Precautions Hemorrhage is the most common complication. Risk factors for bleeding include bacterial endocarditis; congenital or acquired bleeding disorders; active ulcerative or angiodysplastic GI diseases; severe uncontrolled hypertension; hemorrhagic stroke; or use shortly after brain, spinal, or ophthalmology surgery; patient treated concomitantly with platelet inhibitors; conditions associated with increased bleeding tendencies (hemophilia, vascular purpura); recent GI bleeding; thrombocytopenia or platelet defects; severe liver disease; hypertensive or diabetic retinopathy; or in patients undergoing invasive procedures. A higher incidence of bleeding has been reported in women >60 years of age.

Patients who develop thrombocytopenia on heparin may be at risk of developing a new thrombus ("White-clot syndrome"). Hypersensitivity reactions can occur. Heparin should be used cautiously in patients with a documented hypersensitivity reaction and only in life-threatening situations. Osteoporosis can occur following long-term use (>6 months). May cause hyperkalemia due to effects on aldosterone. Discontinue therapy and consider alternatives if platelets are <100,000/mm³. Patients >60 years of age may require lower doses of heparin.

Heparin does not possess fibrinolytic activity and, therefore, cannot lyse established thrombi; discontinue heparin if hemorrhage occurs; severe hemorrhage or overdosage may require protamine.

Drug Interactions

Decreased Effect: Nitroglycerin (I.V.) may decrease heparin's anticoagulant effect. This interaction has not been validated in some studies, and may only occur at high nitroglycerin dosages.

Increased Effect/Toxicity: The risk of hemorrhage associated with heparin may be increased by oral anticoagulants (warfarin), thrombolytics, dextran, and drugs which affect platelet function (eg, aspirin, NSAIDs, dipyridamole, ticlopidine, clopidogrel, IIb/IIIa antagonists). However, heparin is often used in conjunction with thrombolytic therapy or during the initiation of warfarin therapy to assure anticoagulation and to protect against possible transient hypercoagulability. Cephalosporins which contain the MTT side chain and parenteral penicillins (may inhibit platelet aggregation) may increase the risk of hemorrhage. Other drugs reported to increase heparin's anticoagulant effect include antihistamines, tetracycline, quinine, nicotine, and cardiac glycosides (digoxin).

Nutritional/Ethanol Interactions

Food: When taking for >6 months, may interfere with calcium absorption.

Herb/Nutraceutical: Avoid cat's claw, dong quai, evening primrose, feverfew, red clover, horse chestnut, garlic, green tea, ginseng, ginkgo (all have additional antiplatelet activity).

Lab Interactions Increased thyroxine (S) (competitive protein binding methods), PT, PTT, bleeding time. A volume of at least 10 mL of blood should be removed and discarded from a heparinized line before blood samples are sent for coagulation testing.

Adverse Reactions

Cardiovascular: Chest pain, vasospasm (possibly related to thrombosis), hemorrhagic shock

Central nervous system: Fever, headache, chills

Dermatologic: Unexplained bruising, urticaria, alopecia, dysesthesia pedis, purpura, eczema, cutaneous necrosis (following deep SubQ injection), erythematous plaques (case reports)

Endocrine & metabolic: Hyperkalemia (supression of aldosterone), rebound hyperlipidemia on discontinuation

Gastrointestinal: Nausea, vomiting, constipation, hematemesis

Genitourinary: Frequent or persistent erection

Hematologic: Hemorrhage, blood in urine, bleeding from gums, epistaxis, adrenal hemorrhage, ovarian hemorrhage, retroperitoneal hemorrhage, thrombocytopenia (see note)

Hepatic: Elevated liver enzymes (AST/ALT)

Local: Irritation, ulceration, cutaneous necrosis have been rarely reported with deep SubQ injections, I.M. injection (not recommended) is associated with a high incidence of these effects

Neuromuscular & skeletal: Peripheral neuropathy, osteoporosis (chronic therapy effect)

Ocular: Conjunctivitis (allergic reaction)

Respiratory: Hemoptysis, pulmonary hemorrhage, asthma, rhinitis, bronchospasm (case reports)

Miscellaneous: Allergic reactions, anaphylactoid reactions

Note: Thrombocytopenia has been reported to occur at an incidence between 0% and 30%. It is often of no clinical significance. However, immunologically mediated heparin-induced thrombocytopenia has been estimated to occur in 1% to 2% of patients, and is marked by a progressive fall in platelet counts and, in some cases, thromboembolic complications (skin necrosis, pulmonary embolism, gangrene of the extremities, stroke or MI). For recommendations regarding platelet monitoring during heparin therapy, consult "Seventh ACCP Consensus Conference on Antithrombotic and Thrombolytic Therapy."

Overdosage/Toxicology The primary symptom of overdose is bleeding. Antidote is protamine; dose 1 mg neutralizes 1 mg (100 units) of heparin. Discontinue all heparin if evidence of progressive immune thrombocytopenia occurs.

Pharmacodynamics/Kinetics

Onset of Action: Anticoagulation: I.V.: Immediate; SubQ: ~20-30 minutes

Half-Life Elimination: Mean: 1.5 hours; Range: 1-2 hours; affected by obesity, renal function, hepatic function, malignancy, presence of pulmonary embolism, and infections

Metabolism: Hepatic; may be partially metabolized in the reticuloendothelial system

Excretion: Urine (small amounts as unchanged drug)

Available Dosage Forms [DSC] = Discontinued product

Infusion, as sodium [premixed in NaCl 0.45%; porcine intestinal mucosa source]: 12,500 units (250 mL); 25,000 units (250 mL, 500 mL)

Infusion, as sodium [preservative free; premixed in D₅W; porcine intestinal mucosa source]: 10,000 units (100 mL) [contains sodium metabisulfite]; 12,500 units (250 mL) [contains sodium metabisulfite]; 20,000 units (500 mL) [contains sodium metabisulfite]; 25,000 units (250 mL, 500 mL) [contains sodium metabisulfite]

Infusion, as sodium [preservative free; premixed in NaCl 0.9%; porcine intestinal mucosa source]: 1000 units (500 mL); 2000 units (1000 mL)

(Continued)

Heparin *(Continued)*

Injection, solution, as sodium [beef lung source; multidose vial]: 1000 units/mL (10 mL, 30 mL); 5000 units/mL (10 mL), 10,000 units/mL (1 mL, 4 mL) [contains benzyl alcohol] [DSC]

Injection, solution, as sodium [lock flush preparation; porcine intestinal mucosa source; multidose vial]: 10 units/mL (1 mL, 10 mL, 30 mL) [contains parabens]; 100 units/mL (1 mL, 5 mL) [contains parabens]

Injection, solution, as sodium [lock flush preparation; porcine intestinal mucosa source; multidose vial]: 10 units/mL (10 mL, 30 mL); 100 units/mL (10 mL, 30 mL) [contains benzyl alcohol]

Hep-Lock®: 10 units/mL (1 mL, 2 mL, 10 mL, 30 mL); 100 units/mL (1 mL, 2 mL, 10 mL, 30 mL) [contains benzyl alcohol]

Injection, solution, as sodium [lock flush preparation; porcine intestinal mucosa source; prefilled syringe]: 10 units/mL (1 mL, 2 mL, 3 mL, 5 mL); 100 units/mL (1 mL, 2 mL, 3 mL, 5 mL) [contains benzyl alcohol]

Injection, solution, as sodium [preservative free; lock flush preparation; porcine intestinal mucosa source; prefilled syringe]: 100 units/mL (5 mL)

Injection, solution, as sodium [preservative free; lock flush preparation; porcine intestinal mucosa source; vial] (HepFlush®-10): 10 units/mL (10 mL)

Injection, solution, as sodium [porcine intestinal mucosa source; multidose vial]: 1000 units/mL (1 mL, 10 mL, 30 mL) [contains benzyl alcohol]; 1000 units/mL (1 mL, 10 mL, 30 mL) [contains methylparabens]; 5000 units/mL (1 mL, 10 mL) [contains benzyl alcohol]; 5000 units/mL (1 mL) [contains methylparabens]; 10,000 units/mL (1 mL, 4 mL) [contains benzyl alcohol]; 10,000 units/mL (1 mL, 5 mL) [contains methylparabens]; 20,000 units/mL (1 mL) [contains methylparabens]

Injection, solution, as sodium [porcine intestinal mucosa source; prefilled syringe]: 5000 units/mL (1 mL) [contains benzyl alcohol]

Injection, solution, as sodium [preservative free; porcine intestinal mucosa source; prefilled syringe]: 10,000 units/mL (0.5 mL)

Injection, solution, as sodium [preservative free; porcine intestinal mucosa source; vial]: 1000 units/mL (2 mL); 2000 units/mL (5 mL); 2500 units/mL (10 mL)

Dosing

Adults:

DVT Prophylaxis (low-dose heparin): SubQ: 5000 units every 8-12 hours

Systemic anticoagulation: I.V. infusion (weight-based dosing per institutional nomogram recommended):

Acute coronary syndromes or MI: Fibrinolytic therapy: I.V. infusion:

Full-dose alteplase, reteplase, or tenecteplase with dosing as follows: Concurrent bolus of 60 units/kg (maximum: 4000 units), then 12 units/kg/hour (maximum: 1000 units/hour) as continuous infusion. Check aPTT every 4-6 hours; adjust to target of 1.5-2 times the upper limit of control (50-70 seconds in clinical trials); usual range 10-30 units/kg/hour. Duration of heparin therapy depends on concurrent therapy and the specific patient risks for systemic or venous thromboembolism.

Combination regimen (unlabeled): Half-dose tenecteplase (15-25 mg based on weight) and abciximab 0.25 mg/kg bolus then 0.125 mcg/kg/minute (maximum 10 mcg/minute) for 12 hours with heparin dosing as follows: Concurrent bolus of 40 units/kg (maximum 3000 units), then 7 units/kg/hour (maximum: 800 units/hour) as continuous infusion. Adjust to a aPTT target of 50-70 seconds.

Streptokinase: Heparin use optional depending on concurrent therapy and specific patient risks for systemic or venous thromboembolism (anterior MI, CHF, previous embolus, atrial fibrillation, LV thrombus): If heparin is administered, start when aPTT <2 times the upper limit of control; do not use a bolus, but initiate infusion adjusted to a target aPTT of 1.5-2 times the upper limit of control (50-70 seconds in clinical trials). If heparin is not administered by infusion, 7500-12,500 units SubQ every 12 hours (when aPTT <2 times the upper limit of control) is recommended.

Percutaneous coronary intervention: Heparin bolus and infusion may be administered to an activated clotting time (ACT) of 300-350 seconds if no concurrent GPIIb/IIIa receptor antagonist is administered or 200-250 seconds if a GPIIb/IIIa receptor antagonist is administered.

Unstable angina (high-risk and some intermediate-risk patients): Initial bolus of 60-70 units/kg (maximum: 5000 units), followed by an initial infusion of 12-15 units/kg/hour (maximum: 1000 units/hour). The American College of Chest Physicians consensus conference has recommended dosage adjustments to correspond to a therapeutic range equivalent to heparin levels of 0.3-0.7 units/mL by antifactor Xa determinations.

Venous thromboembolism :

DVT/PE: I.V. push: 80 units/kg followed by continuous infusion of 18 units/kg/hour

DVT: SubQ: 17,500 units every 12 hours

Intermittent I.V. Anticoagulation: Intermittent I.V.: Initial: 10,000 units, then 50-70 units/kg (5000-10,000 units) every 4-6 hours

Maintenance of line patency (line flushing): When using daily flushes of heparin to maintain patency of single and double lumen central catheters, 10 units/mL is commonly used for younger infants (eg, <10 kg) while 100 units/mL is used for older infants, children, and adults. Capped PVC catheters and peripheral heparin locks require flushing more frequently (eg, every 6-8 hours). Volume of heparin flush is usually similar to volume of catheter (or slightly greater). Additional flushes should be given when stagnant blood is observed in catheter, after catheter is used for drug or blood administration, and after blood withdrawal from catheter.

Parenteral nutrition: Addition of heparin (0.5-3 unit/mL) to peripheral and central parenteral nutrition has not been shown to decrease catheter-related thrombosis. The final concentration of heparin used for TPN solutions may need to be decreased to 0.5 units/mL in small infants receiving larger amounts of volume in order to avoid approaching therapeutic amounts. Arterial lines are heparinized with a final concentration of 1 unit/mL.

Elderly: Patients >60 years of age may have higher serum levels and clinical response (longer aPTTs) as compared to younger patients receiving similar dosages. Lower dosages may be required.

Pediatrics:

Anticoagulation: Intermittent I.V.: Initial: 50-100 units/kg, then 50-100 units/kg every 4 hours

Anticoagulation: I.V. infusion: Initial: 50 units/kg, then 15-25 units/kg/hour; increase dose by 2-4 units/kg/hour every 6-8 hours as required

Note: Refer to adult dosing for notes on line flushing and TPN.

Administration

I.M.: Do not administer I.M. due to pain, irritation, and hematoma formation.

I.V.:

Continuous infusion: Infuse via infusion pump.

Heparin lock: Inject via injection cap using positive pressure flushing technique. Heparin lock flush solution is intended only to maintain patency of I.V. devices and is **not** to be used for anticoagulant therapy.

I.V. Detail:
Using a standard heparin solution (25,000 units/500 mL D_5W), the following infusion rates can be used to achieve the listed doses.
For a dose of:
400 units/hour: Infuse at 8 mL/hour
500 units/hour: Infuse at 10 mL/hour
600 units/hour: Infuse at 12 mL/hour
700 units/hour: Infuse at 14 mL/hour
800 units/hour: Infuse at 16 mL/hour
900 units/hour: Infuse at 18 mL/hour
1000 units/hour: Infuse at 20 mL/hour
1100 units/hour: Infuse at 22 mL/hour
1200 units/hour: Infuse at 24 mL/hour
1300 units/hour: Infuse at 26 mL/hour
1400 units/hour: Infuse at 28 mL/hour
1500 units/hour: Infuse at 30 mL/hour
1600 units/hour: Infuse at 32 mL/hour
1700 units/hour: Infuse at 34 mL/hour
1800 units/hour: Infuse at 36 mL/hour
1900 units/hour: Infuse at 38 mL/hour
2000 units/hour: Infuse at 40 mL/hour

Other: SubQ: Inject in subcutaneous tissue only (not muscle tissue). Injection sites should be rotated (usually left and right portions of the abdomen, above iliac crest).

Stability
Reconstitution: Stability at room temperature and refrigeration:
Prepared bag: 24 hours
Premixed bag: After seal is broken 4 days
Out of overwrap stability: 30 days
Standard diluent: 25,000 units/500 mL D_5W (premixed)
Minimum volume: 250 mL D_5W

Compatibility: Stable in dextran 6% in dextrose, dextran 6% in NS, D_5LR, $D_5{}^1/_4NS$, $D_5{}^1/_2NS$, $D_{25}W$, fat emulsion 10%, $^1/_2NS$, NS

Y-site administration: Incompatible with alatrofloxacin, alteplase, amiodarone, amphotericin B cholesteryl sulfate complex, amsacrine, ciprofloxacin, clarithromycin, diazepam, doxycycline, ergotamine, filgrastim, gatifloxacin, gentamicin, haloperidol, idarubicin, isosorbide dinitrate, levofloxacin, methotrimeprazine, nicardipine, phenytoin, tobramycin, triflupromazine, vancomycin

Compatibility in syringe: Incompatible with amikacin, amiodarone, chlorpromazine, diazepam, doxorubicin, droperidol, droperidol and fentanyl, erythromycin, erythromycin lactobionate, gentamicin, haloperidol, kanamycin, meperidine, methotrimeprazine, pentazocine, promethazine, streptomycin, tobramycin, triflupromazine, vancomycin, warfarin

Compatibility when admixed: Incompatible with alteplase, amikacin, atracurium, ciprofloxacin, cytarabine, daunorubicin, erythromycin lactobionate, gentamicin, hyaluronidase, kanamycin, levorphanol, meperidine, morphine, polymyxin B sulfate, promethazine, streptomycin

Storage: Heparin solutions are colorless to slightly yellow. Minor color variations do not affect therapeutic efficacy. Heparin should be stored at controlled room temperature and protected from freezing and temperatures >40°C.

Laboratory Monitoring Platelet counts, hemoglobin, hematocrit, signs of bleeding; aPTT or ACT depending upon indication. For intermittent I.V. injections, PTT is measured 3.5-4 hours after I.V. injection. **Note:** Continuous I.V. infusion is preferred vs I.V. intermittent injections. For full-dose heparin (ie, nonlow-dose), the dose should be titrated according to PTT results. For anticoagulation, an aPTT 1.5-2.5 times normal is usually desired; aPTT is usually measured prior to heparin therapy, 6-8 hours after initiation of a continuous infusion (following a loading dose), and 6-8 hours after

changes in the infusion rate; increase or decrease infusion by 2-4 units/kg/hour dependent on PTT.
Heparin infusion dose adjustment:
aPTT >3x control: Decrease infusion rate 50%.
aPTT 2-3x control: Decrease infusion rate 25%.
aPTT 1.5-2x control: No change.
aPTT <1.5x control: Increase rate of infusion 25%; max 2500 units/hour.

Nursing Actions
Physical Assessment: Assess potential for interactions with other pharmacological agents or herbal products patient may be taking (especially anything that will affect coagulation or platelet function). Note specific infusion directions in Administration. Bleeding precautions should be observed at all times during heparin therapy. Monitor laboratory tests for dosing adjustments and therapeutic effectiveness. Monitor patient response closely during therapy (eg, hypersensitivity reaction, bleeding, chest pain, hyperkalemia, peripheral neuropathy). Teach possible side effects/appropriate interventions (eg, bleeding precautions) and adverse symptoms to report.

Patient Education: Do not take any new medication, including over-the-counter and biological products, during therapy unless approved by prescriber. This drug can only be administered by infusion or injection. You may have a tendency to bleed easily while taking this drug (brush teeth with soft brush, floss with waxed floss, use electric razor, avoid scissors or sharp knives, and potentially harmful activities). Report immediately any chest pain; difficulty breathing or unusual cough; bleeding or bruising (bleeding gums, nosebleed, blood in urine, dark stool); pain in joints or back; CNS changes (fever, confusion); unusual fever; persistent nausea or GI upset; change in vision, or swelling, pain, or redness at injection site. **Pregnancy precaution:** Inform prescriber if you are pregnant.

Geriatric Considerations At similar dosages, heparin levels tend to be higher in elderly patients (>60 years of age). In the clinical setting, age has not been shown to be a reliable predictor of a patient's anticoagulant response to heparin. However, it is common for older patients to have a "standard" response for the first 24-48 hours after a loading dose (5000 units) and a maintenance infusion of 800-1000 units/hour. After this period, they then have an exaggerated response (eg, elevated PTT), requiring a lower infusion rate. Hence, monitor closely during this period of therapy. Older women (>60 years of age) are more likely to have bleeding complications and osteoporosis may be a problem when used >3 months or total daily dose exceeds 30,000 units.

Additional Information Heparin lock flush solution is intended only to maintain patency of I.V. devices and is **not** to be used for anticoagulant therapy.

Related Information
Compatibility of Drugs *on page 1370*
Compatibility of Drugs in Syringe *on page 1372*
Overdose and Toxicology *on page 1423*

Hetastarch (HET a starch)

U.S. Brand Names Hespan®; Hextend®
Synonyms HES; Hydroxyethyl Starch
Pharmacologic Category Plasma Volume Expander, Colloid
Medication Safety Issues
Sound-alike/look-alike issues:
Hespan® may be confused with heparin
Pregnancy Risk Factor C
Lactation Excretion in breast milk unknown/use caution
Use Blood volume expander used in treatment of hypovolemia
(Continued)

Hetastarch *(Continued)*

Hespan®: Adjunct in leukapheresis to improve harvesting and increasing the yield of granulocytes by centrifugal means

Unlabeled/Investigational Use Hextend®: Priming fluid in pump oxygenators during cardiopulmonary bypass, and as a plasma volume expander during cardiopulmonary bypass

Mechanism of Action/Effect Produces plasma volume expansion by virtue of its highly colloidal starch structure, similar to albumin

Contraindications Hypersensitivity to hydroxyethyl starch or any component of the formulation; severe bleeding disorders, renal failure with oliguria or anuria, or severe congestive heart failure; per the manufacturer, Hextend® is also contraindicated in the treatment of lactic acidosis and in leukapheresis

Warnings/Precautions Anaphylactoid reactions have occurred; use caution in patients allergic to corn (may have cross allergy to hetastarch); use with caution in patients with thrombocytopenia (may interfere with platelet function); large volume may cause drops in hemoglobin concentrations; use with caution in patients at risk from overexpansion of blood volume, including the very young or aged patients, those with CHF or pulmonary edema; volumes >1500 mL may interfere with platelet function and prolong PT and PTT times; use with caution in patients with history of liver disease; note electrolyte content of Hextend® including calcium, lactate, and potassium; use caution in situations where electrolyte and/or acid-base disturbances may be exacerbated (renal impairment, respiratory alkalosis). Safety and efficacy in pediatric patients have not been established, but limited data available.

Adverse Reactions Frequency not defined.

Cardiovascular: Circulatory overload, heart failure, peripheral edema

Central nervous system: Chills, fever, headache, intracranial bleeding

Dermatologic: Itching, pruritus, rash

Endocrine & metabolic: Amylase levels increased, parotid gland enlargement, indirect bilirubin increased, metabolic acidosis

Gastrointestinal: Vomiting

Hematologic: Bleeding, factor VIII:C plasma levels decreased, decreased plasma aggregation decreased, von Willebrand factor decreased, dilutional coagulopathy; prolongation of PT, PTT, clotting time, and bleeding time; thrombocytopenia, anemia, disseminated intravascular coagulopathy (rare), hemolysis (rare)

Neuromuscular & skeletal: Myalgia

Miscellaneous: Anaphylactoid reactions, hypersensitivity, flu-like symptoms (mild)

Overdosage/Toxicology Symptoms of overdose include heart failure, nausea, vomiting, circulatory overload, and bleeding. Treatment is supportive. Hetastarch is not eliminated by hemodialysis.

Pharmacodynamics/Kinetics

Onset of Action: Volume expansion: I.V.: ~30 minutes

Duration of Action: 24-36 hours

Metabolism: Molecules >50,000 daltons require enzymatic degradation by the reticuloendothelial system or amylases in the blood

Excretion: Urine (~40%) within 24 hours; smaller molecular weight molecules readily excreted

Available Dosage Forms

Infusion [premixed in lactated electrolyte injection] (Hextend®): 6% (500 mL)

Infusion, solution [premixed in NaCl 0.9%] (Hespan®): 6% (500 mL)

Dosing

Adults & Elderly:

Volume expansion: 500-1000 mL (up to 1500 mL/day) or 20 mL/kg/day (up to 1500 mL/day); larger volumes (15,000 mL/24 hours) have been used safely in small numbers of patients

Leukapheresis: 250-700 mL; **Note:** Citrate anticoagulant is added before use.

Pediatrics: Safety and efficacy have not been established.

Renal Impairment: Cl_{cr} <10 mL/minute: Initial dose is the same but subsequent doses should be reduced by 20% to 50% of normal.

Administration

I.V.: Administer I.V. only; infusion pump is required. May administer up to 1.2 g/kg/hour (20 mL/kg/hour). Change I.V. tubing or flush copiously with normal saline before administering blood through the same line. Change I.V. tubing at least every 24 hours. Do not administer Hextend® with blood through the same administration set. Anaphylactoid reactions can occur, have epinephrine and resuscitative equipment available.

I.V. Detail: Do not use if crystalline precipitate forms or is turbid deep brown.

pH: 3.5-7

Other: Leukapheresis: Mix Hespan® and citrate well. Administer to the input line of the centrifuge apparatus at a ration of 1:8 to 1:13 to venous whole blood.

Stability

Reconstitution: Do not use if crystalline precipitate forms or is turbid deep brown.

Compatibility: Stable in NS

Y-site administration: Incompatible with amikacin, cefamandole, cefoperazone, cefotaxime, cefoxitin, gentamicin, ranitidine, theophylline, tobramycin

Storage: Store at room temperature; do not freeze. In leukapheresis, admixtures of 500-560 mL of Hespan® with citrate concentrations up to 2.5% are compatible for 24 hours.

Laboratory Monitoring Hemoglobin, hematocrit

Leukapheresis: CBC, total leukocyte and platelet counts, leukocyte differential count, hemoglobin, hematocrit, PT, PTT

Nursing Actions

Physical Assessment: Assess allergies prior to beginning treatment (patients allergic to corn may have a cross allergy to hetastarch). Patient must be monitored closely for hypersensitivity (anaphylactic reaction) and other major adverse reactions (eg, circulatory overload, cranial bleed, pulmonary edema). Blood pressure, pulse, central venous pressure, and urine output should be monitored every 5-15 minutes for the first hour and closely thereafter. Assess results of laboratory tests during and after treatment. Patient teaching should be appropriate to patient condition.

Patient Education: Report immediately any respiratory difficulty, acute headache, muscle pain, or abdominal cramping. **Pregnancy/breast-feeding precautions:** Inform prescriber if you are pregnant. Consult prescriber if breast-feeding.

Additional Information Hetastarch is a synthetic polymer derived from a waxy starch composed of amylopectin.

Hespan®: 6% hetastarch in 0.9% sodium chloride
Molecular weight: 450,000
Sodium: 154 mEq/L
Chloride: 154 mEq/L

Hextend®: 6% hetastarch in lactated electrolyte injection
Molecular weight: 670,000
Sodium: 143 mEq/L
Chloride: 124 mEq/L
Calcium: 5 mEq/L
Potassium: 3 mEq/L

Magnesium: 0.9 mEq/L
Lactate: 28 mEq/L
Dextrose: 0.99 g/L

HydrALAZINE (hye DRAL a zeen)

Synonyms Apresoline [DSC]; Hydralazine Hydrochloride
Pharmacologic Category Vasodilator
Medication Safety Issues
Sound-alike/look-alike issues:
HydrALAZINE may be confused with hydrOXYzine
Pregnancy Risk Factor C
Lactation Enters breast milk/compatible
Use Management of moderate to severe hypertension, congestive heart failure, hypertension secondary to pre-eclampsia/eclampsia; treatment of primary pulmonary hypertension
Mechanism of Action/Effect Direct vasodilation of arterioles (with little effect on veins) with decreased systemic resistance
Contraindications Hypersensitivity to hydralazine or any component of the formulation; mitral valve rheumatic heart disease
Warnings/Precautions May cause a drug-induced lupus-like syndrome (more likely on larger doses, longer duration). Adjust dose in severe renal dysfunction. Use with caution in CAD (increase in tachycardia may increase myocardial oxygen demand). Use with caution in pulmonary hypertension (may cause hypotension). Titrate cautiously to response. Hypotensive effect after I.V. administration may be delayed and unpredictable in some patients. Hydralazine-induced fluid and sodium retention may require addition or increased dosage of a diuretics.
Drug Interactions
Cytochrome P450 Effect: Inhibits CYP3A4 (weak)
Decreased Effect: NSAIDs (eg, indomethacin) may decrease the hemodynamic effects of hydralazine.
Increased Effect/Toxicity: Hydralazine may increase levels of beta-blockers (metoprolol, propranolol). Some beta-blockers (acebutolol, atenolol, and nadolol) are unlikely to be affected due to limited hepatic metabolism. Concurrent use of hydralazine with MAO inhibitors may cause a significant decrease in blood pressure. Propranolol may increase hydralazine serum concentrations.
Nutritional/Ethanol Interactions
Ethanol: Avoid ethanol (may increase CNS depression).
Food: Food enhances bioavailability of hydralazine.
Herb/Nutraceutical: Avoid dong quai if using for hypertension (has estrogenic activity). Avoid ephedra, yohimbe, ginseng (may worsen hypertension). Avoid garlic (may have increased antihypertensive effect).
Adverse Reactions Frequency not defined.
Cardiovascular: Tachycardia, angina pectoris, orthostatic hypotension (rare), dizziness (rare), paradoxical hypertension, peripheral edema, vascular collapse (rare), flushing
Central nervous system: Increased intracranial pressure (I.V., in patient with pre-existing increased intracranial pressure), fever (rare), chills (rare), anxiety*, disorientation*, depression*, coma*
Dermatologic: Rash (rare), urticaria (rare), pruritus (rare)
Gastrointestinal: Anorexia, nausea, vomiting, diarrhea, constipation, adynamic ileus
Genitourinary: Difficulty in micturition, impotence
Hematologic: Hemolytic anemia (rare), eosinophilia (rare), decreased hemoglobin concentration (rare), reduced erythrocyte count (rare), leukopenia (rare), agranulocytosis (rare), thrombocytopenia (rare)
Neuromuscular & skeletal: Rheumatoid arthritis, muscle cramps, weakness, tremor, peripheral neuritis (rare)
Ocular: Lacrimation, conjunctivitis

Respiratory: Nasal congestion, dyspnea
Miscellaneous: Drug-induced lupus-like syndrome (dose related; fever, arthralgia, splenomegaly, lymphadenopathy, asthenia, myalgia, malaise, pleuritic chest pain, edema, positive ANA, positive LE cells, maculopapular facial rash, positive direct Coombs' test, pericarditis, pericardial tamponade), diaphoresis
*Seen in uremic patients and severe hypertension where rapidly escalating doses may have caused hypotension leading to these effects.
Overdosage/Toxicology Symptoms of overdose include hypotension, tachycardia, and shock. Treatment is supportive and symptomatic.
Pharmacodynamics/Kinetics
Onset of Action: Oral: 20-30 minutes; I.V.: 5-20 minutes
Duration of Action: Oral: Up to 8 hours; I.V.: 1-4 hours; **Note:** May vary depending on acetylator status of patient
Protein Binding: 85% to 90%
Half-Life Elimination: Normal renal function: 2-8 hours; End-stage renal disease: 7-16 hours
Metabolism: Hepatically acetylated; extensive first-pass effect (oral)
Excretion: Urine (14% as unchanged drug)
Available Dosage Forms
Injection, solution, as hydrochloride: 20 mg/mL (1 mL)
Tablet, as hydrochloride: 10 mg, 25 mg, 50 mg, 100 mg
Dosing
Adults:
Hypertension: Oral:
Initial: 10 mg 4 times/day; increase by 10-25 mg/dose every 2-5 days (maximum: 300 mg/day); usual dose range (JNC 7): 25-100 mg/day in 2 divided doses
Acute hypertension: I.M., I.V.: Initial: 10-20 mg/dose every 4-6 hours as needed, may increase to 40 mg/dose; change to oral therapy as soon as possible.
Pre-eclampsia/eclampsia: I.M., I.V.: 5 mg/dose then 5-10 mg every 20-30 minutes as needed
Congestive heart failure: Oral:
Initial dose: 10-25 mg 3-4 times/day
Adjustment: Dosage must be adjusted based on individual response
Target dose: 225-300 mg/day in divided doses; use in combination with isosorbide dinitrate
Elderly: Oral: Initial: 10 mg 2-3 times/day; increase by 10-25 mg/day every 2-5 days.
Pediatrics:
Hypertension: Oral: Initial: 0.75-1 mg/kg/day in 2-4 divided doses; increase over 3-4 weeks to maximum of 7.5 mg/kg/day in 2-4 divided doses; maximum daily dose: 200 mg/day
Acute hypertension: I.M., I.V.: 0.1-0.2 mg/kg/dose (not to exceed 20 mg) every 4-6 hours as needed, up to 1.7-3.5 mg/kg/day in 4-6 divided doses
Renal Impairment:
Cl$_{cr}$ 10-50 mL/minute: Administer every 8 hours.
Cl$_{cr}$ <10 mL/minute: Administer every 8-16 hours in fast acetylators and every 12-24 hours in slow acetylators.
Hemodialysis effects: Supplemental dose is not necessary.
Peritoneal dialysis effects: Supplemental dose is not necessary.
Administration
I.V.: Inject over 1 minute. Hypotensive effect may be delayed and unpredictable in some patients.
I.V. Detail: pH: 3.4-4.0
Stability
Reconstitution: Hydralazine should be diluted in NS for IVPB administration due to decreased stability in D$_5$W. Stability of IVPB solution in NS is 4 days at room temperature.
(Continued)

HydrALAZINE *(Continued)*

Compatibility: Stable in dextran 6% in dextrose, dextran 6% in NS, D_5LR, $D_5\frac{1}{4}NS$, $D_5\frac{1}{2}NS$, D_5NS, $D_{10}W$, LR, $\frac{1}{2}NS$, NS; **incompatible** with D_5W

Y-site administration: Incompatible with aminophylline, ampicillin, diazoxide, furosemide

Compatibility when admixed: Incompatible with aminophylline, ampicillin, chlorothiazide, edetate calcium disodium, ethacrynate, hydrocortisone sodium succinate, mephentermine, methohexital, nitroglycerin, phenobarbital, verapamil

Storage: Intact ampuls/vials of hydralazine should not be stored under refrigeration because of possible precipitation or crystallization.

Laboratory Monitoring ANA titer

Nursing Actions

Physical Assessment: Assess potential for interactions with other pharmacological agents or herbal products patient may be taking (especially anything that may impact blood pressure). For infusion see Administration specifics. Orthostatic precautions should be observed and patient monitored closely during and following infusion. Assess results of laboratory tests, therapeutic effectiveness (decreased blood pressure), and adverse response (eg, hypotension, fluid retention) periodically during therapy. Teach patient proper use (oral), possible side effects/appropriate interventions, and adverse symptoms to report.

Patient Education: Do not take any new medication during therapy unless approved by prescriber. Take as directed, with meals. Avoid alcohol. This medication does not replace other antihypertensive interventions; follow prescriber's instructions for diet and lifestyle changes. Weigh daily at the same time, in the same clothes for the first 2 weeks and weekly thereafter. Report weight gain >5 lb/week or swelling of feet or ankles. May cause postural hypotension, dizziness, or weakness (change position slowly when rising from sitting or lying position, climbing stairs, and avoid driving or activities requiring alertness until response to drug is known); nausea or vomiting (small, frequent meals, frequent mouth care, chewing gum, or sucking lozenges may help); impotence (reversible); diarrhea (boiled milk, buttermilk, or yogurt may help); or constipation (increased exercise, fluids, fruit, or fiber may help). Report chest pain, rapid heartbeat, or palpitations; flu-like symptoms; respiratory difficulty; skin rash; numbness and tingling of extremities; muscle cramps, weakness, or tremors; persistent GI problems; or other adverse reactions. **Pregnancy precaution:** Inform prescriber if you are or intend to become pregnant

Dietary Considerations Administer with meals.

Breast-Feeding Issues Crosses into breast milk in extremely small amounts. Available evidence suggests safe use during breast-feeding. AAP considers **compatible** with breast-feeding.

Pregnancy Issues Crosses the placenta. One report of fetal arrhythmia; transient neonatal thrombocytopenia and fetal distress reported following late 3rd trimester use. A large amount of clinical experience with the use of this drug for management of hypertension during pregnancy is available.

Related Information

FDA Name Differentiation Project: The Use of Tall-Man Letters *on page 12*

Hydralazine and Hydrochlorothiazide
(hye DRAL a zeen & hye droe klor oh THYE a zide)

Synonyms Apresazide [DSC]; Hydrochlorothiazide and Hydralazine

Pharmacologic Category Antihypertensive Agent, Combination

Pregnancy Risk Factor C

Lactation Enters breast milk/compatible

Use Management of moderate to severe hypertension and treatment of congestive heart failure

Available Dosage Forms Capsule:
25/25: Hydralazine hydrochloride 25 mg and hydrochlorothiazide 25 mg
50/50: Hydralazine hydrochloride 50 mg and hydrochlorothiazide 50 mg
100/50: Hydralazine hydrochloride 100 mg and hydrochlorothiazide 50 mg

Dosing
Adults: Hypertension: Oral: 1 capsule twice daily
Elderly: Refer to dosing in individual monographs.

Nursing Actions
Physical Assessment: See individual agents.
Patient Education: See individual agents. **Pregnancy precaution:** Inform prescriber if you are or intend to become pregnant.

Related Information
HydrALAZINE *on page 609*
Hydrochlorothiazide *on page 610*

Hydrochlorothiazide
(hye droe klor oh THYE a zide)

U.S. Brand Names Microzide™

Synonyms HCTZ (error-prone abbreviation)

Pharmacologic Category Diuretic, Thiazide

Medication Safety Issues
Sound-alike/look-alike issues:
Hydrochlorothiazide may be confused with hydrocortisone, hydroflumethiazide
Esidrix may be confused with Lasix®
HCTZ is an error-prone abbreviation (mistaken as hydrocortisone)

Pregnancy Risk Factor B (manufacturer); D (expert analysis)

Lactation Enters breast milk/use caution (AAP rates "compatible")

Use Management of mild to moderate hypertension; treatment of edema in congestive heart failure and nephrotic syndrome

Unlabeled/Investigational Use Treatment of lithium-induced diabetes insipidus

Mechanism of Action/Effect Inhibits sodium reabsorption in the distal tubules causing increased excretion of sodium and water as well as potassium and hydrogen ions

Contraindications Hypersensitivity to hydrochlorothiazide or any component of the formulation, thiazides, or sulfonamide-derived drugs; anuria; renal decompensation; pregnancy

Warnings/Precautions Avoid in severe renal disease (ineffective as a diuretic). Electrolyte disturbances (hypokalemia, hypochloremic alkalosis, hyponatremia) can occur. Use with caution in severe hepatic dysfunction; hepatic encephalopathy can be caused by electrolyte disturbances. Gout may be precipitated in patients with a history of gout, a familial predisposition to gout, or chronic renal failure. Use caution in patients with diabetes; may alter glucose control. May cause SLE exacerbation or activation. Use with caution in patients with moderate or high cholesterol concentrations.

Photosensitization may occur. Correct hypokalemia before initiating therapy.

Chemical similarities are present among sulfonamides, sulfonylureas, carbonic anhydrase inhibitors, thiazides, and loop diuretics (except ethacrynic acid). Use in patients with sulfonamide allergy is specifically contraindicated in product labeling, however, a risk of cross-reaction exists in patients with allergy to any of these compounds; avoid use when previous reaction has been severe.

Drug Interactions

Decreased Effect: Effects of oral hypoglycemics may be decreased. Decreased absorption of hydrochlorothiazide with cholestyramine and colestipol. NSAIDs can decrease the efficacy of thiazides, reducing the diuretic and antihypertensive effects.

Increased Effect/Toxicity: Increased effect of hydrochlorothiazide with furosemide and other loop diuretics. Increased hypotension and/or renal adverse effects of ACE inhibitors may result in aggressively diuresed patients. Beta-blockers increase hyperglycemic effects of thiazides in type 2 diabetes mellitus. Cyclosporine and thiazides can increase the risk of gout or renal toxicity. Digoxin toxicity can be exacerbated if a thiazide induces hypokalemia or hypomagnesemia. Lithium toxicity can occur with thiazides due to reduced renal excretion of lithium. Thiazides may prolong the duration of action with neuromuscular blocking agents.

Nutritional/Ethanol Interactions

Food: Hydrochlorothiazide peak serum levels may be decreased if taken with food. This product may deplete potassium, sodium, and magnesium.

Herb/Nutraceutical: Avoid dong quai if using for hypertension (has estrogenic activity). Dong quai may also cause photosensitization. Avoid ephedra, ginseng, yohimbe (may worsen hypertension). Avoid garlic (may have increased antihypertensive effect).

Lab Interactions Increased creatine phosphokinase [CPK] (S), ammonia (B), amylase (S), calcium (S), chloride (S), cholesterol (S), glucose, acid (S); decreased chloride (S), magnesium, potassium (S), sodium (S); tyramine and phentolamine tests; histamine tests for pheochromocytoma

Adverse Reactions

1% to 10%:
Cardiovascular: Orthostatic hypotension, hypotension
Dermatologic: Photosensitivity
Endocrine & metabolic: Hypokalemia
Gastrointestinal: Anorexia, epigastric distress

Overdosage/Toxicology Symptoms of overdose include hypermotility, diuresis, lethargy, confusion, and muscle weakness. Treatment is supportive.

Pharmacodynamics/Kinetics

Onset of Action: Diuresis: ~2 hours; Peak effect: 4-6 hours

Duration of Action: 6-12 hours

Time to Peak: 1-2.5 hours

Protein Binding: 68%

Half-Life Elimination: 5.6-14.8 hours

Metabolism: Not metabolized

Excretion: Urine (as unchanged drug)

Available Dosage Forms

Capsule (Microzide™): 12.5 mg
Tablet: 25 mg, 50 mg

Dosing

Adults:

Edema (diuresis): Oral: 25-100 mg/day in 1-2 doses; maximum: 200 mg/day

Hypertension: Oral: 12.5-50 mg/day; minimal increase in response and more electrolyte disturbances are seen with doses >50 mg/day

Elderly: Oral: 12.5-25 mg once daily; minimal increase in response and more electrolyte disturbances are seen with doses >50 mg/day (see Geriatric Considerations).

Pediatrics: Hypertension, edema (diuretic): Oral (effect of drug may be decreased when used every day):

Children <6 months: 2-3 mg/kg/day in 2 divided doses

Children >6 months: 2 mg/kg/day in 2 divided doses

Note: In pediatric patients, chlorothiazide may be preferred over hydrochlorothiazide as there are more dosage formulations (eg, suspension) available.

Renal Impairment: Cl_{cr} <10 mL/minute: Avoid use. Usually ineffective with GFR <30 mL/minute. Effective at lower GFR in combination with a loop diuretic.

Administration

Oral: May be taken with food or milk. Take early in day to avoid nocturia. Take the last dose of multiple doses no later than 6 PM unless instructed otherwise.

Laboratory Monitoring Serum electrolytes, BUN, creatinine

Nursing Actions

Physical Assessment: Allergy history should be identified prior to beginning therapy (sulfonamides). Assess potential for interactions with other pharmacological or herbal products patient may be taking (altered affect of oral hypoglycemics, increased risk of hypotension or toxicity). Monitor laboratory tests, therapeutic effectiveness (according to purpose for use), and adverse response (eg, hypotension, hypokalemia, confusion) regularly during therapy. Caution patients with diabetes to monitor glucose levels closely; may alter glucose control. Teach proper use, possible side effects/appropriate interventions, and adverse symptoms to report.

Patient Education: Do not take any new medication during therapy unless approved by prescriber. This medication does not replace other antihypertensive interventions; follow prescriber's instructions for diet and lifestyle changes. Take as directed, with meals, early in the day to avoid nocturia. Your prescriber may prescribe a potassium supplement or recommend that you eat foods high in potassium (include bananas and/or orange juice in daily diet). Do not change your diet on your own while taking this medication, especially if you are taking potassium supplements or medications to reduce potassium loss; too much potassium can be as harmful as too little. If you have diabetes, monitor serum glucose closely; this medication may increase serum glucose levels. May cause dizziness or postural hypotension (use caution when rising from sitting or lying position, when driving, climbing stairs, or engaging in tasks that require alertness until response to drug is known); nausea or vomiting (small, frequent meals, frequent mouth care, sucking lozenges, or chewing gum may help); impotence (reversible); constipation (increased exercise, fluids, fruit, or fiber may help); or photosensitivity (use sunscreen, wear protective clothing and eyewear, and avoid direct sunlight). Report persistent flu-like symptoms, chest pain, palpitations, muscle cramping, respiratory difficulty, skin rash or itching, unusual bruising or easy bleeding, or excessive fatigue. **Pregnancy/breast-feeding precautions:** Inform prescriber if you are pregnant. Consult prescriber if breast-feeding.

Geriatric Considerations Hydrochlorothiazide is not effective in patients with a Cl_{cr} <30 mL/minute, therefore, it may not be a useful agent in many elderly patients.

Pregnancy Issues Although there are no adequate and well-controlled studies using hydrochlorothiazide in pregnancy, thiazide diuretics may cause an increased risk of congenital defects. Hypoglycemia, hypokalemia, hyponatremia, jaundice, and thrombocytopenia are also reported as possible complications to the fetus or newborn.

(Continued)

Hydrochlorothiazide *(Continued)*

Additional Information If given the morning of surgery it may render the patient volume depleted and blood pressure may be labile during general anesthesia. Effect of drug may be decreased when used every day.

Hydrochlorothiazide and Spironolactone

(hye droe klor oh THYE a zide & speer on oh LAK tone)

U.S. Brand Names Aldactazide®
Synonyms Spironolactone and Hydrochlorothiazide
Pharmacologic Category Antihypertensive Agent, Combination
Pregnancy Risk Factor C
Lactation Enters breast milk/use caution
Use Management of mild to moderate hypertension; treatment of edema in congestive heart failure and nephrotic syndrome, and cirrhosis of the liver accompanied by edema and/or ascites

Available Dosage Forms
Tablet: Hydrochlorothiazide 25 mg and spironolactone 25 mg
Aldactazide®:
25/25: Hydrochlorothiazide 25 mg and spironolactone 25 mg
50/50: Hydrochlorothiazide 50 mg and spironolactone 50 mg

Dosing
Adults: Hypertension, edema: Oral:
Hydrochlorothiazide 25 mg and spironolactone 25 mg: ½-8 tablets daily
Hydrochlorothiazide 50 mg and spironolactone 50 mg: ½-4 tablets daily in 1-2 doses
Elderly: Oral: Initial: 1 tablet/day; increase as necessary.
Renal Impairment: Efficacy of hydrochlorothiazide is limited in patients with Cl$_{cr}$ <30 mL/minute.
Nursing Actions
Physical Assessment: See individual agents.
Patient Education: See individual agents. **Pregnancy/breast-feeding precautions:** Inform prescriber if you are or intend to become pregnant. Consult prescriber if breast-feeding.
Related Information
Hydrochlorothiazide *on page 610*
Spironolactone *on page 1142*

Hydrochlorothiazide and Triamterene

(hye droe klor oh THYE a zide & trye AM ter een)

U.S. Brand Names Dyazide®; Maxzide®; Maxzide®-25
Synonyms Triamterene and Hydrochlorothiazide
Pharmacologic Category Antihypertensive Agent, Combination; Diuretic, Potassium-Sparing; Diuretic, Thiazide
Pregnancy Risk Factor C (per manufacturer)
Lactation Excretion in breast milk unknown/use caution
Use Management of mild to moderate hypertension; treatment of edema in congestive heart failure and nephrotic syndrome

Available Dosage Forms
Capsule (Dyazide®): Hydrochlorothiazide 25 mg and triamterene 37.5 mg
Tablet:
Maxzide®: Hydrochlorothiazide 50 mg and triamterene 75 mg
Maxzide®-25: Hydrochlorothiazide 25 mg and triamterene 37.5 mg

Dosing
Adults & Elderly: Hypertension, edema: Oral:
Triamterene 37.5 mg and hydrochlorothiazide 25 mg: 1-2 tablets/capsules once daily
Triamterene 75 mg and hydrochlorothiazide 50 mg: ½-1 tablet daily
Nursing Actions
Physical Assessment: See individual agents.
Patient Education: See individual agents. **Pregnancy/breast-feeding precautions:** Inform prescriber if you are or intend to become pregnant. Consult prescriber if breast-feeding.
Related Information
Hydrochlorothiazide *on page 610*

Hydrocodone and Acetaminophen

(hye droe KOE done & a seet a MIN oh fen)

U.S. Brand Names Anexsia®; Bancap HC®; Ceta-Plus®; Co-Gesic®; hycet™; Lorcet® 10/650; Lorcet®-HD [DSC]; Lorcet® Plus; Lortab®; Margesic® H; Maxidone™; Norco®; Stagesic®; Vicodin®; Vicodin® ES; Vicodin® HP; Zydone®
Synonyms Acetaminophen and Hydrocodone
Restrictions C-III
Pharmacologic Category Analgesic Combination (Narcotic)
Medication Safety Issues
Sound-alike/look-alike issues:
Lorcet® may be confused with Fioricet®
Lortab® may be confused with Cortef®, Lorabid®, Luride®
Vicodin® may be confused with Hycodan®, Hycomine®, Indocin®, Uridon®
Zydone® may be confused with Vytone®
Pregnancy Risk Factor C/D (prolonged use or high doses near term)
Lactation Excretion in breast milk unknown/contraindicated
Use Relief of moderate to severe pain
Contraindications Hypersensitivity to hydrocodone, acetaminophen, or any component of the formulation; CNS depression; severe respiratory depression
Warnings/Precautions Use with caution in patients with hypersensitivity reactions to other phenanthrene derivative opioid agonists (morphine, hydromorphone, levorphanol, oxycodone, oxymorphone); tolerance or drug dependence may result from extended use.

Respiratory depressant effects may be increased with head injuries. Use caution with acute abdominal conditions; clinical course may be obscured. Use caution with thyroid dysfunction, prostatic hyperplasia, hepatic or renal disease, and in the elderly. Causes sedation; caution must be used in performing tasks which require alertness (eg, operating machinery or driving).

Limit acetaminophen to <4 g/day. May cause severe hepatic toxicity in acute overdose; in addition, chronic daily dosing in adults has resulted in liver damage in some patients. Use with caution in patients with alcoholic liver disease; consuming ≥3 alcoholic drinks/day may increase the risk of liver damage. Use caution in patients with known G6PD deficiency.

Drug Interactions
Cytochrome P450 Effect:
Hydrocodone: **Substrate** of CYP2D6 (major)
Acetaminophen: **Substrate** (minor) of CYP1A2, 2A6, 2C8/9, 2D6, 2E1, 3A4; **Inhibits** CYP3A4 (weak)
Increased Effect/Toxicity: Also see Acetaminophen monograph. Hydrocodone with other narcotic analgesics, CNS depressants, antianxiety agents, or antipsychotics may cause enhanced CNS depression. MAO inhibitors or tricyclic antidepressants with hydrocodone may increase the effect of either agent.

Nutritional/Ethanol Interactions

Ethanol: Avoid ethanol (may increase CNS depression); consuming ≥3 alcoholic drinks/day may increase the risk of liver damage

Herb/Nutraceutical: Avoid valerian, St John's wort, SAMe, kava kava (may increase risk of excessive sedation).

Adverse Reactions Frequency not defined.

Cardiovascular: Bradycardia, cardiac arrest, circulatory collapse, coma, hypotension

Central nervous system: anxiety, dizziness, drowsiness, dysphoria, euphoria, fear, lethargy, lightheadedness, malaise, mental clouding, mental impairment, mood changes, physiological dependence, sedation, somnolence, stupor

Dermatologic: Pruritus, rash

Endocrine & metabolic: Hypoglycemic coma

Gastrointestinal: Abdominal pain, constipation, gastric distress, heartburn, nausea, peptic ulcer, vomiting

Genitourinary: Ureteral spasm, urinary retention, vesical sphincter spasm

Hematologic: Agranulocytosis, bleeding time prolonged, hemolytic anemia, iron deficiency anemia, occult blood loss, thrombocytopenia

Hepatic: Hepatic necrosis, hepatitis

Neuromuscular & skeletal: Skeletal muscle rigidity

Otic: Hearing impairment or loss (chronic overdose)

Renal: Renal toxicity, renal tubular necrosis

Respiratory: Acute airway obstruction, apnea, dyspnea, respiratory depression (dose related)

Miscellaneous: Allergic reactions, clamminess, diaphoresis

Overdosage/Toxicology

Symptoms of overdose include hepatic necrosis, blood dyscrasias, and respiratory depression. Treatment consists of acetylcysteine 140 mg/kg orally (loading) followed by 70 mg/kg every 4 hours for 17 doses; therapy should be initiated based upon laboratory analysis suggesting a high probability for hepatotoxic potential. Naloxone, 2 mg I.V. with repeat administration as necessary up to a total of 10 mg, can also be used to reverse toxic effects of the opiate. Activated charcoal is effective at binding certain chemicals, and this is especially true for acetaminophen.

Pharmacodynamics/Kinetics

Onset of Action:

Hydrocodone: Narcotic analgesic: 10-20 minutes

Duration of Action:

Hydrocodone: 4-8 hours

Half-Life Elimination:

Hydrocodone: 3.3-4.4 hours

Metabolism:

Hydrocodone: Hepatic; O-demethylation; N-demethylation and 6-ketosteroid reduction

Excretion:

Hydrocodone: Urine

Pharmacokinetic Note See Acetaminophen monograph.

Available Dosage Forms

Capsule (Bancap HC®, Ceta-Plus®, Margesic® H, Stagesic®): Hydrocodone bitartrate 5 mg and acetaminophen 500 mg

Elixir: Hydrocodone bitartrate 7.5 mg and acetaminophen 500 mg per 15 mL (480 mL)

Lortab®: Hydrocodone bitartrate 7.5 mg and acetaminophen 500 mg per 15 mL (480 mL) [contains alcohol 7%; tropical fruit punch flavor]

Solution, oral (hycet™): Hydrocodone bitartrate 7.5 mg and acetaminophen 325 mg per 15 mL (480 mL) [contains alcohol 7%; tropical fruit punch flavor]

Tablet:

Hydrocodone bitartrate 2.5 mg and acetaminophen 500 mg

Hydrocodone bitartrate 5 mg and acetaminophen 325 mg

Hydrocodone bitartrate 5 mg and acetaminophen 500 mg

Hydrocodone bitartrate 7.5 mg and acetaminophen 325 mg

Hydrocodone bitartrate 7.5 mg and acetaminophen 500 mg

Hydrocodone bitartrate 7.5 mg and acetaminophen 650 mg

Hydrocodone bitartrate 7.5 mg and acetaminophen 750 mg

Hydrocodone bitartrate 10 mg and acetaminophen 325 mg

Hydrocodone bitartrate 10 mg and acetaminophen 500 mg

Hydrocodone bitartrate 10 mg and acetaminophen 650 mg

Hydrocodone bitartrate 10 mg and acetaminophen 660 mg

Anexsia®:

5/500: Hydrocodone bitartrate 5 mg and acetaminophen 500 mg

7.5/650: Hydrocodone bitartrate 7.5 mg and acetaminophen 650 mg

Co-Gesic® 5/500: Hydrocodone bitartrate 5 mg and acetaminophen 500 mg

Lorcet® 10/650: Hydrocodone bitartrate 10 mg and acetaminophen 650 mg

Lorcet® Plus: Hydrocodone bitartrate 7.5 mg and acetaminophen 650 mg

Lortab®:

2.5/500: Hydrocodone bitartrate 2.5 mg and acetaminophen 500 mg

5/500: Hydrocodone bitartrate 5 mg and acetaminophen 500 mg

7.5/500: Hydrocodone bitartrate 7.5 mg and acetaminophen 500 mg

10/500: Hydrocodone bitartrate 10 mg and acetaminophen 500 mg

Maxidone™: Hydrocodone bitartrate 10 mg and acetaminophen 750 mg

Norco®:

Hydrocodone bitartrate 5 mg and acetaminophen 325 mg

Hydrocodone bitartrate 7.5 mg and acetaminophen 325 mg

Hydrocodone bitartrate 10 mg and acetaminophen 325 mg

Vicodin®: Hydrocodone bitartrate 5 mg and acetaminophen 500 mg

Vicodin® ES: Hydrocodone bitartrate 7.5 mg and acetaminophen 750 mg

Vicodin® HP: Hydrocodone bitartrate 10 mg and acetaminophen 660 mg

Zydone®:

Hydrocodone bitartrate 5 mg and acetaminophen 400 mg

Hydrocodone bitartrate 7.5 mg and acetaminophen 400 mg

Hydrocodone bitartrate 10 mg and acetaminophen 400 mg

Dosing

Adults:

Pain management (analgesic): Oral (doses should be titrated to appropriate analgesic effect): Average starting dose in opioid naive patients: Hydrocodone 5-10 mg 4 times/day; the dosage of acetaminophen should be limited to ≤4 g/day (and possibly less in patients with hepatic impairment or ethanol use).

Dosage ranges (based on specific product labeling): Hydrocodone 2.5-10 mg every 4-6 hours; maximum: 60 mg hydrocodone/day (maximum dose of hydrocodone may be limited by the acetaminophen content of specific product)

Elderly: Doses should be titrated to appropriate analgesic effect; 2.5-5 mg of the hydrocodone component every 4-6 hours. Do not exceed 4 g/day of acetaminophen.

(Continued)

Hydrocodone and Acetaminophen
(Continued)

Pediatrics:

Pain management (analgesic): Oral (doses should be titrated to appropriate analgesic effect):

Children 2-13 years or <50 kg: Hydrocodone 0.135 mg/kg/dose every 4-6 hours; do not exceed 6 doses/day or the maximum recommended dose of acetaminophen

Children ≥50 kg: Refer to adult dosing.

Hepatic Impairment: Use with caution. Limited, low-dose therapy usually well tolerated in hepatic disease/cirrhosis; however, cases of hepatotoxicity at daily acetaminophen dosages <4 g/day have been reported. Avoid chronic use in hepatic impairment.

Nursing Actions

Physical Assessment: Assess patient for history of liver disease or ethanol abuse (acetaminophen and excessive ethanol may have adverse liver effects). Assess other medications patient may be taking for additive or adverse interactions. Monitor therapeutic effectiveness (eg, pain relief) and signs and signs of adverse reactions at beginning of therapy and at regular intervals with long-term use. May cause physical and/or psychological dependence. Discontinue slowly after long-term use. For inpatients, implement safety measures (eg, side rails up, call light within reach, instructions to call for assistance). Assess knowledge/teach patient appropriate use, adverse reactions to report, and appropriate interventions to reduce side effects.

Patient Education: If self-administered, use exactly as directed; do not increase dose or frequency. Drug may cause physical and/or psychological dependence. Take with food or milk. While using this medication, do not use alcohol and other prescription or OTC medications (especially sedatives, tranquilizers, antihistamines, or pain medications) without consulting prescriber. Maintain adequate hydration (2-3 L/day of fluids) unless instructed to restrict fluid intake. May cause dizziness, lightheadedness, confusion, or drowsiness (use caution when driving, climbing stairs, or changing position - rising from sitting or lying to standing, or when engaging in tasks requiring alertness until response to drug is known); or nausea or vomiting (frequent mouth care, frequent sips of fluids, chewing gum, or sucking lozenges may help). Report chest pain or palpitations; persistent dizziness, shortness of breath, or respiratory difficulty; unusual bleeding or bruising; or unusual fatigue and weakness. **Pregnancy/breast-feeding precautions:** Inform prescriber if you are or intend to become pregnant. Do not breast-feed.

Geriatric Considerations The elderly may be particularly susceptible to the CNS depressant action (sedation, confusion) and constipating effects of narcotics. If 1 tablet/dose is used, it may be useful to add an additional 325 mg of acetaminophen to maximize analgesic effect and minimize additional risk of narcotic related adverse effects.

Breast-Feeding Issues Acetaminophen is excreted in breast milk. The AAP considers it to be "compatible" with breast-feeding. Information is not available for hydrocodone; codeine and other opioids are excreted in breast milk and the AAP considers codeine to be "compatible" with breast-feeding. The manufacturers recommend discontinuing the medication or to discontinue nursing during therapy.

Pregnancy Issues Animal reproduction studies have not been conducted with this combination product. Opioid analgesics are considered FDA risk category D if used for prolonged periods or in large doses near term. Withdrawal symptoms may be observed in babies born to mothers taking opioids regularly during pregnancy.

Respiratory depression may be observed in the newborn if opioids are given close to delivery.

Related Information

Acetaminophen *on page 30*

Hydrocodone and Aspirin
(hye droe KOE done & AS pir in)

U.S. Brand Names Damason-P®

Synonyms Aspirin and Hydrocodone

Restrictions C-III

Pharmacologic Category Analgesic Combination (Narcotic)

Pregnancy Risk Factor D

Lactation Enters breast milk/contraindicated

Use Relief of moderate to moderately severe pain

Mechanism of Action/Effect

Based on **hydrocodone** component: Binds to opiate receptors in the CNS, altering the perception of and response to pain; suppresses cough in medullary center; produces generalized CNS depression

Based on **aspirin** component: Inhibits prostaglandin synthesis, acts on the hypothalamus heat-regulating center to reduce fever, blocks prostaglandin synthetase action which prevents formation of the platelet-aggregating substance thromboxane A_2

Contraindications

Based on **hydrocodone** component: Hypersensitivity to hydrocodone or any component of the formulation

Based on **aspirin** component: Hypersensitivity to salicylates, other NSAIDs, or any component of the formulation; asthma; rhinitis; nasal polyps; inherited or acquired bleeding disorders (including factor VII and factor IX deficiency); pregnancy (in 3rd trimester especially); do not use in children (<16 years) for viral infections (chickenpox or flu symptoms), with or without fever, due to a potential association with Reye's syndrome

Warnings/Precautions Use with caution in patients with impaired renal function, erosive gastritis, or peptic ulcer disease. Children and teenagers should not use for chickenpox or flu symptoms before a physician is consulted about Reye's syndrome.

Drug Interactions

Cytochrome P450 Effect:

Hydrocodone: **Substrate** of CYP2D6 (major)

Aspirin: **Substrate** of CYP2C8/9 (minor)

Decreased Effect: Based on **aspirin** component: The effects of ACE inhibitors may be blunted by aspirin administration (may be significant only at higher aspirin dosages). Aspirin may decrease the effects of beta-blockers, loop diuretics (furosemide), thiazide diuretics, and probenecid. Aspirin may cause a decrease in NSAIDs serum concentration and decrease the effects of probenecid. Increased serum salicylate levels when taken with with urine acidifiers (ammonium chloride, methionine).

Increased Effect/Toxicity:

Based on **hydrocodone** component: CNS depressants, MAO inhibitors, general anesthetics, and tricyclic antidepressants may potentiate the effects of opiate agonists; dextroamphetamine may enhance the analgesic effect of opiate agonists.

Based on **aspirin** component: May increase methotrexate serum levels/toxicity and may displace valproic acid from binding sites which can result in toxicity. NSAIDs and aspirin increase GI adverse effects (ulceration). Aspirin with oral anticoagulants (warfarin), thrombolytic agents, heparin, low molecular weight heparins, and antiplatelet agents (ticlopidine, clopidogrel, dipyridamole, NSAIDs, and IIb/IIIa antagonists) may increase risk of bleeding. Bleeding times may be additionally prolonged with verapamil. The effects of older sulfonylurea agents (tolazamide, tolbutamide) may be potentiated due to displacement from plasma proteins. This effect does not appear to be clinically significant for newer sulfonylurea agents (glyburide, glipizide, glimepiride).

Nutritional/Ethanol Interactions

Based on **hydrocodone** component: Ethanol: Avoid or limit ethanol (may increase CNS depression). Watch for sedation.

Based on **aspirin** component:

Ethanol: Avoid ethanol (may enhance gastric mucosal damage).

Food: Food may decrease the rate but not the extent of oral absorption. Take with food or large volume of water or milk to minimize GI upset.

Herb/Nutraceutical: Avoid cat's claw, dong quai, evening primrose, feverfew, garlic, ginger, ginkgo, red clover, horse chestnut, green tea, ginseng (all have additional antiplatelet activity).

Lab Interactions Urine glucose, urinary 5-HIAA, serum uric acid

Adverse Reactions

>10%:

Cardiovascular: Hypotension

Central nervous system: Lightheadedness, dizziness, sedation, drowsiness, fatigue

Gastrointestinal: Nausea, heartburn, stomach pain, dyspepsia, epigastric discomfort

Neuromuscular & skeletal: Weakness

1% to 10%:

Cardiovascular: Bradycardia

Central nervous system: Confusion

Dermatologic: Rash

Gastrointestinal: Vomiting, gastrointestinal ulceration

Genitourinary: Decreased urination

Hematologic: Hemolytic anemia

Respiratory: Dyspnea

Miscellaneous: Anaphylactic shock

Overdosage/Toxicology Naloxone is the antidote for hydrocodone. Naloxone, 2 mg I.V. with repeat administration as necessary up to a total of 10 mg, can also be used to reverse toxic effects of the opiate. Nomograms, such as the "Done" nomogram, can be very helpful for estimating the severity of aspirin poisoning and for directing treatment using serum salicylate levels. Treatment can also be based upon symptomatology; symptoms of aspirin overdose include tinnitus, headache, dizziness, confusion, metabolic acidosis, hyperpyrexia, hypoglycemia, and coma.

Pharmacodynamics/Kinetics

Onset of Action:

Hydrocodone: Narcotic analgesic: 10-20 minutes

Duration of Action:

Hydrocodone: 4-8 hours

Half-Life Elimination:

Hydrocodone: 3.3-4.4 hours

Metabolism:

Hydrocodone: Hepatic; O-demethylation; N-demethylation and 6-ketosteroid reduction

Excretion:

Hydrocodone: Urine

Pharmacokinetic Note See Aspirin monograph.

Available Dosage Forms Tablet: Hydrocodone bitartrate 5 mg and aspirin 500 mg

Dosing

Adults: Pain management (analgesic): Oral: 1-2 tablets every 4-6 hours as needed for pain

Elderly: Refer to dosing in individual monographs.

Administration

Oral: Administer with food or a full glass of water to minimize GI distress.

Nursing Actions

Physical Assessment: Do not use for persons with allergic reaction to aspirin or aspirin-containing medications. Assess other medications patient may be taking for additive or adverse interactions. Monitor for effectiveness of pain relief and monitor for signs of overdose. Monitor vital signs and signs of adverse reactions at beginning of therapy and at regular intervals with long-term use. May cause physical and/or psychological dependence. Discontinue slowly after long-term use. For inpatients, implement safety measures (eg, side rails up, call light within reach, instructions to call for assistance). Assess knowledge/teach patient appropriate use if self-administered. Teach patient to monitor for adverse reactions, adverse reactions to report, and appropriate interventions to reduce side effects.

Patient Education: If self-administered, use exactly as directed; do not increase dose or frequency. Drug may cause physical and/or psychological dependence. Take with food or milk. While using this medication, do not use alcohol, excessive amounts of vitamin C, or salicylate-containing foods (curry powder, prunes, raisins, tea, or licorice), other aspirin- or salicylate-containing medications, and other prescription or OTC medications (especially sedatives, tranquilizers, antihistamines, or pain medications) without consulting prescriber. Maintain adequate hydration (2-3 L/day of fluids) unless instructed to restrict fluid intake. May cause hypotension, dizziness, drowsiness, impaired coordination, or blurred vision (use caution when driving, climbing stairs, or changing position - rising from sitting or lying to standing, or when engaging in tasks requiring alertness until response to drug is known); nausea, vomiting, or dry mouth (frequent mouth care, small frequent meals, chewing gum, or sucking lozenges may help); or constipation (increased exercise, fluids, fruit, or fiber may help; if unresolved, consult prescriber about use of stool softeners). Report ringing in ears; persistent stomach pain; unresolved nausea or vomiting; respiratory difficulty or shortness of breath; yellowing of skin or eyes; changes in color of stool or urine; or unusual bruising or bleeding.

Pregnancy/breast-feeding precautions: Use appropriate contraceptive measures; do not get pregnant while taking this drug. Do not breast-feed.

Breast-Feeding Issues

Hydrocodone: No data reported.

Aspirin: Cautious use due to potential adverse effects in nursing infants.

Related Information

Aspirin *on page 114*

Hydrocodone and Ibuprofen
(hye droe KOE done & eye byoo PROE fen)

U.S. Brand Names Reprexain™; Vicoprofen®

Synonyms Ibuprofen and Hydrocodone

Restrictions C-III

Pharmacologic Category Analgesic, Narcotic; Nonsteroidal Anti-inflammatory Drug (NSAID), Oral

Pregnancy Risk Factor C/D (3rd trimester)

Lactation Excretion in breast milk unknown/contraindicated

Use Short-term (generally <10 days) management of moderate to severe acute pain; is not indicated for treatment of such conditions as osteoarthritis or rheumatoid arthritis

Available Dosage Forms

Tablet: Hydrocodone bitartrate 5 mg and ibuprofen 200 mg; hydrocodone bitartrate 7.5 mg and ibuprofen 200 mg

Reprexain™: Hydrocodone bitartrate 5 mg and ibuprofen 200 mg

Vicoprofen®: Hydrocodone bitartrate 7.5 mg and ibuprofen 200 mg

(Continued)

Hydrocodone and Ibuprofen

(Continued)

Dosing

Adults: Analgesic: Oral (Short-term use is recommended, not to exceed 10 days): 1 tablet every 4-6 hours, do not exceed 5 tablets during a 24-hour period.

Elderly: Refer to dosing in individual monographs.

Nursing Actions

Physical Assessment: Assess other medications patient may be taking for additive or adverse interactions. Monitor for effectiveness of pain relief and monitor for signs of overdose. Monitor vital signs and signs of adverse reactions at beginning of therapy and at regular intervals with long-term use. May cause physical and/or psychological dependence. Discontinue slowly after long-term use. For inpatients, implement safety measures (eg, side rails up, call light within reach, instructions to call for assistance). Assess knowledge/teach patient appropriate use if self-administered. Teach patient to monitor for adverse reactions, adverse reactions to report, and appropriate interventions to reduce side effects.

Patient Education: If self-administered, use exactly as directed; do not increase dose or frequency. Drug may cause physical and/or psychological dependence. Take with food or milk. While using this medication, do not use alcohol and other prescription or OTC medications (especially sedatives, tranquilizers, antihistamines, or pain medications) without consulting prescriber. Maintain adequate hydration (2-3 L/day of fluids) unless instructed to restrict fluid intake. May cause dizziness, drowsiness, confusion, nervousness, or anxiety (use caution when driving, climbing stairs, or changing position - rising from sitting or lying to standing, or when engaging in tasks requiring alertness until response to drug is known); nausea, dry mouth, decreased appetite, or gastric distress (frequent mouth care, frequent sips of fluids, chewing gum, or sucking lozenges may help); or constipation (increased exercise, fluids, fruit, or fiber may help; if unresolved, consult prescriber about use of stool softeners). Report chest pain or palpitations; persistent dizziness, shortness of breath, or respiratory difficulty; unusual bleeding (stool, mouth, urine) or bruising; unusual fatigue and weakness; change in elimination patterns; or change in color of urine or stool. **Pregnancy/breast-feeding precautions:** Inform prescriber if you are or intend to become pregnant. Do not breast-feed.

Related Information

Ibuprofen *on page 630*

Hydrocodone, Carbinoxamine, and Pseudoephedrine

(hye droe KOE done, kar bi NOKS a meen, & soo doe e FED rin)

U.S. Brand Names Histex™ HC; Tri-Vent™ HC

Synonyms Carbinoxamine, Pseudoephedrine, and Hydrocodone; Hydrocodone Bitartrate, Carbinoxamine Maleate, and Pseudoephedrine Hydrochloride; Pseudoephedrine, Hydrocodone, and Carbinoxamine

Restrictions C-III

Pharmacologic Category Antihistamine/Decongestant/Antitussive

Pregnancy Risk Factor C

Lactation Excretion in breast milk unknown/use caution

Use Symptomatic relief of cough, congestion, and rhinorrhea associated with the common cold, influenza, bronchitis, or sinusitis

Available Dosage Forms

Liquid: Hydrocodone bitartrate 5 mg, carbinoxamine maleate 2 mg, and pseudoephedrine hydrochloride 30 mg per 5 mL (480 mL)

Histex™ HC, Tri-Vent™ HC: Hydrocodone bitartrate 5 mg, carbinoxamine maleate 2 mg, and pseudoephedrine hydrochloride 30 mg per 5 mL (480 mL) [alcohol free, sugar free; peach flavor]

Dosing

Adults: Relief of cough, congestion, and runny nose: Oral: 5-10 mL every 4-6 hours; maximum dose: 30 mL/24 hours

Pediatrics: Relief of cough, congestion, and runny nose: Oral:

Children *2-10 years:* Dosing based on hydrocodone content: 0.6 mg/kg/day given in 4 divided doses. Alternately, the following dosing may be used based on age:

2-4 years: 1.25 mL every 4-6 hours; maximum dose: 7.5 mL/24 hours

4-10 years: 2.5 mL every 4-6 hours; maximum dose: 15 mL/24 hours

Children *>10 years:* Refer to adult dosing.

Related Information

Pseudoephedrine *on page 1047*

Hydrocodone, Phenylephrine, and Diphenhydramine

(hye droe KOE done, fen il EF rin, & dye fen HYE dra meen)

U.S. Brand Names Endal® HD; Hydro DP; TussiNate™

Synonyms Diphenhydramine, Hydrocodone, and Phenylephrine; Hydrocodone Bitartrate, Phenylephrine Hydrochloride, and Diphenhydramine Hydrochloride; Phenylephrine, Diphenhydramine, and Hydrocodone

Restrictions C-III

Pharmacologic Category Antihistamine/Decongestant/Antitussive; Antitussive; Decongestant; Histamine H₁ Antagonist

Pregnancy Risk Factor C

Lactation Excretion in breast milk unknown/contraindicated

Use Symptomatic relief of cough and congestion associated with the common cold, sinusitis, or acute upper respiratory tract infections

Available Dosage Forms Syrup:

Endal® HD: Hydrocodone bitartrate 2 mg, phenylephrine hydrochloride 7.5 mg, and diphenhydramine hydrochloride 12.5 mg per 5 mL (480 mL) [alcohol free, sugar free; contains sodium benzoate; cherry flavor]

Hydro DP: Hydrocodone bitartrate 2 mg, phenylephrine hydrochloride 7.5 mg, and diphenhydramine hydrochloride 12.5 mg per 5 mL (480 mL) [cherry flavor]

TussiNate™: Hydrocodone bitartrate 3.5 mg, phenylephrine hydrochloride 5 mg, and diphenhydramine hydrochloride 12.5 mg per 5 mL (480 mL) [alcohol free; contains sodium benzoate; black raspberry flavor]

Dosing

Adults: Relief of cough, congestion: Oral: 10 mL every 4 hours (maximum: 40 mL/24 hours)

Pediatrics: Relief of cough, congestion: Oral:

Children 6-12 years: 5 mL every 4 hours (maximum: 20 mL/24 hours)

Children >12 years: Refer to adult dosing.

Related Information

DiphenhydrAMINE *on page 375*
Phenylephrine *on page 980*

Hydrocodone, Phenylephrine, and Guaifenesin

(hye droe KOE done, fen il EF rin, & gwye FEN e sin)

U.S. Brand Names Crantex HC; De-Chlor G; Giltuss HC®; Hydro-GP; Levall 5.0; Quintex HC; Tussafed® HC

Synonyms Guaifenesin, Hydrocodone Bitartrate, and Phenylephrine Hydrochloride; Phenylephrine, Guaifenesin, and Hydrocodone

Restrictions C-III

Pharmacologic Category Antitussive/Decongestant/Expectorant

Pregnancy Risk Factor C

Lactation Excretion in breast milk unknown/use caution

Use Temporary relief of cough, congestion, and other symptoms associated with colds or allergies

Available Dosage Forms

Liquid: Hydrocodone bitartrate 2 mg, phenylephrine hydrochloride 10 mg, and guaifenesin 100 mg per 5 mL (120 mL, 480 mL)

Crantex HC: Hydrocodone bitartrate 5 mg, phenylephrine hydrochloride 7.5 mg, and guaifenesin 100 mg per 5 mL (480 mL) [alcohol free, dye free, sugar free; black cherry flavor]

De-Chlor G: Hydrocodone bitartrate 2 mg, phenylephrine hydrochloride 10 mg, and guaifenesin 100 mg per 5 mL (480 mL) [grape-menthol mint flavor]

Giltuss HC®: Hydrocodone bitartrate 5 mg, phenylephrine hydrochloride 10 mg, and guaifenesin 300 mg per 5 mL (480 mL) [alcohol free, dye free, sugar free; strawberry banana flavor]

Hydro-GP: Hydrocodone bitartrate 2.5 mg, phenylephrine hydrochloride 7.5 mg, and guaifenesin 50 mg per 5 mL (480 mL) [cherry flavor]

Levall 5.0: Hydrocodone bitartrate 5 mg, phenylephrine hydrochloride 15 mg, and guaifenesin 100 mg per 5 mL (480 mL) [grape flavor]

Quintex HC: Hydrocodone bitartrate 5 mg, phenylephrine hydrochloride 7.5 mg, and guaifenesin 100 mg per 5 mL (480 mL) [black cherry flavor]

Syrup (Tussafed® HC): Hydrocodone bitartrate 2.5 mg, phenylephrine hydrochloride 7.5 mg, and guaifenesin 50 mg per 5 mL (480 mL) [alcohol free]

Dosing

Adults: Cough/congestion: Oral:

Crantex HC: 5-10 mL every 4-6 hours (maximum: 40 mL/24 hours)

Giltuss HC®: 5 mL every 6 hours (maximum: 6 doses/24 hours)

Tussafed® HC: 10 mL every 4-6 hours as needed (maximum: 6 doses/24 hours)

Pediatrics: Cough/congestion: Oral: Children:

2-6 years (Crantex HC): 2.5 mL every 4-6 hours (maximum: 10 mL/24 hours)

3-6 years:

Giltuss HC®: 1.25 mL every 6 hours (maximum: 6 doses/24 hours)

Tussafed® HC: 2.5 mL every 4-6 hours as needed (maximum: 6 doses/24 hours)

6-12 years:

Crantex HC: 5 mL every 4-6 hours (maximum: 4 doses/24 hours)

Giltuss HC®: 2.5 mL every 6 hours (maximum: 6 doses/24 hours)

Tussafed® HC: 5 mL every 4-6 hours as needed (maximum: 6 doses/24 hours)

≥12 years: Refer to adult dosing.

Nursing Actions

Physical Assessment: See individual agents.

Hydrocortisone (hye droe KOR ti sone)

U.S. Brand Names Anucort-HC®; Anusol-HC®; Anusol® HC-1 [OTC]; Aquanil™ HC [OTC]; Beta-HC®; Caldecort® [OTC]; Cetacort®; Colocort®; Cortaid® Intensive Therapy [OTC]; Cortaid® Maximum Strength [OTC]; Cortaid® Sensitive Skin [OTC]; Cortef®; Corticool® [OTC]; Cortifoam®; Cortizone®-10 Maximum Strength [OTC]; Cortizone®-10 Plus Maximum Strength [OTC]; Cortizone®-10 Quick Shot [OTC]; Dermarest Dricort® [OTC]; Dermtex® HC [OTC]; EarSol® HC; Encort™; Hemril®-30; HydroZone Plus [OTC]; Hytone®; IvySoothe® [OTC]; Locoid®; Locoid Lipocream® [OTC]; Nupercainal® Hydrocortisone Cream [OTC]; Nutracort®; Pandel®; Post Peel Healing Balm [OTC]; Preparation H® Hydrocortisone [OTC]; Proctocort®; ProctoCream® HC; Procto-Kit™; Procto-Pak™; Proctosert; Proctosol-HC®; Proctozone-HC™; Sarnol®-HC [OTC]; Solu-Cortef®; Summer's Eve® SpecialCare™ Medicated Anti-Itch Cream [OTC]; Texacort®; Tucks® Anti-Itch [OTC]; Westcort®

Synonyms A-hydroCort; Compound F; Cortisol; Hemorrhoidal HC; Hydrocortisone Acetate; Hydrocortisone Butyrate; Hydrocortisone Probutate; Hydrocortisone Sodium Succinate; Hydrocortisone Valerate

Pharmacologic Category Corticosteroid, Rectal; Corticosteroid, Systemic; Corticosteroid, Topical

Medication Safety Issues

Sound-alike/look-alike issues:

Hydrocortisone may be confused with hydrocodone, hydroxychloroquine, hydrochlorothiazide

Anusol® may be confused with Anusol-HC®, Aplisol®, Aquasol®

Anusol-HC® may be confused with Anusol®

Cortef® may be confused with Lortab®

Cortizone® may be confused with cortisone

HCT (occasional abbreviation for hydrocortisone) is an error-prone abbreviation (mistaken as hydrochlorothiazide)

Hytone® may be confused with Vytone®

Proctocort® may be confused with ProctoCream®

ProctoCream® may be confused with Proctocort®

Pregnancy Risk Factor C

Lactation Excretion in breast milk unknown/use caution

Use Management of adrenocortical insufficiency; relief of inflammation of corticosteroid-responsive dermatoses (low and medium potency topical corticosteroid); adjunctive treatment of ulcerative colitis

Mechanism of Action/Effect Decreases inflammation by suppression of migration of polymorphonuclear leukocytes and reversal of increased capillary permeability

Contraindications Hypersensitivity to hydrocortisone or any component of the formulation; serious infections, except septic shock or tuberculous meningitis; viral, fungal, or tubercular skin lesions

Warnings/Precautions Use with caution in patients with hyperthyroidism, cirrhosis, nonspecific ulcerative colitis, hypertension, osteoporosis, thromboembolic tendencies, CHF, convulsive disorders, myasthenia gravis, thrombophlebitis, peptic ulcer, diabetes, glaucoma, cataracts, or tuberculosis. Use caution in hepatic impairment. May cause HPA axis suppression. Acute adrenal insufficiency may occur with abrupt withdrawal after long-term therapy or with stress. Young pediatric patients may be more susceptible to adrenal axis suppression from topical therapy. Avoid use of topical preparations with occlusive dressings or on weeping or exudative lesions. Because of the risk of adverse effects, systemic corticosteroids should be used
(Continued)

Hydrocortisone *(Continued)*

cautiously in the elderly, in the smallest possible dose, and for the shortest possible time.

Drug Interactions

Cytochrome P450 Effect: Substrate of CYP3A4 (minor); **Induces** CYP3A4 (weak)

Decreased Effect: Hydrocortisone may decrease the hypoglycemic effect of insulin. Phenytoin, phenobarbital, ephedrine, and rifampin increase metabolism of hydrocortisone resulting in a decreased steroid blood level.

Increased Effect/Toxicity: Hydrocortisone in combination with oral anticoagulants may increase prothrombin time. Potassium-depleting diuretics increase risk of hypokalemia. Cardiac glycosides increase risk of arrhythmias or digitalis toxicity secondary to hypokalemia.

Nutritional/Ethanol Interactions

Ethanol: Avoid ethanol (may enhance gastric mucosal irritation).

Food: Hydrocortisone interferes with calcium absorption.

Herb/Nutraceutical: St John's wort may decrease hydrocortisone levels. Avoid cat's claw, echinacea (have immunostimulant properties).

Adverse Reactions

Systemic:

>10%:

Central nervous system: Insomnia, nervousness

Gastrointestinal: Increased appetite, indigestion

1% to 10%:

Dermatologic: Hirsutism

Endocrine & metabolic: Diabetes mellitus

Neuromuscular & skeletal: Arthralgia

Ocular: Cataracts

Respiratory: Epistaxis

Topical:

>10%: Dermatologic: Eczema (12.5%)

1% to 10%: Dermatologic: Pruritus (6%), stinging (2%), dry skin (2%)

Overdosage/Toxicology When consumed in high doses for prolonged periods, systemic hypercorticism and adrenal suppression may occur. In those cases, discontinuation of the corticosteroid should be done judiciously.

Pharmacodynamics/Kinetics

Onset of Action:

Hydrocortisone acetate: Slow

Hydrocortisone sodium succinate (water soluble): Rapid

Duration of Action: Hydrocortisone acetate: Long

Half-Life Elimination: Biologic: 8-12 hours

Metabolism: Hepatic

Excretion: Urine (primarily as 17-hydroxysteroids and 17-ketosteroids)

Available Dosage Forms [DSC] = Discontinued product

Aerosol, rectal, as acetate (Cortifoam®): 10% (15 g) [90 mg/applicator]

Cream, rectal, as acetate (Nupercainal® Hydrocortisone Cream): 1% (30 g) [strength expressed as base]

Cream, rectal, as base:

Cortizone®-10: 1% (30 g) [contains aloe]

Preparation H® Hydrocortisone: 1% (27 g)

Cream, topical, as acetate: 0.5% (9 g, 30 g, 60 g) [available with aloe]; 1% (30 g, 454 g) [available with aloe]

Cream, topical, as base: 0.5% (30 g); 1% (1.5 g, 30 g, 114 g, 454 g); 2.5% (20 g, 30 g, 454 g)

Anusol-HC®: 2.5% (30 g) [contains benzyl alcohol]

Caldecort®: 1% (30 g) [contains aloe vera gel]

Cortaid® Intensive Therapy: 1% (60 g)

Cortaid® Maximum Strength: 1% (15 g, 30 g, 40 g, 60 g) [contains aloe vera gel and benzyl alcohol]

Cortaid® Sensitive Skin: 0.5% (15 g) [contains aloe vera gel]

Cortizone®-10 Maximum Strength: 1% (15 g, 30 g, 60 g) [contains aloe]

Cortizone®-10 Plus Maximum Strength: 1% (30 g, 60 g) [contains vitamins A, D, E and aloe]

Dermarest® Dricort®: 1% (15 g, 30 g)

HydroZone Plus, Proctocort®, Procto-Pak™: 1% (30 g)

Hytone®: 2.5% (30 g, 60 g)

IvySoothe®: 1% (30 g) [contains aloe]

Post Peel Healing Balm: 1% (23 g)

ProctoCream® HC: 2.5% (30 g) [contains benzyl alcohol]

Procto-Kit™: 1% (30 g) [packaged with applicator tips and finger cots]; 2.5% (30 g) [packaged with applicator tips and finger cots]

Proctosol-HC®, Proctozone-HC™: 2.5% (30 g)

Summer's Eve® SpecialCare™ Medicated Anti-Itch Cream: 1% (30 g)

Cream, topical, as butyrate (Locoid®, Locoid Lipocream®): 0.1% (15 g, 45 g)

Cream, topical, as probutate (Pandel®): 0.1% (15 g, 45 g, 80 g)

Cream, topical, as valerate (Westcort®): 0.2% (15 g, 45 g, 60 g)

Gel, topical, as base (Corticool®): 1% (45 g)

Injection, powder for reconstitution, as sodium succinate (Solu-Cortef®): 100 mg, 250 mg, 500 mg, 1 g [diluent contains benzyl alcohol; strength expressed as base]

Lotion, topical, as base: 1% (120 mL); 2.5% (60 mL)

Aquanil™ HC: 1% (120 mL)

Beta-HC®, Cetacort®, Sarnol®-HC: 1% (60 mL)

HydroZone Plus: 1% (120 mL)

Hytone®: 2.5% (60 mL)

Nutracort®: 1% (60 mL, 120 mL); 2.5% (60 mL, 120 mL)

Ointment, topical, as acetate: 1% (30 g) [strength expressed as base; available with aloe]

Anusol® HC-1: 1% (21 g) [strength expressed as base]

Cortaid® Maximum Strength: 1% (15 g, 30 g) [strength expressed as base]

Ointment, topical, as base: 0.5% (30 g); 1% (30 g, 454 g); 2.5% (20 g, 30 g, 454 g)

Cortizone®-10 Maximum Strength: 1% (30 g, 60 g)

Hytone®: 2.5% (30 g) [DSC]

Ointment, topical, as butyrate (Locoid®): 0.1% (15 g, 45 g)

Ointment, topical, as valerate (Westcort®): 0.2% (15 g, 45 g, 60 g)

Solution, otic, as base (EarSol® HC): 1% (30 mL) [contains alcohol 44%, benzyl benzoate, yerba santa]

Solution, topical, as base (Texacort®): 2.5% (30 mL) [contains alcohol]

Solution, topical, as butyrate (Locoid®): 0.1% (20 mL, 60 mL) [contains alcohol 50%]

Solution, topical spray, as base:

Cortaid® Intensive Therapy: 1% (60 mL) [contains alcohol]

Cortizone®-10 Quick Shot: 1% (44 mL) [contains benzyl alcohol]

Dermtex® HC: 1% (52 mL) [contains menthol 1%]

Suppository, rectal, as acetate: 25 mg (12s, 24s, 100s)

Anucort-HC®, Tucks® Anti-Itch: 25 mg (12s, 24s, 100s) [strength expressed as base; Anucort-HC® *renamed* Tucks® Anti-Itch]

Anusol-HC®, Proctosol-HC®: 25 mg (12s, 24s)

Encort™: 30 mg (12s)

Hemril®-30, Proctocort®, Proctosert: 30 mg (12s, 24s)

Suspension, rectal, as base: 100 mg/60 mL (7s)

Colocort®: 100 mg/60 mL (1s, 7s)

Tablet, as base: 20 mg

Cortef®: 5 mg, 10 mg, 20 mg

Dosing

Adults & Elderly: Dose should be based on severity of disease and patient response.

Acute adrenal insufficiency: I.M., I.V.: Succinate: 100 mg I.V. bolus, then 300 mg/day in divided doses every 8 hours or as a continuous infusion for

48 hours. Once patient is stable change to oral, 50 mg every 8 hours for 6 doses, then taper to 30-50 mg/day in divided doses.

Chronic adrenal corticoid insufficiency/physiologic replacement: Oral: 20-30 mg/day

Anti-inflammatory or immunosuppressive: Oral, I.M., I.V.: Succinate: 15-240 mg every 12 hours

Congenital adrenal hyperplasia: Oral: Initial: 10-20 mg/m²/day in 3 divided doses; a variety of dosing schedules have been used. **Note:** Inconsistencies have occurred with liquid formulations; tablets may provide more reliable levels. Doses must be individualized by monitoring growth, bone age, and hormonal levels. Mineralocorticoid and sodium supplementation may be required based upon electrolyte regulation and plasma renin activity.

Shock: I.M., I.V.: Succinate: 500 mg to 2 g every 2-6 hours

Status asthmaticus: I.V.: Succinate: 1-2 mg/kg/dose every 6 hours for 24 hours, then maintenance of 0.5-1 mg/kg every 6 hours

Stress dosing (surgery) in patients known to be adrenally-suppressed or on chronic systemic steroids: I.V.:

Minor stress (ie, inguinal herniorrhaphy): 25 mg/day for 1 day

Moderate stress (ie, joint replacement, cholecystectomy): 50-75 mg/day (25 mg every 8-12 hours) for 1-2 days

Major stress (pancreatoduodenectomy, esophagogastrectomy, cardiac surgery): 100-150 mg/day (50 mg every 8-12 hours) for 2-3 days

Rheumatic diseases:

Intralesional, intra-articular, soft tissue injection: Acetate:

Large joints: 25 mg (up to 37.5 mg)

Small joints: 10-25 mg

Tendon sheaths: 5-12.5 mg

Soft tissue infiltration: 25-50 mg (up to 75 mg)

Bursae: 25-37.5 mg

Ganglia: 12.5-25 mg

Dermatosis: Topical: Apply to affected area 2-4 times/day.

Ulcerative colitis: Rectal: 10-100 mg 1-2 times/day for 2-3 weeks

Pediatrics: Dose should be based on severity of disease and patient response.

Acute adrenal insufficiency: I.M., I.V.:

Infants and young Children: Succinate: 1-2 mg/kg/dose bolus, then 25-150 mg/day in divided doses every 6-8 hours

Older Children: Succinate: 1-2 mg/kg bolus then 150-250 mg/day in divided doses every 6-8 hours

Anti-inflammatory or immunosuppressive: .

Infants and Children:

Oral: 2.5-10 mg/kg/day **or** 75-300 mg/m²/day every 6-8 hours

I.M., I.V.: Succinate: 1-5 mg/kg/day **or** 30-150 mg/m²/day divided every 12-24 hours

Adolescents: Oral, I.M., I.V.: Succinate: 15-240 mg every 12 hours

Congenital adrenal hyperplasia: Oral: Initial: 10-20 mg/m²/day in 3 divided doses; a variety of dosing schedules have been used. **Note:** Inconsistencies have occurred with liquid formulations; tablets may provide more reliable levels. Doses must be individualized by monitoring growth, bone age, and hormonal levels. Mineralocorticoid and sodium supplementation may be required based upon electrolyte regulation and plasma renin activity

Physiologic replacement: Children:

Oral: 0.5-0.75 mg/kg/day **or** 20-25 mg/m²/day every 8 hours

I.M.: Succinate: 0.25-0.35 mg/kg/day **or** 12-15 mg/m²/day once daily

Shock: I.M., I.V.: Succinate:

Children: Initial: 50 mg/kg, then repeated in 4 hours and/or every 24 hours as needed

Adolescents: 500 mg to 2 g every 2-6 hours

Status asthmaticus: Children: I.V.: Succinate: 1-2 mg/kg/dose every 6 hours for 24 hours, then maintenance of 0.5-1 mg/kg every 6 hours.

Dermatosis: Topical: Children >2 years: Apply to affected area 2-4 times/day (Buteprate: Apply once or twice daily).

Administration

Oral: Administer with food or milk to decrease GI upset.

I.V.:

Parenteral: Hydrocortisone sodium succinate may be administered by I.M. or I.V. routes.

I.V. bolus: Dilute to 50 mg/mL and give over 30 seconds to several minutes (depending on the dose).

I.V. intermittent infusion: Dilute to 1 mg/mL and give over 20-30 minutes.

Note: Should be administered in a 0.1-1 mg/mL concentration due to stability problems.

I.V. Detail:

pH: Hydrocortisone sodium succinate: 7-8

Topical: Apply a thin film sparingly to clean, dry skin and rub in gently.

Stability

Reconstitution:

Sodium succinate: Reconstitute 100 mg vials with bacteriostatic water (not >2 mL). Act-O-Vial (self-contained powder for injection plus diluent) may be reconstituted by pressing the activator to force diluent into the powder compartment. Following gentle agitation, solution may be withdrawn via syringe through a needle inserted into the center of the stopper. May be administered (I.V. or I.M.) without further dilution.

Solutions for I.V. infusion: Reconstituted solutions may be added to an appropriate volume of compatible solution for infusion. Concentration should generally not exceed 1 mg/mL. However, in cases where administration of a small volume of fluid is desirable, 100-3000 mg may be added to 50 mL of D_5W or NS (stability limited to 4 hours).

Compatibility:

Hydrocortisone sodium phosphate: Stable in D_5W, NS, fat emulsion 10%

Y-site administration: Incompatible with sargramostim

Compatibility in syringe: Incompatible with doxapram

Hydrocortisone sodium succinate: Stable in dextran 6% in dextrose, dextran 6% in NS, D_5LR, $D_5\frac{1}{4}NS$, $D_5\frac{1}{2}NS$, D_5NS, D_5W, $D_{10}W$, $D_{20}W$, LR, $\frac{1}{2}NS$, NS, fat emulsion 10%

Y-site administration: Incompatible with ciprofloxacin, diazepam, ergotamine, idarubicin, midazolam, phenytoin, sargramostim

Compatibility in syringe: Incompatible with doxapram

Compatibility when admixed: Incompatible with aminophylline with cephalothin, bleomycin, colistimethate, ephedrine, hydralazine, nafcillin, pentobarbital, phenobarbital, prochlorperazine edisylate, promethazine

Storage: Store at controlled room temperature 20°C to 25°C (59°F to 86°F). Hydrocortisone sodium phosphate and hydrocortisone sodium succinate are clear, light yellow solutions which are heat labile.

Sodium succinate: After initial reconstitution, hydrocortisone sodium succinate solutions are stable for 3 days at room temperature or under refrigeration when protected from light. Stability of parenteral admixture (Solu-Cortef®) at room temperature

(Continued)

Hydrocortisone *(Continued)*

(25°C) and at refrigeration temperature (4°C) is concentration-dependent:

Stability of concentration 1 mg/mL: 24 hours

Stability of concentration 2 mg/mL to 60 mg/mL: At least 4 hours

Solutions for I.V. infusion: Reconstituted solutions may be added to an appropriate volume of compatible solution for infusion. Concentration should generally not exceed 1 mg/mL. However, in cases where administration of a small volume of fluid is desirable, 100-3000 mg may be added to 50 mL of D₅W or NS (stability limited to 4 hours).

Laboratory Monitoring Serum glucose, electrolytes

Nursing Actions

Physical Assessment: Monitor laboratory results, effects, and interactions of other medications patient may be taking, response to therapy, and adverse effects according to diagnosis, formulation of hydrocortisone, dosage, and extent of time used. Systemic administration and long-term use will require close and frequent monitoring, especially for Cushing's syndrome. Assess for signs of fluid retention. Taper dosage when discontinuing. Assess/teach patient appropriate use, interventions for possible adverse reactions, and symptoms to report. Topical absorption may be minimal.

Patient Education: Systemic: Take as directed; do not increase doses and do not stop abruptly without consulting prescribed. Dosage of systemic hydrocortisone is usually tapered off gradually. Take oral dose with food to reduce GI upset. Avoid alcohol. Hydrocortisone may cause immunosuppression and mask symptoms of infection; avoid exposure to contagion and notify prescriber of any signs of infection (eg, fever, chills, sore throat, injury) and notify dentist or surgeon (if necessary) that you are taking this medication. You may experience increased appetite, indigestion, or increased nervousness. Report any sudden weight gain (>5 lb/week), swelling of extremities or respiratory difficulty, abdominal pain, severe vomiting, black or tarry stools, fatigue, anorexia, weakness, or unusual mood swings. **Pregnancy/ breast-feeding precautions:** Inform prescriber if you are or intend to become pregnant. Consult prescriber if breast-feeding.

Topical: Before applying, wash area gently and thoroughly. Apply a thin film to cleansed area and rub in gently until medication vanishes. Avoid use of occlusive dressings over topical application unless directed by a physician. Avoid use on weeping or exudative lesions. Avoid exposing affected area to sunlight; you will be more sensitive and severe sunburn may occur. Consult prescriber if breast-feeding.

Rectal: Gently insert suppository as high as possible with gloved finger while lying down. Avoid injury with long or sharp fingernails. Remain in resting position for 10 minutes after insertion.

Dietary Considerations Systemic use of corticosteroids may require a diet with increased potassium, vitamins A, B₆, C, D, folate, calcium, zinc, phosphorus, and decreased sodium. Sodium content of 1 g (sodium succinate injection): 47.5 mg (2.07 mEq)

Breast-Feeding Issues It is not known if hydrocortisone is excreted in breast milk, however, other corticosteroids are excreted. Prednisone and prednisolone are excreted in breast milk; the AAP considers them to be "usually compatible" with breast-feeding. Hypertension was reported in a nursing infant when a topical corticosteroid was applied to the nipples of the mother.

Pregnancy Issues There are no adequate and well-controlled studies in pregnant women. Corticosteroid use has been associated with cleft palate, neonatal adrenal suppression, low birth weight, and cataracts in the infant; including cases associated with topical administration. Use only if potential benefit to the mother exceeds the potential risk to the fetus. Avoid high doses or prolonged use.

Additional Information Hydrocortisone base topical cream, lotion, and ointments in concentrations of 0.25%, 0.5%, and 1% may be OTC or prescription depending on the product labeling.

Related Information

Compatibility of Drugs *on page 1370*

Hydromorphone *(hye droe MOR fone)*

U.S. Brand Names Dilaudid®; Dilaudid-HP®; Palladone™ *[Withdrawn]*

Synonyms Dihydromorphinone; Hydromorphone Hydrochloride

Restrictions C-II

Pharmacologic Category Analgesic, Narcotic

Medication Safety Issues

Sound-alike/look-alike issues:

Dilaudid® may be confused with Demerol®, Dilantin®

Hydromorphone may be confused with morphine; significant overdoses have occurred when hydromorphone products have been inadvertently administered instead of morphine sulfate. Commercially available prefilled syringes of both products looks similar and are often stored in close proximity to each other. **Note:** Hydromorphone 1 mg oral is approximately equal to morphine 4 mg oral; hydromorphone 1 mg I.V. is approximately equal to morphine 5 mg I.V.

Dilaudid®, Dilaudid-HP®: Extreme caution should be taken to avoid confusing the highly-concentrated (Dilaudid-HP®) injection with the less-concentrated (Dilaudid®) injectable product.

Pregnancy Risk Factor C/D (prolonged use or high doses at term)

Lactation Excretion in breast milk unknown/not recommended

Use Management of moderate-to-severe pain

Unlabeled/Investigational Use Antitussive

Mechanism of Action/Effect Binds to opiate receptors in the CNS, causing inhibition of ascending pain pathways, altering the perception of and response to pain; causes cough supression by direct central action in the medulla; produces generalized CNS depression

Contraindications Hypersensitivity to hydromorphone, any component of the formulation, or other phenanthrene derivative; increased intracranial pressure; acute or severe asthma, severe respiratory depression (in absence of resuscitative equipment or ventilatory support); severe CNS depression; pregnancy (prolonged use or high doses at term)

Palladone™ is also contraindicated with known or suspected paralytic ileus.

Warnings/Precautions Controlled release capsules should only be used when continuous analgesia is required over an extended period of time. Palladone™ should only be used in opioid tolerant patients requiring doses of hydromorphone >12 mg/day (or equianalgesic dose of another opioid) and who have been at that dose for >7 days. Controlled release products are not to be used on an as needed basis. Hydromorphone shares toxic potential of opiate agonists, and precaution of opiate agonist therapy should be observed; use with caution in patients with hypersensitivity to other phenanthrene opiates, respiratory disease, biliary tract disease, acute pancreatitis, or severe liver or renal failure; tolerance or drug dependence may result from extended use. Those at risk for opioid abuse include patients with a history of substance abuse or mental illness.

An opioid-containing analgesic regimen should be tailored to each patient's needs and based upon the type of pain being treated (acute versus chronic), the route of administration, degree of tolerance for opioids (naive versus chronic user), age, weight, and medical condition. The optimal analgesic dose varies widely among patients. Doses should be titrated to pain relief/prevention. I.M. use may result in variable absorption and a lag time to peak effect.

Some dosage forms contain trace amounts of sodium bisulfite which may cause allergic reactions in susceptible individuals.

Drug Interactions

Decreased Effect: Hydromorphone may diminish the effects of pegvisomant.

Increased Effect/Toxicity: Effects may be additive with CNS depressants; hypotensive effects may be increased with phenothiazines; serotonergic effects may be additive with SSRIs

Nutritional/Ethanol Interactions

Ethanol: Avoid ethanol (may increase CNS depression).

Herb/Nutraceutical: Avoid valerian, St John's wort, kava kava, gotu kola (may increase CNS depression).

Lab Interactions

Some quinolones may produce a false-positive urine screening result for opiates using commercially-available immunoassay kits. This has been demonstrated most consistently for levofloxacin and ofloxacin, but other quinolones have shown cross-reactivity in certain assay kits. Confirmation of positive opiate screens by more specific methods should be considered.

Adverse Reactions Frequency not defined.

Cardiovascular: Palpitations, hypotension, peripheral vasodilation, tachycardia, bradycardia, flushing of face

Central nervous system: CNS depression, increased intracranial pressure, fatigue, headache, nervousness, restlessness, dizziness, lightheadedness, drowsiness, hallucinations, mental depression, seizure

Dermatologic: Pruritus, rash, urticaria

Endocrine & metabolic: Antidiuretic hormone release

Gastrointestinal: Nausea, vomiting, constipation, stomach cramps, xerostomia, anorexia, biliary tract spasm, paralytic ileus

Genitourinary: Decreased urination, ureteral spasm, urinary tract spasm

Hepatic: LFTs increased, AST increased, ALT increased

Local: Pain at injection site (I.M.)

Neuromuscular & skeletal: Trembling, weakness, myoclonus

Ocular: Miosis

Respiratory: Respiratory depression, dyspnea

Miscellaneous: Histamine release, physical and psychological dependence

Overdosage/Toxicology Symptoms of overdose include CNS depression, respiratory depression, miosis, apnea, pulmonary edema, and convulsions. Along with supportive measures, naloxone, 2 mg I.V. with repeat administration as necessary up to a total of 10 mg, can also be used to reverse toxic effects of the opiate.

Pharmacodynamics/Kinetics

Onset of Action: Analgesic: Immediate release formulations: Oral: 15-30 minutes; Peak effect: Oral: 30-60 minutes

Duration of Action: Immediate release formulations: 4-5 hours

Protein Binding: ~20%

Half-Life Elimination: Immediate release formulations: 1-3 hours; Palladone™: 18.6 hours

Metabolism: Hepatic; to inactive metabolites

Excretion: Urine (primarily as glucuronide conjugates)

Available Dosage Forms [CAN] = Canadian brand name

Capsule, controlled release (Hydromorph Contin®) [CAN]: 3 mg, 6 mg, 12 mg, 18 mg, 24 mg, 30 mg [not available in U.S.]

Capsule, extended release, as hydrochloride (Palladone™): 12 mg, 16 mg, 24 mg, 32 mg [withdrawn from market]

Injection, powder for reconstitution, as hydrochloride (Dilaudid-HP®): 250 mg

Injection, solution, as hydrochloride: 1 mg/mL (1 mL); 2 mg/mL (1 mL, 20 mL); 4 mg/mL (1 mL); 10 mg/mL (1 mL, 5 mL, 10 mL)

Dilaudid®: 1 mg/mL (1 mL); 2 mg/mL (1 mL, 20 mL) [20 mL size contains edetate sodium; vial stopper contains latex]; 4 mg/mL (1 mL)

Dilaudid-HP®: 10 mg/mL (1 mL, 5 mL, 50 mL)

Liquid, oral, as hydrochloride (Dilaudid®): 1 mg/mL (480 mL) [may contain trace amounts of sodium bisulfite]

Suppository, rectal, as hydrochloride (Dilaudid®): 3 mg (6s)

Tablet, as hydrochloride (Dilaudid®): 2 mg, 4 mg, 8 mg (8 mg tablets may contain trace amounts of sodium bisulfite)

Dosing

Adults:

Antitussive (unlabeled use): Oral: 1 mg every 3-4 hours as needed

Acute pain (moderate to severe): Note: These are guidelines and do not represent the maximum doses that may be required in all patients. Doses should be titrated to pain relief/prevention. Doses should be titrated to appropriate analgesic effects; when changing routes of administration, note that oral doses are <50% as effective as parenteral doses (may be only one-fifth as effective).

Oral:

Initial: Opiate-naive: 2-4 mg every 3-4 hours as needed; patients with prior opiate exposure may require higher initial doses

Usual dosage range: 2-8 mg every 3-4 hours as needed

I.V.: Initial: Opiate-naive: 0.2-0.6 mg every 2-3 hours as needed; patients with prior opiate exposure may tolerate higher initial doses

Note: More frequent dosing may be required.

Mechanically-ventilated patients (based on 70 kg patient): 0.7-2 mg every 1-2 hours as needed; infusion (based on 70 kg patient): 0.5-1 mg/hour

Patient-controlled analgesia (PCA): (Opiate-naive: Consider lower end of dosing range)

Usual concentration: 0.2 mg/mL

Demand dose: Usual: 0.1-0.2 mg; range: 0.05-0.5 mg

Lockout interval: 5-15 minutes

4-hour limit: 4-6 mg

Epidural:

Bolus dose: 1-1.5 mg

Infusion concentration: 0.05-0.075 mg/mL

Infusion rate: 0.04-0.4 mg/hour

Demand dose: 0.15 mg

Lockout interval: 30 minutes

I.M., SubQ: **Note:** I.M. use may result in variable absorption and a lag time to peak effect.

Initial: Opiate-naive: 0.8-1 mg every 4-6 hours as needed; patients with prior opiate exposure may require higher initial doses

Usual dosage range: 1-2 mg every 3-6 hours as needed

Rectal: 3 mg every 4-8 hours as needed

Chronic pain: Note: Patients taking opioids chronically may become tolerant and require doses higher than the usual dosage range to maintain the desired effect. Tolerance can be managed by appropriate

(Continued)

Hydromorphone *(Continued)*

dose titration. There is no optimal or maximal dose for hydromorphone in chronic pain. The appropriate dose is one that relieves pain throughout its dosing interval without causing unmanageable side effects.

Controlled release formulation (Hydromorph Contin®, not available in U.S.): Oral: 3-30 mg every 12 hours. **Note:** A patient's hydromorphone requirement should be established using prompt release formulations; conversion to long acting products may be considered when chronic, continuous treatment is required. Higher dosages should be reserved for use only in opioid-tolerant patients.

Extended release formulation (Palladone™): Oral: For use only in opioid-tolerant patients requiring extended treatment of pain. Initial Palladone™ dose should be calculated using standard conversion estimates based on previous total daily opioid dose, rounding off to the most appropriate strength available. Doses should be administered once every 24 hours. Discontinue all previous around-the-clock opioids when treatment is initiated. Dose may be adjusted every 2 days as needed.

Conversion from transdermal fentanyl to oral Palladone™ (limited clinical experience): Initiate Palladone™ 18 hours after removal of patch; substitute Palladone™ 12 mg/day for each fentanyl 50 mcg/hour patch; monitor closely

Conversion from opioid combination drugs: Initial dose: Palladone™ 12 mg/day in patients receiving around-the-clock fixed combination-opioid analgesics with a total dose greater than or equal to oxycodone 45 mg/day, hydrocodone 45 mg/day, or codeine 300 mg/day

Elderly: Doses should be titrated to appropriate analgesic effects. When changing routes of administration, note that oral doses are less than half as effective as parenteral doses (may be only 20% as effective).

Pain: Oral: 1-2 mg every 4-6 hours

Antitussive: Refer to adult dosing.

Pediatrics:

Acute pain (moderate to severe): Note: These are guidelines and do not represent the maximum doses that may be required in all patients. Doses should be titrated to pain relief/prevention.

Young Children ≥6 months and <50 kg:

Oral: 0.03-0.08 mg/kg/dose every 3-4 hours as needed

I.V.: 0.015 mg/kg/dose every 3-6 hours as needed

Older Children >50 kg: Refer to adult dosing.

Antitussive: Oral:

Children 6-12 years: 0.5 mg every 3-4 hours as needed

Children >12 years: 1 mg every 3-4 hours as needed

Hepatic Impairment: Dose adjustment should be considered.

Administration

Oral:

Hydromorph Contin®: Capsule should be swallowed whole; do not crush or chew; contents may be sprinkled on soft food and swallowed

Palladone™: Capsule must be swallowed whole; do not break open, crush, chew, dissolve, or sprinkle on food.

I.M.: May be given SubQ or I.M.; vial stopper contains latex

I.V.: For IVP, must be given slowly over 2-3 minutes (rapid IVP has been associated with an increase in side effects, especially respiratory depression and hypotension)

I.V. Detail: pH: 4.0-5.5

Other: May be given SubQ or I.M.

Stability

Compatibility: Stable in D_5LR, D_5W, $D_5\frac{1}{2}NS$, D_5NS, LR, $\frac{1}{2}NS$, NS

Y-site administration: Incompatible with amphotericin B cholesteryl sulfate complex, diazepam, minocycline, phenobarbital, phenytoin, sargramostim, tetracycline, thiopental

Compatibility in syringe: Incompatible with ampicillin, diazepam, hyaluronidase, phenobarbital, phenytoin

Compatibility when admixed: Incompatible with sodium bicarbonate, thiopental

Storage: Store injection and oral dosage forms at 25°C (77°F). Protect tablets from light. A slightly yellowish discoloration has not been associated with a loss of potency.

Nursing Actions

Physical Assessment: Assess other medications patient may be taking for additive or adverse interactions. Monitor for effectiveness of pain relief and for signs of adverse reactions or overdose. Monitor blood pressure, CNS and respiratory status, and degree of sedation at beginning of therapy and at regular intervals with long-term use. May cause physical and/or psychological dependence. For inpatients, implement safety measures (eg, side rails up, call light within reach, instructions to call for assistance). Assess knowledge/teach patient appropriate use (if self-administered). Teach patient to monitor for adverse reactions, adverse reactions to report, and appropriate interventions to reduce side effects. Discontinue slowly after prolonged use.

Patient Education: If self-administered, use exactly as directed; do not increase dose or frequency. Drug may cause physical and/or psychological dependence. Palladone™ must be swallowed whole. While using this medication, do not use alcohol and other prescription or OTC medications (especially sedatives, tranquilizers, antihistamines, or pain medications) without consulting prescriber. Maintain adequate hydration (2-3 L/day of fluids) unless instructed to restrict fluid intake. May cause dizziness, drowsiness, impaired coordination, or blurred vision (use caution when driving, climbing stairs, or changing position - rising from sitting or lying to standing, or when engaging in tasks requiring alertness until response to drug is known); loss of appetite, nausea, or vomiting (frequent mouth care, small frequent meals, chewing gum, or sucking lozenges may help); or constipation (increased exercise, fluids, fruit, or fiber may help; if unresolved, consult prescriber about use of stool softeners). Report chest pain, slow or rapid heartbeat, acute dizziness, or persistent headache; swelling of extremities or unusual weight gain; changes in urinary elimination; acute headache; back or flank pain or spasms; or other adverse reactions. **Pregnancy/breast-feeding precautions:** Inform prescriber if you are or intend to become pregnant. Breast-feeding is not recommended.

Geriatric Considerations Elderly may be particularly susceptible to the CNS depressant and constipating effects of narcotics.

Breast-Feeding Issues Other opioid analgesics can be found in breast milk; specific data for hydromorphone is not available. The possibility of sedation or respiratory depression in the nursing infant should be considered.

Pregnancy Issues Hydromorphone was teratogenic in some, but not all, animal studies; however, maternal toxicity was also reported. Hydromorphone crosses the placenta. Chronic opioid use during pregnancy may lead to a withdrawal syndrome in the neonate. Symptoms include irritability, hyperactivity, loss of sleep pattern,

abnormal crying, tremor, vomiting, diarrhea, weight loss, or failure to gain weight.
Additional Information Equianalgesic doses: Morphine 10 mg I.M. = hydromorphone 1.5 mg I.M.

Hydroquinone (HYE droe kwin one)

U.S. Brand Names Alphaquin HP®; Claripel™; Dermarest® Skin Correction Cream Plus [OTC]; Eldopaque [OTC]; Eldopaque Forte®; Eldoquin® [OTC]; Eldoquin Forte®; EpiQuin™ Micro; Esoterica® Regular [OTC]; Glyquin®; Glyquin-XM™; Lustra®; Lustra-AF™; Melanex®; Melpaque HP®; Melquin-3®; Melquin HP®; NeoStrata® AHA [OTC]; Nuquin HP®; Palmer's® Skin Success Eventone® Fade Cream [OTC]; Solaquin® [OTC]; Solaquin Forte®
Synonyms Hydroquinol; Quinol
Pharmacologic Category Depigmenting Agent
Medication Safety Issues
Sound-alike/look-alike issues:
Eldopaque® may be confused with Eldoquin®
Eldoquin® may be confused with Eldopaque®
Eldopaque Forte® may be confused with Eldoquin Forte®
Eldoquin Forte® may be confused with Eldopaque Forte®

Pregnancy Risk Factor C
Lactation Excretion in breast milk unknown
Use Gradual bleaching of hyperpigmented skin conditions
Mechanism of Action/Effect Produces reversible depigmentation of the skin by suppression of melanocyte metabolic processes, in particular the inhibition of the enzymatic oxidation of tyrosine to DOPA (3,4-dihydroxyphenylalanine); sun exposure reverses this effect and will cause repigmentation.
Contraindications Hypersensitivity to hydroquinone or any component of the formulation; sunburn, depilatory usage
Warnings/Precautions Limit application to area no larger than face and neck or hands and arms.
Adverse Reactions Frequency not defined.
Dermatologic: Dermatitis, dryness, erythema, stinging, inflammatory reaction, sensitization
Local: Irritation
Pharmacodynamics/Kinetics
Onset of Action: Onset of depigmentation produced by hydroquinone varies among individuals
Duration of Action: Onset and duration of depigmentation produced by hydroquinone varies among individuals
Available Dosage Forms
Cream, topical: 4% (30 g) [may contain sodium metabisulfite]
Alphaquin HP®: 4% (30 g, 60 g)
Eldoquin®: 2% (15 g, 30 g)
Eldoquin Forte®: 4% (30 g) [contains sodium metabisulfite]
EpiQuin™ Micro: 4% (30 g) [contains benzyl alcohol and sodium metabisulfite]
Esoterica® Regular: 2% (85 g) [contains sodium bisulfite]
Lustra®: 4% (30 g) [contains sodium metabisulfite]
Melquin HP®: 4% (15 g, 30 g) [contains sodium metabisulfite]
Cream, topical [with sunscreen]: 4% (30 g) [may contain sodium metabisulfite]
Claripel™: 4% (30 g, 45 g) [contains sodium metabisulfite]
Dermarest® Skin Correcting Cream Plus: 2% (85 g) [contains aloe vera, sodium bisulfite]
Eldopaque®: 2% (15 g, 30 g)
Eldopaque Forte®: 4% (30 g) [contains sodium metabisulfite]
Glyquin®: 4% (30 g)

Glyquin-XM™: 4% (30 g)
Lustra-AF™: 4% (30 g, 60 g) [contains sodium metabisulfite]
Melpaque HP®: 4% (15 g, 30 g) [contains sodium metabisulfite; sunblocking cream base]
Nuquin HP®: 4% (15 g, 30 g, 60 g) [contains sodium metabisulfite]
Palmer's® Skin Success Eventone® Fade Cream: 2% (81 g, 132 g) [contains sodium metabisulfite; available in regular, oily skin, and dry skin formulas]
Solaquin®: 2% (30 g)
Solaquin Forte®: 4% (30 g) [contains sodium metabisulfite]
Gel, topical (NeoStrata® AHA): 2% (45 g) [contains glycolic acid 10%, sodium bisulfite, and sodium sulfite]
Gel, topical [with sunscreen]: 4% (30 g)
Nuquin HP: 4% (15 g, 30 g) [contains sodium bisulfite]
Solaquin Forte®: 4% (30 g) [contains sodium metabisulfite]
Solution, topical (Melanex®, Melquin-3®): 3% (30 mL) [contains alcohol]
Dosing
Adults & Elderly: Bleaching: Topical: Apply a thin layer and rub in twice daily.
Pediatrics: Refer to adult dosing.
Administration
Topical: For external use only; avoid contact with eyes
Nursing Actions
Physical Assessment: When applied to large areas or for extensive periods of time, monitor for adverse reactions (eg, skin irritation). Assess knowledge/teach patient appropriate application and use and adverse symptoms to report.
Patient Education: Use exactly as directed; do not overuse. Therapeutic effect may take several weeks. Test response by applying to small area of unbroken skin and check in 24 hours; if irritation or blistering occurs do not use. Avoid contact with eyes. Do not apply to open wounds or weeping areas. Before using, wash and dry area gently. Apply a thin film to affected area and rub in gently. Avoid direct sunlight or use sunblock or protective clothing to prevent repigmentation. Report swelling, redness, rash, itching, signs of infection, worsening of condition, or lack of healing. **Pregnancy/breast-feeding precautions:** Inform prescriber if you are or intend to become pregnant. Consult prescriber if breast-feeding.

Hydroxocobalamin (hye droks oh koe BAL a min)

Synonyms Vitamin B$_{12}$
Pharmacologic Category Vitamin, Water Soluble
Pregnancy Risk Factor A/C (dose exceeding RDA recommendation)
Lactation Enters breast milk/compatible
Use Treatment of pernicious anemia, vitamin B$_{12}$ deficiency, increased B$_{12}$ requirements due to pregnancy, thyrotoxicosis, hemorrhage, malignancy, liver or kidney disease
Unlabeled/Investigational Use Neuropathies, multiple sclerosis
Mechanism of Action/Effect Coenzyme for various metabolic functions, including fat and carbohydrate metabolism and protein synthesis, used in cell replication and hematopoiesis
Contraindications Hypersensitivity to cyanocobalamin or any component of the formulation, cobalt; patients with hereditary optic nerve atrophy
Warnings/Precautions Some products contain benzoyl alcohol. Avoid use in premature infants. An intradermal test dose should be performed for hypersensitivity. Use only if oral supplementation not possible or when treating pernicious anemia.
(Continued)

Hydroxocobalamin *(Continued)*

Adverse Reactions Frequency not defined.
Cardiovascular: Peripheral vascular thrombosis
Dermatologic: Itching, urticaria
Gastrointestinal: Diarrhea
Miscellaneous: Hypersensitivity reactions

Available Dosage Forms Injection, solution: 1000 mcg/mL (30 mL)

Dosing
Adults & Elderly: Vitamin B$_{12}$ deficiency: I.M.: 30 mcg/day for 5-10 days, followed by 100-200 mcg/month
Pediatrics: Vitamin B$_{12}$ deficiency: I.M.: 1-5 mg given in single doses of 100 mcg over 2 or more weeks, followed by 30-50 mcg/month.

Administration
I.M.: Administer I.M. only. May require coadministration of folic acid.

Stability
Storage: Clear pink to red solutions are stable at room temperature; protect from light; incompatible with chlorpromazine, phytonadione, prochlorperazine, warfarin, ascorbic acid, dextrose, heavy metals, oxidizing or reducing agents; avoid freezing

Laboratory Monitoring Reticulocyte count, hematocrit, iron and folic acid, and serum levels before treatment, after first week of treatment, and routinely thereafter

Nursing Actions
Physical Assessment: Monitor laboratory tests at beginning of therapy and periodically with long-term therapy. Assess knowledge/teach patient appropriate administration (injection technique and needle disposal), appropriate nutrition counseling, and adverse symptoms to report.
Patient Education: Use exactly as directed. Pernicious anemia may require monthly injections for life. Report skin rash; swelling, pain, or redness in extremities; or acute persistent diarrhea. **Pregnancy precaution:** Inform prescriber if you are pregnant.
Geriatric Considerations Evidence exists that people, particularly elderly, whose serum cobalamin concentrations are <500 pg/mL, should receive replacement parenteral therapy. This recommendation is based upon neuropsychiatric disorders and cardiovascular disorders associated with lower sodium cobalamin concentrations.

Hydroxychloroquine
(hye droks ee KLOR oh kwin)

U.S. Brand Names Plaquenil®
Synonyms Hydroxychloroquine Sulfate
Pharmacologic Category Aminoquinoline (Antimalarial)
Medication Safety Issues
Sound-alike/look-alike issues:
Hydroxychloroquine may be confused with hydrocortisone
Plaquenil® may be confused with Platinol®
Pregnancy Risk Factor C
Lactation Enters breast milk/compatible
Use Suppression and treatment of acute attacks of malaria; treatment of systemic lupus erythematosus and rheumatoid arthritis
Unlabeled/Investigational Use Porphyria cutanea tarda, polymorphous light eruptions
Mechanism of Action/Effect Interferes with digestive vacuole function within sensitive malarial parasites by increasing the pH and interfering with lysosomal degradation of hemoglobin; inhibits locomotion of neutrophils and chemotaxis of eosinophils; impairs complement-dependent antigen-antibody reactions
Contraindications Hypersensitivity to hydroxychloroquine, 4-aminoquinoline derivatives, or any component

of the formulation; retinal or visual field changes attributable to 4-aminoquinolines
Warnings/Precautions Use with caution in patients with hepatic disease, G6PD deficiency, psoriasis, and porphyria. Long-term use in children is not recommended. Perform baseline and periodic (6 months) ophthalmologic examinations. Test periodically for muscle weakness.
Drug Interactions
Decreased Effect: Chloroquine and other 4-aminoquinolones absorption may be decreased due to GI binding with kaolin or magnesium trisilicate.
Increased Effect/Toxicity: Cimetidine increases levels of chloroquine and probably other 4-aminoquinolones.
Nutritional/Ethanol Interactions Ethanol: Avoid ethanol (due to GI irritation).
Adverse Reactions Frequency not defined.
Cardiovascular: Cardiomyopathy (rare, relationship to hydroxychloroquine unclear)
Central nervous system: Irritability, nervousness, emotional changes, nightmares, psychosis, headache, dizziness, vertigo, seizure, ataxia, lassitude
Dermatologic: Bleaching of hair, alopecia, pigmentation changes (skin and mucosal; black-blue color), rash (urticarial, morbilliform, lichenoid, maculopapular, purpuric, erythema annulare centrifugum, Stevens-Johnson syndrome, acute generalized exanthematous pustulosis, and exfoliative dermatitis)
Endocrine & metabolic: Weight loss
Gastrointestinal: Anorexia, nausea, vomiting, diarrhea, abdominal cramping
Hematologic: Aplastic anemia, agranulocytosis, leukopenia, thrombocytopenia, hemolysis (in patients with glucose-6-phosphate deficiency)
Hepatic: Abnormal liver function/hepatic failure (isolated cases)
Neuromuscular & skeletal: Myopathy, palsy, or neuromyopathy leading to progressive weakness and atrophy of proximal muscle groups (may be associated with mild sensory changes, loss of deep tendon reflexes, and abnormal nerve conduction)
Ocular: Disturbance in accommodation, keratopathy, corneal changes/deposits (visual disturbances, blurred vision, photophobia - reversible on discontinuation), macular edema, atrophy, abnormal pigmentation, retinopathy (early changes reversible - may progress despite discontinuation if advanced), optic disc pallor/atrophy, attenuation of retinal arterioles, pigmentary retinopathy, scotoma, decreased visual acuity, nystagmus
Otic: Tinnitus, deafness
Miscellaneous: Exacerbation of porphyria and nonlight sensitive psoriasis
Overdosage/Toxicology Symptoms of overdose include headache, drowsiness, visual changes, cardiovascular collapse, and seizures followed by respiratory and cardiac arrest. Treatment is symptomatic. Urinary alkalinization will enhance renal elimination.
Pharmacodynamics/Kinetics
Onset of Action: Rheumatic disease: May require 4-6 weeks to respond
Time to Peak: Rheumatic disease: Several months
Protein Binding: 55%
Half-Life Elimination: 32-50 days
Metabolism: Hepatic
Excretion: Urine (as metabolites and unchanged drug); may be enhanced by urinary acidification
Available Dosage Forms Tablet, as sulfate: 200 mg [equivalent to 155 mg base]
Dosing
Adults & Elderly:
Note: Hydroxychloroquine sulfate 200 mg is equivalent to 155 mg hydroxychloroquine base and 250 mg chloroquine phosphate.

Chemoprophylaxis of malaria: 310 mg base weekly on same day each week; begin 2 weeks before exposure. Continue for 4-6 weeks after leaving endemic area; if suppressive therapy is not begun prior to the exposure, double the initial dose and give in 2 doses, 6 hours apart.

Malaria, acute attack: 620 mg first dose day 1; 310 mg in 6 hours day 1; 310 mg in 1 dose day 2; and 310 mg in 1 dose on day 3

Rheumatoid arthritis: 310-465 mg/day to start taken with food or milk; increase dose until optimum response level is reached; usually after 4-12 weeks dose should be reduced by ½ and a maintenance dose of 155-310 mg/day given

Lupus erythematosus: 310 mg every day or twice daily for several weeks depending on response; 155-310 mg/day for prolonged maintenance therapy

Pediatrics:

Note: Hydroxychloroquine sulfate 200 mg is equivalent to 155 mg hydroxychloroquine base and 250 mg chloroquine phosphate.

Chemoprophylaxis of malaria: Oral: 5 mg/kg (base) once weekly; should not exceed the recommended adult dose. Begin 2 weeks before exposure and continue for 4-6 weeks after leaving endemic area. If suppressive therapy is not begun prior to the exposure, double the initial dose and give in 2 doses, 6 hours apart.

Malaria, acute attack: Oral: 10 mg/kg (base) initial dose; followed by 5 mg/kg at 6, 24, and 48 hours.

Juvenile rheumatoid arthritis (JRA) or SLE: Oral: 3-5 mg/kg/day divided 1-2 times/day; avoid exceeding 7 mg/kg/day.

Hepatic Impairment: Use with caution; dosage adjustment may be necessary.

Administration

Oral: Take with food or milk.

Laboratory Monitoring CBC, liver function

Nursing Actions

Physical Assessment: Assess potential for interactions with other pharmacological agents patient may be taking. Assess results of periodic CBC and liver function tests, therapeutic effectiveness (according to purpose for therapy), and adverse response (eg, deep tendon reflexes, muscle weakness). Teach patient appropriate use, possible side effects/interventions (necessity for periodic ophthalmic examinations with long-term therapy), and adverse symptoms to report.

Patient Education: Do not take any new medication during therapy unless approved by prescriber. It is important to complete full course of therapy, which may take up to 6 months for full effect. May be taken with meals to decrease GI upset and bitter aftertaste. Avoid alcohol. You should have regular ophthalmic exams (every 4-6 months) if using this medication over extended periods. You may experience skin discoloration (blue/black), hair bleaching, or skin rash. If you have psoriasis, you may experience exacerbation. You may experience dizziness, headache, nervousness, or lightheadedness (use caution when driving or engaging in tasks requiring alertness until response to drug is known); nausea, vomiting, or loss of appetite (small, frequent meals, frequent mouth care, sucking lozenges, or chewing gum may help); or increased sensitivity to sunlight (wear dark glasses and protective clothing, use sunblock, and avoid direct exposure to sunlight). Report weakness, numbness, tingling or tremors in muscles; vision changes; rash or itching; persistent diarrhea or GI disturbances; change in hearing acuity or ringing in the ears; chest pain or palpitation; CNS changes; unusual fatigue; easy bruising or bleeding; or any other persistent adverse reactions. **Pregnancy precaution:** Inform prescriber if you are or intend to become pregnant.

Dietary Considerations May be taken with food or milk.

Hydroxyurea (hye droks ee yoor EE a)

U.S. Brand Names Droxia®; Hydrea®; Mylocel™

Synonyms Hydroxycarbamide

Pharmacologic Category Antineoplastic Agent, Antimetabolite

Medication Safety Issues

Sound-alike/look-alike issues:

Hydroxyurea may be confused with hydrOXYzine

Pregnancy Risk Factor D

Lactation Enters breast milk/contraindicated

Use Treatment of melanoma, refractory chronic myelocytic leukemia (CML), relapsed and refractory metastatic ovarian cancer; radiosensitizing agent in the treatment of squamous cell head and neck cancer (excluding lip cancer); adjunct in the management of sickle cell patients who have had at least three painful crises in the previous 12 months (to reduce frequency of these crises and the need for blood transfusions)

Unlabeled/Investigational Use Treatment of HIV; treatment of psoriasis, treatment of hematologic conditions such as essential thrombocythemia, polycythemia vera, hypereosinophilia, and hyperleukocytosis due to acute leukemia; treatment of uterine, cervix and nonsmall cell lung cancers; radiosensitizing agent in the treatment of primary brain tumors; has shown activity against renal cell cancer and prostate cancer

Mechanism of Action/Effect Interferes with synthesis of DNA, without interfering with RNA synthesis

Contraindications Hypersensitivity to hydroxyurea or any component of the formulation; severe anemia; severe bone marrow suppression; WBC <2500/mm^3 or platelet count <100,000/mm^3; pregnancy

Warnings/Precautions Hazardous agent — use appropriate precautions for handling and disposal. Patients with a history of prior cytotoxic chemotherapy and radiation therapy are more likely to experience bone marrow depression. Patients with a history of radiation therapy are also at risk for exacerbation of post irradiation erythema. Megaloblastic erythropoiesis may be seen early in hydroxyurea treatment; plasma iron clearance may be delayed and the rate of utilization of iron by erythrocytes may be delayed. HIV-infected patients treated with hydroxyurea and didanosine (with or without stavudine) are at higher risk for pancreatitis, hepatotoxicity, hepatic failure, and severe peripheral neuropathy. Treatment of myeloproliferative disorders (polycythemia vera and thrombocythemia) with long-term hydroxyurea is associated with secondary leukemia; it is unknown if this is drug-related or disease-related. Cutaneous vasculitic toxicities (vasculitic ulceration and gangrene) have been reported with hydroxyurea treatment, most often in patients with a history of or receiving concurrent interferon therapy; discontinue hydroxyurea and consider alternate cytoreductive therapy if cutaneous vasculitic toxicity develops. Use caution with renal dysfunction; may require dose reductions. Safety and efficacy in children have not been established.

Drug Interactions

Increased Effect/Toxicity: Hydroxyurea may increase the toxicity of didanosine.

Adverse Reactions Frequency not defined.

Cardiovascular: Edema

Central nervous system: Chills, disorientation, dizziness, drowsiness (dose-related), fever, hallucinations, headache, malaise, seizure

Dermatologic: Alopecia (rare), cutaneous vasculitic toxicities, dermatomyositis-like skin changes, dry skin, facial erythema, gangrene, hyperpigmentation, maculopapular rash, nail atrophy, nail pigmentation, peripheral erythema, scaling, skin atrophy, skin cancer, vasculitis ulcerations, violet papules

Endocrine & metabolic: Hyperuricemia

(Continued)

Hydroxyurea (Continued)

Gastrointestinal: Anorexia, constipation, diarrhea, gastrointestinal irritation and mucositis, (potentiated with radiation therapy), nausea, pancreatitis, stomatitis, vomiting

Genitourinary: Dysuria (rare)

Hematologic: Myelosuppression (primarily leukopenia; onset: 24-48 hours; nadir: 10 days; recovery: 7 days after stopping drug; reversal of WBC count occurs rapidly but the platelet count may take 7-10 days to recover); thrombocytopenia and anemia, megaloblastic erythropoiesis, macrocytosis, hemolysis, serum iron decreased, persistent cytopenias, secondary leukemias (long-term use)

Hepatic: Hepatic enzymes increased, hepatotoxicity

Neuromuscular & skeletal: Weakness, peripheral neuropathy

Renal: BUN increased, creatinine increased

Respiratory: Acute diffuse pulmonary infiltrates (rare), dyspnea, pulmonary fibrosis (rare)

Overdosage/Toxicology Symptoms of overdose include myelosuppression, facial swelling, hallucinations, disorientation, soreness, violet erythema, edema on palms and soles, scaling on hands and feet, severe generalized hyperpigmentation of the skin, and stomatitis. Treatment is symptom-directed and supportive.

Pharmacodynamics/Kinetics
Time to Peak: 1-4 hours

Half-Life Elimination: 3-4 hours

Metabolism: 60% via hepatic and GI tract

Excretion: Urine (80%, 50% as unchanged drug, 30% as urea); exhaled gases (as CO_2)

Available Dosage Forms
Capsule: 500 mg

Droxia®: 200 mg, 300 mg, 400 mg

Hydrea®: 500 mg

Tablet (Mylocel™): 1000 mg

Dosing
Adults & Elderly: Refer to individual protocols.

Note: Dose should always be titrated to patient response and WBC counts; usual oral doses range from 10-30 mg/kg/day or 500-3000 mg/day; if WBC count falls to <2500 cells/mm^3, or the platelet count to <100,000/mm^3, therapy should be stopped for at least 3 days and resumed when values rise toward normal.

Solid tumors: Oral:

Intermittent therapy: 80 mg/kg as a single dose every third day

Continuous therapy: 20-30 mg/kg/day given as a single dose/day

Concomitant therapy with irradiation: 80 mg/kg as a single dose every third day starting at least 7 days before initiation of irradiation

Resistant chronic myelocytic leukemia: Oral: Continuous therapy: 20-30 mg/kg as a single daily dose

HIV (unlabeled use; in combination with antiretroviral agents): 1000-1500 mg daily in single or divided doses

Psoriasis: 1000-1500 mg daily in single or divided doses

Sickle cell anemia (moderate/severe disease): Initial: 15 mg/kg/day, increased by 5 mg/kg every 12 weeks if blood counts are in an acceptable range until the maximum tolerated dose of 35 mg/kg/day is achieved or the dose that does not produce toxic effects

Pediatrics: Refer to individual protocols. All dosage should be based on ideal or actual body weight, whichever is less: Children (unlabeled use):

Note: No FDA-approved dosage regimens have been established; dosages of 1500-3000 mg/m^2 as a single dose in combination with other agents every

4-6 weeks have been used in the treatment of pediatric astrocytoma, medulloblastoma, and primitive neuroectodermal tumors

CML: Oral: Initial: 10-20 mg/kg/day once daily; adjust dose according to hematologic response

Renal Impairment:
Sickle cell anemia: Cl$_{cr}$ <60 mL/minute or ESRD: Reduce initial dose to 7.5 mg/kg; titrate to response/ avoidance of toxicity (refer to usual dosing).

Other indications:

Cl$_{cr}$ 10-50 mL/minute: Administer 50% of normal dose.

Cl$_{cr}$ <10 mL/minute: Administer 20% of normal dose.

Hemodialysis: Administer dose after dialysis on dialysis days; supplemental dose is not necessary. Hydroxyurea is a low molecular weight compound with high aqueous solubility that may be freely dialyzable, however, clinical studies confirming this hypothesis have not been performed.

CAPD effects: Unknown

CAVH effects: Dose for GFR 10-50 mL/minute.

Dosing Adjustment for Toxicity:
Acceptable range:

Neutrophils ≥2500 cells/mm^3

Platelets ≥95,000/mm^3

Hemoglobin >5.3 g/dL, and

Reticulocytes ≥95,000/mm^3 if the hemoglobin concentration is <9 g/dL

Toxic range:

Neutrophils <2000 cells/mm^3

Platelets <80,000/mm^3

Hemoglobin <4.5 g/dL

Reticulocytes <80,000/mm^3 if the hemoglobin concentration is <9 g/dL

Monitor for toxicity every 2 weeks; if toxicity occurs, stop treatment until the bone marrow recovers; restart at 2.5 mg/kg/day less than the dose at which toxicity occurs; if no toxicity occurs over the next 12 weeks, then the subsequent dose should be increased by 2.5 mg/kg/day; reduced dosage of hydroxyurea alternating with erythropoietin may decrease myelotoxicity and increase levels of fetal hemoglobin in patients who have not been helped by hydroxyurea alone

Administration
Oral: Capsules may be opened and emptied into water (will not dissolve completely); observe proper handling procedures

Stability
Storage: Store at room temperature between 15°C and 30°C (59°F and 86°F).

Laboratory Monitoring CBC with differential and platelets, renal function and liver function tests, serum uric acid

Sickle cell disease: Monitor for toxicity every 2 weeks. If toxicity occurs, stop treatment until the bone marrow recovers; restart at 2.5 mg/kg/day less than the dose at which toxicity occurs. If no toxicity occurs over the next 12 weeks, then the subsequent dose should be increased by 2.5 mg/kg/day. Reduced dosage of hydroxyurea alternating with erythropoietin may decrease myelotoxicity and increase levels of fetal hemoglobin in patients who have not been helped by hydroxyurea alone.

Acceptable range: Neutrophils ≥2500 cells/mm^3, platelets ≥95,000/mm^3, hemoglobin >5.3 g/dL, and reticulocytes ≥95,000/mm^3 if the hemoglobin concentration is <9 g/dL

Toxic range: Neutrophils <2000 cells/mm^3, platelets <80,000/mm^3, hemoglobin <4.5 g/dL, and reticulocytes <80,000/mm^3 if the hemoglobin concentration is <9 g/dL

Nursing Actions
Physical Assessment: Assess potential for interactions with other pharmacological agents patient may

be taking (eg, potential for increased neurotoxicity or hepatotoxicity). Hydroxyurea therapy requires close monitoring of laboratory tests, therapeutic effectiveness, and adverse response (eg, CNS changes, gastrointestinal upset. hepatotoxicity, peripheral neuropathy). Teach proper use and need for frequent monitoring, possible side effects/appropriate interventions, and adverse symptoms to report.

Patient Education: Do not take any new medication during therapy unless approved by prescriber. Take capsules exactly as directed by prescriber (dosage and timing will be specific to purpose of therapy). Contents of capsule may be emptied into a glass of water and taken immediately. You will require frequent monitoring and blood tests while taking this medication to assess effectiveness and monitor adverse reactions. You will be susceptible to infection (avoid crowds and exposure to infection and do not have any vaccinations without consulting prescriber). May cause nausea, vomiting, or loss of appetite (small frequent meals, frequent mouth care, sucking lozenges, or chewing gum may help); constipation (increased exercise, fluid, fruit, or fiber may help); diarrhea (buttermilk, boiled milk, or yogurt may help); or mouth sores (frequent mouth care will help). Report persistent vomiting, diarrhea, constipation, stomach pain, or mouth sores; skin rash, redness, irritation, or sores; painful or difficult urination; anemia (unusual fatigue, lethargy), CNS changes (increased confusion, depression, hallucinations, or seizures); opportunistic infection (persistent fever or chills, white plaques in mouth, vaginal discharge, or unhealed sores); unusual lassitude, muscle tremors or weakness; easy bruising/bleeding; or blood in vomitus, stool, or urine. **Note:** People not taking hydroxyurea should not be exposed to it. If powder from capsule is spilled, wipe up with damp, disposable towel immediately, and discard the towel in a closed container, such as a plastic bag. Wash hands thoroughly. **Pregnancy/breast-feeding precautions:** Do not get pregnant while taking this medication. Consult prescriber for appropriate barrier contraceptive measures. Do not breast-feed.

Geriatric Considerations Elderly may be more sensitive to the effects of this drug. Advance dose slowly and adjust dose for renal function with careful monitoring.

Breast-Feeding Issues Due to the potential for serious adverse reactions, breast-feeding is not recommended.

Pregnancy Issues Animal studies have demonstrated teratogenicity and embryotoxicity. There are no adequate and well-controlled studies in pregnant women. Women of childbearing potential should be advised to avoid pregnancy.

Additional Information Although I.V. use is reported, no parenteral product is commercially available in the U.S.

If WBC decreases to <2500/mm^3 or platelet count to <100,000/mm^3, interrupt therapy until values rise significantly toward normal. Treat anemia with whole blood replacement; do not interrupt therapy. Adequate trial period to determine the antineoplastic effectiveness is 6 weeks. Almost all patients receiving hydroxyurea in clinical trials needed to have their medication stopped for a time to allow their low blood count to return to acceptable levels.

HydrOXYzine (hye DROKS i zeen)

U.S. Brand Names Atarax®; Vistaril®
Synonyms Hydroxyzine Hydrochloride; Hydroxyzine Pamoate
Pharmacologic Category Antiemetic; Antihistamine
Medication Safety Issues
Sound-alike/look-alike issues:
HydrOXYzine may be confused with hydrALAZINE, hydroxyurea
Atarax® may be confused with amoxicillin, Ativan®
Vistaril® may be confused with Restoril®, Versed, Zestril®
Pregnancy Risk Factor C
Lactation Enters breast milk/contraindicated
Use Treatment of anxiety; preoperative sedative; antipruritic
Unlabeled/Investigational Use Antiemetic; ethanol withdrawal symptoms
Mechanism of Action/Effect Competes with histamine for H$_1$-receptor sites on effector cells in the gastrointestinal tract, blood vessels, and respiratory tract. Possesses skeletal muscle relaxing, bronchodilator, antihistamine, antiemetic, and analgesic properties.
Contraindications Hypersensitivity to hydroxyzine or any component of the formulation; early pregnancy
Warnings/Precautions Causes sedation, caution must be used in performing tasks which require alertness (eg, operating machinery or driving). Sedative effects of CNS depressants or ethanol are potentiated. SubQ and intra-arterial administration are not recommended since thrombosis and digital gangrene can occur; should be used with caution in patients with narrow-angle glaucoma, prostatic hyperplasia, and bladder neck obstruction; should also be used with caution in patients with asthma or COPD. Not recommended for use as a sedative or anxiolytic in the elderly.
Drug Interactions
Cytochrome P450 Effect: Inhibits CYP2D6 (weak)
Increased Effect/Toxicity: CNS depressants, anticholinergics, used in combination with hydroxyzine may result in additive effects.
Nutritional/Ethanol Interactions
Ethanol: Avoid ethanol (may increase CNS depression).
Herb/Nutraceutical: Avoid valerian, St John's wort, kava kava, gotu kola (may increase CNS depression).
Adverse Reactions Frequency not defined.
Central nervous system: Drowsiness, headache, fatigue, nervousness, dizziness, hallucination
Dermatologic: Pruritus, rash, urticaria
Gastrointestinal: Xerostomia
Neuromuscular & skeletal: Tremor, paresthesia, seizure, involuntary movements
Ocular: Blurred vision
Respiratory: Thickening of bronchial secretions
Miscellaneous: Allergic reaction
Overdosage/Toxicology Symptoms of overdose include seizures, sedation, and hypotension. There is no specific treatment for antihistamine overdose. Clinical toxicity is due to blockade of cholinergic receptors. For anticholinergic overdose with severe life-threatening symptoms, physostigmine 1-2 mg I.V. slowly, may be given to reverse these effects.
Pharmacodynamics/Kinetics
Onset of Action: 15-30 minutes
Duration of Action: 4-6 hours
Time to Peak: ~2 hours
Half-Life Elimination: 3-7 hours
Metabolism: Exact fate unknown
Available Dosage Forms [DSC] = Discontinued product
Capsule, as pamoate (Vistaril®): 25 mg, 50 mg, 100 mg
Injection, solution, as hydrochloride: 25 mg/mL (1 mL); 50 mg/mL (1 mL, 2 mL, 10 mL)
(Continued)

HydrOXYzine (Continued)

Suspension, oral, as pamoate (Vistaril®): 25 mg/5 mL (120 mL, 480 mL) [lemon flavor]

Syrup, as hydrochloride: 10 mg/5 mL (120 mL, 480 mL)

Atarax®: 10 mg/5 mL (480 mL) [contains alcohol, sodium benzoate; mint flavor] [DSC]

Tablet, as hydrochloride: 10 mg, 25 mg, 50 mg

Atarax®: 10 mg, 25 mg, 50 mg, 100 mg [DSC]

Dosing

Adults:

Antiemetic: I.M.: 25-100 mg/dose every 4-6 hours as needed

Anxiety: Oral: 25-100 mg 4 times/day; maximum: 600 mg/day

Preoperative sedation:

Oral: 50-100 mg

I.M.: 25-100 mg

Management of pruritus: Oral: 25 mg 3-4 times/day

Elderly: Management of pruritus: 10 mg 3-4 times/day; increase to 25 mg 3-4 times/day if necessary.

Pediatrics:

Preoperative sedation:

Oral: 0.6 mg/kg/dose every 6 hours

I.M.: 0.5-1.1 mg/kg/dose every 4-6 hours as needed

Pruritus, anxiety: Manufacturer labeling:

<6 years: 50 mg daily in divided doses

≥6 years: 50-100 mg daily in divided doses

Hepatic Impairment: Change dosing interval to every 24 hours in patients with primary biliary cirrhosis.

Administration

I.M.: Do not administer SubQ or intra-arterially. Administer I.M. deep in large muscle.

I.V.: Irritant. Use caution when administering I.V. Not generally recommended. May be given as a short (30-60 minute) infusion.

I.V. Detail: Extravasation can result in sterile abscess and marked tissue induration.

pH: 3.5-6.0

Stability

Reconstitution: For I.V. infusion, dilute in 50-250 mL NS or D5W.

Compatibility:

Y-site administration: Incompatible with allopurinol, amifostine, amphotericin B cholesteryl sulfate complex, cefepime, doxorubicin liposome, fluconazole, fludarabine, paclitaxel, piperacillin/tazobactam, sargramostim

Compatibility in syringe: Incompatible with dimenhydrinate, haloperidol, ketorolac, pentobarbital, ranitidine

Compatibility when admixed: Incompatible with aminophylline, amobarbital, chloramphenicol, penicillin G potassium, penicillin G sodium, pentobarbital, phenobarbital

Storage: Protect from light. Store at 15°C to 30°C.

Nursing Actions

Physical Assessment: Assess other medications patient may be taking for effectiveness and possible interactions. **Systemic:** Monitor therapeutic response and adverse reactions; ensure patient safety (side rails up, call light within reach); have patient void prior to administration; and ensure adequate hydration and environmental temperature control. **Oral:** Monitor therapeutic response according to purpose for use and adverse reactions (eg, acute atropine toxicity). Assess knowledge/teach patient appropriate use, interventions to reduce side effects, and adverse symptoms to report.

Patient Education: Will cause drowsiness. While using this medication, do not use alcohol and other prescription or OTC medications (especially sedatives, tranquilizers, antihistamines, or pain medications) without consulting prescriber. Use caution when driving or engaging in activities requiring alertness until response to drug is known. **Pregnancy/**

breast-feeding precautions: Inform prescriber if you are or intend to become pregnant. Breast-feeding is contraindicated.

Geriatric Considerations Anticholinergic effects are not well tolerated in the elderly. Hydroxyzine may be useful as a short-term antipruritic, but it is not recommended for use as a sedative or anxiolytic in the elderly.

Pregnancy Issues Hydroxyzine-induced fetal abnormalities at high dosages in animal studies. Use in early pregnancy is contraindicated by the manufacturer.

Additional Information

Hydroxyzine hydrochloride: Atarax®, Vistaril® injection

Hydroxyzine pamoate: Vistaril® capsule and suspension

Related Information

Anxiolytic / Hypnotic Use in Long-Term Care Facilities on page 1418

Compatibility of Drugs on page 1370

Compatibility of Drugs in Syringe on page 1372

FDA Name Differentiation Project: The Use of Tall-Man Letters on page 12

Federal OBRA Regulations Recommended Maximum Doses on page 1421

Hyoscyamine (hye oh SYE a meen)

U.S. Brand Names Anaspaz®; Cystospaz®; Cystospaz-M® [DSC]; Hyosine; Levbid®; Levsin®; Levsinex®; Levsin/SL®; NuLev™; Spacol [DSC]; Spacol T/S [DSC]; Symax SL; Symax SR

Synonyms Hyoscyamine Sulfate; l-Hyoscyamine Sulfate

Pharmacologic Category Anticholinergic Agent

Medication Safety Issues

Sound-alike/look-alike issues:

Anaspaz® may be confused with Anaprox®, Antispas®

Levbid® may be confused with Lithobid®, Lopid®, Lorabid®

Levsinex® may be confused with Lanoxin®

Pregnancy Risk Factor C

Lactation Enters breast milk/not recommended

Use

Oral: Adjunctive therapy for peptic ulcers, irritable bowel, neurogenic bladder/bowel; treatment of infant colic, GI tract disorders caused by spasm; to reduce rigidity, tremors, sialorrhea, and hyperhidrosis associated with parkinsonism; as a drying agent in acute rhinitis

Injection: Preoperative antimuscarinic to reduce secretions and block cardiac vagal inhibitory reflexes; to improve radiologic visibility of the kidneys; symptomatic relief of biliary and renal colic; reduce GI motility to facilitate diagnostic procedures (ie, endoscopy, hypotonic duodenography); reduce pain and hypersecretion in pancreatitis, certain cases of partial heart block associated with vagal activity; reversal of neuromuscular blockade

Mechanism of Action/Effect Blocks the action of acetylcholine at parasympathetic sites in smooth muscle, secretory glands, and the CNS; increases cardiac output, dries secretions, antagonizes histamine and serotonin

Contraindications Hypersensitivity to belladonna alkaloids or any component of the formulation; glaucoma; obstructive uropathy; myasthenia gravis; obstructive GI tract disease, paralytic ileus, intestinal atony of elderly or debilitated patients, severe ulcerative colitis, toxic megacolon complicating ulcerative colitis; unstable cardiovascular status in acute hemorrhage, myocardial ischemia

Warnings/Precautions Heat prostration may occur in hot weather. Diarrhea may be a sign of incomplete intestinal obstruction, treatment should be discontinued if this occurs. May produce side effects as seen with other anticholinergic medications including drowsiness, dizziness, blurred vision, or psychosis. Children and the elderly may be more susceptible to these effects. Use with caution in children with spastic paralysis. Use with caution in patients with autonomic neuropathy, coronary heart disease, CHF, cardiac arrhythmias, prostatic hyperplasia, hyperthyroidism, hypertension, chronic lung disease, renal disease, and hiatal hernia associated with reflux esophagitis. Use with caution in the elderly, may precipitate undiagnosed glaucoma and/or severely impair memory function (especially in those patients with previous memory problems). NuLev™ contains phenylalanine.

Drug Interactions
Decreased Effect: Decreased effect with antacids.

Increased Effect/Toxicity: Increased toxicity with amantadine, antihistamines, antimuscarinics, haloperidol, phenothiazines, tricyclic antidepressants, and MAO inhibitors.

Adverse Reactions Frequency not defined.
Cardiovascular: Palpitations, tachycardia

Central nervous system: Ataxia, dizziness, drowsiness, headache, insomnia, mental confusion/excitement, nervousness, speech disorder

Dermatologic: Urticaria

Endocrine & metabolic: Lactation suppression

Gastrointestinal: Bloating, constipation, dry mouth, loss of taste, nausea, vomiting

Genitourinary: Impotence, urinary hesitancy, urinary retention

Neuromuscular & skeletal: Weakness

Ocular: Blurred vision, cycloplegia, increased ocular tension, mydriasis

Miscellaneous: Allergic reactions, sweating decreased

Overdosage/Toxicology
Symptoms of overdose include dilated, unreactive pupils; blurred vision; hot, dry flushed skin; CNS stimulation; dryness of mucous membranes; difficulty swallowing; foul breath; diminished or absent bowel sounds; urinary retention; tachycardia; hyperthermia; hypertension; and increased respiratory rate. For anticholinergic overdose with severe life-threatening symptoms, physostigmine 0.5-2 mg SubQ or I.V. slowly, may be given to reverse these effects; may repeat as necessary to reverse the effects, up to total of 5 mg. Hyoscyamine sulfate is dialyzable.

Pharmacodynamics/Kinetics
Onset of Action: 2-3 minutes

Duration of Action: 4-6 hours

Protein Binding: 50%

Half-Life Elimination: 3-5 hours

Metabolism: Hepatic

Excretion: Urine

Available Dosage Forms [DSC] = Discontinued product
Capsule, timed release, as sulfate (Cystospaz-M® [DSC], Levsinex®): 0.375 mg

Elixir, as sulfate: 0.125 mg/5 mL (480 mL)
Hyosine: 0.125 mg/5 mL (480 mL) [contains alcohol 20% and sodium benzoate; orange flavor]
Levsin®: 0.125 mg/5 mL (480 mL) [contains alcohol 20%; orange flavor]

Injection, solution, as sulfate (Levsin®): 0.5 mg/mL (1 mL)

Liquid, as sulfate (Spacol [DSC]): 0.125 mg/5 mL (120 mL) [sugar free, alcohol free, simethicone based, bubble gum flavor]

Solution, oral drops, as sulfate: 0.125 mg/mL (15 mL)
Hyosine: 0.125 mg/mL (15 mL) [contains alcohol 5% and sodium benzoate; orange flavor]
Levsin®: 0.125 mg/mL (15 mL) [contains alcohol 5%; orange flavor]

Tablet (Cystospaz®): 0.15 mg

Tablet, as sulfate (Anaspaz®, Levsin®, Spacol [DSC]): 0.125 mg

Tablet, extended release, as sulfate (Levbid®, Symax SR, Spacol T/S [DSC]): 0.375 mg

Tablet, orally disintegrating, as sulfate (NuLev™): 0.125 mg [contains phenylalanine 1.7 mg/tablet, mint flavor]

Tablet, sublingual, as sulfate: 0.125 mg
Levsin/SL®: 0.125 mg [peppermint flavor]
Symax SL: 0.125 mg

Dosing
Adults & Elderly:
Gastrointestinal spasms:
Oral or S.L.: 0.125-0.25 mg every 4 hours or as needed (before meals or food); maximum: 1.5 mg/24 hours
Product-specific dosing: Cystospaz®: 0.15-0.3 mg up to 4 times/day
Oral, timed release: 0.375-0.75 mg every 12 hours; maximum: 1.5 mg/24 hours
I.M., I.V., SubQ: 0.25-0.5 mg; may repeat as needed up to 4 times/day, at 4-hour intervals

Diagnostic procedures: I.V.: 0.25-0.5 mg given 5-10 minutes prior to procedure

Preanesthesia: I.V.: 5 mcg/kg given 30-60 minutes prior to induction of anesthesia or at the time preoperative narcotics or sedatives are administered

To reduce drug-induced bradycardia during surgery: I.V.: 0.125 mg; repeat as needed

Reverse neuromuscular blockade: I.V.: 0.2 mg for every 1 mg neostigmine (or the physostigmine/pyridostigmine equivalent)

Pediatrics:
Gastrointestinal disorders:
Children <2 years: Oral: Dose as listed, based on age and weight (kg) using the 0.125 mg/mL drops. Repeat dose every 4 hours as needed:
3.4 kg: 4 drops; maximum: 24 drops/24 hours
5 kg: 5 drops; maximum: 30 drops/24 hours
7 kg: 6 drops; maximum: 36 drops/24 hours
10 kg: 8 drops; maximum: 48 drops/24 hours
Children 2-12 years: Oral or S.L.: Dose as listed, based on age and weight (kg); repeat dose every 4 hours as needed:
10 kg: 0.031-0.033 mg; maximum: 0.75 mg/24 hours
20 kg: 0.0625 mg; maximum: 0.75 mg/24 hours
40 kg: 0.0938 mg; maximum: 0.75 mg/24 hours
50 kg: 0.125 mg; maximum: 0.75 mg/24 hours

Preanesthesia: Children >2 years: I.V.: Refer to adult dosing.

Administration
Oral: Oral: Tablets should be administered before meals or food.
Levbid®: Tablets are scored and may be broken in half for dose titration; do not crush or chew.
Levsin/SL®: Tablets may be used sublingually, chewed, or swallowed whole.
NuLev™: Tablet is placed on tongue and allowed to disintegrate before swallowing; may take with or without water.
Symax SL: Tablets may be used sublingually or swallowed whole.

I.M.: May be administered without dilution.

I.V.: Inject over at least 1 minute. May be administered without dilution.

I.V. Detail: May be administered undiluted.

Stability
Storage: Store at controlled room temperature. Protect NuLev™ from moisture.

Nursing Actions
Physical Assessment: Assess potential for interactions with other prescriptions, OTC medications, or herbal products patient may be taking (eg, anything that may add to anticholinergic effects). **I.V./I.M.:** Have patient void before administration. Monitor therapeutic effectiveness and adverse response (eg, excessive dryness of eyes, nose, mouth, or throat). Teach patient proper use (according to formulation prescribed), possible side effects/appropriate interventions, and adverse symptoms to report.

Patient Education: Do not take any new medication during therapy unless approved by prescriber. Take (Continued)

Hyoscyamine *(Continued)*

as directed before meals; do not increase dose and do not discontinue without consulting prescriber. Void immediately before taking medication. Do not crush or chew (swallow whole) extended release form. Levbid® and Levsinex® may not completely disintegrate and may be excreted. You may experience dizziness or blurred vision (use caution when driving or engaging in tasks that require alertness until response to drug is known); dry mouth (sucking on lozenges may help); photosensitivity (wear dark glasses in bright sunlight); decreased ability to sweat (use caution in hot weather or hot rooms or when engaging in strenuous activity); or impotence (temporary). Report excessive and persistent anticholinergic effects (blurred vision, headache, flushing, tachycardia, nervousness, constipation, dizziness, insomnia, mental confusion or excitement, dry mouth, altered taste perception, dysphagia, palpitations, bradycardia, urinary hesitancy or retention, impotence, decreased sweating). **Pregnancy/breast-feeding precautions:** Inform prescriber if you are or intend to become pregnant. Breast-feeding is not recommended.

Sublingual tablets: Place tablet under tongue and allow to dissolve.

Orally-disintegrating tablet: Place tablet on tongue and allow to disintegrate before swallowing. Take with or without food.

Dietary Considerations Should be taken before meals or food; NuLev™ contains phenylalanine

Geriatric Considerations Avoid long-term use. The potential for toxic reactions is higher than the potential benefit, elderly are particularly prone to CNS side effects of anticholinergics (eg, confusion, delirium, hallucinations). Side effects often occur before clinical response is obtained. Generally not recommended because of the side effects.

Breast-Feeding Issues Excreted in breast milk in trace amounts. May also suppress lactation. Breast-feeding is not recommended.

Hyoscyamine, Atropine, Scopolamine, and Phenobarbital

(hye oh SYE a meen, A troe peen, skoe POL a meen, & fee noe BAR bi tal)

U.S. Brand Names Donnatal®; Donnatal Extentabs®

Synonyms Atropine, Hyoscyamine, Scopolamine, and Phenobarbital; Belladonna Alkaloids With Phenobarbital; Phenobarbital, Hyoscyamine, Atropine, and Scopolamine; Scopolamine, Hyoscyamine, Atropine, and Phenobarbital

Pharmacologic Category Anticholinergic Agent; Antispasmodic Agent, Gastrointestinal

Pregnancy Risk Factor C

Lactation Excretion in breast milk unknown/use caution

Use Adjunct in treatment of irritable bowel syndrome, acute enterocolitis, duodenal ulcer

Available Dosage Forms

Elixir (Donnatal®): Hyoscyamine sulfate 0.1037 mg, atropine sulfate 0.0194 mg, scopolamine hydrobromide 0.0065 mg, and phenobarbital 16.2 mg per 5 mL (120 mL, 480 mL) [contains alcohol 95%; grape flavor]

Tablet (Donnatal®): Hyoscyamine sulfate 0.1037 mg, atropine sulfate 0.0194 mg, scopolamine hydrobromide 0.0065 mg, and phenobarbital 16.2 mg

Tablet, extended release (Donnatal Extentabs®): Hyoscyamine sulfate 0.3111 mg, atropine sulfate 0.0582 mg, scopolamine hydrobromide 0.0195 mg, and phenobarbital 48.6 mg

---

Dosing

Adults & Elderly: Spasmolytic: Oral:

Donnatal®: 1-2 tablets or 5-10 mL of elixir 3-4 times/day

Donnatal Extentabs®: 1 tablet every 12 hours; may increase to 1 tablet every 8 hours if needed

Pediatrics: Oral: Donnatal® elixir: To be given every 4-6 hours; initial dose based on weight:

4.5 kg: 0.5 mL every 4 hours **or** 0.75 mL every 6 hours

10 kg: 1 mL every 4 hours **or** 1.5 mL every 6 hours

14 kg: 1.5 mL every 4 hours **or** 2 mL every 6 hours

23 kg: 2.5 mL every 4 hours **or** 3.8 mL every 6 hours

34 kg: 3.8 mL every 4 hours **or** 5 mL every 6 hours

≥45 kg: 5 mL every 4 hours **or** 7.5 mL every 6 hours

Nursing Actions

Physical Assessment: See individual agents.

Patient Education: See individual agents. **Pregnancy/breast-feeding precautions:** Inform prescriber if you are or intend to become pregnant. Consult prescriber if breast-feeding.

Related Information

Atropine *on page 126*
Hyoscyamine *on page 628*
Phenobarbital *on page 977*
Scopolamine Derivatives *on page 1112*

Ibuprofen *(eye byoo PROE fen)*

U.S. Brand Names Advil® [OTC]; Advil® Children's [OTC]; Advil® Infants' [OTC]; Advil® Junior [OTC]; Advil® Migraine [OTC]; ElixSure™ IB [OTC]; Genpril® [OTC]; Ibu-200 [OTC]; I-Prin [OTC]; Midol® Cramp and Body Aches [OTC]; Motrin®; Motrin® Children's [OTC]; Motrin® IB [OTC]; Motrin® Infants' [OTC]; Motrin® Junior Strength [OTC]; Proprinal [OTC]; Ultraprin [OTC]

Synonyms *p*-Isobutylhydratropic Acid

Restrictions A medication guide should be dispensed with each prescription. A template for the required MedGuide can be found on the FDA website at: http://www.fda.gov/medwatch/SAFETY/2005/safety05.htm#NSAID

Pharmacologic Category Nonsteroidal Anti-inflammatory Drug (NSAID), Oral

Medication Safety Issues

Sound-alike/look-alike issues:

Haltran® may be confused with Halfprin®

Pregnancy Risk Factor C/D (3rd trimester)

Lactation Enters breast milk/use caution (AAP rates "compatible")

Use Inflammatory diseases and rheumatoid disorders including juvenile rheumatoid arthritis, mild to moderate pain, fever, dysmenorrhea

Unlabeled/Investigational Use Cystic fibrosis, gout, ankylosing spondylitis, acute migraine headache

Mechanism of Action/Effect Inhibits prostaglandin synthesis by decreasing the activity of the enzyme, cyclooxygenase, which results in decreased formation of prostaglandin precursors

Contraindications Hypersensitivity to ibuprofen, aspirin, other NSAIDs, or any component of the formulation; perioperative pain in the setting of coronary artery bypass surgery (CABG); pregnancy (3rd trimester)

Warnings/Precautions NSAIDs are associated with an increased risk of adverse cardiovascular events, including MI, stroke, and new onset or worsening of pre-existing hypertension. Risk may be increased with duration of use or pre-existing cardiovascular risk-factors or disease. Carefully evaluate individual cardiovascular risk profiles prior to prescribing. Use caution with fluid retention, CHF or hypertension.

Use of NSAIDs can compromise existing renal function. Renal toxicity can occur in patient with impaired renal function, dehydration, heart failure, liver dysfunction, those taking diuretics and ACEI and the elderly. Rehydrate patient before starting therapy. Monitor renal function closely. Ibuprofen is not recommended for patients with advanced renal disease.

NSAIDs may increase risk of gastrointestinal irritation, ulceration, bleeding, and perforation. These events may occur at any time during therapy and without warning. Use caution with a history of GI disease (bleeding or ulcers), concurrent therapy with aspirin, anticoagulants and/or corticosteroids, smoking, use of alcohol, the elderly or debilitated patients.

Use the lowest effective dose for the shortest duration of time, consistent with individual patient goals, to reduce risk of cardiovascular or GI adverse events. Alternate therapies should be considered for patients at high risk.

NSAIDs may cause serious skin adverse events including exfoliative dermatitis, Stevens-Johnson syndrome (SJS) and toxic epidermal necrolysis (TEN). Anaphylactoid reactions may occur, even without prior exposure; patients with "aspirin triad" (bronchial asthma, aspirin intolerance, rhinitis) may be at increased risk. Do not use in patients who experience bronchospasm, asthma, rhinitis, or urticaria with NSAID or aspirin therapy.

Use with caution in patients with decreased hepatic function. Closely monitor patients with any abnormal LFT. Severe hepatic reactions (eg, fulminant hepatitis, liver failure) have occurred with NSAID use, rarely; discontinue if signs or symptoms of liver disease develop, or if systemic manifestations occur.

The elderly are at increased risk for adverse effects (especially peptic ulceration, CNS effects, renal toxicity) from NSAIDs even at low doses.

Withhold for at least 4-6 half-lives prior to surgical or dental procedures.

OTC labeling: Prior to self-medication, patients should contact health care provider if they have had recurring stomach pain or upset, ulcers, bleeding problems, high blood pressure, heart or kidney disease, other serious medical problems, are currently taking a diuretic, or are ≥60 years of age. Recommended dosages should not be exceeded, due to an increased risk of GI bleeding. Consuming ≥3 alcoholic beverages/day or taking longer than recommended may increase the risk of GI bleeding. When used for self-medication, patients should contact healthcare provider if used for fever lasting >3 days or for pain lasting >10 days in adults or >3 days in children. In children with a sore throat, do not use for >2 days or administer to children <3 years of age unless instructed by healthcare provider. Consult healthcare provider when sore throat pain is severe, persistent, or accompanied by fever, headache, nausea, and/or vomiting.

Drug Interactions

Cytochrome P450 Effect: Substrate (minor) of CYP2C8/9, 2C19; **Inhibits** CYP2C8/9 (strong)

Decreased Effect: Aspirin may decrease ibuprofen serum concentrations. Ibuprofen may decrease the effect of some antihypertensive agents (including ACE inhibitors and angiotensin antagonists) and diuretics. Ibuprofen and other COX-1 inhibitors, may reduce the cardioprotective effects of aspirin.

Increased Effect/Toxicity: Ibuprofen may increase cyclosporine, digoxin, lithium, and methotrexate serum concentrations. The renal adverse effects of ACE inhibitors may be potentiated by NSAIDs. Corticosteroids may increase the risk of GI ulceration. Ibuprofen may increase the levels/effects of amiodarone, fluoxetine, glimepiride, glipizide, nateglinide, phenytoin, pioglitazone, rosiglitazone, sertraline, warfarin, and other CYP2C8/9 substrates.

Nutritional/Ethanol Interactions

Ethanol: Avoid ethanol (may enhance gastric mucosal irritation).

Food: Ibuprofen peak serum levels may be decreased if taken with food.

Herb/Nutraceutical: Avoid alfalfa, anise, bilberry, bladderwrack, bromelain, cat's claw, celery, coleus, cordyceps, dong quai, evening primrose, feverfew, fenugreek, garlic, ginger, ginkgo biloba, red clover, horse chestnut, grapeseed, green tea, ginseng, guggul, horse chestnut seed, horseradish, licorice, prickly ash, red clover, reishi, SAMe, sweet clover, turmeric, white willow (all have additional antiplatelet activity).

Lab Interactions Increased chloride (S), sodium (S), bleeding time

Adverse Reactions

1% to 10%:

Cardiovascular: Edema (1% to 3%)

Central nervous system: Dizziness (3% to 9%), headache (1% to 3%), nervousness (1% to 3%)

Dermatologic: Itching (1% to 3%), rash (3% to 9%)

Endocrine & metabolic: Fluid retention (1% to 3%)

Gastrointestinal: Dyspepsia (1% to 3%), vomiting (1% to 3%), abdominal pain/cramps/distress (1% to 3%), heartburn (3% to 9%), nausea (3% to 9%), diarrhea (1% to 3%), constipation (1% to 3%), flatulence (1% to 3%), epigastric pain (3% to 9%), appetite decreased (1% to 3%)

Otic: Tinnitus (3% to 9%)

Overdosage/Toxicology Symptoms of overdose include apnea, metabolic acidosis, coma, nystagmus, seizures, leukocytosis, and renal failure. Management of NSAID intoxication is supportive and symptomatic. Since many NSAIDs undergo enterohepatic cycling, multiple doses of charcoal may be needed to reduce the potential for delayed toxicities.

Pharmacodynamics/Kinetics

Onset of Action: Analgesic: 30-60 minutes; Anti-inflammatory: ≤7 days; Peak effect: 1-2 weeks

Duration of Action: 4-6 hours

Time to Peak: ~1-2 hours

Protein Binding: 90% to 99%

Half-Life Elimination: 2-4 hours; End-stage renal disease: Unchanged

Metabolism: Hepatic via oxidation

Excretion: Urine (1% as free drug); some feces

Available Dosage Forms [DSC] = Discontinued product

Caplet: 200 mg [OTC]

Advil®: 200 mg [contains sodium benzoate]

Ibu-200, Motrin® IB: 200 mg

Motrin® Junior Strength: 100 mg

Capsule, liqui-gel:

Advil®: 200 mg

Advil® Migraine: 200 mg [solubilized ibuprofen; contains potassium 20 mg]

Gelcap:

Advil®: 200 mg [contains coconut oil]

Motrin® IB: 200 mg [contains benzyl alcohol] [DSC]

Suspension, oral: 100 mg/5 mL (5 mL, 120 mL, 480 mL)

Advil® Children's: 100 mg/5 mL (60 mL, 120 mL) [contains sodium benzoate; blue raspberry, fruit, and grape flavors]

ElixSure™ IB: 100 mg/5 mL (120 mL) [berry flavor]

Motrin® Children's: 100 mg/5 mL (60 mL, 120 mL) [contains sodium benzoate; berry, dye free berry, bubble gum, and grape flavors]

Suspension, oral drops: 40 mg/mL (15 mL)

Advil® Infants': 40 mg/mL (15 mL) [contains sodium benzoate; fruit and grape flavors]

Motrin® Infants': 40 mg/mL (15 mL, 30 mL) [contains sodium benzoate; berry and dye-free berry flavors]

Tablet: 200 mg [OTC], 400 mg, 600 mg, 800 mg

Advil®: 200 mg [contains sodium benzoate]

(Continued)

Ibuprofen (Continued)

Advil® Junior: 100 mg [contains sodium benzoate; coated tablets]

Genpril®, I-Prin, Midol® Cramp and Body Aches, Motrin® IB, Proprinal, Ultraprin: 200 mg

Motrin®: 400 mg, 600 mg, 800 mg

Tablet, chewable:

Advil® Children's: 50 mg [contains phenylalanine 2.1 mg; grape flavors]

Advil® Junior: 100 mg [contains phenylalanine 4.2 mg; grape flavors]

Motrin® Children's: 50 mg [contains phenylalanine 1.4 mg; grape and orange flavor]

Motrin® Junior Strength: 100 mg [contains phenylalanine 2.1 mg; grape and orange flavors]

Dosing

Adults & Elderly:

Inflammatory disease: Oral: 400-800 mg/dose 3-4 times/day (maximum: 3.2 g/day)

Analgesia/pain/fever/dysmenorrhea: Oral: 200-400 mg/dose every 4-6 hours (maximum daily dose: 1.2 g, unless directed by physician)

OTC labeling (analgesic, antipyretic): Oral: 200 mg every 4-6 hours as needed (maximum: 1200 mg/24 hours)

Pediatrics:

Antipyretic: Oral: 6 months to 12 years: Temperature <102.5°F (39°C): 5 mg/kg/dose; temperature >102.5°F: 10 mg/kg/dose given every 6-8 hours; maximum daily dose: 40 mg/kg/day

Juvenile rheumatoid arthritis: Oral: 30-50 mg/kg/24 hours divided every 8 hours; start at lower end of dosing range and titrate upward (maximum: 2.4 g/day)

Analgesic: Oral: 4-10 mg/kg/dose every 6-8 hours

Cystic fibrosis (unlabeled use): Oral: Chronic (>4 years) twice daily dosing adjusted to maintain serum levels of 50-100 mcg/mL has been associated with slowing of disease progression in younger patients with mild lung disease

OTC labeling (analgesic, antipyretic): Oral:

Children 6 months to 11 years: See table; use of weight to select dose is preferred; doses may be repeated every 6-8 hours (maximum: 4 doses/day)

Children ≥12 years: Refer to adult dosing.

Ibuprofen Dosing

Weight (lb)	Age	Dosage (mg)
12-17	6-11 mo	50
18-23	12-23 mo	75
24-35	2-3 y	100
35-47	4-5 y	150
48-59	6-8 y	200
60-71	9-10 y	250
72-95	11 y	300

Hepatic Impairment: Avoid use in severe hepatic impairment.

Administration

Oral: Administer with food.

Laboratory Monitoring CBC, periodic liver function, renal function (serum BUN and creatinine)

Nursing Actions

Physical Assessment: Assess patient for allergic reaction to salicylates or other NSAIDs. Assess other medications patient may be taking for additive or adverse interactions. Monitor blood pressure at the beginning of therapy and periodically during use. Monitor therapeutic effectiveness and signs of adverse reactions or overdose (especially adverse gastrointestinal response) at beginning of therapy and periodically during long-term therapy. With long-term therapy, periodic ophthalmic exams are recommended. Assess knowledge/teach patient appropriate use. Teach patient to monitor for adverse reactions, adverse reactions to report, and appropriate interventions to reduce side effects.

Patient Education: If self-administered, use exactly as directed; do not increase dose or frequency. Adverse reactions can occur with overuse. Consult your prescriber before use if you have hypertension or heart failure. Do not take longer than 3 days for fever, or 10 days for pain without consulting medical advisor. Take with food or milk. While using this medication, do not use alcohol, excessive amounts of vitamin C, or salicylate-containing foods (curry powder, prunes, raisins, tea, or licorice), other prescription or OTC medications containing aspirin or salicylate, or other NSAIDs without consulting prescriber. Maintain adequate hydration (2-3 L/day of fluids) unless instructed to restrict fluid intake. You may experience nausea, vomiting, gastric discomfort (frequent mouth care, small frequent meals, chewing gum, sucking lozenges may help). GI bleeding, ulceration, or perforation can occur with or without pain. Stop taking medication and report ringing in ears; persistent cramping or stomach pain; unresolved nausea or vomiting; respiratory difficulty or shortness of breath; unusual bruising or bleeding (mouth, urine, stool); skin rash; unusual swelling of extremities; chest pain; or palpitations. **Pregnancy/breast-feeding precautions:** Inform prescriber if you are or intend to become pregnant. This drug should not be used in the 3rd trimester of pregnancy. Consult prescriber if breast-feeding.

Dietary Considerations Should be taken with food. Chewable tablets may contain phenylalanine; amount varies by product, consult manufacturers labeling.

Geriatric Considerations Elderly are at a high risk for adverse effects from NSAIDs. As much as 60% of elderly can develop peptic ulceration and/or hemorrhage asymptomatically. The concomitant use of H_2 blockers, omeprazole, and sucralfate is not effective as prophylaxis with the exception of NSAID-induced duodenal ulcers which may be prevented by the use of ranitidine. Misoprostol is the only prophylactic agent proven effective. Also, concomitant disease and drug use contribute to the risk for GI adverse effects. Use lowest effective dose for shortest period possible. Consider renal function decline with age. Use of NSAIDs can compromise existing renal function especially when Cl_{cr} is ≤30 mL/minute. Tinnitus may be a difficult and unreliable indication of toxicity due to age-related hearing loss or eighth cranial nerve damage. CNS adverse effects such as confusion, agitation, and hallucination are generally seen in overdose or high-dose situations, but elderly may demonstrate these adverse effects at lower doses than younger adults.

Breast-Feeding Issues Limited data suggests minimal excretion in breast milk.

Ibutilide (i BYOO ti lide)

U.S. Brand Names Corvert®

Synonyms Ibutilide Fumarate

Pharmacologic Category Antiarrhythmic Agent, Class III

Pregnancy Risk Factor C

Lactation Enters breast milk/contraindicated

Use Acute termination of atrial fibrillation or flutter of recent onset; the effectiveness of ibutilide has not been determined in patients with arrhythmias >90 days in duration

Mechanism of Action/Effect Exact mechanism of action is unknown; prolongs the action potential in cardiac tissue

Contraindications Hypersensitivity to ibutilide or any component of the formulation; QT_c >440 msec

Warnings/Precautions Potentially fatal arrhythmias (eg, polymorphic ventricular tachycardia) can occur with ibutilide, **usually** in association with torsade de pointes (QT prolongation). The drug should be given in a setting of continuous ECG monitoring and by personnel trained in treating arrhythmias particularly polymorphic ventricular tachycardia. Patients with chronic atrial fibrillation often revert after conversion; the risks of treatment may not be justified when compared to alternative management. Safety and efficacy in children have not been established. Use caution in elderly patients. Avoid concurrent use of any drug that can prolong QT interval. Correct hyperkalemia and hypomagnesemia before using. Monitor for heart block.

Drug Interactions

Increased Effect/Toxicity: Class Ia antiarrhythmic drugs (disopyramide, quinidine, and procainamide) and other class III drugs such as amiodarone and sotalol should not be given concomitantly with ibutilide due to their potential to prolong refractoriness. Signs of digoxin toxicity may be masked when coadministered with ibutilide. Toxicity of ibutilide is potentiated by concurrent administration of other drugs which may prolong QT interval: phenothiazines, tricyclic and tetracyclic antidepressants, cisapride, sparfloxacin, gatifloxacin, moxifloxacin, and erythromycin.

Adverse Reactions 1% to 10%:

Cardiovascular: Sustained polymorphic ventricular tachycardia (ie, torsade de pointes) (1.7%, often requiring cardioversion), nonsustained polymorphic ventricular tachycardia (2.7%), nonsustained monomorphic ventricular tachycardia (4.9%), ventricular extrasystoles (5.1%), nonsustained monomorphic VT (4.9%), tachycardia/supraventricular tachycardia (2.7%), hypotension (2%), bundle branch block (1.9%), AV block (1.5%), bradycardia (1.2%), QT segment prolongation, hypertension (1.2%), palpitation (1%)

Central nervous system: Headache (3.6%)

Gastrointestinal: Nausea (>1%)

Overdosage/Toxicology Symptoms of overdose include CNS depression, rapid gasping breathing, and convulsions. Arrhythmias occur. Treatment is supportive. Antiarrhythmics are generally avoided.

Pharmacodynamics/Kinetics

Onset of Action: ~90 minutes after start of infusion (½ of conversions to sinus rhythm occur during infusion)

Protein Binding: 40%

Half-Life Elimination: 2-12 hours (average: 6 hours)

Metabolism: Extensively hepatic; oxidation

Excretion: Urine (82%, 7% as unchanged drug and metabolites); feces (19%)

Available Dosage Forms Injection, solution, as fumarate: 0.1 mg/mL (10 mL)

Dosing

Adults:

Atrial fibrillation/flutter: I.V.:

<60 kg: 0.01 mg/kg over 10 minutes

≥60 kg: 1 mg over 10 minutes

If the arrhythmia does not terminate within 10 minutes after the end of the initial infusion, a second infusion of equal strength may be infused over a 10-minute period.

Elderly: Refer to adult dosing. Dose selection should be cautious, usually starting at the lower end of the dosing range.

Administration

I.V.: May be administered undiluted or diluted in 50 mL diluent (0.9% NS or D_5W). Infuse over 10 minutes.

I.V. Detail: Observe patient with continuous ECG monitoring for at least 4 hours following infusion or until QT_c has returned to baseline. Skilled personnel and proper equipment should be available during administration of ibutilide and subsequent monitoring of the patient.

Stability

Reconstitution: May be administered undiluted or diluted in 50 mL diluent (0.9% NS or D_5W). Admixtures are chemically and physically stable for 24 hours at room temperature and for 48 hours at refrigerated temperatures.

Laboratory Monitoring Electrolytes

Nursing Actions

Physical Assessment: Assess other medications patient may be taking for effectiveness and interactions. Requires infusion pump and continuous cardiac and hemodynamic monitoring during and for 4 hours following infusion. Monitor laboratory tests, therapeutic response, and adverse reactions. Teach patient adverse symptoms to report.

Patient Education: This drug is only given I.V. and you will be on continuous cardiac monitoring during and for several hours following administration. You may experience headache or irregular heartbeat during infusion. Report chest pain or respiratory difficulty immediately. **Pregnancy/breast-feeding precautions:** Inform prescriber if you are or intend to become pregnant. Do not breast-feed.

Pregnancy Issues Teratogenic and embryocidal in rats; avoid use in pregnancy.

Idarubicin (eye da ROO bi sin)

U.S. Brand Names Idamycin PFS®

Synonyms 4-Demethoxydaunorubicin; 4-DMDR; Idarubicin Hydrochloride; IDR; IMI 30; NSC-256439; SC 33428

Pharmacologic Category Antineoplastic Agent, Anthracycline; Antineoplastic Agent, Antibiotic

Medication Safety Issues

Sound-alike/look-alike issues:

Idarubicin may be confused with DOXOrubicin, DAUNOrubicin, epirubicin

Idamycin PFS® may be confused with Adriamycin

Pregnancy Risk Factor D

Lactation Excretion in breast milk unknown

Use Treatment of acute leukemias (AML, ANLL, ALL), accelerated phase or blast crisis of chronic myelogenous leukemia (CML), breast cancer

Unlabeled/Investigational Use Autologous hematopoietic stem cell transplantation

Mechanism of Action/Effect Similar to daunorubicin, idarubicin exhibits inhibitory effects on DNA and RNA polymerase.

Contraindications Hypersensitivity to idarubicin, other anthracyclines, or any component of the formulation; bilirubin >5 mg/dL; pregnancy

(Continued)

Idarubicin (Continued)

Warnings/Precautions Hazardous agent — use appropriate precautions for handling and disposal. Can cause myocardial toxicity and is more common in patients who have previously received anthracyclines or have pre-existing cardiac disease; reduce dose in patients with impaired hepatic function.

Drug Interactions

Decreased Effect: Patients may experience impaired immune response to vaccines; possible infection after administration of live vaccines in patients receiving immunosuppressants.

Adverse Reactions

>10%:

Cardiovascular: Transient ECG abnormalities (supraventricular tachycardia, S-T wave changes, atrial or ventricular extrasystoles); generally asymptomatic and self-limiting. CHF, dose related. The relative cardiotoxicity of idarubicin compared to doxorubicin is unclear. Some investigators report no increase in cardiac toxicity at cumulative oral idarubicin doses up to 540 mg/m^2; other reports suggest a maximum cumulative intravenous dose of 150 mg/m^2.

Central nervous system: Headache

Dermatologic: Alopecia (25% to 30%), radiation recall, skin rash (11%), urticaria

Gastrointestinal: Nausea, vomiting (30% to 60%); diarrhea (9% to 22%); stomatitis (11%); GI hemorrhage (30%)

Genitourinary: Discoloration of urine (darker yellow)

Hematologic: Myelosuppression, primarily leukopenia; thrombocytopenia and anemia. Effects are generally less severe with oral dosing.

Nadir: 10-15 days

Recovery: 21-28 days

Hepatic: Bilirubin and transaminases increased (44%)

1% to 10%:

Central nervous system: Seizures

Neuromuscular & skeletal: Peripheral neuropathy

Overdosage/Toxicology Symptoms of overdose include severe myelosuppression and increased GI toxicity. Treatment is supportive. It is unlikely that therapeutic efficacy or toxicity would be altered by conventional peritoneal or hemodialysis.

Pharmacodynamics/Kinetics

Time to Peak: Serum: 1-5 hours

Protein Binding: 94% to 97%

Half-Life Elimination: Oral: 14-35 hours; I.V.: 12-27 hours

Metabolism: Hepatic to idarubicinol (pharmacologically active)

Excretion:

Oral: Urine (~5% of dose; 0.5% to 0.7% as unchanged drug, 4% as idarubicinol); hepatic (8%)

I.V.: Urine (13% as idarubicinol, 3% as unchanged drug); hepatic (17%)

Available Dosage Forms Injection, solution, as hydrochloride [preservative free] (Idamycin PFS®): 1 mg/mL (5 mL, 10 mL, 20 mL)

Dosing

Adults & Elderly: Refer to individual protocols.

Leukemia: I.V.:

Induction: 12 mg/m^2/day for 3 days

Consolidation: 10-12 mg/m^2/day for 2 days

Stem cell transplantation (unlabeled use): 20 mg/m^2/24 hours continuous I.V. infusion **or** 21 mg/m^2/24 hours continuous infusion for 48 hours (both with high-dose oral busulfan)

Pediatrics:

Leukemia: I.V.: 10-12 mg/m^2 once daily for 3 days every 3 weeks.

Solid tumors: I.V.: 5 mg/m^2 once daily for 3 days every 3 weeks.

Renal Impairment: Dose reduction is recommended.

Serum creatinine ≥2 mg/dL: Reduce dose by 25%.

Hepatic Impairment:

Bilirubin 1.5-5 mg/dL or AST 60-180 units: Reduce dose 50%.

Bilirubin >5 mg/dL or AST >180 units: Do not administer.

Administration

I.V.: Do not administer I.M. or SubQ; administer as slow push over 3-5 minutes, preferably into the side of a freely-running saline or dextrose infusion **or** as intermittent infusion over 10-15 minutes into a free-flowing I.V. solution of NS or D$_5$W; also occasionally administered as a bladder lavage.

I.V. Detail: Administer into a free-flowing I.V. solution of NS or D$_5$W. Avoid extravasation - potent vesicant. Local erythematous streaking along the vein may indicate rapid administration. Unless specific data is available, do not mix with other drugs.

Extravasation management: Topical cooling may be achieved using ice packs or cooling pad with circulating ice water. Cooling of site for 24 hours as tolerated by the patient. Elevate and rest extremity 24-48 hours, then resume normal activity as tolerated. Application of cold inhibits vesicant's cytotoxicity. **Application of heat can be harmful and is contraindicated.** If pain, erythema, and/or swelling persist beyond 48 hours, refer patient immediately to plastic surgeon for consultation and possible debridement.

pH: 5-7

Stability

Compatibility: Stable in D$_5$NS, D$_5$W, LR, NS, SWFI; **incompatible** with bacteriostatic water

Y-site administration: Incompatible with acyclovir, allopurinol, ampicillin/sulbactam, cefazolin, cefepime, ceftazidime, clindamycin, dexamethasone sodium phosphate, etoposide, fluorouracil, furosemide, gentamicin, heparin, hydrocortisone sodium succinate, lorazepam, meperidine, methotrexate, piperacillin/tazobactam, sodium bicarbonate, teniposide, vancomycin, vincristine

Compatibility when admixed: Incompatible with heparin

Storage: Store intact vials of solution under refrigeration (2°C to 8°C/36°F to 46°F). Protect from light. Solutions diluted in D$_5$W or NS for infusion are stable for 4 weeks at room temperature, protected from light. Syringe and IVPB solutions are stable for 72 hours at room temperature and 7 days under refrigeration.

Laboratory Monitoring CBC with differential, platelet count, cardiac function, serum electrolytes, creatinine, uric acid, ALT, AST, bilirubin

Nursing Actions

Physical Assessment: See Administration for specific infusion directions. Infusion site must be closely monitored; extravasation can cause severe cellulitis or tissue necrosis (eg, do not apply heat). Assess results of laboratory tests prior to each infusion and on a regular basis throughout therapy. Monitor therapeutic effectiveness (symptom relief) and adverse response (eg, cardiac toxicity, myelosuppression, peripheral neuropathy) frequently for full course of therapy. Teach patient possible side effects/appropriate interventions and adverse symptoms to report.

Patient Education: Do not take any new medication during therapy unless approved by prescriber. This medication is only administered by intravenous infusion; report immediately any swelling, pain, burning, redness at infusion site or sudden onset of chest pain, breathing or swallowing difficulty or chills. It is important to maintain adequate hydration (2-3 L/day of fluids unless instructed to restrict fluid intake), and nutrition. You will be more susceptible to infection (avoid crowds and exposure to infection and do not have any vaccinations without consulting prescriber). You may experience nausea or vomiting (small frequent meals, frequent mouth care, sucking lozenges, or chewing gum may help); diarrhea (buttermilk, boiled milk, or yogurt may help); or loss of hair (reversible). Urine may turn darker (normal). Report immediately chest pain, swelling of extremities, respiratory difficulty, palpitations, or rapid heartbeat. Report unresolved nausea, vomiting, or diarrhea; alterations in urinary pattern (increased or decreased); opportunistic infection (eg, fever, chills, unusual bruising or bleeding, signs of infection fatigue, purulent vaginal discharge, unhealed mouth sores); abdominal pain or blood in stools; excessive fatigue; yellowing of eyes or skin; swelling of extremities; respiratory difficulty; or unresolved diarrhea. **Pregnancy/breast-feeding precautions:** Do not get pregnant while taking this medication. Consult prescriber for use appropriate contraceptive measures. Consult prescriber if breast-feeding.

Geriatric Considerations During induction therapy, patients >60 years of age experience CHF, arrhythmias, MI, and decline in LVEF more frequently than younger populations.

Ifosfamide (eye FOSS fa mide)

U.S. Brand Names Ifex®

Synonyms Isophosphamide; NSC-109724; Z4942

Pharmacologic Category Antineoplastic Agent, Alkylating Agent; Antineoplastic Agent, Alkylating Agent (Nitrogen Mustard)

Medication Safety Issues
Sound-alike/look-alike issues:
Ifosfamide may be confused with cyclophosphamide

Pregnancy Risk Factor D

Lactation Enters breast milk/contraindicated

Use Treatment of lung cancer, Hodgkin's and non-Hodgkin's lymphoma, breast cancer, acute and chronic lymphocytic leukemias, ovarian cancer, sarcomas, pancreatic and gastric carcinomas
Orphan drug: Treatment of testicular cancer

Mechanism of Action/Effect Inhibits protein synthesis and DNA synthesis

Contraindications Hypersensitivity to ifosfamide or any component of the formulation; patients with severely depressed bone marrow function; pregnancy

Warnings/Precautions Hazardous agent — use appropriate precautions for handling and disposal. Used in combination with mesna as a prophylactic agent to protect against hemorrhagic cystitis. Use with caution in patients with impaired renal function or those with compromised bone marrow reserve. Carcinogenic in rats.

Drug Interactions
Cytochrome P450 Effect: Substrate of CYP2A6 (minor), 2B6 (minor), 2C8/9 (minor), 2C19 (minor), 3A4 (major); **Inhibits** CYP3A4 (weak); **Induces** CYP2C8/9 (weak)

Decreased Effect: CYP3A4 inhibitors may decrease the levels/effects of acrolein (the active metabolite of ifosfamide); example inhibitors include azole antifungals, clarithromycin, diclofenac, doxycycline, erythromycin, imatinib, isoniazid, nefazodone, nicardipine, propofol, protease inhibitors, quinidine, telithromycin, and verapamil.

Increased Effect/Toxicity: CYP3A4 inducers may increase the levels/effects of acrolein (the active metabolite of ifosfamide); example inducers include aminoglutethimide, carbamazepine, nafcillin, nevirapine, phenobarbital, phenytoin, and rifamycins.

Nutritional/Ethanol Interactions Herb/Nutraceutical: St John's wort may decrease ifosfamide levels.

Adverse Reactions
>10%:
Central nervous system: Somnolence, confusion, hallucinations (12%)
Dermatologic: Alopecia (75% to 100%)
Endocrine & metabolic: Metabolic acidosis (31%)
Gastrointestinal: Nausea and vomiting (58%), may be more common with higher doses or bolus infusions; constipation
Genitourinary: Hemorrhagic cystitis (40% to 50%), patients should be vigorously hydrated (at least 2 L/day) and receive mesna
Hematologic: Myelosuppression, leukopenia (65% to 100%), thrombocytopenia (10%) - dose related
Onset: 7-14 days
Nadir: 21-28 days
Recovery: 21-28 days
Renal: Hematuria (6% to 92%)
1% to 10%:
Central nervous system: Hallucinations, depressive psychoses, polyneuropathy
Dermatologic: Dermatitis, nail banding/ridging, hyperpigmentation
Endocrine & metabolic: SIADH, sterility
Hematologic: Anemia
Hepatic: Transaminases increased (3%)
Local: Phlebitis
Renal: BUN/creatinine increased (6%)
Respiratory: Nasal stuffiness

Overdosage/Toxicology Symptoms of overdose include myelosuppression, nausea, vomiting, diarrhea, and alopecia; direct extensions of the drug's pharmacologic effect. Treatment is supportive.

Pharmacodynamics/Kinetics
Time to Peak: Plasma: Oral: Within 1 hour
Protein Binding: Negligible
Half-Life Elimination: Beta: High dose: 11-15 hours (3800-5000 mg/m^2); Lower dose: 4-7 hours (1800 mg/m^2)
Metabolism: Hepatic to active metabolites phosphoramide mustard, acrolein, and inactive dichloroethylated and carboxy metabolites; acrolein is the agent implicated in development of hemorrhagic cystitis
Excretion: Urine (15% to 50% as unchanged drug, 41% as metabolites)

Pharmacokinetic Note Pharmacokinetics are dose dependent.

Available Dosage Forms
Injection, powder for reconstitution: 1 g
Ifex®: 1 g, 3 g

Dosing
Adults & Elderly: Refer to individual protocols.
Antineoplastic: I.V.:
50 mg/kg/day or 700-2000 mg/m^2 for 5 days every 3-4 weeks
Alternatives: 2400 mg/m^2/day for 3 days or 5000 mg/m^2 as a single dose every 3-4 weeks
Note: To prevent bladder toxicity, ifosfamide should be given with extensive hydration consisting of at least 2 L of oral or I.V. fluid per day. The dose-limiting toxicity is hemorrhagic cystitis and, therefore, ifosfamide should be used in conjunction with a uroprotective agent, such as mesna.
Pediatrics: Refer to individual protocols.
Antineoplastic: I.V.:
1200-1800 mg/m^2/day for 3-5 days every 21-28 days **or**
5 g/m^2 once every 21-28 days **or**
3 g/m^2/day for 2 days every 21-28 days
See "Note" in adult dosing.
Renal Impairment: Limited experience in renal impairment; manufacturer does not provide adjustment. Several published recommendations include dose reductions between 20% and 30% in significant renal impairment. Consult individual protocols.
(Continued)

Ifosfamide *(Continued)*

Hepatic Impairment:
Although no specific guidelines are available from the manufacturer, it is possible that adjusted doses are indicated in hepatic disease. One suggestion in the literature: AST >300 or bilirubin >3.0 mg/dL: Decrease ifosfamide dose by 75%

Administration
I.V.: Administer slow I.V. push, IVPB over 30 minutes to several hours or continuous intravenous infusion over 5 days.

I.V. Detail: Adequate hydration (at least 2 L/day) of the patient before and for 72 hours after therapy is recommended to minimize the risk of hemorrhagic cystitis.

pH: 6

Stability
Reconstitution: Dilute powder with SWI or NS to a concentration of 50 mg/mL. Further dilution in 50-1000 mL D_5W or NS is recommended for I.V. infusion.

Compatibility: Stable in D_5LR, D_5NS, D_5W, LR, 1/2NS, NS; **incompatible** with bacteriostatic SWI or bacteriostatic NS

Y-site administration: Incompatible with cefepime, methotrexate

Compatibility in syringe: Incompatible with mesna with epirubicin

Compatibility when admixed: Incompatible with mesna with epirubicin

Storage: Store intact vials at room temperature. Reconstituted solutions may be stored under refrigeration for up to 21 days. Solutions diluted for administration are stable for 7 days at room temperature and for 6 weeks under refrigeration.

Laboratory Monitoring CBC with differential, platelet count, urinalysis, liver and renal function

Nursing Actions
Physical Assessment: Assess potential for interactions with other pharmacological agents or herbal products patient may be taking (eg, increased or decreased levels/effects of ifosfamide). Note Administration for infusion specifics. To prevent bladder toxicity, maintain adequate hydration for 72 hours prior to infusion to minimize risk of hemorrhagic cystitis (2-3 L/day). Premedication with antiemetic may be ordered. Monitor vital signs and laboratory tests prior to each infusion and regularly during therapy. Monitor therapeutic effectiveness (according to purpose for use) and adverse response (eg, CNS depression or psychoses, hematuria [hemorrhagic cystitis], myelosuppression [anemia]) throughout therapy. Teach patient (or caregiver) possible side effects/appropriate interventions (eg, importance of adequate hydration) and adverse symptoms to report.

Patient Education: Do not take any new medication during therapy unless approved by prescriber. This drug can only be administered by infusion. Report immediately any swelling, redness, or pain at infusion site. Maintain adequate hydration (3-4 L/day of fluids unless instructed to restrict fluid intake) for at least 3 days prior to infusion and each day of therapy. You will be more susceptible to infection (avoid crowds and exposure to infection and do not have any vaccinations without consulting prescriber). May cause loss of hair (reversible, although regrowth hair may be different color or texture); fertility or amenorrhea; nausea or vomiting (small, frequent meals, good mouth care, chewing gum, or sucking lozenges may help - if persistent consult prescriber for antiemetic); headache (consult prescriber for analgesic); or mouth sores (use soft toothbrush or cotton swab for oral care). Report any difficulty or pain with urination; chest pain, rapid heartbeat, or palpitations; CNS changes (eg, hallucinations, confusion, somnolence); unusual rash; persistent nausea or vomiting; swelling of extremities; respiratory difficulty; unusual fatigue; or opportunistic infection (eg, fever, chills, easy bruising or unusual bleeding). **Pregnancy/breast-feeding precautions:** Inform prescriber if you are pregnant. Do not get pregnant during or for 1 month following therapy. Male: Do not cause a female to become pregnant. Male/female: Consult prescriber for instruction on appropriate contraceptive measures. This drug may cause severe fetal defects. Do not breast-feed.

Imatinib *(eye MAT eh nib)*

U.S. Brand Names Gleevec®

Synonyms CGP-57148B; Glivec; Imatinib Mesylate; STI571

Pharmacologic Category Antineoplastic Agent, Tyrosine Kinase Inhibitor

Pregnancy Risk Factor D

Lactation Excretion in breast milk unknown/not recommended

Use Treatment of adult patients with Philadelphia chromosome-positive (Ph+) chronic myeloid leukemia (CML) in chronic phase; treatment of patients with Ph+ CML in blast crisis, accelerated phase or chronic phase after failure of interferon therapy; treatment of pediatric patients with Ph+ CML (chronic phase) recurring following stem cell transplant or who are resistant to interferon-alpha therapy; treatment of Kit-positive (CD117) unresectable and/or (metastatic) malignant gastrointestinal stromal tumors (GIST)

Mechanism of Action/Effect Inhibits a specific enzyme (Bcr-Abl tyrosine kinase) produced by the Philadelphia chromosome found in many patients with chronic myeloid leukemia (CML). Inhibition of this enzyme blocks proliferation and induces cell death in leukemic cells. Also inhibits tyrosine kinase for platelet-derived growth factor (SCF), c-kit, and events mediated by PDGF and SCF.

Contraindications Hypersensitivity to imatinib or any component of the formulation; pregnancy

Warnings/Precautions Hazardous agent - use appropriate precautions for handling and disposal. Often associated with fluid retention, weight gain, and edema; occasionally leading to significant complications, including pleural effusion, pericardial effusion, pulmonary edema, and ascites. Use caution in patients where fluid accumulation may be poorly tolerated, such as in cardiovascular disease (CHF or hypertension) and pulmonary disease. Severe dermatologic reactions have been reported; reintroduction has been attempted following resolution. Successful resumption at a lower dose (with corticosteroids and/or antihistamine) has been described; however, some patients may experience recurrent reactions.

Use with caution in renal impairment, hematologic impairment, or hepatic disease. May cause GI irritation, hemorrhage, hematologic toxicity (neutropenia, or thrombocytopenia), or hepatotoxicity. Hepatotoxic reactions may be severe. Has been associated with development of opportunistic infections. Use with caution in patients receiving concurrent therapy with drugs which alter cytochrome P450 activity or require metabolism by these isoenzymes. Safety and efficacy in patients <3 years of age have not been established.

Drug Interactions
Cytochrome P450 Effect: Substrate of CYP1A2 (minor), 2D6 (minor), 2C8/9 (minor), 2C19 (minor), 3A4 (major), **Inhibits** CYP2C8/9 (weak), 2D6 (weak), 3A4 (strong)

Decreased Effect: The levels/effects of imatinib may be decreased by aminoglutethimide, carbamazepine, nafcillin, nevirapine, phenobarbital, phenytoin, rifamycins, and other CYP3A4 inducers. Dosage of imatinib should be increased by at least 50% (with careful monitoring) when used concurrently with a strong inducer. Imatinib may decrease the absorption of digoxin (tablet formulation). Imatinib may decrease the effects of levothyroxine replacement therapy.

Increased Effect/Toxicity: Note: Drug interaction data are limited. Few clinical studies have been conducted. Many interactions listed here are derived by extrapolation from *in vitro* inhibition of cytochrome P450 isoenzymes. Chronic use of acetaminophen may increase potential for hepatotoxic reaction with imatinib (case report of hepatic failure with concurrent therapy).

Imatinib may increase the levels/effects of amiodarone, selected benzodiazepines, calcium channel blockers, cisapride, cyclosporine, ergot derivatives, fluoxetine, glimepiride, glipizide, HMG-CoA reductase inhibitors, nateglinide, phenytoin, phenytoin, propranolol, sertraline, mirtazapine, nateglinide, nefazodone, pioglitazone, rosiglitazone, sertraline, sildenafil (and other PDE-5 inhibitors), tacrolimus, telithromycin, venlafaxine, warfarin, and other substrates of CYP2C8/9 or 3A4. Selected benzodiazepines (midazolam and triazolam), cisapride, ergot alkaloids, selected HMG-CoA reductase inhibitors (lovastatin and simvastatin), mesoridazine, pimozide, and thioridazine are generally contraindicated with strong CYP3A4 inhibitors. When used with strong CYP3A4 inhibitors, dosage adjustment/limits are recommended for sildenafil and other PDE-5 inhibitors; consult individual monographs.

The levels/effects of imatinib may be increased by azole antifungals, clarithromycin, diclofenac, doxycycline, erythromycin, isoniazid, nefazodone, nicardipine, propofol, protease inhibitors, quinidine, telithromycin, verapamil, and other CYP3A4 inhibitors. Lansoprazole may enhance the dermatologic adverse effects of Imatinib.

Nutritional/Ethanol Interactions
Ethanol: Avoid ethanol.
Food: Food may reduce gastrointestinal irritation.
Herb/Nutraceutical: Avoid St John's wort (may increase metabolism and decrease imatinib plasma concentration).

Adverse Reactions Adverse reactions listed were established in patients with a wide variation in level of illness or specific diagnosis. In many cases, other medications were used concurrently (relationship to imatinib not specific). Effects reported in children were similar to adults, except that musculoskeletal pain was less frequent (21%) and peripheral edema was not reported in children.
>10%:
Cardiovascular: Chest pain (7% to 11%)
Central nervous system: Fatigue (30% to 53%), pyrexia (15% to 41%), headache (27% to 39%), insomnia (10% to 19%), dizziness (11% to 16%), depression (13%), anxiety (7% to 12%)
Dermatologic: Rash (36% to 53%), pruritus (8% to 14%)
Endocrine & metabolic: Fluid retention (7% to 81% includes aggravated edema, anasarca, ascites, pericardial effusion, pleural effusion, pulmonary edema); hypokalemia (6% to 13%)
Gastrointestinal: Nausea (47% to 74%), diarrhea (39% to 70%), vomiting (21% to 58%), abdominal pain (30% to 40%), flatulence (30% to 34%), weight gain (5% to 32%), dyspepsia (12% to 27%), anorexia (7% to 17%), constipation (9% to 16%), sore throat (10% to 15%), loose stools (10% to 12%)
Hematologic: Hemorrhage (24% to 53%; grade 3 or 4: 11% to 19%), neutropenia (grade 3 or 4: 3% to 48%), anemia (grade 3 or 4: <1% to 42%), thrombocytopenia (grade 3 or 4: <1% to 33%)
Hepatic: Hepatotoxicity (6% to 12%)

Neuromuscular & skeletal: Muscle cramps (28% to 62%), musculoskeletal pain (30% to 49%), arthralgia (25% to 40%), joint pain (11 to 30%), myalgia (9% to 27%), back pain (23% to 26%), weakness (15% to 21%), rigors (10% to 12%)
Ocular: Lacrimation increased (16% to 18%)
Respiratory: Cough (14% to 27%), nasopharyngitis (10% to 27%), dyspnea (12% to 21%), upper respiratory tract infection (3% to 19%), pharyngolaryngeal pain (7% to 17%), pneumonia (4% to 13%)
Miscellaneous: Superficial edema (58% to 81%), night sweats (13% to 17%), influenza (1% to 11%)
1% to 10%:
Central nervous system: CNS hemorrhage (1% to 9%), paresthesia
Dermatologic: Alopecia, dry skin
Gastrointestinal: Gastrointestinal hemorrhage (1% to 8%), abdominal distension, gastroesophageal reflux, mouth ulceration
Hepatic: Ascites or pleural effusion (GIST: 4% to 6%), alkaline phosphatase increased (grade 3 or 4: <1% to 6%), ALT increased (grade 3 or 4: <1% to 7%), bilirubin increased (grade 3 or 4: <1% to 3%), AST increased (grade 3 or 4: <1% to 5%)
Neuromuscular & skeletal: Joint swelling
Ocular: Blurred vision, conjunctivitis
Renal: Albumin decreased (grade 3 or 4: 3% to 4%), creatine increased (grade 3 or 4: <1% to 2%)
Miscellaneous: Flu-like syndrome (<1% to 10%)

Overdosage/Toxicology Experience with overdose (>800 mg/day) is limited. Patients taking doses of 1200-1600 mg per day experienced elevated transaminases, elevated bilirubin, and muscle cramps; treatment was interrupted until reversal of abnormalities, then resumed at the normal doses without recurrence of symptoms. Hematologic adverse effects are more common at dosages >750 mg/day. Treatment is symptomatic and supportive

Pharmacodynamics/Kinetics
Time to Peak: 2-4 hours
Protein Binding: 95% to albumin and alpha$_1$-acid glycoprotein
Half-Life Elimination: Parent drug: 18 hours; N-demethyl metabolite: 40 hours
Metabolism: Hepatic via CYP3A4 (minor metabolism via CYP1A2, CYP2D6, CYP2C9, CYP2C19); primary metabolite (active): N-demethylated piperazine derivative; severe hepatic impairment (bilirubin >3-10 times ULN) increases AUC by 45% to 55% for imatinib and its active metabolite, respectively
Excretion: Feces (68% primarily as metabolites, 20% as unchanged drug); urine (13% primarily as metabolites, 5% as unchanged drug)
Clearance: Highly variable; Mean: 8-14 L/hour (for 50 kg and 100 kg male, respectively)

Available Dosage Forms Tablet: 100 mg; 400 mg
Dosing
Adults & Elderly:
CML:
Chronic phase: Oral: 400 mg once daily; may be increased to 600 mg daily
Accelerated phase or blast crisis: 600 mg once daily; may be increased to 800 mg daily (400 mg twice daily)
Gastrointestinal stromal tumors: 400-600 mg/day.
Note: Dosage should be increased by at least 50% when used concurrently with a potent enzyme-inducing agent (ie, rifampin, phenytoin).
Pediatrics:
CML (chronic phase): Oral: 260 mg/m^2/day; may be increased to 340 mg/m^2/day
Note: Dosage should be increased by at least 50% when used concurrently with a potent enzyme-inducing agent (ie, rifampin, phenytoin).
(Continued)

Imatinib *(Continued)*

Dosage adjustment for hepatotoxicity or other nonhematologic adverse reactions: Refer to "Hepatic Impairment" dosing.

Dosage adjustment for hematologic adverse reactions: Refer to adult dosing.

Hepatic Impairment:

Treatment initiation:

Mild-to-moderate impairment: Starting dose 400 mg/day

Severe impairment: Starting dose 300 mg/day

Hepatotoxicity or other nonhematologic adverse reactions: If elevations of bilirubin >3 times upper limit of normal (ULN) or transaminases (ALT/AST) >5 times ULN occur, withhold until bilirubin <1.5 times ULN or transaminases <2.5 times ULN. Resume treatment at a reduced dose:

Children:

If initial dose 260 mg/m^2/day, reduce dose to 200 mg/m^2/day

If initial dose 340 mg/m^2/day, reduce dose to 260 mg/m^2/day

Adults:

If initial dose 400 mg, reduce dose to 300 mg

If initial dose 600 mg, reduce dose to 400 mg

Dosing Adjustment for Toxicity:

Dosage adjustment for hematologic adverse reactions:

Chronic phase (initial dose 400 mg/day in adults or 260 mg/m^2/day in children) or GIST (initial dose 400 mg or 600 mg): If ANC <1.0 x 10^9/L and/or platelets <50 x 10^9/L: Discontinue until ANC ≥1.5 x 10^9/L and platelets ≥75 x 10^9/L; resume treatment at original initial dose of 400 or 600 mg/day (260 mg/m^2/day in children). If depression in neutrophils or platelets recurs, withhold until recovery, and reinstitute treatment at a reduced dose:

Children:

If initial dose 260 mg/m^2/day, reduce dose to 200 mg/m^2/day

If initial dose 340 mg/m^2/day, reduce dose to 260 mg/m^2/day

Adults:

If initial dose 400 mg, reduce dose to 300 mg

If initial dose 600 mg, reduce dose to 400 mg

Accelerated phase or blast crisis: Adults: Check to establish whether cytopenia is related to leukemia (bone marrow aspirate). If unrelated to leukemia, reduce dose of imatinib by 25%. If cytopenia persists for an additional 2 weeks, further reduce dose to 50% of original dose. If cytopenia persists for 4 weeks and is still unrelated to leukemia, stop treatment until ANC ≥1.0 x 10^9/L and platelets ≥20 x 10^9/L, resume treatment at 50% of original dose.

Administration

Oral: Should be administered with food and a large glass of water. Tablets may be dispersed in water or apple juice (using ~50 mL for 100 mg tablet, ~200 mL for 400 mg tablet); stir until dissolved and use immediately.

Stability

Storage: Store at 15°C to 30°C (59°F to 86°F). Protect from moisture.

Laboratory Monitoring CBC (weekly for first month, biweekly for second month, then periodically thereafter), liver function tests (at baseline and monthly or as clinically indicated), renal function, and thyroid function tests

Nursing Actions

Physical Assessment: Monitor closely any other pharmacological agents or herbal products patient may be taking for effectiveness and possible interactions prior to beginning therapy (especially those drugs affected by cytochrome P450 actions). Monitor laboratory tests, therapeutic effectiveness, and adverse reactions at beginning of therapy and periodically during therapy (eg, weight and fluid status, hemorrhage, paresthesia, respiratory or CNS changes). Teach appropriate use, interventions to reduce side effects, and symptoms to report.

Patient Education: Take with food or a large glass of water. Avoid alcohol, chronic use of acetaminophen or aspirin, OTC or prescription medications, or herbal products unless approved by prescriber. Maintain adequate hydration (2-3 L/day of fluids) unless instructed to restrict fluid intake. You will be required to have regularly scheduled laboratory tests while on this medication. You will be more susceptible to infection (avoid crowds and exposure to infection and do not receive any vaccination unless approved by prescriber). You may experience headache or fatigue (use caution when driving or engaging in tasks requiring alertness until response to drug in known); loss of appetite, nausea, vomiting, or mouth sores (small frequent meals, frequent mouth care, chewing gum, or sucking lozenges may help); constipation (increased exercise, fluids, fruit, or fiber may help); or diarrhea (buttermilk, boiled milk, or yogurt may reduce diarrhea). Report chest pain, palpitations, or swelling of extremities; cough, respiratory difficulty, or wheezing; weight gain >5 lb; skin rash; muscle or bone pain, tremors, or cramping; persistent fatigue or weakness; easy bruising or unusual bleeding (eg, tarry stools, blood in vomitus, stool, urine, or mouth); persistent GI problems or pain; or other adverse effects. **Pregnancy/breast-feeding precautions:** Inform prescriber if you are pregnant. Do not get pregnant. Consult prescriber for appropriate contraception while using this medication. Breast-feeding is not recommended.

Dietary Considerations Should be taken with food and a large glass of water to decrease gastrointestinal irritation.

Geriatric Considerations Incidence of edema and edema-related adverse effects is increased in elderly patients.

Additional Information Median time to hematologic response was one month; only short-term studies have been completed. Follow-up is insufficient to estimate duration of cytogenic response.

Imipenem and Cilastatin
(i mi PEN em & sye la STAT in)

U.S. Brand Names Primaxin®

Synonyms Imipemide

Pharmacologic Category Antibiotic, Carbapenem

Medication Safety Issues

Sound-alike/look-alike issues:

Primaxin® may be confused with Premarin®, Primacor®

Pregnancy Risk Factor C

Lactation Enters breast milk (small amounts)/use caution

Use Treatment of respiratory tract, urinary tract, intra-abdominal, gynecologic, bone and joint, skin structure, and polymicrobic infections as well as bacterial septicemia and endocarditis. Antibacterial activity includes resistant gram-negative bacilli (*Pseudomonas aeruginosa* and *Enterobacter* sp), gram-positive bacteria (methicillin-sensitive *Staphylococcus aureus* and *Streptococcus* sp) and anaerobes.

Note: I.M. administration is not intended for severe or life-threatening infections (eg, septicemia, endocarditis, shock)

Mechanism of Action/Effect A carbapenem with broad-spectrum antibacterial activity including resistant gram-negative bacilli (*Pseudomonas aeruginosa* and

Enterococcus sp), gram-positive bacteria (methicillin-sensitive *Staphylococcus aureus* and *Enterococcus* sp) and anaerobes; inhibits cell wall synthesis; cilastatin prevents renal metabolism of imipenem

Contraindications Hypersensitivity to imipenem/cilastatin or any component of the formulation; consult information on Lidocaine for contraindications associated with I.M. dosing

Warnings/Precautions Dosage adjustment is required in patients with impaired renal function. Prolonged use may result in superinfection. Has been associated with CNS adverse events. Use with caution in patients with a history of seizures or hypersensitivity to beta-lactams. Elderly patients often require lower doses (adjust carefully to renal function). Doses for I.M. administration are mixed with lidocaine, consult information on lidocaine for associated warnings/precautions. Two different imipenem/cilastin products are available; due to differences in formulation, the I.V. and I.M. preparations **cannot** be interchanged.

Drug Interactions

Decreased Effect: Imipenem may decrease valproic acid concentrations to subtherapeutic levels; monitor.

Lab Interactions Interferes with urinary glucose determination using Clinitest®

Adverse Reactions 1% to 10%:

Gastrointestinal: Nausea/diarrhea/vomiting (1% to 2%)

Local: Phlebitis (3%), pain at I.M. injection site (1.2%)

Overdosage/Toxicology Symptoms of overdose include neuromuscular hypersensitivity and seizures. Hemodialysis may be helpful to aid in removal of the drug from blood; otherwise, treatment is supportive or symptom-directed.

Pharmacodynamics/Kinetics

Half-Life Elimination: Both drugs: 60 minutes; prolonged with renal impairment

Metabolism: Renally by dehydropeptidase; activity is blocked by cilastatin; cilastatin is partially metabolized renally

Excretion: Both drugs: Urine (~70% as unchanged drug)

Available Dosage Forms

Injection, powder for reconstitution [I.M.]: Imipenem 500 mg and cilastatin 500 mg [contains sodium 32 mg (1.4 mEq)]

Injection, powder for reconstitution [I.V.]: Imipenem 250 mg and cilastatin 250 mg [contains sodium 18.8 mg (0.8 mEq)]; imipenem 500 mg and cilastatin 500 mg [contains sodium 37.5 mg (1.6 mEq)]

Dosing

Adults & Elderly: Dosage based on **imipenem** content: **Note:** For adults weighing <70 kg, refer to Dosing Adjustment in Renal Impairment:

Burkholderia mallei (melioidosis): I.V.: 20 mg/kg every 8 hours for 10 days

Intra-abdominal infections: I.V.: Mild infection: 750 mg every 12 hours; Severe: 500 mg every 6 hours

Liver abscess: I.V.: 500 mg every 6 hours for 2-3 weeks, then appropriate oral therapy for a total of 4-6 weeks

Moderate infections:

I.M.: 750 mg every 12 hours

I.V.:

Fully-susceptible organisms: 500 mg every 6-8 hours

Moderately-susceptible organisms: 500 mg every 6 hours or 1 g every 8 hours

Neutropenic fever, otitis externa, *Pseudomonas* **infections:** I.V.: 500 mg every 6 hours

Severe infections: I.V.: **Note:** I.M. administration is not intended for severe or life-threatening infections (eg, septicemia, endocarditis, shock):

Fully-susceptible organisms: 500 mg every 6 hours

Moderately-susceptible organisms: 1 g every 6-8 hours

Maximum daily dose should not exceed 50 mg/kg or 4 g/day, whichever is lower

Urinary tract infection, uncomplicated: I.V.: 250 mg every 6 hours

Urinary tract infection, complicated: I.V.: 500 mg every 6 hours

Mild infections: Note: Rarely a suitable option in mild infections; normally reserved for moderate-severe cases:

I.M.: 500 mg every 12 hours

I.V.:

Fully-susceptible organisms: 250 mg every 6 hours

Moderately-susceptible organisms: 500 mg every 6 hours

Pediatrics: Dosage based on **imipenem** content:

Non-CNS infections: I.V.:

Neonates:

<1 week: 25 mg/kg every 12 hours

1-4 weeks: 25 mg/kg every 8 hours

4 weeks to 3 months: 25 mg/kg every 6 hours

Children: >3 months: 15-25 mg/kg every 6 hours

Maximum dosage: Susceptible infections: 2 g/day; moderately-susceptible organisms: 4 g/day

Burkholderia mallei (melioidosis): 20 mg/kg every 8 hours for 10 days

Cystic fibrosis: Doses up to 90 mg/kg/day have been used

Renal Impairment: I.V.: **Note:** Adjustments have not been established for I.M. dosing:

Patients with a Cl$_{cr}$ <5 mL/minute/1.73 m^2 should not receive imipenem/cilastatin unless hemodialysis is instituted within 48 hours.

Patients weighing <30 kg with impaired renal function should not receive imipenem/cilastatin.

Hemodialysis: Use the dosing recommendation for patients with a Cl$_{cr}$ 6-20 mL/minute.

Peritoneal dialysis: Dose as for Cl$_{cr}$ <10 mL/minute.

Continuous arteriovenous or venovenous hemofiltration: Dose as for Cl$_{cr}$ 20-30 mL/minute; monitor for seizure activity. Imipenem is well removed by CAVH but cilastatin is not; removes 20 mg of imipenem per liter of filtrate per day.

See table on next page.

Administration

I.M.:

I.M.: Administer by deep injection into a large muscle (gluteal or lateral thigh). Aspiration is necessary to avoid inadvertent injection into a blood vessel. **Only the I.M. formulation can be used for I.M. administration.**

I.V.:

I.V.: Do not administer I.V. push. Infuse doses ≤500 mg over 20-30 minutes; infuse doses ≥750 mg over 40-60 minutes. **Only the I.V. formulation can be used for I.V. administration.**

I.V. Detail: Vial contents must be transferred to 100 mL of infusion solution. If nausea and/or vomiting occur during administration, decrease the rate of I.V. infusion. Do not mix with or physically add to other antibiotics; however, may administer concomitantly.

pH: 6.5-7.5 (buffered)

Stability

Reconstitution:

I.M.: Prepare 500 mg vial with 2 mL 1% lidocaine (do not use lidocaine with epinephrine). The I.V. formulation does not form a stable suspension in lidocaine and cannot be used to prepare an I.M. dose.

I.V.: Prior to use, dilute dose into 100 mL of an appropriate solution. Imipenem is inactivated at acidic or alkaline pH. Final concentration should not exceed 5 mg/mL. The I.M. formulation is not buffered and cannot be used to prepare I.V. solutions.

(Continued)

Imipenem and Cilastatin *(Continued)*

Imipenem and Cilastatin Dosage in Renal Impairment

Reduced I.V. Dosage Regimen Based on Creatinine Clearance (mL/minute/1.73 m²) and/or Body Weight <70 kg				
	Body Weight (kg)			
	≥70	60	50	40	30
Total daily dose for normal renal function: 1 g/day				
Cl_cr ≥71	250 mg q6h	250 mg q8h	125 mg q6h	125 mg q6h	125 mg q8h
Cl_cr 41-70	250 mg q8h	125 mg q6h	125 mg q6h	125 mg q8h	125 mg q8h
Cl_cr 21-40	250 mg q12h	250 mg q12h	125 mg q8h	125 mg q12h	125 mg q12h
Cl_cr 6-20	250 mg q12h	125 mg q12h	125 mg q12h	125 mg q12h	125 mg q12h
Total daily dose for normal renal function: 1.5 g/day				
Cl_cr ≥71	500 mg q8h	250 mg q6h	250 mg q6h	250 mg q8h	125 mg q6h
Cl_cr 41-70	250 mg q6h	250 mg q8h	250 mg q8h	125 mg q6h	125 mg q8h
Cl_cr 21-40	250 mg q8h	250 mg q8h	250 mg q12h	125 mg q8h	125 mg q8h
Cl_cr 6-20	250 mg q12h	250 mg q12h	250 mg q12h	125 mg q12h	125 mg q12h
Total daily dose for normal renal function: 2 g/day				
Cl_cr ≥71	500 mg q6h	500 mg q8h	250 mg q6h	250 mg q6h	250 mg q8h
Cl_cr 41-70	500 mg q8h	250 mg q6h	250 mg q6h	250 mg q8h	125 mg q6h
Cl_cr 21-40	250 mg q6h	250 mg q8h	250 mg q8h	250 mg q12h	125 mg q8h
Cl_cr 6-20	250 mg q12h	250 mg q12h	250 mg q12h	250 mg q12h	125 mg q12h
Total daily dose for normal renal function: 3 g/day				
Cl_cr ≥71	1000 mg q8h	750 mg q8h	500 mg q6h	500 mg q8h	250 mg q6h
Cl_cr 41-70	500 mg q6h	500 mg q8h	500 mg q8h	250 mg q6h	250 mg q8h
Cl_cr 21-40	500 mg q8h	500 mg q8h	250 mg q6h	250 mg q8h	250 mg q8h
Cl_cr 6-20	500 mg q12h	500 mg q12h	250 mg q12h	250 mg q12h	250 mg q12h
Total daily dose for normal renal function: 4 g/day				
Cl_cr ≥71	1000 mg q6h	1000 mg q8h	750 mg q8h	500 mg q6h	500 mg q8h
Cl_cr 41-70	750 mg q8h	750 mg q8h	500 mg q6h	500 mg q8h	250 mg q6h
Cl_cr 21-40	500 mg q6h	500 mg q8h	500 mg q8h	250 mg q6h	250 mg q8h
Cl_cr 6-20	500 mg q12h	500 mg q12h	500 mg q12h	250 mg q12h	250 mg q12h

Compatibility: Y-site administration: Incompatible with allopurinol, amphotericin B cholesteryl sulfate complex, etoposide phosphate, fluconazole, gemcitabine, lorazepam, meperidine, midazolam, sargramostim, sodium bicarbonate

Storage:
Imipenem/cilastatin powder for injection should be stored at <25°C (77°F).
I.M.: The I.M. suspension should be used within 1 hour of reconstitution.
I.V.: Reconstituted I.V. solutions are stable for 4 hours at room temperature and 24 hours when refrigerated.

Laboratory Monitoring Perform culture and sensitivity studies prior to initiating therapy. Periodically monitor renal, hepatic, and hematologic function.

Nursing Actions

Physical Assessment: Results of culture and sensitivity tests and patient's allergy history should be assessed prior to beginning therapy. Note Administration for I.M. and I.V. specifics. Monitor laboratory tests, therapeutic effectiveness (resolution of infection), and adverse response periodically during therapy. Advise patients with diabetes about use of Clinitest®. Teach patient possible side effects/appropriate interventions and adverse symptoms to report.

Patient Education: Do not take any new medication during therapy unless approved by prescriber. This medication can only be administered by injection or infusion. Report immediately any warmth, swelling, pain, or redness at infusion or injection site. Maintain adequate hydration (2-3 L/day of fluids) unless instructed to restrict fluid intake, and nutrition (small, frequent meals). May cause false test results with Clinitest®; use of another type of glucose testing is preferable. Report immediately any CNS changes (dizziness, hallucinations, anxiety, visual disturbances); swelling of throat, tongue, lips, or face; chills or fever; or unusual discharge or foul-smelling urine. **Pregnancy/breast-feeding precautions:** Inform prescriber if you are or intend to become pregnant. Consult prescriber if breast-feeding.

Dietary Considerations Sodium content of 500 mg injection:
I.M.: 32 mg (1.4 mEq)
I.V.: 37.5 mg (1.6 mEq)

Geriatric Considerations Many of the seizures attributed to imipenem/cilastatin were in elderly patients. Dose must be carefully adjusted for creatinine clearance.

Imipramine *(im IP ra meen)*

U.S. Brand Names Tofranil®; Tofranil-PM®

Synonyms Imipramine Hydrochloride; Imipramine Pamoate

Restrictions A medication guide concerning the use of antidepressants in children and teenagers can be found on the FDA website at http://www.fda.gov/cder/Offices/ODS/labeling.htm. It should be dispensed to parents or guardians of children and teenagers receiving this medication.

Pharmacologic Category Antidepressant, Tricyclic (Tertiary Amine)

Medication Safety Issues
Sound-alike/look-alike issues:
Imipramine may be confused with amitriptyline, desipramine, Norpramin®

Pregnancy Risk Factor D

Lactation Enters breast milk/not recommended (AAP rates "of concern")

Use Treatment of depression; treatment of nocturnal enuresis in children

Unlabeled/Investigational Use Analgesic for certain chronic and neuropathic pain; panic disorder; attention-deficit/hyperactivity disorder (ADHD)

Mechanism of Action/Effect Traditionally believed to increase the synaptic concentration of serotonin and/or norepinephrine in the central nervous system by inhibition of their reuptake by the presynaptic neuronal membrane. However, additional receptor effects have been found including desensitization of adenyl cyclase, down regulation of beta-adrenergic receptors, and down regulation of serotonin receptors.

Contraindications Hypersensitivity to imipramine (cross-reactivity with other dibenzodiazepines may occur) or any component of the formulation; concurrent use of MAO inhibitors (within 14 days); in a patient during acute recovery phase of MI; pregnancy

Warnings/Precautions Antidepressants increase the risk of suicidal thinking and behavior in children and adolescents with major depressive disorder (MDD) and other depressive disorders; consider risk prior to prescribing. All patients must be closely monitored for clinical worsening, suicidality, or unusual changes in behavior, especially during the initiation of therapy or following an increase or decrease in dosage. When used in children, the child's family or caregiver should be instructed to closely observe the patient and communicate condition with healthcare provider. A medication guide should be dispensed with each prescription. **Imipramine is FDA approved for the treatment of nocturnal enuresis in children ≥6 years of age.**

The possibility of a suicide attempt is inherent in major depression and may persist until remission occurs. Use caution in high-risk patients. Worsening depression and severe abrupt suicidality that are not part of the presenting symptoms may require discontinuation or modification of drug therapy. The patient's family or caregiver should be alerted to monitor patients for the emergence of suicidality and associated behaviors (such as agitation, irritability, hostility, impulsivity, and hypomania) and notify healthcare provider.

May worsen psychosis in some patients or precipitate a shift to mania or hypomania in patients with bipolar disorder. Patients presenting with depressive symptoms should be screened for bipolar disorder. Monotherapy in patients with bipolar disorder should be avoided. **Imipramine is not FDA approved for the treatment of bipolar depression.**

The degree of sedation, anticholinergic effects, orthostasis, and conduction abnormalities are high relative to other antidepressants. Imipramine often causes drowsiness/sedation, resulting in impaired performance of tasks requiring alertness (eg, operating machinery or driving). Sedative effects may be additive with other CNS depressants and/or ethanol. Use with caution in patients with a history of cardiovascular disease (including previous MI, stroke, tachycardia, or conduction abnormalities). Use with caution in patients with urinary retention, benign prostatic hyperplasia, narrow-angle glaucoma, xerostomia, visual problems, constipation, or a history of bowel obstruction.

Consider discontinuing, when possible, prior to elective surgery. Therapy should not be abruptly discontinued in patients receiving high doses for prolonged periods. May lower seizure threshold - use caution in patients with a previous seizure disorder or condition predisposing to seizures such as brain damage, alcoholism, or concurrent therapy with other drugs which lower the seizure threshold. May increase the risks associated with electroconvulsive therapy. Use with caution in hyperthyroid patients or those receiving thyroid supplementation. Use with caution in patients with hepatic or renal dysfunction and in elderly patients. Has been associated with photosensitization.

Drug Interactions

Cytochrome P450 Effect: Substrate of CYP1A2 (minor), 2B6 (minor), 2C19 (major), 2D6 (major), 3A4 (minor); **Inhibits** CYP1A2 (weak), 2C19 (weak), 2D6 (moderate), 2E1 (weak)

Decreased Effect: CYP2C19 inducers may decrease the levels/effects of imipramine; example inducers include aminoglutethimide, carbamazepine, phenytoin, and rifampin. Imipramine inhibits the antihypertensive response to bethanidine, clonidine, debrisoquin, guanadrel, guanethidine, guanabenz, and guanfacine. Cholestyramine and colestipol may bind TCAs and reduce their absorption; monitor for altered response.

Increased Effect/Toxicity: When used with MAO inhibitors, hyperpyrexia, hypertension, tachycardia, confusion, seizures, and **deaths have been reported** (serotonin syndrome). Serotonin syndrome has also been reported with ritonavir (rare). Use of lithium with a TCA may increase the risk for neurotoxicity.

CYP2C19 inhibitors may increase the levels/effects of imipramine; example inhibitors include delavirdine, fluconazole, fluvoxamine, gemfibrozil, isoniazid, omeprazole, and ticlopidine. Imipramine increases the effects of amphetamines, anticholinergics, other CNS depressants (sedatives, hypnotics, or ethanol), chlorpropamide, tolazamide, and warfarin. CYP2D6 inhibitors may increase the levels/effects of imipramine; example inhibitors include chlorpromazine, delavirdine, fluoxetine, miconazole, paroxetine, pergolide, quinidine, quinine, ritonavir, and ropinirole.

Phenothiazines may increase concentration of some TCAs and TCAs may increase concentration of phenothiazines. Pressor response to I.V. epinephrine, norepinephrine, and phenylephrine may be enhanced in patients receiving TCAs (**Note:** Effect is unlikely with epinephrine or levonordefrin dosages typically administered as infiltration in combination with local anesthetics).

Combined use of beta-agonists or drugs which prolong QT_c (including quinidine, procainamide, disopyramide, cisapride, sparfloxacin, gatifloxacin, moxifloxacin) with TCAs may predispose patients to cardiac arrhythmias.

Nutritional/Ethanol Interactions

Ethanol: Avoid ethanol (may increase CNS depression).

Food: Grapefruit juice may inhibit the metabolism of some TCAs and clinical toxicity may result.

Herb/Nutraceutical: St John's wort may decrease imipramine levels. Avoid valerian, St John's wort, SAMe, kava kava (may increase risk of serotonin syndrome and/or excessive sedation).

Lab Interactions Increased glucose

Adverse Reactions Frequency not defined.

Cardiovascular: Orthostatic hypotension, arrhythmia, tachycardia, hypertension, palpitation, MI, heart block, ECG changes, CHF, stroke

Central nervous system: Dizziness, drowsiness, headache, agitation, insomnia, nightmares, hypomania, psychosis, fatigue, confusion, hallucinations, disorientation, delusions, anxiety, restlessness, seizure

Endocrine & metabolic: Gynecomastia, breast enlargement, galactorrhea, increase or decrease in libido, increase or decrease in blood sugar, SIADH

Gastrointestinal: Nausea, unpleasant taste, weight gain, xerostomia, constipation, ileus, stomatitis, abdominal cramps, vomiting, anorexia, epigastric disorders, diarrhea, black tongue, weight loss

Genitourinary: Urinary retention, impotence

Neuromuscular & skeletal: Weakness, numbness, tingling, paresthesia, incoordination, ataxia, tremor, peripheral neuropathy, extrapyramidal symptoms

Ocular: Blurred vision, disturbances of accommodation, mydriasis

Otic: Tinnitus

Miscellaneous: Diaphoresis

Overdosage/Toxicology Symptoms of overdose include confusion, hallucinations, constipation, cyanosis, tachycardia, urinary retention, ventricular tachycardia, and seizures. Following initiation of essential overdose management, toxic symptoms should be treated. Ventricular arrhythmias often respond to (Continued)

Imipramine (Continued)

concurrent systemic alkalinization (sodium bicarbonate 0.5-2 mEq/kg I.V.) Physostigmine (1-2 mg I.V. slowly for adults) may be indicated to reverse life-threatening cardiac arrhythmias.

Pharmacodynamics/Kinetics

Onset of Action: Peak antidepressant effect: Usually after ≥2 weeks

Half-Life Elimination: 6-18 hours

Metabolism: Hepatic via CYP to desipramine (active) and other metabolites; significant first-pass effect

Excretion: Urine (as metabolites)

Available Dosage Forms

Capsule, as pamoate (Tofranil-PM®): 75 mg, 100 mg, 125 mg, 150 mg

Tablet, as hydrochloride (Tofranil®): 10 mg, 25 mg, 50 mg [generic tablets may contain sodium benzoate]

Dosing

Adults: Antidepressant:

Oral: Initial: 25 mg 3-4 times/day; increase dose gradually, total dose may be given at bedtime; maximum: 300 mg/day.

Note: Maximum antidepressant effect may not be seen for 2 or more weeks after initiation of therapy.

Elderly:

Antidepressant: Initial: 10-25 mg at bedtime; increase by 10-25 mg every 3 days for inpatients and weekly for outpatients if tolerated. Average daily dose to achieve a therapeutic concentration: 100 mg/day; range: 50-150 mg/day.

Urinary incontinence (urge or mixed type): 10-50 mg at bedtime or twice daily

Pediatrics:

Depression: Oral:

Children (unlabeled use): 1.5 mg/kg/day with dosage increments of 1 mg/kg every 3-4

Adolescents: Initial: 30-40 mg/day; increase gradually; maximum: 100 mg/day in single or divided doses. days to a maximum dose of 5 mg/kg/day in 1-4 divided doses; monitor carefully especially with doses ≥3.5 mg/kg/day.

Enuresis: Oral: Children ≥6 years: Initial: 25 mg at bedtime, if inadequate response still seen after 1 week of therapy, increase by 25 mg/day; dose should not exceed 2.5 mg/kg/day or 50 mg at bedtime if 6-12 years of age or 75 mg at bedtime if ≥12 years of age.

Adjunct in the treatment of cancer pain (unlabeled use): Oral: Children: Initial: 0.2-0.4 mg/kg at bedtime; dose may be increased by 50% every 2-3 days up to 1-3 mg/kg/dose at bedtime.

Laboratory Monitoring ECG, CBC

Nursing Actions

Physical Assessment: Assess other medications patient may be taking for effectiveness and interactions. Monitor laboratory tests, therapeutic response (eg, mental status, mood, affect, suicidal ideation), and adverse reactions at beginning of therapy and periodically with long-term use. Taper dosage slowly when discontinuing, if possible. Assess knowledge/ teach patient appropriate use, interventions to reduce side effects, and adverse symptoms to report.

Patient Education: Take exactly as directed; do not increase dose or frequency. It may take 2-3 weeks to achieve desired results. Take in the evening. Avoid alcohol, caffeine, and other prescription or OTC medications not approved by prescriber. Maintain adequate hydration (2-3 L/day of fluids) unless instructed to restrict fluid intake. You may experience drowsiness, lightheadedness, impaired coordination, dizziness, or blurred vision (use caution when driving or engaging in tasks requiring alertness until response to drug is known); nausea, vomiting, altered taste, dry mouth (small frequent meals, frequent mouth care,

chewing gum, or sucking lozenges may help); constipation (increased exercise, fluids, fruit, or fiber may help); diarrhea (buttermilk, yogurt, or boiled milk may help); postural hypotension (use caution when climbing stairs or changing position from lying or sitting to standing); or urinary retention (void before taking medication). Report persistent insomnia; muscle cramping or tremors; chest pain, palpitations, rapid heartbeat, swelling of extremities, or severe dizziness; unresolved urinary retention; rash or skin irritation; yellowing of eyes or skin; pale stools/dark urine; worsening of condition; and suicide ideation.

Pregnancy/breast-feeding precautions: Do not get pregnant while taking this medication; use appropriate contraceptive measures. Breast-feeding is not recommended.

Geriatric Considerations Orthostatic hypotension is a concern with this agent, especially in patients taking other medications that may affect blood pressure. May precipitate arrhythmias in predisposed patients; may aggravate seizures. A less anticholinergic antidepressant may be a better choice. Data from a clinical trial comparing fluoxetine to tricyclics suggests that fluoxetine is significantly less effective than nortriptyline in hospitalized elderly patients with unipolar major affective disorder, especially those with melancholia and concurrent cardiovascular diseases.

Related Information

Antidepressant Medication Guidelines *on page 1414*

Federal OBRA Regulations Recommended Maximum Doses *on page 1421*

Peak and Trough Guidelines *on page 1387*

Imiquimod (i mi KWI mod)

U.S. Brand Names Aldara™

Pharmacologic Category Skin and Mucous Membrane Agent; Topical Skin Product

Medication Safety Issues

Sound-alike/look-alike issues:

Aldara™ may be confused with Alora®

Pregnancy Risk Factor C

Lactation Excretion in breast milk unknown/consult prescriber

Use Treatment of external genital and perianal warts/ condyloma acuminata; nonhyperkeratotic, nonhypertrophic actinic keratosis on face or scalp; superficial basal cell carcinoma (sBCC) with a maximum tumor diameter of 2 cm located on the trunk, neck, or extremities (excluding hands or feet)

Unlabeled/Investigational Use Treatment of common warts

Mechanism of Action/Effect Mechanism of action is unknown; however, induces cytokines, including interferon-alpha and others

Contraindications Hypersensitivity to imiquimod or any component of the formulation

Warnings/Precautions Imiquimod has not been evaluated for the treatment of urethral, intravaginal, cervical, rectal, or intra-anal human papilloma viral disease and is not recommended for these conditions. Topical imiquimod is not intended for ophthalmic use. Topical imiquimod administration is not recommended until genital/perianal tissue is healed from any previous drug or surgical treatment. Imiquimod has the potential to exacerbate inflammatory conditions of the skin. Intense inflammatory reactions may occur, and may be accompanied by systemic symptoms (fever, malaise, myalgia); interruption of therapy should be considered. May increase sunburn susceptibility; patients should protect themselves from the sun. Use in basal cell carcinoma should be limited to superficial carcinomas with a maximum diameter of 2 cm. Efficacy in treatment of SBCC lesions of the face, head, and anogenital area, or other subtypes of basal cell carcinoma, have not been established. Safety and efficacy in immunosuppressed patients have not been established. Treatment of actinic keratosis should be limited to areas ≤5 cm². Safety and efficacy of repeated use in the same 25 cm² area has not been established. Safety and efficacy in patients <12 years of age have not been established.

Drug Interactions
Cytochrome P450 Effect: Substrate (minor) of CYP1A2, 3A4

Adverse Reactions
>10%:

Local: Application site reactions are common. Frequency of reactions vary, and are related to the degree of inflammation associated with the treated disease, number of weekly applications, and individual sensitivity. Symptoms of local reaction include burning, edema, erosion, erythema, excoriation/flaking, pain, pruritus, vesicles, and scabbing. In some cases, systemic symptoms (fever, malaise, myalgia, flu-like symptoms) occur, which should prompt consideration of an interruption of therapy.

Respiratory: Upper respiratory infection (15%)

1% to 10%:

Cardiovascular: Hypertension (1% to 3%), atrial fibrillation (1%)

Central nervous system: Pain (2% to 8%), headache (4% to 8%), fatigue (1% to 2%), fever (1% to 2%), dizziness (1%)

Dermatologic: Hyperkeratosis (2% to 9%), eczema (2%), alopecia (1%), hypopigmentation (1%), rash (<1% to 2%)

Endocrine & metabolic: Hypercholesterolemia (2%), gout (1%)

Gastrointestinal: Diarrhea (3%), dyspepsia (2% to 3%), nausea (1%)

Neuromuscular & skeletal: Myalgia (1%), back pain (<1% to 4%)

Respiratory: Sinusitis (7%), rhinitis (3%), pharyngitis (2%), coughing (2%)

Miscellaneous: Influenza-like symptoms (also see Local reactions; 1% to 3%), squamous cell carcinoma (4%)

Overdosage/Toxicology
Overdosage is unlikely because of minimal percutaneous absorption. Persistent topical overdosing of imiquimod could result in severe local skin reactions. The most clinically serious adverse event reported following multiple oral imiquimod doses ≥200 mg was hypotension that resolved following oral or I.V. fluid administration. Treat symptomatically.

Pharmacodynamics/Kinetics
Excretion: Urine and feces (<0.9%)

Available Dosage Forms
Cream: 5% (12s) [contains benzyl alcohol; single-dose packets]

Dosing
Adults & Elderly:

Perianal warts/condyloma acuminata: Topical: Apply a thin layer 3 times/week on alternative days prior to bedtime and leave on skin for 6-10 hours. Remove by washing with mild soap and water. Continue imiquimod treatment until there is total clearance of the genital/perianal warts for ≤16 weeks. A rest period of several days may be taken if required by the patient's discomfort or severity of the local skin reaction. Treatment may resume once the reaction subsides.

Actinic keratosis: Topical: Apply twice weekly for 16 weeks to a treatment area on face or scalp; apply prior to bedtime and leave on skin for 8 hours. Remove with mild soap and water.

Common warts (unlabeled use): Topical: Apply once daily prior to bedtime.

Superficial basal cell carcinoma: Topical: Apply once daily prior to bedtime, 5 days/week for 6 weeks. Treatment area should include a 1 cm margin of skin around the tumor. Leave on skin for 8 hours. Remove with mild soap and water.

Pediatrics: Perianal warts/condyloma acuminata: Topical: Children ≥12 years: Refer to adult dosing.

Administration
Topical:

Actinic keratosis: Treatment area should be a single contiguous area (approximately 25 cm²) on the face or scalp. Both areas should not be treated concurrently. No more than one packet should eb applied at each application. Apply a thin layer to the wart area and rub in until the cream is no longer visible. Avoid contact with the eyes, lips, and nostrils. Do not occlude the application site. Wash hands following application.

External genital warts: Nonocclusive dressings such as cotton gauze or cotton underwear may be used in the management of skin reactions. Handwashing before and after cream application is recommended. Imiquimod is packaged in single-use packets that contain sufficient cream to cover a wart area of up to 20 cm²; avoid use of excessive amounts of cream. Instruct patients to apply imiquimod to external or perianal warts; not for vaginal use. Apply a thin layer to the wart area and rub in until the cream is no longer visible. Do not occlude the application site. Wash hands following application.

Superficial basal cell carcinoma: Treatment area should have a maximum diameter no more than 2 cm on the trunk, neck, or extremities (excluding the hands and feet). Treatment area should include a 1 cm margin around the tumor. Apply a thin layer to the wart area (and margin) and rub in until the cream is no longer visible. Avoid contact with the eyes, lips, and nostrils. Do not occlude the application site. Wash hands following application.

Stability
Storage: Store below 25°C (77°F). Avoid freezing.

Nursing Actions
Physical Assessment: Teach patient appropriate use, possible side effects/appropriate interventions, and adverse symptoms to report.

Patient Education: This medication will not eliminate nor prevent the transmission of the virus. For external use only; avoid contact with eyes, mouth, or vagina. Use only as frequently as directed and apply as instructed. Exposure to sun should be avoided or minimized. Use sunscreen or wear protective clothing if sun exposure is unavoidable. Sexual contact (vaginal, anal, or oral) should be avoided while cream is on skin. May cause pain, itching, redness, burning, flaking, swelling, or scabbing in treated area. If these effects persist or become severe or open sores develop, stop treatment and notify prescriber. Prescriber may recommend a rest period of several days before resuming treatment. **Pregnancy/breast-feeding precautions:** Inform prescriber if you are or intend to become pregnant. This medication may weaken condoms or vaginal diaphragms; consult prescriber for appropriate forms of protection. Consult prescriber if breast-feeding.

Apply treatment just prior to sleeping and leave on 6-10 hours. Wash hands thoroughly before and after application. Wash and dry area to be treated before applying cream. After treatment period, remove cream with mild soap and water. Apply a thin layer to external warts and rub in until cream is no longer visible. Avoid use of excessive cream. May cover area with light gauze dressing or cotton underwear; do not apply occlusive dressing.

Immune Globulin (Intravenous)
(i MYUN GLOB yoo lin, IN tra VEE nus)

U.S. Brand Names Carimune™ NF; Gammagard®
Liquid; Gammagard® S/D; Gammar®-P I.V.; Gamunex®;
Iveegam EN; Octagam®; Panglobulin® NF; Polygam® S/
D

Synonyms IVIG

Pharmacologic Category Immune Globulin

Medication Safety Issues
Sound-alike/look-alike issues:
Gamimune® N may be confused with CytoGam®

Pregnancy Risk Factor C

Lactation Excretion in breast milk unknown

Use
Treatment of primary immunodeficiency syndromes
(congenital agammaglobulinemia, severe combined
immunodeficiency syndromes [SCIDS], common variable
immunodeficiency, X-linked immunodeficiency,
Wiskott-Aldrich syndrome); idiopathic thrombocytopenic
purpura (ITP); Kawasaki disease (in combination
with aspirin)
Prevention of bacterial infection in B-cell chronic
lymphocytic leukemia (CLL); pediatric HIV infection;
bone marrow transplant (BMT)

Unlabeled/Investigational Use Autoimmune diseases
(myasthenia gravis, SLE, bullous pemphigoid, severe
rheumatoid arthritis), Guillain-Barré syndrome; used in
conjunction with appropriate anti-infective therapy to
prevent or modify acute bacterial or viral infections in
patients with iatrogenically-induced or
disease-associated immunodepression; autoimmune
hemolytic anemia or neutropenia, refractory dermatomyositis/polymyositis

Mechanism of Action/Effect Replacement therapy for
primary and secondary immunodeficiencies; interference
with F_c receptors on the cells of the reticuloendothelial
system for autoimmune cytopenias and ITP;
possible role of contained antiviral-type antibodies

Contraindications Hypersensitivity to immune globulin
or any component of the formulation; selective IgA deficiency

Warnings/Precautions Anaphylactic hypersensitivity
reactions can occur, especially in IgA-deficient patients;
studies indicate that the currently available products
have no discernible risk of transmitting HIV or hepatitis
B; aseptic meningitis may occur with high doses (≥2 g/
kg). Use with caution in the elderly, patients with renal
disease, diabetes mellitus, volume depletion, sepsis,
paraproteinemia, and nephrotoxic medications due to
risk of renal dysfunction. Patients should be adequately
hydrated prior to therapy. Acute renal dysfunction
(increased serum creatinine, oliguria, acute renal
failure) can rarely occur; usually within 7 days of use
(more likely with products stabilized with sucrose). Use
caution in patients with a history of thrombotic events or
cardiovascular disease; there is clinical evidence of a
possible association between thrombotic events and
administration of intravenous immune globulin. For
intravenous administration only.

Drug Interactions
Decreased Effect: Decreased effect of live virus
vaccines (eg, measles, mumps, rubella); separate
administration by at least 3 months

Lab Interactions Octagam® contains maltose.
Falsely-elevated blood glucose levels may occur when
glucose monitoring devices and test strips utilizing the
glucose dehydrogenase pyrroloquinolinequinone
(GDH-PQQ) based methods are used. Glucose monitoring
devices and test strips which utilize the
glucose-specific method are recommended.

Adverse Reactions Frequency not defined.
Cardiovascular: Flushing of the face, tachycardia,
hyper-/hypotension, chest tightness, angioedema,
lightheadedness, chest pain, MI, CHF, pulmonary
embolism
Central nervous system: Anxiety, chills, dizziness,
drowsiness, fatigue, fever, headache, irritability, lethargy,
malaise, aseptic meningitis syndrome
Dermatologic: Pruritus, rash, urticaria
Gastrointestinal: Abdominal cramps, diarrhea, nausea,
sore throat, vomiting
Hematologic: Autoimmune hemolytic anemia, hematocrit
decreased, leukopenia, mild hemolysis
Hepatic: Liver function test increased
Local: Pain or irritation at the infusion site
Neuromuscular & skeletal: Arthralgia, back or hip pain,
myalgia, nuchal rigidity
Ocular: Photophobia, painful eye movements
Renal: Acute renal failure, acute tubular necrosis,
anuria, BUN increased, creatinine increased, nephrotic
syndrome, oliguria, proximal tubular nephropathy,
osmotic nephrosis
Respiratory: Cough, dyspnea, wheezing, nasal congestion,
pharyngeal pain, rhinorrhea, sinusitis
Miscellaneous: Diaphoresis, hypersensitivity reactions,
anaphylaxis

Pharmacodynamics/Kinetics
Onset of Action: I.V.: Provides immediate antibody
levels
Duration of Action: Immune effects: 3-4 weeks (variable)
Half-Life Elimination: IgG (variable among patients):
Healthy subjects: 14-24 days; Patients with congenital
humoral immunodeficiencies: 26-40 days; hypermetabolism
associated with fever and infection have
coincided with a shortened half-life

Available Dosage Forms
Injection, powder for reconstitution [preservative free]:
Gammar®-P I.V.: 5 g, 10 g [stabilized with human
albumin and sucrose]
Iveegam EN: 5 g [stabilized with glucose]
Injection, powder for reconstitution [preservative free,
nanofiltered]:
Carimune™ NF: 3 g, 6 g, 12 g [contains sucrose]
Panglobulin® NF: 6 g, 12 g [contains sucrose]
Injection, powder for reconstitution [preservative free,
solvent detergent-treated]:
Gammagard® S/D: 2.5 g, 5 g, 10 g [stabilized with
human albumin, glycine, glucose, and polyethylene
glycol]
Polygam® S/D: 5 g, 10 g [stabilized with human
albumin, glycine, glucose, and polyethylene glycol]
Injection, solution [preservative free; solvent detergent-treated]:
Gammagard® Liquid: 10% [100 mg/mL] (10 mL, 25
mL, 50 mL, 100 mL, 200 mL) [latex free, sucrose
free; stabilized with glycine]
Octagam®: 5% [50 mg/mL] (20 mL, 50 mL, 100 mL,
200 mL) [sucrose free; contains sodium 30 mmol/L
and maltose]
Injection, solution [preservative free] (Gamunex®): 10%
(10 mL, 25 mL, 50 mL, 100 mL, 200 mL) [caprylate/
chromatography purified]

Dosing
Adults & Elderly: Approved doses and regimens may
vary between brands; check manufacturer guidelines.
Note: Some clinicians dose IVIG on ideal body weight
or an adjusted ideal body weight in morbidly obese
patients.

Primary immunodeficiency disorders: I.V.:
200-400 mg/kg every 4 weeks or as per monitored
serum IgG concentrations
Gammagard® Liquid, Gamunex®, Octagam®:
300-600 mg/kg every 3-4 weeks; adjusted based
on dosage and interval in conjunction with monitored
serum IgG concentrations
B-cell chronic lymphocytic leukemia (CLL): I.V.:
400 mg/kg/dose every 3 weeks

Idiopathic thrombocytopenic purpura (ITP): I.V.:
Acute: 400 mg/kg/day for 5 days or 1000 mg/kg/day for 1-2 days
Chronic: 400 mg/kg as needed to maintain platelet count >30,000/mm³; may increase dose to 800 mg/kg (1000 mg/kg if needed)

Kawasaki disease: Initiate therapy within 10 days of disease onset: I.V.: 2 g/kg as a single dose administered over 10 hours, or 400 mg/kg/day for 4 days.
Note: Must be used in combination with aspirin: 80-100 mg/kg/day in 4 divided doses for 14 days; when fever subsides, dose aspirin at 3-5 mg/kg once daily for ≥6-8 weeks

Acquired immunodeficiency syndrome (patients must be symptomatic) (unlabeled use): I.V.: Various regimens have been used, including:
200-250 mg/kg/dose every 2 weeks
or
400-500 mg/kg/dose every month or every 4 weeks

Autoimmune hemolytic anemia and neutropenia (unlabeled use): I.V.: 1000 mg/kg/dose for 2-3 days

Autoimmune diseases (unlabeled use): I.V.: 400 mg/kg/day for 4 days

Bone marrow transplant: I.V.: 500 mg/kg beginning on days 7 and 2 pretransplant, then 500 mg/kg/week for 90 days post-transplant

Adjuvant to severe cytomegalovirus infections (unlabeled use): I.V.: 500 mg/kg/dose every other day for 7 doses

Guillain-Barré syndrome (unlabeled use): I.V.: Various regimens have been used, including:
400 mg/kg/day for 4 days
or
1000 mg/kg/day for 2 days
or
2000 mg/kg/day for one day

Refractory dermatomyositis (unlabeled use): I.V.: 2 g/kg/dose every month x 3-4 doses

Refractory polymyositis (unlabeled use): I.V.: 1 g/kg/day x 2 days every month x 4 doses

Chronic inflammatory demyelinating polyneuropathy (unlabeled use): I.V.: Various regimens have been used, including:
400 mg/kg/day for 5 doses once each month
or
800 mg/kg/day for 3 doses once each month
or
1000 mg/kg/day for 2 days once each month

Pediatrics: Approved doses and regimens may vary between brands; check manufacturer guidelines.
Note: Some clinicians dose IVIG on ideal body weight or an adjusted ideal body weight in morbidly obese patients.

Pediatric HIV: I.V.: 400 mg/kg every 28 days

Severe systemic viral and bacterial infections: Children: I.V.: 500-1000 mg/kg/week

Prevention of gastroenteritis: Infants and Children: Oral: 50 mg/kg/day divided every 6 hours

For additional indications, refer to adult dosing.

Renal Impairment: Cl$_{cr}$ <10 mL/minute: Avoid use; in patients at risk of renal dysfunction, consider infusion at a rate less than maximum.

Administration

I.V.: For I.V. use only; for initial treatment, a lower concentration and/or a slower rate of infusion should be used. Refrigerated product should be warmed to room temperature prior to infusion.

I.V. Detail: Infuse over 2-24 hours; administer in separate infusion line from other medications; if using primary line, flush with saline prior administration. Decrease dose, rate and/or concentration of infusion in patients who may be at risk of renal failure. Decreasing the rate or stopping the infusion may help relieve some adverse effects (flushing, changes in

pulse rate, changes in blood pressure). Epinephrine should be available during administration.
Carimune™ NF, Panglobulin® NF: pH 6.4-6.8
Gamimune®, Gamunex®: pH 4.0-4.5
Octagam®: pH 5.1-6.0

Stability

Reconstitution: Dilution is dependent upon the manufacturer and brand; do not shake, avoid foaming; discard unused portion:

Carimune™ NF, Panglobulin® NF: Reconstitute with NS, D$_5$W, or SWFI.
Iveegam EN: Reconstitute with SWFI; use immediately after reconstitution
Gammagard® Liquid: May dilute in D$_5$W only.
Gammagard® S/D, Polygam® S/D: Reconstitute with sterile water for injection.
Gammar®-P I.V.: Reconstitute with SWFI.
Gamunex®: Dilute in D$_5$W only.

Compatibility: Stable in D$_5$W, D$_{15}$W, D$_5$¼NS

Storage: Stability and dilution is dependent upon the manufacturer and brand; do not freeze:

Carimune™ NF, Panglobulin® NF: Prior to reconstitution, store at or below 30°C (86°F). Following reconstitution, store under refrigeration; use within 24 hours. Do not freeze.
Gammagard® Liquid: May be stored for up to 9 months at room temperature of 25°C (77°F) within 24 months of manufacture date. May be stored for up to 36 months under refrigeration at 2°C to 8°C (36°F to 46°F). Do not freeze.
Gammar®-P I.V., Gammagard® S/D, Polygam® S/D, Venoglobulin®-S: Store below 25°C (77°F).
Gammagard® S/D, Polygam® S/D: May store diluted solution under refrigeration for up to 24 hours.
Gamunex®: May be stored for up to 5 months at room temperature up to 25°C (up to 77°F) within 18 months of manufacture date.
Iveegam EN: Store at 2°C to 8°C (36°F to 46°F).
Octagam®: Store at 2°C to 8°C (36°F to 46°F) for 24 months or ≤25°C (77°F) for 18 months.
Polygam® S/D: Store at room temperature at or below 25°C (77°F); do not freeze.

Nursing Actions

Physical Assessment: Assess for history of previous allergic reactions. Monitor vital signs during infusion and observe for adverse or allergic reactions. Teach patient adverse symptoms to report.

Patient Education: This medication can only be administered by infusion. You will be monitored closely during the infusion. If you experience nausea ask for assistance, do not get up alone. Do not have any vaccinations for the next 3 months without consulting prescriber. Immediately report chills; chest pain, tightness, or rapid heartbeat; acute back pain; or respiratory difficulty. **Pregnancy/breast-feeding precautions:** Inform prescriber if you are or intend to become pregnant. Consult prescriber if breast-feeding.

Dietary Considerations Octagam® contains sodium 30 mmol/L

Additional Information

Intravenous Immune Globulin Product Comparison:

Carimune™ NF, Panglobulin® NF:
FDA indication: Primary immunodeficiency, ITP
Contraindication: IgA deficiency
IgA content: 720 mcg/mL
Plasma source: Pooled donors
Half-life: 23 days
IgG subclass (%):
IgG1 (60-70): 60.5
IgG2 (19-31): 30.2
IgG3 (5-8.4): 6.6
IgG4 (0.7-4): 2.8
Storage: Room temperature at or below 30°C (86°F); refrigerate after reconstitution

(Continued)

Immune Globulin (Intravenous)
(Continued)

Recommendations for **initial** infusion rate: 0.5-1 mL/minute

Maximum infusion rate: 2 mg/kg/minute

Gammagard® Liquid:
FDA indication: Primary immunodeficiency
Contraindication: IgA deficiency, history of anaphylaxis with immune globulin
IgA content: 37 mcg/mL
Half-life: 35 days
Storage: Room temperature (stable for 9 months) or refrigeration (stable for 36 months)
Recommendations for **initial** infusion rate: 0.5 mL/kg/hour
Maximum infusion rate: 5 mL/kg/hour; <2 mL/kg/hour in patients at risk for renal impairment or thrombosis

Gammagard® SD:
FDA indication: Primary immunodeficiency, ITP, CLL prophylaxis
Contraindication: None (caution with IgA deficiency)
IgA content: 0.92-1.6 mcg/mL
Adverse reactions (%): 6
Plasma source: 4000-5000 paid donors
Half-life: 24 days
IgG subclass (%):
IgG_1 (60-70): 67 (66.8)
IgG_2 (19-31): 25 (25.4)
IgG_3 (5-8.4): 5 (7.4)
IgG_4 (0.7-4): 3 (0.3)
Monomers (%): >95
Gamma globulin (%): >90
Storage: Room temperature
Recommendations for **initial** infusion rate: 0.5 mL/kg/hour
Maximum infusion rate: 4 mL/kg/hour
Maximum concentration for infusion (%): 5

Gammar®-P I.V.:
FDA indication: Primary immunodeficiency
Contraindication: IgA deficiency
IgA content: <20 mcg/mL
Adverse reactions (%): 15
Plasma source: >8000 paid donors
Half-life: 21-24 days
IgG subclass (%):
IgG_1 (60-70): 69
IgG_2 (19-31): 23
IgG_3 (5-8.4): 6
IgG_4 (0.7-4): 2
Monomers (%): >98
Gamma globulin (%): >98
Storage: Room temperature
Recommendations for **initial** infusion rate: 0.01-0.02 mL/kg/minute
Maximum infusion rate: 0.06 mL/kg/minute
Maximum concentration for infusion (%): 5

Gamunex®:
FDA indication: Primary immunodeficiency, ITP
Contraindication: Caution in severe, selective IgA deficiency
IgA content: 40 mcg/mL
IgM content: <2 mcg/mL
Plasma source: Pooled donors
Half-life: 36 days
IgG subclass (%):
IgG_1 (60-70): 65
IgG_2 (19-31): 26
IgG_3 (5-8.4): 5.6
IgG_4 (0.7-4): 2.6
Monomer + dimer (%): 100
Gamma globulin (%): >98
Storage: 2°C to 8°C; may be stored at room temperature for 5 months (only during first 18 months after manufacture)

Recommendations for **initial** infusion rate: 0.01 mL/kg/minute
Maximum infusion rate: 0.08 mL/kg/minute
Maximum concentration for infusion (%): 10

Octagam®:
FDA indication: Primary immunodeficiency
Contraindications: IgA deficiency
IgA content: 100 mcg/mL
Half-life: Immunodeficiency: 40 days
IgG subclass (%):
IgG_1 (60-70): 65
IgG_2 (19-31): 30
IgG_3 (5-8.4): 3
IgG_4 (0.7-4): 2
Monomers (%): ≥90
Gamma globulin (%): 96
Storage: Refrigerated or room temperature
Recommendations for initial infusion rate: 0.6 mL/kg/hour
Maximum infusion rate: 4 mL/kg/hour
Maximum concentration for infusion: 5%

Polygam®:
FDA indication: Primary immunodeficiency, ITP, CLL
Contraindication: None (caution with IgA deficiency)
IgA content: 0.74 ± 0.33 mcg/mL
Adverse reactions (%): 6
Plasma source: 50,000 voluntary donors
Half-life: 21-25 days
IgG subclass (%):
IgG_1 (60-70): 67
IgG_2 (19-31): 25
IgG_3 (5-8.4): 5
IgG_4 (0.7-4): 3
Monomers (%): >95
Gamma globulin (%): >90
Storage: Room temperature
Recommendations for **initial** infusion rate: 0.5 mL/kg/hour
Maximum infusion rate: 4 mL/kg/hour
Maximum concentration for infusion (%): 10

Immune Globulin (Subcutaneous)
(i MYUN GLOB yoo lin sub kyoo TAY nee us)

U.S. Brand Names Vivaglobin®
Synonyms Immune Globulin Subcutaneous (Human); SCIG
Pharmacologic Category Immune Globulin
Pregnancy Risk Factor C
Lactation Excretion in breast milk unknown/use caution
Use Treatment of primary immune deficiency (PID)
Mechanism of Action/Effect Immune globulin replacement therapy
Contraindications Hypersensitivity to immune globulin or any component of the formulation; history of anaphylactic or severe systemic reaction to immune globulin preparations; selective IgA deficiency with known antibody against IgA
Warnings/Precautions For subcutaneous administration only; not for I.V. use. Hypersensitivity reactions and anaphylactic reactions can occur; use caution with initial treatment, when switching brands of immune globulin, and with treatment interruptions of >8 weeks. Patients should be monitored for adverse events during and after the first infusion. Stop infusion with signs of infusion reaction (fever, chills, nausea, vomiting, and rarely shock); medications for the treatment of hypersensitivity reactions should be available for immediate use. Use caution with IgA deficiency; sensitization to IgA may cause anaphylactic reaction. Product of human plasma; may potentially contain infectious agents which could transmit disease. Screening of donors, as well as testing and/or inactivation or removal of certain viruses, reduces this risk. Infections thought to be transmitted by

this product should be reported to ZLB Behring at 1-800-504-5434. Safety and effectiveness for children <2 years of age have not been established.

Drug Interactions
Decreased Effect: Immune globulin may decrease the efficacy of immune response to live vaccines.

Lab Interactions Passively-transferred antibodies may yield false-positive serologic testing results; may yield false-positive direct and indirect Coombs' test

Adverse Reactions Adverse reactions can be expected to be similar to those experienced with other immune globulin products; percentages are reported as adverse events per patient; injection-site reactions decreased with subsequent infusions

>10%:
Central nervous system: Headache (32% to 48%), fever (3% to 25%)
Dermatologic: Rash (6% to 17%)
Gastrointestinal: Gastrointestinal disorder (5% to 37%), nausea (11% to 18%), sore throat (17%)
Local: Injection-site reactions (swelling, redness, itching; 92%)
Miscellaneous: Allergic reaction (11%)
1% to 10%:
Cardiovascular: Tachycardia (3%)
Central nervous system: Pain (10%)
Dermatologic: Skin disorder (3%)
Gastrointestinal: Diarrhea (10%)
Genitourinary: Urine abnormality (3%)
Neuromuscular & skeletal: Weakness (5%)
Respiratory: Cough (10%)

Overdosage/Toxicology Treatment should be symptom directed and supportive.

Pharmacodynamics/Kinetics
Time to Peak: Plasma: 2.5 days

Available Dosage Forms Injection, solution [preservative free]: IgG 160 mg/mL (3 mL, 10 mL, 20 mL)

Dosing
Adults & Elderly: Note: Consider premedicating with acetaminophen and diphenhydramine.

Primary immune deficiency: SubQ infusion: 100-200 mg/kg weekly (maximum rate: 20 mL/hour; doses >15 mL should be divided between sites); adjust the dose over time to achieve desired clinical response or target IgG levels

Conversion from I.V. to SubQ: Multiply previous I.V. dose by 1.37, then divide into a weekly regimen by dividing by the previous I.V. dosing interval (eg, if the dosing interval was every 3 weeks, divide by 3); adjust the dose over time to achieve desired clinical response or target IgG levels. SubQ infusion administration should begin 1 week after the last I.V. dose.

Pediatrics:
Children ≥2 years: Refer to adult dosing.

Administration
I.V. Detail: pH: 6.4-7.2

Other: Subcutaneous: Initial dose should be administered in a healthcare setting capable of providing monitoring and treatment in the event of hypersensitivity. Using aseptic technique, follow the infusion device manufacturer's instructions for filling the reservoir and preparing the pump. Remove air from administration set and needle by priming. Inject via infusion pump into the abdomen, thigh, upper arm, and/or lateral hip. The maximum rate is 20 mL/hour and maximum volume per injection site is 15 mL (doses >15 mL should be divided and infused into several sites). Select the number of required infusion sites; multiple concurrent injection sites may be achieved with the use of Y-site connection tubing; injection sites must be at least 2 inches apart. After the sites are clean and dry, insert subcutaneous needle and prime administration set. Attach sterile needle to administration set, gently pull back on the syringe to assure a blood vessel has not been inadvertently accessed.

Repeat for each injection site; infuse following instructions for the infusion device. Rotate the site(s) weekly. Treatment may be transitioned to the home/home care setting in the absence of adverse reactions.

Stability
Compatibility: Do not mix with other products.

Storage: Store at 2°C to 8°C (36°F to 46°F); do not freeze; do not shake. Store in original box until ready to use. Allow vial(s) to reach room temperature prior to use. The appearance of immune globulin (subcutaneous) may vary from colorless to light brown; do not use if cloudy or contains precipitate.

Laboratory Monitoring IgG levels

Nursing Actions
Physical Assessment: This medication can only be administered via SubQ infusion. Assess for history of previous allergic reaction. Monitor for an allergic reaction during infusion; have anaphylaxis kit available. Assess infusion site periodically during infusion. Observe for redness, swelling, or itching. Teach patient adverse symptoms to report. Teach patient appropriate infusion technique if patient is to self administer.

Patient Education: Do not have any vaccinations for at least 3 months unless approved by prescriber. You may experience headache, fever, rash, nausea, diarrhea, cough, or sore throat. Stop infusion and report signs of infusion reaction (fever, chills, nausea, vomiting, and rarely, shock) immediately. **Pregnancy/breast-feeding precautions:** Inform prescriber if you are or intend to become pregnant. Consult prescriber if breast-feeding.

Pregnancy Issues Animal studies have not been conducted. There are no adequate and well-controlled studies in pregnant women. Use during pregnancy only if clearly needed.

Additional Information Serum IgG levels may be drawn at any time. Subcutaneous weekly treatments provide more constant levels rather than the more pronounced peak and trough patterns observed with I.V. monthly immune globulin treatments.

Indapamide (in DAP a mide)

U.S. Brand Names Lozol®

Pharmacologic Category Diuretic, Thiazide-Related

Medication Safety Issues
Sound-alike/look-alike issues:
Indapamide may be confused with Iopidine®

Pregnancy Risk Factor B (manufacturer); D (expert analysis)

Lactation Excretion in breast milk unknown

Use Management of mild to moderate hypertension; treatment of edema in congestive heart failure and nephrotic syndrome

Mechanism of Action/Effect Enhances sodium, chloride, and water excretion by interfering with the transport of sodium ions across the renal tubular epithelium

Contraindications Hypersensitivity to indapamide or any component of the formulation, thiazides, or sulfonamide-derived drugs; anuria; renal decompensation; pregnancy (based on expert analysis)

Warnings/Precautions Use with caution in severe renal disease. Use with caution in severe hepatic dysfunction; hepatic encephalopathy can be caused by electrolyte disturbances. Gout may be precipitated in patients with a history of gout, a familial predisposition to gout, or chronic renal failure. Use caution in patients with diabetes; may alter glucose control. May cause SLE exacerbation or activation. Use with caution in patients with moderate or high cholesterol concentrations. Photosensitization may occur. Correct hypokalemia
(Continued)

Indapamide *(Continued)*

before initiating therapy. Electrolyte disturbances (hypokalemia, hypochloremic alkalosis, hyponatremia) may occur with use.

Chemical similarities are present among sulfonamides, sulfonylureas, carbonic anhydrase inhibitors, thiazides, and loop diuretics (except ethacrynic acid). Use in patients with thiazide or sulfonamide allergy is specifically contraindicated in product labeling, however, a risk of cross-reaction exists in patients with allergy to any of these compounds; avoid use when previous reaction has been severe.

Drug Interactions

Decreased Effect: Effects of oral hypoglycemics may be decreased. Decreased absorption of indapamide with cholestyramine and colestipol. NSAIDs can decrease the efficacy of thiazide-type diuretics, reducing the diuretic and antihypertensive effects.

Increased Effect/Toxicity: The diuretic effect of indapamide is synergistic with furosemide and other loop diuretics. Increased hypotension and/or renal adverse effects of ACE inhibitors may result in aggressively diuresed patients. Cyclosporine and thiazide-type diuretics can increase the risk of gout or renal toxicity. Digoxin toxicity can be exacerbated if a diuretic induces hypokalemia or hypomagnesemia. Lithium toxicity can occur with thiazide-type diuretics due to reduced renal excretion of lithium. Thiazide-type diuretics may prolong the duration of action of neuromuscular blocking agents.

Nutritional/Ethanol Interactions Herb/Nutraceutical: Avoid dong quai if using for hypertension (has estrogenic activity). Avoid ephedra, yohimbe, ginseng (may worsen hypertension). Avoid garlic (may have increased antihypertensive effect).

Adverse Reactions 1% to 10%:

Cardiovascular: Orthostatic hypotension, palpitation (<5%), flushing

Central nervous system: Dizziness (<5%), lightheadedness (<5%), vertigo (<5%), headache (≥5%), restlessness (<5%), drowsiness (<5%), fatigue, lethargy, malaise, lassitude, anxiety, agitation, depression, nervousness (≥5%)

Dermatologic: Rash (<5%), pruritus (<5%), hives (<5%)

Endocrine & metabolic: Hyperglycemia (<5%), hyperuricemia (<5%)

Gastrointestinal: Anorexia, gastric irritation, nausea, vomiting, abdominal pain, cramping, bloating, diarrhea, constipation, dry mouth, weight loss

Genitourinary: Nocturia, frequent urination, polyuria, impotence (<5%), reduced libido (<5%), glycosuria (<5%)

Neuromuscular & skeletal: Muscle cramps, spasm, weakness (≥5%)

Ocular: Blurred vision (<5%)

Renal: Necrotizing angiitis, vasculitis, cutaneous vasculitis (<5%)

Respiratory: Rhinorrhea (<5%)

Overdosage/Toxicology Symptoms of overdose include lethargy, diuresis, hypermotility, confusion, and muscle weakness. Treatment is supportive.

Pharmacodynamics/Kinetics

Onset of Action: 1-2 hours

Duration of Action: ≤36 hours

Time to Peak: 2-2.5 hours

Protein Binding: Plasma: 71% to 79%

Half-Life Elimination: 14-18 hours

Metabolism: Extensively hepatic

Excretion: Urine (~60%) within 48 hours; feces (~16% to 23%)

Available Dosage Forms

Tablet: 1.25 mg, 2.5 mg

Lozol®: 1.25 mg

Dosing

Adults & Elderly:

Edema (diuretic): Oral: 2.5-5 mg/day. **Note:** There is little therapeutic benefit to increasing the dose >5 mg/day; there is, however, an increased risk of electrolyte disturbances.

Hypertension: Oral: 1.25 mg in the morning, may increase to 5 mg/day by increments of 1.25-2.5 mg; consider adding another antihypertensive and decreasing the dose if response is not adequate.

Administration

Oral: May be taken with food or milk. Take early in day to avoid nocturia. Take the last dose of multiple doses no later than 6 PM unless instructed otherwise.

Laboratory Monitoring Serum electrolytes, renal function

Nursing Actions

Physical Assessment: Allergy history should be assessed prior to beginning therapy (sulfonamides, thiazides). Assess potential for interactions with other pharmacological agents or herbal products patient may be taking (eg, altered effect of oral hypoglycemics, increased risk of hypotension or toxicity). Assess results of laboratory tests, therapeutic effectiveness (according to purpose for use), and adverse response (hypotension, hypokalemia, confusion) at regular intervals during therapy. Instruct patients with diabetes to monitor glucose levels closely; may interfere with oral hypoglycemic medications. Teach patient proper use, possible side effects (eg, orthostatic hypotension, photosensitivity) and appropriate interventions, and adverse symptoms to report.

Patient Education: Do not take any new medication during therapy unless approved by prescriber. Take as directed, early in the day. Do not exceed recommended dosage. This medication does not replace other antihypertensive interventions; follow prescriber's instructions for diet and lifestyle changes. If you have diabetes, monitor serum glucose closely (medication may decrease effect of oral hypoglycemics). Monitor weight on a regular basis. Report sudden or excessive weight gain (>5 lb/week), swelling of ankles or hands, or respiratory difficulty. You may experience dizziness, weakness, or drowsiness (use caution when rising from sitting or lying position, when climbing stairs and when driving or engaging in tasks that require alertness until response to drug is known); sensitivity to sunlight (use sunblock, wear protective clothing or sunglasses); impotence (reversible); or dry mouth or thirst (frequent mouth care, chewing gum, or sucking lozenges may help). Report any changes in visual acuity; unusual bleeding; chest pain or palpitations; or numbness, tingling, cramping of muscles. **Pregnancy/breast-feeding precaution:** Inform prescriber if you are pregnant. Consult prescriber if breast-feeding.

Dietary Considerations May be taken with food or milk to decrease GI adverse effects.

Geriatric Considerations Thiazide diuretics lose efficacy when Cl$_{cr}$ is <30-35 mL/minute. Many elderly may have Cl$_{cr}$ below this limit. Calculate Cl$_{cr}$ for elderly before initiating therapy. Indapamide has the advantage over thiazide diuretics in that it is effective when Cl$_{cr}$ is <30 mL/minute.

Indinavir (in DIN a veer)

U.S. Brand Names Crixivan®

Synonyms Indinavir Sulfate

Pharmacologic Category Antiretroviral Agent, Protease Inhibitor

Medication Safety Issues
Sound-alike/look-alike issues:
Indinavir may be confused with Denavir™

Pregnancy Risk Factor C

Lactation Enters breast milk/contraindicated

Use Treatment of HIV infection; should always be used as part of a multidrug regimen (at least three antiretroviral agents)

Mechanism of Action/Effect Indinavir is a protease inhibitor which prevents cleavage of protein precursors essential for HIV infection of new cells and viral replication.

Contraindications Hypersensitivity to indinavir or any component of the formulation; concurrent use of amiodarone, cisapride, triazolam, midazolam, pimozide, or ergot alkaloids

Warnings/Precautions Because indinavir may cause nephrolithiasis/urolithiasis the drug should be discontinued if signs and symptoms occur. Adequate hydration is recommended. May cause tubulointerstitial nephritis (rare); severe asymptomatic leukocyturia may warrant evaluation. Indinavir should not be administered concurrently with lovastatin or simvastatin (caution with atorvastatin and cerivastatin) because of competition for metabolism of these drugs through the CYP3A4 system, and potential serious or life-threatening events. Use caution with other drugs metabolized by this enzyme (particular caution with phosphodiesterase-5 inhibitors, including sildenafil). Avoid concurrent use of St John's wort. Patients with hepatic insufficiency due to cirrhosis should have dose reduction. Warn patients about fat redistribution that can occur. Indinavir has been associated with hemolytic anemia (discontinue if diagnosed), hepatitis, and hyperglycemia (exacerbation or new-onset diabetes). Treatment may result in immune reconstitution syndrome (acute inflammatory response to indolent or residual opportunistic infections). Use caution in patients with hemophilia; spontaneous bleeding has been reported.

Drug Interactions
Cytochrome P450 Effect: Substrate of CYP2D6 (minor), 3A4 (major); **Inhibits** CYP2C8/9 (weak), 2C19 (weak), 2D6 (weak), 3A4 (strong)

Decreased Effect: The levels/effects of indinavir may be decreased by aminoglutethimide, carbamazepine, nafcillin, nevirapine, phenobarbital, phenytoin, rifamycins, and other CYP3A4 inducers; dosage adjustment may be recommended (see individual agents). Rifampin and/or St John's wort (*Hypericum perforatum*); should not be used with indinavir.

Increased Effect/Toxicity: Indinavir may increase the levels/effects of selected benzodiazepines, calcium channel blockers, cyclosporine, mirtazapine, nateglinide, nefazodone, quinidine, sildenafil (and other PDE-5 inhibitors), tacrolimus, venlafaxine, and other CYP3A4 substrates. Selected benzodiazepines (midazolam, triazolam), cisapride, ergot alkaloids, selected HMG-CoA reductase inhibitors (lovastatin and simvastatin), mesoridazine, pimozide, and thioridazine are generally contraindicated with strong CYP3A4 inhibitors. When used with strong CYP3A4 inhibitors, dosage adjustment/limits are recommended for sildenafil and other PDE-5 inhibitors; refer to individual monographs.

Itraconazole or ketoconazole may increase the serum concentrations of indinavir; dosage adjustment is recommended. The levels/effects of indinavir may be increased by azole antifungals, clarithromycin, diclofenac, doxycycline, erythromycin, imatinib, isoniazid, nefazodone, nicardipine, propofol, protease inhibitors, quinidine, telithromycin, verapamil, and other CYP3A4 inhibitors.

When used with delavirdine, serum levels of indinavir are increased; dosage adjustment of indinavir may be required for this combination. Serum levels of both nelfinavir and indinavir are increased with concurrent use. Serum concentrations of indinavir may be increased by ritonavir; serum levels of ritonavir and saquinavir may be increased; dosage adjustments of indinavir are required during concurrent therapy. Rifabutin serum concentrations has been increased when coadministered with indinavir; dosage adjustments of both agents required. Concurrent use or atazanavir with indinavir may increase the risk of hyperbilirubinemia.

Nutritional/Ethanol Interactions
Food: Indinavir bioavailability may be decreased if taken with food. Meals high in calories, fat, and protein result in a significant decrease in drug levels. Indinavir serum concentrations may be decreased by grapefruit juice.

Herb/Nutraceutical: St John's wort *(Hypericum)* appears to induce CYP3A enzymes and has lead to 57% reductions in indinavir AUCs and 81% reductions in trough serum concentrations, which may lead to treatment failures; should not be used concurrently with indinavir.

Adverse Reactions Protease inhibitors cause dyslipidemia which includes elevated cholesterol and triglycerides and a redistribution of body fat centrally to cause increased abdominal girth, buffalo hump, facial atrophy, and breast enlargement. These agents also cause hyperglycemia (exacerbation or new-onset diabetes).

>10%:
Gastrointestinal: Nausea (12%)
Hepatic: Hyperbilirubinemia (14%)
Renal: Nephrolithiasis/urolithiasis (29%, pediatric patients; 12% adult patients)

1% to 10%:
Central nervous system: Headache (6%), insomnia (3%)
Gastrointestinal: Abdominal pain (9%), diarrhea/vomiting (4% to 5%), taste perversion (3%)
Neuromuscular & skeletal: Weakness (4%), flank pain (3%)
Renal: Hematuria

Pharmacodynamics/Kinetics
Time to Peak: 0.8 ± 0.3 hour
Protein Binding: Plasma: 60%
Half-Life Elimination: 1.8 ± 0.4 hour
Metabolism: Hepatic via CYP3A4 enzymes; seven metabolites of indinavir identified
Excretion: Urine and feces

Available Dosage Forms Capsule: 100 mg, 200 mg, 333 mg, 400 mg

Dosing
Adults & Elderly: HIV Infection: Oral:
Unboosted regimen: 800 mg every 8 hours
Ritonavir-boosted regimens:
Ritonavir 100-200 mg twice daily plus indinavir 800 mg twice daily **or**
Ritonavir 400 mg twice daily plus indinavir 400 mg twice daily
Dosage adjustments for indinavir when administered in combination therapy:
Delavirdine, itraconazole, or ketoconazole: Reduce indinavir dose to 600 mg every 8 hours
Efavirenz: Increase indinavir dose to 1000 mg every 8 hours
Lopinavir and ritonavir (Kaletra™): Indinavir 600 mg twice daily
(Continued)

Indinavir *(Continued)*

Nelfinavir: Increase indinavir dose to 1200 mg twice daily

Nevirapine: Increase indinavir dose to 1000 mg every 8 hours

Rifabutin: Reduce rifabutin to 1/2 the standard dose plus increase indinavir to 1000 mg every 8 hours

Pediatrics: HIV: Children 4-15 years (investigational): 500 mg/m^2 every 8 hours

Hepatic Impairment: 600 mg every 8 hours with mild/medium impairment due to cirrhosis or with ketoconazole coadministration

Administration

Oral: Drink at least 48 oz of water daily. Administer with water, 1 hour before or 2 hours after a meal. Administer around-the-clock to avoid significant fluctuation in serum levels. May be taken with food when administered in combination with ritonavir.

Stability

Storage: Capsules are sensitive to moisture; medication should be stored and used in the original container and the desiccant should remain in the bottle

Laboratory Monitoring Monitor viral load, CD4 count, triglycerides, cholesterol, glucose, liver function tests, CBC, urinalysis (severe leukocyturia should be monitored frequently).

Nursing Actions

Physical Assessment: Assess potential for interactions with other pharmacological agents and herbal products patient may be taking. A list of medications that should not be used is available in each bottle and patients should be provided with this information. Monitor laboratory tests, patient response, and adverse reactions (eg, gastrointestinal disturbance [nausea, vomiting, diarrhea] that can lead to dehydration and weight loss; hyperlipidemia and redistribution of body fat; rash; CNS effects [malaise, insomnia, abnormal thinking]; electrolyte imbalance) at regular intervals during therapy. Teach patient proper use (eg, timing of multiple medications and drugs that should not be used concurrently), possible side effects/appropriate interventions (eg, glucose testing; protease inhibitors may cause hyperglycemia, exacerbation or new-onset diabetes; use of barrier contraceptives; protease inhibitors may decrease effectiveness of oral contraceptives), and adverse symptoms to report.

Patient Education: You will be provided with a list of specific medications that should not be used during therapy; do not take any new prescriptions, over-the-counter medications, or herbal products (even if they are not on the list) without consulting prescriber. This is not a cure for HIV, nor has it been found to reduce transmission of HIV; use appropriate precautions to prevent spread to other persons. Take as directed with meals. Maintain adequate hydration (2-3 L/day of fluids) unless instructed to restrict fluid intake. This medication will be prescribed with a combination of other medications; time these medications as directed by prescriber. You may be advised to check your glucose levels; this class of drug can cause hyperglycemia. Frequent blood tests may be required with prolonged therapy. You may be susceptible to infection; avoid crowds and exposure to known infections and do not have any vaccinations without consulting prescriber. May cause body changes due to redistribution of body fat, facial atrophy, or breast enlargement (normal effects of drug); headache, dizziness, or fatigue (use caution when driving or engaged in potentially hazardous tasks until response to drug is known); nausea or vomiting (small frequent meals, frequent mouth care, chewing gum, or sucking lozenges may help); diarrhea (buttermilk, boiled milk, or yogurt may help); back pain, or arthralgia (consult prescriber for approved analgesic). Inform prescriber if you experience muscle numbness or tingling; unresolved persistent vomiting, diarrhea, or abdominal pain; respiratory difficulty or chest pain; unusual skin rash; change in color of stool or urine; or any persistent adverse effects. **Pregnancy/breast-feeding precautions:** Inform prescriber if you are or intend to become pregnant. Effectiveness of oral contraceptives may be decreased; use of alternative (nonhormonal) forms of contraception is recommended; consult prescriber for appropriate contraceptives. Do not breast-feed.

Dietary Considerations Should be taken without food but with water 1 hour before or 2 hours after a meal. Administration with lighter meals (eg, dry toast, skim milk, corn flakes) resulted in little/no change in indinavir concentration. If taking with ritonavir, may take with food. Patient should drink at least 48 oz of water daily. May be taken with food when administered in combination with ritonavir.

Breast-Feeding Issues Indinavir is minimally excreted in breast milk. HIV-infected mothers are discouraged from breast-feeding to decrease potential transmission of HIV.

Pregnancy Issues Safety and pharmacokinetic studies are currently underway in pregnant women; hyperbilirubinemia may be exacerbated in neonates and indinavir plasma levels may be lower in pregnant women. Pregnancy and protease inhibitors are both associated with an increased risk of hyperglycemia. Glucose levels should be closely monitored. The Perinatal HIV Guidelines Working Group considers indinavir to be an alternative PI if nelfinavir or saquinavir/ritonavir are not able to be used. Healthcare professionals are encouraged to contact the antiretroviral pregnancy registry to monitor outcomes of pregnant women exposed to antiretroviral medications (1-800-258-4263 or www.APRegistry.com).

Indomethacin *(in doe METH a sin)*

U.S. Brand Names Indocin®; Indocin® I.V.; Indocin® SR

Synonyms Indometacin; Indomethacin Sodium Trihydrate

Restrictions A medication guide should be dispensed with each prescription. A template for the required MedGuide can be found on the FDA website at: http://www.fda.gov/medwatch/SAFETY/2005/safety05.htm#NSAID

Pharmacologic Category Nonsteroidal Anti-inflammatory Drug (NSAID), Oral; Nonsteroidal Anti-inflammatory Drug (NSAID), Parenteral

Medication Safety Issues

Sound-alike/look-alike issues:

Indocin® may be confused with Imodium®, Lincocin®, Minocin®, Vicodin®

Pregnancy Risk Factor C/D (3rd trimester)

Lactation Enters breast milk/use caution (AAP rates "compatible")

Use Acute gouty arthritis, acute bursitis/tendonitis, moderate to severe osteoarthritis, rheumatoid arthritis, ankylosing spondylitis; I.V. form used as alternative to surgery for closure of patent ductus arteriosus in neonates

Mechanism of Action/Effect Inhibits prostaglandin synthesis by decreasing the activity of the enzyme, cyclooxygenase, which results in decreased formation of prostaglandin precursors

Contraindications Hypersensitivity to indomethacin, aspirin, other NSAIDs, or any component of the formulation; perioperative pain in the setting of coronary artery bypass surgery (CABG); pregnancy (3rd trimester)

Neonates: Necrotizing enterocolitis, impaired renal function, active bleeding, thrombocytopenia, coagulation defects, untreated infection

Warnings/Precautions NSAIDs are associated with an increased risk of adverse cardiovascular events, including MI, stroke, and new onset or worsening of pre-existing hypertension. Risk may be increased with duration of use or pre-existing cardiovascular risk-factors or disease. Carefully evaluate individual cardiovascular risk profiles prior to prescribing. Use caution with fluid retention, CHF or hypertension.

Use of NSAIDs can compromise existing renal function. Renal toxicity can occur in patient with impaired renal function, dehydration, heart failure, liver dysfunction, those taking diuretics and ACEI and the elderly. Rehydrate patient before starting therapy. Monitor renal function closely. Indomethacin is not recommended for patients with advanced renal disease.

NSAIDs may increase risk of gastrointestinal irritation, ulceration, bleeding, and perforation. These events may occur at any time during therapy and without warning. Use caution with a history of GI disease (bleeding or ulcers), concurrent therapy with aspirin, anticoagulants and/or corticosteroids, smoking, use of alcohol, the elderly or debilitated patients.

Use the lowest effective dose for the shortest duration of time, consistent with individual patient goals, to reduce risk of cardiovascular or GI adverse events. Alternate therapies should be considered for patients at high risk.

NSAIDs may cause serious skin adverse events including exfoliative dermatitis, Stevens-Johnson syndrome (SJS) and toxic epidermal necrolysis (TEN). Anaphylactoid reactions may occur, even without prior exposure; patients with "aspirin triad" (bronchial asthma, aspirin intolerance, rhinitis) may be at increased risk. Do not use in patients who experience bronchospasm, asthma, rhinitis, or urticaria with NSAID or aspirin therapy.

Use with caution in patients with decreased hepatic function. Closely monitor patients with any abnormal LFT. Severe hepatic reactions (eg, fulminant hepatitis, liver failure) have occurred with NSAID use, rarely; discontinue if signs or symptoms of liver disease develop, or if systemic manifestations occur.

Withhold for at least 4-6 half-lives prior to surgical or dental procedures.

Drug Interactions
Cytochrome P450 Effect: Substrate (minor) of CYP2C8/9, 2C19; **Inhibits** CYP2C8/9 (strong), 2C19 (weak)

Decreased Effect: May reduce effect of some diuretics and antihypertensive effect of beta-blockers, ACE inhibitors, angiotensin II inhibitors, hydralazine Cholestyramine and colestipol may reduce absorption of indomethacin.

Increased Effect/Toxicity: Indomethacin may increase effect/toxicity of anticoagulants (bleeding), antiplatelet agents (bleeding), aminoglycosides, biphosphonates (GI irritation), corticosteroids (GI irritation), cyclosporine (nephrotoxicity), lithium, methotrexate, pemetrexed, treprostinil (bleeding), vancomycin. Tilundronate serum concentrations may be increased. CYP2C8/9 substrates (eg, amiodarone, fluoxetine, glimepiride, glipizide, nateglinide, phenytoin, pioglitazone, rosiglitazone, sertraline, and warfarin) serum concentrations may be increased with concurrent use.

Nutritional/Ethanol Interactions
Ethanol: Avoid ethanol (may enhance gastric mucosal irritation).
Food: Food may decrease the rate but not the extent of absorption. Indomethacin peak serum levels may be delayed if taken with food.
Herb/Nutraceutical: Avoid alfalfa, anise, bilberry, bladderwrack, bromelain, cat's claw, celery, coleus, cordyceps, dong quai, evening primrose, feverfew, fenugreek, garlic, ginger, ginkgo biloba, red clover, horse chestnut, grapeseed, green tea, ginseng, guggul, horse chestnut seed, horseradish, licorice, prickly ash, red clover, reishi, SAMe, sweet clover, turmeric, white willow (all have additional antiplatelet activity).

Lab Interactions False-negative dexamethasone suppression test

Adverse Reactions
>10%: Central nervous system: Headache (12%)
1% to 10%:
  Central nervous system: Dizziness (3% to 9%), drowsiness (<1%), fatigue (<3%), vertigo (<3%), depression (<3%), malaise (<3%), somnolence (<3%)
  Gastrointestinal: Nausea (3% to 9%), epigastric pain (3% to 9%), abdominal pain/cramps/distress (<3%), heartburn (3% to 9%), indigestion (3% to 9%), constipation (<3%), diarrhea (<3%), dyspepsia (3% to 9%), vomiting
  Otic: Tinnitus (<3%)

Overdosage/Toxicology Symptoms of overdose include drowsiness, lethargy, nausea, vomiting, seizures, paresthesia, headache, dizziness, GI bleeding, cerebral edema, tinnitus, leukocytosis, and renal failure. Management of NSAID intoxication is supportive and symptomatic.

Pharmacodynamics/Kinetics
Onset of Action: ~30 minutes
Duration of Action: 4-6 hours
Time to Peak: Oral: 2 hours
Protein Binding: 99%
Half-Life Elimination: 4.5 hours; prolonged with neonates
Metabolism: Hepatic; significant enterohepatic recirculation
Excretion: Urine (60%, primarily as glucuronide conjugates); feces (33%, primarily as metabolites)

Available Dosage Forms
Capsule (Indocin®): 25 mg, 50 mg
Capsule, sustained release (Indocin® SR): 75 mg
Injection, powder for reconstitution, as sodium trihydrate (Indocin® I.V.): 1 mg
Suspension, oral (Indocin®): 25 mg/5 mL (237 mL) [contains alcohol 1%; pineapple-coconut-mint flavor]

Dosing
Adults & Elderly:
Inflammatory/rheumatoid disorders (use lowest effective dose): Oral: 25-50 mg/dose 2-3 times/day; maximum dose: 200 mg/day; extended release capsule should be given on a 1-2 times/day schedule; maximum dose for sustained release is 150 mg/day. In patients with arthritis and persistent night pain and/or morning stiffness may give the larger portion (up to 100 mg) of the total daily dose at bedtime.
Bursitis/tendonitis: Oral: Initial dose: 75-150 mg/day in 3-4 divided doses; usual treatment is 7-14 days
Acute gouty arthritis: Oral: 50 mg 3 times daily until pain is tolerable then reduce dose; usual treatment <3-5 days
Pediatrics:
Patent ductus arteriosus:
Neonates: I.V.: Initial: 0.2 mg/kg, followed by 2 doses depending on postnatal age (PNA):
  PNA at time of FIRST dose <48 hours: 0.1 mg/kg at 12- to 24-hour intervals
  PNA at time of FIRST dose 2-7 days: 0.2 mg/kg at 12- to 24-hour intervals
  PNA at time of FIRST dose >7 days: 0.25 mg/kg at 12- to 24-hour intervals
Note: In general, may use 12-hour dosing interval if urine output >1 mL/kg/hour after prior dose; use 24-hour dosing interval if urine output is <1 mL/kg/hour but >0.6 mL/kg/hour; doses should be withheld if patient has oliguria (urine output <0.6 mL/kg/hour) or anuria

(Continued)

Indomethacin (Continued)

Inflammatory/rheumatoid disorders: Children: Oral: 1-2 mg/kg/day in 2-4 divided doses; maximum dose: 4 mg/kg/day; not to exceed 150-200 mg/day

Renal Impairment: Not recommended with advanced renal disease.

Administration

Oral: Administer with food, milk, or antacids to decrease GI adverse effects. Extended release capsules must be swallowed whole, do not crush.

I.V.: Administer over 20-30 minutes at a concentration of 0.5-1 mg/mL in preservative-free sterile water for injection or normal saline. Reconstitute I.V. formulation just prior to administration; discard any unused portion; avoid I.V. bolus administration or infusion via an umbilical catheter into vessels near the superior mesenteric artery as these may cause vasoconstriction and can compromise blood flow to the intestines. Do not administer intra-arterially.

I.V. Detail: pH: 6.0-7.5

Stability

Reconstitution: Reconstitute just prior to administration; discard any unused portion. Do not use preservative-containing diluents for reconstitution.

Compatibility: Stable in NS

Y-site administration: Incompatible with amino acid injection, calcium gluconate, cimetidine, dobutamine, dopamine, gentamicin, levofloxacin, tobramycin, tolazoline

Storage: I.V.: Store below 30°C (86°F). Protect from light.

Laboratory Monitoring Renal function (serum creatinine and BUN), CBC, liver function

Nursing Actions

Physical Assessment: Assess potential for interactions with other prescriptions, OTC medications, or herbal products patient may be taking. Monitor blood pressure at the beginning of therapy and periodically during use. Monitor laboratory tests, therapeutic effectiveness (according to rationale for use), and adverse response when beginning therapy and at regular intervals during treatment. Teach patient proper use, side effects/appropriate interventions (regular ophthalmic evaluations with long-term use), and adverse symptoms to report.

Patient Education: Do not take any new medication during therapy without consulting prescriber. Use exactly as directed; do not increase dose without consulting prescriber. Do not crush, break, or chew capsules. Take with food or milk to reduce GI distress. Maintain adequate hydration (2-3 L/day of fluids) unless instructed to restrict fluid intake. May cause drowsiness, dizziness, nervousness, or headache (use caution when driving or engaging in tasks that require alertness until response to drug is known); anorexia, nausea, vomiting, or heartburn (small frequent meals, frequent mouth care, chewing gum, or sucking lozenges may help); fluid retention (weigh yourself weekly and report unusually weight gain >3-5 lb/week); or may turn urine green (normal). GI bleeding, ulceration, or perforation can occur with or without pain; discontinue medication and contact prescriber if persistent abdominal pain or cramping or blood in stool occurs. Report difficult breathing or unusual cough; chest pain, rapid heartbeat, or palpitations; unusual bruising or bleeding; blood in urine, gums, or vomitus; swollen extremities; skin rash, irritation, or itching; acute persistent fatigue; or vision changes or ringing in ears. **Pregnancy/breast-feeding precautions:** Inform prescriber if you are or intend to become pregnant. This drug should not be used in the 3rd trimester of pregnancy. Consult prescriber if breast-feeding.

Dietary Considerations May cause GI upset; take with food or milk to minimize

Geriatric Considerations Elderly are at high risk for adverse effects from NSAIDs. As much as 60% of elderly can develop peptic ulceration and/or hemorrhage asymptomatically. The concomitant use of H₂ blockers, omeprazole, and sucralfate is not effective as prophylaxis with the exception of NSAID-induced duodenal ulcers which may be prevented by the use of ranitidine. Misoprostol is the only prophylactic agent proven effective. Also, concomitant disease and drug use contribute to the risk for GI adverse effects. Use lowest effective dose for shortest period possible. Consider renal function decline with age. Use of NSAIDs can compromise existing renal function especially when Cl_cr is ≤30 mL/minute. Tinnitus may be a difficult and unreliable indication of toxicity due to age-related hearing loss or eighth cranial nerve damage. CNS adverse effects such as confusion, agitation, and hallucination are generally seen in overdose or high-dose situations, but elderly may demonstrate these adverse effects at lower doses than younger adults. Indomethacin frequently causes confusion at recommended doses in the elderly.

Infliximab (in FLIKS e mab)

U.S. Brand Names Remicade®

Synonyms Infliximab, Recombinant

Pharmacologic Category Antirheumatic, Disease Modifying; Gastrointestinal Agent, Miscellaneous; Monoclonal Antibody; Tumor Necrosis Factor (TNF) Blocking Agent

Medication Safety Issues

Sound-alike/look-alike issues:

Remicade® may be confused with Renacidin®, Rituxan®

Infliximab may be confused with rituximab

Pregnancy Risk Factor B (manufacturer)

Lactation Excretion in breast milk unknown/not recommended

Use

Ankylosing spondylitis: Improving signs and symptoms of disease

Crohn's disease: Induction and maintenance of remission in patients with moderate to severe disease who have an inadequate response to conventional therapy; to reduce the number of draining enterocutaneous and rectovaginal fistulas and to maintain fistula closure

Psoriatic arthritis: Improving signs and symptoms of active arthritis in patients with psoriatic arthritis

Rheumatoid arthritis: Inhibits the progression of structural damage and improves physical function in patients with moderate to severe disease; used with methotrexate

Ulcerative colitis (UC): To reduce signs and symptoms, achieve clinical remission and mucosal healing and eliminate corticosteroid use in moderately to severely active UC inadequately responsive to conventional therapy

Mechanism of Action/Effect Infliximab is a monoclonal antibody that binds to human tumor necrosis factor alpha (TNFα), thereby decreasing inflammatory and other responses.

Contraindications Hypersensitivity to murine proteins or any component of the formulation; doses >5 mg/kg in patients with moderate or severe congestive heart failure (NYHA Class III/IV)

Warnings/Precautions Serious infections (including sepsis, pneumonia, and fatal infections) have been reported in patients receiving TNF-blocking agents. Many of the serious infections in patients treated with infliximab have occurred in patients on concomitant immunosuppressive therapy. Caution should be exercised when considering the use of infliximab in patients with a chronic infection or history of recurrent infection. Infliximab should not be given to patients with a clinically important, active infection. Patients who develop a new infection while undergoing treatment with infliximab should be monitored closely. If a patient develops a serious infection or sepsis, infliximab should be discontinued. Rare reactivation of hepatitis B has occurred in chronic virus carriers; evaluate prior to initiation and during treatment. Patients should be evaluated for latent tuberculosis infection with a tuberculin skin test prior to infliximab therapy. Treatment of latent tuberculosis should be initiated before infliximab is used. Tuberculosis (may be disseminated or extrapulmonary) has been reactivated in patients previously exposed to TB while on infliximab. Most cases have been reported within the first 3-6 months of treatment. Other opportunistic infections (eg, invasive fungal infections, listeriosis, *Pneumocystis*) have occurred during therapy. The risk/benefit ratio should be weighed in patients who have resided in regions where histoplasmosis is endemic.

Impact on the development and course of malignancies is not fully defined. As compared to the general population, an increased risk of lymphoma has been noted in clinical trials; however, rheumatoid arthritis has been previously associated with an increased rate of lymphoma.

Severe hepatic reactions have been reported during treatment. Use caution with CHF; if a decision is made to use with CHF, monitor closely and discontinue if exacerbated or new symptoms occur. Use caution with history of hematologic abnormalities; hematologic toxicities (eg, leukopenia, neutropenia, thrombocytopenia, pancytopenia) have been reported; discontinue if significant abnormalities occur. Autoimmune antibodies and a lupus-like syndrome have been reported. If antibodies to double-stranded DNA are confirmed in a patient with lupus-like symptoms, infliximab should be discontinued. Rare cases of optic neuritis and demyelinating disease have been reported; use with caution in patients with pre-existing or recent onset CNS demyelinating disorders, or seizures; discontinue if significant CNS adverse reactions develop.

Medications for the treatment of hypersensitivity reactions should be available for immediate use. Safety and efficacy for use in juvenile rheumatoid arthritis and in pediatric patients with Crohn's disease have not been established.

Drug Interactions
Decreased Effect: Specific drug interaction studies have not been conducted.

Increased Effect/Toxicity: Specific drug interaction studies have not been conducted. Anti-TNF agents may be associated with increased risk of serious infection when used in combination with anakinra. Abciximab may increase potential for hypersensitivity reaction to infliximab, and may increase risk of thrombocytopenia and/or reduced therapeutic efficacy of infliximab.

Adverse Reactions Note: Although profile is similar, frequency of adverse effects may vary with disease state. Except where noted, percentages reported with rheumatoid arthritis:

>10%:
Central nervous system: Headache (18%)
Dermatologic: Rash (10%)
Gastrointestinal: Nausea (21%), diarrhea (12%), abdominal pain (12%, Crohn's 26%)
Genitourinary: Urinary tract infection (8%)
Hepatic: ALT increased (risk increased with concomitant methotrexate)
Local: Infusion reactions (20%)
Neuromuscular & skeletal: Arthralgia (8%), back pain (8%)
Respiratory: Upper respiratory tract infection (32%), cough (12%), sinusitis (14%), pharyngitis (12%)

Miscellaneous: Development of antinuclear antibodies (~50%), infection (36%), development of antibodies to double-stranded DNA (17%); Crohn's patients with fistulizing disease: Development of new abscess (15%)
5% to 10%:
Cardiovascular: Hypertension (7%)
Central nervous system: Pain (8%), fatigue (9%), fever (7%)
Dermatologic: Pruritus (7%)
Gastrointestinal: Dyspepsia (10%)
Respiratory: Bronchitis (10%), dyspnea (6%), rhinitis (8%)
Miscellaneous: Moniliasis (5%)

Overdosage/Toxicology Doses of up to 20 mg/kg have been given without toxic effects. In case of overdose, treatment should be symptom-directed and supportive.

Pharmacodynamics/Kinetics
Onset of Action: Crohn's disease: ~2 weeks
Half-Life Elimination: 8-9.5 days

Available Dosage Forms Injection, powder for reconstitution [preservative free]: 100 mg

Dosing
Adults & Elderly:
Crohn's disease: I.V.:
Induction regimen: 5 mg/kg at 0, 2, and 6 weeks, followed by 5 mg/kg every 8 weeks; dose may be increased to 10 mg/kg in patients who respond but then lose their response. If no response by week 14, consider discontinuing therapy.
Psoriatic arthritis (with or without methotrexate): 5 mg/kg at 0,2, and 6 weeks, then every 8 weeks
Rheumatoid arthritis: I.V. (in combination with methotrexate therapy): 3 mg/kg at 0, 2, and 6 weeks then every 8 weeks thereafter; doses have ranged from 3-10 mg/kg intravenous infusion repeated at 4- to 8-week intervals
Ankylosing spondylitis: I.V.: 5 mg/kg at 0, 2, and 6 weeks, followed by 5 mg/kg every 6 weeks thereafter
Ulcerative colitis: I.V.: 5 mg/kg at 0, 2, and 6 weeks, followed by 5 mg/kg every 8 weeks thereafter
Dosage adjustment with CHF: Weigh risk versus benefits for individual patient:
NYHA Class III or IV: ≤5 mg/kg
Pediatrics: Safety and efficacy have not been established
Renal Impairment: No adjustment is recommended.
Hepatic Impairment: No adjustment necessary.
Administration
I.V.: Infuse over at least 2 hours.
I.V. Detail: Do not infuse with other agents. Use in-line low protein binding filter (≤ 1.2 micron). pH ~7.2
Stability
Reconstitution: Reconstitute vials with 10 mL sterile water for injection; swirl vial gently to dissolve powder, do not shake, allow solution to stand for 5 minutes; total dose of reconstituted product should be further diluted to 250 mL of 0.9% sodium chloride injection; infusion of dose should begin within 3 hours of preparation
Compatibility: Do not infuse with other agents.
Storage: Store vials at 2°C to 8°C (36°F to 46°F). Do not freeze.
Nursing Actions
Physical Assessment: Monitor therapeutic response and adverse reactions (eg, hypersensitivity, respiratory effects). Monitor for signs or symptoms of infection. Assess for signs of liver dysfunction (eg, unusual fatigue, easy bruising or bleeding, jaundice). Teach patient appropriate interventions to reduce side effects and adverse symptoms to report.
Patient Education: This drug can only be administered by infusion. Avoid receiving immunizations unless approved by prescriber. You will be more (Continued)

Infliximab *(Continued)*

prone to infection. Avoid crowds and wash your hands frequently. Report headache or unusual fatigue; increased nausea or abdominal pain; bruising or bleeding easily; cough, runny nose, respiratory difficulty; chest pain or persistent dizziness; fatigue; muscle pain or weakness, back pain; fever or chills; mouth sores; vaginal itching or discharge; sore throat; unhealed sores; or frequent infections. **Breast-feeding precaution:** Breast-feeding is not recommended.

Breast-Feeding Issues It is not known whether infliximab is secreted in human milk. Because many immunoglobulins are secreted in milk and the potential for serious adverse reactions exists, a decision should be made whether to discontinue nursing or discontinue the drug, taking into account the importance of the drug to the mother.

Pregnancy Issues Reproduction studies have not been conducted. Use during pregnancy only if clearly needed. A Rheumatoid Arthritis and Pregnancy Registry has been established for women exposed to infliximab during pregnancy (Organization of Teratology Information Services, 877-311-8972).

Insulin Aspart *(IN soo lin AS part)*

U.S. Brand Names NovoLog®
Synonyms Aspart Insulin
Pharmacologic Category Antidiabetic Agent, Insulin
Pregnancy Risk Factor C
Lactation Excretion in breast milk unknown/compatible
Use Treatment of type 1 diabetes mellitus (insulin dependent, IDDM); type 2 diabetes mellitus (noninsulin dependent, NIDDM) to control hyperglycemia
Available Dosage Forms Injection, solution (NovoLog®): 100 units/mL (3 mL) [FlexPen® prefilled syringe or PenFill® prefilled cartridge]; (10 mL) [vial]

Dosing
Adults & Elderly: Refer to Insulin Regular *on page 658*. Insulin aspart is a rapid-acting insulin analog which is normally administered as a a premeal component of the insulin regimen. It is normally used along with a long-acting (basal) form of insulin.
Pediatrics: Refer to Insulin Regular *on page 658*.
Renal Impairment: Insulin requirements are reduced due to changes in insulin clearance or metabolism.

Nursing Actions
Physical Assessment: Assess potential for interactions with other prescriptions, OTC medications, or herbal products patient may be taking. Monitor laboratory tests, therapeutic effectiveness, and adverse reactions (eg, hypoglycemia) at regular intervals during therapy. Teach patient proper use, including appropriate injection technique and syringe/needle disposal and monitoring requirements (or refer to diabetic educator), possible side effects/appropriate interventions, and adverse symptoms to report.
Patient Education: Do not take any new medication during therapy unless approved by prescriber. This medication is used to control diabetes; it is not a cure. It is imperative to follow other components of prescribed treatment (eg, diet and exercise regimen). Take exactly as directed. Do not change dose or discontinue unless advised by prescriber. With insulin aspart (NovoLog®), you must start eating within 5-10 minutes after injection. If you experience hypoglycemic reaction, contact prescriber immediately. Always carry quick source of sugar with you. Monitor glucose levels as directed by prescriber. Report adverse side effects, including chest pain or palpitations; persistent fatigue, confusion, headache; skin rash or redness; numbness of mouth, lips, or tongue;

muscle weakness or tremors; vision changes; respiratory difficulty; or nausea, vomiting, or flu-like symptoms. **Pregnancy/breast-feeding precautions:** Inform prescriber if you are or intend to become pregnant. Consult prescriber if breast-feeding.
Related Information
Insulin Regular *on page 658*

Insulin Aspart Protamine and Insulin Aspart *(IN soo lin AS part PROE ta meen & IN soo lin AS part)*

U.S. Brand Names NovoLog® Mix 70/30
Synonyms Insulin Aspart and Insulin Aspart Protamine
Pharmacologic Category Antidiabetic Agent, Insulin
Pregnancy Risk Factor C
Lactation Excretion in breast milk unknown/compatible
Use Treatment of type 1 diabetes mellitus (insulin dependent, IDDM); type 2 diabetes mellitus (noninsulin dependent, NIDDM) to control hyperglycemia
Available Dosage Forms Injection, suspension (NovoLog® Mix 70/30): Insulin aspart protamine suspension 70% [intermediate acting] and insulin aspart solution 30% [rapid acting]: 100 units/mL (3 mL) [PenFill® prefilled cartridge or FlexPen® prefilled syringe]; (10 mL) [vial]

Dosing
Adults & Elderly: Refer to Insulin Regular *on page 658*. Fixed ratio insulins (such as insulin aspart protamine and insulin aspart combination) are normally administered in 2 daily doses.
Renal Impairment: Insulin requirements are reduced due to changes in insulin clearance or metabolism.
Related Information
Insulin Regular *on page 658*

Insulin Detemir *(IN soo lin DE te mir)*

U.S. Brand Names Levemir®
Synonyms Detemir Insulin
Pharmacologic Category Antidiabetic Agent, Insulin
Pregnancy Risk Factor C
Lactation Excretion in breast milk unknown/compatible
Use Treatment of type 1 diabetes mellitus (insulin dependent, IDDM); type 2 diabetes mellitus (noninsulin dependent, NIDDM) to control hyperglycemia
Available Dosage Forms Injection, solution (Levemir®): 100 units/mL (3 mL) [Innolet® prefilled syringe, Penfill® prefilled cartridge, or FlexPen® prefilled syringe]; (10 mL) [vial]

Dosing
Adults & Elderly: Also refer to Insulin Regular *on page 658*.

Note: Duration is dose-dependent. Dosage must be carefully titrated (adjustment of dose and timing. Adjustment of concomitant antidiabetic treatment (short-acting insulins or oral antidiabetic agents) may be required.

Type 1 or type 2 diabetes:
Basal insulin or basal-bolus: May be substituted on a unit-per-unit basis. Adjust dose to achieve glycemic targets.
Insulin-naive patients (type 2 diabetes only): 0.1-0.2 units/kg once daily in the evening or 10 units once or twice daily. Adjust dose to achieve glycemic targets. Note: Canadian labeling recommends 10 units once daily (twice daily dosing is not included).

Pediatrics: Children ≥ 6 years: Refer to adult dosing. Note: In Canada, insulin detemir is not approved for use in children.

Renal Impairment: Insulin requirements are reduced due to changes in insulin clearance or metabolism.

Nursing Actions

Physical Assessment: Assess potential for interactions with other prescriptions, OTC medications, or herbal products patient may be taking. Monitor laboratory tests, therapeutic effectiveness, and adverse reactions (eg, hypoglycemia) at regular intervals during therapy. Teach patient proper use, including appropriate injection technique and syringe/needle disposal and monitoring requirements (or refer to diabetic educator), possible side effects/appropriate interventions, and adverse symptoms to report.

Patient Education: Do not take any new medication during therapy unless approved by prescriber. This medication is used to control diabetes; it is not a cure. It is imperative to follow other components of prescribed treatment (eg, diet and exercise regimen). Take exactly as directed. Do not change dose or discontinue unless advised by prescriber. If you experience hypoglycemic reaction, contact prescriber immediately. Always carry quick source of sugar with you. Monitor glucose levels as directed by prescriber. Report adverse side effects, including chest pain or palpitations; persistent fatigue, confusion, headache; skin rash or redness; numbness of mouth, lips, or tongue; muscle weakness or tremors; vision changes; respiratory difficulty; or nausea, vomiting, or flu-like symptoms. **Pregnancy/breast-feeding precautions:** Inform prescriber if you are or intend to become pregnant. Consult prescriber if breast-feeding.

Related Information
Insulin Regular *on page 658*

Insulin Glargine (IN soo lin GLAR jeen)

U.S. Brand Names Lantus®
Synonyms Glargine Insulin
Pharmacologic Category Antidiabetic Agent, Insulin
Pregnancy Risk Factor C
Lactation Excretion in breast milk unknown/compatible
Use Treatment of type 1 diabetes mellitus (insulin dependent, IDDM); type 2 diabetes mellitus (noninsulin dependent, NIDDM) requiring basal (long-acting) insulin to control hyperglycemia
Available Dosage Forms Injection, solution (Lantus®): 100 units/mL (3 mL) [cartridge]; (10 mL) [vial]
Dosing
Adults & Elderly: SubQ:
Type 1 diabetes: Refer to Insulin Regular *on page 658*.
Type 2 diabetes:
Patient not already on insulin: 10 units once daily, adjusted according to patient response (range in clinical study: 2-100 units/day)
Patient already receiving insulin: In clinical studies, when changing to insulin glargine from once-daily NPH or Ultralente® insulin, the initial dose was not changed; when changing from twice-daily NPH to once-daily insulin glargine, the total daily dose was reduced by 20% and adjusted according to patient response
Pediatrics: Refer to adult dosing.
Renal Impairment: Insulin requirements are reduced due to changes in insulin clearance or metabolism.

Nursing Actions

Physical Assessment: Assess potential for interactions with other prescriptions, OTC medications, or herbal products patient may be taking. Monitor laboratory tests, therapeutic effectiveness, and adverse reactions (eg, hypoglycemia) at regular intervals

during therapy. Teach patient proper use, including appropriate injection technique and syringe/needle disposal and monitoring requirements (or refer to diabetic educator), possible side effects/appropriate interventions, and adverse symptoms to report.

Patient Education: Do not take any new medication during therapy unless approved by prescriber. This medication is used to control diabetes; it is not a cure. It is imperative to follow other components of prescribed treatment (eg, diet and exercise regimen). Take exactly as directed. Do not change dose or discontinue unless advised by prescriber. If you experience hypoglycemic reaction, contact prescriber immediately. Always carry quick source of sugar with you. Monitor glucose levels as directed by prescriber. Report adverse side effects, including chest pain or palpitations; persistent fatigue, confusion, headache; skin rash or redness; numbness of mouth, lips, or tongue; muscle weakness or tremors; vision changes; respiratory difficulty; or nausea, vomiting, or flu-like symptoms. **Pregnancy/breast-feeding precautions:** Inform prescriber if you are or intend to become pregnant. Consult prescriber if breast-feeding.

Related Information
Insulin Regular *on page 658*

Insulin Glulisine (IN soo lin gloo LIS een)

U.S. Brand Names Apidra®
Synonyms Glulisine Insulin
Pharmacologic Category Antidiabetic Agent, Insulin
Pregnancy Risk Factor C
Lactation Excretion in breast milk unknown/compatible
Use Treatment of type 1 diabetes mellitus (insulin dependent, IDDM); type 2 diabetes mellitus (noninsulin dependent, NIDDM) to control hyperglycemia
Available Dosage Forms
Injection, solution:
Apidra®: 100 units/mL (3 mL [cartridge], 10 mL [vial])
Dosing
Adults & Elderly: Refer to Insulin Regular *on page 658*.
Pediatrics: Refer to Insulin Regular *on page 658*.
Renal Impairment: Insulin requirements are reduced due to changes in insulin clearance or metabolism.

Nursing Actions

Physical Assessment: Assess potential for interactions with other prescriptions, OTC medications, or herbal products patient may be taking. Monitor laboratory tests, therapeutic effectiveness, and adverse reactions (eg, hypoglycemia) at regular intervals during therapy. Teach patient proper use, including appropriate injection technique and syringe/needle disposal and monitoring requirements (or refer to diabetic educator), possible side effects/appropriate interventions, and adverse symptoms to report.

Patient Education: Do not take any new medication during therapy unless approved by prescriber. This medication is used to control diabetes; it is not a cure. It is imperative to follow other components of prescribed treatment (eg, diet and exercise regimen). Take exactly as directed. Do not change dose or discontinue unless advised by prescriber. Insulin glulisine (Apidra®) should be administered within 15 minutes before or within 20 minutes after start of a meal. If you experience hypoglycemic reaction, contact prescriber immediately. Always carry quick source of sugar with you. Monitor glucose levels as directed by prescriber. Report adverse side effects, including chest pain or palpitations; persistent fatigue, confusion, headache; skin rash or redness; numbness of mouth, lips, or tongue; muscle weakness or tremors; vision changes; respiratory difficulty; or nausea, vomiting, or flu-like symptoms. **Pregnancy/**
(Continued)

Insulin Glulisine *(Continued)*

breast-feeding precautions: Inform prescriber if you are or intend to become pregnant. Consult prescriber if breast-feeding.

Related Information
Insulin Regular *on page 658*

Insulin Inhalation (IN soo lin in ha LAY shun)

U.S. Brand Names Exubera®
Synonyms Inhaled Insulin
Restrictions A medication guide must be distributed to each patient to whom this medication is dispensed.
Pharmacologic Category Antidiabetic Agent, Insulin
Pregnancy Risk Factor C
Lactation Excretion in breast milk unknown/compatible
Use Treatment of type 1 diabetes mellitus (insulin dependent, IDDM); type 2 diabetes mellitus (noninsulin dependent, NIDDM)

Available Dosage Forms
Powder for oral inhalation [prefilled blister pack]: 1 mg (90s) [purchased with or provided with inhaler and 2 release units]; 3 mg (90s) [purchased with or provided with inhaler and 2 release units]
Combination package [prefilled blister pack]: Powder for inhalation: 1 mg (90s); powder for inhalation: 3 mg (90s)

Dosing
Adults & Elderly: Diabetes mellitus (type 1 or 2): Inhalation:
Initial: 0.05 mg/kg (rounded down to nearest whole milligram) 3 times/daily administered within 10 minutes of a meal
Adjustment: Dosage may be increased or decreased based on serum glucose monitoring, meal size, nutrient composition, time of day, and exercise patterns.

Note: A 1 mg blister is approximately equivalent to 3 units of regular insulin, while a 3 mg blister is approximately equivalent to 8 units of regular insulin administered subcutaneously. Patients should combine 1 mg and 3 mg blisters so that the fewest blisters are required to achieve the prescribed dose. Consecutive inhalation of three 1 mg blisters results in significantly higher insulin levels as compared to inhalation of a single 3 mg blister (do not substitute). In a patient stabilized on a dosage which uses 3 mg blisters, if 3 mg blister is temporarily unavailable, inhalation of two 1 mg blisters may be substituted.

Pediatrics: Diabetes mellitus (type 1 or 2): Inhalation: Children ≥6 years: Refer to adult dosing.

Renal Impairment: Insulin requirements are reduced due to changes in insulin clearance or metabolism.

Nursing Actions
Physical Assessment: Assess potential for interactions with other prescriptions, OTC medications, or herbal products patient may be taking. Monitor laboratory tests, therapeutic effectiveness, and adverse reactions (eg, hypoglycemia) at regular intervals during therapy. Emphasize to patient the need to avoid smoking and secondhand smoke. Teach patient proper use and monitoring requirements (or refer to diabetic educator), possible side effects/appropriate interventions, and adverse symptoms to report.

Patient Education:
Do not smoke; avoid secondhand smoke. Do not take any new medication during therapy unless approved by prescriber. This medication is used to control diabetes; it is not a cure. It is imperative to follow other components of prescribed treatment (eg, diet and exercise regimen). Take exactly as directed. Do not change dose or discontinue unless advised by

prescriber. When used as your mealtime insulin, take within 10 minutes before your meal. If you experience hypoglycemic reaction, contact prescriber immediately. Always carry quick source of sugar with you. Monitor glucose levels as directed by prescriber. You may experience respiratory infections, dry mouth, cough, sore throat, sinus problems, or nasal congestion. Report adverse side effects, including chest pain or palpitations; persistent fatigue, confusion, headache; skin rash or redness; numbness of mouth, lips, or tongue; muscle weakness or tremors; vision changes; respiratory difficulty; or nausea, vomiting, or flu-like symptoms. **Pregnancy/breast-feeding precautions:** Inform prescriber if you are or intend to become pregnant. Consult prescriber if breast-feeding.

Related Information
Insulin Regular *on page 658*

Insulin Lispro (IN soo lin LYE sproe)

U.S. Brand Names Humalog®
Synonyms Lispro Insulin
Pharmacologic Category Antidiabetic Agent, Insulin
Pregnancy Risk Factor B
Lactation Excretion in breast milk unknown/compatible
Use Treatment of type 1 diabetes mellitus (insulin dependent, IDDM); type 2 diabetes mellitus (noninsulin dependent, NIDDM) to control hyperglycemia
Note: In type 1 diabetes mellitus (insulin dependent, IDDM), insulin lispro (Humalog®) should be used in combination with a long-acting insulin. However, in type 2 diabetes mellitus (noninsulin dependent, NIDDM), insulin lispro (Humalog®) may be used without a long-acting insulin when used in combination with a sulfonylurea.

Available Dosage Forms Injection, solution (Humalog®): 100 units/mL (3 mL) [prefilled cartridge or prefilled disposable pen]; (10 mL) [vial]

Dosing
Adults & Elderly: Refer to Insulin Regular *on page 658*. Insulin lispro is equipotent to insulin regular, but has a more rapid onset.
Pediatrics: Refer to Insulin Regular *on page 658*. Insulin lispro is equipotent to insulin regular, but has a more rapid onset.
Renal Impairment: Insulin requirements are reduced due to changes in insulin clearance or metabolism.

Nursing Actions
Physical Assessment: Assess potential for interactions with other prescriptions, OTC medications, or herbal products patient may be taking. Monitor laboratory tests, therapeutic effectiveness, and adverse reactions (eg, hypoglycemia) at regular intervals during therapy. Teach patient proper use, including appropriate injection technique and syringe/needle disposal and monitoring requirements (or refer to diabetic educator), possible side effects/appropriate interventions, and adverse symptoms to report.

Patient Education: Do not take any new medication during therapy unless approved by prescriber. This medication is used to control diabetes; it is not a cure. It is imperative to follow other components of prescribed treatment (eg, diet and exercise regimen). Take exactly as directed. Do not change dose or discontinue unless advised by prescriber. If you experience hypoglycemic reaction, contact prescriber immediately. Always carry quick source of sugar with you. Monitor glucose levels as directed by prescriber. Report adverse side effects, including chest pain or palpitations; persistent fatigue, confusion, headache; skin rash or redness; numbness of mouth, lips, or tongue; muscle weakness or tremors; vision changes; respiratory difficulty; or nausea, vomiting, or flu-like symptoms. **Pregnancy/breast-feeding precautions:** Inform prescriber if you are or intend to become pregnant. Consult prescriber if breast-feeding.

Related Information
Insulin Regular *on page 658*

Insulin Lispro Protamine and Insulin Lispro

(IN soo lin LYE sproe PROE ta meen & IN soo lin LYE sproe)

U.S. Brand Names Humalog® Mix 50/50™; Humalog® Mix 75/25™
Synonyms Insulin Lispro and Insulin Lispro Protamine
Pharmacologic Category Antidiabetic Agent, Insulin
Pregnancy Risk Factor B
Lactation Excretion in breast milk unknown/compatible
Use Treatment of type 1 diabetes mellitus (insulin dependent, IDDM); type 2 diabetes mellitus (noninsulin dependent, NIDDM) to control hyperglycemia
Available Dosage Forms Injection, suspension:
Humalog® Mix 50/50™: Insulin lispro protamine suspension 50% [intermediate acting] and insulin lispro solution 50% [rapid acting]: 100 units/mL (3 mL) [disposable pen]
Humalog® Mix 75/25™: Insulin lispro protamine suspension 75% [intermediate acting] and insulin lispro solution 25% [rapid acting]: 100 units/mL (3 mL) [disposable pen]; (10 mL) [vial]
Dosing
Adults: Refer to Insulin Regular *on page 658*. Fixed ratio insulins (such as insulin lispro protamine and insulin lispro) are normally administered in 2 daily doses.
Renal Impairment: Insulin requirements are reduced due to changes in insulin clearance or metabolism.
Related Information
Insulin Regular *on page 658*

Insulin NPH (IN soo lin N P H)

U.S. Brand Names Humulin® N; Novolin® N
Synonyms Isophane Insulin; NPH Insulin
Pharmacologic Category Antidiabetic Agent, Insulin
Pregnancy Risk Factor B
Lactation Excretion in breast milk unknown/compatible
Use Treatment of type 1 diabetes mellitus (insulin dependent, IDDM); type 2 diabetes mellitus (noninsulin dependent, NIDDM) to control hyperglycemia
Available Dosage Forms [CAN] = Canadian brand name
Injection, suspension:
Humulin® N: 100 units/mL (3 mL) [disposable pen]; (10 mL) [vial]
Novolin® ge NPH [CAN]: 100 units/mL (3 mL) [NovolinSet® prefilled syringe or PenFill® prefilled cartridge]; 10 mL [vial]
Novolin® N: 100 units/mL (3 mL) [InnoLet® prefilled syringe or PenFill® prefilled cartridge]; (10 mL) [vial]
Dosing
Adults & Elderly: Refer to Insulin Regular *on page 658*. Insulin NPH is usually administered 1-2 times daily.
Pediatrics: Refer to Insulin Regular *on page 658*. Insulin NPH is usually administered 1-2 times daily.
Renal Impairment: Insulin requirements are reduced due to changes in insulin clearance or metabolism.
Nursing Actions
Physical Assessment: Assess potential for interactions with other prescriptions, OTC medications, or herbal products patient may be taking. Assess results

of laboratory tests, therapeutic effectiveness, and adverse response (eg, hypoglycemia) at regular intervals during therapy. Teach patient proper use, including appropriate injection technique and syringe/needle disposal and monitoring requirements (or refer to diabetic educator), possible side effects/appropriate interventions, and adverse symptoms to report.

Patient Education: Do not take any new medication during therapy unless approved by prescriber. This medication is used to control diabetes; it is not a cure. It is imperative to follow other components of prescribed treatment (eg, diet and exercise regimen). Take exactly as directed. Do not change dose or discontinue unless advised by prescriber. If you experience hypoglycemic reaction, contact prescriber immediately. Always carry quick source of sugar with you. Monitor glucose levels as directed by prescriber. Report adverse side effects, including chest pain or palpitations; persistent fatigue, confusion, headache; skin rash or redness; numbness of mouth, lips, or tongue; muscle weakness or tremors; vision changes; respiratory difficulty; or nausea, vomiting, or flu-like symptoms. **Pregnancy/breat-feeding precautions:** Inform prescriber if you are or intend to become pregnant. Consult prescriber if breast-feeding.

Related Information
Insulin Regular *on page 658*

Insulin NPH and Insulin Regular

(IN soo lin N P H & IN soo lin REG yoo ler)

U.S. Brand Names Humulin® 50/50; Humulin® 70/30; Novolin® 70/30
Synonyms Insulin Regular and Insulin NPH; Isophane Insulin and Regular Insulin; NPH Insulin and Regular Insulin
Pharmacologic Category Antidiabetic Agent, Insulin
Pregnancy Risk Factor C
Use Treatment of type 1 diabetes mellitus (insulin dependent, IDDM); type 2 diabetes mellitus (noninsulin dependent, NIDDM) to control hyperglycemia
Available Dosage Forms
Injection, suspension:
Humulin® 50/50: Insulin NPH suspension 50% [intermediate acting] and insulin regular solution 50% [short acting]: 100 units/mL (10 mL) [vial]
Humulin® 70/30: Insulin NPH suspension 70% [intermediate acting] and insulin regular solution 30% [short acting]: 100 units/mL (3 mL) [disposable pen]; (10 mL) [vial]
Novolin® 70/30: Insulin NPH suspension 70% [intermediate acting] and insulin regular solution 30% [short acting]: 100 units/mL (3 mL) [InnoLet® prefilled syringe or PenFill® prefilled cartridge]; (10 mL) [vial]

Additional formulations available in Canada: Injection, suspension:
Humulin® 20/80: Insulin regular solution 20% [short acting] and insulin NPH suspension 80% [intermediate acting]: 100 units/mL (3 mL) [PenFill® prefilled cartridge]
Novolin® ge 10/90: Insulin regular solution 10% [short acting] and insulin NPH suspension 90% [intermediate acting]: 100 units/mL (3 mL) [PenFill® prefilled cartridge]
Novolin® ge 20/80: Insulin regular solution 20% [short acting] and insulin NPH suspension 80% [intermediate acting]: 100 units/mL (3 mL) [PenFill® prefilled cartridge]
Novolin® ge 30/70: Insulin regular solution 30% [short acting] and insulin NPH suspension 70% [intermediate acting]: 100 units/mL (3 mL) [prefilled syringe or PenFill® prefilled cartridge]; (10 mL) [vial]
(Continued)

Insulin NPH and Insulin Regular
(Continued)

Novolin® ge 40/60: Insulin regular solution 40% [short acting] and insulin NPH suspension 60% [intermediate acting]: 100 units/mL (3 mL) [PenFill® prefilled cartridge]

Novolin® ge 50/50: Insulin regular solution 50% [short acting] and insulin NPH suspension 50% [intermediate acting]: 100 units/mL (3 mL) [PenFill® prefilled cartridge]

Dosing
Adults & Elderly:
Refer to Insulin Regular *on page 658*. Fixed ratio insulins are normally administered in 1-2 daily doses.

Pediatrics:
Refer to Insulin Regular *on page 658*. Fixed ratio insulins are normally administered in 1-2 daily doses.

Related Information
Insulin Regular *on page 658*

Insulin Regular (IN soo lin REG yoo ler)

U.S. Brand Names Humulin® R; Humulin® R (Concentrated) U-500; Novolin® R

Synonyms Regular Insulin

Pharmacologic Category Antidiabetic Agent, Insulin; Antidote

Medication Safety Issues
Sound-alike/look-alike issues:
Humulin® may be confused with Humalog®, Humira®
Novolin® may be confused with NovoLog®

High alert medication: The Institute for Safe Medication Practices (ISMP) includes this medication among its list of drugs which have a heightened risk of causing significant patient harm when used in error. *Due to the number of insulin preparations, it is essential to identify/clarify the type of insulin to be used.*

Concentrated solutions (eg, U-500) should not be available in patient care areas.

Pregnancy Risk Factor B

Lactation Excretion in breast milk unknown/compatible

Use Treatment of type 1 diabetes mellitus (insulin dependent, IDDM); type 2 diabetes mellitus (noninsulin dependent, NIDDM) unresponsive to treatment with diet and/or oral hypoglycemics, to control hyperglycemia; adjunct to parenteral nutrition; diabetic ketoacidosis (DKA)

Unlabeled/Investigational Use Hyperkalemia (regular insulin only; use with glucose to shift potassium into cells to lower serum potassium levels)

Mechanism of Action/Effect Insulin acts via specific membrane-bound receptors on target tissues to regulate metabolism of carbohydrate, protein, and fats. Target organs for insulin include the liver, skeletal muscle, and adipose tissue. Within the liver, insulin stimulates hepatic glycogen synthesis. Insulin promotes hepatic synthesis of fatty acids, which are released into the circulation as lipoproteins. Skeletal muscle effects of insulin include increased protein synthesis and increased glycogen synthesis. Within adipose tissue, insulin stimulates the processing of circulating lipoproteins to provide free fatty acids, facilitating triglyceride synthesis and storage by adipocytes. Insulin also directly inhibits the hydrolysis of triglycerides. Normally secreted by the pancreas, insulin products are manufactured for pharmacologic use through recombinant DNA technology using either *E. coli* or *Saccharomyces cerevisiae*. Insulins are categorized based on promptness and duration of effect, including rapid-, short-, intermediate- and long-acting insulins.

Contraindications Hypersensitivity to any component of the formulation

Warnings/Precautions Hypoglycemia is the most common adverse effect of insulin. The timing of hypoglycemia differs among various insulin formulations. Any change of insulin should be made cautiously; changing manufacturers, type, and/or method of manufacture may result in the need for a change of dosage. Human insulin differs from animal-source insulin. Regular insulin is the only insulin to be used I.V. Hypoglycemia may result from increased work or exercise without eating; use of long-acting insulin preparations (insulin glargine, Ultralente®, insulin U) may delay recovery from hypoglycemia. Use with caution in renal or hepatic impairment.

The general objective of insulin replacement therapy is to approximate the physiologic pattern of insulin secretion. This requires a basal level of insulin throughout the day, supplemented by additional insulin at mealtimes. Since combinations of agents are frequently used, dosage adjustment must address the individual component of the insulin regimen which most directly influences the blood glucose value in question, based on the known onset and duration of the insulin component. The frequency of doses and monitoring must be individualized in consideration of the patient's ability to manage therapy. Diabetic education and nutritional counseling are essential to maximize the effectiveness of therapy.

In type 1 diabetes mellitus (insulin dependent, IDDM), insulin lispro (Humalog®) and insulin glulisine (Apidra™) should be used in combination with a long-acting insulin. However, in type 2 diabetes mellitus (noninsulin dependent, NIDDM), insulin lispro (Humalog®) may be used without a long-acting insulin when used in combination with a sulfonylurea.

Drug Interactions
Cytochrome P450 Effect: Induces CYP1A2 (weak)
Decreased Effect: Decreased hypoglycemic effect of insulin with corticosteroids, dextrothyroxine, diltiazem, dobutamine, epinephrine, niacin, oral contraceptives, thiazide diuretics, thyroid hormone, and smoking.

Increased Effect/Toxicity: Increased hypoglycemic effect of insulin with alcohol, alpha-blockers, anabolic steroids, beta-blockers (nonselective beta-blockers may delay recovery from hypoglycemic episodes and mask signs/symptoms of hypoglycemia; cardioselective beta-blocker agents may be alternatives), clofibrate, guanethidine, MAO inhibitors, pentamidine, phenylbutazone, salicylates, sulfinpyrazone, and tetracyclines.

Insulin increases the risk of hypoglycemia associated with oral hypoglycemic agents (including sulfonylureas, metformin, pioglitazone, rosiglitazone, and troglitazone).

Nutritional/Ethanol Interactions
Ethanol: Caution with ethanol (may increase hypoglycemia).
Food: Insulin shifts potassium from extracellular to intracellular space. Decreases potassium serum concentration.
Herb/Nutraceutical: Use caution with chromium, garlic, gymnema (may increase hypoglycemia).

Adverse Reactions Frequency not defined.
Cardiovascular: Palpitation, pallor, tachycardia
Central nervous system: Fatigue, headache, hypothermia, loss of consciousness, mental confusion
Dermatologic: Urticaria, redness
Endocrine & metabolic: Hypoglycemia
Gastrointestinal: Hunger, nausea, numbness of mouth
Local: Atrophy or hypertrophy of SubQ fat tissue; edema, itching, pain or warmth at injection site; stinging
Neuromuscular & skeletal: Muscle weakness, paresthesia, tremor
Ocular: Transient presbyopia or blurred vision

Miscellaneous: Anaphylaxis, diaphoresis, local allergy, systemic allergic symptoms

Overdosage/Toxicology Symptoms of overdose include tachycardia, anxiety, hunger, tremor, pallor, headache, motor dysfunction, speech disturbances, sweating, palpitations, coma, and death. Antidote is glucose and glucagon, if necessary.

Pharmacodynamics/Kinetics
Onset of Action: 0.5 hours
Duration of Action: 6-8 hours (may increase with dose)
Time to Peak: 2-4 hours
Excretion: Urine

Available Dosage Forms
Injection, solution:
Humulin® R: 100 units/mL (10 mL) [vial]
Novolin® R: 100 units/mL (3 mL) [InnoLet® prefilled syringe or PenFill® prefilled cartridge]; (10 mL) [vial]
Injection, solution [concentrate] (Humulin® R U-500): 500 units/mL (20 mL vial)

Dosing
Adults & Elderly: SubQ (regular insulin may also be administered I.V.): The number and size of daily doses, time of administration, and diet and exercise require continuous medical supervision. In addition, specific formulations may require distinct administration procedures (see Administration).

Type 1 Diabetes Mellitus: Note: Multiple daily doses guided by blood glucose monitoring are the standard of diabetes care. Combinations of insulin are commonly used.

Initial dose: 0.2-0.6 unit /kg/day in divided doses. Conservative initial doses of 0.2-0.4 units/kg/day are often recommended to avoid the potential for hypoglycemia.

Division of daily insulin requirement: Generally, 50% to 75% of the daily insulin dose is given as an intermediate- or long-acting form of insulin (in 1-2 daily injections). The remaining portion of the 24-hour insulin requirement is divided and administered as a rapid-acting or short-acting form of insulin. These may be given with meals (before or at the time of meals depending on the form of insulin) or at the same time as injections of intermediate forms (some premixed combinations are intended for this purpose).

Adjustment of dose: Dosage must be titrated to achieve glucose control and avoid hypoglycemia. Adjust dose to maintain premeal and bedtime glucose of 80-140 mg/dL (children <5 years: 100-200 mg/dL). Since combinations of agents are frequently used, dosage adjustment must address the individual component of the insulin regimen which most directly influences the blood glucose value in question, based on the known onset and duration of the insulin component. Also see Additional Information.

Usual maintenance range: 0.5-1.2 units/kg/day in divided doses. An estimate of anticipated needs may be based on body weight and/or activity factors as follows:
Adolescents: May require ≤1.5 units/kg/day during growth spurts
Nonobese: 0.4-0.6 units/kg/day
Obese: 0.8-1.2 units/kg/day
Renal failure: Due to alterations in pharmacokinetics of insulin, may require <0.2 units/kg/day

Type 2 Diabetes Mellitus:
Augmentation therapy: Initial dosage of 0.15 (insulin glargine, corresponding to ~10 units) to 0.2 units/kg/day (insulins other than glargine) have been recommended. Dosage must be carefully adjusted.
Note: Administered when residual beta-cell function is present, as a supplemental agent when oral hypoglycemics have not achieved goal

glucose control. Twice daily NPH, or an evening dose of NPH, lente, or glargine insulin may be added to oral therapy with metformin or a sulfonylurea. Augmentation to control postprandial glucose may be accomplished with regular, glulisine, aspart, or lispro insulin.

Monotherapy: Initial dose: Highly variable: See Augmentation therapy dosing.

Note: An empirically-defined scheme for dosage estimation based on fasting plasma glucose and degree of obesity has been published with recommended doses ranging from 6-77 units/day (Holman, 1995). In the setting of glucose toxicity (loss of beta-cell sensitivity to glucose concentrations), insulin therapy may be used for short-term management to restore sensitivity of beta-cells; in these cases, the dose may need to be rapidly reduced/withdrawn when sensitivity is re-established.

Hyperkalemia (unlabeled use): I.V.: Administer dextrose at 0.5-1 mL/kg and regular insulin 1 unit for every 4-5 g dextrose given

Diabetic ketoacidosis:
I.V.: Regular insulin 0.15 units/kg initially followed by an infusion of 0.1 units/kg/hour
SubQ, I.M.: Regular insulin 0.4 units/kg given half as I.V. bolus and half as SubQ or I.M., followed by 0.1 units/kg/hour SubQ or I.M.
If serum glucose does not fall by 50-70 mg/dL in the first hour, double insulin dose hourly until glucose falls at an hourly rate of 50-70 mg/dL. Decrease dose to 0.05-0.1 units/kg/hour once serum glucose reaches 250 mg/dL.
Note: Newly-diagnosed patients with IDDM presenting in DKA and patients with blood sugars <800 mg/dL may be relatively "sensitive" to insulin and should receive loading and initial maintenance doses ~50% of those indicated.
Infusion should continue until reversal of acid-base derangement/ketonemia. Serum glucose is not a direct indicator of these abnormalities, and may decrease more rapidly than correction of the range of metabolic abnormalities.

Pediatrics: Diabetes mellitus: Refer to adult dosing. Adolescents (growth spurts): ≤1.5 units/kg/day in divided doses.

Diabetic ketoacidosis: Children <20 years:
I.V.: Regular insulin infused at 0.1 units/kg/hour; continue until acidosis clears, then decrease to 0.05 units/kg/hour until SubQ replacement dosing can be initiated
SubQ, I.M.: If no I.V. infusion access, regular insulin 0.1 units/kg I.M. bolus followed by 0.1 units/kg/hour SubQ or I.M.; continue until acidosis clears, then decrease to 0.05 units/kg/hour until SubQ replacement dosing can be initiated
If serum glucose does not fall by 50-70 mg/dL in the first hour, double insulin dose hourly until glucose falls at an hourly rate of 50-70 mg/dL. Decrease dose to 0.05-0.1 units/kg/hour once serum glucose reaches 250 mg/dL.
Note: Newly-diagnosed patients with IDDM presenting in DKA and patients with blood sugars <800 mg/dL may be relatively "sensitive" to insulin and should receive loading and initial maintenance doses ~50% of those indicated.

Hyperkalemia (unlabeled use): Refer to adult dosing.

Renal Impairment: Insulin requirements are reduced due to changes in insulin clearance or metabolism.

Cl_{cr} 10-50 mL/minute: Administer 75% of normal dose.
Cl_{cr} <10 mL/minute: Administer 25% to 50% of normal dose and monitor glucose closely.
Hemodialysis: Because of a large molecular weight (6000 daltons), insulin is not significantly removed by either peritoneal or hemodialysis.

(Continued)

Insulin Regular *(Continued)*

Supplemental dose is not necessary.

Peritoneal dialysis: Supplemental dose is not necessary.

Continuous arteriovenous or venovenous hemofiltration effects: Supplemental dose is not necessary.

Administration

I.V.: Regular insulin may be administered by SubQ, I.M., or I.V. routes.

I.V. administration (requires use of an infusion pump): **Only regular insulin** may be administered I.V.

I.V. Detail: I.V. administration (requires use of an infusion pump): **Only regular insulin** may be administered I.V.

I.V. infusions: To minimize adsorption problems to I.V. solution bag:

If new tubing is **not** needed: Wait a minimum of 30 minutes between the preparation of the solution and the initiation of the infusion.

If new tubing is needed: After receiving the insulin drip solution, the administration set should be attached to the I.V. container and the line should be flushed with the insulin solution. The nurse should wait 30 minutes, then flush the line again with the insulin solution prior to initiating the infusion.

If insulin is required prior to the availability of the insulin drip, regular insulin should be administered by I.V. push injection.

Because of adsorption, the actual amount of insulin being administered could be substantially less than the apparent amount. Therefore, adjustment of the insulin drip rate should be based on effect and not solely on the apparent insulin dose. Furthermore, the apparent dose should not be used as the basis for determining the subsequent insulin dose upon discontinuing the insulin drip. Dose requires continuous medical supervision.

pH: Regular insulin: 7.0-7.8

Other: SubQ administration: Cold injections should be avoided. SubQ administration is usually made into the thighs, arms, buttocks, or abdomen, with sites rotated. When mixing regular insulin with other preparations of insulin, regular insulin should be drawn into syringe first. Except for rapid-acting, short-acting, or insulin glargine, gently roll vial or pen in the palms of the hands to resuspend before using. When rapid-acting insulin is mixed with an intermediate or long-acting insulin, it should be administered within 15 minutes before a meal.

Human regular insulin: Should be administered within 30-60 minutes before a meal; may be administered by SubQ, I.M., or I.V. routes

Stability

Reconstitution: Standard diluent for regular insulin: 100 units/100 mL NS; **Note:** All bags should be prepared fresh; tubing should be flushed 30 minutes prior to administration to allow adsorption as time permits. Can be given as a more diluted solution (eg, 100 units/250 mL 0.45% NS).

Compatibility:

Y-site administration: **Incompatible** with dopamine, nafcillin, norepinephrine, ranitidine

Compatibility when admixed: **Incompatible** with aminophylline, amobarbital, chlorothiazide, cytarabine, dobutamine, methylprednisolone sodium succinate, octreotide, pentobarbital, phenobarbital, phenytoin, thiopental

Storage: Insulin, regular (Humulin® R, Novolin® R): Store unopened containers in refrigerator at 2°C to 8°C (36°F to 46°F); do not freeze. Vial in use may be stored under refrigeration or at room temperature; store below 30°C (86°F) away from direct heat or light. Regular insulin should only be used if clear.

Laboratory Monitoring

Urine sugar and acetone, serum glucose, electrolytes, Hb A_{1c}, lipid profile

DKA: Arterial blood gases, CBC with differential, urinalysis, serum glucose (baseline and every hour until reaches 250 mg/dL), BUN, creatinine, electrolytes, anion gap

Hyperkalemia: Serum potassium and glucose must be closely monitored to avoid hypoglycemia and/or hypokalemia.

Nursing Actions

Physical Assessment: Assess potential for interactions with other prescriptions, OTC medications, or herbal products patient may be taking. Monitor laboratory tests, therapeutic effectiveness, and adverse reactions (eg, hypoglycemia) at regular intervals during therapy. Teach patient proper use, including appropriate injection technique and syringe/needle disposal and monitoring requirements (or refer to diabetic educator), possible side effects/appropriate interventions, and adverse symptoms to report.

Patient Education: Do not take any new medication during therapy unless approved by prescriber. This medication is used to control diabetes; it is not a cure. It is imperative to follow other components of prescribed treatment (eg, diet and exercise regimen). Take exactly as directed. Do not change dose or discontinue unless advised by prescriber. With insulin aspart (NovoLog®), you must start eating within 5-10 minutes after injection. Insulin glulisine (Apidra™) should be administered within 15 minutes before or within 20 minutes after start of meal. If you experience hypoglycemic reaction, contact prescriber immediately. Always carry quick source of sugar with you. Monitor glucose levels as directed by prescriber. Report adverse side effects, including chest pain or palpitations; persistent fatigue, confusion, headache; skin rash or redness; numbness of mouth, lips, or tongue; muscle weakness or tremors; vision changes; respiratory difficulty; or nausea, vomiting, or flu-like symptoms. **Pregnancy/breast-feeding precautions:** Inform prescriber if you are or intend to become pregnant. Consult prescriber if breast-feeding.

Dietary Considerations Dietary modification based on ADA recommendations is a part of therapy.

Geriatric Considerations How "tightly" a geriatric patient's blood glucose should be controlled is controversial; however, a fasting blood sugar <150 mg/dL is now an acceptable end point. Such a decision should be based on the patient's functional and cognitive status, how well he/she recognizes hypoglycemic or hyperglycemic symptoms, and how to respond to them and any other disease states. Patients who are unable to accurately draw up their dose will need assistance such as prefilled syringes. Initial doses may require considerations for renal function in the elderly with dosing adjusted subsequently based on blood glucose monitoring.

Breast-Feeding Issues Endogenous insulin can be found in breast milk. The gastrointestinal tract destroys insulin when administered orally; therefore, would not be expected to be absorbed intact by the breast-feeding infant.

Pregnancy Issues Insulin is the drug of choice for the control of diabetes mellitus during pregnancy.

Additional Information

Split-mixed or basal-bolus regimens: Combination regimens which exploit differences in the onset and duration of different insulin products are commonly used to approximate physiologic secretion. In split-mixed regimens, an intermediate-acting insulin (such as NPH insulin) is administered once or twice daily and supplemented by short-acting (regular) or rapid-acting (lispro, aspart, or glulisine) insulin. Blood glucose measurements are completed several times daily. Dosages are adjusted emphasizing the individual component of the regimen which most directly influences the blood sugar in question (either the intermediate-acting component or the shorter-acting component). Fixed-ratio formulations (eg, 70/30 mix) may be used as twice daily injections in this scenario; however, the ability to titrate the dosage of an individual component is limited. A example of a "split-mixed" regimen would be 21 units of NPH plus 9 units of regular insulin in the morning and an evening meal dose consisting of 14 units of NPH plus 6 units of regular insulin.

Basal-bolus regimens are designed to more closely mimic physiologic secretion. These employ a long-acting insulin (eg, glargine) to simulate basal insulin secretion. The basal component is frequently administered at bedtime or in the early morning. This is supplemented by multiple daily injections of very rapid-acting products (lispro or aspart) immediately prior to a meal, which provides insulin at the time when nutrients are absorbed. An example of a basal-bolus regimen would be 30 units of glargine at bedtime and 12 units of lispro insulin prior to each meal.

Estimation of the effect per unit: A "Rule of 1500" has been frequently used as a means to estimate the change in blood sugar relative to each unit of insulin administered. In fact, the recommended values used in these calculations may vary from 1500-2200 (a value of at least 1800 is recommended for lispro). The higher values lead to more conservative estimates of the effect per unit of insulin, and therefore lead to more cautious adjustments. The effect per unit of insulin is approximated by dividing the selected numerical value (eg, 1500-2200) by the number of units/day received by the patient. This may be used as a crude approximation of the patient's insulin sensitivity as adjustments to individual components of the regimen are made. Each additional unit of insulin added to the corresponding insulin dose may be expected to lower the blood glucose by this amount.

To illustrate, in the "basal-bolus" regimen example presented above, the rule of 1800 would indicate an expected change of 27 mg/dL per unit of lispro insulin (the total daily insulin dose is 66 units; using the formula: 1800/66 = 27). A patient may be instructed to add additional insulin if the preprandial glucose is >125 mg/dL. For a prelunch glucose of 195 mg/dL, this would mean the patient would administer the scheduled 12 units of lispro along with an additional "correctional" 3 units for a total of 15 units prior to the meal. If correctional doses are required on a consistent basis, an adjustment of the patients diet and/or scheduled insulin dose may be necessary.

Related Information

Insulin Aspart *on page 654*

Insulin Aspart Protamine and Insulin Aspart *on page 654*

Insulin Detemir *on page 654*

Insulin Glargine *on page 655*

Insulin Glulisine *on page 655*

Insulin Inhalation *on page 656*

Insulin Lispro *on page 656*

Insulin Lispro Protamine and Insulin Lispro *on page 657*

Insulin NPH *on page 657*

Insulin NPH and Insulin Regular *on page 657*

Interferon Alfa-2a (in ter FEER on AL fa too aye)

U.S. Brand Names Roferon-A®
Synonyms IFLrA; rIFN-A
Restrictions An FDA-approved medication guide is available at http://www.fda.gov/cder/Offices/ODS/labeling.htm; distribute to each patient to whom this medication is dispensed.
Pharmacologic Category Interferon
Medication Safety Issues
Sound-alike/look-alike issues:
Interferon alfa-2a may be confused with interferon alfa-2b
Roferon-A® may be confused with Rocephin®
Pregnancy Risk Factor C
Lactation Enters breast milk/contraindicated (AAP rates "compatible")
Use
Patients >18 years of age: Hairy cell leukemia, AIDS-related Kaposi's sarcoma, chronic hepatitis C
Children and Adults: Chronic myelogenous leukemia (CML), Philadelphia chromosome positive, within 1 year of diagnosis (limited experience in children)
Unlabeled/Investigational Use Adjuvant therapy for malignant melanoma, AIDS-related thrombocytopenia, cutaneous ulcerations of Behçet's disease, brain tumors, metastatic ileal carcinoid tumors, cervical and colorectal cancers, genital warts, idiopathic mixed cryoglobulinemia, hemangioma, hepatitis D, hepatocellular carcinoma, idiopathic hypereosinophilic syndrome, mycosis fungoides, Sézary syndrome, low-grade non-Hodgkin's lymphoma, macular degeneration, multiple myeloma, renal cell carcinoma, basal and squamous cell skin cancer, essential thrombocythemia, cutaneous T-cell lymphoma
Mechanism of Action/Effect Alpha interferons are a family of proteins that have antiviral, antiproliferative, and immune-regulating activity. Inhibits cell growth and proliferation and enhances immune response.
Contraindications Hypersensitivity to alfa interferon, benzyl alcohol, or any component of the formulation; autoimmune hepatitis; hepatic decompensation (Child-Pugh class B or C)
Warnings/Precautions Use caution in patients with a history of depression. May cause severe psychiatric adverse events (psychosis, mania, depression, suicidal behavior/ideation) in patients with and without previous psychiatric symptoms; careful neuropsychiatric monitoring is required during therapy. Use with caution in patients with seizure disorders, brain metastases, or compromised CNS function. Higher doses in the elderly or in malignancies other than hairy cell leukemia may result in severe obtundation.

Use caution in patients with autoimmune diseases, pre-existing cardiac disease (ischemic or thromboembolic), arrhythmias, renal impairment (Cl_{cr} <50 mL/minute), mild hepatic impairment, or myelosuppression. Also use caution in patients receiving therapeutic immunosuppression. Use caution in patients with diabetes or pre-existing thyroid disease. Discontinue if persistent unexplained pulmonary infiltrates are noted. Gastrointestinal ischemia, ulcerative colitis and hemorrhage have been associated rarely with alpha interferons; some cases are severe and life-threatening. Ophthalmologic disorders have occurred in patients receiving alpha interferons; close monitoring is warranted.

Treatment should be discontinued in patients with worsening or persistently severe signs/symptoms of autoimmune, infectious, ischemic, or neuropsychiatric disorders (including depression and/or suicidal thoughts/behavior). Discontinue treatment if neutrophils <0.5 x 10^9/L or platelets <25 x 10^9/L. **Due to differences in dosage, patients should not change brands of interferons.** Injection solution contains benzyl
(Continued)

Interferon Alfa-2a *(Continued)*

alcohol; do not use in neonates or infants. Safety and efficacy in children <18 years of age have not been established.

Drug Interactions

Cytochrome P450 Effect: Inhibits CYP1A2 (weak)

Decreased Effect: Prednisone may decrease the therapeutic effects of interferon alpha. A decreased response to erythropoietin has been reported (case reports) in patients receiving interferons. Interferon alpha may decrease the serum concentrations of melphalan (may or may not decrease toxicity of melphalan).

Increased Effect/Toxicity: Note: May exacerbate the toxicity of other agents with respect to CNS, myelotoxicity, or cardiotoxicity. Theophylline clearance has been reported to be decreased in hepatitis patients receiving interferon. Interferons may increase the adverse/toxic effects of ACE inhibitors, specifically the development of granulocytopenia. Agranulocytosis has been reported with concurrent use of clozapine (case report). Interferons may increase the anticoagulant effects of warfarin, and interferons may increase serum levels of zidovudine. Concurrent therapy with ribavirin may increase the risk of hemolytic anemia.

Adverse Reactions Note: A flu-like syndrome (fever, chills, tachycardia, malaise, myalgia, arthralgia, headache) occurs within 1-2 hours of administration; may last up to 24 hours and may be dose-limiting (symptoms in up to 92% of patients). For the listing below, the percentage of incidence noted generally corresponds to highest reported ranges. Incidence depends upon dosage and indication.

>10%:

Cardiovascular: Chest pain (4% to 11%), edema (11%), hypertension (11%)

Central nervous system: Psychiatric disturbances (including depression and suicidal behavior/ideation; reported incidence highly variable, generally >15%), fatigue (90%), headache (52%), dizziness (21%), irritability (15%), insomnia (14%), somnolence, lethargy, confusion, mental impairment, and motor weakness (most frequently seen at high doses [>100 million units], usually reverses within a few days); vertigo (19%); mental status changes (12%)

Dermatologic: Rash (usually maculopapular) on the trunk and extremities (7% to 18%), alopecia (19% to 22%), pruritus (13%), dry skin

Endocrine & metabolic: Hypocalcemia (10% to 51%), hyperglycemia (33% to 39%), transaminases increased (25% to 30%), alkaline phosphatase increased (48%)

Gastrointestinal: Loss of taste, anorexia (30% to 70%), nausea (28% to 53%), vomiting (10% to 30%, usually mild), diarrhea (22% to 34%, may be severe), taste change (13%), dry throat, xerostomia, abdominal cramps, abdominal pain

Hematologic (often due to underlying disease): Myelosuppression; neutropenia (32% to 70%); thrombocytopenia (22% to 70%); anemia (24% to 65%, may be dose-limiting, usually seen only during the first 6 months of therapy)

Onset: 7-10 days

Nadir: 14 days, may be delayed 20-40 days in hairy cell leukemia

Recovery: 21 days

Hepatic: Elevation of AST (SGOT) (77% to 80%), LDH (47%), bilirubin (31%)

Local: Injection site reaction (29%)

Neuromuscular & skeletal: Weakness (may be severe at doses >20,000,000 units/day); arthralgia and myalgia (5% to 73%, usually during the first 72 hours of treatment); rigors

Renal: Proteinuria (15% to 25%)

Respiratory: Cough (27%), irritation of oropharynx (14%)

Miscellaneous: Flu-like syndrome (up to 92% of patients), diaphoresis (15%)

1% to 10%:

Cardiovascular: Hypotension (6%), supraventricular tachyarrhythmia, palpitation (<3%), acute MI (<1% to 1%)

Central nervous system: Confusion (10%), delirium

Dermatologic: Erythema (diffuse), urticaria

Endocrine & metabolic: Hyperphosphatemia (2%)

Gastrointestinal: Stomatitis, pancreatitis (<5%), flatulence, liver pain

Genitourinary: Impotence (6%), menstrual irregularities

Neuromuscular & skeletal: Leg cramps; peripheral neuropathy, paresthesia (7%), and numbness (4%) are more common in patients previously treated with vinca alkaloids or receiving concurrent vinblastine

Ocular: Conjunctivitis (4%)

Respiratory: Dyspnea (7.5%), epistaxis (4%), rhinitis (3%)

Miscellaneous: Antibody production to interferon (10%)

Overdosage/Toxicology Symptoms of overdose include CNS depression, obtundation, flu-like symptoms, and myelosuppression. Treatment is supportive.

Pharmacodynamics/Kinetics

Time to Peak: Serum: I.M., SubQ: ~6-8 hours

Half-Life Elimination: I.V.: 3.7-8.5 hours (mean: ~5 hours)

Metabolism: Primarily renal; filtered through glomeruli and undergoes rapid proteolytic degradation during tubular reabsorption

Available Dosage Forms Injection, solution [single-dose prefilled syringe; SubQ use only]: 3 million units/0.5 mL (0.5 mL); 6 million units/0.5 mL (0.5 mL); 9 million units/0.5 mL (0.5 mL) [contains benzyl alcohol]

Dosing

Adults & Elderly: Refer to individual protocols.

Hairy cell leukemia: SubQ, I.M.: 3 million units/day for 16-24 weeks, then 3 million units 3 times/week for up to 6-24 months

Chronic myelogenous leukemia (CML): SubQ, I.M.: 9 million units/day, continue treatment until disease progression

AIDS-related Kaposi's sarcoma: SubQ, I.M.: 36 million units/day for 10-12 weeks, then 36 million units 3 times/week; to minimize adverse reactions, can use escalating dose (3-, 9-, then 18 million units each day for 3 days, then 36 million units daily thereafter)

Hepatitis C: SubQ, I.M.: 3 million units 3 times/week for 12 months

Pediatrics: Refer to individual protocols. Children (limited data):

Chronic myelogenous leukemia (CML): I.M.: 2.5-5 million units/m^2/day. **Note:** In juveniles, higher dosages (30 million units/m^2/day) have been associated with severe adverse events, including death.

Renal Impairment: Not removed by hemodialysis

Administration

I.M.: Reconstitute with recommended amount of bacteriostatic water and agitate gently; do not shake. **Note:** Different vial strengths require different amounts of diluent.

Other: SubQ administration is suggested for those who are at risk for bleeding or are thrombocytopenic. Rotate SubQ injection site. Patient should be well hydrated. Reconstitute with recommended amount of bacteriostatic water and agitate gently; do not shake. **Note:** Different vial strengths require different amounts of diluent.

Stability

Reconstitution: Reconstitute vial with the diluent provided, or SWFI, NS, or D$_5$W; concentrations ≥3 x 10^6 units/mL are hypertonic.

Storage: Refrigerate (2°C to 8°C/36°F to 46°F); do not freeze; do not shake. After reconstitution, the solution is stable for 24 hours at room temperature and for 1 month when refrigerated.

Laboratory Monitoring Baseline chest x-ray, ECG, CBC with differential, liver function, electrolytes, platelets

Nursing Actions

Physical Assessment: Monitor laboratory results on a regular basis. Monitor for effectiveness of therapy and possible adverse reactions. Monitor for neuropsychiatric changes (psychosis, mania, depression, suicidal behavior/ideation). Monitor for signs of depression or suicidal ideation. Perform eye exam prior to initiating therapy and periodically during treatment. Monitor weight periodically. Assess knowledge/instruct patient/caregiver on appropriate reconstitution, injection and needle disposal, possible side effects, and symptoms to report.

Patient Education: Use as directed; do not change dosage, brand, or schedule of administration without consulting prescriber. Maintain adequate hydration (2-3 L/day of fluids) unless instructed to restrict fluid intake. You may experience flu-like syndrome (acetaminophen may help); nausea, vomiting, dry mouth, or metallic taste (small frequent meals, frequent mouth care, sucking lozenges, or chewing gum may help); or drowsiness, dizziness, agitation, abnormal thinking (use caution when driving or engaging in tasks requiring alertness until response to drug is known). Inform prescriber **immediately** if you feel depressed or have any thoughts of suicide. Report unusual bruising or bleeding; persistent abdominal disturbances; unusual fatigue; muscle pain or tremors; chest pain or palpitation; swelling of extremities or unusual weight gain; respiratory difficulty; pain, swelling, or redness at injection site; change in vision; or other unusual symptoms. **Pregnancy/breast-feeding precautions:** Inform prescriber if you are or intend to become pregnant. Consult prescriber if breast-feeding.

Geriatric Considerations No specific data is available for the elderly; however, pay close attention to Warnings/Precautions since the elderly often have reduced Cl$_{cr}$ (<50 mL/minute), diabetes, and hyper-/hypothyroidism.

Breast-Feeding Issues Women with hepatitis C should be instructed that there is a theoretical risk the virus may be transmitted in breast milk. HIV-infected mothers are discouraged from breast-feeding to decrease potential transmission of HIV.

Pregnancy Issues Safety and efficacy for use during pregnancy have not been established. Interferon alpha has been shown to decrease serum estradiol and progesterone levels in humans. Menstrual irregularities and abortion have been reported in animals. Effective contraception is recommended during treatment.

Interferon Alfa-2b (in ter FEER on AL fa too bee)

U.S. Brand Names Intron® A
Synonyms α-2-interferon; INF-alpha 2; rLFN-α2
Pharmacologic Category Interferon
Medication Safety Issues
Sound-alike/look-alike issues:
Interferon alfa-2b may be confused with interferon alfa-2a

Pregnancy Risk Factor C
Lactation Enters breast milk/not recommended (AAP rates "compatible")

Use

Patients ≥1 year of age: Chronic hepatitis B
Patients ≥18 years of age: Condyloma acuminata, chronic hepatitis C, hairy cell leukemia, malignant melanoma, AIDS-related Kaposi's sarcoma, follicular non-Hodgkin's lymphoma

Unlabeled/Investigational Use AIDS-related thrombocytopenia, cutaneous ulcerations of Behçet's disease, carcinoid syndrome, cervical cancer, lymphomatoid granulomatosis, genital herpes, hepatitis D, chronic myelogenous leukemia (CML), non-Hodgkin's lymphomas (other than follicular lymphoma, see approved use), polycythemia vera, medullary thyroid carcinoma, multiple myeloma, renal cell carcinoma, basal and squamous cell skin cancers, essential thrombocytopenia, thrombocytopenic purpura

Investigational: West Nile virus

Mechanism of Action/Effect Alpha interferons are a family of proteins that have antiviral, antiproliferative, and immune-regulating activity. Inhibits cell growth and proliferation and enhances immune response.

Contraindications Hypersensitivity to interferon alfa or any component of the formulation; decompensated liver disease; autoimmune hepatitis; history of autoimmune disease; immunosuppressed transplant patients

Warnings/Precautions Suicidal ideation or attempts may occur more frequently in pediatric patients when compared to adults. May cause severe psychiatric adverse events (psychosis, mania, depression, suicidal behavior/ideation) in patients with and without previous psychiatric symptoms, avoid use in severe psychiatric disorders or in patients with a history of depression; careful neuropsychiatric monitoring is required during therapy. Use with caution in patients with a history of seizures, brain metastases, multiple sclerosis, cardiac disease (ischemic or thromboembolic), arrhythmias, myelosuppression, hepatic impairment, or renal dysfunction (use is not recommended if Cl$_{cr}$<50 mL/minute). Use caution in patients with a history of pulmonary disease, coagulopathy, thyroid disease (monitor thyroid function), hypertension, or diabetes mellitus (particularly if prone to DKA). Caution in patients receiving drugs that may cause lactic acidosis (eg, nucleoside analogues).

Avoid use in patients with autoimmune disorders; worsening of psoriasis and/or development of autoimmune disorders has been associated with alpha interferons. Higher doses in elderly patients, or diseases other than hairy cell leukemia, may result in increased CNS toxicity. Treatment should be discontinued in patients who develop severe pulmonary symptoms with chest x-ray changes, autoimmune disorders, worsening of hepatic function, psychiatric symptoms (including depression and/or suicidal thoughts/behaviors), ischemic and/or infectious disorders. Ophthalmologic disorders (including retinal hemorrhages, cotton wool spots and retinal artery or vein obstruction) have occurred in patients receiving alpha interferons. Hypertriglyceridemia has been reported (discontinue if severe).

Safety and efficacy in children <1 year of age have not been established. Do not treat patients with visceral AIDS-related Kaposi's sarcoma associated with rapidly-progressing or life-threatening disease. A transient increase in SGOT (>2x baseline) is common in patients treated with interferon alfa-2b for chronic hepatitis. Therapy generally may continue, however, functional indicators (albumin, prothrombin time, bilirubin) should be monitored at 2-week intervals. **Due to differences in dosage, patients should not change brands of interferons without the prescribers knowledge.**

Intron® A may cause bone marrow suppression, including very rarely, aplastic anemia. Hemolytic anemia (hemoglobin <10 g/dL) was observed in up to 10% of treated patients in clinical trials when combined with (Continued)

Interferon Alfa-2b *(Continued)*

ribavirin; anemia occurred within 1-2 weeks of initiation of therapy.

Drug Interactions

Cytochrome P450 Effect: Inhibits CYP1A2 (weak)

Increased Effect/Toxicity: Theophylline clearance has been reported to be decreased in hepatitis patients receiving interferon. Interferons may increase the adverse/toxic effects of ACE inhibitors, specifically the development of granulocytopenia. Agranulocytosis has been reported with concurrent use of clozapine (case report). Interferons may increase the anticoagulant effects of warfarin, and interferons may increase serum levels of zidovudine. Concurrent therapy with ribavirin may increase the risk of hemolytic anemia.

Adverse Reactions Note: In a majority of patients, a flu-like syndrome (fever, chills, tachycardia, malaise, myalgia, headache), occurs within 1-2 hours of administration; may last up to 24 hours and may be dose-limiting.

>10%:
Cardiovascular: Chest pain (2% to 28%)
Central nervous system: Fatigue (8% to 96%), headache (21% to 62%), fever (34% to 94%), depression (4% to 40%), somnolence (1% to 33%), irritability (1% to 22%), paresthesia (1% to 21%, more common in patients previously treated with vinca alkaloids or receiving concurrent vinblastine), dizziness (7% to 23%), confusion (1% to 12%), malaise (3% to 14%), pain (3% to 15%), insomnia (1% to 12%), impaired concentration (1% to 14%, usually reverses within a few days), amnesia (1% to 14%), chills (45% to 54%)
Dermatologic: Alopecia (8% to 38%), rash (usually maculopapular) on the trunk and extremities (1% to 25%), pruritus (3% to 11%), dry skin (1% to 10%)
Endocrine & metabolic: Alkaline phosphatase increased (48%), hypocalcemia (10% to 51%), hyperglycemia (33% to 39%), amenorrhea (up to 12% in lymphoma)
Gastrointestinal: Anorexia (1% to 69%), nausea (19% to 66%), vomiting (2% to 32%, usually mild), diarrhea (2% to 45%, may be severe), taste change (2% to 24%), xerostomia (1% to 28%), abdominal pain (2% to 23%), gingivitis (2% to 14%), constipation (1% to 14%)
Hematologic: Myelosuppression; neutropenia (30% to 66%); thrombocytopenia (5% to 15%); anemia (15% to 32%, may be dose-limiting, usually seen only during the first 6 months of therapy)
Onset: 7-10 days
Nadir: 14 days, may be delayed 20-40 days in hairy cell leukemia
Recovery: 21 days
Hepatic: Right upper quadrant pain (15% in hepatitis C), transaminases increased (increased SGOT in up to 63%)
Local: Injection site reaction (1% to 20%)
Neuromuscular & skeletal: Weakness (5% to 63%) may be severe at doses >20,000,000 units/day; mild arthralgia and myalgia (5% to 75% - usually during the first 72 hours of treatment), rigors (2% to 42%), back pain (1% to 19%), musculoskeletal pain (1% to 21%), paresthesia (1% to 21%)
Renal: Urinary tract infection (up to 5% in hepatitis C)
Respiratory: Dyspnea (1% to 34%), cough (1% to 31%), pharyngitis (1% to 31%)
Miscellaneous: Loss of smell, flu-like symptoms (5% to 79%), diaphoresis (2% to 21%)
5% to 10%:
Cardiovascular: Hypertension (9% in hepatitis C)
Central nervous system: Anxiety (1% to 9%), nervousness (1% to 3%), vertigo (up to 8% in lymphoma)
Dermatologic: Dermatitis (1% to 8%)

Endocrine & metabolic: Decreased libido (1% to 5%)
Gastrointestinal: Loose stools (1% to 21%), dyspepsia (2% to 8%)
Neuromuscular & skeletal: Hypoesthesia (1% to 10%)
Respiratory: Nasal congestion (1% to 10%)

Overdosage/Toxicology Symptoms of overdose include CNS depression, obtundation, flu-like symptoms, and myelosuppression. Treatment is supportive.

Pharmacodynamics/Kinetics

Time to Peak: Serum: I.M., SubQ: ~3-12 hours
Half-Life Elimination: I.M., I.V.: 2 hours; SubQ: 3 hours
Metabolism: Primarily renal

Available Dosage Forms

Injection, powder for reconstitution: 10 million units; 18 million units; 50 million units [contains human albumin]
Injection, solution [multidose prefilled pen]:
Delivers 3 million units/0.2 mL (1.5 mL) [delivers 6 doses; 18 million units]
Delivers 5 million units/0.2 mL (1.5 mL) [delivers 6 doses; 30 million units]
Delivers 10 million units/0.2 mL (1.5 mL) [delivers 6 doses; 60 million units]
Injection, solution [multidose vial]: 6 million units/mL (3 mL); 10 million units/mL (2.5 mL)
Injection, solution [single-dose vial]: 10 million units/ mL (1 mL)

See also Interferon Alfa-2b and Ribavirin Combination Pack monograph.

Dosing

Adults & Elderly: Refer to individual protocols.
Hairy cell leukemia: I.M., SubQ: 2 million units/m^2 3 times/week for 2-6 months
Lymphoma (follicular): SubQ: 5 million units 3 times/week for up to 18 months
Malignant melanoma: 20 million units/m^2 I.V. for 5 consecutive days per week for 4 weeks, then 10 million units/m^2 SubQ 3 times/week for 48 weeks
AIDS-related Kaposi's sarcoma: I.M., SubQ: 30 million units/m^2 3 times/week
Chronic hepatitis B: I.M., SubQ: 5 million units/day or 10 million units 3 times/week for 16 weeks
Chronic hepatitis C: I.M., SubQ: 3 million units 3 times/week for 16 weeks. In patients with normalization of ALT at 16 weeks, continue treatment for 18-24 months; consider discontinuation if normalization does not occur at 16 weeks. **Note:** May be used in combination therapy with ribavirin in previously untreated patients or in patients who relapse following alpha interferon therapy; refer to Interferon Alfa-2b and Ribavirin Combination Pack monograph.
Condyloma acuminata: Intralesionally: 1 million units/lesion (maximum: 5 lesions/treatment) 3 times/week (on alternate days) for 3 weeks. May administer a second course at 12-16 weeks.
Pediatrics: Refer to individual protocols.
Chronic hepatitis B: SubQ: Children 1-17 years: 3 million units/m^2 3 times/week for 1 week; then 6 million units/m^2 3 times/week; maximum: 10 million units 3 times/week; total duration of therapy 16-24 weeks

Renal Impairment:

Combination therapy with ribavirin (hepatitis C) should not be used in patients with reduced renal function (Cl$_{cr}$ <50 mL/minute).

Dosing Adjustment for Toxicity: Manufacturer-recommended adjustments, listed according to indication:
Lymphoma (follicular):
Severe toxicity (neutrophils <1000 cells/mm^3 or platelets <50,000 cells/mm^3): Reduce dose by 50% or temporarily discontinue
AST/ALT >5 times ULN: Permanently discontinue

Hairy cell leukemia:

Severe toxicity: Reduce dose by 50% or temporarily discontinue; permanently discontinue if persistent or recurrent severe toxicity is noted

Hepatitis B or C:

WBC <1500 cells/mm³, granulocytes <750 cells/mm³, or platelet count <50,000 cells/mm³: Reduce dose by 50%

WBC <1000 cells/mm³, granulocytes <500 cells/mm³, or platelet count <25,000 cells/mm³: Permanently discontinue

Kaposi sarcoma: Severe toxicity: Reduce dose by 50% or temporarily discontinue

Malignant melanoma:

Severe toxicity (neutrophils <500 cells/mm³ or AST/ALT >5 times ULN): Reduce dose by 50% or temporarily discontinue

Neutrophils <250 cells/mm³ or AST/ALT >10 times ULN: Permanently discontinue

Administration

I.V. Detail: pH: 6.9-7.5

Other: SubQ administration is suggested for those who are at risk for bleeding or are thrombocytopenic. Rotate SubQ injection site. Patient should be well hydrated. Reconstitute with recommended amount of SWFI and agitate gently; do not shake. **Note:** Different vial strengths require different amounts of diluent. Not every dosage form is appropriate for every indication; refer to manufacturer's labeling.

Stability

Reconstitution: The manufacturer recommends reconstituting vial with the diluent provided (SWFI). To prepare solution for infusion, further dilute appropriate dose in NS 100 mL. Final concentration should not be <10 million units/100 mL.

Compatibility: Stable in LR, NS; **incompatible** with D₅W

Storage: Store powder and solution for injection (vials and pens) under refrigeration (2°C to 8°C).

Powder for injection: Following reconstitution, should be used immediately, but may be stored under refrigeration for up to 24 hours.

Prefilled pens: After first use, discard unused portion after 1 month.

Laboratory Monitoring Baseline chest x-ray, ECG, CBC with differential, liver function, electrolytes, platelets

Nursing Actions

Physical Assessment: Monitor laboratory results on a regular basis. Monitor for effectiveness of therapy and possible adverse reactions. Monitor for neuropsychiatric changes (psychosis, mania, depression, suicidal behavior/ideation). Assess knowledge/instruct patient/caregiver on appropriate reconstitution, injection and needle disposal, possible side effects, and symptoms to report.

Patient Education: Use as directed; do not change dosage or schedule of administration without consulting prescriber. Maintain adequate hydration (2-3 L/day of fluids) unless instructed to restrict fluid intake. You may experience flu-like syndrome (acetaminophen may help); nausea, vomiting, dry mouth, or metallic taste (small frequent meals, frequent mouth care, sucking lozenges, or chewing gum may help); fatigue, drowsiness, insomnia, dizziness, agitation, abnormal thinking (use caution when driving or engaging in tasks requiring alertness until response to drug is known). Inform prescriber **immediately** if you feel depressed or have any thoughts of suicide. Report unusual bruising or bleeding; persistent abdominal disturbances; unusual fatigue; muscle pain or tremors; chest pain or palpitation; swelling of extremities or unusual weight gain; respiratory difficulty; pain, swelling, or redness at injection site; or other unusual symptoms. **Pregnancy/breast-feeding precautions:** Inform prescriber if you are or intend to

become pregnant. Consult prescriber if breast-feeding.

Breast-Feeding Issues Women with hepatitis C should be instructed that there is a theoretical risk the virus may be transmitted in breast milk. HIV-infected mothers are discouraged from breast-feeding to decrease potential transmission of HIV.

Pregnancy Issues Safety and efficacy for use during pregnancy have not been established. Interferon alpha has been shown to decrease serum estradiol and progesterone levels in humans. Menstrual irregularities and abortion have been reported in animals. Effective contraception is recommended during treatment.

Interferon Alfa-2b and Ribavirin
(in ter FEER on AL fa too bee & rye ba VYE rin)

U.S. Brand Names Rebetron®

Synonyms Interferon Alfa-2b and Ribavirin Combination Pack; Ribavirin and Interferon Alfa-2b Combination Pack

Restrictions An FDA-approved medication guide is available at http://www.fda.gov/cder/Offices/ODS/labeling.htm; distribute to each patient to whom this medication is dispensed.

Pharmacologic Category Antiviral Agent; Interferon

Pregnancy Risk Factor X

Lactation Excretion in breast milk unknown/not recommended

Use Combination therapy for the treatment of chronic hepatitis C in patients with compensated liver disease previously untreated with alpha interferon or who have relapsed after alpha interferon therapy

Mechanism of Action/Effect

Interferon Alfa-2b: Alpha interferons are a family of proteins, produced by nucleated cells, that have antiviral, antiproliferative, and immune-regulating activity. There are 16 known subtypes of alpha interferons. Interferons interact with cells through high affinity cell surface receptors. Following activation, multiple effects can be detected including induction of gene transcription. Inhibits cellular growth, alters the state of cellular differentiation, interferes with oncogene expression, alters cell surface antigen expression, increases phagocytic activity of macrophages, and augments cytotoxicity of lymphocytes for target cells

Ribavirin: Inhibits replication of RNA and DNA viruses; inhibits influenza virus RNA polymerase activity and inhibits the initiation and elongation of RNA fragments resulting in inhibition of viral protein synthesis

Contraindications Hypersensitivity to interferon alfa-2b, ribavirin, or any component of the formulation; autoimmune hepatitis; males with a pregnant female partner; pregnancy

Warnings/Precautions

Interferon alfa-2b: Suicidal ideation or attempts may occur more frequently in pediatric patients when compared to adults. May cause severe psychiatric adverse events (psychosis, mania, depression, suicidal behavior/ideation) in patients with and without previous psychiatric symptoms; avoid use in severe psychiatric disorders or in patients with a history of depression; careful neuropsychiatric monitoring is required during therapy. Use with caution in patients with a history of seizures, brain metastases, multiple sclerosis, cardiac disease (ischemic or thromboembolic), arrhythmias, myelosuppression, hepatic impairment, or renal dysfunction (use is not recommended if Cl_cr<50 mL/minute). Use caution in patients with a history of pulmonary disease, coagulopathy, thyroid disease (monitor thyroid function), hypertension, or diabetes mellitus (particularly if prone to DKA). Caution in patients receiving drugs that may cause lactic acidosis (eg, nucleoside analogues). Avoid use in patients with (Continued)

Interferon Alfa-2b and Ribavirin
(Continued)

autoimmune disorders; worsening of psoriasis and/or development of autoimmune disorders has been associated with alpha interferons. Higher doses in elderly patients, or diseases other than hairy cell leukemia, may result in increased CNS toxicity. Treatment should be discontinued in patients who develop severe pulmonary symptoms with chest x-ray changes, autoimmune disorders, worsening of hepatic function, psychiatric symptoms (including depression and/or suicidal thoughts/behaviors), ischemic and/or infectious disorders. Ophthalmologic disorders (including retinal hemorrhages, cotton wool spots and retinal artery or vein obstruction) have occurred in patients receiving alpha interferons. Hypertriglyceridemia has been reported (discontinue if severe).

Safety and efficacy in children <3 years of age have not been established. Do not treat patients with visceral AIDS-related Kaposi's sarcoma associated with rapidly-progressing or life-threatening disease. A transient increase in SGOT (>2x baseline) is common in patients treated with interferon alfa-2b for chronic hepatitis. Therapy generally may continue, however, functional indicators (albumin, prothrombin time, bilirubin) should be monitored at 2-week intervals. **Due to differences in dosage, patients should not change brands of interferons.**

Intron® A may cause bone marrow suppression, including very rarely, aplastic anemia. Hemolytic anemia (hemoglobin <10 g/dL) was observed in up to 10% of treated patients in clinical trials when combined with ribavirin; anemia occurred within 1-2 weeks of initiation of therapy.

Ribavirin: Oral: Anemia has been observed in patients receiving the interferon/ribavirin combination. Severe psychiatric events have also occurred including depression and suicidal behavior during combination therapy; avoid use in patients with a psychiatric history. Hemolytic anemia is a significant toxicity; usually occurring within 1-2 weeks. Assess cardiac disease before initiation. Anemia may worsen underlying cardiac disease; use caution. If any deterioration in cardiovascular status occurs, discontinue therapy. Use caution in pulmonary disease; pulmonary symptoms have been associated with administration. Use caution in patients with sarcoidosis (exacerbation reported). Negative pregnancy test is required before initiation and monthly thereafter. Avoid pregnancy in female patients and female partners of patients during therapy. Discontinue therapy in suspected/confirmed pancreatitis. Use caution in elderly patients; higher frequency of anemia; take renal function into consideration before initiating. Safety and efficacy have not been established in organ transplant patients, decompensated liver disease, concurrent hepatitis B virus or HIV exposure, or pediatric patients <3 years of age. Use caution in patients receiving concurrent medications which may cause lactic acidosis (eg, nucleoside analogues).

Drug Interactions
Cytochrome P450 Effect: Interferon Alfa-2b: Inhibits CYP1A2 (weak)

Decreased Effect:

Interferon alpha: Prednisone may decrease the therapeutic effects of interferon alpha. A decreased response to erythropoietin has been reported (case reports) in patients receiving interferons. Interferon alpha may decrease the serum concentrations of melphalan (may or may not decrease toxicity of melphalan). Thyroid dysfunction has been reported during treatment; monitor response to thyroid hormones.

Ribavirin: Decreased effect of stavudine and zidovudine.

Increased Effect/Toxicity: Interferon alpha: Cimetidine may augment the antitumor effects of interferon in melanoma. Theophylline clearance has been reported to be decreased in hepatitis patients receiving interferon. Vinblastine enhances interferon toxicity in several patients; increased incidence of paresthesia has also been noted. Interferons may increase the adverse/toxic effects of ACE inhibitors, specifically the development of granulocytopenia. Agranulocytosis has been reported with concurrent use of clozapine (case report). Interferons may increase the anticoagulant effects of warfarin, and interferons may increase serum levels of zidovudine. Concurrent therapy with ribavirin may increase the risk of hemolytic anemia. Concomitant use of ribavirin and nucleoside analogues may increase the risk of developing lactic acidosis. Concomitant therapy of interferon (alfa) and ribavirin may increase the risk of hemolytic anemia.

Adverse Reactions Note: Adverse reactions listed are specific to combination regimen in previously untreated hepatitis patients. See individual agents for additional adverse reactions reported with each agent during therapy for other diseases.

>10%:
Central nervous system: Fatigue (children 61%; adults 68%), headache (63%), insomnia (children 14%; adults 39%), fever (children 61%; adults 37%), depression (children 13%; adults 32% to 36%), irritability (children 10%; adults 23% to 32%), dizziness (17% to 23%), emotional lability (children 16%; adults 7% to 11%), impaired concentration (5% to 14%)

Dermatologic: Alopecia (23% to 32%), pruritus (children 12%; adults 19% to 21%), rash (17% to 28%)

Gastrointestinal: Nausea (33% to 46%), anorexia (children 51%; adults 25% to 27%), dyspepsia (children <1%; adults 14% to 16%), vomiting (children 42%; adults 9% to 11%)

Hematologic: Leukopenia, neutropenia (usually recovers within 4 weeks of treatment discontinuation), anemia

Hepatic: Hyperbilirubinemia (27%; only 0.9% to 2% >3.0-6 mg/dL)

Local: Injection site inflammation (13%)

Neuromuscular & skeletal: Myalgia (children 32%; adults 61% to 64%), rigors (40%), arthralgia (children 15%; adults 30% to 33%), musculoskeletal pain (20% to 28%)

Respiratory: Dyspnea (children 5%; adults 18% to 19%)

Miscellaneous: Flu-like syndrome (children 31%; adults 14% to 18%)

1% to 10%:
Cardiovascular: Chest pain (5% to 9%)

Central nervous system: Nervousness (3% to 4%)

Endocrine & metabolic: Thyroid abnormalities (hyper- or hypothyroidism), serum uric acid increased, hyperglycemia

Gastrointestinal: Taste perversion (children <1%; adults 7% to 8%)

Hematologic: Hemolytic anemia (10%), thrombocytopenia, anemia

Local: Injection site reaction (7%)

Neuromuscular & skeletal: Weakness (5% to 9%)

Respiratory: Sinusitis (children <1%; adults 9% to 10%)

Overdosage/Toxicology Interferon Alfa-2b: Signs and symptoms of overdose include CNS depression, obtundation, flu-like symptoms, myelosuppression; treatment is supportive.

Pharmacokinetic Note See individual agents.

Available Dosage Forms Combination package:
For patients ≤75 kg [contains single-dose vials]:
Injection, solution: Interferon alfa-2b (Intron® A): 3 million int. units/0.5 mL (0.5 mL) [6 vials (3 million int. units/vial), 6 syringes, and alcohol swabs]

Capsule: Ribavirin (Rebetol®): 200 mg (70s)

For patients ≤75 kg [contains multidose vials]:

Injection, solution: Interferon alfa-2b (Intron® A): 3 million int. units/0.5 mL (3.8 mL) [1 multidose vial (18 million int. units/vial), 6 syringes, and alcohol swabs]

Capsule: Ribavirin (Rebetol®): 200 mg (70s)

For patients ≤75 kg [contains multidose pen]:

Injection, solution: Interferon alfa-2b (Intron® A): 3 million int. units/0.2 mL (1.5 mL) [1 multidose pen (18 million int. units/pen), 6 needles, and alcohol swabs]

Capsule: Ribavirin (Rebetol®): 200 mg (70s)

For patients >75 kg [contains single-dose vials]:

Injection, solution: Interferon alfa-2b (Intron® A): 3 million int. units/0.5 mL (0.5 mL) [6 vials (3 million int. units/vial), 6 syringes, and alcohol swabs]

Capsule: Ribavirin (Rebetol®): 200 mg (84s)

For patients >75 kg [contains multidose vials]:

Injection, solution: Interferon alfa-2b (Intron® A): 3 million int. units/0.5 mL (3.8 mL) [1 multidose vial (18 million int. units/vial), 6 syringes, and alcohol swabs]

Capsule: Ribavirin (Rebetol®): 200 mg (84s)

For patients >75 kg [contains multidose pen]:

Injection, solution: Interferon alfa-2b (Intron® A): 3 million int. units/0.2 mL (1.5 mL) [1 multidose pen (18 million int. units/pen), 6 needles, and alcohol swabs]

Capsule: Ribavirin (Rebetol®): 200 mg (84s)

For Rebetol® dose reduction [contains single-dose vials]:

Injection, solution: Interferon alfa-2b (Intron® A): 3 million int. units/0.5 mL (0.5 mL) [6 vials (3 million int. units/vial), 6 syringes, and alcohol swabs]

Capsule: Ribavirin (Rebetol®): 200 mg (42s)

For Rebetol® dose reduction [contains multidose vials]:

Injection, solution: Interferon alfa-2b (Intron® A): 3 million int. units/0.5 mL (3.8 mL) [1 multidose vial (18 million int. units/vial), 6 syringes, and alcohol swabs]

Capsule: Ribavirin (Rebetol®): 200 mg (42s)

For Rebetol® dose reduction [contains multidose pen]:

Injection, solution: Interferon alfa-2b (Intron® A): 3 million int. units/0.2 mL (1.5 mL) [1 multidose pen (18 million int. units/pen), 6 needles, and alcohol swabs]

Capsule: Ribavirin (Rebetol®): 200 mg (42s)

Dosing

Adults & Elderly:

Chronic hepatitis C: Recommended dosage of combination therapy:

Intron® A: SubQ: 3 million int. units 3 times/week **and**

Rebetol® capsule: Oral:

≤75 kg (165 pounds): 1000 mg/day (two 200 mg capsules in the morning and three 200 mg capsules in the evening)

>75 kg: 1200 mg/day (three 200 mg capsules in the morning and three 200 mg capsules in the evening)

Pediatrics: Chronic hepatitis C:

Children ≥3 years: **Note:** Duration of therapy: genotype 1: 48 weeks; genotype 2 or 3: 24 weeks. Discontinue treatment in any patient if HCV-RNA is not below the limits of detection of the assay after 24 weeks of therapy. Combination therapy:

Intron® A: SubQ:

25-61 kg: 3 million int. units/m² 3 times/week

>61 kg: Refer to Adults dosing

Rebetol®: Oral: **Note:** Oral solution should be used in children 3-5 years of age, children ≤25 kg, or those unable to swallow capsules.

Capsule/solution: 15 mg/kg/day in 2 divided doses (morning and evening)

Capsule dosing recommendations:

25-36 kg: 400 mg/day (200 mg morning and evening)

37-49 kg: 600 mg/day (200 mg in the morning and two 200 mg capsules in the evening)

50-61 kg: 800 mg/day (two 200 mg capsules morning and evening)

>61 kg: Refer to adult dosing.

Renal Impairment: Patients with Cl_{cr} <50 mL/minutes should not receive ribavirin.

Dosing Adjustment for Toxicity: Note: Recommendations (per manufacturer labeling):

Anemia (RBC depression):

Patient **without** cardiac history:

Hemoglobin <10 g/dL:

Children: Decrease dose by 1/2

Adults: Decrease dose to 600 mg/day

Hemoglobin <8.5 g/dL: Permanently discontinue treatment

Patient **with** cardiac history:

Hemoglobin has ≥2 g/dL decrease during any 4-week period of treatment:

Children: Decrease ribavirin dose by 1/2 **and** decrease interferon alfa-2b to 1.5 million int. units 3 times/week

Adults: Decrease dose to ribavirin to 600 mg/day **and** decrease interferon-alfa 2b dose to 1.5 million int. units 3 times/week.

Hemoglobin <12 g/dL after 4 weeks of reduced dose: Permanently discontinue treatment

WBC, neutrophil, or platelet depression:

WBC <1500 cells/mm³, neutrophils <750 cells/mm³, or platelet count <50,000 cells/ mm³ (<80,000 cells/mm³ in children): Reduce interferon alfa-2b dose to 1.5 million int. units 3 times/week (50% reduction)

WBC <1000 cells/mm³, neutrophils <500 cells/mm³, or platelet count <25,000 cells/mm³ (<50,000 cells/mm³ in children): Permanently discontinue therapy

Administration

Oral: Capsule should not be opened, crushed, chewed, or broken. Capsules are not for use in children <5 years of age. Use oral solution for children 3-5 years, those ≤25 kg, or those who cannot swallow capsules.

Other: See individual agents.

Stability

Storage: Store the Rebetol® capsules plus Intron® A injection combination package refrigerated between 2°C and 8°C (36°F and 46°F)

When separated, the individual carton of Rebetol® capsules should be stored refrigerated between 2°C and 8°C (36°F and 46°F) or at 25°C (77°F); excursions are permitted between 15°C and 30°C (59°F and 86°F)

When separated, the individual carton or vial of Intron® A injection and the Intron® A multidose pen should be stored refrigerated between 2°C and 8°C (36°F and 46°F)

Laboratory Monitoring Obtain pretreatment CBC, liver function tests, TSH, and electrolytes and monitor routinely throughout therapy (at 2 weeks and 4 weeks, more frequently if indicated); discontinue if WBC <1.0 x 10^9/L, neutrophils <0.5 x 10^9/L, platelets <25 x 10^9/L, or if hemoglobin <8.5 g/dL (in cardiac patients, discontinue if hemoglobin <12 g/dL after 4 weeks of dosage reduction). Pretreatment and monthly pregnancy test for women of childbearing age. Reticulocyte count, serum HCV RNA levels

Nursing Actions

Physical Assessment: Assess other medications patient may be taking for increased risk of drug/drug interactions. Monitor laboratory results and adverse reactions on a frequent and regular basis during therapy (see monographs for Interferon Alfa-2b and Ribavirin). Monitor for neuropsychiatric changes (Continued)

Interferon Alfa-2b and Ribavirin
(Continued)

(psychosis, mania, depression, suicidal behavior/ideation). Assess knowledge/teach patient appropriate use (including appropriate injection technique and needle disposal), interventions to reduce side effects, and adverse symptoms to report. **Pregnancy risk factor X:** Determine that patient is not pregnant before beginning treatment and do not give to women of childbearing age or to males who may have intercourse with women of childbearing ages unless both male and female are capable of complying with contraceptive measures for 6 months prior to therapy and for 1 month following therapy. Breast-feeding is not recommended.

Patient Education: This a combination therapy. Both the injections and the oral capsules are necessary for effective therapy. Follow administration directions exactly and dispose of needles as instructed. Do not discontinue, alter dose or frequency without consulting prescriber. Do not crush, chew, or open capsules. Take at the same times each day. Maintain adequate hydration (2-3 L/day of fluids) unless instructed to restrict fluid intake. You may experience flu-like symptoms (consult prescriber for relief); nausea, vomiting, or GI upset (small frequent meals, frequent mouth care, sucking lozenges, or chewing gum may help); or insomnia, drowsiness, lethargy, fatigue, dizziness, abnormal thinking (use caution when driving or engaging in tasks that require alertness until response to drug is known). Report unusual bruising or bleeding, inflammation or pain at injection site, persistent GI disturbances, muscle pain or tremors, chest pain or palpitations, swelling of extremities, unusual weight gain, or rash. Contact prescriber immediately if you experience unusual agitation, nervousness, feelings of depression, or have thoughts of suicide. **Pregnancy/breast-feeding precautions:** This drug will cause severe fetal defects. Inform prescriber if you are pregnant. Females must not get pregnant or males must not cause a pregnancy during therapy, and for 6 months after therapy is completed. Pregnancy tests are required for females. Consult prescriber for instruction on appropriate contraceptive measures. Breast-feeding is not recommended.

Dietary Considerations Take oral formulation without regard to food, but always in a consistent manner with respect to food intake (ie, always take with food or always take on an empty stomach).

Breast-Feeding Issues Women with hepatitis C should be instructed that there is a theoretical risk the virus may be transmitted in breast milk.

Pregnancy Issues Abortifacient and teratogenic effects have been reported. Women of childbearing potential should not be treated unless 2 reliable forms of contraception are used. In addition, male patients and their female partners must also use 2 reliable forms of contraception. Pregnancy must be avoided for 6 months following therapy.

Related Information
Interferon Alfa-2b *on page 663*
Ribavirin *on page 1077*

Interferon Alfacon-1
(in ter FEER on AL fa con one)

U.S. Brand Names Infergen®

Restrictions An FDA-approved medication guide is available at http://www.fda.gov/cder/Offices/ODS/ labeling.htm; distribute to each patient to whom this medication is dispensed.

Pharmacologic Category Interferon

Pregnancy Risk Factor C

Lactation Excretion in breast milk unknown/use caution (AAP rates "compatible")

Use Treatment of chronic hepatitis C virus (HCV) infection in patients ≥18 years of age with compensated liver disease and anti-HCV serum antibodies or HCV RNA.

Mechanism of Action/Effect Alpha interferons are a family of proteins, produced by nucleated cells, that have antiviral, antiproliferative, and immune-regulating activity. There are at least 25 alpha interferons identified. Interferons interact with cells through high affinity cell surface receptors. Following activation, multiple effects can be detected. Interferons induce gene transcription, inhibit cellular growth, alter the state of cellular differentiation, interfere with oncogene expression, alter cell surface antigen expression, increase phagocytic activity of macrophages, and augment cytotoxicity of lymphocytes for target cells. Although all alpha interferons share similar properties, the actual biological effects vary between subtypes.

Contraindications Hypersensitivity to interferon alfacon-1 or any component of the formulation, other alpha interferons, or *E. coli*-derived products

Warnings/Precautions Severe psychiatric adverse effects, including depression, suicidal ideation, and suicide attempt, may occur. Avoid use in severe psychiatric disorders. Use with caution in patients with a history of depression. Use with caution in patients with prior cardiac disease (ischemic or thromboembolic), arrhythmias, patients who are chronically immunosuppressed, and patients with endocrine disorders. Do not use in patients with hepatic decompensation. Ophthalmologic disorders (including retinal hemorrhages, cotton wool spots and retinal artery or vein obstruction) have occurred in patients using other alpha interferons. Prior to start of therapy, visual exams are recommended for patients with diabetes mellitus or hypertension. Treatment should be discontinued in patients with worsening or persistently severe signs/symptoms of autoimmune, infectious, ischemic (including radiographic changes or worsening hepatic function), or neuropsychiatric disorders (including depression and/or suicidal thoughts/behavior). Use caution in patients with autoimmune disorders; type-1 interferon therapy has been reported to exacerbate autoimmune diseases. Do not use interferon alfacon-1 in patients with autoimmune hepatitis. Use caution in patients with low peripheral blood counts or myelosuppression, including concurrent use of myelosuppressive therapy. Safety and efficacy have not been determined for patients <18 years of age.

Drug Interactions

Decreased Effect: Prednisone may decrease the therapeutic effects of interferon alpha. A decreased response to erythropoietin has been reported (case reports) in patients receiving interferons. Interferon alpha may decrease the serum concentrations of melphalan (may or may not decrease toxicity of melphalan).

Increased Effect/Toxicity: Cimetidine may augment the antitumor effects of interferon in melanoma. Theophylline clearance has been reported to be decreased in hepatitis patients receiving interferon. Vinblastine enhances interferon toxicity in several patients; increased incidence of paresthesia has also been noted. Interferons may increase the adverse/toxic effects of ACE inhibitors, specifically the development of granulocytopenia. Agranulocytosis has been reported with concurrent use of clozapine (case report). Interferons may increase the anticoagulant effects of warfarin, and interferons may increase serum levels of zidovudine.

Adverse Reactions Adverse reactions reported using 9 mcg/dose interferon alfacon-1 3 times/week. Reactions listed were reported in ≥5% of patients treated.

>10%:

Central nervous system: Headache (82%), fatigue (69%), fever (61%), insomnia (39%), nervousness (31%), depression (26%), dizziness (22%), anxiety (19%), noncardiac chest pain (13%), emotional lability (12%), malaise (11%)

Dermatologic: Alopecia (14%), pruritus (14%), rash (13%)

Endocrine & metabolic: Hot flashes (13%)

Gastrointestinal: Abdominal pain (41%), nausea (40%), diarrhea (29%), anorexia (24%), dyspepsia (21%), vomiting (12%)

Hematologic: Granulocytopenia (23%), thrombocytopenia (19%), leukopenia (15%)

Local: Injection site erythema (23%)

Neuromuscular & skeletal: Myalgia (58%), body pain (54%), arthralgia (51%), back pain (42%), limb pain (26%), neck pain (14%), skeletal pain (14%), paresthesia (13%)

Respiratory: Pharyngitis (34%), upper respiratory tract infection (31%), cough (22%), sinusitis (17%), rhinitis (13%), respiratory tract congestion (12%)

Miscellaneous: Flu-like syndrome (15%), diaphoresis increased (12%)

1% to 10%:

Cardiovascular: Peripheral edema (9%), hypertension (5%), tachycardia (4%), palpitation (3%)

Central nervous system: Amnesia (10%), hypoesthesia (10%), abnormal thinking (8%), agitation (6%), confusion (4%), somnolence (4%)

Dermatologic: Bruising (6%), erythema (6%), dry skin (6%), wound (4%)

Endocrine & metabolic: Thyroid test abnormalities (9%), dysmenorrhea (9%), increased triglycerides (6%), menstrual disorder (6%), decreased libido (5%), hypothyroidism (4%)

Gastrointestinal: Constipation (9%), flatulence (8%), toothache (7%), decreased salivation (6%), hemorrhoids (6%), weight loss (5%), taste perversion (3%)

Genitourinary: Vaginitis (8%), genital moniliasis (2%)

Hepatic: Hepatomegaly (5%), liver tenderness (5%), increased prothrombin time (3%)

Local: Injection site pain (9%), access pain (8%), injection site bruising (6%)

Neuromuscular & skeletal: Weakness (9%), hypertonia (7%), musculoskeletal disorder (4%)

Ocular: Conjunctivitis (8%), eye pain (5%), vision abnormalities (3%)

Otic: Tinnitus (6%), earache (5%), otitis (2%)

Respiratory: Upper respiratory tract congestion (10%), epistaxis (8%), dyspnea (7%), bronchitis (6%)

Miscellaneous: Allergic reaction (7%), lymphadenopathy (6%), lymphocytosis (5%), infection (3%)

Flu-like symptoms (which included headache, fatigue, fever, myalgia, rigors, arthralgia, and increased diaphoresis) were the most commonly reported adverse reaction. This was reported separately from flu-like syndrome. Most patients were treated symptomatically.

Other adverse reactions associated with interferon therapy include arrhythmia, autoimmune disorders, chest pain, hepatotoxic reactions, lupus erythematosus, MI, neuropsychiatric disorders (including suicidal thoughts/behavior), pneumonia, pneumonitis, severe hypersensitivity reactions (rare), vasculitis

Overdosage/Toxicology One overdose has been reported. A patient received ten times the prescribed dose (150 mcg) for 3 days. In addition to an increase in anorexia, chills, fever, and myalgia, there was also an increase in ALT, AST, and LDH. Laboratory values reportedly returned to baseline within 30 days.

Pharmacodynamics/Kinetics

Time to Peak: Healthy volunteers: 24-36 hours

Pharmacokinetic Note Pharmacokinetic studies have not been conducted on patients with chronic hepatitis C.

Available Dosage Forms Injection, solution [preservative free]: 30 mcg/mL (0.3 mL, 0.5 mL)

Dosing

Adults & Elderly: Chronic HCV infection: SubQ: 9 mcg 3 times/week for 24 weeks; allow 48 hours between doses.

Patients who have previously tolerated interferon therapy but did not respond or relapsed: SubQ: 15 mcg 3 times/week for 6 months

Pediatrics: Not indicated for patients <18 years of age.

Hepatic Impairment: Avoid use in decompensated hepatic disease.

Dosing Adjustment for Toxicity: Dose should be held in patients who experience a severe adverse reaction, and treatment should be stopped or decreased if the reaction does not become tolerable.

Doses were reduced from 9 mcg to 7.5 mcg in the pivotal study.

For patients receiving 15 mcg/dose, doses were reduced in 3 mcg increments. Efficacy is decreased with doses <7.5 mcg.

Administration

I.V.: Interferon alfacon-1 is given by SubQ injection, 3 times/week, with at least 48 hours between doses.

Stability

Storage: Store in refrigerator 2°C to 8°C (36°F to 46°F). Do not freeze. Avoid exposure to direct sunlight. Do not shake vigorously.

Laboratory Monitoring Hemoglobin and hematocrit, white blood cell count, platelets, triglycerides, and thyroid function. Laboratory tests should be taken 2 weeks prior to therapy, after therapy has begun, and periodically during treatment. HCV RNA, and ALT to determine success/response to therapy.

The following guidelines were used during the clinical studies as acceptable baseline values:

Platelet count ≥75 x 10^9/L

Hemoglobin ≥100 g/L

ANC ≥1500 x 10^6/L

S_{cr} <180 μmol/L (<2 mg/dL) or Cl_{cr} >0.83 mL/second (>50 mL/minute)

Serum albumin ≥25 g/L

Bilirubin WNL

TSH and T_4 WNL

Nursing Actions

Physical Assessment: Assess other medications patient may be taking for effectiveness and interactions. Monitor laboratory results on a regular basis during therapy. Monitor for signs of depression and suicidal ideation. Patient with pre-existing diabetes mellitus or hypertension should have an ophthalmic exam prior to beginning treatment. Monitor patient closely for adverse reactions. If self-administered, instruct patient in appropriate storage, injection technique, and syringe disposal. Assess knowledge/teach patient purpose for use, adverse reactions and interventions, and adverse reactions to report.

Patient Education: Use exactly as directed (if self-administered, follow exact instructions for injection and syringe disposal). Do not alter dosage or brand of medication without consulting prescriber. You will need frequent laboratory tests during course of therapy. If you have diabetes or hypertension you should have ophthalmic exam prior to beginning therapy. You may experience headache, dizziness, nervousness, anxiety (use caution when driving or (Continued)

Interferon Alfacon-1 *(Continued)*

engaging in dangerous tasks until response to medication is known); nausea, vomiting, diarrhea, or loss of appetite (small frequent meals, frequent mouth care, sucking hard candy or chewing gum may help); flu-like symptoms such as headache, fatigue, muscle or joint pain, increased perspiration (mild non-narcotic analgesic may help); or hair loss (will probably grow back when treatment is completed). Promptly report any persistent GI upset; insomnia, depression, suicide ideation, anxiety, nervousness; chest pain or palpitations; muscle, bone, or joint pain; respiratory difficulties or congestion; vision changes; or other persistent adverse effects. **Pregnancy/breast-feeding precautions:** Inform prescriber if you are or intend to become pregnant. Consult prescriber if breast-feeding.

Breast-Feeding Issues Women with hepatitis C should be instructed that there is a theoretical risk the virus may be transmitted in breast milk.

Pregnancy Issues There have been no well-controlled studies in pregnant women. Animal studies have shown embryolethal or abortifacient effects. Males and females who are being treated with interferon alfacon-1 should use effective contraception.

Interferon Beta-1a

(in ter FEER on BAY ta won aye)

U.S. Brand Names Avonex®; Rebif®

Synonyms rIFN beta-1a

Restrictions An FDA-approved medication guide is available at http://www.fda.gov/cder/Offices/ODS/labeling.htm; distribute to each patient to whom this medication is dispensed.

Pharmacologic Category Interferon

Medication Safety Issues
Sound-alike/look-alike issues:
Avonex® may be confused with Avelox®

Pregnancy Risk Factor C

Lactation Excretion in breast milk unknown/not recommended

Use Treatment of relapsing forms of multiple sclerosis (MS)

Mechanism of Action/Effect Mechanism in the treatment of MS is unknown; slows the accumulation of physical disability and decreases frequency of clinical MS exacerbations

Contraindications Hypersensitivity to natural or recombinant interferons, human albumin, or any other component of the formulation

Warnings/Precautions Interferons have been associated with severe psychiatric adverse events (psychosis, mania, depression, suicidal behavior/ideation) in patients with and without previous psychiatric symptoms, avoid use in severe psychiatric disorders and use caution in patients with a history of depression; patients exhibiting depressive symptoms should be closely monitored and discontinuation of therapy should be considered.

Allergic reactions, including anaphylaxis, have been reported. Caution should be used in patients with hepatic impairment or in those who abuse alcohol. Rare cases of severe hepatic injury, including hepatic failure, have been reported in patients receiving interferon beta-1a; risk may be increased by ethanol use or concurrent therapy with hepatotoxic drugs. Treatment should be suspended if jaundice or symptoms of hepatic dysfunction occur. Hematologic effects, including pancytopenia (rare) and thrombocytopenia, have been reported. Associated with a high incidence of flu-like adverse effects; use of analgesics and/or antipyretics on treatment days may be helpful. Use caution in patients with pre-existing cardiovascular disease, pulmonary

disease, seizure disorders, myelosuppression, or renal impairment. Safety and efficacy in patients <18 years of age have not been established.

Drug Interactions

Increased Effect/Toxicity: Interferons may increase the adverse/toxic effects of ACE inhibitors, specifically the development of granulocytopenia. Agranulocytosis has been reported with concurrent use of clozapine (case report). Interferons may increase the anticoagulant effects of warfarin, and interferons may increase serum levels of zidovudine. Concurrent use of hepatotoxic drugs may increase the risk of hepatic injury in patients receiving interferon beta-1a.

Adverse Reactions

>10%:
Central nervous system: Headache (Avonex® 58%; Rebif® 65% to 70%), fatigue (Rebif® 33% to 41%), fever (Avonex® 20%; Rebif® 25% to 28%), pain (Avonex® 23%), chills (Avonex® 19%), depression (Avonex® 18%), dizziness (Avonex® 14%)

Gastrointestinal: Nausea (Avonex® 23%), abdominal pain (Avonex® 8%; Rebif® 20% to 22%)

Genitourinary: Urinary tract infection (Avonex® 17%)

Hematologic: Leukopenia (Rebif® 28% to 36%)

Hepatic: ALT increased (Rebif® 20% to 27%), AST increased (Rebif® 10% to 17%)

Local: Injection site reaction (Avonex® 3%; Rebif® 89% to 92%)

Neuromuscular & skeletal: Myalgia (Avonex® 29%; Rebif® 25%), back pain (Rebif® 23% to 25%), weakness (Avonex® 24%), skeletal pain (Rebif® 10% to 15%), rigors (Rebif® 6% to 13%)

Ocular: Vision abnormal (Rebif® 7% to 13%)

Respiratory: Sinusitis (Avonex® 14%), upper respiratory tract infection (Avonex® 14%)

Miscellaneous: Flu-like symptoms (Avonex® 49%; Rebif® 56% to 59%), neutralizing antibodies (significance not known; Avonex® 5%; Rebif® 24%), lymphadenopathy (Rebif® 11% to 12%)

1% to 10% (reported with one or both products):
Cardiovascular: Chest pain, vasodilation

Central nervous system: Convulsions, malaise, migraine, somnolence

Dermatologic: Alopecia, erythematous rash, maculopapular rash, urticaria

Endocrine & metabolic: Thyroid disorder

Gastrointestinal: Toothache, xerostomia

Genitourinary: Micturition frequency, urinary incontinence

Hematologic: Anemia, thrombocytopenia

Hepatic: Bilirubinemia, hepatic function abnormal

Local: Injection site bruising, injection site inflammation, injection site necrosis, injection site pain

Neuromuscular & skeletal: Arthralgia, coordination abnormal, hypertonia

Ocular: Eye disorder, xerophthalmia

Respiratory: Bronchitis

Miscellaneous: Infection

Overdosage/Toxicology Symptoms of overdose include CNS depression, obtundation, flu-like symptoms, myelosuppression. Treatment is supportive.

Pharmacodynamics/Kinetics

Time to Peak: Serum: Avonex® (I.M.): 3-15 hours; Rebif® (SubQ): 16 hours

Half-Life Elimination: Avonex®: 10 hours; Rebif®: 69 hours

Pharmacokinetic Note Limited data due to small doses used.

Available Dosage Forms

Combination package [preservative free] (Rebif® Titration Pack):
Injection, solution: 8.8 mcg/0.2 mL (0.2 mL) [6 prefilled syringes; contains albumin]
Injection, solution: 22 mcg/0.5 mL (0.5 mL) [6 prefilled syringes; contains albumin]

Injection, powder for reconstitution (Avonex®): 33 mcg [6.6 million units; provides 30 mcg/mL following reconstitution] [contains albumin; packaged with SWFI, alcohol wipes, and access pin and needle]

Injection, solution (Avonex®): 30 mcg/0.5 mL (0.5 mL) [albumin free; prefilled syringe; syringe cap contains latex; packaged with alcohol wipes, gauze pad, and adhesive bandages]

Injection, solution [preservative free] (Rebif®): 22 mcg/0.5 mL (0.5 mL) [prefilled syringe; contains albumin]; 44 mcg/0.5 mL (0.5 mL) [prefilled syringe; contains albumin]

Dosing

Adults & Elderly: Multiple sclerosis: **Note:** Analgesics and/or antipyretics may help decrease flu-like symptoms on treatment days:

I.M. (Avonex®): 30 mcg once weekly

SubQ (Rebif®): Doses should be separated by at least 48 hours:

Target dose 44 mcg 3 times/week: 11

Initial: 8.8 mcg (20 % of final dose) 3 times/week for 8 weeks

Titration: 22 mcg (50% of final dose) 3 times/week for 8 weeks

Final dose: 44 mcg 3 times/week

Target dose 22 mcg 3 times/week:

Initial: 4.4 mcg (20 % of final dose) 3 times/week for 8 weeks

Titration: 11 mcg (50% of final dose) 3 times/week for 8 weeks

Final dose: 22 mcg 3 times/week

Hepatic Impairment: Rebif®: If liver function tests increase or in case of leukopenia: Decrease dose 20% to 50% until toxicity resolves

Administration

I.M.: Avonex®: Must be given by I.M. injection.

Other: Rebif®: Administer SubQ at the same time of day on the same 3 days each week (ie, late afternoon/evening Mon, Wed, Fri). Rotate injection sites.

Stability

Reconstitution: Avonex®: Reconstitute with 1.1 mL of diluent and swirl gently to dissolve. Do not shake. The reconstituted product contains no preservative and is for single-use only; discard unused portion.

Storage:

Avonex®:

Prefilled syringe: Store at 2°C to 8°C (36°F to 46°F); do not freeze, protect from light. Allow to warm to room temperature prior to use. Use within 12 hours after removing from refrigerator.

Vial: Store unreconstituted vial at 2°C to 8°C (36°F to 46°F). If refrigeration is not available, may be stored at 25°C (77°F) for up to 30 days. Do not freeze, protect from light. Following reconstitution, use immediately, but may be stored up to 6 hours at 2°C to 8°C (36°F to 46°F); do not freeze.

Rebif®: Store at 2°C to 8°C (36°F to 46°F). Do not freeze, protect from light. May also be stored ≤25°C (77°F) for up to 30 days if protected from heat and light.

Laboratory Monitoring Liver function, blood chemistries, CBC and differential, BUN, creatinine

Avonex®: Frequency of monitoring has not been specifically defined; in clinical trials, monitoring was at 6-month intervals.

Rebif®: CBC and liver function testing at 1-, 3-, and 6 months, then periodically thereafter; thyroid function every 6 months (in patients with pre-existing abnormalities and/or clinical indications)

Nursing Actions

Physical Assessment: Monitor laboratory results on a regular a basis. Monitor for effectiveness of therapy and possible adverse reactions. Monitor for signs of depression and suicidal ideation. Assess knowledge/

instruct patient/caregiver on appropriate reconstitution, injection and needle disposal, possible side effects, and symptoms to report.

Patient Education: This is not a cure for MS; you will continue to receive regular treatment and follow-up for MS. Use as directed; do not change dosage or schedule of administration without consulting prescriber. If self-injecting and you miss a dose, take it as soon as you remember, but two injections should not be given within 48 hours of each other. Maintain adequate hydration (2-3 L/day of fluids) unless instructed to restrict fluid intake. You may experience flu-like syndrome (analgesics and/or antipyretics may help); nausea, vomiting, or loss of appetite (small frequent meals, frequent mouth care, sucking lozenges, or chewing gum may help); or drowsiness, sleep disturbances, dizziness, agitation, or abnormal thinking (use caution when driving or engaging in tasks requiring alertness until response to drug is known). Inform prescriber **immediately** if you feel depressed or have any thoughts of suicide. Report unusual bruising or bleeding; persistent abdominal disturbances; unusual fatigue; muscle pain or tremors; chest pain or palpitations; swelling of extremities; visual disturbances; pain, swelling, or redness at injection site; or other unusual symptoms. **Pregnancy/breast-feeding precautions:** Inform prescriber if you are or intend to become pregnant. Breast-feeding is not recommended.

Breast-Feeding Issues Potential for serious adverse reactions. Because its use has not been evaluated during lactation, a decision should be made to either discontinue breast-feeding or discontinue the drug.

Pregnancy Issues Safety and efficacy in pregnant women have not been established. Treatment should be discontinued if a woman becomes pregnant, or plans to become pregnant during therapy. A dose-related abortifacient activity was reported in Rhesus monkeys.

Interferon Beta-1b
(in ter FEER on BAY ta won bee)

U.S. Brand Names Betaseron®

Synonyms rIFN beta-1b

Pharmacologic Category Interferon

Pregnancy Risk Factor C

Lactation Excretion in breast milk unknown/contraindicated

Use Treatment of relapsing forms of multiple sclerosis (MS)

Mechanism of Action/Effect Alters the expression and response to cell surface antigens and can enhance immune cell activities; mechanism in MS in unknown

Contraindications Hypersensitivity to *E. coli*-derived products, natural or recombinant interferon beta, albumin human or any other component of the formulation

Warnings/Precautions Hepatotoxicity has been reported with all beta interferons, including rare reports of hepatitis (autoimmune) and hepatic failure requiring transplant. Interferons have been associated with severe psychiatric adverse events (psychosis, mania, depression, suicidal behavior/ideation) in patients with and without previous psychiatric symptoms, avoid use in severe psychiatric disorders and use caution in patients with a history of depression; patients exhibiting symptoms of depression should be closely monitored and discontinuation of therapy should be considered. Due to high incidence of flu-like adverse effects, use caution in patients with pre-existing cardiovascular disease, pulmonary disease, seizure disorders, myelosuppression, renal impairment or hepatic impairment. Severe injection site reactions (necrosis) may occur, which may or may not heal with continued therapy; patient and/or (Continued)

Interferon Beta-1b *(Continued)*

caregiver competency in injection technique should be confirmed and periodically re-evaluated. Safety and efficacy in patients <18 years of age have not been established.

Drug Interactions

Increased Effect/Toxicity: Interferons may increase the adverse/toxic effects of ACE inhibitors, specifically the development of granulocytopenia. Risk: Monitor A case report of agranulocytosis has been reported with concurrent use of clozapine. Case reports of decreased hematopoietic effect with erythropoietin. Interferon alpha may decrease the P450 isoenzyme metabolism of theophylline. Interferons may increase the anticoagulant effects of warfarin. Interferons may decrease the metabolism of zidovudine.

Adverse Reactions Note: Flu-like symptoms (including at least two of the following - headache, fever, chills, malaise, diaphoresis, and myalgia) are reported in the majority of patients (60%) and decrease over time (average duration ~1 week).

>10%:
Cardiovascular: Peripheral edema (15%), chest pain (11%)

Central nervous system: Headache (57%), fever (36%), pain (51%), chills (25%), dizziness (24%), insomnia (24%)

Dermatologic: Rash (24%), skin disorder (12%)

Endocrine & metabolic: Metrorrhagia (11%)

Gastrointestinal: Nausea (27%), diarrhea (19%), abdominal pain (19%), constipation (20%), dyspepsia (14%)

Genitourinary: Urinary urgency (13%)

Hematologic: Lymphopenia (88%), neutropenia (14%), leukopenia (14%)

Local: Injection site reaction (85%), inflammation (53%), pain (18%)

Neuromuscular & skeletal: Weakness (61%), myalgia (27%), hypertonia (50%), myasthenia (46%), arthralgia (31%), incoordination (21%)

Miscellaneous: Flu-like symptoms (60%)

1% to 10%:
Cardiovascular: Palpitation (4%), vasodilation (8%), hypertension (7%), tachycardia (4%), peripheral vascular disorder (6%)

Central nervous system: Anxiety (10%), malaise (8%), nervousness (7%)

Dermatologic: Alopecia (4%)

Endocrine & metabolic: Menorrhagia (8%), dysmenorrhea (7%)

Gastrointestinal: Weight gain (7%)

Genitourinary: Impotence (9%), pelvic pain (6%), cystitis (8%), urinary frequency (7%), prostatic disorder (3%)

Hematologic: Lymphadenopathy (8%)

Hepatic: SGPT increased >5x baseline (10%), SGOT increased >5x baseline (3%)

Local: Injection site necrosis (5%), edema (3%), mass (2%)

Neuromuscular & skeletal: Leg cramps (4%)

Respiratory: Dyspnea (7%)

Miscellaneous: Diaphoresis (8%), hypersensitivity (3%)

Overdosage/Toxicology Symptoms of overdose include CNS depression, obtundation, flu-like symptoms, and myelosuppression. Treatment is supportive.

Pharmacodynamics/Kinetics

Time to Peak: 1-8 hours

Half-Life Elimination: 8 minutes to 4.3 hours

Pharmacokinetic Note Limited data due to small doses used.

Available Dosage Forms Injection, powder for reconstitution [preservative free]: 0.3 mg [9.6 million units]

[contains albumin; packaged with prefilled syringe containing diluent]

Dosing

Adults & Elderly: Multiple sclerosis (relapsing-remitting): SubQ: 0.25 mg (8 million units) every other day

Pediatrics: Not recommended in children <18 years of age

Administration

Other: SubQ: Withdraw 1 mL of reconstituted solution from the vial into a sterile syringe fitted with a 27-gauge needle and inject the solution subcutaneously. Sites for self-injection include arms, abdomen, hips, and thighs. SubQ administration is suggested for those who are at risk for bleeding or are thrombocytopenic. Rotate SubQ injection site. Patient should be well hydrated.

Stability

Reconstitution: To reconstitute solution, inject 1.2 mL of diluent (provided); gently swirl to dissolve, do not shake. Reconstituted solution provides 0.25 mg/mL. Use product within 3 hours of reconstitution.

Storage: Store at room temperature of 25°C (77°F); excursions permitted to 15°C to 30°C (59°F to 86°F). If not used immediately following reconstitution, refrigerate solution at 2°C to 8°C (36°F to 46°F); do not freeze or shake solution.

Laboratory Monitoring Hemoglobin, liver function, blood chemistries

Nursing Actions

Physical Assessment: Monitor laboratory results. Monitor closely for adverse reactions, especially patients with psychiatric or suicidal histories (eg, psychosis, mania, depression, suicidal behavior/ideation). Assess patient/caregiver knowledge and teach proper administration for SubQ injections and disposal of needles if appropriate. Teach the need for adequate hydration. Monitor for opportunistic infection.

Patient Education: This is not a cure for MS; you will continue to receive regular treatment and follow-up for MS. Use as directed; do not change dosage or schedule of administration without consulting prescriber. Maintain adequate hydration (2-3 L/day of fluids) unless instructed to restrict fluid intake. You may experience flu-like syndrome (acetaminophen may help); nausea, vomiting, or loss of appetite (small frequent meals, frequent mouth care, sucking lozenges, or chewing gum may help); or drowsiness, sleep disturbances, dizziness, agitation, or abnormal thinking (use caution when driving or engaging in tasks requiring alertness until response to drug is known). Inform prescriber **immediately** if you feel depressed or have any thoughts of suicide. Report any broken skin or black-blue discoloration around the injection site. Report unusual bruising or bleeding; persistent abdominal disturbances; unusual fatigue; muscle pain or tremors; chest pain or palpitations; swelling of extremities; visual disturbances; pain, swelling, or redness at injection site; or other unusual symptoms. **Pregnancy/breast-feeding precautions:** Inform prescriber if you are or intend to become pregnant. Do not breast-feed.

Breast-Feeding Issues Because its use has not been evaluated during lactation, breast-feeding is not recommended

Pregnancy Issues There are no adequate and well-controlled studies in pregnant women. Treatment should be discontinued if a woman becomes pregnant, or plans to become pregnant during therapy.

Interferon Gamma-1b
(in ter FEER on GAM ah won bee)

U.S. Brand Names Actimmune®

Pharmacologic Category Interferon

Pregnancy Risk Factor C

Lactation Excretion in breast milk unknown/contraindicated

Use Reduce frequency and severity of serious infections associated with chronic granulomatous disease; delay time to disease progression in patients with severe, malignant osteopetrosis

Contraindications Hypersensitivity to interferon gamma, E. coli derived proteins, or any component of the formulation

Warnings/Precautions Patients with pre-existing cardiac disease, seizure disorders, CNS disturbances, or myelosuppression should be carefully monitored; long-term effects on growth and development are unknown; safety and efficacy in children <1 year of age have not been established.

Drug Interactions

Cytochrome P450 Effect: Inhibits CYP1A2 (weak), 2E1 (weak)

Increased Effect/Toxicity: Interferon gamma-1b may increase hepatic enzymes or enhance myelosuppression when taken with other myelosuppressive agents. May decrease cytochrome P450 concentrations leading to increased serum concentrations of drugs metabolized by this pathway.

Nutritional/Ethanol Interactions Herb/Nutraceutical: Dietary supplements containing aristolochic acid (found most often in Chinese medicines/herbal therapies); cases of nephropathy and ESRD associated with their use.

Adverse Reactions Based on 50 mcg/m^2 dose administered 3 times weekly for chronic granulomatous disease
>10%:
Central nervous system: Fever (52%), headache (33%), chills (14%), fatigue (14%)
Dermatologic: Rash (17%)
Gastrointestinal: Diarrhea (14%), vomiting (13%)
Local: Injection site erythema or tenderness (14%)
1% to 10%:
Central nervous system: Depression (3%)
Gastrointestinal: Nausea (10%), abdominal pain (8%)
Neuromuscular & skeletal: Myalgia (6%), arthralgia (2%), back pain (2%)

Pharmacodynamics/Kinetics

Time to Peak: Plasma: I.M.: 4 hours (1.5 ng/mL); SubQ: 7 hours (0.6 ng/mL)

Half-Life Elimination: I.V.: 38 minutes; I.M., SubQ: 3-6 hours

Available Dosage Forms Injection, solution [preservative free]: 100 mcg [2 million int. units] (0.5 mL)

Previously, 100 mcg was expressed as 3 million units. This is equivalent to 2 million int. units.

Dosing

Adults & Elderly: If severe reactions occur, modify dose (50% reduction) or therapy should be discontinued until adverse reactions abate.

Chronic granulomatous disease: SubQ:
BSA ≤0.5 m^2: 1.5 mcg/kg/dose 3 times/week
BSA >0.5 m^2: 50 mcg/m^2 (1 million int. units/m^2) 3 times/week

Severe, malignant osteopetrosis: Children >1 year: SubQ:
BSA ≤0.5 m^2: 1.5 mcg/kg/dose 3 times/week
BSA >0.5 m^2: 50 mcg/m^2 (1 million int. units/m^2) 3 times/week

Note: Previously expressed as 1.5 million units/m^2; 50 mcg is equivalent to 1 million int. units/m^2.

Pediatrics: Children >1 year: Refer to adult dosing.

Stability

Storage: Store in refrigerator. Do not freeze. Do not shake. Discard if left unrefrigerated for >12 hours.

Laboratory Monitoring CBC, platelet counts, renal and liver function, urinalysis (at 3-month intervals during treatment)

Nursing Actions

Physical Assessment: Monitor closely for effectiveness and/or interactions. Monitor laboratory results on a regular basis. Monitor for effectiveness of therapy and possible adverse reactions. Assess knowledge and instruct patient/caregiver on appropriate reconstitution, injection and needle disposal, possible side effects, and symptoms to report.

Patient Education: This is not a cure for MS; you will continue to receive regular treatment and follow-up for MS. Use as directed; do not change the dosage or schedule of administration without consulting prescriber. Maintain adequate hydration (2-3 L/day of fluids) unless instructed to restrict fluid intake. You may experience flu-like syndrome (acetaminophen may help); nausea, vomiting, or loss of appetite (small frequent meals, frequent mouth care, sucking lozenges, or chewing gum may help); or drowsiness, dizziness, agitation, or abnormal thinking (use caution when driving or engaging in tasks requiring alertness until response to drug is known). Report unusual bruising or bleeding; persistent abdominal disturbances; unusual fatigue; muscle pain or tremors; chest pain or palpitations; swelling of extremities; visual disturbances; pain, swelling, or redness at injection site; or other unusual symptoms. **Pregnancy/breast-feeding precautions:** Inform prescriber if you are or intend to become pregnant. Do not breast-feed.

Breast-Feeding Issues Potential for serious adverse reactions. Because its use has not been evaluated during lactation, breast-feeding is not recommended

Pregnancy Issues Safety and efficacy in pregnant women has not been established. Treatment should be discontinued if a woman becomes pregnant, or plans to become pregnant during therapy. A dose-related abortifacient activity was reported in Rhesus monkeys.

Iodoquinol (eye oh doe KWIN ole)

U.S. Brand Names Yodoxin®

Synonyms Diiodohydroxyquin

Pharmacologic Category Amebicide

Pregnancy Risk Factor C

Lactation Excretion in breast milk unknown

Use Treatment of acute and chronic intestinal amebiasis; asymptomatic cyst passers; Blastocystis hominis infections; ineffective for amebic hepatitis or hepatic abscess

Mechanism of Action/Effect Contact amebicide that works in the lumen of the intestine by an unknown mechanism

Contraindications Hypersensitivity to iodine or iodoquinol or any component of the formulation; hepatic damage; pre-existing optic neuropathy

Warnings/Precautions Optic neuritis, optic atrophy, and peripheral neuropathy have occurred following prolonged use. Avoid long-term therapy. Use with caution in patients with thyroid disease.

Lab Interactions May increase protein-bound serum iodine concentrations reflecting a decrease in ^{131}I uptake; false-positive ferric chloride test for phenylketonuria

Adverse Reactions Frequency not defined.
Central nervous system: Fever, chills, agitation, retrograde amnesia, headache
Dermatologic: Rash, urticaria, pruritus
Endocrine & metabolic: Thyroid gland enlargement
(Continued)

Iodoquinol *(Continued)*

Gastrointestinal: Diarrhea, nausea, vomiting, stomach pain, abdominal cramps

Neuromuscular & skeletal: Peripheral neuropathy, weakness

Ocular: Optic neuritis, optic atrophy, visual impairment

Miscellaneous: Itching of rectal area

Overdosage/Toxicology Chronic overdose can result in vomiting, diarrhea, abdominal pain, metallic taste, paresthesia, paraplegia, and loss of vision. Can lead to destruction of long fibers of the spinal cord and optic nerve. Acute overdose may cause delirium, stupor, coma, and amnesia. Treatment is symptomatic.

Pharmacodynamics/Kinetics
Metabolism: Hepatic
Excretion: Feces (high percentage)
Available Dosage Forms Tablet: 210 mg, 650 mg
Dosing

Adults: Treatment of susceptible infections: Oral: 650 mg 3 times/day after meals for 20 days; not to exceed 2 g/day

Elderly: This agent is no longer a drug of choice; use only if other therapy is contraindicated or has failed. Due to optic nerve damage, use cautiously in the elderly.

Pediatrics: Treatment of susceptible infections: Oral: Children: 30-40 mg/kg/day (maximum: 650 mg/dose) in 3 divided doses for 20 days; not to exceed 1.95 g/day

Administration

Oral: Tablets may be crushed and mixed with applesauce or chocolate syrup. May take with food or milk to reduce stomach upset. Complete full course of therapy.

Nursing Actions

Physical Assessment: Check allergy history (iodine) prior to beginning therapy. Ophthalmic exams are recommended with long-term use. Teach patient appropriate use, reinfection prevention, possible side effects/interventions, and adverse symptoms to report.

Patient Education: Do not take any new medication during therapy unless approved by prescriber. Take as directed; complete full course of therapy. Maintain adequate hydration (2-3 L/day of fluids) unless instructed to restrict fluid intake and nutrition (small frequent meals may help). You may experience GI upset (small frequent meals, frequent mouth care, sucking lozenges, or chewing gum may help). Report unresolved or severe nausea or vomiting, skin rash, fever, or fatigue. **Pregnancy/breast-feeding precautions:** Inform prescriber if you are or intend to become pregnant. Consult prescriber if breast-feeding.

Dietary Considerations Should be taken after meals.

Ipecac Syrup *(IP e kak SIR up)*

Synonyms Syrup of Ipecac
Pharmacologic Category Antidote
Pregnancy Risk Factor C
Lactation Excretion in breast milk unknown/use caution
Use Treatment of acute oral drug overdosage and in certain poisonings
Mechanism of Action/Effect Irritates the gastric mucosa and stimulates the medullary chemoreceptor trigger zone to induce vomiting
Contraindications Hypersensitivity to ipecac or any component of the formulation; do not use in unconscious patients; patients with no gag reflex; following ingestion of strong bases, acids, or volatile oils; when seizures are likely
Warnings/Precautions Do not confuse ipecac syrup with ipecac fluid extract, which is 14 times more potent.

Use with caution in patients with cardiovascular disease and bulimics. May not be effective in antiemetic overdose.

Drug Interactions

Decreased Effect: Activated charcoal, milk, carbonated beverages decrease the effect of ipecac syrup.

Increased Effect/Toxicity: Phenothiazines (chlorpromazine has been associated with serious dystonic reactions).

Nutritional/Ethanol Interactions Food: Milk, carbonated beverages may decrease effectiveness.

Adverse Reactions Frequency not defined.
Cardiovascular: Cardiotoxicity
Central nervous system: Lethargy
Gastrointestinal: Protracted vomiting, diarrhea
Neuromuscular & skeletal: Myopathy

Overdosage/Toxicology Contains cardiotoxin. Symptoms of overdose include tachycardia, CHF, atrial fibrillation, depressed myocardial contractility, myocarditis, diarrhea, persistent vomiting, and hypotension. Treatment is activated charcoal and gastric lavage.

Pharmacodynamics/Kinetics
Onset of Action: 15-30 minutes
Duration of Action: 20-25 minutes; 60 minutes in some cases
Excretion: Urine; emetine (alkaloid component) may be detected in urine 60 days after excess dose or chronic use
Available Dosage Forms Syrup: 70 mg/mL (30 mL) [contains alcohol]
Dosing

Adults & Elderly: Emetic: Oral: 15-30 mL followed by 200-300 mL of water; repeat dose one time if vomiting does not occur within 20 minutes.

Pediatrics: Emetic: Oral:

6-12 months: 5-10 mL followed by 10-20 mL/kg of water; repeat dose one time if vomiting does not occur within 20 minutes.

1-12 years: 15 mL followed by 10-20 mL/kg of water; repeat dose one time if vomiting does not occur within 20 minutes.

Note: If emesis does not occur within 30 minutes after second dose, ipecac must be removed from stomach by gastric lavage.

Administration

Oral: Do **not** administer to unconscious patients. Patients should be kept active and moving following administration of ipecac. If vomiting does not occur after second dose, gastric lavage may be considered to remove ingested substance.

Nursing Actions

Physical Assessment: The Poison Control Center should be contacted before administration. Administer only to conscious patients. If vomiting does not occur within 30 minutes, contact the Poison Control Center (or prescriber) again. Assess patient's knowledge for home use.

Patient Education: The Poison Control Center should be contacted before administration. Take only as directed; do not take more than recommended or more often than recommended. Follow with 8 oz of water. If vomiting does not occur within 30 minutes, contact the Poison Control Center or emergency services again. Do not administer if vomiting. If vomiting occurs after taking, do not eat or drink until vomiting subsides. **Breast-feeding precaution:** Consult prescriber if breast-feeding.

Additional Information The benefit of ipecac syrup to treat poisoning in children has been questioned. In November 2003, the American Academy of Pediatrics recommended that syrup of ipecac no longer be used routinely for the management of poisonings in the home. They advised parents to dispose of existing supplies of ipecac to help prevent inappropriate use.

Ipratropium (i pra TROE pee um)

U.S. Brand Names Atrovent®; Atrovent® HFA
Synonyms Ipratropium Bromide
Pharmacologic Category Anticholinergic Agent
Medication Safety Issues
Sound-alike/look-alike issues:
Atrovent® may be confused with Alupent®
Pregnancy Risk Factor B
Lactation Excretion in breast milk unknown/use caution
Use Anticholinergic bronchodilator used in bronchospasm associated with COPD, bronchitis, and emphysema; symptomatic relief of rhinorrhea associated with the common cold and allergic and nonallergic rhinitis
Mechanism of Action/Effect Blocks the action of acetylcholine at parasympathetic sites in bronchial smooth muscle causing bronchodilation
Contraindications Hypersensitivity to ipratropium, atropine, its derivatives, or any component of the formulation
In addition, Atrovent® inhalation aerosol is contraindicated in patients with hypersensitivity to soya lecithin or related food products (eg, soybean and peanut). **Note:** Other formulations may include these components; refer to product-specific labeling.
Warnings/Precautions Not indicated for the initial treatment of acute episodes of bronchospasm. Use with caution in patients with myasthenia gravis, narrow-angle glaucoma, benign prostatic hyperplasia (BPH), or bladder neck obstruction.

Drug Interactions
Increased Effect/Toxicity: Increased toxicity with anticholinergics or drugs with anticholinergic properties.

Adverse Reactions
Inhalation aerosol and inhalation solution:
>10%: Bronchitis (10% to 23%), upper respiratory tract infection (13%)
1% to 10%:
Cardiovascular: Palpitation
Central nervous system: Dizziness (2% to 3%)
Dermatologic: Rash (1%)
Gastrointestinal: Nausea, xerostomia, stomach upset, dry mucous membranes
Renal: Urinary tract infection
Respiratory: Nasal congestion, dyspnea (10%), sputum increased (1%), bronchospasm (2%), pharyngitis (3%), rhinitis (2%), sinusitis (5%)
Miscellaneous: Flu-like syndrome

Nasal spray: Respiratory: Epistaxis (8%), nasal dryness (5%), nausea (2%)
Overdosage/Toxicology Symptoms of overdose include dry mouth, drying of respiratory secretions, cough, nausea, GI distress, blurred vision or impaired visual accommodation, headache, and nervousness. Acute overdose with ipratropium by inhalation is unlikely since it is so poorly absorbed. However, if poisoning occurs, it can be treated like any other anticholinergic toxicity. An anticholinergic overdose with severe life-threatening symptoms may be treated with physostigmine 1-2 mg SubQ or I.V. slowly.

Pharmacodynamics/Kinetics
Onset of Action: Bronchodilation: 1-3 minutes; Peak effect: 1.5-2 hours
Duration of Action: ≤4 hours
Available Dosage Forms [DSC] = Discontinued product
Aerosol for oral inhalation, as bromide (Atrovent®): 18 mcg/actuation (14 g) [contains soya lecithin and chlorofluorocarbons] [DSC]
Aerosol for oral inhalation, as bromide (Atrovent® HFA): 17 mcg/actuation (12.9 g)
Solution for nebulization, as bromide: 0.02% (2.5 mL)

Solution, intranasal, as bromide [spray] (Atrovent®): 0.03% (30 mL); 0.06% (15 mL)
Dosing
Adults & Elderly:
Bronchospasm:
Nebulization: 500 mcg (one unit-dose vial), 3-4 times/day with doses 6-8 hours apart
Metered-dose inhaler: 2 inhalations 4 times/day, up to 12 inhalations/24 hours
Colds (symptomatic relief of rhinorrhea): Safety and efficacy of use beyond 4 days not established: Nasal spray (0.06%): 2 sprays in each nostril 3-4 times/day
Allergic/nonallergic rhinitis: Nasal spray (0.03%): 2 sprays in each nostril 2-3 times/day
Pediatrics:
Bronchospasm:
Nebulization:
Infants and Children ≤12 years: 125-250 mcg 3 times/day
Children >12 years: Refer to adult dosing.
Metered-dose inhaler:
Children 3-12 years: 1-2 inhalations 3 times/day, up to 6 inhalations/24 hours
Children >12 years: Refer to adult dosing.
Colds (symptomatic relief of rhinorrhea): Intranasal: Safety and efficacy of use beyond 4 days in patients with the common cold have not been established:
Children 5-11 years: 0.06%: 2 sprays in each nostril 3 times/day
Children ≥5 years and Adults: 0.06%: 2 sprays in each nostril 3-4 times/day
Allergic/nonallergic rhinitis: Intranasal: Children ≥6 years: Refer to adult dosing.

Administration
Inhalation:
Atrovent®: Shake inhaler before each use; rinsing mouth after each use decreases dry mouth side effect
Atrovent® HFA: Prime inhaler by releasing 2 test sprays into the air. If the inhaler has not been used for >3 days, reprime.

Stability
Compatibility: Compatible for 1 hour when mixed with albuterol in a nebulizer
Storage: Store at 15°C to 30°C (59°F to 86°F). Do not store near heat or open flame.

Nursing Actions
Physical Assessment: Assess potential for interactions with other prescriptions, OTC medications, or herbal products patient may be taking (especially anything that may have anticholinergic properties). Monitor patient response on a regular basis throughout therapy. Teach patient proper use, possible side effects/appropriate interventions (eg, importance of adequate hydration), and adverse symptoms to report.
Patient Education: Do not take any new medication during therapy without consulting prescriber. Use exactly as directed (see below). Do not use more often than recommended. Store solution away from light. Maintain adequate hydration (2-3 L/day of fluids) unless instructed to restrict fluid intake. May cause sensitivity to heat (avoid extremes in temperature); nervousness, dizziness, or fatigue (use caution when driving or engaging in tasks requiring alertness until response to drug is known); dry mouth, unpleasant taste, stomach upset (small frequent meals, frequent mouth care, chewing gum, or sucking hard candy may help); or difficulty urinating (always void before treatment). Report unresolved GI upset, dizziness or fatigue, vision changes, palpitations, persistent inability to void, nervousness, or insomnia. **Breast-feeding precaution:** Consult prescriber if breast-feeding
(Continued)

Ipratropium *(Continued)*

Inhaler: Follow instructions for use accompanying the product. Close eyes when administering ipratropium; blurred vision may result if sprayed into eyes. Effects are enhanced by holding breath 10 seconds after inhalation; wait at least 1 full minute between inhalations.

Nebulizer: Wash hands before and after treatment. Wash and dry nebulizer after each treatment. Twist open the top of one unit dose vial and squeeze the contents into the nebulizer reservoir. Connect the nebulizer reservoir to the mouthpiece or face mask. Connect nebulizer to compressor. Sit in a comfortable, upright position. Place mouthpiece in your mouth or put on the face mask and turn on the compressor. If a face mask is used, avoid leakage around the mask (temporary blurring of vision, worsening of narrow-angle glaucoma, or eye pain may occur if mist gets into eyes). Breathe calmly and deeply until no more mist is formed in the nebulizer (about 5 minutes). At this point, treatment is finished.

Dietary Considerations Some dosage forms may contain soya lecithin. Do not use in patients allergic to soya lecithin or related food products such as soybean and peanut.

Geriatric Considerations Older patients may find it difficult to use the metered dose inhaler. A spacer device may be useful. Ipratropium has not been specifically studied in the elderly, but it is poorly absorbed from the airways and appears to be safe in this population.

Ipratropium and Albuterol
(i pra TROE pee um & al BYOO ter ole)

U.S. Brand Names Combivent®; DuoNeb™

Synonyms Albuterol and Ipratropium

Pharmacologic Category Bronchodilator

Pregnancy Risk Factor C

Lactation Excretion in breast milk unknown

Use Treatment of COPD in those patients that are currently on a regular bronchodilator who continue to have bronchospasms and require a second bronchodilator

Available Dosage Forms

Aerosol for oral inhalation (Combivent®): Ipratropium bromide 18 mcg and albuterol sulfate 103 mcg per actuation [200 doses] (14.7 g) [contains soya lecithin]

Solution for nebulization (DuoNeb™): Ipratropium bromide 0.5 mg [0.017%] and albuterol base 2.5 mg [0.083%] per 3 mL vial (30s, 60s)

Dosing

Adults & Elderly:

COPD:

Inhalation: 2 metered-dose inhalations 4 times/day; may receive additional doses as necessary, but total number of doses in 24 hours should not exceed 12 inhalations.

Inhalation via nebulization: Initial: 3 mL every 6 hours (maximum: 3 mL every 4 hours)

Nursing Actions

Physical Assessment: See individual agents.

Patient Education: See individual agents. **Pregnancy/breast-feeding precautions:** Inform prescriber if you are or intend to become pregnant. Consult prescriber if breast-feeding.

Related Information

Albuterol *on page 47*
Ipratropium *on page 675*

Irbesartan *(ir be SAR tan)*

U.S. Brand Names Avapro®

Pharmacologic Category Angiotensin II Receptor Blocker

Medication Safety Issues

Sound-alike/look-alike issues:

Avapro® may be confused with Anaprox®

Pregnancy Risk Factor C/D (2nd and 3rd trimesters)

Lactation Excretion in breast milk unknown/contraindicated

Use Treatment of hypertension alone or in combination with other antihypertensives; treatment of diabetic nephropathy in patients with type 2 diabetes mellitus (noninsulin dependent, NIDDM) and hypertension

Mechanism of Action/Effect Irbesartan is an angiotensin receptor antagonist. Angiotensin II acts as a vasoconstrictor and stimulates the release of aldosterone, which results in reabsorption of sodium and water. These effects result in an elevation in blood pressure. Irbesartan blocks the AT1 angiotensin II receptor, thereby blocking the vasoconstriction and the aldosterone secreting effects of angiotensin II.

Contraindications Hypersensitivity to irbesartan or any component of the formulation; hypersensitivity to other A-II receptor antagonists; bilateral renal artery stenosis; pregnancy (2nd and 3rd trimesters)

Warnings/Precautions Avoid use or use smaller doses in patients who are volume depleted; correct depletion first. Deterioration in renal function can occur with initiation. Use with caution in unilateral renal artery stenosis and pre-existing renal insufficiency; significant aortic/mitral stenosis. Safety and efficacy have not been established in pediatric patients <6 years of age.

Drug Interactions

Cytochrome P450 Effect: Substrate of CYP2C8/9 (minor); **Inhibits** CYP2C8/9 (moderate), 2D6 (weak), 3A4 (weak)

Increased Effect/Toxicity: Potassium salts/supplements, co-trimoxazole (high dose), ACE inhibitors, and potassium-sparing diuretics (amiloride, spironolactone, triamterene) may increase the risk of hyperkalemia. Irbesartan may increase the levels/effects of amiodarone, fluoxetine, glimepiride, glipizide, nateglinide, phenytoin, pioglitazone, rosiglitazone, sertraline, warfarin, and other CYP2C8/9 substrates.

Nutritional/Ethanol Interactions Herb/Nutraceutical: Avoid dong quai if using for hypertension (has estrogenic activity). Avoid ephedra, yohimbe, ginseng (may worsen hypertension). Avoid garlic (may have increased antihypertensive effect).

Adverse Reactions Unless otherwise indicated, percentage of incidence is reported for patients with hypertension.

>10%: Endocrine & metabolic: Hyperkalemia (19%, diabetic nephropathy)

1% to 10%:

Cardiovascular: Orthostatic hypotension (5%, diabetic nephropathy)

Central nervous system: Fatigue (4%), dizziness (10%, diabetic nephropathy)

Gastrointestinal: Diarrhea (3%), dyspepsia (2%)

Respiratory: Upper respiratory infection (9%), cough (2.8% versus 2.7% in placebo)

>1% but frequency ≤ placebo: Abdominal pain, anxiety, chest pain, edema, headache, influenza, musculoskeletal pain, nausea, nervousness, pharyngitis, rash, rhinitis, sinus abnormality, syncope, tachycardia, urinary tract infection, vertigo, vomiting

Overdosage/Toxicology Likely manifestations of overdose include hypotension and tachycardia. Treatment is supportive. Not removed by hemodialysis.

Pharmacodynamics/Kinetics

Onset of Action: Peak levels in 1-2 hours

Duration of Action: >24 hours

Time to Peak: Serum: 1.5-2 hours

Protein Binding: Plasma: 90%

Half-Life Elimination: Terminal: 11-15 hours

Metabolism: Hepatic, primarily CYP2C9

Excretion: Feces (80%); urine (20%)

Available Dosage Forms Tablet: 75 mg, 150 mg, 300 mg

Dosing

Adults & Elderly:

Hypertension: Oral: 150 mg once daily; patients may be titrated to 300 mg once daily. **Note:** Starting dose in volume-depleted patients should be 75 mg.

Nephropathy in patients with type 2 diabetes and hypertension: Oral: Target dose: 300 mg once daily

Pediatrics: Hypertension: Oral:

<6 years: Safety and efficacy have not been established.

≥6-12 years: Initial: 75 mg once daily; may be titrated to a maximum of 150 mg once daily

13-16 years: Refer to adult dosing.

Renal Impairment: No dosage adjustment necessary with mild to severe impairment unless the patient is also volume depleted.

Stability

Storage: Store at room temperature of 15°C to 30°C (59°F to 86°F).

Laboratory Monitoring Electrolytes, serum creatinine, BUN, urinalysis

Nursing Actions

Physical Assessment: Assess potential for interactions with other pharmacological agents or herbal products patient may be taking (risk of hyperkalemia or toxicity). Monitor laboratory tests, therapeutic effectiveness, and adverse response (eg, hypotension) at regular intervals during therapy. Teach patient proper use, possible side effects/appropriate interventions, and adverse symptoms to report.

Patient Education: Do not take any new medication during therapy unless approved by prescriber. Take exactly as directed; do not discontinue without consulting prescriber. May be taken with or without food. Take first dose at bedtime. This medication does not replace other antihypertensive interventions; follow prescriber's instructions for diet and lifestyle changes. May cause dizziness, fainting, or lightheadedness (use caution when driving or engaging in tasks that require alertness until response to drug is known); nausea, vomiting, or abdominal pain (small, frequent meals, frequent mouth care, sucking lozenges, or chewing gum may help); or diarrhea (buttermilk, boiled milk, yogurt may help). Report chest pain or palpitations, skin rash, fluid retention (swelling of extremities), respiratory difficulty or unusual cough, or other persistent adverse reactions. **Pregnancy/breast-feeding precautions:** Inform prescriber if you are or intend to become pregnant. This drug should not be used in the 2nd or 3rd trimester of pregnancy. Consult prescriber for appropriate contraceptive measures if necessary. Do not breast-feed.

Dietary Considerations May be taken with or without food.

Pregnancy Issues The drug should be discontinued as soon as possible after detection of pregnancy. Drugs which act directly on the renin-angiotensin system can cause fetal and neonatal morbidity and death.

Irbesartan and Hydrochlorothiazide
(ir be SAR tan & hye droe klor oh THYE a zide)

U.S. Brand Names Avalide®

Synonyms Avapro® HCT; Hydrochlorothiazide and Irbesartan

Pharmacologic Category Angiotensin II Receptor Blocker Combination; Antihypertensive Agent, Combination; Diuretic, Thiazide

Pregnancy Risk Factor C/D (2nd and 3rd trimesters)

Lactation Enters breast milk/contraindicated

Use Combination therapy for the management of hypertension

Available Dosage Forms Tablet:
Irbesartan 150 mg and hydrochlorothiazide 12.5 mg
Irbesartan 300 mg and hydrochlorothiazide 12.5 mg
Irbesartan 300 mg and hydrochlorothiazide 25 mg

Dosing

Adults & Elderly:

Hypertension: Oral: Dose must be individualized. A patient who is not controlled with either agent alone may be switched to the combination product. Mean effect increases with the dose of each component. The lowest dosage available is irbesartan 150 mg/hydrochlorothiazide 12.5 mg. Dose increases should be made not more frequently than every 2-4 weeks.

Pediatrics: Refer to adult dosing.

Nursing Actions

Physical Assessment: See individual agents.

Patient Education: See individual agents. **Pregnancy/breast-feeding precautions:** Inform prescriber if you are or intend to become pregnant. Do not breast-feed.

Related Information
Hydrochlorothiazide *on page 610*
Irbesartan *on page 676*

Irinotecan (eye rye no TEE kan)

U.S. Brand Names Camptosar®

Synonyms Camptothecin-11; CPT-11; NSC-616348

Pharmacologic Category Antineoplastic Agent, Natural Source (Plant) Derivative

Pregnancy Risk Factor D

Lactation Excretion in breast milk unknown/not recommended

Use Treatment of metastatic carcinoma of the colon or rectum

Unlabeled/Investigational Use Lung cancer (small cell and nonsmall cell), cervical cancer, gastric cancer, pancreatic cancer, leukemia, lymphoma, breast cancer

Mechanism of Action/Effect Irinotecan and its active metabolite (SN-38) bind reversibly to topoisomerase I and stabilize the cleavable complex so that religation of the cleaved DNA strand cannot occur. This results in the accumulation of cleavable complexes and single-strand DNA breaks. This interaction results in single-stranded DNA breaks and cell death consistent with S-phase cell cycle specificity.

Contraindications Hypersensitivity to irinotecan or any component of the formulation; concurrent use of atazanavir, ketoconazole, St John's wort; pregnancy

Warnings/Precautions Hazardous agent — use appropriate precautions for handling and disposal. Severe hypersensitivity reactions have occurred.

Deaths due to sepsis following severe myelosuppression have been reported. Therapy should be temporarily discontinued if neutropenic fever occurs or if the absolute neutrophil count is <1000/mm³. The dose of irinotecan should be reduced if there is a clinically significant decrease in the total WBC (<200/mm³), neutrophil
(Continued)

Irinotecan *(Continued)*

count (<1500/mm^3), hemoglobin (<8 g/dL), or platelet count (<100,000/mm^3). Routine administration of a colony-stimulating factor is generally not necessary, but may be considered for patients experiencing significant neutropenia.

Patients homozygous for the UGT1A1*28 allele are at increased risk of neutropenia; initial one-level dose reduction should be considered for both single-agent and combination regimens. Heterozygous carriers of the UGT1A1*28 allele may also be at increased risk; however, most patients have tolerated normal starting doses.

Patients with even modest elevations in total serum bilirubin levels (1.0-2.0 mg/dL) have a significantly greater likelihood of experiencing first-course grade 3 or 4 neutropenia than those with bilirubin levels that were <1.0 mg/dL. Patients with abnormal glucuronidation of bilirubin, such as those with Gilbert's syndrome, may also be at greater risk of myelosuppression when receiving therapy with irinotecan. Use caution when treating patients with known hepatic dysfunction or hyperbilirubinemia. Dosage adjustments should be considered.

Patients with diarrhea should be carefully monitored and treated promptly. Severe diarrhea may be dose-limiting and potentially fatal; two severe (life-threatening) forms of diarrhea may occur. Early diarrhea occurs during or within 24 hours of receiving irinotecan and is characterized by cholinergic symptoms (eg, increased salivation, diaphoresis, abdominal cramping; it is usually responsive to atropine. Late diarrhea occurs more than 24 hours after treatment which may lead to dehydration, electrolyte imbalance, or sepsis; it should be promptly treated with loperamide.

Hold diuretics during dosing due to potential risk of dehydration secondary to vomiting and/or diarrhea induced by irinotecan.

Use caution in patients who previously received pelvic/abdominal radiation, elderly patients with comorbid conditions, or baseline performance status of 2; close monitoring and dosage adjustments are recommended.

Drug Interactions

Cytochrome P450 Effect: Substrate (major) of CYP2B6, 3A4

Decreased Effect: CYP2B6 inducers may decrease the levels/effects of irinotecan; example inducers include carbamazepine, nevirapine, phenobarbital, phenytoin, and rifampin. CYP3A4 inducers may decrease the levels/effects of irinotecan; example inducers include aminoglutethimide, carbamazepine, nafcillin, nevirapine, phenobarbital, phenytoin, and rifamycins. St John's wort decreases therapeutic effect of irinotecan; discontinue ≥2 weeks prior to irinotecan therapy; **concurrent use is contraindicated.**

Increased Effect/Toxicity: CYP2B6 inhibitors may increase the levels/effects of irinotecan; example inhibitors include desipramine, paroxetine, and sertraline. CYP3A4 inhibitors may increase the levels/effects of irinotecan; example inhibitors include azole antifungals, clarithromycin, diclofenac, doxycycline, erythromycin, imatinib, isoniazid, nefazodone, nicardipine, propofol, protease inhibitors, quinidine, telithromycin, and verapamil. Bevacizumab may increase the adverse effects of irinotecan (eg, diarrhea, neutropenia). Ketoconazole increases the levels/effects of irinotecan and active metabolite; discontinue ketoconazole 1 week prior to irinotecan therapy; **concurrent use is contraindicated.**

Nutritional/Ethanol Interactions Herb/Nutraceutical: St John's wort decreases the efficacy of irinotecan.

Adverse Reactions Frequency of adverse reactions reported for single-agent use of irinotecan only.

Frequencies vary with alternative dosage regimens or combination therapy.

>10%:
  Cardiovascular: Vasodilatation (9% to 11%)
  Central nervous system: Pain (23% to 62%), fever (26% to 45%; neutropenic grade 3/4: <1% to 6%), dizziness (15% to 21%), headache (17%), chills (14%), insomnia (19%)
  Dermatologic: Rash (13% to 14%), alopecia (17% to 60%, grade 2), hand/foot syndrome (13%), cutaneous reactions (20%)
  Gastrointestinal: Diarrhea, early (43% to 51%; grade 3/4: 7% to 22%), diarrhea, late (45% to 88%; grade 3/4: 6% to 31%), nausea (55% to 86%), abdominal pain (17% to 68%), vomiting (32% to 67%), anorexia (19% to 55%), constipation (25% to 32%), mucositis (29% to 30%), flatulence (12%), stomatitis (12%), dyspepsia (10%), abdominal cramping (57%), weight loss (30%), dehydration (15%)
  Hepatic: Bilirubin increased (36% to 84%), alkaline phosphatase increased (13%)
  Neuromuscular & skeletal: Weakness (48% to 76%), back pain (14%)
  Respiratory: Dyspnea (5% to 22%), cough (17% to 20%), rhinitis (16%)
  Miscellaneous: Infection (14% to 34%), diaphoresis (16%)
1% to 10%:
  Cardiovascular: Hypotension (<1% to 6%), thromboembolic events (5% to 6%), edema (10%)
  Central nervous system: Somnolence (9%), confusion (3%)
  Gastrointestinal: Abdominal enlargement (10%)
  Hepatic: SGOT increased (10%), ascites and/or jaundice (9%)
  Respiratory: Pneumonia (4%)
Note: In limited pediatric experience, dehydration (often associated with severe hypokalemia and hyponatremia) was among the most significant grade 3/4 adverse events, with a frequency up to 29%. In addition, grade 3/4 infection was reported in 24%.

Overdosage/Toxicology Symptoms of overdose include bone marrow suppression, leukopenia, thrombocytopenia, nausea, and vomiting. Treatment is supportive.

Pharmacodynamics/Kinetics

Time to Peak: SN-38: Following 90-minute infusion: ~1 hour

Protein Binding: Plasma: Predominantly albumin; Parent drug: 30% to 68%, SN-38 (active drug): ~95%

Half-Life Elimination: SN-38: Mean terminal: 10-20 hours

Metabolism: Primarily hepatic to SN-38 (active metabolite) by carboxylesterase enzymes; SN-38 undergoes conjugation by UDP- glucuronosyl transferase 1A1 (UGT1A1) to form a glucuronide metabolite. SN-38 is increased by UGT1A1*28 polymorphism (10% of North Americans are homozygous for UGT1A1*28 allele). The lactones of both irinotecan and SN-38 undergo hydrolysis to inactive hydroxy acid forms.

Excretion: Within 24 hours:Urine: Irinotecan (11% to 20%), metabolites (SN-38 <1%, SN-38 glucuronide, 3%)

Available Dosage Forms Injection, solution, as hydrochloride: 20 mg/mL (2 mL, 5 mL)

Dosing

Adults & Elderly: Refer to individual protocols. **Note:** A reduction in the starting dose by one dose level should be considered for patients ≥65 years of age, prior pelvic/abdominal radiotherapy, performance status of 2, homozygosity for UGT1A1*28 allele, or increased bilirubin (dosing for patients with a bilirubin >2 mg/dL cannot be recommended based on lack of data per manufacturer).

Single-agent therapy:

I.V.: Weekly regimen: 125 mg/m² over 90 minutes on days 1, 8, 15, and 22, followed by a 2-week rest

Adjusted dose level -1: 100 mg/m²

Adjusted dose level -2: 75 mg/m²

I.V.: Once-every-3-week regimen: 350 mg/m² over 90 minutes, once every 3 weeks

Adjusted dose level -1: 300 mg/m²

Adjusted dose level -2: 250 mg/m²

Depending on the patient's ability to tolerate therapy, doses should be adjusted in increments of 25-50 mg/m². Irinotecan doses may range from 50-150 mg/m² for the weekly regimen. Patients may be dosed as low as 200 mg/m² (in 50 mg/m² decrements) for the once-every-3-week regimen.

Combination therapy with fluorouracil and leucovorin: Six-week (42-day) cycle:

Regimen 1: I.V.: 125 mg/m² over 90 minutes on days 1, 8, 15, and 22; to be given in combination with bolus leucovorin and fluorouracil (leucovorin administered immediately following irinotecan; fluorouracil immediately following leucovorin)

Adjusted dose level -1: 100 mg/m²

Adjusted dose level -2: 75 mg/m²

Regimen 2: 180 mg/m² over 90 minutes on days 1, 15, and 29; to be given in combination with infusional leucovorin and bolus/infusion fluorouracil (leucovorin administered immediately following irinotecan; fluorouracil immediately following leucovorin)

Adjusted dose level -1: 150 mg/m²

Adjusted dose level -2: 120 mg/m²

Note: For all regimens: It is recommended that new courses begin only after the granulocyte count recovers to ≥1500/mm³, the platelet count recovers to ≥100,000/mm³, and treatment-related diarrhea has fully resolved. Treatment should be delayed 1-2 weeks to allow for recovery from treatment-related toxicities. If the patient has not recovered after a 2-week delay, consideration should be given to discontinuing irinotecan.

Hepatic Impairment: The manufacturer recommends that no change in dosage or administration be made for patients with liver metastases and normal hepatic function. Consideration may be given to starting irinotecan at a lower dose (eg, 100 mg/m²) if bilirubin is 1-2 mg/dL; for total serum bilirubin elevations >2.0 mg/dL, specific recommendations are not available.

Dosing Adjustment for Toxicity: It is recommended that new courses begin only after the granulocyte count recovers to ≥1500/mm³, the platelet counts recover to ≥100,000/mm³, and treatment-related diarrhea has fully resolved. Depending on the patient's ability to tolerate therapy, doses should be adjusted in increments of 25-50 mg/m². Treatment should be delayed 1-2 weeks to allow for recovery from treatment-related toxicities. If the patient has not recovered after a 2-week delay, consideration should be given to discontinuing irinotecan. See tables on this page and next.

Administration

I.V.: I.V. infusion, usually over 90 minutes.

I.V. Detail: pH: 3.0-3.8

Stability

Reconstitution: Dilute in 250-500 mL D₅W or NS to a final concentration of 0.12-2.8 mg/mL. Due to the relatively acidic pH, irinotecan appears to be more stable in D₅W than NS.

Compatibility: Stable in D₅W, NS

Y-site administration: Incompatible with gemcitabine

Compatibility when admixed: Incompatible with methylprednisolone sodium succinate

Storage: Store intact vials of injection at room temperature of 15°C to 30°C (59°F to 86°F); protect from light. Solutions diluted in NS may precipitate if refrigerated. Solutions diluted in D₅W are stable for 24 hours at room temperature or 48 hours under refrigeration at 2°C to 8°C.

Laboratory Monitoring CBC with differential and platelet count

Single-Agent Schedule: Recommended Dosage Modifications[1]

Toxicity NCI Grade[2] (Value)	During a Cycle of Therapy	At Start of Subsequent Cycles of Therapy (After Adequate Recovery), Compared to Starting Dose In Previous Cycle[1]	
	Weekly	Weekly	Once Every 3 Weeks
No toxicity	Maintain dose level	↑ 25 mg/m² up to a maximum dose of 150 mg/m²	Maintain dose level
Neutropenia			
1 (1500-1999/ mm³)	Maintain dose level	Maintain dose level	Maintain dose level
2 (1000-1499/ mm³)	↓ 25 mg/m²	Maintain dose level	Maintain dose level
3 (500-999/ mm³)	Omit dose until resolved to ≤ grade 2, then ↓ 25 mg/m²	↓ 25 mg/m²	↓ 50 mg/m²
4 (<500/mm³)	Omit dose until resolved to ≤ grade 2, then ↓ 50 mg/m²	↓ 50 mg/m²	↓ 50 mg/m²
Neutropenic Fever (grade 4 neutropenia and ≥ grade 2 fever)	Omit dose until resolved, then ↓ 50 mg/m²	↓ 50 mg/m²	↓ 50 mg/m²
Other Hematologic Toxicities	Dose modifications for leukopenia, thrombocytopenia, and anemia during a course of therapy and at the start of subsequent courses of therapy are also based on NCI toxicity criteria and are the same as recommended for neutropenia above.		
Diarrhea			
1 (2-3 stools/ day > pretreatment)	Maintain dose level	Maintain dose level	Maintain dose level
2 (4-6 stools/ day > pretreatment)	↓ 25 mg/m²	Maintain dose level	Maintain dose level
3 (7-9 stools/ day > pretreatment)	Omit dose until resolved to ≤ grade 2, then ↓ 25 mg/m²	↓ 25 mg/m²	↓ 50 mg/m²
4 (≥10 stools/ day > pretreatment)	Omit dose until resolved to ≤ grade 2, then ↓ 50 mg/m²	↓ 50 mg/m²	↓ 50 mg/m²
Other Nonhematologic Toxicities[3]			
1	Maintain dose level	Maintain dose level	Maintain dose level
2	↓ 25 mg/m²	↓ 25 mg/m²	↓ 50 mg/m²
3	Omit dose until resolved to ≤ grade 2, then ↓ 25 mg/m²	↓ 25 mg/m²	↓ 50 mg/m²
4	Omit dose until resolved to ≤ grade 2, then ↓ 50 mg/m²	↓ 50 mg/m²	↓ 50 mg/m²

[1]All dose modifications should be based on the worst preceding toxicity.

[2]National Cancer Institute Common Toxicity Criteria (version 1.0).

[3]Excludes alopecia, anorexia, asthenia.

Nursing Actions

Physical Assessment: Assess potential for interactions with other pharmacological agents prescriptions or herbal products patient may be taking (eg, potential for increased or decreased levels/effects of (Continued)

Irinotecan *(Continued)*

irinotecan). Premedication with antiemetic may be ordered (emetic potential moderately high). Monitor infusion site closely to prevent extravasation. Monitor laboratory tests and patient response prior to each infusion and at regular intervals during therapy (eg, acute diarrhea, neutropenia, sepsis, mucositis and/or stomatitis). Teach patient possible side effects/appropriate interventions, and adverse symptoms to report.

Combination Schedules: Recommended Dosage Modifications[1]

Toxicity NCI[2] Grade (Value)	During a Cycle of Therapy	At the Start of Subsequent Cycles of Therapy (After Adequate Recovery), Compared to the Starting Dose in the Previous Cycle[1]
No toxicity	Maintain dose level	Maintain dose level
Neutropenia		
1 (1500-1999/mm^3)	Maintain dose level	Maintain dose level
2 (1000-1499/mm^3)	↓ 1 dose level	Maintain dose level
3 (500-999/mm^3)	Omit dose until resolved to ≤ grade 2, then ↓ 1 dose level	↓ 1 dose level
4 (<500/mm^3)	Omit dose until resolved to ≤ grade 2, then ↓ 2 dose levels	↓ 2 dose levels
Neutropenic Fever (grade 4 neutropenia and ≥ grade 2 fever)	Omit dose until resolved, then ↓ 2 dose levels	
Other Hematologic Toxicities	Dose modifications for leukopenia or thrombocytopenia during a course of therapy and at the start of subsequent courses of therapy are also based on NCI toxicity criteria and are the same as recommended for neutropenia above.	
Diarrhea		
1 (2-3 stools/day > pretreatment)	Delay dose until resolved to baseline, then give same dose	Maintain dose level
2 (4-6 stools/day > pretreatment)	Omit dose until resolved to baseline, then ↓ 1 dose level	Maintain dose level
3 (7-9 stools/day > pretreatment)	Omit dose until resolved to baseline, then ↓ by 1 dose level	↓ 1 dose level
4 (≥10 stools/day > pretreatment)	Omit dose until resolved to baseline, then ↓ 2 dose levels	↓ 2 dose levels
Other Nonhematologic Toxicities[3]		
1	Maintain dose level	Maintain dose level
2	Omit dose until resolved to ≤ grade 1, then ↓ 1 dose level	Maintain dose level
3	Omit dose until resolved to ≤ grade 2, then ↓ 1 dose level	↓ 1 dose level
4	Omit dose until resolved to ≤ grade 2, then ↓ 2 dose levels	↓ 2 dose levels
Mucositis and/or stomatitis	Decrease only 5-FU, not irinotecan	Decrease only 5-FU, not irinotecan

[1]All dose modifications should be based on the worst preceding toxicity.

[2]National Cancer Institute Common Toxicity Criteria (version 1.0).

[3]Excludes alopecia, anorexia, asthenia.

Patient Education: Do not take any new medication during therapy unless approved by prescriber. This drug can only be administered by infusion. Report immediately any burning, pain, redness, or swelling at infusion site. Maintain adequate hydration (3-4 L/day of fluids) unless instructed to restrict fluid intake during therapy. May cause severe diarrhea; follow instructions for taking antidiarrheal medication. Report immediately if diarrhea persists or you experience signs of dehydration (eg, fainting, dizziness, light-headedness). You may be more susceptible to infection (avoid crowds and exposure to infection and do not have any vaccinations without consulting prescriber). You may experience nausea or vomiting (small, frequent meals, frequent mouth care, sucking lozenges, or chewing gum may help); hair loss (will regrow after treatment is completed). Report unresolved nausea, or vomiting, alterations in urinary pattern (increased or decreased); opportunistic infection (fever, chills, unusual bruising or bleeding, fatigue, purulent vaginal discharge, unhealed mouth sores), chest pain or respiratory difficulty. **Pregnancy/breast-feeding precautions:** Inform prescriber if you are pregnant. Do not get pregnant or cause a pregnancy (males) while taking this medication. Consult prescriber for use appropriate contraceptive measures (may cause severe fetal defects). Do not breast-feed.

Pregnancy Issues Has shown to be teratogenic in animals. Teratogenic effects include a variety of external, visceral, and skeletal abnormalities. The patient should be warned of potential hazards to the fetus.

Additional Information Patients who are homozygous for the UGT1A1*28 allele are at increased risk for neutropenia; a decreased dose is recommended. Clinical research of patients who are heterozygous for UGT1A1*28 have been variable for increased neutropenic risk and such patients have tolerated normal starting doses.

Iron Dextran Complex
(EYE ern DEKS tran KOM pleks)

U.S. Brand Names Dexferrum®; INFeD®

Pharmacologic Category Iron Salt

Medication Safety Issues
Sound-alike/look-alike issues:
Dexferrum® may be confused with Desferal®

Pregnancy Risk Factor C

Lactation Enters breast milk/contraindicated

Use Treatment of microcytic hypochromic anemia resulting from iron deficiency in patients in whom oral administration is infeasible or ineffective

Mechanism of Action/Effect The released iron, from the plasma, eventually replenishes the depleted iron stores in the bone marrow where it is incorporated into hemoglobin

Contraindications Hypersensitivity to iron dextran or any component of the formulation; all anemias that are not involved with iron deficiency; hemochromatosis; hemolytic anemia

Warnings/Precautions Use with caution in patients with history of asthma, hepatic impairment, or rheumatoid arthritis. Not recommended in children <4 months of age. Deaths associated with parenteral administration following anaphylactic-type reactions have been reported. Use only in patients where the iron deficient state is not amenable to oral iron therapy. A test dose of 0.5 mL I.V. or I.M. should be given to observe for adverse reactions. I.V. administration of iron dextran is often preferred.

Drug Interactions
Decreased Effect: Decreased effect with chloramphenicol.

Nutritional/Ethanol Interactions Food: Iron bioavailability may be decreased if taken with dairy products.

Lab Interactions May cause falsely elevated values of serum bilirubin and falsely decreased values of serum calcium.

Adverse Reactions
>10%:
Cardiovascular: Flushing

Central nervous system: Dizziness, fever, headache, pain

Gastrointestinal: Nausea, vomiting, metallic taste

Local: Staining of skin at the site of I.M. injection

Miscellaneous: Diaphoresis

1% to 10%:

Cardiovascular: Hypotension (1% to 2%)

Dermatologic: Urticaria (1% to 2%), phlebitis (1% to 2%)

Gastrointestinal: Diarrhea

Genitourinary: Discoloration of urine

Note: Diaphoresis, urticaria, arthralgia, fever, chills, dizziness, headache, and nausea may be delayed 24-48 hours after I.V. administration or 3-4 days after I.M. administration.

Anaphylactoid reactions: Respiratory difficulties and cardiovascular collapse have been reported and occur most frequently within the first several minutes of administration.

Overdosage/Toxicology Symptoms of overdose include erosion of GI mucosa, pulmonary edema, hyperthermia, convulsions, tachycardia, hepatic and renal impairment, coma, hematemesis, lethargy, tachycardia, and acidosis. Serum iron level >300 mcg/mL requires treatment of overdose due to severe toxicity. If severe iron overdose (when the serum iron concentration exceeds the total iron-binding capacity) occurs, it may be treated with deferoxamine. Deferoxamine may be administered I.V. (80 mg/kg over 24 hours) or I.M. (40-90 mg/kg every 8 hours).

Pharmacodynamics/Kinetics

Excretion: Urine and feces via reticuloendothelial system

Available Dosage Forms Note: Strength expressed as elemental iron

Injection, solution:

Dexferrum®: 50 mg/mL (1 mL, 2 mL)

INFeD®: 50 mg/mL (2 mL)

Dosing

Adults & Elderly:

Note: A 0.5 mL test dose should be given prior to starting iron dextran therapy.

Milliliters of Iron Dextran (50 mg/mL) Required for Hemoglobin Restoration and Replacement of Iron Stores

Patient's IBW (kg)	Observed Hemoglobin							
	3 g/dL	4 g/dL	5 g/dL	6 g/dL	7 g/dL	8 g/dL	9 g/dL	10 g/dL
5	3	3	3	3	2	2	2	2
10	7	6	6	5	5	4	4	3
15	10	9	9	8	7	7	6	5
20	16	15	14	13	12	11	10	9
25	20	18	17	16	15	14	13	12
30	23	22	21	19	18	17	15	14
35	27	26	24	23	21	20	18	17
40	31	29	28	26	24	22	21	19
45	35	33	31	29	27	25	23	21
50	39	37	35	32	30	28	26	24
55	43	41	38	36	33	31	28	26
60	47	44	42	39	36	34	31	28
65	51	48	45	42	39	36	34	31
70	55	52	49	45	42	39	36	33
75	59	55	52	49	45	42	39	35
80	63	59	55	52	48	45	41	38
85	66	63	59	55	51	48	44	40
90	70	66	62	58	54	50	46	42
95	74	70	66	62	57	53	49	45
100	78	74	69	65	60	56	52	47

Iron dextran doses calculated for normal adult hemoglobin of 14.8 g/dL for IBW >15 kg, and normal hemoglobin of 12.0 g/dL for IBW ≤15 kg.

Iron-deficiency anemia: I.M., I.V.: (see table)

Dose (mL) = 0.0442 (desired Hgb - observed Hgb) x LBW + (0.26 x LBW)

Desired hemoglobin: Usually 14.8 g/dL

LBW = Lean body weight in kg

IBW (male) = 50 kg + (2.3 kg x inches over 60")

IBW (female) = 45.5 kg + (2.3 kg x inches over 60")

Iron replacement therapy for blood loss: I.M., I.V.:

Replacement iron (mg) = blood loss (mL) x Hct

Maximum daily dosage:

Manufacturer's labeling: **Note:** Replacement of larger estimated iron deficits may be achieved by serial administration of smaller incremental dosages. Daily dosages should be limited to: Adults >50 kg: 100 mg iron (2 mL)

Total dose infusion (unlabeled): The entire dose (estimated iron deficit) may be diluted and administered as a one-time I.V. infusion.

Pediatrics: Note: A 0.5 mL test dose (0.25 mL in infants) should be given prior to starting iron dextran therapy.

Iron-deficiency anemia: I.M., I.V.:

Children 5-15 kg: Should not normally be given in the first 4 months of life:

Dose (mL) = 0.0442 (desired Hgb - observed Hgb) x W + (0.26 x W)

Desired hemoglobin: Usually 12 g/dL

W = Total body weight in kg

Children >15 kg: Refer to adult dosing.

Iron replacement therapy for blood loss: Refer to adult dosing.

Maximum daily dose:

5-10 kg: 50 mg iron (1 mL)

10-50 kg: 100 mg iron (2 mL)

Administration

I.M.: Note: Test dose: A test dose should be given on the first day of therapy; patient should be observed for 1 hour for hypersensitivity reaction, then the remaining dose (dose minus test dose) should be given. Epinephrine should be available.

I.M.: Use Z-track technique (displacement of the skin laterally prior to injection); injection should be deep into the upper outer quadrant of buttock; subsequent injections should be given into alternate buttock.

I.V.: A test dose should be given on the first day of therapy and administer gradually over at least 5 minutes. Subsequent dose(s) may be administered by I.V. bolus at rate of ≤50 mg/minute or diluted in 250-1000 mL NS and infused over 1-6 hours (initial 25 mL should be given slowly and patient should be observed for allergic reactions); avoid dilutions with dextrose (increased incidence of local pain and phlebitis)

I.V. Detail: pH: 5.2-6.5

Stability

Reconstitution: Solutions for infusion should be diluted in 250-1000 mL NS.

Compatibility: Stable in D_5W, NS

Storage: Store at room temperature. Stability of parenteral admixture is 3 months refrigerated.

Laboratory Monitoring Hemoglobin, hematocrit, reticulocyte count, serum ferritin

Nursing Actions

Physical Assessment: Monitor laboratory tests regularly. Monitor patient for adverse reactions. Note that adverse response may occur some time (1-4 days) after administration. Assess patients with rheumatoid arthritis for exacerbated swelling and joint pain; adjust medications as needed.

Patient Education: You will need frequent blood tests while on this therapy. If you have rheumatoid arthritis, you may experience increased swelling or joint pain; consult prescriber for medication adjustment. If you experience dizziness or severe headache, use

(Continued)

Iron Dextran Complex *(Continued)*

caution when driving or engaging in tasks that require alertness until response to drug is known. Small frequent meals, frequent mouth care, sucking lozenges, or chewing gum may relieve nausea and metallic taste. You may experience increased sweating. Report acute GI problems, fever, respiratory difficulty, rapid heartbeat, yellowing of skin or eyes, or swelling of hands and feet. **Pregnancy/breast-feeding precautions:** Inform prescriber if you are or intend to become pregnant. Do not breast-feed.

Geriatric Considerations Anemia in the elderly is most often caused by "anemia of chronic disease", a result of aging effect in bone marrow, or associated with inflammation rather than blood loss. Iron stores are usually normal or increased, with a serum ferritin >50 ng/mL and a decreased total iron binding capacity. Hence, the anemia is not secondary to iron deficiency but the inability of the reticuloendothelial system to use available iron stores. I.V. administration of iron dextran is often preferred over I.M. in the elderly secondary to a decreased muscle mass and the need for daily injections.

Iron Sucrose *(EYE ern SOO krose)*

U.S. Brand Names Venofer®

Pharmacologic Category Iron Salt

Pregnancy Risk Factor B

Lactation Excretion in breast milk unknown/use caution

Use Treatment of iron-deficiency anemia in chronic renal failure, including nondialysis-dependent patients (with or without erythropoietin therapy) and dialysis-dependent patients receiving erythropoietin therapy

Mechanism of Action/Effect Iron sucrose is dissociated by the reticuloendothelial system into iron and sucrose. The released iron increases serum iron concentrations and is incorporated into hemoglobin.

Contraindications Hypersensitivity to iron sucrose or any component of the formulation; evidence of iron overload; anemia not caused by iron deficiency

Warnings/Precautions Rare anaphylactic and anaphylactoid reactions, including serious or life-threatening reactions, have been reported. Facilities (equipment and personnel) for cardiopulmonary resuscitation should be available during initial administration until response/tolerance has been established. Hypotension has been reported frequently in hemodialysis dependent patients. The incidence of hypotension in nondialysis patients is substantially lower. Hypotension may be related to total dose or rate of administration (avoid rapid I.V. injection), follow recommended guidelines. Withhold iron in the presence of tissue iron overload; periodic monitoring of hemoglobin, hematocrit, serum ferritin, and transferrin saturation is recommended. Safety and efficacy in children have not been established.

Drug Interactions

Decreased Effect: Ace inhibitors may enhance the adverse/toxic effects (erythema, abdominal cramps, nausea, vomiting, hypotension) of iron sucrose.

Increased Effect/Toxicity: Iron sucrose injection may reduce the absorption of oral iron preparations.

Adverse Reactions

>10%:

Cardiovascular: Hypotension (1% to 7%; 39% in hemodialysis patients; may be related to total dose or rate of administration); peripheral edema (2% to 13%)

Central nervous system: Headache (3% to 13%)

Gastrointestinal: Nausea (1% to 15%)

Neuromuscular & skeletal: Muscle cramps (1% to 3%; 29% in hemodialysis patients)

1% to 10%:

Cardiovascular: Hypertension (6% to 8%), edema (1% to 7%), chest pain (1% to 6%), murmur (<1% to 3%), CHF

Central nervous system: Dizziness (1% to 10%), fatigue (2% to 5%), fever (1% to 3%), anxiety

Dermatologic: Pruritus (1% to 7%), rash (<1% to 2%)

Endocrine & metabolic: Gout (2% to 7%), hypoglycemia (<1% to 4%), hyperglycemia (3% to 4%), fluid overload (1% to 3%)

Gastrointestinal: Diarrhea (1% to 10%), vomiting (5% to 9%), taste perversion (1% to 9%), peritoneal infection (8%), constipation (1% to 7%), abdominal pain (1% to 4%), positive fecal occult blood (1% to 3%)

Genitourinary: Urinary tract infection (≤1%)

Local: Injection site reaction (2% to 4%), catheter site infection (4%)

Neuromuscular & skeletal: Muscle pain (1% to 7%), extremity pain (3% to 6%), arthralgia (1% to 4%), weakness (1% to 3%), back pain (1% to 3%)

Ocular: Conjunctivitis (<1% to 3%)

Otic: Ear pain (1% to 7%)

Respiratory: Dyspnea (1% to 10%), pharyngitis (<1% to 7%), cough (1% to 7%), sinusitis (1% to 4%), rhinitis (1% to 3%), upper respiratory infection (1% to 3%), nasal congestion (1%)

Miscellaneous: Graft complication (1% to 10%), hypersensitivity, sepsis

Overdosage/Toxicology Symptoms associated with overdose or rapid infusion include hypotension, headache, vomiting, nausea, dizziness, joint aches, paresthesia, abdominal and muscle pain, edema, and cardiovascular collapse. Reducing rate of infusion can alleviate some symptoms. Most symptoms can be treated with I.V. fluids, hydrocortisone, and/or antihistamines.

For severe iron overdose (serum iron concentration exceeds TIBC), deferoxamine may be administered intravenously.

Pharmacodynamics/Kinetics

Half-Life Elimination: Healthy adults: 6 hours

Metabolism: Dissociated into iron and sucrose by the reticuloendothelial system

Excretion: Healthy adults: Urine (5%) within 24 hours

Available Dosage Forms Injection, solution [preservative free]: 20 mg of elemental iron/mL (5 mL)

Dosing

Adults: Doses expressed in mg of **elemental** iron. **Note:** Test dose: Product labeling does not indicate need for a test dose in product-naive patients; test doses were administered in some clinical trials as 50 mg (2.5 mL) in 50 mL 0.9% NaCl administered over 3-10 minutes.

Iron-deficiency anemia in chronic renal disease: I.V.:

Hemodialysis-dependent patient: 100 mg (5 mL of iron sucrose injection) administered 1-3 times/week during dialysis; administer no more than 3 times/week to a cumulative total dose of 1000 mg (10 doses); may continue to administer at lowest dose necessary to maintain target hemoglobin, hematocrit, and iron storage parameters

Peritoneal dialysis-dependent patient: Slow intravenous infusion at the following schedule: Two infusions of 300 mg each over 1½ hours 14 days apart followed by a single 400 mg infusion over 2½ hours 14 days later (total cumulative dose of 1000 mg in 3 divided doses)

Nondialysis-dependent patient: 200 mg slow injection (over 2-5 minutes) on 5 different occasions within a 14-day period. Total cumulative dose: 1000 mg in 14-day period. **Note:** Dosage has also been administered as two infusions of 500 mg in a maximum of 250 mL 0.9% NaCl infused over 3.5-4 hours on day 1 and day 14 (limited experience)

Elderly: Insufficient data to identify differences between elderly and other adults; use caution.

Administration

I.V.: Not for rapid (bolus) I.V. injection; can be administered through dialysis line. Do not mix with other medications or parenteral nutrient solutions.

Slow I.V. injection: 1 mL (20 mg iron) of undiluted solution per minute (100 mg over 2-5 minutes)

Infusion: Dilute 1 vial (100 mg/5 mL) in maximum of 100 mL 0.9% NaCl; infuse over at least 15 minutes; 300 mg/250 mL should be infused over at least $1\frac{1}{2}$ hours; 400 mg/250 mL should be infused over at least $2\frac{1}{2}$ hours; 500 mg/250 mL should be infused over at least $3\frac{1}{2}$ hours.

Stability

Reconstitution: May be administered via the dialysis line as an undiluted solution or by diluting 100 mg (5 mL) in 100 mL normal saline. Doses ≥200mg should be diluted in a maximum of 250 mL normal saline. Do not mix with other medications.

Storage: Store vials at room temperature of 15°C to 30°C (59°F to 86°F); do not freeze. Following dilution, solutions are stable for 48 hours at room temperature or under refrigeration.

Laboratory Monitoring Hematocrit, hemoglobin, serum ferritin, transferrin, percent transferrin saturation, TIBC; takes about 4 weeks of treatment to see increased serum iron and ferritin, and decreased TIBC. Serum iron concentrations should be drawn 48 hours after last dose.

Nursing Actions

Physical Assessment: Assess other medications patient may be taking for effectiveness and interactions. Facilities for cardiopulmonary resuscitation must be available during administration. Monitor blood pressure closely during infusion. Monitor laboratory tests, therapeutic response, and adverse reactions at beginning of therapy and periodically throughout therapy. Assess knowledge/teach patient appropriate use according to product and purpose (dangers of iron overdosing), interventions to reduce side effects, and adverse symptoms to report.

Patient Education: You will be watched closely during infusion. You will need frequent blood tests while on this therapy. You may experience hypotension (use caution when driving or climbing stairs or engaging in tasks requiring alertness until response to drug is known); black tarry stools (normal), nausea, vomiting (taking with meals will reduce this), constipation (adequate fluids and exercise may help, may need a stool softener); or diarrhea (buttermilk, boiled milk, or yogurt may help). Report immediately severe unresolved GI irritation (cramping, nausea, vomiting, diarrhea, constipation); headache, lethargy, fatigue, dizziness, or other CNS changes; rapid respiration; leg cramps; chest pain or palpations; swelling of extremities or unexplained weight gain; vision changes; choking sensation; loss of consciousness; or convulsions. **Breast-feeding precaution:** Consult prescriber if breast-feeding.

Isoniazid (eye soe NYE a zid)

U.S. Brand Names Nydrazid® [DSC]
Synonyms INH; Isonicotinic Acid Hydrazide
Pharmacologic Category Antitubercular Agent
Pregnancy Risk Factor C
Lactation Enters breast milk/compatible
Use Treatment of susceptible tuberculosis infections; treatment of latent tuberculosis infection (LTBI)
Mechanism of Action/Effect Unknown, but may include the inhibition of myocolic acid synthesis resulting in disruption of the bacterial cell wall
Contraindications Hypersensitivity to isoniazid or any component of the formulation; acute liver disease; previous history of hepatic damage during isoniazid therapy
Warnings/Precautions Use with caution in patients with renal impairment and chronic liver disease. Severe and sometimes fatal hepatitis may occur or develop even after many months of treatment. Patients must report any prodromal symptoms of hepatitis, such as fatigue, weakness, malaise, anorexia, nausea, or vomiting. Periodic ophthalmic examinations are recommended even when usual symptoms do not occur. Pyridoxine (10-50 mg/day) is recommended in individuals likely to develop peripheral neuropathies.
Drug Interactions
Cytochrome P450 Effect: Substrate of CYP2E1 (major); **Inhibits** CYP1A2 (weak), 2A6 (moderate), 2C9 (weak), 2C19 (strong), 2D6 (moderate), 2E1 (moderate), 3A4 (strong); **Induces** CYP2E1 (after discontinuation) (weak)
Decreased Effect: Decreased effect/levels of isoniazid with aluminum salts or antacids. Isoniazid may decrease the levels/effects of CYP2D6 prodrug substrates (eg, codeine, hydrocodone, oxycodone, tramadol).
Increased Effect/Toxicity: Concurrent use of disulfiram may result in acute intolerance reactions. Isoniazid may increase the levels/effects of amphetamines, benzodiazepines, beta-blockers, calcium channel blockers, citalopram, dexmedetomidine, dextromethorphan, diazepam, fluoxetine, ifosfamide, inhalational anesthetics, lidocaine, methsuximide, mirtazapine, nateglinide, nefazodone, phenytoin, propranolol, risperidone, ritonavir, sertraline, tacrolimus, theophylline, thioridazine, tricyclic antidepressants, trimethadione, venlafaxine, and other substrates of CYP2A6, 2C19, 2D6, 2E1, or 3A4. Selected benzodiazepines (midazolam and triazolam), cisapride, ergot alkaloids, selected HMG-CoA reductase inhibitors (lovastatin and simvastatin), and pimozide are generally contraindicated with strong CYP3A4 inhibitors. Mesoridazine and thioridazine are generally contraindicated with strong CYP2D6 inhibitors. When used with strong CYP3A4 inhibitors, dosage adjustment/limits are recommended for sildenafil and other PDE-5 inhibitors; consult individual monographs.
Nutritional/Ethanol Interactions
Ethanol: Avoid ethanol (increases the risk of hepatitis).
Food: Isoniazid serum levels may be decreased if taken with food. Has some ability to inhibit tyramine metabolism; several case reports of mild reactions (flushing, palpitations) after ingestion of cheese with or without wine. Isoniazid decreases folic acid absorption. Isoniazid alters pyridoxine metabolism.
Lab Interactions False-positive urinary glucose with Clinitest®
Adverse Reactions Frequency not defined.
Cardiovascular: Hypertension, palpitation, tachycardia, vasculitis
Central nervous system: Dizziness, encephalopathy, memory impairment, slurred speech, lethargy, fever, depression, psychosis, seizure
(Continued)

683

Isoniazid (Continued)

Dermatologic: Rash (morbilliform, maculopapular, pruritic, or exfoliative), flushing

Endocrine & metabolic: Hyperglycemia, metabolic acidosis, gynecomastia, pellagra, pyridoxine deficiency

Gastrointestinal: Anorexia, nausea, vomiting, stomach pain

Hematologic: Agranulocytosis, anemia (sideroblastic, hemolytic, or aplastic), thrombocytopenia, eosinophilia, lymphadenopathy

Hepatic: LFTs mildly increased (10% to 20%); hyperbilirubinemia, jaundice, hepatitis (may involve progressive liver damage; risk increases with age; 2.3% in patients >50 years)

Neuromuscular & skeletal: Weakness, peripheral neuropathy (dose-related incidence, 10% to 20% incidence with 10 mg/kg/day), hyper-reflexia, arthralgia, lupus-like syndrome

Ocular: Blurred vision, loss of vision, optic neuritis and atrophy

Overdosage/Toxicology Symptoms of overdose generally occur within 30 minutes to 3 hours, and may include nausea, vomiting, slurred speech, dizziness, blurred vision, metabolic acidosis, hallucinations, stupor, coma, and intractable seizures. Because of high morbidity and mortality rates with isoniazid overdose, patients who are asymptomatic after an overdose should be monitored for 4-6 hours. Pyridoxine has been shown to be effective in the treatment of intoxication, especially when seizures occur. Pyridoxine I.V. is administered on a milligram to milligram dose. If the amount of isoniazid ingested is unknown, 5 g of pyridoxine should be given over 3-5 minutes and may be followed by an additional 5 g in 30 minutes. Treatment is supportive. Forced diuresis and hemodialysis can result in more rapid removal.

Pharmacodynamics/Kinetics

Time to Peak: Serum: 1-2 hours

Protein Binding: 10% to 15%

Half-Life Elimination: Fast acetylators: 30-100 minutes; Slow acetylators: 2-5 hours; may be prolonged with hepatic or severe renal impairment

Metabolism: Hepatic with decay rate determined genetically by acetylation phenotype

Excretion: Urine (75% to 95%); feces; saliva

Available Dosage Forms

Injection, solution (Nydrazid®): 100 mg/mL (10 mL) [DSC]

Syrup: 50 mg/5 mL (473 mL) [orange flavor]

Tablet: 100 mg, 300 mg

Dosing

Adults & Elderly: Recommendations often change due to resistant strains and newly-developed information; consult *MMWR* for current CDC recommendations. Intramuscular is available in patients who are unable to either take or absorb oral therapy.

Treatment of latent tuberculosis infection (LTBI): 300 mg/day or 900 mg twice weekly for 6-9 months in patients who do not have HIV infection (9 months is optimal, 6 months may be considered to reduce costs of therapy) and 9 months in patients who have HIV infection. Extend to 12 months of therapy if interruptions in treatment occur.

Treatment of active TB infection (drug susceptible):

Daily therapy: 5 mg/kg/day given daily (usual dose: 300 mg/day); 10 mg/kg/day in 1-2 divided doses in patients with disseminated disease

Twice weekly directly observed therapy (DOT): 15 mg/kg (maximum: 900 mg); 3 times/week therapy: 15 mg/kg (maximum: 900 mg)

Note: Treatment may be defined by the number of doses administered (eg, "six-month" therapy involves 192 doses of INH and rifampin, and 56 doses of pyrazinamide). Six months is the shortest interval of time over which these doses may be administered, assuming no interruption of therapy.

Note: Concomitant administration of 6-50 mg/day pyridoxine is recommended in malnourished patients or those prone to neuropathy (eg, alcoholics, diabetics)

Pediatrics: Recommendations often change due to resistant strains and newly-developed information; consult *MMWR* for current CDC recommendations. Intramuscular is available in patients who are unable to either take or absorb oral therapy.

Treatment of latent TB infection (LTBI): Infants and Children: Oral: 10-20 mg/kg/day in 1-2 divided doses (maximum: 300 mg/day) or 20-40 mg/kg (maximum: 900 mg/dose) twice weekly for 9 months

Treatment of active TB infection: Infants and Children: Oral:

Daily therapy: 10-15 mg/kg/day in 1-2 divided doses (maximum: 300 mg/day)

Twice weekly directly observed therapy (DOT): 20-30 mg/kg (maximum: 900 mg)

Renal Impairment:

Cl$_{cr}$ <10 mL/minute: Administer 50% of normal dose

Hemodialysis: Dialyzable (50% to 100%) Administer dose postdialysis

Peritoneal dialysis, continuous arteriovenous or venovenous hemofiltration: Dose for Cl$_{cr}$ <10 mL/minute

Hepatic Impairment: Dose should be reduced in severe hepatic disease.

Administration

Oral: Should be administered 1 hour before or 2 hours after meals on an empty stomach.

Stability

Storage: Protect oral dosage forms from light.

Laboratory Monitoring Transaminase levels at baseline 1, 3, 6, and 9 months

Nursing Actions

Physical Assessment: Assess potential for interactions with other pharmacological agents patient may be taking (eg, risk of toxicity or decreased effects). Assess results of laboratory tests, therapeutic effectiveness, and adverse response (eg, nausea, vomiting, peripheral neuropathy, liver damage, CNS changes). at regular intervals during therapy. Advise patients with diabetes about use of Clinitest®. Teach patient proper use, possible side effects/appropriate interventions (eg, diet [see Tyramine Content of Foods *on page 1406*] and ophthalmic examinations), and adverse symptoms to report.

Patient Education: Do not take any new medication during therapy unless approved by prescriber. Best if taken on an empty stomach, 1 hour before or 2 hours after meals. Avoid missing any dose and do not discontinue without notifying prescriber. Avoid excessive alcohol and tyramine-containing foods (eg, aged cheese, broad beans, dry sausage, preserved meats or sausages, liver pate, fish, soy bean, protein supplements, wine) and increase dietary intake of folate, niacin, magnesium. May cause false test results with Clinitest®; use of another type of glucose testing is preferable. You will need to have frequent ophthalmic exams and periodic medical check-ups to evaluate drug effects. You may experience nausea or vomiting (small frequent meals, frequent mouth care, chewing gum, or sucking lozenges may help). Report tingling or numbness in hands or feet, loss of sensation, unusual weakness, fatigue, nausea or vomiting, dark colored urine, change in urinary pattern, yellowing skin or eyes, or change in color of stool. Prodromal hepatitis, such as fatigue, weakness, malaise, anorexia, nausea, or vomiting. **Pregnancy precaution:** Inform prescriber if you are or intend to become pregnant.

Dietary Considerations Should be taken 1 hour before or 2 hours after meals on an empty stomach; increase dietary intake of folate, niacin, magnesium. No need to restrict tyramine-containing foods.

Geriatric Considerations Age has not been shown to affect the pharmacokinetics of INH since acetylation phenotype determines clearance and half-life, acetylation rate does not change significantly with age. Most strains of *M. tuberculosis* found the elderly should be susceptible to INH since most acquired their initial infection prior to INH's introduction.

Breast-Feeding Issues Small amounts of isoniazid are excreted in breast milk. However, women with tuberculosis should not be discouraged from breast-feeding. Pyridoxine supplementation is recommended for the mother and infant.

Additional Information The AAP recommends that pyridoxine supplementation (1-2 mg/kg/day) should be administered to malnourished patients, children or adolescents on meat or milk-deficient diets, breast-feeding infants, and those predisposed to neuritis to prevent peripheral neuropathy; administration of isoniazid syrup has been associated with diarrhea

Related Information
Overdose and Toxicology *on page 1423*
Tyramine Content of Foods *on page 1406*

Isoproterenol (eye soe proe TER e nole)

U.S. Brand Names Isuprel®
Synonyms Isoproterenol Hydrochloride
Pharmacologic Category Beta$_1$- & Beta$_2$-Adrenergic Agonist Agent
Medication Safety Issues
Sound-alike/look-alike issues:
Isuprel® may be confused with Disophrol®, Ismelin®, Isordil®

Pregnancy Risk Factor C
Lactation Excretion in breast milk unknown
Use Ventricular arrhythmias due to AV nodal block; hemodynamically compromised bradyarrhythmias or atropine- and dopamine-resistant bradyarrhythmias (when transcutaneous/venous pacing is not available); temporary use in third-degree AV block until pacemaker insertion
Unlabeled/Investigational Use Temporizing measure before transvenous pacing for torsade de pointes; diagnostic aid (vasovagal syncope)
Mechanism of Action/Effect Stimulates beta$_1$- and beta$_2$-receptors resulting in relaxation of bronchial, GI, and uterine smooth muscle, increased heart rate and contractility, vasodilation of peripheral vasculature
Contraindications Hypersensitivity to sulfites or isoproterenol, any component of the formulation, or other sympathomimetic amines; angina, pre-existing cardiac arrhythmias (ventricular); tachycardia or AV block caused by cardiac glycoside intoxication
Warnings/Precautions Use with extreme caution; not currently a treatment of choice; use with caution in elderly patients, patients with diabetes, renal or cardiovascular disease, seizure disorder, or hyperthyroidism; excessive or prolonged use may result in decreased effectiveness.
Drug Interactions
Increased Effect/Toxicity: Sympathomimetic agents may cause headaches and elevate blood pressure. General anesthetics may cause arrhythmias.
Nutritional/Ethanol Interactions Herb/Nutraceutical: Avoid ephedra, yohimbe (may cause CNS stimulation).
Adverse Reactions Frequency not defined.
Cardiovascular: Premature ventricular beats, bradycardia, hyper-/hypotension, chest pain, palpitation, tachycardia, ventricular arrhythmia, MI size increased

Central nervous system: Headache, nervousness or restlessness
Endocrine & metabolic: Serum glucose increased, serum potassium decreased, hypokalemia
Gastrointestinal: Nausea, vomiting
Respiratory: Dyspnea

Overdosage/Toxicology Symptoms of overdose include tachycardia, tremor, hypertension or hypotension, angina, and seizures. Hypokalemia also may occur. Cardiac arrest and death may be associated with abuse of beta-agonist bronchodilators. Treatment includes immediate discontinuation and symptomatic and supportive therapies. Cautious use of beta-adrenergic blocking agents may be considered in severe cases.

Pharmacodynamics/Kinetics
Onset of Action: Bronchodilation: I.V.: Immediate
Duration of Action: I.V.: 10-15 minutes
Half-Life Elimination: 2.5-5 minutes
Metabolism: Via conjugation in many tissues including hepatic and pulmonary
Excretion: Urine (primarily as sulfate conjugates)
Available Dosage Forms Injection, solution, as hydrochloride: 0.02 mg/mL (10 mL); 0.2 mg/mL (1:5000) (1 mL, 5 mL) [contains sodium metabisulfite]

Dosing
Adults & Elderly: Cardiac arrhythmias: I.V.: Initial: 2 mcg/minute; titrate to patient response (2-10 mcg/minute)
Pediatrics: Cardiac arrhythmias: I.V.: Start 0.1 mcg/kg/minute (usual effective dose 0.2-2 mcg/kg/minute)
Administration
I.V.: I.V. infusion administration requires the use of an infusion pump. To prepare for infusion: 1 mg isoproterenol to 500 mL D$_5$W, final concentration 2 mcg/mL
I.V. Detail: pH: 2.5-4.5
Stability
Reconstitution: Stability of parenteral admixture at room temperature (25°C) or at refrigeration (4°C) is 24 hours.

Standard diluent: 2 mg/500 mL D$_5$W; 4 mg/500 mL D$_5$W
Minimum volume: 1 mg/100 mL D$_5$W
Compatibility: Stable in dextran 6% in dextrose, dextran 6% in NS, D$_5$LR, D$_5$¼ NS, D$_5$½NS, D$_5$NS, D$_5$W, D$_{10}$W, LR, ½NS, NS; **incompatible** with sodium bicarbonate 5%, and alkaline solutions
Compatibility when admixed: Incompatible with aminophylline, furosemide, sodium bicarbonate
Storage: Isoproterenol solution should be stored at room temperature. It should not be used if a color or precipitate is present. Exposure to air, light, or increased temperature may cause a pink to brownish pink color to develop.
Laboratory Monitoring ECG, arterial blood gas, serum magnesium, serum potassium, serum glucose (in selected patients)
Nursing Actions
Physical Assessment: Monitor laboratory tests, cardiac, respiratory, and hemodynamic status when used in acute or emergency situations. Assess knowledge/teach patient appropriate use and administration procedures and adverse reactions to report.
Patient Education: You may experience nervousness, dizziness, or fatigue (use caution when driving or engaging in tasks requiring alertness until response to drug is known); or dry mouth, nausea, or vomiting (small frequent meals may reduce the incidence of nausea or vomiting). If you have diabetes, check blood sugar; blood glucose level may be increased. Report chest pain, rapid heartbeat or palpitations, unresolved/persistent GI upset, dizziness, fatigue, (Continued)

Isoproterenol *(Continued)*

trembling, increased anxiety, sleeplessness, or respiratory difficulty. **Pregnancy/breast-feeding precautions:** Inform prescriber if you are pregnant. Consult prescriber if breast-feeding.

Isosorbide Dinitrate

(eye soe SOR bide dye NYE trate)

U.S. Brand Names Dilatrate®-SR; Isochron™; Isordil®

Synonyms ISD; ISDN

Pharmacologic Category Vasodilator

Medication Safety Issues

Sound-alike/look-alike issues:

Isordil® may be confused with Inderal®, Isuprel®

Pregnancy Risk Factor C

Lactation Excretion in breast milk unknown

Use Prevention and treatment of angina pectoris; for congestive heart failure; to relieve pain, dysphagia, and spasm in esophageal spasm with GE reflux

Unlabeled/Investigational Use Esophageal spastic disorders

Mechanism of Action/Effect Relaxes vascular smooth muscles, decreases arterial resistance and venous return which reduces cardiac oxygen demand. Additionally, coronary artery dilation improves collateral flow to ischemic regions; esophageal smooth muscle is relaxed via the same mechanism.

Contraindications Hypersensitivity to isosorbide dinitrate or any component of the formulation; hypersensitivity to organic nitrates; concurrent use with phosphodiesterase-5 (PDE-5) inhibitors (sildenafil, tadalafil, or vardenafil); angle-closure glaucoma (intraocular pressure may be increased); head trauma or cerebral hemorrhage (increase intracranial pressure); severe anemia

Warnings/Precautions Use with caution in volume depletion, hypotension, and right ventricular infarctions. Paradoxical bradycardia and increased angina pectoris can accompany hypotension. Postural hypotension may also occur; ethanol may potentiate this effect. Tolerance does develop to nitrates and appropriate dosing is needed to minimize this. Safety and efficacy have not been established in pediatric patients. Nitrate may aggravate angina caused by hypertrophic cardiomyopathy.

Drug Interactions

Cytochrome P450 Effect: Substrate of CYP3A4 (major)

Decreased Effect: CYP3A4 inducers may decrease the levels/effects of isosorbide dinitrate; example inducers include aminoglutethimide, carbamazepine, nafcillin, nevirapine, phenobarbital, phenytoin, and rifamycins.

Increased Effect/Toxicity: CYP3A4 inhibitors may increase the levels/effects of isosorbide dinitrate; example inhibitors include azole antifungals, clarithromycin, diclofenac, doxycycline, erythromycin, imatinib, isoniazid, nefazodone, nicardipine, propofol, protease inhibitors, quinidine, telithromycin, and verapamil. Significant reduction of systolic and diastolic blood pressure with concurrent use of sildenafil, tadalafil, or vardenafil (contraindicated). Do not administer sildenafil, tadalafil, or vardenafil within 24 hours of a nitrate preparation.

Nutritional/Ethanol Interactions Ethanol: Caution with ethanol (may increase risk of hypotension).

Lab Interactions Decreased cholesterol (S)

Adverse Reactions Frequency not defined.

Cardiovascular: Hypotension (infrequent), postural hypotension, crescendo angina (uncommon), rebound hypertension (uncommon), pallor, cardiovascular collapse, tachycardia, shock, flushing, peripheral edema

Central nervous system: Headache (most common), lightheadedness (related to blood pressure changes), syncope (uncommon), dizziness, restlessness

Gastrointestinal: Nausea, vomiting, bowel incontinence, xerostomia

Genitourinary: Urinary incontinence

Hematologic: Methemoglobinemia (rare, overdose)

Neuromuscular & skeletal: Weakness

Ocular: Blurred vision

Miscellaneous: Cold sweat

The incidence of hypotension and adverse cardiovascular events may be increased when used in combination with sildenafil (Viagra®).

Overdosage/Toxicology Symptoms of overdose include hypotension, throbbing headache, palpitations, visual disturbances, tachycardia, methemoglobinemia, flushing, diaphoresis, metabolic acidosis, and coma. High levels or methemoglobinemia can cause signs or symptoms of hypoxemia. Treat symptomatically.

Pharmacodynamics/Kinetics

Onset of Action: Sublingual tablet: 2-10 minutes; Chewable tablet: 3 minutes; Oral tablet: 45-60 minutes

Duration of Action: Sublingual tablet: 1-2 hours; Chewable tablet: 0.5-2 hours; Oral tablet: 4-6 hours

Half-Life Elimination: Parent drug: 1-4 hours; Metabolite (5-mononitrate): 4 hours

Metabolism: Extensively hepatic to conjugated metabolites, including isosorbide 5-mononitrate (active) and 2-mononitrate (active)

Excretion: Urine and feces

Available Dosage Forms [DSC] = Discontinued product

Capsule, sustained release (Dilatrate®-SR): 40 mg

Tablet: 5 mg, 10 mg, 20 mg, 30 mg

Isordil®: 5 mg, 10 mg [DSC], 20 mg [DSC], 30 mg [DSC], 40 mg

Tablet, extended release (Isochron™): 40 mg

Tablet, sublingual: 2.5 mg, 5 mg

Isordil®: 2.5 mg, 5 mg, 10 mg [DSC]

Dosing

Adults:

Angina:

Oral: 5-40 mg 4 times/day or 40 mg every 8-12 hours in sustained released dosage form

Sublingual: 2.5-5 mg every 5-10 minutes for maximum of 3 doses in 15-30 minutes; may also use prophylactically 15 minutes prior to activities which may provoke an attack

Congestive heart failure:

Initial dose: 20 mg 3-4 times/day

Target dose: 120-160 mg/day in divided doses; use in combination with hydralazine

Esophageal spastic disorders (unlabeled use):

Oral: 5-10 mg before meals

Sublingual: 2.5 mg after meals

Note: Tolerance to nitrate effects develops with chronic exposure. Dose escalation does not overcome this effect. Tolerance can only be overcome by short periods of nitrate absence from the body. Short periods (10-12 hours) of nitrate withdrawal help minimize tolerance. General recommendations are to take the last dose of short-acting agents no later than 7 PM; administer 2-3 times/day rather than 4 times/day. Sustained release preparations could be administered at times to allow a 15- to 17-hour interval between first and last daily dose. Example: Administer sustained release at 8 AM and 2 PM for a twice daily regimen.

Elderly: Elderly patients should be given lowest recommended adult daily doses initially and titrate upward.

Renal Impairment: Hemodialysis: During hemodialysis, administer dose postdialysis or administer supplemental 10-20 mg dose. During peritoneal dialysis, supplemental dose is not necessary.

Administration

Oral: Do not administer around-the-clock; the first dose of nitrates should be administered in a physician's office to observe for maximal cardiovascular dynamic effects and adverse effects (orthostatic blood pressure drop, headache); when immediate release products are prescribed twice daily (recommend 7 AM and noon); for 3 times/day dosing (recommend 7 AM, noon, and 5 PM); when sustained-release products are indicated, suggest once a day in morning or via twice daily dosing at 8 AM and 2 PM. Do not crush sublingual tablets.

Nursing Actions

Physical Assessment: Assess potential for interactions with other pharmacological agents patient may be taking (potential for decreased or increased levels/effect of Isosorbide, additive hypotension). Monitor therapeutic effectiveness (blood pressure normalization) and adverse response (eg, hypotension, tolerance) at regular intervals during therapy. When discontinuing, dose should be discontinued gradually. Teach patient proper use, possible side effects/appropriate interventions (eg, importance of maintaining dosing schedule to provide drug-free period), and adverse symptoms to report.

Patient Education: Do not take any new medication during therapy unless approved by prescriber. Take exactly as directed, at the same time each day with last dose in early evening. Do not chew or swallow sublingual tablets; allow them to dissolve under your tongue. Do not crush or chew sustained release capsules, swallow whole with 8 oz water. Do not change brands without consulting prescriber. Do not discontinue abruptly. Keep medication in original container, tightly closed. Avoid excessive alcohol; combination may cause severe hypotension. May cause postural hypotension (take medication while sitting down and use caution when rising from sitting or lying position or climbing stairs until response to drug is known); headache, dizziness, weakness, or blurred vision (use caution when driving or engaging in hazardous activities until response to drug is known); or nausea or vomiting (small frequent meals, frequent mouth care, chewing gum, or sucking lozenges may help). If chest pain occurs, seek emergency medical help at once. Report acute headache, rapid heartbeat, unusual restlessness or dizziness, muscular weakness, or blurring vision. **Pregnancy/breast-feeding precautions:** Inform prescriber if you are or intend to become pregnant. Consult prescriber if breast-feeding.

Isosorbide Dinitrate and Hydralazine
(eye soe SOR bide dye NYE trate & hye DRAL a zeen)

U.S. Brand Names BiDil®

Synonyms Hydralazine and Isosorbide Dinitrate

Pharmacologic Category Vasodilator

Pregnancy Risk Factor C

Lactation See individual agents.

Use Treatment of heart failure, adjunct to standard therapy, in self-identified African-Americans

Mechanism of Action/Effect Both hydralazine and isosorbide dinitrate are vasodilators

Contraindications Hypersensitivity to isosorbide dinitrate, hydralazine, or any component of the formulation; hypersensitivity to organic nitrates; concurrent use with phosphodiesterase-5 inhibitors (sildenafil, tadalafil, or vardenafil); angle-closure glaucoma (intraocular pressure may be increased); head trauma or cerebral hemorrhage (increase intracranial pressure); severe anemia; mitral valve rheumatic heart disease

Warnings/Precautions May cause a drug-induced lupus-like syndrome (more likely on larger doses, longer duration). Adjust dose in severe renal dysfunction. Use with caution in CAD (increase in tachycardia may increase myocardial oxygen demand). Use with caution in pulmonary hypertension; severe hypotension can occur. Use with caution in volume depletion, hypotension, and right ventricular infarctions. Paradoxical bradycardia and increased angina pectoris can accompany hypotension. Postural hypotension can also occur. Nitrates may aggravate angina caused by hypertrophic cardiomyopathy. Tolerance may develop to nitrates and appropriate dosing is needed to minimize this. Safety and efficacy have not been established in pediatric patients.

Drug Interactions

Cytochrome P450 Effect: Hydralazine: **Inhibits** CYP3A4 (weak); Isosorbide dinitrate: **Substrate** of CYP3A4 (major)

Increased Effect/Toxicity: See individual agents.

Adverse Reactions The following events were reported in the A-HeFT Study using the combination isosorbide dinitrate/hydralazine product. See individual drug monographs for additional information.

>10%:
Cardiovascular: Chest pain (16%)
Central nervous system: Headache (50%), dizziness (32%)
Neuromuscular & skeletal: Weakness (14%)

1% to 10%:
Cardiovascular: Hypotension (8%), ventricular tachycardia (4%), palpitations (4%), tachycardia (2%)
Dermatologic: Alopecia (1%), angioedema (1%)
Endocrine & metabolic: Hyperglycemia (4%), hyperlipidemia (3%), hypercholesterolemia (1%)
Gastrointestinal: Nausea (10%), vomiting (4%)
Hepatic: Cholecystitis (1%)
Neuromuscular & skeletal: Paresthesia (4%), arthralgia (1%), myalgia (1%), tendon disorder (1%)
Respiratory: Bronchitis (8%), sinusitis (4%), rhinitis (4%)
Miscellaneous: Allergic reaction (1%), diaphoresis (1%)

Overdosage/Toxicology See individual agents.

Pharmacodynamics/Kinetics

Time to Peak: 1 hour (both agents)

Half-Life Elimination: Hydralazine: 4 hours; Isosorbide dinitrate: 2 hours

Available Dosage Forms Tablet: Isosorbide dinitrate 20 mg and hydralazine 37.5 mg

Dosing

Adults & Elderly: Heart failure: Oral: Initial: 1 tablet 3 times/day; titrate to a maximum dose of 2 tablets 3 times/day

Dosing Adjustment for Toxicity: If patient experiences persistent headache, adjust dosing to twice daily.

Stability

Storage: Store at controlled room temperature of 15°C to 30°C (58°F to 86°F). Protect from light.

Nursing Actions

Physical Assessment: See individual agents.

Geriatric Considerations The pharmacokinetics of hydralazine and isosorbide alone or in combination have not been studied. As with all antihypertensives and nitrate products, caution should be used on initiation of therapy, as hypotension may be encountered. Since many elderly are volume depleted, secondary to their blunted thirst reflex and/or use of diuretics, doses used initially should be at lowest recommended dose. The use of nitrates may occasionally promote reflux esophagitis. Monitor for these effects at start of therapy.

Breast-Feeding Issues See individual agents.

Isosorbide Mononitrate
(eye soe SOR bide mon oh NYE trate)

U.S. Brand Names Imdur®; Ismo®; Monoket®

Synonyms ISMN

Pharmacologic Category Vasodilator

Medication Safety Issues
Sound-alike/look-alike issues:
Imdur® may be confused with Imuran®, Inderal LA®, K-Dur®
Monoket® may be confused with Monopril®

Pregnancy Risk Factor C

Lactation Excretion in breast milk unknown

Use Long-acting metabolite of the vasodilator isosorbide dinitrate used for the prophylactic treatment of angina pectoris

Mechanism of Action/Effect Systemic venodilation, decreasing preload and increasing ejection fractions; improves congestive symptoms in heart failure and improves the myocardial perfusion in patients with coronary artery disease

Contraindications Hypersensitivity to isosorbide or any component of the formulation; hypersensitivity to organic nitrates; concurrent use with phosphodiesterase-5 (PDE-5) inhibitors (sildenafil, tadalafil, or vardenafil); angle-closure glaucoma (intraocular pressure may be increased); head trauma or cerebral hemorrhage (increase intracranial pressure); severe anemia

Warnings/Precautions Use with caution in volume depletion, hypotension, and right ventricular infarctions. Paradoxical bradycardia and increased angina pectoris can accompany hypotension. Orthostatic hypotension can also occur; ethanol can accentuate this. Tolerance does develop to nitrates and appropriate dosing is needed to minimize this (drug-free interval). Safety and efficacy have not been established in pediatric patients. Nitrates may aggravate angina caused by hypertrophic cardiomyopathy.

Drug Interactions
Cytochrome P450 Effect: Substrate of CYP3A4 (major)
Increased Effect/Toxicity: CYP3A4 inhibitors may increase the levels/effects of isosorbide dinitrate; example inhibitors include azole antifungals, clarithromycin, diclofenac, doxycycline, erythromycin, imatinib, isoniazid, nefazodone, nicardipine, propofol, protease inhibitors, quinidine, telithromycin, and verapamil. Significant reduction of systolic and diastolic blood pressure with concurrent use of sildenafil, tadalafil, or vardenafil (contraindicated). Do not administer sildenafil, tadalafil, or vardenafil within 24 hours of a nitrate preparation.

Nutritional/Ethanol Interactions Ethanol: Caution with ethanol (may increase risk of hypotension).

Adverse Reactions
>10%: Central nervous system: Headache (19% to 38%)
1% to 10%:
Central nervous system: Dizziness (3% to 5%)
Gastrointestinal: Nausea/vomiting (2% to 4%)

The incidence of hypotension and adverse cardiovascular events may be increased when used in combination with sildenafil (Viagra®).

Overdosage/Toxicology Symptoms of overdose include hypotension, throbbing headache, palpitations, visual disturbances, tachycardia, methemoglobinemia, flushing, diaphoresis, metabolic acidosis, and coma. High levels or methemoglobinemia can cause signs or symptoms of hypoxemia. Treat symptomatically.

Pharmacodynamics/Kinetics
Onset of Action: 30-60 minutes
Half-Life Elimination: Mononitrate: ~4 hours
Metabolism: Hepatic
Excretion: Urine and feces

Available Dosage Forms
Tablet: 10 mg, 20 mg
Ismo®: 20 mg
Monoket®: 10 mg, 20 mg
Tablet, extended release (Imdur®): 30 mg, 60 mg, 120 mg

Dosing
Adults:
Angina: Oral:
Regular tablet: 5-10 mg twice daily with the two doses given 7 hours apart (eg, 8 AM and 3 PM) to decrease tolerance development; then titrate to 10 mg twice daily in first 2-3 days.
Extended release tablet: Initial: 30-60 mg given in morning as a single dose; titrate upward as needed, giving at least 3 days between increases; maximum daily single dose: 240 mg
Note: Tolerance to nitrate effects develops with chronic exposure. Dose escalation does not overcome this effect. Tolerance can only be overcome by short periods of nitrate absence from the body. Short periods (10-12 hours) of nitrate withdrawal help minimize tolerance. Recommended dosage regimens incorporate this interval. General recommendations are to take the last dose of short-acting agents no later than 7 PM; administer 2 times/day rather than 4 times/day. Administer sustained release tablet once daily in the morning.

Elderly: Start with lowest recommended adult dose.

Renal Impairment: Not necessary for elderly or patients with altered renal or hepatic function. Tolerance to nitrate effects develops with chronic exposure.

Administration
Oral: Do not administer around-the-clock; Monoket® and Ismo® should be scheduled twice daily with doses 7 hours apart (8 AM and 3 PM); Imdur® may be administered once daily. Extended release tablets should not be chewed or crushed. Should be swallowed with a half-glassful of fluid.

Stability
Storage: Tablets should be stored in a tight container at room temperature of 15°C to 30°C (59°F to 86°F).

Laboratory Monitoring Orthostasis

Nursing Actions
Physical Assessment: Assess potential for interactions with other pharmacological agents patient may be taking (potential for decreased or increased levels/ effect of Isosorbide, additive hypotension). Monitor therapeutic effectiveness (blood pressure normalization) and adverse response (eg, hypotension, tolerance) at regular intervals during therapy. When discontinuing, reduce dosage gradually. Teach patient proper use, possible side effects/appropriate interventions (eg, importance of maintaining dosing schedule, drug-free period), and adverse symptoms to report.

Patient Education: Do not take any new medication during therapy unless approved by prescriber. Take exactly as directed, at the same time each day with last dose in early evening. Do not chew or swallow sublingual tablets; allow them to dissolve under your tongue. Do not crush or chew sustained release capsules, swallow whole with ½ glass of water. Do not change brands without consulting prescriber. Do not discontinue abruptly. Keep medication in original container, tightly closed. Avoid excessive alcohol; combination may cause severe hypotension. May cause postural hypotension (take medication while sitting down and use caution when rising from sitting or lying position or climbing stairs until response to drug is known); headache, dizziness, weakness, or blurred vision (use caution when driving or engaging in hazardous activities until response to drug is known); or nausea or vomiting (small frequent meals, frequent mouth care, chewing gum, or sucking lozenges may help). If chest pain occurs, seek emergency medical help at once. Report acute headache, rapid heartbeat, unusual restlessness or dizziness, muscular weakness, or blurring vision. **Pregnancy/breast-feeding precautions:** Inform prescriber if you are or intend to become pregnant. Consult prescriber if breast-feeding.

Geriatric Considerations The first dose of nitrates (sublingual, chewable, oral) should be taken in a physician's office to observe for maximal cardiovascular dynamic effects and adverse effects (orthostatic blood pressure drop, headache). The use of nitrates for angina may occasionally promote reflux esophagitis. This may require dose adjustments or changing therapeutic agents to correct this adverse effect.

Isotretinoin (eye soe TRET i noyn)

U.S. Brand Names Accutane®; Amnesteem™; Claravis™; Sotret®

Synonyms 13-cis-Retinoic Acid

Restrictions A new program for risk minimization (iPLEDGE) is being designed by the FDA and the manufacturers of isotretinoin. The program will be implemented December 31, 2005. Details may be found on the FDA website at Additional details may be found on the FDA website at http://www.fda.gov/cder/drug/infopage/accutane/default.htm, last accessed August 12, 2005.. When implemented, iPLEDGE will strengthen the current prescribing and dispensing requirements. All patients, prescribers, wholesalers and dispensing pharmacists must be registered. Registration will be possible via internet at www.ipledgeprogram.com or by calling 866-495-0654.

Under the current guidelines, prescriptions for isotretinoin may not be dispensed unless they are affixed with a yellow, self-adhesive, qualification sticker filled out by the prescriber. Telephone, fax, or computer-generated prescriptions are no longer valid. Prescriptions may not be written for more than a 1-month supply and must be dispensed with a patient education guide every month. In addition, prescriptions for females must be filled within 7 days of the qualification date noted on the yellow sticker; prescriptions filled after 7 days of the noted date are considered to be expired and cannot be honored. Pharmacists may call the manufacturer to confirm the prescriber's authority to write for this medication; however, this is not mandatory.

Prescribers will be provided with qualification stickers after they have read the details of the program and have signed (and mailed to the manufacturer) their agreement to participate. Audits of pharmacies will be conducted to monitor program compliance.

An FDA-approved medication guide is available at http://www.fda.gov/cder/Offices/ODS/labeling.htm; distribute to each patient to whom this medication is dispensed.

Pharmacologic Category Acne Products; Retinoic Acid Derivative

Medication Safety Issues

Sound-alike/look-alike issues:

Accutane® may be confused with Accolate®, Accupril®

Pregnancy Risk Factor X

Lactation Excretion in breast milk unknown/contraindicated

Use Treatment of severe recalcitrant nodular acne unresponsive to conventional therapy

Unlabeled/Investigational Use Investigational: Treatment of children with metastatic neuroblastoma or leukemia that does not respond to conventional therapy

Mechanism of Action/Effect Reduces sebaceous gland size and reduces sebum production; regulates cell proliferation and differentiation

Contraindications Hypersensitivity to isotretinoin or any component of the formulation; sensitivity to parabens, vitamin A, or other retinoids; pregnancy

Warnings/Precautions This medication should only be prescribed by prescribers competent in treating severe recalcitrant nodular acne, are experienced in the use of systemic retinoids and are participating in the pregnancy prevention programs authorized by the FDA and product manufacturer. Use with caution in patients with diabetes mellitus, hypertriglyceridemia; acute pancreatitis and fatal hemorrhagic pancreatitis (rare) have been reported. Not to be used in women of childbearing potential unless woman is capable of complying with effective contraceptive measures. Patients must select and commit to two forms of contraception. Therapy is begun after two negative pregnancy tests; effective contraception must be used for at least 1 month before beginning therapy, during therapy, and for 1 month after discontinuation of therapy. Prescriptions should be written for no more than a 1-month supply, and pregnancy testing and counseling should be repeated monthly. Because of the high likelihood of teratogenic effects (~20%), do not prescribe isotretinoin for women who are or who are likely to become pregnant while using the drug (see Additional Information for details). Male and female patients must be enrolled in the manufacturer sponsored and FDA approved monitoring programs.

Depression, psychosis, aggressive or violent behavior, and changes in mood. Rarely, suicidal thoughts and actions have been reported during isotretinoin usage. All patients should be observed closely for symptoms of depression or suicidal thoughts. Discontinuation of treatment alone may not be sufficient, further evaluation may be necessary. Cases of pseudotumor cerebri (benign intracranial hypertension) have been reported, some with concomitant use of tetracycline (avoid using together). Patients with papilledema, headache, nausea, vomiting, and visual disturbances should be referred to a neurologist and treatment with isotretinoin discontinued. Hearing impairment, which can continue after therapy is discontinued, may occur. Clinical hepatitis, elevated liver enzymes, inflammatory bowel disease, skeletal hyperostosis, premature epiphyseal closure, vision impairment, corneal opacities, and decreased night vision have also been reported with the use of isotretinoin. Bone mineral density may decrease; use caution in patients with a genetic predisposition to bone disorders (ie osteoporosis, osteomalacia) and with disease states or concomitant medications that can induce bone disorders. Patients may be at risk when participating in activities with repetitive impact (such as sports). Safety of long-term use is not established and is not recommended.

Drug Interactions

Decreased Effect: Isotretinoin may increase clearance of carbamazepine resulting in reduced carbamazepine levels. Retinoic acid derivatives may diminish the therapeutic effect of oral contraceptives (two forms of contraception are recommended in females of childbearing potential during retinoic acid therapy).

Increased Effect/Toxicity: Increased toxicity: Corticosteroids may cause osteoporosis; interactive effect with isotretinoin unknown; use with caution. Phenytoin may cause osteomalacia; interactive effect with isotretinoin unknown; use with caution. Cases of pseudotumor cerebri have been reported in concurrent use with tetracycline; avoid combination.

(Continued)

Isotretinoin *(Continued)*

Nutritional/Ethanol Interactions
Ethanol: Avoid or limit ethanol (may increase triglyceride levels if taken in excess).

Food: Isotretinoin bioavailability increased if taken with food or milk.

Herb/Nutraceutical: Avoid dong quai, St John's wort (may also cause photosensitization and may decrease the effectiveness of oral contraceptives). Additional vitamin A supplements may lead to vitamin A toxicity (dry skin, irritation, arthralgias, myalgias, abdominal pain, hepatic changes); avoid use.

Adverse Reactions Frequency not defined.
Cardiovascular: Palpitation, tachycardia, vascular thrombotic disease, stroke, chest pain, syncope, flushing

Central nervous system: Edema, fatigue, pseudotumor cerebri, dizziness, drowsiness, headache, insomnia, lethargy, malaise, nervousness, paresthesia, seizure, stroke, suicidal ideation, suicide attempts, suicide, depression, psychosis, aggressive or violent behavior, emotional instability

Dermatologic: Cutaneous allergic reactions, purpura, acne fulminans, alopecia, bruising, cheilitis, dry mouth, dry nose, dry skin, epistaxis, eruptive xanthomas, fragility of skin, hair abnormalities, hirsutism, hyperpigmentation, hypopigmentation, peeling of palms, peeling of soles, photoallergic reactions, photosensitizing reactions, pruritus, rash, dystrophy, paronychia, facial erythema, seborrhea, eczema, increased sunburn susceptibility, diaphoresis, urticaria, abnormal wound healing

Endocrine & metabolic: Triglycerides increased (25%), abnormal menses, blood glucose increased, cholesterol increased, HDL decreased

Gastrointestinal: Weight loss, inflammatory bowel disease, regional ileitis, pancreatitis, bleeding and inflammation of the gums, colitis, nausea, nonspecific gastrointestinal symptoms

Genitourinary: Nonspecific urogenital findings

Hematologic: Anemia, thrombocytopenia, neutropenia, agranulocytosis, pyogenic granuloma

Hepatic: Hepatitis

Neuromuscular & skeletal: Skeletal hyperostosis, calcification of tendons and ligaments, premature epiphyseal closure, arthralgia, CPK elevations, arthritis, tendonitis, bone abnormalities, weakness, back pain (29% in pediatric patients), rhabdomyolysis (rare), bone mineral density decreased

Ocular: Corneal opacities, decreased night vision, cataracts, color vision disorder, conjunctivitis, dry eyes, eyelid inflammation, keratitis, optic neuritis, photophobia, visual disturbances

Otic: Hearing impairment, tinnitus

Renal: Vasculitis, glomerulonephritis,

Respiratory: Bronchospasms, respiratory infection, voice alteration, Wegener's granulomatosis

Miscellaneous: Allergic reactions, anaphylactic reactions, lymphadenopathy, infection, disseminated herpes simplex, diaphoresis

Overdosage/Toxicology
Symptoms of overdose include headache, vomiting, flushing, abdominal pain, cheilosis, dizziness, and ataxia. All signs or symptoms have been transient. Patients should not donate blood for at least 30 days following overdose. Male patients should use a condom or avoid sexual activity for 30 days following overdose.

Pharmacodynamics/Kinetics
Time to Peak: Serum: 3-5 hours

Protein Binding: 99% to 100%; primarily albumin

Half-Life Elimination: Terminal: Parent drug: 21 hours; Metabolite: 21-24 hours

Metabolism: Hepatic via CYP2B6, 2C8, 2C9, 2D6, 3A4; forms metabolites; major metabolite: 4-oxo-isotretinoin (active)

Excretion: Urine and feces (equal amounts)

Available Dosage Forms Capsule:
Accutane®: 10 mg, 20 mg, 40 mg [contains soybean oil and parabens]

Amnesteem™: 10 mg, 20 mg, 40 mg [contains soybean oil]

Claravis™: 10 mg, 20 mg, 40 mg

Sotret®: 10 mg, 20 mg, 30 mg, 40 mg [contains soybean oil]

Dosing
Adults & Elderly: Severe recalcitrant nodular acne: Oral: 0.5-2 mg/kg/day in 2 divided doses (dosages as low as 0.05 mg/kg/day have been reported to be beneficial) for 15-20 weeks or until the total cyst count decreases by 70%, whichever is sooner. A second course of therapy may be initiated after a period of ≥2 months off therapy.

Pediatrics:
Neuroblastoma (investigational): Oral: Children: Maintenance therapy for neuroblastoma: 100-250 mg/m²/day in 2 divided doses

Acne (severe recalcitrant nodular): Children: Refer to adult dosing.

Hepatic Impairment: Empiric dose reductions are recommended in patient with hepatitis.

Administration
Oral: Administer with food. Capsules can be swallowed, or chewed and swallowed. The capsule may be opened with a large needle and the contents placed on applesauce or ice cream for patients unable to swallow the capsule. Whole capsules should be swallowed with a full glass of liquid.

Stability
Storage: Store at room temperature and protect from light.

Laboratory Monitoring Must have two negative pregnancy tests prior to beginning therapy, CBC with differential and platelet count, baseline sedimentation rate, serum triglycerides, liver enzymes

Nursing Actions
Physical Assessment: Assess effectiveness and interactions of other medications patient may be taking. Monitor laboratory tests, effectiveness of therapy, and adverse effects at beginning of therapy and regularly with long-term use. Monitor patients with diabetes closely. Observe for depression or suicidal thoughts. Assess knowledge/teach patient appropriate use, possible side effects/interventions, and adverse symptoms to report. **Pregnancy risk factor X:** Determine that patient is not pregnant before beginning treatment and do not give to women of childbearing age unless female is capable of complying with two contraceptive measures 1 month prior to therapy, during therapy, and 1 month following therapy.

Patient Education: A patient information/consent form must be signed before this medication is prescribed. Do not sign (and do not take this medication) if you do not understand any information on the form. Use exactly as directed; do not take more than recommended. Prescriptions will be written for a 1-month supply and must be filled within 7 days; they will not be honored if filled after that time or if they do not have the appropriate yellow qualification sticker attached. Capsule can be chewed and swallowed, swallowed, or opened with a large needle and contents sprinkled on applesauce or ice cream. Whole capsules should be swallowed with a full glass of liquid. Do not take any other vitamin A products, limit vitamin A intake, and increase exercise during therapy. Limit or avoid alcohol intake. Exacerbations of acne may occur during first weeks of therapy. You may experience headache, loss of night vision, lethargy, or visual disturbances (use caution when driving or engaging in tasks requiring alertness until response to drug is known); photosensitivity (use sunscreen, wear protective clothing and eyewear, and avoid direct sunlight); dry mouth or nausea (small frequent meals, sucking hard candy, or chewing gum may help); or dryness, redness, or itching of skin, eye irritation, or increased sensitivity to contact lenses (wear regular glasses). Report depression or suicidal thoughts. Discontinue therapy and report acute vision changes, ringing in the ears or changes in hearing, rectal bleeding, abdominal cramping, or unresolved diarrhea. **Pregnancy/breast-feeding precautions:** Inform prescriber if you are pregnant. Do not get pregnant 1 month before, during, or for 1 month following therapy. This drug may cause severe fetal defects. Two forms of contraception and monthly tests to rule out pregnancy are required during therapy. It is important to note that any type of contraception may fail, it is the responsibility of the patient to be compliant with contraceptive therapy. Do not donate blood during or for 1 month following therapy (same reason). Do not breast-feed.

Dietary Considerations Should be taken with food. Limit intake of vitamin A; avoid use of other vitamin A products. Some formulations may contain soybean oil.

Pregnancy Issues Major fetal abnormalities (both internal and external), spontaneous abortion, premature births and low IQ scores in surviving infants have been reported. This medication is contraindicated in females of childbearing potential unless they are able to comply with the guidelines of pregnancy prevention programs put in place by the FDA and the manufacturer of Accutane®.

Additional Information Females of childbearing potential must receive oral and written information reviewing the hazards of therapy and the effects that isotretinoin can have on a fetus. Therapy should not begin without two negative pregnancy tests, one to be performed in the physician's office when qualifying the patient for treatment, the second test performed on the second day of the next normal menstrual period or 11 days after the last unprotected intercourse, whichever is last. Two forms of contraception (a primary and secondary form as described in the pregnancy prevention program materials) must be used during treatment and limitations to their use must be explained. Prescriptions should be written for no more than a 1-month supply, and pregnancy testing and counseling should be repeated monthly. Urine pregnancy test kits (for monthly pregnancy testing) and a Pregnancy Prevention Program kit (to be given to the patient prior to therapy) are provided by the manufacturer. Any cases of accidental pregnancy should be reported to the manufacturer or the FDA MedWatch Program. All patients (male and female) must read and sign the informed consent material provided in the pregnancy prevention program. Prescriptions will not be honored unless they have the yellow qualification sticker affixed.

The manufacturers of isotretinoin have developed comprehensive educational programs for healthcare providers and patients. Prior to prescribing isotretinoin, healthcare providers must be registered in one of these programs. Additional information for Accutane® and the corresponding S.M.A.R.T. (System To Manage Accutane®-Related Teratogenicity) program may be obtained from Roche Laboratories. Additional information for Amnesteem™ and the S.P.I.R.I.T.™ program (System To Prevent Isotretinoin-Related Issues of Teratogenicity) program maybe obtained from Bertek Pharmaceuticals. Additional information for Sotret® and I.M.P.A.R.T.™ (Isotretinoin Medication Program: Alerting you to the Risks of Teratogenicity) may be obtained from Ranbaxy Pharmaceuticals.

Note: In November 2004, the Food and Drug Administration (FDA) announced an update to the monitoring programs currently implemented to decrease fetal exposures to isotretinoin. The strengthened program, risk minimization action plan (RiskMAP), will include Accutane® as well as all the generic equivalents. When implemented, RiskMAP will replace the SMART program, which is managed by Roche, as well as programs supported by other isotretinoin manufacturers such as S.P.I.R.I.T.™ (Bertek Pharmaceuticals) and I.M.P.A.R.T.™ (Ranbaxy Pharmaceuticals).

Isradipine (iz RA di peen)

U.S. Brand Names DynaCirc® [DSC]; DynaCirc® CR
Pharmacologic Category Calcium Channel Blocker
Medication Safety Issues
Sound-alike/look-alike issues:
DynaCirc® may be confused with Dynabac®, Dynacin®
Pregnancy Risk Factor C
Lactation Excretion in breast milk unknown/not recommended
Use Treatment of hypertension
Mechanism of Action/Effect Inhibits calcium ion from entering the "slow channels" or select voltage-sensitive areas of vascular smooth muscle and myocardium during depolarization
Contraindications Hypersensitivity to isradipine or any component of the formulation; hypotension (<90 mm Hg systolic)
Warnings/Precautions Use cautiously in CHF, hypertropic cardiomyopathy (IHSS), and in hepatic dysfunction. Safety and efficacy have not been established in pediatric patients. Adjust doses at 2- to 4-week intervals.
Drug Interactions
Cytochrome P450 Effect: Substrate of CYP3A4 (major); **Inhibits** CYP3A4 (weak)
Decreased Effect: NSAIDs (diclofenac) may decrease the antihypertensive response of isradipine. Isradipine may cause a decrease in lovastatin effect. CYP3A4 inducers may decrease the levels/effects of isradipine; example inducers include aminoglutethimide, carbamazepine, nafcillin, nevirapine, phenobarbital, phenytoin, and rifamycins.
Increased Effect/Toxicity: Isradipine may increase cardiovascular adverse effects of beta-blockers. Isradipine may minimally increase cyclosporine levels. CYP3A4 inhibitors may increase the levels/effects of isradipine; example inhibitors include azole antifungals, clarithromycin, diclofenac, doxycycline, erythromycin, imatinib, isoniazid, nefazodone, nicardipine, propofol, protease inhibitors, quinidine, telithromycin, and verapamil. Blood pressure-lowering effects may be additive with sildenafil, tadalafil, and vardenafil (use caution).
Nutritional/Ethanol Interactions
Food: Administration with food delays absorption, but does not affect availability
Herb/Nutraceutical: St John's wort may decrease isradipine levels. Avoid dong quai if using for hypertension (has estrogenic activity). Avoid ephedra, yohimbe, ginseng (may worsen hypertension). Avoid garlic (may have increased antihypertensive effect).
Adverse Reactions
>10%: Central nervous system: Headache (dose related 2% to 22%)
1% to 10%:
Cardiovascular: Edema (dose related 1% to 9%), palpitation (dose related 1% to 5%), flushing (dose related 1% to 5%), tachycardia (1% to 3%), chest pain (2% to 3%)
Central nervous system: Dizziness (2% to 8%), fatigue (dose related 1% to 9%), flushing (9%)
Dermatologic: Rash (1.5% to 2%)
Gastrointestinal: Nausea (1% to 5%), abdominal discomfort (≤3%), vomiting (≤1%), diarrhea (≤3%)
(Continued)

Isradipine *(Continued)*

Renal: Urinary frequency (1% to 3%)
Respiratory: Dyspnea (1% to 3%)

Overdosage/Toxicology Primary cardiac symptoms of calcium blocker overdose include hypotension and bradycardia. Hypotension is caused by peripheral vasodilation, myocardial depression, and bradycardia. Bradycardia results from sinus bradycardia, second- or third-degree atrioventricular block, or sinus arrest with junctional rhythm. Intraventricular conduction is usually not affected so QRS duration is normal (verapamil does prolong the PR interval and bepridil prolongs the QT interval and may cause ventricular arrhythmias, including torsade de pointes).

Noncardiac symptoms include confusion, stupor, nausea, vomiting, metabolic acidosis and hyperglycemia. Repeated calcium administration may promptly reverse the depressed cardiac contractility (but not sinus node depression or peripheral vasodilation).

Pharmacodynamics/Kinetics
Onset of Action: Immediate release: 20 minutes
Duration of Action: Immediate release: >12 hours
Time to Peak: Serum: 1-1.5 hours
Protein Binding: 95%
Half-Life Elimination: 8 hours
Metabolism: Hepatic; CYP3A4 substrate (major); extensive first-pass effect
Excretion: Urine (as metabolites)

Available Dosage Forms
Capsule (DynaCirc®): 2.5 mg, 5 mg [DSC]
Tablet, controlled release (DynaCirc® CR): 5 mg, 10 mg

Dosing
Adults & Elderly: Hypertension: Oral: 2.5 mg twice daily; antihypertensive response is seen in 2-3 hours; maximal response in 2-4 weeks; increase dose at 2- to 4-week intervals at 2.5-5 mg increments; usual dose range (JNC 7): 2.5-10 mg/day in 2 divided doses. **Note:** Most patients show no improvement with doses >10 mg/day except adverse reaction rate increases. Therefore, maximal dose in older adults should be 10 mg/day.

Administration
Oral: May open capsule; avoid crushing contents

Nursing Actions
Physical Assessment: Assess potential for interactions with other pharmacological agents or herbal products patient may be taking (eg, potential to increase or decrease levels/effects of isradipine). Assess therapeutic effectiveness (normotensive) and adverse response (eg, tachycardia, hypotension, edema, dyspnea) at regular intervals during therapy. When discontinuing, dose should be tapered slowly. Teach patient proper use, possible side effects/appropriate interventions, and adverse symptoms to report.

Patient Education: Do not take any new medication during therapy unless approved by prescriber. Take as prescribed, with or without food. Do not stop abruptly without consulting prescriber. Do not crush extended release tablets. This medication does not replace other antihypertensive interventions; follow prescriber's instructions for diet and lifestyle changes. You may experience headache (if unrelieved, consult prescriber for approved analgesic); nausea or vomiting (small, frequent meals, frequent mouth care, chewing gum, or sucking lozenges may help); constipation (increased dietary bulk and fluids may help); or dizziness, fatigue, confusion (use caution when driving or engaging in potentially hazardous tasks until response to drug is known). Report unrelieved headache, vomiting, or constipation; chest pain, palpitations, or rapid heartbeat; swelling of hands or feet or sudden weight gain (>5 lb/week); or unusual cramps in legs or feet. **Pregnancy/breast-feeding precautions:** Inform prescriber if you are or intend to become pregnant. Breast-feeding is not recommended.

Dietary Considerations May be taken without regard to meals.
Geriatric Considerations Elderly may experience a greater hypotensive response. Constipation may be more of a problem in the elderly.

Itraconazole (i tra KOE na zole)

U.S. Brand Names Sporanox®
Pharmacologic Category Antifungal Agent, Oral
Medication Safety Issues
Sound-alike/look-alike issues:
Sporanox® may be confused with Suprax®

Pregnancy Risk Factor C
Lactation Enters breast milk/not recommended
Use Treatment of susceptible fungal infections in immunocompromised and immunocompetent patients including blastomycosis and histoplasmosis; indicated for aspergillosis, and onychomycosis of the toenail; treatment of onychomycosis of the fingernail without concomitant toenail infection via a pulse-type dosing regimen; has activity against *Aspergillus, Candida, Coccidioides, Cryptococcus, Sporothrix,* tinea unguium

Oral: Useful in superficial mycoses including dermatophytoses (eg, tinea capitis), pityriasis versicolor, sebopsoriasis, vaginal and chronic mucocutaneous candidiases; systemic mycoses including candidiasis, meningeal and disseminated cryptococcal infections, paracoccidioidomycosis, coccidioidomycoses; miscellaneous mycoses such as sporotrichosis, chromomycosis, leishmaniasis, fungal keratitis, alternariosis, zygomycosis

Oral solution: Treatment of oral and esophageal candidiasis

Intravenous solution: Indicated in the treatment of blastomycosis, histoplasmosis (nonmeningeal), and aspergillosis (in patients intolerant or refractory to amphotericin B therapy); empiric therapy of febrile neutropenic fever

Mechanism of Action/Effect Interferes with cytochrome P450 activity, decreasing ergosterol synthesis (principal sterol in fungal cell membrane) and inhibiting cell membrane formation

Contraindications Hypersensitivity to itraconazole, any component of the formulation, or to other azoles; concurrent administration with cisapride, dofetilide, ergot derivatives, levomethadyl, lovastatin, midazolam, pimozide, quinidine, simvastatin, or triazolam; treatment of onychomycosis in patients with evidence of left ventricular dysfunction, CHF, or a history of CHF

Warnings/Precautions Discontinue if signs or symptoms of CHF or neuropathy occur during treatment. Rare cases of serious cardiovascular adverse events (including death), ventricular tachycardia, and torsade de pointes have been observed due to increased cisapride concentrations induced by itraconazole. Use with caution in patients with left ventricular dysfunction or a history of CHF. Not recommended for use in patients with active liver disease, elevated liver enzymes, or prior hepatotoxic reactions to other drugs. Itraconazole has been associated with rare cases of serious hepatotoxicity (including fatal cases and cases within the first week of treatment); treatment should be discontinued in patients who develop clinical symptoms of liver dysfunction or abnormal liver function tests during itraconazole therapy except in cases where expected benefit exceeds risk. Large differences in itraconazole pharmacokinetic parameters have been observed in cystic fibrosis patients receiving the solution; if a patient with cystic fibrosis does not respond to therapy, alternate therapies should be considered. **Due to differences in bioavailability, oral capsules and oral solution cannot be used interchangeably.** Intravenous formulation should be used with caution in renal impairment; consider conversion to oral therapy if renal dysfunction/toxicity is noted. Initiation of treatment with oral solution is not recommended in patients at immediate risk for systemic candidiasis (eg, patients with severe neutropenia).

Drug Interactions
Cytochrome P450 Effect: Substrate of CYP3A4 (major); **Inhibits** CYP3A4 (strong)

Decreased Effect: Absorption of itraconazole requires gastric acidity; therefore, antacids, H$_2$ antagonists (cimetidine, famotidine, nizatidine, and ranitidine), proton pump inhibitors (omeprazole, lansoprazole, rabeprazole), and sucralfate may significantly reduce bioavailability resulting in treatment failures and should not be administered concomitantly. Antacids may decrease serum concentration of itraconazole; administer antacids 1 hour before or 2 hours after itraconazole capsules. Serum levels of itraconazole may be decreased with didanosine, isoniazid, and nevirapine. The levels/effects of itraconazole may be reduced by aminoglutethimide, carbamazepine, nafcillin, phenobarbital, phenytoin, rifamycins, and other CYP3A4 inducers. Oral contraceptive efficacy may be reduced (limited data).

Increased Effect/Toxicity: Itraconazole is a strong inhibitor of CYP3A4, and is contraindicated with cisapride, dofetilide, ergot derivatives, lovastatin, midazolam, pimozide, quinidine, simvastatin, and triazolam. Itraconazole may also increase the levels of alfentanil, benzodiazepines (alprazolam, diazepam, and others), buspirone, busulfan, calcium channel blockers (felodipine, nifedipine, verapamil), carbamazepine, corticosteroids, cyclosporine, digoxin, docetaxel, eletriptan, HMG-CoA reductase inhibitors (except fluvastatin, pravastatin), indinavir, oral hypoglycemics (sulfonylureas), phenytoin, rifabutin, ritonavir, saquinavir, sirolimus, tacrolimus, trimetrexate, vincristine, vinblastine, warfarin, and zolpidem. Other medications metabolized by CYP3A4 should be used with caution. Serum concentrations of itraconazole may be increased by strong CYP3A4 inhibitors. Serum concentrations of PDE-5 inhibitors (sildenafil, tadalafil, and vardenafil) are increased by itraconazole; specific dosage reductions/limitations are recommended.

Nutritional/Ethanol Interactions
Food:
Capsules: Enhanced by food and possibly by gastric acidity. cola drinks have been shown to increase the absorption of the capsules in patients with achlorhydria or those taking H$_2$-receptor antagonists or other gastric acid suppressors. Avoid grapefruit juice.
Solution: Decreased by food, time to peak concentration prolonged by food.
Herb/Nutraceutical: St John's wort may decrease itraconazole levels.

Adverse Reactions Listed incidences are for higher doses appropriate for systemic fungal infection.

>10%: Gastrointestinal: Nausea (11%)
1% to 10%:
Cardiovascular: Edema (4%), hypertension (3%)
Central nervous system: Headache (4%), fatigue (2% to 3%), malaise (1%), fever (3%), dizziness (2%)
Dermatologic: Rash (9%), pruritus (3%)
Endocrine & metabolic: Decreased libido (1%), hypertriglyceridemia, hypokalemia (2%)
Gastrointestinal: Abdominal pain (2%), anorexia (1%), vomiting (5%), diarrhea (3%)
Hepatic: Abnormal LFTs (3%), hepatitis
Renal: Albuminuria (1%)

Overdosage/Toxicology Overdoses are well tolerated. Treatment is supportive. Dialysis is not effective.

Pharmacodynamics/Kinetics
Protein Binding: Plasma: 99.9%; metabolite hydroxy-itraconazole: 99.5%

Half-Life Elimination: Oral: After single 200 mg dose: 21 ± 5 hours; 64 hours at steady-state; I.V.: steady-state: 35 hours; steady-state concentrations are achieved in 13 days with multiple administration of itraconazole 100-400 mg/day.

Metabolism: Extensively hepatic via CYP3A4 into >30 metabolites including hydroxy-itraconazole (major metabolite); appears to have *in vitro* antifungal activity. Main metabolic pathway is oxidation; may undergo saturation metabolism with multiple dosing.

Excretion: Feces (~3% to 18%); urine (~0.03% as parent drug, 40% as metabolites)

Available Dosage Forms
Capsule: 100 mg
Injection, solution: 10 mg/mL (25 mL) [packaged in a kit containing sodium chloride 0.9% (50 mL); filtered infusion set (1)]
Solution, oral: 100 mg/10 mL (150 mL) [cherry flavor]

Dosing
Adults & Elderly:
Aspergillosis:
Oral: 200-400 mg/day
I.V.: 200 mg twice daily for 4 doses, followed by 200 mg daily

Blastomycosis/histoplasmosis:
Oral: 200 mg once daily, if no obvious improvement or there is evidence of progressive fungal disease, increase the dose in 100 mg increments to a maximum of 400 mg/day. Doses >200 mg/day are given in 2 divided doses. Length of therapy varies from 1 day to >6 months depending on the condition and mycological response.
I.V.: 200 mg twice daily for 4 doses, followed by 200 mg daily

Brain abscess: Cerebral phaeohyphomycosis (dematiaceous): Oral: 200 mg twice daily for at least 6 months with amphotericin

Candidiasis:
Oropharyngeal: Oral (solution): 200 mg once daily for 1-2 weeks; in patients unresponsive or refractory to fluconazole: 100 mg twice daily (clinical response expected in 1-2 weeks)
Esophageal: Oral (solution): 100-200 mg once daily for a minimum of 3 weeks; continue dosing for 2 weeks after resolution of symptoms

Coccidioides: Oral: 200 mg twice daily

Infections, Life-threatening:
Oral: Loading dose: 200 mg 3 times/day (600 mg/day) should be given for the first 3 days of therapy.
I.V.: 200 mg twice daily for 4 doses, followed by 200 mg/day

Meningitis: Oral:
Coccidioides: 400-800 mg/day
Cryptococcal: HIV positive (unlabeled use): Induction: 400 mg/day for 10-12 weeks; maintenance: 200 mg twice daily lifelong

Onychomycosis: Oral: 200 mg once daily for 12 consecutive weeks

Pneumonia:
Coccidioides: Mild to moderate: Oral, I.V.: 200 mg twice daily
Cryptococcal: Mild to moderate (unlabeled use): 200-400 mg/day for 6-12 months (lifelong for HIV positive)

Prototheccal infection: 200 mg once daily for 2 months

Sporotrichosis: Oral:
Lymphocutaneous: 100-200 mg/day for 3-6 months
Osteoarticular and pulmonary: 200 mg twice daily for 1-2 years (may use amphotericin B initially for stabilization)

Pediatrics: Efficacy and safety have not been established; a small number of patients 3-16 years of age have been treated with 100 mg/day for systemic
(Continued)

Itraconazole *(Continued)*

fungal infections with no serious adverse effects reported. A dose of 5 mg/kg once daily was used in a pharmacokinetic study using the oral solution in patients 6 months-12 years; duration of study was 2 weeks.

Renal Impairment: Not necessary. Itraconazole injection is not recommended in patients with a creatinine clearance <30 mL/minute; hydroxypropyl-β-cyclo-dextrin (the excipient) is eliminated primarily by the kidneys.

Not dialyzable

Hepatic Impairment: May be necessary, but specific guidelines are not available. Risk-to-benefit evaluation should be undertaken in patients who develop liver function abnormalities during treatment.

Administration

Oral: Doses >200 mg/day are given in 2 divided doses; do not administer with antacids. Capsule absorption is best if taken with food, therefore, it is best to administer itraconazole after meals; solution should be taken on an empty stomach. When treating oropharyngeal and esophageal candidiasis, solution should be swished vigorously in mouth, then swallowed.

I.V.: Infuse 60 mL of the dilute solution (3.33 mg/mL = 200 mg itraconazole, pH ~4.8) over 60 minutes; flush with 15-20 mL of 0.9% sodium chloride over 30 seconds to 15 minutes

Stability

Reconstitution: Dilute with 0.9% sodium chloride. A precise mixing ratio is required to maintain stability (3.33:1) and avoid precipitate formation. Add 25 mL (1 ampul) to 50 mL 0.9% sodium chloride. Mix and withdraw 15 mL of solution before infusing.

Storage:

Capsule: Store at room temperature, 15°C to 25°C (59°F to 77°F); protect from light and moisture

Oral solution: Store at ≤25°C (77°F); do not freeze

Solution for injection: Store at ≤25°C (77°F); protect from light; do not freeze. Stable for 48 hours at room temperature or under refrigeration.

Laboratory Monitoring Liver function in patients with pre-existing hepatic dysfunction, and in all patients being treated for longer than 1 month.

Nursing Actions

Physical Assessment: Assess potential for interactions with other pharmacological or herbal products patient may be taking (eg, anything that reduces gastric acidity may result in treatment failure of Itraconazole). See Administration for capsule, oral solution and infusion specifics (eg, oral capsules and oral solution cannot be used interchangeably). Assess results of laboratory tests (LFTs), therapeutic effectiveness (resolution of fungal infection), and adverse reactions at regular intervals during therapy. Teach patient proper use (eg, necessity of taking full course of therapy), possible side effects/appropriate interventions, and adverse symptoms to report.

Patient Education: Do not take any new medication during therapy unless approved by prescriber. Use exactly as directed. Take full course of medication even if infections appears to be resolved, do not discontinue without consulting prescriber (treatment for some fungal infections may take several weeks or months). Take capsule immediately after meals; take solution on empty stomach, 1 hour before or 2 hours after meals. Do not take antacids of other medications within 1 hour before or 2 hours after itraconazole. Avoid grapefruit juice while taking this medication. Observe good hygiene measures to prevent reinfection. If you have diabetes, test serum glucose regularly (may affect response to oral hypoglycemics). Frequent blood tests may be required with prolonged therapy. May cause dizziness or drowsiness (use caution when driving or engaging in tasks that require

alertness until response to drug is known); nausea, vomiting, or anorexia (small frequent meals, frequent mouth care, sucking lozenges, or chewing gum may help). Stop therapy and report immediately any signs and symptoms that may suggest liver dysfunction (eg, unusual fatigue, anorexia, nausea and/or vomiting, jaundice [yellowing of skin or sclera], dark urine, or pale stool) so that the appropriate laboratory testing can be done. **Pregnancy/breast-feeding precautions:** Inform prescriber if you are or intend to become pregnant. Consult prescriber about appropriate contraceptive use, efficacy of oral contraceptives may be reduced. Breast-feeding is not recommended.

Dietary Considerations

Capsule: Administer with food.

Solution: Take without food, if possible.

Pregnancy Issues Should not be used to treat onychomycosis during pregnancy. Effective contraception should be used during treatment and for 2 months following treatment. Congenital abnormalities have been reported during postmarketing surveillance, but a causal relationship has not been established.

Additional Information Due to potential toxicity, the manufacturer recommends confirmation of diagnosis testing of nail specimens prior to treatment of onychomycosis.

Ketoconazole *(kee toe KOE na zole)*

U.S. Brand Names Nizoral®; Nizoral® A-D [OTC]

Pharmacologic Category Antifungal Agent, Oral; Antifungal Agent, Topical

Medication Safety Issues

Sound-alike/look-alike issues:

Nizoral® may be confused with Nasarel®, Neoral®, Nitrol®

Pregnancy Risk Factor C

Lactation Enters breast milk/not recommended

Use Treatment of susceptible fungal infections, including candidiasis, oral thrush, blastomycosis, histoplasmosis, paracoccidioidomycosis, coccidioidomycosis, chromomycosis, candiduria, chronic mucocutaneous candidiasis, as well as certain recalcitrant cutaneous dermatophytoses; used topically for treatment of tinea corporis, tinea cruris, tinea versicolor, and cutaneous candidiasis, seborrheic dermatitis

Unlabeled/Investigational Use Treatment of prostate cancer (androgen synthesis inhibitor)

Mechanism of Action/Effect Inhibits several fungal enzymes that results in a build-up of toxic concentrations of hydrogen peroxide resulting in cell death; inhibits androgen synthesis

Contraindications Hypersensitivity to ketoconazole or any component of the formulation; CNS fungal infections (due to poor CNS penetration); coadministration with ergot derivatives or cisapride is contraindicated due to risk of potentially fatal cardiac arrhythmias

Warnings/Precautions Use with caution in patients with impaired hepatic function; has been associated with hepatotoxicity, including some fatalities; perform periodic liver function tests; high doses of ketoconazole may depress adrenocortical function.

Drug Interactions

Cytochrome P450 Effect: Substrate of CYP3A4 (major); **Inhibits** CYP1A2 (strong), 2A6 (moderate), 2B6 (weak), 2C8/9 (strong), 2C19 (moderate), 2D6 (moderate), 3A4 (strong)

Decreased Effect: Oral: Absorption requires gastric acidity; therefore, antacids, H₂ antagonists (cimetidine, famotidine, nizatidine, and ranitidine), proton pump inhibitors (omeprazole, lansoprazole, rabeprazole), and sucralfate may significantly reduce bioavailability resulting in treatment failures and should not be administered concomitantly. Decreased serum levels with didanosine and isoniazid. The levels/effects of ketoconazole may be decreased by aminoglutethimide, carbamazepine, nafcillin, nevirapine, phenobarbital, phenytoin, rifamycins, or other CYP3A4 inducers. **Should not be administered concomitantly with rifampin.** Oral contraceptive efficacy may be reduced (limited data). Ketoconazole may decrease the levels/effects of CYP2D6 prodrug substrates (eg, codeine, hydrocodone, oxycodone, tramadol).

Increased Effect/Toxicity: Due to inhibition of hepatic CYP3A4, ketoconazole use is contraindicated with cisapride, lovastatin, midazolam, simvastatin, and triazolam due to large substantial increases in the toxicity of these agents. Ketoconazole may increase the serum levels/effects of amiodarone, amphetamines, benzodiazepines, beta-blockers, buspirone, busulfan, calcium channel blockers, citalopram, dexmedetomidine, dextromethorphan, diazepam, digoxin, docetaxel, fluoxetine, fluvoxamine, glimepiride, glipizide, ifosfamide, inhalational anesthetics, lidocaine, mesoridazine, methsuximide, mexiletine, mirtazapine, nateglinide, nefazodone, paroxetine, phenytoin, pioglitazone, propranolol, risperidone, ritonavir, ropinirole, rosiglitazone, sertraline, sirolimus, tacrolimus, theophylline, thioridazine, tricyclic antidepressants, trifluoperazine, trimetrexate, venlafaxine, vincristine, vinblastine, warfarin, zolpidem, and other substrates of CYP1A2, 2A6, 2C8/9, 2C19, 2D6, or 3A4. Selected benzodiazepines (midazolam and triazolam), cisapride, ergot alkaloids, selected HMG-CoA reductase inhibitors (lovastatin and simvastatin), and pimozide are generally contraindicated with strong CYP3A4 inhibitors. Mesoridazine and thioridazine are generally contraindicated with strong CYP2D6 inhibitors. When used with strong CYP3A4 inhibitors, dosage adjustment/limits are recommended for sildenafil and other PDE-5 inhibitors; consult individual monographs.

Nutritional/Ethanol Interactions

Food: Ketoconazole peak serum levels may be prolonged if taken with food.

Herb/Nutraceutical: St John's wort may decrease ketoconazole levels.

Adverse Reactions

Oral: 1% to 10%:

Dermatologic: Pruritus (2%)

Gastrointestinal: Nausea/vomiting (3% to 10%), abdominal pain (1%)

Cream: Severe irritation, pruritus, stinging (~5%)

Shampoo: Increases in normal hair loss, irritation (<1%), abnormal hair texture, scalp pustules, mild dryness of skin, itching, oiliness/dryness of hair

Overdosage/Toxicology Oral: Symptoms of overdose include dizziness, headache, nausea, vomiting, diarrhea. Overdoses are well tolerated. Treatment includes supportive measures and gastric decontamination.

Pharmacodynamics/Kinetics

Time to Peak: Serum: 1-2 hours

Protein Binding: 93% to 96%

Half-Life Elimination: Biphasic: Initial: 2 hours; Terminal: 8 hours

Metabolism: Partially hepatic via CYP3A4 to inactive compounds

Excretion: Feces (57%); urine (13%)

Available Dosage Forms

Cream, topical: 2% (15 g, 30 g, 60 g)

Shampoo, topical (Nizoral® A-D): 1% (6 mL, 120 mL, 210 mL)

Tablet (Nizoral®): 200 mg

Dosing

Adults & Elderly:

Fungal infections:

Oral: 200-400 mg/day as a single daily dose

Shampoo: Apply twice weekly for 4 weeks with at least 3 days between each shampoo.

Topical: Rub gently into the affected area once daily to twice daily.

Prostate cancer (unlabeled use): Oral: Adults: 400 mg 3 times/day

Pediatrics:

Fungal infections: Oral:

Children ≥2 years: 3.3-6.6 mg/kg/day as a single dose for 1-2 weeks for candidiasis, for at least 4 weeks in recalcitrant dermatophyte infections, and for up to 6 months for other systemic mycoses

Renal Impairment: Not dialyzable (0% to 5%)

Hepatic Impairment: Dose reductions should be considered in patients with severe liver disease.

Administration

Oral: Do not take with antacids; take at least 2 hours before antacids.

Topical: Cream and shampoo: External use only.

Laboratory Monitoring Liver function

Nursing Actions

Physical Assessment: Assess potential for interactions with other pharmacological agents or herbal products patient may be taking (eg, anything that reduces gastric acidity may result in treatment failures with ketoconazole, concurrent use of ergot derivatives or cisapride increases the risk of potentially fatal cardiac arrhythmias, oral contraceptive efficacy may be reduced). Monitor liver function, therapeutic effect (resolution of viral infection), and adverse reactions on a regular basis. Instruct patients with diabetes to monitor glucose levels closely; may impact effectiveness of oral hypoglycemics. Teach patient proper use (necessity of completely full therapy), possible side effects/appropriate interventions (eg, importance of adequate hydration), and adverse symptoms to report.

Patient Education: Do not take any new medication during therapy without consulting prescriber. Oral formulation may be taken with food, at least 2 hours before any antacids. Take full course of medication as directed; some infections may require long periods of therapy. If you have diabetes, test serum glucose regularly; may impact effectiveness of oral hypoglycemics. May cause nausea and vomiting (small, frequent meals, frequent mouth care, sucking lozenges, or chewing gum may help); headache (mild analgesic may be necessary); or dizziness (use caution when driving). Report unresolved headache, rash or itching, yellowing of eyes or skin, changes in color of urine or stool, chest pain or palpitations, or sense of fullness or ringing in ears. **Pregnancy/breast-feeding precautions:** Inform prescriber if you are or intend to become pregnant. Breast-feeding is not recommended.

Topical: Wash and dry area before applying medication thinly. Do not cover with occlusive dressing. Report severe skin irritation or if condition does not improve.

Shampoo: Allow 3 days between shampoos. You may experience some hair loss, scalp irritations, itching change in hair texture, or scalp pustules. Report severe side effects or if infestation persists.

Dietary Considerations May be taken with food or milk to decrease GI adverse effects.

Ketoprofen (kee toe PROE fen)

U.S. Brand Names Orudis® KT [OTC] [DSC]

Restrictions A medication guide should be dispensed with each prescription. A template for the required MedGuide can be found on the FDA website at: http://www.fda.gov/medwatch/SAFETY/2005/safety05.htm#NSAID

Pharmacologic Category Nonsteroidal Anti-inflammatory Drug (NSAID), Oral

Medication Safety Issues
Sound-alike/look-alike issues:
Oruvail® may be confused with Clinoril®, Elavil®

Pregnancy Risk Factor C/D (3rd trimester)

Lactation Excretion in breast milk unknown/not recommended

Use Acute and long-term treatment of rheumatoid arthritis and osteoarthritis; primary dysmenorrhea; mild to moderate pain

Mechanism of Action/Effect Inhibits prostaglandin synthesis by decreasing the activity of the enzyme, cyclooxygenase, which results in decreased formation of prostaglandin precursors

Contraindications Hypersensitivity to ketoprofen, aspirin, other NSAIDs, or any component of the formulation; perioperative pain in the setting of coronary artery bypass surgery (CABG); pregnancy (3rd trimester)

Warnings/Precautions NSAIDs are associated with an increased risk of adverse cardiovascular events, including MI, stroke, and new onset or worsening of pre-existing hypertension. Risk may be increased with duration of use or pre-existing cardiovascular risk-factors or disease. Carefully evaluate individual cardiovascular risk profiles prior to prescribing. Use caution with fluid retention, CHF or hypertension.

Use of NSAIDs can compromise existing renal function. Renal toxicity can occur in patient with impaired renal function, dehydration, heart failure, liver dysfunction, those taking diuretics and ACEI and the elderly. Rehydrate patient before starting therapy. Monitor renal function closely. Ketoprofen is not recommended for patients with advanced renal disease.

NSAIDs may increase risk of gastrointestinal irritation, ulceration, bleeding, and perforation. These events may occur at any time during therapy and without warning. Use caution with a history of GI disease (bleeding or ulcers), concurrent therapy with aspirin, anticoagulants and/or corticosteroids, smoking, use of alcohol, the elderly or debilitated patients.

Use the lowest effective dose for the shortest duration of time, consistent with individual patient goals, to reduce risk of cardiovascular or GI adverse events. Alternate therapies should be considered for patients at high risk.

NSAIDs may cause serious skin adverse events including exfoliative dermatitis, Stevens-Johnson syndrome (SJS) and toxic epidermal necrolysis (TEN). Anaphylactoid reactions may occur, even without prior exposure; patients with "aspirin triad" (bronchial asthma, aspirin intolerance, rhinitis) may be at increased risk. Do not use in patients who experience bronchospasm, asthma, rhinitis, or urticaria with NSAID or aspirin therapy.

Use with caution in patients with decreased hepatic function. Closely monitor patients with any abnormal LFT. Severe hepatic reactions (eg, fulminant hepatitis, liver failure) have occurred with NSAID use, rarely; discontinue if signs or symptoms of liver disease develop, or if systemic manifestations occur.

Withhold for at least 4-6 half-lives prior to surgical or dental procedures. Safety and efficacy have not been established in pediatric patients.

Drug Interactions

Cytochrome P450 Effect: Inhibits CYP2C8/9 (weak)

Decreased Effect: May reduce effect of some diuretics and antihypertensive effect of beta-blockers, ACE inhibitors, angiotensin II inhibitors, hydralazine. Cholestyramine and colestipol may reduce absorption of ketoprofen.

Increased Effect/Toxicity: Ketoprofen may increase effect/toxicity of anticoagulants (bleeding), antiplatelet agents (bleeding), aminoglycosides, biphosphonates (GI irritation), corticosteroids (GI irritation), cyclosporine (nephrotoxicity), lithium, methotrexate, pemetrexed, treprostinil (bleeding), vancomycin. Probenecid may increase serum concentrations of ketoprofen.

Nutritional/Ethanol Interactions

Ethanol: Avoid ethanol (due to GI irritation).

Food: Food slows rate of absorption resulting in delayed and reduced peak serum concentrations.

Herb/Nutraceutical: Avoid alfalfa, anise, bilberry, bladderwrack, bromelain, cat's claw, celery, coleus, cordyceps, dong quai, evening primrose, feverfew, fenugreek, garlic, ginger, ginkgo biloba, red clover, horse chestnut, grapeseed, green tea, ginseng, guggul, horse chestnut seed, horseradish, licorice, prickly ash, red clover, reishi, SAMe, sweet clover, turmeric, white willow (all have additional antiplatelet activity).

Adverse Reactions

>10%: Gastrointestinal: Dyspepsia (11%)

1% to 10%:
Central nervous system: Headache (3% to 9%), depression, dizziness (>1%), dreams, insomnia, malaise, nervousness, somnolence

Dermatologic: Rash

Gastrointestinal: Abdominal pain (3% to 9%), constipation (3% to 9%), diarrhea (3% to 9%), flatulence (3% to 9%), nausea (3% to 9%), anorexia (>1%), stomatitis (>1%), vomiting (>1%)

Genitourinary: Urinary tract infection (>1%)

Ocular: Visual disturbances

Otic: Tinnitus

Renal: Renal dysfunction (3% to 9%)

Overdosage/Toxicology Common symptoms of acute NSAID overdose include lethargy, drowsiness, nausea, vomiting and epigastric pain. Respiratory depression, coma, convulsions, GI bleeding, or acute renal failure are rare. Management of NSAID intoxication is supportive and symptomatic; multiple dosing of activated charcoal may be effective.

Pharmacodynamics/Kinetics

Time to Peak: Capsule: 0.5-2 hours

Capsule, extended release: 6-7 hours

Protein Binding: >99%, primarily albumin

Half-Life Elimination:
Capsule, immediate release: 2-4 hours; moderate-severe renal impairment: 5-9 hours

Capsule, extended release: ~3-7.5 hours

Metabolism: Hepatic via glucuronidation; metabolite can be converted back to parent compound; may have enterohepatic recirculation

Excretion: Urine (~80%, primarily as glucuronide conjugates)

Available Dosage Forms [DSC] = Discontinued product

Capsule: 50 mg, 75 mg

Capsule, extended release: 200 mg

Tablet (Orudis® KT): 12.5 mg [contains tartrazine and sodium benzoate] [DSC]

Dosing

Adults:

Rheumatoid arthritis or osteoarthritis: Oral:
Capsule: 50-75 mg 3-4 times/day up to a maximum of 300 mg/day
Capsule, extended release: 200 mg once daily

Note: Lower doses may be used in small patients or in the elderly, or debilitated.

Mild to moderate pain: Oral: Capsule: 25-50 mg every 6-8 hours up to a maximum of 300 mg/day
OTC labeling: 12.5 mg every 4-6 hours, up to a maximum of 6 tablets/24 hours

Elderly: Initial: 25-50 mg 3-4 times/day; increase up to 150-300 mg/day (maximum daily dose: 300 mg)

Pediatrics:

Mild to moderate pain, rheumatoid arthritis: Children ≥16 years: Refer to adult dosing.

Renal Impairment: In general, NSAIDs are not recommended for use in patients with advanced renal disease, but the manufacturer of ketoprofen does provide some guidelines for adjustment in renal dysfunction:

Mild impairment: Maximum dose: 150 mg/day

Severe impairment: $Cl_{cr} < 25$ mL/minute: Maximum dose: 100 mg/day

Hepatic Impairment: Hepatic impairment and serum albumin <3.5 g/dL: Maximum dose: 100 mg/day ●

Administration

Oral: May take with food to reduce GI upset. Do not crush or break extended release capsules.

Laboratory Monitoring CBC, occult blood loss, periodic liver function; renal function (urine output, serum BUN, creatinine)

Nursing Actions

Physical Assessment: Assess effectiveness and interactions of other medications patient may be taking. Monitor blood pressure at the beginning of therapy and periodically during use. Monitor laboratory tests and therapeutic response (eg, relief of pain and inflammation, increased activity tolerance), and adverse reactions (eg, GI effects, hepatotoxicity, or ototoxicity) at beginning of therapy and periodically throughout therapy. Schedule ophthalmic evaluations for patients who develop eye complaints during long-term NSAID therapy. Assess knowledge/teach patient appropriate use, interventions to reduce side effects, and adverse symptoms to report.

Patient Education: Take this medication exactly as directed; do not increase dose without consulting prescriber. Do not crush tablets or break capsules. Take with food or milk to reduce GI distress. Maintain adequate hydration (2-3 L/day of fluids) unless instructed to restrict fluid intake. Do not use alcohol, aspirin or aspirin-containing medication, or any other anti-inflammatory medications without consulting prescriber. You may experience drowsiness, dizziness, nervousness, or headache (use caution when driving or engaging in tasks requiring alertness until response to drug is known); anorexia, nausea, vomiting, or heartburn (small frequent meals, frequent mouth care, sucking lozenges, or chewing gum may help); fluid retention (weigh yourself weekly and report unusual (3-5 lb/week) weight gain); GI bleeding, ulceration, or perforation can occur with or without pain; discontinue medication and contact prescriber if persistent abdominal pain or cramping, or blood in stool occurs. Report breathlessness, respiratory difficulty, or unusual cough; chest pain, rapid heartbeat, palpitations; unusual bruising/bleeding; blood in urine, stool, mouth, or vomitus; swollen extremities; skin rash or itching; acute fatigue; hearing changes (ringing in ears); jaundice; right upper quadrant tenderness; or flu-like symptoms. **Pregnancy/breast-feeding precautions:** Inform prescriber if you are or intend to become pregnant. This drug should not be used in the 3rd trimester of pregnancy. Breast-feeding is not recommended.

Dietary Considerations In order to minimize gastrointestinal effects, ketoprofen can be prescribed to be taken with food or milk.

Geriatric Considerations Elderly are at high risk for adverse effects from NSAIDs. As much as 60% of

elderly can develop peptic ulceration and/or hemorrhage asymptomatically. The concomitant use of H_2 blockers, omeprazole, and sucralfate is not effective as prophylaxis with the exception of NSAID-induced duodenal ulcers which may be prevented by the use of ranitidine. Misoprostol is the only prophylactic agent proven effective. Also, concomitant disease and drug use contribute to the risk for GI adverse effects. Use lowest effective dose for shortest period possible. Consider renal function decline with age. Use of NSAIDs can compromise existing renal function especially when Cl_{cr} is ≤30 mL/minute. Tinnitus may be a difficult and unreliable indication of toxicity due to age-related hearing loss or eighth cranial nerve damage. CNS adverse effects such as confusion, agitation, and hallucination are generally seen in overdose or high-dose situations, but elderly may demonstrate these adverse effects at lower doses than younger adults.

Pregnancy Issues Exposure to NSAIDs late in pregnancy may lead to premature closure of the ductus arteriosus and may inhibit uterine contractions. ●

Ketorolac (KEE toe role ak)

U.S. Brand Names Acular®; Acular LS™; Acular® PF; Toradol®

Synonyms Ketorolac Tromethamine

Restrictions A medication guide should be dispensed with each prescription. A template for the required MedGuide can be found on the FDA website at: http://www.fda.gov/medwatch/SAFETY/2005/safety05.htm#NSAID

Pharmacologic Category Nonsteroidal Anti-inflammatory Drug (NSAID), Ophthalmic; Nonsteroidal Anti-inflammatory Drug (NSAID), Oral; Nonsteroidal Anti-inflammatory Drug (NSAID), Parenteral

Medication Safety Issues

Sound-alike/look-alike issues:

Acular® may be confused with Acthar®, Ocular®

Toradol® may be confused with Foradil®, Inderal®, Tegretol®, Torecan®, tramadol

Pregnancy Risk Factor C/D (3rd trimester)

Lactation Enters breast milk/contraindicated (AAP rates "compatible")

Use

Oral, injection: Short-term (≤5 days) management of moderately-severe acute pain requiring analgesia at the opioid level

Ophthalmic: Temporary relief of ocular itching due to seasonal allergic conjunctivitis; postoperative inflammation following cataract extraction; reduction of ocular pain and photophobia following incisional refractive surgery, reduction of ocular pain, burning and stinging following corneal refractive surgery

Mechanism of Action/Effect A potent NSAID; provides analgesia by inhibiting the synthesis of prostaglandin

Contraindications Hypersensitivity to ketorolac, aspirin, other NSAIDs, or any component of the formulation; active or history of peptic ulcer disease; recent or history of GI bleeding or perforation; patients with advanced renal disease or risk of renal failure; labor and delivery; nursing mothers; prophylaxis before major surgery; suspected or confirmed cerebrovascular bleeding; hemorrhagic diathesis; concurrent ASA or other NSAIDs; epidural or intrathecal administration; concomitant probenecid; perioperative pain in the setting of coronary artery bypass surgery (CABG); pregnancy (3rd trimester)

Warnings/Precautions

Systemic: Treatment should be started with I.V./I.M. administration then changed to oral only as a continuation of treatment. Total therapy is not to exceed 5 days. Should not be used for minor or chronic pain.
(Continued)

Ketorolac (Continued)

May prolong bleeding time; do not use when hemostasis is critical. Patients should be euvolemic prior to treatment. Low doses of narcotics may be needed for breakthrough pain.

NSAIDs are associated with an increased risk of adverse cardiovascular events, including MI, stroke, and new onset or worsening of pre-existing hypertension. Risk may be increased with duration of use or pre-existing cardiovascular risk-factors or disease. Carefully evaluate individual cardiovascular risk profiles prior to prescribing. Use caution with fluid retention, CHF or hypertension.

Use of NSAIDs can compromise existing renal function. Renal toxicity can occur in patient with impaired renal function, dehydration, heart failure, liver dysfunction, those taking diuretics and ACEI and the elderly. Rehydrate patient before starting therapy. Monitor renal function closely. Ketorolac is not recommended for patients with advanced renal disease.

NSAIDs may increase risk of gastrointestinal irritation, ulceration, bleeding, and perforation. These events may occur at any time during therapy and without warning. Use caution with a history of GI disease (bleeding or ulcers), concurrent therapy with aspirin, anticoagulants and/or corticosteroids, smoking, use of alcohol, the elderly or debilitated patients.

Use the lowest effective dose for the shortest duration of time, consistent with individual patient goals, to reduce risk of cardiovascular or GI adverse events. Alternate therapies should be considered for patients at high risk.

NSAIDs may cause serious skin adverse events including exfoliative dermatitis, Stevens-Johnson syndrome (SJS) and toxic epidermal necrolysis (TEN). Anaphylactoid reactions may occur, even without prior exposure; patients with "aspirin triad" (bronchial asthma, aspirin intolerance, rhinitis) may be at increased risk. Do not use in patients who experience bronchospasm, asthma, rhinitis, or urticaria with NSAID or aspirin therapy.

Use with caution in patients with decreased hepatic function. Closely monitor patients with any abnormal LFT. Severe hepatic reactions (eg, fulminant hepatitis, liver failure) have occurred with NSAID use, rarely; discontinue if signs or symptoms of liver disease develop, or if systemic manifestations occur.

The elderly are at increased risk for adverse effects (especially peptic ulceration, CNS effects, renal toxicity) from NSAIDs even at low doses.

Withhold for at least 4-6 half-lives prior to surgical or dental procedures.

Ophthalmic: May increase bleeding time associated with ocular surgery. Use with caution in patients with known bleeding tendencies or those receiving anticoagulants. Healing time may be slowed or delayed. Corneal thinning, erosion, or ulceration have been reported with topical NSAIDs; discontinue if corneal epithelial breakdown occurs. Use caution with complicated ocular surgery, corneal denervation, corneal epithelial defects, diabetes, rheumatoid arthritis, ocular surface disease, or ocular surgeries repeated within short periods of time; risk of corneal epithelial breakdown may be increased. Use for >24 hours prior to or for >14 days following surgery also increases risk of corneal adverse effects. Do not administer while wearing soft contact lenses. Safety and efficacy in pediatric patients <3 years of age have not been established.

Drug Interactions

Decreased Effect: Decreased effect: Decreased antihypertensive effect seen with ACE inhibitors and angiotensin II antagonists; decreased antiepileptic effect seen with carbamazepine, phenytoin

Increased Effect/Toxicity: Increased toxicity: Lithium, methotrexate, probenecid increased drug level; increased effect/toxicity with salicylates, probenecid, anticoagulants, nondepolarizing muscle relaxants, alprazolam, fluoxetine, thiothixene

Nutritional/Ethanol Interactions

Ethanol: Avoid ethanol (may enhance gastric mucosal irritation).

Food: Oral: High-fat meals may delay time to peak (by ~1 hour) and decrease peak concentrations.

Herb/Neutraceuticals: Avoid alfalfa, anise, bilberry, bladderwrack, bromelain, cat's claw, celery, coleus, cordyceps, dong quai, evening primrose, feverfew, fenugreek, garlic, ginger, ginkgo biloboa, red clover, horse chestnut, grapeseed, green tea, ginseng, guggul, horse chestnut seed, horseradish, licorice, prickly ash, red clover, reishi, SAMe, sweet clover, turmeric, white willow (all have additional antiplatelet activity).

Lab Interactions Increased chloride (S), sodium (S), bleeding time

Adverse Reactions

Systemic:

>10%:

Central nervous system: Headache (17%)

Gastrointestinal: Gastrointestinal pain (13%), dyspepsia (12%), nausea (12%)

>1% to 10%:

Cardiovascular: Edema (4%), hypertension

Central nervous system: Dizziness (7%), drowsiness (6%)

Dermatologic: Pruritus, purpura, rash

Gastrointestinal: Diarrhea (7%), constipation, flatulence, gastrointestinal fullness, vomiting, stomatitis

Local: Injection site pain (2%)

Miscellaneous: Diaphoresis

Ophthalmic solution:

>10%: Ocular: Transient burning/stinging (Acular®: 40%; Acular® PF: 20%)

>1% to 10%:

Central nervous system: Headache

Ocular: Conjunctival hyperemia, corneal infiltrates, iritis, ocular edema, ocular inflammation, ocular irritation, ocular pain, superficial keratitis, superficial ocular infection

Miscellaneous: Allergic reactions

Overdosage/Toxicology Symptoms of overdose include abdominal pain, peptic ulcers, and metabolic acidosis. Management of NSAID intoxication is supportive and symptomatic. Dialysis is not effective.

Pharmacodynamics/Kinetics

Onset of Action: Analgesic: I.M.: ~10 minutes; Peak effect: Analgesic: 2-3 hours

Duration of Action: Analgesic: 6-8 hours

Time to Peak: Serum: I.M.: 30-60 minutes

Protein Binding: 99%

Half-Life Elimination: 2-8 hours; increased 30% to 50% in elderly

Metabolism: Hepatic

Excretion: Urine (61% as unchanged drug)

Available Dosage Forms [DSC] = Discontinued product

Injection, solution, as tromethamine: 15 mg/mL (1 mL); 30 mg/mL (1 mL, 2 mL, 10 mL) [contains alcohol]

Solution, ophthalmic, as tromethamine:

Acular®: 0.5% (3 mL, 5 mL, 10 mL) [contains benzalkonium chloride]

Acular LS™: 0.4% (5 mL) [contains benzalkonium chloride]

Acular® P.F. [preservative free]: 0.5% (0.4 mL)

Tablet, as tromethamine: 10 mg

Toradol®: 10 mg [DSC]

Dosing

Adults:

Pain management (acute; moderately-severe): Children ≥16 years and Adults:

Note: The maximum combined duration of treatment (for parenteral and oral) is 5 days; do not increase dose or frequency; supplement with low dose opioids if needed for breakthrough pain. For patients <50 kg and/or ≥65 years of age, see Elderly dosing.

I.M.: 60 mg as a single dose or 30 mg every 6 hours (maximum daily dose: 120 mg)

I.V.: 30 mg as a single dose or 30 mg every 6 hours (maximum daily dose: 120 mg)

Oral: 20 mg, followed by 10 mg every 4-6 hours; do not exceed 40 mg/day; oral dosing is intended to be a continuation of I.M. or I.V. therapy only

Ophthalmic uses:

Seasonal allergic conjunctivitis (relief of ocular itching) (Acular®): Ophthalmic: Instill 1 drop (0.25 mg) 4 times/day for seasonal allergic conjunctivitis

Inflammation following cataract extraction (Acular®): Ophthalmic: Instill 1 drop (0.25 mg) to affected eye(s) 4 times/day beginning 24 hours after surgery; continue for 2 weeks

Pain and photophobia following incisional refractive surgery (Acular® PF): Ophthalmic: Instill 1 drop (0.25 mg) 4 times/day to affected eye for up to 3 days

Pain following corneal refractive surgery (Acular LS™): Ophthalmic: Instill 1 drop 4 times/day as needed to affected eye for up to 4 days

Elderly: Elderly >65 years: Renal insufficiency or weight <50 kg: **Note:** Ketorolac has decreased clearance and increased half-life in the elderly. In addition, the elderly have reported increased incidence of GI bleeding, ulceration, and perforation. The maximum combined duration of treatment (for parenteral and oral) is 5 days.

I.M.: 30 mg as a single dose or 15 mg every 6 hours (maximum daily dose: 60 mg)

I.V.: 15 mg as a single dose or 15 mg every 6 hours (maximum daily dose: 60 mg)

Oral: 10 mg every 4-6 hours; do not exceed 40 mg/day; oral dosing is intended to be a continuation of I.M. or I.V. therapy only

Pediatrics: Note: Do not exceed adult doses.

Anti-inflammatory, single-dose treatment: Children 2-16 years:

I.M.: 1 mg/kg (maximum: 30 mg)

I.V.: 0.5 mg/kg (maximum: 15 mg)

Oral (unlabeled): 1 mg/kg as a single dose reported in one study

Anti-inflammatory, multiple-dose treatment (unlabeled): Children 2-16 years: Limited pediatric studies. The maximum combined duration of treatment (for parenteral and oral) is 5 days.

I.V.: Initial dose: 0.5 mg/kg followed by 0.25-1 mg/kg every 6 hours for up to 48 hours; maximum daily dose: 90 mg

Oral: 0.25 mg/kg every 6 hours

Ophthalmic uses: Children ≥3 years: Refer to adult dosing.

Renal Impairment: Do not use in patients with advanced renal impairment. Patients with moderately-elevated serum creatinine should use half the recommended dose, not to exceed 60 mg/day I.M./I.V.

Hepatic Impairment: Use with caution, may cause elevation of liver enzymes.

Administration

Oral: May take with food to reduce GI upset.

I.M.: Administer slowly and deeply into the muscle. Analgesia begins in 30 minutes and maximum effect within 2 hours.

I.V.: Administer I.V. bolus over a minimum of 15 seconds; onset within 30 minutes; peak analgesia within 2 hours.

I.V. Detail: pH: 6.9-7.9

Other: Ophthalmic solution: Contact lenses should be removed before instillation.

Stability

Compatibility: Stable in D_5NS, D_5W, LR, NS

Compatibility when admixed: Incompatible with hydroxyzine, meperidine, morphine, promethazine

Storage: Ketorolac injection and ophthalmic solution should be stored at controlled room temperature and protected from light. Injection is clear and has a slight yellow color. Precipitation may occur at relatively low pH values. Store tablets at controlled room temperature.

Laboratory Monitoring CBC, liver function, platelets; renal function (serum creatinine, BUN, urine output)

Nursing Actions

Physical Assessment: Assess allergy history prior to beginning therapy. Assess potential for interactions with other prescriptions, OTC medications, or herbal products patient may be taking. **I.V./I.M.:** Monitor vital signs on a regular basis during infusion or following injection. **Oral:** Monitor blood pressure at the beginning of therapy and periodically during use. Monitor laboratory tests, therapeutic effectiveness, and adverse response on a regular basis throughout therapy. Teach patient proper use, possible side effects/appropriate interventions (eg, importance of adequate hydration), and adverse symptoms to report.

Patient Education: Do not take any new medication during therapy without consulting prescriber (especially aspirin-containing products or other NSAIDs or any other NSAIDs). Use exactly as directed; do not increase dose or frequency. Adverse reactions can occur with overuse. Oral doses may be taken with food or milk. Avoid alcohol. Maintain adequate hydration (2-3 L/day of fluids) unless instructed to restrict fluid intake. May cause nausea or vomiting (frequent mouth care, small frequent meals, chewing gum, or sucking lozenges may help). Report GI bleeding, ulceration or perforation with or without pain (stop medication and report abdominal pain or blood in urine or stool); ringing in ears; unresolved nausea or vomiting; respiratory difficulty or shortness of breath; skin rash; unusual swelling of extremities; chest pain; or palpitations. **Pregnancy/breast-feeding precautions:** Inform prescriber if you are or intend to become pregnant. This drug should not be used in the 2nd or 3rd trimester of pregnancy. Consult prescriber for appropriate contraceptive measures if necessary. Consult prescriber if breast-feeding.

Ophthalmic: Instill drops as often as recommended. Wash hands before instilling. Sit or lie down to instill. Open eye, look at ceiling, and instill prescribed amount of solution. Close eye and roll eye in all directions. Apply gentle pressure to inner corner of eye for 1-2 minutes after instillation. Do not let tip of applicator touch eye; do not contaminate tip of applicator (may cause eye infection, eye damage, or vision loss). Temporary stinging or blurred vision may occur. Do not wear soft contact lenses. Report persistent pain, burning, double vision, swelling, itching, or worsening of condition.

Dietary Considerations Administer tablet with food or milk to decrease gastrointestinal distress.

Geriatric Considerations Ketorolac is eliminated more slowly in the elderly. It is recommended to use lower doses in the elderly. The elderly are at high risk for adverse effects from NSAIDs. As much as 60% of elderly can develop peptic ulceration and/or hemorrhage asymptomatically. The concomitant use of H_2 blockers, omeprazole, and sucralfate is not effective as prophylaxis with the exception of NSAID-induced (Continued)

Ketorolac *(Continued)*

duodenal ulcers which may be prevented by the use of ranitidine. Misoprostol is the only prophylactic agent proven effective. Also, concomitant disease and drug use contribute to the risk for GI adverse effects. Use lowest effective dose for shortest period possible. Consider renal function decline with age. Use of NSAIDs can compromise existing renal function especially when Cl_{cr} is ≤30 mL/minute. Tinnitus may be a difficult and unreliable indication of toxicity due to age-related hearing loss or eighth cranial nerve damage. CNS adverse effects such as confusion, agitation, and hallucination are generally seen in overdose or high-dose situations, but elderly may demonstrate these adverse effects at lower doses than younger adults.

Pregnancy Issues Ketorolac is contraindicated during labor and delivery (may inhibit uterine contractions and adversely affect fetal circulation). Avoid use of ketorolac ophthalmic solution during late pregnancy.

Additional Information First parenteral NSAID for analgesia; 30 mg provides the analgesia comparable to 12 mg of morphine or 100 mg of meperidine.

Ketotifen (kee toe TYE fen)

U.S. Brand Names Zaditor™
Synonyms Ketotifen Fumarate
Pharmacologic Category Antihistamine, H_1 Blocker, Ophthalmic
Pregnancy Risk Factor C
Lactation Use caution
Use Temporary prevention of eye itching due to allergic conjunctivitis
Contraindications Hypersensitivity to ketotifen or any component of the formulation (the preservative is benzalkonium chloride)
Adverse Reactions 1% to 10%:
Ocular: Allergic reactions, burning or stinging, conjunctivitis, discharge, dry eyes, eye pain, eyelid disorder, itching, keratitis, lacrimation disorder, mydriasis, photophobia, rash
Respiratory: Pharyngitis
Miscellaneous: Flu syndrome
Overdosage/Toxicology No serious signs or symptoms seen after ingestion of up to 20 mg of ketotifen
Pharmacodynamics/Kinetics
Onset of Action: Minutes
Duration of Action: 8-12 hours
Available Dosage Forms Solution, ophthalmic, as fumarate: 0.025% (5 mL) [contains benzalkonium chloride]
Dosing
Adults & Elderly: Allergic conjunctivitis: Ophthalmic: Instill 1 drop into the affected eye(s) twice daily, every 8-12 hours
Pediatrics: Children ≥3 years: Refer to adult dosing.
Stability
Storage: Stable at room temperature.
Nursing Actions
Physical Assessment: Assess potential for interactions with other prescriptions, OTC medications, or herbal products patient may be taking. Monitor patient response and adverse effects. Teach patient proper use, side effects/appropriate interventions, and symptoms to report.
Patient Education: For use in eyes only. Do not let tip of applicator touch eye; do not contaminate tip of applicator (may cause eye infection, eye damage, or vision loss). Not to be used to treat contact lens-related irritation. Wait at least 10 minutes before putting soft contact lenses in. Do not wear contact lenses if eyes are red. Store at room temperature.

Pregnancy/breast-feeding precautions: Inform prescriber if you are pregnant or breast-feeding.
Pregnancy Issues Oral treatment administered to pregnant animals have resulted in retarded ossification of the sternebrae, slight increase in postnatal mortality, and a decrease in weight gain in the first 4 days of life. Topical ocular administration has not been studied.

Labetalol (la BET a lole)

U.S. Brand Names Trandate®
Synonyms Ibidomide Hydrochloride; Labetalol Hydrochloride
Pharmacologic Category Beta Blocker With Alpha-Blocking Activity
Medication Safety Issues
Sound-alike/look-alike issues:
Labetalol may be confused with betaxolol, Hexadrol®, lamotrigine
Trandate® may be confused with tramadol, Trendar®, Trental®, Tridrate®
Pregnancy Risk Factor C (manufacturer); D (2nd and 3rd trimesters - expert analysis)
Lactation Enters breast milk/use caution (AAP rates "compatible")
Use Treatment of mild to severe hypertension; I.V. for hypertensive emergencies
Mechanism of Action/Effect Blocks alpha-, $beta_1$-, and $beta_2$-adrenergic receptor sites; elevated renins are reduced
Contraindications Hypersensitivity to labetalol or any component of the formulation; sinus bradycardia; heart block greater than first degree (except in patients with a functioning artificial pacemaker); cardiogenic shock; bronchial asthma; uncompensated cardiac failure; pregnancy (2nd and 3rd trimesters)
Warnings/Precautions Use only with extreme caution in compensated heart failure and monitor for a worsening of the condition. Use caution with concurrent use of beta-blockers and either verapamil or diltiazem; bradycardia or heart block can occur. Avoid concurrent I.V. use of both agents. Patients with bronchospastic disease should not receive beta-blockers. Labetalol may be used with caution in patients with nonallergic bronchospasm (chronic bronchitis, emphysema). Use cautiously in patients with diabetes because it can mask prominent hypoglycemic symptoms. Can mask signs of thyrotoxicosis. Can cause fetal harm when administered in pregnancy. Use cautiously in hepatic impairment. Use caution when using I.V. labetalol and inhalational anesthetics concurrently (significant myocardial depression). Avoid abrupt discontinuation in patients with a history of CAD.
Drug Interactions
Cytochrome P450 Effect: Substrate of CYP2D6 (major); **Inhibits** CYP2D6 (weak)
Decreased Effect: Decreased effect of beta-blockers with aluminum salts, barbiturates, calcium salts, cholestyramine, colestipol, NSAIDs, penicillins (ampicillin), rifampin, salicylates, and sulfinpyrazone due to decreased bioavailability and plasma levels. Beta-blockers may decrease the effect of sulfonylureas.
Increased Effect/Toxicity: CYP2D6 inhibitors may increase the levels/effects of labetalol; example inhibitors include chlorpromazine, delavirdine, fluoxetine, miconazole, paroxetine, pergolide, quinidine, quinine, ritonavir, and ropinirole. Cimetidine increases the bioavailability of labetalol. Labetalol has additive hypotensive effects with other antihypertensive agents. Concurrent use with alpha-blockers (prazosin, terazosin) and beta-blockers increases the risk of orthostasis. Concurrent use with diltiazem, verapamil, or digoxin may increase the risk of bradycardia with

beta-blocking agents. Halothane, enflurane, isoflurane, and potentially other inhalation anesthetics may cause synergistic hypotension. Beta-blockers may affect the action or levels of ethanol, disopyramide, nondepolarizing muscle relaxants, and theophylline although the effects are difficult to predict.

Nutritional/Ethanol Interactions

Food: Labetalol serum concentrations may be increased if taken with food.

Herb/Nutraceutical: Avoid dong quai if using for hypertension (has estrogenic activity). Avoid ephedra, yohimbe, ginseng (may worsen hypertension). Avoid natural licorice (causes sodium and water retention and increases potassium loss). Avoid garlic (may have increased antihypertensive effect).

Lab Interactions False-positive urine catecholamines, VMA if measured by fluorometric or photometric methods; use HPLC or specific catecholamine radioenzymatic technique

Adverse Reactions

>10%:
Central nervous system: Dizziness (1% to 16%)
Gastrointestinal: Nausea (0% to 19%)

1% to 10%:
Cardiovascular: Edema (0% to 2%), hypotension (1% to 5%); with IV use, hypotension may occur in up to 58%
Central nervous system: Fatigue (1% to 10%), paresthesia (1% to 5%), headache (2%), vertigo (2%)
Dermatologic: Rash (1%), scalp tingling (1% to 5%)
Gastrointestinal: Vomiting (<1% to 3%), dyspepsia (1% to 4%)
Genitourinary: Ejaculatory failure (0% to 5%), impotence (1% to 4%)
Hepatic: Transaminases increased (4%)
Neuromuscular & skeletal: Weakness (1%)
Respiratory: Nasal congestion (1% to 6%), dyspnea (2%)
Miscellaneous: Taste disorder (1%), abnormal vision (1%)

Other adverse reactions noted with beta-adrenergic blocking agents include mental depression, catatonia, disorientation, short-term memory loss, emotional lability, clouded sensorium, intensification of pre-existing AV block, laryngospasm, respiratory distress, agranulocytosis, thrombocytopenic purpura, nonthrombocytopenic purpura, mesenteric artery thrombosis, and ischemic colitis.

Overdosage/Toxicology Symptoms of intoxication include cardiac disturbances, CNS toxicity, bronchospasm, hypoglycemia, and hyperkalemia. The most common cardiac symptoms include hypotension and bradycardia. Atrioventricular block, intraventricular conduction disturbances, cardiogenic shock, and asystole may occur with severe overdose, especially with membrane-depressant drugs (eg, propranolol). CNS effects include convulsions, coma, and respiratory arrest and are commonly seen with propranolol and other membrane-depressant and lipid-soluble drugs. Treatment is symptomatic. Glucagon may be administered to improve cardiac function.

Pharmacodynamics/Kinetics

Onset of Action: Oral: 20 minutes to 2 hours; I.V.: 2-5 minutes; Peak effect: Oral: 1-4 hours; I.V.: 5-15 minutes

Duration of Action: Oral (dose dependent): 8-24 hours; I.V.: 2-4 hours

Protein Binding: 50%

Half-Life Elimination: Normal renal function: 2.5-8 hours

Metabolism: Hepatic, primarily via glucuronide conjugation; extensive first-pass effect

Excretion: Urine (<5% as unchanged drug)
Clearance: Possibly decreased in neonates/infants

Available Dosage Forms

Injection, solution, as hydrochloride: 5 mg/mL (4 mL, 20 mL, 40 mL)
Trandate®: 5 mg/mL (20 mL, 40 mL)
Tablet, as hydrochloride: 100 mg, 200 mg, 300 mg
Trandate®: 100 mg, 200 mg [contains sodium benzoate], 300 mg

Dosing

Adults:

Hypertension: Oral: Initial: 100 mg twice daily, may increase as needed every 2-3 days by 100 mg until desired response is obtained; usual dose: 200-400 mg twice daily; not to exceed 2.4 g/day
Usual dose range (JNC 7): 200-800 mg/day in 2 divided doses

Acute hypertension (hypertensive urgency/emergency):
I.V. bolus: 20 mg or 1-2 mg/kg whichever is lower, IVP over 2 minutes, may give 40-80 mg at 10-minute intervals, up to 300 mg total dose
I.V. infusion: Initial: 2 mg/minute; titrate to response up to 300 mg total dose. Administration requires the use of an infusion pump.
Note: Continuous infusion at low rates (2-4 mg/hour) have been used in some settings for patients unable to transition rapidly to oral medication.

Elderly: Oral: Initial: 100 mg 1-2 times/day increasing as needed

Pediatrics: Note: Due to limited documentation of its use, labetalol should be initiated cautiously in pediatric patients with careful dosage adjustment and blood pressure monitoring.

Hypertension:
Oral: Limited information regarding labetalol use in pediatric patients is currently available in literature. Some centers recommend initial oral doses of 4 mg/kg/day in 2 divided doses. Reported oral doses have started at 3 mg/kg/day and 20 mg/kg/day and have increased up to 40 mg/kg/day.
I.V.: Intermittent bolus doses of 0.3-1 mg/kg/dose have been reported.

Pediatric hypertensive emergencies: Initial continuous infusions of 0.4-1 mg/kg/hour with a maximum of 3 mg/kg/hour have been used; administration requires the use of an infusion pump.

Renal Impairment: Not removed by hemo- or peritoneal dialysis; supplemental dose is not necessary.

Hepatic Impairment: Dosage reduction may be necessary.

Administration

I.V.: Bolus administered over 2 minutes.

I.V. Detail: Loading infusions (2 mg/minute) require close monitoring of heart rate and blood pressure and are terminated after response or cumulative dose of 300 mg. Continuous infusions of 2-6 mg/hour have been used in some settings and should not be confused with loading infusions.

pH: 3-4

Stability

Reconstitution: Stability of parenteral admixture at room temperature (25°C) and refrigeration temperature (4°C) is 3 days.

Standard diluent: 500 mg/250 mL D_5W
Minimum volume: 250 mL D_5W

Compatibility: Stable in D_5LR, $D_5\frac{1}{4}NS$, $D_5\frac{1}{3}NS$, D_5NS, D_5W, LR, NS; most stable at pH of 2-4. **Incompatible** with sodium bicarbonate 5% and alkaline solutions.

Y-site administration: Incompatible with amphotericin B cholesteryl sulfate complex, cefoperazone, ceftriaxone, nafcillin, thiopental, warfarin

Compatibility when admixed: Incompatible with sodium bicarbonate

(Continued)

Labetalol (Continued)

Storage: Labetalol should be stored at room temperature or under refrigeration and should be protected from light and freezing. The solution is clear to slightly yellow.

Nursing Actions

Physical Assessment: Assess potential for interactions with other prescriptions, OTC medications, or herbal products patient may be taking (especially anything that will effect blood pressure). Monitor blood pressure and heart rate prior to and following first dose and with any change in dosage. Caution patients with diabetes to monitor glucose levels closely; beta-blockers may alter glucose tolerance. Monitor laboratory tests, therapeutic effectiveness, and adverse response (eg, CHF). Teach patient proper use, possible side effects/appropriate interventions, and adverse symptoms to report.

Patient Education: Do not take any new medication during therapy unless approved by prescriber. Take as directed, with meals. Do not skip dose or discontinue without consulting prescriber. This medication does not replace other antihypertensive interventions; follow prescriber's instructions for diet and lifestyle changes. If you have diabetes, monitor serum glucose closely and notify prescriber of changes (this medication can alter hypoglycemic requirements). You may experience drowsiness, dizziness, or impaired judgment (use caution when driving or engaging in tasks that require alertness until response to drug is known); postural hypotension (use caution when rising from sitting or lying position or when climbing stairs); dry mouth, nausea, or loss of appetite (frequent mouth care or sucking lozenges may help); or sexual dysfunction (reversible, may resolve with continued use). Report altered CNS status (eg, fatigue, depression, numbness or tingling of fingers, toes, or skin); palpitations or slowed heartbeat; respiratory difficulty; edema or cold extremities; or other persistent side effects. **Pregnancy/breast-feeding precautions:** Inform prescriber if you are or intend to become pregnant. Consult prescriber if breast-feeding.

Geriatric Considerations Due to alterations in the beta-adrenergic autonomic nervous system, beta-adrenergic blockade may result in less hemodynamic response than seen in younger adults.

Breast-Feeding Issues Available evidence suggests safe use during breast-feeding. Monitor breast-fed infant for symptoms of beta-blockade.

Pregnancy Issues Labetalol crosses the placenta. Beta-blockers have been associated with persistent bradycardia, hypotension, and IUGR; IUGR is probably related to maternal hypertension. Available evidence suggests beta-blockers are generally safe during pregnancy (JNC 7). Cases of neonatal hypoglycemia have been reported following maternal use of beta-blockers at parturition or during breast-feeding. Monitor breast-fed infant for symptoms of beta-blockade.

Lactobacillus (lak toe ba SIL us)

U.S. Brand Names Bacid® [OTC]; Culturelle® [OTC]; Dofus [OTC]; Flora-Q™ [OTC]; Kala® [OTC]; Lactinex™ [OTC]; Lacto-Bifidus [OTC]; Lacto-Key [OTC]; Lacto-Pectin [OTC]; Lacto-TriBlend [OTC]; Megadophilus® [OTC]; MoreDophilus® [OTC]; Superdophilus® [OTC]

Synonyms Lactobacillus acidophilus; Lactobacillus bifidus; Lactobacillus bulgaricus; Lactobacillus casei; Lactobacillus paracasei; Lactobacillus reuteri; Lactobacillus rhamnosus GG

Pharmacologic Category Dietary Supplement; Probiotic

Use Promote normal bacterial flora of the intestinal tract

Mechanism of Action/Effect Helps re-establish normal intestinal flora; suppresses the growth of potentially pathogenic microorganisms by producing lactic acid which favors the establishment of an aciduric flora.

Contraindications Hypersensitivity to any component of the formulation

Warnings/Precautions Lactobacillus species have been studied for various gastrointestinal disorders including diarrhea, inflammatory bowel disease, gastrointestinal infection. Effectiveness may be dependant upon actual species used; studies are ongoing. Currently, there are no FDA-approved disease-prevention or therapeutic indications for these products.

Adverse Reactions Gastrointestinal: Flatulence

Pharmacodynamics/Kinetics
Excretion: Feces

Available Dosage Forms
Capsule:

Culturelle®: L. rhamnosus GG 10 billion colony-forming units [contains casein and whey]

Dofus: L. acidophilus and L. bifidus 10:1 ratio [beet root powder base]

Flora-Q™: L. acidophilus and L. paracasei ≥8 billion colony-forming units [also contains Bifidobacterium and S. thermophilus]

Lacto-Key:
100: L. acidophilus 1 billion colony-forming units [milk, soy, and yeast free; rice derived]
600: L. acidophilus 6 billion colony-forming units [milk, soy, and yeast free; rice derived]

Lacto-Bifidus:
100: L. bifidus 1 billion colony-forming units [milk, soy, and yeast free; rice derived]
600: L. bifidus 6 billion colony-forming units [milk, soy, and yeast free; rice derived]

Lacto-Pectin: L. acidophilus and L. casei ≥5 billion colony-forming units [also contains Bifidobacterium lactis and citrus pectin cellulose complex]

Lacto-TriBlend:
100: L. acidophilus, L. bifidus, and L. bulgaricus 1 billion colony-forming units [milk, soy and yeast free; rice derived]
600: L. acidophilus, L. bifidus, and L. bulgaricus 6 billion colony-forming units [milk, soy and yeast free; rice derived]

Megadophilus®, Superdophilus®: L. acidophilus 2 billion units [available in dairy based or dairy free formulations]

Capsule, softgel: L. acidophilus 100 active units

Caplet (Bacid®): L. acidophilus 80% and L. bulgaricus 10% [also contains Bifidobacterium biffidum 5% and S. thermophilus 5%]

Granules (Lactinex™): L. acidophilus and L. bulgaricus 100 million live cells per 1 g packet (12s) [contains whey, evaporated milk, soy peptone, lactose, and beef extract]

Powder:
Lacto-TriBlend: L. acidophilus, L. bifidus, and L. bulgaricus 10 billion colony-forming units per ¼ teaspoon (60 g) [milk, soy, and yeast free; rice derived]
Megadophilus®, Superdophilus®: L. acidophilus 2 billion units per half-teaspoon (49 g, 70 g, 84 g, 126 g) [available in dairy based or dairy free (garbanzo bean) formulations]
MoreDophilus®: L. acidophilus 12.4 billion units per teaspoon (30 g, 120 g) [dairy free, yeast free; soy and carrot derived]

Tablet:
Kala®: L. acidophilus 200 million units [dairy free, yeast free; soy based]

Lactinex™: *L. acidophilus* and *L. bulgaricus* 1 million live cells [contains whey, evaporated milk, soy peptone, lactose, and beef extract; contains sodium 5.6 mg/4 tablets]

Tablet, chewable: *L. reuteri* 100 million organisms

Wafer: *L. acidophilus* 90 mg and *L. bifidus* 25 mg (100s) [provides 1 billion organisms/wafer at time of manufacture; milk free]

Dosing

Adults & Elderly:

Dietary supplement: Oral: Dosing varies by manufacturer; consult product labeling

Bacid®: 2 caplets/day

Culturelle®: 1 capsule daily; may increase to twice daily

Flora-Q™: 1 capsule/day

Lacto-Key 100 or 600: 1-2 capsules/day

Lactinex™: 1 packet or 4 tablets 3-4 times/day

Pediatrics:

Dietary supplement: Oral: Dosing varies by manufacturer; consult product labeling

Culturelle®: 1 capsule daily

Administration

Oral:

Culturelle®: Capsules may be opened and mixed in a cool beverage or sprinkled onto baby food or applesauce.

Flora-Q™: May be taken with or without food.

Lactinex™: Granules may be added to or administered with cereal, food, or milk.

Megadophilus®, Superdophilus®: Administer on an empty stomach; powder should be mixed in unchilled water.

Stability

Storage: Bacid®: Store at room temperature.

Flora-Q™: Store at or below room temperature; do not store in bathroom

Kala®, MoreDophilus®: Refrigeration recommended after opening.

Lactinex™, Dofus: Store in refrigerator.

Nursing Actions

Physical Assessment: Teach patient proper use and adverse symptoms to report (eg, discontinue and notify prescriber if high fever develops).

Patient Education: Use exactly as directed; do not take more than prescribed. Granules in capsules may be added to or taken with cereal, food, milk, fruit juice, or water. You may experience increased flatus while taking this medication. Discontinue and notify prescriber if a high fever develops. Refrigerate Lactinex™ and Bacid®. **Breast-feeding precaution:** Consult prescriber if breast-feeding.

Dietary Considerations

Products may contain whey, evaporated milk, soy peptone casein and/or beef extract; consult individual product labeling. Lactinex™ contains sodium 5.6 mg/4 tablets

---

Lactulose (LAK tyoo lose)

U.S. Brand Names Constulose®; Enulose®; Generlac; Kristalose™

Pharmacologic Category Ammonium Detoxicant; Laxative, Osmotic

Medication Safety Issues

Sound-alike/look-alike issues:

Lactulose may be confused with lactose

Pregnancy Risk Factor B

Lactation Excretion in breast milk unknown

Use Adjunct in the prevention and treatment of portal-systemic encephalopathy; treatment of chronic constipation

Mechanism of Action/Effect The bacterial degradation of lactulose resulting in an acidic pH inhibits the diffusion of NH_3 into the blood by causing the conversion of NH_3 to NH_4+; also enhances the diffusion of NH_3 from the blood into the gut where conversion to NH_4+ occurs; produces an osmotic effect in the colon with resultant distention promoting peristalsis

Contraindications Hypersensitivity to lactulose or any component of the formulation; galactosemia (or patients requiring a low galactose diet)

Warnings/Precautions Use with caution in patients with diabetes mellitus; monitor periodically for electrolyte imbalance when lactulose is used >6 months or in patients predisposed to electrolyte abnormalities (eg, elderly); patients receiving lactulose and an oral anti-infective agent should be monitored for possible inadequate response to lactulose

Drug Interactions

Decreased Effect: Oral neomycin, laxatives, antacids

Adverse Reactions Frequency not defined: Gastrointestinal: Flatulence, diarrhea (excessive dose), abdominal discomfort, nausea, vomiting, cramping

Overdosage/Toxicology Symptoms of overdose include diarrhea, abdominal pain, hypochloremic alkalosis, dehydration, hypotension, and hypokalemia. Treatment includes supportive care.

Pharmacodynamics/Kinetics

Metabolism: Via colonic flora to lactic acid and acetic acid; requires colonic flora for drug activation

Excretion: Primarily feces and urine (~3%)

Available Dosage Forms

Crystals for reconstitution (Kristalose™): 10 g/packet (30s), 20 g/packet (30s)

Syrup: 10 g/15 mL (15 mL, 30 mL, 237 mL, 473 mL, 946 mL, 1890 mL)

Constulose®: 10 g/15 mL (240 mL, 960 mL)

Enulose®: 10 g/15 mL (480 mL)

Generlac: 10 g/15 mL (480 mL, 1920 mL)

Dosing

Adults & Elderly:

Note: Diarrhea may indicate overdosage and responds to dose reduction.

Acute portal-systemic encephalopathy (PSE):

Oral: 20-30 g (30-45 mL) every 1-2 hours to induce rapid laxation; adjust dosage daily to produce 2-3 soft stools; doses of 30-45 mL may be given hourly to cause rapid laxation, then reduce to recommended dose; usual daily dose: 60-100 g (90-150 mL) daily

Rectal: 200 g (300 mL) diluted with 700 mL of H_2O or NS; administer rectally via rectal balloon catheter and retain 30-60 minutes every 4-6 hours.

Constipation: Oral: 10-20 g/day (15-30 mL/day) increased to 60 mL/day in 1-2 divided doses if necessary

Pediatrics: Diarrhea may indicate overdosage and responds to dose reduction.

Prevention of portal systemic encephalopathy (PSE): Oral:

Infants: 2.5-10 mL/day divided 3-4 times/day; adjust dosage to produce 2-3 stools/day.

Older Children: Daily dose of 40-90 mL divided 3-4 times/day; if initial dose causes diarrhea, then reduce it immediately; adjust dosage to produce 2-3 stools/day.

Constipation: Oral: 5 g/day (7.5 mL) after breakfast

Administration

Oral: Dilute lactulose in water, usually 60-120 mL, prior to administering through a gastric or feeding tube.

Other: Syrup formulation has been used in preparation of rectal solution.

Stability

Storage: Keep solution at room temperature to reduce viscosity. Discard solution if cloudy or very dark.

Laboratory Monitoring Serum potassium, serum ammonia

(Continued)

Lactulose *(Continued)*

Nursing Actions

Physical Assessment: Monitor laboratory tests (see above), therapeutic effectiveness (soft formed stools or resolution of CNS status in PSE), and adverse response (eg, CHF). Monitor frequency/consistency of stools; diarrhea may indicate overdose. Teach patient proper use, possible side effects/appropriate interventions, and adverse symptoms to report.

Patient Education: Not for long-term use. Take as directed, alone, or diluted with water, juice or milk, or take with food. Laxative results may not occur for 24-48 hours; do not take more often than recommended or for a longer time than recommended. Do not use any other laxatives while taking lactulose. Increased fiber, fluids, and exercise may also help reduce constipation. Do not use if experiencing abdominal pain, nausea, or vomiting. Diarrhea may indicate overdose. May cause flatulence, belching, or abdominal cramping. Report persistent or severe diarrhea or abdominal cramping. **Breast-feeding precaution:** Consult prescriber if breast-feeding.

Dietary Considerations Contraindicated in patients on galactose-restricted diet; may be mixed with fruit juice, milk, water, or citrus-flavored carbonated beverages.

Geriatric Considerations Elderly are more likely to show CNS signs of dehydration and electrolyte loss than younger adults. Therefore, monitor closely for fluid and electrolyte loss with chronic use. Sorbitol is equally effective as a laxative and less expensive. However, sorbitol **cannot be substituted** in the treatment of hepatic encephalopathy.

Lamivudine *(la MI vyoo deen)*

U.S. Brand Names Epivir®; Epivir-HBV®
Synonyms 3TC
Pharmacologic Category Antiretroviral Agent, Reverse Transcriptase Inhibitor (Nucleoside)
Medication Safety Issues
Sound-alike/look-alike issues:
Lamivudine may be confused with lamotrigine
Epivir® may be confused with Combivir®

Pregnancy Risk Factor C
Lactation Enters breast milk/contraindicated
Use

Epivir®: Treatment of HIV infection when antiretroviral therapy is warranted; should always be used as part of a multidrug regimen (at least three antiretroviral agents)

Epivir-HBV®: Treatment of chronic hepatitis B associated with evidence of hepatitis B viral replication and active liver inflammation

Unlabeled/Investigational Use Prevention of HIV following needlesticks (with or without protease inhibitor)

Mechanism of Action/Effect Lamivudine is a cytosine analog. *In vitro,* lamivudine is phosphorylated to its active 5′-triphosphate metabolite (L-TP), which inhibits HIV reverse transcription via viral DNA chain termination; L-TP also inhibits the RNA- and DNA-dependent DNA polymerase activities of reverse transcriptase. The monophosphate form is incorporated into viral DNA by hepatitis B polymerase, resulting in DNA chain termination.

Contraindications Hypersensitivity to lamivudine or any component of the formulation

Warnings/Precautions A decreased dosage is recommended in patients with renal dysfunction since AUC, C_{max}, and half-life increased with diminishing renal function; use with extreme caution in children with history of pancreatitis or risk factors for development of pancreatitis. Do not use as monotherapy in treatment of HIV.

Treatment of HBV in patients with unrecognized/ untreated HIV may lead to rapid HIV resistance. In addition, treatment of HIV in patients with unrecognized/ untreated HBV may lead to rapid HBV resistance. Patients with HIV infection should receive only dosage forms appropriate for treatment of HIV.

Lactic acidosis and severe hepatomegaly with steatosis have been reported, including fatal cases. Use caution in hepatic impairment. Pregnancy, obesity, and/or prolonged therapy may increase the risk of lactic acidosis and liver damage.

Monitor patients closely for several months following discontinuation of therapy for chronic hepatitis B; clinical exacerbations may occur.

Drug Interactions

Decreased Effect: Zalcitabine and lamivudine may inhibit the intracellular phosphorylation of each other; concomitant use should be avoided.

Increased Effect/Toxicity: Zidovudine concentrations increase significantly (~39%) with lamivudine coadministration. sulfamethoxazole/trimethoprim increases lamivudine's blood levels. Concomitant use of ribavirin and nucleoside analogues may increase the risk of developing lactic acidosis (includes adefovir, didanosine, lamivudine, stavudine, zalcitabine, zidovudine). Trimethoprim (and other drugs excreted by organic cation transport) may increase serum levels/effects of lamivudine.

Nutritional/Ethanol Interactions Food: Food decreases the rate of absorption and C_{max}; however, there is no change in the systemic AUC. Therefore, may be taken with or without food.

Adverse Reactions (As reported in adults treated for HIV infection)

>10%:
Central nervous system: Headache, fatigue
Gastrointestinal: Nausea, diarrhea, vomiting, pancreatitis (range: 0.5% to 18%; higher percentage in pediatric patients)
Neuromuscular & skeletal: Peripheral neuropathy, paresthesia, musculoskeletal pain

1% to 10%:
Central nervous system: Dizziness, depression, fever, chills, insomnia
Dermatologic: Rash
Gastrointestinal: Anorexia, abdominal pain, heartburn, elevated amylase
Hematologic: Neutropenia
Hepatic: Elevated AST, ALT
Neuromuscular & skeletal: Myalgia, arthralgia
Respiratory: Nasal signs and symptoms, cough

Overdosage/Toxicology Limited information is available, although there have been no clinical signs or symptoms noted, and hematologic tests remained normal in overdose. No antidote is available. Limited (negligible) removal following 4-hour hemodialysis. It is not known if continuous 24-hour hemodialysis would be effective.

Pharmacodynamics/Kinetics
Protein Binding: Plasma: <36%
Half-Life Elimination: Children: 2 hours; Adults: 5-7 hours
Metabolism: 5.6% to trans-sulfoxide metabolite
Excretion: Primarily urine (as unchanged drug)

Available Dosage Forms
Solution, oral:
Epivir®: 10 mg/mL (240 mL) [strawberry-banana flavor]
Epivir-HBV®: 5 mg/mL (240 mL) [strawberry-banana flavor]
Tablet:
Epivir®: 150 mg, 300 mg
Epivir-HBV®: 100 mg

Dosing

Adults & Elderly: Note: The formulation and dosage of Epivir-HBV® are not appropriate for patients infected with both HBV and HIV.

HIV: Oral (use with at least two other antiretroviral agents): 150 mg twice daily **or** 300 mg once daily

<50 kg: 4 mg/kg twice daily (maximum: 150 mg twice daily)

Prevention of HIV following needlesticks (unlabeled use): Oral: 150 mg twice daily (with zidovudine with or without a protease inhibitor, depending on risk)

Treatment of hepatitis B (Epivir-HBV®): Oral: 100 mg/day

Pediatrics: Note: The formulation and dosage of Epivir-HBV® are not appropriate for patients infected with both HBV and HIV.

HIV: Oral (use with at least two other antiretroviral agents)

3 months to 16 years: 4 mg/kg twice daily (maximum: 150 mg twice daily)

>16 years: Refer to adult dosing.

Treatment of hepatitis B: Oral: Children 2-17 years: 3 mg/kg once daily (maximum: 100 mg/day)

Renal Impairment: Oral:

Pediatric patients: Insufficient data; however, dose reduction should be considered.

Treatment of HIV patients >16 years:

Cl$_{cr}$ 30-49 mL/minute: Administer 150 mg once daily.

Cl$_{cr}$ 15-29 mL/minute: Administer 150 mg first dose, then 100 mg once daily.

Cl$_{cr}$ 5-14 mL/minute: Administer 150 mg first dose, then 50 mg once daily.

Cl$_{cr}$ <5 mL/minute: Administer 50 mg first dose, then 25 mg once daily.

Dialysis: No data available.

Treatment of hepatitis B patients: Adults:

Cl$_{cr}$ 30-49 mL/minute: Administer 100 mg first dose, then 50 mg once daily.

Cl$_{cr}$ 15-29 mL/minute: Administer 100 mg first dose, then 25 mg once daily.

Cl$_{cr}$ 5-14 mL/minute: Administer 35 mg first dose, then 15 mg once daily.

Cl$_{cr}$ <5 mL/minute: Administer 35 mg first dose, then 10 mg once daily.

Dialysis: Negligible amounts are removed by 4-hour hemodialysis or peritoneal dialysis. Supplemental dosing is not required.

Administration

Oral: May be taken with or without food. Adjust dosage in renal failure.

Stability

Storage: Store at 2°C to 25°C (68°F to 77°F) tightly closed.

Laboratory Monitoring Amylase, bilirubin, liver enzymes, CBC

Nursing Actions

Physical Assessment: Assess potential for interactions with other pharmacological agents patient may be taking. Assess results of laboratory tests, therapeutic effectiveness, and adverse reactions (eg, nausea/vomiting [dehydration]; peripheral neuropathy; hepatitis B [jaundice, fatigue, anorexia]) on a regular basis throughout therapy. Monitor patients closely for several months following discontinuation of therapy for chronic hepatitis B and clinical exacerbations. Teach patient proper use (eg, timing of multiple medications), possible side effects/appropriate interventions, and adverse symptoms to report.

Patient Education: Do not take any new medication during therapy unless approved by prescriber. This is not a cure for HIV, nor has it been found to reduce transmission of HIV; use appropriate precautions to prevent spread to other persons. Maintain adequate hydration (2-3 L/day of fluids) unless instructed to restrict fluid intake. This medication may be prescribed with a combination of other medications; time these medications as directed by prescriber. Take with or without food. Do not take antacids within 1 hour of lamivudine. Frequent blood tests may be required with prolonged therapy. You may be susceptible to infection; avoid crowds and exposure to known infections and do not have any vaccinations without consulting prescriber. May cause loss of appetite or change in taste (sucking on lozenges, chewing gum, or small frequent meals may help); dizziness or numbness (use caution when driving or engaging in tasks that require alertness until response to drug is known); or headache, fever, or muscle pain (an analgesic may be recommended). Report persistent lethargy or unusual fatigue, yellowing of eyes, pale stool and dark urine, acute headache, severe nausea or vomiting, respiratory difficulty, loss of sensation, rash, or other persistent adverse effects. **Pregnancy/breast-feeding precautions:** Inform prescriber if you are or intend to become pregnant. Do not breast-feed.

Dietary Considerations May be taken with or without food. Each 5 mL of oral solution contains 1 g of sucrose.

Breast-Feeding Issues HIV-infected mothers are discouraged from breast-feeding to decrease potential transmission of HIV.

Pregnancy Issues Lamivudine crosses the placenta. The pharmacokinetics of lamivudine during pregnancy are not significantly altered and dosage adjustment is not required. The Perinatal HIV Guidelines Working Group recommends lamivudine for use during pregnancy; the combination of lamivudine with zidovudine is the recommended dual combination NRTI in pregnancy. It may also be used in combination with zidovudine in HIV-infected women who are in labor, but have had no prior antiretroviral therapy, in order to reduce the maternal-fetal transmission of HIV. Cases of lactic acidosis/hepatic steatosis syndrome have been reported in pregnant women receiving nucleoside analogues. It is not known if pregnancy itself potentiates this known side effect; however, pregnant women may be at increased risk of lactic acidosis and liver damage. Hepatic enzymes and electrolytes should be monitored frequently during the 3rd trimester of pregnancy in women receiving nucleoside analogues. Health professionals are encouraged to contact the antiretroviral pregnancy registry to monitor outcomes of pregnant women exposed to antiretroviral medications (1-800-258-4263 or www.APRegistry.com).

Additional Information Lamivudine has been well studied in the treatment of chronic hepatitis B infection. Potential compliance problems, frequency of administration, and adverse effects should be discussed with patients before initiating therapy to help prevent the emergence of resistance.

A high rate of early virologic nonresponse was observed when abacavir, lamivudine and tenofovir were used as the initial regimen in treatment-naive patients. A high rate of early virologic nonresponse was also observed when didanosine, lamivudine, and tenofovir were used as the initial regimen in treatment-naive patients. Use of either of these combinations is not recommended; patients currently on either of these regimens should be closely monitored for modification of therapy.

Lamotrigine (la MOE tri jeen)

U.S. Brand Names Lamictal®
Synonyms BW-430C; LTG
Pharmacologic Category Anticonvulsant, Miscellaneous
Medication Safety Issues
Sound-alike/look-alike issues:
Lamotrigine may be confused with labetalol, Lamisil®, lamivudine, Lomotil®, ludiomil
Lamictal® may be confused with Lamisil®, Lomotil®, ludiomil
Pregnancy Risk Factor C
Lactation Enters breast milk/not recommended (AAP rates "of concern")
Use Adjunctive therapy in the treatment of generalized seizures of Lennox-Gastaut syndrome and partial seizures in adults and children ≥2 years of age; conversion to monotherapy in adults with partial seizures who are receiving treatment with valproate or a single enzyme-inducing antiepileptic drug; maintenance treatment of bipolar disorder
Mechanism of Action/Effect A triazine derivative which inhibits release of glutamate (an excitatory amino acid) and inhibits voltage-sensitive sodium channels, which stabilizes neuronal membranes. Lamotrigine has weak inhibitory effect on the $5HT_3$ receptor; *in vitro* inhibits dihydrofolate reductase.
Contraindications Hypersensitivity to lamotrigine or any component of the formulation
Warnings/Precautions Severe and potentially life-threatening skin rashes requiring hospitalization have been reported (children 0.8%; adults 0.3%); risk may be increased by coadministration with valproic acid, higher than recommended starting doses, and rapid dose titration. The majority of cases occur in the first 8 weeks; however, isolated cases may occur after prolonged treatment. Discontinue at first sign of rash unless rash is clearly not drug related. Use with caution in patients with impaired renal, hepatic, or cardiac function. Avoid abrupt cessation, taper over at least 2 weeks if possible. May cause CNS depression, which may impair physical or mental abilities. Patients must be cautioned about performing tasks which require mental alertness (eg, operating machinery or driving). Effects with other sedative drugs or ethanol may be potentiated. **Use caution in writing and/or interpreting prescriptions/orders; medication dispensing errors have occurred with similar-sounding medications (Lamisil®, ludiomil, lamivudine, labetalol, and Lomotil®).**
Drug Interactions
Decreased Effect: Acetaminophen (chronic administration), carbamazepine, oral contraceptives (estrogens), phenytoin, phenobarbital may decrease concentrations of lamotrigine; dosage adjustments may be needed when adding or withdrawing agent; monitor
Increased Effect/Toxicity: Lamotrigine may increase the epoxide metabolite of carbamazepine resulting in toxicity. Valproic acid increases blood levels of lamotrigine. Valproic acid inhibits the clearance of lamotrigine, dosage adjustment required when adding or withdrawing valproic acid; inhibition appears maximal at valproic acid 250-500 mg/day; the incidence of serious rash may be increased by valproic acid. Toxicity has been reported following addition of sertraline (limited documentation).
Nutritional/Ethanol Interactions
Ethanol: Avoid ethanol (may increase CNS depression).
Food: Has no effect on absorption.
Herb/Nutraceutical: Avoid evening primrose (seizure threshold decreased).
Adverse Reactions Percentages reported in adults receiving adjunctive therapy:

>10%:
Central nervous system: Headache (29%), dizziness (38%), ataxia (22%), somnolence (14%)
Gastrointestinal: Nausea (19%)
Ocular: Diplopia (28%), blurred vision (16%)
Respiratory: Rhinitis (14%)
1% to 10%:
Cardiovascular: Peripheral edema
Central nervous system: Depression (4%), anxiety (4%), irritability (3%), confusion, speech disorder (3%), difficulty concentrating (2%), malaise, seizure (includes exacerbations) (2% to 3%), incoordination (6%), insomnia (6%), pain, amnesia, hostility, memory decreased, nervousness, vertigo
Dermatologic: Hypersensitivity rash (10%; serious rash requiring hospitalization - adults 0.3%, children 0.8%), pruritus (3%)
Gastrointestinal: Abdominal pain (5%), vomiting (9%), diarrhea (6%), dyspepsia (5%), xerostomia, constipation (4%), anorexia (2%), tooth disorder (3%)
Genitourinary: Vaginitis (4%), dysmenorrhea (7%), amenorrhea (2%)
Neuromuscular & skeletal: Tremor (4%), arthralgia (2%), neck pain (2%)
Ocular: Nystagmus (2%), visual abnormality
Respiratory: Epistaxis, bronchitis, dyspnea
Miscellaneous: Flu syndrome (7%), fever (6%)
Overdosage/Toxicology Symptoms of overdose include QRS prolongation, AV block, dizziness, drowsiness, sedation, and ataxia. Enhancement of elimination: Multiple dosing of activated charcoal may be useful.
Pharmacodynamics/Kinetics
Time to Peak: Plasma: 1-4 hours
Protein Binding: 55%
Half-Life Elimination: Adults: 25-33 hours; Concomitant valproic acid therapy: 59-70 hours; Concomitant phenytoin or carbamazepine therapy: 13-14 hours
Metabolism: Hepatic and renal; metabolized by glucuronic acid conjugation to inactive metabolites
Excretion: Urine (94%, ~90% as glucuronide conjugates and ~10% unchanged); feces (2%)
Available Dosage Forms
Tablet: 25 mg, 100 mg, 150 mg, 200 mg [contains lactose]
Tablet, combination package [each unit-dose starter kit contains]:
Lamictal® (blue kit; for patients taking valproate):
Tablet: Lamotrigine 25 mg (35s)
Lamictal® (green kit; for patients taking carbamazepine, phenytoin, phenobarbital, primidone, or rifampin and **not** taking valproate):
Tablet: Lamotrigine 25 mg (84s)
Tablet: Lamotrigine 100 mg (14s)
Lamictal® (orange kit; for patients **not** taking carbamazepine, phenytoin, phenobarbital, primidone, rifampin, or valproate; for use in bipolar patients only):
Tablet: Lamotrigine 25 mg (42s)
Tablet: Lamotrigine 100 mg (7s)
Tablet, dispersible/chewable: 2 mg, 5 mg, 25 mg [black currant flavor]
Dosing
Adults & Elderly: Note: Only whole tablets should be used for dosing, round calculated dose down to the nearest whole tablet:
Lennox-Gastaut (adjunctive) or treatment of partial seizures (adjunctive): Oral:
Patients receiving AED regimens containing valproic acid: Initial dose: 25 mg every other day for 2 weeks, then 25 mg every day for 2 weeks; dose may be increased by 25-50 mg every day for 1-2 weeks in order to achieve maintenance dose. Maintenance dose: 100-400 mg/day in 1-2 divided doses (usual range 100-200 mg/day).
Patients receiving enzyme-inducing AED regimens without valproic acid: Initial dose: 50 mg/day for 2

weeks, then 100 mg in 2 doses for 2 weeks; thereafter, daily dose can be increased by 100 mg every 1-2 weeks to be given in 2 divided doses. Usual maintenance dose: 300-500 mg/day in 2 divided doses; doses as high as 700 mg/day have been reported

Conversion to monotherapy (partial seizures in patients ≥16 years of age):

Adjunctive therapy with valproate: Initiate and titrate as per recommendations to a lamotrigine dose of 200 mg/day. Then taper valproate dose in decrements of not more than 500 mg/day at intervals of one week (or longer) to a valproate dosage of 500 mg/day; this dosage should be maintained for one week. The lamotrigine dosage should then be increased to 300 mg/day while valproate is decreased to 250 mg/day; this dosage should be maintained for one week. Valproate may then be discontinued, while the lamotrigine dose is increased by 100 mg/day at weekly intervals to achieve a lamotrigine maintenance dose of 500 mg/day.

Adjunctive therapy with enzyme-inducing AED: Initiate and titrate as per recommendations to a lamotrigine dose of 500 mg/day. Concomitant enzyme-inducing AED should then be withdrawn by 20% decrements each week over a 4-week period. Patients should be monitored for rash.

Adjunctive therapy with nonenzyme-inducing AED: No specific guidelines available

Bipolar disorder: 25 mg/day for 2 weeks, followed by 50 mg/day for 2 weeks, followed by 100 mg/day for 1 week; thereafter, daily dosage may be increased to 200 mg/day

Patients receiving valproic acid: Initial: 25 mg every other day for 2 weeks, followed by 25 mg/day for 2 weeks, followed by 50 mg/day for 1 week, followed by 100 mg/day (target dose) thereafter. **Note:** If valproate is discontinued, increase daily lamotrigine dose in 50 mg increments at weekly intervals until daily dosage of 200 mg is attained.

Patients receiving enzyme-inducing drugs (eg, carbamazepine): Initial: 50 mg/day for 2 weeks, followed by 100 mg/day (in divided doses) for 2 weeks, followed by 200 mg/day (in divided doses) for 1 week, followed by 300 mg/day (in divided doses) for 1 week. May increase to 400 mg/day (in divided doses) during week 7 and thereafter. **Note:** If carbamazepine (or other enzyme-inducing drug) is discontinued, decrease daily lamotrigine dose in 100 mg increments at weekly intervals until daily dosage of 200 mg is attained.

Discontinuing therapy: Decrease dose by ~50% per week, over at least 2 weeks unless safety concerns require a more rapid withdrawal.

Restarting therapy after discontinuation: If lamotrigine has been withheld for >5 half-lives, consider restarting according to initial dosing recommendations.

Pediatrics: Note: Only whole tablets should be used for dosing, rounded down to the nearest whole tablet.

Lennox-Gastaut (adjunctive) or partial seizures (adjunctive): Oral:

Children 2-12 years: **Note:** Children 2-6 years will likely require maintenance doses at the higher end of recommended range

Patients receiving AED regimens containing valproic acid:

Weeks 1 and 2: 0.15 mg/kg/day in 1-2 divided doses; round dose down to the nearest whole tablet. For patients >6.7 kg and <14 kg, dosing should be 2 mg every other day.

Weeks 3 and 4: 0.3 mg/kg/day in 1-2 divided doses; round dose down to the nearest whole tablet

Maintenance dose: Titrate dose to effect; after week 4, increase dose every 1-2 weeks by a calculated increment; calculate increment as 0.3 mg/kg/day rounded down to the nearest whole tablet; add this amount to the previously administered daily dose; usual maintenance: 1-5 mg/kg/day in 1-2 divided doses; maximum: 200 mg/day

Patients receiving enzyme-inducing AED regimens without valproic acid:

Weeks 1 and 2: 0.6 mg/kg/day in 2 divided doses; round dose down to the nearest whole tablet

Weeks 3 and 4: 1.2 mg/kg/day in 2 divided doses; round dose down to the nearest whole tablet

Maintenance dose: Titrate dose to effect; after week 4, increase dose every 1-2 weeks by a calculated increment; calculate increment as 1.2 mg/kg/day rounded down to the nearest whole tablet; add this amount to the previously administered daily dose; usual maintenance: 5-15 mg/kg/day in 2 divided doses; maximum: 400 mg/day

Children >12 years: Refer to adult dosing.

Conversion from single enzyme-inducing AED regimen to monotherapy: Children ≥16 years: Refer to adult dosing.

Discontinuing therapy: Decrease dose by ~50% per week, over at least 2 weeks unless safety concerns require a more rapid withdrawal.

Restarting therapy after discontinuation: If lamotrigine has been withheld for >5 half-lives, consider restarting according to initial dosing recommendations.

Renal Impairment: Decreased dosage may be effective in patients with significant renal impairment; use with caution.

Hepatic Impairment:

Child-Pugh Grade B: Reduce initial, escalation, and maintenance doses by 50%.

Child-Pugh Grade C: Reduce initial, escalation, and maintenance doses by 75%.

Administration

Oral: Doses should be rounded down to the nearest whole tablet. Dispersible tablets may be chewed, dispersed in water, or swallowed whole. To disperse tablets, add to a small amount of liquid (just enough to cover tablet); let sit ~1 minute until dispersed; swirl solution and consume immediately. Do not administer partial amounts of liquid. If tablets are chewed, a small amount of water or diluted fruit juice should be used to aid in swallowing.

Stability

Storage: Store at 25°C (77°F). Excursions are permitted to 15°C to 30°C (59°F to 86°F). Protect from light.

Laboratory Monitoring Serum levels of concurrent anticonvulsants, LFTs, renal function

Nursing Actions

Physical Assessment: Assess effectiveness and interactions of other medications patient may be taking. Monitor therapeutic response (seizure activity, force, type, duration), laboratory values, and adverse reactions at beginning of therapy and periodically with long-term use. Taper dosage slowly when discontinuing. Observe and teach seizure/safety precautions. Use caution in writing and/or interpreting prescriptions/orders. Confusion between Lamictal® (lamotrigine) and Lamisil® (terbinafine) has occurred. Assess knowledge/teach patient appropriate use, interventions to reduce side effects, and adverse symptoms to report.

Patient Education: Take exactly as directed; do not increase dose or frequency or discontinue without consulting prescriber. Only whole tablets should be

(Continued)

Lamotrigine *(Continued)*

used for dosing, rounded down to the nearest whole tablet. When having the prescription refilled, contact the prescriber if the medicine looks different or the label name has changed. While using this medication, do not use alcohol and other prescription or OTC medications (especially pain medications, sedatives, antihistamines, or hypnotics) without consulting prescriber. Maintain adequate hydration (2-3 L/day of fluids) unless instructed to restrict fluid intake. You may experience drowsiness, dizziness, or blurred vision (use caution when driving or engaging in tasks requiring alertness until response to drug is known); or nausea, vomiting, loss of appetite, heartburn, or dry mouth (small frequent meals, frequent mouth care, chewing gum, or sucking lozenges may help). Wear identification of epileptic status and medications. Report CNS changes, mentation changes, or changes in cognition; persistent GI symptoms (cramping, constipation, vomiting, anorexia); skin rash; swelling of face, lips, or tongue; easy bruising or bleeding (mouth, urine, stool); vision changes; worsening of seizure activity, or loss of seizure control. **Pregnancy/breast-feeding precautions:** Inform prescriber if you are or intend to become pregnant. Breast-feeding is not recommended.

Dietary Considerations Take without regard to meals; drug may cause GI upset.

Geriatric Considerations Use with caution in the elderly with significant renal impairment.

Pregnancy Issues Safety and efficacy in pregnant women have not been established. Healthcare providers may enroll patients in the Lamotrigine Pregnancy Registry by calling (800) 336-2176. Patients may enroll themselves in the North American Antiepileptic Drug Pregnancy Registry by calling (888) 233-2334. Dose of lamotrigine may need adjustment during pregnancy to maintain clinical response; lamotrigine serum levels may decrease during pregnancy and return to prepartum levels following delivery.

Lansoprazole *(lan SOE pra zole)*

U.S. Brand Names Prevacid®; Prevacid® SoluTab™

Pharmacologic Category Proton Pump Inhibitor; Substituted Benzimidazole

Medication Safety Issues
Sound-alike/look-alike issues:
Prevacid® may be confused with Pravachol®, Prevpac®, Prilosec®, Prinivil®

Pregnancy Risk Factor B

Lactation Excretion in breast milk unknown/not recommended

Use
Oral: Short-term treatment of active duodenal ulcers; maintenance treatment of healed duodenal ulcers; as part of a multidrug regimen for *H. pylori* eradication to reduce the risk of duodenal ulcer recurrence; short-term treatment of active benign gastric ulcer; treatment of NSAID-associated gastric ulcer; to reduce the risk of NSAID-associated gastric ulcer in patients with a history of gastric ulcer who require an NSAID; short-term treatment of symptomatic GERD; short-term treatment for all grades of erosive esophagitis; to maintain healing of erosive esophagitis; long-term treatment of pathological hypersecretory conditions, including Zollinger-Ellison syndrome
I.V.: Short-term treatment (≤7 days) of erosive esophagitis in adults unable to take oral medications

Unlabeled/Investigational Use Active ulcer bleeding (parenteral formulation)

Mechanism of Action/Effect A proton pump inhibitor which decreases acid secretion in gastric parietal cells

Contraindications Hypersensitivity to lansoprazole, substituted benzimidazoles (ie, esomeprazole, omeprazole, pantoprazole, rabeprazole), or any component of the formulation

Warnings/Precautions Severe liver dysfunction may require dosage reductions. Symptomatic response does not exclude malignancy. Safety and efficacy have not been established in children <1 year of age.

Drug Interactions
Cytochrome P450 Effect: Substrate of CYP2C8/9 (minor), 2C19 (major), 3A4 (major); **Inhibits** CYP2C8/9 (weak), 2C19 (moderate), 2D6 (weak), 3A4 (weak); **Induces** CYP1A2 (weak)
Decreased Effect: Proton pump inhibitors may decrease the absorption of atazanavir, indinavir, itraconazole, and ketoconazole. The levels/effects of lansoprazole may be decreased by aminoglutethimide, carbamazepine, nafcillin, nevirapine, phenobarbital, phenytoin, rifamycins, and other CYP2C19 or 3A4 inducers.
Increased Effect/Toxicity: Lansoprazole may increase the levels/effects of citalopram, diazepam, methsuximide, phenytoin, propranolol, sertraline, and other CYP2C19 substrates.

Nutritional/Ethanol Interactions
Ethanol: Avoid ethanol (may cause gastric mucosal irritation).
Food: Lansoprazole serum concentrations may be decreased if taken with food.

Adverse Reactions 1% to 10%:
Central nervous system: Headache (children 1-11 years 3%, 12-17 years 7%)
Gastrointestinal: Abdominal pain (children 12-17 years 5%; adults 2%), constipation (children 1-11 years 5%; adults 1%), diarrhea (4%; 4% to 7% at doses of 30-60 mg/day), nausea (children 12-17 years 3%; adults 1%)

Overdosage/Toxicology No symptoms of toxicity were observed in animal studies; limited human experience in overdose. Treatment is symptomatic and supportive. Lansoprazole is not removed by hemodialysis.

Pharmacodynamics/Kinetics
Duration of Action: >1 day
Time to Peak: Plasma: 1.7 hours
Protein Binding: 97%
Half-Life Elimination: 2 hours; Elderly: 2-3 hours; Hepatic impairment: ≤7 hours
Metabolism: Hepatic via CYP2C19 and 3A4, and in parietal cells to two inactive metabolites
Excretion: Feces (67%); urine (33%)

Available Dosage Forms
Capsule, delayed release (Prevacid®): 15 mg, 30 mg
Granules, for oral suspension, delayed release (Prevacid®): 15 mg/packet (30s), 30 mg/packet (30s) [strawberry flavor]
Injection, powder for reconstitution (Prevacid®): 30 mg
Tablet, orally disintegrating (Prevacid® SoluTab™): 15 mg [contains phenylalanine 2.5 mg; strawberry flavor]; 30 mg [contains phenylalanine 5.1 mg; strawberry flavor]

Dosing
Adults & Elderly:
Symptomatic GERD: Oral: Short-term treatment: 15 mg once daily for up to 8 weeks
Erosive esophagitis:
Oral: Short-term treatment: 30 mg once daily for up to 8 weeks; continued treatment for an additional 8 weeks may be considered for recurrence or for patients that do not heal after the first 8 weeks of therapy; maintenance therapy: 15 mg once daily
I.V.: 30 mg once daily for up to 7 days; patients should be switched to an oral formulation as soon as they can take oral medications.
Hypersecretory conditions: Oral: Initial: 60 mg once daily; adjust dose based upon patient response and to reduce acid secretion to <10 mEq/hour (5 mEq/

hour in patients with prior gastric surgery); doses of 90 mg twice daily have been used; administer doses >120 mg/day in divided doses

Duodenal ulcer: Oral: Short-term treatment: 15 mg once daily for 4 weeks; maintenance therapy: 15 mg once daily

Peptic ulcer disease: Eradication of *Helicobacter pylori*: Currently accepted recommendations (may differ from product labeling): Oral: Dose varies with regimen: 30 mg once daily or 60 mg/day in 2 divided doses; requires combination therapy with antibiotics

Gastric ulcer: Oral: Short-term treatment: 30 mg once daily for up to 8 weeks

NSAID-associated gastric ulcer (healing): Oral: 30 mg once daily for 8 weeks; controlled studies did not extend past 8 weeks

NSAID-associated gastric ulcer (to reduce risk): Oral: 15 mg once daily for up to 12 weeks; controlled studies did not extend past 12 weeks

Prevention of rebleeding in peptic ulcer bleed (unlabeled use): I.V.: 60 mg, followed by 6 mg/hour infusion for 72 hours

Pediatrics:

GERD, erosive esophagitis: Oral: Children 1-11 years:

≤30 kg: 15 mg once daily

>30 kg: 30 mg once daily

Note: Doses were increased in some pediatric patients if still symptomatic after 2 or more weeks of treatment (maximum dose: 30 mg twice daily)

Erosive esophagitis: Children 12-17 years: Oral: 30 mg once daily for up to 8 weeks

Nonerosive GERD: Children 12-17 years: Oral: 15 mg once daily for up to 8 weeks

Renal Impairment: No adjustment is necessary.

Hepatic Impairment: May require a dose reduction.

Administration

Oral: Administer before food; best if taken before breakfast. The intact granules should not be chewed or crushed; however, in addition to oral suspension, several options are available for those patients unable to swallow capsules:

Capsules may be opened and the intact granules sprinkled on 1 tablespoon of applesauce, Ensure® pudding, cottage cheese, yogurt, or strained pears. The granules should then be swallowed immediately.

Capsules may be opened and emptied into ~60 mL orange juice, apple juice, or tomato juice; mix and swallow immediately. Rinse the glass with additional juice and swallow to assure complete delivery of the dose.

Capsule granules may be mixed with apple, cranberry, grape, orange, pineapple, prune, tomato and V-8® juice and stored for up to 30 minutes.

Delayed release oral suspension granules should be mixed with 2 tablespoonfuls (30 mL) of water; no other liquid should be used. Stir well and drink immediately. Should not be administered through enteral administration tubes.

Orally-disintegrating tablets: Should not be swallowed whole or chewed. Place tablet on tongue; allow to dissolve (with or without water) until particles can be swallowed. Orally-disintegrating tablets may also be administered via an oral syringe: Place the 15 mg tablet in an oral syringe and draw up ~4 mL water, or place the 30 mg tablet in an oral syringe and draw up ~10 mL water. After tablet has dispersed, administer within 15 minutes. Refill the syringe with water (2 mL for the 15 mg tablet; 4 mL for the 30 mg tablet), shake gently, then administer any remaining contents.

I.V.: Administer over 30 minutes. Use of an in-line filter is required. Before and after administration, flush I.V. line with NS, LR, or D_5W. Do not administer with other medications.

Other: Nasogastric tube administration:

Capsule: Capsule can be opened, the granules mixed (not crushed) with 40 mL of apple juice and then injected through the NG tube into the stomach, then flush tube with additional apple juice. Granules for oral suspension should not be administered through enteral administration tubes.

Orally-disintegrating tablet: Nasogastric tube (≥8 French): Place a 15 mg tablet in a syringe and draw up ~4 mL water, or place the 30 mg tablet in a syringe and draw up ~10 mL water. After tablet has dispersed, administer within 15 minutes. Refill the syringe with ~5 mL water, shake gently, and then flush the nasogastric tube.

Stability

Reconstitution:

Oral suspension: Empty packet into container with 2 tablespoons of water. Do **not** mix with other liquids or food. Stir well and drink immediately.

Powder for injection: Reconstitute with sterile water 5 mL; mix gently until dissolved. Prior to administration, further dilute with 50 mL of NS, LR, or D_5W.

Storage: Store at 15°C to 30°C (59°F to 86°F); protect from light and moisture.

Powder for injection: After reconstitution, the solution may be stored for up to 1 hour at room temperature prior to final dilution. Following final dilution, solutions mixed with NS or LR are stable at room temperature for 24 hours; solutions mixed with D_5W are stable for 12 hours

Laboratory Monitoring CBC, liver function, renal function, and serum gastrin levels. Patients with Zollinger-Ellison syndrome should be monitored for gastric acid output, which should be maintained at ≤10 mEq/hour during the last hour before the next lansoprazole dose.

Nursing Actions

Physical Assessment: Assess periodic laboratory results. Assess effectiveness of medications that require an acid medium for absorption (eg, ketoconazole, itraconazole). Monitor effectiveness of ulcer symptom relief.

Patient Education: Take as directed, before eating. Do not crush or chew granules. Patients who may have difficulty swallowing capsules may open the delayed-release capsules and sprinkle the contents on applesauce, pudding, cottage cheese, or yogurt. Avoid alcohol. Report unresolved diarrhea. **Breast-feeding precaution:** Breast-feeding is not recommended.

Dietary Considerations Should be taken before eating; best if taken before breakfast. Prevacid® SoluTab™ contains phenylalanine 2.5 mg per 15 mg tablet; phenylalanine 5.1 mg per 30 mg tablet.

Geriatric Considerations The clearance of lansoprazole is decreased in the elderly; however, the half-life is only increased by 50% to 100%. This still results in a short half-life and no accumulation is seen in the elderly. The rate of healing and side effects is similar to younger adults; no dosage adjustment is necessary.

Lansoprazole, Amoxicillin, and Clarithromycin

(lan SOE pra zole, a moks i SIL in, & kla RITH roe mye sin)

U.S. Brand Names Prevpac®

Synonyms Amoxicillin, Lansoprazole, and Clarithromycin; Clarithromycin, Lansoprazole, and Amoxicillin

(Continued)

Lansoprazole, Amoxicillin, and Clarithromycin *(Continued)*

Pharmacologic Category Antibiotic, Macrolide Combination; Antibiotic, Penicillin; Gastrointestinal Agent, Miscellaneous

Pregnancy Risk Factor C (clarithromycin)

Lactation Excretion in breast milk unknown/not recommended

Use Eradication of *H. pylori* to reduce the risk of recurrent duodenal ulcer

Available Dosage Forms Combination package (Prevpac®) [each administration card contains]:

Capsule (Trimox®): Amoxicillin 500 mg (4 capsules/day)

Capsule, delayed release (Prevacid®): Lansoprazole 30 mg (2 capsules/day)

Tablet (Biaxin®): Clarithromycin 500 mg (2 tablets/day)

Dosing

Adults & Elderly: *H. pylori* eradication: Oral: Lansoprazole 30 mg, amoxicillin 1 g, and clarithromycin 500 mg taken together twice daily for 10 or 14 days

Renal Impairment:

Cl$_{cr}$ <30 mL/minute: Use is not recommended.

Nursing Actions

Physical Assessment: See individual agents.

Patient Education: See individual agents. **Pregnancy/breast-feeding precautions:** Inform prescriber if you are or intend to become pregnant. Do not breast-feed.

Related Information

Amoxicillin *on page 81*

Clarithromycin *on page 278*

Lansoprazole *on page 708*

Lansoprazole and Naproxen

(lan SOE pra zole & na PROKS en)

U.S. Brand Names Prevacid® NapraPAC™

Synonyms NapraPAC™; Naproxen and Lansoprazole

Pharmacologic Category Nonsteroidal Anti-inflammatory Drug (NSAID), Oral; Proton Pump Inhibitor

Pregnancy Risk Factor B (naproxen: D/third trimester)

Lactation Enters breast milk/not recommended

Use Reduction of the risk of NSAID-associated gastric ulcers in patients with history of gastric ulcer who require an NSAID for the treatment of rheumatoid arthritis, osteoarthritis, and ankylosing spondylitis

Available Dosage Forms [DSC] = Discontinued product

Combination package:

Prevacid® NapraPAC™ 375 [each administration card contains] [DSC]:

Capsule, delayed release (Prevacid®): Lansoprazole 15 mg (7 capsules per card)

Tablet (Naprosyn®): Naproxen 375 mg (14 tablets per card)

Prevacid® NapraPAC™ 500 [each administration card contains]:

Capsule, delayed release (Prevacid®): Lansoprazole 15 mg (7 capsules per card)

Tablet (Naprosyn®): Naproxen 500 mg (14 tablets per card)

Dosing

Adults: Reduce NSAID-associated gastric ulcers during treatment for arthritis: Oral: Lansoprazole 15 mg once daily in the morning; naproxen 375 mg or 500 mg twice daily

Elderly: Naproxen: Dosing adjustment should be considered.

Renal Impairment: Naproxen: Dosing adjustment should be considered.

Hepatic Impairment: Naproxen: Dosing adjustment should be considered.

Related Information

Lansoprazole *on page 708*

Naproxen *on page 863*

Latanoprost (la TA noe prost)

U.S. Brand Names Xalatan®

Pharmacologic Category Ophthalmic Agent, Antiglaucoma; Prostaglandin, Ophthalmic

Medication Safety Issues

Sound-alike/look-alike issues:

Xalatan® may be confused with Travatan®, Zarontin®

Pregnancy Risk Factor C

Use Reduction of elevated intraocular pressure in patients with open-angle glaucoma or ocular hypertension

Contraindications Hypersensitivity to latanoprost or any component of the formulation

Warnings/Precautions Latanoprost may gradually change eye color, increasing the amount of brown pigment in the iris by increasing the number of melanosome in melanocytes. The long-term effects on the melanocytes and the consequences of potential injury to the melanocytes or deposition of pigment granules to other areas of the eye is currently unknown. Patients should be examined regularly, and depending on the clinical situation, treatment may be stopped if increased pigmentation ensues.

There have been reports of bacterial keratitis associated with the use of multiple-dose containers of topical ophthalmic products. Do not administer while wearing contact lenses.

Drug Interactions

Decreased Effect: Precipitation occurs when eye drops containing thimerosal are mixed with latanoprost. If such drugs are used, administer with an interval of at least 5 minutes between applications. May be used concomitantly with other topical ophthalmic drugs if administration is separated by at least 5 minutes.

Increased Effect/Toxicity:

Combination therapy with bimatoprost may result in higher IOP than either agent alone.

Adverse Reactions

>10%: Ocular: Blurred vision, burning and stinging, conjunctival hyperemia, foreign body sensation, itching, increased pigmentation of the iris, and punctate epithelial keratopathy

1% to 10%:

Cardiovascular: Chest pain, angina pectoris

Dermatologic: Rash, allergic skin reaction

Neuromuscular & skeletal: Myalgia, arthralgia, back pain

Ocular: Dry eye, excessive tearing, eye pain, lid crusting, lid edema, lid erythema, lid discomfort/pain, photophobia

Respiratory: Upper respiratory tract infection, cold, flu

Overdosage/Toxicology

Symptoms include ocular irritation and conjunctival or episcleral hyperemia

Treatment should be symptomatic

Pharmacodynamics/Kinetics

Onset of Action: 3-4 hours; Peak effect: Maximum: 8-12 hours

Half-Life Elimination: 17 minutes

Metabolism: Primarily hepatic via fatty acid beta-oxidation

Excretion: Urine (as metabolites)
Available Dosage Forms Solution, ophthalmic: 0.005% (2.5 mL) [contains benzalkonium chloride]
Dosing
Adults & Elderly: Glaucoma: Ophthalmic: 1 drop (1.5 mcg) in the affected eye(s) once daily in the evening; do not exceed the once daily dosage because it has been shown that more frequent administration may decrease the IOP lowering effect
Note: A medication delivery device (Xal-Ease™) is available for use with Xalatan®.
Administration
Other: If more than one topical ophthalmic drug is being used, administer the drugs at least 5 minutes apart. A delivery aid, Xal-Ease™, is available for administering Xalatan®.
Stability
Storage: Protect from light; store intact bottles under refrigeration (2°C to 8°C/36°F to 46°F). Once opened, the container may be stored at room temperature up to 25°C (77°F) for 6 weeks.
Nursing Actions
Physical Assessment: Assess potential for interactions with other prescriptions, OTC medications, or herbal products patient may be taking. Monitor patient response and adverse effects (eg, blurred vision, burning and stinging, conjunctival hyperemia, foreign body sensation, itching, increased pigmentation of the iris, and punctate epithelial keratopathy). Teach patient proper use, side effects/appropriate interventions, and symptoms to report.
Patient Education: For use in eyes only. Iris color may change because of an increase of the brown pigment (cosmetically different eye coloration that may occur). Iris pigmentation changes may be more noticeable in patients with green-brown, blue/gray-brown, or yellow-brown irides. If any ocular reaction develops, particularly conjunctivitis and lid reactions, immediately notify prescriber. If more than one topical ophthalmic drug is being used, administer the drugs at least 5 minutes apart. Latanoprost contains benzalkonium chloride, which may be absorbed by contact lenses. Remove contact lenses prior to administration; lenses may be reinserted after 15 minutes. Do not let tip of applicator touch eye; do not contaminate tip of applicator (may cause eye infection, eye damage, or vision loss). Serious damage to the eye and subsequent loss of vision may result from using contaminated solutions. A delivery aid, Xal-Ease™, is available for administering Xalatan®. **Pregnancy precaution:** Inform prescriber if you are pregnant.

Leflunomide (le FLOO noh mide)

U.S. Brand Names Arava®
Pharmacologic Category Antirheumatic, Disease Modifying
Pregnancy Risk Factor X
Lactation Excretion in breast milk unknown/contraindicated
Use Treatment of active rheumatoid arthritis; indicated to reduce signs and symptoms, and to retard structural damage and improve physical function
Orphan drug: Prevention of acute and chronic rejection in recipients of solid organ transplants
Unlabeled/Investigational Use
Treatment of cytomegalovirus (CMV) disease
Mechanism of Action/Effect Inhibits pyrimidine synthesis, resulting in antiproliferative and anti-inflammatory effects. For CMV, may interfere with virion assembly.
Contraindications Hypersensitivity to leflunomide or any component of the formulation; pregnancy

Warnings/Precautions Leflunomide has been associated with rare reports of hepatotoxicity, hepatic failure, and death. Multiple risk factors for hepatotoxicity including hepatic disease (including seropositive hepatitis B or C patients) and/or concurrent exposure to other hepatotoxins may increase the risk of hepatotoxicity. Most severe cases occur within 6 months of initiation. Monitoring of hepatic function is required.

Not recommended for patients with severe immune deficiency, bone marrow dysplasia, or uncontrolled infection. Has been associated with rare pancytopenia, agranulocytosis, and thrombocytopenia, particularly when given in combination with methotrexate or other immunosuppressive agents. Monitoring of hematologic function is required. Use with caution in patients with a prior history of significant hematologic abnormalities. Discontinue if evidence of bone marrow suppression or severe dermatologic reaction occurs, and begin procedure to accelerate elimination (cholestyramine or activated charcoal, see Overdosage/Toxicology). Interstitial lung disease has been associated (rarely) with leflunomide use. Discontinue in patients who develop new onset or worsening of pulmonary symptoms; accelerated elimination procedures should be considered if interstitial lung disease occurs; fatal outcomes have been reported. Consider interruption of therapy and accelerated elimination in patients who develop serious infections. The use of live vaccines is not recommended.

Women of childbearing potential should not receive leflunomide until pregnancy has been excluded; patients have been counseled concerning fetal risk and reliable contraceptive measures have been confirmed. Caution in renal impairment. Leflunomide will increase uric acid excretion. Immunosuppression may increase the risk of lymphoproliferative disorders or other malignancies.
Drug Interactions
Cytochrome P450 Effect: Inhibits CYP2C8/9 (weak)
Decreased Effect: Bile acid sequestrants (cholestyramine) may interfere with enterohepatic recycling of leflunomide; this is used emergently to remove drug from the circulation, but may decrease levels inadvertently if used concomitantly.

Increased Effect/Toxicity: Leflunomide may increase the risk of hepatotoxicity when combined with drugs which may cause hepatic injury. Concomitant treatment of methotrexate with leflunomide may increase the risk of hepatotoxicity or hematologic toxicity. Rifampin may increase the serum concentration of leflunomide's active metabolite. Leflunomide may increase the effects of warfarin.

Nutritional/Ethanol Interactions Food: No interactions with food have been noted.
Adverse Reactions
>10%:
Gastrointestinal: Diarrhea (17%)
Respiratory: Respiratory tract infection (15%)
1% to 10%:
Cardiovascular: Hypertension (10%), chest pain (2%), palpitation, tachycardia, vasculitis, vasodilation, varicose vein, edema (peripheral)
Central nervous system: Headache (7%), dizziness (4%), pain (2%), fever, malaise, migraine, anxiety, depression, insomnia, sleep disorder
Dermatologic: Alopecia (10%), rash (10%), pruritus (4%), dry skin (2%), eczema (2%), acne, dermatitis, hair discoloration, hematoma, herpes infection, nail disorder, subcutaneous nodule, skin disorder/discoloration, skin ulcer, bruising
Endocrine & metabolic: Hypokalemia (1%), diabetes mellitus, hyperglycemia, hyperlipidemia, hyperthyroidism, menstrual disorder
Gastrointestinal: Nausea (9%), abdominal pain (5%), dyspepsia (5%), weight loss (4%), anorexia (3%), gastroenteritis (3%), stomatitis (3%), vomiting (3%),
(Continued)

Leflunomide *(Continued)*

cholelithiasis, colitis, constipation, esophagitis, flatulence, gastritis, gingivitis, melena, candidiasis (oral), enlarged salivary gland, tooth disorder, xerostomia, taste disturbance

Genitourinary: Urinary tract infection (5%), albuminuria, cystitis, dysuria, hematuria, vaginal candidiasis, prostate disorder, urinary frequency

Hematologic: Anemia

Hepatic: Abnormal LFTs (5%)

Neuromuscular & skeletal: Back pain (5%), joint disorder (4%), weakness (3%), tenosynovitis (3%), synovitis (2%), arthralgia (1%), paresthesia (2%), muscle cramps (1%), neck pain, pelvic pain, increased CPK, arthrosis, bursitis, myalgia, bone necrosis, bone pain, tendon rupture, neuralgia, neuritis

Ocular: Blurred vision, cataract, conjunctivitis, eye disorder

Respiratory: Bronchitis (7%), cough (3%), pharyngitis (3%), pneumonia (2%), rhinitis (2%), sinusitis (2%), asthma, dyspnea, epistaxis

Miscellaneous: Infection (4%), accidental injury (5%), allergic reactions (2%), diaphoresis

Overdosage/Toxicology There is no human experience with overdose. Leflunomide is not dialyzable. Cholestyramine and/or activated charcoal enhance elimination of leflunomide's active metabolite (M1). In cases of significant overdose or toxicity, cholestyramine 8 g every 8 hours for 1-3 days or activated charcoal 50 g every 6 hours for 24 hours may be administered to enhance elimination. Plasma levels are reduced by ~40% in 24 hours and 49% to 65% after 48 hours of cholestyramine dosing. Activated charcoal reduces plasma levels by 37% after 24 hours and 48% after 48 hours of continuous dosing. Activated charcoal without sorbitol should be used.

To reach undetectable levels (recommended in women of childbearing potential who wish to become pregnant), an extended protocol is necessary. Without this procedure, it may take up to 2 years to reach plasma concentrations <0.02 mg/L (a concentration expected to have minimal risk of teratogenicity based on animal models). The procedure consists of the following steps: Administer cholestyramine 8 g 3 times/day for 11 days (the 11 days do not need to be consecutive). Plasma levels <0.02 mg/L should be verified by two separate tests performed at least 14 days apart. If plasma levels are >0.02 mg/L, additional cholestyramine treatment should be considered.

Pharmacodynamics/Kinetics

Time to Peak: 6-12 hours

Half-Life Elimination: Mean: 14-15 days; enterohepatic recycling appears to contribute to the long half-life of this agent, since activated charcoal and cholestyramine substantially reduce plasma half-life

Metabolism: Hepatic to A77 1726 (MI) which accounts for nearly all pharmacologic activity; further metabolism to multiple inactive metabolites; undergoes enterohepatic recirculation

Excretion: Feces (48%); urine (43%)

Available Dosage Forms

Tablet (Arava®): 10 mg, 20 mg

Dosing

Adults & Elderly:

Rheumatoid arthritis: Oral: Initial: 100 mg/day for 3 days, followed by 20 mg/day; dosage may be decreased to 10 mg/day in patients who have difficulty tolerating the 20 mg dose. Due to the long half-life of the active metabolite, plasma levels may require a prolonged period to decline after dosage reduction.

CMV (unlabeled): Some authors recommend 200 mg daily for 7 days, followed by 40-60 mg/day targeting

blood levels of 100 mcg/mL. Others have utilized the standard arthritis dosing.

Renal Impairment: No specific dosage adjustment is recommended. There is no clinical experience in the use of leflunomide in patients with renal impairment. The free fraction of MI is doubled in dialysis patients. Patients should be monitored closely for adverse effects requiring dosage adjustment.

Hepatic Impairment: No specific dosage adjustment is recommended. Since the liver is involved in metabolic activation and subsequent metabolism/elimination of leflunomide, patients with hepatic impairment should be monitored closely for adverse effects requiring dosage adjustment.

Dosing adjustment in hepatic toxicity: Guidelines for dosage adjustment or discontinuation based on the severity and persistence of ALT elevation secondary to leflunomide have been developed. If ALT elevations >2 times but ≤3 times ULN are noted, reduce dose to 10 mg/day, and monitor closely. If elevations persist or if elevations >3 times ULN are observed, discontinue leflunomide and initiate protocol to accelerate elimination. Cholestyramine (8 g 3 times/day for 1-3 days) or activated charcoal (50 g every 6 hours for 24 hours) may be administered to decrease leflunomide concentrations rapidly. If elevations >3 times ULN persist additional cholestyramine and/or activated charcoal may be required.

Dosing Adjustment for Toxicity: Hepatic toxicity: Guidelines for dosage adjustment or discontinuation based on the severity and persistence of ALT elevation secondary to leflunomide have been developed. If ALT elevations >2 times but ≤3 times ULN are noted, reduce dose to 10 mg/day, and monitor closely. If elevations persist or if elevations >3 times ULN are observed, discontinue leflunomide and initiate protocol to accelerate elimination. Cholestyramine (8 g 3 times/day for 1-3 days) or activated charcoal (50 g every 6 hours for 24 hours) may be administered to decrease leflunomide concentrations rapidly. If elevations >3 times ULN persist additional cholestyramine and/or activated charcoal may be required.

Stability

Storage: Protect from light; store at 25°C (77°F).

Laboratory Monitoring A complete blood count (WBC, hemoglobin, hematocrit, and platelet count), serum phosphate, as well as serum transaminase determinations, should be monitored at baseline and monthly during the initial 6 months of treatment; if stable, monitoring frequency may be decreased to every 6-8 weeks thereafter (continue monthly when used in combination with other immunosuppressive agents). If coadministered with methotrexate, monthly transaminase and serum albumin levels are recommended.

Nursing Actions

Physical Assessment: Assess other medications patient may be taking for effectiveness and interactions. Monitor laboratory tests, therapeutic effectiveness (eg, reduction of rheumatoid arthritis signs and symptoms, structural damage), and adverse reactions. Monitor for signs and symptoms of severe infection, hypertension, or hepatic dysfunction. Monitor for new onset or worsening of pulmonary symptoms. **Pregnancy risk factor X:** Determine that patient is not pregnant before starting therapy. Do not give to sexually-active female patients unless capable of complying with contraceptive use. Breast-feeding is contraindicated.

Patient Education: Take as directed; do not increase dose without consulting prescriber. Maintain adequate hydration (2-3 L/day of fluids) unless instructed to restrict fluid intake. Store medication away from light. You may experience diarrhea (buttermilk, boiled milk, or yogurt may help); nausea, vomiting, loss of appetite, and flatulence (small frequent meals, frequent mouth care, chewing gum, or sucking lozenges may help); or dizziness (use caution when driving or engaging in tasks requiring alertness until response to drug is known). If you have diabetes, monitor blood sugars closely; this medication may alter glucose levels. If you experience symptoms such as nausea, vomiting, stomach pain or swelling, jaundice, dark urine, or unusual tiredness, report these to your prescriber **immediately**. Report chest pain, palpitations, rapid heartbeat, or swelling of extremities; persistent GI problems; skin rash, mucus membrane lesions, redness, irritation, acne, ulcers; frequent, painful, or difficult urination; or genital itching or irritation; depression, acute headache, anxiety, or difficulty sleeping; muscle tremors, cramping or weakness, back pain, or altered gait; cough, cold symptoms, wheezing, or respiratory difficulty; easy bruising/bleeding; blood in vomitus, stool, urine; or other unusual effects related to this medication. **Pregnancy/breast-feeding precautions:** Inform prescriber if you are pregnant. Do not get pregnant or have sex unless using appropriate contraception while on this medication. This drug may cause severe fetal defects. Do not breast-feed.

Dietary Considerations Administer without regard to meals.

Breast-Feeding Issues It is not known whether leflunomide is secreted in human milk. Because many immunoglobulins are secreted in milk, and the potential for serious adverse reactions exists, a decision should be made whether to discontinue nursing or discontinue the drug, taking into account the importance of the drug to the mother.

Pregnancy Issues Leflunomide is contraindicated in pregnant women or women of childbearing potential who are not using reliable contraception. Pregnancy must be excluded prior to initiating treatment. Following treatment, pregnancy should be avoided until undetectable plasma levels (< 0.02 mcg/mL) are verified. This may be accomplished by an extended drug elimination procedure: Administer cholestyramine 8 g 3 times/day for 11 days (the 11 days do not need to be consecutive). Plasma levels <0.02 mg/L should be verified by two separate tests performed at least 14 days apart. If plasma levels are >0.02 mg/L, additional cholestyramine treatment should be considered.

Lenalidomide (le na LID oh mide)

U.S. Brand Names Revlimid®

Synonyms CC-5013; IMid-3

Restrictions Lenalidomide is approved for marketing only under a Food and Drug Administration (FDA) approved, restricted distribution program called RevAssist^{SM} (www.REVLIMID.com or 1-888-423-5436). Physicians, pharmacies, and patients must be registered; a maximum 28-day supply may be dispensed; a new prescription is required each time it is filled; pregnancy testing is required for females of childbearing potential.

Pharmacologic Category Angiogenesis Inhibitor; Immunosuppressant Agent; Tumor Necrosis Factor (TNF) Blocking Agent

Pregnancy Risk Factor X

Lactation Excretion in breast milk unknown/not recommended

Use Treatment of transfusion-dependent anemia in myelodysplastic syndrome (MDS) patients with deletion 5q (del 5q) cytogenetic abnormality with or without additional cytogenetic abnormalities

Unlabeled/Investigational Use Treatment of multiple myeloma

Mechanism of Action/Effect Immune system modulator with antiangiogenic properties

Contraindications Hypersensitivity to lenalidomide or any component of the formulation; pregnancy or women capable of becoming pregnant; patients unable to comply with the RevAssist^{SM} program

Warnings/Precautions Hematologic toxicity (neutropenia and thrombocytopenia) occurs in a majority of patients (grade 3/4: 80%) and may require dose reductions and/or delays; the use of blood product support and/or growth factors may be needed. Lenalidomide has been associated with a significant increase in thrombosis and embolism; deep vein thrombosis (DVT) and pulmonary embolism (PE) have occurred; monitor for signs and symptoms of thromboembolism (shortness of breath, chest pain, or arm or leg swelling) and seek prompt medical attention with development of these symptoms. Use caution in renal impairment; may experience an increased rate of toxicities. Distribution of lenalidomide is restricted and all patients must be enrolled in the RevAssist^{SM} program. Safety and effectiveness in children <18 years have not been established.

Drug Interactions

Increased Effect/Toxicity: Abatacept and anakinra may increase the risk of serious infection when used in combination with lenalidomide. Lenalidomide may increase the risk of infections associated with vaccines (live organism).

Adverse Reactions Note: Myelosuppression is dose-dependent and reversible with treatment interruption or dose reduction.

>10%:

Cardiovascular: Edema (peripheral 8% to 20%)

Central nervous system: Fatigue (31%), pyrexia (21%), dizziness (20%), headache (20%)

Dermatologic: Pruritus (42%), rash (36%), dry skin (14%)

Endocrine & metabolic: Hypokalemia (11%)

Gastrointestinal: Diarrhea (49%), constipation (24%), nausea (24%), abdominal pain (8% to 12%)

Genitourinary: Urinary tract infection (11%)

Hematologic: Thrombocytopenia (62%; grades 3/4: 50%), neutropenia (59%; grades 3/4: 53%), anemia (12%)

Neuromuscular & skeletal: Arthralgia (22%), back pain (21%), muscle cramp (18%), weakness (15%), limb pain (11%)

Respiratory: Nasopharyngitis (23%), cough (20%), dyspnea (17%), pharyngitis (16%), epistaxis (15%), upper respiratory infection (15%), pneumonia (12%)

1% to 10%:

Cardiovascular: Hypertension (6%), chest pain (5%), palpitations (5%)

Central nervous system: Insomnia (10%), hypoesthesia (7%), pain (7%), depression (5%)

Dermatologic: Bruising (5% to 8%), cellulitis (5%), erythema (5%)

Endocrine & metabolic: Hypothyroidism (7%), hypomagnesemia (6%)

Gastrointestinal: Anorexia (10%), vomiting (10%), xerostomia (7%), loose stools (6%), taste perversion (6%)

Genitourinary: Dysuria (7%)

Hematologic: Leukopenia (8%), febrile neutropenia (5%)

Hepatic: ALT increased (8%)

Neuromuscular & skeletal: Myalgia (9%), rigors (6%), neuropathy (peripheral 5%)

Respiratory: Sinusitis (8%), dyspnea (on exertion 7%), rhinitis (7%), bronchitis (6%)

Miscellaneous: Night sweats (8%), diaphoresis increased (7%)

Overdosage/Toxicology Treatment is symptomatic and supportive.

(Continued)

Lenalidomide *(Continued)*

Pharmacodynamics/Kinetics
Protein Binding: ~30%
Half-Life Elimination: ~3 hours
Excretion: Urine (~67% as unchanged drug)
Available Dosage Forms Capsule: 5 mg, 10 mg

Dosing
Adults:
Myelodysplastic syndrome (MDS): Oral: 10 mg once daily

Multiple myeloma (unlabeled use): Oral: Doses of 25-30 mg once daily (either daily or for 21 days of a 28-day treatment cycle) have been studied in clinical trials

Elderly: Refer to adult dosing. Due to the potential for decreased renal function in the elderly, select dose carefully and closely monitor renal function.

Renal Impairment: Not studied in renal insufficiency; select dose carefully and closely monitor renal function.

Dosing Adjustment for Toxicity:
Adjustment for thrombocytopenia:
Thrombocytopenia developing within 4 weeks of beginning treatment at 10 mg/day:
Baseline platelets ≥100,000/mcL:
If platelets <50,000/mcL: Hold treatment
When platelets return to ≥50,000/mcL: Resume treatment at 5 mg/day
Baseline platelets <100,000/mcL:
If baseline ≥60,000/mcL and platelet level returns to ≥50,000/mcL: Resume at 5 mg/day
If baseline <60,000/mcL and platelet level returns to ≥30,000/mcL: Resume at 5 mg/day
Thrombocytopenia developing after 4 weeks of beginning treatment at 10 mg/day:
Platelets <30,000/mcL **or** <50,000/mcL with platelet transfusions: Hold treatment
When platelets return to ≥30,000/mcL (without hemostatic failure): Resume at 5 mg/day
Thrombocytopenia developing with treatment at 5 mg/day:
Platelets <30,000/mcL **or** <50,000/mcL with platelet transfusions: Hold treatment
When platelets return to ≥30,000/mcL (without hemostatic failure): Resume at 5 mg every other day

Adjustment for neutropenia:
Neutropenia developing within 4 weeks of beginning treatment at 10 mg/day:
For baseline absolute neutrophil count (ANC) ≥1000/mcL:
ANC <750/mcL: Hold treatment
When ANC returns to ≥1000/mcL: Resume at 5 mg/day
For baseline absolute neutrophil count (ANC) <1000/mcL:
ANC <500/mcL: Hold treatment
When ANC returns to ≥500/mcL: Resume at 5 mg/day
Neutropenia developing after 4 weeks of beginning treatment at 10 mg/day:
ANC <500/mcL for ≥7 days or associated with fever: Hold treatment
When ≥500/mcL: Resume at 5 mg/day
Neutropenia developing with treatment at 5 mg/day:
ANC <500/mcL for ≥7 days or associated with fever: Hold treatment
When ≥500/mcL: Resume at 5 mg every other day

Administration
Oral: Administer with water. Swallow capsule whole; do not break, open, or chew.

Stability
Storage: Store at controlled room temperature between 15°C and 30°C (59°F and 86°F).

Laboratory Monitoring CBC with differential weekly for first 8 weeks, then monthly thereafter; serum creatinine, liver function tests, thyroid function tests. Women of childbearing potential: Pregnancy test 10-14 days **and** 24 hours prior to initiating therapy, then every 2-4 weeks through 4 weeks after therapy discontinued

Nursing Actions
Physical Assessment: Verify that patient is not pregnant prior to initiating therapy. Instruct patient on the need to use two reliable forms of contraception beginning 4 weeks prior to, during, and for 4 weeks after therapy and during therapy interruptions. Monitor for signs of thromboembolism (shortness of breath, chest pain, or arm or leg swelling), infection, or bleeding. Assess knowledge/teach patient appropriate use, side effects, and symptoms to report.

Patient Education:
Do not take any new medication during therapy without consulting prescriber. You will need frequent blood tests while taking this medication. Maintain adequate hydration (2-3 L/day) unless instructed to restrict intake by prescriber. You may be susceptible to infections. Avoid crowds and exposure to infections. Avoid vaccinations unless approved by prescriber. You may experience headache, fever, fatigue, dizziness (use caution when driving or engaging in activities requiring alertness until response to drug is known), swelling of extremities, rash, itching, nausea, diarrhea (buttermilk, boiled milk, or yogurt may help), constipation (increasing exercise, fluids, fruit/fiber may help), abdominal pain, upper respiratory infections, or sore throat. Report shortness of breath; chest pain; arm or leg swelling; extreme weakness or fatigue; muscle cramping; unusual bleeding or bruising; or nose bleeds. **Pregnancy/breast-feeding precautions:** Do not get pregnant while taking this medication. May cause fetal harm. Two forms of contraception are required beginning 4 weeks prior to, during, and for 4 weeks after therapy and during therapy interruptions. Male patients must use a latex condom even if he has undergone a successful vasectomy when having sexual contact with females of childbearing age. Do not breast-feed.

Geriatric Considerations The manufacturer reports that the frequency of serious adverse effects was higher in patients >65 years of age compared to younger patients (54% vs 33%). More older patients withdrew from the clinical studies because of side effects. There was no significant difference in efficacy in older versus younger patients.

Breast-Feeding Issues Due to the potential for adverse reactions, breast-feeding is not recommended.

Pregnancy Issues Lenalidomide is an analogue of the known human teratogen thalidomide and may cause fetal harm when administered to pregnant women. Animal studies with lenalidomide are ongoing; there are no adequate and well-controlled studies in pregnant women. Women of childbearing potential should be treated only if they are able to comply with the conditions of the RevAssist[SM] program. Two forms of effective contraception are required beginning 4 weeks prior to, during, and for 4 weeks after therapy and during therapy interruptions. Pregnancy tests (sensitivity of at least 50 mIU/mL) must be performed 10-14 days and 24 hours prior to beginning therapy; weekly for the first 4 weeks and every 4 weeks (every 2 weeks if menstrual cycle irregular) thereafter and during therapy interruptions. Lenalidomide must be immediately discontinued and the patient referred to a reproductive toxicity specialist if pregnancy occurs during treatment. Males (even those vasectomized) must use a latex condom during any sexual contact with women of childbearing age. Risk to the fetus from semen of male patients is unknown. The parent or legal guardian for patients between 12 and 18 years of age must agree to ensure compliance with the required guidelines. Any suspected fetal exposure should be reported to the FDA via the MedWatch program (1-800-FDA-1088) and to Celgene Corporation (1-888-423-5436).

Additional Information Pregnancy tests are required prior to beginning therapy and throughout treatment for all women of childbearing age. Pregnancy tests are also required during therapy interruptions. The pregnancy test must be verified by the prescriber and the pharmacist prior to dispensing. Effective contraception with at least two reliable forms of contraception (IUD, hormonal contraception, tubal ligation or partner's vasectomy plus latex condom, diaphragm, or cervical cap) must be used for 4 weeks prior to beginning therapy, during therapy, and for 4 weeks following discontinuance of therapy. Women who have undergone a hysterectomy or have been postmenopausal for at least 24 consecutive months are the only exception. Do not prescribe, administer, or dispense to women of childbearing age or males who may have intercourse with women of childbearing age unless both female and male are capable of complying with contraceptive measures. Even males who have undergone vasectomy must acknowledge these risks in writing, and must use a latex condom during any sexual contact with women of childbearing age. Oral and written warnings concerning contraception and the hazards of thalidomide must be conveyed to females and males and they must acknowledge their understanding in writing. Parents or guardians must consent and sign acknowledgment for patients 12-18 years of age following therapy.

Lepirudin (leh puh ROO din)

U.S. Brand Names Refludan®

Synonyms Lepirudin (rDNA); Recombinant Hirudin

Pharmacologic Category Anticoagulant, Thrombin Inhibitor

Pregnancy Risk Factor B

Lactation Enters breast milk/consult prescriber

Use Indicated for anticoagulation in patients with heparin-induced thrombocytopenia (HIT) and associated thromboembolic disease in order to prevent further thromboembolic complications

Unlabeled/Investigational Use Investigational: Prevention or reduction of ischemic complications associated with unstable angina

Mechanism of Action/Effect Lepirudin is a highly specific direct thrombin inhibitor. Each molecule is capable of binding one molecule of thrombin and inhibiting its thrombogenic activity.

Contraindications Hypersensitivity to hirudins or any component of the formulation

Warnings/Precautions Cautiously administer after a thrombolytic episode; risk of intracranial bleeding. Hemorrhage is the most common complication. Patients at increased risk of bleeding include: bacterial endocarditis; congenital or acquired bleeding disorders; recent puncture of large vessels or organ biopsy; recent CVA, stroke, intracerebral surgery, or other neuraxial procedure; severe uncontrolled hypertension; renal impairment; recent major surgery; recent major bleeding (intracranial, GI, intraocular, or pulmonary). With renal impairment, relative overdose might occur even with standard dosage regimen. The bolus dose and rate of infusion must be reduced in patients with known or suspected renal insufficiency. Strict monitoring of aPTT is required; formation of antihirudin antibodies can increase the anticoagulant effect of lepirudin. Use cautiously in cirrhosis. Allergic reactions may occur frequently in patients treated concomitantly with streptokinase; caution is warranted during re-exposure (anaphylaxis has been reported). Potentially may cause hyperkalemia by affecting aldosterone (similar to heparin).

Drug Interactions

Increased Effect/Toxicity: Thrombolytics may enhance anticoagulant properties of lepirudin on aPTT and can increase the risk of bleeding complications. Bleeding risk may also be increased by oral anticoagulants (warfarin) and platelet function inhibitors (NSAIDs, dipyridamole, ticlopidine, clopidogrel, IIb/IIIa antagonists, and aspirin).

Nutritional/Ethanol Interactions Herb/Nutraceutical: Avoid cat's claw, dong quai, evening primrose, feverfew, garlic, ginger, ginkgo, red clover, horse chestnut, green tea, ginseng (all have additional antiplatelet activity)

Adverse Reactions As with all anticoagulants, bleeding is the most common adverse event associated with lepirudin. Hemorrhage may occur at virtually any site. Risk is dependent on multiple variables.

HIT patients:

>10%: Hematologic: Anemia (12%), bleeding from puncture sites (11%), hematoma (11%)

1% to 10%:

Cardiovascular: Heart failure (3%), pericardial effusion (1%), ventricular fibrillation (1%)

Central nervous system: Fever (7%)

Dermatologic: Eczema (3%), maculopapular rash (4%)

Gastrointestinal: GI bleeding/rectal bleeding (5%)

Genitourinary: Vaginal bleeding (2%)

Hepatic: Transaminases increased (6%)

Renal: Hematuria (4%)

Respiratory: Epistaxis (4%)

Non-HIT populations (including those receiving thrombolytics and/or contrast media):

1% to 10%: Respiratory: Bronchospasm/stridor/dyspnea/cough

Overdosage/Toxicology Risk of bleeding is increased, and therefore management is directed towards control of bleeding.

Pharmacodynamics/Kinetics

Half-Life Elimination: Initial: ~10 minutes; Terminal: Healthy volunteers: 1.3 hours; Significant renal impairment (Cl_{cr} <15 mL/minute and on hemodialysis): ≤2 days

Metabolism: Via release of amino acids via catabolic hydrolysis of parent drug

Excretion: Urine (~48%, 35% as unchanged drug and unchanged drug fragments of parent drug); systemic clearance is proportional to glomerular filtration rate or creatinine clearance

Available Dosage Forms Injection, powder for reconstitution: 50 mg

Dosing

Adults & Elderly: Note: Maximum dose: Do not exceed 0.21 mg/kg/hour unless an evaluation of coagulation abnormalities limiting response has been completed. **Dosing is weight-based, however, patients weighing >110 kg should not receive doses greater than the recommended dose for a patient weighing 110 kg (44 mg bolus and initial maximal infusion rate of 16.5 mg/hour).**

Heparin-induced thrombocytopenia: I.V.: Bolus dose: 0.4 mg/kg IVP (over 15-20 seconds), followed by continuous infusion at 0.15 mg/kg/hour; bolus and infusion must be reduced in renal insufficiency

Concomitant use with thrombolytic therapy: I.V.: Bolus dose: 0.2 mg/kg IVP (over 15-20 seconds), followed by continuous infusion at 0.1 mg/kg/hour

Dosing adjustments during infusions: Monitor first aPTT 4 hours after the start of the infusion. Subsequent determinations of aPTT should be obtained at least once daily during treatment. More frequent monitoring is recommended in renally impaired patients. Any aPTT ratio measurement out of range (1.5-2.5) should be confirmed prior to adjusting dose, unless a clinical need for immediate reaction exists. If the aPTT is below target range, increase infusion by 20%. If the aPTT is in excess

(Continued)

Lepirudin (Continued)

of the target range, decrease infusion rate by 50%. A repeat aPTT should be obtained 4 hours after any dosing change.

Transition to oral anticoagulants: Reduce lepirudin dose gradually to reach aPTT ratio just above 1.5 before starting warfarin therapy; as soon as INR reaches 2.0, lepirudin therapy should be discontinued.

Renal Impairment: All patients with Cl_{cr} <60 or serum creatinine >1.5 mg/dL require dosage reduction.

Initial: Bolus dose: 0.2 mg/kg IVP (over 15-20 seconds); see table. Additional bolus doses of 0.1 mg/kg may be administered every other day (only if aPTT falls below lower therapeutic limit).

Lepirudin Infusion Rates in Patients With Renal Impairment

Creatinine Clearance (mL/min)	Serum Creatinine (mg/dL)	Adjusted Infusion Rate	
		% of Standard Initial Infusion Rate	mg/kg/h
45-60	1.6-2.0	50%	0.075
30-44	2.1-3.0	30%	0.045
15-29	3.1-6.0	15%	0.0225
<15	>6.0	Avoid or STOP infusion	

Administration

Oral: Administer **only** intravenously

I.V.: I.V. bolus: Inject slowly for continuous infusion; solutions with 0.2 or 0.4 mg/mL may be used.

Stability

Reconstitution: Reconstitute 50 mg vials with 1 mL water for injection or 0.9% sodium chloride injection. Bolus dose: Prepare 5 mg/mL solution by transferring contents of 1 reconstituted vial to single use, sterile syringe. Dilute to total volume of 10 mL with 0.9 sodium chloride or 5% dextrose injection. To prepare continuous infusion solutions, either 0.9% sodium chloride or 5% dextrose may be used. Add contents of two reconstituted vials to either 250 mL (to prepare 0.4 mg/mL solution) or 500 mL (to prepare 0.2 mg/mL solution). Once reconstituted, use immediately. Reconstituted solutions remain stable for 24 hours (duration of infusion).

Laboratory Monitoring The aPTT ratio should be maintained between 1.5 and 2.5.

Nursing Actions

Physical Assessment: Assess potential for interactions with other pharmacological agents or herbal products patient may be taking (especially anything that will affect coagulation or platelet function). Note Administration for infusion specifics. Bleeding precautions should be observed. Assess results of laboratory tests (see above), therapeutic effectiveness, and adverse response (eg, hypersensitivity reaction, bleeding, chest pain, rash) regularly during therapy. Teach possible side effects/appropriate interventions (eg, bleeding precautions) and adverse symptoms to report.

Patient Education: Do not take any new medication during therapy unless approved by prescriber. This drug can only be administered by infusion. Report immediately any pain, swelling, burning, or bleeding at infusion site. You may have a tendency to bleed easily while taking this drug (brush teeth with soft brush, floss with waxed floss, use electric razor, avoid scissors or sharp knives, and avoid potentially harmful activities). Report unusual bleeding or bruising

(bleeding gums, nosebleed, blood in urine, dark stool); pain in joints or back; CNS changes (fever, confusion); unusual fever; persistent nausea or GI upset; or swelling or pain at injection site. **Breast-feeding precaution:** Consult prescriber if breast-feeding.

Letrozole (LET roe zole)

U.S. Brand Names Femara®
Synonyms CGS-20267; NSC-719345
Pharmacologic Category Antineoplastic Agent, Aromatase Inhibitor
Medication Safety Issues
Sound-alike/look-alike issues:
Femara® may be confused with femhrt®
Pregnancy Risk Factor D
Lactation Excretion in breast milk unknown/use caution
Use First-line treatment of hormone receptor positive or hormone receptor unknown, locally advanced, or metastatic breast cancer in postmenopausal women; treatment of advanced breast cancer in postmenopausal women with disease progression following antiestrogen therapy; adjuvant treatment of postmenopausal hormone receptor positive early breast cancer; extended adjuvant treatment of early breast cancer in postmenopausal women who have received 5 years of adjuvant tamoxifen therapy
Mechanism of Action/Effect Competitive inhibitor of the aromatase enzyme system, which catalyzes conversion of androgens to estrogens. Inhibition leads to a significant reduction in plasma estrogen levels. Does not affect synthesis of adrenal or thyroid hormones, aldosterone, or androgens.
Contraindications Hypersensitivity to letrozole or any component of the formulation; pregnancy
Warnings/Precautions Use caution with hepatic impairment; dose adjustment may be required. Increases in transaminases ≥5 times the upper limit of normal and in bilirubin ≥1.5 times the upper limit of normal were most often, but not always, associated with metastatic liver disease. May cause dizziness, fatigue, and somnolence; patients should be cautioned before performing tasks which require mental alertness (eg, operating machinery or driving). May increase total serum cholesterol. May cause decreases in bone mineral density. For use in postmenopausal women only.
Drug Interactions
Cytochrome P450 Effect: Substrate (minor) of CYP2A6, 3A4; **Inhibits** CYP2A6 (strong), 2C19 (weak)
Increased Effect/Toxicity: Letrozole may increase the levels/effects of CYP2A6 substrates; example substrates include dexmedetomidine and ifosfamide.
Adverse Reactions
>10%:
Central nervous system: Headache (8% to 12%), fatigue (6% to 13%)
Endocrine & metabolic: Hot flashes (5% to 19%)
Gastrointestinal: Nausea (13% to 17%)
Neuromuscular & skeletal: Musculoskeletal pain, bone pain (22%), back pain (18%), arthralgia (8% to 16%)
Respiratory: Dyspnea (7% to 18%), cough (5% to 13%)
2% to 10%:
Cardiovascular: Chest pain (3% to 8%), peripheral edema (5%), hypertension (5% to 8%)
Central nervous system: Pain (5%), insomnia (7%), dizziness (3% to 5%), somnolence (2% to 3%), depression (<5%), anxiety (<5%), vertigo (<5%)
Dermatologic: Rash (4% to 5%), alopecia (<5%), pruritus (1% to 2%)

Endocrine & metabolic: Breast pain (7%), hypercholesterolemia (3%), hypercalcemia (<5%)

Gastrointestinal: Vomiting (7%), constipation (6% to 10%), diarrhea (5% to 8%), abdominal pain (5% to 6%), anorexia (3% to 5%), dyspepsia (3% to 4%), weight loss (7%), weight gain (2%)

Neuromuscular & skeletal: Limb pain (10%), arthritis (7%), myalgia (6% to 7%), bone fractures (6%), bone mineral density decreased (3% to 5%), osteoporosis (2%)

Miscellaneous: Flu (6%)

Overdosage/Toxicology Firm recommendations for treatment are not possible; emesis could be induced if the patient is alert. In general, supportive care and frequent monitoring of vital signs are appropriate.

Pharmacodynamics/Kinetics

Time to Peak: Steady state, plasma: 2-6 weeks

Protein Binding: Plasma: Weak

Half-Life Elimination: Terminal: ~2 days

Metabolism: Hepatic via CYP3A4 and 2A6 to an inactive carbinol metabolite

Excretion: Urine (90%; 6% as unchanged drug, 75% as glucuronide carbinol metabolite, 9% as unidentified metabolites)

Available Dosage Forms Tablet: 2.5 mg

Dosing

Adults & Elderly: Refer to individual protocols.
Breast cancer: Oral: 2.5 mg once daily

Renal Impairment: No dosage adjustment is required in patients with renal impairment if Cl_{cr} is ≥10 mL/minute.

Hepatic Impairment:

Mild-to-moderate impairment: No adjustment recommended

Severe impairment: Child-Pugh class C: 2.5 mg every other day

Stability

Storage: Store at 15°C to 30°C (59°F to 86°F)

Laboratory Monitoring CBC, cholesterol, thyroid function tests, serum electrolytes, serum transaminases, serum creatinine

Nursing Actions

Physical Assessment: For use in postmenopausal women only. Monitor laboratory tests, therapeutic effectiveness (slowing of disease process), and adverse reactions (eg, hypertension, pain, gastrointestinal upset, hot flashes) on a regular basis throughout therapy. Teach patient proper use, possible side effects/appropriate interventions, and adverse symptoms to report.

Patient Education: Do not take any new medication during therapy unless approved by prescriber. Take as directed, without regard to food. You may experience nausea, vomiting, hot flashes, or loss of appetite (frequent mouth care, small, frequent meals, chewing gum, or sucking lozenges may help); musculoskeletal pain or headache (consult prescriber for analgesics relief); sleepiness, fatigue, or dizziness (use caution when driving, climbing stairs, or engaging in tasks that require alertness until response to drug is known); constipation (increased exercise or dietary fruit or fluids may help); diarrhea (buttermilk, boiled milk, or yogurt may help); or loss of hair (will grow back). Report chest pain, pressure, palpitations, or swollen extremities; weakness, severe headache, numbness, or loss of strength in any part of the body; difficulty speaking; vaginal bleeding; unusual signs of bleeding or bruising; respiratory difficulty; severe nausea; or muscle pain; or skin rash.

Dietary Considerations May be taken without regard to meals. Calcium and vitamin D supplementation are recommended.

Pregnancy Issues Letrozole may cause fetal harm when administered to pregnant women. Animal studies have demonstrated embryotoxicity and fetotoxicity. There are no adequate and well-controlled studies in pregnant women. If used in pregnancy, or if patient becomes pregnant during treatment, the patient should be apprised of potential hazard to the fetus. Letrozole is FDA indicated for postmenopausal women only.

Leucovorin (loo koe VOR in)

Synonyms Calcium Leucovorin; Citrovorum Factor; Folinic Acid; 5-Formyl Tetrahydrofolate; Leucovorin Calcium

Pharmacologic Category Antidote; Vitamin, Water Soluble

Medication Safety Issues

Sound-alike/look-alike issues:

Leucovorin may be confused with Leukeran®, Leukine®

Folinic acid may be confused with folic acid

Pregnancy Risk Factor C

Lactation Enters breast milk/compatible

Use Antidote for folic acid antagonists (methotrexate, trimethoprim, pyrimethamine); treatment of megaloblastic anemias when folate is deficient as in infancy, sprue, pregnancy, and nutritional deficiency when oral folate therapy is not possible; in combination with fluorouracil in the treatment of colon cancer

Mechanism of Action/Effect A reduced form of folic acid, leucovorin supplies the necessary cofactor blocked by methotrexate, enters the cells via the same active transport system as methotrexate. Stabilizes the binding of 5-dUMP and thymidylate synthetase, enhancing the activity of fluorouracil.

Contraindications Hypersensitivity to leucovorin or any component of the formulation; pernicious anemia or vitamin B_{12}-deficient megaloblastic anemias

Drug Interactions

Decreased Effect: May decrease efficacy of co-trimoxazole against *Pneumocystis carinii* pneumonitis

Adverse Reactions Frequency not defined.

Dermatologic: Rash, pruritus, erythema, urticaria

Hematologic: Thrombocytosis

Respiratory: Wheezing

Miscellaneous: Anaphylactoid reactions

Pharmacodynamics/Kinetics

Onset of Action: Oral: ~30 minutes; I.V.: ~5 minutes

Half-Life Elimination: Leucovorin: 15 minutes; 5MTHF: 33-35 minutes

Metabolism: Intestinal mucosa and hepatically to 5-methyl-tetrahydrofolate (5MTHF; active)

Excretion: Urine (80% to 90%); feces (5% to 8%)

Available Dosage Forms

Injection, powder for reconstitution, as calcium: 50 mg, 100 mg, 200 mg, 350 mg, 500 mg

Injection, solution, as calcium: 10 mg/mL (50 mL)

Tablet, as calcium: 5 mg, 10 mg, 15 mg, 25 mg

Dosing

Adults & Elderly:

Treatment of folic acid antagonist overdosage: Oral: 2-15 mg/day for 3 days or until blood counts are normal, **or** 5 mg every 3 days; doses of 6 mg/day are needed for patients with platelet counts <100,000/mm³.

Folate-deficient megaloblastic anemia: I.M.: 1 mg/day

Megaloblastic anemia secondary to congenital deficiency of dihydrofolate reductase: I.M.: 3-6 mg/day

Rescue dose: Initial: I.V.: 10 mg/m², then:
Oral, I.M., I.V., SubQ: 10-15 mg/m² every 6 hours until methotrexate level <0.05 micromole/L; if methotrexate level remains >5 micromole/L at 48-72 hours after the end of the methotrexate infusion, increase to 20-100 mg/m² every 6 hours until methotrexate level <0.05 micromole/L

(Continued)

Leucovorin *(Continued)*

Investigational: Post I.T. methotrexate: Oral, I.V.: 12 mg/m^2 as a single dose

Pediatrics: Refer to adult dosing.

Administration

Oral: Doses >25 mg should be administered parenterally.

I.V.: Refer to individual protocols. Leucovorin calcium should be administered I.M. or I.V. Leucovorin should not be administered concurrently with methotrexate. It is commonly initiated 24 hours after the start of methotrexate. Toxicity to normal tissues may be irreversible if leucovorin is not initiated by ~40 hours after the start of methotrexate. **Note:** The manufacturer states that leucovorin should not be given intrathecally/intraventricularly; however, it has been given by these routes.

As a rescue after folate antagonists: Leucovorin may be administered by I.V. bolus injection, I.M. injection, or orally. Doses >25 mg should be administered parenterally.

In combination with fluorouracil: When leucovorin is used to modulate fluorouracil activity, the fluorouracil is usually given after, or at the midpoint, of the leucovorin infusion. Leucovorin is usually administered by I.V. bolus injection or short (10-15 minutes) I.V. infusion. Other administration schedules have been used; refer to individual protocols.

I.V. Detail: pH: 8.1 (vials)

Stability

Reconstitution: Reconstitute with SWFI, bacteriostatic NS, BWFI, NS, or D$_5$W; dilute in 100-1000 mL NS, D$_5$W for infusion

Compatibility: Stable in D$_{10}$NS, D$_5$W, D$_{10}$W, LR, SWFI, bacteriostatic water, NS, bacteriostatic NS

Y-site administration: Incompatible with amphotericin B cholesteryl sulfate complex, droperidol, foscarnet, sodium bicarbonate

Compatibility in syringe: Incompatible with droperidol

Compatibility when admixed: Incompatible with concentrations >2 mg/mL of leucovorin and >25 mg/mL of fluorouracil

Storage: Store at room temperature; protect from light. Reconstituted solution is chemically stable for 7 days; reconstitutions with bacteriostatic water for injection, U.S.P., must be used within 7 days. Parenteral admixture is stable for 24 hours stored at room temperature (25°C) and for 4 days when stored under refrigeration (4°C).

Laboratory Monitoring Plasma methotrexate concentration as a therapeutic guide to high-dose methotrexate therapy with leucovorin factor rescue. Leucovorin is continued until the plasma methotrexate level is <0.05 micromole/L. Each dose of leucovorin is increased if the plasma methotrexate concentration is excessively high. With 4- to 6-hour high-dose methotrexate infusions, plasma drug values in excess of 50 and 1 micromole/L at 24 and 48 hours after starting the infusion, respectively, are often predictive of delayed methotrexate clearance.

Nursing Actions

Physical Assessment: Monitor for adverse reactions.

Patient Education: Take as directed, at evenly spaced intervals around-the-clock. Maintain hydration (2-3 L of water/day while taking for rescue therapy). For folic acid deficiency, eat foods high in folic acid (eg, meat proteins, bran, dried beans, asparagus, green leafy vegetables). Report respiratory difficulty, lethargy, or rash or itching. **Pregnancy precaution:** Inform prescriber if you are or intend to become pregnant.

Leuprolide (loo PROE lide)

U.S. Brand Names Eligard®; Lupron®; Lupron Depot®; Lupron Depot-Ped®; Viadur®

Synonyms Abbott-43818; Leuprolide Acetate; Leuprorelin Acetate; NSC-377526; TAP-144

Pharmacologic Category Gonadotropin Releasing Hormone Agonist

Medication Safety Issues
Sound-alike/look-alike issues:
Lupron® may be confused with Nuprin®
Lupron Depot®-3 Month may be confused with Lupron Depot-Ped®

Pregnancy Risk Factor X

Lactation Excretion in breast milk unknown/contraindicated

Use Palliative treatment of advanced prostate carcinoma; management of endometriosis; treatment of anemia caused by uterine leiomyomata (fibroids); central precocious puberty

Unlabeled/Investigational Use Treatment of breast, ovarian, and endometrial cancer; infertility; prostatic hyperplasia

Mechanism of Action/Effect Potent inhibitor of gonadotropin secretion; continuous daily administration results in suppression of ovarian and testicular steroidogenesis due to decreased levels of LH and FSH with subsequent decrease in testosterone (male) and estrogen (female) levels. Leuprolide may also have a direct inhibitory effect on the testes, and act by a different mechanism not directly related to reduction in serum testosterone.

Contraindications Hypersensitivity to leuprolide, GnRH, GnRH-agonist analogs, or any component of the formulation; spinal cord compression (orchiectomy suggested); undiagnosed abnormal vaginal bleeding; pregnancy; breast-feeding

Warnings/Precautions Transient increases in testosterone serum levels occur at the start of treatment. Tumor flare, bone pain, neuropathy, urinary tract obstruction, and spinal cord compression have been reported when used for prostate cancer; closely observe patients for weakness, paresthesias, hematuria, and urinary tract obstruction in first few weeks of therapy. Observe patients with metastatic vertebral lesions or urinary obstruction closely. Exacerbation of endometriosis or uterine leiomyomata may occur initially. Decreased bone density has been reported when used for ≥6 months. Use caution in patients with a history of psychiatric illness; alteration in mood, memory impairment, and depression have been associated with use. Rare cases of pituitary apoplexy (frequently secondary to pituitary adenoma) have been observed with leuprolide administration (onset from 1 hour to usually <2 weeks); may present as sudden headache, vomiting, visual or mental status changes, and infrequently cardiovascular collapse; immediate medical attention required. Females treated for precocious puberty may experience menses or spotting during the first 2 months of treatment; notify healthcare provider if bleeding continues after the second month.

Lab Interactions Interferes with pituitary gonadotropic and gonadal function tests during and up to 3 months after therapy. Viadur®: Efficacy and stability of product not affected by MRI or radiographic exposure, although device will be visualized during these diagnostic procedures.

Adverse Reactions
Children: 2% to 10%:
Central nervous system: Pain (2%)
Dermatologic: Acne (2%), rash (2% including erythema multiforme), seborrhea (2%)
Genitourinary: Vaginitis (2%), vaginal bleeding (2%), vaginal discharge (2%)
Local: Injection site reaction (5%)

Adults (frequency dependent upon formulation and indication):

Cardiovascular: Angina, atrial fibrillation, CHF, deep vein thrombosis, edema, hot flashes, hypertension, MI, peripheral edema, syncope, tachycardia

Central nervous system: Abnormal thinking, agitation, amnesia, anxiety, chills, confusion, convulsion, dementia, depression, dizziness, fatigue, fever, headache, insomnia, malaise, pain, vertigo

Dermatologic: Alopecia, bruising, burning, cellulitis, pruritus

Endocrine & metabolic: Bone density decreased, breast enlargement, breast tenderness, dehydration, hirsutism, hyperglycemia, hyperlipidemia, hyperphosphatemia, libido decreased, menstrual disorders, potassium decreased

Gastrointestinal: Anorexia, appetite increased, constipation, diarrhea, dry mucous membranes, dysphagia, eructation, GI hemorrhage, gingivitis, gum hemorrhage, intestinal obstruction, nausea, peptic ulcer, vomiting, weight gain/loss

Genitourinary: Balanitis, impotence, nocturia, penile shrinkage, testicular atrophy; urinary disorder (eg, urgency, incontinence, retention); UTI, vaginitis

Hematologic: Anemia, platelets decreased, PT prolonged, WBC increased

Hepatic: Hepatomegaly, liver function tests abnormal

Local: Abscess, injection site reaction

Neuromuscular & skeletal: Arthritis, bone pain, leg cramps, myalgia, paresthesia, tremor, weakness

Renal: BUN increased

Respiratory: Allergic reaction, dyspnea, emphysema, hemoptysis, hypoxia, lung edema, pulmonary embolism

Miscellaneous: Body odor, diaphoresis, flu-like syndrome, neoplasm, night sweats, voice alteration

Overdosage/Toxicology Treatment is supportive.

Pharmacodynamics/Kinetics

Onset of Action: Following transient increase, testosterone suppression occurs in ~2-4 weeks of continued therapy

Protein Binding: 43% to 49%

Half-Life Elimination: I.V.: 3 hours

Metabolism: Major metabolite, pentapeptide (M-1)

Excretion: Urine (<5% as parent and major metabolite)

Available Dosage Forms

Implant (Viadur®): 65 mg [released over 12 months; packaged with administration kit]

Injection, solution, as acetate (Lupron®): 5 mg/mL (2.8 mL) [contains benzyl alcohol; packaged with syringes and alcohol swabs]

Injection, powder for reconstitution, as acetate [depot formulation; prefilled syringe]:

Eligard®:

7.5 mg [released over 1 month]

22.5 mg [released over 3 months]

30 mg [released over 4 months]

45 mg [released over 6 months]

Lupron Depot®: 3.75 mg, 7.5 mg [released over 1 month; contains polysorbate 80]

Lupron Depot®-3 Month: 11.25 mg, 22.5 mg [released over 3 months; contains polysorbate 80]

Lupron Depot®-4 Month: 30 mg [released over 4 months; contains polysorbate 80]

Lupron Depot-Ped®: 7.5 mg, 11.25 mg, 15 mg [released over 1 month; contains polysorbate 80]

Dosing

Adults & Elderly:

Advanced prostatic carcinoma:

SubQ:

Eligard®: 7.5 mg monthly **or** 22.5 mg every 3 months **or** 30 mg every 4 months **or** 45 mg every 6 months

Lupron®: 1 mg/day

Viadur®: 65 mg implanted subcutaneously every 12 months

I.M.:

Lupron Depot®: 7.5 mg/dose given monthly (every 28-33 days) **or**

Lupron Depot®-3: 22.5 mg every 3 months **or**

Lupron Depot®-4: 30 mg every 4 months

Endometriosis: I.M.: Initial therapy may be with leuprolide alone or in combination with norethindrone; if retreatment for an additional 6 months is necessary, norethindrone should be used. Retreatment is not recommended for longer than one additional 6-month course.

Lupron Depot®: 3.75 mg/month for up to 6 months **or**

Lupron Depot®-3: 11.25 mg every 3 months for up to 2 doses (6 months total duration of treatment)

Uterine leiomyomata (fibroids): I.M. (in combination with iron):

Lupron Depot®: 3.75 mg/month for up to 3 months **or**

Lupron Depot®-3: 11.25 mg as a single injection

Pediatrics:

Precocious puberty (consider discontinuing by age 11 for females and by age 12 for males):

SubQ (Lupron®): Initial: 50 mcg/kg/day (per manufacturer, doses of 20-45 mcg/kg/day have also been reported); titrate dose upward by 10 mcg/kg/day if down-regulation is not achieved

I.M. (Lupron Depot-Ped®): 0.3 mg/kg/dose given every 28 days (minimum dose: 7.5 mg)

≤25 kg: 7.5 mg

>25-37.5 kg: 11.25 mg

>37.5 kg: 15 mg

Titrate dose upward in increments of 3.75 mg every 4 weeks if down-regulation is not achieved

Administration

I.M.:

I.M.: Lupron Depot®: Vary injection site periodically

SubQ:

Eligard®: Vary injection site; choose site with adequate subcutaneous tissue (eg, abdomen, upper buttocks)

Lupron®: Vary injection site; if an alternate syringe from the syringe provided is required, insulin syringes should be used; use disposable syringe once only

Other: Viadur® implant: Requires surgical implantation (subcutaneous) and removal at 12-month intervals

Stability

Reconstitution:

Eligard®: Packaged in two syringes; one contains the Atrigel® polymer system and the second contains leuprolide acetate powder; follow package instructions for mixing

Lupron Depot®: Reconstitute only with diluent provided

Storage:

Lupron®: Store unopened vials of injection in refrigerator, vial in use can be kept at room temperature of ≤30°C (86°F) for several months with minimal loss of potency. Protect from light and store vial in carton until use. Do not freeze.

Eligard®: Store at 2°C to 8°C (36°F to 46°C). Allow to reach room temperature prior to using; once mixed, must be administered within 30 minutes.

Lupron Depot® may be stored at room temperature of 25°C, excursions permitted to 15°C to 30°C (59°F to 86°F). Upon reconstitution, the suspension does not contain a preservative and should be used immediately.

Viadur® may be stored at room temperature of 15°C to 30°C (59°F and 86°F).

(Continued)

Leuprolide *(Continued)*

Laboratory Monitoring Precocious puberty: GnRH testing (blood LH and FSH levels), testosterone in males and estradiol in females

Nursing Actions

Physical Assessment: Monitor laboratory tests, therapeutic effectiveness, and adverse reactions (eg, urinary tract obstruction, weakness, paresthesias, and urinary tract obstruction in first few weeks of therapy) on a regular basis throughout therapy. Teach patient (or caregiver) proper use (eg, storage, injection technique, syringe/needle disposal), possible side effects/appropriate interventions, and adverse symptoms to report. **Pregnancy risk factor X:** Determine that patient is not pregnant before beginning treatment and do not give to female of childbearing age unless capable of complying with contraceptive measures 1 month prior to therapy, during therapy, and 1 month following therapy. Instruct patient in appropriate contraceptive measures. Breast-feeding is contraindicated.

Patient Education: Use as directed. Do not discontinue without consulting prescriber. You may experience disease flare (increased bone pain) and urinary retention during early treatment (usually resolves); dizziness, headache, lethargy, or faintness (use caution when driving or engaging in tasks that require alertness until response to drug is known); nausea or vomiting (small frequent meals or analgesics may help); hot flashes, flushing, or redness (cold cloth and cool environment may help); breast swelling or tenderness; or decreased libido. Report irregular or rapid heartbeat, palpitations, chest pain; inability to void or changes in urinary pattern; unresolved nausea or vomiting; numbness of extremities; breast swelling or pain, respiratory difficulty, or redness, swelling or pain at injection sites. **Pregnancy/breast-feeding precautions:** Inform prescriber if you are pregnant. Do not get pregnant. Consult prescriber for appropriate contraceptive use during and for a time following therapy. Do not breast-feed.

Geriatric Considerations Leuprolide has the advantage of not increasing risk of atherosclerotic vascular disease, causing swelling of breasts, fluid retention, and thromboembolism as compared to estrogen therapy.

Pregnancy Issues Pregnancy must be excluded prior to the start of treatment. Although leuprolide usually inhibits ovulation and stops menstruation, contraception is not ensured and a nonhormonal contraceptive should be used. May cause fetal harm if administered to a pregnant woman.

Additional Information

Eligard® Atrigel®: A nongelatin-based, biodegradable, polymer matrix

Viadur®: Leuprolide acetate implant containing 72 mg of leuprolide acetate, equivalent to 65 mg leuprolide free base. One Viadur® implant delivers 120 mcg of leuprolide/day over 12 months.

Levalbuterol *(leve al BYOO ter ole)*

U.S. Brand Names Xopenex®; Xopenex HFA™

Synonyms Levalbuterol Hydrochloride; Levalbuterol Tartrate; R-albuterol

Pharmacologic Category Beta$_2$-Adrenergic Agonist

Medication Safety Issues

Sound-alike/look-alike issues:

Xopenex® may be confused with Xanax®

Pregnancy Risk Factor C

Lactation Excretion in breast milk unknown/use caution

Use Treatment or prevention of bronchospasm in children and adults with reversible obstructive airway disease

Mechanism of Action/Effect Relaxes bronchial smooth muscle by action on beta-2 receptors with little effect on heart rate

Contraindications Hypersensitivity to levalbuterol, albuterol, or any component of the formulation

Warnings/Precautions Optimize anti-inflammatory treatment before initiating maintenance treatment with levalbuterol. Do not use as a component of chronic therapy without an anti-inflammatory agent. Only the mildest form of asthma (Step 1 and/or exercise-induced) would not require concurrent use based upon asthma guidelines. Patient must be instructed to seek medical attention in cases where acute symptoms are not relieved or a previous level of response is diminished. The need to increase frequency of use may indicate deterioration of asthma, and treatment must not be delayed.

Use caution in patients with cardiovascular disease (arrhythmia or hypertension or CHF), convulsive disorders, diabetes, glaucoma, hyperthyroidism, or hypokalemia. Beta agonists may cause elevation in blood pressure, heart rate, and result in CNS stimulation/excitation. Beta$_2$ agonists may increase risk of arrhythmia, increase serum glucose, or decrease serum potassium.

Do not exceed recommended dose; serious adverse events including fatalities, have been associated with excessive use of inhaled sympathomimetics. Rarely, paradoxical bronchospasm may occur with use of inhaled bronchodilating agents; this should be distinguished from inadequate response. Use with caution during labor and delivery. Safety and efficacy have not been established in patients <4 years of age.

Drug Interactions

Decreased Effect: Beta-blockers (particularly nonselective agents) block the effect of levalbuterol. Digoxin levels may be decreased.

Increased Effect/Toxicity: May add to effects of medications which deplete potassium (eg, loop or thiazide diuretics). Cardiac effects of levalbuterol may be potentiated in patients receiving MAO inhibitors, tricyclic antidepressants, sympathomimetics (eg, amphetamine, dobutamine), or inhaled anesthetics (eg, enflurane).

Adverse Reactions

>10%:

Endocrine & metabolic: Serum glucose increased, serum potassium decreased

Respiratory: Viral infection (7% to 12%), rhinitis (3% to 11%)

>2% to 10%:

Central nervous system: Nervousness (3% to 10%), tremor (≤7%), anxiety (≤3%), dizziness (1% to 3%), migraine (≤3%), pain (1% to 3%)

Cardiovascular: Tachycardia (~3%)

Gastrointestinal: Dyspepsia (1% to 3%)

Neuromuscular & skeletal: Leg cramps (≤3%)

Respiratory: Asthma (9%), pharyngitis (8%), cough (1% to 4%), nasal edema (1% to 3%), sinusitis (1% to 4%)

Miscellaneous: Flu-like syndrome (1% to 4%), accidental injury (≤3%)

Overdosage/Toxicology Symptoms of overdose include tachycardia, tremor, hypertension, angina, and seizures. Hypokalemia also may occur. Cardiac arrest and death may be associated with abuse of beta-agonist bronchodilators. Treatment includes immediate discontinuation and symptomatic and supportive therapies. Cautious use of beta-adrenergic blocking agents may be considered in severe cases.

Pharmacodynamics/Kinetics

Onset of Action:

Aerosol: 5.5-10.2 minutes; Peak effect: ~77 minutes

Nebulization: 10-17 minutes (measured as a 15% increase in FEV$_1$); Peak effect: 1.5 hours

Duration of Action:
Aerosol: 3-4 hours (up to 6 hours in some patients)

Nebulization: 5-6 hours (up to 8 hours in some patients)

Time to Peak:
Aerosol: 0.5 hours

Nebulization: 0.2 hours

Half-Life Elimination: 3.3-4 hours

Available Dosage Forms Note: Strength expressed as base.

Aerosol, oral, as tartrate:

Xopenex HFA™: 45 mcg/actuation (15 g) [200 doses; chlorofluorocarbon free]

Solution for nebulization, as hydrochloride:

Xopenex®: 0.31 mg/3 mL (24s); 0.63 mg/3 mL (24s); 1.25 mg/3 mL (24s)

Solution for nebulization, concentrate, as hydrochloride:

Xopenex®: 1.25 mg/0.5 mL (30s)

Dosing
Adults: Bronchospasm:

Metered-dose inhalation: Aerosol: 1-2 puffs every 4-6 hours

Nebulization: 0.63 mg 3 times/day at intervals of 6-8 hours; dosage may be increased to 1.25 mg 3 times/day with close monitoring for adverse effects. Most patients gain optimal benefit from regular use

Elderly: Only a small number of patients have been studied. Although greater sensitivity of some elderly patients cannot be ruled out, no overall differences in safety or effectiveness were observed. An initial dose of 0.63 mg should be used in all patients >65 years of age.

Pediatrics: Bronchospasm:

Metered-dose inhalation: Aerosol: Children ≥4 years: Refer to adult dosing.

Nebulization:

Children 6-11 years: 0.31 mg 3 times/day (maximum dose: 0.63 mg 3 times/day)

Children >12 years: Refer to adult dosing.

Administration
Inhalation: Aerosol: Shake well before use; prime with 4 test sprays prior to first use or if inhaler has not been use of more than 3 days. Clean actuator (mouthpiece) weekly.

Solution for nebulization: Safety and efficacy were established when administered with the following nebulizers: PARI LC Jet™, PARI LC Plus™, as well as the following compressors: PARI Master®, Dura-Neb® 2000, and Dura-Neb® 3000. Concentrated solution should be diluted prior to use.

Stability
Reconstitution: Concentrated solution should be diluted with 2.5 mL NS prior to use.

Storage: Aerosol: Store at room temperature of 20°C to 25°C (68°F to 77°F); protect from freezing and direct sunlight. Store with mouthpiece up. Discard after 200 actuations.

Solution for nebulization: Store in protective foil pouch at room temperature of 20°C to 25°C (68°F to 77°F). Protect from light and excessive heat. Vials should be used within 2 weeks after opening protective pouch. Use within 1 week and protect from light if removed from pouch. Vials of concentrated solution should be used immediately after removing from protective pouch.

Laboratory Monitoring FEV$_1$ and/or peak expiratory flow rate, arterial blood gases (if condition warrants); serum potassium, serum glucose (in selected patients)

Nursing Actions
Physical Assessment: Assess effectiveness and interactions of other medications patient may be taking. Monitor therapeutic effectiveness (relief of asthma effect), adverse reactions (eg, anaphylaxis or hypertension, first dose administered under supervision), or overdose. Patients with diabetes should monitor serum glucose on a regular basis (possibility of hyperglycemia). Assess knowledge/teach patient appropriate use (safe use of nebulizer), interventions to reduce side effects, and adverse reactions to report

Patient Education: Use only when necessary or as prescribed; tolerance may develop with overuse. Do not administer more frequently than prescribed. First dose should not be used when you are alone. Avoid OTC medications without consulting prescriber. Maintain adequate hydration (2-3 L/day of fluids) unless instructed to restrict fluid intake. Stress or excessive exercising may exacerbate wheezing or bronchospasm (controlled breathing or relaxation techniques may help). If you have diabetes, you will need to monitor serum glucose levels closely until response is known; notify diabetic advisor if hyperglycemia occurs. You may experience tremor, anxiety, dizziness (use caution when driving or engaging in hazardous activities until response to drug is known); or temporarily upset stomach, nausea, or vomiting (small frequent meals, frequent mouth care, chewing gum, or sucking hard candy may help). Paradoxical bronchospasm can occur. Stop drug immediately and notify prescriber if any of the following occur: chest pain, tightness, palpitations; severe headache; respiratory difficulty; increased nervousness, restlessness, or trembling; muscle cramps or weakness; or seizures. Report unusual signs of flu or infection, leg or muscle cramps, unusual cough, persistent GI problems, vision changes, or other adverse effects. **Pregnancy/breast-feeding precautions:** Inform prescriber if you are or intend to become pregnant. Consult prescriber if breast-feeding.

Geriatric Considerations For aerosol formulation, start with low end of dosage range. Refer to dosing information for nebulization dosing specifics.

Breast-Feeding Issues It is not known whether levalbuterol is excreted in human milk. Plasma levels following oral inhalation are low. Racemic albuterol was shown to be tumorigenic in animal studies.

Pregnancy Issues Teratogenic effects were not observed in animal studies; however, racemic albuterol was teratogenic in some species. There are no adequate and well-controlled studies in pregnant women. This drug should be used during pregnancy only if benefit exceeds risk. Use caution if needed for bronchospasm during labor and delivery; has potential to interfere with uterine contractions.

Levetiracetam (lee va tye RA se tam)

U.S. Brand Names Keppra®

Pharmacologic Category Anticonvulsant, Miscellaneous

Medication Safety Issues

Sound-alike/look-alike issues:

Potential for dispensing errors between Keppra® and Kaletra™ (lopinavir/ritonavir)

Pregnancy Risk Factor C

Lactation Enters breast milk/not recommended

Use Adjunctive therapy in the treatment of partial onset seizures

Unlabeled/Investigational Use Bipolar disorder

Mechanism of Action/Effect The precise mechanism by which levetiracetam exerts its antiepileptic effect is unknown. However, several studies have suggested the mechanism may involve one or more central pharmacologic effects.

Contraindications Hypersensitivity to levetiracetam or any component of the formulation

Warnings/Precautions Psychotic symptoms (psychosis, hallucinations) and behavioral symptoms (Continued)

Levetiracetam *(Continued)*

(including aggression, anger, anxiety, depersonalization, depression, personality disorder) may occur; incidence may be increased in children. Dose reduction may be required. Levetiracetam should be withdrawn gradually to minimize the potential of increased seizure frequency. There is a potential for dispensing errors between Keppra® and Kaletra™ (lopinavir/ritonavir); use caution when prescribing, dispensing, or administering. Use caution with renal impairment (dosage adjustment may be necessary).

Drug Interactions

Increased Effect/Toxicity: No interaction was observed in pharmacokinetic trials with other anticonvulsants, including phenytoin, carbamazepine, valproic acid, phenobarbital, lamotrigine, gabapentin, and primidone.

Nutritional/Ethanol Interactions

Ethanol: Avoid ethanol (may increase CNS depression).
Food: Food may delay, but does not affect the extent of absorption.

Adverse Reactions

>10%:
Central nervous system: Behavioral symptoms (agitation, aggression, anger, anxiety, apathy, depersonalization, depression, emotional lability, hostility, hyperkinesias, irritability, nervousness, neurosis and personality disorder: adults 13%; children 38%), somnolence (15% to 23%), headache (14%), hostility (2% to 12%)
Gastrointestinal: Vomiting (15%), anorexia (13%)
Neuromuscular & skeletal: Weakness (9% to 15%)
Respiratory: Rhinitis (4% to 13%), cough (2% to 11%)
Miscellaneous: Accidental injury (17%), infection (2% to 13%)

1% to 10%:
Cardiovascular: Facial edema (2%)
Central nervous system: Nervousness (4% to 10%), dizziness (7% to 9%), personality disorder (8%), pain (6% to 7%), agitation (6%), emotional lability (2% to 6%), depression (3% to 4%), ataxia (3%), vertigo (3%), amnesia (2%), anxiety (2%), confusion (2%), psychotic symptoms (1%)
Dermatologic: Bruising (4%), pruritus (2%), rash (2%), skin discoloration (2%)
Gastrointestinal: Diarrhea (8%), gastroenteritis (4%), anorexia (3%), constipation (3%), dehydration (2%)
Hematologic: Decreased leukocytes (2% to 3%)
Neuromuscular & skeletal: Neck pain (2%), paresthesia (2%), reflexes increased (2%)
Ocular: Conjunctivitis (3%), diplopia (2%), amblyopia (2%)
Otic: Ear pain (2%)
Renal: Albuminuria (4%), urine abnormality (2%)
Respiratory: Pharyngitis (6% to 10%), asthma (2%), sinusitis (2%)
Miscellaneous: Flu-like symptoms (3%), viral infection (2%)

Overdosage/Toxicology Limited experience. Symptoms would be expected to include drowsiness, somnolence and ataxia. Treatment is symptomatic and supportive. Hemodialysis may be effective (estimated clearance of ~50% in 4 hours).

Pharmacodynamics/Kinetics

Onset of Action: Peak effect: 1 hour
Protein Binding: <10%
Half-Life Elimination: 6-8 hours
Metabolism: Not extensive; primarily by enzymatic hydrolysis; forms metabolites (inactive)
Excretion: Urine (66% as unchanged drug)

Available Dosage Forms

Solution, oral:
Keppra®: 100 mg/mL (480 mL) [dye free; grape flavor]
Tablet: 250 mg, 500 mg, 750 mg
Keppra®: 250 mg, 500 mg, 750 mg, 1000 mg

Dosing

Adults & Elderly:
Partial onset seizures (adjunctive): Oral: Initial: 500 mg twice daily; may increase every 2 weeks by 500 mg/dose to a maximum of 1500 mg twice daily. Doses >3000 mg/day have been used in trials; however, there is no evidence of increased benefit.
Bipolar disorder (unlabeled use): Initial: 500 mg twice daily; if tolerated, increase to 500 mg twice daily; dose may be increased every 3 days until target dose of 3000 mg/day is reached; maximum: 4000 mg/day

Pediatrics:
Partial onset seizures: Oral:
Children 4-15 years: Partial onset seizures: 10 mg/kg/dose twice daily; may increase every 2 weeks by 10 mg/kg/dose to a maximum of 30 mg/kg/dose twice daily
Children ≥16 years: Refer to adult dosing.
Bipolar disorder (unlabeled use): Oral: Children ≥16 years: Refer to adult dosing.

Renal Impairment: Adults:
Cl_{cr} >80 mL/minute: 500-1500 mg every 12 hours
Cl_{cr} 50-80 mL/minute: 500-1000 mg every 12 hours
Cl_{cr} 30-50 mL/minute: 250-750 mg every 12 hours
Cl_{cr} <30 mL/minute: 250-500 mg every 12 hours
End-stage renal disease patients using dialysis: 500-1000 mg every 24 hours; a supplemental dose of 250-500 mg following dialysis is recommended

Hepatic Impairment: No adjustment necessary.

Administration

Oral: Tablets may be crushed and placed in food if unable to swallow whole (bitter taste may be expected).

Stability

Storage: Store at 25°C (77°F).

Nursing Actions

Physical Assessment: Assess effectiveness and interactions of other medications patient may be taking. Monitor therapeutic response (seizure activity, force, type, duration), laboratory values, and adverse reactions at beginning of therapy and periodically with long-term use. Monitor for CNS depression (somnolence and fatigue), behavioral abnormalities (psychosis, hallucinations, psychotic depression), and other behavioral symptoms (agitation, anger, aggression, irritability, hostility, anxiety, apathy, emotional lability, depersonalization, and depression). Taper dosage slowly when discontinuing. Observe and teach seizure/safety precautions. Assess knowledge/teach patient appropriate use, interventions to reduce side effects, and adverse symptoms to report.

Patient Education: Take exactly as directed; do not increase dose or frequency or discontinue without consulting prescriber. While using this medication, do not use alcohol and other prescription or OTC medications (especially pain medications, sedatives, antihistamines, or hypnotics) without consulting prescriber. Maintain adequate hydration (2-3 L/day of fluids) unless instructed to restrict fluid intake. You may experience drowsiness, dizziness, or blurred vision (use caution when driving or engaging in tasks requiring alertness until response to drug is known); or nausea, vomiting, loss of appetite, or dry mouth (small frequent meals, frequent mouth care, chewing gum, or sucking lozenges may help). Wear identification of epileptic status and medications. Report CNS changes, mentation changes, or changes in cognition; muscle cramping, weakness, tremors, changes in gait; persistent GI symptoms (cramping, constipation, vomiting, anorexia); rash or skin irritations; unusual bruising or bleeding (mouth, urine, stool); or worsening of seizure activity or loss of seizure control.

Pregnancy/breast-feeding precautions: Inform prescriber if you are or intend to become pregnant. Breast-feeding is not recommended.

Dietary Considerations May be taken with or without food.

Pregnancy Issues Developmental toxicities were observed in animal studies. There are no adequate and well-controlled studies in pregnant women. Two registries are available for women exposed to levetiracetam during pregnancy:

Antiepileptic Drug Pregnancy Registry (888-233-2334 or http://www.mgh.harvard.edu/aed/)

Keppra® pregnancy registry (888-537-7734 or http://www.keppra.com)

Levobupivacaine (LEE voe byoo PIV a kane)

U.S. Brand Names Chirocaine® [DSC]

Pharmacologic Category Local Anesthetic

Pregnancy Risk Factor B

Lactation Excretion in breast milk unknown/use caution

Use Production of local or regional anesthesia for surgery and obstetrics, and for postoperative pain management

Mechanism of Action/Effect Blocks both the initiation and transmission of nerve impulses

Contraindications Hypersensitivity to levobupivacaine, any component of the formulation, bupivacaine, or any local anesthetic of the amide type

Warnings/Precautions Local anesthetics should be administered only by clinicians familiar with the use of local anesthetic agents, procedures, and management of drug-related toxicity and other acute emergencies. Resuscitative equipment and medications should be readily available. Not for intravenous injection (cardiac arrest may occur) or obstetrical paracervical block. Risk of cardiac toxicity increases with higher concentration solutions. Avoid use of 0.75% solution with obstetrical patients. Use with caution in patients with hypotension, hypovolemia, heart block, hepatic impairment, cardiac impairment, or those receiving other local anesthetics or structurally-related agents.

Drug Interactions

Cytochrome P450 Effect: Substrate (minor) of CYP1A2, 3A4

Nutritional/Ethanol Interactions Herb/Nutraceutical: St John's wort may decrease levobupivacaine levels.

Adverse Reactions

>10%:
Cardiovascular: Hypotension (20% to 31%)
Central nervous system: Pain (postoperative) (7% to 18%), fever (7% to 17%)
Gastrointestinal: Nausea (12% to 21%), vomiting (8% to 14%)
Hematologic: Anemia (10% to 12%)

1% to 10%:
Cardiovascular: Abnormal ECG (3%), bradycardia (2%), tachycardia (2%), hypertension (1%)
Central nervous system: Pain (4% to 8%), headache (5% to 7%), dizziness (5% to 6%), hypoesthesia (3%), somnolence (1%), anxiety (1%), hypothermia (2%)
Dermatologic: Pruritus (4% to 9%), purpura (1%)
Endocrine & metabolic: Breast pain - female (1%)
Gastrointestinal: Constipation (3% to 7%), enlarged abdomen (3%), flatulence (2%), abdominal pain (2%), dyspepsia (2%), diarrhea (1%)
Genitourinary: Urinary incontinence (1%), urine flow decreased (1%), urinary tract infection (1%)
Hematologic: Leukocytosis (1%)
Local: Anesthesia (1%)
Neuromuscular & skeletal: Back pain (6%), rigors (3%), paresthesia (2%)
Ocular: Diplopia (3%)
Renal: Albuminuria (3%), hematuria (2%)
Respiratory: Cough (1%)
Miscellaneous: Fetal distress (5% to 10%), delayed delivery (6%), hemorrhage in pregnancy (2%), uterine abnormality (2%), increased wound drainage (1%)

Overdosage/Toxicology Related to local concentration or due to unintended intrathecal or intravenous injection. Symptoms may include restlessness, anxiety, incoherent speech, lightheadedness, numbness and tingling of the mouth and lips, metallic taste, tinnitus, dizziness, blurred vision, tremors, respiratory arrest, twitching, depression or drowsiness. In addition, cardiac toxicity, including AV block, bradycardia, arrhythmia, and hypotension may occur. Treatment is symptomatic.

Pharmacodynamics/Kinetics

Onset of Action: Epidural: 10-14 minutes

Duration of Action: Dose dependent: 1-8 hours

Time to Peak: Epidural: 30 minutes

Protein Binding: Plasma: >97%

Half-Life Elimination: 1.3 hours

Metabolism: Extensively hepatic via CYP3A4 and CYP1A2

Excretion: Urine (71%) and feces (24%) as metabolites

Available Dosage Forms [DSC] = Discontinued product

Injection, solution [preservative free]: 2.5 mg/mL (10 mL, 30 mL); 5 mg/mL (10 mL, 30 mL); 7.5 mg/mL (10 mL, 30 mL) [DSC]

Dosing

Adults & Elderly: Note: Rapid injection of a large volume of local anesthetic solution should be avoided. Fractional (incremental) doses are recommended.

Guidelines (individual response varies): See table.

	Concentration	Volume	Dose	Motor Block
Surgical Anesthesia				
Epidural for surgery	0.5%-0.75%	10-20 mL	50-150 mg	Moderate to complete
Epidural for C-section	0.5%	20-30 mL	100-150 mg	Moderate to complete
Peripheral nerve	0.25%-0.5%	0.4 mL/kg (30 mL)	1-2 mg/kg (75-150 mg)	Moderate to complete
Ophthalmic	0.75%	5-15 mL	37.5-112.5 mg	Moderate to complete
Local infiltration	0.25%	60 mL	150 mg	Not applicable
Pain Management				
Levobupivacaine can be used epidurally with fentanyl or clonidine; dilutions for epidural administration should be made with preservative free 0.9% saline according to standard hospital procedures for sterility				
Labor analgesia (epidural bolus)	0.25%	10-20 mL	25-50 mg	Minimal to moderate
Postoperative pain (epidural infusion)	0.125%[1]-0.25%	4-10 mL/h	5-25 mg/h	Minimal to moderate

[1]0.125%: Adjunct therapy with fentanyl or clonidine.

Maximum dosage: Epidural doses up to 375 mg have been administered incrementally to patients during a surgical procedure.

Intraoperative block and postoperative pain: 695 mg in 24 hours

Postoperative epidural infusion over 24 hours: 570 mg

Single-fractionated injection for brachial plexus block: 300 mg

Administration

Other: Isopropyl or ethyl alcohol are recommended to disinfect the surface of the vial. Disinfectants containing heavy metals should not be used for mucous membrane disinfection since they have been related to incidents of swelling and edema. Prior to administration, it is essential that aspiration for blood or cerebrospinal fluid (where applicable) be performed prior to injecting any local anesthetic, both before the original dosage and at all subsequent doses (to avoid (Continued)

723

Levobupivacaine (Continued)

intravascular or intrathecal injection). A negative aspiration does not ensure against intrathecal or intravascular injection. Rapid injection of a large volume of local anesthetic solution should be avoided. Fractional (incremental) doses are recommended. Monitor patient during and after injection for symptoms of CNS or cardiac toxicity.

Stability

Compatibility: Stable in 0.9% NS USP. Stable for 24 hours in PVC bags at room temperature when diluted to 0.625-2.5 mg levobupivacaine per mL.

Incompatible with alkaline pH solutions (pH >8.5)

Storage: Store at room temperature (20°C to 25°C/68°F to 77°F). Disinfectants containing heavy metals should not be used for mucous membrane disinfection since they have been related to incidents of swelling and edema. Isopropyl or ethyl alcohol is recommended. Stability of solution in vial has been demonstrated following an autoclave cycle at 121°C for 15 minutes.

Nursing Actions

Physical Assessment: Monitor for effectiveness of anesthesia according to purpose for use. Monitor closely during and after injection for symptoms of CNS, cardiac toxicity, or hypotension. Monitor for return of sensation. Use appropriate patient safety measures until full return of sensation. Teach patient adverse symptoms to report.

Patient Education: This medication is given to reduce sensation and pain. You will experience decreased sensation to pain, heat, or cold in the area and/or decreased muscle strength (depending on area of application). Until sensation returns, use caution to prevent injury (eg, avoid extremes of heat or cold to area, do not use sharp objects, avoid driving, climbing stairs, or sudden moves if muscle strength is affected). Immediately report chest pain or palpitations; increased restlessness, anxiety, dizziness or lightheadedness; sensation of sudden muscle weakness; swelling or tingling of mouth or lips; metallic taste; vision changes or hearing. **Breast-feeding precaution:** Consult prescriber if breast-feeding.

Pregnancy Issues Local anesthetics rapidly cross the placenta and may cause varying degrees of maternal, fetal, and neonatal toxicity. Close maternal and fetal monitoring (heart rate and electronic fetal monitoring advised) are required during obstetrical use.

Levocabastine (LEE voe kab as teen)

U.S. Brand Names Livostin® [DSC]

Synonyms Levocabastine Hydrochloride

Pharmacologic Category Antihistamine, H₁ Blocker, Ophthalmic

Medication Safety Issues

Sound-alike/look-alike issues:

Levocabastine may be confused with levobunolol, levocarnitine

Livostin® may be confused with lovastatin

Pregnancy Risk Factor C

Use Treatment of allergic conjunctivitis

Contraindications Hypersensitivity to levocabastine any component of product; use while soft contact lenses are being worn

Warnings/Precautions Safety and efficacy in children <12 years of age have not been established. Not for injection. Not for use in patients wearing soft contact lenses during treatment.

Adverse Reactions

>10%: Local: Transient burning, stinging, discomfort

1% to 10%:

Central nervous system: Headache, somnolence, fatigue

Dermatologic: Rash

Gastrointestinal: Xerostomia

Ocular: Blurred vision, eye pain, somnolence, red eyes, eyelid edema

Respiratory: Dyspnea

Available Dosage Forms [DSC] = Discontinued product

Suspension, ophthalmic: 0.05% (5 mL, 10 mL) [contains benzalkonium chloride] [DSC]

Dosing

Adults & Elderly: Allergic conjunctivitis: Ophthalmic: Instill 1 drop in affected eye(s) 4 times/day for up to 2 weeks

Pediatrics: Children ≥12 years: Refer to adult dosing.

Nursing Actions

Physical Assessment: Assess potential for interactions with other prescriptions, OTC medications, or herbal products patient may be taking. Monitor patient response and adverse effects. Teach patient proper use, side effects/appropriate interventions, and symptoms to report.

Patient Education: For use in eyes only. Shake well before using. Do not let tip of applicator touch eye; do not contaminate tip of applicator (may cause eye infection, eye damage, or vision loss). Do not wear contact lenses during treatment. This medication may cause drowsiness in some patients. **Pregnancy precaution:** Inform prescriber if you are pregnant.

Levocarnitine (lee voe KAR ni teen)

U.S. Brand Names Carnitor®

Synonyms L-Carnitine

Pharmacologic Category Dietary Supplement

Medication Safety Issues

Sound-alike/look-alike issues:

Levocarnitine may be confused with levocabastine

Pregnancy Risk Factor B

Lactation Excretion in breast milk unknown/use caution

Use Orphan drug:

Oral: Primary systemic carnitine deficiency; acute and chronic treatment of patients with an inborn error of metabolism which results in secondary carnitine deficiency

I.V.: Acute and chronic treatment of patients with an inborn error of metabolism which results in secondary carnitine deficiency; prevention and treatment of carnitine deficiency in patients with end-stage renal disease (ESRD) who are undergoing hemodialysis.

Mechanism of Action/Effect Carnitine is a naturally occurring metabolic compound which facilitates energy production

Warnings/Precautions Caution in patients with seizure disorders or in those at risk of seizures (CNS mass or medications which may lower seizure threshold). Both new-onset seizure activity as well as an increased frequency of seizures has been observed. Safety and efficacy of oral carnitine have not been established in ESRD. Chronic administration of high oral doses to patients with severely compromised renal function or ESRD patients on dialysis may result in accumulation of metabolites.

Lab Interactions Normal carnitine levels are 40-50 μmol/L; levels should be maintained on therapy between 35-60 μmol/L. therapy between 35-60 μmol/L.

Adverse Reactions Frequencies noted with I.V. therapy (hemodialysis patients):

Cardiovascular: Hypertension (18% to 21%), peripheral edema (3% to 6%)

Central nervous system: Dizziness (10% to 18%), fever (5% to 12%), paresthesia (3% to 12%), depression (5% to 6%)

Endocrine & metabolic: Hypercalcemia (6% to 15%)

Gastrointestinal: Diarrhea (9% to 35%), abdominal pain (5% to 21%), vomiting (9% to 21%), nausea (5% to 12%)

Neuromuscular & skeletal: Weakness (9% to 12%)

Miscellaneous: Allergic reaction (2% to 6%)

Overdosage/Toxicology No reports of overdose. Easily removed by dialysis.

Pharmacodynamics/Kinetics

Time to Peak: Tablet/solution: 3.3 hours

Half-Life Elimination: 17.4 hours

Metabolism: Hepatic (limited with moderate renal impairment), to trimethylamine (TMA) and trimethylamine N-oxide (TMAO)

Excretion: Urine (4% to 9% as unchanged drug); metabolites also eliminated in urine

Available Dosage Forms

Capsule: 250 mg

Injection, solution (Carnitor®): 200 mg/mL (5 mL)

Solution, oral (Carnitor®): 100 mg/mL (118 mL) [cherry flavor]

Tablet: 500 mg

Carnitor®: 330 mg

Dosing

Adults & Elderly:

Carnitine supplementation: Oral: 990 mg (oral tablets) 2-3 times/day or 1-3 g/day (oral solution)

Metabolic disorders: I.V.: 50 mg/kg as a slow 2- to 3-minute I.V. bolus or by I.V. infusion

Severe metabolic crisis: I.V.:

Initial: A loading dose of 50 mg/kg over 2-3 minutes followed by an equivalent dose over the following 24 hours administered as every 3 hours or every 4 hours (never less than every 6 hours either by infusion or by intravenous injection)

Subsequent dosing: All subsequent daily doses are recommended to be in the range of 50 mg/kg or as therapy may require.

Maximum: The highest dose administered has been 300 mg/kg.

It is recommended that a plasma carnitine concentration be obtained prior to beginning parenteral therapy accompanied by weekly and monthly monitoring.

ESRD patients on hemodialysis: I.V.:

Predialysis levocarnitine concentrations below normal (40-50 μmol/L): 10-20 mg/kg dry body weight as a slow 2- to 3-minute bolus after each dialysis session

Adjustment: Dosage adjustments should be guided by predialysis trough levocarnitine concentrations and downward dose adjustments (to 5 mg/kg after dialysis) may be made as early as every 3rd or 4th week of therapy.

Pediatrics:

Carnitine supplementation:

Oral: Infants/Children: Initial: 50 mg/kg/day; titrate to 50-100 mg/kg/day in divided doses with a maximum dose of 3 g/day

I.V.: Refer to adult dosing.

Administration

Oral: Solution may be dissolved in either drink or liquid food. The oral solution should be consumed slowly and spaced evenly throughout the day to improve tolerance. Doses should be spaced every 3 to 4 hours throughout the day, preferably during or following meals.

I.V.: Hemodialysis patients: Injection should be given over 2-3 minutes into the venous return line after each dialysis session.

Stability

Storage: Store at 25°C (77°F). Compatible at concentrations between 0.5-8 mg/mL in 0.9% sodium chloride or lactated Ringer's solution. Stable in PVC bags for 24 hours.

Laboratory Monitoring Plasma concentrations should be obtained prior to beginning parenteral therapy, and should be monitored weekly to monthly. In metabolic disorders: monitor blood chemistry and plasma carnitine levels (maintain between 35-60 μmol/L). In ESRD patients on dialysis: Plasma levels below the normal range should prompt initiation of therapy. Monitor predialysis (trough) plasma carnitine levels.

Nursing Actions

Physical Assessment: Monitor therapeutic response (according to rationale for therapy) and adverse reactions (eg, CNS, hypertension). Oral: Monitor therapeutic response. Assess knowledge and teach patient appropriate use, interventions to reduce side effects, and adverse reactions to report.

Patient Education: I.V.: Report immediately any dizziness, loss of feeling, acute headache, tremors, or nausea.

Oral: Take exactly as directed; do not alter dose or frequency except as directed by prescriber. Dissolve solution in any liquid and drink with or following meals. The oral solution should be consumed slowly and spaced evenly throughout the day to improve tolerance. You may experience abdominal pain, nausea, or vomiting (small frequent meals, chewing gum, or sucking hard candy); diarrhea (yogurt, boiled milk, or buttermilk may help); or dizziness (use caution driving or engaging in hazardous activities until response to drug is known). Report acute headache, chest pain, tremors, or visual changes; muscle or skeletal weakness; skin rash; swelling of extremities; or other adverse effects. **Breast-feeding precaution:** Consult prescriber if breast-feeding.

Breast-Feeding Issues In breast-feeding women, use must be weighed against the potential exposure of the infant to increased carnitine intake. Use caution in breast-feeding women.

Additional Information Although supplemental carnitine has been shown to increase carnitine concentrations, effects on the signs and symptoms of carnitine deficiency have not been determined.

Levodopa and Carbidopa
(lee voe DOE pa & kar bi DOE pa)

U.S. Brand Names Parcopa™; Sinemet®; Sinemet® CR

Synonyms Carbidopa and Levodopa

Pharmacologic Category Anti-Parkinson's Agent, Dopamine Agonist

Pregnancy Risk Factor C

Lactation Excretion in breast milk unknown/use caution

Use Idiopathic Parkinson's disease; postencephalitic parkinsonism; symptomatic parkinsonism

Unlabeled/Investigational Use Restless leg syndrome

Mechanism of Action/Effect Parkinson's symptoms are due to a lack of striatal dopamine; levodopa circulates in the plasma to the blood-brain-barrier (BBB), where it crosses, to be converted by striatal enzymes to dopamine; carbidopa inhibits the peripheral plasma breakdown of levodopa by inhibiting its decarboxylation, and thereby increases available levodopa at the BBB

Contraindications Hypersensitivity to levodopa, carbidopa, or any component of the formulation; narrow-angle glaucoma; use of MAO inhibitors within prior 14 days (however, may be administered concomitantly with the manufacturer's recommended dose of an MAO inhibitor with selectivity for MAO type B); history of melanoma or undiagnosed skin lesions
(Continued)

Levodopa and Carbidopa (Continued)

Warnings/Precautions Use with caution in patients with history of cardiovascular disease (including myocardial infarction and arrhythmias); pulmonary diseases such as asthma, psychosis, wide-angle glaucoma, peptic ulcer disease; as well as in renal, hepatic, or endocrine disease. Sudden discontinuation of levodopa may cause a worsening of Parkinson's disease. Elderly may be more sensitive to CNS effects of levodopa. May cause or exacerbate dyskinesias. May cause orthostatic hypotension; Parkinson's disease patients appear to have an impaired capacity to respond to a postural challenge; use with caution in patients at risk of hypotension (such as those receiving antihypertensive drugs) or where transient hypotensive episodes would be poorly tolerated (cardiovascular disease or cerebrovascular disease). Observe patients closely for development of depression with concomitant suicidal tendencies. Has been associated with a syndrome resembling neuroleptic malignant syndrome on withdrawal or significant dosage reduction after long-term use. Protein in the diet should be distributed throughout the day to avoid fluctuations in levodopa absorption.

Drug Interactions

Decreased Effect: Antipsychotics, benzodiazepines, L-methionine, phenytoin, pyridoxine, spiramycin, and tacrine may inhibit the antiparkinsonian effects of levodopa; monitor for reduced effect. Antipsychotics may inhibit the antiparkinsonian effects of levodopa via dopamine receptor blockade. Use antipsychotics with low dopamine blockade (clozapine, olanzapine, quetiapine). High-protein diets may inhibit levodopa's efficacy; avoid high protein foods. Iron binds levodopa and reduces its bioavailability; separate doses of iron and levodopa.

Increased Effect/Toxicity: Concurrent use of levodopa with nonselective MAO inhibitors may result in hypertensive reactions via an increased storage and release of dopamine, norepinephrine, or both. Use with carbidopa to minimize reactions if combination is necessary; otherwise avoid combination.

Nutritional/Ethanol Interactions

Ethanol: Avoid ethanol (due to CNS depression).

Food: Avoid high protein diets and high intakes of vitamin B_6.

Herb/Nutraceutical: Avoid kava kava (may decrease effects). Pyridoxine in doses >10-25 mg (for levodopa alone) or higher doses >200 mg/day (for levodopa/carbidopa) may decrease efficacy.

Lab Interactions False-positive reaction for urinary glucose with Clinitest®; false-negative reaction using Clinistix®; false-positive urine ketones with Acetest®, Ketostix®, Labstix®

Adverse Reactions Frequency not defined.

Cardiovascular: Orthostatic hypotension, arrhythmia, chest pain, hypertension, syncope, palpitation, phlebitis

Central nervous system: Dizziness, anxiety, confusion, nightmares, headache, hallucinations, on-off phenomenon, decreased mental acuity, memory impairment, disorientation, delusions, euphoria, agitation, somnolence, insomnia, gait abnormalities, nervousness, ataxia, EPS, falling, psychosis, peripheral neuropathy, seizure (causal relationship not established)

Dermatologic: Rash, alopecia, malignant melanoma, hypersensitivity (angioedema, urticaria, pruritus, bullous lesions, Henoch-Schönlein purpura)

Endocrine & metabolic: Increased libido

Gastrointestinal: Anorexia, nausea, vomiting, constipation, GI bleeding, duodenal ulcer, diarrhea, dyspepsia, taste alterations, sialorrhea, heartburn

Genitourinary: Discoloration of urine, urinary frequency

Hematologic: Hemolytic anemia, agranulocytosis, thrombocytopenia, leukopenia; decreased hemoglobin and hematocrit; abnormalities in AST and ALT, LDH, bilirubin, BUN, Coombs' test

Neuromuscular & skeletal: Choreiform and involuntary movements, paresthesia, bone pain, shoulder pain, muscle cramps, weakness

Ocular: Blepharospasm, oculogyric crises (may be associated with acute dystonic reactions)

Renal: Difficult urination

Respiratory: Dyspnea, cough

Miscellaneous: Hiccups, discoloration of sweat, diaphoresis (increased)

Overdosage/Toxicology Symptoms of overdose include palpitations, arrhythmias, spasms; may cause hypertension or hypotension. Treatment is supportive. ECG monitoring is warranted. May precipitate a variety of arrhythmias.

Pharmacokinetic Note See individual agents.

Available Dosage Forms

Tablet immediate release (Sinemet®):
10/100: Carbidopa 10 mg and levodopa 100 mg
25/100: Carbidopa 25 mg and levodopa 100 mg
25/250: Carbidopa 25 mg and levodopa 250 mg

Tablet, immediate release, orally disintegrating (Parcopa™):
10/100: Carbidopa 10 mg and levodopa 100 mg [contains phenylalanine 3.4 mg/tablet; mint flavor]
25/100: Carbidopa 25 mg and levodopa 100 mg [contains phenylalanine 3.4 mg/tablet; mint flavor]
25/250: Carbidopa 25 mg and levodopa 250 mg [contains phenylalanine 8.4 mg/tablet; mint flavor]

Tablet, sustained release (Sinemet® CR):
Carbidopa 25 mg and levodopa 100 mg
Carbidopa 50 mg and levodopa 200 mg

Dosing

Adults:

Parkinson's disease: Oral: Initial:

Immediate release tablet:

Initial: Carbidopa 25 mg/levodopa 100 mg 3 times/day

Dosage adjustment: Alternate tablet strengths may be substituted according to individual carbidopa/levodopa requirements. Increase by 1 tablet every other day as necessary, except when using the carbidopa 25 mg/levodopa 250 mg tablets where increases should be made using 1/2-1 tablet every 1-2 days. Use of more than 1 dosage strength or dosing 4 times/day may be required (maximum: 8 tablets of any strength/day or 200 mg of carbidopa and 2000 mg of levodopa)

Sustained release tablet:

Initial: Carbidopa 50 mg/levodopa 200 mg 2 times/day, at intervals not <6 hours

Dosage adjustment: May adjust every 3 days; intervals should be between 4-8 hours during the waking day (maximum: 8 tablets/day)

Restless leg syndrome (unlabeled use): Oral: Carbidopa 25 mg/levodopa 100 mg given 30-60 minutes before bedtime; may repeat dose once

Elderly: Initial dose: 25/100 twice daily, increase as necessary. Sinemet® CR may be used as initial therapy.

Administration

Oral: Space doses evenly over the waking hours. Give with meals to decrease GI upset. Sustained release product should not be crushed. Orally-disintegrating tablets do not require water; the tablet should disintegrate on the tongue's surface before swallowing.

Stability

Storage: Store at 20°C to 25°C (68°F to 77°F); excursions are allowed between 15°C to 30°C (59°F to 86°F). Protect from light and moisture.

Nursing Actions

Physical Assessment: Assess effectiveness and interactions of other medications patient may be taking. Monitor therapeutic response (eg, mental status, involuntary movements), and adverse reactions (including levodopa toxicity) at beginning of therapy and periodically throughout therapy. Assess knowledge/teach patient appropriate use, interventions to reduce side effects, and adverse symptoms to report.

Patient Education: Take exactly as directed; do not change dosage or discontinue without consulting prescriber. Do not crush sustained release form. Therapeutic effects may take several weeks or months to achieve and you may need frequent monitoring during first weeks of therapy. Take with meals if GI upset occurs, before meals if dry mouth occurs, after eating if drooling or if nausea occurs. Take at the same time each day. Maintain adequate hydration (2-3 L/day of fluids) unless instructed to restrict fluid intake; void before taking medication. Do not use alcohol and prescription or OTC sedatives or CNS depressants without consulting prescriber. Urine or perspiration may appear darker. You may experience drowsiness, dizziness, confusion, or vision changes (use caution when driving, climbing stairs, or engaging in tasks requiring alertness until response to drug is known); orthostatic hypotension (use caution when changing position - rising to standing from sitting or lying); increased susceptibility to heat stroke, decreased perspiration (use caution in hot weather - maintain adequate fluids and reduce exercise activity); constipation (increased exercise, fluids, fruit, or fiber may help); dry skin or nasal passages (consult prescriber for appropriate relief); or nausea, vomiting, loss of appetite, or stomach discomfort (small frequent meals, frequent mouth care, chewing gum, or sucking lozenges may help). Report unresolved constipation or vomiting; chest pain or irregular heartbeat; respiratory difficulty; acute headache or dizziness; CNS changes (hallucination, loss of memory, nervousness, etc); painful or difficult urination; abdominal pain or blood in stool; increased muscle spasticity or rigidity; skin rash; or significant worsening of condition. **Pregnancy/breast-feeding precautions:** Inform prescriber if you are or intend to become pregnant. Consult prescriber if breast-feeding.

Dietary Considerations Levodopa peak serum concentrations may be decreased if taken with food. High protein diets (>2 g/kg) may decrease the efficacy of levodopa via competition with amino acids in crossing the blood-brain barrier.

Parcopa™: Contains phenylalanine 3.4 mg per 10/100 mg and 25/100 mg strengths; phenylalanine 8.4 mg in 25/250 mg strength

Geriatric Considerations The elderly may be more sensitive to the CNS effects of levodopa.

Additional Information 50-100 mg/day of carbidopa is needed to block the peripheral conversion of levodopa to dopamine. "On-off" (a clinical syndrome characterized by sudden periods of drug activity/inactivity), can be managed by giving smaller, more frequent doses of Sinemet® or adding a dopamine agonist or selegiline; when adding a new agent, doses of Sinemet® can usually be decreased. Protein in the diet should be distributed throughout the day to avoid fluctuations in levodopa absorption. Levodopa is the drug of choice when rigidity is the predominant presenting symptom.

Conversion from levodopa to carbidopa/levodopa: **Note:** Levodopa must be discontinued at least 12 hours prior to initiation of levodopa/carbidopa:

Initial dose: Levodopa portion of carbidopa/levodopa should be at least 25% of previous levodopa therapy.

Levodopa <1500 mg/day: Sinemet® or Parcopa™ (levodopa 25 mg/carbidopa 100 mg) 3-4 times/day

Levodopa ≥1500 mg/day: Sinemet® or Parcopa™ (levodopa 25 mg/carbidopa 250 mg) 3-4 times/day

Conversion from immediate release carbidopa/levodopa (Sinemet® or Parcopa™) to Sinemet® CR (50/200):

Sinemet® or Parcopa™ [total daily dose of levodopa]/Sinemet® CR:

Sinemet® or Parcopa™ (levodopa 300-400 mg/day): Sinemet® CR (50/200) 1 tablet twice daily

Sinemet® or Parcopa™ (levodopa 500-600 mg/day): Sinemet® CR (50/200) 1 1/2 tablets twice daily or 1 tablet 3 times/day

Sinemet® or Parcopa™ (levodopa 700-800 mg/day): Sinemet® CR (50/200) 4 tablets in 3 or more divided doses

Sinemet® or Parcopa™ (levodopa 900-1000 mg/day): Sinemet® CR (50/200) 5 tablets in 3 or more divided doses

Intervals between doses of Sinemet® CR should be 4-8 hours while awake; when divided doses are not equal, smaller doses should be given toward the end of the day,

---

Levodopa, Carbidopa, and Entacapone
(lee voe DOE pa, kar bi DOE pa, & en TA ka pone)

U.S. Brand Names Stalevo™

Synonyms Carbidopa, Levodopa, and Entacapone; Entacapone, Carbidopa, and Levodopa

Pharmacologic Category Anti-Parkinson's Agent, COMT Inhibitor; Anti-Parkinson's Agent, Dopamine Agonist

Pregnancy Risk Factor C

Lactation Excretion in breast milk unknown/use caution

Use Treatment of idiopathic Parkinson's disease

Available Dosage Forms Tablet:

50: Carbidopa 12.5 mg, levodopa 50 mg, and entacapone 200 mg

100: Carbidopa 25 mg, levodopa 100 mg, and entacapone 200 mg

150: Carbidopa 37.5 mg, levodopa 150 mg, and entacapone 200 mg

Dosing

Adults & Elderly:

Note: All strengths of Stalevo™ contain a carbidopa/levodopa ratio of 1:4 plus entacapone 200 mg.

Parkinson's disease: Oral: Dose should be individualized based on therapeutic response; doses may be adjusted by changing strength or adjusting interval. Fractionated doses are not recommended and only 1 tablet should be given at each dosing interval; maximum dose: 8 tablets/day (equivalent to entacapone 1600 mg/day)

Patients previously treated with carbidopa/levodopa immediate release tablets (ratio of 1:4):

With current entacapone therapy: May switch directly to corresponding strength of combination tablet. No data available on transferring patients from controlled release preparations or products with a 1:10 ratio of carbidopa/levodopa.

Without entacapone therapy:

If current levodopa dose is >600 mg/day: Levodopa dose reduction may be required when adding entacapone to therapy; therefore, titrate dose using individual products first (carbidopa/levodopa immediate release with a ratio of 1:4 plus entacapone 200 mg); then transfer to combination product once stabilized.

If current levodopa dose is <600 mg without dyskinesias: May transfer to corresponding dose of combination product; monitor, dose reduction of levodopa may be required.

Renal Impairment: Use caution with severe renal impairment; specific dosing recommendations not available.

Hepatic Impairment: Use with caution; specific dosing recommendations not available.
(Continued)

Levodopa, Carbidopa, and Entacapone
(Continued)

Nursing Actions
Physical Assessment: See individual agents.
Patient Education: See individual agents. **Pregnancy/breast-feeding precautions:** Inform prescriber if you are or intend to become pregnant. Consult prescriber if breast-feeding.

Related Information
Entacapone *on page 425*

Levofloxacin (lee voe FLOKS a sin)

U.S. Brand Names Iquix®; Levaquin®; Quixin™
Pharmacologic Category Antibiotic, Quinolone
Pregnancy Risk Factor C
Lactation Excretion in breast milk unknown/not recommended

Use
Systemic: Treatment of mild, moderate, or severe infections caused by susceptible organisms. Includes the treatment of community-acquired pneumonia, including multidrug resistant strains of *S. pneumoniae* (MDRSP); nosocomial pneumonia; chronic bronchitis (acute bacterial exacerbation); acute bacterial sinusitis; urinary tract infection (uncomplicated or complicated), including acute pyelonephritis caused by *E. coli*; prostatitis (chronic bacterial); skin or skin structure infections (uncomplicated or complicated); prevention of inhalational anthrax (postexposure)
Ophthalmic: Treatment of bacterial conjunctivitis caused by susceptible organisms (Quixin™ 0.5% ophthalmic solution); treatment of corneal ulcer caused by susceptible organisms (Iquix® 1.5% ophthalmic solution)

Unlabeled/Investigational Use Diverticulitis, enterocolitis, (*Shigella* sp), gonococcal infections, Legionnaires' disease, peritonitis, PID

Mechanism of Action/Effect Levofloxacin, a fluorinated quinolone, is a pyridine carboxylic acid derivative which exerts a broad spectrum bactericidal effect. It inhibits DNA gyrase inhibitor, an essential bacterial enzyme that maintains the superhelical structure of DNA. DNA gyrase is required for DNA replication and transcription, DNA repair, recombination, and transposition within the bacteria.

Contraindications Hypersensitivity to levofloxacin, any component of the formulation, or other quinolones

Warnings/Precautions Systemic: Not recommended in children <18 years of age; CNS stimulation may occur (tremor, restlessness, confusion, and very rarely hallucinations or seizures); use with caution in patients with known or suspected CNS disorders or renal dysfunction; use caution to avoid possible photosensitivity reactions during and for several days following fluoroquinolone therapy

Rare cases of torsade de pointes have been reported in patients receiving levofloxacin. Risk may be minimized by avoiding use in patients with known prolongation of QT interval, bradycardia, hypokalemia, hypomagnesemia, cardiomyopathy, or in those receiving concurrent therapy with Class Ia or Class III antiarrhythmics.

Severe hypersensitivity reactions, including anaphylaxis, have occurred with quinolone therapy. If an allergic reaction occurs (itching, urticaria, dyspnea or facial edema, loss of consciousness, tingling, cardiovascular collapse), discontinue drug immediately. Prolonged use may result in superinfection; pseudomembranous colitis may occur and should be considered in all patients who present with diarrhea. Tendon inflammation and/or rupture has been reported; risk may be increased with concurrent corticosteroids, particularly in the elderly. Discontinue at first sign of tendon inflammation or pain. Peripheral neuropathies have been linked to levofloxacin use; discontinue if numbness, tingling, or weakness develops. Quinolones may exacerbate myasthenia gravis.

Ophthalmic solution: For topical use only. Do not inject subconjunctivally or introduce into anterior chamber of the eye. Contact lenses should not be worn during treatment for bacterial conjunctivitis. Safety and efficacy in children <1 year of age (Quixin™) or <6 years of age (Iquix®) have not been established. **Note:** Indications for ophthalmic solutions are product concentration-specific and should not be used interchangeably.

Drug Interactions
Decreased Effect: Concurrent administration of metal cations, including most antacids, oral electrolyte supplements, quinapril, sucralfate, some didanosine formulations (chewable/buffered tablets and pediatric powder for oral suspension), and other highly-buffered oral drugs, may decrease quinolone levels; separate doses.
Increased Effect/Toxicity: Levofloxacin may increase the effects/toxicity of glyburide and warfarin. Concomitant use with corticosteroids may increase the risk of tendon rupture. Concomitant use with other QT_c-prolonging agents (eg, Class Ia and Class III antiarrhythmics, erythromycin, cisapride, antipsychotics, and cyclic antidepressants) may result in arrhythmias, such as torsade de pointes. Probenecid may increase levofloxacin levels.

Lab Interactions Some quinolones may produce a false-positive urine screening result for opiates using commercially-available immunoassay kits. This has been demonstrated most consistently for levofloxacin and ofloxacin, but other quinolones have shown cross-reactivity in certain assay kits. Confirmation of positive opiate screens by more specific methods should be considered.

Adverse Reactions 1% to 10%:
Cardiovascular: Chest pain (1%)
Central nervous system: Headache (6%), insomnia (5%), dizziness (2%), fatigue (1%), pain (1%), fever
Dermatologic: Pruritus (1%), rash (1%)
Gastrointestinal: Nausea (7%), diarrhea (5%), abdominal pain (3%), constipation (3%), dyspepsia (2%), vomiting (2%), flatulence (1%)
Genitourinary: Vaginitis (1%)
Hematologic: Lymphopenia (2%)
Ocular (with ophthalmic solution use): Decreased vision (transient), foreign body sensation, transient ocular burning, ocular pain or discomfort, photophobia
Respiratory: Pharyngitis (4%), dyspnea (1%), rhinitis (1%), sinusitis (1%)

Overdosage/Toxicology
Symptoms of overdose include acute renal failure, seizures
Treatment should include GI decontamination and supportive care; not removed by peritoneal or hemodialysis

Pharmacodynamics/Kinetics
Time to Peak: 1-2 hours
Protein Binding: 50%
Half-Life Elimination: 6-8 hours
Metabolism: Minimally hepatic
Excretion: Primarily urine (as unchanged drug)

Available Dosage Forms
Infusion [premixed in D_5W] (Levaquin®): 250 mg (50 mL); 500 mg (100 mL); 750 mg (150 mL)
Injection, solution [preservative free] (Levaquin®): 25 mg/mL (20 mL, 30 mL)
Solution, ophthalmic:
Iquix®: 1.5% (5 mL)
Quixin™: 0.5% (5 mL) [contains benzalkonium chloride]
Solution, oral (Levaquin®): 25 mg/mL (480 mL) [contains benzyl alcohol]

Tablet (Levaquin®): 250 mg, 500 mg, 750 mg
Levaquin® Leva-Pak: 750 mg (5s)

Dosing

Adults & Elderly: Note: Sequential therapy (intravenous to oral) may be instituted based on prescriber's discretion.

Anthrax (inhalational): 500 mg every 24 hours for 60 days, beginning as soon as possible after exposure

Chronic bronchitis (acute bacterial exacerbation):
Oral, I.V.: 500 mg every 24 hours for at least 7 days

Conjunctivitis (0.5% ophthalmic solution):
Ophthalmic:
Treatment day 1 and day 2: Instill 1-2 drops into affected eye(s) every 2 hours while awake, up to 8 times/day
Treatment day 3 through day 7: Instill 1-2 drops into affected eye(s) every 4 hours while awake, up to 4 times/day

Corneal ulceration (1.5% ophthalmic solution):
Ophthalmic: Treatment day 1 through day 3: Instill 1-2 drops into affected eye(s) every 30 minutes to 2 hours while awake and 4-6 hours after retiring.

Diverticulitis, peritonitis (unlabeled use): Oral, I.V.: 750 mg every 24 hours for 7-10 days; use adjunctive metronidazole therapy

Dysenteric enterocolitis, *Shigella spp.* (unlabeled use): Oral, I.V.: 500 mg every 24 hours for 3-5 days

Gonococcal infection (unlabeled use): Oral, I.V.:
Cervicitis, urethritis: 250 mg for one dose with azithromycin or doxycycline
Disseminated infection: 250 mg I.V. once daily; 24 hours after symptoms improve may change to 500 mg orally every 24 hours to complete total therapy of 7 days
Epididymo-orchitis: 750 mg once daily for 10-14 days

Legionella (unlabeled use): Oral, I.V.: 500 mg every 24 hours for 10-21 days or 750 mg every 24 hours for 5 days

Pelvic inflammatory disease (unlabeled use): Oral, I.V.: 500 mg every 24 hours for 14 days with adjunctive metronidazole

Pneumonia: Oral, I.V.:
Community-acquired: 500 mg every 24 hours for 7-14 days or 750 mg every 24 hours for 5 days (efficacy of 5-day regimen for MDRSP not established)
Nosocomial: 750 mg every 24 hours for 7-14 days

Prostatitis (chronic bacterial): Oral, I.V.: 500 mg every 24 hours for 28 days

Sinusitis (bacterial acute): Oral, I.V.: 500 mg every 24 hours for 10-14 days or 750 mg every 24 hours for 5 days

Skin and skin structure infections: Oral, I.V.:
Uncomplicated: 500 mg every 24 hours for 7-10 days
Complicated: 750 mg every 24 hours for 7-14 days

Traveler's diarrhea (unlabeled use): Oral, I.V.: 500 mg for one dose

Urinary tract infections: Oral, I.V.:
Uncomplicated: 250 mg once daily for 3 days
Complicated, including acute pyelonephritis: 250 mg every 24 hours for 10 days

Pediatrics: Not approved for systemic use in children.
Conjunctivitis (bacterial): Ophthalmic: Children ≥1 year: Refer to adult dosing.
Corneal ulceration: Ophthalmic: Children ≥6 years: Refer to adult dosing.

Renal Impairment:
Chronic bronchitis, acute bacterial sinusitis, uncomplicated skin infection, community-acquired pneumonia, chronic bacterial prostatitis, or inhalational anthrax: Initial: 500 mg, then as follows:
Cl$_{cr}$ 20-49 mL/minute: 250 mg every 24 hours
Cl$_{cr}$ 10-19 mL/minute: 250 mg every 48 hours
Hemodialysis/CAPD: 250 mg every 48 hours
Uncomplicated UTI: No dosage adjustment required

Complicated UTI, acute pyelonephritis: Cl$_{cr}$ 10-19 mL/minute: 250 mg every 48 hours

Complicated skin infection, acute bacterial sinusitis, community-acquired pneumonia, or nosocomial pneumonia: Initial: 750 mg, then as follows:
Cl$_{cr}$ 20-49 mL/minute: 750 mg every 48 hours
Cl$_{cr}$ 10-19 mL/minute: 500 mg every 48 hours
Hemodialysis/CAPD: 500 mg every 48 hours

Administration

Oral: Tablets may be administered without regard to meals. Oral solution should be administered 1 hour before or 2 hours after meals.

I.V.: Infuse 250-500 mg I.V. solution over 60 minutes; infuse 750 mg I.V. solution over 90 minutes. Too rapid of infusion can lead to hypotension. Avoid administration through an intravenous line with a solution containing multivalent cations (eg, magnesium, calcium).

I.V. Detail: pH: 3.8-5.8

Stability

Reconstitution: Solution for injection: Single-use vials must be further diluted in compatible solution to a final concentration of 5 mg/mL prior to infusion.

Compatibility: Stable in D$_5$LR, D$_5$NS, D$_5$½NS with 0.15% KCl, D$_5$W, NS, Plasma-Lyte® 56/5% dextrose, sodium lactate (M/6); **incompatible** with mannitol 20%, sodium bicarbonate 5%

Y-site administration: Incompatible with acyclovir, alprostadil, furosemide, heparin, indomethacin, nitroglycerin, sodium nitroprusside

Storage:
Solution for injection:
Vial: Store at room temperature; protect from light. Diluted solution is stable for 72 hours when stored at room temperature; stable for 14 days when stored under refrigeration. When frozen, stable for 6 months; do not refreeze. Do not thaw in microwave or by bath immersion.
Premixed: Store at ≤25°C (77°F); brief exposure to 40°C (104°F) does not affect product; protect from freezing and light.
Tablet, oral solution: Store at 25°C (77°F); excursions permitted to 15°C to 25°C (59°F to 77°F).
Ophthalmic solution: Store at 15°C to 25°C (59°F to 77°F).

Laboratory Monitoring Perform culture and sensitivity studies prior to initiating drug therapy. Monitor CBC periodically during therapy. Monitor renal or hepatic function if therapy is prolonged.

Nursing Actions

Physical Assessment: Results of culture and sensitivity tests and patient's allergy history should be assessed before initiating therapy. Assess potential for interactions with other pharmacological or herbal agents patient may be taking (eg, increased risk of tendon rupture or arrhythmias). See Administration for infusion specifics. Monitor patient closely; if an allergic reaction occurs (itching, urticaria, dyspnea or facial edema, loss of consciousness, tingling, cardiovascular collapse) drug should be discontinued immediately and prescriber notified. Monitor laboratory tests, therapeutic effectiveness (resolution of infection), and adverse reactions (eg, hypersensitivity reaction, diarrhea, opportunistic infection, tendon rupture) regularly during therapy. Teach patient proper use (according to formulation), possible side effects/appropriate interventions, and adverse symptoms to report.

Patient Education: Do not take any new medication during therapy unless approved by prescriber. **Pregnancy/breast-feeding precautions:** Inform prescriber if you are or intend to become pregnant. Breast-feeding is not recommended.

I.V.: Report immediately any chest or back pain, tightness in chest, difficulty swallowing, swelling of face or mouth, or redness, swelling or pain at infusion site. May cause dizziness, lightheadedness, or confusion (Continued)

Levofloxacin *(Continued)*

(use caution to avoid falls or injury); nausea or vomiting (request antiemetic from prescriber). Report any tendon pain, chest pain or palpitations, or other adverse reactions.

Oral: Take exactly as directed; at least 1 hour before or 2 hours after antacids or other drug products containing calcium, iron, or zinc. Take entire prescription even if feeling better. Maintain adequate hydration (2-3 L/day of fluids) unless advised by prescriber to restrict fluid intake. May cause dizziness, lightheadedness, or confusion (use caution when driving or engaging in tasks that require alertness until response to drug is known); nausea or vomiting (small frequent meals, frequent mouth care, sucking lozenges, or chewing gum may help); or photosensitivity (use sunscreen, wear protective clothing and eyewear, and avoid direct sunlight). Discontinue use immediately and report to prescriber if inflammation, tendon pain, or allergic reaction occurs (itching urticaria, respiratory difficulty, facial edema, difficulty swallowing, loss of consciousness, tingling, chest pain, palpitations). Report persistent diarrhea or constipation; signs of infection (unusual fever or chills); vaginal itching or foul-smelling vaginal discharge; or easy bruising or bleeding.

Ophthalmic: Wash hands before instilling solution. Sit or lie down to instill. Open eye, look at ceiling, and instill prescribed amount of solution. Close eye and roll eye in all directions, and apply gentle pressure to inner corner of eye. Do not let tip of applicator touch eye; do not contaminate tip of applicator (may cause eye infection, eye damage, or vision loss). Temporary stinging or blurred vision may occur. Report persistent pain, burning, vision changes, swelling, itching, or worsening of condition. Discontinue medication and contact prescriber immediately if you develop a rash or allergic reaction. Do not wear contact lenses.

Dietary Considerations Tablets may be taken without regard to meals. Oral solution should be administered on an empty stomach (1 hour before or 2 hours after a meal).

Geriatric Considerations The risk of torsade de pointes and tendon inflammation and/or rupture associated with the concomitant use of corticosteroids and quinolones is increased in the elderly population. Adjust dose for renal function.

Breast-Feeding Issues Other quinolones are known to be excreted in breast milk. Based on data from ofloxacin, excretion of levofloxacin would be expected. The manufacturer recommends to discontinue nursing or to discontinue levofloxacin.

Pregnancy Issues Reports of arthropathy (observed in immature animals and reported rarely in humans) have limited the use of fluoroquinolones in pregnancy. Teratogenic effects were not observed with levofloxacin in animal studies; however, decreased body weight and increased fetal mortality were reported. Based on limited data, quinolones are not expected to be a major human teratogen. Although quinolone antibiotics should not be used as first-line agents during pregnancy, when considering treatment for life-threatening infection and/or prolonged duration of therapy, the potential risk to the fetus must be balanced against the severity of the potential illness.

Levonorgestrel *(LEE voe nor jes trel)*

U.S. Brand Names Mirena®; Plan B®
Synonyms LNg 20
Pharmacologic Category Contraceptive; Progestin
Pregnancy Risk Factor X
Lactation Enters breast milk/use caution (AAP rates "compatible")
Use Prevention of pregnancy
Mechanism of Action/Effect Ovulation is inhibited and an insufficient luteal phase has also been demonstrated with levonorgestrel administration.
Contraindications Hypersensitivity to levonorgestrel or any component of the formulation; undiagnosed abnormal uterine bleeding, active hepatic disease or malignant tumors, active thrombophlebitis, or thromboembolic disorders (current or history of), known or suspected carcinoma of the breast; history of intracranial hypertension; renal impairment; pregnancy

Additional product-specific contraindications: Intra-uterine system: Congenital or acquired uterine anomaly, acute pelvic inflammatory disease, history of pelvic inflammatory disease (unless there has been a subsequent intrauterine pregnancy), postpartum endometritis, infected abortion within past 3 months, known or suspected uterine or cervical neoplasia, unresolved/abnormal Pap smear, untreated acute cervicitis or vaginitis, patient or partner with multiple sexual partners, conditions which increase susceptibility to infections (ie, leukemia, AIDS, I.V. drug abuse), unremoved IUD, history of ectopic pregnancy, conditions which predispose to ectopic pregnancy

Warnings/Precautions Menstrual bleeding patterns may be altered, missed menstrual periods should not be used to identify early pregnancy. These products do not protect against HIV infection or other sexually-transmitted diseases. Patients presenting with lower abdominal pain should be evaluated for follicular atresia and ectopic pregnancy. Patients receiving enzyme-inducing medications should be evaluated for an alternative method of contraception. Levonorgestrel may affect glucose tolerance, monitor serum glucose in patients with diabetes. Safety and efficacy for use in renal or hepatic impairment have not been established. Use with caution in conditions that may be aggravated by fluid retention, depression, or history of migraine. Only for use in women of reproductive age.

Use of combination hormonal contraceptives increases the risk of cardiovascular side effects in women who smoke cigarettes, especially those who are >35 years of age; although this may be an estrogen-related effect, the risk with progestin-only contraceptives is not known and women should be strongly advised not to smoke. Combination hormonal contraceptives may lead to increased risk of myocardial infarction and should be used with caution in patients with risk factors for coronary artery disease; the actual risk with progestin-only contraceptives is not known, however, there have been postmarketing reports of myocardial infarction in women using levonorgestrel-only contraception. May increase the risk of thromboembolism; discontinue therapy if this occurs. Combination hormonal contraceptives may have a dose-related risk of vascular disease and hypertension; strokes have also been reported with postmarketing use of levonorgestrel-only contraception. Women with hypertension should be encouraged to use a nonhormonal form of contraception. The use of combination hormonal contraceptives has been associated with a slight increase in frequency of breast cancer (studies are not consistent); studies with progestin only contraceptives have been similar. Retinal thrombosis has been reported (rarely) with combination hormonal contraceptives and may be related to the estrogen component, however, progestin-only therapy should also be discontinued with unexplained partial or complete loss of vision.

Additional formulation-specific warnings:

Intrauterine system: Increased incidence of group A streptococcal sepsis and pelvic inflammatory disease (may be asymptomatic); may perforate uterus or cervix; risk of perforation is increased in lactating women; partial penetration or embedment in the myometrium may decrease effectiveness and lead to difficult removal; postpartum insertion should be delayed until uterine involution is complete; use caution in patients with coagulopathy or receiving anticoagulants

Oral tablet: Not intended to be used for routine contraception and will not terminate an existing pregnancy

Drug Interactions

Cytochrome P450 Effect: Substrate of CYP3A4 (major)

Decreased Effect: CYP3A4 inducers may decrease the levels/effects of levonorgestrel; example inducers include aminoglutethimide, carbamazepine, nafcillin, nevirapine, phenobarbital, phenytoin, and rifamycins.

Nutritional/Ethanol Interactions Herb/Nutraceutical: St John's wort (an enzyme inducer) may decrease serum levels of levonorgestrel.

Lab Interactions Increased triiodothyronine uptake; decreased concentrations of sex hormone-binding globulin, thyroxine concentrations (slight)

Adverse Reactions

Intrauterine system:

>5%:

Cardiovascular: Hypertension

Central nervous system: Headache, depression, nervousness

Dermatologic: Acne

Endocrine & metabolic: Breast pain, dysmenorrhea, decreased libido, abnormal Pap smear, amenorrhea (20% at 1 year), enlarged follicles (12%)

Gastrointestinal: Abdominal pain, nausea, weight gain

Genitourinary: Leukorrhea, vaginitis

Neuromuscular & skeletal: Back pain

Respiratory: Upper respiratory tract infection, sinusitis

<3% and postmarketing reports: Alopecia, anemia, cervicitis, dyspareunia, eczema, failed insertion, migraine, sepsis, vomiting

Oral tablets:

>10%:

Central nervous system: Fatigue (17%), headache (17%), dizziness (11%)

Endocrine & metabolic: Heavier menstrual bleeding (14%), lighter menstrual bleeding (12%), breast tenderness (11%)

Gastrointestinal: Nausea (23%), abdominal pain (18%)

1% to 10%: Gastrointestinal: Vomiting (6%), diarrhea (5%)

Overdosage/Toxicology Can result if >6 capsules are *in situ*. Symptoms include uterine bleeding irregularities and fluid retention.

Pharmacodynamics/Kinetics

Duration of Action: Intrauterine system: Up to 5 years

Protein Binding: Highly bound to albumin and sex hormone-binding globulin

Half-Life Elimination: Oral tablet: ~24 hours

Metabolism: To inactive metabolites

Excretion: Primarily urine

Available Dosage Forms

Intrauterine device (Mirena®): 52 mg levonorgestrel/unit [releases levonorgestrel 20 mcg/day]

Tablet (Plan B®): 0.75 mg

Dosing

Adults & Elderly: Females:

Long-term prevention of pregnancy: Intrauterine system (Mirena®): To be inserted into uterine cavity; should be inserted within 7 days of onset of menstruation or immediately after 1st trimester abortion. Releases 20 mcg levonorgestrel/day over 5 years. May be removed and replaced with a new unit at anytime during menstrual cycle. Do not leave any one system in place for >5 years.

Emergency contraception: Oral tablet (Plan B™): One 0.75 mg tablet as soon as possible within 72 hours of unprotected sexual intercourse. A second 0.75 mg tablet should be taken 12 hours after the first dose; may be used at any time during menstrual cycle.

Administration

Other: Intrauterine system: Inserted in the uterine cavity, to a depth of 6-9 cm, with the provided insertion device; should not be forced into the uterus

Stability

Storage: Store at room temperature of 25°C (77°F).

Nursing Actions

Physical Assessment: Monitor for prolonged menstrual bleeding, amenorrhea, irregularity of menses, and other adverse effects. Caution patient about need for annual medical exams. **Pregnancy risk factor X.**

Patient Education: This drug does not protect against HIV infection or other sexually-transmitted diseases. Cigarette smoking is not recommended. You may experience cramping, headache, abdominal discomfort, hair loss, weight changes, or unusual menses (breakthrough bleeding, irregularity, excessive bleeding). Report sudden acute headache or visual disturbance, unusual nausea or vomiting, any loss of feeling in arms or legs, or lower abdominal pain. **Pregnancy/breast-feeding precautions:** Inform prescriber if you are pregnant. Consult prescriber if breast-feeding

Intrauterine system: This method provides up to 5 years of birth control from a T-shaped device inserted into the uterus. It will be inserted and removed by your prescriber. Notify your prescriber if the system comes out by itself, if you have long-lasting or heavy bleeding, unusual vaginal discharge, low abdominal pain, painful sexual intercourse, chills or fever. There is an increased risk of ectopic pregnancy with this product. Thread placement should be checked following each menstrual cycle; do not pull thread.

Tablet: This method provides emergency contraception. It is used after your normal form of birth control has failed, or following unprotected sexual intercourse. It should be used within 72 hours. Contact prescriber if you vomit within 1 hour of taking either dose.

Breast-Feeding Issues Enters breast milk (infant serum levels of ~7% have been found when using the intrauterine system, 1% to 6% with the oral tablets), use caution; not considered contraception method of first choice for breast-feeding women (AAP considers **compatible** with breast-feeding)

Pregnancy Issues Epidemiologic studies have not shown an increased risk of birth defects when used prior to pregnancy or inadvertently during early pregnancy, although rare reports of congenital anomalies have been reported.

Intrauterine system: Women who become pregnant with an IUD in place risk septic abortion (septic shock and death may occur), removal of IUD may result in pregnancy loss. In addition, miscarriage, premature labor, and premature delivery may occur if pregnancy is continued with IUD in place.

Additional Information Intrauterine system: The cumulative 5-year pregnancy rate is ~0.7 pregnancies/100 users. Over 70% of women in the trials had previously used IUDs. The reported pregnancy rate after 12 months was ≤0.2 pregnancies/100 users. Approximately 80% of women who wish to conceive have become pregnant within 12 months of device removal. The (Continued)

Levonorgestrel *(Continued)*

recommended patient profile for this product: A woman who has at least one child, is in a stable and mutually-monogamous relationship, no history of pelvic inflammatory disease, and no history of ectopic pregnancy or predisposition to ectopic pregnancy.

Oral tablet: When used as directed for emergency contraception, the expected pregnancy rate is decreased from 8% to 1%. Approximately 87% of women have their next menstrual period at approximately the expected time. A rapid return to fertility following use is expected.

Levorphanol *(lee VOR fa nole)*

U.S. Brand Names Levo-Dromoran®
Synonyms Levorphanol Tartrate; Levorphan Tartrate
Restrictions C-II
Pharmacologic Category Analgesic, Narcotic
Pregnancy Risk Factor B/D (prolonged use or high doses at term)
Lactation Excretion in breast milk unknown/not recommended
Use Relief of moderate to severe pain; also used parenterally for preoperative sedation and an adjunct to nitrous oxide/oxygen anesthesia
Mechanism of Action/Effect Levorphanol tartrate is a synthetic opioid agonist that is classified as a morphinan derivative. Opioids interact with stereospecific opioid receptors in various parts of the central nervous system and other tissues.
Contraindications Hypersensitivity to levorphanol or any component of the formulation; pregnancy (prolonged use or high doses at term)
Warnings/Precautions An opioid-containing analgesic regimen should be tailored to each patient's needs and based upon the type of pain being treated (acute versus chronic), the route of administration, degree of tolerance for opioids (naive versus chronic user), age, weight, and medical condition. The optimal analgesic dose varies widely among patients. Doses should be titrated to pain relief/prevention.

Use with caution in patients with hypersensitivity reactions to other phenanthrene derivative opioid agonists (morphine, hydrocodone, hydromorphone, levorphanol, oxycodone, oxymorphone); respiratory diseases including asthma, emphysema, COPD, or severe liver or renal insufficiency. Some preparations contain sulfites which may cause allergic reactions. May be habit-forming. Dextromethorphan has equivalent antitussive activity but has much lower toxicity in accidental overdose. Elderly may be particularly susceptible to the CNS depressant and constipating effects of narcotics.

Drug Interactions
Increased Effect/Toxicity: CNS depression is enhanced with coadministration of other CNS depressants.
Nutritional/Ethanol Interactions
Ethanol: Avoid or limit ethanol (may increase CNS depression). Watch for sedation.
Herb/Nutraceutical: Avoid valerian, St John's wort, kava kava, gotu kola (may increase CNS depression).
Adverse Reactions Frequency not defined.
Cardiovascular: Palpitations, hypotension, bradycardia, peripheral vasodilation, cardiac arrest, shock, tachycardia
Central nervous system: CNS depression, fatigue, drowsiness, dizziness, nervousness, headache, restlessness, anorexia, malaise, confusion, coma, convulsion, insomnia, amnesia, mental depression, hallucinations, paradoxical CNS stimulation, intracranial pressure (increased)
Dermatologic: Pruritus, urticaria, rash

Endocrine & metabolic: Antidiuretic hormone release
Gastrointestinal: Nausea, vomiting, dyspepsia, stomach cramps, xerostomia, constipation, abdominal pain, dry mouth, biliary tract spasm, paralytic ileus
Genitourinary: Decreased urination, urinary tract spasm, urinary retention
Local: Pain at injection site
Neuromuscular & skeletal: Weakness
Ocular: Miosis, diplopia
Respiratory: Respiratory depression, apnea, hypoventilation, cyanosis
Miscellaneous: Histamine release, physical and psychological dependence
Overdosage/Toxicology Symptoms of overdose include CNS depression, respiratory depression, miosis, apnea, pulmonary edema, and convulsions. Naloxone, 2 mg I.V. with repeat administration as necessary up to a total dose of 10 mg, can be used to reverse opiate effects.
Pharmacodynamics/Kinetics
Onset of Action: Oral: 10-60 minutes
Duration of Action: 4-8 hours
Half-Life Elimination: 11-16 hours
Metabolism: Hepatic
Excretion: Urine (as inactive metabolite)
Available Dosage Forms
Injection, solution, as tartrate: 2 mg/mL (1 mL, 10 mL)
Tablet, as tartrate: 2 mg
Dosing
Adults & Elderly: Note: These are guidelines and do not represent the maximum doses that may be required in all patients. Doses should be titrated to pain relief/prevention.
Acute pain (moderate to severe):
Oral: Initial: Opiate-naive: 2 mg every 6-8 hours as needed; patients with prior opiate exposure may require higher initial doses; usual dosage range: 2-4 mg every 6-8 hours as needed
I.M., SubQ: Initial: Opiate-naive: 1 mg every 6-8 hours as needed; patients with prior opiate exposure may require higher initial doses; usual dosage range: 1-2 mg every 6-8 hours as needed
I.V. (slow): Initial: Opiate-naive: Up to 1 mg/dose every 3-6 hours as needed; patients with prior opiate exposure may require higher initial doses
Chronic pain: Patients taking opioids chronically may become tolerant and require doses higher than the usual dosage range to maintain the desired effect. Tolerance can be managed by appropriate dose titration. **There is no optimal or maximal dose for levorphanol in chronic pain. The appropriate dose is one that relieves pain throughout its dosing interval without causing unmanageable side effects.**
Premedication: I.M., SubQ: 1-2 mg/dose 60-90 minutes prior to surgery; older or debilitated patients usually require less drug
Hepatic Impairment: Reduce dose in patients with liver disease.
Administration
Oral: For lactating women, administer 4-6 hours prior to breast-feeding.
I.V.: Inject 3 mg over 4-5 minutes
I.V. Detail: pH: 4.3 (adjusted)
Stability
Compatibility: when admixed: Incompatible with aminophylline, ammonium chloride, amobarbital, chlorothiazide, heparin, pentobarbital, phenobarbital, phenytoin, sodium bicarbonate, thiopental
Storage: Store at room temperature. Protect from freezing.
Nursing Actions
Physical Assessment: Assess other medications patient may be taking for additive or adverse interactions. Monitor for effectiveness of pain relief and monitor for signs of overdose. Monitor blood pressure,

CNS and respiratory status, and degree of sedation at beginning of therapy and at regular intervals with long-term use. May cause physical and/or psychological dependence. For inpatients, implement safety measures (eg, side rails up, call light within reach, instructions to call for assistance). Assess knowledge/ teach patient appropriate use (if self-administered). Teach patient to monitor for adverse reactions, adverse reactions to report, and appropriate interventions to reduce side effects. Discontinue slowly after prolonged use.

Patient Education: If self-administered, use exactly as directed; do not increase dose or frequency. Drug may cause physical and/or psychological dependence. While using this medication, do not use alcohol and other prescription or OTC medications (especially sedatives, tranquilizers, antihistamines, or pain medications) without consulting prescriber. Maintain adequate hydration (2-3 L/day of fluids) unless instructed to restrict fluid intake. May cause hypotension, dizziness, drowsiness, impaired coordination, or blurred vision (use caution when driving, climbing stairs, or changing position - rising from sitting or lying to standing, or when engaging in tasks requiring alertness until response to drug is known); loss of appetite, nausea, or vomiting (frequent mouth care, small frequent meals, chewing gum, or sucking lozenges may help); or constipation (increased exercise, fluids, fruit, or fiber may help; if unresolved, consult prescriber about use of stool softeners). Report chest pain, slow or rapid heartbeat, acute dizziness, or persistent headache; swelling of extremities or unusual weight gain; changes in urinary elimination; acute headache; back or flank pain or spasms; blurred vision; skin rash; or shortness of breath. **Pregnancy/breast-feeding precautions:** Inform prescriber if you are or intend to become pregnant. Breast-feeding is not recommended.

Geriatric Considerations The elderly may be particularly susceptible to the CNS depressant and constipating effects of narcotics.

Levothyroxine (lee voe thye ROKS een)

U.S. Brand Names Levothroid®; Levoxyl®; Synthroid®; Unithroid®

Synonyms Levothyroxine Sodium; L-Thyroxine Sodium; T₄

Pharmacologic Category Thyroid Product

Medication Safety Issues

Sound-alike/look-alike issues:

Levothyroxine may be confused with liothyronine
Levoxyl® may be confused with Lanoxin®, Luvox®
Synthroid® may be confused with Symmetrel®

To avoid errors due to misinterpretation of a decimal point, always express dosage in mcg (**not** mg).

Pregnancy Risk Factor A

Lactation Enters breast milk/compatible

Use Replacement or supplemental therapy in hypothyroidism; pituitary TSH suppression

Mechanism of Action/Effect It is believed the thyroid hormone exerts its many metabolic effects through control of DNA transcription and protein synthesis

Contraindications Hypersensitivity to levothyroxine sodium or any component of the formulation; recent MI or thyrotoxicosis; uncorrected adrenal insufficiency

Warnings/Precautions Ineffective and potentially toxic for weight reduction. High doses may produce serious or even life-threatening toxic effects particularly when used with some anorectic drugs. Use with caution and reduce dosage in patients with angina pectoris or other cardiovascular disease. Use cautiously in the elderly since they may be more likely to have compromised cardiovascular functions. Patients with adrenal insufficiency, myxedema, diabetes mellitus and insipidus may have symptoms exaggerated or aggravated. Thyroid replacement requires periodic assessment of thyroid status. Chronic hypothyroidism predisposes patients to coronary artery disease. Levoxyl® may rapidly swell and disintegrate causing choking or gagging (should be administered with a full glass of water); use caution in patients with dysphagia or other swallowing disorders.

Drug Interactions

Decreased Effect: Also refer to Additional Information. Some medications may decrease absorption of levothyroxine: Cholestyramine, colestipol (separate administration by at least 2 hours); aluminum- and magnesium-containing antacids, iron preparations, sucralfate, Kayexalate® (separate administration by at least 4 hours). Enzyme inducers (phenytoin, phenobarbital, carbamazepine, and rifampin/rifabutin) may decrease levothyroxine levels. Levothyroxine may decrease effect of oral sulfonylureas. Serum levels of digoxin and theophylline may be altered by thyroid function. Estrogens may decrease serum free-thyroxine concentrations. Imatinib may decrease the effects of thyroid replacement therapy.

Increased Effect/Toxicity: Also refer to Additional Information. Levothyroxine may potentiate the hypoprothrombinemic effect of warfarin (and other oral anticoagulants). Tricyclic antidepressants (TCAs) coadministered with levothyroxine may increase potential for toxicity of both drugs. Coadministration with ketamine may lead to hypertension and tachycardia.

Nutritional/Ethanol Interactions Food: Taking levothyroxine with enteral nutrition may cause reduced bioavailability and may lower serum thyroxine levels leading to signs or symptoms of hypothyroidism. Limit intake of goitrogenic foods (eg, asparagus, cabbage, peas, turnip greens, broccoli, spinach, Brussels sprouts, lettuce, soybeans). Soybean flour (infant formula), cottonseed meal, walnuts, and dietary fiber may decrease absorption of levothyroxine from the GI tract.

Lab Interactions Many drugs may have effects on thyroid function tests: para-aminosalicylic acid, aminoglutethimide, amiodarone, barbiturates, carbamazepine, chloral hydrate, clofibrate, colestipol, corticosteroids, danazol, diazepam, estrogens, ethionamide, fluorouracil, I.V. heparin, insulin, lithium, methadone, methimazole, mitotane, nitroprusside, oxyphenbutazone, phenylbutazone, PTU, perphenazine, phenytoin, propranolol, salicylates, sulfonylureas, and thiazides.

Adverse Reactions Frequency not defined.

Cardiovascular: Angina, arrhythmia, blood pressure increased, cardiac arrest, flushing, heart failure, MI, palpitation, pulse increased, tachycardia

Central nervous system: Anxiety, emotional lability, fatigue, fever, headache, hyperactivity, insomnia, irritability, nervousness, pseudotumor cerebri (children), seizure (rare)

Dermatologic: Alopecia

Endocrine & metabolic: Fertility impaired, menstrual irregularities

Gastrointestinal: Abdominal cramps, appetite increased, diarrhea, vomiting, weight loss

Hepatic: Liver function tests increased

Neuromuscular & skeletal: Bone mineral density decreased, muscle weakness, tremor, slipped capital femoral epiphysis (children)

Respiratory: Dyspnea

Miscellaneous: Diaphoresis, heat intolerance, hypersensitivity (to inactive ingredients, symptoms include urticaria, pruritus, rash, flushing, angioedema, GI symptoms, fever, arthralgia, serum sickness, wheezing)

Levoxyl®: Choking, dysphagia, gagging
(Continued)

Levothyroxine *(Continued)*

Overdosage/Toxicology

Chronic: Chronic overdose may cause hyperthyroidism, weight loss, nervousness, sweating, tachycardia, insomnia, heat intolerance, menstrual irregularities, palpitations, psychosis, and fever. Overtreatment of children may result in premature closure of epiphyses or craniosynostosis (infants). Reduce dose or temporarily discontinue therapy. Hypothalamic-pituitary-thyroid axis will return to normal in 6-8 weeks. Serum T_4 levels do not correlate well with toxicity. Provide general supportive care

Acute: Acute overdose may cause fever, hypoglycemia, CHF, and unrecognized adrenal insufficiency. Acute massive overdose may be life-threatening; treatment should be symptomatic and supportive. Massive overdose may be a require beta-blockers for increased sympathomimetic activity.

Pharmacodynamics/Kinetics

Onset of Action: Therapeutic: Oral: 3-5 days; I.V. 6-8 hours; Peak effect: I.V.: ~24 hours

Time to Peak: Serum: 2-4 hours

Protein Binding: >99%

Half-Life Elimination: Euthyroid: 6-7 days; Hypothyroid: 9-10 days; Hyperthyroid: 3-4 days

Metabolism: Hepatic to triiodothyronine (active)

Excretion: Urine and feces; decreases with age

Available Dosage Forms

Injection, powder for reconstitution, as sodium: 0.2 mg, 0.5 mg

Tablet, as sodium: 25 mcg, 50 mcg, 75 mcg, 88 mcg, 100 mcg, 112 mcg, 125 mcg, 150 mcg, 175 mcg, 200 mcg, 300 mcg

Levothroid®: 25 mcg, 50 mcg, 75 mcg, 88 mcg, 100 mcg, 112 mcg, 125 mcg, 150 mcg, 175 mcg, 200 mcg, 300 mcg

Levoxyl®, Synthroid®: 25 mcg, 50 mcg, 75 mcg, 88 mcg, 100 mcg, 112 mcg, 125 mcg, 137 mcg, 150 mcg, 175 mcg, 200 mcg, 300 mcg

Unithroid®: 25 mcg, 50 mcg, 75 mcg, 88 mcg, 100 mcg, 112 mcg, 125 mcg, 150 mcg, 175 mcg, 200 mcg, 300 mcg

Dosing

Adults: Doses should be adjusted based on clinical response and laboratory parameters.

Hypothyroidism:

Oral: 1.7 mcg/kg/day in otherwise healthy adults <50 years old, children in whom growth and puberty are complete, and older adults who have been recently treated for hyperthyroidism or who have been hypothyroid for only a few months. Titrate dose every 6 weeks. Average starting dose ~100 mcg; usual doses are ≤200 mcg/day; doses ≥300 mcg/day are rare (consider poor compliance, malabsorption, and/or drug interactions). **Note:** For patients >50 years or patients with cardiac disease, refer to elderly dosing.

I.M., I.V.: 50% of the oral dose

Severe hypothyroidism: Oral: Initial: 12.5-25 mcg/day; adjust dose by 25 mcg/day every 2-4 weeks as appropriate

Subclinical hypothyroidism (if treated): Oral: 1 mcg/kg/day

TSH suppression: Oral:

Well-differentiated thyroid cancer: Highly individualized; Doses >2 mcg/kg/day may be needed to suppress TSH to <0.1 mU/L.

Benign nodules and nontoxic multinodular goiter: Goal TSH suppression: 0.1-0.3 mU/L

Myxedema coma or stupor: I.V.: 200-500 mcg, then 100-300 mcg the next day if necessary; smaller doses should be considered in patients with cardiovascular disease

Elderly: Doses should be adjusted based on clinical response and laboratory parameters.

Hypothyroidism:

Oral:

>50 years without cardiac disease **or** <50 years with cardiac disease: Initial: 25-50 mcg/day; adjust dose at 6- to 8-week intervals as needed

>50 years with cardiac disease: Initial: 12.5-25 mcg/day; adjust dose by 12.5-25 mcg increments at 4- to 6-week intervals. (**Note:** Many clinicians prefer to adjust at 6- to 8-week intervals.)

Note: Elderly patients may require <1 mcg/kg/day

I.M., I.V.: 50% of the oral dose

Myxedema coma: I.V.: Refer to adult dosing; lower doses may be needed

Pediatrics: Doses should be adjusted based on clinical response and laboratory parameters.

Hypothyroidism:

Oral:

Newborns: Initial: 10-15 mcg/kg/day. Lower doses of 25 mcg/day should be considered in newborns at risk for cardiac failure. Newborns with T_4 levels <5 mcg/dL should be started at 50 mcg/day. Adjust dose at 4- to 6-week intervals.

Infants and Children: Dose based on body weight and age as listed below. Children with severe or chronic hypothyroidism should be started at 25 mcg/day; adjust dose by 25 mcg every 2-4 weeks. In older children, hyperactivity may be decreased by starting with $1/4$ of the recommended dose and increasing by $1/4$ dose each week until the full replacement dose is reached. Refer to adult dosing once growth and puberty are complete.

0-3 months: 10-15 mcg/kg/day

3-6 months: 8-10 mcg/kg/day

6-12 months: 6-8 mcg/kg/day

1-5 years: 5-6 mcg/kg/day

6-12 years: 4-5 mcg/kg/day

12 years: 2-3 mcg/kg/day

I.M., I.V.: 50% of the oral dose

Administration

Oral: Administer in the morning on an empty stomach, at least 30 minutes before food. Tablets may be crushed and suspended in 1-2 teaspoonfuls of water; suspension should be used immediately. Levoxyl® should be administered with a full glass of water to prevent gagging (due to tablet swelling).

I.V.: Dilute vial with 5 mL normal saline; use immediately after reconstitution; do not mix with other IV fluids

I.V. Detail: Dilute vial with 5 mL normal saline. Use immediately after reconstitution. I.V. form must be prepared immediately prior to administration. Should not be admixed with other solutions.

Stability

Reconstitution: Dilute vial with 5 mL normal saline. Shake well and use immediately after reconstitution; discard any unused portions.

Compatibility: Do not mix I.V. solution with other I.V. infusion solutions.

Storage: Store tablets and injection at room temperature of 15°C to 30°C (59°F to 86°F). Protect tablets from light and moisture.

Laboratory Monitoring Thyroid function (serum thyroxine, thyrotropin concentrations), resin triiodothyronine uptake (rT_3U), free thyroxine index (FTI), T_4, TSH, TSH may be elevated during the first few months of thyroid replacement despite patients being clinically euthyroid. In cases where T_4 remains low and TSH is within normal limits, an evaluation of "free" (unbound) T_4 is needed to evaluate further increase in dosage.

Nursing Actions

Physical Assessment: Assess potential for interactions with other pharmacological agents patient may be taking (eg, toxic effects with some anorectic drugs, decreased effect of oral hypoglycemics, decreased or increased effect of levothyroxine and potential toxicities). See Administration for infusion specifics. Monitor results of laboratory tests, therapeutic benefits, and adverse effects on a regular basis during therapy (eg, hypo-/hyperthyroidism). **Important:** Many drugs may have effects on thyroid function tests and results of laboratory tests. Teach patient proper use, possible side effects/appropriate interventions (eg, goitrogenic foods), and adverse symptoms to report.

Patient Education: Consult prescriber before taking new medication or herbal products during therapy; some other medications or herbals may cause adverse effects with levothyroxine. Thyroid replacement therapy is generally for life. Take as directed, in the morning 30 minutes before breakfast. Do not take antacids or iron preparations within 8 hours of thyroid medication. Do not change brands and do not discontinue without consulting prescriber. Do not eat excessive amounts of goitrogenic foods (eg, asparagus, cabbage, peas, turnip greens, broccoli, spinach, brussel sprouts, lettuce, soybeans). Report chest pain, rapid heart rate, palpitations, heat intolerance, excessive sweating, increased nervousness, agitation, or lethargy.

Dietary Considerations Should be taken on an empty stomach, at least 30 minutes before food.

Geriatric Considerations The elderly do not have a change in serum thyroxine (T_4) associated with aging; however, plasma T_3 concentrations are decreased 25% to 40% in the elderly. There is not a compensatory rise in thyrotropin suggesting that lower T_3 is not reacted upon as a deficiency by the pituitary. This indicates a slightly lower than normal dosage of thyroid hormone replacement is usually sufficient in older patients than in younger adult patients. TSH must be monitored since insufficient thyroid replacement (elevated TSH) is a risk for coronary artery disease and excessive replacement (low TSH) may cause signs of hyperthyroidism and excessive bone loss. Some clinicians suggest levothyroxine is the drug of choice for replacement therapy.

Breast-Feeding Issues Minimally excreted in human milk; adequate levels are needed to maintain normal lactation

Pregnancy Issues Untreated maternal hypothyroidism may have adverse effects on fetal growth and development and is associated with higher rate of complications (spontaneous abortion, pre-eclampsia, stillbirth, premature delivery). Treatment should not be discontinued during pregnancy. TSH levels should be monitored during each trimester and 6-8 weeks postpartum. Increased doses may be needed during pregnancy.

Additional Information Equivalent doses: The following statement on relative potency of thyroid products is included in a joint statement by American Thyroid Association (ATA), American Association of Clinical Endocrinologists (AACE) and The Endocrine Society (TES): For purposes of conversion, levothyroxine sodium (T_4) 100 mcg is usually considered equivalent to desiccated thyroid 60 mg, thyroglobulin 60 mg, or liothyronine sodium (T_3) 25 mcg. However, these are rough guidelines only and do not obviate the careful re-evaluation of a patient when switching thyroid hormone preparations, including a change from one brand of levothyroxine to another. Joint position statement is available at http://www.thyroid.org/professionals/advocacy/04_12_08_thyroxine.html.

Note: Several medications have effects on thyroid production or conversion. The impact in thyroid replacement has not been specifically evaluated, but patient response should be monitored:

Methimazole: Decreases thyroid hormone secretion, while propylthiouracil decrease thyroid hormone secretion and decreases conversion of T_4 to T_3.

Beta-adrenergic antagonists: Decrease conversion of T_4 to T_3 (dose related, propranolol ≥160 mg/day); patients may be clinically euthyroid.

Iodide, iodine-containing radiographic contrast agents may decrease thyroid hormone secretion; may also increase thyroid hormone secretion, especially in patients with Graves' disease.

Other agents reported to impact on thyroid production/conversion include aminoglutethimide, amiodarone, chloral hydrate, diazepam, ethionamide, interferon-alpha, interleukin-2, lithium, lovastatin (case report), glucocorticoids (dose-related), mercaptopurine, sulfonamides, thiazide diuretics, and tolbutamide.

In addition, a number of medications have been noted to cause transient depression in TSH secretion, which may complicate interpretation of monitoring tests for levothyroxine, including corticosteroids, octreotide, and dopamine. Metoclopramide may increase TSH secretion

Lidocaine (LYE doe kane)

U.S. Brand Names Anestacon®; Band-Aid® Hurt-Free™ Antiseptic Wash [OTC]; Burnamycin [OTC]; Burn Jel [OTC]; Burn-O-Jel [OTC]; LidaMantle®; Lidoderm®; L-M-X™ 4 [OTC]; L-M-X™ 5 [OTC]; LTA® 360; Premjact® [OTC]; Solarcaine® Aloe Extra Burn Relief [OTC]; Topicaine® [OTC]; Xylocaine®; Xylocaine® MPF; Xylocaine® Viscous; Zilactin-L® [OTC]

Synonyms Lidocaine Hydrochloride; Lignocaine Hydrochloride

Pharmacologic Category Analgesic, Topical; Antiarrhythmic Agent, Class Ib; Local Anesthetic

Medication Safety Issues
High alert medication: The Institute for Safe Medication Practices (ISMP) includes this medication (I.V. formulation) among its list of drugs which have a heightened risk of causing significant patient harm when used in error.

Transdermal patch may contain conducting metal (eg, aluminum); remove patch prior to MRI.

Pregnancy Risk Factor B

Lactation Enters breast milk (small amounts)/use caution (AAP rates "compatible")

Use Local anesthetic and acute treatment of ventricular arrhythmias from myocardial infarction, or cardiac manipulation

Rectal: Temporary relief of pain and itching due to anorectal disorders

Topical: Local anesthetic for use in laser, cosmetic, and outpatient surgeries; minor burns, cuts, and abrasions of the skin

Lidoderm® Patch: Relief of allodynia (painful hypersensitivity) and chronic pain in postherpetic neuralgia

Unlabeled/Investigational Use ACLS guidelines (not considered drug of choice): Stable monomorphic VT (preserved ventricular function), polymorphic VT (preserved ventricular function), drug-induced monomorphic VT

Mechanism of Action/Effect Class Ib antiarrhythmic; suppresses automaticity of conduction tissue by increasing electrical stimulation threshold of ventricles, His-Purkinje system, and spontaneous depolarization of ventricles during diastole by direct action on tissues; blocks both initiation and conduction of nerve impulses by decreasing the neuronal membrane's permeability to sodium ions, which results in inhibition of depolarization with resultant blockade of conduction

Contraindications Hypersensitivity to lidocaine or any component of the formulation; hypersensitivity to another local anesthetic of the amide type; Adam-Stokes syndrome; severe degrees of SA, AV, or intraventricular heart block (except in patients with a (Continued)

Lidocaine *(Continued)*

functioning artificial pacemaker); premixed injection may contain corn-derived dextrose and its use is contraindicated in patients with allergy to corn-related products

Warnings/Precautions

Intravenous: Constant ECG monitoring is necessary during I.V. administration. Use cautiously in hepatic impairment, any degree of heart block, Wolff-Parkinson-White syndrome, CHF, marked hypoxia, severe respiratory depression, hypovolemia, history of malignant hyperthermia, or shock. Increased ventricular rate may be seen when administered to a patient with atrial fibrillation. Correct any underlying causes of ventricular arrhythmias. Monitor closely for signs and symptoms of CNS toxicity. The elderly may be prone to increased CNS and cardiovascular side effects. Reduce dose in hepatic dysfunction and CHF.

Injectable anesthetic: Follow appropriate administration techniques so as not to administer any intravascularly. Solutions containing antimicrobial preservatives should not be used for epidural or spinal anesthesia. Some solutions contain a bisulfite; avoid in patients who are allergic to bisulfite. Resuscitative equipment, medicine and oxygen should be available in case of emergency. Use products containing epinephrine cautiously in patients with significant vascular disease, compromised blood flow, or during or following general anesthesia (increased risk of arrhythmias). Adjust the dose for the elderly, pediatric, acutely ill, and debilitated patients.

Topical: L-M-X™ 4 cream: Do not leave on large body areas for >2 hours. Observe young children closely to prevent accidental ingestion. Not for use ophthalmic use or for use on mucous membranes.

Transdermal patch: May contain conducting metal (eg, aluminum); remove patch prior to MRI.

Drug Interactions

Cytochrome P450 Effect: Substrate of CYP1A2 (minor), 2A6 (minor), 2B6 (minor), 2C8/9 (minor), 2D6 (major), 3A4 (major); **Inhibits** CYP1A2 (strong), 2D6 (moderate), 3A4 (moderate)

Decreased Effect: The levels/effects of lidocaine may be decreased by aminoglutethimide, carbamazepine, nafcillin, nevirapine, phenobarbital, phenytoin, rifamycins and other CYP3A4 inducers. Lidocaine may decrease the levels/effects of CYP2D6 prodrug substrates (eg, codeine, hydrocodone, oxycodone, tramadol).

Increased Effect/Toxicity: The levels/effects of lidocaine may be increased by amphetamines, amiodarone, azole antifungals, beta-blockers, chlorpromazine, clarithromycin, delavirdine, diclofenac, doxycycline, erythromycin, fluoxetine, imatinib, isoniazid, miconazole, nefazodone, nicardipine, paroxetine, pergolide, propofol, protease inhibitors, quinidine, quinine, ritonavir, ropinirole, telithromycin, verapamil, and other CYP2D6 or 3A4 inhibitors. Concomitant cimetidine or propranolol may result in increased serum concentrations of lidocaine resulting in toxicity.

Lidocaine may increase the levels/effects of aminophylline, amphetamines, selected beta-blockers, selected benzodiazepines, calcium channel blockers, cisapride, cyclosporine, dextromethorphan, ergot alkaloids, fluoxetine, fluvoxamine, selected HMG-CoA reductase inhibitors, lidocaine, mesoridazine, mexiletine, mirtazapine, nateglinide, nefazodone, paroxetine, risperidone, ritonavir, ropinirole, sildenafil (and other PDE-5 inhibitors), tacrolimus, theophylline, thioridazine, tricyclic antidepressants, trifluoperazine, venlafaxine, and other substrates of CYP1A2, 2D6 or 3A4. The effect of succinylcholine may be enhanced by lidocaine.

Nutritional/Ethanol Interactions Herb/Nutraceutical: St John's wort may decrease lidocaine levels; avoid concurrent use.

Adverse Reactions Effects vary with route of administration. Many effects are dose related.

Frequency not defined:
  Cardiovascular: Bradycardia, hypotension, heart block, arrhythmia, cardiovascular collapse, sinus node supression, increase defibrillator threshold, vascular insufficiency (periarticular injections), arterial spasms
  Central nervous system: Agitation, anxiety, coma, dizziness, drowsiness, euphoria, hallucinations, lethargy, lightheadedness, paresthesia, psychosis, seizure, slurred speech
  Dermatologic: Angioedema, contact dermatitis, edema of the skin, itching, rash,
  Gastrointestinal: Nausea, vomiting, taste disorder
  Local: Thrombophlebitis
  Neuromuscular & skeletal: Transient radicular pain (subarachnoid administration; up to 1.9%), tremor, twitching
  Ocular: Diplopia, visual changes
  Otic: Tinnitus
  Respiratory: Dyspnea, respiratory depression or arrest, bronchospasm
  Miscellaneous: Allergic reactions, urticaria, edema, anaphylactoid reaction

Following spinal anesthesia: Positional headache (3%), shivering (2%) nausea, peripheral nerve symptoms, respiratory inadequacy and double vision (<1%), hypotension, cauda equina syndrome

Overdosage/Toxicology Lidocaine has a narrow therapeutic index. Severe toxicity may occur at doses slightly above the therapeutic range, especially in conjunction with other antiarrhythmic drugs. Symptoms of overdose include sedation, confusion, coma, seizures, respiratory arrest, and cardiac toxicity (sinus arrest, AV block, asystole, and hypotension). QRS and QT intervals are usually normal, although they may be prolonged after massive overdose. Other effects include dizziness, paresthesia, tremor, ataxia, and GI disturbance. Treatment is supportive.

Pharmacodynamics/Kinetics

Onset of Action: Single bolus dose: 45-90 seconds

Duration of Action: 10-20 minutes

Protein Binding: 60% to 80% to alpha$_1$ acid glycoprotein

Half-Life Elimination: Biphasic: Prolonged with congestive heart failure, liver disease, shock, severe renal disease; Initial: 7-30 minutes; Terminal: Infants, premature: 3.2 hours; Adults: 1.5-2 hours

Metabolism: 90% hepatic; active metabolites monoethylglycinexylidide (MEGX) and glycinexylidide (GX) can accumulate and may cause CNS toxicity

Available Dosage Forms [DSC] = Discontinued product
  Cream, rectal (L-M-X™ 5): 5% (15 g) [contains benzyl alcohol; packaged with applicator]; (30 g) [contains benzyl alcohol]
  Cream, topical (L-M-X™ 4): 4% (5 g) [contains benzyl alcohol; packaged with Tegaderm™ dressing]; (15 g, 30 g) [contains benzyl alcohol]
  Cream, topical, as hydrochloride: 3% (30 g)
    LidaMantle®: 3% (30 g, 85 g)
  Gel, topical:
    Burn-O-Jel: 0.5% (90 g)
    Topicaine®: 4% (10 g, 30 g, 113 g) [contains alcohol 35%, benzyl alcohol, aloe vera, and jojoba]
  Gel, topical, as hydrochloride:
    Burn Jel: 2% (3.5 g, 120 g)
    Solarcaine® Aloe Extra Burn Relief: 0.5% (113 g, 226 g) [contains aloe vera gel and tartrazine]

Infusion, as hydrochloride [premixed in D₅W]: 0.4% [4 mg/mL] (250 mL, 500 mL); 0.8% [8 mg/mL] (250 mL, 500 mL)

Injection, solution, as hydrochloride: 0.5% [5 mg/mL] (50 mL); 1% [10 mg/mL] (2 mL, 10 mL, 20 mL, 30 mL, 50 mL); 2% [20 mg/mL] (2 mL, 5 mL, 20 mL, 50 mL)

Xylocaine®: 0.5% [5 mg/mL] (50 mL); 1% [10 mg/mL] (10 mL, 20 mL, 50 mL); 2% [20 mg/mL] (1.8 mL, 10 mL, 20 mL, 50 mL)

Injection, solution, as hydrochloride [preservative free]: 0.5% [5 mg/mL] (50 mL); 1% [10 mg/mL] (2 mL, 5 mL, 30 mL); 1.5% [15 mg/mL] (20 mL); 2% [20 mg/mL] (2 mL, 5 mL, 10 mL); 4% [40 mg/mL] (5 mL)

Xylocaine®: 10% [100 mg/mL] (5 mL) [for ventricular arrhythmias]

Xylocaine® MPF: 0.5% [5 mg/mL] (50 mL); 1% [10 mg/mL] (2 mL, 5 mL, 10 mL, 30 mL); 1.5% [15 mg/mL] (10 mL, 20 mL); 2% [20 mg/mL] (2 mL, 5 mL, 10 mL); 4% [40 mg/mL] (5 mL)

Injection, solution, as hydrochloride [premixed in D₇.₅W, preservative free]: 5% (2 mL)

Xylocaine® MPF: 1.5% (2 mL) [DSC]

Jelly, topical, as hydrochloride: 2% (5 mL, 30 mL)

Anestacon®: 2% (15 mL) [contains benzalkonium chloride]

Xylocaine®: 2% (5 mL, 30 mL)

Liquid, topical (Zilactin®-L): 2.5% (7.5 mL)

Lotion, topical, as hydrochloride (LidaMantle®): 3% (177 mL)

Ointment, topical: 5% (37 g, 50 g)

Solution, topical, as hydrochloride: 4% [40 mg/mL] (50 mL)

Band-Aid® Hurt-Free™ Antiseptic Wash: 2% (180 mL)

LTA® 360: 4% [40 mg/mL] (4 mL) [packaged with cannula for laryngotracheal administration]

Xylocaine®: 4% [40 mg/mL] (50 mL)

Solution, viscous, as hydrochloride: 2% [20 mg/mL] (20 mL, 100 mL)

Xylocaine® Viscous: 2% [20 mg/mL] (100 mL, 450 mL)

Spray, topical:

Burnamycin: 0.5% (60 mL) [contains aloe vera gel and menthol]

Premjact®: 9.6% (13 mL)

Solarcaine® Aloe Extra Burn Relief: 0.5% (127 g) [contains aloe vera]

Transdermal system, topical (Lidoderm®): 5% (30s)

Dosing

Adults & Elderly:

Antiarrhythmic:

I.V.: 1-1.5 mg/kg bolus over 2-3 minutes; may repeat doses of 0.5-0.75 mg/kg in 5-10 minutes up to a total of 3 mg/kg; continuous infusion: 1-4 mg/minute

Ventricular fibrillation or pulseless ventricular tachycardia (after defibrillation, CPR, and vasopressor administration): I.V.: Initial: 1-1.5 mg/kg. Refractory ventricular tachycardia or ventricular fibrillation, a repeat 0.5-0.75 mg/kg bolus may be given every 5-10 minutes after initial dose for a maximum of 3 doses. Total dose should not exceed 3 mg/kg. Follow with continuous infusion (1-4 mg/minute) after return of perfusion. Reappearance of arrhythmia during constant infusion: 0.5 mg/kg bolus and reassessment of infusion.

E.T. (loading dose only): 2-2.5 times the I.V. dose
Note: Decrease dose in patients with CHF, shock, or hepatic disease.

Anesthetic, topical:
Cream:

LidaMantle®: Skin irritation: Apply to affected area 2-3 times/day as needed

L-M-X™ 4: Apply ¼ inch thick layer to intact skin. Leave on until adequate anesthetic effect is obtained. Remove cream and cleanse area before beginning procedure.

L-M-X™ 5: Relief of anorectal pain and itching: Rectal: Apply topically to clean, dry area **or** using applicator, insert rectally, up to 6 times/day

Gel, ointment, solution: Apply to affected area ≤3 times/day as needed (maximum dose: 4.5 mg/kg, not to exceed 300 mg)

Jelly: Maximum dose: 30 mL (600 mg) in any 12-hour period:

Anesthesia of male urethra: 5-30 mL (100-600 mg)

Anesthesia of female urethra: 3-5 mL (60-100 mg)

Lubrication of endotracheal tube: Apply a moderate amount to external surface only

Liquid: Cold sores and fever blisters: Apply to affected area every 6 hours as needed

Patch: Postherpetic neuralgia: Apply patch to most painful area. Up to 3 patches may be applied in a single application. Patch may remain in place for up to 12 hours in any 24-hour period.

Anesthetic, local injectable: Varies with procedure, degree of anesthesia needed, vascularity of tissue, duration of anesthesia required, and physical condition of patient; maximum: 4.5 mg/kg/dose; do not repeat within 2 hours.

Pediatrics:

Antiarrhythmic:

I.V., I.O.: **Note:** For use in pulseless VT or VF, give after defibrillation, CPR, and epinephrine:

Loading dose: 1 mg/kg (maximum 100 mg); follow with continuous infusion; may administer second bolus of 0.5-1 mg/kg if delay between bolus and start of infusion is >15 minutes

Continuous infusion: 20-50 mcg/kg/minute. Use 20 mcg/kg/minute in patients with shock, hepatic disease, cardiac arrest, mild CHF; moderate-to-severe CHF may require ½ loading dose and lower infusion rates to avoid toxicity.

E.T. (loading dose only): 2-10 times the I.V. bolus dose

Anesthetic, topical:
Cream:

LidaMantle®: Skin irritation: Refer to adult dosing.

L-M-X™ 4: Children ≥2 years: Refer to adult dosing.

L-M-X™ 5: Relief of anorectal pain and itching: Rectal: Children ≥12 years: Refer to adult dosing.

Jelly: Children ≥10 years: Dose varies with age and weight (maximum dose: 4.5 mg/kg)

Liquid: Cold sores and fever blisters: Children ≥5 years: Refer to adult dosing.

Injectable local anesthetic: Refer to adult dosing.

Renal Impairment: Not dialyzable (0% to 5%) by hemo- or peritoneal dialysis; supplemental dose is not necessary.

Hepatic Impairment: Reduce dose in acute hepatitis and decompensated cirrhosis by 50%.

Administration

I.V.: Use microdrip (60 drops/mL) or infusion pump to administer an accurate dose.

Infusion rates: 2 g/250 mL D₅W (infusion pump should be used):

1 mg/minute: 7.5 mL/hour

2 mg/minute: 15 mL/hour

3 mg/minute: 22.5 mL/hour

4 mg/minute: 30 mL/hour

Buffered lidocaine for injectable local anesthetic: Add 2 mL of sodium bicarbonate 8.4% to 18 mL of lidocaine 1%

I.V. Detail: Local thrombophlebitis may occur in patients receiving prolonged I.V. infusions.
(Continued)

Lidocaine *(Continued)*

pH: 5-7 (injection); 3.5-6.0 (premixed infusion solution
. in D₅W)

Topical:

Patch: May be cut to appropriate size. Remove immediately if burning sensation occurs. Wash hands after application.

Gel (Topicaine®): Avoid mucous membranes; remove prior to laser treatment.

Other: Intratracheal: Dilute in NS or distilled water. Absorption is greater with distilled water, but causes more adverse effects on PaO₂. Pass catheter beyond tip of tracheal tube, stop compressions, spray drug quickly down tube. Follow immediately with several quick insufflations and continue chest compressions.

Stability

Reconstitution: Standard diluent: 2 g/250 mL D₅W

Compatibility: Stable in D₅LR, D₅¹/₂NS, D₅NS, D₅W, LR, ¹/₄NS, NS

Y-site administration: Incompatible with amphotericin B cholesteryl sulfate complex, thiopental

Compatibility in syringe: Incompatible with cefazolin

Compatibility when admixed: Incompatible with amphotericin B, dacarbazine, methohexital, phenytoin

Storage: Lidocaine injection is stable at room temperature. Stability of parenteral admixture at room temperature (25°C) is the expiration date on premixed bag; out of overwrap stability is 30 days.

Laboratory Monitoring I.V.: Serum lidocaine levels. Therapeutic levels range from 1.5-5 mcg/mL; >6 mcg/mL is associated with toxicity.

Nursing Actions

Physical Assessment: Assess other medications patient may be taking for adverse interactions. **Local anesthetic:** Monitor for effectiveness of anesthesia and adverse reactions. **Dental/local anesthetic:** Use caution to prevent gagging or choking. Avoid food or drink for 1 hour. **Antiarrhythmic: I.V.:** Monitor ECG, blood pressure, and respirations closely and continually. Keep patient supine to reduce hypotensive effects. Assess frequently for adverse reactions or signs of CNS toxicity (eg, drowsiness, lightheadedness, dizziness, tinnitus, blurred vision, vomiting, twitching, tremor, lethargy, coma, agitation, slurred speech, seizure, anxiety, euphoria, hallucinations, paresthesia, psychosis). Teach patient adverse reactions to report and appropriate interventions to promote safety.

Patient Education: I.V.: You will be monitored during infusion. Do not get up without assistance. Report dizziness, numbness, double vision, nausea, pain or burning at infusion site, nightmares, hearing strange noises, seeing unusual visions, or respiratory difficulty.

Dermatologic: You will experience decreased sensation to pain, heat, or cold in the area and/or decreased muscle strength (depending on area of application) until effects wear off; use necessary caution to reduce incidence of possible injury until full sensation returns. Report irritation, pain, persistent numbness, tingling, swelling; restlessness, dizziness, acute weakness; blurred vision; ringing in ears; or respiratory difficulty.

Dental/local anesthetic: Lidocaine can cause numbness of tongue, cheeks, and throat. Do not eat or drink for 1 hour after use. Take small sips of water at first to ensure that you can swallow without difficulty. Your tongue and mouth may be numb; use caution avoid biting yourself. Immediately report swelling of face, lips, or tongue

Transdermal patch: Patch may be cut to appropriate size. Apply patch to most painful area. Up to 3 patches may be applied in a single application. Patch may remain in place for up to 12 hours in any 24-hour period. Remove immediately if burning sensation occurs. Wash hands after application.

Pregnancy precaution: Inform prescriber if you are pregnant.

Dietary Considerations Premixed injection may contain corn-derived dextrose and its use is contraindicated in patients with allergy to corn-related products.

Geriatric Considerations Due to decreases in Phase I metabolism and possibly decrease in splanchnic perfusion with age, there may be a decreased clearance or increased half-life in the elderly and increased risk for CNS side effects and cardiac effects.

Related Information

Compatibility of Drugs *on page 1370*
Peak and Trough Guidelines *on page 1387*

Lidocaine and Epinephrine

(LYE doe kane & ep i NEF rin)

U.S. Brand Names LidoSite™; Xylocaine® MPF With Epinephrine; Xylocaine® With Epinephrine

Synonyms Epinephrine and Lidocaine

Pharmacologic Category Local Anesthetic

Pregnancy Risk Factor B

Lactation Enters breast milk/compatible

Use Local infiltration anesthesia; AVS for nerve block; topical local analgesia for superficial dermatologic procedures

Available Dosage Forms

Injection, solution:

0.5% / 1:200,000: Lidocaine hydrochloride 0.5% and epinephrine 1:200,000 (50 mL)

1% / 1:100,000: Lidocaine hydrochloride 1% and epinephrine 1:100,000 (20 mL, 30 mL, 50 mL)

1% / 1:200,000: Lidocaine hydrochloride 1% and epinephrine 1:200,000 (30 mL)

1.5% / 1:200,000: Lidocaine hydrochloride 1.5% and epinephrine 1:200,000 (30 mL)

2% / 1:50,000: Lidocaine hydrochloride 2% and epinephrine 1:50,000 (1.8 mL)

2% / 1:100,000: Lidocaine hydrochloride 2% and epinephrine 1:100,000 (1.8 mL, 30 mL, 50 mL)

2% / 1:200,000: Lidocaine hydrochloride 2% and epinephrine 1:200,000 (20 mL)

Xylocaine® with Epinephrine:

0.5% / 1:200,000: Lidocaine hydrochloride 0.5% and epinephrine 1:200,000 (50 mL) [contains methylparaben]

1% / 1:100,000: Lidocaine hydrochloride 1% and epinephrine 1:100,000 (10 mL, 20 mL, 50 mL) [contains methylparaben]

2% / 1:50,000: Lidocaine hydrochloride 2% and epinephrine 1:50,000 (1.8 mL) [contains sodium metabisulfite]

2% / 1:100,000: Lidocaine hydrochloride 2% and epinephrine 1:100,000 (1.8 mL) [contains sodium metabisulfite]; (10 mL, 20 mL, 50 mL) [contains methylparaben]

Xylocaine®-MPF with Epinephrine:

1% / 1:200,000: Lidocaine hydrochloride 1% and epinephrine 1:200,000 (5 mL, 10 mL, 30 mL) [contains sodium metabisulfite]

1.5% / 1:200,000: Lidocaine hydrochloride 1.5% and epinephrine 1:200,000 (5 mL, 10 mL, 30 mL) [contains sodium metabisulfite]

2% / 1:200,000: Lidocaine hydrochloride 2% and epinephrine 1:200,000 (5 mL, 10 mL, 20 mL) [contains sodium metabisulfite]

Transdermal system (LidoSite™): Lidocaine hydrochloride 10% and epinephrine 0.1% (25s) [contains sodium metabisulfite; for use only with LidoSite™ controller]

Dosing

Adults & Elderly: Dosage varies with the anesthetic procedure, degree of anesthesia needed, vascularity of tissue, duration of anesthesia required, and physical condition of patient.

Dental anesthesia, infiltration, or conduction block:

Children <10 years: 20-30 mg (1-1.5 mL) of lidocaine hydrochloride as a 2% solution with epinephrine 1:100,000; maximum: 4-5 mg of lidocaine hydrochloride/kg of body weight or 100-150 mg as a single dose

Children >10 years and Adults: Do not exceed 6.6 mg/kg body weight or 300 mg of lidocaine hydrochloride and 3 mcg (0.003 mg) of epinephrine/kg of body weight or 0.2 mg epinephrine per dental appointment. The effective anesthetic dose varies with procedure, intensity of anesthesia needed, duration of anesthesia required, and physical condition of the patient. Always use the lowest effective dose along with careful aspiration.

The following numbers of dental carpules (1.8 mL) provide the indicated amounts of lidocaine hydrochloride 2% and epinephrine 1:100,000 (see table):

# of Cartridges (1.8 mL)	Lidocaine HCl (2%) (mg)	Epinephrine 1:100,000 (mg)
1	36	0.018
2	72	0.036
3	108	0.054
4	144	0.072
5	180	0.090
6	216	0.108
7	252	0.126
8	288	0.144
9	324	0.162
10	360	0.180

For most routine dental procedures, lidocaine hydrochloride 2% with epinephrine 1:100,000 is preferred. When a more pronounced hemostasis is required, a 1:50,000 epinephrine concentration should be used. The following numbers of dental carpules (1.8 mL) provide the indicated amounts of lidocaine hydrochloride 2% and epinephrine 1:50,000 (see table):

# of Cartridges (1.8 mL)	Lidocaine HCl (2%) (mg)	Epinephrine 1:50,000 (mg)
1	36	0.036
2	72	0.072
3	108	0.108
4	144	0.144
5	180	0.180
6	216	0.216

Dermatologic procedure: Topical: Place 1 transdermal patch over area requiring analgesia; attach patch to iontophoretic controller and leave on for 10 minutes. Remove patch and perform procedure within 10-20 minutes of patch removal. Do not use another patch for 30 minutes.

Pediatrics: Local anesthetic:

Infiltration: Use lidocaine concentrations of 0.5% to 1% (or even more diluted) to decrease possibility of toxicity. Lidocaine dose should not exceed 7 mg/kg/dose; do not repeat within 2 hours.

Dermatologic procedure: Topical: Children ≥5 years: Refer to adult dosing.

Nursing Actions

Physical Assessment: See individual agents.
Patient Education: See individual agents.

Related Information
Epinephrine *on page 427*
Lidocaine *on page 735*

Lindane (LIN dane)

Synonyms Benzene Hexachloride; Gamma Benzene Hexachloride; Hexachlorocyclohexane

Restrictions An FDA-approved medication guide is available at http://www.fda.gov/cder/Offices/ODS/labeling.htm; distribute to each patient to whom this medication is dispensed.

Pharmacologic Category Antiparasitic Agent, Topical; Pediculocide; Scabicidal Agent

Pregnancy Risk Factor C

Lactation Enters breast milk/contraindicated

Use Treatment of *Sarcoptes scabiei* (scabies), *Pediculus capitis* (head lice), and *Phthirus pubis* (crab lice); FDA recommends reserving lindane as a second-line agent or with inadequate response to other therapies

Mechanism of Action/Effect Directly absorbed by parasites and ova through the exoskeleton; stimulates the nervous system resulting in seizures and death of parasitic arthropods

Contraindications Hypersensitivity to lindane or any component of the formulation; uncontrolled seizure disorders; crusted (Norwegian) scabies, acutely-inflamed skin or raw, weeping surfaces or other skin conditions which may increase systemic absorption

Warnings/Precautions Not considered a drug of first choice; seizures and death have been reported with use; use with caution in infants, small children, patients <50 kg, or patients with a history of seizures; use caution with conditions which may increase risk of seizures or medications which decrease seizure threshold; use caution with hepatic impairment; avoid contact with face, eyes, mucous membranes, and urethral meatus. Because of the potential for systemic absorption and CNS side effects, lindane should be used with caution; consider permethrin or crotamiton agent first. Oil-based hair dressing may increase toxic potential. A lindane medication guide must be given to all patients along with instructions for proper use. Should be used as a part of an overall lice management program.

Drug Interactions

Increased Effect/Toxicity: Increased toxicity: Drugs which lower seizure threshold

Adverse Reactions Frequency not defined (includes postmarketing and/or case reports).

Cardiovascular: Cardiac arrhythmia

Central nervous system: Ataxia, dizziness, headache, restlessness, seizure, pain

Dermatologic: Alopecia, contact dermatitis, skin and adipose tissue may act as repositories, eczematous eruptions, pruritus, urticaria

Gastrointestinal: Nausea, vomiting

Hematologic: Aplastic anemia

Hepatic: Hepatitis

Local: Burning and stinging

Neuromuscular & skeletal: Paresthesias

Renal: Hematuria

Respiratory: Pulmonary edema

Overdosage/Toxicology Symptoms of overdose include vomiting, restlessness, ataxia, seizures, arrhythmias, pulmonary edema, hematuria, and hepatitis. The drug is absorbed through the skin, mucous membranes, and GI tract, and has occasionally caused serious CNS, hepatic, and renal toxicity when used excessively for prolonged periods, or with accidental ingestion. If (Continued)

Lindane (Continued)

ingested, perform gastric lavage and general supportive measures.

Pharmacodynamics/Kinetics
Time to Peak: Serum: Children: 6 hours
Half-Life Elimination: Children: 17-22 hours
Metabolism: Hepatic
Excretion: Urine and feces

Available Dosage Forms
Lotion, topical: 1% (60 mL)
Shampoo, topical: 1% (60 mL) [contains alcohol 0.5%]

Dosing
Adults & Elderly:
Scabies: Topical: Apply a thin layer of lotion and massage it on skin from the neck to the toes; after 8-12 hours, bathe and remove the drug
Head lice, crab lice: Topical: Apply shampoo to dry hair and massage into hair for 4 minutes; add small quantities of water to hair until lather forms, then rinse hair thoroughly and comb with a fine tooth comb to remove nits. Amount of shampoo needed is based on length and density of hair; most patients will require 30 mL (maximum: 60 mL).
Pediatrics: Refer to adult dosing.

Administration
Oral: Never administer orally.
Topical: For topical use only. Caregivers should apply with gloves (avoid natural latex, may be permeable to lindane). Rinse off with warm (not hot) water.
Lotion: Apply to dry, cool skin; do not apply to face or eyes. Wait at least 1 hour after bathing or showering (wet or warm skin increases absorption). Skin should be clean and free of any other lotions, creams, or oil prior to lindane application.
Shampoo: Apply to clean, dry hair. Wait at least 1 hour after washing hair before applying lindane shampoo. Hair should be washed with a shampoo not containing a conditioner; hair and skin of head and neck should be free of any lotions, oils, or creams prior to lindane application.

Nursing Actions
Physical Assessment: Assess head, hair, and skin surfaces for presence of lice and nits. Assess knowledge/teach patient appropriate application, use, and adverse symptoms to report.
Patient Education: For external use only. Do not apply to face and avoid getting in eyes. Do not apply immediately after hot, soapy bath. For scabies, Apply from neck to toes. Bathe to remove drug after 8-12 hours. For head lice or crab lice, massage into dry hair for 4 minutes; add water to hair to form lather, then rinse thoroughly. Clothing and bedding must be washed in hot water or dry cleaned to kill nits. Wash combs and brushes with lindane shampoo and thoroughly rinse. May need to treat all members of household and all sexual contacts concurrently. Report if condition persists or infection occurs. **Pregnancy/breast-feeding precautions:** Inform prescriber if you are pregnant. Do not breast-feed.
Geriatric Considerations Safety and efficacy have not been studied in the elderly; deaths following use have been reported.
Breast-Feeding Issues Nursing mothers should interrupt breast-feeding, express and discard milk for at least 24 hours following use.
Pregnancy Issues There are no adequate and well-controlled studies in pregnant women. CDC recommends alternative treatment in pregnant women (pyrethrins with piperonyl butoxide or permethrin for lice, permethrin for scabies). Per manufacturer, should be used no more than twice in a pregnancy. Reapplication of lindane is **not** the appropriate treatment if itching continues after the single treatment.

Linezolid (li NE zoh lid)

U.S. Brand Names Zyvox™
Pharmacologic Category Antibiotic, Oxazolidinone
Medication Safety Issues
Sound-alike/look-alike issues:
Zyvox™ may be confused with Vioxx®, Ziox™, Zosyn®, Zovirax®
Pregnancy Risk Factor C
Lactation Excretion in breast milk unknown/use caution
Use Treatment of vancomycin-resistant *Enterococcus faecium* (VRE) infections, nosocomial pneumonia caused by *Staphylococcus aureus* including MRSA or *Streptococcus pneumoniae* (including multi-drug-resistant strains [MDRSP]), complicated and uncomplicated skin and skin structure infections (including diabetic foot infections without concomitant osteomyelitis), and community-acquired pneumonia caused by susceptible gram-positive organisms
Mechanism of Action/Effect Inhibits bacterial protein synthesis by binding to bacterial 23S ribosomal RNA of the 50S subunit. This prevents the formation of a functional 70S initiation complex that is essential for the bacterial translation process. Linezolid is bacteriostatic against enterococci and staphylococci and bactericidal against most strains of streptococci.
Contraindications Hypersensitivity to linezolid or any other component of the formulation
Warnings/Precautions Myelosuppression has been reported and may be dependent on duration of therapy (generally >2 weeks of treatment); use with caution in patients with pre-existing myelosuppression, in patients receiving other drugs which may cause bone marrow suppression, or in chronic infection (previous or concurrent antibiotic therapy). Weekly CBC monitoring is recommended. Discontinue linezolid in patients developing myelosuppression (or in whom myelosuppression worsens during treatment).

Lactic acidosis has been reported with use. Linezolid exhibits mild MAO inhibitor properties and has the potential to have the same interactions as other MAO inhibitors; use with caution in uncontrolled hypertension, pheochromocytoma, carcinoid syndrome, or untreated hyperthyroidism; avoid use with serotonergic agents such as TCAs, venlafaxine, trazodone, sibutramine, meperidine, dextromethorphan, and SSRIs; concomitant use has been associated with the development of serotonin syndrome. Unnecessary use may lead to the development of resistance to linezolid; consider alternatives before initiating outpatient treatment.

Peripheral and optic neuropathy (with vision loss) has been reported and may occur primarily with extended courses of therapy >28 days; any symptoms of visual change or impairment warrant immediate ophthalmic evaluation and possible discontinuation of therapy.

Due to inconsistent therapeutic concentrations in the CSF, empiric use in pediatric patients with CNS infections is not recommended.

Drug Interactions
Increased Effect/Toxicity: Linezolid is a reversible, nonselective inhibitor of MAO. Serotonergic agents (eg, TCAs, venlafaxine, trazodone, sibutramine, meperidine, dextromethorphan, and SSRIs) may cause a serotonin syndrome (eg, hyperpyrexia, cognitive dysfunction) when used concomitantly. Adrenergic agents (eg, phenylpropanolamine, pseudoephedrine, sympathomimetic agents, vasopressor or dopaminergic agents) may cause hypertension. Tramadol may increase the risk of seizures when used concurrently with linezolid. Myelosuppressive medications may increase risk of myelosuppression when used concurrently with linezolid.

Nutritional/Ethanol Interactions

Ethanol: Avoid ethanol (may contain tyramine, hypertensive crisis may result).

Food: Avoid foods (eg, cheese) and beverages containing tyramine in patients receiving linezolid (hypertensive crisis may result).

Adverse Reactions Percentages as reported in adults; frequency similar in pediatric patients

>10%:
Central nervous system: Headache (<1% to 11%)
Gastrointestinal: Diarrhea (3% to 11%)

1% to 10%:
Central nervous system: Insomnia (3%), dizziness (0.4% to 2%), fever (2%)
Dermatologic: Rash (2%)
Gastrointestinal: Nausea (3% to 10%), vomiting (1% to 4%), pancreatic enzymes increased (<1% to 4%), constipation (2%), taste alteration (1% to 2%), tongue discoloration (0.2% to 1%), oral moniliasis (0.4% to 1%), pancreatitis
Genitourinary: Vaginal moniliasis (1% to 2%)
Hematologic: Thrombocytopenia (0.3% to 10%), hemoglobin decreased (0.9% to 7%), anemia, leukopenia, neutropenia; **Note:** Myelosuppression (including anemia, leukopenia, pancytopenia, and thrombocytopenia) may be more common in patients receiving linezolid for >2 weeks)
Hepatic: Abnormal LFTs (0.4% to 1%)
Renal: BUN increased (<1% to 2%)
Miscellaneous: Fungal infection (0.1% to 2%), lactate dehydrogenase increased (<1% to 2%)

Overdosage/Toxicology Treatment includes supportive care. Hemodialysis may improve elimination (30% of a dose is removed during a 3-hour hemodialysis session).

Pharmacodynamics/Kinetics

Time to Peak: Adults: Oral: 1-2 hours

Protein Binding: Adults: 31%

Half-Life Elimination: Children ≥1 week (full-term) to 11 years: 1.5-3 hours; Adults: 4-5 hours

Metabolism: Hepatic via oxidation of the morpholine ring, resulting in two inactive metabolites (aminoethoxyacetic acid, hydroxyethyl glycine); does not involve CYP

Excretion: Urine (30% as parent drug, 50% as metabolites); feces (9% as metabolites)
Nonrenal clearance: 65%; increased in children ≥1 week to 11 years

Available Dosage Forms

Infusion [premixed]: 200 mg (100 mL) [contains sodium 1.7 mEq]; 400 mg (200 mL) [contains sodium 3.3 mEq]; 600 mg (300 mL) [contains sodium 5 mEq]
Powder for oral suspension: 20 mg/mL (150 mL) [contains phenylalanine 20 mg/5 mL, sodium benzoate, and sodium 0.4 mEq/5 mL; orange flavor]
Tablet: 600 mg [contains sodium 0.1 mEq/tablet]

Dosing

Adults & Elderly:

VRE infections: Oral, I.V.: 600 mg every 12 hours for 14-28 days

Nosocomial pneumonia, complicated skin and skin structure infections, community-acquired pneumonia including concurrent bacteremia: Oral, I.V.: 600 mg every 12 hours for 10-14 days

Uncomplicated skin and skin structure infections: Oral: 400 mg every 12 hours for 10-14 days

Pediatrics:

VRE infections: Oral, I.V.:
Preterm neonates (<34 weeks gestational age): 10 mg/kg every 12 hours; neonates with a suboptimal clinical response can be advanced to 10 mg/kg every 8 hours. By day 7 of life, all neonates should receive 10 mg/kg every 8 hours.
Infants (excluding preterm neonates <1 week) and Children ≤11 years: 10 mg/kg every 8 hours for 14-28 days

Children ≥12 years: Refer to adult dosing.

Nosocomial pneumonia, complicated skin and skin structure infections, community acquired pneumonia including concurrent bacteremia: Oral, I.V.:
Infants (excluding preterm neonates <1 week) and Children ≤11 years: 10 mg/kg every 8 hours for 10-14 days
Children ≥12 years: Refer to adult dosing.

Uncomplicated skin and skin structure infections: Oral:
Infants (excluding preterm neonates <1 week) and Children <5 years: 10 mg/kg every 8 hours for 10-14 days
Children 5-11 years: 10 mg/kg every 12 hours for 10-14 days
Children ≥12-18 years: 600 mg every 12 hours for 10-14 days

Renal Impairment: No adjustment is recommended. The two primary metabolites may accumulate in patients with renal impairment but the clinical significance is unknown. Weigh the risk of accumulation of metabolites versus the benefit of therapy. Both linezolid and the two metabolites are eliminated by dialysis. Linezolid should be given after hemodialysis.

Hepatic Impairment: No dosage adjustment required for mild to moderate hepatic insufficiency (Child-Pugh class A or B). Use in severe hepatic insufficiency has not been adequately evaluated.

Administration

Oral: Oral suspension: Invert gently to mix prior to administration, do not shake

I.V.: Administer intravenous infusion over 30-120 minutes. Do not mix or infuse with other medications. When the same intravenous line is used for sequential infusion of other medications, flush line with D_5W, NS, or LR before and after infusing linezolid. The yellow color of the injection may intensify over time without affecting potency.

Stability

Compatibility:

Y-site administration: Incompatible with amphotericin B, chlorpromazine, diazepam, erythromycin, pentamidine, phenytoin, sulfamethoxazole/trimethoprim

Compatibility when admixed: Incompatible with ceftriaxone

Storage:
Infusion: Store at 25°C (77°F). Protect from light. Keep infusion bags in overwrap until ready for use. Protect infusion bags from freezing.
Oral suspension: Following reconstitution, store at room temperature; use reconstituted suspension within 21 days

Laboratory Monitoring Weekly CBC and platelet counts, particularly in patients at increased risk of bleeding, with pre-existing myelosuppression, on concomitant medications that cause bone marrow suppression, in those who require >2 weeks of therapy, or in those with chronic infection who have received previous or concomitant antibiotic therapy.

Nursing Actions

Physical Assessment: Previous drug allergies should be assessed before administering first dose. Assess other pharmacological agents patient may be taking for effectiveness and interactions (eg, serotonergic agents may increase resistance to linezolid and increase risk of serotonin syndrome, increased risk of hypertension with adrenergic agents). Assess results of laboratory tests, therapeutic effectiveness (resolution of infection), and adverse reactions (eg, myelosuppression, anemia; lactic acidosis) on a regular basis. Teach patient proper use (oral), possible side effects/appropriate interventions (eg, tyramine free diet - see Tyramine Contents of Foods *on page 1406*), and adverse reactions to report.
(Continued)

Linezolid *(Continued)*

Patient Education: Oral: Take exactly as directed. Do not alter dosage without consulting prescriber. Complete full course of therapy even if condition appears controlled. Maintain adequate hydration (2-3 L/day of fluids) unless instructed to restrict fluid intake. Avoid alcohol. Avoid tyramine-containing foods (eg, pickles, aged cheese, wine).

Oral/I.V.: You may experience GI discomfort, nausea, vomiting, taste alteration (small, frequent meals, frequent mouth care, sucking lozenges, or chewing gum may help); mild headache (analgesic may help); or constipation (increase exercise, fluids, fruit, or fiber may help). Report immediately unresolved, liquid diarrhea; white plaques in mouth; skin rash or irritation; acute headache, dizziness, blurred vision; or other persistent adverse reactions. **Pregnancy/breast-feeding precautions:** Inform prescriber if you are or intend to become pregnant. Consult prescriber if breast-feeding.

Dietary Considerations Take with or without food. Avoid foods with high tyramine content (eg, pickled or fermented foods, cheese, beer and wine). Suspension contains 20 mg phenylalanine per teaspoonful. Sodium content: 0.1 mEq/tablet; 0.4 mEq/5 mL; 1.7 mEq/100 mL infusion; 3.3 mEq/200 mL infusion; 5 mEq/300 mL infusion

Lisinopril *(lyse IN oh pril)*

U.S. Brand Names Prinivil®; Zestril®

Pharmacologic Category Angiotensin-Converting Enzyme (ACE) Inhibitor

Medication Safety Issues

Sound-alike/look-alike issues:
Lisinopril may be confused with fosinopril, Lioresal®, Risperdal®
Prinivil® may be confused with Plendil®, Pravachol®, Prevacid®, Prilosec®, Proventil®
Zestril® may be confused with Desyrel®, Restoril®, Vistaril®, Zetia™, Zostrix®

Pregnancy Risk Factor C (1st trimester)/D (2nd and 3rd trimesters)

Lactation Excretion in breast milk unknown/not recommended

Use Treatment of hypertension, either alone or in combination with other antihypertensive agents; adjunctive therapy in treatment of CHF (afterload reduction); treatment of acute myocardial infarction within 24 hours in hemodynamically-stable patients to improve survival; treatment of left ventricular dysfunction after myocardial infarction

Mechanism of Action/Effect Competitive inhibitor of angiotensin-converting enzyme (ACE); prevents conversion of angiotensin I to angiotensin II, a potent vasoconstrictor; results in lower levels of angiotensin II which causes an increase in plasma renin activity and a reduction in aldosterone secretion

Contraindications Hypersensitivity to lisinopril or any component of the formulation; angioedema related to previous treatment with an ACE inhibitor; bilateral renal artery stenosis; pregnancy (2nd and 3rd trimesters)

Warnings/Precautions Anaphylactic reactions can occur. Angioedema can occur at any time during treatment (especially following first dose). It may involve head and neck (potentially affecting the airway) or the intestine (presenting with abdominal pain). Prolonged monitoring may be required especially if tongue, glottis, or larynx are involved as they are associated with airway obstruction. Those with a history of airway surgery in this situation have a higher risk. Careful blood pressure monitoring with first dose (hypotension can occur especially in volume depleted patients). Dosage adjustment needed in renal impairment. Use with caution in hypovolemia; collagen vascular diseases; valvular stenosis (particularly aortic stenosis); hyperkalemia; or before, during, or immediately after anesthesia. Avoid rapid dosage escalation, which may lead to renal insufficiency. Rare toxicities associated with ACE inhibitors include cholestatic jaundice (which may progress to hepatic necrosis) and neutropenia/agranulocytosis with myeloid hyperplasia. If patient has renal impairment then a baseline WBC with differential and serum creatinine should be evaluated and monitored closely during the first 3 months of therapy. Hypersensitivity reactions may be seen during hemodialysis with high-flux dialysis membranes (eg, AN69). Deterioration in renal function can occur with initiation. Use with caution in unilateral renal artery stenosis and pre-existing renal insufficiency. Safety and efficacy have not been established in children <6 years of age.

Drug Interactions

Decreased Effect: Aspirin (high dose) may reduce the therapeutic effects of ACE inhibitors; at low dosages this does not appear to be significant. Rifampin may decrease the effect of ACE inhibitors. Antacids may decrease the bioavailability of ACE inhibitors (may be more likely to occur with captopril); separate administration times by 1-2 hours. NSAIDs, specifically indomethacin, may reduce the hypotensive effects of ACE inhibitors. More likely to occur in low renin or volume dependent hypertensive patients.

Increased Effect/Toxicity: Potassium supplements, co-trimoxazole (high dose), angiotensin II receptor antagonists (eg, candesartan, losartan, irbesartan), or potassium-sparing diuretics (amiloride, spironolactone, triamterene) may result in elevated serum potassium levels when combined with lisinopril. ACE inhibitor effects may be increased by phenothiazines or probenecid (increases levels of captopril). ACE inhibitors may increase serum concentrations/effects of lithium.

Diuretics have additive hypotensive effects with ACE inhibitors, and hypovolemia increases the potential for adverse renal effects of ACE inhibitors. In patients with compromised renal function, coadministration with NSAIDs may result in further deterioration of renal function. Allopurinol and ACE inhibitors may cause a higher risk of hypersensitivity reaction when taken concurrently.

Nutritional/Ethanol Interactions Herb/Nutraceutical: Avoid dong quai if using for hypertension (has estrogenic activity). Avoid ephedra, yohimbe, ginseng (may worsen hypertension). Avoid garlic (may have increased antihypertensive effect).

Lab Interactions May cause false-positive results in urine acetone determinations using sodium nitroprusside reagent; increased potassium (S), serum creatinine/BUN

Adverse Reactions Note: Frequency ranges include data from hypertension and heart failure trials. Higher rates of adverse reactions have generally been noted in patients with CHF. However, the frequency of adverse effects associated with placebo is also increased in this population.

1% to 10%:
Cardiovascular: Orthostatic effects (1%), hypotension (1% to 4%)
Central nervous system: Headache (4% to 6%), dizziness (5% to 12%), fatigue (3%)
Dermatologic: Rash (1% to 2%)
Endocrine & metabolic: Hyperkalemia (2% to 5%)
Gastrointestinal: Diarrhea (3% to 4%), nausea (2%), vomiting (1%), abdominal pain (2%)
Genitourinary: Impotence (1%)
Hematologic: Decreased hemoglobin (small)
Neuromuscular & skeletal: Chest pain (3%), weakness (1%)

Renal: BUN increased (2%); deterioration in renal function (in patients with bilateral renal artery stenosis or hypovolemia); serum creatinine increased (often transient)

Respiratory: Cough (4% to 9%), upper respiratory infection (2% to 2%)

Overdosage/Toxicology Mild hypotension has been the primary toxic effect seen with acute overdose. Bradycardia may also occur; hyperkalemia occurs even with therapeutic doses, especially in patients with renal insufficiency and those taking NSAIDs. Treatment and is symptomatic and supportive.

Pharmacodynamics/Kinetics

Onset of Action: 1 hour; Peak effect: Hypotensive: Oral: ~6 hours

Duration of Action: 24 hours

Protein Binding: 25%

Half-Life Elimination: 11-12 hours

Excretion: Primarily urine (as unchanged drug)

Available Dosage Forms [DSC] = Discontinued product

Tablet: 2.5 mg, 5 mg, 10 mg, 20 mg, 30 mg, 40 mg

Prinivil®: 5 mg, 10 mg, 20 mg, 30 mg; 40 mg [DSC]

Zestril®: 2.5 mg, 5 mg, 10 mg, 20 mg, 30 mg, 40 mg

Dosing

Adults:

Hypertension: Oral: Usual dosage range (JNC 7): 10-40 mg/day

Not maintained on diuretic: Initial: 10 mg/day

Maintained on diuretic: Initial: 5 mg/day

Note: Antihypertensive effect may diminish toward the end of the dosing interval especially with doses of 10 mg/day. An increased dose may aid in extending the duration of antihypertensive effect. Doses up to 80 mg/day have been used, but do not appear to give greater effect (Zesteril® Product Information, 12/04).

Patients taking diuretics should have them discontinued 2-3 days prior to initiating lisinopril if possible. Restart diuretic after blood pressure is stable if needed. If diuretic cannot be discontinued prior to therapy, begin with 5 mg with close supervision until stable blood pressure. In patients with hyponatremia (<130 mEq/L), start dose at 2.5 mg/day.

Congestive heart failure: Oral: Initial: 2.5-5 mg once daily; then increase by no more than 10 mg increments at intervals no less than 2 weeks to a maximum daily dose of 40 mg. Usual maintenance: 5-40 mg/day as a single dose. Target dose: 20-40 mg once daily (ACC/AHA 2005 Heart Failure Guidelines)

Note: If patient has hyponatremia (serum sodium <130 meq/L) or renal impairment (Cl_{cr} <30 mL/ minute or creatinine >3 mg/dL), then initial dose should be 2.5 mg/day

Acute myocardial infarction (within 24 hours in hemodynamically stable patients): Oral: 5 mg immediately, then 5 mg at 24 hours, 10 mg at 48 hours, and 10 mg every day thereafter for 6 weeks. Patients should continue to receive standard treatments such as thrombolytics, aspirin, and beta-blockers.

Elderly: Oral:

Initial: 2.5-5 mg/day; increase doses 2.5-5 mg/day at 1- to 2-week intervals; maximum daily dose: 40 mg

Patients taking diuretics should have them discontinued 2-3 days prior to initiating lisinopril if possible. Restart diuretic after blood pressure is stable if needed. In patients with hyponatremia (<130 mEq/ L), start dose at 2.5 mg/day (see Renal Impairment).

Pediatrics:

Hypertension: Children ≥6 years: Oral: Initial: 0.07 mg/kg once daily (up to 5 mg); increase dose at 1-

to 2-week intervals; doses >0.61 mg/kg or >40 mg have not been evaluated.

Renal Impairment:

Hypertension:

Adults: Initial doses should be modified and upward titration should be cautious, based on response (maximum: 40 mg/day)

Cl_{cr} >30 mL/minute: Initial: 10 mg/day

Cl_{cr} 10-30 mL/minute: Initial: 5 mg/day

Hemodialysis: Initial: 2.5 mg/day; dialyzable (50%)

Children: Use in not recommended in pediatric patients with GFR <30 mL/minute/1.73 m^2

Congestive heart failure: Adults: Cl_{cr} <30 mL/minute or creatinine >3 mg/dL): Initial: 2.5 mg/day

Administration

Oral: Watch for hypotensive effects within 1-3 hours of first dose or new higher dose.

Laboratory Monitoring CBC, renal function tests, electrolytes. If patient has renal impairment, a baseline WBC with differential and serum creatinine should be evaluated and monitored closely during the first 3 months of therapy.

Nursing Actions

Physical Assessment: Assess potential for interactions with other pharmacological agents or herbal products patient is taking that may impact fluid balance or cardiac status. Monitor patient very closely following first dose, following any increase in dose, and regularly during therapy (severe reactions can occur with first dose; eg, angioedema that may potentially affect airway or intestine, hypovolemia, postural hypotension, or anaphylactic reaction). Evaluate results of laboratory tests and therapeutic effectiveness on a (normotensive) regular basis. Teach patient proper use, possible side effects/appropriate interventions, and adverse symptoms to report.

Patient Education: Do not take any new medication during therapy unless approved by prescriber. Take exactly as directed; do not discontinue without consulting prescriber. Take first dose at bedtime. Take all doses on an empty stomach, 1 hour before or 2 hours after meals. Do not use potassium supplement or salt substitutes without consulting prescriber. This drug does not eliminate need for diet or exercise regimen as recommended by prescriber. May cause dizziness, fainting, or lightheadedness (use caution when driving or engaging in tasks that require alertness until response to drug is known); postural hypotension (use caution when rising from lying or sitting position or climbing stairs); or nausea, vomiting, abdominal pain, dry mouth, or transient loss of appetite (small frequent meals, frequent mouth care, sucking lozenges, or chewing gum may help), report if these persist. Report chest pain or palpitations; mouth sores; fever or chills; swelling of extremities, face, mouth, or tongue; skin rash; numbness, tingling, or pain in muscles; respiratory difficulty or unusual cough; other persistent adverse reactions. **Pregnancy/breast-feeding precautions:** Inform prescriber if you are or intend to become pregnant. This drug should not be used in the 2nd or 3rd trimester of pregnancy. Consult prescriber for appropriate contraceptive measures. Breast-feeding is not recommended.

Geriatric Considerations Due to frequent decreases in glomerular filtration (also creatinine clearance) with aging, elderly patients may have exaggerated responses to ACE inhibitors. Differences in clinical response due to hepatic changes are not observed. ACE inhibitors may be preferred agents in elderly patients with congestive heart failure and diabetes mellitus. Diabetic proteinuria is reduced and insulin sensitivity is enhanced. In general, the side effect profile is favorable in the elderly and causes little or no CNS confusion. Use lowest dose recommendations initially. (Continued)

Lisinopril *(Continued)*

Breast-Feeding Issues Lisinopril is not recommended (per manufacturer) in breast-feeding women. A similar drug, captopril, has been rated as compatible.

Pregnancy Issues ACE inhibitors can cause fetal injury or death if taken during the 2nd or 3rd trimester. Discontinue ACE inhibitors as soon as pregnancy is detected.

Lisinopril and Hydrochlorothiazide
(lyse IN oh pril & hye droe klor oh THYE a zide)

U.S. Brand Names Prinzide®; Zestoretic®
Synonyms Hydrochlorothiazide and Lisinopril
Pharmacologic Category Antihypertensive Agent, Combination
Pregnancy Risk Factor C/D (2nd and 3rd trimesters)
Lactation
Hydrochlorothiazide: Compatible
Lisinopril: Excretion in breast milk unknown
Use Treatment of hypertension
Available Dosage Forms Tablet:
Lisinopril 10 mg and hydrochlorothiazide 12.5 mg
Lisinopril 20 mg and hydrochlorothiazide 12.5 mg
Lisinopril 20 mg and hydrochlorothiazide 25 mg
Dosing
Adults & Elderly: Hypertension: Oral: Initial: Lisinopril 10 mg/hydrochlorothiazide 12.5 mg or lisinopril 20 mg/ hydrochlorothiazide 12.5 mg with further increases of either or both components could depend on clinical response. Doses >80 mg/day lisinopril or >50 mg/day hydrochlorothiazide are not recommended.
Renal Impairment: Dosage adjustments should be made with caution. Usual regimens of therapy need not be adjusted as long as patient's Cl$_{cr}$ >30 mL/ minute. In patients with more severe renal impairment, loop diuretics are preferred.
Nursing Actions
Physical Assessment: See individual agents.
Patient Education: See individual agents. **Pregnancy/breast-feeding precautions:** Inform prescriber if you are or intend to become pregnant. Consult prescriber if breast-feeding.
Related Information
Hydrochlorothiazide *on page 610*
Lisinopril *on page 742*

Lithium *(LITH ee um)*

U.S. Brand Names Eskalith® [DSC]; Eskalith CR®; Lithobid®
Synonyms Lithium Carbonate; Lithium Citrate
Pharmacologic Category Lithium
Medication Safety Issues
Sound-alike/look-alike issues:
Eskalith® may be confused with Estratest®
Lithobid® may be confused with Levbid®, Lithostat®
Pregnancy Risk Factor D
Lactation Enters breast milk/contraindicated
Use Management of bipolar disorders; treatment of mania in individuals with bipolar disorder (maintenance treatment prevents or diminishes intensity of subsequent episodes)
Unlabeled/Investigational Use Potential augmenting agent for antidepressants; aggression, post-traumatic stress disorder, conduct disorder in children
Mechanism of Action/Effect Stabilizes mood by actions on nerve cells of the central nervous system; involves serotonin, phosphatidylinositol cycle, and dopamine receptor sensitivity
Contraindications Hypersensitivity to lithium or any component of the formulation; avoid use in patients with severe cardiovascular or renal disease, or with severe debilitation, dehydration, or sodium depletion; pregnancy

Warnings/Precautions Lithium toxicity is closely related to serum levels and can occur at therapeutic doses; serum lithium determinations are required to monitor therapy. Use with caution in patients with thyroid disease, mild-moderate renal impairment, or mild-moderate cardiovascular disease. Use caution in patients receiving medications which alter sodium excretion (eg, diuretics, ACE inhibitors, NSAIDs), or in patients with significant fluid loss (protracted sweating, diarrhea, or prolonged fever); temporary reduction or cessation of therapy may be warranted. Some elderly patients may be extremely sensitive to the effects of lithium, see Dosing. Chronic therapy results in diminished renal concentrating ability (nephrogenic DI); this is usually reversible when lithium is discontinued. Changes in renal function should be monitored, and re-evaluation of treatment may be necessary. Use caution in patients at risk of suicide (suicidal thoughts or behavior).

Use with caution in patients receiving neuroleptic medications - a syndrome resembling NMS has been associated with concurrent therapy. Lithium may impair the patient's alertness, affecting the ability to operate machinery or driving a vehicle. Neuromuscular-blocking agents should be administered with caution; the response may be prolonged.

Higher serum concentrations may be required and tolerated during an acute manic phase; however, the tolerance decreases when symptoms subside. Normal fluid and salt intake must be maintained during therapy.

Safety and efficacy have not been established in children <12 years of age.

Drug Interactions
Decreased Effect: Combined use of lithium and chlorpromazine may lower serum concentrations of both drugs. Lithium may blunt the pressor response to sympathomimetics (epinephrine, norepinephrine). Caffeine (xanthine derivatives) may lower lithium serum concentrations by increasing urinary lithium excretion (monitor).

Increased Effect/Toxicity: Concurrent use of lithium with carbamazepine, diltiazem, SSRIs (fluoxetine, fluvoxamine), haloperidol, methyldopa, metronidazole (rare), phenothiazines, phenytoin, TCAs, and verapamil may increase the risk for neurotoxicity. A rare encephalopathic syndrome has been reported in association with haloperidol (causal relationship not established). Lithium concentrations/toxicity may be increased by diuretics, NSAIDs (sulindac and aspirin may be exceptions), ACE inhibitors, angiotensin receptor antagonists (losartan), tetracyclines, or COX-2 inhibitors (celecoxib).

Lithium and MAO inhibitors should generally be avoided due to use reports of fatal malignant hyperpyrexia; risk with selective MAO type B inhibitors (selegiline) appears to be lower. Potassium iodide may enhance the hypothyroid effects of lithium. Combined use of lithium with tricyclic antidepressants or sibutramine may increase the risk of serotonin syndrome; this combination is best avoided. Lithium may potentiate effect of neuromuscular blockers.

Nutritional/Ethanol Interactions Food: Lithium serum concentrations may be increased if taken with food. Limit caffeine.

Lab Interactions Increased calcium (S), glucose, magnesium, potassium (S); decreased thyroxine (S)

Adverse Reactions Frequency not defined.
Cardiovascular: Cardiac arrhythmia, hypotension, sinus node dysfunction, flattened or inverted T waves (reversible), edema, bradycardia, syncope

Central nervous system: Dizziness, vertigo, slurred speech, blackout spells, seizure, sedation, restlessness, confusion, psychomotor retardation, stupor, coma, dystonia, fatigue, lethargy, headache, pseudotumor cerebri, slowed intellectual functioning, tics

Dermatologic: Dry or thinning of hair, folliculitis, alopecia, exacerbation of psoriasis, rash

Endocrine & metabolic: Euthyroid goiter and/or hypothyroidism, hyperthyroidism, hyperglycemia, diabetes insipidus

Gastrointestinal: Polydipsia, anorexia, nausea, vomiting, diarrhea, xerostomia, metallic taste, weight gain, salivary gland swelling, excessive salivation

Genitourinary: Incontinence, polyuria, glycosuria, oliguria, albuminuria

Hematologic: Leukocytosis

Neuromuscular & skeletal: Tremor, muscle hyperirritability, ataxia, choreoathetoid movements, hyperactive deep tendon reflexes, myasthenia gravis (rare)

Ocular: Nystagmus, blurred vision, transient scotoma

Miscellaneous: Coldness and painful discoloration of fingers and toes

Overdosage/Toxicology Symptoms include sedation, confusion, tremors, joint pain, visual changes, seizures, and coma. There is no specific antidote for lithium poisoning. For acute ingestion, following initiation of essential overdose management, discontinue lithium and remove any unabsorbed lithium via gastric lavage (activated charcoal is ineffective as it does not bind lithium). Correct fluid and electrolyte imbalances, provide supportive care. In severe cases, patient should be dialyzed. Hemodialysis is preferred (and more effective) than peritoneal dialysis. The goal is to decrease serum lithium level to <1 mEq/L on a serum sample drawn 6-8 hours after completion of dialysis. Agents that increase the excretion of lithium are of questionable value.

Pharmacodynamics/Kinetics

Time to Peak: Serum: Nonsustained release: ~0.5-2 hours; slow release: 4-12 hours; syrup: 15-60 minutes

Protein Binding: Not protein bound

Half-Life Elimination: 18-24 hours; can increase to more than 36 hours in elderly or with renal impairment

Metabolism: Not metabolized

Excretion: Urine (90% to 98% as unchanged drug); sweat (4% to 5%); feces (1%)

Clearance: 80% of filtered lithium is reabsorbed in the proximal convoluted tubules; therefore, clearance approximates 20% of GFR or 20-40 mL/minute

Available Dosage Forms

[DSC] = Discontinued product

Capsule, as carbonate: 150 mg, 300 mg, 600 mg
Eskalith®: 300 mg [contains benzyl alcohol] [DSC]

Syrup, as citrate: 300 mg/5 mL (5 mL, 10 mL, 480 mL) [contains alcohol]

Tablet, as carbonate: 300 mg

Tablet, controlled release, as carbonate (Eskalith CR®): 450 mg

Tablet, slow release, as carbonate (Lithobid®): 300 mg

Dosing

Adults:

Bipolar disorders: Oral: 900-2400 mg/day in 3-4 divided doses or 900-1800 mg/day in two divided doses of sustained release

Note: Monitor serum concentrations and clinical response (efficacy and toxicity) to determine proper dose

Elderly: Bipolar disorders: Oral: Initial: 300 mg twice daily; increase weekly in increments of 300 mg/day, monitoring levels; rarely need to go >900-1200 mg/day.

Pediatrics:

Bipolar disorders: Oral: Children 6-12 years: 15-60 mg/kg/day in 3-4 divided doses; dose not to exceed

usual adult dosage. **Note:** Monitor serum concentrations and clinical response (efficacy and toxicity) to determine proper dose.

Conduct disorder (unlabeled use): Oral: Children 6-12 years: 15-30 mg/kg/day in 3-4 divided doses; dose not to exceed usual adult dosage

Renal Impairment:

Cl_{cr} 10-50 mL/minute: Administer 50% to 75% of normal dose.

Cl_{cr} <10 mL/minute: Administer 25% to 50% of normal dose.

Dialyzable (50% to 100%); 4-7 times more efficient than peritoneal dialysis

Administration

Oral: Administer with meals to decrease GI upset. Slow release tablets must be swallowed whole; do not crush or chew.

Laboratory Monitoring Serum lithium every 4-5 days during initial therapy. Monitor renal and thyroid; serum electrolytes; CBC with differential, urinalysis.

Levels should be obtained twice weekly until both patient's clinical status and levels are stable then levels may be obtained every 1-3 months.

Timing of serum samples: Draw trough just before next dose (8-12 hours after previous dose).

Therapeutic levels:

Acute mania: 0.6-1.2 mEq/L (SI: 0.6-1.2 mmol/L)

Protection against future episodes in most patients with bipolar disorder: 0.8-1 mEq/L (SI: 0.8-1.0 mmol/L); a higher rate of relapse is described in subjects who are maintained at <0.4 mEq/L (SI: 0.4 mmol/L).

Elderly patients can usually be maintained at lower end of therapeutic range (0.6-0.8 mEq/L).

Toxic concentration: >1.5 mEq/L (SI: >2 mmol/L)

Adverse effect levels:

GI complaints/tremor: 1.5-2 mEq/L

Confusion/somnolence: 2-2.5 mEq/L

Seizures/death: >2.5 mEq/L

Nursing Actions

Physical Assessment: Assess effectiveness and interactions of other medications patient may be taking. Monitor cardiovascular status; assess for fluid retention. Monitor laboratory results at beginning of therapy, when adjusting dose, and periodically thereafter. Monitor effectiveness of therapy and adverse reactions at beginning of therapy and periodically with long-term use. **Note:** Lithium has a very small window of safety (TI). Assess knowledge/teach patient appropriate use, interventions to reduce side effects, and importance of reporting adverse symptoms promptly.

Patient Education: Take exactly as directed; do not change dosage without consulting prescriber. Do not crush or chew extended or slow release tablets or capsules. Maintain adequate hydration (2-3 L/day of fluids) unless instructed to restrict fluid intake (especially in summer). Avoid changes in sodium content (eg, low sodium diets); reduction of sodium can increase lithium toxicity. Limit caffeine intake (diuresis can increase lithium toxicity). Frequent blood test and monitoring will be necessary. You may experience decreased appetite or altered taste sensation (small frequent meals may help maintain nutrition); or drowsiness or dizziness, especially during early therapy (use caution when driving or engaging in tasks requiring alertness until response to drug is known). Immediately report unresolved diarrhea, abrupt changes in weight, muscular tremors or lack of coordination, fever, or changes in urinary volume. **Pregnancy/breast-feeding precautions:** Do not get pregnant while taking this medication; use appropriate contraceptive measures. Do not breast-feed.

Dietary Considerations May be taken with meals to avoid GI upset; have patient drink 2-3 L of water daily.

Geriatric Considerations Some elderly patients may be extremely sensitive to the effects of lithium. Initial (Continued)

Lithium (Continued)

doses need to be adjusted for renal function in the elderly; thereafter, adjust doses based upon serum concentrations and response.

Pregnancy Issues Cardiac malformations in the infant, including Ebstein's anomaly, are associated with use of lithium during the first trimester of pregnancy. Nontoxic effects to the newborn include shallow respiration, hypotonia, lethargy, cyanosis, diabetes insipidus, thyroid depression, and nontoxic goiter when lithium is used near term. Efforts should be made to avoid lithium use during the first trimester; if an alternative therapy is not appropriate, the lowest possible dose of lithium should be used throughout the pregnancy. Fetal echocardiography and ultrasound to screen for anomalies should be conducted between 16-20 weeks of gestation. Lithium levels should be monitored in the mother and may need adjusted following delivery.

Related Information

Peak and Trough Guidelines *on page 1387*

Lodoxamide (loe DOKS a mide)

U.S. Brand Names Alomide®

Synonyms Lodoxamide Tromethamine

Pharmacologic Category Mast Cell Stabilizer

Pregnancy Risk Factor B

Use Treatment of vernal keratoconjunctivitis, vernal conjunctivitis, and vernal keratitis

Contraindications Hypersensitivity to lodoxamide tromethamine or any component of the formulation

Warnings/Precautions Safety and efficacy in children <2 years of age have not been established. Not for injection. Not for use in patients wearing soft contact lenses during treatment.

Adverse Reactions

>10%: Local: Transient burning, stinging, discomfort

1% to 10%:

Central nervous system: Headache

Ocular: Blurred vision, corneal erosion/ulcer, eye pain, corneal abrasion, blepharitis

Overdosage/Toxicology Symptoms include feeling of warmth of flushing, headache, dizziness, fatigue, sweating, nausea, loose stools, and urinary frequency/urgency; consider emesis in the event of accidental ingestion

Available Dosage Forms Solution, ophthalmic: 0.1% (10 mL) [contains benzalkonium chloride]

Dosing

Adults & Elderly: Vernal conjunctivitis, keratitis: Ophthalmic: Children ≥2 years and Adults: Instill 1-2 drops in eye(s) 4 times/day for up to 3 months

Pediatrics: Children ≥2 years: Refer to adult dosing.

Nursing Actions

Physical Assessment: Assess potential for interactions with other prescriptions, OTC medications, or herbal products patient may be taking. Monitor patient response. Teach patient proper use, side effects/appropriate interventions, and symptoms to report.

Patient Education: For use in eyes only. Avoid wearing soft contact lenses while using this medication. Wash hands before using. Lie down or tilt your head back and look upward. Hold dropper tip as near as possible to your eyelid without touching it. Pull the lower lid of eye down to form a pocket. Drop the prescribed number of drops into the pocket made by the lower lid and the eye. (Placing drops on the surface of the eyeball can cause stinging.) Do not blink or rub eye. Close your eye and press lightly against the inside corner of your eye for about 1 minute. Repeat in other eye if directed by prescriber. Replace and tighten cap right away, do not allow tip of dropper to become contaminated. Wipe off any

excess liquid from cheek. Wash your hands again. Do not use any other eye medication without consulting prescriber. Do not share mediation with anyone else. You may experience temporary stinging or burning in the eyes, headache, increased eye tearing or dry eye, sneezing, or blurred vision. Inform prescriber if you experience eye pain, disturbance of vision; skin rash; swelling in or around the eyes; any other adverse response; or if condition worsens or fails to improve. Store medication at room temperature, away from excess heat and moisture. Do not use if solution has changed color, is cloudy, or contains particles.

Lomefloxacin (loe me FLOKS a sin)

U.S. Brand Names Maxaquin® [DSC]

Synonyms Lomefloxacin Hydrochloride

Pharmacologic Category Antibiotic, Quinolone

Pregnancy Risk Factor C

Lactation Excretion in breast milk unknown/not recommended

Use Acute bacterial exacerbation of chronic bronchitis caused by susceptible gram-negative organisms; urinary tract infections (uncomplicated and complicated) caused by susceptible organisms; surgical prophylaxis (transrectal prostate biopsy or transurethral procedures)

Mechanism of Action/Effect Inhibits DNA-gyrase in susceptible organisms thereby inhibits relaxation of supercoiled DNA and promotes breakage of DNA strands. DNA gyrase (topoisomerase II), is an essential bacterial enzyme that maintains the superhelical structure of DNA and is required for DNA replication and transcription, DNA repair, recombination, and transposition.

Contraindications Hypersensitivity to lomefloxacin, any component of the formulation, or other members of the quinolone group (such as, nalidixic acid, oxolinic acid, cinoxacin, norfloxacin, and ciprofloxacin); avoid use in children <18 years of age due to association of other quinolones with transient arthropathies

Warnings/Precautions CNS stimulation may occur (tremor, restlessness, confusion, and very rarely hallucinations or seizures); use with caution in patients with known or suspected CNS disorders; use caution to avoid possible photosensitivity reactions during and for several days following fluoroquinolone therapy. Use caution in renal impairment; may require dosage adjustment. Severe hypersensitivity reactions, including anaphylaxis, have occurred with quinolone therapy. If an allergic reaction occurs (itching, urticaria, dyspnea or facial edema, loss of consciousness, tingling, cardiovascular collapse), discontinue drug immediately. Prolonged use may result in superinfection; pseudomembranous colitis may occur and should be considered in all patients who present with diarrhea.

Rare incidence of peripheral neuropathy has been documented; discontinue if patient experiences symptoms of neuropathy including pain, burning, tingling, weakness or other sensory abnormalities. Tendon inflammation and/or rupture has been reported. Risk may be increased with concurrent corticosteroids, particularly in the elderly. Discontinue at first sign of tendon inflammation or pain. Quinolones may exacerbate myasthenia gravis; use with caution (rare, potentially life-threatening weakness of respiratory muscles may occur); avoid use in children <18 years of age due to association of other quinolones with transient arthropathies. Safety and efficacy has not been established in pediatric patients and adolescents <18 years of age, pregnant or lactating women.

Drug Interactions

Cytochrome P450 Effect: Inhibits CYP1A2 (weak)

Decreased Effect: Concurrent administration of metal cations, including most antacids, oral electrolyte supplements, quinapril, sucralfate, some didanosine formulations (chewable/buffered tablets and pediatric powder for oral suspension), and other highly-buffered oral drugs, may decrease quinolone level; separate doses.

Increased Effect/Toxicity: Concomitant use with corticosteroids may increase the risk of tendon rupture. Probenecid may increase lomefloxacin levels.

Nutritional/Ethanol Interactions
Food: Lomefloxacin peak serum levels may be prolonged if taken with food.
Herb/Nutraceutical: Avoid dong quai, St John's wort (may cause photosensitization).

Adverse Reactions 1% to 10%:
Central nervous system: Headache (4%), dizziness (2%)
Dermatologic: Photosensitivity (2%)
Gastrointestinal: Nausea (4%), abdominal pain (1%), diarrhea (1%)

Overdosage/Toxicology Symptoms of overdose include acute renal failure and seizures. Treatment is supportive; not removed by peritoneal or hemodialysis.

Pharmacodynamics/Kinetics
Time to Peak: 1.5 hours
Protein Binding: 10%
Half-Life Elimination: 7.8 hours
Excretion: Urine (65% as unchanged drug, 9% as metabolite); feces (10% as unchanged drug)

Available Dosage Forms [DSC] = Discontinued product
Tablet: 400 mg [DSC]

Dosing
Adults & Elderly:
Acute bacterial exacerbation of chronic bronchitis: Oral: 400 mg once daily for 10 days
Urinary tract infection (UTI) due to susceptible organisms: Oral:
Uncomplicated cystitis caused by Escherichia coli: 400 mg once daily for 3 successive days
Uncomplicated cystitis caused by Klebsiella pneumoniae, Proteus mirabilis, **or** *Staphylococcus saprophyticus*: 400 mg once daily for 10 successive days
Complicated UTI caused by Escherichia coli, Klebsiella pneumoniae, Proteus mirabilis, or *Pseudomonas aeruginosa*: 400 mg once daily for 14 successive days
Urologic surgical prophylaxis: Oral:
Transrectal prostate biopsy: 400 mg as a single dose, 1-6 hours before procedure
Transurethral surgical procedure: 400 mg as a single dose, 2-6 hours before procedure
Renal Impairment:
Cl$_{cr}$ 10-40 mL/minute: Initial loading dose = 400 mg; followed by 200 mg once daily maintenance dose
Hemodialysis: Same as for renal impairment.

Administration
Oral: Take 1 hour before or 2 hours after meals.

Laboratory Monitoring Perform culture and sensitivity studies prior to initiating therapy to determine the causative organism and its susceptibility to lomefloxacin. Monitor CBC, renal and hepatic function periodically if therapy is prolonged.

Nursing Actions
Physical Assessment: Results of culture and sensitivity tests and allergy history should be assessed before initiating therapy. Assess potential for interactions with other pharmacological or herbal agents patient may be taking (eg, increased risk of tendon rupture or arrhythmias). Monitor laboratory tests, therapeutic effectiveness (resolution of infection), and adverse reactions (eg, hypersensitivity reactions such as itching, urticaria, dyspnea or facial edema, loss of consciousness, tingling, or cardiovascular collapse which can occur days after therapy has started; diarrhea; opportunistic infection; pseudomembranous

colitis; tendon rupture) regularly during therapy. Teach patient proper use (according to formulation), possible side effects/appropriate interventions, and adverse symptoms to report.

Patient Education: Do not take any new medication during therapy unless approved by prescriber. Take exactly as directed: at least 4 hours before or 8 hours after antacids or other drug products containing calcium, iron, or zinc. Take entire prescription even if feeling better. Maintain adequate hydration (2-3 L/day of fluids) unless instructed to restrict fluid intake. You may experience dizziness, lightheadedness, or confusion (use caution when driving or engaging in tasks that require alertness until response to drug is known); nausea or vomiting (small, frequent meals, frequent mouth care, sucking lozenges, or chewing gum may help); or photosensitivity (use sunscreen, wear protective clothing and eyewear, and avoid direct sunlight). Discontinue use immediately and report to prescriber if inflammation, tendon pain, or allergic reaction occurs (itching urticaria, respiratory difficulty, facial edema, difficulty swallowing, loss of consciousness, tingling, chest pain, palpitations). Report palpitations or chest pain; CNS changes (excitability, seizures); persistent diarrhea or constipation; signs of infection (unusual fever or chills, vaginal itching or foul-smelling vaginal discharge, easy bruising or bleeding). **Pregnancy/breast-feeding precautions:** Inform prescriber if you are or intend to become pregnant. Do not breast-feed.

Dietary Considerations May be taken without regard to meals.

Geriatric Considerations Dosage adjustment is not necessary in patients with normal renal function, Cl$_{cr}$ ≥40 mL/minute; otherwise, follow dosage guidelines for renal impairment. Age-associated increase in half-life and decrease in clearance are thought to be secondary to age-related changes in renal function.

Breast-Feeding Issues Other quinolones are known to be excreted in breast milk. The manufacturer recommends to discontinue nursing or to discontinue the lomefloxacin.

Pregnancy Issues Reports of arthropathy (observed in immature animals and reported rarely in humans) have limited the use of fluoroquinolones in pregnancy. Teratogenic effects were not observed with lomefloxacin in animal studies; however, an increase in fetal loss was observed in one species. Based on limited data, quinolones are not expected to be a major human teratogen. Although quinolone antibiotics should not be used as first-line agents during pregnancy, when considering treatment for life-threatening infection and/or prolonged duration of therapy, the potential risk to the fetus must be balanced against the severity of the potential illness.

Lomustine (loe MUS teen)

U.S. Brand Names CeeNU®
Synonyms CCNU
Pharmacologic Category Antineoplastic Agent, Alkylating Agent
Medication Safety Issues
Sound-alike/look-alike issues:
Lomustine may be confused with carmustine
Pregnancy Risk Factor D
Lactation Enters breast milk/contraindicated
Use Treatment of brain tumors and Hodgkin's disease, non-Hodgkin's lymphoma, melanoma, renal carcinoma, lung cancer, colon cancer
Mechanism of Action/Effect Inhibits DNA and RNA synthesis via carbamylation of DNA polymerase, alkylation of DNA, and alteration of RNA, proteins, and enzymes
(Continued)

Lomustine (Continued)

Contraindications Hypersensitivity to lomustine, any component of the formulation, or other nitrosoureas; pregnancy

Warnings/Precautions The U.S. Food and Drug Administration (FDA) currently recommends that procedures for proper handling and disposal for antineoplastic agents be considered. Use with caution in patients with depressed platelet, leukocyte or erythrocyte counts. Bone marrow depression, notably thrombocytopenia and leukopenia, may lead to bleeding and overwhelming infections in an already compromised patient; will last for at least 6 weeks after a dose, do not give courses more frequently than every 6 weeks because the toxicity is cumulative. Use with caution in patients with liver function abnormalities.

Drug Interactions

Cytochrome P450 Effect: Substrate of CYP2D6 (major); **Inhibits** CYP2D6 (weak), 3A4 (weak)

Decreased Effect: Decreased effect with phenobarbital, resulting in reduced efficacy of both drugs.

Increased Effect/Toxicity: CYP2D6 inhibitors may increase the levels/effects of lomustine; example inhibitors include chlorpromazine, delavirdine, fluoxetine, miconazole, paroxetine, pergolide, quinidine, quinine, ritonavir, and ropinirole. Increased toxicity with cimetidine, reported to cause bone marrow depression or to potentiate the myelosuppressive effects of lomustine.

Nutritional/Ethanol Interactions Ethanol: Avoid ethanol (due to GI irritation).

Lab Interactions Liver function tests

Adverse Reactions

>10%:

Gastrointestinal: Nausea and vomiting, usually within 3-6 hours after oral administration. Administration of the dose at bedtime, with an antiemetic, significantly reduces both the incidence and severity of nausea.

Hematologic: Myelosuppression, common, dose-limiting, may be cumulative and irreversible
Onset: 10-14 days
Nadir: Leukopenia: 6 weeks
Thrombocytopenia: 4 weeks
Recovery: 6-8 weeks

1% to 10%:

Dermatologic: Rash

Gastrointestinal: Anorexia, stomatitis, diarrhea

Genitourinary: Progressive azotemia, renal failure, decrease in kidney size

Hematologic: Anemia

Hepatic: Elevated liver enzymes, transient, reversible

Overdosage/Toxicology Symptoms of overdose include nausea, vomiting, and leukopenia. There are no known antidotes. Treatment is symptomatic and supportive.

Pharmacodynamics/Kinetics

Duration of Action: Marrow recovery: ≤6 weeks

Time to Peak: Serum: Active metabolite: ~3 hours

Protein Binding: 50%

Half-Life Elimination: Parent drug: 16-72 hours; Active metabolite: Terminal: 1.3-2 days

Metabolism: Rapidly hepatic via hydroxylation producing at least two active metabolites; enterohepatically recycled

Excretion: Urine; feces (<5%); expired air (<10%)

Available Dosage Forms

Capsule: 10 mg, 40 mg, 100 mg

Capsule [dose pack]: 10 mg (2s); 40 mg (2s); 100 mg (2s)

Dosing

Adults & Elderly: Refer to individual protocols.

Chemotherapy: Oral: 100-130 mg/m^2 as a single dose every 6 weeks; readjust after initial treatment according to platelet and leukocyte counts

With compromised marrow function: Initial dose: 100 mg/m^2 as a single dose every 6 weeks

Note: Repeat courses should only be administered after adequate recovery: WBC >4000 and platelet counts >100,000

Subsequent dosing adjustment based on nadir:

Leukocytes 2000-2900/mm^3, platelets 25,000-74,999/mm^3: Administer 70% of prior dose

Leukocytes <2000/mm^3, platelets <25,000/mm^3: Administer 50% of prior dose

Pediatrics: Chemotherapy: Oral (refer to individual protocols): Children: 75-150 mg/m^2 as a single dose every 6 weeks; subsequent doses are readjusted after initial treatment according to platelet and leukocyte counts.

Renal Impairment:

Cl$_{cr}$ 10-50 mL/minute: Administer 75% of normal dose.

Cl$_{cr}$ <10 mL/minute: Administer 50% of normal dose.

Hemodialysis effects: Supplemental dose is not necessary.

Administration

Oral: Take with fluids on an empty stomach; no food or drink for 2 hours after administration.

Stability

Storage: Refrigerate (<40°C/<104°F).

Laboratory Monitoring CBC with differential, platelet count, hepatic and renal function, pulmonary function

Nursing Actions

Physical Assessment: Assess potential for interactions with other pharmacological agents patient may be taking (eg, decreased levels/effects of lomustine, increased toxicity). Monitor laboratory tests, therapeutic effectiveness, and adverse reaction prior to each treatment and on a regular basis throughout therapy. Teach patient possible side effects/appropriate interventions and adverse symptoms to report.

Patient Education: Do not take any new medication during therapy unless approved by prescriber. Take with fluids on an empty stomach; do not eat or drink for 2 hours prior to or following administration to reduce nausea and vomiting. Your prescriber may recommend that you take your medication at bedtime with a prescribed antiemetic to reduce the severity of nausea. During therapy, do not use excessive alcohol. It is important to maintain adequate hydration (2-3 L/day of fluids) unless instructed to restrict fluid intake, and nutrition (small, frequent meals may help). You will be more susceptible to infection (avoid crowds and exposure to infection and do not have any vaccinations without consulting prescriber). You may experience hair loss (reversible); nausea or vomiting (small, frequent meals, frequent mouth care, sucking lozenges, or chewing gum may help or consult prescriber for approved antiemetic); mouth sores (frequent mouth care and use of a soft toothbrush or cotton swabs may help); or diarrhea (buttermilk, boiled milk, or yogurt may help reduce diarrhea - consult prescriber for approved medication). Report persistent nausea, vomiting, or diarrhea; bleeding or bruising; fever, chills, sore throat; vaginal discharge; rash; blood in urine, stool, or vomitus; delayed healing of any wounds; yellowing of skin or eyes; or changes in color of urine of stool. **Pregnancy/breast-feeding precautions:** Do not get pregnant while taking this medication and for 1 month following therapy. Consult prescriber for appropriate contraceptives measures. This drug may cause severe fetal birth defects. Do not breast-feed.

Dietary Considerations Should be taken with fluids on an empty stomach; no food or drink for 2 hours after administration to decrease nausea.

Pregnancy Issues May cause fetal harm when administered to a pregnant woman. Women of childbearing potential should be advised to avoid pregnancy and should be advised of the potential harm to the fetus.

Loperamide (loe PER a mide)

U.S. Brand Names Diamode [OTC]; Imodium® A-D [OTC]; Kao-Paverin® [OTC]; K-Pek II [OTC]
Synonyms Loperamide Hydrochloride
Pharmacologic Category Antidiarrheal
Medication Safety Issues
Sound-alike/look-alike issues:
Imodium® A-D may be confused with Indocin®, Ionamin®
Pregnancy Risk Factor C
Lactation Enters breast milk/not recommended.
Use Treatment of chronic diarrhea associated with inflammatory bowel disease; acute nonspecific diarrhea; increased volume of ileostomy discharge
OTC labeling: Control of symptoms of diarrhea, including Traveler's diarrhea
Unlabeled/Investigational Use Cancer treatment-induced diarrhea (eg, irinotecan induced); chronic diarrhea caused by bowel resection
Mechanism of Action/Effect Acts directly on circular and longitudinal intestinal muscles, through the opioid receptor, to inhibit peristalsis and prolong transit time; reduces fecal volume, increases viscosity, and diminishes fluid and electrolyte loss; demonstrates antisecretory activity. Loperamide increases tone on the anal sphincter
Contraindications Hypersensitivity to loperamide or any component of the formulation; abdominal pain without diarrhea; children <2 years
Avoid use as primary therapy in acute dysentery, acute ulcerative colitis, bacterial enterocolitis, pseudomembranous colitis
Warnings/Precautions Should not be used if diarrhea is accompanied by high fever or blood in stool. Use caution in young children as response may be variable because of dehydration. Concurrent fluid and electrolyte replacement is often necessary in all age groups depending upon severity of diarrhea. Should not be used when inhibition of peristalsis is undesirable or dangerous. Discontinue if constipation, abdominal pain, or ileus develop. Use caution in patients with hepatic impairment because of reduced first pass metabolism. Use caution in treatment of AIDS patients; stop therapy at the sign of abdominal distention. Cases of toxic megacolon have occurred in this population. Loperamide is a symptom-directed treatment; if an underlying diagnosis is made, other disease-specific treatment may be indicated. Use caution in patients with hepatic impairment because of reduced first-pass metabolism; monitor for signs of CNS toxicity.

OTC labeling: If diarrhea lasts longer than 2 days, patient should stop taking loperamide and consult healthcare provider.
Drug Interactions
Cytochrome P450 Effect: Substrate (minor) of CYP2B6
Decreased Effect: Loperamide may decrease levels/effects of saquinavir.
Increased Effect/Toxicity: P-glycoprotein Inhibitors may increase CNS depressant effects.
Adverse Reactions 1% to 10%:
Central nervous system: Dizziness (1%)
Gastrointestinal: Constipation (2% to 5%), abdominal cramping (<1% to 3%), nausea (<1% to 3%)
Postmarketing and/or case reports: Abdominal distention, abdominal pain, allergic reactions, anaphylactic shock, anaphylactoid reactions, angioedema, bullous eruption (rare), drowsiness, dry mouth, dyspepsia, erythema multiforme (rare), fatigue, flatulence, paralytic ileus, megacolon, pruritus, rash, Stevens-Johnson syndrome, toxic epidermal necrolysis, toxic megacolon, urinary retention, urticaria, vomiting

Overdosage/Toxicology Symptoms of overdose include CNS depression, urinary retention, and paralytic ileus. Treatment of overdose includes gastric lavage followed by 100 g activated charcoal through a nasogastric tube. Naloxone can be given as an antidote. The prolonged action of loperamide may necessitate naloxone's repeated administration and close patient monitoring for recurrent CNS depression.
Pharmacodynamics/Kinetics
Time to Peak: Liquid: 2.5 hours; Capsule: 5 hours
Half-Life Elimination: 7-14 hours
Metabolism: Hepatic via oxidative N-demethylation
Excretion: Urine and feces (1% as metabolites, 30% to 40% as unchanged drug)
Available Dosage Forms
Caplet, as hydrochloride: 2 mg
Diamode, Imodium® A-D, Kao-Paverin®: 2 mg
Capsule, as hydrochloride: 2 mg
Liquid, oral, as hydrochloride: 1 mg/5 mL (5 mL, 10 mL, 120 mL)
Imodium® A-D: 1 mg/5 mL (60 mL, 120 mL) [contains alcohol, sodium benzoate, benzoic acid; cherry mint flavor]
Imodium® A-D [new formulation]: 1 mg/7.5 mL (60 mL, 120 mL, 360 mL) [contains sodium 10 mg/30 mL, sodium benzoate; creamy mint flavor]
Tablet, as hydrochloride: 2 mg
K-Pek II: 2 mg
Dosing
Adults & Elderly:
Acute diarrhea: Oral: Initial: 4 mg, followed by 2 mg after each loose stool, up to 16 mg/day
Chronic diarrhea: Oral: Initial: Follow acute diarrhea; maintenance dose should be slowly titrated downward to minimum required to control symptoms (typically, 4-8 mg/day in divided doses)
Traveler's diarrhea: Oral: Initial: 4 mg after first loose stool, followed by 2 mg after each subsequent stool (maximum dose: 8 mg/day)
Irinotecan-induced diarrhea (unlabeled use): Oral: 4 mg after first loose or frequent bowel movement, then 2 mg every 2 hours until 12 hours have passed without a bowel movement. If diarrhea recurs, then repeat administration
Pediatrics:
Acute diarrhea: Initial doses (in first 24 hours):
2-5 years (13-20 kg): 1 mg 3 times/day
6-8 years (20-30 kg): 2 mg twice daily
8-12 years (>30 kg): 2 mg 3 times/day
Maintenance: After initial dosing, 0.1 mg/kg doses after each loose stool, but not exceeding initial dosage
Traveler's diarrhea:
6-8 years: 2 mg after first loose stool, followed by 1 mg after each subsequent stool (maximum dose: 4 mg/day)
9-11 years: 2 mg after first loose stool, followed by 1 mg after each subsequent stool (maximum dose: 6 mg/day)
≥12 years: Refer to adult dosing.
Hepatic Impairment: No specific guidelines available.
Stability
Storage: Store at 15°C to 25°C (59°F to 77°F).
Nursing Actions
Physical Assessment: Assess for cause of diarrhea before administering first dose. Teach patient proper use, possible side effects/appropriate interventions, and adverse symptoms to report.
Patient Education: Adults should not take more than 8 capsules or 80 mL in 24 hours. May cause drowsiness; use caution. Increased exercise, identifying and avoiding foods that cause diarrhea, safe food preparation and storage, use of buttermilk, yogurt, or boiled milk may help reduce diarrhea. If acute diarrhea lasts longer than 48 hours, consult prescriber. Do not take if diarrhea is bloody. **Pregnancy/breast-feeding** (Continued)

Loperamide *(Continued)*

precautions: Inform prescriber if you are or intend to be pregnant or breast-feed.

Dietary Considerations
Imodium® A-D [new formulation] contains sodium 10 mg/30 mL.

Geriatric Considerations Elderly are particularly sensitive to fluid and electrolyte loss. This generally results in lethargy, weakness, and confusion. Repletion and maintenance of electrolytes and water are essential in the treatment of diarrhea. Drug therapy must be limited in order to avoid toxicity with this agent.

Lopinavir and Ritonavir
(loe PIN a veer & rit ON uh veer)

U.S. Brand Names Kaletra®
Synonyms Ritonavir and Lopinavir
Pharmacologic Category Antiretroviral Agent, Protease Inhibitor
Pregnancy Risk Factor C
Lactation Excretion in breast milk unknown/contraindicated
Use Treatment of HIV infection in combination with other antiretroviral agents
Available Dosage Forms [DSC] = Discontinued product
Capsule: Lopinavir 133.3 mg and ritonavir 33.3 mg [DSC]
Solution, oral: Lopinavir 80 mg and ritonavir 20 mg per mL (160 mL) [contains alcohol 42.4%]
Tablet: Lopinavir 200 mg and ritonavir 50 mg

Dosing
Adults: Note: Tablet and capsule [DSC] contain differing amounts of drug.
HIV infection (as a component of combination therapy): Oral:
Therapy-naive: Lopinavir 800 mg/ritonavir 200 mg once daily **or** lopinavir 400 mg/ritonavir 100 mg twice daily
Therapy-experienced: Lopinavir 400 mg/ritonavir 100 mg twice daily
Note: Once-daily dosing regimen has not been evaluated with concurrent indinavir or saquinavir and should not be used with concomitant phenytoin, carbamazepine, or phenobarbital therapy.
Dosage adjustment when taken with amprenavir, efavirenz, fosamprenavir, nelfinavir, or nevirapine: Oral:
Therapy-naive: Tablet: Adjustment not needed with twice-daily dosing
Therapy-experienced:
Solution: Lopinavir 533 mg/ritonavir 133 mg twice daily
Tablet: Lopinavir 600 mg/ritonavir 150 mg twice daily
Note: Once-daily dosing regimen should not be used when concomitantly taking amprenavir, efavirenz, nelfinavir, or nevirapine therapy.
Elderly: Initial studies did not include enough elderly patients to determine effects based on age. Use with caution due to possible decreased hepatic, renal, and cardiac function.
Pediatrics: Note: Tablet and capsule [DSC] contain differing amounts of drug.
HIV infection (component of combination therapy): Oral:
Children 6 months to 12 years: Dosage based on weight, presented based on mg of lopinavir (maximum dose: Lopinavir 400 mg/ritonavir 100 mg)
7-<15 kg: 12 mg/kg twice daily
15-40 kg: 10 mg/kg twice daily
>40 kg: Refer to adult dosing.
Children >12 years: Refer to adult dosing. **Note:** Once-daily dosing regimen has not been evaluated in pediatric patients.
Dosage adjustment when taken with amprenavir, efavirenz, fosamprenavir, nelfinavir, or nevirapine:
Note: Once-daily dosing regimen should not be used when concomitantly taking efavirenz or nevirapine therapy.
Children 6 months to 12 years: Solution:
7-<15 kg: 13 mg/kg twice daily
15-45 kg: 11 mg/kg twice daily
>45 kg: Refer to adult dosing.
Note: In the USHHS guidelines, the cutoff for adult dosing is 50 kg. (Pediatric Guidelines - March 24, 2005, are available at http://www.aidsinfo.nih.gov)
Children >12 years: Refer to adult dosing.
Renal Impairment: Has not been studied in patients with renal impairment; however, a decrease in clearance is not expected.
Hepatic Impairment: No specific guidelines available - plasma levels may be increased in patients with mild-to-moderate hepatic impairment. Lopinavir's AUC may be increased by 30%.

Nursing Actions
Physical Assessment: Assess potential for interactions with other pharmacological agents and herbal products patient may be taking. A list of medications that should not be used is available in each bottle and patients should be provided with this information. Monitor laboratory tests, patient response, and adverse reactions (eg, gastrointestinal disturbance, nausea, vomiting, diarrhea that can lead to dehydration and weight loss; hyperlipidemia and redistribution of body fat; rash; CNS effects, malaise, insomnia, abnormal thinking; electrolyte imbalance) at regular intervals during therapy. Teach patient proper use (eg, timing of multiple medications and drugs that should not be used concurrently), possible side effects/appropriate interventions (eg, glucose testing; protease inhibitors may cause hyperglycemia, exacerbation or new-onset diabetes; use of barrier contraceptives; protease inhibitors may decrease effectiveness of oral contraceptives), and adverse symptoms to report.
Patient Education: You will be provided with a list of specific medications that should not be used during therapy; do not take any new prescriptions, over-the-counter medications, or herbal products (even if they are not on the list) without consulting prescriber. This is not a cure for HIV, nor has it been found to reduce transmission of HIV; use appropriate precautions to prevent spread to other persons. Take as directed with meals. Maintain adequate hydration (2-3 L/day of fluids) unless instructed to restrict fluid intake. This medication will be prescribed with a combination of other medications; time these medications as directed by prescriber. You may be advised to check your glucose levels; this class of drugs can cause hyperglycemia. Frequent blood tests may be required with prolonged therapy. You may be susceptible to infection; avoid crowds and exposure to known infections and do not have any vaccinations without consulting prescriber. May cause body changes due to redistribution of body fat, facial atrophy, or breast enlargement (normal effects of drug); headache, dizziness, or fatigue (use caution when driving or engaged in potentially hazardous tasks until response to drug is known); nausea or vomiting (small frequent meals, frequent mouth care, chewing gum, or sucking lozenges may help); diarrhea (buttermilk, boiled milk, or yogurt may help); back pain, or arthralgia (consult prescriber for approved analgesic). Inform prescriber if you experience muscle numbness or tingling; unresolved persistent vomiting, diarrhea, or abdominal

pain; respiratory difficulty or chest pain; unusual skin rash; change in color of stool or urine; or any persistent adverse effects. **Pregnancy/breast-feeding precautions:** Inform prescriber if you are or intend to become pregnant. Effectiveness of oral contraceptives may be decreased, use of alternative (nonhormonal) forms of contraception is recommended; consult prescriber for appropriate contraceptives. Do not breast-feed.

Related Information
Ritonavir *on page 1091*

Loracarbef (lor a KAR bef)

U.S. Brand Names Lorabid®
Pharmacologic Category Antibiotic, Carbacephem
Medication Safety Issues
Sound-alike/look-alike issues:

Lorabid® may be confused with Levbid®, Lopid®, Lortab®, Slo-bid™

Pregnancy Risk Factor B
Lactation Excretion in breast milk unknown/use caution
Use Treatment of infections caused by susceptible organisms involving the upper and lower respiratory tract, uncomplicated skin and skin structure, and urinary tract (including uncomplicated pyelonephritis)

Mechanism of Action/Effect Inhibits bacterial cell wall synthesis by binding to one or more of the penicillin binding proteins (PBPs); inhibits the final transpeptidation step of peptidoglycan synthesis in bacterial cell walls, thus inhibiting cell wall biosynthesis.

Contraindications Hypersensitivity to loracarbef, any component of the formulation, or cephalosporins

Warnings/Precautions Modify dosage in patients with severe renal impairment. Prolonged use may result in superinfection. Use with caution in patients with a previous history of hypersensitivity to other beta-lactam antibiotics (eg, penicillins, cephalosporins). Safety and efficacy in children <6 months of age have not been established.

Drug Interactions
Increased Effect/Toxicity: Loracarbef serum levels are increased with coadministered probenecid.

Nutritional/Ethanol Interactions Food: Administration with food decreases and delays the peak plasma concentration.

Adverse Reactions
1% to 10%:

Central nervous system: Headache (1% to 3%), somnolence (<1% to 2%)

Dermatologic: Rash (1% to 3%)

Gastrointestinal: Diarrhea (4% to 6%), nausea (2% to 3%), vomiting (1% to 3%), anorexia (<1% to 2%), abdominal pain (1%)

Genitourinary: Vaginitis (1%), vaginal moniliasis (1%)

Respiratory: Rhinitis (2% to 6%)

Miscellaneous: Hypersensitivity reactions (1%; eg, urticaria, pruritus, erythema multiforme)

Other adverse reactions observed with beta-lactam antibiotics: Agranulocytosis, allergic reactions, aplastic anemia, hemolytic anemia, hemorrhage, interstitial nephritis, LDH increased, neutropenia, pancytopenia, positive direct Coombs' test, pseudomembranous colitis, seizure (with high doses and renal dysfunction), toxic epidermal necrolysis

Overdosage/Toxicology Symptoms of overdose include nausea and vomiting, abdominal discomfort and diarrhea. Treatment is symptom-directed and supportive.

Pharmacodynamics/Kinetics
Time to Peak: Serum: ~1 hour
Protein Binding: ~25%
Half-Life Elimination: ~1 hour
Excretion: Clearance: Plasma: ~200-300 mL/minute

Available Dosage Forms
Capsule: 200 mg, 400 mg
Powder for oral suspension: 100 mg/5 mL (100 mL); 200 mg/5 mL (100 mL) [strawberry bubble gum flavor]

Dosing
Adults & Elderly:
Bronchitis: Oral: 200-400 mg every 12 hours for 7 days
Pharyngitis/tonsillitis: Oral: 200 mg every 12 hours for 10 days
Pneumonia: Oral: 400 mg every 12 hours for 14 days
Sinusitis: Oral: 400 mg every 12 hours for 10 days
Skin and soft tissue, uncomplicated: Oral: 200 mg every 12 hours for 7 days
Urinary tract infections, uncomplicated: Oral: 200 mg once daily for 7 days
Pyelonephritis, uncomplicated: Oral: 400 mg every 12 hours for 14 days

Pediatrics:
Children 6 months to 12 years:
Acute otitis media, maxillary sinusitis: Oral: 15 mg/kg twice daily for 10 days
Note: Only suspension formulation should be used for otitis media due to attainment of higher peak plasma levels; do not substitute capsules.
Pharyngitis/tonsillitis: Oral: 7.5 mg/kg twice daily for 10 days
Impetigo: Oral: 7.5 mg/kg twice daily for 7 days
Children ≥13 years: Refer to adult dosing.

Renal Impairment:
Cl_{cr} ≥50 mL/minute: Administer usual dose.
Cl_{cr} 10-49 mL/minute: Administer 50% of usual dose at usual interval or usual dose given half as often.
Cl_{cr} <10 mL/minute: Administer usual dose every 3-5 days.
Hemodialysis: Doses should be administered after dialysis sessions.

Administration
Oral: Administer on an empty stomach at least 1 hour before or 2 hours after meals. Finish all medication. Shake suspension well before using.

Stability
Storage:
Capsule: Store at 15°C to 30°C (59°F to 86°F).
Suspension: Prior to reconstitution, store at 15°C to 30°C (59°F to 86°F). After reconstitution, suspension may be kept at room temperature for 14 days.

Laboratory Monitoring Perform culture and sensitivity studies prior to initiating therapy.

Nursing Actions
Physical Assessment: Assess previous history of allergies. Monitor laboratory tests, therapeutic effectiveness, and adverse response on a regular basis during therapy. Teach patient proper use, possible side effects/appropriate interventions, and adverse symptoms to report.

Patient Education: Do not take any new medication during therapy unless approved by prescriber. Take as directed, preferably on an empty stomach, 1 hour before or 2 hours after meals. Take entire prescription even if feeling better. Shake suspension well before using. Maintain adequate hydration (2-3 L/day of fluids) unless instructed to restrict fluid intake. You may experience nausea, vomiting, or anorexia (small, frequent meals, frequent mouth care, sucking lozenges, or chewing gum may help). Report immediately any signs of skin rash, joint or back pain, or respiratory difficulty. Report unusual fever, chills, vaginal itching or foul-smelling vaginal discharge, or easy bruising or bleeding. **Breast-feeding precaution:** Consult prescriber if breast-feeding.

(Continued)

751

Loracarbef *(Continued)*

Dietary Considerations Should be taken on an empty stomach at least 1 hour before or 2 hours after meals.

Geriatric Considerations Half-life is slightly prolonged with age, presumably due to the reduced creatinine clearance related to aging. Adjust dose for renal function.

Pregnancy Issues There are no adequate and well-controlled studies in pregnant women.

Loratadine *(lor AT a deen)*

U.S. Brand Names Alavert® [OTC]; Claritin® 24 Hour Allergy [OTC]; Claritin® Hives Relief [OTC]; Tavist® ND [OTC]; Triaminic® Allerchews™ [OTC]

Pharmacologic Category Antihistamine, Nonsedating

Medication Safety Issues
Sound-alike/look-alike issues:
Dimetapp® may be confused with Dermatop®, Dimetabs®, Dimetane®

Pregnancy Risk Factor B

Lactation Enters breast milk/not recommended (AAP rates "compatible")

Use Relief of nasal and non-nasal symptoms of seasonal allergic rhinitis; treatment of chronic idiopathic urticaria

Mechanism of Action/Effect Long-acting tricyclic antihistamine with selective peripheral histamine H_1 receptor antagonistic properties; management of idiopathic chronic urticaria

Contraindications Hypersensitivity to loratadine or any component of the formulation

Warnings/Precautions Patients with liver or renal impairment should start with a lower dose (10 mg every other day), since their ability to clear the drug will be reduced. Safety in children <6 years of age has not been established.

Drug Interactions
Cytochrome P450 Effect: Substrate (minor) of CYP2D6, 3A4; **Inhibits** CYP2C19 (moderate), 2D6 (weak)
Increased Effect/Toxicity: Increased toxicity with procarbazine, other antihistamines. Protease inhibitors (amprenavir, ritonavir, nelfinavir) may increase the serum levels of loratadine. Loratadine may increase the levels/effects of citalopram, diazepam, methsuximide, phenytoin, propranolol, sertraline, and other CYP2C19 substrates.

Nutritional/Ethanol Interactions
Ethanol: Avoid ethanol (although sedation is limited with loratadine, may increase risk of CNS depression).
Food: Increases bioavailability and delays peak.
Herb/Nutraceutical: St John's wort may decrease loratadine levels.

Adverse Reactions
Adults:
Central nervous system: Headache (12%), somnolence (8%), fatigue (4%)
Gastrointestinal: Xerostomia (3%)
Children:
Central nervous system: Nervousness (4% ages 6-12 years), fatigue (3% ages 6-12 years, 2% to 3% ages 2-5 years), malaise (2% ages 6-12 years)
Dermatologic: Rash (2% to 3% ages 2-5 years)
Gastrointestinal: Abdominal pain (2% ages 6-12 years), stomatitis (2% to 3% ages 2-5 years)
Neuromuscular & skeletal: Hyperkinesia (3% ages 6-12 years)
Ocular: Conjunctivitis (2% ages 6-12 years)
Respiratory: Wheezing (4% ages 6-12 years), dysphonia (2% ages 6-12 years), upper respiratory infection (2% ages 6-12 years), epistaxis (2% to 3% ages 2-5 years), pharyngitis (2% to 3% ages 2-5

years), flu-like symptoms (2% to 3% ages 2-5 years)
Miscellaneous: Viral infection (2% to 3% ages 2-5 years)

Overdosage/Toxicology Symptoms of overdose include somnolence, tachycardia, and headache. No specific antidote is available. Treatment is symptomatic and supportive. Loratadine is not eliminated by dialysis.

Pharmacodynamics/Kinetics
Onset of Action: 1-3 hours; Peak effect: 8-12 hours
Duration of Action: >24 hours
Half-Life Elimination: 12-15 hours
Metabolism: Extensively hepatic via CYP2D6 and 3A4 to active metabolite
Excretion: Urine (40%) and feces (40%) as metabolites

Available Dosage Forms
Syrup: 1 mg/mL (120 mL)
Claritin®: 1 mg/mL (120 mL) [contains sodium benzoate; fruit flavor]; (60 mL, 120 mL) [alcohol free, dye free, sugar free; contains sodium 6 mg/5 mL and sodium benzoate; grape flavor]
Tablet: 10 mg
Alavert®, Claritin®, Claritin® Hives Relief, Claritin® 24 Hour Allergy, Tavist® ND: 10 mg
Tablet, rapidly disintegrating: 10 mg
Alavert®: 10 mg [contains phenylalanine 8.4 mg/tablet]
Claritin® RediTabs®: 10 mg [mint flavor]
Triaminic® Allerchews™: 10 mg

Dosing
Adults & Elderly: Seasonal allergic rhinitis, chronic idiopathic urticaria: Oral: 10 mg/day
Pediatrics:
Children 2-5 years: Seasonal allergic rhinitis, chronic idiopathic urticaria: Oral: 5 mg once daily
Children ≥6 years: Refer to adult dosing.
Renal Impairment:
Cl_{cr} ≤30 mL/minute:
Children 2-5 years: 5 mg every other day
Children ≥6 years and Adults: 10 mg every other day
Hepatic Impairment:
Elimination half-life increases with severity of disease.
Children 2-5 years: 5 mg every other day
Children ≥6 years and Adults: 10 mg every other day

Administration
Oral: Take on an empty stomach.
Stability
Storage: Store at 2°C to 25°C (36°F to 77°F). Rapidly-disintegrating tablets: Use within 6 months of opening foil pouch, and immediately after opening individual tablet blister. Store in a dry place.

Nursing Actions
Physical Assessment: Assess effectiveness and interactions of other medications patient may be taking. Monitor effectiveness of therapy and adverse reactions at beginning of therapy and periodically with long-term use. Assess knowledge/teach patient appropriate use, interventions to reduce side effects, and adverse symptoms to report.

Patient Education: Take as directed; do not exceed recommended dose. Avoid use of other depressants, alcohol, or sleep-inducing medications unless approved by prescriber. You may experience drowsiness or dizziness (use caution when driving or engaging in tasks requiring alertness until response to drug is known); or dry mouth or nausea (small frequent meals, frequent mouth care, chewing gum, or sucking hard candy may help). Report persistent dizziness, sedation, or seizures; chest pain, rapid heartbeat, or palpitations; swelling of face, mouth, lips, or tongue; respiratory difficulty; changes in urinary pattern; yellowing of skin or eyes; dark urine or pale stool; or lack of improvement or worsening or condition. **Breast-feeding precaution:** Consult prescriber if breast-feeding.

Rapidly-disintegrating tablets: Place tablet on tongue; it dissolves rapidly. May be used with or without water. Use within 6 months of opening foil pouch, and immediately after opening individual tablet blister.

Dietary Considerations Take on an empty stomach. Alavert® and Dimetapp® Children's ND contain phenylalanine 8.4 mg per 10 mg tablet.

Geriatric Considerations Loratadine is one of the newer, nonsedating antihistamines. Because of its low incidence of side effects, it seems to be a good choice in the elderly. However, there is a wide variation in loratadine half-life reported in the elderly and this should be kept in mind when initiating dosing.

Loratadine and Pseudoephedrine
(lor AT a deen & soo doe e FED rin)

U.S. Brand Names Alavert™ Allergy and Sinus [OTC]; Claritin-D® 12-Hour [OTC]; Claritin-D® 24-Hour [OTC]
Synonyms Pseudoephedrine and Loratadine
Pharmacologic Category Antihistamine/Decongestant Combination
Pregnancy Risk Factor B
Lactation Enters breast milk/not recommended
Use Temporary relief of symptoms of seasonal allergic rhinitis, other upper respiratory allergies, or the common cold
Available Dosage Forms
Tablet, extended release: Loratadine 10 mg and pseudoephedrine sulfate 240 mg
Alavert™ Allergy and Sinus, Claritin-D® 12-hour: Loratadine 5 mg and pseudoephedrine sulfate 120 mg
Claritin-D® 24-hour: Loratadine 10 mg and pseudoephedrine sulfate 240 mg
Dosing
Adults & Elderly: Seasonal allergic rhinitis/nasal congestion:
Oral: 1 tablet every 12 hours
Extended release: 1 tablet daily
Pediatrics: Seasonal allergic rhinitis/nasal congestion: Children ≥12 years: Refer to adult dosing.
Renal Impairment: Cl$_{cr}$ <30 mL/minute:
Claritin-D® 12-Hour: 1 tablet daily
Claritin-D® 24-Hour: 1 tablet every other day
Hepatic Impairment: Should be avoided.
Nursing Actions
Physical Assessment: See individual agents.
Patient Education: See individual agents. Do not crush, break, or chew tablet. Take with a full glass of water. **Breast-feeding precaution:** Breast-feeding is not recommended.
Related Information
Loratadine *on page 752*
Pseudoephedrine *on page 1047*

Lorazepam (lor A ze pam)

U.S. Brand Names Ativan®; Lorazepam Intensol®
Restrictions C-IV
Pharmacologic Category Benzodiazepine
Medication Safety Issues
Sound-alike/look-alike issues:
Lorazepam may be confused with alprazolam, clonazepam, diazepam, temazepam
Ativan® may be confused with Atarax®, Atgam®, Avitene®
Pregnancy Risk Factor D

Lactation Enters breast milk/contraindicated (AAP rates "of concern")
Use
Oral: Management of anxiety disorders or short-term relief of the symptoms of anxiety or anxiety associated with depressive symptoms
I.V.: Status epilepticus, preanesthesia for desired amnesia, antiemetic adjunct
Unlabeled/Investigational Use Ethanol detoxification; insomnia; psychogenic catatonia; partial complex seizures; agitation (I.V.)
Mechanism of Action/Effect Binds to stereospecific benzodiazepine receptors on the postsynaptic GABA neuron at several sites within the central nervous system, including the limbic system, reticular formation. Enhancement of the inhibitory effect of GABA on neuronal excitability results by increased neuronal membrane permeability to chloride ions. This shift in chloride ions results in hyperpolarization (a less excitable state) and stabilization.
Contraindications Hypersensitivity to lorazepam or any component of the formulation (cross-sensitivity with other benzodiazepines may exist); acute narrow-angle glaucoma; sleep apnea (parenteral); intra-arterial injection of parenteral formulation; severe respiratory insufficiency (except during mechanical ventilation); pregnancy
Warnings/Precautions Causes CNS depression (dose-related) which may impair physical and mental capabilities. Use with caution in patients receiving other CNS depressants or psychoactive agents. Benzodiazepines have been associated with falls and traumatic injury and should be used with extreme caution in patients who are at risk of these events (especially the elderly). Use with caution in patients with a history of drug dependence.

Use with caution in elderly or debilitated patients, patients with hepatic disease (including alcoholics), renal impairment, respiratory disease, impaired gag reflex, or obese patients. Prolonged lorazepam use may have a possible relationship to GI disease, including esophageal dilation. Use is not recommended in patients with depressive disorders or psychoses. Avoid use in patients with sleep apnea.

The parenteral formulation of lorazepam contains polyethylene glycol and propylene glycol. Also contains benzyl alcohol - avoid in neonates.

Benzodiazepines have been associated with anterograde amnesia. Paradoxical reactions, including hyperactive or aggressive behavior, have been reported with benzodiazepines, particularly in adolescent/pediatric and psychiatric patients. Does not have analgesic, antidepressant, or antipsychotic properties.
Drug Interactions
Decreased Effect: Oral contraceptives may increase the clearance of lorazepam. Lorazepam may decrease the antiparkinsonian efficacy of levodopa. Theophylline and other CNS stimulants may antagonize the sedative effects of lorazepam.
Increased Effect/Toxicity: Ethanol and other CNS depressants may increase the CNS effects of lorazepam. Scopolamine in combination with parenteral lorazepam may increase the incidence of sedation, hallucinations, and irrational behavior. There are rare reports of significant respiratory depression, stupor, and/or hypotension with concomitant use of loxapine and lorazepam. Use caution if concomitant administration of loxapine and CNS drugs is required.
Nutritional/Ethanol Interactions
Ethanol: Avoid or limit ethanol (may increase CNS depression).
Herb/Nutraceutical: Avoid valerian, St John's wort, kava kava, gotu kola (may increase CNS depression).
Lab Interactions May result in elevated liver function tests
(Continued)

Lorazepam *(Continued)*

Adverse Reactions

>10%:

Central nervous system: Sedation

Respiratory: Respiratory depression

1% to 10%:

Cardiovascular: Hypotension

Central nervous system: Confusion, dizziness, akathisia, unsteadiness, headache, depression, disorientation, amnesia

Dermatologic: Dermatitis, rash

Gastrointestinal: Weight gain/loss, nausea, changes in appetite

Neuromuscular & skeletal: Weakness

Respiratory: Nasal congestion, hyperventilation, apnea

Overdosage/Toxicology Symptoms of overdose include confusion, coma, hypoactive reflexes, dyspnea, labored breathing. **Note:** Prolonged infusions have been associated with toxicity from propylene glycol and/or polyethylene glycol. Treatment for benzodiazepine overdose is supportive. Flumazenil has been shown to selectively block the binding of benzodiazepines to CNS receptors, resulting in a reversal of benzodiazepine-induced CNS depression but not respiratory depression

Pharmacodynamics/Kinetics

Onset of Action: Hypnosis: I.M.: 20-30 minutes; Sedation: I.V.: 5-20 minutes; Anticonvulsant: I.V.: 5 minutes, oral: 30-60 minutes

Duration of Action: 6-8 hours

Protein Binding: 85%; free fraction may be significantly higher in elderly

Half-Life Elimination: Neonates: 40.2 hours; Older children: 10.5 hours; Adults: 12.9 hours; Elderly: 15.9 hours; End-stage renal disease: 32-70 hours

Metabolism: Hepatic to inactive compounds

Excretion: Urine; feces (minimal)

Available Dosage Forms

Injection, solution (Ativan®): 2 mg/mL (1 mL, 10 mL); 4 mg/mL (1 mL, 10 mL) [contains benzyl alcohol]

Solution, oral concentrate (Lorazepam Intensol®): 2 mg/mL (30 mL) [alcohol free, dye free]

Tablet (Ativan®): 0.5 mg, 1 mg, 2 mg

Dosing

Adults:

Antiemetic: Oral, I.V. (**Note:** May be administered sublingually; not a labeled route): 0.5-2 mg every 4-6 hours as needed

Anxiety and sedation: Oral: 1-10 mg/day in 2-3 divided doses; usual dose: 2-6 mg/day in divided doses; initial dose should not exceed 2 mg in debilitated patients

Insomnia: Oral: 2-4 mg at bedtime

Preoperative:

I.M.: 0.05 mg/kg administered 2 hours before surgery; maximum: 4 mg/dose

I.V.: 0.044 mg/kg 15-20 minutes before surgery; usual maximum: 2 mg/dose

Operative amnesia: I.V.: Up to 0.05 mg/kg; maximum: 4 mg/dose

Status epilepticus: I.V.: 4 mg/dose given slowly over 2-5 minutes; may repeat in 10-15 minutes; usual maximum dose: 8 mg

Rapid tranquilization of agitated patient (administer every 30-60 minutes):

Oral: 1-2 mg

I.M.: 0.5-1 mg

Average total dose for tranquilization: 4-8 mg

Agitation in the ICU patient (unlabeled):

I.V.: 0.02-0.06 mg/kg every 2-6 hours

I.V. infusion: 0.01-0.1 mg/kg/hour

Elderly: Anxiety and sedation: Oral, I.V.: 0.5-4 mg/day; refer to adult dosing for other indications. Dose selection should generally be on the low end of the dosage range (ie, initial dose not to exceed 2 mg)

Pediatrics:

Antiemetic: Children 2-15 years: I.V.: 0.05 mg/kg (up to 2 mg/dose) prior to chemotherapy

Anxiety and sedation: Infants and Children: Oral, I.V.: Usual: 0.05 mg/kg/dose (range: 0.02-0.09 mg/kg) every 4-8 hours

Sedation (preprocedure): Infants and Children:

Oral, I.M., I.V.: Usual: 0.05 mg/kg; range: 0.02-0.09 mg/kg

I.V.: May use smaller doses (eg, 0.01-0.03 mg/kg) and repeat every 20 minutes, as needed to titrate to effect

Status epilepticus: I.V.:

Infants and Children: 0.1 mg/kg slow I.V. over 2-5 minutes, do not exceed 4 mg/single dose; may repeat second dose of 0.05 mg/kg slow I.V. in 10-15 minutes if needed

Adolescents: 0.07 mg/kg slow I.V. over 2-5 minutes; maximum: 4 mg/dose; may repeat in 10-15 minutes

Administration

I.M.: Should be administered deep into the muscle mass.

I.V.: Continuous infusion solutions should have an in-line filter and the solution should be checked frequently for possible precipitation.

I.V. Detail:

Dilute I.V. dose with equal volume of compatible diluent (D₅W, NS, SWI).

Stability

Reconstitution:

I.V.: Dilute with equal volume of compatible diluent (D₅W, NS, SWI).

Infusion: Use 2 mg/mL injectable solution to prepare; dilute ≤1 mg/mL and mix in glass bottle; precipitation may develop; can also be administered undiluted via infusion.

Compatibility:

Y-site administration: Incompatible with aldesleukin, aztreonam, floxacillin, foscarnet, idarubicin, imipenem/cilastatin, omeprazole, ondansetron, sargramostim, sufentanil

Compatibility in syringe: Incompatible with sufentanil

Compatibility when admixed: Incompatible with buprenorphine, dexamethasone sodium phosphate with diphenhydramine and metoclopramide

Storage:

I.V.: Intact vials should be refrigerated, protected from light; do not use discolored or precipitate-containing solutions. May be stored at room temperature for up to 60 days. Parenteral admixture is stable at room temperature (25°C) for 24 hours.

Tablet: Store at room temperature.

Nursing Actions

Physical Assessment: Assess other medications the patient may be taking for effectiveness and interactions. **Oral:** Assess for history of addiction; long-term use can result in dependence, abuse, or tolerance; periodically evaluate need for continued use. For inpatient use, institute safety measures and monitor effectiveness and adverse reactions. For outpatients, monitor therapeutic effectiveness and adverse reactions at beginning of therapy and periodically with long-term use. Taper dosage slowly when discontinuing. Assess knowledge/teach patient appropriate use, interventions to reduce side effects, and adverse symptoms to report. **I.V./I.M.:** Monitor cardiac, respiratory, and CNS status (possible retrograde amnesia with I.V.), and ability to void. Maintain bedrest for 2-3 hours, and observe when up.

Patient Education: Oral: Take exactly as directed; do not increase dose or frequency. Drug may cause physical and/or psychological dependence. Do not use alcohol or other prescription or OTC medications (especially pain medications, sedatives, antihistamines, or hypnotics) without consulting prescriber. Maintain adequate hydration (2-3 L/day of fluids) unless instructed to restrict fluid intake. You may experience drowsiness, lightheadedness, impaired coordination, dizziness, or blurred vision (use caution when driving or engaging in tasks requiring alertness until response to drug is known); nausea, vomiting, or dry mouth (small frequent meals, frequent mouth care, chewing gum, or sucking lozenges may help); constipation (increased exercise, fluids, fruit, or fiber may help); altered sexual drive or ability (reversible); or photosensitivity (use sunscreen, wear protective clothing and eyewear, and avoid direct sunlight). Report persistent CNS effects (eg, confusion, depression, increased sedation, excitation, headache, agitation, insomnia or nightmares, dizziness, fatigue, impaired coordination, changes in personality, or changes in cognition); changes in urinary pattern; chest pain, palpitations, or rapid heartbeat; muscle cramping, weakness, tremors, or rigidity; ringing in ears or visual disturbances; excessive perspiration; excessive GI symptoms (cramping, constipation, vomiting, anorexia); or worsening of condition. **Pregnancy/breast-feeding precautions:** Do not get pregnant while taking this medication; use appropriate contraceptive measures. Do not breast-feed.

Geriatric Considerations Because lorazepam is relatively short-acting with an inactive metabolite, it is a preferred agent to use in elderly patients when a benzodiazepine is indicated. Use with caution since elderly patients have decreased pulmonary reserve and are more prone to hypoxia.

Breast-Feeding Issues Crosses into breast milk and no data on clinical effects on the infant. AAP states MAY BE OF CONCERN.

Pregnancy Issues Benzodiazepines cross the placenta. The association between benzodiazepine exposure and malformations remains controversial. A number of types of malformation have been reported (oral cleft, inguinal hernia, cardiac defects, spina bifida, dysmorphic facial features, skeletal defects); however, confounding factors make a clear association difficult. Overall, the risk to the fetus may be low. Nonteratogenic effects (including neonatal flaccidity, respiratory and feeding problems, and withdrawal symptoms) during the postnatal period have also been reported with benzodiazepine use.

Other Issues Taper dosage gradually after long-term therapy, especially in epileptic patients. Abrupt withdrawal may cause tremors, nausea, vomiting, abdominal and/or muscle cramps.

Additional Information Oral doses >0.09 mg/kg produced increased ataxia without increased sedative benefit vs lower doses; preferred anxiolytic when I.M. route needed. Abrupt discontinuation after sustained use (generally >10 days) may cause withdrawal symptoms.

Related Information

Anxiolytic / Hypnotic Use in Long-Term Care Facilities *on page 1418*

Federal OBRA Regulations Recommended Maximum Doses *on page 1421*

Losartan (loe SAR tan)

U.S. Brand Names Cozaar®

Synonyms DuP 753; Losartan Potassium; MK594

Pharmacologic Category Angiotensin II Receptor Blocker

Medication Safety Issues
Sound-alike/look-alike issues:
Losartan may be confused with valsartan
Cozaar® may be confused with Hyzaar®, Zocor®

Pregnancy Risk Factor C/D (2nd and 3rd trimesters)

Lactation Excretion in breast milk unknown/not recommended

Use Treatment of hypertension (HTN); treatment of diabetic nephropathy in patients with type 2 diabetes mellitus (noninsulin dependent, NIDDM) and a history of hypertension; stroke risk reduction in patients with HTN and left ventricular hypertrophy (LVH)

Mechanism of Action/Effect As a selective and competitive, nonpeptide angiotensin II receptor antagonist, losartan blocks the vasoconstrictor and aldosterone-secreting effects of angiotensin II. Losartan increases urinary flow rate and in addition to being natriuretic and kaliuretic, increases excretion of chloride, magnesium, uric acid, calcium, and phosphate.

Contraindications Hypersensitivity to losartan or any component of the formulation; hypersensitivity to other A-II receptor antagonists; bilateral renal artery stenosis; pregnancy (2nd and 3rd trimesters)

Warnings/Precautions Avoid use or use a smaller dose in patients who are volume depleted. Deterioration in renal function can occur with initiation. May cause hyperkalemia; avoid potassium supplementation unless specifically required by healthcare provider. Use with caution in unilateral renal artery stenosis and pre-existing renal insufficiency; significant aortic/mitral stenosis. When used to reduce the risk of stroke in patients with HTN and LVH, may not be effective in African-American population. Use caution with hepatic dysfunction, dose adjustment may be needed. Safety and efficacy in children <6 years of age have not been established.

Drug Interactions
Cytochrome P450 Effect: Substrate (major) of CYP2C8/9, 3A4; Inhibits CYP1A2 (weak), 2C8/9 (moderate), 2C19 (weak), 3A4 (weak)
Decreased Effect: The levels/effects of losartan may be decreased by aminoglutethimide, carbamazepine, nafcillin, nevirapine, phenobarbital, phenytoin, rifampin, rifapentine, secobarbital, and other CYP2C8/9 or 3A4 inducers. NSAIDs may decrease the efficacy of losartan.
Increased Effect/Toxicity: Cimetidine may increase the absorption of losartan by 18% (clinical effect is unknown). Potassium salts/supplements, co-trimoxazole (high dose), ACE inhibitors, and potassium-sparing diuretics (amiloride, spironolactone, triamterene) may increase the risk of hyperkalemia. Risk of lithium toxicity may be increased by losartan. Losartan may increase the levels/effects of amiodarone, fluoxetine, glimepiride, glipizide, nateglinide, phenytoin, pioglitazone, rosiglitazone, sertraline, warfarin, and other CYP2C8/9 substrates. Fluconazole may increase the levels/effects of losartan.

Nutritional/Ethanol Interactions Herb/Nutraceutical: St John's wort may decrease levels. Avoid dong quai if using for hypertension (has estrogenic activity). Avoid ephedra, yohimbe, ginseng (may worsen hypertension). Avoid garlic (may have increased antihypertensive effect).

Adverse Reactions
>10%:
Cardiovascular: Chest pain (12% diabetic nephropathy)
(Continued)

Losartan *(Continued)*

Central nervous system: Fatigue (14% diabetic nephropathy)

Endocrine: Hypoglycemia (14% diabetic nephropathy)

Gastrointestinal: Diarrhea (2% hypertension to 15% diabetic nephropathy)

Genitourinary: Urinary tract infection (13% diabetic nephropathy)

Hematologic: Anemia (14% diabetic nephropathy)

Neuromuscular & skeletal: Weakness (14% diabetic nephropathy), back pain (2% hypertension to 12% diabetic nephropathy)

Respiratory: Cough (≤3% to 11%; similar to placebo; incidence higher in patients with previous cough related to ACE inhibitor therapy)

1% to 10%:

Cardiovascular: Hypotension (7% diabetic nephropathy), orthostatic hypotension (4% hypertension to 4% diabetic nephropathy), first-dose hypotension (dose related: <1% with 50 mg, 2% with 100 mg)

Central nervous system: Dizziness (4%), hypoesthesia (5% diabetic nephropathy), fever (4% diabetic nephropathy), insomnia (1%)

Dermatology: Cellulitis (7% diabetic nephropathy)

Endocrine: Hyperkalemia (<1% hypertension to 7% diabetic nephropathy)

Gastrointestinal: Gastritis (5% diabetic nephropathy), weight gain (4% diabetic nephropathy), dyspepsia (1% to 4%), abdominal pain (2%), nausea (2%)

Neuromuscular & skeletal: Muscular weakness (7% diabetic nephropathy), knee pain (5% diabetic nephropathy), leg pain (1% to 5%), muscle cramps (1%), myalgia (1%)

Respiratory: Bronchitis (10% diabetic nephropathy), upper respiratory infection (8%), nasal congestion (2%), sinusitis (1% hypertension to 6% diabetic nephropathy)

Miscellaneous: Infection (5% diabetic nephropathy), flu-like syndrome (10% diabetic nephropathy)

Overdosage/Toxicology Hypotension and tachycardia may occur with significant overdose. Treatment should be supportive. Not removed via hemodialysis.

Pharmacodynamics/Kinetics

Onset of Action: 6 hours

Time to Peak: Serum: Losartan: 1 hour; E-3174: 3-4 hours

Protein Binding: Plasma: High

Half-Life Elimination: Losartan: 1.5-2 hours; E-3174: 6-9 hours

Metabolism: Hepatic (14%) via CYP2C9 and 3A4 to an active metabolite E-3174 (40 times more potent than losartan); extensive first-pass effect

Excretion: Excretion: Urine (4% as unchanged drug, 6% as active metabolite)

Clearance: Plasma: Losartan: 600 mL/minute; Active metabolite: 50 mL/minute

Available Dosage Forms Tablet, as potassium: 25 mg, 50 mg, 100 mg

Dosing

Adults & Elderly:

Hypertension: Oral: Initial: 25-50 mg once daily; can be administered once or twice daily with total daily doses ranging from 25-100 mg

Usual initial doses in patients receiving diuretics or those with intravascular volume depletion: 25 mg

Nephropathy in patients with type 2 diabetes and hypertension: Oral: Initial: 50 mg once daily; can be increased to 100 mg once daily based on blood pressure response

Stroke reduction (HTN with LVH): Oral: 50 mg once daily (maximum daily dose: 100 mg); may be used in combination with a thiazide diuretic

Pediatrics:

Hypertension: Oral: Children 6-16 years: 0.7 mg/kg once daily (maximum: 50 mg/day); adjust dose based on response; doses >1.4 mg/kg (maximum: 100 mg) have not been studied.

Renal Impairment:

Children: Use is not recommended if Cl_{cr} <30 mL/minute.

Adults: No adjustment necessary.

Hepatic Impairment: Reduce the initial dose to 25 mg/day; divide dosage intervals into two.

Administration

Oral: May be administered with or without food.

Stability

Storage: Store at 15°C to 30°C (59°F to 86°F). Protect from light.

Laboratory Monitoring Electrolytes, serum creatinine, BUN, urinalysis, CBC

Nursing Actions

Physical Assessment: Use caution in presence of impaired renal function, significant aortic/mitral stenosis. Assess potential for interactions with pharmacological or herbal products patient may be taking (eg, decreased or increased levels/effects of losartan, risk of toxicities). Monitor laboratory tests, therapeutic effectiveness (normotensive), and adverse response (eg, hypotension) on a regular basis during therapy. Teach patient proper use, possible side effects/appropriate interventions, and adverse symptoms to report.

Patient Education: Do not take any new medication during therapy unless approved by prescriber. Take exactly as directed and do not discontinue without consulting prescriber. Preferable to take at same time each day; without regard to meals. This drug does not eliminate need for diet or exercise regimen as recommended by prescriber. Do not use potassium supplement or salt substitutes without consulting prescriber. May cause dizziness, fainting, or lightheadedness (use caution when driving or engaging in tasks that require alertness until response to drug is known); postural hypotension (use caution when rising from lying or sitting position or climbing stairs); diarrhea (boiled milk, buttermilk, or yogurt may help). Report chest pain or palpitations; unrelenting headache; back or muscle pain or weakness; CNS changes (delusions or depression); swelling of face mouth, tongue or throat; or other persistent adverse reactions. **Pregnancy/breast-feeding precautions:** Inform prescriber if you are or intend to become pregnant. This drug should not be used in the 2nd or 3rd trimester of pregnancy. Consult prescriber for appropriate contraceptive measures. Breast-feeding is not recommended.

Dietary Considerations May be taken with or without food.

Geriatric Considerations Serum concentrations of losartan and its metabolites are not significantly different in the elderly patient and no initial dose adjustment is necessary even in low creatinine clearance states (<30 mL/minute).

Breast-Feeding Issues Avoid use in the nursing mother, if possible, since it is postulated that losartan is excreted in breast milk. Recommend discontinuing drug or discontinuing nursing based on the importance of the drug to the mother.

Pregnancy Issues Discontinue as soon as possible when pregnancy is detected. Drugs which act directly on renin-angiotensin can cause fetal and neonatal morbidity and death.

Losartan and Hydrochlorothiazide
(loe SAR tan & hye droe klor oh THYE a zide)

U.S. Brand Names Hyzaar®
Synonyms Hydrochlorothiazide and Losartan
Pharmacologic Category Angiotensin II Receptor Blocker Combination; Antihypertensive Agent, Combination; Diuretic, Thiazide
Pregnancy Risk Factor C/D (2nd and 3rd trimesters)
Lactation Enters breast milk/contraindicated
Use Treatment of hypertension; stroke risk reduction in patients with HTN and left ventricular hypertrophy (LVH)
Available Dosage Forms Tablet:
  50-12.5: Losartan potassium 50 mg and hydrochlorothiazide 12.5 mg
  100-12.5: Losartan potassium 100 mg and hydrochlorothiazide 12.5 mg
  100-25: Losartan potassium 100 mg and hydrochlorothiazide 25 mg
Dosing
  Adults: Hypertension (dosage must be individualized): Oral: 1 tablet/day
  Elderly: Refer to dosing in individual monographs.
  Renal Impairment: Cl_{cr} ≤30 mL/minute: Use of combination formulation is not recommended.
  Hepatic Impairment: Use is not recommended.
Nursing Actions
  Physical Assessment: See individual agents.
  Patient Education: See individual agents. **Pregnancy/breast-feeding precautions:** Inform prescriber if you are or intend to become pregnant. Do not breast-feed.
Related Information
  Hydrochlorothiazide on page 610
  Losartan on page 755

Loteprednol (loe te PRED nol)

U.S. Brand Names Alrex®; Lotemax®
Synonyms Loteprednol Etabonate
Pharmacologic Category Corticosteroid, Ophthalmic
Pregnancy Risk Factor C
Lactation Excretion in breast milk unknown/use caution
Use
  Suspension, 0.2% (Alrex®): Temporary relief of signs and symptoms of seasonal allergic conjunctivitis
  Suspension, 0.5% (Lotemax®): Inflammatory conditions (treatment of steroid-responsive inflammatory conditions of the palpebral and bulbar conjunctiva, cornea, and anterior segment of the globe such as allergic conjunctivitis, acne rosacea, superficial punctate keratitis, herpes zoster keratitis, iritis, cyclitis, selected infective conjunctivitis, when the inherent hazard of steroid use is accepted to obtain an advisable diminution in edema and inflammation) and treatment of postoperative inflammation following ocular surgery
Contraindications Hypersensitivity to loteprednol, other corticosteroids, and any component of the formulation; viral diseases of the cornea and conjunctiva; mycobacterial infection of the eye; fungal diseases of ocular structures
Warnings/Precautions For ophthalmic use only; patients should be re-evaluated if symptoms fail to improve after 2 days. Intraocular pressure should be monitored if this product is used >10 days. Prolonged use may result in glaucoma and injury to the optic nerve. Visual defects in acuity and field of vision may occur. Posterior subcapsular cataracts may form after long-term use. Use with caution in presence of glaucoma (steroids increase intraocular pressure). Perforation may occur with topical steroids in diseases which thin the cornea or sclera. Steroids may mask infection or

enhance existing infection. Steroid use may delay healing after cataract surgery.
Adverse Reactions
  >10%:
    Central nervous system: Headache
    Respiratory: Rhinitis, pharyngitis
  1% to 10%: Ocular: Abnormal vision/blurring, burning on instillation, chemosis, dry eyes, itching, injection, conjunctivitis/irritation, corneal abnormalities, eyelid erythema, papillae uveitis
Available Dosage Forms Suspension, ophthalmic, as etabonate:
  Alrex®: 0.2% (5 mL, 10 mL) [contains benzalkonium chloride]
  Lotemax®: 0.5% (2.5 mL, 5 mL, 10 mL, 15 mL) [contains benzalkonium chloride]
Dosing
  Adults & Elderly:
    Seasonal allergic conjunctivitis: Ophthalmic: 0.2% suspension (Alrex®): Instill 1 drop into affected eye(s) 4 times/day.
    Inflammatory conditions: Ophthalmic: 0.5% suspension (Lotemax®): Apply 1-2 drops into the conjunctival sac of the affected eye(s) 4 times/day. During the initial treatment within the first week, the dosing may be increased up to 1 drop every hour. Advise patients not to discontinue therapy prematurely. If signs and symptoms fail to improve after 2 days, re-evaluate the patient.
    Postoperative inflammation: Ophthalmic: 0.5% suspension (Lotemax®): Apply 1-2 drops into the conjunctival sac of the operated eye(s) 4 times/day beginning 24 hours after surgery and continuing throughout the first 2 weeks of the postoperative period.
Nursing Actions
  Physical Assessment: Assess potential for interactions with other prescriptions, OTC medications, or herbal products patient may be taking. Monitor patient response and adverse effects. Teach patient proper use, side effects/appropriate interventions, and symptoms to report.
  Patient Education: For use in eyes only. Store in a cool place. Shake well before using. Do not let tip of applicator touch eye; do not contaminate tip of applicator (may cause eye infection, eye damage, or vision loss). Tilt head back, place medication in conjunctival sac, and close eyes. Apply finger pressure at corner of eye for 1 minute following application. May cause temporary sensitivity to bright light, blurring or stinging, changes in visual acuity, headache, runny nose, or sore throat. Do not discontinue therapy prematurely. If improvement is not noted within 2 days, notify prescriber. Report persistent vision changes, signs of increased infection, swollen eyelids, extreme itching, or if inflammation does not improve. **Pregnancy precaution:** Inform prescriber if you are pregnant.

Loteprednol and Tobramycin
(loe te PRED nol & toe bra MYE sin)

U.S. Brand Names Zylet™
Synonyms Loteprednol Etabonate and Tobramycin; Tobramycin and Loteprednol Etabonate
Pharmacologic Category Antibiotic/Corticosteroid, Ophthalmic
Pregnancy Risk Factor C
Lactation Excretion in breast milk unknown/use caution
Use Treatment of steroid-responsive ocular inflammatory conditions where either a superficial bacterial ocular infection or the risk of a superficial bacterial ocular infection exists
(Continued)

Loteprednol and Tobramycin
(Continued)

Available Dosage Forms Suspension, ophthalmic: Loteprednol 0.5% and tobramycin 0.3% (2.5 mL, 5 mL, 10 mL) [contains benzalkonium chloride]

Dosing

Adults & Elderly: Ophthalmic: Instill 1-2 drops into the affected eye(s) every 4-6 hours; may increase frequency during the first 24-48 hours to every 1-2 hours. Interval should increase as signs and symptoms improve. Further evaluation should occur for use of greater than 20 mL.

Nursing Actions

Physical Assessment: See individual agents.

Lovastatin (LOE va sta tin)

U.S. Brand Names Altoprev™; Mevacor®

Synonyms Mevinolin; Monacolin K

Pharmacologic Category Antilipemic Agent, HMG-CoA Reductase Inhibitor

Medication Safety Issues

Sound-alike/look-alike issues:

Lovastatin may be confused with Leustatin®, Livostin®, Lotensin®

Mevacor® may be confused with Mivacron®

Pregnancy Risk Factor X

Lactation Excretion unknown/contraindicated

Use

Adjunct to dietary therapy to decrease elevated serum total and LDL-cholesterol concentrations in primary hypercholesterolemia

Primary prevention of coronary artery disease (patients without symptomatic disease with average to moderately elevated total and LDL-cholesterol and below average HDL-cholesterol); slow progression of coronary atherosclerosis in patients with coronary heart disease

Adjunct to dietary therapy in adolescent patients (10-17 years of age, females >1 year postmenarche) with heterozygous familial hypercholesterolemia having LDL >189 mg/dL, **or** LDL >160 mg/dL with positive family history of premature cardiovascular disease (CVD), **or** LDL >160 mg/dL with the presence of at least two other CVD risk factors

Mechanism of Action/Effect Lovastatin acts by competitively inhibiting 3-hydroxyl-3-methylglutaryl-coenzyme A (HMG-CoA) reductase, the enzyme that catalyzes the rate-limiting step in cholesterol biosynthesis.

Contraindications Hypersensitivity to lovastatin or any component of the formulation; active liver disease; unexplained persistent elevations of serum transaminases; pregnancy; breast-feeding

Warnings/Precautions Liver function tests should be assessed before initiation of therapy in patients with a history of liver disease, prior to upwards dosage adjustment to ≥40 mg daily or when otherwise indicated; enzyme levels should be followed periodically thereafter as clinically warranted. Rhabdomyolysis with or without acute renal failure has occurred. Risk is dose-related and is increased with concurrent use of lipid-lowering agents which may cause rhabdomyolysis (gemfibrozil, fibric acid derivatives, or niacin at doses ≥1 g/day) or during concurrent use with potent CYP3A4 inhibitors. Avoid concurrent use of azole antifungals, macrolide antibiotics, and protease inhibitors. Use caution/limit dose with amiodarone, cyclosporine, danazol, gemfibrozil (or other fibrates), lipid-lowering doses of niacin, or verapamil. Patients should be instructed to report unexplained muscle pain or weakness; lovastatin should be discontinued if myopathy is suspected/confirmed. Temporarily discontinue in any patient experiencing an acute or serious condition predisposing to renal failure secondary to rhabdomyolysis. Use with caution in patients who consume large amounts of ethanol or have a history of liver disease. Safety and efficacy of the immediate release tablet have not been evaluated in prepubertal patients, patients <10 years of age, or doses >40 mg/day in appropriately-selected adolescents; extended release tablets have not been studied in patients <20 years of age.

Drug Interactions

Cytochrome P450 Effect: Substrate of CYP3A4 (major); **Inhibits** CYP2C8/9 (weak), 2D6 (weak), 3A4 (weak)

Decreased Effect: Cholestyramine taken with lovastatin reduces lovastatin absorption and effect.

Increased Effect/Toxicity: CYP3A4 inhibitors may increase the levels/effects of lovastatin; example inhibitors include azole antifungals, clarithromycin, diclofenac, doxycycline, erythromycin, imatinib, isoniazid, nefazodone, nicardipine, propofol, protease inhibitors, quinidine, telithromycin, and verapamil. Suspend lovastatin therapy during concurrent clarithromycin, erythromycin, itraconazole, or ketoconazole therapy. Concurrent use of danazol may increase risk of myopathy (limit dose of lovastatin). Cyclosporine, clofibrate, fenofibrate, gemfibrozil, and niacin also may increase the risk of myopathy and rhabdomyolysis. The effect/toxicity of warfarin (elevated PT) and levothyroxine may be increased by lovastatin. Digoxin, norethindrone, and ethinyl estradiol levels may be increased. Effects are additive with other lipid-lowering therapies.

Nutritional/Ethanol Interactions

Ethanol: Avoid excessive ethanol consumption (due to potential hepatic effects).

Food: Food **decreases** the bioavailability of lovastatin extended release tablets and **increases** the bioavailability of lovastatin immediate release tablets. Lovastatin serum concentrations may be increased if taken with grapefruit juice; avoid concurrent intake of large quantities (>1 quart/day). Red yeast rice contains an estimated 2.4 mg lovastatin per 600 mg rice.

Herb/Nutraceutical: St John's wort may decrease lovastatin levels.

Lab Interactions Altered thyroid function tests

Adverse Reactions Percentages as reported with immediate release tablets; similar adverse reactions seen with extended release tablets.

>10%: Neuromuscular & skeletal: Increased CPK (>2x normal) (11%)

1% to 10%:

Central nervous system: Headache (2% to 3%), dizziness (0.5% to 1%)

Dermatologic: Rash (0.8% to 1%)

Gastrointestinal: Abdominal pain (2% to 3%), constipation (2% to 4%), diarrhea (2% to 3%), dyspepsia (1% to 2%), flatulence (4% to 5%), nausea (2% to 3%)

Neuromuscular & skeletal: Myalgia (2% to 3%), weakness (1% to 2%), muscle cramps (0.6% to 1%)

Ocular: Blurred vision (0.8% to 1%)

Overdosage/Toxicology Few adverse events have been reported. Treatment is symptomatic.

Pharmacodynamics/Kinetics

Onset of Action: LDL-cholesterol reductions: 3 days

Time to Peak: Serum: 2-4 hours

Protein Binding: 95%

Half-Life Elimination: 1.1-1.7 hours

Metabolism: Hepatic; extensive first-pass effect; hydrolyzed to B-hydroxy acid (active)

Excretion: Feces (~80% to 85%); urine (10%)

Available Dosage Forms

Tablet: 10 mg, 20 mg, 40 mg

Mevacor®: 20 mg, 40 mg

Tablet, extended release (Altoprev™): 10 mg, 20 mg, 40 mg, 60 mg

Dosing

Adults & Elderly:

Dyslipidemia and primary prevention of CAD:
Oral: Initial: 20 mg with evening meal, then adjust at 4-week intervals; maximum: 80 mg/day immediate release tablet **or** 60 mg/day extended release tablet.

Dosage modification/limits based on concurrent therapy:

Cyclosporine and other immunosuppressant drugs: Initial dose: 10 mg/day with a maximum recommended dose of 20 mg/day

Concurrent therapy with fibrates, danazol, and/or lipid-lowering doses of niacin (>1 g/day): Maximum recommended dose: 20 mg/day. Concurrent use with fibrates should be avoided unless risk to benefit favors use.

Concurrent therapy with amiodarone or verapamil: Maximum recommended dose: 40 mg/day of regular release or 20 mg/day with extended release.

Dosage adjustment in renal impairment: Cl_{cr} <30 mL/minute: Use doses >20 mg/day with caution.

Pediatrics:

Heterozygous familial hypercholesterolemia: Oral (immediate release tablet): Adolescents 10-17 years:

LDL reduction <20%: Initial: 10 mg/day with evening meal

LDL reduction ≥20%: Initial: 20 mg/day with evening meal

Usual range: 10-40 mg with evening meal, then adjust dose at 4-week intervals

Renal Impairment: Cl_{cr} <30 mL/minute: Use with caution and carefully consider doses >20 mg/day.

Administration

Oral: Administer immediate release tablet with meals. Administer extended release tablet at bedtime; do not crush or chew.

Stability

Storage:

Tablet, immediate release: Store between 5°C to 30°C (41°F to 86°F). Protect from light.

Tablet, extended release: Store between 20°C to 25°C (68°F to 77°F). Avoid excessive heat and humidity.

Laboratory Monitoring Obtain baseline LFTs and total cholesterol profile. LFTs should be performed before initiation of therapy, at 6 and 12 weeks after initiation or first dose, and periodically thereafter.

Nursing Actions

Physical Assessment: Assess potential for interactions with other pharmacological agents or herbal products patient may be taking (eg, increased risk of myopathy or rhabdomyolysis). Monitor laboratory tests and patient response (eg, rash, myalgia, blurred vision, abdominal pain, hepatic function) on a regular basis throughout therapy. Teach patient proper use, possible side effects/appropriate interventions, and adverse symptoms to report. **Pregnancy risk factor X:** Determine that patient is not pregnant before starting therapy. Do not give to women of childbearing age unless they are capable of complying with effective contraceptive use. Instruct patient in appropriate contraceptive measures.

Patient Education: Inform prescriber of all prescriptions, OTC medications, or herbal products you are taking, and any allergies you have. Do not take any new medication during therapy unless approved by prescriber. Take as directed, with food at evening meal. Follow diet and exercise regimen as prescribed. You will have periodic blood tests to assess effectiveness. You may experience nausea or dyspepsia (small, frequent meals, frequent mouth care, chewing gum, or sucking lozenges may help); diarrhea (buttermilk, boiled milk, or yogurt may help); or headache

(see prescriber for analgesic). Report muscle pain or cramping; tremor; CNS changes (eg, memory loss, depression, personality changes; numbness, weakness, tingling or pain in extremities). **Pregnancy/breast-feeding precautions:** Inform prescriber if you are pregnant. Consult prescriber for appropriate barrier contraceptive measures to use during and for 1 month following therapy. This drug may cause severe fetal defects. Do not donate blood during or for 1 month following therapy. Do not breast-feed.

Dietary Considerations Before initiation of therapy, patients should be placed on a standard cholesterol-lowering diet for 6 weeks and the diet should be continued during drug therapy. Avoid intake of large quantities of grapefruit juice (≥1 quart/day); may increase toxicity. Red yeast rice contains an estimated 2.4 mg lovastatin per 600 mg rice.

Geriatric Considerations The definition of and, therefore, when to treat hyperlipidemia in the elderly is a controversial issue. The National Cholesterol Education Program recommends that all adults maintain a plasma cholesterol <160 mg/dL. In elderly patients with one additional risk factor, goal LDL would decrease to <130 mg/dL. Pharmacologic treatment should be reserved for those who are unable to obtain a desirable plasma cholesterol concentration by diet alone and for whom the benefits of treatment are believed to outweigh the potential adverse effects, drug interactions, and cost of treatment.

Pregnancy Issues Cholesterol biosynthesis may be important in fetal development. Contraindicated in pregnancy. Administer to women of childbearing potential only when conception is highly unlikely and patients have been informed of potential hazards.

Lutropin Alfa (LOO troe pin AL fa)

U.S. Brand Names Luveris®

Synonyms Recombinant Human Luteinizing Hormone; r-hLH

Pharmacologic Category Gonadotropin; Ovulation Stimulator

Pregnancy Risk Factor X

Lactation Excretion in breast milk unknown/use caution

Use Stimulation of follicular development in infertile hypogonadotropic hypogonadal (HH) women with profound luteinizing hormone (LH) deficiency; to be used in combination with follitropin alfa

Mechanism of Action/Effect Replaces endogenously secreted luteinizing hormone. Stimulates development of the follicle and prepares reproductive tract for implantation and pregnancy.

Contraindications Hypersensitivity to lutropin alfa or any component of the formulation; primary ovarian failure; uncontrolled thyroid or adrenal dysfunction; uncontrolled organic intracranial lesion; abnormal uterine bleeding of undetermined origin; ovarian cyst or enlargement of undetermined origin; sex hormone-dependent tumors of the reproductive tract and accessory organs; pregnancy

Warnings/Precautions For use by infertility specialists. May cause ovarian hyperstimulation syndrome (OHSS); if severe, treatment should be discontinued and patient should be hospitalized. OHSS results in a rapid (<24 hours to 7 days) accumulation of fluid in the peritoneal cavity, thorax, and possibly the pericardium, which may become more severe if pregnancy occurs; monitor for ovarian enlargement. Patients should be advised of the potential risk for multiple births before beginning therapy. Safety and efficacy have not been established with hepatic or renal dysfunction. Not for use in children or postmenopausal women.
(Continued)

Lutropin Alfa *(Continued)*

Adverse Reactions
1% to 10%:
Central nervous system: Headache (10%), fatigue (2% to 3%)
Endocrine & metabolic: Ovarian hyperstimulation (6%)
Gastrointestinal: Nausea (7%), constipation (2% to 3%), diarrhea (2% to 3%)
Adverse events reported with gonadotropin or menotropin therapy: Adnexal torsion, arterial thromboembolism, congenital abnormalities, ectopic pregnancy, hemoperitoneum, ovarian enlargement (mild-to-moderate), ovarian neoplasms (infrequent), postpartum fever, premature labor, pulmonary complications, spontaneous abortion, vascular complications

Overdosage/Toxicology Multiple gestations and ovarian hyperstimulation may occur following overdose.

Pharmacodynamics/Kinetics
Time to Peak: 4-16 hours
Half-Life Elimination: Terminal: ~18 hours
Excretion: Urine (<5% unchanged)

Available Dosage Forms Injection, powder for reconstitution: 75 int. units [contains sucrose; packaged with SWFI]

Dosing
Adults: Infertility: Female: SubQ: 75 units daily until adequate follicular development is noted; maximum duration of treatment: 14 days; to be used concomitantly with follitropin alfa

Administration
Other: SubQ: Administer on the stomach, a few inches above or below the navel.

Stability
Reconstitution: Reconstitute with SWFI; mix gently, do not shake.
Storage: Store under refrigeration or at room temperature of 2°C to 25°C (36°F to 77°F). Protect from light. Use immediately after reconstitution.

Nursing Actions
Physical Assessment: For subcutaneous use only. Administer around navel area. Instruct patient in appropriate administration technique and disposal of used needles and syringes. **Pregnancy risk factor X:** Pregnancy must be excluded before starting medication. Consult prescriber if breast-feeding.
Patient Education: For subcutaneous injection only. Follow administration schedule as directed by prescriber. Do not alter dosage or miss a dose. If a dose is missed, notify prescriber. You may experience headache, nausea (small frequent meals, frequent oral care, sucking lozenges, or chewing gum may help), fatigue, constipation, or diarrhea. Report immediately abdominal pain/distension, persistent nausea. **Pregnancy/breast-feeding precautions:** Pregnancy must be excluded before starting medication. Consult prescriber if breast-feeding.

Magaldrate and Simethicone
(MAG al drate & sye METH i kone)

U.S. Brand Names Riopan Plus® [OTC] [DSC]; Riopan Plus® Double Strength [OTC] [DSC]
Synonyms Simethicone and Magaldrate
Pharmacologic Category Antacid; Antiflatulent
Pregnancy Risk Factor C
Lactation Excretion in breast milk unknown/incompatible
Use Relief of hyperacidity associated with peptic ulcer, gastritis, peptic esophagitis and hiatal hernia which are accompanied by symptoms of gas
Available Dosage Forms [DSC] = Discontinued product

Suspension, oral: Magaldrate 540 mg and simethicone 20 mg per 5 mL (360 mL)
Riopan Plus®: Magaldrate 540 mg and simethicone 20 mg per 5 mL (360 mL) [DSC]
Riopan Plus® Double Strength: Magaldrate 1080 mg and simethicone 40 mg per 5 mL (360 mL) [DSC]

Dosing
Adults & Elderly: Hyperacidity/gas: Oral: 5-10 mL between meals and at bedtime

Nursing Actions
Physical Assessment: See individual agents.
Patient Education: See individual agents. **Pregnancy precaution:** Inform prescriber if you are or intend to become pregnant.

Magnesium Chloride
(mag NEE zhum KLOR ide)

U.S. Brand Names Chloromag®; Mag Delay® [OTC]; Mag-SR® [OTC]; Slow-Mag® [OTC]
Pharmacologic Category Magnesium Salt
Pregnancy Risk Factor D
Use Correction or prevention of hypomagnesemia
Available Dosage Forms
Injection, solution (Chloromag®): 200 mg/mL [1.97 mEq/mL] (50 mL)
Tablet [enteric coated] (Slow-Mag®): Elemental magnesium 64 mg [contains elemental calcium 106 mg]
Tablet, extended release (Mag Delay®, Mag-SR®): Magnesium chloride hexahydrate 535 mg [equivalent to elemental magnesium 64 mg]

Dosing
Adults & Elderly: Dietary supplement: Oral: Dietary supplement: 54-283 mg/day in divided doses
In TPN: I.V.: 8-24 mEq/day
Pediatrics:
In TPN: I.V.: Children: 2-10 mEq/day
Note: The usual recommended pediatric maintenance intake of magnesium ranges from 0.2-0.6 mEq/kg/day. The dose of magnesium may also be based on the caloric intake; on that basis, 3-10 mEq/day of magnesium are needed; maximum maintenance dose: 8-16 mEq/day
Renal Impairment: Patients in severe renal failure should not receive magnesium due to toxicity from accumulation. Patients with a Cl_{cr} <25 mL/minute should be monitored by serum magnesium levels.

Magnesium Citrate *(mag NEE zhum SIT rate)*

Synonyms Citrate of Magnesia
Pharmacologic Category Laxative, Saline; Magnesium Salt
Pregnancy Risk Factor B
Use Evacuation of bowel prior to certain surgical and diagnostic procedures or overdose situations
Contraindications Renal failure, appendicitis, abdominal pain, intestinal impaction, obstruction or perforation, diabetes mellitus, complications in gastrointestinal tract, patients with colostomy or ileostomy, ulcerative colitis or diverticulitis
Warnings/Precautions Use with caution in patients with impaired renal function, especially if Cl_{cr} <30 mL/minute (accumulation of magnesium which may lead to magnesium intoxication. Use caution in patients receiving a cardiac glycoside; may increase the AV-blocking effects. Use with caution in patients with lithium administration; use with caution with neuromuscular-blocking agents, and CNS depressants.
Lab Interactions Increased magnesium; decreased protein, decreased calcium (S), decreased potassium (S)

Adverse Reactions 1% to 10%:
Cardiovascular: Hypotension
Endocrine & metabolic: Hypermagnesemia
Gastrointestinal: Abdominal cramps, diarrhea, gas formation
Respiratory: Respiratory depression

Overdosage/Toxicology
Serious, potentially life-threatening electrolyte disturbances may occur with long-term use or overdosage due to diarrhea; hypermagnesemia may occur. CNS depression, confusion, hypotension, muscle weakness, blockage of peripheral neuromuscular transmission.
Serum level >4 mEq/L (4.8 mg/dL): Deep tendon reflexes may be depressed
Serum level ≥10 mEq/L (12 mg/dL): Deep tendon reflexes may disappear, respiratory paralysis may occur, heart block may occur
I.V. calcium (5-10 mEq) will reverse respiratory depression or heart block; in extreme cases, peritoneal dialysis or hemodialysis may be required.
Serum level >12 mEq/L may be fatal, serum level ≥10 mEq/L may cause complete heart block

Pharmacodynamics/Kinetics
Excretion: Urine

Available Dosage Forms
Solution, oral: 290 mg/5 mL (300 mL) [cherry and lemon flavors]
Tablet: 100 mg [as elemental magnesium]

Dosing
Adults & Elderly: Cathartic: Oral: Adults: ½ to 1 full bottle (120-300 mL)
Pediatrics: Cathartic: Oral: Children:
<6 years: 0.5 mL/kg up to a maximum of 200 mL repeated every 4-6 hours until stools are clear
6-12 years: 100-150 mL
≥12 years: Refer to adult dosing.
Renal Impairment: Patients in severe renal failure should not receive magnesium due to toxicity from accumulation. Patients with a Cl_cr <25 mL/minute should be monitored by serum magnesium levels.

Administration
Oral: To increase palatability, chill the solution prior to administration.

Nursing Actions
Physical Assessment: Monitor patient response and adverse effects.
Patient Education: Take with a glass of water, fruit juice, or citrus-flavored carbonated beverage to improve taste. Chill before using. Report severe abdominal pain to physician.
Dietary Considerations Magnesium content of 5 mL: 3.85-4.71 mEq

Magnesium Gluconate
(mag NEE zhum GLOO koe nate)

U.S. Brand Names Almora® [OTC]; Mag G® [OTC]; Magonate® [OTC]; Magonate® Sport [OTC] [DSC]; Magtrate® [OTC]
Pharmacologic Category Magnesium Salt
Use Dietary supplement for treatment of magnesium deficiencies
Available Dosage Forms [DSC] = Discontinued product
Solution:
Magonate®: 1000 mg/5 mL (480 mL) [magnesium 4.8 mEq/5 mL; equivalent to elemental magnesium 54 mg/5 mL; contains sodium benzoate]
Magonate® Sport: 1000 mg/5 mL (30 mL) [magnesium 4.8 mEq/5 mL; equivalent to elemental magnesium 54 mg/5 mL; contains sodium benzoate; fruit flavor] [DSC]

Tablet (Almora®, Mag G®, Magonate®, Magtrate®): 500 mg [magnesium 2.4 mEq; equivalent to elemental magnesium 27 mg]

Dosing
Adults & Elderly: The recommended dietary allowance (RDA) of magnesium is 4.5 mg/kg which is a total daily allowance of 350-400 mg for adult men and 280-300 mg for adult women. During pregnancy the RDA is 300 mg and during lactation the RDA is 355 mg.
Dietary supplement: Oral: 54-483 mg/day in divided doses; refer to product labeling
Pediatrics: Dietary supplement: Oral: Children: 3-6 mg/kg/day in divided doses 3-4 times/day; maximum: 400 mg/day
Renal Impairment: Patients in severe renal failure should not receive magnesium due to toxicity from accumulation. Patients with a Cl_cr <25 mL/minute should be monitored by serum magnesium levels.

Magnesium Hydroxide
(mag NEE zhum hye DROKS ide)

U.S. Brand Names Dulcolax® Milk of Magnesia [OTC]; Phillips'® Milk of Magnesia [OTC]
Synonyms Magnesia Magma; Milk of Magnesia; MOM
Pharmacologic Category Antacid; Magnesium Salt
Pregnancy Risk Factor B
Use Short-term treatment of occasional constipation and symptoms of hyperacidity, magnesium replacement therapy

Available Dosage Forms
Liquid, oral: 400 mg/5 mL (360 mL, 480 mL, 960 mL, 3780 mL)
Dulcolax® Milk of Magnesia: 400 mg/5 mL (360 mL, 780 mL) [regular and mint flavors]
Phillips'® Milk of Magnesia: 400 mg/5 mL (120 mL, 360 mL, 780 mL) [original, French vanilla, cherry, and mint flavors]
Liquid, oral concentrate: 800 mg/5 mL (100 mL, 400 mL)
Phillips'® Milk of Magnesia [concentrate]: 800 mg/5 mL (240 mL) [strawberry créme flavor]
Tablet, chewable (Phillips'® Milk of Magnesia): 311 mg [mint flavor]

Dosing
Adults & Elderly:
Laxative: Oral: ≥12 years: 30-60 mL/day or in divided doses
Antacid: Oral: 5-15 mL up to 4 times/day as needed
Pediatrics:
Laxative: Oral:
<2 years: 0.5 mL/kg/dose
2-5 years: 5-15 mL/day or in divided doses
6-12 years: 15-30 mL/day or in divided doses
≥12 years: 30-60 mL/day or in divided doses
Antacid: Oral:
Children: 2.5-5 mL as needed up to 4 times/day
Renal Impairment: Patients in severe renal failure should not receive magnesium due to toxicity from accumulation. Patients with a Cl_cr <25 mL/minute should be monitored by serum magnesium levels.

Magnesium Oxide (mag NEE zhum OKS ide)

U.S. Brand Names Mag-Ox® 400 [OTC]; Uro-Mag® [OTC]
Pharmacologic Category Electrolyte Supplement, Oral
Pregnancy Risk Factor B
Use Electrolyte replacement
Contraindications Patients with colostomy or an ileostomy, appendicitis, ulcerative colitis, diverticulitis, heart
(Continued)

Magnesium Oxide *(Continued)*

block, myocardial damage, serious renal impairment, hepatitis, Addison's disease, hypersensitivity to any component

Warnings/Precautions Hypermagnesemia and toxicity may occur due to decreased renal clearance (Cl_{cr} <30 mL/minute) of absorbed magnesium; monitor serum magnesium level, respiratory rate, deep tendon reflex, renal function when magnesium sulfate is administered parenterally. Use caution in patients receiving a cardiac glycoside; may increase the AV-blocking effects. Use with caution in patients with lithium administration; elderly, due to disease or drug therapy, may be predisposed to diarrhea; diarrhea may result in electrolyte imbalance; monitor for toxicity.

Drug Interactions

Decreased Effect: Decreased absorption of aminoquinolones, digoxin, nitrofurantoin, penicillamine, and tetracyclines may occur with magnesium salts

Increased Effect/Toxicity: Nondepolarizing neuromuscular blockers

Lab Interactions Increased magnesium; decreased protein, calcium (S), decreased potassium (S)

Adverse Reactions

>10%: Gastrointestinal: Diarrhea

1% to 10%:
Cardiovascular: Hypotension, ECG changes
Central nervous system: Mental depression, coma
Gastrointestinal: Nausea, vomiting
Respiratory: Respiratory depression

Overdosage/Toxicology

Magnesium antacids are also laxative and may cause diarrhea and hypokalemia. In patients with renal failure, magnesium may accumulate to toxic levels.

Serious, potentially life-threatening electrolyte disturbances may occur with long-term use or overdosage due to diarrhea; hypermagnesemia may occur. CNS depression, confusion, hypotension, muscle weakness, blockage of peripheral neuromuscular transmission.

Serum level >4 mEq/L (4.8 mg/dL): Deep tendon reflexes may be depressed

Serum level ≥10 mEq/L (12 mg/dL): Deep tendon reflexes may disappear, respiratory paralysis may occur, heart block may occur

I.V. calcium (5-10 mEq) will reverse respiratory depression or heart block; in extreme cases, peritoneal dialysis or hemodialysis may be required.

Serum level >12 mEq/L may be fatal, serum level ≥10 mEq/L may cause complete heart block

Pharmacodynamics/Kinetics

Onset of Action: Laxative: 4-8 hours

Excretion: Urine (up to 30% as absorbed magnesium ions); feces (as unabsorbed drug)

Available Dosage Forms

Capsule (Uro-Mag®): 140 mg [magnesium 7 mEq; equivalent to elemental magnesium 84 mg]

Tablet (Mag-Ox® 400): 400 mg [magnesium 20 mEq; equivalent to elemental magnesium 242 mg]

Dosing

Adults & Elderly:

Dietary supplement: Oral: 20-40 mEq (1-2 tablets) 2-3 times/day

Product labeling:

Mag-Ox 400®: 1-2 tablets daily with food

Uro-Mag®: 1-2 tablets 3 times/day with food

Note: Oral magnesium is not generally adequate for repletion in patients with serum magnesium concentrations <1.5 mEq/L

Renal Impairment: Patients in severe renal failure should not receive magnesium due to toxicity from accumulation. Patients with a Cl_{cr} <25 mL/minute should be monitored by serum magnesium levels.

Physical Assessment: Monitor patient response and adverse effects.

Dietary Considerations Should be taken with food. Contains 60% elemental magnesium; 49.6 mEq magnesium/g; 25 mmol magnesium/g.

Magnesium Sulfate *(mag NEE zhum SUL fate)*

Synonyms Epsom Salts; $MgSO_4$ (error-prone abbreviation)

Pharmacologic Category Antacid; Anticonvulsant, Miscellaneous; Electrolyte Supplement, Parenteral; Laxative, Saline; Magnesium Salt

Pregnancy Risk Factor B

Use Treatment and prevention of hypomagnesemia; seizure prevention in severe pre-eclampsia or eclampsia, pediatric acute nephritis; short-term treatment torsade de pointes; treatment of cardiac arrhythmias (VT/VF) caused by hypomagnesemia; short-term treatment of constipation or soaking aid

Available Dosage Forms

Infusion [premixed in D_5W]: 10 mg/mL (100 mL); 20 mg/mL (500 mL, 1000 mL)

Infusion [premixed in water for injection]: 40 mg/mL (100 mL, 500 mL, 1000 mL); 80 mg/mL (50 mL)

Injection, solution: 125 mg/mL (8 mL); 500 mg/mL (2 mL, 5 mL, 10 mL, 20 mL, 50 mL)

Powder: Magnesium sulfate USP (480 g, 1810 g, 1920 g)

Dosing

Adults & Elderly:

Daily allowance: The recommended dietary allowance (RDA) of magnesium is 4.5 mg/kg which is a total daily allowance of 350-400 mg for adult men and 280-300 mg for adult women. During pregnancy the RDA is 300 mg and during lactation the RDA is 355 mg. Average daily intakes of dietary magnesium have declined in recent years due to processing of food. The latest estimate of the average American dietary intake was 349 mg/day. Dose represented as magnesium sulfate unless stated otherwise.

Note: Serum magnesium is poor reflection of repletional status as the majority of magnesium is intracellular; serum levels may be transiently normal for a few hours after a dose is given, therefore, aim for consistently high normal serum levels in patients with normal renal function for most efficient repletion

Hypomagnesemia:

Oral: 3 g every 6 hours for 4 doses as needed

I.M., I.V.: 1 g every 6 hours for 4 doses; for severe hypomagnesemia: 8-12 g magnesium sulfate/day in divided doses has been used

Eclampsia, pre-eclampsia:

I.M.: 1-4 g every 4 hours

I.V.: Initial: 4 g, then switch to I.M. or 1-4 g/hour by continuous infusion

Note: Maximum dose not to exceed 30-40 g/day; maximum rate of infusion: 1-2 g/hour

Life-threatening arrhythmia: I.V.: 1-2 g (8-16 mEq) in 100 mL D_5W, administered over 5-60 minutes followed by an infusion of 0.5-1 g/hour, **or** 1-6 g administered over several minutes, followed by (in some cases) I.V. infusion of 3-20 mg/minute for 5-48 hours (depending on patient response and serum magnesium levels)

Maintenance electrolyte requirements:

Daily requirements: 0.2-0.5 mEq/kg/24 hours or 3-10 mEq/1000 kcal/24 hours

Maximum: 8-16 mEq/24 hours

Cathartic: Oral: 10-30 g/day in a single or divided doses

Soaking aid: Topical: Dissolve 2 capfuls of powder per gallon of warm water

Pediatrics:

Note: Serum magnesium is poor reflection of repletional status as the majority of magnesium is intracellular; serum levels may be transiently normal for a few hours after a dose is given, therefore, aim for consistently high normal serum levels in patients with normal renal function for most efficient repletion

Hypomagnesemia:

Children: I.M., I.V.: 25-50 mg/kg/dose (0.2-0.4 mEq/kg/dose) every 4-6 hours for 3-4 doses, maximum single dose: 2000 mg (16 mEq), may repeat if hypomagnesemia persists (higher dosage up to 100 mg/kg/dose magnesium sulfate I.V. has been used)

Maintenance: I.V.: 30-60 mg/kg/day (0.25-0.5 mEq/kg/day)

Management of seizures and hypertension: I.M., I.V.: 20-100 mg/kg/dose every 4-6 hours as needed; in severe cases doses as high as 200 mg/kg/dose have been used

Cathartic: Oral: Children:

2-5 years: 2.5-5 g/kg/day in a single or divided doses

6-11 years: 5-10 g/day in a single or divided doses

≥12 years: Refer to adult dosing.

Renal Impairment: Patients in severe renal failure should not receive magnesium due to toxicity from accumulation. Patients with a Cl$_{cr}$ <25 mL/minute should be monitored by serum magnesium levels.

Nursing Actions

Physical Assessment:

Assess other medications patient may be taking for effectiveness and interactions. Assess results of laboratory tests, therapeutic effect, and adverse/toxic effects. Assess knowledge/teach patient proper use, appropriate interventions to reduce side effects, and adverse symptoms to report.

When administered parenterally, monitor serum magnesium level, respiratory rate, deep tendon reflex, renal function. Hypermagnesemia and toxicity may occur due to decreased renal clearance of magnesium when Clcr <30 mL/minute.

Patient Education: Take in divided doses. Report diarrhea (>5 stools/day) or changes in mental function to prescriber.

Mannitol (MAN i tole)

U.S. Brand Names Osmitrol®; Resectisol®

Synonyms *D*-Mannitol

Pharmacologic Category Diuretic, Osmotic

Medication Safety Issues

Sound-alike/look-alike issues:

Osmitrol® may be confused with esmolol

Pregnancy Risk Factor C

Lactation Excretion in breast milk unknown/use caution

Use Reduction of increased intracranial pressure associated with cerebral edema; promotion of diuresis in the prevention and/or treatment of oliguria or anuria due to acute renal failure; reduction of increased intraocular pressure; promoting urinary excretion of toxic substances; genitourinary irrigant in transurethral prostatic resection or other transurethral surgical procedures

Mechanism of Action/Effect Increases the osmotic pressure of glomerular filtrate, which inhibits tubular reabsorption of water and electrolytes and increases urinary output

Contraindications Hypersensitivity to mannitol or any component or the formulation; severe renal disease (anuria); severe dehydration; active intracranial bleeding except during craniotomy; progressive heart failure,

pulmonary congestion, or renal dysfunction after mannitol administration; severe pulmonary edema or congestion

Warnings/Precautions Should not be administered until adequacy of renal function and urine flow is established; use 1-2 test doses to assess renal response. Diuretic effects may mask and intensify underlying dehydration; excessive loss of water and electrolytes may lead to imbalances and aggravate preexisting hyponatremia. May cause renal dysfunction especially with high doses; use caution in patients taking other nephrotoxic agents, with sepsis or preexisting renal disease. To minimize adverse renal effects, adjust to keep serum osmolality less than 320 mOsm/L. Discontinue if evidence of acute tubular necrosis.

In patients being treated for cerebral edema, mannitol may accumulate in the brain (causing rebound increases in intracranial pressure) if circulating for long periods of time as with continuous infusion; intermittent boluses preferred. Cardiovascular status should also be evaluated; do not administer electrolyte-free mannitol solutions with blood. If hypotension occurs monitor cerebral perfusion pressure to insure adequate.

Drug Interactions

Increased Effect/Toxicity: Lithium toxicity (with diuretic-induced hyponatremia).

Adverse Reactions Frequency not defined.

Cardiovascular: Chest pain, CHF, circulatory overload, hyper-/hypotension, tachycardia

Central nervous system: Chills, convulsions, dizziness, headache

Dermatologic: Rash, urticaria

Endocrine & metabolic: Fluid and electrolyte imbalance, dehydration and hypovolemia secondary to rapid diuresis, hyperglycemia, hypernatremia, hyponatremia (dilutional), hyperosmolality-induced hyperkalemia, metabolic acidosis (dilutional), osmolar gap increased, water intoxication

Gastrointestinal: Nausea, vomiting, xerostomia

Genitourinary: Dysuria, polyuria

Local: Pain, thrombophlebitis, tissue necrosis

Ocular: Blurred vision

Renal: Acute renal failure, acute tubular necrosis (>200 g/day; serum osmolality >320 mOsm/L)

Respiratory: Pulmonary edema, rhinitis

Miscellaneous: Allergic reactions

Overdosage/Toxicology Symptoms of overdose include acute renal failure, polyuria, hypotension, cardiovascular collapse, pulmonary edema, hyponatremia, hypokalemia, oliguria, and seizures. Increased electrolyte excretion and fluid overload can occur. Hemodialysis will clear mannitol and reduce osmolality.

Pharmacodynamics/Kinetics

Onset of Action: Diuresis: Injection: 1-3 hours; Reduction in intracranial pressure: ~15-30 minutes

Duration of Action: Reduction in intracranial pressure: 3-6 hours

Half-Life Elimination: 1.1-1.6 hours

Metabolism: Minimally hepatic to glycogen

Excretion: Primarily urine (as unchanged drug)

Available Dosage Forms

Injection, solution: 5% [50 mg/mL] (1000 mL); 10% [100 mg/mL] (500 mL, 1000 mL); 15% [150 mg/mL] (500 mL); 20% [200 mg/mL] (150 mL, 250 mL, 500 mL); 25% [250 mg/mL] (50 mL)

Osmitrol®: 5% [50 mg/mL] (1000 mL); 10% [100 mg/mL] (500 mL, 1000 mL); 15% [150 mg/mL] (500 mL); 20% [200 mg/mL] (250 mL, 500 mL)

Solution, urogenital (Resectisol®): 5% [50 mg/mL] (2000 mL, 4000 mL)

Dosing

Adults:

Test dose (to assess adequate renal function): I.V.: 12.5 g (200 mg/kg) over 3-5 minutes to produce a urine flow of at least 30-50 mL of urine per hour. If urine flow does not increase, a second

(Continued)

763

Mannitol *(Continued)*

test dose may be given. If test dose does not produce an acceptable urine output, then need to reassess management.

Initial: 0.5-1 g/kg

Maintenance: 0.25-0.5 g/kg every 4-6 hours; usual daily dose: 20-200 g/24 hours

Edema (osmotic diuretic): Initial: 0.5-1 g/kg; Maintenance: 0.25-0.5 g/kg every 4-6 hours; usual adult dose: 20-200 g/24 hours

Intracranial pressure/Cerebral edema: I.V.: 0.25-1.5 g/kg/dose I.V. as a 15% to 20% solution over ≥30 minutes; maintain serum osmolality 310 to <320 mOsm/kg.

Prevention of acute renal failure (oliguria): 50-100 g dose

Treatment of oliguria: 100 g dose

Preoperative for neurosurgery: I.V.: 1.5-2 g/kg administered 1-1.5 hours prior to surgery.

Transurethral: Irrigation: Use urogenital solution as required for irrigation.

Elderly: Refer to adult dosing. Consider initiation at lower end of dosing range.

Pediatrics:

Test dose (to assess adequate renal function): I.V.: Children: 200 mg/kg over 3-5 minutes to produce a urine flow of at least 1 mL/kg for 1-3 hours

Edema (osmotic diuretic): I.V.: Children: Initial: 0.5-1 g/kg; Maintenance: 0.25-0.5 g/kg given every 4-6 hours

Renal Impairment:

Contraindicated in severe renal impairment. If test dose does not produce adequate urine output reassess options. Use caution in patients with underlying renal disease.

Hepatic Impairment:

No adjustment required.

Administration

I.V.: Vesicant. Do not administer with blood. Crenation and agglutination of red blood cells may occur if administered with whole blood. Inspect for crystals prior to administration. If crystals present redissolve by warming solution. Use filter-type administration set.

I.V. Detail: Avoid extravasation.

pH: 4.5-7

Stability

Compatibility:

Y-site administration: Incompatible with cefepime, doxorubicin liposome, filgrastim

Compatibility when admixed: Incompatible with imipenem/cilastatin, meropenem

Storage: Should be stored at room temperature (15°C to 30°C) and protected from freezing. Crystallization may occur at low temperatures. Do not use solutions that contain crystals, heating in a hot water bath and vigorous shaking may be utilized for resolubilization. Cool solutions to body temperature before using.

Laboratory Monitoring Renal function, serum electrolytes, serum and urine osmolality. For treatment of elevated intracranial pressure, maintain serum osmolality 310-320 mOsm/kg

Nursing Actions

Physical Assessment: Adequate renal function and urine flow should be present prior to administration. Lithium toxicity is increased with concurrent use, and concurrent use of other nephrotic agents may increase potential for renal dysfunction. Monitor infusion site closely for extravasation; this is a vesicant. Monitor renal and cardiovascular status during infusion. Assess results of laboratory tests, therapeutic effectiveness (according to purpose for use), and adverse response (eg, circulatory overload, CHF, rash, water intoxication). Patient teaching should be appropriate to patient condition.

Patient Education: Report immediately any muscle weakness, numbness, tingling, acute headache, nausea, dizziness, blurred vision, eye pain, respiratory difficulty, chest pain, or pain at infusion site. **Pregnancy/breast-feeding precautions:** Inform prescriber if you are pregnant. Consult prescriber if breast-feeding.

Additional Information May autoclave or heat to redissolve crystals; mannitol 20% has an approximate osmolarity of 1100 mOsm/L and mannitol 25% has an approximate osmolarity of 1375 mOsm/L

Mebendazole *(me BEN da zole)*

U.S. Brand Names Vermox® [DSC]

Pharmacologic Category Anthelmintic

Pregnancy Risk Factor C

Lactation Excretion in breast milk unknown/use caution

Use Treatment of pinworms (*Enterobius vermicularis*), whipworms (*Trichuris trichiura*), roundworms (*Ascaris lumbricoides*), and hookworms (*Ancylostoma duodenale*)

Mechanism of Action/Effect Selectively and irreversibly blocks glucose uptake and other nutrients in susceptible adult intestine-dwelling helminths

Contraindications Hypersensitivity to mebendazole or any component of the formulation

Warnings/Precautions Pregnancy and children <2 years of age are relative contraindications since safety has not been established. Not effective for hydatid disease.

Drug Interactions

Decreased Effect: Anticonvulsants such as carbamazepine and phenytoin may increase metabolism of mebendazole

Nutritional/Ethanol Interactions Food: Mebendazole serum levels may be increased if taken with food.

Lab Interactions Increased LFTs

Adverse Reactions Frequency not defined.

Cardiovascular: Angioedema

Central nervous system: Fever, dizziness, headache, seizure

Dermatologic: Rash, itching, alopecia (with high doses)

Gastrointestinal: Abdominal pain, diarrhea, nausea, vomiting

Hematologic: Neutropenia (sore throat, unusual fatigue)

Neuromuscular & skeletal: Unusual weakness

Overdosage/Toxicology Symptoms of overdose include abdominal pain and altered mental status. Treatment is supportive.

Pharmacodynamics/Kinetics

Time to Peak: Serum: 2-4 hours

Protein Binding: 95%

Half-Life Elimination: 1-11.5 hours

Metabolism: Extensively hepatic

Excretion: Primarily feces; urine (5% to 10%)

Available Dosage Forms Tablet, chewable: 100 mg

Dosing

Adults & Elderly:

Pinworms: Oral: 100 mg as a single dose; may need to repeat after 2 weeks; treatment should include family members in close contact with patient.

Whipworms, roundworms, hookworms: Oral: 1 tablet twice daily, morning and evening on 3 consecutive days; if patient is not cured within 3-4 weeks, a second course of treatment may be administered.

Capillariasis: Oral: 200 mg twice daily for 20 days

Pediatrics: Refer to adult dosing.

Renal Impairment: Not dialyzable (0% to 5%)

Hepatic Impairment: Dosage reduction may be necessary in patients with liver dysfunction.

Administration

Oral: Tablets may be chewed, swallowed whole, or crushed and mixed with food.

Laboratory Monitoring Check for helminth ova in feces within 3-4 weeks following the initial therapy. Periodically assess hematologic and hepatic function.

Nursing Actions

Physical Assessment: Since worm infestations are easily transmitted, all persons sharing same household should be treated. Teach proper use, transmission prevention, side effects/appropriate interventions, and adverse reactions to report.

Patient Education: Do not take any new medication during therapy unless approved by prescriber. Take exactly as directed for full course of medication. Tablets may be chewed, swallowed whole, or crushed and mixed with food. Increase dietary intake of fruit juices. All family members and close friends should also be treated. To reduce possibility of reinfection, wash hands and scrub nails carefully with soap and hot water before handling food, before eating, and before and after toileting. Keep hands out of mouth. Disinfect toilet daily and launder bed linens, undergarments, and nightclothes daily with hot water and soap. Do not go barefoot and do not sit directly on grass or ground. May cause abdominal pain, nausea, or vomiting (small, frequent meals, frequent mouth care, sucking lozenges, or chewing gum may help); or hair loss (reversible). Report skin rash or itching, unusual fatigue or sore throat, unresolved diarrhea or vomiting, or CNS changes. **Pregnancy/breast-feeding precautions:** Inform prescriber if you are or intend to become pregnant. Consult prescriber if breast-feeding.

Dietary Considerations Tablet can be crushed and mixed with food, swallowed whole, or chewed.

Breast-Feeding Issues Since only 2% to 10% of mebendazole is absorbed, it is unlikely that it is excreted in breast milk in significant quantities.

Mechlorethamine (me klor ETH a meen)

U.S. Brand Names Mustargen®

Synonyms Chlorethazine; Chlorethazine Mustard; HN₂; Mechlorethamine Hydrochloride; Mustine; Nitrogen Mustard; NSC-762

Pharmacologic Category Antineoplastic Agent, Alkylating Agent (Nitrogen Mustard)

Pregnancy Risk Factor D

Lactation Excretion in breast milk unknown/not recommended

Use Hodgkin's disease; non-Hodgkin's lymphoma; intracavitary injection for treatment of metastatic tumors; pleural and other malignant effusions; topical treatment of mycosis fungoides

Mechanism of Action/Effect Bifunctional alkylating agent that inhibits DNA and RNA synthesis via formation of carbonium ions; produces interstrand and intrastrand cross-links in DNA resulting in miscoding, breakage, and failure of replication. Although not cell phase-specific *per se*, mechlorethamine effect is most pronounced in the S phase, and cell proliferation is arrested in the G₂ phase.

Contraindications Hypersensitivity to mechlorethamine or any component of the formulation; pre-existing profound myelosuppression or infection; pregnancy

Warnings/Precautions Hazardous agent — use appropriate precautions for handling and disposal. Mechlorethamine is a potent vesicant; if extravasation occurs, severe tissue damage (leading to ulceration and necrosis) and pain may occur. Urate precipitation should be anticipated especially with lymphomas.

Drug Interactions

Decreased Effect: Patients may experience impaired immune response to vaccines; possible infection after administration of live vaccines in patients receiving immunosuppressants.

Nutritional/Ethanol Interactions Ethanol: Avoid ethanol (due to GI irritation).

Adverse Reactions

>10%:

Dermatologic: Alopecia; hyperpigmentation of veins; contact and allergic dermatitis (50% with topical use)

Endocrine & metabolic: Chromosomal abnormalities, delayed menses, oligomenorrhea, amenorrhea, impaired spermatogenesis

Gastrointestinal: Nausea and vomiting (almost 100%), onset may be within minutes of drug administration

Genitourinary: Azoospermia

Hematologic: Myelosuppression, leukopenia, and thrombocytopenia

Onset: 4-7 days

Nadir: 14 days

Recovery: 21 days

1% to 10%:

Central nervous system: Fever

Gastrointestinal: Diarrhea, anorexia, metallic taste

Otic: Tinnitus

Overdosage/Toxicology Suppression of all formed elements of blood, uric acid crystals, nausea, vomiting, and diarrhea. Sodium thiosulfate is the specific antidote for nitrogen mustard extravasations. Treatment of systemic overdose is supportive.

Pharmacodynamics/Kinetics

Duration of Action: Unchanged drug is undetectable in blood within a few minutes

Half-Life Elimination: <1 minute

Metabolism: Rapid hydrolysis and demethylation, possibly in plasma

Excretion: Urine (50% as metabolites, <0.01% as unchanged drug)

Available Dosage Forms Injection, powder for reconstitution, as hydrochloride: 10 mg

Dosing

Adults & Elderly: Refer to individual protocols. Dosage should be based on ideal dry weight. The presence of edema or ascites must be considered so that dosage will be based on actual weight unaugmented by these conditions.

MOPP: I.V.: 6 mg/m² on days 1 and 8 of a 28-day cycle

Typical dose: I.V.: 0.4 mg/kg or 12-16 mg/m² for one dose or divided into 0.1 mg/kg/day for 4 days, repeated at 4- to 6-week intervals

Intracavitary: 10-20 mg diluted in 10 mL of SWI or 0.9% sodium chloride

Intrapericardially: 0.2-0.4 mg/kg diluted in up to 100 mL of 0.9% sodium chloride

Mycosis fungoides: Topical mechlorethamine has been used in the treatment of cutaneous lesions of mycosis fungoides. A skin test should be performed prior to treatment with the topical preparation to detect sensitivity and possible irritation (use fresh mechlorethamine 0.1 mg/mL and apply over a 3 x 5 cm area of normal skin).

Pediatrics: Refer to individual protocols. Dosage should be based on ideal dry weight; the presence of edema or ascites must be considered so that dosage will be based on actual weight unaugmented by these conditions.

MOPP: Children: I.V.: 6 mg/m² on days 1 and 8 of a 28-day cycle

Renal Impairment:

Hemodialysis: Not removed; supplemental dosing is not necessary.

(Continued)

Mechlorethamine *(Continued)*

Peritoneal dialysis: Not removed; supplemental dosing is not necessary.

Administration

I.V.: Vesicant. Margin of error is very slight. Check dosage carefully before administration. Administer with caution. Administer I.V. push through a free-flowing I.V. over 1-3 minutes at a concentration not to exceed 1 mg/mL.

I.V. Detail: Mechlorethamine may cause extravasation. Use within 1 hour of preparation. Avoid extravasation since mechlorethamine is a potent vesicant.

Extravasation management: Sodium thiosulfate $^1/_6$ molar solution is the specific antidote for nitrogen mustard extravasations and should be used as follows: Mix 4 mL of 10% sodium thiosulfate with 6 mL of sterile water for injection. Inject 5-6 mL of this solution into the existing I.V. line. Remove the needle. Inject 2-3 mL of the solution SubQ clockwise into the infiltrated area using a 25-gauge needle. Change the needle with each new injection. Apply ice immediately for 6-12 hours.

pH: 3-5

Stability

Reconstitution: Must be prepared immediately before use; solution is stable for only 15-60 minutes after dilution. Dilute powder with 10 mL SWI to a final concentration of 1 mg/mL. May be diluted in up to 100 mL NS for intracavitary administration.

Compatibility: Stable in sterile water for injection; **incompatible** with D_5W.

Y-site administration: Incompatible with allopurinol, cefepime

Compatibility when admixed: Incompatible with methohexital

Storage: Store intact vials at room temperature.

Laboratory Monitoring CBC with differential and platelet count

Nursing Actions

Physical Assessment: This is a powerful vesicant; see Administration for infusion specifics. Premedication with antiemetic recommended (highly emetogenic; emesis may begin within minutes of beginning infusion). Monitor infusion site closely; extravasation can cause severe sloughing or tissue necrosis. Assess results of laboratory tests prior to each treatment and on a regular basis throughout therapy. Monitor patient closely during infusion and between treatments (eg, adverse reactions can be severe and involve several systems). Teach patient possible side effects/appropriate interventions (eg, importance of adequate hydration) and adverse symptoms to report.

Patient Education: This medication can only be given by infusion. Report immediately any swelling, redness, pain, or burning at infusion site. Do not use alcohol during treatment; may increase gastric irritation. Maintain adequate fluid balance (2-3 L/day) unless instructed to restrict fluid intake, and adequate nutrition (small, frequent meals, frequent mouth care, sucking lozenges, or chewing gum may reduce anorexia and nausea). May cause discoloration (brown color) of veins used for infusion; hair loss (reversible); easy bleeding or bruising (use soft toothbrush or cotton swabs and frequent mouth care, use electric razor, avoid sharp knives or scissors); or increased susceptibility to infection (avoid crowds and exposure to infection and do not have any vaccinations unless approved by prescriber). This drug may cause menstrual irregularities, permanent sterility, and birth defects. Report changes in auditory or visual acuity; unusual bleeding or bruising or persistent fever or sore throat; blood in urine, stool, or vomitus; delayed healing of any wounds; skin rash; yellowing of skin or eyes; changes in color of urine of stool; acute or unresolved nausea or vomiting; diarrhea; or

loss of appetite. **Pregnancy/breast-feeding precautions:** Inform prescriber if you are pregnant. Do not get pregnant while taking this medication and for 1 month following therapy; consult prescriber for appropriate barrier contraceptives. Breast-feeding is not recommended.

Meclizine *(MEK li zeen)*

U.S. Brand Names Antivert®; Bonine® [OTC]; Dramamine® Less Drowsy Formula [OTC]

Synonyms Meclizine Hydrochloride; Meclozine Hydrochloride

Pharmacologic Category Antiemetic; Antihistamine

Medication Safety Issues

Sound-alike/look-alike issues:

Antivert® may be confused with Axert™

Pregnancy Risk Factor B

Lactation Excretion in breast milk unknown/not recommended

Use Prevention and treatment of symptoms of motion sickness; management of vertigo with diseases affecting the vestibular system

Mechanism of Action/Effect Has central anticholinergic action by blocking chemoreceptor trigger zone; decreases excitability of the middle ear labyrinth and blocks conduction in the middle ear vestibular-cerebellar pathways

Contraindications Hypersensitivity to meclizine or any component of the formulation

Warnings/Precautions Use with caution in patients with angle-closure glaucoma, prostatic hyperplasia, pyloric or duodenal obstruction, or bladder neck obstruction. Use with caution in hot weather, and during exercise. Elderly may be at risk for anticholinergic side effects such as glaucoma, prostatic hyperplasia, constipation, GI obstructive disease. If vertigo does not respond in 1-2 weeks, it is advised to discontinue use.

Drug Interactions

Increased Effect/Toxicity: Increased toxicity with CNS depressants, neuroleptics, and anticholinergics.

Nutritional/Ethanol Interactions Ethanol: Avoid ethanol (may increase CNS depression).

Adverse Reactions

>10%:

Central nervous system: Slight to moderate drowsiness

Respiratory: Thickening of bronchial secretions

1% to 10%:

Central nervous system: Headache, fatigue, nervousness, dizziness

Gastrointestinal: Appetite increase, weight gain, nausea, diarrhea, abdominal pain, xerostomia

Neuromuscular & skeletal: Arthralgia

Respiratory: Pharyngitis

Overdosage/Toxicology Symptoms of overdose include CNS depression, confusion, nervousness, hallucinations, dizziness, blurred vision, nausea, vomiting, and hyperthermia. There is no specific treatment for antihistamine overdose. Clinical toxicity is due to blockade of cholinergic receptors. For anticholinergic overdose with severe life-threatening symptoms, physostigmine 1-2 mg I.V. slowly, may be given to reverse these effects.

Pharmacodynamics/Kinetics

Onset of Action: ~1 hour

Duration of Action: 8-24 hours

Half-Life Elimination: 6 hours

Metabolism: Hepatic

Excretion: Urine (as metabolites); feces (as unchanged drug)

Available Dosage Forms

Tablet, as hydrochloride: 12.5 mg, 25 mg

Antivert®: 12.5 mg, 25 mg, 50 mg
Dramamine® Less Drowsy Formula: 25 mg
Tablet, chewable, as hydrochloride (Bonine®): 25 mg

Dosing

Adults & Elderly:

Motion sickness: Oral: 12.5-25 mg 1 hour before travel, repeat dose every 12-24 hours if needed; doses up to 50 mg may be needed

Vertigo: Oral: 25-100 mg/day in divided doses

Pediatrics: Children >12 years: Refer to adult dosing.

Nursing Actions

Physical Assessment: Determine cause of vomiting before beginning therapy. Assess effectiveness and interactions of other medications patient may be taking. **Inpatients:** Observe safety precautions (eg, bed rails up, call bell at hand). Monitor effectiveness of therapy and adverse response. Assess knowledge/teach patient possible side effects/appropriate interventions and adverse symptoms to report.

Patient Education: Take exactly as prescribed; do not increase dose. Avoid alcohol, other CNS depressants, sleeping aids without consulting prescriber. You may experience dizziness, drowsiness, or blurred vision (use caution when driving or engaging in tasks that require alertness until response to drug is known); dry mouth (frequent mouth care, sucking lozenges, or chewing gum may help); constipation (increased exercise, fluids, fruit, or may help); or heat intolerance (avoid excessive exercise, hot environments, maintain adequate hydration). Report CNS change (hallucination, confusion, nervousness); sudden or unusual weight gain; unresolved nausea or diarrhea; chest pain or palpitations; muscle pain; or changes in urinary pattern. **Breast-feeding precaution:** Breast-feeding is not recommended.

Geriatric Considerations Due to anticholinergic action, use lowest dose in divided doses to avoid side effects and their inconvenience. Limit use if possible. May cause confusion or aggravate symptoms of confusion in those with dementia.

MedroxyPROGESTERone
(me DROKS ee proe JES te rone)

U.S. Brand Names Depo-Provera®; Depo-Provera® Contraceptive; depo-subQ provera 104™; Provera®

Synonyms Acetoxymethylprogesterone; Medroxyprogesterone Acetate; Methylacetoxyprogesterone; MPA

Pharmacologic Category Contraceptive; Progestin

Medication Safety Issues

Sound-alike/look-alike issues:

MedroxyPROGESTERone may be confused with hydroxyprogesterone, methylPREDNISolone, methylTESTOSTERone

Provera® may be confused with Covera®, Parlodel®, Premarin®

Pregnancy Risk Factor X

Lactation Enters breast milk/compatible

Use Endometrial carcinoma or renal carcinoma; secondary amenorrhea or abnormal uterine bleeding due to hormonal imbalance; reduction of endometrial hyperplasia in nonhysterectomized postmenopausal women receiving conjugated estrogens; prevention of pregnancy; management of endometriosis-associated pain

Mechanism of Action/Effect Inhibits secretion of pituitary gonadotropins, which prevents follicular maturation and ovulation; causes endometrial thinning

Contraindications Hypersensitivity to medroxyprogesterone or any component of the formulation; history of or current thrombophlebitis or venous thromboembolic disorders (including DVT, PE); cerebral vascular disease; severe hepatic dysfunction or disease; carcinoma of the breast or genital organs, undiagnosed

vaginal bleeding; missed abortion, diagnostic test for pregnancy, pregnancy

Warnings/Precautions Prolonged use of medroxyprogesterone contraceptive injection may result in a loss of bone mineral density (BMD). Loss is related to the duration of use, and may not be completely reversible on discontinuation of the drug. The impact on peak bone mass in adolescents should be considered in treatment decisions. Long-term use (ie, >2 years) should be limited to situations where other birth control methods are inadequate. Consider other methods of birth control in women with (or at risk for) osteoporosis.

Use caution with cardiovascular disease or dysfunction. MPA used in combination with estrogen may increase the risks of hypertension, myocardial infarction (MI), stroke, pulmonary emboli (PE), and deep vein thrombosis; incidence of these effects was shown to be significantly increased in postmenopausal women using conjugated equine estrogens (CEE) in combination with MPA. MPA in combination with estrogens should not be used to prevent coronary heart disease.

The risk of dementia may be increased in postmenopausal women; increased incidence was observed in women ≥65 years of age taking MPA in combination with CEE. An increased risk of invasive breast cancer was observed in postmenopausal women using MPA in combination with CEE. An increase in abnormal mammograms has also been reported with estrogen and progestin therapy.

Discontinue pending examination in cases of sudden partial or complete vision loss, sudden onset of proptosis, diplopia, or migraine; discontinue permanently if papilledema or retinal vascular lesions are observed on examination. Use with caution in patients with diseases that may be exacerbated by fluid retention (including asthma, epilepsy, migraine, diabetes, or renal dysfunction). Use caution with history of depression. Whenever possible, progestins in combination with estrogens should be discontinued at least 4-6 weeks prior to surgeries associated with an increased risk of thromboembolism or during periods of prolonged immobilization. Progestins used in combination with estrogen should be used for shortest duration possible consistent with treatment goals. Conduct periodic risk:benefit assessments.

Drug Interactions

Cytochrome P450 Effect: Substrate of CYP3A4 (major); **Induces** CYP3A4 (weak)

Decreased Effect: Acitretin, and griseofulvin may diminish the therapeutic effect of progestin contraceptives (contraceptive failure is possible). CYP3A4 inducers may decrease the levels/effects of medroxyprogesterone; example inducers include aminoglutethimide, carbamazepine, nafcillin, nevirapine, phenobarbital, phenytoin, and rifamycins. Progestins may diminish the anticoagulant effect of coumarin derivatives; and in contrast, enhanced anticoagulant effects have also been noted with some products.

Nutritional/Ethanol Interactions

Ethanol: Avoid ethanol (may increase risk of osteoporosis).

Food: Bioavailability of the oral tablet is increased when taken with food; half-life is unchanged.

Herb/Nutraceutical: St John's wort may diminish the therapeutic effect of progestin contraceptives (contraceptive failure is possible).

Lab Interactions

The following tests may be decreased: Steroid levels (plasma and urinary), gonadotropin levels, SHBG concentration, T_3 uptake

The following tests may be increased: Protein-bound iodine, butanol extractable protein-bound iodine, Factors II, VII, VIII, IX, X

Pathologist should be advised of estrogen/progesterone therapy when specimens are submitted.

(Continued)

MedroxyPROGESTERone *(Continued)*

Adverse Reactions Adverse effects as reported with any dosage form; percent ranges presented are noted with the MPA contraceptive injection:

>5%:

Central nervous system: Dizziness, headache, nervousness

Endocrine & metabolic: Libido decreased, menstrual irregularities (includes bleeding, amenorrhea, or both)

Gastrointestinal: Abdominal pain/discomfort, weight changes (average 3-5 pounds after 1 year, 8 pounds after 2 years)

Neuromuscular & skeletal: Weakness

1% to 5%:

Cardiovascular: Edema

Central nervous system: Depression, fatigue, insomnia, irritability, pain

Dermatologic: Acne, alopecia, rash

Endocrine & metabolic: Anorgasmia, breast pain, hot flashes

Gastrointestinal: Bloating, nausea

Genitourinary: Cervical smear abnormal, leukorrhea, menometrorrhagia, menorrhagia, pelvic pain, urinary tract infection, vaginitis, vaginal infection, vaginal hemorrhage

Local: Injection site atrophy, injection site reaction, injection site pain

Neuromuscular & skeletal: Arthralgia, backache, leg cramp

Respiratory: Respiratory tract infections

Overdosage/Toxicology Toxicity is unlikely following single exposure of excessive doses. Supportive treatment is adequate in most cases.

Pharmacodynamics/Kinetics

Time to Peak: Oral: 2-4 hours

Protein Binding: 86% to 90% primarily to albumin; does not bind to sex hormone-binding globulin

Half-Life Elimination: Oral: 12-17 hours; I.M. (Depo-Provera® Contraceptive): 50 days; SubQ: ~40 days

Metabolism: Extensively hepatic via hydroxylation and conjugation; forms metabolites

Excretion: Urine

Available Dosage Forms

Injection, suspension, as acetate: 150 mg/mL (1 mL)

Depo-Provera®: 400 mg/mL (2.5 mL)

Depo-Provera® Contraceptive: 150 mg/mL (1 mL) [prefilled syringe or vial]

depo-subQ provera 104™: 104 mg/0.65 mL (0.65 mL) [prefilled syringe]

Tablet, as acetate (Provera®): 2.5 mg, 5 mg, 10 mg

Dosing

Adults & Elderly:

Amenorrhea: Oral: 5-10 mg/day for 5-10 days

Abnormal uterine bleeding: Oral: 5-10 mg for 5-10 days starting on day 16 or 21 of cycle

Contraception:

Depo-Provera® Contraceptive: I.M.: 150 mg every 3 months

depo-subQ provera 104™: SubQ: 104 mg every 3 months (every 12-14 weeks)

Endometriosis: depo-subQ provera 104™: SubQ: 104 mg every 3 months (every 12-14 weeks)

Endometrial or renal carcinoma (Depo-Provera®): I.M.: 400-1000 mg/week

Accompanying cyclic estrogen therapy, postmenopausal: Oral: 5-10 mg for 12-14 consecutive days each month, starting on day 1 or day 16 of the cycle; lower doses may be used if given with estrogen continuously throughout the cycle

Pediatrics: Adolescents:

Amenorrhea: Refer to adult dosing.

Abnormal uterine bleeding: Refer to adult dosing.

Contraception: Refer to adult dosing.

Endometriosis: Refer to adult dosing.

Hepatic Impairment: Use is contraindicated with severe impairment. Consider lower dose or less frequent administration with mild-to-moderate impairment. Use of the contraceptive injection has not been studied in patients with hepatic impairment; consideration should be given to not readminister if jaundice develops

Administration

I.M.: Depo-Provera® Contraceptive: Administer first dose during the first 5 days of menstrual period, or within the first 5 days postpartum if not breast-feeding, or at the sixth week postpartum if breast feeding exclusively. Shake vigorously prior to administration. Administer by deep I.M. injection in the gluteal or deltoid muscle.

Other: SubQ: depo-subQ provera 104™: Administer first dose during the first 5 days of menstrual period, or at the sixth week postpartum if breast-feeding. Shake vigorously prior to administration. Administer by SubQ injection in the upper thigh or abdomen; avoid boney areas and the umbilicus. Administer over 5-7 seconds. Do not rub the injection area. When switching from combined hormonal contraceptives (estrogen plus progestin), the first injection should be within 7 days after the last active pill, or removal of patch or ring. If switching from the I.M. to SubQ formulation, the next dose should be given within the prescribed dosing period for the I.M. injection.

Stability

Storage: Store at controlled room temperature.

Laboratory Monitoring Must have pregnancy test prior to beginning therapy.

Nursing Actions

Physical Assessment: Monitor for effectiveness of therapy and adverse effects. Instruct patient on appropriate dose scheduling (according to purpose of therapy), possible side effects, and symptoms to report. **Pregnancy risk factor X:** Determine that patient is not pregnant before starting therapy. Do not give to sexually-active female patients unless capable of complying with contraceptive use.

Patient Education: Follow dosage schedule and do not take more than prescribed. You may experience sensitivity to sunlight (use sunblock, wear protective clothing and eyewear, and avoid extensive exposure to direct sunlight); dizziness, anxiety, depression (use caution when driving or engaging in tasks that require alertness until response to drug is known); changes in appetite; maintain adequate hydration (2-3 L/day of fluids) unless instructed to restrict fluid intake and diet; decreased libido or increased body hair (reversible when drug is discontinued); hot flashes (cool clothes and environment may help). May cause discoloration of stool (green). Report swelling of face, lips, or mouth; absence or altered menses; abdominal pain; vaginal itching, irritation, or discharge; heat, warmth, redness, or swelling of extremities; or sudden onset change in vision. **Pregnancy precaution:** Inform prescriber if you are pregnant. Consult prescriber for instruction on appropriate contraceptive measures.

Injection for contraception: This product does not protect against HIV or other sexually-transmitted diseases.

Dietary Considerations Ensure adequate calcium and vitamin D intake when used for the prevention of pregnancy

Geriatric Considerations No specific recommendations for dosage adjustments. Monitor closely for adverse effects when starting therapy.

Breast-Feeding Issues Composition, quality and quantity of breast milk are not affected; adverse developmental and behavioral effects have not been noted following exposure of infant to MPA while breast-feeding.

Endometriosis: Refer to adult dosing.

Pregnancy Issues There is an increased risk of minor birth defects in children whose mothers take progesterones during the first 4 months of pregnancy. Hypospadias has been reported in male and mild masculinization of the external genitalia has been reported in female babies exposed during the first trimester. High doses are used to impair fertility. Low birth weight has been reported in neonates from unexpected pregnancies which occurred 1-2 months following injection of medroxyprogesterone (MPA) contraceptive. Ectopic pregnancies have been reported with use of the MPA contraceptive injection. When therapy is discontinued, fertility returns sooner in women of lower body weight. Median time to conception/return to ovulation following discontinuation of MPA contraceptive injection is 10 months following the last injection.

Related Information
FDA Name Differentiation Project: The Use of Tall-Man Letters *on page 12*

Medrysone (ME dri sone)

U.S. Brand Names HMS Liquifilm® [DSC]
Pharmacologic Category Corticosteroid, Ophthalmic
Pregnancy Risk Factor C
Lactation Excretion in breast milk unknown/use caution
Use Treatment of allergic conjunctivitis, vernal conjunctivitis, episcleritis, ophthalmic epinephrine sensitivity reaction
Mechanism of Action/Effect Decreases inflammation by suppression of migration of polymorphonuclear leukocytes and reversal of increased capillary permeability
Contraindications Hypersensitivity to medrysone or any component of the formulation; fungal, viral, or untreated pus-forming bacterial ocular infections; not for use in iritis and uveitis
Warnings/Precautions Prolonged use has been associated with the development of corneal or scleral perforation and posterior subcapsular cataracts. May mask or enhance the establishment of acute purulent untreated infections of the eye. Use caution in patients with glaucoma. Medrysone is a synthetic corticosteroid; structurally related to progesterone; if no improvement after several days of treatment, discontinue medrysone and institute other therapy. Duration of therapy: 3-4 days to several weeks dependent on type and severity of disease. Taper dose to avoid disease exacerbation. Safety and efficacy have not been established in children <3 years of age.
Adverse Reactions Frequency not defined: Ocular: Acute anterior uveitis, allergic reactions, blurred vision (mild, temporary), burning, cataracts, conjunctivitis, corneal thinning, corneal ulcers, delayed wound healing, foreign body sensation, glaucoma, IOP increased, keratitis, mydriasis, optic nerve damage, ptosis, secondary ocular infection stinging, visual activity defects
Overdosage/Toxicology Systemic toxicity is unlikely from the ophthalmic preparation.
Pharmacodynamics/Kinetics
Metabolism: Hepatic if absorbed
Excretion: Urine and feces
Available Dosage Forms [DSC] = Discontinued product
Solution, ophthalmic: 1% (5 mL, 10 mL) [contains benzalkonium chloride] [DSC]
Dosing
Adults & Elderly: Conjunctivitis: Ophthalmic: Instill 1 drop in conjunctival sac 2-4 times/day up to every 4 hours; may use every 1-2 hours during first 1-2 days.
Pediatrics: Children ≥3 years: Refer to adult dosing.
Administration
Other: Ophthalmic: Shake well before using. Do not touch dropper to the eye.

Stability
Storage: Store at room temperature of 25°C (77°F). Protect from freezing.
Nursing Actions
Physical Assessment: Assess knowledge/teach patient appropriate use, possible side effects/appropriate interventions, and adverse symptoms to report.
Patient Education: This medication is only for use in your eyes. Use exactly as directed. Wash hands thoroughly before using. Shake well before using. Do not allow applicator tip to touch eye. Gently pull down lower lid and put drop(s) into inner corner of eye. Close eye and roll eyeball in all directions. Do not blink for 30 seconds. Apply gentle pressure to inner corner of eye for 30 seconds. Gently wipe away any excess from skin around eye. Do not use any other eye medication for 10-15 minutes. May cause sensitivity to light (dark glasses may help); or temporary stinging, burning, or blurred vision. Report pain, swelling, scratchiness, itching, watering, or dryness of eye; drainage, redness, or sign of eye infection; change in vision (eg, double vision, reduced visual field, halo around lights); or worsening of condition or lack of improvement in 3-4 days. **Pregnancy/breast-feeding precautions:** Inform prescriber if you are pregnant. Consult prescriber if breast-feeding.

Mefloquine (ME floe kwin)

U.S. Brand Names Lariam®
Synonyms Mefloquine Hydrochloride
Restrictions A medication guide and wallet card must be provided to patients when mefloquine is dispensed for malaria. An FDA-approved medication guide is available at http://www.fda.gov/cder/Offices/ODS/labeling.htm.
Pharmacologic Category Antimalarial Agent
Pregnancy Risk Factor C
Lactation Enters breast milk/not recommended
Use Treatment of acute malarial infections and prevention of malaria
Mechanism of Action/Effect Mefloquine is a quinoline-methanol compound structurally similar to quinine; mefloquine's effectiveness in the treatment and prophylaxis of malaria is due to the destruction of the asexual blood forms of the malarial pathogens that affect humans, *Plasmodium falciparum*, *P. vivax*, *P. malariae*, *P. ovale*
Contraindications Hypersensitivity mefloquine, related compounds (such as quinine and quinidine), or any component of the formulation; history of convulsions; cardiac conduction abnormalities; severe psychiatric disorder (including active or recent history of depression, generalized anxiety disorder, psychosis, or schizophrenia); use with halofantrine
Warnings/Precautions Use with caution in patients with a previous history of depression (see Contraindications regarding severe psychiatric illness, including active/recent depression). May cause a range of psychiatric symptoms (anxiety, paranoia, depression, hallucinations and psychosis). Occasionally, symptoms have been reported to persist long after mefloquine has been discontinued. Rare cases of suicidal ideation and suicide have been reported (no causal relationship established). The appearance of psychiatric symptoms such as acute anxiety, depression, restlessness or confusion may be considered a prodrome to more serious events. When used as prophylaxis, substitute an alternative medication. Discontinue if unexplained neuropsychiatric disturbances occur. Use caution in patients with significant cardiac disease. If mefloquine is to be used for a prolonged period, periodic evaluations including liver function tests and ophthalmic examinations should be performed. (Retinal abnormalities have not been observed with mefloquine in humans; (Continued)

Mefloquine *(Continued)*

however, it has with long-term administration to rats.) In cases of life-threatening, serious, or overwhelming malaria infections due to *Plasmodium falciparum*, patients should be treated with intravenous antimalarial drug. Mefloquine may be given orally to complete the course. Dizziness, loss of balance, and other CNS disorders have been reported; due to long half-life, effects may persist after mefloquine is discontinued. Use caution in activities requiring alertness and fine motor coordination (driving, piloting planes, operating machinery, deep sea diving, etc).

Drug Interactions

Cytochrome P450 Effect: Substrate of CYP3A4 (major); **Inhibits** CYP2D6 (weak), 3A4 (weak)

Decreased Effect: Mefloquine may decrease the effect of valproic acid, carbamazepine, phenobarbital, and phenytoin. CYP3A4 inducers may decrease the levels/effects of mefloquine; example inducers include aminoglutethimide, carbamazepine, nafcillin, nevirapine, phenobarbital, phenytoin, and rifamycins. Vaccination with oral live attenuated Ty21a vaccine should be delayed for at least 24 hours after the administration of mefloquine.

Increased Effect/Toxicity: Use caution with drugs that alter cardiac conduction; increased toxicity with chloroquine, quinine, and quinidine (hold treatment until at least 12 hours after these later drugs); increased toxicity with halofantrine (concurrent use is contraindicated). CYP3A4 inhibitors may increase the levels/effects of mefloquine; example inhibitors include azole antifungals, clarithromycin, diclofenac, doxycycline, erythromycin, imatinib, isoniazid, nefazodone, nicardipine, propofol, protease inhibitors, quinidine, telithromycin, and verapamil.

Nutritional/Ethanol Interactions Food: Food increases bioavailability by ~40%.

Adverse Reactions

Frequency not defined: Neuropsychiatric events

1% to 10%:

Central nervous system: Headache, fever, chills, fatigue

Dermatologic: Rash

Gastrointestinal: Vomiting (3%), diarrhea, stomach pain, nausea, appetite decreased

Neuromuscular & skeletal: Myalgia

Otic: Tinnitus

Overdosage/Toxicology Treatment is supportive. Monitor cardiac function and psychiatric status for at least 24 hours.

Pharmacodynamics/Kinetics

Time to Peak: Plasma: 6-24 hours (median: ~17 hours)

Protein Binding: 98%

Half-Life Elimination: 21-22 days

Metabolism: Extensively hepatic; main metabolite is inactive

Excretion: Primarily bile and feces; urine (9% as unchanged drug, 4% as primary metabolite)

Available Dosage Forms Tablet, as hydrochloride: 250 mg [equivalent to 228 mg base]

Dosing

Adults & Elderly: Dose expressed as mg of mefloquine hydrochloride:

Malaria treatment (mild to moderate infection): Oral: 5 tablets (1250 mg) as a single dose. Take with food and at least 8 oz of water. If clinical improvement is not seen within 48-72 hours, an alternative therapy should be used for retreatment.

Malaria prophylaxis: Oral: 1 tablet (250 mg) weekly starting 1 week before, arrival in endemic area, continuing weekly during travel and for 4 weeks after leaving endemic area. Take with food and at least 8 oz of water.

Pediatrics: Dose expressed as mg of mefloquine hydrochloride: Children ≥6 months and >5 kg:

Malaria treatment: Oral: 20-25 mg/kg in 2 divided doses, taken 6-8 hours apart (maximum: 1250 mg) Take with food and an ample amount of water. If clinical improvement is not seen within 48-72 hours, an alternative therapy should be used for retreatment.

Malaria prophylaxis: Oral: 5 mg/kg/once weekly (maximum dose: 250 mg) starting 1 week before, arrival in endemic area, continuing weekly during travel and for 4 weeks after leaving endemic area. Take with food and an ample amount of water.

Renal Impairment: No dosage adjustment needed in patients with renal impairment or on dialysis.

Hepatic Impairment: Half-life may be prolonged and plasma levels may be higher.

Administration

Oral: Administer with food and with at least 8 oz of water. When used for malaria prophylaxis, dose should be taken once weekly on the same day each week. If vomiting occurs within 30-60 minutes after dose, an additional half-dose should be given. Tablets may be crushed and suspended in a small amount of water, milk, or another beverage for persons unable to swallow tablets.

Stability

Storage: Store at 25°C (77°F); excursions permitted to 15°C to 30°C (59°F to 86°F)

Laboratory Monitoring When use is prolonged, periodically monitor liver function tests.

Nursing Actions

Physical Assessment: Prior to beginning therapy, assess potential for interactions with pharmacological or herbal products patient may be taking. Monitor therapeutic effects and adverse reactions (eg, hypertension, cardiomyopathy, hyperglycemia, hepatotoxicity) on a regular basis throughout therapy. Monitor patient closely for any development of psychiatric symptoms (anxiety, paranoia, depression, hallucinations, and psychosis); may persist long after mefloquine has been discontinued. Advise patient about the importance of carrying medication guide and wallet provided when mefloquine is dispensed for malaria. Teach patient proper use, possible side effects/appropriate interventions (eg, importance of adequate hydration), and adverse symptoms to report.

Patient Education: Do not take any new medication during therapy unless approved by prescriber. Follow exact dosage schedule and do not take more than prescribed. Take with food and at least 8 oz of water. Maintain adequate nutrition and maintain adequate hydration (2-3 L/day of fluids unless instructed to restrict fluid intake). Carry drug information card in wallet for as long as you are taking this drug. May cause dizziness, anxiety, loss of balance (use caution when driving or engaging in tasks that require alertness until response to drug is known); nausea, vomiting, or decreased appetite (small, frequent meals, frequent mouth care, or chewing gum may help). Report immediately any anxiety, confusion, agitation, restlessness, paranoia, depression, hallucinations, suicidal ideation. **Pregnancy/breast-feeding precautions:** Inform prescriber if you are or intend to be pregnant or breast-feeding.

Dietary Considerations Take with food and with at least 8 oz of water.

Breast-Feeding Issues Excreted in small quantities; effect to nursing infant is unknown. Breast-feeding is not recommended during therapy and the long half-life of mefloquine should also be considered once therapy is complete.

Megestrol (me JES trole)

U.S. Brand Names Megace®; Megace® ES
Synonyms 5071-1DL(6); Megestrol Acetate; NSC-10363
Pharmacologic Category Antineoplastic Agent, Hormone; Appetite Stimulant; Progestin
Medication Safety Issues
Sound-alike/look-alike issues:
Megace® may be confused with Reglan®
Pregnancy Risk Factor X
Lactation Enters breast milk/contraindicated
Use Palliative treatment of breast and endometrial carcinoma; treatment of anorexia, cachexia, or unexplained significant weight loss in patients with AIDS
Mechanism of Action/Effect A synthetic progestin with antiestrogenic properties which disrupt the estrogen receptor cycle. May also have a direct effect on the endometrium. Megestrol is an antineoplastic progestin thought to act through an antileutenizing effect mediated via the pituitary. May stimulate appetite by antagonizing the metabolic effects of catabolic cytokines.
Contraindications Hypersensitivity to megestrol or any component of the formulation; pregnancy
Warnings/Precautions Use with caution in patients with a history of thrombophlebitis. Elderly females may have vaginal bleeding or discharge. May suppress hypothalamic-pituitary-adrenal (HPA) axis during chronic administration. Consider the possibility of adrenal suppression in any patient receiving or being withdrawn from chronic therapy when signs/symptoms suggestive of hypoadrenalism are noted (during stress or in unstressed state). Laboratory evaluation and replacement/stress doses of rapid-acting glucocorticoid should be considered.
Nutritional/Ethanol Interactions Herb/Nutraceutical: Avoid black cohosh, dong quai in estrogen-dependent tumors.
Lab Interactions Altered thyroid and liver function tests
Adverse Reactions
Cardiovascular: Edema, hypertension (≤8%), cardiomyopathy, palpitation
Central nervous system: Insomnia, fever (2% to 6%), headache (≤10%), pain (≤6%, similar to placebo), confusion (1% to 3%), convulsions (1% to 3%), depression (1% to 3%)
Dermatologic: Allergic rash (2% to 12%) with or without pruritus, alopecia
Endocrine & metabolic: Breakthrough bleeding and amenorrhea, spotting, changes in menstrual flow, changes in cervical erosion and secretions, increased breast tenderness, changes in vaginal bleeding pattern, edema, fluid retention, hyperglycemia (≤6%), diabetes, HPA axis suppression, adrenal insufficiency, Cushing's syndrome
Gastrointestinal: Weight gain (not attributed to edema or fluid retention), nausea, vomiting (7%), diarrhea (8% to 15%, similar to placebo), flatulence (≤10%), constipation (1% to 3%)
Genitourinary: Impotence (4% to 14%), decreased libido (≤5%)
Hepatic: Cholestatic jaundice, hepatotoxicity, hepatomegaly (1% to 3%)
Local: Thrombophlebitis
Neuromuscular & skeletal: Carpal tunnel syndrome, weakness, paresthesia (1% to 3%)
Respiratory: Hyperpnea, dyspnea (1% to 3%), cough (1% to 3%)
Miscellaneous: Diaphoresis
Overdosage/Toxicology Toxicity is unlikely following single exposure of excessive doses.
Pharmacodynamics/Kinetics
Time to Peak: Serum: 1-3 hours
Half-Life Elimination: 15-100 hours
Metabolism: Completely hepatic to free steroids and glucuronide conjugates

Excretion: Urine (57% to 78% as steroid metabolites and inactive compound); feces (8% to 30%)
Available Dosage Forms
Suspension, oral, as acetate: 40 mg/mL (240 mL, 480 mL)
Megace®: 40 mg/mL (240 mL) [contains alcohol 0.06% and sodium benzoate; lemon-lime flavor]
Megace® ES: 125 mg/mL (150 mL) [contains alcohol 0.06% and sodium benzoate; lemon-lime flavor]
Tablet, as acetate: 20 mg, 40 mg
Dosing
Adults & Elderly:
Breast carcinoma (female): Refer to individual protocols: Oral: 40 mg 4 times/day
Endometrial carcinoma: Refer to individual protocols: Oral: 40-320 mg/day in divided doses; use for 2 months to determine efficacy; maximum doses used have been up to 800 mg/day
HIV-related cachexia (male/female): Oral:
Megace®: Initial dose: 800 mg/day; daily doses of 400 and 800 mg/day were found to be clinically effective
Megace ES®: 625 mg/day
Renal Impairment: No data available; however, the urinary excretion of megestrol acetate administered in doses of 4-90 mg ranged from 56% to 78% within 10 days.
Hemodialysis: Megestrol acetate has not been tested for dialyzability; however, due to its low solubility, it is postulated that dialysis would not be an effective means of treating an overdose.

Administration
Oral: Megestrol acetate (Megace®) oral suspension is compatible with water, orange juice, apple juice, or Sustacal H.C. for immediate consumption.

Stability
Storage: Store at 25°C (77°F); excursions permitted at 15°C to 30°C (59°F to 86°F)

Nursing Actions
Physical Assessment: Prior to beginning therapy, assess potential for interactions with herbal products patient may be taking. Monitor therapeutic effects (according to purpose for use) and adverse reactions (eg, hypertension, CNS changes [confusion, convulsions, insomnia], rash, changes in menses, gastrointestinal upset, jaundice, thrombophlebitis) regularly during therapy. Teach patient proper use, possible side effects/appropriate interventions (eg, importance of adequate hydration), and adverse symptoms to report.
Patient Education: Do not take any new medication during therapy unless approved by prescriber. Follow dosage schedule and do not take more than prescribed. May cause sensitivity to sunlight (use sunblock, wear protective clothing, and avoid extended exposure to direct sunlight); dizziness, anxiety, depression (use caution when driving or engaging in tasks that require alertness until response to drug is known); change in appetite (maintain adequate hydration [2-3 L/day of fluids, unless instructed to restrict fluid intake] and diet); decreased libido or increased body hair (reversible when drug is discontinued); or hot flashes (cool clothes and environment may help). Report swelling of face, lips, or mouth; absent or altered menses; abdominal pain; vaginal itching, irritation, or discharge; heat, warmth, redness, or swelling of extremities; or sudden onset change in vision. **Pregnancy/breast-feeding precautions:** Do not get pregnant while taking this medication and for 1 month following therapy; consult prescriber for appropriate contraceptives. This drug may cause fetal defects. Do not donate blood during or for 1 month following therapy. Do not breast-feed.
Geriatric Considerations Elderly females may have vaginal bleeding or discharge and need to be forewarned of this side effect and inconvenience. No (Continued)

Megestrol *(Continued)*

specific changes in dose are required for elderly. Megestrol has been used in the treatment of the failure to thrive syndrome in cachectic elderly in addition to proper nutrition.

Meloxicam *(mel OKS i kam)*

U.S. Brand Names Mobic®

Restrictions A medication guide should be dispensed with each prescription. A template for the required MedGuide can be found on the FDA website at: http://www.fda.gov/medwatch/SAFETY/2005/safety05.htm#NSAID

Pharmacologic Category Nonsteroidal Anti-inflammatory Drug (NSAID), Oral

Pregnancy Risk Factor C/D (3rd trimester)

Lactation Excretion in breast milk unknown/not recommended

Use Relief of signs and symptoms of osteoarthritis, rheumatoid arthritis, and juvenile rheumatoid arthritis (JRA)

Mechanism of Action/Effect Inhibits prostaglandin synthesis by decreasing the activity of the enzyme, cyclooxygenase, which results in decreased formation of prostaglandin precursors

Contraindications Hypersensitivity to meloxicam, aspirin, other NSAIDs, or any component of the formulation; perioperative pain in the setting of coronary artery bypass surgery (CABG); pregnancy (3rd trimester)

Warnings/Precautions NSAIDs are associated with an increased risk of adverse cardiovascular events, including MI, stroke, and new onset or worsening of pre-existing hypertension. Risk may be increased with duration of use or pre-existing cardiovascular risk-factors or disease. Carefully evaluate individual cardiovascular risk profiles prior to prescribing. Use caution with fluid retention, CHF or hypertension.

Use of NSAIDs can compromise existing renal function. Renal toxicity can occur in patient with impaired renal function, dehydration, heart failure, liver dysfunction, those taking diuretics and ACEI and the elderly. Rehydrate patient before starting therapy. Monitor renal function closely. Meloxicam is not recommended for patients with advanced renal disease

NSAIDs may increase risk of gastrointestinal irritation, ulceration, bleeding, and perforation. These events may occur at any time during therapy and without warning. Use caution with a history of GI disease (bleeding or ulcers), concurrent therapy with aspirin, anticoagulants and/or corticosteroids, smoking, use of alcohol, the elderly or debilitated patients.

Use the lowest effective dose for the shortest duration of time, consistent with individual patient goals, to reduce risk of cardiovascular or GI adverse events. Alternate therapies should be considered for patients at high risk.

NSAIDs may cause serious skin adverse events including exfoliative dermatitis, Stevens-Johnson syndrome (SJS) and toxic epidermal necrolysis (TEN). Anaphylactoid reactions may occur, even without prior exposure; patients with "aspirin triad" (bronchial asthma, aspirin intolerance, rhinitis) may be at increased risk. Do not use in patients who experience bronchospasm, asthma, rhinitis, or urticaria with NSAID or aspirin therapy.

Use with caution in patients with decreased hepatic function. Closely monitor patients with any abnormal LFT. Severe hepatic reactions (eg, fulminant hepatitis, liver failure) have occurred with NSAID use, rarely; discontinue if signs or symptoms of liver disease develop, or if systemic manifestations occur.

The elderly are at increased risk for adverse effects (especially peptic ulceration, CNS effects, renal toxicity) from NSAIDs even at low doses.

Withhold for at least 4-6 half-lives prior to surgical or dental procedures. Safety and efficacy have not been established in pediatric patients <2 years of age.

Drug Interactions

Cytochrome P450 Effect: Substrate (minor) of CYP2C8/9, 3A4; **Inhibits** CYP2C8/9 (weak)

Decreased Effect: Cholestyramine (and possibly colestipol) increases the clearance of meloxicam. Hydralazine's antihypertensive effect is decreased; avoid concurrent use. Loop diuretic efficacy (diuretic and antihypertensive effect) may be reduced by NSAIDs. Antihypertensive effects of thiazide diuretics are decreased; avoid concurrent use.

Increased Effect/Toxicity: Anticoagulants (warfarin, heparin, LMWHs) in combination with NSAIDs can cause increased risk of bleeding. Antiplatelet drugs (ticlopidine, clopidogrel, aspirin, abciximab, dipyridamole, eptifibatide, tirofiban) can cause an increased risk of bleeding. Aspirin increases serum concentrations (AUC) of meloxicam (in addition to potential for additive adverse effects); concurrent use is not recommended. Corticosteroids may increase the risk of GI ulceration; avoid concurrent use. NSAIDs may increase serum creatinine, potassium, blood pressure, and cyclosporine levels; monitor cyclosporine levels and renal function carefully. Lithium levels can be increased; avoid concurrent use if possible or monitor lithium levels and adjust dose. When NSAID is stopped, lithium will need adjustment again. Serum concentration/toxicity of methotrexate may be increased. Warfarin INRs may be increased by meloxicam. Monitor INR closely, particularly during initiation or change in dose. May increase risk of bleeding. Use lowest possible dose for shortest duration possible.

Nutritional/Ethanol Interactions

Ethanol: Avoid ethanol (may enhance gastric mucosal irritation).

Herb/Nutraceutical: Avoid alfalfa, anise, bilberry, bladderwrack, bromelain, cat's claw, celery, coleus, cordyceps, dong quai, evening primrose, feverfew, fenugreek, garlic, ginger, ginkgo biloboa, red clover, horse chestnut, grapeseed, green tea, ginseng, guggul, horse chestnut seed, horseradish, licorice, prickly ash, red clover, reishi, SAMe, sweet clover, turmeric, white willow (all have additional antiplatelet activity).

Adverse Reactions Percentages reported in adult patients; abdominal pain, diarrhea, headache, pyrexia, and vomiting were reported more commonly in pediatric patients

2% to 10%:

Cardiovascular: Edema (<1% to 4%)

Central nervous system: Headache (2% to 8%), dizziness (<1% to 4%), insomnia (<1% to 4%)

Dermatologic: Pruritus (<1% to 2%), rash (<1% to 3%)

Gastrointestinal: Diarrhea (3% to 8%), dyspepsia (4% to 9%), abdominal pain (2% to 5%), nausea (2% to 7%), constipation (<1% to 3%), flatulence (<1% to 3%), vomiting (<1% to 3%)

Hematologic: Anemia (<1% to 4%)

Neuromuscular & skeletal: Arthralgia (<1% to 5%), back pain (<1% to 3%)

Respiratory: Cough (<1% to 2%), pharyngitis (<1% to 3%), upper respiratory infection (2% to 8%)

Miscellaneous: Flu-like symptoms (2% to 6%), falls (3%)

Overdosage/Toxicology Symptoms of overdose include lethargy, drowsiness, nausea, vomiting, and epigastric pain. Rarely, severe symptoms have been associated with NSAID overdose including apnea, metabolic acidosis, coma, nystagmus, seizures, leukocytosis, and renal failure. Management of NSAID intoxication is supportive and symptomatic. Since meloxicam undergoes enterohepatic cycling, multiple doses of charcoal may be needed to reduce the potential for delayed toxicities. Cholestyramine has been shown to increase meloxicam clearance. Meloxicam is not dialyzable.

Pharmacodynamics/Kinetics
Time to Peak: Initial: 5-10 hours; Secondary: 12-14 hours
Protein Binding: 99.4%
Half-Life Elimination: Adults: 15-20 hours
Metabolism: Hepatic via CYP2C9 and CYP3A4 (minor); forms 4 metabolites (inactive)
Excretion: Urine and feces (as inactive metabolites)

Available Dosage Forms
Suspension: 7.5 mg/5 mL (100 mL) [contains sodium benzoate; raspberry flavor]
Tablet: 7.5 mg, 15 mg

Dosing
Adults & Elderly: Osteoarthritis, rheumatoid arthritis: Oral: Initial: 7.5 mg once daily; some patients may receive additional benefit from an increased dose of 15 mg once daily.
Pediatrics: JRA: Oral: Children ≥2 years: 0.125 mg/kg/day; maximum dose: 7.5 mg/day
Renal Impairment:
Mild to moderate impairment: No specific dosage recommendations
Significant impairment (Cl_{cr} ≤15 mL/minute): Avoid use
Hemodialysis: Supplemental dose after dialysis not necessary.
Hepatic Impairment:
Mild (Child-Pugh class A) to moderate (Child-Pugh class B) hepatic dysfunction: No dosage adjustment is necessary
Severe hepatic impairment: Patients with severe hepatic impairment have not been adequately studied

Stability
Storage: Store at 25°C (77°F).
Laboratory Monitoring CBC, periodic liver function, renal function (serum BUN, and creatinine)

Nursing Actions
Physical Assessment: Assess effectiveness and interactions of other medications patient may be taking. Monitor blood pressure at the beginning of therapy and periodically during use. Monitor laboratory tests and therapeutic response (eg, relief of pain and inflammation, activity tolerance), and adverse reactions (eg, gastrointestinal effects or ototoxicity) at beginning of therapy and periodically throughout therapy. Assess knowledge/teach patient appropriate use, interventions to reduce side effects, and adverse symptoms to report.

Patient Education: Take this medication exactly as directed; do not increase dose without consulting prescriber. Take with food or milk to reduce GI distress. Maintain adequate hydration (2-3 L/day of fluids) unless instructed to restrict fluid intake. Avoid alcohol, excessive vitamin C intake, or salicylate-containing foods (eg, curry powder, prunes, raisins, tea, or licorice). Do not use aspirin or aspirin-containing medication, or any other anti-inflammatory medications without consulting prescriber. You may experience anorexia, nausea, vomiting, or heartburn (small frequent meals, frequent mouth care, sucking lozenges, or chewing gum may help); drowsiness, dizziness, nervousness, or headache (use caution when driving or engaging in tasks requiring alertness until response to drug is known); or fluid retention (weigh yourself weekly and report unusual (3-5 lb/week) weight gain). GI bleeding, ulceration, or perforation can occur with or without pain; discontinue medication and contact prescriber if persistent abdominal pain or cramping, or blood in

stool occurs. Report breathlessness, respiratory difficulty, or unusual cough; chest pain, rapid heartbeat, palpitations; slurring of speech; unusual bruising/bleeding; blood in urine, stool, mouth, or vomitus; swollen extremities; skin blisters, rash, or itching; acute fatigue, jaundice, flu-like symptoms, hearing changes (ringing in ears); or other adverse reactions.
Pregnancy/breast-feeding precautions: Inform prescriber if you are or intend to become pregnant. This drug should not be used in the 3rd trimester of pregnancy. Do not breast-feed.
Dietary Considerations Should be taken with food or milk to minimize gastrointestinal irritation.

Geriatric Considerations
The elderly are at increased risk for adverse effects from NSAIDs. As many as 60% of elderly can develop peptic ulceration and/or hemorrhage asymptomatically. CNS adverse effects such as confusion, agitation, and hallucination are generally seen in overdose or high-dose situations; however, elderly patients may demonstrate these adverse effects at lower doses than younger adults. The elderly are also at increased risk of renal toxicity.
Breast-Feeding Issues It is not known whether meloxicam is excreted in human milk. Due to a potential for serious adverse reactions, the manufacturer recommends that a decision be made whether to discontinue nursing or discontinue the drug, taking into account the importance of the drug to the mother.
Pregnancy Issues May cause premature closure of the ductus arteriosus in the 3rd trimester of pregnancy.

Melphalan (MEL fa lan)

U.S. Brand Names Alkeran®
Synonyms L-PAM; L-Sarcolysin; Phenylalanine Mustard
Pharmacologic Category Antineoplastic Agent, Alkylating Agent
Medication Safety Issues
Sound-alike/look-alike issues:
Melphalan may be confused with Mephyton®, Myleran®
Alkeran® may be confused with Alferon®, Leukeran®
Pregnancy Risk Factor D
Lactation Excretion in breast milk unknown/not recommended
Use Palliative treatment of multiple myeloma and nonresectable epithelial ovarian carcinoma; neuroblastoma, rhabdomyosarcoma, breast cancer
Mechanism of Action/Effect Alkylating agent which is a derivative of mechlorethamine that inhibits DNA and RNA synthesis via formation of carbonium ions; cross-links strands of DNA
Contraindications Hypersensitivity to melphalan or any component of the formulation; severe bone marrow suppression; patients whose disease was resistant to prior therapy; pregnancy
Warnings/Precautions Hazardous agent - use appropriate precautions for handling and disposal. Melphalan is potentially mutagenic, carcinogenic, and teratogenic; produces amenorrhea. Discontinue therapy if leukocyte count is <3000/mm^3 or platelet count is <100,000/mm^3; use with caution in patients with bone marrow suppression, impaired renal function, or who have received prior chemotherapy or irradiation; will cause amenorrhea. Toxicity to immunosuppressives is increased in the elderly. Start with lowest recommended adult doses. Signs of infection, such as fever and WBC rise, may not occur. Lethargy and confusion may be more prominent signs of infection.
Drug Interactions
Decreased Effect: Cimetidine and other H_2 antagonists: The reduction in gastric pH has been reported to decrease bioavailability of melphalan by 30%.
(Continued)

Melphalan *(Continued)*

Increased Effect/Toxicity: Risk of nephrotoxicity of cyclosporine is increased by melphalan. Concomitant use of I.V. melphalan may cause serious GI toxicity.

Nutritional/Ethanol Interactions
Ethanol: Avoid ethanol (due to GI irritation).
Food: Food interferes with oral absorption.

Lab Interactions False-positive Coombs' test [direct]

Adverse Reactions
>10%: Hematologic: Myelosuppressive: Leukopenia and thrombocytopenia are the most common effects of melphalan; irreversible bone marrow failure has been reported
WBC: Moderate
Platelets: Moderate
Onset: 7 days
Nadir: 8-10 days and 27-32 days
Recovery: 42-50 days
1% to 10%:
Cardiovascular: Vasculitis
Dermatologic: Vesiculation of skin, alopecia, pruritus, rash
Endocrine & metabolic: SIADH, sterility, amenorrhea
Gastrointestinal: Nausea and vomiting are mild; stomatitis and diarrhea are infrequent
Genitourinary: Hemorrhagic cystitis, bladder irritation
Hematologic: Anemia, agranulocytosis, hemolytic anemia
Hepatic: Transaminases increased (hepatitis, jaundice have been reported)
Respiratory: Pulmonary fibrosis, interstitial pneumonitis
Miscellaneous: Hypersensitivity, secondary malignancy

Overdosage/Toxicology Symptoms of overdose include hypocalcemia, pulmonary fibrosis, nausea and vomiting, and bone marrow suppression. Treatment is symptomatic and supportive.

Pharmacodynamics/Kinetics
Time to Peak: Serum: ~2 hours
Half-Life Elimination: Terminal: 1.5 hours
Excretion: Oral: Feces (20% to 50%); urine (10% to 30% as unchanged drug)

Available Dosage Forms
Injection, powder for reconstitution: 50 mg [diluent contains ethanol and propylene glycol]
Tablet: 2 mg

Dosing
Adults & Elderly: Refer to individual protocols; dose should always be adjusted to patient response and weekly blood counts.

Multiple myeloma:
Oral: 6 mg/day initially adjusted as indicated **or** 0.15 mg/kg/day for 7 days **or** 0.25 mg/kg/day for 4 days; repeat at 4- to 6-week intervals.
I.V.: 16 mg/m^2 administered at 2-week intervals for 4 doses, then repeat monthly as per protocol for multiple myeloma.
Ovarian carcinoma: Oral: 0.2 mg/kg/day for 5 days, repeat every 4-5 weeks
High dose BMT: I.V.: 140-240 mg/m^2 as a single dose or divided into 2-5 daily doses. Infuse over 20-60 minutes.

Pediatrics: Oral (refer to individual protocols); dose should always be adjusted to patient response and weekly blood counts.

Various protocols: Oral: 4-20 mg/m^2/day for 1-21 days
Pediatric rhabdomyosarcoma: I.V.: 10-35 mg/m^2/dose every 21-28 days
High-dose melphalan with bone marrow transplantation for neuroblastoma: I.V.: 70-100 mg/m^2/day on day 7 and 6 before BMT **or**
140-220 mg/m^2 single dose before BMT **or**

50 mg/m^2/day for 4 days **or**
70 mg/m^2/day for 3 days

Renal Impairment:
Cl$_{cr}$ 10-50 mL/minute: Administer 75% of normal dose.
Cl$_{cr}$ <10 mL/minute: Administer 50% of normal dose.
or
BUN >30 mg/dL: Reduce dose by 50%.
Serum creatinine >1.5 mg/dL: Reduce dose by 50%.
Hemodialysis effects: Unknown
CAPD effects: Unknown
CAVH effects: Unknown

Administration
Oral: Administer on an empty stomach.
I.V.: Due to limited stability, complete administration of I.V. dose should occur within 60 minutes of reconstitution
I.V. infusion: Infuse over 15-20 minutes
I.V. bolus:
Central line: I.V. bolus doses of 17-200 mg/m^2 (reconstituted and not diluted) have been infused over 2-20 minutes
Peripheral line: I.V. bolus doses of 2-23 mg/m^2 (reconstituted and not diluted) have been infused over 1-4 minutes

I.V. Detail: Avoid skin contact with I.V. formulation.

BMT only: Saline-based hydration (100-125 mg/m^2/hour) preceding (2-4 hours), during, and following (6-12 hours) administration reduces risk of drug precipitation in renal tubules. Hydrolysis causes loss of 1% melphalan injection per 10 minutes. Infusion of admixture must be completed within 100 minutes of preparation to deliver ordered dose. Reconstitute dose to 5 mg/mL in diluent provided by manufacturer. Dose may be infused via central or peripheral venous access without further dilution to minimize volume of infusion.

pH: 6.5-7.0

Stability
Reconstitution:
Injection must be prepared fresh. **The time between reconstitution/dilution and administration of parenteral melphalan must be kept to a minimum (<60 minutes) because reconstituted and diluted solutions are unstable.** Dissolve powder initially with 10 mL of diluent to a concentration of 5 mg/mL. Shake vigorously to dissolve. **Immediately** dilute dose in 250-500 mL NS to a concentration of 0.1-0.45 mg/mL.

Compatibility: Incompatible with D$_5$W, LR
Y-site administration: Incompatible with amphotericin B, chlorpromazine

Storage:
Tablet: Store in refrigerator at 2°C to 8°C (36°F to 46°F). Protect from light.
Injection: Store at room temperature (15°C to 30°C). Protect from light. Reconstituted solution is chemically and physically stable for at least 90 minutes when stored at 25°C (77°F). Diluted solution is physically and chemically stable for at least 60 minutes at 25°C (77°F).

Laboratory Monitoring CBC with differential, platelet count, serum electrolytes, serum uric acid

Nursing Actions
Physical Assessment: Assess potential for interactions with other pharmacological agents patient may be taking (eg, cimetidine, cyclosporine). For intravenous infusion see Administration and Reconstitution specifics. Monitor laboratory tests, patient response, and adverse reactions (eg, myelosuppression [leukopenia], SIADH, diarrhea, bladder irritation [hematuria], interstitial pneumonitis) regularly during therapy. Teach patient proper use (oral), possible side effects/appropriate interventions, and adverse symptoms to report.

Patient Education: I.V.: Report immediately any burning, swelling, pain, or redness at infusion or injection site: **Oral:** Take on an empty stomach, if possible, 1 hour before or 2 hours after meals. Avoid excessive alcohol (may increase gastric irritation). Maintain adequate nutrition (small, frequent meals may help) and adequate hydration (2-3 L/day of fluids) unless instructed to restrict fluid intake. You may be more susceptible to infection (avoid crowds and exposure to infection and do not have any vaccinations unless approved by prescriber). May cause hair loss (reversible); easy bleeding or bruising (use soft toothbrush or cotton swabs and frequent mouth care, use electric razor, avoid sharp knives or scissors); or nausea or vomiting (small, frequent meals, frequent mouth care, chewing gum, or sucking lozenges may help). Report chest pain or palpitations; unusual fatigue; difficulty or pain on urination; unusual bruising/bleeding; respiratory difficulty; or other adverse reactions. **Pregnancy/breast-feeding precautions:** Inform prescriber if you are pregnant. Do not get pregnant during or for 1 month following therapy. Consult prescriber for instruction on appropriate contraceptive measures. This drug may cause severe fetal defects. Breast-feeding is not recommended.

Dietary Considerations Should be taken on an empty stomach (1 hour prior to or 2 hours after meals).

Geriatric Considerations Toxicity to immunosuppressives is increased in the elderly. Start with lowest recommended adult doses. Signs of infection, such as fever and WBC rise, may not occur. Lethargy and confusion may be more prominent signs of infection.

Memantine (me MAN teen)

U.S. Brand Names Namenda™

Synonyms Memantine Hydrochloride

Pharmacologic Category N-Methyl-D-Aspartate Receptor Antagonist

Pregnancy Risk Factor B

Lactation Excretion in breast milk unknown/use caution

Use Treatment of moderate-to-severe dementia of the Alzheimer's type

Unlabeled/Investigational Use Treatment of mild-to-moderate vascular dementia

Mechanism of Action/Effect Memantine reduces the decline in function in Alzheimer's disease; it has not been shown to prevent or slow neurodegeneration associated with this disease.

Contraindications Hypersensitivity to memantine or any component of the formulation

Warnings/Precautions Use caution with seizure disorders or hepatic impairment. Caution with use in severe renal impairment; dose adjustment recommended. Clearance is significantly reduced by alkaline urine; use caution with medications, dietary changes, or patient conditions which may alter urine pH.

Drug Interactions

Increased Effect/Toxicity: Clearance of memantine is decreased 80% at urinary pH 8; use caution with medications (carbonic anhydrase inhibitors, sodium bicarbonate) which may increase urinary pH.

Adverse Reactions

1% to 10%:

Cardiovascular: Hypertension (4%), cardiac failure, syncope, cerebrovascular accident, transient ischemic attack

Central nervous system: Dizziness (7%), confusion (6%), headache (6%), hallucinations (3%), pain (3%), somnolence (3%), fatigue (2%), aggressive reaction, ataxia, vertigo

Dermatologic: Rash

Gastrointestinal: Constipation (5%), vomiting (3%), weight loss

Genitourinary: Micturition

Hematologic: Anemia

Hepatic: Alkaline phosphatase increased

Neuromuscular & skeletal: Back pain (3%), hypokinesia

Ocular: Cataract, conjunctivitis

Respiratory: Cough (4%), dyspnea (2%), pneumonia

Overdosage/Toxicology Loss of consciousness, psychosis, restlessness, somnolence, stupor, and visual hallucinations were reported following ingestion of memantine 400 mg. In case of overdose, treatment should be symptomatic and supportive. Elimination may be increased by acidifying the urine.

Pharmacodynamics/Kinetics

Time to Peak: Serum: 3-7 hours

Protein Binding: 45%

Half-Life Elimination: Terminal: 60-80 hours; severe renal impairment (Cl_{cr} 5-29 mL/minute): 117-156 hours

Metabolism: Forms 3 metabolites (minimal activity)

Excretion: Urine (57% to 82% unchanged); excretion reduced by alkaline urine pH

Available Dosage Forms

Solution, oral: 2 mg/mL (360 mL) [alcohol free, dye free, sugar free; peppermint flavor]

Tablet, as hydrochloride: 5 mg, 10 mg

Combination package [titration pack contains two separate tablet formulations]: Memantine hydrochloride 5 mg (28s) and memantine hydrochloride 10 mg (21s)

Dosing

Adults & Elderly:

Alzheimer's disease: Oral: Initial: 5 mg/day; increase dose by 5 mg/day to a target dose of 20 mg/day; wait at least 1 week between dosage changes. Doses >5 mg/day should be given in 2 divided doses.

Suggested titration: 5 mg/day for ≥1 week; 5 mg twice daily for ≥1 week; 15 mg/day given in 5 mg and 10 mg separated doses for ≥1 week; then 10 mg twice daily.

Mild-to-moderate vascular dementia (unlabeled use): Oral: 10 mg twice daily

Renal Impairment:

Mild-to-moderate impairment: No adjustment required.

Severe impairment: Cl_{cr} 5-29 mL/minute): 5 mg twice daily

Stability

Storage: Store at controlled room temperature of 15°C to 30°C (59°F to 86°F).

Nursing Actions

Physical Assessment: Assess therapeutic effectiveness and adverse reactions (eg, hypertension, CNS changes, rash, constipation) on a regular basis throughout therapy. Teach patient possible side effects/appropriate interventions and adverse symptoms to report.

Patient Education: Take as directed with or without food. May cause hypertension (monitor if recommended); headache (consult prescriber for analgesic). Report increase or changes in CNS symptoms (confusion, hallucinations, fatigue, aggressive reaction); chest pain or palpitations, dizziness or fainting; difficulty breathing of tightness in chest; rash; alteration in elimination patterns, or other persistent adverse reactions. **Breast-feeding precaution:** Consult prescriber if breast-feeding.

Dietary Considerations May be taken with or without food.

Geriatric Considerations In clinical trials, patients on memantine had less of a decline in cognitive function and activities of daily living (ADL) as compared to placebo. This was true for monotherapy with memantine, as well as combination therapy with donepezil, an acetylcholinesterase inhibitor.

Menotropins (men oh TROE pins)

U.S. Brand Names Menopur®; Pergonal® [DSC]; Repronex®

Pharmacologic Category Gonadotropin; Ovulation Stimulator

Medication Safety Issues
Sound-alike/look-alike issues:
Repronex® may be confused with Regranex®

Pregnancy Risk Factor X

Lactation Excretion in breast milk unknown/use caution

Use
Female:
In conjunction with hCG to induce ovulation and pregnancy in infertile females experiencing oligoanovulation or anovulation when the cause of anovulation is functional and not caused by primary ovarian failure (Pergonal®, Repronex®)
Stimulation of multiple follicle development in ovulatory patients as part of an assisted reproductive technology (ART) (Menopur®, Pergonal®, Repronex®)
Male: Stimulation of spermatogenesis in primary or secondary hypogonadotropic hypogonadism (Pergonal®)

Mechanism of Action/Effect Actions occur as a result of both follicle stimulating hormone (FSH) effects and luteinizing hormone (LH) effects; menotropins stimulate the development and maturation of the ovarian follicle (FSH), cause ovulation (LH), and stimulate the development of the corpus luteum (LH); in males it stimulates spermatogenesis (LH)

Contraindications Hypersensitivity to menotropins or any component of the formulation; primary ovarian failure as indicated by a high follicle-stimulating hormone (FSH) level; uncontrolled thyroid and adrenal dysfunction; abnormal bleeding of undetermined origin; intracranial lesion (ie, pituitary tumor); ovarian cyst or enlargement not due to polycystic ovary syndrome; infertility due to any cause other than anovulation (except candidates for *in vitro* fertilization); men with normal urinary gonadotropin concentrations, elevated gonadotropin levels indicating primary testicular failure; sex hormone-dependent tumors of the reproductive tract and accessory organs; pregnancy

Warnings/Precautions Advise patient of frequency and potential hazards of multiple pregnancy. To minimize the hazard of abnormal ovarian enlargement, use the lowest possible dose. Safety and efficacy have not been established in renal or hepatic impairment, or in pediatric and geriatric patients.

Adverse Reactions Adverse effects may vary according to specific product, route, and/or dosage.

Male:
>10%: Endocrine & metabolic: Gynecomastia
1% to 10%: Erythrocytosis (dyspnea, dizziness, anorexia, syncope, epistaxis)

Female:
>10%:
Central nervous system: Headache (up to 34%)
Gastrointestinal: Abdominal pain (up to 18%), nausea (up to 12%)
Genitourinary: OHSS (up to 13%, dose related)
Local: Injection site reaction (4% to 12%)
1% to 10%:
Cardiovascular: Flushing
Central nervous system: Dizziness, malaise, migraine
Endocrine & metabolic: Breast tenderness, hot flashes, menstrual irregularities
Gastrointestinal: Abdominal cramping, abdominal fullness, constipation, diarrhea, enlarged abdomen, vomiting
Genitourinary: Ectopic pregnancy, ovarian disease, vaginal hemorrhage
Local: Injection site edema/pain

Neuromuscular & skeletal: Back pain
Respiratory: Cough increased, respiratory disorder
Miscellaneous: Infection, flu-like syndrome

Frequency not defined:
Cardiovascular: Stroke, tachycardia, thrombosis (venous or arterial)
Central nervous system: Dizziness
Dermatologic: Angioedema, urticaria
Genitourinary: Adnexal torsion, hemoperitoneum, ovarian enlargement
Neuromuscular & skeletal: Limb necrosis
Respiratory: Acute respiratory distress syndrome, atelectasis, dyspnea, embolism, laryngeal edema pulmonary infarction tachypnea
Miscellaneous: Allergic reaction, anaphylaxis, rash

Overdosage/Toxicology Symptoms of overdose include ovarian hyperstimulation.

Pharmacodynamics/Kinetics
Excretion: Urine (~10% as unchanged drug)

Available Dosage Forms [DSC] = Discontinued product
Injection, powder for reconstitution:
Menopur®: Follicle stimulating hormone activity 75 int. units and luteinizing hormone activity 75 int. units [packaged with diluent; contains lactose 21 mg]
Pergonal®: Follicle stimulating hormone activity 75 int. units and luteinizing hormone activity 75 int. units [packaged with diluent; contains lactose 10 mg] [DSC]
Repronex®: Follicle stimulating hormone activity 75 int. units and luteinizing hormone activity 75 int. units [packaged with diluent]

Dosing
Adults:
Pergonal®: I.M.
Spermatogenesis (Male): Following pretreatment with hCG: 75 int. units 3 times/week and hCG 2000 units twice weekly until sperm is detected in the ejaculate (4-6 months); may then be increased to menotropins 150 int. units 3 times/week
Induction of ovulation (Female): 75 int. units for 7-12 days, followed by 10,000 units hCG one day after the last dose; repeated at least twice at same level before increasing dosage to 150 int. units

Repronex®: I.M., SubQ:
Induction of ovulation in patients with oligoanovulation (Female): Initial: 150 int. units daily for the first 5 days of treatment. Adjustments should not be made more frequently than once every 2 days and should not exceed 75-150 int. units per adjustment. Maximum daily dose should not exceed 450 int. units and dosing beyond 12 days is not recommended. If patient's response is appropriate, hCG 5000-10,000 units should be given one day following the last dose of Repronex®. Hold dose if serum estradiol is >2000 pg/mL, if the ovaries are abnormally enlarged, or if abdominal pain occurs; the patient should also be advised to refrain from intercourse. May repeat process if follicular development is inadequate or if pregnancy does not occur.
Assisted reproductive technologies (Female): Initial (in patients who have received GnRH agonist or antagonist pituitary suppression): 225 int. units; adjustments in dose should not be made more frequently than once every 2 days and should not exceed more than 75-150 int. units per adjustment. The maximum daily doses of Repronex® given should not exceed 450 int. units and dosing beyond 12 days is not recommended. Once adequate follicular development is evident, hCG (5000-10,000 units) should be administered to induce final follicular maturation in preparation for oocyte retrieval. Withhold treatment when ovaries

are abnormally enlarged on last day of therapy (to reduce chance of developing OHSS).

Menopur®: SubQ:

Assisted reproductive technologies (ART): Initial (in patients who have received GnRH agonist for pituitary suppression): 225 int. units; adjustments in dose should not be made more frequently than once every 2 days and should not exceed more than 150 int. units per adjustment. The maximum daily dose given should not exceed 450 int. units and dosing beyond 20 days is not recommended. Once adequate follicular development is evident, hCG should be administered to induce final follicular maturation in preparation for oocyte retrieval. Withhold treatment when ovaries are abnormally enlarged on last day of therapy (to reduce chance of developing OHSS).

Administration

I.M.: Pergonal®, Repronex®: Administer deep in a large muscle.

Other: SubQ:

Menopur®: Administer to alternating sites of the abdomen. When administration to the lower abdomen is not possible, the injection may be given into the thigh.

Repronex®: Administer to alternating sites of the lower abdomen.

Stability

Reconstitution: After reconstitution inject immediately, discard any unused portion.

Storage: Lyophilized powder may be refrigerated or stored at room temperature.

Nursing Actions

Physical Assessment: Female: Assess knowledge/teach appropriate method for measuring basal body temperature to indicate ovulation. Stress importance of following prescriber's instructions for timing intercourse. If self-administered, assess/teach appropriate injection technique and needle disposal. **Pregnancy risk factor X:** Determine pregnancy status prior to beginning therapy.

Patient Education: Self injection: Follow prescriber's recommended schedule for injections. Multiple ovulations resulting in multiple pregnancies have been reported. Male infertility and/or breast enlargement may occur. You may experience headache, nausea, abdominal pain, flushing, dizziness, or menstrual irregularities. Report pain at injection site; enlarged breasts (male); respiratory difficulty; nosebleeds; acute abdominal discomfort; abdominal distention; fever; or warmth, swelling, weight gain, pain, or redness in calves.

Pregnancy Issues Ectopic pregnancy and congenital abnormalities have been reported. The incidence of congenital abnormality is similar during natural conception.

Meperidine (me PER i deen)

U.S. Brand Names Demerol®; Meperitab®
Synonyms Isonipecaine Hydrochloride; Meperidine Hydrochloride; Pethidine Hydrochloride
Restrictions C-II
Pharmacologic Category Analgesic, Narcotic
Medication Safety Issues
Sound-alike/look-alike issues:
Meperidine may be confused with meprobamate
Demerol® may be confused with Demulen®, Desyrel®, dicumarol, Dilaudid®, Dymelor®, Pamelor®
Pregnancy Risk Factor C/D (prolonged use or high doses at term)
Lactation Enters breast milk/contraindicated (AAP rates "compatible")

Use Management of moderate to severe pain; adjunct to anesthesia and preoperative sedation
Unlabeled/Investigational Use
Reduce postoperative shivering; reduce rigors from amphotericin
Mechanism of Action/Effect Binds to opiate receptors in the CNS, causing inhibition of ascending pain pathways, altering the perception of and response to pain; produces generalized CNS depression
Contraindications Hypersensitivity to meperidine or any component of the formulation; use with or within 14 days of MAO inhibitors; pregnancy (prolonged use or high doses near term)
Warnings/Precautions Meperidine is not recommended for the management of chronic pain. When used for acute pain (in patients without renal or CNS disease), treatment should be limited to 48 hours and doses should not exceed 600 mg/24 hours. Oral meperidine is not recommended for acute pain management. Normeperidine (an active metabolite and CNS stimulant) may accumulate and precipitate anxiety, tremors, or seizures; risk increases with renal dysfunction and cumulative dose.

Use only with extreme caution (if at all) in patients with head injury or increased intracranial pressure (ICP); potential to elevate ICP may be greatly exaggerated in these patients. Use caution with pulmonary, hepatic, or renal disorders, supraventricular tachycardias, acute abdominal conditions, hypothyroidism, Addison's disease, BPH, or urethral stricture.

An opioid-containing analgesic regimen should be tailored to each patient's needs and based upon the type of pain being treated (acute versus chronic), the route of administration, degree of tolerance for opioids (naive versus chronic user), age, weight, and medical condition. The optimal analgesic dose varies widely among patients. Doses should be titrated to pain relief/prevention.

Some preparations contain sulfites which may cause allergic reaction. Tolerance or drug dependence may result from extended use.

Drug Interactions
Cytochrome P450 Effect: Substrate (minor) of CYP2B6, 2C19, 3A4
Decreased Effect: Barbiturates may decrease the analgesic efficacy and increase the sedative effects of meperidine. Phenytoin may decrease the analgesic effects of meperidine.
Increased Effect/Toxicity: MAO inhibitors may enhance the serotonergic effect of meperidine, which may cause serotonin syndrome; concurrent use with or within 14 days of an MAO inhibitor is contraindicated. CNS depressants may potentiate the sedative effects of meperidine or increase respiratory depression. Phenothiazines may potentiate the sedative effects of meperidine and may increase the incidence of hypotension. Serotonin agonists, serotonin reuptake inhibitors, sibutramine, and tricyclic antidepressants may potentiate the effects of meperidine. In addition, concurrent therapy with these drugs potentially may increase the risk of serotonin syndrome. A number of drugs may increase meperidine metabolite concentrations (including acyclovir, cimetidine, and ritonavir).
Nutritional/Ethanol Interactions
Ethanol: Avoid or limit ethanol (may increase CNS depression). Watch for sedation.
Herb/Nutraceutical: Avoid valerian, St John's wort, kava kava, gotu kola (may increase CNS depression).
Lab Interactions Increased amylase (S), BSP retention, CPK (I.M. injections)
Adverse Reactions Frequency not defined.
Cardiovascular: Hypotension
Central nervous system: Fatigue, drowsiness, dizziness, nervousness, headache, restlessness, malaise, (Continued)

Meperidine *(Continued)*

confusion, mental depression, hallucinations, paradoxical CNS stimulation, increased intracranial pressure, seizure (associated with metabolite accumulation), serotonin syndrome

Dermatologic: Rash, urticaria

Gastrointestinal: Nausea, vomiting, constipation, anorexia, stomach cramps, xerostomia, biliary spasm, paralytic ileus, sphincter of Oddi spasm

Genitourinary: Ureteral spasms, decreased urination

Local: Pain at injection site

Neuromuscular & skeletal: Weakness

Respiratory: Dyspnea

Miscellaneous: Histamine release, physical and psychological dependence

Overdosage/Toxicology Symptoms of overdose include CNS depression, respiratory depression, mydriasis, bradycardia, pulmonary edema, chronic tremor, CNS excitability, and seizures. Treatment is symptomatic. Naloxone, 2 mg I.V. with repeat administration as necessary up to a total dose of 10 mg, can be used to reverse opiate effects. Naloxone should not be used to treat meperidine-induced seizures. Naloxone does not reverse the adverse effects of normeperidine.

Pharmacodynamics/Kinetics

Onset of Action: Onset of action: Analgesic: Oral, SubQ: 10-15 minutes; I.V.: ~5 minutes. Peak effect: SubQ.: ~1 hour; Oral: 2 hours

Duration of Action: Oral, SubQ.: 2-4 hours

Protein Binding: 65% to 75%

Half-Life Elimination:

Parent drug: Terminal phase: Adults: 2.5-4 hours, Liver disease: 7-11 hours

Normeperidine (active metabolite): 15-30 hours; can accumulate with high doses or renal impairment

Metabolism: Hepatic; hydrolyzed to meperidinic acid (inactive) or undergoes N-demethylation to normeperidine (active; has ½ the analgesic effect and 2-3 times the CNS effects of meperidine)

Excretion: Urine (as metabolites)

Available Dosage Forms

Injection, solution, as hydrochloride [ampul]: 25 mg/0.5 mL (0.5 mL); 25 mg/mL (1 mL); 50 mg/mL (1 mL, 1.5 mL, 2 mL); 75 mg/mL (1 mL); 100 mg/mL (1 mL)

Injection, solution, as hydrochloride [prefilled syringe]: 25 mg/mL (1 mL); 50 mg/mL (1 mL); 75 mg/mL (1 mL); 100 mg/mL (1 mL)

Injection, solution, as hydrochloride [for PCA pump]: 10 mg/mL (30 mL, 50 mL, 60 mL)

Injection, solution, as hydrochloride [vial]: 25 mg/mL (1 mL); 50 mg/mL (1 mL, 30 mL); 75 mg/mL (1 mL); 100 mg/mL (1 mL, 20 mL) [may contain sodium metabisulfite]

Syrup, as hydrochloride: 50 mg/5 mL (500 mL) [contains sodium benzoate]

Demerol®: 50 mg/5 mL (480 mL) [contains benzoic acid; banana flavor]

Tablet, as hydrochloride (Demerol®, Meperitab®): 50 mg, 100 mg

Dosing

Adults: Note: Doses should be titrated to necessary analgesic effect. When changing route of administration, note that oral doses are about half as effective as parenteral dose. Not recommended for chronic pain. These are guidelines and do not represent the maximum doses that may be required in all patients. In patients with normal renal function, doses of ≤600 mg/24 hours and use for ≤48 hours are recommended (American Pain Society, 1999).

Pain (analgesic):

Oral: Initial: Opiate-naive: 50 mg every 3-4 hours as needed; usual dosage range: 50-150 mg every 2-4 hours as needed (manufacturers recommendation; oral route is not recommended for acute pain)

I.M., SubQ: Initial: Opiate-naive: 50-75 mg every 3-4 hours as needed; patients with prior opiate exposure may require higher initial doses.

Preoperatively: 50-100 mg given 30-90 minutes before the beginning of anesthesia

Slow I.V.: Initial: 5-10 mg every 5 minutes as needed

Patient-controlled analgesia (PCA): Usual concentration: 10 mg/mL

Initial dose: 10 mg

Demand dose: 1-5 mg (manufacturer recommendations); range 5-25 mg (American Pain Society, 1999).

Lockout interval: 5-10 minutes

Elderly: Note: Doses should be titrated to necessary analgesic effect. When changing route of administration, note that oral doses are about half as effective as parenteral dose. Oral route not recommended for chronic pain. These are guidelines and do not represent the maximum doses that may be required in all patients.

Oral: 50 mg every 4 hours

I.M.: 25 mg every 4 hours

Pediatrics: Pain (analgesic): Refer to "Note" in adult dosing.

Oral, I.M., I.V., SubQ: Children: 1-1.5 mg/kg/dose every 3-4 hours as needed; 1-2 mg/kg as a single dose preoperative medication may be used; maximum 100 mg/dose. (Oral route is not recommended for acute pain.)

Renal Impairment:

Cl_{cr} 10-50 mL/minute: Administer 75% of normal dose.

Cl_{cr} <10 mL/minute: Administer 50% of normal dose.

Note: Repeated use in renal impairment **should be avoided** due to potential accumulation of neuroexcitatory metabolite.

Hepatic Impairment: Increased narcotic effect in cirrhosis; reduction in dose is more important for oral than I.V. route.

Administration

Oral: Administer syrup diluted in ½ glass of water; undiluted syrup may exert topical anesthetic effect on mucous membranes

I.V.: Meperidine may be administered I.M., SubQ, or I.V. IVP should be given slowly, use of a 10 mg/mL concentration has been recommended. For continuous I.V. infusions, a more dilute solution (eg, 1 mg/mL) should be used.

I.V. Detail: pH: 3.5-6.0 (adjusted)

Stability

Compatibility: Stable in dextran 6% in dextrose, dextran 6% in NS, D_5LR, $D_5\frac{1}{4}NS$, $D_5\frac{1}{2}NS$, D_5NS, D_5W, $D_{10}W$, LR, ½NS, NS

Y-site administration: Incompatible with allopurinol, amphotericin B cholesteryl sulfate complex, cefepime, cefoperazone, doxorubicin liposome, idarubicin, imipenem/cilastatin, minocycline

Compatibility in syringe: Incompatible with heparin, morphine, pentobarbital

Compatibility when admixed: Incompatible with aminophylline, amobarbital, floxacillin, furosemide, heparin, morphine, phenobarbital, phenytoin, thiopental

Storage: Meperidine injection should be stored at room temperature and protected from light and freezing. Protect oral dosage forms from light.

Nursing Actions

Physical Assessment: Assess other medications patient may be taking for additive or adverse interactions. Monitor for effectiveness of pain relief and monitor for signs of overdose. Monitor blood pressure, CNS and respiratory status, and degree of sedation at beginning of therapy and at regular intervals with long-term use. May cause physical and/or psychological dependence. For inpatients, implement safety measures (eg, side rails up, call light within reach, instructions to call for assistance). Assess knowledge/ teach patient appropriate use (if self-administered). Teach patient to monitor for adverse reactions, adverse reactions to report, and appropriate interventions to reduce side effects. Discontinue slowly after prolonged use.

Patient Education: If self-administered, use exactly as directed; do not increase dose or frequency. Drug may cause physical and/or psychological dependence. While using this medication, do not use alcohol and other prescription or OTC medications (especially sedatives, tranquilizers, antihistamines, or pain medications) without consulting prescriber. Maintain adequate hydration (2-3 L/day of fluids) unless instructed to restrict fluid intake. May cause hypotension, dizziness, drowsiness, impaired coordination, or blurred vision (use caution when driving, climbing stairs, or changing position - rising from sitting or lying to standing, or when engaging in tasks requiring alertness until response to drug is known); loss of appetite, nausea, or vomiting (frequent mouth care, small frequent meals, chewing gum, or sucking lozenges may help); or constipation (increased exercise, fluids, fruit, or fiber may help; if unresolved, consult prescriber about use of stool softeners). Report chest pain, slow or rapid heartbeat, acute dizziness or persistent headache; changes in mental status; seizures; swelling of extremities or unusual weight gain; changes in urinary elimination; acute headache; back or flank pain or muscle spasms; blurred vision; skin rash; or shortness of breath. **Pregnancy/ breast-feeding precautions:** Inform prescriber if you are or intend to become pregnant. Consult prescriber if breast-feeding.

Geriatric Considerations Meperidine is not recommended as a drug of first choice for the treatment of chronic pain in the elderly due to the accumulation of its metabolite, normeperidine, which leads to serious CNS side effects (eg, tremor, seizures). For acute pain, its use should be limited to 1-2 doses.

Breast-Feeding Issues Meperidine is excreted in breast milk and may cause CNS and/or respiratory depression in the nursing infant.

Pregnancy Issues Meperidine is known to cross the placenta, which may result in respiratory or CNS depression in the newborn.

Related Information
Compatibility of Drugs *on page 1370*
Compatibility of Drugs in Syringe *on page 1372*

Meprobamate (me proe BA mate)

U.S. Brand Names Miltown® [DSC]
Synonyms Equanil
Restrictions C-IV
Pharmacologic Category Antianxiety Agent, Miscellaneous
Medication Safety Issues
Sound-alike/look-alike issues:
Meprobamate may be confused with Mepergan, meperidine
Equanil may be confused with Elavil®
Pregnancy Risk Factor D
Lactation Enters breast milk/not recommended
Use Management of anxiety disorders
Unlabeled/Investigational Use Demonstrated value for muscle contraction, headache, premenstrual tension, external sphincter spasticity, muscle rigidity, opisthotonos-associated with tetanus
Mechanism of Action/Effect Affects the thalamus and limbic system; also appears to inhibit multineuronal spinal reflexes
Contraindications Hypersensitivity to meprobamate, related compounds (including carisoprodol), or any

component of the formulation; acute intermittent porphyria; pre-existing CNS depression; narrow-angle glaucoma; severe uncontrolled pain; pregnancy

Warnings/Precautions Physical and psychological dependence and abuse may occur; abrupt cessation may precipitate withdrawal. Use with caution in patients with depression or suicidal tendencies, or in patients with a history of drug abuse. May cause CNS depression, which may impair physical or mental abilities. Patients must be cautioned about performing tasks which require mental alertness (eg, operating machinery or driving). Effects with other sedative drugs or ethanol may be potentiated. Not recommended in children <6 years of age; allergic reaction may occur in patients with history of dermatological condition (usually by fourth dose). Use with caution in patients with renal or hepatic impairment, or with a history of seizures. Use caution in the elderly as it may cause confusion, cognitive impairment, or excessive sedation.

Drug Interactions
Increased Effect/Toxicity: CNS depressants (ethanol) may increase CNS depression.
Nutritional/Ethanol Interactions
Ethanol: Avoid ethanol (may increase CNS depression).
Herb/Nutraceutical: Avoid valerian, St John's wort, kava kava, gotu kola (may increase CNS depression).
Adverse Reactions Frequency not defined.
Cardiovascular: Syncope, peripheral edema, palpitation, tachycardia, arrhythmia
Central nervous system: Drowsiness, ataxia, dizziness, paradoxical excitement, confusion, slurred speech, headache, euphoria, chills, vertigo, paresthesia, overstimulation
Dermatologic: Rashes, purpura, dermatitis, Stevens-Johnson syndrome, petechiae, ecchymosis
Gastrointestinal: Diarrhea, vomiting, nausea
Hematologic: Leukopenia, eosinophilia, agranulocytosis, aplastic anemia
Neuromuscular & skeletal: Weakness
Ocular: Blurred vision, impairment of accommodation
Renal: Renal failure
Respiratory: Wheezing, dyspnea, bronchospasm, angioneurotic edema

Overdosage/Toxicology Symptoms of overdose include drowsiness, lethargy, ataxia, coma, hypotension, shock, and death. Treatment is supportive following attempts to enhance drug elimination.

Pharmacodynamics/Kinetics
Onset of Action: Sedation: ~1 hour
Half-Life Elimination: 10 hours
Metabolism: Hepatic
Excretion: Urine (8% to 20% as unchanged drug); feces (10% as metabolites)

Available Dosage Forms
[DSC] = Discontinued product
Tablet: 200 mg, 400 mg
Miltown®: 200 mg, 400 mg [DSC]

Dosing
Adults: Oral: 400 mg 3-4 times/day, up to 2400 mg/day
Elderly: Oral (use lowest effective dose): Initial: 200 mg 2-3 times/day
Pediatrics: Oral: 6-12 years: 100-200 mg 2-3 times/day
Renal Impairment:
Cl_{cr} 10-50 mL/minute: Administer every 9-12 hours.
Cl_{cr} 10-50 mL/minute: Administer every 9-12 hours.
Cl_{cr} <10 mL/minute: Administer every 12-18 hours.
Moderately dialyzable (20% to 50%)
Hepatic Impairment: Probably necessary in patients with liver disease; no specific recommendations.

Nursing Actions
Physical Assessment: Assess other medications the patient may be taking for effectiveness and interactions. Assess for history of addiction; long-term use can result in dependence, abuse, or tolerance; periodically evaluate need for continued use. Monitor therapeutic response (eg, mood, affect, anxiety level, (Continued)

Meprobamate (Continued)

sleep pattern, CNS depression) and adverse reactions at beginning of therapy and periodically with long-term use. Taper dosage slowly when discontinuing. Assess knowledge/teach patient appropriate use, interventions to reduce side effects, and adverse symptoms to report.

Patient Education: Take exactly as directed; do not increase dose or frequency. Drug may cause physical and/or psychological dependence. Do not use alcohol or other prescription or OTC medications (especially pain medications, sedatives, antihistamines, or hypnotics) without consulting prescriber. Maintain adequate hydration (2-3 L/day of fluids) unless instructed to restrict fluid intake. You may experience drowsiness, lightheadedness, impaired coordination, dizziness, or blurred vision (use caution when driving or engaging in tasks requiring alertness until response to drug is known); nausea, vomiting, or dry mouth (small frequent meals, frequent mouth care, chewing gum, or sucking lozenges may help); or diarrhea (boiled milk, yogurt, or buttermilk may help). Report persistent CNS effects, skin rash or irritation, changes in urinary pattern, wheezing or respiratory difficulty, or worsening of condition. **Pregnancy/breast-feeding precautions:** Do not get pregnant while taking this medication; use appropriate contraceptive measures. Breast-feeding is not recommended.

Geriatric Considerations Meprobamate is not considered a drug of choice in the elderly because of its potential to cause physical and psychological dependence. Interpretive guidelines from the Centers for Medicare and Medicaid Services (CMS) strongly discourage the use of meprobamate in residents of long-term care facilities.

Breast-Feeding Issues Breast milk concentrations are higher than plasma; effects are unknown.

Additional Information Withdrawal should be gradual over 1-2 weeks. Benzodiazepine and buspirone are better choices for treatment of anxiety disorders.

Related Information
Anxiolytic / Hypnotic Use in Long-Term Care Facilities on page 1418
Federal OBRA Regulations Recommended Maximum Doses on page 1421

Mequinol and Tretinoin
(ME kwi nole & TRET i noyn)

U.S. Brand Names Solagé™
Synonyms Tretinoin and Mequinol
Pharmacologic Category Retinoic Acid Derivative; Vitamin A Derivative; Vitamin, Topical
Pregnancy Risk Factor X
Lactation Excretion in breast milk unknown/use caution
Use Treatment of solar lentigines; the efficacy of using Solagé™ daily for >24 weeks has not been established. The local cutaneous safety of Solagé™ in non-Caucasians has not been adequately established.
Available Dosage Forms Liquid, topical: Mequinol 2% and tretinoin 0.01% (30 mL) [contains alcohol 78%; dispensed in applicator bottle]

Dosing
Adults & Elderly: Solar lentigines: Topical: Apply twice daily to solar lentigines using the applicator tip while avoiding application to the surrounding skin. Separate application by at least 8 hours or as directed by physician.

Nursing Actions
Physical Assessment: Assess effectiveness and interactions of other medications. Monitor effectiveness of therapy, and adverse effects at beginning of therapy and regularly with long-term use. Assess

knowledge/teach patient appropriate use, possible side effects/interventions, and adverse symptoms to report. **Pregnancy risk factor X:** Determine that patient is not pregnant before beginning treatment and do not give to women of childbearing age unless female is capable of complying with contraceptive measures 1 month prior to therapy, during therapy, and 1 month following therapy

Patient Education: Use exactly as directed. Use applicator tip; avoid application to surrounding skin, eyes, mouth, nose creases, or mucous membranes. Separate applications by at least 8 hours. Wait 30 minutes after application before applying make-up and do not bath or shower for 6 hours after application). Do not use more frequently than recommended. Do not use other vitamin A topical products; limit vitamin A intake. Avoid topical products with skin-drying effects (eg, those containing alcohol, astringents, spices, lime, medicated soaps or shampoos, permanent wave solutions, depilatories or other hair removal products). You will be very sensitive to direct sunlight or sunlamps (use sunscreen, wear protective clothing and eyewear, and avoid direct exposure to sunlight or sunlamps). You may experience stinging, burning, or irritation after application. If skin reactions are severe or persistent, discontinue use and contact prescriber. **Pregnancy/breast-feeding precautions:** Inform prescriber if you are pregnant. Do not get pregnant 1 month before, during, or for 1 month following therapy. Consult prescriber for instruction on appropriate contraceptive measures. This drug may cause severe fetal defects. Do not donate blood during or for 1 month following therapy (same reason). Consult prescriber if breast-feeding.

Related Information
Tretinoin (Oral) on page 1245
Tretinoin (Topical) on page 1247

Mercaptopurine (mer kap toe PYOOR een)

U.S. Brand Names Purinethol®
Synonyms 6-Mercaptopurine; 6-MP; NSC-755
Restrictions Note: I.V. formulation is not commercially available in the U.S.
Pharmacologic Category Antineoplastic Agent, Antimetabolite
Medication Safety Issues
Sound-alike/look-alike issues:
Purinethol® may be confused with propylthiouracil

To avoid potentially serious dosage errors, the terms "6-mercaptopurine" or "6-MP" should be avoided; use of these terms has been associated with sixfold overdosages.

Pregnancy Risk Factor D
Lactation Enters breast milk/contraindicated
Use Treatment (maintenance and induction) of acute lymphoblastic leukemia (ALL)
Mechanism of Action/Effect Purine antagonist which inhibits DNA and RNA synthesis
Contraindications Hypersensitivity to mercaptopurine or any component of the formulation; patients whose disease showed prior resistance to mercaptopurine or thioguanine; severe liver disease, severe bone marrow suppression; pregnancy
Warnings/Precautions Hazardous agent — use appropriate precautions for handling and disposal. Mercaptopurine is potentially carcinogenic, and may be teratogenic; use with caution in patients with prior bone marrow suppression. Common signs of infection, such as fever and leukocytosis may not occur; lethargy and confusion may be more prominent signs of infection. Use caution with other hepatotoxic drugs or in dosages >2.5 mg/kg/day; hepatotoxicity may occur. Patients with

genetic deficiency of thiopurine methyltransferase (TPMT) or concurrent therapy with drugs which may inhibit TPMT (eg, olsalazine) or xanthine oxidase (eg, allopurinol) may be sensitive to myelosuppressive effects.

To avoid potentially serious dosage errors, the terms "6-mercaptopurine" or "6-MP" should be avoided; use of these terms has been associated with sixfold overdosages.

Drug Interactions
Decreased Effect: Mercaptopurine inhibits the anticoagulation effect of warfarin by an unknown mechanism.

Increased Effect/Toxicity: Allopurinol can cause increased levels of mercaptopurine by inhibition of xanthine oxidase. Decrease dose of mercaptopurine by 75% when both drugs are used concomitantly. Seen only with oral mercaptopurine usage, not with I.V. May potentiate effect of bone marrow suppression (reduce mercaptopurine to 25% of dose). Synergistic liver toxicity between doxorubicin and mercaptopurine has been reported. Any agent which could potentially alter the metabolic function of the liver could produce higher drug levels and greater toxicities from either mercaptopurine or thioguanine (6-TG). Aminosalicylates (eg, olsalazine, mesalamine, sulfasalazine) may inhibit TPMT, increasing toxicity/myelosuppression of mercaptopurine.

Adverse Reactions
>10%:
Hematologic: Myelosuppression; leukopenia, thrombocytopenia, anemia
Onset: 7-10 days
Nadir: 14-16 days
Recovery: 21-28 days
Hepatic: Intrahepatic cholestasis and focal centralobular necrosis (40%), characterized by hyperbilirubinemia, increased alkaline phosphatase and AST, jaundice, ascites, encephalopathy; more common at doses >2.5 mg/kg/day. Usually occurs within 2 months of therapy but may occur within 1 week, or be delayed up to 8 years.
1% to 10%:
Central nervous system: Drug fever
Dermatologic: Hyperpigmentation, rash
Endocrine & metabolic: Hyperuricemia
Gastrointestinal: Nausea, vomiting, diarrhea, stomatitis, anorexia, stomach pain, mucositis
Renal: Renal toxicity

Overdosage/Toxicology
Symptoms of overdose include nausea and vomiting (immediate); bone marrow suppression, hepatic necrosis, and gastroenteritis (delayed). Treatment is supportive. Efforts to minimize absorption (charcoal, gastric lavage) may be ineffective unless instituted within 60 minutes of ingestion.

Pharmacodynamics/Kinetics
Time to Peak: Serum: ~2 hours
Protein Binding: 19%
Half-Life Elimination: Age dependent: Children: 21 minutes; Adults: 47 minutes
Metabolism: Hepatic and via GI mucosa; hepatically via xanthine oxidase and methylation via TPMT to sulfate conjugates, 6-thiouric acid, and other inactive compounds; first-pass effect
Excretion: Urine; following high (1 g/m^2) I.V. doses, 20% to 40% as unchanged urine; at lower doses renal elimination minor

Available Dosage Forms
Tablet [scored]: 50 mg

Dosing
Adults: Antineoplastic: Refer to individual protocols.
Induction: Oral: 2.5-5 mg/kg/day (100-200 mg)
Maintenance: Oral: 1.5-2.5 mg/kg/day or 80-100 mg/m^2/day given once daily
Note: In ALL, administration in the evening (vs morning administration) may lower the risk of relapse.

Dosage adjustment with concurrent allopurinol: Reduce mercaptopurine dosage to $\frac{1}{3}$ to $\frac{1}{2}$ the usual dose.

Dosage adjustment in TPMT-deficiency: Not established; substantial reductions are generally required only in homozygous deficiency.

Elderly: Due to renal decline with age, start with lower recommended doses for adults.

Pediatrics: Antineoplastic: Refer to individual protocols: Oral:
Induction: 2.5-5 mg/kg/day or 70-100 mg/m^2/day given once daily
Maintenance: 1.5-2.5 mg/kg/day or 50-75 mg/m^2/day given once daily
Note: In ALL, administration in the evening (vs morning administration) may lower the risk of relapse.

Renal Impairment: Dose should be reduced to avoid accumulation, but specific guidelines are not available.
Hemodialysis: Removed; supplemental dosing is usually required

Hepatic Impairment: Dose should be reduced to avoid accumulation, but specific guidelines are not available.

Administration
I.V.: Administer by slow I.V. continuous infusion.

Stability
Reconstitution: Further dilute the 10 mg/mL reconstituted solution in normal saline or D$_5$W to a final concentration for administration of 1-2 mg/mL.

Storage: Store at room temperature.

Laboratory Monitoring
CBC with differential, platelet count, liver function, uric acid, renal function

Nursing Actions
Physical Assessment: Assess potential for interactions with other pharmacological agents patient may be taking (increased potential for liver toxicity or mercaptopurine toxicity). Monitor laboratory tests, therapeutic response, and adverse reactions (eg, hepatic function, jaundice, ascites, encephalopathy can occur some time following therapy; nutritional status, dehydration; myelosuppression, anemia, leukopenia; and renal status) on a regular basis throughout therapy. Teach patient proper use, possible side effects/appropriate interventions (eg, importance of adequate hydration), and adverse symptoms to report.

Patient Education: Do not take any new medication during therapy unless approved by prescriber. Take daily dose at the same time each day. Preferable to take an on empty stomach, 1 hour before or 2 hours after meals. Maintain adequate hydration (2-3 L/day of fluids) unless instructed to restrict fluid intake. You may be more susceptible to infection (avoid crowds and exposure to infection and do not have any vaccinations without consulting prescriber). May cause nausea and vomiting, diarrhea, or loss of appetite (small, frequent meals may help/request medication); weakness or lethargy (use caution when driving or engaging in tasks that require alertness until response to drug is known); mouth sores; or headache (consult prescriber for approved medications). Report signs of persistent fever; opportunistic infection (eg, fever, chills, sore throat, burning urination, fatigue); bleeding (eg, tarry stools, easy bruising); unresolved mouth sores; nausea or vomiting; swelling of extremities; respiratory difficulty; unusual weight gain; or changes in urinary pattern. **Pregnancy/breast-feeding precautions:** Inform prescriber if you are pregnant. Do not get pregnant while taking this medication. Consult prescriber for appropriate contraceptive measures. Do not breast-feed.

Dietary Considerations Should not be administered with meals.
(Continued)

Mercaptopurine *(Continued)*

Geriatric Considerations Toxicity to immunosuppressives is increased in the elderly. Start with lowest recommended adult doses. Signs of infection, such as fever and WBC rise, may not occur. Lethargy and confusion may be more prominent signs of infection.

Meropenem *(mer oh PEN em)*

U.S. Brand Names Merrem® I.V.
Pharmacologic Category Antibiotic, Carbapenem
Pregnancy Risk Factor B
Lactation Excretion in breast milk unknown/use caution
Use Treatment of intra-abdominal infections (complicated appendicitis and peritonitis); treatment of bacterial meningitis in pediatric patients ≥3 months of age caused by *S. pneumoniae, H. influenzae,* and *N. meningitidis;* treatment of complicated skin and skin structure infections caused by susceptible organisms
Unlabeled/Investigational Use
Febrile neutropenia, urinary tract infections
Mechanism of Action/Effect Inhibits cell wall synthesis in susceptible bacteria
Contraindications Hypersensitivity to meropenem, any component of the formulation, or other carbapenems (eg, imipenem); patients who have experienced anaphylactic reactions to other beta-lactams
Warnings/Precautions
Hypersensitivity reactions, including anaphylaxis, have occurred and often require immediate drug discontinuation. Seizures and other CNS adverse reactions have occurred, most commonly in patients with renal impairment and/or underlying neurologic disorders (less frequent than with Primaxin®). Use with caution in renal impairment; dose adjustment is necessary. Thrombocytopenia has been reported in patients with significant renal dysfunction. Pseudomembranous colitis has been associated with meropenem use. Superinfection is possible with long courses of therapy. Safety and efficacy have not been established for children <3 months of age
Drug Interactions
Decreased Effect: Meropenem may decrease valproic acid serum concentrations to subtherapeutic levels.
Increased Effect/Toxicity: Probenecid may increase meropenem serum concentrations.
Lab Interactions Increased SGPT, SGOT, alkaline phosphatase, LDH, bilirubin, platelets, eosinophils, BUN, creatinine; decreased platelets, hemoglobin/hematocrit, WBC; prolonged or shortened PT; prolonged PTT; positive direct or indirect Coombs' test; presence of urine red blood cells
Adverse Reactions
1% to 10%:
Cardiovascular: Peripheral vascular disorder (<1%)
Central nervous system: Headache (2% to 8%), pain (5%)
Dermatologic: Rash (2% to 3%, includes diaper-area moniliasis in pediatrics), pruritus (1%)
Gastrointestinal: Diarrhea (4% to 5%), nausea/vomiting (1% to 8%), constipation (1% to 7%), oral moniliasis (up to 2% in pediatric patients), glossitis (1%)
Hematologic: Anemia (up to 6%)
Local: Inflammation at the injection site (2%), phlebitis/thrombophlebitis (1%), injection site reaction (1%)
Respiratory: Apnea (1%)
Miscellaneous: Sepsis (2%), septic shock (1%)
Overdosage/Toxicology No cases of acute overdosage are reported which have resulted in symptoms. Accidental overdose is possible with the use of large doses in patients with renal impairment. Supportive

therapy is recommended. Meropenem and its metabolite are removable by dialysis.
Pharmacodynamics/Kinetics
Time to Peak: Tissue: 1 hour following infusion
Protein Binding: 2%
Half-Life Elimination:
Normal renal function: 1-1.5 hours
Cl_{cr} 30-80 mL/minute: 1.9-3.3 hours
Cl_{cr} 2-30 mL/minute: 3.82-5.7 hours
Metabolism: Hepatic; metabolized to open beta-lactam form (inactive)
Excretion: Urine (~25% as inactive metabolites)
Available Dosage Forms Injection, powder for reconstitution: 500 mg [contains sodium 45.1 mg as sodium carbonate (1.96 mEq)]; 1 g [contains sodium 90.2 mg as sodium carbonate (3.92 mEq)]
Dosing
Adults & Elderly:
Cholangitis, intra-abdominal infections, otitis externa and septic lateral sinus thrombosis: I.V.: 1 g every 8 hours
Febrile neutropenia, pneumonia, other severe infections (unlabeled use): I.V.: 1 g every 8 hours
Liver abscess: I.V.: 1 g every 8 hours for 2-3 weeks, then oral therapy for duration of 4-6 weeks
Meningitis: I.V.: 2 g every 8 hours
Skin and skin structure infections (complicated): I.V.: 500 mg every 8 hours; diabetic foot: 1 g every 8 hours
Urinary tract infections, complicated (unlabeled use): I.V.: 500 mg to 1 g every 8 hours
Pediatrics:
Febrile neutropenia (unlabeled use): I.V.:
Children >3 months (<50 kg): 20 mg/kg every 8 hours (maximum dose: 1 g every 8 hours)
Children >50 kg: Refer to adult dosing.
Intra-abdominal infections: I.V.:
Children >3 months (<50 kg): 20 mg/kg every 8 hours (maximum dose: 1 g every 8 hours)
Children >50 kg: 1 g every 8 hours
Meningitis: I.V.:
Children >3 months (<50 kg): 40 mg/kg every 8 hours (maximum dose: 2 g every 8 hours)
Children >50 kg: 2 g every 8 hours
Skin and skin structure infections (complicated): I.V.:
Children >3 months (<50 kg): 10 mg/kg every 8 hours (maximum dose: 500 mg every 8 hours)
Children >50 kg: Refer to adult dosing.
Renal Impairment:
Cl_{cr} 26-50 mL/minute: Administer recommended dose based on indication every 12 hours
Cl_{cr} 10-25 mL/minute: Administer one-half recommended dose every 12 hours
Cl_{cr} <10 mL/minute: Administer one-half recommended dose every 24 hours
Dialysis: Meropenem and its metabolites are readily dialyzable
Continuous arteriovenous or venovenous hemodiafiltration effects: Dose as Cl_{cr} 10-50 mL/minute
Administration
I.V.: Administer I.V. infusion over 15-30 minutes; I.V. bolus injection over 3-5 minutes.
I.V. Detail: pH: 7.3-8.3
Stability
Reconstitution: Meropenem infusion vials may be reconstituted with SWFI or a compatible diluent (eg, NS). The 500 mg vials should be reconstituted with 10 mL, and 1 g vials with 20 mL. May be further diluted with compatible solutions for infusion. Consult detailed reference/product labeling for compatibility.
Compatibility:
Y-site administration: **Incompatible** with amphotericin B, diazepam, metronidazole
Compatibility when admixed: **Incompatible** with amphotericin B, metronidazole, multivitamins

Storage: Dry powder should be stored at controlled room temperature 20°C to 25°C (68°F to 77°F).

Injection reconstitution: Stability in vial when constituted (up to 50 mg/mL) with:

SWFI: Stable for up to 2 hours at room temperature and for up to 12 hours under refrigeration

Sodium chloride: Stable for up to 2 hours at room temperature or for up to 18 hours under refrigeration.

Dextrose 5% injection: Stable for 1 hour at room temperature or for 8 hours under refrigeration

Infusion admixture (1-20 mg/mL): Solution stability when diluted in NS is 4 hours at room temperature or 24 hours under refrigeration. Stability in D_5W is 1 hour at room temperature and 4 hours under refrigeration.

Laboratory Monitoring Perform culture and sensitivity testing prior to initiating therapy. Monitor renal function, liver function, CBC.

Nursing Actions

Physical Assessment: Results of culture and sensitivity tests and patient's allergy history should be assessed prior to beginning treatment. See Administration for infusion specifics. Infusion site should be monitored closely to prevent phlebitis/thrombophlebitis. Monitor laboratory tests, therapeutic effectiveness (resolution of infection), and adverse reactions. Teach patient proper use (according to formulation), possible side effects/appropriate interventions (eg, importance of adequate hydration), and adverse symptoms to report.

Patient Education: This medication can only be given by infusion. Report immediately any burning, pain, swelling, or redness at infusion site. Maintain adequate hydration (2-3 L/day of fluids) unless instructed to restrict fluid intake. May cause nausea or vomiting (small, frequent meals, frequent mouth care, chewing gum, or sucking lozenges may help); diarrhea (boiled milk, buttermilk, or yogurt may help); or headache. Report persistent GI distress, diarrhea, mouth sores, respiratory difficulty, headache, or CNS changes (agitation, delirium). **Breast-feeding precaution:** Consult prescriber if breast-feeding.

Dietary Considerations 1 g of meropenem contains 90.2 mg of sodium as sodium carbonate (3.92 mEq)

Geriatric Considerations Adjust dose based on renal function.

Mesalamine (me SAL a meen)

U.S. Brand Names Asacol®; Canasa™; Pentasa®; Rowasa®

Synonyms 5-Aminosalicylic Acid; 5-ASA; Fisalamine; Mesalazine

Pharmacologic Category 5-Aminosalicylic Acid Derivative

Medication Safety Issues

Sound-alike/look-alike issues:

Mesalamine may be confused with mecamylamine

Asacol® may be confused with Ansaid®, Os-Cal®

Pregnancy Risk Factor B

Lactation Excretion in breast milk unknown/use caution

Use

Oral: Treatment and maintenance of remission of mildly to moderately active ulcerative colitis

Rectal: Treatment of active mild to moderate distal ulcerative colitis, proctosigmoiditis, or proctitis

Mechanism of Action/Effect Mesalamine (5-aminosalicylic acid) is the active component of sulfasalazine; the specific mechanism of action of mesalamine is unknown; however, it is thought that it modulates local chemical mediators of the inflammatory response, especially leukotrienes, and is also postulated to be a free radical scavenger or an inhibitor of tumor necrosis factor (TNF); action appears topical rather than systemic

Contraindications Hypersensitivity to mesalamine, sulfasalazine, salicylates, or any component of the formulation; Canasa™ suppositories contain saturated vegetable fatty acid esters (contraindicated in patients with allergy to these components)

Warnings/Precautions May cause an acute intolerance syndrome. Pericarditis should be considered in patients with chest pain; pancreatitis should be considered in patients with new abdominal complaints. Symptomatic worsening of colitis/IBD may occur following initiation of therapy. Oligospermia (rare) has been reported in males. Use with caution in patients with impaired hepatic or renal function. Postmarketing reports suggest an increased incidence of blood dyscrasias in patients >65 years of age. In addition, elderly may have difficulty administering and retaining rectal suppositories and decreased renal function; use with caution and monitor. Safety and efficacy in pediatric patients have not been established.

Rowasa® enema: Contains potassium metabisulfite; may cause anaphylactic reactions in patients with sulfite allergies.

Drug Interactions

Decreased Effect: Decreased digoxin bioavailability.

Increased Effect/Toxicity: Mesalamine may increase the risk of myelosuppression from azathioprine, mercaptopurine, and thioguanine.

Nutritional/Ethanol Interactions Food: Oral: Mesalamine serum levels may be decreased if taken with food.

Adverse Reactions Adverse effects vary depending upon dosage form. Effects as reported with tablets, unless otherwise noted:

>10%:

Central nervous system: Headache (suppository 14%), pain (14%)

Gastrointestinal: Abdominal pain (18%; enema 8%)

Genitourinary: Eructation (16%)

Respiratory: Pharyngitis (11%)

1% to 10%:

Cardiovascular: Chest pain (3%), peripheral edema (3%)

Central nervous system: Chills (3%), dizziness (suppository 3%), fever (enema 3%; suppository 1%), insomnia (2%), malaise (2%)

Dermatologic: Rash (6%; suppository 1%), pruritus (3%; enema 1%), acne (2%; suppository 1%)

Gastrointestinal: Abdominal pain (enema 8%; suppository 5%), colitis exacerbation (3%; suppository 1%), constipation (5%), diarrhea (suppository 3%), dyspepsia (6%), flatulence (enema 6%; suppository 5%), hemorrhoids (enema 1%), nausea (capsule/suppository 3%), nausea and vomiting (capsule 1%), rectal pain (enema 1%; suppository 2%), vomiting (5%)

Local: Pain on insertion of enema tip (enema 1%)

Neuromuscular & skeletal: Back pain (7%; enema 1%), arthralgia (5%), hypertonia (5%), myalgia (3%), arthritis (2%), leg/joint pain (enema 2%)

Ocular: Conjunctivitis (2%)

Respiratory: Flu-like syndrome (3%; enema 5%), cough increased (2%)

Miscellaneous: Diaphoresis (3%)

Overdosage/Toxicology Symptoms of overdose include decreased motor activity, diarrhea, vomiting, and renal function impairment. Treatment is supportive; emesis, gastric lavage, and follow with activated charcoal slurry.

Pharmacodynamics/Kinetics

Time to Peak: Serum: 4-7 hours

Half-Life Elimination: 5-ASA: 0.5-1.5 hours; acetyl-5-ASA: 5-10 hours

Metabolism: Hepatic and via GI tract to acetyl-5-aminosalicylic acid

(Continued)

Mesalamine *(Continued)*

Excretion: Urine (as metabolites); feces (<2%)

Available Dosage Forms

Capsule, controlled release (Pentasa®): 250 mg, 500 mg

Suppository, rectal (Canasa™): 500 mg [DSC], 1000 mg [contains saturated vegetable fatty acid esters]

Suspension, rectal: 4 g/60 mL (7s, 28s) [contains potassium metabisulfite and sodium benzoate]

Rowasa®: 4 g/60 mL (7s, 28s) [contains potassium metabisulfite and sodium benzoate]

Tablet, delayed release [enteric coated] (Asacol®): 400 mg

Dosing

Adults & Elderly:

Treatment of ulcerative colitis: Oral:

Capsule: 1 g 4 times/day

Tablet: 800 mg 3 times/day for 6 weeks

Maintenance of remission of ulcerative colitis: Oral:

Capsule: 1 g 4 times/day

Tablet: 1.6 g/day in divided doses

Distal ulcerative colitis, proctosigmoiditis, or proctitis: Rectal: Retention enema: 60 mL (4 g) at bedtime, retained overnight, approximately 8 hours

Active ulcerative proctitis: Rectal: Rectal suppository (Canasa™):

500 mg: Insert 1 suppository in rectum twice daily; may increase to 3 times/day if inadequate response is seen after 2 weeks

1000 mg: Insert 1 suppository in rectum daily at bedtime

Note: Suppositories should be retained for at least 1-3 hours to achieve maximum benefit.

Note: Some patients may require rectal and oral therapy concurrently.

Administration

Oral: Swallow capsules or tablets whole, do not chew or crush.

Other:

Rectal enema: Shake bottle well. Retain enemas for 8 hours or as long as practical.

Suppository: Remove foil wrapper; avoid excessive handling. Should be retained for at least 1-3 hours to achieve maximum benefit.

Stability

Storage:

Enema: Store at controlled room temperature. Use promptly once foil wrap is removed; contents may darken with time (do not use if dark brown)

Suppository: Store at controlled room temperature away from direct heat, light, and humidity; do not refrigerate

Tablet: Store at controlled room temperature

Laboratory Monitoring CBC and renal function, particularly in elderly patients

Nursing Actions

Physical Assessment: Assess history of allergies prior to beginning treatment. Monitor laboratory tests (see above), therapeutic effectiveness, and adverse reactions on a regular basis throughout therapy. Teach patient proper use (according to formulation), possible side effects/appropriate interventions (eg, importance of adequate hydration), and adverse symptoms to report.

Patient Education: Inform prescriber of all prescriptions, OTC medications, or herbal products you are taking, and any allergies you have. Do not take any new medication during therapy unless approved by prescriber. Take as directed.

Oral: Do not chew or break tablets or capsules. Notify prescriber if whole or partial tablets are repeatedly found in stool.

Enemas: Shake well before using, retain for 8 hours or as long as possible. May cause staining of clothing, undergarments.

Suppository: Do not refrigerate. After removing foil wrapper, insert high in rectum without excessive handling (warmth will melt suppository). Retain suppositories for at least 1-3 hours to achieve maximum benefit. Report severe abdominal pain, unresolved diarrhea, jaundice, severe headache, any unusual pain (back, joint, muscle, swelling of extremities, or chest pain). May cause staining of clothing, undergarments; lubricating gel may be used if needed to assist insertion.

Enema and suppository: May cause staining of clothing, undergarments; lubricating gel may be used if needed to assist insertion.

Breast-feeding precaution: Consult prescriber if breast-feeding.

Dietary Considerations Canasa™ rectal suppository contains saturated vegetable fatty acid esters.

Geriatric Considerations Elderly may have difficulty administering and retaining rectal suppositories. Given renal function decline with aging, monitor serum creatinine often during therapy.

Breast-Feeding Issues Adverse effects (diarrhea) in a nursing infant have been reported while the mother received rectal administration of mesalamine within 12 hours after the first dose. The AAP recommends to monitor the infant stool for consistency and to use with caution.

Mesna *(MES na)*

U.S. Brand Names Mesnex®

Synonyms Sodium 2-Mercaptoethane Sulfonate

Pharmacologic Category Antidote

Pregnancy Risk Factor B

Lactation Excretion in breast milk unknown/not recommended

Use Orphan drug: Prevention of hemorrhagic cystitis induced by ifosfamide

Unlabeled/Investigational Use Prevention of hemorrhagic cystitis induced by cyclophosphamide

Mechanism of Action/Effect Binds with and detoxifies urotoxic metabolites of ifosfamide and cyclophosphamide to prevent hemorrhagic cystitis induced by ifosfamide and cyclophosphamide

Contraindications Hypersensitivity to mesna or other thiol compounds, or any component of the formulation

Warnings/Precautions Examine morning urine specimen for hematuria prior to ifosfamide or cyclophosphamide treatment; if hematuria (>50 RBC/HPF) develops, reduce the ifosfamide/cyclophosphamide dose or discontinue the drug; will not prevent or alleviate other toxicities associated with ifosfamide or cyclophosphamide and will not prevent hemorrhagic cystitis in all patients. Allergic reactions have been reported; patients with autoimmune disorders may be at increased risk. Symptoms ranged from mild hypersensitivity to systemic anaphylactic reactions. I.V. formulation contains benzyl alcohol; do not use in neonates or infants.

Drug Interactions

Decreased Effect: Warfarin: Questionable alterations in coagulation control.

Lab Interactions False-positive urinary ketones with Multistix® or Labstix®

Adverse Reactions It is difficult to distinguish reactions from those caused by concomitant chemotherapy.

>10%: Gastrointestinal: Bad taste in mouth with oral administration (100%), vomiting (secondary to the bad taste after oral administration, or with high I.V. doses)

Pharmacodynamics/Kinetics

Time to Peak: Plasma: 2-3 hours

Protein Binding: 69% to 75%

Half-Life Elimination: Parent drug: 24 minutes; Mesna disulfide: 72 minutes

Metabolism: Rapidly oxidized intravascularly to mesna disulfide; mesna disulfide is reduced in renal tubules back to mesna following glomerular filtration.

Excretion: Urine; as unchanged drug (18% to 26%) and metabolites

Available Dosage Forms

Injection, solution: 100 mg/mL (10 mL) [contains benzyl alcohol]

Tablet: 400 mg

Dosing

Adults & Elderly: Prevention of toxicity: Refer to individual protocols.

I.V.: Recommended dose is 60% of the ifosfamide dose given in 3 divided doses (0, 4, and 8 hours after the start of ifosfamide)

Note: Alternative I.V. regimens include 80% of the ifosfamide dose given in 4 divided doses (0, 3, 6, and 9 hours after the start of ifosfamide) and continuous infusions

I.V./Oral: Recommended dose is 100% of the ifosfamide dose, given as 20% of the ifosfamide dose I.V. at hour 0, followed by 40% of the ifosfamide dose given orally 2 and 6 hours after start of ifosfamide

Pediatrics: Refer to adult dosing.

Administration

Oral: Administer orally in tablet formulation or parenteral solution diluted in water, milk, juice, or carbonated beverages; patients who vomit within 2 hours of taking oral mesna should repeat the dose or receive I.V. mesna

I.V.: Administer by short (15-30 minutes) infusion or continuous (24 hour) infusion

I.V. Detail: pH: 6.5-8.5

Stability

Reconstitution: Dilute in 50-1000 mL NS, D$_5$W, or lactated Ringer's.

Compatibility: Stable in D$_5$¼NS, D$_5$⅓NS, D$_5$½NS, D$_5$W, LR, NS

Y-site administration: Incompatible with amphotericin B cholesteryl sulfate complex

Compatibility in syringe: Incompatible with ifosfamide/epirubicin

Compatibility when admixed: Incompatible with carboplatin, cisplatin, ifosfamide/epirubicin

Storage: Store intact vials and tablets at controlled room temperature of 20°C to 25°C (68°F to 77°F). Opened multidose vials may be stored and used for use to 8 days after opening. Infusion solutions diluted in D$_5$W or lactated Ringer's are stable for at least 48 hours at room temperature. Solutions in NS are stable for at least 24 hours at room temperature. Solutions in plastic syringes are stable for 9 days under refrigeration, or at room or body temperature. Solutions of mesna and ifosfamide in lactated Ringer's are stable for 7 days in a PVC ambulatory infusion pump reservoir. Mesna injection is stable for at least 7 days when diluted 1:2 or 1:5 with grape- and orange-flavored syrups or 11:1 to 1:100 in carbonated beverages for oral administration.

Laboratory Monitoring Urinalysis

Nursing Actions

Physical Assessment: Monitor laboratory results and assess frequently for hematuria/bladder hemorrhage.

Patient Education: This drug is given to help prevent side effects of other chemotherapeutic agents you are taking. Report blood in urine. **Breast-feeding precaution:** Do not breast-feed.

Additional Information A parenteral formulation without benzyl alcohol can be requested directly from the manufacturer.

Mesoridazine (mez oh RID a zeen)

U.S. Brand Names Serentil® [DSC]

Synonyms Mesoridazine Besylate

Pharmacologic Category Antipsychotic Agent, Typical, Phenothiazine

Medication Safety Issues

Sound-alike/look-alike issues:

Serentil® may be confused with selegiline, Serevent®, Seroquel®, sertraline, Serzone®, Sinequan®, Surgicel®

Pregnancy Risk Factor C

Lactation Enters breast milk/contraindicated (AAP rates "of concern")

Use Management of schizophrenic patients who fail to respond adequately to treatment with other antipsychotic drugs, either because of insufficient effectiveness or the inability to achieve an effective dose due to intolerable adverse effects from these drugs

Unlabeled/Investigational Use Psychosis

Mechanism of Action/Effect Mesoridazine is a piperidine phenothiazine antipsychotic which blocks of postsynaptic CNS dopamine$_2$ receptors in the mesolimbic and mesocortical areas

Contraindications Hypersensitivity to mesoridazine or any component of the formulation (cross-reactivity between phenothiazines may occur); severe CNS depression and coma; prolonged QT interval (>450 msec), including prolongation due to congenital causes; history of arrhythmias; concurrent use of medications which prolong QT$_c$ (including type Ia and type III antiarrhythmics, cyclic antidepressants, some fluoroquinolones, cisapride)

Warnings/Precautions Has been shown to prolong QT$_c$ interval in a dose-dependent manner (associated with an increased risk of torsade de pointes). Patients should have a baseline ECG prior to initiation, and should not receive mesoridazine if baseline QT$_c$ >450 msec. Mesoridazine should be discontinued in patients with a QT$_c$ interval >500 msec. Potassium levels must be evaluated and normalized prior to and throughout treatment.

May cause hypotension, particularly with I.M. administration. Highly sedating, use with caution in disorders where CNS depression is a feature. Use with caution in Parkinson's disease. Caution in patients with hemodynamic instability; bone marrow suppression; predisposition to seizures; subcortical brain damage; severe cardiac, hepatic, renal, or respiratory disease. Esophageal dysmotility and aspiration have been associated with antipsychotic use; use with caution in patients at risk of pneumonia (ie, Alzheimer's disease). Caution in breast cancer or other prolactin-dependent tumors (may elevate prolactin levels). May alter temperature regulation or mask toxicity of other drugs due to antiemetic effects. May cause orthostatic hypotension - use with caution in patients at risk of this effect or those who would tolerate transient hypotensive episodes (cerebrovascular disease, cardiovascular disease, or other medications which may predispose).

Phenothiazines may cause anticholinergic effects (confusion, agitation, constipation, xerostomia, blurred vision, urinary retention). Therefore, they should be used with caution in patients with decreased gastrointestinal motility, urinary retention, BPH, xerostomia, or visual problems. Conditions which also may be exacerbated by cholinergic blockade include narrow-angle glaucoma (screening is recommended) and worsening of myasthenia gravis. Relative to other antipsychotics, (Continued)

Mesoridazine *(Continued)*

mesoridazine has a high potency of cholinergic blockade.

May cause extrapyramidal symptoms, including pseudoparkinsonism, acute dystonic reactions, akathisia, and tardive dyskinesia (risk of these reactions is low relative to other neuroleptics). May be associated with neuroleptic malignant syndrome (NMS) or pigmentary retinopathy (particularly at doses >1 g/day).

Drug Interactions

Decreased Effect: Mesoridazine may inhibit the activity of bromocriptine and levodopa. Benztropine (and other anticholinergics) may inhibit the therapeutic response to mesoridazine and excess anticholinergic effects may occur. Mesoridazine and possibly other low potency antipsychotic may reverse the pressor effects of epinephrine.

Increased Effect/Toxicity: Use of mesoridazine with other agents known to prolong QT_c may increase the risk of malignant arrhythmias; concurrent use is contraindicated - includes type I and type III antiarrhythmics, TCAs, and some quinolone antibiotics (sparfloxacin, moxifloxacin, gatifloxacin). Mesoridazine may increase the effect and/or toxicity of antihypertensives, anticholinergics, lithium, CNS depressants (ethanol, narcotics), and trazodone. Metoclopramide may increase risk of extrapyramidal symptoms (EPS). Acetylcholinesterase inhibitors (central) may increase the risk of antipsychotic-related EPS.

Nutritional/Ethanol Interactions

Ethanol: Avoid ethanol (may increase CNS depression).

Herb/Nutraceutical: Avoid valerian, St John's wort, kava kava, gotu kola (may increase CNS depression).

Lab Interactions Increased cholesterol (S), glucose; decreased uric acid (S)

Adverse Reactions Frequency not defined.

Cardiovascular: Hypotension, orthostatic hypotension, tachycardia, QT prolongation (dose dependent, up to 100% of patients at higher dosages), syncope, edema

Central nervous system: Pseudoparkinsonism, akathisia, dystonias, tardive dyskinesia, dizziness, drowsiness, restlessness, ataxia, slurred speech, neuroleptic malignant syndrome (NMS), impairment of temperature regulation, lowering of seizure threshold

Dermatologic: Increased sensitivity to sun, rash, itching, angioneurotic edema, dermatitis, discoloration of skin (blue-gray)

Endocrine & metabolic: Changes in menstrual cycle, libido (changes in), gynecomastia, lactation, galactorrhea

Gastrointestinal: Constipation, xerostomia, weight gain, nausea, vomiting, stomach pain

Genitourinary: Difficulty in urination, ejaculatory disturbances, impotence, enuresis, incontinence, priapism, urinary retention

Hematologic: Agranulocytosis, leukopenia, eosinophilia, thrombocytopenia, anemia, aplastic anemia

Hepatic: Cholestatic jaundice, hepatotoxicity

Neuromuscular & skeletal: Weakness, tremor, rigidity

Ocular: Pigmentary retinopathy, photophobia, blurred vision, cornea and lens changes

Respiratory: Nasal congestion

Miscellaneous: Diaphoresis (decreased), lupus-like syndrome

Overdosage/Toxicology Symptoms of overdose include deep sleep, coma, extrapyramidal symptoms, abnormal involuntary muscle movements, and hypotension. Monitor for cardiac arrhythmias and avoid use of drugs which prolong QT interval. Treatment is symptomatic and supportive.

Pharmacodynamics/Kinetics

Duration of Action: 4-6 hours

Time to Peak: Serum: 2-4 hours; Steady-state serum: 4-7 days

Protein Binding: 91% to 99%

Half-Life Elimination: 24-48 hours

Excretion: Urine

Available Dosage Forms [DSC] = Discontinued product

Injection, solution, as besylate [DSC]: 25 mg/mL (1 mL)

Liquid, oral, as besylate [DSC]: 25 mg/mL (118 mL) [contains alcohol 0.61%]

Tablet, as besylate [DSC]: 10 mg, 25 mg, 50 mg, 100 mg

Dosing

Adults:

Schizophrenia/psychoses:

Oral: 25-50 mg 3 times/day; maximum: 100-400 mg/day

Note: Concentrate may be diluted just prior to administration with distilled water, acidified tap water, orange or grape juice. Do not prepare and store bulk dilutions.

I.M.: Initial: 25 mg, repeat in 30-60 minutes as needed; optimal dosage range: 25-200 mg/day

Elderly: Behavioral symptoms associated with dementia:

Oral: Initial: 10 mg 1-2 times/day; if <10 mg/day is desired, consider administering 10 mg every other day. Increase dose at 4- to 7-day intervals by 10-25 mg/day; increase dose intervals (eg, twice daily, 3 times/day) as necessary to control response or side effects. Maximum daily dose: 250 mg. Gradual increases (titration) may prevent some side effects or decrease their severity.

I.M.: Initial: 25 mg; repeat doses in 30-60 minutes if necessary. Dose range: 25-200 mg/day. Elderly usually require less than maximal daily dose.

Renal Impairment: Not dialyzable (0% to 5%)

Oral: Dilute oral concentrate just prior to administration with distilled water, acidified tap water, orange or grape juice. Do not prepare and store bulk dilutions. Do not mix oral solutions of mesoridazine and lithium, these oral liquids are incompatible when mixed. **Note:** Avoid skin contact with oral medication; may cause contact dermatitis.

I.M.: Watch for hypotension when administering I.M.

I.V.: Watch for hypotension when administering I.V.

Stability

Reconstitution: Solutions may be diluted or mixed with fruit juices or other liquids but must be administered immediately after mixing; do not prepare bulk dilutions or store bulk dilutions.

Storage: Protect all dosage forms from light; clear or slightly yellow solutions may be used; should be dispensed in amber or opaque vials/bottles.

Laboratory Monitoring Baseline potassium, baseline liver and kidney function, lipid profile, CBC prior to and periodically during therapy, fasting blood glucose/Hgb A_{1c}, baseline (and periodic) serum potassium; BMI; monitor hepatic function (especially if fever with flu-like symptoms); baseline (and periodic) ECG; do not initiate if QT_c >450 msec (discontinue in QT_c 500 msec)

Physical Assessment: Assess other medications patient is taking for effectiveness and interactions. Review ophthalmic screening and monitor laboratory results, therapeutic response (mental status, mood, affect, depression), and adverse reactions at beginning of therapy and periodically with long-term use (eg, orthostatic hypotension, fluid balance, anticholinergic response, extrapyramidal symptoms, pigmentary retinopathy). With I.M. or I.V. use, monitor closely for hypotension. **Note:** Avoid skin contact with oral or injection medication; may cause contact dermatitis (wash immediately with warm, soapy water). Initiate at lower doses and taper dosage slowly when discontinuing. Assess knowledge/teach patient appropriate use, interventions to reduce side effects, and adverse symptoms to report.

Patient Education: Use exactly as directed; do not increase dose or frequency. It may take 2-3 weeks to achieve desired results; do not discontinue without consulting prescriber. Dilute oral concentration with water, orange or grape juice. Do not take within 2 hours of any antacid. Avoid alcohol or caffeine and other prescription or OTC medications not approved by prescriber. Maintain adequate hydration (2-3 L/day of fluids) unless instructed to restrict fluid intake. Avoid skin contact with medication; may cause contact dermatitis (wash immediately with warm, soapy water). You may experience excess drowsiness, restlessness, dizziness, or blurred vision (use caution driving or when engaging in tasks requiring alertness until response to drug is known); dry mouth, nausea, vomiting (small frequent meals, frequent mouth care, chewing gum, or sucking lozenges may help); constipation (increased exercise, fluids, fruit, or fiber may help); postural hypotension (use caution climbing stairs or when changing position from lying or sitting to standing); urinary retention (void before taking medication); photosensitivity (use sunscreen, wear protective clothing and eyewear, and avoid direct sunlight); decreased perspiration (avoid strenuous exercise in hot environments); or changes in menstrual cycle, libido, ejaculation (will resolve when medication is discontinued). Report persistent CNS effects (eg, trembling fingers, altered gait or balance, excessive sedation, seizures, unusual movements, anxiety, abnormal thoughts, confusion, personality changes); chest pain, palpitations, rapid heartbeat, severe dizziness; unresolved urinary retention or changes in urinary pattern; menstrual pattern, change in libido, swelling or pain in breasts (male or female); vision changes; skin rash or yellowing of skin; respiratory difficulty; or worsening of condition. **Pregnancy/breast-feeding precautions:** Inform prescriber if you are or intend to become pregnant. Do not breast-feed.

Geriatric Considerations (See Warnings/Precautions, Adverse Reactions, and Overdose/Toxicology.) Elderly patients have an increased risk of adverse response to side effects or adverse reactions to antipsychotics.

Related Information
Antipsychotic Medication Guidelines *on page 1415*
Federal OBRA Regulations Recommended Maximum Doses *on page 1421*

Mestranol and Norethindrone
(MES tra nole & nor eth IN drone)

U.S. Brand Names Necon® 1/50; Norinyl® 1+50; Ortho-Novum® 1/50

Synonyms Norethindrone and Mestranol; Ortho Novum 1/50

Pharmacologic Category Contraceptive; Estrogen and Progestin Combination

Medication Safety Issues
Sound-alike/look-alike issues:
Norinyl® may be confused with Nardil®

Pregnancy Risk Factor X

Lactation Enters breast milk/not recommended (AAP rates "compatible")

Use Prevention of pregnancy

Unlabeled/Investigational Use Treatment of hypermenorrhea (menorrhagia); pain associated with endometriosis; dysmenorrhea; dysfunctional uterine bleeding

Mechanism of Action/Effect Combination hormonal contraceptives inhibit ovulation and also produce changes in the cervical mucus and endometrium creating an unfavorable environment for sperm penetration and nidation.

Contraindications Hypersensitivity to mestranol, norethindrone, or any component of the formulation; history of or current thrombophlebitis or venous thromboembolic disorders (including DVT, PE); active or recent (within 1 year) arterial thromboembolic disease (eg, stroke, MI); cerebral vascular disease, coronary artery disease, valvular heart disease with complications, severe hypertension; diabetes mellitus with vascular involvement; severe headache with focal neurological symptoms; known or suspected breast carcinoma, endometrial cancer, estrogen-dependent neoplasms, undiagnosed abnormal genital bleeding; hepatic dysfunction or tumor, cholestatic jaundice of pregnancy, jaundice with prior combination hormonal contraceptive use; major surgery with prolonged immobilization; heavy smoking (≥15 cigarettes/day) in patients >35 years of age; pregnancy

Warnings/Precautions Combination hormonal contraceptives do not protect against HIV infection or other sexually-transmitted diseases. The risk of cardiovascular side effects increases in women who smoke cigarettes, especially those who are >35 years of age; women who use combination hormonal contraceptives should be strongly advised not to smoke. Combination hormonal contraceptives may lead to increased risk of myocardial infarction, use with caution in patients with risk factors for coronary artery disease. May increase the risk of thromboembolism. Whenever possible, combination hormonal contraceptives should be discontinued at least 4 weeks prior to and for 2 weeks following elective surgery associated with an increased risk of thromboembolism or during periods of prolonged immobilization. Combination hormonal contraceptives may have a dose-related risk of vascular disease, hypertension, and gallbladder disease. Women with hypertension or renal disease should be encouraged to use a nonhormonal form of contraception. The use of combination hormonal contraceptives has been associated with a slight increase in frequency of breast cancer, however, studies are not consistent. Combination hormonal contraceptives may cause glucose intolerance. Retinal thrombosis has been reported (rarely). Use caution with conditions that may be aggravated by fluid retention, depression, or history of migraine. Not for use prior to menarche.

The minimum dosage combination of estrogen/progestin that will effectively treat the individual patient should be used. New patients should be started on products containing ≤0.035 mg of estrogen per tablet.

Drug Interactions
Cytochrome P450 Effect:
Mestranol: **Substrate** of CYP2C19 (major); Based on active metabolite ethinyl estradiol: **Substrate** of CYP3A4 (major), 3A5-7 (minor); **Inhibits** CYP1A2 (weak), 2B6 (weak), 2C19 (weak), 3A4 (weak)
Norethindrone: **Substrate** of CYP3A4 (major); **Induces** CYP2C19 (weak)

Decreased Effect: CYP2C8/9 inhibitors may decrease the levels of ethinyl estradiol (active metabolite of mestranol); example inhibitors include delavirdine, fluconazole, gemfibrozil, ketoconazole, nicardipine, NSAIDs, pioglitazone, and sulfonamides. CYP3A4 inducers may decrease the levels of ethinyl estradiol (active metabolite of mestranol); example inducers include aminoglutethimide, carbamazepine, nafcillin, nevirapine, phenobarbital, phenytoin, and rifamycins. Combination hormonal contraceptives may decrease plasma levels of acetaminophen, clofibric acid, lorazepam, morphine, oxazepam, salicylic acid, temazepam. Contraceptive effect decreased by acitretin, aminoglutethimide, amprenavir, griseofulvin, lopinavir, nelfinavir, nevirapine, penicillins (effect not consistent), ritonavir, tetracyclines (effect not consistent) troglitazone. Combination hormonal contraceptives may decrease (or increase) the effects of coumarin derivatives.

(Continued)

Mestranol and Norethindrone

(Continued)

Increased Effect/Toxicity: Acetaminophen and ascorbic acid may increase plasma levels of estrogen component. Atorvastatin and indinavir increase plasma levels of combination hormonal contraceptives. Combination hormonal contraceptives increase the plasma levels of alprazolam, chlordiazepoxide, cyclosporine, diazepam, prednisolone, selegiline, theophylline, tricyclic antidepressants. Combination hormonal contraceptives may increase (or decrease) the effects of coumarin derivatives.

Nutritional/Ethanol Interactions

Food: CNS effects of caffeine may be enhanced if oral contraceptives are used concurrently with caffeine. Grapefruit juice increases ethinyl estradiol concentrations and would be expected to increase progesterone serum levels as well; clinical implications are unclear.

Herb/Nutraceutical: St John's wort may decrease the effectiveness of combination hormonal contraceptives by inducing hepatic enzymes. Avoid dong quai and black cohosh (have estrogen activity). Avoid saw palmetto, red clover, ginseng.

Adverse Reactions Frequency not defined.

Cardiovascular: Arterial thromboembolism, cerebral hemorrhage, cerebral thrombosis, edema, hypertension, mesenteric thrombosis, MI

Central nervous system: Depression, dizziness, headache, migraine, nervousness, premenstrual syndrome, stroke

Dermatologic: Acne, erythema multiforme, erythema nodosum, hirsutism, loss of scalp hair, melasma (may persist), rash (allergic)

Endocrine & metabolic: Amenorrhea, breakthrough bleeding, breast enlargement, breast secretion, breast tenderness, carbohydrate intolerance, lactation decreased (postpartum), glucose tolerance decreased, libido changes, menstrual flow changes, sex hormone-binding globulins (SHBG) increased, spotting, temporary infertility (following discontinuation), thyroid-binding globulin increased, triglycerides increased

Gastrointestinal: Abdominal cramps, appetite changes, bloating, cholestasis, colitis, gallbladder disease, jaundice, nausea, vomiting, weight gain/loss

Genitourinary: Cervical erosion changes, cervical secretion changes, cystitis-like syndrome, vaginal candidiasis, vaginitis

Hematologic: Antithrombin III decreased, folate levels decreased, hemolytic uremic syndrome, norepinephrine induced platelet aggregability increased, porphyria, prothrombin increased; factors VII, VIII, IX, and X increased

Hepatic: Benign liver tumors, Budd-Chiari syndrome, cholestatic jaundice, hepatic adenomas

Local: Thrombophlebitis

Ocular: Cataracts, change in corneal curvature (steepening), contact lens intolerance, optic neuritis, retinal thrombosis

Renal: Impaired renal function

Respiratory: Pulmonary thromboembolism

Miscellaneous: Hemorrhagic eruption

Overdosage/Toxicology Toxicity is unlikely following single exposures of excessive doses. May cause withdrawal bleeding in females. Any treatment following emesis and charcoal administration should be supportive and symptomatic.

Pharmacodynamics/Kinetics

Metabolism:

Mestranol: Hepatic via demethylation to ethinyl estradiol

Pharmacokinetic Note See Norethindrone monograph for additional information.

Available Dosage Forms Tablet, monophasic formulations:

Necon® 1/50: Norethindrone 1 mg and mestranol 0.05 mg [21 light blue tablets and 7 white inactive tablets] (28s)

Norinyl® 1+50: Norethindrone 1 mg and mestranol 0.05 mg [21 white tablets and 7 orange inactive tablets] (28s)

Ortho-Novum® 1/50: Norethindrone 1 mg and mestranol 0.05 mg [21 yellow tablets and 7 green inactive tablets] (28s)

Dosing

Adults: Female: Contraception: Oral:

Schedule 1 (Sunday starter): Dose begins on first Sunday after onset of menstruation; if the menstrual period starts on Sunday, take first tablet that very same day. **With a Sunday start, an additional method of contraception should be used until after the first 7 days of consecutive administration.**

For 21-tablet package: Dosage is 1 tablet daily for 21 consecutive days, followed by 7 days off of the medication; a new course begins on the 8th day after the last tablet is taken.

For 28-tablet package: Dosage is 1 tablet daily without interruption.

Schedule 2 (Day 1 starter): Dose starts on first day of menstrual cycle taking 1 tablet daily.

For 21-tablet package: Dosage is 1 tablet daily for 21 consecutive days, followed by 7 days off of the medication; a new course begins on the 8th day after the last tablet is taken.

For 28-tablet package: Dosage is 1 tablet daily without interruption.

Note: If all doses have been taken on schedule and one menstrual period is missed, continue dosing cycle. If two consecutive menstrual periods are missed, pregnancy test is required before new dosing cycle is started.

Missed doses: Monophasic formulations (refer to package insert for complete information):

One dose missed: Take as soon as remembered or take 2 tablets next day

Two consecutive doses missed in the first 2 weeks: Take 2 tablets as soon as remembered or 2 tablets next 2 days. **An additional method of contraception should be used for 7 days after missed dose.**

Two consecutive doses missed in week 3 or three consecutive doses missed at any time: **An additional method of contraception must be used for 7 days after a missed dose:**

Schedule 1 (Sunday starter): Continue dose of 1 tablet daily until Sunday, then discard the rest of the pack, and a new pack should be started that same day.

Schedule 2 (Day 1 starter): Current pack should be discarded, and a new pack should be started that same day.

Pediatrics: Female: Contraception: Oral: See adult dosing; not to be used prior to menarche.

Renal Impairment: Specific guidelines not available; use with caution and monitor blood pressure closely. Consider other forms of contraception.

Hepatic Impairment: Contraindicated in patients with hepatic impairment.

Administration

Oral: Administer at the same time each day. Administer at bedtime to minimize occurrence of adverse effects.

Stability

Storage: Store at controlled room temperature of 25°C (77°F).

Nursing Actions

Physical Assessment: Monitor or teach patient to monitor blood pressure on a regular basis. Monitor or teach patient to monitor for occurrence of adverse effects and symptoms to report (eg, thromboembolic disease, visual changes, neuromuscular weakness). Assess knowledge/teach importance of regular (monthly) blood pressure checks and annual physical assessment, Pap smear, and vision assessment. Teach importance of maintaining prescribed schedule of dosing. **Pregnancy risk factor X:** Do not use if patient is pregnant.

Patient Education: Oral contraceptives do not protect against HIV or other sexually-transmitted disease. Take exactly as directed by prescriber (also see package insert). Take at the same time each day. You are at risk of becoming pregnant if doses are missed. Detailed and complete information on dosing and missed doses can be found in the package insert. Be aware that some medications may reduce the effectiveness of oral contraceptives; an alternate form of contraception may be needed. Check all medicines (prescription and OTC), herbal, and alternative products with prescriber. It is important that you check your blood pressure monthly (on same day each month) and that you have an annual physical assessment, Pap smear, and vision assessment while taking this medication. Avoid smoking while taking this medication; smoking increases risk of adverse effects, including thromboembolic events and heart attacks. You may experience loss of appetite (small frequent meals will help); or constipation (increased exercise, fluids, fruit, fiber, or stool softeners may help). If you have diabetes, use accurate serum glucose testing to identify any changes in glucose tolerance; notify prescriber of significant changes so antidiabetic medication can be adjusted if necessary. Report immediately pain or muscle soreness; warmth, swelling, pain, or redness in calves; shortness of breath; sudden loss of vision; unresolved leg or foot swelling; change in menstrual pattern (unusual bleeding, amenorrhea, breakthrough spotting); breast tenderness that does not go away; acute abdominal cramping; signs of vaginal infection (drainage, pain, itching); CNS changes (blurred vision, confusion, acute anxiety, or unresolved depression); or significant weight gain (>5 lb/week). Notify prescriber of changes in contact lens tolerance. **Pregnancy/breast-feeding precautions:** This medication should not be used during pregnancy. If you suspect you may become pregnant, contact prescriber immediately. Consult prescriber if breast-feeding.

Dietary Considerations Should be taken at same time each day.

Breast-Feeding Issues Jaundice and breast enlargement in the nursing infant have been reported following the use of combination hormonal contraceptives. May decrease the quality and quantity of breast milk; a nonhormonal form of contraception is recommended.

Pregnancy Issues Pregnancy should be ruled out prior to treatment and discontinued if pregnancy occurs. In general, the use of combination hormonal contraceptives when inadvertently taken early in pregnancy have not been associated with teratogenic effects. Due to increased risk of thromboembolism postpartum, combination hormonal contraceptives should not be started earlier than 4-6 weeks following delivery. Hormonal contraceptives may be less effective in obese patients. An increase in oral contraceptive failure was noted in women with a BMI >27.3. Similar findings were noted in patients weighing ≥90 kg (198 lb) using the contraceptive patch.

Additional Information The World Health Organization (WHO) has issued revised management recommendations for missed combined oral contraceptive pills. Refer to the following reference for a complete presentation and discussion of the guidelines:

Faculty of Family Planning and Reproductive Health Care Clinical Effectiveness Unit, "Faculty Statement from the CEU on a New Publication: WHO Selected Practice Recommendations for Contraceptive Use

Update. Missed Pills: New Recommendations," *J Fam Plann Reprod Health Care*, 2005, 31(2):153-5.
Related Information
Norethindrone *on page 896*

Metformin (met FOR min)

U.S. Brand Names Fortamet™; Glucophage®; Glucophage® XR; Riomet™
Synonyms Metformin Hydrochloride
Pharmacologic Category Antidiabetic Agent, Biguanide
Medication Safety Issues
Sound-alike/look-alike issues:
Metformin may be confused with metronidazole
Glucophage® may be confused with Glucotrol®, Glutofac®
Pregnancy Risk Factor B
Lactation Excretion in breast milk unknown/not recommended
Use Management of type 2 diabetes mellitus (noninsulin dependent, NIDDM) as monotherapy when hyperglycemia cannot be managed on diet alone. May be used concomitantly with a sulfonylurea or insulin to improve glycemic control.
Unlabeled/Investigational Use Treatment of HIV lipodystrophy syndrome
Mechanism of Action/Effect Decreases hepatic glucose production, decreasing intestinal absorption of glucose and improves insulin sensitivity (increases peripheral glucose uptake and utilization)
Contraindications Hypersensitivity to metformin or any component of the formulation; renal disease or renal dysfunction (serum creatinine ≥1.5 mg/dL in males or ≥1.4 mg/dL in females or abnormal creatinine clearance from any cause, including shock, acute myocardial infarction, or septicemia); congestive heart failure requiring pharmacological management; acute or chronic metabolic acidosis with or without coma (including diabetic ketoacidosis)

Note: Temporarily discontinue in patients undergoing radiologic studies in which intravascular iodinated contrast materials are utilized.

Warnings/Precautions Lactic acidosis is a rare, but potentially severe consequence of therapy with metformin. Lactic acidosis should be suspected in any diabetic patient receiving metformin who has evidence of acidosis when evidence of ketoacidosis is lacking. Discontinue metformin in clinical situations predisposing to hypoxemia, including conditions such as cardiovascular collapse, respiratory failure, acute myocardial infarction, acute congestive heart failure, and septicemia.

Metformin is substantially excreted by the kidney. The risk of accumulation and lactic acidosis increases with the degree of impairment of renal function. Patients with renal function below the limit of normal for their age should not receive metformin. In elderly patients, renal function should be monitored regularly; should not be used in any patient ≥80 years of age unless measurement of creatinine clearance verifies normal renal function. Use of concomitant medications that may affect renal function (ie, affect tubular secretion) may also affect metformin disposition. Metformin should be suspended in patients with dehydration and/or prerenal azotemia. Therapy should be suspended for any surgical procedures (resume only after normal intake resumed and normal renal function is verified). Metformin should also be temporarily discontinued for 48 hours in patients undergoing radiologic studies involving the intravascular administration of iodinated contrast materials (potential for acute alteration in renal function).
(Continued)

Metformin *(Continued)*

Avoid use in patients with impaired liver function. Patient must be instructed to avoid excessive acute or chronic ethanol use. Administration of oral antidiabetic drugs has been reported to be associated with increased cardiovascular mortality; metformin does not appear to share this risk. Safety and efficacy of metformin have been established for use in children ≥10 years of age; the extended release preparation is for use in patients ≥17 years of age.

Drug Interactions
Decreased Effect: Drugs which tend to produce hyperglycemia (eg, diuretics, corticosteroids, phenothiazines, thyroid products, estrogens, oral contraceptives, phenytoin, nicotinic acid, sympathomimetics, calcium channel blocking drugs, isoniazid) may lead to a loss of glucose control.

Increased Effect/Toxicity: Furosemide and cimetidine may increase metformin blood levels. Cationic drugs (eg, amiloride, digoxin, morphine, procainamide, quinidine, quinine, ranitidine, triamterene, trimethoprim, and vancomycin) which are eliminated by renal tubular secretion have the potential to increase metformin levels by competing for common renal tubular transport systems. Contrast agents may increase the risk of metformin-induced lactic acidosis; discontinue metformin prior to exposure and withhold for 48 hours.

Nutritional/Ethanol Interactions
Ethanol: Avoid or limit ethanol (incidence of lactic acidosis may be increased; may cause hypoglycemia).

Food: Food decreases the extent and slightly delays the absorption. May decrease absorption of vitamin B_{12} and/or folic acid.

Herb/Nutraceutical: Caution with chromium, garlic, gymnema (may cause hypoglycemia).

Adverse Reactions
>10%:
Gastrointestinal: Nausea/vomiting (6% to 25%), diarrhea (10% to 53%), flatulence (12%)
Neuromuscular & skeletal: Weakness (9%)

1% to 10%:
Cardiovascular: Chest discomfort, flushing, palpitation
Central nervous system: Headache (6%), chills, dizziness, lightheadedness
Dermatologic: Rash
Endocrine & metabolic: Hypoglycemia
Gastrointestinal: Indigestion (7%), abdominal discomfort (6%), abdominal distention, abnormal stools, constipation, dyspepsia/ heartburn, taste disorder
Neuromuscular & skeletal: Myalgia
Respiratory: Dyspnea, upper respiratory tract infection
Miscellaneous: Decreased vitamin B_{12} levels (7%), increased diaphoresis, flu-like syndrome, nail disorder

Overdosage/Toxicology Hypoglycemia (10% of cases) or lactic acidosis (~32% of cases) may occur. Metformin is dialyzable with a clearance of up to 170 mL/minute. Hemodialysis may be useful for removal of accumulated drug from patients in whom metformin overdose is suspected. Treatment is supportive.

Pharmacodynamics/Kinetics
Onset of Action: Within days; maximum effects up to 2 weeks

Protein Binding: Negligible

Half-Life Elimination: Plasma: 6.2 hours

Excretion: Urine (90% as unchanged drug)

Available Dosage Forms
Solution, oral, as hydrochloride (Riomet™): 100 mg/mL (118 mL, 473 mL) [contains saccharin; cherry flavor]
Tablet, as hydrochloride (Glucophage®): 500 mg, 850 mg, 1000 mg
Tablet, extended release, as hydrochloride: 500 mg
Fortamet™: 500 mg, 1000 mg
Glucophage® XR: 500 mg, 750 mg

Dosing
Adults: **Note:** Oral (allow 1-2 weeks between dose titrations): Generally, clinically significant responses are not seen at doses <1500 mg daily; however, a lower recommended starting dose and gradual increased dosage is recommended to minimize gastrointestinal symptoms

Management of type 2 diabetes mellitus: Oral:
Immediate release tablet or oral solution: Initial: 500 mg twice daily (give with the morning and evening meals) **or** 850 mg once daily; increase dosage incrementally.
Adjustment: Incremental dosing recommendations are based on dosage form:
500 mg tablet: One tablet/day at weekly intervals
850 mg tablet: One tablet/day every other week
Oral solution: 500 mg twice daily every other week
Note: Doses of up to 2000 mg/day may be given twice daily. If a dose >2000 mg/day is required, it may be better tolerated in three divided doses. Maximum recommended dose 2550 mg/day.
Extended release tablet: Initial: 500 mg once daily (with the evening meal); dosage may be increased by 500 mg weekly; maximum dose: 2000 mg once daily. If glycemic control is not achieved at maximum dose, may divide dose to 1000 mg twice daily. If doses >2000 mg/day are needed, switch to regular release tablets and titrate to maximum dose of 2550 mg/day.

Transfer from other antidiabetic agents: No transition period is generally necessary except when transferring from chlorpropamide. When transferring from chlorpropamide, care should be exercised during the first 2 weeks because of the prolonged retention of chlorpropamide in the body, leading to overlapping drug effects and possible hypoglycemia.

Concomitant metformin and oral sulfonylurea therapy: If patients have not responded to 4 weeks of the maximum dose of metformin monotherapy, consider a gradual addition of an oral sulfonylurea, even if prior primary or secondary failure to a sulfonylurea has occurred. Continue metformin at the maximum dose.

Failed sulfonylurea therapy: Patients with prior failure on glyburide may be treated by gradual addition of metformin. Initiate with glyburide 20 mg and metformin 500 mg daily. Metformin dosage may be increased by 500 mg/day at weekly intervals, up to a maximum of 2500 mg/day (dosage of glyburide maintained at 20 mg/day).

Concomitant metformin and insulin therapy:
Initial: 500 mg metformin once daily, continue current insulin dose; increase by 500 mg metformin weekly until adequate glycemic control is achieved
Maximum dose: 2500 mg metformin; 2000 mg metformin extended release
Note: Decrease insulin dose 10% to 25% when FPG <120 mg/dL; monitor and make further adjustments as needed

Elderly: The initial and maintenance dosing should be conservative, due to the potential for decreased renal function. Generally, elderly patients should **not** be titrated to the maximum dose of metformin. See Geriatric Considerations.

Pediatrics: **Note:** Allow 1-2 weeks between dose titrations: Generally, clinically significant responses are not seen at doses <1500 mg daily; however, a lower recommended starting dose and gradual increased dosage is recommended to minimize gastrointestinal symptoms

Management of type 2 diabetes mellitus: Children 10-16 years: Oral (500 mg tablet or oral solution): Initial: 500 mg twice daily (given with the morning and evening meals); increases in daily dosage should be made in increments of 500 mg at weekly intervals, given in divided doses, up to a maximum of 2000 mg/day

Renal Impairment: The plasma and blood half-life of metformin is prolonged and the renal clearance is decreased in proportion to the decrease in creatinine clearance. Per the manufacturer, metformin is contra-indicated in the presence of renal dysfunction defined as a serum creatinine >1.5 mg/dL in males, or >1.4 mg/dL in females and in patients with abnormal clearance. Clinically, it has been recommended that metformin be avoided in patients with Cl_{cr} <60-70 mL/ minute (DeFronzo, 1999).

Hepatic Impairment: Avoid metformin; liver disease is a risk factor for the development of lactic acidosis during metformin therapy.

Administration

Oral: Extended release dosage form should be swallowed whole; do not crush, break, or chew. Patients who are anorexic or NPO may need to have their dose held to avoid hypoglycemia.

Stability

Storage: Store tablets and oral solution at 20°C to 25°C (68°F to 77°F).

Laboratory Monitoring Urine for glucose and ketones, fasting blood glucose, hemoglobin A_{1c}, and fructosamine. Initial and periodic monitoring of hematologic parameters (eg, hemoglobin/hematocrit and red blood cell indices) and renal function should be performed, at least annually. While megaloblastic anemia has been rarely seen with metformin, if suspected, vitamin B_{12} deficiency should be excluded.

Nursing Actions

Physical Assessment: Assess potential for interactions with other prescriptions, OTC medications, or herbal products patient may be taking (eg, anything that may effect glucose levels). Monitor laboratory tests, therapeutic effectiveness, and adverse reactions (eg, assess for signs and symptoms of vitamin B_{12} and/or folic acid deficiency; supplementation may be required) during therapy. Teach patient (or refer patient to diabetic educator for instruction) in appropriate use, possible side effects/appropriate interventions, and adverse symptoms to report.

Patient Education: Do not take any new medication during therapy unless approved by prescriber. Take as directed (may take with food to reduce GI upset). Do not chew or crush tablets. Parts of extended-release tablets may be excreted in the stool (normal). Do not change dosage or discontinue without consulting prescriber. Avoid overuse of alcohol (could cause severe reaction). It is important to follow dietary and lifestyle recommendations of prescriber. You will be instructed in signs of hypo- or hyperglycemia by prescriber or diabetic educator. May cause drowsiness or dizziness (use caution driving or engaging in potentially hazardous tasks until response to drug is known); nausea or vomiting (taking with meals, eating small frequent meals, frequent mouth care, or sucking lozenges may help); or abdominal distention, flatulence, diarrhea, constipation, or heartburn (if these persist consult prescriber for approved medication). Report immediately unusual weakness or fatigue; unusual muscle pain; persistent GI discomfort; dizziness or lightheadedness; sudden respiratory difficulty, chest discomfort, slow or irregular heartbeat; or other adverse reactions. **Breast-feeding precaution:** Breast-feeding is not recommended.

Dietary Considerations Drug may cause GI upset; take with food (to decrease GI upset). Take at the same time

each day. Dietary modification based on ADA recommendations is a part of therapy. Monitor for signs and symptoms of vitamin B_{12} and/or folic acid deficiency; supplementation may be required.

Geriatric Considerations Limited data suggests that metformin's total body clearance may be decreased and AUC and half-life increased in older patients; presumably due to decreased renal clearance. Metformin has been well tolerated by the elderly but lower doses and frequent monitoring are recommended.

Breast-Feeding Issues It is not known if metformin is excreted in human breast milk (excretion occurs in animal models); insulin therapy should be considered in breast-feeding women.

Pregnancy Issues Abnormal blood glucose levels are associated with a higher incidence of congenital abnormalities. Insulin is the drug of choice for the control of diabetes mellitus during pregnancy.

Methadone (METH a done)

U.S. Brand Names Dolophine®; Methadone Diskets®; Methadone Intensol™; Methadose®

Synonyms Methadone Hydrochloride

Restrictions C-II

When used for treatment of narcotic addiction: May only be dispensed in accordance to guidelines established by the Substance Abuse and Mental Health Services Administration's (SAMHSA) Center for Substance Abuse Treatment (CSAT).

Pharmacologic Category Analgesic, Narcotic

Medication Safety Issues

Sound-alike/look-alike issues:

Methadone may be confused with Mephyton®, methylphenidate

Pregnancy Risk Factor C/D (prolonged use or high doses at term)

Lactation Enters breast milk/not recommended (AAP rates "compatible")

Use Management of severe pain; detoxification and maintenance treatment of narcotic addiction (if used for detoxification and maintenance treatment of narcotic addiction, it must be part of an FDA-approved program)

Mechanism of Action/Effect Binds to opiate receptors in the CNS, causing inhibition of ascending pain pathways, altering the perception of and response to pain; produces generalized CNS depression

Contraindications Hypersensitivity to methadone or any component of the formulation; respiratory depression (in the absence of resuscitative equipment or in an unmonitored setting); acute bronchial asthma or hypercarbia; pregnancy (prolonged use or high doses near term)

Warnings/Precautions An opioid-containing analgesic regimen should be tailored to each patient's needs and based upon the type of pain being treated (acute versus chronic), the route of administration, degree of tolerance for opioids (naive versus chronic user), age, weight, and medical condition. The optimal analgesic dose varies widely among patients. Doses should be titrated to pain relief/prevention. Patients maintained on stable doses of methadone may need higher and/or more frequent doses in case of acute pain (eg, postoperative pain, physical trauma). Methadone is ineffective for the relief of anxiety.

May prolong the QT interval; use caution in patients at risk for QT prolongation, with medications known to prolong the QT interval, or history of conduction abnormalities. QT interval prolongation and torsade de pointes may be associated with doses >200 mg/day, but have also been observed with lower doses. May cause severe hypotension; use caution with severe volume depletion or other conditions which may compromise (Continued)

Methadone (Continued)

maintenance of normal blood pressure. Use caution with cardiovascular disease or patients predisposed to dysrhythmias.

May cause respiratory depression. Use caution in patients with respiratory disease or pre-existing respiratory conditions (eg, severe obesity, asthma, COPD, sleep apnea, CNS depression). Because the respiratory effects last longer than the analgesic effects, slow titration is required. Abrupt cessation may precipitate withdrawal symptoms.

May cause CNS depression, which may impair physical or mental abilities. Patients must be cautioned about performing tasks which require mental alertness (eg, operating machinery or driving). Effects with other sedative drugs or ethanol may be potentiated. Use with caution in patients with depression or suicidal tendencies, or in patients with a history of drug abuse. Tolerance or psychological and physical dependence may occur with prolonged use.

Use with caution in patients with head injury or increased intracranial pressure. May obscure diagnosis or clinical course of patients with acute abdominal conditions. Elderly may be more susceptible to adverse effects (eg, CNS, respiratory, gastrointestinal). Decrease initial dose and use caution in the elderly or debilitated; with hyper/hypothyroidism, prostatic hypertrophy, or urethral stricture; or with severe renal or hepatic failure. Safety and efficacy have not been established in patients <18 years of age. Tablets contain excipients to deter use by injection.

Drug Interactions

Cytochrome P450 Effect: Substrate of CYP2C8/9 (minor), 2C19 (minor), 2D6 (minor), 3A4 (major); **Inhibits** CYP2D6 (moderate), 3A4 (weak)

Decreased Effect: Agonist/antagonist analgesics (buprenorphine, butorphanol, nalbuphine, pentazocine) may decrease analgesic effect of methadone and precipitate withdrawal symptoms; use is not recommended. Efavirenz and nevirapine may decrease levels of methadone (opioid withdrawal syndrome has been reported). Methadone may decrease bioavailability of didanosine and stavudine. Ritonavir (and combinations) may decrease levels of methadone; withdrawal symptoms have inconsistently been observed, monitor. CYP3A4 inducers may decrease the levels/effects of methadone (eg, aminoglutethimide, carbamazepine, nafcillin, nevirapine, phenobarbital, phenytoin, rifamycins). Monitor for methadone withdrawal. Larger doses of methadone may be required. Methadone may decrease the levels/effects of CYP2D6 prodrug substrates (eg, codeine, hydrocodone, oxycodone, tramadol). Ritonavir may decrease levels/effects of methadone with continued dosing.

Increased Effect/Toxicity: CYP3A4 inhibitors may increase the levels/effects of methadone (eg, azole antifungals, clarithromycin, diclofenac, doxycycline, erythromycin, imatinib, isoniazid, nefazodone, nicardipine, propofol, protease inhibitors, quinidine, telithromycin, verapamil). Methadone may increase the levels/effects of CYP2D6 substrates (eg, amphetamines, selected beta-blockers, dextromethorphan, fluoxetine, lidocaine, mirtazapine, nefazodone, paroxetine, risperidone, ritonavir, thioridazine, tricyclic antidepressants, venlafaxine). Methadone may increase bioavailability and toxic effects of zidovudine. CNS depressants (including but not limited to opioid analgesics, general anesthetics, sedatives, hypnotics, ethanol) may cause respiratory depression, hypotension, profound sedation, or coma. Levels of desipramine may be increased by methadone. Effects/toxicity of QT$_c$ interval-prolonging agents may be increased; use with caution (including but may not be limited to amitriptyline, astemizole, bepridil, disopyramide, erythromycin, haloperidol, imipramine, quinidine, pimozide, procainamide, sotalol, thioridazine). Ritonavir may increase levels/effects of methadone shortly after initiation.

Nutritional/Ethanol Interactions

Ethanol: Avoid ethanol (may increase CNS effects). Watch for sedation.

Herb/Nutraceutical: Avoid St John's wort (may decrease methadone levels; may increase CNS depression). Avoid valerian, kava kava, gotu kola (may increase CNS depression). Methadone is metabolized by CYP3A4 in the intestines; avoid concurrent use of grapefruit juice.

Lab Interactions

Some quinolones may produce a false-positive urine screening result for opiates using commercially-available immunoassay kits. This has been demonstrated most consistently for levofloxacin and ofloxacin, but other quinolones have shown cross-reactivity in certain assay kits. Confirmation of positive opiate screens by more specific methods should be considered.

Adverse Reactions Frequency not defined. During prolonged administration, adverse effects may decrease over several weeks; however, constipation and sweating may persist.

Cardiovascular: Bradycardia, peripheral vasodilation, cardiac arrest, syncope, faintness, shock, hypotension, edema, arrhythmia, bigeminal rhythms, extrasystoles, tachycardia, torsade de pointes, ventricular fibrillation, ventricular tachycardia, ECG changes, QT interval prolonged, T-wave inversion, cardiomyopathy, flushing, heart failure, palpitation, phlebitis, orthostatic hypotension

Central nervous system: Euphoria, dysphoria, headache, insomnia, agitation, disorientation, drowsiness, dizziness, lightheadedness, sedation, confusion, seizure

Dermatologic: Pruritus, urticaria, rash, hemorrhagic urticaria

Endocrine & metabolic: Libido decreased, hypokalemia, hypomagnesemia, antidiuretic effect, amenorrhea

Gastrointestinal: Nausea, vomiting, constipation, anorexia, stomach cramps, xerostomia, biliary tract spasm, abdominal pain, glossitis, weight gain

Genitourinary: Urinary retention or hesitancy, impotence

Hematologic: Thrombocytopenia (reversible, reported in patients with chronic hepatitis)

Neuromuscular & skeletal: Weakness

Local: I.M./SubQ injection: Pain, erythema, swelling; I.V. injection: pruritus, urticaria, rash, hemorrhagic urticaria (rare)

Ocular: Miosis, visual disturbances

Respiratory: Respiratory depression, respiratory arrest, pulmonary edema

Miscellaneous: Physical and psychological dependence, death, diaphoresis

Overdosage/Toxicology Symptoms include respiratory depression, CNS depression, miosis, hypothermia, circulatory collapse, and convulsions. Treatment includes naloxone 2 mg I.V. (0.01 mg/kg for children), with repeat administration as necessary, up to a total of 10 mg, or as a continuous infusion. Nalmefene may also be used to reverse signs of intoxication. Patient should be monitored for depressant effects of methadone for 36-48 hours and other supportive measures should be employed as needed. Forced diuresis, peritoneal dialysis, hemodialysis, or charcoal hemoperfusion have not been established as beneficial for increasing methadone or metabolite elimination.

Pharmacodynamics/Kinetics

Onset of Action: Oral: Analgesic: 0.5-1 hour; Parenteral: 10-20 minutes; Peak effect: Parenteral: 1-2 hours

Duration of Action: Oral: 4-8 hours, increases to 22-48 hours with repeated doses

Protein Binding: 85% to 90%

Half-Life Elimination: 8-59 hours; may be prolonged with alkaline pH, decreased during pregnancy

Metabolism: Hepatic; N-demethylation primarily via CYP3A4, CYP2B6, and CYP2C19 to inactive metabolites

Excretion: Urine (<10% as unchanged drug); increased with urine pH <6

Available Dosage Forms

Injection, solution, as hydrochloride: 10 mg/mL (20 mL)

Solution, oral, as hydrochloride: 5 mg/5 mL (500 mL); 10 mg/5 mL (500 mL) [contains alcohol 8%; citrus flavor]

Solution, oral concentrate, as hydrochloride: 10 mg/mL (946 mL)

Methadone Intensol™: 10 mg/mL (30 mL)

Methadose®: 10 mg/mL (1000 mL) [cherry flavor]

Methadose®: 10 mg/mL (1000 mL) [dye free, sugar free, unflavored]

Tablet, as hydrochloride (Dolophine®, Methadose®): 5 mg, 10 mg

Tablet, dispersible, as hydrochloride:

Methadose®: 40 mg

Methadone Diskets®: 40 mg [orange-pineapple flavor]

Dosing

Adults: Regulations regarding methadone use may vary by state and/or country. Obtain advice from appropriate regulatory agencies and/or consult with pain management/palliative care specialists. **Note:** These are guidelines and do not represent the maximum doses that may be required in all patients. Methadone accumulates with repeated doses and dosage may need reduction after 3-5 days to prevent CNS depressant effects. Some patients may benefit from every 8-12 hour dosing interval for chronic pain management. Doses should be titrated to appropriate effects.

Pain (analgesia):

Oral: Initial: 5-10 mg; dosing interval may range from 4-12 hours during initial therapy; decrease in dose or frequency may be required (~days 2-5) due to accumulation with repeated doses

Manufacturer's labeling: 2.5-10 mg every 3-4 hours as needed

I.V.: Manufacturers labeling: Initial: 2.5-10 mg every 8-12 hours in opioid-naive patients; titrate slowly to effect; may also be administered by SubQ or I.M. injection

Note: Conversion from oral to parenteral dose: Initial dose: Oral: parenteral: 2:1 ratio

Detoxification: *Oral:*

Initial: Should not exceed 30 mg; lower doses should be considered in patients with low tolerance at initiation (eg, absence of opioids ≥5 days); an additional 5-10 mg of methadone may be provided if withdrawal symptoms have not been suppressed or if symptoms reappear after 2-4 hours; total daily dose on the first day should not exceed 40 mg, unless the program physician documents in the patient's record that 40 mg did not control opiate abstinence symptoms.

Maintenance: Usual range: 80-120 mg/day (titration should occur cautiously)

Withdrawal: Dose reductions should be <10% of the maintenance dose, every 10-14 days

Detoxification (short-term): *Oral:*

Initial: Titrate to 40 mg/day in 2 divided doses

Maintenance: Continue 40 mg dose for 2-3 days

Withdrawal: Decrease daily or every other day, keeping withdrawal symptoms tolerable; hospitalized patients may tolerate a 20% reduction/day; ambulatory patients may require a slower reduction

Dosage adjustment during pregnancy: Methadone dose may need to be increased, or the dosing interval decreased; see Pregnancy Issues —

use should be reserved for cases where the benefits clearly outweigh the risks

Elderly: Oral, I.M.: 2.5 mg every 8-12 hours; refer to adult dosing.

Pediatrics: Regulations regarding methadone use may vary by state and/or country. Obtain advice from appropriate regulatory agencies and/or consult with pain management/palliative care specialists. **Note:** These are guidelines and do not represent the maximum doses that may be required in all patients. Methadone accumulates with repeated doses and dosage may need reduction after 3-5 days to prevent CNS depressant effects. Some patients may benefit from every 8-12 hour dosing interval for chronic pain management. Doses should be titrated to appropriate effects.

Pain (analgesia):

Oral (unlabeled use): Initial: 0.1-0.2 mg/kg 4-8 hours initially for 2-3 doses, then every 6-12 hours as needed. Dosing interval may range from 4-12 hours during initial therapy; decrease in dose or frequency may be required (~ days 2-5) due to accumulation with repeated doses (maximum dose: 5-10 mg)

I.V. (unlabeled use): 0.1 mg/kg every 4-8 hours initially for 2-3 doses, then every 6-12 hours as needed. Dosing interval may range from 4-12 hours during initial therapy; decrease in dose or frequency may be required (~ days 2-5) due to accumulation with repeated doses (maximum dose: 5-8 mg)

Iatrogenic narcotic dependency (unlabeled): Oral: General guidelines: Initial: 0.05-0.1 mg/kg/dose every 6 hours; increase by 0.05 mg/kg/dose until withdrawal symptoms are controlled; after 24-48 hours, the dosing interval can be lengthened to every 12-24 hours; to taper dose, wean by 0.05 mg/kg/day; if withdrawal symptoms recur, taper at a slower rate

Renal Impairment: Cl$_{cr}$ <10 mL/minute: Administer 50% to 75% of normal dose.

Hepatic Impairment: Avoid in severe liver disease.

Administration

Oral: Oral dose for detoxification and maintenance may be administered in fruit juice or water.

I.V. Detail: pH: 4.5-6.5

Stability

Compatibility: Stable in NS

Storage:

Injection: Store at controlled room temperature of 15°C to 30°C (59°F to 86°F). Protect from light.

Oral concentrate, oral solution, tablet: Store at controlled room temperature of 15°C to 30°C (59°F to 86°F).

Nursing Actions

Physical Assessment: Assess other medications patient may be taking for additive or adverse interactions. Monitor for effectiveness of pain relief and monitor for signs of overdose. Monitor blood pressure, CNS and respiratory status, and degree of sedation at beginning of therapy and at regular intervals with long-term use. May cause physical and/or psychological dependence. For inpatients, implement safety measures (eg, side rails up, call light within reach, instructions to call for assistance). Assess knowledge/teach patient appropriate use (if self-administered). Teach patient to monitor for adverse reactions, adverse reactions to report, and appropriate interventions to reduce side effects. Discontinue slowly after prolonged use.

Patient Education: If self-administered, use exactly as directed; do not increase dose or frequency. Drug may cause physical and/or psychological dependence. While using this medication, do not use alcohol and other prescription or OTC medications (especially sedatives, tranquilizers, antihistamines, or (Continued)

Methadone *(Continued)*

pain medications) without consulting prescriber. Maintain adequate hydration (2-3 L/day of fluids) unless instructed to restrict fluid intake. May cause hypotension, dizziness, drowsiness, impaired coordination, or blurred vision (use caution when driving, climbing stairs, or changing position - rising from sitting or lying to standing, or when engaging in tasks requiring alertness until response to drug is known); loss of appetite, nausea, or vomiting (frequent mouth care, small frequent meals, chewing gum, or sucking lozenges may help); or constipation (increased exercise, fluids, fruit, or fiber may help; if unresolved, consult prescriber about use of stool softeners). Report chest pain, slow or rapid heartbeat, acute dizziness or persistent headache; changes in mental status; swelling of extremities or unusual weight gain; changes in urinary elimination; acute headache; back or flank pain or muscle spasms; blurred vision; skin rash; or shortness of breath. **Pregnancy/breast-feeding precautions:** Inform prescriber if you are or intend to become pregnant. If you are breast-feeding, consult prescriber.

Geriatric Considerations Because of its long half-life and risk of accumulation, methadone is not considered a drug of first choice in the elderly. The elderly may be particularly susceptible to the CNS depressant and constipating effects of narcotics. Adjust dose for renal function.

Breast-Feeding Issues Peak methadone levels appear in breast milk 4-5 hours after an oral dose. Methadone has been detected in the plasma of some breast-fed infants whose mothers are taking methadone. Use during breast-feeding is not recommended, and the manufacturer recommends that women on high dose methadone maintenance who already are breast-feeding be instructed to wean breast-feeding gradually to avoid neonatal abstinence syndrome. Unless otherwise contraindicated (concurrent medical conditions, other medications of abuse), the AAP rates methadone "compatible" with breast-feeding.

Pregnancy Issues Teratogenic effects have been observed in some, but not all, animal studies. Data collected by the Teratogen Information System are complicated by maternal use of illicit drugs, nutrition, infection, and psychosocial circumstances. However, pregnant women in methadone treatment programs are reported to have improved fetal outcomes compared to pregnant women using illicit drugs. Methadone can be detected in the amniotic fluid, cord plasma, and newborn urine. Fetal growth, birth weight, length, and/or head circumference may be decreased in infants born to narcotic-addicted mothers treated with methadone during pregnancy. Growth deficits do not appear to persist; however, decreased performance on psychometric and behavioral tests has been found to continue into childhood. Abnormal fetal nonstress tests have also been reported. Withdrawal symptoms in the neonate may be observed up to 2-4 weeks after delivery. The manufacturer states that methadone should be used during pregnancy only if clearly needed. Because methadone clearance in pregnant women is increased and half-life is decreased during the 2nd and 3rd trimesters of pregnancy, withdrawal symptoms may be observed in the mother; dosage of methadone may need increased or dosing interval decreased during pregnancy.

Methenamine *(meth EN a meen)*

U.S. Brand Names Hiprex®; Mandelamine®; Urex®

Synonyms Hexamethylenetetramine; Methenamine Hippurate; Methenamine Mandelate

Pharmacologic Category Antibiotic, Miscellaneous

Medication Safety Issues
Sound-alike/look-alike issues:
Methenamine may be confused with methazolamide, methionine
Urex® may be confused with Eurax®, Serax®

Pregnancy Risk Factor C

Lactation Enters breast milk/compatible

Use Prophylaxis or suppression of recurrent urinary tract infections; urinary tract discomfort secondary to hypermotility

Mechanism of Action/Effect Methenamine is hydrolyzed to formaldehyde and ammonia in acidic urine; formaldehyde has nonspecific bactericidal action

Contraindications Hypersensitivity to methenamine or any component of the formulation; severe dehydration, renal insufficiency, hepatic insufficiency in patients receiving hippurate salt; concurrent treatment with sulfonamides

Warnings/Precautions Methenamine should not be used to treat infections outside of the lower urinary tract. Use with caution in patients with hepatic disease, gout, and the elderly; doses of 8 g/day for 3-4 weeks may cause bladder irritation. Use care to maintain an acid pH of the urine, especially when treating infections due to urea splitting organisms (eg, *Proteus* and strains of *Pseudomonas*); reversible increases in LFTs have occurred during therapy especially in patients with hepatic dysfunction. Hiprex® contains tartrazine dye.

Drug Interactions
Decreased Effect: Sodium bicarbonate and acetazolamide will decrease effect secondary to alkalinization of urine.
Increased Effect/Toxicity: Sulfonamides may precipitate in the urine; concurrent use is contraindicated.

Nutritional/Ethanol Interactions Food: Foods/diets which alkalinize urine pH >5.5 decrease therapeutic effect of methenamine.

Lab Interactions Increased catecholamines and VMA (U); decreased HIAA (U)

Adverse Reactions 1% to 10%:
Dermatologic: Rash (<4%)
Gastrointestinal: Nausea, dyspepsia (<4%)
Genitourinary: Dysuria (<4%)

Overdosage/Toxicology The drug is well tolerated. Treatment is supportive.

Pharmacodynamics/Kinetics
Half-Life Elimination: 3-6 hours
Metabolism: Gastric juices: Hydrolyze 10% to 30% unless protected via enteric coating; Hepatic: ~10% to 25%
Excretion: Urine (~70% to 90% as unchanged drug) within 24 hours

Available Dosage Forms
Tablet, as hippurate (Hiprex®, Urex®): 1 g [Hiprex® contains tartrazine dye]
Tablet, enteric coated, as mandelate (Mandelamine®): 500 mg, 1 g

Dosing
Adults & Elderly: Urinary tract infection: Oral:
Hippurate: 0.5-1 g twice daily
Mandelate: 1 g 4 times/day after meals and at bedtime
Pediatrics: Oral:
>2-6 years: *Mandelate:* 50-75 mg/kg/day in 3-4 doses or 0.25 g/30 lb 4 times/day
6-12 years:
Hippurate: 0.5-1 g twice daily

Mandelate: 50-75 mg/kg/day in 3-4 doses or 0.5 g 4 times/day

>12 years: Refer to adult dosing.

Renal Impairment: Cl_{cr} <50 mL/minute: Avoid use.

Administration
Oral: Administer around-the-clock to promote less variation in effect. Foods/diets which alkalinize urine pH >5.5 decrease activity of methenamine.

Stability
Storage: Protect from excessive heat

Laboratory Monitoring Urinalysis, periodic liver function

Nursing Actions
Physical Assessment: Assess potential for interactions with other pharmacological agents patient may be taking (eg, anything that alkalizes urine or sulfonamides). Monitor therapeutic effectiveness (urinalysis — indicates resolution of infection) and adverse response. Teach patient proper use, possible side effects/appropriate interventions, and adverse symptoms to report.

Patient Education: Do not take any new medication during therapy unless approved by prescriber. Take per recommended schedule, at regular intervals around-the-clock. Complete full course of therapy; do not skip doses. Maintain adequate hydration (2-3 L/day of fluids) unless instructed to restrict fluid intake. Avoid excessive citrus fruits, milk, or alkalizing medications. May cause nausea or vomiting or GI upset (small, frequent meals, frequent mouth care, sucking lozenges, or chewing gum may help). Report pain on urination or blood in urine, skin rash, other persistent adverse effects, or if condition does not improve. **Pregnancy precaution:** Inform prescriber if you are or intend to become pregnant.

Dietary Considerations Foods/diets which alkalinize urine pH >5.5 decrease activity of methenamine; cranberry juice can be used to acidify urine and increase activity of methenamine. Hiprex® contains tartrazine dye.

Geriatric Considerations Methenamine has little, if any, role in the treatment or prevention of infections in patients with indwelling urinary (Foley) catheters. Furthermore, in noncatheterized patients, more effective antibiotics are available for the prevention or treatment of urinary tract infections. The influence of decreased renal function on the pharmacologic effects of methenamine results are unknown.

Breast-Feeding Issues The concentration of methenamine hippurate in breast milk is approximately the same as that in the maternal plasma. The amount ingested by a breast-feeding infant is considered to be below a therapeutic dose.

Additional Information Should not be used to treat infections outside of the lower urinary tract. Methenamine has little, if any, role in the treatment or prevention of infections in patients with indwelling urinary (Foley) catheters. Furthermore, in noncatheterized patients, more effective antibiotics are available for the prevention or treatment of urinary tract infections. The influence of decreased renal function on the pharmacologic effects of methenamine results are unknown.

Methimazole (meth IM a zole)

U.S. Brand Names Tapazole®

Synonyms Thiamazole

Pharmacologic Category Antithyroid Agent

Medication Safety Issues
Sound-alike/look-alike issues:
Methimazole may be confused with metolazone

Pregnancy Risk Factor D

Lactation Enters breast milk/contraindicated (AAP rates "compatible")

Use Palliative treatment of hyperthyroidism, return the hyperthyroid patient to a normal metabolic state prior to thyroidectomy, and to control thyrotoxic crisis that may accompany thyroidectomy. The use of antithyroid thioamides is as effective in elderly as they are in younger adults; however, the expense, potential adverse effects, and inconvenience (compliance, monitoring) make them undesirable. The use of radioiodine due to ease of administration and less concern for long-term side effects and reproduction problems (some older males) makes it a more appropriate therapy.

Mechanism of Action/Effect Inhibits the synthesis of thyroid hormones by blocking the oxidation of iodine in the thyroid gland, blocking iodine's ability to combine with tyrosine to form thyroxine and triiodothyronine (T_3), does not inactivate circulating T_4 and T_3

Contraindications Hypersensitivity to methimazole or any component of the formulation; nursing mothers (per manufacturer; however, expert analysis and the AAP state this drug may be used with caution in nursing mothers); pregnancy

Warnings/Precautions Use with extreme caution in patients receiving other drugs known to cause myelosuppression particularly agranulocytosis, patients >40 years of age. Avoid doses >40 mg/day (increased myelosuppression). May cause acneiform eruptions or worsen the condition of the thyroid.

Drug Interactions

Cytochrome P450 Effect: Inhibits CYP1A2 (weak), 2A6 (weak), 2B6 (weak), 2C8/9 (weak), 2C19 (weak), 2D6 (moderate), 2E1 (weak), 3A4 (weak)

Decreased Effect: Anticoagulant effect of warfarin may be decreased. Methimazole may decrease the levels/effects of CYP2D6 prodrug substrates (eg, codeine, hydrocodone, oxycodone, tramadol).

Increased Effect/Toxicity: Dosage of some drugs (including beta-blockers, digoxin, and theophylline) require adjustment during treatment of hyperthyroidism. Methimazole may increase the levels/effects of CYP2D6 substrates (eg, amphetamines, selected beta-blockers, dextromethorphan, fluoxetine, lidocaine, mirtazapine, nefazodone, paroxetine, risperidone, ritonavir, thioridazine, tricyclic antidepressants, venlafaxine).

Adverse Reactions Frequency not defined.

Cardiovascular: Edema

Central nervous system: Headache, vertigo, drowsiness, CNS stimulation, depression

Dermatologic: Skin rash, urticaria, pruritus, erythema nodosum, skin pigmentation, exfoliative dermatitis, alopecia

Endocrine & metabolic: Goiter

Gastrointestinal: Nausea, vomiting, stomach pain, abnormal taste, constipation, weight gain, salivary gland swelling

Hematologic: Leukopenia, agranulocytosis, granulocytopenia, thrombocytopenia, aplastic anemia, hypoprothrombinemia

Hepatic: Cholestatic jaundice, jaundice, hepatitis

Neuromuscular & skeletal: Arthralgia, paresthesia

Renal: Nephrotic syndrome

Miscellaneous: SLE-like syndrome

Overdosage/Toxicology Symptoms of overdose include nausea, vomiting, epigastric distress, headache, fever, arthralgia, pruritus, edema, pancytopenia, and signs of hypothyroidism. Management of overdose is supportive.

Pharmacodynamics/Kinetics

Onset of Action: Antithyroid: Oral: 12-18 hours

Duration of Action: 36-72 hours

Protein Binding: Plasma: None

Half-Life Elimination: 4-13 hours

Metabolism: Hepatic

Excretion: Urine (80%)

Available Dosage Forms
Tablet: 5 mg, 10 mg, 20 mg
(Continued)

Methimazole (Continued)

Tapazole® 5 mg, 10 mg

Dosing

Adults & Elderly:

Hyperthyroidism: Oral: Administer in 3 equally divided doses at approximately 8-hour intervals

Initial: 15 mg/day for mild hyperthyroidism; 30-40 mg/day in moderately severe hyperthyroidism; 60 mg/day in severe hyperthyroidism; maintenance: 5-15 mg/day

Adjustment: Adjust dosage as required to achieve and maintain serum T_3, T_4, and TSH levels in the normal range. An elevated T_3 may be the sole indicator of inadequate treatment. An elevated TSH indicates excessive antithyroid treatment.

Pediatrics: Note: Administer in 3 equally divided doses at ~8-hour intervals.

Hyperthyroidism: Oral:

Initial: 0.4 mg/kg/day in 3 divided doses; maintenance: 0.2 mg/kg/day in 3 divided doses up to 30 mg/24 hours maximum

Alternatively: Initial: 0.5-0.7 mg/kg/day **or** 15-20 mg/m²/day in 3 divided doses

Maintenance: 1/3 to 2/3 of the initial dose beginning when the patient is euthyroid

Maximum: 30 mg/24 hours

Stability

Storage: Protect from light.

Laboratory Monitoring T_4, T_3, CBC with differential, liver function (baseline and as needed), serum thyroxine, free thyroxine index

Nursing Actions

Physical Assessment: Assess potential for interactions with other pharmacological agents patient may be taking (eg, extreme caution with anything that may cause myelosuppression; may increase or decrease levels/effects of other agents). Assess results of laboratory tests at baseline and periodically. Evaluate therapeutic effectiveness (clinical and laboratory indicators) and adverse reactions (eg, hyper-/hypothyroidism, rash, gastrointestinal upset, leukopenia, anemia, arthralgia) during therapy. Teach patient proper use, possible side effects/appropriate interventions, and adverse symptoms to report.

Patient Education: Do not take any new medication during therapy unless approved by prescriber. Take as directed, at the same time each day, around-the-clock (eg, every 8 hours). Do not miss doses or make up missed doses. This drug will need to be taken for an extended period of time to achieve appropriate results. May cause nausea or vomiting (small, frequent meals may help); or dizziness or drowsiness (use caution when driving or engaging in tasks that require alertness until response to drug is known). Report rash, fever, unusual bleeding or bruising, unresolved headache, yellowing of eyes or skin, changes in color of urine or feces, or unresolved malaise. **Pregnancy/breast-feeding precautions:** Inform prescriber if you are pregnant and do not get pregnant while taking this medicine. Consult prescriber for appropriate contraceptive measures. Consult prescriber if breast-feeding.

Dietary Considerations Should be taken consistently in relation to meals every day.

Geriatric Considerations The use of antithyroid thioamides is as effective in the elderly as in younger adults; however, the expense, potential adverse effects, and inconvenience (compliance, monitoring) make them undesirable.

Breast-Feeding Issues Use with caution; consider monitoring thyroid function in the infant (weekly or biweekly)

Pregnancy Issues Hypothyroidism and congenital defects (rare) may occur.

Methocarbamol (meth oh KAR ba mole)

U.S. Brand Names Robaxin®

Pharmacologic Category Skeletal Muscle Relaxant

Medication Safety Issues

Sound-alike/look-alike issues:

Methocarbamol may be confused with mephobarbital

Robaxin® may be confused with Rubex®

Pregnancy Risk Factor C

Lactation Excretion in breast milk unknown/use caution

Use Treatment of muscle spasm associated with acute painful musculoskeletal conditions; supportive therapy in tetanus

Mechanism of Action/Effect Causes skeletal muscle relaxation by general CNS depression

Contraindications Hypersensitivity to methocarbamol or any component of the formulation; renal impairment (injection formulation)

Warnings/Precautions

Oral: Use caution with renal or hepatic impairment.

Injection: Rate of injection should not exceed 3 mL/minute; solution is hypertonic; avoid extravasation. Use with caution in patients with a history of seizures. Use caution with hepatic impairment.

Drug Interactions

Increased Effect/Toxicity: Increased effect/toxicity with CNS depressants.

Nutritional/Ethanol Interactions

Ethanol: Avoid ethanol (may increase CNS depression).

Herb/Nutraceutical: Avoid valerian, St John's wort, kava kava, gotu kola (may increase CNS depression).

Lab Interactions May cause color interference in certain screening tests for 5-HIAA using nitrosonaphthol reagent and in screening tests for urinary VMA using the Gitlow method.

Adverse Reactions Frequency not defined.

Cardiovascular: Flushing of face, bradycardia, hypotension, syncope

Central nervous system: Drowsiness, dizziness, lightheadedness, convulsion, vertigo, headache, fever, amnesia, confusion, insomnia, sedation, coordination impaired (mild)

Dermatologic: Allergic dermatitis, urticaria, pruritus, rash, angioneurotic edema

Gastrointestinal: Nausea, vomiting, metallic taste, dyspepsia

Hematologic: Leukopenia

Hepatic: Jaundice

Local: Pain at injection site, thrombophlebitis

Ocular: Nystagmus, blurred vision, diplopia, conjunctivitis

Renal: Renal impairment

Respiratory: Nasal congestion

Miscellaneous: Allergic manifestations, anaphylactic reaction

Overdosage/Toxicology Symptoms of overdose include cardiac arrhythmias, nausea, vomiting, drowsiness, and coma. Treatment is supportive.

Pharmacodynamics/Kinetics

Onset of Action: Muscle relaxation: Oral: ~30 minutes

Time to Peak: Serum: ~2 hours

Protein Binding: 46% to 50%

Half-Life Elimination: 1-2 hours

Metabolism: Hepatic via dealkylation and hydroxylation

Excretion: Urine (as metabolites)

Available Dosage Forms

Injection, solution: 100 mg/mL (10 mL) [in polyethylene glycol; vial stopper contains latex]

Tablet: 500 mg, 750 mg

Dosing

Adults:

Muscle spasm:

Oral: 1.5 g 4 times/day for 2-3 days (up to 8 g/day may be given in severe conditions), then decrease to 4-4.5 g/day in 3-6 divided doses

I.M., I.V.: 1 g every 8 hours if oral not possible; injection should not be used for more than 3 consecutive days. If condition persists, may repeat course of therapy after a drug-free interval of 48 hours.

Tetanus: I.V.: Initial dose: 1-3 g; may repeat dose every 6 hours until oral dosing is possible; injection should not be used for more than 3 consecutive days

Elderly: Muscle spasm: Oral: Initial: 500 mg 4 times/day; titrate to response

Pediatrics:

Tetanus (recommended **only** for use in tetanus): I.V.: 15 mg/kg/dose or 500 mg/m²/dose, may repeat every 6 hours if needed; maximum dose: 1.8 g/m²/day for 3 days only

Muscle spasm: Children ≥16 years: Refer to adult dosing.

Renal Impairment: Do not administer parenteral formulation to patients with renal dysfunction.

Hepatic Impairment: Specific dosing guidelines are not available. Plasma protein binding and clearance are decreased; half-life is increased.

Administration

Oral: Tablets may be crushed and mixed with food or liquid if needed. Avoid alcohol.

I.M.: A maximum of 5 mL can be administered into each gluteal region.

I.V.: Maximum rate: 3 mL/minute; injection should not be used for more than 3 consecutive days; may be administered undiluted

I.V. Detail: Monitor closely for extravasation. Administer I.V. while in recumbent position. Maintain position 15-30 minutes following infusion.

Stability

Reconstitution: Injection may be diluted to 4 mg/mL in sterile water, 5% dextrose, or 0.9% saline.

Storage:

Injection: Prior to dilution, store at controlled room temperature of 20°C to 25°C (68°F to 77°F). Injection when diluted to 4 mg/mL in sterile water, 5% dextrose, or 0.9% saline is stable for 6 days at room temperature; do **not** refrigerate after dilution

Tablet: Store at controlled room temperature of 20°C to 25°C (68°F to 77°F).

Nursing Actions

Physical Assessment: Assess other medications for excess CNS depression. Monitor effectiveness of therapy (according to rationale for therapy) and adverse reactions at beginning and periodically during therapy. Monitor I.V. site closely to prevent extravasation. Assess knowledge/teach patient appropriate use, interventions to reduce side effects (postural hypotension precautions), and adverse symptoms to report.

Patient Education: Take exactly as directed. Do not increase dose or discontinue without consulting prescriber. Do not use alcohol, prescriptive or OTC antidepressants, sedatives, or pain medications without consulting prescriber. You may experience drowsiness, dizziness, lightheadedness (avoid driving or engaging in tasks requiring alertness until response to drug is known); or nausea or vomiting (small frequent meals, frequent mouth care, or sucking hard candy may help). Report excessive drowsiness or mental agitation, chest pain, skin rash, swelling of mouth/face, difficulty speaking, or vision changes. **Pregnancy/breast-feeding precautions:** Inform prescriber if you are or intend to become pregnant. Consult prescriber if breast-feeding.

Geriatric Considerations There is no specific information on the use of skeletal muscle relaxants in the elderly. Methocarbamol has a short half-life, so it may be considered one of the safer agents in this class.

Methotrexate (meth oh TREKS ate)

U.S. Brand Names Rheumatrex®; Trexall™

Synonyms Amethopterin; Methotrexate Sodium; MTX (error-prone abbreviation); NSC-740

Pharmacologic Category Antineoplastic Agent, Antimetabolite (Antifolate)

Medication Safety Issues

Sound-alike/look-alike issues:

Methotrexate may be confused with metolazone, mitoxantrone

MTX is an error-prone abbreviation (mistaken as mitoxantrone)

High alert medication: The Institute for Safe Medication Practices (ISMP) includes this medication among its list of drugs which have a heightened risk of causing significant patient harm when used in error.

Errors have occurred (resulting in death) when oral methotrexate was administered as "daily" dose instead of the recommended "weekly" dose.

Pregnancy Risk Factor X (psoriasis, rheumatoid arthritis)

Lactation Enters breast milk/contraindicated

Use Treatment of trophoblastic neoplasms; leukemias; psoriasis; rheumatoid arthritis (RA), including polyarticular-course juvenile rheumatoid arthritis (JRA); breast, head and neck, and lung carcinomas; osteosarcoma; soft-tissue sarcomas; carcinoma of gastrointestinal tract, esophagus, testes; lymphomas

Unlabeled/Investigational Use

Treatment and maintenance of remission in Crohn's disease

Mechanism of Action/Effect Methotrexate is a folate antimetabolite that inhibits DNA synthesis. Methotrexate irreversibly binds to dihydrofolate reductase, inhibiting the formation of reduced folates, and thymidylate synthetase, resulting in inhibition of purine and thymidylic acid synthesis. Methotrexate is cell cycle specific for the S phase of the cycle.

The MOA in the treatment of rheumatoid arthritis is unknown, but may affect immune function. In psoriasis, methotrexate is thought to target rapidly proliferating epithelial cells in the skin.

In Crohn's disease, it may have immune modulator and anti-inflammatory activity

Contraindications Hypersensitivity to methotrexate or any component of the formulation; severe renal or hepatic impairment; pre-existing profound bone marrow suppression in patients with psoriasis or rheumatoid arthritis, alcoholic liver disease, AIDS, pre-existing blood dyscrasias; pregnancy (in patients with psoriasis or rheumatoid arthritis); breast-feeding

Warnings/Precautions Hazardous agent - use appropriate precautions for handling and disposal. May cause potentially life-threatening pneumonitis (may occur at any time during therapy and at any dosage); monitor closely for pulmonary symptoms, particularly dry, nonproductive cough. Methotrexate may cause photosensitivity and/or severe dermatologic reactions which are not dose-related. Methotrexate has been associated with acute and chronic hepatotoxicity, fibrosis, and cirrhosis. Risk is related to cumulative dose and prolonged exposure. Ethanol abuse, obesity, advanced age, and diabetes may increase the risk of hepatotoxic reactions.

Methotrexate may cause renal failure, gastrointestinal toxicity, or bone marrow depression. Use with caution in (Continued)

Methotrexate *(Continued)*

patients with renal impairment, peptic ulcer disease, ulcerative colitis, or pre-existing bone marrow suppression. Diarrhea and ulcerative stomatitis may require interruption of therapy; death from hemorrhagic enteritis or intestinal perforation has been reported. Methotrexate penetrates slowly into 3rd space fluids, such as pleural effusions or ascites, and exits slowly from these compartments (slower than from plasma). Dosage reduction may be necessary in patients with renal or hepatic impairment, ascites, and pleural effusion. Toxicity from methotrexate or any immunosuppressive is increased in the elderly.

Severe bone marrow suppression, aplastic anemia, and GI toxicity have occurred during concomitant administration with NSAIDs. Use caution when used with other hepatotoxic agents (azathioprine, retinoids, sulfasalazine). Methotrexate given concomitantly with radiotherapy may increase the risk of soft tissue necrosis and osteonecrosis. Immune suppression may lead to opportunistic infections.

For rheumatoid arthritis and psoriasis, immunosuppressive therapy should only be used when disease is active and less toxic; traditional therapy is ineffective. Discontinue therapy in RA or psoriasis if a significant decrease in hematologic components is noted. Methotrexate formulations and/or diluents containing preservatives should not be used for intrathecal or high-dose therapy. Methotrexate injection may contain benzyl alcohol and should not be used in neonates.

Drug Interactions

Decreased Effect: Cholestyramine may decrease levels of methotrexate. Corticosteroids may decrease uptake of methotrexate into leukemia cells. Administration of these drugs should be separated by 12 hours. Dexamethasone has been reported to not affect methotrexate influx into cells.

Increased Effect/Toxicity: Concurrent therapy with NSAIDs has resulted in severe bone marrow suppression, aplastic anemia, and GI toxicity. NSAIDs should not be used during moderate or high-dose methotrexate due to increased and prolonged methotrexate levels (may increase toxicity); NSAID use during treatment of rheumatoid arthritis has not been fully explored, but continuation of prior regimen has been allowed in some circumstances, with cautious monitoring. Salicylates may increase methotrexate levels, however salicylate doses used for prophylaxis of cardiovascular events are not likely to be of concern.

Penicillins, probenecid, sulfonamides, tetracyclines may increase methotrexate concentrations due to a reduction in renal tubular secretion; primarily a concern with high doses of methotrexate. Hepatotoxic agents (acitretin, azathioprine, retinoids, sulfasalazine) may increase the risk of hepatotoxic reactions with methotrexate.

Concomitant administration of cyclosporine with methotrexate may increase levels and toxicity of each. Methotrexate may increase mercaptopurine or theophylline levels. Methotrexate, when administered prior to cytarabine, may enhance the efficacy and toxicity of cytarabine; some combination treatment regimens (eg, hyper-CVAD) have been designed to take advantage of this interaction.

Concurrent use of live virus vaccines may result in infections.

Nutritional/Ethanol Interactions

Ethanol: Avoid ethanol (may be associated with increased liver injury).

Food: Methotrexate peak serum levels may be decreased if taken with food. Milk-rich foods may decrease methotrexate absorption. Folate may decrease drug response.

Herb/Nutraceutical: Avoid echinacea (has immunostimulant properties).

Adverse Reactions Note: Adverse reactions vary by route and dosage. Hematologic and/or gastrointestinal toxicities may be common at dosages used in chemotherapy; these reactions are much less frequent when used at typical dosages for rheumatic diseases.

>10%:

Central nervous system (with I.T. administration or very high-dose therapy):

Arachnoiditis: Acute reaction manifested as severe headache, nuchal rigidity, vomiting, and fever; may be alleviated by reducing the dose

Subacute toxicity: 10% of patients treated with 12-15 mg/m^2 of I.T. methotrexate may develop this in the second or third week of therapy; consists of motor paralysis of extremities, cranial nerve palsy, seizure, or coma. This has also been seen in pediatric cases receiving very high-dose I.V. methotrexate.

Demyelinating encephalopathy: Seen months or years after receiving methotrexate; usually in association with cranial irradiation or other systemic chemotherapy

Dermatologic: Reddening of skin

Endocrine & metabolic: Hyperuricemia, defective oogenesis or spermatogenesis

Gastrointestinal: Ulcerative stomatitis, glossitis, gingivitis, nausea, vomiting, diarrhea, anorexia, intestinal perforation, mucositis (dose dependent; appears in 3-7 days after therapy, resolving within 2 weeks)

Hematologic: Leukopenia, thrombocytopenia

Renal: Renal failure, azotemia, nephropathy

Respiratory: Pharyngitis

1% to 10%:

Cardiovascular: Vasculitis

Central nervous system: Dizziness, malaise, encephalopathy, seizure, fever, chills

Dermatologic: Alopecia, rash, photosensitivity, depigmentation or hyperpigmentation of skin

Endocrine & metabolic: Diabetes

Genitourinary: Cystitis

Hematologic: Hemorrhage

Myelosuppressive: This is the primary dose-limiting factor (along with mucositis) of methotrexate; occurs about 5-7 days after methotrexate therapy, and should resolve within 2 weeks

WBC: Mild

Platelets: Moderate

Onset: 7 days

Nadir: 10 days

Recovery: 21 days

Hepatic: Cirrhosis and portal fibrosis have been associated with chronic methotrexate therapy; acute elevation of liver enzymes are common after high-dose methotrexate, and usually resolve within 10 days.

Neuromuscular & skeletal: Arthralgia

Ocular: Blurred vision

Renal: Renal dysfunction: Manifested by an abrupt rise in serum creatinine and BUN and a fall in urine output; more common with high-dose methotrexate, and may be due to precipitation of the drug.

Respiratory: Pneumonitis: Associated with fever, cough, and interstitial pulmonary infiltrates; treatment is to withhold methotrexate during the acute reaction; interstitial pneumonitis has been reported to occur with an incidence of 1% in patients with RA (dose 7.5-15 mg/week)

Overdosage/Toxicology Symptoms of overdose include nausea, vomiting, alopecia, melena, and renal failure. Administer leucovorin (see Dosing).

Hydration and alkalinization may be used to prevent precipitation of methotrexate or methotrexate metabolites in the renal tubules. Severe bone marrow toxicity can result from overdose. Generally, neither peritoneal nor hemodialysis have been shown to increase elimination. However, effective clearance of methotrexate has been reported with acute, intermittent hemodialysis using a high-flux dialyzer.

Pharmacodynamics/Kinetics

Onset of Action: Antirheumatic: 3-6 weeks; additional improvement may continue longer than 12 weeks

Time to Peak: Serum: Oral: 1-2 hours; I.M.: 30-60 minutes

Protein Binding: 50%

Half-Life Elimination: Low dose: 3-10 hours; High dose: 8-12 hours

Metabolism: <10%; degraded by intestinal flora to DAMPA by carboxypeptidase; hepatic aldehyde oxidase converts methotrexate to 7-OH methotrexate; polyglutamates are produced intracellularly and are just as potent as methotrexate; their production is dose- and duration-dependent and they are slowly eliminated by the cell once formed

Excretion: Urine (44% to 100%); feces (small amounts)

Available Dosage Forms

Injection, powder for reconstitution [preservative free]: 20 mg, 1 g

Injection, solution: 25 mg/mL (2 mL, 10 mL) [contains benzyl alcohol]

Injection, solution [preservative free]: 25 mg/mL (2 mL, 4 mL, 8 mL, 10 mL)

Tablet: 2.5 mg

Trexall™: 5 mg, 7.5 mg, 10 mg, 15 mg

Tablet, as sodium [dose pack] (Rheumatrex® Dose Pack): 2.5 mg (4 cards with 2, 3, 4, 5, or 6 tablets each)

Dosing

Adults: Refer to individual protocols.

Note: Doses between 100-500 mg/m² **may require** leucovorin rescue. Doses >500 mg/m² **require** leucovorin rescue: I.V., I.M., Oral: Leucovorin 10-15 mg/m² every 6 hours for 8 or 10 doses, starting 24 hours after the start of methotrexate infusion. Continue until the methotrexate level is ≤0.1 micromolar (10⁻⁷M). Some clinicians continue leucovorin until the methotrexate level is <0.05 micromolar (5 x 10⁻⁸M) or 0.01 micromolar (10⁻⁸M).

If the 48-hour methotrexate level is >1 micromolar (10⁻⁷M) or the 72-hour methotrexate level is >0.2 micromolar (2 x 10⁻⁷M): I.V., I.M, Oral: Leucovorin 100 mg/m² every 6 hours until the methotrexate level is ≤0.1 micromolar (10⁻⁷M). Some clinicians continue leucovorin until the methotrexate level is <0.05 micromolar (5 x 10⁻⁸M) or 0.01 micromolar (10⁻⁸M).

Antineoplastic dosage range: I.V.: Range is wide from 30-40 mg/m²/week to 100-12,000 mg/m² with leucovorin rescue

Trophoblastic neoplasms:

Oral, I.M.: 15-30 mg/day for 5 days; repeat in 7 days for 3-5 courses

I.V.: 11 mg/m² days 1 through 5 every 3 weeks

Head and neck cancer: Oral, I.M., I.V.: 25-50 mg/m² once weekly

Mycosis fungoides (cutaneous T-cell lymphoma):

Oral, I.M.: Initial (early stages):

5-50 mg once weekly **or**

15-37.5 mg twice weekly

Bladder cancer: I.V.:

30 mg/m² day 1 and 8 every 3 weeks **or**

30 mg/m² day 1, 15, and 22 every 4 weeks

Breast cancer: I.V.: 30-60 mg/m² Day 1 and 8 every 3-4 weeks

Gastric cancer: I.V.:1500 mg/m² every 4 weeks

Lymphoma, non-Hodgkin's: I.V.:

30 mg/m² days 3 and 10 every 3 weeks **or**

120 mg/m² day 8 and 15 every 3 weeks **or**

200 mg/m² day 8 and 15 every 3 weeks **or**

400 mg/m² every 4 weeks for 3 cycles **or**

1 g/m² every 3 weeks **or**

1.5 g/m² every 4 weeks

Sarcoma: I.V.: 8-12 g/m² weekly for 2-4 weeks

Rheumatoid arthritis: Oral: 7.5 mg once weekly **or** 2.5 mg every 12 hours for 3 doses/week, not to exceed 20 mg/week

Psoriasis: Oral: 2.5-5 mg/dose every 12 hours for 3 doses given weekly **or** Oral, I.M.: 10-25 mg/dose given once weekly

Ectopic pregnancy: I.M., I.V.: 50 mg/m² single-dose

Active Crohn's disease (unlabeled use): Induction of remission: I.M., SubQ: 15-25 mg once weekly; remission maintenance: 15 mg once weekly

Note: Oral dosing has been reported as effective but oral absorption is highly variable. If patient relapses after a switch to oral, may consider returning to injectable.

Elderly: Refer to individual protocols; adjust for renal impairment.

Rheumatoid arthritis/psoriasis: Oral: Initial: 5-7.5 mg/week, not to exceed 20 mg/week

Pediatrics: Refer to individual protocols.

Note: Doses between 100-500 mg/m² **may require** leucovorin rescue. Doses >500 mg/m² **require** leucovorin rescue: I.V., I.M., Oral: Leucovorin 10-15 mg/m² every 6 hours for 8 or 10 doses, starting 24 hours after the start of methotrexate infusion. Continue until the methotrexate level is ≤0.1 micromolar (10⁻⁷M). Some clinicians continue leucovorin until the methotrexate level is <0.05 micromolar (5 x 10⁻⁸M) or 0.01 micromolar (10⁻⁸M).

If the 48-hour methotrexate level is >1 micromolar (10⁻⁷M) or the 72-hour methotrexate level is >0.2 micromolar (2 x 10⁻⁷M): I.V., I.M, Oral: Leucovorin 100 mg/m² every 6 hours until the methotrexate level is ≤0.1 micromolar (10⁻⁷M). Some clinicians continue leucovorin until the methotrexate level is <0.05 micromolar (5 x 10⁻⁸M) or 0.01 micromolar (10⁻⁸M).

Dermatomyositis: Oral: 15-20 mg/m²/week as a single dose once weekly **or** 0.3-1 mg/kg/dose once weekly

Juvenile rheumatoid arthritis: Oral, I.M.:10 mg/m² once weekly, then 5-15 mg/m²/week as a single dose **or** as 3 divided doses given 12 hours apart

Antineoplastic dosage range:

Oral, I.M.: 7.5-30 mg/m²/week **or** every 2 weeks

I.V.: 10-18,000 mg/m² bolus dosing **or** continuous infusion over 6-42 hours

For dosing schedules, see table.

Methotrexate Dosing Schedules

Dose	Route	Frequency
Conventional		
15-20 mg/m²	P.O.	Twice weekly
30-50 mg/m²	P.O., I.V.	Weekly
15 mg/day for 5 days	P.O., I.M.	Every 2-3 weeks
Intermediate		
50-150 mg/m²*	I.V. push	Every 2-3 weeks
240 mg/m²*	I.V. infusion	Every 4-7 days
0.5-1 g/m²**	I.V. infusion	Every 2-3 weeks
High		
1-25 g/m²*	I.V. infusion	Every 1-3 weeks

*Doses between 100-500 mg/m² may require leucovorin rescue in some patients.

**Followed with leucovorin rescue - refer to Leucovorin monograph for details.

Pediatric solid tumors (high-dose): I.V.:

<12 years: 12-25 g/m²

≥12 years: 8 g/m²

(Continued)

Methotrexate *(Continued)*

Acute lymphocytic leukemia (intermediate-dose):
I.V.: Loading: 100 mg/m² bolus dose, followed by 900 mg/m²/day infusion over 23-41 hours.

Meningeal leukemia: I.T.: 10-15 mg/m² (maximum dose: 15 mg) **or** an age-based dosing regimen; one possible system is:

≤3 months: 3 mg/dose
4-11 months: 6 mg/dose
1 year: 8 mg/dose
2 years: 10 mg/dose
≥3 years: 12 mg/dose

Renal Impairment:

Cl$_{cr}$ 61-80 mL/minute: Reduce dose to 75%.
Cl$_{cr}$ 51-60 mL/minute: Reduce dose to 70%.
Cl$_{cr}$ 10-50 mL/minute: Reduce dose to 30% to 50%.
Cl$_{cr}$ <10 mL/minute: Avoid use.
Hemodialysis effects: Not dialyzable (0% to 5%)
Supplemental dose is not necessary.
Peritoneal dialysis effects: Supplemental dose is not necessary.
CAVH effects: Unknown

Hepatic Impairment:

Bilirubin 3.1-5 mg/dL or AST >180 units: Administer 75% of dose.
Bilirubin >5 mg/dL: Do not use.

Administration

I.M.: May be administered I.M.

I.V.: May be administered I.V.; I.V. administration may be as slow push, short bolus infusion, or 24- to 42-hour continuous infusion

Specific dosing schemes vary, but high dose should be followed by leucovorin calcium to prevent toxicity; refer to Leucovorin monograph *on page 717*

Other: May be administered I.T.

Stability

Reconstitution: Dilute powder with D₅W or NS to a concentration of ≤25 mg/mL (20 mg and 50 mg vials) and 50 mg/mL (1 g vial). Intrathecal solutions may be reconstituted to 2.5-5 mg/mL with NS, D₅W, lactated Ringer's, or Elliott's B solution. **Use preservative free preparations for intrathecal or high-dose administration.**

Compatibility: Stable in D₅NS, D₅W, NS

Y-site administration: Incompatible with chlorpromazine, gemcitabine, idarubicin, ifosfamide, midazolam, nalbuphine, promethazine, propofol

Compatibility when admixed: Incompatible with bleomycin

Storage: Store tablets and intact vials at room temperature (15°C to 25°C); protect from light. Solution diluted in D₅W or NS is stable for 24 hours at room temperature (21°C to 25°C). Reconstituted solutions with a preservative may be stored under refrigeration for up to 3 months, and up to 4 weeks at room temperature. Intrathecal dilutions are stable at room temperature for 7 days, but it is generally recommended that they be used within 4-8 hours.

Laboratory Monitoring For prolonged use (especially rheumatoid arthritis, psoriasis) a baseline liver biopsy, repeated at each 1-1.5 g cumulative dose interval, should be performed; WBC and platelet counts every 4 weeks; CBC and creatinine, LFTs every 3-4 months; chest x-ray

Nursing Actions

Physical Assessment: Assess potential for interactions with other pharmacological agents and herbal products patient may be using (eg, NSAIDs and salicylates or other hepatotoxic agents, or drugs that may effect the levels/effects of methotrexate). Monitor laboratory tests and adverse reactions frequently (eg, hyper- or hypothyroidism, pneumonitis [dry, nonproductive cough], gastrointestinal disturbance [ulcerative stomatitis, pain, intestinal perforation], renal failure [decreased urine output]). Monitor effectiveness at regular intervals (according to purpose for use). Teach patient proper use, possible side effects/appropriate interventions, and adverse symptoms to report. **Pregnancy risk factor X:** Determine that patient is not pregnant before beginning treatment. Instruct patient of childbearing age (or males who may have intercourse with women of childbearing age) in appropriate use of contraceptive measures during therapy and for 3 months following treatment of males or 1 ovulatory cycle in females.

Patient Education: Do not take any new medication during therapy unless approved by prescriber. **Infusion/injection:** Report immediately any redness, swelling, pain, or burning at infusion/injection site. It is very important to maintain adequate hydration (2-3 L/day of fluids) unless instructed to restrict fluid intake and nutrition (small frequent meals may help). Avoid alcohol to prevent serious side effects. You will be more susceptible to infection (avoid crowds and exposure to infection and do not have any vaccinations without consulting prescriber). May cause sensitivity to sunlight (use sunscreen, wear protective clothing, and eyewear); nausea or vomiting (small frequent meals, frequent mouth care, sucking lozenges, or chewing gum may help; if unresolved, contact prescriber); drowsiness, dizziness, numbness, or blurred vision (use caution when driving or engaging in tasks that require alertness until response to drug is known); loss of hair (may be reversible); color change of skin; permanent sterility; or mouth sores (frequent mouth care with soft toothbrush or cotton swabs and frequent rinses may help). Report immediately any rash, excessive or unusual fatigue, or respiratory difficulty. Report rapid heartbeat or palpitations, black or tarry stools, fever, chills, unusual bleeding or bruising, shortness of breath, persistent GI disturbances, diarrhea, constipation, pain on urination or change in urinary patterns, or any other persistent adverse effects. **Pregnancy/breast-feeding precautions:** Do not get pregnant while taking this medication. Consult prescriber for appropriate contraceptive measures. This drug may cause birth defects. Do not breast-feed.

Dietary Considerations

Sodium content of 100 mg injection: 20 mg (0.86 mEq)
Sodium content of 100 mg (low sodium) injection: 15 mg (0.65 mEq)

Geriatric Considerations Toxicity to methotrexate or any immunosuppressive is increased in the elderly. Must monitor carefully. For rheumatoid arthritis and psoriasis, immunosuppressive therapy should only be used when disease is active and less toxic, traditional therapy is ineffective. Recommended doses should be reduced when initiating therapy in the elderly due to possible decreased metabolism, reduced renal function, and presence of interacting diseases and drugs. Adjust dose as needed for renal function (Cl$_{cr}$).

Additional Information Latex-free products: 50 mg/2 mL, 100 mg/4 mL, and 250 mg/10 mL vials with and without preservatives by Immunex

---

Methoxsalen *(meth OKS a len)*

U.S. Brand Names 8-MOP®; Oxsoralen®; Oxsoralen-Ultra®; Uvadex®

Synonyms Methoxypsoralen; 8-Methoxypsoralen; 8-MOP

Pharmacologic Category Psoralen

Pregnancy Risk Factor C/D (Uvadex®)

Lactation Excretion in breast milk unknown/not recommended

Use

Oral: Symptomatic control of severe, recalcitrant disabling psoriasis; repigmentation of idiopathic vitiligo; palliative treatment of skin manifestations of cutaneous T-cell lymphoma (CTCL)

Topical: Repigmentation of idiopathic vitiligo

Extracorporeal: Palliative treatment of skin manifestations of CTCL

Mechanism of Action/Effect Bonds covalently to pyrimidine bases in DNA, inhibits the synthesis of DNA, and suppresses cell division. The augmented sunburn reaction involves excitation of the methoxsalen molecule by radiation in the long-wave ultraviolet light (UVA), resulting in transference of energy to the methoxsalen molecule producing an excited state ("triplet electronic state"). The molecule, in this "triplet state", then reacts with cutaneous DNA.

Contraindications Hypersensitivity to methoxsalen (psoralens) or any component of the formulation; diseases associated with photosensitivity; cataract; invasive squamous cell cancer; aphakia; melanoma; pregnancy (Uvadex®)

Warnings/Precautions Serious burns may occur from ultraviolet radiation or sunlight even if exposed through glass if dose and/or exposure schedule is not maintained. Therapy may lead to increased risk of melanoma; this risk may be increased with fair skin or prior exposure to prolonged tar and UVB treatment, ionizing radiation, or arsenic. Methoxsalen concentrates in the lens; eyes should be shielded from light for 24 hours to prevent possible formation of cataracts. Soft-gelatin capsules and hard-gelatin capsule are not interchangeable. Use caution with basal cell carcinoma, hepatic, kidney, cardiac disease, or in the elderly. Use caution with other agents that may cause photosensitivity.

CTCL: For use only if inadequate response to other forms of therapy. Used in conjunction with long wave radiation of white blood cells using the UVAR® photopheresis system. Safety and efficacy in pediatric patients have not been established.

Psoriasis: For use only if inadequate response to other therapies when the diagnosis is biopsy proven. Administer only in conjunction with scheduled controlled doses of long wave ultraviolet (UVA) radiation (combination referred to as PUVA). Safety and efficacy in pediatric patients have not been established.

Vitiligo: Used in conjunction with controlled doses of long wave ultraviolet radiation or sunlight. Lotion should only be applied under direct supervision of prescriber and should not be dispensed to the patient. Safety and efficacy in children <12 years of age have not been established.

Drug Interactions

Cytochrome P450 Effect: Substrate of CYP2A6 (minor); **Inhibits** CYP1A2 (strong), 2A6 (strong), 2C8/9 (weak), 2C19 (weak), 2D6 (weak), 2E1 (weak), 3A4 (weak)

Increased Effect/Toxicity: Methoxsalen may increase the levels/effects of CYP1A2 substrates (eg, aminophylline, fluvoxamine, mexiletine, mirtazapine, ropinirole, theophylline, trifluoperazine) and CYP2A6 substrates (eg, dexmedetomidine, ifosfamide).

Nutritional/Ethanol Interactions Food: Methoxsalen serum concentrations may be increased if taken with food. Avoid furocoumarin-containing foods (limes, figs, parsley, celery, cloves, lemon, mustard, carrots).

Adverse Reactions Frequency not always defined.

Cardiovascular: Severe edema, hypotension

Central nervous system: Nervousness, vertigo, depression, dizziness, headache, malaise

Dermatologic: Painful blistering, burning, and peeling of skin; pruritus (10%), freckling, hypopigmentation, rash, cheilitis, erythema, itching, urticaria

Gastrointestinal: Nausea (10%)

Neuromuscular & skeletal: Loss of muscle coordination, leg cramps

Miscellaneous: Miliaria

Overdosage/Toxicology Symptoms of overdose include nausea and severe burns. Follow accepted treatment of severe burns. Keep room darkened until reaction subsides (8-24 hours or more).

Pharmacodynamics/Kinetics

Time to Peak: Time to peak, serum:
Hard-gelatin capsules: 1.5-6 hours (peak photosensitivity: ~4 hours)
Soft-gelatin capsules: 0.5-4 hours (peak photosensitivity: 1.5-2 hours)

Protein Binding: Reversibly bound to albumin

Half-Life Elimination: ~2 hours

Metabolism: Hepatic; forms metabolites

Excretion: Urine (~95% as metabolites)

Available Dosage Forms

Capsule:
8-MOP®: 10 mg [hard-gelatin capsule]
Oxsoralen-Ultra®: 10 mg [soft-gelatin capsule]
Lotion (Oxsoralen®): 1% (30 mL) [contains alcohol 71%]
Solution, for extracorporeal administration (Uvadex®): 20 mcg/mL (10 mL) **[not for injection]**

Dosing

Adults & Elderly: Note: Refer to treatment protocols for UVA exposure guidelines.

Psoriasis: Oral: 10-70 mg 11/2-2 hours before exposure to UVA light; dose may be repeated 2-3 times per week, based on UVA exposure; doses must be given at least 48 hours apart; dosage is based upon patient's body weight and skin type:
<30 kg: 10 mg
30-50 kg: 20 mg
51-65 kg: 30 mg
66-80 kg: 40 mg
81-90 kg: 50 mg
91-115 kg: 60 mg
>115 kg: 70 mg

Vitiligo:
Oral (8-MOP®): 20 mg 2-4 hours before exposure to UVA light; dose may be repeated based on erythema and tenderness of skin; do not give on 2 consecutive days
Topical: Apply lotion 1-2 hours before exposure to UVA light, no more than once weekly

CTCL: Extracorporeal (Uvadex®): 200 mcg injected into the photoactivation bag during the collection cycle using the UVAR® photopheresis system (consult user's guide). Treatment schedule: Two consecutive days every 4 weeks for a minimum of 7 treatment cycles

Pediatrics: Vitiligo: Topical: Children >12 years: Refer to adult dosing.

Administration

Topical: Hands and fingers of person applying the lotion should be protected to prevent possible photosensitization and/or burns.

Nursing Actions

Physical Assessment: Note: This drug is administered in conjunction with ultraviolet light or ultraviolet radiation therapy. Teach patient proper use, side effects/appropriate interventions (eg, sunlight precautions), and adverse reactions to report.

Patient Education: Do not take any new medication during therapy unless approved by prescriber. This medication is used in conjunction with specific ultraviolet treatment. Take as directed, with food or milk to reduce nausea. Consult prescriber for specific dietary instructions. Avoid use of any other skin treatments unless approved by prescriber. Control exposure to direct sunlight as per prescriber's instructions. If sunlight cannot be avoided, use sunblock (consult prescriber for specific SPF level); wear protective clothing and wraparound protective eyewear. Consult prescriber immediately if burning, blistering, or skin (Continued)

Methoxsalen *(Continued)*

irritation occur. **Pregnancy/breast-feeding precautions:** Inform prescriber if you are or intend to become pregnant. Breast-feeding is not recommended.

Dietary Considerations To reduce nausea, oral drug can be administered with food or milk or in 2 divided doses 30 minutes apart.

Pregnancy Issues Fetal toxicity has been observed in animal studies, however, there are no adequate and well-controlled studies in pregnant women. Use during pregnancy is not recommended. Women of childbearing potential should be advised to avoid pregnancy.

Methyldopa *(meth il DOE pa)*

Synonyms Aldomet; Methyldopate Hydrochloride

Pharmacologic Category Alpha-Adrenergic Inhibitor

Medication Safety Issues
Sound-alike/look-alike issues:
Methyldopa may be confused with L-dopa, levodopa

Pregnancy Risk Factor B

Lactation Enters breast milk/compatible

Use Management of moderate to severe hypertension

Mechanism of Action/Effect Stimulation of central alpha-adrenergic receptors by a false transmitter that results in a decreased sympathetic outflow to the heart, kidneys, and peripheral vasculature

Contraindications Hypersensitivity to methyldopa or any component of the formulation; active hepatic disease; liver disorders previously associated with use of methyldopa; on MAO inhibitors; bisulfite allergy if using oral suspension or injectable

Warnings/Precautions May rarely produce hemolytic anemia and liver disorders; positive Coombs' test occurs in 10% to 20% of patients (perform periodic CBCs); sedation usually transient may occur during initial therapy or whenever the dose is increased. Use with caution in patients with previous liver disease or dysfunction, the active metabolites of methyldopa accumulate in uremia. Patients with impaired renal function may respond to smaller doses. Elderly patients may experience syncope (avoid by giving smaller doses). Tolerance may occur usually between the second and third month of therapy. Adding a diuretic or increasing the dosage of methyldopa frequently restores blood pressure control. Because of its CNS effects, methyldopa is not considered a drug of first choice in the elderly. Often considered the drug of choice for treatment of hypertension in pregnancy. Do not use injectable if bisulfite allergy.

Drug Interactions
Decreased Effect: Iron supplements can interact and cause a significant **increase** in blood pressure. Ferrous sulfate and ferrous gluconate decrease bioavailability. Barbiturates and TCAs may reduce response to methyldopa.

Increased Effect/Toxicity: Beta-blockers, MAO inhibitors, phenothiazines, and sympathomimetics (including epinephrine) may result in hypertension (sometimes severe) when combined with methyldopa. Methyldopa may increase lithium serum levels resulting in lithium toxicity. Levodopa may cause enhanced blood pressure lowering; methyldopa may also potentiate the effect of levodopa. Tolbutamide, haloperidol, and anesthetics effects/toxicity are increased with methyldopa.

Nutritional/Ethanol Interactions Herb/Nutraceutical: Avoid dong quai if using for hypertension (has estrogenic activity). Avoid ephedra, yohimbe, ginseng (may worsen hypertension). Avoid valerian, St John's wort, kava kava, gotu kola (may increase CNS depression).

Avoid natural licorice (causes sodium and water retention and increases potassium loss). Avoid garlic (may have increased antihypertensive effect).

Lab Interactions Methyldopa interferes with the following laboratory tests: urinary uric acid, serum creatinine (alkaline picrate method), AST (colorimetric method), and urinary catecholamines (falsely high levels)

Adverse Reactions
>10%: Cardiovascular: Peripheral edema
1% to 10%:
Central nervous system: Drug fever, mental depression, anxiety, nightmares, drowsiness, headache
Gastrointestinal: Dry mouth

Overdosage/Toxicology Symptoms of overdose include hypotension, sedation, bradycardia, dizziness, constipation or diarrhea, flatus, nausea, and vomiting. Treatment is supportive and symptomatic. Can be removed by hemodialysis.

Pharmacodynamics/Kinetics
Onset of Action: Peak effect: Hypotensive: Oral/parenteral: 3-6 hours
Duration of Action: 12-24 hours
Protein Binding: <15%
Half-Life Elimination: 75-80 minutes; End-stage renal disease: 6-16 hours
Metabolism: Intestinal and hepatic
Excretion: Urine (85% as metabolites) within 24 hours

Available Dosage Forms
Injection, solution, as methyldopate hydrochloride: 50 mg/mL (5 mL) [contains sodium bisulfite]
Tablet: 250 mg, 500 mg

Dosing
Adults: Hypertension:
Oral: Initial: 250 mg 2-3 times/day; increase every 2 days as needed (maximum dose: 3 g/day); usual dose range (JNC 7): 250-1000 mg/day in 2 divided doses
I.V.: 250-1000 mg every 6-8 hours; maximum: 1 g every 6 hours
Elderly: Oral: Initial: 125 mg 1-2 times/day; increase by 125 mg every 2-3 days as needed. Adjust for renal impairment. See Geriatric Considerations.
Pediatrics: Hypertension:
Oral: Initial: 10 mg/kg/day in 2-4 divided doses; increase every 2 days as needed to maximum dose of 65 mg/kg/day. Do not exceed 3 g/day.
I.V.: 5-10 mg/kg/dose every 6-8 hours up to a total dose of 65 mg/kg/24 hours or 3 g/24 hours
Renal Impairment:
Cl_{cr} >50 mL/minute: Administer every 8 hours.
Cl_{cr} 10-50 mL/minute: Administer every 8-12 hours.
Cl_{cr} <10 mL/minute: Administer every 12-24 hours.
Slightly dialyzable (5% to 20%)

Administration
I.V.: Infuse over 30 minutes.

Stability
Compatibility: Stable in dextran 6% in NS, D_5NS, D_5W, sodium bicarbonate 5%, NS
Compatibility when admixed: Incompatible with amphotericin B, methohexital
Storage: Injectable dosage form is most stable at acid to neutral pH. Stability of parenteral admixture at room temperature (25°C) is 24 hours. Stability of parenteral admixture at refrigeration temperature (4°C) is 4 days.
Standard diluent: 250-500 mg/100 mL D_5W

Laboratory Monitoring CBC, liver enzymes, Coombs' test (direct)

Nursing Actions
Physical Assessment: Assess potential for interactions with other pharmacological agents or herbal products patient may be taking (eg, anything that affects blood pressure). See Administration for infusion specifics (eg, do not use injectable in presence of bisulfite allergy). Monitor laboratory tests at baseline

and regularly during therapy. Monitor therapeutic effectiveness (normotensive), and adverse reactions (eg, hypotension, bradycardia, CNS changes) on a regular basis. Teach patient proper use, possible side effects/appropriate interventions, and adverse symptoms to report.

Patient Education: Do not take any new medication during therapy unless approved by prescriber (especially any cough or cold remedies, diet pills, stay-awake medications). **Oral:** Take as directed. Do not skip dose or discontinue without consulting prescriber. Follow recommended diet and exercise program. Periodic laboratory tests may be required. This medication may cause altered color of urine (normal); drowsiness, dizziness, or impaired judgment (use caution when driving or engaging in tasks that require alertness until response to drug is known); postural hypotension (use caution when rising from sitting or lying position or when climbing stairs); or dry mouth or nausea (frequent mouth care or sucking lozenges may help). Report altered CNS status (eg, nightmares, depression, anxiety, increased nervousness); sudden weight gain (weigh yourself in the same clothes at the same time of day once a week); unusual or persistent swelling of ankles, feet, or extremities; palpitations or rapid heartbeat; persistent weakness, fatigue, or unusual bleeding; or other persistent side effects.

Dietary Considerations Dietary requirements for vitamin B_{12} and folate may be increased with high doses of methyldopa.

Geriatric Considerations Because of its CNS effects, methyldopa is not considered a drug of first choice in the elderly. Adjust dose for renal function.

Breast-Feeding Issues Crosses into breast milk at extremely low levels. AAP considers **compatible** with breast-feeding.

Pregnancy Issues Crosses the placenta. Hypotension reported. A large amount of clinical experience with the use of these drugs for the management of hypertension during pregnancy is available. Available evidence suggests safe use during pregnancy.

Methyldopa and Hydrochlorothiazide
(meth il DOE pa & hye droe klor oh THYE a zide)

U.S. Brand Names Aldoril®
Synonyms Hydrochlorothiazide and Methyldopa
Pharmacologic Category Antihypertensive Agent, Combination
Pregnancy Risk Factor C
Lactation Enters breast milk/compatible
Use Management of moderate to severe hypertension
Available Dosage Forms
Tablet:
Methyldopa 250 mg and hydrochlorothiazide 15 mg
Methyldopa 250 mg and hydrochlorothiazide 25 mg
Aldoril® 25: Methyldopa 250 mg and hydrochlorothiazide 25 mg

Dosing
Adults: Hypertension: Oral: 1 tablet 2-3 times/day for first 48 hours, then decrease or increase at intervals of not less than 2 days until an adequate response is achieved. Patients requiring higher doses may receive Aldoril® D30 once daily. Hydrochlorothiazide doses greater than 50 mg daily should be avoided.
Elderly: Refer to dosing in individual monographs.
Renal Impairment: Cl_{cr} 30 mL/minute: Thiazides are recommended; loop diuretics are preferred.

Nursing Actions
Physical Assessment: See individual agents.
Patient Education: See individual agents. **Pregnancy precaution:** Inform prescriber if you are or intend to become pregnant.

Related Information
Hydrochlorothiazide *on page 610*
Methyldopa *on page 802*

Methylergonovine (meth il er goe NOE veen)

U.S. Brand Names Methergine®
Synonyms Methylergometrine Maleate; Methylergonovine Maleate
Pharmacologic Category Ergot Derivative
Medication Safety Issues
Sound-alike/look-alike issues:
Methylergonovine and terbutaline parenteral dosage forms look similar. Due to their contrasting indications, use care when administering these agents.
Pregnancy Risk Factor C
Lactation Enters breast milk/use caution
Use Prevention and treatment of postpartum and postabortion hemorrhage caused by uterine atony or subinvolution
Mechanism of Action/Effect Similar smooth muscle actions as seen with ergotamine; however, it affects primarily uterine smooth muscles producing sustained contractions and thereby shortens the third stage of labor
Contraindications Hypersensitivity to methylergonovine or any component of the formulation; ergot alkaloids are contraindicated with potent inhibitors of CYP3A4 (includes protease inhibitors, azole antifungals, and some macrolide antibiotics); hypertension; toxemia; pregnancy
Warnings/Precautions Use caution in patients with sepsis, obliterative vascular disease, hepatic, or renal involvement, or second stage of labor; administer with extreme caution if using intravenously. Pleural and peritoneal fibrosis have been reported with prolonged daily use. Cardiac valvular fibrosis has also been associated with ergot alkaloids.
Drug Interactions
Cytochrome P450 Effect: Substrate of CYP3A4 (major)
Decreased Effect: Effects of methylergonovine may be diminished by antipsychotics, metoclopramide/
Increased Effect/Toxicity: CYP3A4 inhibitors may increase the levels/effects of methylergonovine; example inhibitors include azole antifungals, clarithromycin, diclofenac, doxycycline, erythromycin, imatinib, isoniazid, nefazodone, nicardipine, propofol, protease inhibitors, quinidine, telithromycin, and verapamil. Ergot alkaloids are contraindicated with potent CYP3A4 inhibitors. Methylergonovine may increase the effects of 5-HT_1 agonists (eg, sumatriptan), MAO inhibitors, sibutramine, and other serotonin agonists (serotonin syndrome). Severe vasoconstriction may occur when peripheral vasoconstrictors or beta-blockers are used in patients receiving ergot alkaloids; concurrent use is contraindicated.
Adverse Reactions Frequency not defined.
Cardiovascular: Acute MI, hypertension, temporary chest pain, palpitation
Central nervous system: Hallucinations, dizziness, seizure, headache
Endocrine & metabolic: Water intoxication
Gastrointestinal: Nausea, vomiting, diarrhea, foul taste
Local: Thrombophlebitis
Neuromuscular & skeletal: Leg cramps
Otic: Tinnitus
Renal: Hematuria
Respiratory: Dyspnea, nasal congestion
Miscellaneous: Diaphoresis
Overdosage/Toxicology Symptoms of overdose include prolonged gangrene, numbness in extremities, acute nausea, vomiting, abdominal pain, respiratory *(Continued)*

Methylergonovine *(Continued)*

depression, hypotension, and seizures. Treatment is symptomatic and supportive.

Pharmacodynamics/Kinetics

Onset of Action: Oxytocic: Oral: 5-10 minutes; I.M.: 2-5 minutes; I.V.: Immediately

Duration of Action: Oral: ~3 hours; I.M.: ~3 hours; I.V.: 45 minutes

Time to Peak: Serum: Oral: 0.3-2 hours; I.M.: 0.2-0.6 hours

Half-Life Elimination: Biphasic: Initial: 1-5 minutes; Terminal: 0.5-2 hours

Metabolism: Hepatic

Excretion: Urine and feces

Available Dosage Forms

Injection, solution, as maleate: 0.2 mg/mL (1 mL)

Tablet, as maleate: 0.2 mg

Dosing

Adults & Elderly: Prevention of hemorrhage:

Oral: 0.2 mg 3-4 times/day for 2-7 days

I.M., I.V.: 0.2 mg after delivery of anterior shoulder, after delivery of placenta, or during puerperium; may be repeated as required at intervals of 2-4 hours

Administration

I.V.: Administer over ≥60 seconds. Should not be routinely administered I.V. because of possibility of inducing sudden hypertension and cerebrovascular accident.

I.V. Detail: pH: 2.7-3.5

Stability

Compatibility: Stable in NS

Storage:

Ampul: Store under refrigeration at 2°C to 8°C (36°F to 46°F). Protect from light.

Tablet: Store below 25°C (77°F).

Nursing Actions

Physical Assessment: Monitor blood pressure, CNS status, and vaginal bleeding on a regular basis - especially with infusion or injection. Monitor therapeutic effectiveness and adverse reactions (eg, ergotamine toxicity [headache, ringing in ears, nausea and vomiting, diarrhea, numbness or coldness of extremities, confusion, hallucinations, dyspnea, chest pain, convulsions]). Teach patient proper use (when self-administered), possible side effects/appropriate interventions, and adverse symptoms to report.

Patient Education: This drug will generally not be needed for more than a week. May cause nausea and vomiting (small, frequent meals may help), dizziness, headache, or ringing in the ears (will reverse when drug is discontinued). Report immediately any chest pain or tightness, jaw, shoulder or midback pain; difficulty breathing; acute headache; numb, cold, or cramping extremities; or severe abdominal cramping. **Breast-feeding precaution:** Consult prescriber if breast-feeding.

Pregnancy Issues Prolonged constriction of the uterine vessels and/or increased myometrial tone may lead to reduced placental blood flow. This has contributed to fetal growth retardation in animals. Methylergonovine is intended for use after delivery of the infant.

Methylphenidate *(meth il FEN i date)*

U.S. Brand Names Concerta®; Daytrana™; Metadate® CD; Metadate® ER; Methylin®; Methylin® ER; Ritalin®; Ritalin® LA; Ritalin-SR®

Synonyms Methylphenidate Hydrochloride

Restrictions C-II

Pharmacologic Category Central Nervous System Stimulant

Medication Safety Issues

Sound-alike/look-alike issues:

Methylphenidate may be confused with methadone

Ritalin® may be confused with Ismelin®, Rifadin®

Pregnancy Risk Factor C

Lactation Excretion in breast milk unknown/use caution

Use Treatment of attention-deficit/hyperactivity disorder (ADHD); symptomatic management of narcolepsy

Unlabeled/Investigational Use Depression (especially elderly or medically ill)

Mechanism of Action/Effect Mild CNS stimulant; blocks the reuptake of norepinephrine and dopamine into presynaptic neurons; appears to stimulate the cerebral cortex and subcortical structures similar to amphetamines

Contraindications Hypersensitivity to methylphenidate, any component of the formulation, or idiosyncratic reactions to sympathomimetic amines; marked anxiety, tension, and agitation; glaucoma; use during or within 14 days following MAO inhibitor therapy; Tourette's syndrome or tics

Warnings/Precautions Has demonstrated value as part of a comprehensive treatment program for ADHD. Safety and efficacy in children <6 years of age not established. Use with caution in patients with bipolar disorder, diabetes mellitus, cardiovascular disease, hyperthyroidism, seizure disorders, insomnia, porphyria, or hypertension. Do not use in patients with known structural cardiac abnormalities; sudden death associated with CNS stimulant use has been reported in these patients. Use caution in patients with history of ethanol or drug abuse. May exacerbate symptoms of behavior and thought disorder in psychotic patients. Do not use to treat severe depression or fatigue states. Potential for drug dependency exists - avoid abrupt discontinuation in patients who have received for prolonged periods. Visual disturbances have been reported (rare). Stimulant use has been associated with growth suppression. Growth should be monitored during treatment. Stimulants may unmask tics in individuals with coexisting Tourette's syndrome. Concerta® should not be used in patients with esophageal motility disorders or pre-existing severe gastrointestinal narrowing (small bowel disease, short gut syndrome, history of peritonitis, cystic fibrosis, chronic intestinal pseudo-obstruction, Meckel's diverticulum). Transdermal system may cause allergic contact sensitization, characterized by intense local reactions (edema, papules); sensitization may subsequently manifest systemically with other routes of methylphenidate administration; monitor closely. Efficacy of transdermal methylphenidate therapy for >7 weeks has not been established.

Drug Interactions

Cytochrome P450 Effect: Substrate of CYP2D6 (major); Inhibits CYP2D6 (weak)

Decreased Effect: Effectiveness of antihypertensive agents may be decreased. Carbamazepine may decrease the effect of methylphenidate.

Increased Effect/Toxicity: Methylphenidate may cause hypertensive effects when used in combination with MAO inhibitors or drugs with MAO-inhibiting activity (linezolid). Risk may be less with selegiline (MAO type B selective at low doses); it is best to avoid this combination. CYP2D6 inhibitors may increase the levels/effects of methylphenidate; example inhibitors include chlorpromazine, delavirdine, fluoxetine, miconazole, paroxetine, pergolide, quinidine, quinine, ritonavir, and ropinirole. Methylphenidate may increase levels of phenytoin, phenobarbital, and TCAs. Increased toxicity with clonidine and sibutramine.

Nutritional/Ethanol Interactions

Ethanol: Avoid ethanol (may cause CNS depression).

Food: Food may increase oral absorption; Concerta® formulation is not affected. Food delays early peak and high-fat meals increase C_{max} and AUC of Metadate® CD formulation.

Herb/Nutraceutical: Avoid ephedra (may cause hypertension or arrhythmias) and yohimbe (also has CNS stimulatory activity).

Adverse Reactions

Transdermal system: Frequency of adverse events as reported in trials of 7-week duration. Incidence of some events reportedly higher with extended use.

>10%:

Central nervous system: Insomnia (13%)

Endocrine and metabolic: Appetite decreased (26%)

Gastrointestinal: Nausea (12%)

1% to 10%:

Central nervous system: Tic (7%), emotional instability (6%)

Gastrointestinal: Vomiting (10%), anorexia (5%)

Respiratory: Nasal congestion (6%), nasopharyngitis (5%)

Endocrine and metabolic: Weight loss (9%)

All dosage forms: Frequency not defined:

Cardiovascular: Angina, cardiac arrhythmia, cerebral arteritis, cerebral occlusion, hyper-/hypotension, MI, necrotizing vasculitis, palpitation, pulse increase/decrease, tachycardia

Central nervous system: Depression, dizziness, drowsiness, fever, headache, insomnia, nervousness, neuroleptic malignant syndrome (NMS), Tourette's syndrome, toxic psychosis

Dermatologic: Erythema multiforme, exfoliative dermatitis, hair loss, rash, urticaria

Endocrine & metabolic: Growth retardation

Gastrointestinal: Abdominal pain, anorexia, diarrhea, nausea, vomiting, weight loss

Hematologic: Anemia, leukopenia, thrombocytopenic purpura

Hepatic: Liver function tests abnormal, hepatic coma, transaminases increased

Neuromuscular & skeletal: Arthralgia, dyskinesia

Ocular: Blurred vision

Renal: Necrotizing vasculitis

Respiratory: Cough increased, pharyngitis, sinusitis, upper respiratory tract infection

Miscellaneous: Accidental injury, hypersensitivity reactions

Overdosage/Toxicology Symptoms of overdose include vomiting, agitation, tremor, hyperpyrexia, muscle twitching, hallucinations, tachycardia, mydriasis, sweating, and palpitations. There is no specific antidote; treatment is symptom-directed and supportive. Transdermal system: Remove patch and thoroughly cleanse area; consider that absorption may continue in absence of patch.

Pharmacodynamics/Kinetics

Onset of Action: Peak effect:

Immediate release tablet: Cerebral stimulation: ~2 hours

Extended release capsule (Metadate® CD): Biphasic; initial peak similar to immediate release product, followed by second rising portion (corresponding to extended release portion)

Sustained release tablet: 4-7 hours

Osmotic release tablet (Concerta®): Initial: 1-2 hours

Transdermal: ~2 hours

Duration of Action: Immediate release tablet: 3-6 hours; Sustained release tablet: 8 hours

Time to Peak: Concerta®: C_{max}: 6-8 hours

Half-Life Elimination: d-methylphenidate: 3-4 hours; l-methylphenidate: 1-3 hours

Metabolism: Hepatic via de-esterification to minimally active metabolite

Excretion: Urine (90%; 80% as metabolite)

Available Dosage Forms

Capsule, extended release, as hydrochloride:

Metadate® CD: 10 mg, 20 mg, 30 mg

Ritalin® LA: 10 mg, 20 mg, 30 mg, 40 mg

Solution, oral, as hydrochloride:

Methylin®: 5 mg/5 mL (500 mL) [grape flavor]; 10 mg/5 mL (500 mL) [grape flavor]

Tablet, as hydrochloride: 5 mg, 10 mg, 20 mg

Methylin®, Ritalin®: 5 mg, 10 mg, 20 mg

Tablet, chewable, as hydrochloride:

Methylin®: 2.5 mg [contains phenylalanine 0.42 mg; grape flavor]; 5 mg [contains phenylalanine 0.84 mg; grape flavor]; 10 mg [contains phenylalanine 1.68 mg; grape flavor]

Tablet, extended release, as hydrochloride: 20 mg

Concerta®: 18 mg, 27 mg, 36 mg, 54 mg [osmotic controlled release]

Metadate® ER, Methylin® ER: 10 mg, 20 mg

Tablet, sustained release, as hydrochloride:

Ritalin-SR®: 20 mg

Transdermal system [once-daily patch]:

Daytrana™: 10 mg/9 hours (10s, 30s) [12.5 cm², total methylphenidate 27.5 mg]; 15 mg/9 hours (10s, 30s) [18.75 cm², total methylphenidate 41.3 mg]; 20 mg/9 hours (10s, 30s) [25 cm², total methylphenidate 55 mg]; 30 mg/9 hours (10s, 30s) [37.5 cm², total methylphenidate 82.5 mg]

Dosing

Adults & Elderly:

Narcolepsy: Oral: 10 mg 2-3 times/day, up to 60 mg/day

Depression: Oral: Initial: 2.5 mg every morning before 9 AM; dosage may be increased by 2.5-5 mg every 2-3 days as tolerated to a maximum of 20 mg/day. May be divided (eg, 7 AM and 12 noon), but should not be given after noon. Do not use sustained release product.

ADHD: Oral: Refer to pediatric dosing.

Note: Discontinue periodically to re-evaluate or if no improvement occurs within 1 month.

Pediatrics:

ADHD:

Oral: Children ≥6 years: Initial: 0.3 mg/kg/dose or 2.5-5 mg/dose given before breakfast and lunch; increase by 0.1 mg/kg/dose or by 5-10 mg/day at weekly intervals; usual dose: 0.5-1 mg/kg/day; maximum dose: 2 mg/kg/day or 90 mg/day. **Note:** Oral: Discontinue periodically to re-evaluate or if no improvement occurs within 1 month.

Extended release products:

Metadate® ER, Methylin® ER, Ritalin® SR: Duration of action is 8 hours. May be given in place of regular tablets, once the daily dose is titrated using the regular tablets and the titrated 8-hour dosage corresponds to sustained release tablet size.

Metadate® CD, Ritalin® LA: Initial: 20 mg once daily; may be adjusted in 10-20 mg increments at weekly intervals; maximum: 60 mg/day

Concerta®:

Initial dose:

Children not currently taking methylphenidate: 18 mg once daily in the morning

Children currently taking methylphenidate: **Note:** Dosing based on current regimen and clinical judgment; suggested dosing listed below:

Patients taking methylphenidate 5 mg 2-3 times/day or 20 mg/day sustained release formulation: 18 mg once every morning

(Continued)

Methylphenidate *(Continued)*

Patients taking methylphenidate 10 mg 2-3 times/day or 40 mg/day sustained release formulation: 36 mg once every morning

Patients taking methylphenidate 15 mg 2-3 times/day or 60 mg/day sustained release formulation: 54 mg once every morning

Dose adjustment: May increase dose in increments of 18 mg; dose may be adjusted at weekly intervals. A dosage strength of 27 mg is available for situations in which a dosage between 18-36 mg is desired. Maximum dose should not exceed 2 mg/kg/day **or** 54 mg/day in children 6-12 years or 72 mg/day in children 13-17 years.

Transdermal (Daytrana™): Children 6-12 years: Initial: 10 mg patch once daily; remove up to 9 hours after application. Titrate based on response and tolerability; may increase to next transdermal dose no more frequently than every week; Note: Application should occur 2 hours prior to desired effect. Drug absorption may continue for a period of time after patch removal.

Administration

Oral: Do not crush or allow patient to chew sustained release dosage form. To effectively avoid insomnia, dosing should be completed by noon.

Concerta®: Administer dose once daily in the morning. May be taken with or without food, but must be taken with water, milk, or juice.

Metadate® CD, Ritalin® LA: Capsules may be opened and the contents sprinkled onto a small amount (equal to 1 tablespoon) of applesauce. Swallow applesauce without chewing. Do not crush or chew capsule contents.

Methylin® chewable tablet: Administer with at least 8 ounces of water or other fluid.

Topical: Transdermal (Daytrana™): Apply to clean, dry, non-oily, intact skin to the hip area, avoiding the waistline. Apply at the same time each day to alternating hips. Press firmly for 30 seconds to ensure proper adherence. Avoid exposure of application site to external heat source, which may increase the amount of drug absorbed. If patch should dislodge, may replace with new patch (to different site) but total wear time should not exceed 9 hours. Patch may be removed early if a shorter duration of effect is desired or if late day side effects occur. Wash hands with soap and water after handling. Avoid touching the sticky side of the patch. Dispose of used patch by folding adhesive side onto itself, and discard in toilet or appropriate lidded container.

Stability

Storage:

Chewable tablet: Store at room temperature of 20°C to 25°C (68°F to 77°F). Protect from moisture.

Extended release capsule: Store in dose pack provided at 25°C (77°F).

Immediate release tablet: Do not store above 30°C (86°F). Protect from light .

Osmotic controlled release tablet (Concerta®): Store at 25°C (77°F). Protect from humidity.

Solution: Store at room temperature of 20°C to 25°C (68°F to 77°F).

Sustained release tablet: Do not store above 30°C (86°F). Protect from moisture.

Transdermal system: Store at 15°C to 30°C (59°F to 86°F). Keep patches stored in protective pouch. Once tray is opened, use patches within 2 months.

Nursing Actions

Physical Assessment: Assess effectiveness and interactions of other medications patient may be taking. Assess for history of addiction; long-term use can result in dependence, abuse, or tolerance. Evaluate periodically for need for continued use. After long-term use, taper dosage slowly when discontinuing. Monitor growth pattern in children. Monitor laboratory tests, effectiveness of therapy, and adverse reactions at beginning of therapy and periodically with long-term use. Monitor blood pressure and pulse periodically. Assess knowledge/teach patient appropriate use, interventions to reduce side effects, and importance of reporting adverse symptoms promptly.

Patient Education: Take exactly as directed. Do not change dosage or discontinue without consulting prescriber. Response may take some time. Do not crush or chew sustained release dosage forms. Tablets and sustained release tablets should be taken 30-45 minutes before meals. Concerta® may be taken with or without food, but must be taken with water, milk, or juice. Metadate® CD and Ritalin® LA capsules may be opened and the contents sprinkled onto a small amount (equal to 1 tablespoon) of applesauce; swallow applesauce without chewing. Do not crush or chew capsule contents. Avoid alcohol, caffeine, or other stimulants. Maintain adequate hydration (2-3 L/day of fluids) unless instructed to restrict fluid intake. You may experience decreased appetite or weight loss (small frequent meals may help maintain adequate nutrition); or restlessness, impaired judgment, or dizziness, especially during early therapy (use caution when driving or engaging in tasks requiring alertness until response to drug is known). Report unresolved rapid heartbeat; excessive agitation, nervousness, insomnia, tremors, or dizziness; change in vision; blackened stool; skin rash or irritation; or altered gait or movement. Concerta® tablet shell may appear intact in stool; this is normal. Pediatrics: Monitor growth. **Pregnancy/breast-feeding precautions:** Inform prescriber if you are or intend to become pregnant. Consult prescriber if breast-feeding.

Transdermal: Apply to clean, dry skin, immediately after removing from package. Firmly press in place and hold for 30 seconds. Avoid exposing application site to external heat sources (eg, heating pad, electric blanket, hot tub, heat lamp).

Dietary Considerations Should be taken 30-45 minutes before meals. Concerta® is not affected by food and should be taken with water, milk, or juice. Metadate® CD should be taken before breakfast. Metadate™ ER should be taken before breakfast and lunch.

Geriatric Considerations Methylphenidate is often useful in treating elderly patients who are discouraged, withdrawn, apathetic, or disinterested in their activities. In particular, it is useful in patients who are starting a rehabilitation program but have resigned themselves to fail; these patients may not have a major depressive disorder; will not improve memory or cognitive function; use with caution in patients with dementia who may have increased agitation and confusion (see Dosing and Adverse Reactions).

Additional Information Treatment with methylphenidate may include "drug holidays" or periodic discontinuation in order to assess the patient's requirements and to decrease tolerance and limit suppression of linear growth and weight. Specific patients may require 3 doses/day for treatment of ADHD (ie, additional dose at 4 PM).

Concerta® is an osmotic controlled release formulation (OROS®) of methylphenidate. The tablet has an immediate-release overcoat that provides an initial dose of methylphenidate within 1 hour. The overcoat covers a trilayer core. The trilayer core is composed of two layers containing the drug and excipients, and one layer of osmotic components. As water from the gastrointestinal tract enters the core, the osmotic components expand and methylphenidate is released.

Metadate® CD capsules contain a mixture of immediate release and extended release beads, designed to release 30% of the dose (6 mg) immediately and 70% (14 mg) over an extended period.

Ritalin® LA uses a combination of immediate release and enteric coated, delayed release beads.

MethylPREDNISolone
(meth il pred NIS oh lone)

U.S. Brand Names Depo-Medrol®; Medrol®; Solu-Medrol®

Synonyms 6-α-Methylprednisolone; A-Methapred; Methylprednisolone Acetate; Methylprednisolone Sodium Succinate

Pharmacologic Category Corticosteroid, Systemic

Medication Safety Issues
Sound-alike/look-alike issues:
MethylPREDNISolone may be confused with medroxyPROGESTERone, predniSONE
Depo-Medrol® may be confused with Solu-Medrol®
Medrol® may be confused with Mebaral®
Solu-Medrol® may be confused with Depo-Medrol®

Pregnancy Risk Factor C

Lactation Excretion in breast milk unknown

Use Primarily as an anti-inflammatory or immunosuppressant agent in the treatment of a variety of diseases including those of hematologic, allergic, inflammatory, neoplastic, and autoimmune origin. Prevention and treatment of graft-versus-host disease following allogeneic bone marrow transplantation.

Unlabeled/Investigational Use Treatment of fibrosing-alveolitis phase of adult respiratory distress syndrome (ARDS)

Mechanism of Action/Effect In a tissue-specific manner, corticosteroids regulate gene expression subsequent to binding specific intracellular receptors and translocation into the nucleus. Corticosteroids exert a wide array of physiologic effects, including modulation of carbohydrate, protein, and lipid metabolism, and maintenance of fluid and electrolyte homeostasis. Moreover, cardiovascular, immunologic, musculoskeletal, endocrine, and neurologic physiology are influenced by corticosteroids.

Contraindications Hypersensitivity to methylprednisolone or any component of the formulation; viral, fungal, or tubercular skin lesions; administration of live virus vaccines; serious infections, except septic shock or tuberculous meningitis. Methylprednisolone formulations containing benzyl alcohol preservative are contraindicated in infants.

Warnings/Precautions Use with caution in patients with hyperthyroidism, cirrhosis, nonspecific ulcerative colitis, hypertension, osteoporosis, thromboembolic tendencies, CHF, convulsive disorders, myasthenia gravis, thrombophlebitis, peptic ulcer, diabetes, glaucoma, cataracts, or tuberculosis. Use caution in hepatic impairment. Acute adrenal insufficiency may occur with abrupt withdrawal after long-term therapy or with stress. Because of the risk of adverse effects, systemic corticosteroids should be used cautiously in the elderly, in the smallest possible dose, and for the shortest possible time.

Drug Interactions
Cytochrome P450 Effect: Substrate of CYP3A4 (minor); **Inhibits** CYP3A4 (weak)

Decreased Effect: Phenytoin, phenobarbital, rifampin increase clearance of methylprednisolone. Potassium-depleting diuretics enhance potassium depletion. Skin test antigens, immunizations decrease antibody response and increase potential infections.

Increased Effect/Toxicity: Methylprednisolone may increase circulating glucose levels; may need adjustments of insulin or oral hypoglycemics. Methylprednisolone increases cyclosporine and tacrolimus blood levels. Itraconazole increases corticosteroid levels.

Nutritional/Ethanol Interactions
Ethanol: Avoid ethanol (may increase gastric mucosal irritation).
Food: Methylprednisolone interferes with calcium absorption. Limit caffeine.
Herb/Nutraceutical: St John's wort may decrease methylprednisolone levels. Avoid cat's claw, echinacea (have immunostimulant properties).

Lab Interactions Interferes with skin tests

Adverse Reactions Frequency not defined.
Cardiovascular: Edema, hypertension, arrhythmia
Central nervous system: Insomnia, nervousness, vertigo, seizure, psychoses, pseudotumor cerebri, headache, mood swings, delirium, hallucinations, euphoria
Dermatologic: Hirsutism, acne, skin atrophy, bruising, hyperpigmentation
Endocrine & metabolic: Diabetes mellitus, adrenal suppression, hyperlipidemia, Cushing's syndrome, pituitary-adrenal axis suppression, growth suppression, glucose intolerance, hypokalemia, alkalosis, amenorrhea, sodium and water retention, hyperglycemia
Gastrointestinal: Increased appetite, indigestion, peptic ulcer, nausea, vomiting, abdominal distention, ulcerative esophagitis, pancreatitis
Hematologic: Transient leukocytosis
Neuromuscular & skeletal: Arthralgia, muscle weakness, osteoporosis, fractures
Ocular: Cataracts, glaucoma
Miscellaneous: Infections, hypersensitivity reactions, avascular necrosis, secondary malignancy, intractable hiccups

Overdosage/Toxicology When consumed in high doses for prolonged periods, systemic hypercorticism and adrenal suppression may occur. In these cases, discontinuation should be done judiciously. Arrhythmias and cardiovascular collapse are possible with rapid intravenous infusion of high-dose methylprednisolone. May mask signs and symptoms of infection.

Pharmacodynamics/Kinetics
Onset of Action: Peak effect (route dependent): Oral: 1-2 hours; I.M.: 4-8 days; Intra-articular: 1 week; methylprednisolone sodium succinate is highly soluble and has a rapid effect by I.M. and I.V. routes

Duration of Action: Route dependent: Oral: 30-36 hours; I.M.: 1-4 weeks; Intra-articular: 1-5 weeks; methylprednisolone acetate has a low solubility and has a sustained I.M. effect

Half-Life Elimination: 3-3.5 hours; reduced in obese

Excretion: Clearance: Reduced in obese

Available Dosage Forms
Injection, powder for reconstitution, as sodium succinate: 125 mg [strength expressed as base]
Solu-Medrol®: 40 mg, 125 mg, 500 mg, 1 g, 2 g [packaged with diluent; diluent contains benzyl alcohol; strength expressed as base]
Solu-Medrol®: 500 mg, 1 g
Injection, suspension, as acetate (Depo-Medrol®): 20 mg/mL (5 mL); 40 mg/mL (5 mL); 80 mg/mL (5 mL) [contains benzyl alcohol; strength expressed as base]
Injection, suspension, as acetate [single-dose vial] (Depo-Medrol®): 40 mg/mL (1 mL, 10 mL); 80 mg/mL (1 mL)
Tablet: 4 mg
Medrol®: 2 mg, 4 mg, 8 mg, 16 mg, 32 mg
Tablet, dose-pack: 4 mg (21s)
Medrol® Dosepack™: 4 mg (21s)

Dosing
Adults: Only sodium succinate may be given I.V.; methylprednisolone sodium succinate is highly soluble and has a rapid effect by I.M. and I.V. routes. Methylprednisolone acetate has a low solubility and has a sustained I.M. effect.
(Continued)

MethylPREDNISolone *(Continued)*

Anti-inflammatory or immunosuppressive:

Oral: 2-60 mg/day in 1-4 divided doses to start, followed by gradual reduction in dosage to the lowest possible level consistent with maintaining an adequate clinical response.

I.M. (sodium succinate): 10-80 mg/day once daily

I.M. (acetate): 10-80 mg every 1-2 weeks

I.V. (sodium succinate): 10-40 mg over a period of several minutes and repeated I.V. or I.M. at intervals depending on clinical response; when high dosages are needed, give 30 mg/kg over a period ≥30 minutes and may be repeated every 4-6 hours for 48 hours.

Status asthmaticus: I.V. (sodium succinate): Loading dose: 2 mg/kg/dose, then 0.5-1 mg/kg/dose every 6 hours for up to 5 days

Acute spinal cord injury: I.V. (sodium succinate): 30 mg/kg over 15 minutes, followed in 45 minutes by a continuous infusion of 5.4 mg/kg/hour for 23 hours

Lupus nephritis: High-dose "pulse" therapy: I.V. (sodium succinate): 1 g/day for 3 days

Aplastic anemia: I.V. (sodium succinate): 1 mg/kg/day or 40 mg/day (whichever dose is higher), for 4 days. After 4 days, change to oral and continue until day 10 or until symptoms of serum sickness resolve, then rapidly reduce over approximately 2 weeks.

Pneumonia in AIDS patients due to *Pneumocystis*: I.V.: 40-60 mg every 6 hours for 7-10 days

Arthritis: Intra-articular (acetate): Administer every 1-5 weeks.

Large joints: 20-80 mg

Small joints: 4-10 mg

Intralesional (acetate): 20-60 mg every 1-5 weeks

Elderly: Only sodium succinate salt may be given I.V. Use the lowest effective adult dose.

Pediatrics: Dosing should be based on the lesser of ideal body weight or actual body weight. **Only sodium succinate may be given I.V.;** methylprednisolone sodium succinate is highly soluble and has a rapid effect by I.M. and I.V. routes. Methylprednisolone acetate has a low solubility and has a sustained I.M. effect.

Anti-inflammatory or immunosuppressive: Oral, I.M., I.V. (sodium succinate): Children: 0.5-1.7 mg/kg/day **or** 5-25 mg/m^2/day in divided doses every 6-12 hours; "Pulse" therapy: 15-30 mg/kg/dose over ≥30 minutes given once daily for 3 days

Status asthmaticus: Children: I.V. (sodium succinate): Loading dose: 2 mg/kg/dose, then 0.5-1 mg/kg/dose every 6 hours for up to 5 days

Acute spinal cord injury: I.V. (sodium succinate): 30 mg/kg over 15 minutes, followed in 45 minutes by a continuous infusion of 5.4 mg/kg/hour for 23 hours

Lupus nephritis: I.V. (sodium succinate): 30 mg/kg over ≥30 minutes every other day for 6 doses

Renal Impairment:

Hemodialysis effects: Slightly dialyzable (5% to 20%) Administer dose posthemodialysis.

Administration

Oral: Give oral formulation with meals to decrease GI upset. Give daily dose in the morning to mimic normal peak blood levels.

I.V.: Only sodium succinate formulation may be given I.V. Acetate salt should not be given I.V.

Parenteral: Methylprednisolone sodium succinate may be administered I.M. or I.V.; I.V. administration may be IVP over one to several minutes or IVPB or continuous I.V. infusion.

I.V.: Succinate:

Low dose: ≤1.8 mg/kg or ≤125 mg/dose: I.V. push over 3-15 minutes

Moderate dose: ≥2 mg/kg or 250 mg/dose: I.V. over 15-30 minutes

High dose: 15 mg/kg or ≥500 mg/dose: I.V. over ≥30 minutes

Doses >15 mg/kg or ≥1 g: Administer over 1 hour

Do **not** administer high-dose I.V. push; hypotension, cardiac arrhythmia, and sudden death have been reported in patients given high-dose methylprednisolone I.V. push over <20 minutes. Intermittent infusion over 15-60 minutes; maximum concentration: I.V. push 125 mg/mL.

I.V. Detail: pH: 7-8 (adjusted with sodium hydroxide)

Topical: For external use only. Apply sparingly.

Stability

Reconstitution:

Standard diluent (Solu-Medrol®): 40 mg/50 mL D$_5$W; 125 mg/50 mL D$_5$W

Minimum volume (Solu-Medrol®): 50 mL D$_5$W

Compatibility: Incompatible with D$_5$½NS

Y-site administration: Incompatible with allopurinol, amsacrine, ciprofloxacin, docetaxel, etoposide phosphate, filgrastim, gemcitabine, ondansetron, paclitaxel, propofol, sargramostim, vinorelbine

Compatibility in syringe: Incompatible with doxapram

Compatibility when admixed: Incompatible with calcium gluconate, glycopyrrolate, insulin (regular), metaraminol, nafcillin, penicillin G sodium

Storage: Intact vials of methylprednisolone sodium succinate should be stored at controlled room temperature. Reconstituted solutions of methylprednisolone sodium succinate should be stored at room temperature (15°C to 30°C) and used within 48 hours. Stability of parenteral admixture at room temperature (25°C) and at refrigeration temperature (4°C) is 48 hours.

Laboratory Monitoring Blood glucose, electrolytes

Nursing Actions

Physical Assessment: Assess effectiveness and interactions of other medications patient may be taking. Monitor for effectiveness of therapy and adverse reactions according to dose, route, and length of therapy (especially with systemic administration). Assess knowledge/teach patient appropriate use, possible side effects/interventions, and adverse symptoms to report (ie, opportunistic infection, adrenal suppression). Instruct patients with diabetes to monitor serum glucose levels closely; corticosteroids can alter glycemic response. Dose may need to be increased if patient is experiencing higher than normal levels of stress. When discontinuing, taper dose and frequency slowly.

Patient Education: Maintain adequate nutritional intake; consult prescriber for possibility of special dietary instructions. If you have diabetes, monitor serum glucose closely and notify prescriber of any changes; this medication can alter glycemic response. Avoid alcohol. Inform prescriber if you are experiencing unusual stress; dosage may need to be adjusted. You will be susceptible to infection (avoid crowds and and exposure to infection). You may experience insomnia or nervousness; use caution when driving or engaging in tasks requiring alertness until response to drug is known. Report increased pain, swelling, or redness in area being treated; excessive or sudden weight gain; swelling of extremities; respiratory difficulty; muscle pain or weakness; change in menstrual pattern; vision changes; signs of hyperglycemia; signs of infection (eg, fever, chills, mouth sores, perianal itching, vaginal discharge); blackened stool; other persistent side effects; or worsening of condition. **Pregnancy/breast-feeding precautions:** Inform prescriber if you are or intend to become pregnant. Consult prescriber if breast-feeding.

Oral: Take as directed, with food or milk. Take once-a-day dose in the morning. Do not take more than prescribed or discontinue without consulting prescriber.

Intra-articular: Refrain from excessive use of joint following therapy, even if pain is gone.

Dietary Considerations Should be taken after meals or with food or milk; need diet rich in pyridoxine, vitamin C, vitamin D, folate, calcium, phosphorus, and protein.

Sodium content of 1 g sodium succinate injection: 2.01 mEq; 53 mg of sodium succinate salt is equivalent to 40 mg of methylprednisolone base

Methylprednisolone acetate: Depo-Medrol®

Methylprednisolone sodium succinate: Solu-Medrol®

Geriatric Considerations Because of the risk of adverse effects, systemic corticosteroids should be used cautiously in the elderly, in the smallest possible dose, and for the shortest possible time.

Additional Information Sodium content of 1 g sodium succinate injection: 2.01 mEq; 53 mg of sodium succinate salt is equivalent to 40 mg of methylprednisolone base

Methylprednisolone acetate: Depo-Medrol®

Methylprednisolone sodium succinate: Solu-Medrol®

Related Information
FDA Name Differentiation Project: The Use of Tall-Man Letters on page 12

MethylTESTOSTERone
(meth il tes TOS te rone)

U.S. Brand Names Android®; Methitest™; Testred®; Virilon®

Restrictions C-III

Pharmacologic Category Androgen

Medication Safety Issues
Sound-alike/look-alike issues:
MethylTESTOSTERone may be confused with medroxyPROGESTERone
Virilon® may be confused with Verelan®

Pregnancy Risk Factor X

Lactation Excretion in breast milk unknown/contraindicated

Use
Male: Hypogonadism; delayed puberty; impotence and climacteric symptoms
Female: Palliative treatment of metastatic breast cancer

Mechanism of Action/Effect Male: Stimulates receptors in organs and tissues to promote growth and development of male sex organs and maintains secondary sex characteristics in androgen-deficient males.

Contraindications Hypersensitivity to methyltestosterone or any component of the formulation; in males, known or suspected carcinoma of the breast or the prostate; pregnancy

Warnings/Precautions Use with extreme caution in patients with liver or kidney disease or serious heart disease. May accelerate bone maturation without producing compensatory gain in linear growth.

Drug Interactions
Decreased Effect: Decreased oral anticoagulant effect

Increased Effect/Toxicity: Effects of oral anticoagulants and hypoglycemic agents may be increased. Toxicity may occur with cyclosporine; avoid concurrent use.

Adverse Reactions Frequency not defined.
Male: Virilism, priapism, prostatic hyperplasia, prostatic carcinoma, impotence, testicular atrophy, gynecomastia
Female: Virilism, menstrual problems (amenorrhea), breast soreness, hirsutism (increase in pubic hair growth) atrophy
Cardiovascular: Edema
Central nervous system: Headache, anxiety, depression
Dermatologic: Acne, "male pattern" baldness, seborrhea
Endocrine & metabolic: Hypercalcemia, hypercholesterolemia

Gastrointestinal: GI irritation, nausea, vomiting
Hematologic: Leukopenia, polycythemia
Hepatic: Hepatic dysfunction, hepatic necrosis, cholestatic hepatitis
Miscellaneous: Hypersensitivity reactions

Overdosage/Toxicology Abnormal liver function tests

Pharmacodynamics/Kinetics
Metabolism: Hepatic
Excretion: Urine

Available Dosage Forms
Capsule (Android®, Testred®, Virilon®): 10 mg
Tablet (Methitest™): 10 mg

Dosing
Adults & Elderly: Note: Buccal absorption produces twice the androgenic activity of oral tablets.

Hypogonadism; delayed puberty; impotence and climacteric symptoms (males):
Oral: 10-40 mg/day
Buccal: 5-25 mg/day

Breast pain/engorgement (Female):
Oral: 80 mg/day for 3-5 days
Buccal: 40 mg/day for 3-5 days

Breast cancer (Female):
Oral: 50-200 mg/day
Buccal: 25-100 mg/day

Nursing Actions
Physical Assessment: Assess potential for interactions with other pharmacological agents patient may be taking (eg, effects of hypoglycemic agents may be increased). Monitor therapeutic effects (according to purpose for use) and adverse response (eg, virilism [male and female], edema, CNS changes [anxiety, depression], acne, baldness, GI irritation, leukopenia, hepatic dysfunction) frequently during therapy. Caution patients with diabetes; effects of hypoglycemic agents may be increased. Teach patient proper use, possible side effects/appropriate interventions, and adverse symptoms to report. **Pregnancy risk factor X** - determine that patient is not pregnant before beginning treatment. Instruct patients of childbearing age or males who may have intercourse with women of childbearing age on appropriate contraceptive measures. Breast-feeding is contraindicated.

Patient Education: Take as directed; do not discontinue without consulting prescriber. If you have diabetes, monitor serum glucose closely and notify prescriber of changes; this medication can alter hypoglycemic requirements. May cause acne, growth of body hair, loss of libido, impotence, or menstrual irregularity (usually reversible); or nausea or vomiting (small, frequent meals, frequent mouth care, sucking lozenges, or chewing gum may help). Report changes in menstrual pattern; deepening of voice or unusual growth of body hair; gynecomastia or breast soreness; priapism; fluid retention (swelling of ankles, feet, or hands, respiratory difficulty, or sudden weight gain); change in color of urine or stool; yellowing of eyes or skin; unusual bruising or bleeding; unusual fatigue or weakness; or other adverse reactions. **Pregnancy/breast-feeding precautions:** Inform prescriber if you are pregnant. Do not get pregnant or cause a pregnancy (males) during or for 1 month following therapy. Consult prescriber for instruction on appropriate barrier contraceptive measures. This drug may cause severe fetal defects. Do not breast-feed.

Geriatric Considerations Since elderly males have prostate changes with age, it would be best to obtain a PSA initially and periodically. Retention of sodium and water could be a problem in patients with CHF and hypertension.

Related Information
FDA Name Differentiation Project: The Use of Tall-Man Letters on page 12

Metoclopramide (met oh kloe PRA mide)

U.S. Brand Names Reglan®

Pharmacologic Category Antiemetic; Gastrointestinal Agent, Prokinetic

Medication Safety Issues
Sound-alike/look-alike issues:
Metoclopramide may be confused with metolazone
Reglan® may be confused with Megace®, Regonol®, Renagel®

Pregnancy Risk Factor B

Lactation Enters breast milk/use caution

Use
Oral: Symptomatic treatment of diabetic gastric stasis; gastroesophageal reflux

I.V., I.M.: Symptomatic treatment of diabetic gastric stasis; postpyloric placement of enteral feeding tubes; prevention and/or treatment of nausea and vomiting associated with chemotherapy, or postsurgery; to stimulate gastric emptying and intestinal transit of barium during radiological examination

Mechanism of Action/Effect Blocks dopamine receptors and (when given in higher doses) also blocks serotonin receptors in chemoreceptor trigger zone of the CNS; enhances the response to acetylcholine of tissue in upper GI tract causing enhanced motility and accelerated gastric emptying without stimulating gastric, biliary, or pancreatic secretions; increases lower esophageal sphincter tone

Contraindications Hypersensitivity to metoclopramide or any component of the formulation; GI obstruction, perforation or hemorrhage; pheochromocytoma; history of seizures

Warnings/Precautions Use caution with a history of mental illness; has been associated with extrapyramidal symptoms (EPS) and depression. The frequency of EPS is higher in pediatric patients and adults <30 years of age; risk is increased at higher dosages. Extrapyramidal reactions typically occur within the initial 24-48 hours of treatment. Use caution with concurrent use of other drugs associated with EPS. Use caution in the elderly and with Parkinson's disease; may have increased risk of tardive dyskinesia. Use caution in patients with a history of seizures; risk of metoclopramide-associated seizures is increased. Neuroleptic malignant syndrome (NMS) has been reported (rarely) with metoclopramide. Use lowest recommended doses initially; may cause transient increase in serum aldosterone; use caution in patients who are at risk of fluid overload (CHF, cirrhosis). Use caution in patients with hypertension or following surgical anastomosis/closure. Patients with NADH-cytochrome b5 reductase deficiency are at increased risk of methemoglobinemia and/or sulfhemoglobinemia. Abrupt discontinuation may (rarely) result in withdrawal symptoms (dizziness, headache, nervousness). Use caution and adjust dose in renal impairment.

Drug Interactions
Cytochrome P450 Effect: Substrate (minor) of CYP1A2, 2D6; **Inhibits** CYP2D6 (weak)

Decreased Effect: Anticholinergic agents antagonize metoclopramide's actions.

Increased Effect/Toxicity: Opiate analgesics may increase CNS depression. Metoclopramide may increase extrapyramidal symptoms (EPS) or risk when used concurrently with antipsychotic agents. Metoclopramide may increase cyclosporine levels.

Nutritional/Ethanol Interactions Ethanol: Avoid ethanol (may increase CNS depression).

Lab Interactions Increased aminotransferase [ALT (SGPT)/AST (SGOT)] (S), amylase (S)

Adverse Reactions Frequency not always defined.
Cardiovascular: AV block, bradycardia, CHF, fluid retention, flushing (following high I.V. doses), hyper-/hypotension, supraventricular tachycardia

Central nervous system: Drowsiness (~10% to 70%; dose related), fatigue (~10%), restlessness (~10%), acute dystonic reactions (<1% to 25%; dose and age related), akathisia, confusion, depression, dizziness, hallucinations (rare), headache, insomnia, neuroleptic malignant syndrome (rare), Parkinsonian-like symptoms, suicidal ideation, seizures, tardive dyskinesia

Dermatologic: Angioneurotic edema (rare), rash, urticaria

Endocrine & metabolic: Amenorrhea, galactorrhea, gynecomastia, impotence

Gastrointestinal: Diarrhea, nausea

Genitourinary: Incontinence, urinary frequency

Hematologic: Agranulocytosis, leukopenia, neutropenia, porphyria

Hepatic: Hepatotoxicity (rare)

Ocular: Visual disturbance

Respiratory: Bronchospasm, laryngeal edema (rare)

Miscellaneous: Allergic reactions, methemoglobinemia, sulfhemoglobinemia

Overdosage/Toxicology Symptoms of overdose include drowsiness, ataxia, extrapyramidal symptoms, seizures, methemoglobinemia (in infants). Disorientation, muscle hypertonia, irritability, and agitation are common. Metoclopramide often causes extrapyramidal symptoms (eg, dystonic reactions) requiring management with diphenhydramine 1-2 mg/kg (adults) up to a maximum of 50-100 mg I.M. or I.V. slow push followed by a maintenance dose (25-50 mg orally every 4-6 hours) for 48-72 hours. When these reactions are unresponsive to diphenhydramine, benztropine mesylate I.V. 1-2 mg (adults) may be effective. These agents are generally effective within 2-5 minutes. Methylene blue is not recommended in patients with G6PD deficiency who experience methemoglobinemia due to metoclopramide.

Pharmacodynamics/Kinetics
Onset of Action: Oral: 0.5-1 hour; I.V.: 1-3 minutes; I.M.: 10-15 minutes

Duration of Action: Therapeutic: 1-2 hours, regardless of route

Time to Peak: Serum: Oral: 1-2 hours

Protein Binding: 30%

Half-Life Elimination: May be dose dependent: Normal renal function: 4-6 hours

Excretion: Urine (~85%)

Available Dosage Forms
Injection, solution (Reglan®): 5 mg/mL (2 mL, 10 mL, 30 mL)

Syrup: 5 mg/5 mL (10 mL, 480 mL)

Tablet (Reglan®): 5 mg, 10 mg

Dosing
Adults:
Gastroesophageal reflux: Oral: 10-15 mg/dose up to 4 times/day 30 minutes before meals or food and at bedtime; single doses of 20 mg are occasionally needed for provoking situations. Treatment >12 weeks has not been evaluated.

Diabetic gastric stasis:
Oral: 10 mg 30 minutes before each meal and at bedtime

I.M., I.V. (for severe symptoms): 10 mg over 1-2 minutes; 10 days of I.V. therapy may be necessary for best response

Chemotherapy-induced emesis:
I.V.: 1-2 mg/kg 30 minutes before chemotherapy and repeated every 2 hours for 2 doses, then every 3 hours for 3 doses (manufacturer labeling)

Alternate dosing (with or without diphenhydramine):
Moderate emetic risk chemotherapy: 0.5 mg/kg every 6 hours on days 2-4

Low and minimal risk chemotherapy: 1-2 mg/kg every 3-4 hours

Breakthrough treatment: 1-2 mg/kg every 3-4 hours

Oral (unlabeled use; with or without diphenhydramine):

Moderate emetic risk chemotherapy: 0.5 mg/kg every 6 hours or 20 mg 4 times/day on days 2-4

Low and minimal risk chemotherapy: 20-40 mg every 4-6 hours

Breakthrough treatment: 20-40 mg every 4-6 hours

Postoperative nausea and vomiting: I.M., I.V.: 10-20 mg near end of surgery

Postpyloric feeding tube placement, radiological exam: I.V.: 10 mg

Elderly:

Gastroesophageal reflux: Oral: 5 mg 4 times/day (30 minutes before meals or food and at bedtime); increase dose to 10 mg 4 times/day if no response at lower dose

Gastrointestinal hypomotility:

Oral: Initial: 5 mg 30 minutes before meals and at bedtime; increase if necessary to 10 mg doses

I.V.: Initiate at 5 mg over 1-2 minutes; increase to 10 mg if necessary

Postoperative nausea and vomiting: I.M., I.V.: 5 mg near end of surgery; may repeat dose if necessary

Pediatrics:

Gastroesophageal reflux (unlabeled use): Oral: 0.1-0.2 mg/kg/dose 4 times/day

Chemotherapy-induced emesis (unlabeled use): I.V.: 1-2 mg/kg 30 minutes before chemotherapy and every 2-4 hours

Postpyloric feeding tube placement: I.V.:

<6 years: 0.1 mg/kg

6-14 years: 2.5-5 mg

>14 years: Refer to Adults dosing.

Renal Impairment:

Cl_{cr} <40 mL/minute: Administer 50% of normal dose. Not dialyzable (0% to 5%); supplemental dose is not necessary.

Administration

I.M.: May be administered I.M.

I.V.: Injection solution may be given I.M., direct I.V. push, short infusion (15-30 minutes), or continuous infusion; lower doses (≤10 mg) of metoclopramide can be given I.V. push undiluted over 1-2 minutes; higher doses to be given IVPB over at least 15 minutes; continuous SubQ infusion and rectal administration have been reported. **Note:** Rapid I.V. administration may be associated with a transient (but intense) feeling of anxiety and restlessness, followed by drowsiness.

I.V. Detail: pH: 3.0-6.5

Other: Continuous SubQ infusion and rectal administration have been reported

Stability

Compatibility: Stable in $D_5\frac{1}{2}NS$, D_5W, mannitol 20%, LR, NS

Y-site administration: Incompatible with allopurinol, amphotericin B cholesteryl sulfate complex, amsacrine, cefepime, doxorubicin liposome, furosemide, propofol

Compatibility in syringe: Incompatible with ampicillin, calcium gluconate, chloramphenicol, furosemide, penicillin G potassium, sodium bicarbonate

Compatibility when admixed: Incompatible with dexamethasone sodium phosphate with lorazepam and diphenhydramine, erythromycin lactobionate, floxacillin, fluorouracil, furosemide

Storage:

Injection: Store intact vial at controlled room temperature; injection is photosensitive and should be protected from light during storage; parenteral admixtures in D_5W or NS are stable for at least 24 hours, and do not require light protection if used within 24 hours.

Tablet: Store at controlled room temperature.

Laboratory Monitoring Periodic renal function

Nursing Actions

Physical Assessment: Assess potential for interactions with other pharmacological agents patient may be taking (eg, any antipsychotic agents, opioids, anticholinergics). Monitor vital signs during intravenous administration. Inpatients should use safety measures (eg, side rails up, call light within reach) and caution patient to call for assistance with ambulation. Monitor laboratory tests, therapeutic effectiveness (relief of symptoms), and adverse reactions (eg, extrapyramidal effects, parkinsonian-like reactions, seizures, fluid retention, adverse CNS changes). Teach patient proper use, possible side effects/appropriate interventions, and adverse symptoms to report (eg, CNS restlessness, drowsiness, depression, rash).

Patient Education: Do not take any new medication during therapy unless approved by prescriber. Oral: Take this drug as prescribed, 30 minutes prior to eating. Do not increase dosage. Avoid alcohol; may increase adverse effects. May cause dizziness, drowsiness, or blurred vision (use caution when driving or engaging in tasks that require alertness until response to drug is known); cause restlessness, anxiety, depression, or insomnia (will reverse when medication is discontinued). Report any CNS changes, spasticity or involuntary movements, unresolved diarrhea, fluid retention (swelling of extremities, weight gain); visual disturbances; palpitations or rapid heart beat; or any other persistent adverse effects. **Breast-feeding precaution:** Breast-feeding is not recommended.

Geriatric Considerations Elderly are more likely to develop tardive dyskinesia syndrome (especially elderly females) reactions than younger adults. Use lowest recommended doses initially. Must consider renal function (estimate creatinine clearance). It is recommended to do involuntary movement assessments on elderly using this medication at high doses and for long-term therapy.

Breast-Feeding Issues Enters breast milk; may increase milk production

Pregnancy Issues Crosses the placenta; available evidence suggests safe use during pregnancy.

Related Information

Compatibility of Drugs in Syringe *on page 1372*

Metolazone (me TOLE a zone)

U.S. Brand Names Zaroxolyn®

Pharmacologic Category Diuretic, Thiazide-Related

Medication Safety Issues

Sound-alike/look-alike issues:

Metolazone may be confused with metaxalone, methazolamide, methimazole, methotrexate, metoclopramide, metoprolol, minoxidil

Zaroxolyn® may be confused with Zarontin®

Pregnancy Risk Factor B (manufacturer); D (expert analysis)

Lactation Enters breast milk/use caution

Use Management of mild to moderate hypertension; treatment of edema in congestive heart failure and nephrotic syndrome, impaired renal function

Mechanism of Action/Effect Inhibits sodium reabsorption in the distal tubules causing increased excretion of sodium and water, as well as, potassium and hydrogen ions

Contraindications Hypersensitivity to metolazone, any component of the formulation, other thiazides, and sulfonamide derivatives; anuria; hepatic coma; pregnancy (expert analysis)

Warnings/Precautions Electrolyte disturbances (hypokalemia, hypochloremic alkalosis, hyponatremia) can occur. Use with caution in severe hepatic dysfunction; *(Continued)*

Metolazone *(Continued)*

hepatic encephalopathy can be caused by electrolyte disturbances. Gout can be precipitate in certain patients with a history of gout, a familial predisposition to gout, or chronic renal failure. Cautious use in patients with diabetes; may see a change in glucose control. Hypersensitivity reactions can occur. Can cause SLE exacerbation or activation. Use caution in severe renal impairment. Orthostatic hypotension may occur (potentiated by alcohol, barbiturates, narcotics, other antihypertensive drugs). Mykrox® tablets are not interchangeable with Zaroxolyn® tablets. Use with caution in patients with moderate or high cholesterol concentrations. Photosensitization may occur.

Chemical similarities are present among sulfonamides, sulfonylureas, carbonic anhydrase inhibitors, thiazides, and loop diuretics (except ethacrynic acid). Use in patients with thiazide or sulfonamide allergy is specifically contraindicated in product labeling, however, a risk of cross-reaction exists in patients with allergy to any of these compounds; avoid use when previous reaction has been severe.

Drug Interactions

Decreased Effect: Decreased absorption of metolazone with cholestyramine and colestipol. NSAIDs can decrease the efficacy of thiazide-type diuretics, reducing the diuretic and antihypertensive effects.

Increased Effect/Toxicity: Increased diuretic effect of metolazone with furosemide and other loop diuretics. Increased hypotension and/or renal adverse effects of ACE inhibitors may result in aggressively diuresed patients. Cyclosporine and thiazide-type diuretics can increase the risk of gout or renal toxicity. Digoxin toxicity can be exacerbated if a diuretic induces hypokalemia or hypomagnesemia. Lithium toxicity can occur with thiazide-type diuretics due to reduced renal excretion of lithium. Thiazide-type diuretics may prolong the duration of action of neuromuscular blocking agents.

Nutritional/Ethanol Interactions Herb/Nutraceutical: Avoid dong quai if using for hypertension (has estrogenic activity). Avoid dong quai, St John's wort (may also cause photosensitization). Avoid ephedra, yohimbe, ginseng (may worsen hypertension). Avoid natural licorice. Avoid garlic (may have increased antihypertensive effect).

Adverse Reactions

>10%: Central nervous system: Dizziness

1% to 10%:

Cardiovascular: Orthostatic hypotension, palpitation, chest pain, cold extremities (rapidly acting), edema (rapidly acting), venous thrombosis (slow acting), syncope (slow acting)

Central nervous system: Headache, fatigue, lethargy, malaise, lassitude, anxiety, depression, nervousness, "weird" feeling (rapidly acting), chills (slow acting)

Dermatologic: Rash, pruritus, dry skin (rapidly acting)

Endocrine & metabolic: Hypokalemia, impotence, reduced libido, excessive volume depletion (slow acting), hemoconcentration (slow acting), acute gouty attach (slow acting)

Gastrointestinal: Nausea, vomiting, abdominal pain, cramping, bloating, diarrhea or constipation, dry mouth

Genitourinary: Nocturia

Neuromuscular & skeletal: Muscle cramps, spasm, weakness

Ocular: Eye itching (rapidly acting)

Otic: Tinnitus (rapidly acting)

Respiratory: Cough (rapidly acting), epistaxis (rapidly acting), sinus congestion (rapidly acting), sore throat (rapidly acting)

Overdosage/Toxicology Symptoms of overdose include orthostatic hypotension, dizziness, drowsiness, syncope, hemoconcentration and hemodynamic changes due to plasma volume depletion. Treatment is symptomatic and supportive.

Pharmacodynamics/Kinetics

Onset of Action: Diuresis: ~60 minutes

Duration of Action: 12-24 hours

Protein Binding: 95%

Half-Life Elimination: Dependent upon renal function: 6-20 hours

Metabolism: Undergoes enterohepatic recirculation

Excretion: Urine (80% to 95%)

Available Dosage Forms Tablet, slow acting: 2.5 mg, 5 mg, 10 mg

Dosing

Adults:

Edema: Oral: 2.5-20 mg/dose every 24 hours (ACC/AHA 2005 Heart Failure Guidelines)

Hypertension:

Zaroxolyn®: Oral: 2.5-5 mg/dose every 24 hours

Mykrox®: Oral: 0.5 mg/day; if response is not adequate, increase dose to maximum of 1 mg/day.

Elderly: Oral:

Zaroxolyn®: Initial: 2.5 mg/day or every other day

Mykrox®: 0.5 mg once daily; may increase to 1 mg if response is inadequate; do not use more than 1 mg/day.

Pediatrics: Limited experience in pediatric patients. Doses used have generally ranged from 0.05 to 0.1 mg/kg administered once daily. Prolonged use is not recommended.

Renal Impairment: Not dialyzable (0% to 5%)

Administration

Oral: May be taken with food or milk. Take early in day to avoid nocturia. Take the last dose of multiple doses no later than 6 PM unless instructed otherwise.

Laboratory Monitoring Serum electrolytes (potassium, sodium, chloride, bicarbonate), renal function

Nursing Actions

Physical Assessment: Patient's renal status and allergy history (thiazides and sulfonamide derivatives) should be assessed prior to beginning therapy. Assess potential for interactions with other pharmacological agents and herbal products patient may be taking (eg, especially anything that will affect blood pressure). Monitor electrolytes and renal function, therapeutic effectiveness, and adverse reactions (eg, hypersensitivity reactions, electrolyte imbalance, hypotension). Caution patients with diabetes (may see a change in glucose control). Teach patient proper use, possible side effects/appropriate interventions (eg, orthostatic hypotension precautions), and adverse symptoms to report.

Patient Education: Do not take any new medication during therapy unless approved by prescriber. Take exactly as directed, after breakfast. Include bananas or orange juice in daily diet but do not take potassium supplements without advice of prescriber. This medication does not replace other antihypertensive interventions; follow prescriber's instructions for diet and lifestyle changes. Weigh yourself weekly at the same time, in the same clothes. Report weight gain >5 lb/week. May cause dizziness or weakness (change position slowly when rising from sitting or lying, avoid driving or tasks requiring alertness until response to drug is known); nausea or loss of appetite (small, frequent meals, frequent mouth care, chewing gum, or sucking lozenges may help); impotence (reversible); constipation (increased exercise, fluids, fruit, or fiber may help); or photosensitivity (use sunscreen, wear protective clothing and eyewear, and avoid direct sunlight). Report flu-like symptoms, headache, joint soreness or weakness, respiratory difficulty, skin rash, excessive fatigue, or swelling of extremities.

Pregnancy/breast-feeding precautions: Inform prescriber if you are pregnant. Do not get pregnant while taking this medication. Consult prescriber for appropriate contraceptives. Consult prescriber if breast-feeding.

Dietary Considerations Should be taken after breakfast; may require potassium supplementation

Geriatric Considerations When metolazone is used in combination with other diuretics, there is an increased risk of azotemia and electrolyte depletion, particularly in the elderly, monitor closely. May be effective in patients with glomerular filtration rate <20 mL/minute. Metolazone is often used in combination with a loop diuretic in patients who are unresponsive to the loop diuretic alone.

Additional Information Metolazone 5 mg is approximately equivalent to hydrochlorothiazide 50 mg. When taken the day of surgery, it may cause hypovolemia and the hypertensive patient undergoing general anesthesia to have labile blood pressure; use with caution prior to surgery or perioperatively.

Metoprolol (me toe PROE lole)

U.S. Brand Names Lopressor®; Toprol-XL®
Synonyms Metoprolol Succinate; Metoprolol Tartrate
Pharmacologic Category Beta Blocker, Beta₁ Selective

Medication Safety Issues
Sound-alike/look-alike issues:
Metoprolol may be confused with metaproterenol, metolazone, misoprostol
Toprol-XL® may be confused with Tegretol®, Tegretol®-XR, Topamax®

Pregnancy Risk Factor C (manufacturer); D (2nd and 3rd trimesters - expert analysis)

Lactation Enters breast milk/use caution (AAP rates "compatible")

Use Treatment of hypertension and angina pectoris; prevention of myocardial infarction, atrial fibrillation, flutter, symptomatic treatment of hypertrophic subaortic stenosis; to reduce mortality/hospitalization in patients with congestive heart failure (stable NYHA Class II or III) in patients already receiving ACE inhibitors, diuretics, and/or digoxin (sustained-release only)

Unlabeled/Investigational Use Treatment of ventricular arrhythmias, atrial ectopy, migraine prophylaxis, essential tremor, aggressive behavior

Mechanism of Action/Effect Selective inhibitor of beta₁-adrenergic receptors; competitively blocks beta₁-receptors, with little or no effect on beta₂-receptors at doses <100 mg; does not exhibit any membrane stabilizing or intrinsic sympathomimetic activity

Contraindications Hypersensitivity to metoprolol or any component of the formulation; sinus bradycardia; heart block greater than first degree (except in patients with a functioning artificial pacemaker); cardiogenic shock; uncompensated cardiac failure; pregnancy (2nd and 3rd trimesters)

Warnings/Precautions Use with caution in compensated heart failure; monitor closely for a worsening of the condition (efficacy has been demonstrated for metoprolol). Use caution in patients with PVD (can aggravate arterial insufficiency). Use caution with concurrent use of beta-blockers and either verapamil or diltiazem; bradycardia or heart block can occur. Avoid concurrent I.V. use of both agents. In general, beta-blockers should be avoided in patients with bronchospastic disease. Metoprolol, with B1 selectivity, should be used cautiously in bronchospastic disease with close monitoring. Beta-blockers may increase the risk of anaphylaxis (in predisposed patients) and blunt response to epinephrine. Use cautiously in patients with diabetes because it can mask prominent hypoglycemic symptoms. Can mask signs of thyrotoxicosis. Can cause fetal harm when administered in pregnancy. Use cautiously in the hepatically impaired. Use care with anesthetic agents which decrease myocardial function. Beta-blocker therapy should not be withdrawn abruptly (particularly in patients with CAD), but gradually tapered to avoid acute tachycardia, hypertension, and/or ischemia. Avoid use of extended release tablets (Toprol-XL®) in patients with known stricture/narrowing of the GI tract.

Drug Interactions
Cytochrome P450 Effect: Substrate of CYP2C19 (minor), 2D6 (major); Inhibits CYP2D6 (weak)

Decreased Effect: Decreased effect of beta-blockers with aluminum salts, barbiturates, calcium salts, cholestyramine, colestipol, NSAIDs, penicillins (ampicillin), rifampin, salicylates, and sulfinpyrazone due to decreased bioavailability and plasma levels. Beta-blockers may decrease the effect of sulfonylureas.

Increased Effect/Toxicity: CYP2D6 inhibitors may increase the levels/effects of metoprolol; example inhibitors include chlorpromazine, delavirdine, fluoxetine, miconazole, paroxetine, pergolide, quinidine, quinine, ritonavir, and ropinirole. Metoprolol may increase the effects of other drugs which slow AV conduction (digoxin, verapamil, diltiazem), alpha-blockers (prazosin, terazosin), and alpha-adrenergic stimulants (epinephrine, phenylephrine). Metoprolol may mask the tachycardia from hypoglycemia caused by insulin and oral hypoglycemics. In patients receiving concurrent therapy, the risk of hypertensive crisis is increased when either clonidine or the beta-blocker is withdrawn. Reserpine has been shown to enhance the effect of beta-blockers. Beta-blockers may increase the action or levels of ethanol, disopyramide, nondepolarizing muscle relaxants, and theophylline although the effects are difficult to predict.

Nutritional/Ethanol Interactions
Food: Food increases absorption. Metoprolol serum levels may be increased if taken with food.
Herb/Nutraceutical: Avoid dong quai if using for hypertension (has estrogenic activity). Avoid ephedra, yohimbe, ginseng (may worsen hypertension). Avoid garlic (may have increased antihypertensive effect).

Adverse Reactions
>10%:
Central nervous system: Drowsiness, insomnia
Endocrine & metabolic: Decreased sexual ability
1% to 10%:
Cardiovascular: Bradycardia, palpitation, edema, CHF, reduced peripheral circulation
Central nervous system: Mental depression
Gastrointestinal: Diarrhea or constipation, nausea, stomach discomfort
Respiratory: Bronchospasm
Miscellaneous: Cold extremities

Overdosage/Toxicology Symptoms of intoxication include cardiac disturbances, CNS toxicity, bronchospasm, hypoglycemia and hyperkalemia. The most common cardiac symptoms include hypotension and bradycardia. Atrioventricular block, intraventricular conduction disturbances, cardiogenic shock, and asystole may occur with severe overdose, especially with membrane-depressant drugs (eg, propranolol). CNS effects include convulsions, coma, and respiratory arrest. Treatment is symptom-directed and supportive.

Pharmacodynamics/Kinetics
Onset of Action: Peak effect: Antihypertensive: Oral: 1.5-4 hours
Duration of Action: 10-20 hours
Protein Binding: 8%
Half-Life Elimination: 3-4 hours; End-stage renal disease: 2.5-4.5 hours
Metabolism: Extensively hepatic; significant first-pass effect
(Continued)

Metoprolol *(Continued)*

Excretion: Urine (3% to 10% as unchanged drug)

Available Dosage Forms

Injection, solution, as tartrate (Lopressor®): 1 mg/mL (5 mL)

Tablet, as tartrate: 25 mg, 50 mg, 100 mg

Lopressor®: 50 mg, 100 mg

Tablet, extended release, as succinate (Toprol-XL®): 25 mg, 50 mg, 100 mg, 200 mg [expressed as mg equivalent to tartrate]

Dosing

Adults:

Hypertension: Oral: 100-450 mg/day in 2-3 divided doses, begin with 50 mg twice daily and increase doses at weekly intervals to desired effect; usual dosage range (JNC 7): 50-100 mg/day

> *Extended release:* Initial: 25-100 mg/day (maximum: 400 mg/day)

Angina, SVT, MI prophylaxis: Oral: 100-450 mg/day in 2-3 divided doses, begin with 50 mg twice daily and increase doses at weekly intervals to desired effect

> *Extended release:* Initial: 100 mg/day (maximum: 400 mg/day)

Hypertension/ventricular rate control: I.V. (in patients having nonfunctioning GI tract): Initial: 1.25-5 mg every 6-12 hours; titrate initial dose to response. Initially, low doses may be appropriate to establish response; however, up to 15 mg every 3-6 hours has been employed.

Congestive heart failure: Oral (extended release): Initial: 25 mg once daily (reduce to 12.5 mg once daily in NYHA class higher than class II); may double dosage every 2 weeks as tolerated, up to 200 mg/day

Myocardial infarction (acute): I.V.: 5 mg every 2 minutes for 3 doses in early treatment of myocardial infarction; thereafter give 50 mg orally every 6 hours 15 minutes after last I.V. dose and continue for 48 hours; then administer a maintenance dose of 100 mg twice daily.

Elderly: Oral: Initial: 25 mg/day; usual dose range: 25-300 mg/day; increase at 1- to 2-week intervals.

Extended release: 25-50 mg/day initially as a single dose; increase at 1- to 2-week intervals.

Pediatrics:

Hypertension, arrhythmia: Oral: Children: 1-5 mg/kg/24 hours divided twice daily; allow 3 days between dose adjustments.

Renal Impairment: Hemodialysis: Administer dose posthemodialysis or administer 50 mg supplemental dose. Supplemental dose is not necessary following peritoneal dialysis.

Hepatic Impairment: Reduced dose is probably necessary.

Administration

Oral: Extended release tablets may be divided in half; do not crush or chew.

I.V.: When administered acutely for cardiac treatment, monitor ECG and blood pressure. May administer by rapid infusion (I.V. push) over 1 minute or by slow infusion (ie, 5-10 mg of metoprolol in 50 mL of fluid) over ~30 minutes. Necessary monitoring for surgical patients who are unable to take oral beta-blockers (prolonged ileus) has not been defined. Some institutions require monitoring of baseline and postinfusion heart rate and blood pressure when a patient's response to beta-blockade has not been characterized (ie, the patient's initial dose or following a change in dose). Consult individual institutional policies and procedures.

I.V. Detail: pH: 7.5

Stability

Compatibility: Stable in D_5W, NS

Y-site administration: Incompatible with amphotericin B cholesteryl sulfate complex

Storage:

Injection: Do not store above 30°C (86°F). Protect from light.

Tablet: Store between 15°C to 30°C (59°F to 86°F).

Nursing Actions

Physical Assessment: Assess potential for interactions with other prescriptions, OTC medications, or herbal products patient may be taking. I.V.: Monitor blood pressure and cardiac status. Monitor patient response and adverse reactions (eg, fluid balance, CHF, postural hypotension). Caution patients with diabetes to monitor serum glucose closely; may decrease the effect of sulfonylureas and can mask prominent hypoglycemic symptoms. Teach patient proper use (oral), possible side effects/appropriate interventions, and adverse symptoms to report.

Patient Education: I.V. use in emergency situations: Patient information is appropriate to patient condition.

Oral: Do not take any new medication during therapy unless approved by prescriber. Take exactly as directed. Do not change dosage or discontinue without consulting prescriber. Take pulse daily, prior to medication and follow prescriber's instruction about holding medication. Do not take with antacids. If you have diabetes, monitor serum sugar closely (drug may alter glucose tolerance or mask signs of hypoglycemia). May cause fatigue, dizziness, or postural hypotension (use caution when changing position from lying or sitting to standing, when driving, or when climbing stairs until response to medication is known); or alteration in sexual performance (reversible). Report unresolved swelling of extremities, respiratory difficulty or new cough, unresolved fatigue, unusual weight gain, unresolved constipation, or unusual muscle weakness. **Pregnancy/breast-feeding precautions:** Inform prescriber if you are or intend to become pregnant. Consult prescriber if breast-feeding.

Dietary Considerations Regular tablets should be taken with food. Extended release tablets may be taken without regard to meals.

Geriatric Considerations Due to alterations in the beta-adrenergic autonomic nervous system, beta-adrenergic blockade may result in less hemodynamic response than seen in younger adults.

Breast-Feeding Issues Metoprolol is considered compatible by the AAP. However, monitor the infant for signs of beta-blockade (hypotension, bradycardia, etc) with long-term use.

Pregnancy Issues Metoprolol crosses the placenta. Beta-blockers have been associated with bradycardia, hypotension, and IUGR; IUGR is probably related to maternal hypertension. Available evidence suggests beta-blockers are generally safe during pregnancy (JNC 7). Cases of neonatal hypoglycemia have been reported following maternal use of beta-blockers at parturition or during breast-feeding. Monitor breast-fed infant for symptoms of beta-blockade.

Metronidazole (me troe NI da zole)

U.S. Brand Names Flagyl®; Flagyl ER®; Flagyl® I.V. RTU™; MetroCream®; MetroGel®; MetroGel-Vaginal®; MetroLotion®; Noritate®; Vandazole™

Synonyms Metronidazole Hydrochloride

Pharmacologic Category Amebicide; Antibiotic, Miscellaneous; Antibiotic, Topical; Antiprotozoal, Nitroimidazole

Medication Safety Issues
Sound-alike/look-alike issues:
Metronidazole may be confused with metformin.

Pregnancy Risk Factor B (may be contraindicated in 1st trimester)

Lactation Enters breast milk/not recommended (AAP rates "of concern")

Use Treatment of susceptible anaerobic bacterial and protozoal infections in the following conditions: Amebiasis, symptomatic and asymptomatic trichomoniasis; skin and skin structure infections; CNS infections; intra-abdominal infections (as part of combination regimen); systemic anaerobic infections; treatment of antibiotic-associated pseudomembranous colitis (AAPC), bacterial vaginosis; as part of a multidrug regimen for *H. pylori* eradication to reduce the risk of duodenal ulcer recurrence
Topical: Treatment of inflammatory lesions and erythema of rosacea

Unlabeled/Investigational Use Crohn's disease

Mechanism of Action/Effect Inhibits DNA synthesis in susceptible organisms

Contraindications Hypersensitivity to metronidazole, nitroimidazole derivatives, or any component of the formulation; pregnancy (1st trimester - found to be carcinogenic in rats)

Warnings/Precautions Use with caution in patients with liver impairment due to potential accumulation, blood dyscrasias; history of seizures, CHF, or other sodium retaining states; reduce dosage in patients with severe liver impairment, CNS disease, and severe renal failure (Cl$_{cr}$ <10 mL/minute); if *H. pylori* is not eradicated in patients being treated with metronidazole in a regimen, it should be assumed that metronidazole-resistance has occurred and it should not again be used; seizures and neuropathies have been reported especially with increased doses and chronic treatment; if this occurs, discontinue therapy

Drug Interactions
Cytochrome P450 Effect: Inhibits CYP2C8/9 (weak), 3A4 (moderate)
Decreased Effect: Phenytoin, phenobarbital (potentially other enzyme inducers) may decrease metronidazole half-life and effects.
Increased Effect/Toxicity: Ethanol may cause a disulfiram-like reaction. Warfarin and metronidazole may increase bleeding times (PT) which may result in bleeding. Cimetidine may increase metronidazole levels. Metronidazole may inhibit metabolism of cisapride, causing potential arrhythmias; avoid concurrent use. Metronidazole may increase lithium levels/toxicity. Metronidazole may increase the levels/effects of selected benzodiazepines, calcium channel blockers, cyclosporine, ergot derivatives, selected HMG-CoA reductase inhibitors, mirtazapine, nateglinide, nefazodone, sildenafil (and other PDE-5 inhibitors), tacrolimus, venlafaxine, and other CYP3A4 substrates.

Nutritional/Ethanol Interactions
Ethanol: The manufacturer recommends to avoid all ethanol or any ethanol-containing drugs (may cause disulfiram-like reaction characterized by flushing, headache, nausea, vomiting, sweating or tachycardia).
Food: Peak antibiotic serum concentration lowered and delayed, but total drug absorbed not affected.

Lab Interactions May cause falsely decreased AST and ALT levels.

Adverse Reactions
Systemic: Frequency not defined:
Cardiovascular: Flattening of the T-wave, flushing
Central nervous system: Ataxia, confusion, coordination impaired, dizziness, fever, headache, insomnia, irritability, seizure, vertigo
Dermatologic: Erythematous rash, urticaria
Endocrine & metabolic: Disulfiram-like reaction, dysmenorrhea, libido decreased
Gastrointestinal: Nausea (~12%), anorexia, abdominal cramping, constipation, diarrhea, furry tongue, glossitis, proctitis, stomatitis, unusual/metallic taste, vomiting, xerostomia
Genitourinary: Cystitis, darkened urine (rare), dysuria, incontinence, polyuria, vaginitis
Hematologic: Neutropenia (reversible), thrombocytopenia (reversible, rare)
Neuromuscular & skeletal: Peripheral neuropathy, weakness
Respiratory: Nasal congestion, rhinitis, sinusitis, pharyngitis
Miscellaneous: Flu-like syndrome, moniliasis

Topical: Frequency not defined:
Central nervous system: Headache
Dermatologic: Burning, contact dermatitis, dryness, erythema, irritation, pruritus, rash
Gastrointestinal: Unusual/metallic taste, nausea, constipation
Local: Local allergic reaction
Neuromuscular & skeletal: Tingling/numbness of extremities
Ocular: Eye irritation

Vaginal:
>10%: Genitourinary: Vaginal discharge (12%)
1% to 10%:
Central nervous system: Headache (5%), dizziness (2%)
Gastrointestinal: Gastrointestinal discomfort (7%), nausea and/or vomiting (4%), unusual/metallic taste (2%), diarrhea (1%)
Genitourinary: Vaginitis (10%), vulva/vaginal irritation (9%), pelvic discomfort (3%)
Hematologic: WBC increased (2%)

Overdosage/Toxicology Symptoms of overdose include nausea, vomiting, ataxia, seizures, and peripheral neuropathy. Treatment is symptomatic and supportive.

Pharmacodynamics/Kinetics
Time to Peak: Serum: Oral: Immediate release: 1-2 hours
Protein Binding: <20%
Half-Life Elimination: Neonates: 25-75 hours; Others: 6-8 hours, prolonged with hepatic impairment; End-stage renal disease: 21 hours
Metabolism: Hepatic (30% to 60%)
Excretion: Urine (20% to 40% as unchanged drug); feces (6% to 15%)

Available Dosage Forms [DSC] = Discontinued product
Capsule (Flagyl®): 375 mg
Cream, topical: 0.75% (45 g)
MetroCream®: 0.75% (45 g) [contains benzyl alcohol]
Noritate®: 1% (60 g)
Gel, topical (MetroGel®): 0.75% (45 g) [DSC], 1% (45 g)
Gel, vaginal (MetroGel-Vaginal®, Vandazole™): 0.75% (70 g)
Infusion (Flagyl® I.V. RTU™) [premixed iso-osmotic sodium chloride solution]: 500 mg (100 mL) [contains sodium 14 mEq]
Lotion, topical (MetroLotion®): 0.75% (60 mL) [contains benzyl alcohol]
Tablet (Flagyl®): 250 mg, 500 mg
Tablet, extended release (Flagyl® ER): 750 mg
(Continued)

Metronidazole *(Continued)*

Dosing

Adults:

Anaerobic infections (diverticulitis, intra-abdominal, peritonitis, cholangitis, or abscess): Oral, I.V.: 500 mg every 6-8 hours, not to exceed 4 g/day

Acne rosacea: Topical:

0.75%: Apply and rub a thin film twice daily, morning and evening, to entire affected areas after washing. Significant therapeutic results should be noticed within 3 weeks. Clinical studies have demonstrated continuing improvement through 9 weeks of therapy.

1%: Apply thin film to affected area once daily

Amebiasis: Oral: 500-750 mg every 8 hours for 5-10 days

Antibiotic-associated pseudomembranous colitis: Oral: 250-500 mg 3-4 times/day for 10-14 days

Giardiasis: 500 mg twice daily for 5-7 days

Peptic ulcer disease: *Helicobacter pylori* **eradication:** Oral: 250-500 mg with meals and at bedtime for 14 days; requires combination therapy with at least one other antibiotic and an acid-suppressing agent (proton pump inhibitor or H_2 blocker)

Bacterial vaginosis or vaginitis due to *Gardnerella, Mobiluncus*:

Oral: 500 mg twice daily (regular release) or 750 mg once daily (extended release tablet) for 7 days

Vaginal: 1 applicatorful (~37.5 mg metronidazole) intravaginally once or twice daily for 5 days; apply once in morning and evening if using twice daily, if daily, use at bedtime

Trichomoniasis: Oral: 250 mg every 8 hours for 7 days **or** 375 mg twice daily for 7 days **or** 2 g as a single dose

Elderly: Use the lower end of the dosing recommendations for adults; do not administer as single dose as efficacy has not been established.

Pediatrics:

Anaerobic infections: Oral, I.V.:

Postnatal age >7 days:

1200-2000 g: 15 mg/kg/day in divided doses every 12 hours

>2000 g: 30 mg/kg/day in divided doses every 12 hours

Infants and Children:

Oral: 15-35 mg/kg/day in divided doses every 8 hours

I.V.: 30 mg/kg/day in divided doses every 6 hours

Colitis due to *Clostridium difficile*: Oral: 20 mg/kg/day divided every 6 hours. Maximum dose: 2 g/day

Amebiasis: Infants and Children: Oral: 35-50 mg/kg/day in divided doses every 8 hours for 10 days

Trichomoniasis: Infants and Children: Oral: 15-30 mg/kg/day in divided doses every 8 hours for 7 days

Renal Impairment:

Cl_{cr} <10 mL/minute: Administer 50% of dose or every 12 hours.

Hemodialysis effects: Extensively removed by hemodialysis and peritoneal dialysis (50% to 100%). Administer dose posthemodialysis. During peritoneal dialysis, dose as for Cl_{cr} <10 mL/minute.

Continuous arteriovenous or venovenous hemofiltration: Dose as for normal renal function

Hepatic Impairment: Unchanged in mild liver disease; reduce dosage in severe liver disease.

Administration

Oral: May be taken with food to minimize stomach upset. Extended release tablets should be taken on an empty stomach (1 hour before or 2 hours after meals).

I.V. Detail: pH: 5-7 (ready to use); 0.5-2.0 (reconstituted); 6-7 (further dilution)

Topical: No disulfiram-like reactions have been reported after **topical** application, although metronidazole can be detected in the blood. Apply to clean, dry skin. Cosmetics may be used after application (wait at least 5 minutes after using lotion).

Stability

Reconstitution: Standard diluent: 500 mg/100 mL NS

Compatibility: Stable in D_5W, NS

Y-site administration: Incompatible with amphotericin B cholesteryl sulfate complex, aztreonam, filgrastim, meropenem, warfarin

Compatibility when admixed: Incompatible with aztreonam, dopamine, meropenem

Storage: Metronidazole injection should be stored at 15°C to 30°C and protected from light. Product may be refrigerated but crystals may form; crystals redissolve on warming to room temperature. Prolonged exposure to light will cause a darkening of the product. However, short-term exposure to normal room light does not adversely affect metronidazole stability. Direct sunlight should be avoided. Stability of parenteral admixture at room temperature (25°C): Out of overwrap stability: 30 days.

Nursing Actions

Physical Assessment: Assess effectiveness and interactions of other medications patient may be taking. Monitor laboratory tests, therapeutic response, and adverse reactions (eg, CNS, neuromuscular, and dermatologic reactions) according to dose, route of administration, and purpose of therapy. Assess knowledge/teach patient appropriate use, interventions to reduce side effects, and adverse symptoms to report.

Patient Education: Take exactly as directed. May take with or without food. Take with food if medication causes upset stomach. Avoid alcohol during and for 72 hours after last dose. With alcohol you may experience severe flushing, headache, nausea, vomiting, or chest and abdominal pain. May discolor urine (brown/black/dark) (normal). You may experience "metallic" taste disturbance or nausea or vomiting (small frequent meals, frequent mouth care, chewing gum, or sucking lozenges may help). Refrain from intercourse or use a contraceptive if being treated for trichomoniasis. Report unresolved or severe fatigue; weakness; fever or chills; mouth or vaginal sores; numbness, tingling, or swelling of extremities; respiratory difficulty; or lack of improvement or worsening of condition. **Pregnancy/breast-feeding precautions:** Inform prescriber if you are pregnant. Breast-feeding is not recommended.

Topical: Wash hands and area before applying. Apply medication thinly. Wash hands after applying. Avoid contact with eyes. Do not cover with occlusive dressing. Report severe skin irritation or if condition does not improve.

Dietary Considerations Take on an empty stomach. Drug may cause GI upset; if GI upset occurs, take with food. Extended release tablets should be taken on an empty stomach (1 hour before or 2 hours after meals). Sodium content of 500 mg (I.V.): 322 mg (14 mEq). The manufacturer recommends that ethanol be avoided during treatment and for 3 days after therapy is complete.

Geriatric Considerations Adjust dose based on renal function.

Breast-Feeding Issues It is suggested to stop breast-feeding for 12-24 hours following single dose therapy to allow excretion of dose.

Pregnancy Issues Crosses the placenta; contraindicated for the treatment of trichomoniasis during the first trimester of pregnancy, unless alternative treatment is inadequate. Until safety and efficacy for other indications have been established, use only during pregnancy when the benefit to the mother outweighs the potential risk to the fetus.

Mexiletine (MEKS i le teen)

U.S. Brand Names Mexitil® [DSC]

Pharmacologic Category Antiarrhythmic Agent, Class Ib

Pregnancy Risk Factor C

Lactation Enters breast milk/compatible

Use Management of serious ventricular arrhythmias; suppression of PVCs

Unlabeled/Investigational Use Diabetic neuropathy

Mechanism of Action/Effect Class IB antiarrhythmic, structurally related to lidocaine, which inhibits inward sodium current, decreases rate of rise of Phase 0, increases effective refractory period/action potential duration ratio

Contraindications Hypersensitivity to mexiletine or any component of the formulation; cardiogenic shock; second- or third-degree AV block (except in patients with a functioning artificial pacemaker)

Warnings/Precautions Can be proarrhythmic. May cause acute hepatic injury. Use cautiously in patients with first-degree block, pre-existing sinus node dysfunction, intraventricular conduction delays, significant hepatic dysfunction, hypotension, or severe CHF. Electrolytes disturbances alter response. Alterations in urinary pH may change urinary excretion. Rare hepatic toxicity may occur. Electrolyte abnormalities should be corrected before initiating therapy (can worsen CHF).

Drug Interactions

Cytochrome P450 Effect: Substrate (major) of CYP1A2, 2D6; **Inhibits** CYP1A2 (strong)

Decreased Effect: The levels/effects of mexiletine may be decreased by aminoglutethimide, carbamazepine, phenobarbital, rifampin, and other CYP1A2 inducers. Urinary acidifying agents may decrease mexiletine levels.

Increased Effect/Toxicity: Mexiletine may increase the levels/effects of aminophylline, fluvoxamine, mirtazapine, ropinirole, trifluoperazine, or other CYP1A2 substrates. The levels/effects of mexiletine may be increased by inhibitors of CYP1A2 or 2D6; example inhibitors include amiodarone, chlorpromazine, ciprofloxacin, delavirdine, fluoxetine, fluvoxamine, ketoconazole, miconazole, norfloxacin, ofloxacin, paroxetine, pergolide, quinidine, quinine, ritonavir, rofecoxib, ropinirole, and other CYP1A2 or 2D6 inhibitors. Mexiletine may increase levels of theophylline and caffeine. Quinidine and urinary alkalinizers (antacids, sodium bicarbonate, acetazolamide) may increase mexiletine blood levels.

Nutritional/Ethanol Interactions Food: Food may decrease the rate, but not the extent of oral absorption; diets which affect urine pH can increase or decrease excretion of mexiletine. Avoid dietary changes that alter urine pH.

Lab Interactions Abnormal liver function test, positive ANA, thrombocytopenia

Adverse Reactions

>10%:

Central nervous system: Lightheadedness (11% to 25%), dizziness (20% to 25%), nervousness (5% to 10%), incoordination (10%)

Gastrointestinal: GI distress (41%), nausea/vomiting (40%)

Neuromuscular & skeletal: Trembling, unsteady gait, tremor (13%), ataxia (10% to 20%)

1% to 10%:

Cardiovascular: Chest pain (3% to 8%), premature ventricular contractions (1% to 2%), palpitation (4% to 8%), angina (2%), proarrhythmic (10% to 15% in patients with malignant arrhythmia)

Central nervous system: Confusion, headache, insomnia (5% to 7%), depression (2%)

Dermatologic: Rash (4%)

Gastrointestinal: Constipation or diarrhea (4% to 5%), xerostomia (3%), abdominal pain (1%)

Neuromuscular & skeletal: Weakness (5%), numbness of fingers or toes (2% to 4%), paresthesia (2%), arthralgia (1%)

Ocular: Blurred vision (5% to 7%), nystagmus (6%)

Otic: Tinnitus (2% to 3%)

Respiratory: Dyspnea (3%)

Overdosage/Toxicology Has a narrow therapeutic index and severe toxicity may occur slightly above the therapeutic range, especially with other antiarrhythmic drugs. Acute ingestion of twice the daily therapeutic dose is potentially life-threatening. Symptoms of overdose include sedation, confusion, coma, seizures, respiratory arrest and cardiac toxicity (sinus arrest, AV block, asystole, and hypotension). The QRS and QT intervals are usually normal, although they may be prolonged after massive overdose. Other effects include dizziness, paresthesia, tremor, ataxia, and GI disturbance. Treatment is symptomatic and supportive.

Pharmacodynamics/Kinetics

Time to Peak: 2-3 hours

Protein Binding: 50% to 70%

Half-Life Elimination: Adults: 10-14 hours (average: 14.4 hours elderly, 12 hours younger adults); prolonged with hepatic impairment or heart failure

Metabolism: Hepatic; low first-pass effect

Excretion: Urine (10% to 15% as unchanged drug); urinary acidification increases excretion, alkalinization decreases excretion

Available Dosage Forms [DSC] = Discontinued product

Capsule, as hydrochloride: 150 mg, 200 mg, 250 mg

Mexitil®: 150 mg, 200 mg, 250 mg [DSC]

Dosing

Adults & Elderly: Arrhythmias: Oral: Initial: 200 mg every 8 hours (may load with 400 mg if necessary); adjust dose every 2-3 days; usual dose: 200-300 mg every 8 hours; maximum: 1.2 g/day (some patients respond to every 12-hour dosing). When switching from another antiarrhythmic, initiate a 200 mg dose 6-12 hours after stopping former agents, 3-6 hours after stopping procainamide.

Hepatic Impairment: Patients with hepatic impairment or CHF may require dose reduction; reduce dose to 25% to 30% of usual dose

Administration

Oral: Administer with food. Administer around-the-clock to promote less variation in peak and trough serum levels.

I.V. Detail: pH: 3-4 (adjusted with hydrochloric acid)

Laboratory Monitoring Regular serum levels

Nursing Actions

Physical Assessment: Assess other medications patient may be taking for effectiveness and interactions. Monitor cardiac status. Assess for CNS changes (trembling, unsteady gait, ataxia, lightheadedness, dizziness, or nervousness). Monitor laboratory tests, therapeutic response (cardiac status), and adverse reactions at beginning of therapy, when titrating dosage, and on a regular basis with long-term therapy. **Note:** Mexiletine has a low toxic:therapeutic ratio and overdose may easily produce severe and life-threatening reactions. Assess knowledge/teach patient appropriate use, interventions to reduce side effects, and adverse symptoms to report.

Patient Education: Take exactly as directed with food or antacids, around-the-clock. Do not take additional doses or discontinue without consulting prescriber. Do not change diet without consulting prescriber. You will need regular cardiac checkups and blood tests while taking this medication. You may experience drowsiness or dizziness, numbness, or visual changes (use caution when driving or engaging in tasks requiring alertness until response to drug is known); nausea, vomiting, or heartburn (small frequent meals, frequent (Continued)

Mexiletine *(Continued)*

mouth care, chewing gum, or sucking lozenges may help); or headaches or sleep disturbances (usually temporary, if persistent consult prescriber). Report chest pain, palpitation, or erratic heartbeat; increased weight or swelling of hands or feet; chills, fever, or persistent sore throat; numbness, weakness, trembling, or unsteady gait; blurred vision or ringing in ears; or respiratory difficulty. **Pregnancy precaution:** Inform prescriber if you are or intend to become pregnant.

Miconazole *(mi KON a zole)*

U.S. Brand Names Aloe Vesta® 2-n-1 Antifungal [OTC]; Baza® Antifungal [OTC]; Carrington Antifungal [OTC]; DermaFungal [OTC]; Dermagran® AF [OTC]; DiabetAid™ Antifungal Foot Bath [OTC]; Fungoid® Tincture [OTC]; Lotrimin® AF Jock Itch Powder Spray [OTC]; Lotrimin® AF Powder/Spray [OTC]; Micaderm® [OTC]; Micatin® Athlete's Foot [OTC]; Micatin® Jock Itch [OTC]; Micro-Guard® [OTC]; Mitrazol™ [OTC]; Monistat® 1 Combination Pack [OTC]; Monistat® 3 [OTC]; Monistat® 7 [OTC]; Monistat-Derm®; Neosporin® AF [OTC]; Podactin Cream [OTC]; Secura® Antifungal [OTC]; Zeasorb®-AF [OTC]

Synonyms Miconazole Nitrate

Pharmacologic Category Antifungal Agent, Topical; Antifungal Agent, Vaginal

Medication Safety Issues

Sound-alike/look-alike issues:

Miconazole may be confused with Micronase®, Micronor®

Lotrimin® may be confused with Lotrisone®, Otrivin®

Micatin® may be confused with Miacalcin®

Pregnancy Risk Factor C

Lactation Excretion in breast milk unknown/use caution

Use Treatment of vulvovaginal candidiasis and a variety of skin and mucous membrane fungal infections

Mechanism of Action/Effect Inhibits biosynthesis of ergosterol, damaging the fungal cell wall membrane, which increases permeability causing leaking of nutrients

Contraindications Hypersensitivity to miconazole or any component of the formulation

Warnings/Precautions For external use only; discontinue if sensitivity or irritation develop. Petrolatum-based vaginal products may damage rubber or latex condoms or diaphragms. Separate use by 3 days.

Drug Interactions

Cytochrome P450 Effect: Substrate of CYP3A4 (major); **Inhibits** CYP1A2 (moderate), 2A6 (strong), 2B6 (weak), 2C8/9 (strong), 2C19 (strong), 2D6 (strong), 2E1 (moderate), 3A4 (strong)

Decreased Effect: Amphotericin B may decrease antifungal effect of both agents. The levels/effects of miconazole may be decreased by aminoglutethimide, carbamazepine, nafcillin, nevirapine, phenobarbital, phenytoin, rifamycins or other CYP3A4 inducers. Miconazole may decrease the levels/effects of CYP2D6 prodrug substrates (eg, codeine, hydrocodone, oxycodone, tramadol).

Increased Effect/Toxicity: Note: The majority of reported drug interactions were observed following intravenous miconazole administration. Although systemic absorption following topical and/or vaginal administration is low, potential interactions due to CYP isoenzyme inhibition may occur (rarely). This may be particularly true in situations where topical absorption may be increased (ie, inflamed tissue).

Miconazole coadministered with warfarin has increased the anticoagulant effect of warfarin (including reports associated with vaginal miconazole

therapy of as little as 3 days). Concurrent administration of cisapride is contraindicated due to an increased risk of cardiotoxicity. Miconazole may increase the serum levels/effects of amiodarone, amphetamines, benzodiazepines, beta-blockers, buspirone, busulfan, calcium channel blockers, citalopram, dexmedetomidine, dextromethorphan, diazepam, digoxin, docetaxel, fluoxetine, fluvoxamine, glimepiride, glipizide, ifosfamide, inhalational anesthetics, lidocaine, mesoridazine, methsuximide, mexiletine, mirtazapine, nateglinide, nefazodone, paroxetine, phenytoin, pioglitazone, propranolol, risperidone, ritonavir, ropinirole, rosiglitazone, sertraline, sirolimus, tacrolimus, theophylline, thioridazine, tricyclic antidepressants, trifluoperazine, trimetrexate, venlafaxine, vincristine, vinblastine, warfarin, zolpidem, and other substrates of CYP1A2, 2A6, 2C8/9, 2C19, 2D6, or 3A4. Selected benzodiazepines (midazolam and triazolam), cisapride, ergot alkaloids, selected HMG-CoA reductase inhibitors (lovastatin and simvastatin), and pimozide are generally contraindicated with strong CYP3A4 inhibitors. Mesoridazine and thioridazine are generally contraindicated with strong CYP2D6 inhibitors. When used with strong CYP3A4 inhibitors, dosage adjustment/limits are recommended for sildenafil and other PDE-5 inhibitors; consult individual monographs.

Nutritional/Ethanol Interactions Herb/Nutraceutical: St John's wort may decrease miconazole levels.

Lab Interactions Increased protein

Adverse Reactions Frequency not defined.

Topical: Allergic contact dermatitis, burning, maceration

Vaginal: Abdominal cramps, burning, irritation, itching

Pharmacodynamics/Kinetics

Protein Binding: 91% to 93%

Half-Life Elimination: Multiphasic: Initial: 40 minutes; Secondary: 126 minutes; Terminal: 24 hours

Metabolism: Hepatic

Excretion: Feces (~50%); urine (<1% as unchanged drug)

Available Dosage Forms [DSC] = Discontinued product

Combination products: Miconazole nitrate vaginal suppository 200 mg (3s) and miconazole nitrate external cream 2%

Monistat® 1 Combination Pack: Miconazole nitrate vaginal insert 1200 mg (1) and miconazole nitrate external cream 2% (5 g) [Note: Do not confuse with 1-Day™ (formerly Monistat® 1) which contains tioconazole]

Monistat® 3 Combination Pack:

Miconazole nitrate vaginal suppository 200 mg (3s) and miconazole nitrate external cream 2%

Miconazole nitrate vaginal cream 4% and miconazole nitrate external cream 2%

Monistat® 7 Combination Pack:

Miconazole nitrate vaginal suppository 100 mg (7s) and miconazole nitrate external cream 2%

Miconazole nitrate vaginal cream 2% (7 prefilled applicators) and miconazole nitrate external cream 2%

Cream, topical, as nitrate: 2% (15 g, 30 g, 45 g)

Baza® Antifungal: 2% (4 g, 57 g, 142 g) [zinc oxide based formula]

Carrington Antifungal: 2% (150 g)

Micaderm®, Neosporin® AF, Podactin: 2% (30 g)

Micatin® Athlete's Foot, Micatin® Jock Itch: 2% (15 g)

Micro-Guard®, Mitrazol™: 2% (60 g)

Monistat-Derm®: 2% (15 g, 30 g, 85 g)

Secura® Antifungal: 2% (60 g, 98 g)

Cream, vaginal, as nitrate [prefilled or refillable applicator]: 2% (45 g)

Monistat® 3: 4% (15 g, 25 g)

Monistat® 7: 2% (45 g)

Liquid, spray, topical, as nitrate:

Micatin® Athlete's Foot: 2% (90 mL) [contains alcohol]

Neosporin AF®: 2% (105 mL)

Lotion, powder, as nitrate (Zeasorb®-AF): 2% (56 g) [contains alcohol 36%]

Ointment, topical, as nitrate:
Aloe Vesta® 2-n-1 Antifungal: 2% (60 g, 150 g)
DermaFungal: 2% (113 g)
Dermagran® AF: (113 g) [contains vitamin A and zinc]

Powder, topical, as nitrate:
Lotrimin® AF: 2% (160 g)
Micro-Guard®: 2% (90 g)
Mitrazol™: 2% (30 g)
Zeasorb®-AF: 2% (70 g)

Powder spray, topical, as nitrate:
Lotrimin® AF, Lotrimin® AF Jock Itch: 2% (140 g)
Micatin® Athlete's Foot, Micatin® Jock Itch: 2% (90 g) [contains alcohol]
Neosporin® AF: 2% (85 g)

Suppository, vaginal, as nitrate: 100 mg (7s); 200 mg (3s)
Monistat® 3: 200 mg (3s)
Monistat® 7: 100 mg (7s)

Tablet, effervescent, topical, as nitrate (DiabetAid™ Antifungal Foot Bath): 2% (10s)

Tincture, topical, as nitrate (Fungoid®): 2% (30 mL, 473 mL) [contains isopropyl alcohol 30%]; 30 mL size also available in a treatment kit which contains nail scrub and nail brush]

Dosing

Adults & Elderly:

Tinea corporis: Topical: Apply twice daily for 4 weeks

Tinea pedis: Topical: Apply twice daily for 4 weeks
Effervescent tablet: Dissolve 1 tablet in ~1 gallon of water; soak feet for 15-30 minutes; pat dry

Tinea cruris: Topical: Apply twice daily for 2 weeks

Vulvovaginal candidiasis: Vaginal:
Cream, 2%: Insert 1 applicatorful at bedtime for 7 days
Cream, 4%: Insert 1 applicatorful at bedtime for 3 days
Suppository, 100 mg: Insert 1 suppository at bedtime for 7 days
Suppository, 200 mg: Insert 1 suppository at bedtime for 3 days
Suppository, 1200 mg: Insert 1 suppository (a one-time dose); may be used at bedtime or during the day

Note: Many products are available as a combination pack, with a suppository for vaginal instillation and cream to relieve external symptoms. External cream may be used twice daily, as needed, for up to 7 days.

Pediatrics: Refer to adult dosing. **Note:** Not for OTC use in children <2 years.

Nursing Actions

Physical Assessment: Assess potential for interactions with other prescriptions, OTC medications, or herbal products patient may be taking. Caution patients with diabetes to test serum glucose regularly; may inhibit the metabolism of oral sulfonylureas. Teach patient proper use, possible side effects/appropriate interventions (eg, bleeding precautions), and adverse symptoms to report.

Patient Education: Inform prescriber of all prescriptions, OTC medications, or herbal products you are taking, and any allergies you have. Do not take any new medication during therapy. Use full course of therapy as directed; do not discontinue without consulting prescriber. Some infections may require long periods of therapy. Practice good hygiene measures to prevent reinfection. If you have diabetes, you should test serum glucose regularly - this medication may inhibit the metabolism of oral sulfonylureas. Report persistent burning, itching, or irritation to healthcare provider. **Pregnancy/breast-feeding precautions:** Inform prescriber if you are or intend to

become pregnant. Consult prescriber if breast-feeding.

Topical: Wash and dry area before applying medication; apply thinly. Do not get in or near eyes. Not for OTC use in children <2 years of age.

Vaginal: Consult with healthcare provider if using for a vaginal yeast infection for the first time. Insert high in vagina. Refrain from intercourse during treatment. Condoms and diaphragms may not be effective during therapy. Do not use tampons, douches, spermicides, or other vaginal products during treatment. Deodorant-free pads or panty shields may be used to protect clothing during use.

Geriatric Considerations Assess patient's ability to self administer, may be difficult in patients with arthritis or limited range of motion.

Midazolam (MID aye zoe lam)

Synonyms Midazolam Hydrochloride; Versed
Restrictions C-IV
Pharmacologic Category Benzodiazepine
Medication Safety Issues
Sound-alike/look-alike issues:
Versed may be confused with VePesid®, Vistaril®

Pregnancy Risk Factor D
Lactation Enters breast milk/not recommended (AAP rates "of concern")
Use Preoperative sedation and provides conscious sedation prior to diagnostic or radiographic procedures; ICU sedation (continuous infusion); intravenous anesthesia (induction); intravenous anesthesia (maintenance)
Unlabeled/Investigational Use Anxiety, status epilepticus
Mechanism of Action/Effect Binds to stereospecific benzodiazepine receptors on the postsynaptic GABA neuron at several sites within the central nervous system, including the limbic system, reticular formation. Enhancement of the inhibitory effect of GABA on neuronal excitability results by increased neuronal membrane permeability to chloride ions. This shift in chloride ions results in hyperpolarization (a less excitable state) and stabilization.
Contraindications Hypersensitivity to midazolam or any component of the formulation, including benzyl alcohol (cross-sensitivity with other benzodiazepines may exist); parenteral form is not for intrathecal or epidural injection; narrow-angle glaucoma; concurrent use of potent inhibitors of CYP3A4 (amprenavir, atazanavir, or ritonavir); pregnancy
Warnings/Precautions May cause severe respiratory depression, respiratory arrest, or apnea. Use with extreme caution, particularly in noncritical care settings. Appropriate resuscitative equipment and qualified personnel must be available for administration and monitoring. Initial dosing must be cautiously titrated and individualized, particularly in elderly or debilitated patients, hepatic impairment, or renal impairment, particularly if other CNS depressants (including opiates) are used concurrently. Initial doses in elderly or debilitated patients should not exceed 2.5 mg. Use with caution in patients with respiratory disease or impaired gag reflex. Use during upper airway procedures may increase risk of hypoventilation. Prolonged responses have been noted following extended administration by continuous infusion (possibly due to metabolite accumulation) or in the presence of drugs which inhibit midazolam metabolism.

May cause hypotension - hemodynamic events are more common in pediatric patients or patients with hemodynamic instability. Hypotension and/or respiratory depression may occur more frequently in patients who have received narcotic analgesics. Use with caution in (Continued)

Midazolam *(Continued)*

obese patients, chronic renal failure, and CHF. Parenteral form contains benzyl alcohol - avoid rapid injection in neonates or prolonged infusions. Should not be used in shock, coma, or acute alcohol intoxication. Avoid intra-arterial administration or extravasation of parenteral formulation.

Causes CNS depression (dose-related) resulting in sedation, dizziness, confusion, or ataxia which may impair physical and mental capabilities. A minimum of 1 day should elapse after midazolam administration before attempting to drive or operate machinery. Use with caution in patients receiving other CNS depressants or psychoactive agents. Effects with other sedative drugs or ethanol may be potentiated. Benzodiazepines have been associated with falls and traumatic injury and should be used with extreme caution in patients who are at risk of these events (especially the elderly).

Midazolam causes anterograde amnesia. Paradoxical reactions, including hyperactive or aggressive behavior have been reported with benzodiazepines, particularly in adolescent/pediatric or psychiatric patients. Does not have analgesic, antidepressant, or antipsychotic properties.

Benzodiazepines have been associated with dependence and acute withdrawal symptoms on discontinuation or reduction in dose. Acute withdrawal, including seizures, may be precipitated after administration of flumazenil to patients receiving long-term benzodiazepine therapy.

Drug Interactions

Cytochrome P450 Effect: Substrate of CYP2B6 (minor), 3A4 (major); **Inhibits** CYP2C8/9 (weak), 3A4 (weak)

Decreased Effect: CYP3A4 inducers may decrease the levels/effects of midazolam; example inducers include aminoglutethimide, carbamazepine, nafcillin, nevirapine, phenobarbital, phenytoin, and rifamycins.

Increased Effect/Toxicity: CYP3A4 inhibitors may increase the levels/effects of midazolam; example inhibitors include azole antifungals, clarithromycin, diclofenac, doxycycline, erythromycin, imatinib, isoniazid, nefazodone, nicardipine, propofol, protease inhibitors, quinidine, telithromycin, and verapamil. Use is contraindicated with amprenavir, atazanavir, and ritonavir. **If narcotics or other CNS depressants are administered concomitantly, the midazolam dose should be reduced by 30% if <65 years of age, or by at least 50% if >65 years of age.**

Nutritional/Ethanol Interactions

Ethanol: Avoid ethanol (may increase CNS depression).

Food: Grapefruit juice may increase serum concentrations of midazolam; avoid concurrent use with oral form.

Herb/Nutraceutical: Avoid concurrent use with St John's wort (may decrease midazolam levels, may increase CNS depression). Avoid concurrent use with valerian, kava kava, gotu kola (may increase CNS depression).

Adverse Reactions As reported in adults unless otherwise noted:

>10%: Respiratory: Decreased tidal volume and/or respiratory rate decrease, apnea (3% children)

1% to 10%:

Cardiovascular: Hypotension (3% children)

Central nervous system: Drowsiness (1%), oversedation, headache (1%), seizure-like activity (1% children)

Gastrointestinal: Nausea (3%), vomiting (3%)

Local: Pain and local reactions at injection site (4% I.M., 5% I.V.; severity less than diazepam)

Ocular: Nystagmus (1% children)

Respiratory: Cough (1%)

Miscellaneous: Physical and psychological dependence with prolonged use, hiccups (4%, 1% children), paradoxical reaction (2% children)

Overdosage/Toxicology Symptoms of overdose include respiratory depression, hypotension, coma, stupor, confusion, and apnea. Treatment for benzodiazepine overdose is supportive. Flumazenil has been shown to selectively block the binding of benzodiazepines to its receptor, resulting in reversal of CNS depression but not always respiratory depression.

Pharmacodynamics/Kinetics

Onset of Action: I.M.: Sedation: ~15 minutes; I.V.: 1-5 minutes; Peak effect: I.M.: 0.5-1 hour

Duration of Action: I.M.: Up to 6 hours; Mean: 2 hours

Protein Binding: 95%

Half-Life Elimination: 1-4 hours; prolonged with cirrhosis, congestive heart failure, obesity, elderly

Metabolism: Extensively hepatic via CYP3A4

Excretion: Urine (as glucuronide conjugated metabolites); feces (~2% to 10%)

Available Dosage Forms

Injection, solution: 1 mg/mL (2 mL, 5 mL, 10 mL); 5 mg/mL (1 mL, 2 mL, 5 mL, 10 mL) [contains benzyl alcohol 1%]

Injection, solution [preservative free]: 1 mg/mL (2 mL, 5 mL); 5 mg/mL (1 mL, 2 mL)

Syrup: 2 mg/mL (118 mL) [contains sodium benzoate; cherry flavor]

Dosing

Adults:

Note: The dose of midazolam needs to be individualized based on the patient's age, underlying diseases, and concurrent medications. Decrease dose (by ~30%) if narcotics or other CNS depressants are administered concomitantly. **Personnel and equipment needed for standard respiratory resuscitation should be immediately available during midazolam administration.**

Preoperative sedation:

I.M.: 0.07-0.08 mg/kg 30-60 minutes prior to surgery/procedure; usual dose: 5 mg; **Note:** Reduce dose in patients with COPD, high-risk patients, patients ≥60 years of age, and patients receiving other narcotics or CNS depressants

I.V.: 0.02-0.04 mg/kg; repeat every 5 minutes as needed to desired effect or up to 0.1-0.2 mg/kg

Intranasal (not an approved route): 0.2 mg/kg (up to 0.4 mg/kg in some studies); administer 30-45 minutes prior to surgery/procedure

Conscious sedation: I.V.: Initial: 0.5-2 mg slow I.V. over at least 2 minutes; slowly titrate to effect by repeating doses every 2-3 minutes if needed; usual total dose: 2.5-5 mg; use decreased doses in elderly.

Healthy Adults <60 years:

Initial: Some patients respond to doses as low as 1 mg; no more than 2.5 mg should be administered over a period of 2 minutes. Additional doses of midazolam may be administered after a 2-minute waiting period and evaluation of sedation after each dose increment. A total dose >5 mg is generally not needed. If narcotics or other CNS depressants are administered concomitantly, the midazolam dose should be reduced by 30%. *Refer to elderly dosing for patients ≥60 years, debilitated, or chronically ill.*

Maintenance: 25% of dose used to reach sedative effect

Anesthesia: I.V.:

Induction:

Unpremedicated patients: 0.3-0.35 mg/kg (up to 0.6 mg/kg in resistant cases)

Premedicated patients: 0.15-0.35 mg/kg

Maintenance: 0.05-0.3 mg/kg as needed, or continuous infusion 0.25-1.5 mcg/kg/minute

Sedation in mechanically-ventilated patients: I.V. continuous infusion: 100 mg in 250 mL D$_5$W or NS (if patient is fluid-restricted, may concentrate up to a maximum of 0.5 mg/mL); initial dose: 0.02-0.08 mg/kg (~1 mg to 5 mg in 70 kg adult) initially and either repeated at 5-15 minute intervals until adequate sedation is achieved or continuous infusion rates of 0.04-0.2 mg/kg/hour and titrate to reach desired level of sedation

Elderly: The dose of midazolam needs to be individualized based on the patient's age, underlying diseases, and concurrent medications. Decrease dose (by ~30%) if narcotics or other CNS depressants are administered concomitantly. **Personnel and equipment needed for standard respiratory resuscitation should be immediately available during midazolam administration.**

I.V.: Conscious sedation: Initial: 0.5 mg slow I.V.; give no more than 1.5 mg in a 2-minute period. If additional titration is needed, give no more than 1 mg over 2 minutes, waiting another 2 or more minutes to evaluate sedative effect. A total dose >3.5 mg is rarely necessary.

Pediatrics:

Notes: The dose of midazolam needs to be individualized based on the patient's age, underlying diseases, and concurrent medications. Decrease dose (by ~30%) if narcotics or other CNS depressants are administered concomitantly. **Personnel and equipment needed for standard respiratory resuscitation should be immediately available during midazolam administration.** Children <6 years may require higher doses and closer monitoring than older children; calculate dose on ideal body weight

Conscious sedation for procedures or preoperative sedation:

Oral: 0.25-0.5 mg/kg as a single dose preprocedure, up to a maximum of 20 mg; administer 30-40 minutes prior to procedure. Children <6 years, or less cooperative patients may require as much as 1 mg/kg as a single dose; 0.25 mg/kg may suffice for children 6-16 years of age.

Intranasal (not an approved route): 0.2 mg/kg (up to 0.4 mg/kg in some studies), administered 30-45 minutes prior to procedure

I.M.: 0.1-0.15 mg/kg 30-60 minutes before surgery or procedure; range 0.05-0.15 mg/kg; doses up to 0.5 mg/kg have been used in more anxious patients; maximum total dose: 10 mg

I.V.:

Infants <6 months: Limited information is available in nonintubated infants; dosing recommendations not clear; infants <6 months are at higher risk for airway obstruction and hypoventilation; titrate dose in small increments to desired effect; monitor carefully

Infants 6 months to Children 5 years: Initial: 0.05-0.1 mg/kg; titrate dose carefully; total dose of 0.6 mg/kg may be required; usual maximum total dose: 6 mg

Children 6-12 years: Initial: 0.025-0.05 mg/kg; titrate dose carefully; total doses of 0.4 mg/kg may be required; usual maximum total dose: 10 mg

Children 12-16 years: Dose as adults; usual maximum total dose: 10 mg

Conscious sedation during mechanical ventilation: I.V.: Children: Loading dose: 0.05-0.2 mg/kg, followed by initial continuous infusion: 1-2 mcg/kg/minute; titrate to the desired effect; usual range: 0.4-6 mcg/kg/minute

Status epilepticus refractory to standard therapy: I.V.: Infants >2 months and Children: Loading dose: 0.15 mg/kg followed by a continuous infusion of 1 mcg/kg/minute; titrate dose upward every 5 minutes until clinical seizure activity is controlled; mean infusion rate required in 24 children was 2.3 mcg/kg/minute with a range of 1-18 mcg/kg/minute

Renal Impairment:
Hemodialysis: Supplemental dose is not necessary.
Peritoneal dialysis: Significant drug removal is unlikely based on physiochemical characteristics.

Administration
Oral: Do not mix with any liquid (such as grapefruit juice) prior to administration.
I.M.: Give deep I.M. into large muscle.
I.V.: Administer by slow I.V. injection over at least 2-5 minutes at a concentration of 1-5 mg/mL or by I.V. infusion. Continuous infusions should be administered via an infusion pump.
I.V. Detail: pH: 3 (adjusted)
Other: Intranasal: Administer using a 1 mL needleless syringe into the nares over 15 seconds; use the 5 mg/mL injection; $^1/_2$ of the dose may be administered to each nare

Stability
Compatibility: Stable in D$_5$NS, D$_5$W, NS; **incompatible** with LR
Y-site administration: Incompatible with albumin, amphotericin B cholesteryl sulfate complex, ampicillin, bumetanide, butorphanol, ceftazidime, cefuroxime, clonidine, dexamethasone sodium succinate, floxacillin, foscarnet, fosphenytoin, furosemide, hydrocortisone sodium succinate, imipenem/cilastatin, methotrexate, nafcillin, omeprazole, sodium bicarbonate, thiopental, trimethoprim/sulfamethoxazole
Compatibility in syringe: Incompatible with dimenhydrinate, pentobarbital, perphenazine, prochlorperazine edisylate, ranitidine
Storage: Stable for 24 hours at room temperature/refrigeration; at a final concentration of 0.5 mg/mL, stable for up to 24 hours when diluted with D$_5$W or NS, or for up to 4 hours when diluted with lactated Ringer's; admixtures do not require protection from light for short-term storage

Nursing Actions
Physical Assessment: Assess other medications the patient may be taking for effectiveness and interactions **I.V.:** Monitor cardiac and respiratory status continuously. Monitor I.V. infusion site carefully for extravasation. For inpatient use, institute safety measures and monitor effectiveness and adverse reactions. For outpatients, monitor therapeutic effectiveness and adverse reactions at beginning of therapy and periodically with long-term use. **I.V./I.M.:** Monitor closely following administration. Provide bedrest and assistance with ambulation for several hours. **Note:** Full recovery usually occurs within 2-3 hours, but may take 6 hours.

Patient Education: Avoid use of alcohol, prescription or OTC sedatives, or hypnotics for a minimum of 24 hours after administration. Avoid driving or engaging in any tasks that require alertness for 24 hours following administration. You may experience some loss of memory following administration. **Pregnancy/breast-feeding precautions:** Advise prescriber if you are pregnant; this medication is contraindicated for pregnant women. Breast-feeding is not recommended.

Dietary Considerations Injection: Sodium content of 1 mL: 0.14 mEq

Geriatric Considerations If concomitant CNS depressant medications are used in the elderly, the midazolam dose will be at least 50% less than doses used in healthy, young, unpremedicated patients (see Warnings/Precautions and Pharmacodynamics/Kinetics). (Continued)

Midazolam (Continued)

Pregnancy Issues Benzodiazepines cross the placenta. The association between benzodiazepine exposure and malformations remains controversial. A number of types of malformation have been reported (oral cleft, inguinal hernia, cardiac defects, spina bifida, dysmorphic facial features, skeletal defects); however, confounding factors make a clear association difficult. Overall, the risk to the fetus may be low. Nonteratogenic effects (including neonatal flaccidity, respiratory and feeding problems, and withdrawal symptoms) during the post-natal period have also been reported with benzodiazepine use.

Additional Information Abrupt discontinuation after sustained use (generally >10 days) may cause withdrawal symptoms. For neonates, since both concentrations of the injection contain 1% benzyl alcohol, use the 5 mg/mL injection and dilute to 0.5 mg/mL with SWI without preservatives to decrease the amount of benzyl alcohol delivered to the neonate; with continuous infusion, midazolam may accumulate in peripheral tissues; use lowest effective infusion rate to reduce accumulation effects; midazolam is 3-4 times as potent as diazepam; paradoxical reactions associated with midazolam use in children (eg, agitation, restlessness, combativeness) have been successfully treated with flumazenil (see Massanari, 1997).

Related Information
Compatibility of Drugs in Syringe *on page 1372*

Midodrine (MI doe dreen)

U.S. Brand Names Orvaten™; ProAmatine®
Synonyms Midodrine Hydrochloride
Pharmacologic Category Alpha$_1$ Agonist
Medication Safety Issues
Sound-alike/look-alike issues:
ProAmatine® may be confused with protamine
Pregnancy Risk Factor C
Lactation Excretion in breast milk is unknown/use caution
Use Orphan drug: Treatment of symptomatic orthostatic hypotension
Unlabeled/Investigational Use Investigational: Management of urinary incontinence
Mechanism of Action/Effect Midodrine forms an active metabolite, desglymidodrine that is an alpha$_1$-agonist. This agent increases arteriolar and venous tone resulting in a rise in standing, sitting, and supine systolic and diastolic blood pressure in patient with orthostatic hypotension.
Contraindications Hypersensitivity to midodrine or any component of the formulation; severe organic heart disease; urinary retention; pheochromocytoma; thyrotoxicosis; persistent and significant supine hypertension
Warnings/Precautions Indicated for patients for whom orthostatic hypotension significantly impairs their daily life despite standard clinical care. Use is not recommended with supine hypertension. Caution should be exercised in patients with diabetes, visual problems (especially if receiving fludrocortisone), urinary retention (reduce initial dose), or hepatic dysfunction; monitor renal and hepatic function prior to and periodically during therapy; safety and efficacy has not been established in children; discontinue and re-evaluate therapy if signs of bradycardia occur.
Drug Interactions
Increased Effect/Toxicity: Concomitant fludrocortisone results in hypernatremia or an increase in intraocular pressure and glaucoma. Bradycardia may be accentuated with concomitant administration of cardiac glycosides, psychotherapeutics, and

beta-blockers. Alpha agonists may increase the pressure effects and alpha antagonists may negate the effects of midodrine.

Adverse Reactions
>10%:
Cardiovascular: Supine hypertension (7% to 13%)
Dermatologic: Piloerection (13%), pruritus (12%)
Genitourinary: Urinary urgency, retention, or polyuria, dysuria (up to 13%)
Neuromuscular & skeletal: Paresthesia (18%)
1% to 10%:
Central nervous system: Chills (5%), pain (5%)
Dermatologic: Rash (2%)
Gastrointestinal: Abdominal pain

Overdosage/Toxicology
Symptoms of overdose include hypertension, piloerection, urinary retention
Treatment is symptomatic following gastric decontamination; alpha-sympatholytics and/or dialysis may be helpful

Pharmacodynamics/Kinetics
Onset of Action: ~1 hour
Duration of Action: 2-3 hours
Time to Peak: Desglymidodrine: 1-2 hours; Midodrine: 30 minutes
Protein Binding: Minimal
Half-Life Elimination: Desglymidodrine: ~3-4 hours; Midodrine: 25 minutes
Metabolism: Hepatic; midodrine is a prodrug which undergoes rapid deglycination to desglymidodrine (active metabolite); metabolism occurs in many tissues and plasma
Excretion: Urine (2% to 4%)
Clearance: Desglymidodrine: 385 mL/minute (predominantly by renal secretion)

Available Dosage Forms Tablet, as hydrochloride: 2.5 mg, 5 mg, 10 mg

Dosing
Adults & Elderly: Orthostatic hypotension: Oral: 10 mg 3 times/day during daytime hours (every 3-4 hours) when patient is upright (maximum: 40 mg/day)
Renal Impairment: 2.5 mg 3 times/day; gradually increase as tolerated.
Hemodialysis: Dialyzable

Administration
Oral: Doses may be given in approximately 3- to 4-hour intervals (eg, shortly before or upon rising in the morning, at midday, in the late afternoon not later than 6 PM). Avoid dosing after the evening meal or within 4 hours of bedtime. Continue therapy only in patients who appear to attain symptomatic improvement during initial treatment. Standing systolic blood pressure may be elevated 15-30 mm Hg at 1 hour after a 10 mg dose. Some effect may persist for 2-3 hours.

Laboratory Monitoring Kidney and liver function tests

Nursing Actions
Physical Assessment: Assess potential for interactions with other pharmacological agents and herbal products patient may be taking (eg, risk for increased bradycardia with cardiac glycosides, psychotherapeutics, beta blockers). Monitor therapeutic effectiveness (reduction of hypotension) and adverse reactions (eg, supine hypertension, urinary urgency/retention, rash) at beginning of therapy and periodically thereafter. Note: Standing blood pressure may be elevated 1 hour after administration and remain slightly elevated 3-4 hours. Teach patient possible side effects/appropriate interventions and adverse symptoms to report.

Patient Education: Do not take any new medication during therapy unless approved by prescriber (especially anything that may affect blood pressure; cough or cold medications, diet, weight reduction, stay-awake products). Take exactly as directed; take when sitting upright. Do not take within 4 hours of bedtime or when lying down for any length of time. Follow instructions for checking blood pressure and pulse routinely (same time of day; for 1 week at least). May cause urinary urgency or retention (void before taking or consult prescriber if difficulty persists); or dizziness, drowsiness, or headache (use caution when driving or engaging in tasks that require alertness until response to drug is known). Report skin rash, severe gastric upset or pain, muscle weakness or pain, or other persistent side effects. **Pregnancy/breast-feeding precautions:** Inform prescriber if you are or intend to become pregnant. Consult prescriber if breast-feeding.

Mifepristone (mi FE pris tone)

U.S. Brand Names Mifeprex®
Synonyms RU-486; RU-38486
Restrictions Investigators wishing to obtain the agent for use in oncology patients must apply for a patient-specific IND from the FDA. Mifepristone will be supplied only to licensed physicians who sign and return a "Prescriber's Agreement." Distribution of mifepristone will be subject to specific requirements imposed by the distributor. Mifepristone will **not** be available to the public through licensed pharmacies. A patient medication guide is available and must be dispensed with the medication; the FDA-approved medication guide is available at http://www.fda.gov/cder/Offices/ODS/labeling.htm.

Not available in Canada
Pharmacologic Category Abortifacient; Antineoplastic Agent; Hormone Antagonist; Antiprogestin
Medication Safety Issues
　Sound-alike/look-alike issues:
　Mifeprex® may be confused with Mirapex®
Pregnancy Risk Factor X
Lactation Excretion in breast milk unknown/contraindicated
Use Medical termination of intrauterine pregnancy, through day 49 of pregnancy. Patients may need treatment with misoprostol and possibly surgery to complete therapy
Unlabeled/Investigational Use Treatment of unresectable meningioma; has been studied in the treatment of breast cancer, ovarian cancer, and adrenal cortical carcinoma
Mechanism of Action/Effect Mifepristone, a synthetic steroid, competitively binds to the intracellular progesterone receptor, blocking the effects of progesterone. When used for the termination of pregnancy, this leads to contraction-inducing activity in the myometrium. In the absence of progesterone, mifepristone acts as a partial progesterone agonist. Mifepristone also has weak antiglucocorticoid and antiandrogenic properties; it blocks the feedback effect of cortisol on corticotropin secretion.
Contraindications Hypersensitivity to mifepristone, misoprostol, other prostaglandins, or any component of the formulation; chronic adrenal failure; porphyrias; hemorrhagic disorder or concurrent anticoagulant therapy; pregnancy termination >49 days; intrauterine device (IUD) in place; ectopic pregnancy or undiagnosed adnexal mass; concurrent long-term corticosteroid therapy; inadequate or lack of access to emergency medical services; inability to understand effects and/or comply with treatment
Warnings/Precautions Patient must be instructed of the treatment procedure and expected effects. A signed agreement form must be kept in the patient's file. Physicians may obtain patient agreement forms, physician enrollment forms, and medical consultation directly from Danco Laboratories at 1-877-432-7596. Adverse effects (including blood transfusions, hospitalization, ongoing pregnancy, and other major complications) must be reported in writing to the medication distributor. To be

administered only by physicians who can date pregnancy, diagnose ectopic pregnancies, provide access to surgical abortion (if needed), and can provide access to emergency care. Medication will be distributed directly to these physicians following signed agreement with the distributor. Must be administered under supervision by the qualified physician. Pregnancy is dated from day 1 of last menstrual period (presuming a 28-day cycle, ovulation occurring midcycle). Pregnancy duration can be determined using menstrual history and clinical examination. Ultrasound should be used if an ectopic pregnancy is suspected or if duration of pregnancy is uncertain. Ultrasonography may not identify all ectopic pregnancies, and healthcare providers should be alert for signs and symptoms which may be related to undiagnosed ectopic pregnancy in any patient who receives mifepristone

Bleeding occurs and should be expected (average 9-16 days, may be ≥30 days). In some cases, bleeding may be prolonged and heavy, potentially leading to hypovolemic shock. Patients should be counseled to seek medical attention in cases of excessive bleeding; the manufacturer cites soaking through two thick sanitary pads per hour for two consecutive hours as an example of excessive bleeding. Bleeding may require blood transfusion (rare), curettage, saline infusions, and/or vasoconstrictors. Use caution in patients with severe anemia. Confirmation of pregnancy termination by clinical exam or ultrasound must be made 14 days following treatment. Manufacturer recommends surgical termination of pregnancy when medical termination fails or is not complete. Prescriber should determine in advance whether they will provide such care themselves or through other providers. Preventative measures to prevent rhesus immunization must be taken prior to surgical abortion. Prescriber should also give the patient clear instructions on whom to call and what to do in the event of an emergency following administration of mifepristone.

Bacterial infections have been reported following use of this product. In rare cases, these infections may be serious and/or fatal, with septic shock as a potential complication. A causal relationship has not been established. Sustained fever, abdominal pain, or pelvic tenderness should prompt evaluation; however, healthcare professionals are warned that atypical presentations of serious infection without these symptoms have also been noted. Patients presenting with nausea, vomiting, diarrhea, or weakness, with or without abdominal pain or fever, should be evaluated for serious bacterial infection when symptoms occur >24 hours after taking misoprostol. Treatment with antibiotics, including coverage for anaerobic bacteria (eg, *Clostridium sordellii*) should be initiated. Patients undergoing treatment with mifepristone should be instructed to bring their Medication Guide with them when an obtaining treatment from an emergency room or healthcare provider that did not prescribe the medication initially in order to identify that they are undergoing a medical abortion.

Safety and efficacy have not been established for use in women with chronic cardiovascular, hypertensive, hepatic, respiratory, or renal disease, insulin-dependent diabetes mellitus, severe anemia, or heavy smokers. Women >35 years of age and smokers (>10 cigarettes/day) were excluded from clinical trials. Safety and efficacy in pediatric patients have not been established.

Drug Interactions
Cytochrome P450 Effect: Substrate of CYP3A4 (minor); **Inhibits** CYP2D6 (weak), 3A4 (weak)
Increased Effect/Toxicity: There are no reported interactions. It might be anticipated that the concurrent administration of mifepristone and a progestin would result in an attenuation of the effects of one or both agents.
(Continued)

Mifepristone (Continued)

Nutritional/Ethanol Interactions

Food: Do not take with grapefruit juice; grapefruit juice may inhibit mifepristone metabolism leading to increased levels.

Herb/Nutraceutical: Avoid St John's wort (may induce mifepristone metabolism, leading to decreased levels).

Lab Interactions hCG levels will not be useful to confirm pregnancy termination until at least 10 days following mifepristone treatment.

Adverse Reactions Vaginal bleeding and uterine cramping are expected to occur when this medication is used to terminate a pregnancy; 90% of women using this medication for this purpose also report adverse reactions. Bleeding or spotting occurs in most women for a period of 9-16 days. Up to 8% of women will experience some degree of bleeding or spotting for 30 days or more. In some cases, bleeding may be prolonged and heavy, potentially leading to hypovolemic shock.

>10%:

Central nervous system: Headache (2% to 31%), dizziness (1% to 12%)

Gastrointestinal: Abdominal pain (cramping) (96%), nausea (43% to 61%), vomiting (18% to 26%), diarrhea (12% to 20%)

Genitourinary: Uterine cramping (83%)

1% to 10%:

Cardiovascular: Syncope (1%)

Central nervous system: Fatigue (10%), fever (4%), insomnia (3%), anxiety (2%), fainting (2%)

Gastrointestinal: Dyspepsia (3%)

Genitourinary: Uterine hemorrhage (5%), vaginitis (3%), pelvic pain (2%), endometriosis/salpingitis/pelvic inflammatory disease (1%)

Hematologic: Decreased hemoglobin >2 g/dL (6%), anemia (2%), leukorrhea (2%)

Neuromuscular & skeletal: Back pain (9%), rigors (3%), leg pain (2%), weakness (2%)

Respiratory: Sinusitis (2%)

Miscellaneous: Viral infection (4%)

Overdosage/Toxicology In studies using 3 times the recommended dose for termination of pregnancy, no serious maternal adverse effects were reported. This medication is supplied in single-dose containers to be given under physician supervision, therefore, the risk of overdose should be low. In case of massive ingestion, treat symptomatically and monitor for signs of adrenal failure.

Pharmacodynamics/Kinetics

Time to Peak: Oral: 90 minutes

Protein Binding: 98% to albumin and α_1-acid glycoprotein

Half-Life Elimination: Terminal: 18 hours following a slower phase where 50% eliminated between 12-72 hours

Metabolism: Hepatic via CYP3A4 to three metabolites (may possess some antiprogestin and antiglucocorticoid activity)

Excretion: Feces (83%); urine (9%)

Available Dosage Forms Tablet: 200 mg

Dosing

Adults:

Termination of pregnancy: Oral: Treatment consists of three office visits by the patient; the patient must read medication guide and sign patient agreement prior to treatment:

Day 1: 600 mg (three 200 mg tablets) taken as a single dose under physician supervision

Day 3: Patient must return to the healthcare provider 2 days following administration of mifepristone; unless abortion has occurred (confirmed using ultrasound or clinical examination): 400 mcg (two 200 mcg tablets) of misoprostol; patient

may need treatment for cramps or gastrointestinal symptoms at this time

Day 14: Patient must return to the healthcare provider ~14 days after administration of mifepristone; confirm complete termination of pregnancy by ultrasound or clinical exam. Surgical termination is recommended to manage treatment failures.

Dosing for unlabeled uses: Refer to individual protocols. The dose used in meningioma is usually 200 mg/day, continued based on toxicity and response.

Elderly: Safety and efficacy have not been established.

Renal Impairment: Safety and efficacy have not been established.

Hepatic Impairment: Safety and efficacy have not been established; use with caution due to CYP3A4 metabolism.

Stability

Storage: Store at room temperature of 25°C (77°F).

Laboratory Monitoring

Consider CBC in any patient who reports nausea, vomiting, or diarrhea and weakness with or without abdominal pain, and without fever or other signs of infection more than 24 hours after administration of misoprostol.

Nursing Actions

Physical Assessment: May only be administered under supervision of a qualified physician. Patient must be instructed in procedure and sign patient agreement forms. Monitor response and adverse reactions. Monitor for excessive bleeding. Monitor vital signs. Assess knowledge/teach patient interventions to reduce side effects, and adverse reactions to report. **Pregnancy risk factor X:** This medication is used to terminate pregnancy.

Patient Education: This medication is used to terminate pregnancy under 7 weeks. It must be administered under direction of a qualified physician. You will need follow-up visits as directed by your prescriber (approximately 3 days and 14 days after treatment). Surgical termination of pregnancy may be required if medication fails; there is a risk of fetal malformation if treatment fails. You may experience vaginal bleeding and cramping that is heavier than a normal menstrual period; report immediately if severe or persistent. You may experience nausea, vomiting, and diarrhea. It is possible to get pregnant before your next period. Once the pregnancy has proved to be ended, contraception should be started before having sexual intercourse. Read carefully all information about this medication provided by your prescriber. **Pregnancy/breast-feeding precautions:** Your physician will give you a phone number to call for problems, questions, or emergencies; you should not use this medication if you do not have access to emergency care. You will be given a medication guide to help you understand this medication and its effects. It is important to review this carefully. Ask any questions you may have. You will also be required to sign a form saying that you understand the effects of this treatment and are able to return to the physician for follow-up appointments. Do not breast-feed. Discard breast milk for a few days following use of this medication.

Breast-Feeding Issues Breast milk should be discarded for a few days following use of this medication.

Pregnancy Issues This medication is used to terminate pregnancy; there are no approved treatment indications for its use during pregnancy. Prostaglandins (including mifepristone and misoprostol) may have teratogenic effects when used during pregnancy. If treatment fails, there is a risk of fetal malformation. In sexually active women, pregnancy can occur prior to the first menstrual period following treatment. Appropriate contraception can be started as soon as termination of pregnancy is confirmed or before sexual intercourse is resumed.

Additional Information Medication will be distributed directly to qualified physicians following signed agreement with the distributor, Danco Laboratories. It will not be available through pharmacies. Major adverse reactions (hospitalization, blood transfusion, ongoing pregnancy, etc) should be reported to Danco Laboratories.

Miglitol (MIG li tol)

U.S. Brand Names Glyset®

Pharmacologic Category Antidiabetic Agent, Alpha-Glucosidase Inhibitor

Pregnancy Risk Factor B

Lactation Enters breast milk (small amounts)/not recommended

Use Type 2 diabetes mellitus (noninsulin-dependent, NIDDM):

Monotherapy adjunct to diet to improve glycemic control in patients with type 2 diabetes mellitus (noninsulin-dependent, NIDDM) whose hyperglycemia cannot be managed with diet alone

Combination therapy with a sulfonylurea when diet plus either miglitol or a sulfonylurea alone do not result in adequate glycemic control. The effect of miglitol to enhance glycemic control is additive to that of sulfonylureas when used in combination.

Mechanism of Action/Effect In contrast to sulfonylureas, miglitol does not enhance insulin secretion. The antihyperglycemic action of miglitol results from a reversible inhibition of membrane-bound intestinal alpha-glucosidases which hydrolyze oligosaccharides and disaccharides to glucose and other monosaccharides in the brush border of the small intestine. In diabetic patients, this enzyme inhibition results in delayed glucose absorption and lowering of postprandial hyperglycemia.

Contraindications Hypersensitivity to miglitol or any component of the formulation; diabetic ketoacidosis; inflammatory bowel disease; colonic ulceration; partial intestinal obstruction or predisposition to intestinal obstruction; chronic intestinal diseases associated with marked disorders of digestion or absorption or with conditions that may deteriorate as a result of increased gas formation in the intestine

Warnings/Precautions GI symptoms are the most common reactions. The incidence of abdominal pain and diarrhea tend to diminish considerably with continued treatment. Long-term clinical trials in diabetic patients with significant renal dysfunction (serum creatinine >2 mg/dL) have not been conducted. Treatment of these patients is not recommended. Because of its mechanism of action, miglitol administered alone should not cause hypoglycemia in the fasting of postprandial state. In combination with a sulfonylurea will cause a further lowering of blood glucose and may increase the hypoglycemic potential of the sulfonylurea.

Drug Interactions

Decreased Effect: Miglitol may decrease the absorption and bioavailability of digoxin, propranolol, and ranitidine. Digestive enzymes (amylase, pancreatin, charcoal) may reduce the effect of miglitol and should **not** be taken concomitantly.

Adverse Reactions

>10%: Gastrointestinal: Flatulence (42%), diarrhea (29%), abdominal pain (12%)

1% to 10%: Dermatologic: Rash

Overdosage/Toxicology An overdose of miglitol will not result in hypoglycemia. An overdose may result in transient increases in flatulence, diarrhea, and abdominal discomfort. No serious systemic reactions are expected in the event of an overdose.

Pharmacodynamics/Kinetics
Time to Peak: 2-3 hours
Protein Binding: <4%
Half-Life Elimination: ~2 hours
Metabolism: None
Excretion: Urine (as unchanged drug)

Available Dosage Forms Tablet: 25 mg, 50 mg, 100 mg

Dosing
Adults & Elderly: Type 2 diabetes (noninsulin dependent, NIDDM): Oral: 25 mg 3 times/day with the first bite of food at each meal; the dose may be increased to 50 mg 3 times/day after 4-8 weeks; maximum recommended dose: 100 mg 3 times/day

Renal Impairment: Miglitol is primarily excreted by the kidneys; there is little information of miglitol in patients with a Cl_{cr} <25 mL/minute.

Hepatic Impairment: No adjustment necessary.

Administration

Oral: Should be taken orally at the start (with the first bite) of each main meal.

Laboratory Monitoring Blood glucose tests; measurement of glycosylated hemoglobin is recommended for the monitoring of long-term glycemic control.

Nursing Actions

Physical Assessment: Monitor laboratory tests, therapeutic effectiveness, and adverse reactions on a regular basis throughout therapy. Teach patient proper use (or refer patient to diabetic educator), possible side effects/appropriate interventions (eg, importance of adequate hydration), and adverse symptoms to report.

Patient Education: Inform prescriber of all prescriptions, OTC medications, or herbal products you are taking, and any allergies you have. Do not take any new medication during therapy unless approved by prescriber. Take exactly as directed, with the first bite of each main meal. Do not change dosage or discontinue without first consulting prescriber. Avoid alcohol. It is important to follow dietary and lifestyle recommendations of prescriber. You will be instructed in signs of hypo- or hyperglycemia by prescriber or diabetic educator. If combining this medication with other diabetic medication (eg, sulfonylureas, insulin), keep source of glucose (sugar) on hand in case hypoglycemia occurs. May cause mild side effects during first weeks of therapy (eg, bloating, flatulence, diarrhea, abdominal discomfort); these should diminish over time. Report severe or persistent side effects, fever, extended vomiting or flu, or change in color of urine or stool. **Breast-feeding precaution:** Breast-feeding is not recommended.

Pregnancy Issues Abnormal blood glucose levels are associated with a higher incidence of congenital abnormalities. Insulin is the drug of choice for the control of diabetes mellitus during pregnancy.

Miglustat (MIG loo stat)

U.S. Brand Names Zavesca®

Synonyms OGT-918

Pharmacologic Category Enzyme Inhibitor

Pregnancy Risk Factor X

Lactation Excretion in breast milk unknown/not recommended

Use Treatment of mild-to-moderate type 1 Gaucher disease when enzyme replacement therapy is not a therapeutic option

Mechanism of Action/Effect Miglustat inhibits the enzyme needed to produce glycosphingolipids and decreases the rate of glycosphingolipid glucosylceramide formation.
(Continued)

Miglustat (Continued)

Contraindications Hypersensitivity to miglustat or any component of the formulation; pregnancy

Warnings/Precautions Peripheral neuropathy has been reported with use and neurologic monitoring is required. Tremor or exacerbations of existing tremor may occur; may resolve over time or respond to dosage reduction. Weigh risk versus benefit of therapy if patient develops numbness and tingling. Use caution in renal impairment. Safety and efficacy in severe type 1 Gaucher disease have not been established. Safety and efficacy in patients <18 or >65 years of age have not been established.

Drug Interactions

Decreased Effect: Miglustat increases the clearance of imiglucerase; combination therapy is not indicated.

Nutritional/Ethanol Interactions

Food: Food decreases the rate, but not the extent, of absorption.

Adverse Reactions Percentages reported from open-label, uncontrolled monotherapy trials.

>10%:

Central nervous system: Headache (21% to 22%), dizziness (up to 11%)

Gastrointestinal: Diarrhea (89%; up to 100% in other studies), weight loss (39% to 67%), abdominal pain (18% to 50%), flatulence (29% to 44%), nausea (14% to 22%), vomiting (4% to 11%), cramps (up to 11%)

Neuromuscular & skeletal: Tremor (11%; up to 30% in other studies), leg cramps (4% to 11%),

Ocular: visual disturbances (up to 17%)

1% to 10%:

Central nervous system: headache (up to 6%)

Endocrine & metabolic: Menstrual disorder (up to 6%)

Gastrointestinal: Anorexia (up to 7%), dyspepsia (up to 7%), epigastric pain (up to 6%)

Hematologic: Thrombocytopenia (6% to 7%)

Neuromuscular & skeletal: Paresthesia (up to 7%)

Overdosage/Toxicology Doses of up to 3000 mg/day were used in HIV-positive patients during clinical development. Dizziness, granulocytopenia, leukopenia, neutropenia, and paresthesia were observed.

Pharmacodynamics/Kinetics

Time to Peak: Plasma: 2-2.5 hours

Protein Binding: No binding to plasma proteins

Half-Life Elimination: 6-7 hours

Excretion: Urine (as unchanged drug)

Available Dosage Forms Capsule: 100 mg

Dosing

Adults: Type 1 Gaucher disease: Oral: 100 mg 3 times/day; dose may be reduced to 100 mg 1-2 times/day in patients with adverse effects (ie, tremor, GI distress)

Renal Impairment:

Cl_{cr} 50-75 mL/minute: 100 mg twice daily

Cl_{cr} 30-50 mL/minute: 100 mg once daily

Cl_{cr} <30 mL/minute: Not recommended

Administration

Oral: Capsules should be swallowed whole and taken at the same time each day. May be taken with or without food.

Stability

Storage: Store at 20°C to 25°C (68°F to 77°F).

Nursing Actions

Physical Assessment: Monitor neurological status at beginning of therapy and every 6 months during therapy. Teach patient proper use, possible side effects/appropriate interventions, and adverse symptoms to report (tremor, peripheral neuropathy). **Pregnancy risk factor X** - determine that patient is not pregnant before beginning treatment. Do not give to women of childbearing age or males who may have intercourse with childbearing age females unless they are capable of complying with effective contraceptive measures during therapy. Men should continue contraceptive measures for 3 months following treatment.

Patient Education: Capsules should be swallowed whole and taken at the same time each day, with or without food. May cause headache and dizziness (use caution when driving or engaging in hazardous tasks until response to drug is known); nausea, vomiting, or loss of appetite (small, frequent meals and good mouth care may help); or diarrhea (buttermilk, boiled milk, or yogurt may help). Notify prescriber at once of persistent diarrhea, numbness or tingling in extremities, change in vision, or other adverse effects. **Pregnancy/breast-feeding precautions:** Inform prescriber if you are pregnant. This drug can cause fetal abnormalities. Both females and males should use (consult prescriber) appropriate contraception during therapy. Males should continue contraceptive use for 3 months following therapy. Breast-feeding is not recommended.

Dietary Considerations May be take, with or without food. Patients with diarrhea should avoid foods with high carbohydrate content.

Pregnancy Issues Decreased fetus weight, fetal loss, and difficult or delayed births were observed in animal studies. Women with reproduction potential should use effective contraception during therapy. In addition, adverse effects on spermatogenesis and reduced fertility were observed in male animal studies. The manufacturer recommends that male patients use reliable contraception during therapy and for 3 months following treatment.

Milrinone (MIL ri none)

U.S. Brand Names Primacor®

Synonyms Milrinone Lactate

Pharmacologic Category Phosphodiesterase Enzyme Inhibitor

Medication Safety Issues

Sound-alike/look-alike issues:

Primacor® may be confused with Primaxin®

Pregnancy Risk Factor C

Lactation Excretion in breast milk unknown

Use Short-term I.V. therapy of congestive heart failure; calcium antagonist intoxication

Mechanism of Action/Effect Phosphodiesterase inhibitor resulting in vasodilation

Contraindications Hypersensitivity to milrinone, inamrinone, or any component of the formulation; concurrent use of inamrinone

Warnings/Precautions Avoid in severe obstructive aortic or pulmonic valvular disease. Milrinone may aggravate outflow tract obstruction in hypertrophic subaortic stenosis. Supraventricular and ventricular arrhythmias have developed in high-risk patients. Ensure that ventricular rate controlled in atrial fibrillation/flutter prior to initiating milrinone. Not recommended for use in acute MI patients. Monitor and correct fluid and electrolyte problems. Adjust dose in renal dysfunction. Has not been demonstrated to be safe or effective for longer than 48 hours.

Adverse Reactions

>10%: Cardiovascular: Ventricular arrhythmia (ectopy 9%, NSVT 3%, sustained ventricular tachycardia 1%, ventricular fibrillation <1%); life-threatening arrhythmia are infrequent, often associated with underlying factors (eg, pre-existing arrhythmia, electrolyte disturbances, catheter insertion)

1% to 10%:

Cardiovascular: Supraventricular arrhythmia (4%), hypotension

Central nervous system: Headache

Overdosage/Toxicology Treatment is supportive and symptomatic.

Pharmacodynamics/Kinetics

Onset of Action: I.V.: 5-15 minutes

Serum level: I.V.: Following a 125 mcg/kg dose, peak plasma concentrations ~1000 ng/mL were observed at 2 minutes postinjection, decreasing to <100 ng/mL in 2 hours

Drug concentration levels:

Therapeutic:

Serum levels of 166 ng/mL, achieved during I.V. infusions of 0.25-1 mcg/kg/minute, were associated with sustained hemodynamic benefit in severe congestive heart failure patients over a 24-hour period

Maximum beneficial effects on cardiac output and pulmonary capillary wedge pressure following I.V. infusion have been associated with plasma milrinone concentrations of 150-250 ng/mL

Toxic: Serum concentrations >250-300 ng/mL have been associated with marked reductions in mean arterial pressure and tachycardia; however, more studies are required to determine the toxic serum levels for milrinone

Protein Binding: Plasma: ~70%

Half-Life Elimination: I.V.: 136 minutes in patients with congestive heart failure (CHF); patients with severe CHF have a more prolonged half-life, with values ranging from 1.7-2.7 hours. Patients with CHF have a reduction in the systemic clearance of milrinone, resulting in a prolonged elimination half-life. Alternatively, one study reported that 1 month of therapy with milrinone did not change the pharmacokinetic parameters for patients with CHF despite improvement in cardiac function.

Metabolism: Hepatic (12%)

Excretion: I.V.: Urine (85% as unchanged drug) within 24 hours; active tubular secretion is a major elimination pathway for milrinone

Clearance: I.V. bolus: 25.9 ± 5.7 L/hour (0.37 L/hour/kg); Severe congestive heart failure: 0.11-0.13 L/hour/kg. The reduction in clearance may be a result of reduced renal function. Creatinine clearance values were ½ those reported for healthy adults in patients with severe congestive heart failure (52 vs 119 mL/minute).

Available Dosage Forms [DSC] = Discontinued product

Infusion [premixed in D_5W] (Primacor®): 200 mcg/mL (100 mL, 200 mL)

Injection, solution: 1 mg/mL (10 mL, 20 mL, 50 mL)

Primacor®: 1 mg/mL (10 mL, 20 mL; 50 mL [DSC])

Dosing

Adults & Elderly: CHF/Hemodynamic support: I.V.: Loading dose: 50 mcg/kg administered over 10 minutes followed by a maintenance dose titrated according to the hemodynamic and clinical response, see table.

Maintenance Dosage	Dose Rate (mcg/kg/min)	Total Dose (mg/kg/24 h)
Minimum	0.375	0.59
Standard	0.500	0.77
Maximum	0.750	1.13

Renal Impairment:

Cl_{cr} 50 mL/minute/1.73 m²: Administer 0.43 mcg/kg/minute.

Cl_{cr} 40 mL/minute/1.73 m²: Administer 0.38 mcg/kg/minute.

Cl_{cr} 30 mL/minute/1.73 m²: Administer 0.33 mcg/kg/minute.

Cl_{cr} 20 mL/minute/1.73 m²: Administer 0.28 mcg/kg/minute.

Cl_{cr} 10 mL/minute/1.73 m²: Administer 0.23 mcg/kg/minute.

Cl_{cr} 5 mL/minute/1.73 m²: Administer 0.2 mcg/kg/minute.

Administration

I.V.: Infuse via infusion pump.

I.V. Detail: pH: 3.2-4.0

Stability

Reconstitution: Stable at 0.2 mg/mL in 0.9% sodium chloride or D_5W for 72 hours at room temperature in normal light.

Standard dilution: For a final concentration of 0.2 mg/mL: Dilute Primacor® 1 mg/mL (20 mL) with 80 mL diluent (final volume: 100 mL); may also dilute 1 mg/mL (10 mL) with 40 mL diluent (final volume: 50 mL)

Compatibility: Stable in D_5W, LR, ½NS, NS

Y-site administration: Incompatible with furosemide, procainamide

Compatibility in syringe: Incompatible with furosemide

Compatibility when admixed: Incompatible with bumetanide, furosemide, procainamide

Storage: Colorless to pale yellow solution. Store at room temperature and protect from light.

Laboratory Monitoring Serum potassium

Nursing Actions

Physical Assessment: Use infusion pump. Monitor cardiac/hemodynamic status continuously during therapy and serum potassium at regular intervals. Monitor for fluid retention.

Patient Education: This drug can only be given intravenously. If you experience increased voiding call for assistance. Report pain at infusion site, numbness or tingling of extremities, or respiratory difficulty. **Pregnancy/breast-feeding precautions:** Inform prescriber if you are pregnant. Consult prescriber if breast-feeding.

Minocycline (mi noe SYE kleen)

U.S. Brand Names Dynacin®; Minocin®; myrac™

Synonyms Minocycline Hydrochloride

Pharmacologic Category Antibiotic, Tetracycline Derivative

Medication Safety Issues

Sound-alike/look-alike issues:

Dynacin® may be confused with Dyazide®, Dynabac®, DynaCirc®, Dynapen®

Minocin® may be confused with Indocin®, Lincocin®, Minizide®, Mithracin®, niacin

Pregnancy Risk Factor D

Lactation Enters breast milk/not recommended (AAP rates "compatible")

Use Treatment of susceptible bacterial infections of both gram-negative and gram-positive organisms; treatment of anthrax (inhalational, cutaneous, and gastrointestinal); acne; meningococcal (asymptomatic) carrier state; Rickettsial diseases (including Rocky Mountain spotted fever, Q fever); nongonococcal urethritis, gonorrhea; acute intestinal amebiasis

Mechanism of Action/Effect Inhibits bacterial protein synthesis by binding with the 30S and possibly the 50S ribosomal subunit(s) of susceptible bacteria; cell wall synthesis is not affected

Contraindications Hypersensitivity to minocycline, other tetracyclines, or any component of the formulation; pregnancy

Warnings/Precautions May cause permanent tooth discoloration; avoid use during tooth development (children ≤8 years of age) unless other drugs are not likely to be effective or are contraindicated. May be associated with increases in BUN secondary to antianabolic effects; (Continued)

Minocycline *(Continued)*

use caution in patients with renal impairment. Hepatotoxicity has been reported; use caution in patients with hepatic insufficiency. CNS effects (lightheadedness, vertigo) may occur; patients must be cautioned about performing tasks which require mental alertness (eg, operating machinery or driving). Has been associated (rarely) with pseudotumor cerebri. May cause photosensitivity; discontinue if skin erythema occurs. May cause overgrowth of nonsusceptible organisms, including fungi; discontinue if superinfection occurs. Avoid use in children ≤8 years of age.

Drug Interactions

Decreased Effect: Although anecdotal reports suggest oral contraceptive efficacy could be reduced by tetracyclines, this has been refuted by more rigorous scientific and clinical data. Calcium-, magnesium-, or aluminum-containing antacids, bile acid sequestrants, bismuth, oral contraceptives, iron, zinc, sodium bicarbonate, penicillins, cimetidine, quinapril may decrease absorption of tetracyclines. Methoxyflurane anesthesia (when concurrent with tetracyclines) may cause fatal nephrotoxicity. Tetracyclines may reduce bactericidal efficacy of penicillins and cephalosporins. Tetracycline may reduce the efficacy of the live, attenuated typhoid vaccine (Ty21a).

Increased Effect/Toxicity: Minocycline may increase the effect of warfarin. Retinoic acid derivatives may increase risk of pseudotumor cerebri.

Nutritional/Ethanol Interactions

Food: Minocycline serum concentrations are not significantly altered if taken with food or dairy products.

Herb/Nutraceutical: Avoid dong quai, St John's wort (may also cause photosensitization).

Lab Interactions May cause interference with fluorescence test for urinary catecholamines (false elevations)

Adverse Reactions Frequency not defined.

Cardiovascular: Myocarditis, pericarditis, vasculitis

Central nervous system: Bulging fontanels, dizziness, fever, headache, hypoesthesia, paresthesia, pseudotumor cerebri, sedation, seizure, vertigo

Dermatologic: Alopecia, angioedema, erythema multiforme, erythema nodosum, erythematous rash, exfoliative dermatitis, hyperpigmentation of nails, maculopapular rash, photosensitivity, pigmentation of the skin and mucous membranes, pruritus, Stevens-Johnson syndrome, toxic epidermal necrolysis, urticaria

Endocrine & metabolic: Thyroid dysfunction

Gastrointestinal: Anorexia, diarrhea, dyspepsia, dysphagia, enamel hypoplasia, enterocolitis, esophageal ulcerations, esophagitis, glossitis, inflammatory lesions (oral/anogenital), moniliasis, nausea, oral cavity discoloration, pancreatitis, pseudomembranous colitis, stomatitis, tooth discoloration, vomiting

Genitourinary: Balanitis, vulvovaginitis

Hematologic: Agranulocytosis, eosinophilia, hemolytic anemia, leukopenia, neutropenia, pancytopenia, thrombocytopenia

Hepatic: Hepatic cholestasis, hepatic failure, hepatitis, hyperbilirubinemia, jaundice, liver enzyme increases

Neuromuscular & skeletal: Arthralgia, arthritis, bone discoloration, joint stiffness, joint swelling, myalgia

Otic: Hearing loss, tinnitus

Renal: Acute renal failure, BUN increased, interstitial nephritis

Respiratory: Asthma, bronchospasm, cough, dyspnea, pneumonitis, pulmonary infiltrate

Miscellaneous: Anaphylaxis, lupus erythematosus, serum sickness

Overdosage/Toxicology Symptoms of overdose include diabetes insipidus, nausea, anorexia, dizziness, vomiting, and diarrhea. Treatment is supportive. Not dialyzable (0% to 5%).

Pharmacodynamics/Kinetics

Protein Binding: 70% to 75%

Half-Life Elimination: 16 hours (range: 11-23 hours)

Excretion: Urine

Available Dosage Forms [DSC] = Discontinued product

Capsule: 50 mg, 75 mg, 100 mg

Dynacin®: 50 mg [DSC], 75 mg, 100 mg

Capsule, pellet filled (Minocin®): 50 mg, 100 mg

Tablet (Dynacin®, myrac™): 50 mg, 75 mg, 100 mg

Dosing

Adults & Elderly:

Usual dosage (general): Oral: 200 mg initially, followed by 100 mg every 12 hours, not to exceed 400 mg/24 hours

Acne: Oral: 50-100 mg daily

Chlamydial or *Ureaplasma urealyticum* infection, uncomplicated: Urethral, endocervical, or rectal: 100 mg every 12 hours for at least 7 days

Gonococcal infection, uncomplicated (males): Without urethritis or anorectal infection: 200 mg initially, followed by 100 mg every 12 hours for at least 4 days (cultures 2-3 days post-therapy)

Gonococcal infection, uncomplicated urethritis: 100 mg every 12 hours for 5 days

Meningococcal carrier state: 100 mg every 12 hours for 5 days

Mycobacterium marinum: 100 mg every 12 hours for 6-8 weeks

Syphilis: 200 mg initially, followed by 100 mg every 12 hours for 10-15 days

Pediatrics: Children >8 years: Oral: Initial: 4 mg/kg followed by 2 mg/kg/dose every 12 hours

Renal Impairment: Consider decreasing dose or increasing dosing interval; total daily dose should not exceed 200 mg.

Administration

Oral: May be taken with food or milk. Administer with adequate fluid to decrease the risk of esophageal irritation and ulceration.

Stability

Storage: Store at 20°C to 25°C (68°F to 77°F). Protect from light and moisture.

Laboratory Monitoring Perform culture and sensitivity testing prior to initiating therapy.

Nursing Actions

Physical Assessment: Results of culture and sensitivity tests and allergy history before beginning therapy. Assess potential for interactions with other pharmacological agents or herbal products patient may be taking (eg, warfarin, antacids, hydantoins, carbamazepine). Monitor therapeutic effectiveness (resolution of infection) and adverse reactions on a regular basis during therapy. Teach patient proper use, possible side effects/appropriate interventions (eg, importance of adequate hydration), and adverse symptoms to report.

Patient Education: Do not take any new medication during therapy unless approved by prescriber. Take at intervals around-the-clock; may be taken with food. Complete full course of therapy; do not discontinue even if condition is resolved. May cause photosensitivity reaction (avoid sun, use sunblock, or wear protective clothing); nausea (small, frequent meals, frequent mouth care, chewing gum, or sucking lozenges may help); or diarrhea (boiled milk, buttermilk, or yogurt may help). Report rash or itching, unresolved nausea or diarrhea, change in urinary output (excess); or opportunistic infection (eg, fever, chills, sore throat, burning urination, fatigue). **Pregnancy/ breast-feeding precautions:** Do not get pregnant while taking this medication. Consult prescriber for appropriate contraceptive measures. Consult prescriber if breast-feeding.

Dietary Considerations May be taken with food or milk.

Geriatric Considerations Minocycline has not been studied in the elderly but its CNS effects may limit its use (see Adverse Reactions). Dose reduction for renal function not necessary.

Breast-Feeding Issues Although tetracyclines are excreted in limited amounts, the potential for staining of unerupted teeth has led some experts to recommend against breast-feeding. The AAP identified tetracyclines as "compatible" with breast-feeding.

Pregnancy Issues May cause permanent discoloration (brown-gray) of teeth. Animal studies indicate possible tumorigenicity and impairment of fertility. Congenital anomalies have been reported postmarketing.

Mirtazapine (mir TAZ a peen)

U.S. Brand Names Remeron®; Remeron SolTab®

Restrictions A medication guide concerning the use of antidepressants in children and teenagers can be found on the FDA website at http://www.fda.gov/cder/Offices/ODS/labeling.htm. It should be dispensed to parents or guardians of children and teenagers receiving this medication.

Pharmacologic Category Antidepressant, Alpha-2 Antagonist

Medication Safety Issues
Sound-alike/look-alike issues:
Remeron® may be confused with Premarin®, Zemuron®

Pregnancy Risk Factor C

Lactation Excretion in breast milk unknown/not recommended

Use Treatment of depression

Mechanism of Action/Effect Mirtazapine is a tetracyclic antidepressant that works by its central presynaptic alpha$_2$-adrenergic antagonist effects, which results in increased release of norepinephrine and serotonin. It is also a potent antagonist of 5-HT$_2$ and 5-HT$_3$ serotonin receptors and H1 histamine receptors and a moderate peripheral alpha$_1$-adrenergic and muscarinic antagonist; it does not inhibit the reuptake of norepinephrine or serotonin.

Contraindications Hypersensitivity to mirtazapine or any component of the formulation; use of MAO inhibitors within 14 days

Warnings/Precautions Antidepressants increase the risk of suicidal thinking and behavior in children and adolescents with major depressive disorder (MDD) and other depressive disorders; consider risk prior to prescribing. All patients must be closely monitored for clinical worsening, suicidality, or unusual changes in behavior, especially during the initiation of therapy or following an increase or decrease in dosage. When used in children, the child's family or caregiver should be instructed to closely observe the patient and communicate condition with healthcare provider. A medication guide should be dispensed with each prescription. **Mirtazapine is not FDA approved for use in children.**

The possibility of a suicide attempt is inherent in major depression and may persist until remission occurs. Use caution in high-risk patients. Worsening depression and severe abrupt suicidality that are not part of the presenting symptoms may require discontinuation or modification of drug therapy. The patient's family or caregiver should be alerted to monitor patients for the emergence of suicidality and associated behaviors (such as agitation, irritability, hostility, impulsivity, and hypomania) and call healthcare provider.

May worsen psychosis in some patients or precipitate a shift to mania or hypomania in patients with bipolar disorder. Patients presenting with depressive symptoms should be screened for bipolar disorder. Monotherapy in patients with bipolar disorder should be avoided.

Mirtazapine is not FDA approved for the treatment of bipolar depression.

Discontinue immediately if signs and symptoms of neutropenia/agranulocytosis occur. May cause sedation, resulting in impaired performance of tasks requiring alertness (eg, operating machinery or driving). Sedative effects may be additive with other CNS depressants and/or ethanol. The degree of sedation is moderate-high relative to other antidepressants. The risks of orthostatic hypotension or anticholinergic effects are low relative to other antidepressants. The incidence of sexual dysfunction with mirtazapine is generally lower than with SSRIs.

May increase appetite and stimulate weight gain. Weight gain of >7% of body weight reported in 7.5% of patients treated with mirtazapine compared to 0% for placebo; 8% of patients receiving mirtazapine discontinued treatment due to the weight gain. In an 8-week pediatric clinical trial, 49% of mirtazapine-treated patients had a weight gain of at least 7% (mean increase 4 kg) as compared to 5.7% of placebo-treated patients (mean increase 1 kg). May increase serum cholesterol and triglyceride levels.

Use caution in patients with a previous seizure disorder or condition predisposing to seizures such as brain damage, alcoholism, or concurrent therapy with other drugs which lower the seizure threshold. Use with caution in patients with hepatic or renal dysfunction and in elderly patients. SolTab® formulation contains phenylalanine.

Drug Interactions
Cytochrome P450 Effect: Substrate of CYP1A2 (major), 2C8/9 (minor), 2D6 (major), 3A4 (major); **Inhibits** CYP1A2 (weak), 3A4 (weak)

Decreased Effect: CYP1A2 inducers may decrease the levels/effects of mirtazapine; example inducers include aminoglutethimide, carbamazepine, phenobarbital, and rifampin. Decreased effect seen with clonidine. CYP3A4 inducers may decrease the levels/effects of mirtazapine; example inducers include aminoglutethimide, carbamazepine, nafcillin, nevirapine, phenobarbital, phenytoin, and rifamycins.

Increased Effect/Toxicity: Contraindicated with drugs which inhibit MAO (including linezolid, selegiline, sibutramine, and MAOIs); severe/fatal reactions may occur. CYP1A2 inhibitors may increase the levels/effects of mirtazapine; example inhibitors include amiodarone, ciprofloxacin, fluvoxamine, ketoconazole, norfloxacin, ofloxacin, and rofecoxib. CYP2D6 inhibitors may increase the levels/effects of mirtazapine; example inhibitors include chlorpromazine, delavirdine, fluoxetine, miconazole, paroxetine, pergolide, quinidine, quinine, ritonavir, and ropinirole. CYP3A4 inhibitors may increase the levels/effects of mirtazapine; example inhibitors include azole antifungals, clarithromycin, diclofenac, doxycycline, erythromycin, imatinib, isoniazid, nefazodone, nicardipine, propofol, protease inhibitors, quinidine, telithromycin, and verapamil. Increased sedative effect seen with CNS depressants.

Nutritional/Ethanol Interactions
Ethanol: Avoid ethanol (may increase CNS depression).
Herb/Nutraceutical: Avoid St John's wort (may decrease mirtazapine levels). Avoid valerian, St John's wort, SAMe, kava kava (may increase CNS depression).

Adverse Reactions
>10%:
Central nervous system: Somnolence (54%)
Endocrine & metabolic: Increased cholesterol
Gastrointestinal: Constipation (13%), xerostomia (25%), increased appetite (17%), weight gain (12%; weight gain of >7% reported in 8% of adults, ≤49% of pediatric patients)
1% to 10%:
Cardiovascular: Hypertension, vasodilatation, peripheral edema (2%), edema (1%)
(Continued)

Mirtazapine *(Continued)*

Central nervous system: Dizziness (7%), abnormal dreams (4%), abnormal thoughts (3%), confusion (2%), malaise

Endocrine & metabolic: Increased triglycerides

Gastrointestinal: Vomiting, anorexia, abdominal pain

Genitourinary: Urinary frequency (2%)

Neuromuscular & skeletal: Myalgia (2%), back pain (2%), arthralgia, tremor (2%), weakness (8%)

Respiratory: Dyspnea (1%)

Miscellaneous: Flu-like symptoms (5%), thirst

Overdosage/Toxicology Experience with overdose is limited. Signs and symptoms have included disorientation, drowsiness, impaired memory, and tachycardia. Treatment should be symptomatic and supportive. Activated charcoal should be administered. Emesis is not recommended; however, gastric lavage with airway protection may be used in symptomatic patients or if performed soon after ingestion. Consider the possibility of multiple drug involvement.

Pharmacodynamics/Kinetics

Time to Peak: Serum: 2 hours

Protein Binding: 85%

Half-Life Elimination: 20-40 hours; hampered with renal or hepatic impairment

Metabolism: Extensively hepatic via CYP1A2, 2C9, 2D6, 3A4 and via demethylation and hydroxylation

Excretion: Urine (75%) and feces (15%) as metabolites

Available Dosage Forms

Tablet (Remeron®): 15 mg, 30 mg, 45 mg

Tablet, orally disintegrating: 15 mg, 30 mg

Remeron SolTab®:

15 mg [contains phenylalanine 2.6 mg/tablet; orange flavor]

30 mg [contains phenylalanine 5.2 mg/tablet; orange flavor]

45 mg [contains phenylalanine 7.8 mg/tablet; orange flavor]

Dosing

Adults: Depression: Oral: Initial: 15 mg nightly, titrate up to 15-45 mg/day with dose increases made no more frequently than every 1-2 weeks. There is an inverse relationship between dose and sedation.

Elderly: Initial: 7.5 mg/day as a single bedtime dose; increase by 7.5-15 mg/day every 1-2 weeks; usual dose: 15-30 mg/day; maximum dose: 45 mg/day

Renal Impairment:

Cl_{cr} 11-39 mL/minute: 30% decreased clearance

Cl_{cr} <10 mL/minute: 50% decreased clearance

Hepatic Impairment: Clearance is decreased by 30%.

Stability

Storage: Store at controlled room temperature

SolTab®: Protect from light and moisture; use immediately upon opening tablet blister

Laboratory Monitoring

CBC

Nursing Actions

Physical Assessment: Assess other medications patient may be taking for effectiveness and interactions. Has potential for psychological or physiological dependence, abuse, or tolerance. Monitor therapeutic response (ie, mood, affect, mental status) and adverse reactions at beginning of therapy and periodically with long-term use. Monitor for CNS depression/sedation. Monitor for clinical worsening and suicidal ideation. Taper dosage slowly when discontinuing. Assess knowledge/teach patient appropriate use, interventions to reduce side effects, and adverse symptoms to report.

Patient Education: Take exactly as directed; do not increase dose or frequency. It may take 2-3 weeks to achieve desired results. Take once-a-day dose at bedtime. Avoid alcohol, caffeine, and other prescription or OTC medications not approved by prescriber. Maintain adequate hydration (2-3 L/day of fluids) unless instructed to restrict fluid intake. You may experience drowsiness, dizziness, or lightheadedness (use caution when driving or engaging in tasks requiring alertness until response to drug is known); nausea, vomiting, anorexia, or dry mouth (small frequent meals, frequent mouth care, chewing gum, or sucking lozenges may help); or orthostatic hypotension (use caution when climbing stairs or changing position from lying or sitting to standing). Report persistent insomnia, agitation, or confusion; suicidal ideation; muscle cramping, tremors, weakness, or change in gait; breathlessness or respiratory difficulty; chest pain, palpitations, or rapid heartbeat; change in urinary pattern; vision changes or eye pain; yellowing of eyes or skin; pale stools/dark urine; or worsening of condition.

SolTab®: Open blister pack and place tablet on the tongue. Do not split tablet. Tablet is formulated to dissolve on the tongue without water.

Pregnancy/breast-feeding precautions: Inform prescriber if you are or intend to become pregnant. Breast-feeding is not recommended.

Dietary Considerations Remeron SolTab® contains phenylalanine: 2.6 mg per 15 mg tablet; 5.2 mg per 30 mg tablet; 7.8 mg per 45 mg tablet

Additional Information Note: At least 14 days should elapse between discontinuation of an MAO inhibitor and initiation of therapy with mirtazapine; at least 14 days should be allowed after discontinuing mirtazapine before starting an MAO inhibitor.

Related Information

Antidepressant Medication Guidelines *on page 1414*

Misoprostol *(mye soe PROST ole)*

U.S. Brand Names Cytotec®

Pharmacologic Category Prostaglandin

Medication Safety Issues

Sound-alike/look-alike issues:

Misoprostol may be confused with metoprolol

Cytotec® may be confused with Cytoxan®, Sytobex®

Pregnancy Risk Factor X

Lactation Excretion in breast milk unknown/contraindicated

Use Prevention of NSAID-induced gastric ulcers; medical termination of pregnancy of ≤49 days (in conjunction with mifepristone)

Unlabeled/Investigational Use Cervical ripening and labor induction; NSAID-induced nephropathy; fat malabsorption in cystic fibrosis

Mechanism of Action/Effect Misoprostol is a synthetic prostaglandin E_1 analog that replaces the protective prostaglandins consumed with prostaglandin-inhibiting therapies (eg, NSAIDs); has been shown to induce uterine contractions

Contraindications Hypersensitivity to misoprostol, prostaglandins, or any component of the formulation; pregnancy (when used to reduce NSAID-induced ulcers)

Warnings/Precautions Safety and efficacy have not been established in children <18 years of age. Use with caution in patients with renal impairment and the elderly. Not to be used in pregnant women or women of childbearing potential unless woman is capable of complying with effective contraceptive measures; therapy is normally begun on the second or third day of next normal menstrual period. Uterine perforation and/or rupture have been reported in association with intravaginal use to induce labor or with combined oral/intravaginal use to induce abortion. The manufacturer states that Cytotec® should not be used as a cervical-ripening agent for induction of labor. However, The American College of Obstetricians and Gynecologists (ACOG) continues to support this off-label use.

Drug Interactions

Increased Effect/Toxicity: Misoprostol may increase the effect of oxytocin; wait 6-12 hours after misoprostol administration before initiating oxytocin.

Nutritional/Ethanol Interactions Food: Misoprostol peak serum concentrations may be decreased if taken with food (not clinically significant).

Adverse Reactions

>10%: Gastrointestinal: Diarrhea, abdominal pain

1% to 10%:

Central nervous system: Headache

Gastrointestinal: Constipation, flatulence, nausea, dyspepsia, vomiting

Overdosage/Toxicology Symptoms of overdose include sedation, tremor, convulsions, dyspnea, abdominal pain, diarrhea, hypotension, and bradycardia. Treatment is symptom-directed and supportive.

Pharmacodynamics/Kinetics

Time to Peak: Serum: Active metabolite: Fasting: 15-30 minutes

Half-Life Elimination: Metabolite: 20-40 minutes

Metabolism: Hepatic; rapidly de-esterified to misoprostol acid (active)

Excretion: Urine (64% to 73%) and feces (15%) within 24 hours

Available Dosage Forms Tablet: 100 mcg, 200 mcg

Dosing

Adults:

Prevention of NSAID-induced ulcers: Oral: 200 mcg 4 times/day with food; if not tolerated, may decrease dose to 100 mcg 4 times/day with food or 200 mcg twice daily with food. Last dose of the day should be taken at bedtime.

Labor induction or cervical ripening (unlabeled uses): Intravaginal: 25 mcg (¹/₄ of 100 mcg tablet); may repeat at intervals no more frequent than every 3-6 hours. Do not use in patients with previous cesarean delivery or prior medical uterine surgery.

Medical termination of pregnancy: Oral: Refer to Mifepristone monograph.

Elderly: Oral: 100-200 mcg 4 times/day with food; if 200 mcg 4 times/day not tolerated, reduce to 100 mcg 4 times/day or 200 mcg twice daily with food. **Note:** To avoid the diarrhea potential, doses can be initiated at 100 mcg/day and increased 100 mcg/day at 3-day intervals until desired dose is achieved; also, recommend administering with food to decrease diarrhea incidence.

Pediatrics: Children 8-16 years: Oral: Fat absorption in cystic fibrosis (unlabeled use): 100 mcg 4 times/day

Administration

Oral: Incidence of diarrhea may be lessened by having patient take dose right after meals. Therapy is usually begun on the second or third day of the next normal menstrual period.

Stability

Storage: Store at or below 25°C (77°F).

Nursing Actions

Physical Assessment: Assess knowledge/teach appropriate antiulcer diet and lifestyle. Monitor renal function and fluid balance (I & O, weight gain, edema). **Pregnancy risk factor X:** Determine that patient is not pregnant before beginning treatment and do not give to women of childbearing age or to males who may have intercourse with women of childbearing age unless both male and female are capable of complying with contraceptive measures during therapy and for 1 month following therapy.

Patient Education: Take as directed; continue taking your NSAIDs while taking this medication. Take with meals or after meals to prevent nausea, diarrhea, and flatulence. Avoid using antacids. You may experience

increased menstrual pain, or cramping; request analgesics. Report abnormal menstrual periods, spotting (may occur even in postmenstrual women), or severe menstrual bleeding. **Pregnancy/breast-feeding precautions:** When used to prevent NSAID-induced ulcers: Inform prescriber if you are pregnant. Do not get pregnant during or for 1 month following therapy. Male: Do not cause a female to become pregnant. Male/female: Consult prescriber for instruction on appropriate contraceptive measures. This drug may cause severe fetal defects, miscarriage, or abortion; do not share medication with others. Do not breast-feed.

Dietary Considerations Should be taken with food; incidence of diarrhea may be lessened by having patient take dose right after meals.

Geriatric Considerations Elderly, due to extensive use of NSAIDs and the high percentage of asymptomatic hemorrhage and perforation from NSAIDs, are at risk for NSAID-induced ulcers and may be candidates for misoprostol use. However, routine use for prophylaxis is not justified. Patients must be selected upon demonstration that they are at risk for NSAID-induced lesions. Misoprostol should not be used as a first-line therapy for gastric or duodenal ulcers.

Breast-Feeding Issues It is not known if misoprostol is excreted in human milk, however, because significant diarrhea may occur in a nursing infant, breast-feeding is contraindicated

Pregnancy Issues Misoprostol is an abortifacient. During pregnancy, use to prevent NSAID-induced ulcers is contraindicated. Reports of fetal death, congenital anomalies, uterine perforation, and abortion have been received after the use of misoprostol in pregnancy.

Mitomycin (mye toe MYE sin)

U.S. Brand Names Mutamycin®

Synonyms Mitomycin-C; Mitomycin-X; MTC; NSC-26980

Pharmacologic Category Antineoplastic Agent, Antibiotic

Medication Safety Issues

Sound-alike/look-alike issues:

Mitomycin may be confused with mithramycin, mitotane, mitoxantrone, Mutamycin®

Mutamycin® may be confused with mitomycin

Pregnancy Risk Factor D

Lactation Enters breast milk/contraindicated

Use Treatment of adenocarcinoma of stomach or pancreas, bladder cancer, breast cancer, or colorectal cancer

Unlabeled/Investigational Use Prevention of excess scarring in glaucoma filtration procedures in patients at high risk of bleb failure

Mechanism of Action/Effect Acts like an alkylating agent and produces DNA cross-linking (primarily with guanine and cytosine pairs); cell-cycle nonspecific; inhibits DNA and RNA synthesis; degrades preformed DNA, causes nuclear lysis and formation of giant cells. While not phase-specific *per se*, mitomycin has its maximum effect against cells in late G and early S phases.

Contraindications Hypersensitivity to mitomycin or any component of the formulation; thrombocytopenia; coagulation disorders, increased bleeding tendency; pregnancy

Warnings/Precautions Hazardous agent - use appropriate precautions for handling and disposal. Use with caution in patients who have received radiation therapy or in the presence of hepatobiliary dysfunction; reduce dosage in patients who are receiving radiation therapy simultaneously. Hemolytic-uremic syndrome, potentially fatal, occurs in some patients receiving long-term (Continued)

Mitomycin (Continued)

therapy. It is correlated with total dose (single doses ≥60 mg or cumulative doses ≥50 mg/m^2) and total duration of therapy (>5-11 months). **Mitomycin is a potent vesicant, may cause ulceration, necrosis, cellulitis, and tissue sloughing if infiltrated.**

Drug Interactions

Increased Effect/Toxicity: *Vinca* alkaloids or doxorubicin may enhance cardiac toxicity when coadministered with mitomycin.

Nutritional/Ethanol Interactions Herb/Nutraceutical: Avoid black cohosh, dong quai in estrogen-dependent tumors.

Adverse Reactions

>10%:
  Cardiovascular: CHF (3% to 15%) (doses >30 mg/m^2)
  Central nervous system: Fever (14%)
  Dermatologic: Alopecia, nail banding/discoloration
  Gastrointestinal: Nausea, vomiting and anorexia (14%)
  Hematologic: Anemia (19% to 24%); myelosuppression, common, dose-limiting, delayed
    Onset: 3 weeks
    Nadir: 4-6 weeks
    Recovery: 6-8 weeks
1% to 10%:
  Dermatologic: Rash
  Gastrointestinal: Stomatitis
  Neuromuscular: Paresthesias
  Renal: Creatinine increase (2%)
  Respiratory: Interstitial pneumonitis, infiltrates, dyspnea, cough (7%)

Overdosage/Toxicology Symptoms of overdose include bone marrow suppression, nausea, vomiting, and alopecia. Treatment is symptom-directed and supportive.

Pharmacodynamics/Kinetics

Half-Life Elimination: 23-78 minutes; Terminal: 50 minutes

Metabolism: Hepatic

Excretion: Urine (<10% as unchanged drug), with elevated serum concentrations

Available Dosage Forms Injection, powder for reconstitution: 5 mg, 20 mg, 40 mg

Dosing

Adults & Elderly: Refer to individual protocols:
  Single-agent therapy: I.V.: 20 mg/m^2 every 6-8 weeks
  Combination therapy: I.V.: 10 mg/m^2 every 6-8 weeks
  Bladder carcinoma: Intravesicular instillations (unapproved route): 20-40 mg/dose instilled into the bladder for 3 hours repeated up to 3 times/week for up to 20 procedures per course.
  Glaucoma surgery (unlabeled use): Dosages and techniques vary; 0.2-0.5 mg may be applied to a pledget (using a 0.2-0.5 mg/mL solution), and placed in contact with the surgical wound for 2-5 minutes; other protocols have been reported

Pediatrics: Refer to adult dosing.

Renal Impairment: Varying approaches to dosing adjustments have been published; one representative recommendation: Cl$_{cr}$ <10 mL/minute: Administer 75% of normal dose
  Note: The manufacturers state that products should not be given to patients with serum creatinine >1.7 mg/dL.
  Hemodialysis: Unknown
  CAPD effects: Unknown
  CAVH effects: Unknown

Hepatic Impairment: Although some mitomycin may be excreted in the bile, no specific guidelines regarding dosage adjustment in hepatic impairment can be made.

Administration

I.V.: Vesicant. Administer slow I.V. push or by slow (15-30 minute) infusion via a freely-running dextrose or saline infusion. Consider using a central venous catheter.

I.V. Detail:

Extravasation management: Care should be taken to avoid extravasation. If extravasation occurs, the site should be observed closely. These injuries frequently cause necrosis. A plastic surgery consult may be required. Few agents have been effective as antidotes, but there are reports in the literature of some benefit with dimethylsulfoxide (DSMO). Delayed dermal reactions with mitomycin are possible, even in patients who are asymptomatic at time of drug administration.

pH: 6-8

Stability

Reconstitution: Dilute powder with SWFI or 0.9% sodium chloride to a concentration of 0.5-1 mg/mL.

Compatibility: Stable in LR
  Y-site administration: Incompatible with aztreonam, cefepime, etoposide phosphate, filgrastim, gemcitabine, piperacillin/tazobactam, sargramostim, topotecan, vinorelbine
  Compatibility when admixed: Incompatible with bleomycin

Storage: Store intact vials at controlled room temperature. Mitomycin solution is stable for 7 days at room temperature and 14 days when refrigerated if protected from light. Solution of 0.5 mg/mL in a syringe is stable for 7 days at room temperature and 14 days when refrigerated and protected from light.

Further dilution to 20-40 mcg/mL:
  In normal saline: Stable for 12 hours at room temperature.
  In sodium lactate: Stable for 24 hours at room temperature.

Laboratory Monitoring Platelet count, CBC with differential, prothrombin time, renal and pulmonary function

Nursing Actions

Physical Assessment: Assess potential for interactions with other pharmacological and herbal products patient may be taking. See Administration for infusion specifics; infusion site must be closely monitored to prevent extravasation. Mitomycin is a potent vesicant; may cause ulceration, necrosis, cellulitis, and tissue sloughing if infiltrated. Monitor laboratory tests, therapeutic response, and adverse reactions (eg, signs of CHF, hydration and nutritional status, and opportunistic infection) on a regular basis throughout therapy. Teach patient possible side effects/appropriate interventions and adverse symptoms to report.

Patient Education: Do not take any new medication during therapy unless approved by prescriber. This drug is administered intravenously; report immediately any redness, swelling, burning, or pain at infusion site. Maintain adequate hydration (2-3 L/day of fluids) unless instructed to restrict fluid intake, and nutrition. You may be more susceptible to infection (avoid crowds and exposure to infection and do not have any vaccinations unless approved by prescriber). May cause nausea, vomiting, or anorexia (small, frequent meals, frequent mouth care, chewing gum, or sucking lozenges may help); mouth sores (use soft toothbrush, waxed dental floss, and frequent mouth rinses); or loss of hair or discoloration of nails (may be reversible when therapy is discontinued). Report rash or itching, unresolved nausea or diarrhea; respiratory difficulty, swelling of extremities, sudden weight gain, or unusual cough; any numbness, tingling, or loss of sensation; or opportunistic infection (fever, chills, sore throat, burning urination, fatigue). **Pregnancy/breast-feeding precautions:** Do not get pregnant while taking this medication. Consult prescriber for appropriate contraceptive measures. Do not breast-feed.

Pregnancy Issues Mitomycin can cause fetal harm in humans. Animal studies show delayed fetal development, fetal external anomalies, and neonatal anomalies.

Mitotane (MYE toe tane)

U.S. Brand Names Lysodren®

Synonyms NSC-38721; o,p'-DDD

Pharmacologic Category Antineoplastic Agent, Miscellaneous

Medication Safety Issues
Sound-alike/look-alike issues:
Mitotane may be confused with mitomycin

Pregnancy Risk Factor C

Lactation Enters breast milk/contraindicated

Use Treatment of adrenocortical carcinoma

Unlabeled/Investigational Use Treatment of Cushing's syndrome

Mechanism of Action/Effect Causes adrenal cortical atrophy; drug affects mitochondria in adrenal cortical cells and decreases production of cortisol; also alters the peripheral metabolism of steroids

Contraindications Hypersensitivity to mitotane or any component of the formulation

Warnings/Precautions Hazardous agent - use appropriate precautions for handling and disposal. Steroid replacement with glucocorticoid, and sometimes mineralocorticoid, is necessary. It has been recommended that replacement therapy be initiated at the start of therapy, rather than waiting for evidence of adrenal insufficiency. Because mitotane can increase the metabolism of hydrocortisone, higher than usual replacement doses of the latter may be required. Acute adrenal insufficiency may occur in the face of shock, trauma, or infection. Mitotane should be discontinued temporarily in this setting and appropriate steroid coverage should be administered.

Drug Interactions
Decreased Effect: Mitotane may enhance the clearance of barbiturates and warfarin by induction of the hepatic microsomal enzyme system resulting in a decreased effect. Coadministration of spironolactone has resulted in negation of mitotane's effect. Mitotane may increase clearance of phenytoin by microsomal enzyme stimulation.

Increased Effect/Toxicity: CNS depressants taken with mitotane may enhance CNS depression.

Nutritional/Ethanol Interactions Ethanol: Avoid ethanol (may increase CNS depression).

Adverse Reactions
>10%:
Central nervous system: CNS depression (32%), dizziness (15%)
Dermatologic: Skin rash (12%)
Gastrointestinal: Anorexia (24%), nausea (39%), vomiting (37%), diarrhea (13%)
Neuromuscular & skeletal: Weakness (12%)
1% to 10%:
Central nervous system: Headache (5%), confusion (3%)
Neuromuscular & skeletal: Muscle tremor (3%)

Overdosage/Toxicology Symptoms of overdose include diarrhea, vomiting, numbness of limbs, and weakness. Treatment is symptom-directed and supportive.

Pharmacodynamics/Kinetics
Time to Peak: Serum: 3-5 hours
Half-Life Elimination: 18-159 days
Metabolism: Hepatic and other tissues
Excretion: Urine and feces (as metabolites)

Available Dosage Forms Tablet [scored]: 500 mg

Dosing
Adults & Elderly: Adrenal carcinoma: Oral: Start at 1-6 g/day in divided doses, then increase incrementally to 8-10 g/day in 3-4 divided doses (maximum daily dose: 18 g)

Pediatrics: Adrenal carcinoma: Oral: Children: 0.1-0.5 mg/kg or 1-2 g/day in divided doses increasing gradually to a maximum of 5-7 g/day

Hepatic Impairment: Dose may need to be decreased in patients with liver disease.

Stability
Storage: Protect from light. Store at room temperature.

Nursing Actions
Physical Assessment: Assess potential for interactions with other pharmacological and herbal products patient may be taking. Evaluate therapeutic response and adverse reactions on a regular basis throughout therapy. Teach patient possible side effects/appropriate interventions and adverse symptoms to report.

Patient Education: Take as directed; do not alter dose or discontinue without consulting prescriber. Desired effects of this drug may not be seen for 2-3 months. Wear identification that alerts medical personnel that you are taking this drug in event of shock or trauma. Maintain adequate hydration (2-3 L/day of fluids) unless instructed to restrict fluid intake, and nutrition. Avoid alcohol. May cause dizziness, headache, confusion (avoid driving or performing tasks requiring alertness until response to drug is known); nausea, vomiting, or loss of appetite (small, frequent meals, frequent mouth care, sucking lozenges, or chewing gum may help); or diarrhea (buttermilk, boiled milk, or yogurt may help). Report severe vomiting or diarrhea; or muscular twitching, tremor, numbness, or weakness. **Pregnancy/breast-feeding precautions:** Inform prescriber if you are or intend to become pregnant. Do not breast-feed.

Mitoxantrone (mye toe ZAN trone)

U.S. Brand Names Novantrone®

Synonyms DAD; DHAD; DHAQ; Dihydroxyanthracenedione Dihydrochloride; Mitoxantrone Hydrochloride CL-232315; Mitozantrone; NSC-301739

Pharmacologic Category Antineoplastic Agent, Anthracenedione

Medication Safety Issues
Sound-alike/look-alike issues:
Mitoxantrone may be confused with methotrexate, mitomycin

Pregnancy Risk Factor D

Lactation Enters breast milk/contraindicated

Use Treatment of acute leukemias, lymphoma, breast cancer, pediatric sarcoma, progressive or relapsing-remitting multiple sclerosis, prostate cancer

Mechanism of Action/Effect Analogue of the anthracyclines, but different in mechanism of action, cardiac toxicity, and potential for tissue necrosis; inhibits DNA and RNA synthesis

Contraindications Hypersensitivity to mitoxantrone or any component of the formulation; multiple sclerosis with left ventricular ejection fraction (LVEF) <50% or clinically significant decrease in LVEF; pregnancy

Warnings/Precautions Hazardous agent - use appropriate precautions for handling and disposal.

Dosage should be reduced in patients with impaired hepatobiliary function; not for treatment of multiple sclerosis in patients with concurrent hepatic impairment. Treatment may lead to severe myelosuppression; use with caution in patients with pre-existing myelosuppression. Do not use if baseline neutrophil count <1500 cells/mm^3 (except for treatment of ANLL).
(Continued)

Mitoxantrone (Continued)

May cause myocardial toxicity and potentially-fatal CHF; risk increases with cumulative dosing. Predisposing factors for mitoxantrone-induced cardiotoxicity include prior anthracycline therapy, prior cardiovascular disease, and mediastinal irradiation. Not recommended for use when left ventricular ejection fraction (LVEF) <50%. Use in multiple sclerosis should be limited to a cumulative dose of ≤140 mg/m², and discontinued if a significant decrease in LVEF is observed. Not for treatment of primary progressive multiple sclerosis. Has been associated with the development of secondary acute myelogenous leukemia and myelodysplasia. May cause urine, saliva, tears, and sweat to turn blue-green for 24 hours postinfusion. Whites of eyes may have blue-green tinge.

Drug Interactions
Cytochrome P450 Effect: Inhibits CYP3A4 (weak)

Decreased Effect: Patients may experience impaired immune response to vaccines; possible infection after administration of live vaccines in patients receiving immunosuppressants.

Nutritional/Ethanol Interactions Herb/Nutraceutical: Avoid black cohosh, dong quai in estrogen-dependent tumors.

Adverse Reactions Reported with any indication; incidence varies based on treatment/dose
>10%:
Cardiovascular: Arrhythmia (3% to 18%), edema (10% to 31%), nail bed changes (11%)
Central nervous system: Fatigue (up to 39%), fever (7% to 78%), headache (6% to 13%)
Dermatologic: Alopecia (22% to 61%)
Endocrine & metabolic: Amenorrhea (28% to 53%), menstrual disorder (26% to 61%)
Gastrointestinal: Abdominal pain (9% to 15%), anorexia (24% to 25%), nausea (29% to 76%), constipation (10% to 16%), diarrhea (16% to 47%), GI bleeding (2% to 16%), mucositis (10% to 29%), stomatitis (8% to 29%), vomiting (6% to 12%), weight gain/loss (13% to 18%)
Genitourinary: Abnormal urine (6% to 11%), urinary tract infection (7% to 32%)
Hematologic: Hemoglobin decreased, leukopenia, lymphopenia, petechiae/bruising; myelosuppressive effects of chemotherapy:
WBC: Mild
Platelets: Mild
Onset: 7-10 days
Nadir: 14 days
Recovery: 21 days
Hepatic: GGT increased (3% to 15%)
Neuromuscular & skeletal: Weakness (24%)
Respiratory: Cough (5% to 13%), dyspnea (6% to 18%), upper respiratory tract infection (7% to 53%)
Miscellaneous: Fungal infection (9% to 15%), infection (4% to 18%), sepsis (ANLL 31% to 34%)
1% to 10%:
Cardiovascular: CHF (2% to 3%; risk is much lower with anthracyclines, some reports suggest cumulative doses >160 mg/mL cause CHF in ~10% of patients), ECG changes, hypertension, ischemia, LVEF decreased (≤5%)
Central nervous system: Chills, anxiety, depression, seizure
Dermatologic: Skin infection
Endocrine & metabolic: Hypocalcemia, hypokalemia, hyponatremia, hyperglycemia
Gastrointestinal: Dyspepsia, aphthosis
Genitourinary: Impotence, proteinuria, renal failure, sterility
Hematologic: Anemia, granulocytopenia, hemorrhage
Hepatic: Jaundice, increased SGOT, increased SGPT
Neuromuscular & skeletal: Back pain, myalgia, arthralgia
Ocular: Blurred vision, conjunctivitis

Renal: Hematuria
Respiratory: Pneumonia, rhinitis, sinusitis
Miscellaneous: Systemic infection, sweats, development of secondary leukemia

Overdosage/Toxicology Symptoms of overdose include leukopenia, tachycardia, and marrow hypoplasia. No known antidote. Treatment is symptom-directed and supportive.

Pharmacodynamics/Kinetics
Protein Binding: >95%, 76% to albumin
Half-Life Elimination: Terminal: 23-215 hours; may be prolonged with hepatic impairment
Metabolism: Hepatic; pathway not determined
Excretion: Urine (6% to 11%) and feces as unchanged drug and metabolites

Available Dosage Forms
Injection, solution: 2 mg/mL (10 mL, 12.5 mL, 15 mL)
Novantrone®: 2 mg/mL (10 mL, 12.5 mL, 15 mL)

Dosing
Adults & Elderly: Refer to individual protocols. I.V. (may dilute in D₅W or NS):
Acute leukemias: I.V.: 8-12 mg/m²/day once daily for 4-5 days
Solid tumors: I.V.: 12-14 mg/m² every 3-4 weeks **or** 2-4 mg/m²/day for 5 days
Hormone-refractory prostate cancer: I.V.: 12-14 mg/m²
Multiple sclerosis: I.V.: 12 mg/m² every 3 months (maximum lifetime cumulative dose: 140 mg/m²
BMT high dose: I.V.: 24-48 mg/m² as a single dose; duration of infusion is 1-4 hours; generally combined with other high-dose chemotherapeutic drugs.

Pediatrics: Refer to individual protocols.
Acute leukemias: I.V. (may dilute in D₅W or NS):
Children ≤2 years: 0.4 mg/kg/day once daily for 3-5 days
Children >2 years: Refer to adult dosing.
Solid tumors: I.V.: Children: 18-20 mg/m² every 3-4 weeks **or** 5-8 mg/m² every week

Hepatic Impairment: Official dosage adjustment recommendations have not been established.
Moderate dysfunction (bilirubin 1.5-3 mg/dL): Some clinicians recommend a 50% dosage reduction.
Severe dysfunction (bilirubin >3.0 mg/dL) may require a dosage adjustment to 8 mg/m²; some clinicians recommend a dosage reduction to 25% of dose.

Administration
I.V.: Irritant. Administered as a short (15-30 minutes) I.V. infusion; continuous 24-hour infusions are occasionally used. Although not generally recommended, mitoxantrone has been given as a rapid bolus over 1-3 minutes. High doses for bone marrow transplant are usually given as 1- to 4-hour infusions.

I.V. Detail: Avoid extravasation - although has not generally been proven to be a vesicant.

BMT only: Extensive pretreatment with anthracyclines increases risk of cardiac toxicity.

pH: 3.0-4.5

Stability
Reconstitution: Dilute in at least 50 mL of NS or D₅W.
Compatibility: Stable in in D₅NS, D₅W, NS
Y-site administration: Incompatible with amphotericin B cholesteryl sulfate complex, aztreonam, cefepime, doxorubicin liposome, paclitaxel, piperacillin/tazobactam, propofol
Compatibility when admixed: Incompatible with heparin

Storage: Store intact vials at 15°C to 25°C (59°F to 77°F); do not freeze. Opened vials may be stored at room temperature for 7 days or under refrigeration for up to 14 days. Solutions diluted for administration are stable for 7 days at room temperature or under refrigeration.

Laboratory Monitoring CBC, serum uric acid, liver function, echocardiogram

Nursing Actions

Physical Assessment: Note Administration for infusion specifics. Infusion site must be monitored closely to prevent extravasation. Monitor laboratory tests, therapeutic effectiveness, and adverse reactions (eg, arrhythmia, hypersensitivity reactions, myelosuppression [anemia], gastrointestinal upset [nutritional and hydration status], opportunistic infection, gout, CHF [rales, dyspnea, edema]). Teach patient possible side effects/appropriate interventions (eg, avoid crowds, maintain hydration) and adverse symptoms to report (eg, symptoms of cardiotoxicity).

Patient Education: Do not take any new medication during therapy unless approved by prescriber. This drug is only administered by infusion; report immediately any redness, swelling, burning, or pain at infusion site. Maintain adequate hydration (2-3 L/day of fluids) unless instructed to restrict fluid intake, and nutrition. You will be more susceptible to infection (avoid crowds and exposure to infection and do not have any vaccinations without consulting prescriber). May cause urine, saliva, tears, sweat, and whites of eyes to turn blue-green for 24 hours postinfusion (this is normal); nausea, vomiting, or GI upset (small, frequent meals, frequent mouth care, chewing gum, or sucking lozenges may help); mouth sores (use soft toothbrush or cotton swabs, waxed dental floss, and frequent mouth rinses); headache, dizziness, or blurred vision (use caution when driving or engaging in tasks that are potentially hazardous until response to drug is known); or loss of hair (may be reversible). Report chest pain or palpitations; rapid or erratic heartbeat; difficulty breathing or constant cough; swelling of extremities or sudden weight gain; persistent fever or chills; or opportunistic infection (eg, fever, chills, sore throat, burning urination, fatigue); changed or decreased urine output. **Pregnancy/breast-feeding precautions:** Do not get pregnant while taking this medication. Consult prescriber for appropriate contraceptive measures. Do not breast-feed.

Breast-Feeding Issues Mitoxantrone is excreted in human milk and significant concentrations (180 mg/mL) have been reported for 28 days after the last administration. Because of the potential for serious adverse reactions in infants from mitoxantrone, breast-feeding should be discontinued before starting treatment.

Pregnancy Issues May cause fetal harm if administered to a pregnant woman. Women with multiple sclerosis and who are biologically capable of becoming pregnant should have a pregnancy test prior to each dose. Mitoxantrone is excreted in human milk and significant concentrations (180 mg/mL) have been reported for 28 days after the last administration.

Mivacurium (mye va KYOO ree um)

U.S. Brand Names Mivacron®

Synonyms Mivacurium Chloride

Pharmacologic Category Neuromuscular Blocker Agent, Nondepolarizing

Medication Safety Issues
Sound-alike/look-alike issues:
Mivacron® may be confused with Mevacor®

Pregnancy Risk Factor C

Lactation Excretion in breast milk unknown/use caution

Use Adjunct to general anesthesia to facilitate endotracheal intubation and to relax skeletal muscles during surgery; to facilitate mechanical ventilation in ICU patients; does not relieve pain or produce sedation

Contraindications Hypersensitivity to mivacurium chloride, any component of the formulation, or other benzylisoquinolinium agents; use of multidose vials in patients with allergy to benzyl alcohol; pre-existing tachycardia

Warnings/Precautions Ventilation must be supported during neuromuscular blockade; does not counteract bradycardia produced by anesthetics/vagal stimulation; prolonged neuromuscular block may be seen in patients with reduced or atypical plasma cholinesterase activity (eg, pregnancy, liver or kidney disease, infections, peptic ulcer, anemia); patients homozygous for the atypical plasma cholinesterase gene are extremely sensitive to the neuromuscular blocking effect of mivacurium (use extreme caution if at all in those patients); duration prolonged in patients with renal and/or hepatic impairment; reduce initial dosage and inject slowly (over 60 seconds) in patients in whom substantial histamine release would be potentially hazardous; certain clinical conditions may result in potentiation or antagonism of neuromuscular blockade (such as, potentiation by electrolyte abnormalities, neuromuscular diseases, or acidosis; antagonism with demyelinating lesions).

Increased sensitivity in patients with myasthenia gravis, Eaton-Lambert syndrome, resistance in burn patients (>30% of body) for period of 5-70 days postinjury; resistance in patients with muscle trauma, denervation, immobilization, infection. Cross-sensitivity with other neuromuscular-blocking agents may occur; use extreme caution in patients with previous anaphylactic reactions.

Drug Interactions

Decreased Effect: Effect of nondepolarizing neuromuscular blockers may be reduced by carbamazepine (chronic use), corticosteroids (also associated with myopathy - see increased effect), phenytoin (chronic use), sympathomimetics, and theophylline.

Increased Effect/Toxicity: Increased effects are possible with aminoglycosides, beta-blockers, clindamycin, calcium channel blockers, halogenated anesthetics, imipenem, ketamine, lidocaine, loop diuretics (furosemide), macrolides (case reports), magnesium sulfate, procainamide, quinidine, quinolones, tetracyclines, and vancomycin. May increase risk of myopathy when used with high-dose corticosteroids for extended periods. Drugs which inhibit acetylcholinesterase may prolong effect of mivacurium.

Adverse Reactions
>10%: Cardiovascular: Flushing of face
1% to 10%: Cardiovascular: Hypotension

Pharmacodynamics/Kinetics

Onset of Action: Neuromuscular blockade: I.V. (dose dependent): 1.5-3 minutes

Duration of Action: Short due to rapid hydrolysis by plasma cholinesterases; clinically effective block may last for 12-20 minutes; spontaneous recovery may be 95% complete in 25-30 minutes; duration shorter in children and may be slightly longer in elderly

Half-Life Elimination: 2 minutes (more active isomers only)

Metabolism: Via plasma cholinesterase, inactive metabolites

Excretion: Urine (<10%)

Available Dosage Forms
Injection, solution [preservative free]: 2 mg/mL (5 mL, 10 mL)
Injection, solution: 2 mg/mL (20 mL, 50 mL) [with benzyl alcohol]

Dosing

Adults & Elderly: Note: Continuous infusion requires an infusion pump; dose should be based on ideal body weight

Neuromuscular blockade: Initial: I.V.: 0.15-0.25 mg/kg bolus followed by maintenance doses of 0.1 mg/kg at approximately 15-minute intervals; for prolonged neuromuscular block, initial infusion of 9-10 mcg/kg/minute is used upon evidence of spontaneous recovery from initial dose, usual infusion
(Continued)

Mivacurium *(Continued)*

rate of 6-7 mcg/kg/minute (1-15 mcg/kg/minute) under balanced anesthesia; initial dose after succinylcholine for intubation (balanced anesthesia): Adults: 0.1 mg/kg

Pretreatment/priming: 10% of intubating dose given 3-5 minutes before initial dose

Pediatrics: Note: Continuous infusion requires an infusion pump; dose should be based on ideal body weight

Neuromuscular blockade: I.V.: Children 2-12 years (duration of action is shorter and dosage requirements are higher): 0.2 mg/kg followed by average infusion rate of 14 mcg/kg/minute (range: 5-31 mcg/kg/minute) upon evidence of spontaneous recovery from initial dose

Renal Impairment: 150 mcg/kg I.V. bolus; duration of action of blockade: 1.5 times longer in ESRD, may decrease infusion rates by as much as 50%, dependent on degree of renal impairment

Hepatic Impairment: 150 mcg/kg I.V. bolus; duration of blockade: 3 times longer in ESLD, may decrease rate of infusion by as much as 50% in ESLD, dependent on the degree of impairment

Administration

I.V.: Children require higher mivacurium infusion rates than adults; during opioid/nitrous oxide/oxygen anesthesia, the infusion rate required to maintain 89% to 99% neuromuscular block averages 14 mcg/kg/minute (range: 5-31). For adults and children, the amount of infusion solution required per hour depends upon the clinical requirements of the patient, the concentration of mivacurium in the infusion solution, and the patient's weight. The contribution of the infusion solution to the fluid requirements of the patient must be considered.

Stability

Compatibility: Stable in D₅LR, D₅NS, D₅W, LR, NS

Storage: Store at room temperature of 15°C to 25°C (59°F to 77°F); protect from direct ultraviolet light.

Nursing Actions

Physical Assessment: Only clinicians experienced in the use of neuromuscular-blocking agents should administer and/or manage the use of mivacurium. Assess potential for interactions with other prescriptions, OTC medications, or herbal products patient may be taking (eg, other drugs that affect neuromuscular activity may increase/decrease neuromuscular block induced by mivacurium). Ventilatory support must be instituted and maintained until adequate respiratory muscle function and/or airway protection are assured. This drug does not cause anesthesia or analgesia; pain must be treated with appropriate agents. Continuous monitoring of vital signs, cardiac and respiratory status, and neuromuscular block (objective assessment with peripheral external nerve stimulator) are mandatory until full muscle tone has returned. Safety precautions must be maintained until full muscle tone has returned. **Note:** It may take longer for return of muscle tone in elderly persons or patients with myasthenia gravis, myopathy, other neuromuscular diseases, dehydration, electrolyte imbalance, or severe acid/base imbalance. Provide appropriate teaching/support prior to, during, and following administration.

Long-term use: Monitor vital signs and fluid levels regularly during treatment. Every 2- to 3-hour repositioning, and skin, mouth, and eye care is necessary while patient is sedated. Emotional and sensory support (auditory and environmental) should be provided.

Patient Education: Patient education should be appropriate for patient condition. Reassurance of constant monitoring and emotional support should precede and follow administration. Patients should be

reminded as muscle tone returns not to attempt to change position or rise from bed without assistance and to report any skin rash, hives, pounding heartbeat, respiratory difficulty, or muscle tremors. **Pregnancy/breast-feeding precaution:** Inform prescriber if you are pregnant. Consult prescriber if breast-feeding.

Additional Information Mivacurium is classified as a short-duration neuromuscular-blocking agent. Do not mix with barbiturates in the same syringe. Mivacurium does not appear to have a cumulative effect on the duration of blockade. It does not relieve pain or produce sedation.

Modafinil *(moe DAF i nil)*

U.S. Brand Names Provigil®

Restrictions C-IV

Pharmacologic Category Stimulant

Pregnancy Risk Factor C

Lactation Excretion in breast milk unknown/use caution

Use Improve wakefulness in patients with excessive daytime sleepiness associated with narcolepsy and shift work sleep disorder (SWSD); adjunctive therapy for obstructive sleep apnea/hypopnea syndrome (OSAHS)

Unlabeled/Investigational Use Attention-deficit/hyperactivity disorder (ADHD); treatment of fatigue in MS and other disorders

Mechanism of Action/Effect The exact mechanism of action is unclear, it does not appear to alter the release of dopamine or norepinephrine, it may exert its stimulant effects by decreasing GABA-mediated neurotransmission, although this theory has not yet been fully evaluated; several studies also suggest that an intact central alpha-adrenergic system is required for modafinil's activity; the drug increases high-frequency alpha waves while decreasing both delta and theta wave activity, and these effects are consistent with generalized increases in mental alertness

Contraindications Hypersensitivity to modafinil or any component of the formulation

Warnings/Precautions Use is not recommended with a history of angina, cardiac ischemia, recent history of myocardial infarction, left ventricular hypertrophy, or patients with mitral valve prolapse who have developed mitral valve prolapse syndrome with previous CNS stimulant use. Caution should be exercised when modafinil is given to patients with a history of psychosis; caution is warranted when operating machinery or driving, although functional impairment has not been demonstrated with modafinil, all CNS-active agents may alter judgment, thinking and/or motor skills. Stimulants may unmask tics in individuals with coexisting Tourette's syndrome. Use caution with renal or hepatic impairment. Safety and efficacy in children ≤16 years of age have not been established.

Drug Interactions

Cytochrome P450 Effect: Substrate of CYP3A4 (major); **Inhibits** CYP1A2 (weak), 2A6 (weak), 2C8/9 (weak), 2C19 (strong), 2E1 (weak), 3A4 (weak); **Induces** CYP1A2 (weak), 2B6 (weak), 3A4 (weak)

Decreased Effect: Modafinil may decrease serum concentrations of oral contraceptives, cyclosporine, and to a lesser degree, theophylline. The levels/effects of modafinil may be decreased by aminoglutethimide, carbamazepine, nafcillin, nevirapine, phenobarbital, phenytoin, rifamycins, and other CYP3A4 inducers. There is also evidence to suggest that modafinil may induce its own metabolism.

Increased Effect/Toxicity: Modafinil may increase the levels/effects of citalopram, diazepam, methsuximide, phenytoin, propranolol, sertraline, or other CYP2C19 substrates. Modafinil may increase levels of warfarin. In populations deficient in the CYP2D6

isoenzyme, where CYP2C19 acts as a secondary metabolic pathway, concentrations of tricyclic antidepressants and selective serotonin reuptake inhibitors may be increased during coadministration. The levels/effects of modafinil may be increased by azole antifungals, clarithromycin, diclofenac, doxycycline, erythromycin, imatinib, isoniazid, nefazodone, nicardipine, propofol, protease inhibitors, quinidine, telithromycin, verapamil, or other CYP3A4 inhibitors.

Nutritional/Ethanol Interactions
Ethanol: Avoid or limit ethanol.
Food: Delays absorption, but does not affect bioavailability.

Adverse Reactions
>10%:
Central nervous system: Headache (34%, dose related)
Gastrointestinal: Nausea (11%)
1% to 10%:
Cardiovascular: Chest pain (3%), hypertension (3%), palpitation (2%), tachycardia (2%), vasodilation (2%), edema (1%)
Central nervous system: Nervousness (7%), dizziness (5%), depression (2%), anxiety (5%, dose related), insomnia (5%), somnolence (2%), chills (1%), agitation (1%), confusion (1%), emotional lability (1%), vertigo (1%)
Gastrointestinal: Diarrhea (6%), dyspepsia (5%), xerostomia (4%), anorexia (4%), constipation (2%), flatulence (1%), mouth ulceration (1%), taste perversion (1%)
Genitourinary: Abnormal urine (1%), hematuria (1%), pyuria (1%)
Hematologic: Eosinophilia (1%)
Hepatic: Abnormal LFTs (2%)
Neuromuscular & skeletal: Back pain (6%), paresthesia (2%), dyskinesia (1%), hyperkinesia (1%), hypertonia (1%), neck rigidity (1%), tremor (1%)
Ocular: Amblyopia (1%), abnormal vision (1%), eye pain (1%)
Respiratory: Pharyngitis (4%), rhinitis (7%), lung disorder (2%), asthma (1%), epistaxis (1%)
Miscellaneous: Diaphoresis
Postmarketing and/or case reports: Agranulocytosis, mania, psychosis

Overdosage/Toxicology Symptoms of overdose include agitation, irritability, aggressiveness, confusion, nervousness, tremor, insomnia, palpitations, and elevations in hemodynamic parameters. Treatment is symptomatic and supportive. Cardiac monitoring is warranted.

Pharmacodynamics/Kinetics
Time to Peak: Serum: 2-4 hours
Protein Binding: 60%, primarily to albumin
Half-Life Elimination: Effective half-life: 15 hours; Steady-state: 2-4 days
Metabolism: Hepatic; multiple pathways including CYP3A4
Excretion: Urine (as metabolites, <10% as unchanged drug)
Pharmacokinetic Note Modafinil is a racemic compound (10% d-isomer and 90% l-isomer at steady state), whose enantiomers have different pharmacokinetics.

Available Dosage Forms Tablet: 100 mg, 200 mg
Dosing
Adults:
ADHD (unlabeled use): Oral: 100-300 mg once daily
Narcolepsy, OSAHS: Oral: Initial: 200 mg as a single daily dose in the morning.
SWSD: Oral: Initial: 200 mg as a single dose taken ~1 hour prior to start of work shift.
Note: Doses of 400 mg/day, given as a single dose, have been well tolerated, but there is no consistent evidence that this dose confers additional benefit.

Elderly: Elimination of modafinil and its metabolites may be reduced as a consequence of aging and as a result, lower doses should be considered.
Pediatrics:
ADHD (unlabeled use): Oral: 50-100 mg once daily
Renal Impairment: Inadequate data to determine safety and efficacy in severe renal impairment.
Hepatic Impairment: Dose should be reduced to one-half of that recommended for patients with normal liver function.

Nursing Actions
Physical Assessment: Assess effectiveness and interactions of other medications, especially those that are metabolized by P450 enzymes. Note that modafinil has potential for abuse; caution patient about inappropriate or overuse. Assess knowledge/teach patient possible side effects/interventions, and adverse symptoms to report
Patient Education: Take exactly as prescribed; do not exceed recommended dosage without consulting prescriber. Avoid drinking alcohol. Do not share medication with anyone else. Void before taking medication. You may experience headache, nervousness, confusion, or dizziness (use caution when driving or engaging in tasks requiring alertness until response to drug is known); diarrhea (yogurt or buttermilk may help); or dry mouth or sore mouth, loss of appetite, or vomiting (small frequent meals, frequent mouth care, chewing gum, or sucking lozenges may help). If you have diabetes, monitor glucose levels closely. Report chest pain or palpitations; respiratory difficulty; excessive insomnia, CNS agitation, depression, or memory disturbances; vision changes; changes in urinary pattern or ejaculation disturbances; or persistent joint pain or stiffness. **Pregnancy/breast-feeding precautions:** Inform prescriber if you are or intend to become pregnant. Consult prescriber if breast-feeding.
Pregnancy Issues Embryotoxic effects have been observed in some, but not all animal studies. There are no adequate and well-controlled studies in pregnant women; use only when the potential risk of drug therapy is outweighed by the drug's benefits. Efficacy of steroidal contraceptives may be decreased; alternate means of contraception should be considered during therapy and for 1 month after modafinil is discontinued.

Moexipril (mo EKS i pril)

U.S. Brand Names Univasc®
Synonyms Moexipril Hydrochloride
Pharmacologic Category Angiotensin-Converting Enzyme (ACE) Inhibitor
Medication Safety Issues
Sound-alike/look-alike issues:
Moexipril may be confused with Monopril®
Pregnancy Risk Factor C (1st trimester)/D (2nd and 3rd trimesters)
Lactation Excretion in breast milk unknown/use caution
Use Treatment of hypertension, alone or in combination with thiazide diuretics; treatment of left ventricular dysfunction after myocardial infarction
Mechanism of Action/Effect Competitive inhibitor of angiotensin-converting enzyme (ACE); prevents conversion of angiotensin I to angiotensin II, a potent vasoconstrictor; results in lower levels of angiotensin II which causes an increase in plasma renin activity and a reduction in aldosterone secretion
Contraindications Hypersensitivity to moexipril, moexiprilat, or any component of the formulation; hypersensitivity or allergic reactions or angioedema related to previous treatment with an ACE inhibitor; pregnancy (2nd or 3rd trimester)
(Continued)

Moexipril (Continued)

Warnings/Precautions Anaphylactic reactions can occur. Angioedema can occur at any time during treatment (especially following first dose). It may involve head and neck (potentially affecting the airway) or the intestine (presenting with abdominal pain). Prolonged monitoring may be required especially if tongue, glottis, or larynx are involved as they are associated with airway obstruction. Those with a history of airway surgery in this situation have a higher risk. Careful blood pressure monitoring with first dose (hypotension can occur especially in volume-depleted patients). Dosage adjustment needed in renal impairment. Use with caution in hypovolemia; collagen vascular diseases; valvular stenosis (particularly aortic stenosis); hyperkalemia; or before, during, or immediately after anesthesia. Avoid rapid dosage escalation which may lead to renal insufficiency. Rare toxicities associated with ACE inhibitors include cholestatic jaundice (which may progress to hepatic necrosis) and neutropenia/agranulocytosis with myeloid hyperplasia. Hypersensitivity reactions may be seen during hemodialysis with high-flux dialysis membranes (eg, AN69). Deterioration in renal function can occur with initiation. Use with caution in unilateral renal artery stenosis and pre-existing renal insufficiency.

Drug Interactions
Decreased Effect: Aspirin (high dose) may reduce the therapeutic effects of ACE inhibitors; at low dosages this does not appear to be significant. Rifampin may decrease the effect of ACE inhibitors. Antacids may decrease the bioavailability of ACE inhibitors (may be more likely to occur with captopril); separate administration times by 1-2 hours. NSAIDs, specifically indomethacin, may reduce the hypotensive effects of ACE inhibitors. More likely to occur in low renin or volume dependent hypertensive patients.

Increased Effect/Toxicity: Potassium supplements, co-trimoxazole (high dose), angiotensin II receptor antagonists (eg, candesartan, losartan, irbesartan), or potassium-sparing diuretics (amiloride, spironolactone, triamterene) may result in elevated serum potassium levels when combined with moexipril. ACE inhibitor effects may be increased by probenecid (increases levels of captopril). ACE inhibitors may increase serum concentrations/effects of lithium.

Diuretics have additive hypotensive effects with ACE inhibitors, and hypovolemia increases the potential for adverse renal effects of ACE inhibitors. In patients with compromised renal function, coadministration with NSAIDs may result in further deterioration of renal function. Allopurinol and ACE inhibitors may cause a higher risk of hypersensitivity reaction when taken concurrently.

Nutritional/Ethanol Interactions
Food: Food may delay and reduce peak serum levels.
Herb/Nutraceutical: Avoid dong quai if using for hypertension (has estrogenic activity). Avoid ephedra, yohimbe, ginseng (may worsen hypertension). Avoid garlic (may have increased antihypertensive effect).

Lab Interactions Increased BUN, creatinine, potassium, positive Coombs' [direct]; decreased cholesterol (S); may cause false-positive results in urine acetone determinations using sodium nitroprusside reagent

Adverse Reactions 1% to 10%:
Cardiovascular: Hypotension, peripheral edema
Central nervous system: Headache, dizziness, fatigue
Dermatologic: Rash, alopecia, flushing, rash
Endocrine & metabolic: Hyperkalemia, hyponatremia
Gastrointestinal: Diarrhea, nausea, heartburn
Genitourinary: Polyuria
Neuromuscular & skeletal: Myalgia
Renal: Reversible increases in creatinine or BUN
Respiratory: Cough, pharyngitis, upper respiratory infection, sinusitis

Overdosage/Toxicology Mild hypotension has been the primary toxic effect seen with acute overdose. Bradycardia may also occur. Hyperkalemia occurs even with therapeutic doses, especially in patients with renal insufficiency and those taking NSAIDs. Treatment is symptom-directed and supportive.

Pharmacodynamics/Kinetics
Onset of Action: Peak effect: 1-2 hours
Duration of Action: >24 hours
Time to Peak: 1.5 hours
Protein Binding: Plasma: Moexipril: 90%; Moexiprilat: 50% to 70%
Half-Life Elimination: Moexipril: 1 hour; Moexiprilat: 2-9 hours
Metabolism: Parent drug: Hepatic and via GI tract to moexiprilat, 1000 times more potent than parent
Excretion: Feces (50%)

Available Dosage Forms Tablet, as hydrochloride [scored]: 7.5 mg, 15 mg

Dosing
Adults: Hypertension, LV dysfunction (post MI): Oral: Initial: 7.5 mg once daily (in patients **not** receiving diuretics), 1 hour prior to a meal **or** 3.75 mg once daily (when combined with thiazide diuretics); maintenance dose: 7.5-30 mg/day in 1 or 2 divided doses 1 hour before meals
Elderly: Dose the same as adults; adjust for renal impairment. Tablet may be cut in half (3.75 mg) for starting therapy (see Renal Impairment).
Renal Impairment: Cl$_{cr}$ ≤40 mL/minute: Patients may be cautiously placed on 3.75 mg once daily, then upwardly titrated to a maximum of 15 mg/day.

Laboratory Monitoring Electrolytes, CBC, renal function. If patient has renal impairment, a baseline WBC with differential and serum creatinine should be evaluated and monitored closely during the first 3 months of therapy.

Nursing Actions
Physical Assessment: Assess potential for interactions with other pharmacological agents or herbal products patient may be taking (especially anything that may impact fluid balance or cardiac status). Monitor laboratory tests on a regular basis during therapy. Patient should be monitored closely for anaphylactic reaction or angioedema which can occur at any time during treatment and may involve head and neck. Monitor therapeutic effectiveness (blood pressure) and adverse responses (eg, hypotension, rash, diarrhea, myalgia, electrolyte imbalance) regularly during therapy. Teach patient proper use, possible side effects/appropriate interventions, and adverse symptoms to report.

Patient Education: Do not take any new medication during therapy unless approved by prescriber. Do not use potassium supplements or salt substitutes without consulting prescriber. Take exactly as directed; do not discontinue without consulting prescriber. Take first dose at bedtime. Take all doses on an empty stomach, 1 hour before or 2 hours after meals. This drug does not eliminate need for diet or exercise regimen as recommended by prescriber. May cause dizziness, fainting, or lightheadedness (use caution when driving or engaging in tasks that require alertness until response to drug is known); postural hypotension (use caution when rising from lying or sitting position or climbing stairs); nausea, vomiting, abdominal pain, dry mouth, or transient loss of appetite (small, frequent meals, frequent mouth care, sucking lozenges, or chewing gum may help). Report immediately unusual swelling of mouth, tongue, face, throat. Report respiratory difficulty or unusual cough, rash, excessive urination, chest pain or palpitations, mouth sores, fever or chills, numbness, tingling or pain in muscles, or other persistent adverse reactions. **Pregnancy/breast-feeding precautions:** Inform prescriber if you are or intend to become pregnant.

This drug should not be used in the 2nd or 3rd trimester of pregnancy. Consult prescriber for appropriate contraceptive measures if necessary. Consult prescriber if breast-feeding.

Dietary Considerations Administer on an empty stomach.

Geriatric Considerations Due to frequent decreases in glomerular filtration (also creatinine clearance) with aging, elderly patients may have exaggerated responses to ACE inhibitors. Differences in clinical response due to hepatic changes are not observed.

Pregnancy Issues ACE inhibitors can cause fetal injury or death if taken during the 2nd or 3rd trimester. Discontinue ACE inhibitors as soon as pregnancy is detected.

Moexipril and Hydrochlorothiazide
(mo EKS i pril & hye droe klor oh THYE a zide)

U.S. Brand Names Uniretic®
Synonyms Hydrochlorothiazide and Moexipril
Pharmacologic Category Antihypertensive Agent, Combination
Pregnancy Risk Factor C/D (2nd and 3rd trimesters)
Lactation Enters breast milk/use caution
Use Combination therapy for hypertension, however, not indicated for initial treatment of hypertension; replacement therapy in patients receiving separate dosage forms (for patient convenience); when monotherapy with one component fails to achieve desired antihypertensive effect, or when dose-limiting adverse effects limit upward titration of monotherapy
Available Dosage Forms Tablet [scored]:
7.5/12.5: Moexipril hydrochloride 7.5 mg and hydrochlorothiazide 12.5 mg
15/12.5: Moexipril hydrochloride 15 mg and hydrochlorothiazide 12.5 mg
15/25: Moexipril hydrochloride 15 mg and hydrochlorothiazide 25 mg
Dosing
Adults: Adults: Oral: 7.5-30 mg of moexipril, taken either in a single or divided dose one hour before meals; hydrochlorothiazide dose should be ≤50 mg/day
Elderly: Overall safety and efficacy are not different in elderly patients, although a higher moexipril AUC was observed in elderly patients. Greater sensitivity to effects may be observed in some older individuals. Refer to adult dosing.
Nursing Actions
Physical Assessment: See individual agents.
Patient Education: See individual agents. **Pregnancy/breast-feeding precautions:** Inform prescriber if you are or intend to become pregnant. Consult prescriber if breast-feeding.
Related Information
Hydrochlorothiazide *on page 610*
Moexipril *on page 837*

Mometasone Furoate
(moe MET a sone FYOOR oh ate)

U.S. Brand Names Asmanex® Twisthaler®; Elocon®; Nasonex®
Pharmacologic Category Corticosteroid, Inhalant (Oral); Corticosteroid, Nasal; Corticosteroid, Topical
Medication Safety Issues
Sound-alike/look-alike issues:
Elocon® lotion may be confused with ophthalmic solutions. Manufacturer's labeling emphasizes the product is **NOT** for use in the eyes.
Pregnancy Risk Factor C
Lactation Excretion in breast milk unknown/use caution

Use Relief of the inflammatory and pruritic manifestations of corticosteroid-responsive dermatoses (medium potency topical corticosteroid); treatment of nasal symptoms of seasonal and perennial allergic rhinitis; prevention of nasal symptoms associated with seasonal allergic rhinitis; treatment of nasal polyps in adults; maintenance treatment of asthma as prophylactic therapy or as a supplement in asthma patients requiring oral corticosteroids for the purpose of decreasing or eliminating the oral corticosteroid requirement

Mechanism of Action/Effect Corticosteroid with medium range potency. Reverses capillary permeability and release of inflammatory mediators (leukotrienes and prostaglandins); suppresses migration of polymorphonuclear leukocytes.

Contraindications Hypersensitivity to mometasone or any component of the formulation; treatment of acute bronchospasm (oral inhaler)

Warnings/Precautions
May cause suppression of hypothalamic-pituitary-adrenal (HPA) axis, particularly in younger children, or in patients receiving high doses for prolonged periods, or when used topically on large areas of the body, denuded areas, or with an occlusive dressing. Use caution if replacing systemic corticosteroid with nasal or oral inhaler; may cause symptoms of withdrawal or acute adrenal insufficiency. Transfer to oral inhaler may unmask previously-suppressed allergic conditions (rhinitis, conjunctivitis, eczema).

Controlled clinical studies have shown that corticosteroids may cause a reduction in growth velocity in pediatric patients; titrate to the lowest effective dose. Decreases in bone mineral density have been observed. May suppress the immune system, patients may be more susceptible to infection; monitor for signs of oropharyngeal candidiasis. Use with caution, if at all, in patients with systemic infections, active or quiescent tuberculosis infection, or ocular herpes simplex. Avoid exposure to chickenpox and measles. Rare instances of glaucoma have been reported with inhaled steroids.

Drug Interactions
Cytochrome P450 Effect: Substrate of CYP3A4 (minor)
Increased Effect/Toxicity:
Concomitant use with ketoconazole may result in increased mometasone furoate plasma levels.

Adverse Reactions
Nasal/oral inhalation:
>10%:
Central nervous system: Headache (17% to 22%), fatigue (oral inhalation 1% to 13%), depression (oral inhalation 11%)
Neuromuscular & skeletal: Musculoskeletal pain (1% to 22%), arthralgia (oral inhalation 13%)
Respiratory: Sinusitis (oral inhalation 22%), rhinitis (2% to 20%), upper respiratory infection (8% to 15%), pharyngitis (8% to 13%), cough (nasal inhalation 7% to 13%), epistaxis (1% to 11%)
Miscellaneous: Viral infection (nasal inhalation 8% to 14%), oral candidiasis (oral inhalation 4% to 22%)
1% to 10%:
Cardiovascular: Chest pain
Gastrointestinal: Abdominal pain, dry throat (oral inhalation), vomiting (1% to 5%), diarrhea, dyspepsia, flatulence, gastroenteritis, nausea, vomiting
Genitourinary: Dysmenorrhea
Neuromuscular & skeletal: Back pain, myalgia
Ocular: Conjunctivitis
Otic: Earache, otitis media
Respiratory: Asthma, bronchitis, dysphonia, epistaxis, nasal irritation, rhinitis, wheezing
Miscellaneous: Accidental injury, flu-like symptoms

Topical:
1% to 10%: Dermatologic: Bacterial skin infection, burning, furunculosis, pruritus, skin atrophy, tingling/stinging
(Continued)

Mometasone Furoate *(Continued)*

Cataract formation, reduction in growth velocity, and HPA axis suppression have been reported with other corticosteroids

Pharmacodynamics/Kinetics

Protein Binding: Mometasone furoate: 98% to 99%

Half-Life Elimination: Oral inhalation: 5 hours

Metabolism: Mometasone furoate: Hepatic via CYP3A4; forms metabolite

Excretion: Feces, bile, urine

Available Dosage Forms

Cream, topical:
Elocon®: 0.1% (15 g, 45 g)

Lotion, topical:
Elocon®: 0.1% (30 mL, 60 mL) [contains isopropyl alcohol 40%]

Ointment, topical: 0.1% (15 g, 45 g)
Elocon®: 0.1% (15 g, 45 g)

Powder for oral inhalation:
Asmanex® Twisthaler®: 220 mcg (14 units, 30 units, 60 units, 120 units) [contains lactose]

Suspension, intranasal [spray]:
Nasonex®: 50 mcg/spray (17 g) [delivers 120 sprays; contains benzalkonium chloride]

Dosing

Adults & Elderly:

Treatment of seasonal and perennial allergic rhinitis: Nasal spray: 2 sprays (100 mcg) in each nostril daily

Prevention of seasonal and perennial allergic rhinitis: Nasal spray: 2 sprays (100 mcg) in each nostril daily beginning 2-4 weeks prior to pollen season

Treatment of corticosteroid-responsive dermatoses: Topical: Apply sparingly, do not use occlusive dressings. Therapy should be discontinued when control is achieved; if no improvement is seen in 2 weeks, reassessment of diagnosis may be necessary.

Cream, ointment: Apply a thin film to affected area once daily

Lotion: Apply a few drops to affected area once daily

Treatment of nasal polyps: Nasal spray: 2 sprays (100 mcg) in each nostril twice daily; 2 sprays (100 mcg) once daily may be effective in some patients

Asthma: Oral inhalation:

Bronchodilators or inhaled corticosteroids: Initial: 1 inhalation (220 mcg) daily (maximum 2 inhalations or 440 mcg/day); may be given in the evening or in divided doses twice daily

Oral corticosteroids: Initial: 440 mcg twice daily (maximum 880 mcg/day); prednisone should be reduced no faster than 2.5 mg/day on a weekly basis, beginning after at least 1 week of mometasone furoate use

Note: Maximum effects may not be evident for 1-2 weeks or longer; dose should be titrated to effect, using the lowest possible dose

Pediatrics:

Treatment of seasonal and perennial allergic rhinitis treatment:

Nasal spray:

Children 2-11 years: 1 spray (50 mcg) in each nostril daily

Children ≥12 years: Refer to adult dosing.

Treatment of corticosteroid-responsive dermatoses: Topical:

Cream, ointment: Children ≥2 years: Refer to adult dosing. Do not use in pediatric patients for longer than 3 weeks.

Lotion: Children ≥12 years: Refer to adult dosing.

Asthma: Oral inhalation: Children ≥12 years: Refer to adult dosing.

Administration

Inhalation:

Nasal spray: Prior to first use, prime pump by actuating 10 times or until fine spray appears; may store for a maximum of 1 week without repriming. Spray should be administered once or twice daily, at a regular interval. Shake well prior to use.

Oral inhalation: Exhale fully prior to bringing the Twisthaler® up to the mouth. Place between lips and inhale quickly and deeply. Do not breath out through the inhaler. Remove inhaler and hold breath for 10 seconds if possible.

Topical: Apply sparingly; avoid eyes, face, underarms, and groin. Do not wrap or bandage affected area.

Stability

Storage:

Cream: Store between 2°C to 25°C (36°F to 77°F).

Lotion: Store between 2°C to 30°C (36°F to 86°F).

Nasal spray: Store at room temperature of 15°C to 30°C (59°F to 86°F). Protect from light.

Ointment: Store at room temperature of 15°C to 30°C (59°F to 86°F).

Oral Inhaler: Store at room temperature of 15°C to 30°C (59°F to 86°F). Discard when oral dose counter reads "0" (or 45 days after opening the foil pouch).

Nursing Actions

Physical Assessment: Assess potential for interactions with other prescriptions, OTC medications, or herbal products patient may be taking. Monitor patient response. Teach patient proper use (according to formulation), side effects/appropriate interventions, and symptoms to report.

Patient Education: For external use only. Do not take anything new during treatment without consulting prescriber. Use exactly as directed and for no longer than the period prescribed. **Pregnancy/breast-feeding precautions:** Inform prescriber if you are or intend to become pregnant. Consult prescriber if breast-feeding.

Nasal: Read complete instructions in package. Prime the pump as directed. Gently blow your nose to clear nostrils. Close one nostril. Tilt your head forward slightly and, keeping the bottle upright, carefully insert the nasal applicator into the other nostril. After the spray, breath gently inward through the nostril, then breath out through the mouth. Repeat in other nostril. You may experience headache, cough, or nosebleed. Report unusual chest pain, gastrointestinal upset, muscle pain, flu-like symptoms, other persistent adverse reactions, worsening of condition or failure to improve. Store at room temperature, away from light.

Topical: Do not use for eyes, mucous membranes, or open wounds. Use exactly as directed and for no longer than the period prescribed. Before using, wash and dry area gently. Apply in a thin layer (cream, ointment) or a few drops (lotion) and rub in lightly. Apply light dressing (if necessary) to area being treated. Do not use occlusive dressing unless so advised by prescriber. Avoid prolonged or excessive use around sensitive tissues, underarms, genital, or rectal areas. Avoid exposing treated area to direct sunlight (severe sunburn may occur). Inform prescriber if condition worsens (redness, swelling, irritation, signs of infection, or open sores) or fails to improve.

Dietary Considerations

Asmanex® Twisthaler® contains lactose.

Breast-Feeding Issues Systemic corticosteroids are excreted in human milk. The extent of topical absorption is variable. Use with caution while breast-feeding; do not apply topical products to nipples.

Pregnancy Issues

There are no adequate and well-controlled studies using topical mometasone during pregnancy. However, teratogenicity and intrauterine growth retardation has been reported in animal studies with some topical steroids. Avoid use of large amounts for long periods of time during pregnancy. Hypoadrenalism may occur in infants born to women receiving corticosteroids during pregnancy. Monitor these infants closely after birth.

Montelukast (mon te LOO kast)

U.S. Brand Names Singulair®

Synonyms Montelukast Sodium

Pharmacologic Category Leukotriene-Receptor Antagonist

Medication Safety Issues
Sound-alike/look-alike issues:
Singulair® may be confused with Sinequan®

Pregnancy Risk Factor B

Lactation Excretion in breast milk unknown/use caution

Use Prophylaxis and chronic treatment of asthma; relief of symptoms of seasonal allergic rhinitis and perennial allergic rhinitis

Unlabeled/Investigational Use Acute asthma

Mechanism of Action/Effect Montelukast is a selective leukotriene receptor antagonist which inhibits cysteinyl leukotriene that is responsible for edema, smooth muscle contraction that is felt to be associated with the signs and symptoms of asthma.

Contraindications Hypersensitivity to montelukast or any component of the formulation

Warnings/Precautions Inform phenylketonuric patients that the chewable tablet contains phenylalanine. Montelukast is not FDA approved for use in the reversal of bronchospasm in acute asthma attacks; some clinicians, however, support its use (Cylly, 2003; Camargo, 2003; Ferreira, 2001). Should not be used as monotherapy for the treatment and management of exercise-induced bronchospasm. Has been associated with eosinophilic vasculitis (Churg-Strauss syndrome), usually following reduction or withdrawal of oral corticosteroids. Healthcare providers should be alert to eosinophilia, vasculitic rash, worsening pulmonary symptoms, cardiac complications, and/or neuropathy presenting in their patients. A casual association between montelukast and these underlying conditions has not been established. Safety and efficacy in children <6 months of age have not been established.

Drug Interactions

Cytochrome P450 Effect: Substrate (major) of CYP2C8/9, 3A4; **Inhibits** CYP2C8/9 (weak)

Decreased Effect: CYP2C8/9 inducers may decrease the levels/effects of montelukast; example inducers include carbamazepine, phenobarbital, phenytoin, rifampin, rifapentine, and secobarbital. CYP3A4 inducers may decrease the levels/effects of montelukast; example inducers include aminoglutethimide, carbamazepine, nafcillin, nevirapine, phenobarbital, phenytoin, and rifamycins.

Nutritional/Ethanol Interactions Herb/Nutraceutical: St John's wort may decrease montelukast levels.

Adverse Reactions (As reported in adults)
1% to 10%:
Central nervous system: Dizziness (2%), fatigue (2%), fever (2%)
Dermatologic: Rash (2%)
Gastrointestinal: Abdominal pain (3%), dyspepsia (2%), dental pain (2%), gastroenteritis (2%)
Neuromuscular & skeletal: Weakness (2%)
Respiratory: Cough (3%), nasal congestion (2%), upper respiratory infection (2%)
Miscellaneous: Flu-like symptoms (4%), trauma (1%)

Overdosage/Toxicology No specific antidote

Remove unabsorbed material from the GI tract, employ clinical monitoring and institute supportive therapy if required. Abdominal pain, hyperkinesia, mydriasis, somnolence, and thirst have been reported with acute overdose of ≥150 mg/day.

Pharmacodynamics/Kinetics

Duration of Action: >24 hours

Time to Peak: Serum: Tablet: 10 mg: 3-4 hours; 5 mg: 2-2.5 hours; 4 mg: 2 hours

Protein Binding: Plasma: >99%

Half-Life Elimination: Plasma: Mean: 2.7-5.5 hours

Metabolism: Extensively hepatic via CYP3A4 and 2C8/9

Excretion: Feces (86%); urine (<0.2%)

Available Dosage Forms

Granules: 4 mg/packet
Tablet: 10 mg
Tablet, chewable: 4 mg [contains phenylalanine 0.674 mg; cherry flavor]; 5 mg [contains phenylalanine 0.842 mg; cherry flavor]

Dosing

Adults & Elderly:
Asthma, allergic seasonal or perennial rhinitis: Oral: One 10 mg tablet daily in the evening
Asthma, acute (unlabeled use): 10 mg as a single dose administered with first-line therapy

Pediatrics:
Asthma: Oral:
6-11 months (unlabeled use): 4 mg (oral granules) once daily, taken in the evening
12-23 months: 4 mg (oral granules) once daily, taken in the evening
Seasonal or perennial allergic rhinitis: Oral: *6-23 months:* 4 mg (oral granules) once daily
Asthma, seasonal or perennial allergic rhinitis: Oral:
2-5 years: 4 mg (chewable tablet or oral granules) once daily, taken in the evening
6-14 years: Chew one 5 mg chewable tablet/day, taken in the evening
≥15 years: Refer to adult dosing.

Renal Impairment: No adjustment is necessary.

Hepatic Impairment: No adjustment necessary in mild-to-moderate hepatic disease. Patients with severe hepatic disease were **not** studied.

Administration

Oral: When treating asthma, administer dose in the evening. Granules may be administered directly in the mouth or mixed with applesauce, carrots, rice, ice cream, baby formula, or breast milk; do not add to any other liquids. Administer within 15 minutes of opening packet.

Stability

Storage: Store at room temperature of 15°C to 30°C (59°F to 86°F). Protect from moisture and light.
Granules: Use within 15 minutes of opening packet.

Nursing Actions

Physical Assessment: Not for use in acute asthma attacks, including status asthmaticus. Assess effectiveness and interactions of other medications patient may be taking. Monitor effectiveness of therapy and adverse reactions at beginning of therapy and periodically with long-term use. Assess knowledge/teach patient appropriate use, interventions to reduce side effects, and adverse symptoms to report.

Patient Education: Do not stop other asthma medication unless advised by prescriber. Chewable tablet contains phenylalanine. Take every evening on a continuous basis; do not discontinue even if feeling better (this medication may help reduce incidence of acute attacks). Granules may be administered directly in the mouth or mixed with applesauce, carrots, rice, ice cream, baby formula, or breast milk (do not add to any other liquids); administer within 15 minutes of opening packet. You may experience mild headache (mild analgesic may help); or fatigue or dizziness (use (Continued)

Montelukast *(Continued)*

caution when driving). Report skin rash or itching, abdominal pain or persistent GI upset, unusual cough or congestion, feeling of numbness in arms or legs, flu-like illness, or worsening of asthmatic condition. **Breast-feeding precaution:** Consult prescriber if breast-feeding.

Dietary Considerations Tablet, chewable: 4 mg strength contains phenylalanine 0.674 mg; 5 mg strength contains phenylalanine 0.842 mg

Breast-Feeding Issues Zafirlukast, another leukotriene receptor antagonist, is excreted in breast milk and use while breast-feeding is not recommended.

Moricizine (mor I siz een)

U.S. Brand Names Ethmozine®
Synonyms Moricizine Hydrochloride
Pharmacologic Category Antiarrhythmic Agent, Class I
Medication Safety Issues
Sound-alike/look-alike issues:
Ethmozine® may be confused with Erythrocin®, erythromycin

Pregnancy Risk Factor B
Lactation Enters breast milk/not recommended
Use Treatment of ventricular tachycardia and life-threatening ventricular arrhythmias
Unlabeled/Investigational Use PVCs, complete and nonsustained ventricular tachycardia, atrial arrhythmias
Mechanism of Action/Effect Class I antiarrhythmic agent; reduces the fast inward current carried by sodium ions, shortens Phase I and Phase II repolarization, resulting in decreased action potential duration and effective refractory period

Contraindications Hypersensitivity to moricizine or any component of the formulation; pre-existing second- or third-degree AV block (except in patients with a functioning artificial pacemaker); right bundle branch block when associated with left hemiblock or bifascicular block (unless functional pacemaker in place); cardiogenic shock

Warnings/Precautions Can be proarrhythmic; watch for new rhythm disturbances or existing arrhythmias that worsen. Use cautiously in CAD, previous history of MI, CHF, and cardiomegaly. The CAST II trial demonstrated a decreased trend in survival for patients receiving moricizine. Dose-related increases in PR and QRS intervals occur. Use cautiously in patients with pre-existing conduction abnormalities, and significant hepatic impairment. Safety and efficacy have not been established in pediatric patients.

Drug Interactions
Cytochrome P450 Effect: Substrate of CYP3A4 (major); **Induces** CYP1A2 (weak), 3A4 (weak)
Decreased Effect: Moricizine may decrease levels of theophylline (50%) and diltiazem. CYP3A4 inducers may decrease the levels/effects of moricizine; example inducers include aminoglethimide, carbamazepine, nafcillin, nevirapine, phenobarbital, phenytoin, and rifamycins.
Increased Effect/Toxicity: CYP3A4 inhibitors may increase the levels/effects of moricizine; example inhibitors include azole antifungals, clarithromycin, diclofenac, doxycycline, erythromycin, imatinib, isoniazid, nefazodone, nicardipine, propofol, protease inhibitors, quinidine, telithromycin, and verapamil. Moricizine levels may be increased by cimetidine and diltiazem. Digoxin may result in additive prolongation of the PR interval when combined with moricizine (but not rate of second- and third-degree AV block). Drugs which may prolong QT interval (including cisapride, erythromycin, phenothiazines, cyclic antidepressants,

and some quinolones) are contraindicated with type Ia antiarrhythmics. Moricizine has some type Ia activity, and caution should be used.

Nutritional/Ethanol Interactions Food: Moricizine peak serum concentrations may be decreased if taken with food.

Adverse Reactions
>10%: Central nervous system: Dizziness
1% to 10%:
Cardiovascular: Proarrhythmia, palpitation, cardiac death, ECG abnormalities, CHF
Central nervous system: Headache, fatigue, insomnia
Endocrine & metabolic: Decreased libido
Gastrointestinal: Nausea, diarrhea, ileus
Ocular: Blurred vision, periorbital edema
Respiratory: Dyspnea

Overdosage/Toxicology Has a narrow therapeutic index and severe toxicity may occur slightly above the therapeutic range, especially if combined with other antiarrhythmic drugs. Acute single ingestion of twice the daily therapeutic dose is life-threatening. Symptoms of overdose include increases in PR, QRS, QT intervals and amplitude of the T wave, AV block, bradycardia, hypotension, ventricular arrhythmias (monomorphic or polymorphic ventricular tachycardia), and asystole. Other symptoms include dizziness, blurred vision, headache, and GI upset.

Treatment is symptom-directed and supportive. **Note:** Type Ia antiarrhythmic agents should not be used to treat cardiotoxicity caused by type Ic drugs.

Pharmacodynamics/Kinetics
Protein Binding: Plasma: 95%
Half-Life Elimination: Healthy volunteers: 3-4 hours; Cardiac disease: 6-13 hours
Metabolism: Significant first-pass effect; some enterohepatic recycling
Excretion: Feces (56%); urine (39%)
Available Dosage Forms Tablet, as hydrochloride: 200 mg, 250 mg, 300 mg
Dosing
Adults & Elderly: Ventricular arrhythmias: Oral: 200-300 mg every 8 hours, adjust dosage at 150 mg/day at 3-day intervals. See table for dosage recommendations of transferring from other antiarrhythmic agents to Ethmozine®. Hospitalization required to start therapy.

Moricizine

Transferred From	Start Ethmozine®
Encainide, propafenone, tocainide, or mexiletine	8-12 hours after last dose
Flecainide	12-24 hours after last dose
Procainamide	3-6 hours after last dose
Quinidine, disopyramide	6-12 hours after last dose

Renal Impairment: Start at 600 mg/day or less.
Hepatic Impairment: Start at 600 mg/day or less.
Laboratory Monitoring Electrolytes (correct any imbalance) prior to beginning therapy
Nursing Actions
Physical Assessment: Assess other medications patient may be taking for effectiveness and interactions. Monitor laboratory tests, therapeutic response (cardiac status), and adverse reactions at beginning of therapy, when titrating dosage, and on a regular basis with long-term therapy. **Note:** Moricizine has a low toxic:therapeutic ratio and overdose may easily produce severe and life-threatening reactions. Assess knowledge/teach patient appropriate use, interventions to reduce side effects, and adverse symptoms to report.

Patient Education: Take exactly as directed; do not take additional doses or discontinue without consulting prescriber. You will need regular cardiac checkups and blood tests while taking this medication. You may experience dizziness or visual changes (use caution when driving or engaging in tasks requiring alertness until response to drug is known); nausea or vomiting (small frequent meals, frequent mouth care, chewing gum, or sucking lozenges may help); or headaches, sleep disturbances, or decreased libido (usually temporary, if persistent consult prescriber). Report chest pain, palpitation, or erratic heartbeat; increased weight or swelling of hands or feet; blurred vision or facial swelling; acute diarrhea; changes in bowel or bladder patterns; or respiratory difficulty. **Breast-feeding precaution:** Breast-feeding is not recommended.

Dietary Considerations Best if taken on an empty stomach.

Geriatric Considerations Due to moricizine binding to plasma albumin and alpha-glycoprotein, other highly bound drugs may displace moricizine. Since elderly may require multiple drugs, caution with highly bound drugs is necessary. Consider changes in renal and hepatic function with age and monitor closely since half-life may be prolonged.

Morphine Sulfate (MOR feen SUL fate)

U.S. Brand Names Astramorph/PF™; Avinza®; DepoDur™; Duramorph®; Infumorph®; Kadian®; MS Contin®; Oramorph SR®; RMS®; Roxanol™; Roxanol 100™; Roxanol™-T [DSC]

Synonyms MSO₄ (error-prone abbreviation and should not be used)

Restrictions C-II

Pharmacologic Category Analgesic, Narcotic

Medication Safety Issues
Sound-alike/look-alike issues:
Morphine may be confused with hydromorphone
Morphine sulfate may be confused with magnesium sulfate
MSO₄ is an error-prone abbreviation (mistaken as magnesium sulfate)
Avinza® may be confused with Evista®, Invanz®
Roxanol™ may be confused with OxyFast®, Roxicet™

Use care when prescribing and/or administering morphine solutions. These products are available in different concentrations. Always prescribe dosage in mg; **not** by volume (mL).

Pregnancy Risk Factor C/D (prolonged use or high doses at term)

Lactation Enters breast milk/use caution (AAP rates "compatible")

Use Relief of moderate to severe acute and chronic pain; relief of pain of myocardial infarction; relief of dyspnea of acute left ventricular failure and pulmonary edema; preanesthetic medication
DepoDur™: Epidural (lumbar) single-dose management of surgical pain
Infumorph®: Used in microinfusion devices for intraspinal administration in treatment of intractable chronic pain

Mechanism of Action/Effect Binds to opiate receptors in the CNS, causing inhibition of ascending pain pathways, altering the perception of and response to pain; produces generalized CNS depression

Contraindications Hypersensitivity to morphine sulfate or any component of the formulation; increased intracranial pressure; severe respiratory depression; acute or severe asthma; known or suspected paralytic ileus; sustained release products are not recommended with gastrointestinal obstruction or in acute/postoperative pain; pregnancy (prolonged use or high doses at term)

Warnings/Precautions An opioid-containing analgesic regimen should be tailored to each patient's needs and based upon the type of pain being treated (acute versus chronic), the route of administration, degree of tolerance for opioids (naive versus chronic user), age, weight, and medical condition. The optimal analgesic dose varies widely among patients. Doses should be titrated to pain relief/prevention. When used as an epidural injection, monitor for delayed sedation.

May cause respiratory depression; use with caution in patients (particularly elderly or debilitated) with impaired respiratory function or severe hepatic dysfunction and in patients with hypersensitivity reactions to other phenanthrene derivative opioid agonists (codeine, hydrocodone, hydromorphone, levorphanol, oxycodone, oxymorphone). Infants <3 months of age are more susceptible to respiratory depression, use with caution and generally in reduced doses in this age group. May cause hypotension in patients with acute myocardial infarction, volume depletion, or concurrent drug therapy which may exaggerate vasodilation. Tolerance or drug dependence may result from extended use. MS Contin® 200 mg tablets are for use only in opioid-tolerant patients requiring >400 mg/day. Infumorph® solutions are **for use in microinfusion devices only**; not for I.V., I.M., or SubQ administration.

Use caution in CNS depression, toxic psychosis, delirium tremens, or convulsive disorders. Sedation and psychomotor impairment are likely, and are additive with other CNS depressants or ethanol. Use caution in renal impairment, gastrointestinal motility disturbances, biliary tract disease (including acute pancreatitis), prostatic hyperplasia, urethral stricture, thyroid disorders (Addison's disease, myxedema, or hypothyroidism). Extended or sustained release dosage forms should not be crushed or chewed. Do not administer Avinza® with alcoholic beverages or ethanol-containing products, which may disrupt extended-release characteristic of product. Controlled-, extended-, or sustained-release products are not intended for "as needed (PRN)" use. Some preparations contain sulfites which may cause allergic reactions.

Elderly and/or debilitated may be particularly susceptible to the CNS depressant and constipating effects of narcotics. May mask diagnosis or clinical course in patients with acute abdominal conditions.

Drug Interactions
Cytochrome P450 Effect: Substrate of CYP2D6 (minor)
Decreased Effect: The therapeutic efficacy of pegvisomant may be decreased by concomitant opiates, possibly requiring dosage adjustment of pegvisomant. Rifamycin derivatives may decrease levels or effects of morphine.
Increased Effect/Toxicity: Antipsychotic agents may increase the hypotensive effects of morphine. Use of selective serotonin reuptake inhibitors (SSRIs) or meperidine may lead to additive serotonergic effects with concomitant morphine, possibly precipitating serotonin syndrome. CNS depressants and tricyclic antidepressants may potentiate the effects of morphine. Concurrent use of MAO inhibitors and meperidine has been associated with significant adverse effects; use caution with morphine. Some manufacturers recommend avoiding use within 14 days of MAO inhibitors.

Nutritional/Ethanol Interactions
Ethanol: Avoid ethanol (may increase CNS depression).
Avinza®: Alcoholic beverages or ethanol-containing products may disrupt extended-release formulation resulting in rapid release of entire morphine dose.
Food: Administration of oral morphine solution with food may increase bioavailability (ie, a report of 34% increase in morphine AUC when morphine oral solution followed a high-fat meal). The bioavailability of
(Continued)

Morphine Sulfate *(Continued)*

Oramorph SR® or Kadian® does not appear to be affected by food.

Herb/Nutraceutical: Avoid valerian, St John's wort, kava kava, gotu kola (may increase CNS depression).

Lab Interactions

Some quinolones may produce a false-positive urine screening result for opiates using commercially-available immunoassay kits. This has been demonstrated most consistently for levofloxacin and ofloxacin, but other quinolones have shown cross-reactivity in certain assay kits. Confirmation of positive opiate screens by more specific methods should be considered.

Adverse Reactions Note: Individual patient differences are unpredictable, and percentage may differ in acute pain (surgical) treatment.

Frequency not defined: Flushing, CNS depression, sedation, antidiuretic hormone release, physical and psychological dependence, diaphoresis

>10%:

Cardiovascular: Palpitations, hypotension, bradycardia

Central nervous system: Drowsiness (48%, tolerance usually develops to drowsiness with regular dosing for 1-2 weeks); dizziness (20%), confusion, headache (following epidural or intrathecal use)

Dermatologic: Pruritus (may be secondary to histamine release)

Note: Pruritus may be dose-related, but not confined to the site of administration.

Gastrointestinal: Nausea (28%, tolerance usually develops to nausea and vomiting with chronic use); constipation (40%, tolerance develops very slowly if at all); xerostomia (78%)

Genitourinary: Urinary retention (16%; may be prolonged, up to 20 hours, following epidural or intrathecal use)

Local: Pain at injection site

Neuromuscular & skeletal: Weakness

Miscellaneous: Histamine release

1% to 10%:

Cardiovascular: Atrial fibrillation (<3%), chest pain (<3%), edema (<3%), syncope (<3%), tachycardia (<3%)

Central nervous system: Amnesia, anxiety, apathy, ataxia, chills, depression, euphoria, false feeling of well being, fever, headache, hypoesthesia, insomnia, lethargy, malaise, restlessness, seizure, vertigo

Endocrine & metabolic: Gynecomastia (<3%), hyponatremia (<3%)

Gastrointestinal: Anorexia, biliary colic, dyspepsia, dysphagia, GERD, GI irritation, paralytic ileus, vomiting (9%)

Genitourinary: Decreased urination

Hematologic: Anemia (<3%), leukopenia (<3%), thrombocytopenia (<3%)

Neuromuscular & skeletal: Arthralgia, back pain, bone pain, paresthesia, trembling

Ocular: Vision problems

Respiratory: Asthma, atelectasis, dyspnea, hiccups, hypoxia, noncardiogenic pulmonary edema, respiratory depression, rhinitis

Miscellaneous: Diaphoresis, flu-like syndrome, withdrawal syndrome

Overdosage/Toxicology Symptoms of overdose include respiratory depression, miosis, hypotension, bradycardia, apnea, and pulmonary edema. Treatment is symptomatic. Naloxone, 2 mg I.V. with repeat administration as necessary up to a total dose of 10 mg, can be used to reverse opiate effects.

Pharmacodynamics/Kinetics

Onset of Action: Oral (immediate release): ~30 minutes; I.V.: 5-10 minutes

Duration of Action: Pain relief: Immediate release formulations: 4 hours; extended release epidural injection (DepoDur™): >48 hours

Time to Peak: Kadian®: ~10 hours

Protein Binding: 30% to 35%

Half-Life Elimination: Adults: 2-4 hours (immediate release forms)

Metabolism: Hepatic via conjugation with glucuronic acid to morphine-3-glucuronide (inactive), morphine-6-glucuronide (active), and in lesser amounts, morphine-3-6-diglucuronide; other minor metabolites include normorphine (active) and the 3-ethereal sulfate

Excretion: Urine (primarily as morphine-3-glucuronide, ~2% to 12% excreted unchanged); feces (~7% to 10%). It has been suggested that accumulation of morphine-6-glucuronide might cause toxicity with renal insufficiency. All of the metabolites (ie, morphine-3-glucuronide, morphine-6-glucuronide, and normorphine) have been suggested as possible causes of neurotoxicity (eg, myoclonus).

Available Dosage Forms

[DSC] = Discontinued product

Capsule, extended release (Avinza®): 30 mg, 60 mg, 90 mg, 120 mg

Capsule, sustained release (Kadian®): 20 mg, 30 mg, 50 mg, 60 mg, 100 mg

Infusion [premixed in D₅W]: 1 mg/mL (100 mL, 250 mL)

Injection, extended release liposomal suspension [lumbar epidural injection, preservative free] (DepoDur™): 10 mg/mL (1 mL, 1.5 mL, 2 mL)

Injection, solution: 2 mg/mL (1 mL); 4 mg/mL (1 mL); 5 mg/mL (1 mL); 8 mg/mL (1 mL); 10 mg/mL (1 mL, 10 mL); 15 mg/mL (1 mL, 20 mL); 25 mg/mL (4 mL, 10 mL, 20 mL, 40 mL, 50 mL, 100 mL, 250 mL); 50 mg/mL (20 mL, 40 mL) [some preparations contain sodium metabisulfite]

Injection, solution [epidural, intrathecal, or I.V. infusion; preservative free]:

Astramorph/PF™: 0.5 mg/mL (2 mL, 10 mL); 1 mg/mL (2 mL, 10 mL)

Duramorph®: 0.5 mg/mL (10 mL); 1 mg/mL (10 mL)

Injection, solution [epidural or intrathecal infusion via microinfusion device; preservative free] (Infumorph®): 10 mg/mL (20 mL); 25 mg/mL (20 mL)

Injection, solution [I.V. infusion via PCA pump]: 0.5 mg/mL (30 mL); 1 mg/mL (30 mL, 50 mL); 2 mg/mL (30 mL); 5 mg/mL (30 mL, 50 mL)

Injection, solution [preservative free]: 0.5 mg/mL (10 mL); 1 mg/mL (10 mL); 25 mg/mL (4 mL, 10 mL, 20 mL)

Solution, oral: 10 mg/5 mL (5 mL, 10 mL, 100 mL, 500 mL); 20 mg/5 mL (100 mL, 500 mL); 20 mg/mL (30 mL, 120 mL, 240 mL)

Roxanol™: 20 mg/mL (30 mL, 120 mL)

Roxanol 100™: 100 mg/5 mL (240 mL) [with calibrated spoon]

Roxanol™-T: 20 mg/mL (30 mL, 120 mL) [tinted, flavored] [DSC]

Suppository, rectal (RMS®): 5 mg (12s), 10 mg (12s), 20 mg (12s), 30 mg (12s)

Tablet: 15 mg, 30 mg

Tablet, controlled release (MS Contin®): 15 mg, 30 mg, 60 mg, 100 mg, 200 mg

Tablet, extended release: 15 mg, 30 mg, 60 mg, 100 mg, 200 mg

Tablet, sustained release (Oramorph SR®): 15 mg, 30 mg, 60 mg, 100 mg

Dosing

Adults: Note: These are guidelines and do not represent the doses that may be required in all patients. Doses should be titrated to pain relief/prevention.

Acute pain (moderate-to-severe):

Oral: Prompt release formulations: Opiate-naive: Initial: 10 mg every 3 to 4 hours as needed; patients with prior opiate exposure may require higher initial doses: usual dosage range: 10-30 mg every 3-4 hours as needed

I.M., SubQ: Note: Repeated SubQ administration causes local tissue irritation, pain, and induration.
Initial: Opiate-naive: 5-10 mg every 3-4 hours as needed; patients with prior opiate exposure may require higher initial doses; usual dosage range: 5-20 mg every 3-4 hours as needed

Rectal: 10-20 mg every 3-4 hours

I.V.: Initial: Opiate-naive: 2.5-5 mg every 3 to 4 hours; patients with prior opiate exposure may require higher initial doses. **Note:** Repeated doses (up to every 5 minutes if needed) in small increments (eg, 1-4 mg) may be preferred to larger and less frequent doses.

I.V., SubQ continuous infusion: 0.8-10 mg/hour; usual range: Up to 80 mg/hour
Mechanically-ventilated patients (based on 70 kg patient): 0.7-10 mg every 1-2 hours as needed; infusion: 5-35 mg/hour

Patient-controlled analgesia (PCA): (Opiate-naive: Consider lower end of dosing range):
Usual concentration: 1 mg/mL
Demand dose: Usual: 1 mg; range: 0.5-2.5 mg
Lockout interval: 5-10 minutes

Intrathecal (I.T.): **Note:** Administer with extreme caution and in reduced dosage to geriatric or debilitated patients.
Opioid-naive: 0.2-0.25 mg/dose (may provide adequate relief for 24 hours); repeat doses are **not** recommended.

Epidural: **Note:** Administer with extreme caution and in reduced dosage to geriatric or debilitated patients. Vigilant monitoring is particularly important in these patients.
Pain management:
Single-dose (Duramorph®): Initial: 3-5 mg
Infusion:
Bolus dose: 1-6 mg
Infusion rate: 0.1-0.2 mg/hour
Maximum dose: 10 mg/24 hours

Surgical anesthesia: Epidural: Single-dose (extended release, Depo-Dur™): Lumbar epidural only; not recommended in patients <18 years of age:
Cesarean section: 10 mg
Lower abdominal/pelvic surgery: 10-15 mg
Major orthopedic surgery of lower extremity: 15 mg
For Depo-Dur™: To minimize the pharmacokinetic interaction resulting in higher peak serum concentrations of morphine, administer the test dose of the local anesthetic at least 15 minutes prior to Depo-Dur™ administration. Use of Depo-Dur™ with epidural local anesthetics has not been studied.
Note: Some patients may benefit from a 20 mg dose, however, the incidence of adverse effects may be increased.

Chronic pain: Note: Patients taking opioids chronically may become tolerant and require doses higher than the usual dosage range to maintain the desired effect. Tolerance can be managed by appropriate dose titration. There is no optimal or maximal dose for morphine in chronic pain. The appropriate dose is one that relieves pain throughout its dosing interval without causing unmanageable side effects.

Oral: Controlled-, extended-, or sustained-release formulations: A patient's morphine requirement should be established using prompt-release formulations. Conversion to long-acting products may be considered when chronic, continuous treatment is required. Higher dosages should be reserved for use only in opioid-tolerant patients.

Capsules, extended release (Avinza™): Daily dose administered once daily (for best results, administer at same time each day)

Capsules, sustained release (Kadian®): Daily dose administered once daily or in 2 divided doses daily (every 12 hours)

Tablets, controlled release (MS Contin®), sustained release (Oramorph SR®), or extended release: Daily dose divided and administered every 8 or every 12 hours

Elderly: Refer to adult dosing. Use with caution; may require reduced dosage in the elderly and debilitated patients.

Pediatrics: Note: These are guidelines and do not represent the doses that may be required in all patients. Doses should be titrated to pain relief/prevention.
Acute pain (moderate-to-severe): Children >6 months and <50 kg:
Oral (prompt release): 0.15-0.3 mg/kg every 3-4 hours as needed
I.M.: 0.1 mg/kg every 3-4 hours as needed
I.V.: 0.05-0.1 mg/kg every 3-4 hours as needed
I.V. infusion: Range: 10-30 mcg/kg/hour
Sedation/analgesia for procedures: Adolescents >12 years: I.V.: 3-4 mg and repeat in 5 minutes if necessary

Renal Impairment:
Cl$_{cr}$ 10-50 mL/minute: Administer 75% of normal dose.
Cl$_{cr}$ <10 mL/minute: Administer 50% of normal dose.

Hepatic Impairment: Unchanged in mild liver disease; substantial extrahepatic metabolism may occur. Excessive sedation may occur in cirrhosis.

Administration

Oral: Do not crush controlled release drug product, swallow whole. Kadian® and Avinza™ can be opened and sprinkled on applesauce; do not crush or chew the beads. Contents of Kadian® capsules may be opened and sprinkled over 10 mL water and flushed through prewetted 16F gastrostomy tube; do not administer Kadian® through nasogastric tube. Administration of oral morphine solution with food may increase bioavailability (not observed with Oramorph SR®).

I.V.: When giving morphine I.V. push, it is best to first dilute in 4-5 mL of sterile water, and then to administer slowly (eg, 15 mg over 3-5 minutes).

I.V. Detail: pH: 2.5-6.0

Other: Use preservative-free solutions for intrathecal or epidural use.
Epidural, extended release liposomal suspension (DepoDur™): May be administered undiluted or diluted up to 5 mL total volume in preservative-free NS. Do not use an in-line filter during administration. Not for I.V. or I.M. administration.
Resedation may occur following epidural administration; this may be delayed ≥48 hours in patients receiving extended-release (DepoDur™) injections.
Administration of an epidural test dose (lidocaine 1.5% and epinephrine 1:200,000) may affect the release of morphine from the liposomal preparation. Delaying the dose for an interval of at least 15 minutes following the test dose minimizes this pharmacokinetic interaction. Except for a test dose, other epidural local anesthetics should not be used before or after this product.

Stability

Reconstitution: Usual concentration for continuous I.V. infusion: 0.1-1 mg/mL in D$_5$W. DepoDur™ may be diluted in preservative-free NS to a volume of 5 mL.

Compatibility: Stable in dextran 6% in dextrose, dextran 6% in NS, D$_5$LR, D$_5$¼NS, D$_5$½NS, D$_5$NS, D$_5$W, D$_{10}$W, LR, ½NS, NS
Y-site administration: Incompatible with alatrofloxacin, amphotericin B cholesteryl sulfate complex, cefepime, doxorubicin liposome, minocycline, sargramostim

(Continued)

Morphine Sulfate *(Continued)*

Compatibility in syringe: Incompatible with meperidine, thiopental

Compatibility when admixed: Incompatible with aminophylline, amobarbital, chlorothiazide, floxacillin, fluorouracil, heparin, meperidine, phenobarbital, phenytoin, sodium bicarbonate, thiopental

DepoDur™: Do not mix with other medications.

Storage:

Capsule, sustained release (Kadian®): Store at controlled room temperature 15°C to 30°C (59°F to 86°F). Protect from light and moisture.

Suppositories: Store at controlled room temperature 25°C (77°F). Protect from light.

Injection: Store at controlled room temperature. Protect from light. Degradation depends on pH and presence of oxygen; relatively stable in pH ≤4; darkening of solutions indicate degradation.

DepoDur™: Store under refrigeration, 2°C to 8°C (36°F to 46°F). Do not freeze. May store at room temperature for up to 7 days. Once vial is opened, use within 4 hours.

Nursing Actions

Physical Assessment: Assess other medications patient may be taking for additive or adverse interactions. Monitor for effectiveness of pain relief and monitor for signs of adverse reactions or overdose. Monitor blood pressure, CNS and respiratory status, and degree of sedation at beginning of therapy and at regular intervals with long-term use. May cause physical and/or psychological dependence. For inpatients, implement safety measures (eg, side rails up, call light within reach, instructions to call for assistance). Assess knowledge/teach patient appropriate use (if self-administered), adverse reactions to report, and appropriate interventions to reduce side effects. Discontinue slowly after prolonged use.

Patient Education: If self-administered, use exactly as directed; do not increase dose or frequency. Do not crush or chew controlled release tablet or capsule. If using Avinza®, do not take with alcohol. May cause physical and/or psychological dependence. While using this medication, do not use alcohol and other prescription or OTC medications (especially sedatives, tranquilizers, antihistamines, or pain medications) without consulting prescriber. Maintain adequate hydration (2-3 L/day of fluids) unless instructed to restrict fluid intake. May cause hypotension, dizziness, drowsiness, impaired coordination, or blurred vision (use caution when driving, climbing stairs, or changing position - rising from sitting or lying to standing, or when engaging in tasks requiring alertness until response to drug is known); loss of appetite, nausea, or vomiting (frequent mouth care, small frequent meals, chewing gum, or sucking lozenges may help); or constipation (increased exercise, fluids, fruit, or fiber may help; if unresolved, consult prescriber about use of stool softeners and/or laxatives). Report chest pain, slow or rapid heartbeat, acute dizziness, or persistent headache; changes in mental status; swelling of extremities or unusual weight gain; changes in urinary elimination or pain on urination; acute headache; back or flank pain; muscle spasms; blurred vision; skin rash; or shortness of breath. **Pregnancy/breast-feeding precautions:** Inform prescriber if you are or intend to become pregnant. If you are breast-feeding, consult prescriber.

Dietary Considerations Morphine may cause GI upset; take with food if GI upset occurs. Be consistent when taking morphine with or without meals.

Geriatric Considerations The elderly may be particularly susceptible to the CNS depressant and constipating effects of narcotics. For chronic administration of narcotic analgesics, morphine is preferable in the elderly due to its pharmacokinetics and side effect profile as compared to meperidine and methadone.

Breast-Feeding Issues Morphine concentrates in breast milk, with a milk to plasma ratio of 2.5:1. Detectable serum levels of morphine can be found in infants following morphine administration to nursing mothers. Treatment of the mother with single doses of morphine is not expected to cause detrimental effects in nursing infants. Breast-feeding following chronic use or in neonates with hepatic or renal dysfunction may lead to higher levels of morphine in the infant and a risk of adverse effects. Some clinicians recommend administering morphine immediately after breast-feeding or 3-4 hours prior to the next feeding. Breast-feeding should be delayed for 48 hours after DepoDur™ administration.

Pregnancy Issues Morphine crosses the placenta. The frequency of congenital malformations has not been reported to be greater than expected in children from mothers treated with morphine during pregnancy. Reduced growth and behavioral abnormalities in offspring have been observed in animal studies. Neonates born to mothers receiving chronic opioids during pregnancy should be monitored for neonatal withdrawal syndrome.

DepoDur™ may be used in women undergoing cesarean section following clamping of the umbilical cord; not for use in vaginal labor and delivery.

Related Information

Compatibility of Drugs *on page 1370*
Compatibility of Drugs in Syringe *on page 1372*

Moxifloxacin *(moxs i FLOKS a sin)*

U.S. Brand Names Avelox®; Avelox® I.V.; Vigamox™

Synonyms Moxifloxacin Hydrochloride

Pharmacologic Category Antibiotic, Ophthalmic; Antibiotic, Quinolone

Medication Safety Issues

Sound-alike/look-alike issues:
Avelox® may be confused with Avonex®

Pregnancy Risk Factor C

Lactation Excretion in breast milk unknown/not recommended

Use Treatment of mild-to-moderate community-acquired pneumonia, including multidrug-resistant *Streptococcus pneumoniae* (MDRSP); acute bacterial exacerbation of chronic bronchitis; acute bacterial sinusitis; complicated and uncomplicated skin and skin structure infections; complicated intra-abdominal infections; bacterial conjunctivitis (ophthalmic formulation)

Unlabeled/Investigational Use *Legionella*

Mechanism of Action/Effect Moxifloxacin is a quinolone antibiotic with bactericidal activity against susceptible gram negative and gram positive microorganisms.

Contraindications Hypersensitivity to moxifloxacin, other quinolone antibiotics, or any component of the formulation

Warnings/Precautions Use with caution in patients with significant bradycardia or acute myocardial ischemia. Moxifloxacin causes a concentration-dependent QT prolongation. Do not exceed recommended dose or infusion rate. Avoid use with uncorrected hypokalemia, with other drugs that prolong the QT interval or induce bradycardia, or with class IA or III antiarrhythmic agents. Use with caution in individuals at risk of seizures (CNS disorders or concurrent therapy with medications which may lower seizure threshold). Discontinue in patients who experience significant CNS adverse effects (dizziness, hallucinations, suicidal ideation or actions). Not recommended in patients with moderate to severe hepatic insufficiency. Use with caution in diabetes; glucose regulation may be altered. Tendon inflammation and/or rupture have been reported with quinolone antibiotics. Risk may be increased with concurrent corticosteroids, particularly in the elderly. Discontinue at first signs or symptoms of tendon pain.

Severe hypersensitivity reactions, including anaphylaxis, have occurred with quinolone therapy. If an allergic reaction occurs (itching, urticaria, dyspnea or facial edema, loss of consciousness, tingling, cardiovascular collapse) discontinue drug immediately. May cause photosensitivity. Prolonged use may result in superinfection; pseudomembranous colitis may occur and should be considered in all patients who present with diarrhea. Quinolones may exacerbate myasthenia gravis, use with caution (rare, potentially life-threatening weakness of respiratory muscles may occur). Peripheral neuropathy may rarely occur. Safety and efficacy of systemically administered moxifloxacin (oral, intravenous) in patients <18 years of age have not been established.

Ophthalmic: Eye drops should not be injected subconjunctivally or introduced directly into the anterior chamber of the eye. Contact lenses should not be worn during therapy.

Drug Interactions

Decreased Effect: Concurrent administration of metal cations, including most antacids, oral electrolyte supplements, quinapril, sucralfate, some didanosine formulations (chewable/buffered tablets and pediatric powder for oral suspension), and other higly-buffered oral drugs, may decrease quinolone levels; separate doses.

Increased Effect/Toxicity: Moxifloxacin may increase the effects/toxicity of glyburide and warfarin. Concomitant use with corticosteroids may increase the risk of tendon rupture. Concomitant use with other QT_c-prolonging agents (eg, Class Ia and Class III antiarrhythmics, erythromycin, cisapride, antipsychotics, and cyclic antidepressants) may result in arrhythmias, such as torsade de pointes.

Nutritional/Ethanol Interactions Food: Absorption is not affected by administration with a high-fat meal or yogurt.

Lab Interactions Some quinolones may produce a false-positive urine screening result for opiates using commercially-available immunoassay kits. This has been demonstrated most consistently for levofloxacin and ofloxacin, but other quinolones have shown cross-reactivity in certain assay kits. Confirmation of positive opiate screens by more specific methods should be considered.

Adverse Reactions

Systemic:

3% to 10%: Gastrointestinal: Nausea (6%), diarrhea (5%)

0.1% to 3%:
Cardiovascular: Hypertension, palpitation, QT_c prolongation, tachycardia, vasodilation
Central nervous system: Anxiety, chills, dizziness, headache, insomnia, nervousness, pain, somnolence, tremor, vertigo
Dermatologic: Dry skin, pruritus, rash (maculopapular, purpuric, pustular)
Endocrine & metabolic: Serum chloride increased (≥2%), serum ionized calcium increased (≥2%), serum glucose decreased (≥2%)
Gastrointestinal: Abdominal pain, amylase increased, amylase decreased (≥2%), anorexia, constipation, dry mouth, dyspepsia, flatulence, glossitis, lactic dehydrogenase increased, stomatitis, taste perversion, vomiting
Genitourinary: Vaginal moniliasis, vaginitis
Hematologic: Eosinophilia, leukopenia, prothrombin time prolonged, increased INR, thrombocythemia
Increased serum levels of the following (≥2%): MCH, neutrophils, WBC
Decreased serum levels of the following (≥2%): Basophils, eosinophils, hemoglobin, RBC, neutrophils

Hepatic: Bilirubin decreased or increased (≥2%), GGTP increased, liver function test abnormal
Local: Injection site reaction
Neuromuscular & skeletal: Arthralgia, myalgia, weakness
Renal: Kidney function abnormal, serum albumin increased (≥2%)
Respiratory: Pharyngitis, pneumonia, rhinitis, sinusitis, pO_2 increased (≥2%)

Additional reactions with **ophthalmic** preparation: 1% to 6%: Conjunctivitis, dry eye, ocular discomfort, ocular hyperemia, ocular pain, ocular pruritus, subconjunctival hemorrhage, tearing, visual acuity decreased

Overdosage/Toxicology Potential symptoms of overdose may include CNS excitation, seizures, QT prolongation, and arrhythmias (including torsade de pointes). Patients should be monitored by continuous ECG in the event of an overdose. Management is supportive and symptomatic. Hemodialysis only removes ~9% of dose.

Pharmacodynamics/Kinetics
Protein Binding: 30% to 50%
Half-Life Elimination: Oral: 12 hours; I.V.: 15 hours
Metabolism: Hepatic (52% of dose) via glucuronide (14%) and sulfate (38%) conjugation
Excretion: Excretion: Approximately 45% of a dose is excreted in feces (25%) and urine (20%) as unchanged drug; Metabolites: Sulfate conjugates in feces, glucuronide conjugates in urine

Available Dosage Forms
Infusion [premixed in sodium chloride 0.8%] (Avelox® I.V.): 400 mg (250 mL)
Solution, ophthalmic (Vigamox™): 0.5% (3 mL)
Tablet:
Avelox®: 400 mg
Avelox® ABC Pack [unit-dose pack]: 400 mg (5s)

Dosing
Adults & Elderly:
Acute bacterial sinusitis: Oral, I.V.: 400 mg every 24 hours for 10 days
Bacterial conjunctivitis: Ophthalmic: Instill 1 drop into affected eye(s) 3 times/day for 7 days
Chronic bronchitis, acute bacterial exacerbation: Oral, I.V.: 400 mg every 24 hours for 5 days
Note: Avelox® ABC Pack™ (Avelox® Bronchitis Course) contains five tablets of 400 mg each.
Intra-abdominal infections, complicated: Oral, I.V.: 400 mg every 24 hours for 5-14 days (initiate with I.V.)
***Legionella* (unlabeled use):** Oral, I.V.: 400 mg every 24 hours for 10-21 days
Pneumonia, community-acquired (including MDRSP): Oral, I.V.: 400 mg every 24 hours for 7-14 days
Skin and skin structure infections: Oral, I.V.:
Complicated: 400 mg every 24 hours for 7-21 days
Uncomplicated: 400 mg every 24 hours for 7 days
Pediatrics: Bacterial conjunctivitis: Ophthalmic: Children ≥1 year: Refer to adult dosing.
Renal Impairment: No adjustment is necessary, including patients on hemodialysis or CAPD.
Hepatic Impairment: No dosage adjustment is required in mild to moderate hepatic insufficiency (Child-Pugh Classes A and B). Not recommended in patients with severe hepatic insufficiency.

Administration
I.V.: Infuse over 60 minutes; do not infuse by rapid or bolus intravenous infusion

Stability
Compatibility: Stable in NS, D_5W, $D_{10}W$, SWFI, LR
Do not add other medications to intravenous solution
Storage: Store at 15°C to 30°C (59°F to 86°F). Do not refrigerate infusion solution.

Laboratory Monitoring WBC
(Continued)

Moxifloxacin (Continued)

Nursing Actions

Physical Assessment: Results of culture and sensitivity tests and patient's allergy history should be assessed before initiating therapy. Assess potential for interactions with other pharmacological agents or herbal products patient is taking that may increase risk of tendon rupture or arrhythmias. I.V.: See Administration for infusion specifics. If allergic reaction occurs (itching, urticaria, dyspnea or facial edema, loss of consciousness, tingling, cardiovascular collapse) infusion should be discontinued immediately and prescriber notified. Monitor laboratory tests, therapeutic effectiveness (resolution of infection), and adverse effects. Teach patient proper use, possible side effects/appropriate interventions, and adverse symptoms to report (eg, allergic reaction, tendon rupture).

Patient Education: Inform prescriber of all prescriptions, OTC medications, or herbal products you are taking, and any allergies you have. Do not take any new medication during therapy unless approved by prescriber. **Pregnancy/breast-feeding precautions:** Inform prescriber if you are or intend to become pregnant. Breast-feeding is not recommended.

I.V.: Report any redness, swelling, or pain at infusion site; any swelling of mouth, lips, tongue, or throat; chest pain or tightness; respiratory difficulty; back pain; itching; skin rash; tingling; tendon pain; dizziness; abnormal thinking; or anxiety.

Oral: Take exactly as directed with or without food. Do not take antacids 4 hours before or 8 hours after taking this medication. Do not miss a dose (take a missed dose as soon as possible, unless it is almost time for your next dose). Take entire prescription even if feeling better. Maintain adequate hydration (2-3 L/day of fluids) unless instructed to restrict fluid intake. May cause nausea, vomiting, taste perversion (small, frequent meals, good mouth care, chewing gum, or sucking hard candy may help); headache, dizziness, insomnia, anxiety (use caution when driving or engaging in tasks requiring alertness until response to drug is known). Report immediately any swelling of mouth, lips, tongue or throat; chest pain or tightness; respiratory difficulty; back pain; itching; skin rash; tingling; tendon pain; pain or numbness (loss of sensation) in extremities; confusion, dizziness, abnormal thinking, or anxiety; or insomnia. Report changes in voiding pattern; vaginal itching, burning, or discharge; vision changes or hearing; abnormal bruising or bleeding or blood in urine; or other adverse reactions.

Ophthalmic: Wash hands before instilling solution. Sit or lie down to instill. Open eye, look at ceiling, and instill prescribed amount of solution as directed. Do not touch tip of applicator or let tip of applicator touch eye. Do not wear contact lenses during therapy. Temporary stinging or blurred vision, or dry eyes may occur. Report persistent pain, burning, excessive tearing, decreased visual acuity, swelling, itching, or worsening of condition.

Dietary Considerations May be taken with or without food. Take 4 hours before or 8 hours after multiple vitamins, antacids, or other products containing magnesium, aluminum, iron, or zinc.

Breast-Feeding Issues Other quinolones are known to be excreted in breast milk. The manufacturer recommends to discontinue nursing or to discontinue moxifloxacin.

Pregnancy Issues Reports of arthropathy (observed in immature animals and reported rarely in humans) have limited the use of fluoroquinolones during pregnancy. Teratogenic effects were not observed with moxifloxacin in animal studies; however, delayed skeletal development and smaller fetuses were observed in some species. There are no adequate and well-controlled studies in pregnant women. Based on limited data, quinolones are not expected to be a major human teratogen. Although quinolone antibiotics should not be used as first-line agents during pregnancy, when considering treatment for life-threatening infection and/or prolonged duration of therapy, the potential risk to the fetus must be balanced against the severity of the potential illness.

Mupirocin (myoo PEER oh sin)

U.S. Brand Names Bactroban®; Bactroban® Nasal; Centany™

Synonyms Mupirocin Calcium; Pseudomonic Acid A

Pharmacologic Category Antibiotic, Topical

Medication Safety Issues

Sound-alike/look-alike issues:
Bactroban® may be confused with bacitracin, baclofen

Pregnancy Risk Factor B

Lactation Excretion in breast milk unknown/use caution

Use

Intranasal: Eradication of nasal colonization with MRSA in adult patients and healthcare workers

Topical treatment of impetigo due to *Staphylococcus aureus*, beta-hemolytic *Streptococcus*, and *S. pyogenes*

Unlabeled/Investigational Use Intranasal: Surgical prophylaxis to prevent wound infections

Mechanism of Action/Effect Binds to bacterial isoleucyl transfer-RNA synthetase resulting in the inhibition of protein and RNA synthesis

Contraindications Hypersensitivity to mupirocin, polyethylene glycol, or any component of the formulation

Warnings/Precautions Potentially toxic amounts of polyethylene glycol contained in the vehicle may be absorbed percutaneously in patients with extensive burns or open wounds. Prolonged use may result in over growth of nonsusceptible organisms. For external use only. Not for treatment of pressure sores.

Adverse Reactions Frequency not defined.

Central nervous system: Dizziness, headache

Dermatologic: Pruritus, rash, erythema, dry skin, cellulitis, dermatitis

Gastrointestinal: Nausea, taste perversion

Local: Burning, stinging, tenderness, edema, pain

Respiratory: Rhinitis, upper respiratory tract infection, pharyngitis, cough

Pharmacodynamics/Kinetics

Protein Binding: 95%

Half-Life Elimination: 17-36 minutes

Metabolism: Skin: 3% to monic acid

Excretion: Urine

Available Dosage Forms

Cream, topical, as calcium (Bactroban®): 2% (15 g, 30 g) [contains benzyl alcohol]

Ointment, intranasal, topical, as calcium (Bactroban® Nasal): 2% (1 g) [single-use tube]

Ointment, topical: 2% (0.9 g, 22 g)
Bactroban®: 2% (22 g)
Centany™: 2% (15 g, 30 g)

Dosing

Adults & Elderly:

Impetigo: Topical: Apply small amount to affected area 2-5 times/day for 5-14 days.

Elimination of MRSA colonization: Nasal: Approximately one-half of the ointment from the single-use tube should be applied into one nostril and the other half into the other nostril twice daily for 5 days.

Pediatrics:

Topical: Children: Refer to adult dosing.

Nasal: ≥12 years: Refer to adult dosing.

Administration
Topical: For external use only.

Stability
Compatibility: Do not mix with Aquaphor®, coal tar solution, or salicylic acid.

Nursing Actions
Physical Assessment: Monitor effectiveness of therapy and symptoms of infection. Assess knowledge/teach patient appropriate application and use and adverse symptoms to report.

Patient Education: For external use only. Wash hands before and after application. Apply thin film over affected areas exactly as directed. Avoid getting in eyes. Report rash, persistent burning, stinging, swelling, itching, or pain. Contact prescriber if no improvement is seen in 3-5 days. **Breast-feeding precaution:** Consult prescriber if breast-feeding.

Additional Information Not for treatment of pressure sores; contains polyethylene glycol vehicle.

Muromonab-CD3
(myoo roe MOE nab see dee three)

U.S. Brand Names Orthoclone OKT® 3
Synonyms Monoclonal Antibody; OKT3
Pharmacologic Category Immunosuppressant Agent
Pregnancy Risk Factor C
Lactation Excretion in breast milk unknown/contraindicated
Use Treatment of acute allograft rejection in renal transplant patients; treatment of acute hepatic, kidney, and pancreas rejection episodes resistant to conventional treatment. Acute graft-versus-host disease following bone marrow transplantation resistant to conventional treatment.
Mechanism of Action/Effect Reverses graft rejection by binding to T cells and interfering with their function
Contraindications Hypersensitivity to OKT3 or any murine product; patients in fluid overload or those with >3% weight gain within 1 week prior to start of OKT3; mouse antibody titers >1:1000
Warnings/Precautions It is imperative, especially prior to the first few doses, that there be no clinical evidence

Suggested Prevention/Treatment of Muromonab-CD3 First-Dose Effects

Adverse Reaction	Effective Prevention or Palliation	Supportive Treatment
Severe pulmonary edema	Clear chest x-ray within 24 hours preinjection; weight restriction to ≤3% gain over 7 days preinjection	Prompt intubation and oxygenation; 24 hours close observation
Fever, chills	15 mg/kg methylprednisolone sodium succinate 1 hour preinjection; fever reduction to <37.8°C (100°F) 1 hour preinjection; acetaminophen (1 g orally) and diphenhydramine (50 mg orally) 1 hour preinjection	Cooling blanket Acetaminophen prn
Respiratory effects	100 mg hydrocortisone sodium succinate 30 minutes postinjection	Additional 100 mg hydrocortisone sodium succinate prn for wheezing; if respiratory distress, give epinephrine 1:1000 (0.3 mL SubQ)

of volume overload, uncontrolled hypertension, or uncompensated heart failure, including a clear chest x-ray and weight restriction of ≤3% above the patient's minimum weight during the week prior to injection.

May result in an increased susceptibility to infection; dosage of concomitant immunosuppressants should be reduced during OKT3 therapy; cyclosporine should be decreased to 50% usual maintenance dose and maintenance therapy resumed about 4 days before stopping OKT3.

Severe pulmonary edema has occurred in patients with fluid overload.

First dose effect (flu-like symptoms, anaphylactic-type reaction): may occur within 30 minutes to 6 hours up to 24 hours after the first dose and may be minimized by using the recommended regimens. See table.

Cardiopulmonary resuscitation may be needed. If the patient's temperature is >37.8°C, reduce before administering OKT3

Drug Interactions
Decreased Effect: Decreased effect with immunosuppressive drugs.

Increased Effect/Toxicity: Recommend decreasing dose of prednisone to 0.5 mg/kg, azathioprine to 0.5 mg/kg (approximate 50% decrease in dose), and discontinuing cyclosporine while patient is receiving OKT3.

Adverse Reactions Note: Signs and symptoms of Cytokine Release Syndrome (characterized by pyrexia, chills, dyspnea, nausea, vomiting, chest pain, diarrhea, tremor, wheezing, headache, tachycardia, rigor, hypertension, pulmonary edema and/or other cardiorespiratory manifestations) occurs in a significant proportion of patients following the first couple of doses of muromonab-CD3. See Warnings/Precautions. Additionally, some patients have experienced immediate hypersensitivity reactions to muromonab-CD3 (characterized by cardiovascular collapse, cardiorespiratory arrest, loss of consciousness, hypotension/shock, tachycardia, tingling, angioedema (including laryngeal, pharyngeal, or facial edema), airway obstruction, bronchospasm, dyspnea, urticaria, and/or pruritus) upon initial exposure and re-exposure.

>10%:
   Cardiovascular: Tachycardia (26%), hypotension (25%), hypertension (19%), edema (12%)
   Central nervous system: Pyrexia (77%), chills (43%), headache (28%)
   Dermatologic: Rash (14%; erythematous 2%)
   Gastrointestinal: Diarrhea (37%), nausea (32%), vomiting (25%)
   Respiratory: Dyspnea (16%)
1% to 10%:
   Cardiovascular: Chest pain (9%), vasodilation (7%), arrhythmia (4%), bradycardia (4%), vascular occlusion (2%)
   Central nervous system: Fatigue (9%), confusion (6%), dizziness (6%), lethargy (6%), pain trunk (6%), malaise (5%), nervousness (5%), depression (3%), somnolence (2%), meningitis (1%), seizures (1%)
   Dermatologic: Pruritus (7%)
   Gastrointestinal: Gastrointestinal pain (7%), abdominal pain (6%), anorexia (4%)
   Hematologic: Leukopenia (7%), anemia (2%), thrombocytopenia (2%), leukocytosis (1%)
   Neuromuscular & skeletal: Weakness (10%), arthralgia (7%), myalgia (1%), tremor (14%)
   Ocular: Photophobia (1%)
   Otic: Tinnitus (1%)
   Renal: Renal dysfunction (3%)
   Respiratory: Abnormal chest sound (10%), hyperventilation (7%), wheezing (6%), respiratory congestion (4%), pulmonary edema (2%), hypoxia (1%), pneumonia (1%)
(Continued)

Muromonab-CD3 *(Continued)*

Miscellaneous: Diaphoresis (7%), infections (various)

Pharmacodynamics/Kinetics

Duration of Action: 7 days after discontinuation

Time to Peak: Steady-state: Trough: 3-14 days

Available Dosage Forms Injection, solution: 1 mg/mL (5 mL) [contains sodium 43 mg/5 mL]

Dosing

Adults & Elderly: Treatment of acute allograft rejection or acute graft-versus-host disease: I.V. (refer to individual protocols): 5 mg/day once daily for 10-14 days

Pediatrics: Refer to individual protocols.

Treatment of acute allograft rejection or acute graft-versus-host disease: I.V.

Children <30 kg: 2.5 mg/day once daily for 7-14 days

Children >30 kg: 5 mg/day once daily for 7-14 days

or

Children <12 years: 0.1 mg/kg/day once daily for 10-14 days

Children ≥12 years: Refer to adult dosing.

Renal Impairment: Removal by dialysis: Molecular size of OKT3 is 150,000 daltons. Not dialyzed by most standard dialyzers; however, may be dialyzed by high flux dialysis. OKT3 will be removed by plasmapheresis. Administer following dialysis treatments.

Administration

I.V.: Not for I.M. administration. Give I.V. push over <1 minute at a final concentration of 1 mg/mL. Methylprednisolone sodium succinate 1 mg/kg I.V. given prior to first muromonab-CD3 administration, and I.V. hydrocortisone sodium succinate 50-100 mg, given 30 minutes after administration are strongly recommended to decrease the incidence of reactions to the first dose.

I.V. Detail: Filter each dose through a low protein-binding 0.22 micron filter (Millex GV) before administration. Patient temperature should not exceed 37.8°C (100°F) at time of administration.

Stability

Storage: Refrigerate; do not shake or freeze. Stable in Becton Dickinson syringe for 16 hours at room temperature or refrigeration.

Laboratory Monitoring Chest x-ray, CBC with differential, immunologic monitoring of T cells, serum levels of OKT3

Nursing Actions

Physical Assessment: Monitor pretreatment laboratory results prior to beginning therapy. Monitor closely for acute adverse pulmonary and cardiac effects, and anaphylactic-type effects during and for 24 hours following first infusion. Monitor vital signs, cardiac status, and respiratory status on a regular basis. Monitor/instruct patient on appropriate interventions to reduce side effects, to monitor for signs of opportunistic infection (eg, persistent fever, malaise, sore throat, unusual bleeding or bruising), and reactions to report.

Patient Education: There may be a severe reaction to the first infusion of this medication. You may experience high fever, chills, respiratory difficulty, or congestion. You will be closely monitored and comfort measures provided. Effects are substantially reduced with subsequent infusions. During the period of therapy and for some time after the regimen of infusions you will be susceptible to infection. People may wear masks and gloves while caring for you to protect you as much as possible from infection (avoid crowds and exposure to infection). You may experience dizziness, faintness, or trembling (use caution until response to medication is known); nausea or vomiting (small frequent meals, frequent mouth care); or sensitivity to direct sunlight (wear dark glasses, and protective clothing, use sunscreen, or avoid exposure to direct sunlight). Report chest pain or tightness; symptoms of respiratory infection, wheezing, or respiratory difficulty; vision change; or muscular trembling. **Pregnancy/breast-feeding precautions:** Inform prescriber if you are or intend to become pregnant. Do not breast-feed.

Dietary Considerations Injection solution contains sodium 43 mg/5 mL.

Mycophenolate *(mye koe FEN oh late)*

U.S. Brand Names CellCept®; Myfortic®

Synonyms MMF; MPA; Mycophenolate Mofetil; Mycophenolate Sodium; Mycophenolic Acid

Pharmacologic Category Immunosuppressant Agent

Pregnancy Risk Factor C (manufacturer)

Lactation Excretion in breast milk unknown/not recommended

Use Prophylaxis of organ rejection concomitantly with cyclosporine and corticosteroids in patients receiving allogenic renal (CellCept®, Myfortic®), cardiac (CellCept®), or hepatic (CellCept®) transplants

Unlabeled/Investigational Use Treatment of rejection in liver transplant patients unable to tolerate tacrolimus or cyclosporine due to neurotoxicity; mild rejection in heart transplant patients; treatment of moderate-severe psoriasis; treatment of proliferative lupus nephritis; treatment of myasthenia gravis

Mechanism of Action/Effect Inhibition of purine synthesis of human lymphocytes and proliferation of human lymphocytes

Contraindications Hypersensitivity to mycophenolate mofetil, mycophenolic acid, mycophenolate sodium, or any component of the formulation; intravenous formulation is contraindicated in patients who are allergic to polysorbate 80

Warnings/Precautions Hazardous agent — use appropriate precautions for handling and disposal. Risk for infection and development of lymphoproliferative disorders (particularly of the skin) is increased. Patients should be monitored appropriately, instructed to limit exposure to sunlight/UV light, and given supportive treatment should these conditions occur. Severe neutropenia may occur, requiring interruption of treatment (risk greater from day 31-180 post-transplant). Use caution with active peptic ulcer disease; may be associated with GI bleeding and/or perforation. Use caution in renal impairment as toxicity may be increased; may require dosage adjustment in severe impairment. Patients may be at increased risk of infection.

Mycophenolate mofetil is a potential teratogen; tablets should not be crushed, and capsules should not be opened or crushed. Avoid inhalation or direct contact with skin or mucous membranes of the powder contained in the capsules and the powder for oral suspension. Caution should be exercised in the handling and preparation of solutions of intravenous mycophenolate. Avoid skin contact with the intravenous solution and reconstituted suspension. If such contact occurs, wash thoroughly with soap and water, rinse eyes with plain water.

Theoretically, use should be avoided in patients with the rare hereditary deficiency of hypoxanthine-guanine phosphoribosyltransferase (such as Lesch-Nyhan or Kelley-Seegmiller syndrome). Intravenous solutions should be given over at least 2 hours; **never** administer intravenous solution by rapid or bolus injection.

Note: CellCept® and Myfortic® dosage forms should not be used interchangeably due to differences in absorption.

Drug Interactions

Decreased Effect: Antacids decrease serum levels (C_{max} and AUC); **do not administer together**. Cholestyramine resin decreases serum levels; **do not administer together**. Avoid use of live vaccines; vaccinations may be less effective. Influenza vaccine may be of value. During concurrent use of oral contraceptives, progesterone levels are not significantly affected, however, effect on estrogen component varies; an additional form of contraception should be used.

Increased Effect/Toxicity: Acyclovir, valacyclovir, ganciclovir, and valganciclovir levels may increase due to competition for tubular secretion of these drugs. Probenecid may increase mycophenolate levels due to inhibition of tubular secretion. High doses of salicylates may increase free fraction of mycophenolic acid. Azathioprine's bone marrow suppression may be potentiated; do not administer together.

Nutritional/Ethanol Interactions

Food: Decreases C_{max} of MPA by 40% following CellCept® administration and 33% following Myfortic® use; the extent of absorption is not changed

Herb/Nutraceutical: Avoid cat's claw, echinacea (have immunostimulant properties)

Adverse Reactions As reported in adults following oral dosing of CellCept® alone in renal, cardiac, and hepatic allograft rejection studies. In general, lower doses used in renal rejection patients had less adverse effects than higher doses. Rates of adverse effects were similar for each indication, except for those unique to the specific organ involved. The type of adverse effects observed in pediatric patients was similar to those seen in adults; abdominal pain, anemia, diarrhea, fever, hypertension, infection, pharyngitis, respiratory tract infection, sepsis, and vomiting were seen in higher proportion; lymphoproliferative disorder was the only type of malignancy observed. Percentages of adverse reactions were similar in studies comparing CellCept® to Myfortic® in patients following renal transplant.

>20%:

Cardiovascular: Hypertension (28% to 77%), hypotension (up to 33%), peripheral edema (27% to 64%), edema (27% to 28%), tachycardia (20% to 22%)

Central nervous system: Pain (31% to 76%), headache (16% to 54%), insomnia (41% to 52%), fever (21% to 52%), dizziness (up to 29%), anxiety (28%)

Dermatologic: Rash (up to 22%)

Endocrine & metabolic: Hyperglycemia (44% to 47%), hypercholesterolemia (41%), hypokalemia (32% to 37%), hypocalcemia (up to 30%), hypomagnesemia (up to 39%), hyperkalemia (up to 22%)

Gastrointestinal: Abdominal pain (25% to 62%), nausea (20% to 54%), diarrhea (31% to 52%), constipation (18% to 41%), vomiting (33% to 34%), anorexia (up to 25%), dyspepsia (22%)

Genitourinary: Urinary tract infection (37%)

Hematologic: Leukopenia (23% to 46%), leukocytosis (22% to 40%), hypochromic anemia (26% to 43%), thrombocytopenia (24% to 36%)

Hepatic: Liver function tests abnormal (up to 25%), ascites (24%)

Neuromuscular & skeletal: Back pain (35% to 47%), weakness (35% to 43%), tremor (24% to 34%), paresthesia (21%)

Renal: BUN increased (up to 35%), creatinine increased (up to 39%)

Respiratory: Dyspnea (31% to 37%), respiratory tract infection (22% to 37%), cough (31%), lung disorder (22% to 30%)

Miscellaneous: Infection (18% to 27%), *Candida* (11% to 22%), herpes simplex (10% to 21%)

3% to <20%:

Cardiovascular: Angina, arrhythmia, arterial thrombosis, atrial fibrillation, atrial flutter, bradycardia, cardiac arrest, cardiac failure, CHF, extrasystole, facial edema, hypervolemia, pallor, palpitation, pericardial effusion, peripheral vascular disorder, postural hypotension, supraventricular extrasystoles, supraventricular tachycardia, syncope, thrombosis, vasodilation, vasospasm, venous pressure increased, ventricular extrasystole, ventricular tachycardia

Central nervous system: Agitation, chills with fever, confusion, convulsion, delirium, depression, emotional lability, hallucinations, hypoesthesia, malaise, nervousness, psychosis, somnolence, thinking abnormal, vertigo

Dermatologic: Acne, alopecia, bruising, cellulitis, hirsutism, petechia, pruritus, skin carcinoma, skin hypertrophy, skin ulcer, vesiculobullous rash

Endocrine & metabolic: Acidosis, Cushing's syndrome, dehydration, diabetes mellitus, gout, hypercalcemia, hyperlipemia, hyperphosphatemia, hyperuricemia, hypochloremia, hypoglycemia, hyponatremia, hypoproteinemia, hypothyroidism, parathyroid disorder, weight gain/loss

Gastrointestinal: Abdomen enlarged, dry mouth, dysphagia, esophagitis, flatulence, gastritis, gastroenteritis, gastrointestinal hemorrhage, gastrointestinal moniliasis, gingivitis, gum hyperplasia, ileus, melena, mouth ulceration, oral moniliasis, stomach disorder, stomatitis

Genitourinary: Impotence, nocturia, pelvic pain, prostatic disorder, scrotal edema, urinary frequency, urinary incontinence, urinary retention, urinary tract disorder

Hematologic: Coagulation disorder, hemorrhage, neutropenia, pancytopenia, polycythemia, prothrombin time increased, thromboplastin increased

Hepatic: Alkaline phosphatase increased, alkalosis, bilirubinemia, cholangitis, cholestatic jaundice, GGT increased, hepatitis, jaundice, liver damage, transaminases increased

Local: Abscess

Neuromuscular & skeletal: Arthralgia, hypertonia, joint disorder, leg cramps, myalgia, myasthenia, neck pain, neuropathy, osteoporosis

Ocular: Amblyopia, cataract, conjunctivitis, eye hemorrhage, lacrimation disorder, vision abnormal

Otic: Deafness, ear disorder, ear pain, tinnitus

Renal: Albuminuria, creatinine increased, dysuria, hematuria, hydronephrosis, kidney failure, kidney tubular necrosis, oliguria

Respiratory: Apnea, asthma, atelectasis, bronchitis, epistaxis, hemoptysis, hiccup, hyperventilation, hypoxia, respiratory acidosis, lung edema, pharyngitis, pleural effusion, pneumonia, pneumothorax, pulmonary hypertension, respiratory moniliasis, rhinitis, sinusitis, sputum increased, voice alteration

Miscellaneous: *Candida* (mucocutaneous 15% to 18%), CMV viremia/syndrome (12% to 14%), CMV tissue invasive disease (6% to 11%), herpes zoster cutaneous disease (4% to 10%), cyst, diaphoresis, flu-like syndrome, fungal dermatitis, healing abnormal, hernia, ileus infection, lactic dehydrogenase increased, peritonitis, pyelonephritis, thirst

Overdosage/Toxicology There are no reported overdoses with mycophenolate. At plasma concentrations >100 mcg/mL, small amounts of the inactive metabolite MPAG are removed by hemodialysis. Excretion of the active metabolite, MPA, may be increased by using bile acid sequestrants (cholestyramine).

Pharmacodynamics/Kinetics

Onset of Action: Peak effect: Correlation of toxicity or efficacy is still being developed, however, one study indicated that 12-hour AUCs >40 mcg/mL/hour were correlated with efficacy and decreased episodes of rejection

T_{max}: Oral: MPA:

CellCept®: 1-1.5 hours

(Continued)

Mycophenolate *(Continued)*

Myfortic®: 1.5-2.5 hours

Protein Binding: MPA: 97%, MPAG 82%

Half-Life Elimination:

CellCept®: MPA: Oral: 18 hours; I.V.: 17 hours

Myfortic®: MPA: Oral: 8-16 hours; MPAG: 13-17 hours

Metabolism: Hepatic and via GI tract; CellCept® is completely hydrolyzed in the liver to mycophenolic acid (MPA; active metabolite); enterohepatic recirculation of MPA may occur; MPA is glucuronidated to MPAG (inactive metabolite)

Excretion:

CellCept®: MPA: Urine (<1%), feces (6%); MPAG: Urine (87%)

Myfortic®: MPA: Urine (3%), feces; MPAG: Urine (>60%)

Available Dosage Forms

Capsule, as mofetil (CellCept®): 250 mg

Injection, powder for reconstitution, as mofetil hydrochloride (CellCept®): 500 mg [contains polysorbate 80]

Powder for oral suspension, as mofetil (CellCept®): 200 mg/mL (225 mL) [provides 175 mL suspension following reconstitution; contains phenylalanine 0.56 mg/mL; mixed fruit flavor]

Tablet, as mofetil (CellCept®): 500 mg [may contain ethyl alcohol]

Tablet, delayed release, as mycophenolic acid (Myfortic®): 180 mg, 360 mg [formulated as a sodium salt]

Dosing

Adults:

Renal transplant:

CellCept®:

Oral: 1 g twice daily. Doses >2 g/day are not recommended.

I.V.: 1 g twice daily

Myfortic®: Oral: 720 mg twice daily (1440 mg/day)

Cardiac transplantation:

Oral (CellCept®): 1.5 g twice daily

I.V. (CellCept®): 1.5 g twice daily

Hepatic transplantation:

Oral (CellCept®): 1.5 g twice daily

I.V. (CellCept®): 1 g twice daily

Myasthenia gravis (unlabeled use): Oral (CellCept®): 1 g twice daily (range 1-3 g/day)

Dosing adjustment for toxicity (neutropenia): ANC <1.3 x 10^3/µL: Dosing should be interrupted or the dose reduced, appropriate diagnostic tests performed and patients managed appropriately

Elderly: Dosage is the same as younger patients, however, dosing should be cautious due to possibility of increased hepatic, renal, or cardiac dysfunction. Elderly patients may be at an increased risk of certain infections, gastrointestinal hemorrhage, and pulmonary edema, as compared to younger patients.

Pediatrics:

Renal transplant: Oral:

CellCept® suspension: 600 mg/m²/dose twice daily; maximum dose: 1 g twice daily

Alternatively, may use solid dosage forms according to BSA as follows:

BSA 1.25-1.5 m²: 750 mg capsule twice daily

BSA >1.5 m²: 1 g capsule or tablet twice daily

Myfortic®: 400 mg/m²/dose twice daily; maximum dose: 720 mg twice daily

BSA <1.19 m²: Use of this formulation is not recommended

BSA 1.19-1.58 m²: 540 mg twice daily (maximum: 1080 mg/day)

BSA >1.58 m²: 720 mg twice daily (maximum: 1440 mg/day)

Renal Impairment:

Renal transplant: GFR <25 mL/minute in patients outside the immediate post-transplant period:

CellCept®: Doses of >1 g administered twice daily should be avoided; patients should also be carefully observed; no dose adjustments are needed in renal transplant patients experiencing delayed graft function postoperatively

Myfortic®: Cl$_{cr}$ <25 mL/minute: Monitor carefully

Cardiac or liver transplant: No data available; mycophenolate may be used in cardiac or hepatic transplant patients with severe chronic renal impairment if the potential benefit outweighs the potential risk.

Hemodialysis: Not removed; supplemental dose is not necessary.

Peritoneal dialysis: Supplemental dose is not necessary.

Hepatic Impairment: No dosage adjustment is recommended for renal patients with severe hepatic parenchymal disease; however, it is not currently known whether dosage adjustments are necessary for hepatic disease with other etiologies.

Administration

Oral: Oral dosage formulations (tablet, capsule, suspension) should be administered on an empty stomach to avoid variability in MPA absorption. The oral solution may be administered via a nasogastric tube (minimum 8 French, 1.7 mm interior diameter); oral suspension should not be mixed with other medications. Delayed release tablets should not be crushed, cut, or chewed.

I.V.: Intravenous solutions should be given over at least 2 hours. Do not administer intravenous solution by rapid or bolus injection.

I.V. Detail:

Reconstituted solution: pH 2.4-4.1

Stability

Reconstitution:

Oral suspension: Should be constituted prior to dispensing to the patient and **not** mixed with any other medication. Add 47 mL of water to the bottle and shake well for ~1 minute. Add another 47 mL of water to the bottle and shake well for an additional minute. Final concentration is 200 mg/mL of mycophenolate mofetil.

I.V.: Reconstitute the contents of each vial with 14 mL of 5% dextrose injection; dilute the contents of a vial with 5% dextrose in water to a final concentration of 6 mg mycophenolate mofetil per mL.

Storage:

Capsules: Store at room temperature of 15°C to 39°C (59°F to 86°F).

Tablets: Store at room temperature of 15°C to 39°C (59°F to 86°F). Protect from light.

Oral suspension: Store powder for oral suspension at room temperature of 15°C to 39°C (59°F to 86°F). Once reconstituted, the oral solution may be stored at room temperature or under refrigeration. Do not freeze. The mixed suspension is stable for 60 days.

Injection: Store intact vials at room temperature 15°C to 30°C (59°F to 86°F). Stability of the infusion solution: 4 hours from reconstitution and dilution of the product. Store solutions at 15°C to 30°C (59°F to 86°F).

Laboratory Monitoring Renal and liver function, CBC

Nursing Actions

Physical Assessment: Assess other medications patient may be taking for effectiveness and interactions. Monitor laboratory tests, response to therapy, and adverse reactions. Patients with diabetes should monitor glucose levels closely (this medication may alter glucose levels). Monitor/instruct patient on appropriate interventions to reduce side effects, to monitor for signs of opportunistic infection (eg, persistent fever, malaise, sore throat, unusual bleeding or bruising), and adverse reactions to report.

Patient Education: Take oral formulations as directed, preferably 1 hour before or 2 hours after meals. Do not take within 1 hour before or 2 hours after antacids or cholestyramine medications. Do not alter dose and do not discontinue without consulting prescriber. Maintain adequate hydration (2-3 L/day of fluids) during entire course of therapy unless instructed to restrict fluid intake. You will be susceptible to infection (avoid crowds and exposure to infection). May be at increased risk for skin cancer, wear protective clothing and use sunscreen with high protective factor to help limit exposure to sunlight and UV light. If you have diabetes, monitor glucose levels closely (drug may alter glucose levels). You may experience dizziness or trembling (use caution until response to medication is known); nausea or vomiting (small frequent meals, frequent mouth care may help); diarrhea (boiled milk, yogurt, or buttermilk may help); sores or white plaques in mouth (frequent rinsing of mouth and frequent mouth care may help); or muscle or back pain (mild analgesics may be recommended). Report chest pain, acute headache or dizziness; symptoms of respiratory infection, cough, or respiratory difficulty; unresolved GI effects; fatigue, chills, fever unhealed sores, white plaques in mouth; irritation in genital area or unusual discharge; unusual bruising or bleeding; or other unusual effects related to this medication. **Pregnancy/breast-feeding precautions:** Inform prescriber if you are or intend to become pregnant. Two reliable forms of contraception should be used prior to, during, and for 6 weeks after therapy. Breast-feeding is not recommended.

Dietary Considerations Oral dosage formulations should be taken on an empty stomach to avoid variability in MPA absorption. However, in stable renal transplant patients, may be administered with food if necessary. Oral suspension contains 0.56 mg phenylalanine/mL; use caution if administered to patients with phenylketonuria.

Breast-Feeding Issues It is unknown if mycophenolate is excreted in human milk. Due to potentially serious adverse reactions, the decision to discontinue the drug or discontinue breast-feeding should be considered. Breast-feeding is not recommended during therapy or for 6 weeks after treatment is complete.

Pregnancy Issues There are no adequate and well-controlled studies using mycophenolate in pregnant women, however, it may cause fetal harm. Women of childbearing potential should have a negative pregnancy test within 1 week prior to beginning therapy. Two reliable forms of contraception should be used prior to, during, and for 6 weeks after therapy.

Nabumetone (na BYOO me tone)

U.S. Brand Names Relafen®

Restrictions A medication guide should be dispensed with each prescription. A template for the required MedGuide can be found on the FDA website at: http://www.fda.gov/medwatch/SAFETY/2005/safety05.htm#NSAID

Pharmacologic Category Nonsteroidal Anti-inflammatory Drug (NSAID), Oral

Pregnancy Risk Factor C/D (3rd trimester)

Lactation Excretion in breast milk unknown/not recommended

Use Management of osteoarthritis and rheumatoid arthritis

Unlabeled/Investigational Use Moderate pain

Mechanism of Action/Effect Nabumetone is a nonacidic NSAID that inhibits the production of inflammation and pain during arthritis. The active metabolite of nabumetone is felt to be the compound primarily responsible for therapeutic effect. Comparatively, the parent drug is a poor inhibitor of prostaglandin synthesis.

Contraindications Hypersensitivity to nabumetone, aspirin, other NSAIDs, or any component of the formulation; perioperative pain in the setting of coronary artery bypass surgery (CABG); pregnancy (3rd trimester)

Warnings/Precautions NSAIDs are associated with an increased risk of adverse cardiovascular events, including MI, stroke, and new onset or worsening of pre-existing hypertension. Risk may be increased with duration of use or pre-existing cardiovascular risk-factors or disease. Carefully evaluate individual cardiovascular risk profiles prior to prescribing. Use caution with fluid retention, CHF or hypertension.

Use of NSAIDs can compromise existing renal function. Renal toxicity can occur in patient with impaired renal function, dehydration, heart failure, liver dysfunction, those taking diuretics and ACEI and the elderly. Rehydrate patient before starting therapy. Monitor renal function closely. Not recommended for use in patients with advanced renal disease.

NSAIDs may increase risk of gastrointestinal irritation, ulceration, bleeding, and perforation. These events may occur at any time during therapy and without warning. Use caution with a history of GI disease (bleeding or ulcers), concurrent therapy with aspirin, anticoagulants and/or corticosteroids, smoking, use of alcohol, the elderly or debilitated patients.

Use the lowest effective dose for the shortest duration of time, consistent with individual patient goals, to reduce risk of cardiovascular or GI adverse events. Alternate therapies should be considered for patients at high risk.

NSAIDs may cause serious skin adverse events including exfoliative dermatitis, Stevens-Johnson syndrome (SJS) and toxic epidermal necrolysis (TEN). Anaphylactoid reactions may occur, even without prior exposure; patients with "aspirin triad" (bronchial asthma, aspirin intolerance, rhinitis) may be at increased risk. Do not use in patients who experience bronchospasm, asthma, rhinitis, or urticaria with NSAID or aspirin therapy.

Use with caution in patients with decreased hepatic function. Closely monitor patients with any abnormal LFT. Severe hepatic reactions (eg, fulminant hepatitis, liver failure) have occurred with NSAID use, rarely; discontinue if signs or symptoms of liver disease develop, or if systemic manifestations occur.

The elderly are at increased risk for adverse effects (especially peptic ulceration, CNS effects, renal toxicity) from NSAIDs even at low doses

Withhold for at least 4-6 half-lives prior to surgical or dental procedures. May cause photosensitivity reactions. Safety and efficacy have not been established in pediatric patients.

Drug Interactions

Decreased Effect: NSAIDs may decrease the effect of some antihypertensive agents, including ACE inhibitors, angiotensin receptor antagonists, and hydralazine. The efficacy of diuretics (loop and/or thiazide) may be decreased.

Increased Effect/Toxicity: NSAIDs may increase digoxin, methotrexate, and lithium serum concentrations. The renal adverse effects of ACE inhibitors may be potentiated by NSAIDs. Potential for bleeding may be increased with anticoagulants or antiplatelet agents. Concurrent use of corticosteroids may increase the risk of GI ulceration.
(Continued)

Nabumetone *(Continued)*

Nutritional/Ethanol Interactions

Ethanol: Avoid ethanol (may enhance gastric mucosal irritation).

Food: Nabumetone peak serum concentrations may be increased if taken with food or dairy products.

Herb/Nutraceutical: Avoid alfalfa, anise, bilberry, bladderwrack, bromelain, cat's claw, celery, coleus, cordyceps, dong quai, evening primrose, feverfew, fenugreek, garlic, ginger, ginkgo biloboa, red clover, horse chestnut, grapeseed, green tea, ginseng, guggul, horse chestnut seed, horseradish, licorice, prickly ash, red clover, reishi, SAMe, sweet clover, turmeric, white willow (all have additional antiplatelet activity).

Adverse Reactions

>10%: Gastrointestinal: Abdominal pain (12%), diarrhea (14%), dyspepsia (13%)

1% to 10%:

Cardiovascular: Edema (3% to 9%)

Central nervous system: Dizziness (3% to 9%), headache (3% to 9%), fatigue (1% to 3%), insomnia (1% to 3%), nervousness (1% to 3%), somnolence (1% to 3%)

Dermatologic: Pruritus (3% to 9%), rash (3% to 9%)

Gastrointestinal: Constipation (3% to 9%), flatulence (3% to 9%), guaic positive (3% to 9%), nausea (3% to 9%), gastritis (1% to 3%), stomatitis (1% to 3%), vomiting (1% to 3%), xerostomia (1% to 3%)

Otic: Tinnitus

Miscellaneous: Diaphoresis (1% to 3%)

Overdosage/Toxicology

Symptoms of overdose include drowsiness, epigastric pain, lethargy, nausea and vomiting. Acute renal failure, coma, hypertension and respiratory depression may also rarely occur. Management of NSAID intoxication is supportive and symptomatic. 6-Methoxy-2-naphthylacetic acid (6MNA) is not dialyzable.

Pharmacodynamics/Kinetics

Onset of Action: Several days

Time to Peak: Serum: 6MNA: Oral: 2.5-4 hours; Synovial fluid: 4-12 hours

Protein Binding: 6MNA: >99%

Half-Life Elimination: 6MNA: ~24 hours

Metabolism: Prodrug, rapidly metabolized in the liver to an active metabolite [6-methoxy-2-naphthylacetic acid (6MNA)] and inactive metabolites; extensive first-pass effect

Excretion: 6MNA: Urine (80%) and feces (9%)

Available Dosage Forms
Tablet: 500 mg, 750 mg

Dosing

Adults: Osteoarthritis, rheumatoid arthritis: Oral: 1000 mg/day; an additional 500-1000 mg may be needed in some patients to obtain more symptomatic relief; may be administered once or twice daily; maximum dose: 2000 mg/day

Note: Patients <50 kg are less likely to require doses >1000 mg/day.

Elderly: Refer to adult dosing; do not exceed 2000 mg/ day.

Renal Impairment: In general, NSAIDs are not recommended for use in patients with advanced renal disease, but the manufacturer of nabumetone does provide some guidelines for adjustment in renal dysfunction:

Moderate impairment (Cl_{cr} 30-49 mL/minute): Initial dose: 750 mg/day; maximum dose: 1500 mg/day

Severe impairment (Cl_{cr} <30 mL/minute): Initial dose: 500 mg/day; maximum dose: 1000 mg/day

Laboratory Monitoring Patients with renal insufficiency: Baseline renal function followed by repeat test within weeks (to determine if renal function has deteriorated)

Nursing Actions

Physical Assessment: Assess effectiveness and interactions of other medications patient may be taking. Monitor blood pressure at the beginning of therapy and periodically during use. Monitor laboratory tests and therapeutic response (eg, relief of pain and inflammation, increased activity tolerance), and adverse reactions (eg, GI effects, hepatotoxicity, or ototoxicity) at beginning of therapy and periodically throughout therapy. Schedule ophthalmic evaluations for patients who develop eye complaints during long-term NSAID therapy. Assess knowledge/teach patient appropriate use, interventions to reduce side effects, and adverse symptoms to report.

Patient Education: Take this medication exactly as directed; do not increase dose without consulting prescriber. Do not crush tablets. Take with food or milk to reduce GI distress. Maintain adequate hydration (2-3 L/day of fluids) unless instructed to restrict fluid intake. Do not use alcohol, aspirin or aspirin-containing medication, or any other anti-inflammatory medications without consulting healthcare prescriber. You may experience drowsiness, dizziness, nervousness, or headache (use caution when driving or engaging in tasks requiring alertness until response to drug is known); anorexia, nausea, vomiting, or heartburn (small frequent meals, frequent oral care, sucking lozenges, or chewing gum may help); fluid retention (weigh yourself weekly and report unusual [3-5 lb/week] weight gain). GI bleeding, ulceration, or perforation can occur with or without pain; discontinue medication and contact prescriber if persistent abdominal pain or cramping, or blood in stool occurs. Report breathlessness, respiratory difficulty, or unusual cough; chest pain, rapid heartbeat, palpitations; unusual bruising/bleeding; blood in urine, stool, mouth, or vomitus; swollen extremities; skin rash or itching; acute fatigue; or hearing changes (ringing in ears). **Pregnancy/breast-feeding precautions:** Inform prescriber if you are pregnant. Breast-feeding is not recommended.

Geriatric Considerations In trials with nabumetone, no significant differences were noted between young and elderly in regards to efficacy and safety. However, elderly are at high risk for adverse effects from NSAIDs. As much as 60% of elderly can develop peptic ulceration and/or hemorrhage asymptomatically. The concomitant use of H_2 blockers, omeprazole, and sucralfate is not effective as prophylaxis with the exception of NSAID-induced duodenal ulcers which may be prevented by the use of ranitidine. Misoprostol is the only prophylactic agent proven effective. Also, concomitant disease and drug use contribute to the risk for GI adverse effects. Use lowest effective dose for shortest period possible. Consider renal function decline with age. Use of NSAIDs can compromise existing renal function especially when Cl_{cr} is ≤30 mL/minute. Tinnitus may be a difficult and unreliable indication of toxicity due to age-related hearing loss or eighth cranial nerve damage. CNS adverse effects such as confusion, agitation, and hallucination are generally seen in overdose or high-dose situations, but elderly may demonstrate these adverse effects at lower doses than younger adults.

Nadolol *(nay DOE lole)*

U.S. Brand Names Corgard®

Pharmacologic Category Beta-Adrenergic Blocker, Nonselective

Medication Safety Issues

Sound-alike/look-alike issues:

Nadolol may be confused with Mandol®

Corgard® may be confused with Cognex®

Pregnancy Risk Factor C

Lactation Enters breast milk/use caution (AAP rates "compatible")

Use Treatment of hypertension and angina pectoris; prophylaxis of migraine headaches

Mechanism of Action/Effect Competitively blocks response to beta$_1$- and beta$_2$-adrenergic stimulation; does not exhibit any membrane stabilizing or intrinsic sympathomimetic activity

Contraindications Hypersensitivity to nadolol or any component of the formulation; bronchial asthma; sinus bradycardia; sinus node dysfunction; heart block greater than first degree (except in patients with a functioning artificial pacemaker); cardiogenic shock; uncompensated cardiac failure

Warnings/Precautions Administer only with extreme caution in patients with compensated heart failure, monitor for a worsening of the condition. Efficacy in heart failure has not been established for nadolol. Use caution with concurrent use of beta-blockers and either verapamil or diltiazem; bradycardia or heart block can occur. In general, patients with bronchospastic disease should not receive beta-blockers. Nadolol, if used at all, should be used cautiously in bronchospastic disease with close monitoring. Use cautiously in patients with diabetes because it can mask prominent hypoglycemic symptoms. Can mask signs of thyrotoxicosis. Can cause fetal harm when administered in pregnancy. Use cautiously in the renally impaired (dosage adjustments are required). Use care with anesthetic agents which decrease myocardial function. Beta-blocker therapy should not be withdrawn abruptly (particularly in patients with CAD), but gradually tapered to avoid acute tachycardia, hypertension, and/or ischemia.

Drug Interactions

Decreased Effect: Decreased effect of beta-blockers with aluminum salts, barbiturates, calcium salts, cholestyramine, colestipol, NSAIDs, penicillins (ampicillin), rifampin, salicylates, and sulfinpyrazone due to decreased bioavailability and plasma levels. Beta-blockers may decrease the effect of sulfonylureas (possibly hyperglycemia). Nonselective beta-blockers blunt the effect of beta-2 adrenergic agonists (albuterol).

Increased Effect/Toxicity: The heart rate lowering effects of nadolol are additive with other drugs which slow AV conduction (digoxin, verapamil, diltiazem). Concurrent use of alpha-blockers (prazosin, terazosin) with beta-blockers may increase risk of orthostasis. Nadolol may mask the tachycardia from hypoglycemia caused by insulin and oral hypoglycemics. In patients receiving concurrent therapy, the risk of hypertensive crisis is increased when either clonidine or the beta-blocker is withdrawn. Reserpine has been shown to enhance the effect of beta-blockers. Avoid using with alpha-adrenergic stimulants (phenylephrine, epinephrine, etc) which may have exaggerated hypertensive responses. Beta-blockers may affect the action or levels of ethanol, disopyramide, nondepolarizing muscle relaxants, and theophylline although the effects are difficult to predict. The vasoconstrictive effects of ergot alkaloids may be enhanced.

Nutritional/Ethanol Interactions Herb/Nutraceutical: Avoid dong quai if using for hypertension (has estrogenic activity). Avoid ephedra, garlic, yohimbe, ginseng (may worsen hypertension). Avoid natural licorice (causes sodium and water retention and increases potassium loss).

Adverse Reactions

>10%:

Central nervous system: Drowsiness, insomnia

Endocrine & metabolic: Decreased sexual ability

1% to 10%:

Cardiovascular: Bradycardia, palpitation, edema, CHF, reduced peripheral circulation

Central nervous system: Mental depression

Gastrointestinal: Diarrhea or constipation, nausea, vomiting, stomach discomfort

Respiratory: Bronchospasm

Miscellaneous: Cold extremities

Overdosage/Toxicology Symptoms of intoxication include cardiac disturbances, CNS toxicity, bronchospasm, hypoglycemia and hyperkalemia. The most common cardiac symptoms include hypotension and bradycardia. Atrioventricular block, intraventricular conduction disturbances, cardiogenic shock, and asystole may occur with severe overdose. CNS effects include convulsions, coma, and respiratory arrest. Treatment is symptom-directed and supportive. Glucagon has been used to reverse cardiac depression.

Pharmacodynamics/Kinetics

Duration of Action: 17-24 hours

Time to Peak: Serum: 2-4 hours

Protein Binding: 28%

Half-Life Elimination: Adults: 10-24 hours, prolonged with renal impairment; End-stage renal disease: 45 hours

Excretion: Urine (as unchanged drug)

Available Dosage Forms [DSC] = Discontinued product

Tablet: 20 mg, 40 mg, 80 mg, 120 mg, 160 mg

Corgard®: 20 mg, 40 mg, 80 mg, 120 mg [DSC], 160 mg [DSC]

Dosing

Adults:

Hypertension, angina: Oral: Initial: 40-80 mg/day, increase dosage gradually by 40-80 mg increments at 3- to 7-day intervals until optimum clinical response is obtained with profound slowing of heart rate. Doses up to 160-240 mg/day in angina and 240-320 mg/day in hypertension may be necessary. Doses as high as 640 mg/day have been used.

Usual dosage range (JNC 7): 40-120 mg once daily

Elderly: Oral: Initial: 20 mg/day; increase doses by 20 mg increments at 3- to 7-day intervals; usual dosage range: 20-240 mg/day. Adjust for renal impairment.

Renal Impairment:

Cl$_{cr}$ 31-40 mL/minute: Administer every 24-36 hours or administer 50% of normal dose.

Cl$_{cr}$ 10-30 mL/minute: Administer every 24-48 hours or administer 50% of normal dose.

Cl$_{cr}$ <10 mL/minute: Administer every 40-60 hours or administer 25% of normal dose.

Hemodialysis effects: Moderately dialyzable (20% to 50%) via hemodialysis. Administer dose postdialysis or administer 40 mg supplemental dose. Supplemental dose is not necessary following peritoneal dialysis.

Hepatic Impairment: Reduced dose is probably necessary.

Nursing Actions

Physical Assessment: Assess other medications the patient may taking for effectiveness and interactions. Assess blood pressure and heart rate prior to and following first dose, any change in dosage, and periodically thereafter. Monitor or advise patient to monitor weight and fluid balance (I & O), assess for signs of CHF (edema, new cough or dyspnea, unresolved fatigue), and assess therapeutic effectiveness. Monitor serum glucose levels of patients with diabetes since beta-blockers may alter glucose tolerance. Use/teach postural hypotension precautions.

Patient Education: Check pulse daily prior to taking medication. If pulse is <50, hold medication and consult prescriber. Take exactly as directed; do not adjust dosage or discontinue without consulting prescriber. May cause dizziness, fatigue, blurred vision; change position slowly (lying/sitting to standing) and use caution when driving or engaging in tasks that require alertness until response to drug is known. Exercise and increasing bulk or fiber in diet may help resolve constipation. If you have diabetes, (Continued)

Nadolol *(Continued)*

monitor serum glucose closely (the drug may mask symptoms of hypoglycemia). Report swelling in feet or legs, respiratory difficulty or persistent cough, unresolved fatigue, unusual weight gain >5 lb/week, or unresolved constipation. **Pregnancy/breast-feeding precautions:** Inform prescriber if you are or intend to become pregnant. Consult prescriber if breast-feeding.

Dietary Considerations May be taken without regard to meals.

Geriatric Considerations Due to alterations in the beta-adrenergic autonomic nervous system, beta-adrenergic blockade may result in less hemodynamic response than seen in younger adults. Studies indicate that despite decreased sensitivity to the chronotropic effects of beta blockade with age, there appears to be an increased myocardial sensitivity to the negative inotropic effect during stress (eg, exercise). See Warnings/Precautions.

Breast-Feeding Issues Considered compatible by the AAP. However, monitor the infant for signs of beta-blockade (hypotension, bradycardia, etc) with long-term use.

Pregnancy Issues No data available on crossing the placenta. Beta-blockers have been associated with bradycardia, hypotension, and IUGR; IUGR is probably related to maternal hypertension. Alternative beta-blockers are preferred for use during pregnancy due to limited data and prolonged half-life. Cases of neonatal hypoglycemia have been reported following maternal use of beta-blockers at parturition or during breast-feeding. Monitor breast-fed infant for symptoms of beta-blockade.

Nafarelin *(NAF a re lin)*

U.S. Brand Names Synarel®

Synonyms Nafarelin Acetate

Pharmacologic Category Gonadotropin Releasing Hormone Agonist

Medication Safety Issues

Sound-alike/look-alike issues:

Nafarelin may be confused with Anafranil®, enalapril

Pregnancy Risk Factor X

Lactation Enters breast milk/contraindicated

Use Treatment of endometriosis, including pain and reduction of lesions; treatment of central precocious puberty (gonadotropin-dependent precocious puberty) in children of both sexes

Mechanism of Action/Effect Potent synthetic decapeptide analogue of gonadotropin-releasing hormone (GnRH; LHRH) which is approximately 200 times more potent than GnRH in terms of pituitary release of luteinizing hormone (LH) and follicle-stimulating hormone (FSH)

Contraindications Hypersensitivity to GnRH, GnRH-agonist analogs, or any component of the formulation; undiagnosed abnormal vaginal bleeding; pregnancy

Warnings/Precautions Use with caution in patients with risk factors for decreased bone mineral content. Nafarelin therapy may pose an additional risk. Hypersensitivity reactions occur in 0.2% of the patients.

Adverse Reactions

>10%:

Central nervous system: Headache, emotional lability

Dermatologic: Acne

Endocrine & metabolic: Hot flashes, decreased libido, decreased breast size

Genitourinary: Vaginal dryness

Neuromuscular & skeletal: Myalgia

Respiratory: Nasal irritation

1% to 10%:

Cardiovascular: Edema, chest pain

Central nervous system: Insomnia

Dermatologic: Urticaria, rash, pruritus, seborrhea

Respiratory: Dyspnea

Pharmacodynamics/Kinetics

Time to Peak: Serum: 10-45 minutes

Protein Binding: Plasma: 80%

Available Dosage Forms Solution, intranasal spray: 2 mg/mL (8 mL) [200 mcg/spray; 60 metered doses; contains benzalkonium chloride]

Dosing

Adults & Elderly: Endometriosis: Nasal: 1 spray (200 mcg) in 1 nostril each morning and the other nostril each evening starting on days 2-4 of menstrual cycle for 6 months

Pediatrics: Central precocious puberty: Nasal: 2 sprays (400 mcg) into each nostril in the morning 2 sprays (400 mcg) into each nostril in the evening. If inadequate suppression, may increase dose to 3 sprays (600 mcg) into alternating nostrils 3 times/day.

Administration

Inhalation: Nasal spray: Do not use topical nasal decongestant for at least 30 minutes after nafarelin use.

Stability

Storage: Store at room temperature. Protect from light.

Nursing Actions

Physical Assessment: For treatment of precocious puberty, consult appropriate pediatric reference. Monitor therapeutic effectiveness and adverse response. Teach patient (caregiver) proper use (correct timing and administration of nasal spray), possible side effects/appropriate interventions, and adverse symptoms to report. **Pregnancy risk factor X:** Determine that female patient is not pregnant before beginning therapy. Do not give to childbearing age female unless capable of complying with contraceptive use.

Patient Education: Endometriosis: You will begin this treatment between days 2-4 of your regular menstrual cycle. Use as directed, daily at the same time (arising and bedtime), and rotate nostrils. Maintain regular follow-up schedule. May cause hot flashes, flushing, or redness (cold cloth and cool environment may help); decreased or increased libido; emotional lability; weight gain; decreased breast size; or hirsutism. Report any breakthrough bleeding or continuing menstruation or musculoskeletal pain. Do not use a nasal decongestant within 30 minutes after nafarelin. **Pregnancy/breast-feeding precautions:** Inform prescriber if you are pregnant. Do not get pregnant while taking this medication. Consult prescriber for instruction on appropriate contraceptive measures. Do not breast-feed.

Additional Information Each spray delivers 200 mcg

Nafcillin *(naf SIL in)*

Synonyms Ethoxynaphthamido Penicillin Sodium; Nafcillin Sodium; Nallpen; Sodium Nafcillin

Pharmacologic Category Antibiotic, Penicillin

Pregnancy Risk Factor B

Lactation Enters breast milk/use caution

Use Treatment of infections such as osteomyelitis, septicemia, endocarditis, and CNS infections caused by susceptible strains of staphylococci species

Mechanism of Action/Effect Interferes with bacterial cell wall synthesis during active multiplication, causing cell wall death and resultant bactericidal activity against susceptible bacteria

Contraindications Hypersensitivity to nafcillin, or any component of the formulation, or penicillins

Warnings/Precautions Extravasation of I.V. infusions should be avoided. Modification of dosage is necessary in patients with both severe renal and hepatic impairment. Elimination rate will be slow in neonates.

Drug Interactions

Cytochrome P450 Effect: Induces CYP3A4 (strong)

Decreased Effect: Chloramphenicol may decrease nafcillin efficacy. If taken concomitantly with warfarin, nafcillin may inhibit the anticoagulant response to warfarin. This effect may persist for up to 30 days after nafcillin has been discontinued. Subtherapeutic cyclosporine levels may result when taken concomitantly with nafcillin. Although anecdotal reports suggest oral contraceptive efficacy could be reduced by penicillins, this has been refuted by more rigorous scientific and clinical data. Nafcillin may decrease the levels/effects of benzodiazepines, calcium channel blockers, clarithromycin, cyclosporine, erythromycin, estrogens, mirtazapine, nateglinide, nefazodone, nevirapine, protease inhibitors, tacrolimus, venlafaxine, and other CYP3A4 substrates.

Increased Effect/Toxicity: Probenecid may cause an increase in nafcillin levels. Penicillins may increase the exposure to methotrexate during concurrent therapy; monitor.

Lab Interactions Positive Coombs' test (direct)

Adverse Reactions Frequency not defined.

Central nervous system: Pain, fever

Dermatologic: Rash

Gastrointestinal: Nausea, diarrhea

Hematologic: Agranulocytosis, bone marrow depression, neutropenia

Local: Pain, swelling, inflammation, phlebitis, skin sloughing, and thrombophlebitis at the injection site; oxacillin (less likely to cause phlebitis) is often preferred in pediatric patients

Renal: Interstitial nephritis (acute)

Miscellaneous: Hypersensitivity reactions

Overdosage/Toxicology Symptoms of penicillin overdose include neuromuscular hypersensitivity (eg, agitation, hallucinations, asterixis, encephalopathy, confusion, and seizures). Electrolyte imbalance may occur if the preparation contains potassium or sodium salts, especially in renal failure. Treatment is supportive or symptom-directed.

Pharmacodynamics/Kinetics

Time to Peak: Serum: I.M.: 30-60 minutes

Protein Binding: 70% to 90%

Half-Life Elimination:

Neonates: <3 weeks: 2.2-5.5 hours; 4-9 weeks: 1.2-2.3 hours

Children 3 months to 14 years: 0.75-1.9 hours

Adults: Normal renal/hepatic function: 30 minutes to 1.5 hours

Metabolism: Primarily hepatic; undergoes enterohepatic recirculation

Excretion: Primarily feces; urine (10% to 30% as unchanged drug)

Available Dosage Forms

Infusion [premixed iso-osmotic dextrose solution]: 1 g (50 mL); 2 g (100 mL)

Injection, powder for reconstitution, as sodium: 1 g, 2 g, 10 g

Dosing

Adults & Elderly:

Susceptible infections:

I.M.: 500 mg every 4-6 hours

I.V.: 500-2000 mg every 4-6 hours

Endocarditis: MSSA:

Native valve: I.V.: 2 g every 4 hours

Prosthetic valve: I.V.: 1 g every 4 hours with rifampin for 6 weeks with gentamicin for 2 weeks

Tricuspid valve: I.V.: 2 g every 4 hours with gentamicin for 2 weeks

Joint:

Bursitis, septic: I.V.: 2 g every 4 hours

Prosthetic: I.V.: 2 g every 4-6 hours with rifampin for 6 weeks

***Staphylococcus aureus*, methicillin-susceptible infections, including brain abscess, empyema, erysipelas, mastitis, myositis, osteomyelitis, pneumonia, toxic shock, urinary tract (perinephric abscess):** I.V.: 2 g every 4 hours

Toxic epidermal necrolysis: I.V.: 2 g every 4 hours

Pediatrics:

Neonates:

Arthritis, septic: I.V.:

<2000 g, <7 days: 50 mg/kg/day divided every 12 hours

>2000 g, <7 days: 75 mg/kg/day divided every 8 hours

<2000 g, >7 days: 75 mg/kg/day divided every 8 hours

>2000 g, >7 days: 222 mg/kg/day divided every 6 hours

Children:

I.M.: 25 mg/kg twice daily

I.V.:

Epiglottitis: 150-200 mg/kg/day divided in 4 doses

Mild to moderate infections: 50-100 mg/kg/day in divided doses every 6 hours

Severe infections: 100-200 mg/kg/day in divided doses every 4-6 hours (maximum: 12 g/day)

Toxic epidermal necrolysis: I.V.: 150 mg/kg/day divided every 6 hours for 5-7 days

Renal Impairment: No adjustment is necessary.

Hemodialysis effects: Not dialyzable (0% to 5%) via hemodialysis. Supplemental dose is not necessary with hemo- or peritoneal dialysis or continuous arteriovenous or venovenous hemofiltration.

Hepatic Impairment: In patients with both hepatic and renal impairment, modification of dosage may be necessary; no data available.

Administration

I.M.: Rotate injection sites.

I.V.: Vesicant. Administer around-the-clock to promote less variation in peak and trough serum levels. Infuse over 30-60 minutes.

I.V. Detail: Extravasation management: Use cold packs.

Hyaluronidase: Add 1 mL NS to 150 unit vial to make 150 units/mL of concentration; mix 0.1 mL of above with 0.9 mL NS in 1 mL syringe to make final concentration = 15 units/mL.

pH: 6.0-8.5

Stability

Compatibility: Stable in dextran 40 10% in dextrose, D_5LR, $D_5^1/_4NS$, $D_5^1/_2NS$, D_5NS, D_5W, $D_{10}NS$, $D_{10}W$, LR, NS

Y-site administration: Incompatible with droperidol, fentanyl and droperidol, insulin (regular), labetalol, midazolam, nalbuphine, pentazocine, verapamil

Compatibility when admixed: Incompatible with ascorbic acid injection, aztreonam, bleomycin, cytarabine, gentamicin, hydrocortisone sodium succinate, methylprednisolone sodium succinate, promazine

Storage: Reconstituted parenteral solution is stable for 3 days at room temperature, 7 days when refrigerated, or 12 weeks when frozen. For I.V. infusion in NS or D_5W, solution is stable for 24 hours at room temperature and 96 hours when refrigerated.

Laboratory Monitoring Perform culture and sensitivity studies prior to initiating drug therapy. Monitor renal, hepatic, CBC with prolonged therapy.

Nursing Actions

Physical Assessment: Assess results of culture and sensitivity tests and allergy history prior to starting therapy. Assess potential for interactions with other pharmacological agents patient may be taking (eg, Increased [toxic] or decreased [subtherapeutic] levels/ (Continued)

857

Nafcillin (Continued)

effects. Infusion/Injection site must be monitored closely to prevent extravasation (use ice packs). Assess for therapeutic effect (resolution of infection) and adverse reactions (eg, hypersensitivity, opportunistic infection [eg, fever, chills, unhealed sores, white plaques in mouth or vagina, purulent vaginal discharge, fatigue]). Teach patient possible side effects/appropriate interventions and adverse symptoms to report.

Patient Education: Do not take any new medication during therapy unless approved by prescriber. This medication can only be administered by infusion or injection. Report immediately any redness, swelling, burning, or pain at injection/infusion site; respiratory difficulty or swallowing; chest pain; or rash. May cause nausea (small, frequent meals, frequent mouth care, chewing gum, or sucking lozenges may help); or opportunistic infection (eg, fever, chills, sore throat, burning urination, fatigue). Report persistent side effects or if condition does not respond to treatment. **Breast-feeding precaution:** Consult prescriber if breast-feeding.

Dietary Considerations Sodium content of 1 g: 76.6 mg (3.33 mEq)

Geriatric Considerations Nafcillin has not been studied exclusively in the elderly, however, given its route of elimination, dosage adjustments based upon age and renal function are not necessary. Consider sodium content in patients who may be sensitive to volume expansion (ie, CHF).

Nalbuphine (NAL byoo feen)

U.S. Brand Names Nubain®

Synonyms Nalbuphine Hydrochloride

Pharmacologic Category Analgesic, Narcotic

Medication Safety Issues
Sound-alike/look-alike issues:
Nubain® may be confused with Navane®, Nebcin®

Pregnancy Risk Factor B/D (prolonged use or high doses at term)

Lactation Enters breast milk/use caution

Use Relief of moderate to severe pain; preoperative analgesia, postoperative and surgical anesthesia, and obstetrical analgesia during labor and delivery

Mechanism of Action/Effect Binds to opiate receptors in the CNS, causing inhibition of ascending pain pathways, altering the perception of and response to pain; produces generalized CNS depression

Contraindications Hypersensitivity to nalbuphine or any component of the formulation

Warnings/Precautions Use caution in CNS depression. Sedation and psychomotor impairment are likely, and are additive with other CNS depressants or ethanol. May cause respiratory depression. Ambulatory patients must be cautioned about performing tasks which require mental alertness (eg, operating machinery or driving). Use with caution in patients with recent myocardial infarction, biliary tract surgery, head trauma, or increased intracranial pressure. Use caution in patients with decreased hepatic or renal function. May result in tolerance and/or drug dependence with chronic use; use with caution in patients with a history of drug dependence. Abrupt discontinuation following prolonged use may lead to withdrawal symptoms. May precipitate withdrawal symptoms in patients following prolonged therapy with mu opiod agonists. Use with caution in pregnancy (close neonatal monitoring required when used in labor and delivery). Safety and efficacy in pediatric patients (<18 years of age) have not been established.

Drug Interactions
Increased Effect/Toxicity: Barbiturate anesthetics may increase CNS depression.

Nutritional/Ethanol Interactions
Ethanol: Avoid ethanol (may increase CNS depression).
Herb/Nutraceutical: Avoid valerian, St John's wort, kava kava, gotu kola (may increase CNS depression).

Adverse Reactions
>10%: Central nervous system: Sedation (36%)
1% to 10%:
Central nervous system: Dizziness (5%), headache (3%)
Gastrointestinal: Nausea/vomiting (6%), xerostomia (4%)
Miscellaneous: Clamminess (9%)

Overdosage/Toxicology Symptoms of overdose include CNS depression, respiratory depression, miosis, hypotension, and bradycardia. Treatment is symptomatic. Naloxone, 2 mg I.V. with repeat administration as necessary up to a total dose of 10 mg, can be used to reverse opiate effects.

Pharmacodynamics/Kinetics
Onset of Action: Peak effect: SubQ, I.M.: <15 minutes; I.V.: 2-3 minutes
Half-Life Elimination: 5 hours
Metabolism: Hepatic
Excretion: Feces; urine (~7% as metabolites)

Available Dosage Forms [DSC] = Discontinued product
Injection, solution, as hydrochloride: 10 mg/mL (10 mL); 20 mg/mL (10 mL)
Nubain®: 10 mg/mL (10 mL) [DSC]; 20 mg/mL (10 mL)
Injection, solution, as hydrochloride [preservative free]: 10 mg/mL (1 mL); 20 mg/mL (1 mL)
Nubain®: 10 mg/mL (1 mL); 20 mg/mL (1 mL)

Dosing
Adults:
Pain management: I.M., I.V., SubQ: 10 mg/70 kg every 3-6 hours; maximum single dose in nonopioid-tolerant patients: 20 mg; maximum daily dose: 160 mg
Surgical anesthesia supplement: I.V.: Induction: 0.3-3 mg/kg over 10-15 minutes; maintenance doses of 0.25-0.5 mg/kg may be given as required
Elderly: Refer to adult dosing; use with caution.
Pediatrics: Pain management (unlabeled use): Children ≥1 year: I.M., I.V., SubQ: 0.1-0.2 mg/kg every 3-4 hours as needed; maximum: 20 mg/dose and/or 160 mg/day
Renal Impairment: Use with caution and reduce dose. Monitor.
Hepatic Impairment: Use with caution and reduce dose.

Administration
I.V. Detail: pH: 3.5-3.7 (adjusted)

Stability
Compatibility: Stable in D₅NS, D₁₀W, LR, NS
Y-site administration: Incompatible with allopurinol, amphotericin B cholesteryl sulfate complex, cefepime, docetaxel, ketorolac, methotrexate, nafcillin, piperacillin/tazobactam, sargramostim, sodium bicarbonate
Compatibility in syringe: Incompatible with diazepam, ketorolac, pentobarbital
Storage: Store at room temperature of 15°C to 30°C (59°F to 86°F). Protect from light.

Nursing Actions
Physical Assessment: Monitor for effectiveness of pain relief and monitor for signs of overdose. Monitor blood pressure, CNS and respiratory status, and degree of sedation at beginning of therapy and at regular intervals during use. For inpatients, implement safety measures (eg, side rails up, call light within reach, instructions to call for assistance). Generally

used in conjunction with surgical anesthesia or during labor and delivery; however, if self-administered for relief of pain, assess knowledge/teach patient appropriate use. Teach patient to monitor for adverse reactions, adverse reactions to report, and appropriate interventions to reduce side effects.

Patient Education: If self-administered, use exactly as directed; do not increase dose or frequency. Drug may cause physical and/or psychological dependence. While using this medication, do not use alcohol and other prescription or OTC medications (especially sedatives, tranquilizers, antihistamines, or pain medications) without consulting prescriber. Maintain adequate hydration (2-3 L/day of fluids) unless instructed to restrict fluid intake. May cause hypotension, dizziness, drowsiness, impaired coordination, or blurred vision (use caution when driving, climbing stairs, or changing position - rising from sitting or lying to standing, or when engaging in tasks requiring alertness until response to drug is known); loss of appetite, nausea, or vomiting (frequent mouth care, small frequent meals, chewing gum, or sucking lozenges may help); or constipation (increased exercise, fluids, fruit, or fiber may help; if unresolved, consult prescriber about use of stool softeners). Report chest pain, slow or rapid heartbeat, acute dizziness or persistent headache; changes in mental status; swelling of extremities or unusual weight gain; changes in urinary elimination or pain on urination; acute headache; back or flank pain or muscle spasms; blurred vision; skin rash; or shortness of breath. **Pregnancy/breast-feeding precautions:** Inform prescriber if you are or intend to become pregnant. If you are breast-feeding, take medication immediately after breast-feeding or 3-4 hours prior to next feeding.

Geriatric Considerations The elderly may be particularly susceptible to CNS effects; monitor closely.

Pregnancy Issues Severe fetal bradycardia has been reported following use in labor/delivery. Fetal bradycardia may occur when administered earlier in pregnancy (not documented). Use only if clearly needed, with monitoring to detect and manage possible adverse fetal effects. Naloxone has been reported to reverse bradycardia. Newborn should be monitored for respiratory depression or bradycardia following nalbuphine use in labor.

Related Information
Compatibility of Drugs in Syringe *on page 1372*

Nalmefene (NAL me feen)

U.S. Brand Names Revex®
Synonyms Nalmefene Hydrochloride
Pharmacologic Category Antidote
Medication Safety Issues
Sound-alike/look-alike issues:
Revex® may be confused with Nimbex®, ReVia®
Pregnancy Risk Factor B
Lactation Enters breast milk/use caution
Use Complete or partial reversal of opioid drug effects, including respiratory depression induced by natural or synthetic opioids; reversal of postoperative opioid depression; management of known or suspected opioid overdose
Mechanism of Action/Effect Nalmefene acts as a competitive antagonist at opioid receptor sites, preventing or reversing the respiratory depression, sedation, and hypotension induced by opiates; no pharmacologic activity of its own (eg, opioid agonist activity) has been demonstrated
Contraindications Hypersensitivity to nalmefene, naltrexone, or any component of the formulation

Warnings/Precautions May induce symptoms of acute withdrawal in opioid-dependent patients; recurrence of respiratory depression is possible if the opioid involved is long-acting; observe patients until there is no reasonable risk of recurrent respiratory depression. Safety and efficacy have not been established in children. Avoid abrupt reversal of opioid effects in patients of high cardiovascular risk or who have received potentially cardiotoxic drugs. Pulmonary edema and cardiovascular instability have been reported in association with abrupt reversal with other narcotic antagonists. Animal studies indicate nalmefene may not completely reverse buprenorphine-induced respiratory depression.

Drug Interactions
Increased Effect/Toxicity: Potential increased risk of seizures may exist with use of flumazenil and nalmefene coadministration.

Adverse Reactions
>10%: Gastrointestinal: Nausea
1% to 10%:
Cardiovascular: Tachycardia, hyper-/hypotension, vasodilation
Central nervous system: Fever, dizziness, headache, chills
Gastrointestinal: Vomiting
Miscellaneous: Postoperative pain

Overdosage/Toxicology No reported symptoms with significant overdose. Large doses of opioids administered to overcome a full blockade of opioid antagonists, however, have resulted in adverse respiratory and circulatory reactions.

Pharmacodynamics/Kinetics
Onset of Action: I.M., SubQ: 5-15 minutes
Time to Peak: Serum: I.M.: 2.3 hours; I.V.: <2 minutes; SubQ: 1.5 hours
Protein Binding: 45%
Half-Life Elimination: 10.8 hours
Metabolism: Hepatic via glucuronide conjugation to metabolites with little or no activity
Excretion: Feces (17%); urine (<5% as unchanged drug)
Clearance: 0.8 L/hour/kg

Available Dosage Forms Injection, solution: 100 mcg/mL (1 mL) [blue label]; 1000 mcg/mL (2 mL) [green label]

Dosing
Adults & Elderly:
Reversal of postoperative opioid depression: I.V.: Blue labeled product (100 mcg/mL): Titrate to reverse the undesired effects of opioids; initial dose for nonopioid dependent patient: 0.25 mcg/kg followed by 0.25 mcg/kg incremental doses at 2- to 5-minute intervals. After a total dose >1 mcg/kg, further therapeutic response is unlikely.
Management of known/suspected opioid overdose: I.V.: Green labeled product (1000 mcg/mL): Initial: 0.5 mg/70 kg; may repeat with 1 mg/70 kg in 2-5 minutes. Further increase beyond a total dose of 1.5 mg/70 kg will not likely result in improved response and may result in cardiovascular stress and precipitated withdrawal syndrome. (If opioid dependency is suspected, administer a challenge dose of 0.1 mg/70 kg; if no withdrawal symptoms are observed in 2 minutes, the recommended doses can be administered).
Recurrence of respiratory depression: If noted, dose may again be titrated to clinical effect using incremental doses.
Loss of I.V. access: If I.V. access is lost or not readily obtainable, a single SubQ or I.M. dose of 1 mg may be effective in 5-15 minutes.
Renal Impairment: Not necessary with single uses, however, slow administration (over 60 seconds) of incremental doses is recommended to minimize hypertension and dizziness.
(Continued)

Nalmefene (Continued)

Hepatic Impairment: Not necessary with single uses, however, slow administration (over 60 seconds) of incremental doses is recommended to minimize hypertension and dizziness.

Administration

I.M.: If I.V. access is lost or not readily obtainable, a single SubQ or I.M. dose of 1 mg may be effective in 5-15 minutes.

I.V.: Slow administration (over 60 seconds) of incremental doses is recommended to minimize hypertension and dizziness.

I.V. Detail: Check dosage strength carefully before use to avoid error. Dilute drug (1:1) with diluent and use smaller doses in patients known to be at increased cardiovascular risk. May be administered via I.M. or SubQ routes if I.V. access is not feasible.

pH: 3.9 (adjusted)

Stability

Compatibility: Stable in D$_5$LR, D$_5$¹/$_2$NS, D$_5$W, LR, sodium bicarbonate 5%, ¹/$_2$NS, NS

Nursing Actions

Physical Assessment: Assess patient for opioid dependency. Monitor vital signs, respiratory, and cardiac status carefully during infusion and for some time thereafter (effects may continue for several days; use nonopioid analgesics for pain).

Patient Education: This drug can only be administered I.V. You may experience drowsiness, dizziness, or blurred vision for several days; use caution when driving or engaging in tasks requiring alertness until response to drug is known. Small frequent meals and good mouth care may reduce any nausea or vomiting. Report yellowing of eyes or skin, unusual bleeding, dark or tarry stools, acute headache, or palpitations. **Breast-feeding precaution:** Consult prescriber if breast-feeding.

Breast-Feeding Issues Limited information available; do not use in lactating women if possible.

Pregnancy Issues Limited information available

Additional Information Proper steps should be used to prevent use of the incorrect dosage strength. The goal of treatment in the postoperative setting is to achieve reversal of excessive opioid effects without inducing a complete reversal and acute pain.

If opioid dependence is suspected, nalmefene should only be used in opioid overdose if the likelihood of overdose is high based on history or the clinical presentation of respiratory depression with concurrent pupillary constriction is present.

Naloxone (nal OKS one)

U.S. Brand Names Narcan® [DSC]

Synonyms N-allylnoroxymorphine Hydrochloride; Naloxone Hydrochloride

Pharmacologic Category Antidote

Medication Safety Issues

Sound-alike/look-alike issues:

Naloxone may be confused with naltrexone

Narcan® may be confused with Marcaine®, Norcuron®

Pregnancy Risk Factor C

Lactation Excretion in breast milk unknown/not recommended

Use

Complete or partial reversal of opioid depression, including respiratory depression, induced by natural and synthetic opioids, including propoxyphene, methadone, and certain mixed agonist-antagonist analgesics: nalbuphine, pentazocine, and butorphanol

Diagnosis of suspected opioid tolerance or acute opioid overdose

Adjunctive agent to increase blood pressure in the management of septic shock

Unlabeled/Investigational Use PCP and ethanol ingestion

Mechanism of Action/Effect Pure opioid antagonist that competes and displaces narcotics at opioid receptor sites

Contraindications Hypersensitivity to naloxone or any component of the formulation

Warnings/Precautions Due to an association between naloxone and acute pulmonary edema, use with caution in patients with cardiovascular disease or in patients receiving medications with potential adverse cardiovascular effects (eg, hypotension, pulmonary edema or arrhythmias). Excessive dosages should be avoided after use of opiates in surgery. Abrupt postoperative reversal may result in nausea, vomiting, sweating, tachycardia, hypertension, seizures, and other cardiovascular events (including pulmonary edema and arrhythmias). May precipitate withdrawal symptoms in patients addicted to opiates, including pain, hypertension, sweating, agitation, irritability; in neonates: shrill cry, failure to feed. Recurrence of respiratory depression is possible if the opioid involved is long-acting; observe patients until there is no reasonable risk of recurrent respiratory depression.

Drug Interactions

Decreased Effect: Decreased effect of narcotic analgesics.

Adverse Reactions Frequency not defined.

Cardiovascular: Hyper-/hypotension, tachycardia, ventricular arrhythmia, cardiac arrest

Central nervous system: Irritability, anxiety, narcotic withdrawal, restlessness, seizure

Gastrointestinal: Nausea, vomiting, diarrhea

Neuromuscular & skeletal: Tremulousness

Respiratory: Dyspnea, pulmonary edema, runny nose, sneezing

Miscellaneous: Diaphoresis

Overdosage/Toxicology Naloxone is the drug of choice for respiratory depression that is known or suspected to be caused by overdose of an opiate or opioid. **Caution:** Naloxone's effects are due to its action on narcotic reversal, not due to any direct effect upon opiate receptors. Therefore, adverse events occur secondarily to reversal (withdrawal) of narcotic analgesia and sedation, which can cause severe reactions.

Pharmacodynamics/Kinetics

Onset of Action: Endotracheal, I.M., SubQ: 2-5 minutes; I.V.: ~2 minutes

Duration of Action: 20-60 minutes; since shorter than that of most opioids, repeated doses are usually needed

Half-Life Elimination: Neonates: 1.2-3 hours; Adults: 1-1.5 hours

Metabolism: Primarily hepatic via glucuronidation

Excretion: Urine (as metabolites)

Available Dosage Forms

Injection, solution, as hydrochloride: 0.4 mg/mL (1 mL, 10 mL)

Narcan®: 0.4 mg/mL (1 mL) [DSC]

Dosing

Adults & Elderly:

Narcotic overdose:

I.V. (preferred), I.M., intratracheal, SubQ: 0.4-2 mg every 2-3 minutes as needed; may need to repeat doses every 20-60 minutes. If no response is observed after 10 mg, question the diagnosis. **Note:** Use 0.1-0.2 mg increments in patients who are opioid dependent and in postoperative patients to avoid large cardiovascular changes.

Continuous infusion: I.V.: If continuous infusion is required, calculate dosage/hour based on effective intermittent dose used and duration of adequate response seen; adult dose typically 0.25-6.25 mg/hour (short-term infusions as high as 2.4 mg/kg/hour have been tolerated in adults during treatment for septic shock); alternatively, continuous infusion utilizes $^2/_3$ of the initial naloxone bolus on an hourly basis; add 10 times this dose to each liter of D_5W and infuse at a rate of 100 mL/hour; $^1/_2$ of the initial bolus dose should be readministered 15 minutes after initiation of the continuous infusion to prevent a drop in naloxone levels; increase infusion rate as needed to assure adequate ventilation

Pediatrics:

Postanesthesia narcotic reversal: I.M., I.V. (preferred), intratracheal, SubQ: Infants and Children: 0.01 mg/kg; may repeat every 2-3 minutes as needed based on response

Narcotic overdose:

I.M., I.V. (preferred), intratracheal, SubQ:

Birth (including premature infants) to 5 years or <20 kg: 0.1 mg/kg; repeat every 2-3 minutes if needed; may need to repeat doses every 20-60 minutes

>5 years or ≥20 kg: 2 mg/dose; if no response, repeat every 2-3 minutes; may need to repeat doses every 20-60 minutes

Continuous infusion: I.V.: Refer to adult dosing.

Administration

I.V.:

I.V. push: Administer over 30 seconds as undiluted preparation

I.V. continuous infusion: Dilute to 4 mcg/mL in D_5W or normal saline

Other: Intratracheal: Dilute to 1-2 mL with normal saline

Stability

Reconstitution: Stable in 0.9% sodium chloride and D_5W at 4 mcg/mL for 24 hours.

Compatibility: Stable in D_5W, NS

Y-site administration: Incompatible with amphotericin B cholesteryl sulfate complex

Storage: Store at 25°C (77°F). Protect from light.

Nursing Actions

Physical Assessment: Assess patient for opioid dependency. Monitor vital signs and cardiorespiratory status continuously during infusion, maintain patent airway.

Patient Education: This drug can only be administered I.V.; if patient is responsive, instructions are individualized. Report respiratory difficulty, palpitations, or tremors. **Breast-feeding precaution:** Breast-feeding is not recommended.

Geriatric Considerations In small trials, naloxone has shown temporary improvement in Alzheimer's disease; however, is not recommended for treatment.

Breast-Feeding Issues No data reported. Since naloxone is used for opiate reversal the concern should be on opiate drug levels in a breast-feeding mother and transfer to the infant rather than naloxone exposure. The safest approach would be **not** to breast-feed.

Pregnancy Issues Consider benefit to the mother and the risk to the fetus before administering to a pregnant woman who is known or suspected to be opioid dependent. May precipitate withdrawal in both the mother and fetus.

Additional Information May contain methyl and propylparabens

Naltrexone (nal TREKS one)

U.S. Brand Names Depade®; ReVia®
Synonyms Naltrexone Hydrochloride
Pharmacologic Category Antidote
Medication Safety Issues
Sound-alike/look-alike issues:
Naltrexone may be confused with naloxone
ReVia® may be confused with Revex®
Pregnancy Risk Factor C
Lactation Excretion in breast milk unknown
Use Treatment of ethanol dependence; blockade of the effects of exogenously administered opioids
Mechanism of Action/Effect Naltrexone (a pure opioid antagonist) is a cyclopropyl derivative of oxymorphone similar in structure to naloxone and nalorphine (a morphine derivative); it acts as a competitive antagonist at opioid receptor sites
Contraindications Hypersensitivity to naltrexone or any component of the formulation; narcotic dependence or current use of opioid analgesics; acute opioid withdrawal; failure to pass Narcan® challenge or positive urine screen for opioids; acute hepatitis; liver failure
Warnings/Precautions Dose-related hepatocellular injury is possible; the margin of separation between the apparent safe and hepatotoxic doses appear to be only fivefold or less. May precipitate withdrawal symptoms in patients addicted to opiates, including pain, hypertension, sweating, agitation, irritability; in neonates; shrill cry, failure to feed. Use with caution in patients with hepatic or renal impairment.

Patients who had been treated with naltrexone may respond to lower opioid doses than previously used. This could result in potentially life-threatening opioid intoxication. Patients should be aware that they may be more sensitive to lower doses of opioids after naltrexone treatment is discontinued. Use of naltrexone does not eliminate or diminish withdrawal symptoms.
Drug Interactions
Decreased Effect: Naltrexone decreases effects of opioid-containing products.
Increased Effect/Toxicity: Lethargy and somnolence have been reported with the combination of naltrexone and thioridazine.
Adverse Reactions
>10%:
Central nervous system: Insomnia, nervousness, headache, low energy
Gastrointestinal: Abdominal cramping, nausea, vomiting
Neuromuscular & skeletal: Arthralgia
1% to 10%:
Central nervous system: Increased energy, feeling down, irritability, dizziness, anxiety, somnolence
Dermatologic: Rash
Endocrine & metabolic: Polydipsia
Gastrointestinal: Diarrhea, constipation
Genitourinary: Delayed ejaculation, impotency
Overdosage/Toxicology Symptoms of overdose include clonic-tonic convulsions and respiratory failure. Patients receiving up to 800 mg/day for 1 week have shown no toxicity. Seizures and respiratory failure have been seen in animals.
Pharmacodynamics/Kinetics
Duration of Action: 50 mg: 24 hours; 100 mg: 48 hours; 150 mg: 72 hours
Time to Peak: Serum: ~60 minutes
Protein Binding: 21%
Half-Life Elimination: 4 hours; 6-β-naltrexol: 13 hours
Metabolism: Extensive first-pass effect to 6-β-naltrexol
Excretion: Primarily urine (as metabolites and unchanged drug)
(Continued)

Naltrexone (Continued)

Available Dosage Forms
Tablet, as hydrochloride: 50 mg

Depade®: 25 mg, 50 mg, 100 mg

ReVia®: 50 mg

Dosing
Adults & Elderly: Opioid dependence or alcoholism (Do not give until patient is opioid-free for 7-10 days as required by urine analysis): Oral: 25 mg; if no withdrawal signs within 1 hour give another 25 mg; maintenance regimen is flexible, variable and individualized (50 mg/day to 100-150 mg 3 times/ week).

Renal Impairment: Use caution.

Hepatic Impairment: Use caution. An increase in naltrexone AUC of approximately five- and 10-fold in patients with compensated or decompensated liver cirrhosis respectively, compared with normal liver function has been reported.

Laboratory Monitoring Periodic LFTs

Nursing Actions
Physical Assessment: Do not use until patient has been opioid-free for 7-10 days. Assess carefully for several days following start of therapy for narcotic withdrawal symptoms or severe adverse reactions. Use non-narcotic analgesics for pain.

Patient Education: This medication will help you achieve abstinence from opiates if taken as directed. Do not increase or change dose. Do not use opiates or any medications not approved by your prescriber during naltrexone therapy. You may experience drowsiness, dizziness, or blurred vision (use caution when driving or engaging in tasks requiring alertness until response to drug is known); abdominal cramping, nausea or vomiting (small frequent meals, frequent mouth care, chewing gum, or sucking lozenges may help); low energy; or decreased sexual function (reversible when drug is discontinued). Report yellowing of skin or eyes, change in color of stool or urine, increased perspiration or chills, acute headache, palpitations, or unusual joint pain. **Pregnancy/ breast-feeding precautions:** Inform prescriber if you are or intend to become pregnant. Consult prescriber if breast-feeding.

Nandrolone (NAN droe lone)

Synonyms Nandrolone Decanoate; Nandrolone Phenpropionate

Restrictions C-III

Pharmacologic Category Androgen

Pregnancy Risk Factor X

Lactation Excretion in breast milk unknown/contraindicated

Use Control of metastatic breast cancer; management of anemia of renal insufficiency

Mechanism of Action/Effect Promotes tissue-building processes, increases production of erythropoietin, causes protein anabolism; increases hemoglobin and red blood cell volume

Contraindications Hypersensitivity to nandrolone or any component of the formulation; carcinoma of breast or prostate; nephrosis; pregnancy; not for use in infants

Warnings/Precautions Monitor diabetic patients carefully. Anabolic steroids may cause peliosis hepatis, liver cell tumors, and blood lipid changes with increased risk of arteriosclerosis. Use with caution in elderly patients, they may be at greater risk for prostatic hyperplasia. Use with caution in patients with cardiac, renal, or hepatic disease or epilepsy.

Drug Interactions
Increased Effect/Toxicity: Nandrolone may increase the effect of oral anticoagulants, insulin, oral hypoglycemic agents, adrenal steroids, or ACTH when taken together.

Lab Interactions Altered glucose tolerance tests

Adverse Reactions
Male:
Postpubertal:
>10%:
Dermatologic: Acne
Endocrine & metabolic: Gynecomastia
Genitourinary: Bladder irritability, priapism
1% to 10%:
Central nervous system: Insomnia, chills
Endocrine & metabolic: Decreased libido, hepatic dysfunction
Gastrointestinal: Nausea, diarrhea
Genitourinary: Prostatic hyperplasia (elderly)
Hematologic: Iron deficiency anemia, suppression of clotting factors
Prepubertal:
>10%:
Dermatologic: Acne
Endocrine & metabolic: Virilism
1% to 10%:
Central nervous system: Chills, insomnia
Dermatologic: Hyperpigmentation
Gastrointestinal: Diarrhea, nausea
Hematologic: Iron deficiency anemia, suppression of clotting
Female:
>10%: Endocrine & metabolic: Virilism
1% to 10%:
Central nervous system: Chills, insomnia
Endocrine & metabolic: Hypercalcemia
Gastrointestinal: Nausea, diarrhea
Hematologic: Iron deficiency anemia, suppression of clotting factors
Hepatic: Hepatic dysfunction

Pharmacodynamics/Kinetics
Onset of Action: 3-6 months

Duration of Action: Up to 30 days

Metabolism: Hepatic

Excretion: Urine

Available Dosage Forms Injection, solution, as decanoate [in sesame oil]: 100 mg/mL (2 mL); 200 mg/mL (1 mL) [contains benzyl alcohol]

Dosing
Adults & Elderly:
Breast cancer, male/female (phenpropionate):
I.M.: 50-100 mg/week
Anemia of renal insufficiency (decanoate): I.M.:
Male: 100-200 mg/week
Female: 50-100 mg/week
Note: Deep I.M. (into gluteal muscle):
Pediatrics: Deep I.M. (into gluteal muscle): Children 2-13 years (decanoate): 25-50 mg every 3-4 weeks

Administration
I.M.: Inject deeply I.M., preferably into the gluteal muscle.

Laboratory Monitoring LFTs on a regular basis

Nursing Actions
Physical Assessment: Use caution in presence of cardiac, renal, or hepatic disease or epilepsy. Assess potential for interactions with other pharmacological agents. Monitor laboratory tests, therapeutic effectiveness (according to purpose of use), and adverse response on a regular basis (adverse reactions may differ according to gender and age). Caution patients with diabetes to monitor serum glucose closely (may increase the effect of hypoglycemic agents). Teach patient possible side effects/appropriate interventions and adverse symptoms to report. **Pregnancy risk factor X:** Determine that patient is not pregnant before starting therapy. Do not give to females of

childbearing age unless patient is capable of complying with barrier contraceptive use.

Patient Education: Do not take any new medication during therapy unless approved by prescriber. This drug can only be given injection. Report immediately any redness, swelling, burning, or pain at injection site. If you have diabetes, monitor serum glucose closely and notify prescriber of significant changes (nandrolone may increase the effect of insulin and oral hypoglycemic agents). May cause nausea or vomiting (small, frequent meals, frequent mouth care, sucking lozenges, or chewing gum may help); diarrhea (buttermilk, boiled milk, yogurt may help). **Male:** acne, swelling of breasts, loss of libido, impotence. **Female:** virilism, menstrual irregularity (usually reversible). Report changes in menstrual pattern; enlarged or painful breasts; deepening of voice or unusual growth of body hair; fluid retention (eg, swelling of ankles, feet, or hands, respiratory difficulty, or sudden weight gain); bladder irritability; unresolved CNS changes (eg, nervousness, chills, insomnia); change in color of urine or stool; yellowing of eyes or skin; unusual bruising or bleeding; or other adverse reactions. **Pregnancy/breast-feeding precautions:** Inform prescriber if you are pregnant. Do not get pregnant during or for 1 month following therapy. Consult prescriber for instruction on appropriate contraceptive measures. This drug may cause severe fetal defects. Do not breast-feed.

Additional Information Both phenpropionate and decanoate are injections in oil.

Naproxen (na PROKS en)

U.S. Brand Names Aleve® [OTC]; Anaprox®; Anaprox® DS; EC-Naprosyn®; Midol® Extended Relief; Naprelan®; Naprosyn®; Pamprin® Maximum Strength All Day Relief [OTC]

Synonyms Naproxen Sodium

Restrictions A medication guide should be dispensed with each prescription. A template for the required MedGuide can be found on the FDA website at: http://www.fda.gov/medwatch/SAFETY/2005/safety05.htm#NSAID

Pharmacologic Category Nonsteroidal Anti-inflammatory Drug (NSAID), Oral

Medication Safety Issues
Sound-alike/look-alike issues:
Naproxen may be confused with Natacyn®, Nebcin®
Aleve® may be confused with Alesse®
Anaprox® may be confused with Anaspaz®, Avapro®
Naprelan® may be confused with Naprosyn®
Naprosyn® may be confused with Naprelan®, Natacyn®, Nebcin®

Pregnancy Risk Factor C/D (3rd trimester)

Lactation Enters breast milk/not recommended (AAP rates "compatible")

Use Management of ankylosing spondylitis, osteoarthritis, and rheumatoid disorders (including juvenile rheumatoid arthritis); acute gout; mild to moderate pain; tendonitis, bursitis; dysmenorrhea; fever, migraine headache

Mechanism of Action/Effect Inhibits prostaglandin synthesis by decreasing the activity of the enzyme, cyclooxygenase, which results in decreased formation of prostaglandin precursors

Contraindications Hypersensitivity to naproxen, aspirin, other NSAIDs, or any component of the formulation; perioperative pain in the setting of coronary artery bypass surgery (CABG); pregnancy (3rd trimester)

Warnings/Precautions NSAIDs are associated with an increased risk of adverse cardiovascular events, including MI, stroke, and new onset or worsening of pre-existing hypertension. Risk may be increased with duration of use or pre-existing cardiovascular

risk-factors or disease. Carefully evaluate individual cardiovascular risk profiles prior to prescribing. Use caution with fluid retention, CHF or hypertension.

Use of NSAIDs can compromise existing renal function. Renal toxicity can occur in patient with impaired renal function, dehydration, heart failure, liver dysfunction, those taking diuretics and ACEI and the elderly. Rehydrate patient before starting therapy. Monitor renal function closely. Naproxen is not recommended for patients with advanced renal disease.

NSAIDs may increase risk of gastrointestinal irritation, ulceration, bleeding, and perforation. These events may occur at any time during therapy and without warning. Use caution with a history of GI disease (bleeding or ulcers), concurrent therapy with aspirin, anticoagulants and/or corticosteroids, smoking, use of alcohol, the elderly or debilitated patients.

Use the lowest effective dose for the shortest duration of time, consistent with individual patient goals, to reduce risk of cardiovascular or GI adverse events. Alternate therapies should be considered for patients at high risk.

NSAIDs may cause serious skin adverse events including exfoliative dermatitis, Stevens-Johnson Syndrome (SJS) and toxic epidermal necrolysis (TEN). Anaphylactoid reactions may occur, even without prior exposure; patients with "aspirin triad" (bronchial asthma, aspirin intolerance, rhinitis) may be at increased risk. Do not use in patients who experience bronchospasm, asthma, rhinitis, or urticaria with NSAID or aspirin therapy.

Use with caution in patients with decreased hepatic function. Closely monitor patients with any abnormal LFT. Severe hepatic reactions (eg, fulminant hepatitis, liver failure) have occurred with NSAID use, rarely; discontinue if signs or symptoms of liver disease develop, or if systemic manifestations occur.

The elderly are at increased risk for adverse effects (especially peptic ulceration, CNS effects, renal toxicity) from NSAIDs even at low doses.

Withhold for at least 4-6 half-lives prior to surgical or dental procedures. Safety and efficacy have not been established in children <2 years of age.

OTC labeling: Prior to self-medication, patients should contact health care provider if they have had recurring stomach pain or upset, ulcers, bleeding problems, high blood pressure, heart or kidney disease, other serious medical problems, are currently taking a diuretic, or are ≥60 years of age. Recommended dosages should not be exceeded, due to an increased risk of GI bleeding. Consuming ≥3 alcoholic beverages/day or taking longer than recommended may increase the risk of GI bleeding. When used for self-medication, patients should be instructed to contact healthcare provider if used for fever lasting >3 days or for pain lasting >10 days in adults or >3 days in children. Not for self-medication (OTC use) in children <12 years of age.

Drug Interactions

Cytochrome P450 Effect: Substrate (minor) of CYP1A2, 2C8/9

Decreased Effect: NSAIDs may decrease the effect of some antihypertensive agents, including ACE inhibitors, angiotensin receptor antagonists, and hydralazine. The efficacy of diuretics (loop and/or thiazide) may be decreased.

Increased Effect/Toxicity: Naproxen could displace other highly protein-bound drugs, increasing the effect of oral anticoagulants, hydantoins, salicylates, sulfonamides, and first-generation sulfonylureas. Naproxen and warfarin may cause a slight increase in free warfarin. Naproxen and probenecid may cause increased levels of naproxen. Naproxen and methotrexate may significantly increase and prolong blood methotrexate concentration, which may be severe or (Continued)

Naproxen *(Continued)*

fatal. May increase lithium or cyclosporine levels. Corticosteroids may increase risk of GI ulceration.

Nutritional/Ethanol Interactions
Ethanol: Avoid ethanol (may enhance gastric mucosal irritation).

Food: Naproxen absorption ratelevels may be decreased if taken with food.

Herb/Nutraceutical: Avoid alfalfa, anise, bilberry, bladderwrack, bromelain, cat's claw, celery, coleus, cordyceps, dong quai, evening primrose, feverfew, fenugreek, garlic, ginger, ginkgo biloboa, red clover, horse chestnut, grapeseed, green tea, ginseng, guggul, horse chestnut seed, horseradish, licorice, prickly ash, red clover, reishi, SAMe, sweet clover, turmeric, white willow (all have additional antiplatelet activity).

Lab Interactions Increased chloride (S), sodium (S), bleeding time

Adverse Reactions 1% to 10%:
Cardiovascular: Edema (3% to 9%), palpitations (<3%)
Central nervous system: Dizziness (3% to 9%), drowsiness (3% to 9%), headache (3% to 9%), lightheadedness (<3%), vertigo (<3%)
Dermatologic: Pruritus (3% to 9%), skin eruption (3% to 9%), rash, ecchymosis (3% to 9%), purpura (<3%)
Endocrine & metabolic: Fluid retention (3% to 9%)
Gastrointestinal: Abdominal pain (3% to 9%), constipation (3% to 9%), nausea (3% to 9%), heartburn (3% to 9%), diarrhea (<3%), dyspepsia (<3%), stomatitis (<3%), heartburn (<3%), flatulence, gross bleeding/perforation, indigestion, ulcers, vomiting
Genitourinary: Abnormal renal function
Hematologic: Hemolysis (3% to 9%), ecchymosis (3% to 9%), anemia, bleeding time increased
Hepatic: LFTS increased
Ocular: Visual disturbances (<3%)
Otic: Tinnitus (3% to 9%), hearing disturbances (<3%)
Respiratory: Dyspnea (3% to 9%)
Miscellaneous: Diaphoresis (<3%), thirst (<3%)

Overdosage/Toxicology Symptoms of overdose include drowsiness, heartburn, vomiting, CNS depression, leukocytosis, and renal failure. Management is supportive and symptomatic. Seizures tend to be very short-lived and often do not require drug treatment.

Pharmacodynamics/Kinetics
Onset of Action: Analgesic: 1 hour; Anti-inflammatory: ~2 weeks; Peak effect: Anti-inflammatory: 2-4 weeks
Duration of Action: Analgesic: ≤7 hours; Anti-inflammatory: ≤12 hours
Time to Peak: Serum: 1-4 hours
Protein Binding: >99%; increased free fraction in elderly
Half-Life Elimination: Normal renal function: 12-17 hours; End-stage renal disease: No change
Excretion: Urine (95%)

Available Dosage Forms
Caplet, as sodium (Aleve®, Midol® Extended Relief, Pamprin® Maximum Strength All Day Relief): 220 mg [equivalent to naproxen 200 mg and sodium 20 mg]
Gelcap, as sodium (Aleve®): 220 mg [equivalent to naproxen 200 mg and sodium 20 mg]
Suspension, oral (Naprosyn®): 125 mg/5 mL (480 mL) [contains sodium 0.3 mEq/mL; orange-pineapple flavor]
Tablet (Naprosyn®): 250 mg, 375 mg, 500 mg
Tablet, as sodium: 220 mg [equivalent to naproxen 200 mg and sodium 20 mg]; 275 mg [equivalent to naproxen 250 mg and sodium 25 mg]; 550 mg [equivalent to naproxen 500 mg and sodium 50 mg]
Aleve®: 220 mg [equivalent to naproxen 200 mg and sodium 20 mg]
Anaprox®: 275 mg [equivalent to naproxen 250 mg and sodium 25 mg]

Anaprox® DS: 550 mg [equivalent to naproxen 500 mg and sodium 50 mg]
Tablet, controlled release, as sodium: 550 mg [equivalent to naproxen 500 mg and sodium 50 mg]
Naprelan®: 421.5 mg [equivalent to naproxen 375 mg and sodium 37.5 mg]; 550 mg [equivalent to naproxen 500 mg and sodium 50 mg]
Tablet, delayed release (EC-Naprosyn®): 375 mg, 500 mg

Dosing
Adults: Note: Dosage expressed as naproxen base; 200 mg naproxen base is equivalent to 220 mg naproxen sodium.
Acute gout: Oral: Initial: 750 mg, followed by 250 mg every 8 hours until attack subsides; **Note:** EC-Naprosyn® is not recommended
Rheumatoid arthritis, osteoarthritis, and ankylosing spondylitis: 500-1000 mg/day in 2 divided doses; may increase to 1.5 g/day of naproxen base for limited time period
Mild-to-moderate pain, dysmenorrhea, acute tendonitis, bursitis: Oral: Initial: 500 mg, then 250 mg every 6-8 hours; maximum: 1250 mg/day naproxen base
OTC labeling: Pain/fever:
Adults ≤65 years: 200 mg naproxen base every 8-12 hours; if needed, may take 400 mg naproxen base for the initial dose; maximum: 600 mg naproxen base/24 hours
Adults >65 years: Refer to elderly dosing.
Elderly: Refer to adult dosing and Geriatric Considerations.
OTC labeling: Pain/fever: Adults >65 years: 200 mg naproxen base every 12 hours
Pediatrics: Note: Dosage expressed as naproxen base; 200 mg naproxen base is equivalent to 220 mg naproxen sodium.
Fever: Oral: Children >2 years: 2.5-10 mg/kg/dose; maximum: 10 mg/kg/day
Juvenile arthritis: Oral: Children >2 years: 10 mg/kg/day in 2 divided doses
OTC labeling: Pain/fever: Oral: Children ≥12 years: Refer to adult dosing.
Renal Impairment: Cl$_{cr}$ <30 mL/minute: use is not recommended

Administration
Oral: Administer with food, milk, or antacids to decrease GI adverse effects
Suspension: Shake suspension well before administration.
Tablet, extended release: Swallow tablet whole; do not break, crush, or chew.

Stability
Storage: Store oral suspension and tablet at 15°C to 30°C (59°F to 86°F).
Laboratory Monitoring Periodic liver function, CBC, BUN, serum creatinine

Nursing Actions
Physical Assessment: Assess effectiveness and interactions of other medications patient may be taking. Monitor blood pressure at the beginning of therapy and periodically during use. Monitor laboratory tests, therapeutic response (eg, relief of pain and inflammation, increased activity tolerance), and adverse reactions (eg, GI effects, hepatotoxicity, or ototoxicity) at beginning of therapy and periodically throughout therapy. Schedule ophthalmic evaluations for patients who develop eye complaints during long-term NSAID therapy. Assess knowledge/teach patient appropriate use, interventions to reduce side effects, and adverse symptoms to report.

Patient Education: Take this medication exactly as directed; do not increase dose without consulting prescriber. Do not crush tablets. Take with food or milk to reduce GI distress. Maintain adequate hydration (2-3 L/day of fluids) unless instructed to restrict fluid intake. Do not use alcohol, aspirin or aspirin-containing medication, or any other anti-inflammatory medications without consulting prescriber. You may experience drowsiness, dizziness, lightheadedness, or headache (use caution when driving or engaging in tasks requiring alertness until response to drug is known); anorexia, nausea, vomiting, or heartburn (small frequent meals, frequent mouth care, sucking lozenges, or chewing gum may help); or fluid retention (weigh yourself weekly and report unusual [3-5 lb/week] weight gain), GI bleeding, ulceration, or perforation can occur with or without pain; or discontinue medication and contact prescriber if persistent abdominal pain or cramping, or blood in stool occurs. Report breathlessness, respiratory difficulty, or unusual cough; chest pain, rapid heartbeat, palpitations; unusual bruising/bleeding; blood in urine, stool, mouth, or vomitus; swollen extremities; skin rash or itching; acute fatigue; or changes in eyesight (double vision, color changes, blurred vision), hearing, or ringing in ears. **Breast-feeding precautions:** Notify prescriber if you are or intend to become pregnant. Do not take this drug during last trimester of pregnancy.

Dietary Considerations Drug may cause GI upset, bleeding, ulceration, perforation; take with food or milk to minimize GI upset.

Geriatric Considerations Elderly are at high risk for adverse effects from NSAIDs. As much as 60% of elderly can develop peptic ulceration and/or hemorrhage asymptomatically. The concomitant use of H_2 blockers, omeprazole, and sucralfate is not effective as prophylaxis with the exception of NSAID-induced duodenal ulcers which may be prevented by the use of ranitidine. Misoprostol is the only prophylactic agent proven effective. Also, concomitant disease and drug use contribute to the risk for GI adverse effects. Use lowest effective dose for shortest period possible. Consider renal function decline with age. Use of NSAIDs can compromise existing renal function especially when Cl_{cr} is ≤30 mL/minute. Tinnitus may be a difficult and unreliable indication of toxicity due to age-related hearing loss or eighth cranial nerve damage. CNS adverse effects such as confusion, agitation, and hallucination are generally seen in overdose or high-dose situations, but elderly may demonstrate these adverse effects at lower doses than younger adults.

Naratriptan (NAR a trip tan)

U.S. Brand Names Amerge®
Synonyms Naratriptan Hydrochloride
Pharmacologic Category Serotonin 5-HT$_{1D}$ Receptor Agonist
Medication Safety Issues
Sound-alike/look-alike issues:
Amerge® may be confused with Altace®, Amaryl®
Pregnancy Risk Factor C
Lactation Excretion in breast milk unknown/use caution
Use Treatment of acute migraine headache with or without aura
Mechanism of Action/Effect The therapeutic effect for migraine is due to serotonin agonist activity.
Contraindications Hypersensitivity to naratriptan or any component of the formulation; cerebrovascular, peripheral vascular disease (ischemic bowel disease), ischemic heart disease (angina pectoris, history of myocardial infarction, or proven silent ischemia); or in patients with symptoms consistent with ischemic heart disease, coronary artery vasospasm, or Prinzmetal's angina; uncontrolled hypertension or patients who have received within 24 hours another 5-HT agonist (sumatriptan, zolmitriptan) or ergotamine-containing product;

patients with known risk factors associated with coronary artery disease; patients with severe hepatic or renal disease (Cl_{cr} <15 mL/minute); do not administer naratriptan to patients with hemiplegic or basilar migraine

Warnings/Precautions Use only if there is a clear diagnosis of migraine. May cause vasospastic reactions resulting in colonic, peripheral, or coronary ischemia. Monitor closely, especially after the first dose. Patients who are at risk of CAD (based on risk factor evaluation) but have had a satisfactory cardiovascular evaluation may receive naratriptan, but extreme caution should be used; administration of the first dose in a setting with medical staff and equipment (ie, in a physician's office) is recommended, and ECG monitoring after the first dose should be considered. Periodically re-evaluate risk factors for CAD in patients receiving long-term intermittent treatment. Blood pressure may increase with the administration of naratriptan. If the patient does not respond to the first dose, re-evaluate the diagnosis of migraine before trying a second dose.

Drug Interactions
Decreased Effect: Smoking increases the clearance of naratriptan.

Increased Effect/Toxicity: Ergot-containing drugs (dihydroergotamine or methysergide) may cause vasospastic reactions when taken with naratriptan. Avoid concomitant use with ergots; separate dose of naratriptan and ergots by at least 24 hours. Oral contraceptives taken with naratriptan reduced the clearance of naratriptan ~30% which may contribute to adverse effects. Selective serotonin reuptake inhibitors (SSRIs) (eg, fluoxetine, fluvoxamine, paroxetine, sertraline) may cause lack of coordination, hyper-reflexia, or weakness and should be avoided when taking naratriptan.

Adverse Reactions 1% to 10%:
Central nervous system: Dizziness, drowsiness, malaise/fatigue
Gastrointestinal: Nausea, vomiting
Neuromuscular & skeletal: Paresthesias
Miscellaneous: Pain or pressure in throat or neck

Pharmacodynamics/Kinetics
Onset of Action: 30 minutes
Time to Peak: 2-3 hours
Protein Binding: Plasma: 28% to 31%
Metabolism: Hepatic via CYP
Excretion: Urine
Available Dosage Forms Tablet: 1 mg, 2.5 mg
Dosing
Adults: Migraine: Oral: 1 mg to 2.5 mg at the onset of headache. It is recommended to use the lowest possible dose to minimize adverse effects. If headache returns or does not fully resolve, the dose may be repeated after 4 hours. Do not exceed 5 mg in 24 hours.
Elderly: Not recommended for use in the elderly.
Renal Impairment:
Cl_{cr} 18-39 mL/minute: Initial: 1 mg; do not exceed 2.5 mg in 24 hours.
Cl_{cr} <15 mL/minute: Do not use.
Hepatic Impairment: Contraindicated in patients with severe liver failure. The maximum dose is 2.5 mg in 24 hours for patients with mild or moderate liver failure. The recommended starting dose is 1 mg.
Administration
Oral: Do **not** crush or chew tablet; swallow whole with water.
Nursing Actions
Physical Assessment: Assess potential for interactions with other pharmacological agents patient may be taking (eg, ergot-containing drugs, SSRIs). Monitor closely, especially after the first dose. Monitor therapeutic effectiveness and adverse response (eg, (Continued)

Naratriptan *(Continued)*

drowsiness, nausea/vomiting, paresthesias, hypertension). Teach patient proper use, possible side effects/appropriate interventions, and adverse symptoms to report.

Patient Education: Do not take any new medication during therapy unless approved by prescriber. Do not crush or chew tablet; swallow whole with water. This drug is to be used to reduce your migraine, not to prevent or reduce the number of attacks. If headache returns or is not fully resolved, the dose may be repeated after 4 hours. If you have no relief with first dose, do not take a second dose without consulting prescriber. **Do not exceed 5 mg in 24 hours. Do not take within 24 hours of any other migraine medication without first consulting prescriber.** May cause dizziness, fatigue, or drowsiness (use caution when driving or engaging in tasks that require alertness until response to drug is known); or nausea or vomiting (small, frequent meals, frequent mouth care, chewing gum, or sucking lozenges may help). Report immediately any chest pain, palpitations, or rapid heartbeat; tightness in throat or neck; or rash, itching, or hives. **Pregnancy/breast-feeding precautions:** Inform prescriber if you are or intend to become pregnant. Breast-feeding is not recommended.

Geriatric Considerations Naratriptan was not studied in patients >65 years of age. Use in elderly patients is not recommended because of the presence of risk factors associated with adverse effects. These include the presence of coronary artery disease, decreased liver or renal function, and the risk of pronounced blood pressure increases.

Natalizumab *(na ta LIZ u mab)*

U.S. Brand Names Tysabri®

Synonyms AN100226; Anti-4 Alpha Integrin; IgG4-Kappa Monoclonal Antibody

Pharmacologic Category Monoclonal Antibody, Selective Adhesion-Molecule Inhibitor

Pregnancy Risk Factor C

Lactation Excretion in breast milk unknown/not recommended

Use Treatment of relapsing forms of multiple sclerosis

Unlabeled/Investigational Use Crohn's disease

Mechanism of Action/Effect Natalizumab inhibits the movement of white blood cells such as T-lymphocytes from the blood into areas of inflamed tissue. Treatment results in decreased frequency of relapse in multiple sclerosis.

Contraindications Hypersensitivity to natalizumab, murine proteins, or any component of the formulation; pregnancy

Warnings/Precautions During clinical studies, ~22% of patients experienced an infusion-related reaction; serious systemic hypersensitivity reactions occurred in <1% of patients. Severe reactions, including anaphylaxis, occur rarely; upon presentation, the infusion should be discontinued immediately. Retreatment is not recommended. Infusion-related reactions may occur more frequently in patients with antibody to natalizumab. Antibody formation (which occurs in about 10% of patients) is associated with a decrease in natalizumab levels and a decrease in the efficacy of natalizumab. Use caution in patients with a history of depression; closely monitor. Safety and efficacy have not been established in chronic progressive multiple sclerosis and in children (<18 years of age).

Drug Interactions

Increased Effect/Toxicity: Concomitant immunosuppressant therapy may increase the risk of infection.

Interferon beta-1a may increase the levels of natalizumab (no dosage adjustment necessary).

Adverse Reactions

>10%:
Central nervous system: Headache (35%), fatigue (24%), depression (17%)
Genitourinary: Urinary tract infection (18%)
Neuromuscular & skeletal: Arthralgia (15%)
Respiratory: Lower respiratory infection (15%)
Miscellaneous: Infusion-related reaction (22%)

1% to 10%:
Cardiovascular: Chest discomfort (4%),
Central nervous system: Syncope (2%), suicidal ideation (1%)
Dermatologic: Rash (9%), dermatitis (5%), pruritus (4%), urticaria (2%)
Endocrine & metabolic: Menstrual irregularities (7%), amenorrhea (2%)
Gastrointestinal: Abdominal discomfort (10%), gastroenteritis (9%), cholelithiasis (1%)
Genitourinary: Urinary frequency (7%), vaginitis (8%)
Hepatic: Transaminase abnormal (5%)
Local: Bleeding at injection site (3%)
Neuromuscular & skeletal: Rigors (3%), tremor (3%)
Respiratory: Tonsillitis (5%), pneumonia (1%)
Miscellaneous: Allergic reaction (7%), infection (2%), anaphylaxis (1%)

Overdosage/Toxicology Safety of doses >300 mg has not been evaluated.

Pharmacodynamics/Kinetics

Half-Life Elimination: 7-15 days

Excretion: Clearance: 11-21 mL/hour

Available Dosage Forms Injection, solution [preservative free]: 300 mg/15 mL (15 mL) [contains polysorbate-80]

Dosing

Adults & Elderly:

Multiple sclerosis: I.V.: 300 mg infused over 1 hour every 4 weeks

Crohn's disease (unlabeled use): I.V.: 3-6 mg/kg, followed by a second infusion 4 weeks later

Renal Impairment: No adjustment recommended.

Hepatic Impairment: Not studied

Administration

I.V.: Solution may be warmed to room temperature prior to administration. Diluted solution should be infused over 1 hour; do not administer by I.V. bolus or push. Patients should be closely monitored for signs and symptoms of hypersensitivity during the infusion and for at least 1 hour after the infusion is complete. The infusion should be discontinued if a reaction occurs, and treatment of the reaction should be instituted. Following infusion, flush line with NS.

I.V. Detail: pH: 6.1

Stability

Reconstitution: Dilute natalizumab 300 mg in NS 100 mL. Gently invert to mix; do not shake.

Storage: Store concentrated solution under refrigeration between 2°C to 8°C (36°F to 46°F). Protect from light. Do not shake or freeze. Following dilution, may store refrigerated for use within up to 8 hours.

Nursing Actions

Physical Assessment: Monitor patient closely for infusion-related reactions (eg, urticaria, dizziness, fever, rash, rigors, pruritus, nausea, flushing, hypotension, dyspnea, chest pain) during and for 1 hour following infusion. If hypersensitivity reaction occurs, promptly discontinue infusion and notify prescriber. See Administration specifics. Monitor patient response (reduction in relapses of MS) and adverse effects (eg, opportunistic infection, excessive fatigue, depression or suicidal ideation). Teach patient/caregiver possible side effects, appropriate interventions, and adverse symptoms to report.

Patient Education: This drug can only be administered by intravenous infusion. You will be monitored closely during and following infusion. Report immediately any skin rash, dizziness, nausea, flushing, difficulty breathing, chest pain or pain, redness, swelling at infusion site. Following infusion, you may experience headache or joint pain (consult prescriber for appropriate analgesic); unusual fatigue (adequate and frequent rest periods may help). Report any signs of urinary tract infection (itching, pain, discolored urine, or frequency of urination); lower respiratory infection (cough, difficulty breathing, chest tightness); chest discomfort or pain; unusual depression or suicidal ideation; or other persistent adverse effects. **Pregnancy/breast-feeding precautions:** Inform prescriber if you are or intend to be pregnant or breast-feed.

Breast-Feeding Issues Immunoglobulin may be excreted in breast milk. Effects on infant are unknown. Manufacturer recommends that consideration be given to discontinuing breast-feeding during treatment.

Nateglinide (na te GLYE nide)

U.S. Brand Names Starlix®
Pharmacologic Category Antidiabetic Agent, Meglitinide Derivative
Pregnancy Risk Factor C
Lactation Excretion in breast milk unknown/not recommended
Use Management of type 2 diabetes mellitus (noninsulin dependent, NIDDM) as monotherapy when hyperglycemia cannot be managed by diet and exercise alone; in combination with metformin or a thiazolidinedione to lower blood glucose in patients whose hyperglycemia cannot be controlled by exercise, diet, or a single agent alone
Mechanism of Action/Effect Increases insulin release from pancreatic beta cells; decreases postprandial hyperglycemia; not a sulfonylurea
Contraindications Hypersensitivity to nateglinide or any component of the formulation; diabetic ketoacidosis, with or without coma (treat with insulin); type 1 diabetes mellitus (insulin dependent, IDDM)
Warnings/Precautions Use with caution in patients with moderate-to-severe hepatic impairment. Use caution in severe renal dysfunction, elderly, malnourished, or patients with adrenal/pituitary dysfunction; may be more susceptible to glucose-lowering effects. All oral hypoglycemic agents are capable of producing hypoglycemia. Proper patient selection, dosage, and instructions to the patients are important to avoid hypoglycemic episodes. It may be necessary to discontinue nateglinide and administer insulin if the patient is exposed to stress (ie, fever, trauma, infection, surgery). Indicated for adjunctive therapy with metformin; not to be used as a substitute for metformin monotherapy. Combination treatment with sulfonylureas is not recommended (no additional benefit). Patients not adequately controlled on oral agents which stimulate insulin release (eg, glyburide) should not be switched to nateglinide or have nateglinide added to therapy. Safety and efficacy in pediatric patients have not been established.
Drug Interactions
Cytochrome P450 Effect: Substrate (major) of CYP2C8/9, 3A4; **Inhibits** CYP2C8/9 (weak)
Decreased Effect: CYP2C8/9 inducers may decrease the levels/effects of nateglinide; example inducers include carbamazepine, phenobarbital, phenytoin, rifampin, rifapentine, and secobarbital. CYP3A4 inducers may decrease the levels/effects of nateglinide; example inducers include aminoglutethimide, carbamazepine, nafcillin, nevirapine, phenobarbital, phenytoin, and rifamycins. Possible decreased hypoglycemic effect may be seen with thiazides, corticosteroids, thyroid products, and sympathomimetic

drugs; monitor glucose closely when agents are initiated, modified, or discontinued.
Increased Effect/Toxicity: CYP2C8/9 inhibitors may increase the levels/effects of nateglinide; example inhibitors include delavirdine, fluconazole, gemfibrozil, ketoconazole, nicardipine, NSAIDs, pioglitazone, and sulfonamides. CYP3A4 inhibitors may increase the levels/effects of nateglinide; example inhibitors include azole antifungals, clarithromycin, diclofenac, doxycycline, erythromycin, imatinib, isoniazid, nefazodone, nicardipine, propofol, protease inhibitors, quinidine, telithromycin, and verapamil. Possible increased hypoglycemic effect may be seen with salicylates, MAO inhibitors, and nonselective beta-adrenergic blocking agents; monitor glucose closely when agents are initiated, modified, or discontinued.
Nutritional/Ethanol Interactions
Ethanol: Avoid ethanol (increased risk of hypoglycemia).
Food: Rate of absorption is decreased and time to T_{max} is delayed when taken with food. Food does not affect AUC. Multiple peak plasma concentrations may be observed if fasting. Not affected by composition of meal.
Adverse Reactions As reported with nateglinide monotherapy:
1% to 10%:
Central nervous system: Dizziness (4%)
Endocrine & metabolic: Hypoglycemia (2%), increased uric acid
Gastrointestinal: Weight gain
Neuromuscular & skeletal: Arthropathy (3%)
Respiratory: Upper respiratory infection (10%)
Miscellaneous: Flu-like symptoms (4%)
Overdosage/Toxicology In case of overdose, hypoglycemic symptoms would be expected. Severe hypoglycemic reactions should be treated with intravenous glucose. Dialysis is not effective.
Pharmacodynamics/Kinetics
Onset of Action: Insulin secretion: ~20 minutes; Peak effect: 1 hour
Duration of Action: 4 hours
Time to Peak: ≤1 hour
Protein Binding: 98%, primarily to albumin
Half-Life Elimination: 1.5 hours
Metabolism: Hepatic via hydroxylation followed by glucuronide conjugation via CYP2C9 (70%) and CYP3A4 (30%) to metabolites
Excretion: Urine (83%, 16% as unchanged drug); feces (10%)
Available Dosage Forms Tablet: 60 mg, 120 mg
Dosing
Adults & Elderly: Management of type 2 diabetes mellitus: Oral: Initial and maintenance dose: 120 mg 3 times/day, 1-30 minutes before meals; may be given alone or in combination with metformin or a thiazolidinedione; patients close to Hb A_{1c} goal may be started at 60 mg 3 times/day
Renal Impairment: No specific dosage adjustment is recommended for patients with mild-to-severe renal disease. Patients on dialysis showed reduced medication exposure and plasma protein binding. Patients with severe renal dysfunction are more susceptible to glucose-lowering effect; use with caution.
Hepatic Impairment: Increased serum levels are seen with mild hepatic insufficiency; no dosage adjustment is needed. Has not been studied in patients with moderate to severe liver disease; use with caution.
Stability
Storage: Store at 25°C (77°F).
Laboratory Monitoring Glucose and Hb A_{1c} levels, lipid profile
(Continued)

Nateglinide *(Continued)*

Nursing Actions

Physical Assessment: Assess potential for interactions with other prescriptions, OTC medications, or herbal products patient may be taking. Monitor laboratory tests, therapeutic effectiveness, and adverse response on a regular basis throughout therapy. Teach patient proper use (or refer patient to diabetic educator), possible side effects/appropriate interventions (eg, importance of adequate hydration), and adverse symptoms to report.

Patient Education: Do not take any new medication during therapy unless approved by prescriber. Take this medication exactly as directed, 1-30 minutes before a meal. If you skip a meal (or add an extra meal),skip a dose for that meal. Do not change dosage or discontinue without first consulting prescriber. Follow dietary and lifestyle recommendations of provider. You will be instructed in signs of hypo- or hyperglycemia by prescriber or diabetic educator; be alert for adverse hypoglycemia (tachycardia, profuse perspiration, tingling of lips and tongue, seizures, or change in sensorium) and follow prescriber's instructions for intervention. Note that unusual strenuous exercise, excessive alcohol intake, or acute reduction in caloric intake may increase risk of hypoglycemia. Persistent nausea or vomiting, or severely decreased dietary intake may increase risk of hyperglycemia. May cause mild side effects during first weeks of therapy (dizziness, weight gain, mild muscle aches or pain, or flu-like symptoms); if these do not diminish, notify prescriber. Report signs of respiratory infection or other persistent adverse effects. **Pregnancy/breast-feeding precautions:** Inform prescriber if you are or intend to become pregnant. Breast-feeding is not recommended.

Dietary Considerations Nateglinide should be taken 1-30 minutes prior to meals. Scheduled dose should not be taken if meal is missed. Dietary modification based on ADA recommendations is a part of therapy. Decreases blood glucose concentration. Hypoglycemia may occur. Must be able to recognize symptoms of hypoglycemia (palpitations, sweaty palms, lightheadedness).

Pregnancy Issues Safety and efficacy in pregnant women have not been established. Do not use during pregnancy. Abnormal blood glucose levels are associated with a higher incidence of congenital abnormalities. Insulin is the drug of choice for the control of diabetes mellitus during pregnancy.

Additional Information An increase in weight was seen in nateglinide monotherapy, which was not seen when used in combination with metformin.

Nedocromil *(ne doe KROE mil)*

U.S. Brand Names Alocril®; Tilade®
Synonyms Nedocromil Sodium
Pharmacologic Category Mast Cell Stabilizer
Pregnancy Risk Factor B
Lactation Excretion in breast milk unknown/use caution
Use
Aerosol: Maintenance therapy in patients with mild to moderate bronchial asthma
Ophthalmic: Treatment of itching associated with allergic conjunctivitis

Mechanism of Action/Effect Inhibits the activation of and mediator release from a variety of inflammatory cell types associated with asthma including eosinophils, neutrophils, macrophages, mast cells, monocytes, and platelets; it inhibits the release of histamine, leukotrienes, and slow-reacting substance of anaphylaxis; it inhibits the development of early and late bronchoconstriction responses to inhaled antigen

Contraindications Hypersensitivity to nedocromil or any component of the formulation

Warnings/Precautions
Aerosol: Safety and efficacy in children <6 years of age have not been established. If systemic or inhaled steroid therapy is at all reduced, monitor patients carefully. Nedocromil is **not** a bronchodilator and, therefore, should not be used for reversal of acute bronchospasm.
Ophthalmic solution: Users of contact lenses should not wear them during periods of symptomatic allergic conjunctivitis

Adverse Reactions
Inhalation aerosol:
>10%: Gastrointestinal: Unpleasant taste
1% to 10%:
Cardiovascular: Chest pain
Central nervous system: Dizziness, dysphonia, headache, fatigue
Dermatologic: Rash
Gastrointestinal: Nausea, vomiting, dyspepsia, diarrhea, abdominal pain, xerostomia, unpleasant taste
Hepatic: Increased ALT
Neuromuscular & skeletal: Arthritis, tremor
Respiratory: Cough, pharyngitis, rhinitis, bronchitis, upper respiratory infection, bronchospasm, increased sputum production
Ophthalmic solution:
>10%:
Central nervous system: Headache (40%)
Gastrointestinal: Unpleasant taste
Ocular: Burning, irritation, stinging
Respiratory: Nasal congestion
1% to 10%:
Ocular: Conjunctivitis, eye redness, photophobia
Respiratory: Asthma, rhinitis

Pharmacodynamics/Kinetics
Duration of Action: Therapeutic effect: 2 hours
Protein Binding: Plasma: 89%
Half-Life Elimination: 1.5-2 hours
Excretion: Urine (as unchanged drug)

Available Dosage Forms
Aerosol for oral inhalation, as sodium (Tilade®): 1.75 mg/activation (16.2 g)
Solution, ophthalmic, as sodium (Alocril®): 2% (5 mL) [contains benzalkonium chloride]

Dosing
Adults & Elderly:
Asthma: Inhalation: 2 inhalations 4 times/day; may reduce dosage to 2-3 times/day once desired clinical response to initial dose is observed. Drug has no known therapeutic systemic activity when delivered by inhalation.
Allergic conjunctivitis: Ophthalmic: 1-2 drops in each eye twice daily
Pediatrics: Children ≥6 years: Refer to adult dosing.

Stability
Storage: Store at 2°C to 30°C/36°F to 86°F. Do not freeze.

Nursing Actions

Physical Assessment: Not for use during acute bronchospasm. Monitor effectiveness of therapy and adverse reactions at beginning of therapy and periodically with long-term use. Assess knowledge/teach patient appropriate use, interventions to reduce side effects, and adverse symptoms to report.

Patient Education: Aerosol: Do not use during acute bronchospasm. Use exactly as directed; do not use more often than instructed or discontinue without consulting prescriber. You may experience drowsiness, dizziness, fatigue, especially during early therapy (use caution when driving or engaging in tasks requiring alertness until response to drug is known); dry mouth, nausea, or vomiting (small frequent meals, frequent mouth care, chewing gum, or sucking lozenges may help). Report persistent runny nose, cough, cold symptoms; unresolved GI effects; skin rash; joint pain or tremor; or if breathing difficulty persists or worsens. **Breast-feeding precaution:** Consult prescriber if breast-feeding.

Inhaler: Review use with prescriber or follow package insert for directions. Prime with 3 activations prior to first use or if unused more than 7 days. Keep inhaler clean and unobstructed. Always rinse mouth and throat after use of inhaler to prevent advantageous infection. If you are also using a steroid bronchodilator, wait 10 minutes before using this aerosol.

Ophthalmic: Do not wear contact lenses with allergic conjunctivitis. For the eye only. Open eyes, look up, and pull lower lid down. Squeeze medicine into lower eyelid and close eye. Do not touch bottle tip to eye, eyelid, or other skin.

Geriatric Considerations Elderly may have difficulty using inhaler delivery system, especially if they have physical or medical impairment (eg, Parkinson's disease, stroke). If this prophylactic modality is desired but patient cannot tolerate nedocromil inhalations, consider cromolyn sodium solution for nebulizer use.

Additional Information Nedocromil has no known therapeutic systemic activity when delivered by inhalation.

Nefazodone (nef AY zoe done)

Synonyms Nefazodone Hydrochloride; Serzone

Restrictions A medication guide concerning the use of antidepressants in children and teenagers can be found on the FDA website at http://www.fda.gov/cder/Offices/ODS/labeling.htm. It should be dispensed to parents or guardians of children and teenagers receiving this medication.

Pharmacologic Category Antidepressant, Serotonin Reuptake Inhibitor/Antagonist

Medication Safety Issues
Sound-alike/look-alike issues:
Serzone® may be confused with selegiline, Serentil®, Seroquel®, sertraline

Pregnancy Risk Factor C

Lactation Enters breast milk/not recommended

Use Treatment of depression

Unlabeled/Investigational Use Post-traumatic stress disorder

Mechanism of Action/Effect Inhibits neuronal reuptake of serotonin and norepinephrine; also blocks 5-HT$_2$ and alpha$_1$ receptors; has no significant affinity for alpha$_2$, beta-adrenergic, 5-HT$_{1A}$, cholinergic, dopaminergic, or benzodiazepine receptors

Contraindications Hypersensitivity to nefazodone, related compounds (phenylpiperazines), or any component of the formulation; liver injury due to previous nefazodone treatment, active liver disease, or elevated serum transaminases; concurrent use or use of MAO inhibitors within previous 14 days; use in a patient during the acute recovery phase of MI; concurrent use with carbamazepine, cisapride, or pimozide; concurrent therapy with triazolam or alprazolam is generally contraindicated (dosage must be reduced by 75% for triazolam and 50% for alprazolam; such reductions may not be possible with available dosage forms).

Warnings/Precautions Antidepressants increase the risk of suicidal thinking and behavior in children and adolescents with major depressive disorder (MDD) and other depressive disorders; consider risk prior to prescribing. All patients must be closely monitored for clinical worsening, suicidality, or unusual changes in behavior, especially during the initiation of therapy or following an increase or decrease in dosage. When used in children, the child's family or caregiver should be instructed to closely observe the patient and communicate condition with healthcare provider. A medication

guide should be dispensed with each prescription. **Nefazodone is not FDA approved for use in children.**

The possibility of a suicide attempt is inherent in major depression and may persist until remission occurs. Use caution in high-risk patients. Worsening depression and severe abrupt suicidality that are not part of the presenting symptoms may require discontinuation or modification of drug therapy. The patient's family or caregiver should be alerted to monitor patients for the emergence of suicidality and associated behaviors (such as agitation, irritability, hostility, impulsivity, and hypomania) and call healthcare provider.

May worsen psychosis in some patients or precipitate a shift to mania or hypomania in patients with bipolar disorder. Patients presenting with depressive symptoms should be screened for bipolar disorder. Monotherapy in patients with bipolar disorder should be avoided. **Nefazodone is not FDA approved for the treatment of bipolar depression.**

Cases of life-threatening hepatic failure have been reported (risk should be considered when choosing an agent for the treatment of depression); discontinue if clinical signs or symptoms suggest liver failure. May cause sedation, resulting in impaired performance of tasks requiring alertness (eg, operating machinery or driving). May increase the risks associated with electroconvulsive therapy. Consider discontinuing, when possible, prior to elective surgery. Therapy should not be abruptly discontinued in patients receiving high doses for prolonged periods. Rare reports of priapism have occurred. The incidence of sexual dysfunction with nefazodone is generally lower than with SSRIs.

The risk of sedation, conduction disturbances, orthostatic hypotension, or anticholinergic effects are very low relative to other antidepressants. Use with caution in patients with a history of cardiovascular disease (including previous MI, stroke, tachycardia, or conduction abnormalities). Use with caution in patients with urinary retention, benign prostatic hyperplasia, narrow-angle glaucoma, xerostomia, visual problems, constipation, or history of bowel obstruction (due to anticholinergic effects).

Use caution in patients with a previous seizure disorder or condition predisposing to seizures such as brain damage, alcoholism, or concurrent therapy with other drugs which lower the seizure threshold. Use with caution in patients with renal dysfunction and in elderly patients.

Drug Interactions

Cytochrome P450 Effect: Substrate (major) of CYP2D6, 3A4; **Inhibits** CYP1A2 (weak), 2B6 (weak), 2D6 (weak), 3A4 (strong)

Decreased Effect: Carbamazepine may reduce serum concentrations of nefazodone; concurrent administration should be avoided. The levels/effects of nefazodone may be decreased by aminoglutethimide, nafcillin, nevirapine, phenobarbital, phenytoin, and rifamycins and other CYP3A4 inducers.

Increased Effect/Toxicity: Concurrent use of carbamazepine, cisapride, or pimozide is contraindicated. Concurrent therapy with triazolam or alprazolam is generally contraindicated (dosage must be reduced by 75% for triazolam and 50% for alprazolam; such reductions may not be possible with available dosage forms). Concurrent use of ergot alkaloids and/or selected HMG-CoA reductase inhibitors (lovastatin and simvastatin) is generally contraindicated with strong CYP3A4 inhibitors.

Concurrent use of MAO inhibitors may lead to serotonin syndrome; avoid concurrent use or use within 14 days (includes phenelzine, isocarboxazid, and linezolid). Selegiline may increase the risk of serotonin syndrome, particularly at higher doses (>10 mg/day, where selectivity for MAO type B is decreased). (Continued)

Nefazodone *(Continued)*

Theoretically, concurrent use of buspirone, meperidine, serotonin agonists (sumatriptan and rizatriptan), SSRIs, and venlafaxine may result in serotonin syndrome.

Nefazodone may increase the serum levels/effects of antiarrhythmics (amiodarone, lidocaine, propafenone, quinidine), some antipsychotics (clozapine, haloperidol, mesoridazine, quetiapine, and risperidone), some benzodiazepines (triazolam is contraindicated; decrease alprazolam dose by 50%), buspirone (limit buspirone dose to <2.5 mg/day), Nefazodone may increase the levels/effects of calcium channel blockers, cyclosporine, mirtazapine, nateglinide, nefazodone, quinidine, sildenafil (and other PDE-5 inhibitors), tacrolimus, venlafaxine, and other CYP3A4 substrates. When used with strong CYP3A4 inhibitors, dosage adjustment/limits are recommended for sildenafil and other PDE-5 inhibitors; refer to individual monographs.

The levels/effects of nefazodone may be increased by azole antifungals, chlorpromazine, clarithromycin, delavirdine, diclofenac, doxycycline, erythromycin, fluoxetine, imatinib, isoniazid, miconazole, nicardipine, paroxetine, pergolide, propofol, protease inhibitors, quinidine, quinine, ritonavir, ropinirole, telithromycin, verapamil, and other CYP2D6 or 3A4 inhibitors.

Nutritional/Ethanol Interactions

Ethanol: Avoid ethanol (may increase CNS depression).

Food: Nefazodone absorption may be delayed and bioavailability may be decreased if taken with food.

Herb/Nutraceutical: Avoid valerian, St John's wort, SAMe, kava kava (may increase risk of serotonin syndrome and/or excessive sedation).

Adverse Reactions

>10%:

Central nervous system: Headache, drowsiness, insomnia, agitation, dizziness

Gastrointestinal: Xerostomia, nausea, constipation

Neuromuscular & skeletal: Weakness

1% to 10%:

Cardiovascular: Bradycardia, hypotension, peripheral edema, postural hypotension, vasodilation

Central nervous system: Chills, fever, incoordination, lightheadedness, confusion, memory impairment, abnormal dreams, decreased concentration, ataxia, psychomotor retardation, tremor

Dermatologic: Pruritus, rash

Endocrine & metabolic: Breast pain, impotence, libido decreased

Gastrointestinal: Gastroenteritis, vomiting, dyspepsia, diarrhea, increased appetite, thirst, taste perversion

Genitourinary: Urinary frequency, urinary retention

Hematologic: Hematocrit decreased

Neuromuscular & skeletal: Arthralgia, hypertonia, paresthesia, neck rigidity, tremor

Ocular: Blurred vision (9%), abnormal vision (7%), eye pain, visual field defect

Otic: Tinnitus

Respiratory: Bronchitis, cough, dyspnea, pharyngitis

Miscellaneous: Flu syndrome, infection

Overdosage/Toxicology

Symptoms of overdose include drowsiness, vomiting, hypotension, tachycardia, incontinence, and coma. Following initiation of essential overdose management, toxic symptoms should be treated.

Pharmacodynamics/Kinetics

Onset of Action: Therapeutic: Up to 6 weeks

Time to Peak: Serum: 1 hour, prolonged in presence of food

Half-Life Elimination: Parent drug: 2-4 hours; active metabolites persist longer

Metabolism: Hepatic to three active metabolites: Triazoledione, hydroxynefazodone, and m-chlorophenylpiperazine (mCPP)

Excretion: Primarily urine (as metabolites); feces

Available Dosage Forms Tablet, as hydrochloride: 50 mg, 100 mg, 150 mg, 200 mg, 250 mg

Dosing

Adults: Depression: Oral: 200 mg/day, administered in two divided doses initially, with a range of 300-600 mg/day in two divided doses thereafter.

Elderly: Oral: Initial: 50 mg twice daily; increase dose to 100 mg twice daily in 2 weeks; usual maintenance dose: 200-400 mg/day

Pediatrics: Children and Adolescents: Depression (unlabeled use): Oral: Target dose: 300-400 mg/day (mean: 3.4 mg/kg)

Administration

Oral: Dosing after meals may decrease lightheadedness and postural hypotension, but may also decrease absorption and therefore effectiveness.

Stability

Storage: Store at room temperature, below 40°C (104°F) in a tight container.

Laboratory Monitoring If AST/ALT increase >3 times ULN, the drug should be discontinued and not reintroduced.

Nursing Actions

Physical Assessment: Assess other medications patient may be taking for effectiveness and interactions. Monitor therapeutic response (ie, mental status, mood, affect, suicidal ideation), and adverse reactions at beginning of therapy and periodically with long-term use. Monitor for clinical worsening and suicidal ideation. Taper dosage slowly when discontinuing. Assess knowledge/teach patient appropriate use, interventions to reduce side effects, and adverse symptoms to report.

Patient Education: Take exactly as directed; do not increase dose or frequency. It may take 2-3 weeks to achieve desired results. Avoid alcohol, caffeine, and other prescription or OTC medications not approved by prescriber. Maintain adequate hydration (2-3 L/day of fluids) unless instructed to restrict fluid intake. You may experience drowsiness, dizziness, or lightheadedness (use caution when driving or engaging in tasks requiring alertness until response to drug is known); nausea or vomiting (small frequent meals, frequent mouth care, chewing gum, or sucking lozenges may help); or orthostatic hypotension (use caution when climbing stairs or changing position from lying or sitting to standing). Report persistent insomnia or excessive daytime sedation; suicidal ideation; muscle cramping, tremors, weakness, tiredness, or change in gait; chest pain, palpitations, or rapid heartbeat; vision changes or eye pain; respiratory difficulty or breathlessness; malaise, loss of appetite, GI complaints, abdominal pain, or blood in stool; yellowing of skin or eyes (jaundice); or worsening of condition. Pregnancy/breast-feeding precautions: Inform prescriber if you are or intend to become pregnant. Breast-feeding is not recommended.

Geriatric Considerations Data on nefazodone in the elderly is limited, specifically regarding efficacy. Clinical trials in adult patients have found it superior to placebo and similar to imipramine. Nefazodone's C_{max} and AUC have been reported to be increased twofold in the elderly and women after a single dose compared to younger patients, however, these differences were markedly reduced with multiple dosing.

Breast-Feeding Issues Drowsiness, lethargy, poor feeding, and failure to maintain body temperature have been reported in a nursing infant.

Additional Information May cause less sexual dysfunction than other antidepressants. Women and elderly receiving single doses attain significant higher peak concentrations than male volunteers.

Related Information
Antidepressant Medication Guidelines *on page 1414*

Nelfinavir (nel FIN a veer)

U.S. Brand Names Viracept®
Synonyms NFV
Pharmacologic Category Antiretroviral Agent, Protease Inhibitor
Medication Safety Issues
Sound-alike/look-alike issues:
Nelfinavir may be confused with nevirapine
Viracept® may be confused with Viramune®
Pregnancy Risk Factor B
Lactation Excretion in breast milk unknown/contraindicated
Use In combination with other antiretroviral therapy in the treatment of HIV infection
Mechanism of Action/Effect Inhibits HIV-1 protease enzyme; inhibition of the viral protease prevents cleavage of the gag-pol polyprotein resulting in the production of immature, noninfectious virions; cross-resistance with other protease inhibitors is possible, although, not known at this time
Contraindications Hypersensitivity to nelfinavir or any component of the formulation; concurrent therapy with amiodarone, ergot derivatives, midazolam, pimozide, quinidine, triazolam; additional medications which should not be coadministered (per manufacturer) include lovastatin and simvastatin
Warnings/Precautions Nelfinavir is hepatically metabolized and has multiple drug interactions. A listing of medications that should not be used is available with each bottle and patients should be provided with this information. Use caution with hepatic impairment. Warn patients that redistribution of body fat can occur. New onset diabetes mellitus, exacerbation of diabetes, and hyperglycemia have been reported in HIV-infected patients receiving protease inhibitors. Immune reconstitution syndrome has been reported; may require additional evaluation and treatment. The oral powder contains phenylalanine; use caution in patients with phenylketonuria.
Drug Interactions
Cytochrome P450 Effect: Substrate of CYP2C8/9 (minor), 2C19 (major), 2D6 (minor), 3A4 (major); **Inhibits** CYP1A2 (weak), 2B6 (weak), 2C8/9 (weak), 2C19 (weak), 2D6 (weak), 3A4 (strong)
Decreased Effect: The levels/effects of nelfinavir may be decreased by aminoglutethimide, carbamazepine, nafcillin, nevirapine, phenobarbital, phenytoin, rifamycins, or other inducers of CYP2C19 or 3A4. Nelfinavir effects may be decreased by St John's wort. Nelfinavir may decrease the effects of delavirdine, methadone, and oral contraceptives
Increased Effect/Toxicity: Nelfinavir effects may be increased by azithromycin, delavirdine, and protease inhibitors. Nelfinavir may increase the levels/effects of selected benzodiazepines, calcium channel blockers, corticosteroids (eg, fluticasone), cyclosporine, mirtazapine, nateglinide, nefazodone, quinidine, sildenafil (and other PDE-5 inhibitors), tacrolimus, venlafaxine, and other CYP3A4 substrates. Selected benzodiazepines (midazolam, triazolam), cisapride, ergot alkaloids, selected HMG-CoA reductase inhibitors (lovastatin and simvastatin), and pimozide are generally contraindicated with strong CYP3A4 inhibitors. When used with strong CYP3A4 inhibitors, dosage adjustment/limits are recommended for sildenafil and other PDE-5 inhibitors; refer to individual monographs.
Nutritional/Ethanol Interactions
Food: Nelfinavir taken with food increases plasma concentration time curve (AUC) by two- to threefold.

Do not administer with acidic food or juice (orange juice, apple juice, or applesauce) since the combination may have a bitter taste.
Herb/Nutraceutical: St John's wort may decrease nelfinavir serum concentrations; avoid concurrent use.
Adverse Reactions
>10%: Gastrointestinal: Diarrhea
2% to 10%:
Dermatologic: Rash
Gastrointestinal: Nausea, flatulence
Hematologic: Abnormal creatine kinase, hemoglobin, lymphocytes, neutrophils
Hepatic: Abnormal ALT, AST
Overdosage/Toxicology Limited data available; however, unabsorbed drug should be removed via gastric lavage and activated charcoal; significant symptoms beyond gastrointestinal disturbances are likely following acute overdose; hemodialysis will not be effective due to high protein binding of nelfinavir
Pharmacodynamics/Kinetics
Time to Peak: Serum: 2-4 hours
Protein Binding: 98%
Half-Life Elimination: 3.5-5 hours
Metabolism: Hepatic via CYP2C19 and 3A4; major metabolite has activity comparable to parent drug
Excretion: Feces (98% to 99%, 78% as metabolites, 22% as unchanged drug); urine (1% to 2%)
Available Dosage Forms
Powder, oral: 50 mg/g (144 g) [contains phenylalanine 11.2 mg/g]
Tablet: 250 mg, 625 mg
Dosing
Adults & Elderly: HIV infection: Oral: 750 mg 3 times/day with meals or 1250 mg twice daily with meals in combination with other antiretroviral therapies
Pediatrics: HIV infection: Oral: Children 2-13 years: 45-55 mg/kg twice daily **or** 25-35 mg/kg 3 times/day (maximum: 2500 mg/day); all doses should be taken with a meal. If tablets are unable to be taken, use oral powder in small amount of water, milk, formula, or dietary supplements; do not use acidic food/juice or store for >6 hours.
Renal Impairment: No adjustment is necessary.
Hepatic Impairment: Use caution.
Administration
Oral: Mix powder or tablets in a small amount of water, milk, formula, soy milk, soy formula, or dietary supplement. Be sure entire contents is consumed to receive full dose. Do not use acidic food/juice to dilute due to bitter taste. One mixed, solution should be used immediately, but may be stored for up to 6 hours if refrigerated.
Stability
Storage: Store at room temperature of 15°C to 30°C (59°F to 86°F). Oral powder (or dissolved tablets) diluted in nonacidic liquid is stable for 6 hours under refrigeration.
Laboratory Monitoring Liver function tests, blood glucose levels, CBC with differential, CD4 cell count, plasma levels of HIV RNA
Nursing Actions
Physical Assessment: Assess potential for interactions with other pharmacological agents and herbal products patient may be taking. A list of medications that should not be used is available in each bottle and patients should be provided with this information. Monitor laboratory tests, patient response, and adverse reactions (eg, gastrointestinal disturbance, nausea, vomiting, diarrhea that can lead to dehydration and weight loss; hyperlipidemia and redistribution of body fat; rash; CNS effects, malaise, insomnia, abnormal thinking; electrolyte imbalance) at regular intervals during therapy. Teach patient proper use (eg, timing of multiple medications and drugs that should not be used concurrently), possible side (Continued)

Nelfinavir (Continued)

effects/appropriate interventions (eg, use of barrier contraceptives, protease inhibitors may decrease effectiveness of oral contraceptives), and adverse symptoms to report.

Patient Education: You will be provided with a list of specific medications that should not be used during therapy; do not take any new prescription, over-the-counter medications, or herbal products (even if they are not on the list) without consulting prescriber. This is not a cure for HIV, nor has it been found to reduce transmission of HIV; use appropriate precautions to prevent spread to other persons. Take exactly as directed with food. Mix powder with nonacid, noncitric fluids (orange juice, apple juice, or applesauce) and do not store reconstituted powder mixture for longer than 6 hours. If unable to swallow tablets whole, the tablet may be dissolved in water or crushed in food. Mixed or dissolved tablets must be consumed within 6 hours. If you miss a dose, take as soon as possible and return to your regular schedule (never take a double dose). This medication will be prescribed with a combination of other medications; time these medications as directed by prescriber. You may be advised to check your glucose levels; this class of drugs can cause hyperglycemia. Frequent blood tests may be required with prolonged therapy. You may be susceptible to infection (avoid crowds and exposure to known infections and do not have any vaccinations without consulting prescriber). May cause body changes due to redistribution of body fat, facial atrophy, or breast enlargement (normal effects of drug); headache, dizziness, or fatigue (use caution when driving or engaging in potentially hazardous tasks until response to drug is known); nausea or vomiting (small frequent meals, frequent mouth care, chewing gum, or sucking lozenges may help); diarrhea (buttermilk, boiled milk, or yogurt may help); back pain; or arthralgia (consult prescriber for approved analgesic). Inform prescriber if you experience muscle numbness or tingling; unresolved, persistent vomiting, diarrhea, or abdominal pain; respiratory difficulty or chest pain; unusual skin rash; change in color of stool or urine; or any persistent adverse effects. **Pregnancy/breast-feeding precautions:** Inform prescriber if you are or intend to become pregnant. Effectiveness of oral contraceptives may be decreased; use of alternative (nonhormonal) forms of contraception is recommended; consult prescriber for appropriate contraceptives. Do not breast-feed.

Dietary Considerations Should be taken as scheduled with food. Oral powder contains phenylalanine 11.2 mg/g.

Breast-Feeding Issues Nelfinavir is minimally excreted in breast milk. HIV-infected mothers are discouraged from breast-feeding to decrease potential transmission of HIV.

Pregnancy Issues The Perinatal HIV Guidelines Working Group recommends nelfinavir as the preferred PI in combination regimens during pregnancy, especially with HAART for perinatal prophylaxis. A dose of 1250 mg twice daily has been shown to provide adequate plasma levels; 750 mg 3 times/day produced low and variable levels. Pregnancy and protease inhibitors are both associated with an increased risk of hyperglycemia. Glucose levels should be closely monitored. Health professionals are encouraged to contact the antiretroviral pregnancy registry to monitor outcomes of pregnant women exposed to antiretroviral medications (1-800-258-4263 or www.APRegistry.com).

Neomycin (nee oh MYE sin)

U.S. Brand Names Neo-Fradin™; Neo-Rx
Synonyms Neomycin Sulfate
Pharmacologic Category Ammonium Detoxicant; Antibiotic, Aminoglycoside; Antibiotic, Topical
Medication Safety Issues
Sound-alike/look-alike issues:
Myciguent may be confused with Mycitracin®
Pregnancy Risk Factor D
Lactation Excretion in breast milk unknown
Use Orally to prepare GI tract for surgery; topically to treat minor skin infections; treatment of diarrhea caused by *E. coli*; adjunct in the treatment of hepatic encephalopathy; bladder irrigation; ocular infections
Mechanism of Action/Effect Interferes with bacterial protein synthesis by binding to 30S ribosomal subunits
Contraindications Hypersensitivity to neomycin or any component of the formulation, or other aminoglycosides; intestinal obstruction
Warnings/Precautions Use with caution in patients with renal impairment, pre-existing hearing impairment (ototoxicity), neuromuscular disorders. Topical neomycin is a contact sensitizer with sensitivity occurring in 5% to 15% of patients treated with the drug. Symptoms include itching, reddening, edema, and failure to heal. Do not use as peritoneal lavage.
Drug Interactions
Decreased Effect: May decrease GI absorption of digoxin and methotrexate.
Increased Effect/Toxicity: Oral neomycin may potentiate the effects of oral anticoagulants. Neomycin may increase the adverse effects with other neurotoxic, ototoxic, or nephrotoxic drugs.
Adverse Reactions
Oral: >10%: Gastrointestinal: Nausea, diarrhea, vomiting, irritation or soreness of the mouth or rectal area
Topical: >10%: Dermatologic: Contact dermatitis
Overdosage/Toxicology Symptoms of overdose (rare due to poor oral bioavailability) include ototoxicity, nephrotoxicity, and neuromuscular toxicity. The treatment of choice following a single acute overdose appears to be maintenance of urine output of at least 3 mL/kg/hour during the acute treatment phase. Dialysis is of questionable value in enhancing aminoglycoside elimination. If required, hemodialysis is preferred over peritoneal dialysis in patients with normal renal function. Chelation with penicillin may be of benefit.
Pharmacodynamics/Kinetics
Time to Peak: Serum: Oral: 1-4 hours
Half-Life Elimination: Age and renal function dependent: 3 hours
Metabolism: Slightly hepatic
Excretion: Feces (97% of oral dose as unchanged drug); urine (30% to 50% of absorbed drug as unchanged drug)
Available Dosage Forms
Powder, micronized, as sulfate [for prescription compounding] (Neo-Rx): (10 g, 100 g)
Solution, oral, as sulfate (Neo-Fradin™): 125 mg/5 mL (60 mL, 480 mL) [contains benzoic acid; cherry flavor]
Tablet, as sulfate: 500 mg
Dosing
Adults & Elderly:
Dermatologic infections: Topical: Topical solutions containing 0.1% to 1% neomycin have been used for irrigation
Preoperative intestinal antisepsis: Oral: 1 g each hour for 4 doses then 1 g every 4 hours for 5 doses; or 1 g at 1 PM, 2 PM, and 11 PM on day preceding surgery as an adjunct to mechanical cleansing of the bowel and oral erythromycin; or 6 g/day divided every 4 hours for 2-3 days

Hepatic encephalopathy: Oral: 500-2000 mg every 6-8 hours or 4-12 g/day divided every 4-6 hours for 5-6 days

Chronic hepatic insufficiency: Oral: 4 g/day for an indefinite period

Pediatrics:

Preoperative intestinal antisepsis: Oral: Children: 90 mg/kg/day divided every 4 hours for 2 days; or 25 mg/kg at 1 PM, 2 PM, and 11 PM on the day preceding surgery as an adjunct to mechanical cleansing of the intestine and in combination with erythromycin base

Hepatic encephalopathy: Oral: Children: 50-100 mg/kg/day in divided doses every 6-8 hours or 2.5-7 g/m^2/day divided every 4-6 hours for 5-6 days not to exceed 12 g/day

Dermatologic infections: Topical: Children: Refer to adult dosing.

Laboratory Monitoring Renal function; perform culture and sensitivity prior to initiating therapy.

Nursing Actions

Physical Assessment: Assess effectiveness and interactions of other medications patient may be taking. Monitor effectiveness of therapy, laboratory tests, and adverse response (eg, ototoxicity, nephrotoxicity, neurotoxicity). Assess knowledge/teach patient appropriate use (application of cream/ointment), possible side effects/interventions, and adverse symptoms to report. Minimal absorption across GI mucosa or skin surfaces, however with ulceration, open or burned surfaces (especially large surfaces) absorption is possible.

Patient Education: Oral: Take as directed. Maintain adequate hydration (2-3 L/day of fluids) unless instructed to restrict fluid intake. You may experience nausea or vomiting (small frequent meals, frequent mouth care, sucking lozenges, or chewing gum may help); constipation (increased exercise, fluids, fruit, or fiber may help, or consult prescriber); or diarrhea (buttermilk, boiled milk, or yogurt may help). Report immediately any change in hearing; ringing or sense of fullness in ears; persistent diarrhea; changes in voiding patterns; or numbness, tingling, or pain in any extremity. **Pregnancy/breast-feeding precautions:** Inform prescriber if you are or intend to become pregnant. Consult prescriber if breast-feeding.

Neomycin and Polymyxin B
(nee oh MYE sin & pol i MIKS in bee)

U.S. Brand Names Neosporin® G.U. Irrigant

Synonyms Polymyxin B and Neomycin

Pharmacologic Category Antibiotic, Topical

Pregnancy Risk Factor C/D (for G.U. irrigant)

Lactation Excretion in breast milk unknown

Use Short-term as a continuous irrigant or rinse in the urinary bladder to prevent bacteriuria and gram-negative rod septicemia associated with the use of indwelling catheters; to help prevent infection in minor cuts, scrapes, and burns

Available Dosage Forms Solution, irrigant: Neomycin 40 mg and polymyxin B sulfate 200,000 units per mL (1 mL, 20 mL)

Dosing

Adults & Elderly: Bladder irrigation: **Not for I.V. injection**; add 1 mL irrigant to 1 liter isotonic saline solution and connect container to the inflow of lumen of 3-way catheter. Continuous irrigant or rinse in the urinary bladder for up to a maximum of 10 days with administration rate adjusted to patient's urine output; usually no more than 1 L of irrigant is used per day.

Pediatrics: Refer to adult dosing.

Nursing Actions

Physical Assessment: See individual agents.

Patient Education: See individual agents. **Pregnancy/breast-feeding precautions:** Inform prescriber if you are or intend to become pregnant. Consult prescriber if breast-feeding.

Related Information
Neomycin *on page 872*
Polymyxin B *on page 1005*

Neomycin, Colistin, Hydrocortisone, and Thonzonium
(nee oh MYE sin, koe LIS tin, hye droe KOR ti sone, & thon ZOE nee um)

U.S. Brand Names Coly-Mycin® S; Cortisporin®-TC

Synonyms Colistin, Neomycin, Hydrocortisone, and Thonzonium; Hydrocortisone, Neomycin, Colistin, and Thonzonium; Thonzonium, Neomycin, Colistin, and Hydrocortisone

Pharmacologic Category Antibiotic/Corticosteroid, Otic

Use Treatment of superficial and susceptible bacterial infections of the external auditory canal; for treatment of susceptible bacterial infections of mastoidectomy and fenestration cavities

Available Dosage Forms Suspension, otic [drops]:

Coly-Mycin® S: Neomycin 0.33%, colistin 0.3%, hydrocortisone acetate 1%, and thonzonium bromide 0.05% (5 mL) [contains thimerosal; packaged with dropper]

Cortisporin®-TC: Neomycin 0.33%, colistin 0.3%, hydrocortisone acetate 1%, and thonzonium bromide 0.05% (10 mL) [contains thimerosal; packaged with dropper]

Dosing

Adults & Elderly: Ear inflammation/infection: Otic:

Calibrated dropper: 5 drops in affected ear 3-4 times/day
Dropper bottle: 4 drops in affected ear 3-4 times/day

Note: Alternatively, a cotton wick may be inserted in the ear canal and saturated with suspension every 4 hours; wick should be replaced at least every 24 hours

Pediatrics: Ear inflammation/infection: Otic:

Calibrated dropper: 4 drops in affected ear 3-4 times/day
Dropper bottle: 3 drops in affected ear 3-4 times/day

Note: Alternatively, a cotton wick may be inserted in the ear canal and saturated with suspension every 4 hours; wick should be replaced at least every 24 hours

Nursing Actions

Physical Assessment: See individual agents.

Patient Education: Shake well before using.

Related Information
Hydrocortisone *on page 617*
Neomycin *on page 872*

Neomycin, Polymyxin B, and Hydrocortisone
(nee oh MYE sin, pol i MIKS in bee, & hye droe KOR ti sone)

U.S. Brand Names Cortisporin® Cream; Cortisporin® Ophthalmic; Cortisporin® Otic; PediOtic®

Synonyms Hydrocortisone, Neomycin, and Polymyxin B; Polymyxin B, Neomycin, and Hydrocortisone
(Continued)

Neomycin, Polymyxin B, and Hydrocortisone *(Continued)*

Pharmacologic Category Antibiotic/Corticosteroid, Ophthalmic; Antibiotic/Corticosteroid, Otic; Topical Skin Product

Pregnancy Risk Factor C

Use Steroid-responsive inflammatory condition for which a corticosteroid is indicated and where bacterial infection or a risk of bacterial infection exists

Available Dosage Forms

Cream, topical (Cortisporin®): Neomycin 3.5 mg, polymyxin B 10,000 units, and hydrocortisone acetate 5 mg per g (7.5 g)

Solution, otic (Cortisporin®): Neomycin 3.5 mg, polymyxin B 10,000 units, and hydrocortisone 10 mg per mL (10 mL) [contains potassium metabisulfite]

Suspension, ophthalmic (Cortisporin®): Neomycin 3.5 mg, polymyxin B 10,000 units, and hydrocortisone 10 mg per mL (7.5 mL) [contains thimerosal]

Suspension, otic: Neomycin 3.5 mg, polymyxin B 10,000 units, and hydrocortisone 10 mg per mL (10 mL)

Cortisporin®: Neomycin 3.5 mg, polymyxin B 10,000 units, and hydrocortisone 10 mg per mL (10 mL) [contains thimerosal]

PediOtic®: Neomycin 3.5 mg, polymyxin B 10,000 units, and hydrocortisone 10 mg per mL (7.5 mL) [contains thimerosal]

Dosing

Adults & Elderly:

Note: Duration of use should be limited to 10 days unless otherwise directed by the physician. Otic solution is used **only** for swimmer's ear (infections of external auditory canal)

Auditory canal inflammation/infection: Otic: Instill 4 drops 3-4 times/day; otic suspension is the preferred otic preparation

Ocular inflammation/infection: Ophthalmic: Instill 1-2 drops 2-4 times/day, or more frequently as required for severe infections; in acute infections, instill 1-2 drops every 15-30 minutes gradually reducing the frequency of administration as the infection is controlled

Dermatologic inflammation/infection: Topical: Apply a thin layer 1-4 times/day. Therapy should be discontinued when control is achieved; if no improvement is seen, reassessment of diagnosis may be necessary.

Pediatrics:

Note: Duration of use should be limited to 10 days unless otherwise directed by the physician. Otic solution is used **only** for swimmer's ear (infections of external auditory canal).

Auditory canal inflammation/infection: Otic: Children: Instill 3 drops into affected ear 3-4 times/day.

Ocular inflammation/infection: Children: Refer to adult dosing.

Dermatologic inflammation/infection: Children: Refer to adult dosing.

Nursing Actions

Physical Assessment: See individual agents.

Patient Education:

Otic: Hold container in hand to warm; if drops are in suspension form, shake well for approximately 10 seconds, lie on your side with affected ear up; for adults hold the ear lobe up and back, for children hold the ear lobe down and back; instill drops in ear without inserting dropper into ear; maintain tilted ear for 2 minutes.

Ophthalmic: May cause sensitivity to bright light; may cause temporary blurring of vision or stinging following administration, but discontinue product

and see prescriber if problems persist or increase; to use, tilt head back and place medication in conjunctival sac and close eyes; apply light pressure on lacrimal sac for 1 minute.

Cream: Discontinue product if irritation persists or increases.

Related Information

Hydrocortisone *on page 617*
Neomycin *on page 872*
Polymyxin B *on page 1005*

Neostigmine *(nee oh STIG meen)*

U.S. Brand Names Prostigmin®

Synonyms Neostigmine Bromide; Neostigmine Methylsulfate

Pharmacologic Category Acetylcholinesterase Inhibitor

Medication Safety Issues

Sound-alike/look-alike issues:

Prostigmin® may be confused with physostigmine

Pregnancy Risk Factor C

Lactation Excretion in breast milk unknown/not recommended

Use Diagnosis and treatment of myasthenia gravis; prevention and treatment of postoperative bladder distention and urinary retention; reversal of the effects of nondepolarizing neuromuscular-blocking agents after surgery

Mechanism of Action/Effect Inhibits destruction of acetylcholine by acetylcholinesterase which facilitates transmission of impulses across myoneural junction

Contraindications Hypersensitivity to neostigmine, bromides, or any component of the formulation; GI or GU obstruction

Warnings/Precautions Does **not** antagonize and may prolong the Phase I block of depolarizing muscle relaxants (eg, succinylcholine). Use with caution in patients with epilepsy, asthma, bradycardia, hyperthyroidism, cardiac arrhythmias, or peptic ulcer. Adequate facilities should be available for cardiopulmonary resuscitation when testing and adjusting dose for myasthenia gravis. Have atropine and epinephrine ready to treat hypersensitivity reactions. Overdosage may result in cholinergic crisis, this must be distinguished from myasthenic crisis. Anticholinesterase insensitivity can develop for brief or prolonged periods.

Drug Interactions

Decreased Effect: Antagonizes effects of nondepolarizing muscle relaxants (eg, pancuronium, tubocurarine). Atropine antagonizes the muscarinic effects of neostigmine.

Increased Effect/Toxicity: Neuromuscular blocking agent effects are increased when combined with neostigmine.

Lab Interactions Increased aminotransferase [ALT (SGPT)/AST (SGOT)] (S), amylase (S)

Adverse Reactions Frequency not defined.

Cardiovascular: Arrhythmias (especially bradycardia), hypotension, decreased carbon monoxide, tachycardia, AV block, nodal rhythm, nonspecific ECG changes, cardiac arrest, syncope, flushing

Central nervous system: Convulsions, dysarthria, dysphonia, dizziness, loss of consciousness, drowsiness, headache

Dermatologic: Skin rash, thrombophlebitis (I.V.), urticaria

Gastrointestinal: Hyperperistalsis, nausea, vomiting, salivation, diarrhea, stomach cramps, dysphagia, flatulence

Genitourinary: Urinary urgency

Neuromuscular & skeletal: Weakness, fasciculations, muscle cramps, spasms, arthralgia

Ocular: Small pupils, lacrimation

Respiratory: Increased bronchial secretions, laryngospasm, bronchiolar constriction, respiratory muscle paralysis, dyspnea, respiratory depression, respiratory arrest, bronchospasm

Miscellaneous: Diaphoresis (increased), anaphylaxis, allergic reactions

Overdosage/Toxicology Symptoms of overdose include muscle weakness, blurred vision, excessive sweating, tearing and salivation, nausea, vomiting, diarrhea, hypertension, bradycardia, muscle weakness, and paralysis. Atropine sulfate injection should be readily available as an antagonist for the effects of neostigmine.

Pharmacodynamics/Kinetics

Onset of Action: I.M.: 20-30 minutes; I.V.: 1-20 minutes

Duration of Action: I.M.: 2.5-4 hours; I.V.: 1-2 hours

Half-Life Elimination: Normal renal function: 0.5-2.1 hours; End-stage renal disease: Prolonged

Metabolism: Hepatic

Excretion: Urine (50% as unchanged drug)

Available Dosage Forms

Injection, solution, as methylsulfate: 0.5 mg/mL (1 mL, 10 mL); 1 mg/mL (10 mL)

Tablet, as bromide: 15 mg

Dosing

Adults & Elderly:

Myasthenia gravis, diagnosis: I.M.: 0.02 mg/kg as a single dose

Myasthenia gravis, treatment:

Oral: 15 mg/dose every 3-4 hours up to 375 mg/day maximum

I.M., I.V., SubQ: 0.5-2.5 mg every 1-3 hours up to 10 mg/24 hours maximum

Reversal of nondepolarizing neuromuscular blockade after surgery in conjunction with atropine: I.V.: 0.5-2.5 mg; total dose not to exceed 5 mg; must administer atropine several minutes prior to neostigmine

Bladder atony: I.M., SubQ:

Prevention: 0.25 mg every 4-6 hours for 2-3 days

Treatment: 0.5-1 mg every 3 hours for 5 doses after bladder has emptied

Pediatrics:

Myasthenia gravis, diagnosis: I.M.: Children: 0.04 mg/kg as a single dose

Myasthenia gravis, treatment: Children:

Oral: 2 mg/kg/day divided every 3-4 hours

I.M., I.V., SubQ: 0.01-0.04 mg/kg every 2-4 hours

Reversal of nondepolarizing neuromuscular blockade after surgery in conjunction with atropine (must administer atropine several minutes prior to neostigmine): I.V.:

Infants: 0.025-0.1 mg/kg/dose

Children: 0.025-0.08 mg/kg/dose

Renal Impairment:

Cl_{cr} 10-50 mL/minute: Administer 50% of normal dose.

Cl_{cr} <10 mL/minute: Administer 25% of normal dose.

Administration

I.M.: In the diagnosis of myasthenia gravis, all anticholinesterase medications should be discontinued for at least 8 hours before administering neostigmine.

I.V. Detail: pH: 5.9 (adjusted)

Stability

Compatibility: Stable in NS

Nursing Actions

Physical Assessment: Used for MG diagnosis by physicians. **Bladder atony:** Assess bladder adequacy prior to administering medication. Monitor therapeutic response, adverse effects (eg, vital signs, respiratory and CNS response), and cholinergic crisis (DUMBELS - diarrhea, urination, miosis, bronchospasm/bradycardia, excitability, lacrimation, and salivation/excessive sweating). Teach patient symptoms to report.

Patient Education: Take this drug exactly as prescribed. You may experience visual difficulty (eg, blurring and dark adaptation, use caution at night) or urinary frequency. Promptly report any muscle weakness, respiratory difficulty, severe or unresolved diarrhea, persistent abdominal cramping or vomiting, sweating, or tearing. **Pregnancy/breast-feeding precautions:** Inform prescriber if you are pregnant. Breast-feeding is not recommended.

Geriatric Considerations Many elderly will have diseases which may influence the use of neostigmine. Also, many elderly will need doses reduced 50% due to creatinine clearances in the 10-50 mL/minute range (common in the aged). Side effects or concomitant disease may warrant use of pyridostigmine.

Additional Information In the diagnosis of myasthenia gravis, all anticholinesterase medications should be discontinued for at least 8 hours before administering neostigmine.

Nepafenac (ne pa FEN ak)

U.S. Brand Names Nevanac™

Pharmacologic Category Nonsteroidal Anti-inflammatory Drug (NSAID), Ophthalmic

Pregnancy Risk Factor C/D (3rd trimester)

Lactation Excretion in breast milk unknown/use caution

Use Treatment of pain and inflammation associated with cataract surgery

Mechanism of Action/Effect Nepafenac is a prodrug which once converted to amfenac inhibits prostaglandin synthesis by decreasing the activity of the enzyme, cyclooxygenase, which results in decreased formation of prostaglandin precursors.

Contraindications Hypersensitivity to nepafenac, other NSAIDs, or any component of the formulation

Warnings/Precautions Use caution in patients with previous sensitivity to acetylsalicylic acid and phenylacetic acid derivatives, including patients who experience bronchospasm, asthma, rhinitis, or urticaria following NSAID or aspirin. May slow/delay healing or prolong bleeding time following surgery. Use caution in patients with a predisposition to bleeding (bleeding tendencies or medications which interfere with coagulation).

May cause keratitis; continued use of nepafenac in a patient with keratitis may cause severe corneal adverse reactions, potentially resulting in loss of vision. Immediately discontinue use in patients with evidence of corneal epithelial damage.

Use caution in patients with complicated ocular surgeries, corneal denervation, corneal epithelial defects, diabetes mellitus, ocular surface disease, rheumatoid arthritis, or repeat ocular surgeries (within a short timeframe); may be at risk of corneal adverse events, potentially resulting in loss of vision. Use more than 1 day prior to surgery or for 14 days beyond surgery may increase risk and severity of corneal adverse events. Patients using ophthalmic drops should not wear soft contact lenses.

Safety and efficacy have not been established in children <10 years of age.

Adverse Reactions 1% to 10%:

Cardiovascular: Hypertension (1% to 4%)

Central nervous system: Headache (1% to 4%)

Gastrointestinal: Nausea (1% to 4%), vomiting (1% to 4%)

Ocular: Capsular opacity (5% to 10%), foreign body sensation (5% to 10%), intraocular pressure increased (5% to 10%), sticky sensation (5% to 10%), visual acuity decreased (5% to 10%), conjunctival edema (1% to 5%), corneal edema (1% to 5%), dry eye (1% to 5%), lid margin crusting (1% to 5%), ocular discomfort (1% to 5%), ocular hyperemia (1% to 5%), ocular pain (1% to 5%), ocular pruritus (1% to 5%), (Continued)

Nepafenac *(Continued)*

photophobia (1% to 5%), tearing (1% to 5%), vitreous detachment (1% to 5%)

Respiratory: Sinusitis (1% to 4%)

Pharmacodynamics/Kinetics

Metabolism: Hydrolyzed in ocular tissue to amfenac (active)

Available Dosage Forms Suspension, ophthalmic: 0.1% (3 mL) [contains benzalkonium chloride]

Dosing

Adults & Elderly: Pain, inflammation associated with cataract surgery: Ophthalmic: Instill 1 drop into affected eye(s) 3 times/day, beginning 1 day prior to surgery, the day of surgery, and through the first 2 weeks of the postoperative period

Pediatrics: Pain, inflammation associated with cataract surgery: Ophthalmic: Children ≥10 years: Refer to adult dosing.

Administration

Other:

Ophthalmic: Shake well prior to use.

Stability

Storage: Store at 2°C o 25°C (36°F to 77°F).

Nursing Actions

Physical Assessment: Assess other prescription and OTC medications the patient may be taking to avoid duplications and interactions. Assess knowledge/ teach patient appropriate use, side effects, and symptoms to report.

Patient Education: Ophthalmic: Instill drops as often as recommended. Wash hands before instilling. Sit or lie down to instill. Open eye, look at the ceiling, and instill prescribed amount. Close eye and roll eye in all directions. Apply gentle pressure to inner corner of eye for 1-2 minutes after instillation. Do not wear soft contract lenses while using this medication. **Pregnancy/breast-feeding precautions:** Inform prescriber if you are or intend to become pregnant. Consult prescriber if breast-feeding.

Pregnancy Issues Teratogenic events were not observed in animal studies. Safety and efficacy in pregnant women have not been established. Exposure to nonsteroidal anti-inflammatory drugs late in pregnancy may lead to premature closure of the ductus arteriosus.

Nesiritide *(ni SIR i tide)*

U.S. Brand Names Natrecor®

Synonyms B-type Natriuretic Peptide (Human); hBNP; Natriuretic Peptide

Pharmacologic Category Natriuretic Peptide, B-Type, Human; Vasodilator

Medication Safety Issues

High alert medication: The Institute for Safe Medication Practices (ISMP) includes this medication among its list of drugs which have a heightened risk of causing significant patient harm when used in error.

Pregnancy Risk Factor C

Lactation Excretion in breast milk unknown/use caution

Use Treatment of acutely decompensated congestive heart failure (CHF) in patients with dyspnea at rest or with minimal activity

Mechanism of Action/Effect Binds to cell surface receptors in vasculature, resulting in smooth muscle cell relaxation. Has been shown to produce dose-dependent reductions in pulmonary capillary wedge pressure (PCWP) and systemic arterial pressure providing symptomatic improvements (dyspnea decreased) for several days.

Contraindications Hypersensitivity to natriuretic peptide or any component of the formulation; cardiogenic shock (when used as primary therapy); hypotension (systolic blood pressure <90 mm Hg)

Warnings/Precautions May cause hypotension; administer in clinical situations when blood pressure may be closely monitored. Use caution in patients systolic blood pressure <100 mm Hg (contraindicated if <90 mm Hg); more likely to experience hypotension. Effects may be additive with other agents capable of causing hypotension. Hypotensive effects may last for several hours.

Should not be used in patients with low filling pressures, or in patients with conditions which depend on venous return including significant valvular stenosis, restrictive or obstructive cardiomyopathy, constrictive pericarditis, and pericardial tamponade. May be associated with development of azotemia; use caution in patients with renal impairment or in patients where renal perfusion is dependent on renin-angiotensin-aldosterone system.

Monitor for allergic or anaphylactic reactions. Use caution with prolonged infusions; limited experience for infusions >48 hours. Safety and efficacy in pediatric patients have not been established.

Drug Interactions

Increased Effect/Toxicity: An increased frequency of symptomatic hypotension was observed with concurrent administration of ACE inhibitors. Other hypotensive agents are likely to have additive effects on hypotension. In patients receiving diuretic therapy leading to depletion of intravascular volume, the risk of hypotension and/or renal impairment may be increased. Nesiritide should be avoided in patients with low filling pressures.

Adverse Reactions Note: Frequencies cited below were recorded in VMAC trial at dosages similar to approved labeling. Higher frequencies have been observed in trials using higher dosages of nesiritide.

>10%:

Cardiovascular: Hypotension (total: 11%; symptomatic: 4% at recommended dose, up to 17% at higher doses)

Renal: Increased serum creatinine (28% with >0.5 mg/dL increase over baseline)

1% to 10%:

Cardiovascular: Ventricular tachycardia (3%)*, ventricular extrasystoles (3%)*, angina (2%)*, bradycardia (1%), tachycardia, atrial fibrillation, AV node conduction abnormalities

Central nervous system: Headache (8%)*, dizziness (3%)*, insomnia (2%), anxiety (3%), fever, confusion, paresthesia, somnolence, tremor

Dermatologic: Pruritus, rash

Gastrointestinal: Nausea (4%)*, abdominal pain (1%)*, vomiting (1%)*

Hematologic: Anemia

Local: Injection site reaction

Neuromuscular & skeletal: Back pain (4%), leg cramps

Ocular: Amblyopia

Respiratory: Cough (increased), hemoptysis, apnea

Miscellaneous: Increased diaphoresis

*Frequency less than or equal to placebo or other standard therapy

Overdosage/Toxicology No data. Symptoms of overdose would be expected to include excessive and/or prolonged hypotension. Treatment is symptomatic and supportive. Drug discontinuation and/or dosage reduction may be required.

Pharmacodynamics/Kinetics

Onset of Action: 15 minutes (60% of 3-hour effect achieved)

Duration of Action: >60 minutes (up to several hours) for systolic blood pressure; hemodynamic effects persist longer than serum half-life would predict

Time to Peak: 1 hour

Half-Life Elimination: Initial (distribution) 2 minutes; Terminal: 18 minutes

Metabolism: Proteolytic cleavage by vascular endopeptidases and proteolysis following receptor binding and cellular internalization

Excretion: Urine

Available Dosage Forms Injection, powder for reconstitution: 1.5 mg

Dosing

Adults & Elderly:

Congestive heart failure: I.V.: Initial: 2 mcg/kg (bolus); followed by continuous infusion at 0.01 mcg/kg/minute; **Note:** Should not be initiated at a dosage higher than initial recommended dose. At intervals of ≥3 hours, the dosage may be increased by 0.005 mcg/kg/minute (preceded by a bolus of 1 mcg/kg), up to a maximum of 0.03 mcg/kg/minute. Increases beyond the initial infusion rate should be limited to selected patients and accompanied by hemodynamic monitoring.

Patients experiencing hypotension during the infusion: Infusion should be interrupted. May attempt to restart at a lower dose (reduce initial infusion dose by 30% and omit bolus).

Renal Impairment: No adjustment required

Administration

I.V.: Do not administer through a heparin-coated catheter (concurrent administration of heparin via a separate catheter is acceptable, per manufacturer).

I.V. Detail: Prime I.V. tubing with 25 mL of infusion prior to connection with vascular access port and prior to administering bolus or starting the infusion. Withdraw bolus from the prepared infusion bag and administer over 60 seconds. Begin infusion immediately following administration of the bolus. Using a standard 6 mcg/mL concentration, bolus volume in mL = patient weight in kg x 0.33.

Stability

Reconstitution: Reconstitute 1.5 mg vial with 5 mL of diluent removed from a premixed plastic I.V. bag (compatible with 5% dextrose, 0.9% sodium chloride, 5% dextrose and 0.45% sodium chloride, or 5% dextrose and 0.2% sodium chloride). Do not shake vial to dissolve (roll gently). Withdraw entire contents of vial and add to 250 mL I.V. bag. Resultant concentration of solution approximately 6 mcg/mL.

Compatibility: Incompatible with heparin, insulin, ethacrynate sodium, bumetanide, enalaprilat, hydralazine, and furosemide. Do not administer through the same catheter. Do not administer with any solution containing sodium metabisulfite. Catheter must be flushed between administration of nesiritide and physically incompatible drugs.

Storage: Vials may be stored at controlled room temperature of 20°C to 25°C (68°F to 77 °F) or under refrigeration at 2°C to 8°C (36°F to 46°F). Following reconstitution, vials are stable under these conditions for up to 24 hours.

Nursing Actions

Physical Assessment: Assess potential for interactions with other prescriptions, OTC medications, or herbal products patient may be taking (eg, other hypotensive agents or diuretics). Monitor blood pressure and cardiac function before and at frequent intervals during and for 24 hours following (hemodynamic monitoring with larger doses). Monitor laboratory tests, renal function, and patient response on a regular basis throughout therapy (eg, hypersensitivity reaction). Teach patient possible side effects/appropriate interventions and adverse symptoms to report.

Patient Education: This medication can only be administered by infusion; you will be monitored closely during and following infusion. Report immediately any pain, burning, swelling at infusion site, or any signs of allergic reaction (eg, respiratory or swallowing difficulty, back pain, chest tightness, rash, hives, swelling of lips or mouth). Remain in bed until advised otherwise; call for assistance with turning or changing position. Report any chest pain, respiratory difficulty, confusion, nausea, leg cramps, swelling of extremities, sudden or excessive weight gain, or any other adverse effects. **Pregnancy/breast-feeding precautions:** Inform prescriber if you are or intend to become pregnant. Consult prescriber if breast-feeding.

Geriatric Considerations No specific data to date; elderly are liable to have hypotension, see Warnings/Precautions for blood pressure criteria. Elderly with reduced renal function should be monitored closely.

Additional Information The duration of symptomatic improvement with nesiritide following discontinuation of the infusion has been limited (generally lasting several days). Atrial natriuretic peptide, which is related to nesiritide, has been associated with increased vascular permeability. This has not been observed in clinical trials with nesiritide, but patients should be monitored for this effect.

Nevirapine (ne VYE ra peen)

U.S. Brand Names Viramune®

Synonyms NVP

Restrictions An FDA-approved medication guide is available at http://www.fda.gov/cder/Offices/ODS/labeling.htm

Pharmacologic Category Antiretroviral Agent, Reverse Transcriptase Inhibitor (Non-nucleoside)

Medication Safety Issues

Sound-alike/look-alike issues:

Nevirapine may be confused with nelfinavir

Viramune® may be confused with Viracept®

Pregnancy Risk Factor C

Lactation Enters breast milk/contraindicated

Use In combination therapy with other antiretroviral agents for the treatment of HIV-1

Mechanism of Action/Effect Blocks the RNA-dependent DNA polymerase activity

Contraindications Hypersensitivity to nevirapine or any component of the formulation

Warnings/Precautions Severe hepatotoxic reactions may occur (fulminant and cholestatic hepatitis, hepatic necrosis) and, in some cases, have resulted in hepatic failure and death. Intensive monitoring is required during the initial 18 weeks of therapy to detect potentially life-threatening dermatologic, hypersensitivity, and hepatic reactions. The greatest risk of these reactions is within the initial 6 weeks of treatment. Patients with a history of chronic hepatitis (B or C) or increased baseline transaminase levels may be at increased risk of hepatotoxic reactions. Female gender and patients with increased CD4$^+$-cell counts may be at substantially greater risk of hepatic events (often associated with rash). Therapy should not be started with elevated CD4$^+$-cell counts unless the benefit of therapy outweighs the risk of serious hepatotoxicity (adult females: CD4$^+$-cell counts >250 cells/mm^3; adult males: CD4$^+$-cell counts >400 cells/mm^3).

Severe life-threatening skin reactions (eg, Stevens-Johnson syndrome, toxic epidermal necrolysis, hypersensitivity reactions with rash and organ dysfunction) have occurred. Nevirapine must be initiated with a 14-day lead-in dosing period to decrease the incidence of adverse effects.

If a severe dermatologic or hypersensitivity reaction occurs, or if signs and symptoms of hepatitis occur, nevirapine should be permanently discontinued. These may include a severe rash, or a rash associated with fever, blisters, oral lesions, conjunctivitis, facial edema, muscle or joint aches, general malaise, hepatitis, eosinophilia, granulocytopenia, lymphadenopathy, or renal dysfunction.

(Continued)

Nevirapine *(Continued)*

Consider alteration of antiretroviral therapies if disease progression occurs while patients are receiving nevirapine. Safety and efficacy have not been established in neonates.

Drug Interactions

Cytochrome P450 Effect: Substrate of CYP2B6 (minor), 2D6 (minor), 3A4 (major); **Inhibits** CYP1A2 (weak), 2D6 (weak), 3A4 (weak); **Induces** CYP2B6 (strong), 3A4 (strong)

Decreased Effect: The levels/effects of nevirapine may be decreased by aminoglutethimide, carbamazepine, nafcillin, nevirapine, phenobarbital, phenytoin, and rifamycins, and other CYP3A4 inducers; avoid concurrent use. Nevirapine may decrease the levels/effects of benzodiazepines, bupropion, calcium channel blockers, clarithromycin, cyclosporine, efavirenz, erythromycin, estrogens, mirtazapine, nateglinide, nefazodone, promethazine, selegiline, sertraline, tacrolimus, venlafaxine, and other CYP2B6 or 3A4 substrates. Nevirapine may decrease serum concentrations of some protease inhibitors (AUC of indinavir, lopinavir, nelfinavir, and saquinavir may be decreased, however, no effect noted with ritonavir); specific dosage adjustments have not been recommended; no adjustment recommended for ritonavir, unless combined with lopinavir (Kaletra™). Nevirapine may decrease the effectiveness of oral contraceptives; suggest alternate method or additional form of birth control. Nevirapine also decreases the effect of ketoconazole and methadone.

Increased Effect/Toxicity: Cimetidine, itraconazole, ketoconazole, and some macrolide antibiotics may increase nevirapine plasma concentrations. Concurrent administration of prednisone for the initial 14 days of nevirapine therapy was associated with an increased incidence and severity of rash. Rifabutin concentrations are increased by nevirapine.

Nutritional/Ethanol Interactions

Herb/Nutraceutical: Nevirapine serum concentration may be decreased by St John's wort; avoid concurrent use.

Adverse Reactions

Note: Potentially life-threatening nevirapine-associated adverse effects may present with the following symptoms: Abrupt onset of flu-like symptoms, abdominal pain, jaundice, or fever with or without rash; may progress to hepatic failure with encephalopathy. Skin rash is present in ~50% of cases.

Percentages of adverse effects vary by clinical trial:

>10%:

Dermatologic: Rash (grade 1/2: 13%; grade 3/4: 1.5%) is the most common toxicity; occurs most frequently within the first 6 weeks of therapy; women may be at higher risk than men

Hepatic: ALT >250 units/L (5% to 14%); symptomatic hepatic events (4%, range: up to 11%) are more common in women, women with CD4+ cell counts >250 cells/mm^3, and men with CD4+ cell counts >400 cells/mm^3

1% to 10%:

Central nervous system: Headache (1% to 4%), fatigue (up to 5%)

Gastrointestinal: Nausea (<1% to 9%), abdominal pain (<1% to 2%), diarrhea (up to 2%)

Hepatic: AST >250 units/L (4% to 8%); coinfection with hepatitis B or C and/or increased liver function tests at the beginning of therapy are associated with a greater risk of asymptomatic transaminase elevations (ALT or AST >5 times ULN: 6%, range: up to 9%) or symptomatic events occurring ≥6 weeks after beginning treatment

Overdosage/Toxicology Edema, erythema nodosum, fatigue, fever, headache, insomnia, nausea, pulmonary infiltrates, rash, vertigo, and weight loss have been reported following large doses.

Pharmacodynamics/Kinetics

Time to Peak: Serum: 2-4 hours

Protein Binding: Plasma: 60%

Half-Life Elimination: Decreases over 2- to 4-week time with chronic dosing due to autoinduction (ie, half-life = 45 hours initially and decreases to 25-30 hours)

Metabolism: Extensively hepatic via CYP3A4 (hydroxylation to inactive compounds); may undergo enterohepatic recycling

Excretion: Urine (~81%, primarily as metabolites, <3% as unchanged drug); feces (~10%)

Available Dosage Forms

Suspension, oral: 50 mg/5 mL (240 mL)

Tablet: 200 mg

Dosing

Adults & Elderly:

HIV infection: Oral: Initial: 200 mg once daily for 14 days; maintenance: 200 mg twice daily (in combination with an additional antiretroviral agents).

Note: If patient experiences a rash during the 14-day lead-in period, dose should not be increased until the rash has resolved. Discontinue if severe rash, or rash with constitutional symptoms, is noted. If a therapy is interrupted for >7 days, restart with initial dose for 14 days. Use of prednisone to prevent nevirapine-associated rash is not recommended. Permanently discontinue if symptomatic hepatic events occur.

Prevention of maternal-fetal HIV transmission in women with no prior antiretroviral therapy (AIDS information guidelines): Oral:

Mother: 200 mg as a single dose at onset of labor. May be used in combination with zidovudine.

Infant: 2 mg/kg as a single dose at age 48-72 hours. If a maternal dose was given <1 hour prior to delivery, administer a 2 mg/kg dose as soon as possible after birth and repeat at 48-72 hours. May be used in combination with zidovudine.

Pediatrics:

HIV infection: Oral:

Children 2 months to <8 years: Initial: 4 mg/kg/dose once daily for 14 days; increase dose to 7 mg/kg/dose every 12 hours if no rash or other adverse effects occur; maximum dose: 200 mg/dose every 12 hours

Children ≥8 years: Initial: 4 mg/kg/dose once daily for 14 days; increase dose to 4 mg/kg/dose every 12 hours if no rash or other adverse effects occur; maximum dose: 200 mg/dose every 12 hours

Alternative pediatric dosing (AIDSinfo guidelines): 120-200 mg/m^2 every 12 hours; this dosing has been proposed due to the fact that dosing based on mg/kg may result in an abrupt decrease in dose at the 8th birthday, which may be inappropriate.

Note: If patient experiences a rash during the 14-day lead-in period, dose should not be increased until the rash has resolved. Discontinue if severe rash, or rash with constitutional symptoms, is noted. If therapy is interrupted for >7 days, restart with initial dose for 14 days. Use of prednisone to prevent nevirapine-associated rash is not recommended. Permanently discontinue if symptomatic hepatic events occur.

Renal Impairment:

Cl$_{cr}$ ≥20 mL/minute: No adjustment required

Hemodialysis: An additional 200 mg dose is recommended following dialysis.

Hepatic Impairment:

Use not recommended with moderate-to-severe hepatic impairment. Permanently discontinue if symptomatic hepatic events occur.

Administration

Oral: May be administered with or without food. May be administered with an antacid or didanosine. Shake suspension gently prior to administration.

Laboratory Monitoring Monitor CBC and viral load. Liver function tests should be monitored at baseline, and intensively during the first 18 weeks of therapy (optimal frequency not established, some practitioners recommend more often than once a month, including prior to dose escalation, and at 2 weeks following dose escalation), then periodically throughout therapy; observe for CNS side effects. Assess/evaluate AST/ALT in any patients with a rash. Permanently discontinue if patient experiences severe rash, constitutional symptoms associated with rash, rash with elevated AST/ALT, or clinical hepatitis, Mild-to-moderate rash without AST/ALT elevation may continue treatment per discretion of prescriber. If mild-to-moderate urticarial rash, do not restart if treatment is interrupted.

Nursing Actions

Physical Assessment: Assess potential for interactions with extensive list of other pharmacological agents and herbal products. Monitor laboratory tests (especially LFTs at baseline and frequently during therapy). Monitor patient closely for any signs of hypersensitivity during 14 days of lead-in dosing. Monitor regularly and frequently during initial 18 weeks of therapy for symptoms of hypersensitivity/dermatologic reactions (which may include severe rash, rash with fever, blisters, oral lesions, conjunctivitis, facial edema, muscle or joint aches, general malaise, jaundice, hepatitis, or renal dysfunction). Teach patient proper use, possible side effects/appropriate interventions, and adverse symptoms to report (refer to Patient Education).

Patient Education: Do not take any new prescription, over-the-counter medications, or herbal products during therapy (without consulting prescriber). This is not a cure for HIV, nor has it been found to reduce transmission of HIV; use appropriate precautions to prevent spread to other persons. Take as directed, with food. Shake suspension gently prior to use. When using dosing cups, rinse cup with water and drink. If you miss a dose, take as soon as possible and return to regular schedule (never take a double dose). Frequent blood tests may be required with prolonged therapy. If rash, blisters, or facial edema develops, stop medicine and contact prescriber immediately. Report any change in urinary pattern, dark urine or light stool, easy bleeding, unusual fatigue, flu-like symptoms, abdominal pain, or other persistent adverse effects. **Pregnancy/breast-feeding precautions:** Inform prescriber if you are or intend to become pregnant. Effectiveness of oral contraceptives may be decreased, use of alternative (nonhormonal) forms of contraception is recommended; consult prescriber for appropriate contraceptives. Do not breast-feed.

Breast-Feeding Issues HIV-infected mothers are discouraged from breast-feeding to decrease potential transmission of HIV.

Pregnancy Issues Nevirapine crosses the placenta. Pharmacokinetics are not altered during pregnancy and dose adjustment is not needed. The Perinatal HIV Guidelines Working Group recommends nevirapine as the NNRTI for use during pregnancy. When used to prevent perinatal transmission in women who do not need therapy for their own health, use is not recommended if CD4+ lymphocyte counts >250/mm³ (monitor for liver toxicity during first 18 weeks of therapy). It may also be used in combination with zidovudine in HIV-infected women who are in labor, but have had no prior antiretroviral therapy, in order to reduce the maternal-fetal transmission of HIV; consider adding intrapartum and postpartum zidovudine and lamivudine to reduce nevirapine resistance. Health professionals are encouraged to contact the antiretroviral pregnancy registry to monitor outcomes of pregnant women exposed to antiretroviral medications (1-800-258-4263 or www.APRegistry.com).

Additional Information Potential compliance problems, frequency of administration, and adverse effects should be discussed with patients before initiating therapy to help prevent the emergence of resistance. Early virologic failure was observed with tenofovir and didanosine delayed release capsules, plus either efavirenz or nevirapine; use caution in treatment-naive patients with high baseline viral loads.

Niacin (NYE a sin)

U.S. Brand Names Niacor®; Niaspan®; Slo-Niacin® [OTC]

Synonyms Nicotinic Acid; Vitamin B₃

Pharmacologic Category Antilipemic Agent, Miscellaneous; Vitamin, Water Soluble

Medication Safety Issues

Sound-alike/look-alike issues:

Niacin may be confused with Minocin®, Niaspan®, Nispan®

Niaspan® may be confused with niacin

Nicobid® may be confused with Nitro-Bid®

Pregnancy Risk Factor A/C (dose exceeding RDA recommendation)

Lactation Enters breast milk/consult prescriber

Use Adjunctive treatment of dyslipidemias (types IIa and IIb or primary hypercholesterolemia) to lower the risk of recurrent MI and/or slow progression of coronary artery disease, including combination therapy with other antidyslipidemic agents when additional triglyceride-lowering or HDL-increasing effects are desired; treatment of hypertriglyceridemia in patients at risk of pancreatitis; treatment of peripheral vascular disease and circulatory disorders; treatment of pellagra; dietary supplement

Mechanism of Action/Effect Component of two coenzymes which is necessary for tissue respiration, lipid metabolism, and glycogenolysis; inhibits the synthesis of very low density lipoproteins

Contraindications Hypersensitivity to niacin, niacinamide, or any component of the formulation; active hepatic disease; active peptic ulcer; arterial hemorrhage

Warnings/Precautions Use caution in heavy ethanol users, unstable angina or MI, diabetes (interferes with glucose control), renal disease, active gallbladder disease (can exacerbate), gout, past history of hepatic disease, or with anticoagulants. Monitor glucose and liver function tests. Rare cases of rhabdomyolysis have occurred during concomitant use with HMG-CoA reductase inhibitors. With concurrent use or if symptoms suggestive of myopathy occur, monitor creatinine phosphokinase (CPK) and potassium. Immediate and extended or sustained release products should not be interchanged. Flushing is common and can be attenuated with a gradual increase in dose, and/or by taking aspirin 30-60 minutes before dosing. Compliance is enhanced with twice daily dosing.

Niaspan®: 500 mg and 750 mg tablets are not interchangeable (eg, three 500 mg tablets are not equivalent to two 750 mg tablets).

Nutritional/Ethanol Interactions Ethanol: Avoid heavy use; avoid use around niacin dose.

Lab Interactions False elevations in some fluorometric determinations of urinary catecholamines; false-positive urine glucose (Benedict's reagent)

Adverse Reactions Frequency not defined.

Cardiovascular: Arrhythmias, atrial fibrillation, edema, flushing, hypotension, orthostasis, palpitation, syncope (rare), tachycardia

Central nervous system: Chills, dizziness, insomnia, migraine

Dermatologic: Acanthosis nigricans, dry skin, hyperpigmentation, maculopapular rash, pruritus, rash, urticaria

(Continued)

Niacin *(Continued)*

Endocrine & metabolic: Glucose tolerance decreased, gout, phosphorous levels decreased, uric acid level increased

Gastrointestinal: Abdominal pain, dyspepsia, eructation, flatulence, nausea, peptic ulcers, vomiting

Hematologic: Platelet counts decreased, prothrombin time increased

Hepatic: Hepatic necrosis (rare), jaundice, liver enzymes increased

Neuromuscular & skeletal: Leg cramps, myalgia, myasthenia, myopathy (with concurrent HMG-CoA reductase inhibitor), pain, rhabdomyolysis (with concurrent HMG-CoA reductase inhibitor; rare), weakness

Ocular: Cystoid macular edema, toxic amblyopia

Respiratory: Dyspnea

Miscellaneous: Diaphoresis, hypersensitivity reactions (rare)

Overdosage/Toxicology Symptoms of acute overdose include flushing, GI distress, and pruritus. Chronic excessive use has been associated with hepatitis. Antihistamines may relieve niacin-induced histamine release; otherwise treatment is symptomatic.

Pharmacodynamics/Kinetics

Time to Peak: Serum: Immediate release formulation: ~45 minutes; extended release formulation: 4-5 hours

Half-Life Elimination: 45 minutes

Metabolism: Extensive first-pass effects; converted to nicotinamide adenine dinucleotide, nicotinuric acid, and other metabolites

Excretion: Urine 60% to 88% (unchanged drug and metabolites)

Available Dosage Forms

Capsule, extended release: 125 mg, 250 mg, 400 mg, 500 mg

Capsule, timed release: 250 mg

Tablet: 50 mg, 100 mg, 250 mg, 500 mg

Niacor®: 500 mg

Tablet, controlled release (Slo-Niacin®): 250 mg, 500 mg, 750 mg

Tablet, extended release (Niaspan®): 500 mg, 750 mg, 1000 mg

Note: 500 mg and 750 mg tablets are not interchangeable (eg, three 500 mg tablets are not equivalent to two 750 mg tablets)

Tablet, timed release: 250 mg, 500 mg, 750 mg, 1000 mg

Dosing

Adults & Elderly:

Recommended daily allowances:

Male: 25-50 years: 19 mg/day; >51 years: 15 mg/day

Female: 25-50 years: 15 mg/day; >51 years: 13 mg/day

Hyperlipidemia: Oral: Usual target dose: 1.5-6 g/day in 3 divided doses with or after meals using a dosage titration schedule; extended release: 375 mg to 2 g once daily at bedtime

Regular release formulation (Niacor®): Initial: 250 mg once daily (with evening meal); increase frequency and/or dose every 4-7 days to desired response or first-level therapeutic dose (1.5-2 g/day in 2-3 divided doses); after 2 months, may increase at 2- to 4-week intervals to 3 g/day in 3 divided doses

Extended release formulation (Niaspan®): 500 mg at bedtime for 4 weeks, then 1 g at bedtime for 4 weeks; adjust dose to response and tolerance; can increase to a maximum of 2 g/day, but only at 500 mg/day at 4-week intervals

Pellagra: Oral: 50-100 mg 3-4 times/day, maximum: 500 mg/day

Niacin deficiency: Oral: 10-20 mg/day, maximum: 100 mg/day

Pediatrics:

Pellagra: Oral: Children: 50-100 mg/dose 3 times/day

Recommended daily allowances:

0-0.5 years: 5 mg/day

0.5-1 year: 6 mg/day

1-3 years: 9 mg/day

4-6 years: 12 mg/day

7-10 years: 13 mg/day

RDA: Children and Adolescents:

Male:

11-14 years: 17 mg/day

15-18 years: 20 mg/day

19-24 years: 19 mg/day

Female: 11-24 years: 15 mg/day

Renal Impairment: Use with caution.

Hepatic Impairment: Not recommended for use in patients with significant or unexplained hepatic dysfunction.

Dosing Adjustment for Toxicity: Transaminases rise to 3 times ULN: Discontinue therapy.

Administration

Oral: Administer with food. Administer Niaspan® at bedtime. Niaspan® tablet strengths are not interchangeable. When switching from immediate release tablet, initiate Niaspan® at lower dose and titrate. Long-acting forms should not be crushed, broken, or chewed. Do not substitute long-acting forms for immediate release ones.

Laboratory Monitoring Blood glucose; liver function tests (dyslipidemia, high dose, prolonged therapy) pretreatment and every 6-12 weeks for first year then periodically; lipid profile

Nursing Actions

Physical Assessment: Assess other medications patient may be taking for increased risk of drug/drug interactions. Teach patient appropriate use, interventions to reduce side effects, and adverse symptoms to report.

Patient Education: Take exactly as directed; do not exceed recommended dosage. Take with food to reduce incidence of GI upset. Do not crush sustained release capsules. You may experience flushing, sensation of heat, or headache; these reactions may be decreased by increasing dose slowly or by taking aspirin (consult prescriber) 30 minutes prior to taking niacin. Avoid alcohol or hot drinks around time of taking medication to minimize flushing. Taking at bedtime is also recommended. You may experience dizziness, lightheadedness (use caution when driving or engaging in tasks requiring alertness until response to drug is known). Report persistent GI disturbance or changes in color of urine or stool. **Pregnancy/breast-feeding precautions:** Inform prescriber if you are pregnant. Consult prescriber if breast-feeding

Dietary Considerations Should be taken with meal; low-fat meal if treating hyperlipidemia. Avoid hot drinks around the time of niacin dose.

NICARdipine *(nye KAR de peen)*

U.S. Brand Names Cardene®; Cardene® I.V.; Cardene® SR

Synonyms Nicardipine Hydrochloride

Pharmacologic Category Calcium Channel Blocker

Medication Safety Issues

Sound-alike/look-alike issues:

NICARdipine may be confused with niacinamide, NIFEdipine, nimodipine

Cardene® may be confused with Cardizem®, Cardura®, codeine

Pregnancy Risk Factor C

Lactation Enters breast milk/not recommended

Use Chronic stable angina (immediate-release product only); management of essential hypertension (immediate and sustained release; parenteral only for short time that oral treatment is not feasible)

Unlabeled/Investigational Use Congestive heart failure

Mechanism of Action/Effect Inhibits calcium ion from entering the "slow channels" or select voltage-sensitive areas of vascular smooth muscle and myocardium during depolarization, producing a relaxation of coronary vascular smooth muscle and coronary vasodilation; increases myocardial oxygen delivery in patients with vasospastic angina

Contraindications Hypersensitivity to nicardipine or any component of the formulation; advanced aortic stenosis; severe hypotension; cardiogenic shock; ventricular tachycardia

Warnings/Precautions Blood pressure lowering should be done at a rate appropriate for the patient's condition. Rapid drops in blood pressure can lead to arterial insufficiency. Use with caution in CAD (can cause increase in angina), CHF (can worsen heart failure symptoms), and pheochromocytoma (limited clinical experience). Peripheral infusion sites (for I.V. therapy) should be changed ever 12 hours. Titrate I.V. dose cautiously in patients with CHF, renal, or hepatic dysfunction. Use the I.V. form cautiously in patients with portal hypertension (can cause increase in hepatic pressure gradient). Safety and efficacy have not been demonstrated in pediatric patients. Abrupt withdrawal may cause rebound angina in patients with CAD.

Drug Interactions

Cytochrome P450 Effect: Substrate of CYP1A2 (minor), 2C8/9 (minor), 2D6 (minor), 2E1 (minor), 3A4 (major); **Inhibits** CYP2C8/9 (strong), 2C19 (moderate), 2D6 (moderate), 3A4 (strong)

Decreased Effect: The levels/effects of nicardipine may be decreased by aminoglutethimide, carbamazepine, nafcillin, nevirapine, phenobarbital, phenytoin, rifamycins, and other CYP3A4 inducers. Nicardipine may decrease the levels/effects of CYP2D6 prodrug substrates (eg, codeine, hydrocodone, oxycodone, tramadol). Calcium may reduce the calcium channel blocker's effects, particularly hypotension.

Increased Effect/Toxicity: H_2 blockers (cimetidine) may increase the bioavailability of nicardipine. The levels/effects of nicardipine may be increased by azole antifungals, clarithromycin, diclofenac, doxycycline, erythromycin, imatinib, isoniazid, nefazodone, propofol, protease inhibitors, quinidine, telithromycin, verapamil and other CYP3A4 inhibitors.

Nicardipine may increase the effect of vecuronium (reduce dose 25%). Nicardipine increase the levels/effects of amiodarone, amphetamines, selected benzodiazepines, selected beta-blockers, calcium channel blockers, cisapride, citalopram, cyclosporine, dextromethorphan, diazepam, ergot derivatives, fluoxetine, glimepiride, glipizide, HMG-CoA reductase inhibitors, lidocaine, methsuximide, mirtazapine, nateglinide, nefazodone, paroxetine, phenytoin, pioglitazone, propranolol, risperidone, ritonavir, rosiglitazone, sertraline, sildenafil (and other PDE-5 inhibitors), tacrolimus, thioridazine, tricyclic antidepressants, venlafaxine, warfarin, and other substrates of CYP2C8/9, 2C19, 2D6, or 3A4.

Nutritional/Ethanol Interactions

Ethanol: Avoid ethanol (may increase CNS depression).

Food: Nicardipine average peak concentrations may be decreased if taken with food. Serum concentrations/toxicity of nicardipine may be increased by grapefruit juice; avoid concurrent use.

Herb/Nutraceutical: St John's wort may decrease levels. Avoid dong quai if using for hypertension (has estrogenic activity). Avoid ephedra, yohimbe, ginseng (may worsen hypertension). Avoid garlic (may have increased antihypertensive effect).

Adverse Reactions

1% to 10%:

Cardiovascular: Flushing (6% to 10%), palpitation (3% to 4%), tachycardia (1% to 4%), peripheral edema (dose related 7% to 8%), increased angina (dose related 6%), hypotension (I.V. 6%), orthostasis (I.V. 1%)

Central nervous system: Headache (6% to 15%), dizziness (4% to 7%), somnolence (4% to 6%), paresthesia (1%)

Dermatologic: Rash (1%)

Gastrointestinal: Nausea (2% to 5%), dry mouth (1%)

Genitourinary: Polyuria (1%)

Local: Injection site reaction (I.V. 1%)

Neuromuscular & skeletal: Weakness (4% to 6%), myalgia (1%)

Miscellaneous: Diaphoresis

Overdosage/Toxicology The primary cardiac symptoms of calcium blocker overdose include hypotension and bradycardia. Noncardiac symptoms include confusion, stupor, nausea, vomiting, metabolic acidosis, and hyperglycemia. Following initial gastric decontamination, if possible, repeated calcium administration may promptly reverse the depressed cardiac contractility (but not sinus node depression or peripheral vasodilation). Glucagon and epinephrine may treat refractory hypotension. Glucagon and epinephrine also increase the heart rate (outside the U.S., 4-aminopyridine may be available as an antidote). Dialysis and hemoperfusion are not effective in enhancing elimination although repeat-dose activated charcoal may serve as an adjunct with sustained-release preparations.

Pharmacodynamics/Kinetics

Onset of Action: Oral: 0.5-2 hours; I.V.: 10 minutes; Hypotension: ~20 minutes

Duration of Action: ≤8 hours

Time to Peak: Serum: 30-120 minutes

Protein Binding: >95%

Half-Life Elimination: 2-4 hours

Metabolism: Hepatic; CYP3A4 substrate (major); extensive first-pass effect (saturable)

Excretion: Urine (60% as metabolites); feces (35%)

Available Dosage Forms

Capsule (Cardene®): 20 mg, 30 mg

Capsule, sustained release (Cardene® SR): 30 mg, 45 mg, 60 mg

Injection, solution (Cardene® IV): 2.5 mg/mL (10 mL)

Dosing

Adults & Elderly:

Angina: Immediate release: Oral: 20 mg 3 times/day; usual range: 60-120 mg/day; increase dose at 3-day intervals

Hypertension: Oral:

Immediate release: Initial: 20 mg 3 times/day; usual: 20-40 mg 3 times/day (allow 3 days between dose increases)

Sustained release: Initial: 30 mg twice daily, titrate up to 60 mg twice daily

Note: The total daily dose of immediate-release product may not automatically be equivalent to the daily sustained-release dose; use caution in converting.

Acute hypertension: I.V. (dilute to 0.1 mg/mL): Initial: 5 mg/hour increased by 2.5 mg/hour every 15 minutes to a maximum of 15 mg/hour; consider reduction to 3 mg/hour after response is achieved. Monitor and titrate to lowest dose necessary to maintain stable blood pressure.

Substitution for oral therapy (approximate equivalents):

20 mg every 8 hours oral, equivalent to 0.5 mg/hour I.V. infusion

30 mg every 8 hours oral, equivalent to 1.2 mg/hour I.V. infusion

40 mg every 8 hours oral, equivalent to 2.2 mg/hour I.V. infusion

Renal Impairment: Titrate dose beginning with 20 mg 3 times/day (immediate release) or 30 mg twice daily (sustained release). Specific guidelines for adjustment (Continued)

NiCARdipine *(Continued)*

of I.V. nicardipine are not available, but careful monitoring/adjustment is warranted.

Hepatic Impairment: Starting dose: 20 mg twice daily (immediate release) with titration. Refer to "Note" in adult dosing. Specific guidelines for adjustment of I.V. nicardipine are not available, but careful monitoring/adjustment is warranted.

Administration

Oral: Do not chew or crush the sustained release formulation, swallow whole. Do not open or cut capsules.

I.V.: Ampuls must be diluted before use. Administer as a slow continuous infusion.

I.V. Detail: Avoid extravasation.

pH: 3.5 (buffered)

Stability

Compatibility: Stable in D_5W with KCl 40 mEq, $D_5^{1}/_2NS$, D_5NS, D_5W, $^{1}/_2NS$, NS; **incompatible** with sodium bicarbonate 5%, LR

Y-site administration: Incompatible with furosemide, heparin, thiopental

Storage: I.V.: Store at room temperature. Protect from light. Freezing does not affect stability.

Nursing Actions

Physical Assessment: Assess potential for interactions with other pharmacological agents or herbal products patient may be taking (eg, increased risk for toxicity). See Administration for infusion specifics; infusion site must be monitored closely to prevent extravasation; peripheral infusion sites should be changed ever 12 hours. Monitor effectiveness (cardiac status and blood pressure) and adverse reactions (eg, rash, hypotension, bradycardia, confusion, nausea) when starting, adjusting dose, or discontinuing. Teach patient proper use, possible side effects/appropriate interventions (eg, orthostatic precautions), and adverse symptoms to report.

Patient Education: This medication may be administered by intravenous infusion; report immediately any swelling, redness, burning, or pain at infusion site. **Oral:** Take as directed; do not alter dose or decrease without consulting prescriber. Do not crush or chew sustained release forms; swallow whole. Take with nonfatty food. Avoid caffeine and alcohol. Consult prescriber before increasing exercise routine (decreased angina does not mean it is safe to increase exercise). May cause orthostatic hypotension (change position slowly from sitting or lying to standing, or when climbing stairs); sore mouth (inspect gums for swelling or redness, use soft toothbrush, waxed dental floss, and frequent mouth rinses); dizziness or fatigue (use caution when driving or engaging in tasks that require alertness until response to drug is known); or nausea and dry mouth (small frequent meals, frequent mouth care, chewing gum, or sucking lozenges may help). Report chest pain, palpitations, rapid heartbeat; swelling of extremities; muscle weakness or pain; respiratory difficulty; or nervousness. **Pregnancy/breast-feeding precautions:** Inform prescriber if you are or intend to become pregnant. Breast-feeding is not recommended.

Geriatric Considerations Elderly may experience a greater hypotensive response. Constipation may be more of a problem in the elderly.

Related Information

FDA Name Differentiation Project: The Use of Tall-Man Letters *on page 12*

Nicotine *(nik oh TEEN)*

U.S. Brand Names Commit™ [OTC]; NicoDerm® CQ® [OTC]; Nicorette® [OTC]; Nicotrol® Inhaler; Nicotrol® NS; Nicotrol® Patch [OTC]

Synonyms Habitrol

Pharmacologic Category Smoking Cessation Aid

Medication Safety Issues

Sound-alike/look-alike issues:

NicoDerm® may be confused with Nitroderm

Nicorette® may be confused with Nordette®

Transdermal patch may contain conducting metal (eg, aluminum); remove patch prior to MRI.

Pregnancy Risk Factor D (nasal)

Lactation Excretion in breast milk unknown/use caution

Use Treatment to aid smoking cessation for the relief of nicotine withdrawal symptoms (including nicotine craving)

Unlabeled/Investigational Use Management of ulcerative colitis (transdermal)

Mechanism of Action/Effect Nicotine is one of two naturally-occurring alkaloids which exhibit their primary effects via autonomic ganglia stimulation. Nicotine is a potent ganglionic and central nervous system stimulant, the actions of which are mediated via nicotine-specific receptors. Stimulation of the central nervous system (CNS) is characterized by tremors and respiratory excitation. However, convulsions may occur with higher doses, along with respiratory failure secondary to both central paralysis and peripheral blockade to respiratory muscles.

Contraindications Hypersensitivity to nicotine or any component of the formulation; patients who are smoking during the postmyocardial infarction period; patients with life-threatening arrhythmias, or severe or worsening angina pectoris; active temporomandibular joint disease (gum); pregnancy; not for use in nonsmokers

Warnings/Precautions The risk versus the benefits must be weighed for each of these groups: patients with CAD, serious cardiac arrhythmias, vasospastic disease. Use caution in patients with hyperthyroidism, pheochromocytoma, or insulin-dependent diabetes. Use with caution in oropharyngeal inflammation and in patients with history of esophagitis, peptic ulcer, coronary artery disease, vasospastic disease, angina, hypertension, pheochromocytoma, severe renal dysfunction, and hepatic dysfunction. The inhaler should be used with caution in patients with bronchospastic disease (other forms of nicotine replacement may be preferred). Use of nasal product is not recommended with chronic nasal disorders (eg, allergy, rhinitis, nasal polyps, and sinusitis). Transdermal patch may contain conducting metal (eg, aluminum); remove patch prior to MRI. Cautious use of topical nicotine in patients with certain skin diseases. Hypersensitivity to the topical products can occur. Dental problems may be worsened by chewing the gum. Urge patients to stop smoking completely when initiating therapy. Safety and efficacy have not been established in pediatric patients.

Drug Interactions

Cytochrome P450 Effect: Substrate (minor) of CYP1A2, 2A6, 2B6, 2C8/9, 2C19, 2D6, 2E1, 3A4; **Inhibits** CYP2A6 (weak), 2E1 (weak)

Increased Effect/Toxicity: Nicotine increases the hemodynamic and AV blocking effects of adenosine; monitor. Cimetidine increases nicotine concentrations; therefore, may decrease amount of gum or patches needed. Monitor for treatment-emergent hypertension in patients treated with the combination of nicotine patch and bupropion.

Nutritional/Ethanol Interactions Food: Lozenge: Acidic foods/beverages decrease absorption of nicotine.

Adverse Reactions

Nasal spray/inhaler:

>10%:

Central nervous system: Headache (18% to 26%)

Gastrointestinal: Inhaler: Mouth/throat irritation (66%), dyspepsia (18%)

Respiratory: Inhaler: Cough (32%), rhinitis (23%)

1% to 10%:

Dermatologic: Acne (3%)

Endocrine & metabolic: Dysmenorrhea (3%)

Gastrointestinal: Flatulence (4%), gum problems (4%), diarrhea, hiccup, nausea, taste disturbance, tooth disorder

Neuromuscular & skeletal: Back pain (6%), arthralgia (5%), jaw/neck pain

Respiratory: Sinusitis

Miscellaneous: Withdrawal symptoms

Adverse events previously reported in prescription labeling for chewing gum, lozenge and/or transdermal systems. Frequency not defined; may be product or dose specific:

Central nervous system: Concentration impaired, depression, dizziness, headache, insomnia, nervousness, pain

Gastrointestinal: Aphthous stomatitis, constipation, cough, diarrhea, dyspepsia, flatulence, gingival bleeding, glossitis, hiccups, jaw pain, nausea, salivation increased, stomatitis, taste perversion, tooth disorder, ulcerative stomatitis, xerostomia

Dermatologic: Rash

Local: Application site reaction, local edema, local erythema

Neuromuscular & skeletal: Arthralgia, myalgia, paresthesia

Respiratory: Cough, sinusitis

Miscellaneous: Allergic reaction, diaphoresis

Overdosage/Toxicology Symptoms of overdose include nausea, vomiting, abdominal pain, mental confusion, diarrhea, salivation, tachycardia, respiratory and cardiovascular collapse. Treatment is symptomatic and supportive. Remove patch, rinse area with water, and dry. Do not use soap as this may increase absorption.

Pharmacodynamics/Kinetics

Onset of Action: Intranasal: More closely approximate the time course of plasma nicotine levels observed after cigarette smoking than other dosage forms

Duration of Action: Transdermal: 24 hours

Time to Peak: Serum: Transdermal: 8-9 hours

Half-Life Elimination: 4 hours

Metabolism: Hepatic, primarily to cotinine ($\frac{1}{5}$ as active)

Excretion: Urine

Clearance: Renal: pH dependent

Available Dosage Forms

Gum, chewing, as polacrilex: 2 mg (48s, 108s); 4 mg (48s, 108s)

Nicorette®: 2 mg (48s, 50s, 110s, 168s, 170s, 192s, 200s, 216s); 4 mg (48s, 108s, 168s) [mint, fresh mint, orange, and original flavors]

Lozenge, as polacrilex (Commit™): 2 mg (48s, 72s) [contains phenylalanine 3.4 mg/lozenge; mint flavor]; 4 mg (48s, 72s) [contains phenylalanine 3.4 mg/lozenge; mint flavor]

Oral inhalation system (Nicotrol® Inhaler): 10 mg cartridge [delivering 4 mg nicotine] (168s) [each unit consists of 5 mouthpieces, 28 storage trays each containing 6 cartridges, and 1 storage case]

Patch, transdermal: 7 mg/24 (30s); 14 mg/24 hours (30s); 21 mg/24 hours (30s)

NicoDerm® CQ®: 7 mg/24 hours (14s); 14 mg/24 hours (14s); 21 mg/24 hours (14s) [available in tan or clear patch]

Nicotrol®: 15 mg/16 hours (7s, 14s) [step 1]; 10 mg/16 hours (14s) [step 2]; 5 mg/16 hours (14s) [step 3]

Solution, intranasal spray (Nicotrol® NS): 10 mg/mL (10 mL) [delivers 0.5 mg/spray; 200 sprays]

Dosing

Adults & Elderly:

Tobacco cessation (patients should be advised to completely stop smoking upon initiation of therapy):

Gum: Oral: Chew 1 piece of gum when urge to smoke, up to 30 pieces/day; most patients require 10-12 pieces of gum/day

Inhaler: Oral: Usually 6 to 16 cartridges per day; best effect was achieved by frequent continuous puffing (20 minutes); recommended duration of treatment is 3 months, after which patients may be weaned from the inhaler by gradual reduction of the daily dose over 6-12 weeks

Lozenge: Oral: Patients who smoke their first cigarette within 30 minutes of waking should use the 4 mg strength; otherwise the 2 mg strength is recommended.

Weeks 1-6: One lozenge every 1-2 hours

Weeks 7-9: One lozenge every 2-4 hours

Weeks 10-12: One lozenge every 4-8 hours

Note: Use at least 9 lozenges/day during first 6 weeks to improve chances of quitting; do not use more than one lozenge at a time (maximum: 5 lozenges every 6 hours, 20 lozenges/day)

Spray: Nasal: 1-2 sprays/hour; do not exceed more than 5 doses (10 sprays) per hour [maximum: 40 doses/day (80 sprays); each dose (2 sprays) contains 1 mg of nicotine

Transdermal patch: Topical: Apply new patch every 24 hours to nonhairy, clean, dry skin on the upper body or upper outer arm; each patch should be applied to a different site. **Note:** Adjustment may be required during initial treatment (move to higher dose if experiencing withdrawal symptoms; lower dose if side effects are experienced).

NicoDerm CQ®:

Patients smoking ≥10 cigarettes/day: Begin with step 1 (21 mg/day) for 4-6 weeks, **followed by** step 2 (14 mg/day) for 2 weeks; **finish with** step 3 (7 mg/day) for 2 weeks

Patients smoking <10 cigarettes/day: Begin with step 2 (14 mg/day) for 6 weeks, **followed by** step 3 (7 mg/day) for 2 weeks

Note: Initial starting dose for patients <100 pounds, history of cardiovascular disease: 14 mg/day for 4-6 weeks, **followed by** 7 mg/day for 2-4 weeks

Note: Patients who are receiving >600 mg/day of cimetidine: Decrease to the next lower patch size

Nicotrol®: One patch daily for 6 weeks

Benefits of use of nicotine transdermal patches beyond 3 months have not been demonstrated

Ulcerative colitis (unlabeled use): Topical: Transdermal: Titrated to 22-25 mg/day

Administration

Oral:

Gum: Should be chewed slowly to avoid jaw ache and to maximize benefit.

Lozenge: Should not be chewed or swallowed.

Topical: Do not cut patch; causes rapid evaporation, rendering the patch useless. Use of an aerosol corticosteroid may diminish local irritation under patches.

Stability

Storage: Nicotrol®: Store inhaler cartridge at room temperature not to exceed 30°C (86°F); protect cartridges from light

Nursing Actions

Physical Assessment: Monitor cardiac status and vital signs prior to, when beginning, and periodically during therapy. Monitor effectiveness of therapy

(Continued)

Nicotine *(Continued)*

(according to rationale for therapy), and adverse reactions at beginning and periodically during therapy. Assess knowledge/teach patient appropriate use, interventions to reduce side effects, and adverse symptoms to report for prescribed form of drug.

Patient Education: Use exactly as directed; do not use more often than prescribed. Stop smoking completely during therapy. Do not smoke, chew tobacco, use snuff, nicotine gum, or any other form of nicotine. Nicotine overdose could occur.

Gum: Chew slowly for 30 minutes. Discard chewed gum away from access by children.

Lozenge: Allow to dissolve slowly in the mouth. Do not chew or swallow lozenge whole. Avoid food or drink 15 minutes prior to, during, or after lozenge.

Transdermal patch: Follow directions in package for dosing schedule and use. Do not cut patches or wear more than one patch at a time. Remove backing from patch and press immediately on skin. Hold for 10 seconds. Apply to clean, dry skin in different site each day. Do not touch eyes; wash hands after application. You may experience vivid dreams and sleep disturbances, dizziness or lightheadedness (use caution driving or when engaging in tasks requiring alertness until response to drug is known). For nausea, vomiting or GI upset, small frequent meals, chewing gum, and frequent oral care may help. Report persistent vomiting, diarrhea, chills, sweating, chest pain or palpitations, or burning or redness at application site.

Spray: Follow directions in package. Blow nose gently before use. Use 1-2 sprays/hour; do not exceed 5 doses (10 sprays) per hour. Excessive use can result in severe (even life-threatening) reactions. You may experience temporary stinging or burning after spray.

Pregnancy/breast-feeding precautions: Inform prescriber if you are pregnant. Consult prescriber for instruction on appropriate contraceptive measures.

Dietary Considerations Commit™: Each lozenge contains phenylalanine 3.4 mg.

Geriatric Considerations Must evaluate benefit in the elderly who may have chronic diseases mentioned (see Warnings/Precautions and Contraindications). The transdermal systems are as effective in the elderly as they are in younger adults; however, complaints of body aches, dizziness, and asthenia were reported more often in the elderly.

Breast-Feeding Issues Nicotine from cigarette smoke is found in breast milk at 1.5-3 times the maternal plasma concentrations. The amount from nicotine replacement products is not known. Women who are breastfeeding are encouraged not to smoke.

Pregnancy Issues Nicotine is teratogenic in animal studies. Nicotine exposure via cigarette smoke may cause increased ectopic pregnancy, low birth weight, increased risk of spontaneous abortion, increased perinatal mortality; increased aortic blood flow, increased heart rate, decreased uterine blood flow, and decreased breathing have been reported in the fetus. Smoking during pregnancy is associated with sudden infant death syndrome (SIDS), an increased risk of asthma, infantile colic, and childhood obesity. Women who are pregnant should be encouraged not to smoke. The use of nicotine replacement products to aid in smoking cessation has not been adequately studied in pregnant women (amount of nicotine exposure is varied). Nonpharmacologic treatments are recommended. If the benefits of nicotine replacement therapy outweigh the unknown risks, products with intermittent dosing are suggested to be tried first. If a patch is used, it is suggested to remove it overnight while sleeping to decrease fetal exposure.

Additional Information A cigarette has 10-25 mg nicotine.

NIFEdipine *(nye FED i peen)*

U.S. Brand Names Adalat® CC; Afeditab™ CR; Nifediac™ CC; Nifedical™ XL; Procardia®; Procardia XL®

Pharmacologic Category Calcium Channel Blocker

Medication Safety Issues

Sound-alike/look-alike issues:

NIFEdipine may be confused with niCARdipine, nimodipine, nisoldipine

Procardia XL® may be confused with Cartia® XT

Pregnancy Risk Factor C

Lactation Enters breast milk/compatible

Use Angina and hypertension (sustained release only), pulmonary hypertension

Mechanism of Action/Effect Inhibits calcium ion from entering the "slow channels" or select voltage-sensitive areas of vascular smooth muscle and myocardium during depolarization, producing a relaxation of coronary vascular smooth muscle and coronary vasodilation; increases myocardial oxygen delivery in patients with vasospastic angina

Contraindications Hypersensitivity to nifedipine or any component of the formulation; immediate release preparation for treatment of urgent or emergent hypertension; acute MI

Warnings/Precautions The use of sublingual short-acting nifedipine in hypertensive emergencies and pseudoemergencies is neither safe nor effective and SHOULD BE ABANDONED! Serious adverse events (cerebrovascular ischemia, syncope, heart block, stroke, sinus arrest, severe hypotension, acute myocardial infarction, ECG changes, and fetal distress) have been reported in relation to such use.

Blood pressure lowering should be done at a rate appropriate for the patient's condition. Rapid drops in blood pressure can lead to arterial insufficiency. Increased angina and/or MI has occurred with initiation or dosage titration of calcium channel blockers. Severe hypotension may occur in patients taking immediate release nifepine concurrently with beta blockers when undergoing CABG with high dose fentanyl anesthesia. When considering surgery with high dose fentanyl, may consider withdrawing nifedipine (>36 hours) before surgery if possible.

Use caution in severe aortic stenosis. Use caution in patients with severe hepatic impairment (may need dosage adjustment). Abrupt withdrawal may cause rebound angina in patients with CAD. Use caution in CHF (may cause worsening of symptoms). Avoid use of extended release tablets (Procardia XL®) in patients with known stricture/narrowing of the GI tract. Avoid grapefruit juice during treatment with nifedipine.

Drug Interactions

Cytochrome P450 Effect: Substrate of CYP2D6 (minor), 3A4 (major); **Inhibits** CYP1A2 (moderate), 2C8/9 (weak), 2D6 (weak), 3A4 (weak)

Decreased Effect: Nifedipine may decrease quinidine serum levels. Calcium may reduce the hypotension from of calcium channel blockers. The levels/effects of nifedipine may be decreased by aminoglutethimide, barbiturates, carbamazepine, nafcillin, nevirapine, phenobarbital, phenytoin, rifamycins, and other CYP3A4 inducers.

Increased Effect/Toxicity: The levels/effects of nifedipine may be increased by alpha-1 blockers, azole antifungals, cisapride, clarithromycin, cyclosporine, diclofenac, doxycycline, erythromycin, grapefruit juice, imatinib, isoniazid, nefazodone, nicardipine, propofol, protease inhibitors, quinidine, quinupristin/dalfopristin, telithromycin, verapamil, and other CYP3A4 inhibitors. Cimetidine may also increase nifedipine levels. Nifedipine may increase the levels/

effects of aminophylline, digoxin, fluvoxamine, mexiletine, mirtazapine, ropinirole, trifluoperazine, vincristine, and other CYP1A2 substrates. Digoxin, phenytoin, and vincristine levels may also be increased by nifedipine.

Blood pressure-lowering effects may be additive with sildenafil, tadalafil, and vardenafil (use caution). Concurrent use with magnesium salts may enhance the adverse/toxic effects of magnesium and enhance the hypotensive effects of the calcium channel blocker. Calcium channel blockers may enhance the neuromuscular blocking effect from nondepolarizing neuromuscular blockers. Calcium channel blocker (nondihydropyridine) may enhance the hypotensive effects of calcium channel blocker (dihydropyridine).

Nutritional/Ethanol Interactions

Ethanol: Avoid ethanol (may increase CNS depression and may increase the effects of nifedipine). Monitor.

Food: Nifedipine serum levels may be decreased if taken with food. Food may decrease the rate but not the extent of absorption of Procardia XL®. Increased therapeutic and vasodilator side effects, including severe hypotension and myocardial ischemia, may occur if nifedipine is taken by patients ingesting grapefruit.

Herb/Nutraceutical: St John's wort may decrease nifedipine levels. Avoid dong quai if using for hypertension (has estrogenic activity). Avoid ephedra, yohimbe, ginseng (may worsen hypertension). Avoid garlic (may have increased antihypertensive effect).

Adverse Reactions

>10%:

Cardiovascular: Flushing (10% to 25%), peripheral edema (dose related 7% to 10%; up to 50%)

Central nervous system: Dizziness/lightheadedness/giddiness (10% to 27%), headache (10% to 23%)

Gastrointestinal: Nausea/heartburn (10% to 11%)

Neuromuscular & skeletal: Weakness (10% to 12%)

≥1% to 10%:

Cardiovascular: Palpitations (≤2% to 7%), transient hypotension (dose related 5%), CHF (2%)

Central nervous system: Nervousness/mood changes (≤2% to 7%), shakiness (≤2%), jitteriness (≤2%), sleep disturbances (≤2%), difficulties in balance (≤2%), fever (≤2%), chills (≤2%)

Dermatologic: Dermatitis (≤2%), pruritus (≤2%), urticaria (≤2%)

Endocrine & metabolic: Sexual difficulties (≤2%)

Gastrointestinal: Diarrhea (≤2%), constipation (≤2%), cramps (≤2%), flatulence (≤2%), gingival hyperplasia (≤10%)

Neuromuscular & skeletal: Muscle cramps/tremor (≤2% to 8%), weakness (10%), inflammation (≤2%), joint stiffness (≤2%)

Ocular: Blurred vision (≤2%)

Respiratory: Dyspnea/cough/wheezing (6%), nasal congestion/sore throat (≤2% to 6%), chest congestion (≤2%), dyspnea (≤2%)

Miscellaneous: Diaphoresis (≤2%)

Overdosage/Toxicology Primary cardiac symptoms of calcium blocker overdose include hypotension and bradycardia. Noncardiac symptoms include confusion, stupor, nausea, vomiting, metabolic acidosis, and hyperglycemia. Following initial gastric decontamination, treat symptomatically.

Pharmacodynamics/Kinetics

Onset of Action: Immediate release: ~20 minutes

Protein Binding: Concentration dependent: 92% to 98%

Half-Life Elimination: Adults: Healthy: 2-5 hours, Cirrhosis: 7 hours; Elderly: 6.7 hours

Metabolism: Hepatic to inactive metabolites

Excretion: Urine (as metabolites)

Available Dosage Forms

Capsule, softgel: 10 mg, 20 mg

Procardia®: 10 mg

Tablet, extended release: 30 mg, 60 mg, 90 mg

Adalat® CC, Procardia XL®: 30 mg, 60 mg, 90 mg

Afeditab™ CR, Nifedical™ XL: 30 mg, 60 mg

Nifediac™ CC: 30 mg, 60 mg, 90 mg [90 mg tablet contains tartrazine]

Dosing

Adults & Elderly:

Hypertension: Oral: Initial: 10 mg 3 times/day as capsules or 30 mg once daily as sustained release

Usual dose: 10-30 mg 3 times/day as capsules or 30-60 mg once daily as sustained release

Maximum: 120-180 mg/day

Note: Adjustment of sustained release formulations should be made at 7- to 14-day intervals

Pediatrics:

Hypertrophic cardiomyopathy (unlabeled use): Oral: Children: 0.6-0.9 mg/kg/24 hours in 3-4 divided doses

Hypertension: Oral: Adolescents: Refer to adult dosing.

Hepatic Impairment: Reduce oral dose by 50% to 60% in patients with cirrhosis.

Administration

Oral: Extended release tablets should be swallowed whole; do not crush or chew.

Nursing Actions

Physical Assessment: Assess potential for interactions with other pharmacological agents or herbal products patient is taking that may increase risk of hypotension or toxicity. Assess therapeutic effectiveness (blood pressure and cardiac status) and adverse reactions (eg, hypotension, peripheral edema, gastrointestinal upset, CNS changes) when starting, adjusting dose, or discontinuing. Teach patient proper use, possible side effects/appropriate interventions (eg, orthostatic precautions), and adverse symptoms to report.

Patient Education: Do not take any new medication during therapy unless approved by prescriber (especially anything that may act as a stimulant or depressant). Take as directed; do not alter dose or decrease without consulting prescriber. Do not crush or chew sustained release forms, swallow whole. Take with nonfatty food. Avoid caffeine, alcohol, and grapefruit juice. Consult prescriber before increasing exercise routine (decreased angina does not mean it is safe to increase exercise). May cause orthostatic hypotension (change position slowly from sitting or lying to standing, or when climbing stairs); sore mouth (inspect gums for swelling or redness, use soft toothbrush, waxed dental floss, and frequent mouth rinses); dizziness, difficulties in balance, or fatigue (use caution when driving or engaging in tasks that require alertness until response to drug is known); or nausea or heartburn (small frequent meals, frequent mouth care, chewing gum, or sucking lozenges may help). Report chest pain, palpitations, rapid heartbeat; swelling of extremities; muscle weakness or pain; respiratory difficulty; nervousness or mood change, rash; or vision changes. **Pregnancy precaution:** Inform prescriber if you are or intend to become pregnant.

Dietary Considerations Capsule is rapidly absorbed orally if it is administered without food, but may result in vasodilator side effects; administration with low-fat meals may decrease flushing. Avoid grapefruit juice.

Geriatric Considerations Elderly may experience a greater hypotensive response. Theoretically, constipation may be more of a problem in elderly patients. The half-life of nifedipine is extended in elderly patients (6.7 hours) as compared to younger subjects (3.8 hours).

Breast-Feeding Issues Crosses into breast milk. Available evidence suggests safe use during breast-feeding. AAP considers **compatible** with breast-feeding. (Continued)

NIFEdipine (Continued)

Pregnancy Issues Hypotension, IUGR reported. IUGR probably related to maternal hypertension. May exhibit tocolytic effects.

Additional Information When measuring smaller doses from the liquid-filled capsules, consider the following concentrations (for Procardia®) 10 mg capsule = 10 mg/0.34 mL; 20 mg capsule = 20 mg/0.45 mL; may be used preoperative to treat hypertensive urgency.

Considerable attention has been directed to potential increases in mortality and morbidity when short-acting nifedipine is used in treating hypertension. The rapid reduction in blood pressure may precipitate adverse cardiovascular events. At this time, there is no indication for the use of short-acting calcium channel blocker therapy. Nifedipine also has potent negative inotropic effects and can worsen heart failure.

Related Information
FDA Name Differentiation Project: The Use of Tall-Man Letters on page 12

Nilutamide (ni LOO ta mide)

U.S. Brand Names Nilandron®
Synonyms RU-23908
Pharmacologic Category Antiandrogen; Antineoplastic Agent, Antiandrogen
Pregnancy Risk Factor C
Lactation Not indicated for use in women
Use Treatment of metastatic prostate cancer
Mechanism of Action/Effect Nonsteroidal antiandrogen that inhibits androgen uptake or inhibits binding of androgen in target tissues
Contraindications Hypersensitivity to nilutamide or any component of the formulation; severe hepatic impairment; severe respiratory insufficiency
Warnings/Precautions Hazardous agent - use appropriate precautions for handling and disposal. May cause interstitial pneumonitis; the suggestive signs of pneumonitis most often occurred within the first 3 months of nilutamide treatment. Has been associated with severe hepatitis, which has resulted in fatality. In addition, foreign postmarketing surveillance has revealed isolated cases of aplastic anemia (a causal relationship with nilutamide could not be ascertained).

May alter time for visual adaptation to darkness, ranging from seconds to a few minutes. This effect sometimes does not abate as drug treatment is continued. Caution patients who experience this effect about driving at night or through tunnels. This effect can be alleviated by wearing tinted glasses.

Drug Interactions
Cytochrome P450 Effect: Substrate of CYP2C19 (major); **Inhibits** CYP2C19 (weak)
Decreased Effect: CYP2C19 inducers may decrease the levels/effects of nilutamide; example inducers include aminoglutethimide, carbamazepine, phenytoin, and rifampin.
Increased Effect/Toxicity: CYP2C19 inhibitors may increase the levels/effects of nilutamide; example inhibitors include delavirdine, fluconazole, fluvoxamine, gemfibrozil, isoniazid, omeprazole, and ticlopidine.

Nutritional/Ethanol Interactions
Ethanol: Avoid ethanol. Up to 5% of patients may experience a systemic reaction (flushing, hypotension, malaise) when combined with nilutamide.
Herb/Nutraceutical: St John's wort may decrease nilutamide levels.

Adverse Reactions
>10%:
Central nervous system: Headache, insomnia

Endocrine & metabolic: Hot flashes (30% to 67%), gynecomastia (10%)
Gastrointestinal: Nausea (mild - 10% to 32%), abdominal pain (10%), constipation, anorexia
Genitourinary: Testicular atrophy (16%), libido decreased
Hepatic: Transaminases increased (8% to 13%; transient)
Ocular: Impaired dark adaptation (13% to 57%), usually reversible with dose reduction, may require discontinuation of the drug in 1% to 2% of patients
Respiratory: Dyspnea (11%)
1% to 10%:
Cardiovascular: Chest pain, edema, heart failure, hypertension, syncope
Central nervous system: Dizziness, drowsiness, malaise, hypoesthesia, depression
Dermatologic: Pruritus, alopecia, dry skin, rash
Endocrine & metabolic: Disulfiram-like reaction (hot flashes, rash) (5%); Flu-like syndrome, fever
Gastrointestinal: Vomiting, diarrhea, dyspepsia, GI hemorrhage, melena, weight loss, xerostomia
Genitourinary: Hematuria, nocturia
Hematologic: Anemia
Hepatic: Hepatitis (1%)
Neuromuscular & skeletal: Arthritis, paresthesia
Ocular: Chromatopsia (9%), abnormal vision (6% to 7%), cataracts, photophobia
Respiratory: Interstitial pneumonitis (2% - typically exertional dyspnea, cough, chest pain, and fever; most often occurring within the first 3 months of treatment); rhinitis
Miscellaneous: Diaphoresis
Overdosage/Toxicology Symptoms of overdose may include nausea, vomiting, malaise, headache, dizziness, and elevated liver enzymes. Management is supportive. Dialysis is of no benefit.
Pharmacodynamics/Kinetics
Protein Binding: 72% to 85%
Half-Life Elimination: Terminal: 23-87 hours; Metabolites: 35-137 hours
Metabolism: Hepatic, forms active metabolites
Excretion: Urine (up to 78% at 120 hours; <1% as unchanged drug); feces (1% to 7%)
Available Dosage Forms Tablet: 150 mg
Dosing
Adults & Elderly: Refer to individual protocols. Prostate cancer: Oral: 300 mg daily for 30 days starting the same day or day after surgical castration, then 150 mg/day
Stability
Storage: Store at room temperature of 15°C to 30°C (59°F to 86°F). Protect from light.
Laboratory Monitoring Chest x-rays prior to and regularly during treatment. Measure serum hepatic enzyme levels at baseline and at regular intervals (3 months). If transaminases increase over 2-3 times the upper limit of normal, discontinue treatment. Perform appropriate laboratory testing at the first symptom/sign of liver injury (eg, jaundice, dark urine, fatigue, abdominal pain, or unexplained GI symptoms).

Nursing Actions
Physical Assessment: Assess potential for interactions with other prescriptions, OTC medications, or herbal products patient may be taking. Assess results of laboratory tests prior to and regularly during therapy. Assess therapeutic effectiveness and adverse response. Teach patient proper use, possible side effects/appropriate interventions (eg, orthostatic precautions), and adverse symptoms to report.
Patient Education: Do not take any new medication during therapy unless approved by prescriber. Take as prescribed; do not change dosing schedule or stop taking without consulting prescriber. Avoid alcohol while taking this medication; may cause severe

adverse reaction. Periodic laboratory tests are necessary while taking this medication. May cause loss of light accommodation (avoid night driving and use caution in poorly lighted or changing light situations such as tunnels); dizziness, confusion, or blurred vision (avoid driving or engaging in tasks that are potentially hazardous until response to drug is known); nausea or anorexia (small frequent meals, frequent mouth care, chewing gum, or sucking lozenges may help); or hot flashes, gynecomastia, decreased libido, impotence or sexual dysfunction (consult prescriber). Report any decreased respiratory function (eg, dyspnea, increased cough); unexplained fever; difficulty or painful voiding or blood in urine; or other persistent adverse effects.

Dietary Considerations May be taken without regard to food.

Nimodipine (nye MOE di peen)

U.S. Brand Names Nimotop®
Pharmacologic Category Calcium Channel Blocker
Medication Safety Issues
Sound-alike/look-alike issues:
Nimodipine may be confused with niCARdipine, NIFEdipine
Nimodipine has inadvertently been administered I.V. when withdrawn from capsules into a syringe for subsequent nasogastric administration. Severe cardiovascular adverse events, including fatalities, have resulted. Employ precautions against such an event.

Pregnancy Risk Factor C
Lactation Enters breast milk/not recommended
Use Spasm following subarachnoid hemorrhage from ruptured intracranial aneurysms regardless of the patients neurological condition postictus (Hunt and Hess grades I-V)
Mechanism of Action/Effect Nimodipine shares the pharmacology of other calcium channel blockers; animal studies indicate that nimodipine has a greater effect on cerebral arterials than other arterials; inhibits calcium ion from entering the "slow channels" or select voltage sensitive areas of vascular smooth muscle and myocardium during depolarization
Contraindications Hypersensitivity to nimodipine or any component of the formulation
Warnings/Precautions May cause reductions in blood pressure. Use caution in hepatic impairment. Intestinal pseudo-obstruction and ileus have been reported during the use of nimodipine. Use caution in patients with decreased GI motility of a history of bowel obstruction. Use caution when treating patients with increased intracranial pressure.

Nimodipine has inadvertently been administered I.V. when withdrawn from capsules into a syringe for subsequent nasogastric administration. Severe cardiovascular adverse events, including fatalities, have resulted; precautions should be employed against such an event.

Drug Interactions
Cytochrome P450 Effect: Substrate of CYP3A4 (major)
Decreased Effect: CYP3A4 inducers may decrease the levels/effects of nimodipine; example inducers include aminoglutethimide, carbamazepine, nafcillin, nevirapine, phenobarbital, phenytoin, and rifamycins.
Increased Effect/Toxicity: Calcium channel blockers and nimodipine may result in enhanced cardiovascular effects of other calcium channel blockers. Cimetidine, omeprazole, and valproic acid may increase serum nimodipine levels. The effects of antihypertensive agents may be increased by nimodipine. Blood pressure-lowering effects may be additive with sildenafil, tadalafil, and vardenafil (use caution).

CYP3A4 inhibitors may increase the levels/effects of nimodipine; example inhibitors include azole antifungals, clarithromycin, diclofenac, doxycycline, erythromycin, imatinib, isoniazid, nefazodone, nicardipine, propofol, protease inhibitors, quinidine, telithromycin, and verapamil.

Nutritional/Ethanol Interactions
Food: Nimodipine has shown a 1.5-fold increase in bioavailability when taken with grapefruit juice; avoid concurrent use.
Herb/Nutraceutical: St John's wort may decrease levels. Avoid dong quai if using for hypertension (has estrogenic activity). Avoid ephedra, yohimbe, ginseng (may worsen hypertension). Avoid garlic (may have increased antihypertensive effect).
Adverse Reactions 1% to 10%:
Cardiovascular: Reductions in systemic blood pressure (1% to 8%)
Central nervous system: Headache (1% to 4%)
Dermatologic: Rash (1% to 2%)
Gastrointestinal: Diarrhea (2% to 4%), abdominal discomfort (2%)
Overdosage/Toxicology Primary cardiac symptoms of calcium blocker overdose include hypotension and bradycardia. Noncardiac symptoms include confusion, stupor, nausea, vomiting, metabolic acidosis and hyperglycemia. Treat symptomatically.
Pharmacodynamics/Kinetics
Time to Peak: Serum: ~1 hour
Protein Binding: >95%
Half-Life Elimination: 1-2 hours; prolonged with renal impairment
Metabolism: Extensively hepatic
Excretion: Urine (50%) and feces (32%) within 4 days
Available Dosage Forms Capsule, liquid filled: 30 mg
Dosing
Adults & Elderly: Note: Capsules and contents are for oral administration **ONLY.**
Subarachnoid hemorrhage: Oral: 60 mg every 4 hours for 21 days, start therapy within 96 hours after subarachnoid hemorrhage.
Renal Impairment: Not removed by hemo- or peritoneal dialysis; supplemental dose is not necessary.
Hepatic Impairment: Reduce dosage to 30 mg every 4 hours in patients with liver failure.
Administration
Oral: For oral administration **ONLY.** If the capsules cannot be swallowed, the liquid may be removed by making a hole in each end of the capsule with an 18-gauge needle and extracting the contents into a syringe. If given via NG tube, follow with a flush of 30 mL NS.
Nursing Actions
Physical Assessment: Assess potential for interactions with other pharmacological agents and herbal products patient may be taking (eg, increased risk of hypotension with other antihypertensives). Monitor therapeutic effectiveness (blood pressure and cardiac status) and adverse response (eg, rash, hypotension, diarrhea, confusion) when starting or adjusting dose and periodically during long-term therapy. Teach patient proper use, possible side effects/appropriate interventions, and adverse symptoms to report.
Patient Education: Do not take any new medication during therapy unless approved by prescriber. Take as directed; do not alter dose or decrease without consulting prescriber. Avoid grapefruit juice while taking this medication. May cause orthostatic hypotension (change position slowly from sitting or lying to standing, or when climbing stairs); headache (consult prescriber for approved analgesic); or diarrhea (buttermilk, boiled milk, or yogurt may help). Report chest pain, palpitations, slow heartbeat, respiratory difficulty, or other persistent adverse effects. **Pregnancy/breast-feeding precautions:** Inform

(Continued)

Nimodipine *(Continued)*

prescriber if you are or intend to become pregnant. Breast-feeding is not recommended.

Geriatric Considerations Elderly may experience a greater hypotensive response. Constipation may be more of a problem in the elderly.

Nisoldipine *(NYE sole di peen)*

U.S. Brand Names Sular®

Pharmacologic Category Calcium Channel Blocker

Medication Safety Issues
Sound-alike/look-alike issues:
Nisoldipine may be confused with NIFEdipine

Pregnancy Risk Factor C

Lactation Excretion in breast milk unknown

Use Management of hypertension, alone or in combination with other antihypertensive agents

Mechanism of Action/Effect As a dihydropyridine calcium channel blocker, structurally similar to nifedipine, nisoldipine impedes the movement of calcium ions into vascular smooth muscle and cardiac muscle. Dihydropyridines are potent vasodilators and are not as likely to suppress cardiac contractility and slow cardiac conduction as other calcium antagonists such as verapamil and diltiazem; nisoldipine is 5-10 times as potent a vasodilator as nifedipine.

Contraindications Hypersensitivity to nisoldipine, any component of the formulation, or other dihydropyridine calcium channel blockers

Warnings/Precautions May cause increased angina and/or myocardial infarction in patients with coronary artery disease (rare). Use with caution in patients with hypotension, CHF, and hepatic impairment. Blood pressure lowering must be done at a rate appropriate for the patient's condition.

Drug Interactions
Cytochrome P450 Effect: Substrate of CYP3A4 (major); **Inhibits** CYP1A2 (weak), 3A4 (weak)
Decreased Effect: CYP3A4 inducers may decrease the levels/effects of nisoldipine; example inducers include aminoglutethimide, carbamazepine, nafcillin, nevirapine, phenobarbital, phenytoin, and rifamycins. Calcium may decrease the hypotension from calcium channel blockers.
Increased Effect/Toxicity: CYP3A4 inhibitors may increase the levels/effects of nisoldipine; example inhibitors include azole antifungals, clarithromycin, diclofenac, doxycycline, erythromycin, imatinib, isoniazid, nefazodone, nicardipine, propofol, protease inhibitors, quinidine, telithromycin, and verapamil. Calcium may reduce the calcium channel blocker's effects, particularly hypotension. Blood pressure-lowering effects may be additive with sildenafil, tadalafil, and vardenafil (use caution). Digoxin and nisoldipine may increase digoxin effect.

Nutritional/Ethanol Interactions
Food: Nisoldipine bioavailability may be increased if taken with high-lipid foods or with grapefruit juice. Avoid grapefruit products before and after dosing.
Herb/Nutraceutical: St John's wort may decrease nisoldipine levels. Avoid dong quai if using for hypertension (has estrogenic activity). Avoid ephedra, yohimbe, ginseng (may worsen hypertension). Avoid garlic (may have increased antihypertensive effect).

Adverse Reactions
>10%:
Cardiovascular: Peripheral edema (dose related 7% to 29%)
Central nervous system: Headache (22%)
1% to 10%:
Cardiovascular: Chest pain (2%), palpitation (3%), vasodilation (4%)

Central nervous system: Dizziness (3% to 10%)
Dermatologic: Rash (2%)
Gastrointestinal: Nausea (2%)
Respiratory: Pharyngitis (5%), sinusitis (3%), dyspnea (3%), cough (5%)

Overdosage/Toxicology Primary cardiac symptoms of calcium blocker overdose include hypotension and bradycardia. Noncardiac symptoms include confusion, stupor, nausea, vomiting, metabolic acidosis and hyperglycemia. Treat symptomatically.

Pharmacodynamics/Kinetics
Duration of Action: >24 hours
Time to Peak: 6-12 hours
Protein Binding: >99%
Half-Life Elimination: 7-12 hours
Metabolism: Extensively hepatic; 1 active metabolite (10% of parent); first-pass effect
Excretion: Urine (as metabolites)

Available Dosage Forms Tablet, extended release: 10 mg, 20 mg, 30 mg, 40 mg

Dosing
Adults:
Hypertension: Oral: Initial: 20 mg once daily, then increase by 10 mg/week (or longer intervals) to attain adequate control of blood pressure
Usual dose range (JNC 7): 10-40 mg once daily; doses >60 mg once daily are not recommended.
Elderly: Initial dose: 10 mg/day, increase by 10 mg/week (or longer intervals) to attain adequate blood pressure control. Those with hepatic disease should be started with 10 mg/day.
Hepatic Impairment: A starting dose not exceeding 10 mg/day is recommended for patients with hepatic impairment.

Administration
Oral: Administer at the same time each day to ensure minimal fluctuation of serum levels. Avoid high-fat diet.

Nursing Actions
Physical Assessment: Assess potential for interactions with other pharmacological agents and herbal products patient may be taking (eg, increased potential for hypotension with other antihypertensives). Monitor therapeutic effectiveness (cardiac status and blood pressure) and adverse response (eg, chest pain, dyspnea, cough, edema, rash, nausea, confusion) when starting or adjusting dose and periodically during long-term therapy. Dose should be tapered gradually (over 2 weeks) when discontinuing. Teach patient proper use, possible side effects/appropriate interventions, and adverse symptoms to report.
Patient Education: Do not take any new medication during therapy unless approved by prescriber. Take exactly as directed; do not alter dose or decrease without consulting prescriber. Do not crush or chew capsules; swallow whole. Take with food, but avoid fatty food and grapefruit juice. This drug does not replace diet and other exercise recommendations of prescriber. May cause orthostatic hypotension (change position slowly when rising from sitting or lying, or when climbing stairs); headache (consult prescriber for approved analgesic); dizziness (use caution when driving or engaging in tasks that require alertness until response to drug is known); or nausea (small, frequent meals, frequent mouth care, chewing gum, or sucking lozenges may help). Report chest pain, palpitations, irregular heartbeat; respiratory difficulty; unusual cough; rash; vision changes; anxiety, confusion, depression, or other CNS changes; or other persistent adverse reactions. **Pregnancy/breast-feeding precautions:** Inform prescriber if you are or intend to become pregnant. Consult prescriber if breast-feeding.
Geriatric Considerations Elderly may experience a greater hypotensive response. Constipation may be more of a problem in the elderly. Calcium channel

blockers are no more effective in the elderly than other therapies; however, they do not cause significant CNS effects which is an advantage over some antihypertensive agents.

Nitazoxanide (nye ta ZOX a nide)

U.S. Brand Names Alinia®

Synonyms NTZ

Pharmacologic Category Antiprotozoal

Pregnancy Risk Factor B

Lactation Excretion in breast milk unknown/use caution

Use Treatment of diarrhea caused by *Cryptosporidium parvum* or *Giardia lamblia*

Mechanism of Action/Effect Nitazoxanide is rapidly metabolized to the active metabolite tizoxanide *in vivo*. Nitazoxanide and its metabolite inhibit the growth of sporozoites and oocysts of *Cryptosporidium parvum* and trophozoites of *Giardia lamblia*.

Contraindications Hypersensitivity to nitazoxanide or any component of the formulation

Warnings/Precautions Use caution with renal or hepatic impairment. Safety and efficacy have not been established with HIV infection, immunodeficiency, or in children <1 year of age.

Nutritional/Ethanol Interactions Food: Food increases AUC.

Adverse Reactions Rates of adverse effects were similar to those reported with placebo.

1% to 10%:

Central nervous system: Headache (1% to 3%)

Gastrointestinal: Abdominal pain (7% to 8%), diarrhea (2% to 4%), nausea (3%), vomiting (1%)

Overdosage/Toxicology Treatment should be symptomatic and supportive.

Pharmacodynamics/Kinetics

Time to Peak: Plasma: Tizoxanide and tizoxanide glucuronide: 1-4 hours

Protein Binding: Tizoxanide: >99%

Metabolism: Hepatic, to an active metabolite, tizoxanide. Tizoxanide undergoes conjugation to form tizoxanide glucuronide. Nitazoxanide is not detectable in the serum following oral administration.

Excretion: Tizoxanide: Urine, bile, and feces; Tizoxanide glucuronide: Urine and bile

Available Dosage Forms

Powder for oral suspension: 100 mg/5 mL (60 mL) [contains sucrose 1.48 g/5 mL, sodium benzoate; strawberry flavor]

Tablet: 500 mg

Alinia® 3-Day Therapy Packs™ [unit-dose pack]: 500 mg (6s)

Dosing

Adults: Diarrhea caused by *Cryptosporidium parvum* or *Giardia lamblia*: Oral: 500 mg every 12 hours for 3 days

Pediatrics: Diarrhea caused by *Cryptosporidium parvum* or *Giardia lamblia*: Oral:

Children 1-3 years: 100 mg every 12 hours for 3 days

Children 4-11 years: 200 mg every 12 hours for 3 days

Children ≥12 years: Refer to adult dosing.

Renal Impairment: Specific recommendations are not available; use with caution.

Hepatic Impairment: Specific recommendations are not available; use with caution.

Administration

Oral: Administer with food. Shake suspension well prior to administration.

Stability

Reconstitution: For preparation at time of dispensing, add 48 mL incrementally to 60 mL bottle; shake vigorously; resulting suspension is 20 mg/mL (100 mg per 5 mL).

Storage:

Suspension: Prior to and following reconstitution, store at room temperature of 15°C to 30°C (59°F to 86°F). Following reconstitution, discard unused portion of suspension after 7 days.

Tablet: Store at room temperature.

Nursing Actions

Patient Education: Administer exactly as directed. Do not alter dose; administer with food. Shake suspension well before using. Store at room temperature and discard any unused portion of suspension after 7 days. May cause headache, abdominal pain, diarrhea, or vomiting. If severe or persistent, contact prescriber. **Breast-feeding precaution:** Consult prescriber if breast-feeding.

Dietary Considerations Should be taken with food. Suspension contains sucrose 1.48 g/5 mL.

Nitrofurantoin (nye troe fyoor AN toyn)

U.S. Brand Names Furadantin®; Macrobid®; Macrodantin®

Pharmacologic Category Antibiotic, Miscellaneous

Pregnancy Risk Factor B (contraindicated at term)

Lactation Enters breast milk/not recommended (infants <1 month); AAP rates "compatible"

Use Prevention and treatment of urinary tract infections caused by susceptible gram-negative and some gram-positive organisms; *Pseudomonas*, *Serratia*, and most species of *Proteus* are generally resistant to nitrofurantoin

Mechanism of Action/Effect Inhibits several bacterial enzyme systems including acetyl coenzyme A interfering with metabolism and possibly cell wall synthesis

Contraindications Hypersensitivity to nitrofurantoin or any component of the formulation; renal impairment (anuria, oliguria, significantly elevated serum creatinine, or Cl_{cr}< 60 mL/minute); infants <1 month (due to the possibility of hemolytic anemia); pregnancy at term (38-42 weeks gestation), during labor and delivery, or when the onset of labor is imminent

Warnings/Precautions Use with caution in patients with G6PD deficiency or in patients with anemia. Therapeutic concentrations of nitrofurantoin are not attained in urine of patients with Cl_{cr}<60 mL/minute. Use with caution if prolonged therapy is anticipated due to possible pulmonary toxicity. Acute, subacute, or chronic (usually after 6 months of therapy) pulmonary reactions have been observed in patients treated with nitrofurantoin; if these occur, discontinue therapy immediately; monitor closely for malaise, dyspnea, cough, fever, radiologic evidence of diffuse interstitial pneumonitis or fibrosis. Rare, but severe hepatic reactions have been associated with nitrofurantoin (onset may be insidious); discontinue immediately if hepatitis occurs. Has been associated with peripheral neuropathy (rare); risk may be increased by renal impairment, diabetes, vitamin B deficiency, or electrolyte imbalance; use caution.

Drug Interactions

Decreased Effect: Antacids decrease absorption of nitrofurantoin.

Increased Effect/Toxicity: Probenecid decreases renal excretion of nitrofurantoin.

Nutritional/Ethanol Interactions

Ethanol: Avoid ethanol (may increase CNS depression).

Food: Nitrofurantoin serum concentrations may be increased if taken with food.

(Continued)

Nitrofurantoin *(Continued)*

Lab Interactions False-positive urine glucose (Benedict's and Fehling's methods); no false positives with enzymatic tests

Adverse Reactions Frequency not defined.

Cardiovascular: Chest pain, cyanosis, ECG changes (associated with pulmonary toxicity)

Central nervous system: Chills, depression, dizziness, drowsiness, fatigue, fever, headache, pseudotumor cerebri, psychotic reaction

Dermatologic: Alopecia, erythema multiforme, exfoliative dermatitis, pruritus, rash, Stevens-Johnson syndrome

Gastrointestinal: Abdominal pain, *C. difficile*-colitis, constipation, diarrhea, dyspepsia, loss of appetite, nausea (most common), pancreatitis, sore throat, vomiting

Hematologic: Agranulocytosis, aplastic anemia, eosinophilia, hemolytic anemia, methemoglobinemia, thrombocytopenia

Hepatic: Cholestasis, hepatitis, hepatic necrosis, transaminases increased, jaundice (cholestatic)

Neuromuscular & skeletal: Arthralgia, numbness, paresthesia, peripheral neuropathy, weakness

Ocular: Amblyopia, nystagmus, optic neuritis (rare)

Respiratory: Cough, dyspnea, pneumonitis, pulmonary fibrosis

Miscellaneous: Hypersensitivity (including acute pulmonary hypersensitivity), lupus-like syndrome

Overdosage/Toxicology Symptoms of overdose include vomiting. Treatment is supportive.

Pharmacodynamics/Kinetics

Protein Binding: 60% to 90%

Half-Life Elimination: 20-60 minutes; prolonged with renal impairment

Metabolism: Body tissues (except plasma) metabolize 60% of drug to inactive metabolites

Excretion:

Suspension: Urine (40%) and feces (small amounts) as metabolites and unchanged drug

Macrocrystals: Urine (20% to 25% as unchanged drug)

Available Dosage Forms

Capsule, macrocrystal: 50 mg, 100 mg

Macrodantin®: 25 mg, 50 mg, 100 mg

Capsule, macrocrystal/monohydrate (Macrobid®): 100 mg

Suspension, oral (Furadantin®): 25 mg/5 mL (470 mL)

Dosing

Adults:

Treatment of UTI: Oral: 50-100 mg/dose every 6 hours (not to exceed 400 mg/24 hours)

Prophylaxis of UTI: Oral: 50-100 mg/dose at bedtime

Elderly: Refer to adult dosing (see Geriatric Considerations).

Pediatrics:

Treatment of UTI: Oral: Children >1 month: 5-7 mg/kg/day in divided doses every 6 hours; maximum: 400 mg/day

Chronic therapy: Oral: 1-2 mg/kg/day in divided doses every 12-24 hours; maximum: 100 mg/day

Renal Impairment:

Cl_{cr} <60 mL/minute: Contraindicated

Contraindicated in hemo- and peritoneal dialysis and continuous arteriovenous or venovenous hemofiltration.

Administration

Oral: Suspension: Shake well before use. Higher peak serum levels may cause increased GI upset. Give with meals to slow the rate of absorption and decrease adverse effects.

Stability

Storage: Store at room temperature 15°C to 30°C (59°F to 86°F).

Laboratory Monitoring CBC, periodic liver function. Perform culture and sensitivity prior to initiating therapy.

Nursing Actions

Physical Assessment: Assess results of laboratory tests, therapeutic effectiveness, and adverse response. Advise patients with diabetes about use of Clinitest® (may cause false-positive urine glucose). Teach patient proper use, possible side effects/appropriate interventions, and adverse symptoms to report.

Patient Education: Do not take any new medication during therapy unless approved by prescriber. Take entire prescription, even if you are feeling better. Take with food. Maintain adequate hydration (2-3 L/day of fluids) unless instructed to restrict fluid intake. If you have diabetes, drug may cause false test results with Clinitest® urine glucose monitoring; use of another type of glucose monitoring is preferable. May cause nausea or vomiting (small, frequent meals, frequent mouth care, sucking lozenges, or chewing gum may help); or diarrhea (buttermilk, boiled milk, or yogurt may help). Report immediately and rash; swelling of face, tongue, mouth, or throat; or chest tightness. Report if condition being treated worsens or does not improve by the time prescription is completed.

Geriatric Considerations Because of nitrofurantoin's decreased efficacy in patients with a Cl_{cr} <60 mL/minute and its side effect profile, it is not an antibiotic of choice for acute or prophylactic treatment of urinary tract infections in the elderly. An increased rate of severe hepatic toxicity has been suggested by postmarketing reports.

Breast-Feeding Issues Excreted in trace amounts in breast milk; may cause hyperbilirubinemia or hemolytic anemia in infants (<1 month of age). AAP rates "compatible." Use caution in G6PD deficiency.

Pregnancy Issues Teratogenic effects have not been observed, however may cause hemolytic anemia in infants. Use of nitrofurantoin is contraindicated at term (38-42 weeks gestation), during labor and delivery, or when the onset of labor is imminent.

Nitroglycerin *(nye troe GLI ser in)*

U.S. Brand Names Minitran™; Nitrek®; Nitro-Bid®; Nitro-Dur®; Nitrolingual®; NitroQuick®; Nitrostat®; Nitro-Tab®; NitroTime®

Synonyms Glyceryl Trinitrate; Nitroglycerol; NTG

Pharmacologic Category Vasodilator

Medication Safety Issues

Sound-alike/look-alike issues:

Nitroglycerin may be confused with nitroprusside

Nitro-Bid® may be confused with Nicobid®

Nitroderm may be confused with NicoDerm®

Nitrol® may be confused with Nizoral®

Nitrostat® may be confused with Hyperstat®, Nilstat®, nystatin

Nitroglycerin transdermal patches should be removed prior to defibrillation or MRI study.

Pregnancy Risk Factor C

Lactation Excretion in breast milk unknown/use caution

Use Treatment of angina pectoris; I.V. for congestive heart failure (especially when associated with acute myocardial infarction); pulmonary hypertension; hypertensive emergencies occurring perioperatively (especially during cardiovascular surgery)

Unlabeled/Investigational Use Esophageal spastic disorders (sublingual)

Mechanism of Action/Effect Works by relaxation of smooth muscle, producing a vasodilator effect on the peripheral veins and arteries with more prominent effects on the veins. Primarily reduces cardiac oxygen demand by decreasing preload (left ventricular end-diastolic pressure); may modestly reduce afterload; dilates coronary arteries and improves collateral flow to ischemic regions

Contraindications Hypersensitivity to organic nitrates; hypersensitivity to isosorbide, nitroglycerin, or any component of the formulation; concurrent use with phosphodiesterase-5 (PDE-5) inhibitors (sildenafil, tadalafil, or vardenafil); angle-closure glaucoma (intraocular pressure may be increased); head trauma or cerebral hemorrhage (increase intracranial pressure); severe anemia; allergy to adhesive (transdermal product)

Additional contraindications for I.V. product: Hypotension; uncorrected hypovolemia; inadequate cerebral circulation; constrictive pericarditis; pericardial tamponade

Warnings/Precautions Severe hypotension can occur. Use with caution in volume depletion, hypotension, and right ventricular infarctions. Paradoxical bradycardia and increased angina pectoris can accompany hypotension. Orthostatic hypotension can also occur. Ethanol can accentuate this. Tolerance does develop to nitrates and appropriate dosing is needed to minimize this (drug-free interval). Safety and efficacy have not been established in pediatric patients. Avoid use of long-acting agents in acute MI or CHF; cannot easily reverse. Nitrate may aggravate angina caused by hypertrophic cardiomyopathy. Nitroglycerin transdermal patches should be removed prior to defibrillation or MRI study.

Drug Interactions

Decreased Effect: I.V. nitroglycerin may antagonize the anticoagulant effect of heparin (possibly only at high nitroglycerin dosages); monitor closely. May need to decrease heparin dosage when nitroglycerin is discontinued. Alteplase (tissue plasminogen activator) has a lesser effect when used with I.V. nitroglycerin; avoid concurrent use. Ergot alkaloids may cause an increase in blood pressure and decrease in antianginal effects; avoid concurrent use.

Increased Effect/Toxicity: Significant reduction of systolic and diastolic blood pressure with concurrent use of sildenafil, tadalafil, or vardenafil (contraindicated); do not administer sildenafil, tadalafil, or vardenafil within 24 hours of a nitrate preparation. Ethanol can cause hypotension when nitrates are taken 1 hour or more after ethanol ingestion.

Adverse Reactions

Spray or patch:

>10%: Central nervous system: Headache (patch 63%, spray 50%)

1% to 10%:

Cardiovascular: Hypotension (patch 4%), increased angina (patch 2%)

Central nervous system: Lightheadedness (patch 6%), syncope (patch 4%)

Topical, sublingual, intravenous: Frequency not defined:

Cardiovascular: Hypotension (infrequent), postural hypotension, crescendo angina (uncommon), rebound hypertension (uncommon), pallor, cardiovascular collapse, tachycardia, shock, flushing, peripheral edema

Central nervous system: Headache (most common), lightheadedness (related to blood pressure changes), syncope (uncommon), dizziness, restlessness

Gastrointestinal: Nausea, vomiting, bowel incontinence, xerostomia

Genitourinary: Urinary incontinence

Hematologic: Methemoglobinemia (rare, overdose)

Neuromuscular & skeletal: Weakness

Ocular: Blurred vision

Miscellaneous: Cold sweat

The incidence of hypotension and adverse cardiovascular events may be increased when used in combination with sildenafil (Viagra®).

Overdosage/Toxicology Symptoms of overdose include hypotension, throbbing headache, palpitations, bloody diarrhea, bradycardia, cyanosis, tissue hypoxia, metabolic acidosis, clonic convulsions, circulatory collapse, and methemoglobinemia with extremely large overdoses. Treatment is supportive and symptomatic. Methemoglobinemia should be treated with methylene blue (1-2 mg/kg over 5 minutes). Additional doses may be necessary (0.5-1 mg/kg) based on follow-up methemoglobin levels (obtained after 30 minutes).

Pharmacodynamics/Kinetics

Onset of Action: Sublingual tablet: 1-3 minutes; Translingual spray: 2 minutes; Sustained release: 20-45 minutes; Topical: 15-60 minutes; Transdermal: 40-60 minutes; I.V. drip: Immediate

Peak effect: Sublingual tablet: 4-8 minutes; Translingual spray: 4-10 minutes; Sustained release: 45-120 minutes; Topical: 30-120 minutes; Transdermal: 60-180 minutes; I.V. drip: Immediate

Duration of Action: Sublingual tablet: 30-60 minutes; Translingual spray: 30-60 minutes; Sustained release: 4-8 hours; Topical: 2-12 hours; Transdermal: 18-24 hours; I.V. drip: 3-5 minutes

Protein Binding: 60%

Half-Life Elimination: 1-4 minutes

Metabolism: Extensive first-pass effect

Excretion: Urine (as inactive metabolites)

Available Dosage Forms

Capsule, extended release (Nitro-Time®): 2.5 mg, 6.5 mg, 9 mg

Infusion [premixed in D_5W]: 25 mg (250 mL) [0.1 mg/mL]; 50 mg (250 mL) [0.2 mg/mL]; 50 mg (500 mL) [0.1 mg/mL]; 100 mg (250 mL) [0.4 mg/mL]; 200 mg (500 mL) [0.4 mg/mL]

Injection, solution: 5 mg/mL (5 mL, 10 mL) [contains alcohol and propylene glycol]

Ointment, topical (Nitro-Bid®): 2% [20 mg/g] (1 g, 30 g, 60 g)

Solution, translingual spray (Nitrolingual®): 0.4 mg/metered spray (4.9 g) [contains alcohol 20%; 60 metered sprays]; (12 g) [contains alcohol 20%; 200 metered sprays]

Tablet, sublingual (NitroQuick®, Nitrostat®, Nitro-Tab®): 0.3 mg, 0.4 mg, 0.6 mg

Transdermal system [once daily patch]: 0.1 mg/hour (30s); 0.2 mg/hour (30s); 0.4 mg/hour (30s); 0.6 mg/hour (30s)

Minitran™: 0.1 mg/hour (30s); 0.2 mg/hour (30s); 0.4 mg/hour (30s); 0.6 mg/hour (30s)

Nitrek®: 0.2 mg/hour (30s); 0.4 mg/hour (30s); 0.6 mg/hour (30s)

Nitro-Dur®: 0.1 mg/hour (30s); 0.2 mg/hour (30s); 0.3 mg/hour (30s); 0.4 mg/hour (30s); 0.6 mg/hour (30s); 0.8 mg/hour (30s)

Dosing

Adults & Elderly: Note: Hemodynamic and antianginal tolerance often develop within 24-48 hours of continuous nitrate administration. Nitrate-free interval (10-12 hours/day) is recommended to avoid tolerance development; gradually decrease dose in patients receiving NTG for prolonged period to avoid withdrawal reaction.

Angina/coronary artery disease:

Oral: 2.5-9 mg 2-4 times/day (up to 26 mg 4 times/day)

I.V.: 5 mcg/minute, increase by 5 mcg/minute every 3-5 minutes to 20 mcg/minute. If no response at 20 mcg/minute increase by 10 mcg/minute every 3-5 minutes, up to 200 mcg/minute.

Topical ointment: Include a nitrate free interval, ~10 to 12 hours; Apply 0.5" to 2" every 6 hours with a nitrate free interval.

Topical patch, transdermal: 0.2-0.4 mg/hour initially and titrate to doses of 0.4-0.8 mg/hour. Tolerance is minimized by using a patch-on period of 12-14 hours and patch-off period of 10-12 hours.

Sublingual: 0.2-0.6 mg every 5 minutes for maximum of 3 doses in 15 minutes; may also use prophylactically 5-10 minutes prior to activities which may provoke an attack.

(Continued)

Nitroglycerin (Continued)

Esophageal spastic disorders (unlabeled use): 0.3-0.4 mg 5 minutes before meals

Translingual: 1-2 sprays into mouth under tongue every 3-5 minutes for maximum of 3 doses in 15 minutes, may also be used 5-10 minutes prior to activities which may provoke an attack prophylactically.

Pediatrics:

Pulmonary hypertension: I.V. Continuous infusion: Children: Start 0.25-0.5 mcg/kg/minute and titrate by 1 mcg/kg/minute at 20- to 60-minute intervals to desired effect; usual dose: 1-3 mcg/kg/minute; maximum: 5 mcg/kg/minute

Note: Hemodynamic and antianginal tolerance often develop within 24-48 hours of continuous nitrate administration.

Administration

Oral: Do not crush sublingual drug product.

I.V.: I.V. must be prepared in glass bottles and use special sets intended for nitroglycerin. glass I.V. bottles and administration sets provided by manufacturer.

I.V. Detail: Nitroglycerin can be absorbed by plastic (polyvinyl chloride) tubing or containers. Infusion pump may not infuse accurately with different tubing. Be alert to potential for unregulated flow.

pH: 3.0-6.5

Stability

Reconstitution: Doses should be made in glass bottles, Excel® or PAB® containers; adsorption occurs to soft plastic (eg, PVC). Nitroglycerin diluted in D_5W or NS in glass containers is physically and chemically stable for 48 hours at room temperature and 7 days under refrigeration. In D_5W or NS in Excel®/PAB® containers is physically and chemically stable for 24 hours at room temperature and 14 days under refrigeration.

Standard diluent: 50 mg/250 mL D_5W; 50 mg/500 mL D_5W

Minimum volume: 100 mg/250 mL D_5W; concentration should not exceed 400 mcg/mL.

Compatibility: Stable in D_5LR, $D_5\frac{1}{2}NS$, D_5NS, LR, $\frac{1}{2}NS$

Y-site administration: Incompatible with alteplase, levofloxacin

Compatibility when admixed: Dose is variable and may require titration, therefore it is not advisable to mix with other agents. **Incompatible** with hydralazine, phenytoin

Storage: Doses should be made in glass bottles, Excel® or PAB® containers. Adsorption occurs to soft plastic (eg, PVC). Premixed bottles are stable according to the manufacturer's expiration dating. Store sublingual tablets and ointment in tightly closed containers at 15°C to 30°C. Store spray and transdermal patch at 25°C, excursions permitted to 15°C to 30°C (59°F to 86°F).

Nursing Actions

Physical Assessment: Assess potential for interactions with other pharmacological agents patient may be taking (eg, heparin, ergot alkaloids, sildenafil, tadalafil, or vardenafil). See Administration specifics for different formulations. Monitor therapeutic effectiveness (cardiac status) and adverse response (eg, hypotension, arrhythmias, CNS changes, GI disturbances). Dose should be reduced gradually when discontinuing after long-term therapy. Teach patient proper use (according to purpose and formulation), possible side effects/appropriate interventions (eg, drug-free intervals; remove transdermal patches for specific periods of time), and adverse symptoms to report.

Patient Education: Do not take any new medication during therapy unless approved by prescriber. Take as per directions (see below). Do not change brands without consulting prescriber. Do not discontinue abruptly. Keep medication in original container, tightly closed. If anginal chest pain is unresolved in 15 minutes, seek emergency medical help at once. Daily use may cause dizziness or lightheadedness (use caution when driving or engaging in hazardous activities until response to drug is known); headache (consult prescriber for approved analgesic); hypotension (use care when changing position from sitting or lying to standing, when climbing stairs or when engaging in tasks that are potentially hazardous until response to drug is known); GI disturbances (small, frequent meals, frequent mouth care, chewing gum, or sucking lozenges may help). Report acute headache, rapid heartbeat, unusual restlessness or dizziness, muscular weakness, or blurred vision or seeing abnormal colors. **Pregnancy/breast-feeding precautions:** Inform prescriber if you are or intend to become pregnant. Consult prescriber if breast-feeding.

Oral: Take as directed. Do not chew or swallow sublingual tablets; allow to dissolve under tongue. Sit down before using sublingual or buccal tablet or spray form. Do not chew or crush extended release capsules; swallow with 8 oz of water.

Spray: Spray directly on mucous membranes; do not inhale.

Topical: Spread prescribed amount thinly on applicator; rotate application sites.

Transdermal: Use as directed; place on hair-free area of skin, rotate sites (usually, patches will be removed for a period each day)

Geriatric Considerations Caution should be used when using nitrate therapy in the elderly due to hypotension. Hypotension is enhanced in the elderly due to decreased baroreceptor response, decreased venous tone, and often hypovolemia (dehydration) or other hypotensive drugs. Elderly patients may be at greater risk of falling due to nitroglycerin-associated hypotension/orthostasis.

Additional Information I.V. preparations contain alcohol and/or propylene glycol; may need to use nitrate-free interval (10-12 hours/day) to avoid tolerance development. Tolerance may possibly be reversed with acetylcysteine; gradually decrease dose in patients receiving NTG for prolonged period to avoid withdrawal reaction.

Concomitant use of sildenafil (Viagra®) or other phosphodiesterase-5 enzyme inhibitors (PDE-5) may precipitate acute hypotension, myocardial infarction, or death. Nitrates used in right ventricular infarction may induce acute hypotension. Nitrate use in severe pericardial effusion may reduce cardiac filling pressure and precipitate cardiac tamponade. In the management of heart failure, the combination of isosorbide dinitrate and hydralazine confers beneficial effects on disease progression and cardiac outcomes.

Related Information

Compatibility of Drugs *on page 1370*

Nitroprusside (nye troe PRUS ide)

U.S. Brand Names Nitropress®

Synonyms Nitroprusside Sodium; Sodium Nitroferricyanide; Sodium Nitroprusside

Pharmacologic Category Vasodilator

Medication Safety Issues

Sound-alike/look-alike issues:
Nitroprusside may be confused with nitroglycerin

High alert medication: The Institute for Safe Medication Practices (ISMP) includes this medication among its list of drugs which have a heightened risk of causing significant patient harm when used in error.

Pregnancy Risk Factor C

Lactation Excretion in breast milk unknown

Use Management of hypertensive crises; congestive heart failure; used for controlled hypotension to reduce bleeding during surgery

Mechanism of Action/Effect Causes peripheral vaso-dilation by direct action on venous and arteriolar smooth muscle, thus reducing peripheral resistance; will increase cardiac output by decreasing afterload; reduces aortal and left ventricular impedance

Contraindications Hypersensitivity to nitroprusside or any component of the formulation; treatment of compensatory hypertension (aortic coarctation, arteriovenous shunting); high output failure; congenital optic atrophy or tobacco amblyopia

Warnings/Precautions Except when used briefly or at low (<2 mcg/kg/minute) infusion rates, nitroprusside gives rise to large cyanide quantities. Do not use the maximum dose for more than 10 minutes. Use with extreme caution in patients with elevated intracranial pressure. Use extreme caution in patients with hepatic or renal dysfunction. Watch for cyanide toxicity in patients with impaired hepatic function. Use the lowest end of the dosage range with renal impairment. Thiocyanate toxicity occurs in patients with renal impairment or those on prolonged infusions. Continuous blood pressure monitoring is needed.

Adverse Reactions 1% to 10%:

Cardiovascular: Excessive hypotensive response, palpitation, substernal distress

Central nervous system: Disorientation, psychosis, headache, restlessness

Endocrine & metabolic: Thyroid suppression

Gastrointestinal: Nausea, vomiting

Neuromuscular & skeletal: Weakness, muscle spasm

Otic: Tinnitus

Respiratory: Hypoxia

Miscellaneous: Diaphoresis, thiocyanate toxicity

Overdosage/Toxicology Symptoms of overdose include hypotension, vomiting, hyperventilation, tachycardia, muscular twitching, hypothyroidism, cyanide or thiocyanate toxicity. Thiocyanate toxicity includes psychosis, hyper-reflexia, confusion, weakness, tinnitus, seizures, and coma; cyanide toxicity includes acidosis (decreased HCO_3, decreased pH, increased lactate), increase in mixed venous blood oxygen tension, tachycardia, altered consciousness, coma, convulsions, and almond smell on breath.

Nitroprusside has been shown to release cyanide *in vivo* with hemoglobin. Cyanide toxicity does not usually occur because of the rapid uptake of cyanide by erythrocytes and its eventual incorporation into thiocyanate in the liver. However, high doses, prolonged administration of nitroprusside, or reduced elimination can lead to cyanide poisoning or thiocyanate intoxication. Anemia and liver impairment pose a risk for cyanide accumulation, while renal impairment predisposes thiocyanate accumulation. If toxicity develops, airway support with oxygen therapy is appropriate, followed closely with antidotal therapy of amyl nitrate perles, sodium nitrate 300 mg I.V. for adults (range based on hemoglobin concentration: 6-12 mg/kg for children) and sodium thio-sulfate 12.5 g I.V. for adults (range based on hemoglobin concentration: 0.95-1.95 mL/kg of the 25% solution for children); nitrates should not be administered to neonates and small children. Thiocyanate is dialyzable. May be mixed with sodium thiosulfate in I.V. to prevent cyanide toxicity.

Pharmacodynamics/Kinetics

Onset of Action: BP reduction <2 minutes

Duration of Action: 1-10 minutes

Half-Life Elimination: Parent drug: <10 minutes; Thiocyanate: 2.7-7 days

Metabolism: Nitroprusside is converted to cyanide ions in the bloodstream; decomposes to prussic acid which in the presence of sulfur donor is converted to thiocyanate (hepatic and renal rhodanase systems)

Excretion: Urine (as thiocyanate)

Available Dosage Forms Injection, solution, as sodium: 25 mg/mL (2 mL)

Dosing

Adults & Elderly:

Acute hypertension: I.V.: Initial: 0.3-0.5 mcg/kg/minute; increase in increments of 0.5 mcg/kg/minute, titrating to the desired hemodynamic effect or the appearance of headache or nausea; usual dose: 3 mcg/kg/minute; rarely need >4 mcg/kg/minute; maximum: 10 mcg/kg/minute. When >500 mcg/kg is administered by prolonged infusion of faster than 2 mcg/kg/minute, cyanide is generated faster than an unaided patient can handle.

Note: Administration requires the use of an infusion pump. Average dose: 5 mcg/kg/minute.

Pediatrics:

Pulmonary hypertension: I.V.: Children: Initial: 1 mcg/kg/minute by continuous I.V. infusion; increase in increments of 1 mcg/kg/minute at intervals of 20-60 minutes; titrating to the desired response; usual dose: 3 mcg/kg/minute, rarely need >4 mcg/kg/minute; maximum: 5 mcg/kg/minute.

Note: Administration requires the use of an infusion pump. Average dose: 5 mcg/kg/minute.

Renal Impairment: Limit use; accumulation of thiocyanate may occur.

Hepatic Impairment: Limit use; risk of cyanide toxicity.

Administration

I.V.: I.V. infusion only, use only as an infusion with 5% dextrose in water. Infusion pump required. Not for direct injection.

I.V. Detail: Continuously monitor patient's blood pressure.

pH: 3.5-6.0

Stability

Reconstitution: Brownish solution is usable, discard if bluish in color. Nitroprusside sodium should be reconstituted freshly by diluting 50 mg in 250-1000 mL of D_5W. Use only clear solutions; solutions of nitroprusside exhibit a color described as brownish, brown, brownish-pink, light orange, and straw. Solutions are highly sensitive to light. Exposure to light causes decomposition, resulting in a highly colored solution of orange, dark brown or blue. **A blue color indicates almost complete degradation and breakdown to cyanide. Solutions should be wrapped with aluminum foil or other opaque material to protect from light (do as soon as possible).** Stability of parenteral admixture at room temperature (25°C) and at refrigeration temperature (4°C) is 24 hours.

Compatibility: Stable in LR

Y-site administration: Incompatible with levofloxacin

Compatibility when admixed: Incompatible with atracurium

Storage:

Use only clear solutions; solutions of nitroprusside exhibit a color described as brownish, brown, brownish-pink, light orange, and straw. Solutions are highly sensitive to light. Exposure to light causes decomposition, resulting in a highly colored solution of orange, dark brown or blue. **A blue color indicates almost complete degradation and breakdown to cyanide.**

Solutions should be wrapped with aluminum foil or other opaque material to protect from light (do as soon as possible)

Stability of parenteral admixture at room temperature (25°C) and at refrigeration temperature (4°C): 24 hours

(Continued)

Nitroprusside *(Continued)*

Nursing Actions

Physical Assessment: See Administration and Reconstitution for infusion specifics and warnings. Monitor infusion site closely to prevent extravasation. Monitor patient blood pressure continuously. Monitor patient response and adverse reactions (eg, acid/base balance [metabolic acidosis is early sign of cyanide toxicity], disorientation, hypoxia, muscular twitching). Provide patient teaching according to patient condition.

Patient Education: Patient condition should indicate extent of education and instruction needed. This drug can only be given I.V. You will be monitored at all times during infusion. Promptly report any chest pain or pain/burning at site of infusion. **Breast-feeding precaution:** Consult prescriber if breast-feeding.

Geriatric Considerations Elderly patients may have an increased sensitivity to nitroprusside possibly due to a decreased baroreceptor reflex, altered sensitivity to vasodilating effects or a resistance of cardiac adrenergic receptors to stimulation by catecholamines.

Nizatidine *(ni ZA ti deen)*

U.S. Brand Names Axid®; Axid® AR [OTC]

Pharmacologic Category Histamine H$_2$ Antagonist

Medication Safety Issues

Sound-alike/look-alike issues:

Axid® may be confused with Ansaid®

Pregnancy Risk Factor B

Lactation Enters breast milk/may be compatible

Use Treatment and maintenance of duodenal ulcer; treatment of benign gastric ulcer; treatment of gastroesophageal reflux disease (GERD); OTC tablet used for the prevention of meal-induced heartburn, acid indigestion, and sour stomach

Unlabeled/Investigational Use Part of a multidrug regimen for *H. pylori* eradication to reduce the risk of duodenal ulcer recurrence

Mechanism of Action/Effect Nizatidine is an H$_2$-receptor antagonist.

Contraindications Hypersensitivity to nizatidine or any component of the formulation; hypersensitivity to other H$_2$ antagonists (cross-sensitivity has been observed)

Warnings/Precautions Use with caution in children <12 years of age. Use with caution in patients with liver and renal impairment. Dosage modification required in patients with renal impairment.

Drug Interactions

Cytochrome P450 Effect: Inhibits 3A4 (weak)

Decreased Effect: May decrease the absorption of itraconazole or ketoconazole.

Nutritional/Ethanol Interactions

Ethanol: Avoid ethanol (may cause gastric mucosal irritation).

Food: Administration with apple juice may decrease absorption.

Lab Interactions False-positive urine protein using Multistix®, gastric acid secretion test, skin tests allergen extracts, serum creatinine and serum transaminase concentrations, urine protein test

Adverse Reactions

>10%: Central nervous system: Headache (16%)

1% to 10%:

Central nervous system: Anxiety, dizziness, fever (reported in children), insomnia, irritability (reported in children), somnolence, nervousness

Dermatologic: Pruritus, rash

Gastrointestinal: Abdominal pain, anorexia, constipation, diarrhea, dry mouth, flatulence, heartburn, nausea, vomiting

Respiratory: Reported in children: Cough, nasal congestion, nasopharyngitis

Overdosage/Toxicology Symptoms of overdose include muscular tremor, vomiting, and rapid respiration. LD$_{50}$ ~80 mg/kg. Treatment is symptomatic and supportive.

Pharmacodynamics/Kinetics

Time to Peak: Plasma: 0.5-3.0 hours

Protein Binding: 35% to α$_1$-acid glycoprotein

Half-Life Elimination: 1-2 hours; prolonged with renal impairment

Metabolism: Partially hepatic; forms metabolites

Excretion: Urine (90%; ~60% as unchanged drug); feces (<6%)

Available Dosage Forms

Capsule (Axid®): 150 mg, 300 mg

Solution, oral (Axid®): 15 mg/mL (120 mL, 480 mL) [bubble gum flavor]

Tablet (Axid® AR): 75 mg

Dosing

Adults & Elderly:

Duodenal ulcer: Oral:

Treatment of active ulcer: 300 mg at bedtime or 150 mg twice daily

Maintenance of healed ulcer: 150 mg/day at bedtime

Gastric ulcer: Oral: 150 mg twice daily or 300 mg at bedtime

GERD: Oral: 150 mg twice daily

Meal-induced heartburn, acid indigestion, and sour stomach (OTC labeling): Oral: 75 mg tablet [OTC] twice daily, 30-60 minutes prior to consuming food or beverages

Eradication of *Helicobacter pylori* (unlabeled use): Oral: 150 mg twice daily; requires combination therapy

Pediatrics:

GERD (unlabeled use): Oral:

Children <12 years: 10 mg/kg/day in divided doses given twice daily; may not be as effective in children <12 years

Children ≥12 years: Refer to adult dosing.

Meal-induced heartburn, acid indigestion and sour stomach: Oral: Children ≥12 years: Refer to adult dosing.

Renal Impairment:

Active treatment:

Cl$_{cr}$ 20-50 mL/minute: 150 mg/day

Cl$_{cr}$ <20 mL/minute: 150 mg every other day

Maintenance treatment:

Cl$_{cr}$ 20-50 mL/minute: 150 mg every other day

Cl$_{cr}$ <20 mL/minute: 150 mg every 3 days

Nursing Actions

Physical Assessment: Monitor patient response. Teach patient proper use, possible side effects/appropriate interventions, and adverse symptoms to report.

Patient Education: Do not take any new medication during therapy unless approved by prescriber. Take as directed; do not change dose or discontinue without consulting prescriber. Do not take within 1 hour of any antacids. Follow diet instructions of prescriber. May cause drowsiness; use caution when driving or engaging in tasks that require alertness until response to drug is known. Report fever, sore throat, tarry stools, CNS changes, or muscle or joint pain. **Pregnancy precaution:** Inform prescriber if you are or intend to become pregnant.

Geriatric Considerations H$_2$ blockers are the preferred drugs for treating peptic ulcer disorder (PUD) in the elderly due to cost and ease of administration. These agents are no less or more effective than any other therapy. The preferred agents (due to side effects and drug interaction profile and pharmacokinetics) are ranitidine, famotidine, and nizatidine. Treatment for PUD in the elderly is recommended for 12 weeks since their lesions are larger, and therefore, take longer to heal. Always adjust dose based upon creatinine clearance.

Breast-Feeding Issues The amount of nizatidine excreted in breast milk is 0.1%.

Additional Information Giving dose at 6 PM (rather than 10 PM) may better suppress nocturnal acid secretion

---

Norepinephrine (nor ep i NEF rin)

U.S. Brand Names Levophed®

Synonyms Levarterenol Bitartrate; Noradrenaline; Noradrenaline Acid Tartrate; Norepinephrine Bitartrate

Pharmacologic Category Alpha/Beta Agonist

Pregnancy Risk Factor C

Lactation Excretion in breast milk unknown

Use Treatment of shock which persists after adequate fluid volume replacement

Mechanism of Action/Effect Stimulates beta$_1$-adrenergic receptors and alpha-adrenergic receptors causing increased contractility and heart rate as well as vasoconstriction, thereby increasing systemic blood pressure and coronary blood flow; clinically alpha effects (vasoconstriction) are greater than beta effects (inotropic and chronotropic effects)

Contraindications Hypersensitivity to norepinephrine, bisulfites (contains metabisulfite), or any component of the formulation; hypotension from hypovolemia except as an emergency measure to maintain coronary and cerebral perfusion until volume could be replaced; mesenteric or peripheral vascular thrombosis unless it is a lifesaving procedure; during anesthesia with cyclopropane or halothane anesthesia (risk of ventricular arrhythmias)

Warnings/Precautions Assure adequate circulatory volume to minimize need for vasoconstrictors. Avoid hypertension; monitor blood pressure closely and adjust infusion rate. Infuse into a large vein if possible. Avoid infusion into leg veins. Watch I.V. site closely. Avoid extravasation. Never use leg veins for infusion sites.

Drug Interactions

Decreased Effect: Alpha-blockers may blunt response to norepinephrine.

Increased Effect/Toxicity: The effects of norepinephrine may be increased by tricyclic antidepressants, MAO inhibitors, antihistamines (diphenhydramine, tripelennamine), beta-blockers (nonselective), guanethidine, ergot alkaloids, reserpine, and methyldopa. Atropine sulfate may block the reflex bradycardia caused by norepinephrine and enhances the vasopressor response.

Adverse Reactions Frequency not defined.

Cardiovascular: Bradycardia, arrhythmia, peripheral (digital) ischemia

Central nervous system: Headache (transient), anxiety

Local: Skin necrosis (with extravasation)

Respiratory: Dyspnea, respiratory difficulty

Overdosage/Toxicology Symptoms of overdose include hypertension, sweating, cerebral hemorrhage, and convulsions. Infiltrate the area of extravasation with phentolamine 5-10 mg in 10-15 mL of saline solution; inject a small amount of this dilution into extravasated area; blanching should reverse immediately. Monitor site; if blanching should recur, additional injections of phentolamine may be needed.

Pharmacodynamics/Kinetics

Onset of Action: I.V.: Very rapid-acting

Duration of Action: Limited

Metabolism: Via catechol-o-methyltransferase (COMT) and monoamine oxidase (MAO)

Excretion: Urine (84% to 96% as inactive metabolites)

Available Dosage Forms Injection, solution, as bitartrate: 1 mg/mL (4 mL) [contains sodium metabisulfite]

Dosing

Adults & Elderly: Note: Norepinephrine dosage is stated in terms of norepinephrine base and intravenous formulation is norepinephrine bitartrate.

Norepinephrine bitartrate 2 mg = norepinephrine base 1 mg

Hypotension/shock: Continuous I.V. infusion:

Adults: Initial: 0.5-1 mcg/minute and titrate to desired response; 8-30 mcg/minute is usual range; range used in clinical trials: 0.01-3 mcg/kg/minute;

ACLS dosing range: 0.5-30 mcg/minute

Rate of infusion: 4 mg in 500 mL D$_5$W

2 mcg/minute = 15 mL/hour

4 mcg/minute = 30 mL/hour

6 mcg/minute = 45 mL/hour

8 mcg/minute = 60 mL/hour

10 mcg/minute = 75 mL/hour

Pediatrics: Administration requires the use of an infusion pump

Note: Norepinephrine dosage is stated in terms of norepinephrine base and intravenous formulation is norepinephrine bitartrate.

Norepinephrine bitartrate 2 mg = Norepinephrine base 1 mg

Hypotension/shock: Continuous I.V. infusion: Children: Initial: 0.05-0.1 mcg/kg/minute; titrate to desired effect; maximum dose: 1-2 mcg/kg/minute

Administration

I.V.: Administer into large vein to avoid the potential for extravasation; potent drug, must be diluted prior to use; do not administer NaHCO$_3$ through an I.V. line containing norepinephrine. Central line administration is required. Do not administer NaHCO$_3$ through an I.V. line containing norepinephrine.

I.V. Detail: Administer into large vein to avoid the potential for extravasation. Potent drug, must be diluted prior to use.

Extravasation management: Use phentolamine as antidote. Mix 5 mg with 9 mL of NS. Inject a small amount of this dilution into extravasated area. Blanching should reverse immediately. Monitor site; if blanching should recur, additional injections of phentolamine may be needed.

pH: 3.0-4.5

Stability

Reconstitution: Dilute with D$_5$W or D$_5$NS, but not recommended to dilute in normal saline. Stability of parenteral admixture at room temperature (25°C) is 24 hours.

Compatibility: Stable in D$_5$NS, D$_5$W, LR; may dilute with D$_5$W or D$_5$NS, but not recommended to dilute in normal saline; not stable in alkaline solutions. Stability of parenteral admixture at room temperature (25°C) is 24 hours.

Y-site administration: Incompatible with insulin (regular), thiopental

Compatibility when admixed: Incompatible with aminophylline, amobarbital, chlorothiazide, chlorpheniramine, pentobarbital, phenobarbital, phenytoin, sodium bicarbonate, streptomycin, thiopental

Storage: Readily oxidized; protect from light. Do not use if brown coloration.

Nursing Actions

Physical Assessment: Assess other medications patient may be taking. Monitor blood pressure and cardiac status, CNS status, skin temperature and color during and following infusion. Monitor fluid status (I & O). Assess infusion site frequently for extravasation. Blanching along vein pathway is a preliminary sign of extravasation.

Patient Education: This drug is used in emergency situations. Patient information is based on patient condition.

(Continued)

Norepinephrine *(Continued)*

Related Information

Compatibility of Drugs *on page 1370*

Norethindrone *(nor eth IN drone)*

U.S. Brand Names Aygestin®; Camila™; Errin™; Jolivette™; Micronor®; Nora-BE™; Nor-QD®

Synonyms Norethindrone Acetate; Norethisterone

Pharmacologic Category Contraceptive; Progestin

Medication Safety Issues

Sound-alike/look-alike issues:

Micronor® may be confused with miconazole, Micronase®

Pregnancy Risk Factor X

Lactation Enters breast milk/use caution

Use Treatment of amenorrhea; abnormal uterine bleeding; endometriosis, oral contraceptive; **higher rate of failure with progestin only contraceptives**

Mechanism of Action/Effect Inhibits secretion of pituitary gonadotropin (LH) which prevents follicular maturation and ovulation; in the presence of adequate endogenous estrogen, transforms a proliferative endometrium to a secretory one

Contraindications Hypersensitivity to norethindrone or any component of the formulation; thromboembolic disorders; severe hepatic disease; breast cancer; undiagnosed vaginal bleeding; pregnancy

Warnings/Precautions Use of any progestin during the first 4 months of pregnancy is not recommended. Discontinue if sudden partial or complete loss of vision, proptosis, diplopia, or migraine occur. **There is a higher rate of failure with progestin only contraceptives.** Progestin-induced withdrawal bleeding occurs within 3-7 days after discontinuation of drug. Use with caution in patients with asthma, diabetes, seizure disorder, hyperlipidemias, migraine, cardiac or renal dysfunction, or psychic depression.

Drug Interactions

Cytochrome P450 Effect: Substrate of CYP3A4 (major); **Induces** CYP2C19 (weak)

Decreased Effect: Nelfinavir decreases the pharmacologic effect of norethindrone. CYP3A4 inducers may decrease the levels/effects of norethindrone; example inducers include aminoglutethimide, carbamazepine, nafcillin, nevirapine, phenobarbital, phenytoin, and rifamycins.

Nutritional/Ethanol Interactions

Food; Limit caffeine.

Herb/Nutraceutical: High-dose vitamin C (1 g/day) may increase adverse effects. Avoid St John's wort.

Lab Interactions Thyroid function test, metyrapone test, liver function tests, coagulation tests (prothrombin time, factors VII, VIII, IX, X)

Adverse Reactions

>10%:

Cardiovascular: Edema

Endocrine & metabolic: Breakthrough bleeding, spotting, changes in menstrual flow, amenorrhea

Gastrointestinal: Anorexia

Local: Pain at injection site

Neuromuscular & skeletal: Weakness

1% to 10%:

Cardiovascular: Edema

Central nervous system: Mental depression, fever, insomnia

Dermatologic: Melasma or chloasma, allergic rash with or without pruritus

Endocrine & metabolic: Increased breast tenderness

Gastrointestinal: Weight gain/loss

Genitourinary: Changes in cervical erosion and secretions

Hepatic: Cholestatic jaundice

Pharmacodynamics/Kinetics

Time to Peak: 1-2 hours

Protein Binding: 61% to albumin, 36% to sex hormone-binding globulin (SHBG); SHBG capacity affected by plasma ethinyl estradiol levels

Half-Life Elimination: 5-14 hours

Metabolism: Oral: Hepatic via reduction and conjugation; first-pass effect

Excretion: Primarily urine (as metabolites)

Available Dosage Forms

Tablet (Camila™, Errin™, Jolivette™, Micronor®, Nora-BE™, Nor-QD®): 0.35 mg

Tablet, as acetate (Aygestin®): 5 mg

Dosing

Adults:

Contraception (Females): Oral: Progesterone only: Norethindrone 0.35 mg every day of the year starting on first day of menstruation; if one dose is missed take as soon as remembered; then next tablet at regular time; if two doses are missed, take one of the missed doses, discard the other, and take daily dose at usual time; if three doses are missed, use another form of birth control until menses appear or pregnancy is ruled out

Amenorrhea and abnormal uterine bleeding: Oral:

Norethindrone: 5-20 mg/day on days 5-25 of menstrual cycle

Acetate salt (Aygestin®): 2.5-10 mg on days 5-25 of menstrual cycle

Endometriosis: Oral:

Norethindrone: 10 mg/day for 2 weeks; increase at increments of 5 mg/day every 2 weeks until 30 mg/day; continue for 6-9 months or until breakthrough bleeding demands temporary termination

Acetate salt (Aygestin®): 5 mg/day for 14 days; increase at increments of 2.5 mg/day every 2 weeks up to 15 mg/day; continue for 6-9 months or until breakthrough bleeding demands temporary termination

Pediatrics: Adolescents: Refer to adult dosing

Administration

Oral: Administer with food.

Laboratory Monitoring Long-term therapy, annual Pap tests, mammogram

Nursing Actions

Physical Assessment: Assess patient knowledge/teach appropriate administration schedule and adverse signs to report. Teach appropriate breast self-exam and the need for regular breast self-exam and necessity of annual physical check-up with long-term use. **Pregnancy risk factor X:** Determine that patient is not pregnant before beginning treatment.

Patient Education: Take according to prescribed schedule. Follow instructions for regular self-breast exam. You may experience dizziness or lightheadedness; use caution when driving or engaging in tasks that require alertness until response to drug is known. Limit intake of caffeine. Avoid high-dose vitamin C. You may experience photosensitivity; use sunscreen, wear protective clothing and eyewear, and avoid direct sunlight. You may experience loss of hair (reversible), swelling of hands or feet, weight gain or loss. Report sudden severe headache or vomiting, disturbances of vision or speech, sudden blindness, numbness of weakness in an extremity, chest pain, calf pain, respiratory difficulty, weight gain >5 lb/week, depression or acute fatigue, unusual bleeding, spotting, or changes in menstrual flow. **Pregnancy/breast-feeding precautions:** Inform prescriber if you are pregnant. Consult prescriber if breast-feeding.

Dietary Considerations Should be taken with food at same time each day.

Breast-Feeding Issues Norethindrone can cause changes in milk production in the mother. Monitor infant growth. Use lowest possible dose of norethindrone for less effect on milk production.

Norgestrel (nor JES trel)

U.S. Brand Names Ovrette® [DSC]

Pharmacologic Category Contraceptive; Progestin

Pregnancy Risk Factor X

Lactation Enters breast milk/use caution

Use Prevention of pregnancy; **progestin only products have higher risk of failure in contraceptive use**

Mechanism of Action/Effect Inhibits secretion of pituitary gonadotropin (LH) which prevents follicular maturation and ovulation

Contraindications Hypersensitivity to norgestrel or any component of the formulation; hypersensitivity to tartrazine; thromboembolic disorders; severe hepatic disease; breast cancer; undiagnosed vaginal bleeding; pregnancy

Warnings/Precautions Discontinue if sudden loss of vision or if diplopia or proptosis occur. Use with caution in patients with a history of mental depression.

Drug Interactions

Cytochrome P450 Effect: Substrate of CYP3A4 (major)

Decreased Effect: CYP3A4 inducers may decrease the levels/effects of norgestrel; example inducers include aminoglutethimide, carbamazepine, nafcillin, nevirapine, phenobarbital, phenytoin, and rifamycins. Antibiotics (penicillins, tetracyclines, griseofulvin) were reported to decrease efficacy of oral contraceptives, but this has not been validated in more rigorous investigations.

Increased Effect/Toxicity: Oral contraceptives may increase toxicity of acetaminophen, anticoagulants, benzodiazepines, caffeine, corticosteroids, metoprolol, theophylline, and tricyclic antidepressants.

Nutritional/Ethanol Interactions

Food: CNS effects of caffeine may be enhanced if oral contraceptives are used concurrently with caffeine.

Herb/Nutraceutical: St John's wort may decrease levels. Avoid dong quai and black cohosh (have estrogen activity). Avoid saw palmetto, red clover, ginseng.

Lab Interactions Thyroid function tests, metyrapone test, liver function tests

Adverse Reactions Frequency not defined.

Cardiovascular: Embolism, cerebral thrombosis, edema

Central nervous system: Mental depression, fever, insomnia

Dermatologic: Melasma or chloasma, allergic rash with or without pruritus

Endocrine & metabolic: Breakthrough bleeding, spotting, changes in menstrual flow, amenorrhea, changes in cervical erosion and secretions, increased breast tenderness

Gastrointestinal: Weight gain/loss, anorexia

Hepatic: Cholestatic jaundice

Local: Thrombophlebitis

Neuromuscular & skeletal: Weakness

Overdosage/Toxicology

Toxicity is unlikely following single exposures of excessive doses.

Supportive treatment is adequate in most cases.

Pharmacodynamics/Kinetics

Protein Binding: >97% to sex hormone-binding globulin

Half-Life Elimination: ~20 hours

Metabolism: Primarily hepatic via reduction and conjugation

Excretion: Urine (as metabolites)

Available Dosage Forms [DSC] = Discontinued product

Tablet: 0.075 mg [contains tartrazine] [DSC]

Dosing

Adults: Contraception: Oral: Administer daily, starting the first day of menstruation, take 1 tablet at the same time each day, every day of the year. If one dose is missed, take as soon as remembered, then next tablet at regular time; if two doses are missed, take 1 tablet as soon as it is remembered, followed by an additional dose that same day at the usual time. When one or two doses are missed, additional contraceptive measures should be used until 14 consecutive tablets have been taken. If three doses are missed, discontinue norgestrel and use an additional form of birth control until menses or pregnancy is ruled out.

Nursing Actions

Physical Assessment: Monitor or teach patient to monitor blood pressure on a regular basis. Monitor or teach patient to monitor for occurrence of adverse effects and symptoms to report (eg, thromboembolic disease, visual changes, neuromuscular weakness). Assess knowledge/teach importance of regular (monthly) blood pressure checks, annual physical assessment, Pap smear, and vision assessment. Teach importance of maintaining prescribed schedule of dosing (see Dosing for dosing and missed dose information). **Pregnancy risk factor X:** Do not use if patient is pregnant.

Patient Education: Take exactly as directed by prescriber (also see package insert). You are at risk of becoming pregnant if doses are missed. If you miss a dose, take as soon as possible or double the dose next day. If more than three doses are missed, contact prescriber for restarting directions. Use additional form of contraception during first week of taking this medication. Detailed and complete information on dosing and missed doses can be found in the package insert. Be aware that some medications may reduce the effectiveness of oral contraceptives; an alternate form of contraception may be needed. It is important that you check your blood pressure monthly (on same day each month) and that you have an annual physical assessment, Pap smear, and vision assessment while taking this medication. Avoid smoking while taking this medication; smoking increases risk of adverse effects, including thromboembolic events and heart attacks. You may experience loss of appetite (small frequent meals will help); or constipation (increased exercise, fluids, fruit, fiber, or stool softeners may help). If you have diabetes, use accurate serum glucose testing to identify any changes in glucose tolerance; notify prescriber of significant changes so antidiabetic medication can be adjusted if necessary. Report immediately pain or muscle soreness; warmth, swelling, or redness in calves; shortness of breath; sudden loss of vision; unresolved leg or foot swelling; change in menstrual pattern (unusual bleeding, amenorrhea, breakthrough spotting); breast tenderness that does not go away; acute abdominal cramping; signs of vaginal infection (drainage, pain, itching); CNS changes (blurred vision, confusion, acute anxiety, or unresolved depression); or significant weight gain (>5 lb/week). **Pregnancy/breast-feeding precautions:** This drug may cause severe fetal complication. If you suspect you may become pregnant, contact prescriber immediately. Consult prescriber if breast-feeding.

Dietary Considerations Should be taken with food at same time each day.

Nortriptyline (nor TRIP ti leen)

U.S. Brand Names Pamelor®

Synonyms Nortriptyline Hydrochloride

Restrictions A medication guide concerning the use of antidepressants in children and teenagers can be found on the FDA website at http://www.fda.gov/cder/Offices/ODS/labeling.htm. It should be dispensed to parents or guardians of children and teenagers receiving this medication.

Pharmacologic Category Antidepressant, Tricyclic (Secondary Amine)

Medication Safety Issues

Sound-alike/look-alike issues:

Nortriptyline may be confused with amitriptyline, desipramine, Norpramin®

Aventyl® HCl may be confused with Bentyl®

Pamelor® may be confused with Demerol®, Dymelor®

Pregnancy Risk Factor D

Lactation Enters breast milk/contraindicated (AAP rates "of concern")

Use Treatment of symptoms of depression

Unlabeled/Investigational Use Chronic pain, anxiety disorders, enuresis, attention-deficit/hyperactivity disorder (ADHD); adjunctive therapy for smoking cessation

Mechanism of Action/Effect Traditionally believed to increase the synaptic concentration of serotonin and/or norepinephrine in the central nervous system by inhibition of their reuptake by the presynaptic neuronal membrane. However, additional receptor effects have been found including desensitization of adenyl cyclase, down regulation of beta-adrenergic receptors, and down regulation of serotonin receptors.

Contraindications Hypersensitivity to nortriptyline and similar chemical class, or any component of the formulation; use of MAO inhibitors within 14 days; use in a patient during the acute recovery phase of MI; pregnancy

Warnings/Precautions Antidepressants increase the risk of suicidal thinking and behavior in children and adolescents with major depressive disorder (MDD) and other depressive disorders; consider risk prior to prescribing. All patients must be closely monitored for clinical worsening, suicidality, or unusual changes in behavior, especially during the initiation of therapy or following an increase or decrease in dosage. When used in children, the child's family or caregiver should be instructed to closely observe the patient and communicate condition with healthcare provider. A medication guide should be dispensed with each prescription. **Nortriptyline is not FDA approved for use in children.**

The possibility of a suicide attempt is inherent in major depression and may persist until remission occurs. Use caution in high-risk patients. Worsening depression and severe abrupt suicidality that are not part of the presenting symptoms may require discontinuation or modification of drug therapy. The patient's family or caregiver should be alerted to monitor patients for the emergence of suicidality and associated behaviors (such as agitation, irritability, hostility, impulsivity, and hypomania) and call healthcare provider.

May worsen psychosis in some patients or precipitate a shift to mania or hypomania in patients with bipolar disorder. Patients presenting with depressive symptoms should be screened for bipolar disorder. Monotherapy in patients with bipolar disorder should be avoided. **Nortriptyline is not FDA approved for the treatment of bipolar depression.**

The risk of sedation and orthostatic effects are low relative to other antidepressants. However, nortriptyline may result in impaired performance of tasks requiring alertness (eg, operating machinery or driving). Sedative effects may be additive with other CNS depressants and/or ethanol. The degree of anticholinergic blockade produced by this agent is moderate relative to other cyclic antidepressants, however, caution should still be used in patients with urinary retention, benign prostatic hyperplasia, narrow-angle glaucoma, xerostomia, visual problems, constipation, or history of bowel obstruction. May cause orthostatic hypotension (risk is low relative to other antidepressants) or conduction disturbances. Use with caution in patients with a history of cardiovascular disease (including previous MI, stroke, tachycardia, or conduction abnormalities). The risk conduction abnormalities with this agent is moderate relative to other antidepressants.

Consider discontinuing, when possible, prior to elective surgery. Therapy should not be abruptly discontinued in patients receiving high doses for prolonged periods. May alter glucose regulation - use caution in patients with diabetes. Use caution in patients with a previous seizure disorder or condition predisposing to seizures such as brain damage, alcoholism, or concurrent therapy with other drugs which lower the seizure threshold. May increase the risks associated with electroconvulsive therapy. Use with caution in hyperthyroid patients or those receiving thyroid supplementation. Use with caution in patients with hepatic or renal dysfunction and in elderly patients.

Drug Interactions

Cytochrome P450 Effect: Substrate of CYP1A2 (minor), 2C19 (minor), 2D6 (major), 3A4 (minor); **Inhibits** CYP2D6 (weak), 2E1 (weak)

Decreased Effect: Carbamazepine, phenobarbital, and rifampin may increase the metabolism of nortriptyline resulting in decreased effect of nortriptyline. Nortriptyline inhibits the antihypertensive response to bethanidine, clonidine, debrisoquin, guanadrel, guanethidine, guanabenz, or guanfacine. Cholestyramine and colestipol may bind TCAs and reduce their absorption; monitor for altered response.

Increased Effect/Toxicity: Nortriptyline increases the effects of amphetamines, anticholinergics, other CNS depressants (sedatives, hypnotics, ethanol), chlorpropamide, tolazamide, and warfarin. When used with MAO inhibitors, hyperpyrexia, hypertension, tachycardia, confusion, seizures, and **deaths have been reported** (serotonin syndrome). Serotonin syndrome has also been reported with ritonavir (rare). CYP2D6 inhibitors may increase the levels/effects of nortriptyline; example inhibitors include chlorpromazine, delavirdine, fluoxetine, miconazole, paroxetine, pergolide, quinidine, quinine, ritonavir, and ropinirole. Cimetidine, grapefruit juice, indinavir, methylphenidate, diltiazem, and verapamil may increase the serum concentrations of TCAs. Use of lithium with a TCA may increase the risk for neurotoxicity. Phenothiazines may increase concentration of some TCAs and TCAs may increase concentration of phenothiazines. Pressor response to I.V. epinephrine, norepinephrine, and phenylephrine may be enhanced in patients receiving TCAs (**Note:** Effect is unlikely with epinephrine or levonordefrin dosages typically administered as infiltration in combination with local anesthetics). Combined use of beta-agonists or drugs which prolong QT$_c$ (including quinidine, procainamide, disopyramide, cisapride, sparfloxacin, gatifloxacin, moxifloxacin) with TCAs may predispose patients to cardiac arrhythmias. Use with altretamine may cause orthostatic hypotension.

Nutritional/Ethanol Interactions

Ethanol: Avoid ethanol (may increase CNS depression).

Food: Grapefruit juice may inhibit the metabolism of some TCAs and clinical toxicity may result.

Herb/Nutraceutical: Avoid valerian, St John's wort, SAMe, kava kava (may increase risk of serotonin syndrome and/or excessive sedation).

Lab Interactions Increased glucose

Adverse Reactions Frequency not defined.

Cardiovascular: Postural hypotension, arrhythmia, hypertension, heart block, tachycardia, palpitation, MI

Central nervous system: Confusion, delirium, hallucinations, restlessness, insomnia, disorientation, delusions, anxiety, agitation, panic, nightmares, hypomania, exacerbation of psychosis, incoordination, ataxia, extrapyramidal symptoms, seizure

Dermatologic: Alopecia, photosensitivity, rash, petechiae, urticaria, itching

Endocrine & metabolic: Sexual dysfunction, gynecomastia, breast enlargement, galactorrhea, increase or decrease in libido, increase in blood sugar, SIADH

Gastrointestinal: Xerostomia, constipation, vomiting, anorexia, diarrhea, abdominal cramps, black tongue, nausea, unpleasant taste, weight gain/loss

Genitourinary: Urinary retention, delayed micturition, impotence, testicular edema

Hematologic: Rarely agranulocytosis, eosinophilia, purpura, thrombocytopenia

Hepatic: Increased liver enzymes, cholestatic jaundice

Neuromuscular & skeletal: Tremor, numbness, tingling, paresthesia, peripheral neuropathy

Ocular: Blurred vision, eye pain, disturbances in accommodation, mydriasis

Otic: Tinnitus

Miscellaneous: Diaphoresis (excessive), allergic reactions

Overdosage/Toxicology Symptoms of overdose include agitation, confusion, hallucinations, urinary retention, hypothermia, hypotension, seizures, and ventricular tachycardia. Treatment is symptomatic and supportive. Alkalinization by sodium bicarbonate and/or hyperventilation may limit cardiac toxicity.

Pharmacodynamics/Kinetics

Onset of Action: Therapeutic: 1-3 weeks

Time to Peak: Serum: 7-8.5 hours

Protein Binding: 93% to 95%

Half-Life Elimination: 28-31 hours

Metabolism: Primarily hepatic; extensive first-pass effect

Excretion: Urine (as metabolites and small amounts of unchanged drug); feces (small amounts)

Available Dosage Forms

Capsule, as hydrochloride: 10 mg, 25 mg, 50 mg, 75 mg

Pamelor®: 10 mg, 25 mg, 50 mg, 75 mg [may contain benzyl alcohol; 50 mg may also contain sodium bisulfite]

Solution, as hydrochloride (Pamelor®): 10 mg/5 mL (473 mL) [contains alcohol 4% and benzoic acid]

Dosing

Adults:

Depression: Oral: 25 mg 3-4 times/day up to 150 mg/day

Chronic urticaria, angioedema, nocturnal pruritus (unlabeled use): Oral: 75 mg/day

Smoking cessation (unlabeled use): Oral: 25-75 mg/day beginning 10-14 days before "quit" day; continue therapy for ≥12 weeks after "quit" day

Elderly: Note: Nortriptyline is one of the best tolerated TCAs in the elderly.

Initial: 10-25 mg at bedtime

Dosage can be increased by 25 mg every 3 days for inpatients and weekly for outpatients if tolerated.

Usual maintenance dose: 75 mg as a single bedtime dose or 2 divided doses; however, lower or higher doses may be required to stay within the therapeutic window.

Pediatrics:

Nocturnal enuresis (unlabeled use): Oral: 10-20 mg/day; titrate to a maximum of 40 mg/day

Depression (unlabeled use): Oral: 1-3 mg/kg/day

Hepatic Impairment: Lower doses and slower titration are recommended dependent on individualization of dosage.

Stability

Storage: Protect from light.

Nursing Actions

Physical Assessment: Assess potential for interactions with other prescriptions, OTC medications, or herbal products patient may be taking. Assess for suicidal tendencies before beginning therapy. May cause physiological or psychological dependence, tolerance, or abuse; periodically evaluate need for continued use. Assess therapeutic response (mental status, mood, affect) and adverse reactions (eg, suicidal ideation) at beginning of therapy and periodically with long-term use. Dosage should be tapered slowly when discontinuing (allow 3-4 weeks between discontinuing this medication and starting another antidepressant). Caution patients with diabetes to monitor glucose levels closely; may increase or decrease serum glucose levels. Teach patient appropriate use, interventions to reduce side effects, and adverse symptoms to report.

Patient Education: Do not take any new medication during therapy unless approved by prescriber. Take exactly as directed; take once-a-day dose at bedtime. Do not increase dose or frequency; may take 2-3 weeks to achieve desired results. This drug may cause physical and/or psychological dependence. Avoid alcohol and grapefruit juice. Maintain adequate hydration (2-3 L/day of fluids) unless instructed to restrict fluid intake. May cause drowsiness, lightheadedness, impaired coordination, dizziness, or blurred vision (use caution when driving or engaging in tasks requiring alertness until response to drug is known); nausea, vomiting, loss of appetite, or disturbed taste (small frequent meals, good mouth care, chewing gum, or sucking lozenges may help); constipation (increased exercise, fluids, fruit, or fiber may help); urinary retention (void before taking medication); postural hypotension (use caution climbing stairs or when changing position from lying or sitting to standing); altered sexual drive or ability (reversible); or photosensitivity (use sunscreen, wear protective clothing and eyewear, and avoid direct sunlight). Report chest pain, palpitations, or rapid heartbeat; persistent adverse CNS effects (eg, suicidal ideation, nervousness, restlessness, insomnia, anxiety, excitation, headache, agitation, impaired coordination, changes in cognition); muscle cramping, weakness, tremors, or rigidity; blurred vision or eye pain; breast enlargement or swelling; yellowing of skin or eyes; or worsening of condition. **Pregnancy/breast-feeding precautions:** Inform prescriber if you pregnant. Do not get pregnant while taking this medication. Consult prescriber for appropriate contraceptive measures. Do not breast-feed.

Geriatric Considerations Since nortriptyline is the least likely of the tricyclic antidepressants (TCAs) to cause orthostatic hypotension and one of the least anticholinergic and sedating TCAs, it is a preferred agent when a TCA is indicated. Data from a clinical trial comparing fluoxetine to tricyclics suggests that fluoxetine is significantly less effective than nortriptyline in hospitalized elderly patients with unipolar affective disorder, especially those with melancholia and concurrent cardiovascular disease.

Related Information

Antidepressant Medication Guidelines *on page 1414*
Federal OBRA Regulations Recommended Maximum Doses *on page 1421*
Peak and Trough Guidelines *on page 1387*

Nystatin (nye STAT in)

U.S. Brand Names Bio-Statin®; Mycostatin®; Nyamyc™; Nystat-Rx®; Nystop®; Pedi-Dri®

Pharmacologic Category Antifungal Agent, Oral Nonabsorbed; Antifungal Agent, Topical; Antifungal Agent, Vaginal

Medication Safety Issues

Sound-alike/look-alike issues:

Nystatin may be confused with Nilstat®, Nitrostat® Nilstat may be confused with Nitrostat®, nystatin

Pregnancy Risk Factor B/C (oral)

Lactation Does not enter breast milk/compatible (not absorbed orally)

Use Treatment of susceptible cutaneous, mucocutaneous, and oral cavity fungal infections normally caused by the *Candida* species

Mechanism of Action/Effect Binds to sterols in fungal cell membrane, changing the cell wall permeability allowing for leakage of cellular contents and cell death

Contraindications Hypersensitivity to nystatin or any component of the formulation

Adverse Reactions

Frequency not defined: Dermatologic: Contact dermatitis, Stevens-Johnson syndrome

1% to 10%: Gastrointestinal: Nausea, vomiting, diarrhea, stomach pain

Overdosage/Toxicology Symptoms of overdose include nausea, vomiting, and diarrhea. Treatment is supportive.

Pharmacodynamics/Kinetics

Onset of Action: Symptomatic relief from candidiasis: 24-72 hours

Excretion: Feces (as unchanged drug)

Available Dosage Forms

Capsule (Bio-Statin®): 500,000 units, 1 million units

Cream: 100,000 units/g (15 g, 30 g)

Mycostatin®: 100,000 units/g (30 g)

Ointment, topical: 100,000 units/g (15 g, 30 g)

Powder, for prescription compounding: 50 million units (10 g); 150 million units (30 g); 500 million units (100 g); 2 billion units (400 g)

Nystat-Rx®: 50 million units (10 g); 150 million units (30 g); 500 million units (100 g); 1 billion units (190 g); 2 billion units (350 g)

Powder, topical:

Mycostatin®: 100,000 units/g (15 g)

Nyamyc™: 100,000 units/g (15 g, 30 g)

Nystop®: 100,000 units/g (15 g, 30 g, 60 g)

Pedi-Dri®: 100,000 units/g (56.7 g)

Suspension, oral: 100,000 units/mL (5 mL, 60 mL, 480 mL)

Tablet: 500,000 units

Tablet, vaginal: 100,000 units (15s) [packaged with applicator]

Dosing

Adults & Elderly:

Oral candidiasis: Suspension (swish and swallow orally): 400,000-600,000 units 4 times/day

Mucocutaneous infections: Topical: Apply 2-3 times/day to affected areas; very moist topical lesions are treated best with powder.

Intestinal infections: Oral tablets: 500,000-1,000,000 units every 8 hours

Vaginal infections: Vaginal tablets: Insert 1 tablet/day at bedtime for 2 weeks. (May also be given orally.)

Note: Powder for compounding: ¹/₈ teaspoon (500,000 units) to equal approximately ¹/₂ cup of water; give 4 times/day

Pediatrics:

Oral candidiasis:

Suspension (swish and swallow orally):

Premature infants: 100,000 units 4 times/day

Infants: 200,000 units 4 times/day or 100,000 units to each side of mouth 4 times/day

Children: 400,000-600,000 units 4 times/day

Powder for compounding: Children: Refer to adult dosing.

Mucocutaneous infections: Children: Refer to adult dosing.

Administration

Oral: Suspension: Shake well before using. Should be swished about the mouth and retained in the mouth for as long as possible (several minutes) before swallowing.

Stability

Storage:

Vaginal insert: Store in refrigerator. Protect from temperature extremes, moisture, and light.

Oral tablet, ointment, topical powder, and oral suspension: Store at controlled room temperature 15°C to 25°C (59°F to 77°F).

Nursing Actions

Physical Assessment: Determine that cause of infection is fungal. Avoid skin contact when applying. Monitor therapeutic response, adverse reactions at beginning of therapy and periodically throughout therapy. Assess knowledge/teach patient appropriate use, interventions to reduce side effects, and adverse symptoms to report.

Patient Education: Take as directed. Maintain adequate hydration (2-3 L/day of fluids) unless instructed to restrict fluid intake. Do not allow medication to come in contact with eyes. Report persistent nausea, vomiting, or diarrhea; or if condition being treated worsens or does not improve. **Pregnancy precaution:** Inform prescriber if you are pregnant.

Oral tablet: Swallow whole; do not crush or chew.

Oral suspension: Shake well before using. Remove dentures, clean mouth (do not replace dentures until after using medications). Swish suspension in mouth for several minutes before swallowing

Oral troche: Remove dentures, clean mouth (do not replace dentures until after using medication). Allow troche to dissolve in mouth; do not chew or swallow whole.

Topical: Wash and dry area before applying (do not reuse towels without washing, apply clean clothing after use). Report unresolved burning, redness, or swelling in treated areas.

Vaginal tablet: Wash hands before using. Lie down to insert high into vagina at bedtime.

Geriatric Considerations For oral infections, patients who wear dentures must have them removed and cleaned in order to eliminate source of reinfection.

Nystatin and Triamcinolone
(nye STAT in & trye am SIN oh lone)

U.S. Brand Names Mycolog®-II [DSC]

Synonyms Triamcinolone and Nystatin

Pharmacologic Category Antifungal Agent, Topical; Corticosteroid, Topical

Pregnancy Risk Factor C

Lactation Excretion in breast milk unknown

Use Treatment of cutaneous candidiasis

Available Dosage Forms [DSC] = Discontinued product

Cream (Mycolog®-II [DSC]): Nystatin 100,000 units and triamcinolone acetonide 0.1% (15 g, 30 g, 60 g)

Ointment: Nystatin 100,000 units and triamcinolone acetonide 0.1% (15 g, 30 g, 60 g)

Mycolog®-II: Nystatin 100,000 units and triamcinolone acetonide 0.1% (15 g, 30 g, 60 g) [DSC]

Dosing

Adults & Elderly: Cutaneous *Candida*: Topical: Apply sparingly 2-4 times/day,

Pediatrics: Refer to adult dosing.

Nursing Actions

Physical Assessment: See individual agents.

Patient Education: See individual agents. **Pregnancy/breast-feeding precautions:** Inform prescriber if you are or intend to become pregnant. Consult prescriber if breast-feeding.

Related Information

Nystatin *on page 900*
Triamcinolone *on page 1248*

Octreotide (ok TREE oh tide)

U.S. Brand Names Sandostatin®; Sandostatin LAR®

Synonyms Octreotide Acetate

Pharmacologic Category Antidiarrheal; Somatostatin Analog

Medication Safety Issues

Sound-alike/look-alike issues:
Sandostatin® may be confused with Sandimmune®

Pregnancy Risk Factor B

Lactation Excretion in breast milk unknown/use caution

Use Control of symptoms in patients with metastatic carcinoid and vasoactive intestinal peptide-secreting tumors (VIPomas); acromegaly

Unlabeled/Investigational Use AIDS-associated secretory diarrhea (including *Cryptosporidiosis*), control of bleeding of esophageal varices, breast cancer, cryptosporidiosis, Cushing's syndrome (ectopic), insulinomas, small bowel fistulas, pancreatic tumors, gastrinoma, postgastrectomy dumping syndrome, chemotherapy-induced diarrhea, graft-versus-host disease (GVHD) induced diarrhea, Zollinger-Ellison syndrome, congenital hyperinsulinism

Mechanism of Action/Effect Mimics natural somatostatin by inhibiting serotonin release, and the secretion of gastrin, VIP, insulin, glucagon, secretin, motilin, and pancreatic polypeptide. Decreases growth hormone and IGF-1 in acromegaly.

Contraindications Hypersensitivity to octreotide or any component of the formulation

Warnings/Precautions May impair gall bladder function; monitor patients for cholelithiasis. Use with caution in patients with renal impairment. Somatostatin analogs may affect glucose regulation; in type I diabetes, severe hypoglycemia may occur; in type II diabetes or nondiabetic patients, hyperglycemia may occur. Insulin and other hypoglycemic medication requirements may change. Bradycardia, conduction abnormalities, and arrhythmia have been observed in acromegalic patients; use caution with CHF or concomitant medications that alter heart rate or rhythm. May alter absorption of dietary fats; monitor for pancreatitis. Chronic treatment has been associated with abnormal Schillings test; monitor vitamin B$_{12}$ levels.

Drug Interactions

Decreased Effect: Octreotide may lower cyclosporine serum levels (case reports of transplant rejection due to reduction of serum cyclosporine levels when cyclosporine was given orally in conjunction with a somatostatin analogue).

Adverse Reactions Adverse reactions vary by route of administration. Frequency of cardiac, endocrine, and gastrointestinal adverse reactions were generally higher in acromegalics.

>16%:

Cardiovascular: Sinus bradycardia (19% to 25%), chest pain (16% to 20%)

Central nervous system: Fatigue (1% to 20%), malaise (16% to 20%), dizziness (5% to 20%), headache (6% to 20%), fever (16% to 20%)

Endocrine & metabolic: Hyperglycemia (2% to 27%)

Gastrointestinal: Diarrhea (5% to 61%), abdominal discomfort (5% to 61%), flatulence (<10% to 38%), constipation (9% to 21%), nausea (5% to 61%), cholelithiasis (27%; length of therapy dependent), biliary duct dilatation (12%; biliary sludge (24%; length of therapy dependent), loose stools (5% to 61%), vomiting (4% to 21%)

Hematologic: Antibodies to octreotide (up to 25%; no efficacy change)

Local: Injection pain (2% to 50%; dose- and formulation-related)

Neuromuscular & skeletal: Backache (1% to 20%), arthropathy (16% to 20%)

Respiratory: Dyspnea (16% to 20%), upper respiratory infection (16% to 20%)

Miscellaneous: Flu symptoms (1% to 20%)

5% to 15%:

Cardiovascular: Conduction abnormalities (9% to 10%), arrhythmia (3% to 9%), hypertension, palpitations, peripheral edema

Central nervous system: Anxiety, confusion, depression, hypoesthesia, insomnia, vertigo

Dermatologic: Pruritus, rash

Endocrine & metabolic: Hypothyroidism (2% to 12%), goiter (2% to 8%)

Gastrointestinal: Abdominal pain, anorexia, cramping, dehydration, discomfort, hemorrhoids, tenesmus (4% to 6%), dyspepsia (4% to 6%), steatorrhea (4% to 6%), feces discoloration (4% to 6%), weight loss

Genitourinary: UTI

Hematologic: Anemia

Hepatic: Hepatitis

Neuromuscular & skeletal: Arthralgia, leg cramps, myalgia, paresthesia, rigors, weakness

Otic: Ear ache, otitis media

Renal: Renal calculus

Respiratory: coughing, pharyngitis, sinusitis, rhinitis

Miscellaneous: Allergy, diaphoresis

1% to 4%:

Cardiovascular: Angina, cardiac failure, cerebral vascular disorder, edema, flushing, hematoma, phlebitis, tachycardia

Central nervous system: Abnormal gait, amnesia, dysphonia, hallucinations, nervousness, neuralgia, neuropathy, somnolence, tremor, vertigo

Dermatologic: Acne, alopecia, bruising, cellulitis, urticaria

Endocrine & metabolic: Hypoglycemia (2% to 4%), hypokalemia, hypoproteinemia, gout, cachexia, menstrual irregularities, breast pain, impotence

Gastrointestinal: Colitis, diverticulitis, dysphagia, fat malabsorption, gastritis, gastroenteritis, gingivitis, glossitis, melena, rectal bleeding, stomatitis, taste perversion, xerostomia

Genitourinary: Incontinence

Hematologic: Epistaxis

Hepatic: Ascites, jaundice

Local: Injection hematoma

Neuromuscular & skeletal: Hyperkinesia, hypertonia, joint pain

Ocular: Blurred vision, visual disturbance

Otic: Tinnitus

Renal: Albuminuria, renal abscess

Respiratory: Bronchitis, pleural effusion, pneumonia, pulmonary embolism

Miscellaneous: Bacterial infection, cold symptoms, moniliasis

Overdosage/Toxicology Symptoms of overdose include hypo- or hyperglycemia, blurred vision, dizziness, drowsiness, and loss of motor function. Well tolerated bolus doses up to 1000 mcg have failed to produce adverse effects.

Pharmacodynamics/Kinetics

Duration of Action: SubQ: 6-12 hours

Time to Peak: SubQ: 0.4 hours (0.7 hours acromegaly)

(Continued)

Octreotide *(Continued)*

Protein Binding: 65%

Half-Life Elimination: 1.7-1.9 hours; up to 3.7 hours with cirrhosis

Metabolism: Extensively hepatic

Excretion: Urine (32%)

Available Dosage Forms

Injection, microspheres for suspension, as acetate [depot formulation] (Sandostatin LAR®): 10 mg, 20 mg, 30 mg [with diluent and syringe]

Injection, solution, as acetate (Sandostatin®): 0.05 mg/mL (1 mL); 0.1 mg/mL (1 mL); 0.2 mg/mL (5 mL); 0.5 mg/mL (1 mL); 1 mg/mL (5 mL)

Dosing

Adults & Elderly: SubQ, I.V.: Initial: 50 mcg 2-3 times/day; titrate dose based on response, tolerance, and indication

Carcinoid tumors:

SubQ, I.V.: Initial 2 weeks: 100-600 mcg/day in 2-4 divided doses; usual range 50-1500 mcg/day

I.M. Depot injection: Patients must be stabilized on subcutaneous octreotide for at least 2 weeks before switching to the long-acting depot: Upon switch: 20 mg I.M. intragluteally every 4 weeks for 2-3 months, then the dose may be modified based upon response

Dosage adjustment: See dosing for VIPomas.

VIPomas:

SubQ, I.V.: Initial 2 weeks: 200-300 mcg/day in 2-4 divided doses; titrate dose based on response/tolerance. Range: 150-750 mcg/day (doses >450 mcg/day are rarely required)

I.M. Depot injection: Patients must be stabilized on subcutaneous octreotide for at least 2 weeks before switching to the long-acting depot: Upon switch: 20 mg I.M. intragluteally every 4 weeks for 2-3 months, then the dose may be modified based upon response

Dosage adjustment for carcinoid tumors and VIPomas: After 2 months of depot injections the dosage may be continued or modified as follows:

Increase to 30 mg I.M. every 4 weeks if symptoms are inadequately controlled

Decrease to 10 mg I.M. every 4 weeks, for a trial period, if initially responsive to 20 mg dose

Dosage >30 mg is not recommended

Diarrhea: I.V.: Initial: 50-100 mcg every 8 hours; increase by 100 mcg/dose at 48-hour intervals; maximum dose: 500 mcg every 8 hours

Esophageal varices bleeding (unlabeled use): I.V. bolus: 25-50 mcg followed by continuous I.V. infusion of 25-50 mcg/hour

Acromegaly:

SubQ, I.V.: Initial: 50 mcg 3 times/day; titrate to achieve growth hormone levels <5 ng/mL or IGF-I (somatomedin C) levels <1.9 U/mL in males and <2.2 U/mL in females. Usual effective dose 100 mcg 3 times/day. Range 300-1500 mcg/day. **Note:** Should be withdrawn yearly for a 4 week interval (8 weeks for depot injection) in patients who have received irradiation. Resume if levels increase and signs/symptoms recur.

I.M. Depot injection: Patients must be stabilized on subcutaneous octreotide for at least 2 weeks before switching to the long-acting depot: Upon switch: 20 mg I.M. intragluteally every 4 weeks for 2-3 months, then the dose may be modified based upon response

Dosage adjustment for acromegaly: After 3 months of depot injections the dosage may be continued or modified as follows:

GH ≤1 ng/mL, IGF-1 is normal, symptoms controlled: Reduce octreotide LAR® to 10 mg I.M. every 4 weeks

GH ≤2.5 ng/mL, IGF-1 is normal, symptoms controlled: Maintain octreotide LAR® at 20 mg I.M. every 4 weeks

GH >2.5 ng/mL, IGF-1 is elevated, or symptoms uncontrolled: Increase octreotide LAR® to 30 mg I.M. every 4 weeks

Dosages >40 mg are not recommended

Pediatrics: Infants and Children:

Secretory diarrhea (unlabeled use): I.V., SubQ: Doses of 1-10 mcg/kg every 12 hours have been used in children beginning at the low end of the range and increasing by 0.3 mcg/kg/dose at 3-day intervals. Suppression of growth hormone (animal data) is of concern when used as long-term therapy.

Congenital hyperinsulinism (unlabeled use): SubQ: Doses of 3-40 mcg/kg/day have been used.

Renal Impairment: Half-life may be increased, requiring adjustment of maintenance dose.

Administration

I.M.: Depot formulation: Administer I.M. intragluteal (avoid deltoid administration); do not administer Sandostatin LAR® intravenously or subcutaneously; must be administered immediately after mixing

I.V.: Regular injection only (not suspension): IVP should be administered undiluted over 3 minutes. IVPB should be administered over 15-30 minutes. Continuous I.V. infusion rates have ranged from 25-50 mcg/hour for the treatment of esophageal variceal bleeding.

I.V. Detail: Do not use if solution contains particles or is discolored. I.V. administration may be IVP, IVPB, or continuous I.V. infusion.

pH: 4.0-4.6

Other: Regular injection formulation (not depot) can be administered SubQ

Stability

Compatibility: Stable in D$_5$W, NS; **incompatible** with fat emulsion 10%.

The manufacturer states that octreotide solution is not compatible in TPN solutions due to the formation of a glycosyl octreotide conjugate which may have decreased activity; other sources give it limited compatibility.

Storage:

Solution: Octreotide is a clear solution and should be stored under refrigeration; may be stored at room temperature for up to 14 days when protected from light. Stability of parenteral admixture is stable in NS for 96 hours at room temperature (25°C) and in D$_5$W for 24 hours.

Suspension: Prior to dilution, store under refrigeration and protect from light; may be at room temperature for 30-60 minutes prior to use; use suspension immediately after preparation.

Laboratory Monitoring Blood glucose

Acromegaly: Growth hormone, somatomedin C (IGF-1), heart rate, EKG

Carcinoid: 5-HIAA, plasma serotonin and plasma substance P

VIPomas: Vasoactive intestinal peptide

Chronic therapy: Thyroid function (baseline and periodic), vitamin B$_{12}$ level

Nursing Actions

Physical Assessment: Assess potential for interactions with other pharmacological agents patient may be taking (eg, may increase effect of insulin or sulfonylureas). See Administration for I.V. and I.M. specifics. Monitor laboratory tests with long-term therapy. Monitor therapeutic effectiveness according to purpose for use and adverse effects (eg, hypo-/hyperglycemia, bradycardia, diarrhea, GI disturbance, CNS changes, jaundice, blurred vision). Caution patients with diabetes to monitor serum glucose closely; may increase the effect of insulin or sulfonylureas, which may result in hypoglycemia. Teach patient proper use if self-administered (appropriate injection technique and syringe/needle disposal), possible side effects/appropriate interventions, and adverse symptoms to report.

Patient Education: Do not take any new medication during therapy unless approved by prescriber (especially any other antidiarrheals or "stomach" medications). If self-administered, follow instructions for injection and syringe/needle disposal. Schedule injections between meals to decrease GI effects. Consult prescriber about appropriate diet. If you have diabetes, monitor serum glucose closely and notify prescriber of significant changes (this drug may increase the effects of insulin or sulfonylureas). May cause skin flushing; nausea or vomiting (small frequent meals, frequent mouth care, sucking lozenges, or chewing gum may help); or dizziness, fatigue, or drowsiness (use caution when driving or engaging in tasks that require alertness until response to drug is known). Report unusual weight gain, swelling of extremities, or respiratory difficulty; acute or persistent GI distress (eg, diarrhea, vomiting, constipation, abdominal pain); muscle weakness or tremors or loss of motor function; chest pain or palpitations; blurred vision; depression; or redness, swelling, burning, or pain at injection site.

Breast-feeding precaution: Do not breast-feed.

Dietary Considerations Schedule injections between meals to decrease GI effects. May alter absorption of dietary fats.

Ofloxacin (oh FLOKS a sin)

U.S. Brand Names Floxin®; Ocuflox®

Synonyms Floxin Otic Singles

Pharmacologic Category Antibiotic, Quinolone

Medication Safety Issues
Sound-alike/look-alike issues:
Floxin® may be confused with Flexeril®
Ocuflox® may be confused with Ocufen®

Pregnancy Risk Factor C

Lactation Enters breast milk/not recommended (AAP rates "compatible")

Use Quinolone antibiotic for the treatment of acute exacerbations of chronic bronchitis, community-acquired pneumonia, skin and skin structure infections (uncomplicated), urethral and cervical gonorrhea (acute, uncomplicated), urethritis and cervicitis (nongonococcal), mixed infections of the urethra and cervix, pelvic inflammatory disease (acute), cystitis (uncomplicated), urinary tract infections (complicated), prostatitis

Ophthalmic: Treatment of superficial ocular infections involving the conjunctiva or cornea due to strains of susceptible organisms

Otic: Otitis externa, chronic suppurative otitis media, acute otitis media

Unlabeled/Investigational Use Epididymitis (gonorrhea), leprosy, Traveler's diarrhea

Mechanism of Action/Effect Ofloxacin, a fluorinated quinolone, is a pyridine carboxylic acid derivative which exerts a broad spectrum bactericidal effect. It inhibits DNA gyrase inhibitor, an essential bacterial enzyme that maintains the superhelical structure of DNA. DNA gyrase is required for DNA replication and transcription, DNA repair, recombination, and transposition within the bacteria.

Contraindications Hypersensitivity to ofloxacin or other members of the quinolone group such as nalidixic acid, oxolinic acid, cinoxacin, norfloxacin, and ciprofloxacin; hypersensitivity to any component of the formulation

Warnings/Precautions Use with caution in patients with epilepsy or other CNS diseases which could predispose seizures. Use with caution in patients with renal or hepatic impairment. Has been associated with rare tendonitis or ruptured tendons (discontinue immediately with signs of inflammation or tendon pain). Risk may be increased with concurrent corticosteroids, particularly in the elderly. Discontinue at first sign of tendon inflammation or pain. Peripheral neuropathies have been linked to ofloxacin use; discontinue if numbness, tingling, or weakness develops.

Rare cases of torsade de pointes have been reported in patients receiving ofloxacin and other quinolones. Risk may be minimized by avoiding use in patients with known prolongation of the QT interval, bradycardia, hypokalemia, hypomagnesemia, cardiomyopathy, or in those receiving concurrent therapy with Class Ia or Class III antiarrhythmics.

Severe hypersensitivity reactions, including anaphylaxis, have occurred with quinolone therapy. Discontinue immediately if an allergic reaction occurs. Prolonged use may result in superinfection; pseudomembranous colitis may occur and should be considered in all patients who present with diarrhea. Quinolones may exacerbate myasthenia gravis.

Drug Interactions

Cytochrome P450 Effect: Inhibits CYP1A2 (strong)

Decreased Effect: Concurrent administration of metal cations, including most antacids, oral electrolyte supplements, quinapril, sucralfate, some didanosine formulations (chewable/buffered tablets and pediatric powder for oral suspension), and other highly-buffered oral drugs, may decrease quinolone levels; separate doses.

Increased Effect/Toxicity: Ofloxacin may increase the effects/toxicity of CYP1A2 substrates (eg, aminophylline, fluvoxamine, mexiletine, mirtazapine, ropinirole, and trifluoperazine), glyburide, theophylline and warfarin. Concomitant use with corticosteroids may increase the risk of tendon rupture. Concomitant use with other QT_c-prolonging agents (eg, Class Ia and Class III antiarrhythmics, erythromycin, cisapride, antipsychotics, and cyclic antidepressants) may result in arrhythmias such as torsade de pointes. Probenecid may increase ofloxacin levels.

Nutritional/Ethanol Interactions

Food: Ofloxacin average peak serum concentrations may be decreased by 20% if taken with food.

Herb/Nutraceutical: Avoid dong quai, St John's wort (may also cause photosensitization).

Lab Interactions Some quinolones may produce a false-positive urine screening result for opiates using commercially-available immunoassay kits. This has been demonstrated most consistently for levofloxacin and ofloxacin, but other quinolones have shown cross-reactivity in certain assay kits. Confirmation of positive opiate screens by more specific methods should be considered.

Adverse Reactions

Systemic:

1% to 10%:
Cardiovascular: Chest pain (1% to 3%)
Central nervous system: Headache (1% to 9%), insomnia (3% to 7%), dizziness (1% to 5%), fatigue (1% to 3%), somnolence (1% to 3%), sleep disorders (1% to 3%), nervousness (1% to 3%), pyrexia (1% to 3%)
Dermatologic: Rash/pruritus (1% to 3%)
Gastrointestinal: Diarrhea (1% to 4%), vomiting (1% to 4%), GI distress (1% to 3%), abdominal cramps (1% to 3%), flatulence (1% to 3%), abnormal taste (1% to 3%), xerostomia (1% to 3%), decreased appetite (1% to 3%), nausea (3% to 10%), constipation (1% to 3%)
Genitourinary: Vaginitis (1% to 5%), external genital pruritus in women (1% to 3%)
Ocular: Visual disturbances (1% to 3%)
Respiratory: Pharyngitis (1% to 3%)
Miscellaneous: Trunk pain

(Continued)

Ofloxacin *(Continued)*

Ophthalmic: Frequency not defined:

Central nervous system: Dizziness

Gastrointestinal: Nausea

Ocular: Blurred vision, burning, chemical conjunctivitis/keratitis, discomfort, dryness, edema, eye pain, foreign body sensation, itching, photophobia, redness, stinging, tearing

Otic:

>10%: Local: Application site reaction (<1% to 17%)

1% to 10%:

Central nervous system: Dizziness (≤1%), vertigo (≤1%)

Dermatologic: Pruritus (1% to 4%), rash (1%)

Gastrointestinal: Taste perversion (7%)

Neuromuscular & skeletal: Paresthesia (1%)

Overdosage/Toxicology Symptoms of overdose include acute renal failure, seizures, nausea, and vomiting. Treatment includes GI decontamination, if possible, and supportive care. Not removed by peritoneal or hemodialysis.

Pharmacodynamics/Kinetics

Protein Binding: 20%

Half-Life Elimination: Biphasic: 5-7.5 hours and 20-25 hours (accounts for <5%); prolonged with renal impairment

Excretion: Primarily urine (as unchanged drug)

Available Dosage Forms [DSC] = Discontinued product

Solution, ophthalmic (Ocuflox®): 0.3% (5 mL; 10 mL [DSC]) [contains benzalkonium chloride]

Solution, otic:

Floxin®: 0.3% (5 mL, 10 mL) [contains benzalkonium chloride]

Floxin® Otic Singles™: 0.3% (0.25 mL) [contains benzalkonium chloride; packaged as 2 single-dose containers per pouch, 10 pouches per carton, total net volume 5 mL]

Tablet (Floxin®): 200 mg, 300 mg, 400 mg

Dosing

Adults:

Cervicitis/urethritis (nongonococcal) due to *C. trachomatis,* mixed infection of urethra and cervix due to *C. trachomatis* and *N. gonorrhoea*: 300 mg every 12 hours for 7 days

Chronic bronchitis (acute exacerbation), community-acquired pneumonia, skin and skin structure infections (uncomplicated): 400 mg every 12 hours for 10 days

Conjunctivitis: Ophthalmic: Instill 1-2 drops in affected eye(s) every 2-4 hours for the first 2 days, then use 4 times/day for an additional 5 days.

Corneal ulcer: Ophthalmic: Instill 1-2 drops every 30 minutes while awake and every 4-6 hours after retiring for the first 2 days; beginning on day 3, instill 1-2 drops every hour while awake for 4-6 additional days; thereafter, 1-2 drops 4 times/day until clinical cure.

Cystitis (uncomplicated), *E. coli* or *K. pneumoniae*: 200 mg every 12 hours for 3 days or up to 7 days for other organisms

Epididymitis, gonococcal (unlabeled use): 300 mg twice daily for 10 days

Leprosy (unlabeled use): 400 mg once daily

Otitis media, chronic suppurative with perforated tympanic membranes: Otic: Instill 10 drops (or the contents of 2 single-dose containers) into affected ear twice daily for 14 days

Otitis externa: Otic: Instill 10 drops (or the contents of 2 single-dose containers) into affected ear(s) once daily for 7 days

Pelvic inflammatory disease (acute): 400 mg every 12 hours for 10-14 days

Prostatitis:

Acute: 400 mg for 1 dose, then 300 mg twice daily for 10 days

Chronic: 200 mg every 12 hours for 6 weeks

Traveler's diarrhea (unlabeled use): 300 mg twice daily for 3 days

Urethral and cervical gonorrhea (acute, uncomplicated): 400 mg as a single dose

UTI (complicated): 200 mg every 12 hours for 10 days

Elderly: Oral: 200-400 mg every 12-24 hours (based on estimated renal function) for 7 days to 6 weeks depending on indication.

Pediatrics: Not for systemic use

Acute otitis media with tympanotomy tubes: Otic: Children 1-12 years: Instill 5 drops (or the contents of 1 single-dose container) into affected ear twice daily for 10 days.

Conjunctivitis: Ophthalmic: Children ≥1 year: Refer to adult dosing.

Corneal ulcer: Ophthalmic: Children ≥1 year: Refer to adult dosing.

Otitis externa: Otic:

Children 6 months to 13 years: Instill 5 drops (or the contents of 1 single-dose container) into affected ear(s) once daily for 7 days

Children ≥13 years: Refer to adult dosing.

Otitis media, chronic suppurative with perforated tympanic membranes: Otic: Children >12 years: Refer to adult dosing.

Renal Impairment: Adults: Oral: After a normal initial dose, adjust as follows:

Cl_{cr} 20-50 mL/minute: Administer usual dose every 24 hours

Cl_{cr} <20 mL/minute: Administer half the usual dose every 24 hours

Continuous arteriovenous or venovenous hemodiafiltration effects: Administer 300 mg every 24 hours

Hepatic Impairment: Severe impairment: Maximum dose: 400 mg/day

Administration

Oral: Do not take within 2 hours of food or any antacids which contain zinc, magnesium, or aluminum.

Other:

Ophthalmic: For ophthalmic use only; avoid touching tip of applicator to eye or other surfaces.

Otic: Prior to use, warm solution by holding container in hands for 1-2 minutes. Patient should lie down with affected ear upward and medication instilled. Pump tragus 4 times to ensure penetration of medication. Patient should remain in this position for 5 minutes.

Stability

Storage:

Ophthalmic and otic solution: Store between 15°C to 25°C (59°F to 77°F).

Otic Singles™: Store between 15°C to 30°C (59°F to 86°F). Store in pouch to protect from light.

Tablet: Store below 30°C (86°F).

Laboratory Monitoring Perform culture and sensitivity studies before initiating therapy. Monitor CBC, renal and hepatic function periodically if therapy is prolonged.

Nursing Actions

Physical Assessment: Results of culture and sensitivity tests and patient's allergy history should be assessed before initiating therapy. Assess potential for interactions with other pharmacological agents and herbal products patient may be taking (eg, increased risk of tendon rupture or arrhythmias). See Administration specifics for different formulations (otic, ophthalmic, oral). Monitor laboratory tests, renal function, and hepatic function with long-term therapy. Patient should be monitored for an allergic reaction (itching, urticaria, dyspnea or facial edema, loss of consciousness, tingling, cardiovascular collapse). If allergic reaction or tendon inflammation or pain occurs, drug should be discontinued. Monitor therapeutic effectiveness (resolution of infection) and adverse reactions. Teach patient appropriate use (according to formulation), possible side effects/appropriate interventions, and adverse symptoms to report (eg, allergic reaction, tendon pain).

Patient Education: Do not take any new medication during therapy unless approved by prescriber. Take as directed; on an empty stomach (1 hour before or 2 hours after meals, dairy products, antacids, or other medication). Complete full course of therapy, even if symptoms resolve. Maintain adequate hydration (2-3 L/day of fluids) unless instructed to restrict fluid intake. May cause dizziness, lightheadedness, or headache (use caution when driving or engaging in tasks that require alertness until response to drug is known); nausea, vomiting, or taste perversion (small frequent meals, frequent mouth care, sucking lozenges, or chewing gum may help). If inflammation or tendon pain occurs discontinue use immediately and report to prescriber. If sign of allergic reaction (eg, itching, urticaria, respiratory difficulty, facial edema or difficulty swallowing, loss of consciousness, tingling, chest pain, palpitations) occurs, discontinue use immediately and report to prescriber. Report GI disturbances; CNS changes (eg, excessive sleepiness, agitation, or tremors); skin rash; vision changes; respiratory difficulty; signs of opportunistic infection (eg, sore throat, chills, fever, burning, itching on urination, vaginal discharge, white plaques in mouth); or worsening of condition. **Pregnancy/breast-feeding precautions:** Inform prescriber if you are or intend to become pregnant. Breast-feeding is not recommended.

Ophthalmic: Wash hands before instilling solution. Sit or lie down to instill. Open eye, look at ceiling, and instill prescribed amount of solution as directed. Close eye and roll eye in all directions, and apply gentle pressure to inner corner of eye. Do not touch tip of applicator or let tip of applicator touch eye (may cause eye infection, eye damage, or vision loss). Do not wear contact lenses during therapy. Temporary stinging, blurred vision, dry eyes or a bad taste in your mouth may occur after installation. Report persistent pain, burning, excessive tearing, decreased visual acuity, swelling, itching, or worsening of condition.

Otic: Wash hands before and after applying drops. Lie with affected ear up and instill prescribed number of drops into ear. Remain on side with ear up for 5 minutes.

Geriatric Considerations The risk of torsade de pointes and tendon inflammation and/or rupture associated with the concomitant use of corticosteroids and quinolones is increased in the elderly population. Dosage must be carefully adjusted to renal function. The half-life of ofloxacin may be prolonged, and serum concentrations are elevated in elderly patients even in the absence of overt renal impairment.

Breast-Feeding Issues Following oral use, levels of ofloxacin in breast milk are similar to those in plasma. The manufacturer recommends to discontinue nursing or to discontinue ofloxacin.

Pregnancy Issues Reports of arthropathy (observed in immature animals and reported rarely in humans) have limited the use of fluoroquinolones in pregnancy. Teratogenic effects were not observed with ofloxacin in animal studies; however, decreased fetal body weight and increased fetal mortality were observed in some species. Ofloxacin crosses the placenta. Although quinolone antibiotics should not be used as first-line agents during pregnancy, when considering treatment for life-threatening infection and/or prolonged duration of therapy, the potential risk to the fetus must be balanced against the severity of the potential illness.

Olanzapine (oh LAN za peen)

U.S. Brand Names Zyprexa®; Zyprexa® Zydis®
Synonyms LY170053; Zyprexa Zydis
Pharmacologic Category Antipsychotic Agent, Atypical
Medication Safety Issues
Sound-alike/look-alike issues:
Olanzapine may be confused with olsalazine
Zyprexa® may be confused with Celexa™, Zyrtec®
Pregnancy Risk Factor C
Lactation Enters breast milk/not recommended
Use Treatment of the manifestations of schizophrenia; treatment of acute or mixed mania episodes associated with Bipolar I Disorder (as monotherapy or in combination with lithium or valproate); maintenance treatment of bipolar disorder; acute agitation (patients with schizophrenia or bipolar mania)
Unlabeled/Investigational Use Treatment of psychotic symptoms; chronic pain
Mechanism of Action/Effect The efficacy of olanzapine in schizophrenia and bipolar disorder is thought to be mediated through combined antagonism of dopamine and serotonin type 2 receptor sites.
Contraindications Hypersensitivity to olanzapine or any component of the formulation
Warnings/Precautions Patients with dementia-related behavioral disorders treated with atypical antipsychotics are at an increased risk of cerebrovascular adverse events and death compared to placebo. Olanzapine is not approved for this indication.

Moderate to highly sedating, use with caution in disorders where CNS depression is a feature; patients must be cautioned about performing tasks which require mental alertness (eg, operating machinery or driving). Use with caution in Parkinson's disease; in patients with bone marrow suppression; predisposition to seizures; subcortical brain damage; severe hepatic, renal, or respiratory disease. Life-threatening arrhythmias have occurred some neuroleptics. May induce orthostatic hypotension; use caution with history of cardiovascular disease. Esophageal dysmotility and aspiration have been associated with antipsychotic use; use with caution in patients at risk of aspiration pneumonia. Caution in breast cancer or other prolactin-dependent tumors. Significant weight gain may occur. Impaired core body temperature regulation may occur; caution with strenuous exercise, heat exposure, dehydration, and concomitant medication possessing anticholinergic effects.

May cause anticholinergic effects; use with caution in patients with decreased gastrointestinal motility, urinary retention, BPH, xerostomia, glaucoma, or myasthenia gravis. Relative to other neuroleptics, olanzapine has a moderate potency of cholinergic blockade.

May cause extrapyramidal symptoms, although risk of these reactions is lower relative to other neuroleptics). May be associated with neuroleptic malignant syndrome (NMS). May cause extreme and life-threatening hyperglycemia; use with caution in patients with diabetes or other disorders of glucose regulation; monitor. Olanzapine levels may be lower in patients who smoke, requiring dosage adjustment.

The possibility of a suicide attempt is inherent in psychotic illness or bipolar disorder; use caution in high-risk patients during initiation of therapy. Prescriptions should be written for the smallest quantity consistent with good patient care. Safety and efficacy in pediatric patients have not been established.

Drug Interactions
Cytochrome P450 Effect: Substrate of CYP1A2 (major), 2D6 (minor); **Inhibits** CYP1A2 (weak), 2C8/9 (weak), 2C19 (weak), 2D6 (weak), 3A4 (weak)
(Continued)

Olanzapine *(Continued)*

Decreased Effect: Olanzapine levels may be decreased by CYP1A2 inducers such as rifampin, omeprazole, and carbamazepine (also cigarette smoking).

Increased Effect/Toxicity: Olanzapine levels may be increased by CYP1A2 inhibitors such as cimetidine and fluvoxamine. Sedation from olanzapine is increased with ethanol or other CNS depressants. Concomitant use with pramlintide and other anticholinergic agents may result in increased anticholinergic adverse effects. Concomitant use with ciprofloxacin may increase the levels/effects of olanzapine. Use of acetylcholinesterase inhibitors (central) or lithium may increase the risk of antipsychotic-related EPS.

Nutritional/Ethanol Interactions

Ethanol: Avoid ethanol (may increase CNS depression).

Herb/Nutraceutical: Avoid dong quai, St John's wort (may also cause photosensitization). Avoid kava kava, gotu kola, valerian, St John's wort (may increase CNS depression).

Adverse Reactions

>10%:

Central nervous system: Somnolence (6% to 39% dose-dependent), extrapyramidal symptoms (15% to 32% dose-dependent), insomnia (up to 12%), dizziness (4% to 18%)

Gastrointestinal: Dyspepsia (7% to 11%), constipation (9% to 11%), weight gain (5% to 6%, has been reported as high as 40%), xerostomia (9% to 22% dose-dependent)

Neuromuscular & skeletal: Weakness (2% to 20% dose-dependent)

Miscellaneous: Accidental injury (12%)

1% to 10%:

Cardiovascular: Postural hypotension (1% to 5%), tachycardia (up to 3%), peripheral edema (up to 3%), chest pain (up to 3%), hyper-/hypotension (up to 2%)

Central nervous system: Personality changes (8%), speech disorder (7%), fever (up to 6%), abnormal dreams, euphoria, amnesia, delusions, emotional lability, mania, schizophrenia

Dermatologic: Bruising (up to 5%)

Endocrine & metabolic: Cholesterol increased, prolactin increased

Gastrointestinal: Nausea (up to 9% dose-dependent), appetite increased (3% to 6%), vomiting (up to 4%), flatulence, salivation increased, thirst

Genitourinary: Incontinence (up to 2%), UTI (up to 2%), vaginitis

Local: Injection site pain (I.M. administration)

Neuromuscular & skeletal: Twitching, hypertonia (up to 3%), tremor (up to 7% dose-dependent), back pain (up to 5%), abnormal gait (6%), joint/extremity pain (up to 5%), akathisia (3% to 5%), articulation impairment (up to 2%), falling (particularly in older patients), joint stiffness

Ocular: Amblyopia (up to 3%), conjunctivitis

Respiratory: Rhinitis (up to 7%), cough (up to 6%), pharyngitis (up to 4%), dyspnea

Miscellaneous: Dental pain, diaphoresis, flu-like symptoms

Overdosage/Toxicology Signs and symptoms of overdose include CNS depression (ranging from drowsiness to coma), extrapyramidal movements, fasciculations, hypotension (possible, though not described), miosis, respiratory depression, rhinitis (10%), slurred speech, tachycardia, trismus, and possible NMS. Treatment is symptom-directed and supportive. Cardiac monitoring should be initiated, inclusing continuous EEG monitoring. Activated charcoal (1 g) may reduce the C_{max} and AUC of olanzapine by ~60%.

Pharmacodynamics/Kinetics

Time to Peak: Oral: ~6 hours; I.M.: 15-45 minutes

Maximum plasma concentrations after I.M. administration are 5 times higher than maximum plasma concentrations produced by an oral dose.

Protein Binding: Plasma: 93%, bound to albumin and alpha$_1$-glycoprotein

Half-Life Elimination: 21-54 hours; approximately 1.5 times greater in elderly

Metabolism: Highly metabolized via direct glucuronidation and cytochrome P450 mediated oxidation (CYP1A2, CYP2D6); 40% removed via first pass metabolism

Excretion: Urine (57%, 7% as unchanged drug); feces (30%)

Clearance: 40% increase in olanzapine clearance in smokers; 30% decrease in females

Pharmacokinetic Note Tablets and orally-disintegrating tablets are bioequivalent.

Available Dosage Forms

Injection, powder for reconstitution (Zyprexa® IntraMuscular): 10 mg [contains lactose 50 mg]

Tablet (Zyprexa®): 2.5 mg, 5 mg, 7.5 mg, 10 mg, 15 mg, 20 mg

Tablet, orally disintegrating (Zyprexa® Zydis®): 5 mg [contains phenylalanine 0.34 mg/tablet], 10 mg [contains phenylalanine 0.45 mg/tablet], 15 mg [contains phenylalanine 0.67 mg/tablet], 20 mg [contains phenylalanine 0.9 mg/tablet]

Dosing

Adults:

Schizophrenia: Initial: 5-10 mg once daily (increase to 10 mg once daily within 5-7 days); thereafter, adjust by 5 mg/day at 1-week intervals, up to a recommended maximum of 20 mg/day. Maintenance: 10-20 mg once daily. **Note:** Doses of 30-50 mg/day have been used; however, doses >10 mg/day have not demonstrated better efficacy, and safety and efficacy of doses >20 mg/day have not been evaluated.

Acute mania associated with bipolar disorder: Oral:

Monotherapy: Initial: 10-15 mg once daily; increase by 5 mg/day at intervals of not less than 24 hours. Maintenance: 5-20 mg/day; recommended maximum dose: 20 mg/day

Combination therapy (with lithium or valproate): Initial: 10 mg once daily; dosing range: 5-20 mg/day

Agitation (acute, associated with bipolar disorder or schizophrenia): I.M.: Initial dose: 5-10 mg (a lower dose of 2.5 mg may be considered when clinical factors warrant); additional doses (2.5-10 mg) may be considered; however, 2-4 hours should be allowed between doses to evaluate response (maximum total daily dose: 30 mg, per manufacturer's recommendation)

Elderly: Refer to adult dosing. Consider lower starting dose of 2.5-5 mg/day for elderly or debilitated patients; may increase as clinically indicated and tolerated with close monitoring of orthostatic blood pressure.

Pediatrics:

Schizophrenia/bipolar disorder: Oral: Initial: 2.5 mg/day; titrate as necessary to 20 mg/day (0.12-0.29 mg/kg/day)

Renal Impairment: No dosage adjustment required. Not removed by dialysis

Hepatic Impairment: Dosage adjustment may be necessary, however, there are no specific recommendations. Monitor closely.

Administration

Oral:

Tablet: May be administered with or without food/meals.

Orally-disintegrating tablet: Remove from foil blister by peeling back (do not push tablet through the foil). Place tablet in mouth immediately upon removal. Tablet dissolves rapidly in saliva and may be swallowed with or without liquid. May be administered with or without food/meals.

I.M.: Injection: For I.M. administration only; inject slowly, deep into muscle. If dizziness and/or drowsiness are noted, patient should remain recumbent until examination indicates postural hypotension and/or bradycardia are not a problem.

I.V.: Do not administer injection intravenously.

Stability

Reconstitution: Injection, powder for reconstitution: Reconstitute 10 mg vial with 2.1 mL SWFI; resulting solution is ~5 mg/mL. Use immediately (within 1 hour) following reconstitution. Discard any unused portion.

Storage:

Injection, powder for reconstitution: Store at room temperature 15°C to 30°C (59°F to 86°F). Protect from light. Do not freeze.

Tablet and orally-disintegrating tablet: Store at room temperature of 15°C to 30°C (59°F to 86°F). Protect from light and moisture.

Laboratory Monitoring Fasting lipid profile and fasting blood glucose/Hgb A_{1c} (prior to treatment, at 3 months, then annually); periodic assessment of hepatic transaminases (in patients with hepatic disease)

Nursing Actions

Physical Assessment: Assess other medications patient is taking for effectiveness and interactions (especially with drugs that alter P450 enzymes). Monitor therapeutic response (eg, mental status, mood, affect) and adverse reactions at beginning of therapy and periodically with long-term use (sedation, CNS changes, extrapyramidal symptoms, neuroleptic malignant syndrome). Monitor weight prior to initiating therapy and at least monthly. Assess knowledge/teach patient appropriate use, interventions to reduce side effects, and adverse symptoms to report.

Patient Education: Do not take any new medication during therapy unless approved by prescriber. Use exactly as directed; do not increase dose or frequency. It may take 2-3 weeks to achieve desired results; do not discontinue without consulting prescriber. Avoid alcohol or caffeine and other prescription or OTC medications not approved by prescriber. Maintain adequate hydration (2-3 L/day of fluids) unless instructed to restrict fluid intake. If diabetic, you may experience increased blood sugars. Monitor blood sugars closely. If you have glaucoma, periodic ophthalmic exams are recommended. You may experience excess drowsiness, restlessness, weakness, dizziness, or blurred vision (use caution driving or when engaging in tasks requiring alertness until response to drug is known); constipation (increased exercise, fluids, fruit, or fiber may help); heartburn; dry mouth; or weight gain. Report persistent CNS effects (eg, trembling fingers, altered gait or balance, excessive sedation, seizures, unusual movements, anxiety, abnormal thoughts, confusion, personality changes); unresolved constipation or GI effects; vision changes; respiratory difficulty; unusual cough or flu-like symptoms; or worsening of condition. **Pregnancy/breast-feeding precautions:** Inform prescriber if you are or intend to become pregnant. Breast-feeding is not recommended.

Orally-disintegrating tablet: Remove from foil blister by peeling back (do not push tablet through the foil). Place tablet in mouth immediately upon removal. Tablet dissolves rapidly in saliva and may be swallowed with or without liquid.

Dietary Considerations Tablets may be taken with or without food/meals. Zyprexa® Zydis®: 5 mg tablet contains phenylalanine 0.34 mg; 10 mg tablet contains

phenylalanine 0.45 mg; 15 mg tablet contains phenylalanine 0.67 mg; 20 mg tablet contains phenylalanine 0.9 mg

Geriatric Considerations Elderly patients have an increased risk of adverse response to side effects or adverse reactions to antipsychotics. A higher incidence of falls has been reported in elderly patients, particularly in debilitated patients. Olanzapine half-life that was 1.5 times that of younger (<65 years of age) adults; therefore, lower initial doses are recommended.

Breast-Feeding Issues At steady-state concentrations, it is estimated that a breast-fed infant may be exposed to ~2% of the maternal dose.

Pregnancy Issues No evidence of teratogenicity reported in animal studies. However, fetal toxicity and prolonged gestation have been observed. There are no adequate and well-controlled studies in pregnant women.

Related Information
Antipsychotic Medication Guidelines *on page 1415*

Olanzapine and Fluoxetine
(oh LAN za peen & floo OKS e teen)

U.S. Brand Names Symbyax™

Synonyms Fluoxetine and Olanzapine; Olanzapine and Fluoxetine Hydrochloride

Restrictions A medication guide concerning the use of antidepressants in children and teenagers can be found on the FDA website at http://www.fda.gov/cder/Offices/ODS/labeling.htm. It should be dispensed to parents or guardians of children and teenagers receiving this medication.

Pharmacologic Category Antidepressant, Selective Serotonin Reuptake Inhibitor; Antipsychotic Agent, Atypical

Pregnancy Risk Factor C

Lactation Enters breast milk/not recommended

Use Treatment of depressive episodes associated with bipolar disorder

Available Dosage Forms Capsule:
6/25: Olanzapine 6 mg and fluoxetine 25 mg
6/50: Olanzapine 6 mg and fluoxetine 50 mg
12/25: Olanzapine 12 mg and fluoxetine 25 mg
12/50: Olanzapine 12 mg and fluoxetine 50 mg

Dosing

Adults: Depression associated with bipolar disorder: Oral: Initial: Olanzapine 6 mg/fluoxetine 25 mg once daily in the evening. Dosing range: Olanzapine 6-12 mg/fluoxetine 25-50 mg. Use caution adjusting dose in patients predisposed to hypotension, in females, and in nonsmokers (metabolism may be decreased). Safety of daily doses of olanzapine >18 mg/fluoxetine >75 mg have not been evaluated.

Elderly: Oral: Initial: Olanzapine 6 mg/fluoxetine 25 mg once daily in the evening; use caution adjusting dose (metabolism may be decreased). Safety and efficacy have not been established in patients >65 years of age.

Hepatic Impairment: Initial: Olanzapine 6 mg/fluoxetine 25 mg once daily in the evening; use caution adjusting dose (metabolism may be decreased).

Nursing Actions
Physical Assessment: See individual agents.
Patient Education: See individual agents. **Pregnancy/breast-feeding precautions:** Inform prescriber if you are pregnant. Breast-feeding is not recommended.

Related Information
Fluoxetine *on page 531*
Olanzapine *on page 905*

Olmesartan (ole me SAR tan)

U.S. Brand Names Benicar®

Synonyms Olmesartan Medoxomil

Pharmacologic Category Angiotensin II Receptor Blocker

Pregnancy Risk Factor C/D (2nd and 3rd trimesters)

Lactation Excretion in breast milk unknown/contraindicated

Use Treatment of hypertension with or without concurrent use of other antihypertensive agents

Mechanism of Action/Effect As a selective and competitive, nonpeptide angiotensin II receptor antagonist, olmesartan blocks the vasoconstrictor and aldosterone-secreting effects of angiotensin II. Olmesartan increases urinary flow rate and in addition to being natriuretic and kaliuretic, increases excretion of chloride, magnesium, uric acid, calcium, and phosphate.

Contraindications Hypersensitivity to olmesartan or any component of the formulation; hypersensitivity to other A-II receptor antagonists; bilateral renal artery stenosis; pregnancy (2nd and 3rd trimesters)

Warnings/Precautions Avoid use or use a smaller dose in patients who are volume depleted; correct depletion first. Deterioration in renal function can occur with initiation. Use with caution in unilateral renal artery stenosis and pre-existing renal insufficiency; significant aortic/mitral stenosis. Safety and efficacy in pediatric patients have not been established.

Drug Interactions

Decreased Effect: NSAIDs may decrease the efficacy of olmesartan.

Increased Effect/Toxicity: The risk of hyperkalemia may be increased during concomitant use with potassium-sparing diuretics, potassium supplements, and trimethoprim; may increase risk of lithium toxicity.

Nutritional/Ethanol Interactions

Food: Does not affect olmesartan bioavailability.

Herb/Nutraceutical: Avoid ephedra, yohimbe, ginseng (may worsen hypertension). Avoid garlic (may have increased antihypertensive effect).

Adverse Reactions 1% to 10%:

Central nervous system: Dizziness (3%), headache

Endocrine & metabolic: Hyperglycemia, hypertriglyceridemia

Gastrointestinal: Diarrhea

Neuromuscular & skeletal: Back pain, CPK increased

Renal: Hematuria

Respiratory: Bronchitis, pharyngitis, rhinitis, sinusitis

Miscellaneous: Flu-like syndrome

Overdosage/Toxicology Hypotension and tachycardia may occur with significant overdose. Bradycardia is possible if vagal stimulation occurs. Treatment should be supportive.

Pharmacodynamics/Kinetics

Time to Peak: 1-2 hours

Protein Binding: 99%

Half-Life Elimination: Terminal: 13 hours

Metabolism: Olmesartan medoxomil is hydrolyzed in the GI tract to active olmesartan. No further metabolism occurs.

Excretion: All as unchanged drug: Feces (50% to 65%); urine (35% to 50%)

Available Dosage Forms Tablet, as medoxomil: 5 mg, 20 mg, 40 mg

Dosing

Adults: Antihypertensive: Oral: Initial: Usual starting dose is 20 mg once daily; if initial response is inadequate, may be increased to 40 mg once daily after 2 weeks. May administer with other antihypertensive agents if blood pressure inadequately controlled with olmesartan. Consider lower starting dose in patients with possible depletion of intravascular volume (eg, patients receiving diuretics).

Elderly: Initial: May start at 5-10 mg/day (due to concomitant disease or age changes).

Renal Impairment: No specific guidelines for dosage adjustment; patients undergoing hemodialysis have not been studied.

Hepatic Impairment: No adjustment necessary.

Administration

Oral: May be administered with or without food.

Stability

Storage: Store at 20°C to 25°C (68°F to 77°F).

Nursing Actions

Physical Assessment: Assess potential for interactions with other pharmacological agents and herbal products patient may be taking. Monitor therapeutic effectiveness (blood pressure) and adverse response (eg, tachycardia, hypotension, diarrhea, bronchitis) on a regular basis throughout therapy. Instruct patients with diabetes to monitor glucose levels closely (may cause hyperglycemia). Teach patient proper use, possible side effects/appropriate interventions, and adverse symptoms to report.

Patient Education: Do not take any new medication during therapy unless approved by prescriber. Do not use potassium supplement or salt substitutes without consulting prescriber. Take exactly as directed. Do not alter dose or discontinue without consulting prescriber. May be taken with or without food. This drug does not eliminate the need for diet or exercise regimen as recommended by prescriber. If you have diabetes, check glucose levels closely (drug may alter glucose levels). May cause headache or dizziness (use caution when driving or engaging in tasks that require alertness until response to drug is known); diarrhea (boiled milk, buttermilk, or yogurt may help); or back or joint pain (consult prescriber for approved analgesic). Report chest pain or palpitations; unrelieved headache; flu-like symptoms or upper respiratory infection; or other persistent adverse reactions. **Pregnancy/breast-feeding precautions:** Inform prescriber if you are or intend to become pregnant. This drug should not be used in the 2nd or 3rd trimester of pregnancy. Consult prescriber for appropriate contraceptive measures if necessary. Do not breast-feed.

Dietary Considerations May be taken with or without food.

Pregnancy Issues The drug should be discontinued as soon as possible when pregnancy is detected. Drugs which act directly on renin-angiotensin can cause fetal and neonatal morbidity and death.

Olmesartan and Hydrochlorothiazide (ole me SAR tan & hye droe klor oh THYE a zide)

U.S. Brand Names Benicar HCT®

Synonyms Hydrochlorothiazide and Olmesartan Medoxomil; Olmesartan Medoxomil and Hydrochlorothiazide

Pharmacologic Category Angiotensin II Receptor Blocker Combination; Antihypertensive Agent, Combination; Diuretic, Thiazide

Pregnancy Risk Factor C/D (2nd and 3rd trimesters)

Lactation Excretion in breast milk unknown/contraindicated

Use Treatment of hypertension (not recommended for initial treatment)

Available Dosage Forms Tablet:

20/12.5: Olmesartan medoxomil 20 mg and hydrochlorothiazide 12.5 mg

40/12.5: Olmesartan medoxomil 40 mg and hydrochlorothiazide 12.5 mg

40/25: Olmesartan medoxomil 40 mg and hydrochlorothiazide 25 mg

Dosing

Adults & Elderly:

Hypertension: Oral: Dosage must be individualized; may be titrated at 2- to 4-week intervals.

Replacement therapy: May be substituted for titrated components.

Patients not controlled with single-agent therapy: Initiate by adding the lowest available dose of the alternative component (hydrochlorothiazide 12.5 mg or olmesartan 20 mg). Titrate to effect (maximum hydrochlorothiazide dose: 25 mg, maximum olmesartan dose: 40 mg).

Renal Impairment: Not recommended in patients with Cl$_{cr}$ <30 mL/minute.

Nursing Actions

Physical Assessment: See individual agents.

Patient Education: See individual agents. **Pregnancy/breast-feeding precautions:** Inform prescriber if you are or intend to become pregnant. Do not breast-feed.

Related Information

Hydrochlorothiazide *on page 610*
Olmesartan *on page 908*

Olopatadine (oh loe pa TA deen)

U.S. Brand Names Patanol®

Pharmacologic Category Antihistamine; Ophthalmic Agent, Miscellaneous

Medication Safety Issues

Sound-alike/look-alike issues:

Patanol® may be confused with Platinol®

Pregnancy Risk Factor C

Use Treatment of the signs and symptoms of allergic conjunctivitis

Contraindications Hypersensitivity to olopatadine hydrochloride or any component of the formulation

Warnings/Precautions Contains benzalkonium chloride which may be absorbed by contact lenses; do not wear contact lenses if eyes are red. Safety and efficacy in children <3 years of age have not been established.

Adverse Reactions

>5%: Central nervous system: Headache (7%)

<5%:

Central nervous system: Cold syndrome

Gastrointestinal: Nausea, taste perversion

Neuromuscular & skeletal: Weakness

Ocular: Blurred vision, burning, stinging, dry eyes, foreign body sensation, hyperemia, keratitis, eyelid edema, itching

Respiratory: Pharyngitis, rhinitis, sinusitis

Pharmacodynamics/Kinetics

Half-Life Elimination: ~3 hours

Excretion: Urine (60% to 70%)

Available Dosage Forms Solution, ophthalmic: 0.1% (5 mL) [contains benzalkonium chloride]

Dosing

Adults & Elderly: Allergic conjunctivitis: Ophthalmic: Instill 1 to 2 drops into affected eye(s) twice daily (allowing 6-8 hours between doses); results from an environmental study demonstrated that olopatadine was effective when dosed twice daily for up to 6 weeks

Administration

Other: After instilling drops, wait at least 10 minutes before inserting contact lenses. Do not insert contacts if eyes are red.

Nursing Actions

Physical Assessment: Monitor patient response and adverse effects. Teach patient proper use, side effects/appropriate interventions, and symptoms to report.

Patient Education: For use in eyes only. Do not let tip of applicator touch eye; do not contaminate tip of applicator (may cause eye infection, eye damage, or vision loss). **Pregnancy precaution:** Inform prescriber if you are pregnant.

Olsalazine (ole SAL a zeen)

U.S. Brand Names Dipentum®

Synonyms Olsalazine Sodium

Pharmacologic Category 5-Aminosalicylic Acid Derivative

Medication Safety Issues

Sound-alike/look-alike issues:

Olsalazine may be confused with olanzapine

Dipentum® may be confused with Dilantin®

Pregnancy Risk Factor C

Lactation Enters breast milk/use caution (monitor for diarrhea)

Use Maintenance of remission of ulcerative colitis in patients intolerant to sulfasalazine

Mechanism of Action/Effect The mechanism of action appears to be localized in the colon rather than systemic

Contraindications Hypersensitivity to olsalazine, salicylates, or any component of the formulation

Warnings/Precautions Diarrhea is a common adverse effect of olsalazine. Use with caution in patients with hypersensitivity to salicylates, sulfasalazine, or mesalamine.

Drug Interactions

Increased Effect/Toxicity: Olsalazine has been reported to increase the prothrombin time in patients taking warfarin. Olsalazine may increase the risk of myelosuppression with azathioprine, mesalamine, or sulfasalazine.

Lab Interactions Increased ALT, AST (S)

Adverse Reactions

>10%: Gastrointestinal: Diarrhea, cramps, abdominal pain

1% to 10%:

Central nervous system: Headache, fatigue, depression

Dermatologic: Rash, itching

Gastrointestinal: Nausea, heartburn, bloating, anorexia

Neuromuscular & skeletal: Arthralgia

Overdosage/Toxicology Symptoms of overdose include decreased motor activity and diarrhea. Treatment is supportive.

Pharmacodynamics/Kinetics

Time to Peak: ~1 hour

Protein Binding: Plasma: >99%

Half-Life Elimination: 56 minutes

Metabolism: Primarily via colonic bacteria to active drug, 5-aminosalicylic acid

Excretion: Primarily feces

Available Dosage Forms Capsule, as sodium: 250 mg

Dosing

Adults & Elderly: Ulcerative colitis: Oral: 1 g/day in 2 divided doses

Administration

Oral: Take with food in evenly divided doses.

Nursing Actions

Physical Assessment: Assess allergy history before initiating therapy (salicylates, sulfasalazine, or mesalamine). Monitor effectiveness (reduction of clinical signs of ulcerative colitis) and adverse effects (eg, diarrhea). Teach patient proper use, possible side effects/appropriate interventions, and adverse symptoms to report.

Patient Education: Do not take any other medication during therapy unless approved by prescriber. Take as directed, with meals, in evenly divided doses. May
(Continued)

Olsalazine (Continued)

cause flu-like symptoms or muscle pain (consult prescriber for approved analgesic); diarrhea (buttermilk, boiled milk, or yogurt may help); or nausea or loss of appetite (small, frequent meals, frequent mouth care, sucking lozenges, or chewing gum may help). Report persistent diarrhea or abdominal cramping, skin rash or itching, or other adverse reactions. **Pregnancy/breast-feeding precautions:** Inform prescriber if you are or intend to become pregnant. Consult prescriber if breast-feeding.

Dietary Considerations Administer with food, increases residence of drug in body.

Geriatric Considerations No specific data is available on elderly to suggest the drug needs alterations in dose. Since so little is absorbed, dosing should not be changed for reasons of age. Diarrhea may pose a serious problem for elderly in that it may cause dehydration, electrolyte imbalance, hypotension, and confusion.

Omalizumab (oh mah lye ZOO mab)

U.S. Brand Names Xolair®

Synonyms rhuMAb-E25

Pharmacologic Category Monoclonal Antibody, Anti-Asthmatic

Pregnancy Risk Factor B

Lactation Excretion in breast milk unknown/use caution

Use Treatment of moderate-to-severe, persistent allergic asthma not adequately controlled with inhaled corticosteroids

Mechanism of Action/Effect Blocks the binding of IgE to mast cells and basophils, decreasing the allergic response, corticosteroid usage, and asthma exacerbations.

Contraindications Hypersensitivity to omalizumab or any component of the formulation; acute bronchospasm, status asthmaticus

Warnings/Precautions For use in patients with a documented reactivity to a perennial aeroallergen and with symptoms uncontrolled using inhaled corticosteroids; not used to control acute asthma symptoms. Dosing is based on pretreatment IgE serum levels and body weight. IgE levels remain elevated up to 1 year following treatment, therefore, levels taken during treatment can not be used as a dosage guide. Corticosteroid therapy should be tapered gradually, do not discontinue abruptly. Anaphylactic reactions have been reported within 2 hours of initial dose; appropriate medications for the treatment of hypersensitivity reactions should be available. Malignant neoplasm have been reported with use (<1%) in short-term studies; impact of long-term use is not known. Safety and efficacy in children <12 years of age have not been established.

Lab Interactions Total IgE levels are elevated for up to 1 year following treatment. Total serum IgE may be retested after interruption of therapy for 1 year or more.

Adverse Reactions

>10%:
Central nervous system: Headache (15%)
Local: Injection site reaction (45%; placebo 43%), severe injection site reactions (12%; placebo 9%). Most reactions occurred within 1 hour, lasted <8 days, and decreased in frequency with additional dosing.
Respiratory: Upper respiratory tract infection (23%), sinusitis (16%), pharyngitis (11%)
Miscellaneous: Viral infection (23%)

1% to 10%:
Central nervous system: Pain (7%), fatigue (3%), dizziness (3%)
Dermatologic: Dermatitis (2%), pruritus (2%)

Neuromuscular & skeletal: Arthralgia (8%), leg pain (4%), arm pain (2%), fracture (2%)
Otic: Earache (2%)

Overdosage/Toxicology Limited data; single doses up to 4000 mg and cumulative doses up to 44,000 mg (over 20 weeks) have not been associated with toxicity.

Pharmacodynamics/Kinetics
Time to Peak: 7-8 days
Half-Life Elimination: 26 days
Metabolism: Hepatic; IgG degradation by reticuloendothelial system and endothelial cells
Excretion: Primarily via hepatic degradation; intact IgG may be secreted in bile

Available Dosage Forms Injection, powder for reconstitution [preservative free]: 150 mg [contains sucrose 145.5 g]

Dosing
Adults & Elderly: Asthma: SubQ: Dose is based on pretreatment IgE serum levels and body weight. Dosing should not be adjusted based on IgE levels taken during treatment or <1 year following therapy; doses should be adjusted during treatment for significant changes in body weight
IgE ≥30-100 int. units/mL:
30-90 kg: 150 mg every 4 weeks
>90-150 kg: 300 mg every 4 weeks
IgE >100-200 int. units/mL:
30-90 kg: 300 mg every 4 weeks
>90-150 kg: 225 mg every 2 weeks
IgE >200-300 int. units/mL:
30-60 kg: 300 mg every 4 weeks
>60-90 kg: 225 mg every 2 weeks
>90-150 kg: 300 mg every 2 weeks
IgE >300-400 int. units/mL:
30-70 kg: 225 mg every 2 weeks
>70-90 kg: 300 mg every 2 weeks
>90 kg: Do not administer dose
IgE >400-500 int. units/mL:
30-70 kg: 300 mg every 2 weeks
>70-90 kg: 375 mg every 2 weeks
>90 kg: Do not administer dose
IgE >500-600 int. units/mL:
30-60 kg: 300 mg every 2 weeks
>60-70 kg: 375 mg every 2 weeks
>70 kg: Do not administer dose
IgE >600-700 int. units/mL:
30-60 kg: 375 mg every 2 weeks
>60 kg: Do not administer dose

Pediatrics: Asthma: Children ≥12 years: SubQ: Refer to adult dosing.

Administration
Other: For SubQ injection only; doses >150 mg should divided over more than one site. Injections may take 5-10 seconds to administer.

Stability
Reconstitution: Prepare using SWFI, USP only; add to upright vial and swirl gently for 5-10 seconds every 5 minutes until dissolved, may take >20 minutes to dissolve completely. Do not use if powder takes >40 minutes to dissolve.
Storage: Prior to reconstitution, store under refrigeration at 2°C to 8°C (36°F to 46°F); product may be shipped at room temperature. Following reconstitution, protect from direct sunlight. May be stored for up to 8 hours if refrigerated or 4 hours if stored at room temperature.

Laboratory Monitoring Baseline IgE; FEV_1, peak flow, and/or other pulmonary function tests

Nursing Actions
Physical Assessment: For SubQ use only. Monitor laboratory tests and pulmonary function at baseline and as necessary with treatment. Anaphylactic reactions have been reported within 2 hours of initial dose; appropriate medications for the treatment of hypersensitivity reactions should be available. Monitor patient response (relief of asthmatic symptoms) and

adverse reactions (eg, hypersensitivity reaction, upper respiratory tract infection, viral infection, dermatitis, arthralgia) at beginning and periodically during therapy. Teach patient proper use if self-administered (storage, reconstitution, administration, needle/ syringe disposal), possible side effects/interventions, and adverse symptoms to report.

Patient Education: If self-administered, follow exact directions for storage, reconstitution, administration, and needle/syringe disposal. Report immediately any reaction at injection site (eg, redness, swelling, itching) or signs of allergic response (eg, chest pain, respiratory difficulty, skin rash). May cause headache or dizziness (use caution when driving or engaging in hazardous tasks until response to drug is known); or joint or bone pain, earache (consult prescriber for analgesic). Report unusual or increased respiratory difficulty, signs of infection, or skin rash. **Pregnancy/ breast-feeding precautions:** Inform prescriber if you are or intend to become pregnant. Consult prescriber if you are breast-feeding.

Breast-Feeding Issues IgG is excreted in human milk and excretion of omalizumab is expected. Effects to nursing infant are not known; use with caution.

Omega-3-Acid Ethyl Esters

(oh MEG a three AS id ETH il ES ters)

U.S. Brand Names Omacor®
Synonyms Ethyl Esters of Omega-3 Fatty Acids; Fish Oil
Pharmacologic Category Antilipemic Agent, Miscellaneous
Medication Safety Issues
Sound-alike/look-alike issues:
Omacor® may be confused with Amicar®

Pregnancy Risk Factor C
Lactation Excretion in breast milk unknown/use caution
Use Omacor®: Treatment of hypertriglyceridemia (≥500 mg/dL)

Note: A number of OTC formulations containing omega-3 fatty acids are marketed as nutritional supplements; these do not have FDA-approved indications.

Unlabeled/Investigational Use Omacor®: Treatment of IgA nephropathy

Mechanism of Action/Effect Lowers serum triglycerides; possibly by increased metabolism or decreased synthesis of triglycerides

Contraindications Hypersensitivity to omega-3-acid ethyl esters or any component of the formulation

Warnings/Precautions Use with caution in patients with known allergy to fish. Should be used as an adjunct to diet and exercise only in those with very high triglyceride levels. Treatment of primary metabolic disorders (eg, diabetes, thyroid disease) and/or evaluation of the patient's medication regimen for possible etiologic agents should be completed prior to a decision to initiate therapy. If triglyceride levels do not adequately respond after 2 months of treatment with omega-3-acid ethyl esters, discontinue treatment. Prolongation of bleeding time has been observed in some clinical studies. Use caution in patients with coagulopathy or in those receiving therapeutic anticoagulation. Safety and efficacy have not been established in children (<18 years of age).

Drug Interactions
Decreased Effect: Beta-blockers, estrogens, and thiazide diuretics may decrease the therapeutic effect of omega-3-acid ethyl esters.

Increased Effect/Toxicity: Omega-3-acid ethyl esters may prolong bleeding time; effect of concurrent anticoagulant therapy or concurrent medications which may alter platelet function has not been evaluated. Thiazide diuretics may increase serum triglycerides. Omega-3-acid ethyl esters may augment the antihypertensive effect of beta blockers and thiazide diuretics.

Nutritional/Ethanol Interactions
Ethanol: Monitor ethanol use (alcohol use may increase triglycerides).

Adverse Reactions
Cardiovascular: Angina (1%)
Central nervous system: Pain (2%)
Dermatologic: Rash (2%)
Gastrointestinal: Eructation (5%), dyspepsia (3%), taste perversion (3%)
Neuromuscular and skeletal: Back pain (2%)
Miscellaneous: Flu-like syndrome (4%), infection (4%)

Available Dosage Forms Capsule: 1 g [contains EPA ~465 mg and DHA ~375 mg]

Dosing
Adults & Elderly:
Hypertriglyceridemia: Oral: 4 g/day as a single daily dose or in 2 divided doses.
Treatment of IgA nephropathy (unlabeled use): Oral: 4 g/day

Renal Impairment: No dosage adjustment required.

Administration
Oral: May be administered with meals.

Stability
Storage: Store at 25°C (77°F); excursions permitted to 15°C to 30°C (59°F to 86°F). Do not freeze.

Laboratory Monitoring Triglycerides and other lipids (LDL-C) should be monitored at baseline and periodically. Hepatic transaminase levels, particularly ALT, should be monitored periodically.

Nursing Actions
Physical Assessment: Do not use if allergic to fish. Encourage diet and exercise along with use of this medication.

Patient Education: Do not use if allergic to fish. This medication should be used in addition to diet and exercise. Avoid alcohol use. You may experience flu-like syndrome, fever, burping, or an "upset stomach". Report any significant or continued problems to prescriber. **Pregnancy/breast-feeding precautions:** Inform prescriber if you are or intend to become pregnant. Consult prescriber before breast-feeding.

Dietary Considerations May be taken with meals. Dietary modification is important in the control of severe hypertriglyceridemia. Maintain dietary restrictions during therapy.

Geriatric Considerations Specific information about the safety and efficacy of omega-3-acid ethyl esters is limited. The manufacturer states there were no apparent differences between persons <60 and >60 years of age.

Omeprazole (oh ME pray zol)

U.S. Brand Names Prilosec®; Prilosec OTC™ [OTC]
Pharmacologic Category Proton Pump Inhibitor; Substituted Benzimidazole
Medication Safety Issues
Sound-alike/look-alike issues:
Prilosec® may be confused with Plendil®, Prevacid®, predniSONE, prilocaine, Prinivil®, Proventil®, Prozac®

Pregnancy Risk Factor C
Lactation Enters breast milk/not recommended
Use Short-term (4-8 weeks) treatment of active duodenal ulcer disease or active benign gastric ulcer; treatment of heartburn and other symptoms associated with gastroesophageal reflux disease (GERD); short-term (4-8 weeks) treatment of endoscopically-diagnosed erosive
(Continued)

Omeprazole *(Continued)*

esophagitis; maintenance healing of erosive esophagitis; long-term treatment of pathological hypersecretory conditions; as part of a multidrug regimen for *H. pylori* eradication to reduce the risk of duodenal ulcer recurrence

OTC labeling: Short-term treatment of frequent, uncomplicated heartburn occurring ≥2 days/week

Unlabeled/Investigational Use Healing NSAID-induced ulcers; prevention of NSAID-induced ulcers

Mechanism of Action/Effect Suppresses gastric basal and stimulated acid secretion by inhibiting the parietal cell H+/K+ ATP pump

Contraindications Hypersensitivity to omeprazole, substituted benzimidazoles (ie, esomeprazole, lansoprazole, pantoprazole, rabeprazole), or any component of the formulation

Warnings/Precautions In long-term (2-year) studies in rats, omeprazole produced a dose-related increase in gastric carcinoid tumors. While available endoscopic evaluations and histologic examinations of biopsy specimens from human stomachs have not detected a risk from short-term exposure to omeprazole, further human data on the effect of sustained hypochlorhydria and hypergastrinemia is needed to rule out the possibility of an increased risk for the development of tumors in humans receiving long-term therapy. Bioavailability may be increased in the elderly, Asian population, and with hepatic dysfunction. Safety and efficacy have not been established in children <2 years of age. When used for self-medication (OTC), do not use for >14 days; treatment should not be repeated more than once every 4 months; OTC and oral suspension are not approved for use in children <18 years of age

Drug Interactions

Cytochrome P450 Effect: Substrate of CYP2A6 (minor), 2C9 (minor), 2C19 (major), 2D6 (minor), 3A4 (minor); **Inhibits** CYP1A2 (weak), 2C9 (moderate), 2C19 (strong), 2D6 (weak), 3A4 (weak); **Induces** CYP1A2 (weak)

Decreased Effect: Proton pump inhibitors may decrease the absorption of atazanavir, indinavir, itraconazole, and ketoconazole. The levels/effects of omeprazole may be decreased by aminoglutethimide, carbamazepine, phenytoin, rifampin, and other CYP2C19 inducers. Omeprazole may alter the concentrations/effects of clozapine.

Increased Effect/Toxicity: Esomeprazole and omeprazole may increase the levels of benzodiazepines metabolized by oxidation (eg, diazepam, midazolam, triazolam), methotrexate, and carbamazepine. Elimination of phenytoin or warfarin may be prolonged when used concomitantly with omeprazole. Omeprazole may increase the levels/effects of amiodarone, citalopram, diazepam, fluoxetine, glimepiride, glipizide, methsuximide, nateglinide, phenytoin, pioglitazone, propranolol, rosiglitazone, sertraline, warfarin, and other CYP2C9 or 2C19 substrates. Omeprazole may alter the concentrations/effects of clozapine.

Nutritional/Ethanol Interactions

Ethanol: Avoid ethanol (may cause gastric mucosal irritation).

Food: Food delays absorption.

Herb/Nutraceutical: St John's wort may decrease omeprazole levels.

Adverse Reactions 1% to 10%:

Central nervous system: Headache (3% to 7%), dizziness (2%)

Dermatologic: Rash (2%)

Gastrointestinal: Diarrhea (3% to 4%), abdominal pain (2% to 5 %), nausea (2% to 4%), vomiting (2% to 3%), flatulence (3%), acid regurgitation (2%), constipation (1% to 2%), taste perversion

Neuromuscular & skeletal: Weakness (1%), back pain (1%)

Respiratory: Upper respiratory infection (2%), cough (1%)

Overdosage/Toxicology Limited experience with overdose in humans. Doses up to 2400 mg have been reported. Symptoms include confusion, drowsiness, blurred vision, tachycardia, nausea, flushing, diaphoresis, headache, and dry mouth. Treatment is symptom-directed and supportive. Not dialyzable.

Pharmacodynamics/Kinetics

Onset of Action: Antisecretory: ~1 hour; Peak effect: 2 hours

Duration of Action: 72 hours

Protein Binding: 95%

Half-Life Elimination: Delayed release capsule: 0.5-1 hour

Metabolism: Extensively hepatic to inactive metabolites

Excretion: Urine (77% as metabolites, very small amount as unchanged drug); feces

Available Dosage Forms

Capsule, delayed release: 10 mg, 20 mg
Prilosec®: 10 mg, 20 mg, 40 mg

Tablet, delayed release:
Prilosec OTC™: 20 mg

Dosing

Adults & Elderly:

Active duodenal ulcer: Oral: 20 mg/day for 4-8 weeks

Gastric ulcers: Oral: 40 mg/day for 4-8 weeks

Symptomatic GERD: Oral: 20 mg/day for up to 4 weeks

Erosive esophagitis: Oral: 20 mg/day for 4-8 weeks; maintenance of healing: 20 mg/day for up to 12 months total therapy (including treatment period of 4-8 weeks)

Peptic ulcer disease: Eradication of *Helicobacter pylori*: Oral: Dose varies with regimen: 20 mg once daily **or** 40 mg/day as single dose or in 2 divided doses; requires combination therapy with antibiotics

Pathological hypersecretory conditions: Oral: Initial: 60 mg once daily; doses up to 120 mg 3 times/day have been administered; administer daily doses >80 mg in divided doses

Frequent heartburn (OTC labeling): Oral: 20 mg/day for 14 days; treatment may be repeated after 4 months if needed

Pediatrics:

GERD or other acid-related disorders: Oral: Children ≥2 years:
<20 kg: 10 mg once daily
≥20 kg: 20 mg once daily

Renal Impairment: No adjustment is necessary.

Hepatic Impairment: Specific guidelines are not available; bioavailability is increased with chronic liver disease.

Administration

Oral:

Capsule: Should be swallowed whole; do not chew or crush. Best if taken before breakfast. Delayed release capsule may be opened and contents added to applesauce. Administration via NG tube should be in an acidic juice.

Tablet: Should be swallowed whole; do not crush or chew.

Stability

Storage: Store at 15°C to 30°C (59°F to 86°F).

Nursing Actions

Physical Assessment: Assess other medications patient may be taking for effectiveness and interactions (especially those dependent on cytochrome P450 metabolism or those dependent on a acid environment for absorption). Monitor effectiveness of therapeutic response and adverse reactions at beginning of therapy and periodically throughout therapy.

Assess knowledge/teach appropriate use of this medication, interventions to reduce side effects, and adverse symptoms to report.

Patient Education: Take as directed, before eating. Do not crush or chew capsules. Delayed release capsule may be opened and contents added to applesauce. Avoid alcohol. You may experience anorexia; small frequent meals may help to maintain adequate nutrition. Report changes in urination or pain on urination, unresolved severe diarrhea, testicular pain, or changes in respiratory status. **Pregnancy/breast-feeding precautions:** Inform prescriber if you are or intend to become pregnant. Breast-feeding is not recommended.

Dietary Considerations Should be taken on an empty stomach; best if taken before breakfast.

Geriatric Considerations The incidence of side effects in the elderly is no different than that of younger adults (≤65 years) despite slight decrease in elimination and increase in bioavailability. Bioavailability may be increased in the elderly (≥65 years of age), however, dosage adjustments are not necessary.

Pregnancy Issues Crosses the placenta; congenital abnormalities have been reported sporadically following omeprazole use during pregnancy. Based on data collected by the Teratogen Information System (TERIS), it was concluded that therapeutic doses used during pregnancy would be unlikely to pose a substantial teratogenic risk (quantity/quality of data: fair). Because the possibility of harm still exists, the manufacturer recommends use during pregnancy only if the potential benefit to the mother outweighs the possible risk to the fetus.

Ondansetron (on DAN se tron)

U.S. Brand Names Zofran®; Zofran® ODT

Synonyms GR38032R; Ondansetron Hydrochloride

Pharmacologic Category Antiemetic; Selective 5-HT$_3$ Receptor Antagonist

Medication Safety Issues
Sound-alike/look-alike issues:
Ondansetron may be confused with dolasetron, granisetron, palonosetron
Zofran® may be confused with Zantac®, Zosyn®

Pregnancy Risk Factor B

Lactation Excretion in breast milk unknown/use caution

Use Prevention of nausea and vomiting associated with moderately- to highly-emetogenic cancer chemotherapy [not recommended for treatment of **existing** chemotherapy-induced emesis (CIE)]; radiotherapy in patients receiving total body irradiation or fractions to the abdomen; prevention of postoperative nausea and vomiting (PONV); treatment of PONV if no prophylactic dose received

Unlabeled/Investigational Use Treatment of early-onset alcoholism; hyperemesis gravidarum

Mechanism of Action/Effect Selective 5-HT$_3$ receptor antagonist, blocking serotonin, both peripherally on vagal nerve terminals and centrally in the chemoreceptor trigger zone

Contraindications Hypersensitivity to ondansetron, other selective 5-HT$_3$ antagonists, or any component of the formulation

Warnings/Precautions Ondansetron should be used on a scheduled basis, not on an "as needed" (PRN) basis, since data support the use of this drug only in the prevention of nausea and vomiting (due to antineoplastic therapy) and not in the rescue of nausea and vomiting. Ondansetron should only be used in the first 24-48 hours of chemotherapy. Data do not support any increased efficacy of ondansetron in delayed nausea and vomiting. Does not stimulate gastric or intestinal peristalsis; may mask progressive ileus and/or gastric

distension. Orally-disintegrating tablets contain phenylalanine. Safety and efficacy for children <1 month of age have not been established.

Drug Interactions

Cytochrome P450 Effect: Substrate of CYP1A2 (minor), 2C8/9 (minor), 2D6 (minor), 2E1 (minor), 3A4 (major); **Inhibits** CYP1A2 (weak), 2C8/9 (weak), 2D6 (weak)

Decreased Effect: CYP3A4 inducers may decrease the levels/effects of ondansetron; example inducers include aminoglutethimide, carbamazepine, nafcillin, nevirapine, phenobarbital, phenytoin, and rifamycins. The manufacturer does not recommend dosage adjustment in patients receiving CYP3A4 inducers.

Increased Effect/Toxicity: Ondansetron may enhance the hypotensive effect of apomorphine; concurrent use is contraindicated.

Nutritional/Ethanol Interactions
Food: Food increases the extent of absorption. The C_{max} and T_{max} do not change much.
Herb/Nutraceutical: St John's wort may decrease ondansetron levels.

Adverse Reactions
Note: Percentages reported in adult patients.
>10%:
Central nervous system: Headache (9% to 27%), malaise/fatigue (9% to 13%)
Gastrointestinal: Constipation (6% to 11%)
1% to 10%:
Central nervous system: Drowsiness (8%), fever (2% to 8%), dizziness (4% to 7%), anxiety (6%), cold sensation (2%)
Dermatologic: Pruritus (2% to 5%), rash (1%)
Gastrointestinal: Diarrhea (2% to 7%)
Genitourinary: Gynecological disorder (7%), urinary retention (5%)
Hepatic: ALT/AST increased (1% to 5%)
Local: Injection site reaction (4%; pain, redness, burning)
Neuromuscular & skeletal: Paresthesia (2%)
Respiratory: Hypoxia (9%)

Overdosage/Toxicology Sudden transient blindness, severe constipation, hypotension, and vasovagal episode with transient secondary heart block have been reported in some cases of overdose. I.V. doses of up to 252 mg/day have been inadvertently given without adverse effects. There is no specific antidote. Treatment is symptom-directed and supportive.

Pharmacodynamics/Kinetics
Onset of Action: ~30 minutes
Time to Peak: Oral: ~2 hours
Protein Binding: Plasma: 70% to 76%
Half-Life Elimination:
Children <15 years: 2-7 hours; Adults: 3-6 hours
Mild-to-moderate hepatic impairment: Adults: 12 hours
Severe hepatic impairment (Child-Pugh C): Adults: 20 hours
Metabolism: Extensively hepatic via hydroxylation, followed by glucuronide or sulfate conjugation; CYP1A2, CYP2D6, and CYP3A4 substrate, some demethylation occurs
Excretion: Urine (44% to 60% as metabolites, 5% to 10% as unchanged drug); feces (~25%)

Available Dosage Forms [DSC] = Discontinued product
Infusion [premixed in D$_5$W, preservative free]:
Zofran®: 32 mg (50 mL)
Injection, solution:
Zofran®: 2 mg/mL (2 mL, 20 mL)
Solution, oral:
Zofran®: 4 mg/5 mL (50 mL) [contains sodium benzoate; strawberry flavor]
Tablet:
Zofran®: 4 mg; 8 mg; 24 mg [DSC]
(Continued)

Ondansetron (Continued)

Tablet, orally disintegrating:
Zofran® ODT: 4 mg, 8 mg [each strength contains phenylalanine <0.03 mg/tablet; strawberry flavor]

Dosing

Adults & Elderly: Note: Studies in adults have shown a single daily dose of 8-12 mg I.V. or 8-24 mg orally to be as effective as mg/kg dosing, and should be considered for all patients whose mg/kg dose exceeds 8-12 mg I.V.; oral solution and ODT formulations are bioequivalent to corresponding doses of tablet formulation.

Prevention of chemotherapy-induced emesis:
I.V.:
0.15 mg/kg 3 times/day beginning 30 minutes prior to chemotherapy **or**
0.45 mg/kg once daily **or**
8-10 mg 1-2 times/day **or**
24 mg or 32 mg once daily

Highly-emetogenic agents/single-day therapy: Oral: 24 mg given 30 minutes prior to the start of therapy

Moderately-emetogenic agents: Oral: 8 mg every 12 hours beginning 30 minutes before chemotherapy, continuously for 1-2 days after chemotherapy completed

Total body irradiation: Oral: 8 mg 1-2 hours before each daily fraction of radiotherapy

Single high-dose fraction radiotherapy to abdomen: Oral: 8 mg 1-2 hours before irradiation, then 8 mg every 8 hours after first dose for 1-2 days after completion of radiotherapy

Daily fractionated radiotherapy to abdomen: 8 mg 1-2 hours before irradiation, then 8 mg 8 hours after first dose for each day of radiotherapy

Postoperative nausea and vomiting (PONV):
Oral: 16 mg given one hour prior to induction of anesthesia
I.M., I.V.: 4 mg as a single dose immediately before induction of anesthesia, or shortly following procedure if vomiting occurs
Note: Repeat doses given in response to inadequate control of nausea/vomiting from preoperative doses are generally ineffective.

Treatment of hyperemesis gravidum (unlabeled use):
Oral: 8 mg every 12 hours
I.V.: 8 mg administered over 15 minutes every 12 hours or 1 mg/hour infused continuously for up to 24 hours

Pediatrics: Note: Studies in adults have shown a single daily dose of 8-12 mg I.V. or 8-24 mg orally to be as effective as mg/kg dosing, and should be considered for all patients whose mg/kg dose exceeds 8-12 mg I.V.; oral solution and ODT formulations are bioequivalent to corresponding doses of tablet formulation.

Prevention of chemotherapy-induced emesis:
I.V.: Children 6 months to 18 years: 0.15 mg/kg/dose administered 30 minutes prior to chemotherapy, 4 and 8 hours after the first dose **or** 0.45 mg/kg/day as a single dose

Oral:
4-11 years: 4 mg 30 minutes before chemotherapy; repeat 4 and 8 hours after initial dose, then 4 mg every 8 hours for 1-2 days after chemotherapy completed
≥12 years: Refer to adult dosing.

Prevention of postoperative nausea and vomiting (PONV): I.V.: Children 1 month to 12 years:
≤40 kg: 0.1 mg/kg as a single dose
>40 kg: 4 mg as a single dose

Renal Impairment: No adjustment is necessary.

Hepatic Impairment: Severe liver disease (Child-Pugh C): Maximum daily dose: 8 mg

Administration

Oral: Oral dosage forms should be given 30 minutes prior to chemotherapy; 1-2 hours before radiotherapy; 1 hour prior to the induction of anesthesia
Orally-disintegrating tablets: Do not remove from blister until needed. Peel backing off the blister, do not push tablet through. Using dry hands, place tablet on tongue and allow to dissolve. Swallow with saliva.
The I.V. preparation has been successful when administered orally.

I.M.: Should be given undiluted

I.V.: Give first dose 30 minutes prior to beginning chemotherapy; the I.V. preparation has been successful when administered orally
I.V. injection: Single doses for prevention of postoperative nausea and vomiting may be administered I.V. over 2-5 minutes as undiluted solution
IVPB: Dilute in 50 mL D_5W or NS. Infuse over 15-30 minutes; 24-hour continuous infusions have been reported, but are rarely used

I.V. Detail: pH: 3-4

Stability

Reconstitution: Prior to I.V. infusion, dilute in 50 mL D_5W or NS.

Compatibility: Stable in $D_5^{1}/_2NS$, D_5NS, D_5W, mannitol 10%, LR, NS, NS 3%; do not mix injection with alkaline solutions
Y-site administration: Incompatible with acyclovir, allopurinol, aminophylline, amphotericin B, amphotericin B cholesteryl sulfate complex, ampicillin, ampicillin/sulbactam, amsacrine, cefepime, cefoperazone, furosemide, ganciclovir, lorazepam, methylprednisolone sodium succinate, piperacillin, sargramostim, sodium bicarbonate

Storage:
Oral solution: Store between 15°C and 30°C (59°F and 86°F). Protect from light.
Premixed bag: Store between 2°C and 30°C (36°F and 86°F). Protect from light.
Tablet: Store between 2°C and 30°C (36°F and 86°F)
Vial: Store between 2°C and 30°C (36°F and 86°F). Protect from light. Stable when mixed in D_5W or NS for 48 hours at room temperature.

Nursing Actions

Physical Assessment: To be used on a scheduled basis, not on an "as needed" (PRN) basis for prevention of nausea and vomiting associated with moderately- to highly-emetogenic cancer chemotherapy; not recommended for treatment of existing chemotherapy-induced emesis. Assess potential for interactions with other pharmacological agents and herbal products patient may be taking (eg, increase or decrease levels/effects of ondansetron). See Administration for specifics according to formulation. Monitor effectiveness (avoidance of nausea and vomiting) and adverse effects (dizziness, constipation, diarrhea, urinary retention, hypoxia). Teach patient possible side effects/appropriate interventions, and adverse symptoms to report.

Patient Education: This drug is given to reduce the incidence of nausea and vomiting. Do not take any other medication for nausea and vomiting with this medication unless approved by prescriber. If self-administered, take as directed. May cause headache, drowsiness, or dizziness (do not change position rapidly, request assistance when getting up or changing position and do not perform activities requiring alertness) or diarrhea (request appropriate treatment from prescriber). Report persistent headache, excessive drowsiness, fever, numbness or tingling, or changes in elimination patterns (constipation or diarrhea); and chest pain or palpitations.

Orally-disintegrating tablets: Do not remove from blister until needed. Peel backing off the blister, do not push tablet through. Using dry hands, place tablet on tongue and allow to dissolve. Swallow with saliva. Contains <0.03 mg phenylalanine/tablet.

Dietary Considerations Take without regard to meals. Orally-disintegrating tablet contains <0.03 mg phenylalanine

Geriatric Considerations Elderly have a slightly decreased hepatic clearance rate. This does not, however, require a dose adjustment.

Opium Tincture (OH pee um TING chur)

Synonyms DTO (error-prone abbreviation); Opium Tincture, Deodorized

Restrictions C-II

Pharmacologic Category Analgesic, Narcotic; Antidiarrheal

Medication Safety Issues
Sound-alike/look-alike issues:
Opium tincture may be confused with camphorated tincture of opium (paregoric)

Use care when prescribing opium tincture; each mL contains the equivalent of morphine 10 mg; paregoric contains the equivalent of morphine 0.4 mg/mL

DTO is an error-prone abbreviation (mistaken as Diluted Tincture of Opium; dose equivalency of paregoric)

Pregnancy Risk Factor B/D (prolonged use or high doses at term)

Lactation Enters breast milk/use caution

Use Treatment of diarrhea or relief of pain

Mechanism of Action/Effect Contains many narcotic alkaloids including morphine; its mechanism for gastric motility inhibition is primarily due to this morphine content; it results in a decrease in digestive secretions, an increase in GI muscle tone, and therefore a reduction in GI propulsion

Contraindications Hypersensitivity to morphine sulfate or any component of the formulation; increased intracranial pressure; severe respiratory depression; severe hepatic or renal insufficiency; pregnancy (prolonged use or high dosages near term)

Warnings/Precautions Opium shares the toxic potential of opiate agonists, and usual precautions of opiate agonist therapy should be observed; some preparations contain sulfites which may cause allergic reactions; infants <3 months of age are more susceptible to respiratory depression, use with caution and generally in reduced doses in this age group; this is **not** paregoric, dose accordingly

Drug Interactions
Increased Effect/Toxicity: Opium tincture and CNS depressants, MAO inhibitors, tricyclic antidepressants may potentiate the effects of opiate agonists (eg, codeine, morphine). Dextroamphetamine may enhance the analgesic effect of opiate agonists.

Nutritional/Ethanol Interactions Ethanol: Avoid ethanol (may increase CNS depression).

Lab Interactions Increased aminotransferase [ALT (SGPT)/AST (SGOT)] (S)

Adverse Reactions Frequency not defined.
Cardiovascular: Palpitations, hypotension, bradycardia, peripheral vasodilation
Central nervous system: Drowsiness, dizziness, restlessness, headache, malaise, CNS depression, increased intracranial pressure, insomnia, mental depression
Gastrointestinal: Nausea, vomiting, constipation, anorexia, stomach cramps, biliary tract spasm
Genitourinary: Decreased urination, urinary tract spasm
Neuromuscular & skeletal: Weakness
Ocular: Miosis
Respiratory: Respiratory depression
Miscellaneous: Histamine release, physical and psychological dependence

Overdosage/Toxicology Primary attention should be directed to ensuring adequate respiratory exchange. Naloxone, 2 mg I.V. with repeat administration as necessary up to a total of 10 mg, can also be used to reverse toxic effects of the opiate.

Pharmacodynamics/Kinetics
Duration of Action: 4-5 hours
Metabolism: Hepatic
Excretion: Urine

Available Dosage Forms Liquid: 10% (120 mL, 480 mL) [0.6 mL equivalent to morphine 6 mg; contains alcohol 19%]

Dosing
Adults & Elderly:
Diarrhea: Oral: 0.3-1 mL/dose every 2-6 hours to maximum of 6 mL/24 hours
Analgesia: Oral: 0.6-1.5 mL/dose every 3-4 hours
Pediatrics:
Diarrhea: Oral: Children: 0.005-0.01 mL/kg/dose every 3-4 hours for a maximum of 6 doses/24 hours
Analgesia: Oral: Children: 0.01-0.02 mL/kg/dose every 3-4 hours

Stability
Storage: Protect from light

Nursing Actions
Physical Assessment: Assess other medications patient may be taking for additive or adverse interactions. Monitor for effectiveness of pain relief and monitor for signs of overdose. Monitor blood pressure, CNS and respiratory status, and degree of sedation at beginning of therapy and at regular intervals with long-term use. May cause physical and or psychological dependence. For inpatients, implement safety measures (eg, side rails up, call light within reach, instructions to call for assistance). Assess knowledge/teach patient appropriate use (if self-administered). Teach patient to monitor for adverse reactions, adverse reactions to report, and appropriate interventions to reduce side effects.

Patient Education: If self-administered, use exactly as directed; do not increase dose or frequency. Drug may cause physical and/or psychological dependence. While using this medication, do not use alcohol and other prescription or OTC medications (especially sedatives, tranquilizers, antihistamines, or pain medications) without consulting prescriber. Maintain adequate hydration (2-3 L/day of fluids). May cause hypotension, dizziness, drowsiness, impaired coordination, or blurred vision (use caution when driving, climbing stairs, or changing position - rising from sitting or lying to standing, or when engaging in tasks requiring alertness until response to drug is known); or dry mouth (frequent mouth care, small frequent meals, chewing gum, or sucking lozenges may help). Report slow or rapid heartbeat, acute dizziness, or persistent headache; changes in mental status; swelling of extremities or unusual weight gain; changes in urinary elimination or pain on urination; acute headache; trembling or muscle spasms; blurred vision; skin rash; or shortness of breath. **Pregnancy/breast-feeding precautions:** Inform prescriber if you are or intend to become pregnant.

Orlistat (OR li stat)

U.S. Brand Names Xenical®
Pharmacologic Category Lipase Inhibitor
Medication Safety Issues
Sound-alike/look-alike issues:
Xenical® may be confused with Xeloda®
Pregnancy Risk Factor B
Lactation Excretion in breast milk unknown/not recommended
(Continued)

Orlistat *(Continued)*

Use Management of obesity, including weight loss and weight management when used in conjunction with a reduced-calorie diet; reduce the risk of weight regain after prior weight loss; indicated for obese patients with an initial body mass index (BMI) ≥ 30 kg/m^2 or ≥ 27 kg/m^2 in the presence of other risk factors

Mechanism of Action/Effect Inhibits gastric and pancreatic lipases, thus inhibiting the absorption of dietary fats (by 30% at doses of 120 mg 3 times/day)

Contraindications Hypersensitivity to orlistat or any component of the formulation; chronic malabsorption syndrome or cholestasis

Warnings/Precautions Patients should be advised to adhere to dietary guidelines; gastrointestinal adverse events may increase if taken with a diet high in fat (>30% total daily calories from fat). The daily intake of fat should be distributed over three main meals. If taken with any one meal very high in fat, the possibility of gastrointestinal effects increases. Patients should be counseled to take a multivitamin supplement that contains fat-soluble vitamins to ensure adequate nutrition because orlistat has been shown to reduce the absorption of some fat-soluble vitamins and beta-carotene. Some patients may develop increased levels of urinary oxalate following treatment; caution should be exercised when prescribing it to patients with a history of hyperoxaluria or calcium oxalate nephrolithiasis. As with any weight-loss agent, the potential exists for misuse in appropriate patient populations (eg, patients with anorexia nervosa or bulimia). Safety and efficacy have not been established in children <12 years of age. **Note:** Dispensing errors have been made between Xenical® (orlistat) and Xeloda® (capecitabine).

Drug Interactions
Decreased Effect: Orlistat may decrease amiodarone absorption (monitor). Coadministration with cyclosporine may decrease plasma levels of cyclosporine (administer cyclosporine 2 hours before or after orlistat and monitor). Orlistat does not alter the pharmacokinetics of warfarin, however, vitamin K absorption may be decreased during orlistat therapy (patients stabilized on warfarin should be monitored for changes in warfarin effects).

Nutritional/Ethanol Interactions
Fat-soluble vitamins: Absorption of vitamins A, D, E, and K may be decreased by orlistat. A multivitamin containing the fat-soluble vitamins (A, D, E, and K) should be administered once daily at least 2 hours before or after orlistat.

Adverse Reactions
>10%:
Central nervous system: Headache (31%)
Gastrointestinal: Oily spotting (27%), abdominal pain/discomfort (26%), flatus with discharge (24%), fatty/oily stool (20%), fecal urgency (22%), oily evacuation (12%), increased defecation (11%)
Neuromuscular & skeletal: Back pain (14%)
Respiratory: Upper respiratory infection (38%)
1% to 10%:
Central nervous system: Fatigue (7%), anxiety (5%), sleep disorder (4%)
Dermatologic: Dry skin (2%)
Endocrine & metabolic: Menstrual irregularities (10%)
Gastrointestinal: Fecal incontinence (8%), nausea (8%), infectious diarrhea (5%), rectal pain/discomfort (5%), vomiting (4%)
Neuromuscular & skeletal: Arthritis (5%), myalgia (4%)
Otic: Otitis (4%)

Overdosage/Toxicology Single doses of 800 mg and multiple doses of up to 400 mg 3 times daily for 15 days have been studied in normal weight and obese patients without significant adverse findings. In case of significant overdose, it is recommended that the patient be observed for 24 hours.

Pharmacodynamics/Kinetics
Metabolism: Metabolized within the gastrointestinal wall; forms inactive metabolites
Excretion: Feces (83% as unchanged drug)
Available Dosage Forms Capsule: 120 mg
Dosing
Adults & Elderly: Obesity: Oral: 120 mg 3 times daily with each main meal containing fat (during or up to 1 hour after the meal); omit dose if meal is occasionally missed or contains no fat.
Pediatrics: Obesity: Children ≥ 12 years: Refer to adult dosing.

Nursing Actions
Physical Assessment: Assess effectiveness of other medications patient may be taking (especially anticoagulants). Monitor effectiveness of therapy, laboratory results, and adverse reactions at beginning of therapy and periodically during therapy. Assess knowledge/teach patient appropriate use, possible side effects/appropriate interventions, and adverse symptoms to report.

Patient Education: Take this medication exactly as ordered; do not alter prescribed dose without consulting prescriber. Maintain prescribed diet (high-fat meals may result in GI distress), exercise regimen, and vitamin supplements as prescribed. You may experience dizziness or lightheadedness (use caution when driving or engaging in tasks requiring alertness until response to drug is known) or increased flatus and fecal urgency (this may lessen with continued use). Report persistent back, muscle, or joint pain; signs of respiratory tract infection or flu-like symptoms; skin rash or irritation; or other reactions. **Breast-feeding precaution:** Breast-feeding is not recommended.

Dietary Considerations Multivitamin supplements that contain fat-soluble vitamins should be taken once daily at least 2 hours before or after the administration of orlistat (ie, bedtime). Distribute the daily intake of fat over 3 main meals. Gastrointestinal effects of orlistat may increase if taken with any 1 meal very high in fat.

Orphenadrine *(or FEN a dreen)*

U.S. Brand Names Norflex™
Synonyms Orphenadrine Citrate
Pharmacologic Category Anti-Parkinson's Agent, Anticholinergic; Skeletal Muscle Relaxant
Medication Safety Issues
Sound-alike/look-alike issues:
Norflex™ may be confused with norfloxacin, Noroxin®
Pregnancy Risk Factor C
Lactation Excretion in breast milk unknown
Use Treatment of muscle spasm associated with acute painful musculoskeletal conditions; supportive therapy in tetanus
Mechanism of Action/Effect Indirect skeletal muscle relaxant thought to work by central atropine-like effects; has some euphorogenic and analgesic properties
Contraindications Hypersensitivity to orphenadrine or any component of the formulation; glaucoma; GI obstruction; cardiospasm; myasthenia gravis
Warnings/Precautions Use with caution in patients with CHF or cardiac arrhythmias. Some products contain sulfites.
Drug Interactions
Cytochrome P450 Effect: Substrate (minor) of CYP1A2, 2B6, 2D6, 3A4; **Inhibits** CYP1A2 (weak), 2A6 (weak), 2B6 (weak), 2C8/9 (weak), 2C19 (weak), 2D6 (weak), 2E1 (weak), 3A4 (weak)
Increased Effect/Toxicity: Orphenadrine may increase potential for anticholinergic adverse effects of anticholinergic agents; includes drugs with high

anticholinergic activity (diphenhydramine, TCAs, phenothiazines). Sedative effects of may be additive in concurrent use of orphenadrine and CNS depressants (monitor). Effects of levodopa may be decreased by orphenadrine. Monitor.

Nutritional/Ethanol Interactions
Ethanol: Avoid ethanol (may increase CNS depression). Herb/Nutraceutical: St John's wort may decrease orphenadrine levels. Avoid valerian, St John's wort, kava kava, gotu kola (may increase CNS depression).

Adverse Reactions
>10%:
Central nervous system: Drowsiness, dizziness
Ocular: Blurred vision
1% to 10%:
Cardiovascular: Flushing of face, tachycardia, syncope
Dermatologic: Rash
Gastrointestinal: Nausea, vomiting, constipation
Genitourinary: Decreased urination
Neuromuscular & skeletal: Weakness
Ocular: Nystagmus, increased intraocular pressure
Respiratory: Nasal congestion

Overdosage/Toxicology Symptoms of overdose include blurred vision, tachycardia, confusion, seizures, respiratory arrest, and dysrhythmias. There is no specific treatment for antihistamine overdose. Clinical toxicity is due to blockade of cholinergic receptors. Lethal dose is 2-3 g; treatment is generally symptomatic. For anticholinergic overdose with severe life-threatening symptoms, physostigmine 1-2 mg I.V. slowly, may be given to reverse these effects.

Pharmacodynamics/Kinetics
Onset of Action: Peak effect: Oral: Within 2-4 hours
Duration of Action: 4-6 hours
Protein Binding: 20%
Half-Life Elimination: 14-16 hours
Metabolism: Extensively hepatic
Excretion: Primarily urine (8% as unchanged drug)

Available Dosage Forms
Injection, solution, as citrate: 30 mg/mL (2 mL)
Norflex™: 30 mg/mL (2 mL) [contains sodium bisulfite]
Tablet, extended release, as citrate: 100 mg
Norflex™: 100 mg

Dosing
Adults: Muscle spasms:
Oral: 100 mg twice daily
I.M., I.V.: 60 mg every 12 hours
Elderly: Not recommended for use in the elderly (see Geriatric Considerations).

Administration
Oral: Do not crush sustained release drug product.

Nursing Actions
Physical Assessment: Monitor effectiveness of therapy (according to rationale for therapy) and adverse reactions at beginning of therapy and periodically with long-term use. Do not discontinue abruptly; taper dosage slowly. Assess knowledge/teach patient appropriate use, interventions to reduce side effects (postural hypotension precautions), and adverse symptoms to report.

Patient Education: Take exactly as directed. Do not increase dose or discontinue without consulting prescriber. Do not chew or crush sustained release tablets. Do not use alcohol, prescriptive or OTC antidepressants, sedatives, or pain medications without consulting prescriber. You may experience drowsiness, dizziness, lightheadedness (avoid driving or engaging in tasks requiring alertness until response to drug is known); nausea or vomiting (small frequent meals, frequent mouth care, or sucking hard candy may help); constipation (increased exercise, fluids, fruit, or fibers may help); or decreased urination (void before taking medication). Report excessive drowsiness or mental agitation, chest pain, skin rash, swelling of mouth/face, difficulty speaking, or vision changes. **Pregnancy/breast-feeding precautions:** Inform prescriber if you are or intend to become pregnant. Consult prescriber if breast-feeding.

Geriatric Considerations Because of its anticholinergic side effects, orphenadrine is not a drug of choice in the elderly.

Orphenadrine, Aspirin, and Caffeine
(or FEN a dreen, AS pir in, & KAF een)

U.S. Brand Names Norgesic™ [DSC]; Norgesic™ Forte [DSC]; Orphengesic [DSC]; Orphengesic Forte [DSC]
Synonyms Aspirin, Orphenadrine, and Caffeine; Caffeine, Orphenadrine, and Aspirin
Pharmacologic Category Skeletal Muscle Relaxant
Pregnancy Risk Factor D
Lactation Enters breast milk/use caution due to aspirin content
Use Relief of discomfort associated with skeletal muscular conditions
Available Dosage Forms [DSC] = Discontinued product
Tablet: Orphenadrine citrate 25 mg, aspirin 385 mg, and caffeine 30 mg; orphenadrine citrate 50 mg, aspirin 770 mg, and caffeine 60 mg
Norgesic™, Orphengesic: Orphenadrine citrate 25 mg, aspirin 385 mg, and caffeine 30 mg [DSC]
Norgesic™ Forte, Orphengesic Forte: Orphenadrine citrate 50 mg, aspirin 770 mg, and caffeine 60 mg [DSC]

Dosing
Adults: Muscular pain/spasms: Oral: 1-2 tablets 3-4 times/day
Elderly: Not recommended for use in the elderly; see individual agents

Nursing Actions
Physical Assessment: See individual agents.
Patient Education: See individual agents. **Pregnancy/breast-feeding precautions:** Inform prescriber if you are or intend to become pregnant. Consult prescriber if breast-feeding.

Related Information
Aspirin on page 114
Orphenadrine on page 916

Oseltamivir (oh sel TAM i vir)

U.S. Brand Names Tamiflu®
Pharmacologic Category Antiviral Agent; Neuraminidase Inhibitor
Medication Safety Issues
Sound-alike/look-alike issues:
Tamiflu® may be confused with Thera-Flu®
Pregnancy Risk Factor C
Lactation Excretion in breast milk unknown/not recommended
Use Treatment of uncomplicated acute illness due to influenza (A or B) infection in children ≥1 year of age and adults who have been symptomatic for no more than 2 days; prophylaxis against influenza (A or B) infection in children ≥1 year of age and adults
Mechanism of Action/Effect Thought to inhibit influenza virus by altering virus particle aggregation and release
Contraindications Hypersensitivity to oseltamivir or any component of the formulation
Warnings/Precautions Oseltamivir is not a substitute for the influenza virus vaccine. Use caution with renal impairment; dosage adjustment is required for creatinine clearance between 10-30 mL/minute. Also consider primary or concomitant bacterial infections. Safety and (Continued)

Oseltamivir *(Continued)*

efficacy for use in hepatic impairment or for treatment or prophylaxis in immunocompromised patients have not been established. Efficacy has not been established if treatment begins >40 hours after the onset of symptoms or in the treatment of patients with chronic cardiac and/ or respiratory disease. Rare but severe hypersensitivity reactions (anaphylaxis, severe dermatologic reactions) have been associated with use. Safety and efficacy in children (<1 year of age) have not been established.

Drug Interactions

Decreased Effect: Influenza virus vaccine nasal spray (fluMist™): Safety and efficacy for use with influenza virus vaccine nasal spray have not been established. Do not administer nasal spray until 48 hours after stopping antiviral; do not administer antiviral for 2 weeks after receiving influenza virus vaccine nasal spray.

Adverse Reactions

>10%: Gastrointestinal: Vomiting (2% to 15%)

1% to 10%: Gastrointestinal: Nausea (3% to 10%), abdominal pain (2% to 5%)

Overdosage/Toxicology Single doses of 1000 mg resulted in nausea and vomiting.

Pharmacodynamics/Kinetics

Protein Binding: Plasma: Oseltamivir carboxylate: 3%; Oseltamivir: 42%

Half-Life Elimination: Oseltamivir: 1-3 hours; Oseltamivir carboxylate: 6-10 hours

Metabolism: Hepatic (90%) to oseltamivir carboxylate; neither the parent drug nor active metabolite has any effect on CYP.

Excretion: Urine (>90% as oseltamivir carboxylate); feces

Available Dosage Forms

Capsule, as phosphate: 75 mg

Powder for oral suspension: 12 mg/mL (25 mL) [contains sodium benzoate; tutti-frutti flavor]

Dosing

Adults & Elderly:

Influenza prophylaxis: Oral: 75 mg once daily; initiate treatment within 2 days of contact with an infected individual; duration of treatment: 10 days. During community outbreaks, dosing is 75 mg once daily. May be used for up to 6 weeks; duration of protection lasts for length of dosing period.

Influenza treatment: Oral: 75 mg twice daily initiated within 2 days of onset of symptoms; duration of treatment: 5 days

Pediatrics:

Influenza prophylaxis: Oral: Initiate treatment within 2 days of contact with an infected individual; duration of treatment: 10 days:

Children: 1-12 years:

≤15 kg: 30 mg twice daily

>15 kg to ≤23 kg: 45 mg twice daily

>23 kg to ≤40 kg: 60 mg twice daily

>40 kg: 75 mg twice daily

Influenza treatment: Oral: Initiate treatment within 2 days of onset of symptoms; duration of treatment: 5 days:

Children: 1-12 years:

≤15 kg: 30 mg twice daily

>15 kg - ≤23 kg: 45 mg twice daily

>23 kg - ≤40 kg: 60 mg twice daily

>40 kg: 75 mg twice daily

Adolescents ≥13 years: Refer to adult dosing.

Renal Impairment: Adults:

Cl_{cr} 10-30 mL/minute:

Treatment: Reduce dose to 75 mg once daily for 5 days.

Prophylaxis: Administer 75 mg every other day or 30 mg once daily.

Cl_{cr} <10 mL/minute: Dosing recommendations are not available.

Hepatic Impairment: Dosing recommendations are not available.

Stability

Reconstitution: Oral suspension: Reconstitute with 23 mL of water (to make 25 mL total suspension).

Storage:

Capsules: Store at 25°C (77°F).

Oral suspension: Store powder for suspension at 25°C (77°F). Once reconstituted, store suspension under refrigeration at 2°C to 8°C (36°F to 46°F); do not freeze. Use within 10 days of preparation.

Nursing Actions

Physical Assessment: Teach patient appropriate use, interventions to reduce side effects, and adverse reactions to report.

Patient Education: This is not a substitute for the flu shot. Must be taken within 2 days of onset of flu symptoms (eg, fever, cough, headache, fatigue, muscular weakness, and sore throat). Take as directed; do not increase dose or frequency, and do not miss a dose. You may experience nausea or vomiting (small frequent meals, good mouth care, chewing gum, or sucking hard candy may help). Report significant adverse effects to your prescriber. **Pregnancy/breast-feeding precautions:** Inform prescriber if you are or intend to become pregnant. Breast-feeding is not recommended.

Dietary Considerations Take with or without food; take with food to improve tolerance.

Breast-Feeding Issues Oseltamivir and its metabolite are excreted in the breast milk of lactating rats. It is unknown if they appear in human milk.

Additional Information In clinical studies of the influenza virus, 1.3% of post-treatment isolates in adults and adolescents and 8.6% of isolates in children had decreased neuraminidase susceptibility *in vitro* to oseltamivir carboxylate.

Oxacillin *(oks a SIL in)*

Synonyms Methylphenyl Isoxazolyl Penicillin; Oxacillin Sodium

Pharmacologic Category Antibiotic, Penicillin

Pregnancy Risk Factor B

Lactation Enters breast milk/compatible

Use Treatment of infections such as osteomyelitis, septicemia, endocarditis, and CNS infections caused by susceptible strains of *Staphylococcus*

Mechanism of Action/Effect Inhibits bacterial cell wall synthesis by binding to one or more of the penicillin binding proteins (PBPs); which in turn inhibits the final transpeptidation step of peptidoglycan synthesis in bacterial cell walls, thus inhibiting cell wall biosynthesis. Bacteria eventually lyse due to ongoing activity of cell wall autolytic enzymes (autolysins and murein hydrolases) while cell wall assembly is arrested.

Contraindications Hypersensitivity to oxacillin or other penicillins or any component of the formulation

Warnings/Precautions Elimination rate will be slow in neonates; modify dosage in patients with renal impairment and in the elderly; use with caution in patients with cephalosporin hypersensitivity

Drug Interactions

Decreased Effect: Although anecdotal reports suggest oral contraceptive efficacy could be reduced by penicillins, this has been refuted by more rigorous scientific and clinical data.

Increased Effect/Toxicity: Probenecid increases penicillin levels. Penicillins and anticoagulants may increase the effect of anticoagulants. Penicillins may increase the exposure to methotrexate during concurrent therapy; monitor.

Lab Interactions May interfere with urinary glucose tests using cupric sulfate (Benedict's solution, Clinitest®); may inactivate aminoglycosides *in vitro*; false-positive urinary and serum proteins

Adverse Reactions Frequency not defined.
Central nervous system: Fever
Dermatologic: Rash
Gastrointestinal: Nausea, diarrhea, vomiting
Hematologic: Eosinophilia, leukopenia, neutropenia, thrombocytopenia, agranulocytosis
Hepatic: Hepatotoxicity, AST increased
Renal: Acute interstitial nephritis, hematuria
Miscellaneous: Serum sickness-like reactions

Overdosage/Toxicology Symptoms of penicillin overdose include neuromuscular hypersensitivity (eg, agitation, hallucinations, asterixis, encephalopathy, confusion, and seizures). Electrolyte imbalance may occur if the preparation contains potassium or sodium salts, especially in renal failure. Hemodialysis may be helpful to aid in removal of the drug from blood; otherwise, treatment is supportive or symptom-directed.

Pharmacodynamics/Kinetics
Time to Peak: I.M.: 30-60 minutes
Protein Binding: ~94%
Half-Life Elimination: Children 1 week to 2 years: 0.9-1.8 hours; Adults: 23-60 minutes; prolonged with renal impairment and in neonates
Metabolism: Hepatic to active metabolites
Excretion: Urine and feces (small amounts as unchanged drug and metabolites)

Available Dosage Forms
Infusion [premixed iso-osmotic dextrose solution]: 1 g (50 mL); 2 g (50 mL)
Injection, powder for reconstitution, as sodium: 1 g, 2 g, 10 g

Dosing
Adults & Elderly:
Endocarditis: I.V.: 2 g every 4 hours with gentamicin
Mild-to-moderate infections: I.M., I.V.: 250-500 mg every 4-6 hours
Prosthetic joint infection: I.V.: 2 g every 4 hours with rifampin
Severe infections: I.M., I.V.: 1-2 g every 4-6 hours
Staphylococcus aureus, methicillin-susceptible infections, including brain abscess, bursitis, erysipelas, mastitis, mastoiditis, osteomyelitis, perinephric abscess, pneumonia, pyomyositis, scalded skin syndrome, toxic shock syndrome: I.V.: 2 g every 4 hours
Pediatrics:
Arthritis (septic): I.V.: 37 mg/kg every 6 hours
Epiglottitis: I.V.: 150-200 mg/kg/day divided every 6 hours
Mild-to-moderate infections: I.M., I.V.: 100-150 mg/kg/day in divided doses every 6 hours (maximum: 4 g/day)
Severe infections: I.M., I.V.: 150-200 mg/kg/day in divided doses every 6 hours (maximum: 12 g/day)
Staphylococcal scalded-skin syndrome: I.V.: 150 mg/kg/day divided every 6 hours for 5-7 days
Renal Impairment:
Cl_{cr} <10 mL/minute: Clinical practice varies; some clinicians recommend adjustment to the lower range of the usual dosage as based on severity of infection.
Not dialyzable (0% to 5%)

Administration
I.V.: Administer around-the-clock to promote less variation in peak and trough serum levels. Administer IVP over 10 minutes. Administer IVPB over 30 minutes.
I.V. Detail: Rapid administration may result in seizures.
Stability
Compatibility: Stable in dextran 70 6% in dextrose, dextran 40 10% in dextrose, D_5LR, $D_{10}W$, hetastarch 6%, LR

Y-site administration: Incompatible with sodium bicarbonate, verapamil
Compatibility when admixed: Incompatible with cytarabine
Storage: Reconstituted parenteral solution is stable for 3 days at room temperature and 7 days when refrigerated. For I.V. infusion in NS or D_5W, solution is stable for 6 hours at room temperature.
Laboratory Monitoring Perform culture and sensitivity studies prior to initiating therapy.

Nursing Actions
Physical Assessment: Assess patient reports of allergy or sensitivity before administering. I.V. - monitor infusion site for extravasation. Monitor response to therapy; if no response, therapy should be re-evaluated.
Patient Education: Complete course of treatment as prescribed. You may experience nausea or vomiting; small, frequent meals and good mouth care may help. If you have diabetes, drug may cause false test results with Clinitest® urine glucose monitoring; use of glucose oxidase methods (Clinistix®) or serum glucose monitoring is preferable. Report persistent fever, sore throat, sores in mouth, diarrhea, unusual bleeding or bruising, respiratory difficulty, or skin rash. Notify prescriber if condition does not respond to treatment.
Dietary Considerations Sodium content of 1 g: 92.4 mg (4.02 mEq)
Geriatric Considerations Oxacillin has not been studied in the elderly. Dosing adjustments are not necessary except in renal failure (eg, Cl_{cr} <10 mL/minute). Consider sodium content in patients who may be sensitive to volume expansion (ie, CHF).
Breast-Feeding Issues No adverse effects have been reported in the nursing infant. Theoretically, the antibiotic effect of oxacillin may appear in the infant and change the bowel flora or affect culture results.

Oxaliplatin (ox AL i pla tin)

U.S. Brand Names Eloxatin™
Synonyms Diaminocyclohexane Oxalatoplatinum; L-OHP; NSC-266046
Pharmacologic Category Antineoplastic Agent, Alkylating Agent
Medication Safety Issues
Sound-alike/look-alike issues:
Oxaliplatin may be confused with Aloxi™
Pregnancy Risk Factor D
Lactation Excretion in breast milk unknown/not recommended
Use Treatment of advanced colon cancer and advanced rectal carcinoma
Unlabeled/Investigational Use Head and neck cancer, nonsmall cell lung cancer, non-Hodgkin's lymphoma, ovarian cancer
Mechanism of Action/Effect Oxaliplatin is an alkylating agent. It binds to DNA, RNA, or proteins, disrupting DNA function. Cytotoxicity is cell-cycle nonspecific.
Contraindications Hypersensitivity to oxaliplatin, other platinum-containing compounds, or any component of the formulation; pregnancy
Warnings/Precautions The U.S. Food and Drug Administration (FDA) currently recommends that procedures for proper handling and disposal of antineoplastic agents be considered. Anaphylactic-like reaction may occur within minutes of oxaliplatin administration. Two different types of neuropathy may occur: First, acute (within first 2 days), reversible (resolves within 14 days), primarily peripheral symptoms that are often exacerbated by cold (may include pharyngolaryngeal dysesthesia); and secondly, a more persistent (>14 days) (Continued)

Oxaliplatin *(Continued)*

presentation that often interferes with daily activities (eg, writing, buttoning, swallowing), these symptoms may improve upon discontinuing treatment. May cause pulmonary fibrosis or hepatotoxicity. The presence of hepatic vascular disorders (including veno-occlusive disease) should be considered, especially in individuals developing portal hypertension or who present with increased liver function tests. Caution in renal dysfunction. Safety and efficacy in pediatric patients have not been established.

Drug Interactions

Increased Effect/Toxicity: Taxane derivatives may increase oxaliplatin toxicity if administered before the platin as a sequential infusion. Nephrotoxic agents may increase oxaliplatin toxicity. Prolonged prothrombin time and increased INR associated with hemorrhage have been reported in patients receiving oxaliplatin/fluorouracil/leucovorin concomitantly with oral anticoagulants.

Adverse Reactions Based on clinical trial data using oxaliplatin alone. Some adverse effects (eg, thrombocytopenia, hemorrhagic events, neutropenia) may be increased when therapy is combined with fluorouracil/leucovorin.

>10%:

Central nervous system: Fatigue (61%), fever (25%), pain (14%), headache (13%), insomnia (11%)

Gastrointestinal: Nausea (64%), diarrhea (46%), vomiting (37%), abdominal pain (31%), constipation (31%), anorexia (20%), stomatitis (14%)

Hematologic: Anemia (64%), thrombocytopenia (30%), leukopenia (13%)

Hepatic: SGOT increased (54%), SGPT increased (36%), total bilirubin increased (13%)

Neuromuscular & skeletal: Neuropathy (may be dose-limiting), peripheral (acute 56%, persistent 48%), back pain (11%)

Respiratory: Dyspnea (13%), cough (11%)

1% to 10%:

Cardiovascular: Edema (10%), chest pain (5%), flushing (3%), thrombosis (2% to 6%), thromboembolism (6% to 9%)

Central nervous system: Rigors (9%), dizziness (7%), hand-foot syndrome (1%)

Dermatologic: Rash (5%), alopecia (3%)

Endocrine & metabolic: Dehydration (5%), hypokalemia (3%)

Gastrointestinal: Dyspepsia (7%), taste perversion (5%), flatulence (3%), mucositis (2%), gastroesophageal reflux (1%), dysphagia (acute 1% to 2%)

Genitourinary: Dysuria (1%)

Hematologic: Neutropenia (7%)

Local: Injection site reaction (9%)

Neuromuscular & skeletal: Arthralgia (7%)

Ocular: Abnormal lacrimation (1%)

Renal: Serum creatinine increased (10%)

Respiratory: URI (7%), rhinitis (6%), epistaxis (2%), pharyngitis (2%), pharyngolaryngeal dysesthesia (1% to 2%)

Miscellaneous: Allergic reactions (3%), hiccup (2%)

Overdosage/Toxicology Overdose symptoms are extensions of known side effects (eg, thrombocytopenia, myelosuppression, nausea, vomiting, neurotoxicity, respiratory symptoms). Treatment should be supportive.

Pharmacodynamics/Kinetics

Protein Binding: >90% primarily albumin and gamma globulin (irreversible binding to platinum)

Half-Life Elimination: Distribution: Alpha phase: 0.4, Beta phase: 16.8 hours

Metabolism: Nonenzymatic (rapid and extensive), forms active and inactive derivatives

Excretion: Primarily urine

Available Dosage Forms

Injection, powder for reconstitution: 50 mg, 100 mg [contains lactose]

Injection, solution [preservative free]: 5 mg/mL (10 mL, 20 mL)

Dosing

Adults:

Colorectal cancer (labeled dosing): Refer to individual protocols. I.V.:

85 mg/m^2 every 2 weeks **or**

20-25 mg/m^2 days 1-5 every 3 weeks **or**

100-130 mg/m^2 every 2-3 weeks

Elderly: No dosing adjustment recommended.

Renal Impairment: Consider omitting dose or changing chemotherapy regimen if Cl$_{cr}$ ≤19 mL/minute.

Dosing Adjustment for Toxicity: Longer infusion times (over 6 hours instead of 2 hours) may mitigate acute toxicities. In patients experiencing persistent neurosensory events (grade 2) which do not resolve, a dose reduction may be considered. Grade 3 neurosensory events may prompt consideration to discontinue oxaliplatin (while fluorouracil/leucovorin are continued or decreased). After recovery from grade 3/4 gastrointestinal toxicity, grade 4 neutropenia, or grade 3/4 thrombocytopenia, a dosage reduction is recommended.

Administration

I.V.: Administer as I.V. infusion over 2-6 hours. Longer infusion times (eg, those approaching or equal to 6 hours) may mitigate signs/symptoms of acute reactions. Flush infusion line with D$_5$W prior to administration of any concomitant medication.

Stability

Reconstitution: Do not reconstitute using a chloride-containing solution (eg, NaCl). Further dilution with D$_5$W (250 or 500 mL) is required prior to administration. Reconstituted solution does not require protection from light.

Compatibility: Incompatible with alkaline solutions (eg, fluorouracil) and chloride-containing solutions. Flush infusion line with D$_5$W prior to, and following, administration of concomitant medications via same I.V. line.

Storage: Store in original outer carton at room temperature of 15°C to 30°C (59°F to 86°F); do not freeze. Protect from light. Diluted solution is stable up to 6 hours at room temperature of 20°C to 25°C (68°F to 77°F) or up to 24 hours under refrigeration at 2°C to 8°C (36°F to 46°F).

Nursing Actions

Physical Assessment: Assess potential for interactions with other pharmacological agents (eg, increased toxicity with taxane derivatives or nephrotoxic agents). See Administration for infusion specifics. Patient must be observed closely for anaphylactic-like reactions (which can occur within minutes of administration). Monitor for adverse reactions during and between each infusion (eg, pulmonary and hepatic toxicity, neuropathy, GI disturbance, anemia, chest pain, thromboembolism). Teach patient possible side effects/appropriate interventions and adverse symptoms to report.

Patient Education: Do not take any new medication during therapy without consulting prescriber. This medication can only be administered by infusion; you will be monitored closely during and following infusion. Report immediately any rash, pain, burning, swelling at infusion site, or any signs of allergic reaction (eg, respiratory difficulty or swallowing, back pain, chest tightness, rash, hives, swelling of lips or mouth). It is important that you maintain adequate nutrition (small, frequent meals may help) and adequate hydration (2-3 L/day of fluids) unless instructed to restrict fluid intake. You will be susceptible to infection (avoid crowds and exposure to infection and do not have any vaccinations without consulting prescriber). May cause nausea, vomiting, loss of appetite, or taste perversion (small, frequent meals, frequent mouth care, chewing gum, or sucking lozenges may help - if nausea/vomiting is unresolved, consult prescriber for approved antiemetic); mouth sores (use soft tooth-brush or cotton swabs for mouth care); diarrhea (boiled milk, buttermilk, or yogurt may help); or loss of hair (reversible). Report any numbness, pain, tingling, or loss of sensation of extremities; chest pain or palpi-tations; swelling, pain, or hot areas in legs; unusual fatigue; unusual bruising or bleeding; respiratory diffi-culty; muscle cramps or twitching; change in hearing acuity; or other persistent adverse effects. **Preg-nancy/breast-feeding precautions:** Do not get preg-nant while taking this medication; use appropriate barrier contraceptive measures. Breast-feeding is not recommended.

Oxaprozin (oks a PROE zin)

U.S. Brand Names Daypro®

Restrictions A medication guide should be dispensed with each prescription. A template for the required MedGuide can be found on the FDA website at: http://www.fda.gov/medwatch/SAFETY/2005/safety05.htm#NSAID

Pharmacologic Category Nonsteroidal Anti-inflammatory Drug (NSAID), Oral

Medication Safety Issues

Sound-alike/look-alike issues:

Daypro® may be confused with Diupres®

Oxaprozin may be confused with oxazepam

Pregnancy Risk Factor C/D (3rd trimester)

Lactation Excretion in breast milk unknown/not recom-mended

Use Acute and long-term use in the management of signs and symptoms of osteoarthritis and rheumatoid arthritis; juvenile rheumatoid arthritis

Mechanism of Action/Effect Inhibits prostaglandin synthesis by decreasing the activity of the enzyme, cyclooxygenase, which results in decreased formation of prostaglandin precursors

Contraindications Hypersensitivity to oxaprozin, aspirin, other NSAIDs, or any component of the formula-tion; perioperative pain in the setting of coronary artery bypass surgery (CABG); pregnancy (3rd trimester)

Warnings/Precautions NSAIDs are associated with an increased risk of adverse cardiovascular events, including MI, stroke, and new onset or worsening of pre-existing hypertension. Risk may be increased with duration of use or pre-existing cardiovascular risk-factors or disease. Carefully evaluate individual cardiovascular risk profiles prior to prescribing. Use caution with fluid retention, CHF or hypertension.

Use of NSAIDs can compromise existing renal function. Renal toxicity can occur in patient with impaired renal function, dehydration, heart failure, liver dysfunction, those taking diuretics and ACEI and the elderly. Rehy-drate patient before starting therapy. Monitor renal func-tion closely. Oxaprozin is not recommended for patients with advanced renal disease.

NSAIDs may increase risk of gastrointestinal irritation, ulceration, bleeding, and perforation. These events may occur at any time during therapy and without warning. Use caution with a history of GI disease (bleeding or ulcers), concurrent therapy with aspirin, anticoagulants and/or corticosteroids, smoking, use of alcohol, the elderly or debilitated patients.

Use the lowest effective dose for the shortest duration of time, consistent with individual patient goals, to reduce risk of cardiovascular or GI adverse events. Alternate therapies should be considered for patients at high risk.

NSAIDs may cause serious skin adverse events including exfoliative dermatitis, Stevens-Johnson syndrome (SJS) and toxic epidermal necrolysis (TEN). Anaphylactoid reactions may occur, even without prior exposure; patients with "aspirin triad" (bronchial asthma, aspirin intolerance, rhinitis) may be at increased risk. Do not use in patients who experience bronchospasm, asthma, rhinitis, or urticaria with NSAID or aspirin therapy.

Use with caution in patients with decreased hepatic function. Closely monitor patients with any abnormal LFT. Severe hepatic reactions (eg, fulminant hepatitis, liver failure) have occurred with NSAID use, rarely; discontinue if signs or symptoms of liver disease develop, or if systemic manifestations occur.

The elderly are at increased risk for adverse effects (especially peptic ulceration, CNS effects, renal toxicity) from NSAIDs even at low doses.

Withhold for at least 4-6 half-lives prior to surgical or dental procedures. May cause mild photosensitivity reactions. Safety and efficacy have not been estab-lished in children <6 years of age.

Drug Interactions

Decreased Effect: Oxaprozin may decrease the effect of some antihypertensive agents (including ACE inhibitors and angiotensin antagonists) and diuretics.

Increased Effect/Toxicity: Oxaprozin may increase cyclosporine, digoxin, lithium, and methotrexate serum concentrations. The renal adverse effects of ACE inhibitors may be potentiated by NSAIDs. Corti-costeroids may increase the risk of GI ulceration. The risk of bleeding with anticoagulants (warfarin, anti-platelet agents, low molecular weight heparins) may be increased.

Nutritional/Ethanol Interactions

Ethanol: Avoid ethanol (may enhance gastric mucosal irritation).

Herb/Nutraceutical: Avoid alfalfa, anise, bilberry, blad-derwrack, bromelain, cat's claw, celery, coleus, cordy-ceps, dong quai, evening primrose, feverfew, fenugreek, garlic, ginger, ginkgo biloboa, red clover, horse chestnut, grapeseed, green tea, ginseng, guggul, horse chestnut seed, horseradish, licorice, prickly ash, red clover, reishi, SAMe, sweet clover, turmeric, white willow (all have additional antiplatelet activity).

Lab Interactions False-positive urine immunoassay screening tests for benzodiazepines have been reported and may occur several days after discontinuing oxaprozin.

Adverse Reactions

1% to 10%:

Cardiovascular: Edema

Central nervous system: Confusion, depression, dizzi-ness, headache, sedation, sleep disturbance, somnolence

Dermatologic: Pruritus, rash

Gastrointestinal: Abdominal distress, abdominal pain, anorexia, constipation, diarrhea, flatulence, gastro-intestinal ulcer, gross bleeding with perforation, heartburn, nausea, vomiting

Hematologic: Anemia, bleeding time increased

Hepatic: Liver enzyme elevation

Otic: Tinnitus

Renal: Dysuria, renal function abnormal, urinary frequency

Overdosage/Toxicology Symptoms of overdose include acute renal failure, vomiting, drowsiness, and leukocytes. Management of NSAID intoxication is supportive and symptomatic. Since many NSAIDs undergo enterohepatic cycling, multiple doses of char-coal may be needed to reduce the potential for delayed toxicities.

(Continued)

Oxaprozin *(Continued)*

Pharmacodynamics/Kinetics
Onset of Action: Steady-state 4-7 days
Time to Peak: 2-4 hours
Protein Binding: >99%
Half-Life Elimination: 40-50 hours
Metabolism: Hepatic via oxidation and glucuronidation; no active metabolites
Excretion: Urine (5% unchanged, 65% as metabolites); feces (35% as metabolites)

Available Dosage Forms Tablet: 600 mg

Dosing
Adults & Elderly:
Osteoarthritis: Oral: 600-1200 mg once daily; patients should be titrated to lowest dose possible; patients with low body weight should start with 600 mg daily
Rheumatoid arthritis: Oral: 1200 mg once daily; a one-time loading dose of up to 1800 mg/day or 26 mg/kg (whichever is lower) may be given
Maximun doses:
Patient <50 kg: Maximum: 1200 mg/day
Patient >50 kg with normal renal/hepatic function and low risk of peptic ulcer: Maximum: 1800 mg or 26 mg/kg (whichever is lower) in divided doses

Pediatrics:
Juvenile rheumatoid arthritis: Oral:
Note: Individualize to lowest effective dose.
Children 6-16 years:
22-31 kg: 600 mg once daily
32-54 kg: 900 mg once daily
≥55 kg: 1200 mg once daily

Renal Impairment: In general NSAIDs are not recommended for use in patients with advanced renal disease but the manufacturer of oxaprozin does provide some guidelines for adjustment in renal dysfunction.
Severe renal impairment or on dialysis: 600 mg once daily, may increase cautiously to 1200 mg/day with close monitoring.

Hepatic Impairment: Use caution in patients with severe dysfunction.

Stability
Storage: Store at 25°C (77°F). Protect from light. Keep bottle tightly closed.

Laboratory Monitoring CBC; hepatic, renal function

Nursing Actions
Physical Assessment: Assess effectiveness and interactions of other medications patient may be taking. Monitor blood pressure at the beginning of therapy and periodically during use. Monitor laboratory tests, therapeutic response (eg, relief of pain and inflammation, increased activity tolerance), and adverse reactions (eg, GI effects, hepatotoxicity, or ototoxicity) at beginning of therapy and periodically throughout therapy. Schedule ophthalmic evaluations for patients who develop eye complaints during long-term NSAID therapy. Assess knowledge/teach patient appropriate use, interventions to reduce side effects, and adverse symptoms to report

Patient Education: Take this medication exactly as directed; do not increase dose without consulting prescriber. Do not crush tablets. Take with food or milk to reduce GI distress. Maintain adequate hydration (2-3 L/day of fluids) unless instructed to restrict fluid intake. Do not use alcohol, aspirin or aspirin-containing medication, or any other anti-inflammatory medications without consulting prescriber. You may experience drowsiness, dizziness, or nervousness (use caution when driving or engaging in tasks requiring alertness until response to drug is known); anorexia, nausea, vomiting, or heartburn (small frequent meals, frequent mouth care, sucking lozenges, or chewing gum may help). GI bleeding, ulceration, or perforation can occur with or without pain. Discontinue medication and contact prescriber if persistent abdominal pain, cramping, or blood in stool occurs. Report vaginal bleeding; breathlessness, respiratory difficulty, or unusual cough; chest pain, rapid heartbeat, palpitations; unusual bruising or bleeding (blood in urine, mouth, or vomitus); swollen extremities; skin rash or itching; acute fatigue; or swelling of face, lips, tongue, or throat. **Pregnancy/breast-feeding precautions:** Inform prescriber if you are or intend to become pregnant. This drug should not be used in the 3rd trimester of pregnancy. Breast-feeding is not recommended.

Geriatric Considerations Elderly are at high risk for adverse effects from NSAIDs. As much as 60% of elderly can develop peptic ulceration and/or hemorrhage asymptomatically. The concomitant use of H₂ blockers, omeprazole, and sucralfate is not generally effective as prophylaxis with the exception of NSAID-induced duodenal ulcers which may be prevented by the use of ranitidine. Misoprostol is the only prophylactic agent proven effective. Also, concomitant disease and drug use contribute to the risk for GI adverse effects. Use lowest effective dose for shortest period possible. Consider renal function decline with age. Use of NSAIDs can compromise existing renal function especially when Cl$_{cr}$ is ≤30 mL/minute. Tinnitus may be a difficult and unreliable indication of toxicity due to age-related hearing loss or eighth cranial nerve damage. CNS adverse effects such as confusion, agitation, and hallucination are generally seen in overdose or high-dose situations, but elderly may demonstrate these adverse effects at lower doses than younger adults.

Pregnancy Issues Safety and efficacy in pregnant women have not been established. Exposure late in pregnancy may lead to premature closure of the ductus arteriosus and may inhibit uterine contractions.

Oxazepam *(oks A ze pam)*

U.S. Brand Names Serax®
Restrictions C-IV
Pharmacologic Category Benzodiazepine
Medication Safety Issues
Sound-alike/look-alike issues:
Oxazepam may be confused with oxaprozin, quazepam
Serax® may be confused with Eurax®, Urex®, Zyrtec®

Pregnancy Risk Factor D
Lactation Enters breast milk/not recommended
Use Treatment of anxiety; management of ethanol withdrawal
Unlabeled/Investigational Use Anticonvulsant in management of simple partial seizures; hypnotic
Mechanism of Action/Effect Binds to stereospecific benzodiazepine receptors on the postsynaptic GABA neuron at several sites within the central nervous system, including the limbic system, reticular formation. Enhancement of the inhibitory effect of GABA on neuronal excitability results by increased neuronal membrane permeability to chloride ions. This shift in chloride ions results in hyperpolarization (a less excitable state) and stabilization.
Contraindications Hypersensitivity to oxazepam or any component of the formulation (cross-sensitivity with other benzodiazepines may exist); narrow-angle glaucoma (not in product labeling, however, benzodiazepines are contraindicated); not indicated for use in the treatment of psychosis; pregnancy
Warnings/Precautions May cause hypotension (rare) - use with caution in patients with cardiovascular or cerebrovascular disease, or in patients who would not tolerate transient decreases in blood pressure. Serax®

15 mg tablet contains tartrazine; use is not recommended in pediatric patients <6 years of age; dose has not been established between 6-12 years of age.

Use with caution in elderly or debilitated patients, patients with hepatic disease (including alcoholics), or renal impairment. Use with caution in patients with respiratory disease or impaired gag reflex. Avoid use in patients with sleep apnea.

Causes CNS depression (dose-related) resulting in sedation, dizziness, confusion, or ataxia which may impair physical and mental capabilities. Use with caution in patients receiving other CNS depressants or psychoactive agents. Benzodiazepines have been associated with falls and traumatic injury and should be used with extreme caution in patients who are at risk of these events (especially the elderly).

Use caution in patients with depression, particularly if suicidal risk may be present. Use with caution in patients with a history of drug dependence. Benzodiazepines have been associated with dependence and acute withdrawal symptoms on discontinuation or reduction in dose.

Benzodiazepines have been associated with anterograde amnesia. Paradoxical reactions, including hyperactive or aggressive behavior have been reported with benzodiazepines, particularly in adolescent/pediatric or psychiatric patients. Does not have analgesic, antidepressant, or antipsychotic properties.

Drug Interactions
Decreased Effect: Oral contraceptives may increase the clearance of oxazepam. Theophylline and other CNS stimulants may antagonize the sedative effects of oxazepam. Phenytoin may increase the clearance of oxazepam.

Increased Effect/Toxicity: Ethanol and other CNS depressants may increase the CNS effects of oxazepam. Oxazepam may decrease the antiparkinsonian efficacy of levodopa. Flumazenil may cause seizures if administered following long-term benzodiazepine treatment.

Nutritional/Ethanol Interactions

Ethanol: Avoid ethanol (may increase CNS depression).

Herb/Nutraceutical: Avoid valerian, St John's wort, kava kava, gotu kola (may increase CNS depression).

Adverse Reactions Frequency not defined.

Cardiovascular: Syncope (rare), edema

Central nervous system: Drowsiness, ataxia, dizziness, vertigo, memory impairment, headache, paradoxical reactions (excitement, stimulation of effect), lethargy, amnesia, euphoria

Dermatologic: Rash

Endocrine & metabolic: Decreased libido, menstrual irregularities

Genitourinary: Incontinence

Hematologic: Leukopenia, blood dyscrasias

Hepatic: Jaundice

Neuromuscular & skeletal: Dysarthria, tremor, reflex slowing

Ocular: Blurred vision, diplopia

Miscellaneous: Drug dependence

Overdosage/Toxicology Symptoms of overdose include somnolence, confusion, coma, hypoactive reflexes, dyspnea, hypotension, slurred speech, and impaired coordination. Treatment for benzodiazepine overdose is supportive. Flumazenil has been shown to selectively block the binding of benzodiazepines to CNS receptors, resulting in a reversal of benzodiazepine-induced CNS depression, but not respiratory depression due to toxicity.

Pharmacodynamics/Kinetics
Time to Peak: Serum: 2-4 hours
Protein Binding: 86% to 99%
Half-Life Elimination: 2.8-5.7 hours
Metabolism: Hepatic to inactive compounds (primarily as glucuronides)
Excretion: Urine (as unchanged drug (50%) and metabolites)
Available Dosage Forms
Capsule: 10 mg, 15 mg, 30 mg
Tablet: 15 mg [contains tartrazine]
Dosing
Adults:
Anxiety: Oral: 10-30 mg 3-4 times/day
Ethanol withdrawal: Oral: 15-30 mg 3-4 times/day
Hypnotic: Oral: 15-30 mg
Elderly: Oral: Anxiety: 10 mg 2-3 times/day; increase gradually as needed to a total of 30-45 mg/day. Dose titration should be slow to evaluate sensitivity.
Pediatrics:
Anxiety: Oral: Children: 1 mg/kg/day has been administered
Renal Impairment: Not dialyzable (0% to 5%)
Administration
Oral: Give orally in divided doses
Nursing Actions
Physical Assessment: Assess other medications the patient may be taking for effectiveness and interactions. Assess for history of addiction; long-term use can result in dependence, abuse, or tolerance; periodically evaluate need for continued use. For inpatient use, institute safety measures and monitor effectiveness and adverse reactions. For outpatients, monitor therapeutic effectiveness and adverse reactions at beginning of therapy and periodically with long-term use. Can cause CNS depression (dose-related), monitor for sedation, dizziness, confusion, or ataxia which may impair physical and mental capabilities. Be alert to the possibility of suicide ideation. Assess knowledge/teach patient appropriate use, interventions to reduce side effects, and adverse symptoms to report.

Patient Education: Take exactly as directed; do not increase dose or frequency. It may take 2-3 weeks to achieve desired results. Drug may cause physical and/or psychological dependence. Do not use alcohol or other prescription or OTC medications (especially pain medications, sedatives, antihistamines, or hypnotics) without consulting prescriber. Maintain adequate hydration (2-3 L/day of fluids) unless instructed to restrict fluid intake. You may experience drowsiness, lightheadedness, impaired coordination, dizziness, or blurred vision (use caution when driving or engaging in tasks requiring alertness until response to drug is known); nausea, vomiting, or dry mouth (small frequent meals, frequent mouth care, chewing gum, or sucking lozenges may help); constipation (increased exercise, fluids, fruit, or fiber may help); altered sexual drive or ability (reversible); or photosensitivity (use sunscreen, wear protective clothing and eyewear, and avoid direct sunlight). Report persistent CNS effects (eg, confusion, depression, thoughts of suicide, increased sedation, excitation, headache, agitation, insomnia or nightmares, dizziness, fatigue, impaired coordination, changes in personality, or changes in cognition); changes in urinary pattern; muscle cramping, weakness, tremors, or rigidity; ringing in ears or visual disturbances; chest pain, palpitations, or rapid heartbeat; excessive perspiration; excessive GI symptoms (cramping, constipation, vomiting, anorexia); or worsening of condition.
Pregnancy/breast-feeding precautions: Do not get pregnant while taking this medication; use appropriate contraceptive measures. Breast-feeding is not recommended.
(Continued)

Oxazepam *(Continued)*

Geriatric Considerations Because of its relatively short half-life and its lack of active metabolites, oxazepam is recommended for use in the elderly when a benzodiazepine is indicated.

Pregnancy Issues Benzodiazepines cross the placenta. The association between benzodiazepine exposure and malformations remains controversial. A number of types of malformation have been reported (oral cleft, inguinal hernia, cardiac defects, spina bifida, dysmorphic facial features, skeletal defects); however, confounding factors make a clear association difficult. Overall, the risk to the fetus may be low. Nonteratogenic effects (including neonatal flaccidity, respiratory and feeding problems, and withdrawal symptoms) during the postnatal period have also been reported with benzodiazepine use.

Other Issues Taper dosage gradually after long-term therapy, especially in epileptic patients. Abrupt withdrawal may cause tremors, nausea, vomiting, abdominal and/or muscle cramps.

Additional Information Not intended for management of anxieties and minor distresses associated with everyday life. Treatment longer than 4 months should be re-evaluated to determine the patient's need for the drug. Abrupt discontinuation after sustained use (generally >10 days) may cause withdrawal symptoms.

Related Information

Anxiolytic / Hypnotic Use in Long-Term Care Facilities *on page 1418*

Federal OBRA Regulations Recommended Maximum Doses *on page 1421*

Oxcarbazepine *(ox car BAZ e peen)*

U.S. Brand Names Trileptal®

Synonyms GP 47680; OCBZ

Pharmacologic Category Anticonvulsant, Miscellaneous

Pregnancy Risk Factor C

Lactation Enters breast milk/not recommended

Use Monotherapy or adjunctive therapy in the treatment of partial seizures in adults and children ≥4 years of age with epilepsy; adjunctive therapy in the treatment of partial seizures in children ≥2 years of age with epilepsy.

Unlabeled/Investigational Use Bipolar disorder; treatment of neuropathic pain

Mechanism of Action/Effect Precise mechanism of action has not been determined. Believed to prevent the spread of seizures by decreasing propagation of synaptic impulses.

Contraindications Hypersensitivity to oxcarbazepine or any component of the formulation

Warnings/Precautions Clinically-significant hyponatremia (sodium <125 mmol/L) can develop during oxcarbazepine use; monitor serum sodium, particularly during the first 3 months of therapy or in patients at risk for hyponatremia. Potentially serious, sometimes fatal, dermatologic reactions (eg, Stevens-Johnson, toxic epidermal necrolysis) and hypersensitivity reactions have been reported in adults and children; monitor for signs and symptoms of skin reactions and possible disparate manifestations associated with lymphatic, hepatic, renal and/or hematologic organ systems; gradual discontinuation and conversion to alternate therapy may be required. As with all antiepileptic drugs, oxcarbazepine should be withdrawn gradually to minimize the potential of increased seizure frequency. Use of oxcarbazepine has been associated with CNS related adverse events, most significant of these were cognitive symptoms including psychomotor slowing, difficulty with concentration, and speech or language problems, somnolence or fatigue, and coordination abnormalities, including ataxia and gait disturbances. Use caution in patients with previous hypersensitivity to carbamazepine (cross-sensitivity occurs in 25% to 30%). May reduce the efficacy of oral contraceptives (nonhormonal contraceptive measures are recommended).

Drug Interactions

Cytochrome P450 Effect: Inhibits CYP2C19 (weak); **Induces** CYP3A4 (strong)

Decreased Effect: Oxcarbazepine serum concentrations may be reduced by carbamazepine, phenytoin, phenobarbital, valproic acid and verapamil (decreases levels of active oxcarbazepine metabolite). Oxcarbazepine reduces the serum concentrations of hormonal contraceptives; use alternative contraceptive measures. Oxcarbazepine may decrease the levels/effects of benzodiazepines, calcium channel blockers, clarithromycin, cyclosporine, erythromycin, estrogens, mirtazapine, nateglinide, nefazodone, nevirapine, protease inhibitors, tacrolimus, venlafaxine, and other CYP3A4 substrates.

Increased Effect/Toxicity: Serum concentrations of phenytoin and phenobarbital are increased by oxcarbazepine.

Nutritional/Ethanol Interactions

Ethanol: Avoid ethanol (may increase CNS depression).

Herb/Nutraceutical: St John's wort may decrease oxcarbazepine levels. Avoid evening primrose (seizure threshold decreased). Avoid valerian, St John's wort, kava kava, gotu kola.

Lab Interactions Thyroid function tests may depress serum T_4 without affecting T_3 levels or TSH.

Adverse Reactions As reported in adults with doses of up to 2400 mg/day (includes patients on monotherapy, adjunctive therapy, and those not previously on AEDs); incidence in children was similar.

>10%:

Central nervous system: Dizziness (22% to 49%), somnolence (20% to 36%), headache (13% to 32%, placebo 23%), ataxia (5% to 31%), fatigue (12% to 15%), vertigo (6% to 15%)

Gastrointestinal: Vomiting (7% to 36%), nausea (15% to 29%), abdominal pain (10% to 13%)

Neuromuscular & skeletal: Abnormal gait (5% to 17%), tremor (3% to 16%)

Ocular: Diplopia (14% to 40%), nystagmus (7% to 26%), abnormal vision (4% to 14%)

1% to 10%:

Cardiovascular: Hypotension (1% to 2%), leg edema (1% to 2%, placebo 1%)

Central nervous system: Nervousness (2% to 5%, placebo 1% to 2%), amnesia (4%), abnormal thinking (2% to 4%), insomnia (2% to 4%), speech disorder (1% to 3%), EEG abnormalities (2%), abnormal feelings (1% to 2%), agitation (1% to 2%, placebo 1%), confusion (1% to 2%, placebo 1%)

Dermatologic: Rash (4%), acne (1% to 2%)

Endocrine & metabolic: Hyponatremia (1% to 3%, placebo 1%)

Gastrointestinal: Diarrhea (5% to 7%), dyspepsia (5% to 6%), constipation (2% to 6%, placebo 0% to 4%), gastritis (1% to 2%, placebo 1%), weight gain (1% to 2%, placebo 1%)

Neuromuscular & skeletal: Weakness (3% to 6%, placebo 5%), back pain (4%), falling down (4%), abnormal coordination (1% to 4%, placebo 1% to 2%), dysmetria (1% to 3%), sprains/strains (2%), muscle weakness (1% to 2%)

Ocular: Abnormal accommodation (2%)

Respiratory: Upper respiratory tract infection (7%), rhinitis (2% to 5%, placebo 4%), chest infection (4%), epistaxis (4%), sinusitis (4%)

Overdosage/Toxicology Symptoms may include CNS depression (somnolence, ataxia). Treatment is symptomatic and supportive.

Pharmacodynamics/Kinetics

Time to Peak: Serum: 4.5 hours (3-13 hours)

Protein Binding: Serum: MHD: 40%

Half-Life Elimination: Parent drug: 2 hours; MHD: 9 hours; renal impairment (Cl_{cr} 30 mL/minute): MHD: 19 hours

Clearance of MHD is increased in younger children (~80% in children 2-4 years of age) and approaches that of adults by ~13 years of age

Metabolism: Hepatic to 10-monohydroxy metabolite (MHD; active); MHD is further conjugated to DHD (inactive)

Excretion: Urine (95%, <1% as unchanged oxcarbazepine, 27% as unchanged MHD, 49% as MHD glucuronides); feces (<4%)

Available Dosage Forms

Suspension, oral: 300 mg/5 mL (250 mL) [contains ethanol; packaged with oral syringe]

Tablet: 150 mg, 300 mg, 600 mg

Dosing

Adults & Elderly:

Adjunctive therapy, partial seizures (epilepsy): Oral: Initial: 300 mg twice daily; dosage may be increased by 600 mg/day at approximate weekly intervals. Recommended daily dose is 1200 mg/day in 2 divided doses. Although daily doses >1200 mg/day demonstrated greater efficacy, most patients were unable to tolerate 2400 mg/day (due to CNS effects).

Conversion to monotherapy, partial seizures (epilepsy): Oral: Patients receiving concomitant antiepileptic drugs (AEDs): Initial: 300 mg twice daily while simultaneously reducing the dose of concomitant AEDs. Withdraw concomitant AEDs completely over 3-6 weeks, while increasing the oxcarbazine dose in increments of 600 mg/day at weekly intervals, reaching the maximum oxcarbazine dose (2400 mg/day) in about 2-4 weeks (lower doses have been effective in patients in whom monotherapy has been initiated).

Initiation of monotherapy, partial seizures (epilepsy): Oral: Patients not receiving prior AEDs: 300 mg twice daily (total dose 600 mg/day). Increase dose by 300 mg/day every third day to a dose of 1200 mg/day. Higher dosages (2400 mg/day) have been shown to be effective in patients converted to monotherapy from other AEDs.

Pediatrics:

Adjunctive treatment, partial seizures (epilepsy): Oral: Children 2-3 years:

Initial: 8-10 mg/kg/day (not to exceed 600 mg/day) given in a twice daily regimen.

Maintenance: The target maintenance dose should be achieved over 2 weeks, and depends on weight of the child:

<20 kg: 600 mg/day in 2 divided doses; consider initiating dose at 16-20 mg/kg/day; maximum maintenance dose should be achieved over 2-4 weeks and should not exceed 60 mg/kg/day

Adjunctive treatment, partial seizures (epilepsy): Oral: Children 4-16 years:

Initial: 8-10 mg/kg/day (not to exceed 600 mg/day) given in a twice daily regimen.

Maintenance: The target maintenance dose should be achieved over 2 weeks, and depends on weight of the child:

20-29 kg: 900 mg/day in 2 divided doses

29.1-39 kg: 1200 mg/day in 2 divided doses

>39 kg: 1800 mg/day in 2 divided doses

Conversion to monotherapy: Children 4-16 years: Oxcarbazepine 8-10 mg/kg/day in twice daily divided doses, while simultaneously initiating the reduction of the dose of the concomitant antiepileptic drug; the concomitant drug should be withdrawn over 3-6 weeks. Oxcarbazepine dose may be increased by a maximum of 10 mg/kg/day at

weekly intervals. See below for recommended total daily dose by weight.

Initiation of monotherapy: Children 4-16 years: Oxcarbazepine should be initiated at 8-10 mg/kg/day in twice daily divided doses; doses may be titrated by 5 mg/kg/day every third day. See below for recommended total daily dose by weight.

Range of maintenance doses by weight during monotherapy:

20 kg: 600-900 mg/day

25-30 kg: 900-1200 mg/day

35-40 kg: 900-1500 mg/day

45 kg: 1200-1500 mg/day

50-55 kg: 1200-1800 mg/day

60-65 kg: 1200-2100 mg/day

70 kg: 1500-2100 mg/day

Renal Impairment: Cl_{cr} <30 mL/minute: Therapy should be initiated at one-half the usual starting dose (300 mg/day in adults) and increased slowly to achieve the desired clinical response

Hepatic Impairment: No dosage adjustment recommended in mild to moderate hepatic impairment. Patients with severe hepatic impairment have not been evaluated.

Administration

Oral: Suspension: Prior to using for the first time, firmly insert the plastic adapter provided with the bottle. Cover adapter with child-resistant cap when not in use. Shake bottle for at least 10 seconds, remove child-resistant cap and insert the oral dosing syringe provided to withdraw appropriate dose. Dose may be taken directly from oral syringe or may be mixed in a small glass of water immediately prior to swallowing. Rinse syringe with warm water after use and allow to dry thoroughly. Discard any unused portion after 7 weeks of first opening bottle.

Stability

Storage: Store tablets and suspension at 25°C (77°F). Use suspension within 7 weeks of first opening container.

Laboratory Monitoring Serum sodium (particularly during first 3 months of therapy); additional serum sodium monitoring is recommended during maintenance treatment in patients receiving other medications known to decrease sodium levels, in patients with signs/symptoms of hyponatremia, and in patients with an increase in seizure frequency or severity.

Nursing Actions

Physical Assessment: Determine absence of any allergic reactions to other anticonvulsants (carbamazepine). Assess effectiveness and interactions of other medications. Monitor therapeutic effectiveness (seizure activity, frequency, duration, type), laboratory results, and adverse reactions (eg, sedation, CNS changes, visual changes). Monitor for skin reactions. Dosage should be tapered when discontinuing to reduce risk of increased seizures. Assess knowledge/teach patient appropriate use, interventions to reduce side effects, and adverse reactions to report. **Note:** Oxcarbazepine may reduce the effectiveness of oral contraceptives, nonhormonal contraception is recommended.

Patient Education: Do not increase dose or frequency or discontinue without consulting prescriber. While using the medication do not use alcohol and other prescription or OTC medications (especially medications to relieve pain, induce sleep, reduce anxiety, treat or prevent cold, coughs, or allergies) unless approved by prescriber. Maintain adequate hydration (2-3 L/day of fluids) unless instructed to restrict fluid intake. You may experience drowsiness, dizziness, or blurred vision (use caution when driving or engaging in tasks requiring alertness until response to drug is known); nausea or vomiting (small frequent meals, good mouth care, chewing gum, or sucking hard candy may help, or contact

(Continued)

Oxcarbazepine *(Continued)*

prescriber). Report CNS changes, increase in seizure frequency or severity, mentation changes, changes in cognition or memory, acute fatigue or weakness, or insomnia; muscle cramping, weakness, or pain; rash or skin irritations; unusual bruising or bleeding (mouth, urine, stool); swelling of extremities; or other adverse response. **Pregnancy/breast-feeding precautions:** Inform prescriber if you are or intend to become pregnant. **Note:** Oxcarbazepine may reduce the effectiveness of oral contraceptives, nonhormonal contraception is recommended. Breast-feeding is not recommended.

Dietary Considerations May be taken with or without food.

Geriatric Considerations Studies in elderly volunteers (60-82 years of age) with both single dose (300 mg) and multiple doses (600 mg/day) reported maximum plasma concentrations and AUC as being 30% to 60% higher than younger volunteers (18-32 years of age). These results were due to differences in creatinine clearance between the two groups. Since elderly may have Cl_{cr} <30 mL/minute, dose reductions may be needed. See dosing information.

Breast-Feeding Issues Oxcarbazepine and its active metabolite (MHD) are excreted in human breast milk. A milk-to-plasma concentration ratio of 0.5 was found for both. Because of the potential for serious adverse reactions to oxcarbazepine in nursing infants, a decision should be made whether to discontinue nursing or to discontinue the drug in nursing women.

Pregnancy Issues Although many epidemiological studies of congenital anomalies in infants born to women treated with various anticonvulsants during pregnancy have been reported, none of these investigations includes enough women treated with oxcarbazepine to assess possible teratogenic effects of this drug. Given that teratogenic effects have been observed in animal studies, and that oxcarbazepine is structurally related to carbamazepine (teratogenic in humans), use during pregnancy only if the benefit to the mother outweighs the potential risk to the fetus.

Oxybutynin *(oks i BYOO ti nin)*

U.S. Brand Names Ditropan®; Ditropan® XL; Oxytrol®
Synonyms Oxybutynin Chloride
Pharmacologic Category Antispasmodic Agent, Urinary
Medication Safety Issues
Sound-alike/look-alike issues:
Oxybutynin may be confused with OxyContin®
Ditropan® may be confused with Detrol®, diazepam, Diprivan®, dithranol

Transdermal patch may contain conducting metal (eg, aluminum); remove patch prior to MRI.
Pregnancy Risk Factor B
Lactation Excretion in breast milk unknown/use caution
Use Antispasmodic for neurogenic bladder (urgency, frequency, urge incontinence) and uninhibited bladder
Mechanism of Action/Effect Direct antispasmodic effect on smooth muscle, also inhibits the action of acetylcholine on smooth muscle (exhibits $\frac{1}{5}$ the anticholinergic activity of atropine, but is 4-10 times the antispasmodic activity); does not block effects at skeletal muscle or at autonomic ganglia; increases bladder capacity, decreases uninhibited contractions, and delays desire to void; therefore, decreases urgency and frequency
Contraindications Hypersensitivity to oxybutynin or any component of the formulation; untreated glaucoma; partial or complete GI obstruction; GU obstruction; urinary retention; megacolon; toxic megacolon

Warnings/Precautions Use with caution in patients with urinary tract obstruction, angle-closure glaucoma (treated), hyperthyroidism, reflux esophagitis (including concurrent therapy with oral bisphosphonates or drugs which may increase the risk of esophagitis), heart disease, hepatic or renal disease, prostatic hyperplasia, autonomic neuropathy, ulcerative colitis (may cause ileus and toxic megacolon), hypertension, hiatal hernia, myasthenia gravis, ulcerative colitis, or intestinal atony. Transdermal patch may contain conducting metal (eg, aluminum); remove patch prior to MRI. Avoid use of extended release tablets (Ditropan® XL) in patients with known stricture/narrowing of the GI tract. Caution should be used in elderly due to anticholinergic activity (eg, confusion, constipation, blurred vision, and tachycardia). May increase the risk of heat prostration.

Drug Interactions
Cytochrome P450 Effect: Substrate of CYP3A4 (minor); **Inhibits** CYP2D6 (weak), 3A4 (weak)
Increased Effect/Toxicity: Additive sedation with CNS depressants and ethanol. Additive anticholinergic effects with antihistamines and anticholinergic agents.
Nutritional/Ethanol Interactions Ethanol: Use ethanol with caution (may increase CNS depression and toxicity). Watch for sedation.
Lab Interactions May suppress the wheal and flare reactions to skin test antigens.
Adverse Reactions
Oral:
>10%:
Central nervous system: Dizziness (6% to 16%), somnolence (12% to 13%)
Gastrointestinal: Xerostomia (61% to 71%), constipation (13%)
Genitourinary: Urination impaired (11%)
1% to 10%:
Cardiovascular: Palpitation (2% to <5%), peripheral edema (2% to <5%), hypertension (2% to <5%), vasodilation (2% to <5%)
Central nervous system: Headache (6% to 10%), pain (7%), confusion (2% to <5%), insomnia (2% to <5%), nervousness (2% to <5%)
Dermatologic: Dry skin (2% to <5%), skin rash (2% to <5%)
Gastrointestinal: Nausea (9% to 10%), dyspepsia (7%), abdominal pain (2% to 6%), diarrhea (5% to 9%), flatulence (2% to <5%), gastrointestinal reflux (2% to <5%), taste perversion (2% to <5%)
Genitourinary: Postvoid residuals increased (2% to 9%), urinary tract infection (5%)
Neuromuscular & skeletal: Weakness (2% to 7%)
Ocular: Blurred vision (8% to 9%), dry eyes (2% to 6%)
Respiratory: Rhinitis (6%), dry nasal and sinus membranes (2% to <5%)
Transdermal:
>10%: Local: Application site reaction (17%), pruritus (14%)
1% to 10%:
Gastrointestinal: Xerostomia (4% to 10%), diarrhea (3%), constipation (3%)
Genitourinary: Dysuria (2%)
Local: Erythema (6% to 8%), vesicles (3%), rash (3%)
Ocular: Vision changes (3%)
Overdosage/Toxicology Symptoms of overdose include hypotension, circulatory failure, psychotic behavior, flushing, respiratory failure, paralysis, tremor, irritability, seizures, delirium, hallucinations, and coma. Treatment is symptomatic and supportive. For anticholinergic overdose with severe life-threatening symptoms, physostigmine 1-2 mg I.V. slowly, may be given to reverse these effects.
Pharmacodynamics/Kinetics
Onset of Action: Onset of action: Oral: 30-60 minutes; Peak effect: 3-6 hours

Duration of Action: 6-10 hours (up to 24 hours for extended release oral formulation)

Time to Peak: Serum: Oral: ~60 minutes; Transdermal: 24-48 hours

Half-Life Elimination: I.V.: ~2 hours (parent drug), 7-8 hours (metabolites)

Metabolism: Hepatic via CYP3A4; Oral: High first-pass metabolism; I.V.: Forms active and inactive metabolites

Excretion: Urine (<0.1%)

Available Dosage Forms

Syrup, as chloride: 5 mg/5 mL (473 mL)
  Ditropan®: 5 mg/5 mL (473 ml)
Tablet, as chloride: 5 mg
  Ditropan®: 5 mg
Tablet, extended release, as chloride:
  Ditropan® XL: 5 mg, 10 mg, 15 mg
Transdermal system:
  Oxytrol®: 3.9 mg/day (8s) [39 cm²; total oxybutynin 36 mg]

Dosing

Adults:

Bladder spasms:

Oral:
  Regular release: 5 mg 2-3 times/day up to maximum of 5 mg 4 times/day
  Extended release: Initial: 5-10 mg once daily, may increase in 5-10 mg increments; maximum: 30 mg daily

Transdermal: Apply one 3.9 mg/day patch twice weekly (every 3-4 days)

Note: Should be discontinued periodically to determine whether the patient can manage without the drug and to minimize resistance to the drug.

Elderly:

Oral: 2.5-5 mg 2-3 times/day

Transdermal: Refer to adult dosing. **Note:** Should be discontinued periodically to determine whether the patient can manage without the drug and to minimize resistance to the drug.

Pediatrics:

Bladder spasms: Oral: Children:
  1-5 years (unlabeled use): 0.2 mg/kg/dose 2-4 times/day
  >5 years: 5 mg twice daily, up to 5 mg 3 times/day maximum
  >6 years: Extended release: 5 mg once daily; maximum dose: 20 mg/day

Administration

Oral: Immediate release tablets and solution should be administered on an empty stomach with water. Extended release tablets may be taken with or without food and must be swallowed whole; do not crush, divide, or chew.

Other: Transdermal: Apply to clean, dry skin on abdomen, hip, or buttock. Select a new site for each new system (avoid reapplication to same site within 7 days).

Stability

Storage: Store at controlled room temperature. Protect syrup from light. Keep transdermal patch in sealed pouch.

Nursing Actions

Physical Assessment: Assess other medications patient may be taking for interactions. Assess voiding pattern, incontinent episodes, frequency, urgency, distention, and urinary retention prior to beginning therapy and periodically with long-term use. Assess knowledge/teach patient appropriate use, possible side effects, and symptoms to report.

Patient Education: Take prescribed oral dose preferably on an empty stomach, 1 hour before or 2 hours after meals. Swallow extended-release tablets whole, do not chew or crush. You may experience dizziness, lightheadedness, or drowsiness (use caution when driving or engaging in tasks requiring alertness until

response to drug is known); dry mouth or changes in appetite (small frequent meals, frequent mouth care, sucking lozenges, or chewing gum may help); constipation (increased exercise, fluids, fruit, fiber, or stool softener may help); decreased sexual ability (reversible with discontinuance of drug); or decreased sweating (use caution in hot weather, avoid extreme exercise or activity). Use alcohol with caution; may increase drowsiness. Report rapid heartbeat, palpitations, or chest pain; difficulty voiding; or vision changes.

Dietary Considerations Food causes a slight delay in the absorption of the oral solution and bioavailability is deceased by ~25%. Absorption of the extended release tablet is not affected by food.

Geriatric Considerations Caution should be used in the elderly due to anticholinergic activity (eg, confusion, constipation, blurred vision, and tachycardia). Start with lower doses. Transdermal dosage form may have less potential for these effects. Oxybutynin may cause memory problems in the elderly. A study of 12 healthy volunteers with an average age of 69 showed cognitive decline while taking the drug (*J Am Geriatr Soc*, 1998, L46:8-13).

Breast-Feeding Issues Suppression of lactation has been reported (rarely).

Oxycodone (oks i KOE done)

U.S. Brand Names OxyContin®; Oxydose™; OxyFast®; OxyIR®; Roxicodone™; Roxicodone™ Intensol™

Synonyms Dihydrohydroxycodeinone; Oxycodone Hydrochloride

Restrictions C-II

Pharmacologic Category Analgesic, Narcotic

Medication Safety Issues

Sound-alike/look-alike issues:
  Oxycodone may be confused with OxyContin®
  OxyContin® may be confused with oxybutynin, oxycodone
  OxyFast® may be confused with Roxanol™

Pregnancy Risk Factor B/D (prolonged use or high doses at term)

Lactation Enters breast milk/use caution

Use Management of moderate to severe pain, normally used in combination with non-narcotic analgesics

OxyContin® is indicated for around-the-clock management of moderate to severe pain when an analgesic is needed for an extended period of time. **Note:** OxyContin® is not intended for use as an "as needed" analgesic or for immediately-postoperative pain management (should be used postoperatively only if the patient has received it prior to surgery or if severe, persistent pain is anticipated).

Mechanism of Action/Effect Binds to opiate receptors in the CNS, causing inhibition of ascending pain pathways, altering the perception of and response to pain; produces generalized CNS depression

Contraindications Hypersensitivity to oxycodone or any component of the formulation; significant respiratory depression; hypercarbia; acute or severe bronchial asthma; OxyContin® is also contraindicated in paralytic ileus (known or suspected); pregnancy (prolonged use or high doses at term)

Warnings/Precautions Use with caution in patients with hypersensitivity reactions to other phenanthrene derivative opioid agonists (morphine, hydrocodone, hydromorphone, levorphanol, oxycodone, oxymorphone), respiratory diseases including asthma, emphysema, or COPD. Use with caution in pancreatitis or biliary tract disease, acute alcoholism (including delirium tremens), adrenocortical insufficiency, CNS depression/coma, kyphoscoliosis (or other skeletal disorder which may alter respiratory function), hypothyroidism (Continued)

927

Oxycodone *(Continued)*

(including myxedema), prostatic hyperplasia, urethral stricture, and toxic psychosis.

Use with caution in the elderly, debilitated, severe hepatic or renal function. Hemodynamic effects (hypotension, orthostasis) may be exaggerated in patients with hypovolemia, concurrent vasodilating drugs, or in patients with head injury. Respiratory depressant effects and capacity to elevate CSF pressure may be exaggerated in presence of head injury, other intracranial lesion, or pre-existing intracranial pressure. Tolerance or drug dependence may result from extended use. Healthcare provider should be alert to problems of abuse, misuse, and diversion. Do **not** crush controlled-release tablets. Some preparations contain sulfites which may cause allergic reactions. OxyContin® 80 mg and 160 mg strengths are for use only in opioid-tolerant patients requiring high daily dosages >160 mg (80 mg formulation) or >320 mg (160 mg formulation).

Drug Interactions

Cytochrome P450 Effect: Substrate of CYP2D6 (major)

Increased Effect/Toxicity: MAO inhibitors may increase adverse symptoms. Cimetidine may increase narcotic analgesic serum levels resulting in toxicity. CNS depressants (barbiturates, ethanol) and TCAs may potentiate the sedative and respiratory depressive effects of morphine and other opiate agonists. Dextroamphetamine may enhance the analgesic effect of morphine and other opiate agonists.

Nutritional/Ethanol Interactions

Ethanol: Avoid ethanol (may increase CNS depression).

Food: When taken with a high-fat meal, peak concentration is 25% greater following a single OxyContin® 160 mg tablet as compared to two 80 mg tablets.

Herb/Nutraceutical: Avoid valerian, St John's wort, kava kava, gotu kola (may increase CNS depression).

Lab Interactions

Some quinolones may produce a false-positive urine screening result for opiates using commercially-available immunoassay kits. This has been demonstrated most consistently for levofloxacin and ofloxacin, but other quinolones have shown cross-reactivity in certain assay kits. Confirmation of positive opiate screens by more specific methods should be considered.

Adverse Reactions

>10%:

Central nervous system: Fatigue, drowsiness, dizziness, somnolence

Dermatologic: Pruritus

Gastrointestinal: Nausea, vomiting, constipation

Neuromuscular & skeletal: Weakness

1% to 10%:

Cardiovascular: Postural hypotension

Central nervous system: Nervousness, headache, restlessness, malaise, confusion, anxiety, abnormal dreams, euphoria, thought abnormalities

Dermatologic: Rash

Gastrointestinal: Anorexia, stomach cramps, xerostomia, biliary spasm, abdominal pain, dyspepsia, gastritis

Genitourinary: Ureteral spasms, decreased urination

Local: Pain at injection site

Respiratory: Dyspnea, hiccups

Miscellaneous: Diaphoresis

Overdosage/Toxicology Symptoms of toxicity include CNS depression, respiratory depression, and miosis. Naloxone, 2 mg I.V. with repeat administration as necessary up to a total of 10 mg, can also be used to reverse toxic effects of the opiate.

Pharmacodynamics/Kinetics

Onset of Action: Pain relief: 10-15 minutes; Peak effect: 0.5-1 hour

Duration of Action: 3-6 hours; Controlled release: ≤12 hours

Half-Life Elimination: 2-3 hours

Metabolism: Hepatic

Excretion: Urine

Available Dosage Forms

Capsule, immediate release, as hydrochloride (OxyIR®): 5 mg

Solution, oral, as hydrochloride: 5 mg/5 mL (500 mL)

Roxicodone™: 5 mg/5 mL (5 mL, 500 mL) [contains alcohol]

Solution, oral concentrate, as hydrochloride: 20 mg/mL (30 mL)

Oxydose™: 20 mg/mL (30 mL) [contains sodium benzoate; berry flavor]

OxyFast®, Roxicodone™ Intensol™: 20 mg/mL (30 mL) [contains sodium benzoate]

Tablet, as hydrochloride: 5 mg, 15 mg, 30 mg

Roxicodone™: 5 mg, 15 mg, 30 mg

Tablet, controlled release, as hydrochloride (OxyContin®): 10 mg, 20 mg, 40 mg, 80 mg, 160 mg

Tablet, extended release, as hydrochloride: 10 mg, 20 mg, 40 mg, 80 mg

Dosing

Adults & Elderly: Management of pain: Oral:

Regular or immediate release formulations: 2.5-5 mg every 6 hours as needed

Controlled release:

Opioid naive (not currently on opioid): 10 mg every 12 hours

Currently on opioid/ASA or acetaminophen or NSAID combination:

1-5 tablets: 10-20 mg every 12 hours

6-9 tablets: 20-30 mg every 12 hours

10-12 tablets: 30-40 mg every 12 hours

May continue the nonopioid as a separate drug.

Currently on opioids: Use standard conversion chart to convert daily dose to oxycodone equivalent. Divide daily dose in 2 (for every 12-hour dosing) and round down to nearest dosage form.

Note: 80 mg or 160 mg tablets are for use **only** in opioid-tolerant patients. Special safety considerations must be addressed when converting to OxyContin® doses ≥160 mg every 12 hours. Dietary caution must be taken when patients are initially titrated to 160 mg tablets.

Pediatrics: Oral: Regular or immediate release formulations:

6-12 years: 1.25 mg every 6 hours as needed

>12 years: 2.5 mg every 6 hours as needed

Hepatic Impairment: Reduce dosage in patients with severe liver disease.

Administration

Oral: Do not crush controlled-release tablets; 80 mg and 160 mg tablets are for use **only** in opioid-tolerant patients. Do not administer OxyContin® 160 mg tablet with a high-fat meal.

Stability

Storage: Tablets should be stored at room temperature.

Nursing Actions

Physical Assessment: Assess other medications patient may be taking for additive or adverse interactions . Monitor for effectiveness of pain relief and monitor for signs of overdose. Monitor blood pressure, CNS and respiratory status, and degree of sedation at beginning of therapy and at regular intervals with long-term use. May cause physical and/or psychological dependence. For inpatients, implement safety measures (eg, side rails up, call light within reach, instructions to call for assistance). Assess knowledge/teach patient appropriate use (if self-administered). Teach patient to monitor for adverse reactions, adverse reactions to report, and appropriate interventions to reduce side effects.

Patient Education: If self-administered, use exactly as directed; do not increase dose or frequency. Drug may cause physical and/or psychological dependence. Do not crush or chew controlled-release tablets. While using this medication, do not use alcohol and other prescription or OTC medications (especially sedatives, tranquilizers, antihistamines, or pain medications) without consulting prescriber. Maintain adequate hydration (2-3 L/day of fluids) unless instructed to restrict fluid intake. May cause hypotension, dizziness, drowsiness, impaired coordination, or blurred vision (use caution when driving, climbing stairs, or changing position - rising from sitting or lying to standing, or when engaging in tasks requiring alertness until response to drug is known); nausea, vomiting, or dry mouth (frequent mouth care, small frequent meals, chewing gum, or sucking lozenges may help); or constipation (increased exercise, fluids, fruit, or fiber may help; if unresolved, consult prescriber about use of stool softeners). Report persistent dizziness or headache; excessive fatigue or sedation; changes in mental status; changes in urinary elimination or pain on urination; weakness or trembling; blurred vision; or shortness of breath. **Pregnancy/breast-feeding precautions:** Inform prescriber if you are or intend to become pregnant. If you are breast-feeding, take medication immediately after breast-feeding or 3-4 hours prior to next feeding.

Dietary Considerations Instruct patient to avoid high-fat meals when taking OxyContin® 160 mg tablets.

Geriatric Considerations The elderly may be particularly susceptible to the CNS depressant and constipating effects of narcotics. Serum levels at a given dose may also be increased relative to concentrations in younger patients.

Pregnancy Issues Use of narcotics during pregnancy may produce physical dependence in the neonate; respiratory depression may occur in the newborn if narcotics are used prior to delivery (especially high doses).

Additional Information Prophylactic use of a laxative should be considered. OxyContin® 80 mg and 160 mg tablets are for use in opioid-tolerant patients only.

Oxycodone and Acetaminophen
(oks i KOE done & a seet a MIN oh fen)

U.S. Brand Names Endocet®; Percocet®; Roxicet™; Roxicet™ 5/500; Tylox®

Synonyms Acetaminophen and Oxycodone

Restrictions C-II

Pharmacologic Category Analgesic, Narcotic

Pregnancy Risk Factor C/D (prolonged periods or high doses at term)

Lactation Enters breast milk/use caution

Use Management of moderate to severe pain

Available Dosage Forms
Caplet:
Roxicet™ 5/500: Oxycodone hydrochloride 5 mg and acetaminophen 500 mg
Capsule: 5/500: Oxycodone hydrochloride 5 mg and acetaminophen 500 mg
Tylox®: 5/500: Oxycodone hydrochloride 5 mg and acetaminophen 500 mg [contains sodium benzoate and sodium metabisulfite]
Solution, oral:
Roxicet™: Oxycodone hydrochloride 5 mg and acetaminophen 325 mg per 5 mL (5 mL, 500 mL) [contains alcohol <0.5%]
Tablet: 5/325: Oxycodone hydrochloride 5 mg and acetaminophen 325 mg; 7.5/325: Oxycodone hydrochloride 7.5 mg and acetaminophen 325 mg; 7.5/500:

Oxycodone hydrochloride 7.5 mg and acetaminophen 500 mg; 10/325: Oxycodone hydrochloride 10 mg and acetaminophen 325 mg; 10/650: Oxycodone hydrochloride 10 mg and acetaminophen 650 mg
Endocet® 5/325 [scored]: Oxycodone hydrochloride 5 mg and acetaminophen 325 mg
Endocet® 7.5/325: Oxycodone hydrochloride 7.5 mg and acetaminophen 325 mg
Endocet® 7.5/500: Oxycodone hydrochloride 7.5 mg and acetaminophen 500 mg
Endocet® 10/325: Oxycodone hydrochloride 10 mg and acetaminophen 325 mg
Endocet® 10/650: Oxycodone hydrochloride 10 mg and acetaminophen 650 mg
Percocet® 2.5/325: Oxycodone hydrochloride 2.5 mg and acetaminophen 325 mg
Percocet® 5/325 [scored]: Oxycodone hydrochloride 5 mg and acetaminophen 325 mg
Percocet® 7.5/325: Oxycodone hydrochloride 7.5 mg and acetaminophen 325 mg
Percocet® 7.5/500: Oxycodone hydrochloride 7.5 mg and acetaminophen 500 mg
Percocet® 10/325: Oxycodone hydrochloride 10 mg and acetaminophen 325 mg
Percocet® 10/650: Oxycodone hydrochloride 10 mg and acetaminophen 650 mg
Roxicet™ [scored]: Oxycodone hydrochloride 5 mg and acetaminophen 325 mg

Dosing
Adults:
Note: Initial dose is based on the **oxycodone** content; however, the maximum daily dose is based on the **acetaminophen** content.
Management of pain: Doses should be given every 4-6 hours as needed and titrated to appropriate analgesic effects.
Maximum daily dose, based on acetaminophen content: Oral: 4 g/day.
Mild to moderate pain: Oral: Initial dose, **based on oxycodone content:** 5 mg
Severe pain: Oral: Initial dose, **based on oxycodone content:** 15-30 mg

Elderly: Doses should be titrated to appropriate analgesic effects: Oral: Initial dose, **based on oxycodone content:** 2.5-5 mg every 6 hours. Do not exceed 4 g/day of acetaminophen.

Pediatrics:
Note: Initial dose is based on the **oxycodone** content; however, the maximum daily dose is based on the **acetaminophen** content.
Management of pain: Doses should be given every 4-6 hours as needed and titrated to appropriate analgesic effects.
Mild to moderate pain: Oral: Initial dose, **based on oxycodone content:** 0.05-0.1 mg/kg/dose
Severe pain: Oral: Initial dose, **based on oxycodone content:** 0.3 mg/kg/dose

Maximum dose, based on acetaminophen content: Oral: Children <45 kg: 90 mg/kg/day; children >45 kg: 4 g/day

Hepatic Impairment: Dose should be reduced in patients with severe liver disease.

Nursing Actions
Physical Assessment: See individual agents.
Patient Education: See individual agents. **Pregnancy/breast-feeding precautions:** Inform prescriber if you are or intend to become pregnant. Consult prescriber if breast-feeding.

Related Information
Acetaminophen *on page 30*
Oxycodone *on page 927*

Oxycodone and Aspirin
(oks i KOE done & AS pir in)

U.S. Brand Names Endodan® [DSC]; Percodan®
Synonyms Aspirin and Oxycodone
Restrictions C-II
Pharmacologic Category Analgesic, Narcotic
Pregnancy Risk Factor D
Lactation Enters breast milk/use caution
Use Management of moderate to severe pain
Available Dosage Forms [DSC] = Discontinued product
  Tablet: Oxycodone hydrochloride 4.5 mg, oxycodone terephthalate 0.38 mg, and aspirin 325 mg
  Endodan® [DSC], Percodan®: Oxycodone hydrochloride 4.5 mg, oxycodone terephthalate 0.38 mg, and aspirin 325 mg
Dosing
  Adults & Elderly: Analgesic: Oral (based on oxycodone combined salts): Percodan®: 1 tablet every 6 hours as needed for pain; maximum aspirin dose should not exceed 4 g/day.
  Pediatrics: Analgesic: Oral (based on oxycodone combined salts): Maximum oxycodone: 5 mg/dose; maximum aspirin dose should not exceed 4 g/day. Doses should be given every 6 hours as needed.
  Mild-to-moderate pain: Initial dose, **based on oxycodone content:** 0.05-0.1 mg/kg/dose
  Severe pain: Initial dose, **based on oxycodone content:** 0.3 mg/kg/dose
  Hepatic Impairment: Dose should be reduced in patients with severe liver disease.
Nursing Actions
  Physical Assessment: See individual agents.
  Patient Education: See individual agents. **Pregnancy/breast-feeding precautions:** Inform prescriber if you are or intend to become pregnant. Consult prescriber if breast-feeding.
Related Information
  Aspirin *on page 114*
  Oxycodone *on page 927*

Oxycodone and Ibuprofen
(oks i KOE done & eye byoo PROE fen)

U.S. Brand Names Combunox™
Synonyms Ibuprofen and Oxycodone
Restrictions C-II
Pharmacologic Category Analgesic, Narcotic; Nonsteroidal Anti-inflammatory Drug (NSAID), Oral
Pregnancy Risk Factor C/D (3rd trimester)
Lactation Enters breast milk/contraindicated
Use Short-term (≤7 days) management of acute, moderate-to-severe pain
Mechanism of Action/Effect
  Based on **oxycodone** component: Binds to opiate receptors in the CNS, altering the perception of and response to pain; suppresses cough in medullary center; produces generalized CNS depression
  Based on **ibuprofen** component: Inhibits prostaglandin synthesis by decreasing the activity of the enzyme, cyclooxygenase, which results in decreased formation of prostaglandin precursors
Contraindications Hypersensitivity to oxycodone, other opioids, ibuprofen, aspirin, other NSAIDs, or any component of the formulation; patients with suspected paralytic ileus; pregnancy (3rd trimester)
Warnings/Precautions Use with caution in elderly or debilitated patients, and those with severe hepatic or renal dysfunction, hypothyroidism, Addison's disease, prostatic hyperplasia, or urethral stricture. Respiratory depression is possible; use with caution in patients with underlying respiratory depression, acute or severe asthma, or hypercarbia. Oxycodone suppresses the cough reflex; use caution postoperatively and in patients with pulmonary disease. Patients with head injury, increased intracranial pressure, acute abdominal condition, or impaired thyroid function should use this agent cautiously. Tolerance or drug dependence may result from extended use.

NSAIDs are associated with an increased risk of adverse cardiovascular events, including MI, stroke, and new onset or worsening of pre-existing hypertension. Risk may be increased with duration of use or pre-existing cardiovascular risk-factors or disease. Use caution with fluid retention, CHF, or hypertension. Use of NSAIDs can compromise existing renal function. Rehydrate patient before starting therapy. Monitor renal function closely. Ibuprofen is not recommended for patients with advanced renal disease.NSAIDs may increase risk of gastrointestinal irritation, ulceration, bleeding, and perforation. Use caution with a history of GI disease (bleeding or ulcers), concurrent therapy with aspirin, anticoagulants and/or corticosteroids, smoking, use of alcohol, the elderly or debilitated patients. NSAIDs may cause serious skin adverse events. Anaphylactoid reactions may occur, even without prior exposure. Do not use in patients who experience bronchospasm, asthma, rhinitis, or urticaria with NSAID or aspirin therapy. The elderly are at increased risk for adverse effects (especially peptic ulceration, CNS effects, renal toxicity) from NSAIDs even at low doses.

Safety and efficacy in pediatric patients have not been established.
Drug Interactions
  Cytochrome P450 Effect:
    Oxycodone: **Substrate** of CYP2D6
    Ibuprofen: **Substrate** (minor) of CYP2C8/9, 2C19; **Inhibits** CYP2C8/9 (strong)
  Decreased Effect: See individual agents.
  Increased Effect/Toxicity: See individual agents.
Nutritional/Ethanol Interactions
  Based on **oxycodone** component:
    Ethanol: Avoid or limit ethanol (may increase CNS depression). Watch for sedation.
  Based on **ibuprofen** component:
    Ethanol: Avoid ethanol (may enhance gastric mucosal irritation).
    Food: Food or milk are recommended to decrease gastric irritation.
    Herb/Nutraceutical: Avoid alfalfa, anise, bilberry, bladderwrack, bromelain, cat's claw, celery, coleus, cordyceps, dong quai, evening primrose, feverfew, fenugreek, garlic, ginger, ginkgo biloboa, red clover, horse chestnut, grapeseed, green tea, ginseng, guggul, horse chestnut seed, horseradish, licorice, prickly ash, red clover, reishi, SAMe, sweet clover, turmeric, white willow (all have additional antiplatelet activity).
Adverse Reactions
  >10%:
    Central nervous system: Dizziness (5% to 19%), somnolence (7% to 17%)
    Gastrointestinal: Nausea (9% to 25%)
  2% to 10%:
    Cardiovascular: Vasodilation (<1% to 3%)
    Central nervous system: Headache (10%), fever (3%)
    Gastrointestinal: Constipation (<1% to 5%), vomiting (5%), diarrhea (2%), dyspepsia (<1% to 2%), flatulence (1%)
    Neuromuscular & skeletal: Weakness (3%)
    Miscellaneous: Diaphoresis (2%)
Overdosage/Toxicology Symptoms of toxicity may include respiratory depression, CNS depression, metabolic acidosis, seizures, hypotension, blood loss, coma, miosis, and renal failure. In cases of acute overdose, ipecac-induced emesis or gastric lavage may be used to empty the stomach. Emesis is most effective if within 30

minutes of ingestion, and is not recommended in patients who are not fully conscious or who have ingested >400 mg/kg of the ibuprofen component. Naloxone is the antidote for oxycodone. Repeat administration as necessary up to a total of 10 mg may be used to reverse toxic effects of the opiate. Treatment of NSAID overdose is supportive with symptomatic management as necessary; activated charcoal may be used to reduce the absorption and reabsorption of ibuprofen.

Pharmacodynamics/Kinetics
Time to Peak: Ibuprofen: 1.6-3.1 hours; Oxycodone 1.3-2.1 hours

Protein Binding: Ibuprofen: 99%; Oxycodone: 45%

Half-Life Elimination: Ibuprofen: 1.8-2.6 hours; Oxycodone: 3.1-3.7 hours

Metabolism: Oxycodone: Hepatic to metabolites, noroxycodone (major), and oxymorphone (minor)

Excretion: Ibuprofen: Urine (<0.2% unchanged); Oxycodone: Urine (~4 % unchanged)

Pharmacokinetic Note See individual agents.

Available Dosage Forms
Tablet:
Combunox™: 5/400: Oxycodone 5 mg and ibuprofen 400 mg

Dosing
Adults: Pain: Oral: Take 1 tablet every 6 hours as needed (maximum: 4 tablets/24 hours); do not take for longer than 7 days

Stability
Storage: Store between 15°C to 30°C (59°F to 86°F).

Nursing Actions
Physical Assessment:
Assess other medications patient may be taking for additive or adverse interactions. Monitor for effectiveness of pain relief and monitor for signs of overdose. Monitor blood pressure, CNS and respiratory status, and degree of sedation at beginning of therapy and at regular intervals with long-term use. May cause physical and/or psychological dependence. For inpatients, implement safety measures (eg, side rails up, call light within reach, instructions to call for assistance). Assess knowledge/teach patient appropriate use (if self-administered). Teach patient to monitor for adverse reactions, adverse reactions to report, and appropriate interventions to reduce side effects.

Patient Education:
If self-administered, use exactly as directed; do not increase dose or frequency. Drug may cause physical and/or psychological dependence. While using this medication, do not use alcohol and other prescription or OTC medications (especially sedatives, tranquilizers, antihistamines, or pain medications) without consulting prescriber. Maintain adequate hydration (2-3 L/day of fluids) unless instructed to restrict fluid intake. May cause hypotension, dizziness, drowsiness, impaired coordination, or blurred vision (use caution when driving, climbing stairs, or changing position - rising from sitting or lying to standing, or when engaging in tasks requiring alertness until response to drug is known); nausea, vomiting, (frequent mouth care, small frequent meals, chewing gum, or sucking lozenges may help); or constipation (increased exercise, fluids, fruit, or fiber may help; if unresolved, consult prescriber about use of stool softeners). Report persistent dizziness or headache; excessive fatigue or sedation; changes in mental status; gastrointestinal bleeding, unexplained weight gain, edema, blurred vision; or shortness of breath. **Pregnancy/breast-feeding precautions:** Inform prescriber if you are or intend to become pregnant. If you are breast-feeding, take medication immediately after breast-feeding or 3-4 hours prior to next feeding.

Dietary Considerations Take with or without food.

Geriatric Considerations The elderly are at increased risk for adverse effects from NSAIDs. As many as 60%

of elderly can develop peptic ulceration and/or hemorrhage asymptomatically. CNS adverse effects such as confusion, agitation, and hallucination are generally seen in overdose or high-dose situations; however, elderly patients may demonstrate these adverse effects at lower doses than younger adults. The elderly are also at increased risk of renal toxicity.

Breast-Feeding Issues Ibuprofen is not transferred to milk in significant quantities and is considered compatible with breast-feeding by AAP Oxycodone, however, is excreted in breast milk and withdrawal may occur in breast-fed infants when maternal opioid administration is discontinued. Discontinuation of either the opioid-containing medication (Combunox™) or breast-feeding is recommended.

Oxymorphone (oks i MOR fone)

U.S. Brand Names Numorphan®

Synonyms Oxymorphone Hydrochloride

Restrictions C-II

Pharmacologic Category Analgesic, Narcotic

Medication Safety Issues
Sound-alike/look-alike issues:
Oxymorphone may be confused with oxymetholone

Pregnancy Risk Factor B/D (prolonged use or high doses at term)

Lactation Excretion in breast milk unknown/use caution

Use Management of moderate to severe pain and preoperatively as a sedative and a supplement to anesthesia

Mechanism of Action/Effect Oxymorphone hydrochloride (Numorphan®) is a potent narcotic analgesic with uses similar to those of morphine. The drug is a semisynthetic derivative of morphine (phenanthrene derivative) and is closely related to hydromorphone chemically (Dilaudid®).

Contraindications Hypersensitivity to oxymorphone or any component of the formulation; increased intracranial pressure; severe respiratory depression; pregnancy (prolonged use or high doses at term)

Warnings/Precautions Some preparations contain sulfites which may cause allergic reactions; infants <3 months of age are more susceptible to respiratory depression, use with caution and generally in reduced doses in this age group; use with caution in patients with impaired respiratory function or severe hepatic dysfunction and in patients with hypersensitivity reactions to other phenanthrene derivative opioid agonists (codeine, hydrocodone, hydromorphone, levorphanol, oxycodone, oxymorphone); tolerance or drug dependence may result from extended use

Drug Interactions
Decreased Effect: Decreased effect with phenothiazines.

Increased Effect/Toxicity: Increased effect/toxicity with CNS depressants (phenothiazines, tranquilizers, anxiolytics, sedatives, hypnotics, alcohol), tricyclic antidepressants, and dextroamphetamine.

Nutritional/Ethanol Interactions
Ethanol: Avoid ethanol (may increase CNS depression).
Herb/Nutraceutical: Avoid valerian, St John's wort, kava kava, gotu kola (may increase CNS depression).

Lab Interactions
Some quinolones may produce a false-positive urine screening result for opiates using commercially-available immunoassay kits. This has been demonstrated most consistently for levofloxacin and ofloxacin, but other quinolones have shown cross-reactivity in certain assay kits. Confirmation of positive opiate screens by more specific methods should be considered.

Adverse Reactions
>10%:
Cardiovascular: Hypotension
(Continued)

Oxymorphone *(Continued)*

Central nervous system: Fatigue, drowsiness, dizziness

Gastrointestinal: Nausea, vomiting, constipation

Neuromuscular & skeletal: Weakness

Miscellaneous: Histamine release

1% to 10%:

Central nervous system: Nervousness, headache, restlessness, malaise, confusion

Gastrointestinal: Anorexia, stomach cramps, xerostomia, biliary spasm

Genitourinary: Decreased urination, ureteral spasms

Local: Pain at injection site

Respiratory: Dyspnea

Overdosage/Toxicology Symptoms of overdose include respiratory depression, miosis, hypotension, bradycardia, apnea, and pulmonary edema. Treatment of overdose includes maintaining patent airway and establishing an I.V. line. Naloxone, 2 mg I.V., with repeat administration as necessary up to a total of 10 mg, can also be used to reverse toxic effects of the opiate.

Pharmacodynamics/Kinetics

Onset of Action: Analgesic: I.V., I.M., SubQ: 5-10 minutes; Rectal: 15-30 minutes

Duration of Action: Analgesic: Parenteral, rectal: 3-4 hours

Metabolism: Hepatic via glucuronidation

Excretion: Urine

Available Dosage Forms

Injection, solution, as hydrochloride: 1 mg (1 mL); 1.5 mg/mL (10 mL)

Suppository, rectal, as hydrochloride: 5 mg

Dosing

Adults & Elderly: Analgesia: **Note:** More frequent dosing may be required.

I.M., SubQ: 0.5 mg initially, 1-1.5 mg every 4-6 hours as needed

I.V.: 0.5 mg initially

Rectal: 5 mg every 4-6 hours

Administration

I.V. Detail: pH: 2.7-4.5

Stability

Storage: Refrigerate suppository.

Nursing Actions

Physical Assessment: Assess other medications patient may be taking for additive or adverse interactions. Monitor for effectiveness of pain relief and monitor for signs of overdose. Monitor blood pressure, CNS and respiratory status, and degree of sedation at beginning of therapy and at regular intervals with long-term use. May cause physical and/or psychological dependence. For inpatients, implement safety measures (eg, side rails up, call light within reach, instructions to call for assistance). Assess knowledge/teach patient appropriate use (if self-administered). Teach patient to monitor for adverse reactions, adverse reactions to report, and appropriate interventions to reduce side effects.

Patient Education: If self-administered, use exactly as directed; do not increase dose or frequency or discontinue without consulting prescriber. Drug may cause physical and/or psychological dependence. While using this medication, do not use alcohol and other prescription or OTC medications (especially sedatives, tranquilizers, antihistamines, or pain medications) without consulting prescriber. Maintain adequate hydration (2-3 L/day of fluids) unless instructed to restrict fluid intake. May cause hypotension, dizziness, drowsiness, impaired coordination, or blurred vision (use caution when driving, climbing stairs, or changing position - rising from sitting or lying to standing, or when engaging in tasks requiring alertness until response to drug is known); nausea, vomiting or dry mouth (frequent mouth care, small frequent meals, chewing gum, or sucking lozenges may help); or constipation (increased exercise, fluids, fruit, or fiber may help; if unresolved, consult prescriber about use of stool softeners). Report persistent dizziness or headache; excessive fatigue or sedation; changes in mental status; changes in urinary elimination or pain on urination; weakness or trembling; blurred vision; or shortness of breath. **Pregnancy/breast-feeding precautions:** Inform prescriber if you are or intend to become pregnant.

Geriatric Considerations The elderly may be particularly susceptible to the CNS depressant and constipating effects of narcotics.

Oxytocin *(oks i TOE sin)*

U.S. Brand Names Pitocin®

Synonyms Pit

Pharmacologic Category Oxytocic Agent

Medication Safety Issues

Sound-alike/look-alike issues:

Pitocin® may be confused with Pitressin®

Pregnancy Risk Factor X

Lactation Excretion in breast milk unknown/use caution

Use Induction of labor at term; control of postpartum bleeding; adjunctive therapy in management of abortion

Mechanism of Action/Effect Produces rhythmic uterine contractions characteristic of delivery and stimulates breast milk flow during nursing

Contraindications Hypersensitivity to oxytocin or any component of the formulation; significant cephalopelvic disproportion; unfavorable fetal positions; fetal distress; hypertonic or hyperactive uterus; contraindicated vaginal delivery (invasive cervical cancer, active genital herpes, prolapse of the cord, cord presentation, total placenta previa, or vasa previa)

Warnings/Precautions To be used for medical rather than elective induction of labor. May produce antidiuretic effect (ie, water intoxication and excess uterine contractions). High doses or hypersensitivity to oxytocin may cause uterine hypertonicity, spasm, tetanic contraction, or rupture of the uterus. Severe water intoxication with convulsions, coma, and death has been associated with a slow oxytocin infusion over 24 hours.

Drug Interactions

Increased Effect/Toxicity: Dinoprostone and misoprostol may increase the effect of oxytocin; wait 6-12 hours after dinoprostone or misoprostol administration before initiating oxytocin.

Adverse Reactions Frequency not defined.

Fetus or neonate:

Cardiovascular: Arrhythmias (including premature ventricular contractions), bradycardia

Central nervous system: Brain or CNS damage (permanent), neonatal seizure

Hepatic: Neonatal jaundice

Ocular: Neonatal retinal hemorrhage

Miscellaneous: Fetal death, low Apgar score (5 minute)

Mother:

Cardiovascular: Arrhythmias, hypertensive episodes, premature ventricular contractions

Gastrointestinal: Nausea, vomiting

Genitourinary: Pelvic hematoma, postpartum hemorrhage, uterine hypertonicity, tetanic contraction of the uterus, uterine rupture, uterine spasm

Hematologic: Afibrinogenemia (fatal)

Miscellaneous: Anaphylactic reaction, subarachnoid hemorrhage

Overdosage/Toxicology Symptoms of overdose include tetanic uterine contractions, impaired uterine blood flow, amniotic fluid embolism, uterine rupture, SIADH, and seizures. Treatment is symptom-directed and supportive.

Pharmacodynamics/Kinetics

Onset of Action: Uterine contractions: I.M.: 3-5 minutes; I.V.: ~1 minute

Duration of Action: I.M.: 2-3 hour; I.V.: 1 hour

Half-Life Elimination: 1-5 minutes

Metabolism: Rapidly hepatic and via plasma (by oxytocinase) and to a smaller degree the mammary gland

Excretion: Urine

Available Dosage Forms

Injection, solution: 10 units/mL (1 mL, 10 mL)

Pitocin®: 10 units/mL (1 mL)

Dosing

Adults: Note: I.V. administration requires the use of an infusion pump.

Induction of labor: I.V.: 0.5-1 milliunits/minute; gradually increase dose in increments of 1-2 milliunits/minute until desired contraction pattern is established; dose may be decreased after desired frequency of contractions is reached and labor has progressed to 5-6 cm dilation. Infusion rates of 6 milliunits/minute provide oxytocin levels similar to those at spontaneous labor; rates of >9-10 milliunits/minute are rarely required.

Postpartum bleeding:

I.M.: Total dose of 10 units after delivery

I.V.: 10-40 units by I.V. infusion in 1000 mL of intravenous fluid at a rate sufficient to control uterine atony

Adjunctive treatment of abortion: I.V.: 10-20 milliunits/minute; maximum total dose: 30 units/12 hours

Administration

I.V.: Refer to Reconstitution for dilution information. An infusion pump is required for administration.

Stability

Reconstitution: I.V.

Induction or stimulation of labor: Add oxytocin 10 units to NS or LR 1000 mL to yield a solution containing oxytocin 10 milliunits/mL; rotate solution to mix

Postpartum uterine bleeding: Add oxytocin 10-40 units to running I.V. infusion; maximum: 40 units/1000 mL

Adjunctive management of abortion: Add oxytocin 10 units to 500 mL of a physiologic saline solution or D_5W

Compatibility: Stable in dextran 6% in dextrose, dextran 6% in NS, D_5LR, $D_5^{1}/_4NS$, $D_5^{1}/_2NS$, D_5NS, D_5W, $D_{10}W$, LR, $^{1}/_2NS$, NS

Compatibility when admixed: Incompatible with fibrinolysin (human), norepinephrine, prochlorperazine edisylate, warfarin

Storage: Store oxytocin at 2°C to 8°C (36°F to 46°F); protect from freezing. Pitocin® may also be stored at 15°C to 25°C (59°F to 77°F) for up to 30 days.

Nursing Actions

Physical Assessment: Monitor blood pressure, fluid intake and output, and labor closely if using oxytocin for induction; fetal monitoring is strongly recommended. **Pregnancy risk factor X.**

Patient Education: I.V./I.M.: Generally used in emergency situations. Drug teaching should be incorporated in other situational teaching. **Breast-feeding precaution:** Use caution.

Breast-Feeding Issues Endogenous levels of oxytocin naturally increase during breast-feeding.

Pregnancy Issues Reproduction studies have not been conducted. When used as indicated, teratogenic effects would not be expected. Nonteratogenic adverse reactions are reported in the neonate as well as the mother.

Paclitaxel (PAK li taks el)

U.S. Brand Names Onxol™; Taxol®

Synonyms NSC-125973; NSC-673089

Pharmacologic Category Antineoplastic Agent, Antimicrotubular; Antineoplastic Agent, Natural Source (Plant) Derivative

Medication Safety Issues

Sound-alike/look-alike issues:

Paclitaxel may be confused with paroxetine, Paxil®

Paclitaxel (conventional) may be confused with paclitaxel (protein-bound)

Taxol® may be confused with Abraxane™, Paxil®, Taxotere®

Pregnancy Risk Factor D

Lactation Excretion in breast milk unknown/contraindicated

Use Treatment of breast, lung (small cell and nonsmall cell), and ovarian cancers; treatment of AIDS-related Kaposi's sarcoma (KS)

Unlabeled/Investigational Use Treatment of bladder, cervical, prostate, and head and neck cancers

Mechanism of Action/Effect Paclitaxel promotes microtubule assembly by enhancing the action of tubulin dimers, stabilizing existing microtubules, and inhibiting their disassembly, interfering with the late G_2 mitotic phase, and inhibiting cell replication. In addition, the drug can distort mitotic spindles, resulting in the breakage of chromosomes. Paclitaxel may also suppress cell proliferation and modulate immune response.

Contraindications Hypersensitivity to paclitaxel, Cremophor® EL (polyoxyethylated castor oil), or any component of the formulation; pregnancy

Warnings/Precautions Hazardous agent - use appropriate precautions for handling and disposal. Severe hypersensitivity reactions have been reported; prolongation of the infusion (to ≥6 hours) plus premedication may minimize this effect. Stop infusion and do not rechallenge for severe hypersensitivity reactions (hypotension requiring treatment, dyspnea requiring bronchodilators, angioedema, urticaria). Minor hypersensitivity reactions (flushing, skin reactions, dyspnea, hypotension, or tachycardia) do not require interruption of treatment. Bone marrow suppression is the dose-limiting toxicity; do not administer if baseline absolute neutrophil count (ANC) is <1500 cells/mm³ (<1000 cells/mm³ for patients with AIDS-related KS); reduce future doses by 20% for severe neutropenia (<500 cells/mm³ for 7 days or more) and consider the use of supportive therapy, including growth factor treatment.

Use extreme caution with hepatic dysfunction (myelotoxicity may be worsened); dose reductions are recommended. Peripheral neuropathy may occur; patients with pre-existing neuropathies from chemotherapy or coexisting conditions (eg, diabetes mellitus) may be at a higher risk; reduce dose by 20% for severe neuropathy. Paclitaxel formulations contain dehydrated alcohol; may cause adverse CNS effects. Hypotension, bradycardia, and hypertension may occur; frequent monitoring of vital signs is recommended, especially during the first hour of the infusion. Rare but severe conduction abnormalities have been reported; conduct cardiac monitoring during subsequent infusions for these patients. When administered as sequential infusions, taxane derivatives (docetaxel, paclitaxel) should be administered before platinum derivatives (carboplatin, cisplatin) to limit myelosuppression. Elderly patients have an increased risk of toxicity (neutropenia, neuropathy). Safety and efficacy in children have not been established.

Drug Interactions

Cytochrome P450 Effect: Substrate (major) of CYP2C8/9, 3A4; **Induces** CYP3A4 (weak)

(Continued)

Paclitaxel *(Continued)*

Decreased Effect: CYP2C8/9 inducers may decrease the levels/effects of paclitaxel; example inducers include carbamazepine, phenobarbital, phenytoin, rifampin, rifapentine, and secobarbital. CYP3A4 inducers may decrease the levels/effects of paclitaxel; example inducers include aminoglutethimide, carbamazepine, nafcillin, nevirapine, phenobarbital, phenytoin, and rifamycins.

Increased Effect/Toxicity: CYP2C8/9 inhibitors may increase the levels/effects of paclitaxel; example inhibitors include delavirdine, fluconazole, gemfibrozil, ketoconazole, nicardipine, NSAIDs, pioglitazone, and sulfonamides. CYP3A4 inhibitors may increase the levels/effects of paclitaxel; example inhibitors include azole antifungals, clarithromycin, diclofenac, doxycycline, erythromycin, imatinib, isoniazid, nefazodone, nicardipine, propofol, protease inhibitors, quinidine, telithromycin, and verapamil. In Phase I trials, myelosuppression was more profound when given after cisplatin than with alternative sequence. administered as sequential infusions, studies indicate a potential for increased toxicity when platinum derivatives (carboplatin, cisplatin) are administered before taxane derivatives (docetaxel, paclitaxel). Paclitaxel may increase doxorubicin levels/toxicity.

Nutritional/Ethanol Interactions Herb/Nutraceutical: Avoid black cohosh, dong quai in estrogen-dependent tumors. Avoid valerian, St John's wort, kava kava, gotu kola (may increase CNS depression).

Adverse Reactions Percentages reported with single-agent therapy, first- or second-line treatment. **Note:** Myelosuppression is dose related, schedule related, and infusion-rate dependent (increased incidences with higher doses, more frequent doses, and longer infusion times) and, in general, rapidly reversible upon discontinuation.

>10%:
Cardiovascular: Flushing (28%), ECG abnormal (14% to 23%), edema (21%), hypotension (4% to 12%),
Dermatologic: Alopecia (87%), rash (12%)
Gastrointestinal: Nausea/vomiting (52%), diarrhea (38%), mucositis (17% to 35%; grades 3/4: up to 3%), stomatitis (15%; most common at doses >390 mg/m^2), abdominal pain (with intraperitoneal paclitaxel)
Hematologic: Neutropenia (78% to 98%; grade 4: 14% to 75%; onset 8-10 days, median nadir 11 days, recovery 15-21 days), leukopenia (90%; grade 4: 17%), anemia (47% to 90%; grades 3/4: 2% to 16%), thrombocytopenia (4% to 20%; grades 3/4: 1% to 7%), bleeding (14%)
Hepatic: Alkaline Phosphatase increased (22%), AST increased (19%)
Local: Injection site reaction (erythema, tenderness, skin discoloration, swelling; 13%)
Neuromuscular & skeletal: Peripheral neuropathy (42% to 70%; grades 3/4: up to 7%), arthralgia/myalgia (60%), weakness (17%)
Renal: Creatinine increased (observed in KS patients only: 18% to 34%; severe: 5% to 7%)
Miscellaneous: Hypersensitivity reaction (31% to 45%; grades 3/4: up to 2%), infection (15% to 30%)
1% to 10%:
Cardiovascular: Bradycardia (3%), tachycardia (2%), hypertension (1%), rhythm abnormalities (1%), syncope (1%), venous thrombosis (1%)
Dermatologic: Nail changes (2%)
Hematologic: Febrile neutropenia (2%)
Hepatic: Bilirubin increased (7%)
Respiratory: Dyspnea (2%)
Overdosage/Toxicology Potential symptoms of overdose would include bone marrow suppression, peripheral neurotoxicity, and mucositis. Overdoses in children would be associated with acute ethanol toxicity. There is no known antidote; treatment is symptom-directed and supportive.

Pharmacodynamics/Kinetics

Protein Binding: 89% to 98%

Half-Life Elimination:
1- to 6-hour infusion: Mean (beta): 6.4 hours
3-hour infusion: Mean (terminal): 13.1-20.2 hours
24-hour infusion: Mean (terminal): 15.7-52.7 hours

Metabolism: Hepatic via CYP2C8 and 3A4; forms metabolites (primarily 6α-hydroxypaclitaxel)

Excretion: Feces (~70%, 5% as unchanged drug); urine (14%)
Clearance: Mean: Total body: After 1- and 6-hour infusions: 5.8-16.3 L/hour/m^2; After 24-hour infusions: 14.2-17.2 L/hour/m^2

Available Dosage Forms

Injection, solution: 6 mg/mL (5 mL, 16.7 mL, 50 mL) [contains alcohol and purified Cremophor® EL (polyoxyethylated castor oil)]
Onxol™: 6 mg/mL (5 mL, 25 mL, 50 mL) [contains alcohol] [contains alcohol and purified Cremophor® EL (polyoxyethylated castor oil)]
Taxol®: 6 mg/mL (5 mL, 16.7 mL, 50 mL) [contains alcohol and purified Cremophor® EL (polyoxyethylated castor oil)]

Dosing

Adults & Elderly: Note: Premedication with dexamethasone (20 mg orally or I.V. at 12 and 6 hours or 14 and 7 hours before the dose; reduce dexamethasone dose to 10 mg orally with advanced HIV disease), diphenhydramine (50 mg I.V. 30-60 minutes prior to the dose), and cimetidine, famotidine or ranitidine (I.V. 30-60 minutes prior to the dose) is recommended.

Ovarian carcinoma:
I.V.: 135-175 mg/m^2 over 3 hours every 3 weeks **or**
135 mg/m^2 over 24 hours every 3 weeks **or**
50-80 mg/m^2 over 1-3 hours weekly **or**
1.4-4 mg/m^2/day continuous infusion for 14 days every 4 weeks
Intraperitoneal (unlabeled route): 60 mg on day 8 of a 21-day treatment cycle for 6 cycles, in combination with I.V. paclitaxel and intraperitoneal cisplatin. **Note:** Administration of intraperitoneal paclitaxel should include the standard paclitaxel premedication regimen.

Metastatic breast cancer: I.V.: 175-250 mg/m^2 over 3 hours every 3 weeks **or**
50-80 mg/m^2 weekly **or**
1.4-4 mg/m^2/day continuous infusion for 14 days every 4 weeks

Nonsmall cell lung carcinoma: I.V.: 135 mg/m^2 over 24 hours every 3 weeks

AIDS-related Kaposi's sarcoma: I.V.: 135 mg/m^2 over 3 hours every 3 weeks
or 100 mg/m^2 over 3 hours every 2 weeks

Hepatic Impairment:

Note: These recommendations are based upon the patient's first course of therapy where the usual dose would be 135 mg/m^2 dose over 24 hours or the 175 mg/m^2 dose over 3 hours in patients with normal hepatic function. Dosage in subsequent courses should be based upon individual tolerance. Adjustments for other regimens are not available.
24-hour infusion:
If transaminase levels <2 times upper limit of normal (ULN) and bilirubin level ≤1.5 mg/dL: 135 mg/m^2
If transaminase levels 2-<10 times ULN and bilirubin level ≤1.5 mg/dL: 100 mg/m^2
If transaminase levels <10 times ULN and bilirubin level 1.6-7.5 mg/dL: 50 mg/m^2
If transaminase levels ≥10 times ULN and bilirubin level >7.5 mg/dL: Avoid use

3-hour infusion:

If transaminase levels <10 times ULN and bilirubin level ≤1.25 times ULN: 175 mg/m²

If transaminase levels <10 times ULN and bilirubin level 1.26-2 times ULN: 135 mg/m²

If transaminase levels <10 times ULN and bilirubin level 2.01-5 times ULN: 90 mg/m²

If transaminase levels ≥10 times ULN and bilirubin level >5 times ULN: Avoid use

Dosing Adjustment for Toxicity:

Dosage modification for toxicity (solid tumors, including ovary, breast, and lung carcinoma): Courses of paclitaxel should not be repeated until the neutrophil count is ≥1500 cells/mm³ and the platelet count is ≥100,000 cells/mm³; reduce dosage by 20% for patients experiencing severe peripheral neuropathy or severe neutropenia (neutrophil <500 cells/mm³ for a week or longer)

Dosage modification for immunosuppression in advanced HIV disease: Paclitaxel should not be given to patients with HIV if the baseline or subsequent neutrophil count is <1000 cells/mm³. Additional modifications include: Reduce dosage of dexamethasone in premedication to 10 mg orally; reduce dosage by 20% in patients experiencing severe peripheral neuropathy or severe neutropenia (neutrophil <500 cells/mm³ for a week or longer); initiate concurrent hematopoietic growth factor (G-CSF) as clinically indicated

Administration

I.V.: Irritant. Manufacturer recommends administration over 1-24 hours. Other routes are being studied. When administered as sequential infusions, taxane derivatives should be administered before platinum derivatives (cisplatin, carboplatin) to limit myelosuppression and to enhance efficacy.

Premedication with dexamethasone (20 mg orally or I.V. at 12 and 6 hours **or** 14 and 7 hours before the dose; reduce to 10 mg with advanced HIV disease), diphenhydramine (50 mg I.V. 30-60 minutes prior to the dose), and cimetidine 300 mg, famotidine 20 mg, or ranitidine 50 mg (I.V. 30-60 minutes prior to the dose) is recommended.

Administer I.V. infusion over 1-24 hours; use of a 0.22 micron in-line filter and nonsorbing administration set is recommended during the infusion.

Nonpolyvinyl (non-PVC) tubing (eg, polyethylene) should be used to minimize leaching. Formulated in a vehicle known as Cremophor® EL (polyoxyethylated castor oil). Cremophor® EL has been found to leach the plasticizer DEHP from polyvinyl chloride infusion bags or administration sets. Contact of the undiluted concentrate with plasticized polyvinyl chloride (PVC) equipment or devices is not recommended. Administer through I.V. tubing containing an in-line (NOT >0.22 μ) filter; administration through IVEX-2® filters (which incorporate short inlet and outlet polyvinyl chloride-coated tubing) has not resulted in significant leaching of DEHP.

I.V. Detail: Should be dispensed in either glass or Excel®/PAB®. Should also use non-PVC tubing (eg, polyethylene) to minimize leaching. Administer through I.V. tubing containing an in-line (0.22 micron) filter. Formulated in a vehicle known as Cremophor® EL (polyoxyethylated castor oil). Cremophor® EL has been found to leach the plasticizer DEHP from polyvinyl chloride infusion bags or administration sets. Contact of the undiluted concentrate with plasticized polyvinyl chloride (PVC) equipment or devices is not recommended. Administration through IVEX-2® filters (which incorporate short inlet and outlet polyvinyl chloride-coated tubing) has not resulted in significant leaching of DEHP.

pH: 4.4-5.6

Stability

Reconstitution: Dilute in 250-1000 mL D₅W, D₅LR, D₅NS, or NS to a concentration of 0.3-1.2 mg/mL. Chemotherapy dispensing devices (eg, Chemo Dispensing Pin™) should not be used to withdraw paclitaxel from the vial.

Compatibility: Stable in D₅W, D₅NS, D₅LR, NS

Y-site administration: Incompatible with amphotericin B, amphotericin B cholesteryl sulfate complex, chlorpromazine, doxorubicin liposome, hydroxyzine, methylprednisolone sodium succinate, mitoxantrone

Storage: Store intact vials at room temperature of 20°C to 25°C (68°F to 77°F). Protect from light. Per the manufacturer, reconstituted solution is stable for up to 27 hours at room temperature (25°C) and ambient light conditions. Other sources report that solutions in D₅W and NS are stable for up to 3 days at room temperature (25°C).

Paclitaxel should be dispensed in either glass or Excel™/PAB™ containers. Should also use **nonpolyvinyl** (non-PVC) tubing (eg, polyethylene) to minimize leaching. Formulated in a vehicle known as Cremophor® EL (polyoxyethylated castor oil). Cremophor® EL has been found to leach the plasticizer DEHP from polyvinyl chloride infusion bags or administration sets. Contact of the undiluted concentrate with plasticized polyvinyl chloride (PVC) equipment or devices is not recommended.

Laboratory Monitoring CBC with differential and platelet count, liver and kidney function

Nursing Actions

Physical Assessment: Note sequencing specifics: Taxane derivatives should be administered before platinum derivatives to limit myelosuppression. Assess potential for interactions with other pharmacological agents and herbal products patient may be taking (eg, risk of increased or decrease levels/effects of paclitaxel). See Administration for specific infusion directions. Premedication with dexamethasone, diphenhydramine and an H₂ blocker may be ordered to reduce severe hypersensitivity reactions. Monitor infusion site closely monitored to prevent extravasation. Monitor laboratory tests and assess adverse response prior to, during, and between each infusion (eg, hypersensitivity reactions, peripheral neuropathy [numbness, tingling, burning pain], myelosuppression [anemia, opportunistic infection], GI irritation [nausea, vomiting, mucositis, stomatitis]). Teach patient possible side effects/appropriate interventions and adverse symptoms to report.

Patient Education: Do not take any new medication during therapy unless approved by prescriber. This drug can only be given by infusion. Report immediately any redness, swelling, burning, pain at infusion site or signs of allergic' reaction (eg, respiratory difficulty or swallowing, chest tightness, rash, hives, swelling of lips or mouth). Maintain adequate hydration (2-3 L/day of fluids) unless instructed to restrict fluid intake, and nutrition. You will be more susceptible to infection (avoid crowds and exposure to infection and do not have any vaccinations without consulting prescriber). May cause loss of hair (will grow back after therapy); experience nausea or vomiting (consult prescriber for approved antiemetic); feel weak or lethargic (use caution when driving or engaging in tasks that require alertness until response to drug is known); or mouth sores (sucking ice chips may help; use good oral care with soft toothbrush and waxed dental floss; consult prescriber if severe or infection developes). Report numbness or tingling in fingers or toes (use care to prevent injury); signs of opportunistic infection (fever, chills, sore throat, burning urination, fatigue); unusual bleeding (tarry stools, easy bruising, or blood in stool, urine, or mouth); unresolved mouth sores; nausea or vomiting; (Continued)

Paclitaxel *(Continued)*

or skin rash or itching. **Pregnancy/breast-feeding precautions:** Do not get pregnant while taking this medication. Consult prescriber for appropriate barrier contraceptive measures. Do not breast-feed.

Geriatric Considerations Elderly patients may have a higher incidence of severe neuropathy, severe myelosuppression, or cardiovascular events as compared to younger patients.

Breast-Feeding Issues Due to the potential for serious adverse reactions, breast-feeding is contraindicated.

Pregnancy Issues Animal studies have demonstrated embryotoxicity, fetal toxicity, and maternal toxicity. There are no adequate and well-controlled studies in pregnant women. Women of childbearing potential should be advised to avoid becoming pregnant.

Additional Information Sensory neuropathy is almost universal at doses >250 mg/m^2; motor neuropathy is uncommon at doses <250 mg/m^2. Myopathic effects are common with doses >200 mg/m^2, generally occur within 2-3 days of treatment, and resolve over 5-6 days. Intraperitoneal administration of paclitaxel is associated with a higher incidence of chemotherapy related toxicity.

Paclitaxel (Protein Bound)
(PAK li taks el PROE teen bownd)

U.S. Brand Names Abraxane™

Synonyms BI-007; NAB-Paclitaxel; Protein-Bound Paclitaxel

Pharmacologic Category Antineoplastic Agent, Antimicrotubular; Antineoplastic Agent, Natural Source (Plant) Derivative

Medication Safety Issues
Sound-alike/look-alike issues:
Paclitaxel (protein bound) may be confused with paclitaxel (conventional)
Abraxane™ may be confused with Paxil®, Taxol®, Taxotere®

Pregnancy Risk Factor D

Lactation Excretion in breast milk unknown/not recommended

Use Treatment of breast cancer (second-line)

Mechanism of Action/Effect Paclitaxel promotes microtubule assembly by enhancing the action of tubulin dimers, stabilizing existing microtubules, and inhibiting their disassembly, interfering with the late G$_2$ mitotic phase, and inhibiting cell replication. In addition, the drug can distort mitotic spindles, resulting in the breakage of chromosomes. Paclitaxel may also suppress cell proliferation and modulate immune response.

Contraindications Hypersensitivity to paclitaxel or any component of the formulation

Warnings/Precautions Hazardous agent — use appropriate precautions for handling and disposal.

Paclitaxel (protein-bound) is not interchangeable with Cremophor®-based paclitaxel. Severe sensory neuropathy may occur. Use caution in hepatic and renal dysfunction. When administered as sequential infusions, taxane derivatives (docetaxel, paclitaxel) should be administered before platinum derivatives (carboplatin, cisplatin) to limit myelosuppression.

Drug Interactions
Cytochrome P450 Effect: Substrate (major) of CYP2C8/9, 3A4; **Induces** CYP3A4 (weak)

Decreased Effect: CYP2C8/9 inducers may decrease the levels/effects of paclitaxel; example inducers include carbamazepine, phenobarbital, phenytoin, rifampin, rifapentine, and secobarbital. CYP3A4 inducers may decrease the levels/effects of paclitaxel;

example inducers include aminoglutethimide, carbamazepine, nafcillin, nevirapine, phenobarbital, phenytoin, and rifamycins.

Increased Effect/Toxicity: CYP2C8/9 inhibitors may increase the levels/effects of paclitaxel; example inhibitors include delavirdine, fluconazole, gemfibrozil, ketoconazole, nicardipine, NSAIDs, pioglitazone, and sulfonamides. CYP3A4 inhibitors may increase the levels/effects of paclitaxel; example inhibitors include azole antifungals, clarithromycin, diclofenac, doxycycline, erythromycin, imatinib, isoniazid, nefazodone, nicardipine, propofol, protease inhibitors, quinidine, telithromycin, and verapamil. In Phase I trials, myelosuppression was more profound when given after cisplatin than with alternative sequence. administered as sequential infusions, studies indicate a potential for increased toxicity when platinum derivatives (carboplatin, cisplatin) are administered before taxane derivatives (docetaxel, paclitaxel). Paclitaxel may increase doxorubicin levels/toxicity.

Nutritional/Ethanol Interactions
Herb/Nutraceutical: Avoid black cohosh, dong quai in estrogen-dependent tumors. Avoid valerian, St John's wort, kava kava, gotu kola (may increase CNS depression).

Adverse Reactions
>10%:
Cardiovascular: EKG abnormal (60%)
Dermatologic: Alopecia (90%)
Gastrointestinal: Nausea (30%; severe 3%), diarrhea (26%; severe <1%), vomiting (18%; severe 4%)
Hematologic: Neutropenia (80%; grade 4 - 9%), anemia (33%; severe 1%)
Hepatic: AST increased (39%), alkaline phosphatase increased (36%)
Neuromuscular & skeletal: Sensory neuropathy (71%; severe 10%), asthenia (47%; severe 8%), myalgia/arthralgia (44%; severe 8%)
Ocular: Vision disturbance (13%; severe 1%)
Respiratory: Dyspnea (12%)
Miscellaneous: Infections (24%; primarily included oral candidiasis, respiratory tract infections, and pneumonia)
1% to 10%:
Cardiovascular: Edema (10%; severe 0%), hypotension (5%), cardiovascular events (grade 3 - 3%; included chest pain, cardiac arrest, supraventricular tachycardia, edema, thrombosis, pulmonary thromboembolism, pulmonary emboli, and hypertension)
Central nervous system: Febrile neutropenia (2%)
Gastrointestinal: Mucositis (7%; severe <1%)
Hematologic: Thrombocytopenia (2%), bleeding (2%)
Hepatic: Bilirubin increased (7%)
Local: Injection site reaction (1%)
Renal: Creatinine increased (11%; severe 1%)
Respiratory: Cough (6%)
Miscellaneous: Hypersensitivity reaction (4%)

Overdosage/Toxicology Overdose would likely result in severe bone marrow suppression, sensory neuropathy, and mucositis. Treatment should be supportive.

Pharmacodynamics/Kinetics
Protein Binding: 89% to 98%
Half-Life Elimination: Terminal: 27 hours
Metabolism: Hepatic via CYP3A4 and 2C8
Excretion: Urine (4% as unchanged drug, 1% as metabolites); feces (20%)
Clearance 15 L/hour/m^2

Available Dosage Forms Injection, powder for reconstitution: 100 mg [contains human albumin 900 mg]

Dosing
Adults: Breast cancer: I.V.: 260 mg/m^2 every 3 weeks
Renal Impairment: Safety not established for serum creatinine >2 mg/dL; use with caution.
Hepatic Impairment: Effects of hepatic dysfunction (serum bilirubin >1.5 mg/dL) unknown; dosage adjustment recommendations are not available.

Dosing Adjustment for Toxicity:

Severe neutropenia (<500 cells/mm^3) ≥1 week: Reduce dose to 220 mg/m^2 for subsequent courses

Recurrent severe neutropenia: Reduce dose to 180 mg/m^2

Severe sensory neuropathy: Reduce dose to 180 mg/m^2

Sensory neuropathy grade 3 or 4: Hold treatment until resolved to grade 1 or 2, then resume with reduced dose

Administration

I.V.: Administer over 30 minutes. Do not use an in-line filter.

Stability

Reconstitution: Reconstitute vial with 20 mL NS to achieve 5 mg/mL solution. Inject dose for infusion into empty sterile container. **Note:** Use of DEHP-free containers or administration sets is not necessary. **Do not use an in-line filter.**

Compatibility: Stable in NS. Formulation contains albumin; do not mix with other drugs.

Storage: Store intact vial at room temperature of 20°C to 25°C (68°F to 77°F) and protect from bright light. Reconstituted solution may be stored under refrigeration 2°C to 8°C (36°F to 46°F) for up to 8 hours. The solution for administration is stable for up to 8 hours at room temperature and ambient light.

Laboratory Monitoring CBC, BP (during infusion)

Nursing Actions

Physical Assessment: Note: Paclitaxel (protein bound) is not interchangeable with paclitaxel. Taxane derivatives should be administered before platinum derivatives to limit myelosuppression. Assess potential for interactions with other pharmacological agents and herbal products patient may be taking (eg, risk of increased or decrease levels/effects of paclitaxel). See Administration for specific infusion directions. Monitor laboratory tests and adverse response prior to, during, and between each infusion (eg, cardiovascular abnormalities; sensory neuropathy [numbness, tingling, burning pain], myelosuppression [anemia, opportunistic infection], GI irritation [nausea, vomiting, mucositis, stomatitis]). Teach patient possible side effects/appropriate interventions and adverse symptoms to report.

Patient Education: This drug can only be administered by intravenous infusion; you will be monitored closely during and following infusions. Immediately report any burning, pain, or swelling at infusion site; any unusual chest pain or tightness, rapid heartbeat or palpitations; difficulty breathing; difficulty swallowing; nausea or vomiting; or other adverse symptoms during infusion. Do not take any new medications during therapy without consulting prescriber. You will be more susceptible to infection (avoid crowds and exposure to infection and do not have any vaccinations unless approved by prescriber. It is important that you maintain adequate nutrition and fluid intake (2-3 L/day of fluids, unless instructed to restrict fluid intake). May cause nausea or vomiting (small frequent meals, and frequent mouth care may help); mouth sores (sucking ice chip may be beneficial, use good mouth care with a soft toothbrush and waxed dental floss; if severe or infection occurs consult prescriber for appropriate treatment); diarrhea (buttermilk or yogurt may help); loss of hair (will grow back after therapy). Report chest pain, palpitations; swelling of extremities; difficult breathing; pain or decreased sensation in extremities; unusual sign of weakness, fatigue, lethargy, persistent gastrointestinal disturbances (nausea, vomiting, diarrhea); or other adverse reactions. **Pregnancy/breast-feeding precautions:** Inform prescriber if you are pregnant. Females should not get pregnant while taking this medication and males should not father a child while

receiving treatment. This drug may cause fetal deformities or loss of pregnancy; consult prescriber for appropriate contraceptives. Consult prescriber if breast-feeding.

Breast-Feeding Issues The manufacturer recommends that nursing be discontinued during paclitaxel (protein-bound) therapy.

Palonosetron (pal oh NOE se tron)

U.S. Brand Names Aloxi®

Synonyms Palonosetron Hydrochloride; RS-25259; RS-25259-197

Pharmacologic Category Antiemetic; Selective 5-HT$_3$ Receptor Antagonist

Medication Safety Issues

Sound-alike/look-alike issues:

Aloxi® may be confused with oxaliplatin

Palonosetron may be confused with dolasetron, granisetron, ondansetron

Pregnancy Risk Factor B

Lactation Excretion in breast milk unknown/not recommended

Use Prevention of acute (within 24 hours) and delayed (2-5 days) chemotherapy-induced nausea and vomiting

Note: Not recommended for treatment of existing chemotherapy-induced emesis (CIE)

Unlabeled/Investigational Use Prevention of postoperative vomiting

Mechanism of Action/Effect Selective 5-HT$_3$ receptor antagonist, blocking serotonin, both peripherally on vagal nerve terminals and centrally in the chemoreceptor trigger zone

Contraindications Hypersensitivity to palonosetron or any component of the formulation

Warnings/Precautions Use caution in patients allergic to other 5-HT$_3$ receptor antagonists; cross-reactivity is possible. Caution in patients with congenital QT syndrome or other risk factors for QT prolongation (eg, drugs, electrolyte abnormalities). Not intended for treatment of nausea and vomiting or for chronic continuous therapy. **For chemotherapy, should be used on a scheduled basis, not on an "as needed" (PRN) basis,** since data support the use of this drug only in the prevention of nausea and vomiting (due to antineoplastic therapy) and not in the rescue of nausea and vomiting. Safety and efficacy in pediatric patients (<18 years of age) have not been established.

Drug Interactions

Cytochrome P450 Effect: Substrate (minor) of CYP1A2, 2D6, 3A4

Increased Effect/Toxicity: Palonosetron may enhance the hypotensive effect of apomorphine; concurrent use is contraindicated.

Adverse Reactions

>10%: Dermatologic: Pruritus (8% to 22%)

1% to 10%:

Cardiovascular: Bradycardia (1%), hypotension (1%), tachycardia (nonsustained) (1%)

Central nervous system: Headache (6% to 9%), anxiety (1% to 5%), dizziness (1%)

Endocrine & metabolic: Hyperkalemia (1%)

Gastrointestinal: Constipation (5% to 10%), diarrhea (1%)

Neuromuscular & skeletal: Weakness (1%)

Overdosage/Toxicology Dose-ranging studies in humans using doses up to 25 times the recommended dose of 0.25 mg revealed no increase in the incidence of adverse effects compared to lower dose groups. Due to the large volume of distribution, dialysis would not be effective in the event of an overdose. Treatment should be symptom-directed and supportive.

(Continued)

Palonosetron *(Continued)*

Pharmacodynamics/Kinetics

Protein Binding: 62%

Half-Life Elimination: Terminal: 40 hours

Metabolism: ~50% metabolized via CYP enzymes (and likely other pathways) to relatively inactive metabolites (N-oxide-palonosetron and 6-S-hydroxy-palonosetron); CYP1A2, 2D6, and 3A4 contribute to its metabolism

Excretion: Urine (80%, 40% as unchanged drug)

Available Dosage Forms

Injection, solution:

Aloxi®: 0.05 mg/mL (5 mL) [contains disodium edetate]

Dosing

Adults:

Chemotherapy-induced nausea and vomiting: I.V.: 0.25 mg 30 minutes prior to chemotherapy administration, day 1 of each cycle (doses should not be given more than once weekly)

Breakthrough: Palonosetron has not been shown to be effective in terminating nausea or vomiting once it occurs and should not be used for this purpose.

Postoperative nausea and vomiting (unlabeled use): I.V.: 30 mcg/kg (used in hysterectomy, lower doses ineffective; no significant reduction in nausea at any dose)

Elderly: No dosage adjustment necessary.

Renal Impairment: No dosage adjustment necessary.

Hepatic Impairment: No dosage adjustment necessary.

Administration

I.V.: Infuse over 30 seconds; flush I.V. line with NS prior to and following administration.

I.V. Detail: pH: 4.5-5.5

Stability

Compatibility: Stable in D_5W, NS, $D_51/2NS$, and D_5LR

Y-site administration: Compatible: Doxorubicin, epirubicin

Storage: Store intact vials at controlled room temperature of 20°C to 25°C (68°F to 77°F); protect from freezing and light. Solutions of 5 mcg/mL and 30 mcg/mL in NS, D_5W, $D_51/2NS$, and D_5LR injection are stable for 48 hours at room temperature and 14 days under refrigeration.

Nursing Actions

Physical Assessment: Assess allergy history (5-HT$_3$ receptor antagonists) prior to administering. To be used on a scheduled basis (not on a "PRN" basis). Follow infusion specifics. Assess patient response and adverse reactions at beginning and periodically during therapy.

Patient Education: This medication can only be given by intravenous infusion. You will be monitored during infusion. Report immediately any chest pain, respiratory difficulty, pain or itching at infusion site. May cause dizziness, headache, or weakness (use caution to avoid falls or injury when driving or engaging in hazardous tasks until response to drug is known). Report rash or any unusual or persistent adverse effects. **Pregnancy/breast-feeding precautions:** Inform prescriber if you are or intend to become pregnant. Breast-feeding is not recommended.

Breast-Feeding Issues The extent to which palonosetron is excreted in breast milk, if at all, is unknown. Use in nursing women only if potential risks outweigh benefits.

Pamidronate (pa mi DROE nate)

U.S. Brand Names Aredia®

Synonyms Pamidronate Disodium

Pharmacologic Category Antidote; Bisphosphonate Derivative

Medication Safety Issues

Sound-alike/look-alike issues:

Aredia® may be confused with Adriamycin

Pregnancy Risk Factor D

Lactation Excretion in breast milk unknown/use caution

Use Treatment of hypercalcemia associated with malignancy; treatment of osteolytic bone lesions associated with multiple myeloma or metastatic breast cancer; moderate to severe Paget's disease of bone

Unlabeled/Investigational Use Treatment of pediatric osteoporosis, treatment of osteogenesis imperfecta

Mechanism of Action/Effect A bisphosphonate which inhibits bone resorption via actions on osteoclasts or on osteoclast precursors. Does not appear to produce any significant effects on renal tubular calcium handling and is poorly absorbed following oral administration (high oral doses have been reported effective); therefore, I.V. therapy is preferred.

Contraindications Hypersensitivity to pamidronate, other bisphosphonates, or any component of the formulation; pregnancy

Warnings/Precautions Bisphosphonate therapy has been associated with osteonecrosis, primarily of the jaw; this has been observed mostly in cancer patients, but also in patients with postmenopausal osteoporosis and other diagnoses. Dental exams and preventative dentistry should be performed prior to placing patients with risk factors on chronic bisphosphonate therapy. Invasive dental procedures should be avoided during treatment.

May cause deterioration in renal function. Use caution in patients with renal impairment and avoid in severe renal impairment. Assess serum creatinine prior to each dose; withhold dose in patients with bone metastases who experience deterioration in renal function. Leukopenia has been observed with oral pamidronate and monitoring of white blood cell counts is suggested. Patients with pre-existing anemia, leukopenia, or thrombocytopenia should be closely monitored during the first 2 weeks of treatment.

Vein irritation and thrombophlebitis may occur with infusions. Monitor serum electrolytes, especially in the elderly.

Severe (and occasionally debilitating) bone, joint, and/or muscle pain have been reported infrequently during bisphosphonate treatment. Onset of pain ranged from a single day to several months, with relief in most cases upon discontinuation of the drug. Patients may experience recurrence when rechallenged with the same drug or another bisphosphonate.

Drug Interactions

Decreased Effect: The following agents may decrease the absorption of oral bisphosphonate derivatives: Antacids (aluminum, calcium, magnesium), oral calcium salts, oral iron salts, and oral magnesium salts.

Increased Effect/Toxicity: Aminoglycosides may lower serum calcium levels with prolonged administration; concomitant use may have an additive hypocalcemic effect. NSAIDs may enhance the gastrointestinal adverse/toxic effects (increased incidence of GI ulcers) of bisphosphonate derivatives. Bisphosphonate derivatives may enhance the hypocalcemic effect of phosphate supplements.

Lab Interactions Bisphosphonates may interfere with diagnostic imaging agents such as technetium-99m-diphosphonate in bone scans.

Adverse Reactions Percentage of adverse effect varies upon dose and duration of infusion.

>10%:

Central nervous system: Fatigue (12% to 40%), fever (18% to 39%), headache (24% to 27%), anxiety (8% to 18%), insomnia (1% to 25%), pain (13% to 15%)

Endocrine & metabolic: Hypophosphatemia (9% to 18%), hypokalemia (4% to 18%), hypomagnesemia (4% to 12%), hypocalcemia (1% to 12%)

Gastrointestinal: Nausea (4% to 64%), vomiting (4% to 46%), anorexia (1% to 31%), abdominal pain (1% to 24%), dyspepsia (4% to 23%)

Genitourinary: Urinary tract infection (15% to 20%)

Hematologic: Anemia (6% to 48%), leukopenia (4% to 21%)

Local: Infusion site reaction (4% to 18%)

Neuromuscular & skeletal: Weakness (16% to 26%), myalgia (1% to 26%), arthralgia (11% to 15%)

Renal: Serum creatinine increased (19%)

Respiratory: Dyspnea (22% to 35%), cough (25% to 26%), upper respiratory tract infection (3% to 20%), sinusitis (15% to 16%), pleural effusion (3% to 15%)

1% to 10%:

Cardiovascular: Atrial fibrillation (6%), hypertension (6%), syncope (6%), tachycardia (6%), atrial flutter (1%), cardiac failure (1%), edema (1%)

Central nervous system: Somnolence (1% to 6%), psychosis (4%)

Endocrine & metabolic: Hypothyroidism (6%)

Gastrointestinal: Constipation (4% to 6%), gastrointestinal hemorrhage (6%), diarrhea (1%), stomatitis (1%)

Hematologic: Neutropenia (1%), thrombocytopenia (1%)

Neuromuscular & skeletal: Back pain (5%), bone pain (5%)

Renal: Uremia (4%)

Respiratory: Rales (6%), rhinitis (6%)

Miscellaneous: Moniliasis (6%)

Overdosage/Toxicology Symptoms of overdose include hypocalcemia, hypotension, ECG changes, seizures, bleeding, paresthesia, carpopedal spasm, and fever. Treat with I.V. calcium gluconate, and general supportive care; fever and hypotension can be treated with corticosteroids.

Pharmacodynamics/Kinetics

Onset of Action: 24-48 hours; Peak effect: Maximum: 5-7 days

Half-Life Elimination: 21-35 hours

Metabolism: Not metabolized

Excretion: Biphasic; urine (~50% as unchanged drug) within 120 hours

Available Dosage Forms

Injection, powder for reconstitution, as disodium (Aredia®): 30 mg, 90 mg

Injection, solution: 3 mg/mL (10 mL); 6 mg/mL (10 mL); 9 mg/mL (10 mL)

Dosing

Adults: Note: Drug must be diluted properly before administration and infused intravenously slowly. Due to risk of nephrotoxicity, doses should not exceed 90 mg.

Hypercalcemia of malignancy: I.V.:

Moderate cancer-related hypercalcemia (corrected serum calcium: 12-13.5 mg/dL): 60-90 mg, as a single dose

Severe cancer-related hypercalcemia (corrected serum calcium: >13.5 mg/dL): 90 mg, as a single dose

Repeat dosing: A period of 7 days should elapse before the use of second course; repeat infusions every 2-3 weeks have been suggested, however, could be administered every 2-3 months according to the degree and of severity of hypercalcemia and/or the type of malignancy.

Osteolytic bone lesions with multiple myeloma: I.V.: 90 mg monthly

Osteolytic bone lesions with metastatic breast cancer: I.V.: 90 mg repeated every 3-4 weeks

Paget's disease: I.V.: 30 mg for 3 consecutive days

Elderly: Refer to adult dosing. Begin at lower end of adult dosing range.

Renal Impairment: Not recommended in severe renal impairment (patients with bone metastases). Safety and efficacy have not been established in patients with serum creatinine >5 mg/dL. Studies are limited in multiple myeloma patients with serum creatinine ≥3 mg/dL.

Dosing adjustment in renal toxicity: In patients with bone metastases, treatment should be withheld in patients who experience deterioration in renal function (increase of serum creatinine ≥0.5 mg/dL in patients with normal baseline or ≥1.0 mg/dL in patients with abnormal baseline). Resumption of therapy may be considered when serum creatinine returns to within 10% of baseline.

Administration

I.V.: I.V. infusion over 2-24 hours.

I.V. Detail: pH: 6-7.4

Stability

Reconstitution: Powder for injection: Reconstitute by adding 10 mL of SWFI to each vial of lyophilized pamidronate disodium powder, the resulting solution will be 30 mg/10 mL or 90 mg/10 mL.

Pamidronate may be further diluted in 250-1000 mL of 0.45% or 0.9% sodium chloride or 5% dextrose.

Compatibility: Incompatible with calcium-containing infusion solutions such as lactated Ringer's

Storage:

Powder for reconstitution: Store below 30°C (86°F). The reconstituted solution is stable for 24 hours stored under refrigeration at 2°C to 8°C (36°F to 46°F).

Solution for injection: Store below 25°C (77°F).

Pamidronate solution for infusion is stable at room temperature for up to 24 hours.

Laboratory Monitoring Serum calcium, electrolytes, phosphate, magnesium, CBC with differential; monitor for hypocalcemia for at least 2 weeks after therapy; monitor serum creatinine prior to each dose; patients with pre-existing anemia, leukopenia or thrombocytopenia should be closely monitored during the first 2 weeks of treatment

Nursing Actions

Physical Assessment: Monitor laboratory results and assess for signs of hypocalcemia. Ensure adequate hydration. Teach patient lifestyle and dietary changes that will be beneficial, possible side effects, interventions to reduce side effects, and adverse reactions to report.

Patient Education: Do not take any new medication during therapy unless approved by prescriber. This medication can only be administered intravenously; report immediately any difficulty breathing, chest tightness, difficulty swallowing, redness, swelling, or pain at infusion site. You may experience nausea or vomiting (small frequent meals and good mouth care may help); loss of appetite; abdominal pain; heartburn; recurrent bone pain (consult prescriber for analgesic); fever; headache; anxiety; insomnia; increased fatigue (adequate rest is important); dizziness (use caution when driving or engaged in potentially dangerous tasks until response to drug is known). Report palpitations or rapid heart beat, unusual muscle twitching or spasms, persistent diarrhea/constipation, or acute bone pain, respiratory difficulty, or other persistent adverse effects. **Pregnancy/breast-feeding precautions:** Inform prescriber if you are pregnant. Do not get pregnant while taking this (Continued)

Pamidronate *(Continued)*

medication. Consult prescriber for appropriate contraceptive measures. Consult prescriber if breast-feeding.

Geriatric Considerations No overall differences in safety for the elderly were observed in studies. The elderly may be more sensitive to the effects of pamidronate. Consider initiating doses for the elderly at the lower end of the dosing range. Monitor serum electrolytes periodically since elderly are often receiving diuretics which can result in decreases in serum calcium, potassium, and magnesium.

Pregnancy Issues Pamidronate has been shown to cross the placenta and cause nonteratogenic embryo/fetal effects in animals. There are no adequate and well-controlled studies in pregnant women; manufacturer states pamidronate should not be used in pregnancy. Based on limited case reports, serum calcium levels in the newborn may be altered if pamidronate is administered during pregnancy. Bisphosphonates are incorporated into the bone matrix and gradually released over time. Theoretically, there may be a risk of fetal harm when pregnancy follows the completion of therapy. Women of childbearing potential should be advised to use effective contraception and avoid becoming pregnant during therapy.

Pancrelipase *(pan kre LI pase)*

U.S. Brand Names Creon®; Dygase; ku-zyme® HP; Lapase; Lipram 4500; Lipram-CR; Lipram-PN; Lipram-UL; Pancrease® [DSC]; Pancrease® MT; Pancrecarb MS®; Pangestyme™ CN; Pangestyme™ EC; Pangestyme™ MT; Pangestyme™ UL; Panokase®; Panokase® 16; Plaretase® 8000; Ultrase®; Ultrase® MT; Viokase®

Synonyms Lipancreatin

Pharmacologic Category Enzyme

Pregnancy Risk Factor B/C (product specific)

Lactation Excretion in breast milk unknown/use caution

Use Replacement therapy in symptomatic treatment of malabsorption syndrome caused by pancreatic insufficiency

Unlabeled/Investigational Use Treatment of occluded feeding tubes

Mechanism of Action/Effect Replaces endogenous pancreatic enzymes to assist in digestion of protein, starch and fats

Contraindications Hypersensitivity to pork protein or any component of the formulation; acute pancreatitis or acute exacerbations of chronic pancreatic disease

Warnings/Precautions Pancrelipase is inactivated by acids. Use microencapsulated products whenever possible, since these products permit better dissolution of enzymes in the duodenum and protect the enzyme preparations from acid degradation in the stomach. Fibrotic strictures in the colon, some requiring surgery, have been reported with high doses; use caution, especially in children with cystic fibrosis. Use caution when adjusting doses or changing brands. Avoid inhalation of powder, may cause nasal and respiratory tract irritation.

Nutritional/Ethanol Interactions Food: Avoid placing contents of opened capsules on alkaline food (pH >5.5); pancrelipase may impair absorption of oral iron and folic acid.

Adverse Reactions Frequency not defined; occurrence of events may be dose related.

Central nervous system: Pain

Dermatologic: Rash

Endocrine & metabolic: Hyperuricemia

Gastrointestinal: Nausea, cramps, constipation, diarrhea, perianal irritation/inflammation (large doses), irritation of the mouth, abdominal pain, intestinal obstruction, vomiting, flatulence, melena, weight loss, fibrotic strictures, greasy stools

Ocular: Lacrimation

Renal: Hyperuricosuria

Respiratory: Sneezing, dyspnea, bronchospasm

Miscellaneous: Allergic reactions

Overdosage/Toxicology Symptoms of overdose include diarrhea, other transient intestinal upset, hyperuricosuria, and hyperuricemia. Treatment is supportive.

Pharmacodynamics/Kinetics

Excretion: Feces

Available Dosage Forms [DSC] = Discontinued product

Capsule:

Dygase: Lipase 2400 units, protease 30,000 units, and amylase 30,000 units

ku-zyme® HP: Lipase 8000 units, protease 30,000 units, and amylase 30,000 units

Lapase: Lipase 1200 units, protease 15,000 units, and amylase 15,000 units [contains tartrazine]

Capsule, delayed release, enteric coated granules:

Pangestyme™ CN-10: Lipase 10,000 units, protease 37,500 units, amylase 33,200 units

Pangestyme™ CN-20: Lipase 20,000 units, protease 75,000 units, amylase 66,400 units

Pangestyme™ EC: Lipase 4500 units, protease 25,000 units, and amylase 20,000 units

Pangestyme™ MT16: Lipase 16,000 units, protease 48,000 units, and amylase 48,000 units

Pangestyme™ UL 12: Lipase 12,000 units, protease 39,000 units, and amylase 39,000 units

Pangestyme™ UL 18: Lipase 18,000 units, protease 58,500 units, and amylase 58,500 units

Pangestyme™ UL 20: Lipase 20,000 units, protease 65,000 units, and amylase 65,000 units

Capsule, delayed release, enteric coated microspheres:

Lipase 4500 units, protease 25,000 units, and amylase 25,000 units

Creon® 5: Lipase 5000 units, protease 18,750 units, and amylase 16,600 units

Creon® 10: Lipase 10,000 units, protease 37,500 units, and amylase 33,200 units

Creon® 20: Lipase 20,000 units, protease 75,000 units, and amylase 66,400 units

Lipram 4500: Lipase 4500 units, protease 25,000 units, and amylase 20,000 units

Lipram-CR5: Lipase 5000 units, protease 18,750 units, and amylase 16,600 units [DSC]

Lipram-CR10: Lipase 10,000 units, protease 37,500 units, and amylase 33,200 units

Lipram-CR20: Lipase 20,000 units, protease 75,000 units, and amylase 66,400 units

Lipram-PN10: Lipase 10,000 units, protease 30,000 units, and amylase 30,000 units

Lipram-PN16: Lipase 16,000 units, protease 48,000 units, and amylase 48,000 units

Lipram-PN20: Lipase 20,000 units, protease 44,000 units, and amylase 56,000 units

Lipram-UL12: Lipase 12,000 units, protease 39,000 units, and amylase 39,000 units

Lipram-UL18: Lipase 18,000 units, protease 58,500 units, and amylase 58,500 units

Lipram-UL20: Lipase 20,000 units, protease 65,000 units, and amylase 65,000 units

Pancrecarb MS-4®: Lipase 4000 units, protease 25,000 units, and amylase 25,000 units [buffered]

Pancrecarb MS-8®: Lipase 8000 units, protease 45,000 units, and amylase 40,000 units [buffered]

Capsule, enteric coated microspheres:

Pancrease® [DSC], Ultrase®: Lipase 4500 units, protease 25,000 units, and amylase 20,000 units

Capsule, enteric coated microtablets:

Pancrease® MT 4: Lipase 4000 units, protease 12,000 units, and amylase 12,000 units

Pancrease® MT 10: Lipase 10,000 units, protease 30,000 units, and amylase 30,000 units

Pancrease® MT 16: Lipase 16,000 units, protease 48,000 units, and amylase 48,000 units
Pancrease® MT 20: Lipase 20,000 units, protease 44,000 units, and amylase 56,000 units

Capsule, enteric coated minitablets:
Ultrase® MT12: Lipase 12,000 units, protease 39,000 units, and amylase 39,000 units
Ultrase® MT18: Lipase 18,000 units, protease 58,500 units, and amylase 58,500 units
Ultrase® MT20: Lipase 20,000 units, protease 65,000 units, and amylase 65,000 units

Powder (Viokase®): Lipase 16,800 units, protease 70,000 units, and amylase 70,000 units per 0.7 g (227 g)

Tablet: Lipase 8000 units, protease 30,000 units, and amylase 30,000 units

Panokase®: Lipase 8000 units, protease 30,000 units, and amylase 30,000 units

Panokase® 16: Lipase 16,000 units, protease 60,000 units, and amylase 60,000 units

Plaretase™ 8000: Lipase 8000 units, protease 30,000 units, and amylase 30,000 units

Viokase® 8: Lipase 8000 units, protease 30,000 units, and amylase 30,000 units

Viokase® 16: Lipase 16,000 units, protease 60,000 units, and amylase 60,000 units

Dosing

Adults & Elderly:

Malabsorption: Oral:

Powder: Actual dose depends on the condition being treated and the digestive requirements of the patient: 0.7 g (¼ teaspoonful) with meals

Capsules/tablets: The following dosage recommendations are only an approximation for initial dosages. The actual dosage will depend on the condition being treated and the digestive requirements of the individual patient.

Note: Dosage adjustment: Adjust dose based on body weight and stool fat content. Total daily dose reflects ~3 meals/day and 2-3 snacks/day, with half the mealtime dose given with a snack. Older patients may need less units/kg due to increased weight, but decreased ingestion of fat/kg. Maximum dose: 2500 units of lipase/kg/meal (10,000 units of lipase/kg/day): 4000-48,000 units of lipase with meals and with snacks

Occluded feeding tubes (unlabeled use): One tablet of Viokase® crushed with one 325 mg tablet of sodium bicarbonate (to activate the Viokase®) in 5 mL of water can be instilled into the nasogastric tube and clamped for 5 minutes; then, flushed with 50 mL of tap water

Pediatrics:

Malabsorption: Oral:

Powder: Actual dose depends on the condition being treated and the digestive requirements of the patient: Children <1 year: Start with ⅛ teaspoonful with feedings

Capsules/tablets: Children: Approximate initial dosages; actual dosage will depend on the condition being treated and the digestive requirements of the individual patient.

<1 year: 2000 units of lipase with meals
1-6 years: 4000-8000 units of lipase with meals and 4000 units with snacks
7-12 years: 4000-12,000 units of lipase with meals and snacks

Note: Dosage adjustment: Adjust dose based on body weight and stool fat content. Total daily dose reflects ~3 meals/day and 2-3 snacks/day, with half the mealtime dose given with a snack.

Administration

Oral: Oral: Administer with meals or snacks and swallow whole with a generous amount of liquid. Do not crush or chew; retention in the mouth before swallowing may cause mucosal irritation and stomatitis. Delayed-release capsules containing enteric-coated microspheres or microtablets may also be opened and the contents sprinkled on soft food with a low pH that does not require chewing, such as applesauce, gelatin; apricot, banana, or sweet potato baby food; baby formula. Dairy products such as milk, custard, or ice cream may have a high pH and should be avoided. Avoid inhalation of powder, may cause nasal and respiratory tract irritation.

Stability

Storage: Store between 15°C to 25°C (59°F to 77°F). Keep in a dry place. Do not refrigerate.

Nursing Actions

Physical Assessment: Dosing and administration depends on purpose for use. Use caution preparing powder. If powder spills on skin, wash off immediately. Do not inhale powder. Teach patient possible side effects/appropriate interventions and adverse symptoms to report

Patient Education: Do not take any new medication during therapy unless approved by prescriber. Take right before or with foods and swallow whole with a generous amount of liquid. Dairy products, such as milk, custard, or ice cream, may have a high pH and should not taken together with this medication. Do not crush or chew tablets or regular capsules. Delayed-release capsules containing enteric coated microspheres or microtablets may be opened and the contents sprinkled on soft food with a low pH such as applesauce, gelatin, apricot, banana, or sweet potato baby food. **Powder:** If powder spills on skin, wash off immediately, do not inhale powder when preparing. You may experience some gastric discomfort. Report unusual rash, persistent GI upset; or respiratory difficulty. **Pregnancy/breast-feeding precautions:** Inform prescriber if you are or intend to become pregnant. Consult prescriber if breast-feeding.

Dietary Considerations Should be used as part of a high-calorie diet, appropriate for age and clinical status. Administer with meals or snacks and swallow whole with a generous amount of liquid. Do not crush or chew. Delayed-release capsules containing enteric coated microspheres or microtablets may also be opened and the contents sprinkled on soft food with a low pH such as applesauce, gelatin; apricot, banana, or sweet potato baby food; baby formula. Dairy products such as milk, custard or ice cream may have a high pH and should be avoided.

Geriatric Considerations No special considerations are necessary since drug is dosed to response; however, drug-induced diarrhea can result in unwanted side effects (confusion, hypotension, lethargy, fluid and electrolyte loss).

Breast-Feeding Issues Systemic absorption and concentration in the breast milk is unlikely, but unknown.

Pancuronium (pan kyoo ROE nee um)

Synonyms Pancuronium Bromide; Pavulon [DSC]

Pharmacologic Category Neuromuscular Blocker Agent, Nondepolarizing

Medication Safety Issues

Sound-alike/look-alike issues:
Pancuronium may be confused with pipecuronium

Pregnancy Risk Factor C

Lactation Excretion in breast milk unknown/not recommended

Use Adjunct to general anesthesia to facilitate endotracheal intubation and to relax skeletal muscles during surgery; to facilitate mechanical ventilation in ICU patients; does not relieve pain or produce sedation

Drug of choice for neuromuscular blockade except in patients with renal failure, hepatic failure, or cardiovascular instability or in situations not suited for pancuronium's long duration of action

(Continued)

Pancuronium (Continued)

Mechanism of Action/Effect Blocks neural transmission at the myoneural junction by binding with cholinergic receptor sites

Contraindications Hypersensitivity to pancuronium, bromide, or any component of the formulation

Warnings/Precautions Ventilation must be supported during neuromuscular blockade; use with caution in patients with renal and/or hepatic impairment (adjust dose appropriately); certain clinical conditions may result in potentiation or antagonism of neuromuscular blockade:

Potentiation: Electrolyte abnormalities, severe hyponatremia, severe hypocalcemia, severe hypokalemia, hypermagnesemia, neuromuscular diseases, acidosis, acute intermittent porphyria, renal failure, hepatic failure

Antagonism: Alkalosis, hypercalcemia, demyelinating lesions, peripheral neuropathies, diabetes mellitus

Increased sensitivity in patients with myasthenia gravis, Eaton-Lambert syndrome; resistance in burn patients (>30% of body) for period of 5-70 days postinjury; resistance in patients with muscle trauma, denervation, immobilization, infection. Cross-sensitivity with other neuromuscular-blocking agents may occur; use extreme caution in patients with previous anaphylactic reactions.

Drug Interactions

Decreased Effect: Effect of nondepolarizing neuromuscular blockers may be reduced by carbamazepine (chronic use), corticosteroids (also associated with myopathy - see increased effect), phenytoin (chronic use), sympathomimetics, and theophylline.

Increased Effect/Toxicity: Increased effects are possible with aminoglycosides, beta-blockers, clindamycin, calcium channel blockers, halogenated anesthetics, imipenem, ketamine, lidocaine, loop diuretics (furosemide), macrolides (case reports), magnesium sulfate, procainamide, quinidine, quinolones, tetracyclines, and vancomycin. May increase risk of myopathy when used with high-dose corticosteroids for extended periods.

Adverse Reactions Frequency not defined.

Cardiovascular: Elevation in pulse rate, elevated blood pressure and cardiac output, tachycardia, edema, skin flushing, circulatory collapse

Dermatologic: Rash, itching, erythema, burning sensation along the vein

Gastrointestinal: Excessive salivation

Neuromuscular & skeletal: Profound muscle weakness

Respiratory: Wheezing, bronchospasm

Miscellaneous: Hypersensitivity reaction

Causes of prolonged neuromuscular blockade: Excessive drug administration; cumulative drug effect, decreased metabolism/excretion (hepatic and/or renal impairment); accumulation of active metabolites; electrolyte imbalance (hypokalemia, hypocalcemia, hypermagnesemia, hypernatremia); hypothermia; drug interactions; increased sensitivity to muscle relaxants (eg, neuromuscular disorders such as myasthenia gravis or polymyositis)

Overdosage/Toxicology Symptoms of overdose include apnea, respiratory depression, and cardiovascular collapse. Pyridostigmine, neostigmine, or edrophonium in conjunction with atropine will usually antagonize the action of pancuronium.

Pharmacodynamics/Kinetics

Onset of Action: Peak effect: I.V.: 2-3 minutes

Duration of Action: Dose dependent: 60-100 minutes

Half-Life Elimination: 110 minutes

Metabolism: Hepatic (30% to 45%); active metabolite 3-hydroxypancuronium ($\frac{1}{3}$ to $\frac{1}{2}$ the activity of parent drug)

Excretion: Urine (55% to 70% as unchanged drug)

Available Dosage Forms Injection, solution, as bromide: 1 mg/mL (10 mL); 2 mg/mL (2 mL, 5 mL) [may contain benzyl alcohol]

Dosing

Adults & Elderly: Administer I.V.; dose to effect; doses will vary due to interpatient variability; use ideal body weight for obese patients

Neuromuscular blockade: Initial: 0.06-0.1 mg/kg or 0.05 mg/kg after initial dose of succinylcholine for intubation; maintenance dose: 0.01 mg/kg 60-100 minutes after initial dose and then 0.01 mg/kg every 25-60 minutes

Pretreatment/priming: 10% of intubating dose given 3-5 minutes before initial dose

Neuromuscular blockade in the ICU: 0.05-0.1 mg/kg bolus followed by 0.8-1.7 mcg/kg/minute once initial recovery from bolus observed or 0.1-0.2 mg/kg every 1-3 hours

Pediatrics: Infants >1 month and Children: Refer to adult dosing.

Renal Impairment: Elimination half-life is doubled, plasma clearance is reduced, and rate of recovery is sometimes much slower.

Cl$_{cr}$ 10-50 mL/minute: Administer 50% of normal dose.

Cl$_{cr}$ <10 mL/minute: Do not use.

Hepatic Impairment: Elimination half-life is doubled, plasma clearance is doubled, recovery time is prolonged, volume of distribution is increased (50%) and results in a slower onset, higher total dosage, and prolongation of neuromuscular blockade. Patients with liver disease may develop slow resistance to nondepolarizing muscle relaxant. Large doses may be required and problems may arise in antagonism.

Administration

I.V.: May be administered undiluted by rapid I.V. injection.

I.V. Detail: pH: 4 (adjusted)

Stability

Compatibility: Stable in D$_5$NS, D$_5$W, LR, NS

Y-site administration: Incompatible with diazepam, thiopental

Storage: Refrigerate; however, is stable for up to 6 months at room temperature.

Nursing Actions

Physical Assessment: Only clinicians experienced in the use of neuromuscular blocking drugs should administer and/or manage the use of pancuronium. Ventilatory support must be instituted and maintained until adequate respiratory muscle function and/or airway protection are assured. Assess other medications for effectiveness and safety. Other drugs that affect neuromuscular activity may increase/decrease neuromuscular block induced by pancuronium. This drug does not cause anesthesia or analgesia; pain must be treated with appropriate analgesic agents. Continuous monitoring of vital signs, cardiac status, respiratory status, and degree of neuromuscular block (objective assessment with peripheral external nerve stimulator) is mandatory and until full muscle tone has returned. Muscle tone returns in a predictable pattern, starting with diaphragm, abdomen, chest, limbs, and finally muscles of the neck, face, and eyes. Safety precautions must be maintained until full muscle tone has returned. **Note:** It may take longer for return of muscle tone in obese or elderly patients or patients with renal or hepatic disease, myasthenia gravis, myopathy, other neuromuscular disease, dehydration, electrolyte imbalance, or severe acid/base imbalance. Provide appropriate patient teaching/support prior to and following administration.

Long-term use: Monitor fluid levels (intake and output) during and following infusion. Reposition patient and provide appropriate skin care, mouth care, and care of patient's eyes every 2-3 hours while sedated. Provide appropriate emotional and sensory support (auditory and environmental).

Patient Education: Patient will usually be unconscious prior to administration. Patient education should be appropriate to individual situation. Reassurance of constant monitoring and emotional support to reduce fear and anxiety should precede and follow administration. Following return of muscle tone, do not attempt to change position or rise from bed without assistance. Report immediately any skin rash or hives, pounding heartbeat, respiratory difficulty, or muscle tremors. **Pregnancy/breast-feeding precautions:** Inform prescriber if you are pregnant. Breast-feeding is not recommended.

Additional Information Pancuronium is classified as a long-duration neuromuscular-blocking agent. Neuromuscular blockade will be prolonged in patients with decreased renal function. Pancuronium does not relieve pain or produce sedation. It may produce cumulative effect on duration of blockade. It produces tachycardia secondary to vagolytic activity and sympathetic stimulation.

Pantoprazole (pan TOE pra zole)

U.S. Brand Names Protonix®

Pharmacologic Category Proton Pump Inhibitor; Substituted Benzimidazole

Medication Safety Issues
Sound-alike/look-alike issues:
Protonix® may be confused with Lotronex®, Lovenox®, protamine

Vials containing Protonix® I.V. for injection are not recommended for use with spiked I.V. system adaptors. Nurses and pharmacists have reported breakage of the glass vials during attempts to connect spiked I.V. system adaptors, which may potentially result in injury to healthcare professionals.

Pregnancy Risk Factor B

Lactation Enters breast milk/not recommended

Use
Oral: Treatment and maintenance of healing of erosive esophagitis associated with GERD; reduction in relapse rates of daytime and nighttime heartburn symptoms in GERD; hypersecretory disorders associated with Zollinger-Ellison syndrome or other neoplastic disorders

I.V.: Short-term treatment (7-10 days) of patients with gastroesophageal reflux disease (GERD) and a history of erosive esophagitis; hypersecretory disorders associated with Zollinger-Ellison syndrome or other neoplastic disorders

Unlabeled/Investigational Use Peptic ulcer disease, active ulcer bleeding (parenteral formulation); adjunct treatment with antibiotics for *Helicobacter pylori* eradication

Mechanism of Action/Effect Suppresses gastric acid secretion by inhibiting the parietal cell H^+/K^+ ATP pump

Contraindications Hypersensitivity to pantoprazole, substituted benzamidazoles (ie, esomeprazole, lansoprazole, omeprazole, rabeprazole), or any component of the formulation

Warnings/Precautions Symptomatic response does not preclude gastric malignancy. Not indicated for maintenance therapy; safety and efficacy for use beyond 16 weeks have not been established. Prolonged treatment (typically >3 years) may lead to vitamin B_{12} malabsorption. Intravenous preparation contains edetate sodium (EDTA); use caution in patients who are risk for zinc deficiency if other EDTA-containing solutions are coadministered. Safety and efficacy in pediatric patients have not been established.

Drug Interactions

Cytochrome P450 Effect: Substrate of CYP2C19 (major), 3A4 (minor); **Inhibits** 2C8/9 (moderate); **Induces** CYP1A2 (weak), 3A4 (weak)

Decreased Effect: Proton pump inhibitors may decrease the absorption of atazanavir, indinavir, iron salts, itraconazole, and ketoconazole. The levels/effects of pantoprazole may be decreased by aminoglutethimide, carbamazepine, phenytoin, rifampin, and other CYP2C19 inducers.

Increased Effect/Toxicity: Pantoprazole may increase the levels/effects of amiodarone, fluoxetine, glimepiride, glipizide, nateglinide, phenytoin, pioglitazone, rosiglitazone, sertraline, warfarin, and other CYP2C8/9 substrates.

Nutritional/Ethanol Interactions
Ethanol: Avoid ethanol (may cause gastric mucosal irritation).
Herb/Nutraceutical: Prolonged treatment (typically >3 years) may lead to vitamin B_{12} malabsorption.

Lab Interactions False-positive urine screening tests for tetrahydrocannabinol (THC) have been reported in patients receiving proton pump inhibitors, including pantoprazole.

Adverse Reactions
≥1%:
Cardiovascular: Chest pain
Central nervous system: Headache (5% to 9%), insomnia (<1% to 1%), dizziness, migraine, anxiety
Dermatologic: Rash (<1% to 2%)
Endocrine and metabolic: Hyperglycemia (<1% to 1%), hyperlipidemia
Gastrointestinal: Diarrhea (4% to 6%), flatulence (2% to 4%), abdominal pain (1% to 4%), nausea (≤2%), vomiting (≤2%), eructation (≤1%), constipation, dyspepsia, gastroenteritis, rectal disorder
Genitourinary: Urinary frequency, UTI
Hepatic: Liver function abnormal (up to 2%)
Local: Injection site reaction (includes thrombophlebitis and abscess)
Neuromuscular & skeletal: Arthralgia, back pain, hypertonia, neck pain, weakness
Respiratory: Bronchitis, cough, dyspnea, pharyngitis, rhinitis, sinusitis, upper respiratory tract infection
Miscellaneous: Flu syndrome, infection, pain

Overdosage/Toxicology Treatment of an overdose would include appropriate supportive treatment. No adverse events were seen with ingestions of 400 and 600 mg doses. Pantoprazole is not removed by hemodialysis.

Pharmacodynamics/Kinetics
Time to Peak: Oral: 2.5 hours
Protein Binding: 98%, primarily to albumin
Half-Life Elimination: 1 hour; increased to 3.5-10 hours with CYP2C19 deficiency
Metabolism: Extensively hepatic; CYP2C19 (demethylation), CYP3A4; no evidence that metabolites have pharmacologic activity
Excretion: Urine (71%); feces (18%)

Available Dosage Forms [DSC] = Discontinued product; **Note:** Strength expressed as base
Injection, powder for reconstitution, as sodium: 40 mg [original formulation] [DSC]
Injection, powder for reconstitution, as sodium: 40 mg [contains edetate sodium 1 mg]
Tablet, delayed release, as sodium: 20 mg, 40 mg

Dosing
Adults & Elderly:
Erosive esophagitis associated with GERD:
Oral:
Treatment: 40 mg once daily for up to 8 weeks; an additional 8 weeks may be used in patients who have not healed after an 8-week course
Maintenance of healing: 40 mg once daily

(Continued)

Pantoprazole *(Continued)*

Note: Lower doses (20 mg once daily) have been used successfully in mild GERD treatment and maintenance of healing

I.V.: 40 mg once daily for 7-10 days

Peptic ulcer disease: Eradication of *Helicobacter pylori* (unlabeled use): Oral: Doses up to 40 mg twice daily have been used as part of combination therapy

Hypersecretory disorders (including Zollinger-Ellison):

Oral: Initial: 40 mg twice daily; adjust dose based on patient needs; doses up to 240 mg/day have been administered

I.V.: 80 mg twice daily; adjust dose based on acid output measurements; 160-240 mg/day in divided doses has been used for a limited period (up to 7 days)

Prevention of rebleeding in peptic ulcer bleed (unlabeled use): I.V.: 80 mg, followed by 8 mg/hour infusion for 72 hours. **Note:** A daily infusion of 40 mg does not raise gastric pH sufficiently to enhance coagulation in active GI bleeds.

Renal Impairment: No adjustment is required. Pantoprazole is not removed by hemodialysis.

Hepatic Impairment: No adjustment is required.

Administration

Oral: Tablets should be swallowed whole, do not crush or chew. Best if taken before breakfast.

I.V.: Flush I.V. line before and after administration. Solutions prepared from original formulation must be infused through an inline filter. Solutions prepared from the EDTA-stabilized formulation do not require an in-line filter (per manufacturer).

2-minute infusion: The volume of reconstituted solution (4 mg/mL) to be injected may be administered intravenously over at least 2 minutes.

15-minute infusion: Infuse over 15 minutes at a rate not to exceed 7 mL/minute (3 mg/minute).

Stability

Reconstitution: Reconstitute with 10 mL NS (final concentration 4 mg/mL). Reconstituted solution may be given intravenously (over 2 minutes) or may be added to 100 mL D_5W, NS, or LR (for 15-minute infusion).

Compatibility: Y-site administration: Incompatible: Midazolam, zinc

Storage:

Oral: Store tablet at 15°C to 30°C (59°F to 77°F)

I.V.:

EDTA-stabilized formulation: Prior to use: Store at 15°C to 30°C (59°F to 86°F). Protect from light. When reconstituted with 10 mL NS (final concentration 4 mg/mL), solution is stable up to 24 hours at room temperature. Diluted solution is stable at room temperature for up to 24 hours from the time of initial reconstitution; potection from light not required.

Original formulation (discontinued): Store at 2°C to 8°C (36°F to 46°F). Protect from light. When reconstituted with 10 mL NS (final concentration 4 mg/mL), solution is stable up to 2 hours at room temperature; protection from light not required. When diluted in 100 mL D_5W, LR, or NS, may be stored at room temperature for up to 12 hours.

Nursing Actions

Physical Assessment: Assess other medications for effectiveness and interactions. Monitor therapeutic effectiveness (reduction in symptoms) and adverse effects at beginning of therapy and regularly with long-term use. Monitor therapeutic effectiveness and adverse effects at beginning of therapy and regularly with long-term use. Assess knowledge/teach patient appropriate use, possible side effects/interventions, and adverse symptoms to report.

Patient Education: Take as directed; do not alter dosage without consulting prescriber. Take at similar time each day. Swallow tablet whole (do not crush or chew). Avoid alcohol. You may experience dizziness, headache, or anxiety (use caution when driving or engaging in dangerous activities until response to medication is known); vomiting or loss of appetite (small frequent meals, frequent mouth care, sucking lozenges, or chewing gum may help); or diarrhea (boiled milk, yogurt, or buttermilk may help). Report persistent abdominal discomfort; chest pain or palpitations; acute headache; unresolved diarrhea; excessive fatigue; increased muscle, joint, or body pain; shortness of breath or wheezing; cold or flu symptoms; changes in urinary pattern; or other persistent adverse reactions. **Pregnancy/breast-feeding precautions:** Inform prescriber if you are pregnant. Breast-feeding is not recommended.

Dietary Considerations

Oral: May be taken with or without food; best if taken before breakfast.

I.V.: Due to EDTA in preparation, zinc supplementation may be needed in patients prone to zinc deficiency.

Breast-Feeding Issues Not recommended due to carcinogenicity in animal studies.

Papain and Urea *(pa PAY in & yoor EE a)*

U.S. Brand Names Accuzyme®; Ethezyme™; Ethezyme™ 830; Gladase®; Kovia®

Pharmacologic Category Enzyme, Topical Debridement

Use Debridement of necrotic tissue and liquefaction of slough in acute and chronic lesions such as pressure ulcers, varicose and diabetic ulcers, burns, postoperative wounds, pilonidal cyst wounds, carbuncles, and miscellaneous traumatic or infected wounds

Available Dosage Forms

Ointment, topical:

Accuzyme®: Papain 6.5 x 10^5 units/g and urea 10% (6 g, 30 g)

Ethezyme™: Papain 1.1 x 10^6 units and urea 10% (30 g)

Ethezyme™ 830: Papain 8.3 x 10^5 units/g and urea 10% (30 g)

Gladase®: Papain 8.3 x 10^5 units/g and urea 10% (6 g, 30 g)

Kovia®: Papain 8.3 x 10^5 units/g and urea 10% (3.5 g) [single-dose packet]; 30 g

Spray, topical:

Accuzyme®: Papain 6.5 x 10^5 units/g and urea 10% (33 mL)

Dosing

Adults & Elderly: Topical: Apply with each dressing change. Daily or twice daily dressing changes are preferred, but may be every 2-3 days. Cover with dressing following application.

Ointment: Apply 1/8- inch thickness over the wound with clean applicator

Spray: Completely cover the wound site so that the wound is not visible

Nursing Actions

Physical Assessment: Monitor therapeutic response and adverse reactions at the beginning and periodically throughout therapy.

Patient Education: For external use only. Skin should be cleansed or irrigated prior to use. Hydrogen peroxide should not be used (may inactivate papain). Apply to entire wound area so that wound is not visible. Dressing changes are recommended once to twice daily. Do not use near eyes. **Pregnancy/breast-feeding precautions:** Inform prescriber if you are or intend to become pregnant. Consult prescriber if breast-feeding.

Papaverine (pa PAV er een)

U.S. Brand Names Para-Time SR®
Synonyms Papaverine Hydrochloride; Pavabid [DSC]
Pharmacologic Category Vasodilator
Pregnancy Risk Factor C
Lactation Excretion in breast milk unknown/not recommended
Use Oral: Relief of peripheral and cerebral ischemia associated with arterial spasm and myocardial ischemia complicated by arrhythmias
Unlabeled/Investigational Use Investigational: Parenteral: Various vascular spasms associated with muscle spasms as in myocardial infarction, angina, peripheral and pulmonary embolism, peripheral vascular disease, angiospastic states, and visceral spasm (ureteral, biliary, and GI colic); testing for impotence
Mechanism of Action/Effect Smooth muscle spasmolytic producing a generalized smooth muscle relaxation including: vasodilatation, GI sphincter relaxation, bronchiolar muscle relaxation, and potentially a depressed myocardium (with large doses); muscle relaxation may occur due to inhibition or cyclic nucleotide phosphodiesterase, increasing cyclic AMP; muscle relaxation is unrelated to nerve innervation; papaverine increases cerebral blood flow in normal subjects; oxygen uptake is unaltered
Contraindications Hypersensitivity to papaverine or any component of the formulation
Warnings/Precautions Use with caution in patients with glaucoma. Administer I.V. cautiously since apnea and arrhythmias may result. May, in large doses, depress cardiac conduction (eg, AV node) leading to arrhythmias. May interfere with levodopa therapy of Parkinson's disease. Hepatic hypersensitivity has been noted with jaundice, eosinophilia, and abnormal LFTs.
Drug Interactions
  Decreased Effect: Papaverine decreases the effects of levodopa.
Nutritional/Ethanol Interactions Ethanol: Avoid ethanol (may increase CNS depression).
Adverse Reactions Frequency not defined.
  Cardiovascular: Arrhythmias (with rapid I.V. use), flushing of the face, mild hypertension, tachycardia
  Central nervous system: Drowsiness, headache, lethargy, sedation, vertigo
  Gastrointestinal: Abdominal distress, anorexia, constipation, diarrhea, nausea
  Hepatic: Chronic hepatitis, hepatic hypersensitivity
  Respiratory: Apnea (with rapid I.V. use)
Overdosage/Toxicology Symptoms of overdose include nausea, vomiting, weakness, gastric distress, ataxia, hepatic dysfunction, drowsiness, nystagmus, hyperventilation, hypotension, and hypokalemia. Treatment is supportive.
Pharmacodynamics/Kinetics
  Onset of Action: Oral: Rapid
  Protein Binding: 90%
  Half-Life Elimination: 0.5-1.5 hours
  Metabolism: Rapidly hepatic
  Excretion: Primarily urine (as metabolites)
Available Dosage Forms
  Capsule, sustained release, as hydrochloride (Para-Time SR®): 150 mg
  Injection, solution, as hydrochloride: 30 mg/mL (2 mL, 10 mL)
Dosing
  Adults & Elderly: Arterial spasm:
    Oral, sustained release: 150-300 mg every 12 hours; in difficult cases: 150 mg every 8 hours
    I.M., I.V.: 30-65 mg (rarely up to 120 mg); may repeat every 3 hours
  Pediatrics: Arterial spasm: I.M., I.V.: 6 mg/kg/day in 4 divided doses

  I.V.: Rapid I.V. administration may result in arrhythmias and fatal apnea; administer no faster than over 1-2 minutes.
  I.V. Detail: pH: Not <3; 3-4 (2% solution in water)
Stability
  Reconstitution: Solutions should be clear to pale yellow. Precipitates with lactated Ringer's.
  Compatibility: Stable in dextran 6% in dextrose, dextran 6% in NS, D₅LR, D₅¼NS, D₅½NS, D₅NS, D₅W, D₁₀W, ½NS, NS; **incompatible** with LR
    Compatibility in syringe: Incompatible with diatrizoate meglumine 52%, diatrizoate sodium 8%
    Compatibility when admixed: Incompatible with aminophylline with trimecaine
  Storage: Protect from heat or freezing. Refrigerate injection at 2°C to 8°C (35°F to 46°F).
Nursing Actions
  Physical Assessment: I.V., I.M.: Blood pressure and heart rate should be monitored. **I.V.:** Should be administered slowly (over 1-2 minutes) to avoid apnea or arrhythmias. **Oral:** Blood pressure and heart rate should be monitored prior to therapy and at frequent intervals thereafter. Monitor therapeutic effectiveness and adverse response (eg, arrhythmias, tachycardia, hypertension, GI disturbance). Teach patient proper use, possible side effects/appropriate interventions, and adverse symptoms to report.
  Patient Education: Do not take any new medication during therapy unless approved by prescriber. Take as directed; do not alter dose or discontinue without consulting prescriber. Swallow extended release capsules whole; do not chew, crush, or dissolve. May cause dizziness, confusion, or blurred vision (avoid driving or engaging in tasks that require alertness until response to drug is known); or constipation (increased exercise, fluids, fruit, or fiber may help). Report rapid heartbeat or palpitations and CNS changes (eg, depression, persistent sedation or lethargy, or acute headache). **Pregnancy/breast-feeding precautions:** Inform prescriber if you are or intend to become pregnant. Breast-feeding is not recommended.
  Dietary Considerations May be taken with food.
  Geriatric Considerations Vasodilators have been used to treat dementia upon the premise that dementia is secondary to a cerebral blood flow insufficiency. The hypothesis is that if blood flow could be increased, cognitive function would be increased. This hypothesis is no longer valid. The use of vasodilators for cognitive dysfunction is not recommended or proven by appropriate scientific study.

Paregoric (par e GOR ik)

Synonyms Camphorated Tincture of Opium (error-prone synonym)
Restrictions C-III
Pharmacologic Category Analgesic, Narcotic
Medication Safety Issues
  Sound-alike/look-alike issues:
    Camphorated tincture of opium is an error-prone synonym (mistaken as opium tincture)
    Paregoric may be confused with Percogesic®

  Use care when prescribing opium tincture; each mL contains the equivalent of morphine 10 mg; paregoric contains the equivalent of morphine 0.4 mg/mL
Pregnancy Risk Factor B/D (prolonged use or high doses)
Lactation Enters breast milk/use caution
Use Treatment of diarrhea or relief of pain; neonatal opiate withdrawal
(Continued)

Paregoric (Continued)

Mechanism of Action/Effect Increases smooth muscle tone in GI tract, decreases motility and peristalsis, diminishes digestive secretions

Contraindications Hypersensitivity to opium or any component of the formulation; diarrhea caused by poisoning until the toxic material has been removed; pregnancy (prolonged use or high doses)

Warnings/Precautions Use with caution in patients with respiratory, hepatic or renal dysfunction, severe prostatic hyperplasia, or history of narcotic abuse. Opium shares the toxic potential of opiate agonists, and usual precautions of opiate agonist therapy should be observed. Some preparations contain sulfites which may cause allergic reactions.

Drug Interactions
Increased Effect/Toxicity: Increased effect/toxicity with CNS depressants (eg, alcohol, narcotics, benzodiazepines, tricyclic antidepressants, MAO inhibitors, phenothiazine).

Nutritional/Ethanol Interactions Ethanol: Avoid ethanol (may increase CNS depression).

Lab Interactions Increased aminotransferase [ALT (SGPT)/AST (SGOT)] (S)

Adverse Reactions Frequency not defined.
Cardiovascular: Hypotension, peripheral vasodilation
Central nervous system: Drowsiness, dizziness, insomnia, CNS depression, mental depression, increased intracranial pressure, restlessness, headache, malaise
Gastrointestinal: Constipation, anorexia, stomach cramps, nausea, vomiting, biliary tract spasm
Genitourinary: Ureteral spasms, decreased urination, urinary tract spasm
Hepatic: Increased liver function tests
Neuromuscular & skeletal: Weakness
Ocular: Miosis
Respiratory: Respiratory depression
Miscellaneous: Physical and psychological dependence, histamine release

Overdosage/Toxicology Symptoms of overdose include hypotension, drowsiness, seizures, and respiratory depression. Naloxone, 2 mg I.V. with repeat administration as necessary up to a total of 10 mg, can be used to reverse opiate effects.

Pharmacodynamics/Kinetics
Metabolism: In terms of opium: Hepatic
Excretion: In terms of opium: Urine (primarily as morphine glucuronide conjugates and unchanged drug - morphine, codeine, papaverine, etc)

Available Dosage Forms Liquid, oral: Morphine equivalent 2 mg/5 mL (473 mL) [equivalent to opium 20 mg powder; contains alcohol 45% and benzoic acid]

Dosing
Adults & Elderly: Diarrhea: Oral: 5-10 mL 1-4 times/day

Pediatrics:
Neonatal opiate withdrawal: Oral: 3-6 drops every 3-6 hours as needed, or initially 0.2 mL every 3 hours; increase dosage by approximately 0.05 mL every 3 hours until withdrawal symptoms are controlled; it is rare to exceed 0.7 mL/dose. Stabilize withdrawal symptoms for 3-5 days, then gradually decrease dosage over a 2- to 4-week period.
Diarrhea: Oral: Children: 0.25-0.5 mL/kg 1-4 times/day

Stability
Storage: Store in light-resistant, tightly closed container

Physical Assessment: Monitor for excessive sedation, respiratory depression, or hypotension. For inpatients, implement safety measures (eg, side rails up, call light within reach, patient instructions to call for

assistance). Has potential for psychological or physiological dependence.

Patient Education: Take exactly as directed; do not increase dosage. May cause dependence with prolonged or excessive use. Avoid alcohol or any other prescription and OTC medications that may cause sedation (sleeping medications, some cough/cold remedies, antihistamines, etc). You may experience drowsiness, dizziness, or impaired judgment (use caution when driving or engaging in tasks that require alertness until response to drug is known) or postural hypotension (use caution when rising from sitting or lying position or when climbing stairs). You may experience nausea or loss of appetite (small frequent meals may help) or constipation (a laxative may be necessary). Report unresolved nausea, vomiting, respiratory difficulty (shortness of breath or decreased respirations), chest pain, or palpitations. **Pregnancy/breast-feeding precautions:** Inform prescriber if you are pregnant. If breast-feeding, take immediately after feeding or 4-6 hour before next feeding.

Breast-Feeding Issues Information regarding use while breast-feeding is based on experience with morphine. Probably safe with low doses and by administering dose after breast-feeding to further minimize exposure to the drug. Monitor the infant for possible side effects related to opiates.

Additional Information Contains morphine 0.4 mg/mL and alcohol 45%. Do **not** confuse this product with opium tincture which is 25 times **more** potent; each 5 mL of paregoric contains 2 mg morphine equivalent, 0.02 mL anise oil, 20 mg benzoic acid, 20 mg camphor, 0.2 mL glycerin and alcohol; final alcohol content 45%; paregoric also contains papaverine and noscapine; because all of these additives may be harmful to neonates, **a 25-fold dilution of opium tincture** is often preferred for treatment of neonatal abstinence syndrome (opiate withdrawal).

Paricalcitol (pah ri KAL si tole)

U.S. Brand Names Zemplar®

Pharmacologic Category Vitamin D Analog

Pregnancy Risk Factor C

Lactation Excretion in breast milk unknown/not recommended

Use
I.V.: Prevention and treatment of secondary hyperparathyroidism associated with stage 5 chronic kidney disease (CKD)
Oral: Prevention and treatment of secondary hyperparathyroidism associated with stage 3 and 4 CKD

Mechanism of Action/Effect Vitamin D analog which suppresses parathyroid hormone release, improving calcium and phosphate homeostasis

Contraindications Hypersensitivity to paricalcitol or any component of the formulation; patients with evidence of vitamin D toxicity; hypercalcemia

Warnings/Precautions Excessive administration may lead to over suppression of PTH, hypercalcemia, hypercalciuria, hyperphosphatemia and adynamic bone disease. Acute hypercalcemia may increase risk of cardiac arrhythmias and seizures; use caution with cardiac glycosides as toxicity may be increased. Chronic hypercalcemia may lead to generalized vascular and other soft-tissue calcification. Phosphate and vitamin D (and its derivatives) should be withheld during therapy to avoid hypercalcemia. Safety and efficacy in pediatric patients (oral formulation) and in children <5 years of age (I.V. formulation) have not been established.

Drug Interactions
Cytochrome P450 Effect:
Substrate of CYP3A4 (major)
Increased Effect/Toxicity:
CYP3A4 inhibitors (strong) may increase the levels/effects of paricalcitol; example CYP3A4 inhibitors include azole antifungals, ciprofloxacin, clarithromycin, diclofenac, doxycycline, erythromycin, imatinib, isoniazid, nefazodone, nicardipine, propofol, protease inhibitors, quinidine, and verapamil. Ketoconazole may increase paricalcitol levels/effects.

Adverse Reactions
>10%: Gastrointestinal: Nausea (6% to 13%)
1% to 10%:
Cardiovascular: Edema (7%), hypertension (7%), hypotension (5%), palpitation (3%), chest pain (3%), syncope (3%), cardiomyopathy (2%), MI (2%), postural hypotension (2%)
Central nervous system: Pain (8%), chills (5%), dizziness (5%), headache (5%), lightheadedness (5%), vertigo (5%), fever (3% to 5%), depression (3%), insomnia (2%)
Dermatologic: Rash (2% to 6%), skin ulcer (3%), pruritus (3%), skin hypertrophy (2%)
Endocrine & metabolic: Dehydration (3%), acidosis (2%), hypokalemia (2%)
Gastrointestinal: Vomiting (6% to 8%), diarrhea (7%), GI bleeding (5%), abdominal pain (4%), xerostomia (3%), constipation (4%), gastroenteritis (3%), dyspepsia (2%), gastritis (2%), rectal disorder (2%)
Genitourinary: Urinary tract infection (3%), kidney function abnormal (2%)
Neuromuscular & skeletal: Arthritis (5%), back pain (4%), leg cramps (3%), weakness (3%), neuropathy (2%)
Ocular: Amblyopia (2%), retinal disorder (2%)
Respiratory: Pneumonia (2% to 5%), rhinitis (5%), sinusitis (3%), bronchitis (3%), cough (3%), epistaxis (2%)
Miscellaneous: Infection (bacterial, fungal, viral: 2% to 8%); allergic reaction (6%), flu-like syndrome (2% to 5%), sepsis (5%), cyst (2%)

Overdosage/Toxicology
Acute overdose may cause hypercalcemia, hypercalciuria, and hyperphosphatemia. Monitor serum calcium and phosphorus closely during titration of paricalcitol. Dosage reduction/interruption may be required if hypercalcemia develops. Chronic use may predispose to metastatic calcification. Bone lesions may develop if parathyroid hormone is suppressed below normal.

Pharmacodynamics/Kinetics
Protein Binding: >99%
Half-Life Elimination:
Healthy subjects: Oral: 4-6 hours
Stage 3 and 4 CKD: Oral: 17-20 hours
Stage 5 CKD: I.V.: 14-15 hours
Metabolism:
Hydroxylation and glucuronidation via hepatic and nonhepatic enzymes, including CYP24, CYP3A4, UGT1A4; forms metabolites (at least one active)
Excretion: Healthy subjects: Feces (oral: 70% to 74%; I.V.: 63%); urine (oral: 16% to 18%, I.V.: 19%); 51% to 59% as metabolites

Available Dosage Forms
Capsule, gelatin: 1 mcg, 2 mcg, 4 mcg [contains alcohol and coconut or palm kernel oil]
Injection, solution: 2 mcg/mL (1 mL); 5 mcg/mL (1 mL, 2 mL) [contains alcohol 20% v/v and propylene glycol 30% v/v]

Dosing
Adults & Elderly: Note: If hypercalcemia or Ca x P >75 is observed, reduce or interrupt dosing until parameters are normalized.
Secondary hyperparathyroidism associated with chronic renal failure (stage 5 CKD): Children ≥5 years and Adults: I.V.: 0.04-0.1 mcg/kg (2.8-7 mcg)

given as a bolus dose no more frequently than every other day at any time during dialysis; dose may be increased by 2-4 mcg every 2-4 weeks; doses as high as 0.24 mcg/kg (16.8 mcg) have been administered safely; the dose of paricalcitol should be adjusted based on serum intact PTH (iPTH) levels, as follows:
Same or increasing iPTH level: Increase paricalcitol dose
iPTH level decreased by <30%: Increase paricalcitol dose
iPTH level decreased by >30% and <60%: Maintain paricalcitol dose
iPTH level decrease by >60%: Decrease paricalcitol dose
iPTH level 1.5-3 times upper limit of normal: Maintain paricalcitol dose

Secondary hyperparathyroidism associated with stage 3 and 4 CKD: Adults: Oral: Initial dose based on baseline serum iPTH:
iPTH ≤500 pg/mL: 1 mcg/day or 2 mcg 3 times/week
iPTH >500 pg/mL: 2 mcg/day or 4 mcg 3 times/week

Dosage adjustment based on iPTH level relative to baseline, adjust dose at 2-4 week intervals:
iPTH same or increased: Increase paricalcitol dose by 1 mcg/day or 2 mcg 3 times/week
iPTH decreased by <30%: Increase paricalcitol dose by 1 mcg/day or 2 mcg 3 times//week
iPTH decreased by ≥30% or ≤60%: Maintain paricalcitol dose
iPTH decreased by >60%: Decrease paricalcitol dose by 1 mcg/day* or 2 mcg 3 times/week
iPTH <60 pg/mL: Decrease paricalcitol dose by 1 mcg/day* or 2 mcg 3 times/week
*If patient is taking the lowest dose on a once-daily regimen, but further dose reduction is needed, decrease dose to 1 mcg 3 times/week. If further dose reduction is required, withhold drug as needed and restart at a lower dose. If applicable, calcium-phosphate binder dosing may also be adjusted or withheld, or switch to noncalcium-based binder

Pediatrics: Secondary hyperparathyroidism associated with chronic renal failure (stage 5 CKD): I.V.: Children ≥5 years: Refer to adult dosing.
Renal Impairment: Refer to adult dosing.
Hepatic Impairment: Adjustment not needed for mild-to-moderate impairment. Paricalcitol has not been evaluated in severe hepatic impairment.

Administration
Oral:
May be administered with or without food. With the 3 times/week dosing schedule, doses should not be given more frequently than every other day.
I.V.:
Administered as a bolus dose at anytime during dialysis. Doses should not be administered more often than every other day.
Laboratory Monitoring Serum calcium and phosphorus should be monitored closely (eg, twice weekly) during dose titration. Monitor serum PTH. In trials, a mean PTH level reduction of 30% was achieved within 6 weeks.

Nursing Actions
Physical Assessment: Monitor laboratory results. Monitor patient response and adverse effects. Monitor for signs and symptoms of vitamin D intoxication and hypercalcemia. Assess knowledge/instruct patient on safe and appropriate use of paricalcitol and dietary requirements.
Patient Education: Take as directed; do not increase dosage without consulting prescriber. Adhere to diet as recommended (do not take any other phosphate or (Continued)

Paricalcitol (Continued)

vitamin D related compounds while taking paricalcitol). You may experience nausea or vomiting (small frequent meals, frequent mouth care, chewing gums, or sucking lozenges may help); swelling of extremities (elevate feet when sitting); or lightheadedness or dizziness (use caution when driving or engaging in tasks requiring alertness until response to drug is known). Report persistent fever, gastric disturbances, abdominal pain or blood in stool, chest pain or palpitations, bone pain, irritability, muscular twitching, weakness, or signs of respiratory infection or flu. **Pregnancy/breast-feeding precautions:** Inform prescriber if you are or intend to become pregnant. Consult prescriber if breast-feeding.

Dietary Considerations
The capsules may contain coconut or palm kernel oil.

Geriatric Considerations Kinetics have not been investigated in geriatric patients. No specific dose changes necessary. Monitor closely. It may be advised to obtain baseline electrolytes, calcium, phosphorous, and digoxin serum concentrations, if applicable.

Paroxetine (pa ROKS e teen)

U.S. Brand Names Paxil®; Paxil CR®; Pexeva®
Synonyms Paroxetine Hydrochloride; Paroxetine Mesylate
Restrictions A medication guide concerning the use of antidepressants in children and teenagers can be found on the FDA website at http://www.fda.gov/cder/Offices/ODS/labeling.htm. It should be dispensed to parents or guardians of children and teenagers receiving this medication.
Pharmacologic Category Antidepressant, Selective Serotonin Reuptake Inhibitor
Medication Safety Issues
Sound-alike/look-alike issues:
Paroxetine may be confused with paclitaxel, pyridoxine
Paxil® may be confused with Doxil®, paclitaxel, Plavix®, Taxol®
Pregnancy Risk Factor D
Lactation Enters breast milk/use caution (AAP rates "of concern")
Use Treatment of depression in adults; treatment of panic disorder with or without agoraphobia; obsessive-compulsive disorder (OCD) in adults; social anxiety disorder (social phobia); generalized anxiety disorder (GAD); post-traumatic stress disorder (PTSD)

Paxil CR®: Treatment of depression; panic disorder; premenstrual dysphoric disorder (PMDD); social anxiety disorder (social phobia)
Unlabeled/Investigational Use May be useful in eating disorders, impulse control disorders, self-injurious behavior; premenstrual disorders, vasomotor symptoms of menopause; treatment of depression and obsessive-compulsive disorder (OCD) in children
Mechanism of Action/Effect Paroxetine is a selective serotonin reuptake inhibitor, chemically unrelated to tricyclic, tetracyclic, or other antidepressants; presumably, the inhibition of serotonin reuptake from brain synapse stimulated serotonin activity in the brain
Contraindications Hypersensitivity to paroxetine or any component of the formulation; use of MAO inhibitors or within 14 days; concurrent use with thioridazine or pimozide
Warnings/Precautions Antidepressants increase the risk of suicidal thinking and behavior in children and adolescents with major depressive disorder (MDD) and other depressive disorders; consider risk prior to prescribing. All patients must be closely monitored for clinical worsening, suicidality, or unusual changes in behavior, especially during the initiation of therapy or following an increase or decrease in dosage. When used in children, the child's family or caregiver should be instructed to closely observe the patient and communicate condition with healthcare provider. A medication guide should be dispensed with each prescription. **Paroxetine is not FDA approved for use in children.**

The possibility of a suicide attempt is inherent in major depression and may persist until remission occurs. Use caution in high-risk patients. Worsening depression and severe abrupt suicidality that are not part of the presenting symptoms may require discontinuation or modification of drug therapy. The patient's family or caregiver should be alerted to monitor patients for the emergence of suicidality and associated behaviors (such as agitation, irritability, hostility, impulsivity, and hypomania) and call healthcare provider.

May worsen psychosis in some patients or precipitate a shift to mania or hypomania in patients with bipolar disorder. Patients presenting with depressive symptoms should be screened for bipolar disorder. Monotherapy in patients with bipolar disorder should be avoided. **Paroxetine is not FDA approved for the treatment of bipolar depression.**

The potential for severe reaction exists when used with MAO inhibitors - serotonin syndrome (hyperthermia, muscular rigidity, mental status changes/agitation, autonomic instability) may occur; concurrent use contraindicated. May increase the risks associated with electroconvulsive therapy. Has a low potential to impair cognitive or motor performance - caution operating hazardous machinery or driving. Symptoms of agitation and/or restlessness may occur during initial few weeks of therapy. Low potential for sedation or anticholinergic effects relative to cyclic antidepressants.

Use caution in patients with a previous seizure disorder or condition predisposing to seizures such as brain damage, alcoholism, or concurrent therapy with other drugs which lower the seizure threshold. Use with caution in patients with hepatic dysfunction and in elderly patients. May cause hyponatremia/SIADH. Use with caution in patients at risk of bleeding or receiving anticoagulant therapy - may cause impairment in platelet aggregation. Use with caution in patients with renal insufficiency or other concurrent illness (due to limited experience); dose reduction recommended with severe renal impairment. May cause or exacerbate sexual dysfunction. Use caution in patients with narrow-angle glaucoma. Avoid use in the first trimester of pregnancy.

Upon discontinuation of paroxetine therapy, gradually taper dose and monitor for discontinuation symptoms (eg, dizziness, dysphoric mood, irritability, agitation, confusion, paresthesias). If intolerable symptoms occur following a decrease in dosage or upon discontinuation of therapy, then resuming the previous dose with a more gradual taper should be considered.

Drug Interactions
Cytochrome P450 Effect: Substrate of CYP2D6 (major); **Inhibits** CYP1A2 (weak), 2B6 (moderate), 2C8/9 (weak), 2C19 (weak), 2D6 (strong), 3A4 (weak)
Decreased Effect: Cyproheptadine, a serotonin antagonist, may inhibit the effects of serotonin reuptake inhibitors (paroxetine). Paroxetine may decrease the levels/effects of CYP2D6 prodrug substrates (eg, codeine, hydrocodone, oxycodone, tramadol).
Increased Effect/Toxicity: Paroxetine should not be used with nonselective MAO inhibitors (phenelzine, isocarboxazid) or other drugs with MAO inhibition (linezolid); fatal reactions have been reported. Wait 5 weeks after stopping fluoxetine before starting a nonselective MAO inhibitor and 2 weeks after stopping an MAO inhibitor before starting paroxetine. Concurrent selegiline has been associated with

mania, hypertension, or serotonin syndrome (risk may be reduced relative to nonselective MAO inhibitors). Serum levels of atomoxetine, carbamazepine, and galantamine may be increased by paroxetine.

Paroxetine may inhibit the metabolism of thioridazine or mesoridazine, resulting in increased plasma levels and increasing the risk of QT_c interval prolongation. This may lead to serious ventricular arrhythmias, such as torsade de pointes-type arrhythmias and sudden death. Do not use together. Wait at least 5 weeks after discontinuing paroxetine prior to starting thioridazine.

The levels/effects of paroxetine may be increased by chlorpromazine, delavirdine, fluoxetine, miconazole, pergolide, quinidine, quinine, ritonavir, ropinirole, and other CYP2D6 inhibitors. Paroxetine may increase the levels/effects of amphetamines, selected beta-blockers, bupropion, dextromethorphan, fluoxetine, lidocaine, mirtazapine, nefazodone, promethazine, propofol, risperidone, ritonavir, sertraline, tricyclic antidepressants, venlafaxine, and other CYP2B6 or 2D6 substrates.

Concomitant use of paroxetine and NSAIDs, aspirin, or other drugs affecting coagulation has been associated with an increased risk of bleeding. Paroxetine may increase the hypoprothrombinemic response to warfarin. Paroxetine increases levels of procyclidine; this may result in increased anticholinergic effects; procyclidine dose reduction may be necessary.

Combined use of SSRIs and amphetamines, buspirone, meperidine, nefazodone, serotonin agonists (such as sumatriptan), sibutramine, other SSRIs, sympathomimetics, ritonavir, tramadol, and venlafaxine may increase the risk of serotonin syndrome. Combined use of sumatriptan (and other serotonin agonists) may result in toxicity; weakness, hyper-reflexia, and incoordination have been observed with sumatriptan and SSRIs. In addition, concurrent use may theoretically increase the risk of serotonin syndrome; includes sumatriptan, naratriptan, rizatriptan, and zolmitriptan. Concurrent lithium may increase risk of nephrotoxicity. Risk of hyponatremia may increase with concurrent use of loop diuretics (bumetanide, furosemide, torsemide).

Nutritional/Ethanol Interactions
Ethanol: Avoid ethanol.

Food: Peak concentration is increased, but bioavailability is not significantly altered by food.

Herb/Nutraceutical: Avoid valerian, St John's wort, SAMe, kava kava.

Lab Interactions Increased LFTs

Adverse Reactions
Frequency varies by dose and indication. Adverse reactions reported as a composite of all indications.

>10%:
 Central nervous system: Somnolence (15% to 24%), insomnia (11% to 24%), headache (17% to 18%), dizziness (6% to 14%)
 Endocrine & metabolic: Libido decreased (6% to 15%)
 Gastrointestinal: Nausea (19% to 26%), xerostomia (9% to 18%), constipation (5% to 16%), diarrhea (9% to 12%)
 Genitourinary: Ejaculatory disturbances (10% to 28%)
 Neuromuscular & skeletal: Weakness (12% to 22%), tremor (4% to 11%)
 Miscellaneous: Diaphoresis (5% to 14%)

1% to 10%:
 Cardiovascular: Vasodilation (2% to 4%), chest pain (3%), palpitations (2% to 3%), hypertension (≥1%), tachycardia (≥1%)
 Central nervous system: Nervousness (4% to 9%), anxiety (5%), agitation (3% to 5%), abnormal dreams (3% to 4%), concentration impaired (3% to 4%), yawning (2% to 4%), depersonalization (up to

3%), amnesia (2%), emotional lability (≥1%), vertigo (≥1%), confusion (1%), chills (2%)
 Dermatologic: Rash (2% to 3%), pruritus (≥1%)
 Endocrine & metabolic: Orgasmic disturbance (2% to 9%), dysmenorrhea (5%)
 Gastrointestinal: Anorexia, appetite decreased (5% to 9%), dyspepsia (2% to 5%), flatulence (4%), abdominal pain (4%), appetite increased (2% to 4%), vomiting (2% to 3%), taste perversion (2%), weight gain (≥1%)
 Genitourinary: Impotence (2% to 9%), genital disorder (female 2% to 9%), urinary frequency (2% to 3%), urinary tract infection (2%)
 Neuromuscular & skeletal: Paresthesia (4%), myalgia (2% to 4%), back pain (3%), myoclonus (2% to 3%), myopathy (2%), myasthenia (1%), arthralgia (≥1%)
 Ocular: Blurred vision (4%), abnormal vision (2% to 3%)
 Otic: Tinnitus (≥1%)
 Respiratory: Respiratory disorder (up to 7%), pharyngitis (4%), sinusitis (up to 4%), rhinitis (3%)
 Miscellaneous: Infection (5% to 6%)

Overdosage/Toxicology Symptoms of overdose include somnolence, nausea, vomiting, hepatic dysfunction, drowsiness, sinus tachycardia, urinary retention, renal failure (acute), and dilated pupils. Convulsions, status epilepticus, and ventricular arrhythmias (including torsade de pointes) have been reported, as well as serotonin syndrome and manic reaction. There are no specific antidotes, following attempts at decontamination, treatment is supportive and symptom-directed. Forced diuresis, dialysis, and hemoperfusion are unlikely to be beneficial.

Pharmacodynamics/Kinetics
Time to Peak: Immediate release: 5.2 hours; controlled release: 6-10 hours

Protein Binding: 93% to 95%

Half-Life Elimination: 21 hours (3-65 hours)

Metabolism: Extensively hepatic via CYP enzymes via oxidation and methylation; nonlinear pharmacokinetics may be seen with higher doses and longer duration of therapy. Saturation of CYP2D6 appears to account for the nonlinearity. C_{min} concentrations 70% to 80% greater in the elderly compared to nonelderly patients; clearance is also decreased.

Excretion: Urine (64%, 2% as unchanged drug); feces (36% primarily via bile)

Available Dosage Forms Note: Available as paroxetine hydrochloride or mesylate; mg strength refers to paroxetine

Suspension, oral, as hydrochloride (Paxil®): 10 mg/5 mL (250 mL) [orange flavor]

Tablet, as hydrochloride (Paxil®): 10 mg, 20 mg, 30 mg, 40 mg

Tablet, as mesylate (Pexeva®): 10 mg, 20 mg, 30 mg, 40 mg

Tablet, controlled release, as hydrochloride (Paxil CR®): 12.5 mg, 25 mg, 37.5 mg

Dosing
Adults:
 Depression: Oral:
  Paxil®, Pexeva®: Initial: 20 mg once daily, preferably in the morning; increase if needed by 10 mg/day increments at intervals of at least 1 week; maximum dose: 50 mg/day
  Paxil CR®: Initial: 25 mg once daily; increase if needed by 12.5 mg/day increments at intervals of at least 1 week; maximum dose: 62.5 mg/day
 GAD (Paxil®): Oral: Initial: 20 mg once daily, preferably in the morning; doses of 20-50 mg/day were used in clinical trials, however, no greater benefit was seen with doses >20 mg. If dose is increased, adjust in increments of 10 mg/day at 1-week intervals.
 OCD (Paxil®, Pexeva®): Oral: Initial: 20 mg once daily, preferably in the morning; increase if needed
(Continued)

Paroxetine *(Continued)*

by 10 mg/day increments at intervals of at least 1 week; recommended dose: 40 mg/day; range: 20-60 mg/day; maximum dose: 60 mg/day

Panic disorder: Oral:

Paxil®, Pexeva®: Initial: 10 mg once daily, preferably in the morning; increase if needed by 10 mg/day increments at intervals of at least 1 week; recommended dose: 40 mg/day; range: 10-60 mg/day; maximum dose: 60 mg/day

Paxil CR®: Initial: 12.5 mg once daily; increase if needed by 12.5 mg/day at intervals of at least 1 week; maximum dose: 75 mg/day

PMDD (Paxil CR®): Oral: Initial: 12.5 mg once daily in the morning; may be increased to 25 mg/day; dosing changes should occur at intervals of at least 1 week. May be given daily throughout the menstrual cycle or limited to the luteal phase.

PTSD (Paxil®): Oral: Initial: 20 mg once daily, preferably in the morning; increase if needed by 10 mg/day increments at intervals of at least 1 week; range: 20-50 mg. Limited data suggest doses of 40 mg/day were not more efficacious than 20 mg/day.

Social anxiety disorder: Oral:

Paxil®: Initial: 20 mg once daily, preferably in the morning; recommended dose: 20 mg/day; range: 20-60 mg/day; doses >20 mg may not have additional benefit

Paxil CR®: Initial: 12.5 mg once daily, preferably in the morning; may be increased by 12.5 mg/day at intervals of at least 1 week; maximum dose: 37.5 mg/day

Menopause-associated vasomotor symptoms (unlabeled use, Paxil CR®): Oral: 12.5-25 mg/day

Elderly:

Depression, obsessive compulsive disorder, panic attack, social anxiety disorder:

Paxil®, Pexeva®: Oral: Initial: 10 mg/day; increase if needed by 10 mg/day increments at intervals of at least 1 week; maximum dose: 40 mg/day

Paxil CR®: Initial: 12.5 mg/day; increase if needed by 12.5 mg/day increments at intervals of at least 1 week; maximum dose: 50 mg/day

Pediatrics:

Depression (unlabeled use; not recommended by FDA): Oral: Initial: 10 mg/day and adjusted upward on an individual basis to 20 mg/day

OCD (unlabeled use): Oral: Initial: 10 mg/day and titrate up as necessary to 60 mg/day

Self-Injurious behavior (unlabeled use): Oral: 20 mg/day

Social phobia (unlabeled use): Oral: 2.5-15 mg/day

Renal Impairment:

Cl_{cr} <30 mL/minute: Mean plasma concentrations ~4 times that seen in normal function.

Cl_{cr} 30-60 mL/minute: Plasma concentrations 2 times that seen in normal function.

Paxil®, Pexeva®: Adults: Initial: 10 mg/day; increase if needed by 10 mg/day increments at intervals of at least 1 week; maximum dose: 40 mg/day

Paxil CR®: Initial: 12.5 mg/day; increase if needed by 12.5 mg/day increments at intervals of at least 1 week; maximum dose: 50 mg/day

Hepatic Impairment: In hepatic dysfunction, plasma concentration is 2 times that seen in normal function.

Paxil®, Pexeva®: Adults: Initial: 10 mg/day; increase if needed by 10 mg/day increments at intervals of at least 1 week; maximum dose: 40 mg/day

Paxil CR®: Initial: 12.5 mg/day; increase if needed by 12.5 mg/day increments at intervals of at least 1 week; maximum dose: 50 mg/day

Administration

Oral: May be administered with or without food. Do not crush, break, or chew controlled release tablets.

Stability

Storage:

Suspension: Store at ≤25°C (≤77°F)

Tablet: Store at 15°C to 30°C (59°F to 86°F)

Laboratory Monitoring Hepatic and renal function

Nursing Actions

Physical Assessment: Assess potential for interactions with other prescription or OTC medications or herbal products patient may be taking. Monitor laboratory tests, therapeutic response (according to rationale for prescribing), and adverse reactions at beginning of therapy and frequently with long-term use. Monitor for clinical worsening and suicidal ideation. Taper dosage slowly when discontinuing. Assess knowledge/teach patient appropriate use, interventions to reduce side effects, and adverse symptoms to report.

Patient Education: Take exactly as directed; do not increase dose or frequency or discontinue without consulting prescriber. It may take 2-3 weeks to achieve desired results. Take in the morning to reduce the incidence of insomnia (may be taken with or without food). Do not crush, break, or chew controlled release (Paxil CR®) tablets. Avoid alcohol, caffeine, and other prescription or OTC medications not approved by prescriber. Maintain adequate hydration (2-3 L/day of fluids) unless instructed to restrict fluid intake. You may experience drowsiness, dizziness, or lightheadedness (use caution when driving or engaging in tasks requiring alertness until response to drug is known); nausea, vomiting, anorexia, or dry mouth (small frequent meals, frequent mouth care, chewing gum, or sucking lozenges may help); or orthostatic hypotension (use caution when climbing stairs or changing position from lying or sitting to standing). Report persistent insomnia or excessive daytime sedation; muscle cramping, tremors, weakness, or change in gait; chest pain, palpitations, or rapid heartbeat; vision changes or eye pain; respiratory difficulty or breathlessness; abdominal pain or blood in stool; change in affect or thought processes, unusual agitation, or abnormal dreams; worsening of condition; or suicidal ideation. **Pregnancy/breast-feeding precautions:** Inform prescriber if you are or intend to become pregnant. Consult prescriber if breast-feeding.

Dietary Considerations May be taken with or without food.

Geriatric Considerations Paroxetine's favorable side effect profile make it a useful alternative to traditional tricyclic antidepressants. Paroxetine is the most sedating of the currently available selective serotonin reuptake inhibitors. Paroxetine's half-life is approximately 21 hours and it has no active metabolites.

Pregnancy Issues Teratogenic effects were not observed in animal studies. Preliminary results from a retrospective epidemiologic studies in humans show the risk of congenital malformations, specifically atrial or ventricular septal defects, may be increased with paroxetine relative to other antidepressants. Nonteratogenic effects including respiratory distress, cyanosis, apnea, seizures, temperature instability, feeding difficulty, vomiting, hypoglycemia, hypo- or hypertonia, hyper-reflexia, jitteriness, irritability, constant crying, and tremor have been reported in the neonate immediately following delivery after exposure late in the third trimester. Adverse effects may be due to toxic effects of SSRI or drug discontinuation. There are no adequate and well-controlled studies in pregnant women. Use during pregnancy only if the potential benefit to the mother outweighs the possible risk to the fetus. If treatment during pregnancy is required, consider tapering therapy during the third trimester.

Additional Information Paxil CR® incorporates a degradable polymeric matrix (Geomatrix™) to control dissolution rate over a period of 4-5 hours. An enteric coating delays the start of drug release until tablets have left the stomach.

Related Information
Antidepressant Medication Guidelines *on page 1414*

Pegaspargase (peg AS par jase)

U.S. Brand Names Oncaspar®
Synonyms NSC-644954; PEG-L-asparaginase
Pharmacologic Category Antineoplastic Agent, Miscellaneous
Medication Safety Issues
Sound-alike/look-alike issues:
Pegaspargase may be confused with asparaginase
Pregnancy Risk Factor C
Lactation Excretion in breast milk unknown/not recommended
Use Treatment of acute lymphocytic leukemia when L-asparaginase is required in treatment regimen but previous hypersensitivity to native L-asparaginase exists
Mechanism of Action/Effect Pegaspargase is a modified version of asparaginase. Leukemic cells, especially lymphoblasts, require exogenous asparagine; normal cells can synthesize asparagine. Asparaginase contains L-asparaginase amidohydrolase type EC-2 which inhibits protein synthesis by deaminating asparagine to aspartic acid and ammonia in the plasma and extracellular fluid and therefore deprives tumor cells of the amino acid for protein synthesis. Asparaginase is cycle-specific for the G_1 phase of the cell cycle.
Contraindications Hypersensitivity to pegaspargase or any component of the formulation; pancreatitis or a history of pancreatitis; previous serious allergic reactions (urticaria, bronchospasm, laryngeal edema, hypotension) or other unacceptable adverse reactions to pegaspargase; previous hemorrhagic event with L-asparaginase
Warnings/Precautions Hazardous agent — use appropriate precautions for handling and disposal. Monitor for severe allergic reactions. Use cautiously in patients with an underlying coagulopathy or previous hematologic complications from asparaginase, hepatic dysfunction, hyperglycemia or diabetes. May be used cautiously in patients who have had hypersensitivity reactions to *E. coli* asparaginase; however, up to 32% of patients who have an allergic reaction to *E. coli* asparaginase will also react to pegaspargase.
Adverse Reactions In general, pegaspargase toxicities tend to be less frequent and appear somewhat later than comparable toxicities of asparaginase. Intramuscular rather than intravenous injection may decrease the incidence of coagulopathy, GI, hepatic, and renal toxicity. Except for hypersensitivity reactions, adults tend to have a higher incidence than children.
>10%:
Cardiovascular: Edema
Central nervous system: Fever, malaise
Gastrointestinal: Nausea, vomiting (50% to 60%), generally mild to moderate, but may be severe and protracted in some patients; anorexia (33%); abdominal pain (38%); diarrhea (28%); increased serum lipase and amylase
Hematologic: Hypofibrinogenemia and depression of clotting factors V and VII, variable decreases in factors VII and IX, severe protein C deficiency and decrease in antithrombin III - overt bleeding is uncommon, but may be dose-limiting, or fatal in some patients
Hypersensitivity: Acute allergic reactions, including fever, rash, urticaria, arthralgia, hypotension, angioedema, bronchospasm, anaphylaxis (10% to 30%) - dose-limiting in some patients
Neuromuscular & skeletal: Weakness (33%)

1% to 10%:
Cardiovascular: Hypotension, tachycardia, thrombosis
Dermatologic: Urticaria, erythema, lip edema
Endocrine & metabolic: Hyperglycemia (3%)
Gastrointestinal: Acute pancreatitis (1%)
Overdosage/Toxicology Symptoms of overdose include nausea, diarrhea, rash, and increased liver enzymes.
Pharmacodynamics/Kinetics
Duration of Action: Asparaginase was measurable for at least 15 days following initial treatment with pegaspargase
Half-Life Elimination: 5.7 days; unaffected by age, renal or hepatic function; half life decreased to 3.2 days in patients with previous hypersensitivity to native L-asparaginase
Metabolism: Systemically degraded
Excretion: Urine (trace amounts)
Available Dosage Forms Injection, solution [preservative free]: 750 units/mL (5 mL)
Dosing
Adults & Elderly: Usually administered as part of a combination chemotherapy regimen.
I.M. administration is **preferred** over I.V. administration due to lower incidence of hepatotoxicity, coagulopathy, gastrointestinal and renal disorders with I.M. administration.
Acute lymphoblastic leukemia (ALL): I.M., I.V.: 2500 int. units/m² every 14 days
Pediatrics: Usually administered as part of a combination chemotherapy regimen.
I.M. administration is **preferred** over I.V. administration due to lower incidence of hepatotoxicity, coagulopathy, gastrointestinal and renal disorders with I.M. administration.
Acute lymphoblastic leukemia: I.M., I.V.:
Body surface area <0.6 m²: 82.5 int. units/kg every 14 days
Body surface area ≥0.6 m²: 2500 int. units/m² every 14 days
Administration
I.M.: Must only be administered as a deep intramuscular injection into a large muscle; if I.M. injection volume is >2 mL, use multiple injection sites.
I.V.: May be administered as a 1- to 2-hour I.V. infusion; **do not administer I.V. push.**
I.V. Detail: Do not filter solution. Have available appropriate agents for maintenance of an adequate airway and treatment of a hypersensitivity reaction (antihistamine, epinephrine, oxygen, I.V. corticosteroids). Be prepared to treat anaphylaxis at each administration. Administer through an infusion that is already running.
pH: 7.3
Stability
Reconstitution: Avoid excessive agitation; do **not** shake.
Standard I.M. dilution: Do not exceed 2 mL volume per injection site
Standard I.V. dilution: Dilute in 100 mL NS or D_5W; stable for 48 hours at room temperature.
Storage: Refrigerate at 2°C to 8°C (36°F to 46°F). Do not use of cloudy or if precipitate is present. Do not use if stored at room temperature for >48 hours. Do **not** freeze. Do not use product if it is known to have been frozen.
Laboratory Monitoring CBC with differential, platelets, amylase, liver enzymes, fibrinogen, PT, PTT, renal function tests, urine dipstick for glucose, blood glucose
Nursing Actions
Physical Assessment: See Administration for infusion specifics and anaphylactic precautions (have a freely-running I.V. in place and emergency medications at hand). Monitor patient closely during and for 1 hour following each infusion (anaphylactic reactions (Continued)

Pegaspargase *(Continued)*

can occur with each dose, including fever, rash, urticaria, arthralgia, hypotension, angioedema, bronchospasm, anaphylaxis). Monitor laboratory tests and patient response with each dose (eg, GI disturbance, nausea, vomiting, hypotension). **Note:** I.M. rather than I.V. administration may decrease the incidence of coagulopathy and GI, hepatic, and renal toxicity. Teach patient possible side effects/appropriate interventions and adverse symptoms to report.

Patient Education: This drug is given by infusion or injection; report immediately any redness, swelling, burning, or pain at infusion/injection site or any signs of allergic reaction (eg, respiratory difficulty or swallowing, chest tightness, rash, hives, swelling of lips or mouth). Maintain adequate hydration (2-3 L/day of fluids) unless instructed to restrict fluid intake and nutrition (small frequent meals will help). You may be more susceptible to infection (avoid crowds and exposure to infection and do not have vaccinations without consulting prescriber). May cause nausea, vomiting, or loss of appetite (frequent mouth care, chewing gum, or sucking lozenges may help); mouth sores (use soft toothbrush, waxed dental floss, and frequent mouth rinses); diarrhea (buttermilk, boiled milk, or yogurt may help); dizziness, drowsiness, syncope, or blurred vision (use caution when driving or engaging in tasks that require alertness until response to drug is known); increased sweating; decreased sexual drive; or cough. Report immediately any unusual bleeding or bruising, nose bleeds, bleeding gums, black tarry stools, blood in urine or stool, pinpoint red spots on your skin; persistent nausea or vomiting; allergic reaction (fever, rash, swelling around mouth, chest pain, rapid heart beat); weakness or fatigue, edema (swelling of extremities or sudden weight gain); or other adverse reactions. **Pregnancy/breast-feeding precautions:** Inform prescriber if you are or intend to become pregnant. Do not breast-feed.

Breast-Feeding Issues Due to the potential for serious adverse reactions, breast-feeding is not recommended.

Pregnancy Issues Reproduction studies have not been conducted with pegaspargase.

Peginterferon Alfa-2a
(peg in ter FEER on AL fa too aye)

U.S. Brand Names Pegasys®

Synonyms Interferon Alfa-2a (PEG Conjugate); Pegylated Interferon Alfa-2a

Restrictions An FDA-approved medication guide is available at http://www.fda.gov/cder/Offices/ODS/labeling.htm; distribute to each patient to whom this medication is dispensed.

Pharmacologic Category Interferon

Pregnancy Risk Factor C; X when used with ribavirin

Lactation Excretion in breast milk unknown/not recommended

Use Treatment of chronic hepatitis C (CHC), alone or in combination with ribavirin, in patients with compensated liver disease and histological evidence of cirrhosis (Child-Pugh class A) and patients with clinically-stable HIV disease; treatment of patients with HBeAg positive and HBeAg negative chronic hepatitis B with compensated liver disease and evidence of viral replication and liver inflammation

Mechanism of Action/Effect Alpha interferons are a family of proteins, produced by nucleated cells, that have antiviral, antiproliferative, and immune-regulating activity. There are 16 known subtypes of alpha interferons. Interferons interact with cells through high affinity cell surface receptors. Following activation, multiple effects can be detected including induction of gene transcription. Inhibits cellular growth, alters the state of cellular differentiation, interferes with oncogene expression, alters cell surface antigen expression, increases phagocytic activity of macrophages, and augments cytotoxicity of lymphocytes for target cells.

Contraindications Hypersensitivity to polyethylene glycol (PEG), interferon alfa, or any component of the formulation; autoimmune hepatitis; decompensated liver disease in cirrhotic patients (Child-Pugh score >6); decompensated liver disease (Child-Pugh score ≥6, class B and C) in CHC coinfected with HIV; neonates and infants

Warnings/Precautions Severe acute hypersensitivity reactions have occurred rarely. Use caution with prior cardiovascular disease, endocrine disorders, autoimmune disorders, and pulmonary dysfunction. Discontinue treatment with worsening or persistently severe signs/symptoms of autoimmune, infectious, respiratory, or neuropsychiatric disorders (including depression and/or suicidal thoughts/behavior). Severe psychiatric adverse effects (including depression, suicidal ideation, and suicide attempt) may occur. Avoid use in severe psychiatric disorders; use caution in patients with a history of depression.

Hepatic decompensation and death have been associated with the use of alpha interferons including Pegasys®, in cirrhotic chronic hepatitis C patients; patients coinfected with HIV and receiving highly active antiretroviral therapy have shown an increased risk. Monitor hepatic function. In hepatitis B patients, flares (transient and potentially severe increases in serum ALT) may occur during or after treatment; more frequent monitoring of LFTs and a dose reduction are recommended. Discontinue if ALT elevation continues despite dose reduction or if increased bilirubin or hepatic decompensation occur.

May cause myelosuppression (including neutropenia, lymphopenia, aplastic anemia); use caution with renal dysfunction (Cl_{cr} <50 mL/minute). Patients with renal dysfunction should be monitored for signs/symptoms of toxicity (dosage adjustment required if toxicity occurs). Discontinue if new or worsening ophthalmologic disorders occur visual exams are recommended.

Use caution with baseline neutrophil count <1500/mm^3, platelet count <90,000/mm^3 or hemoglobin <10 g/dL. Discontinue therapy (at least temporarily) if ANC <500/mm^3 or platelet count <25,000/mm^3, colitis develops, or if known or suspected pancreatitis develops. Use caution in patients with an increased risk for severe anemia (eg, spherocytosis, history of GI bleeding).

Use caution in geriatric patients. Safety and efficacy have not been established in patients who have failed other alpha interferon therapy, received organ transplants, been coinfected with HBV and HCV or HIV; or with HCV and HIV with a CD4$^+$ cell count <100 cells/microL, or been treated for >48 weeks. Due to differences in dosage, patients should not change brands of interferon. Safety and efficacy have not been established in children.

Drug Interactions

Cytochrome P450 Effect: Inhibits CYP1A2 (weak)

Decreased Effect: Prednisone may decrease the therapeutic effects of interferon alfa; interferon alfa may decrease the serum concentrations of melphalan

Increased Effect/Toxicity: Interferons may increase the risk of neutropenia when used with ACE inhibitors; fluorouracil concentrations doubled with interferon alfa-2b; interferon alfa may decrease the metabolism of theophylline and zidovudine; interferons may increase the anticoagulant effects of warfarin. Concurrent therapy with ribavirin may increase the risk of hemolytic anemia.

Nutritional/Ethanol Interactions Ethanol: Avoid use in patients with hepatitis C virus.

Adverse Reactions Note: Percentages are reported for peginterferon alfa-2a in chronic hepatitis C (CHC)

patients. Other percentages indicated as "with ribavirin" or "in HIV/CHC" are those which significantly exceed incidence reported for peginterferon monotherapy in CHC patients.

>10%:

Central nervous system: Headache (54%), fatigue (50%), pyrexia (37%; 41% with ribavirin; 54% in hepatitis B), insomnia (19%; 30% with ribavirin), depression (18%), dizziness (16%), irritability/anxiety/nervousness (19%; 33% with ribavirin), pain (11%)

Dermatologic: Alopecia (23%; 28% with ribavirin), pruritus (12%; 19% with ribavirin), dermatitis (16% with ribavirin)

Gastrointestinal: Nausea/vomiting (24%), anorexia (17%; 24% with ribavirin), diarrhea (16%), weight loss (16% in HIV/CHC), abdominal pain (15%)

Hematologic: Neutropenia (21%; 27% with ribavirin; 40% in HIV/CHC), lymphopenia (14% with ribavirin), anemia (11% with ribavirin; 14% in HIV/CHC)

Hepatic: ALT increases 5-10 x ULN during treatment (25% to 27% in hepatitis B); ALT increases >10 x ULN during treatment (12% to 18% in hepatitis B); ALT increases 5-10 x ULN after treatment (13% to 16% in hepatitis B); ALT increases >10 x ULN after treatment (7% to 12% in hepatitis B)

Local: Injection site reaction (22%)

Neuromuscular & skeletal: Weakness (56%; 65% with ribavirin), myalgia (37%), rigors (32%; 25% to 27% in hepatitis B), arthralgia (28%)

Respiratory: Dyspnea (13% with ribavirin)

1% to 10%:

Central nervous system: Concentration impaired (8%), memory impaired (5%), mood alteration (3%; 9% in HIV/CHC)

Dermatologic: Dermatitis (8%), rash (5%), dry skin (4%; 10% with ribavirin), eczema (5% with ribavirin)

Endocrine & metabolic: Hypothyroidism (4%), hyperthyroidism (1%)

Gastrointestinal: Xerostomia (6%), dyspepsia (6% with ribavirin), weight loss (4%; 10% with ribavirin)

Hematologic: Thrombocytopenia (5%), platelets decreased <50,000/mm³ (5%), lymphopenia (3%), anemia (2%)

Hepatic: Hepatic decompensation (2% CHC/HIV patients)

Neuromuscular & skeletal: Back pain (9%)

Ocular: Blurred vision (4%)

Respiratory: Cough (4%; 10% with ribavirin), dyspnea (4%), exertional dyspnea (4% with ribavirin)

Miscellaneous: Diaphoresis (6%), bacterial infection (3%; 5% in HIV/CHC)

Overdosage/Toxicology Experience with overdosage is limited and no serious reactions have been reported. Dose-limiting toxicities include fatigue, elevated liver enzymes, neutropenia and thrombocytopenia. In case of overdose, treatment should be symptom-directed and supportive. Hemodialysis and peritoneal dialysis are not effective.

Pharmacodynamics/Kinetics

Time to Peak: Serum: 72-96 hours

Half-Life Elimination: Terminal: 50-140 hours; increased with renal dysfunction

Available Dosage Forms Injection, solution:

180 mcg/0.5 mL (0.5 mL) [prefilled syringe; contains benzyl alcohol; packaged with needles and alcohol swabs]

180 mcg/mL (1 mL) [contains benzyl alcohol]

Dosing

Adults:

Chronic hepatitis C (monoinfection or coinfection with HIV): SubQ:

Monotherapy: 180 mcg once weekly for 48 weeks

Combination therapy with ribavirin: Recommended dosage: 180 mcg once/week with ribavirin (Copegus®)

Duration of therapy: Monoinfection (based on genotype):

Genotype 1,4: 48 weeks

Genotype 2,3: 24 weeks

Duration of therapy: Coinfection: 48 weeks

Chronic hepatitis B: SubQ: 180 mcg once weekly for 48 weeks

Dose modifications for adverse events/toxicity:

For moderate to severe adverse reactions: Initial: 135 mcg/week; may need decreased to 90 mcg/week in some cases

Based on hematologic parameters:

ANC <750/mm³: 135 mcg/week

ANC <500/mm³: Suspend therapy until >1000/mm³, then restart at 90 mcg/week and monitor

Platelet count <50,000/mm³: 90 mcg/week

Platelet count <25,000/mm³: Discontinue therapy

Depression (severity based on DSM-IV criteria):

Mild depression: No dosage adjustment required; evaluate once weekly by visit/phone call. If depression remains stable, continue weekly visits. If depression improves, resume normal visit schedule

Moderate depression: Decrease interferon dose to 90-135 mcg once/week; evaluate once weekly with an office visit at least every other week. If depression remains stable, consider psychiatric evaluation and continue with reduced dosing. If symptoms improve and remain stable for 4 weeks, resume normal visit schedule; continue reduced dosing or return to normal dose.

Severe depression: Discontinue interferon permanently. Obtain immediate psychiatric consultation. Discontinue ribavirin if using concurrently.

Renal Impairment:

Cl_cr <50 mL/minute: Use caution; monitor for toxicity

End-stage renal disease requiring hemodialysis: 135 mcg/week; monitor for toxicity

Hepatic Impairment:

HCV: ALT progressively rising above baseline: Decrease dose to 135 mcg/week. If ALT continues to rise or is accompanied by increased bilirubin or hepatic decompensation, discontinue therapy immediately.

HBV:

ALT >5 x ULN: Monitor LFTs more frequently; consider decreasing dose to 135 mcg/week or temporarily discontinuing (may resume after ALT flare subsides).

ALT >10 x ULN: Consider discontinuing.

Administration

Other: SubQ: Administer in the abdomen or thigh. Rotate injection site. Do not use if solution contains particulate matter or is discolored. Discard unused solution. Administration should be done on the same day and at approximately the same time each week.

Stability

Storage: Store in refrigerator at 2°C to 8°C (36°F to 46°F). Do not freeze or shake; protect from light. Discard unused solution.

Laboratory Monitoring Standard hematological tests should be performed prior to therapy, at week 2, and periodically. Standard biochemical tests should be performed prior to therapy, at week 4, and periodically. Baseline eye examination and periodically in patients with baseline disorders; baseline echocardiogram in patients with cardiac disease; serum HCV RNA levels after 12 weeks of treatment

Clinical studies tested as follows: CBC (including hemoglobin, WBC, and platelets) and chemistries (including liver function tests and uric acid) measured at weeks 1, 2, 4, 6, and 8, and then every 4 weeks; TSH measured every 12 weeks

(Continued)

Peginterferon Alfa-2a *(Continued)*

In addition, the following baseline values were used as entrance criteria:

Platelet count ≥ 90,000/mm³ (as low as 75,000/mm³ in patients with cirrhosis or transition to cirrhosis)

ANC ≥ 1500/mm³

Serum creatinine <1.5 times ULN

TSH and T₄ within normal limits or adequately controlled

Consider discontinuing treatment if virologic tests indicate no response by week 12.

Nursing Actions

Physical Assessment: Assess potential for interactions with other prescriptions, OTC medications, or herbal products patient may be taking. Monitor laboratory tests prior to and periodically during therapy. Evaluate for depression and other psychiatric symptoms before and during therapy; baseline eye examination and periodically in patients with baseline disorders; baseline echocardiogram in patients with cardiac disease. Monitor patient for therapeutic effectiveness and adverse response at beginning of and at regular intervals during therapy. Teach patient proper use if self-administered (appropriate injection technique and syringe/needle disposal), possible side effects/appropriate interventions, and adverse symptoms to report.

Patient Education: Inform prescriber of all prescriptions, OTC medications, or herbal products you are taking, and any allergies you have. Do not take any new medication during therapy without consulting prescriber. This medication must be given by injection; if self-administered, follow exact instructions for injection and syringe/needle disposal. Avoid alcohol. You will need laboratory tests and ophthalmic exams prior to and during therapy. May cause headache, insomnia, dizziness (use caution when driving or engaging in potentially hazardous tasks until response to drug is known); loss of hair (will grow back after therapy); nausea or anorexia (small frequent meals or frequent mouth care may help); diarrhea (boiled milk, buttermilk, or yogurt may help); weakness, fatigue; muscle, skeletal, or joint pain; or increased perspiration. Report any severe or persistent adverse effects, including nausea, vomiting, or abdominal pain; severe depression, anxiety, or suicidal ideation; skin rash; pain, redness, or swelling at injection site; signs of infection, unusual bleeding or bruising, changes in vision, chest pain, palpitations, or respiratory difficulty. **Pregnancy/breast-feeding precautions:** Inform prescriber if you are or intend to become pregnant. Consult prescriber for appropriate contraceptive measures. Breast-feeding is not recommended.

Dietary Considerations Avoid ethanol use in patients with hepatitis C virus.

Pregnancy Issues Animal teratogenicity studies have not been conducted; very high doses are abortifacient in Rhesus monkeys. Assumed to have abortifacient potential in humans. There are no adequate and well-controlled studies in pregnant women; use during pregnancy only if the potential benefit to the mother outweighs the possible risk to the fetus. Risk of maternal-infant transmission of hepatitis C is <5%. Reliable contraception should be used in women of childbearing potential.

Pegvisomant *(peg VI soe mant)*

U.S. Brand Names Somavert®

Synonyms B2036-PEG

Pharmacologic Category Growth Hormone Receptor Antagonist

Pregnancy Risk Factor B

Lactation Excretion in breast milk unknown/use caution

Use Treatment of acromegaly in patients resistant to or unable to tolerate other therapies

Mechanism of Action/Effect A recombinant human growth hormone (GH) antagonist that binds to GH receptors, leading to decreased serum concentrations of insulin-like growth factor-I (IGF-I) and other GH-responsive proteins.

Contraindications Hypersensitivity to polyethylene glycol or any component of the formulation

Warnings/Precautions Use caution with hepatic or renal disease, or in the elderly. Growth hormone (GH)-secreting tumor size and liver function should be carefully monitored. Interferes with commercially available GH assays; IGF-I levels not GH levels, should be used to adjust therapy. The manufacturer recommends the initial dose be administered under the supervision of prescribing health care provider. Safety and efficacy in pediatric patients have not been established.

Drug Interactions

Decreased Effect: Pegvisomant may increase glucose tolerance; dose reduction of hypoglycemic agents may be needed.

Increased Effect/Toxicity: Increased doses of pegvisomant may be needed when used with opioids.

Lab Interactions Interferes with measurement of serum GH concentrations by available GH assays.

Adverse Reactions

>10%:

Central nervous system: Pain (4% to 14%; placebo: 6%)

Gastrointestinal: Diarrhea (4% to 14%), nausea (8% to 14%)

Hepatic: Liver function tests abnormal (4% to 12%)

Local: Injection site reaction (4% to 11%)

Miscellaneous: Infection (23%), non-neutralizing anti-GH antibodies (17%; relevance unknown), flu-like syndrome (4% to 12%)

1% to 10%:

Cardiovascular: Hypertension (8%), chest pain (4% to 8%), peripheral edema (4% to 8%)

Central nervous system: Dizziness (4% to 8%; placebo: 6%)

Neuromuscular & skeletal: Back pain (4% to 8%), paresthesia (7%)

Respiratory: Sinusitis (4% to 8%)

Overdosage/Toxicology No specific experience with overdose. Fatigue reported at a dose of 80 mg/day for 7 days. In case of overdose, discontinue until IGF-I levels return to normal.

Pharmacodynamics/Kinetics

Time to Peak: Serum: 33-77 hours

Half-Life Elimination: 6 days

Excretion: Urine (<1%)

Available Dosage Forms Injection, powder for reconstitution [preservative free]: 10 mg, 15 mg, 20 mg [vial stopper contains latex; packaged with SWFI]

Dosing

Adults & Elderly: Acromegaly: SubQ: Initial loading dose: 40 mg; maintenance dose: 10 mg once daily; doses may be adjusted by 5 mg in 4- to 6-week intervals based on IGF-I concentrations (maximum dose: 30 mg/day)

Hepatic Impairment:

Baseline liver function tests (LFT) >3 times ULN: Do not initiate treatment without comprehensive work-up to determine cause; monitor closely if treatment is started.

LFT ≥3 times but <5 times ULN: Continue treatment, but monitor weekly if no signs or symptoms of hepatitis or liver injury; perform comprehensive hepatic work-up

LFT ≥5 times ULN or transaminase >3 times ULN associated with any increase in total bilirubin: Discontinue immediately and perform comprehensive hepatic work-up. If LFTs return to normal, may cautiously consider restarting therapy with frequent monitoring.

Signs or symptoms of hepatitis or hepatic injury: Evaluate liver function tests; discontinue if liver injury is confirmed

Administration

Other: For SubQ administration only; rotate injection site daily; may administer in upper arm, upper thigh, abdomen, or buttocks; do not rub injection site. The manufacturer recommends the initial dose be administered under the supervision of prescribing healthcare provider.

Stability

Reconstitution: Reconstitute with SWFI; gently roll, do not shake, in order to dissolve powder.

Storage: Store intact vials under refrigeration at 2°C to 8°C (36°F to 46°F); protect from freezing. Following reconstitution, use within 6 hours. Do not use solution if cloudy.

Laboratory Monitoring Serum glucose, serum IGF-I (every 4-6 weeks after initial dose and dosage change, every 6 months when normalized)

Liver function tests:

Normal at baseline: Monthly for first 6 months, quarterly for next 6 months, biannually for the next year

Elevated, but ≤ 3 times ULN: Monitor monthly for at least 1 year, then biannually the next year

Nursing Actions

Physical Assessment: Assess potential for interactions with other prescriptions, OTC medications, and herbal products patient may be taking Monitor results of laboratory tests at beginning and periodically during therapy. **Note:** First dose should be administered under supervision of prescriber. Monitor therapeutic effectiveness and adverse reactions. Teach patient proper use (storage, reconstitution, injection technique, site rotation, and disposal of syringes/needles), possible side effects/appropriate interventions, and adverse symptoms to report. Instruct patients with diabetes on need to monitor glucose levels regularly; dose adjustment of hypoglycemic agent may be needed.

Patient Education: Inform prescriber of all prescriptions, OTC medications, or herbal products you are taking, and any allergies you have. This medication may only be administered by injection. If instructed in self-injection, follow instructions exactly. Report immediately any reaction at injection site (redness, swelling, itching). May cause diarrhea (buttermilk, boiled milk, or yogurt may help); nausea (frequent small meals and good mouth care may help); or signs of allergic response (chest pain, respiratory difficulty, skin rash). **Breast-feeding precaution:** Consult prescriber if breast-feeding.

Pemetrexed (pem e TREKS ed)

U.S. Brand Names Alimta®

Synonyms LY231514; MTA; Multitargeted Antifolate; NSC-698037; Pemetrexed Disodium

Pharmacologic Category Antineoplastic Agent, Antimetabolite; Antineoplastic Agent, Antimetabolite (Antifolate)

Pregnancy Risk Factor D

Lactation Excretion in breast milk unknown/not recommended

Use Treatment of malignant pleural mesothelioma in combination with cisplatin; treatment of nonsmall cell lung cancer

Unlabeled/Investigational Use Bladder, breast, cervical, colorectal, esophageal, gastric, head and neck, ovarian, pancreatic, and renal cell cancers

Mechanism of Action/Effect Disrupts folate-dependent metabolic processes essential for cell replication.

Contraindications Hypersensitivity to pemetrexed or any component of the formulation

Warnings/Precautions Hazardous agent - use appropriate precautions for handling and disposal. Prophylactic folic acid and vitamin B_{12} supplements are necessary to reduce hematologic and gastrointestinal toxicity. Folic acid and vitamin B_{12} should be started 1 week before the first dose of pemetrexed. Pretreatment with corticosteroids reduces the incidence and severity of cutaneous reactions. Use caution with hepatic dysfunction not due to metastases and in patients receiving concurrent nephrotoxins. Safety and efficacy have not been established in pediatric patients.

Drug Interactions

Increased Effect/Toxicity: NSAIDs may increase the toxicity of pemetrexed.

Nutritional/Ethanol Interactions Lower ANC nadirs occur in patients with elevated baseline cystathionine or homocysteine concentrations. Levels of these substances can be reduced by folic acid and vitamin B_{12} supplementation.

Adverse Reactions Note: Reported frequencies of adverse effects vary by indication/population and concurrent therapy.

>10%:

Cardiovascular: Chest pain (38% to 40%), edema (19%)

Central nervous system: Fatigue (80% to 87%), fever (17% to 26%), depression (11% to 14%)

Dermatologic: Rash (17% to 22%), alopecia (11%)

Gastrointestinal: Nausea (39% to 84%; grade 3/4 in 12%), vomiting (25% to 58%; grade 3/4 in 11%), constipation (30% to 44%), anorexia (35% to 62%), stomatitis/pharyngitis (20% to 28%), diarrhea (21% to 26%)

Hematologic: Neutropenia (11% to 58%), leukopenia (13% to 55%), anemia (33%), thrombocytopenia (9% to 27%)

Nadir: 8-10 days

Recovery: 12-17 days

Neuromuscular & skeletal: Neuropathy (17% to 29%), myalgia (13%)

Renal: Creatinine increased (3% to 16%)

Respiratory: Dyspnea (66%)

Miscellaneous: Infection (17% to 23%)

1% to 10%:

Cardiovascular: Thrombosis/embolism (4% to 7%), cardiac ischemia (3%)

Endocrine & metabolic: Dehydration (3% to 7%)

Gastrointestinal: Dysphagia/esophagitis/odynophagia (5% to 6%)

Renal: Renal failure (<1% to 2%)

Miscellaneous: Allergic reaction (2% to 8%)

Neuromuscular & skeletal: Arthralgia (8%)

(Continued)

Pemetrexed (Continued)

Overdosage/Toxicology Toxicities include neutropenia, anemia, thrombocytopenia, mucositis, rash, infection, and diarrhea. Treatment is supportive and symptom-directed. Continuing leucovorin may help minimize additional hematologic toxicity. The intravenous leucovorin doses used in clinical trials were 100 mg/m^2 once, followed by 50 mg/m^2 every 6 hours for 8 days. It is unknown if pemetrexed is removed by hemodialysis.

Pharmacodynamics/Kinetics

Duration of Action: V_{dss}: 16.1 L

Protein Binding: ~81%

Half-Life Elimination: Normal renal function: 3.5 hours

Metabolism: Minimal

Excretion: Urine (70% to 90% as unchanged drug)

Available Dosage Forms Injection, powder for reconstitution: 500 mg

Dosing

Adults:

Nonsmall cell lung cancer: 500 mg/m^2 on day 1 of each 21-day cycle

Malignant pleural mesothelioma: I.V.: 500-600 mg/m^2 on day 1 of each 21-day cycle

Note: Start vitamin supplements 1 week before initial dose of pemetrexed. Folic acid 350-1000 mcg/day orally (continuing for 21 days after last dose of pemetrexed) and vitamin B$_{12}$ 1000 mcg I.M. every 9 weeks. Dexamethasone 4 mg twice daily can be started the day before therapy, and continued the day of and the day after to minimize cutaneous reactions.

Renal Impairment:

Cl$_{cr}$ <45 mL/minute: No dosage adjustment guidelines are available; manufacturer recommends not using the drug.

Cl$_{cr}$ ≥45 mL/minute: No dosage adjustment required.

Hepatic Impairment: No dosage adjustment required.

Dosing Adjustment for Toxicity:

Toxicity: Discontinue if patient has any grade 3 or 4 toxicity after two dose reductions (except grade 3 transaminase elevations) or immediately if grade 3 or 4 neurotoxicity develops

Hematologic toxicity: Upon recovery, reinitiate therapy
Nadir ANC <500/mm^3 and nadir platelets ≥50,000/mm^3: Reduce dose to 75% of previous dose of pemetrexed and cisplatin

Nadir platelets <50,000/mm^3: Reduce dose to 50% of previous dose of pemetrexed and cisplatin

Nonhematologic toxicity (excluding neurotoxicity or ≥ grade 3 transaminase elevations): Upon recovery, reinitiate therapy

Grade 3 or 4 toxicity (excluding mucositis or transaminase elevations): Reduce dose to 75% of previous dose of pemetrexed and cisplatin

Diarrhea requiring hospitalization: Reduce dose to 75% of previous dose of pemetrexed and cisplatin

Grade 3 or 4 mucositis: Reduce dose to 50% of previous dose of pemetrexed; continue cisplatin at 100% of previous dose

Neurotoxicity:

Common Toxicity Criteria (CTC) Grade 0-1: Continue at previous dose of pemetrexed and cisplatin.

CTC Grade 2: Continue at previous dose of pemetrexed; Reduce dose to 50% of previous dose of cisplatin.

Administration

I.V.: Infuse over 10 minutes.

Stability

Reconstitution: Add 20 mL of 0.9% preservative free sodium chloride injection to make a 25 mg/mL solution. Gently swirl. Solution may be colorless to green-yellow. Further dilute in 50-200 mL of 0.9% sodium chloride for administration.

Compatibility: Physically **incompatible** with calcium-containing products.

Y-site administration: Incompatible: Amphotericin B, calcium gluconate, cefazolin sodium, cefotaxime sodium, cefotetan disodium, cefoxitin sodium, ceftazidime, chlorpromazine hydrochloride, ciprofloxacin, dobutamine hydrochloride, doxorubicin hydrochloride, doxycycline hyclate, droperidol, gemcitabine hydrochloride, gentamicin sulfate, irinotecan hydrochloride, metronidazole, minocycline hydrochloride, mitoxantrone hydrochloride, nalbuphine hydrochloride, ondansetron hydrochloride, prochlorperazine edisylate, tobramycin sulfate, topotecan hydrochloride

Storage: Store unopened vials at 25°C (77°F). Reconstituted and infusion solutions are stable for 24 hours when refrigerated or stored at room temperature.

Laboratory Monitoring CBC (before each dose); serum creatinine, total bilirubin, ALT, AST (day 1 of each, or every other, cycle)

Nursing Actions

Physical Assessment: Premedication may be prescribed. (eg, folic acid and vitamin B$_{12}$ one week before first dose of pemetrexed). Corticosteroids may be ordered to reduce cutaneous reactions. Assess potential for interactions with other pharmacological agents (eg, NSAIDs and other agents with nephrotoxic potential). Monitor laboratory tests on a regular schedule and assess adverse response at frequent intervals during treatment (eg, chest pain, CNS changes, GI upset [nausea, vomiting, diarrhea, constipation], anemia, neuropathy, rash, infection). Teach patient appropriate interventions to reduce side effects and adverse symptoms to report.

Patient Education: This medication is only administered intravenously (with your cisplatin). Report immediately any burning, pain, itching, or redness at infusion site or any sudden feelings of anxiety, difficulty breathing, chest or back pain. It is important that you maintain adequate hydration (2-3 L/day of fluids, unless instructed to restrict fluid intake) and adequate nutrition (frequent small meals may help). Maintain regularly scheduled dietary supplements (vitamin B$_{12}$ and folic acid) as prescribed. May cause severe nausea, vomiting, constipation or diarrhea (small frequent meals, and good mouth care are important - if persistent, consult prescriber for medication); mouth sores (use soft toothbrush or cotton swabs for mouth care). Report promptly any chest pain, skin rash, tingling or loss of sensation in extremities, difficulty breathing, fever, chills, unusual fatigue, or any other unusual symptoms. **Pregnancy/breast-feeding precautions:** Inform prescriber if you are pregnant. Do not get pregnant during therapy. Consult prescriber for instruction on appropriate contraceptive measures. This drug may cause severe fetal defects. Do not breast-feed.

Dietary Considerations Initiate folic acid supplementation 1 week before first dose of pemetrexed, continue for full course of therapy, and for 21 days after last dose. Institute vitamin B$_{12}$ 1 week before the first dose; administer every 9 weeks thereafter.

Pregnancy Issues In animal studies, was associated with fetotoxicity and teratogenicity when given on gestation days 6-15. Embryotoxicity also occurred. There are no adequate or well-controlled studies in pregnant women. Patients should avoid becoming pregnant while using this drug. If used during pregnancy or if patient becomes pregnant during therapy, patient should be educated about the potential hazards to the fetus.

Pemoline (PEM oh leen)

U.S. Brand Names Cylert® [DSC]; PemADD® [DSC]; PemADD® CT [DSC]

Synonyms Phenylisohydantoin; PIO

Restrictions C-IV

Pharmacologic Category Stimulant

Pregnancy Risk Factor B

Lactation Excretion in breast milk unknown/not recommended

Use Treatment of attention-deficit/hyperactivity disorder (ADHD) (not first-line)

Unlabeled/Investigational Use Narcolepsy

Mechanism of Action/Effect Blocks the reuptake mechanism of dopaminergic neurons, appears to act at the cerebral cortex and subcortical structures; CNS and respiratory stimulant with weak sympathomimetic effects; actions may be mediated via increase in CNS dopamine

Contraindications Hypersensitivity to pemoline or any component of the formulation; hepatic impairment (including abnormalities on baseline liver function tests); children <6 years of age; Tourette's syndrome; psychosis

Warnings/Precautions Not considered first-line therapy for ADHD due to association with hepatic failure. The manufacturer has recommended that signed informed consent following a discussion of risks and benefits must or should be obtained prior to the initiation of therapy. Therapy should be discontinued if a response is not evident after 3 weeks of therapy. Pemoline should not be started in patients with abnormalities in baseline liver function tests, and should be discontinued if clinically significant liver function test abnormalities are revealed at any time during therapy. Use with caution in patients with renal dysfunction or psychosis. In general, stimulant medications should be used with caution in patients with bipolar disorder, diabetes mellitus, cardiovascular disease, seizure disorders, insomnia, porphyria, or hypertension (although pemoline has been demonstrated to have a low potential to elevate blood pressure relative to other stimulants). May exacerbate symptoms of behavior and thought disorder in psychotic patients. Potential for drug dependency exists - avoid abrupt discontinuation in patients who have received for prolonged periods. Stimulant use has been associated with growth suppression, and careful monitoring is recommended.

Drug Interactions
Decreased Effect: Pemoline in combination with antiepileptic medications may decrease seizure threshold.

Increased Effect/Toxicity: Use caution when pemoline is used with other CNS-acting medications.

Nutritional/Ethanol Interactions Ethanol: Avoid ethanol (may increase CNS depression).

Adverse Reactions Frequency not defined.

Central nervous system: Insomnia, dizziness, drowsiness, mental depression, increased irritability, seizure, precipitation of Tourette's syndrome, hallucinations, headache, movement disorders

Dermatologic: Rash

Endocrine & metabolic: Suppression of growth in children

Gastrointestinal: Anorexia, weight loss, stomach pain, nausea

Hematologic: Aplastic anemia

Hepatic: Increased liver enzyme (usually reversible upon discontinuation), hepatitis, jaundice, hepatic failure

Overdosage/Toxicology Symptoms of overdose include tachycardia, hallucinations, and agitation. There is no specific antidote for intoxication and treatment is primarily supportive.

Pharmacodynamics/Kinetics
Onset of Action: Peak effect: 4 hours

Duration of Action: 8 hours

Time to Peak: Serum: 2-4 hours

Protein Binding: 50%

Half-Life Elimination: Children: 7-8.6 hours; Adults: 12 hours

Metabolism: Partially hepatic

Excretion: Urine; feces (negligible amounts)

Available Dosage Forms [DSC] = Discontinued product

Tablet (Cylert® [DSC], PemADD® [DSC]): 18.75 mg, 37.5 mg, 75 mg

Tablet, chewable (Cylert® [DSC], PemADD® CT [DSC]): 37.5 mg

Dosing
Adults & Elderly: ADHD: Oral: Initial: 37.5 mg given once daily in the morning, increase by 18.75 mg/day at weekly intervals; usual effective dose range: 56.25-75 mg/day; maximum: 112.5 mg/day; dosage range: 0.5-3 mg/kg/24 hours; significant benefit may not be evident until third or fourth week of administration.

Pediatrics: Children ≥6 years: Refer to adult dosing.

Renal Impairment: Cl_{cr} <50 mL/minute: Avoid use.

Administration
Oral: Administer medication in the morning.

Laboratory Monitoring Liver enzymes (baseline and every 2 weeks)

Nursing Actions
Physical Assessment: Assess effectiveness and interactions of other medications patient may be taking. After long-term use, taper dosage slowly when discontinuing. Monitor laboratory results, effectiveness of therapy, and adverse reactions at beginning of therapy and periodically with long-term use. Assess knowledge/teach patient appropriate use, interventions to reduce side effects, and adverse symptoms to report.

Patient Education: Take exactly as directed; do not change dosage or discontinue without consulting prescriber. Response may take some time. Avoid alcohol, caffeine, or other stimulants. Maintain adequate hydration (2-3 L/day of fluids) unless instructed to restrict fluid intake. You may experience nausea, decreased appetite, or altered taste sensation (small frequent meals may help maintain adequate nutrition); or drowsiness, dizziness, or mental depression, especially during early therapy (use caution when driving or engaging in tasks requiring alertness until response to drug is known). Report unresolved rapid heartbeat; excessive agitation, nervousness, insomnia, tremors, dizziness, or seizures; skin rash or irritation; altered gait or movement; unusual mouth movements or vocalizations (Tourette's syndrome); yellowing of skin or eyes; or dark urine or pale stools. **Breast-feeding precaution:** Breast-feeding is not recommended.

Additional Information Treatment of ADHD should include "Drug Holidays" or periodic discontinuation of stimulant medication in order to assess the patient's requirements and to decrease tolerance and limit suppression of linear growth and weight. The labeling for Cylert® includes recommendations for liver function monitoring and a Patient Information Consent Form.

Penciclovir (pen SYE kloe veer)

U.S. Brand Names Denavir®

Pharmacologic Category Antiviral Agent

Medication Safety Issues

Sound-alike/look-alike issues:

Denavir® may be confused with indinavir

Pregnancy Risk Factor B

Lactation Excretion in breast milk unknown

Use Topical treatment of herpes simplex labialis (cold sores)

Mechanism of Action/Effect Phosphorylated in the virus-infected cells to penciclovir triphosphate, which competitively inhibits DNA polymerase in HSV-1 and HSV-2 strains. This prevents viral replication by inhibition of viral DNA synthesis. Some activity has been demonstrated against Epstein-Barr and varicella-zoster virus (VZV).

Contraindications Hypersensitivity to the penciclovir or any component of the formulation; previous and significant adverse reactions to famciclovir

Warnings/Precautions Apply only to herpes labialis on lips and face. Application to mucous membranes is not recommended. Effect has not been evaluated in immunocompromised patients.

Adverse Reactions

>10%: Dermatologic: Mild erythema (50%)

1% to 10%: Central nervous system: Headache (5.3%)

Overdosage/Toxicology Penciclovir is poorly absorbed if ingested orally. Adverse reactions related to oral ingestion are unlikely.

Available Dosage Forms Cream: 1% (1.5 g)

Dosing

Adults & Elderly: Herpes simplex labialis (cold sores): Topical: Apply cream at the first sign or symptom of cold sore (eg, tingling, swelling); apply every 2 hours during waking hours for 4 days.

Pediatrics: Herpes simplex labialis (cold sores): Children ≥12 years: Refer to adult dosing.

Stability

Storage: Store at controlled room temperature of 20°C to 25°C (68°F to 77°F).

Nursing Actions

Physical Assessment: Monitor effectiveness of therapy. Teach patient appropriate application and use and adverse symptoms to report.

Patient Education: This is not a cure for herpes (recurrences tend to appear within 3 months of original infection), nor will this medication reduce the risk of transmission to others when lesions are present. For external use only. Wash hands before and after application. Apply this film over affected areas at first sign of cold sore. Avoid use of other topical creams, lotions, or ointments unless approved by prescriber. You may experience headache, mild rash, or taste disturbances. **Breast-feeding precaution:** Consult prescriber if breast-feeding.

Additional Information Penciclovir is the active metabolite of the prodrug famciclovir. Penciclovir is an alternative to topical acyclovir for HSV-1 and HSV-2 infections. Neither drug will prevent recurring HSV attacks.

Penicillin G Benzathine (pen i SIL in jee BENZ a theen)

U.S. Brand Names Bicillin® L-A

Synonyms Benzathine Benzylpenicillin; Benzathine Penicillin G; Benzylpenicillin Benzathine

Pharmacologic Category Antibiotic, Penicillin

Medication Safety Issues

Sound-alike/look-alike issues:

Penicillin may be confused with penicillamine

Bicillin® may be confused with Wycillin®

Bicillin® C-R (penicillin G benzathine and penicillin G procaine) may be confused with Bicillin® L-A (penicillin G benzathine). Penicillin G benzathine is the only product currently approved for the treatment of syphilis. Administration of penicillin G benzathine and penicillin G procaine combination instead of Bicillin® L-A may result in inadequate treatment response.

Penicillin G benzathine may only be administered by deep intramuscular injection; intravenous administration of penicillin G benzathine has been associated with cardiopulmonary arrest and death.

Pregnancy Risk Factor B

Lactation Enters breast milk/compatible

Use Active against some gram-positive organisms, few gram-negative organisms such as *Neisseria gonorrhoeae*, and some anaerobes and spirochetes; used in the treatment of syphilis; used only for the treatment of mild to moderately severe infections caused by organisms susceptible to low concentrations of penicillin G or for prophylaxis of infections caused by these organisms

Mechanism of Action/Effect Interferes with bacterial cell wall synthesis during active multiplication, causing cell wall death and resultant bactericidal activity against susceptible bacteria

Contraindications Hypersensitivity to penicillin or any component of the formulation

Warnings/Precautions Use with caution in patients with impaired renal function, seizure disorder. CDC and AAP do not currently recommend the use of penicillin G benzathine to treat congenital syphilis or neurosyphilis due to reported treatment failures and lack of published clinical data on its efficacy.

Drug Interactions

Decreased Effect: Tetracyclines may decrease penicillin effectiveness. Although anecdotal reports suggest oral contraceptive efficacy could be reduced by penicillins, this has been refuted by more rigorous scientific and clinical data.

Increased Effect/Toxicity: Probenecid increases penicillin levels. Aminoglycosides may lead to synergistic efficacy. Penicillins may increase the exposure to methotrexate during concurrent therapy; monitor.

Lab Interactions Positive Coombs' [direct], false-positive urinary and/or serum proteins; false-positive or negative urinary glucose using Clinitest®

Adverse Reactions Frequency not defined.

Central nervous system: Convulsions, confusion, drowsiness, myoclonus, fever

Dermatologic: Rash

Endocrine & metabolic: Electrolyte imbalance

Hematologic: Positive Coombs' reaction, hemolytic anemia

Local: Pain, thrombophlebitis

Renal: Acute interstitial nephritis

Miscellaneous: Anaphylaxis, hypersensitivity reactions, Jarisch-Herxheimer reaction

Overdosage/Toxicology Symptoms of penicillin overdose include neuromuscular hypersensitivity (eg, agitation, hallucinations, asterixis, encephalopathy, confusion, and seizures). Electrolyte imbalance may occur if the preparation contains potassium or sodium salts, especially in renal failure. Hemodialysis may be helpful to aid in removal of the drug from blood; otherwise, treatment is supportive or symptom-directed.

Pharmacodynamics/Kinetics
Duration of Action: Dose dependent: 1-4 weeks; larger doses result in more sustained levels

Time to Peak: Serum: 12-24 hours

Available Dosage Forms Injection, suspension [prefilled syringe]: 600,000 units/mL (1 mL, 2 mL, 4 mL)

Dosing
Adults & Elderly: Note: Not indicated as single drug therapy for neurosyphilis, but may be given 1 time/week for 3 weeks following I.V. treatment (refer to Penicillin G monograph for dosing)

Group A streptococcal upper respiratory infection: I.M.: 1.2 million units as a single dose

Prophylaxis of recurrent rheumatic fever: I.M.: 1.2 million units every 3-4 weeks or 600,000 units twice monthly

Syphilis:
Early: I.M.: 2.4 million units as a single dose in 2 injection sites

More than 1-year duration: I.M.: 2.4 million units in 2 injection sites once weekly for 3 doses

Neurosyphilis: Not indicated as single-drug therapy, but may be given once weekly for 3 weeks following I.V. treatment; refer to Penicillin G Parenteral/Aqueous monograph for dosing

Pediatrics:
Congenital syphilis (asymptomatic): I.M.: Neonates >1200g: 50,000 units/kg as a single dose

Group A streptococcal upper respiratory infection: I.M.: Infants and Children: 25,000-50,000 units/kg as a single dose (maximum: 1.2 million units)

Prophylaxis of recurrent rheumatic fever: I.M.: Infants and Children: 25,000-50,000 units/kg every 3-4 weeks (maximum: 1.2 million units/dose)

Syphilis:
Early: I.M.: Infants and Children: 50,000 units/kg as a single injection (maximum: 2.4 million units)

More than 1-year duration: I.M.: Infants and Children: 50,000 units/kg every week for 3 doses (maximum: 2.4 million units/dose)

Administration
I.M.: Administer by deep I.M. injection in the upper outer quadrant of the buttock. Do **not** give I.V., intra-arterially, or SubQ. When doses are repeated, rotate the injection site.

Stability
Storage: Store in refrigerator.

Laboratory Monitoring Perform culture and sensitivity before administering first dose.

Nursing Actions
Physical Assessment: Results of culture and sensitivity tests and patient's allergy history should be assessed prior to starting therapy. Assess potential for interactions with other pharmacological agents patient may be taking (eg, increase or decrease levels/effect of penicillin). Advise patients with diabetes about use of Clinitest®; may cause false readings. Monitor for therapeutic effectiveness (resolution of infection) and adverse reactions (eg, hypersensitivity reactions, opportunistic infection). Teach patient possible side effects/appropriate interventions and adverse symptoms to report.

Patient Education: This drug can only be given by injection. Report immediately any redness, swelling, burning, or pain at injection site or any signs of allergic reaction (eg, respiratory difficulty or swallowing, chest tightness, rash, hives, swelling of lips or mouth). Maintain adequate hydration (2-3 L/day of fluids) unless instructed to restrict fluid intake. If being treated for sexually-transmitted disease, partner will also need to be treated. If you have diabetes, drug may cause false test results with Clinitest®; consult prescriber for alternative method of glucose monitoring. May cause confusion or drowsiness (use caution when driving or engaging in tasks that require alertness until response to drug is known). Report persistent adverse effects or signs of opportunistic infection (eg, fever, chills, unhealed sores, white plaques in mouth or vagina, purulent vaginal discharge, fatigue).

Penicillin G (Parenteral/Aqueous)
(pen i SIL in jee, pa REN ter al, AYE kwee us)

U.S. Brand Names Pfizerpen®

Synonyms Benzylpenicillin Potassium; Benzylpenicillin Sodium; Crystalline Penicillin; Penicillin G Potassium; Penicillin G Sodium

Pharmacologic Category Antibiotic, Penicillin

Medication Safety Issues
Sound-alike/look-alike issues:
Penicillin may be confused with penicillamine

Pregnancy Risk Factor B

Lactation Enters breast milk/compatible

Use Active against some gram-positive organisms, generally not *Staphylococcus aureus*; some gram-negative organisms such as *Neisseria gonorrhoeae*, and some anaerobes and spirochetes

Mechanism of Action/Effect Interferes with bacterial cell wall synthesis during active multiplication, causing cell wall death and resultant bactericidal activity against susceptible bacteria

Contraindications Hypersensitivity to penicillin or any component of the formulation

Warnings/Precautions Avoid intravascular or intra-arterial administration or injection into or near major peripheral nerves or blood vessels since such injections may cause severe and/or permanent neurovascular damage. Use with caution in patients with renal impairment (dosage reduction required), pre-existing seizure disorders.

Drug Interactions
Decreased Effect: Tetracyclines may decrease penicillin effectiveness. Although anecdotal reports suggest oral contraceptive efficacy could be reduced by penicillins, this has been refuted by more rigorous scientific and clinical data.

Increased Effect/Toxicity: Probenecid increases penicillin levels. Aminoglycosides may lead to synergistic efficacy. Penicillins may increase the exposure to methotrexate during concurrent therapy; monitor.

Lab Interactions False-positive or negative urinary glucose determination using Clinitest®; positive Coombs' [direct]; false-positive urinary and/or serum proteins

Adverse Reactions Frequency not defined.
Central nervous system: Convulsions, confusion, drowsiness, myoclonus, fever

Dermatologic: Rash

Endocrine & metabolic: Electrolyte imbalance

Hematologic: Positive Coombs' reaction, hemolytic anemia

Local: Injection site reaction, thrombophlebitis

Renal: Acute interstitial nephritis

Miscellaneous: Anaphylaxis, hypersensitivity reactions, Jarisch-Herxheimer reaction

Overdosage/Toxicology Symptoms of penicillin overdose include neuromuscular hypersensitivity (eg, agitation, hallucinations, asterixis, encephalopathy, confusion, and seizures). Electrolyte imbalance may occur if the preparation contains potassium or sodium salts, especially in renal failure. Treatment is supportive or symptom-directed.
(Continued)

Penicillin G (Parenteral/Aqueous)
(Continued)

Pharmacodynamics/Kinetics
Time to Peak: Serum: I.M.: ~30 minutes; I.V. ~1 hour
Protein Binding: 65%
Half-Life Elimination:
Neonates: <6 days old: 3.2-3.4 hours; 7-13 days old: 1.2-2.2 hours; >14 days old: 0.9-1.9 hours
Children and Adults: Normal renal function: 20-50 minutes
End-stage renal disease: 3.3-5.1 hours
Metabolism: Hepatic (30%) to penicilloic acid
Excretion: Urine

Available Dosage Forms
Infusion, as potassium [premixed iso-osmotic dextrose solution, frozen]: 1 million units (50 mL), 2 million units (50 mL), 3 million units (50 mL) [contains sodium 1.02 mEq and potassium 1.7 mEq per 1 million units]
Injection, powder for reconstitution, as potassium (Pfizerpen®): 5 million units, 20 million units [contains sodium 6.8 mg (0.3 mEq) and potassium 65.6 mg (1.68 mEq) per 1 million units]
Injection, powder for reconstitution, as sodium: 5 million units [contains sodium 1.68 mEq per 1 million units]

Dosing
Adults & Elderly:
Actinomyces species: I.V.: 10-20 million units/day divided every 4-6 hours for 4-6 weeks
Anthrax (cutaneous): I.V.: 2 million units every 3 hours for 5-7 days
Clostridium perfringens: I.V.: 24 million units/day divided every 4-6 hours with clindamycin
Corynebacterium diptheriae: I.V.: 25,000-50,000 units/kg to maximum 1.2 million units every 12 hours, until oral therapy tolerated
Erysipelas: I.V.: 1-2 million units every 4-6 hours
Erysipelothrix: I.V.: 2-4 million units every 4 hours
Fascial space infections: I.V.: 2-4 million units every 4-6 hours with metronidazole
Leptospirosis: I.V.: 1.5 million units every 6 hours for 7 days
Listeria: I.V.: 300,000 units/kg/day every 4 hours
Lyme disease (meningitis): I.V.: 20 million units/day in divided doses
Neurosyphilis: I.M., I.V.: 18-24 million units/day in divided doses every 4 hours (or by continuous infusion) for 10-14 days
Streptococcus:
Brain abscess: I.V.: 20-24 million units/day in divided doses with metronidazole
Endocarditis or osteomyelitis: I.V.: 3-4 million units every 4 hours for at least 4 weeks
Meningitis: I.V.: 3-4 million units every 4 hours for 2-3 weeks
Pregnancy (prophylaxis GBS): I.V.: 5-6 million units x 1 dose, then 2.5-3 million units every 4 hours until delivery
Skin and soft tissue: I.V.: 3-4 million units every 4 hours for 10 days
Toxic shock: I.V.: 24 million units/day in divided doses with clindamycin
Streptococcal pneumonia:
Meningitis: I.V.: 2-4 million units every 2-4 hours
Nonmeningitis: I.V.: 2-3 million units every 4 hours
Whipple's disease: I.V.: 2 million units every 4 hours (with streptomycin) for 10-14 days, followed by oral trimethoprim/sulfamethoxazole or doxycycline for 1 year

Pediatrics:
Susceptible infections: I.M., I.V.:
Neonates:
<7 days, <2000 g: 25,000-50,000 units/kg every 12 hours
<7 days, >2000 g: 25,000-50,000 units/kg every 8 hours

>7 days, <2000 g: 25,000-50,000 units/kg every 8 hours
>7 days, >2000 g: 25,000-50,000 units/kg every 6 hours
Infants and Children: I.M., I.V.: 250,000 to 400,000 units/kg/day in divided doses every 4-6 hours (maximum dose: 24 million units/day)
Gonococcal:
Disseminated or ophthalmia: I.V.: 100,000 units/kg/day in 2 divided doses (>1 week of age: 4 divided doses)
Meningitis: I.V.: 150,000 units/kg in 2 divided doses (>1 week of age: 4 divided doses)
Mild-to-moderate infections: I.M., I.V.: 25,000-50,000 units/kg/day in 4 divided doses
Severe infections: I.M., I.V.: 250,000-400,000 units/kg/day in divided doses every 4-6 hours (maximum dose: 24 million units/day)
Syphilis (congenital):
Neonates:
≤7 days: 50,000 units/kg I.V. every 12 hours for a total of 10 days
>7 days: 50,000 units/kg I.V. every 8 hours for a total of 10 days
Infants: I.V.: 50,000 units/kg every 4-6 hours for 10 days

Renal Impairment: Dosage modification is required in patients with renal insufficiency.
Cl_{cr} >10 mL/minute: Administer full loading dose followed by 1/2 loading dose given every 4-5 hours
Cl_{cr} <10 mL/minute: Administer full loading dose followed by 1/2 loading dose given every 8-10 hours

Administration
I.M.: Administer I.M. by deep injection in the upper outer quadrant of the buttock. Administer injection around-the-clock to promote less variation in peak and trough levels.
I.V.: While I.M. route is preferred route of administration, large doses should be administered by continuous I.V. infusion. Determine volume and rate of fluid administration required in a 24-hour period. Add appropriate daily dosage to this fluid. Rapid administration or excessive dosage can cause electrolyte imbalance, cardiac arrhythmias, and/or seizures.
I.V. Detail: pH: 6-7.5

Stability
Compatibility: Inactivated in acidic or alkaline solutions
Penicillin G potassium: Stable in dextran 6% in dextrose, dextran 6% in NS, D_5LR, $D_5^1/_4NS$, $D_5^1/_2NS$, D_5NS, D_5W, $D_{10}W$, LR, $^1/_2NS$, NS, hetastarch 6%; **incompatible** with dextran 70 6% in dextrose, dextran 40 10% in dextrose
Compatibility in syringe: Incompatible with metoclopramide
Compatibility when admixed: Incompatible with aminoglycosides, aminophylline, amphotericin B, chlorpromazine, dopamine, floxacillin, hydroxyzine, metaraminol, pentobarbital, phenytoin, prochlorperazine mesylate, promazine, thiopental, vancomycin, vitamin B complex with C with oxytetracycline
Penicillin G sodium: Stable in dextran 40 10%; **incompatible** with fat emulsion 10%
Compatibility when admixed: Incompatible with amphotericin B, bleomycin, chlorpromazine, cytarabine, floxacillin, hydroxyzine, methylprednisolone sodium succinate, prochlorperazine mesylate, promethazine, vancomycin
Storage:
Penicillin G potassium powder for injection should be stored below 86°F (30°C); following reconstitution, solution may be stored for up to 7 days under refrigeration. Premixed bags for infusion should be stored in the freezer (-20°C to -4°F); frozen bags

may be thawed at room temperature or in refrigerator. Once thawed, solution is stable for 14 days if stored in refrigerator or for 24 hours when stored at room temperature. Do not re-freeze once thawed.

Penicillin G sodium powder for injection should be stored at controlled room temperature; reconstituted solution may be stored under refrigeration for up to 3 days.

Laboratory Monitoring Perform culture and sensitivity before administering first dose.

Nursing Actions

Physical Assessment: Results of culture and sensitivity tests and patient's allergy history should be assessed prior to starting therapy. Assess potential for interactions with other pharmacological agents (eg, decreased or increased levels/effects of penicillin G). Avoid intravascular or intra-arterial administration or injection into or near major peripheral nerves or blood vessels; may cause severe and/or permanent neurovascular damage. Advise patients with diabetes about use of Clinitest®; may cause false positive or negative. Monitor effectiveness (resolution of infections) and adverse reactions (eg, hypersensitivity reactions, opportunistic infection [fever, chills, unhealed sores, white plaques in mouth or vagina, purulent vaginal discharge, fatigue], CNS changes, thrombophlebitis). Teach patient possible side effects/appropriate interventions and adverse symptoms to report.

Patient Education: This drug can only be given by injection or infusion. Report immediately any redness, swelling, burning, or pain at infusion site or any signs of allergic reaction (eg, respiratory or swallowing difficulty, chest tightness, rash, hives, swelling of lips or mouth). Maintain adequate hydration (2-3 L/day of fluids) unless instructed to restrict fluid intake. If being treated for sexually-transmitted disease, partner will also need to be treated. If you have diabetes, drug may cause false test results with Clinitest®, consult prescriber for alternative method of glucose monitoring. May cause confusion or drowsiness (use caution when driving or engaging in tasks that require alertness until response to drug is known). Report persistent adverse effects or signs of opportunistic infection (eg, fever, chills, unhealed sores, white plaques in mouth or vagina, purulent vaginal discharge, fatigue).

Dietary Considerations
Injection powder for reconstitution as potassium contains sodium 6.8 mg (0.3 mEq) and potassium 65.6 mg (1.68 mEq) per 1 million units

Geriatric Considerations Despite a reported prolonged half-life, it is usually not necessary to adjust the dose of penicillin G or VK in the elderly to account for renal function changes with age, however, it is advised to calculate an estimated creatinine clearance and adjust dose accordingly. Consider sodium content in patients who may be sensitive to volume expansion (ie, CHF).

Additional Information 1 million units is approximately equal to 625 mg.

Penicillin G Procaine
(pen i SIL in jee PROE kane)

Synonyms APPG; Aqueous Procaine Penicillin G; Procaine Benzylpenicillin; Procaine Penicillin G; Wycillin [DSC]

Pharmacologic Category Antibiotic, Penicillin

Medication Safety Issues
Sound-alike/look-alike issues:
Penicillin G procaine may be confused with penicillin V potassium
Wycillin® may be confused with Bicillin®

Pregnancy Risk Factor B

Lactation Enters breast milk/compatible

Use Moderately severe infections due to *Treponema pallidum* and other penicillin G-sensitive microorganisms that are susceptible to low, but prolonged serum penicillin concentrations; anthrax due to *Bacillus anthracis* (postexposure) to reduce the incidence or progression of disease following exposure to aerolized *Bacillus anthracis*

Mechanism of Action/Effect Inhibits bacterial cell wall synthesis by binding to one or more of the penicillin binding proteins (PBPs); which in turn inhibits the final transpeptidation step of peptidoglycan synthesis in bacterial cell walls, thus inhibiting cell wall biosynthesis. Bacteria eventually lyse due to ongoing activity of cell wall autolytic enzymes (autolysins and murein hydrolases) while cell wall assembly is arrested.

Contraindications Hypersensitivity to penicillin, procaine, or any component of the formulation

Warnings/Precautions May need to modify dosage in patients with severe renal impairment, seizure disorders. Avoid intravascular, intravenous, or intra-arterial administration of penicillin G procaine since severe and/or permanent neurovascular damage may occur. Use of penicillin for longer than 2 weeks may be associated with an increased risk for some adverse reactions (neutropenia, serum sickness).

Drug Interactions
Decreased Effect: Tetracyclines may decrease penicillin effectiveness. Although anecdotal reports suggest oral contraceptive efficacy could be reduced by penicillins, this has been refuted by more rigorous scientific and clinical data.

Increased Effect/Toxicity: Probenecid increases penicillin levels. Aminoglycosides may lead to synergistic efficacy. Penicillins may increase the exposure to methotrexate during concurrent therapy; monitor.

Lab Interactions Positive Coombs' [direct], false-positive urinary and/or serum proteins

Adverse Reactions Frequency not defined.
Cardiovascular: Myocardial depression, vasodilation, conduction disturbances
Central nervous system: Confusion, drowsiness, myoclonus, CNS stimulation, seizure
Hematologic: Positive Coombs' reaction, hemolytic anemia, neutropenia
Local: Pain at injection site, thrombophlebitis, sterile abscess at injection site
Renal: Interstitial nephritis
Miscellaneous: Pseudoanaphylactic reactions, hypersensitivity reactions, Jarisch-Herxheimer reaction, serum sickness

Overdosage/Toxicology Symptoms of penicillin overdose include neuromuscular hypersensitivity (eg, agitation, hallucinations, asterixis, encephalopathy, confusion, and seizures). Electrolyte imbalance may occur if the preparation contains potassium or sodium salts, especially in renal failure. Hemodialysis may be helpful to aid in removal of the drug from blood; otherwise, treatment is supportive or symptom-directed.

Pharmacodynamics/Kinetics
Duration of Action: Therapeutic: 15-24 hours
Time to Peak: Serum: 1-4 hours
Protein Binding: 65%
Metabolism: ~30% hepatically inactivated
Excretion: Urine (60% to 90% as unchanged drug)
Clearance: Renal: Delayed in neonates, young infants, and renal impairment

Available Dosage Forms Injection, suspension: 600,000 units/mL (1 mL, 2 mL)

Dosing
Adults & Elderly:
Anthrax:
Inhalational (postexposure prophylaxis): I.M.: 1,200,000 units every 12 hours
Note: Overall treatment duration should be 60 days. Available safety data suggest continued
(Continued)

Penicillin G Procaine *(Continued)*

administration of penicillin G procaine for longer than 2 weeks may incur additional risk of adverse reactions. Clinicians may consider switching to effective alternative treatment for completion of therapy beyond 2 weeks.

Cutaneous (treatment): I.M.: 600,000-1,200,000 units/day; alternative therapy is recommended in severe cutaneous or other forms of anthrax infection

Endocarditis caused by susceptible viridans *Streptococcus* (when used in conjunction with an aminoglycoside): I.M.: 1.2 million units every 6 hours for 2-4 weeks

Gonorrhea (uncomplicated): 4.8 million units as a single dose divided in 2 sites given 30 minutes after probenecid 1 g orally

Neurosyphilis: I.M.: 2.4 million units/day with 500 mg probenecid by mouth 4 times/day for 10-14 days; **penicillin G aqueous I.V. is the preferred agent**

Whipple's disease: I.M.: 1.2 million units/day (with streptomycin) for 10-14 days, followed by oral trimethoprim/sulfamethoxazole or doxycycline for 1 year

Pediatrics:

Susceptible infections: I.M.: Infants and Children: 25,000-50,000 units/kg/day in divided doses 1-2 times/day; not to exceed 4.8 million units/24 hours

Anthrax, inhalational (postexposure prophylaxis): I.M.: 25,000 units/kg every 12 hours (maximum: 1,200,000 units every 12 hours).

Note: Overall treatment duration should be 60 days. Available safety data suggest continued administration of penicillin G procaine for longer than 2 weeks may incur additional risk for adverse reactions. Clinicians may consider switching to effective alternative treatment for completion of therapy beyond 2 weeks.

Syphilis (congenital): I.M.: 50,000 units/kg/day once daily for 10 days; if more than 1 day of therapy is missed, the entire course should be restarted

Renal Impairment:

Cl_{cr} 10-30 mL/minute: Administer every 8-12 hours.
Cl_{cr} <10 mL/minute: Administer every 12-18 hours.
Moderately dialyzable (20% to 50%)

Administration

I.M.: Procaine suspension is for deep I.M. injection only. Rotate the injection site. Do not inject in gluteal muscle in children <2 years of age.

Stability

Storage: Store in refrigerator.

Laboratory Monitoring Periodic renal and hematologic function with prolonged therapy; WBC count; perform culture and sensitivity before administering first dose.

Nursing Actions

Physical Assessment: Results of culture and sensitivity tests and patient's allergy history should be assessed prior to starting therapy. Assess potential for interactions with other pharmacological agents (eg, decreased or increased levels/effects of penicillin G). Avoid intravascular or intra-arterial administration or injection into or near major peripheral nerves or blood vessels; may cause severe and/or permanent neurovascular damage. Advise patients with diabetes about use of Clinitest®; may cause false positive or negative. Monitor effectiveness (resolution of infections) and adverse reactions (eg, hypersensitivity reactions, opportunistic infection [fever, chills, unhealed sores, white plaques in mouth or vagina, purulent vaginal discharge, fatigue], CNS changes, thrombophlebitis). Teach patient possible side effects/appropriate interventions and adverse symptoms to report.

Patient Education: This drug can only be given by injection. Report immediately any redness, swelling, burning, or pain at injection site or any signs of allergic reaction (eg, respiratory or swallowing difficulty, chest tightness, rash, hives, swelling of lips or mouth). Maintain adequate hydration (2-3 L/day of fluids) unless instructed to restrict fluid intake. If being treated for sexually-transmitted disease, partner will also need to be treated. If you have diabetes, drug may cause false test results with Clinitest®, consult prescriber for alternative method of glucose monitoring. May cause confusion or drowsiness (use caution when driving or engaging in tasks that require alertness until response to drug is known). Report persistent adverse effects or signs of opportunistic infection (eg, fever, chills, unhealed sores, white plaques in mouth or vagina, purulent vaginal discharge, fatigue).

Geriatric Considerations Dosage does not usually need to be adjusted in the elderly, however, if multiple doses are to be given, adjust dose for renal function.

Penicillin V Potassium

(pen i SIL in vee poe TASS ee um)

U.S. Brand Names Veetids®

Synonyms Pen VK; Phenoxymethyl Penicillin

Pharmacologic Category Antibiotic, Penicillin

Medication Safety Issues

Sound-alike/look-alike issues:

Penicillin V procaine may be confused with penicillin G potassium

Pregnancy Risk Factor B

Lactation Enters breast milk (other penicillins are compatible with breast-feeding)

Use Treatment of infections caused by susceptible organisms involving the respiratory tract, otitis media, sinusitis, skin, and urinary tract; prophylaxis in rheumatic fever

Mechanism of Action/Effect Inhibits bacterial cell wall synthesis by binding to one or more of the penicillin binding proteins (PBPs); which in turn inhibits the final transpeptidation step of peptidoglycan synthesis in bacterial cell walls, thus inhibiting cell wall biosynthesis. Bacteria eventually lyse due to ongoing activity of cell wall autolytic enzymes (autolysins and murein hydrolases) while cell wall assembly is arrested.

Contraindications Hypersensitivity to penicillin or any component of the formulation

Warnings/Precautions Use with caution in patients with severe renal impairment (modify dosage).

Drug Interactions

Decreased Effect: Tetracyclines may decrease penicillin effectiveness. Although anecdotal reports suggest oral contraceptive efficacy could be reduced by penicillins, this has been refuted by more rigorous scientific and clinical data.

Increased Effect/Toxicity: Probenecid increases penicillin levels. Aminoglycosides may cause synergistic efficacy. Penicillins may increase the exposure to methotrexate during concurrent therapy; monitor.

Nutritional/Ethanol Interactions Food: Decreases drug absorption rate; decreases drug serum concentration.

Lab Interactions False-positive or negative urinary glucose determination using Clinitest®; positive Coombs' [direct]; false-positive urinary and/or serum proteins

Adverse Reactions >10%: Gastrointestinal: Mild diarrhea, vomiting, nausea, oral candidiasis

Overdosage/Toxicology Symptoms of penicillin overdose include neuromuscular hypersensitivity (eg, agitation, hallucinations, asterixis, encephalopathy, confusion, and seizures). Electrolyte imbalance may occur if the preparation contains potassium or sodium salts, especially in renal failure. Hemodialysis may be helpful to aid in removal of the drug from blood; otherwise, treatment is supportive or symptom-directed.

Pharmacodynamics/Kinetics
Time to Peak: Serum: 0.5-1 hour
Protein Binding: Plasma: 80%
Half-Life Elimination: 30 minutes; prolonged with renal impairment
Excretion: Urine (as unchanged drug and metabolites)
Available Dosage Forms Note: 250 mg = 400,000 units
Powder for oral solution: 125 mg/5 mL (100 mL, 200 mL); 250 mg/5 mL (100 mL, 200 mL)
Tablet: 250 mg, 500 mg

Dosing
Adults & Elderly:
Acintomycosis:
Mild: 2-4 g/day in 4 divided doses for 8 weeks
Surgical: 2-4 g/day in 4 divided doses for 6-12 months (after I.V. penicillin G therapy of 4-6 weeks)
Erysipelas: 500 mg 4 times/day
Pharyngitis (streptococcal): 500 mg 3-4 times/day for 10 days
Prophylaxis of pneumococcal or recurrent rheumatic fever infections: 250 mg twice daily
Pediatrics:
Pharyngitis (streptococcal): 250 mg 2-3 times/day for 10 days
Prophylaxis of pneumococcal infections:
Children <5 years: 125 mg twice daily
Children ≥5 years: 250 mg twice daily
Prophylaxis of recurrent rheumatic fever:
Children <5 years: 125 mg twice daily
Children ≥5 years: 250 mg twice daily
Renal Impairment:
Cl_{cr} 10-50 mL/minute: Administer every 8-12 hours.
Cl_{cr} <10 mL/minute: Administer every 12-16 hours.

Administration
Oral: Administer around-the-clock to promote less variation in peak and trough serum levels. Take on an empty stomach 1 hour before or 2 hours after meals, to enhance absorption, take until gone, do not skip doses.
I.V. Detail: pH: 6.0-8.5

Stability
Storage: Refrigerate suspension after reconstitution; discard after 14 days.
Laboratory Monitoring Periodic renal and hematologic function during prolonged therapy; perform culture and sensitivity before administering first dose.

Nursing Actions
Physical Assessment: Results of culture and sensitivity tests and patient's allergy history should be assessed prior to starting therapy. Assess potential for interactions with other pharmacological agents (eg. decreased or increased levels/effects of penicillin V). Monitor laboratory tests, effectiveness (resolution of infection), and adverse reactions (eg, hypersensitivity reactions, opportunistic infection [fever, chills, unhealed sores, white plaques in mouth or vagina, purulent vaginal discharge, fatigue]). Advise patients with diabetes about use of Clinitest®; may cause false readings. Teach patient possible side effects/appropriate interventions and adverse symptoms to report.
Patient Education: Take as directed at intervals around-the-clock, preferable on an empty stomach (1 hour before or 2 hours after a meal). Take entire prescription; do not skip doses or discontinue without consulting prescriber. Take a missed dose as soon as possible. If almost time for next dose, skip the missed dose and return to your regular schedule. Do not take a double dose. Maintain adequate hydration (2-3 L/day of fluids) unless instructed to restrict fluid intake. If you have diabetes, drug may cause false test results with Clinitest®, consult prescriber for alternative method of glucose monitoring. May cause nausea or vomiting (small, frequent meals, frequent mouth care,

chewing gum, or sucking lozenges may help); or diarrhea (buttermilk, boiled milk, or yogurt may help). Report persistent adverse effects; signs of opportunistic infection (eg, fever, chills, unhealed sores, white plaques in mouth or vagina, purulent vaginal discharge, fatigue); or signs of hypersensitivity reaction (rash, hives, itching, swelling of lips, tongue, mouth, or throat).
Dietary Considerations Take on an empty stomach 1 hour before or 2 hours after meals.
Breast-Feeding Issues No data reported; however, other penicillins may be taken while breast-feeding.
Additional Information 0.7 mEq of potassium per 250 mg penicillin V; 250 mg equals 400,000 units of penicillin

---

Pentamidine (pen TAM i deen)

U.S. Brand Names NebuPent®; Pentam-300®
Synonyms Pentamidine Isethionate
Pharmacologic Category Antibiotic, Miscellaneous
Pregnancy Risk Factor C
Lactation Excretion in breast milk unknown/contraindicated
Use Treatment and prevention of pneumonia caused by *Pneumocystis carinii* (PCP)
Unlabeled/Investigational Use Treatment of trypanosomiasis and visceral leishmaniasis
Mechanism of Action/Effect Interferes with RNA/DNA synthesis and phospholipids leading to cell death in protozoa.
Contraindications Hypersensitivity to pentamidine isethionate or any component of the formulation (inhalation and injection)
Warnings/Precautions Use with caution in patients with diabetes mellitus, renal or hepatic dysfunction, hyper-/hypotension, leukopenia, thrombocytopenia, asthma, or hypo-/hyperglycemia.
Drug Interactions
Cytochrome P450 Effect: Substrate of CYP2C19 (major); **Inhibits** CYP2C8/9 (weak), 2C19 (weak), 2D6 (weak), 3A4 (weak)
Decreased Effect: CYP2C19 inducers may decrease the levels/effects of pentamidine; example inducers include aminoglutethimide, carbamazepine, phenytoin, and rifampin.
Increased Effect/Toxicity: CYP2C19 inhibitors may increase the levels/effects of pentamidine; example inhibitors include delavirdine, fluconazole, fluvoxamine, gemfibrozil, isoniazid, omeprazole, and ticlopidine. Pentamidine may potentiate the effect of other drugs which prolong QT interval (cisapride, sparfloxacin, gatifloxacin, moxifloxacin, pimozide, and type Ia and type III antiarrhythmics).
Nutritional/Ethanol Interactions Ethanol: Avoid ethanol (may increase CNS depression or aggravate hypoglycemia).
Adverse Reactions Injection (I); Aerosol (A)
>10%:
Cardiovascular: Chest pain (A - 10% to 23%)
Central nervous system: Fatigue (A - 50% to 70%); dizziness (A - 31% to 47%)
Dermatologic: Rash (31% to 47%)
Endocrine & metabolic: Hyperkalemia
Gastrointestinal: Anorexia (A - 50% to 70%), nausea (A - 10% to 23%)
Local: Local reactions at injection site
Renal: Increased creatinine (I - 23%)
Respiratory: Wheezing (A - 10% to 23%), dyspnea (A - 50% to 70%), cough (A - 31% to 47%), pharyngitis (10% to 23%)
1% to 10%:
Cardiovascular: Hypotension (I - 4%)
(Continued)

Pentamidine (Continued)

Central nervous system: Confusion/hallucinations (1% to 2%), headache (A - 1% to 5%)

Dermatologic: Rash (I - 3.3%)

Endocrine & metabolic: Hypoglycemia <25 mg/dL (I - 2.4%)

Gastrointestinal: Nausea/anorexia (I - 6%), diarrhea (A - 1% to 5%), vomiting

Hematologic: Severe leukopenia (I - 2.8%), thrombocytopenia <20,000/mm^3 (I - 1.7%), anemia (A - 1% to 5%)

Hepatic: Increased LFTs (I - 8.7%)

Overdosage/Toxicology Symptoms of overdose include hypotension, hypoglycemia, and cardiac arrhythmias. Treatment is supportive.

Pharmacodynamics/Kinetics

Half-Life Elimination: Terminal: 6.4-9.4 hours; may be prolonged with severe renal impairment

Excretion: Urine (33% to 66% as unchanged drug)

Available Dosage Forms

Injection, powder for reconstitution, as isethionate (Pentam-300®): 300 mg

Powder for nebulization, as isethionate (NebuPent®): 300 mg

Dosing

Adults & Elderly:

Treatment of PCP pneumonia: I.M., I.V. (I.V. preferred): 4 mg/kg/day once daily for 14 days

Prevention of PCP pneumonia: Inhalation: 300 mg every 4 weeks via Respirgard® II nebulizer

Pediatrics:

Treatment of PCP pneumonia: I.M., I.V. (I.V. preferred): Children: 4 mg/kg/day once daily for 10-14 days

Prevention of PCP pneumonia: Children:

I.M., I.V.: 4 mg/kg monthly or every 2 weeks

Inhalation (aerosolized pentamidine in children ≥5 years): 300 mg/dose given every 3-4 weeks via Respirgard® II inhaler (8 mg/kg dose has also been used in children <5 years)

Treatment of trypanosomiasis (unlabeled use): I.V.: 4 mg/kg/day once daily for 10 days

Renal Impairment:

Cl$_{cr}$ 10-50 mL/minute: Administer dose every 24-36 hours.

Cl$_{cr}$ <10 mL/minute: Administer dose every 48 hours.

Not removed by hemo- or peritoneal dialysis or continuous arteriovenous or venovenous hemofiltration. Supplemental dose is not necessary.

Administration

I.M.: Deep I.M.

I.V.: Do not use NS as a diluent. Infuse I.V. slowly over a period of at least 60 minutes or administer deep I.M.

I.V. Detail: pH: 5.4 (sterile water); 4.09-4.38 (D$_5$W)

Inhalation: Deliver until nebulizer is gone (30-45 minutes). Virtually undetectable amounts are transferred to healthcare personnel during aerosol administration.

Stability

Reconstitution: Powder for inhalation should be reconstituted with sterile water for injection (6 mL per 300 mg vial). Powder for injection may be reconstituted with sterile water for injection or D$_5$W (SWFI should be used for I.M. injections). **Do not use NS as a diluent.**

Compatibility: Reconstituted vials with SWFI (60-100 mg/mL) are stable for 48 hours at room temperature protected from light. Solutions for injection (1-2.5 mg/mL) in D$_5$W are stable for at least 24 hours at room temperature.

Y-site administration: Incompatible: Aldesleukin, cefazolin, cefoperazone, cefotaxime, cefoxitin, ceftazidime, ceftriaxone, fluconazole, foscarnet, linezolid

Storage: Store intact vials at controlled room temperature and protect from light. Reconstituted vials with SWFI (60-100 mg/mL) are stable for 48 hours at room temperature and do not require light protection. Diluted solutions in 50-250 mL D$_5$W for infusion (1-2.5 mg/mL) are stable for at least 24 hours at room temperature.

Laboratory Monitoring Liver and renal function, blood glucose, serum potassium and calcium, ECG, CBC with platelets

Nursing Actions

Physical Assessment: Assess potential for interactions with other pharmacological agents patient may be taking (eg, increase or decrease levels/effects of pentamidine). **I.V., I.M.:** Patients should be lying down. Blood pressure, cardiac status, and respiratory function should be monitored closely during I.V. administration or following I.M. injection. Monitor laboratory tests, effectiveness, and adverse reactions (eg, chest pain, hypotension, rash, confusion, hallucinations, hypoglycemia, dyspnea, cough) Teach patient proper use (eg, nebulizer if self-administered), possible side effects/appropriate interventions, and adverse symptoms to report.

Patient Education: Do not take any new medication during therapy without consulting prescriber. I.V. or I.M. preparations must be given every day (if I.M. is self-administered follow exact directions for injection and disposal of syringe/needle). Inhalant drug must be prepared and used with a nebulizer exactly as directed once every 4 weeks. Frequent blood tests and blood pressure checks will be required while using this drug. PCP pneumonia may still occur despite pentamidine use. Maintain adequate hydration (2-3 L/day of fluids) unless instructed to restrict fluid intake. Avoid excessive alcohol (may exacerbate adverse effects). If you have diabetes, monitor glucose levels closely and frequently. May cause hypotension (use caution when rising from sitting or lying position or when climbing stairs); or metallic taste, nausea, vomiting, or anorexia (small, frequent meals, frequent mouth care, chewing gum, or sucking lozenges may help). Report chest pain or irregular heartbeat; unusual confusion or hallucinations; rash; or unusual wheezing, coughing, or respiratory difficulty. **Pregnancy/breast-feeding precautions:** Inform prescriber if you are or intend to become pregnant. Do not breast-feed.

Geriatric Considerations Ten percent of acquired immunodeficiency syndrome (AIDS) cases are in the elderly and this figure is expected to increase. Pentamidine has not as yet been studied exclusively in this population. Adjust dose for renal function.

Additional Information Virtually undetectable amounts are transferred to healthcare personnel during aerosol administration.

Pentazocine (pen TAZ oh seen)

U.S. Brand Names Talwin®; Talwin® NX

Synonyms Naloxone Hydrochloride and Pentazocine Hydrochloride; Pentazocine Hydrochloride; Pentazocine Hydrochloride and Naloxone Hydrochloride; Pentazocine Lactate

Restrictions C-IV

Pharmacologic Category Analgesic, Narcotic

Pregnancy Risk Factor C/D (prolonged use or high doses at term)

Lactation Excretion in breast milk unknown/use caution

Use Relief of moderate to severe pain; has also been used as a sedative prior to surgery and as a supplement to surgical anesthesia

Mechanism of Action/Effect Binds to opiate receptors in the CNS, causing inhibition of ascending pain pathways, altering the perception of and response to pain;

produces generalized CNS depression; partial agonist-antagonist

Contraindications Hypersensitivity to pentazocine, naloxone, or any component of the formulation; increased intracranial pressure (unless the patient is mechanically ventilated); pregnancy (prolonged use or high doses at term)

Warnings/Precautions Use with caution in seizure-prone patients, acute myocardial infarction, patients undergoing biliary tract surgery, patients with renal and hepatic dysfunction, head trauma, increased intracranial pressure, and patients with a history of prior opioid dependence or abuse; pentazocine may precipitate opiate withdrawal symptoms in patients who have been receiving opiates regularly; injection contains sulfites which may cause allergic reaction; tolerance or drug dependence may result from extended use. Severe vascular complications have resulted from misuse (injection) of Talwin® tablet formulations.

Drug Interactions
Decreased Effect: May potentiate or reduce analgesic effect of opiate agonist (eg, morphine) depending on patients tolerance to opiates; can precipitate withdrawal in narcotic addicts.

Increased Effect/Toxicity: Increased effect/toxicity with tripelennamine (can be lethal), CNS depressants (eg, phenothiazines, tranquilizers, anxiolytics, sedatives, hypnotics, alcohol).

Nutritional/Ethanol Interactions Ethanol: Avoid ethanol (may increase CNS depression).

Adverse Reactions Frequency not defined.
Cardiovascular: Hypotension, circulatory depression, shock, tachycardia, syncope, flushing
Central nervous system: Malaise, headache, nightmares, insomnia, CNS depression, sedation, hallucinations, confusion, disorientation, dizziness, euphoria, drowsiness, lightheadedness, irritability, chills, excitement
Dermatologic: Rash, pruritus, dermatitis, urticaria, Stevens-Johnson syndrome, toxic epidermal necrolysis, erythema multiforme
Gastrointestinal: Nausea, vomiting, xerostomia, constipation, anorexia, diarrhea, abdominal distress
Genitourinary: Urinary retention
Hematologic: WBCs decreased, eosinophilia
Local: Tissue damage and irritation with I.M./SubQ use
Neuromuscular & skeletal: Weakness, tremor, paresthesia
Ocular: Blurred vision, miosis
Otic: Tinnitus
Respiratory: Dyspnea, respiratory depression (rare)
Miscellaneous: Physical and psychological dependence, facial edema, diaphoresis, anaphylaxis

Overdosage/Toxicology Symptoms of overdose include drowsiness, sedation, respiratory depression, and coma. Naloxone, 2 mg I.V., with repeat administration as necessary up to a total of 10 mg, can also be used to reverse toxic effects of the opiate.

Pharmacodynamics/Kinetics
Onset of Action: Oral, I.M., SubQ: 15-30 minutes; I.V.: 2-3 minutes
Duration of Action: Oral: 4-5 hours; Parenteral: 2-3 hours
Protein Binding: 60%
Half-Life Elimination: 2-3 hours; prolonged with hepatic impairment
Metabolism: Hepatic via oxidative and glucuronide conjugation pathways; extensive first-pass effect
Excretion: Urine (small amounts as unchanged drug)

Available Dosage Forms
Injection, solution (Talwin®): 30 mg/mL (1 mL, 10 mL) [10 mL size contains sodium bisulfite]
Tablet (Talwin® NX): Pentazocine 50 mg and naloxone 0.5 mg

Dosing
Adults: Analgesic:
Oral: 50 mg every 3-4 hours; may increase to 100 mg/dose if needed, but should not exceed 600 mg/day
I.M., SubQ: 30-60 mg every 3-4 hours; do **not** exceed 30 mg/dose (maximum: 360 mg/day)
I.V.: 30 mg every 3-4 hours; do **not** exceed 30 mg/dose (maximum: 360 mg/day)
Elderly: See Geriatric Considerations. Initial dose:
Oral: 50 mg every 4 hours
I.M.: 30 mg every 4 hours
Pediatrics:
Analgesia:
I.M.: Children:
5-8 years: 15 mg
8-14 years: 30 mg
Oral: Children >12 years: Refer to adult dosing.
Preoperative/preanesthetic: Children 1-16 years: 0.5 mg/kg
Renal Impairment:
Cl_{cr} 10-50 mL/minute: Administer 75% of normal dose.
Cl_{cr} <10 mL/minute: Administer 50% of normal dose.
Hepatic Impairment: Reduce dose or avoid use in patients with liver disease.

Administration
I.M.: Rotate injection site; avoid intra-arterial injection
I.V. Detail: pH: 4-5 (adjusted with lactic acid or sodium hydroxide)
Other: Rotate injection site for SubQ use; avoid SubQ use unless absolutely necessary (may cause tissue damage); avoid intra-arterial injection

Stability
Compatibility:
Y-site administration: **Incompatible** with nafcillin
Compatibility in syringe: **Incompatible** with glycopyrrolate, heparin, pentobarbital
Compatibility when admixed: **Incompatible** with aminophylline, amobarbital, pentobarbital, phenobarbital, sodium bicarbonate
Storage: Injection: Store at room temperature, protect from heat and from freezing.

Nursing Actions
Physical Assessment: Assess other medications patient may be taking for additive or adverse interactions. Monitor for effectiveness of pain relief and monitor for signs of overdose. Monitor blood pressure, CNS and respiratory status, and degree of sedation at beginning of therapy and at regular intervals with long-term use. May cause physical and/or psychological dependence. For inpatients, implement safety measures (eg, side rails up, call light within reach, instructions to call for assistance). Assess knowledge/teach patient appropriate use (if self-administered), adverse reactions to report, and appropriate interventions to reduce side effects.

Patient Education: If self-administered, use exactly as directed; do not increase dose or frequency. Drug may cause physical and/or psychological dependence. While using this medication, do not use alcohol and other prescription or OTC medications (especially sedatives, tranquilizers, antihistamines, or pain medications) without consulting prescriber. Maintain adequate hydration (2-3 L/day of fluids) unless instructed to restrict fluid intake. May cause hypotension, dizziness, drowsiness, impaired coordination, or blurred vision (use caution when driving, climbing stairs, or changing position - rising from sitting or lying to standing, or when engaging in tasks requiring alertness until response to drug is known); nausea, vomiting, loss of appetite, or dry mouth (frequent mouth care, small frequent meals, chewing gum, or sucking lozenges may help); or constipation (increased exercise, fluids, fruit, or fiber may help; if unresolved, consult prescriber about use of stool softeners). Report persistent dizziness or headache; excessive fatigue or sedation; changes in mental
(Continued)

Pentazocine *(Continued)*

status; changes in urinary elimination or pain on urination; weakness or trembling; blurred vision; or shortness of breath. **Pregnancy/breast-feeding precautions:** Inform prescriber if you are or intend to become pregnant. Consult prescriber if breast-feeding.

Geriatric Considerations Pentazocine is not recommended for use in the elderly because of its propensity to cause delirium and agitation. If pentazocine must be used, be sure to adjust dose for renal function.

Breast-Feeding Issues Excretion of pentazocine in breast milk is unknown; no data available for naloxone

Pregnancy Issues Pentazocine was not found to be teratogenic in animal studies. Pentazocine and naloxone have been shown to cross the human placenta. Use should be avoided during labor and delivery of premature infants. Abstinence syndromes in the newborn have been reported after long-term use of pentazocine during pregnancy. Other adverse effects in the newborn have been reported following abuse of pentazocine during pregnancy; these effects may be due to pentazocine, other drugs abused, the mother's lifestyle, or a combination of all factors.

Additional Information Pentazocine hydrochloride: Talwin® NX tablet (with naloxone); naloxone is used to prevent abuse by dissolving tablets in water and using as injection.

Related Information
Compatibility of Drugs in Syringe *on page 1372*

Pentazocine and Acetaminophen
(pen TAZ oh seen & a seet a MIN oh fen)

U.S. Brand Names Talacen®

Synonyms Acetaminophen and Pentazocine; Pentazocine Hydrochloride and Acetaminophen

Restrictions C-IV

Pharmacologic Category Analgesic Combination (Narcotic)

Pregnancy Risk Factor C/D (prolonged use or high doses at term)

Lactation Excretion in breast milk unknown/use caution

Use Relief of mild to moderate pain

Available Dosage Forms Caplet: Pentazocine 25 mg and acetaminophen 650 mg [contains sodium metabisulfite]

Dosing
Adults & Elderly: Analgesic: Oral: 1 caplet every 4 hours up to maximum of 6 caplets

Nursing Actions
Physical Assessment: Assess patient for history of liver disease or ethanol abuse (acetaminophen and excessive ethanol may have adverse liver effects). Assess other medications patient may be taking for additive or adverse interactions. Monitor vital signs, effectiveness of pain relief, adverse reactions, and signs of overdose at beginning of therapy and at regular intervals with long-term use. May cause physical and/or psychological dependence. For inpatients, implement safety measures (eg, side rails up, call light within reach, instructions to call for assistance). Assess knowledge/teach patient appropriate use (if self-administered), adverse reactions to report, and appropriate interventions to reduce side effects.

Patient Education: If self-administered, use exactly as directed; do not increase dose or frequency. Drug may cause physical and/or psychological dependence. Take with food or milk. While using this medication, do not use alcohol and other prescription or OTC medications (especially sedatives, tranquilizers, antihistamines, or pain medications) without consulting prescriber. Maintain adequate hydration

(2-3 L/day of fluids) unless instructed to restrict fluid intake. May cause hypotension, dizziness, drowsiness, confusion, or nervousness (use caution when driving, climbing stairs, or changing position - rising from sitting or lying to standing, or when engaging in tasks requiring alertness until response to drug is known); nausea, dry mouth, decreased appetite, or gastric distress (frequent mouth care, frequent sips of fluids, chewing gum, or sucking lozenges may help); or constipation (increased exercise, fluids, fruit, or fiber may help; if unresolved, consult prescriber about use of stool softeners). Report chest pain, rapid heartbeat, or palpitations; persistent dizziness; change in mental status; shortness of breath or respiratory difficulty; unusual bleeding (stool, mouth, urine) or bruising; unusual fatigue and weakness; pain on urination; change in elimination patterns or change in color of urine or stool; or unresolved nausea or vomiting. **Pregnancy/breast-feeding precautions:** Inform prescriber if you are or intend to become pregnant. Consult prescriber if breast-feeding.

Related Information
Acetaminophen *on page 30*
Pentazocine *on page 964*

Pentobarbital *(pen toe BAR bi tal)*

U.S. Brand Names Nembutal®

Synonyms Pentobarbital Sodium

Restrictions C-II

Pharmacologic Category Anticonvulsant, Barbiturate; Barbiturate

Medication Safety Issues
Sound-alike/look-alike issues:
Pentobarbital may be confused with phenobarbital
Nembutal® may be confused with Myambutol®

Pregnancy Risk Factor D

Lactation Enters breast milk/contraindicated

Use Sedative/hypnotic; preanesthetic; high-dose barbiturate coma for treatment of increased intracranial pressure or status epilepticus unresponsive to other therapy

Mechanism of Action/Effect Short-acting barbiturate with sedative, hypnotic, and anticonvulsant properties. Barbiturates depress the sensory cortex, decrease motor activity, alter cerebellar function, and produce drowsiness, sedation, and hypnosis. In high doses, barbiturates exhibit anticonvulsant activity; barbiturates produce dose-dependent respiratory depression.

Contraindications Hypersensitivity to barbiturates or any component of the formulation; marked hepatic impairment; dyspnea or airway obstruction; porphyria; pregnancy

Warnings/Precautions Tolerance to hypnotic effect can occur; do not use for >2 weeks to treat insomnia. Potential for drug dependency exists, abrupt cessation may precipitate withdrawal, including status epilepticus in epileptic patients. Do not administer to patients in acute pain. Use caution in elderly, debilitated, renally impaired, hepatic dysfunction, or pediatric patients. May cause paradoxical responses, including agitation and hyperactivity, particularly in acute pain and pediatric patients. Use with caution in patients with depression or suicidal tendencies, or in patients with a history of drug abuse. Tolerance, psychological and physical dependence may occur with prolonged use.

May cause CNS depression, which may impair physical or mental abilities. Patients must cautioned about performing tasks which require mental alertness (eg, operating machinery or driving). Effects with other sedative drugs or ethanol may be potentiated. Use of this agent as a hypnotic in the elderly is not recommended due to its long half-life and potential for physical and psychological dependence.

May cause respiratory depression or hypotension, particularly when administered intravenously. Use with caution in hemodynamically unstable patients or patients with respiratory disease. High doses (loading doses of 15-35 mg/kg given over 1-2 hours) have been utilized to induce pentobarbital coma, but these higher doses often cause hypotension requiring vasopressor therapy.

Drug Interactions

Cytochrome P450 Effect: Induces CYP2A6 (strong), 3A4 (strong)

Decreased Effect: Pentobarbital may decrease the levels/effects of benzodiazepines, calcium channel blockers, clarithromycin, cyclosporine, erythromycin, ifosfamide, mirtazapine, nateglinide, nefazodone, nevirapine, protease inhibitors, rifampin, tacrolimus, venlafaxine, and other CYP2A6 or 3A4 substrates. Barbiturates may increase the metabolism of estrogens and reduce the efficacy of oral contraceptives; an alternative method of contraception should be considered. Barbiturates inhibit the hypoprothrombinemic effects of oral anticoagulants via increased metabolism. Barbiturates may enhance the metabolism of methadone resulting in methadone withdrawal.

Increased Effect/Toxicity: When combined with other CNS depressants, ethanol, narcotic analgesics, antidepressants, or benzodiazepines, additive respiratory and CNS depression may occur. Barbiturates may enhance the hepatotoxic potential of acetaminophen overdoses. Chloramphenicol, MAO inhibitors, valproic acid, and felbamate may inhibit barbiturate metabolism. Barbiturates may impair the absorption of griseofulvin, and may enhance the nephrotoxic effects of methoxyflurane.

Nutritional/Ethanol Interactions Ethanol: Avoid ethanol (may increase CNS depression).

Lab Interactions Increased ammonia (B); decreased bilirubin (S)

Adverse Reactions Frequency not defined.
Cardiovascular: Bradycardia, hypotension, syncope
Central nervous system: Drowsiness, lethargy, CNS excitation or depression, impaired judgment, "hangover" effect, confusion, somnolence, agitation, hyperkinesia, ataxia, nervousness, headache, insomnia, nightmares, hallucinations, anxiety, dizziness
Dermatologic: Rash, exfoliative dermatitis, Stevens-Johnson syndrome
Gastrointestinal: Nausea, vomiting, constipation
Hematologic: Agranulocytosis, thrombocytopenia, megaloblastic anemia
Local: Pain at injection site, thrombophlebitis with I.V. use
Renal: Oliguria
Respiratory: Laryngospasm, respiratory depression, apnea (especially with rapid I.V. use), hypoventilation, apnea
Miscellaneous: Gangrene with inadvertent intra-arterial injection

Overdosage/Toxicology Symptoms of overdose include unsteady gait, slurred speech, confusion, jaundice, hypothermia, hypotension, respiratory depression, and coma. Treat symptomatically. Charcoal hemoperfusion may be beneficial in stage IV coma due to high serum concentration.

Pharmacodynamics/Kinetics
Onset of Action: I.M.: 10-15 minutes; I.V.: ~1 minute
Duration of Action: I.V.: 15 minutes
Protein Binding: 35% to 55%
Half-Life Elimination: Terminal: Children: 25 hours; Adults, healthy: 22 hours (range: 15-50 hours)
Metabolism: Extensively hepatic via hydroxylation and oxidation pathways
Excretion: Urine (<1% as unchanged drug)

Available Dosage Forms Injection, solution, as sodium: 50 mg/mL (20 mL, 50 mL) [contains alcohol 10% and propylene glycol 40%]

Dosing
Adults:
Hypnotic:
I.M.: 150-200 mg
I.V.: Initial: 100 mg, may repeat every 1-3 minutes up to 200-500 mg total dose
Preoperative sedation: I.M.: 150-200 mg
Barbiturate coma in head injury patients or status epilepticus: I.V.: Loading dose: 5-10 mg/kg given slowly over 1-2 hours; monitor blood pressure and respiratory rate; maintenance infusion: initial: 1 mg/kg/hour; may increase to 2-3 mg/kg/hour; maintain burst suppression on EEG
Status epilepticus: I.V.: Loading dose: 2-15 mg/kg given slowly over 1-2 hours; maintenance infusion: 0.5-3 mg/kg/hour. **Note:** Intubation required; monitor hemodynamics
Elderly: Not recommended for use in the elderly (see Geriatric Considerations).

Pediatrics:
Hypnotic: I.M.: 2-6 mg/kg; maximum: 100 mg/dose
Preoperative/preprocedure sedation: ≥6 months:
Note: Limited information is available for infants <6 months of age.
I.M.: 2-6 mg/kg; maximum: 100 mg/dose
I.V.: 1-3 mg/kg to a maximum of 100 mg until asleep
Conscious sedation prior to a procedure: I.V.:
Children 5-12 years: I.V.: 2 mg/kg 5-10 minutes before procedures, may repeat one time
Adolescents: 100 mg prior to a procedure
Barbiturate coma in head injury patients: I.V.: Loading dose: 5-10 mg/kg given slowly over 1-2 hours; monitor blood pressure and respiratory rate; Maintenance infusion: Initial: 1 mg/kg/hour; may increase to 2-3 mg/kg/hour; maintain burst suppression on EEG
Status epilepticus: I.V.: **Note**: Intubation required; monitor hemodynamics: Loading dose: 5-15 mg/kg given slowly over 1-2 hours; maintenance infusion: 0.5-5 mg/kg/hour

Hepatic Impairment: Reduce dosage in patients with severe liver dysfunction.

Administration
I.M.: Pentobarbital may be administered by deep I.M.: No more than 5 mL (250 mg) should be injected at any one site because of possible tissue irritation.
I.V.: Pentobarbital must be administered by slow I.V. injection. I.V. push doses can be given undiluted, but should be administered no faster than 50 mg/minute. Avoid intra-arterial injection. Has many incompatibilities when given I.V.
I.V. Detail: Avoid extravasation. Institute safety measures to avoid injuries. Parenteral solutions are highly alkaline. Avoid rapid I.V. administration >50 mg/minute.

pH: 9.5

Stability
Compatibility: Stable in dextran 6% in dextrose, dextran 6% in NS, D_5LR, $D_5^1/_4NS$, $D_5^1/_2NS$, D_5NS, $D_{10}W$, LR, $^1/_2NS$
Y-site administration: Incompatible with amphotericin B cholesteryl sulfate complex
Compatibility in syringe: Incompatible with atropine with cimetidine, butorphanol, chlorpromazine, cimetidine, dimenhydrinate, diphenhydramine, droperidol, fentanyl, glycopyrrolate, hydroxyzine, meperidine, midazolam, nalbuphine, pentazocine, perphenazine, prochlorperazine edisylate, promazine, promethazine, ranitidine
Compatibility when admixed: Incompatible with cefazolin, chlorpheniramine, cimetidine, clindamycin, droperidol, ephedrine, fentanyl, hydrocortisone sodium succinate, hydroxyzine, insulin

(Continued)

Pentobarbital *(Continued)*

(regular), levorphanol, norepinephrine, pancuronium, penicillin G potassium, pentazocine, phenytoin, promazine, promethazine, streptomycin, triflupromazine, vancomycin

Storage: Protect from freezing. Aqueous solutions are not stable; a commercially available vehicle (containing propylene glycol) is more stable. When mixed with an acidic solution, precipitate may form. Use only clear solution.

Nursing Actions

Physical Assessment: Assess effectiveness and interactions of other medications patient may be taking. Assess for history of addiction; long-term use can result in dependence, abuse, or tolerance. Periodically evaluate the need for continued use. **I.V.:** Keep patient under observation (vital signs, CNS, cardiac and respiratory status), use safety precautions. Monitor effectiveness of therapy and adverse reactions. Assess knowledge/teach patient appropriate use, possible side effects, and symptoms to report.

Patient Education: Patient instructions and information are determined by patient condition and therapeutic purpose. Drug may cause physical and/or psychological dependence. While using this medication, do not use alcohol and other prescription or OTC medications (especially pain medications, sedatives, antihistamines, or hypnotics) without consulting prescriber. Maintain adequate hydration (2-3 L/day of fluids) unless instructed to restrict fluid intake. You may experience drowsiness, dizziness, or blurred vision (use caution when driving or engaging in tasks requiring alertness until response to drug is known); nausea, vomiting, or loss of appetite (small frequent meals, frequent mouth care, chewing gum, or sucking lozenges may help); or constipation (increased exercise, fluids, fruit, or fiber may help). Report skin rash or irritation; CNS changes (confusion, depression, increased sedation, excitation, headache, insomnia, or nightmares); respiratory difficulty or shortness of breath; changes in urinary pattern or menstrual pattern; muscle weakness or tremors; or difficulty swallowing or feeling of tightness in throat. **Pregnancy/breast-feeding precautions:** Do not get pregnant; use appropriate contraceptive measures to prevent possible harm to the fetus. Do not breast-feed.

Geriatric Considerations Use of this agent as a hypnotic in the elderly is not recommended due to its long half-life and addiction potential.

Related Information

Anxiolytic / Hypnotic Use in Long-Term Care Facilities *on page 1418*
Compatibility of Drugs *on page 1370*
Compatibility of Drugs in Syringe *on page 1372*
Federal OBRA Regulations Recommended Maximum Doses *on page 1421*

Pentostatin *(PEN toe stat in)*

U.S. Brand Names Nipent®

Synonyms CL-825; Co-Vidarabine; dCF; Deoxycoformycin; NSC-218321; 2'-Deoxycoformycin

Pharmacologic Category Antineoplastic Agent, Antibiotic; Antineoplastic Agent, Antimetabolite (Purine Antagonist)

Medication Safety Issues
Sound-alike/look-alike issues:
Pentostatin may be confused with pentosan

Pregnancy Risk Factor D

Lactation Excretion in breast milk unknown/contraindicated

Use Treatment of hairy cell leukemia; non-Hodgkin's lymphoma, cutaneous T-cell lymphoma

Mechanism of Action/Effect Results in cell death, probably through inhibiting DNA or RNA synthesis. Following a single dose, pentostatin has the ability to inhibit ADA for periods exceeding 1 week.

Contraindications Hypersensitivity to pentostatin or any component; pregnancy

Warnings/Precautions Hazardous agent - use appropriate precautions for handling and disposal. Use cautiously in patients with bone marrow suppression, renal or hepatic dysfunction.

Drug Interactions

Increased Effect/Toxicity: Increased toxicity with vidarabine and allopurinol; combined use with fludarabine may lead to severe, even fatal, pulmonary toxicity

Adverse Reactions

>10%:
Central nervous system: Fever, chills, headache
Dermatologic: Skin rash (25% to 30%), alopecia (10%)
Gastrointestinal: Mild to moderate nausea, vomiting (60%), stomatitis, diarrhea (13%), anorexia
Genitourinary: Acute renal failure (35%)
Hematologic: Thrombocytopenia (50%), dose-limiting in 25% of patients; anemia (40% to 45%), neutropenia, mild to moderate, not dose-limiting (11%)
Nadir: 7 days
Recovery: 10-14 days
Hepatic: Transaminases increased, mild-moderate, usually transient (30%); hepatitis (19%), usually reversible
Respiratory: Pulmonary edema (15%), may be exacerbated by fludarabine
Miscellaneous: Infection (57%; 35% severe, life-threatening)
1% to 10%:
Cardiovascular: Chest pain, arrhythmia, peripheral edema
Central nervous system: Opportunistic infection (8%); anxiety, confusion, depression, dizziness, insomnia, nervousness, somnolence, myalgia, malaise
Dermatologic: Dry skin, eczema, pruritus
Gastrointestinal: Constipation, flatulence, weight loss
Neuromuscular & skeletal: Paresthesia, weakness
Ocular: Moderate to severe keratoconjunctivitis, abnormal vision, eye pain
Otic: Ear pain
Respiratory: Dyspnea, pneumonia, bronchitis, pharyngitis, rhinitis, epistaxis, sinusitis (3% to 7%)

Overdosage/Toxicology Symptoms of overdose include severe renal, hepatic, pulmonary, and CNS toxicity. Treatment is supportive.

Pharmacodynamics/Kinetics

Half-Life Elimination: Distribution half-life: 30-85 minutes; Terminal: 5-15 hours

Excretion: Urine (~50% to 96%) within 24 hours (30% to 90% as unchanged drug)

Available Dosage Forms Injection, powder for reconstitution: 10 mg

Dosing

Adults & Elderly: Refer to individual protocols.
Refractory hairy cell leukemia:
4 mg/m² every other week or
4 mg/m² weekly for 3 weeks, then every 2 weeks or
5 mg/m² daily for 3 days every 3 weeks
Renal Impairment:
Cl_cr <60 mL/minute: Use extreme caution.
Cl_cr 50-60 mL/minute: Administer 2 mg/m²/dose.
Hepatic Impairment:
Bilirubin 1.5-3 mg/dL or AST 60-180 units/L: Administer 75% of normal dose.
Bilirubin 3-5 mg/dL or AST >180 units/L: Administer 50% of normal dose.
Bilirubin >5 mg/dL: Do not administer.

Administration

I.V.: Administer I.V. as a 15- to 30-minute infusion; continuous infusion regimens have been reported, but are not commonly used

I.V. bolus over ≥3-5 minutes

I.V. Detail: pH: 7.0-8.5

Stability

Reconstitution: Reconstitute with SWFI to a concentration of 2 mg/mL. The injection may be further diluted with 25-50 mL NS or D_5W for infusion.

Compatibility: Stable in LR, NS

Storage: Vials are stable under refrigeration at 2°C to 8°C; reconstituted vials, or further dilutions are stable at room temperature for 24 hours in D_5W or 48 hours in NS or lactated Ringer's.

Laboratory Monitoring CBC with differential, platelet count, liver function, serum uric acid, renal function

Nursing Actions

Physical Assessment: Assess potential for adverse interactions with other pharmacological agent patient is taking. Note Administration for infusion specifics. Assess results of laboratory tests prior to and regularly during therapy. Monitor patient response closely (eg, nutritional status, renal function, myelosuppression [anemia], pulmonary edema, opportunistic infection). Teach patient possible side effects/appropriate interventions and adverse reactions to report.

Patient Education: Do not take any new medication during therapy unless approved by prescriber. This drug can only be given by infusion on a specific schedule. Report immediately any redness, swelling, burning, or pain at infusion site; or signs of hypersensitivity (eg, respiratory difficulty or swallowing, chest tightness, rash, hives, swelling of lips or mouth). Maintain adequate hydration (2-3 L/day of fluids) unless instructed to restrict fluid intake. You may be more susceptible to infection (avoid crowds and exposure to infection and do not have any vaccinations without consulting prescriber. May cause nausea and vomiting, or loss of appetite (small, frequent meals or frequent mouth care may help - or request medication from prescriber); headache (consult prescriber for approved analgesic); dizziness, confusion or lethargy (use caution when driving); or mouth sores (use frequent oral care with soft toothbrush or cotton swabs). Report signs of infection (eg, fever, chills, sore throat, mouth sores, burning urination, perianal itching, or vaginal discharge); unusual bruising or bleeding (eg, tarry stools, blood in urine, stool, or vomitus); vision changes or hearing; muscle tremors, weakness, or pain; CNS changes (eg, hallucinations, confusion, insomnia, seizures); or respiratory difficulty. **Pregnancy/breast-feeding precautions:** Do not get pregnant while taking this medication. Consult prescriber for appropriate contraceptive measures. Do not breast-feed.

Pentoxifylline (pen toks I fi leen)

U.S. Brand Names Pentoxil®; Trental®

Synonyms Oxpentifylline

Pharmacologic Category Blood Viscosity Reducer Agent

Medication Safety Issues

Sound-alike/look-alike issues:

Pentoxifylline may be confused with tamoxifen

Trental® may be confused with Bentyl®, Tegretol®, Trandate®

Pregnancy Risk Factor C

Lactation Enters breast milk/not recommended

Use Treatment of intermittent claudication on the basis of chronic occlusive arterial disease of the limbs; may improve function and symptoms, but not intended to replace more definitive therapy

Unlabeled/Investigational Use AIDS patients with increased TNF, CVA, cerebrovascular diseases, diabetic atherosclerosis, diabetic neuropathy, gangrene, hemodialysis shunt thrombosis, vascular impotence, cerebral malaria, septic shock, sickle cell syndromes, and vasculitis

Mechanism of Action/Effect Reduces blood viscosity improves tissue oxygenation through enhanced blood flow

Contraindications Hypersensitivity to pentoxifylline, xanthines (eg, caffeine, theophylline), or any component of the formulation; recent cerebral and/or retinal hemorrhage

Warnings/Precautions Use with caution in patients with renal and hepatic impairment; start with lower doses in elderly patients and monitor renal function. Use caution in patients receiving anticoagulant therapy or at risk for bleeding complications; monitor PT/INR, hematocrit and/or hemoglobin as necessary. May lower blood pressure; monitor with concomitant antihypertensive agent use. Safety and efficacy in pediatric patients have not been established.

Drug Interactions

Cytochrome P450 Effect: Inhibits CYP1A2 (weak)

Increased Effect/Toxicity:

Pentoxifylline may increase the serum levels of theophylline.

Nutritional/Ethanol Interactions Food: Food may decrease rate but not extent of absorption. Pentoxifylline peak serum levels may be decreased if taken with food.

Lab Interactions Decreased calcium (S), magnesium (S); false-positive theophylline levels

Adverse Reactions

1% to 10%: Gastrointestinal: Nausea (2%), vomiting (1%)

Overdosage/Toxicology Symptoms of overdose have been reported to occur 4-5 hours postingestion and last approximately 12 hours. Symptoms may include hypotension, flushing, convulsions, deep sleep, agitation, bradycardia, and AV block. Treatment should be symptom-directed and supportive.

Pharmacodynamics/Kinetics

Time to Peak: Serum: 2-4 hours

Half-Life Elimination: Parent drug: 24-48 minutes; Metabolites: 60-96 minutes

Metabolism: Hepatic and via erythrocytes; extensive first-pass effect

Excretion: Primarily urine (active metabolites); feces (4%)

Available Dosage Forms Tablet, extended release (Pentoxil®, Trental®): 400 mg

Dosing

Adults & Elderly: Peripheral vascular disease: Oral: 400 mg 3 times/day with meals; maximal therapeutic benefit may take 2-4 weeks to develop; recommended to maintain therapy for at least 8 weeks. May reduce to 400 mg twice daily if GI or CNS side effects occur.

Administration

Oral: Tablets should be swallowed whole; do not chew, break, or crush.

Stability

Storage:

Store between 15°C to 30°C (59°F to 86°F).

Nursing Actions

Physical Assessment: Assess potential for interactions with other prescriptions, OTC medications, or herbal products patient may be taking. Monitor patient response at regular intervals during therapy (eg, cardiac status and blood pressure). Teach patient proper use, possible side effects/appropriate interventions, and adverse symptoms to report.

Patient Education: Do not take any new medication during therapy unless approved by prescriber. This may relieve pain of claudication, but additional (Continued)

Pentoxifylline *(Continued)*

therapy may be recommended. Take as prescribed for full length of prescription. May cause dizziness (use caution when driving or engaging in tasks that are potentially hazardous until response to drug is known); or heartburn, nausea, or vomiting (small frequent meals, frequent mouth care, chewing gum, or sucking lozenges may help). Report chest pain; swelling of lips, mouth, or tongue; persistent headache; respiratory difficulty; rash; or unrelieved nausea or vomiting. **Pregnancy/breast-feeding precautions:** Inform prescriber if you are or intend to become pregnant. Consult prescriber if breast-feeding.

Dietary Considerations May be taken with meals or food.

Geriatric Considerations Pentoxifylline's value in the treatment of intermittent claudication is controversial. Walking distance improved statistically in some clinical trials, but the actual distance was minimal when applied to improving physical activity.

Pergolide *(PER go lide)*

U.S. Brand Names Permax®

Synonyms Pergolide Mesylate

Pharmacologic Category Anti-Parkinson's Agent, Dopamine Agonist; Ergot Derivative

Medication Safety Issues
Sound-alike/look-alike issues:
Permax® may be confused with Bumex®, Pentrax®, Pernox®

Pregnancy Risk Factor B

Lactation Excretion in breast milk unknown/not recommended

Use Adjunctive treatment to levodopa/carbidopa in the management of Parkinson's disease

Unlabeled/Investigational Use Tourette's disorder, chronic motor or vocal tic disorder

Mechanism of Action/Effect Pergolide is a semisynthetic ergot alkaloid similar to bromocriptine but stated to be more potent (10-1000 times) and longer-acting; it is a centrally-active dopamine agonist stimulating both D_1 and D_2 receptors. Pergolide is believed to exert its therapeutic effect by directly stimulating postsynaptic dopamine receptors in the nigrostriatal system.

Contraindications Hypersensitivity to pergolide mesylate, other ergot derivatives, or any component of the formulation; ergot alkaloids are contraindicated with potent inhibitors of CYP3A4 (includes protease inhibitors, azole antifungals, and some macrolide antibiotics)

Warnings/Precautions Symptomatic hypotension occurs in 10% of patients. Use with caution in patients with a history of cardiac arrhythmias, hallucinations, or mental illness. Cardiac valvular, pleural, and peritoneal fibrosis have been reported with prolonged daily use. Avoid rapid dose reduction or abrupt discontinuation.

Pergolide has been associated with somnolence. Some patients have been reported to fall asleep during activities of daily living, including driving, while taking this medication. Not all patients exhibited somnolence prior to these events.

Drug Interactions
Cytochrome P450 Effect: Substrate of CYP3A4 (major); **Inhibits** CYP2D6 (strong), 3A4 (weak)

Decreased Effect: Effects of pergolide may be diminished by antipsychotics, metoclopramide. Pergolide may decrease the levels/effects of CYP2D6 prodrug substrates (eg, codeine, hydrocodone, oxycodone, tramadol).

Increased Effect/Toxicity: Effects of pergolide may be increased by levodopa (hallucinations) and MAO inhibitors. Pergolide may increase the levels/effects of amphetamines, selected beta-blockers, dextromethorphan, fluoxetine, lidocaine, mirtazapine, nefazodone, paroxetine, risperidone, ritonavir, thioridazine, tricyclic antidepressants, venlafaxine, and other CYP2D6 substrates. Pergolide may increase the levels/effects of sibutramine and other serotonin agonists (serotonin syndrome). Macrolide antibiotics may increase the effects of pergolide. The levels/effects of pergolide may be increased by azole antifungals, clarithromycin, diclofenac, doxycycline, erythromycin, imatinib, isoniazid, nefazodone, nicardipine, propofol, protease inhibitors, quinidine, telithromycin, verapamil, and other CYP3A4 inhibitors.

Nutritional/Ethanol Interactions Ethanol: Avoid ethanol (may cause CNS depression).

Adverse Reactions
>10%:
Central nervous system: Dizziness (19%), hallucinations (14%), dystonia (12%), somnolence (10%), confusion (10%)
Gastrointestinal: Nausea (24%), constipation (11%)
Neuromuscular & skeletal: Dyskinesia (62%)
Respiratory: Rhinitis (12%)
1% to 10%:
Cardiovascular: Hypotension or postural hypotension (10%), peripheral edema (7%), chest pain (4%), vasodilation (3%), palpitation (2%), syncope (2%), arrhythmia (1%), hypertension (2%), MI (1%)
Central nervous system: Insomnia (8%), pain (7%), anxiety (6%), psychosis (2%), EPS (2%), incoordination (2%), chills (1%)
Dermatologic: Rash (3%)
Gastrointestinal: Diarrhea (6%), dyspepsia (6%), abdominal pain (6%), anorexia (5%), xerostomia (4%), vomiting (3%), dysphagia (1%), nausea (1%)
Hematologic: Anemia (1%)
Neuromuscular & skeletal: Myalgia (1%), neuralgia (1%)
Ocular: Abnormal vision (6%), diplopia (2%)
Respiratory: Dyspnea (5%), epistaxis (2%)
Miscellaneous: Flu syndrome (3%), hiccups (1%)

Overdosage/Toxicology Symptoms of overdose include vomiting, hypotension, agitation, hallucinations, ventricular extrasystoles, and possible seizures. Data on overdose is limited. Treatment is supportive.

Pharmacodynamics/Kinetics
Protein Binding: Plasma: 90%
Half-Life Elimination: 27 hours
Metabolism: Extensively hepatic
Excretion: Urine (~50%); feces (50%)

Available Dosage Forms Tablet: 0.05 mg, 0.25 mg, 1 mg

Dosing
Adults & Elderly:
Parkinson's disease: Oral: Start with 0.05 mg/day for 2 days, then increase dosage by 0.1 or 0.15 mg/day every 3 days over next 12 days, increase dose by 0.25 mg/day every 3 days until optimal therapeutic dose is achieved, up to 5 mg/day maximum; usual dosage range: 2-3 mg/day in 3 divided doses
Note: When adding pergolide to levodopa/carbidopa, the dose of the latter can usually and should be decreased. Patients no longer responsive to bromocriptine may benefit by being switched to pergolide.
Pediatrics: Children and Adolescents: Tourette's disorder, chronic motor or vocal disorder (unlabeled uses): Oral: Up to 300 mcg/day

Nursing Actions
Physical Assessment: Assess effectiveness and interactions of other medications patient may be taking. Monitor therapeutic response (eg, mental status, involuntary movements) and adverse reactions at beginning of therapy and periodically throughout therapy. Monitor blood pressure and level of sedation. Assess knowledge/teach patient appropriate use,

interventions to reduce side effects, and adverse symptoms to report.

Patient Education: Take exactly as directed (may be prescribed in conjunction with levodopa/carbidopa); do not change dosage or discontinue without consulting prescriber. Therapeutic effects may take several weeks or months to achieve and you may need frequent monitoring during first weeks of therapy. Take with meals if GI upset occurs, before meals if dry mouth occurs, or after eating if drooling or if nausea occurs. Take at the same time each day. Maintain adequate hydration (2-3 L/day of fluids) unless instructed to restrict fluid intake; void before taking medication. Do not use alcohol and prescription or OTC sedatives or CNS depressants without consulting prescriber. You may experience drowsiness, dizziness, confusion, or vision changes (use caution when driving, climbing stairs, or engaging in tasks requiring alertness until response to drug is known); orthostatic hypotension (use caution when changing position - rising to standing from sitting or lying); constipation (increased exercise, fluids, fruit, or fiber may help); runny nose or flu-like symptoms (consult prescriber for appropriate relief); nausea, vomiting, loss of appetite, or stomach discomfort (small frequent meals, frequent mouth care, chewing gum, or sucking lozenges may help); or photosensitivity (use sunscreen, wear protective clothing and eyewear, and avoid direct sunlight). Report unresolved constipation or vomiting; chest pain, palpitations, irregular heartbeat; ringing in ears; CNS changes (hallucination, loss of memory, seizures, acute headache, nervousness, etc); painful or difficult urination; increased muscle spasticity, rigidity, or involuntary movements; skin rash; or significant worsening of condition. **Breast-feeding precaution:** Breast-feeding is not recommended.

Geriatric Considerations High incidence of syncope and orthostatic hypotension upon initiation of therapy. Use with caution in patients prone to cardiac dysrhythmias and in patients with a history of confusion or hallucinations.

Perindopril Erbumine
(per IN doe pril er BYOO meen)

U.S. Brand Names Aceon®

Pharmacologic Category Angiotensin-Converting Enzyme (ACE) Inhibitor

Pregnancy Risk Factor C (1st trimester) / D (2nd and 3rd trimesters)

Lactation Excretion in breast milk unknown/use caution

Use Treatment of essential hypertension; reduction of cardiovascular mortality or nonfatal myocardial infarction in patients with stable coronary artery disease

Unlabeled/Investigational Use As a class, ACE inhibitors are recommended in the treatment of congestive heart failure with left ventricular dysfunction.

Mechanism of Action/Effect Perindopril is a prodrug for perindoprilat, which acts as a competitive inhibitor of angiotensin-converting enzyme (ACE); prevents conversion of angiotensin I to angiotensin II, a potent vasoconstrictor; results in lower levels of angiotensin II which, in turn, causes an increase in plasma renin activity and a reduction in aldosterone secretion

Contraindications Hypersensitivity to perindopril or any component of the formulation; angioedema related to previous treatment with an ACE inhibitor; bilateral renal artery stenosis; pregnancy (2nd and 3rd trimesters)

Warnings/Precautions Anaphylactic reactions can occur. Angioedema can occur at any time during treatment (especially following first dose). It may involve head and neck (potentially affecting the airway) or the intestine (presenting with abdominal pain). Prolonged

monitoring may be required especially if tongue, glottis, or larynx are involved as they are associated with airway obstruction. Those with a history of airway surgery in this situation have a higher risk. Careful blood pressure monitoring with first dose (hypotension can occur especially in volume- and/or salt-depleted patients); caution in patients receiving hypotensive-inducing anesthesia. Dosage adjustment needed in renal impairment. Avoid rapid dosage escalation, which may lead to renal insufficiency. Use with caution in unilateral renal artery stenosis and pre-existing renal insufficiency.

Use with caution in hypovolemia; collagen vascular diseases; valvular stenosis (particularly aortic stenosis); concomitant use with potassium-sparing agents, potassium supplements or salt substitutes not recommended; risk of hyperkalemia may be increased with renal insufficiency. Rare toxicities associated with ACE inhibitors include cholestatic jaundice (which may progress to hepatic necrosis) and neutropenia/agranulocytosis with myeloid hyperplasia. If patient has renal impairment then a baseline WBC with differential and serum creatinine should be evaluated and monitored closely during the first 3 months of therapy. Hypersensitivity reactions may be seen during hemodialysis with high-flux dialysis membranes (eg, AN69). Safety and efficacy in pediatric patients have not been established.

Drug Interactions

Decreased Effect: Aspirin (high dose) may reduce the therapeutic effects of ACE inhibitors; at low dosages this does not appear to be significant. Rifampin may decrease the effect of ACE inhibitors. Antacids may decrease the bioavailability of ACE inhibitors (may be more likely to occur with captopril); separate administration times by 1-2 hours. NSAIDs, specifically indomethacin, may reduce the hypotensive effects of ACE inhibitors. More likely to occur in low renin or volume dependent hypertensive patients.

Increased Effect/Toxicity: Potassium supplements, co-trimoxazole (high dose), angiotensin II receptor antagonists (eg, candesartan, losartan, irbesartan), or potassium-sparing diuretics (amiloride, eplerenone, spironolactone, triamterene) may result in elevated serum potassium levels when combined with perindopril. ACE inhibitor effects may be increased by phenothiazines or probenecid (increases levels of captopril). ACE inhibitors may increase serum concentrations/effects of lithium.

Diuretics have additive hypotensive effects with ACE inhibitors, and hypovolemia increases the potential for adverse renal effects of ACE inhibitors. ACE inhibitors may increase nephrotoxicity of cyclosporine. In patients with compromised renal function, coadministration with NSAIDs may result in further deterioration of renal function. Allopurinol and ACE inhibitors may cause a higher risk of hypersensitivity reaction when taken concurrently.

Nutritional/Ethanol Interactions

Food: Perindopril active metabolite concentrations may be lowered if taken with food.

Herb/Nutraceutical: Avoid dong quai if using for hypertension (has estrogenic activity). Avoid ephedra, yohimbe, ginseng (may worsen hypertension). Avoid garlic (may have increased antihypertensive effect).

Adverse Reactions

>10%:

Central nervous system: Headache (24%)

Respiratory: Cough (incidence is higher in women, 3:1) (12%)

1% to 10%:

Cardiovascular: Edema (4%), chest pain (2%)), ECG abnormal (2%), palpitation (1%)

Central nervous system: Dizziness (8%, less than placebo), sleep disorders (3%), depression (2%), fever (2%), nervousness (1%), somnolence (1%)

Dermatologic: Rash (2%)

(Continued)

Perindopril Erbumine *(Continued)*

Endocrine & metabolic: Hyperkalemia (1%, less than placebo), triglycerides increased (1%), menstrual disorder (1%)

Gastrointestinal: Nausea (2%), diarrhea (4%), vomiting (2%), dyspepsia (2%), abdominal pain (3%), flatulence (1%)

Genitourinary: Urinary tract infection (3%), sexual dysfunction (male 1%)

Hepatic: Increased ALT (2%)

Neuromuscular & skeletal: Weakness (8%), back pain (6%), lower extremity pain (5%), upper extremity pain (3%), hypertonia (3%), paresthesia (2%), joint pain (1%), myalgia (1%), arthritis (1%), neck pain (1%)

Renal: Proteinuria (2%)

Respiratory: Upper respiratory tract infection (9%), sinusitis (5%), rhinitis (5%), pharyngitis (3%)

Otic: Tinnitus (2%), ear infection (1%)

Miscellaneous: Viral infection (3%%), allergy (2%)

Note: Some reactions occurred at an incidence >1% but ≤ placebo.

Additional adverse effects that have been reported with **ACE inhibitors** include agranulocytosis (especially in patients with renal impairment or collagen vascular disease), neutropenia, anemia, bullous pemphigus, cardiac arrest, eosinophilic pneumonitis, exfoliative dermatitis, hepatic failure, hyponatremia, jaundice, pancreatitis (acute), pancytopenia, thrombocytopenia; decreases in creatinine clearance in some elderly hypertensive patients or those with chronic renal failure, and worsening of renal function in patients with bilateral renal artery stenosis or hypovolemic patients (diuretic therapy). In addition, a syndrome which may include fever, myalgia, arthralgia, interstitial nephritis, vasculitis, rash, eosinophilia and positive ANA, and elevated ESR has been reported with ACE inhibitors.

Overdosage/Toxicology Mild hypotension has been the primary toxic effect seen with acute overdose. Bradycardia may also occur. Hyperkalemia occurs even with therapeutic doses, especially in patients with renal insufficiency and those taking NSAIDs. Treatment is symptom-directed and supportive. Hemodialysis may be beneficial.

Pharmacodynamics/Kinetics

Onset of Action: Peak effect: 1-2 hours

Time to Peak: Chronic therapy: Perindopril: 1 hour; Perindoprilat: 3-7 hours (maximum perindoprilat serum levels are 2-3 times higher and T_{max} is shorter following chronic therapy); CHF: Perindoprilat: 6 hours

Protein Binding: Perindopril: 60%; Perindoprilat: 10% to 20%

Half-Life Elimination: Parent drug: 1.5-3 hours; Metabolite: Effective: 3-10 hours, Terminal: 30-120 hours

Metabolism: Hydrolyzed hepatically to active metabolite, perindoprilat (~17% to 20% of a dose) and other inactive metabolites

Excretion: Urine (75%, 4% to 12% as unchanged drug)

Available Dosage Forms Tablet: 2 mg, 4 mg, 8 mg

Dosing

Adults:

Essential hypertension: Oral: Initial: 4 mg/day but may be titrated to response; usual range: 4-8 mg/day (may be given in 2 divided doses); increase at 1- to 2-week intervals (maximum: 16 mg/day)

Concomitant therapy with diuretics: To reduce the risk of hypotension, discontinue diuretic, if possible, 2-3 days prior to initiating perindopril. If unable to stop diuretic, initiate perindopril at 2-4 mg/day and monitor blood pressure closely for the first 2 weeks of therapy, and after any dose adjustment of perindopril or diuretic.

Stable coronary artery disease: Oral: Initial: 4 mg once daily for 2 weeks; increase as tolerated to 8 mg once daily.

Congestive heart failure (unlabeled use): Oral: Initial: 2 mg once daily; increase at 1- to 2-week intervals; target dose: 8-16 mg once daily (ACC/AHA 2005 Heart Failure Guidelines)

Elderly:

Essential hypertension: >65 years of age: Initial: 4 mg/day; maintenance: 8 mg/day

Stable coronary artery disease: >70 years of age: Initial: 2 mg/day for 1 week; increase as tolerated to 4 mg/day for 1 week; then increase as tolerated to 8 mg/day

Renal Impairment:

Cl_{cr} >30 mL/minute: Initial: 2 mg/day; maintenance dosing not to exceed 8 mg/day

Cl_{cr} <30 mL/minute: Safety and efficacy not established.

Hemodialysis: Perindopril and its metabolites are dialyzable

Hepatic Impairment: No adjustment required.

Stability

Storage: Store at room temperature of 20°C to 25°C (68°F to 77°F). Protect from moisture.

Laboratory Monitoring Serum creatinine, electrolytes, and WBC with differential initially and repeated at 2-week intervals for at least 90 days (particularly important in patients with renal impairment at baseline).

Nursing Actions

Physical Assessment: Assess potential for interactions with other pharmacological agents and herbal products patient may be taking (eg, other drugs may effect blood pressure or increase risk of toxicities). It is recommended that dose is administered in prescriber's office with careful blood pressure monitoring (hypotension can occur, especially with first dose; angioedema can occur at any time during treatment, especially following first dose). Monitor laboratory tests and patient response at beginning of therapy, when adjusting dose, and periodically with long-term therapy (eg, BP [standing and sitting], cardiac status, and fluid balance). Teach patient appropriate use, possible side effects/appropriate interventions, and adverse symptoms to report.

Patient Education: Do not take any new medication during therapy without consulting prescriber. Take as directed; do not alter dose or discontinue without consulting prescriber. Take first dose at bedtime. Do not take potassium supplements or salt substitutes containing potassium without consulting prescriber. This drug does not eliminate need for diet or exercise regimen as recommended by prescriber. May cause increased cough (if persistent or bothersome, contact prescriber); headache (consult prescriber for approved analgesic); postural hypotension (use caution when rising from lying or sitting position or climbing stairs); dizziness (use caution when driving or engaging in tasks that require alertness until response to drug is known); nausea or vomiting (small frequent meals, frequent mouth care, sucking lozenges, or chewing gum may help); or diarrhea (buttermilk, boiled milk, or yogurt may help). Report chest pain, respiratory difficulty or persistent cough, painful muscles or joints, rash, ringing in ears, or other persistent adverse reactions. **Pregnancy/breast-feeding precautions:** Inform prescriber if you are or intend to become pregnant. This drug should not be used in the 2nd or 3rd trimester of pregnancy. Consult prescriber for appropriate contraceptive measures if necessary. Consult prescriber if breast-feeding.

Pregnancy Issues ACE inhibitors can cause fetal injury or death if taken during the 2nd or 3rd trimester. Discontinue ACE inhibitors as soon as pregnancy is detected.

Permethrin (per METH rin)

U.S. Brand Names A200® Lice [OTC]; Acticin®; Elimite®; Nix® [OTC]; Rid® Spray [OTC]

Pharmacologic Category Antiparasitic Agent, Topical; Scabicidal Agent

Pregnancy Risk Factor B

Lactation Effect on infant unknown

Use Single-application treatment of infestation with *Pediculus humanus capitis* (head louse) and its nits or *Sarcoptes scabiei* (scabies); indicated for prophylactic use during epidemics of lice

Mechanism of Action/Effect Inhibits sodium ion influx through nerve cell membrane channels in parasites resulting in delayed repolarization and thus paralysis and death of the pest

Contraindications Hypersensitivity to pyrethyroid, pyrethrins, chrysanthemums, or any component of the formulation; lotion is contraindicated for use in infants <2 months of age

Warnings/Precautions Treatment may temporarily exacerbate the symptoms of itching, redness, and swelling. For external use only.

Adverse Reactions 1% to 10%:
Dermatologic: Pruritus, erythema, rash of the scalp
Local: Burning, stinging, tingling, numbness or scalp discomfort, edema

Pharmacodynamics/Kinetics
Metabolism: Hepatic via ester hydrolysis to inactive metabolites
Excretion: Urine

Available Dosage Forms
Cream, topical (Acticin®, Elimite®): 5% (60 g) [contains coconut oil]
Lotion, topical: 1% (59 mL)
Liquid, topical [creme rinse formulation] (Nix®): 1% (60 mL) [contains isopropyl alcohol 20%]
Solution, spray [for bedding and furniture]:
A200® Lice: 0.5% (180 mL)
Nix®: 0.25% (148 mL)
Rid®: 0.5% (150 mL)

Dosing
Adults & Elderly:
Head lice: Topical: After hair has been washed with shampoo, rinsed with water and towel dried, apply a sufficient volume of creme rinse to saturate the hair and scalp; also apply behind the ears and at the base of the neck; leave on hair for 10 minutes before rinsing off with water; remove remaining nits. May repeat in 1 week if lice or nits still present; in areas of head lice resistance to 1% permethrin, 5% permethrin has been applied to clean, dry hair and left on overnight (8-14 hours) under a shower cap.
Scabies: Topical: Apply cream from head to toe; leave on for 8-14 hours before washing off with water; may reapply in 1 week if live mites appear. Time of application was limited to 6 hours before rinsing with soap and water.
Pediatrics:
Head lice: Topical: Children >2 months: Refer to adult dosing.
Scabies: Topical: Apply cream from head to toe; leave on for 8-14 hours before washing off with water; for infants, also apply on the hairline, neck, scalp, temple, and forehead; may reapply in 1 week if live mites appear. Permethrin 5% cream was shown to be safe and effective when applied to an infant <1 month of age with neonatal scabies; time of application was limited to 6 hours before rinsing with soap and water.

Administration
Topical: Avoid contact with eyes and mucous membranes during application. Because scabies and lice are so contagious, use caution to avoid spreading or infecting oneself; wear gloves when applying

Cream rinse/lotion: Shake cream rinse well before using. Apply immediately after hair is shampooed, rinsed, and towel-dried. Apply enough to saturate hair and scalp (especially behind ears and on nape of neck). Leave on hair for 10 minutes before rinsing with water. Remove nits with fine-tooth comb. May repeat in 1 week if lice or nits are still present.

Cream: Apply from neck to toes. Bathe to remove drug after 8-14 hours. Repeat in 7 days if lice or nits are still present. Report if condition persists or infection occurs.

Nursing Actions
Physical Assessment: Assess head, hair, and skin surfaces for presence of lice and nits. Assess knowledge/teach patient appropriate application and use and adverse symptoms to report.
Patient Education: For external use only. Do not apply to face and avoid contact with eyes or mucous membrane. Clothing and bedding must be washed in hot water or dry cleaned to kill nits. May need to treat all members of household and all sexual contacts concurrently. Wash all combs and brushes with permethrin and thoroughly rinse. **Breast-feeding precaution:** Consult prescriber if breast-feeding.

Cream rinse/lotion: Apply immediately after hair is shampooed, rinsed, and towel-dried. Apply enough to saturate hair and scalp (especially behind ears and on nape of neck). Leave on hair for 10 minutes before rinsing with water. Remove nits with fine-tooth comb. May repeat in 1 week if lice or nits are still present.

Cream: Apply from neck to toes. Bathe to remove drug after 8-14 hours. Repeat in 7 days if lice or nits are still present. Report if condition persists or infection occurs.

Geriatric Considerations Because of its minimal absorption, permethrin is a drug of choice and is preferred over lindane.

Perphenazine (per FEN a zeen)

Pharmacologic Category Antipsychotic Agent, Typical, Phenothiazine

Medication Safety Issues
Sound-alike/look-alike issues:
Trilafon® may be confused with Tri-Levlen®

Pregnancy Risk Factor C

Lactation Enters breast milk/not recommended (AAP rates "of concern")

Use Treatment of schizophrenia; nausea and vomiting

Unlabeled/Investigational Use Ethanol withdrawal; dementia in elderly; Tourette's syndrome; Huntington's chorea; spasmodic torticollis; Reye's syndrome; psychosis

Mechanism of Action/Effect Perphenazine is a piperazine phenothiazine antipsychotic which blocks postsynaptic mesolimbic dopaminergic receptors in the brain; exhibits alpha-adrenergic blocking effect and depresses the release of hypothalamic and hypophyseal hormones

Contraindications Hypersensitivity to perphenazine or any component of the formulation (cross-reactivity between phenothiazines may occur); severe CNS depression; subcortical brain damage; bone marrow suppression; blood dyscrasias; coma

Warnings/Precautions May cause hypotension. May be sedating, use with caution in disorders where CNS depression is a feature. Use with caution in Parkinson's disease. Caution in patients with hemodynamic instability; predisposition to seizures; severe cardiac, hepatic, renal, or respiratory disease. Esophageal dysmotility and aspiration have been associated with antipsychotic use - use with caution in patients at risk of pneumonia (ie, Alzheimer's disease). Caution in breast cancer or other prolactin-dependent tumors (may
(Continued)

Perphenazine *(Continued)*

elevate prolactin levels). May alter temperature regulation or mask toxicity of other drugs due to antiemetic effects. May alter cardiac conduction - life-threatening arrhythmias have occurred with therapeutic doses of phenothiazines. May cause orthostatic hypotension - use with caution in patients at risk of this effect or those who would tolerate transient hypotensive episodes (cerebrovascular disease, cardiovascular disease, or other medications which may predispose).

Due to anticholinergic effects, use with caution in patients with decreased gastrointestinal motility, urinary retention, BPH, xerostomia, visual problems, narrow-angle glaucoma (screening is recommended) and myasthenia gravis. Relative to other neuroleptics, perphenazine has a low potency of cholinergic blockade.

May cause extrapyramidal symptoms, including pseudoparkinsonism, acute dystonic reactions, akathisia, and tardive dyskinesia (risk of these reactions is moderate-high relative to other neuroleptics). May be associated with neuroleptic malignant syndrome (NMS) or pigmentary retinopathy.

Drug Interactions

Cytochrome P450 Effect: Substrate of CYP1A2 (minor), 2C8/9 (minor), 2C19 (minor), 2D6 (major), 3A4 (minor); **Inhibits** CYP1A2 (weak), 2D6 (weak)

Decreased Effect: Phenothiazines inhibit the ability of bromocriptine to lower serum prolactin concentrations. Benztropine (and other anticholinergics) may inhibit the therapeutic response to perphenazine and excess anticholinergic effects may occur. Cigarette smoking and barbiturates may enhance the hepatic metabolism of chlorpromazine. Antihypertensive effects of guanethidine and guanadrel may be inhibited by perphenazine. Perphenazine may inhibit the antiparkinsonian effect of levodopa. Perphenazine and possibly other low potency antipsychotics may reverse the pressor effects of epinephrine.

Increased Effect/Toxicity: CYP2D6 inhibitors may increase the levels/effects of perphenazine; example inhibitors include chlorpromazine, delavirdine, fluoxetine, miconazole, paroxetine, pergolide, quinidine, quinine, ritonavir, and ropinirole. Effects on CNS depression may be additive when perphenazine is combined with CNS depressants (narcotic analgesics, ethanol, barbiturates, cyclic antidepressants, antihistamines, or sedative-hypnotics). Perphenazine may increase the effects/toxicity of anticholinergics, antihypertensives, lithium (rare neurotoxicity), trazodone, or valproic acid. Concurrent use with TCA may produce increased toxicity or altered therapeutic response. Chloroquine and propranolol may increase perphenazine concentrations. Hypotension may occur when perphenazine is combined with epinephrine. May increase the risk of arrhythmia when combined with antiarrhythmics, cisapride, pimozide, sparfloxacin, or other drugs which prolong QT interval. Metoclopramide may increase risk of extrapyramidal symptoms (EPS). Acetylcholinesterase inhibitors (central) may increase the risk of antipsychotic-related EPS.

Nutritional/Ethanol Interactions

Ethanol: Avoid ethanol (may increase CNS depression).

Herb/Nutraceutical: Avoid kava kava, gotu kola, valerian, St John's wort (may increase CNS depression).

Adverse Reactions Frequency not defined.

Cardiovascular: Hyper-/hypotension, orthostatic hypotension, tachycardia, bradycardia, dizziness, cardiac arrest

Central nervous system: Extrapyramidal symptoms (pseudoparkinsonism, akathisia, dystonias, tardive dyskinesia), dizziness, cerebral edema, seizure, headache, drowsiness, paradoxical excitement, restlessness, hyperactivity, insomnia, neuroleptic malignant syndrome (NMS), impairment of temperature regulation

Dermatologic: Rash, discoloration of skin (blue-gray), photosensitivity

Endocrine & metabolic: Hypoglycemia, hyperglycemia, galactorrhea, lactation, breast enlargement, gynecomastia, menstrual irregularity, amenorrhea, SIADH, libido (changes in)

Gastrointestinal: Constipation, weight gain, vomiting, stomach pain, nausea, xerostomia, salivation, diarrhea, anorexia, ileus

Genitourinary: Difficulty in urination, ejaculatory disturbances, incontinence, polyuria, ejaculating dysfunction, priapism

Hematologic: Agranulocytosis, leukopenia, eosinophilia, hemolytic anemia, thrombocytopenic purpura, pancytopenia

Hepatic: Cholestatic jaundice, hepatotoxicity

Neuromuscular & skeletal: Tremor

Ocular: Pigmentary retinopathy, blurred vision, cornea and lens changes

Respiratory: Nasal congestion

Miscellaneous: Diaphoresis

Overdosage/Toxicology Symptoms of overdose include deep sleep, dystonia, agitation, coma, abnormal involuntary muscle movements, hypotension, and arrhythmias (QT$_c$ prolongation, AV block, torsade de pointes, ventricular tachycardia/fibrillation). Children may have convulsive seizures.

Treatment is symptom-directed and supportive. Induction of emesis is not recommended. Peritoneal dialysis and hemodialysis are of no value. Gastric lavage and administration of activated charcoal together with a laxative should be considered. Cardiac function should be monitored for at least 5 days. Norepinephrine may be used to treat hypotension, but epinephrine should **not** be used.

Pharmacodynamics/Kinetics

Time to Peak: Serum: Perphenazine: 1-3 hours; 7-hydroxyperphenazine: 2-4 hours

Half-Life Elimination: Perphenazine: 9-12 hours; 7-hydroxyperphenazine: 11.3 hours

Metabolism: Extensively hepatic to metabolites via sulfoxidation, hydroxylation, dealkylation, and glucuronidation

Excretion: Urine and feces

Available Dosage Forms Tablet: 2 mg, 4 mg, 8 mg, 16 mg

Dosing

Adults:

Schizophrenia/psychoses: Oral: 4-16 mg 2-4 times/day not to exceed 64 mg/day

Nausea/vomiting: Oral: 8-16 mg/day in divided doses up to 24 mg/day

Elderly: Behavioral symptoms associated with dementia: Oral: Initial: 2-4 mg 1-2 times/day; increase at 4- to 7-day intervals by 2-4 mg/day. Increase dose intervals (bid, tid, etc) as necessary to control behavior response or side effects. Maximum daily dose: 32 mg; gradual increase (titration) and bedtime administration may prevent some side effects or decrease their severity.

Pediatrics:

Schizophrenia/psychoses: Oral:

1-6 years: 4-6 mg/day in divided doses

6-12 years: 6 mg/day in divided doses

>12 years: 4-16 mg 2-4 times/day

Renal Impairment: Not dialyzable (0% to 5%)

Hepatic Impairment: Dosage reductions should be considered in patients with liver disease although no specific guidelines are available.

Stability

Storage: Store at 2°C to 25°C (36°F to 77°F). Protect from light.

Laboratory Monitoring Baseline liver and kidney function, CBC prior to and periodically during therapy, lipid profile, fasting blood glucose/Hgb A_{1c}; BMI

Nursing Actions

Physical Assessment: Assess other medications patient is taking for effectiveness and interactions. Monitor blood pressure, laboratory results, therapeutic response (mental status, mood, affect), and adverse reactions at beginning of therapy and periodically with long-term use (orthostatic hypotension, anticholinergic response, extrapyramidal symptoms, pigmentary retinopathy). Assess knowledge/teach patient appropriate use, interventions to reduce side effects, and adverse symptoms to report.

Patient Education: Use exactly as directed; do not increase dose or frequency. It may take 2-3 weeks to achieve desired results; do not discontinue without consulting prescriber. Do not take within 2 hours of any antacid. Avoid alcohol or caffeine and other prescription or OTC medications not approved by prescriber. Maintain adequate hydration (2-3 L/day of fluids) unless instructed to restrict fluid intake. Avoid skin contact with medication; may cause contact dermatitis (wash immediately with warm, soapy water). You may experience excess drowsiness, restlessness, dizziness, or blurred vision (use caution driving or when engaging in tasks requiring alertness until response to drug is known); dry mouth, nausea, vomiting (small frequent meals, frequent mouth care, chewing gum, or sucking lozenges may help); constipation (increased exercise, fluids, fruit, or fiber may help); postural hypotension (use caution climbing stairs or when changing position from lying or sitting to standing); urinary retention (void before taking medication); photosensitivity (use sunscreen, wear protective clothing and eyewear, and avoid direct sunlight); or decreased perspiration (avoid strenuous exercise in hot environments). Report persistent CNS effects (eg, trembling fingers, altered gait or balance, excessive sedation, seizures, unusual movements, anxiety, abnormal thoughts, confusion, personality changes); chest pain, palpitations, rapid heartbeat, severe dizziness; unresolved urinary retention or changes in urinary pattern; menstrual pattern, change in libido, or ejaculatory difficulty; vision changes; skin rash or yellowing of skin; respiratory difficulty; or worsening of condition. **Pregnancy/breast-feeding precautions:** Inform prescriber if you are or intend to become pregnant. Breast-feeding is not recommended.

Geriatric Considerations (See Warnings/Precautions, Adverse Reactions, and Overdose/Toxicology.) Elderly patients have an increased risk of adverse response to side effects or adverse reactions to antipsychotics. Plasma levels at a given dose are increased in elderly patients. Older patients are also at higher risk of tardive dyskinesia, and prescribing should be approached in a manner which minimizes the development of this effect.

Related Information

Antipsychotic Medication Guidelines *on page 1415*

Federal OBRA Regulations Recommended Maximum Doses *on page 1421*

Phenazopyridine (fen az oh PEER i deen)

U.S. Brand Names AZO-Gesic® [OTC]; AZO-Standard® [OTC]; Baridium® [OTC]; Pyridium®; ReAzo [OTC]; Uristat® [OTC]; UTI Relief® [OTC]

Synonyms Phenazopyridine Hydrochloride; Phenylazo Diamino Pyridine Hydrochloride

Pharmacologic Category Analgesic, Urinary

Medication Safety Issues
Sound-alike/look-alike issues:
Pyridium® may be confused with Dyrenium®, Perdiem®, pyridoxine, pyrithione

Pregnancy Risk Factor B

Lactation Excretion in breast milk unknown

Use Symptomatic relief of urinary burning, itching, frequency and urgency in association with urinary tract infection or following urologic procedures

Mechanism of Action/Effect An azo dye which exerts local anesthetic or analgesic action on urinary tract mucosa through an unknown mechanism

Contraindications Hypersensitivity to phenazopyridine or any component of the formulation; kidney or liver disease; patients with a Cl_{cr} <50 mL/minute

Warnings/Precautions Does not treat infection, acts only as an analgesic; drug should be discontinued if skin or sclera develop a yellow color; use with caution in patients with renal impairment. Use of this agent in the elderly is limited since accumulation of phenazopyridine can occur in patients with renal insufficiency. Use is contraindicated in patients with a Cl_{cr} <50 mL/minute.

Lab Interactions Phenazopyridine may cause delayed reactions with glucose oxidase reagents (Clinistix®); cupric sulfate tests (Clinitest®) are not affected; interference may also occur with urine ketone tests (Acetest®, Ketostix®) and urinary protein tests; tests for urinary steroids and porphyrins may also occur

Adverse Reactions 1% to 10%:
Central nervous system: Headache, dizziness
Gastrointestinal: Stomach cramps

Overdosage/Toxicology Symptoms of overdose include methemoglobinemia, hemolytic anemia, skin pigmentation, and renal and hepatic impairment. For methemoglobinemia, the antidote is methylene blue 1-2 mg/kg I.V.

Pharmacodynamics/Kinetics
Metabolism: Hepatic and via other tissues
Excretion: Urine (65% as unchanged drug)

Available Dosage Forms
Tablet, as hydrochloride: 100 mg, 200 mg
AZO-Gesic®, AZO-Standard®, Uristat®: 95 mg
Baridium®: 97.2 mg
ReAzo: 95 mg
Pyridium®: 100 mg, 200 mg
UTI Relief®: 97.2 mg

Dosing
Adults & Elderly: Urinary analgesic: Oral: 100-200 mg 3 times/day after meals for 2 days when used concomitantly with an antibacterial agent
Pediatrics: Urinary analgesic: Oral: Children: 12 mg/kg/day in 3 divided doses administered after meals for 2 days
Renal Impairment:
Cl_{cr} 50-80 mL/minute: Administer every 8-16 hours.
Cl_{cr} <50 mL/minute: Avoid use.

Nursing Actions

Physical Assessment: Assess therapeutic effectiveness (according to rationale for use). Instruct patients with diabetes to use serum glucose monitoring (phenazopyridine may interfere with certain urine testing reagents). Teach patient appropriate use, side effects/appropriate interventions, and adverse symptoms to report.

Patient Education: Take exactly as directed. May discolor urine (orange/yellow); this is normal, but will
(Continued)

Phenazopyridine *(Continued)*

also stain fabric. If you have diabetes, use serum glucose tests; this medication may interfere with accuracy of urine testing. Report persistent headache, dizziness, or stomach cramping. **Breast-feeding precaution:** Consult prescriber if breast-feeding.

Dietary Considerations Should be taken after meals.

Geriatric Considerations Use of this agent in the elderly is limited since accumulation of phenazopyridine can occur in patients with renal insufficiency. It should not be used in patients with a Cl$_{cr}$ <50 mL/minute.

Phenelzine *(FEN el zeen)*

U.S. Brand Names Nardil®

Synonyms Phenelzine Sulfate

Restrictions A medication guide concerning the use of antidepressants in children and teenagers can be found on the FDA website at http://www.fda.gov/cder/Offices/ODS/labeling.htm. It should be dispensed to parents or guardians of children and teenagers receiving this medication.

Pharmacologic Category Antidepressant, Monoamine Oxidase Inhibitor

Medication Safety Issues
Sound-alike/look-alike issues:
Phenelzine may be confused with phenytoin
Nardil® may be confused with Norinyl®

Pregnancy Risk Factor C

Lactation Excretion in breast milk unknown/not recommended

Use Symptomatic treatment of atypical, nonendogenous, or neurotic depression

Unlabeled/Investigational Use Selective mutism

Mechanism of Action/Effect Thought to act by increasing endogenous concentrations of norepinephrine, dopamine, and serotonin through inhibition of the enzyme (monoamine oxidase) responsible for the breakdown of these neurotransmitters

Contraindications Hypersensitivity to phenelzine or any component of the formulation; uncontrolled hypertension; pheochromocytoma; hepatic disease; congestive heart failure; concurrent use of sympathomimetics (and related compounds), CNS depressants, ethanol, meperidine, bupropion, buspirone, guanethidine, serotonergic drugs (including SSRIs) - do not use within 5 weeks of fluoxetine discontinuation or 2 weeks of other antidepressant discontinuation; general anesthesia, local vasoconstrictors; spinal anesthesia (hypotension may be exaggerated); foods with a high content of tyramine, tryptophan, or dopamine, chocolate, or caffeine (may cause hypertensive crisis)

Warnings/Precautions Antidepressants increase the risk of suicidal thinking and behavior in children and adolescents with major depressive disorder (MDD) and other depressive disorders; consider risk prior to prescribing. All patients must be closely monitored for clinical worsening, suicidality, or unusual changes in behavior, especially during the initiation of therapy or following an increase or decrease in dosage. When used in children, the child's family or caregiver should be instructed to closely observe the patient and communicate condition with healthcare provider. A medication guide should be dispensed with each prescription. **Phenelzine is FDA approved for the treatment of depression in children ≥16 years of age.**

The possibility of a suicide attempt is inherent in major depression and may persist until remission occurs. Use caution in high-risk patients. Worsening depression and severe abrupt suicidality that are not part of the presenting symptoms may require discontinuation or modification of drug therapy. The patient's family or caregiver should be alerted to monitor patients for the emergence of suicidality and associated behaviors (such as agitation, irritability, hostility, impulsivity, and hypomania) and call healthcare provider.

May worsen psychosis in some patients or precipitate a shift to mania or hypomania in patients with bipolar disorder. Patients presenting with depressive symptoms should be screened for bipolar disorder. Monotherapy in patients with bipolar disorder should be avoided. **Phenelzine is not FDA approved for the treatment of bipolar depression.**

Use with caution in patients who are hyperactive, hyperexcitable, or who have glaucoma, hyperthyroidism, suicidal tendencies, or diabetes. Hypertensive crisis may occur with tyramine, tryptophan, or dopamine-containing foods. Should not be used in combination with other antidepressants. Hypotensive effects of antihypertensives (beta-blockers, thiazides) may be exaggerated. May cause orthostatic hypotension - use with caution in patients with hypotension or patients who would not tolerate transient hypotensive episodes (cardiovascular or cerebrovascular disease) - effects may be additive with other agents which cause orthostasis. Use with caution in patients at risk of seizures, or in patients receiving other drugs which may lower seizure threshold. Toxic reactions have occurred with dextromethorphan. Discontinue at least 48 hours prior to myelography. May increase the risks associated with electroconvulsive therapy. Consider discontinuing, when possible, prior to elective surgery.

Drug Interactions

Decreased Effect: Phenelzine (and other MAO inhibitors) inhibits the antihypertensive response to guanadrel or guanethidine; concurrent use is contraindicated.

Increased Effect/Toxicity: In general, the combined use of phenelzine with TCAs, venlafaxine, trazodone, dexfenfluramine, sibutramine, lithium, meperidine, fenfluramine, dextromethorphan, and SSRIs should be avoided due to the potential for severe adverse reactions (serotonin syndrome, death); avoid meperidine within 2 weeks of phenelzine use, allow 5 weeks between discontinuing fluoxetine and starting MAO inhibitors, allow at least 10 days after discontinuing MAO inhibitors and starting fluoxetine; concurrent use with dextromethorphan is contraindicated. MAO inhibitors (including phenelzine) may inhibit the metabolism of barbiturates and prolong their effect. Phenelzine in combination with amphetamines, other stimulants (methylphenidate), levodopa, metaraminol, reserpine, and decongestants (pseudoephedrine) may result in severe hypertensive reactions. Concurrent use with amphetamines, methylphenidate, metaraminol, and pseudoephedrine is contraindicated.

Foods (eg, cheese) and beverages (eg, ethanol) containing tyramine should be avoided; hypertensive crisis may result. Phenelzine may increase the pressor response of norepinephrine and may prolong neuromuscular blockade produced by succinylcholine. Tramadol may increase the risk of seizures and serotonin syndrome in patients receiving an MAO inhibitor. Phenelzine may produce additive hypoglycemic effect in patients receiving hypoglycemic agents and may produce delirium in patients receiving disulfiram. Concurrent use with bupropion is contraindicated; allow at least 14 days between discontinuing MAO inhibitors and starting bupropion. Concurrent use with buspirone may cause hypertension; wait at least 14 days between discontinuing one agent and starting the other.

Nutritional/Ethanol Interactions

Ethanol: Avoid ethanol (alcoholic beverages containing tyramine may induce a severe hypertensive response).

Food: Clinically-severe elevated blood pressure may occur if phenelzine is taken with tyramine-containing foods. Avoid foods containing tryptophan, dopamine, chocolate, or caffeine.

Lab Interactions Decreased glucose

Adverse Reactions Frequency not defined.

Cardiovascular: Orthostatic hypotension, edema

Central nervous system: Dizziness, headache, drowsiness, sleep disturbances, fatigue, hyper-reflexia, twitching, ataxia, mania

Dermatologic: Rash, pruritus

Endocrine & metabolic: Decreased sexual ability (anorgasmia, ejaculatory disturbances, impotence), hypernatremia, hypermetabolic syndrome

Gastrointestinal: Xerostomia, constipation, weight gain

Genitourinary: Urinary retention

Hematologic: Leukopenia

Hepatic: Hepatitis

Neuromuscular & skeletal: Weakness, tremor, myoclonus

Ocular: Blurred vision, glaucoma

Miscellaneous: Diaphoresis

Overdosage/Toxicology Symptoms of overdose include tachycardia, palpitations, muscle twitching, seizures, insomnia, restlessness, transient hypertension, hypotension, drowsiness, hyperpyrexia, and coma. Treatment is symptom-directed and supportive.

Pharmacodynamics/Kinetics

Onset of Action: Therapeutic: 2-4 weeks; geriatric patients receiving an average of 55 mg/day developed a mean platelet MAO activity inhibition of about 85%.

Duration of Action: May continue to have a therapeutic effect and interactions 2 weeks after discontinuing therapy

Half-Life Elimination: 11 hours

Metabolism: Oxidized via monoamine oxidase (primary pathway) and acetylation (minor pathway)

Excretion: Urine (primarily as metabolites and unchanged drug)

Available Dosage Forms Tablet: 15 mg

Dosing

Adults: Depression: Oral: 15 mg 3 times/day; may increase to 60-90 mg/day during early phase of treatment, then reduce dose for maintenance therapy slowly after maximum benefit is obtained. Takes 2-4 weeks for a significant response to occur.

Elderly: Oral: Initial: 7.5 mg/day; increase by 7.5-15 mg/day every 3-4 days as tolerated; usual therapeutic dose: 15-60 mg/day in 3-4 divided doses.

Pediatrics: Selective mutism (unlabeled use): Oral: 30-60 mg/day

Stability

Storage: Protect from light

Nursing Actions

Physical Assessment: Assess other medications patient may be taking for effectiveness and interactions Monitor therapeutic response (ie, blood pressure, mental status, mood, affect, suicidal ideation), and adverse reactions at beginning of therapy and periodically with long-term use. Observe for clinical worsening, suicidality, and unusual behavior changes, especially during the initial few months of therapy or during dosage changes. Patients with diabetes should monitor serum glucose closely (phenelzine may lower glucose level). Assess knowledge/teach patient appropriate use, interventions to reduce side effects (including tyramine-free diet; see Tyramine Contents of Foods *on page 1406* list), and adverse symptoms to report.

Patient Education: Take exactly as directed; do not increase dose or frequency. It may take 2-3 weeks to achieve desired results. Avoid alcohol, caffeine, and other prescription or OTC medications not approved by prescriber. Avoid tyramine-containing foods (eg, pickles, aged cheese, wine). Maintain adequate hydration (2-3 L/day of fluids) unless instructed to restrict fluid intake. You may experience postural

hypotension (use caution when climbing stairs or changing position from lying or sitting to standing); drowsiness, lightheadedness, dizziness (use caution when driving or engaging in tasks requiring alertness until response to drug is known); anorexia, dry mouth (small frequent meals, frequent mouth care, chewing gum, or sucking lozenges may help); constipation (increased exercise, fluids, fruit, or fiber may help); or diarrhea (buttermilk, yogurt, or boiled milk may help). If you have diabetes, monitor serum glucose closely (Nardil® may effect glucose levels). Report persistent insomnia; chest pain, palpitations, irregular or rapid heartbeat, or swelling of extremities; muscle cramping, tremors, or altered gait; blurred vision or eye pain; yellowing of eyes or skin; pale stools/dark urine; suicide ideation; or worsening of condition. **Pregnancy/breast-feeding precautions:** Inform prescriber if you are or intend to become pregnant. Breast-feeding is not recommended.

Geriatric Considerations MAO inhibitors are effective and generally well tolerated by older patients. Potential interactions with tyramine- or tryptophan-containing foods (see Warnings/Precautions) and other drugs, and adverse effects on blood pressure have limited the use of MAO inhibitors. They are usually reserved for patients who do not tolerate or respond to traditional "cyclic" or "second generation" antidepressants. Brain activity due to monoamine oxidase increases with age and even more so in patients with Alzheimer's disease. Therefore, MAO inhibitors may have an increased role in treating depressed patients with Alzheimer's disease. Phenelzine is less stimulating than tranylcypromine.

Additional Information Pyridoxine deficiency has occurred; symptoms include numbness and edema of hands; may respond to supplementation.

The MAO inhibitors are usually reserved for patients who do not tolerate or respond to other antidepressants. The brain activity of monoamine oxidase increases with age and even more so in patients with Alzheimer's disease. Therefore, the MAO inhibitors may have an increased role in patients with Alzheimer's disease who are depressed. Phenelzine is less stimulating than tranylcypromine.

Related Information

Antidepressant Medication Guidelines *on page 1414*
Tyramine Content of Foods *on page 1406*

Phenobarbital *(fee noe BAR bi tal)*

U.S. Brand Names Luminal® Sodium

Synonyms Phenobarbital Sodium; Phenobarbitone; Phenylethylmalonylurea

Restrictions C-IV

Pharmacologic Category Anticonvulsant, Barbiturate; Barbiturate

Medication Safety Issues

Sound-alike/look-alike issues:

Phenobarbital may be confused with pentobarbital

Luminal® may be confused with Tuinal®

Pregnancy Risk Factor D

Lactation Enters breast milk/not recommended (AAP recommends use "with caution")

Use Management of generalized tonic-clonic (grand mal) and partial seizures; sedative

Unlabeled/Investigational Use Febrile seizures in children; may also be used for prevention and treatment of neonatal hyperbilirubinemia and lowering of bilirubin in chronic cholestasis; neonatal seizures; management of sedative/hypnotic withdrawal

Mechanism of Action/Effect Short-acting barbiturate with sedative, hypnotic, and anticonvulsant properties. Barbiturates depress the sensory cortex, decrease motor activity, alter cerebellar function, and produce drowsiness, sedation, and hypnosis. In high doses, (Continued)

Phenobarbital *(Continued)*

barbiturates exhibit anticonvulsant activity; barbiturates produce dose-dependent respiratory depression.

Contraindications Hypersensitivity to barbiturates or any component of the formulation; marked hepatic impairment; dyspnea or airway obstruction; porphyria; pregnancy

Warnings/Precautions Potential for drug dependency exists, abrupt cessation may precipitate withdrawal, including status epilepticus in epileptic patients. Do not administer to patients in acute pain. Use caution in elderly, debilitated, renally or hepatic dysfunction, and pediatric patients. May cause paradoxical responses, including agitation and hyperactivity, particularly in acute pain and pediatric patients. Use with caution in patients with depression or suicidal tendencies, or in patients with a history of drug abuse. Tolerance, psychological and physical dependence may occur with prolonged use. May cause CNS depression, which may impair physical or mental abilities. Effects with other sedative drugs or ethanol may be potentiated. May cause respiratory depression or hypotension, particularly when administered intravenously. Use with caution in hemodynamically unstable patients (hypovolemic shock, CHF) or patients with respiratory disease. Due to its long half-life and risk of dependence, phenobarbital is not recommended as a sedative in the elderly. Use has been associated with cognitive deficits in children. Use with caution in patients with hypoadrenalism.

Drug Interactions

Cytochrome P450 Effect: Substrate of CYP2C8/9 (minor), 2C19 (major), 2E1 (minor); **Induces** CYP1A2 (strong), 2A6 (strong), 2B6 (strong), 2C8/9 (strong), 3A4 (strong)

Decreased Effect: Barbiturates may increase the metabolism of estrogens and reduce the efficacy of oral contraceptives; an alternative method of contraception should be considered. Barbiturates inhibit the hypoprothrombinemic effects of oral anticoagulants via increased metabolism. Barbiturates may enhance the metabolism of methadone resulting in methadone withdrawal. The levels/effects of phenobarbital may be decreased by aminoglutethimide, carbamazepine, phenytoin, rifampin, and other CYP2C19 inducers.

Phenobarbital may decrease the levels/effects of aminophylline, amiodarone, benzodiazepines, bupropion, calcium channel blockers, carbamazepine, citalopram, clarithromycin, cyclosporine, diazepam, efavirenz, erythromycin, estrogens, fluoxetine, fluvoxamine, glimepiride, glipizide, ifosfamide, losartan, methsuximide, mirtazapine, nateglinide, nefazodone, nevirapine, phenytoin, pioglitazone, promethazine, propranolol, protease inhibitors, proton pump inhibitors, rifampin, ropinirole, rosiglitazone, selegiline, sertraline, sulfonamides, tacrolimus, theophylline, venlafaxine, voriconazole, warfarin, zafirlukast, and other CYP1A2, 2A6, 2B6, 2C8/9, or 3A4 substrates.

Increased Effect/Toxicity: When combined with other CNS depressants, ethanol, narcotic analgesics, antidepressants, or benzodiazepines, additive respiratory and CNS depression may occur. Barbiturates may enhance the hepatotoxic potential of acetaminophen overdoses. Chloramphenicol, MAO inhibitors, valproic acid, and felbamate may inhibit barbiturate metabolism. Barbiturates may impair the absorption of griseofulvin, and may enhance the nephrotoxic effects of methoxyflurane. Concurrent use of phenobarbital with meperidine may result in increased CNS depression. Concurrent use of phenobarbital with primidone may result in elevated phenobarbital serum concentrations. The levels/effects of phenobarbital may be increased by delavirdine, fluconazole, fluvoxamine, gemfibrozil, isoniazid, omeprazole, ticlopidine, and other CYP2C19 inhibitors.

Nutritional/Ethanol Interactions

Ethanol: Avoid ethanol (may increase CNS depression).

Food: May cause decrease in vitamin D and calcium.

Herb/Nutraceutical: Avoid evening primrose (seizure threshold decreased). Avoid valerian, St John's wort, kava kava, gotu kola (may increase CNS depression).

Lab Interactions Increased ammonia (B), LFTs, copper (serum); decreased bilirubin (S); assay interference of LDH

Adverse Reactions Frequency not defined.

Cardiovascular: Bradycardia, hypotension, syncope

Central nervous system: Drowsiness, lethargy, CNS excitation or depression, impaired judgment, "hangover" effect, confusion, somnolence, agitation, hyperkinesia, ataxia, nervousness, headache, insomnia, nightmares, hallucinations, anxiety, dizziness

Dermatologic: Rash, exfoliative dermatitis, Stevens-Johnson syndrome

Gastrointestinal: Nausea, vomiting, constipation

Hematologic: Agranulocytosis, thrombocytopenia, megaloblastic anemia

Local: Pain at injection site, thrombophlebitis with I.V. use

Renal: Oliguria

Respiratory: Laryngospasm, respiratory depression, apnea (especially with rapid I.V. use), hypoventilation

Miscellaneous: Gangrene with inadvertent intra-arterial injection

Overdosage/Toxicology Symptoms of overdose include unsteady gait, slurred speech, confusion, jaundice, hypothermia, hypotension, respiratory depression, and coma. In severe overdose, charcoal hemoperfusion may accelerate removal. Treatment is symptom-directed and supportive.

Pharmacodynamics/Kinetics

Onset of Action: Oral: Hypnosis: 20-60 minutes; I.V.: ~5 minutes; Peak effect: I.V.: ~30 minutes

Duration of Action: Oral: 6-10 hours; I.V.: 4-10 hours

Time to Peak: Serum: Oral: 1-6 hours

Protein Binding: 20% to 45%; decreased in neonates

Half-Life Elimination: Neonates: 45-500 hours; Infants: 20-133 hours; Children: 37-73 hours; Adults: 53-140 hours

Metabolism: Hepatic via hydroxylation and glucuronide conjugation

Excretion: Urine (20% to 50% as unchanged drug)

Available Dosage Forms

Elixir: 20 mg/5 mL (473 mL) [contains alcohol]

Injection, solution, as sodium: 65 mg/mL (1 mL); 130 mg/mL (1 mL) [contains alcohol and propylene glycol]

Luminal® Sodium: 60 mg/mL (1 mL); 130 mg/mL (1 mL) [contains alcohol 10% and propylene glycol]

Tablet: 15 mg, 30 mg, 32 mg, 60 mg, 65 mg, 100 mg

Dosing

Adults:

Sedation: Oral, I.M.: 30-120 mg/day in 2-3 divided doses

Hypnotic: Oral, I.M., I.V., SubQ: 100-320 mg at bedtime

Preoperative sedation: I.M.: 100-200 mg 1-1.5 hours before procedure

Anticonvulsant/status epilepticus:

Loading dose: I.V.: 300-800 mg initially followed by 120-240 mg/dose at 20-minute intervals until seizures are controlled or a total dose of 1-2 g

Maintenance dose: Oral, I.V.: 1-3 mg/kg/day in divided doses or 50-100 mg 2-3 times/day

Sedative/hypnotic withdrawal (unlabeled use): Initial daily requirement is determined by substituting phenobarbital 30 mg for every 100 mg pentobarbital used during tolerance testing; then daily requirement is decreased by 10% of initial dose.

Elderly: Geriatric patients should be started at the lowest recommended dose. Refer to adult dosing.

Pediatrics:

Sedation: Oral: Children: 2 mg/kg 3 times/day

Hypnotic: I.M., I.V., SubQ: Children: 3-5 mg/kg at bedtime

Preoperative sedation: Oral, I.M., I.V.: Children: 1-3 mg/kg 1-1.5 hours before procedure

Anticonvulsant/Status epilepticus (Loading dose):
I.V.: Infants and Children: 10-20 mg/kg in a single or divided dose; in select patients may administer additional 5 mg/kg/dose every 15-30 minutes until seizure is controlled or a total dose of 40 mg/kg is reached

Anticonvulsant maintenance dose: Oral, I.V.:
Infants: 5-8 mg/kg/day in 1-2 divided doses
Children:
1-5 years: 6-8 mg/kg/day in 1-2 divided doses
5-12 years: 4-6 mg/kg/day in 1-2 divided doses
>12 years: 1-3 mg/kg/day in divided doses or 50-100 mg 2-3 times/day

Renal Impairment:
Cl_{cr} <10 mL/minute: Administer every 12-16 hours. Moderately dialyzable (20% to 50%)

Hepatic Impairment: Increased side effects may occur in severe liver disease. Monitor plasma levels and adjust dose accordingly.

Administration

I.V.: Avoid rapid I.V. administration >50 mg/minute. Avoid intra-arterial injection.

I.V. Detail: Parenteral solutions are highly alkaline. Avoid extravasation.

pH: 9.2-10.2

Stability

Compatibility: Stable in dextran 6% in dextrose, dextran 6% in NS, D_5LR, $D_5^1/_4NS$, $D_5^1/_2NS$, D_5NS, D_5W, $D_{10}W$, LR, $^1/_2NS$, NS

Y-site administration: Incompatible with amphotericin B cholesteryl sulfate complex, hydromorphone

Compatibility in syringe: Incompatible with hydromorphone, pentazocine, ranitidine, sufentanil

Compatibility when admixed: Incompatible with chlorpromazine, cimetidine, clindamycin, dimenhydrinate, diphenhydramine, droperidol, ephedrine, hydralazine, hydrocortisone sodium succinate, hydroxyzine, insulin (regular), kanamycin, levorphanol, meperidine, morphine, norepinephrine, pancuronium, penicillin G, pentazocine, phenytoin, procaine, prochlorperazine edisylate, prochlorperazine mesylate, promazine, promethazine, streptomycin, succinylcholine, vancomycin

Storage: Protect elixir from light. Not stable in aqueous solutions. Use only clear solutions. Do not add to acidic solutions; precipitation may occur.

Laboratory Monitoring Phenobarbital serum concentrations, CBC, LFTs

Nursing Actions

Physical Assessment: Assess effectiveness and interactions of other medications patient may be taking. Assess for history of addiction; long-term use can result in dependence, abuse, or tolerance. **I.V.:** Keep patient under observation (vital signs, neurologic, cardiac, and respiratory status); use safety precautions. Monitor effectiveness of therapy and adverse reactions. **Oral:** Monitor therapeutic response and adverse reactions at beginning of therapy and periodically with long-term use. Assess knowledge/teach patient appropriate use, possible side effects, and symptoms to report.

Patient Education: I.M./I.V.: Patient instructions and information are determined by patient condition and therapeutic purpose. If self-administered, use exactly as directed; do not increase dose or frequency. Drug may cause physical and/or psychological dependence. While using this medication, do not use alcohol and other prescription or OTC medications (especially pain medications, sedatives, antihistamines, or hypnotics) without consulting prescriber. Maintain adequate hydration (2-3 L/day of fluids) unless instructed to restrict fluid intake. You may experience drowsiness, dizziness, or blurred vision (use caution when driving or engaging in tasks requiring alertness until response to drug is known); nausea, vomiting, or loss of appetite (small frequent meals, frequent mouth care, chewing gum, or sucking lozenges may help); or constipation (increased exercise, fluids, fruit, or fiber may help). Report skin rash or irritation; CNS changes (confusion, depression, increased sedation, excitation, headache, insomnia, or nightmares); respiratory difficulty or shortness of breath; changes in urinary pattern or menstrual pattern; muscle weakness or tremors; or difficulty swallowing or feeling of tightness in throat. **Pregnancy/breast-feeding precautions:** Do not get pregnant while taking this medication; use appropriate contraceptive measures. Breast-feeding is not recommended.

Dietary Considerations Vitamin D: Loss in vitamin D due to malabsorption; increase intake of foods rich in vitamin D. Supplementation of vitamin D and/or calcium may be necessary. Sodium content of injection (65 mg, 1 mL): 6 mg (0.3 mEq).

Geriatric Considerations Due to its long half-life and risk of dependence, phenobarbital is not recommended as a sedative or hypnotic in the elderly. Interpretive guidelines from the Health Care Financing Administration discourage the use of this agent as a sedative/hypnotic in long-term care residents.

Breast-Feeding Issues Sedation has been reported in nursing infants; infantile spasms may occur after weaning from breast milk. AAP recommends USE WITH CAUTION.

Pregnancy Issues Crosses the placenta. Cardiac defect reported; hemorrhagic disease of newborn due to fetal vitamin K depletion may occur; may induce maternal folic acid deficiency; withdrawal symptoms observed in infant following delivery. Epilepsy itself, number of medications, genetic factors, or a combination of these probably influence the teratogenicity of anticonvulsant therapy. Benefit:risk ratio usually favors continued use during pregnancy.

Additional Information Injectable solutions contain propylene glycol.

Related Information
Compatibility of Drugs *on page 1370*
Peak and Trough Guidelines *on page 1387*

Phentolamine (fen TOLE a meen)

Synonyms Phentolamine Mesylate; Regitine [DSC]
Pharmacologic Category Alpha$_1$ Blocker
Medication Safety Issues
Sound-alike/look-alike issues:
Phentolamine may be confused with phentermine, Ventolin®

Pregnancy Risk Factor C
Lactation Excretion in breast milk unknown
Use Diagnosis of pheochromocytoma and treatment of hypertension associated with pheochromocytoma or other forms of hypertension caused by excess sympathomimetic amines; as treatment of dermal necrosis after extravasation of drugs with alpha-adrenergic effects (norepinephrine, dopamine, epinephrine)

Unlabeled/Investigational Use Treatment of pralidoxime-induced hypertension

Mechanism of Action/Effect Competitively blocks alpha-adrenergic receptors to produce brief antagonism of circulating epinephrine and norepinephrine to reduce hypertension caused by alpha effects of these catecholamines; also has a positive inotropic and chronotropic effect on the heart

Contraindications Hypersensitivity to phentolamine or any component of the formulation; renal impairment; coronary or cerebral arteriosclerosis; concurrent use
(Continued)

Phentolamine *(Continued)*

with phosphodiesterase-5 (PDE-5) inhibitors including sildenafil (>25 mg), tadalafil, or vardenafil

Warnings/Precautions Myocardial infarction, cerebrovascular spasm and cerebrovascular occlusion have occurred following administration. Use with caution in patients with gastritis or peptic ulcer, tachycardia, or a history of cardiac arrhythmias.

Drug Interactions

Decreased Effect: Decreased effect of phentolamine with epinephrine and ephedrine.

Increased Effect/Toxicity: Phentolamine's toxicity is increased with ethanol (disulfiram reaction). Blood pressure-lowering effects are additive with sildenafil (use with extreme caution at a dose ≤25 mg), tadalafil (use is contraindicated by the manufacturer), and vardenafil (use is contraindicated by the manufacturer).

Lab Interactions Increased LFTs rarely

Adverse Reactions Frequency not defined.

Cardiovascular: Hypotension, tachycardia, arrhythmia, flushing, orthostatic hypotension

Central nervous system: Dizziness

Gastrointestinal: Nausea, vomiting, diarrhea

Neuromuscular & skeletal: Weakness

Respiratory: Nasal congestion

Case report: Pulmonary hypertension

Overdosage/Toxicology Symptoms of overdose include tachycardia, shock, vomiting, and dizziness. If fluid replacement is inadequate to treat hypotension, only alpha-adrenergic vasopressors such as norepinephrine should be used. Mixed agents such as epinephrine may cause more hypotension.

Pharmacodynamics/Kinetics

Onset of Action: I.M.: 15-20 minutes; I.V.: Immediate

Duration of Action: I.M.: 30-45 minutes; I.V.: 15-30 minutes

Half-Life Elimination: 19 minutes

Metabolism: Hepatic

Excretion: Urine (10% as unchanged drug)

Available Dosage Forms Injection, powder for reconstitution, as mesylate: 5 mg

Dosing

Adults & Elderly:

Treatment of alpha-adrenergic drug extravasation: SubQ:

Infiltrate area with a small amount (eg, 1 mL) of solution (made by diluting 5-10 mg in 10 mL of NS) within 12 hours of extravasation; do not exceed 0.1-0.2 mg/kg or 5 mg total

If dose is effective, normal skin color should return to the blanched area within 1 hour.

Diagnosis of pheochromocytoma: I.M., I.V.: 5 mg

Surgery for pheochromocytoma: Hypertension: I.M., I.V.: 5 mg given 1-2 hours before procedure and repeated as needed every 2-4 hours

Hypertensive crisis: I.V.: 5-20 mg

Treatment of pralidoxime-induced hypertension (unlabeled use): I.V.: 5 mg

Pediatrics:

Treatment of alpha-adrenergic drug extravasation: SubQ: Infiltrate area with a small amount (eg, 1 mL) of solution (made by diluting 5-10 mg in 10 mL of NS) within 12 hours of extravasation; do not exceed 0.1-0.2 mg/kg or 5 mg total

Diagnosis of pheochromocytoma: I.M., I.V.: 0.05-0.1 mg/kg/dose, maximum single dose: 5 mg

Surgery for pheochromocytoma: Hypertension: I.M., I.V.: 0.05-0.1 mg/kg/dose given 1-2 hours before procedure; repeat as needed every 2-4 hours until hypertension is controlled; maximum single dose: 5 mg.

Treatment of pralidoxime-induced hypertension (unlabeled use): I.V.: 1 mg

Administration

I.V.:

Vasoconstrictor (alpha-adrenergic agonist) extravasation: Infiltrate the area of extravasation with multiple small injections using only 27- or 30-gauge needles and changing the needle between each skin entry. Be careful not to cause so much swelling of the extremity or digit that a compartment syndrome occurs. If infiltration is severe, may also need to consult vascular surgeon.

Pheochromocytoma: Inject each 5 mg over 1 minute.

I.V. Detail: pH: 4.5-6.5

Stability

Reconstitution: Reconstituted solution is stable for 48 hours at room temperature and 1 week when refrigerated.

Compatibility: Stable in NS

Nursing Actions

Physical Assessment: See Administration for specifics according to purpose for use. When used to treat dermal necrosis after extravasation of drugs with alpha-adrenergic effects, monitor effectiveness of treatment closely. Monitor patient response. Teach patient adverse symptoms to report.

Patient Education: This medication can only be administered by infusion or injection. Report immediately any pain at infusion/injection site. May cause orthostatic hypotension (use caution when changing position or call for assistance). Report dizziness, rapid heartbeat, feelings of weakness, or nausea/vomiting. **Pregnancy/breast-feeding precautions:** Inform prescriber if you are or intend to become pregnant. Consult prescriber if breast-feeding.

Phenylephrine *(fen il EF rin)*

U.S. Brand Names AH-chew® D [OTC] [DSC]; AK-Dilate®; Altafrin; Anu-Med [OTC]; Formulation R™ [OTC]; Medicone® [OTC]; Mydfrin®; NäSop™; Neo-Synephrine® Extra Strength [OTC]; Neo-Synephrine® Mild [OTC]; Neo-Synephrine® Ophthalmic [DSC]; Neo-Synephrine® Regular Strength [OTC]; Rectacaine [OTC]; Relief® [OTC]; Rhinall [OTC]; Sudafed PE™ [OTC]; Tronolane® Suppository [OTC]; Vicks® Sinex® Nasal Spray [OTC]; Vicks® Sinex® UltraFine Mist [OTC]

Synonyms Phenylephrine Hydrochloride; Phenylephrine Tannate

Pharmacologic Category Alpha/Beta Agonist; Ophthalmic Agent, Antiglaucoma; Ophthalmic Agent, Mydriatic

Medication Safety Issues

Sound-alike/look-alike issues:

Mydfrin® may be confused with Midrin®

Pregnancy Risk Factor C

Lactation Excretion in breast milk unknown/not recommended

Use Treatment of hypotension, vascular failure in shock; as a vasoconstrictor in regional analgesia; as a mydriatic in ophthalmic procedures and treatment of wide-angle glaucoma; supraventricular tachycardia

For OTC use as symptomatic relief of nasal and nasopharyngeal mucosal congestion, treatment of hemorrhoids, relief of redness of the eye due to irritation

Mechanism of Action/Effect Potent, direct-acting alpha-adrenergic stimulator with weak beta-adrenergic activity; causes vasoconstriction of the arterioles of the nasal mucosa and conjunctiva; activates the dilator muscle of the pupil to cause contraction; produces vasoconstriction of arterioles in the body; produces systemic arterial vasoconstriction

Contraindications Hypersensitivity to phenylephrine or any component of the formulation; hypertension; ventricular tachycardia

Oral: Use with or within 14 days of MAO inhibitor therapy

Ophthalmic: Narrow-angle glaucoma

Warnings/Precautions Some products contain sulfites which may cause allergic reactions in susceptible individuals.

Intravenous: Use with caution in the elderly, patients with hyperthyroidism, bradycardia, partial heart block, myocardial disease, or severe CAD. Not a substitute for volume replacement. Avoid hypertension; monitor blood pressure closely and adjust infusion rate. Infuse into a large vein if possible. Watch I.V. site closely. Avoid extravasation.

Nasal, oral, rectal: Use caution with hyperthyroidism, diabetes mellitus, cardiovascular disease, ischemic heart disease, increased intraocular pressure, prostatic hyperplasia or in the elderly. Rebound congestion may occur when nasal products are discontinued after chronic use. When used for self-medication (OTC), notify healthcare provider if symptoms do not improve within 7 days (oral, rectal) or 3 days (nasal), are accompanied by fever (oral), or if bleeding occurs (rectal).

Ophthalmic: Use caution with or within 21 days of MAO inhibitor therapy. When used for self-medication (OTC), notify healthcare provider in case of vision changes, continued redness, or if symptoms worsen or do not improve within 3 days.

Drug Interactions

Increased Effect/Toxicity: Phenylephrine, taken with sympathomimetics, may induce tachycardia or arrhythmias. If taken with MAO inhibitors or oxytocic agents, actions may be potentiated. Nonselective beta-blockers may increase hypertensive effects; MAO inhibitors may potentiate hypertension and hypertensive crisis; TCAs may enhance vasopressor effect; avoid concurrent use with these agents. Methyldopa may increase pressor response.

Nutritional/Ethanol Interactions Herb/Nutraceutical: Avoid ephedra, yohimbe (may cause CNS stimulation).

Adverse Reactions Frequency not defined.

Cardiovascular: Reflex bradycardia, excitability, restlessness, arrhythmia (rare), precordial pain or discomfort, pallor, hypertension, severe peripheral and visceral vasoconstriction, decreased cardiac output

Central nervous system: Headache, anxiety, dizziness, tremor, paresthesia, restlessness

Endocrine & metabolic: Metabolic acidosis

Local: I.V.: Extravasation which may lead to necrosis and sloughing of surrounding tissue, blanching of skin

Neuromuscular & skeletal: Pilomotor response, weakness

Renal: Decreased renal perfusion, reduced urine output, reduced urine output

Respiratory: Respiratory distress

Overdosage/Toxicology Symptoms of overdose include vomiting, hypertension, palpitations, paresthesia, and ventricular extrasystoles. Treatment is supportive. In extreme cases, I.V. phentolamine may be used.

Pharmacodynamics/Kinetics

Onset of Action: I.M., SubQ: 10-15 minutes; I.V.: Immediate; Ophthalmic: 10-15 minutes

Duration of Action: I.M.: 0.5-2 hours; I.V.: 15-30 minutes; SubQ: 1 hour; Ophthalmic: Maximal mydriasis: 1 hour, recover time: 3-6 hours

Metabolism: Hepatic, via intestinal monoamine oxidase to phenolic conjugates

Excretion: Urine (90%)

Available Dosage Forms [DSC] = Discontinued product

Cream, rectal, as hydrochloride (Formulation R™): 0.25% (54 g) [contains sodium benzoate]

Injection, solution, as hydrochloride: 1% [10 mg/mL] (1 mL, 5 mL) [may contain sodium metabisulfite]

Neo-Synephrine®: 1% (1 mL) [contains sodium metabisulfite]

Ointment, rectal, as hydrochloride:

Formulation R™: 0.25% (30 g, 60 g) [contains benzoic acid]

Rectacaine: 0.25% (30 g) [contains shark liver oil]

Solution, intranasal drops, as hydrochloride:

Neo-Synephrine® Extra Strength: 1% (15 mL) [contains benzalkonium chloride]

Neo-Synephrine® Regular Strength: 0.5% (15 mL) [contains benzalkonium chloride]

Rhinall: 0.25% (30 mL) [contains benzalkonium chloride and sodium bisulfite]

Solution, intranasal spray, as hydrochloride:

Neo-Synephrine® Extra Strength: 1% (15 mL) [contains benzalkonium chloride]

Neo-Synephrine® Mild: 0.25% (15 mL) [contains benzalkonium chloride]

Neo-Synephrine® Regular Strength: 0.5% (15 mL) [contains benzalkonium chloride]

Rhinall: 0.25% (40 mL) [contains benzalkonium chloride and sodium bisulfite]

Vicks® Sinex®, Vicks® Sinex® UltraFine Mist: 0.5% (15 mL) [contains benzalkonium chloride]

Solution, ophthalmic, as hydrochloride: 2.5% (1 mL, 2 mL, 3 mL, 5 mL, 15 mL) [may contain sodium bisulfite]

AK-Dilate®: 2.5% (2 mL, 15 mL); 10% (5 mL)

Altrafrin: 0.12% (15 mL) [OTC]; 2.5% (5 mL, 15 mL) [RX; contains benzalkonium chloride]; 10% (5 mL) [RX; contains benzalkonium chloride]

Mydfrin®: 2.5% (3 mL, 5 mL) [contains sodium bisulfite]

Neo-Synephrine®: 2.5% (15 mL); 10% (5 mL) [contains benzalkonium chloride] [DSC]

Neo-Synephrine® Viscous: 10% (5 mL) [contains benzalkonium chloride] [DSC]

Suppository, rectal, as hydrochloride: 0.25% (12s)

Anu-Med, Tronolane®: 0.25% (12s)

Medicone®: 0.25% (18s, 24s)

Rectacaine: 0.25% (12s) [contains shark liver oil]

Suspension, oral, as tannate (NāSop™): 7.5 mg/5 mL (120 mL) [orange flavor]

Tablet, as hydrochloride (Sudafed PE™): 10 mg

Tablet, chewable, as hydrochloride:

AH-chew® D: 10 mg [DSC]

Tablet, orally dissolving, as hydrochloride (NāSop™): 10 mg [contains phenylalanine 4 mg/tablet; bubble gum flavor]

Dosing

Adults:

Hemorrhoids: Rectal:

Cream/ointment: Apply to clean dry area, up to 4 times/day; may be used externally or inserted rectally using applicator.

Suppository: Insert 1 suppository rectally, up to 4 times/day

Hypotension/shock:

I.V. bolus: 0.1-0.5 mg/dose every 10-15 minutes as needed (initial dose should not exceed 0.5 mg)

I.V. infusion: Initial dose: 100-180 mcg/minute; when blood pressure is stabilized, maintenance rate: 40-60 mcg/minute; rates up to 360 mcg/minute have been reported; dosing range: 0.4-9.1 mcg/kg/minute

Nasal congestion:

Intranasal: Instill 1-2 sprays or instill 1-2 drops every 4 hours of 0.25% to 0.5% solution as needed; 1% solution may be used in adult in cases of extreme nasal congestion; do not use nasal solutions more than 3 days

Oral:

Hydrochloride salt: 10-20 mg every 4 hours

Tannate salt (NāSop™ suspension): 7.5-15 mg every 12 hours

(Continued)

Phenylephrine *(Continued)*

Ocular procedures: Ophthalmic: Instill 1 drop of 2.5% or 10% solution, may repeat in 10-60 minutes as needed.

Paroxysmal supraventricular tachycardia: I.V.: 0.25-0.5 mg/dose over 20-30 seconds

Reduction in ocular redness (OTC formulation): Ophthalmic: Instill 1-2 drops 0.12% solution into affected eye, up to 4 times/day; do not use for >72 hours

Elderly:

Nasal decongestant: Administer 2-3 drops or 1-2 sprays every 4 hours of 0.125% to 0.25% solution as needed; do not use more than 3 days.

Ophthalmic preparations for pupil dilation: Instill 1 drop of 2.5% solution, may repeat in 1 hour if necessary.

Refer to adult dosing for other uses and Geriatric Considerations for cautions on I.V. use.

Pediatrics:

Hemorrhoids: Children >12 years: Refer to adult dosing.

Hypotension/shock: Children:

I.V. bolus: 5-20 mcg/kg/dose every 10-15 minutes as needed

I.V. infusion: 0.1-0.5 mcg/kg/minute

Nasal congestion:

2-6 years:

Intranasal: Instill 1 drop every 2-4 hours of 0.125% solution as needed. **(Note:** Therapy should not exceed 3 continuous days.)

Oral: Tannate salt (NāSop™ suspension): 1.87-3.75 mg every 12 hours

6-12 years:

Intranasal: Instill 1-2 sprays or instill 1-2 drops every 4 hours of 0.25% solution as needed. **(Note:** Therapy should not exceed 3 continuous days.)

Oral:

Hydrochloride salt: 10 mg every 4 hours

Tannate salt (NāSop™ suspension): 3.75-7.5 mg every 12 hours

>12 years: Refer to adult dosing.

Ocular procedures: Ophthalmic:

Infants <1 year: Instill 1 drop of 2.5% 15-30 minutes before procedures

Children: Refer to adult dosing.

Paroxysmal supraventricular tachycardia: I.V.: Children: 5-10 mcg/kg/dose over 20-30 seconds

Administration

Oral: NāSop™: Place tablet on tongue and allow to dissolve

I.V. Detail: May cause necrosis or sloughing tissue if extravasation occurs during I.V. administration or SubQ administration.

Extravasation management: Use phentolamine as antidote; mix 5 mg with 9 mL of NS. Inject a small amount of this dilution into extravasated area. Blanching should reverse immediately. Monitor site. If blanching should recur, additional injections of phentolamine may be needed.

pH: 3.0-6.5

Stability

Reconstitution: Solution for injection:

I.V. infusion: May dilute 10 mg in 500 mL NS or D_5W.

I.V. injection: Dilute with SWFI to a concentration of 1 mg/mL.

Compatibility: Stable in dextran 6% in dextrose, dextran 6% in NS, D_5LR, $D_5^1/_4NS$, $D_5^1/_2NS$, D_5NS, D_5W, $D_{10}W$, LR, $^1/_2NS$, NS, sodium bicarbonate 5%

Y-site administration: Incompatible with thiopental

Storage:

Solution for injection: Store vials at controlled room temperature of 15°C to 30°C (59°F to 86°F). Protect from light. Do not use solution if brown or contains a precipitate.

Ophthalmic solution:

0.12%: Store at controlled room temperature. Protect from light and excessive heat.

2.5% and 10%: Refer to product labeling. Some products are labeled to store at room temperature, others should be stored under refrigeration at 2°C to 8°C (36°F to 46°F); do not use solution if brown or contains a precipitate.

Nursing Actions

Physical Assessment: Assess other medications patient may be taking for effectiveness and interactions This drug has multiple uses/doses. Monitor therapeutic response and adverse reactions according to use. **Parenteral:** Monitor arterial blood gases, vital signs, adverse reactions and monitor infusion site frequently for patency. **Nasal/ophthalmic:** Assess knowledge/teach patient appropriate use, interventions to reduce side effects, and adverse symptoms to report. Systemic absorption from ophthalmic instillation is minimal.

Patient Education:

Nasal decongestant: Do not use for more than 3 days in a row. Clear nose as much as possible before use. Tilt head back and instill recommended dose of drops or spray. Do not blow nose for 5-10 minutes. You may experience transient stinging or burning.

Ophthalmic: Do not let tip of applicator touch eye; do not contaminate tip of applicator (may cause eye infection, eye damage, or vision loss). Open eye, look at ceiling, and instill prescribed amount of solution. Close eye and roll eye in all directions, and apply gentle pressure to inner corner of eye for 1-2 minutes after instillation. Temporary stinging or blurred vision may occur. Report persistent pain, burning, double vision, severe headache, or if condition worsens.

Pregnancy/breast-feeding precautions: Inform prescriber if you are pregnant. Consult prescriber if breast-feeding.

Dietary Considerations NāSop™ contains phenylalanine 4 mg/tablet.

Geriatric Considerations Older adults are more predisposed to the adverse effects of sympathomimetics since they frequently have cardiovascular disease and diabetes mellitus, and are on multiple medications. Since oral and topical phenylephrine can be obtained OTC, elderly patients should be counseled about their proper use and in what disease states they should be avoided (see Warnings/Precautions). Phenylephrine I.V. should be used with extreme caution in the elderly. The 10% ophthalmic solution has caused increased blood pressure in elderly patients and its use should, therefore, be avoided.

Additional Information Phenylephrine allows for close titration of blood pressure and should be used in patients with hypotension or shock due to peripheral vasodilation. Phenylephrine should not constitute sole therapy in patients with hypotension due to aortic dysfunction or hypovolemia. An important benefit of this drug is the short half-life, allowing rapid changes in dosage with prompt appropriate blood pressure responses. When administered intravenously, it should be used in intensive care settings or under very close monitoring.

Phenylephrine and Pyrilamine
(fen il EF rin & peer IL a meen)

U.S. Brand Names Pyrilafen Tannate-12™; Ryna-12™; Ryna-12 S™; Ry-T 12; Viravan®; V-Tann

Synonyms Pyrilamine Tannate and Phenylephrine Tannate

Pharmacologic Category Antihistamine; Antihistamine/Decongestant Combination; Sympathomimetic

Pregnancy Risk Factor C

Lactation Excretion in breast milk unknown/contraindicated

Use Symptomatic relief of nasal congestion and discharge associated with the common cold, sinusitis, allergic rhinitis, and other respiratory tract conditions

Available Dosage Forms
Suspension:
Pyrilafen Tannate-12™: Phenylephrine tannate 5 mg and pyrilamine tannate 30 mg per 5 mL (120 mL, 480 mL) [strawberry-black currant flavor]
Ryna-12 S™: Phenylephrine tannate 5 mg and pyrilamine tannate 30 mg per 5 mL (120 mL) [contains benzoic acid; strawberry-currant flavor]
Ry-T 12: Phenylephrine tannate 5 mg and pyrilamine tannate 30 mg per 5 mL (120 mL, 480 mL)
Viravan®, V-Tann: Phenylephrine tannate 12.5 mg and pyrilamine tannate 30 mg per 5 mL (120 mL, 480 mL) [contains sodium benzoate; grape flavor]
Tablet (Ryna-12™): Phenylephrine tannate 25 mg and pyrilamine tannate 60 mg
Tablet, chewable (Viravan®): Phenylephrine tannate 25 mg and pyrilamine tannate 30 mg [dye free; grape flavor]

Dosing
Adults: Relief of cough, congestion (Viravan®): Oral: 5-10 mL of the suspension or 1-2 tablets every 12 hours
Pediatrics: Relief of cough, congestion (Viravan®): Oral:
Children 2-6 years: 2.5 mL of the suspension or ½ tablet every 12 hours
Children 6-12 years: 5 mL of the suspension or ½ to 1 tablet every 12 hours
Children >12 years: Refer to adult dosing.

Related Information
Phenylephrine *on page 980*

Phenylephrine, Hydrocodone, and Chlorpheniramine
(fen il EF rin, hye droe KOE done, & klor fen IR a meen)

U.S. Brand Names Coughtuss; Cytuss HC; De-Chlor HC; De-Chlor HD; Endagen™-HD; Endal® HD Plus; H-C Tussive; Histinex® HC; Histussin® HC; Hydron CP; Hydro-PC II; Hydro PC II Plus; Maxi-Tuss HC®; Maxi-Tuss HCX; Mintuss HC; Mintuss HD; Mintuss MS; Relacon-HC; Rindal HD Plus; Uni-Tricof HC; Uni-Tuss HC; Vanex-HD®; Z-Cof HC

Synonyms Chlorpheniramine, Phenylephrine, and Hydrocodone; Dihydrocodeine Bitartrate, Phenylephrine Hydrochloride, and Chlorpheniramine Maleate; Hydrocodone, Phenylephrine, and Chlorpheniramine; Phenylephrine Hydrochloride, Hydrocodone Bitartrate, and Chlorpheniramine Maleate

Restrictions C-III

Pharmacologic Category Antihistamine; Antihistamine/Decongestant/Antitussive; Antitussive; Decongestant

Pregnancy Risk Factor C

Lactation See individual agents.

Use Symptomatic relief of cough and congestion associated with the common cold, sinusitis, or acute upper respiratory tract infections

Available Dosage Forms
Liquid: Phenylephrine hydrochloride 5 mg, hydrocodone bitartrate 5 mg, and chlorpheniramine maleate 2 mg per 5 mL (480 mL); phenylephrine hydrochloride 10 mg, hydrocodone bitartrate 2.5 mg, and chlorpheniramine maleate 4 mg per 5 mL (480 mL); phenylephrine hydrochloride 10 mg, hydrocodone bitartrate 5 mg, and chlorpheniramine maleate 2 mg per 5 mL (480 mL)
Coughtuss: Phenylephrine hydrochloride 5 mg, hydrocodone bitartrate 5 mg, and chlorpheniramine maleate 2 mg per 5 mL (480 mL) [alcohol free, sugar free]
De-Chlor HC: Phenylephrine hydrochloride 10 mg, hydrocodone bitartrate 2.5 mg, and chlorpheniramine maleate 2 mg per 5 mL (480 mL) [cherry flavor]
De-Chlor HD: Phenylephrine hydrochloride 10 mg, hydrocodone bitartrate 2.5 mg, and chlorpheniramine maleate 4 mg per 5 mL (480 mL) [cherry flavor]
Endal® HD Plus: Phenylephrine hydrochloride 7.5 mg, hydrocodone bitartrate 3.5 mg, and chlorpheniramine maleate 2 mg per 5 mL (480 mL) [alcohol free, sugar free; black raspberry flavor]
Hydron CP: Phenylephrine hydrochloride 10 mg, hydrocodone bitartrate 5 mg, and chlorpheniramine maleate 2 mg per 5 mL (480 mL) [pineapple-orange flavor]
Hydro PC II Plus: Phenylephrine hydrochloride 7.5 mg, hydrocodone bitartrate 3.5 mg, and chlorpheniramine maleate 2 mg per 5 mL (480 mL) [strawberry flavor]
Maxi-Tuss HCX: Phenylephrine hydrochloride 12 mg, hydrocodone bitartrate 6 mg and chlorpheniramine maleate 2 mg per 5 mL (480 mL) [alcohol free, sugar free; contains aspartame; vanilla bean flavor]
Relacon-HC: Phenylephrine hydrochloride 10 mg, hydrocodone bitartrate 3.5 mg, and chlorpheniramine maleate 2.5 mg per 5 mL (480 mL) [raspberry flavor]
Uni-Tricof HC: Phenylephrine hydrochloride 5 mg, hydrocodone bitartrate 1.67 mg, and chlorpheniramine maleate 2 mg per 5 mL (480 mL) [strawberry flavor]
Vanex-HD®: Phenylephrine hydrochloride 5 mg, hydrocodone bitartrate 1.7 mg, and chlorpheniramine maleate 2 mg per 5 mL (480 mL) [dye free; cherry flavor]
Z-Cof HC: Phenylephrine hydrochloride 10 mg, hydrocodone bitartrate 3.5 mg, and chlorpheniramine maleate 2.5 mg per 5 mL (480 mL) [alcohol free, sugar free; raspberry flavor]
Syrup:
Cytuss HC: Phenylephrine hydrochloride 5 mg, hydrocodone bitartrate 2.5 mg, and chlorpheniramine maleate 2 mg per 5 mL (480 mL) [peach flavor]
Endagen™-HD: Phenylephrine hydrochloride 5 mg, hydrocodone bitartrate 1.7 mg, and chlorpheniramine maleate 2 mg per 5 mL (480 mL) [cherry flavor]
H-C Tussive: Phenylephrine hydrochloride 5 mg, hydrocodone bitartrate 2.5 mg, and chlorpheniramine maleate 2 mg per 5 mL (120 mL, 480 mL, 4000 mL) [orange-pineapple flavor]
Histinex® HC: Phenylephrine hydrochloride 5 mg, hydrocodone bitartrate 2.5 mg, and chlorpheniramine maleate 2 mg per 5 mL (480 mL, 960 mL) [alcohol free, sugar free; contains sodium benzoate]
Histussin® HC: Phenylephrine hydrochloride 5 mg, hydrocodone bitartrate 2.5 mg, and chlorpheniramine maleate 2 mg per 5 mL (480 mL) [alcohol free, sugar free; orange-pineapple flavor]

(Continued)

Phenylephrine, Hydrocodone, and Chlorpheniramine *(Continued)*

Hydro-PC II: Phenylephrine hydrochloride 7.5 mg, hydrocodone bitartrate 2 mg, and chlorpheniramine maleate 2 mg per 5 mL (480 mL) [strawberry flavor]

Maxi-Tuss HC®: Phenylephrine hydrochloride 10 mg, hydrocodone bitartrate 2.5 mg, and chlorpheniramine maleate 4 mg per 5 mL (480 mL) [orange flavor]

Mintuss HC: Phenylephrine hydrochloride 10 mg, hydrocodone bitartrate 2.5 mg, and chlorpheniramine maleate 2 mg per 5 mL (480 mL) [alcohol free; contains sodium benzoate; black cherry flavor]

Mintuss HD: Phenylephrine hydrochloride 10 mg, hydrocodone bitartrate 2.5 mg, and chlorpheniramine maleate 4 mg per 5 mL (480 mL) [alcohol free; contains sodium benzoate; cherry flavor]

Mintuss MS: Phenylephrine hydrochloride 10 mg, hydrocodone bitartrate 5 mg, and chlorpheniramine maleate 2 mg per 5 mL (480 mL) [alcohol free; contains sodium benzoate; orange flavor]

Rindal HD Plus: Phenylephrine hydrochloride 7.5 mg, hydrocodone bitartrate 3.5 mg, and chlorpheniramine maleate 2 mg per 5 mL (480 mL) [alcohol free, sugar free; contains sodium benzoate; black raspberry flavor]

Uni-Tuss HC: Phenylephrine hydrochloride 5 mg, hydrocodone bitartrate 1.67 mg, and chlorpheniramine maleate 2 mg per 5 mL (480 mL) [sugar free; orange flavor]

Dosing

Adults: Cough and congestion: Oral:

Endagen™-HD, Vanex-HD®: 10 mL 3-4 times/day (maximum: 40 mL/24 hours)

Histinex® HC, Cytuss HC, Endal® HD Plus: 10 mL every 4 hours (maximum: 40 mL/24 hours)

Maxi-Tuss HC®, Maxi-Tuss HCX: 5 mL every 4 hours (maximum: 30 mL/24 hours)

Z-Cof HC: 5-10 mL every 4-6 hours (maximum: 40 mL/24 hours)

Pediatrics: Cough and congestion: Oral:

Children 2-6 years: *Z-Cof HC:* 1.25-2.5 mL every 4-6 hours (maximum: 10 mL/24 hours)

Children 6-12 years:

Endagen™-HD, Vanex-HD®: 5 mL 3-4 times/day (maximum: 20 mL/24 hours)

Histinex® HC, Cytuss HC, Endal® HD Plus: 5 mL every 4 hours (maximum: 20 mL/24 hours)

Maxi-Tuss HC®, Maxi-Tuss HCX: 2.5 mL every 4 hours (maximum: 15 mL/24 hours)

Z-Cof HC: 2.5-5 mL every 4-6 hours as needed (maximum: 20 mL/24 hours)

Related Information

Phenylephrine *on page 980*

Phenylephrine, Pyrilamine, and Dextromethorphan

(fen il EF rin, peer IL a meen, & deks troe meth OR fan)

U.S. Brand Names Codal-DM [OTC]; Codimal® DM [OTC]; Codituss DM [OTC]; Viravan®-DM

Synonyms Dextromethorphan Tannate, Pyrilamine Tannate, and Phenylephrine Tannate; Pyrilamine Maleate, Dextromethorphan Hydrobromide, and Phenylephrine Hydrochloride

Pharmacologic Category Antihistamine; Antihistamine/Decongestant/Antitussive; Antitussive; Sympathomimetic

Pregnancy Risk Factor C

Lactation Excretion in breast milk unknown/contraindicated

Use Symptomatic relief of cough, nasal congestion, and discharge associated with the common cold, sinusitis, allergic rhinitis, and other respiratory tract conditions

Available Dosage Forms

Suspension (Viravan®-DM): Phenylephrine tannate 12.5 mg, pyrilamine tannate 30 mg, and dextromethorphan tannate 25 mg per 5 mL (480 mL) [contains sodium benzoate; grape flavor]

Syrup:

Codal-DM: Phenylephrine hydrochloride 5 mg, pyrilamine maleate 8.33 mg, and dextromethorphan hydrobromide 10 mg (480 mL) [cherry flavor]

Codimal® DM: Phenylephrine hydrochloride 5 mg, pyrilamine maleate 8.33 mg, and dextromethorphan hydrobromide 10 mg (120 mL, 480 mL) [alcohol free, dye free, sugar free; contains benzoic acid]

Codituss DM: Phenylephrine hydrochloride 5 mg, pyrilamine maleate 8.33 mg, and dextromethorphan hydrobromide 10 mg (120 mL, 480 mL) [alcohol free, dye free, sugar free; cherry punch flavor]

Tablet, chewable (Viravan®-DM): Phenylephrine tannate 25 mg, pyrilamine tannate 30 mg, and dextromethorphan tannate 25 mg [dye free; grape flavor]

Dosing

Adults: Relief of cough, congestion: Oral:

Codimal® DM: 10 mL every 4 hours; maximum: 60 mL/24 hours

Viravan®-DM: 5-10 mL of the suspension or 1-2 tablets every 12 hours

Pediatrics: Relief of cough, congestion: Oral:

Children 2-6 years (Viravan®-DM): 2.5 mL of the suspension or ½ tablet every 12 hours

Children 6-12 years:

Codimal® DM: 5 mL every 4 hours; maximum: 30 mL/24 hours

Viravan®-DM: 5 mL of the suspension or ½ to 1 tablet every 12 hours

Children >12 years: Refer to adult dosing.

Related Information

Phenylephrine *on page 980*

Phenytoin *(FEN i toyn)*

U.S. Brand Names Dilantin®; Phenytek™

Synonyms Diphenylhydantoin; DPH; Phenytoin Sodium; Phenytoin Sodium, Extended; Phenytoin Sodium, Prompt

Pharmacologic Category Antiarrhythmic Agent, Class Ib; Anticonvulsant, Hydantoin

Medication Safety Issues

Sound-alike/look-alike issues:

Phenytoin may be confused with phenelzine, phentermine

Dilantin® may be confused with Dilaudid®, diltiazem, Dipentum®

Pregnancy Risk Factor D

Lactation Enters breast milk/not recommended (AAP rates "compatible")

Use Management of generalized tonic-clonic (grand mal), complex partial seizures; prevention of seizures following head trauma/neurosurgery

Unlabeled/Investigational Use Ventricular arrhythmias, including those associated with digitalis intoxication, prolonged QT interval and surgical repair of congenital heart diseases in children; epidermolysis bullosa

Mechanism of Action/Effect Stabilizes neuronal membranes and decreases seizure activity by increasing efflux or decreasing influx of sodium ions across cell membranes in the motor cortex during generation of nerve impulses; prolongs effective refractory period and suppresses ventricular pacemaker automaticity, shortens action potential in the heart

Contraindications Hypersensitivity to phenytoin, other hydantoins, or any component of the formulation; pregnancy

Warnings/Precautions May increase frequency of petit mal seizures; I.V. form may cause hypotension, skin necrosis at I.V. site; avoid I.V. administration in small veins; use with caution in patients with porphyria; discontinue if rash or lymphadenopathy occurs; use with caution in patients with hepatic dysfunction, sinus bradycardia, SA block, or AV block; use with caution in elderly or debilitated patients, or in any condition associated with low serum albumin levels, which will increase the free fraction of phenytoin in the serum and, therefore, the pharmacologic response. Sedation, confusional states, or cerebellar dysfunction (loss of motor coordination) may occur at higher total serum concentrations, or at lower total serum concentrations when the free fraction of phenytoin is increased. Abrupt withdrawal may precipitate status epilepticus.

Drug Interactions

Cytochrome P450 Effect: Substrate of CYP2C8/9 (major), 2C19 (major), 3A4 (minor); **Induces** CYP2B6 (strong), 2C8/9 (strong), 2C19 (strong), 3A4 (strong)

Decreased Effect: Phenytoin may enhance the metabolism of estrogen and/or oral contraceptives, decreasing their clinical effect; an alternative method of contraception should be considered. Phenytoin may increase the metabolism of anticonvulsants including barbiturates, carbamazepine, ethosuximide, felbamate, lamotrigine, tiagabine, topiramate, and zonisamide. Valproic acid may increase, decrease, or have no effect on phenytoin serum concentrations. Phenytoin may also decrease the serum concentrations/effects of some antiarrhythmics (disopyramide, propafenone, quinidine, quetiapine) and tricyclic antidepressants may be reduced by phenytoin. Phenytoin may enhance the metabolism of doxycycline, decreasing its clinical effect; higher dosages may be required. Phenytoin may increase the metabolism of chloramphenicol or itraconazole.

Phenytoin may decrease the levels/effects of amiodarone, benzodiazepines, bupropion, calcium channel blockers, carbamazepine, citalopram, clarithromycin, clozapine, cyclosporine, efavirenz, erythromycin, estrogens, fluoxetine, glimepiride, glipizide, losartan, methsuximide, mirtazapine, nateglinide, nefazodone, nevirapine, phenytoin, pioglitazone, promethazine, propranolol, protease inhibitors, proton pump inhibitors, rosiglitazone, selegiline, sertraline, sulfonamides, tacrolimus, venlafaxine, voriconazole, warfarin, zafirlukast, and other CYP2B6, 2C8/9, 2C19, or 3A4 substrates.

The levels/effects of phenytoin may be decreased by aminoglutethimide, carbamazepine, phenobarbital, rifampin, rifapentine, secobarbital, and other CYP2C8/9 or 2C19 inducers. Clozapine and vigabatrin may reduce phenytoin serum concentrations. Ciprofloxacin may decrease serum phenytoin concentrations. Dexamethasone may decrease serum phenytoin concentrations. Replacement of folic acid has been reported to increase the metabolism of phenytoin, decreasing its serum concentrations and/or increasing seizures.

Initially, phenytoin increases the response to warfarin; this is followed by a decrease in response to warfarin. Phenytoin may inhibit the anti-Parkinson effect of levodopa. The duration of neuromuscular blockade from neuromuscular-blocking agents may be decreased by phenytoin. Phenytoin may enhance the metabolism of methadone resulting in methadone withdrawal. Phenytoin may decrease serum levels/effects of digitalis glycosides, theophylline, and thyroid hormones.

Several chemotherapeutic agents have been associated with a decrease in serum phenytoin levels;

includes cisplatin, bleomycin, carmustine, methotrexate, and vinblastine. Enzyme-inducing anticonvulsant therapy may reduce the effectiveness of some chemotherapy regimens (specifically in ALL). Teniposide and methotrexate may be cleared more rapidly in these patients.

Increased Effect/Toxicity: The sedative effects of phenytoin may be additive with other CNS depressants including ethanol, barbiturates, sedatives, antidepressants, narcotic analgesics, and benzodiazepines. Selected anticonvulsants (felbamate, gabapentin, and topiramate) have been reported to increase phenytoin levels/effects. In addition, serum phenytoin concentrations may be increased by allopurinol, amiodarone, calcium channel blockers (including diltiazem and nifedipine), cimetidine, disulfiram, methylphenidate, metronidazole, omeprazole, selective serotonin reuptake inhibitors (SSRIs), ticlopidine, tricyclic antidepressants, trazodone, and trimethoprim.

The levels/effects of phenytoin may be increased by delavirdine, fluconazole, fluvoxamine, gemfibrozil, isoniazid, ketoconazole, nicardipine, NSAIDs, omeprazole, pioglitazone, sulfonamides, ticlopidine, and other CYP2C8/9 or 2C19 inhibitors.

Phenytoin enhances the conversion of primidone to phenobarbital resulting in elevated phenobarbital serum concentrations. Concurrent use of acetazolamide with phenytoin may result in an increased risk of osteomalacia. Concurrent use of phenytoin and lithium has resulted in lithium intoxication. Valproic acid (and sulfisoxazole) may displace phenytoin from binding sites; valproic acid may increase, decrease, or have no effect on phenytoin serum concentrations. Phenytoin transiently increased the response to warfarin initially; this is followed by an inhibition of the hypoprothrombinemic response. Phenytoin may enhance the hepatotoxic potential of acetaminophen overdoses. Concurrent use of dopamine and intravenous phenytoin may lead to an increased risk of hypotension.

Nutritional/Ethanol Interactions

Ethanol:
Acute use: Avoid or limit ethanol (inhibits metabolism of phenytoin). Watch for sedation.
Chronic use: Avoid or limit ethanol (stimulates metabolism of phenytoin).

Food: Phenytoin serum concentrations may be altered if taken with food. If taken with enteral nutrition, phenytoin serum concentrations may be decreased. Tube feedings decrease bioavailability; hold tube feedings 2 hours before and 2 hours after phenytoin administration. May decrease calcium, folic acid, and vitamin D levels.

Herb/Nutraceutical: Avoid evening primrose (seizure threshold decreased). Avoid valerian, St John's wort, kava kava, gotu kola (may increase CNS depression).

Lab Interactions Increased glucose, alkaline phosphatase (S); decreased thyroxine (S), calcium (S)

Adverse Reactions I.V. effects: Hypotension, bradycardia, cardiac arrhythmia, cardiovascular collapse (especially with rapid I.V. use), venous irritation and pain, thrombophlebitis

Effects not related to plasma phenytoin concentrations: Hypertrichosis, gingival hypertrophy, thickening of facial features, carbohydrate intolerance, folic acid deficiency, peripheral neuropathy, vitamin D deficiency, osteomalacia, systemic lupus erythematosus

Concentration-related effects: Nystagmus, blurred vision, diplopia, ataxia, slurred speech, dizziness, drowsiness, lethargy, coma, rash, fever, nausea, vomiting, gum tenderness, confusion, mood changes, folic acid depletion, osteomalacia, hyperglycemia

Related to elevated concentrations:
>20 mcg/mL: Far lateral nystagmus
(Continued)

Phenytoin *(Continued)*

>30 mcg/mL: 45° lateral gaze nystagmus and ataxia
>40 mcg/mL: Decreased mentation
>100 mcg/mL: Death
Cardiovascular: Hypotension, bradycardia, cardiac arrhythmia, cardiovascular collapse
Central nervous system: Psychiatric changes, slurred speech, dizziness, drowsiness, headache, insomnia
Dermatologic: Rash
Gastrointestinal: Constipation, nausea, vomiting, gingival hyperplasia, enlargement of lips
Hematologic: Leukopenia, thrombocytopenia, agranulocytosis
Hepatic: Hepatitis
Local: Thrombophlebitis
Neuromuscular & skeletal: Tremor, peripheral neuropathy, paresthesia
Ocular: Diplopia, nystagmus, blurred vision
Rarely seen effects: SLE-like syndrome, lymphadenopathy, hepatitis, Stevens-Johnson syndrome, blood dyscrasias, dyskinesias, pseudolymphoma, lymphoma, venous irritation and pain, coarsening of the facial features, hypertrichosis

Overdosage/Toxicology Symptoms of overdose include unsteady gait, slurred speech, confusion, nausea, hypothermia, fever, hypotension, respiratory depression, coma. Treatment is symptomatic.

Pharmacodynamics/Kinetics
Onset of Action: I.V.: ~0.5-1 hour
Time to Peak: Serum (form dependent): Oral: Extended-release capsule: 4-12 hours; Immediate release preparation: 2-3 hours
Protein Binding:
Neonates: ≥80% (≤20% free)
Infants: ≥85% (≤15% free)
Adults: 90% to 95%
Others: Decreased protein binding
Disease states resulting in a decrease in serum albumin concentration: Burns, hepatic cirrhosis, nephrotic syndrome, pregnancy, cystic fibrosis
Disease states resulting in an apparent decrease in affinity of phenytoin for serum albumin: Renal failure, jaundice (severe), other drugs (displacers), hyperbilirubinemia (total bilirubin >15 mg/dL), Cl_{cr} <25 mL/minute (unbound fraction is increased two- to threefold in uremia)
Half-Life Elimination: Oral: 22 hours (range: 7-42 hours)
Metabolism: Follows dose-dependent capacity-limited (Michaelis-Menten) pharmacokinetics with increased V_{max} in infants >6 months of age and children versus adults; major metabolite (via oxidation), HPPA, undergoes enterohepatic recirculation
Excretion: Urine (<5% as unchanged drug); as glucuronides
Clearance: Highly variable, dependent upon intrinsic hepatic function and dose administered; increased clearance and decreased serum concentrations with febrile illness

Available Dosage Forms
Capsule, extended release, as sodium: 100 mg
Dilantin®: 30 mg [contains sodium benzoate], 100 mg
Phenytek™: 200 mg, 300 mg
Capsule, prompt release, as sodium: 100 mg
Injection, solution, as sodium: 50 mg/mL (2 mL, 5 mL) [contains alcohol and propylene glycol]
Suspension, oral: 125 mg/5 mL (240 mL)
Dilantin®: 125 mg/5 mL (240 mL) [contains alcohol <0.6%, sodium benzoate; orange vanilla flavor]
Tablet, chewable:
Dilantin®: 50 mg

Dosing
Adults & Elderly:
Status epilepticus: I.V.: Loading dose: Manufacturer recommends 10-15 mg/kg, however, 15-25 mg/kg

has been used clinically; maintenance dose: 300 mg/day or 5-6 mg/kg/day in 3 divided doses or 1-2 divided doses using extended release
Anticonvulsant: Oral: Loading dose: 15-20 mg/kg; based on phenytoin serum concentrations and recent dosing history; administer oral loading dose in 3 divided doses given every 2-4 hours to decrease GI adverse effects and to ensure complete oral absorption; maintenance dose: 300 mg/day or 5-6 mg/kg/day in 3 divided doses or 1-2 divided doses using extended release (range 200-1200 mg/day)

Pediatrics:
Status epilepticus: I.V.:
Infants and Children: Loading dose: 15-20 mg/kg in a single or divided dose; maintenance dose: Initial: 5 mg/kg/day in 2 divided doses, usual doses:
6 months to 3 years: 8-10 mg/kg/day
4-6 years: 7.5-9 mg/kg/day
7-9 years: 7-8 mg/kg/day
10-16 years: 6-7 mg/kg/day, some patients may require every 8 hours dosing
Anticonvulsant: Children: Oral: Refer to adult dosing.

Renal Impairment: Phenytoin level in serum may be difficult to interpret in renal failure. Monitoring of free (unbound) concentrations or adjustment to allow interpretation is recommended.
Hepatic Impairment: Safe in usual doses in mild liver disease; clearance may be substantially reduced in cirrhosis and plasma level monitoring with dose adjustment advisable. Free phenytoin levels should be monitored closely.

Administration
Oral: Suspension: Shake well prior to use. Absorption is impaired when phenytoin suspension is given concurrently to patients who are receiving continuous nasogastric feedings. A method to resolve this interaction is to divide the daily dose of phenytoin and withhold the administration of nutritional supplements for 1-2 hours before and after each phenytoin dose.
I.M.: Although approved for I.M. use, I.M. administration is not recommended due to erratic absorption and pain on injection. Fosphenytoin may be considered.
I.V.: Vesicant. Fosphenytoin may be considered for loading in patients who are in status epilepticus, hemodynamically unstable or develop hypotension/ bradycardia with I.V. administration of phenytoin. Phenytoin may be administered by IVP or IVPB administration. The maximum rate of I.V. administration is 50 mg/minute. Highly sensitive patients (eg, elderly, patients with pre-existing cardiovascular conditions) should receive phenytoin more slowly (eg, 20 mg/minute).
I.V. Detail: An in-line 0.22-5 micron filter is recommended for IVPB solutions due to the high potential for precipitation of the solution. Avoid extravasation. Following I.V. administration, NS should be injected through the same needle or I.V. catheter to prevent irritation.
pH: 10.0-12.3
Other: SubQ administration is not recommended because of the possibility of local tissue damage.

Stability
Reconstitution: I.V.: Further dilution of the solution for I.V. infusion is controversial and no consensus exists as to the optimal concentration and length of stability. Stability is concentration and pH dependent. Based on limited clinical consensus, NS or LR are recommended diluents; dilutions of 1-10 mg/mL have been used and should be administered as soon as possible after preparation (some recommend to discard if not used within 4 hours). Do not refrigerate.
Compatibility: Incompatible with D_5NS, D_5W, fat emulsion 10%, LR, ½NS

Compatibility in syringe: Incompatible with hydromorphone, sufentanil

Compatibility when admixed: Incompatible with amikacin, aminophylline, bretylium, chloramphenicol, dimenhydrinate, diphenhydramine, dobutamine, hydroxyzine, insulin (regular), kanamycin, levorphanol, lidocaine, lincomycin, meperidine, metaraminol, morphine, nitroglycerin, norepinephrine, penicillin G potassium, pentobarbital, phenobarbital, phenylephrine, phytonadione, procainamide, procaine, prochlorperazine edisylate, promazine, promethazine, streptomycin, vancomycin, vitamin B complex with C

Storage:

Capsule, tablet: Store below 30°C (86°F); protect from light and moisture

Oral suspension: Store at room temperature of 20°C to 25°C (68°F to 77°F); protect from freezing and light.

Solution for injection: Store at room temperature of 15°C to 30°C (59°F to 86°F); use only clear solutions free of precipitate and haziness, slightly yellow solutions may be used. Precipitation may occur if solution is refrigerated and may dissolve at room temperature.

Laboratory Monitoring Plasma phenytoin level, CBC, liver function. **Note:** Serum phenytoin concentrations should be interpreted in terms of the unbound concentration. Adjustment should be made in patients with renal impairment and/or hypoalbuminemia.

Nursing Actions

Physical Assessment: Assess potential for interactions with other prescriptions, OTC medications, or herbal products patient may be taking. Monitor laboratory tests, therapeutic effectiveness (according to rationale for use), and adverse response when beginning therapy and at regular intervals during treatment. When oral phenytoin is discontinued, dose should be tapered gradually; abrupt discontinuance can cause status epilepticus. Teach patient proper use (oral), side effects/appropriate interventions, and adverse symptoms to report. **I.V.:** Monitor blood pressure. Monitor infusion site closely to prevent extravasation (vesicant, alkaline irritation). Monitor patient closely for adverse/toxic results (eg, cardiorespiratory and CNS status).

Patient Education: Do not take any new medication during therapy without consulting prescriber. Take exactly as directed, preferably on an empty stomach. Do not alter dose or discontinue without consulting prescriber. Do not crush, break, or chew extended release capsules. Shake liquid suspension well before using. Follow recommended diet, avoid alcohol, and maintain adequate hydration (2-3 L/day of fluids) unless instructed to restrict fluid intake. May cause gum or mouth soreness (use good oral hygiene and have frequent dental exams); drowsiness, dizziness, nervousness, or headache (use caution when driving or engaging in tasks that require alertness until response to drug is known); or nausea or vomiting (small frequent meals, frequent mouth care, chewing gum, or sucking lozenges may help). Report chest pain, irregular heartbeat, or palpitations; slurred speech, unsteady gait, coordination difficulties, or change in mentation; skin rash; unresolved nausea, vomiting, or constipation; swollen glands; swollen, sore, or bleeding gums; unusual bruising or bleeding; acute persistent fatigue; vision changes; or other persistent adverse effects. **Pregnancy/breast-feeding precautions:** Do not get pregnant; use contraceptive measures to prevent possible harm to the fetus (effectiveness of oral contraceptives may be affected by phenytoin). Consult prescriber if breast-feeding.

Dietary Considerations

Folic acid: Phenytoin may decrease mucosal uptake of folic acid; to avoid folic acid deficiency and megaloblastic anemia, some clinicians recommend giving patients on anticonvulsants prophylactic doses of folic acid and cyanocobalamin. However, folate supplementation may increase seizures in some patients (dose dependent). Discuss with healthcare provider prior to using any supplements.

Calcium: Hypocalcemia has been reported in patients taking prolonged high-dose therapy with an anticonvulsant. Some clinicians have given an additional 4000 units/week of vitamin D (especially in those receiving poor nutrition and getting no sun exposure) to prevent hypocalcemia.

Vitamin D: Phenytoin interferes with vitamin D metabolism and osteomalacia may result; may need to supplement with vitamin D

Tube feedings: Tube feedings decrease phenytoin absorption. To avoid decreased serum levels with continuous NG feeds, hold feedings for 2 hours prior to and 2 hours after phenytoin administration, if possible. There is a variety of opinions on how to administer phenytoin with enteral feedings. Be **consistent** throughout therapy.

Sodium content of 1 g injection: 88 mg (3.8 mEq)

Geriatric Considerations Elderly may have low albumin which will increase free fraction and increase drug response. Monitor closely in those who are hypoalbuminemic. Free fraction measurements advised, also elderly may display a higher incidence of adverse effects (cardiovascular) when using the I.V. loading regimen; therefore, recommended to decrease loading I.V. dose to 25 mg/minute (see Warnings/Precautions).

Breast-Feeding Issues Phenytoin is excreted in breast milk; however, the amount to which the infant is exposed is considered small. The manufacturers of phenytoin do not recommend breast-feeding during therapy, however, the AAP considers it to be usually compatible. Women should be counseled of the possible risks and benefits associated with breast-feeding while on phenytoin.

Pregnancy Issues Phenytoin crosses the placenta. Congenital malformations (including a pattern of malformations termed the "fetal hydantoin syndrome" or "fetal anticonvulsant syndrome") have been reported in infants. Isolated cases of malignancies (including neuroblastoma) and coagulation defects in the neonate following delivery have also been reported. Epilepsy itself, the number of medications, genetic factors, or a combination of these probably influence the teratogenicity of anticonvulsant therapy.

Total plasma concentrations of phenytoin are decreased by 56% in the mother during pregnancy; unbound plasma (free) concentrations are decreased by 31%. Because protein binding is decreased, monitoring of unbound plasma concentrations is recommended. Concentrations should be monitored through the 8th week postpartum. The use of folic acid throughout pregnancy and vitamin K during the last month of pregnancy is recommended.

A pregnancy registry is available for women exposed to antiepileptic drug (including phenytoin) at the Genetics and Teratology Unit Massachusetts General Hospital, 1-888-233-2334.

Related Information

Peak and Trough Guidelines *on page 1387*

Physostigmine (fye zoe STIG meen)

Synonyms Eserine Salicylate; Physostigmine Salicylate; Physostigmine Sulfate

Pharmacologic Category Acetylcholinesterase Inhibitor

Medication Safety Issues
Sound-alike/look-alike issues:
Physostigmine may be confused with Prostigmin®, pyridostigmine

Pregnancy Risk Factor C

Lactation Excretion in breast milk unknown

Use Reverse toxic CNS effects caused by anticholinergic drugs

Mechanism of Action/Effect Inhibits destruction of acetylcholine by acetylcholinesterase which facilitates transmission of impulses across myoneural junction and prolongs the central and peripheral effects of acetylcholine

Contraindications Hypersensitivity to physostigmine or any component of the formulation; GI or GU obstruction; physostigmine therapy of drug intoxications should be used with extreme caution in patients with asthma, gangrene, severe cardiovascular disease, or mechanical obstruction of the GI tract or urogenital tract. In these patients, physostigmine should be used only to treat life-threatening conditions.

Warnings/Precautions Use with caution in patients with epilepsy, asthma, diabetes, gangrene, cardiovascular disease, bradycardia. Discontinue if excessive salivation or emesis, frequent urination or diarrhea occur. Reduce dosage if excessive sweating or nausea occurs. Administer I.V. slowly or at a controlled rate not faster than 1 mg/minute. Due to the possibility of hypersensitivity or overdose/cholinergic effect, atropine should be readily available; not intended as a first-line agent for anticholinergic toxicity or Parkinson's disease.

Drug Interactions
Increased Effect/Toxicity: Increased toxicity with bethanechol, methacholine. Succinylcholine may increase neuromuscular blockade with systemic administration.

Lab Interactions Increased aminotransferase [ALT (SGPT)/AST (SGOT)] (S), amylase (S)

Adverse Reactions Frequency not defined.
Cardiovascular: Palpitations, bradycardia
Central nervous system: Restlessness, nervousness, hallucinations, seizure
Gastrointestinal: Nausea, salivation, diarrhea, stomach pain
Genitourinary: Frequent urge to urinate
Neuromuscular & skeletal: Muscle twitching
Ocular: Lacrimation, miosis
Respiratory: Dyspnea, bronchospasm, respiratory paralysis, pulmonary edema
Miscellaneous: Diaphoresis

Overdosage/Toxicology Symptoms of overdose include muscle weakness, blurred vision, excessive sweating, tearing and salivation, nausea, vomiting, bronchospasm, and seizures. If physostigmine is used in excess or in the absence of an anticholinergic overdose, patients may manifest signs of cholinergic toxicity. At this point, an anticholinergic agent (eg, atropine 0.015-0.05 mg/kg) may be necessary.

Pharmacodynamics/Kinetics
Onset of Action: ~5 minutes
Duration of Action: 0.5-5 hours
Half-Life Elimination: 15-40 minutes
Metabolism: Hepatic and via hydrolysis by cholinesterases

Available Dosage Forms Injection, solution, as salicylate: 1 mg/mL (2 mL) [contains benzyl alcohol and sodium metabisulfite]

Dosing
Adults & Elderly:
Anticholinergic drug overdose:
I.M., I.V., SubQ: 0.5-2 mg to start; repeat every 20 minutes until response occurs or adverse effect occurs.

Repeat 1-4 mg every 30-60 minutes as life-threatening signs (arrhythmias, seizures, deep coma) recur; maximum I.V. rate: 1 mg/minute.

Pediatrics: Anticholinergic drug overdose (Reserve for life-threatening situations only): children: I.V.: 0.01-0.03 mg/kg/dose (maximum: 0.5 mg/minute). May repeat after 5-10 minutes to a maximum total dose of 2 mg or until response occurs or adverse cholinergic effects occur,

Administration
I.V.: Infuse slowly I.V. at a maximum rate of 0.5 mg/minute in children or 1 mg/minute in adults. Too rapid administration (I.V. rate not to exceed 1 mg/minute) can cause bradycardia, hypersalivation leading to respiratory difficulties and seizures.

Stability
Compatibility: Stable in dextran 6% in dextrose, dextran 6% in NS, D5W, D10W, D5LR, D5¼NS, D5½NS, D5NS, fat emulsion 10%, LR, ½NS, NS

Y-site administration: Incompatible with dobutamine

Compatibility when admixed: Incompatible with phenytoin, ranitidine

Storage: Do not use solution if cloudy or dark brown.

Nursing Actions
Physical Assessment: When used to reverse neuromuscular block (anesthesia or acetylcholine toxicity), monitor patient safety until full return of neuromuscular functioning. Assess bladder and sphincter adequacy prior to administering medication. Assess other medications patient may be taking for effectiveness and interactions. Monitor therapeutic effectiveness and adverse reactions: cholinergic crisis (DUMBELS - diarrhea, urination, miosis, bronchospasm/bradycardia, excitability, lacrimation, and salivation/excessive sweating). Assess knowledge/teach patient appropriate use of ophthalmic forms, interventions to reduce side effects, and adverse symptoms to report.

Patient Education: Maintain adequate hydration (2-3 L/day of fluids) unless instructed to restrict fluid intake. May cause dizziness, drowsiness, or hypotension (rise slowly from sitting or lying position and use caution when driving or climbing stairs); vomiting or loss of appetite (small frequent meals, frequent mouth care, chewing gum, or sucking lozenges may help); or diarrhea (boiled milk, yogurt, or buttermilk may help). Report persistent abdominal discomfort; significantly increased salivation, sweating, tearing, or urination; flushed skin; chest pain or palpitations; acute headache; unresolved diarrhea; excessive fatigue, insomnia, dizziness, or depression; increased muscle, joint, or body pain; vision changes or blurred vision; or shortness of breath or wheezing. **Pregnancy/breast-feeding precautions:** Inform prescriber if you are or intend to become pregnant. Consult prescriber if breast-feeding.

Geriatric Considerations Studies on the use of physostigmine in Alzheimer's disease have reported variable results. Doses generally were in the range of 2-4 mg 4 times/day. Limitations to the use of physostigmine include a short half-life requiring frequent dosing, variable absorption from the GI tract, and no commercially available oral product; therefore, not recommended for treatment of Alzheimer's disease.

Phytonadione (fye toe na DYE one)

U.S. Brand Names Mephyton®

Synonyms Methylphytyl Napthoquinone; Phylloquinone; Phytomenadione; Vitamin K_1

Pharmacologic Category Vitamin, Fat Soluble

Medication Safety Issues

Sound-alike/look-alike issues:

Mephyton® may be confused with melphalan, methadone

Pregnancy Risk Factor C

Lactation Enters breast milk/use caution (APP rates "compatible")

Use Prevention and treatment of hypoprothrombinemia caused by coumarin derivative-induced or other drug-induced vitamin K deficiency, hypoprothrombinemia caused by malabsorption or inability to synthesize vitamin K; hemorrhagic disease of the newborn

Mechanism of Action/Effect Promotes liver synthesis of clotting factors (II, VII, IX, X); however, the exact mechanism as to this stimulation is unknown. Menadiol is a water soluble form of vitamin K; phytonadione has a more rapid and prolonged effect than menadione; menadiol sodium diphosphate (K_4) is half as potent as menadione (K_3).

Contraindications Hypersensitivity to phytonadione or any component of the formulation

Warnings/Precautions Severe reactions resembling hypersensitivity (eg, anaphylaxis) reactions have occurred rarely during or immediately after I.V. administration. Allergic reactions have also occurred with I.M. and SubQ injections; oral administration is the safest. In obstructive jaundice or with biliary fistulas concurrent administration of bile salts is necessary. Manufacturers recommend the SubQ route over other parenteral routes. SubQ is less predictable when compared to the oral route. The American College of Chest Physicians recommends the I.V. route in patients with serious or life-threatening bleeding secondary to warfarin. The I.V. route should be restricted to emergency situations where oral phytonadione cannot be used. Efficacy is delayed regardless of route of administration; patient management may require other treatments in the interim. Administer a dose that will quickly lower the INR into a safe range without causing resistance to warfarin. Use caution in newborns especially premature infants; hemolysis, jaundice and hyperbilirubinemia have been reported with larger than recommended doses. Some dosage forms contain benzyl alcohol. In liver disease, if initial doses do not reverse coagulopathy then higher doses are unlikely to have any effect. Ineffective in hereditary hypoprothrombinemia. Use caution with renal dysfunction (including premature infants). Injectable products may contain aluminum.

Drug Interactions

Decreased Effect:

Phytonadione may diminish the anticoagulant effect of coumarin derivatives (monitor INR). Phytonadione (oral) may not be properly absorbed when administered concurrently with orlistat (separate doses by at least 2 hours).

Adverse Reactions Parenteral administration: Frequency not defined.

Cardiovascular: Cyanosis, flushing, hypotension

Central nervous system: Dizziness

Dermatologic: Scleroderma-like lesions

Endocrine & metabolic: Hyperbilirubinemia (newborn; greater than recommended doses)

Gastrointestinal: Abnormal taste

Local: Injection site reactions

Respiratory: Dyspnea

Miscellaneous: Anaphylactoid reactions, diaphoresis, hypersensitivity reactions

Pharmacodynamics/Kinetics

Onset of Action:

Onset of action: Increased coagulation factors: Oral: 6-10 hours; I.V.: 1-2 hours

Peak effect: INR values return to normal: Oral: 24-48 hours; I.V.: 12-14 hours

Metabolism: Rapidly hepatic

Excretion: Urine and feces

Available Dosage Forms

Injection, aqueous colloidal: 2 mg/mL (0.5 mL); 10 mg/mL (1 mL) [contains benzyl alcohol]

Tablet: 5 mg

Dosing

Adults & Elderly:

Adequate intake: Males: 120 mcg/day; Females: 90 mcg/day

Hypoprothrombinemia due to drugs (other than coumarin derivatives) or factors limiting absorption or synthesis: Oral, SubQ, I.M., I.V.: Initial: 2.5-25 mg (rarely up to 50 mg)

Vitamin K deficiency secondary to coumarin derivative: See table on next page.

Pediatrics:

Adequate intake:

1-3 years: 30 mcg/day

4-8 years: 55 mcg/day

9-13 years: 60 mcg/day

14-18 years: 75 mcg/day

Hemorrhagic disease of the newborn:

Prophylaxis: I.M.: 0.5-1 mg within 1 hour of birth

Treatment: I.M., SubQ: 1 mg/dose/day; higher doses may be necessary if mother has been receiving oral anticoagulants

Administration

Oral: The parenteral preparation has been administered orally to neonates.

I.V.: Infuse slowly; rate of infusion should not exceed 1 mg/minute. The injectable route should be used only if the oral route is not feasible or there is a greater urgency to reverse anticoagulation.

I.V. Detail: pH: 3.5-7.0

Stability

Reconstitution: Dilute injection solution in preservative-free NS, D_5W, or D_5NS.

Storage:

Injection: Store at 15°C to 30°C (59°F to 86°F). **Note:** Store Hospira product at 20°C to 25°C (68°F to 77°F).

Oral: Store tablets at 15°C to 30°C (59°F to 86°F); protect from light.

Laboratory Monitoring PT, INR

Nursing Actions

Physical Assessment: Note dosing specifics according to purpose for use. Monitor laboratory tests and patient response (degree of bleeding). Teach patient proper use, possible side effects/appropriate interventions, and adverse symptoms to report.

Patient Education: Do not take any new medication during therapy (especially any aspirin-containing products or NSAIDs) without consulting prescriber. Oral: Take only as directed; do not take more or more often than prescribed. Consult prescriber for recommended diet. Report bleeding gums; blood in urine, stool, or vomitus; unusual bruising or bleeding; or abdominal cramping. **Pregnancy/breast-feeding precautions:** Inform prescriber if you are or intend to become pregnant. Consult prescriber if breast-feeding.

Management of Elevated INR

INR	Symptom	Action
Above therapeutic range to <5	No significant bleeding	Lower or hold the next dose and monitor frequently; when INR approaches desired range, may resume dosing with a lower dose if INR was significantly above therapeutic range.
≥5 and <9	No significant bleeding	Omit the next 1or 2 doses; monitor INR and resume with a lower dose when the INR approaches the desired range.
		Alternatively, if there are other risk factors for bleeding, omit the next dose and give vitamin K₁ orally ≤5 mg; resume with a lower dose when the INR approaches the desired range.
		If rapid reversal is required for surgery, then given vitamin K₁ orally 2-4 mg and hold warfarin. Expect a response within 24 hours; another 1-2 mg may be given orally if needed.
≥9	No significant bleeding	Hold warfarin, give vitamin K₁ orally 5-10 mg, expect the INR to be reduced within 24-48 hours; monitor INR and administer additional K if necessary. Resume warfarin at lower doses when INR is in the desired range.
Any INR elevation	Serious bleeding	Hold warfarin, give vitamin K₁ (10 mg by slow I.V. infusion), and supplement with fresh plasma transfusion or prothrombin complex concentrate (Factor X complex); recombinant factor VIIa is an alternative to prothrombin complex concentrate. Vitamin K₁ injection can be repeated every 12 hours.
Any INR elevation	Life-threatening bleeding	Hold warfarin, give prothrombin complex concentrate, supplemented with vitamin K₁ (10 mg by slow I.V. infusion); repeat if necessary. Recombinant factor VIIa is an alternative to prothrombin complex concentrate.

Note: Use of high doses of vitamin K₁ (10-15 mg) may cause resistance to warfarin for up to a week. Heparin or low molecular weight heparin can be given until the patient becomes responsive to warfarin. **Reference:** Ansell J, Hirsh J, Poller L et al. "The Pharmacology and Management of the Vitamin K Antagonists", *Chest*, 2004, 126 (3 Suppl):204-33.

Pilocarpine (pye loe KAR peen)

U.S. Brand Names Isopto® Carpine; Pilopine HS®; Salagen®
Synonyms Pilocarpine Hydrochloride
Pharmacologic Category Cholinergic Agonist; Ophthalmic Agent, Antiglaucoma; Ophthalmic Agent, Miotic
Medication Safety Issues
Sound-alike/look-alike issues:
Isopto® Carpine may be confused with Isopto® Carbachol
Salagen® may be confused with Salacid®, selegiline
Pregnancy Risk Factor C
Lactation Excretion in breast milk unknown/not recommended
Use
Ophthalmic: Management of chronic simple glaucoma, chronic and acute angle-closure glaucoma
Oral: Symptomatic treatment of xerostomia caused by salivary gland hypofunction resulting from radiotherapy for cancer of the head and neck or Sjögren's syndrome
Unlabeled/Investigational Use Counter effects of cycloplegics
Mechanism of Action/Effect Directly stimulates cholinergic receptors in the eye causing miosis (by contraction of the iris sphincter), loss of accommodation (by constriction of ciliary muscle), and lowering of intraocular pressure (with decreased resistance to aqueous humor outflow)
Contraindications Hypersensitivity to pilocarpine or any component of the formulation; acute inflammatory disease of the anterior chamber of the eye; in addition, tablets are also contraindicated in patients with uncontrolled asthma, angle-closure glaucoma, severe hepatic impairment

Warnings/Precautions Use caution with cardiovascular disease; patients may have difficulty compensating for transient changes in hemodynamics or rhythm induced by pilocarpine.

Ophthalmic products: May cause decreased visual acuity, especially at night or with reduced lighting.

Oral tablets: Use caution with controlled asthma, chronic bronchitis or COPD; may increase airway resistance, bronchial smooth muscle tone, and bronchial secretions. Use caution with cholelithiasis, biliary tract disease, nephrolithiasis; adjust dose with moderate hepatic impairment.

Drug Interactions
Cytochrome P450 Effect: Inhibits CYP2A6 (weak), 2E1 (weak), 3A4 (weak)
Decreased Effect: May decrease effects of anticholinergic drugs (atropine, ipratropium).
Increased Effect/Toxicity: Concurrent use with beta-blockers may cause conduction disturbances.

Nutritional/Ethanol Interactions Food: Avoid administering oral formulation with high-fat meal; fat decreases the rate of absorption, maximum concentration and increases the time it takes to reach maximum concentration.

Adverse Reactions
Ophthalmic: Frequency not defined:
Cardiovascular: Hypertension, tachycardia
Gastrointestinal: Diarrhea, nausea, salivation, vomiting
Ocular: Burning, ciliary spasm, conjunctival vascular congestion, corneal granularity (gel 10%), lacrimation, lens opacity, myopia, retinal detachment, supraorbital or temporal headache, visual acuity decreased
Respiratory: Bronchial spasm, pulmonary edema
Miscellaneous: Diaphoresis

Oral (frequency varies by indication and dose):
>10%:
  Cardiovascular: Flushing (8% to 13%)
  Central nervous system: Chills (3% to 15%), dizziness (5% to 12%), headache (11%)
  Gastrointestinal: Nausea (6% to 15%)
  Genitourinary: Urinary frequency (9% to 12%)
  Neuromuscular & skeletal: Weakness (2% to 12%)
  Respiratory: Rhinitis (5% to 14%)
  Miscellaneous: Diaphoresis (29% to 68%)
1% to 10%:
  Cardiovascular: Edema (<1% to 5%), facial edema, hypertension (3%), palpitation, tachycardia
  Central nervous system: Pain (4%), fever, somnolence
  Dermatologic: Pruritus, rash
  Gastrointestinal: Diarrhea (4% to 7%), dyspepsia (7%), vomiting (3% to 4%), constipation, flatulence, glossitis, salivation increased, stomatitis, taste perversion
  Genitourinary: Vaginitis, urinary incontinence
  Neuromuscular & skeletal: Myalgias, tremor
  Ocular: Lacrimation (6%), amblyopia (4%), abnormal vision, blurred vision, conjunctivitis
  Otic: Tinnitus
  Respiratory: Cough increased, dysphagia, epistaxis, sinusitis
  Miscellaneous: Allergic reaction, voice alteration

Overdosage/Toxicology Symptoms of overdose include bronchospasm, bradycardia, involuntary urination, vomiting, hypotension, and tremor. Atropine is the treatment of choice for intoxications manifesting with significant muscarinic symptoms. Atropine I.V. 2-4 mg every 3-60 minutes should be repeated to control symptoms and then continued as needed for 1-2 days following acute ingestion. Epinephrine 0.1-1 mg SubQ may be useful for reversing severe cardiovascular or pulmonary sequelae.

Pharmacodynamics/Kinetics
Onset of Action:
  Ophthalmic: Miosis: 10-30 minutes; Intraocular pressure reduction: 1 hour
  Oral: 20 minutes
Duration of Action:
  Ophthalmic: Miosis: 4-8 hours; Intraocular pressure reduction: 4-12 hours
  Oral: 3-5 hours
Half-Life Elimination: Oral: 0.76-1.35 hours; increased with hepatic impairment
Excretion: Urine

Available Dosage Forms
Gel, ophthalmic, as hydrochloride (Pilopine HS®): 4% (4 g) [contains benzalkonium chloride]
Solution, ophthalmic, as hydrochloride: 0.5% (15 mL); 1% (2 mL, 15 mL); 2% (2 mL, 15 mL); 3% (15 mL); 4% (2 mL, 15 mL); 6% (15 mL) [may contain benzalkonium chloride]
  Isopto® Carpine: 1% (15 mL); 2% (15 mL); 4% (15 mL) [contains benzalkonium chloride]
Tablet, as hydrochloride: 5 mg
Salagen®: 5 mg, 7.5 mg

Dosing
Adults & Elderly:
Glaucoma: Ophthalmic
  Solution: Instill 1-2 drops up to 6 times/day; adjust the concentration and frequency as required to control elevated intraocular pressure.
  Gel: Instill 0.5" ribbon into lower conjunctival sac once daily at bedtime.
To counteract the mydriatic effects of sympathomimetic agents (unlabeled use): Ophthalmic solution: Instill 1 drop of a 1% solution in the affected eye.

Xerostomia: Oral:
  Following head and neck cancer: 5 mg 3 times/day, titration up to 10 mg 3 times/day may be considered for patients who have not responded adequately; do not exceed 2 tablets/dose
  Sjögren's syndrome: 5 mg 4 times/day
Hepatic Impairment: Oral: Patients with moderate impairment: 5 mg 2 times/day regardless of indication; adjust dose based on response and tolerability. Do not use with severe impairment (Child-Pugh score 10-15)

Administration
Oral: Avoid administering with high-fat meal. Fat decreases the rate of absorption, maximum concentration, and increases the time it takes to reach maximum concentration.
Other: Ophthalmic: If both solution and gel are used, the solution should be applied first, then the gel at least 5 minutes later. Following administration of the solution, finger pressure should be applied on the lacrimal sac for 1-2 minutes.

Stability
Storage:
  Gel: Store at room temperature of 2°C to 27°C (36°F to 80°F). Do not freeze; avoid excessive heat.
  Tablets: Store at controlled room temperature of 15°C to 30°C (59°F to 86°F).

Nursing Actions
Physical Assessment: Monitor for adverse effects and response to treatment. Monitor results of intraocular pressure testing and visual field testing on a periodic basis. Teach patient appropriate administration of ophthalmic solution.
Patient Education: Use as often as recommended. Avoid taking oral medication with a high fat meal.

Ophthalmic: Wash hands before using. Do not let tip of applicator touch eye; do not contaminate tip of applicator (may cause eye infection, eye damage, or vision loss). Sit or lie down. Open eye, look at ceiling, and instill prescribed amount of solution. Do not blink for 30 seconds, close eye and roll eye in all directions, and apply gentle pressure to inner corner of eye for 1-2 minutes. Temporary stinging or blurred vision may occur. You may experience altered dark adaptation; use caution when driving at night or in poorly lit environments. Report persistent pain, redness, burning, double vision, or severe headache. **Pregnancy/breast-feeding precautions:** Inform prescriber if you are pregnant. Breast-feeding is not recommended
Geriatric Considerations Assure the patient or a caregiver can adequately administer ophthalmic medication dosage form.

Pimecrolimus (pim e KROE li mus)

U.S. Brand Names Elidel®

Restrictions An FDA-approved medication guide is available at http://www.fda.gov/cder/Offices/ODS/labeling.htm; distribute to each patient to whom this medication is dispensed.

Pharmacologic Category Immunosuppressant Agent; Topical Skin Product

Pregnancy Risk Factor C

Lactation Excretion in breast milk unknown/not recommended

Use Short-term and intermittent long-term treatment of mild to moderate atopic dermatitis in patients not responsive to conventional therapy or when conventional therapy is not appropriate

Mechanism of Action/Effect Inhibits T cell activation by blocking proinflammatory cytokine secretion.
(Continued)

Pimecrolimus (Continued)

Contraindications Hypersensitivity to pimecrolimus or any component of the formulation; Netherton's syndrome

Warnings/Precautions Topical calcineurin inhibitors have been associated with rare cases of malignancy. Avoid use on malignant or premalignant skin conditions (eg, cutaneous T-cell lymphoma). Topical calcineurin agents are considered second-line therapies in the treatment of atopic dermatitis/eczema, and should be limited to use in patients who have failed treatment with other therapies. They should be used for short-term and intermittent treatment using the minimum amount necessary for the control of symptoms should be used. Application should be limited to involved areas. Safety of intermittent use for >1 year has not been established.

Should not be used in immunocompromised patients. Do not apply to areas of active viral infection; infections at the treatment site should be cleared prior to therapy. Patients with atopic dermatitis are predisposed to skin infections, and tacrolimus therapy has been associated with risk of developing eczema herpeticum, varicella zoster, and herpes simplex. May be associated with development of lymphadenopathy; possible infectious causes should be investigated. Discontinue use in patients with unknown cause of lymphadenopathy or acute infectious mononucleosis. Not recommended for use in patients with skin disease which may increase systemic absorption (eg, Netherton's syndrome). Avoid artificial or natural sunlight exposure, even when Elidel® is not on the skin. Safety not established in patients with generalized erythroderma. The use of Elidel® in children <2 years of age is not recommended, particularly since the effect on immune system development is unknown.

Drug Interactions
Cytochrome P450 Effect: Substrate of CYP3A4 (minor)

Increased Effect/Toxicity: CYP3A inhibitors may increase pimecrolimus levels in patients where increased absorption expected.

Adverse Reactions
>10%:
Central nervous system: Headache (7% to 25%), pyrexia (1% to 13%)
Local: Burning at application site (2% to 26%; tends to resolve/improve as lesions resolve)
Respiratory: Nasopharyngitis (8% to 27%), cough (2% to 16%), upper respiratory tract infection (4% to 19%), bronchitis (0.4% to 11%)
Miscellaneous: Influenza (3% to 13%)
1% to 10%:
Dermatologic: Skin papilloma (warts) (up to 3%), molluscum contagiosum (0.7% to 2%), herpes simplex dermatitis (up to 2%)
Gastrointestinal: Diarrhea (0.6% to 8%), constipation (up to 4%)
Local: Irritation at application site (0.4% to 6%), erythema at application site (0.4% to 2%), pruritus at application site (0.6% to 6%)
Ocular: Eye infection (up to 1%)
Otic: Ear infection (0.6% to 6%)
Respiratory: Pharyngitis (0.7% to 8%), sinusitis (0.6% to 3%), nasal congestion (0.6% to 3%)
Miscellaneous: Viral infection (up to 7%), herpes simplex infection (0.4% to 4%), tonsillitis (0.4% to 6%)

Overdosage/Toxicology No experience with overdose reported.

Available Dosage Forms Cream, topical: 1% (30 g, 60 g, 100 g)

Dosing
Adults & Elderly:
Mild to moderate atopic dermatitis: Topical: Apply thin layer to affected area twice daily; rub in gently and completely. **Note:** Limit application to involved

areas. Continue as long as signs and symptoms persist; discontinue if resolution occurs; re-evaluate if symptoms persist >6 weeks.
Pediatrics: Children ≥2 years: Topical: Refer to adult dosing.

Administration
Topical: Do not use with occlusive dressings. Burning at the application site is most common in first few days; improves as atopic dermatitis improves. Limit application to areas of involvement. Continue as long as signs and symptoms persist; discontinue if resolution occurs; re-evaluate if symptoms persist >6 weeks.

Stability
Storage: Store at 25°C (77°F); excursions permitted to 15°C to 30°C (59°F to 86°F). Do not freeze.

Nursing Actions
Physical Assessment: Assess knowledge/teach patient appropriate use, interventions to reduce side effects, and adverse symptoms to report.

Patient Education: This medication is for external use only. Do not use for any skin disorder except that for which it was prescribed. Avoid getting any medication in or close to eyes. Apply as often as directed by prescriber, in thin film to affected area. Do not cover with bandages or occlusive dressings. Wash and dry hands thoroughly before applying. Wash hands thoroughly after applying (if affected area is not on hands). Avoid artificial or natural sunlight even when drug not applied to skin. Discontinue therapy after signs and symptoms have disappeared; restart treatment at first sign of recurrence. You may experience burning at site of application, this will usually last less than 5 days, and go away as skin condition improves. You may experience headache, fever, cough, nasal or throat irritation, flu-like symptoms, diarrhea, or constipation; contact prescriber if these persist. Contact prescriber if skin condition worsens or if symptoms persist longer than 6 weeks. **Pregnancy/breast-feeding precautions:** Inform prescriber if you are or intend to become pregnant. Breast-feeding is not recommended.

Pimozide (PI moe zide)

U.S. Brand Names Orap®
Pharmacologic Category Antipsychotic Agent, Typical
Pregnancy Risk Factor C
Lactation Excretion in breast milk unknown
Use Suppression of severe motor and phonic tics in patients with Tourette's disorder who have failed to respond satisfactorily to standard treatment
Unlabeled/Investigational Use Psychosis; reported use in individuals with delusions focused on physical symptoms (ie, preoccupation with parasitic infestation); Huntington's chorea
Mechanism of Action/Effect Pimozide, a diphenylbutylperidine antipsychotic, is a potent centrally-acting dopamine-receptor antagonist resulting in its characteristic neuroleptic effects
Contraindications Hypersensitivity to pimozide or any component of the formulation; severe CNS depression; coma; history of dysrhythmia; prolonged QT syndrome; concurrent use with QT$_c$-prolonging agents; hypokalemia or hypomagnesemia; concurrent use of drugs that are inhibitors of CYP3A4, including concurrent use of azole antifungals, fluvoxamine, macrolide antibiotics (such as clarithromycin or erythromycin), mesoridazine, nefazodone, protease inhibitors (ie, atazanavir, indinavir, nelfinavir, ritonavir, saquinavir), sertraline, thioridazine, zileuton, and ziprasidone; simple tics other than Tourette's
Warnings/Precautions May cause hypotension, use with caution in patients with autonomic instability.

Moderately sedating, use with caution in disorders where CNS depression is a feature. Use with caution in Parkinson's disease. Caution in patients with hemodynamic instability; bone marrow suppression; predisposition to seizures; subcortical brain damage; severe cardiac, hepatic, renal, or respiratory disease. Esophageal dysmotility and aspiration have been associated with antipsychotic use - use with caution in patients at risk of pneumonia (ie, Alzheimer's disease). Caution in breast cancer or other prolactin-dependent tumors (may elevate prolactin levels). May alter temperature regulation or mask toxicity of other drugs due to antiemetic effects. May alter cardiac conduction - life-threatening arrhythmias have occurred with high doses (>10 mg). May prolong QT interval predisposing patients to ventricular arrhythmias. Monitor ECG at baseline and periodically during dosage titration. May cause orthostatic hypotension - use with caution in patients at risk of this effect or those who would tolerate transient hypotensive episodes (cerebrovascular disease, cardiovascular disease, or other medications which may predispose).

May cause anticholinergic effects (confusion, agitation, constipation, xerostomia, blurred vision, urinary retention); therefore, they should be used with caution in patients with decreased gastrointestinal motility, urinary retention, BPH, xerostomia, or visual problems. Conditions which also may be exacerbated by cholinergic blockade include narrow-angle glaucoma (screening is recommended) and worsening of myasthenia gravis. Relative to neuroleptics, pimozide has a moderate potency of cholinergic blockade.

May cause extrapyramidal symptoms, including pseudoparkinsonism, acute dystonic reactions, akathisia, and tardive dyskinesia (risk of these reactions is high relative to other neuroleptics). May be associated with neuroleptic malignant syndrome (NMS) or pigmentary retinopathy.

Avoid grapefruit juice due to potential inhibition of pimozide metabolism.

Drug Interactions

Cytochrome P450 Effect: Substrate (major) of CYP1A2, 3A4; **Inhibits** CYP2C19 (weak), 2D6 (weak), 2E1 (weak), 3A4 (weak)

Decreased Effect: CYP1A2 inducers may decrease the levels/effects of pimozide; example inducers include aminoglutethimide, carbamazepine, phenobarbital, and rifampin. CYP3A4 inducers may decrease the levels/effects of pimozide; example inducers include aminoglutethimide, carbamazepine, nafcillin, nevirapine, phenobarbital, phenytoin, and rifamycins. Benztropine (and other anticholinergics) may inhibit the therapeutic response to pimozide. Antipsychotics such as pimozide inhibit the ability of bromocriptine to lower serum prolactin concentrations. The antihypertensive effects of guanethidine and guanadrel may be inhibited by pimozide. Pimozide may inhibit the antiparkinsonian effect of levodopa. Pimozide (and possibly other low potency antipsychotics) may reverse the pressor effects of epinephrine.

Increased Effect/Toxicity: Concurrent use with QT$_c$-prolonging agents is contraindicated including Class Ia and Class III antiarrhythmics, arsenic trioxide, chlorpromazine, dolasetron, droperidol, halofantrine, levomethadyl, mefloquine, pentamidine, probucol, tacrolimus, ziprasidone, mesoridazine, thioridazine, tricyclic antidepressants, and some quinolone antibiotics (sparfloxacin, moxifloxacin, and gatifloxacin).

CYP1A2 inhibitors may increase the levels/effects of pimozide; example inhibitors include amiodarone, ciprofloxacin, fluvoxamine, ketoconazole, norfloxacin, ofloxacin, and rofecoxib. Chloroquine, propranolol, and sulfadoxine-pyrimethamine also may increase pimozide concentrations. Concurrent use with TCA may produce increased toxicity or altered therapeutic response. Pimozide plus lithium may (rarely) produce neurotoxicity. Pimozide and CNS depressants (ethanol, narcotics) may produce additive CNS depressant effects. Pimozide with fluoxetine has been associated with the development of bradycardia (case report). Metoclopramide may increase risk of extrapyramidal symptoms (EPS). Acetylcholinesterase inhibitors (central) may increase the risk of antipsychotic-related EPS. Macrolide antibiotics may increase the effects of pimozide.

CYP3A4 inhibitors may increase the levels/effects of pimozide; example inhibitors include azole antifungals, clarithromycin, diclofenac, doxycycline, erythromycin, imatinib, isoniazid, nefazodone, nicardipine, propofol, protease inhibitors, quinidine, telithromycin, and verapamil. Concurrent use of strong CYP3A4 inhibitors with pimozide is contraindicated.

Nutritional/Ethanol Interactions
Ethanol: Avoid ethanol (may increase CNS depression).
Food: Pimozide serum concentration may be increased when taken with grapefruit juice; avoid concurrent use.
Herb/Nutraceutical: St John's wort may decrease pimozide levels. Avoid kava kava, gotu kola, valerian, St John's wort (may increase CNS depression).

Lab Interactions Increased prolactin (S)

Adverse Reactions
Frequencies >1% reported in adults (limited data) and/or children with Tourette's disorder:
Cardiovascular: Abnormal ECG (3%)
Central nervous system: Somnolence (up to 28% in children), sedation (14%), akathisia (8%), drowsiness (7%), hyperkinesias (6%), insomnia (2%), depression (2%), headache (1%), nervousness (1% to 8%)
Dermatologic: Rash (8%)
Gastrointestinal: Xerostomia (25%), constipation (20%), increased salivation (14%), diarrhea (5%), thirst (5%), appetite increased (5%), taste disturbance (5%), dysphagia (3%)
Genitourinary: Impotence (15%)
Neuromuscular & skeletal: Weakness (22%), muscle tightness (15%), rigidity (10%), myalgia (3%), torticollis (3%), tremor (3%)
Ocular: Visual disturbance (6% to 20%), accommodation decreased (20%)
Miscellaneous: Speech disorder (10%)
Frequency not established (reported in disorders other than Tourette's disorder): Blood dyscrasias, breast edema, chest pain, dizziness, extrapyramidal symptoms (akathisia, akinesia, dystonia, pseudoparkinsonism, tardive dyskinesia); facial edema, gingival hyperplasia (case report), hyper-/hypotension, hyponatremia, jaundice, libido decreased, neuroleptic malignant syndrome, orthostatic hypotension, palpitation, periorbital edema, postural hypotension, QT$_c$ prolongation, seizure, tachycardia, ventricular arrhythmia, vomiting, weight gain/loss

Overdosage/Toxicology Symptoms of overdose include hypotension, respiratory depression, ECG abnormalities, extrapyramidal symptoms. Treatment is supportive and symptomatic. Epinephrine should not be used (consider norepinephrine or phenylephrine for hypotension).

Pharmacodynamics/Kinetics
Time to Peak: Serum: 6-8 hours
Protein Binding: 99%
Half-Life Elimination: 50 hours
Metabolism: Hepatic; significant first-pass effect
Excretion: Urine
Available Dosage Forms Tablet: 1 mg, 2 mg
(Continued)

Pimozide *(Continued)*

Dosing

Adults:

Tourette's disorder: Oral: Initial: 1-2 mg/day, then increase dosage as needed every other day; range is usually 7-16 mg/day; maximum: 10 mg/day or 0.2 mg/kg/day are not generally recommended.

Note: Sudden unexpected deaths have occurred in patients taking doses >10 mg.

Note: An ECG should be performed baseline and periodically thereafter, especially during dosage adjustment.

Elderly: Recommend initial dose of 1 mg/day; periodically attempt gradual reduction of dose to determine if tic persists; follow up for 1-2 weeks before concluding the tic is a persistent disease phenomenon and not a manifestation of drug withdrawal. **Note:** An ECG should be performed baseline and periodically thereafter, especially during dosage adjustment.

Pediatrics:

Tourette's disorder: Oral:

Children ≤12 years: Initial: 0.05 mg/kg preferably once at bedtime; may be increased every third day; usual range: 2-4 mg/day; do not exceed 10 mg/day (0.2 mg/kg/day)

Children >12 years: Refer to adult dosing.

Note: An ECG should be performed baseline and periodically thereafter, especially during dosage adjustment.

Hepatic Impairment: Reduced dose is necessary.

Laboratory Monitoring Lipid profile, fasting blood glucose/Hgb A_{1c}; BMI

Nursing Actions

Physical Assessment: Assess other medications patient is taking for effectiveness and interactions. Review ophthalmic exam, monitor laboratory tests, monitor blood pressure, therapeutic response (mental status, mood, affect), and adverse reactions at beginning of therapy and periodically with long-term use (endocrine changes, extrapyramidal symptoms, neuroleptic malignant syndrome). Conduct baseline ECG and periodically during therapy (especially during dosage adjustment). Assess knowledge/teach patient appropriate use, interventions to reduce side effects, and adverse symptoms to report

Patient Education: Use exactly as directed; do not increase dose or frequency. It may take 2-3 weeks to achieve desired results; do not discontinue without consulting prescriber. Avoid alcohol or caffeine and other prescription or OTC medications not approved by prescriber. Avoid grapefruit juice. Maintain adequate hydration (2-3 L/day of fluids) unless instructed to restrict fluid intake. You may experience excess drowsiness, restlessness, dizziness, or blurred vision (use caution driving or when engaging in tasks requiring alertness until response to drug is known); or constipation, dry mouth, anorexia (increased exercise, fluids, fruit, or fiber may help). Report persistent CNS effects (eg, trembling fingers, altered gait or balance, excessive sedation, seizures, unusual muscle or facial movements, anxiety, abnormal thoughts, confusion, personality changes); unresolved constipation or GI effects; breast swelling (male and female) or decreased sexual ability; vision changes; respiratory difficulty; unusual cough or flu-like symptoms; or worsening of condition. **Pregnancy/breast-feeding precautions:** Inform prescriber if you are or intend to become pregnant. Consult prescriber if breast-feeding.

Geriatric Considerations (See Warnings/Precautions, Adverse Reactions, and Overdose/Toxicology.) Elderly patients have an increased risk of adverse response to side effects or adverse reactions to antipsychotics.

Additional Information Less sedation, but pimozide is more likely to cause acute extrapyramidal symptoms than chlorpromazine.

Related Information

Antipsychotic Medication Guidelines *on page 1415*

Pindolol *(PIN doe lole)*

Pharmacologic Category Beta Blocker With Intrinsic Sympathomimetic Activity

Medication Safety Issues

Sound-alike/look-alike issues:

Pindolol may be confused with Parlodel®, Plendil®

Visken® may be confused with Visine®

Pregnancy Risk Factor B

Lactation Enters breast milk/use caution

Use Management of hypertension

Unlabeled/Investigational Use Potential augmenting agent for antidepressants; ventricular arrhythmias/tachycardia, antipsychotic-induced akathisia, situational anxiety; aggressive behavior associated with dementia

Mechanism of Action/Effect Blocks both beta$_1$- and beta$_2$-receptors and has mild intrinsic sympathomimetic activity; pindolol has negative inotropic and chronotropic effects and can significantly slow AV nodal conduction. Augmentive action of antidepressants thought to be mediated via a serotonin 1A autoreceptor antagonism.

Contraindications Hypersensitivity to pindolol, beta-blockers, or any component of the formulation; uncompensated congestive heart failure; cardiogenic shock; bradycardia, sinus node dysfunction, or heart block (2nd or 3rd degree) except in patients with a functioning artificial pacemaker; pulmonary edema; severe hyperactive airway disease (asthma or COPD); Raynaud's disease

Warnings/Precautions Administer very cautiously to patients with CHF, asthma, diabetes mellitus, hyperthyroidism. May mask signs and symptoms of thyrotoxicosis. Abrupt withdrawal of the drug should be avoided, drug should be discontinued over 1-2 weeks. Do not use in pregnant or nursing women. May potentiate hypoglycemia in a diabetic patient and mask signs and symptoms. Use with caution in patients with myasthenia gravis or peripheral vascular disease. May cause CNS depression; use caution in patients with a history of psychiatric illness. May potentiate anaphylactic reactions and/or blunt response to epinephrine treatment. Beta-blockers with intrinsic sympathomimetic activity (including pindolol) do not appear to be of benefit in CHF.

Drug Interactions

Cytochrome P450 Effect: Substrate of CYP2D6 (major); **Inhibits** CYP2D6 (weak)

Decreased Effect: Decreased levels/effect of pindolol with aluminum salts, barbiturates, calcium salts, cholestyramine, colestipol, NSAIDs, penicillins (ampicillin), rifampin, salicylates, and sulfinpyrazone due to decreased bioavailability and plasma levels. Beta-blockers may decrease the effect of sulfonylureas (possibly hyperglycemia). Nonselective beta-blockers blunt the effect of beta-2 adrenergic agonists (albuterol).

Increased Effect/Toxicity: CYP2D6 inhibitors may increase the levels/effects of pindolol; example inhibitors include chlorpromazine, delavirdine, fluoxetine, miconazole, paroxetine, pergolide, quinidine, quinine, ritonavir, and ropinirole. Pindolol may increase the effects of other drugs which slow AV conduction (digoxin, verapamil, diltiazem), alpha-blockers (prazosin, terazosin), and alpha-adrenergic stimulants (epinephrine, phenylephrine). Pindolol may mask the tachycardia from hypoglycemia caused by insulin and oral hypoglycemics. In patients receiving concurrent therapy, the risk of hypertensive crisis is increased when either clonidine or the beta-blocker is withdrawn. Reserpine has been shown to enhance the effect of beta-blockers. Beta-blockers may increase the action or levels of ethanol, disopyramide, nonde-polarizing muscle relaxants, and theophylline although the effects are difficult to predict.

Nutritional/Ethanol Interactions Herb/Nutraceutical: Avoid dong quai if using for hypertension (has estrogenic activity). Avoid ephedra, yohimbe, ginseng (may worsen hypertension).

Adverse Reactions 1% to 10%:
Cardiovascular: Chest pain (3%), edema (6%)
Central nervous system: Nightmares/vivid dreams (5%), dizziness (9%), insomnia (10%), fatigue (8%), nervousness (7%), anxiety (<2%)
Dermatologic: Rash, itching (4%)
Gastrointestinal: Nausea (5%), abdominal discomfort (4%)
Neuromuscular & skeletal: Weakness (4%), paresthesia (3%), arthralgia (7%), muscle pain (10%)
Respiratory: Dyspnea (5%)

Overdosage/Toxicology Symptoms of intoxication include cardiac disturbances, CNS toxicity, bronchospasm, hypoglycemia, and hyperkalemia. The most common cardiac symptoms include hypotension and bradycardia. Atrioventricular block, intraventricular conduction disturbances, cardiogenic shock, and asystole may occur with severe overdose, especially with membrane-depressant drugs (eg, propranolol). CNS effects include convulsions, and coma. Respiratory arrest is commonly seen with propranolol and other membrane-depressant and lipid-soluble drugs. Treatment includes symptomatic treatment of seizures, hypotension, hyperkalemia, and hypoglycemia.

Pharmacodynamics/Kinetics
Time to Peak: Serum: 1-2 hours
Protein Binding: 50%
Half-Life Elimination: 2.5-4 hours; prolonged with renal impairment, age, and cirrhosis
Metabolism: Hepatic (60% to 65%) to conjugates
Excretion: Urine (35% to 50% as unchanged drug)
Available Dosage Forms Tablet: 5 mg, 10 mg
Dosing
Adults:
Hypertension: Oral: Initial: 5 mg twice daily, increase as necessary by 10 mg/day every 3-4 weeks (maximum daily dose: 60 mg); usual dose range (JNC 7): 10-40 mg twice daily.
Antidepressant augmentation (unlabeled use): Oral: 2.5 mg 3 times/day
Elderly: Oral: Initial: 5 mg once daily; increase as necessary by 5 mg/day every 3-4 weeks.
Renal Impairment: Reduction is necessary in severe impairment.
Hepatic Impairment: Reduce dose in severely impaired.

Nursing Actions
Physical Assessment: Assess potential for interactions with other prescriptions, OTC medications, or herbal products patient may be taking. Monitor patient response at beginning of therapy, when adjusting dosage, and periodically with long-term therapy (eg, cardiac, respiratory, hemodynamic status). Caution patient to monitor serum glucose levels closely (may alter glucose tolerance, potentiate hypoglycemia, or mask symptoms of hypoglycemia). Teach patient appropriate use, possible side effects/appropriate interventions, and adverse symptoms to report.
Patient Education: Do not take any new medication during therapy unless approved by prescriber. Take exactly as directed. Do not alter dose or discontinue without consulting prescriber. If you have diabetes, monitor serum glucose closely (drug may alter glucose tolerance or mask signs of hypoglycemia). May cause nervousness, fatigue, dizziness, insomnia, or postural hypotension (use caution when changing position from lying or sitting to standing, when driving, or climbing stairs until response to medication is known); or nausea or abdominal discomfort (small

frequent meals, frequent mouth care, chewing gum, or sucking lozenges may help). Report chest pain or swelling of extremities or unusual weight gain (>5 lb/week), unusual muscle weakness or pain; or other persistent adverse effects. **Breast-feeding precaution:** Consult prescriber if breast-feeding.

Dietary Considerations May be taken without regard to meals.

Geriatric Considerations Due to alterations in the beta-adrenergic autonomic nervous system, beta-adrenergic blockade may result in less hemodynamic response than seen in younger adults. Studies indicate that despite decreased sensitivity to the chronotropic effects of beta blockade with age, there appears to be an increased myocardial sensitivity to the negative inotropic effect during stress (eg, exercise). Controlled trials have shown the overall response rate for propranolol to be only 20% to 50% in elderly populations. Therefore, all beta-adrenergic blocking drugs may result in a decreased response as compared to younger adults (see Pharmacodynamics/Kinetics).

Breast-Feeding Issues There is limited experience with pindolol; however, other beta-blockers like metoprolol are considered compatible by the AAP. Monitor the infant for signs of beta-blockade (hypotension, bradycardia, etc) with long-term use.

Pregnancy Issues Pindolol crosses the placenta. Beta-blockers have been associated with bradycardia, hypotension, and IUGR; IUGR is probably related to maternal hypertension. Available evidence suggests beta-blockers are generally safe during pregnancy (JNC 7). Cases of neonatal hypoglycemia have been reported following maternal use of beta-blockers at parturition or during breast-feeding. Monitor breast-fed infant for symptoms of beta-blockade.

Pioglitazone (pye oh GLI ta zone)

U.S. Brand Names Actos®
Pharmacologic Category Antidiabetic Agent, Thiazolidinedione
Medication Safety Issues
Sound-alike/look-alike issues:
Actos® may be confused with Actidose®, Actonel®
Pregnancy Risk Factor C
Lactation Excretion in breast milk unknown/not recommended
Use
Type 2 diabetes mellitus (noninsulin dependent, NIDDM), monotherapy: Adjunct to diet and exercise, to improve glycemic control
Type 2 diabetes mellitus (noninsulin dependent, NIDDM), combination therapy with sulfonylurea, metformin, or insulin: When diet, exercise, and a single agent alone does not result in adequate glycemic control
Mechanism of Action/Effect Thiazolidinedione antidiabetic agent that lowers blood glucose by improving target cell response to insulin, without increasing pancreatic insulin secretion. It has a mechanism of action that is dependent on the presence of insulin for activity. Pioglitazone is a potent and selective agonist for peroxisome proliferator-activated receptor-gamma (PPARgamma). Activation of nuclear PPARgamma receptors influences the production of a number of gene products involved in glucose and lipid metabolism.
Contraindications Hypersensitivity to pioglitazone or any component of the formulation; active liver disease (transaminases >2.5 times the upper limit of normal at baseline); patients who have experienced jaundice during troglitazone therapy
Warnings/Precautions Should not be used in diabetic ketoacidosis. Mechanism requires the presence of insulin, therefore use in type 1 diabetes (insulin

(Continued)

Pioglitazone *(Continued)*

dependent, IDDM) is not recommended. May potentiate hypoglycemia when used in combination with sulfonylureas or insulin. Use with caution in premenopausal, anovulatory women - may result in a resumption of ovulation, increasing the risk of pregnancy. Use with caution in patients with anemia (may reduce hemoglobin and hematocrit). May increase plasma volume and/or increase cardiac hypertrophy. Use with caution in patients with edema. Monitor closely for signs and symptoms of heart failure (including weight gain, edema, or dyspnea). Not recommended for use in patients with NYHA Class III or IV heart failure, unless serum glucose control outweighs the risk of excessive fluid retention. Discontinue if heart failure develops. Use with caution in patients with minor elevations in transaminases (AST or ALT). Idiosyncratic hepatotoxicity has been reported with another thiazolidinedione agent (troglitazone) and postmarketing case reports of hepatitis (with rare hepatic failure) have been received for pioglitazone. Monitoring should include periodic determinations of liver function. Not for use in children <18 years of age.

Drug Interactions

Cytochrome P450 Effect: Substrate (major) of CYP2C8/9, 3A4; **Inhibits** CYP2C8/9 (strong), 2C19 (weak), 2D6 (moderate); **Induces** CYP3A4 (weak)

Decreased Effect: The levels/effects of pioglitazone may be decreased by aminoglutethimide, carbamazepine, nafcillin, nevirapine, phenobarbital, phenytoin, rifamycins, secobarbital, and other CYP2C8/9 or CYP3A4 inducers. Pioglitazone may decrease the levels/effects of CYP2D6 prodrug substrates (eg, codeine, hydrocodone, oxycodone, tramadol). Effects of oral contraceptives (hormonal) may be decreased, based on data from a related compound. This has not been specifically evaluated for pioglitazone. Bile acid sequestrants may decrease pioglitazone levels.

Increased Effect/Toxicity: Concomitant use with thioridazine is contraindicated, due to a risk of arrhythmias. The levels/effects of pioglitazone may be increased by azole antifungals, clarithromycin, delavirdine, diclofenac, doxycycline, erythromycin, fluconazole, gemfibrozil, imatinib, isoniazid, itraconazole, ketoconazole, nefazodone, nicardipine, NSAIDs, propofol, protease inhibitors, quinidine, sulfonamides, telithromycin, verapamil, and other CYP2C8/9 or 3A4 inhibitors.

Pioglitazone may increase the levels/effects of amiodarone, amphetamines, selected beta-blockers, dextromethorphan, fluoxetine, glimepiride, glipizide, lidocaine, mirtazapine, nateglinide, nefazodone, paroxetine, phenytoin, risperidone, ritonavir, rosiglitazone, sertraline, thioridazine, warfarin, and other CYP2D6 or 2C8/9 substrates.

Nutritional/Ethanol Interactions

Ethanol: Caution with ethanol (may cause hypoglycemia).

Food: Peak concentrations are delayed when administered with food, but the extent of absorption is not affected. Pioglitazone may be taken without regard to meals.

Herb/Nutraceutical: St John's wort may decrease levels. Caution with chromium, garlic, gymnema (may cause hypoglycemia).

Adverse Reactions

>10%:

Endocrine & metabolic: Serum triglycerides decreased, HDL-cholesterol increased

Gastrointestinal: Weight gain

Respiratory: Upper respiratory tract infection (13%)

1% to 10%:

Cardiovascular: Edema (5%) (in combination trials with sulfonylureas or insulin, the incidence of edema was as high as 15%)

Central nervous system: Headache (9%), fatigue (4%)

Endocrine & metabolic: Aggravation of diabetes mellitus (5%), hypoglycemia (range 2% to 15% when used in combination with sulfonylureas or insulin)

Hematologic: Anemia (1%)

Neuromuscular & skeletal: Myalgia (5%)

Respiratory: Sinusitis (6%), pharyngitis (5%)

Overdosage/Toxicology Experience in overdose is limited. Symptoms may include hypoglycemia. Treatment is supportive.

Pharmacodynamics/Kinetics

Onset of Action: Delayed; Peak effect: Glucose control: Several weeks

Time to Peak: ~2 hours

Protein Binding: 99.8%

Half-Life Elimination: Parent drug: 3-7 hours; Total: 16-24 hours

Metabolism: Hepatic (99%) via CYP2C8/9 and 3A4 to both active and inactive metabolites

Excretion: Urine (15% to 30%) and feces as metabolites

Available Dosage Forms Tablet: 15 mg, 30 mg, 45 mg

Dosing

Adults & Elderly: Type 2 diabetes: Oral:

Monotherapy: Initial: 15-30 mg once daily; if response is inadequate, the dosage may be increased in increments up to 45 mg once daily; maximum recommended dose: 45 mg once daily

Combination therapy:

Note: Maximum recommended dose: 45 mg/day

With sulfonylureas: Initial: 15-30 mg once daily; dose of sulfonylurea should be reduced if the patient reports hypoglycemia

With metformin: Initial: 15-30 mg once daily; it is unlikely that the dose of metformin will need to be reduced due to hypoglycemia

With insulin: Initial: 15-30 mg once daily; dose of insulin should be reduced by 10% to 25% if the patient reports hypoglycemia or if the plasma glucose falls to below 100 mg/dL.

Dosage adjustment in patients with CHF (NYHA Class II) in mono- or combination therapy: Oral: Initial: 15 mg once daily; may be increased after several months of treatment, with close attention to heart failure symptoms

Renal Impairment: No adjustment is necessary.

Hepatic Impairment: Clearance is significantly lower in hepatic impairment. Therapy should not be initiated if the patient exhibits active liver disease or increased transaminases (>2.5 times the upper limit of normal) at baseline.

Administration

Oral: May be administered without regard to meals.

Laboratory Monitoring Hemoglobin A_{1c}, serum glucose, liver enzymes prior to initiation and periodically during treatment (per clinician judgment); if the ALT is increased to >2.5 times ULN, liver function testing should be performed more frequently until the levels return to normal or pretreatment values. Patients with an elevation in ALT >3 times ULN should be rechecked as soon as possible. If the ALT levels remain >3 times ULN, therapy with pioglitazone should be discontinued.

Nursing Actions

Physical Assessment: Assess other medications patient may be taking. Monitor laboratory results and response to therapy frequently until patient is stable. Monitor for adverse response Assess knowledge/ teach risks of hyper-/hypoglycemia, symptoms, and treatment. Refer patient to a diabetic educator, if available.

Patient Education: Use exactly as directed; do not increase dose or frequency or discontinue without consulting prescriber. May be taken without regard to meals. Avoid or use caution with alcohol while taking this medication. If dose is missed, take as soon as possible. If dose is missed completely one day, do not double dose the next day. Follow dietary, exercise, and glucose monitoring instructions of prescriber (more frequent monitoring may be advised in periods of stress, trauma, surgery, increased exercise etc). Report respiratory infection, unusual weight gain, aggravation of hyper-/hypoglycemic condition, unusual swelling of extremities, shortness of breath, fatigue, yellowing of skin or eyes, dark urine, pale stool, nausea/vomiting, or muscle pain. **Pregnancy/breast-feeding precautions:** Inform prescriber if you are or intend to become pregnant. Use alternate means of contraception if using oral contraceptives. You may be at increased risk of pregnancy while taking this medication. Breast-feeding is not recommended.

Dietary Considerations Management of type 2 diabetes mellitus (noninsulin dependent, NIDDM) should include diet control. May be taken without regard to meals.

Breast-Feeding Issues In animal studies, pioglitazone has been found to be excreted in milk. It is not known whether pioglitazone is excreted in human milk. Should not be administered to a nursing woman.

Pregnancy Issues Treatment during mid-late gestation was associated with delayed parturition, embryotoxicity and postnatal growth retardation in animal models. Abnormal blood glucose levels are associated with a higher incidence of congenital abnormalities. Insulin is the drug of choice for the control of diabetes mellitus during pregnancy.

Piperacillin (pi PER a sil in)

Synonyms Piperacillin Sodium
Pharmacologic Category Antibiotic, Penicillin
Pregnancy Risk Factor B
Lactation Enters breast milk (small amounts - other penicillins are compatible with breast-feeding)
Use Treatment of susceptible infections such as septicemia, acute and chronic respiratory tract infections, skin and soft tissue infections, and urinary tract infections due to susceptible strains of *Pseudomonas*, *Proteus*, and *Escherichia coli* and *Enterobacter*; active against some streptococci and some anaerobic bacteria; febrile neutropenia (as part of combination regimen)

Mechanism of Action/Effect Inhibits bacterial cell wall synthesis by binding to one or more of the penicillin binding proteins (PBPs); which in turn inhibits the final transpeptidation step of peptidoglycan synthesis in bacterial cell walls, thus inhibiting cell wall biosynthesis. Bacteria eventually lyse due to ongoing activity of cell wall autolytic enzymes (autolysins and murein hydrolases) while cell wall assembly is arrested.

Contraindications Hypersensitivity to piperacillin, other beta-lactam antibiotics (penicillins or cephalosporins), or any component of the formulation

Warnings/Precautions Dosage modification required in patients with impaired renal function. Use caution in patients with history of seizure activity. Leukopenia and neutropenia have been reported (during prolonged therapy). An increased frequency of fever and rash has been reported in patients with cystic fibrosis.

Drug Interactions
Decreased Effect: Tetracyclines may decrease penicillin effectiveness. High concentrations of piperacillin may cause physical inactivation of aminoglycosides and lead to potential toxicity in patients with mild-moderate renal dysfunction. Although anecdotal reports suggest oral contraceptive efficacy could be reduced by penicillins, this has been refuted by more rigorous scientific and clinical data.

Increased Effect/Toxicity: Probenecid may increase penicillin levels. Neuromuscular blockers may increase duration of blockade. Penicillins may increase the exposure to methotrexate during concurrent therapy; monitor.

Lab Interactions May interfere with urinary glucose tests using cupric sulfate (Benedict's solution, Clinitest®); false-positive urinary and serum proteins, positive Coombs' test [direct]. False-positive Platelia® *Aspergillus* EIA test (Bio-Rad Laboratories) has been reported.

Some penicillin derivatives may cause the degradation of aminoglycosides *in vitro*, leading to a potential underestimation of aminoglycoside serum concentration.

Adverse Reactions Frequency not defined.
Central nervous system: Confusion, convulsions, drowsiness, fever, Jarisch-Herxheimer reaction
Dermatologic: Rash, toxic epidermal necrolysis, urticaria
Endocrine & metabolic: Electrolyte imbalance, hypokalemia
Hematologic: Abnormal platelet aggregation and prolonged PT (high doses), agranulocytosis, Coombs' reaction (positive), hemolytic anemia, pancytopenia
Local: Thrombophlebitis
Neuromuscular & skeletal: Myoclonus
Renal: Acute interstitial nephritis, acute renal failure
Miscellaneous: Anaphylaxis, hypersensitivity reactions

Overdosage/Toxicology Symptoms of penicillin overdose include neuromuscular hypersensitivity (eg, agitation, hallucinations, asterixis, encephalopathy, confusion, and seizures). Electrolyte imbalance may occur if the preparation contains potassium or sodium salts, especially in renal failure. Hemodialysis may be helpful to aid in removal of the drug from blood; otherwise, treatment is supportive or symptom-directed.

Pharmacodynamics/Kinetics
Time to Peak: Serum: I.M.: 30-50 minutes
Protein Binding: 22%
Half-Life Elimination: Dose dependent; prolonged with moderately severe renal or hepatic impairment:
Neonates: 1-5 days old: 3.6 hours; >6 days old: 2.1-2.7 hours
Children: 1-6 months: 0.79 hour; 6 months to 12 years: 0.39-0.5 hour
Adults: 36-80 minutes
Excretion: Primarily urine; partially feces
Available Dosage Forms Injection, powder for reconstitution: 2 g, 3 g, 4 g, 40 g
Dosing
Adults:
Usual dosage range:
I.M.: 2-3 g/dose every 6-12 hours; maximum: 24 g/24 hours
I.V.: 3-4 g/dose every 4-6 hours; maximum: 24 g/24 hours
Burn wound sepsis: I.V.: 4 g every 4 hours with vancomycin and amikacin
Cholangitis, acute: I.V.: 4 g every 6 hours
Keratitis *(Pseudomonas):* Ophthalmic: 6-12 mg/mL every 15-60 minutes around the clock for 24-72 hours, then slow reduction
Malignant otitis externa: I.V.: 4-6 g every 4-6 hours with tobramycin
Moderate infections: I.M., I.V.: 2-3 g/dose every 6-12 hours (maximum: 2 g I.M./site)
Prosthetic joint *(Pseudomonas):* I.V.: 3 g every 6 hours with aminoglycoside
***Pseudomonas* infections:** I.V.: 4 g every 4 hours
Severe infections: I.M., I.V.: 3-4 g/dose every 4-6 hours (maximum: 24 g/24 hours)
Urinary tract infections: I.V.: 2-3 g/dose every 6-12 hours
Uncomplicated gonorrhea: I.M.: 2 g in a single dose accompanied by 1 g probenecid 30 minutes prior to injection
(Continued)

Piperacillin *(Continued)*

Elderly: Adjust dose for renal impairment:
I.M.: 1-2 g every 8-12 hours
I.V.: 2-4 g every 6-8 hours

Pediatrics:
Usual dosage range:
Neonates: I.M., I.V.: 100 mg/kg every 12 hours
Infants and Children: I.M., I.V.: 200-300 mg/kg/day in divided doses every 4-6 hours
Cystic fibrosis: I.M., I.V.: 350-500 mg/kg/day in divided doses every 4-6 hours

Renal Impairment:
Cl_{cr} 10-50 mL/minute: Administer every 6-8 hours.
Cl_{cr} <10 mL/minute: Administer every 8 hours.
Moderately dialyzable (20% to 50%)
Continuous arteriovenous or venovenous hemofiltration: Dose as for Cl_{cr} 10-50 mL/minute.

Administration
I.M.: Do not administer more than 2 g per injection site.
I.V.: Administer around-the-clock to promote less variation in peak and trough serum levels. Give at least 1 hour apart from aminoglycosides. Rapid administration can lead to seizures. Administer direct I.V. over 3-5 minutes. Intermittently infusion over 30 minutes.
Some penicillins (eg, carbenicillin, ticarcillin and piperacillin) have been shown to inactivate aminoglycosides *in vitro*. This has been observed to a greater extent with tobramycin and gentamicin, while amikacin has shown greater stability against inactivation. Concurrent use of these agents may pose a risk of reduced antibacterial efficacy *in vivo*, particularly in the setting of profound renal impairment. However, definitive clinical evidence is lacking. If combination penicillin/aminoglycoside therapy is desired in a patient with renal dysfunction, separation of doses (if feasible), and routine monitoring of aminoglycoside levels, CBC, and clinical response should be considered.

I.V. Detail: pH: 5.5-7.5

Stability
Compatibility: Stable in dextran 6% in NS, D_5NS, D_5W, LR, NS, SWFI, bacteriostatic water
Y-site administration: Incompatible with amphotericin B cholesteryl sulfate complex, filgrastim, fluconazole, gatifloxacin, gemcitabine, ondansetron, sargramostim, vinorelbine
Compatibility when admixed: Incompatible with aminoglycosides
Storage: Reconstituted solution is stable (I.V. infusion) in NS or D_5W for 24 hours at room temperature, 7 days when refrigerated, or 4 weeks when frozen. After freezing, thawed solution is stable for 24 hours at room temperature or 48 hours when refrigerated. 40 g bulk vial should **not** be frozen after reconstitution.

Laboratory Monitoring Perform culture and sensitivity before administering first dose.

Nursing Actions
Physical Assessment: Results of culture and sensitivity tests and patient's allergy history should be assessed prior to starting therapy. Assess potential for interactions with other pharmacological agents patient may be taking (eg, increase or decrease levels/effect of penicillin or increase risk of toxicity [aminoglycosides]). See Administration for infusion specifics. Monitor effectiveness (resolution of infection) and adverse reactions (eg, hypersensitivity reactions, opportunistic infection [fever, chills, unhealed sores, white plaques in mouth or vagina, purulent vaginal discharge, fatigue], confusion, convulsions, rash, thrombophlebitis, renal failure). Advise patients with diabetes about use of Clinitest®; may cause false positive rest results. Teach patient possible side effects/appropriate interventions and adverse symptoms to report.

Patient Education: Do not take any new medication during therapy unless approved by prescriber. This drug can only be given by injection or infusion. Report immediately any redness, swelling, burning, or pain at infusion/injection site or any signs of allergic reaction (eg, respiratory difficulty or swallowing, chest tightness, rash, hives, swelling of lips or mouth). Maintain adequate hydration (2-3 L/day of fluids) unless instructed to restrict fluid intake. If you have diabetes, drug may cause false test results with Clinitest®, consult prescriber for alternative method of glucose monitoring. May cause confusion or drowsiness (use caution when driving or engaging in tasks that require alertness until response to drug is known). Report chest pain, palpitations, or irregular heartbeat; unusual confusion, pain, swelling or heat in legs, changes in urinary pattern, signs of an opportunistic infection (fever, chills, unhealed sores, white plaques in mouth or vagina, purulent vaginal discharge, fatigue) or persistent adverse effects.

Dietary Considerations Sodium content of 1 g: 1.85 mEq

Geriatric Considerations Antipseudomonal penicillins should not be used alone and are often combined with an aminoglycoside as empiric therapy for lower respiratory infection and sepsis in which gram-negative (including *Pseudomonas*) and/or anaerobes are of a high probability. Because of piperacillin's lower sodium content, it is preferred over ticarcillin in patients with a history of heart failure and/or renal or hepatic disease. Adjust dose for renal function.

Piperacillin and Tazobactam Sodium
(pi PER a sil in & ta zoe BAK tam SOW dee um)

U.S. Brand Names Zosyn®
Synonyms Piperacillin Sodium and Tazobactam Sodium
Pharmacologic Category Antibiotic, Penicillin
Medication Safety Issues
Sound-alike/look-alike issues:
Zosyn® may be confused with Zofran®, Zyvox™
Pregnancy Risk Factor B
Lactation Enters breast milk/use caution
Use Treatment of moderate-to-severe infections caused by susceptible organisms, including infections of the lower respiratory tract (community-acquired pneumonia, nosocomial pneumonia); urinary tract; uncomplicated and complicated skin and skin structures; gynecologic (endometritis, pelvic inflammatory disease); bone and joint infections; intra-abdominal infections (appendicitis with rupture/abscess, peritonitis); and septicemia. Tazobactam expands activity of piperacillin to include beta-lactamase producing strains of *S. aureus*, *H. influenzae*, *Bacteroides*, and other gram-negative bacteria.

Mechanism of Action/Effect Piperacillin interferes with bacterial cell wall synthesis during active multiplication, causing cell wall death and resultant bactericidal activity against susceptible bacteria; tazobactam prevents degradation of piperacillin by binding to the active side on beta-lactamase; tazobactam inhibits many beta-lactamases, including staphylococcal penicillinase and Richmond and Sykes Types II, III, IV, and V, including extended spectrum enzymes; it has only limited activity against Class I beta-lactamases other than Class 1C

Contraindications Hypersensitivity to penicillins, beta-lactamase inhibitors, or any component of the formulation

Warnings/Precautions Bleeding disorders have been observed, particularly in patients with renal impairment; discontinue if thrombocytopenia or bleeding occurs. Due to sodium load and to the adverse effects of high serum concentrations of penicillins, dosage modification is required in patients with impaired or underdeveloped renal function; use with caution in patients with seizures or in patients with history of beta-lactam allergy; associated with an increased incidence of rash and fever in cystic fibrosis patients. Prolonged use may result in superinfection, including pseudomembranous colitis. Safety and efficacy have not been established in children.

Drug Interactions

Decreased Effect: Tetracyclines may decrease penicillin effectiveness. Aminoglycosides may cause physical inactivation of aminoglycosides in the presence of high concentrations of piperacillin and potential toxicity in patients with mild-moderate renal dysfunction. Although anecdotal reports suggest oral contraceptive efficacy could be reduced by penicillins, this has been refuted by more rigorous scientific and clinical data.

Increased Effect/Toxicity: Probenecid may increase penicillin levels. Neuromuscular blockers may increase duration of blockade. Penicillins may increase methotrexate exposure; clinical significance has not been established.

Lab Interactions Positive Coombs' [direct] test; false positive reaction for urine glucose using copper-reduction method (Clinitest®); may result in false positive results with the Platelia® *Aspergillus* enzyme immunoassay (EIA)

Some penicillin derivatives may accelerate the degradation of aminoglycosides *in vitro*, leading to a potential underestimation of aminoglycoside serum concentration.

Adverse Reactions

>10%: Gastrointestinal: Diarrhea (11%)

>1% to 10%:

Cardiovascular: Hypertension (2%), chest pain, edema

Central nervous system: Insomnia (7%), headache (7% to 8%), agitation (2%), fever (2%), pain (2%), anxiety, dizziness

Dermatologic: Rash (4%), pruritus (3%)

Gastrointestinal: Constipation (7% to 8%), nausea (7%), vomiting (3%), dyspepsia (3%), stool changes (2%), abdominal pain

Hepatic: Transaminases increased

Respiratory: Dyspnea, rhinitis

Miscellaneous: Moniliasis (2%)

Overdosage/Toxicology Symptoms of penicillin overdose include neuromuscular hypersensitivity (eg, agitation, hallucinations, asterixis, encephalopathy, confusion, and seizures). Electrolyte imbalance may occur if the preparation contains potassium or sodium salts, especially in renal dysfunction. Hemodialysis may be helpful to aid in removal of the drug from blood; otherwise, treatment is supportive or symptom-directed.

Pharmacodynamics/Kinetics

Time to Peak: Immediately following infusion of 30 minutes

Protein Binding: Piperacillin and tazobactam: ~30%

Half-Life Elimination: Piperacillin and tazobactam: 0.7-1.2 hours

Metabolism:

Piperacillin: 6% to 9% to desethyl metabolite (weak activity)

Tazobactam: ~26% to inactive metabolite

Excretion: Clearance of both piperacillin and tazobactam are directly proportional to renal function

Piperacillin: Urine (68% as unchanged drug); feces (10% to 20%)

Tazobactam: Urine (80% as inactive metabolite)

Pharmacokinetic Note Both AUC and peak concentrations are dose proportional. Hepatic impairment does not affect the kinetics of piperacillin or tazobactam significantly.

Available Dosage Forms Note: 8:1 ratio of piperacillin sodium/tazobactam sodium

Infusion [premixed iso-osmotic solution, frozen]:

2.25 g: Piperacillin 2 g and tazobactam 0.25 g (50 mL) [contains sodium 5.58 mEq (128 mg) and EDTA]

3.375 g: Piperacillin 3 g and tazobactam 0.375 g (50 mL) [contains sodium 8.38 mEq (192 mg) and EDTA]

4.5 g: Piperacillin 4 g and tazobactam 0.5 g (50 mL) [contains sodium 11.17 mEq (256 mg) and EDTA]

Injection, powder for reconstitution:

2.25 g: Piperacillin 2 g and tazobactam 0.25 g [contains sodium 5.58 mEq (128 mg) and EDTA]

3.375 g: Piperacillin 3 g and tazobactam 0.375 g [contains sodium 8.38 mEq (192 mg) and EDTA]

4.5 g: Piperacillin 4 g and tazobactam 0.5 g [contains sodium 11.17 mEq (256 mg) and EDTA]

40.5 g: Piperacillin 36 g and tazobactam 4.5 g [contains sodium 100.4 mEq (2304 mg) and EDTA; bulk pharmacy vial]

Dosing

Adults & Elderly:

Diverticulitis, intra-abdominal abscess, peritonitis: I.V.: 4.5 g every 8 hours or 3.375 g every 6 hours

Moderate infections: I.M.: 2.25 g every 6-8 hours; treatment should be continued for ≥7-10 days depending on severity of disease (**Note:** I.M. route not FDA-approved)

Pneumonia (nosocomial): I.V.: 4.5 g every 6 hours for 7-14 days (when used empirically, combination with an aminoglycoside is recommended; consider discontinuation of aminoglycoside if *P. aeruginosa* is not isolated)

Severe infections: I.V.: 4.5 g every 8 hours or 3.375 g every 6 hours for 7-10 days

Pediatrics:

Children ≥6 months and ≤50 kg (unlabeled use): I.V.: 240-450 mg of piperacillin component/kg/day in divided doses every 4-6 hours for severe infections

Cystic fibrosis, pseudomonal infections: Children ≥6 months an ≤50 kg (unlabeled use): I.V.: 300-450 mg of piperacillin component/kg/day in divided doses every 6-8 hours have been used

Renal Impairment:

Cl$_{cr}$ 20-40 mL/minute: Administer 2.25 g every 6 hours (3.375 g every 6 hours for nosocomial pneumonia)

Cl$_{cr}$ <20 mL/minute: Administer 2.25 g every 8 hours (2.25 g every 6 hours for nosocomial pneumonia)

Hemodialysis/CAPD: Administer 2.25 g every 12 hours (every 8 hours for nosocomial pneumonia) with an additional dose of 0.75 g after each dialysis

Continuous arteriovenous or venovenous hemodiafiltration effects: Dose as for Cl$_{cr}$ 10-50 mL/minute

Hepatic Impairment: Hepatic impairment does not affect the kinetics of piperacillin or tazobactam significantly.

Administration

I.V.: Administer by I.V. infusion over 30 minutes.

Some penicillins (eg, carbenicillin, ticarcillin and piperacillin) have been shown to inactivate aminoglycosides *in vitro*. This has been observed to a greater extent with tobramycin and gentamicin, while amikacin has shown greater stability against inactivation. Concurrent use of these agents may pose a risk of reduced antibacterial efficacy *in vivo*, particularly in the setting of profound renal impairment. However, definitive clinical evidence is lacking. If combination penicillin/aminoglycoside therapy is desired in a patient with renal dysfunction, separation of doses (if feasible), and routine monitoring of aminoglycoside levels, CBC, and clinical response should be considered.

Stability

Reconstitution: Reconstitute with 5 mL of diluent per 1 g of piperacillin and then further dilute.

Compatibility: Stable in dextran 6% in NS, D$_5$W, NS, SWFI **incompatible** with LR

(Continued)

Piperacillin and Tazobactam Sodium
(Continued)

Y-site administration: Incompatible with acyclovir, alatrofloxacin, amphotericin B, amphotericin B cholesteryl sulfate complex, chlorpromazine, cisplatin, dacarbazine, daunorubicin, dobutamine, doxorubicin, doxorubicin liposome, doxycycline, droperidol, famotidine, ganciclovir, gatifloxacin, gemcitabine, haloperidol, hydroxyzine, idarubicin, minocycline, mitomycin, mitoxantrone, nalbuphine, prochlorperazine edisylate, promethazine, streptozocin

Compatibility when admixed: Incompatible: Aminoglycosides

Storage:

Vials: Store at controlled room temperature of 20°C to 25°C (68°F to 77°F). Use single-dose vials immediately after reconstitution (discard unused portions after 24 hours at room temperature and 48 hours if refrigerated). After reconstitution, vials or solution are stable in NS or D_5W for 24 hours at room temperature and 48 hours (vials) or 7 days (solution) when refrigerated.

Premixed solution: Store frozen at -20°C (-4°F). Thawed solution is stable for 24 hours at room temperature or 14 days under refrigeration; do not refreeze.

Laboratory Monitoring LFTs, creatinine, BUN, CBC with differential, serum electrolytes, urinalysis, PT, PTT; perform culture and sensitivity before administering first dose.

Nursing Actions

Physical Assessment: Assess results of culture and sensitivity tests and patient's allergy history prior to starting therapy. Assess potential for interactions with other pharmacological agents patient may be taking (eg, increase or decrease levels/effect of penicillin or increase risk of toxicity [aminoglycosides]). Should be infused over 30 minutes. Assess effectiveness (resolution of infection) and adverse reactions (eg, hypersensitivity reactions, opportunistic infection [fever, chills, unhealed sores, white plaques in mouth or vagina, purulent vaginal discharge, fatigue], confusion, convulsions, rash, thrombophlebitis). Advise patients with diabetes about use of Clinitest® (may cause false positive test results). Teach patient possible side effects/appropriate interventions and adverse symptoms to report.

Patient Education: This drug can only be given by injection or infusion; report immediately any redness, swelling, burning, or pain at infusion site or any signs of allergic reaction (eg, respiratory or swallowing difficulty, chest tightness, rash, hives, swelling of lips or mouth). Maintain adequate hydration (2-3 L/day of fluids) unless instructed to restrict fluid intake. If you have diabetes, drug may cause false test results with Clinitest®, consult prescriber for alternative method of glucose monitoring. May cause diarrhea (consult prescriber for approved medication); nausea or vomiting (small frequent meals, frequent mouth care, chewing gum, or sucking lozenges may help); or constipation (increased exercise, fluids, fruit, or fiber may help). Report acute or persistent headache; rash; CNS changes (eg, agitation, confusion, hallucinations, or seizures); persistent abdominal pain, cramping or diarrhea; unusual fever; or other persistent adverse effects. **Breast-feeding precaution:** Consult prescriber if breast-feeding.

Dietary Considerations

Infusion, premixed: 2.25 g contains sodium 5.58 mEq (128 mg); 3.375 g contains sodium 8.38 mEq (192 mg); 4.5 g contains sodium 11.17 mEq (256 mg)

Injection, powder for reconstitution: 2.25 g contains sodium 5.58 mEq (128 mg); 3.375 g contains sodium 8.38 mEq (192 mg); 4.5 g contains sodium 11.17 mEq (256 mg); 40.5 g contains sodium 100.4 mEq (2304 mg, bulk pharmacy vial)

Geriatric Considerations Has not been studied exclusively in the elderly.

Breast-Feeding Issues Piperacillin is excreted in breast milk.

Related Information

Piperacillin *on page 997*

Pirbuterol *(peer BYOO ter ole)*

U.S. Brand Names Maxair™ Autohaler™

Synonyms Pirbuterol Acetate

Pharmacologic Category Beta$_2$-Adrenergic Agonist

Pregnancy Risk Factor C

Lactation Excretion in breast milk unknown

Use Prevention and treatment of reversible bronchospasm including asthma

Mechanism of Action/Effect Pirbuterol is a beta$_2$-adrenergic agonist with a similar structure to albuterol, specifically a pyridine ring has been substituted for the benzene ring in albuterol. The increased beta$_2$ selectivity of pirbuterol results from the substitution of a tertiary butyl group on the nitrogen of the side chain, which additionally imparts resistance of pirbuterol to degradation by monoamine oxidase and provides a lengthened duration of action in comparison to the less selective previous beta-agonist agents.

Contraindications Hypersensitivity to pirbuterol, albuterol, or any component of the formulation

Warnings/Precautions Optimize anti-inflammatory treatment before initiating maintenance treatment with pirbuterol. Do not use as a component of chronic therapy without an anti-inflammatory agent. Only the mildest form of asthma (Step 1 and/or exercise-induced) would not require concurrent use based upon asthma guidelines. Patient must be instructed to seek medical attention in cases where acute symptoms are not relieved or a previous level of response is diminished. The need to increase frequency of use may indicate deterioration of asthma, and treatment must not be delayed.

Use caution in patients with cardiovascular disease (arrhythmia or hypertension or CHF), convulsive disorders, diabetes, glaucoma, hyperthyroidism, or hypokalemia. Beta agonists may cause elevation in blood pressure, heart rate, and result in CNS stimulation/excitation. Beta$_2$ agonists may increase risk of arrhythmia, increase serum glucose, or decrease serum potassium.

Do not exceed recommended dose; serious adverse events including fatalities, have been associated with excessive use of inhaled sympathomimetics. Rarely, paradoxical bronchospasm may occur with use of inhaled bronchodilating agents; this should be distinguished from inadequate response. All patients should utilize a spacer device when using a metered-dose inhaler. Safety and efficacy have not been established in children <12 years of age.

Drug Interactions

Decreased Effect: Decreased effect with beta-blockers.

Increased Effect/Toxicity: Increased toxicity with other beta agonists, MAO inhibitors, tricyclic antidepressants.

Adverse Reactions

>10%:

Central nervous system: Nervousness (7%)

Endocrine & metabolic: Serum glucose increased, serum potassium decreased

Neuromuscular & skeletal: Trembling (6%)

1% to 10%:

Cardiovascular: Palpitations (2%), tachycardia (1%)

Central nervous system: Headache (2%), dizziness (1%)

Gastrointestinal: Nausea (2%)

Respiratory: Cough (1%)

Overdosage/Toxicology Symptoms of overdose include tachycardia, tremor, hypertension, angina, and seizures. Hypokalemia also may occur. Cardiac arrest and death may be associated with abuse of beta-agonist bronchodilators. Treatment includes immediate discontinuation and symptomatic and supportive therapies. Cautious use of beta-adrenergic blocking agents may be considered in severe cases.

Pharmacodynamics/Kinetics

Onset of Action: Peak effect: Therapeutic: Oral: 2-3 hours with peak serum concentration of 6.2-9.8 mcg/L; Inhalation: 0.5-1 hour

Half-Life Elimination: 2-3 hours

Metabolism: Hepatic

Excretion: Urine (10% as unchanged drug)

Available Dosage Forms Aerosol for oral inhalation, as acetate:

Maxair™ Autohaler™: 14 g [400 inhalations; contains chlorofluorocarbons]

Dosing

Adults & Elderly: Bronchospasm: Inhalation: 2 inhalations every 4-6 hours for prevention; 2 inhalations at an interval of at least 1-3 minutes, followed by a third inhalation in treatment of bronchospasm, not to exceed 12 inhalations/day

Pediatrics: Children ≥12 years: Refer to adult dosing.

Administration

Inhalation: Shake inhaler well before use.

Stability

Storage: Store between 15°C and 30°C (59°F and 86°F).

Laboratory Monitoring FEV$_1$, peak flow, and/or other pulmonary function tests; serum potassium, serum glucose (in selected patients)

Nursing Actions

Physical Assessment: Assess effectiveness and interactions of other medications patient may be taking. Monitor effectiveness of therapy (relief of airway obstruction) and adverse reactions (eg, cardiac and CNS changes) at beginning of therapy and periodically with long-term use. For inpatient care, monitor vital signs and lung sounds prior to and periodically during therapy. Assess knowledge/teach patient appropriate use, interventions to reduce side effects, and adverse symptoms to report.

Patient Education: Use exactly as directed. Do not use more often than recommended. Maintain adequate hydration (2-3 L/day of fluids) unless instructed to restrict fluid intake. You may experience nervousness, dizziness, or fatigue (use caution when driving or engaging in tasks requiring alertness until response to drug is known); or dry mouth or stomach upset (small frequent meals, frequent mouth care, chewing gum, or sucking hard candy may help). If you have diabetes, check blood sugar; blood glucose levels may be increased. Report unresolved GI upset; dizziness or fatigue; vision changes; chest pain, rapid heartbeat, or palpitations; nervousness or insomnia; muscle cramping or tremor; or unusual cough. **Pregnancy/breast-feeding precautions:** Inform prescriber if you are or intend to become pregnant. Consult prescriber if breast-feeding.

Aerosol: Store canister upside down; do not freeze. Shake canister before using. Sit when using medication. Close eyes when administering pirbuterol to avoid spray getting into eyes. Exhale slowly and completely through nose; inhale deeply through mouth while administering aerosol. Hold breath for 5-10 seconds after inhalation. Wait at least 1 full minute between inhalations. Wash mouthpiece

between use. If more than one inhalation medication is used, use bronchodilator first and wait 5 minutes between medications

Maxair™ Autohaler™: Hold upright. Raise lever so that it stays up and snaps into place. Shake well. Exhale. Seal lips tightly around mouthpiece, inhale deeply. A "click" will be heard and you will feel a soft puff when the medication has been triggered. Continue to take a full, deep breath. Remove inhaler from mouth, hold breath for 10 seconds, then exhale slowly. **Note:** A test-fire slide has been added to the bottom of the Autohaler™ actuator/mouthpiece. The inhaler should be primed prior to using for the first time or if it has not been used in 48 hours. To prime, remove mouthpiece; point mouthpiece away from yourself or others, and push the lever so that it stays up. Push the white test-fire slide located on the bottom of the mouthpiece to release the priming spray. In order to release a second priming spray, push lever to "down" position, then repeat steps. When two priming sprays have been done, return lever to "down" position.

Geriatric Considerations Elderly patients may find it beneficial to utilize a spacer device when using a metered dose inhaler. Difficulty in using the inhaler often limits its effectiveness. The Maxair™ Autohaler™ may be easier for the elderly to use.

Piroxicam (peer OKS i kam)

U.S. Brand Names Feldene®

Restrictions A medication guide should be dispensed with each prescription. A template for the required MedGuide can be found on the FDA website at: http://www.fda.gov/medwatch/SAFETY/2005/safety05.htm#NSAID

Pharmacologic Category Nonsteroidal Anti-inflammatory Drug (NSAID), Oral

Pregnancy Risk Factor C/D (3rd trimester)

Lactation Enters breast milk (small amounts)/not recommended (AAP rates "compatible")

Use Symptomatic treatment of acute and chronic rheumatoid arthritis and osteoarthritis

Unlabeled/Investigational Use Ankylosing spondylitis

Mechanism of Action/Effect Inhibits prostaglandin synthesis, acts on the hypothalamus heat-regulating center to reduce fever, blocks prostaglandin synthetase action which prevents formation of the platelet-aggregating substance thromboxane A$_2$; decreases pain receptor sensitivity. Other proposed mechanisms of action for salicylate anti-inflammatory action are lysosomal stabilization, kinin and leukotriene production, alteration of chemotactic factors, and inhibition of neutrophil activation. This latter mechanism may be the most significant pharmacologic action to reduce inflammation.

Contraindications Hypersensitivity to piroxicam, aspirin, other NSAIDs or any component of the formulation; perioperative pain in the setting of coronary artery bypass surgery (CABG); pregnancy (3rd trimester or near term)

Warnings/Precautions NSAIDs are associated with an increased risk of adverse cardiovascular events, including MI, stroke, and new onset or worsening of pre-existing hypertension. Risk may be increased with duration of use or pre-existing cardiovascular risk-factors or disease. Carefully evaluate individual cardiovascular risk profiles prior to prescribing. Use caution with fluid retention, CHF or hypertension.

Use of NSAIDs can compromise existing renal function. Renal toxicity can occur in patient with impaired renal function, dehydration, heart failure, liver dysfunction, (Continued)

Piroxicam *(Continued)*

those taking diuretics and ACEI and the elderly. Rehydrate patient before starting therapy. Monitor renal function closely. Not recommended for use in patients with advanced renal disease.

NSAIDs may increase risk of gastrointestinal irritation, ulceration, bleeding, and perforation. These events may occur at any time during therapy and without warning. Use caution with a history of GI disease (bleeding or ulcers), concurrent therapy with aspirin, anticoagulants and/or corticosteroids, smoking, use of alcohol, the elderly or debilitated patients.

Use the lowest effective dose for the shortest duration of time, consistent with individual patient goals, to reduce risk of cardiovascular or GI adverse events. Alternate therapies should be considered for patients at high risk.

NSAIDs may cause serious skin adverse events including exfoliative dermatitis, Stevens-Johnson syndrome (SJS) and toxic epidermal necrolysis (TEN). Anaphylactoid reactions may occur, even without prior exposure; patients with "aspirin triad" (bronchial asthma, aspirin intolerance, rhinitis) may be at increased risk. Do not use in patients who experience bronchospasm, asthma, rhinitis, or urticaria with NSAID or aspirin therapy. A serum sickness-like reaction can rarely occur; watch for arthralgias, pruritus, fever, fatigue, and rash.

Use with caution in patients with decreased hepatic function. Closely monitor patients with any abnormal LFT. Severe hepatic reactions (eg, fulminant hepatitis, liver failure) have occurred with NSAID use, rarely; discontinue if signs or symptoms of liver disease develop, or if systemic manifestations occur.

The elderly are at increased risk for adverse effects (especially peptic ulceration, CNS effects, renal toxicity) from NSAIDs even at low doses

Withhold for at least 4-6 half-lives prior to surgical or dental procedures.

Drug Interactions

Cytochrome P450 Effect: Substrate of CYP2C8/9 (minor); **Inhibits** CYP2C8/9 (strong)

Decreased Effect: Decreased effect of diuretics, beta-blockers. Decreased effect with aspirin, antacids, and cholestyramine.

Increased Effect/Toxicity: Increased effect/toxicity of lithium and methotrexate (controversial). Piroxicam may increase the levels/effects of amiodarone, fluoxetine, glimepiride, glipizide, nateglinide, phenytoin, pioglitazone, rosiglitazone, sertraline, warfarin, and other CYP2C8/9 substrates.

Nutritional/Ethanol Interactions

Ethanol: Avoid ethanol (may enhance gastric mucosal irritation).

Food: Onset of effect may be delayed if piroxicam is taken with food.

Herb/Nutraceutical: Avoid alfalfa, anise, bilberry, bladderwrack, bromelain, cat's claw, celery, coleus, cordyceps, dong quai, evening primrose, feverfew, fenugreek, garlic, ginger, ginkgo biloboa, red clover, horse chestnut, grapeseed, green tea, ginseng, guggul, horse chestnut seed, horseradish, licorice, prickly ash, red clover, reishi, SAMe, sweet clover, turmeric, white willow (all have additional antiplatelet activity).

Lab Interactions Increased chloride (S), sodium (S), bleeding time

Adverse Reactions

>10%:

Central nervous system: Dizziness

Dermatologic: Rash

Gastrointestinal: Abdominal cramps, heartburn, indigestion, nausea

1% to 10%:

Central nervous system: Headache, nervousness

Dermatologic: Itching

Endocrine & metabolic: Fluid retention

Gastrointestinal: Vomiting

Otic: Tinnitus

Overdosage/Toxicology Symptoms of overdose include nausea, epigastric distress, CNS depression, leukocytosis, and renal failure. Management of NSAID intoxication is supportive and symptomatic. Multiple doses of activated charcoal may interrupt enterohepatic recycling of some NSAIDs.

Pharmacodynamics/Kinetics

Onset of Action: Analgesic: ~1 hour; Peak effect: 3-5 hours

Protein Binding: 99%

Half-Life Elimination: 45-50 hours

Metabolism: Hepatic

Excretion: Primarily urine and feces (small amounts) as unchanged drug (5%) and metabolites

Available Dosage Forms Capsule: 10 mg, 20 mg

Dosing

Adults: Inflammation, rheumatoid arthritis: Oral: 10-20 mg/day once daily; although associated with increase in GI adverse effects, doses >20 mg/day have been used (ie, 30-40 mg/day); maximum dose: 20 mg/day

Elderly: Refer to adult dosing. **Note:** Some clinicians have used 10 mg every other day to initiate therapy in the elderly to help avoid side effects and produce therapeutic effect at minimal dose. Maximum dose: 20 mg/day.

Pediatrics: Oral: Children (unlabeled use): 0.2-0.3 mg/kg/day once daily; maximum dose: 15 mg/day

Renal Impairment: Not recommended in patients with advanced renal disease.

Hepatic Impairment: Reduced dose is necessary.

Laboratory Monitoring Occult blood loss, hemoglobin, hematocrit, and periodic renal and hepatic function tests

Nursing Actions

Physical Assessment: Assess effectiveness and interactions of other medications patient may be taking. Monitor blood pressure at the beginning of therapy and periodically during use. Monitor laboratory tests and therapeutic response (eg, relief of pain and inflammation, increased activity tolerance), and adverse reactions (eg, GI effects, hepatotoxicity, ototoxicity) at beginning of therapy and periodically throughout therapy. Schedule ophthalmic evaluations for patients who develop eye complaints during long-term NSAID therapy. Advise patients with diabetes to use serum glucose testing. Assess knowledge/teach patient appropriate use, interventions to reduce side effects, and adverse symptoms to report.

Patient Education: Take this medication exactly as directed; do not increase dose without consulting prescriber. Do not break capsules. Take with food or milk to reduce GI distress. Maintain adequate hydration (2-3 L/day of fluids) unless instructed to restrict fluid intake. Do not use alcohol, aspirin or aspirin-containing medication, or any other anti-inflammatory medications without consulting prescriber. You may experience drowsiness, dizziness, or nervousness (use caution when driving or engaging in tasks requiring alertness until response to drug is known); anorexia, nausea, vomiting, flatulence, or heartburn (small frequent meals, frequent mouth care, sucking lozenges, or chewing gum may help); or fluid retention (weigh yourself weekly and report unusual weight gain [3-5 lb/week]). GI bleeding, ulceration, or perforation can occur with or without pain; discontinue medication and contact prescriber if persistent abdominal pain or cramping, or blood in stool occurs. Report unusual swelling of extremities or unusual weight gain; breathlessness, respiratory difficulty, or unusual cough; chest pain, rapid heartbeat, palpitations; unusual bruising/bleeding; blood in urine, stool, mouth, or vomitus; unusual fatigue; changes in urinary pattern (polyuria or anuria); skin rash or itching; or change in hearing or ringing in ears. **Pregnancy precaution:** Inform prescriber if you are or intend to become pregnant. This drug should not be used in the 3rd trimester of pregnancy.

Dietary Considerations May be taken with food to decrease GI adverse effect.

Geriatric Considerations Elderly are at high risk for adverse effects from NSAIDs. As much as 60% of elderly can develop peptic ulceration and/or hemorrhage asymptomatically. The concomitant use of H_2 blockers, omeprazole, and sucralfate is not generally effective as prophylaxis with the exception of NSAID-induced duodenal ulcers which may be prevented by the use of ranitidine. Misoprostol is the only prophylactic agent proven effective. Also, concomitant disease and drug use contribute to the risk for GI adverse effects. Use lowest effective dose for shortest period possible. Consider renal function decline with age. Use of NSAIDs can compromise existing renal function especially when Cl_{cr} is ≤30 mL/minute. Tinnitus may be a difficult and unreliable indication of toxicity due to age-related hearing loss or eighth cranial nerve damage. CNS adverse effects such as confusion, agitation, and hallucination are generally seen in overdose or high-dose situations, but elderly may demonstrate these adverse effects at lower doses than younger adults.

Podophyllum Resin (po DOF fil um REZ in)

U.S. Brand Names Podocon-25®

Synonyms Mandrake; May Apple; Podophyllin

Pharmacologic Category Keratolytic Agent

Pregnancy Risk Factor X

Lactation Enters breast milk/contraindicated

Use Topical treatment of benign growths including external genital and perianal warts, papillomas, fibroids; compound benzoin tincture generally is used as the medium for topical application

Mechanism of Action/Effect Directly affects epithelial cell metabolism by arresting mitosis through binding to a protein subunit of spindle microtubules (tubulin)

Contraindications Not to be used on birthmarks, moles, or warts with hair growth; cervical, urethral, oral warts; not to be used by diabetic patient or patient with poor circulation; pregnancy

Warnings/Precautions Use of large amounts of drug should be avoided. Avoid contact with the eyes as it can cause severe corneal damage; do not apply to moles, birthmarks, or unusual warts. To be applied by prescriber only. For external use only; 25% solution should not be applied to or near mucous membranes.

Adverse Reactions 1% to 10%:

Dermatologic: Pruritus

Gastrointestinal: Nausea, vomiting, abdominal pain, diarrhea

Available Dosage Forms Liquid, topical: 25% (15 mL) [in benzoin tincture]

Dosing

Adults & Elderly: Treatment of benign growths (warts, papillomas, fibroids): Topical: 10% to 25% solution in compound benzoin tincture; apply drug to dry surface, use 1 drop at a time allowing drying between drops until area is covered. Total volume should be limited to <0.5 mL per treatment session.

Condylomata acuminatum: 25% solution is applied daily. Use a 10% solution when applied to or near mucous membranes.

Verrucae: 25% solution is applied 3-5 times/day directly to the wart.

Pediatrics: Refer to adult dosing.

Administration

Topical: Shake well before using. **Only to be applied by physician.** Solution should be washed off within 1-4 hours for genital and perianal warts and within 1-2 hours for accessible meatal warts. Use protective occlusive dressing around warts to prevent contact with unaffected skin. For external use only.

Nursing Actions

Physical Assessment: Pregnancy risk factor X: Determine that patient is not pregnant before starting therapy. Do not give to sexually-active female patients unless capable of complying with contraceptive use. Breast-feeding is contraindicated.

Patient Education: Cover with occlusive dressing to prevent contact with unaffected skin. Wash off medication as instructed by professional who applied the treatment. **Pregnancy/breast-feeding precautions:** Inform prescriber if you are pregnant. Do not get pregnant during or for 1 month following therapy. Consult prescriber for instruction on appropriate contraceptive measures. This drug may cause severe fetal defects. Do not breast-feed.

Polyethylene Glycol-Electrolyte Solution

(pol i ETH i leen GLY kol ee LEK troe lite soe LOO shun)

U.S. Brand Names Colyte®; GoLYTELY®; NuLYTELY®; TriLyte™

Synonyms Electrolyte Lavage Solution

Pharmacologic Category Laxative, Osmotic

Medication Safety Issues

Sound-alike/look-alike issues:

GoLYTELY® may be confused with NuLYTELY®

NuLYTELY® may be confused with GoLYTELY®

Pregnancy Risk Factor C

Lactation Excretion in breast milk unknown/use caution

Use Bowel cleansing prior to GI examination or following toxic ingestion

Mechanism of Action/Effect Induces catharsis by strong electrolyte and osmotic effects

Contraindications Hypersensitivity to polyethylene glycol or any component of the formulation; gastrointestinal obstruction, gastric retention, bowel perforation, toxic colitis, megacolon

Warnings/Precautions Do not add flavorings as additional ingredients before use. Observe unconscious or semiconscious patients with impaired gag reflex or those who are otherwise prone to regurgitation or aspiration during administration. Use with caution in ulcerative colitis. Caution against the use of hot loop polypectomy.

Drug Interactions

Decreased Effect: Oral medications should not be administered within 1 hour of start of therapy.

Adverse Reactions Frequency not defined.

Dermatologic: Dermatitis, rash, urticaria

Gastrointestinal: Nausea, abdominal fullness, bloating, abdominal cramps, vomiting, anal irritation, diarrhea, flatulence

Pharmacodynamics/Kinetics

Onset of Action: Oral: ~1-2 hours

Available Dosage Forms

Powder, for oral solution: PEG 3350 240 g, sodium sulfate 22.72 g, sodium bicarbonate 6.72 g, sodium chloride 5.84 g, and potassium chloride 2.98 g (4000 mL)

Colyte®:

PEG 3350 240 g, sodium sulfate 22.72 g, sodium bicarbonate 6.72 g, sodium chloride 5.84 g, and potassium chloride 2.98 g (4000 mL) [available

(Continued)

Polyethylene Glycol-Electrolyte Solution *(Continued)*

with citrus berry, lemon lime, cherry, and pineapple flavor packets]

PEG 3350 227.1 g, sodium sulfate 21.5 g, sodium bicarbonate 6.36 g, sodium chloride 5.53 g, and potassium chloride 2.82 g (4000 mL) [regular and pineapple flavor]

GoLYTELY®:

Disposable jug: PEG 3350 236 g, sodium sulfate 22.74 g, sodium bicarbonate 6.74 g, sodium chloride 5.86 g, and potassium chloride 2.97 g (4000 mL) [regular and pineapple flavor]

Packets: PEG 3350 227.1 g, sodium sulfate 21.5 g, sodium bicarbonate 6.36 g, sodium chloride 5.53 g, and potassium chloride 2.82 g (4000 mL) [regular flavor]

NuLYTELY®: PEG 3350 420 g, sodium bicarbonate 5.72 g, sodium chloride 11.2 g, and potassium chloride 1.48 (4000 mL) [cherry, lemon-lime, and orange flavors]

TriLyte™: PEG 3350 420 g, sodium bicarbonate 5.72 g, sodium chloride 11.2 g, and potassium chloride 1.48 (4000 mL) [supplied with flavor packets]

Dosing

Adults & Elderly: Bowel cleansing prior to GI exam: Ideally, patients should fast for ~3-4 hours prior to administration; absolutely no solid food for at least 2 hours before the solution is given. The solution may be given via nasogastric tube to patients who are unwilling or unable to drink the solution.

Oral: 240 mL (8 oz) every 10 minutes, until 4 L are consumed or the rectal effluent is clear; rapid drinking of each portion is preferred to drinking small amounts continuously.

Nasogastric tube: 20-30 mL/minute (1.2-1.8 L/hour); the first bowel movement should occur ~1 hour after the start of administration.

Pediatrics: Bowel cleansing prior to GI exam: Children ≥6 months: Ideally, patients should fast for ~3-4 hours prior to administration; absolutely no solid food for at least 2 hours before the solution is given.

Oral: 25-40 mL/kg/hour for 4-10 hours until rectal effluent is clear

Nasogastric tube: 25 mL/kg/hour until rectal effluent is clear

Administration

Oral: Oral: Rapid drinking of each portion is preferred to drinking small amounts continuously. Do not add flavorings as additional ingredients before use. Chilled solution often more palatable.

Stability

Reconstitution:

Powder for solution (with electrolytes): Use within 48 hours of preparation; refrigerate reconstituted solution; tap water may be used for preparation of the solution; shake container vigorously several times to ensure dissolution of powder. Do not add additional flavorings to solution.

Storage: Store at 15°C to 30°C (59°F to 86°F) before reconstitution.

Laboratory Monitoring Electrolytes, serum glucose, BUN, urine osmolality

Nursing Actions

Physical Assessment: Instruct patient in appropriate use according to formulation and purpose for use.

Patient Education: Follow instructions exactly; directions will differ according to the formulation and the purpose for which this medication is taken. Do not eat any solid foods for at least 2 -3 hours before taking and do not take any other oral medication for 1 hour before taking. For bowel cleansing prior to GI exam, take 240 mL (8 oz) every 10 minutes, until 4 L is consumed or the rectal effluent is clear. Rapid drinking of each portion is preferred to drinking small

amounts continuously. The first bowel movement should occur approximately 1 hour after the start of administration. May cause abdominal bloating and distention before bowel starts to move. If severe discomfort or distention occurs, stop drinking temporarily or drink each portion at longer intervals until these symptoms disappear. Continue drinking until the watery stool is clear and free of solid matter. This usually requires at least 3 L. It is best to drink all of the solutions. Discard any unused portion. **Pregnancy/breast-feeding precautions:** Inform prescriber if you are or intend to become pregnant. Consult prescriber if breast-feeding.

Dietary Considerations Ideally, the patient should fast for ~3-4 hours prior to administration, but in no case should solid food be given for at least 2 hours before the solution is given.

Breast-Feeding Issues Significant changes in the mother's fluid or electrolyte balance would not be expected.

Polyethylene Glycol-Electrolyte Solution and Bisacodyl

(pol i ETH i leen GLY kol ee LEK troe lite soe LOO shun & bis a KOE dil)

U.S. Brand Names HalfLytely® and Bisacodyl

Synonyms Electrolyte Lavage Solution

Pharmacologic Category Laxative, Bowel Evacuant; Laxative, Stimulant

Pregnancy Risk Factor C

Lactation Excretion in breast milk unknown/use caution

Use Bowel cleansing prior to GI examination

Available Dosage Forms Kit (HalfLytely® and Bisacodyl) [each kit contains]:

Powder for oral solution (HalfLytely®): PEG 3350 210 g, sodium bicarbonate 2.86 g, sodium chloride 5.6 g, potassium chloride 0.74 g (2000 mL) [sulfate-free, regular, cherry, lemon-lime, orange flavor]

Tablet, delayed release (Bisacodyl): 5 mg (4s)

Dosing

Adults & Elderly: Bowel cleansing: Oral:

Bisacodyl: 4 tablets as a single dose. After bowel movement or 6 hours (whichever occurs first), initiate polyethylene glycol-electrolyte solution

Polyethylene glycol-electrolyte solution: 8 ounces every 10 minutes until 2 L are consumed

Nursing Actions

Physical Assessment: Instruct patient in appropriate use and preparation.

Patient Education: This preparation is intended to produce a watery stool which cleanses the bowel before examination. For best results, consume only clear liquids on the day of the examination unless otherwise directed by prescriber. Do not take antacids within 1 hour of taking the bisacodyl delayed-release tablets. Swallow all tablets (4) whole with water. Do not chew or crush. Expect the first bowel movement in approximately 1-6 hours after taking tablets. Wait for bowel movement (or maximum 6 hours), then drink the solution. Drink 8 ounces every 10 minutes. Drink all of the solution. Rapid drinking of each portion is better than drinking small amounts. A bowel movement should occur in approximately 1 hour after drinking the solution. You may experience bloating or abdominal distention before the bowels start to move. If severe discomfort or distention occurs, stop drinking the solution temporarily or drink each portion at longer intervals until symptoms disappear. **Pregnancy/breast-feeding precaution:** Inform prescriber if you are or intend to become pregnant. Consult prescriber if breast-feeding.

Polymyxin B (pol i MIKS in bee)

U.S. Brand Names Poly-Rx
Synonyms Polymyxin B Sulfate
Pharmacologic Category Antibiotic, Irrigation; Antibiotic, Miscellaneous
Pregnancy Risk Factor B (per expert opinion)
Lactation Excretion in breast milk unknown/use caution
Use Treatment of acute infections caused by susceptible strains of *Pseudomonas aeruginosa*; used occasionally for gut decontamination; parenteral use of polymyxin B has mainly been replaced by less toxic antibiotics, reserved for life-threatening infections caused by organisms resistant to the preferred drugs (eg, pseudomonal meningitis - intrathecal administration)
Mechanism of Action/Effect Binds to phospholipids, alters permeability, and damages the bacterial cytoplasmic membrane permitting leakage of intracellular constituents
Contraindications Hypersensitivity to polymyxin B or any component of the formulation; concurrent use of neuromuscular blockers
Warnings/Precautions Use with caution in patients with impaired renal function (modify dosage) neurotoxic reactions are usually associated with high serum levels, found in patients with impaired renal function. Avoid concurrent or sequential use of other nephrotoxic and neurotoxic drugs, particularly bacitracin, colistin, and the aminoglycosides. The drug's neurotoxicity can result in respiratory paralysis from neuromuscular blockade, especially when the drug is given soon after anesthesia or muscle relaxants. Polymyxin B sulfate is toxic when given parenterally; avoid parenteral use whenever possible.

Drug Interactions

Increased Effect/Toxicity: Increased/prolonged effect of neuromuscular blocking agents.

Adverse Reactions Frequency not defined.
Cardiovascular: Facial flushing
Central nervous system: Neurotoxicity (irritability, drowsiness, ataxia, perioral paresthesia, numbness of the extremities, and blurred vision); dizziness, drug fever, meningeal irritation with intrathecal administration
Dermatologic: Urticarial rash
Endocrine & metabolic: Hypocalcemia, hyponatremia, hypokalemia, hypochloremia
Local: Pain at injection site
Neuromuscular & skeletal: Neuromuscular blockade, weakness
Renal: Nephrotoxicity
Respiratory: Respiratory arrest
Miscellaneous: Anaphylactoid reaction

Overdosage/Toxicology Symptoms of overdose include respiratory paralysis, ototoxicity, and nephrotoxicity. Supportive care is indicated as treatment.

Pharmacodynamics/Kinetics

Time to Peak: Serum: I.M.: ~2 hours
Half-Life Elimination: 4.5-6 hours; prolonged with renal impairment
Excretion: Urine (>60% primarily as unchanged drug)

Available Dosage Forms
Injection, powder for reconstitution: 500,000 units
Powder [for prescription compounding] (Poly-Rx): 100 million units (13 g)

Dosing

Adults & Elderly:
Ear canal infections (external): Otic (in combination with other drugs): Instill 1-2 drops, 3-4 times/day; should be used sparingly to avoid accumulation of excess debris.
Systemic infections:
I.M.: 25,000-30,000 units/kg/day divided every 4-6 hours

I.V.: 15,000-25,000 units/kg/day divided every 12 hours
Intrathecal: 50,000 units/day for 3-4 days, then every other day for at least 2 weeks
Note: Total daily dose should not exceed 2,000,000 units/day.
Bladder irrigation (in combination with 57 mg neomycin sulfate): Continuous irrigant or rinse in the urinary bladder for up to 10 days using 20 mg (equal to 200,000 units) added to 1 L of normal saline; usually no more than 1 L of irrigant is used per day unless urine flow rate is high; administration rate is adjusted to patient's urine output.
Topical irrigation or topical solution: 500,000 units/ L of normal saline; topical irrigation should not exceed 2 million units/day in adults.
Ocular infections: Ophthalmic: A concentration of 0.1% to 0.25% is administered as 1-3 drops every hour, then increasing the interval as response indicates to 1-2 drops 4-6 times/day.

Pediatrics:
Ear canal infections (external): Otic (in combination with other drugs): 1-2 drops, 3-4 times/day; should be used sparingly to avoid accumulation of excess debris
Systemic infections: Infants <2 years:
I.M.: Up to 40,000 units/kg/day divided every 6 hours (not routinely recommended due to pain at injection sites)
I.V.: Up to 40,000 units/kg/day divided every 12 hours
Intrathecal: 20,000 units/day for 3-4 days, then 25,000 units every other day for at least 2 weeks after CSF cultures are negative and CSF (glucose) has returned to within normal limits
Children ≥2 years: Refer to adult dosing.
Renal Impairment:
Cl$_{cr}$ 20-50 mL/minute: Administer 75% to 100% of normal dose every 12 hours.
Cl$_{cr}$ 5-20 mL/minute: Administer 50% of normal dose every 12 hours.
Cl$_{cr}$ <5 mL/minute: Administer 15% of normal dose every 12 hours.

Administration

I.M.: Administer into upper outer quadrant of gluteal muscle; however, I.M. route is not recommended due to severe pain at injection site.
I.V.: Infuse over 60-90 minutes.
I.V. Detail: Extravasation management: Monitor I.V. site closely; extravasation may cause serious injury with possible necrosis and tissue sloughing. Rotate infusion site frequently.

pH: 5.0-7.5

Stability

Compatibility: Compatibility when admixed: Incompatible with amphotericin B, calcium chloride, calcium gluconate, cefazolin, chloramphenicol, chlorothiazide, heparin, magnesium sulfate
Storage: Prior to reconstitution, store at room temperature of 15°C to 30°C (59°F to 86°F) and protect from light. After reconstitution, store under refrigeration at 2°C to 8°C (36°F to 46°F). Discard any unused solution after 72 hours. **Incompatible** with strong acids/ alkalies, calcium, magnesium, cephalothin, cefazolin, chloramphenicol, heparin, penicillins.

Laboratory Monitoring Perform culture and sensitivity prior to beginning therapy. Establish baseline renal function prior to initiating therapy. Monitor renal function closely.

Nursing Actions

Physical Assessment: Results of culture and sensitivity tests and patient's allergy history should be assessed prior to starting therapy. Assess potential for interactions with other pharmacological agents patient may be taking (eg. nephrotoxic and neurotoxic
(Continued)

Polymyxin B (Continued)

drugs, neuromuscular blocking agents). See Administration for I.V. and I.M. specifics. Monitor infusion site closely to prevent extravasation; extravasation may cause serious injury with possible necrosis and tissue sloughing (rotate infusion site should be rotated frequently). Monitor effectiveness (resolution of infection) and adverse reactions (eg, renal function, neurotoxicity [irritability, drowsiness, ataxia, perioral paresthesia, numbness of the extremities, and blurring of vision]; neuromuscular blockade, rash, respiratory paralysis, ototoxicity). Teach patient possible side effects/appropriate interventions and adverse symptoms to report.

Patient Education: Wound irrigation/bladder irrigation/gut sterilization/I.V.: Immediately report numbness or tingling of mouth, tongue, or extremities; constant blurring of vision; increased nervousness or irritability; excessive drowsiness; or respiratory difficulty. For I.V. immediately report swelling, redness, burning, or pain at infusion site.

Ophthalmic: Tilt head back, place medication into eyes (as frequently as prescribed), close eyes, apply light pressure over inside corner of the eye for 1 minute. Do not let tip of applicator touch eye; do not contaminate tip of applicator (may cause eye infection, eye damage, or vision loss). You may experience some stinging or burning or temporary blurring of vision; use caution driving or when engaging in hazardous tasks until vision clears. Report any adverse effects including respiratory difficulty or unusual numbness or tingling of mouth or tongue, increased nervousness or irritability, or excessive drowsiness.

Breast-feeding precaution: Consult prescriber if breast-feeding.

Additional Information 1 mg = 10,000 units

Porfimer (POR fi mer)

U.S. Brand Names Photofrin®

Synonyms CL-184116; Dihematoporphyrin Ether; Porfimer Sodium

Pharmacologic Category Antineoplastic Agent, Miscellaneous

Pregnancy Risk Factor C

Lactation Excretion in breast milk unknown/contraindicated

Use Adjunct to laser light therapy for obstructing esophageal cancer, obstructing endobronchial nonsmall cell lung cancer (NSCLC), ablation of high-grade dysplasia in Barrett's esophagus

Unlabeled/Investigational Use Transitional cell carcinoma in situ of the urinary bladder; gastric and rectal cancers

Mechanism of Action/Effect Photosensitizing agent used in the photodynamic therapy (PDT) of tumors: cytotoxic and antitumor actions of porfimer are light and oxygen dependent. Cellular damage caused by porfimer PDT is a consequence of the propagation of radical reactions.

Contraindications Hypersensitivity to porfimer, porphyrins, or any component of the formulation; porphyria; tracheoesophageal or bronchoesophageal fistula; tumors eroding into a major blood vessel

Warnings/Precautions Hazardous agent - use appropriate precautions for handling and disposal. Photosensitivity reactions are common is patients are exposed to direct sunlight or bright indoor light (eg fluorescent lights, unshaded light bulbs, examination/operating lights). Photosensitivity may last 30-90 days. Ocular discomfort has been reported; for at least 30 days, when

outdoors, patients should wear dark sunglasses which have an average white light transmittance of <4%. When treating endobronchial tumors, use caution if treatment-induced inflammation may obstruct airway.

Drug Interactions

Decreased Effect: Compounds that quench active oxygen species or scavenge radicals (eg, dimethyl sulfoxide, beta-carotene, ethanol, mannitol) would be expected to decrease photodynamic therapy (PDT) activity. Allopurinol, calcium channel blockers, and some prostaglandin synthesis inhibitors could interfere with porfimer. Drugs that decrease clotting, vasoconstriction, or platelet aggregation could decrease the efficacy of PDT. Glucocorticoid hormones may decrease the efficacy of the treatment.

Increased Effect/Toxicity: Concomitant administration of other photosensitizing agents (eg, tetracyclines, sulfonamides, phenothiazines, sulfonylureas, thiazide diuretics, griseofulvin) could increase the photosensitivity reaction.

Adverse Reactions

>10%:
Cardiovascular: Atrial fibrillation (10%), chest pain (5% to 22%)
Central nervous system: Insomnia (14%), hyperthermia (31%)
Dermatologic: Photosensitivity reaction (10% to 80%, minor reactions may occur in up to 100%)
Gastrointestinal: Abdominal pain (20%), constipation (23%), dysphagia, nausea (24%), vomiting (17%)
Genitourinary: Urinary tract irritation including frequency, urgency, nocturia, painful urination, or bladder spasm (~100% of bladder cancer patients)
Hematologic: Anemia (26% of esophageal cancer patients)
Neuromuscular & skeletal: Back pain
Respiratory: Dyspnea (20%), pharyngitis (11%), pleural effusion (32% of esophageal cancer patients), pneumonia (18%), respiratory insufficiency
Miscellaneous: Mild-moderate allergic-type reactions (34% of lung cancer patients)

1% to 10%:
Cardiovascular: Hyper-/hypotension (6% to 7%), edema, cardiac failure (6% to 7%), tachycardia (6%), chest pain (substernal)
Central nervous system: Anxiety (7%), confusion (8%)
Dermatologic: Increased hair growth, skin discoloration, skin wrinkles, skin nodules, increased skin fragility
Endocrine & metabolic: Dehydration
Gastrointestinal: Diarrhea (5%), dyspepsia (6%), eructation (5%), esophageal edema (8%), esophageal tumor bleeding, esophageal stricture, esophagitis, hematemesis, melena, weight loss, anorexia
Genitourinary: Urinary tract infection
Neuromuscular & skeletal: Weakness
Respiratory: Coughing, tracheoesophageal fistula
Miscellaneous: Moniliasis, surgical complication

Overdosage/Toxicology Laser treatment should not be given if an overdose of porfimer is administered. In the event of overdose, patients should protect their eyes and skin from direct sunlight or bright indoor lights for 30 days. Patients should be tested for residual photosensitivity. Porfimer is not dialyzable.

Pharmacodynamics/Kinetics

Time to Peak: Serum: ~2 hours

Protein Binding: Plasma: 90%

Half-Life Elimination: Mean: 21.5 days (range: 11-28 days)

Excretion: Feces

Clearance: Plasma: Total: 0.051 mL/minute/kg

Available Dosage Forms Injection, powder for reconstitution, as sodium: 75 mg

Dosing

Adults & Elderly: Cancer photodynamic therapy: I.V.: 2 mg/kg, followed by exposure to the appropriate laser light

Pediatrics: I.V. (refer to individual protocols): Children: Safety and efficacy have not been established.

Administration

I.V.: Administer slow I.V. injection over 3-5 minutes.

I.V. Detail: Avoid extravasation. Eye protection is recommended.

pH: 7-8

Stability

Reconstitution: Reconstitute each vial of porfimer with 31.8 mL of either D₅W or NS injection resulting in a final concentration of 2.5 mg/mL. Shake well until dissolved. Protect the reconstituted product from bright light and use immediately.

Compatibility: Do not mix porfimer with other drugs in the same solution.

Storage: Store intact vials at controlled room temperature of 20°C to 25°C (68°F to 77°F). Reconstituted solutions are stable for 24 hours under refrigeration and protected from light.

Nursing Actions

Physical Assessment: Assess potential for interactions with other pharmacological agents patient may be taking (eg, drugs the decrease the effect of PDT or porfimer or increase photosensitivity reaction). See Administration specifics; infusion site must be monitored closely to prevent extravasation. Patients will be photosensitive and must be protected from direct sunlight or bright indoor light for 30"60 days after treatment. Ambient indoor light is, however, beneficial (should not stay in dark rooms). Assess patient response (eg, atrial fibrillation, hyper-/hypotension, hyperthermia, GI pain or upset, anemia, dyspnea, respiratory insufficiency, dehydration). Teach patient (caregiver) possible side effects/appropriate interventions and adverse symptoms to report.

Patient Education: This drug can only be given by injection or infusion. Report immediately any redness, swelling, burning, or pain at infusion site. The infusion will be followed by laser light therapy. Maintain adequate hydration (2-3 L/day of fluids) unless instructed to restrict fluid intake. You will be highly sensitive to bright light. Avoid exposure to sunlight or bright indoor light for at least 30 days following treatment (cover skin with protective clothing and wear dark sunglasses with light transmittance <4% when outdoors - severe blistering, burning, and skin/eye damage can result). Conventional sunscreens do not protect against photosensitization. After 30 days, test small area of skin (not face) for remaining sensitivity. Retest sensitivity if traveling to a different geographic area with greater sunshine. Exposure to indoor normal light is beneficial since it will help dissipate photosensitivity gradually. May cause nausea or vomiting (small, frequent meals, frequent mouth care, sucking lozenges, or chewing gum may help); or constipation (increased exercise, fluids, fruit, or fiber may help). Report rapid heart rate, chest pain or palpitations, respiratory difficulty or air hunger, persistent fever or chills, foul-smelling urine or burning on urination, swelling of extremities, increased anxiety, confusion, or hallucination. **Pregnancy/breast-feeding precautions:** Inform prescriber if you are pregnant. Do not breast-feed.

Pregnancy Issues Animal studies have shown maternal and fetal toxicity, but no major malformations. Effective contraception is recommended for women of childbearing potential.

Potassium Acetate (poe TASS ee um AS e tate)

Pharmacologic Category Electrolyte Supplement, Parenteral

Pregnancy Risk Factor C

Use Potassium deficiency; to avoid chloride when high concentration of potassium is needed, source of bicarbonate

Available Dosage Forms Injection, solution: 2 mEq/mL (20 mL, 50 mL, 100 mL); 4 mEq/mL (50 mL) [contains aluminum ≤200 mcg/mL]

Dosing

Adults & Elderly: I.V. doses should be incorporated into the patient's maintenance I.V. fluids, intermittent I.V. potassium administration should be reserved for severe depletion situations and requires ECG monitoring; doses listed as mEq of potassium

Treatment of hypokalemia: I.V.: 40-100 mEq/day

I.V. intermittent infusion (must be diluted prior to administration):

5-10 mEq/dose (maximum: 40 mEq/dose) to infuse over 2-3 hours (maximum: 40 mEq over 1 hour)

Note: Continuous cardiac monitor recommended for rates >0.5 mEq/hour

Potassium dosage/rate of infusion guidelines:

Serum potassium >2.5 mEq/L: Maximum infusion rate: 10 mEq/hour; maximum concentration: 40 mEq/L; maximum 24-hour dose: 200 mEq

Serum potassium <2.5 mEq/L: Maximum infusion rate: 40 mEq/hour; maximum concentration: 80 mEq/L; maximum 24-hour dose: 400 mEq

Pediatrics: I.V. doses should be incorporated into the patient's maintenance I.V. fluids, intermittent I.V. potassium administration should be reserved for severe depletion situations and requires ECG monitoring; doses listed as mEq of potassium.

Note: Use caution in premature neonates; potassium acetate for injection contains aluminum.

Treatment of hypokalemia: I.V.: 2-5 mEq/kg/day

I.V. intermittent infusion (must be diluted prior to administration): 0.5-1 mEq/kg/dose (maximum: 30 mEq/dose) to infuse at 0.3-0.5 mEq/kg/hour (maximum: 1 mEq/kg/hour)

Note: Continuous cardiac monitor recommended for rates >0.5 mEq/hour

Potassium dosage/rate of infusion guidelines:

Serum potassium >2.5 mEq/L: Maximum infusion rate: 10 mEq/hour; maximum concentration: 40 mEq/L; maximum 24-hour dose: 200 mEq

Serum potassium <2.5 mEq/L: Maximum infusion rate: 40 mEq/hour; maximum concentration: 80 mEq/L; maximum 24-hour dose: 400 mEq

Renal Impairment: Use caution; potassium acetate injection contains aluminum.

Nursing Actions

Patient Education: This form of potassium may only be given I.V. Report immediately any burning or pain at infusion site, chest pain, palpitations, unusual weakness in muscles, tarry stools, or easy bruising.

Potassium Acetate, Potassium Bicarbonate, and Potassium Citrate
(poe TASS ee um AS e tate, poe TASS ee um bye KAR bun ate, & poe TASS ee um SIT rate)

U.S. Brand Names Tri-K®

Synonyms Potassium Acetate, Potassium Citrate, and Potassium Bicarbonate; Potassium Bicarbonate, Potassium Acetate, and Potassium Citrate; Potassium Bicarbonate, Potassium Citrate, and Potassium Acetate; Potassium Citrate, Potassium Acetate, and Potassium Bicarbonate; Potassium Citrate, Potassium Bicarbonate, and Potassium Acetate

Pharmacologic Category Electrolyte Supplement, Oral

Pregnancy Risk Factor C

Use Treatment or prevention of hypokalemia

Available Dosage Forms Solution, oral: Potassium 45 mEq/15 mL (480 mL) [from potassium acetate 1500 mg, potassium bicarbonate 1500 mg, and potassium citrate 1500 mg per 15 mL]

Dosing
Adults & Elderly: Hypokalemia: Oral:
Prevention: 16-24 mEq/day in 2-4 divided doses
Treatment: 40-100 mEq/day in 2-4 divided doses
Pediatrics: Hypokalemia: Oral:
Children: 1-4 mEq/kg/24 hours in divided doses as required to maintain normal serum potassium

Related Information
Potassium Acetate *on page 1007*
Potassium Bicarbonate *on page 1008*
Potassium Citrate *on page 1010*

Potassium Acid Phosphate
(poe TASS ee um AS id FOS fate)

U.S. Brand Names K-Phos® Original

Pharmacologic Category Urinary Acidifying Agent

Pregnancy Risk Factor C

Use Acidifies urine and lowers urinary calcium concentration; reduces odor and rash caused by ammoniacal urine; increases the antibacterial activity of methenamine

Available Dosage Forms Tablet [scored]: 500 mg [phosphorus 114 mg and potassium 144 mg (3.7 mEq) per tablet; sodium free]

Dosing
Adults & Elderly: Urine acidification: Oral: 1000 mg dissolved in 6-8 oz of water 4 times/day with meals and at bedtime; for best results, soak tablets in water for 2-5 minutes, then stir and swallow

Nursing Actions
Patient Education: Dissolve tablets completely before drinking. Avoid taking magnesium, calcium, or aluminum antacids at the same time. Patients may pass old kidney stones when starting therapy. Notify physician if experiencing nausea, vomiting, or abdominal pain.

Potassium Bicarbonate
(poe TASS ee um bye KAR bun ate)

Pharmacologic Category Electrolyte Supplement, Oral

Pregnancy Risk Factor C

Use Potassium deficiency, hypokalemia

Available Dosage Forms Tablet for oral solution, effervescent: Potassium 25 mEq

Dosing
Adults & Elderly: Hypokalemia: Oral: 25 mEq 2-4 times/day

Pediatrics: Hypokalemia: Oral: Children: 1-4 mEq/kg/day

Nursing Actions
Patient Education: Dissolve completely in 3-8 oz cold water, juice, or other suitable beverage and drink slowly.

Potassium Bicarbonate and Potassium Chloride
(poe TASS ee um bye KAR bun ate & poe TASS ee um KLOR ide)

U.S. Brand Names K-Lyte/Cl®; K-Lyte/Cl® 50 [DSC]

Synonyms Potassium Bicarbonate and Potassium Chloride (Effervescent)

Pharmacologic Category Electrolyte Supplement, Oral

Pregnancy Risk Factor C

Lactation Enters breast milk/compatible

Use Treatment or prevention of hypokalemia

Available Dosage Forms [DSC] = Discontinued product
Tablet for oral solution, effervescent:
K-Lyte/Cl®: Potassium chloride 25 mEq [potassium chloride 1.5 g and potassium bicarbonate 0.5 g; citrus or fruit punch flavor]
K-Lyte/Cl® 50: Potassium chloride 50 mEq [potassium chloride 2.24 g and potassium bicarbonate 2 g; citrus flavor] [DSC]

Dosing
Adults & Elderly: Hypokalemia: Oral:
Prevention: 16-24 mEq/day in 2-4 divided doses
Treatment: 40-100 mEq/day in 2-4 divided doses

Nursing Actions
Physical Assessment: Assess for adequate kidney function, use of ACE inhibitors, or potassium-sparing diuretics prior to starting therapy. Monitor cardiac status and serum potassium levels on a regular basis with long-term therapy. Instruct patient on appropriate diet and administration.

Patient Education: Take as directed; do not take more than directed. Dissolve tablets in water or juice and stir before drinking. Do not take on an empty stomach; take with or after meals. Consult prescriber about increasing dietary potassium intake (eg, salt substitutes, orange juice, bananas). Report tingling of hands or feet, unresolved nausea or vomiting, chest pain, palpitations, persistent abdominal pain, muscle cramping or weakness, tarry stools, easy bruising, or unusual bleeding. **Pregnancy precaution:** Inform prescriber if you are pregnant.

Related Information
Potassium Bicarbonate *on page 1008*
Potassium Chloride *on page 1009*

Potassium Bicarbonate and Potassium Citrate
(poe TASS ee um bye KAR bun ate & poe TASS ee um SIT rate)

U.S. Brand Names Effer-K™; Klor-Con®/EF; K-Lyte®; K-Lyte® DS

Synonyms Potassium Bicarbonate and Potassium Citrate (Effervescent)

Pharmacologic Category Electrolyte Supplement, Oral

Pregnancy Risk Factor C

Use Treatment or prevention of hypokalemia

Available Dosage Forms
Tablet, effervescent: Potassium 25 mEq
Effer-K™: Potassium 25 mEq

Klor-Con®/EF: Potassium 25 mEq [orange flavor]
K-Lyte®: Potassium 25 mEq [orange flavor]
K-Lyte® DS: Potassium 50 mEq [lime or orange flavor]

Dosing

Adults & Elderly: Hypokalemia: Oral:
Prevention: 16-24 mEq/day in 2-4 divided doses
Treatment: 40-100 mEq/day in 2-4 divided doses

Pediatrics: Hypokalemia: Oral: Children: 1-4 mEq/kg/24 hours in divided doses as required to maintain normal serum potassium

Nursing Actions

Patient Education: Dissolve completely in 3-8 oz cold water, juice, or other suitable beverage and drink slowly.

Related Information

Potassium Bicarbonate *on page 1008*
Potassium Citrate *on page 1010*

Potassium Chloride
(poe TASS ee um KLOR ide)

U.S. Brand Names Kaon-Cl-10®; Kaon-Cl® 20; Kay Ciel®; K-Dur® 10; K-Dur® 20; K-Lor®; Klor-Con®; Klor-Con® 8; Klor-Con® 10; Klor-Con®/25; Klor-Con® M; K+ Potassium; K-Tab®; microK®; microK® 10; Rum-K®

Synonyms KCl

Pharmacologic Category Electrolyte Supplement, Oral; Electrolyte Supplement, Parenteral

Medication Safety Issues
Sound-alike/look-alike issues:
Kaon-Cl-10® may be confused with kaolin
KCl may be confused with HCl
K-Dur® may be confused with Cardura®, Imdur®
K-Lor® may be confused with Kaochlor®, Klor-Con®
Klor-Con® may be confused with Klaron®, K-Lor®
Klotrix® may be confused with liotrix
microK® may be confused with Micronase®

High alert medication: The Institute for Safe Medication Practices (ISMP) includes this medication (I.V. formulation) among its list of drugs which have a heightened risk of causing significant patient harm when used in error.

Per JCAHO recommendations, concentrated electrolyte solutions should not be available in patient care areas.

Consider special storage requirements for intravenous potassium salts; I.V. potassium salts have been administered IVP in error, leading to fatal outcomes.

Pregnancy Risk Factor A

Use Treatment or prevention of hypokalemia

Contraindications Severe renal impairment, untreated Addison's disease, heat cramps, hyperkalemia, severe tissue trauma; solid oral dosage forms are contraindicated in patients in whom there is a structural, pathological, and/or pharmacologic cause for delay or arrest in passage through the GI tract; an oral liquid potassium preparation should be used in patients with esophageal compression or delayed gastric emptying time

Warnings/Precautions Use with caution in patients with cardiac disease, severe renal impairment, hyperkalemia.

Drug Interactions
Increased Effect/Toxicity: Potassium-sparing diuretics, salt substitutes, ACE inhibitors

Adverse Reactions
>10%: Gastrointestinal: Diarrhea, nausea, stomach pain, flatulence, vomiting (oral)
1% to 10%:
Cardiovascular: Bradycardia
Endocrine & metabolic: Hyperkalemia
Local: Local tissue necrosis with extravasation, pain at the site of injection
Neuromuscular & skeletal: Weakness

Respiratory: Dyspnea

Overdosage/Toxicology
Symptoms of overdose include muscle weakness, paralysis, peaked T waves, flattened P waves, prolongation of QRS complex, ventricular arrhythmias

Removal of potassium can be accomplished by various means; removal through the GI tract with Kayexalate® administration; by way of the kidney through diuresis, mineralocorticoid administration or increased sodium intake; by hemodialysis or peritoneal dialysis; or by shifting potassium back into the cells by insulin and glucose infusion or sodium bicarbonate; calcium chloride reverses cardiac effects.

Pharmacodynamics/Kinetics
Excretion: Primarily urine; skin and feces (small amounts); most intestinal potassium reabsorbed

Available Dosage Forms [DSC] = Discontinued product

Capsule, extended release: 10 mEq [750 mg]
microK® [microencapsulated]: 8 mEq [600 mg]
microK® 10 [microencapsulated]: 10 mEq [750 mg]
Infusion [premixed in D_5W]: 20 mEq (1000 mL); 30 mEq (1000 mL); 40 mEq (1000 mL)
Infusion [premixed in D_5W and LR]: 20 mEq (1000 mL); 30 mEq (1000 mL); 40 mEq (1000 mL)
Infusion [premixed in D_5W and 1/4NS]: 10 mEq (500 mL, 1000 mL); 20 mEq (250 mL, 500 mL, 1000 mL); 30 mEq (1000 mL); 40 mEq (1000 mL)
Infusion [premixed in D_5W and 1/2NS]: 10 mEq (500 mL, 1000 mL); 20 mEq (500 mL, 1000 mL); 30 mEq (1000 mL); 40 mEq (1000 mL)
Infusion [premixed in D_5 and NS]: 20 mEq (1000 mL); 40 mEq (1000 mL)
Infusion [premixed in D_5W and sodium chloride 0.3%]: 10 mEq (500 mL); 20 mEq (1000 mL); 30 mEq (1000 mL); 40 mEq (1000 mL)
Infusion [premixed in $D_{10}W$ and sodium chloride 0.2%]: 20 mEq (250 mL)
Infusion [premixed in NS]: 20 mEq (1000 mL); 40 mEq (1000 mL)
Infusion [premixed in SWFI; concentrate]: 10 mEq (50 mL, 100 mL); 20 mEq (50 mL, 100 mL); 30 mEq (100 mL); 40 mEq (100 mL)
Injection, solution [concentrate]: 2 mEq/mL (5 mL, 10 mL, 15 mL, 20 mL, 30 mL, 250 mL, 500 mL)
Powder, for oral solution: 20 mEq/packet (30s, 100s, 1000s)
K-Lor™: 20 mEq/packet (30s, 100s) [fruit flavor]
K+ Potassium: 20 mEq/packet (30s) [orange flavor]
Kay Ciel® 10%: 20 mEq/packet (30s, 100s) [sugar free]
Klor-Con®: 20 mEq/packet (30s, 100s) [sugar free; fruit flavor]
Klor-Con®/25: 25 mEq/packet (30s, 100s) [sugar free; fruit flavor]
Solution, oral: 20 mEq/15 mL (480 mL, 3840 mL); 40 mEq/15 mL (480 mL)
Kaon-Cl® 20: 40 mEq/15 mL (480 mL) [sugar free; contains alcohol; cherry flavor]
Kay Ciel®: 10%: 20 mEq/15 mL (480 mL) [sugar free; contains alcohol] [DSC]
Rum-K®: 20 mEq/10 mL (480 mL) [alcohol free, sugar free; butter/rum flavor]
Tablet, extended release: 8 mEq [600 mg]; 10 mEq [750 mg]; 20 mEq [1500 mg]
K-Dur® 10 [microencapsulated]: 10 mEq [750 mg]
K-Dur® 20 [microencapsulated]: 20 mEq [1500 mg; scored]
K-Tab®: 10 mEq [750 mg]
Kaon-Cl® 10: 10 mEq [750 mg]
Klor-Con® 8: 8 mEq [600 mg; wax matrix]
Klor-Con® 10: 10 mEq [750 mg; wax matrix]
Klor-Con® M10 [microencapsulated]: 10 mEq [750 mg]
Klor-Con® M15 [microencapsulated]: 15 mEq [1125 mg; scored]

(Continued)

Potassium Chloride *(Continued)*

Klor-Con® M20 [microencapsulated]: 20 mEq [1500 mg; scored]

Dosing

Adults & Elderly: I.V. doses should be incorporated into the patient's maintenance I.V. fluids; intermittent I.V. potassium administration should be reserved for severe depletion situations in patients undergoing ECG monitoring.

Normal daily requirements: Oral, I.V.: 40-80 mEq/ day

Prevention of hypokalemia during diuretic therapy: Oral: 20-40 mEq/day in 1-2 divided doses

Treatment of hypokalemia (guidelines):

Potassium >2.5 mEq/L:

Oral: 60-80 mEq/day plus additional amounts if needed

I.V.: 10 mEq over 1 hour with additional doses if needed

Potassium <2.5 mEq/L:

Oral: Up to 40-60 mEq initial dose, followed by further doses based on lab values

I.V.: Up to 40 mEq over 1 hour, with doses based on frequent lab monitoring; deficits at a plasma level of 2 mEq/L may be as high as 400-800 mEq of potassium

Acute hypokalemia:

I.V. intermittent infusion: 5-10 mEq/hour (continuous cardiac monitor recommended for rates >5 mEq/hour), not to exceed 40 mEq/hour; usual adult maximum per 24 hours: 400 mEq/day.

Potassium dosage/rate of infusion guidelines:

Serum potassium >2.5 mEq/L: Maximum infusion rate: 10 mEq/hour; maximum concentration: 40 mEq/L; maximum 24-hour dose: 200 mEq

Serum potassium <2.5 mEq/L: Maximum infusion rate: 40 mEq/hour; maximum concentration: 80 mEq/L; maximum 24-hour dose: 400 mEq

Pediatrics: I.V. doses should be incorporated into the patient's maintenance I.V. fluids; intermittent I.V. potassium administration should be reserved for severe depletion situations in patients undergoing ECG monitoring.

Normal daily requirements: Oral, I.V.:

Premature infants: 2-6 mEq/kg/24 hours

Term infants 0-24 hours: 0-2 mEq/kg/24 hours

Infants >24 hours: 1-2 mEq/kg/24 hours

Children: 2-3 mEq/kg/day

Prevention of hypokalemia during diuretic therapy: Oral: Children: 1-2 mEq/kg/day in 1-2 divided doses

Treatment of hypokalemia: Children:

Oral: 1-2 mEq/kg initially, then as needed based on frequently obtained lab values. If deficits are severe or ongoing losses are great, I.V. route should be considered.

I.V.: 1 mEq/kg over 1-2 hours initially, then repeated as needed based on frequently obtained lab values; severe depletion or ongoing losses may require >200% of normal limit needs

I.V. intermittent infusion: Dose should not exceed 1 mEq/kg/hour, or 40 mEq/hour; if it exceeds 0.5 mEq/kg/hour, physician should be at bedside and patient should have continuous ECG monitoring; usual pediatric maximum: 3 mEq/kg/day or 40 mEq/m²/day

Administration

Oral: Wax matrix tablets must be swallowed and not allowed to dissolve in mouth.

I.V.: Potassium must be diluted prior to parenteral administration; maximum recommended concentration (peripheral line): 80 mEq/L; maximum recommended concentration (central line): 150 mEq/L or 15

mEq/100 mL; in severely fluid-restricted patients (with central lines): 200 mEq/L or 20 mEq/100 mL has been used; maximum rate of infusion, see Dosing, I.V. intermittent infusion

Stability

Compatibility: Stable in dextran 6% in dextrose, dextran 6% in NS, D₅LR, D₅¼NS, D₅½NS, D₅NS, D₅W, D₁₀W, D₂₀W, LR, ½NS, NS, sodium chloride 3%

Y-site administration: Incompatible with amphotericin B cholesteryl sulfate complex, diazepam, ergotamine, phenytoin

Compatibility when admixed: Incompatible with amphotericin B

Storage: Store at room temperature, protect from freezing; use only clear solutions; use admixtures within 24 hours

Laboratory Monitoring Serum potassium

Nursing Actions

Physical Assessment: Monitor patient response and adverse effects.

Patient Education: Long-acting and wax matrix tablets should be swallowed whole; do not crush or chew. Powder must be dissolved in water before use. Take with food. Liquid can be diluted or dissolved in water or juice.

Dietary Considerations Administer with plenty of fluid and/or food because of stomach irritation and discomfort.

Related Information

Compatibility of Drugs *on page 1370*

Potassium Citrate *(poe TASS ee um SIT rate)*

U.S. Brand Names Urocit®-K

Pharmacologic Category Alkalinizing Agent, Oral

Pregnancy Risk Factor Not available

Lactation Enters breast milk/compatible

Use Prevention of uric acid nephrolithiasis; prevention of calcium renal stones in patients with hypocitraturia; urinary alkalinizer when sodium citrate is contraindicated

Available Dosage Forms Tablet: 540 mg [5 mEq]; 1080 mg [10 mEq]

Dosing

Adults & Elderly: Alkalinizer, bicarbonate precursor: Oral: 10-20 mEq 3 times/day with meals up to 100 mEq/day

Nursing Actions

Physical Assessment: Assess effectiveness and interactions of other medications patient may be taking. Assess kidney function prior to starting therapy. Monitor cardiac status and serum potassium at beginning of therapy and at regular intervals with long-term therapy. Assess knowledge/teach patient appropriate use, recommended diet, and adverse symptoms to report.

Patient Education: Take as directed; do not take more than directed. Swallow tablet whole with full glass of water or juice and stir before sipping slowly, with or after meals (do not take on an empty stomach). Take any antacids 2 hours before or after potassium. Consult prescriber about advisability of increasing dietary potassium. Report tingling of hands or feet; unresolved nausea or vomiting; chest pain or palpitations; persistent abdominal pain; feelings of weakness, dizziness, listlessness, confusion; acute muscle weakness or cramping; blood in stool or tarry stools; or easy bruising or unusual bleeding.

Potassium Citrate and Citric Acid
(poe TASS ee um SIT rate & SI trik AS id)

U.S. Brand Names Cytra-K; Polycitra®-K
Synonyms Citric Acid and Potassium Citrate
Pharmacologic Category Alkalinizing Agent, Oral
Pregnancy Risk Factor A
Lactation Excretion in breast milk unknown/compatible
Use Treatment of metabolic acidosis; alkalinizing agent in conditions where long-term maintenance of an alkaline urine is desirable
Available Dosage Forms Note: Equivalent to potassium 2 mEq/mL and bicarbonate 2 mEq/mL
Powder:
Cytra-K: Potassium citrate 3300 mg and citric acid 1002 mg per packet (100s) [sugar free; fruit flavor]
Polycitra®-K: Potassium citrate 3300 mg and citric acid 1002 mg per packet (100s) [sugar free]
Solution:
Cytra-K: Potassium citrate 1100 mg and citric acid monohydrate 334 mg per 5 mL (480 mL) [alcohol free, sugar free; contains sodium benzoate; cherry flavor]
Polycitra®-K: Potassium citrate 1100 mg and citric acid monohydrate 334 mg per 5 mL (480 mL) [alcohol free, sugar free]
Dosing
Adults & Elderly: Urine alkalizing agent: Oral:
Powder: One packet dissolved in water after meals and at bedtime; adjust dose to urinary pH
Solution: 15-30 mL after meals and at bedtime; adjust dose based on urinary pH
Pediatrics: Urine alkalizing agent: Oral: Solution: 5-15 mL after meals and at bedtime; adjust dose based on urinary pH
Nursing Actions
Physical Assessment: Assess kidney function prior to starting therapy. Monitor cardiac status and serum potassium at beginning of therapy and at regular intervals with long-term therapy. Assess knowledge/teach patient appropriate use, recommended diet, and adverse symptoms to report.
Patient Education: Take as directed; do not take more than directed. Dilute powder or solution in at least 6 oz of juice or water; stir and drink. May drink additional water or juice after dose. Take with or after meals (do not take on an empty stomach). Take any antacids 2 hours before or after potassium. Consult prescriber about advisability of increasing dietary potassium. Report tingling of hands or feet; unresolved nausea or vomiting; chest pain or palpitations; persistent abdominal pain; feelings of weakness, dizziness, listlessness, or confusion; acute muscle weakness or cramping; blood in stool or tarry stools; or easy bruising or unusual bleeding.
Related Information
Potassium Citrate *on page 1010*

Potassium Gluconate
(poe TASS ee um GLOO coe nate)

U.S. Brand Names Glu-K® [OTC]
Pharmacologic Category Electrolyte Supplement, Oral
Pregnancy Risk Factor A
Use Treatment or prevention of hypokalemia
Available Dosage Forms
Tablet: 500 mg, 610 mg
Glu-K®: 486 mg
Tablet, timed release: 595 mg

Dosing
Adults & Elderly: Note: Doses listed as mEq of potassium:
Normal daily requirement: Oral: 40-80 mEq/day
Prevention of hypokalemia during diuretic therapy: Oral: 16-24 mEq/day in 1-2 divided doses
Treatment of hypokalemia: Oral: 40-100 mEq/day in 2-4 divided doses
Pediatrics: Note: Doses listed as mEq of potassium:
Normal daily requirement: Oral: 2-3 mEq/kg/day
Prevention of hypokalemia during diuretic therapy: Oral: 1-2 mEq/kg/day in 1-2 divided doses
Treatment of hypokalemia: Oral: 2-5 mEq/kg/day in 2-4 divided doses
Nursing Actions
Patient Education: Take with food, water, or fruit juice. Swallow tablets whole; do not crush or chew.

Potassium Iodide
(poe TASS ee um EYE oh dide)

U.S. Brand Names Iosat™ [OTC]; Pima®; SSKI®; ThyroSafe™ [OTC]; ThyroShield™ [OTC]
Synonyms KI
Pharmacologic Category Antithyroid Agent; Expectorant
Pregnancy Risk Factor D
Lactation Enters breast milk/use caution (AAP rates "compatible")
Use Expectorant for the symptomatic treatment of chronic pulmonary diseases complicated by mucous; reduce thyroid vascularity prior to thyroidectomy and management of thyrotoxic crisis; block thyroidal uptake of radioactive isotopes of iodine in a radiation emergency or other exposure to radioactive iodine
Unlabeled/Investigational Use Lymphocutaneous and cutaneous sporotrichosis
Available Dosage Forms
Solution, oral:
SSKI®: 1 g/mL (30 mL, 240 mL) [contains sodium thiosulfate]
ThyroShield™: 65 mg/mL (30 mL) [black raspberry flavor]
Syrup (Pima®): 325 mg/5 mL (473 mL) [equivalent to iodide 249 mg/5 mL; black raspberry flavor]
Tablet:
Iosat™: 130 mg
ThyroSafe™: 65 mg [equivalent to iodine 50 mg]
Dosing
Adults & Elderly:
RDA: 150 mcg (iodine)
Expectorant: Oral:
Pima®: 325-650 mg 3 times/day
SSKI®: 300-600 mg 3-4 times/day
Preoperative thyroidectomy: Oral: 50-250 mg (1-5 drops SSKI®) 3 times/day; administer for 10 days before surgery
Radiation protectant to radioactive isotopes of iodine (Pima®): Oral: 195 mg once daily for 10 days; start 24 hours prior to exposure
To reduce risk of thyroid cancer following nuclear accident (Iosat™, ThyroSafe™, ThyroShield™): Oral: Children >68 kg and Adults (including pregnant/lactating women): Oral: 130 mg once daily. **Note:** Dosing should continue until risk of exposure has passed or other measures have are implemented.
Thyrotoxic crisis: Oral: 300-500 mg (6-10 drops SSKI®) 3 times/day
Sporotrichosis (cutaneous, lymphocutaneous; unlabeled use): Oral: Initial: 5 drops (SSKI®) 3 times/day; increase to 40-50 drops (SSKI®) 3 times/day as tolerated for 3-6 months
(Continued)

Potassium Iodide *(Continued)*

Pediatrics:

Expectorant: Oral *(Pima®):*

Children <3 years: 162 mg 3 times day

Children >3 years: 325 mg 3 times/day

Preoperative thyroidectomy: Refer to adult dosing.

Radiation protectant to radioactive isotopes of iodine (Pima®): Oral:

Infants up to 1 year: 65 mg once daily for 10 days; start 24 hours prior to exposure

Children >1 year: 130 mg once daily for 10 days; start 24 hours prior to exposure

To reduce risk of thyroid cancer following nuclear accident (Iosat™, ThyroSafe™, ThyroShield™): Oral:

Infants <1 month: 16.25 mg once daily

Children 1 month to 3 years: 32.5 mg once daily

Children 3-18 years: 65 mg once daily

Children >68 kg: Refer to adult dosing

Note: Dosing should continue until risk of exposure has passed or other measures are implemented.

Thyrotoxic crisis: Oral:

Infants <1 year: 150-250 mg (3-5 drops SSKI®) 3 times/day

Children: Refer to adult dosing.

Nursing Actions

Physical Assessment: Assess potential for interactions with other pharmacological agents or herbal products patient is taking that may increase risk of hyperkalemia, hypokalemia, or additive hypothyroid effects. Monitor laboratory tests, therapeutic effects (according to purpose for use), and adverse reactions. Teach patient purpose for use, necessity for contraception, possible side effects/appropriate interventions, and adverse symptoms to report.

Patient Education: Take this medication exactly as directed; do not exceed recommended dosage. Take Pima® with at least 4-6 ounces of water; dilute SSKI® in glassful of water, fruit juice, or milk with meals to reduce gastric irritation. May cause metallic taste, nausea, or vomiting (small frequent meals, frequent mouth care, chewing gum, or sucking lozenges may help); soreness of teeth, gums, or glands (use soft toothbrush and frequent mouth rinses); fever, headache or sore joints (consult prescriber for approved analgesic); confusion or tiredness (use caution when driving or engaged in potential hazardous tasks until response to medication is known). Discontinue and report any swelling of lips, mouth, or tongue; difficulty swallowing; chest pain or irregular heartbeat; unusual muscle weakness; eye irritation or eyelid swelling; skin rash or other persistent adverse effects. **Pregnancy/breast-feeding precautions:** Inform prescriber if you are pregnant. Do not get pregnant during therapy. Consult prescriber for instruction on appropriate contraceptive measures. This drug may cause fetal defects. Consult prescriber if breast-feeding.

Potassium Phosphate

(poe TASS ee um FOS fate)

U.S. Brand Names Neutra-Phos®-K [OTC]

Synonyms Phosphate, Potassium

Pharmacologic Category Electrolyte Supplement, Oral; Electrolyte Supplement, Parenteral

Medication Safety Issues

Sound-alike/look-alike issues:

Neutra-Phos®-K may be confused with K-Phos Neutral®

High alert medication: The Institute for Safe Medication Practices (ISMP) includes this medication (I.V. formulation) among its list of drugs which have a heightened risk of causing significant patient harm when used in error.

Per JCAHO recommendations, concentrated electrolyte solutions should not be available in patient care areas.

Consider special storage requirements for intravenous potassium salts; I.V. potassium salts have been administered IVP in error, leading to fatal outcomes.

Pregnancy Risk Factor C

Use Treatment and prevention of hypophosphatemia or hypokalemia

Contraindications Hyperphosphatemia, hyperkalemia, hypocalcemia, hypomagnesemia, renal failure

Warnings/Precautions Use with caution in patients with renal insufficiency, cardiac disease, metabolic alkalosis; admixture of phosphate and calcium in I.V. fluids can result in calcium phosphate precipitation.

Drug Interactions

Decreased Effect: Aluminum and magnesium-containing antacids or sucralfate can act as phosphate binders

Increased Effect/Toxicity: Potassium-sparing diuretics, salt substitutes, or ACE inhibitors; increased effect of digitalis

Nutritional/Ethanol Interactions Food: Avoid administering with oxalate (berries, nuts, chocolate, beans, celery, tomato) or phytate-containing foods (bran, whole wheat).

Lab Interactions Decreased ammonia (B)

Adverse Reactions

>10%: Gastrointestinal: Diarrhea, nausea, stomach pain, flatulence, vomiting

1% to 10%:

Cardiovascular: Bradycardia

Endocrine & metabolic: Hyperkalemia

Neuromuscular & skeletal: Weakness

Respiratory: Dyspnea

Overdosage/Toxicology

Symptoms of overdose include muscle weakness, paralysis, peaked T waves, flattened P waves, prolongation of QRS complex, ventricular arrhythmias, tetany, calcium-phosphate precipitation

Removal of potassium can be accomplished by various means; removal through the GI tract with Kayexalate® administration; by way of the kidney through diuresis, mineralocorticoid administration or increased sodium intake; by hemodialysis or peritoneal dialysis; or by shifting potassium back into the cells by insulin, glucose infusion, or sodium bicarbonate; calcium chloride reverses cardiac effects.

Available Dosage Forms

Injection, solution: Phosphate 3 mmol and potassium 4.4 mEq per mL (5 mL, 15 mL, 50 mL) [equivalent to phosphate 285 mg and potassium 170 mg per mL]

Powder for oral solution [packet] (Neutra-Phos®-K): Monobasic potassium phosphate and dibasic potassium phosphate/packet (100s) [equivalent to elemental phosphorus 250 mg and potassium 556 mg (14.2 mEq) per packet; sodium free]

Dosing

Adults & Elderly: I.V. doses should be incorporated into the patient's maintenance I.V. fluids; intermittent I.V. infusion should be reserved for severe depletion situations in patients undergoing continuous ECG monitoring. It is difficult to determine total body phosphorus deficit; the following dosages are empiric guidelines:

Normal requirements elemental phosphorus: Oral:

Pregnancy lactation: Additional 400 mg/day

Adults: 800 mg

Treatment of hypophosphatemia: It is difficult to provide concrete guidelines for the treatment of severe hypophosphatemia because the extent of total body deficits and response to therapy are difficult to predict. Aggressive doses of phosphate may result in a transient serum elevation followed by redistribution into intracellular compartments or bone tissue. It is recommended that repletion of severe hypophosphatemia (<1 mg/dL in adults) be done I.V. because large doses of oral phosphate may cause diarrhea and intestinal absorption may be unreliable

Adult I.V. phosphate repletion:

Initial dose: 0.08 mmol/kg if recent uncomplicated hypophosphatemia

Initial dose: 0.16 mmol/kg if prolonged hypophosphatemia with presumed total body deficits; increase dose by 25% to 50% if patient symptomatic with severe hypophosphatemia

Do not exceed 0.24 mmol/kg/dose; administer over 6-12 hours by I.V. infusion. Some investigators have used more rapid infusions.

Note: With orders for I.V. phosphate, there is considerable confusion associated with the use of millimoles (mmol) versus milliequivalents (mEq) to express the phosphate requirement. Because inorganic phosphate exists as monobasic and dibasic anions, with the mixture of valences dependent on pH, ordering by mEq amounts is unreliable and may lead to large dosing errors. In addition, I.V. phosphate is available in the sodium and potassium salt; therefore, the content of these cations must be considered when ordering phosphate. The most reliable method of ordering I.V. phosphate is by millimoles, then specifying the potassium or sodium salt. For example, an order for 15 mmol of phosphate as potassium phosphate in one liter of normal saline. The dosing of phosphate should be 0.2-0.3 mmol/kg with a usual daily requirement of 30-60 mmol/day or 15 mmol of phosphate per liter of TPN or 15 mmol phosphate per 1000 calories of dextrose. Would also provide 22 mEq of potassium.

Maintenance:

I.V. solutions: 15-30 mmol/24 hours I.V. or 50-150 mmol/24 hours orally in divided doses

Oral: 1-2 capsules (250-500 mg phosphorus/8-16 mmol) 4 times/day; dilute as instructed

Pediatrics: I.V. doses should be incorporated into the patient's maintenance I.V. fluids; intermittent I.V. infusion should be reserved for severe depletion situations in patients undergoing continuous ECG monitoring. It is difficult to determine total body phosphorus deficit; the following are empiric guidelines

Note: Refer to notes under Adult dosing

Pediatric I.V. phosphate repletion:

Children: 0.25-0.5 mmol/kg **administer over 4-6 hours and repeat if symptomatic hypophosphatemia persists**; to assess the need for further phosphate administration, obtain serum inorganic phosphate after administration of the first dose and base further doses on serum levels and clinical status

Maintenance:

I.V. solutions: Children: 0.5-1.5 mmol/kg/24 hours I.V. or 2-3 mmol/kg/24 hours orally in divided doses

Oral:

Children <4 years: 1 capsule (250 mg phosphorus/8 mmol) 4 times/day; dilute as instructed

Children >4 years: Refer to adult dosing.

Stability

Compatibility: Stable in dextran 6% in dextrose, dextran 6% in NS, D$_{10}$LR, D$_5$¼NS, D$_5$½NS, D$_5$NS, D$_5$W, D$_{10}$W, ½NS, NS; **incompatible** with D$_5$LR, D$_{10}$NS, LR

Y-site administration: Incompatible with gatifloxacin

Compatibility when admixed: Incompatible with dobutamine

Laboratory Monitoring Serum potassium, phosphate

Physical Assessment: Monitor patient response and adverse effects.

Patient Education: Empty contents of packet into 3-4 oz of water. Take with food to reduce the risk of diarrhea.

Potassium Phosphate and Sodium Phosphate

(poe TASS ee um FOS fate & SOW dee um FOS fate)

U.S. Brand Names K-Phos® MF; K-Phos® Neutral; K-Phos® No. 2; Neutra-Phos® [OTC]; Phos-NaK; Phospha 250™ Neutral; Uro-KP-Neutral®

Synonyms Sodium Phosphate and Potassium Phosphate

Pharmacologic Category Electrolyte Supplement, Oral

Pregnancy Risk Factor C

Use Treatment of conditions associated with excessive renal phosphate loss or inadequate GI absorption of phosphate; to acidify the urine to lower calcium concentrations; to increase the antibacterial activity of methenamine; reduce odor and rash caused by ammonia in urine

Available Dosage Forms

Powder, for oral solution (Neutra-Phos®, Phos-NaK): Monobasic sodium, dibasic sodium, and potassium phosphate/packet (100s) [equivalent to elemental phosphorus 250 mg, sodium 164 mg (7.1 mEq), and potassium 278 mg (7.1 mEq) per packet]

Tablet:

K-Phos® MF: Potassium acid phosphate 155 mg and sodium acid phosphate 350 mg [equivalent to elemental phosphorus 125.6 mg, sodium 67 mg (2.9 mEq), and potassium 44.5 mg (1.1 mEq)]

K-Phos® Neutral: Dibasic sodium phosphate 852 mg, monobasic potassium phosphate 155 mg, and monobasic sodium phosphate 130 mg [equivalent to elemental phosphorus 250 mg, sodium 298 mg (13 mEq), and potassium 45 mg (1.1 mEq)]

K-Phos® No. 2: Potassium acid phosphate 305 mg and sodium acid phosphate 700 mg [equivalent to elemental phosphorus 250 mg, sodium 134 mg (5.8 mEq), and potassium 88 mg (2.3 mEq)]

Phospha 250™ Neutral: Dibasic sodium phosphate 852 mg, monobasic potassium phosphate 155 mg, and monobasic sodium phosphate 130 mg [equivalent to elemental phosphorus 250 mg, sodium 298 mg (13 mEq), and potassium 45 mg (1.1 mEq)]

Uro-KP-Neutral®: Sodium phosphate monobasic, dipotassium phosphate, and disodium phosphate [equivalent to elemental phosphorus 258 mg, sodium 262.4 mg (10.8 mEq), and potassium 49.4 mg (1.3 mEq)]

Dosing

Adults & Elderly: Note: All dosage forms to be mixed in 6-8 oz of water prior to administration

Phosphate supplement: Oral: Elemental phosphorus 250-500 mg 4 times/day after meals and at bedtime

Pediatrics: Note: All dosage forms to be mixed in 6-8 oz of water prior to administration

Phosphate supplement: Oral: Children ≥4 years: Elemental phosphorus 250 mg 4 times/day after meals and at bedtime

Patient Education: Powder packets are to be mixed in 6-8 oz of water; following dilution, solution may be chilled to increase palatability. Tablets should be taken with a full glass of water.

Related Information

Potassium Phosphate *on page 1012*

Pramipexole (pra mi PEKS ole)

U.S. Brand Names Mirapex®

Pharmacologic Category Anti-Parkinson's Agent, Dopamine Agonist

Medication Safety Issues

Sound-alike/look-alike issues:

Mirapex® may be confused with Mifeprex®, MiraLax™

Pregnancy Risk Factor C

Lactation Excretion in breast milk unknown/not recommended

Use Treatment of the signs and symptoms of idiopathic Parkinson's disease

Unlabeled/Investigational Use Treatment of depression

Mechanism of Action/Effect Pramipexole is a nonergot dopamine agonist with specificity for the D_2 subfamily dopamine receptor, and has also been shown to bind to D_3 and D_4 receptors. By binding to these receptors, it is thought that pramipexole can stimulate dopamine activity on the nerves of the striatum and substantia nigra.

Contraindications Hypersensitivity to pramipexole or any component of the formulation

Warnings/Precautions Caution should be taken in patients with renal insufficiency and in patients with pre-existing dyskinesias. May cause orthostatic hypotension; Parkinson's disease patients appear to have an impaired capacity to respond to a postural challenge. Use with caution in patients at risk of hypotension (such as those receiving antihypertensive drugs) or where transient hypotensive episodes would be poorly tolerated (cardiovascular disease or cerebrovascular disease). May cause hallucinations, particularly in older patients.

Although not reported for pramipexole, other dopaminergic agents have been associated with a syndrome resembling neuroleptic malignant syndrome on withdrawal or significant dosage reduction after long-term use. Dopaminergic agents from the ergot class have also been associated with fibrotic complications, such as retroperitoneum, lungs, and pleura.

Pramipexole has been associated with somnolence, particularly at higher dosages (>1.5 mg/day). In addition, patients have been reported to fall asleep during activities of daily living, including driving, while taking this medication. Patients should be advised of this issue, cautioned against driving or performing activities requiring alertness, and advised of factors which may increase risk (sleep disorders, other sedating medications, or concomitant medications which increase pramipexole concentrations). Patients should be instructed to report daytime somnolence or sleepiness to the prescriber.

Drug Interactions

Decreased Effect: Dopamine antagonists (antipsychotics, metoclopramide) may decrease the efficiency of pramipexole.

Increased Effect/Toxicity: Cimetidine in combination with pramipexole produced a 50% increase in AUC and a 40% increase in half-life. Drugs secreted by the cationic transport system (diltiazem, triamterene, verapamil, quinidine, quinine, ranitidine) decrease the clearance of pramipexole by ~20%.

Nutritional/Ethanol Interactions

Ethanol: Avoid ethanol (may increase CNS depression).

Food: Food intake does not affect the extent of drug absorption, although the time to maximal plasma concentration is delayed by 60 minutes when taken with a meal.

Herb/Nutraceutical: Avoid valerian, St John's wort, SAMe, kava kava (may increase risk of serotonin syndrome and/or excessive sedation).

Adverse Reactions

>10%:

Cardiovascular: Postural hypotension

Central nervous system: Asthenia, dizziness, somnolence, insomnia, hallucinations, abnormal dreams

Gastrointestinal: Nausea, constipation

Neuromuscular & skeletal: Weakness, dyskinesia, EPS

1% to 10%:

Cardiovascular: Edema, syncope, tachycardia, chest pain

Central nervous system: Malaise, confusion, amnesia, dystonias, akathisia, thinking abnormalities, myoclonus, hyperesthesia, paranoia, fever

Endocrine & metabolic: Decreased libido

Gastrointestinal: Anorexia, weight loss, xerostomia, dysphagia

Genitourinary: Urinary frequency, impotence, urinary incontinence

Neuromuscular & skeletal: Muscle twitching, leg cramps, arthritis, bursitis, myasthenia, gait abnormalities, hypertonia

Ocular: Vision abnormalities

Respiratory: Dyspnea, rhinitis

Pharmacodynamics/Kinetics

Time to Peak: Serum: ~2 hours

Protein Binding: 15%

Half-Life Elimination: ~8 hours; Elderly: 12-14 hours

Excretion: Urine (90% as unchanged drug)

Available Dosage Forms Tablet, as dihydrochloride monohydrate: 0.125 mg, 0.25 mg, 0.5 mg, 1 mg, 1.5 mg

Dosing

Adults & Elderly: Parkinson's disease: Oral: Initial: 0.375 mg/day given in 3 divided doses; increase gradually by 0.125 mg/dose every 5-7 days; range: 1.5-4.5 mg/day.

Renal Impairment:

Cl_{cr} 35-59 mL/minute: Initial: 0.125 mg twice daily (maximum dose: 1.5 mg twice daily)

Cl_{cr} 15-34 mL/minute: Initial: 0.125 mg once daily (maximum dose: 1.5 mg once daily)

Cl_{cr} <15 mL/minute (or hemodialysis patients): Not adequately studied.

Administration

Oral: Doses should be titrated gradually in all patients to avoid the onset of intolerable side effects. The dosage should be increased to achieve a maximum therapeutic effect, balanced against the side effects of dyskinesia, hallucinations, somnolence, and dry mouth.

Nursing Actions

Physical Assessment: Assess potential for interactions with other prescriptions, OTC medications, or herbal products patient may be taking. Monitor blood pressure. Assess degree of somnolence. Assess for therapeutic effectiveness (improvement of symptoms) and adverse response. Teach patient appropriate use, interventions to reduce side effects, and adverse symptoms to report.

Patient Education: Do not take any new medication during therapy unless approved by prescriber. Take exactly as directed. Avoid alcohol. May cause drowsiness and extreme sedation or somnolence (use caution when driving or engaging in hazardous activities until response to drug is known); postural hypotension (use caution when changing position - rise slowly from sitting or lying position to standing and use caution when climbing stairs); constipation (increased exercise, fluids, fruit, or fiber may help); or urinary frequency. Consult prescriber about persistent adverse effects. **Pregnancy/breast-feeding precautions:** Inform prescriber if you are or intend to become pregnant. Breast-feeding is not recommended.

Dietary Considerations May be taken with food to decrease nausea.

Breast-Feeding Issues Prolactin secretion may be inhibited.

Pravastatin (PRA va stat in)

U.S. Brand Names Pravachol®

Synonyms Pravastatin Sodium

Pharmacologic Category Antilipemic Agent, HMG-CoA Reductase Inhibitor

Medication Safety Issues
Sound-alike/look-alike issues:
Pravachol® may be confused with Prevacid®, Prinivil®, propranolol

Pregnancy Risk Factor X

Lactation Enters breast milk/contraindicated

Use Use with dietary therapy for the following:

Primary prevention of coronary events: In hypercholesterolemic patients without established coronary heart disease to reduce cardiovascular morbidity (myocardial infarction, coronary revascularization procedures) and mortality.

Secondary prevention of cardiovascular events in patients with established coronary heart disease: To slow the progression of coronary atherosclerosis; to reduce cardiovascular morbidity (myocardial infarction, coronary vascular procedures) and to reduce mortality; to reduce the risk of stroke and transient ischemic attacks

Hyperlipidemias: Reduce elevations in total cholesterol, LDL-C, apolipoprotein B, and triglycerides (elevations of 1 or more components are present in Fredrickson type IIa, IIb, III, and IV hyperlipidemias)

Heterozygous familial hypercholesterolemia (HeFH): In pediatric patients, 8-18 years of age, with HeFH having LDL-C ≥190 mg/dL **or** LDL ≥160 mg/dL with positive family history of premature cardiovascular disease (CVD) or 2 or more CVD risk factors in the pediatric patient

Mechanism of Action/Effect Pravastatin is a competitive inhibitor of 3-hydroxy-3-methylglutaryl coenzyme A (HMG-CoA) reductase, which is the rate-limiting enzyme involved in *de novo* cholesterol synthesis.

Contraindications Hypersensitivity to pravastatin or any component of the formulation; active liver disease; unexplained persistent elevations of serum transaminases; pregnancy; breast-feeding

Warnings/Precautions Secondary causes of hyperlipidemia should be ruled out prior to therapy. Liver function must be monitored by periodic laboratory assessment. Rhabdomyolysis with acute renal failure has occurred. Risk may be increased with concurrent use of other drugs which may cause rhabdomyolysis (including gemfibrozil, fibric acid derivatives, or niacin at doses ≥1 g/day). Temporarily discontinue in any patient experiencing an acute or serious condition predisposing to renal failure secondary to rhabdomyolysis. Use caution in patients with previous liver disease or heavy ethanol use. Treatment in patients <8 years of age is not recommended.

Drug Interactions

Cytochrome P450 Effect: Substrate of CYP3A4 (minor); **Inhibits** CYP2C8/9 (weak), 2D6 (weak), 3A4 (weak)

Decreased Effect: Concurrent administration of cholestyramine or colestipol can decrease pravastatin absorption.

Increased Effect/Toxicity: Clofibrate, cyclosporine, fenofibrate, gemfibrozil, and niacin may increase the risk of myopathy and rhabdomyolysis. Imidazole antifungals (itraconazole, ketoconazole), P-glycoprotein inhibitors may increase pravastatin concentrations.

Nutritional/Ethanol Interactions
Ethanol: Consumption of large amounts of ethanol may increase the risk of liver damage with HMG-CoA reductase inhibitors.
Food: Red yeast rice contains an estimated 2.4 mg lovastatin per 600 mg rice.
Herb/Nutraceutical: St John's wort may decrease pravastatin levels.

Adverse Reactions As reported in short-term trials; safety and tolerability with long-term use were similar to placebo
1% to 10%:
Cardiovascular: Chest pain (4%)
Central nervous system: Headache (2% to 6%), fatigue (4%), dizziness (1% to 3%)
Dermatologic: Rash (4%)
Gastrointestinal: Nausea/vomiting (7%), diarrhea (6%), heartburn (3%)
Hepatic: Transaminases increased (>3x normal on two occasions - 1%)
Neuromuscular & skeletal: Myalgia (2%)
Respiratory: Cough (3%)
Miscellaneous: Influenza (2%)
Additional class-related events or case reports (not necessarily reported with pravastatin therapy): Angioedema, cataracts, depression, dyspnea, eosinophilia, erectile dysfunction, facial paresis, hypersensitivity reaction, impaired extraocular muscle movement, impotence, leukopenia, malaise, memory loss, ophthalmoplegia, paresthesia, peripheral neuropathy, photosensitivity, psychic disturbance, skin discoloration, thrombocytopenia, thyroid dysfunction, toxic epidermal necrolysis, transaminases increased, vomiting

Overdosage/Toxicology Treatment is symptomatic.

Pharmacodynamics/Kinetics
Onset of Action: Several days; Peak effect: 4 weeks
Time to Peak: Serum: 1-1.5 hours
Protein Binding: 50%
Half-Life Elimination: ~2-3 hours
Metabolism: Hepatic to at least two metabolites
Excretion: Feces (70%); urine (≤20%, 8% as unchanged drug)

Available Dosage Forms Tablet, as sodium: 10 mg, 20 mg, 40 mg, 80 mg

Dosing
Adults & Elderly:
Hyperlipidemias, primary prevention of coronary events, secondary prevention of cardiovascular events: Oral: Initial: 40 mg once daily; titrate dosage to response (usual range: 10-80 mg) (maximum dose: 80 mg once daily)
Dosage adjustment based on concomitant immunosuppressants (ie, cyclosporine): Oral: Initial: 10 mg/day, titrate with caution (maximum dose: 20 mg/day)
Note: Doses should be individualized according to the baseline LDL-cholesterol levels, the recommended goal of therapy, and patient response; adjustments should be made at intervals of 4 weeks or more; doses may need adjusted based on concomitant medications

Pediatrics:
Heterozygous familial hypercholesterolemia (HeFH): Oral: Children:
8-13 years: 20 mg/day
14-18 years: 40 mg/day
Dosage adjustment based on concomitant immunosuppressants (ie, cyclosporine): Refer to adult dosing.
Note: Doses should be individualized according to the baseline LDL-cholesterol levels, the recommended goal of therapy, and patient response; adjustments should be made at intervals of 4 weeks or more; doses may need adjusted based on concomitant medications

(Continued)

Pravastatin *(Continued)*

Renal Impairment: Initial: 10 mg/day

Hepatic Impairment: Initial: 10 mg/day

Administration

Oral: May be taken without regard to meals.

Stability

Storage: Store at 25°C (77°F); excursions permitted to 15°C to 30°C (59°F to 86°F). Protect from moisture and light.

Laboratory Monitoring Obtain baseline LFTs and total cholesterol profile; creatine phosphokinase due to possibility of myopathy. Repeat LFTs prior to elevation of dose. May be measured when clinically indicated and/or periodically thereafter.

Nursing Actions

Physical Assessment: Assess potential for interactions with other pharmacological agents or herbal products patient may be taking (eg, gemfibrozil, fibric acid derivatives, niacin may increase risk of myopathy or rhabdomyolysis). Monitor laboratory tests and patient response on a regular basis throughout therapy (eg, rash, myalgia, blurred vision, abdominal pain, cough). Teach patient proper use (as addition to diet and exercise regimen), possible side effects/appropriate interventions, and adverse symptoms to report. **Pregnancy risk factor X:** Determine that patient is not pregnant before starting therapy. Do not give to women of childbearing age unless they are capable of complying with effective contraceptive use. Instruct patient in appropriate contraceptive measures.

Patient Education: Do not take any new medication during therapy unless approved by prescriber. Take at same time each day. Follow diet and exercise regimen as prescribed. Avoid excess alcohol. You will have periodic blood tests to assess effectiveness. May cause mild nausea or vomiting (small, frequent meals, frequent mouth care, chewing gum, or sucking lozenges may help); diarrhea (buttermilk, boiled milk, or yogurt may help); or headache (see prescriber for analgesic). Report chest pain; CNS changes (memory loss, depression, personality changes); numbness, weakness, tingling, pain, or cramping in extremities or muscles; vision changes; rash; or other persistent adverse reactions. **Pregnancy/breast-feeding precautions:** Inform prescriber if you are pregnant. Consult prescriber for appropriate barrier contraceptive measures to use during and for 1 month following therapy. This drug may cause severe fetal defects. Do not donate blood during or for 1 month following therapy. Do not breast-feed.

Dietary Considerations May be taken without regard to meals. Before initiation of therapy, patients should be placed on a standard cholesterol-lowering diet for 6 weeks and the diet should be continued during drug therapy. Red yeast rice contains an estimated 2.4 mg lovastatin per 600 mg rice.

Geriatric Considerations Effective and well tolerated in the elderly. No specific dosage recommendations. Clearance is reduced in older adults, resulting in an increase in AUC between 25% to 50%. However, substantial accumulation is not expected.

The definition of and, therefore, when to treat hyperlipidemia in older adults is a controversial issue. The National Cholesterol Education Program recommends that all adults maintain a plasma cholesterol <160 mg/dL. In elderly patients with one additional risk factor, goal LDL would decrease to <130 mg/dL. Pharmacologic treatment should be reserved for those who are unable to obtain a desirable plasma cholesterol concentration by diet alone and for whom the benefits of treatment are believed to outweigh the potential adverse effects, drug interactions, and cost of treatment.

Pregnancy Issues Cholesterol biosynthesis may be important in fetal development. Contraindicated in pregnancy. Administer to women of childbearing potential only when conception is highly unlikely and patients have been informed of potential hazards.

Prazosin *(PRA zoe sin)*

U.S. Brand Names Minipress®

Synonyms Furazosin; Prazosin Hydrochloride

Pharmacologic Category Alpha₁ Blocker

Medication Safety Issues

Sound-alike/look-alike issues:

Prazosin may be confused with prazepam, predniSONE

Pregnancy Risk Factor C

Lactation Excretion in breast milk unknown/use caution

Use Treatment of hypertension

Unlabeled/Investigational Use Benign prostatic hyperplasia; Raynaud's syndrome

Mechanism of Action/Effect Competitively inhibits postsynaptic alpha-adrenergic receptors which results in vasodilation of veins and arterioles and a decrease in total peripheral resistance and blood pressure

Contraindications Hypersensitivity to quinazolines (doxazosin, prazosin, terazosin) or any component of the formulation; concurrent use with phosphodiesterase-5 (PDE-5) inhibitors including sildenafil (>25 mg), tadalafil, or vardenafil

Warnings/Precautions May cause significant orthostatic hypotension and syncope, especially with first dose. Risk is increased at doses >1 mg, hypovolemia, or in patients receiving concurrent beta-blocker therapy. Anticipate a similar effect if therapy is interrupted for a few days, if dosage is rapidly increased, or if another antihypertensive drug is introduced.

Drug Interactions

Decreased Effect: Decreased antihypertensive effect if taken with NSAIDs.

Increased Effect/Toxicity: Prazosin's hypotensive effect may be increased with beta-blockers, diuretics, ACE inhibitors, calcium channel blockers, other antihypertensive medications, sildenafil (use with extreme caution at a dose ≤25 mg), tadalafil (use is contraindicated by the manufacturer), and vardenafil (use is contraindicated by the manufacturer). Concurrent use with tricyclic antidepressants (TCAs) and low-potency antipsychotics may increase risk of orthostasis.

Nutritional/Ethanol Interactions

Ethanol: Avoid ethanol (may increase vasodilation).

Food: Food has variable effects on absorption.

Herb/Nutraceutical: Avoid dong quai if using for hypertension (has estrogenic activity). Avoid ephedra, yohimbe, ginseng (may worsen hypertension). Avoid saw palmetto (due to limited experience with this combination). Avoid garlic (may have increased antihypertensive effect).

Lab Interactions Increased urinary VMA 17%, norepinephrine metabolite 42%

Adverse Reactions

>10%: Central nervous system: Dizziness (10%)

1% to 10%:

Cardiovascular: Palpitations (5%), edema, orthostatic hypotension, syncope (1%)

Central nervous system: Headache (8%), drowsiness (8%), weakness (7%), vertigo, depression, nervousness

Dermatologic: Rash (1% to 4%)

Endocrine & metabolic: Decreased energy (7%)

Gastrointestinal: Nausea (5%), vomiting, diarrhea, constipation

Genitourinary: Urinary frequency (1% to 5%)

Ocular: Blurred vision, reddened sclera, xerostomia

Respiratory: Dyspnea, epistaxis, nasal congestion

Overdosage/Toxicology Symptoms of overdose include hypotension and drowsiness. Treatment is otherwise supportive and symptomatic.

Pharmacodynamics/Kinetics

Onset of Action: BP reduction: ~2 hours; Maximum decrease: 2-4 hours

Duration of Action: 10-24 hours

Protein Binding: 92% to 97%

Half-Life Elimination: 2-4 hours; prolonged with congestive heart failure

Metabolism: Extensively hepatic

Excretion: Urine (6% to 10% as unchanged drug)

Available Dosage Forms Capsule, as hydrochloride: 1 mg, 2 mg, 5 mg

Dosing

Adults:

Hypertension: Oral: Initial: 1 mg/dose 2-3 times/day; usual maintenance dose: 3-15 mg/day in divided doses 2-4 times/day; maximum daily dose: 20 mg

Hypertensive urgency: Oral: 10-20 mg once, may repeat in 30 minutes

Raynaud's (unlabeled use): Oral: 0.5-3 mg twice daily

Benign prostatic hyperplasia (unlabeled use): Oral: 2 mg twice daily

Elderly: Oral (first dose given at bedtime): Initial: 1 mg 1-2 times/day

Pediatrics: Oral: Children: Initial: 5 mcg/kg/dose (to assess hypotensive effects); usual dosing interval: every 6 hours; increase dosage gradually up to maximum of 25 mcg/kg/dose every 6 hours.

Stability

Storage: Store in airtight container. Protect from light.

Nursing Actions

Physical Assessment: Assess potential for interactions with other pharmacological agents and herbal products patient may be taking (eg, anything that may increase hypotension (beta-blockers, diuretics, ACE inhibitors, calcium channel blockers, dong quai) and any PDE-5 inhibitors (sildenafil, tadalafil, vardenafil). Monitor effectiveness (cardiac status and blood pressure) and adverse reactions (eg, orthostatic hypotension, rash, drowsiness, nausea, vomiting) at beginning of therapy and on a regular basis with long-term therapy. When discontinuing, monitor blood pressure and taper dose slowly over 1 week or more. Teach patient proper use, possible side effects/appropriate interventions, and adverse symptoms to report.

Patient Education: Inform prescriber of all prescriptions, OTC medications, or herbal products you are taking, and any allergies you have. Do not take any new medication during therapy unless approved by prescriber. Take as directed with or without meals; do not skip dose or discontinue without consulting prescriber. Avoid alcohol. Follow recommended diet and exercise program. May cause drowsiness, dizziness, or impaired judgment (use caution when driving or engaging in tasks that require alertness until response to drug is known); postural hypotension (use caution when rising from sitting or lying position or when climbing stairs); or dry mouth or nausea (frequent mouth care or sucking lozenges may help). Report increased nervousness or depression; sudden weight gain (weigh yourself in the same clothes at the same time of day once a week); palpitations or rapid heartbeat; respiratory difficulty; muscle weakness, fatigue, or pain; vision changes or hearing; rash; changes in urinary pattern (void before taking medications); or other persistent side effects. **Pregnancy/breast-feeding precautions:** Inform prescriber if you are or intend to become pregnant. Consult prescriber if breast-feeding.

Geriatric Considerations See Warnings/Precautions and Pharmacodynamics/Kinetics. Adverse effects such as dry mouth and urinary problems can be particularly bothersome in the elderly.

Prazosin and Polythiazide
(PRA zoe sin & pol i THYE a zide)

U.S. Brand Names Minizide®

Synonyms Polythiazide and Prazosin

Pharmacologic Category Antihypertensive Agent, Combination

Pregnancy Risk Factor C

Lactation Excretion in breast milk unknown

Use Management of mild to moderate hypertension

Available Dosage Forms Capsule:

Minizide® 1: Prazosin 1 mg and polythiazide 0.5 mg
Minizide® 2: Prazosin 2 mg and polythiazide 0.5 mg
Minizide® 5: Prazosin 5 mg and polythiazide 0.5 mg

Dosing

Adults & Elderly: Hypertension: Oral: Initial: 1 capsule 2-3 times/day; maintenance: May be slowly increased to a total daily dose of 20 mg. Therapeutic dosages often used range from 6-15 mg in divided doses.

Nursing Actions

Physical Assessment: See individual agents.

Patient Education: See individual agents. **Pregnancy/breast-feeding precautions:** Inform prescriber if you are or intend to become pregnant. Consult prescriber if breast-feeding.

Related Information

Prazosin *on page 1016*

PrednisoLONE (pred NISS oh lone)

U.S. Brand Names AK-Pred®; Bubbli-Pred™ [DSC]; Econopred® Plus; Orapred®; Pediapred®; Pred Forte®; Pred Mild®; Prelone®

Synonyms Deltahydrocortisone; Metacortandralone; Prednisolone Acetate; Prednisolone Acetate, Ophthalmic; Prednisolone Sodium Phosphate; Prednisolone Sodium Phosphate, Ophthalmic

Pharmacologic Category Corticosteroid, Ophthalmic; Corticosteroid, Systemic

Medication Safety Issues

Sound-alike/look-alike issues:
PrednisoLONE may be confused with predniSONE
Pediapred® may be confused with Pediazole®

Pregnancy Risk Factor C

Lactation Enters breast milk/use caution (AAP rates "compatible")

Use Treatment of palpebral and bulbar conjunctivitis; corneal injury from chemical, radiation, thermal burns, or foreign body penetration; endocrine disorders, rheumatic disorders, collagen diseases, dermatologic diseases, allergic states, ophthalmic diseases, respiratory diseases, hematologic disorders, neoplastic diseases, edematous states, and gastrointestinal diseases; resolution of acute exacerbations of multiple sclerosis

Mechanism of Action/Effect Decreases inflammation by suppression of migration of polymorphonuclear leukocytes and reversal of increased capillary permeability; suppresses the immune system by reducing activity and volume of the lymphatic system

Contraindications Hypersensitivity to prednisolone or any component of the formulation; acute superficial herpes simplex keratitis; live or attenuated virus vaccines; systemic fungal infections; varicella

Warnings/Precautions Use with caution in patients with hyperthyroidism, cirrhosis, nonspecific ulcerative colitis, hypertension, osteoporosis, thromboembolic tendencies, CHF, convulsive disorders, myasthenia gravis, thrombophlebitis, peptic ulcer, diabetes, or tuberculosis; acute adrenal insufficiency may occur with abrupt withdrawal after long-term therapy or with stress; (Continued)

PrednisoLONE (Continued)

young pediatric patients may be more susceptible to adrenal axis suppression from topical therapy.

Prolonged use of corticosteroids may result in glaucoma; damage to the optic nerve (not for treatment of optic neuritis), defects in visual acuity and fields of vision, and posterior subcapsular cataract formation may occur. Prolonged use may increase the incidence of secondary infection, mask acute infection (including fungal) or prolong or exacerbate viral infections. Avoid exposure to chickenpox. Corticosteroids should not treat ocular herpes simplex. Use following cataract surgery may delay healing or increase the incidence of bleb formation.

Corticosteroids should not be used for cerebral malaria. Use cautiously in the elderly.

Drug Interactions
Cytochrome P450 Effect: Substrate of CYP3A4 (minor); **Inhibits** CYP3A4 (weak)

Decreased Effect: Effects of prednisolone may be decreased by aminoglutethimide, antacids, barbiturates, CYP34 inducers, carbamazepine, nafcillin, nevirapine, phenobarbital, phenytoin, rifampin. Prednisolone may decrease the effects of isoniazid, skin tests, toxoids, warfarin, vaccines.

Increased Effect/Toxicity: Effects of prednisolone may be increased by azole antifungals, calcium channel blockers, cyclosporine, estrogens, ketoconazole, salicylates.

Nutritional/Ethanol Interactions
Ethanol: Avoid ethanol (may increase gastric mucosal irritation).

Food: Prednisolone interferes with calcium absorption. Limit caffeine.

Herb/Nutraceutical: St John's wort may decrease prednisolone levels. Avoid cat's claw, echinacea (have immunostimulant properties).

Lab Interactions
Response to skin tests

Adverse Reactions
Frequency not defined.

Ophthalmic formulation:
Endocrine & metabolic: Hypercorticoidism (rare)
Ocular: Conjunctival hyperemia, conjunctivitis, corneal ulcers, delayed wound healing, glaucoma, intraocular pressure increased, keratitis, loss of accommodation, optic nerve damage, mydriasis, posterior subcapsular cataract formation, ptosis, secondary ocular infection

Oral formulation:
Cardiovascular: CHF, edema, hypertension
Central nervous system: Convulsions, headache, insomnia, malaise, nervousness, psychic disorders, vertigo
Dermatologic: Bruising, diaphoresis increased, facial erythema, hirsutism, petechiae, skin test reaction suppression, thin fragile skin, urticaria
Endocrine & metabolic: Carbohydrate tolerance decreased, Cushing's syndrome, diabetes mellitus, growth suppression, hyperglycemia, hypokalemic alkalosis, menstrual irregularities, negative nitrogen balance, pituitary adrenal axis suppression, potassium loss
Gastrointestinal: Abdominal distention, increased appetite, indigestion, nausea, peptic ulcer, ulcerative esophagitis, weight gain
Hepatic: LFTs increased (usually reversible)
Neuromuscular & skeletal: Arthralgia, fractures, intracranial pressure with papilledema (usually after discontinuation), muscle mass decreased, muscle weakness, osteoporosis, steroid myopathy, tendon rupture, weakness
Ocular: Cataracts, exophthalmus, glaucoma, intraocular pressure increased
Respiratory: Epistaxis
Miscellaneous: Impaired wound healing

Overdosage/Toxicology When consumed in high doses for prolonged periods, systemic hypercorticism and adrenal suppression may occur, in those cases discontinuation of the corticosteroid should be done judiciously.

Pharmacodynamics/Kinetics
Duration of Action: 18-36 hours
Protein Binding: Concentration dependent: 65% to 91%; decreased in elderly
Half-Life Elimination: 3.6 hours; End-stage renal disease: 3-5 hours
Metabolism: Primarily hepatic, but also metabolized in most tissues, to inactive compounds
Excretion: Primarily urine (as glucuronides, sulfates, and unconjugated metabolites)

Available Dosage Forms [DSC] = Discontinued product
Solution, ophthalmic, as sodium phosphate: 1% (5 mL, 10 mL, 15 mL) [contains benzalkonium chloride]
AK-Pred®: 1% (5 mL, 15 mL) [contains benzalkonium chloride]
Solution, oral, as sodium phosphate: Prednisolone base 5 mg/5 mL (120 mL)
Bubbli-Pred™: Prednisolone base 5 mg/5 mL (120 mL) [bubble gum flavor] [DSC]
Orapred®: 20 mg/5 mL (240 mL) [equivalent to prednisolone base 15 mg/5 mL; dye free; contains alcohol 2%, sodium benzoate; grape flavor]
Pediapred®: 6.7 mg/5 mL (120 mL) [equivalent to prednisolone base 5 mg/5 mL; dye free; raspberry flavor]
Suspension, ophthalmic, as acetate: 1% (5 mL, 10 mL, 15 mL) [contains benzalkonium chloride]
Econopred® Plus: 1% (5 mL, 10 mL) [contains benzalkonium chloride]
Pred Forte®: 1% (1 mL, 5 mL, 10 mL, 15 mL) [contains benzalkonium chloride and sodium bisulfite]
Pred Mild®: 0.12% (5 mL, 10 mL) [contains benzalkonium chloride and sodium bisulfite]
Syrup, as base: 5 mg/5 mL (120 mL); 15 mg/5 mL (240 mL, 480 mL)
Prelone®: 15 mg/5 mL (240 mL, 480 mL) [contains alcohol 5%, benzoic acid; cherry flavor]
Tablet, as base: 5 mg

Dosing
Adults: Dose depends upon condition being treated and response of patient. Consider alternate day therapy for long-term therapy. Discontinuation of long-term therapy requires gradual withdrawal by tapering the dose. Patients undergoing unusual stress while receiving corticosteroids, should receive increased doses prior to, during, and after the stressful situation.

Usual dose (range): Oral: 5-60 mg/day
Rheumatoid arthritis: Oral: Initial: 5-7.5 mg/day, adjust dose as necessary
Multiple sclerosis: Oral: 200 mg/day for 1 week followed by 80 mg every other day for 1 month
Conjunctivitis: Ophthalmic (suspension/solution): Instill 1-2 drops into conjunctival sac every hour during day, every 2 hours at night until favorable response is obtained, then use 1 drop every 4 hours.
Dosing adjustment in hyperthyroidism: Prednisolone dose may need to be increased to achieve adequate therapeutic effects.

Elderly: Use lowest effective adult dose. Dose depends upon condition being treated and response of patient; alternate day dosing may be attempted in some disease states.

Pediatrics: Dose depends upon condition being treated and response of patient; dosage for infants and children should be based on severity of the disease and response of the patient rather than on strict adherence to dosage indicated by age, weight, or body surface area. Consider alternate day therapy for long-term therapy. Discontinuation of long-term therapy requires gradual withdrawal by tapering the dose. Patients undergoing unusual stress while receiving corticosteroids, should receive increased doses prior to, during, and after the stressful situation.

Acute asthma: Oral: 1-2 mg/kg/day in divided doses 1-2 times/day for 3-5 days

Anti-inflammatory or immunosuppressive dose: Oral: 0.1-2 mg/kg/day in divided doses 1-4 times/ day

Nephrotic syndrome: Oral:

Initial (first 3 episodes): 2 mg/kg/day **or** 60 mg/m²/ day (maximum: 80 mg/day) in divided doses 3-4 times/day until urine is protein free for 3 consecutive days (maximum: 28 days); followed by 1-1.5 mg/kg/dose **or** 40 mg/m²/dose given every other day for 4 weeks

Maintenance (for frequent relapses): 0.5-1 mg/kg/ dose given every other day for 3-6 months

Conjunctivitis: Ophthalmic (suspension/solution): Children: Refer to adult dosing.

Dosing adjustment in hyperthyroidism: Refer to adult dosing.

Renal Impairment: Slightly dialyzable (5% to 20%)

Administration

Oral: Give oral formulation with food or milk to decrease GI effects.

Laboratory Monitoring Blood glucose, electrolytes

Nursing Actions

Physical Assessment: Assess other medications patient may be taking for effectiveness and interactions. Monitor laboratory tests, therapeutic response, and adverse effects according to indications for therapy, dose, route (systemic or topical), and duration of therapy. With systemic administration, patients with diabetes should monitor glucose levels closely (corticosteroids may alter glucose levels). Assess knowledge/teach patient appropriate use, interventions to reduce side effects, and adverse symptoms to report. When used for long-term therapy (>10-14 days), dosages should not be discontinued abruptly.

Patient Education: Take exactly as directed; do not increase dose or discontinue abruptly without consulting prescriber. Avoid alcohol. Limit intake of caffeine or stimulants. Prescriber may recommend increased dietary vitamins, minerals, or iron. If you have diabetes, monitor glucose levels closely (antidiabetic medication may need to be adjusted). Inform prescriber if you are experiencing greater-than-normal levels of stress (medication may need adjustment). Some forms of this medication may cause GI upset (oral medication should be taken with meals to reduce GI upset; small frequent meals and frequent mouth care may reduce GI upset). You may be more susceptible to infection (avoid crowds and exposure to infection). Report promptly excessive nervousness or sleep disturbances; any signs of infection (sore throat, unhealed injuries); excessive growth of body hair or loss of skin color; vision changes; excessive or sudden weight gain (>3 lb/week); swelling of face or extremities; respiratory difficulty; muscle weakness; change in color of stools (black or tarry) or persistent abdominal pain; or worsening of condition or failure to improve. **Pregnancy precaution:** Inform prescriber if you are or intend to become pregnant.

Ophthalmic: For ophthalmic use only. Wash hands before using. Tilt head back and look upward. Put drops of suspension inside lower eyelid. Close eye and roll eyeball in all directions. Do not blink for 1/2 minute. Apply gentle pressure to inner corner of eye for 30 seconds. Do not use any other eye preparation for at least 10 minutes. Do not let tip of applicator touch eye; do not contaminate tip of applicator (may cause eye infection, eye damage, or vision loss). Do not share medication with anyone else. Wear sunglasses when in sunlight; you may be more sensitive to bright light. Inform prescriber if condition worsens or fails to improve or if you experience eye pain, disturbances of vision, or other adverse eye response.

Dietary Considerations Should be taken after meals or with food or milk to decrease GI effects; increase dietary intake of pyridoxine, vitamin C, vitamin D, folate, calcium, and phosphorus.

Geriatric Considerations Useful in patients with inability to activate prednisone (liver disease). Because of the risk of adverse effects, systemic corticosteroids should be used cautiously in the elderly, in the smallest possible dose, and for the shortest possible time. For long-term use, monitor bone mineral density and institute fracture prevention strategies. See Pharmacodynamics/kinetics.

Related Information

FDA Name Differentiation Project: The Use of Tall-Man Letters on page 12

PredniSONE (PRED ni sone)

U.S. Brand Names Prednisone Intensol™; Sterapred®; Sterapred® DS

Synonyms Deltacortisone; Deltadehydrocortisone

Pharmacologic Category Corticosteroid, Systemic

Medication Safety Issues

Sound-alike/look-alike issues:

PredniSONE may be confused with methylPREDNISolone, Pramosone®, prazosin, prednisoLONE, Prilosec®, primidone, promethazine

Pregnancy Risk Factor B

Lactation Enters breast milk/compatible

Use Treatment of a variety of diseases including adrenocortical insufficiency, hypercalcemia, rheumatic, and collagen disorders; dermatologic, ocular, respiratory, gastrointestinal, and neoplastic diseases; organ transplantation and a variety of diseases including those of hematologic, allergic, inflammatory, and autoimmune in origin; not available in injectable form, prednisolone must be used

Unlabeled/Investigational Use Investigational: Prevention of postherpetic neuralgia and relief of acute pain in the early stages

Mechanism of Action/Effect Decreases inflammation by suppression of migration of polymorphonuclear leukocytes and reversal of increased capillary permeability; suppresses the immune system by reducing activity and volume of the lymphatic system; suppresses adrenal function at high doses

Contraindications Hypersensitivity to prednisone or any component of the formulation; serious infections, except tuberculous meningitis; systemic fungal infections; varicella

Warnings/Precautions Use with caution in patients with hypothyroidism, cirrhosis, CHF, ulcerative colitis, thromboembolic disorders, and patients with an increased risk for peptic ulcer disease. Corticosteroids should be used with caution in patients with diabetes, hypertension, osteoporosis, glaucoma, cataracts, or tuberculosis. Use caution in hepatic impairment. May retard bone growth. Gradually taper dose to withdraw therapy. Because of the risk of adverse effects, systemic corticosteroids should be used cautiously in the elderly, in the smallest possible dose, and for the shortest possible time.

Drug Interactions

Cytochrome P450 Effect: Substrate of CYP3A4 (minor); **Induces** CYP2C19 (weak), 3A4 (weak)

Decreased Effect: Decreased effect with barbiturates, phenytoin, rifampin; decreased effect of salicylates, vaccines, and toxoids.

(Continued)

PredniSONE (Continued)

Increased Effect/Toxicity: Concurrent use with NSAIDs may increase the risk of GI ulceration.

Nutritional/Ethanol Interactions

Ethanol: Avoid ethanol (may increase gastric mucosal irritation)

Food: Prednisone interferes with calcium absorption, Limit caffeine.

Herb/Nutraceutical: St John's wort may decrease prednisone levels. Avoid cat's claw, echinacea (have immunostimulant properties).

Lab Interactions Response to skin tests

Adverse Reactions

>10%:

Central nervous system: Insomnia, nervousness
Gastrointestinal: Increased appetite, indigestion

1% to 10%:

Dermatologic: Hirsutism
Endocrine & metabolic: Diabetes mellitus, glucose intolerance, hyperglycemia
Neuromuscular & skeletal: Arthralgia
Ocular: Cataracts, glaucoma
Respiratory: Epistaxis

Overdosage/Toxicology When consumed in high doses for prolonged periods, systemic hypercorticism and adrenal suppression may occur. In those cases, discontinuation of the corticosteroid should be done judiciously.

Pharmacodynamics/Kinetics

Protein Binding: Concentration dependent: 65% to 91%

Half-Life Elimination: Normal renal function: 2.5-3.5 hours

Metabolism: Hepatically converted from prednisone (inactive) to prednisolone (active); may be impaired with hepatic dysfunction

Pharmacokinetic Note See Prednisolone monograph for complete information.

Available Dosage Forms

Solution, oral: 1 mg/mL (5 mL, 120 mL, 500 mL) [contains alcohol 5%, sodium benzoate; vanilla flavor]

Solution, oral concentrate (Prednisone Intensol™): 5 mg/mL (30 mL) [contains alcohol 30%]

Tablet: 1 mg, 2.5 mg, 5 mg, 10 mg, 20 mg, 50 mg

Sterapred®: 5 mg [supplied as 21 tablet 6-day unit-dose package or 48 tablet 12-day unit-dose package]

Sterapred® DS: 10 mg [supplied as 21 tablet 6-day unit-dose package or 48 tablet 12-day unit-dose package]

Dosing

Adults: Dose depends upon condition being treated and response of patient; consider alternate day therapy for long-term therapy. Discontinuation of long-term therapy requires gradual withdrawal by tapering the dose.

Physiologic replacement: Oral: 4-5 mg/m²/day

Immunosuppression/chemotherapy adjunct: Oral: Range: 5-60 mg/day in divided doses 1-4 times/day

Allergic reaction (contact dermatitis): Oral:

Day 1: 30 mg divided as 10 mg before breakfast, 5 mg at lunch, 5 mg at dinner, 10 mg at bedtime

Day 2: 5 mg at breakfast, 5 mg at lunch, 5 mg at dinner, 10 mg at bedtime

Day 3: 5 mg 4 times/day (with meals and at bedtime)

Day 4: 5 mg 3 times/day (breakfast, lunch, bedtime)

Day 5: 5 mg 2 times/day (breakfast, bedtime)

Day 6: 5 mg before breakfast

Acute asthma: Oral: 1-2 mg/kg/day in divided doses 1-2 times/day for 3-5 days

Asthma maintenance:

Moderate persistent: Inhaled corticosteroid (medium dose) or inhaled corticosteroid (low-medium dose) with a long-acting bronchodilator

Severe persistent: Inhaled corticosteroid (high dose) and corticosteroid tablets or syrup long term: 2 mg/kg/day, generally not to exceed 60 mg/day

Pneumonia due to *Pneumocystis carinii*: Oral:

40 mg twice daily for 5 days **followed by**

40 mg once daily for 5 days **followed by**

20 mg once daily for 11 days or until antimicrobial regimen is completed

Thyrotoxicosis: Oral: 60 mg/day

Note: Dosing adjustment in hyperthyroidism: Prednisone dose may need to be increased to achieve adequate therapeutic effects

Chemotherapy (refer to individual protocols): Oral: Range: 20 mg/day to 100 mg/m²/day

Rheumatoid arthritis: Oral: Use lowest possible daily dose (often ≤7.5 mg/day)

Idiopathic thrombocytopenia purpura (ITP): Oral: 60 mg daily for 4-6 weeks, gradually tapered over several weeks

Systemic lupus erythematosus (SLE): Oral:

Acute: 1-2 mg/kg/day in 2-3 divided doses

Maintenance: Reduce to lowest possible dose, usually <1 mg/kg/day as single dose (morning)

Elderly: Refer to adult dosing; use the lowest effective dose. Oral dose depends upon condition being treated and response of patient. Alternate day dosing may be attempted.

Pediatrics: Note: Dose depends upon condition being treated and response of patient; dosage for infants and children should be based on severity of the disease and response of the patient rather than on strict adherence to dosage indicated by age, weight, or body surface area. Consider alternate day therapy for long-term therapy. Discontinuation of long-term therapy requires gradual withdrawal by tapering the dose.

Physiologic replacement: Oral: Children: 4-5 mg/m²/day

Anti-inflammatory or immunosuppressive dose: Oral: 0.05-2 mg/kg/day divided 1-4 times/day

Acute asthma: Oral: 1-2 mg/kg/day in divided doses 1-2 times/day for 3-5 days

Alternatively (for 3- to 5-day "burst"):

<1 year: 10 mg every 12 hours

1-4 years: 20 mg every 12 hours

5-13 years: 30 mg every 12 hours

>13 years: 40 mg every 12 hours

Asthma long-term therapy (alternative dosing by age): Oral:

<1 year: 10 mg every other day

1-4 years: 20 mg every other day

5-13 years: 30 mg every other day

>13 years: 40 mg every other day

Asthma maintenance: Children ≥5 years: Refer to adult dosing.

Nephrotic syndrome: Oral:

Initial (first 3 episodes): 2 mg/kg/day or 60 mg/m²/day (maximum: 80 mg/day) in divided doses 3-4 times/day until urine is protein free for 3 consecutive days (maximum: 28 days); followed by 1-1.5 mg/kg/dose or 40 mg/m²/dose given every other day for 4 weeks

Maintenance dose (for frequent relapses): 0.5-1 mg/kg/dose given every other day for 3-6 months

Renal Impairment: Hemodialysis effects: Supplemental dose is not necessary.

Administration

Oral: Take with food to decrease GI upset.

Laboratory Monitoring Blood glucose, electrolytes

Nursing Actions

Physical Assessment: Assess effectiveness and interactions of other medications patient may be taking. Monitor for effectiveness of therapy and adverse reactions according to dose and length of therapy. Assess knowledge/teach patient appropriate use, possible side effects/interventions, and adverse symptoms to report (ie, opportunistic infection, adrenal suppression). Instruct patients with diabetes to monitor serum glucose levels closely; corticosteroids can alter glucose tolerance. Dose may need to be increased if patient is experiencing higher than normal levels of stress. When discontinuing, taper dose and frequency slowly

Patient Education: Take exactly as directed. Do not take more than prescribed dose and do not discontinue abruptly; consult prescriber. Take with or after meals. Take once-a-day dose with food in the morning. Avoid alcohol. Limit intake of caffeine or stimulants. Maintain adequate nutrition; consult prescriber for possibility of special dietary recommendations. If you have diabetes, monitor serum glucose closely and notify prescriber of changes; this medication can alter hypoglycemic requirements. Notify prescriber if you are experiencing higher than normal levels of stress; medication may need adjustment. Periodic ophthalmic examinations will be necessary with long-term use. You will be susceptible to infection (avoid crowds and exposure to infection). You may experience insomnia or nervousness; use caution when driving or engaging in tasks requiring alertness until response to drug is known. Report weakness, change in menstrual pattern, vision changes, signs of hyperglycemia, signs of infection (eg, fever, chills, mouth sores, perianal itching, vaginal discharge), other persistent side effects, or worsening of condition.

Dietary Considerations Should be taken after meals or with food or milk; increase dietary intake of pyridoxine, vitamin C, vitamin D, folate, calcium, and phosphorus.

Geriatric Considerations Because of the risk of adverse effects, systemic corticosteroids should be used cautiously in the elderly, in the smallest possible dose, and for the shortest possible time.

Breast-Feeding Issues Crosses into breast milk. No data on clinical effects on the infant. AAP considers **compatible** with breast-feeding.

Pregnancy Issues Crosses the placenta. Immunosuppression reported in 1 infant exposed to high-dose prednisone plus azathioprine throughout gestation. One report of congenital cataracts. Available evidence suggests safe use during pregnancy.

Additional Information Tapering of corticosteroids after a short course of therapy (<7-10 days) is generally not required unless the disease/inflammatory process is slow to respond. Tapering after prolonged exposure is dependent upon the individual patient, duration of corticosteroid treatments, and size of steroid dose. Recovery of the HPA axis may require several months. Subtle but important HPA axis suppression may be present for as long as several months after a course of as few as 10-14 days duration. Testing of HPA axis (cosyntropin) may be required, and signs/symptoms of adrenal insufficiency should be monitored in patients with a history of use.

Related Information

FDA Name Differentiation Project: The Use of Tall-Man Letters *on page 12*

Pregabalin (pre GAB a lin)

U.S. Brand Names Lyrica®
Synonyms CI-1008; S-(+)-3-isobutylgaba
Restrictions C-V
Pharmacologic Category Analgesic, Miscellaneous; Anticonvulsant, Miscellaneous
Pregnancy Risk Factor C
Lactation Excretion in breast milk unknown/not recommended
Use Management of pain associated with diabetic peripheral neuropathy; management of postherpetic neuralgia; adjunctive therapy for partial-onset seizure disorder in adults
Mechanism of Action/Effect Decreases symptoms of painful peripheral neuropathies and, as adjunctive therapy in partial seizures, decreases the frequency of seizures
Contraindications Hypersensitivity to pregabalin or any component of the formulation
Warnings/Precautions May cause CNS depression and/or dizziness, which may impair physical or mental abilities. Patients must be cautioned about performing tasks which require mental alertness (eg, operating machinery or driving). Effects with other sedative drugs or ethanol may be potentiated. Visual disturbances (blurred vision, decreased acuity and visual field changes) have been associated with pregabalin therapy; patients should be instructed to notify their physician if these effects are noted.

Pregabalin has been associated with increases in CPK and rare cases of rhabdomyolysis. Patients should be instructed to notify their prescriber if unexplained muscle pain, tenderness, or weakness, particularly if fever and/or malaise are associated with these symptoms. Use may be associated with weight gain and peripheral edema; use caution in patients with congestive heart failure, hypertension, or diabetes. Effect on weight gain/edema may be additive to thiazolidinedione antidiabetic agent; particularly in patients with prior cardiovascular disease. May decrease platelet count or prolong PR interval.

Has been noted to be tumorigenic (increased incidence of hemangiosarcoma) in animal studies; significance of these findings in humans is unknown. Pregabalin has been associated with discontinuation symptoms following abrupt cessation, and increases in seizure frequency (when used as an antiepileptic) may occur. Should not be discontinued abruptly; dosage tapering over at least 1 week is recommended. Use caution in renal impairment; dosage adjustment required. Safety and efficacy have not been established in pediatric patients.

Drug Interactions
Increased Effect/Toxicity:
Sedative effects may be additive with CNS depressants (includes ethanol, barbiturates, narcotic analgesics, and other sedative agents). Pregabalin's effect on weight gain/edema may be additive with thiazolidinedione antidiabetic agents (includes pioglitazone, rosiglitazone).

Nutritional/Ethanol Interactions
Ethanol: Avoid ethanol (may increase CNS depression).
Herb/Nutraceutical: Avoid valerian, St John's wort, kava kava, gotu kola (may increase CNS depression).

Adverse Reactions Note: Frequency of adverse effects may be influenced by dose or concurrent therapy. In add-on trials in epilepsy, frequency of CNS and visual adverse effects were higher than those reported in pain management trials. Range noted below is inclusive of all trials.
>10%:
Cardiovascular: Peripheral edema (up to 16%)
(Continued)

Pregabalin (Continued)

Central nervous system: Dizziness (8% to 38%), somnolence (4% to 28%), ataxia (1% to 20%)

Gastrointestinal: Weight gain (up to 16%), xerostomia (1% to 15%)

Neuromuscular & skeletal: Tremor (1% to 11%)

Ocular: Blurred vision (1% to 12%), diplopia (up to 12%)

Miscellaneous: Infection (up to 14%), accidental injury (2% to 11%)

1% to 10%:

Cardiovascular: Chest pain (up to 4%), edema (up to 6%)

Central nervous system: Neuropathy (up to 9%), headache (up to 9%), thinking abnormal (up to 9%), confusion (up to 7%), speech disorder (up to 7%), incoordination (up to 6%), amnesia (up to 6%), pain (up to 5%), vertigo (up to 4%), nervousness (>2%), euphoria (up to 3%), fever (≥1%), anxiety (≥1%), depersonalization (≥1%), hypertonia (≥1%), hypoesthesia (≥1%), stupor (≥1%)

Dermatologic: Facial edema (up to 3%), ecchymosis (≥1%), pruritus (≥1%)

Endocrine & metabolic: Appetite increased (up to 6%), hypoglycemia (up to 3%), libido decreased (≥1%)

Gastrointestinal: Constipation (up to 7%), flatulence (up to 3%), vomiting (up to 3%), abdominal pain (≥1%), gastroenteritis (≥1%)

Genitourinary: Anorgasmia (≥1%), impotence (≥1%), urinary frequency (≥1%), incontinence (≥1%)

Neuromuscular & skeletal: Abnormal gait (up to 8%), weakness (up to 7%), twitching (up to 5%), myoclonus (up to 4%), back pain (up to 2%), paresthesia (>2%), CPK increased (2%), arthralgia (≥1%), leg cramps (≥1%), myalgia (≥1%), myasthenia (≥1%)

Ocular: Visual abnormalities (up to 5%), visual field defect (≥2%), eye disorder (up to 2%), nystagmus (>2%), conjunctivitis (≥1%)

Otic: Otitis media (≥1%), tinnitus (≥1%)

Respiratory: Dyspnea (up to 3%), bronchitis (up to 3%)

Miscellaneous: Flu-like syndrome (up to 2%), allergic reaction (≥1%)

Overdosage/Toxicology Symptoms are similar to those experienced at therapeutic doses (somnolence). Treatment is symptom-directed and supportive. A 4-hour hemodialysis procedure reduces plasma concentrations by ~50%.

Pharmacodynamics/Kinetics

Onset of Action: Pain management: Effects may be noted as early as the first week of therapy

Time to Peak: 1.5 hours (3 hours with food)

Protein Binding: 0%

Half-Life Elimination: 6.3 hours

Metabolism: Negligible

Excretion: Urine (90% as unchanged drug; minor metabolites)

Available Dosage Forms Capsule: 25 mg, 50 mg, 75 mg, 100 mg, 150 mg, 200 mg, 225 mg, 300 mg

Dosing

Adults & Elderly:

Neuropathic pain (diabetes-associated): Oral: Initial: 150 mg/day in divided doses (50 mg 3 times/day); may be increased within 1 week based on tolerability and effect; maximum dose: 300 mg/day (dosages up to 600 mg/day were evaluated with no significant additional benefit and an increase in adverse effects)

Postherpetic neuralgia: Oral: Initial: 150 mg/day in divided doses (75 mg 2 times/day or 50 mg 3 times/day); may be increased to 300 mg/day within 1 week based on tolerability and effect; further titration (to 600 mg/day) after 2-4 weeks may be considered in patients who do not experience sufficient relief of pain provided they are able to tolerate pregabalin. Maximum dose: 600 mg/day

Partial onset seizures (adjunctive therapy): Oral: Initial: 150 mg per day in divided doses (75 mg 2 times/day or 50 mg 3 times/day); may be increased based on tolerability and effect (optimal titration schedule has not been defined). Maximum dose: 600 mg/day

Note: Discontinuing therapy: Pregabalin should not be abruptly discontinued; taper dosage over at least 1 week

Renal Impairment: Cl_{cr} ≥60 mL/minute: No dosage adjustment required. In renally-impaired patients, dosage adjustment depends on renal function and daily dosage:

Cl_{cr} 30-60 mL/minute: Total daily dose:
75 mg in 2-3 divided doses **or**
150 mg in 2-3 divided doses **or**
300 mg in 2-3 divided doses

Cl_{cr} 15-30 mL/minute: Total daily dose:
25-50 mg in once daily or in 2 divided doses **or**
75 mg once daily or in 2 divided doses **or**
150 mg once daily or in 2 divided doses

Cl_{cr} <15 mL/minute: Total daily dose:
25 mg once daily **or**
25-50 mg once daily **or**
75 mg once daily

Hemodialysis: Total daily dose:
25 mg: Single supplementary dose of 25 mg **or** 50 mg
25-50 mg: Single supplementary dose of 50 mg **or** 75 mg
75 mg: Single supplementary dose of 100 mg **or** 150 mg

Administration

Oral: May be administered with or without food.

Stability

Storage: Store at 25°C (77°F). Excursions permitted to 15°C to 30°C (59°F to 86°F).

Laboratory Monitoring CPK

Nursing Actions

Physical Assessment: Monitor therapeutic response and adverse reactions at the beginning and periodically throughout therapy. Taper dosage over at least one week when discontinuing. Do not discontinue abruptly. Assess other prescription and OTC medications the patient may be taking to avoid duplications and interactions. Assess knowledge/teach patient appropriate use, side effects, and symptoms to report.

Patient Education: Inform prescriber of all prescription medications, OTC medications, or herbal products you are taking. Avoid alcohol; may increase drowsiness/CNS depression. Taper dosage slowly when discontinuing. Do not discontinue abruptly. Maintain adequate hydration (2-3 L/day of fluids) unless instructed to restrict fluid intake by prescriber. May cause CNS depression and/or dizziness (use caution when driving or engaging in activities requiring alertness until response to drug is known), weight gain, or fluid retention. Report immediately any visual disturbances. Report unexplained muscle pain, tenderness, or weakness, especially if accompanied by unexplained fever and malaise, dizziness, confusion or abnormal thinking, weight gain >5 lbs/week, excessively dry mouth, and drowsiness. **Pregnancy/breast-feeding precautions:** Inform prescriber if you are or intend to become pregnant. Breast-feeding is not recommended.

Dietary Considerations May be taken with or without food.

Pregnancy Issues There are no adequate and well-controlled studies in pregnant women. Use only when potential benefit to the mother outweighs possible risk to the fetus.

Primaquine (PRIM a kween)

Synonyms Primaquine Phosphate; Prymaccone
Pharmacologic Category Aminoquinoline (Antimalarial)
Pregnancy Risk Factor C
Lactation Excretion in breast milk unknown
Use Treatment of malaria
Unlabeled/Investigational Use Prevention of malaria; treatment *Pneumocystis carinii* pneumonia
Mechanism of Action/Effect Eliminates the primary tissue exoerythrocytic forms of *P. falciparum*; disrupts mitochondria and binds to DNA
Contraindications Hypersensitivity to primaquine, similar alkaloids, or any component of the formulation; acutely ill patients who have a tendency to develop granulocytopenia (rheumatoid arthritis, SLE); patients receiving other drugs capable of depressing the bone marrow (eg, quinacrine and primaquine)
Warnings/Precautions Use with caution in patients with G6PD deficiency, NADH methemoglobin reductase deficiency. Do not exceed recommended dosage.
Drug Interactions
　Cytochrome P450 Effect: Substrate of CYP3A4 (major); **Inhibits** CYP1A2 (strong), 2D6 (weak), 3A4 (weak); **Induces** CYP1A2 (weak)
　Decreased Effect: The levels/effects of primaquine may be decreased by aminoglutethimide, carbamazepine, nafcillin, nevirapine, phenobarbital, phenytoin, rifamycins, and other CYP3A4 inducers.
　Increased Effect/Toxicity: Increased toxicity/levels with quinacrine. Primaquine may increase the levels/effects of aminophylline, fluvoxamine, mexiletine, mirtazapine, ropinirole, theophylline, trifluoperazine, and other CYP1A2 substrates.
Nutritional/Ethanol Interactions Ethanol: Avoid ethanol (due to GI irritation).
Adverse Reactions Frequency not defined.
　Cardiovascular: Arrhythmias
　Central nervous system: Headache
　Dermatologic: Pruritus
　Gastrointestinal: Abdominal pain, nausea, vomiting
　Hematologic: Agranulocytosis, hemolytic anemia in G6PD deficiency, leukopenia, leukocytosis, methemoglobinemia in NADH-methemoglobin reductase-deficient individuals
　Ocular: Interference with visual accommodation
Overdosage/Toxicology Symptoms of acute overdose include abdominal cramps, vomiting, cyanosis, methemoglobinemia (possibly severe), leukopenia, acute hemolytic anemia (often significant), and granulocytopenia. With chronic overdose, symptoms include ototoxicity and retinopathy. Treatment is supportive.
Pharmacodynamics/Kinetics
　Time to Peak: Serum: 1-2 hours
　Half-Life Elimination: 3.7-9.6 hours
　Metabolism: Hepatic to carboxyprimaquine (active)
　Excretion: Urine (small amounts as unchanged drug)
Available Dosage Forms Tablet, as phosphate: 26.3 mg [15 mg base]
Dosing
　Adults & Elderly: Dosage expressed as mg of base (15 mg base = 26.3 mg primaquine phosphate)
　　Treatment of malaria: To decrease risk of delayed primary attacks and prevent relapse: Oral: 15 mg/day (base) once daily for 14 days or 45 mg base once weekly for 8 weeks
　　　CDC treatment recommendations: Begin therapy during last 2 weeks of, or following a course of, suppression with chloroquine or a comparable drug
　　　Note: A second course (30 mg/day) for 14 days may be required in patients with relapse. Higher initial doses (30 mg/day) have also been used following exposure in S.E. Asia or Somalia.
　　Prevention of malaria (unlabeled use): Initiate prior to travel and continue for 7 days after departure from malaria-endemic area: Oral: 30 mg once daily
　　Pneumonia due to *Pneumocystis carinii* (unlabeled use): Oral: 30 mg once daily for 21 days (in conjunction with clindamycin)
　Pediatrics: Dosage expressed as mg of base (15 mg base = 26.3 mg primaquine phosphate)
　　Treatment of malaria: To Decrease risk of delayed primary attacks and prevent relapse: Oral: 0.3 mg base/kg/day once daily for 14 days (not to exceed 15 mg/day) or 0.9 mg base/kg once weekly for 8 weeks (not to exceed 45 mg base/week
　　　CDC treatment recommendations: Begin therapy during last 2 weeks of, or following a course of, suppression with chloroquine or a comparable drug
　　　Note: A second course (30 mg/day) for 14 days may be required in patients with relapse. Higher initial doses (30 mg/day) have also been used following exposure in S.E. Asia or Somalia.
　　Prevention of malaria (unlabeled use): Oral: Initiate prior to travel and continue for 7 days after departure from malaria-endemic area: 0.5 mg/kg once daily
Administration
　Oral: Take with meals to decrease adverse GI effects. Drug has a bitter taste.
Laboratory Monitoring Periodic CBC, visual color check of urine, glucose, electrolytes; if hemolysis suspected - CBC, haptoglobin, peripheral smear, urinalysis dipstick for occult blood
Nursing Actions
　Physical Assessment: Prior to beginning therapy, assess potential for interactions with pharmacological or herbal products patient may be taking. Monitor therapeutic effects and adverse reactions (eg, arrhythmias, pruritus, gastrointestinal upset, hematological changes) on a regular basis throughout therapy. Teach patient proper use, possible side effects/appropriate interventions (eg, importance of adequate hydration and periodic ophthalmic examinations with long term therapy), and adverse symptoms to report.
　Patient Education: Do not take any new medication during therapy unless approved by prescriber. It is important to complete full course of therapy for full effect. May be taken with meals to decrease GI upset and bitter aftertaste. Avoid alcohol. You should have regular ophthalmic exams (every 4-6 months) if using this medication over extended periods. May cause nausea, vomiting, or loss of appetite (small, frequent meals, frequent mouth care, sucking lozenges, or chewing gum may help). Report persistent GI disturbance, chest pain or palpitation, unusual fatigue, easy bruising or bleeding, visual or hearing disturbances, changes in urine (darkening, tinged with red, decreased volume), or any other persistent adverse reactions. **Pregnancy/breast-feeding precautions:** Inform prescriber if you are or intend to become pregnant. Consult prescriber if breast-feeding.

Primidone (PRI mi done)

U.S. Brand Names Mysoline®
Synonyms Desoxyphenobarbital; Primaclone
Pharmacologic Category Anticonvulsant, Miscellaneous; Barbiturate
Medication Safety Issues
　Sound-alike/look-alike issues:
　　Primidone may be confused with predniSONE
Pregnancy Risk Factor D
(Continued)

Primidone (Continued)

Lactation Enters breast milk/not recommended (AAP recommends use "with caution")

Use Management of grand mal, psychomotor, and focal seizures

Unlabeled/Investigational Use Benign familial tremor (essential tremor)

Mechanism of Action/Effect Decreases neuron excitability, raises seizure threshold similar to phenobarbital; primidone has two active metabolites, phenobarbital and phenylethylmalonamide (PEMA); PEMA may enhance the activity of phenobarbital

Contraindications Hypersensitivity to primidone, phenobarbital, or any component of the formulation; porphyria; pregnancy

Warnings/Precautions Use with caution in patients with renal or hepatic impairment, pulmonary insufficiency; abrupt withdrawal may precipitate status epilepticus. Potential for drug dependency exists. Do not administer to patients in acute pain. Use caution in elderly, debilitated, or pediatric patients - may cause paradoxical responses. May cause CNS depression, which may impair physical or mental abilities. Patients must cautioned about performing tasks which require mental alertness (eg, operating machinery or driving). Effects with other sedative drugs or ethanol may be potentiated. Use with caution in patients with depression or suicidal tendencies, or in patients with a history of drug abuse. Tolerance or psychological and physical dependence may occur with prolonged use. Primidone's metabolite, phenobarbital, has been associated with cognitive deficits in children. Use with caution in patients with hypoadrenalism.

Drug Interactions

Cytochrome P450 Effect: Metabolized to phenobarbital; Induces CYP1A2 (strong), 2B6 (strong), 2C8/9 (strong), 3A4 (strong)

Decreased Effect: Barbiturates may increase the metabolism of estrogens and reduce the efficacy of oral contraceptives; an alternative method of contraception should be considered. Barbiturates inhibit the hypoprothrombinemic effects of oral anticoagulants via increased metabolism. Barbiturates may enhance the metabolism of methadone resulting in methadone withdrawal. The levels/effects of primidone may be decreased by aminoglutethimide, carbamazepine, phenytoin, rifampin, and other CYP2C19 inducers.

Primidone may decrease the levels/effects of aminophylline, amiodarone, benzodiazepines, bupropion, calcium channel blockers, carbamazepine, citalopram, clarithromycin, cyclosporine, diazepam, efavirenz, erythromycin, estrogens, fluoxetine, fluvoxamine, glimepiride, glipizide, ifosfamide, losartan, methsuximide, mirtazapine, nateglinide, nefazodone, nevirapine, phenytoin, pioglitazone, promethazine, propranolol, protease inhibitors, proton pump inhibitors, rifampin, ropinirole, rosiglitazone, selegiline, sertraline, sulfonamides, tacrolimus, theophylline, venlafaxine. voriconazole, warfarin, zafirlukast, and other CYP1A2, 2A6, 2B6, 2C8/9, or 3A4 substrates.

Increased Effect/Toxicity: When combined with other CNS depressants, ethanol, narcotic analgesics, antidepressants, or benzodiazepines, additive respiratory and CNS depression may occur. Barbiturates may enhance the hepatotoxic potential of acetaminophen overdoses. Chloramphenicol, MAO inhibitors, valproic acid, and felbamate may inhibit barbiturate metabolism. Barbiturates may impair the absorption of griseofulvin, and may enhance the nephrotoxic effects of methoxyflurane. Concurrent use of phenobarbital with meperidine may result in increased CNS depression. Concurrent use of phenobarbital with primidone may result in elevated phenobarbital serum concentrations. CYP2C19 inhibitors may increase the levels/effects of primidone; example inhibitors include delavirdine, fluconazole, fluvoxamine, gemfibrozil, isoniazid, omeprazole, and ticlopidine.

Nutritional/Ethanol Interactions

Ethanol: Avoid ethanol (may increase CNS depression).

Food: Protein-deficient diets increase duration of action of primidone.

Herb/Nutraceutical: Avoid valerian, St John's wort, kava kava, gotu kola (may increase CNS depression).

Lab Interactions Increased alkaline phosphatase (S); decreased calcium (S)

Adverse Reactions Frequency not defined.

Central nervous system: Drowsiness, vertigo, ataxia, lethargy, behavior change, fatigue, hyperirritability

Dermatologic: Rash

Gastrointestinal: Nausea, vomiting, anorexia

Genitourinary: Impotence

Hematologic: Agranulocytopenia, agranulocytosis, anemia

Ocular: Diplopia, nystagmus

Overdosage/Toxicology Symptoms of overdose include unsteady gait, slurred speech, confusion, jaundice, hypothermia, fever, hypotension, coma, and respiratory arrest. Assure adequate hydration and renal function. Urinary alkalinization with I.V. sodium bicarbonate also helps to enhance elimination. Repeat oral doses of activated charcoal significantly reduce the half-life of primidone through nonrenal elimination. Hemodialysis or hemoperfusion is of uncertain value. Patients in stage IV coma due to high serum drug levels may require charcoal hemoperfusion.

Pharmacodynamics/Kinetics

Time to Peak: Serum: ~4 hours

Protein Binding: 99%

Half-Life Elimination: Age dependent: Primidone: 10-12 hours; PEMA: 16 hours; Phenobarbital: 52-118 hours

Metabolism: Hepatic to phenobarbital (active) and phenylethylmalonamide (PEMA)

Excretion: Urine (15% to 25% as unchanged drug and active metabolites)

Available Dosage Forms Tablet: 50 mg, 250 mg [generic tablet may contain sodium benzoate]

Dosing

Adults & Elderly:

Essential tremor (unlabeled use): 750 mg early in divided doses

Seizure disorders (grand mal, psychomotor, and focal): Oral: Initial: 125-250 mg/day at bedtime; increase by 125-250 mg/day every 3-7 days; usual dose: 750-1500 mg/day in divided doses 3-4 times/day with maximum dosage of 2 g/day.

Pediatrics: Seizure disorders (grand mal, psychomotor, and focal): Oral:

Children <8 years: Initial: 50-125 mg/day given at bedtime; increase by 50-125 mg/day increments every 3-7 days; usual dose: 10-25 mg/kg/day in divided doses 3-4 times/day.

Children ≥8 years: Refer to adult dosing.

Renal Impairment:

Cl$_{cr}$ 50-80 mL/minute: Administer every 8 hours.

Cl$_{cr}$ 10-50 mL/minute: Administer every 8-12 hours.

Cl$_{cr}$ <10 mL/minute: Administer every 12-24 hours.

Moderately dialyzable (20% to 50%)

Administer dose postdialysis or administer supplemental 30% dose.

Hepatic Impairment: Increased side effects may occur in severe liver disease. Monitor plasma levels and adjust dose accordingly.

Stability

Storage: Protect from light.

Laboratory Monitoring Serum primidone and phenobarbital concentration, CBC. Monitor CBC at 6-month intervals to compare with baseline obtained at start of therapy. Since elderly patients metabolize phenobarbital at a slower rate than younger adults, it is suggested to measure both primidone and phenobarbital levels together.

Nursing Actions

Physical Assessment: Assess effectiveness and interactions of other medications patient may be taking. Monitor therapeutic response (seizure activity, force, type, duration), laboratory values, and adverse reactions at beginning of therapy and periodically with long-term use. Observe and teach seizure/safety precautions. Assess knowledge/teach patient appropriate use, interventions to reduce side effects, and adverse symptoms to report.

Patient Education: Take exactly as directed; do not increase dose or frequency or discontinue without consulting prescriber. Drug may cause physical and/or psychological dependence. While using this medication, do not use alcohol and other prescription or OTC medications (especially pain medications, sedatives, antihistamines, or hypnotics) without consulting prescriber. Maintain adequate hydration (2-3 L/day of fluids) unless instructed to restrict fluid intake. You may experience drowsiness, dizziness, or blurred vision (use caution when driving or engaging in tasks requiring alertness until response to drug is known); nausea, vomiting, or loss of appetite (small frequent meals, frequent mouth care, chewing gum, or sucking lozenges may help); or impotence (reversible). Wear identification of epileptic status and medications. Report behavioral or CNS changes (confusion, depression, increased sedation, excitation, headache, insomnia, or lethargy); muscle weakness, or tremors; unusual bruising or bleeding (mouth, urine, stool); or worsening of seizure activity or loss of seizure control. **Pregnancy/breast-feeding precautions:** Do not get pregnant while taking this drug; use appropriate contraceptive measures. Consult prescriber if breast-feeding.

Dietary Considerations Folic acid: Low erythrocyte and CSF folate concentrations. Megaloblastic anemia has been reported. To avoid folic acid deficiency and megaloblastic anemia, some clinicians recommend giving patients on anticonvulsants prophylactic doses of folic acid and cyanocobalamin.

Geriatric Considerations Due to CNS effects, monitor closely when initiating drug in the elderly. Since elderly metabolize phenobarbital at a slower rate than younger adults, it is suggested to measure both primidone and phenobarbital levels together. Adjust dose for renal function in the elderly when initiating or changing dose.

Breast-Feeding Issues Sedation and feeding problems may occur in nursing infants. AAP recommends USE WITH CAUTION.

Pregnancy Issues Crosses the placenta. Dysmorphic facial features; hemorrhagic disease of newborn due to fetal vitamin K depletion, maternal folic acid deficiency may occur. Epilepsy itself, number of medications, genetic factors, or a combination of these probably influence the teratogenicity of anticonvulsant therapy. Benefit:risk ratio usually favors continued use during pregnancy.

Related Information
Peak and Trough Guidelines *on page 1387*

Probenecid (proe BEN e sid)

Synonyms Benemid [DSC]
Pharmacologic Category Uricosuric Agent
Medication Safety Issues
Sound-alike/look-alike issues:
Probenecid may be confused with Procanbid®
Pregnancy Risk Factor B
Lactation Excretion in breast milk unknown
Use Prevention of gouty arthritis; hyperuricemia; prolongation of beta-lactam effect (ie, serum levels)

Mechanism of Action/Effect Competitively inhibits the reabsorption of uric acid at the proximal convoluted tubule, thereby promoting its excretion and reducing serum uric acid levels; increases plasma levels of weak organic acids (penicillins, cephalosporins, or other beta-lactam antibiotics) by competitively inhibiting their renal tubular secretion

Contraindications Hypersensitivity to probenecid or any component of the formulation; high-dose aspirin therapy; moderate to severe renal impairment; children <2 years of age

Warnings/Precautions Use with caution in patients with peptic ulcer. Use extreme caution in the use of probenecid with penicillin in patients with renal insufficiency. Probenecid may not be effective in patients with a creatinine clearance <30-50 mL/minute. May cause exacerbation of acute gouty attack.

Drug Interactions
Cytochrome P450 Effect: Inhibits CYP2C19 (weak)
Decreased Effect: Salicylates (high-dose) may decrease uricosuria. Decreased urinary levels of nitrofurantoin may decrease efficacy.
Increased Effect/Toxicity: Increases methotrexate toxic potential. Probenecid increases the serum concentrations of quinolones and beta-lactams such as penicillins and cephalosporins. Also increases levels/toxicity of acyclovir, diflunisal, ketorolac, thiopental, benzodiazepines, dapsone, fluoroquinolones, methotrexate, NSAIDs, sulfonylureas, zidovudine.

Lab Interactions False-positive glucosuria with Clinitest®

Adverse Reactions Frequency not defined.
Cardiovascular: Flushing of face
Central nervous system: Headache, dizziness
Dermatologic: Rash, itching
Gastrointestinal: Anorexia, nausea, vomiting, sore gums
Genitourinary: Painful urination
Hematologic: Aplastic anemia, hemolytic anemia, leukopenia
Hepatic: Hepatic necrosis
Neuromuscular & skeletal: Gouty arthritis (acute)
Renal: Renal calculi, nephrotic syndrome, urate nephropathy
Miscellaneous: Anaphylaxis

Overdosage/Toxicology Symptoms of overdose include nausea, vomiting, tonic-clonic seizures, and coma. Activated charcoal is especially effective at binding probenecid, for GI decontamination.

Pharmacodynamics/Kinetics
Onset of Action: Effect on penicillin levels: 2 hours
Time to Peak: Serum: 2-4 hours
Half-Life Elimination: Dose dependent: Normal renal function: 6-12 hours
Metabolism: Hepatic
Excretion: Urine
Available Dosage Forms Tablet: 500 mg
Dosing
Adults & Elderly:
Hyperuricemia with gout: Oral: 250 mg twice daily for 1 week; increase to 250-500 mg/day; may increase by 500 mg/month, if needed, to maximum of 2-3 g/day (dosages may be increased by 500 mg every 6 months if serum urate concentrations are controlled)
Prolong penicillin serum levels: Oral: 500 mg 4 times/day
Gonorrhea: Oral: 1 g 30 minutes before penicillin, ampicillin, or amoxicillin
Neurosyphilis: Oral: Aqueous procaine penicillin 2.4 million units/day I.M. plus probenecid 500 mg 4 times/day for 10-14 days
Pediatrics:
Note: Note recommended in children <2 years of age.
Prolong penicillin serum levels: Oral: Children 2-14 years: 25 mg/kg starting dose, then 40 mg/kg/day given 4 times/day

(Continued)

Probenecid *(Continued)*

Treatment of gonorrhea: Oral: Children <45 kg: 25 mg/kg x 1 (maximum: 1 g/dose) 30 minutes before penicillin, ampicillin, or amoxicillin

Renal Impairment: Cl_{cr} <50 mL/minute: Avoid use.

Laboratory Monitoring Uric acid, renal function, CBC

Nursing Actions

Physical Assessment: Assess effectiveness and interactions of other medications patient may be taking. Monitor therapeutic response (eg, frequency and severity of gouty attacks), laboratory values, and adverse reactions at beginning of therapy and periodically with long-term use. Assess knowledge/teach patient appropriate use, interventions to reduce side effects, and adverse symptoms to report.

Patient Education: Take as directed; do not discontinue without consulting prescriber. May take 6-12 months to reduce gouty attacks (attacks may increase in frequency and severity for first few months of therapy). Take with food or antacids or alkaline ash foods (milk, nuts, beets, spinach, turnip greens). Maintain adequate hydration (2-3 L/day of fluids) unless instructed to restrict fluid intake. Avoid aspirin or aspirin-containing substances. If you have diabetes, use serum glucose monitoring. If you experience severe headache, contact prescriber for medication. You may experience dizziness or lightheadedness (use caution when driving, changing position, or engaging in tasks requiring alertness until response to drug is known); or nausea, vomiting, indigestion, or loss of appetite (small frequent meals, frequent mouth care, chewing gum, or sucking lozenges may help). Report skin rash or itching, persistent headache, blood in urine or painful urination, excessive tiredness or easy bruising or bleeding, or sore gums. **Breast-feeding precaution:** Consult prescriber if breast-feeding.

Dietary Considerations Drug may cause GI upset; take with food if GI upset. Drink plenty of fluids.

Geriatric Considerations Since probenecid loses its effectiveness when the Cl_{cr} is <30 mL/minute, its usefulness in the elderly is limited.

Additional Information Avoid fluctuation in uric acid (increase or decrease); may precipitate gout attack. Use of sodium bicarbonate or potassium citrate is suggested until serum uric acid normalizes and tophaceous deposits disappear.

Procainamide *(proe kane A mide)*

U.S. Brand Names Procanbid®

Synonyms PCA (error-prone abbreviation); Procainamide Hydrochloride; Procaine Amide Hydrochloride

Pharmacologic Category Antiarrhythmic Agent, Class Ia

Medication Safety Issues

Sound-alike/look-alike issues:

Procanbid® may be confused with probenecid

Pronestyl® may be confused with Ponstel®

PCA is an error-prone abbreviation (mistaken as patient controlled analgesia)

Pregnancy Risk Factor C

Lactation Enters breast milk/use caution (AAP rates "compatible")

Use Treatment of ventricular tachycardia (VT), premature ventricular contractions, paroxysmal atrial tachycardia (PSVT), and atrial fibrillation (AF); prevent recurrence of ventricular tachycardia, paroxysmal supraventricular tachycardia, atrial fibrillation or flutter

Unlabeled/Investigational Use ACLS guidelines:

Stable monomorphic VT (EF >40%, no CHF)

Stable wide complex tachycardia, likely VT (EF >40%, no CHF, patient stable)

Atrial fibrillation or flutter, including pre-excitation syndrome (EF >40%, no CHF)

AV reentrant, narrow complex tachycardia (eg, reentrant SVT) [preserved ventricular function]

PALS guidelines: Tachycardia with pulses and poor perfusion (possible VT)

Mechanism of Action/Effect Decreases myocardial excitability and conduction velocity and may depress myocardial contractility, by increasing the electrical stimulation threshold of ventricle, His-Purkinje system and through direct cardiac effects

Contraindications Hypersensitivity to procaine, other ester-type local anesthetics, or any component of the formulation; complete heart block (except in patients with a functioning artificial pacemaker); second-degree AV block (without a functional pacemaker); various types of hemiblock (without a functional pacemaker); SLE; torsade de pointes; concurrent cisapride; QT prolongation

Warnings/Precautions Monitor and adjust dose to prevent QT_c prolongation. Watch for proarrhythmic effects. May precipitate or exacerbate CHF. Reduce dosage in renal impairment. May increase ventricular response rate in patients with atrial fibrillation or flutter; control AV conduction before initiating. Correct hypokalemia before initiating therapy; hypokalemia may worsen toxicity. Use caution in digoxin-induced toxicity (can further depress AV conduction). Reduce dose if first-degree heart block occurs. Use caution with concurrent use of other antiarrhythmics. Avoid use in myasthenia gravis (may worsen condition). Hypersensitivity reactions can occur.

Potentially fatal blood dyscrasias have occurred with therapeutic doses; close monitoring is recommended during the first 3 months of therapy.

Long-term administration leads to the development of a positive antinuclear antibody (ANA) test in 50% of patients which may result in a drug-induced lupus erythematosus-like syndrome (in 20% to 30% of patients); discontinue procainamide with SLE symptoms and choose an alternative agent

Drug Interactions

Cytochrome P450 Effect: Substrate of CYP2D6 (major)

Increased Effect/Toxicity: Amiodarone, cimetidine, ofloxacin (and potentially other renally eliminated quinolones), ranitidine, and trimethoprim increase procainamide and NAPA blood levels; consider reducing procainamide dosage by 25% with concurrent use. Cisapride and procainamide may increase the risk of malignant arrhythmia; concurrent use is contraindicated. Procainamide may potentiate neuromuscular blockade of neuromuscular-blocking agents. CYP2D6 inhibitors may increase the levels/effects of procainamide; example inhibitors include chlorpromazine, delavirdine, fluoxetine, miconazole, paroxetine, pergolide, quinidine, quinine, ritonavir, and ropinirole.

Drugs which may prolong the QT interval include amiodarone, amitriptyline, bepridil, cisapride, disopyramide, erythromycin, haloperidol, imipramine, pimozide, quinidine, sotalol, mesoridazine, thioridazine, and some quinolone antibiotics (sparfloxacin, gatifloxacin, moxifloxacin); concurrent use may result in additional prolongation of the QT interval.

Nutritional/Ethanol Interactions

Ethanol: Avoid ethanol (acute ethanol administration reduces procainamide serum concentrations).

Herb/Nutraceutical: Avoid ephedra (may worsen arrhythmia).

Adverse Reactions >1%:

Cardiovascular: Hypotension (I.V., up to 5%)

Dermatologic: Rash

Gastrointestinal: Diarrhea (3% to 4%), nausea, vomiting, taste disorder, GI complaints (3% to 4%)

Overdosage/Toxicology
Procainamide has a low toxic:therapeutic ratio and may easily produce fatal intoxication (acute toxic dose: 5 g in adults). Symptoms of overdose include sinus bradycardia, sinus node arrest or asystole, P-R, QRS, or QT interval prolongation, torsade de pointes (polymorphous ventricular tachycardia), and depressed myocardial contractility, which along with alpha-adrenergic or ganglionic blockade, may result in hypotension and pulmonary edema. Other effects are seizures, coma, and respiratory arrest. Treatment is symptomatic and effects usually respond to conventional therapies. **Note:** Do not use other Type 1A or 1C antiarrhythmic agents to treat ventricular tachycardia. Sodium bicarbonate may treat wide QRS intervals or hypotension. Markedly impaired conduction or high degree AV block, unresponsive to bicarbonate, indicates consideration of a pacemaker.

Pharmacodynamics/Kinetics
Onset of Action: I.M. 10-30 minutes

Time to Peak: Serum: Capsule: 45 minutes to 2.5 hours; I.M.: 15-60 minutes

Protein Binding: 15% to 20%

Half-Life Elimination:
Procainamide (hepatic acetylator, phenotype, cardiac and renal function dependent):
Children: 1.7 hours; Adults: 2.5-4.7 hours; Anephric: 11 hours
NAPA (renal function dependent):
Children: 6 hours; Adults: 6-8 hours; Anephric: 42 hours

Metabolism: Hepatic via acetylation to produce N-acetyl procainamide (NAPA) (active metabolite)

Excretion: Urine (25% as NAPA)

Available Dosage Forms
Capsule, as hydrochloride: 250 mg, 500 mg
Injection, solution, as hydrochloride: 100 mg/mL (10 mL); 500 mg/mL (2 mL) [contains sodium metabisulfite]
Tablet, extended release, as hydrochloride: 500 mg, 750 mg, 1000 mg
Procanbid®: 500 mg, 1000 mg

Dosing
Adults & Elderly: Dose must be titrated to patient's response.

Antiarrhythmic:
Oral: Usual dose: 50 mg/kg/24 hours; maximum: 5 g/24 hours (**Note:** Twice-daily dosing approved for Procanbid®.)
Immediate release formulation: 250-500 mg/dose every 3-6 hours
Extended release formulation: 500 mg to 1 g every 6 hours; Procanbid®: 1000-2500 mg every 12 hours
I.M.: 0.5-1 g every 4-8 hours until oral therapy is possible
I.V. (infusion requires use of an infusion pump):
Loading dose: 15-18 mg/kg administered as slow infusion over 25-30 minutes **or** 100-200 mg/dose repeated every 5 minutes as needed to a total dose of 1 g. Reduce loading dose to 12 mg/kg in severe renal or cardiac impairment.
Maintenance dose: 1-4 mg/minute by continuous infusion. Maintenance infusions should be reduced by one-third in patients with moderate renal or cardiac impairment and by two-thirds in patients with severe renal or cardiac impairment.
ACLS guidelines: Infuse 20 mg/minute until arrhythmia is controlled, hypotension occurs, QRS complex widens by 50% of its original width, or total of 17 mg/kg is given.

Pediatrics: Must be titrated to patient's response:
Arrhythmias:
Oral: 15-50 mg/kg/24 hours divided every 3-6 hours

I.M.: 50 mg/kg/24 hours divided into doses of 1/8 to 1/4 every 3-6 hours in divided doses until oral therapy is possible
I.V. (infusion requires use of an infusion pump):
Load: 3-6 mg/kg/dose over 5 minutes not to exceed 100 mg/dose; may repeat every 5-10 minutes to maximum of 15 mg/kg/load
Maintenance as continuous I.V. infusion: 20-80 mcg/kg/minute; maximum: 2 g/24 hours

Renal Impairment:
Oral:
Cl$_{cr}$ 10-50 mL/minute: Administer every 6-12 hours.
Cl$_{cr}$ <10 mL/minute: Administer every 8-24 hours.
I.V.:
Loading dose: Reduce dose to 12 mg/kg in severe renal impairment.
Maintenance infusion: Reduce dose by one-third in patients with mild renal impairment. Reduce dose by two-thirds in patients with severe renal impairment.
Dialysis:
Procainamide: Moderately hemodialyzable (20% to 50%): 200 mg supplemental dose posthemodialysis is recommended.
N-acetylprocainamide: Not dialyzable (0% to 5%)
Procainamide/N-acetylprocainamide: Not peritoneal dialyzable (0% to 5%)
Procainamide/N-acetylprocainamide: Replace by blood level during continuous arteriovenous or venovenous hemofiltration

Hepatic Impairment: Reduce dose by 50%.

Administration
Oral: Do **not** crush or chew extended release drug products.

I.V.: Must dilute prior to I.V. administration; maximum rate: 50 mg/minute; give around-the-clock to promote less variation in peak and trough serum levels.
Infusion rate: **2 g/250 mL** (I.V. infusion requires use of an infusion pump):
1 mg/minute: 7.5 mL/hour
2 mg/minute: 15 mL/hour
3 mg/minute: 22.5 mL/hour
4 mg/minute: 30 mL/hour
5 mg/minute: 37.5 mL/hour
6 mg/minute: 45 mL/hour

I.V. Detail: pH: 4-6

Stability
Reconstitution: Minimum volume: 1 g/250 mL NS/D$_5$W
Stability of admixture at room temperature in D$_5$W or NS is 24 hours. Some information indicates that procainamide may be subject to greater decomposition in D$_5$W unless the admixture is refrigerated or the pH is adjusted. Procainamide is believed to form an association complex with dextrose - the bioavailability of procainamide in this complex is not known and the complex formation is reversible.

Compatibility: Stable in 1/2NS, NS, SWFI

Y-site administration: Incompatible with milrinone

Compatibility when admixed: Incompatible with esmolol, ethacrynate, milrinone, phenytoin

Storage: Procainamide may be stored at room temperature up to 27°C; however, refrigeration retards oxidation, which causes color formation. The solution is initially colorless but may turn slightly yellow on standing. Injection of air into the vial causes the solution to darken. Solutions darker than a light amber should be discarded.

Laboratory Monitoring CBC with differential, platelet count

Nursing Actions
Physical Assessment: Assess other medications patient may be taking for effectiveness and interactions. I.V. requires use of infusion pump and continuous cardiac and hemodynamic monitoring. Monitor laboratory tests, therapeutic response (cardiac (Continued)

Procainamide *(Continued)*

status), and adverse reactions at beginning of therapy, when titrating dosage, and on a regular basis with long-term therapy. **Note:** Procainamide has a low toxic:therapeutic ratio and overdose may easily produce severe and life-threatening reactions. Assess knowledge/teach patient appropriate use, interventions to reduce side effects, and adverse symptoms to report.

Patient Education: Oral: Take exactly as directed; do not take additional doses or discontinue without consulting prescriber. Avoid alcohol. You will need regular cardiac checkups and blood tests while taking this medication. You may experience dizziness, light-headedness, or visual changes (use caution when driving or engaging in tasks requiring alertness until response to drug is known); loss of appetite (small frequent meals, frequent mouth care, chewing gum, or sucking lozenges may help); headaches (prescriber may recommend mild analgesic); or diarrhea (yogurt or boiled milk may help; if persistent consult prescriber). Report chest pain, palpitation, or erratic heartbeat; increased weight or swelling of hands or feet; acute diarrhea; or unusual fatigue and tiredness. **Pregnancy/breast-feeding precautions:** Inform prescriber if you are or intend to become pregnant. Consult prescriber if breast-feeding.

Dietary Considerations Should be taken with water on an empty stomach.

Geriatric Considerations Monitor closely since clearance is reduced in those >60 years of age. If clinically possible, start doses at lowest recommended dose. Also, elderly frequently have drug therapy which may interfere with the use of procainamide. Adjust dose for renal function in the elderly.

Breast-Feeding Issues Considered compatible by the AAP. However, the AAP stated concern regarding long-term effects and potential for infant toxicity. Use caution and monitor closely if continuing to breast-feed while taking procainamide.

Related Information
Peak and Trough Guidelines *on page 1387*

Procaine *(PROE kane)*

U.S. Brand Names Novocain®

Synonyms Procaine Hydrochloride

Pharmacologic Category Local Anesthetic

Pregnancy Risk Factor C

Lactation Excretion in breast milk unknown

Use Produces spinal anesthesia and epidural and peripheral nerve block by injection and infiltration methods

Mechanism of Action/Effect Blocks both the initiation and conduction of nerve impulses by decreasing the neuronal membrane's permeability to sodium ions, which results in inhibition of depolarization with resultant blockade of conduction

Contraindications Hypersensitivity to procaine, PABA, parabens, other ester local anesthetics, or any component of the formulation

Warnings/Precautions Patients with cardiac diseases, hyperthyroidism, or other endocrine diseases may be more susceptible to toxic effects of local anesthetics. Some preparations contain metabisulfite.

Drug Interactions
Decreased Effect: Decreased effect of sulfonamides with the PABA metabolite of procaine, chloroprocaine, and tetracaine. Decreased/increased effect of vasopressors, ergot alkaloids, and MAO inhibitors on blood pressure when using anesthetic solutions with a vasoconstrictor.

Adverse Reactions 1% to 10%: Local: Burning sensation at site of injection, tissue irritation, pain at injection site

Overdosage/Toxicology Treatment is symptomatic and supportive. Termination of anesthesia by pneumatic tourniquet inflation should be attempted when procaine is administered by infiltration or regional injection.

Pharmacodynamics/Kinetics
Onset of Action: 2-5 minutes

Duration of Action: Patient, type of block, concentration, and method of anesthesia dependent: 0.5-1.5 hours

Half-Life Elimination: 7.7 minutes

Metabolism: Rapidly hydrolyzed by plasma enzymes to para-aminobenzoic acid and diethylaminoethanol (80% conjugated before elimination)

Excretion: Urine (as metabolites and some unchanged drug)

Available Dosage Forms Injection, solution, as hydrochloride: 1% [10 mg/mL] (2 mL) [contains sodium bisulfite]; 10% (2 mL) [contains sodium bisulfite]

Dosing
Adults & Elderly: Spinal anesthesia, epidural and peripheral nerve block: Injection and infiltration methods: Dose varies with procedure, desired depth, and duration of anesthesia, desired muscle relaxation, vascularity of tissues, physical condition, and age of patient.

Pediatrics: Dose varies with procedure, desired depth, and duration of anesthesia, desired muscle relaxation, vascularity of tissues, physical condition, and age of patient.

Administration
I.V. Detail: pH: 3.0-5.5

Other: Prior to instillation of anesthetic agent, withdraw plunger to ensure needle is not in artery or vein; resuscitative equipment should be available when local anesthetics are administered

Stability
Compatibility: Stable in dextran 6% in dextrose, dextran 6% in NS, D_5LR, $D_5^{1}/_4NS$, $D_5^{1}/_2NS$, D_5NS, D_5W, $D_{10}W$, LR, $^{1}/_2NS$, NS

Compatibility when admixed: Incompatible with amobarbital, amphotericin B, chlorothiazide, magnesium sulfate, phenobarbital, phenytoin, sodium bicarbonate

Nursing Actions
Physical Assessment: Monitor response and degree of pain sensation. Monitor site of injection for adverse reaction. **Epidural:** Monitor CNS status.

Patient Education: The purpose of this medication is to reduce pain sensation. Report local burning or pain at injection site. **Pregnancy/breast-feeding precautions:** Inform prescriber if you are or intend to become pregnant. Consult prescriber if breast-feeding.

Procarbazine *(proe KAR ba zeen)*

U.S. Brand Names Matulane®

Synonyms Benzmethyzin; N-Methylhydrazine; NSC-77213; Procarbazine Hydrochloride

Pharmacologic Category Antineoplastic Agent, Alkylating Agent

Medication Safety Issues
Sound-alike/look-alike issues:
Procarbazine may be confused with dacarbazine
Matulane® may be confused with Modane®

Pregnancy Risk Factor D

Lactation Excretion in breast milk unknown/not recommended

Use Treatment of Hodgkin's disease

Unlabeled/Investigational Use Treatment of non-Hodgkin's lymphoma, brain tumors, melanoma, lung cancer, multiple myeloma

Mechanism of Action/Effect Mechanism of action is not clear, methylating of nucleic acids; inhibits DNA, RNA, and protein synthesis; may damage DNA directly and suppresses mitosis; metabolic activation required by host

Contraindications Hypersensitivity to procarbazine or any component of the formulation; pre-existing bone marrow aplasia; ethanol ingestion; pregnancy

Warnings/Precautions Hazardous agent - use appropriate precautions for handling and disposal. Use with caution in patients with pre-existing renal or hepatic impairment. Procarbazine possesses MAO inhibitor activity. Procarbazine is a carcinogen which may cause acute leukemia. Procarbazine may cause infertility.

Drug Interactions
Increased Effect/Toxicity: Procarbazine exhibits weak MAO inhibitor activity. Foods containing high amounts of tyramine should, therefore, be avoided. When an MAO inhibitor is given with food high in tyramine, hypertensive crisis, intracranial bleeding, and headache have been reported.

Sympathomimetic amines (epinephrine and amphetamines) and antidepressants (tricyclics) should be used cautiously with procarbazine. Barbiturates, narcotics, phenothiazines, and other CNS depressants can cause somnolence, ataxia, and other symptoms of CNS depression. Ethanol has caused a disulfiram-like reaction with procarbazine. May result in headache, respiratory difficulties, nausea, vomiting, sweating, thirst, hypotension, and flushing.

Nutritional/Ethanol Interactions
Ethanol: Use ethanol and ethanol-containing products cautiously.
Food: Clinically severe and possibly life-threatening elevations in blood pressure may occur if procarbazine is taken with tyramine-containing foods.

Adverse Reactions Frequency not defined.
Central nervous system: Reports of neurotoxicity with procarbazine generally originate from early usage with single agent oral (continuous) or I.V. dosing; CNS depression is commonly reported to be additive with other CNS depressants
Hematologic: Myelosuppression, hemolysis in patients with G6PD deficiency
Gastrointestinal: Nausea and vomiting (60% to 90%); increasing the dose in a stepwise fashion over several days may minimize this
Genitourinary: Reproductive dysfunction >10% (in animals, hormone treatment has prevented azoospermia)
Respiratory: Pulmonary toxicity (<1%); the most commonly reported pulmonary toxicity is a hypersensitivity pneumonitis which responds to steroids and discontinuation of the drug. At least one report of persistent pulmonary fibrosis has been reported, however, a higher incidence (18%) of pulmonary toxicity (fibrosis) was reported when procarbazine was given prior to BCNU (BCNU alone does cause pulmonary fibrosis).
Miscellaneous: Second malignancies (cumulative incidence 2% to 15% reported with MOPP combination therapy)

Overdosage/Toxicology Symptoms of overdose include arthralgia, alopecia, paresthesia, bone marrow suppression, hallucinations, nausea, vomiting, diarrhea, seizures, and coma. Treatment is supportive. Adverse effects such as marrow toxicity may begin as late as 2 weeks after exposure.

Pharmacodynamics/Kinetics
Half-Life Elimination: 1 hour
Metabolism: Hepatic and renal
Excretion: Urine and respiratory tract (<5% as unchanged drug, 70% as metabolites)

Available Dosage Forms Capsule, as hydrochloride: 50 mg

Dosing
Adults: Refer to individual protocols.
Chemotherapy: Oral: Initial: 2-4 mg/kg/day in single or divided doses for 7 days then increase dose to 4-6 mg/kg/day until response is obtained or leukocyte count decreased <4000/mm^3 or the platelet count decreased <100,000/mm^3; maintenance: 1-2 mg/kg/day

Elderly: Refer to adult dosing; use with caution. Adjust for renal impairment.

Pediatrics: Refer to individual protocols. Manufacturer states that the dose is based on patient's ideal weight if the patient is obese or has abnormal fluid retention. Other studies suggest that ideal body weight may not be necessary. Oral (may be given as a single daily dose or in 2-3 divided doses): Children:

BMT aplastic anemia conditioning regimen: 12.5 mg/kg/day every other day for 4 doses
Hodgkin's disease: MOPP/IC-MOPP regimens: 100 mg/m^2/day for 14 days and repeated every 4 weeks
Neuroblastoma and medulloblastoma: Doses as high as 100-200 mg/m^2/day once daily have been used.

Renal Impairment: Use with caution, may result in increased toxicity; decrease dose if serum creatinine >2 mg/dL

Hepatic Impairment: Use with caution; may result in increased toxicity; decrease dose if total bilirubin >3 mg/dL

Stability
Storage: Protect from light

Laboratory Monitoring CBC with differential, platelet and reticulocyte count, urinalysis, liver and renal function

Nursing Actions
Physical Assessment: Assess potential for interactions with other pharmacological agents patient may be taking (eg, CNS depressants increase risk of adverse reactions). Emetic potential is high; antiemetic is generally required. Monitor laboratory tests and patient response frequently (eg, neurotoxicity, nausea and vomiting, pneumonitis, arthralgia, paresthesia). Instruct patient about dietary and alcohol cautions (procarbazine has some MAO inhibitory effects, can result in life-threatening hypertension with tyramine [see Tyramine Content of Foods on page 1406]; alcohol may cause disulfiram like reaction). Teach patient proper use, possible side effects/appropriate interventions, and adverse symptoms to report.

Patient Education: Do not take any new medication during therapy unless approved by prescriber. Take as directed. Avoid alcohol; may cause acute disulfiram reaction (headache, respiratory difficulties, nausea, vomiting, sweating, thirst, hypotension, and flushing). Avoid tyramine-containing foods (aged cheese, chocolate, pickles, aged meat, wine, etc), could cause serious hypertensive effects. Maintain adequate hydration (2-3 L/day of fluids) unless instructed to restrict fluid intake. You will be more sensitive to infection (avoid crowds and exposure to infection and do not have any vaccinations without consulting prescriber). May cause considerable nausea or vomiting (consult prescriber for approved antiemetic); mental depression, nervousness, insomnia, nightmares, dizziness, confusion, or lethargy (use caution when driving or engaging in tasks that require alertness until response to drug is known); rash, hair loss, or hyperpigmentation (reversible), loss of libido, sterility, or amenorrhea. Report persistent fever; chills, sore throat; unusual bleeding; blood in urine, stool (black stool), or vomitus; unresolved depression; mania; hallucinations; nightmares; disorientation; seizures; chest pain or palpitations; (Continued)

Procarbazine *(Continued)*

respiratory difficulty; or vision changes. **Pregnancy/ breast-feeding precautions:** Inform prescriber if you are pregnant. Do not get pregnant during or for 1 month following therapy. Male: Do not cause a female to become pregnant. Male/female: Consult prescriber for instruction on appropriate contraceptive measures. This drug may cause severe fetal defects. Breast-feeding is not recommended.

Related Information
Tyramine Content of Foods *on page 1406*

Prochlorperazine *(proe klor PER a zeen)*

U.S. Brand Names Compro™

Synonyms Chlormeprazine; Compazine; Prochlorperazine Edisylate; Prochlorperazine Maleate

Pharmacologic Category Antiemetic; Antipsychotic Agent, Typical, Phenothiazine

Medication Safety Issues
Sound-alike/look-alike issues:
Prochlorperazine may be confused with chlorproMAZINE
Compazine® may be confused with Copaxone®, Coumadin®

CPZ (occasional abbreviation for Compazine®) is an error-prone abbreviation (mistaken as chlorpromazine)

Lactation Excretion in breast milk unknown/use caution

Use Management of nausea and vomiting; psychotic disorders including schizophrenia; anxiety

Unlabeled/Investigational Use Behavioral syndromes in dementia

Mechanism of Action/Effect Prochlorperazine is a piperazine phenothiazine antipsychotic which blocks postsynaptic mesolimbic dopaminergic D_1 and D_2 receptors in the brain, including the chemoreceptor trigger zone; exhibits a strong alpha-adrenergic and anticholinergic blocking effect and depresses the release of hypothalamic and hypophyseal hormones; believed to depress the reticular activating system, thus affecting basal metabolism, body temperature, wakefulness, vasomotor tone and emesis

Contraindications Hypersensitivity to prochlorperazine or any component of the formulation (cross-reactivity between phenothiazines may occur); severe CNS depression; coma; pediatric surgery; Reye's syndrome; should not be used in children <2 years of age or <9 kg

Warnings/Precautions May be sedating; use with caution in disorders where CNS depression is a feature. May obscure intestinal obstruction or brain tumor. May impair physical or mental abilities; patients must be cautioned about performing tasks which require mental alertness (eg, operating machinery or driving). Effects with other sedative drugs or ethanol may be potentiated. Use with caution in Parkinson's disease; hemodynamic instability; bone marrow suppression; predisposition to seizures; subcortical brain damage; and in severe cardiac, hepatic, renal or respiratory disease. Caution in breast cancer or other prolactin-dependent tumors (may elevate prolactin levels). May alter temperature regulation or mask toxicity of other drugs. Use caution with exposure to heat. May alter cardiac conduction - life threatening arrhythmias have occurred with therapeutic doses of phenothiazines. May cause orthostatic hypotension; use with caution in patients at risk of hypotension or where transient hypotensive episodes would be poorly tolerated (cardiovascular disease or cerebrovascular disease). Hypotension may occur following administration, particularly when parenteral form is used or in high dosages.

Phenothiazines may cause anticholinergic effects (eg, constipation, xerostomia, blurred vision, urinary retention); therefore, they should be used with caution in patients with decreased gastrointestinal motility, urinary retention, BPH, xerostomia, or visual problems. Conditions which also may be exacerbated by cholinergic blockade include narrow-angle glaucoma (screening is recommended) and worsening of myasthenia gravis. May cause extrapyramidal symptoms, including pseudoparkinsonism, acute dystonic reactions, akathisia, and tardive dyskinesia (TD). Use caution in the elderly; incidence of TD may be increased. Children with acute illness or dehydration are more susceptible to neuromuscular reactions (eg, dystonias); use cautiously. May be associated with neuroleptic malignant syndrome (NMS).

Drug Interactions
Decreased Effect: The antihypertensive effects of methyldopa and guanadrel may be inhibited by prochlorperazine. Prochlorperazine may inhibit the antiparkinsonian effect of levodopa. Prochlorperazine may reverse the pressor effects of epinephrine. Antacids and attapulgite may decreased absorption of phenothiazines. Anticholinertics may decrease the therapeutic response to phenothiazines.

Increased Effect/Toxicity: Prochlorperazine plus lithium may rarely produce neurotoxicity. Prochlorperazing may produce additive CNS depressant effects with other CNS depressants. Acetylcholinesterase inhibitors may increase the risk of EPS. Alpha-/ beta-agonists, antihistamines, QT_c-prolonging agents may enhance the arrhythmogenic effects of phenothiazines. Concurrent use may enhance the hypotensive effects of narcotics and beta blockers. SSRIs may increase risk of hypotension. Antimalarials and beta blockers may increase serum levels of prochlorperazine.Pramlintide may increase anticholinergic effects of prochlorperazine.

Nutritional/Ethanol Interactions
Ethanol: Avoid ethanol (may increase CNS depression).
Food: Limit caffeine.
Herb/Nutraceutical: Avoid dong quai, St John's wort (may also cause photosensitization). Avoid kava kava, gotu kola, valerian, St John's wort (may increase CNS depression).

Lab Interactions False-positives for phenylketonuria, pregnancy, urinary amylase, uroporphyrins, urobilinogen

Adverse Reactions Reported with prochlorperazine or other phenothiazines. Frequency not defined
Cardiovascular: Cardiac arrest, hypotension, peripheral edema, Q-wave distortions, T-wave distortions
Central nervous system: Agitation, catatonia, cerebral edema, cough reflex suppressed, dizziness, drowsiness, fever (mild — I.M.), headache, hyperactivity, hyperpyrexia, impairment of temperature regulation, insomnia, neuroleptic malignant syndrome (NMS), paradoxical excitement, restlessness, seizure
Dermatologic: Angioedema, contact dermatitis, discoloration of skin (blue-gray), epithelial keratopathy, erythema, eczema, exfoliative dermatitis (injectable), itching, photosensitivity, rash, skin pigmentation, urticaria
Endocrine & metabolic: Amenorrhea, breast enlargement, galactorrhea, gynecomastia, glucosuria, hyperglycemia, hypoglycemia, lactation, libido (changes in), menstrual irregularity, SIADH
Gastrointestinal: Appetite increased, atonic colon, constipation, ileus, nausea, weight gain, xerostomia
Genitourinary: Ejaculating dysfunction, ejaculatory disturbances, impotence, incontinence, polyuria, priapism, urinary retention, urination difficulty
Hematologic: Agranulocytosis, aplastic anemia, eosinophilia, hemolytic anemia, leukopenia, pancytopenia, thrombocytopenic purpura

Hepatic: Biliary stasis, cholestatic jaundice, hepatotoxicity

Neuromuscular & skeletal: Dystonias (torticollis, opisthotonos, carpopedal spasm, trismus, oculogyric crisis, protusion of tongue); extrapyramidal symptoms (pseudoparkinsonism, akathisia, dystonias, tardive dyskinesia); SLE-like syndrome, tremor

Ocular: blurred vision, cornea and lens changes, lenticular/corneal deposits, miosis, mydriasis, pigmentary retinopathy

Respiratory: Asthma, laryngeal edema, nasal congestion

Miscellaneous: Allergic reactions, diaphoresis

Overdosage/Toxicology Symptoms of overdose include deep sleep, coma, extrapyramidal symptoms, abnormal involuntary muscle movements, seizures, and hypotension. Treatment is symptom-directed and supportive. Do not induce emesis because of risk of aspiriation if acute dystonic reaction occurred. Extrapyramidal symptoms may be treated with an anticholinergic such as diphenydramine or benzetropine. Treat hypotension with norephinephrine or phenylephrine. Phenothiazines are not dialyzable.

Pharmacodynamics/Kinetics
Onset of Action: Oral: 30-40 minutes; I.M.: 10-20 minutes; Rectal: ~60 minutes
Peak antiemetic effect: I.V.: 30-60 minutes

Duration of Action: Rectal: 12 hours; Oral: 3-4 hours; I.M., I.V.: Adults: 4-6 hours; I.M.: Children: 12 hours

Half-Life Elimination: Oral: 3-5 hours; I.V.: ~7 hours

Metabolism: Primarily hepatic; N-desmethyl prochlorperazine (major active metabolite)

Available Dosage Forms
Injection, solution, as edisylate: 5 mg/mL (2 mL, 10 mL) [contains benzyl alcohol]
Suppository, rectal: 2.5 mg (12s), 5 mg (12s), 25 mg (12s) [may contain coconut and palm oil]
Compro™: 25 mg (12s) [contains coconut and palm oils]
Tablet, as maleate: 5 mg, 10 mg

Dosing
Adults:
Antiemetic:
Oral (tablet): 5-10 mg 3-4 times/day; usual maximum: 40 mg/day; larger doses may rarely be required
I.M. (deep): 5-10 mg every 3-4 hours; usual maximum: 40 mg/day
I.V.: 2.5-10 mg; maximum 10 mg/dose or 40 mg/day; may repeat dose every 3-4 hours as needed
Rectal: 25 mg twice daily
Surgical nausea/vomiting: Note: Should not exceed 40 mg/day
I.M.: 5-10 mg 1-2 hours before induction or to control symptoms during or after surgery; may repeat once if necessary
I.V. (administer slow IVP <5 mg/minute): 5-10 mg 15-30 minutes before induction or to control symptoms during or after surgery; may repeat once if necessary
Rectal (unlabeled use): 25 mg
Antipsychotic:
Oral: 5-10 mg 3-4 times/day; titrate dose slowly every 2-3 days; doses up to 150 mg/day may be required in some patients for treatment of severe disturbances
I.M.: Initial: 10-20 mg; if necessary repeat initial dose every 1-4 hours to gain control; more than 3-4 doses are rarely needed. If parenteral administration is still required; give 10-20 mg every 4-6 hours; change to oral as soon as possible.
Nonpsychotic anxiety: *Oral (tablet):* Usual dose: 15-20 mg/day in divided doses; do not give doses >20 mg/day or for longer than 12 weeks
Elderly: Dementia behavior (nonpsychotic, unlabeled use): Initial: 2.5-5 mg 1-2 times/day; increase dose at 4- to 7-day intervals by 2.5-5 mg/day. Increase dosing intervals (twice daily, 3 times/day, etc) as necessary to control response or side effects. Maximum daily dose should probably not exceed 75 mg in the elderly. Gradual increases (titration) may prevent some side effects or decrease their severity. See Geriatric Considerations.

Pediatrics: Not recommended in children <10 kg or <2 years.
Antiemetic:
Oral, rectal: >9 kg: 0.4 mg/kg/24 hours in 3-4 divided doses; **or**
9-13 kg: 2.5 mg every 12-24 hours as needed; maximum: 7.5 mg/day
13.1-17 kg: 2.5 mg every 8-12 hours as needed; maximum: 10 mg/day
17.1-37 kg: 2.5 mg every 8 hours or 5 mg every 12 hours as needed; maximum: 15 mg/day
I.M.: 0.13 mg/kg/dose; change to oral as soon as possible
Antipsychotic: Children 2-12 years (not recommended in children <9 kg or <2 years):
Oral, rectal: 2.5 mg 2-3 times/day; do not give more than 10 mg the first day; increase dosage as needed to maximum daily dose of 20 mg for 2-5 years and 25 mg for 6-12 years
I.M.: 0.13 mg/kg/dose; change to oral as soon as possible

Administration
I.M.:
Inject by deep IM into outer quadrant of buttocks.
I.V.: I.V.: Doses should be given as a short (~30 minute) infusion to avoid orthostatic hypotension; administer at ≤5 mg/minute
I.V. Detail: Do not dilute with any diluent containing parabens as a preservative. Avoid skin contact with injection solution, contact dermatitis has occurred. I.V. may be administered IVP or IVPB.

pH: 4.2-6.2
Stability
Compatibility: Stable in dextran 6% in dextrose, dextran 6% in NS, D_5W, $D_{10}W$, D_5LR, $D_5^{1}/_4NS$, $D_5^{1}/_2NS$, D_5NS, LR, $^{1}/_2NS$, NS
Y-site administration: Incompatible with aldesleukin, allopurinol, amifostine, amphotericin B cholesteryl sulfate complex, aztreonam, cefepime, etoposide phosphate, fludarabine, foscarnet, filgrastim, gemcitabine, piperacillin/tazobactam
Compatibility in syringe: Incompatible with dimenhydrinate, ketorolac, midazolam, morphine tartrate, pentobarbital, thiopental
Compatibility when admixed: Incompatible with aminophylline, amphotericin B, ampicillin, calcium salts, cephalothin, foscarnet, chloramphenicol, chlorothiazide, floxacillin, furosemide, heparin, hydrocortisone sodium succinate, methohexital, midazolam, penicillin G sodium, phenobarbital, phenytoin, thiopental
Storage:
Injection: Store at <30°C (<86°F). Do not freeze. Protect from light. Clear or slightly yellow solutions may be used.
I.V. infusion: Injection may be diluted in 50-100 mL NS or D_5W.
Suppository, tablet: Store at 15°C to 30°C (59°F to 86°F). Protect from light.
Laboratory Monitoring Baseline liver and kidney function, CBC prior to and periodically during therapy, lipid profile, fasting blood glucose/Hgb A_{1c}; BMI
Nursing Actions
Physical Assessment: Assess all other medications patient may be taking. For I.V., continuously monitor blood pressure and heart rate during administration. Monitor blood pressure and heart rate, fluid balance (I & O ratio), and dehydration. Monitor for seizures, especially with known seizure disorder. Monitor for
(Continued)

Prochlorperazine *(Continued)*

excessive sedation, neuromuscular malignant syndrome, autonomic instability (eg, anticholinergic effects, such as flushing, excessive sweating, constipation, urinary retention), and extrapyramidal symptoms (eg, tardive dyskinesia, akathisia, pseudoparkinsonism).

Patient Education: Take exact amount as prescribed. Do not change brand names. Do not crush or chew tablets. Do not discontinue without consulting prescriber. Avoid alcohol or other sedatives or sleep-inducing drugs. Avoid skin contact with drug; wash immediately with warm soapy water. You may experience appetite changes; small frequent meals may help. Maintain adequate hydration (2-3 L/day of fluids) unless instructed to restrict fluid intake. May cause dizziness, tremors, or visual disturbance (especially during early therapy); use caution when driving or engaging in tasks that require alertness until response to drug is known. Do not change position rapidly (rise slowly). May cause photosensitivity reaction; use sunscreen, wear protective clothing and eyewear, and avoid direct sunlight. Report immediately any changes in gait or muscular tremors. Report unresolved changes in voiding or elimination (constipation or diarrhea), acute dizziness or unresolved sedation, vision changes, palpitations, yellowing of skin or eyes, or changes in color of urine or stool (pink or red brown urine is expected). **Pregnancy/breast-feeding precautions:** Inform prescriber if you are or intend to become pregnant. Breast-feeding is not recommended.

Dietary Considerations Increase dietary intake of riboflavin; should be administered with food or water. Rectal suppositories may contain coconut and palm oil.

Geriatric Considerations Due to side effect profile (dystonias, EPS) this is not a preferred drug in the elderly for antiemetic therapy.

Breast-Feeding Issues Other phenothiazines are excreted in human milk; excretion of prochlorperazine is not known.

Pregnancy Issues Crosses the placenta. Isolated reports of congenital anomalies, however, some included exposures to other drugs. Jaundice, extrapyramidal signs, hyper-/hyporeflexes have been noted in newborns. Available evidence with use of occasional low doses suggests safe use during pregnancy.

Additional Information Not recommended as an antipsychotic due to inferior efficacy compared to other phenothiazines.

Related Information
Antipsychotic Medication Guidelines *on page 1415*
Compatibility of Drugs in Syringe *on page 1372*

Procyclidine *(proe SYE kli deen)*

U.S. Brand Names Kemadrin®
Synonyms Procyclidine Hydrochloride
Pharmacologic Category Anti-Parkinson's Agent, Anticholinergic; Anticholinergic Agent
Medication Safety Issues
Sound-alike/look-alike issues:
Kemadrin® may be confused with Coumadin®
Pregnancy Risk Factor C
Lactation Excretion in breast milk unknown/not recommended
Use Relieves symptoms of parkinsonian syndrome and drug-induced extrapyramidal symptoms
Mechanism of Action/Effect Thought to act by blocking excess acetylcholine at cerebral synapses; many of its effects are due to its pharmacologic similarities with atropine; it exerts an antispasmodic effect on smooth muscle, is a potent mydriatic; inhibits salivation

Contraindications Hypersensitivity to procyclidine or any component of the formulation; angle-closure glaucoma; myasthenia gravis; safe use in children not established

Warnings/Precautions Use with caution in hot weather or during exercise. Elderly patients frequently develop increased sensitivity and require strict dosage regulation - side effects may be more severe in elderly patients with atherosclerotic changes. Use with caution in patients with tachycardia, cardiac arrhythmias, hypertension, hypotension, prostatic hyperplasia (especially in the elderly) or any tendency toward urinary retention, liver or kidney disorders and obstructive disease of the GI or GU tract. When given in large doses or to susceptible patients, may cause weakness and inability to move particular muscle groups.

Drug Interactions

Decreased Effect: May increase gastric degradation of levodopa and decrease the amount of levodopa absorbed by delaying gastric emptying; the opposite may be true for digoxin. Therapeutic effects of cholinergic agents (tacrine, donepezil) and neuroleptics may be antagonized.

Increased Effect/Toxicity: Central and/or peripheral anticholinergic syndrome can occur when administered with amantadine, rimantadine, narcotic analgesics, phenothiazines and other antipsychotics (especially with high anticholinergic activity), tricyclic antidepressants, quinidine and some other antiarrhythmics, and antihistamines.

Nutritional/Ethanol Interactions Ethanol: Avoid ethanol.

Adverse Reactions Frequency not defined.
Cardiovascular: Tachycardia, palpitation
Central nervous system: Confusion, drowsiness, headache, loss of memory, fatigue, ataxia, giddiness, lightheadedness
Dermatologic: Dry skin, increased sensitivity to light, rash
Gastrointestinal: Constipation, xerostomia, dry throat, nausea, vomiting, epigastric distress
Genitourinary: Difficult urination
Neuromuscular & skeletal: Weakness
Ocular: Increased intraocular pain, blurred vision, mydriasis
Respiratory: Dry nose
Miscellaneous: Diaphoresis (decreased)

Overdosage/Toxicology Symptoms of overdose include disorientation, hallucinations, delusions, blurred vision, dysphagia, absent bowel sounds, hyperthermia, hypertension, and urinary retention. For anticholinergic overdose with severe life-threatening symptoms, physostigmine 1-2 mg SubQ or I.V. slowly, may be given to reverse these effects.

Pharmacodynamics/Kinetics
Onset of Action: 30-40 minutes
Duration of Action: 4-6 hours
Available Dosage Forms Tablet, as hydrochloride [scored]: 5 mg
Dosing
Adults: Parkinson's disease or treatment of EPS: Oral: 2.5 mg 3 times/day after meals; if tolerated, gradually increase dose, to a maximum of 20 mg/day if necessary.
Elderly: Oral: Initial: 2.5 mg once or twice daily, gradually increasing as necessary. Avoid use if possible (see Geriatric Considerations).
Hepatic Impairment: Decrease dose to a twice daily dosing regimen.
Administration
Oral: Should be administered after meals to minimize stomach upset.
Nursing Actions
Physical Assessment: Assess effectiveness and interactions of other medications patient may be taking. Monitor renal function, therapeutic response

(eg, Parkinsonian symptoms), and adverse reactions such as anticholinergic syndrome (dry mouth and mucous membranes, constipation, epigastric distress, CNS disturbances, paralytic ileus) at beginning of therapy and periodically throughout therapy. Assess knowledge/teach patient appropriate use, interventions to reduce side effects, and adverse symptoms to report.

Patient Education: Take exactly as directed (after meals); do not increase, decrease, or discontinue without consulting prescriber. Take at the same time each day. Do not use alcohol, prescription or OTC sedatives, or CNS depressants without consulting prescriber. You may experience drowsiness, dizziness, confusion, and blurred vision (use caution when driving, climbing stairs, or engaging in tasks requiring alertness until response to drug is known); increased susceptibility to heat stroke, decreased perspiration (use caution in hot weather, maintain adequate fluids and reduce exercise activity); constipation (increased exercise, fluids, fruit, or fiber may help); or dry skin or nasal passages (consult prescriber for appropriate relief). Report unresolved constipation, chest pain or palpitations, respiratory difficulty, CNS changes (hallucination, loss of memory, nervousness, etc), painful or difficult urination, increased muscle spasticity or rigidity, skin rash, or significant worsening of condition. **Pregnancy/breast-feeding precautions:** Inform prescriber if you are or intend to become pregnant. Breast-feeding is not recommended.

Dietary Considerations Should be taken after meals to minimize stomach upset.

Geriatric Considerations Anticholinergic agents are generally not well tolerated in the elderly and their use should be avoided when possible (see Warnings/Precautions, Adverse Reactions). In the elderly, anticholinergic agents should not be used as prophylaxis against extrapyramidal symptoms. Elderly patients frequently develop increased sensitivity and require strict dosage regulation - side effects may be more severe in elderly patients with atherosclerotic changes.

Progesterone (proe JES ter one)

U.S. Brand Names Crinone®; Prochieve™; Prometrium®

Synonyms Pregnenedione; Progestin

Pharmacologic Category Progestin

Pregnancy Risk Factor B (Prometrium®, per manufacturer); none established for vaginal gel or injection (contraindicated)

Lactation Enters breast milk/use caution (AAP rates "compatible")

Use

Oral: Prevention of endometrial hyperplasia in nonhysterectomized, postmenopausal women who are receiving conjugated estrogen tablets; secondary amenorrhea

I.M.: Amenorrhea; abnormal uterine bleeding due to hormonal imbalance

Intravaginal gel: Part of assisted reproductive technology (ART) for infertile women with progesterone deficiency; secondary amenorrhea

Mechanism of Action/Effect Natural steroid hormone that induces secretory changes in the endometrium, promotes mammary gland development, relaxes uterine smooth muscle, blocks follicular maturation and ovulation, and maintains pregnancy

Contraindications Hypersensitivity to progesterone or any component of the formulation; undiagnosed abnormal vaginal bleeding; history of or current thrombophlebitis or venous thromboembolic disorders (including DVT, PE); active or recent (within 1 year)

arterial thromboembolic disease (eg, stroke, MI); carcinoma of the breast or genital organs; hepatic dysfunction or disease; missed abortion; diagnostic test for pregnancy; pregnancy (see Pregnancy Implications)

The following are also contraindicated in patients with allergies to their inactive ingredient:
Crinone® and Prochieve™ vaginal gels contain palm oil
Prometrium® capsules contain peanut oil
Oil for injection contains sesame oil

Warnings/Precautions Use caution with cardiovascular disease or dysfunction. Progestins used in combination with estrogen may increase the risks of hypertension, myocardial infarction (MI), stroke, pulmonary emboli (PE), and deep vein thrombosis; incidence of these effects was shown to be significantly increased in postmenopausal women using conjugated equine estrogens (CEE) in combination with medroxyprogesterone acetate (MPA). Similar risk should be assumed with other progestins. Progestins in combination with estrogens should not be used to prevent coronary heart disease.

The risk of dementia may be increased in postmenopausal women; increased incidence was observed in women ≥65 years of age taking CEE in combination with MPA. An increased risk of invasive breast cancer was observed in postmenopausal women using CEE in combination with MPA. An increase in abnormal mammograms has also been reported with estrogen and progestin therapy.

Discontinue pending examination in cases of sudden partial or complete vision loss, sudden onset of proptosis, diplopia, or migraine; discontinue permanently if papilledema or retinal vascular lesions are observed on examination. Use with caution in patients with diseases that may be exacerbated by fluid retention, including asthma, epilepsy, migraine, diabetes or renal dysfunction. Use caution with history of depression. Patients should be warned that progesterone might cause transient dizziness or drowsiness during initial therapy. Whenever possible, progestins in combination with estrogens should be discontinued at least 4-6 weeks prior to surgeries associated with an increased risk of thromboembolism or during periods of prolonged immobilization. Progestins used in combination with estrogen should be used for shortest duration possible consistent with treatment goals. Conduct periodic risk:benefit assessments.

Drug Interactions

Cytochrome P450 Effect: Substrate of CYP1A2 (minor), 2A6 (minor), 2C8/9 (minor), 2C19 (major), 2D6 (minor), 3A4 (major); **Inhibits** CYP2C8/9 (weak), 2C19 (weak), 3A4 (weak)

Decreased Effect: CYP2C19 inducers may decrease the levels/effects of progesterone; example inducers include aminoglutethimide, carbamazepine, phenytoin, and rifampin. CYP3A4 inducers may decrease the levels/effects of progesterone; example inducers include aminoglutethimide, carbamazepine, nafcillin, nevirapine, phenobarbital, phenytoin, and rifamycins.

Increased Effect/Toxicity: Ketoconazole may increase the bioavailability of progesterone. Progesterone may increase concentrations of estrogenic compounds during concurrent therapy with conjugated estrogens.

Nutritional/Ethanol Interactions
Food: Food increases oral bioavailability.
Herb/Nutraceutical: St John's wort may decrease progesterone levels.

Lab Interactions Thyroid function, metyrapone, liver function, coagulation tests, endocrine function tests

Adverse Reactions

Injection (I.M.):
Cardiovascular: Edema
Central nervous system: Depression, fever, insomnia, somnolence
(Continued)

Progesterone *(Continued)*

Dermatologic: Acne, allergic rash (rare), alopecia, hirsutism, pruritus, rash, urticaria

Endocrine & metabolic: Amenorrhea, breakthrough bleeding, breast tenderness, galactorrhea, menstrual flow changes, spotting

Gastrointestinal: Nausea, weight gain, weight loss

Genitourinary: Cervical erosion changes, cervical secretion changes

Hepatic: Cholestatic jaundice

Local: Pain at the injection site

Miscellaneous: Anaphylactoid reactions

Oral capsule (percentages reported when used in combination with or cycled with conjugated estrogens):

>10%:

Central nervous system: Headache (10% to 31%), dizziness (15% to 24%), depression (19%)

Endocrine & metabolic: Breast tenderness (27%), breast pain (6% to 16%)

Gastrointestinal: Abdominal pain (6% to 12%), abdominal bloating (10% to 20%)

Genitourinary: Urinary problems (11%)

Neuromuscular & skeletal: Joint pain (20%), musculoskeletal pain (6% to 12%)

Miscellaneous: Viral infection (7% to 12%)

5% to 10%:

Cardiovascular: Chest pain (7%)

Central nervous system: Fatigue (8% to 9%), emotional lability (6%), irritability (5% to 8%), worry (8%)

Gastrointestinal: Nausea/vomiting (8%), diarrhea (8%)

Respiratory: Upper respiratory tract infection (5%), cough (8%)

Miscellaneous: Night sweats (7%)

Vaginal gel (percentages reported with ART); also refer to oral capsule reactions listing for additional effects noted with progesterone:

>10%:

Central nervous system: Somnolence (27%), headache (13% to 17%), nervousness (16%), depression (11%)

Endocrine & metabolic: Breast enlargement (40%), breast pain (13%), libido decreased (11%)

Gastrointestinal: Constipation (27%), nausea (7% to 22%), cramps (15%), abdominal pain (12%)

Genitourinary: Perineal pain (17%), nocturia (13%)

5% to 10%:

Central nervous system: Pain (8%), dizziness (5%)

Gastrointestinal: Diarrhea (8%), bloating (7%), vomiting (5%)

Genitourinary: Vaginal discharge (7%), dyspareunia (6%), genital moniliasis (5%), genital pruritus (5%)

Neuromuscular & skeletal: Arthralgia (8%)

Overdosage/Toxicology Toxicity is unlikely following single exposure of excessive doses. Supportive treatment is adequate in most cases.

Pharmacodynamics/Kinetics

Time to Peak: Oral: Within 3 hours

Protein Binding: 96% to 99%

Half-Life Elimination: Vaginal gel: 5-20 minutes

Metabolism: Hepatic

Excretion: Urine, bile, feces

Available Dosage Forms

Capsule (Prometrium®): 100 mg, 200 mg [contains peanut oil]

Gel, vaginal (Crinone®, Prochieve™): 4% (45 mg); 8% (90 mg) [contains palm oil; prefilled applicators]

Injection, oil: 50 mg/mL (10 mL) [contains benzyl alcohol 10%, sesame oil]

Dosing

Adults & Elderly: Female:

Amenorrhea: I.M.: 5-10 mg/day for 6-8 consecutive days

Amenorrhea, secondary:

Intravaginal gel: 45 mg (4% gel) every other day for 6 doses; if response is inadequate, may increase to 90 mg (8% gel) at same schedule

Oral: 400 mg every evening for 10 days

ART in patients who require progesterone supplementation:

Intravaginal gel: 90 mg (8% gel) once daily. If pregnancy occurs, may continue treatment for 10-12 weeks.

ART in patients with partial or complete ovarian failure:

Intravaginal gel: 90 mg (8% gel) twice daily. If pregnancy occurs, continue treatment for 10-12 weeks.

Endometrial hyperplasia prevention (in postmenopausal women with a uterus who are receiving daily conjugated estrogen tablets): Oral: 200 mg as a single daily dose every evening for 12 days sequentially per 28-day cycle

Functional uterine bleeding: I.M.: 5-10 mg/day for 6 doses

Administration

I.M.: Administer deep I.M. only

Other: Vaginal gel: (A small amount of gel will remain in the applicator following insertion): Administer into the vagina directly from sealed applicator. Remove applicator from wrapper; holding applicator by thickest end, shake down to move contents to thin end; while holding applicator by flat section of thick end, twist off tab; gently insert into vagina and squeeze thick end of applicator.

For use at altitudes above 2500 feet: Remove applicator from wrapper; hold applicator on both sides of bubble in the thick end; using a lancet, make a single puncture in the bubble to relieve air pressure; holding applicator by thickest end, shake down to move contents to thin end; while holding applicator by flat section of thick end, twist off tab; gently insert into vagina and squeeze thick end of applicator.

Stability

Storage: Store at controlled room temperature.

Nursing Actions

Physical Assessment: Assess potential for interactions with other prescriptions, OTC medications, or herbal products patient may be taking. Monitor patient response (eg, blood pressure, mammogram, and results of Pap smears and pregnancy tests before beginning treatment and at least annually). Teach patient proper use according to formulation, possible side effects/appropriate interventions (eg, annual physicals, Pap smears, and vision assessment), and adverse symptoms to report.

Patient Education: Do not take any new medication during therapy unless approved by prescriber. Use exactly as directed. It is important that you have an annual physical assessment, Pap smear, and vision assessment while taking this medication. May cause temporary dizziness or drowsiness (use caution when driving or engaging in tasks that are potentially hazardous until response to drug is known). Report immediately muscle pain or soreness; warmth, swelling, or redness in calves; shortness of breath; sudden loss or change in vision; change in menstrual pattern (unusual bleeding, amenorrhea, breakthrough spotting); breast tenderness that does not go away; acute abdominal cramping; signs of vaginal infection (drainage, pain, itching); or CNS changes (eg, blurred vision, confusion, acute anxiety, or unresolved depression).

Vaginal gel: A small amount of gel will remain in the applicator following insertion. Administer into the vagina directly from sealed applicator. Remove applicator from wrapper; holding applicator by thickest end, shake down to move contents to thin end; while holding applicator by flat section of thick end, twist off tab; gently insert into vagina and squeeze thick end of applicator.

Geriatric Considerations Not a progestin of choice in the elderly for hormonal cycling.

Pregnancy Issues There is an increased risk of minor birth defects in children whose mothers take progesterones during the first 4 months of pregnancy. Hypospadias has been reported in male and mild masculinization of the external genitalia has been reported in female babies exposed during the first trimester. Cleft lip, cleft palate, congenital heart disease, patent ductus arteriosus, ventricular septal defect, intrauterine death, and spontaneous abortion have been noted in case reports following use of oral progesterone during pregnancy. High doses of progesterone would be expected to impair fertility. According to the American College of Obstetricians and Gynecologists, additional studies are needed to evaluate the use of progesterone to reduce the risk of preterm birth. If needed, use should be restricted to women with history of previous spontaneous abortion at <37 weeks. The vaginal gel is indicated for use in ART.

Promethazine (proe METH a zeen)

U.S. Brand Names Phenadoz™; Phenergan®; Promethegan™

Synonyms Promethazine Hydrochloride

Pharmacologic Category Antiemetic; Antihistamine; Phenothiazine Derivative; Sedative

Medication Safety Issues
Sound-alike/look-alike issues:
Promethazine may be confused with chlorproMAZINE, predniSONE, promazine
Phenergan® may be confused with Phenaphen®, Phrenilin®, Theragran®

Pregnancy Risk Factor C

Lactation Excretion in breast milk unknown/not recommended

Use Symptomatic treatment of various allergic conditions; antiemetic; motion sickness; sedative; postoperative pain (adjunctive therapy); anesthetic (adjunctive therapy); anaphylactic reactions (adjunctive therapy)

Mechanism of Action/Effect Blocks postsynaptic mesolimbic dopaminergic receptors in the brain; exhibits a strong alpha-adrenergic blocking effect and depresses the release of hypothalamic and hypophyseal hormones; competes with histamine for the H_1-receptor; reduces stimuli to the brainstem reticular system

Contraindications Hypersensitivity to promethazine or any component of the formulation (cross-reactivity between phenothiazines may occur); coma; treatment of lower respiratory tract symptoms, including asthma; children <2 years of age

Warnings/Precautions Do not give SubQ or intra-arterially, necrotic lesions may occur. Injection may contain sulfites which may cause allergic reactions in some patients. Rapid I.V. administration may produce a transient fall in blood pressure; rate of administration should not exceed 25 mg/minute. Slow I.V. administration may produce a slightly elevated blood pressure. Not considered an antihistamine of choice in the elderly.

May be sedating and may impair physical or mental abilities. Use with caution in Parkinson's disease, hemodynamic instability, bone marrow suppression, subcortical brain damage, and in severe cardiac, hepatic, renal, or respiratory disease. Avoid use in Reye's syndrome. Respiratory fatalities have been reported in children <2 years of age. In children ≥2 years, use the lowest possible dose; other drugs with respiratory depressant effects should be avoided. May lower seizure threshold; use caution in persons with seizure disorders or in persons using narcotics or local anesthetics which may also affect seizure threshold. May

alter temperature regulation or mask toxicity of other drugs due to antiemetic effects. May alter cardiac conduction (life-threatening arrhythmias have occurred with therapeutic doses of phenothiazines). May cause orthostatic hypotension. Use caution in cardiovascular or cerebrovascular disease.

Due to anticholinergic effects, use caution in patients with decreased gastrointestinal motility, urinary retention, BPH, xerostomia, visual problems, narrow-angle glaucoma, and myasthenia gravis. May cause extrapyramidal symptoms, including pseudoparkinsonism, acute dystonic reactions, akathisia, and tardive dyskinesia. May be associated with neuroleptic malignant syndrome (NMS). Ampuls contain sodium metabisulfite.

Drug Interactions
Cytochrome P450 Effect: Substrate (major) of CYP2B6, 2D6; **Inhibits** CYP2D6 (weak)

Decreased Effect: CYP2B6 inducers may decrease the levels/effects of promethazine; example inducers include carbamazepine, nevirapine, phenobarbital, phenytoin, and rifampin. Benztropine (and other anticholinergics) may inhibit the therapeutic response to promethazine. Promethazine may inhibit the ability of bromocriptine to lower serum prolactin concentrations. The antihypertensive effects of guanethidine and guanadrel may be inhibited by promethazine. Promethazine may inhibit the antiparkinsonian effect of levodopa. Promethazine (and possibly other low potency antipsychotics) may reverse the pressor effects of epinephrine.

Increased Effect/Toxicity: CYP2B6 inhibitors may increase the levels/effects of promethazine; example inhibitors include desipramine, paroxetine, and sertraline. CYP2D6 inhibitors may increase the levels/effects of promethazine; example inhibitors include chlorpromazine, delavirdine, fluoxetine, miconazole, paroxetine, pergolide, quinidine, quinine, ritonavir, and ropinirole. Chloroquine, propranolol, and sulfadoxine-pyrimethamine also may increase promethazine concentrations. Concurrent use with TCA may produce increased toxicity or altered therapeutic response. Promethazine plus lithium may rarely produce neurotoxicity. Concurrent use of promethazine and CNS depressants (ethanol, narcotics) may produce additive depressant effects.

Nutritional/Ethanol Interactions
Ethanol: Avoid ethanol (may increase CNS depression).
Herb/Nutraceutical: Avoid valerian, St John's wort, kava kava, gotu kola (may increase CNS depression).

Lab Interactions Alters the flare response in intradermal allergen tests

Adverse Reactions
Cardiovascular: Bradycardia, hypertension, nonspecific QT changes, postural hypotension, tachycardia

Central nervous system: Akathisia, catatonic states, confusion, delirium, disorientation, dizziness, drowsiness, dystonias, euphoria, excitation, extrapyramidal symptoms, fatigue, hallucinations, hysteria, insomnia, lassitude, nervousness, neuroleptic malignant syndrome, nightmares, pseudoparkinsonism, sedation, seizure, somnolence, tardive dyskinesia

Dermatologic: Angioneurotic edema, dermatitis, photosensitivity, skin pigmentation (slate gray), urticaria

Endocrine & metabolic: Amenorrhea, breast engorgement, gynecomastia, hyper-/hypoglycemia, lactation

Gastrointestinal: Constipation, nausea, vomiting, xerostomia

Genitourinary: Ejaculatory disorder, impotence, urinary retention

Hematologic: Agranulocytosis, aplastic anemia, eosinophilia, hemolytic anemia, leukopenia, thrombocytopenia, thrombocytopenic purpura

Hepatic: Jaundice

Neuromuscular & skeletal: Incoordination, tremor
(Continued)

Promethazine (Continued)

Ocular: Blurred vision, corneal and lenticular changes, diplopia, epithelial keratopathy, pigmentary retinopathy

Otic: Tinnitus

Respiratory: Apnea, asthma, nasal congestion, respiratory depression

Overdosage/Toxicology Symptoms of overdose include CNS depression, respiratory depression, possible CNS stimulation, dry mouth, fixed and dilated pupils, and hypotension. Treatment is symptom-directed and supportive. Epinephrine should not be used. Hemodialysis: Not dialyzable (0% to 5%)

Pharmacodynamics/Kinetics

Onset of Action: I.M.: ~20 minutes; I.V.: 3-5 minutes

Peak effect: C_{max}: 9.04 ng/mL (suppository); 19.3 ng/mL (syrup)

Duration of Action: 2-6 hours

Time to Peak: Maximum serum concentration: 4.4 hours (syrup); 6.7-8.6 hours (suppositories)

Protein Binding: 93%

Half-Life Elimination: 9-16 hours

Metabolism: Hepatic; primarily oxidation; forms metabolites

Excretion: Primarily urine and feces (as inactive metabolites)

Available Dosage Forms [DSC] = Discontinued product

Injection, solution, as hydrochloride: 25 mg/mL (1 mL); 50 mg/mL (1 mL)

Phenergan®: 25 mg/mL (1 mL); 50 mg/mL (1 mL) [contains sodium metabisulfite]

Suppository, rectal, as hydrochloride: 12.5 mg, 25 mg, 50 mg

Phenadoz™: 12.5 mg, 25 mg

Phenergan®: 25 mg, 50 mg [DSC]

Promethegan™: 12.5 mg, 25 mg, 50 mg

Syrup, as hydrochloride: 6.25 mg/5 mL (120 mL, 480 mL) [contains alcohol]

Tablet, as hydrochloride: 12.5 mg, 25 mg, 50 mg

Phenergan®: 25 mg [DSC]

Dosing

Adults & Elderly:

Allergic conditions (including allergic reactions to blood or plasma):

Oral, rectal: 25 mg at bedtime **or** 12.5 mg before meals and at bedtime (range: 6.25-12.5 mg 3 times/day)

I.M., I.V.: 25 mg, may repeat in 2 hours when necessary; switch to oral route as soon as feasible

Antiemetic: Oral, I.M., I.V., rectal: 12.5-25 mg every 4-6 hours as needed

Motion sickness: Oral, rectal: 25 mg 30-60 minutes before departure, then every 12 hours as needed

Sedation: Oral, I.M., I.V., rectal: 12.5-50 mg/dose

Pediatrics:

Allergic conditions: Children ≥2 years: Oral, rectal: 0.1 mg/kg/dose (maximum: 12.5 mg) every 6 hours during the day and 0.5 mg/kg/dose (maximum: 25 mg) at bedtime as needed

Antiemetic: Children ≥2 years: Oral, I.M., I.V., rectal: 0.25-1 mg/kg 4-6 times/day as needed (maximum: 25 mg/dose)

Motion sickness: Children ≥2 years: Oral, rectal: 0.5 mg/kg/dose 30 minutes to 1 hour before departure, then every 12 hours as needed (maximum dose: 25 mg twice daily)

Sedation: Children ≥2 years: Oral, I.M., I.V., rectal: 0.5-1 mg/kg/dose every 6 hours as needed (maximum: 50 mg/dose)

Administration

I.M.: Preferred route of administration; administer into deep muscle

I.V.: I.V. administration is not the preferred route. Solution for injection may be diluted in 25-100 mL NS or D_5W (maximum concentration of 25 mg/mL) and infused over 15-30 minutes at a rate ≤25 mg/minute.

I.V. Detail: Rapid I.V. administration may produce a transient fall in blood pressure.

pH: 4.0-5.5

Other: Not for SubQ or intra-arterial administration.

Stability

Compatibility: Stable in dextran 6% in dextrose, dextran 6% in NS, D_5W, $D_{10}W$, D_5LR, $D_5\frac{1}{4}NS$, $D_5\frac{1}{2}NS$, D_5NS, LR, $\frac{1}{2}NS$, NS

Y-site administration: Incompatible with aldesleukin, allopurinol, amphotericin B cholesteryl sulfate complex, cefazolin, cefepime, cefoperazone, cefotetan, doxorubicin liposome, foscarnet, methotrexate, piperacillin/tazobactam

Compatibility in syringe: Incompatible with cefotetan, chloroquine, diatrizoate sodium 75%, diatrizoate meglumine 52% with diatrizoate sodium 8%, diatrizoate meglumine 34.3% with diatrizoate sodium 35%, dimenhydrinate, heparin, iodipamide meglumine 52%, iothalamate meglumine 60%, iothalamate sodium 80%, ketorolac, pentobarbital, thiopental

Compatibility when admixed: Incompatible with aminophylline, chloramphenicol, chlorothiazide, dimenhydrinate, floxacillin, furosemide, heparin, hydrocortisone sodium succinate, methohexital, penicillin G sodium, pentobarbital, phenobarbital, phenytoin, thiopental

Storage:

Injection: Prior to dilution, store at room temperature; protect from light. Solutions in NS or D_5W are stable for 24 hours at room temperature.

Suppositories: Store refrigerated at 2°C to 8°C (36°F to 46°F).

Tablets: Store at room temperature. Protect from light.

Nursing Actions

Physical Assessment: Assess potential for interactions with other pharmacological agents and herbal products patient may be taking. Note Administration specifics for I.V. and I.M. use (do not give SubQ or intra-arterially; necrotic lesions may occur). Monitor for effectiveness (according to purpose for use) and adverse response (eg. sedation, bradycardia, akathisia, delirium, extrapyramidal symptoms, dermatitis, gastrointestinal upset, urinary retention, blurred vision, respiratory depression). May be sedating and impair physical or mental abilities; use and teach sedation safety measures (eg, side rails up, call light within reach). Teach patient appropriate use (oral), interventions to reduce side effects, and adverse symptoms to report.

Patient Education: Do not take any new medication during therapy unless approved by prescriber (especially anything that may cause CNS depression). Take this drug as prescribed; do not increase dosage. Avoid alcohol; may increase CNS depression. May cause dizziness, drowsiness, or blurred vision (use caution when driving or engaging in tasks requiring alertness until response to drug is known); or nausea, dry mouth, appetite disturbances (small frequent meals, frequent mouth care, chewing gum, or sucking lozenges may help). Report unusual weight gain, unresolved nausea or diarrhea, chest pain or palpitations, excess sedation or stimulation, or sore throat or respiratory difficulty. **Pregnancy/breast-feeding precautions:** Inform prescriber if you are or intend to become pregnant. Breast-feeding is not recommended.

Dietary Considerations Increase dietary intake of riboflavin.

Geriatric Considerations Because promethazine is a phenothiazine (and can, therefore, cause side effects such as extrapyramidal symptoms), it is not considered an antihistamine of choice in the elderly.

Pregnancy Issues Crosses the placenta. Possible respiratory depression if drug is administered near time of delivery; behavioral changes, EEG alterations, impaired platelet aggregation reported with use during labor. Available evidence with use of occasional low doses suggests safe use during pregnancy.

Related Information
Compatibility of Drugs in Syringe *on page 1372*

Promethazine and Codeine
(proe METH a zeen & KOE deen)

Synonyms Codeine and Promethazine
Restrictions C-V
Pharmacologic Category Antihistamine/Antitussive
Pregnancy Risk Factor C
Lactation Enters breast milk (codeine)/not recommended
Use Temporary relief of coughs and upper respiratory symptoms associated with allergy or the common cold
Available Dosage Forms Syrup: Promethazine hydrochloride 6.25 mg and codeine phosphate 10 mg per 5 mL (120 mL, 473 mL, 3840 mL) [contains alcohol]
Dosing
Adults: Upper respiratory symptoms: Oral: 10-20 mg/dose every 4-6 hours as needed; maximum: 120 mg codeine/day; or 5-10 mL every 4-6 hours as needed
Elderly: Refer to dosing in individual monographs.
Pediatrics: Upper respiratory symptoms: Oral (in terms of codeine):
Children: 1-1.5 mg/kg/day every 4 hours as needed; maximum: 30 mg/day **or**
2-6 years: 1.25-2.5 mL every 4-6 hours or 2.5-5 mg/dose every 4-6 hours as needed; maximum: 30 mg codeine/day
6-12 years: 2.5-5 mL every 4-6 hours as needed or 5-10 mg/dose every 4-6 hours as needed; maximum: 60 mg codeine/day
Nursing Actions
Physical Assessment: See individual agents.
Patient Education: See individual agents. **Pregnancy/breast-feeding precautions:** Inform prescriber if you are or intend to become pregnant. Breast-feeding is not recommended.
Related Information
Codeine *on page 296*
Promethazine *on page 1035*

Promethazine and Dextromethorphan
(proe METH a zeen & deks troe meth OR fan)

Synonyms Dextromethorphan and Promethazine
Pharmacologic Category Antihistamine/Antitussive
Pregnancy Risk Factor C
Lactation Excretion in breast milk unknown/not recommended
Use Temporary relief of coughs and upper respiratory symptoms associated with allergy or the common cold
Available Dosage Forms Syrup: Promethazine hydrochloride 6.25 mg and dextromethorphan hydrobromide 15 mg per 5 mL (120 mL, 480 mL, 4000 mL) [contains alcohol 7%]
Dosing
Adults: Cough and upper respiratory symptoms: Oral: 5 mL every 4-6 hours, up to 30 mL in 24 hours
Elderly: Refer to dosing in individual monographs.
Pediatrics: Cough and upper respiratory symptoms: Oral: Children:

2-6 years: 1.25-2.5 mL every 4-6 hours up to 10 mL in 24 hours
6-12 years: 2.5-5 mL every 4-6 hours up to 20 mL in 24 hours
Nursing Actions
Physical Assessment: See individual agents.
Patient Education: See individual agents. **Pregnancy/breast-feeding precautions:** Inform prescriber if you are or intend to become pregnant. Breast-feeding is not recommended.
Related Information
Promethazine *on page 1035*

Promethazine and Phenylephrine
(proe METH a zeen & fen il EF rin)

Synonyms Phenylephrine and Promethazine
Pharmacologic Category Antihistamine/Decongestant Combination
Pregnancy Risk Factor C
Lactation Excretion in breast milk unknown/not recommended
Use Temporary relief of upper respiratory symptoms associated with allergy or the common cold
Available Dosage Forms Syrup: Promethazine hydrochloride 6.25 mg and phenylephrine hydrochloride 5 mg per 5 mL (120 mL, 473 mL) [contains alcohol]
Dosing
Adults: Upper respiratory symptoms: Oral: 5 mL every 4-6 hours, not to exceed 30 mL in 24 hours
Elderly: Refer to dosing in individual monographs.
Pediatrics: Upper respiratory symptoms: Oral: Children:
2-6 years: 1.25 mL every 4-6 hours, not to exceed 7.5 mL in 24 hours
6-12 years: 2.5 mL every 4-6 hours, not to exceed 15 mL in 24 hours
>12 years: Refer to adult dosing.
Nursing Actions
Physical Assessment: See individual agents.
Patient Education: See individual agents. **Pregnancy/breast-feeding precautions:** Inform prescriber if you are or intend to become pregnant. Breast-feeding is not recommended.
Related Information
Phenylephrine *on page 980*
Promethazine *on page 1035*

Promethazine, Phenylephrine, and Codeine
(proe METH a zeen, fen il EF rin, & KOE deen)

Synonyms Codeine, Promethazine, and Phenylephrine; Phenylephrine, Promethazine, and Codeine
Restrictions C-V
Pharmacologic Category Antihistamine/Decongestant/Antitussive
Pregnancy Risk Factor C
Lactation Enters breast milk/not recommended
Use Temporary relief of coughs and upper respiratory symptoms including nasal congestion
Available Dosage Forms Syrup: Promethazine hydrochloride 6.25 mg, phenylephrine hydrochloride 5 mg, and codeine phosphate 10 mg per 5 mL with alcohol 7% (120 mL, 480 mL) [contains alcohol]
Dosing
Adults: Cough and upper respiratory symptoms: Oral: 5 mL every 4-6 hours, not to exceed 30 mL/24 hours
Elderly: Refer to dosing in individual monographs.
(Continued)

Promethazine, Phenylephrine, and Codeine *(Continued)*

Pediatrics: Cough and upper respiratory symptoms: Oral:
Children (expressed in terms of codeine dosage):
1-1.5 mg/kg/day every 4 hours, maximum: 30 mg/day **or**

<2 years: Not recommended

2-6 years:

Weight 25 lb: 1.25-2.5 mL every 4-6 hours, not >6 mL/24 hours

Weight 30 lb: 1.25-2.5 mL every 4-6 hours, not >7 mL/24 hours

Weight 35 lb: 1.25-2.5 mL every 4-6 hours, not >8 mL/24 hours

Weight 40 lb: 1.25-2.5 mL every 4-6 hours, not >9 mL/24 hours

6 to <12 years: 2.5-5 mL every 4-6 hours, not >15 mL/24 hours

Nursing Actions

Physical Assessment: See individual agents.

Patient Education: See individual agents. **Pregnancy/breast-feeding precautions:** Inform prescriber if you are or intend to become pregnant. Breast-feeding is not recommended.

Related Information

Codeine *on page 296*

Phenylephrine *on page 980*

Promethazine *on page 1035*

Propafenone *(proe pa FEEN one)*

U.S. Brand Names Rythmol®; Rythmol® SR

Synonyms Propafenone Hydrochloride

Pharmacologic Category Antiarrhythmic Agent, Class Ic

Pregnancy Risk Factor C

Lactation Enters breast milk/use caution

Use Treatment of life-threatening ventricular arrhythmias

Rythmol® SR: Maintenance of normal sinus rhythm in patients with symptomatic atrial fibrillation

Unlabeled/Investigational Use Supraventricular tachycardias, including those patients with Wolff-Parkinson-White syndrome

Mechanism of Action/Effect Propafenone is a class 1c antiarrhythmic agent which possesses local anesthetic properties, blocks the fast inward sodium current, and slows the rate of increase of the action potential. Prolongs conduction and refractoriness in all areas of the myocardium, with a slightly more pronounced effect on intraventricular conduction; it prolongs effective refractory period, reduces spontaneous automaticity and exhibits some beta-blockade activity.

Contraindications Hypersensitivity to propafenone or any component of the formulation; sinoatrial, AV, and intraventricular disorders of impulse generation and/or conduction (except in patients with a functioning artificial pacemaker); sinus bradycardia; cardiogenic shock; uncompensated cardiac failure; hypotension; bronchospastic disorders; uncorrected electrolyte abnormalities; concurrent use of ritonavir (see Drug Interactions)

Warnings/Precautions Patients with bronchospastic disease should generally not receive this drug. May worsen CHF in some patients. May cause or unmask a variety of conduction disturbances, or lead to the development of new arrhythmias (proarrhythmic events). May alter pacing and sensing thresholds of artificial pacemakers. May prolong QT_c interval; use caution with other QT_c-prolonging drugs. Administer cautiously in significant hepatic dysfunction.

Drug Interactions

Cytochrome P450 Effect: Substrate of CYP1A2 (minor), 2D6 (major), 3A4 (minor); **Inhibits** CYP1A2 (weak), 2C8/9 (weak), 2D6 (weak)

Decreased Effect: Enzyme inducers (phenobarbital, phenytoin, rifabutin, rifampin) may decrease propafenone blood levels.

Increased Effect/Toxicity: Cimetidine and quinidine may increase propafenone levels. Ritonavir may increase propafenone levels; concurrent use is contraindicated. CYP2D6 inhibitors may increase the levels/effects of propafenone; example inhibitors include chlorpromazine, delavirdine, fluoxetine, miconazole, paroxetine, pergolide, quinine, and ropinirole. Digoxin (reduce dose by 25%), metoprolol, propranolol, theophylline, and warfarin blood levels are increased by propafenone. Use caution with Class Ia and Class III antiarrhythmics, erythromycin, cisapride, antipsychotics, and cyclic antidepressants; QT_c-prolonging effects may be additive with propafenone.

Nutritional/Ethanol Interactions

Food: Propafenone serum concentrations may be increased if taken with food.

Herb/Nutraceutical: St John's wort may decrease propafenone levels. Avoid ephedra (may worsen arrhythmia).

Adverse Reactions 1% to 10%:

Cardiovascular: New or worsened arrhythmia (proarrhythmic effect) (2% to 10%), angina (2% to 5%), CHF (1% to 4%), ventricular tachycardia (1% to 3%), palpitation (1% to 3%), AV block (first-degree) (1% to 3%), syncope (1% to 2%), increased QRS interval (1% to 2%), chest pain (1% to 2%), PVCs (1% to 2%), bradycardia (1% to 2%), edema (0% to 1%), bundle branch block (0% to 1%), atrial fibrillation (1%), hypotension (0% to 1%), intraventricular conduction delay (0% to 1%)

Central nervous system: Dizziness (4% to 15%), fatigue (2% to 6%), headache (2% to 5%), ataxia (0% to 2%), insomnia (0% to 2%), anxiety (1% to 2%), drowsiness (1%)

Dermatologic: Rash (1% to 3%)

Gastrointestinal: Nausea/vomiting (2% to 11%), unusual taste (3% to 23%), constipation (2% to 7%), dyspepsia (1% to 3%), diarrhea (1% to 3%), xerostomia (1% to 2%), anorexia (1% to 2%), abdominal pain (1% to 2%), flatulence (0% to 1%)

Neuromuscular & skeletal: Tremor (0% to 1%), arthralgia (0% to 1%), weakness (1% to 2%)

Ocular: Blurred vision (1% to 6%)

Respiratory: Dyspnea (2% to 5%)

Miscellaneous: Diaphoresis (1%)

Overdosage/Toxicology Propafenone has a narrow therapeutic index and severe toxicity may occur slightly above the therapeutic range, especially if combined with other antiarrhythmic drugs. Acute single ingestion of twice the daily therapeutic dose is life-threatening. Symptoms of overdose include increased P-R, QRS, or QT intervals and amplitude of the T wave, AV block, bradycardia, hypotension, ventricular arrhythmias (monomorphic or polymorphic ventricular tachycardia), and asystole. Other symptoms include dizziness, blurred vision, headache, and GI upset. Treatment is supportive. **Note:** Class 1A antiarrhythmic agents should not be used to treat cardiotoxicity caused by Class 1C drugs. Sodium bicarbonate may reverse QRS prolongation, bradycardia, and hypotension. Ventricular pacing may be needed.

Pharmacodynamics/Kinetics

Time to Peak: 150 mg dose: 2 hours; 300 mg dose: 3 hours

Half-Life Elimination: Single dose (100-300 mg): 2-8 hours; Chronic dosing: 10-32 hours

Metabolism: Hepatic; two genetically determined metabolism groups exist: fast or slow metabolizers; 10% of Caucasians are slow metabolizers; exhibits nonlinear pharmacokinetics; when dose is increased from 300-900 mg/day, serum concentrations increase tenfold; this nonlinearity is thought to be due to saturable first-pass effect

Available Dosage Forms

Capsule, extended release, as hydrochloride (Rythmol® SR): 225 mg, 325 mg, 425 mg [contains soy lecithin]

Tablet, as hydrochloride (Rythmol®): 150 mg, 225 mg, 300 mg

Dosing

Adults & Elderly: Note: Patients who exhibit significant widening of QRS complex or second- or third-degree AV block may need dose reduction.

Ventricular arrhythmias: Oral:

Immediate release tablet: Initial: 150 mg every 8 hours, increase at 3- to 4-day intervals up to 300 mg every 8 hours.

Extended release capsule: Initial: 225 mg every 12 hours; dosage increase may be made at a minimum of 5-day intervals; may increase to 325 mg every 12 hours; if further increase is necessary, may increase to 425 mg every 12 hours

Hepatic Impairment: Reduction is necessary; however, specific guidelines are not available.

Administration

Oral: Capsules should be swallowed whole; do not crush or chew.

Stability

Storage: Store at 25°C (77°F). Excursions permitted to 15°C to 30°C (59°F to 86°F).

Nursing Actions

Physical Assessment: Assess other medications patient may be taking for effectiveness and interactions. Monitor therapeutic response and adverse reactions at beginning of therapy, when titrating dosage, and on a regular basis with long-term therapy. Monitor cardiac status (BP, pulse) closely. **Note:** Propafenone has a low toxic:therapeutic ratio and overdose may easily produce severe and life-threatening reactions. Assess knowledge/teach patient appropriate use, interventions to reduce side effects, and adverse symptoms to report.

Patient Education: Take exactly as directed; do not take additional doses or discontinue without consulting prescriber. You will need regular cardiac checkups. You may experience dizziness, drowsiness, or visual changes (use caution when driving or engaging in tasks requiring alertness until response to drug is known); abnormal taste, nausea or vomiting, or loss of appetite (small frequent meals, frequent mouth care, chewing gum, or sucking lozenges may help); headaches (prescriber may recommend mild analgesic); or diarrhea (yogurt or boiled milk may help; if persistent consult prescriber). Report chest pain, palpitation, or erratic heartbeat; respiratory difficulty, increased weight or swelling of hands or feet; acute persistent diarrhea or constipation; or vision changes.

Dietary Considerations

Capsule: May be taken without regard to food.

Rythmol® SR capsules contain soy lecithin.

Tablet: Should be taken at the same time in relation to meals each day, either always with meals or always between meals.

Geriatric Considerations Elderly may have age-related decreases in hepatic Phase I metabolism. Propafenone is dependent upon liver metabolism, therefore, monitor closely in the elderly and adjust dose more gradually during initial treatment (see Warnings/Precautions). No differences in clearance noted with impaired renal function and, therefore, no adjustment for renal function in the elderly is necessary.

Propoxyphene (proe POKS i feen)

U.S. Brand Names Darvon®; Darvon-N®

Synonyms Dextropropoxyphene; Propoxyphene Hydrochloride; Propoxyphene Napsylate

Restrictions C-IV

Pharmacologic Category Analgesic, Narcotic

Medication Safety Issues

Sound-alike/look-alike issues:

Propoxyphene may be confused with proparacaine

Darvon® may be confused with Devrom®, Diovan®

Darvon-N® may be confused with Darvocet-N®

Pregnancy Risk Factor C/D (prolonged use)

Lactation Enters breast milk/use caution (AAP rates "compatible")

Use Management of mild to moderate pain

Mechanism of Action/Effect Binds to opiate receptors in the CNS, causing inhibition of ascending pain pathways, altering the perception of and response to pain; produces generalized CNS depression

Contraindications Hypersensitivity to propoxyphene or any component of the formulation

Warnings/Precautions When given in excessive doses, either alone or in combination with other CNS depressants, propoxyphene is a major cause of drug-related deaths; do not exceed recommended dosage; give with caution in patients dependent on opiates, substitution may result in acute opiate withdrawal symptoms. Avoid use in severely depressed or suicidal patients. Tolerance or drug dependence may result from extended use. Propoxyphene should be used with caution in patients with renal or hepatic dysfunction or in the elderly; consider dosing adjustment.

Drug Interactions

Cytochrome P450 Effect: Inhibits CYP2C8/9 (weak), 2D6 (weak), 3A4 (weak)

Decreased Effect: Decreased effect with cigarette smoking.

Increased Effect/Toxicity: CNS depressants (phenothiazines, tranquilizers, anxiolytics, sedatives, hypnotics, or alcohol) may potentiate pharmacologic effects. Propoxyphene may inhibit the metabolism and increase the serum concentrations of carbamazepine, phenobarbital, MAO inhibitors, tricyclic antidepressants, and warfarin.

Nutritional/Ethanol Interactions

Ethanol: Avoid or limit ethanol (may increase CNS depression). Watch for sedation.

Food: May decrease rate of absorption, but may slightly increase bioavailability.

Lab Interactions False-positive methadone test; increased LFTs; decreased glucose (S), 17-OHCS (U)

Adverse Reactions Frequency not defined.

Cardiovascular: Hypotension, bundle branch block

Central nervous system: Dizziness, lightheadedness, sedation, paradoxical excitement and insomnia, fatigue, drowsiness, mental depression, hallucinations, paradoxical CNS stimulation, increased intracranial pressure, nervousness, headache, restlessness, malaise, confusion, dysphoria, vertigo

Dermatologic: Rash, urticaria

Endocrine & metabolic: Hypoglycemia, urinary 17-OHCS decreased

Gastrointestinal: Anorexia, stomach cramps, xerostomia, biliary spasm, nausea, vomiting, constipation, paralytic ileus, abdominal pain

Genitourinary: Urination decreased, ureteral spasms

Hepatic: LFTs increased, jaundice

Neuromuscular & skeletal: Weakness

Ocular: Visual disturbances

Respiratory: Dyspnea

Miscellaneous: Psychologic and physical dependence with prolonged use, histamine release, hypersensitivity reaction

(Continued)

Propoxyphene *(Continued)*

Overdosage/Toxicology Symptoms of overdose include CNS disturbances, respiratory depression, hypotension, pulmonary edema, and seizures. Naloxone, 2 mg I.V. with repeat administration as necessary up to a total of 10 mg, can also be used to reverse toxic effects of the opiate. Charcoal is very effective (>95%) at binding propoxyphene.

Pharmacodynamics/Kinetics
Onset of Action: 0.5-1 hour

Duration of Action: 4-6 hours

Half-Life Elimination: Adults: Parent drug: 6-12 hours; Norpropoxyphene: 30-36 hours

Metabolism: Hepatic to active metabolite (norpropoxyphene) and inactive metabolites; first-pass effect

Excretion: Urine (primarily as metabolites)

Available Dosage Forms
Capsule, as hydrochloride (Darvon®): 65 mg
Tablet, as napsylate (Darvon-N®): 100 mg

Dosing
Adults: Pain management: Oral:
Hydrochloride: 65 mg every 3-4 hours as needed for pain; maximum: 390 mg/day
Napsylate: 100 mg every 4 hours as needed for pain; maximum: 600 mg/day

Elderly: Pain management: Oral:
Hydrochloride: 65 mg every 4-6 hours as needed for pain
Napsylate: 100 mg every 4-6 hours as needed for pain

Pediatrics: Pain management: Oral: Children: Doses for children are not well established; doses of the hydrochloride of 2-3 mg/kg/d divided every 6 hours have been used.

Renal Impairment: Serum concentrations of propoxyphene may be increased or elimination may be delayed. Avoid use in Cl$_{cr}$ <10 mL/minute. Specific dosing recommendations not available for less severe impairment.
Not dialyzable (0% to 5%)

Hepatic Impairment: Serum concentrations of propoxyphene may be increased or elimination may be delayed. Specific dosing recommendations not available.

Administration
Oral: Should be administered with glass of water on an empty stomach. Food may decrease rate of absorption, but may slightly increase bioavailability.

Stability
Storage: Store at controlled room temperature of 15°C to 30°C (59°F to 86°F).

Nursing Actions
Physical Assessment: Assess other medications patient may be taking for effectiveness and interactions. Monitor for effectiveness of pain relief. Monitor blood pressure, mental and respiratory status, degree of sedation, and CNS changes. Monitor for signs of overdose. Assess knowledge/teach patient appropriate use, interventions to reduce side effects, and adverse symptoms to report.

Patient Education: Take as directed; do not take a larger dose or more often than prescribed. Do not use alcohol, other prescription or OTC sedatives, tranquilizers, antihistamines, or pain medications without consulting prescriber. May cause dizziness, drowsiness, or impaired judgment; avoid driving or engaging in tasks requiring alertness until response to drug is known. If you experience vomiting or loss of appetite, frequent mouth care, small frequent meals, chewing gum, or sucking lozenges may help. Increased fluid intake, exercise, fiber in diet may help with constipation (if unresolved consult prescriber). Report unresolved nausea or vomiting, respiratory difficulty or shortness of breath, or unusual weakness. **Pregnancy/breast-feeding precautions:** Inform prescriber if you are or intend to become pregnant.

Dietary Considerations May administer with food if gastrointestinal distress occurs.

Geriatric Considerations The elderly may be particularly susceptible to the CNS depressant effects of narcotics.

Breast-Feeding Issues Propoxyphene and norpropoxyphene are excreted in breast milk.

Pregnancy Issues Withdrawal symptoms have been reported in the neonate following propoxyphene use during pregnancy. Teratogenic effects have also been noted in case reports. Opioid analgesics are considered pregnancy risk factor D if used for prolonged periods or in large doses near term.

Additional Information 100 mg of napsylate = 65 mg of hydrochloride
Propoxyphene hydrochloride: Darvon®
Propoxyphene napsylate: Darvon-N®

Propoxyphene and Acetaminophen
(proe POKS i feen & a seet a MIN oh fen)

U.S. Brand Names Balacet 325™; Darvocet A500™; Darvocet-N® 50; Darvocet-N® 100; Pronap-100®

Synonyms Acetaminophen and Propoxyphene; Propoxyphene Hydrochloride and Acetaminophen; Propoxyphene Napsylate and Acetaminophen

Restrictions C-IV

Pharmacologic Category Analgesic Combination (Narcotic)

Pregnancy Risk Factor C

Lactation Enters breast milk/compatible

Use Management of mild to moderate pain

Available Dosage Forms
Tablet: Propoxyphene hydrochloride 65 mg and acetaminophen 650 mg, propoxyphene napsylate 100 mg, and acetaminophen 650 mg
Balacet 325™: Propoxyphene napsylate 100 mg and acetaminophen 325 mg
Darvocet A500™: Propoxyphene napsylate 100 mg and acetaminophen 500 mg [contains lactose]
Darvocet-N® 50: Propoxyphene napsylate 50 mg and acetaminophen 325 mg
Darvocet-N® 100, Pronap-100®: Propoxyphene napsylate 100 mg and acetaminophen 650 mg

Dosing
Adults & Elderly:
Pain management: Oral:
Darvocet A500™, Darvocet-N® 100: 1 tablet every 4 hours as needed; maximum: 600 mg propoxyphene napsylate/day
Darvocet-N® 50: 1-2 tablets every 4 hours as needed; maximum: 600 mg propoxyphene napsylate/day
Note: Formulations contain significant amounts of acetaminophen; intake should be limited to <4 g acetaminophen/day (less in patients with hepatic impairment/ethanol abuse)

Renal Impairment: Serum concentrations of propoxyphene may be increased or elimination may be delayed; specific dosing recommendations not available.

Hepatic Impairment: Serum concentrations of propoxyphene may be increased or elimination may be delayed; specific dosing recommendations not available.

Nursing Actions
Physical Assessment: See individual agents.
Patient Education: See individual agents. **Pregnancy precaution:** Inform prescriber if you are or intend to become pregnant.

Related Information
Acetaminophen *on page 30*
Propoxyphene *on page 1039*

Propoxyphene, Aspirin, and Caffeine
(proe POKS i feen, AS pir in, & KAF een)

U.S. Brand Names Darvon® Compound [DSC]
Synonyms Aspirin, Caffeine, and Propoxyphene; Caffeine, Propoxyphene, and Aspirin; Propoxyphene Hydrochloride, Aspirin, and Caffeine
Restrictions C-IV
Pharmacologic Category Analgesic Combination (Narcotic)
Pregnancy Risk Factor C
Lactation Enters breast milk/use caution
Use Treatment of mild-to-moderate pain
Available Dosage Forms [DSC] = Discontinued product
Capsule (Darvon® Compound 65): Propoxyphene hydrochloride 65 mg, aspirin 389 mg, and caffeine 32.4 mg [DSC]
Dosing
Adults: Pain: Oral: One capsule (providing propoxyphene 65 mg) every 4 hours as needed; maximum propoxyphene 390 mg/day. This will also provide aspirin 389 mg and caffeine 32.4 mg per capsule.
Elderly: Refer to adult dosing. Consider increasing dosing interval.
Renal Impairment: Serum concentrations of propoxyphene may be increased or elimination may be delayed; specific dosing recommendations not available. Avoid use with Cl_{cr} <10 mL/minute.
Hepatic Impairment: Serum concentrations or propoxyphene may be increased or elimination may be delayed; specific dosing recommendations not available.
Nursing Actions
Physical Assessment: See individual agents.
Related Information
Aspirin *on page 114*
Propoxyphene *on page 1039*

Propranolol (proe PRAN oh lole)

U.S. Brand Names Inderal®; Inderal® LA; InnoPran XL™
Synonyms Propranolol Hydrochloride
Pharmacologic Category Antiarrhythmic Agent, Class II; Beta-Adrenergic Blocker, Nonselective
Medication Safety Issues
Sound-alike/look-alike issues:
Propranolol may be confused with Pravachol®, Propulsid®
Inderal® may be confused with Adderall®, Enduron®, Enduronyl®, Imdur®, Imuran®, Inderide®, Isordil®, Toradol®
Inderal® 40 may be confused with Enduronyl® Forte
Pregnancy Risk Factor C (manufacturer); D (2nd and 3rd trimesters - expert analysis)
Lactation Enters breast milk/use caution (AAP rates "compatible")
Use Management of hypertension; angina pectoris; pheochromocytoma; essential tremor; tetralogy of Fallot cyanotic spells; arrhythmias (such as atrial fibrillation and flutter, AV nodal re-entrant tachycardias, and catecholamine-induced arrhythmias); prevention of myocardial infarction; migraine headache; symptomatic treatment of hypertrophic subaortic stenosis
Unlabeled/Investigational Use Tremor due to Parkinson's disease; ethanol withdrawal; aggressive behavior; antipsychotic-induced akathisia; prevention of

bleeding esophageal varices; anxiety; schizophrenia; acute panic; gastric bleeding in portal hypertension; thyrotoxicosis
Mechanism of Action/Effect Nonselective beta-adrenergic blocker (class II antiarrhythmic); competitively blocks response to beta$_1$- and beta$_2$-adrenergic stimulation which results in decreases in heart rate, myocardial contractility, blood pressure, and myocardial oxygen demand
Contraindications Hypersensitivity to propranolol, beta-blockers, or any component of the formulation; uncompensated congestive heart failure (unless the failure is due to tachyarrhythmias being treated with propranolol); cardiogenic shock, bradycardia or heart block (2nd or 3rd degree), pulmonary edema, severe hyperactive airway disease (asthma or COPD), Raynaud's disease; pregnancy (2nd and 3rd trimesters)
Warnings/Precautions Administer cautiously in compensated heart failure and monitor for a worsening of the condition (efficacy of propranolol in CHF has not been demonstrated). Beta-blocker therapy should not be withdrawn abruptly (particularly in patients with CAD), but gradually tapered (over 2 weeks) to avoid acute tachycardia, hypertension, and/or ischemia. Use caution in patient with peripheral vascular disease. Use caution with concurrent use of beta-blockers and either verapamil or diltiazem; bradycardia or heart block can occur. Avoid concurrent I.V. use of both agents. Use cautiously in patients with diabetes; may mask prominent hypoglycemic symptoms. May mask signs of thyrotoxicosis. Can cause fetal harm when administered in pregnancy. Use cautiously in hepatic dysfunction (dosage adjustment required). Use care with anesthetic agents which decrease myocardial function. Not indicated for hypertensive emergencies.
Drug Interactions
Cytochrome P450 Effect: Substrate of CYP1A2 (major), 2C19 (minor), 2D6 (major), 3A4 (minor); **Inhibits** CYP1A2 (weak), 2D6 (weak)
Decreased Effect: CYP1A2 inducers may decrease the levels/effects of propranolol; example inducers include aminoglutethimide, carbamazepine, phenobarbital, and rifampin. Aluminum salts, calcium salts, cholestyramine, colestipol, NSAIDs, penicillins (ampicillin), salicylates, and sulfinpyrazone decrease effect of beta-blockers due to decreased bioavailability and plasma levels. Beta-blockers may decrease the effect of sulfonylureas. Ascorbic acid decreases propranolol Cp_{max} and AUC and increases the T_{max} significantly resulting in a greater decrease in the reduction of heart rate, possibly due to decreased absorption and first pass metabolism (n=5). Nefazodone decreased peak plasma levels and AUC of propranolol and increases time to reach steady-state; monitoring of clinical response is recommended. Nonselective beta-blockers blunt the response to beta-2 adrenergic agonists (albuterol).
Increased Effect/Toxicity: CYP1A2 inhibitors may increase the levels/effects of propranolol; example inhibitors include amiodarone, ciprofloxacin, fluvoxamine, ketoconazole, norfloxacin, ofloxacin, and rofecoxib. CYP2D6 inhibitors may increase the levels/effects of propranolol; example inhibitors include chlorpromazine, delavirdine, fluoxetine, miconazole, paroxetine, pergolide, quinidine, quinine, ritonavir, and ropinirole. The heart rate-lowering effects of propranolol are additive with other drugs which slow AV conduction (digoxin, verapamil, diltiazem). Reserpine increases the effects of propranolol. Concurrent use of propranolol may increase the effects of alpha-blockers (prazosin, terazosin), alpha-adrenergic stimulants (epinephrine, phenylephrine), and the vasoconstrictive effects of ergot alkaloids. Propranolol may mask the tachycardia from hypoglycemia caused by insulin and oral hypoglycemics. In patients receiving concurrent therapy, the risk of hypertensive (Continued)

Propranolol *(Continued)*

crisis is increased when either clonidine or the beta-blocker is withdrawn. Beta-blockers may increase the action or levels of ethanol, disopyramide, nondepolarizing muscle relaxants, and theophylline although the effects are difficult to predict. Propranolol may increase the bioavailability of serotonin 5-HT$_{1D}$ receptor agonists. Propranolol may decrease the metabolism of lidocaine.

Beta-blocker effects may be enhanced by oral contraceptives, flecainide, haloperidol (hypotensive effects), cimetidine, hydralazine, phenothiazines, propafenone, thyroid hormones (when hypothyroid patient is converted to euthyroid state). Beta-blockers may increase the effect/toxicity of flecainide, haloperidol (hypotensive effects), hydralazine, phenothiazines, acetaminophen, anticoagulants (warfarin), and benzodiazepines.

Nutritional/Ethanol Interactions

Ethanol: Ethanol may decrease plasma levels of propranolol by increasing metabolism.

Food: Propranolol serum levels may be increased if taken with food. Protein-rich foods may increase bioavailability; a change in diet from high carbohydrate/low protein to low carbohydrate/high protein may result in increased oral clearance.

Cigarette: Smoking may decrease plasma levels of propranolol by increasing metabolism.

Herb/Nutraceutical: Avoid dong quai if using for hypertension (has estrogenic activity). Avoid ephedra, yohimbe, ginseng (may worsen hypertension or arrhythmia). Avoid natural licorice (causes sodium and water retention and increases potassium loss). Avoid garlic (may have increased antihypertensive effect).

Lab Interactions Increased thyroxine (S)

Adverse Reactions Frequency not defined.

Cardiovascular: Bradycardia, CHF, reduced peripheral circulation, chest pain, hypotension, impaired myocardial contractility, worsening of AV conduction disturbance, cardiogenic shock, Raynaud's syndrome, mesenteric thrombosis (rare)

Central nervous system: Mental depression, lightheadedness, amnesia, emotional lability, confusion, hallucinations, dizziness, insomnia, fatigue, vivid dreams, lethargy, cold extremities, vertigo, syncope, cognitive dysfunction, psychosis, hypersomnolence

Dermatologic: Alopecia, contact dermatitis, eczematous eruptions, erythema multiforme, exfoliative dermatitis, hyperkeratosis, nail changes, pruritus, psoriasiform eruptions, rash, ulcerative lichenoid, urticaria, Stevens-Johnson syndrome, toxic epidermal necrolysis

Endocrine & metabolic: Hypoglycemia, hyperglycemia, hyperlipidemia, hyperkalemia

Gastrointestinal: Diarrhea, nausea, vomiting, stomach discomfort, constipation, anorexia

Genitourinary: Impotence, proteinuria (rare), oliguria (rare), interstitial nephritis (rare), Peyronie's disease

Hematologic: Agranulocytosis, thrombocytopenia, thrombocytopenic purpura

Neuromuscular & skeletal: Weakness, carpal tunnel syndrome (rare), paresthesia, myotonus, polyarthritis, arthropathy

Ocular: Hyperemia of the conjunctiva, decreased tear production, decreased visual acuity, mydriasis

Respiratory: Wheezing, pharyngitis, bronchospasm, pulmonary edema, respiratory distress, laryngospasm

Miscellaneous: Lupus-like syndrome (rare), anaphylactic/anaphylactoid allergic reaction

Overdosage/Toxicology Symptoms of intoxication include cardiac disturbances, CNS toxicity, bronchospasm, hypoglycemia, and hyperkalemia. The most common cardiac symptoms include hypotension and bradycardia. Atrioventricular block, intraventricular conduction disturbances, cardiogenic shock, and asystole may occur with severe overdose, especially with membrane-depressant drugs (eg, propranolol). CNS effects include convulsions and coma. Respiratory arrest is commonly seen with propranolol and other membrane-depressant and lipid-soluble drugs. Treatment is symptom-directed and supportive.

Pharmacodynamics/Kinetics

Onset of Action: Beta-blockade: Oral: 1-2 hours

Duration of Action: ~6 hours

Protein Binding: Newborns: 68%; Adults: 93%

Half-Life Elimination: Neonates and Infants: Possible increased half-life; Children: 3.9-6.4 hours; Adults: 4-6 hours

Metabolism: Hepatic to active and inactive compounds; extensive first-pass effect

Excretion: Urine (96% to 99%)

Available Dosage Forms

Capsule, extended release, as hydrochloride (InnoPran XL™): 80 mg, 120 mg

Capsule, sustained release, as hydrochloride (Inderal® LA): 60 mg, 80 mg, 120 mg, 160 mg

Injection, solution, as hydrochloride (Inderal®): 1 mg/mL (1 mL)

Solution, oral, as hydrochloride: 4 mg/mL (5 mL, 500 mL); 8 mg/mL (500 mL) [strawberry-mint flavor; contains alcohol 0.6%]

Tablet, as hydrochloride (Inderal®): 10 mg, 20 mg, 40 mg, 60 mg, 80 mg

Dosing

Adults:

Akathisia: Oral: 30-120 mg/day in 2-3 divided doses

Angina: Oral: 80-320 mg/day in doses divided 2-4 times/day

Long-acting formulation: Initial: 80 mg once daily; maximum dose: 320 mg once daily

Essential tremor: Oral: 20-40 mg twice daily initially; maintenance doses: usually 120-320 mg/day

Hypertension: Initial: 40 mg twice daily; increase dosage every 3-7 days; usual dose: ≤320 mg divided in 2-3 doses/day; maximum dose: 640 mg; usual dosage range (JNC 7): 40-160 mg/day in 2 divided doses

Long-acting formulation: Initial: 80 mg once daily; usual maintenance: 120-160 mg once daily; maximum daily dose: 640 mg; usual dosage range (JNC 7): 60-180 mg/day once daily

Hypertrophic subaortic stenosis: Oral: 20-40 mg 3-4 times/day

Long-acting formulation: 80-160 mg once daily

Migraine headache prophylaxis: Oral: Initial: 80 mg/day divided every 6-8 hours; increase by 20-40 mg/dose every 3-4 weeks to a maximum of 160-240 mg/day given in divided doses every 6-8 hours; if satisfactory response not achieved within 6 weeks of starting therapy, drug should be withdrawn gradually over several weeks

Long-acting formulation: Initial: 80 mg once daily; effective dose range: 160-240 mg once daily

Myocardial infarction prophylaxis: Oral: 180-240 mg/day in 3-4 divided doses

Pheochromocytoma: Oral: 30-60 mg/day in divided doses

Tachyarrhythmias:

Oral: 10-30 mg/dose every 6-8 hours

I.V. (in patients having nonfunctional GI tract): 1 mg/dose slow IVP; repeat every 5 minutes up to a total of 5 mg; titrate initial dose to desired response

Thyrotoxicosis:

Oral: 10-40 mg/dose every 6 hours

I.V.: 1-3 mg/dose slow IVP as a single dose

Elderly: Tachyarrhythmias: Initial: 10 mg twice daily; increase dosage every 3-7 days; usual dose range: 10-320 mg given 1-2 times/day. Refer to adult dosing for additional uses.

Pediatrics:

Hypertension:

Oral: Initial: 0.5-1 mg/kg/day in divided doses every 6-12 hours; increase gradually every 5-7 days; maximum: 16 mg/kg/24 hours

I.V.: 0.01-0.05 mg/kg over 1 hour; maximum dose: 10 mg

Migraine headache prophylaxis: Oral: Initial: 2-4 mg/kg/day **or**

≤35 kg: 10-20 mg 3 times/day

>35 kg: 20-40 mg 3 times/day

Tachyarrhythmias:

Oral: Initial: 0.5-1 mg/kg/day in divided doses every 6-8 hours; titrate dosage upward every 3-7 days; usual dose: 2-6 mg/kg/day; higher doses may be needed; do not exceed 16 mg/kg/day or 60 mg/day

I.V.: 0.01-0.1 mg/kg/dose slow IVP over 10 minutes; maximum dose: 1 mg for infants; 3 mg for children

Tetralogy spells:

Oral: Palliation: Initial: 1 mg/kg/day every 6 hours; if ineffective, may increase dose after 1 week by 1 mg/kg/day to a maximum of 5 mg/kg/day, if patient becomes refractory, may increase slowly to a maximum of 10-15 mg/kg/day. Allow 24 hours between dosing changes.

I.V.: 0.01-0.2 mg/kg/dose infused over 10 minutes; maximum initial dose: 1 mg

Thyrotoxicosis: Oral:

2 mg/kg/day, divided every 6-8 hours, titrate to effective dose

Adolescents: Refer to adult dosing.

Renal Impairment:

Not dialyzable (0% to 5%); supplemental dose is not necessary.

Peritoneal dialysis effects: Supplemental dose is not necessary.

Hepatic Impairment: Marked slowing of heart rate may occur in cirrhosis with conventional doses; low initial dose and regular heart rate monitoring.

Administration

Oral: Do not crush long-acting forms.

I.V.: I.V. dose is much smaller than oral dose. When administered acutely for cardiac treatment, monitor ECG and blood pressure. May administer by rapid infusion (I.V. push) at a rate of 1 mg/minute or by slow infusion over ~30 minutes. Necessary monitoring for surgical patients who are unable to take oral beta-blockers (prolonged ileus) has not been defined. Some institutions require monitoring of baseline and postinfusion heart rate and blood pressure when a patient's response to beta-blockade has not been characterized (ie, the patient's initial dose or following a change in dose). Consult individual institutional policies and procedures.

I.V. Detail: pH: 2.8-3.5

Stability

Compatibility: Stable in $D_5{}^1\!/_2NS$, D_5NS, D_5W, LR, $^1\!/_2NS$, NS

Y-site administration: Incompatible with amphotericin B cholesteryl sulfate complex, diazoxide

Compatibility in syringe: Incompatible with HCO_3

Compatibility when admixed: Incompatible with HCO_3

Storage: Protect injection from light. Solutions have maximum stability at pH of 3 and decompose rapidly in alkaline pH. Propranolol is stable for 24 hours at room temperature in D_5W or NS.

Nursing Actions

Physical Assessment: Assess effectiveness and interactions of other medications patient may be taking. Monitor therapeutic response and adverse reactions (cardiac status, vital signs, fluid status) when starting or adjusting dosage. I.V. infusion requires hemodynamic monitoring. Monitor serum glucose closely in patients with diabetes. Beta-blockers may alter serum glucose levels. Use and teach orthostatic precautions. Assess knowledge/teach patient appropriate use, interventions to reduce side effects, and adverse symptoms to report.

Patient Education: Take exactly as directed; do not increase, decrease, or discontinue without consulting prescriber. Tablets may be crushed and taken with liquids. Do not chew or crush long-acting forms; take whole. Take at the same time each day. Do not alter dietary intake of protein or carbohydrates without consulting prescriber. You may experience orthostatic hypotension, dizziness, drowsiness, or blurred vision (use caution when driving, climbing stairs, or changing position - rising from sitting or lying to standing; or engaging in tasks requiring alertness until response to drug is known); nausea, vomiting, or stomach discomfort (small frequent meals, frequent mouth care, chewing gum, or sucking lozenges may help); or decreased sexual ability (reversible). If you have diabetes, monitor serum glucose closely. Report unusual swelling of extremities, respiratory difficulty, unresolved cough, unusual weight gain, cold extremities, persistent diarrhea, confusion, hallucinations, headache, nervousness, lack of improvement, or worsening of condition. **Pregnancy/breast-feeding precautions:** Inform prescriber if you are or intend to become pregnant. Consult prescriber if breast-feeding.

Dietary Considerations Tablets should be taken on an empty stomach; capsules may be taken with or without food, but should always be taken consistently (with food or on an empty stomach)

Geriatric Considerations Since bioavailability increased in the elderly, about twofold geriatric patients may require lower maintenance doses, therefore, as serum and tissue concentrations increase beta$_1$ selectivity diminishes; due to alterations in the beta-adrenergic autonomic nervous system, beta-adrenergic blockade may result in less hemodynamic response than seen in younger adults.

Breast-Feeding Issues Propranolol is excreted in breast milk and is considered compatible by the AAP. It is recommended that the infant be monitored for signs or symptoms of beta-blockade (hypotension, bradycardia, etc) with long-term use.

Pregnancy Issues Propranolol crosses the placenta. Beta-blockers have been associated with bradycardia, hypotension, and IUGR. IUGR is probably related to maternal hypertension. Available evidence suggests beta-blockers are generally safe during pregnancy (JNC 7). Cases of neonatal hypoglycemia have been reported following maternal use of beta-blockers at parturition or during breast-feeding. Monitor breast-fed infant for symptoms of beta-blockade.

Propranolol and Hydrochlorothiazide

(proe PRAN oh lole & hye droe klor oh THYE a zide)

U.S. Brand Names Inderide®

Synonyms Hydrochlorothiazide and Propranolol

Pharmacologic Category Antihypertensive Agent, Combination

Pregnancy Risk Factor C

Lactation Enters breast milk/compatible

Use Management of hypertension

Available Dosage Forms [DSC] = Discontinued product

Tablet: Propranolol hydrochloride 40 mg and hydrochlorothiazide 25 mg; propranolol hydrochloride 80 mg and hydrochlorothiazide 25 mg

Inderide®:

40/25: Propranolol hydrochloride 40 mg and hydrochlorothiazide 25 mg

(Continued)

Propranolol and Hydrochlorothiazide

(Continued)

80/25: Propranolol hydrochloride 80 mg and hydrochlorothiazide 25 mg [DSC]

Dosing

Adults & Elderly:

Hypertension: Oral: Dose is individualized; typical dosages of **hydrochlorothiazide:** 12.5-50 mg/day; initial dose of **propranolol** 80 mg/day

Note: Daily dose of tablet form should be divided into 2 daily doses; may be used to maximum dosage of up to 160 mg of propranolol; higher dosages would result in higher than optimal thiazide dosages.

Nursing Actions

Physical Assessment: See individual agents.

Patient Education: See individual agents. **Pregnancy precaution:** Inform prescriber if you are or intend to become pregnant.

Related Information

Hydrochlorothiazide *on page 610*

Propranolol *on page 1041*

Propylthiouracil (proe pil thye oh YOOR a sil)

Synonyms PTU (error-prone abbreviation)

Pharmacologic Category Antithyroid Agent

Medication Safety Issues

Sound-alike/look-alike issues:

Propylthiouracil may be confused with Purinethol®

PTU is an error-prone abbreviation (mistaken as mercaptopurine [Purinethol®; 6-MP])

Pregnancy Risk Factor D

Lactation Enters breast milk/use caution (AAP rates "compatible")

Use Palliative treatment of hyperthyroidism as an adjunct to ameliorate hyperthyroidism in preparation for surgical treatment or radioactive iodine therapy; management of thyrotoxic crisis

Mechanism of Action/Effect Inhibits the synthesis of thyroid hormones by blocking the oxidation of iodine in the thyroid gland; blocks synthesis of thyroxine and triiodothyronine

Contraindications Hypersensitivity to propylthiouracil or any component of the formulation; pregnancy

Warnings/Precautions Use with caution in patients >40 years of age because PTU may cause hypoprothrombinemia and bleeding. Use with extreme caution in patients receiving other drugs known to cause agranulocytosis; may cause agranulocytosis, thyroid hyperplasia, thyroid carcinoma (usage >1 year). Discontinue in the presence of agranulocytosis, aplastic anemia, ANCA-positive vasculitis, hepatitis, unexplained fever, or exfoliative dermatitis. Safety and efficacy have not been established in children <6 years of age.

Drug Interactions

Decreased Effect: Oral anticoagulant activity is increased only until metabolic effect stabilizes. Anticoagulants may be potentiated by antivitamin K effect of propylthiouracil. Correction of hyperthyroidism may alter disposition of beta-blockers, digoxin, and theophylline, necessitating a dose reduction of these agents.

Increased Effect/Toxicity: Propylthiouracil may increase the anticoagulant activity of warfarin.

Nutritional/Ethanol Interactions Food: Propylthiouracil serum levels may be altered if taken with food.

Adverse Reactions Frequency not defined.

Cardiovascular: Edema, cutaneous vasculitis, leukocytoclastic vasculitis, ANCA-positive vasculitis

Central nervous system: Fever, drowsiness, vertigo, headache, drug fever, dizziness, neuritis

Dermatologic: Skin rash, urticaria, pruritus, exfoliative dermatitis, alopecia, erythema nodosum

Endocrine & metabolic: Goiter, weight gain, swollen salivary glands

Gastrointestinal: Nausea, vomiting, loss of taste perception, stomach pain, constipation

Hematologic: Leukopenia, agranulocytosis, thrombocytopenia, bleeding, aplastic anemia

Hepatic: Cholestatic jaundice, hepatitis

Neuromuscular & skeletal: Arthralgia, paresthesia

Renal: Nephritis, glomerulonephritis, acute renal failure

Respiratory: Interstitial pneumonitis, alveolar hemorrhage

Miscellaneous: SLE-like syndrome

Overdosage/Toxicology Symptoms of overdose include nausea, vomiting, epigastric pain, headache, fever, arthralgia, pruritus, edema, pancytopenia, epigastric distress, headache, fever, CNS stimulation, or depression. Treatment is supportive. Monitor bone marrow response. Forced diuresis, dialysis, and charcoal hemoperfusion have been used to enhance elimination.

Pharmacodynamics/Kinetics

Onset of Action: Therapeutic: 24-36 hours; Peak effect: Remission: 4 months of continued therapy

Duration of Action: 2-3 hours

Time to Peak: Serum: ~1 hour

Protein Binding: 75% to 80%

Half-Life Elimination: 1.5-5 hours; End-stage renal disease: 8.5 hours

Metabolism: Hepatic

Excretion: Urine (35%)

Available Dosage Forms Tablet: 50 mg

Dosing

Adults:

Hyperthyroidism: Oral: Initial: 300-450 mg/day in divided doses every 8 hours (severe hyperthyroidism may require 600-1200 mg/day); maintenance: 100-150 mg/day in divided doses every 8-12 hours

Note: Administer in 3 equally divided doses at approximately 8-hour intervals. Adjust dosage to maintain T_3, T_4, and TSH levels in normal range; elevated T_3 may be sole indicator of inadequate treatment. Elevated TSH indicates excessive antithyroid treatment.

Elderly: Use lower dose recommendations; adjust for renal impairment.

Initial: 150-300 mg/day in divided doses every 8 hours

Maintenance: 100-150 mg/day in divided doses every 8-12 hours

Pediatrics:

Hyperthyroidism: Oral: Children: Initial: 5-7 mg/kg/day **or** 150-200 mg/m²/day in divided doses every 8 hours **or**

6-10 years: 50-150 mg/day

>10 years: 150-300 mg/day

Maintenance: Determined by patient response **or** $^1/_3$ to $^2/_3$ of the initial dose in divided doses every 8-12 hours. This usually begins after 2 months on an effective initial dose.

Note: Administer in 3 equally divided doses at approximately 8-hour intervals. Adjust dosage to maintain T_3, T_4, and TSH levels in normal range; elevated T_3 may be sole indicator of inadequate treatment. Elevated TSH indicates excessive antithyroid treatment.

Renal Impairment:

Cl_{cr} 10-50 mL/minute: Administer 75% of normal dose.

Cl_{cr} <10 mL/minute: Administer 50% of normal dose.

Laboratory Monitoring CBC with differential, prothrombin time, liver and thyroid function (T_4, T_3, TSH); periodic blood counts are recommended for chronic therapy.

Nursing Actions

Physical Assessment: Assess potential for interactions with other pharmacological agents and herbal products patient may be taking (eg, anticoagulant activity increased). Monitor laboratory tests, therapeutic effectiveness according to use, and adverse response (eg, rash, goiter, nausea, vomiting, leucopenia, agranulocytosis, anemia, jaundice, arthralgia, CNS stimulation or depression). Teach patient proper use, possible side effects/appropriate interventions, and adverse symptoms to report.

Patient Education: Take as directed, at the same time each day at around-the-clock intervals; at the same time in relation to meals, either always with meals or always between meals. Do not miss doses or make up missed doses. This drug may need to be taken for an extended period of time to achieve appropriate results and you may need periodic blood tests to assess effectiveness of therapy. May cause nausea or vomiting (small, frequent meals may help); constipation (increased exercise, fluids, fruit, or fiber may help); or dizziness or drowsiness (use caution when driving or engaging in tasks that require alertness until response to drug is known). Report rash, skin eruptions, or loss of hair; fever; unusual bleeding or bruising; unusual weight gain (>5 lb/week); unresolved headache or fever; yellowing of eyes or skin; changes in color of urine or feces; or joint or muscle pain or weakness. **Pregnancy/breast-feeding precautions:** Inform prescriber if you are pregnant. Do not get pregnant while taking this medication. Consult prescriber for appropriate contraceptive measures. Consult prescriber if breast-feeding.

Dietary Considerations Administer at the same time in relation to meals each day, either always with meals or always between meals.

Geriatric Considerations The use of antithyroid thioamides is as effective in the elderly as they are in younger adults; however, the expense, potential adverse effects, and inconvenience (compliance, monitoring) make them undesirable. The use of radioiodine, due to ease of administration and less concern for long-term side effects and reproduction problems, makes it a more appropriate therapy.

Pregnancy Issues Crosses the placenta and may induce goiter and hypothyroidism in the developing fetus (cretinism). May need to monitor infant's thyroid function periodically.

Additional Information Preferred over methimazole in thyroid storm due to inhibition of peripheral conversion as well as synthesis of thyroid hormone.

Protamine Sulfate (PROE ta meen SUL fate)

Pharmacologic Category Antidote

Medication Safety Issues
Sound-alike/look-alike issues:
Protamine may be confused with ProAmatine®, protamine, Protopam®, Protropin®

Pregnancy Risk Factor C

Lactation Excretion in breast milk unknown

Use Treatment of heparin overdosage; neutralize heparin during surgery or dialysis procedures

Unlabeled/Investigational Use Treatment of low molecular weight heparin (LMWH) overdose

Mechanism of Action/Effect Combines with strongly acidic heparin to form a stable complex (salt) neutralizing the anticoagulant activity of both drugs

Contraindications Hypersensitivity to protamine or any component of the formulation

Warnings/Precautions For I.V. use only. May not be totally effective in some patients following cardiac surgery despite adequate doses. May cause hypersensitivity reaction in patients with a history of allergy to fish (have epinephrine 1:1000 available) and in patients sensitized to protamine (via protamine zinc insulin). Rapid administration can cause severe hypotensive and anaphylactoid-like reactions. Heparin rebound associated with anticoagulation and bleeding has been reported to occur occasionally. Symptoms typically occur 8-9 hours after protamine administration, but may occur as long as 18 hours later.

Adverse Reactions Frequency not defined.
Cardiovascular: Sudden fall in blood pressure, bradycardia, flushing, hypotension
Central nervous system: Lassitude
Gastrointestinal: Nausea, vomiting
Hematologic: Hemorrhage
Respiratory: Dyspnea, pulmonary hypertension
Miscellaneous: Hypersensitivity reactions

Overdosage/Toxicology Symptoms of overdose include hypertension. May cause hemorrhage. Doses exceeding 100 mg may cause paradoxical anticoagulation.

Pharmacodynamics/Kinetics
Duration of Action: Onset of action: I.V.: Heparin neutralization: ~5 minutes

Available Dosage Forms Injection, solution, as sulfate [preservative free]: 10 mg/mL (5 mL, 25 mL)

Dosing
Adults & Elderly:
Heparin neutralization: I.V.: Protamine dosage is determined by the dosage of heparin; 1 mg of protamine neutralizes 90 USP units of heparin (lung) and 115 USP units of heparin (intestinal); maximum dose: 50 mg

Heparin overdosage, following intravenous administration: I.V.: Since blood heparin concentrations decrease rapidly **after** administration, adjust the protamine dosage depending upon the duration of time since heparin administration as follows: See table.

Time Elapsed	Dose of Protamine (mg) to Neutralize 100 units of Heparin
Immediate	1-1.5
30-60 min	0.5-0.75
>2 h	0.25-0.375

Heparin overdosage, following SubQ injection: I.V.: 1-1.5 mg protamine per 100 units heparin; this may be done by a portion of the dose (eg, 25-50 mg) given slowly I.V. followed by the remaining portion as a continuous infusion over 8-16 hours (the expected absorption time of the SubQ heparin dose)

LMWH overdose (unlabeled use):
Enoxaparin: 1 mg protamine for each mg of enoxaparin; if PTT prolonged 2-4 hours after first dose, consider additional dose of 0.5 mg for each mg of enoxaparin.
Dalteparin or tinzaparin: 1 mg protamine for each 100 anti-Xa int. units of dalteparin or tinzaparin; if PTT prolonged 2-4 hours after first dose, consider additional dose of 0.5 mg for each 100 anti-Xa int. units of dalteparin or tinzaparin.
Note: Antifactor Xa activity never completely neutralized (maximum: ~60% to 75%). Excessive protamine doses may worsen bleeding potential.

Pediatrics: Refer to adult dosing.

Administration
I.V.: For I.V. use only. Administer slow IVP (50 mg over 10 minutes). Rapid I.V. infusion causes hypotension. Reconstitute vial with 5 mL sterile water. Resulting solution equals 10 mg/mL. Inject without further dilution over 1-3 minutes; maximum of 50 mg in any 10-minute period.

I.V. Detail: pH: 6-7

Stability
Reconstitution: Reconstitute vial with 5 mL sterile water; if using protamine in neonates, reconstitute

(Continued)

Protamine Sulfate *(Continued)*

with preservative-free sterile water for injection; resulting solution equals 10 mg/mL.

Compatibility: Stable in D₅W, NS

   Compatibility in syringe: Incompatible with diatrizoate meglumine 52%, diatrizoate sodium 8%, diatrizoate sodium 60%, ioxaglate meglumine 39.3%, ioxaglate sodium 19.6%

   Compatibility when admixed: Incompatible with cephalosporins, penicillins

Storage: Refrigerate; avoid freezing. Remains stable for at least 2 weeks at room temperature; preservative-free formulation does not require refrigeration.

Laboratory Monitoring Coagulation test, aPTT or ACT

Nursing Actions

Physical Assessment: Monitor effectiveness of therapy by monitoring laboratory tests frequently during therapy. Monitor closely for adverse response (eg, sudden hemodynamic changes). Assess knowledge/teach patient possible side effects and adverse symptoms to report.

Patient Education: Report any respiratory difficulty, rash or flushing, feeling of warmth, tingling or numbness, dizziness, or disorientation. **Pregnancy/breast-feeding precautions:** Inform prescriber if you are pregnant. Consult prescriber if breast-feeding.

Protriptyline *(proe TRIP ti leen)*

U.S. Brand Names Vivactil®

Synonyms Protriptyline Hydrochloride

Restrictions A medication guide concerning the use of antidepressants in children and teenagers can be found on the FDA website at http://www.fda.gov/cder/Offices/ODS/labeling.htm. It should be dispensed to parents or guardians of children and teenagers receiving this medication.

Pharmacologic Category Antidepressant, Tricyclic (Secondary Amine)

Pregnancy Risk Factor C

Lactation Excretion in breast milk unknown/not recommended

Use Treatment of depression

Mechanism of Action/Effect Increases the synaptic concentration of serotonin and/or norepinephrine in the central nervous system by inhibition of their reuptake by the presynaptic neuronal membrane

Contraindications Hypersensitivity to protriptyline (cross-reactivity to other cyclic antidepressants may occur) or any component of the formulation; use of MAO inhibitors within 14 days; use of cisapride; use in a patient during the acute recovery phase of MI

Warnings/Precautions Antidepressants increase the risk of suicidal thinking and behavior in children and adolescents with major depressive disorder (MDD) and other depressive disorders; consider risk prior to prescribing. All patients must be closely monitored for clinical worsening, suicidality, or unusual changes in behavior, especially during the initiation of therapy or following an increase or decrease in dosage. When used in children, the child's family or caregiver should be instructed to closely observe the patient and communicate condition with healthcare provider. A medication guide should be dispensed with each prescription. **Protriptyline is FDA approved for the treatment of depression in adolescents.**

The possibility of a suicide attempt is inherent in major depression and may persist until remission occurs. Use caution in high-risk patients. Worsening depression and severe abrupt suicidality that are not part of the presenting symptoms may require discontinuation or modification of drug therapy. The patient's family or caregiver should be alerted to monitor patients for the emergence of suicidality and associated behaviors (such as agitation, irritability, hostility, impulsivity, and hypomania) and call healthcare provider.

May worsen psychosis in some patients or precipitate a shift to mania or hypomania in patients with bipolar disorder. Patients presenting with depressive symptoms should be screened for bipolar disorder. Monotherapy in patients with bipolar disorder should be avoided. **Protriptyline is not FDA approved for the treatment of bipolar depression.**

Although the degree of sedation is low relative to other antidepressant agents, protriptyline may cause sedation, resulting in impaired performance of tasks requiring alertness (eg, operating machinery or driving). Sedative effects may be additive with other CNS depressants and/or ethanol. Protriptyline may aggravate aggressive behavior. Consider discontinuing, when possible, prior to elective surgery. Therapy should not be abruptly discontinued in patients receiving high doses for prolonged periods. May alter glucose regulation - use with caution in patients with diabetes.

May cause orthostatic hypotension or conduction abnormalities (risks are moderate relative to other antidepressants). Use with caution in patients with a history of cardiovascular disease (including previous MI, stroke, tachycardia, or conduction abnormalities). The degree of anticholinergic blockade produced by this agent is moderate relative to other cyclic antidepressants, however, caution should still be used in patients with urinary retention, benign prostatic hyperplasia, narrow-angle glaucoma, xerostomia, visual problems, constipation, or history of bowel obstruction.

Use caution in patients with a previous seizure disorder or condition predisposing to seizures such as brain damage, alcoholism, or concurrent therapy with other drugs which lower the seizure threshold. May increase the risks associated with electroconvulsive therapy. Use with caution in hyperthyroid patients or those receiving thyroid supplementation. Use with caution in patients with hepatic or renal dysfunction and in elderly patients.

Drug Interactions

Cytochrome P450 Effect: Substrate of CYP2D6 (major)

Decreased Effect: Carbamazepine, phenobarbital, and rifampin may increase the metabolism of protriptyline, decreasing its effects. Protriptyline inhibits the antihypertensive response to bethanidine, clonidine, debrisoquin, guanadrel, guanethidine, guanabenz, guanfacine. Cimetidine and methylphenidate may decrease the metabolism of protriptyline. Cholestyramine and colestipol may bind TCAs and reduce their absorption.

Increased Effect/Toxicity: Protriptyline increases the effects of amphetamines, anticholinergics, other CNS depressants (sedatives, hypnotics, or ethanol), chlorpropamide, tolazamide, and warfarin. When used with MAO inhibitors, hyperpyrexia, hypertension, tachycardia, confusion, seizures, and **deaths have been reported** (serotonin syndrome). The SSRIs (to varying degrees), cimetidine, grapefruit juice, indinavir, methylphenidate, ritonavir, quinidine, diltiazem, and verapamil inhibit the metabolism of TCAs. Levels/effects of protriptyline may be increased by chlorpromazine, delavirdine, fluoxetine, miconazole, paroxetine, pergolide, quinidine, quinine, ritonavir, ropinirole, and other CYP2D6 inhibitors. Use of lithium with a TCA may increase the risk for neurotoxicity. Phenothiazines may increase concentration of some TCAs and TCAs may increase concentration of phenothiazines. Pressor response to I.V. epinephrine, norepinephrine, and phenylephrine may be enhanced in patients receiving TCAs (**Note:** Effect is unlikely with epinephrine or levonordefrin dosages typically administered as infiltration in combination with local anesthetics). Combined use of beta-agonists or drugs which prolong QT$_c$ (including quinidine, procainamide, disopyramide, cisapride, sparfloxacin, gatifloxacin, moxifloxacin) with TCAs may predispose patients to cardiac arrhythmias.

Nutritional/Ethanol Interactions

Ethanol: Avoid ethanol (may increase CNS depression).

Food: Grapefruit juice may inhibit the metabolism of some TCAs and clinical toxicity may result.

Herb/Nutraceutical: Avoid valerian, St John's wort, SAMe, kava kava (may increase risk of serotonin syndrome and/or excessive sedation).

Lab Interactions Increased glucose

Adverse Reactions Frequency not defined.

Cardiovascular: Arrhythmias, hyper-/hypotension, MI, stroke, heart block, tachycardia, palpitation

Central nervous system: Dizziness, drowsiness, headache, confusion, delirium, hallucinations, restlessness, insomnia, nightmares, fatigue, delusions, anxiety, agitation, hypomania, exacerbation of psychosis, panic, seizure, incoordination, ataxia, EPS

Dermatologic: Alopecia, photosensitivity, rash, petechiae, urticaria, itching

Endocrine & metabolic: Breast enlargement, galactorrhea, SIADH, gynecomastia, increased or decreased libido

Gastrointestinal: Xerostomia, constipation, unpleasant taste, weight gain/loss, increased appetite, nausea, diarrhea, heartburn, vomiting, anorexia, trouble with gums, decreased lower esophageal sphincter tone may cause GE reflux

Genitourinary: Difficult urination, impotence, testicular edema

Hematologic: Agranulocytosis, leukopenia, eosinophilia, thrombocytopenia, purpura

Hepatic: Cholestatic jaundice, increased liver enzymes

Neuromuscular & skeletal: Fine muscle tremor, weakness, tremor, numbness, tingling

Ocular: Blurred vision, eye pain, increased intraocular pressure

Otic: Tinnitus

Miscellaneous: Diaphoresis (excessive), allergic reactions

Overdosage/Toxicology Symptoms of overdose include confusion, hallucinations, urinary retention, hypotension, tachycardia, seizures, and hyperthermia. Following initiation of essential overdose management, toxic symptoms should be treated. Ventricular arrhythmias often respond to systemic alkalinization (sodium bicarbonate 0.5-2 mEq/kg I.V.) Physostigmine (1-2 mg I.V. slowly for adults) may be indicated for reversing life-threatening cardiac arrhythmias.

Pharmacodynamics/Kinetics

Time to Peak: Serum: 24-30 hours

Protein Binding: 92%

Half-Life Elimination: 54-92 hours (average: 74 hours)

Metabolism: Extensively hepatic via N-oxidation, hydroxylation, and glucuronidation; first-pass effect (10% to 25%)

Excretion: Urine

Available Dosage Forms Tablet, as hydrochloride: 5 mg, 10 mg

Dosing

Adults: Depression: Oral: 15-60 mg in 3-4 divided doses

Elderly: Oral: Initial: 5-10 mg/day; increase every 3-7 days by 5-10 mg; usual dose: 15-20 mg/day

Pediatrics: Depression: Oral: Adolescents: 15-20 mg/day

Nursing Actions

Physical Assessment: Assess potential for interactions with other prescriptions, OTC medications, or herbal products patient may be taking (see extensive list of Drug Interactions). Assess for suicidal tendencies before beginning therapy. May cause physiological or psychological dependence, tolerance, or

abuse; periodically evaluate need for continued use. Assess therapeutic response (mental status, mood, affect) and adverse reactions (eg, suicidal ideation) at beginning of therapy and periodically with long-term use. Dosage should be tapered slowly when discontinuing (allow 3-4 weeks between discontinuing this medication and starting another antidepressant). Caution patients with diabetes to monitor glucose levels closely; may increase or decrease serum glucose levels. Teach patient appropriate use, interventions to reduce side effects, and adverse symptoms to report.

Patient Education: Do not take any new medication during therapy unless approved by prescriber. Take exactly as directed; take once-a-day dose at bedtime. Do not increase dose or frequency; may take 2-3 weeks to achieve desired results. This drug may cause physical and/or psychological dependence. Avoid alcohol and grapefruit juice. Maintain adequate hydration (2-3 L/day of fluids) unless instructed to restrict fluid intake. May cause drowsiness, lightheadedness, impaired coordination, dizziness, or blurred vision (use caution when driving or engaging in tasks requiring alertness until response to drug is known); nausea, vomiting, loss of appetite, or disturbed taste (small frequent meals, good mouth care, chewing gum, or sucking lozenges may help); constipation (increased exercise, fluids, fruit, or fiber may help); urinary retention (void before taking medication); postural hypotension (use caution climbing stairs or when changing position from lying or sitting to standing); altered sexual drive or ability (reversible); or photosensitivity (use sunscreen, wear protective clothing and eyewear, and avoid direct sunlight). Report chest pain, palpitations, or rapid heartbeat; persistent adverse CNS effects (eg, suicidal ideation, nervousness, restlessness, insomnia, anxiety, excitation, headache, agitation, impaired coordination, changes in cognition); muscle cramping, weakness, tremors, or rigidity; blurred vision or eye pain; breast enlargement or swelling; yellowing of skin or eyes; or worsening of condition. **Pregnancy/breast-feeding precautions:** Inform prescriber if you are or intend to become pregnant. Breast-feeding is not recommended.

Dietary Considerations May be taken with food to decrease GI distress.

Geriatric Considerations Little data on use in the elderly. Strong anticholinergic properties which may limit protriptyline's use; more often stimulating rather than sedating effects.

Related Information

Antidepressant Medication Guidelines *on page 1414*

Federal OBRA Regulations Recommended Maximum Doses *on page 1421*

Pseudoephedrine (soo doe e FED rin)

U.S. Brand Names Biofed [OTC]; Contact® Cold [OTC]; Dimetapp® 12-Hour Non-Drowsy Extentabs® [OTC]; Dimetapp® Decongestant Infant [OTC]; ElixSure™ Congestion [OTC]; Genaphed® [OTC]; Kidkare Decongestant [OTC]; Kodet SE [OTC]; Oranyl [OTC]; PediaCare® Decongestant Infants [OTC]; Silfedrine Children's [OTC]; Simply Stuffy™ [OTC]; Sudafed® [OTC]; Sudafed® 12 Hour [OTC]; Sudafed® 24 Hour [OTC]; Sudafed® Children's [OTC]; Sudodrin [OTC]; SudoGest [OTC]; Sudo-Tab® [OTC]

Synonyms *d*-Isoephedrine Hydrochloride; Pseudoephedrine Hydrochloride; Pseudoephedrine Sulfate
(Continued)

Pseudoephedrine *(Continued)*

Pharmacologic Category Alpha/Beta Agonist

Medication Safety Issues
Sound-alike/look-alike issues:
Dimetapp® may be confused with Dermatop®, Dimetabs®, Dimetane®
Sudafed® may be confused with Sufenta®

Pregnancy Risk Factor C

Lactation Enters breast milk/use caution (AAP rates "compatible")

Use Temporary symptomatic relief of nasal congestion due to common cold, upper respiratory allergies, and sinusitis; also promotes nasal or sinus drainage

Mechanism of Action/Effect Directly stimulates alpha-adrenergic receptors of respiratory mucosa causing vasoconstriction; directly stimulates beta-adrenergic receptors causing bronchial relaxation, increased heart rate and contractility

Contraindications Hypersensitivity to pseudoephedrine or any component of the formulation; with or within 14 days of MAO inhibitor therapy

Warnings/Precautions Use with caution in patients >60 years of age. Administer with caution to patients with hypertension, hyperthyroidism, diabetes mellitus, cardiovascular disease, ischemic heart disease, increased intraocular pressure, or prostatic hyperplasia. Elderly patients are more likely to experience adverse reactions to sympathomimetics. Overdosage may cause hallucinations, seizures, CNS depression, and death. When used for self-medication (OTC), notify prescriber if symptoms do not improve within 7 days or are accompanied by fever.

Drug Interactions
Decreased Effect: Decreased effect of methyldopa, reserpine.
Increased Effect/Toxicity: MAO inhibitors may increase blood pressure effects of pseudoephedrine. Sympathomimetic agents may increase toxicity.

Nutritional/Ethanol Interactions
Food: Onset of effect may be delayed if pseudoephedrine is taken with food.
Herb/Nutraceutical: Avoid ephedra, yohimbe (may cause hypertension).

Lab Interactions Interferes with urine detection of amphetamine (false-positive)

Adverse Reactions Frequency not defined.
Cardiovascular: Tachycardia, palpitation, arrhythmia
Central nervous system: Nervousness, transient stimulation, insomnia, excitability, dizziness, drowsiness, convulsions, hallucinations, headache
Gastrointestinal: Nausea, vomiting
Genitourinary: Dysuria
Neuromuscular & skeletal: Weakness, tremor
Respiratory: Dyspnea
Miscellaneous: Diaphoresis

Overdosage/Toxicology Symptoms of overdose include seizures, nausea, vomiting, cardiac arrhythmias, hypertension, agitation, hallucinations, and death. There is no specific antidote for pseudoephedrine intoxication. Treatment is primarily supportive.

Pharmacodynamics/Kinetics
Onset of Action: Decongestant: Oral: 15-30 minutes
Duration of Action: Immediate release tablet: 4-6 hours; Extended release: ≤12 hours
Half-Life Elimination: 9-16 hours
Metabolism: Partially hepatic
Excretion: Urine (70% to 90% as unchanged drug, 1% to 6% as active norpseudoephedrine); dependent on urine pH and flow rate; alkaline urine decreases renal elimination of pseudoephedrine

Available Dosage Forms
Caplet, extended release, as hydrochloride (Contact® Cold, Sudafed® 12 Hour): 120 mg
Liquid, as hydrochloride: 30 mg/5 mL (120 mL, 480 mL)

Silfedrine Children's: 15 mg/5 mL (120 mL, 480 mL) [alcohol and sugar free; grape flavor]
Simply Stuffy™: 15 mg/5 mL (120 mL) [alcohol free; contains sodium benzoate; cherry berry flavor]
Sudafed® Children's: 15 mg/5 mL (120 mL) [alcohol and sugar free; contains sodium benzoate; grape flavor]
Liquid, oral drops, as hydrochloride:
Dimetapp® Decongestant Infant Drops: 7.5 mg/0.8 mL (15 mL) [alcohol free; contains sodium benzoate; grape flavor]
Kidkare Decongestant: 7.5 mg/0.8 mL (30 mL) [alcohol free; contains benzoic acid and sodium benzoate; cherry flavor]
PediaCare® Decongestant: 7.5 mg/0.8 mL (15 mL) [alcohol free, dye free; contains benzoic acid, sodium benzoate; fruit flavor]
Syrup, as hydrochloride:
Biofed: 30 mg/5 mL (120 mL, 240 mL, 480 mL, 3840 mL) [alcohol free; contains sodium benzoate]
ElixSure™ Congestion: 15 mg/5 mL (120 mL) [grape bubble gum flavor]
Tablet, as hydrochloride: 30 mg, 60 mg
Genaphed®, Kodet SE, Oranyl, Sudafed®, Sudodrin, Sudo-Tab®: 30 mg
SudoGest: 30 mg, 60 mg
Tablet, chewable, as hydrochloride (Sudafed® Children's): 15 mg [sugar free; contains phenylalanine 0.78 mg/tablet; orange flavor]
Tablet, extended release, as hydrochloride:
Dimetapp® 12-Hour Non-Drowsy Extentabs®: 120 mg
Sudafed® 24 Hour: 240 mg

Dosing
Adults: Nasal congestion: Oral: 30-60 mg every 4-6 hours, sustained release: 120 mg every 12 hours; maximum: 240 mg/24 hours
Elderly: Nasal congestion: 30-60 mg every 6 hours as needed
Pediatrics: Nasal congestion: Oral: General dosing guidelines:
<2 years: 4 mg/kg/day in divided doses every 6 hours
2-5 years: 15 mg every 4-6 hours; maximum: 60 mg/24 hours
6-12 years: 30 mg every 4-6 hours; maximum: 120 mg/24 hours
Renal Impairment: Reduce dose.

Administration
Oral: Do not crush extended release drug product, swallow whole.

Nursing Actions
Physical Assessment: Assess effectiveness and interactions of other medications patient may be taking. Monitor effectiveness of therapy (relief of cough, lung sounds, and respiratory pattern) and adverse reactions (eg, cardiac and CNS changes) at beginning of therapy and periodically with long-term use. Assess knowledge/teach patient appropriate use, interventions to reduce side effects, and adverse symptoms to report.

Patient Education: Take only as prescribed; do not exceed prescribed dose or frequency. Do not chew or crush timed release forms. Maintain adequate hydration (2-3 L/day of fluids) unless instructed to restrict fluid intake. You may experience nervousness, insomnia, dizziness, or drowsiness (use caution when driving or engaging in tasks requiring alertness until response to drug is known). Report persistent CNS changes (dizziness, tremor, agitation, or convulsions); respiratory difficulty; chest pain, palpitations, or rapid heartbeat; muscle tremor; or lack of improvement or worsening of condition. **Pregnancy/breast-feeding precautions:** Inform prescriber if you are or intend to become pregnant. Consult prescriber if breast-feeding.

Dietary Considerations Should be taken with water or milk to decrease GI distress.

Geriatric Considerations Elderly patients should be counseled about the proper use of over-the-counter cough and cold preparations. Elderly are more predisposed to adverse effects of sympathomimetics since they frequently have cardiovascular diseases and diabetes mellitus as well as multiple drug therapies. It may be advisable to treat with a short-acting/immediate-release formulation before initiating sustained-release/long-acting formulations.

Pseudoephedrine, Hydrocodone, and Chlorpheniramine
(soo doe e FED rin, hye droe KOE done, & klor fen IR a meen)

U.S. Brand Names Coldcough HC; Cordron-HC; Detuss; Histinex® PV; Hydron PSC; Hydro-Tussin™ HC; Hyphed; Pediatex™ HC; P-V-Tussin® Syrup; Q-V Tussin; Tussend® Syrup; Tussend® Tablet

Synonyms Chlorpheniramine, Pseudoephedrine, and Hydrocodone; Hydrocodone, Chlorpheniramine, and Pseudoephedrine; Pseudoephedrine Hydrochloride, Hydrocodone Bitartrate, and Chlorpheniramine Maleate

Restrictions C-III

Pharmacologic Category Antihistamine; Antihistamine/Decongestant/Antitussive; Antitussive; Decongestant

Pregnancy Risk Factor C

Lactation Enters breast milk/contraindicated

Use Temporary relief of cough, congestion, and sneezing due to colds, respiratory infections, or hay fever

Available Dosage Forms
Liquid:
Cordron-HC: Pseudoephedrine hydrochloride 20 mg, hydrocodone bitartrate 1.67 mg, and chlorpheniramine maleate 2.5 mg per 5 mL (480 mL) [vanilla mint flavor]
Detuss: Pseudoephedrine hydrochloride 30 mg, hydrocodone bitartrate 5 mg, and chlorpheniramine maleate 2 mg per 5 mL (480 mL) [alcohol free; vanilla flavor]
Hydron PSC: Pseudoephedrine hydrochloride 30 mg, hydrocodone bitartrate 5 mg, and chlorpheniramine maleate 2 mg per 5 mL (480 mL) [vanilla flavor]
Pediatex™ HC: Pseudoephedrine hydrochloride 20 mg, hydrocodone bitartrate 1.67 mg, and chlorpheniramine maleate 2.5 mg per 5 mL (480 mL) [alcohol free, sugar free; vanilla mint flavor]
Syrup:
Coldcough HC: Pseudoephedrine hydrochloride 15 mg, hydrocodone bitartrate 3 mg, and chlorpheniramine maleate 2 mg per 5 mL (480 mL) [alcohol free, dye free, sugar free; grape flavor]
Histinex® PV: Pseudoephedrine hydrochloride 30 mg, hydrocodone bitartrate 2.5 mg, and chlorpheniramine maleate 2 mg per 5 mL (480 mL) [alcohol free, sugar free; apricot flavor]
Hydro-Tussin™ HC: Pseudoephedrine hydrochloride 15 mg, hydrocodone bitartrate 3 mg, and chlorpheniramine maleate 2 mg per 5 mL (480 mL) [alcohol free, dye free, sugar free]
Hyphed: Pseudoephedrine hydrochloride 30 mg, hydrocodone bitartrate 2.5 mg, and chlorpheniramine maleate 2 mg per 5 mL (480 mL) [contains alcohol 5%; raspberry flavor]
P-V-Tussin®, Q-V Tussin, Tussend®: Pseudoephedrine hydrochloride 30 mg, hydrocodone bitartrate 2.5 mg, and chlorpheniramine maleate 2 mg per 5 mL (480 mL) [contains alcohol 5%; banana flavor]
Tablet [scored] (Tussend®): Pseudoephedrine hydrochloride 60 mg, hydrocodone bitartrate 5 mg, and chlorpheniramine maleate 4 mg

Dosing
Adults: Cough and congestion: Oral:
Histinex® PV, Pediatex™ HC, P-V-Tussin®, Tussend®: 10 mL or 1 tablet every 4-6 hours; do not exceed 4 doses in 24 hours
Hydro-Tussin™ HC: 5-10 mL or 1 tablet every 4-6 hours; do not exceed 4 doses in 24 hours
Pediatrics: Cough and congestion: Oral: Children:
2-6 years:
Hydro-Tussin™ HC: 1.25-2.5 mL every 4-6 hours; do not exceed 4 doses in 24 hours
Histinex® PV, Pediatex™ HC, P-V-Tussin®: 2.5 mL every 4-6 hours; do not exceed 4 doses in 24 hours
6-12 years:
Histinex® PV, Pediatex™ HC, P-V-Tussin®, Tussend®: 5 mL or ½ tablet every 4-6 hours; do not exceed 4 doses in 24 hours
Hydro-Tussin™ HC: 2.5-5 mL or ½ tablet every 4-6 hours; do not exceed 4 doses in 24 hours
>12 years: Refer to adult dosing.

Nursing Actions
Physical Assessment: See individual agents.
Related Information
Pseudoephedrine on page 1047

Psyllium (SIL i yum)

U.S. Brand Names Fiberall®; Fibro-Lax [OTC]; Fibro-XL [OTC]; Genfiber® [OTC]; Hydrocil® Instant [OTC]; Konsyl® [OTC]; Konsyl-D® [OTC]; Konsyl® Easy Mix [OTC]; Konsyl® Orange [OTC]; Metamucil® [OTC]; Metamucil® Plus Calcium [OTC]; Metamucil® Smooth Texture [OTC]; Modane® Bulk [OTC]; Natural Fiber Therapy [OTC]; Reguloid® [OTC]; Serutan® [OTC]

Synonyms Plantago Seed; Plantain Seed; Psyllium Hydrophilic Mucilloid

Pharmacologic Category Antidiarrheal; Laxative, Bulk-Producing

Medication Safety Issues
Sound-alike/look-alike issues:
Fiberall® may be confused with Feverall®
Hydrocil® may be confused with Hydrocet®
Modane® may be confused with Matulane®, Moban®
Perdiem® may be confused with Pyridium®

Pregnancy Risk Factor B

Lactation Excretion in breast milk unknown/compatible

Use Treatment of chronic atonic or spastic constipation and in constipation associated with rectal disorders; management of irritable bowel syndrome; labeled for OTC use as fiber supplement, treatment of constipation

Mechanism of Action/Effect Adsorbs water in the intestine to form a viscous liquid which promotes peristalsis and reduces transit time

Contraindications Hypersensitivity to psyllium or any component of the formulation; fecal impaction; GI obstruction

Warnings/Precautions Products must be taken with adequate fluid. Use with caution in patients with esophageal strictures, ulcers, stenosis, or intestinal adhesions. Elderly may have insufficient fluid intake which may predispose them to fecal impaction and bowel obstruction.

Drug Interactions
Decreased Effect: Decreased effect of warfarin, digitalis, potassium-sparing diuretics, salicylates, tetracyclines, nitrofurantoin when taken together. Separate administration times to reduce potential for drug-drug interaction.

Adverse Reactions Frequency not defined.
Gastrointestinal: Esophageal or bowel obstruction, diarrhea, constipation, abdominal cramps
Respiratory: Bronchospasm
(Continued)

Psyllium *(Continued)*

Miscellaneous: Anaphylaxis upon inhalation in susceptible individuals, rhinoconjunctivitis

Overdosage/Toxicology Symptoms of overdose include abdominal pain, diarrhea, and constipation.

Pharmacodynamics/Kinetics
Onset of Action: 12-24 hours; Peak effect: 2-3 days

Available Dosage Forms
Capsule:
Fibro XL: 675 mg
Metamucil®: 0.52 g [contains potassium 5 mg/capsule; provides 3 g dietary fiber 2.4 g per 6 capsules]
Metamucil® Plus Calcium: 0.42 g [contains potassium 6 mg/capsule; provides dietary fiber 2.1 g and calcium 300 mg per 5 capsules]
Granules (Serutan®): 2.5 g/teaspoon (510 g) [contains sodium benzoate]
Powder: 3.4 g/dose (390 g, 570 g)
Bulk-K: 4.725 g/dose (392 g)
Fiberall®: 3.5 g/dose (454 g) [sugar free; contains phenylalanine; orange flavor]
Fibro-Lax: 4.725 g /dose (140 g, 392g)
Genfiber®: 3.4 g/dose (397 g, 595 g) [regular flavor]
Genfiber®: 3.5 g/dose (283 g) [sugar free; orange flavor]
Hydrocil® Instant: 3.5 g/dose (3.7 g unit-dose packets, 300 g) [sugar free]
Konsyl®: 6 g/dose (6 g unit-dose packets, 300 g, 450 g) [sugar free; contains sodium 4.1 mg/dose; regular flavor]
Konsyl-D®: 3.4 g/dose (6.5 g unit-dose packets, 325 g, 397 g, 500 g) [contains sodium 2.3 mg/dose and dextrose]
Konsyl® Easy Mix: 6 g/dose (6 g unit-dose packets, 250 g) [sugar free; contains sodium 4.4 mg/dose]
Konsyl® Orange: 3.4 g/dose (12 g unit-dose packets, 538 g) [contains sodium 2.3 mg/dose and sucrose; orange flavor]
Konsyl® Orange: 3.4 g/dose (425 g) [sugar free; contains sodium 2.3 mg/dose; orange flavor]
Metamucil®: 3.4 g/dose:
(390 g, 570 g, 870 g) [contains sodium 3 mg and potassium 30 mg per dose; regular flavor]
(570 g, 870 g, 1254 g) [contains sodium 5 mg and potassium 30 mg per dose; orange flavor]
Metamucil® Smooth Texture: 3.4 g/dose:
(unit-dose packets, 609 g, 912 g, 1446 g) [contains sodium 5 mg and potassium 30 mg per dose; orange flavor]
(300 g, 450 g, 690 g) [contains sodium 4 mg and potassium 30 mg per dose; regular flavor]
(unit-dose packets, 183 g, 300 g, 450 g, 699 g, 1104 g) [sugar free; contains phenylalanine 25 mg, sodium 5 mg, and potassium 30 mg per dose; orange flavor]
Modane® Bulk: 3.4 g/dose (390 g) [contains dextrose; flavor free]
Natural Fiber Therapy: 3.4 g/dose (369 g, 539 g) [natural and orange flavors]
Reguloid®: 3.4 g/dose (300 g, 450 g) [sugar free; regular or orange flavors]; (390 g, 570g) [regular or orange flavors]
Wafers (Metamucil®): 3.4 g/dose (24s) [one dose = 2 wafers; contains sodium 20 mg and potassium 60 mg per dose; apple crisp and cinnamon spice flavors]

Dosing
Adults & Elderly:
Constipation, IBS: Oral (administer at least 2 hours before or after other drugs): Take 1 dose up to 3 times/day; all doses should be followed with 8 oz of water or liquid
Capsule: 4 capsules/dose (range: 2-6); swallow capsules one at a time

Powder: 1 rounded tablespoonful/dose (1 teaspoonful/dose for many sugar free or select concentrated products) mixed in 8 oz liquid
Tablet: 1 tablet/dose
Wafer: 2 wafers/dose

Pediatrics:
Constipation: Oral (administer at least 2 hours before or after other drugs):
Children 6-11 years: Approximately ½ adult dosage
Children ≥12 years: Refer to adult dosing.

Administration
Oral: Inhalation of psyllium dust may cause sensitivity to psyllium (eg, runny nose, watery eyes, wheezing). Drink a full glass of liquid with each dose. Powder must be mixed in a glass of water or juice. Separate dose from other drug therapies.

Nursing Actions
Physical Assessment: Teach patient proper use (according to formulation), possible side effects/appropriate interventions, and adverse symptoms to report.
Patient Education: Take as directed. Granules/powder: Mix in large glass of water or juice (8 oz or more) and drink immediately. Maintain adequate hydration (2-3 L/day of fluids), unless instructed to restrict fluid intake. Mix carefully; do not inhale powder. Separate this medication from other medications by at least 1 hour. Results may begin in 12 hours; full results may take 2-3 days. Do not increase dose. Report persistent constipation; watery diarrhea; difficulty, pain, or choking with swallowing; respiratory difficulty; or unusual coughing.
Dietary Considerations Products should be taken with large amount of fluids. Some products contain aspartame, dextrose, or sucrose, as well as additional ingredients. Check individual product information for caloric and nutritional value.
Fiberall® (sugar free formulation) contains phenylalanine.
Metamucil® Smooth Texture (sugar free formulation) contains phenylalanine 25 mg per teaspoonful.
Geriatric Considerations Elderly may have insufficient fluid intake which may predispose them to fecal impaction and bowel obstruction. Patients should have a 1 month trial, with at least 14 g/day, before effects in bowel function are determined. Bloating and flatulence are mostly a problem in first 4 weeks of therapy.

Pyrazinamide *(peer a ZIN a mide)*

Synonyms Pyrazinoic Acid Amide
Pharmacologic Category Antitubercular Agent
Pregnancy Risk Factor C
Lactation Enters breast milk/use caution
Use Adjunctive treatment of tuberculosis in combination with other antituberculosis agents
Mechanism of Action/Effect Converted to pyrazinoic acid in susceptible strains of *Mycobacterium* which lowers the pH of the environment; bacteriostatic or bactericidal depending on the drug's concentration at the site of infection
Contraindications Hypersensitivity to pyrazinamide or any component of the formulation; acute gout; severe hepatic damage
Warnings/Precautions Administer with at least one other effective agent for tuberculosis; use with caution in patients with renal failure, chronic gout, diabetes mellitus, or porphyria. Use with caution in patients receiving concurrent medications associated with hepatotoxicity (particularly with rifampin), or in patients with a history of alcoholism (even if ethanol consumption is discontinued during therapy).

Drug Interactions

Increased Effect/Toxicity: Combination therapy with rifampin and pyrazinamide has been associated with severe and fatal hepatotoxic reactions.

Lab Interactions Reacts with Acetest® and Ketostix® to produce pinkish-brown color.

Adverse Reactions 1% to 10%:
Central nervous system: Malaise
Gastrointestinal: Nausea, vomiting, anorexia
Neuromuscular & skeletal: Arthralgia, myalgia

Overdosage/Toxicology Symptoms of overdose include gout, gastric upset, and hepatic damage (mild). Treatment is supportive.

Pharmacodynamics/Kinetics

Time to Peak: Serum: Within 2 hours
Protein Binding: 50%
Half-Life Elimination: 9-10 hours
Metabolism: Hepatic
Excretion: Urine (4% as unchanged drug)

Pharmacokinetic Note Bacteriostatic or bactericidal depending on drug's concentration at infection site.

Available Dosage Forms Tablet: 500 mg

Dosing

Adults:

Tuberculosis treatment: Oral (dosing is based on lean body weight):
Daily therapy: 15-30 mg/kg/day
40-55 kg: 1000 mg
56-75 kg: 1500 mg
76-90 kg: 2000 mg (maximum dose regardless of weight)
Twice weekly directly observed therapy (DOT): 50 mg/kg
40-55 kg: 2000 mg
56-75 kg: 3000 mg
76-90 kg: 4000 mg (maximum dose regardless of weight)
Three times/week DOT: 25-30 mg/kg (maximum: 2.5 g)
40-55 kg: 1500 mg
56-75 kg: 2500 mg
76-90 kg: 3000 mg (maximum dose regardless of weight)

Note: Used as part of a multidrug regimen. Treatment regimens consist of an initial 2-month phase, followed by a continuation phase of 4 or 7 additional months; frequency of dosing may differ depending on phase of therapy.

Elderly: Start with a lower daily dose (15 mg/kg) and increase as tolerated.

Pediatrics:

Tuberculosis treatment: Oral:
Daily therapy: 15-30 mg/kg/day (maximum: 2 g/day)
Twice weekly directly observed therapy (DOT): 50 mg/kg/dose (maximum: 4 g/dose)
See "Note" in adult dosing.

Renal Impairment:
Cl$_{cr}$ <50 mL/minute: Avoid use or reduce dose to 12-20 mg/kg/day.
Avoid use in hemo- and peritoneal dialysis as well as continuous arteriovenous or venovenous hemofiltration.

Hepatic Impairment: Reduce dose.

Laboratory Monitoring Periodic liver function, serum uric acid, sputum culture, chest x-ray 2-3 months into treatment and at completion

Nursing Actions

Physical Assessment: Assess patient history for use cautions and evaluate any history of alcohol intake prior to beginning treatment. Assess for potential interactions with pharmacological or herbal products patient is taking (especially anything associated with hepatotoxicity). Monitor laboratory tests and chest x-ray regularly, therapeutic effectiveness, and adverse reactions. Teach patient proper use and necessity of scheduled laboratory tests, possible side effects/appropriate interventions, and adverse symptoms to report.

Patient Education: Take as directed, with food. It is imperative to take for full length of therapy; do not miss doses and do not discontinue without consulting prescriber. You will need regular medical follow-up and laboratory tests while taking this medication. May cause nausea or loss of appetite (small, frequent meals, frequent mouth care, sucking lozenges, or chewing gum may help). Report change in color of urine, pale stools, easy bruising or bleeding, blood in urine or difficulty urinating, yellowing of skin or eyes, extreme joint pain, unusual fever, or unresolved nausea or vomiting. **Pregnancy precaution:** Inform prescriber if you are or intend to become pregnant.

Geriatric Considerations Pyrazinamide is used in the 2-month intensive treatment phase of a 6-month treatment plan. Most elderly acquired their *Mycobacterium tuberculosis* infection before effective chemotherapy was available; however, older persons with new infections (not reactivation), or who are from areas where drug-resistant *M. tuberculosis* is endemic, or who are HIV-infected should receive 3-4 drug therapies including pyrazinamide.

Pyridostigmine (peer id oh STIG meen)

U.S. Brand Names Mestinon®; Mestinon® Timespan®; Regonol®

Synonyms Pyridostigmine Bromide

Pharmacologic Category Acetylcholinesterase Inhibitor

Medication Safety Issues
Sound-alike/look-alike issues:
Pyridostigmine may be confused with physostigmine
Mestinon® may be confused with Metatensin®
Regonol® may be confused with Reglan®, Renagel®

Pregnancy Risk Factor B

Lactation Enters breast milk/compatible

Use Symptomatic treatment of myasthenia gravis; antidote for nondepolarizing neuromuscular blockers
Military use: Pretreatment for Soman nerve gas exposure

Mechanism of Action/Effect Inhibits destruction of acetylcholine by acetylcholinesterase which facilitates transmission of impulses across myoneural junction

Contraindications Hypersensitivity to pyridostigmine, bromides, or any component of the formulation; GI or GU obstruction

Warnings/Precautions Use with caution in patients with epilepsy, asthma, bradycardia, hyperthyroidism, cardiac arrhythmias, or peptic ulcer. Use with caution in renal impairment (lower dosages may be required). Adequate facilities should be available for cardiopulmonary resuscitation when testing and adjusting dose for myasthenia gravis. Have atropine and epinephrine ready to treat hypersensitivity reactions. Overdosage may result in cholinergic crisis, this must be distinguished from myasthenic crisis. Anticholinesterase insensitivity can develop for brief or prolonged periods. Safety and efficacy in pediatric patients have not been established. Regonol® injection contains 1% benzyl alcohol as the preservative (not intended for use in newborns).

Drug Interactions

Decreased Effect: Neuromuscular blockade reversal effect of pyridostigmine may be decreased by aminoglycosides, quinolones, tetracyclines, bacitracin, colistin, polymyxin B, sodium colistimethate, quinidine, elevated serum magnesium concentrations.

Increased Effect/Toxicity: Increased effect of depolarizing neuromuscular blockers (succinylcholine). Increased toxicity with edrophonium. Increased bradycardia/hypotension with beta-blockers.

(Continued)

Pyridostigmine (Continued)

Lab Interactions Increased aminotransferase [ALT (SGPT)/AST (SGOT)] (S), amylase (S)

Adverse Reactions Frequency not defined.

Cardiovascular: Arrhythmias (especially bradycardia), hypotension, decreased carbon monoxide, tachycardia, AV block, nodal rhythm, nonspecific ECG changes, cardiac arrest, syncope, flushing

Central nervous system: Convulsions, dysarthria, dysphonia, dizziness, loss of consciousness, drowsiness, headache

Dermatologic: Skin rash, thrombophlebitis (I.V.), urticaria

Gastrointestinal: Hyperperistalsis, nausea, vomiting, salivation, diarrhea, stomach cramps, dysphagia, flatulence, abdominal pain

Genitourinary: Urinary urgency

Neuromuscular & skeletal: Weakness, fasciculations, muscle cramps, spasms, arthralgia, myalgia

Ocular: Small pupils, lacrimation, amblyopia

Respiratory: Increased bronchial secretions, laryngospasm, bronchiolar constriction, respiratory muscle paralysis, dyspnea, respiratory depression, respiratory arrest, bronchospasm

Miscellaneous: Diaphoresis (increased), anaphylaxis, allergic reactions

Overdosage/Toxicology Symptoms of overdose include muscle weakness, blurred vision, excessive sweating, tearing and salivation, nausea, vomiting, diarrhea, hypertension, bradycardia, and paralysis. Atropine is the treatment of choice for intoxications manifesting significant muscarinic symptoms. Atropine I.V. 2-4 mg every 3-60 minutes should be repeated to control symptoms and then continued as needed for 1-2 days following acute ingestion. Monitor cardiac function and support ventilation.

Pharmacodynamics/Kinetics

Onset of Action: Oral, I.M.: 15-30 minutes; I.V. injection: 2-5 minutes

Duration of Action: Oral: Up to 6-8 hours (due to slow absorption); I.V.: 2-3 hours

Half-Life Elimination: 1-2 hours; Renal failure: ≤6 hours

Metabolism: Hepatic

Excretion: Urine (80% to 90% as unchanged drug)

Available Dosage Forms

Injection, solution, as bromide:

Mestinon®: 5 mg/mL (2 mL)

Regonol®: 5 mg/mL (2 mL) [contains benzyl alcohol]

Syrup, as bromide (Mestinon®): 60 mg/5 mL (480 mL) [raspberry flavor; contains alcohol 5%, sodium benzoate]

Tablet, as bromide (Mestinon®): 60 mg

Tablet, sustained release, as bromide (Mestinon® Timespan®): 180 mg

Dosing

Adults & Elderly:

Myasthenia gravis:

Oral: Highly individualized dosing ranges: 60-1500 mg/day, usually 600 mg/day divided into 5-6 doses, spaced to provide maximum relief

Sustained release formulation: Highly individualized dosing ranges: 180-540 mg once or twice daily (doses separated by at least 6 hours); **Note:** Most clinicians reserve sustained release dosage form for bedtime dose only.

I.M. or slow I.V. Push: To supplement oral dosage pre- and postoperatively during labor and postpartum, during myasthenic crisis, or when oral therapy is impractical): ~1/30th of oral dose; observe patient closely for cholinergic reactions

I.V. infusion: To supplement oral dosage pre- and postoperatively, during labor and postpartum, during myasthenic crisis, or when oral therapy is

impractical): Initial: 2 mg/hour with gradual titration in increments of 0.5-1 mg/hour, up to a maximum rate of 4 mg/hour

Pretreatment for Soman nerve gas exposure (military use): Oral: 30 mg every 8 hours beginning several hours prior to exposure; discontinue at first sign of nerve agent exposure, then begin atropine and pralidoxime

Reversal of nondepolarizing muscle relaxants: I.V.: 0.1-0.25 mg/kg/dose; 10-20 mg is usually sufficient (full recovery usually occurs ≤15 minutes, but ≥30 minutes may be required).

Note: Atropine sulfate (0.6-1.2 mg) I.V. immediately prior to pyridostigmine to minimize side effects:

Pediatrics:

Myasthenia gravis:

Oral: Children: 7 mg/kg/24 hours divided into 5-6 doses. Most clinicians reserve sustained release dosage form for bedtime dose only.

I.M., slow I.V. push: Children: 0.05-0.15 mg/kg/dose

Reversal of nondepolarizing muscle relaxants: I.V.: Children: Dosing range: 0.1-0.25 mg/kg/dose (full recovery usually occurs ≤15 minutes, but ≥30 minutes may be required).

Note: Atropine sulfate (0.6-1.2 mg) I.V. immediately prior to pyridostigmine to minimize side effects:

Renal Impairment: Lower dosages may be required due to prolonged elimination; no specific recommendations have been published.

Administration

Oral: Do **not** crush sustained release tablet.

I.V. Detail: pH: 5

Stability

Storage:

Injection: Protect from light.

Tablet:

30 mg: Store under refrigeration at 2°C to 8°C (36°F to 46°F) and protect from light. Stable at room temperature for up to 3 months.

Mestinon®: Store at 25°C (77°F). Protect from moisture.

Nursing Actions

Physical Assessment: When used to reverse neuromuscular block (anesthesia or excessive acetylcholine), monitor patient safety until full return of neuromuscular functioning. Assess bladder and sphincter adequacy prior to administering medication. Monitor therapeutic effectiveness and adverse reactions (eg, cholinergic crisis - **DUMBELS** - **d**iarrhea, **u**rination, **m**iosis, **b**ronchospasm/bradycardia, **e**xcitability, **l**acrimation, and **s**alivation/excessive sweating). Assess knowledge/teach patient appropriate use (self injections, oral), interventions to reduce side effects, and adverse symptoms to report.

Patient Education: This drug will not cure myasthenia gravis, but may help reduce symptoms. Use as directed; do not increase dose or discontinue without consulting prescriber. Take extended release tablets at bedtime; do not chew or crush extended release tablets. Maintain adequate hydration (2-3 L/day of fluids) unless instructed to restrict fluid intake. May cause dizziness, drowsiness, or hypotension (rise slowly from sitting or lying position and use caution when driving or climbing stairs); vomiting or loss of appetite (small frequent meals, frequent mouth care, chewing gum, or sucking lozenges may help); or diarrhea (boiled milk, yogurt, or buttermilk may help). Report persistent abdominal discomfort; significantly increased salivation, sweating, tearing, or urination; flushed skin; chest pain or palpitations; acute headache; unresolved diarrhea; excessive fatigue, insomnia, dizziness, or depression; increased muscle, joint, or body pain; vision changes or blurred vision; or shortness of breath or wheezing.

Geriatric Considerations See Warnings/Precautions and Adverse Reactions.

Breast-Feeding Issues Neonates of myasthenia gravis mothers may have difficulty in sucking and swallowing (as well as breathing). Neonatal pyridostigmine may be indicated by symptoms (confirmed by edrophonium test).

Pregnancy Issues Safety has not been established for use during pregnancy. The potential benefit to the mother should outweigh the potential risk to the fetus. When pyridostigmine is needed in myasthenic mothers, giving dose parenterally 1 hour before completion of the second stage of labor may facilitate delivery and protect the neonate during the immediate postnatal state.

Pyridoxine (peer i DOKS een)

U.S. Brand Names Aminoxin® [OTC]
Synonyms Pyridoxine Hydrochloride; Vitamin B$_6$
Pharmacologic Category Vitamin, Water Soluble
Medication Safety Issues
Sound-alike/look-alike issues:
Pyridoxine may be confused with paroxetine, pralidoxime, Pyridium®
Pregnancy Risk Factor A/C (dose exceeding RDA recommendation)
Lactation Enters breast milk/compatible
Use Prevention and treatment of vitamin B$_6$ deficiency, pyridoxine-dependent seizures in infants; adjunct to treatment of acute toxicity from isoniazid, cycloserine, or hydrazine overdose
Mechanism of Action/Effect Precursor to pyridoxal, which functions in the metabolism of proteins, carbohydrates, and fats; pyridoxal also aids in the release of liver and muscle-stored glycogen and in the synthesis of GABA (within the central nervous system) and heme
Contraindications Hypersensitivity to pyridoxine or any component of the formulation
Warnings/Precautions Dependence and withdrawal may occur with doses >200 mg/day.
Drug Interactions
Decreased Effect: Pyridoxine may decrease serum levels of levodopa, phenobarbital, and phenytoin (patients taking levodopa without carbidopa should avoid supplemental vitamin B$_6$ >5 mg per day, which includes multivitamin preparations).
Lab Interactions Urobilinogen
Adverse Reactions Frequency not defined.
Central nervous system: Headache, seizure (following very large I.V. doses), sensory neuropathy
Endocrine & metabolic: Decreased serum folic acid secretions
Gastrointestinal: Nausea
Hepatic: Increased AST
Neuromuscular & skeletal: Paresthesia
Miscellaneous: Allergic reactions
Overdosage/Toxicology Symptoms of overdose include ataxia and sensory neuropathy with doses of 50 mg to 2 g daily over prolonged periods.
Pharmacodynamics/Kinetics
Half-Life Elimination: 15-20 days
Metabolism: Via 4-pyridoxic acid (active form) and other metabolites
Excretion: Urine
Available Dosage Forms
Capsule, as hydrochloride: 250 mg
Injection, solution, as hydrochloride: 100 mg/mL (1 mL)
Tablet, as hydrochloride: 25 mg, 50 mg, 100 mg, 200 mg, 250 mg, 500 mg
Tablet, enteric coated, as hydrochloride (Aminoxin®): 20 mg
Dosing
Adults & Elderly:
Recommended daily allowance (RDA):
Male: 1.7-2.0 mg

Female: 1.4-1.6 mg
Dietary deficiency: Oral: 10-20 mg/day for 3 weeks
Drug-induced neuritis (eg, isoniazid, hydralazine, penicillamine, cycloserine): Oral:
Treatment: 100-200 mg/24 hours
Prophylaxis: 25-100 mg/24 hours
Treatment of seizures and/or coma from acute isoniazid toxicity: A dose of pyridoxine hydrochloride equal to the amount of INH ingested can be given I.M./I.V. in divided doses together with other anticonvulsants; if the amount INH ingested is not known, administer 5 g I.V. pyridoxine.
Treatment of acute hydrazine toxicity: A pyridoxine dose of 25 mg/kg in divided doses I.M./I.V. has been used.
Pediatrics:
Recommended daily allowance (RDA):
1-3 years: 0.9 mg
4-6 years: 1.3 mg
7-10 years: 1.6 mg
Pyridoxine-dependent Infants:
Oral: 2-100 mg/day
I.M., I.V., SubQ: 10-100 mg
Dietary deficiency: Oral: Children: 5-25 mg/24 hours for 3 weeks, then 1.5-2.5 mg/day in multiple vitamin product
Drug-induced neuritis (eg, isoniazid, hydralazine, penicillamine, cycloserine): Oral: Children:
Treatment: 10-50 mg/24 hours
Prophylaxis: 1-2 mg/kg/24 hours
Treatment of seizures and/or coma from acute isoniazid toxicity: A dose of pyridoxine hydrochloride equal to the amount of INH ingested can be given I.M./I.V. in divided doses together with other anticonvulsants. If the amount INH ingested is not known, administer 5 g I.V. pyridoxine.
Treatment of acute hydrazine toxicity: A pyridoxine dose of 25 mg/kg in divided doses I.M./I.V. has been used.
Administration
I.M.: Burning may occur at the injection site after I.M. or SubQ administration.
I.V.: Seizures have occurred following I.V. administration of very large doses.
I.V. Detail: pH: 2.0-3.8
Stability
Compatibility: Stable in fat emulsion 10%
Storage: Protect from light.
Nursing Actions
Physical Assessment: Assess effectiveness and interactions of other medications patient may be taking. Monitor effectiveness of therapy and adverse effects at beginning of therapy and regularly with long-term use. Assess knowledge/teach patient appropriate use, dietary instructions, interventions to reduce side effects, and adverse symptoms to report.

Patient Education: Take exactly as directed. Do not take more than recommended. Do not exceed recommended intake of dietary B$_6$ (eg, red meat, bananas, potatoes, yeast, lima beans, and whole grain cereals). You may experience burning or pain at injection site; notify prescriber if this persists. **Pregnancy precaution:** Inform prescriber if you are pregnant.

Geriatric Considerations Use with caution in patients with Parkinson's disease treated with levodopa.

Breast-Feeding Issues Crosses into breast milk; possible inhibition of lactation at doses >600 mg/day. AAP considers **compatible** with breast-feeding.

Pyrimethamine (peer i METH a meen)

U.S. Brand Names Daraprim®

Pharmacologic Category Antimalarial Agent

Medication Safety Issues

Sound-alike/look-alike issues:

Daraprim® may be confused with Dantrium®, Daranide®

Pregnancy Risk Factor C

Lactation Enters breast milk/not recommended (AAP rates "compatible")

Use Prophylaxis of malaria due to susceptible strains of plasmodia; used in conjunction with quinine and sulfadiazine for the treatment of uncomplicated attacks of chloroquine-resistant *P. falciparum* malaria; used in conjunction with fast-acting schizonticide to initiate transmission control and suppression cure; synergistic combination with sulfonamide in treatment of toxoplasmosis

Mechanism of Action/Effect Inhibits parasitic dihydrofolate reductase, resulting in inhibition of vital tetrahydrofolic acid synthesis

Contraindications Hypersensitivity to pyrimethamine or any component of the formulation; chloroguanide; resistant malaria; megaloblastic anemia secondary to folate deficiency

Warnings/Precautions When used for more than 3-4 days, it may be advisable to give leucovorin to prevent hematologic complications. Use with caution in patients with impaired renal or hepatic function or with possible G6PD. Use caution in patients with seizure disorders or possible folate deficiency (eg, malabsorption syndrome, pregnancy, alcoholism).

Drug Interactions

Cytochrome P450 Effect: Inhibits CYP2C8/9 (moderate), 2D6 (moderate)

Decreased Effect: Pyrimethamine may decrease the levels/effects of CYP2D6 prodrug substrates (eg, codeine, hydrocodone, oxycodone, tramadol).

Increased Effect/Toxicity: Serum levels of antipsychotic agents may be increased by pyrimethamine. Sulfonamides (synergy), methotrexate, TMP/SMZ, and zidovudine may increase the risk of bone marrow suppression. Pyrimethamine may increase the levels/effects of amiodarone, amphetamines, selected beta-blockers, dextromethorphan, fluoxetine, glimepiride, glipizide, lidocaine, mirtazapine, nateglinide, nefazodone, paroxetine, phenytoin, pioglitazone, risperidone, ritonavir, rosiglitazone, sertraline, thioridazine, tricyclic antidepressants, venlafaxine, warfarin, and other CYP2C8/9 or 2D6 substrates.

Adverse Reactions Frequency not defined.

Cardiovascular: Arrhythmias (large doses)

Central nervous system: Depression, fever, insomnia, lightheadedness, malaise, seizure

Dermatologic: Abnormal skin pigmentation, dermatitis, erythema multiforme, rash, Stevens-Johnson syndrome, toxic epidermal necrolysis

Gastrointestinal: Anorexia, abdominal cramps, vomiting, diarrhea, xerostomia, atrophic glossitis

Genitourinary: Hematuria

Hematologic: Megaloblastic anemia, leukopenia, pancytopenia, thrombocytopenia, pulmonary eosinophilia

Miscellaneous: Anaphylaxis

Overdosage/Toxicology Symptoms of overdose include megaloblastic anemia, leukopenia, thrombocytopenia, anorexia, CNS stimulation, seizures, nausea, vomiting, and hematemesis. Following GI decontamination, leucovorin should be administered in an I.M. or I.V. dosage of 5-15 mg/day or orally for 5-7 days, or as required to reverse symptoms of folic acid deficiency. Provide other supportive treatment as required.

Pharmacodynamics/Kinetics

Onset of Action: ~1 hour

Time to Peak: Serum: 1.5-8 hours

Protein Binding: 80% to 87%

Half-Life Elimination: 80-95 hours

Metabolism: Hepatic

Excretion: Urine (20% to 30% as unchanged drug)

Available Dosage Forms Tablet: 25 mg

Dosing

Adults & Elderly:

Malaria chemoprophylaxis (for areas of chloroquine-resistant *P. falciparum*): Oral: Begin prophylaxis 2 weeks before entering endemic area: 25 mg once weekly. Dosage should be continued for all age groups for at least 6-10 weeks after leaving endemic areas

Chloroquine-resistant *P. falciparum* malaria (when used in conjunction with quinine and sulfadiazine): Oral: 25 mg twice daily for 3 days

Toxoplasmosis: Oral: 50-75 mg/day together with 1-4 g of a sulfonamide for 1-3 weeks depending on patient's tolerance and response, then reduce dose by 50% and continue for 4-5 weeks **or** 25-50 mg/day for 3-4 weeks

Prophylaxis for first episode of *Toxoplasma gondii*: Oral: 50 mg once weekly with dapsone, plus oral folinic acid 25 mg once weekly

Prophylaxis to prevent recurrence of *Toxoplasma gondii*: Oral: 25-50 mg once daily in combination with sulfadiazine or clindamycin, plus oral folinic acid 10-25 mg daily. Atovaquone plus oral folinic acid 10 mg daily has also been used in combination with pyrimethamine.

Pediatrics:

Malaria chemoprophylaxis (for areas with chloroquine-resistant *P. falciparum*): Oral: Begin prophylaxis 2 weeks before entering endemic area: *Children:* 0.5 mg/kg once weekly, not to exceed 25 mg/dose

or

<4 years: 6.25 mg once weekly

4-10 years: 12.5 mg once weekly

Children >10 years: Refer to adult dosing

Note: Dosage should be continued for all age groups for at least 6-10 weeks after leaving endemic areas.

Chloroquine-resistant *P. falciparum* malaria (when used in conjunction with quinine and sulfadiazine): Oral:

Children:

<10 kg: 6.25 mg/day once daily for 3 days

10-20 kg: 12.5 mg/day once daily for 3 days

20-40 kg: 25 mg/day once daily for 3 days

Toxoplasmosis:

Infants (congenital toxoplasmosis): Oral: 1 mg/kg once daily for 6 months with sulfadiazine then every other month with sulfa, alternating with spiramycin.

Children: Loading dose: 2 mg/kg/day divided into 2 equal daily doses for 1-3 days (maximum: 100 mg/day) followed by 1 mg/kg/day divided into 2 doses for 4 weeks; maximum: 25 mg/day

With sulfadiazine or trisulfapyrimidines: 2 mg/kg/day divided every 12 hours for 3 days, followed by 1 mg/kg/day once daily or divided twice daily for 4 weeks given with trisulfapyrimidines or sulfadiazine

Prophylaxis for first episode of *Toxoplasma gondii*: Oral:

Children ≥1 month of age: 1 mg/kg/day once daily with dapsone, plus oral folinic acid 5 mg every 3 days ·

Adolescents: Refer to adult dosing.

Prophylaxis to prevent recurrence of *Toxoplasma gondii*: Oral:

Children ≥1 month of age: 1 mg/kg/day once daily given with sulfadiazine or clindamycin, plus oral folinic acid 5 mg every 3 days

Adolescents: Refer to adult dosing.

Administration

Oral: Administer with meals to minimize GI distress.

Stability

Storage: Store at 15°C to 25°C (59°F to 77°F). Protect from light.

Laboratory Monitoring CBC, including platelet counts twice weekly; liver and renal function

Nursing Actions

Physical Assessment: Evaluate any patient history of renal or hepatic impairment or seizures prior to beginning therapy. When used for more than 3-4 days leucovorin may be ordered to prevent hematologic complications. Assess potential for interactions with other pharmacological agent patient may be taking (eg, increased potential for toxicities). Monitor laboratory tests, therapeutic effectiveness according to purpose for use, and adverse reactions (eg, arrhythmias, rash, GI disturbance, hematuria, megoblastic anemia) periodically during therapy. Teach patient appropriate use, possible side effects/interventions, and adverse symptoms to report.

Patient Education: Do not take any new medication during therapy unless approved by prescriber. Take with meals. Tablets may be crushed to prepare oral suspensions of the drug in water, cherry syrup, or sucrose-containing solutions at a concentration of 1 mg drug/mL of liquid. It is important to complete full course of therapy for full effect. Regular blood tests will be necessary during therapy. If used for prophylaxis, consult with prescriber in order to begin 2 weeks before traveling to endemic areas, continue during travel period, and for 6-10 weeks following return. May cause GI distress or loss of appetite (small, frequent meals, frequent mouth care, sucking lozenges, or chewing gum may help); dizziness, lightheadedness, insomnia, or changes in mentation (use caution when driving or with tasks that require alertness until response to drug is known); or changes in skin pigmentation or rash. Report persistent GI disturbance (nausea, vomiting, diarrhea, cramping); chest pain or palpitation; unusual fatigue, easy bruising, bleeding, or bloody emesis; or other adverse reactions. **Pregnancy/breast-feeding precautions:** Inform prescriber if you are or intend to become pregnant. Consult prescriber if breast-feeding.

Breast-Feeding Issues Pyrimethamine enters breast milk and may result in significant systemic concentrations in breast-fed infants. AAP rates as "compatible" (although the manufacturer does not recommend its use during breast-feeding). The effect of concurrent therapy with sulfonamide or dapsone (frequently used with pyrimethamine as combination treatment) must be considered.

Pregnancy Issues There are no adequate or well-controlled studies in pregnant women. If administered during pregnancy (ie, for toxoplasmosis), supplementation of folate (or folinic acid) is strongly recommended (5 mg/day). Pregnancy should be avoided during therapy.

Additional Information Leucovorin may be administered in a dosage of 3-9 mg/day for 3 days or 5 mg every 3 days or as required to reverse symptoms of or to prevent hematologic problems due to folic acid deficiency

Quetiapine (kwe TYE a peen)

U.S. Brand Names Seroquel®
Synonyms Quetiapine Fumarate
Pharmacologic Category Antipsychotic Agent, Atypical
Medication Safety Issues
Sound-alike/look-alike issues:
Seroquel® may be confused with Serentil®, Serzone®, Sinequan®
Pregnancy Risk Factor C
Lactation Excretion in breast milk unknown/not recommended
Use Treatment of schizophrenia; treatment of acute manic episodes associated with bipolar disorder (as monotherapy or in combination with lithium or valproate)
Unlabeled/Investigational Use Autism, psychosis (children)
Mechanism of Action/Effect Mechanism of action of quetiapine (dibenzothiazepine antipsychotic), as with other antipsychotic drugs, is unknown. However, it has been proposed that this drug's antipsychotic activity is mediated through a combination of dopamine type 2 and serotonin type 2 antagonism.

Antagonism at receptors other than dopamine and 5-HT$_2$ with similar receptor affinities may explain some of the other effects of quetiapine. The drug's antagonism of histamine H$_1$-receptors may explain the somnolence observed with it. The drug's antagonism of adrenergic alpha$_1$-receptors may explain the orthostatic hypotension observed with it.

Contraindications Hypersensitivity to quetiapine or any component of the formulation; severe CNS depression; bone marrow suppression; blood dyscrasias; severe hepatic disease, coma

Warnings/Precautions Patients with dementia-related behavioral disorders treated with atypical antipsychotics are at an increased risk of death compared to placebo. Quetiapine is not approved for this indication.

May be sedating, use with caution in disorders where CNS depression is a feature. Use with caution in Parkinson's disease. May cause orthostatic hypotension; use caution in patients predisposed to hypotension or with hemodynamic instability; prior myocardial infarction, cerebrovascular disease or ischemic heart disease. Caution in patients with hypercholesterolemia; thyroid disease; predisposition to seizures; subcortical brain damage; hepatic impairment; or severe cardiac, renal, or respiratory disease. May alter temperature regulation or mask toxicity of other drugs due to antiemetic effects. May alter cardiac conduction - life-threatening arrhythmias have occurred with therapeutic doses of neuroleptics.

Due to anticholinergic effects, use with caution in patients with decreased gastrointestinal motility, urinary retention, BPH, xerostomia, visual problems, narrow-angle glaucoma (screening is recommended), and myasthenia gravis. Relative to other antipsychotics, quetiapine has a moderate potency of cholinergic blockade. Risk of neuroleptic malignant syndrome (NMS), extrapyramidal symptoms or tardive dyskinesias appears to be very low relative to other antipsychotics. May cause hyperglycemia; in some cases may be extreme and associated with ketoacidosis, hyperosmolar coma, or death. Use with caution in patients with diabetes or other disorders of glucose regulation; monitor for worsening of glucose control.

Has been noted to cause cataracts in animals, lens examination on initiation of therapy and every 6 months is recommended.

The possibility of a suicide attempt is inherent in psychotic illness or bipolar disorder; use caution in (Continued)

Quetiapine *(Continued)*

high-risk patients during initiation of therapy. Prescriptions should be written for the smallest quantity consistent with good patient care.

Drug Interactions

Cytochrome P450 Effect: Substrate of CYP2D6 (minor), 3A4 (major)

Decreased Effect: Thioridazine increases quetiapine's clearance (by 65%), decreasing serum levels. CYP3A4 inducers may decrease the levels/effects of quetiapine. Example inducers include aminoglutethimide, carbamazepine, nafcillin, nevirapine, phenobarbital, phenytoin, and rifamycins.

Increased Effect/Toxicity: Quetiapine increases levels of lorazepam. The effects of other centrally-acting drugs, sedatives, or ethanol may be potentiated by quetiapine. Quetiapine may enhance the effects of antihypertensive agents. CYP3A4 inhibitors may increase the levels/effects of quetiapine; example inhibitors include azole antifungals, clarithromycin, diclofenac, doxycycline, erythromycin, imatinib, isoniazid, nefazodone, nicardipine, propofol, protease inhibitors, quinidine, telithromycin, and verapamil; ketoconazole increased serum concentrations of quetiapine by 335%. Concomitant use of quetiapine and divalproex increased the mean maximum plasma concentration of quetiapine at by 17% at steady state (the mean oral clearance of valproic acid was increased by 11%). Cimetidine increases blood levels of quetiapine (quetiapine's clearance is reduced by by 20%). Metoclopramide may increase risk of extrapyramidal symptoms (EPS). Acetylcholinesterase inhibitors (central) may increase the risk of antipsychotic-related EPS.

Nutritional/Ethanol Interactions

Ethanol: Avoid ethanol (may cause excessive impairment in cognition/motor function).

Food: In healthy volunteers, administration of quetiapine with food resulted in an increase in the peak serum concentration and AUC (each by ~15%) compared to the fasting state.

Herb/Nutraceutical: St John's wort may decrease quetiapine levels. Avoid valerian, St John's wort, kava kava, gotu kola (may increase CNS depression).

Adverse Reactions

>10%:

Central nervous system: Agitation, dizziness, headache, somnolence

Endocrine & metabolic: Cholesterol increased (11%), triglycerides increased (17%)

Gastrointestinal: Weight gain (≥7% body weight, dose related), xerostomia

1% to 10%:

Cardiovascular: Postural hypotension, tachycardia, palpitation, peripheral edema

Central nervous system: Anxiety, fever, pain

Dermatologic: Rash

Gastrointestinal: Abdominal pain (dose related), constipation, dyspepsia (dose related), anorexia, vomiting, gastroenteritis

Hematologic: Leukopenia

Hepatic: AST increased, ALT increased, GGT increased

Neuromuscular & skeletal: Dysarthria, back pain, weakness, tremor, hypertonia, dysarthria

Ocular: Amblyopia

Respiratory: Rhinitis, pharyngitis, cough, dyspnea

Miscellaneous: Diaphoresis, flu-like syndrome

Pharmacodynamics/Kinetics

Time to Peak: Plasma: 1.5 hours

Protein Binding: Plasma: 83%

Half-Life Elimination: Mean: Terminal: ~6 hours

Metabolism: Primarily hepatic; via CYP3A4; forms two inactive metabolites

Excretion: Urine (73% as metabolites, <1% as unchanged drug); feces (20%)

Available Dosage Forms

Tablet, as fumarate:

Seroquel®: 25 mg, 50 mg, 100 mg, 200 mg, 300 mg, 400 mg

Dosing

Adults:

Schizophrenia/psychosis: Oral: 25-100 mg 2-3 times/day; usual starting dose 25 mg twice daily, increased in increments of 25-50 mg 2-3 times/day on the second or third day. By the fourth day, the dose should be in the range of 300-400 mg/day in 2-3 divided doses. Further adjustments may be made, as needed, at intervals of at least 2 days in adjustments of 25-50 mg twice daily. Usual maintenance range: 150-750 mg/day.

Mania: Oral: Initial: 50 mg twice daily on day 1, increase dose in increments of 100 mg/day to 200 mg twice daily on day 4; may increase to a target dose of 800 mg/day by day 6 at increments of ≤200 mg/day. Usual dosage range: 400-800 mg/day

Note: Dose reductions should be attempted periodically to establish lowest effective dose in patients with psychosis or to establish need to continue treating agitated symptoms in demented older adults. Patients being restarted after 1 week of no drug need to be titrated as above.

Elderly: Lower clearance in elderly patients (40%), resulting in higher concentrations. Dosage adjustment may be required.

Pediatrics: Children and Adolescents:

Autism (unlabeled use): Oral: 100-350 mg/day (1.6-5.2 mg/kg/day)

Psychosis and mania (unlabeled use): Oral: Initial: 25 mg twice daily; titrate as necessary to 450 mg/day

Renal Impairment: No dosage adjustment required: 25% lower mean oral clearance of quetiapine than normal subjects; however, plasma concentrations similar to normal subjects receiving the same dose.

Hepatic Impairment: Lower clearance in hepatic impairment (30%), may result in higher concentrations. Dosage adjustment may be required.

Oral: Initial: 25 mg/day, increase dose by 25-50 mg/day to effective dose, based on clinical response and tolerability to patient

Laboratory Monitoring Fasting lipid profile and fasting blood glucose/Hgb A_{1c} (prior to treatment, at 3 months, then annually)

Nursing Actions

Physical Assessment: Assess other medications patient is taking for effectiveness and interactions (especially drugs affected by P450 enzymes). Review ophthalmic exam and monitor laboratory results, therapeutic response (mental status, mood, affect), and adverse reactions at beginning of therapy and periodically with long-term use (CNS responses, orthostatic hypotension, seizure threshold). Evaluate for cataracts before initiating treatment and every 6 months during chronic treatment. Monitor weight prior to initiating therapy and at least monthly. Assess knowledge/teach patient appropriate use, interventions to reduce side effects, and adverse symptoms to report.

Patient Education: Use exactly as directed; do not increase dose or frequency. It may take 2-3 weeks to achieve desired results; do not discontinue without consulting prescriber. Avoid alcohol or caffeine and other prescriptions or OTC medications not approved by prescriber. Maintain adequate hydration (2-3 L/day of fluids) unless instructed to restrict fluid intake. If diabetic, you may experience increased blood sugars. Monitor blood closely. You may experience excess drowsiness, restlessness, dizziness, or blurred vision (use caution driving or when engaging in tasks requiring alertness until response to drug is known);

mouth sores or GI upset (small frequent meals, frequent mouth care, chewing gum, or sucking lozenges may help); constipation (increased exercise, fluids, fruit, or fiber may help); or postural hypotension (use caution climbing stairs or when changing position from lying or sitting to standing). Report persistent CNS effects (eg, somnolence, agitation, insomnia); severe dizziness; vision changes; respiratory difficulty; or worsening of condition. **Pregnancy/breast-feeding precautions:** Inform prescriber if you are or intend to become pregnant. Breast-feeding is not recommended.

Dietary Considerations May be taken with or without food.

Geriatric Considerations (See Warnings/Precautions, Adverse Reactions, and Overdose/Toxicology.) Elderly patients have an increased risk of adverse response to side effects or adverse reactions to antipsychotics.

Related Information

Antipsychotic Medication Guidelines *on page 1415*
Federal OBRA Regulations Recommended Maximum Doses *on page 1421*

Quinapril (KWIN a pril)

U.S. Brand Names Accupril®
Synonyms Quinapril Hydrochloride
Pharmacologic Category Angiotensin-Converting Enzyme (ACE) Inhibitor
Medication Safety Issues
Sound-alike/look-alike issues:
Accupril® may be confused with Accolate®, Accutane®, AcipHex®, Monopril®

Pregnancy Risk Factor C (1st trimester)/D (2nd and 3rd trimesters)
Lactation Enters breast milk/use caution
Use Management of hypertension; treatment of congestive heart failure
Unlabeled/Investigational Use Treatment of left ventricular dysfunction after myocardial infarction
Mechanism of Action/Effect Competitive inhibitor of angiotensin-converting enzyme (ACE); prevents conversion of angiotensin I to angiotensin II, a potent vasoconstrictor; results in lower levels of angiotensin II which causes an increase in plasma renin activity and a reduction in aldosterone secretion
Contraindications Hypersensitivity to quinapril or any component of the formulation; angioedema related to previous treatment with an ACE inhibitor; bilateral renal artery stenosis; patients with idiopathic or hereditary angioedema; pregnancy (2nd and 3rd trimesters)
Warnings/Precautions Anaphylactic reactions can occur. Angioedema can occur at any time during treatment (especially following first dose). It may involve head and neck (potentially affecting the airway) or the intestine (presenting with abdominal pain). Prolonged monitoring may be required especially if tongue, glottis, or larynx are involved as they are associated with airway obstruction. Those with a history of airway surgery in this situation have a higher risk. Careful blood pressure monitoring with first dose (hypotension can occur especially in volume-depleted patients). Dosage adjustment needed in renal impairment. Use with caution in hypovolemia; collagen vascular diseases; valvular stenosis (particularly aortic stenosis); hyperkalemia; or before, during, or immediately after anesthesia. Avoid rapid dosage escalation, which may lead to renal insufficiency. Rare toxicities associated with ACE inhibitors include cholestatic jaundice (which may progress to hepatic necrosis) and neutropenia/agranulocytosis with myeloid hyperplasia. Hypersensitivity reactions may be seen during hemodialysis with high-flux dialysis membranes (eg, AN69). Use with caution in unilateral renal artery stenosis and pre-existing renal insufficiency.

Deterioration in renal function can occur with initiation. Due to rare hepatotoxic reactions, discontinue if jaundice or marked elevation of transaminases occurs.

Drug Interactions

Decreased Effect: Quinapril may reduce the absorption of quinolones and tetracycline antibiotics. Aspirin (high dose) may reduce the therapeutic effects of ACE inhibitors; at low dosages this does not appear to be significant. Rifampin may decrease the effect of ACE inhibitors. Antacids may decrease the bioavailability of ACE inhibitors (may be more likely to occur with captopril); separate administration times by 1-2 hours. NSAIDs, specifically indomethacin, may reduce the hypotensive effects of ACE inhibitors.

Increased Effect/Toxicity: Potassium supplements, co-trimoxazole (high dose), angiotensin II receptor antagonists (eg, candesartan, losartan, irbesartan), or potassium-sparing diuretics (amiloride, spironolactone, triamterene) may result in elevated serum potassium levels when combined with quinapril. ACE inhibitor effects may be increased by phenothiazines or probenecid (increases levels of captopril). ACE inhibitors may increase serum concentrations/effects of lithium.

Diuretics have additive hypotensive effects with ACE inhibitors, and hypovolemia increases the potential for adverse renal effects of ACE inhibitors. In patients with compromised renal function, coadministration with NSAIDs may result in further deterioration of renal function. Allopurinol and ACE inhibitors may cause a higher risk of hypersensitivity reaction when taken concurrently.

Nutritional/Ethanol Interactions Herb/Nutraceutical: Avoid dong quai if using for hypertension (has estrogenic activity). Avoid ephedra, yohimbe, ginseng (may worsen hypertension). Avoid garlic (may have increased antihypertensive effect).

Adverse Reactions Note: Frequency ranges include data from hypertension and heart failure trials. Higher rates of adverse reactions have generally been noted in patients with CHF. However, the frequency of adverse effects associated with placebo is also increased in this population.

1% to 10%:
Cardiovascular: Hypotension (3%), chest pain (2%), first-dose hypotension (up to 3%)
Central nervous system: Dizziness (4% to 8%), headache (2% to 6%), fatigue (3%)
Dermatologic: Rash (1%)
Endocrine & metabolic: Hyperkalemia (2%)
Gastrointestinal: Vomiting/nausea (1% to 2%), diarrhea (2%)
Neuromuscular & skeletal: Myalgias (2% to 5%), back pain (1%)
Renal: Increased BUN/serum creatinine (2%, transient elevations may occur with a higher frequency), worsening of renal function (in patients with bilateral renal artery stenosis or hypovolemia)
Respiratory: Upper respiratory symptoms, cough (2% to 4%; up to 13% in some studies), dyspnea (2%)

Overdosage/Toxicology Mild hypotension has been the primary toxic effect seen with acute overdose. Bradycardia may also occur. Hyperkalemia occurs even with therapeutic doses, especially in patients with renal insufficiency and those taking NSAIDs. Treatment is symptom-directed and supportive.

Pharmacodynamics/Kinetics

Onset of Action: 1 hour
Duration of Action: 24 hours
Time to Peak: Serum: Quinapril: 1 hour; Quinaprilat: ~2 hours
Protein Binding: Quinapril: 97%; Quinaprilat: 97%
Half-Life Elimination: Quinapril: 0.8 hours; Quinaprilat: 3 hours; increases as Cl_cr decreases
(Continued)

Quinapril *(Continued)*

Metabolism: Rapidly hydrolyzed to quinaprilat, the active metabolite

Excretion: Urine (50% to 60% primarily as quinaprilat)

Available Dosage Forms Tablet, as hydrochloride: 5 mg, 10 mg, 20 mg, 40 mg

Dosing

Adults:

Hypertension: Oral: Initial: 10-20 mg once daily, adjust according to blood pressure response at peak and trough blood levels; initial dose may be reduced to 5 mg in patients receiving diuretic therapy if the diuretic is continued.

Usual dose range (JNC 7): 10-40 mg once daily

Congestive heart failure or post-MI: Oral: Initial: 5 mg once or twice daily, titrated at weekly intervals to 20-40 mg daily in 2 divided doses; target dose (heart failure): 20 mg twice daily (ACC/AHA 2005 Heart Failure Guidelines)

Elderly: Oral: Initial: 2.5-5 mg/day; increase dosage at increments of 2.5-5 mg at 1- to 2-week intervals; adjust for renal impairment.

Renal Impairment: Lower initial doses should be used; after initial dose (if tolerated), administer initial dose twice daily; may be increased at weekly intervals to optimal response:

Hypertension: Oral: Initial:

Cl_{cr} >60 mL/minute: Administer 10 mg/day

Cl_{cr} 30-60 mL/minute: Administer 5 mg/day

Cl_{cr} 10-30 mL/minute: Administer 2.5 mg/day

Congestive heart failure: Oral: Initial:

Cl_{cr} >30 mL/minute: Administer 5 mg/day

Cl_{cr} 10-30 mL/minute: Administer 2.5 mg/day

Hepatic Impairment: In patients with alcoholic cirrhosis, hydrolysis of quinapril to quinaprilat is impaired; however, the subsequent elimination of quinaprilat is unaltered.

Stability

Reconstitution: Unstable in aqueous solutions. To prepare solution for oral administration, mix prior to administration and use within 10 minutes.

Storage: Store at room temperature.

Laboratory Monitoring CBC, renal function tests, electrolytes If patient has renal impairment, a baseline WBC with differential and serum creatinine should be evaluated and monitored closely during the first 3 months of therapy.

Nursing Actions

Physical Assessment: Assess potential for interactions with other pharmacological agents or herbal products patient may be taking (especially anything that may impact fluid balance or cardiac status). May be advisable to administer first dose in prescriber's office with careful blood pressure monitoring (hypotension or angioedema can occur at any time during treatment, especially following first dose). Monitor laboratory tests, effectiveness (cardiac status and blood pressure), and adverse response (eg, hypovolemia, angioedema, postural hypotension) on a regular basis during therapy. Teach patient proper use, possible side effects/appropriate interventions, and adverse symptoms to report.

Patient Education: Do not take any new medication during therapy unless approved by prescriber. Take as directed; do not alter dose or discontinue without consulting prescriber. Take first dose at bedtime or when sitting down (hypotension may occur). This drug does not eliminate need for diet or exercise regimen as recommended by prescriber. May cause increased cough (if persistent or bothersome, contact prescriber); postural hypotension (use caution when rising from lying or sitting position or climbing stairs); headache (consult prescriber for approved analgesic); dizziness (use caution when driving or engaging in tasks that require alertness until response to drug is known); nausea or vomiting (small, frequent meals, frequent mouth care, sucking lozenges, or chewing gum may help); or muscle or back pain (consult prescriber for approved analgesic). Immediately report swelling of face, mouth, lips, tongue or throat; chest pain or respiratory difficulty. Report persistent cough; persistent pain in muscles, joints, or back; skin rash; or other persistent adverse reactions. **Pregnancy/breast-feeding precautions:** Inform prescriber if you are or intend to become pregnant. This drug should not be used in the 2nd or 3rd trimester of pregnancy. Consult prescriber for appropriate contraceptive measures if necessary. Consult prescriber if breast-feeding.

Geriatric Considerations Due to frequent decreases in glomerular filtration (also creatinine clearance) with aging, elderly patients may have exaggerated responses to ACE inhibitors. Differences in clinical response due to hepatic changes are not observed.

Pregnancy Issues ACE inhibitors can cause fetal injury or death if taken during the 2nd or 3rd trimester. Discontinue ACE inhibitors as soon as pregnancy is detected.

Quinapril and Hydrochlorothiazide

(KWIN a pril & hye droe klor oh THYE a zide)

U.S. Brand Names Accuretic®; Quinaretic

Synonyms Hydrochlorothiazide and Quinapril

Pharmacologic Category Angiotensin-Converting Enzyme (ACE) Inhibitor; Antihypertensive; Diuretic, Thiazide

Pregnancy Risk Factor C (1st trimester); D (2nd and 3rd trimesters)

Lactation Enters breast milk/use caution

Use Treatment of hypertension (not for initial therapy)

Available Dosage Forms Tablet:

10/12.5: Quinapril 10 mg and hydrochlorothiazide 12.5 mg

20/12.5: Quinapril 20 mg and hydrochlorothiazide 12.5 mg

20/25: Quinapril 20 mg and hydrochlorothiazide 25 mg

Dosing

Adults:

Hypertension: Oral:

Patients with inadequate response to quinapril monotherapy: Quinapril 10 mg/ hydrochlorothiazide 12.5 mg **or** quinapril 20 mg/hydrochlorothiazide 12.5 mg once daily

Patients with adequate blood pressure control on hydrochlorothiazide 25 mg/day, but significant potassium loss: Quinapril 10 mg/hydrochlorothiazide 12.5 mg **or** quinapril 20 mg/hydrochlorothiazide 12.5 mg once daily

Note: Clinical trials of quinapril/hydrochlorothiazide combinations used quinapril doses of 2.5-40 mg/day and hydrochlorothiazide doses of 6.25-25 mg/day.

Elderly: If previous response to individual components is unknown, initial dose selection should be cautious, at the low end of adult dosage range; titration should occur at 1- to 2-week intervals.

Pediatrics: Safety and efficacy have not been established.

Renal Impairment: Cl_{cr} <30 mL/minute/1.73 m^2 or serum creatinine ≤3 mg/dL: Use is not recommended.

Nursing Actions

Physical Assessment: See individual agents.

Patient Education: See individual agents. **Pregnancy/breast-feeding precautions:** Do not get pregnant while taking this medication. Consult prescriber for appropriate contraceptive measures. Consult prescriber if breast-feeding.

Related Information

Hydrochlorothiazide *on page 610*

Quinapril *on page 1057*

Quinidine (KWIN i deen)

Synonyms Quinidine Gluconate; Quinidine Polygalacturonate; Quinidine Sulfate

Pharmacologic Category Antiarrhythmic Agent, Class Ia

Medication Safety Issues
Sound-alike/look-alike issues:
Quinidine may be confused with clonidine, quinine, Quinora®

Pregnancy Risk Factor C

Lactation Enters breast milk/compatible

Use Prophylaxis after cardioversion of atrial fibrillation and/or flutter to maintain normal sinus rhythm; prevent recurrence of paroxysmal supraventricular tachycardia, paroxysmal AV junctional rhythm, paroxysmal ventricular tachycardia, paroxysmal atrial fibrillation, and atrial or ventricular premature contractions; has activity against *Plasmodium falciparum* malaria

Mechanism of Action/Effect Class 1a antiarrhythmic agent; depresses phase O of the action potential; decreases myocardial excitability and conduction velocity, and myocardial contractility by decreasing sodium influx during depolarization and potassium efflux in repolarization; also reduces calcium transport across cell membrane

Contraindications Hypersensitivity to quinidine or any component of the formulation; thrombocytopenia; thrombocytopenic purpura; myasthenia gravis; heart block greater than first degree; idioventricular conduction delays (except in patients with a functioning artificial pacemaker); those adversely affected by anticholinergic activity; concurrent use of quinolone antibiotics which prolong QT interval, cisapride, amprenavir, or ritonavir

Warnings/Precautions Monitor and adjust dose to prevent excessive QT$_c$ prolongation. May cause new or worsened arrhythmia (proarrhythmic effect). May precipitate or exacerbate CHF. Reduce dosage in hepatic impairment. In patients with atrial fibrillation or flutter, block the AV node before initiating. Correct hypokalemia before initiating therapy; hypokalemia may worsen toxicity. Use may cause digoxin-induced toxicity (adjust digoxin's dose). Use caution with concurrent use of other antiarrhythmics. Hypersensitivity reactions can occur. Can unmask sick sinus syndrome (causes bradycardia). Has been associated with severe hepatotoxic reactions, including granulomatous hepatitis. Hemolysis may occur in patients with G6PD (glucose-6-phosphate dehydrogenase) deficiency.

Drug Interactions

Cytochrome P450 Effect: Substrate of CYP2C8/9 (minor), 2E1 (minor), 3A4 (major); **Inhibits** CYP2C8/9 (weak), 2D6 (strong), 3A4 (strong)

Decreased Effect: The levels/effects of quinidine may be decreased by aminoglutethimide, carbamazepine, nafcillin, nevirapine, phenobarbital, phenytoin, rifamycins, and other CYP3A4 inducers. Quinidine may decrease the levels/effects of CYP2D6 prodrug substrates (eg, codeine, hydrocodone, oxycodone, tramadol).

Increased Effect/Toxicity: Effects may be additive with drugs which prolong the QT interval, including amiodarone, amitriptyline, bepridil, cisapride (use is contraindicated), disopyramide, erythromycin, haloperidol, imipramine, pimozide, procainamide, sotalol, thioridazine, and some quinolones (sparfloxacin, gatifloxacin, moxifloxacin - concurrent use is contraindicated). Concurrent use of amprenavir, or ritonavir is contraindicated. Quinidine increases digoxin serum concentrations; digoxin dosage may need to be reduced (by 50%) when quinidine is initiated; new

steady-state digoxin plasma concentrations occur in 5-7 days.

Quinidine may increase the levels/effects of amphetamines, selected beta-blockers, selected benzodiazepines, calcium channel blockers, cisapride, cyclosporine, dextromethorphan, ergot alkaloids, fluoxetine, selected HMG-CoA reductase inhibitors, lidocaine, mesoridazine, mirtazapine, nateglinide, nefazodone, paroxetine, risperidone, ritonavir, sildenafil (and other PDE-5 inhibitors), tacrolimus, thioridazine, tricyclic antidepressants, venlafaxine, and other substrates of CYP2D6 or 3A4. Selected benzodiazepines (midazolam and triazolam), cisapride, ergot alkaloids, selected HMG-CoA reductase inhibitors (lovastatin and simvastatin), mesoridazine, pimozide, and thioridazine are generally contraindicated with strong CYP3A4 inhibitors. When used with strong CYP3A4 inhibitors, dosage adjustment/limits are recommended for sildenafil and other PDE-5 inhibitors; refer to individual monographs.

The levels/effects of quinidine may be increased by azole antifungals, clarithromycin, diclofenac, doxycycline, erythromycin, imatinib, isoniazid, nefazodone, nicardipine, propofol, protease inhibitors (amprenavir and ritonavir are contraindicated), telithromycin, verapamil, and other CYP3A4 inhibitors. Quinidine potentiates nondepolarizing and depolarizing muscle relaxants. When combined with quinidine, amiloride may cause prolonged ventricular conduction leading to arrhythmias. Urinary alkalinizers (antacids, sodium bicarbonate, acetazolamide) increase quinidine blood levels. Warfarin effects may be increased by quinidine.

Nutritional/Ethanol Interactions
Food: Dietary salt intake may alter the rate and extent of quinidine absorption. A decrease in dietary salt may lead to an increase in quinidine serum concentrations. Avoid changes in dietary salt intake. Quinidine serum levels may be increased if taken with food. Food has a variable effect on absorption of sustained release formulation. The rate of absorption of quinidine may be decreased following the ingestion of grapefruit juice. In addition, CYP3A4 metabolism of quinidine may be reduced by grapefruit juice. Grapefruit juice should be avoided. Excessive intake of fruit juices or vitamin C may decrease urine pH and result in increased clearance of quinidine with decreased serum concentration. Alkaline foods may result in increased quinidine serum concentrations.
Herb/Nutraceutical: St John's wort may decrease quinidine levels. Avoid ephedra (may worsen arrhythmia).

Adverse Reactions
Frequency not defined: Hypotension, syncope
>10%:
Cardiovascular: QT$_c$ prolongation (modest prolongation is common, however, excessive prolongation is rare and indicates toxicity)
Central nervous system: Lightheadedness (15%)
Gastrointestinal: Diarrhea (35%), upper GI distress, bitter taste, diarrhea, anorexia, nausea, vomiting, stomach cramping (22%)
1% to 10%:
Cardiovascular: Angina (6%), palpitation (7%), new or worsened arrhythmia (proarrhythmic effect)
Central nervous system: Syncope (1% to 8%), headache (7%), fatigue (7%), sleep disturbance (3%), tremor (2%), nervousness (2%), incoordination (1%)
Dermatologic: Rash (5%)
Neuromuscular & skeletal: Weakness (5%)
Ocular: Blurred vision
Otic: Tinnitus
Respiratory: Wheezing

Note: Cinchonism, a syndrome which may include tinnitus, high-frequency hearing loss, deafness, vertigo, (Continued)

Quinidine (Continued)

blurred vision, diplopia, photophobia, headache, confusion, and delirium has been associated with quinidine use. Usually associated with chronic toxicity, this syndrome has also been described after brief exposure to a moderate dose in sensitive patients. Vomiting and diarrhea may also occur as isolated reactions to therapeutic quinidine levels.

Overdosage/Toxicology Has a low toxic:therapeutic ratio and may easily produce fatal intoxication (acute toxic dose: 1 g in adults). Symptoms of overdose include sinus bradycardia, sinus node arrest or asystole, P-R, QRS, or QT interval prolongation, torsade de pointes (polymorphous ventricular tachycardia), and depressed myocardial contractility, which along with alpha-adrenergic or ganglionic blockade, may result in hypotension and pulmonary edema. Other effects are anticholinergic (dry mouth, dilated pupils, and delirium) as well as seizures, coma, and respiratory arrest. Treatment is symptomatic and effects usually respond to conventional therapies. **Note:** Do not use other Class 1A or 1C antiarrhythmic agents to treat ventricular tachycardia. Sodium bicarbonate may treat wide QRS intervals or hypotension. Markedly impaired conduction or high degree AV block, unresponsive to bicarbonate, indicates consideration of a pacemaker.

Pharmacodynamics/Kinetics
Protein Binding:
Newborns: 60% to 70%; decreased protein binding with cyanotic congenital heart disease, cirrhosis, or acute myocardial infarction
Adults: 80% to 90%
Half-Life Elimination: Plasma: Children: 2.5-6.7 hours; Adults: 6-8 hours; prolonged with elderly, cirrhosis, and congestive heart failure
Metabolism: Extensively hepatic (50% to 90%) to inactive compounds
Excretion: Urine (15% to 25% as unchanged drug)

Available Dosage Forms
Injection, solution, as gluconate: 80 mg/mL (10 mL) [equivalent to quinidine base 50 mg]
Tablet, as sulfate: 200 mg, 300 mg
Tablet, extended release, as gluconate: 324 mg [equivalent to quinidine base 202 mg]
Tablet, extended release, as sulfate: 300 mg [equivalent to quinidine base 249 mg]

Dosing
Adults & Elderly:
Note: Dosage expressed in terms of the salt: 267 mg of quinidine gluconate = 275 mg of quinidine polygalacturonate = 200 mg of quinidine sulfate.

Test dose for idiosyncratic reaction: Oral, I.M.: 200 mg administered several hours before full dosage (to determine possibility of idiosyncratic reaction)
Antiarrhythmic:
Oral:
Sulfate: 100-600 mg/dose every 4-6 hours; begin at 200 mg/dose and titrate to desired effect (maximum daily dose: 3-4 g)
Gluconate: 324-972 mg every 8-12 hours
I.M.: 400 mg/dose every 4-6 hours
I.V.: 200-400 mg/dose diluted and given at a rate ≤10 mg/minute
Pediatrics:
Note: Dosage expressed in terms of the salt: 267 mg of quinidine gluconate = 200 mg of quinidine sulfate.

Test dose for idiosyncratic reaction (sulfate, oral or gluconate, I.M.): Children: 2 mg/kg or 60 mg/m²
Antiarrhythmic: Oral (quinidine sulfate): Children: 15-60 mg/kg/day in 4-5 divided doses or 6 mg/kg every 4-6 hours; usual 30 mg/kg/day or 900 mg/m²/day given in 5 daily doses

I.V. **not** recommended (quinidine gluconate): Children: 2-10 mg/kg/dose given at a rate ≤10 mg/minute every 3-6 hours as needed
Renal Impairment:
Cl_{cr} <10 mL/minute: Administer 75% of normal dose.
Hemodialysis effects: Slightly hemodialyzable (5% to 20%); 200 mg supplemental dose posthemodialysis is recommended; not dialyzable (0% to 5%) by peritoneal dialysis.
Hepatic Impairment: Larger loading dose may be indicated; reduce maintenance doses by 50% and monitor serum levels closely.

Administration
Oral: Do not crush, chew, or break sustained release dosage forms. Give around-the-clock to promote less variation in peak and trough serum levels.
I.V.: Give around-the-clock to promote less variation in peak and trough serum levels. Maximum I.V. infusion rate: 10 mg/minute. Minimize use of PVC tubing to enhance bioavailability.
I.V. Detail: pH: 5.5-7.0 (injection)

Stability
Compatibility: Stable in D_5W, NS
Y-site administration: Incompatible with furosemide
Compatibility when admixed: Incompatible with atracurium
Storage: Do not use discolored parenteral solution.
Laboratory Monitoring Routine CBC, liver and renal function during long-term administration

Nursing Actions
Physical Assessment: Assess other medications patient may be taking for effectiveness and interactions. I.V. requires use of infusion pump and continuous cardiac and hemodynamic monitoring. Monitor laboratory tests, therapeutic response (cardiac status), and adverse reactions at beginning of therapy, when titrating dosage, and on a regular basis with long-term therapy. **Note:** Quinidine has a low toxic:therapeutic ratio and overdose may easily produce severe and life-threatening reactions. Assess knowledge/teach patient appropriate use, interventions to reduce side effects, and adverse symptoms to report.
Patient Education: Take exactly as directed, around-the-clock; do not take additional doses or discontinue without consulting prescriber. Do not crush, chew, or break sustained release dosage forms. Do not take with grapefruit juice. You will need regular cardiac checkups and blood tests while taking this medication. You may experience dizziness, drowsiness, or visual changes (use caution when driving or engaging in tasks requiring alertness until response to drug is known); abnormal taste, nausea or vomiting, or loss of appetite (small frequent meals, frequent mouth care, chewing gum, or sucking lozenges may help); headaches (prescriber may recommend mild analgesic); or diarrhea (yogurt or boiled milk may help; if persistent consult prescriber). Report chest pain, palpitation, or erratic heartbeat; respiratory difficulty or wheezing; CNS changes (confusion, delirium, fever, consistent dizziness); skin rash; sense of fullness or ringing in ears; or vision changes. **Pregnancy precaution:** Inform prescriber if you are or intend to become pregnant.
Dietary Considerations Administer with food or milk to decrease gastrointestinal irritation. Avoid changes in dietary salt intake.
Geriatric Considerations Clearance may be decreased with a resultant increased half-life. Must individualize dose. Bioavailability and half-life are increased in the elderly due to decreases in both renal and hepatic function with age.
Related Information
Peak and Trough Guidelines on page 1387

Quinine (KWYE nine)

Synonyms Quinine Sulfate
Pharmacologic Category Antimalarial Agent
Medication Safety Issues
Sound-alike/look-alike issues:
Quinine may be confused with quinidine
Pregnancy Risk Factor X
Lactation Enters breast milk/compatible
Use In conjunction with other antimalarial agents, suppression or treatment of chloroquine-resistant *P. falciparum* malaria; treatment of *Babesia microti* infection in conjunction with clindamycin
Unlabeled/Investigational Use Prevention and treatment of nocturnal recumbency leg muscle cramps
Mechanism of Action/Effect Depresses oxygen uptake and carbohydrate metabolism; intercalates into DNA, disrupting the parasite's replication and transcription; affects calcium distribution within muscle fibers and decreases the excitability of the motor end-plate region; cardiovascular effects similar to quinidine
Contraindications Hypersensitivity to quinine or any component of the formulation; tinnitus, optic neuritis, G6PD deficiency; history of black water fever; thrombocytopenia with quinine or quinidine; pregnancy
Warnings/Precautions Use with caution in patients with cardiac arrhythmias (quinine has quinidine-like activity) and in patients with myasthenia gravis.
Drug Interactions
Cytochrome P450 Effect: Substrate (minor) of CYP1A2, 2C19, 3A4; **Inhibits** CYP2C8/9 (moderate), 2D6 (strong), 3A4 (weak)
Decreased Effect: Phenobarbital, phenytoin, and rifampin may decrease quinine serum concentrations. Quinine may decrease the levels/effects of CYP2D6 prodrug substrates (eg, codeine, hydrocodone, oxycodone, tramadol).
Increased Effect/Toxicity: Quinine may increase the levels/effects of CYP2D6 substrates (eg, amphetamines, selected beta-blockers, dextromethorphan, fluoxetine, lidocaine, mirtazapine, nefazodone, paroxetine, risperidone, ritonavir, thioridazine, tricyclic antidepressants, venlafaxine). Beta-blockers with quinine may increase bradycardia. Quinine may enhance warfarin anticoagulant effect. Quinine potentiates nondepolarizing and depolarizing muscle relaxants. Quinine may increase plasma concentration of digoxin. Closely monitor digoxin concentrations. Digoxin dosage may need to be reduced (by one-half) when quinine is initiated. New steady-state digoxin plasma concentrations occur in 5-7 days. Verapamil, amiodarone, alkalinizing agents, and cimetidine may increase quinine serum concentrations.
Nutritional/Ethanol Interactions Herb/Nutraceutical: St John's wort may decrease quinine levels.
Lab Interactions Positive Coombs' [direct]
Adverse Reactions Frequency not defined.
Central nervous system: Severe headache
Gastrointestinal: Nausea, vomiting, diarrhea
Ocular: Blurred vision
Otic: Tinnitus
Miscellaneous: Cinchonism (risk of cinchonism is directly related to dose and duration of therapy)
Overdosage/Toxicology Symptoms of mild toxicity include nausea, vomiting, and cinchonism. Severe intoxication may cause ataxia, obtundation, convulsions, coma, and respiratory arrest. With massive intoxication quinidine-like cardiotoxicity (hypotension, QRS and QT interval prolongation, AV block, and ventricular arrhythmias) may be fatal. Retinal toxicity occurs 9-10 hours after ingestion (blurred vision, impaired color perception, constriction of visual fields and blindness). Other toxic effects include hypokalemia, hypoglycemia, hemolysis, and congenital malformations when taken during pregnancy. Treatment includes symptomatic therapy with conventional agents. **Note:** Avoid Type 1A and 1C antiarrhythmic drugs. Treat cardiotoxicity with sodium bicarbonate. Dialysis and hemoperfusion procedures are ineffective in enhancing elimination.

Pharmacodynamics/Kinetics
Time to Peak: Serum: 1-3 hours
Protein Binding: 70% to 95%
Half-Life Elimination: Children: 6-12 hours; Adults: 8-14 hours
Metabolism: Primarily hepatic
Excretion: Feces and saliva; urine (<5% as unchanged drug)
Available Dosage Forms
Capsule, as sulfate: 200 mg, 325 mg
Tablet, as sulfate: 260 mg
Dosing
Adults & Elderly:
Treatment of chloroquine-resistant malaria: Oral: 650 mg every 8 hours for 3-7 days with tetracycline
Suppression of malaria: Oral: 325 mg twice daily and continued for 6 weeks after exposure
Babesiosis: Oral: 650 mg every 6-8 hours for 7 days
Leg cramps: Oral: 200-300 mg at bedtime
Pediatrics:
Treatment of chloroquine-resistant malaria: Oral: Children: 25-30 mg/kg/day in divided doses every 8 hours for 3-7 days with tetracycline (consider risk versus benefit in children <8 years of age)
Babesiosis: Oral: Children: 25 mg/kg/day divided every 8 hours for 7 days
Renal Impairment:
Cl_{cr} 10-50 mL/minute: Administer every 8-12 hours or 75% of normal dose.
Cl_{cr} <10 mL/minute: Administer every 24 hours or 30% to 50% of normal dose.
Not removed by hemo- or peritoneal dialysis; dose for Cl_{cr} <10 mL/minute.
Continuous arteriovenous or venovenous hemofiltration: Dose as for Cl_{cr} 10-50 mL/minute.
Administration
Oral: Avoid use of aluminum-containing antacids because of drug absorption problems. Swallow dose whole to avoid bitter taste. May be administered with food.
Stability
Storage: Protect from light.
Nursing Actions
Physical Assessment: Allergy history should be assessed prior to beginning therapy. Assess for potential interactions with other pharmacological agents patient may be taking (eg, increased or decreased level/effects and toxicity [digoxin, beta blockers, warfarin, oxycodone, lidocaine, etc]). Monitor effectiveness (according to purpose for therapy) and adverse reactions. Teach patient appropriate use, possible side effects/interventions, and adverse symptoms to report. **Pregnancy risk factor X:** Determine that patient is not pregnant before starting therapy. Do not give to females of child-bearing age unless patient is capable of complying with contraceptive use during and for 2 months following therapy.
Patient Education: Do not take any new medication during therapy unless approved by prescriber (avoid use of any aluminum-containing antacids). Take on schedule as directed, with full 8 oz of water with or without food. Do not open, crush, or chew sustained release preparations. Do not increase dose without consulting prescriber; overdose can cause severe systemic effects. You will need to return for follow-up blood tests. May cause severe headache (consult prescriber for approved analgesic); nausea or vomiting (small frequent meals, frequent mouth care, chewing gum, or sucking lozenges may help); or diarrhea (buttermilk, boiled milk, or yogurt may help). Report any vision changes (blurring, night-blindness, (Continued)

Quinine *(Continued)*

double vision, etc); ringing in ears; or other persistent side effects. Seek emergency help for chest pain, respiratory difficulty, or seizures. **Pregnancy precautions:** Inform prescriber if you are pregnant. Consult prescriber for appropriate barrier contraceptive measures to use during and for 2 months following therapy. This drug may cause fetal defects. Do not donate blood during or for 1 month following therapy.

Dietary Considerations May be taken with food.

Geriatric Considerations Efficacy in nocturnal leg cramps is not well supported in the medical and pharmacy literature, however, some patients do respond. Nonresponders should be evaluated for other possible etiologies.

Quinupristin and Dalfopristin
(kwi NYOO pris tin & dal FOE pris tin)

U.S. Brand Names Synercid®

Synonyms Pristinamycin; RP-59500

Pharmacologic Category Antibiotic, Streptogramin

Pregnancy Risk Factor B

Lactation Excretion in breast milk unknown/use caution

Use Treatment of serious or life-threatening infections associated with vancomycin-resistant *Enterococcus faecium* bacteremia; treatment of complicated skin and skin structure infections caused by methcillin-susceptible *Staphylococcus aureus* or *Streptococcus pyogenes*

Has been studied in the treatment of a variety of infections caused by *Enterococcus faecium* (not *E. fecalis*) including vancomycin-resistant strains. May also be effective in the treatment of serious infections caused by *Staphylococcus* species including those resistant to methicillin.

Mechanism of Action/Effect Quinupristin/dalfopristin inhibits bacterial protein synthesis by binding to different sites on the 50S bacterial ribosomal subunit thereby inhibiting protein synthesis.

Contraindications Hypersensitivity to quinupristin, dalfopristin, pristinamycin, or virginiamycin, or any component of the formulation

Warnings/Precautions Use with caution in patients with hepatic or renal dysfunction. May cause pain and phlebitis when infused through a peripheral line (not relieved by hydrocortisone or diphenhydramine). May inhibit the metabolism of many drugs metabolized by CYP3A4. Concurrent therapy with cisapride (which may prolong QT_c interval and lead to arrhythmias) should be avoided. Superinfection may occur. As with many antibiotics, antibiotic-associated colitis and pseudomembranous colitis may occur. May cause arthralgias, myalgias, and hyperbilirubinemia.

Drug Interactions

Cytochrome P450 Effect: Quinupristin: **Inhibits** CYP3A4 (weak)

Increased Effect/Toxicity: The manufacturer states that quinupristin/dalfopristin may increase cisapride concentrations and cause QT_c prolongation, and recommends to avoid concurrent use with cisapride. Quinupristin/dalfopristin may increase cyclosporine concentrations; monitor.

Adverse Reactions

>10%:

Hepatic: Hyperbilirubinemia (3% to 35%)

Local: Inflammation at infusion site (38% to 42%), local pain (40% to 44%), local edema (17% to 18%), infusion site reaction (12% to 13%)

Neuromuscular & skeletal: Arthralgia (up to 47%), myalgia (up to 47%)

1% to 10%:

Central nervous system: Pain (2% to 3%), headache (2%)

Dermatologic: Pruritus (2%), rash (3%)

Endocrine & metabolic: Hyperglycemia (1%)

Gastrointestinal: Nausea (3% to 5%), diarrhea (3%), vomiting (3% to 4%)

Hematologic: Anemia (3%)

Hepatic: GGT increased (2%), LDH increased (3%)

Local: Thrombophlebitis (2%)

Neuromuscular & skeletal: CPK increased (2%)

Overdosage/Toxicology Symptoms may include dyspnea, emesis, tremors and ataxia. Treatment is supportive. Not removed by hemodialysis or peritoneal dialysis.

Pharmacodynamics/Kinetics

Protein Binding: Moderate

Half-Life Elimination: Quinupristin: 0.85 hour; Dalfopristin: 0.7 hour (mean elimination half-lives, including metabolites: 3 and 1 hours, respectively)

Metabolism: To active metabolites via nonenzymatic reactions

Excretion: Feces (75% to 77% as unchanged drug and metabolites); urine (15% to 19%)

Available Dosage Forms Injection, powder for reconstitution:

500 mg: Quinupristin 150 mg and dalfopristin 350 mg

600 mg: Quinupristin 180 mg and dalfopristin 420 mg

Dosing

Adults & Elderly:

Vancomycin-resistant *Enterococcus faecium*: I.V.: 7.5 mg/kg every 8 hours

Complicated skin and skin structure infection: I.V.: 7.5 mg/kg every 12 hours

Pediatrics: Limited information: Dosages similar to adult dosing have been used in the treatment of complicated skin/soft tissue infections and infections caused by vancomycin-resistant *Enterococcus faecium*

CNS shunt infection due to vancomycin-resistant *Enterococcus faecium*: I.V.: 7.5 mg/kg/dose every 8 hours. Concurrent intrathecal doses of 1-2 mg/day have been administered for up to 68 days.

Renal Impairment: No adjustment is necessary in renal failure, hemodialysis, or peritoneal dialysis.

Hepatic Impairment: Pharmacokinetic data suggest dosage adjustment may be necessary; however, specific recommendations have not been proposed.

Administration

I.V.: Line should be flushed with 5% dextrose in water prior to and following administration. Incompatible with saline. Infusion should be completed over 60 minutes (toxicity may be increased with shorter infusion). Compatible (Y-site injection) with aztreonam, ciprofloxacin, haloperidol, metoclopramide or potassium chloride when admixed in 5% dextrose in water. Also compatible (Y-site injection) with fluconazole (used as undiluted solution). If severe venous irritation occurs following peripheral administration of quinupristin/dalfopristin diluted in 250 mL 5% dextrose in water, consideration should be given to increasing the infusion volume to 500 mL or 750 mL, changing the infusion site, or infusing by a peripherally inserted central catheter (PICC) or a central venous catheter.

Stability

Reconstitution: Reconstitute single dose vial with 5 mL of 5% dextrose in water or sterile water for injection. Swirl gentle to dissolve - do not shake (to limit foam formation). The reconstituted solution should be diluted within 30 minutes. Stability of the diluted solution prior to the infusion is established as 5 hours at room temperature or 54 hours if refrigerated at 2°C to 8°C. Reconstituted solution should be added to at least 250 mL of 5% dextrose in water for peripheral administration (increase to 500 mL or 750 mL if necessary to limit venous irritation). An infusion volume of 100 mL may be used for central line infusions. Do not freeze solution.

Storage: Store unopened vials under refrigeration (2°C to 8°C/36°F to 46°F).

Laboratory Monitoring Culture and sensitivity

Physical Assessment: Assess effectiveness and interactions of other pharmacological agents (eg, cisapride). See Administration for exact infusion protocols to prevent severe venous irritation. Infusion site must be closely monitored. Monitor effectiveness (reduction of infection) and adverse reactions (eg, arthralgia, headache, rash, hyperglycemia, opportunistic infection [fever, chills, sore throat, burning urination, fatigue], pseudomembranous colitis, hyperbilirubinemia, dyspnea, ataxia). Teach patient possible side effects/interventions, and adverse symptoms to report.

Patient Education: This drug can only be administered by intravenous infusion. Report immediately any pain, irritation, redness, burning, swelling at infusion site. You may experience other side effects. Report headache, rash, nausea, vomiting, diarrhea, pain, heat or swelling in muscle areas, especially in lower extremities; respiratory difficulty, tremors, or difficulty speaking. **Breast-feeding precaution:** Consult prescriber if breast-feeding.

Rabeprazole (ra BE pray zole)

U.S. Brand Names AcipHex®

Synonyms Pariprazole

Pharmacologic Category Proton Pump Inhibitor; Substituted Benzimidazole

Medication Safety Issues
Sound-alike/look-alike issues:
AcipHex® may be confused with Acephen®, Accupril®, Aricept®
Rabeprazole may be confused with aripiprazole

Pregnancy Risk Factor B

Lactation Excretion in breast milk unknown/not recommended

Use Short-term (4-8 weeks) treatment and maintenance of erosive or ulcerative gastroesophageal reflux disease (GERD); symptomatic GERD; short-term (up to 4 weeks) treatment of duodenal ulcers; long-term treatment of pathological hypersecretory conditions, including Zollinger-Ellison syndrome; *H. pylori* eradication (in combination with amoxicillin and clarithromycin)

Unlabeled/Investigational Use Maintenance of duodenal ulcer

Mechanism of Action/Effect Suppresses gastric acid secretion by inhibiting the parietal cell H+/K+ ATP pump

Contraindications Hypersensitivity to rabeprazole, substituted benzimidazoles (ie, esomeprazole, lansoprazole, omeprazole, pantoprazole), or any component of the formulation

Warnings/Precautions Use caution in severe hepatic impairment. Relief of symptoms with rabeprazole does not preclude the presence of a gastric malignancy

Drug Interactions
Cytochrome P450 Effect: Substrate (major) of CYP2C19, 3A4; **Inhibits** CYP2C19 (moderate), 2DC (weak), 3A4 (weak)
Decreased Effect: Proton pump inhibitors may decrease the absorption of atazanavir, indinavir, itraconazole, and ketoconazole. The levels/effects of rabeprazole may be decreased by aminoglutethimide, carbamazepine, nafcillin, nevirapine, phenobarbital, phenytoin, rifampin, and other CYP2C19 or 3A4 inducers.
Increased Effect/Toxicity: Rabeprazole may increase the levels/effects of citalopram, diazepam,

methsuximide, phenytoin, propranolol, sertraline, or other CYP2C19 substrates.

Nutritional/Ethanol Interactions
Ethanol: Avoid ethanol (may cause gastric mucosal irritation).
Food: High-fat meals may delay absorption, but C_{max} and AUC are not altered.

Adverse Reactions 1% to 10%: Central nervous system: Headache

Overdosage/Toxicology No experience with large overdose; rabeprazole is not dialyzable. Treatment of overdosage should be symptomatic and supportive.

Pharmacodynamics/Kinetics
Onset of Action: 1 hour
Duration of Action: 24 hours
Time to Peak: Plasma: 2-5 hours
Protein Binding: Serum: 94.8% to 97.5%
Half-Life Elimination: Dose dependent: 0.85-2 hours
Metabolism: Hepatic via CYP3A and 2C19 to inactive metabolites
Excretion: Urine (90% primarily as thioether carboxylic acid); remainder in feces

Available Dosage Forms Tablet, delayed release, enteric coated, as sodium: 20 mg

Dosing
Adults & Elderly:
GERD: Oral: 20 mg once daily for 4-8 weeks; maintenance: 20 mg once daily
Duodenal ulcer: Oral: 20 mg/day before breakfast for 4 weeks
Eradication of *H. pylori*: Oral: 20 mg twice daily for 7 days; to be administered with amoxicillin 1000 mg and clarithromycin 500 mg, also given twice daily for 7 days.
Hypersecretory conditions: Oral: 60 mg once daily; dose may need to be adjusted as necessary. Doses as high as 100 mg once daily and 60 mg twice daily have been used.

Renal Impairment: No dosage adjustment required.

Hepatic Impairment:
Mild to moderate: Elimination decreased; no dosage adjustment required.
Severe: Use caution.

Oral: May be administered with or without food; best if taken before breakfast. Do not crush, split, or chew tablet. May be administered with an antacid.

Stability
Storage: Rapidly degraded in acid conditions.

Physical Assessment: Assess other medications, especially those dependent on cytochrome P450 metabolism (eg, digoxin) and those requiring acid environment for absorption (eg, ketoconazole, ampicillin). Monitor therapeutic effectiveness (reduction in symptoms), adverse reactions, and toxicity. Assess knowledge/teach patient appropriate use, interventions to reduce side effects, and adverse reactions to report.

Patient Education: Take as directed. Swallow whole, do not crush, split, or chew. Follow recommended diet and activity instructions. Avoid alcohol. You may experience headache (use of mild analgesic may help) or other side effects. Report these to prescriber if they persist. **Breast-feeding precaution:** Breast-feeding is not recommended.

Dietary Considerations May be taken with or without food; best if taken before breakfast.

Geriatric Considerations No difference in efficacy or safety was noted in elderly subjects as compared to younger subjects. No dosage adjustment is necessary in the elderly.

Raloxifene (ral OKS i feen)

U.S. Brand Names Evista®

Synonyms Keoxifene Hydrochloride; Raloxifene Hydrochloride

Pharmacologic Category Selective Estrogen Receptor Modulator (SERM)

Medication Safety Issues
Sound-alike/look-alike issues:
Evista® may be confused with Avinza™

Pregnancy Risk Factor X

Lactation Contraindicated

Use Prevention and treatment of osteoporosis in postmenopausal women

Mechanism of Action/Effect A selective estrogen receptor modulator, meaning that it affects some of the same receptors that estrogen does, but not all, and in some instances, it antagonizes or blocks estrogen; it acts like estrogen to prevent bone loss and improve lipid profiles (decreases total and LDL-cholesterol but does not raise triglycerides), but it has the potential to block some estrogen effects such as those that lead to breast cancer and uterine cancer

Contraindications Hypersensitivity to raloxifene or any component of the formulation; active thromboembolic disorder; pregnancy (not intended for use in premenopausal women)

Warnings/Precautions Use caution in patients with history of or at high risk for venous thromboembolism/pulmonary embolism; patients with cardiovascular disease; history of cervical/uterine carcinoma; renal/hepatic insufficiency (however, pharmacokinetic data are lacking); concurrent use of estrogens; women with a history of elevated triglycerides in response to treatment with oral estrogens (or estrogen/progestin). Discontinue at least 72 hours prior to and during prolonged immobilization (postoperative recovery or prolonged bedrest).

Drug Interactions
Decreased Effect: Ampicillin and cholestyramine reduce raloxifene absorption/blood levels.

Increased Effect/Toxicity: Raloxifene has the potential to interact with highly protein-bound drugs (increase effects of either agent). Use caution with highly protein-bound drugs, warfarin, clofibrate, indomethacin, naproxen, ibuprofen, diazepam, phenytoin, or tamoxifen.

Nutritional/Ethanol Interactions Ethanol: Avoid ethanol (may increase risk of osteoporosis).

Adverse Reactions Note: Has been associated with increased risk of thromboembolism (DVT, PE) and superficial thrombophlebitis; risk is similar to reported risk of HRT

≥2%:
Cardiovascular: Chest pain

Central nervous system: Migraine, depression, insomnia, fever

Dermatologic: Rash

Endocrine & metabolic: Hot flashes

Gastrointestinal: Nausea, dyspepsia, vomiting, flatulence, gastroenteritis, weight gain

Genitourinary: Vaginitis, urinary tract infection, cystitis, leukorrhea

Neuromuscular & skeletal: Leg cramps, arthralgia, myalgia, arthritis

Respiratory: Sinusitis, pharyngitis, cough, pneumonia, laryngitis

Miscellaneous: Infection, flu syndrome, diaphoresis

Overdosage/Toxicology Incidence of overdose in humans has not been reported. In an 8-week study of postmenopausal women, a dose of raloxifene 600 mg/day was safely tolerated. No mortality was seen after a single oral dose in rats or mice at 810 times the human dose for rats and 405 times the human dose for mice. There is no specific antidote for raloxifene.

Pharmacodynamics/Kinetics
Onset of Action: 8 weeks

Protein Binding: >95% to albumin and α-glycoprotein

Half-Life Elimination: 27.7-32.5 hours

Metabolism: Extensive first-pass effect

Excretion: Primarily feces; urine (0.2%)

Available Dosage Forms Tablet, as hydrochloride: 60 mg

Dosing
Adults & Elderly: Osteoporosis prevention or treatment (postmenopausal women): Oral: 1 tablet (60 mg) daily; may be administered any time of the day without regard to meals.

Hepatic Impairment: Avoid use; safety has not been established.

Laboratory Monitoring Monitor lipid profile, bone mineral density

Nursing Actions
Physical Assessment: Assess potential for interactions with other pharmacological agents (eg, highly protein-bound drugs, warfarin, clofibrate, indomethacin, naproxen, ibuprofen, diazepam, phenytoin, or tamoxifen). Monitor laboratory tests, therapeutic effectiveness (repeat BMI is best measure of osteoporosis treatment), and adverse response (eg, DVT, PE, chest pain, migraine, rash, hot flashes, vaginitis, UTI, myalgia, cough) on a regular basis during therapy. Teach patient appropriate use, possible side effects/appropriate interventions, and adverse symptoms to report (eg, thromboembolism). **Pregnancy risk factor X** Determine that patient is not pregnant before starting therapy. For use in postmenopausal women only.

Patient Education: Do not take any new medication during therapy unless approved by prescriber. Avoid excessive use of alcohol (ethanol may increase risk of osteoporosis). May be taken at any time of day without regard to meals. This medication is given to reduce incidence of osteoporosis; it will not reduce menopausal hot flashes or flushing (cool environment may reduce hot flashes). May cause flu-like symptoms at beginning of therapy (these will resolve with use); GI disturbances (eg, nausea, vomiting, dyspepsia - small, frequent meals, frequent mouth care, chewing gum, or sucking lozenges may help); or joint pain (consult prescriber for approved analgesic). Report immediately any pain, redness, warmth, or cramping in leg muscles; sudden chest pain; or respiratory difficulty. Report fever, acute migraine, insomnia or emotional depression, unusual weight gain (>5 lb/week), unresolved gastric distress, urinary infection or vaginal burning or itching, or unusual cough. **Pregnancy/breast-feeding precautions:** Inform prescriber if you are pregnant. For use in postmenopausal women only. Do not breast-feed.

Geriatric Considerations No need to cycle with progesterone.

Pregnancy Issues Raloxifene should not be used by pregnant women or by women planning to become pregnant in the immediate future.

Additional Information The decrease in estrogen-related adverse effects with the selective estrogen-receptor modulators in general and raloxifene in particular should improve compliance and decrease the incidence of cardiovascular events and fractures while not increasing breast cancer.

Ramelteon (ra MEL tee on)

U.S. Brand Names Rozerem™
Synonyms TAK-375
Pharmacologic Category Hypnotic, Nonbenzodiazepine
Pregnancy Risk Factor C
Lactation Excretion in breast milk unknown/not recommended
Use Treatment of insomnia characterized by difficulty with sleep onset
Mechanism of Action/Effect Activates melatonin receptors within an area of the CNS controlling circadian rhythms and sleep-wake cycle.
Contraindications Hypersensitivity to ramelteon or any component of the formulation; severe hepatic impairment; concurrent use with fluvoxamine
Warnings/Precautions Use caution with pre-existing depression or other psychiatric conditions. Caution when using with other CNS depressants; avoid engaging in hazardous activities or activities requiring mental alertness. Not recommended for use in patients with severe sleep apnea or COPD. Use caution with moderate hepatic impairment. Do not take with a high-fat meal. May cause disturbances of hormonal regulation. Use caution when administered concomitantly with strong CYP1A2 inhibitors. Safety and efficacy in pediatric patients have not been established.
Drug Interactions
Cytochrome P450 Effect: Substrate of CYP1A2 (major), CYP3A4 (minor), CYP2C family (minor)
Decreased Effect: Rifampin may decrease the levels/effects of ramelteon.
Increased Effect/Toxicity: The following agents may increase the levels/effects of ramelteon: CNS depressants, CYP1A2 inhibitors (example inhibitors include amiodarone, ciprofloxacin, fluvoxamine (concomitant use not recommended), ketoconazole, norfloxacin, ofloxacin, and rofecoxib), fluvoxamine, fluconazole, and ketoconazole.
Nutritional/Ethanol Interactions
Ethanol: Avoid ethanol (may increase CNS depression).
Adverse Reactions 1% to 10%:
Central nervous system: Headache (7%, same as placebo), somnolence (5%), dizziness (5%), fatigue (4%), insomnia worsened (3%), depression (2%)
Endocrine & metabolic: Serum cortisol decreased (1%)
Gastrointestinal: Nausea (3%), diarrhea (2%, same as placebo), taste perversion (2%)
Neuromuscular & skeletal: Myalgia (2%), arthralgia (2%)
Respiratory: Upper respiratory infection (3%; 2 % with placebo)
Miscellaneous: Influenza (1%)
Overdosage/Toxicology Single doses of up to 160 mg have been administered, with no safety or tolerability concerns noted. Treatment should be symptom-directed and supportive. Hemodialysis is not effective in removing ramelteon.
Pharmacodynamics/Kinetics
Onset of Action: 30 minutes
Time to Peak: Median: 0.5-1.5 hours
Protein Binding: 82%
Half-Life Elimination: Ramelteon: 1-2.6 hours; M-II: 2-5 hours
Metabolism:
Extensive first-pass effect; oxidative metabolism primarily through CYP1A2 and to a lesser extent through CYP2C and CYP3A4; forms active metabolite (M-II)
Excretion: Primarily as metabolites: Urine (84%); feces (4%)
Available Dosage Forms Tablet: 8 mg

Dosing
Adults: Insomnia: Oral: One 8 mg tablet within 30 minutes of bedtime
Elderly:
Refer to adult dosing.
Renal Impairment: No dosage adjustment required
Hepatic Impairment: No adjustment required for mild-to-moderate impairment. Avoid use with severe impairment.
Stability
Storage: Store at 15°C to 30°C (59°F to 86°F).
Physical Assessment: Monitor therapeutic response and adverse reactions. Assess effectiveness and interactions of other medications patient may be taking. Assess knowledge/teach patient appropriate use, possible side effects/interventions, and adverse symptoms to report.
Patient Education: Take approximately 30 minutes before desiring to go to sleep. Avoid alcohol and other CNS depressants. You may experience dizziness or lightheadedness (use caution when driving or engaging in activities requiring alertness until response to drug is known). Avoid meal high in fat prior to taking this medication. **Pregnancy/breast-feeding precautions:** Inform prescriber if you are or intend to become pregnant. Breast-feeding is not recommended.
Dietary Considerations Taking with high-fat meal delays T_{max} and increases AUC (~31%); do not take with high-fat meal.
Geriatric Considerations Although the C_{max} and AUC of ramelteon were increased in elderly patients, in clinical trials there were no significant differences in safety or efficacy between elderly and younger adult subjects.
Pregnancy Issues Animal studies have demonstrated teratogenic effects. May cause disturbances of reproductive hormonal regulation (eg, disruption of menses or decreased libido). There are no adequate and well-controlled studies in pregnant women.

Ramipril (ra MI pril)

U.S. Brand Names Altace®
Pharmacologic Category Angiotensin-Converting Enzyme (ACE) Inhibitor
Medication Safety Issues
Sound-alike/look-alike issues:
Ramipril may be confused with enalapril, Monopril® Altace® may be confused with alteplase, Amaryl®, Amerge®, Artane®
Pregnancy Risk Factor C (1st trimester)/D (2nd and 3rd trimesters)
Lactation Excretion in breast milk unknown/not recommended
Use Treatment of hypertension, alone or in combination with thiazide diuretics; treatment of left ventricular dysfunction after myocardial infarction; to reduce risk of heart attack, stroke, and death in patients at increased risk for these problems
Unlabeled/Investigational Use Treatment of heart failure
Mechanism of Action/Effect Ramipril is an ACE inhibitor which prevents the formation of angiotensin II from angiotensin I and exhibits pharmacologic effects that are similar to captopril. Ramipril must undergo conversion in the liver to its biologically active metabolite, ramiprilat. The pharmacodynamic effects of ramipril result from the high-affinity, competitive, reversible binding of ramiprilat to angiotensin-converting enzyme thus preventing the formation of the potent vasoconstrictor angiotensin II.
Contraindications Hypersensitivity to ramipril or any component of the formulation; prior hypersensitivity (Continued)

Ramipril (Continued)

(including angioedema) to ACE inhibitors; bilateral renal artery stenosis; pregnancy (2nd and 3rd trimesters)

Warnings/Precautions Angioedema can occur at any time during treatment (especially following first dose). It may involve head and neck (potentially affecting the airway) or the intestine (presenting with abdominal pain). Prolonged monitoring may be required especially if tongue, glottis, or larynx are involved as they are associated with airway obstruction. Those with a history of airway surgery in this situation have a higher risk. Careful blood pressure monitoring with first dose (hypotension can occur especially in volume-depleted patients). Dosage adjustment needed in renal impairment. Use with caution in hypovolemia; collagen vascular diseases; valvular stenosis (particularly aortic stenosis); hyperkalemia; or before, during, or immediately after anesthesia. Avoid rapid dosage escalation, which may lead to renal insufficiency. Rare toxicities associated with ACE inhibitors include cholestatic jaundice (which may progress to hepatic necrosis) and neutropenia/agranulocytosis with myeloid hyperplasia. Hypersensitivity reactions may be seen during hemodialysis with high-flux dialysis membranes (eg, AN69). Use with caution in unilateral renal artery stenosis and pre-existing renal insufficiency.

Drug Interactions

Decreased Effect: Aspirin (high dose) may reduce the therapeutic effects of ACE inhibitors; at low dosages this does not appear to be significant. Rifampin may decrease the effect of ACE inhibitors. Antacids may decrease the bioavailability of ACE inhibitors (may be more likely to occur with captopril); separate administration times by 1-2 hours. NSAIDs, specifically indomethacin, may reduce the hypotensive effects of ACE inhibitors. More likely to occur in low renin or volume dependent hypertensive patients.

Increased Effect/Toxicity: Potassium supplements, co-trimoxazole (high dose), angiotensin II receptor antagonists (eg, candesartan, losartan, irbesartan), or potassium-sparing diuretics (amiloride, spironolactone, triamterene) may result in elevated serum potassium levels when combined with ramipril. ACE inhibitor effects may be increased by phenothiazines or probenecid (increases levels of captopril). ACE inhibitors may increase serum concentrations/effects of lithium.

Diuretics have additive hypotensive effects with ACE inhibitors, and hypovolemia increases the potential for adverse renal effects of ACE inhibitors. In patients with compromised renal function, coadministration with NSAIDs may result in further deterioration of renal function. Allopurinol and ACE inhibitors may cause a higher risk of hypersensitivity reaction when taken concurrently.

Nutritional/Ethanol Interactions Herb/Nutraceutical: Avoid dong quai if using for hypertension (has estrogenic activity). Avoid ephedra, yohimbe, ginseng (may worsen hypertension). Avoid garlic (may have increased antihypertensive effect).

Lab Interactions Increases BUN, creatinine, potassium, positive Coombs' [direct]; decreases cholesterol (S); may cause false-positive results in urine acetone determinations using sodium nitroprusside reagent

Adverse Reactions Note: Frequency ranges include data from hypertension and heart failure trials. Higher rates of adverse reactions have generally been noted in patients with CHF. However, the frequency of adverse effects associated with placebo is also increased in this population.

>10%: Respiratory: Cough (increased) (7% to 12%)
1% to 10%:
Cardiovascular: Hypotension (11%), angina (3%), postural hypotension (2%), syncope (2%)

Central nervous system: Headache (1% to 5%), dizziness (2% to 4%), fatigue (2%), vertigo (2%)
Endocrine & metabolic: Hyperkalemia (1% to 10%)
Gastrointestinal: Nausea/vomiting (1% to 2%)
Neuromuscular & skeletal: Chest pain (noncardiac) (1%)
Renal: Renal dysfunction (1%), elevation in serum creatinine (1% to 2%), increased BUN (<1% to 3%); transient elevations of creatinine and/or BUN may occur more frequently
Respiratory: Cough (estimated 1% to 10%)
Worsening of renal function may occur in patients with bilateral renal artery stenosis or in hypovolemia. In addition, a syndrome which may include fever, myalgia, arthralgia, interstitial nephritis, vasculitis, rash, eosinophilia and positive ANA, and elevated ESR has been reported with ACE inhibitors. Risk of pancreatitis and agranulocytosis may be increased in patients with collagen vascular disease or renal impairment.

Overdosage/Toxicology Mild hypotension has been the primary toxic effect seen with acute overdose. Bradycardia may also occur. Hyperkalemia occurs even with therapeutic doses, especially in patients with renal insufficiency and those taking NSAIDs. Treatment is symptom-directed and supportive.

Pharmacodynamics/Kinetics

Onset of Action: 1-2 hours
Duration of Action: 24 hours
Time to Peak: Serum: ~1 hour
Half-Life Elimination: Ramiprilat: Effective: 13-17 hours; Terminal: >50 hours
Metabolism: Hepatic to the active form, ramiprilat
Excretion: Urine (60%) and feces (40%) as parent drug and metabolites
Available Dosage Forms Capsule: 1.25 mg, 2.5 mg, 5 mg, 10 mg

Dosing

Adults:
Hypertension: Oral: 2.5-5 mg once daily, maximum: 20 mg/day
To reduce the risk of MI, stroke, and death from cardiovascular causes: Oral: Initial: 2.5 mg once daily for 1 week, then 5 mg once daily for the next 3 weeks, then increase as tolerated to 10 mg once daily (may be given as divided dose)
Left ventricular dysfunction postmyocardial infarction: Oral: Initial: 2.5 mg twice daily titrated upward, if possible, to 5 mg twice daily.
Heart failure (unlabeled use): Initial: 1.25-2.5 mg once daily; target dose: 10 mg once daily (ACC/AHA 2005 Heart Failure Guidelines)
Note: The dose of any concomitant diuretic should be reduced. If the diuretic cannot be discontinued, initiate therapy with 1.25 mg. After the initial dose, the patient should be monitored carefully until blood pressure has stabilized.

Elderly: Refer to adult dosing (see Geriatric Considerations). Adjust for renal function for elderly since glomerular filtration rates are decreased; may see exaggerated hypotensive effects if renal clearance is not considered.

Renal Impairment:
Cl_{cr} <40 mL/minute: Administer 25% of normal dose.
Renal failure and hypertension: Administer 1.25 mg once daily, titrated upward as possible.
Renal failure and heart failure: Administer 1.25 mg once daily, increasing to 1.25 mg twice daily up to 2.5 mg twice daily as tolerated.

Administration

Oral: Capsule is usually swallowed whole, but may be may be mixed in water, apple juice, or applesauce.

Stability

Storage: Store at controlled room temperature.
Laboratory Monitoring CBC, renal function tests, electrolytes; if patient has renal impairment, a baseline WBC

with differential and serum creatinine should be evaluated and monitored closely during the first 3 months of therapy.

Nursing Actions

Physical Assessment: Assess potential for interactions with other pharmacological agents or herbal products patient may be taking (especially anything that may impact fluid balance or cardiac status). May be advisable to administer first dose in prescriber's office with careful blood pressure monitoring (hypotension or angioedema can occur at any time during treatment, especially following first dose). Monitor laboratory tests, effectiveness (blood pressure and cardiac status), and adverse response (eg, cough, renal dysfunction, nausea/vomiting, hypovolemia, angioedema, postural hypotension) reactions on a regular basis during therapy. Teach patient proper use, possible side effects/appropriate interventions, and adverse symptoms to report.

Patient Education: Do not take any new medication during therapy without consulting prescriber. Take as directed; do not alter dose or discontinue without consulting prescriber. Take first dose at bedtime or when sitting down (hypotension may occur). This drug does not eliminate need for diet or exercise regimen as recommended by prescriber. May cause increased cough (if persistent or bothersome, contact prescriber); headache (consult prescriber for approved analgesic); postural hypotension (use caution when rising from lying or sitting position or climbing stairs); dizziness (use caution when driving or engaging in tasks that require alertness until response to drug is known); or nausea or vomiting (small, frequent meals, frequent mouth care, sucking lozenges, or chewing gum may help). Immediately report swelling of face, mouth, lips, tongue or throat; chest pain or irregular heartbeat. Report respiratory difficulty or persistent cough; persistent pain in muscles, joints, or back; or other persistent adverse reactions. **Pregnancy/breast-feeding precautions:** Inform prescriber if you are or intend to become pregnant. This drug should not be used in the 2nd or 3rd trimester of pregnancy. Consult prescriber for appropriate contraceptive measures if necessary. Breast-feeding is not recommended.

Geriatric Considerations Due to frequent decreases in glomerular filtration (also creatinine clearance) with aging, elderly patients may have exaggerated responses to ACE inhibitors. Differences in clinical response due to hepatic changes are not observed.

Breast-Feeding Issues The manufacturer states that after single dose studies, ramipril was not excreted in breast milk; however, since the amount excreted with daily dosing is unknown, nursing while taking ramipril is not recommended.

Pregnancy Issues ACE inhibitors can cause fetal injury or death if taken during the 2nd or 3rd trimester. Discontinue ACE inhibitors as soon as pregnancy is detected.

Ranitidine (ra NI ti deen)

U.S. Brand Names Zantac®; Zantac 75® [OTC]; Zantac 150™ [OTC]; Zantac® EFFERdose®

Synonyms Ranitidine Hydrochloride

Pharmacologic Category Histamine H_2 Antagonist

Medication Safety Issues

Sound-alike/look-alike issues:

Ranitidine may be confused with amantadine, rimantadine

Zantac® may be confused with Xanax®, Zarontin®, Zofran®, Zyrtec®

Pregnancy Risk Factor B

Lactation Enters breast milk/use caution

Use

Zantac®: Short-term and maintenance therapy of duodenal ulcer, gastric ulcer, gastroesophageal reflux, active benign ulcer, erosive esophagitis, and pathological hypersecretory conditions; as part of a multidrug regimen for *H. pylori* eradication to reduce the risk of duodenal ulcer recurrence

Zantac® 75 [OTC]: Relief of heartburn, acid indigestion, and sour stomach

Unlabeled/Investigational Use Recurrent postoperative ulcer, upper GI bleeding, prevention of acid-aspiration pneumonitis during surgery, and prevention of stress-induced ulcers

Mechanism of Action/Effect Competitive inhibition of histamine at H_2-receptors, gastric acid secretion, gastric volume and hydrogen ion concentration are reduced

Contraindications Hypersensitivity to ranitidine or any component of the formulation

Warnings/Precautions Use with caution in patients with hepatic impairment; dosage modification required in patients with renal impairment; long-term therapy may be associated with vitamin B_{12} deficiency

Drug Interactions

Cytochrome P450 Effect: Substrate (minor) of CYP1A2, 2C19, 2D6; **Inhibits** CYP1A2 (weak), 2D6 (weak)

Decreased Effect:

Decreased effect: Variable effects on warfarin; antacids may decrease absorption of ranitidine; ketoconazole and itraconazole absorptions are decreased; may produce altered serum levels of procainamide and ferrous sulfate; decreased effect of nondepolarizing muscle relaxants, cefpodoxime, cyanocobalamin (decreased absorption), diazepam, oxaprozin

Decreased toxicity of atropine

Increased Effect/Toxicity: Increased the effect/toxicity of cyclosporine (increased serum creatinine), gentamicin (neuromuscular blockade), glipizide, glyburide, midazolam (increased concentrations), metoprolol, pentoxifylline, phenytoin, quinidine, and triazolam.

Nutritional/Ethanol Interactions

Ethanol: Avoid ethanol (may cause gastric mucosal irritation).

Food: Does not interfere with absorption of ranitidine.

Lab Interactions False-positive urine protein using Multistix®, gastric acid secretion test, skin test allergen extracts, serum creatinine and serum transaminase concentrations, urine protein test

Adverse Reactions Frequency not defined.

Cardiovascular: Atrioventricular block, bradycardia, premature ventricular beats, tachycardia, vasculitis

Central nervous system: Agitation, dizziness, depression, hallucinations, headache, insomnia, malaise, mental confusion, somnolence, vertigo

Dermatologic: Alopecia, erythema multiforme, rash

Endocrine & metabolic: Gynecomastia, impotence, increased prolactin levels, loss of libido

Gastrointestinal: Abdominal discomfort/pain, constipation, diarrhea, nausea, pancreatitis, vomiting

Hematologic: Acquired hemolytic anemia, agranulocytosis, aplastic anemia, granulocytopenia, leukopenia, pancytopenia, thrombocytopenia

Hepatic: Hepatic failure, hepatitis

Local: Transient pain, burning or itching at the injection site

Neuromuscular & skeletal: Arthralgia, involuntary motor disturbance, myalgia

Ocular: Blurred vision

Renal: Increased serum creatinine

Miscellaneous: Anaphylaxis, angioneurotic edema, hypersensitivity reactions

Overdosage/Toxicology Symptoms of overdose include abnormal gait, hypotension, and adverse effects (Continued)

Ranitidine *(Continued)*

seen with normal use. Treatment is primarily symptomatic and supportive.

Pharmacodynamics/Kinetics
Time to Peak: Serum: Oral: 2-3 hours; I.M.: ≤15 minutes

Protein Binding: 15%

Half-Life Elimination:
Oral: Normal renal function: 2.5-3 hours; Cl_{cr} 25-35 mL/minute: 4.8 hours
I.V.: Normal renal function: 2-2.5 hours

Metabolism: Hepatic to N-oxide, S-oxide, and N-desmethyl metabolites

Excretion: Urine: Oral: 30%, I.V.: 70% (as unchanged drug); feces (as metabolites)

Available Dosage Forms
Capsule, as hydrochloride: 150 mg, 300 mg
Infusion, as hydrochloride [premixed in NaCl 0.45%; preservative free] (Zantac®): 50 mg (50 mL)
Injection, solution, as hydrochloride: 25 mg/mL (2 mL, 6 mL)
Zantac®: 25 mg/mL (2 mL, 6 mL, 40 mL) [contains phenol 0.5% as preservative]
Syrup, as hydrochloride: 15 mg/mL (10 mL) [contains alcohol 7.5%; peppermint flavor]
Zantac®: 15 mg/mL (473 mL) [contains alcohol 7.5%; peppermint flavor]
Tablet, as hydrochloride: 75 mg [OTC], 150 mg, 300 mg
Zantac®: 150 mg, 300 mg
Zantac 75®: 75 mg
Zantac 150™: 150 mg
Tablet, effervescent, as hydrochloride (Zantac® EFFERdose®): 25 mg [contains sodium 1.33 mEq/tablet, phenylalanine 2.81 mg/tablet, and sodium benzoate]; 150 mg [contains sodium 7.96 mEq/tablet, phenylalanine 16.84 mg/tablet, and sodium benzoate]

Dosing
Adults & Elderly:
Duodenal ulcer: Oral: Treatment: 150 mg twice daily, or 300 mg once daily after the evening meal or at bedtime; maintenance: 150 mg once daily at bedtime

Eradication of *Helicobacter pylori*: Oral: 150 mg twice daily; requires combination therapy

Pathological hypersecretory conditions:
Oral: 150 mg twice daily; adjust dose or frequency as clinically indicated; doses of up to 6 g/day have been used
I.V.: Continuous infusion for Zollinger-Ellison: 1 mg/kg/hour; measure gastric acid output at 4 hours, if >10 mEq or if patient is symptomatic, increase dose in increments of 0.5 mg/kg/hour; doses of up to 2.5 mg/kg/hour have been used

Gastric ulcer, benign: *Oral:* 150 mg twice daily; maintenance: 150 mg once daily at bedtime

Erosive esophagitis: *Oral:* Treatment: 150 mg 4 times/day; maintenance: 150 mg twice daily

Prevention of heartburn: *Oral:* Zantac®75 [OTC]: 75 mg 30-60 minutes before eating food or drinking beverages which cause heartburn; maximum: 150 mg in 24 hours; do not use for more than 14 days

Patients not able to take oral medication:
I.M.: 50 mg every 6-8 hours
I.V.: Intermittent bolus or infusion: 50 mg every 6-8 hours
Continuous I.V. infusion: 6.25 mg/hour

Pediatrics:
Duodenal and gastric ulcer:
Oral: Children 1 month to 16 years:
Treatment: 2-4 mg/kg/day divided twice daily; maximum treatment dose: 300 mg/day
Maintenance: 2-4 mg/kg once daily; maximum maintenance dose: 150 mg/day
I.V.: 2-4 mg/kg/day divided every 6-8 hours; maximum: 150 mg/day

GERD and erosive esophagitis: Children 1 month to 16 years:
Oral: 5-10 mg/kg/day divided twice daily; maximum: GERD: 300 mg/day, erosive esophagitis: 600 mg/day
I.V.: 2-4 mg/kg/day divided every 6-8 hours; maximum: 150 mg/day **or as an alternative**
Continuous infusion: Initial: 1 mg/kg/dose for one dose followed by infusion of 0.08-0.17 mg/kg/hour or 2-4 mg/kg/day

Prevention of heartburn: *Oral:* Children ≥12 years: Zantac® 75 [OTC]: 75 mg 30-60 minutes before eating food or drinking beverages which cause heartburn; maximum: 150 mg/24 hours; do not use for more than 14 days

Renal Impairment: Adults: Cl_{cr} <50 mL/minute:
Oral: 150 mg every 24 hours; adjust dose cautiously if needed
I.V.: 50 mg every 18-24 hours; adjust dose cautiously if needed
Hemodialysis: Adjust dosing schedule so that dose coincides with the end of hemodialysis.

Hepatic Impairment: Patients with hepatic impairment may have minor changes in ranitidine half-life, distribution, clearance, and bioavailability; dosing adjustments are not necessary; monitor patient.

Oral: EFFERdose®: Should not be chewed, swallowed whole, or dissolved on tongue:
25 mg tablet: Dissolve in at least 5 mL (1 teaspoonful) of water; wait until completely dissolved before administering
150 mg tablet: Dissolve each dose in 6-8 ounces of water before drinking

I.M.: No dilution is needed

I.V.:
Intermittent bolus: Dilute vials to 2.5 mg/mL; infuse at 4 mL/minute (5 minutes)
Intermittent infusion: Dilute vials to 0.5 mg/mL; infuse at 5-7 mL/minute (15-20 minutes)
Continuous I.V. infusion: Administer at 6.25 mg/hour and titrate dosage based on gastric pH by continuous infusion over 24 hours

I.V. Detail: I.V. must be diluted and may be administered IVP or IVPB or continuous I.V. infusion.

pH: 6.7-7.3

Stability
Reconstitution: Vials can be mixed with NS or D_5W; solutions are stable for 48 hours at room temperature
Intermittent bolus injection: Dilute to maximum of 2.5 mg/mL
Intermittent infusion: Dilute to maximum of 0.5 mg/mL

Compatibility: Injection: Do not add other medications to premixed bag. Stable in $D_5^1/_2NS$, D_5W, $D_{10}W$, fat emulsion 10%, LR, NS, sodium bicarbonate 5%

Y-site administration: Incompatible with amphotericin B cholesteryl sulfate complex, hetastarch, insulin (regular)

Compatibility in syringe: Incompatible with hydroxyzine, methotrimeprazine, midazolam, pentobarbital, phenobarbital

Compatibility when admixed: Incompatible with amphotericin B, atracurium, cefamandole, cefazolin, cefoxitin, ceftazidime, cefuroxime, ethacrynate, metaraminol, phytonadione

Storage:
Injection: Vials; Store between 4°C to 30°C (39°F to 86°F); protect from light. Solution is a clear, colorless to yellow solution; slight darkening does not affect potency.
Premixed bag: Store between 2°C to 25°C (36°F to 77°F); protect from light.
EFFERdose® formulations: Store between 2°C to 30°C (36°F to 86°F).
Syrup; Store between 4°C to 25°C (39°F to 77°F); protect from light.

Tablets; Store in dry place, between 15°C to 30°C (59°F to 86°F); protect from light.

Laboratory Monitoring AST, ALT, serum creatinine; when used to prevent stress-related GI bleeding, measure the intragastric pH and try to maintain pH >4; occult blood with GI bleeding; monitor renal function and adjust dosage as indicated.

Nursing Actions

Physical Assessment: Assess potential for interactions with other pharmacological agents patient may be taking (eg, increased or decreased levels/effects and toxicity). Monitor laboratory tests, effectiveness, and adverse reactions (eg, bradycardia, PVCs, tachycardia, CNS changes [depression, hallucinations, confusion, malaise], rash, gynecomastia, GI disturbance, hepatic failure). Teach patient appropriate use, possible side effects/appropriate interventions, and adverse symptoms to report.

Patient Education: Do not take any new medication during therapy without consulting prescriber. Take exactly as directed; do not increase dose - may take several days before you notice relief. Allow 1 hour between any other antacids (if approved by prescriber) and ranitidine. Avoid excessive alcohol. Follow diet as prescriber recommends. May cause drowsiness, dizziness, or fatigue (use caution when driving or engaging in tasks requiring alertness until response to drug is known). Report chest pain or irregular heartbeat; skin rash; CNS changes (mental confusion, hallucinations, somnolence); unusual persistent weakness or lethargy; yellowing of skin or eyes; or change in color of urine or stool. **Breast-feeding precaution:** Consult prescriber if breast-feeding.

Dietary Considerations Oral dosage forms may be taken with or without food.
Zantac® EFFERdose®:
Effervescent tablet 25 mg contains sodium 1.33 mEq/tablet and phenylalanine 2.81 mg/tablet
Effervescent tablet 150 mg contains sodium 7.96 mEq/tablet and phenylalanine 16.84 mg/tablet

Geriatric Considerations H$_2$ blockers are the preferred drugs for treating PUD in elderly due to cost and ease of administration. These agents are no less or more effective than any other therapy. The preferred agents, due to side effects and drug interaction profile and pharmacokinetics are ranitidine, famotidine, and nizatidine. Treatment for PUD in elderly is recommended for 12 weeks since their lesions are larger; therefore, take longer to heal. Always adjust dose based upon creatinine clearance. Serum half-life is increased to 3-4 hours in elderly patients.

Pregnancy Issues Ranitidine crosses the placenta, teratogenic effects to the fetus have not been reported. Use with caution during pregnancy.

Related Information
Compatibility of Drugs in Syringe *on page 1372*

Ranolazine (ra NOE la zeen)

U.S. Brand Names Ranexa™
Pharmacologic Category Cardiovascular Agent, Miscellaneous
Lactation Excretion in breast milk unknown/not recommended
Use Treatment of chronic angina in combination with amlodipine, beta-blockers, or nitrates
Mechanism of Action/Effect May improve energy supply during ischemia
Contraindications Hypersensitivity to ranolazine or any component of the formulation; pre-existing QT prolongation (including congenital long-QT syndrome, uncorrected hypokalemia); known history of ventricular tachycardia; hepatic dysfunction (of any degree); concurrent QT$_c$-prolonging drugs; concurrent strong or moderate CYP3A4 inhibitors (including diltiazem and grapefruit juice)

Warnings/Precautions Ranolazine will not relieve acute angina attacks. Has been shown to prolong QT$_c$ interval in a dose/plasma concentration-related manner. Hepatically-impaired patients may have a more significant increase in QT$_c$. Use caution in patients ≥75 years of age; they may experience more adverse events. Use caution in patients with renal dysfunction. In general, avoid use in severe renal dysfunction. Monitor blood pressure in patients with renal dysfunction. Safety and efficacy in children have not been established.

Drug Interactions
Cytochrome P450 Effect: Substrate of CYP3A4 (major), 2D6 (minor); **Inhibits** CYP3A4 (weak), 2D6 (weak)
Decreased Effect: CYP3A4 inducers may decrease the effect of ranolazine.
Increased Effect/Toxicity: CYP3A4 inhibitors (eg, diltiazem, ketoconazole, verapamil) may increase the effects of ranolazine. Ranolazine may increase the effects of simvastatin and digoxin. Concurrent use of QT$_c$ -prolonging agents may further increase QT interval.

Adverse Reactions
>10%: Gastrointestinal: Constipation (5% to 8%; 19% in the elderly)
>0.5% to 10%:
Cardiovascular: Syncope (0.7%), palpitations, peripheral edema
Central nervous system: Dizziness (5% to 6%), headache (3% to 6%), vertigo
Gastrointestinal: Nausea (4% to 6%), abdominal pain, vomiting, xerostomia
Hematologic: Hematocrit decreased
Neuromuscular & skeletal: Weakness
Respiratory: Dyspnea

Overdosage/Toxicology Symptoms of overdose may include dizziness, nausea, vomiting, diplopia, paresthesias, confusion, syncope, and prolonged loss of consciousness. QT prolongation may occur and continuous ECG monitoring may be warranted. Treatment is symptom-directed and supportive. Complete clearance of ranolazine by hemodialysis is unlikely.

Pharmacodynamics/Kinetics
Time to Peak: 2-5 hours
Protein Binding: 62%
Half-Life Elimination: Terminal: 7 hours
Metabolism: Hepatic via CYP3A (major) and 2D6 (minor)
Excretion: Primarily urine (75% mostly as metabolites, <5% to 7% excreted unchanged); feces (25% mostly as metabolites)

Available Dosage Forms Tablet, extended release: 500 mg

Dosing
Adults: Chronic angina: Oral: Initial: 500 mg twice daily; maximum recommended dose: 1000 mg twice daily
Elderly: Refer to adult dosing. Select dose cautiously, starting at the lower end of the dosing range.
Renal Impairment: Dosage adjustment recommendations have not been established. However, plasma ranolazine levels increased ~50% in patients with varying degrees of renal dysfunction. Patients with severe renal dysfunction had an increase in mean diastolic blood pressure of 10-15 mm Hg. Monitor blood pressure closely in these patients. Patients on dialysis have not been studied. Avoid use in severe renal dysfunction.
Hepatic Impairment: Use is contraindicated.

Administration

Oral: May be taken with or without meals. Swallow tablet whole; do not crush, break, or chew.
(Continued)

Ranolazine *(Continued)*

Stability
Storage: Store at 15°C to 30°C (59°F to 86°F).

Laboratory Monitoring Baseline and follow up ECG to evaluate QT interval; correct and maintain serum potassium in normal limits

Nursing Actions
Physical Assessment: Assess other prescription and OTC medications patient may be taking to avoid duplications and interactions. Stress that this medication is not intended to treat an acute angina episode. Instruct them in appropriate measures to take if an acute episode occurs. Assess knowledge/teach patient appropriate use, side effects, and symptoms to report.

Patient Education:
This medication is not intended to be used to treat an acute angina episode. Follow instructions provided by prescriber for acute management. Swallow tablets whole; do not crush, break, or chew the tablets. Avoid grapefruit juice or grapefruit products while taking this medication. You may experience dizziness, lightheadedness (use caution when driving or engaging in activities requiring alertness until response to drug is known), or constipation (increasing exercise, fluids, fruit/fiber may help). Report palpitations, fainting spells, or chest pain that does not respond to recommended interventions. **Pregnancy/breast-feeding precautions:** Inform prescriber if you are or intend to become pregnant. Breast-feeding is not recommended.

Dietary Considerations May be taken with or without food. Concurrent consumption of grapefruit or grapefruit juice is contraindicated.

Rasburicase *(ras BYOOR i kayse)*

U.S. Brand Names Elitek™

Pharmacologic Category Enzyme; Enzyme, Urate-Oxidase (Recombinant)

Pregnancy Risk Factor C

Lactation Excretion in breast milk unknown/not recommended

Use Initial management of uric acid levels in pediatric patients with leukemia, lymphoma, and solid tumor malignancies receiving anticancer therapy expected to result in tumor lysis and elevation of plasma uric acid

Mechanism of Action/Effect Converts uric acid to allantoin (an inactive and soluble metabolite of uric acid); it does not inhibit the formation of uric acid.

Contraindications Hypersensitivity, hemolytic or methemoglobinemia reactions to rasburicase or any component of the formulation; glucose-6-phosphatase dehydrogenase (G6PD) deficiency

Warnings/Precautions Hypersensitivity reactions (including anaphylaxis), methemoglobinemia, and severe hemolysis have been reported; reactions may occur at any time during treatment (including the initial dose); discontinue **immediately and permanently** in patients developing any of these reactions. Hemolysis may be associated with G6PD deficiency; patients at higher risk for G6PD deficiency should be screened prior to therapy. Enzymatic degradation of uric acid in blood samples will occur if left at room temperature; specific guidelines for the collection of plasma uric acid samples must be followed. Rasburicase is immunogenic and can elicit an antibody response; administration of more than one course is not recommended. Efficacy in adults has not been established.

Lab Interactions Specific handling procedures must be followed to prevent the degradation of uric acid in plasma samples. Blood must be collected in prechilled tubes containing heparin anticoagulant. Samples must then be **immediately** immersed in an ice water bath.

Prepare samples by centrifugation in a precooled centrifuge (4°C). Samples must be kept in ice water bath and analyzed within 4 hours of collection.

Adverse Reactions As reported in patients receiving rasburicase with antitumor therapy versus active-control:

>10%:
Central nervous system: Fever (5% to 46%), headache (26%)
Dermatologic: Rash (13%)
Gastrointestinal: Vomiting (50%), nausea (27%), abdominal pain (20%), constipation (20%), mucositis (2% to 15%), diarrhea (≤1% to 20%)
1% to 10%:
Hematologic: Neutropenia with fever (4%), neutropenia (2%)
Respiratory: Respiratory distress (3%)
Miscellaneous: Sepsis (3%)

Overdosage/Toxicology No cases of overdose have been reported; low or undetectable serum levels of uric acid would be expected. Treatment should be symptom-directed and supportive.

Pharmacodynamics/Kinetics
Half-Life Elimination: Elimination: Pediatric patients: 18 hours

Available Dosage Forms Injection, powder for reconstitution: 1.5 mg [packaged with three 1 mL ampuls of diluent]

Dosing
Adults: Refer to pediatric dosing. Insufficient data collected in adult patients to determine response to treatment.

Elderly: Refer to pediatric dosing. Insufficient data collected in geriatric patients to determine response to treatment.

Pediatrics:
Management of uric acid levels: I.V.: Children: 0.15 mg/kg or 0.2 mg/kg once daily for 5 days (manufacturer-recommended duration); begin chemotherapy 4-24 hours after the first dose
Note: Limited data suggest that a single prechemotherapy dose (versus multiple-day administration) may be sufficiently efficacious. Monitoring electrolytes, hydration status, and uric acid concentrations are necessary to identify the need for additional doses. Other clinical manifestations of tumor lysis syndrome (eg, hyperphosphatemia, hypocalcemia, and hyperkalemia) may occur.

Administration
I.V.: I.V. infusion over 30 minutes; do **not** administer as a bolus infusion. Do **not** filter during infusion. If not possible to administer through a separate line, I.V. line should be flushed with at least 15 mL saline prior to and following rasburicase infusion.

Stability
Reconstitution: Reconstitute each vial with 1 mL of the provided diluent. Mix by gently swirling; do **not** shake or vortex. Discard if discolored or containing particulate matter. Total dose should be further diluted in NS to a final volume of 50 mL.

Storage: Prior to reconstitution, store with diluent at 2°C to 8°C (36°F to 46°F). Do not freeze; protect from light. Reconstituted and final solution may be stored up to 24 hours at 2°C to 8°C (36°F to 46°F). Discard unused product.

Nursing Actions
Physical Assessment: See I.V. Administration and Reconstitution for specifics. Monitor patient closely for hypersensitivity reaction (which can occur within minutes of administration). Monitor laboratory tests, therapeutic effectiveness, and adverse reactions prior to initiating therapy and on a regular basis throughout therapy. Teach patient possible side effects/appropriate interventions and adverse symptoms to report.

Patient Education: This medication can only be administered by infusion; you will be monitored closely during and following infusion. Report immediately any pain, burning, swelling at infusion site, or any signs of allergic reaction (eg, respiratory difficulty or swallowing, back pain, chest tightness, rash, hives, swelling of lips or mouth). Report headache, nausea, or respiratory difficulty.

Repaglinide (re pa GLI nide)

U.S. Brand Names Prandin®

Pharmacologic Category Antidiabetic Agent, Meglitinide Derivative

Medication Safety Issues
Sound-alike/look-alike issues:
Prandin® may be confused with Avandia®

Pregnancy Risk Factor C

Lactation Excretion in breast milk unknown/not recommended

Use Management of type 2 diabetes mellitus (noninsulin dependent, NIDDM); may be used in combination with metformin or thiazolidinediones

Mechanism of Action/Effect Nonsulfonylurea hypoglycemic agent which blocks ATP-dependent potassium channels, depolarizing the membrane and facilitating calcium entry through calcium channels. Increased intracellular calcium stimulates insulin release from the pancreatic beta cells.

Contraindications Hypersensitivity to repaglinide or any component of the formulation; diabetic ketoacidosis, with or without coma (treat with insulin); type 1 diabetes (insulin dependent, IDDM)

Warnings/Precautions Use with caution in patients with hepatic or renal impairment. May cause hypoglycemia; appropriate patient selection, dosage, and patient education are important to avoid hypoglycemic episodes. It may be necessary to discontinue repaglinide and administer insulin if the patient is exposed to stress (fever, trauma, infection, surgery). Safety and efficacy have not been established in pediatric patients. Not indicated for use in combination with NPH insulin due to potential cardiovascular events.

Drug Interactions

Cytochrome P450 Effect: Substrate of CYP2C8/9 (major), 3A4 (major)

Decreased Effect: CYP2C8/9 inducers may decrease the levels/effects of repaglinide; example inducers include carbamazepine, phenobarbital, phenytoin, rifampin, rifapentine, and secobarbital. CYP3A4 inducers may decrease the levels/effects of repaglinide; example inducers include aminoglutethimide, carbamazepine, nafcillin, nevirapine, phenobarbital, phenytoin, and rifamycins.

Increased Effect/Toxicity: Concurrent use of other hypoglycemic agents may increase risk of hypoglycemia. Gemfibrozil may increase the serum concentration of repaglinide (resulting in severe, prolonged hypoglycemia), and the addition of itraconazole may augment the effects of gemfibrozil on repaglinide. Macrolide antibiotics may increase the effects of repaglinide. CYP2C8/9 inhibitors may increase the levels/effects of repaglinide; example inhibitors include delavirdine, fluconazole, gemfibrozil, ketoconazole, nicardipine, NSAIDs, pioglitazone, and sulfonamides. CYP3A4 inhibitors may increase the levels/effects of repaglinide; example inhibitors include azole antifungals, clarithromycin, diclofenac, doxycycline, erythromycin, imatinib, isoniazid, nefazodone, nicardipine, propofol, protease inhibitors, quinidine, telithromycin, and verapamil.

Nutritional/Ethanol Interactions
Ethanol: Avoid ethanol (may cause hypoglycemia).

Food: When given with food, the AUC of repaglinide is decreased.

Herb/Nutraceutical: St John's wort may decrease repaglinide levels. Avoid gymnema, garlic (may cause hypoglycemia).

Adverse Reactions
>10%:
Central nervous system: Headache (9% to 11%)
Endocrine & metabolic: Hypoglycemia (16% to 31%)
Respiratory: Upper respiratory tract infection (10% to 16%)
1% to 10%:
Cardiovascular: Chest pain (2% to 3%), ischemia (4%)
Gastrointestinal: Nausea (3% to 5%), heartburn (2% to 4%), vomiting (2% to 3%) constipation (2% to 3%), diarrhea (4% to 5%), tooth disorder (<1% to 2%)
Genitourinary: Urinary tract infection (2% to 3%)
Neuromuscular & skeletal: Arthralgia (3% to 6%), back pain (5% to 6%), paresthesia (2% to 3%)
Respiratory: Sinusitis (3% to 6%), rhinitis (3% to 7%), bronchitis (2% to 6%)
Miscellaneous: Allergy (1% to 2%)

Overdosage/Toxicology Symptoms of severe hypoglycemia include seizures, cerebral damage, tingling of lips and tongue, nausea, yawning, confusion, agitation, tachycardia, sweating, convulsions, stupor, and coma. Management includes glucose administration (oral for milder hypoglycemia or by injection in more severe forms) and symptomatic treatment.

Pharmacodynamics/Kinetics
Onset of Action: Single dose: Increased insulin levels: ~15-60 minutes
Duration of Action: 4-6 hours
Time to Peak: Plasma: ~1 hour
Protein Binding: Plasma: >98%
Half-Life Elimination: 1 hour
Metabolism: Hepatic via CYP3A4 isoenzyme and glucuronidation to inactive metabolites
Excretion: Within 96 hours: Feces (~90%, <2% as parent drug); Urine (~8%)

Available Dosage Forms Tablet: 0.5 mg, 1 mg, 2 mg

Dosing
Adults & Elderly:
Type 2 diabetes: Oral:
Note: Doses should be taken within 15 minutes of the meal, but time may vary from immediately preceding the meal to as long as 30 minutes before the meal
Patients not previously treated or whose Hb A$_{1c}$ is <8%: Initial: 0.5 mg before each meal
Patients previously treated with blood glucose-lowering agents whose Hb A$_{1c}$ is ≥8%: Initial: 1 or 2 mg before each meal.
Dose adjustment: Determine dosing adjustments by blood glucose response, usually fasting blood glucose. Double the preprandial dose up to 4 mg until satisfactory blood glucose response is achieved. At least 1 week should elapse to assess response after each dose adjustment.
Dose range: 0.5-4 mg taken with meals. Repaglinide may be dosed preprandial 2, 3 or 4 times/day in response to changes in the patient's meal pattern. Maximum recommended daily dose: 16 mg.
Patients receiving other oral hypoglycemic agents: When repaglinide is used to replace therapy with other oral hypoglycemic agents, it may be started the day after the final dose is given. Observe patients carefully for hypoglycemia because of potential overlapping of drug effects. When transferred from longer half-life sulfonylureas (eg, chlorpropamide), close monitoring may be indicated for up to ≥1 week.

(Continued)

Repaglinide *(Continued)*

Note: Combination therapy: If repaglinide monotherapy does not result in adequate glycemic control, metformin or a thiazolidinedione may be added. Or, if metformin or thiazolidinedione therapy does not provide adequate control, repaglinide may be added. The starting dose and dose adjustments for combination therapy are the same as repaglinide monotherapy. Carefully adjust the dose of each drug to determine the minimal dose required to achieve the desired pharmacologic effect. Failure to do so could result in an increase in the incidence of hypoglycemic episodes. Use appropriate monitoring of FPG and Hb A$_{1c}$ measurements to ensure that the patient is not subjected to excessive drug exposure or increased probability of secondary drug failure. If glucose is not achieved after a suitable trial of combination therapy, consider discontinuing these drugs and using insulin.

Renal Impairment:
Cl$_{cr}$ 40-80 mL/minute (mild to moderate renal dysfunction): Initial dosage adjustment does not appear to be necessary.

Cl$_{cr}$ 20-40 mL/minute: Initiate 0.5 mg with meals; titrate carefully.

Hepatic Impairment: Use conservative initial and maintenance doses. Use longer intervals between dosage adjustments.

Administration
Oral: Administer repaglinide 15-30 minutes before meals. Patients who are anorexic or NPO, may need to have their dose held to avoid hypoglycemia.

Stability
Storage: Do not store above 25°C (77°F). Protect from moisture.

Laboratory Monitoring
Fasting blood glucose and glycosylated hemoglobin (Hb A$_{1c}$) levels

Nursing Actions
Physical Assessment: Assess potential for interactions with other prescriptions, OTC medications, or herbal products patient may be taking (especially anything that is metabolized via the cytochrome P450 isoenzyme 3A4 route). Monitor laboratory tests and patient response on a regular basis throughout therapy. Teach patient proper use (or refer patient to diabetic educator), possible side effects/appropriate interventions, and adverse symptoms to report (eg, signs of hypoglycemia).

Patient Education: Do not take any new medication during therapy without consulting prescriber. Take this medication exactly as directed (3-4 times a day) 15-30 minutes prior to a meal. If you skip a meal (or add an extra meal), skip (or add) a dose for that meal. Do not change dosage or discontinue without consulting prescriber. Follow dietary and lifestyle directions of prescriber or diabetic educator. Avoid alcohol. You will be instructed in signs of hypo- or hyperglycemia by prescriber or diabetic educator; be alert for adverse hypoglycemia (lightheadedness, tachycardia or palpitations, sweaty palms or profuse perspiration, yawning, tingling of lips and tongue, seizures, or change in sensorium) and follow prescriber's instructions for intervention. May cause headache or mild GI effects during first weeks of therapy (nausea, vomiting, diarrhea, constipation, heartburn), if these do not diminish, consult prescriber for approved medication. Report chest pain; respiratory difficulty or symptoms of upper respiratory infection; urinary tract infection (burning or itching on urination); muscle pain or back pain; or other adverse effects. **Pregnancy/breast-feeding precautions:** Inform prescriber if you are or intend to become pregnant. Breast-feeding is not recommended.

Dietary Considerations
Administer repaglinide 15-30 minutes before meals. Dietary modification based on ADA recommendations is a part of therapy. May cause hypoglycemia. Must be able to recognize symptoms of hypoglycemia (palpitations, tachycardia, sweaty palms, diaphoresis, lightheadedness).

Geriatric Considerations Repaglinide has not been studied exclusively in the elderly; information from the manufacturer states that no differences in its effectiveness or adverse effects had been identified between persons younger than and older than 65 years of age. How "tightly" a geriatric patient's blood glucose should be controlled is controversial; however, a fasting blood glucose <150 mg/dL is now an acceptable endpoint. Such a decision should be based on the patient's functional status, how well he/she recognizes hypoglycemic or hyperglycemic symptoms, and how to respond to them and their other disease states.

Breast-Feeding Issues It is not known whether repaglinide is excreted in breast milk. Because the potential for hypoglycemia in nursing infants may exist, decide whether to discontinue repaglinide or discontinue breast-feeding. If repaglinide is discontinued and if diet alone is inadequate for controlling blood glucose, consider insulin therapy.

Pregnancy Issues Safety in pregnant women has not been established. Use during pregnancy only if clearly needed. Abnormal blood glucose levels are associated with a higher incidence of congenital abnormalities. Insulin is the drug of choice for the control of diabetes mellitus during pregnancy.

Reserpine *(re SER peen)*

Pharmacologic Category Central Monoamine-Depleting Agent; Rauwolfia Alkaloid

Medication Safety Issues
Sound-alike/look-alike issues:
Reserpine may be confused with Risperdal®, risperidone

Pregnancy Risk Factor C

Lactation Enters breast milk/use caution

Use Management of mild-to-moderate hypertension; treatment of agitated psychotic states (schizophrenia)

Unlabeled/Investigational Use Management of tardive dyskinesia

Mechanism of Action/Effect Reduces blood pressure via depletion of sympathetic biogenic amines (norepinephrine and dopamine); this also commonly results in sedative effects

Contraindications Hypersensitivity to reserpine or any component of the formulation; active peptic ulcer disease, ulcerative colitis; history of mental depression (especially with suicidal tendencies); patients receiving electroconvulsive therapy (ECT)

Warnings/Precautions Use with caution in patients with impaired renal function, inflammatory bowel disease, asthma, Parkinson's disease, gallstones, or history of peptic ulcer disease, and the elderly. At high doses, significant mental depression, anxiety, or psychosis may occur (uncommon at dosages <0.25 mg/day). May cause orthostatic hypotension; use with caution in patients at risk of hypotension or in patients where transient hypotensive episodes would be poorly tolerated (cardiovascular disease or cerebrovascular disease). Avoid concurrent use of MAO inhibitors and/or drugs with MAO-inhibiting properties. Some products may contain tartrazine.

Drug Interactions
Decreased Effect: Tricyclic antidepressants may increase antihypertensive effect.

Increased Effect/Toxicity: Reserpine may cause hypertensive reactions in patients receiving an MAO inhibitor; use an alternative antihypertensive. Reserpine may increase the effect of beta-blockers. May increase effects of CNS depressants and/or ethanol.

May increase the effects/toxicity of levodopa, quinidine, procainamide, and digitalis glycosides.

Nutritional/Ethanol Interactions

Ethanol: Avoid ethanol (may increase CNS depression).

Herb/Nutraceutical: Avoid dong quai if using for hypertension (has estrogenic activity). Avoid ephedra, yohimbe (may worsen hypertension). Avoid valerian, St John's wort, kava kava, gotu kola (may increase CNS depression). Avoid garlic (may have increased antihypertensive effect).

Lab Interactions Decreased catecholamines (U)

Adverse Reactions Frequency not defined.

Cardiovascular: Peripheral edema, arrhythmia, bradycardia, chest pain, PVC, hypotension, syncope

Central nervous system: Dizziness, headache, nightmares, nervousness, drowsiness, fatigue, mental depression, parkinsonism, dull sensorium, paradoxical anxiety

Dermatologic: Rash, pruritus, flushing of skin, purpura

Endocrine & metabolic: Gynecomastia, weight gain

Gastrointestinal: Anorexia, diarrhea, dry mouth, nausea, vomiting, increased salivation, increased gastric acid secretion

Genitourinary: Impotence, decreased libido

Hematologic: Thrombocytopenia purpura

Neuromuscular & skeletal: Muscle ache

Ocular: Blurred vision, optic atrophy

Respiratory: Nasal congestion, dyspnea, epistaxis

Overdosage/Toxicology Symptoms of overdose include hypotension, bradycardia, CNS depression, sedation, coma, hypothermia, miosis, tremor, diarrhea, and vomiting. Treatment is symptom-directed and supportive. Anticholinergic agents may be useful in reducing parkinsonian effects and bradycardia.

Pharmacodynamics/Kinetics

Onset of Action: Antihypertensive: 3-6 days

Duration of Action: 2-6 weeks

Protein Binding: 96%

Half-Life Elimination: 50-100 hours

Metabolism: Extensively hepatic (>90%)

Excretion: Feces (30% to 60%); urine (10%)

Available Dosage Forms Tablet: 0.1 mg, 0.25 mg

Dosing

Adults:

Hypertension:

Manufacturer's labeling: Initial: 0.5 mg/day for 1-2 weeks; maintenance: 0.1-0.25 mg/day

Note: Clinically, the need for a "loading" period (as recommended by the manufacturer) is not well supported, and alternative dosing is preferred.

Alternative dosing (unlabeled): Initial: 0.1 mg once daily; adjust as necessary based on response.

Usual dose range (JNC 7): 0.05-0.25 mg once daily; 0.1 mg every other day may be given to achieve 0.05 mg once daily

Schizophrenia (labeled use) or tardive dyskinesia (unlabeled use): Dosing recommendations vary; initial dose recommendations generally range from 0.05-0.25 mg (although manufacturer recommends 0.5 mg once daily initially in schizophrenia). May be increased in increments of 0.1-0.25 mg; maximum dose in tardive dyskinesia: 5 mg/day.

Elderly: Oral: Initial: 0.05 mg once daily increasing by 0.05 mg every week as necessary (full antihypertensive effects may take as long as 3 weeks).

Pediatrics: Children: Hypertension: 0.01-0.02 mg/kg/24 hours divided every 12 hours; maximum dose: 0.25 mg/day (not recommended in children)

Renal Impairment:

Cl$_{cr}$ <10 mL/minute: Avoid use.

Not removed by hemo- or peritoneal dialysis; supplemental dose is not necessary.

Stability

Storage: Protect oral dosage forms from light.

Nursing Actions

Physical Assessment: Assess potential for interactions with other pharmacological agents and herbal products patient may be taking (eg, increase hypotensive effect (TCAs), hypertensive reaction (MAOIs, ephedra, yohimbe), increased effects of toxicity (CNS depressants). Monitor blood pressure and cardiac status prior to starting therapy, during first doses, when changing dose, and regularly thereafter (eg, arrhythmia, hypotension, CNS changes [nervousness, depression], Parkinsonism, rash, diarrhea, nausea, vomiting). Teach patient proper use, possible side effects/appropriate interventions, and adverse symptoms to report.

Patient Education: Do not take any new medication during therapy without consulting prescriber (especially any sleep remedies or stimulants). Take as directed; do not alter dose or discontinue without consulting prescriber. May take up to 2 weeks to see effects of therapy. Avoid alcohol and maintain recommended diet. May cause mild nervousness, dizziness, or fatigue (use caution when driving or engaging in hazardous activities until response to drug is known); orthostatic hypotension (use caution when rising from sitting or lying position or when climbing stairs until response to therapy is known): nausea or loss of appetite (small frequent meals or sucking lozenges may help); constipation (increased exercise, fluids, fruit, or fiber may help); nasal stuffiness (avoid OTC medications and consult prescriber for approved medication); or impotence (will resolve when medication is discontinued). Report chest pain, rapid heartbeat, or palpitations; respiratory difficulty; sudden increase in weight; swelling in ankles or hands; black tarry stools; or unusual feelings of depression, alteration in gait or balance, or other adverse reactions.

Pregnancy/breast-feeding precautions: Inform prescriber if you are or intend to become pregnant. Consult prescriber if breast-feeding.

Geriatric Considerations Some studies advocate the use of reserpine because of its low cost, long half-life, and efficacy, but it is generally not considered a first-line drug. If it is to be used, doses should not exceed 0.25 mg and the patient should be monitored for depressed mood.

Additional Information Adverse effects are usually dose related, mild, and infrequent when administered for the management of hypertension.

Reteplase (RE ta plase)

U.S. Brand Names Retavase®

Synonyms Recombinant Plasminogen Activator; r-PA

Pharmacologic Category Thrombolytic Agent

Pregnancy Risk Factor C

Lactation Excretion in breast milk unknown/use caution

Use Management of acute myocardial infarction (AMI); improvement of ventricular function; reduction of the incidence of CHF and the reduction of mortality following AMI

Mechanism of Action/Effect Reteplase initiates local fibrinolysis by binding to fibrin in a thrombus (clot) and converting entrapped plasminogen to plasmin. Dissolution of thrombus occluding a coronary artery restores perfusion to ischemic myocardium. Reteplase is manufactured by recombinant DNA technology using *E. coli*.

Contraindications Hypersensitivity to reteplase or any component of the formulation; active internal bleeding; history of cerebrovascular accident; recent intracranial or intraspinal surgery or trauma; intracranial neoplasm, arteriovenous malformations, or aneurysm; known bleeding diathesis; severe uncontrolled hypertension (Continued)

Reteplase *(Continued)*

Warnings/Precautions Concurrent heparin anticoagulation can contribute to bleeding; careful attention to all potential bleeding sites. I.M. injections and nonessential handling of the patient should be avoided. Venipunctures should be performed carefully and only when necessary. If arterial puncture is necessary, use an upper extremity vessel that can be manually compressed. If serious bleeding occurs then the infusion of anistreplase and heparin should be stopped.

For the following conditions the risk of bleeding is higher with use of reteplase and should be weighed against the benefits of therapy: recent major surgery (eg, CABG, obstetrical delivery, organ biopsy, previous puncture of noncompressible vessels), cerebrovascular disease, recent gastrointestinal or genitourinary bleeding, recent trauma including CPR, hypertension (systolic BP >180 mm Hg and/or diastolic BP >110 mm Hg), high likelihood of left heart thrombus (eg, mitral stenosis with atrial fibrillation), acute pericarditis, subacute bacterial endocarditis, hemostatic defects including ones caused by severe renal or hepatic dysfunction, significant hepatic dysfunction, pregnancy, diabetic hemorrhagic retinopathy or other hemorrhagic ophthalmic conditions, septic thrombophlebitis or occluded AV cannula at seriously infected site, advanced age (eg, >75 years), patients receiving oral anticoagulants, any other condition in which bleeding constitutes a significant hazard or would be particularly difficult to manage because of location.

Coronary thrombolysis may result in reperfusion arrhythmias. Follow standard MI management. Rare anaphylactic reactions can occur. Safety and efficacy in pediatric patients have not been established.

Drug Interactions
  Decreased Effect: Aminocaproic acid (antifibrinolytic agent) may decrease effectiveness of thrombolytic agents.
  Increased Effect/Toxicity: The risk of bleeding associated with reteplase may be increased by oral anticoagulants (warfarin), heparin, low molecular weight heparins, and drugs which affect platelet function (eg, NSAIDs, dipyridamole, ticlopidine, clopidogrel, IIb/IIIa antagonists). Concurrent use with aspirin and heparin may increase the risk of bleeding; however, aspirin and heparin were used concomitantly with reteplase in the majority of patients in clinical studies.

Adverse Reactions Bleeding is the most frequent adverse effect associated with reteplase. Heparin and aspirin have been administered concurrently with reteplase in clinical trials. The incidence of adverse events is a reflection of these combined therapies, and are comparable with comparison thrombolytics.

>10%: Local: Injection site bleeding (4.6% to 48.6%)
1% to 10%:
  Gastrointestinal: Bleeding (1.8% to 9.0%)
  Genitourinary: Bleeding (0.9% to 9.5%)
  Hematologic: Anemia (0.9% to 2.6%)
Other adverse effects noted are frequently associated with MI (and therefore may or may not be attributable to Retavase®) and include arrhythmia, hypotension, cardiogenic shock, pulmonary edema, cardiac arrest, reinfarction, pericarditis, tamponade, thrombosis, and embolism.

Overdosage/Toxicology Symptoms of overdose include increased incidence of intracranial bleeding. Treatment is supportive.

Pharmacodynamics/Kinetics
  Onset of Action: Thrombolysis: 30-90 minutes
  Half-Life Elimination: 13-16 minutes
  Excretion: Feces and urine
    Clearance: Plasma: 250-450 mL/minute
Available Dosage Forms Injection, powder for reconstitution [preservative free]: 10.4 units [equivalent to reteplase 18.1 mg; contains sucrose and polysorbate 80; packaged with sterile water for injection]

Dosing
  Adults & Elderly:
    Acute MI (thrombolysis): I.V.: 10 units I.V. over 2 minutes, followed by a second dose 30 minutes later of 10 units I.V. over 2 minutes; withhold second dose if serious bleeding or anaphylaxis occurs.
  Pediatrics: Not recommended
Administration
  I.V.: Infuse over 2 minutes.
  I.V. Detail: No other medications should be added to the injection solution.
Stability
  Reconstitution: Reteplase should be reconstituted using the diluent, syringe, needle, and dispensing pin provided with each kit.
  Storage: Dosage kits should be stored at 2°C to 25°C (36°F to 77°F) and remain sealed until use in order to protect from light.
Laboratory Monitoring CBC, PTT, signs and symptoms of bleeding, ECG monitoring
Nursing Actions
  Physical Assessment: Use caution when there is significant risk of bleeding (see Warnings/Precautions for specific use cautions). Assess potential risk interactions with other pharmacological and herbal products patient may be taking (especially those medications that may affect coagulation or platelet function). See Administration for infusion specifics. Monitor patient closely for bleeding during and following treatment: infusion site, neurological status (eg, intracranial hemorrhage), vital signs, and ECG. Maintain bleeding precautions; avoid I.M. injections, venipunctures (unless absolutely necessary), and nonessential handling of the patient. If arterial puncture is necessary, use an upper extremity vessel that can be manually compressed. Patient instructions determined by patient condition.
  Patient Education: This medication can only be administered by infusion; you will be monitored closely during and after treatment. You will have a tendency to bleed easily; use caution to prevent injury (use electric razor, soft toothbrush, and caution with knives, needles, or anything sharp). Follow instructions for strict bedrest to reduce the risk of injury. If bleeding occurs, report immediately and apply pressure to bleeding spot until bleeding stops completely. Report unusual pain (acute headache, joint pain, chest pain); unusual bruising or bleeding; blood in urine, stool, or vomitus; bleeding gums; vision changes; or respiratory difficulty. **Pregnancy/breast-feeding precautions:** Inform prescriber if you are or intend to become pregnant. Consult prescriber if breast-feeding.

Rh₀(D) Immune Globulin
(ar aych oh (dee) i MYUN GLOB yoo lin)

U.S. Brand Names BayRho-D® Full-Dose; BayRho-D® Mini-Dose; MICRhoGAM®; RhoGAM®; Rhophylac®; WinRho® SDF
Synonyms RhIG; Rho(D) Immune Globulin (Human); RhoIGIV; RhoIVIM
Pharmacologic Category Immune Globulin
Pregnancy Risk Factor C
Lactation Does not enter breast milk
Use
  Suppression of Rh isoimmunization: Use in the following situations when an Rh₀(D)-negative individual is exposed to Rh₀(D)-positive blood: During delivery of an Rh₀(D)-positive infant; abortion; amniocentesis; chorionic villus sampling; ruptured tubal pregnancy;

abdominal trauma; transplacental hemorrhage. Used when the mother is Rh$_o$(D) negative, the father of the child is either Rh$_o$(D) positive or Rh$_o$(D) unknown, the baby is either Rh$_o$(D) positive or Rh$_o$(D) unknown.

Transfusion: Suppression of Rh isoimmunization in Rh$_o$(D)-negative female children and female adults in their childbearing years transfused with Rh$_o$(D) antigen-positive RBCs or blood components containing Rh$_o$(D) antigen-positive RBCs

Treatment of idiopathic thrombocytopenic purpura (ITP): Used in the following nonsplenectomized Rh$_o$(D) positive individuals: Children with acute or chronic ITP, adults with chronic ITP, children and adults with ITP secondary to HIV infection

Mechanism of Action/Effect

Rh suppression: Suppresses the immune response and antibody formation of Rh$_o$(D) negative individuals to Rh$_o$(D) positive red blood cells.

ITP: Coats the patients Rh$_o$(D) positive red blood cells with antibody, so that as they are cleared by the spleen, the spleens ability to clear antibody-coated cells is saturated, sparing the platelets.

Contraindications Hypersensitivity to immune globulins or any component of the formulation; prior sensitization to Rh$_o$(D)

Warnings/Precautions Rare but serious signs and symptoms (eg, back pain, shaking, chills, fever, discolored urine; onset within 4 hours of infusion) of intravascular hemolysis (IVH) have been reported in postmarketing experience in patients treated for ITP. Clinically-compromising anemia, acute renal insufficiency and disseminated intravascular coagulation (DIC) have also been reported. ITP patients should be advised of the signs and symptoms of IVH and instructed to report them immediately.

As a product of human plasma, may potentially transmit disease; screening of donors, as well as testing and/or inactivation of certain viruses reduces this risk. Not for replacement therapy in immune globulin deficiency syndromes. Use caution with IgA deficiency, may contain trace amounts of IgA; patients who are IgA deficient may have the potential for developing IgA antibodies, anaphylactic reactions may occur. Administer I.M. injections with caution in patients with thrombocytopenia or coagulation disorders. Some products may contain maltose, which may result in falsely-elevated blood glucose readings. Use caution with renal dysfunction; may require an infusion rate reduction or discontinuation.

Do not administer I.M. or SubQ for the treatment of ITP; administer dose I.V. only. Safety and efficacy not established in Rh$_o$(D) negative, non-ITP thrombocytopenia, or splenectomized patients. Decrease dose with hemoglobin <10 g/dL; use with extreme caution if hemoglobin <8 g/dL

Rh$_o$(D) suppression: For use in the mother; do not administer to the neonate.

Drug Interactions

Decreased Effect: Rh$_o$(D) immune globulin may interfere with the response of live vaccines; vaccines should not be administered within 3 months after Rh$_o$(D)

Lab Interactions Some infants born to women given Rh$_o$(D) antepartum have a weakly positive Coombs' test at birth. Fetal-maternal hemorrhage may cause false blood-typing result in the mother; when there is any doubt to the patients' Rh type, Rh$_o$(D) immune globulin should be administered. WinRho® SDF liquid contains maltose; may result in falsely elevated blood glucose levels with dehydrogenase pyrroloquinolinequinone or glucose-dye-oxidoreductase testing methods. WinRho® SDF contains trace amounts of anti-A, B, C and E; may alter Coombs' tests following administration.

Adverse Reactions Frequency not defined.

Cardiovascular: Hyper-/hypotension, pallor, tachycardia, vasodilation

Central nervous system: Chills, dizziness, fever, headache, malaise, somnolence

Dermatologic: Pruritus, rash

Gastrointestinal: Abdominal pain, diarrhea, nausea, vomiting

Hematologic: Hemoglobin decreased (patients with ITP), intravascular hemolysis (patients with ITP)

Hepatic: LDH increased

Local: Injection site reaction: Discomfort, induration, mild pain, redness, swelling

Neuromuscular & skeletal: Arthralgia, back pain, hyperkinesia, myalgia, weakness

Renal: Acute renal insufficiency

Miscellaneous: Anaphylaxis, diaphoresis, infusion-related reactions

Overdosage/Toxicology No symptoms are likely, however, high doses have been associated with a mild, transient hemolytic anemia. Treatment should be symptom-directed and supportive.

Pharmacodynamics/Kinetics

Onset of Action: Onset of platelet increase: ITP: Platelets should rise within 1-2 days

Peak effect: In 7-14 days

Duration of Action: Suppression of Rh isoimmunization: ~12 weeks; Treatment of ITP: 30 days (variable)

Time to Peak: Plasma: I.M.: 5-10 days; I.V. (WinRho® SDF): ≤2 hours

Half-Life Elimination: 21-30 days

Available Dosage Forms

Injection, solution [preservative free]:

BayRho-D® Full-Dose, RhoGAM®: 300 mcg [for I.M. use only]

BayRho-D® Mini-Dose, MICRhoGAM®: 50 mcg [for I.M. use only]

Rhophylac®: 300 mcg/2 mL (2 mL) [1500 int. units; for I.M. or I.V. use]

WinRho® SDF:

120 mcg/~0.5 mL (~0.5 mL) [600 int. units; contains maltose; for I.M. or I.V. use]

300 mcg/~1.3 mL (~1.3 mL) [1500 int. units; contains maltose; for I.M. or I.V. use]

500 mcg/~2.2 mL (~2.2 mL) [2500 int. units; contains maltose; for I.M. or I.V. use]

1000 mcg/~4.4 mL (~4.4 mL) [5000 int. units; contains maltose; for I.M. or I.V. use]

3000 mcg/~13 mL (~13 mL) [15,000 int. units; contains maltose; for I.M. or I.V. use]

Injection, powder for reconstitution [preservative free] (WinRho® SDF):

120 mcg [600 int. units; for I.M. or I.V. use]

300 mcg [1500 int. units; for I.M. or I.V. use]

1000 mcg [5000 int. units; for I.M. or I.V. use]

Dosing

Adults:

ITP: WinRho® SDF: I.V.:

Initial: 50 mcg/kg as a single injection, or can be given as a divided dose on separate days. If hemoglobin is <10 g/dL: Dose should be reduced to 25-40 mcg/kg

Subsequent dosing: 25-60 mcg/kg can be used if required to elevate platelet count

Maintenance dosing if patient **did respond** to initial dosing: 25-60 mcg/kg based on platelet and hemoglobin levels:

Maintenance dosing if patient **did not respond** to initial dosing:

Hemoglobin 8-10 g/dL: Redose between 25-40 mcg/kg

Hemoglobin >10 g/dL: Redose between 50-60 mcg/kg

Hemoglobin <8 g/dL: Use with caution

Rh$_o$(D) suppression: Note: One "full dose" (300 mcg) provides enough antibody to prevent Rh sensitization if the volume of RBC entering the

(Continued)

Rh₀(D) Immune Globulin (Continued)

circulation is ≤15 mL. When >15 mL is suspected, a fetal red cell count should be performed to determine the appropriate dose.

Pregnancy:

Antepartum prophylaxis: In general, dose is given at 28 weeks. If given early in pregnancy, administer every 12 weeks to ensure adequate levels of passively acquired anti-Rh

BayRho-D® Full Dose, RhoGAM®: I.M.: 300 mcg

Rhophylac®, WinRho® SDF: I.M., I.V.: 300 mcg

Postpartum prophylaxis: In general, dose is administered as soon as possible after delivery, preferably within 72 hours. Can be given up to 28 days following delivery

BayRho-D® Full Dose, RhoGAM®: I.M.: 300 mcg

Rhophylac®: I.M., I.V.: 300 mcg

WinRho® SDF: I.M., I.V.: 120 mcg

Threatened abortion, any time during pregnancy (with continuation of pregnancy):

BayRho-D® Full Dose, RhoGAM®: I.M.: 300 mcg; administer as soon as possible

Rhophylac®, WinRho® SDF: I.M./I.V.: 300 mcg; administer as soon as possible

Abortion, miscarriage, termination of ectopic pregnancy:

BayRho-D®, RhoGAM®: I.M.: ≥13 weeks gestation: 300 mcg.

BayRho-D® Mini Dose, MICRhoGAM®: <13 weeks gestation: I.M.: 50 mcg

Rhophylac®: I.M., I.V.: 300 mcg

WinRho® SDF: I.M., I.V.: After 34 weeks gestation: 120 mcg; administer immediately or within 72 hours

Amniocentesis, chorionic villus sampling:

BayRho-D®, RhoGAM®: I.M.: At 15-18 weeks gestation or during the 3rd trimester: 300 mcg. If dose is given between 13-18 weeks, repeat at 26-28 weeks and within 72 hours of delivery.

Rhophylac®: I.M., I.V.: 300 mcg

WinRho® SDF: I.M., I.V.:

Before 34 weeks gestation: 300 mcg; administer immediately, repeat dose every 12 weeks during pregnancy

After 34 weeks gestation: 120 mcg, administered immediately or within 72 hours

Abdominal trauma, manipulation:

BayRho-D®, RhoGAM®: I.M.: 2nd or 3rd trimester: 300 mcg. If dose is given between 13-18 weeks, repeat at 26-28 weeks and within 72 hours of delivery.

Rhophylac®: I.M., I.V.: 300 mcg

WinRho® SDF: I.M., I.V.: After 34 weeks gestation: 120 mcg; administer immediately or within 72 hours

Transfusion:

BayRho-D®, RhoGAM®: I.M.: Multiply the volume of Rh positive whole blood administered by the hematocrit of the donor unit to equal the volume of RBCs transfused. The volume of RBCs is then divided by 15 mL, providing the number of 300 mcg doses (vials/syringes) to administer. If the dose calculated results in a fraction, round up to the next higher whole 300 mcg dose (vial/syringe).

WinRho® SDF: Administer within 72 hours after exposure of incompatible blood transfusions or massive fetal hemorrhage.

I.V.: Calculate dose as follows; administer 600 mcg every 8 hours until the total dose is administered:

Exposure to Rh₀(D) positive whole blood: 9 mcg/mL blood

Exposure to Rh₀(D) positive red blood cells: 18 mcg/mL cells

I.M.: Calculate dose as follows; administer 1200 mcg every 12 hours until the total dose is administered:

Exposure to Rh₀(D) positive whole blood: 12 mcg/mL blood

Exposure to Rh₀(D) positive red blood cells: 24 mcg/mL cells

Rhophylac®: I.M., I.V.:20 mcg per 2 mL transfused blood or 1 mL erythrocyte concentrate

Pediatrics: ITP, transfusion: WinRho® SDF: Refer to adult dosing.

Renal Impairment: I.V. infusion: Use caution; may require infusion rate reduction or discontinuation.

Administration

I.M.: Administer into the deltoid muscle of the upper arm or anterolateral aspect of the upper thigh. Avoid gluteal region due to risk of sciatic nerve injury. If large doses (>5 mL) are needed, administration in divided doses at different sites is recommended. **Note:** Do not administer I.M. Rho(D) immune globulin for ITP.

I.V.: WinRho® SDF: Infuse over at least 3-5 minutes; do not administer with other medications

I.V. Detail: Note: If preparing dose using liquid formulation, withdraw the entire contents of the vial to ensure accurate calculation of the dosage requirement.

Stability

Reconstitution: WinRho® SDF lyophilized powder: Dilute with provided NS only with volumes specified below. Inject diluent slowly into vial and gently swirl until dissolved; do not shake.

I.V. administration:

600 units (120 mcg) vial: 2.5 mL diluent

1500 units (300 mcg) vial: 2.5 mL diluent

5000 units (1000 mcg) vial: 8.5 mL diluent

I.M. administration:

600 units (120 mcg) vial: 1.25 mL diluent

1500 units (300 mcg) vial: 1.25 mL diluent

5000 units (1000 mcg) vial: 8.5 mL diluent (administer into several sites)

Storage: Store at 2°C to 8°C (35°F to 46°F). Do not freeze.

Rhophylac®: Stored at this temperature, Rhophylac® has a shelf life of 36 months. Protect from light.

WinRho® SDF lyophilized powder: Following reconstitution, may store at room temperature for up to 12 hours.

Laboratory Monitoring Patients with suspected IVH should have CBC, haptoglobulin, plasma hemoglobin, urine dipstick, BUN, serum creatinine, liver function tests, DIC-specific tests (D-dimer, fibrin degradation products [FDP] or fibrin split products [FSP]) for differential diagnosis. Clinical response may be determined by monitoring platelets, red blood cell (RBC) counts, hemoglobulin, and reticulocyte levels.

Nursing Actions

Physical Assessment:

Assess results of laboratory tests, therapeutic effectiveness, and adverse reactions. Monitor blood pressure; may cause hyper- or hypotension. Teach patient possible side effects, interventions to reduce side effects, and adverse reactions to report.

Patient Education: Do not have live virus vaccinations within 3 months of receiving this medication. This medication can only be administered by injection or infusion; report immediately any difficulty breathing, chills, rapid heart beat, back rash, pain, or redness, swelling, pain at injection site, discolored urine, decreased urine output, sudden weight gain, or swelling of extremities. You may experience headache or mild headache (consult prescriber for appropriate analgesic); or sleepiness or dizziness (avoid driving or engaging in activities requiring alertness until response to medication is known). Report any acute or persistent adverse effects. **Pregnancy precautions:** Inform prescriber if you are pregnant or plan to become pregnant.

Pregnancy Issues Animal studies have not been conducted. Available evidence suggests that Rh₀(D) immune globulin administration during pregnancy does not harm the fetus or affect future pregnancies.

Additional Information A "full dose" of Rh₀(D) immune globulin has previously been referred to as a 300 mcg dose. It is not the actual anti-D content. Although dosing has traditionally been expressed in mcg, potency is listed in int. units (1 mcg = 5 int. units). ITP patients requiring transfusions should be transfused with Rho-negative blood cells to avoid exacerbating hemolysis; platelet products may contain red blood cells; caution should be exercised if platelets are from Rh₀-positive donors.

Ribavirin (rye ba VYE rin)

U.S. Brand Names Copegus®; Rebetol®; Ribasphere™; Virazole®

Synonyms RTCA; Tribavirin

Restrictions An FDA-approved medication guide is available at http://www.fda.gov/cder/Offices/ODS/labeling.htm; distribute to each patient to whom this medication is dispensed for the treatment of hepatitis C.

Pharmacologic Category Antiviral Agent

Medication Safety Issues
Sound-alike/look-alike issues:
Ribavirin may be confused with riboflavin

Pregnancy Risk Factor X

Lactation Excretion in breast milk unknown/not recommended

Use
Inhalation: Treatment of patients with respiratory syncytial virus (RSV) infections; specially indicated for treatment of severe lower respiratory tract RSV infections in patients with an underlying compromising condition (prematurity, bronchopulmonary dysplasia and other chronic lung conditions, congenital heart disease, immunodeficiency, immunosuppression), and recent transplant recipients

Oral capsule:
In combination with interferon alfa-2b (Intron® A) injection for the treatment of chronic hepatitis C in patients with compensated liver disease who have relapsed after alpha interferon therapy or were previously untreated with alpha interferons

In combination with peginterferon alfa-2b (PEG-Intron®) injection for the treatment of chronic hepatitis C in patients with compensated liver disease who were previously untreated with alpha interferons

Oral solution: In combination with interferon alfa 2b (Intron® A) injection for the treatment of chronic hepatitis C in patients ≥3 years of age with compensated liver disease who were previously untreated with alpha interferons or patients ≥18 years of age who have relapsed after alpha interferon therapy

Oral tablet: In combination with peginterferon alfa-2a (Pegasys®) injection for the treatment of chronic hepatitis C in patients with compensated liver disease who were previously untreated with alpha interferons (includes patients with histological evidence of cirrhosis [Child-Pugh class A] and patients with clinically-stable HIV disease)

Unlabeled/Investigational Use Used in other viral infections including influenza A and B and adenovirus

Mechanism of Action/Effect Inhibits viral protein synthesis

Contraindications Hypersensitivity to ribavirin or any component of the formulation; women of childbearing age who will not use contraception reliably; pregnancy

Additional contraindications for oral formulation: Male partners of pregnant women; Cl_cr < 50 mL/minute; hemoglobinopathies (eg, thalassemia major, sickle cell anemia); as monotherapy for treatment of chronic hepatitis C; patients with autoimmune hepatitis, anemia, severe heart disease

Refer to individual monographs for Interferon Alfa-2b (Intron® A) and Peginterferon Alfa-2a (Pegasys®) for additional contraindication information.

Warnings/Precautions Negative pregnancy test is required before initiation and monthly thereafter. Avoid pregnancy in female patients and female partners of male patients, during therapy, and for at least 6 months after treatment; two forms of contraception should be used. Elderly patients are more susceptible to adverse effects; use caution. Safety and efficacy have not been established in patients who have failed other alpha interferon therapy, received organ transplants, or been coinfected with hepatitis B or HIV (Copegus® may be used in HIV coinfected patients unless CD4+ cell count is <100 cells/microL). Safety and efficacy have not been established in patients <3 years of age.

Inhalation: Use with caution in patients requiring assisted ventilation because precipitation of the drug in the respiratory equipment may interfere with safe and effective patient ventilation; monitor carefully in patients with COPD and asthma for deterioration of respiratory function. Ribavirin is potentially mutagenic, tumor-promoting, and gonadotoxic. Although anemia has not been reported with inhalation therapy, consider monitoring for anemia 1-2 weeks post-treatment. Pregnant healthcare workers may consider unnecessary occupational exposure; ribavirin has been detected in healthcare workers' urine. Healthcare professionals or family members who are pregnant (or may become pregnant) should be counseled about potential risks of exposure and counseled about risk reduction strategies.

Oral: Severe psychiatric events have occurred including depression and suicidal behavior during combination therapy. Avoid use in patients with a psychiatric history; discontinue if severe psychiatric symptoms occur. Hemolytic anemia is a significant toxicity; usually occurring within 1-2 weeks. Assess cardiac disease before initiation. Anemia may worsen underlying cardiac disease; use caution. If any deterioration in cardiovascular status occurs, discontinue therapy. Use caution in pulmonary disease; pulmonary symptoms have been associated with administration. Discontinue therapy in suspected/confirmed pancreatitis or if hepatic decompensation occurs. Use caution in patients with sarcoidosis (exacerbation reported).

Hemolytic anemia (hemoglobin <10 g/dL) was observed in up to 10% of treated patients in clinical trials when alfa interferons were combined with ribavirin; anemia occurred within 1-2 weeks of initiation of therapy.

Drug Interactions
Decreased Effect: Decreased effect of lamivudine, stavudine, and zidovudine (in vitro).

Increased Effect/Toxicity: Concomitant use of ribavirin and nucleoside analogues may increase the risk of developing lactic acidosis (includes adefovir, didanosine, lamivudine, stavudine, zalcitabine, zidovudine). Concurrent therapy of zidovudine with ribavirin/interferon alfa-2a may cause increased risk of severe anemia and/or severe neutropenia. Concurrent use with didanosine has been noted to increase the risk of pancreatitis and/or peripheral neuropathy in addition to lactic acidosis. Suspend therapy if signs/symptoms of toxicity are present. Concurrent therapy with Interferons (alfa) may increase the risk of hemolytic anemia.

(Continued)

Ribavirin *(Continued)*

Nutritional/Ethanol Interactions Food: Oral: High-fat meal increases the AUC and C_{max}.

Adverse Reactions

Inhalation:

1% to 10%:
Central nervous system: Fatigue, headache, insomnia
Gastrointestinal: Nausea, anorexia
Hematologic: Anemia

Note: Incidence of adverse effects (approximate) in healthcare workers: Headache (51%); conjunctivitis (32%); rhinitis, nausea, rash, dizziness, pharyngitis, and lacrimation (10% to 20%)

Oral (all adverse reactions are documented while receiving combination therapy with interferon alpha-2b or interferon alpha-2a; percentages as reported in adults):

>10%:
Central nervous system: Fatigue (60% to 70%)*, headache (43% to 66%)*, fever (32% to 46%)*, insomnia (26% to 41%), depression (20% to 36%)*, irritability (23% to 32%), dizziness (14% to 26%), impaired concentration (10% to 14%)*, emotional lability (7% to 12%)*
Dermatologic: Alopecia (27% to 36%), pruritus (13% to 29%), dry skin (13% to 24%), rash (5% to 28%), dermatitis (up to 16%)
Gastrointestinal: Nausea (33% to 47%), anorexia (21% to 32%), weight decrease (10% to 29%), diarrhea (10% to 22%), dyspepsia (8% to 16%), vomiting (9% to 14%)*, abdominal pain (8% to 13%), xerostomia (up to 12%), RUQ pain (up to 12%)
Hematologic: Neutropenia (8% to 27%; 40% with HIV coinfection), hemoglobin decreased (25% to 36%), hyperbilirubinemia (24% to 34%), anemia (11% to 17%), lymphopenia (12% to 14%), absolute neutrophil count <0.5 x 10^9/L (5% to 11%), thrombocytopenia (<1% to 14%), hemolytic anemia (10% to 13%), WBC decreased
Neuromuscular & skeletal: Myalgia (40% to 64%)*, rigors (40% to 48%), arthralgia (22% to 34%)*, musculoskeletal pain (19% to 28%)
Respiratory: Dyspnea (13% to 26%), cough (7% to 23%), pharyngitis (up to 13%), sinusitis (up to 12%)*, nasal congestion
Miscellaneous: Flu-like syndrome (13% to 18%)*, viral infection (up to 12%), diaphoresis increased (up to 11%)
*Similar to interferon alone

1% to 10%:
Cardiovascular: Chest pain (5% to 9%)*, flushing (up to 4%)
Central nervous system: Mood alteration (up to 6%; 9% with HIV coinfection), memory impairment (up to 6%), malaise (up to 6%), nervousness (~5%)*
Dermatologic: Eczema (4% to 5%)
Endocrine & metabolic: Hypothyroidism (up to 5%)
Gastrointestinal: Taste perversion (4% to 9%), constipation (up to 5%)
Genitourinary: Menstrual disorder (up to 7%)
Hepatic: Hepatomegaly (up to 4%)
Neuromuscular & skeletal: Weakness (9% to 10%), back pain (5%)
Ocular: Conjunctivitis (up to 6%), blurred vision (up to 5%)
Respiratory: Rhinitis (up to 8%), exertional dyspnea (up to 7%)
Miscellaneous: Fungal infection (up to 6%)
*Similar to interferon alone

Note: Incidence of anorexia, headache, fever, suicidal ideation, and vomiting are higher in children.

Overdosage/Toxicology
Treatment is symptom-directed and supportive. Not effectively removed by hemodialysis.

Pharmacodynamics/Kinetics

Time to Peak: Serum: Inhalation: At end of inhalation period; Oral capsule: Multiple doses: 3 hours; Tablet: 2 hours

Protein Binding: Oral: None

Half-Life Elimination: Plasma:
Children: Inhalation: 6.5-11 hours
Adults: Oral:
Capsule, single dose (Rebetol®, Ribasphere™): 24 hours in healthy adults, 44 hours with chronic hepatitis C infection (increases to ~298 hours at steady state)
Tablet, single dose (Copegus®): 120-170 hours

Metabolism: Hepatically and intracellularly (forms active metabolites); may be necessary for drug action

Excretion: Inhalation: Urine (40% as unchanged drug and metabolites); Oral capsule: Urine (61%), feces (12%)

Available Dosage Forms

Capsule (Rebetol®, Ribasphere™): 200 mg
Powder for aerosol (Virazole®): 6 g
Powder for solution, inhalation [for aerosol administration] (Virazole®): 6 g [reconstituted product provides 20 mg/mL]
Tablet (Copegus®): 200 mg

Dosing

Adults & Elderly:

Chronic hepatitis C (in combination with peginterferon alfa-2a): Oral tablet (Copegus®):
Monoinfection, genotype 1,4:
<75 kg: 1000 mg/day, in 2 divided doses for 48 weeks
≥75 kg: 1200 mg/day, in 2 divided doses for 48 weeks
Monoinfection, genotype 2,3: 800 mg/day, in 2 divided doses, for 24 weeks
Coinfection with HIV: 800 mg/day in 2 divided doses for 48 weeks
Note: Also refer to Peginterferon Alfa-2a monograph

Chronic hepatitis C (in combination with interferon alfa-2b): Oral capsule (Rebetol®, Ribasphere™):
Note: Also refer to Interferon Alfa-2b/Ribavirin combination pack monograph
≤75 kg: 400 mg in the morning, then 600 mg in the evening
>75 kg: 600 mg in the morning, then 600 mg in the evening
Note: If HCV-RNA is undetectable at 24 weeks, duration of therapy is 48 weeks. In patients who relapse following interferon therapy, duration of dual therapy is 24 weeks.

Chronic hepatitis C (in combination with peginterferon alfa-2b): Oral capsule (Rebetol®, Ribasphere™): 400 mg twice daily; duration of therapy is 1 year; after 24 weeks of treatment, if serum HCV-RNA is not below the limit of detection of the assay, consider discontinuation.

Pediatrics:

RSV infection: Infants and Children:
Aerosol inhalation: Use with Viratek® small particle aerosol generator (SPAG-2): A concentration of 20 mg/mL (6 g reconstituted with 300 mL of sterile water without preservatives)
Aerosol only: 12-18 hours/day for 3 days, up to 7 days in length

Chronic hepatitis C (in combination with interferon alfa-2b): Oral solution should be used in children 3-5 years of age, children ≤25 kg, or those unable to swallow capsules.
Capsule/oral solution: Children ≥3 years: 15 mg/kg/day in 2 divided doses.
Capsule dosing recommendations:
25-36 kg: 400 mg/day (200 mg morning and evening)

37-49 kg: 600 mg/day (200 mg in the morning and two 200 mg capsules in the evening)

50-61 kg: 800 mg/day (two 200 mg capsules morning and evening)

>61 kg: Refer to adult dosing.

Note: Duration of therapy is 48 weeks in pediatric patients with genotype 1 and 24 weeks in patients with genotype 2,3. Discontinue treatment in any patient if HCV-RNA is not below the limit of detection of the assay after 24 weeks of therapy.

Note: Also refer to Interferon Alfa-2b/Ribavirin combination pack monograph.

Dosage adjustment for toxicity: Oral (capsule, solution, tablet):

Patient without cardiac history:

Hemoglobin <10 g/dL: 7.5 mg/kg/day

Hemoglobin <8.5 g/dL: Refer to adult dosing.

Patient with cardiac history:

Hemoglobin has decreased ≥2 g/dL during any 4-week period of treatment: 7.5 mg/kg/day

Hemoglobin <12 g/dL after 4 weeks of reduced dose: Refer to adult dosing.

Renal Impairment: Cl_{cr} <50 mL/minute: Oral is route contraindicated.

Dosing Adjustment for Toxicity: Oral: Capsule, solution, tablet:

Patient **without** cardiac history:

Hemoglobin <10 g/dL:

Children: 7.5 mg/kg/day

Adults: Decrease dose to 600 mg/day

Hemoglobin <8.5 g/dL: Children and Adults: Permanently discontinue treatment

Patient **with** cardiac history:

Hemoglobin has decreased ≥2 g/dL during any 4-week period of treatment:

Children: 7.5 mg/kg/day

Adults: Decrease dose to 600 mg/day

Hemoglobin <12 g/dL after 4 weeks of reduced dose: Children and Adults: Permanently discontinue treatment

Administration

Oral: Administer concurrently with interferon alfa injection. Capsule should not be opened, crushed, chewed, or broken. Capsules are not for use in children <5 years of age. Use oral solution for children 3-5 years, those ≤25 kg, or those who cannot swallow capsules.

Capsule, in combination with interferon alfa-2b: May be administered with or without food, but always in a consistent manner in regard to food intake.

Capsule, in combination with peginterferon alfa 2b: Administer with food.

Solution, in combination with interferon alfa-2b: May be administered with or without food, but always in a consistent manner in regard to food intake.

Tablet: Should be administered with food.

Inhalation: Ribavirin should be administered in well-ventilated rooms (at least 6 air changes/hour). In mechanically-ventilated patients, ribavirin can potentially be deposited in the ventilator delivery system depending on temperature, humidity, and electrostatic forces; this deposition can lead to malfunction or obstruction of the expiratory valve, resulting in inadvertently high positive end-expiratory pressures. The use of one-way valves in the inspiratory lines, a breathing circuit filter in the expiratory line, and frequent monitoring and filter replacement have been effective in preventing these problems. Solutions in SPAG-2 unit should be discarded at least every 24 hours and when the liquid level is low before adding newly reconstituted solution. Should not be mixed with other aerosolized medication.

Stability

Reconstitution: Inhalation: Do not use any water containing an antimicrobial agent to reconstitute drug.

Reconstituted solution is stable for 24 hours at room temperature.

Compatibility: Inhalation: Should not be mixed with other aerosolized medication

Storage:

Inhalation: Store vials in a dry place at 15°C to 25°C (59°F to 78°F).

Oral: Store at 15°C to 30°C (59°F to 86°F). Solution may also be refrigerated at 2°C to 8°C (36°F to 46°F).

Laboratory Monitoring

Inhalation: Respiratory function, CBC

Oral: CBC with differential (pretreatment, 2- and 4 weeks after initiation); pretreatment and monthly pregnancy test for women of childbearing age; LFTs, TSH, HCV-RNA after 24 weeks of therapy; ECG in patients with pre-existing cardiac disease

Nursing Actions

Physical Assessment: Note specific cautions for healthcare professionals' exposure risks with inhalation formulation. Monitor results of laboratory tests, therapeutic effectiveness and adverse reactions on a regular basis with long term therapy. Teach patient proper use (according to formulation), possible side effects/appropriate interventions, and adverse symptoms to report (eg, CNS effects [headache, fatigue, irritability, impaired concentration], GI disturbance [nausea, vomiting, anorexia], hematologic [anemia], myalgia, rigors, dyspnea). An FDA-approved medication guide is available at www.fda.gov/cder/Offices/ODS/labeling.htm; distribute to each patient to whom this medication is dispensed for the treatment of hepatitis C. **Pregnancy risk factor X:** Determine that patient is not pregnant before beginning treatment. Do not give to women of childbearing age or males who may have intercourse with childbearing women unless both male and female are capable of complying with using two effective forms of contraception during therapy and 6 months following therapy.

Patient Education: For oral administration, take as directed (capsules with food, solution with or without food, but always in a consistent manner in regard to food intake). For aerosol use, follow exact directions for use of aerosol device. Do not allow pregnant women or women of childbearing age to come in any contact with this medication. If prescribed in conjunction with other medications (injections); maintain schedule as directed. Maintain adequate hydration (2-3 L/day of fluids) unless instructed to restrict fluid intake. You will need regular blood tests while taking this drug. You may experience increased susceptibility to infection (avoid crowds and exposure to infection and do not have any vaccinations without consulting prescriber). May cause confusion, impaired concentration, or headache (use cautions when driving or engaging in potentially hazardous tasks until response to drug is known); nausea, vomiting, or anorexia (small frequent meals, frequent mouth care, chewing gum, or sucking lozenges may help); diarrhea (buttermilk, boiled milk, or yogurt may relieve diarrhea); or loss of hair (reversible). Report rash, infection (fever, chills, unusual bleeding or bruising, infection, or unhealed sores or white plaques in mouth); tingling, weakness, or pain in extremities; or other persistent adverse effects. **Pregnancy/breast-feeding precautions:** Inform prescriber if you are pregnant. Both males and females should use appropriate barrier contraceptive measures during and for 60-90 days following end of therapy. Do not allow family members or friends who are pregnant (or may become pregnant) to handle inhalation powder. This drug may cause serious fetal defects. Consult prescriber for appropriate barrier contraceptive measures. Do not donate blood during or for 6 months following therapy. Breast-feeding is not recommended.

(Continued)

Ribavirin *(Continued)*

Dietary Considerations When used in combination with interferon alfa-2b, capsules and solution may be taken with or without food, but always in a consistent manner in regard to food intake (ie, always take with food or always take on an empty stomach). When used in combination with peginterferon alfa 2b, capsules should be taken with food. Tablets should be taken with food.

Pregnancy Issues Produced significant embryocidal and/or teratogenic effects in all animal studies at ~0.01 times the maximum recommended daily human dose. Use is contraindicated in pregnancy. Negative pregnancy test is required before initiation and monthly thereafter. Avoid pregnancy in female patients and female partners of male patients during therapy by using two effective forms of contraception; continue contraceptive measures for at least 6 months after completion of therapy. If patient or female partner becomes pregnant during treatment, she should be counseled about potential risks of exposure. If pregnancy occurs during use or within 6 months after treatment, report to company (800-593-2214).

Riboflavin *(RYE boe flay vin)*

U.S. Brand Names Ribo-100
Synonyms Lactoflavin; Vitamin B_2; Vitamin G
Pharmacologic Category Vitamin, Water Soluble
Medication Safety Issues
Sound-alike/look-alike issues:
Riboflavin may be confused with ribavirin
Pregnancy Risk Factor A/C (dose exceeding RDA recommendation)
Lactation Enters breast milk/compatible
Use Prevention of riboflavin deficiency and treatment of ariboflavinosis
Mechanism of Action/Effect Component of flavoprotein enzymes that work together, which are necessary for normal tissue respiration; also needed for activation of pyridoxine and conversion of tryptophan to niacin
Warnings/Precautions Riboflavin deficiency often occurs in the presence of other B vitamin deficiencies.
Drug Interactions
Decreased Effect: Decreased absorption with probenecid.
Lab Interactions Large doses may interfere with urinalysis based on spectrometry. May cause false elevations in fluorometric determinations of catecholamines and urobilinogen.
Adverse Reactions Frequency not defined: Genitourinary: Discoloration of urine (yellow-orange)
Pharmacodynamics/Kinetics
Half-Life Elimination: Biologic: 66-84 minutes
Metabolism: None
Excretion: Urine (9%) as unchanged drug
Available Dosage Forms
Tablet: 25 mg, 50 mg, 100 mg
Ribo-100: 100 mg
Dosing
Adults & Elderly:
Riboflavin deficiency: Oral: 5-30 mg/day in divided doses
Recommended daily allowance: Oral: 1.2-1.7 mg
Pediatrics:
Riboflavin deficiency: Oral: Children: 2.5-10 mg/day in divided doses
Recommended daily allowance: Oral: Children: 0.4-1.8 mg
Nursing Actions
Physical Assessment: Assess knowledge/teach patient appropriate use, dietary instruction, possible side effects, and adverse symptoms to report

Patient Education: Take with food. Large doses may cause bright yellow or orange urine.
Additional Information Dietary sources of riboflavin include liver, kidney, dairy products, green vegetables, eggs, whole grain cereals, yeast, and mushroom.

Rifabutin *(rif a BYOO tin)*

U.S. Brand Names Mycobutin®
Synonyms Ansamycin
Pharmacologic Category Antibiotic, Miscellaneous; Antitubercular Agent
Medication Safety Issues
Sound-alike/look-alike issues:
Rifabutin may be confused with rifampin
Pregnancy Risk Factor B
Lactation Excretion in breast milk unknown
Use Prevention of disseminated *Mycobacterium avium* complex (MAC) in patients with advanced HIV infection
Unlabeled/Investigational Use Utilized in multidrug regimens for treatment of MAC
Mechanism of Action/Effect Inhibits DNA-dependent RNA polymerase at the beta subunit which prevents chain initiation
Contraindications Hypersensitivity to rifabutin, any other rifamycins, or any component of the formulation; rifabutin is contraindicated in patients with a WBC <1000/mm³ or a platelet count <50,000/mm³
Warnings/Precautions Rifabutin as a single agent must not be administered to patients with active tuberculosis since its use may lead to the development of tuberculosis that is resistant to both rifabutin and rifampin. Rifabutin should be discontinued in patients with AST >500 units/L or if total bilirubin is >3 mg/dL. Use with caution in patients with liver impairment. Modification of dosage should be considered in patients with renal impairment.
Drug Interactions
Cytochrome P450 Effect: Substrate of CYP3A4 (major); **Induces** CYP3A4 (strong)
Decreased Effect: Rifabutin may decrease the levels/effects of alfentanil, amiodarone, angiotensin II receptor blockers (irbesartan, losartan), CYP3A4 substrates (eg, clarithromycin, erythromycin, mirtazapine, nefazodone, venlafaxine), 5-HT₃ antagonists, imidazole antifungals, aprepitant, barbiturates, benzodiazepines (metabolized by oxidation), beta blockers, buspirone, calcium channel blockers, chloramphenicol, corticosteroids, cyclosporine, dapsone, disopyramide, estrogen and progestin contraceptives, fluconazole, gefitinib, HMG-CoA reductase inhibitors, methadone, morphine, phenytoin, propafenone, protease inhibitors, quinidine, repaglinide, reverse transcriptase inhibitors (non-nucleoside), tacrolimus, tamoxifen, terbinafine, tocainide, tricyclic antidepressants, warfarin, zaleplon, zolpidem. The effects of rifabutin may be decreased by CYP3A4 inducers (eg, aminoglutethimide, carbamazepine, nafcillin, nevirapine, phenobarbital, phenytoin).
Increased Effect/Toxicity: Rifabutin may increase the therapeutic effect of clopidogrel; concurrent use with isoniazid may increase risk of hepatotoxicity; the levels/toxicity of rifabutin may be increased by imidazole antifungals, macrolide antibiotics, and protease inhibitors
Nutritional/Ethanol Interactions Food: High-fat meal may decrease the rate but not the extent of absorption.
Adverse Reactions
>10%:
Dermatologic: Rash (11%)
Genitourinary: Discoloration of urine (30%)
Hematologic: Neutropenia (25%), leukopenia (17%)
1% to 10%:
Central nervous system: Headache (3%)

Gastrointestinal: Vomiting/nausea (3%), abdominal pain (4%), diarrhea (3%), anorexia (2%), flatulence (2%), eructation (3%)

Hematologic: Anemia, thrombocytopenia (5%)

Hepatic: Increased AST/ALT (7% to 9%)

Neuromuscular & skeletal: Myalgia

Overdosage/Toxicology Symptoms of overdose include nausea, vomiting, hepatotoxicity, lethargy, CNS disturbances, and depression. Treatment is supportive. Hemodialysis will remove rifabutin; however, its effect on outcome is unknown.

Pharmacodynamics/Kinetics

Time to Peak: Serum: 2-4 hours

Protein Binding: 85%

Half-Life Elimination: Terminal: 45 hours (range: 16-69 hours)

Metabolism: To active and inactive metabolites

Excretion: Urine (10% as unchanged drug, 53% as metabolites); feces (10% as unchanged drug, 30% as metabolites)

Available Dosage Forms Capsule: 150 mg

Dosing

Adults & Elderly:

Disseminated MAC in advanced HIV infection:

Prophylaxis: Oral: 300 mg once daily (alone or in combination with azithromycin)

Treatment (unlabeled use): Oral:

Patients not receiving NNRTIs or protease inhibitors:

Initial phase: 5 mg/kg daily (maximum: 300 mg)

Second phase: 5 mg/kg daily or twice weekly

Patients receiving nelfinavir, amprenavir, indinavir: Reduce dose to 150 mg/day; no change in dose if administered twice weekly

Pediatrics:

Disseminated MAC in advanced HIV infection:

Children >1 year:

Prophylaxis: Oral: 5 mg/kg daily; higher dosages have been used in limited trials

Treatment (unlabeled use): Oral: Patients not receiving NNRTIs or protease inhibitors:

Initial phase (2 weeks to 2 months): 10-20 mg/kg daily (maximum: 300 mg).

Second phase: 10-20 mg/kg daily (maximum: 300 mg) or twice weekly

Renal Impairment: Cl_{cr} <30 mL/minute: Reduce dose by 50%

Administration

Oral: Should be administered on an empty stomach, but may be taken with meals to minimize nausea or vomiting.

Laboratory Monitoring Periodic liver function, CBC with differential, platelet count

Nursing Actions

Physical Assessment: Assess potential for interactions with other pharmacological agents patient may be taking (eg, decreased levels/effects of multiple other agents). Caution females using hormone contraceptive about potential for decreased contraceptive effects. Monitor laboratory tests, therapeutic effectiveness (prevention of MAC in patients with HIV), and adverse response (eg, anemia, neutropenia, GI disturbance). Teach patient proper use, possible side effects/appropriate interventions, and adverse symptoms to report.

Patient Education: Do not take any new medication during therapy without consulting prescriber. Take as directed, with or without food. Complete full course of therapy; do not skip doses. Will discolor urine, stool, saliva, tears, sweat, and other body fluid a red-brown color. Stains on clothing or contact lenses are permanent. Report skin rash; persistent vomiting or diarrhea; fever, chills, or flu-like symptoms; dark urine or pale stools; unusual bleeding or bruising; or unusual confusion, depression, or fatigue. **Breast-feeding precaution:** Consult prescriber if breast-feeding.

Dietary Considerations May be taken with meals or without food or mix with applesauce.

Rifampin (RIF am pin)

U.S. Brand Names Rifadin®

Synonyms Rifampicin

Pharmacologic Category Antibiotic, Miscellaneous; Antitubercular Agent

Medication Safety Issues

Sound-alike/look-alike issues:

Rifampin may be confused with rifabutin, Rifamate®, rifapentine, rifaximin

Rifadin® may be confused with Ritalin®

Pregnancy Risk Factor C

Lactation Enters breast milk/not recommended (AAP rates "compatible")

Use Management of active tuberculosis in combination with other agents; elimination of meningococci from the nasopharynx in asymptomatic carriers

Unlabeled/Investigational Use Prophylaxis of *Haemophilus influenzae* type b infection; *Legionella* pneumonia; used in combination with other anti-infectives in the treatment of staphylococcal infections; treatment of *M. leprae* infections

Mechanism of Action/Effect Inhibits bacterial RNA synthesis by binding to the beta subunit of DNA-dependent RNA polymerase, blocking RNA transcription

Contraindications Hypersensitivity to rifampin, any rifamycins, or any component of the formulation; concurrent use of amprenavir, saquinavir/ritonavir (possibly other protease inhibitors)

Warnings/Precautions Use with caution and modify dosage in patients with liver impairment. Discontinue therapy if clinical symptoms or any signs of significant hepatocellular damage develop. Use with caution in patients with porphyria. Not for use in meningococcal disease, only for short-term treatment of asymptomatic carrier states. Use with caution in patients receiving concurrent medications associated with hepatotoxicity (particularly with pyrazinamide), or in patients with a history of alcoholism (even if ethanol consumption is discontinued during therapy).

Monitor for compliance and effects including hypersensitivity, thrombocytopenia in patients on intermittent therapy. May discolor urine, feces, saliva, sweat, tears, and CSF (red/orange); remove soft contact lenses during therapy. Regimens of 600 mg once or twice weekly have been associated with a high incidence of adverse reactions including a flu-like syndrome. I.V. formulation is not intended for I.M. or SubQ administration.

Drug Interactions

Cytochrome P450 Effect: Induces CYP1A2 (strong), 2A6 (strong), 2B6 (strong), 2C8 (strong), 2C9 (strong), 2C19 (strong), 3A4 (strong)

Decreased Effect: Rifampin may decrease the levels/effects of the following drugs: Acetaminophen, alfentanil, amiodarone, angiotensin II receptor blockers (irbesartan and losartan), 5-HT₃ antagonists, imidazole antifungals, aprepitant, barbiturates, benzodiazepines (metabolized by oxidation), beta blockers, buspirone, calcium channel blockers, chloramphenicol, corticosteroids, cyclosporine; CYP1A2, 2A6, 2B6, 2C8, 2C9, 2C19, and 3A4 substrates (eg, aminophylline, amiodarone, bupropion, fluoxetine, fluvoxamine, ifosfamide, methsuximide, mirtazapine, nateglinide, pioglitazone, promethazine, proton pump inhibitors, ropinirole, rosiglitazone, selegiline, sertraline, theophylline, venlafaxine, and zafirlukast); dapsone, disopyramide, estrogen and progestin contraceptives, fexofenadine, fluconazole, fusidic acid, gefitinib, HMG-CoA reductase inhibitors, methadone, (Continued)

Rifampin (Continued)

morphine, phenytoin, propafenone, protease inhibitors, quinidine, repaglinide, reverse transcriptase inhibitors (non-nucleoside), sulfonylureas, tacrolimus, tamoxifen, terbinafine, tocainide, tricyclic antidepressants, warfarin, zaleplon, zidovudine, zolpidem.

Increased Effect/Toxicity: Rifampin may increase the therapeutic effect of clopidogrel; concurrent use with isoniazid, pyrazinamide, or protease inhibitors (amprenavir, saquinavir/ritonavir) may increase risk of hepatotoxicity; macrolide antibiotics may increase levels/toxicity of rifampin

Nutritional/Ethanol Interactions

Ethanol: Avoid ethanol (may increase risk of hepatotoxicity).

Food: Food decreases the extent of absorption; rifampin concentrations may be decreased if taken with food.

Herb/Nutraceutical: St John's wort may decrease rifampin levels.

Lab Interactions

Positive Coombs' reaction [direct], inhibit standard assay's ability to measure serum folate and B_{12}

Adverse Reactions

Frequency not defined:

Cardiovascular: Edema, flushing

Central nervous system: Ataxia, behavioral changes, concentration impaired, confusion, dizziness, drowsiness, fatigue, fever, headache, numbness, psychosis

Dermatologic: Pemphigoid reaction, pruritus, urticaria

Endocrine & metabolic: Adrenal insufficiency, menstrual disorders

Hematologic: Agranulocytosis (rare), DIC, eosinophilia, hemoglobin decreased, hemolysis, hemolytic anemia, leukopenia, thrombocytopenia (especially with high-dose therapy)

Hepatic: Hepatitis (rare), jaundice

Neuromuscular & skeletal: Myalgia, osteomalacia, weakness

Ocular: Exudative conjunctivitis, visual changes

Renal: Acute renal failure, BUN increased, hemoglobinuria, hematuria, interstitial nephritis, uric acid increased

Miscellaneous: Flu-like syndrome

1% to 10%:

Dermatologic: Rash (1% to 5%)

Gastrointestinal (1% to 2%): Anorexia, cramps, diarrhea, epigastric distress, flatulence, heartburn, nausea, pseudomembranous colitis, pancreatitis vomiting

Hepatic: LFTs increased (up to 14%)

Overdosage/Toxicology

Symptoms of overdose include nausea, vomiting, hepatotoxicity, lethargy, discoloration of bodily fluids, skin, and/or feces, and CNS depression. Treatment is supportive. Plasma rifampin concentrations are not significantly affected by hemodialysis or peritoneal dialysis.

Pharmacodynamics/Kinetics

Duration of Action: ≤24 hours

Time to Peak: Serum: Oral: 2-4 hours

Protein Binding: 80%

Half-Life Elimination: 3-4 hours, prolonged with hepatic impairment; End-stage renal disease: 1.8-11 hours

Metabolism: Hepatic; undergoes enterohepatic recirculation

Excretion: Feces (60% to 65%) and urine (~30%) as unchanged drug

Available Dosage Forms

Capsule: 150 mg, 300 mg

Injection, powder for reconstitution: 600 mg

Dosing

Adults & Elderly:

Tuberculosis therapy (drug susceptible): Oral, I.V.:

Note: A four-drug regimen (isoniazid, rifampin, pyrazinamide, and ethambutol) is preferred for the initial, empiric treatment of TB. When the drug susceptibility results are available, the regimen should be altered as appropriate.

Daily therapy: 10 mg/kg/day (maximum: 600 mg/day)

Twice weekly directly observed therapy (DOT): 10 mg/kg (maximum: 600 mg); 3 times/week: 10 mg/kg (maximum: 600 mg)

Latent tuberculosis infection (LTBI): As an alternative to isoniazid: Oral, I.V.: 10 mg/kg/day (maximum: 600 mg/day) for 4 months. Note: Combination with pyrazinamide should not generally be offered (MMWR, Aug 8, 2003).

H. influenzae prophylaxis (unlabeled use): Oral, I.V.: 600 mg every 24 hours for 4 days

Leprosy (unlabeled use): Oral, I.V.:

Multibacillary: 600 mg once monthly for 24 months in combination with ofloxacin and minocycline

Paucibacillary: 600 mg once monthly for 6 months in combination with dapsone

Single lesion: 600 mg as a single dose in combination with ofloxacin 400 mg and minocycline 100 mg

Meningococcal meningitis prophylaxis: Oral, I.V.: 600 mg every 12 hours for 2 days

Meningitis (Pneumococcus or Staphylococcus): I.V.: 600 mg once daily

Nasal carriers of Staphylococcus aureus (unlabeled use): Oral, I.V.: 600 mg/day for 5-10 days in combination with other antibiotics

Synergy for Staphylococcus aureus infections (unlabeled use): Oral, I.V.: 300-600 mg twice daily with other antibiotics

Pediatrics:

Tuberculosis therapy (drug susceptible): Oral, I.V.: Infants and Children <12 years:

Daily therapy: 10-20 mg/kg/day usually as a single dose (maximum: 600 mg/day)

Twice weekly directly observed therapy (DOT): 10-20 mg/kg (maximum: 600 mg)

See "Note" in adult dosing.

Latent tuberculosis infection (LTBI): As an alternative to isoniazid: Children: 10-20 mg/kg/day (maximum: 600 mg/day) for 6 months

H. influenzae prophylaxis (unlabeled use): Oral, I.V.: Infants and Children: 20 mg/kg/day every 24 hours for 4 days, not to exceed 600 mg/dose

Meningococcal prophylaxis: Oral:

<1 month: 10 mg/kg/day in divided doses every 12 hours for 2 days

Infants and Children: 20 mg/kg/day in divided doses every 12 hours for 2 days (maximum: 600 mg/dose)

Nasal carriers of Staphylococcus aureus (unlabeled use): Oral, I.V.: 15 mg/kg/day divided every 12 hours for 5-10 days in combination with other antibiotics

Renal Impairment: Plasma rifampin concentrations are not significantly affected by hemodialysis or peritoneal dialysis.

Hepatic Impairment: Dose reductions are necessary to reduce hepatotoxicity.

Administration

Oral: Administer on an empty stomach with a glass of water (ie, 1 hour prior to, or 2 hours after meals or antacids) to increase total absorption (food may delay and reduce the amount of rifampin absorbed). The compounded oral suspension must be shaken well before using. May mix contents of capsule with applesauce or jelly.

I.M.: Do not administer I.M. or SubQ

I.V.: Administer I.V. preparation once daily by slow I.V. infusion over 30 minutes to 3 hours at a final concentration not to exceed 6 mg/mL.

I.V. Detail: Avoid extravasation.

pH: 7.8-8.8

Stability

Reconstitution: Reconstitute powder for injection with SWFI; prior to injection, dilute in appropriate volume of compatible diluent (eg, 100 mL D_5W).

Compatibility:

Y-site administration: Incompatible with diltiazem

Compatibility when admixed: Incompatible with minocycline

Storage: Rifampin powder is reddish brown. Intact vials should be stored at room temperature and protected from excessive heat and light. Reconstituted vials are stable for 24 hours at room temperature

Stability of parenteral admixture at room temperature (25°C) is 4 hours for D_5W and 24 hours for NS

Laboratory Monitoring Periodic monitoring of liver function (AST, ALT), CBC; sputum culture, chest x-ray 2-3 months into treatment

Nursing Actions

Physical Assessment: Assess potential for interactions with other pharmacological agents patient may be taking (eg, concurrent use with rifampin may decrease levels/effects of multiple other drugs, including some oral contraceptives, anticoagulants, hypoglycemics and beta-blockers). See Administration for infusion specifics; infusion site must be monitored to prevent extravasation. Monitor periodic laboratory tests and chest x-ray, therapeutic effectiveness, and adverse reactions (eg, hypersensitivity reactions, hepatotoxicity, CNS changes, hematologic changes, visual disturbances, and gastrointestinal upset) on a regular basis during therapy. Monitor patient compliance with treatment regimen. Teach patient proper use, possible side effects/appropriate interventions, and adverse symptoms to report.

Patient Education: Do not take any new medication during therapy without consulting prescriber. Rifampin may be prescribed in conjunction with another medication; maintain dosing schedule of both drugs as directed. Take rifampin on an empty stomach, 1 hour before or 2 hours after meals. It is extremely important that you complete full course of therapy and do not skip doses. Keep appointments for scheduled laboratory tests and chest x-rays. This medication will discolor urine, stool, saliva, tears, sweat, and other body fluid a red-brown color. Stains on contact lenses and clothing are permanent. Report persistent vomiting or diarrhea; rash; fever, chills, or flu-like symptoms; unusual bruising or bleeding; or other persistent adverse effects. **Pregnancy precaution:** Inform prescriber if you are or intend to become pregnant. This drug may interfere with effectiveness of oral/systemic contraceptives; consult prescriber for alternative contraceptive measures.

Dietary Considerations Rifampin should be taken on an empty stomach.

Geriatric Considerations Rifampin, in combination with isoniazid, is the foundation of tuberculosis treatment. Since most older patients acquired their *Mycobacterium tuberculosis* infection before effective chemotherapy was available, either a 9-month regimen of isoniazid and rifampin or a 6-month regimen of isoniazid and rifampin with pyrazinamide (the first 2 months) should be effective.

Rifampin and Isoniazid

(RIF am pin & eye soe NYE a zid)

U.S. Brand Names Rifamate®
Synonyms Isoniazid and Rifampin
Pharmacologic Category Antibiotic, Miscellaneous
Pregnancy Risk Factor C
Lactation Enters breast milk/compatible
Use Management of active tuberculosis; see individual agents for additional information
Available Dosage Forms Capsule: Rifampin 300 mg and isoniazid 150 mg
Dosing
Adults: Tuberculosis: Oral: 2 capsules/day
Elderly: Refer to dosing in individual monographs.
Nursing Actions
Physical Assessment: See individual agents.
Patient Education: See individual agents. **Pregnancy precaution:** Inform prescriber if you are or intend to become pregnant.
Related Information
Isoniazid *on page 683*
Rifampin *on page 1081*

Rifampin, Isoniazid, and Pyrazinamide

(RIF am pin, eye soe NYE a zid, & peer a ZIN a mide)

U.S. Brand Names Rifater®
Synonyms Isoniazid, Rifampin, and Pyrazinamide; Pyrazinamide, Rifampin, and Isoniazid
Pharmacologic Category Antibiotic, Miscellaneous
Pregnancy Risk Factor C
Lactation Enters breast milk/use caution
Use Initial phase, short-course treatment of pulmonary tuberculosis; see individual agents for additional information
Available Dosage Forms Tablet: Rifampin 120 mg, isoniazid 50 mg, and pyrazinamide 300 mg
Dosing
Adults: Tuberculosis: Oral: Patients weighing:
≤44 kg: 4 tablets
45-54 kg: 5 tablets
≥55 kg: 6 tablets
Doses should be administered in a single daily dose.
Elderly: Refer to dosing in individual monographs.
Nursing Actions
Physical Assessment: See individual agents.
Patient Education: See individual agents. **Pregnancy/breast-feeding precautions:** Inform prescriber if you are or intend to become pregnant. Consult prescriber if breast-feeding.
Related Information
Isoniazid *on page 683*
Pyrazinamide *on page 1050*
Rifampin *on page 1081*

Rifapentine (RIF a pen teen)

U.S. Brand Names Priftin®
Pharmacologic Category Antitubercular Agent
Medication Safety Issues
Sound-alike/look-alike issues:
Rifapentine may be confused with rifampin
Pregnancy Risk Factor C
Lactation Excretion in breast milk unknown/contraindicated
Use Treatment of pulmonary tuberculosis; rifapentine must always be used in conjunction with at least one other antituberculosis drug to which the isolate is
(Continued)

Rifapentine *(Continued)*

susceptible; it may also be necessary to add a third agent (either streptomycin or ethambutol) until susceptibility is known.

Mechanism of Action/Effect Inhibits DNA-dependent RNA polymerase in susceptible strains of *Mycobacterium tuberculosis* (but not in mammalian cells). Rifapentine is bactericidal against both intracellular and extracellular MTB organisms. Strains which are resistant to other rifamycins including rifampin are likely to be resistant to rifapentine. Cross-resistance does not appear between rifapentine and other nonrifamycin antimycobacterial agents.

Contraindications Hypersensitivity to rifapentine, rifampin, rifabutin, any rifamycin analog, or any component of the formulation

Warnings/Precautions Compliance with dosing regimen is absolutely necessary for successful drug therapy. Patients with abnormal liver tests and/or liver disease should only be given rifapentine when absolutely necessary and under strict medical supervision. Monitoring of liver function tests should be carried out prior to therapy and then every 2-4 weeks during therapy if signs of liver disease occur or worsen, rifapentine should be discontinued. Pseudomembranous colitis has been reported to occur with various antibiotics including other rifamycins. If this is suspected, rifapentine should be stopped and the patient treated with specific and supportive treatment. Experience in treating TB in HIV-infected patients is limited.

Rifapentine may produce a red-orange discoloration of body tissues/fluids including skin, teeth, tongue, urine, feces, saliva, sputum, tears, sweat, and cerebral spinal fluid. Contact lenses may become permanently stained.

Drug Interactions

Cytochrome P450 Effect: Induces CYP2C8/9 (strong), 3A4 (strong)

Decreased Effect: Rifapentine may decrease the levels/effects of the following drugs: alfentanil, amiodarone, angiotensin II receptor blockers (irbesartan, losartan), 5-HT$_3$ antagonists, imidazole antifungals, aprepitant, barbiturates, benzodiazepines (metabolized by oxidation), beta blockers, buspirone, calcium channel blockers, corticosteroids, cyclosporine; CYP2C8/9 and 3A4 substrates (eg, amiodarone, clarithromycin, erythromycin, fluoxetine, mirtazapine, nateglinide, nefazodone, nevirapine, pioglitazone, rosiglitazone, sertraline, venlafaxine, and zafirlukast); dapsone, disopyramide, estrogen and progestin contraceptives, fluconazole, gefitinib, HMG-CoA reductase inhibitors, methadone, morphine, phenytoin, propafenone, protease inhibitors, quinidine, repaglinide, reverse transcriptase inhibitors (non-nucleoside), tacrolimus, tamoxifen, terbinafine, tocainide, tricyclic antidepressants, warfarin, zaleplon, zidovudine, and zolpidem.

Increased Effect/Toxicity: Rifapentine may increase the therapeutic effect of clopidogrel; concurrent use with isoniazid may increase risk of hepatotoxicity

Nutritional/Ethanol Interactions Food: Food increases AUC and maximum serum concentration by 43% and 44% respectively as compared to fasting conditions.

Lab Interactions Rifampin has been shown to inhibit standard microbiological assays for serum folate and vitamin B$_{12}$. This should be considered for rifapentine; therefore, alternative assay methods should be considered.

Adverse Reactions

>10%: Endocrine & metabolic: Hyperuricemia (most likely due to pyrazinamide from initiation phase combination therapy)

1% to 10%:

Cardiovascular: Hypertension

Central nervous system: Headache, dizziness

Dermatologic: Rash, pruritus, acne

Gastrointestinal: Anorexia, nausea, vomiting, dyspepsia, diarrhea

Hematologic: Neutropenia, lymphopenia, anemia, leukopenia, thrombocytosis

Hepatic: Increased ALT/AST

Neuromuscular & skeletal: Arthralgia, pain

Renal: Pyuria, proteinuria, hematuria, urinary casts

Respiratory: Hemoptysis

Overdosage/Toxicology There is no experience with treatment of acute overdose with rifapentine; experience with other rifamycins suggests that gastric lavage followed by activated charcoal may help adsorb any remaining drug from the GI tract. Hemodialysis or forced diuresis is not expected to enhance elimination of unchanged rifapentine in an overdose.

Pharmacodynamics/Kinetics

Time to Peak: Serum: 5-6 hours

Protein Binding: Rifapentine and 25-desacetyl metabolite: 97.7% and 93.2%, primarily to albumin

Half-Life Elimination: Rifapentine: 14-17 hours; 25-desacetyl rifapentine: 13 hours

Metabolism: Hepatic; hydrolyzed by an esterase and esterase enzyme to form the active metabolite 25-desacetyl rifapentine

Excretion: Urine (17% primarily as metabolites)

Available Dosage Forms Tablet: 150 mg

Dosing

Adults & Elderly: Note: Rifapentine should not be used alone; initial phase should include a 3- to 4-drug regimen.

Tuberculosis, intensive phase (initial 2 months) of short-term therapy: 600 mg (four 150 mg tablets) given twice weekly (with an interval of not less than 72 hours between doses); following the intensive phase, treatment should continue with rifapentine 600 mg once weekly for 4 months in combination with INH or appropriate agent for susceptible organisms.

Stability

Storage: Store at room temperature (15°C to 30°C; 59°F to 86°F). Protect from excessive heat and humidity.

Laboratory Monitoring Perform baseline liver function tests at beginning of therapy. Patients with pre-existing hepatic problems should have liver function tests monitored every 2-4 weeks during therapy. Perform CBC monthly.

Nursing Actions

Physical Assessment: For use in combination with other antitubercular medications. Assess potential for interactions with other pharmacological agents patient may be taking (eg, concurrent use with rifapentine may decrease levels/effects of multiple other drugs, including some oral contraceptives, anticoagulants, hypoglycemics, and beta-blockers). Monitor periodic laboratory tests and chest x-ray, therapeutic effectiveness, and adverse reactions (eg, hepatotoxicity, CNS changes, hematologic changes, visual disturbances, and gastrointestinal upset) on a regular basis during therapy. Monitor patient compliance with treatment regimen. Teach patient proper use, possible side effects/appropriate interventions, and adverse symptoms to report.

Patient Education: Do not take any new medication during therapy without consulting prescriber. Rifapentine will be prescribed in conjunction with other medications; maintain dosing schedule as directed. It is extremely important that you complete full course of therapy and do not skip doses. Keep appointments for scheduled laboratory tests and chest x-rays. This medication will discolor urine, stool, saliva, tears, sweat, breast milk, and other body fluids a red-brown color. Stains on contact lenses and clothing are permanent. Report persistent vomiting or diarrhea;

rash; fever, chills, or flu-like symptoms; unusual bruising or bleeding; yellowing of skin or sclera, pale stool, or other persistent adverse effects. **Pregnancy precaution:** Inform prescriber is you are or intend to become pregnant. This drug may interfere with effectiveness of oral/systemic contraceptives; consult prescriber for alternative contraceptive measures.

Breast-Feeding Issues May discolor breast milk

Additional Information Rifapentine has only been studied in patients with tuberculosis receiving a 6-month short-course intensive regimen approval. Outcomes have been based on 6-month follow-up treatment observed in clinical trial 008 as a surrogate for the 2-year follow-up generally accepted as evidence for efficacy in the treatment of pulmonary tuberculosis.

Riluzole (RIL yoo zole)

U.S. Brand Names Rilutek®

Synonyms 2-Amino-6-Trifluoromethoxy-benzothiazole; RP-54274

Pharmacologic Category Glutamate Inhibitor

Pregnancy Risk Factor C

Lactation Excretion in breast milk unknown/not recommended

Use Treatment of amyotrophic lateral sclerosis (ALS); riluzole can extend survival or time to tracheostomy

Mechanism of Action/Effect Mechanism of action is not known. Pharmacologic properties include inhibitory effect on glutamate release, inactivation of voltage-dependent sodium channels; and ability to interfere with intracellular events that follow transmitter binding at excitatory amino acid receptors

Contraindications Severe hypersensitivity reactions to riluzole or any component of the formulation

Warnings/Precautions Among 4000 patients given riluzole for ALS, there were 3 cases of marked neutropenia (ANC <500/mm³), all seen within the first 2 months of treatment. Use with caution in patients with concomitant renal insufficiency. Use with caution in patients with current evidence or history of abnormal liver function; do not administer if baseline liver function tests are elevated. The elderly, female, or Japanese patients may have decreased clearance of riluzole; use with caution. May cause dizziness or somnolence; caution should be used performing tasks which require alertness (operating machinery or driving).

Drug Interactions

Cytochrome P450 Effect: Substrate of CYP1A2 (major)

Decreased Effect: CYP1A2 inducers may decrease the levels/effects of riluzole; example inducers include aminoglutethimide, carbamazepine, phenobarbital, and rifampin.

Increased Effect/Toxicity: CYP1A2 inhibitors may increase the levels/effects of riluzole; example inhibitors include amiodarone, ciprofloxacin, fluvoxamine, ketoconazole, norfloxacin, ofloxacin, and rofecoxib.

Nutritional/Ethanol Interactions

Ethanol: Avoid ethanol (due to CNS depression and possible risk of liver toxicity).

Food: A high-fat meal decreases absorption of riluzole (decreasing AUC by 20% and peak blood levels by 45%). Charbroiled food may increase riluzole elimination.

Adverse Reactions

>10%:

Gastrointestinal: Nausea (12% to 21%)

Neuromuscular & skeletal: Weakness (15% to 20%)

Respiratory: Lung function decreased (10% to 16%)

1% to 10%:

Cardiovascular: Edema, hypertension, tachycardia

Central nervous system: Agitation, circumoral paresthesia, depression, dizziness, headache, insomnia, malaise, somnolence, tremor, vertigo

Dermatologic: Alopecia, eczema, pruritus

Gastrointestinal: Abdominal pain, anorexia, diarrhea, dyspepsia, flatulence, oral moniliasis, stomatitis, vomiting

Hepatic: Liver function tests increased

Neuromuscular & skeletal: Arthralgia, back pain

Respiratory: Cough increased, rhinitis, sinusitis

Miscellaneous: Aggravation reaction

Overdosage/Toxicology Methemoglobinemia has been reported with overdose. No specific antidote or treatment information is available. Treatment should be supportive and directed toward alleviating symptoms.

Pharmacodynamics/Kinetics

Protein Binding: Plasma: 96%, primarily to albumin and lipoproteins

Half-Life Elimination: 12 hours

Metabolism: Extensively hepatic to six major and a number of minor metabolites via CYP1A2 dependent hydroxylation and glucuronidation

Excretion: Urine (90%; 85% as metabolites, 2% as unchanged drug) and feces (5%) within 7 days

Available Dosage Forms Tablet: 50 mg

Dosing

Adults & Elderly:

ALS treatment: Oral: 50 mg every 12 hours; no increased benefit can be expected from higher daily doses, but adverse events are increased.

Dosage adjustment in smoking: Cigarette smoking is known to induce CYP1A2; patients who smoke cigarettes would be expected to eliminate riluzole faster. There is no information, however, on the effect of, or need for, dosage adjustment in these patients.

Dosage adjustment in special populations: Females and Japanese patients may possess a lower metabolic capacity to eliminate riluzole compared with male and Caucasian subjects, respectively.

Renal Impairment: Use with caution in patients with concomitant renal insufficiency.

Hepatic Impairment: Use with caution in patients with current evidence or history of abnormal liver function indicated by significant abnormalities in serum transaminase, bilirubin or GGT levels. Baseline elevations of several LFTs (especially elevated bilirubin) should preclude use of riluzole.

Administration

Oral: Administer at the same time each day, 1 hour before or 2 hours after a meal.

Stability

Storage: Store at 20°C to 25°C (68°F to 77°F). Protect from bright light.

Laboratory Monitoring Monitor serum aminotransferases (including ALT levels) before and during therapy. Evaluate serum ALT levels every month during the first 3 months of therapy, every 3 months during the remainder of the first year, and periodically thereafter. Evaluate ALT levels more frequently in patients who develop elevations. Maximum increases in serum ALT usually occurred within 3 months after the start of therapy and were usually transient when <5 times ULN.

In trials, if ALT levels were <5 times ULN, treatment continued and ALT levels usually returned to below 2 times ULN within 2-6 months. Treatment in studies was discontinued, however, if ALT levels exceed 5 times ULN, so that there is no experience with continued treatment of ALS patients once ALT values exceed 5 times ULN.

If a decision is made to continue treatment in patients when the ALT exceeds 5 times ULN, frequent monitoring (at least weekly) of complete liver function is (Continued)

Riluzole *(Continued)*

recommended. Discontinue treatment if ALT exceeds 10 times ULN or if clinical jaundice develops.

Nursing Actions

Physical Assessment: Assess effectiveness and interactions of other medications patient may be taking. Monitor laboratory tests, therapeutic response, and adverse reactions at beginning of therapy and periodically throughout therapy. Assess knowledge/teach patient appropriate use, interventions to reduce side effects, and adverse symptoms to report.

Patient Education: This drug will not cure or stop disease but it may slow progression. Take as directed, at the same time each day, preferably on an empty stomach, 1 hour before or 2 hours after meals. Avoid alcohol. You may experience increased spasticity, dizziness or sleepiness; use caution when driving or engaging in tasks requiring alertness until response to drug is known. Small frequent meals, frequent mouth care, chewing gum, or sucking lozenges may reduce nausea, vomiting, or anorexia. Report fever; severe vomiting, diarrhea, or constipation; change in color of urine or stool; yellowing of skin or eyes; acute back pain or muscle pain; or worsening of condition. **Pregnancy/breast-feeding precautions:** Inform prescriber if you are or intend to become pregnant. Consult prescriber if breast-feeding.

Dietary Considerations Take at least 1 hour before, or 2 hours after, a meal.

Geriatric Considerations In clinical trials, no difference was demonstrated between elderly and younger adults. However, renal and hepatic changes with age can be expected to result in higher serum concentrations of the parent drug and its metabolites.

Rimantadine *(ri MAN ta deen)*

U.S. Brand Names Flumadine®

Synonyms Rimantadine Hydrochloride

Pharmacologic Category Antiviral Agent, Adamantane

Medication Safety Issues

Sound-alike/look-alike issues:

Rimantadine may be confused with amantadine, ranitidine, Rimactane®

Flumadine® may be confused with fludarabine, flunisolide, flutamide

Pregnancy Risk Factor C

Lactation Excretion in breast milk unknown/ not recommended

Use Prophylaxis (adults and children >1 year of age) and treatment (adults) of influenza A viral infection

Unlabeled/Investigational Use Treatment of influenza A viral infection in children ≥13 years of age

Mechanism of Action/Effect Exerts its inhibitory effect on three antigenic subtypes of influenza A virus (H1N1, H2N2, H3N2) early in the viral replicative cycle, possibly inhibiting the uncoating process; it has no activity against influenza B virus and is two- to eightfold more active than amantadine

Contraindications Hypersensitivity to drugs of the adamantane class, including rimantadine and amantadine, or any component of the formulation

Warnings/Precautions Use with caution in patients with renal and hepatic dysfunction; avoid use, if possible, in patients with recurrent and eczematoid dermatitis, uncontrolled psychosis, or severe psychoneurosis. An increase in seizure incidence may occur in patients with seizure disorders; discontinue drug if seizures occur; resistance may develop during treatment; viruses exhibit cross-resistance between amantadine and rimantadine.

Drug Interactions

Decreased Effect: Acetaminophen may cause a small reduction in AUC and peak concentration of rimantadine. Peak plasma and AUC concentrations of rimantadine are slightly reduced by aspirin.

Increased Effect/Toxicity: Cimetidine increases blood levels/toxicity of rimantadine.

Nutritional/Ethanol Interactions Food: Food does not affect rate or extent of absorption

Adverse Reactions 1% to 10%:

Central nervous system: Dizziness (2%), insomnia (2%), anxiety (1%), fatigue (1%), headache (1%), nervousness (1%)

Gastrointestinal: Nausea (3%), anorexia (2%), vomiting (2%), xerostomia (2%), abdominal pain (1%)

Neuromuscular and skeletal: Weakness (1%)

Overdosage/Toxicology Agitation, hallucinations, ventricular cardiac arrhythmias (torsade de pointes and PVCs), slurred speech, anticholinergic effects (dry mouth, urinary retention and mydriasis), ataxia, tremor, myoclonus, seizures, and death have been reported with amantadine (a related drug). Treatment is symptomatic (do not use physostigmine). Tachyarrhythmias may be treated with beta-blockers such as propranolol. Dialysis is not recommended except possibly in renal failure.

Pharmacodynamics/Kinetics

Onset of Action: Antiviral activity: No data exist establishing a correlation between plasma concentration and antiviral effect

Time to Peak: 6 hours

Half-Life Elimination: 25.4 hours; prolonged with elderly

Metabolism: Extensively hepatic

Excretion: Urine (<25% as unchanged drug)

Clearance: Hemodialysis does not contribute to clearance

Available Dosage Forms

Syrup, as hydrochloride: 50 mg/5 mL (240 mL) [raspberry flavor]

Tablet, as hydrochloride: 100 mg

Dosing

Adults:

Prophylaxis of influenza A: Oral: 100 mg twice daily

Treatment of influenza A: Oral: 100 mg twice daily

Elderly:

Prophylaxis of influenza A: Oral: 100 mg/day in nursing home patients or all elderly patients who may experience adverse effects using the adult dose

Treatment of influenza A: Oral: 100 mg once daily in patients ≥65 years

Pediatrics:

Prophylaxis of influenza A: Oral:

Children <10 years: 5 mg/kg once daily; maximum: 150 mg

Children >10 years: Refer to adult dosing.

Treatment of influenza A: Oral: Children ≥13 years (unlabeled use): 100 mg twice daily; children <40 kg should receive 5 mg/kg/day in divided doses, maximum dose 200 mg/day

Renal Impairment:

Cl_{cr} >10 mL/minute: Dose adjustment not required

Cl_{cr} ≤10 mL/minute: 100 mg/day

Hepatic Impairment: Severe dysfunction: 100 mg/day

Administration

Oral: Initiation of rimantadine within 48 hours of the onset of influenza A illness halves the duration of illness and significantly reduces the duration of viral shedding and increased peripheral airways resistance. Continue therapy for 5-7 days after symptoms begin.

Nursing Actions

Physical Assessment: Assess effectiveness (resolution of infection) and adverse reactions (eg, hypotension, CNS changes [confusion, anxiety, agitation], gastrointestinal upset, anticholinergic effects [dry mouth, urinary retention, mydriases]). Teach patient appropriate use, possible side effects/interventions (eg, postural hypotension), and adverse symptoms to report.

Patient Education: Do not take any new medication during therapy unless approved by prescriber. Take as directed. Complete full course of therapy even if feeling better. Take a missed dose as soon as possible. If almost time for next dose, skip the missed dose and return to your regular schedule. Do not take a double dose. May cause dizziness, insomnia, fatigue, nervousness (use caution when driving or engaged in potentially hazardous tasks until response to medication is known); gastrointestinal upset (small frequent meals, frequent mouth care, chewing gum, or sucking lozenges may help). Report rash, palpitations; severe nausea or vomiting; persistent CNS changes (eg, confusion, insomnia, anxiety, restlessness, irritability, hallucinations) or other persistent adverse reactions. **Pregnancy/breast-feeding precautions:** Inform prescriber if you are or intend to become pregnant. Do not breast-feed.

Geriatric Considerations Adverse CNS and GI effects occur frequently if dosage is not adjusted. Monitor GI effects in the elderly or patients with renal or hepatic impairment. Dosing must be individualized (100 mg 1-2 times/day). It is recommended that nursing home patients receive 100 mg/day (see Pharmacodynamics/Kinetics).

Breast-Feeding Issues Do not use in nursing mothers due to potential adverse effect in infants.

Risedronate (ris ED roe nate)

U.S. Brand Names Actonel®

Synonyms Risedronate Sodium

Pharmacologic Category Bisphosphonate Derivative

Pregnancy Risk Factor C

Lactation Excretion in breast milk unknown/not recommended

Use Paget's disease of the bone; treatment and prevention of glucocorticoid-induced osteoporosis; treatment and prevention of osteoporosis in postmenopausal women

Mechanism of Action/Effect A bisphosphonate which inhibits bone resorption via actions on osteoclasts or on osteoclast precursors; decreases the rate of bone resorption, leading to an indirect increase in bone mineral density. In Paget's disease, characterized by disordered resorption and formation of bone, inhibition of resorption leads to an indirect decrease in bone formation; but the newly-formed bone has a more normal architecture.

Contraindications Hypersensitivity to risedronate, bisphosphonates, or any component of the formulation; hypocalcemia; abnormalities of the esophagus which delay esophageal emptying such as stricture or achalasia; inability to stand or sit upright for at least 30 minutes; severe renal impairment (Cl$_{cr}$ <30 mL/minute)

Warnings/Precautions Bisphosphonates may cause upper gastrointestinal disorders such as dysphagia, esophageal ulcer, and gastric ulcer. Use caution in patients with renal impairment. Hypocalcemia must be corrected before therapy initiation with risedronate. Ensure adequate calcium and vitamin D intake, especially for patients with Paget's disease in whom the pretreatment rate of bone turnover may be greatly elevated.

Bisphosphonate therapy has been associated with osteonecrosis, primarily of the jaw; this has been observed mostly in cancer patients, but also in patients with postmenopausal osteoporosis and other diagnoses. There are no data addressing whether discontinuation of therapy reduces the risk of developing osteonecrosis. However, as a precautionary measure, dental exams and preventative dentistry should be performed prior to placing patients with risk factors (eg, chemotherapy, corticosteroids, poor oral hygiene) on chronic bisphosphonate therapy. Invasive dental procedures should be avoided during treatment.

Severe and potentially incapacitating musculoskeletal pain has been observed, with onset ranging from one day to several months after beginning therapy. Symptoms usually abate upon discontinuation, but may recur upon reinitiation of bisphosphonate treatment.

Safety and efficacy in pediatric patients have not been established.

Drug Interactions

Decreased Effect: The following agents may decrease the absorption of oral bisphosphonate derivatives: Antacids (aluminum, calcium, magnesium), oral calcium salts, oral iron salts, and oral magnesium salts

Increased Effect/Toxicity:
Aminoglycosides may lower serum calcium levels with prolonged administration; concomitant use may have an additive hypocalcemic effect. NSAIDs may enhance the gastrointestinal adverse/toxic effects (increased incidence of GI ulcers) of bisphosphonate derivatives. Bisphosphonate derivatives may enhance the hypocalcemic effect of phosphate supplements.

Nutritional/Ethanol Interactions
Ethanol: Avoid ethanol (may increase risk of osteoporosis).
Food: Food may reduce absorption (similar to other bisphosphonates); mean oral bioavailability is decreased when given with food.

Lab Interactions Bisphosphonates may interfere with diagnostic imaging agents such as technetium-99m-diphosphonate in bone scans.

Adverse Reactions Frequency may vary with dose and indication.

>10%:
Central nervous system: Headache (18%), pain (14%)
Dermatologic: Rash (8% to 12%)
Gastrointestinal: Diarrhea (11% to 20%), abdominal pain (12%), nausea (10% to 12%)
Genitourinary: Urinary tract infection (11%)
Neuromuscular & skeletal: Arthralgia (24% to 33%), back pain (26%)

1% to 10%:
Cardiovascular: Hypertension (10%), peripheral edema (8%), chest pain (5% to 7%), cardiovascular disorder (3%), angina (3%)
Central nervous system: Depression (7%), dizziness (6% to 7%), insomnia (5%), anxiety (4%), vertigo (3%)
Dermatologic: Bruising (4%), pruritus (3%), skin carcinoma (2%)
Gastrointestinal: Constipation (7%), flatulence (5%), belching (3%), colitis (3%), gastritis (3%), gastrointestinal disorder (2%), rectal disorder (2%), tooth disorder (2%)
Genitourinary: Cystitis (4%)
Hematologic: Anemia (2%)
Neuromuscular & skeletal: Joint disorder (7%), myalgia (7%), neck pain (5%), asthenia (5%), bone pain (5%), weakness (5%), bone disorder (4%), neuralgia (4%), leg cramps (4%), bursitis (3%), myasthenia (3%), tendon disorder (3%), hypertonia (2%), paresthesia (2%)
Ocular: Cataract (6%), conjunctivitis (3%), amblyopia (3%), dry eyes (3%)
Otic: Otitis media (3%), tinnitus (3%)
(Continued)

Risedronate *(Continued)*

Respiratory: Pharyngitis (6%), rhinitis (6%), sinusitis (5%), dyspnea (4%), bronchitis (3%), pneumonia (3%)

Miscellaneous: Flu symptoms (10%), neoplasm (3%), hernia (3%)

Overdosage/Toxicology Symptoms of overdose include hypocalcemia, hypophosphatemia, and upper GI adverse events (upset stomach, heartburn, esophagitis, gastritis, or ulcer). Milk or antacids containing calcium should be given to bind and reduce absorption. In substantial overdoses, use of gastric lavage to remove unabsorbed drug and I.V. calcium may be required. Dialysis would not be beneficial.

Pharmacodynamics/Kinetics

Onset of Action: May require weeks

Protein Binding: ~24%

Half-Life Elimination: Initial: 1.5 hours; Terminal: 480 hours

Metabolism: None

Excretion: Urine (up to 85%); feces (as unabsorbed drug)

Available Dosage Forms Tablet, as sodium: 5 mg, 30 mg, 35 mg

Dosing

Adults & Elderly:

Paget's disease of bone: Oral: 30 mg once daily for 2 months

Note: Retreatment may be considered (following post-treatment observation of at least 2 months) if relapse occurs, or if treatment fails to normalize serum alkaline phosphatase. For retreatment, the dose and duration of therapy are the same as for initial treatment. No data are available on more than one course of retreatment.

Osteoporosis (postmenopausal) prevention and treatment: Oral: 5 mg once daily or 35 mg once weekly

Osteoporosis (glucocorticoid-induced) prevention and treatment: Oral: 5 mg once daily

Renal Impairment: Cl$_{cr}$ <30 mL/minute: Not recommended

Administration

Oral: Risedronate should be administered 30 or more minutes before the first food or drink of the day other than water. Risedronate should be taken in an upright position with a full glass (6-8 oz) of plain water and the patient should avoid lying down for 30 minutes to minimize the possibility of GI side effects.

Stability

Storage: Store at room temperature of 20°C to 25°C (68°F to 77°F).

Laboratory Monitoring Alkaline phosphatase should be periodically measured; serum calcium, phosphorus, and possibly potassium due to its drug class. Use of absorptiometry may assist in noting benefit in osteoporosis.

Nursing Actions

Physical Assessment: Ascertain that patient is capable of complying with administration directions before starting treatment (eg, remain in standing or sitting position for 30 minutes). Renal status should be assessed (dosage may need to be adjusted in presence of renal impairment) and any hypocalcemia corrected before beginning treatment. Patients with cancer should have dental exams and necessary preventive dentistry should be done before beginning bisphosphonate therapy. Evaluate results of laboratory tests (alkaline phosphatase, serum calcium, phosphorous) and therapeutic effectiveness (according to purpose for use) on a regular basis. Monitor for adverse reactions (eg, rash, diarrhea, arthralgia, peripheral edema, gastrointestinal disturbance [nausea, vomiting, diarrhea], visual changes, hypocalcemia, hypophosphatemia). Teach patient appropriate administration, lifestyle and dietary changes that will have a beneficial impact on Paget's disease or osteoporosis, possible side effects/appropriate interventions (eg, patients with cancer should avoid invasive dental procedures during treatment) and adverse reactions to report.

Patient Education: In order to be effective, this medication must be taken exactly as directed, with a full glass of water first thing in the morning, at least 30 minutes before the first food or beverage of the day. Wait at least 30 minutes after taking this medication before taking anything else. Stay in sitting or standing position for 30 minutes following administration and until after the first food of the day to reduce potential for esophageal irritation. If you have cancer, you may be advised to have a dental exam and necessary preventive dentistry prior to beginning treatment; and you should avoid invasive dental procedures during treatment. Consult prescriber to determine necessity of lifestyle changes (eg, decreased smoking, decreased alcohol intake, dietary supplements of calcium, or increased dietary vitamin D). Avoid alcohol (ethanol may increase risk of osteoporosis). You may experience GI upset such as flatulence, bloating, nausea, or acid regurgitation (small frequent meals may help). Report unresolved muscle twitching, bone pain or leg cramps; acute abdominal pain; rash; chest pain, palpitations, or swollen extremities; disturbed vision or excessively dry eyes; ringing in the ears; rash; or persistent flu-like symptoms. Notify prescriber immediately if you experience difficulty swallowing, pain when swallowing, or severe or persistent heartburn. **Pregnancy/breast-feeding precautions:** Inform prescriber if you are or intend to become pregnant or if you are breast-feeding.

Dietary Considerations Take ≥30 minutes before the first food or drink of the day other than water. Supplemental calcium or vitamin D may be required if dietary intake is not adequate.

Geriatric Considerations No dosage adjustment required if Cl$_{cr}$ ≥30 mL/minute. Since elderly often receive diuretics, evaluate electrolyte status periodically due to the drug class (bisphosphonates). Should assure that immobile patients are sitting up for at least 30 minutes after swallowing tablets.

Breast-Feeding Issues The manufacturer recommends discontinuing nursing or discontinuing risedronate.

Pregnancy Issues Teratogenic and nonteratogenic embryo/fetal effects have been reported in animal studies. There are no adequate and well-controlled studies in pregnant women. Bisphosphonates are incorporated into the bone matrix and gradually released over time. Theoretically, there may be a risk of fetal harm when pregnancy follows the completion of therapy. Based on limited case reports with pamidronate, serum calcium levels in the newborn may be altered if administered during pregnancy.

Risperidone (ris PER i done)

U.S. Brand Names Risperdal®; Risperdal® Consta™; Risperdal® M-Tab®

Synonyms Risperdal M-Tab®

Pharmacologic Category Antipsychotic Agent, Atypical

Medication Safety Issues

Sound-alike/look-alike issues:

Risperidone may be confused with reserpine

Risperdal® may be confused with lisinopril, reserpine

Pregnancy Risk Factor C

Lactation Enters breast milk/not recommended

Use Treatment of schizophrenia; treatment of acute mania or mixed episodes associated with bipolar I disorder (as monotherapy or in combination with lithium or valproate)

Unlabeled/Investigational Use Behavioral symptoms associated with dementia in elderly; treatment of Tourette's disorder; treatment of pervasive developmental disorder and autism in children and adolescents

Mechanism of Action/Effect Risperidone is a benzisoxazole atypical antipsychotic with mixed serotonin-dopamine antagonist activity that binds to 5-HT$_2$-receptors in the CNS and in the periphery with a very high affinity; binds to dopamine-D$_2$ receptors with less affinity. The binding affinity to the dopamine-D$_2$ receptor is 20 times lower than the 5-HT$_2$ affinity. The addition of serotonin antagonism to dopamine antagonism (classic neuroleptic mechanism) is thought to improve negative symptoms of psychoses and reduce the incidence of extrapyramidal side effects. Alpha$_1$, alpha$_2$ adrenergic, and histaminergic receptors are also antagonized with high affinity. Risperidone has low to moderate affinity for 5-HT$_{1C}$, 5-HT$_{1D}$, and 5-HT$_{1A}$ receptors, weak affinity for D$_1$ and no affinity for muscarinics or beta$_1$ and beta$_2$ receptors

Contraindications Hypersensitivity to risperidone or any component of the formulation

Warnings/Precautions Elderly patients with dementia-related behavioral disorders treated with atypical antipsychotics are at an increased risk of cerebrovascular adverse events and death compared to placebo; risk may be increased with dehydration (increased risk of death observed with concurrent furosemide). Risperidone is not approved for the treatment of dementia-related psychosis.

Low to moderately sedating, use with caution in disorders where CNS depression is a feature. Use with caution in Parkinson's disease. Caution in patients with hemodynamic instability; bone marrow suppression; predisposition to seizures; subcortical brain damage; severe cardiac, hepatic, or respiratory disease. Use with caution in renal dysfunction. Esophageal dysmotility and aspiration have been associated with antipsychotic use; use with caution in patients at risk of aspiration pneumonia (ie, Alzheimer's disease). Caution in breast cancer or other prolactin-dependent tumors (elevates prolactin levels). May alter temperature regulation or mask toxicity of other drugs due to antiemetic effects.

May cause orthostasis. Use with caution in patients with cardiovascular diseases (eg, heart failure, history of myocardial infarction or ischemia, cerebrovascular disease, conduction abnormalities). Use caution in patients receiving medications for hypertension (orthostatic effects may be exacerbated) or in patients with hypovolemia or dehydration. May alter cardiac conduction (low risk relative to other neuroleptics); life-threatening arrhythmias have occurred with therapeutic doses of neuroleptics.

May cause anticholinergic effects (confusion, agitation, constipation, xerostomia, blurred vision, urinary retention); therefore, they should be used with caution in patients with decreased gastrointestinal motility, urinary retention, BPH, xerostomia, or visual problems. Conditions which also may be exacerbated by cholinergic blockade include narrow-angle glaucoma (screening is recommended) and worsening of myasthenia gravis. Relative to other neuroleptics, risperidone has a low potency of cholinergic blockade.

May cause extrapyramidal symptoms, including pseudoparkinsonism, acute dystonic reactions, akathisia, and tardive dyskinesia (risk of these reactions is low relative to other neuroleptics, and is dose dependent). Risk of neuroleptic malignant syndrome (NMS) may be increased in patients with Parkinson's disease or Lewy Body Dementia; monitor for symptoms of confusion, obtundation, postural instability and extrapyramidal symptoms. May cause hyperglycemia; in

some cases may be extreme and associated with ketoacidosis, hyperosmolar coma, or death. Use with caution in patients with diabetes or other disorders of glucose regulation; monitor for worsening of glucose control.

The possibility of a suicide attempt is inherent in psychotic illness or bipolar disorder; use caution in high-risk patients during initiation of therapy. Prescriptions should be written for the smallest quantity consistent with good patient care.

Drug Interactions

Cytochrome P450 Effect: Substrate of CYP2D6 (major), 3A4 (minor); **Inhibits** CYP2D6 (weak), 3A4 (weak)

Decreased Effect: Risperidone may antagonize effects of levodopa. Carbamazepine decreases risperidone serum concentrations.

Increased Effect/Toxicity: CYP2D6 inhibitors may increase the levels/effects of risperidone; example inhibitors include chlorpromazine, delavirdine, fluoxetine, miconazole, paroxetine, pergolide, quinidine, quinine, ritonavir, and ropinirole. Risperidone may enhance the hypotensive effects of antihypertensive agents. Clozapine decreases clearance of risperidone. Metoclopramide may increase risk of extrapyramidal symptoms (EPS). Acetylcholinesterase inhibitors (central) may increase the risk of antipsychotic-related EPS. Verapamil may increase the levels and effects of risperidone.

Nutritional/Ethanol Interactions

Ethanol: Avoid ethanol (may increase CNS depression).

Herb/Nutraceutical: Avoid kava kava, gotu kola, valerian, St John's wort (may increase CNS depression).

Adverse Reactions

Frequency not defined: Gastrointestinal: Dysphagia, esophageal dysmotility

>10%:

Central nervous system: Insomnia, agitation, anxiety, headache, extrapyramidal symptoms (dose dependent), dizziness (I.M. injection)

Gastrointestinal: Weight gain

Respiratory: Rhinitis (I.M. injection)

1% to 10%:

Cardiovascular: Hypotension (especially orthostatic), tachycardia

Central nervous system: Sedation, dizziness (oral formulation), restlessness, dystonic reactions, pseudoparkinsonism, tardive dyskinesia, neuroleptic malignant syndrome, altered central temperature regulation, nervousness, fatigue, somnolence, hallucination, tremor, hypoesthesia, akathisia

Dermatologic: Photosensitivity (rare), rash, dry skin, seborrhea, acne

Endocrine & metabolic: Amenorrhea, galactorrhea, gynecomastia, sexual dysfunction

Gastrointestinal: Constipation, GI upset, xerostomia, dyspepsia, vomiting, abdominal pain, nausea, anorexia, diarrhea, weight changes

Genitourinary: Polyuria

Neuromuscular & skeletal: Myalgia

Ocular: Abnormal vision

Respiratory: Rhinitis (oral formulation), cough, sinusitis, pharyngitis, dyspnea

Overdosage/Toxicology Symptoms of overdose include drowsiness, sedation, tachycardia, hypotension, extrapyramidal symptoms (EPS), torsade de pointes, prolonged QT interval, seizures, and cardiopulmonary arrest. Treatment should be symptom-directed and supportive. Gastric decontamination and cardiac monitoring should be initiated. Consider risk of aspiration. Avoid antiarrhythmic therapy known to prolong the QT interval. Avoid vasopressors which may worsen hypotensive effects.
(Continued)

Risperidone *(Continued)*

Pharmacodynamics/Kinetics

Time to Peak: Plasma: Oral: Risperidone: Within 1 hour; 9-hydroxyrisperidone: Extensive metabolizers: 3 hours; Poor metabolizers: 17 hours

Protein Binding: Plasma: Risperidone 90%; 9-hydroxyrisperidone: 77%

Half-Life Elimination: Active moiety (risperidone and its active metabolite 9-hydroxyrisperidone)

Oral: 20 hours (mean)

Extensive metabolizers: Risperidone: 3 hours; 9-hydroxyrisperidone: 21 hours

Poor metabolizers: Risperidone: 20 hours; 9-hydroxyrisperidone: 30 hours

Injection: 3-6 days; related to microsphere erosion and subsequent absorption of risperidone

Metabolism: Extensively hepatic via CYP2D6 to 9-hydroxyrisperidone (similar pharmacological activity as risperidone); *N*-dealkylation is a second minor pathway

Excretion: Urine (70%); feces (15%)

Available Dosage Forms

Injection, microspheres for reconstitution, extended release (Risperdal® Consta™): 25 mg, 37.5 mg, 50 mg [supplied in a dose-pack containing vial with active ingredient in microsphere formulation, prefilled syringe with diluent, needle-free vial access device, and safety needle]

Solution, oral: 1 mg/mL (30 mL) [contains benzoic acid]

Tablet: 0.25 mg, 0.5 mg, 1 mg, 2 mg, 3 mg, 4 mg

Tablet, orally disintegrating (Risperdal® M-Tabs™): 0.5 mg [contains phenylalanine 0.14 mg]; 1 mg [contains phenylalanine 0.28 mg]; 2 mg [contains phenylalanine 0.56 mg]

Dosing

Adults:

Bipolar mania: Oral: Recommended starting dose: 2-3 mg once daily; if needed, adjust dose by 1 mg/day in intervals ≥24 hours; dosing range: 1-6 mg/day.

Schizophrenia:

Oral: Initial: 1 mg twice daily; may be increased by 2 mg/day to a target dose of 6 mg/day; usual range: 4-8 mg/day; may be given as a single daily dose once maintenance dose is achieved; daily dosages >6 mg do not appear to confer any additional benefit, and the incidence of extrapyramidal symptoms is higher than with lower doses. Further dose adjustments should be made in increments/decrements of 1-2 mg/day on a weekly basis. Dose range studied in clinical trials: 4-16 mg/day. Maintenance: Target dose: 4 mg once daily (range 2-8 mg/day)

I.M. (Risperdal® Consta™): 25 mg every 2 weeks; some patients may benefit from larger doses; maximum dose not to exceed 50 mg every 2 weeks. Dosage adjustments should not be made more frequently than every 4 weeks.

Note: Oral risperidone (or other antipsychotic) should be administered with the initial injection of Risperdal® Consta™ and continued for 3 weeks (then discontinued) to maintain adequate therapeutic plasma concentrations prior to main release phase of risperidone from injection site.

Tourette's disorder (unlabeled use): Oral: Initial: 0.5 mg; titrate to 2-4 mg/day

Elderly: A starting dose of 0.5 mg twice daily, and titration should progress slowly in increments of no more than 0.5 mg twice daily; increases to dosages >1.5 mg twice daily should occur at intervals of ≥1 week.

Additional monitoring of renal function and orthostatic blood pressure may be warranted. If once-a-day dosing in the elderly or debilitated patient is considered, a twice daily regimen should be used to titrate to the target dose, and this dose should be maintained for 2-3 days prior to attempts to switch to a once-daily regimen.

Pediatrics: Children and Adolescents:

Autism (unlabeled use): Oral: Initial: 0.25 mg at bedtime; titrate to 1 mg/day (0.1 mg/kg/day)

Bipolar disorder (unlabeled use): Oral: Initial: 0.5 mg; titrate to 0.5-3 mg/day

Pervasive developmental disorder (unlabeled use): Oral: Initial: 0.25 mg twice daily; titrate up 0.25 mg/day every 5-7 days; optimal dose range: 0.75-3 mg/day

Schizophrenia (unlabeled use): Oral: Initial: 0.5 mg once or twice daily; titrate as necessary up to 2-6 mg/day

Tourette's disorder (unlabeled use): Refer to adult dosing.

Renal Impairment: Oral: Starting dose of 0.5 mg twice daily; clearance of the active moiety is decreased by 60% in patients with moderate to severe renal disease compared to healthy subjects.

Hepatic Impairment: Oral: Starting dose of 0.5 mg twice daily; the mean free fraction of risperidone in plasma was increased by 35% compared to healthy subjects.

Administration

Oral: Oral solution can be mixed with water, coffee, orange juice, or low-fat milk, but is **not compatible** with cola or tea. May be administered with or without food.

Risperdal® M-Tabs™ should not be removed from blister pack until administered. Using dry hands, place immediately on tongue. Tablet will dissolve within seconds, and may be swallowed with or without liquid. Do not split or chew.

I.M.: Risperdal® Consta™ should be administered I.M. into the upper outer quadrant of the gluteal area. Injection should alternate between the two buttocks. Do not combine two different dosage strengths into one single administration. Do not substitute any components of the dose-pack; administer with needle provided.

Stability

Reconstitution: Risperdal® Consta™: Bring to room temperature prior to reconstitution. Reconstitute with provided diluent only. Shake vigorously to mix; will form thick, milky suspension. Following reconstitution, store at room temperature and use within 6 hours. If suspension settles prior to use, shake vigorously to resuspend.

Storage: Risperdal® Consta™: Store in refrigerator at 2°C to 8°C (36°F to 46°F) and protect from light. May be stored at room temperature of 25°C (77°F) for up to 7 days prior to administration.

Laboratory Monitoring Fasting lipid profile and fasting blood glucose/Hgb A_{1c} (prior to treatment, at 3 months, then annually)

Nursing Actions

Physical Assessment: Assess other medications patient is taking for effectiveness and interactions. Review ophthalmic exam and monitor therapeutic response (mental status, mood, affect), and adverse reactions at beginning of therapy and periodically with long-term use (CNS responses, anticholinergic and extrapyramidal symptoms, orthostatic hypotension). Monitor weight prior to initiating therapy and at least monthly. Assess knowledge/teach patient appropriate use, interventions to reduce side effects, and adverse symptoms to report.

Patient Education: Do not take any new medication during therapy unless approved by prescriber. Use exactly as directed; do not increase dose or frequency. It may take several weeks to achieve desired results; do not discontinue without consulting prescriber. Dilute solution with water, milk, or orange juice; do not dilute with beverages containing tannin or pectinate (eg, colas, tea). Avoid alcohol or caffeine unless approved by prescriber. Maintain adequate hydration (2-3 L/day of fluids) unless instructed to restrict fluid intake. If diabetic, you may experience increased blood sugars. Monitor blood sugars closely. You may experience excess sedation, drowsiness, restlessness, dizziness, or blurred vision (use caution driving or when engaging in tasks requiring alertness until response to drug is known); dry mouth, nausea, or GI upset (small frequent meals, frequent mouth care, chewing gum, or sucking lozenges may help); postural hypotension (use caution climbing stairs or when changing position from lying or sitting to standing); or urinary retention (void before taking medication). Report persistent CNS effects (eg, trembling fingers, altered gait or balance, excessive sedation, seizures, unusual muscle or skeletal movements, anxiety, abnormal thoughts, confusion, personality changes); chest pain, palpitations, rapid heartbeat, severe dizziness; swelling or pain in breasts (male and female), altered menstrual pattern, sexual dysfunction; pain or difficulty on urination; vision changes; skin rash or yellowing of skin; respiratory difficulty; or worsening of condition. **Pregnancy/ breast-feeding precautions:** Inform prescriber if you are or intend to become pregnant. Do not breast-feed.

Dietary Considerations May be taken with or without food. Risperdal® M-Tabs™ contain phenylalanine.

Geriatric Considerations (See Warnings/Precautions, Adverse Reactions, Elderly Dosing, and Overdose/Toxicology.) Elderly patients have an increased risk of adverse response to side effects or adverse reactions to antipsychotics.

Breast-Feeding Issues Risperidone and its metabolite are excreted in breast milk; it is recommended that women not breast feed during therapy or for 12 weeks after the last injection if using Risperdal® Consta™.

Additional Information Risperdal® Consta™ is an injectable formulation of risperidone using the extended release Medisorb® drug-delivery system; small polymeric microspheres degrade slowly, releasing the medication at a controlled rate.

Related Information
Antipsychotic Medication Guidelines *on page 1415*
Federal OBRA Regulations Recommended Maximum Doses *on page 1421*

Ritonavir (ri TOE na veer)

U.S. Brand Names Norvir®

Pharmacologic Category Antiretroviral Agent, Protease Inhibitor

Medication Safety Issues
Sound-alike/look-alike issues:
Ritonavir may be confused with Retrovir®
Norvir® may be confused with Norvasc®

Pregnancy Risk Factor B

Lactation Excretion in breast milk unknown/not recommended

Use Treatment of HIV infection; should always be used as part of a multidrug regimen (at least three antiretroviral agents); may be used as a pharmacokinetic "booster" for other protease inhibitors

Mechanism of Action/Effect Ritonavir prevents cleavage of protein precursors essential for HIV infection of new cells and viral replication. Saquinavir- and zidovudine-resistant HIV isolates are generally susceptible to ritonavir.

Contraindications Hypersensitivity to ritonavir or any component of the formulation; concurrent alfuzosin, amiodarone, cisapride, dihydroergotamine, ergonovine, ergotamine, flecainide, methylergonovine, midazolam, pimozide, propafenone, quinidine, triazolam, and voriconazole (when ritonavir ≥800 mg/day)

Warnings/Precautions Ritonavir may interact with many medications. Careful review is required. A listing of medications that should not be used is available with each bottle and patients should be provided with this information. Avoid concurrent use with lovastatin, simvastatin, and St John's wort; atorvastatin should be used at the lowest possible dose, while fluvastatin or pravastatin may be safer alternatives. Cushing's syndrome and adrenal suppression have been reported in patients receiving concomitant ritonavir and fluticasone; avoid concurrent use unless benefit outweighs risk. Dosage adjustment is required for combination therapy with amprenavir and ritonavir; in addition, the risk of hyperlipidemia may be increased during concurrent therapy. Cardiac and neurological events have been reported with concurrent use of disopyramide, mexiletine, nefazodone, fluoxetine or beta blockers. Pancreatitis has been observed; use with caution in patients with increased triglycerides; monitor serum lipase and amylase.

Use with caution in patients with hemophilia A or B; increased bleeding during protease inhibitor therapy has been reported. Changes in glucose tolerance, hyperglycemia, exacerbation of diabetes, DKA, and new-onset diabetes mellitus have been reported in patients receiving protease inhibitors. May be associated with fat redistribution (buffalo hump, increased abdominal girth, breast engorgement, facial atrophy, and dyslipidemia). Immune reconstitution syndrome may develop resulting in the occurrence of an inflammatory response to an indolent or residual opportunistic infection; further evaluation and treatment may be required. May cause hepatitis or exacerbate pre-existing hepatic dysfunction; use with caution in patients with hepatitis B or C and in hepatic disease. Safety and efficacy have not been established in children <1 month of age.

Drug Interactions
Cytochrome P450 Effect: Substrate of CYP1A2 (minor), 2B6 (minor), 2D6 (major), 3A4 (major); **Inhibits** CYP2C8 (strong), 2C9 (weak), 2C19 (weak), 2D6 (strong), 2E1 (weak), 3A4 (strong); **Induces** CYP1A2 (weak), 2C8 (weak), 2C9 (weak), 3A4 (weak)

Decreased Effect: The administration of didanosine (buffered formulation) should be separated from ritonavir by 2.5 hours to limit interaction with ritonavir. Concurrent use of rifampin, rifabutin, dexamethasone, and many anticonvulsants may lower serum concentration of ritonavir. Ritonavir may reduce the concentration of ethinyl estradiol which may result in loss of contraception (including combination products). Theophylline concentrations may be reduced in concurrent therapy. Levels of didanosine and zidovudine may be decreased by ritonavir, however, no dosage adjustment is necessary. Voriconazole serum levels are reduced by ritonavir (when ritonavir dose ≥800 mg/day). In addition, ritonavir may decrease the serum concentrations of the following drugs: Atovaquone, divalproex, lamotrigine, methadone, phenytoin. The levels/effects of ritonavir may be decreased by aminoglutethimide, carbamazepine, nafcillin, nevirapine, phenobarbital, phenytoin, rifamycins, and other CYP3A4 inducers. Ritonavir may decrease the levels/effects of CYP2D6 prodrug substrates (eg, codeine, hydrocodone, oxycodone, tramadol).

Increased Effect/Toxicity: Concurrent use of alfuzosin, amiodarone, cisapride, ergot alkaloids (including dihydroergotamine, ergonovine, methylergonovine), flecainide, midazolam, pimozide, propafenone, quinidine, and triazolam is contraindicated.

Saquinavir's serum concentrations are increased by ritonavir; the dosage of both agents should be reduced to 400 mg twice daily. Concurrent therapy with amprenavir may result in increased serum concentrations: dosage adjustment is recommended. Metronidazole or disulfiram may cause disulfiram (Continued)

Ritonavir *(Continued)*

reaction (oral solution contains 43% ethanol). Serum levels/effects of corticosteroids (eg, budesonide, fluticasone) and immunosuppressants (cyclosporine, sirolimus, tacrolimus; monitor) may be increased by ritonavir. Serum concentrations of the parent drug and/or metabolite(s) of several analgesics (eg, tramadol, meperidine, propoxyphene) may be increased by ritonavir; increased levels of normeperidine may increase the risk of CNS toxicity/seizures. Rifabutin and rifabutin metabolite serum concentrations may be increased by ritonavir; reduce rifabutin dose to 150 mg every day.

Ritonavir may increase the levels/effects of amiodarone, amphetamines, selected beta-blockers, selected benzodiazepines (midazolam and triazolam contraindicated), calcium channel blockers, bupropion, carbamazepine, cisapride (contraindicated), delavirdine, dextromethorphan, digoxin, eplerenone, ergot alkaloids (contraindicated), ethosuximide, fentanyl, fluoxetine, lidocaine, HMG-CoA reductase inhibitors, mirtazapine, nateglinide, nefazodone, paclitaxel, paroxetine, perphenazine, pimozide (contraindicated), propafenone (contraindicated), repaglinide, risperidone, rosiglitazone, sildenafil (and other PDE-5 inhibitors), thioridazine, trazodone, tricyclic antidepressants, venlafaxine, zolpidem, and other substrates of CYP2D6 or 3A4. Thioridazine is generally contraindicated with strong CYP2D6 inhibitors. When used with strong CYP3A4 inhibitors, dosage adjustment/limits are recommended for sildenafil and other PDE-5 inhibitors; refer to individual monographs.

Nutritional/Ethanol Interactions

Food: Food enhances absorption.

Herb/Nutraceutical: St John's wort may decrease ritonavir serum levels. Avoid use.

Adverse Reactions
Protease inhibitors cause dyslipidemia which includes elevated cholesterol and triglycerides and a redistribution of body fat centrally to cause increased abdominal girth, buffalo hump, facial atrophy, and breast enlargement. These agents also cause hyperglycemia. Percentages as reported in adults:

>10%:

Endocrine & metabolic: Hypercholesterolemia (>240 mg/dL: 37% to 45%), triglycerides increased (>800 mg/dL: 17% to 34%; >1500 mg/dL: 1% to 13%)

Gastrointestinal: Nausea (26% to 30%), diarrhea (15% to 23%), vomiting (14% to 17%), taste perversion (7% to 11%)

Hematologic: WBCs decreased

Hepatic: GGT increased (5% to 20%)

Neuromuscular & skeletal: Weakness (10% to 15%), creatine phosphokinase increased (9% to 12%)

2% to 10%:

Cardiovascular: Syncope (<1% to 2%), vasodilation (2%)

Central nervous system: Fever (4% to 5%), dizziness (3% to 4%), insomnia (2% to 3%), somnolence (2% to 3%), anxiety (2%),

Dermatologic: Rash

Endocrine & metabolic: Uric acid increased (up to 4%)

Gastrointestinal: Abdominal pain (6% to 8%), anorexia (2% to 8%), dyspepsia (up to 6%), local throat irritation (2% to 3%)

Hematologic: Eosinophilia, neutropenia, neutrophilia

Hepatic: LFTs increased (6% to 10%)

Neuromuscular & skeletal: Paresthesia (3% to 7%), arthralgia (up to 2%), myalgia (2%)

Respiratory: Pharyngitis

Miscellaneous: Circumoral paresthesia, diaphoresis (2% to 3%)

Overdosage/Toxicology
Human experience is limited; there is no specific antidote for overdose with ritonavir.

Oral solution contains 43% ethanol by volume, potentially causing significant ethanol-related toxicity in younger patients. Dialysis is unlikely to be beneficial in significant removal of the drug. Charcoal or gastric lavage may be useful to remove unabsorbed drug.

Pharmacodynamics/Kinetics

Time to Peak: 2 hours (fasted); 4 hours (nonfasted)

Protein Binding: 98% to 99%

Half-Life Elimination: 3-5 hours

Metabolism: Hepatic via CYP3A4 and 2D6; five metabolites, low concentration of an active metabolite achieved in plasma (oxidative)

Excretion: Urine (~11%); feces (~86%)

Available Dosage Forms

Capsule: 100 mg [contains ethanol and polyoxyl 35 castor oil]

Solution: 80 mg/mL (240 mL) [contains ethanol and polyoxyl 35 castor oil; peppermint and caramel flavor]

Dosing

Adults & Elderly:

Treatment of HIV infection: Oral: 600 mg twice daily; dose escalation tends to avoid nausea that many patients experience upon initiation of full dosing. Escalate the dose as follows: 300 mg twice daily for 1 day, 400 mg twice daily for 2 days, 500 mg twice daily for 1 day, then 600 mg twice daily. Ritonavir may be better tolerated when used in combination with other antiretrovirals by initiating the drug alone and subsequently adding the second agent within 2 weeks.

Pharmacokinetic "booster" in combination with other protease inhibitors: 100-400 mg/day

Refer to individual monographs; specific dosage recommendations often require adjustment of both agents.

Dosage adjustments for ritonavir when administered in combination therapy:

Amprenavir: Adjustments necessary for each agent:

Amprenavir 1200 mg with ritonavir 200 mg once daily **or**

Amprenavir 600 mg with ritonavir 100 mg twice daily

Amprenavir plus efavirenz (3-drug regimen): Amprenavir 1200 mg twice daily plus ritonavir 200 mg twice daily plus efavirenz at standard dose

Indinavir: Adjustments necessary for agent:

Indinavir 800 mg twice daily plus ritonavir 100-200 mg twice daily **or**

Indinavir 400 mg twice daily plus ritonavir 400 mg twice daily

Nelfinavir: Ritonavir 400 mg twice daily

Rifabutin: Decrease rifabutin dose to 150 mg every other day

Saquinavir: Ritonavir 400 mg twice daily

Pediatrics:

HIV infection: Oral: Children >1 month: 350-400 mg/m^2 twice daily (maximum dose: 600 mg twice daily). Initiate dose at 250 mg/m^2 twice daily; titrate dose upward every 2-3 days by 50 mg/m^2 twice daily.

Hepatic Impairment: No adjustment required in mild or moderate impairment; however, careful monitoring is required in moderate hepatic impairment (levels may be decreased); caution advised with severe impairment (no data available).

Administration

Oral: Administer with food. Liquid formulations usually have an unpleasant taste. Consider mixing it with chocolate milk or a liquid nutritional supplement. Whenever possible, administer oral solution with calibrated dosing syringe.

Stability

Storage:

Capsule: Store under refrigeration at 2°C to 8°C (36°F to 46°F); may be left out at room temperature of

<25°C (<77°F) if used within 30 days. Protect from light. Avoid exposure to excessive heat.

Solution: Store at room temperature at 20°C to 25°C (68°F to 77°F). Do not refrigerate.

Laboratory Monitoring Triglycerides, cholesterol, LFTs, CBC, CPK, uric acid, viral load, CD4 count, glucose, serum amylase and lipase

Nursing Actions

Physical Assessment: Assess potential for interactions with other pharmacological agents and herbal products patient may be taking. A list of medications that should not be used is available in each bottle and patients should be provided with this information. Monitor laboratory tests, patient response, and adverse reactions at regular intervals during therapy (eg, gastrointestinal disturbance [nausea, vomiting, diarrhea] that can lead to dehydration and weight loss, hyperlipidemia and redistribution of body fat, rash, CNS effects [malaise, insomnia, abnormal thinking], electrolyte imbalance). Teach patient proper use (eg, timing of multiple medications and drugs that should not be used concurrently), possible side effects/ appropriate interventions (eg, glucose testing [protease inhibitors may cause hyperglycemia; exacerbation or new-onset diabetes], use of barrier contraceptives [protease inhibitors may decrease effectiveness of oral contraceptives]), and adverse symptoms to report.

Patient Education: You will be provided with a list of specific medications that should not be used during therapy; do not take any new prescription or over-the-counter medications, or herbal products during therapy (even if they are not on the list) without consulting prescriber. This is not a cure for HIV, nor has it been found to reduce transmission of HIV; use appropriate precautions to prevent spread to other persons. Take exactly as directed with meals. Mix liquid formulation with chocolate milk or liquid nutritional supplement. Capsules may be stored in refrigerator (do not freeze or expose to excessive heat) or stored at room temperature if used within 30 days. Protect from light. Solution should be stored at room temperature. Do not refrigerate. Maintain adequate hydration (2-3 L/day of fluids), unless instructed to restrict fluid intake. If you miss a dose, take as soon as possible and return to your regular schedule (never take a double dose). Frequent blood tests may be required with prolonged therapy. You may be advised to check your glucose levels (this drug can cause exacerbation or new-onset diabetes). May cause body changes due to redistribution of body fat, facial atrophy, or breast enlargement (normal effects of drug). May cause dizziness, insomnia, abnormal thinking (use caution when driving or engaging in potentially hazardous tasks until response to drug is known); nausea, vomiting, or taste perversion (small frequent meals, frequent mouth care, chewing gum, or sucking lozenges may help); muscle weakness (consult prescriber for approved analgesic); or headache (consult prescriber for medication). Inform prescriber if you experience muscle numbness or tingling; unresolved persistent vomiting, diarrhea, or abdominal pain; respiratory difficulty or chest pain; unusual skin rash; or change in color of stool or urine. or any persistent adverse effects. **Pregnancy/ breast-feeding precautions:** Inform prescriber if you are or intend to become pregnant. Effectiveness of oral contraceptives may be decreased, use of alternative (nonhormonal) forms of contraception is recommended, consult prescriber for appropriate measures.

Dietary Considerations Should be taken with food. Oral solution contains 43% ethanol by volume.

Breast-Feeding Issues HIV-infected mothers are discouraged from breast-feeding to decrease potential transmission of HIV.

Pregnancy Issues Early studies have shown lower plasma levels during pregnancy compared to postpartum. If needed during pregnancy, use in combination with another PI to boost levels of second PI. Pregnancy and protease inhibitors are both associated with an increased risk of hyperglycemia. Glucose levels should be closely monitored. The Perinatal HIV Guidelines Working Group considers ritonavir to be an alternative PI for use during pregnancy. Healthcare professionals are encouraged to contact the antiretroviral pregnancy registry to monitor outcomes of pregnant women exposed to antiretroviral medications (1-800-258-4263 or www.APRegistry.com).

Additional Information Potential compliance problems, frequency of administration and adverse effects should be discussed with patients before initiating therapy to help prevent the emergence of resistance.

Rituximab (ri TUK si mab)

U.S. Brand Names Rituxan®

Synonyms Anti-CD20 Monoclonal Antibody; C2B8; C2B8 Monoclonal Antibody; IDEC-C2B8; NSC-687451; Pan-B Antibody

Pharmacologic Category Antineoplastic Agent, Monoclonal Antibody; Monoclonal Antibody

Medication Safety Issues
Sound-alike/look-alike issues:
Rituxan® may be confused with Remicade®
Rituximab may be confused with infliximab

Pregnancy Risk Factor C

Lactation Excretion in breast milk unknown/contraindicated

Use Treatment of relapsed or refractory low-grade or follicular CD20-positive, B-cell non-Hodgkin's lymphoma (NHL); treatment of diffuse large B-cell CD20-positive NHL in combination with chemotherapy; treatment of rheumatoid arthritis (RA) in combination with methotrexate

Unlabeled/Investigational Use Treatment of autoimmune hemolytic anemia (AIHA) in children; chronic immune thrombocytopenic purpura (ITP); chronic lymphocytic leukemia (CLL) (in combination with chemotherapy); Waldenström's macroglobulinemia (WM)

Investigational: Treatment of systemic autoimmune diseases (in addition to rheumatoid arthritis)

Mechanism of Action/Effect Binds to the CD20 antigen on B-lymphocytes and recruits immune effector functions to mediate B-cell lysis *in vitro*. The antibody induces cell death in the DHL-4 human B-cell lymphoma line.

Contraindications Type I hypersensitivity or anaphylactic reactions to murine proteins or any component of the formulation

Warnings/Precautions Severe and occasionally fatal infusion-related reactions (including hypotension, angioedema, bronchospasm, hypoxia, and in more severe cases pulmonary infiltrates, acute respiratory distress syndrome, myocardial infarction, ventricular fibrillation, or cardiogenic shock) have been reported during the first 30-120 minutes of the first infusion. Risk factors associated with fatal outcomes include chronic lymphocytic leukemia, female gender, mantle cell lymphoma, or pulmonary infiltrates. Discontinue infusion for severe reactions; treatment is symptomatic. Medications for the treatment of hypersensitivity reactions (eg, epinephrine, antihistamines, corticosteroids) should be available for immediate use. Infusion may be resumed at a 50% infusion rate reduction upon resolution of symptoms. Discontinue infusion for serious or life-threatening cardiac arrhythmias; subsequent doses should include cardiac monitoring during and after the infusion. Mild-to-moderate infusion-related reactions (eg, chills, (Continued)

Rituximab *(Continued)*

fever, rigors) occur frequently and are managed through slowing or interrupting the infusion.

Tumor lysis syndrome leading to acute renal failure requiring dialysis may occur 12-24 hours following the first dose. Consider prophylaxis in patients at high risk (high numbers of circulating malignant cells ≥25,000/mm^3 or high tumor burden). Severe and sometimes fatal mucocutaneous reactions (lichenoid dermatitis, paraneoplastic pemphigus, Stevens-Johnson syndrome, toxic epidermal necrolysis and vesiculobullous dermatitis) have been reported, occurring from 1-13 weeks following exposure. Patients experiencing severe mucocutaneous skin reactions should not receive further rituximab infusions and should seek prompt medical evaluation. Use caution with cardiac or pulmonary disease and prior cardiopulmonary events; patients with pre-existing cardiac conditions (arrhythmias, coronary artery disease) and patients treated for rheumatoid arthritis should be monitored during and after each infusion. Elderly patients are at higher risk for cardiac and pulmonary adverse events. May cause hypotension; consider withholding antihypertensives 12 hours prior to treatment. Reactivation of hepatitis B has been reported in association with rituximab (rare); consider screening in high-risk patients. May cause renal toxicity; consider discontinuation with increasing serum creatinine or oliguria. Bowel obstruction and perforation have been reported; complaints of abdominal pain should be evaluated. Safety and efficacy of rituximab in combination with biologic agents or disease-modifying antirheumatic drugs (DMARD) other than methotrexate have not been established. Safety and efficacy of retreatment for RA have not been established. Safety and efficacy in children have not been established.

Drug Interactions

Decreased Effect: Currently recommended not to administer live vaccines during rituximab treatment.

Increased Effect/Toxicity: Monoclonal antibodies may increase the risk for allergic reactions to rituximab due to the presence of HACA antibody.

Nutritional/Ethanol Interactions

Herb/Nutraceutical: Avoid hypoglycemic herbs, including alfalfa, bilberry, bitter melon, burdock, celery, damiana, fenugreek, garcinai, garlic, ginger, ginseng, gymnema, marshmallow, and stinging nettle (may enhance the hypoglycemic effect of rituximab). Monitor.

Adverse Reactions Note: Abdominal pain, anemia, dyspnea, hypotension, and neutropenia are more common in patients with bulky disease; percentages reported as monotherapy in NHL patients.

>10%:

Central nervous system: Fever (53%), chills (33%), headache (19%), pain (12%)

Dermatologic: Rash (15%), pruritus (14%), angioedema (11%)

Gastrointestinal: Nausea (23%), abdominal pain (14%)

Hematologic: Lymphopenia (48%; grade 3/4: 40%; median duration 14 days), leukopenia (14%; grade 3/4: 4%), neutropenia (14%; grade 3/4: 6%; median duration 13 days), thrombocytopenia (12%; grade 3/4: 2%)

Neuromuscular & skeletal: Weakness (26%)

Respiratory: Cough (13%), rhinitis (12%)

Miscellaneous: Infection (31%; grade 3/4: 2%), night sweats (15%)

Mild-to-moderate infusion-related reactions: Chills, fever, rigors, dizziness, hypertension, myalgia, nausea, pruritus, rash, and vomiting (lymphoma: first dose 77%; fourth dose 30%; eighth dose 14%); infusion-related reactions reported are lower in RA

1% to 10%:

Cardiovascular: Hypotension (10%), peripheral edema (8%), hypertension (6%), flushing (5%), edema (<5%)

Central nervous system: Dizziness (10%), anxiety (5%), agitation (<5%), depression (<5%), hypoesthesia (<5%), insomnia (<5%), malaise (<5%), nervousness (<5%), neuritis (<5%), somnolence (<5%), vertigo (<5%)

Dermatologic: Urticaria (8%)

Endocrine & metabolic: Hyperglycemia (9%), hypoglycemia (<5%)

Gastrointestinal: Diarrhea (10%), vomiting (10%), anorexia (<5%), dyspepsia (<5%), weight loss (<5%)

Hematologic: Anemia (8%; grade 3/4: 3%)

Local: Pain at the injection site (<5%)

Neuromuscular & skeletal: Arthralgia (10%), back pain (10%), myalgia (10%), arthritis (<5%), hyperkinesia (<5%), hypertonia (<5%), neuropathy (<5%), paresthesia (<5%)

Ocular: Conjunctivitis (<5%), lacrimation disorder (<5%)

Respiratory: Throat irritation (9%), bronchospasm (8%), dyspnea (7%), sinusitis (6%)

Miscellaneous: LDH increased (7%)

Overdosage/Toxicology There has been no experience with overdosage in human clinical trials; single doses higher than 500 mg/m^2 have not been tested. Treatment is symptom-directed and supportive.

Pharmacodynamics/Kinetics

Duration of Action: Detectable in serum 3-6 months after completion of treatment; B-cell recovery begins ~6 months following completion of treatment; median B-cell levels return to normal by 12 months following completion of treatment

Half-Life Elimination:

Cancer: Proportional to dose; wide ranges reflect variable tumor burden and changes in CD20 positive B-cell populations with repeated doses:

>100 mg/m^2: 4.4 days (range 1.6-10.5 days)

375 mg/m^2:

Following first dose: Mean half-life: 3.2 days (range 1.3-6.4 days)

Following fourth dose: Mean half-life: 8.6 days (range 3.5-17 days)

RA: Mean terminal half-life: 19 days

Excretion: Uncertain; may undergo phagocytosis and catabolism in the reticuloendothelial system (RES)

Available Dosage Forms Injection, solution [preservative free]: 10 mg/mL (10 mL, 50 mL)

Dosing

Adults & Elderly:

Refer to individual protocols: **Note:** Pretreatment with acetaminophen and diphenhydramine is recommended.

NHL: I.V. infusion: 375 mg/m^2 once weekly for 4 or 8 doses

or

100 mg/m^2 I.V. day 1, then 375 mg/m^2 3 times/week for 11 doses has also been reported (cycles may be repeated in patients with refractory or relapsed disease)

Retreatment following disease progression: I.V. infusion: 375 mg/m^2 once weekly for 4 doses

Diffuse large B-cell NHL: 375 mg/m^2 given on day 1 of each chemotherapy cycle for up to 8 doses; chemotherapy may be CHOP or other anthracycline-based regimen

Rheumatoid arthritis: 1000 mg on days 1 and 15 in combination with methotrexate; premedication with a corticosteroid (eg, methylprednisolone 100 mg I.V.) prior to each rituximab dose is recommended. In clinical trials, patients received oral corticosteroids on a tapering schedule from baseline through day 16.

Waldenström's macroglobulinemia (unlabeled use): 375 mg/m² once weekly for 4 weeks

Combination therapy with ibritumomab: 250 mg/m² I.V. day 1; repeat in 7-9 days with ibritumomab (also see Ibritumomab monograph):

Pediatrics: Note: Pretreatment with acetaminophen and diphenhydramine is recommended.

AIHA, chronic ITP (unlabeled uses): I.V.: 375 mg/m² once weekly for 2-4 doses

Administration

I.V.: Do **not** administer I.V. push or bolus.

Initial infusion: Start rate of 50 mg/hour; if there is no reaction, increase the rate 50 mg/hour every 30 minutes, to a maximum of 400 mg/hour.

Subsequent infusions: If patient did not tolerate initial infusion follow initial infusion guidelines. If patient tolerated initial infusion, start at 100 mg/hour; if there is no reaction, increase the rate 100 mg/hour every 30 minutes, to a maximum of 400 mg/hour.

Note: If a reaction occurs, slow or stop the infusion. If the reaction abates, restart infusion at 50% of the previous rate.

I.V. Detail: Discontinue infusions in the event of serious or life-threatening cardiac arrhythmias.

pH: 6.5

Stability

Reconstitution: Withdraw necessary amount of rituximab and dilute to a final concentration of 1-4 mg/mL with 0.9% sodium chloride or 5% dextrose in water. Gently invert the bag to mix the solution. Do not shake.

Storage: Store vials at refrigeration at 2°C to 8°C (36°F to 46°F); protect vials from direct sunlight. Do not freeze; do not shake. Solutions for infusion are stable at 2°C to 8°C (36°F to 46°F) for 24 hours and at room temperature for an additional 24 hours.

Laboratory Monitoring CBC with differential and platelets, peripheral CD20+ cells. Patients with elevated HAMA/HACA titers may have an allergic reaction when treated with rituximab or other antibodies from a mouse genetic source.

Nursing Actions

Physical Assessment: Patient history with mouse antibodies should be assessed prior to beginning therapy. Monitor patient closely during and following each infusion. Severe infusion-related reactions can include chills, fever, rigors, dizziness, hypo- or hypertension, angioedema, respiratory distress, myalgia, nausea, pruritus, rash and vomiting. Emergency equipment and medications (epinephrine, antihistamines, corticosteroids) should be immediately available during infusion. In the event of severe infusion reaction, infusion should be stopped and prescriber notified immediately. Acute tumor lysis syndrome leading to acute renal failure 12-24 hours after first dose; severe mucocutaneous reactions can occur from 1-13 weeks following treatment (prescriber should be notified immediately before further infusions). Monitor laboratory tests prior to, during, and following therapy. Teach patient possible side effects/appropriate interventions and importance of reporting adverse reactions.

Patient Education: This medication is only administered by infusion. You may experience a reaction during the infusion of this medication including high fever, chills, respiratory difficulty, or congestion. You will be closely monitored and comfort measures provided. Maintain adequate hydration (2-3 L/day of fluids during entire course of therapy) unless instructed to restrict fluid intake. You will be susceptible to infection and people may wear masks and gloves while caring for you to protect you as much as possible (avoid crowds and exposure to infection and

do not have any vaccinations without consulting prescriber). May cause dizziness or trembling (use caution until response to medication is known); nausea, vomiting or loss of appetite (small, frequent meals, frequent mouth care may help); diarrhea (increase dietary fiber, buttermilk, or yogurt); bone or muscle pain (ask prescriber for appropriate analgesic). Report immediately any unusual skin rash or redness, any persistent dizziness, swelling of extremities, unusual weight gain, respiratory difficulty, chest pain or tightness; symptoms of respiratory infection (wheezing, bronchospasms, or difficulty breathing); unresolved GI disturbance (nausea, vomiting); opportunistic infection (sore or irritated throat; unusual and persistent fatigue, chills, fever, unhealed sores, white plaques in mouth or genital area; unusual bruising or bleeding); or other unusual effects related to this medication. **Pregnancy/breast-feeding precautions:** Inform prescriber if you are or intend to become pregnant. Do not breast-feed.

Breast-Feeding Issues The manufacturer recommends discontinuing breast-feeding until circulating levels of rituximab are no longer detectable.

Pregnancy Issues Animal studies have demonstrated adverse effects including decreased (reversible) B-cells and immunosuppression. There are no adequate and well-controlled studies in pregnant women. Rituximab administration during pregnancy could potentially cause fetal B-cell depletion. Use during pregnancy only if clearly needed. Effective contraception is recommended during treatment and for up to 12 months following treatment.

Rivastigmine (ri va STIG meen)

U.S. Brand Names Exelon®

Synonyms ENA 713; Rivastigmine Tartrate; SDZ ENA 713

Pharmacologic Category Acetylcholinesterase Inhibitor (Central)

Pregnancy Risk Factor B

Lactation Excretion in breast milk unknown/use caution

Use Mild to moderate dementia from Alzheimer's disease

Mechanism of Action/Effect A deficiency of cortical acetylcholine is thought to account for some of the symptoms of Alzheimer's disease; rivastigmine increases acetylcholine in the central nervous system through reversible inhibition of its hydrolysis by cholinesterase

Contraindications Hypersensitivity to rivastigmine, other carbamate derivatives, or any component of the formulation

Warnings/Precautions Significant nausea, vomiting, anorexia, and weight loss are associated with use, occurring more frequently in women and during the titration phase. Use caution in patients with a history of peptic ulcer disease or concurrent NSAID use. Caution in patients undergoing anesthesia who will receive succinylcholine-type muscle relaxation, patients with sick sinus syndrome, bradycardia or supraventricular conduction conditions, urinary obstruction, seizure disorders, or pulmonary conditions such as asthma or COPD. There are no trials evaluating the safety and efficacy in children.

Drug Interactions

Decreased Effect: Anticholinergic agents effects may be reduced with rivastigmine.

Increased Effect/Toxicity:

Acetylcholinesterase inhibitors (central) may increase the risk of antipsychotic-related extrapyramidal symptoms. Beta-blockers without ISA activity may increase risk of bradycardia. Calcium channel blockers (diltiazem or verapamil) may increase risk of bradycardia. Cholinergic agonists effects may be (Continued)

Rivastigmine *(Continued)*

increased with rivastigmine. Cigarette use increases the clearance of rivastigmine by 23%. Depolarizing neuromuscular blocking agents effects may be increased with rivastigmine. Digoxin may increase risk of bradycardia.

Nutritional/Ethanol Interactions
Cigarette use: Increases the clearance of rivastigmine by 23%.
Ethanol: Avoid ethanol (due to risk of sedation; may increase GI irritation).
Food: Food delays absorption by 90 minutes, lowers C_{max} by 30% and increases AUC by 30%.

Adverse Reactions
>10%:
Central nervous system: Dizziness (21%), headache (17%)
Gastrointestinal: Nausea (47%), vomiting (31%), diarrhea (19%), anorexia (17%), abdominal pain (13%)
2% to 10%:
Cardiovascular: Syncope (3%), hypertension (3%)
Central nervous system: Fatigue (9%), insomnia (9%), confusion (8%), depression (6%), anxiety (5%), malaise (5%), somnolence (5%), hallucinations (4%), aggressiveness (3%)
Gastrointestinal: Dyspepsia (9%), constipation (5%), flatulence (4%), weight loss (3%), eructation (2%)
Genitourinary: Urinary tract infection (7%)
Neuromuscular & skeletal: Weakness (6%), tremor (4%)
Respiratory: Rhinitis (4%)
Miscellaneous: Increased diaphoresis (4%), flu-like syndrome (3%)
>2% (but frequency equal to placebo): Chest pain, peripheral edema, vertigo, back pain, arthralgia, pain, bone fracture, agitation, nervousness, delusion, paranoid reaction, upper respiratory tract infection, infection, cough, pharyngitis, bronchitis, rash, urinary incontinence.
<2% (Limited to important or life-threatening symptoms; reactions may be at a similar frequency to placebo): Fever, edema, allergy, periorbital or facial edema, hypothermia, hypotension, postural hypotension, cardiac failure, ataxia, convulsions, apraxia, aphasia, dysphonia, hyperkinesia, hypertonia, hypokinesia, migraine, neuralgia, peripheral neuropathy, hypothyroidism, peptic ulcer, gastroesophageal reflux, GI hemorrhage, intestinal obstruction, pancreatitis, colitis, atrial fibrillation, bradycardia, AV block, bundle branch block, sick sinus syndrome, cardiac arrest, supraventricular tachycardia, tachycardia, abnormal hepatic function, cholecystitis, dehydration, arthritis, angina pectoris, MI, epistaxis, hematoma, thrombocytopenia, purpura, delirium, emotional lability, psychosis, anemia, bronchospasm, apnea, rash (maculopapular, eczema, bullous, exfoliative, psoriaform, erythematous), urticaria, acute renal failure, peripheral ischemia, pulmonary embolism, thrombosis, thrombophlebitis, intracranial hemorrhage, conjunctival hemorrhage, diplopia, glaucoma, lymphadenopathy, leukocytosis.

Overdosage/Toxicology In cases of asymptomatic overdoses, rivastigmine should be held for 24 hours. Cholinergic crisis, caused by significant acetylcholinesterase inhibition, is characterized by severe nausea, vomiting, salivation, sweating, bradycardia, hypotension, respiratory depression, collapse, and convulsions. Treatment is supportive and symptomatic. Dialysis would not be helpful.

Pharmacodynamics/Kinetics
Time to Peak: 1 hour
Protein Binding: 40%
Half-Life Elimination: 1.5 hours
Metabolism: Extensively via cholinesterase-mediated hydrolysis in the brain; metabolite undergoes

N-demethylation and/or sulfate conjugation hepatically; minimal CYP involvement; linear kinetics at 3 mg twice daily, but nonlinear at higher doses
Excretion: Urine (97% as metabolites); feces (0.4%)
Available Dosage Forms
Capsule: 1.5 mg, 3 mg, 4.5 mg, 6 mg
Solution, oral: 2 mg/mL (120 mL) [contains sodium benzoate]
Dosing
Adults & Elderly: Alzheimer's dementia: Oral: Initial: 1.5 mg twice daily for 2 weeks; if tolerated, may be increased to 3 mg twice daily; further increases may be attempted no more frequently than every 2 weeks, to 4.5 mg twice daily and then to 6 mg twice daily; maximum dose: 6 mg twice daily. If gastrointestinal adverse events occur, the patient should be instructed to discontinue treatment for several doses then restart at the same or next lower dosage level; antiemetics have been used to control GI symptoms. If treatment is interrupted for longer than several days, restart the treatment at the lowest dose and titrate as previously described.
Renal Impairment: Dosage adjustments are not recommended, however, titrate the dose to the individual's tolerance.
Hepatic Impairment: Clearance is significantly reduced in mild to moderately impaired patients. Although dosage adjustments are not recommended, use lowest possible dose and titrate according to individual's tolerance. May consider waiting >2 weeks between dosage adjustments.
Administration
Oral: Should be administered with meals (breakfast or dinner). Capsule should be swallowed whole. Liquid form is available for patients who cannot swallow capsules (can be swallowed directly from syringe or mixed with water, milk, or juice). Stir well and drink within 4 hours of mixing.
Stability
Storage: Store below 77°F (25°C). Store solution in an upright position and protect from freezing.
Laboratory Monitoring Cognitive function at periodic intervals
Nursing Actions
Physical Assessment: Assess bladder and sphincter adequacy prior to administering medication. Assess other medications for effectiveness and interactions. Monitor therapeutic effectiveness and adverse reactions (eg, cholinergic crisis: DUMBELS - diarrhea, urination, miosis, bronchospasm/bradycardia, excitability, lacrimation, and salivation/excessive sweating) at beginning of therapy and regularly with long-term use. Assess cognitive function at periodic intervals. Assess knowledge/teach patient appropriate use, possible side effects/appropriate interventions, and adverse symptoms to report.
Patient Education: This drug is not a cure for Alzheimer's disease, but it may reduce the symptoms. Use as directed; do not increase dose or discontinue without consulting prescriber. Swallow capsule whole with meals (do not crush or chew). Liquid can be swallowed directly from syringe or mixed with water, milk, or juice; stir well and drink within 4 hours of mixing. Maintain adequate hydration (2-3 L/day of fluids) unless instructed to restrict fluid intake. Avoid alcohol. May cause dizziness, drowsiness, or postural hypotension (rise slowly from sitting or lying position and use caution when driving or climbing stairs); vomiting or loss of appetite (small frequent meals, frequent mouth care, sucking lozenges, or chewing gum may help); diarrhea (buttermilk, boiled milk, or yogurt may help); or constipation (increased exercise, fluids, fruit, or fiber may help); or urinary frequency. Report persistent abdominal discomfort, diarrhea, or constipation; significantly increased salivation,

sweating, tearing, or urination; chest pain, palpitations, acute headache; CNS changes (eg, excessive fatigue, agitation, insomnia, dizziness, confusion, aggressiveness, depression); increased muscle, joint, or body pain; vision changes or blurred vision; shortness of breath, coughing, or wheezing; skin rash; or other persistent adverse reactions. **Breast-feeding precaution:** Consult prescriber if breast-feeding.

Dietary Considerations Should be taken with meals.

Rizatriptan (rye za TRIP tan)

U.S. Brand Names Maxalt®; Maxalt-MLT®
Synonyms MK462
Pharmacologic Category Serotonin 5-HT$_{1D}$ Receptor Agonist
Pregnancy Risk Factor C
Lactation Excretion in breast milk unknown/use caution
Use Acute treatment of migraine with or without aura
Mechanism of Action/Effect Selective agonist for serotonin (5-HT$_{1D}$ receptor) in cranial arteries to cause vasoconstriction and reduce sterile inflammation associated with antidromic neuronal transmission correlating with relief of migraine
Contraindications Hypersensitivity to rizatriptan or any component of the formulation; documented ischemic heart disease or Prinzmetal's angina; uncontrolled hypertension; basilar or hemiplegic migraine; during or within 2 weeks of MAO inhibitors; during or within 24 hours of treatment with another 5-HT$_1$ agonist, or an ergot-containing or ergot-type medication (eg, methysergide, dihydroergotamine)
Warnings/Precautions Use only in patients with a clear diagnosis of migraine. May cause vasospastic reactions resulting in colonic, peripheral, or coronary ischemia. Use with caution in elderly or patients with hepatic or renal impairment (including dialysis patients), history of hypersensitivity to sumatriptan or adverse effects from sumatriptan, and in patients at risk of coronary artery disease. (as predicted by presence of risk factors); establish absence of cardiovascular disease and administer initial dose in appropriately staffed setting (physician's office). Do not use with ergotamines. May increase blood pressure transiently; may cause coronary vasospasm (less than sumatriptan); avoid in patients with signs/symptoms suggestive of reduced arterial flow (ischemic bowel, Raynaud's) which could be exacerbated by vasospasm.

Patients who experience sensations of chest pain/pressure/tightness or symptoms suggestive of angina following dosing should be evaluated for coronary artery disease or Prinzmetal's angina before receiving additional doses.

Reconsider diagnosis of migraine if no response to initial dose. Long-term effects on vision have not been evaluated.

Drug Interactions
Increased Effect/Toxicity: Use within 24 hours of another selective 5-HT$_1$ antagonist or ergot-containing drug should be avoided due to possible additive vasoconstriction. Use with propranolol increased plasma concentration of rizatriptan by 70%. Rarely, concurrent use with SSRIs results in weakness and incoordination; monitor closely. MAO inhibitors and nonselective MAO inhibitors increase concentration of rizatriptan.

Nutritional/Ethanol Interactions Food: Food delays absorption.

Adverse Reactions 1% to 10%:
Cardiovascular: Systolic/diastolic blood pressure increases (5-10 mm Hg), chest pain (5%), palpitation

Central nervous system: Dizziness, drowsiness, fatigue (13% to 30%, dose related)

Dermatologic: Skin flushing

Endocrine & metabolic: Mild increase in growth hormone, hot flashes

Gastrointestinal: Nausea, abdominal pain, dry mouth (<5%)

Respiratory: Dyspnea

Pharmacodynamics/Kinetics
Onset of Action: ~30 minutes
Duration of Action: 14-16 hours
Time to Peak: 1-1.5 hours
Protein Binding: 14%
Half-Life Elimination: 2-3 hours
Metabolism: Via monoamine oxidase-A; first-pass effect
Excretion: Urine (82%, 8% to 16% as unchanged drug); feces (12%)

Available Dosage Forms
Tablet, as benzoate (Maxalt®): 5 mg, 10 mg
Tablet, orally disintegrating, as benzoate (Maxalt-MLT®): 5 mg [contains phenylalanine 1.05 mg/tablet; peppermint flavor]; 10 mg [contains phenylalanine 2.1 mg/tablet; peppermint flavor]

Dosing
Adults & Elderly: Note: In patients with risk factors for coronary artery disease, following adequate evaluation to establish the absence of coronary artery disease, the initial dose should be administered in a setting where response may be evaluated (physician's office or similarly staffed setting). ECG monitoring may be considered.

Migraine: Oral: 5-10 mg, repeat after 2 hours if significant relief is not attained; maximum: 30 mg in a 24-hour period (use 5 mg dose in patients receiving propranolol with a maximum of 15 mg in 24 hours)
Note: For orally-disintegrating tablets (Maxalt-MLT®): Patient should be instructed to place tablet on tongue and allow to dissolve. Dissolved tablet will be swallowed with saliva.

Stability
Storage: Store in blister pack until administration.

Laboratory Monitoring Consider monitoring vital signs and ECG with first dose in patients with unrecognized coronary disease, such as patients with significant hypertension, hypercholesterolemia, obese patients, patients with diabetes, smokers with other risk factors or strong family history of coronary artery disease

Nursing Actions
Physical Assessment: For use only with clear diagnosis of migraine. Presence of or at risk for coronary disease should be assessed prior to beginning therapy. Initial dose should be administered in a setting where response may be evaluated and ECG monitoring may be considered. Assess potential for interactions with other pharmacological agents patient may be taking (eg, ergot containing drugs, SSRIs). Monitor effectiveness (relief of migraine) and adverse response (eg, drowsiness, nausea/vomiting, chest pain, palpitations). Teach patient proper use, possible side effects/appropriate interventions, and adverse symptoms to report.

Patient Education: This drug is to be used to reduce your migraine, not to prevent or reduce the number of attacks. Follow exact instructions for use. For orally-disintegrating tablets (Maxalt-MLT®), do not open blister pack before using. Open with dry hands, place on tongue, and allow to dissolve (dissolved tablet will be swallowed with saliva). Do not crush, break, or chew. Do not take within 24 hours of any other migraine medication without first consulting prescriber. If first dose brings relief, second dose may be taken anytime after 2 hours if migraine returns. Do not take more than two doses without consulting prescriber. May cause dizziness or drowsiness (use caution when driving or engaging in tasks requiring alertness until response to drug is known); dry mouth (Continued)

Rizatriptan *(Continued)*

(frequent mouth care and sucking on lozenges may help); skin flushing or hot flashes (cool clothes or a cool environment may help); or mild abdominal discomfort or nausea or vomiting. Report immediately any chest pain, palpitations, or irregular heartbeat; severe dizziness, acute headache, stiff or painful neck or facial swelling; muscle weakness or pain; changes in mental acuity; blurred vision or eye pain; or excessive perspiration or urination. **Pregnancy/ breast-feeding precautions:** Inform prescriber if you are or intend to become pregnant. Breast-feeding is not recommended.

Dietary Considerations Orally-disintegrating tablet contains phenylalanine (1.05 mg per 5 mg tablet, 2.10 mg per 10 mg tablet).

Rocuronium *(roe kyoor OH nee um)*

U.S. Brand Names Zemuron®

Synonyms ORG 946; Rocuronium Bromide

Pharmacologic Category Neuromuscular Blocker Agent, Nondepolarizing

Medication Safety Issues

Sound-alike/look-alike issues:

Zemuron® may be confused with Remeron®

Pregnancy Risk Factor C

Lactation Excretion in breast milk unknown/use caution

Use Adjunct to general anesthesia to facilitate both rapid sequence and routine endotracheal intubation and to relax skeletal muscles during surgery; to facilitate mechanical ventilation in ICU patients; does not relieve pain or produce sedation

Contraindications Hypersensitivity to rocuronium or any component of the formulation

Warnings/Precautions Use with caution in patients with valvular heart disease, pulmonary disease, hepatic impairment; ventilation must be supported during neuromuscular blockade; certain clinical conditions may result in potentiation or antagonism of neuromuscular blockade:

Potentiation: Electrolyte abnormalities, severe hyponatremia, severe hypocalcemia, severe hypokalemia, hypermagnesemia, neuromuscular diseases, acidosis, acute intermittent porphyria, renal failure, hepatic failure

Antagonism: Alkalosis, hypercalcemia, demyelinating lesions, peripheral neuropathies, diabetes mellitus

Increased sensitivity in patients with myasthenia gravis, Eaton-Lambert syndrome; resistance in burn patients (>30% of body) for period of 5-70 days postinjury; resistance in patients with muscle trauma, denervation, immobilization, infection. Cross-sensitivity with other neuromuscular-blocking agents may occur; use extreme caution in patients with previous anaphylactic reactions.

Drug Interactions

Decreased Effect: Effect of nondepolarizing neuromuscular blockers may be reduced by carbamazepine (chronic use), corticosteroids (also associated with myopathy - see increased effect), phenytoin (chronic use), sympathomimetics, and theophylline.

Increased Effect/Toxicity: Increased effects are possible with aminoglycosides, beta-blockers, clindamycin, calcium channel blockers, halogenated anesthetics, imipenem, ketamine, lidocaine, loop diuretics (furosemide), macrolides (case reports), magnesium sulfate, procainamide, quinidine, quinolones, tetracyclines, and vancomycin. May increase risk of myopathy when used with high- dose corticosteroids for extended periods.

Adverse Reactions >1%: Cardiovascular: Transient hypotension and hypertension

Overdosage/Toxicology

Symptoms of overdose include prolonged skeletal muscle block, muscle weakness and apnea

Treatment is maintenance of a patent airway and controlled ventilation until recovery of normal neuromuscular block is observed, further recovery may be facilitated by administering an anticholinesterase agent (eg, neostigmine, edrophonium, or pyridostigmine) with atropine, to antagonize the skeletal muscle relaxation; support of the cardiovascular system with fluids and pressors may be necessary

Pharmacodynamics/Kinetics

Onset of Action: Good intubation conditions in 1-2 minutes; maximum neuromuscular blockade within 4 minutes

Duration of Action: ~30 minutes (with standard doses, increases with higher doses)

Half-Life Elimination: 60-70 minutes

Metabolism: Minimally hepatic; 17-desacetylrocuronium (5% to 10% activity of parent drug)

Excretion: Feces (50%); urine (30%)

Available Dosage Forms Injection, solution, as bromide: 10 mg/mL (5 mL, 10 mL)

Dosing

Adults & Elderly: Administer I.V.; dose to effect; doses will vary due to interpatient variability; use ideal body weight for obese patients

Tracheal intubation: I.V.:

Initial: 0.6 mg/kg is expected to provide approximately 31 minutes of clinical relaxation under opioid/nitrous oxide/oxygen anesthesia with neuromuscular block sufficient for intubation attained in 1-2 minutes; lower doses (0.45 mg/kg) may be used to provide 22 minutes of clinical relaxation with median time to neuromuscular block of 1-3 minutes; maximum blockade is achieved in <4 minutes

Maximum: 0.9-1.2 mg/kg may be given during surgery under opioid/nitrous oxide/oxygen anesthesia without adverse cardiovascular effects and is expected to provide 58-67 minutes of clinical relaxation; neuromuscular blockade sufficient for intubation is achieved in <2 minutes with maximum blockade in <3 minutes

Maintenance: 0.1, 0.15, and 0.2 mg/kg administered at 25% recovery of control T_1 (defined as 3 twitches of train-of-four) provides a median of 12, 17, and 24 minutes of clinical duration under anesthesia

Rapid sequence intubation: 0.6-1.2 mg/kg in appropriately premedicated and anesthetized patients with excellent or good intubating conditions within 2 minutes

Continuous infusion: Initial: 0.01-0.012 mg/kg/ minute only after early evidence of spontaneous recovery of neuromuscular function is evident; infusion rates have ranged from 0.004-0.016 mg/kg/ minute.

ICU neuromuscular blockade: 10 mcg/kg/minute; adjust dose to maintain appropriate degree of neuromuscular blockade (eg, 1 or 2 twitches on train-of-four)

Pediatrics: Administer I.V.; dose to effect; doses will vary due to interpatient variability; use ideal body weight for obese patients

Tracheal intubation: I.V.: Children:

Initial: 0.6 mg/kg under halothane anesthesia produce excellent to good intubating conditions within 1 minute and will provide a median time of 41 minutes of clinical relaxation in children 3 months to 1 year of age, and 27 minutes in children 1-12 years

Maintenance: 0.075-0.125 mg/kg administered upon return of T_1 to 25% of control provides clinical relaxation for 7-10 minutes

Administration

I.V.: Administer I.V. only; may be given undiluted as a bolus injection or via a continuous infusion using an infusion pump

Stability

Storage: Store under refrigeration (2°C to 8°C), do not freeze; when stored at room temperature, it is stable for 30 days; unlike vecuronium, it is stable in 0.9% sodium chloride and 5% dextrose in water, this mixture should be used within 24 hours of preparation

Nursing Actions

Physical Assessment: Only clinicians experienced in the use of neuromuscular blocking agents should administer and/or manage the use of rocuronium. Assess potential for interactions with other prescriptions, OTC medications, or herbal products patient may be taking (eg, other drugs that affect neuromuscular activity may increase/decrease neuromuscular block induced by rocuronium). Ventilatory support must be instituted and maintained until adequate respiratory muscle function and/or airway protection are assured. This drug does not cause anesthesia or analgesia; pain must be treated with appropriate agents. Continuous monitoring of vital signs, cardiac and respiratory status, and neuromuscular block (objective assessment with peripheral external nerve stimulator) are mandatory until full muscle tone has returned. Safety precautions must be maintained until full muscle tone has returned. Muscle tone returns in a predictable pattern; starting with diaphragm, abdomen, chest, limbs, and finally muscles of the neck, face, and eyes. **Note:** It may take longer for return of muscle tone in obese or elderly persons or patients with renal or hepatic disease, myasthenia gravis, myopathy, other neuromuscular diseases, dehydration, electrolyte imbalance, or severe acid/base imbalance. Provide appropriate teaching/support prior to, during, and following administration.

Long-term use: Monitor vital sign and fluid levels regularly during treatment. Every 2- to 3-hour repositioning, and skin, mouth, and eye care is necessary while patient is sedated. Emotional and sensory support (auditory and environmental) should be provided

Patient Education: Patient education should be appropriate for patient condition. Reassurance of constant monitoring and emotional support should precede and follow administration. Patients should be reminded as muscle tone returns not to attempt to change position or rise from bed without assistance and to report and skin rash, hives, pounding heartbeat, respiratory difficulty, or muscle tremors. **Pregnancy/breast-feeding precautions:** Inform prescriber if you are pregnant. Consult prescriber if breast-feeding.

Additional Information Rocuronium is classified as an intermediate-duration neuromuscular-blocking agent. Do not mix in the same syringe with barbiturates. Rocuronium does not relieve pain or produce sedation.

Ropinirole (roe PIN i role)

U.S. Brand Names Requip®
Synonyms Ropinirole Hydrochloride
Pharmacologic Category Anti-Parkinson's Agent, Dopamine Agonist
Medication Safety Issues
Sound-alike/look-alike issues:
Ropinirole may be confused with ropivacaine
Pregnancy Risk Factor C
Lactation Excretion in breast milk unknown/not recommended
Use Treatment of idiopathic Parkinson's disease; in patients with early Parkinson's disease who were not receiving concomitant levodopa therapy as well as in patients with advanced disease on concomitant levodopa; treatment of moderate-to-severe primary Restless Legs Syndrome (RLS)

Contraindications Hypersensitivity to ropinirole or any component of the formulation

Warnings/Precautions Syncope, sometimes associated with bradycardia, was observed in association with ropinirole in both early Parkinson's disease (without levodopa) patients and advanced Parkinson's disease (with levodopa) patients. Dopamine agonists appear to impair the systemic regulation of blood pressure resulting in postural hypotension, especially during dose escalation. Parkinson's disease patients appear to have an impaired capacity to respond to a postural challenge; use with caution in patients at risk of hypotension (ie, those receiving antihypertensive drugs) or where transient hypotensive episodes would be poorly tolerated (cardiovascular disease or cerebrovascular disease). Parkinson's patients being treated with dopaminergic agonists ordinarily require careful monitoring for signs and symptoms of postural hypotension, especially during dose escalation, and should be informed of this risk. May cause hallucinations. Use with caution in patients with pre-existing dyskinesia, severe hepatic or renal dysfunction.

Patients treated with ropinirole have reported falling asleep while engaging in activities of daily living; this has been reported to occur without significant warning signs. Monitor for daytime somnolence or pre-existing sleep disorder; caution with concomitant sedating medication; discontinue if significant daytime sleepiness or episodes of falling asleep occur. Patients must be cautioned about performing tasks which require mental alertness (eg, operating machinery or driving). Use with caution in patients receiving other CNS depressants or psychoactive agents. Effects with other sedative drugs or ethanol may be potentiated.

Some patients treated for RLS may experience worsening of symptoms in the early morning hours (rebound) or an increase and/or spread of daytime symptoms (augmentation); clinical management of these phenomena has not been evaluated in controlled clinical trials. Pathologic degenerative changes were observed in the retinas of albino rats during studies with this agent, but were not observed in the retinas of albino mice or in other species. The significance of these data for humans remains uncertain.

Other dopaminergic agents have been associated with a syndrome resembling neuroleptic malignant syndrome on withdrawal or significant dosage reduction after long-term use. Risk of fibrotic complications (eg, pleural effusion/fibrosis, interstitial lung disease) and melanoma has been reported in patients receiving ropinirole; drug causation has not been established.

Drug Interactions

Cytochrome P450 Effect: Substrate of CYP1A2 (major), 3A4 (minor); **Inhibits** CYP1A2 (weak), 2D6 (strong)

Decreased Effect: The levels/effects of ropinirole may be decreased by aminoglutethimide, carbamazepine, phenobarbital, rifampin, and other CYP1A2 inducers. Antipsychotics, cigarette smoking, and metoclopramide may reduce the effect or serum concentrations of ropinirole. Ropinirole may decrease the levels/effects of CYP2D6 prodrug substrates (eg, codeine, hydrocodone, oxycodone, tramadol).

Increased Effect/Toxicity: The levels/effects of ropinirole may be increased by amiodarone, ciprofloxacin, fluvoxamine, ketoconazole, norfloxacin, ofloxacin, rofecoxib, and other CYP1A2 inhibitors. Estrogens may also reduce the metabolism of ropinirole; dosage adjustments may be needed. Ropinirole may increase the levels/effects of amphetamines, selected beta-blockers, dextromethorphan, (Continued)

Ropinirole *(Continued)*

fluoxetine, lidocaine, mirtazapine, nefazodone, paroxetine, risperidone, ritonavir, thioridazine, tricyclic antidepressants, venlafaxine, and other CYP2D6 substrates.

Nutritional/Ethanol Interactions

Ethanol: Avoid ethanol (may increase CNS depression).

Herb/Nutraceutical: Avoid kava kava, gotu kola, valerian, St John's wort (may increase CNS depression).

Adverse Reactions

Data inclusive of trials in early Parkinson's disease (without levodopa) and Restless Legs Syndrome:

>10%:

Cardiovascular: Syncope (1% to 12%)

Central nervous system: Somnolence (12% to 40%), dizziness (11% to 40%), fatigue (8% to 11%)

Gastrointestinal: Nausea (40% to 60%), vomiting (12%)

Miscellaneous: Viral infection (11%)

1% to 10%:

Cardiovascular: Dependent/leg edema (2% to 7%), orthostasis (1% to 6%), hypertension (5%), chest pain (4%), flushing (3%), palpitation (3%), peripheral ischemia (3%), hypotension (2%), tachycardia (2%)

Central nervous system: Pain (3% to 8%), confusion (5%), hallucinations (up to 5%, dose related), hypoesthesia (4%), amnesia (3%), malaise (3%), paresthesia (3%), vertigo (2%), yawning (3%)

Gastrointestinal: Constipation (>5%), dyspepsia (4% to 10%), abdominal pain (3% to 6%), xerostomia (3% to 5%), diarrhea (5%), anorexia (4%), flatulence (3%)

Genitourinary: Urinary tract infection (5%), impotence (3%)

Hepatic: Alkaline phosphatase increased (3%)

Neuromuscular & skeletal: Weakness (6%), arthralgia (4%), muscle cramps (3%)

Ocular: Abnormal vision (6%), xerophthalmia (2%)

Respiratory: Pharyngitis (6% to 9%), rhinitis (4%), sinusitis (4%), dyspnea (3%), influenza (3%), cough (3%), nasal congestion (2%)

Miscellaneous: Diaphoresis increased (3% to 6%)

Advanced Parkinson's disease (with levodopa):

>10%:

Central nervous system: Dizziness (26%), somnolence (20%), headache (17%)

Gastrointestinal: Nausea (30%)

Neuromuscular & skeletal: Dyskinesias (34%)

1% to 10%:

Cardiovascular: Syncope (3%), hypotension (2%)

Central nervous system: Hallucinations (10%, dose related), aggravated parkinsonism, confusion (9%), pain (5%), paresis (3%), amnesia (5%), anxiety (6%), abnormal dreaming (3%), insomnia

Gastrointestinal: Abdominal pain (9%), vomiting (7%), constipation (6%), diarrhea (5%), dysphagia (2%), flatulence (2%), increased salivation (2%), xerostomia, weight loss (2%)

Genitourinary: Urinary tract infection

Hematologic: Anemia (2%)

Neuromuscular & skeletal: Falls (10%), arthralgia (7%), tremor (6%), hypokinesia (5%), paresthesia (5%), arthritis (3%)

Respiratory: Upper respiratory tract infection (9%), dyspnea (3%)

Miscellaneous: Injury, diaphoresis increased (7%), viral infection, increased drug level (7%)

Other adverse effects (all phase 2/3 trials):

1% to 10%:

Central nervous system: Neuralgia (>1%)

Renal: BUN increased (>1%)

Overdosage/Toxicology No reports of intentional overdose; symptoms reported with accidental overdosage were agitation, increased dyskinesia, sedation, orthostatic hypotension, chest pain, confusion, nausea, and vomiting. It is anticipated that the symptoms of overdose will be related to its dopaminergic activity. General supportive measures are recommended. Vital signs should be maintained, if necessary. Removal of any unabsorbed material (eg, by gastric lavage) should be considered. Removal by hemodialysis is unlikely.

Pharmacodynamics/Kinetics

Time to Peak: ~1-2 hours; T_{max} increased by 2.5 hours when taken with food

Half-Life Elimination: ~6 hours

Metabolism: Extensively hepatic via CYP1A2 to inactive metabolites; first-pass effect

Excretion: Clearance: Reduced by 30% in patients >65 years of age

Available Dosage Forms

Combination package:

Requip® [starter kit; contents per each administration card]: Tablet: 0.25 mg (2s), 0.5 mg (5s), 1 mg (7s)

Tablet:

Requip®: 0.25 mg, 0.5 mg, 1 mg, 2 mg, 3 mg, 4 mg, 5 mg

Dosing

Adults & Elderly:

Parkinson's disease: Oral: The dosage should be increased to achieve a maximum therapeutic effect, balanced against the principal side effects of nausea, dizziness, somnolence and dyskinesia. Recommended starting dose is 0.25 mg 3 times/day; based on individual patient response, the dosage should be titrated with weekly increments as described below:

- Week 1: 0.25 mg 3 times/day; total daily dose: 0.75 mg

- Week 2: 0.5 mg 3 times/day; total daily dose: 1.5 mg

- Week 3: 0.75 mg 3 times/day; total daily dose: 2.25 mg

- Week 4: 1 mg 3 times/day; total daily dose: 3 mg

  Note: After week 4, if necessary, daily dosage may be increased by 1.5 mg per day on a weekly basis up to a dose of 9 mg/day, and then by up to 3 mg/day weekly to a total of 24 mg/day

Parkinson's disease discontinuation taper: Ropinirole should be gradually tapered over 7 days as follows: reduce frequency of administration from 3 times daily to twice daily for 4 days, then reduce to once daily for remaining 3 days.

Restless Legs Syndrome: Initial: 0.25 mg once daily 1-3 hours before bedtime. Dose may be increased after 2 days to 0.5 mg daily, and after 7 days to 1 mg daily. Dose may be further titrated upward in 0.5 mg increments every week until reaching a daily dose of 3 mg during week 6. If symptoms persist or reappear, the daily dose may be increased to a maximum of 4 mg beginning week 7.

Note: Doses up to 4 mg per day may be discontinued without tapering.

Renal Impairment: Removal by hemodialysis is unlikely.

Nursing Actions

Physical Assessment: Assess potential for interactions with other prescriptions, OTC medications, or herbal products patient may be taking. Monitor patient response on a regular basis during therapy Monitor for CNS depression/somnolence. Teach patient proper use, side effects/appropriate interventions, and adverse reactions to report

Patient Education: Take exactly as directed, without regard to food. May cause dizziness, sudden, overwhelming sleepiness (use caution when driving or engaging in tasks that require alertness until response to drug is known); postural hypotension (use caution and avoid quick moves when rising from sitting or lying position, when climbing stairs, or engaging in activities that require quick movements); or nausea, vomiting, lack of appetite, or mouth sores (small frequent meals, frequent mouth care, chewing gum, or sucking lozenges may help). Report unusual and persistent sleepiness; chest pain or palpitations; CNS changes (confusion, hallucinations, amnesia, abnormal dreaming, insomnia); skeletal weakness or increased random tremors or movements, gait changes, or difficulty walking; signs of urinary tract or respiratory infection (pain or burning on urination, pus or blood in urine, or unusual cough and chest tightness); or unusual persistent adverse reactions. **Pregnancy/breast-feeding precautions:** Inform prescriber if you are or intend to become pregnant. Breast-feeding is not recommended.

Dietary Considerations May be taken with or without food.

Additional Information If therapy with a drug known to be a potent inhibitor of CYP1A2 is stopped or started during treatment with ropinirole, adjustment of ropinirole dose may be required. Ropinirole binds to melanin-containing tissues (ie, eyes, skin) in pigmented rats. After a single dose, long-term retention of drug was demonstrated, with a half-life in the eye of 20 days; not known if ropinirole accumulates in these tissues over time.

Rosiglitazone (roh si GLI ta zone)

U.S. Brand Names Avandia®

Pharmacologic Category Antidiabetic Agent, Thiazolidinedione

Medication Safety Issues

Sound-alike/look-alike issues:

Avandia® may be confused with Avalide®, Coumadin®, Prandin®

Pregnancy Risk Factor C

Lactation Excretion in breast milk unknown/not recommended

Use Type 2 diabetes mellitus (noninsulin dependent, NIDDM):

Monotherapy: Improve glycemic control as an adjunct to diet and exercise

Combination therapy: In combination with a sulfonylurea, metformin, or insulin, or sulfonylurea plus metformin when diet, exercise, and a single agent do not result in adequate glycemic control

Mechanism of Action/Effect Thiazolidinedione antidiabetic agent that lowers blood glucose by improving target cell response to insulin, without increasing pancreatic insulin secretion. It has a mechanism of action that is dependent on the presence of insulin for activity.

Contraindications Hypersensitivity to rosiglitazone or any component of the formulation; active liver disease (transaminases >2.5 times the upper limit of normal at baseline); contraindicated in patients who previously experienced jaundice during troglitazone therapy

Warnings/Precautions Should not be used in diabetic ketoacidosis. Mechanism requires the presence of insulin, therefore use in type 1 diabetes (insulin dependent, IDDM) is not recommended. Use with caution in premenopausal, anovulatory women; may result in resumption of ovulation, increasing the risk of pregnancy. May result in hormonal imbalance; development of menstrual irregularities should prompt reconsideration of therapy. Use with caution in patients with anemia or depressed leukocyte counts (may reduce hemoglobin, hematocrit, and/or WBC). May increase plasma volume and/or increase cardiac hypertrophy. Assess for fluid accumulation in patients with unusually rapid weight gain. Use with caution in patients with edema. Monitor closely for signs and symptoms of heart failure, unless serum glucose control outweighs the risk of excessive fluid retention. Not recommended for use in patients with NYHA Class III or IV heart failure, unless serum glucose control outweighs the risk of excessive fluid retention. Discontinue if heart failure develops. Use with caution in patients with elevated transaminases (AST or ALT). Idiosyncratic hepatotoxicity has been reported with another thiazolidinedione agent (troglitazone) and (rarely) with rosiglitazone; discontinue if jaundice occurs. Monitoring should include periodic determinations of liver function. Rosiglitazone has been associated with new onset and/or worsening of macular edema in diabetic patients. Rosiglitazone should be used with caution in patients with a pre-existing macular edema or diabetic retinopathy. Discontinuation of rosiglitazone should be considered in any patient who reports visual deterioration. In addition, ophthalmological consultation should be initiated in these patients. Safety and efficacy in pediatric patients have not been established.

Drug Interactions

Cytochrome P450 Effect: Substrate of CYP2C8/9 (major); **Inhibits** CYP2C8/9 (moderate), 2C19 (weak), 2D6 (weak)

Decreased Effect: The levels/effects of rosiglitazone may be decreased by carbamazepine, phenobarbital, phenytoin, rifampin, rifapentine, and secobarbital, and other CYP2C8/9 inducers. Bile acid sequestrants may decrease rosiglitazone levels.

Increased Effect/Toxicity: The levels/effects of rosiglitazone may be increased by delavirdine, fluconazole, gemfibrozil, ketoconazole, nicardipine, NSAIDs, pioglitazone, sulfonamides, and other CYP2C8/9 inhibitors. Gemfibrozil may increase rosiglitazone levels; severe hypoglycemic episodes have been reported. Rosiglitazone may increase the levels/effects of amiodarone, fluoxetine, glimepiride, glipizide, nateglinide, phenytoin, pioglitazone, sertraline, warfarin, and other CYP2C8/9 substrates.

Nutritional/Ethanol Interactions

Ethanol: Avoid ethanol (may cause hypoglycemia).

Food: Peak concentrations are lower by 28% and delayed when administered with food, but these effects are not believed to be clinically significant.

Herb/Nutraceutical: Avoid garlic, gymnema (may cause hypoglycemia).

Adverse Reactions Rare cases of hepatocellular injury have been reported in men in their 60s within 2-3 weeks after initiation of rosiglitazone therapy. LFTs in these patients revealed severe hepatocellular injury which responded with rapid improvement of liver function and resolution of symptoms upon discontinuation of rosiglitazone. Patients were also receiving other potentially hepatotoxic medications (*Ann Intern Med*, 2000, 132:121-4; 132:164-6). The rate of certain adverse reactions (eg, anemia, edema, hypoglycemia) may be higher with some combination therapies.

>10%: Endocrine & metabolic: Weight gain, increase in total cholesterol, increased LDL-cholesterol, increased HDL-cholesterol

1% to 10%:

Cardiovascular: Edema (5%)

Central nervous system: Headache (6%), fatigue (4%)

Endocrine & metabolic: Hyperglycemia (4%), hypoglycemia (1%; increased with insulin to 12% to 14%)

Gastrointestinal: Diarrhea (2%)

Hematologic: Anemia (2%)

Neuromuscular & skeletal: Back pain (4%)

Respiratory: Upper respiratory tract infection (10%), sinusitis (3%)

Miscellaneous: Injury (8%)

Overdosage/Toxicology Experience in overdose is limited. Symptoms may include hypoglycemia. Treatment is supportive.

(Continued)

Rosiglitazone *(Continued)*

Pharmacodynamics/Kinetics

Onset of Action: Delayed; Maximum effect: Up to 12 weeks

Time to Peak: 1 hour; delayed with food

Protein Binding: 99.8%

Half-Life Elimination: 3-4 hours

Metabolism: Hepatic (99%) via CYP2C8; minor metabolism via CYP2C9

Excretion: Urine (64%) and feces (23%) as metabolites

Available Dosage Forms Tablet: 2 mg, 4 mg, 8 mg

Dosing

Adults & Elderly: Type 2 diabetes: Oral:

Monotherapy: Initial: 4 mg daily as a single daily dose or in divided doses twice daily. If response is inadequate after 8-12 weeks of treatment, the dosage may be increased to 8 mg daily as a single daily dose or in divided doses twice daily. In clinical trials, the 4 mg twice-daily regimen resulted in the greatest reduction in fasting plasma glucose and Hb A_{1c}.

Combination therapy: When adding rosiglitazone to existing therapy, continue current dose(s) of previous agents:

With sulfonylureas or metformin (or sulfonylurea plus metformin): Initial: 4 mg daily as a single daily dose or in divided doses twice daily. If response is inadequate after 8-12 weeks of treatment, the dosage may be increased to 8 mg daily as a single daily dose or in divided doses twice daily. Reduce dose of sulfonylurea if hypoglycemia occurs. It is unlikely that the dose of metformin will need to be reduced to hypoglycemia.

With insulin: Initial: 4 mg daily as a single daily dose or in divided doses twice daily. Dose of insulin should be reduced by 10% to 25% if the patient reports hypoglycemia or if the plasma glucose falls to <100 mg/dL. Doses of rosiglitazone >4 mg/day are not indicated in combination with insulin.

Renal Impairment: No adjustment is necessary.

Hepatic Impairment: Clearance is significantly lower in hepatic impairment. Therapy should not be initiated if the patient exhibits active liver disease of increased transaminases (>2.5 times the upper limit of normal) at baseline.

Stability

Storage: Store at 25°C (77°F); excursions permitted to 15°C to 30°C (59°F to 86°F). Protect from light.

Laboratory Monitoring Hemoglobin A_{1c}, serum glucose; liver enzymes (prior to initiation of therapy, then periodically thereafter). Patients with an elevation in ALT >3 times ULN should be rechecked as soon as possible. If the ALT levels remain >3 times ULN, therapy with rosiglitazone should be discontinued.

Nursing Actions

Physical Assessment: Monitor laboratory results closely. Assess other prescriptions, OTC medications, or herbal products patient may be taking. Assess for signs of fluid retention and congestive heart failure. Monitor weight. Monitor response to therapy closely until response is stable. Advise women using oral contraceptives about need for alternative method of contraception. Assess knowledge/teach risks of hyper-/hypoglycemia, its symptoms, treatment, and predisposing conditions. Refer patient to a diabetic educator, if possible. Teach appropriate use of medication, interventions to reduce side effects, and adverse reactions to report.

Patient Education: May be taken without regard to meals. Follow directions of prescriber. If dose is missed at the usual meal, take it with next meal. Do not double dose if daily dose is missed completely. Monitor urine or serum glucose as recommended by prescriber. More frequent monitoring is required during periods of stress, trauma, surgery, pregnancy, increased activity or exercise. Avoid alcohol. Report chest pain, rapid heartbeat or palpitations, abdominal pain, fever, rash, hypoglycemia reactions, yellowing of skin or eyes, dark urine or light stool, or unusual fatigue or nausea/vomiting. Report unusually rapid weight gain; swelling of ankles, legs, or abdomen; or weakness or shortness of breath. **Pregnancy/breast-feeding precautions:** In anovulatory, premenopausal women, ovulation may occur, increasing the risk of pregnancy. Adequate contraception is recommended. Use alternate means of contraception if using oral contraceptives. Breast-feeding is not recommended.

Dietary Considerations Management of type 2 diabetes mellitus (noninsulin dependent, NIDDM) should include diet control. May be taken without regard to meals.

Breast-Feeding Issues In animal studies, rosiglitazone has been found to be excreted in milk. It is not known whether rosiglitazone is excreted in human milk. Should not be administered to a nursing woman.

Pregnancy Issues Treatment during mid to late gestation was associated with fetal death and growth retardation in animal models. Abnormal blood glucose levels are associated with a higher incidence of congenital abnormalities. Insulin is the drug of choice for the control of diabetes mellitus during pregnancy. In anovulatory, premenopausal women, ovulation may occur, increasing the risk of pregnancy; adequate contraception is recommended.

Rosiglitazone and Glimepiride
(roh si GLI ta zone & GLYE me pye ride)

U.S. Brand Names Avandaryl™

Synonyms Glimepiride and Rosiglitazone Maleate

Pharmacologic Category Antidiabetic Agent, Sulfonylurea; Antidiabetic Agent, Thiazolidinedione

Pregnancy Risk Factor C

Lactation Excretion in breast milk unknown/not recommended

Use Management of type 2 diabetes mellitus (noninsulin dependent, NIDDM) in patients who are already treated with the combination of rosiglitazone and a sulfonylurea, or who are not adequately controlled on a sulfonylurea alone, or who initially responded to rosiglitazone alone and require additional glycemic control; used as an adjunct to diet and exercise to lower the blood glucose when hyperglycemia cannot be controlled satisfactorily by diet and exercise alone

Available Dosage Forms Tablet (Avandaryl™):

4 mg/1 mg: Rosiglitazone 4 mg and glimepiride 1 mg

4 mg/2 mg: Rosiglitazone 4 mg and glimepiride 2 mg

4 mg/4 mg: Rosiglitazone 4 mg and glimepiride 4 mg

Dosing

Adults: Type 2 diabetes mellitus: Oral:

Patients inadequately controlled on sulfonylurea monotherapy:

Initial: Rosiglitazone 4 mg and glimepiride 1 mg **or** rosiglitazone 4 mg and glimepiride 2 mg once daily

Dose adjustment: May take 2 weeks to observe decreased blood glucose and 2-3 months to see full effects. If additional glucose control is needed, increase daily dose of glimepiride component.

Maximum: Rosiglitazone 8 mg and glimepiride 4 mg per day

Patients who initially responded to rosiglitazone alone and require additional glucose control:

Initial: Rosiglitazone 4 mg and glimepiride 1 mg **or** rosiglitazone 4 mg and glimepiride 2 mg once daily

Dose adjustment: If not adequately controlled after 1-2 weeks, increase daily dose of glimepiride component in ≤2 mg increments in 1-2 week intervals.

Maximum: Rosiglitazone 8 mg and glimepiride 4 mg per day

Patients switching from combination rosiglitazone and glimepiride as separate tablets: Use current dose. Maximum: Rosiglitazone 8 mg and glimepiride 4 mg per day.

Elderly: Rosiglitazone 4 mg and glimepiride 1 mg once daily. Carefully titrate dose.

Renal Impairment: Rosiglitazone 4 mg and glimepiride 1 mg once daily. Carefully titrate dose.

Hepatic Impairment: Rosiglitazone 4 mg and glimepiride 1 mg once daily. Carefully titrate dose.

ALT ≤2.5 times ULN: Use with caution.

ALT >2.5 times ULN: Do not initiate therapy.

ALT >3 times ULN or jaundice: Discontinue.

Nursing Actions

Physical Assessment: Assess other prescription and OTC medications patient may be taking to avoid duplications and interactions. Assess for signs of fluid retention and congestive heart failure. Monitor weight. Monitor response to therapy closely until response is known. Advise women using oral contraceptives about the need for alternative method of contraception. Assess knowledge/teach patient signs of hypo-/hyperglycemia, its symptoms and treatment, and predisposing condition. Refer patient to diabetic educator if possible. Teach patient appropriate use of medication, intervention to reduce side effects, and adverse reactions to report.

Patient Education: Inform prescriber of all prescription medications, OTC medications, or herbal products you are taking. Do not take any new medications without consulting prescriber. This medication is used to control diabetes; it is not a cure. Take exactly as directed, usually with the first meal of the day. Avoid alcohol; may cause severe reaction. Monitor glucose as directed by prescriber. Maintain regular dietary intake and exercise routine (consult prescriber or diabetic educator). Always carry a quick source of glucose. Contact prescriber immediately if you experience hypoglycemia. May cause headache, nausea, or diarrhea during the first weeks of therapy. Consult prescriber if these persist. Report chest pain, rapid heartbeat or palpitations; hypo-/hyperglycemia reactions; persistent, unusual fatigue; muscle pain or weakness; persistent nausea or vomiting; abdominal pain; loss of appetite; dark urine; rapid weight gain; swelling of the extremities; or respiratory difficulty. **Pregnancy/breast-feeding precautions:** Inform prescriber if you are or intend to become pregnant. Use alternate means of contraception if using oral contraceptives. Do not breast-feed.

Related Information

Glimepiride *on page 584*
Rosiglitazone *on page 1101*

Rosiglitazone and Metformin
(roh si GLI ta zone & met FOR min)

U.S. Brand Names Avandamet™
Synonyms Metformin and Rosiglitazone; Metformin

Hydrochloride and Rosiglitazone Maleate; Rosiglitazone Maleate and Metformin Hydrochloride

Pharmacologic Category Antidiabetic Agent, Biguanide; Antidiabetic Agent, Thiazolidinedione

Pregnancy Risk Factor C

Lactation Excretion in breast milk unknown/not recommended

Use Management of type 2 diabetes mellitus (noninsulin dependent, NIDDM) in patients who are already treated with the combination of rosiglitazone and metformin, or who are not adequately controlled on metformin alone. Used as an adjunct to diet and exercise to lower the blood glucose when hyperglycemia cannot be controlled satisfactorily by diet and exercise alone

Available Dosage Forms Tablet:

1/500: Rosiglitazone 1 mg and metformin hydrochloride 500 mg

2/500: Rosiglitazone 2 mg and metformin hydrochloride 500 mg

4/500: Rosiglitazone 4 mg and metformin hydrochloride 500 mg

2/1000: Rosiglitazone 2 mg and metformin hydrochloride 1000 mg

4/1000: Rosiglitazone 4 mg and metformin hydrochloride 1000 mg

Dosing

Adults: Type 2 diabetes mellitus: Oral: Initial dose should be based on current dose of rosiglitazone and/or metformin; daily dose should be divided and given with meals

Patients inadequately controlled on metformin alone: Initial dose: Rosiglitazone 4 mg/day plus current dose of metformin

Patients inadequately controlled on rosiglitazone alone: Initial dose: Metformin 1000 mg/day plus current dose of rosiglitazone

Note: When switching from combination rosiglitazone and metformin as separate tablets: Use current dose

Dose adjustment: Doses may be increased as increments of rosiglitazone 4 mg and/or metformin 500 mg, up to the maximum dose; doses should be titrated gradually.

After a change in the metformin dosage, titration can be done after 1-2 weeks

After a change in the rosiglitazone dosage, titration can be done after 8-12 weeks

Maximum dose: Rosiglitazone 8 mg/metformin 2000 mg daily

Elderly: The initial and maintenance dosing should be conservative, due to the potential for decreased renal function (monitor). Generally, elderly patients should not be titrated to the maximum. Do not use in patients ≥80 years unless normal renal function has been established.

Renal Impairment: Do not use with renal disease or renal dysfunction (serum creatinine ≥1.5 mg/dL in males or ≥1.4 mg/dL in females or abnormal clearance).

Hepatic Impairment: Do not use with active liver disease or ALT >2.5 times the upper limit of normal.

Nursing Actions

Physical Assessment: Allergy history should be assessed prior to beginning therapy. Assess potential for interactions with other prescriptions, OTC medications, or herbal products patient may be taking (eg, anything that may affect glucose levels). Monitor results of laboratory tests, therapeutic effectiveness, and adverse response (eg, hypoglycemia, vitamin B_{12} and/or folic acid deficiency) at regular intervals during (Continued)

Rosiglitazone and Metformin
(Continued)

therapy. Teach patient proper use, possible side effects/appropriate interventions, and adverse symptoms to report.

Patient Education: Do not take any new medication during therapy without consulting prescriber. This medication is used to control diabetes; it is not a cure. Take exactly as directed with a meal at the same time(s) each day. Avoid excessive alcohol; may cause severe reaction. Monitor glucose as recommended by prescriber. Maintain regular prescribed dietary intake and exercise routine (consult prescriber or diabetic educator) and always carry a quick source of sugar with you. Contact prescriber immediately if you experience a hypoglycemic reaction. May cause headache, nausea, or diarrhea during first weeks of therapy; consult prescriber if these persist. Report chest pain, rapid heartbeat, or palpitations; hypo- or hyperglycemic reactions; persistent, unusual fatigue; changes in visual acuity; muscle pain or weakness; nausea or vomiting; rapid weight gain; swelling of extremities; or respiratory difficulty. **Pregnancy/breast-feeding precautions:** Inform prescriber if you are or intend to become pregnant. Use alternate means of contraception if using oral contraceptives. Breast-feeding is not recommended.

Related Information
Metformin *on page 789*
Rosiglitazone *on page 1101*

Rosuvastatin (roe SOO va sta tin)

U.S. Brand Names Crestor®

Synonyms Rosuvastatin Calcium

Pharmacologic Category Antilipemic Agent, HMG-CoA Reductase Inhibitor

Pregnancy Risk Factor X

Lactation Excretion in breast milk unknown/contraindicated

Use Used with dietary therapy for hyperlipidemias to reduce elevations in total cholesterol (TC), LDL-C, apolipoprotein B, and triglycerides (TG) in patients with primary hypercholesterolemia (elevations of 1 or more components are present in Fredrickson type IIa, IIb, and IV hyperlipidemias); treatment of homozygous familial hypercholesterolemia (FH)

Mechanism of Action/Effect Inhibitor of 3-hydroxy-3-methylglutaryl coenzyme A (HMG-CoA) reductase, the rate limiting enzyme in cholesterol synthesis (reduces the production of mevalonic acid from HMG-CoA); lowers TC, LDL-C, TG and improves HDL:LDL ratio

Contraindications Hypersensitivity to rosuvastatin or any component of the formulation; active liver disease; unexplained persistent elevations of serum transaminases (>3 times ULN); pregnancy; breast-feeding

Warnings/Precautions Secondary causes of hyperlipidemia should be ruled out prior to therapy. Liver function must be monitored by periodic laboratory assessment. Use with caution in patients who consume large amounts of ethanol or have a history of liver disease. Rhabdomyolysis with acute renal failure has occurred. Discontinue in any patient in which CPK levels are markedly elevated (>10 times ULN) or if myopathy is suspected/diagnosed. An increased incidence of rosuvastatin-associated myopathy has been reported during concomitant therapy with fibric acid derivatives, niacin, cyclosporine, and in certain subgroups of the Asian population. Risk is also elevated at higher dosages of rosuvastatin. Patients should be instructed to report unexplained muscle pain, tenderness, or weakness, particularly if associated with fever and/or malaise. Use caution in patients predisposed to myopathy (eg, renal failure, advanced age, inadequately treated hypothyroidism). Temporarily withhold in patients experiencing an acute or serious condition predisposing to renal failure secondary to rhabdomyolysis (sepsis, hypotension, major surgery, trauma, severe metabolic or endocrine or electrolyte disorders, uncontrolled seizures). Safety and efficacy have not been established in children (limited experience with homozygous FH in patients >8 years of age).

Drug Interactions
Cytochrome P450 Effect: Substrate (minor) of CYP2C9, 3A4

Decreased Effect: Plasma concentrations of rosuvastatin may be decreased when given with magnesium/aluminum hydroxide-containing antacids; antacids should be administered at least 2 hours after rosuvastatin. Cholestyramine and colestipol (bile acid sequestrants) may reduce absorption of several HMG-CoA reductase inhibitors; separate administration times by at least 4 hours; cholesterol-lowering effects are additive.

Increased Effect/Toxicity: Cyclosporine may increase serum concentrations of rosuvastatin (up to 10-fold); limit dose to 5 mg/day. Serum concentrations of rosuvastatin may be increased (doubled) during concurrent administration of gemfibrozil; combination should be avoided; limit dose to 10 mg/day. Clofibrate, fenofibrate, or niacin may increase the risk of myopathy and rhabdomyolysis with HMG-CoA reductase inhibitors; the effects on lipids may be additive. The anticoagulant effects of warfarin may be increased by rosuvastatin (monitor). Rosuvastatin increases serum concentrations of hormonal contraceptives (ethinyl estradiol and norgestrel).

Nutritional/Ethanol Interactions Ethanol: Avoid excessive ethanol consumption (due to potential hepatic effects).

Food: Red yeast rice contains an estimated 2.4 mg lovastatin per 600 mg rice.

Adverse Reactions
1% to 10%:
Cardiovascular: Chest pain, hypertension, peripheral edema, palpitation

Central nervous system: Headache (6%), depression, dizziness, insomnia, pain, anxiety, neuralgia, vertigo

Dermatologic: Rash

Gastrointestinal: Pharyngitis (9%), diarrhea, dyspepsia, nausea, abdominal pain, constipation, gastroenteritis, vomiting

Hematologic: Anemia, bruising

Neuromuscular & skeletal: Myalgia (3%), weakness, back pain, arthritis, arthralgia, hypertonia, paresthesia

Respiratory: Bronchitis, rhinitis, sinusitis, cough

Miscellaneous: Flu-like syndrome

Adverse reactions reported with other HMG-CoA reductase inhibitors include a hypersensitivity syndrome (symptoms may include anaphylaxis, angioedema, arthralgia, erythema multiforme, eosinophilia, hemolytic anemia, lupus syndrome, photosensitivity, polymyalgia rheumatica, positive ANA, purpura, Stevens-Johnson syndrome, toxic epidermal necrolysis, urticaria, vasculitis)

Overdosage/Toxicology No specific experience in overdose. Treatment is supportive. Rosuvastatin is not removed by hemodialysis. CNS vascular lesions and corneal opacities have been reported following high-dose, long-term exposure to HMG-CoA reductase inhibitors in animal studies. The relationship to human exposures has not been established.

Pharmacodynamics/Kinetics

Onset of Action: Within 1 week; maximal at 4 weeks

Time to Peak: Plasma: 3-5 hours

Protein Binding: 90%

Half-Life Elimination: 19 hours

Metabolism: Hepatic (10%), via CYP2C9 (1 active metabolite identified)

Excretion: Feces (90%), primarily as unchanged drug

Pharmacokinetic Note Asian patients have been noted to have increased bioavailability.

Available Dosage Forms Tablet, as calcium: 5 mg, 10 mg, 20 mg, 40 mg

Dosing

Adults & Elderly:

Heterozygous familial and nonfamilial hypercholesterolemia; mixed dyslipidemia: Oral:

Initial dose:

General dosing: 10 mg once daily (20 mg in patients with severe hypercholesterolemia)

Conservative dosing: Patients requiring less aggressive treatment or predisposed to myopathy (including patients of Asian descent): 5 mg once daily

Titration: After 2 weeks, may be increased by 5-10 mg once daily; dosing range: 5-40 mg/day (maximum dose: 40 mg once daily)

Note: The 40 mg dose should be reserved for patients who have not achieved goal cholesterol levels on a dose of 20 mg/day, including patients switched from another HMG-CoA reductase inhibitor.

Homozygous familial hypercholesterolemia (HFH): Oral: Initial: 20 mg once daily (maximum dose: 40 mg/day)

Dosage adjustment with concomitant medications: Oral:

Cyclosporine: Rosuvastatin dose should not exceed 5 mg/day

Gemfibrozil: Rosuvastatin dose should not exceed 10 mg/day

Dosage adjustment for persistent, unexplained proteinuria while on 40 mg/day: Reduce dose and evaluate causes.

Renal Impairment:

Mild to moderate impairment: No dosage adjustment required.

Cl_{cr} <30 mL/minute/1.73 m^2: Initial: 5 mg/day; do not exceed 10 mg once daily

Administration

Oral: May be administered with or without food.

Stability

Storage: Store between 20°C and 25°C (68°F to 77°F). Protect from moisture.

Laboratory Monitoring Total cholesterol, LDL, and HDL cholesterol; liver function tests should be determined at baseline (prior to initiation), 3 months following initiation, and 3 months after any increase in dose; baseline CPK (recheck CPK in any patient with symptoms suggestive of myopathy)

Nursing Actions

Physical Assessment: Assess potential for interactions with other pharmacological agents or herbal products patient may be taking (eg, gemfibrozil, fibric acid derivatives, niacin may increase risk of myopathy or rhabdomyolysis). Monitor laboratory tests, therapeutic effectiveness and adverse reactions (eg, rash, myalgia, blurred vision, abdominal pain, cough) on a regular basis throughout therapy. Teach patient proper use (as adjunct to diet and exercise program), possible side effects/appropriate interventions, and adverse symptoms to report. **Pregnancy risk factor X:** Determine that patient is not pregnant before starting therapy. Do not give to women of childbearing age unless they are capable of complying with effective contraceptive use. Instruct patient in appropriate contraceptive measures.

Patient Education: Take at same time each day with or without food. Follow cholesterol-lowering diet and exercise regimen as prescribed. Avoid excess alcohol. You will have periodic blood tests to assess effectiveness. You may experience constipation (increased exercise, fluids, fiber, and fruit may help); headache, dressing, dizziness, insomnia (use caution when driving or engaged in potentially hazardous tasks until response to drug is known). Report unusual chest pain, swelling of extremities, weight gain of >5 lb/week, or persistent cough. Contact prescriber immediately with persistent muscle or skeletal pain, joint pain, or numbness, or any sign of allergic reactions (skin rash, difficulty breathing, tightness in throat, choking sensation, swelling of mouth or face). **Pregnancy/breast-feeding precautions:** Inform prescriber if you are pregnant. Do not get pregnant during and for 1 month following therapy. Consult prescriber for appropriate contraceptive measures. This drug may cause severe fetal defects. Do not donate blood during or for 1 month following therapy. Do not breast feed.

Dietary Considerations May be taken with or without food. Red yeast rice contains an estimated 2.4 mg lovastatin per 600 mg rice.

Pregnancy Issues Cholesterol biosynthesis may be important in fetal development. Contraindicated in pregnancy. Administer to women of childbearing potential only when conception is highly unlikely and patients have been informed of potential hazards.

Sacrosidase (sak ROE si dase)

U.S. Brand Names Sucraid®

Pharmacologic Category Enzyme, Gastrointestinal

Pregnancy Risk Factor C

Lactation Enters breast milk/compatible

Use Orphan drug: Oral replacement therapy in sucrase deficiency, as seen in congenital sucrase-isomaltase deficiency (CSID)

Mechanism of Action/Effect Sacrosidase is a naturally-occurring gastrointestinal enzyme which breaks down the disaccharide sucrose to its monosaccharide components. Hydrolysis is necessary to allow absorption of these nutrients.

Contraindications Hypersensitivity to yeast, yeast products, or glycerin

Warnings/Precautions Hypersensitivity reactions to sacrosidase, including bronchospasm, have been reported. Administer initial doses in a setting where acute hypersensitivity reactions may be treated within a few minutes. Skin testing for hypersensitivity may be performed prior to administration to identify patients at risk.

Drug Interactions

Increased Effect/Toxicity: Drug-drug interactions have not been evaluated.

Nutritional/Ethanol Interactions Food: May be inactivated or denatured if administered with fruit juice, warm or hot food or liquids. Since isomaltase deficiency is not addressed by supplementation of sacrosidase, adherence to a low-starch diet may be required.

Adverse Reactions 1% to 10%: Gastrointestinal: Abdominal pain, vomiting, nausea, diarrhea, constipation

Overdosage/Toxicology Symptoms may include epigastric pain, drowsiness, lethargy, nausea, and vomiting. Gastrointestinal bleeding may occur. Rare manifestations include hypertension, respiratory depression, coma, and acute renal failure. Treatment is symptomatic and supportive. Forced diuresis, hemodialysis and/or urinary alkalinization are not likely to be useful. (Continued)

Sacrosidase *(Continued)*

Pharmacodynamics/Kinetics
Metabolism: GI tract to individual amino acids

Available Dosage Forms Solution, oral: 8500 int. units per mL (118 mL)

Dosing
Adults & Elderly: Sucrase deficiency: Oral: 17,000 int. units (2 mL) per meal or snack. Doses should be diluted with 2-4 ounces of water, milk or formula with each meal or snack. Approximately one-half of the dose may be taken before, and the remainder of a dose taken at the completion of each meal or snack.

Pediatrics:
Infants ≥5 months and Children <15 kg: Oral: 8500 int. units (1 mL) per meal or snack
Children >15 kg: Refer to adult dosing.

Stability
Storage: Store under refrigeration at 4°C to 8°C (36°F to 46°F). Protect from heat or light.

Nursing Actions
Physical Assessment: Hypersensitivity reactions can occur (including bronchospasm), administer initial dose where adverse reactions can be treated immediately; skin testing for hypersensitivity may be performed prior to administering first dose to identify patients at risk. Monitor effectiveness of therapy and adverse reactions at beginning of therapy and periodically with long-term use. Assess knowledge/teach patient appropriate use, interventions to reduce side effects, and adverse symptoms to report.

Patient Education: Use exactly as directed. Dilute dose in 2-4 oz of water, milk, or formula; do not dilute with fruit juice or warm or cold liquids. Take half the dose at beginning of meal and half the dose at end of meal. Maintain adequate hydration (2-3 L/day of fluids) unless instructed to restrict fluid intake. Follow prescribers recommended diet exactly. You may experience headache or nervousness (use caution when driving or engaging in tasks requiring alertness until response to drug is known); or nausea, vomiting, or GI disturbance (frequent mouth care, chewing gum, or sucking hard candy may help). Report immediately skin rash or respiratory difficulty; persistent vomiting, abdominal pain, or blood in stools; change in CNS status (depression, agitation, lethargy); or other adverse response. **Pregnancy precaution:** Inform prescriber if you are or intend to become pregnant.

Additional Information Oral solution contains 50% glycerol.

Salmeterol *(sal ME te role)*

U.S. Brand Names Serevent® Diskus®
Synonyms Salmeterol Xinafoate
Restrictions An FDA-approved medication guide is available at http://www.fda.gov/cder/Offices/ODS/labeling.htm; distribute to each patient to whom this medication is dispensed.
Pharmacologic Category Beta₂-Adrenergic Agonist
Medication Safety Issues
Sound-alike/look-alike issues:
Salmeterol may be confused with Salbutamol
Serevent® may be confused with Serentil®
Pregnancy Risk Factor C
Lactation Enters breast milk/use caution
Use Maintenance treatment of asthma and in prevention of bronchospasm with reversible obstructive airway disease, including patients with symptoms of nocturnal asthma; prevention of exercise-induced bronchospasm; maintenance treatment of bronchospasm associated with COPD
Mechanism of Action/Effect Relaxes bronchial smooth muscle by selective action on beta₂-receptors with little effect on heart rate; because salmeterol acts locally in the lung, therapeutic effect is not predicted by plasma levels

Contraindications Hypersensitivity to salmeterol, adrenergic amines, or any component of the formulation; need for acute bronchodilation

Warnings/Precautions
Asthma treatment: Long-acting beta₂ agonists may increase the risk of asthma-related deaths. Should only be used as adjuvant therapy in patients not adequately controlled on inhaled corticosteroids or whose disease requires two maintenance therapies. Salmeterol is not meant to relieve acute asthmatic symptoms, should not be initiated in patients with significantly worsening or acutely deteriorating asthma, and is not a substitute for inhaled or oral corticosteroids. Short-acting beta₂ agonist should be used for acute symptoms and symptoms occurring between treatments. Corticosteroids should not be stopped or reduced when salmeterol is initiated. During the initiation of salmeterol watch for signs of worsening asthma.

Concurrent diseases: Use caution in patients with cardiovascular disease (eg, arrhythmia, hypertension, or CHF), seizure disorders, diabetes, glaucoma, hyperthyroidism, hepatic impairment, or hypokalemia. Beta agonists may cause elevation in blood pressure, heart rate, CNS stimulation/excitation, increased risk of arrhythmia, increase serum glucose, or decrease serum potassium.

Adverse events: Salmeterol should not be used more than twice daily; do not exceed recommended dose; do not use with other long-acting beta₂ agonists; serious adverse events have been associated with excessive use of inhaled sympathomimetics. Rarely, paradoxical bronchospasm may occur with use of inhaled bronchodilating agents; this should be distinguished from inadequate response. Powder for oral inhalation contains lactose; very rare anaphylactic reactions have been reported in patients with severe milk protein allergy.

Safety and efficacy have not been established in children <4 years of age.

Drug Interactions
Cytochrome P450 Effect: Substrate of CYP3A4 (major)

Decreased Effect: Beta₂-agonists may diminish the bradycardia effect of beta-blockers (beta₁ selective). Beta-blockers (nonselective) may diminish the bronchodilator effect of beta₂-agonists.

Increased Effect/Toxicity: CYP3A4 inhibitors may increase the levels/effects of fluticasone and salmeterol; example inhibitors include amprenavir, atazanavir, clarithromycin, delavirdine, diclofenac, fosamprenavir, imatinib, indinavir, isoniazid, itraconazole, ketoconazole, miconazole, nefazodone, nelfinavir, nicardipine, propofol, quinidine, ritonavir, and telithromycin. Atomoxetine may enhance the tachycardia effect of beta₂-agonists. Sympathomimetics may enhance the adverse/toxic effect of salmeterol.

Adverse Reactions
>10%:
Central nervous system: Headache (13% to 17%)
Neuromuscular & skeletal: Pain (1% to 12%)
1% to 10%:
Cardiovascular: Hypertension (4%), edema (1% to <3%)
Central nervous system: Dizziness (4%), sleep disturbance (1% to 3%), fever (1% to 3%), anxiety (1% to <3%), migraine (1% to <3%)
Dermatologic: Rash (1% to 4%), contact dermatitis (1% to 3%), eczema (1% to 3%), urticaria (3%), photodermatitis (1% to 2%)
Endocrine & metabolic: Hyperglycemia (1% to <3%)

Gastrointestinal: Nausea (1% to 3%), dyspepsia (1% to <3%), dental pain (1% to <3%), infections (1% to <3%), oropharyngeal candidiasis (1% to <3%), xerostomia (1% to <3%)

Neuromuscular & skeletal: Muscular cramps/spasm (3%), paresthesia (1% to 3%), arthralgia (1% to <3%), muscular stiffness, rigidity (1% to <3%)

Ocular: Keratitis/conjunctivitis (1% to <3%)

Respiratory: Tracheitis/bronchitis (7%), pharyngitis (up to 6%), cough (5%), influenza (5%), infection (5%), sinusitis (4% to 5%), rhinitis (4% to 5%), nasal congestion (4%), asthma (3% to 4%)

Overdosage/Toxicology Symptoms of overdose include tachycardia, tremor, hypertension, angina, and seizures. Hypokalemia also may occur. Cardiac arrest and death may be associated with abuse of beta-agonist bronchodilators. Treatment includes immediate discontinuation and symptomatic and supportive therapies. Cautious use of beta-adrenergic blocking agents may be considered in severe cases.

Pharmacodynamics/Kinetics
Onset of Action: Asthma: 30-48 minutes, COPD: 2 hours; Peak effect: 2-4 hours, COPD: 3.27-4.75 hours
Duration of Action: 12 hours
Protein Binding: 96%
Half-Life Elimination: 5.5 hours
Metabolism: Hepatically hydroxylated
Excretion: Feces (60%), urine (25%)

Available Dosage Forms Powder for oral inhalation: 50 mcg (28s, 60s) [delivers 50 mcg/inhalation; contains lactose]

Dosing
Adults & Elderly:
Asthma, maintenance and prevention: Inhalation, powder (Serevent® Diskus®): One inhalation (50 mcg) twice daily (~12 hours apart); maximum: 1 inhalation twice daily

Exercise-induced asthma, prevention: One inhalation (50 mcg) at least 30 minutes prior to exercise; additional doses should not be used for 12 hours; should not be used in individuals already receiving salmeterol twice daily

COPD (maintenance treatment of associated bronchospasm): One inhalation (50 mcg) twice daily (~12 hours apart); maximum: 1 inhalation twice daily

Pediatrics: Asthma (maintenance/prevention) and exercise-induced asthma (prevention): Inhalation, powder (Serevent® Diskus®): Children ≥4 years: Refer to adult dosing.

Administration
Inhalation: Not to be used for the relief of acute attacks. Not for use with a spacer device. Administer with Diskus® in a level, horizontal position. Do not wash mouthpiece; Diskus® should be kept dry.

Stability
Storage: Inhalation powder (Serevent® Diskus®): Store at controlled room temperature 20°C to 25°C (68°F to 77°F) in a dry place away from direct heat or sunlight. Stable for 6 weeks after removal from foil pouch.

Laboratory Monitoring FEV₁, peak flow, and/or other pulmonary function tests

Nursing Actions
Physical Assessment: Not for use to relieve acute asthmatic attacks. Assess effectiveness and interactions of other medications patient may be taking. Monitor effectiveness of therapy (relief of airway obstruction) and adverse reactions (eg, cardiac and CNS changes) at beginning of therapy and periodically with long-term use. Monitor for increased use of short-acting beta₂-agonist inhalers; may be marker of a deteriorating asthma condition. For inpatient care, monitor vital signs and lung sounds prior to and periodically during therapy. Assess knowledge/teach patient appropriate use, interventions to reduce side effects, and adverse symptoms to report.

Patient Education: Use exactly as directed (see Administration). Do not use more often than recommended (excessive use may result in tolerance, overdose may result in serious adverse effects) and do not discontinue without consulting prescriber. Do not use for acute attacks. Maintain adequate hydration (2-3 L/day of fluids) unless instructed to restrict fluid intake. You may experience nervousness, dizziness, or fatigue (use caution when driving or engaging in tasks requiring alertness until response to drug is known); or dry mouth, stomach upset (small frequent meals, frequent mouth care, chewing gum, or sucking hard candy may help). If you have diabetes, check blood sugar; blood glucose level may be increased. Report unresolved GI upset; dizziness or fatigue; vision changes; chest pain, rapid heartbeat, or palpitations; insomnia; nervousness or hyperactivity; muscle cramping, tremors, or pain; unusual cough; or skin rash. **Pregnancy/breast-feeding precautions:** Inform prescriber if you are or intend to become pregnant. Consult prescriber if breast-feeding.

Dietary Considerations Powder for oral inhalation contains lactose; very rare anaphylactic reactions have been reported in patients with severe milk protein allergy.

Geriatric Considerations Geriatric patients were included in four clinical studies of salmeterol; no apparent differences in efficacy and safety were noted in geriatric patients compared to younger adults. Because salmeterol is only to be used for prevention of bronchospasm, patients also need a short-acting beta-agonist to treat acute attacks. Elderly patients should be carefully counseled about which inhaler to use and the proper scheduling of doses; a spacer device may be utilized to maximize effectiveness.

Pregnancy Issues Animal studies have demonstrated (? dose-dependent) teratogenicity. There are no adequate and well-controlled studies in pregnant women. Beta-agonists may interfere with uterine contractility if administered during labor. Use only if clearly needed.

Salsalate (SAL sa late)

U.S. Brand Names Amigesic®
Synonyms Disalicylic Acid; Salicylsalicylic Acid
Pharmacologic Category Salicylate
Medication Safety Issues
Sound-alike/look-alike issues:
Salsalate may be confused with sucralfate, sulfasalazine

Pregnancy Risk Factor C/D (3rd trimester)
Lactation Enters breast milk/contraindicated
Use Treatment of minor pain or fever; arthritis
Mechanism of Action/Effect Inhibits prostaglandin synthesis, acts on the hypothalamus heat-regulating center to reduce fever, blocks prostaglandin synthetase action which prevents formation of the platelet-aggregating substance thromboxane A₂

Contraindications Hypersensitivity to salsalate or any component of the formulation; GI ulcer or bleeding; pregnancy (3rd trimester)

Warnings/Precautions Use with caution in patients with platelet and bleeding disorders, renal dysfunction, erosive gastritis, or peptic ulcer disease, dehydration, previous nonreaction does not guarantee future safe taking of medication.

Drug Interactions
Decreased Effect: Decreased effect with urinary alkalinizers, antacids, and corticosteroids. Decreased effect of uricosurics and spironolactone.

Increased Effect/Toxicity: Increased effect/toxicity of oral anticoagulants, hypoglycemics, and methotrexate.
(Continued)

Salsalate *(Continued)*

Nutritional/Ethanol Interactions

Ethanol: Avoid ethanol (may enhance gastric mucosal irritation).

Food: Salsalate peak serum levels may be delayed if taken with food.

Herb/Nutraceutical: Avoid cat's claw, dong quai, evening primrose, feverfew, garlic, ginger, ginkgo, red clover, horse chestnut, green tea, ginseng (all have additional antiplatelet activity).

Lab Interactions
False-negative results for glucose oxidase urinary glucose tests (Clinistix®); false-positives using the cupric sulfate method (Clinitest®); also, interferes with Gerhardt test, VMA determination; 5-HIAA, xylose tolerance test and T_3 and T_4

Adverse Reactions

>10%: Gastrointestinal: Nausea, heartburn, stomach pain, dyspepsia

1% to 10%:
Central nervous system: Fatigue
Dermatologic: Rash
Gastrointestinal: Gastrointestinal ulceration
Hematologic: Hemolytic anemia
Neuromuscular & skeletal: Weakness
Respiratory: Dyspnea
Miscellaneous: Anaphylactic shock

Overdosage/Toxicology
Symptoms of overdose include respiratory alkalosis, hyperpnea, tachypnea, tinnitus, headache, hyperpyrexia, metabolic acidosis, hypoglycemia, and coma. Nomograms, such as the "Done" nomogram, can be very helpful for estimating the severity of aspirin poisoning and for directing treatment using serum salicylate levels. Treatment can also be based upon symptomatology.

Pharmacodynamics/Kinetics

Onset of Action: Therapeutic: 3-4 days of continuous dosing

Half-Life Elimination: 7-8 hours

Metabolism: Hepatically hydrolyzed to two moles of salicylic acid (active)

Excretion: Primarily urine

Available Dosage Forms

Tablet: 500 mg, 750 mg
Amigesic®: 500 mg, 750 mg

Dosing

Adults & Elderly: Pain, inflammation (arthritis): Oral: 3 g/day in 2-3 divided doses

Renal Impairment: Patients with end-stage renal disease undergoing hemodialysis: Administer 750 mg twice daily with an additional 500 mg after dialysis.

Nursing Actions

Physical Assessment: Assess effectiveness and interactions of other medications patient may be taking. Monitor blood pressure at the beginning of therapy and periodically during use. Monitor laboratory tests and therapeutic response (eg, relief of pain and inflammation, increased activity tolerance), and adverse reactions (eg, GI effects, unusual bleeding, hepatotoxicity) at beginning of therapy and periodically throughout therapy. Schedule ophthalmic evaluations for patients who are on long-term NSAID therapy. Assess knowledge/teach patient appropriate use, interventions to reduce side effects, and adverse symptoms to report.

Patient Education: Take this medication exactly as directed; do not increase dose without consulting prescriber. Do not crush tablets. Take with food or milk to reduce GI distress. Maintain adequate hydration (2-3 L/day of fluids) unless instructed to restrict fluid intake. Do not use alcohol, aspirin or aspirin-containing medication, or any other anti-inflammatory medications without consulting prescriber. You may experience drowsiness (use caution when driving or engaging in tasks requiring alertness until response to drug is known); or nausea

or heartburn (small frequent meals, frequent mouth care, sucking lozenges, or chewing gum may help). GI bleeding, ulceration, or perforation can occur with or without pain; discontinue medication and contact prescriber if persistent abdominal pain or cramping, or blood in stool occurs. Report breathlessness or respiratory difficulty; chest pain; unusual bruising or bleeding; blood in urine, stool, mouth, or vomitus; unusual fatigue; skin rash or itching; change in urinary pattern; or change in hearing or ringing in ears. **Pregnancy/breast-feeding precautions:** Inform prescriber if you are or intend to become pregnant. This drug should not be used in the 3rd trimester of pregnancy. Do not breast-feed.

Dietary Considerations May be taken with food to decrease GI distress.

Geriatric Considerations Elderly are at high risk for adverse effects from NSAIDs. As much as 60% of elderly can develop peptic ulceration and/or hemorrhage asymptomatically. The concomitant use of H_2 blockers, omeprazole, and sucralfate is not effective as prophylaxis with the exception of NSAID-induced duodenal ulcers which may be prevented by the use of ranitidine. Misoprostol is the only prophylactic agent proven effective. Also, concomitant disease and drug use contribute to the risk for GI adverse effects. Use lowest effective dose for shortest period possible. Consider renal function decline with age. Use of NSAIDs can compromise existing renal function especially when Cl_{cr} is ≤30 mL/minute. Tinnitus may be a difficult and unreliable indication of toxicity due to age-related hearing loss or eighth cranial nerve damage. CNS adverse effects such as confusion, agitation, and hallucinations are generally seen in overdose or high-dose situations, but elderly may demonstrate these adverse effects at lower doses than younger adults.

Breast-Feeding Issues Salsalate is metabolized to salicylate which is contraindicated while breast-feeding.

Additional Information Does not appear to inhibit platelet aggregation

---

Saquinavir *(sa KWIN a veer)*

U.S. Brand Names Fortovase® [DSC]; Invirase®

Synonyms Saquinavir Mesylate

Pharmacologic Category Antiretroviral Agent, Protease Inhibitor

Medication Safety Issues

Sound-alike/look-alike issues:
Saquinavir may be confused with Sinequan®
Fortovase® may be confused with Invirase®
Invirase® may be confused with Fortovase®

Pregnancy Risk Factor B

Lactation Excretion in breast milk unknown/contraindicated

Use Treatment of HIV infection; used in combination with at least two other antiretroviral agents

Mechanism of Action/Effect As an inhibitor of HIV protease, saquinavir prevents the cleavage of viral polyprotein precursors which are needed to generate functional proteins in and maturation of HIV-infected cells

Contraindications Hypersensitivity to saquinavir or any component of the formulation; exposure to direct sunlight without sunscreen or protective clothing; severe hepatic impairment; coadministration with amiodarone, bepridil, cisapride, flecainide, midazolam, pimozide, propafenone, quinidine, rifampin, triazolam, or ergot derivatives

Warnings/Precautions Use caution in patients with hepatic insufficiency. May exacerbate pre-existing hepatic dysfunction; use with caution in patients with hepatitis B or C and in cirrhosis. May be associated with fat redistribution (buffalo hump, increased abdominal girth, breast engorgement, facial atrophy). Use caution in hemophilia. May increase cholesterol and/or triglycerides; hypertriglyceridemia may increase risk of pancreatitis.

Saquinavir interacts with multiple medications (including herbal products) when given concurrently; refer to Drug Interactions. Fortovase® and Invirase® are not bioequivalent and should not be used interchangeably; only Fortovase® should be used to initiate therapy. Fortovase® is recommended when saquinavir will be given as the sole protease inhibitor; Invirase® may be used only if combined with ritonavir. Safety and efficacy have not been established in children <16 years of age.

Drug Interactions

Cytochrome P450 Effect: Substrate of CYP2D6 (minor), 3A4 (major); **Inhibits** CYP2C8/9 (weak), 2C19 (weak), 2D6 (weak), 3A4 (moderate)

Decreased Effect: The levels/effects of saquinavir may be reduced by aminoglutethimide, carbamazepine, nafcillin, nevirapine, phenobarbital, phenytoin, rifamycins, and other CYP3A4 inducers. Loss of efficacy and potential resistance may occur. Concurrent use with rifampin is contraindicated.

Serum concentrations of methadone may be decreased; an increased dose may be needed when administered with saquinavir. Serum levels of the hormones in oral contraceptives may decrease significantly with administration of saquinavir. Patients should use alternative methods of contraceptives during saquinavir therapy.

Serum levels of saquinavir and efavirenz may be decreased with concurrent use; saquinavir should not be used as the sole protease inhibitor with efavirenz or nevirapine.

Dexamethasone may decrease serum concentrations of saquinavir; use with caution. Serum concentrations of saquinavir are decreased and levels of rifabutin are increased when used together. Saquinavir should not be used as the sole protease inhibitor when given with rifabutin.

Increased Effect/Toxicity: Concurrent use of amiodarone, bepridil, cisapride, flecainide, midazolam, pimozide, propafenone, quinidine, rifampin, triazolam, or ergot derivatives is contraindicated.

Saquinavir may increase the levels/effects of selected benzodiazepines, calcium channel blockers, cisapride, cyclosporine, ergot alkaloids, selected HMG-CoA reductase inhibitors, mirtazapine, nateglinide, nefazodone, pimozide, quinidine, sildenafil (and other PDE-5 inhibitors), tacrolimus, venlafaxine, and other CYP3A4 substrates. The effects of warfarin may also be increased.

Serum concentrations of saquinavir may be increased by azole antifungals (itraconazole, ketoconazole); dose adjustment was not needed at the study dose when used for a limited time (ketoconazole 400 mg once daily and Fortovase® 1200 mg 3 times/day). Saquinavir serum concentrations may be increased by delavirdine. Atazanavir, indinavir, and ritonavir may increase serum levels of saquinavir. Serum levels of saquinavir and nelfinavir may be increased with concurrent use. Lopinavir/ritonavir (combination product) may increase serum levels of saquinavir. Refer to Dosage (dosage adjustment recommendations with atazanavir have not been established).

Serum concentrations of saquinavir and clarithromycin may both be increased. Dose adjustment was not needed at the study dose when used for 7 days (clarithromycin 500 mg twice daily and Fortovase® 1200 mg 3 times/day); dosage adjustment of clarithromycin is recommended in patients with renal impairment.

Serum concentrations of saquinavir are decreased and levels of rifabutin are increased when used together. Saquinavir should not be used as the sole protease inhibitor when given with rifabutin.

Nutritional/Ethanol Interactions

Food: A high-fat meal maximizes bioavailability. Saquinavir levels may increase if taken with grapefruit juice.

Herb/Nutraceutical: Saquinavir serum concentrations may be decreased by St John's wort; avoid concurrent use. Garlic capsules may decrease saquinavir serum concentrations; avoid use if saquinavir is the only protease inhibitor.

Adverse Reactions Protease inhibitors cause dyslipidemia which includes elevated cholesterol and triglycerides and a redistribution of body fat centrally to cause increased abdominal girth, buffalo hump, facial atrophy, and breast enlargement. These agents also cause hyperglycemia.

10%: Gastrointestinal: Diarrhea, nausea

1% to 10%:

Cardiovascular: Chest pain

Central nervous system: Anxiety, depression, fatigue, headache, insomnia, pain

Dermatologic: Rash, verruca

Endocrine & metabolic: Hyperglycemia, hypoglycemia, hyperkalemia, libido disorder, serum amylase increased

Gastrointestinal: Abdominal discomfort, abdominal pain, appetite decreased, buccal mucosa ulceration, constipation, dyspepsia, flatulence, taste alteration, vomiting

Hepatic: AST increased, ALT increased, bilirubin increased

Neuromuscular & skeletal: Paresthesia, weakness, CPK increased

Renal: Creatinine kinase increased

Pharmacodynamics/Kinetics

Protein Binding: Plasma: ~98%

Metabolism: Extensively hepatic via CYP3A4; extensive first-pass effect

Excretion: Feces (81% to 88%), urine (1% to 3%) within 5 days

Available Dosage Forms Note: Strength expressed as base; [DSC] = Discontinued product

Capsule, as mesylate:

Invirase®: 200 mg [contains lactose 63.3 mg/capsule]

Capsule, soft gelatin, as base:

Fortovase®: 200 mg [DSC]

Tablet, as mesylate:

Invirase®: 500 mg

Dosing

Adults: HIV infection:

Note: Fortovase® and Invirase® are not bioequivalent and should not be used interchangeably; only Fortovase® should be used to initiate therapy:

Unboosted regimen: Fortovase®: 1200 mg (six 200 mg capsules) 3 times/day or 1600 mg twice daily within 2 hours after a meal in combination with a nucleoside analog

Note: Saquinavir hard-gel capsules (Invirase®) should not be used in "unboosted regimens."

Ritonavir-boosted regimens:

Fortovase®: 1000 mg (five 200 mg capsules) twice daily in combination with ritonavir 100 mg twice daily

Invirase®: 1000 mg (five 200 mg capsules or two 500 mg tablets) twice daily given in combination with ritonavir 100 mg twice daily. This combination should be given together and within 2 hours after a full meal in combination with a nucleoside analog.

Dosage adjustments of Fortovase® when administered in combination therapy:

Delavirdine: Fortovase® 800 mg 3 times/day

(Continued)

Saquinavir (Continued)

Lopinavir and ritonavir (Kaletra™): Fortovase® or Invirase® 1000 mg twice daily

Nelfinavir: Fortovase®: 1200 mg twice daily

Elderly: Clinical studies did not include sufficient numbers of patients ≥65 years of age. Use caution due to increased frequency of organ dysfunction.

Pediatrics:

HIV infection: Oral: Children ≥16 years: Refer to adult dosing.

Administration

Oral: Take saquinavir within 2 hours after a full meal. Avoid direct sunlight when taking saquinavir. When used with ritonavir, saquinavir and ritonavir should be administered at the same time.

Stability

Storage:

Fortovase®: Store in refrigerator. Stable for 3 months when stored at room temperature.

Invirase®: Store at room temperature.

Laboratory Monitoring CBC, renal and liver function, electrolytes, triglycerides, cholesterol, glucose, CD4 cell count, plasma levels of HIV RNA

Nursing Actions

Physical Assessment: Assess potential for interactions with other pharmacological agents and herbal products patient may be taking. A list of medications that should not be used is available in each bottle and patients should be provided with this information. Monitor laboratory tests, patient response, and adverse reactions (gastrointestinal disturbance, nausea, vomiting, diarrhea that can lead to dehydration and weight loss; hyperlipidemia and redistribution of body fat; rash; CNS effects, malaise, insomnia, abnormal thinking, electrolyte imbalance) at regular intervals during therapy. Teach patient proper use (eg, timing of multiple medications and drugs that should not be used concurrently), possible side effects/appropriate interventions (eg, glucose testing; protease inhibitors may cause hyperglycemia, exacerbation or new-onset diabetes; use of barrier contraceptives; protease inhibitors may decrease effectiveness of oral contraceptives), and adverse symptoms to report.

Patient Education: You will be provided with a list of specific medications that should not be used during therapy; do not take any new prescriptions, over-the-counter medications, or herbal products (even if they are not on the list) without consulting prescriber. This is not a cure for HIV, nor has it been found to reduce transmission of HIV; use appropriate precautions to prevent spread to other persons. Take exactly as directed. Maintain adequate hydration (2-3 L/day of fluids) unless instructed to restrict fluid intake. If you miss a dose, take as soon as possible and return to your regular schedule (never take a double dose). Frequent blood tests may be required with prolonged therapy. You may be advised to check your glucose levels (this drug can cause exacerbation or new-onset diabetes). May cause body changes due to redistribution of body fat, facial atrophy, or breast enlargement (normal effects of drug). May cause dizziness, insomnia, abnormal thinking (use caution when driving or engaging in potentially hazardous tasks until response to drug is known); nausea, vomiting, or taste perversion (small frequent meals, frequent mouth care, chewing gum, or sucking lozenges may help); muscle weakness (consult prescriber for approved analgesic); or headache or insomnia (consult prescriber for medication). Inform prescriber if you experience muscle numbness or tingling; unresolved persistent vomiting, diarrhea, or abdominal pain; respiratory difficulty or chest pain; unusual skin rash; change in color of stool or urine; or any persistent adverse effects. **Pregnancy/breast-feeding precautions:** Inform prescriber if you are or intend to become pregnant. Effectiveness of oral contraceptives may be decreased, use of alternative (nonhormonal) forms of contraception is recommended; consult prescriber for appropriate contraceptives. Do not breast-feed.

Dietary Considerations Administer within 2 hours of a meal. Invirase® capsules contain lactose 63.3 mg/capsule (not expected to induce symptoms of intolerance).

Breast-Feeding Issues HIV-infected mothers are discouraged from breast-feeding to decrease postnatal transmission of HIV.

Pregnancy Issues Saquinavir soft gelatin capsules (Fortovase®) provide adequate levels when used in normal doses during pregnancy; pharmacokinetic data not available for Invirase®. The Perinatal HIV Guidelines Working Group considers Fortovase® and ritonavir to be a preferred combination for use during pregnancy. Pregnancy and protease inhibitors are both associated with an increased risk of hyperglycemia. Glucose levels should be closely monitored. Health professionals are encouraged to contact the antiretroviral pregnancy registry to monitor outcomes of pregnant women exposed to antiretroviral medications (1-800-258-4263 or www.APRegistry.com).

Additional Information The indication for saquinavir for the treatment of HIV infection is based on changes in surrogate markers. At present, there are no results from controlled clinical trials evaluating the effect of regimens containing saquinavir on patient survival or the clinical progression of HIV infection, such as the occurrence of opportunistic infections or malignancies; in cell culture, saquinavir is additive to synergistic with AZT, ddC, and DDI without enhanced toxicity. According to the manufacturer, Invirase® will be phased out over time and completely replaced by Fortovase®. Potential compliance problems, frequency of administration and adverse effects should be discussed with patients before initiating therapy to help prevent the emergence of resistance.

Sargramostim (sar GRAM oh stim)

U.S. Brand Names Leukine®

Synonyms GM-CSF; Granulocyte-Macrophage Colony Stimulating Factor; rGM-CSF

Pharmacologic Category Colony Stimulating Factor

Medication Safety Issues

Sound-alike/look-alike issues:

Leukine® may be confused with Leukeran®

Pregnancy Risk Factor C

Lactation Excretion in breast milk unknown

Use

Myeloid reconstitution after autologous bone marrow transplantation: Non-Hodgkin's lymphoma (NHL), acute lymphoblastic leukemia (ALL), Hodgkin's lymphoma, metastatic breast cancer

Myeloid reconstitution after allogeneic bone marrow transplantation

Peripheral stem cell transplantation: Metastatic breast cancer, non-Hodgkin's lymphoma, Hodgkin's lymphoma, multiple myeloma

Orphan drug:

Acute myelogenous leukemia (AML) following induction chemotherapy in older adults to shorten time to neutrophil recovery and to reduce the incidence of severe and life-threatening infections and infections resulting in death

Bone marrow transplant (allogeneic or autologous) failure or engraftment delay

Safety and efficacy of GM-CSF given simultaneously with cytotoxic chemotherapy have not been established. Concurrent treatment may increase myelosuppression.

Mechanism of Action/Effect Stimulates proliferation, differentiation and functional activity of neutrophils, eosinophils, monocytes, and macrophages; see table.

Comparative Effects — G-CSF vs GM-CSF

Proliferation/ Differentiation	G-CSF (Filgrastim)	GM-CSF (Sargramostim)
Neutrophils	Yes	Yes
Eosinophils	No	Yes
Macrophages	No	Yes
Neutrophil migration	Enhanced	Inhibited

Contraindications Hypersensitivity to sargramostim, yeast-derived products, or any component of the formulation; concurrent myelosuppressive chemotherapy or radiation therapy. The solution for injection contains benzyl alcohol and should not be used in neonates.

Warnings/Precautions Simultaneous administration, or administration 24 hours preceding/following cytotoxic chemotherapy or radiotherapy is not recommended. Use with caution in patients with pre-existing cardiac problems, hypoxia, fluid retention, pulmonary infiltrates or CHF, renal or hepatic impairment. rapid increase in peripheral blood counts. If ANC is >20,000/mm³, or platelets >500,000/mm³ decrease dose by 50% or discontinue drug (counts will fall to normal within 3-7 days after discontinuing drug). The manufacturer recommends that precaution be exercised in the usage of sargramostim in any malignancy with myeloid characteristics. Sargramostim can potentially act as a growth factor for any tumor type, particularly myeloid malignancies. Tumors of nonhematopoietic origin may have surface receptors for sargramostim.

Drug Interactions
Increased Effect/Toxicity: Lithium, corticosteroids may potentiate myeloproliferative effects.

Adverse Reactions
>10%:
Cardiovascular: Hypotension, tachycardia, flushing, and syncope may occur with the first dose of a cycle ("first-dose effect"); peripheral edema (11%)
Central nervous system: Headache (26%)
Dermatologic: Rash, alopecia
Endocrine & metabolic: Polydypsia
Gastrointestinal: Diarrhea (52% to 89%), stomatitis, mucositis
Local: Local reactions at the injection site (~50%)
Neuromuscular & skeletal: Myalgia (18%), arthralgia (21%), bone pain
Renal: Increased serum creatinine (14%)
Respiratory: Dyspnea (28%)
1% to 10%:
Cardiovascular: Transient supraventricular arrhythmia; chest pain; capillary leak syndrome; pericardial effusion (4%)
Central nervous system: Headache
Gastrointestinal: Nausea, vomiting
Hematologic: Leukocytosis, thrombocytopenia
Neuromuscular & skeletal: Weakness
Respiratory: Cough; pleural effusion (1%)

Overdosage/Toxicology Symptoms of overdose include dyspnea, malaise, nausea, fever, headache, and chills. Discontinue drug and wait for levels to fall. Treatment is supportive. Monitor CBC, respiratory symptoms, and fluid status. Discontinue drug and wait for levels to fall, monitor for pulmonary edema. Toxicity of GM-CSF is dose dependent. Severe reactions such as capillary leak syndrome are seen at higher doses (>15 mcg/kg/day).

Pharmacodynamics/Kinetics
Onset of Action: Increase in WBC: 7-14 days
Duration of Action: WBCs return to baseline within 1 week of discontinuing drug

Time to Peak: Serum: SubQ: 1-2 hours
Half-Life Elimination: 2 hours
Available Dosage Forms
Injection, powder for reconstitution:
Leukine®: 250 mcg [contains sucrose 10 mg/mL]
Injection, solution:
Leukine®: 500 mcg/mL (1 mL) [contains benzyl alcohol, disodium edetate and sucrose 10 mg/mL]
Dosing
Adults & Elderly:
I.V. infusion over ≥2 hours or SubQ: **Rounding the dose to the nearest vial size enhances patient convenience and reduces costs without clinical detriment.**

Myeloid reconstitution after peripheral stem cell, allogeneic or autologous bone marrow transplant: I.V.: 250 mcg/m²/day for 21 days to begin 2-4 hours after the marrow infusion or ≥24 hours after chemotherapy or 12 hours after last dose of radiotherapy.
If a severe adverse reaction occurs, reduce or temporarily discontinue the dose until the reaction abates.
If blast cells appear or progression of the underlying disease occurs, disrupt treatment.
Interrupt or reduce the dose by half if ANC is >20,000 cells/mm³
Patients should not receive sargramostim until the postmarrow infusion ANC is <500 cells/mm³.

Neutrophil recovery following chemotherapy in AML: I.V.: 250 mcg/m²/day over a 4-hour period starting approximately day 11 or 4 days following the completion of induction chemotherapy, if day 10 bone marrow is hypoblastic with <5% blasts.
If a second cycle of chemotherapy is necessary, administer ~4 days after the completion of chemotherapy if the bone marrow is hypoblastic with <5% blasts.
Continue sargramostim until ANC is >1500 cells/mm³ for consecutive days or a maximum of 42 days.
Discontinue sargramostim immediately if leukemic regrowth occurs.
If a severe adverse reaction occurs, reduce the dose by 50% or temporarily discontinue the dose until the reaction abates.

Mobilization of peripheral blood progenitor cells: I.V.: 250 mcg/m²/day over 24 hours or SubQ once daily.
Continue the same dose through the period of PBPC collection.
The optimal schedule for PBPC collection has not been established (usually begun by day 5 and performed daily until protocol specified targets are achieved).
If WBC >50,000 cells/mm³, reduce the dose by 50%.
If adequate numbers of progenitor cells are not collected, consider other mobilization therapy.

Postperipheral blood progenitor cell transplantation: I.V.: 250 mcg/m²/day or SubQ once daily beginning immediately following infusion of progenitor cells and continuing until ANC is >1500 for 3 consecutive days is attained.

BMT failure or engraftment delay: I.V.: 250 mcg/m²/day for 14 days
The dose can be repeated after 7 days off therapy if engraftment has not occurred.
If engraftment still has not occurred, a third course of 500 mcg/m²/day for 14 days may be tried after another 7 days off therapy; if there is still no improvement, it is unlikely that further dose escalation will be beneficial.
If a severe adverse reaction occurs, reduce or temporarily discontinue the dose until the reaction abates.

(Continued)

Sargramostim *(Continued)*

If blast cells appear or disease progression occurs, discontinue treatment.

Pediatrics: Refer to adult dosing.

Administration

I.V.: Can premedicate with analgesics and antipyretics; control bone pain with non-narcotic analgesics. I.V. infusion should be over at least 2 hours; incompatible with dextrose-containing solutions. An in-line membrane filter should not be used for intravenous injection.

I.V. Detail: pH: 7.1-7.7

Other: Administer by SubQ (undiluted). Do not shake solution. When administering GM-CSF subcutaneously, rotate injection sites.

Stability

Reconstitution:

Powder for injection: May be reconstituted with preservative free SWFI or bacteriostatic water for injection (with benzyl alcohol 0.9%). Gently swirl to reconstitute; do not shake.

Sargramostim may also be further diluted in 0.9% sodium chloride to a concentration of ≥10 mcg/mL for I.V. infusion administration.

If the final concentration of sargramostim is <10 mcg/mL, 1 mg of human albumin/1 mL of 0.9% sodium chloride (eg, 1 mL of 5% human albumin/50 mL of 0.9% sodium chloride) should be added.

Standard diluent: 25-100 mL NS

Compatibility: Stable in NS, SWFI, bacteriostatic water; **incompatible** with dextrose-containing solutions

Y-site administration: Incompatible with acyclovir, ampicillin, ampicillin/sulbactam, cefoperazone, chlorpromazine, ganciclovir, haloperidol, hydrocortisone sodium phosphate, hydrocortisone sodium succinate, hydromorphone, hydroxyzine, imipenem/cilastatin, lorazepam, methylprednisolone sodium succinate, mitomycin, morphine, nalbuphine, ondansetron, piperacillin, sodium bicarbonate, tobramycin

Storage: Sargramostim should be stored at 2°C to 8°C (36°F to 46°F). Vials should not be frozen or shaken.

Solution for injection: May be stored for up to 20 days at 2°C to 8°C (36°F to 46°F) once the vial has been entered. Discard remaining solution after 20 days.

Powder for injection: Preparations made with SWFI should be administered as soon as possible, and discarded within 6 hours of reconstitution. Preparations made with bacteriostatic water may be stored for up to 20 days at 2°C to 8°C (36°F to 46°F).

I.V. infusion administration: Preparations diluted with NS are stable for 48 hours at room temperature and refrigeration.

Standard diluent: 25-100 mL NS

Laboratory Monitoring To avoid potential complications of excessive leukocytosis (WBC >50,000 cells/mm³, ANC >20,000 cells/mm³) a CBC with differential is recommended twice per week during therapy. Sargramostim therapy should be interrupted or the dose reduced by half if the ANC is >20,000 cells/mm³. Monitoring of renal and hepatic function in patients displaying renal or hepatic dysfunction prior to initiation of treatment is recommended and at least biweekly during sargramostim administration.

Nursing Actions

Physical Assessment: Monitor laboratory tests, patient response and adverse reactions frequently during therapy (eg, fluid balance [I & O], rash, hypotension, tachycardia, GI disturbance [diarrhea, stomatitis, mucositis], myalgia, bone pain). Teach patient use if self-administered SubQ (eg, appropriate injection technique and syringe/needle disposal), possible

side effects/appropriate interventions, and adverse symptoms to report.

Patient Education: Do not take any new medication during therapy without consulting prescriber. If administered by infusion report any redness, swelling, pain, or burning at infusion site. SubQ (self injection): Follow exact direction for injection and disposal of syringe/needle; report redness, pain, or signs of infections at injection site. You will require frequent blood tests during treatment. May cause bone, joint, or muscle pain (request analgesic); nausea and vomiting (small, frequent meals may help); or hair loss (reversible); diarrhea (buttermilk, boiled milk, or yogurt may help). Report chest pain or palpitations, signs or symptoms of edema (eg, swollen extremities, difficulty breathing, rapid weight gain); onset of severe headache; acute back or chest pain; muscular tremors or seizure activity; or other persistent adverse effects. **Pregnancy/breast-feeding precautions:** Inform prescriber if you are or intend to become pregnant. Consult prescriber if breast-feeding.

Additional Information Reimbursement Hotline (Leukine®): 1-800-321-4669

Scopolamine Derivatives

(skoe POL a meen dah RIV ah tives)

U.S. Brand Names Isopto® Hyoscine; Scopace™; Transderm Scōp®

Synonyms Hyoscine Butylbromide; Hyoscine Hydrobromide; Scopolamine Butylbromide; Scopolamine Hydrobromide

Pharmacologic Category Anticholinergic Agent

Medication Safety Issues

Transdermal patch may contain conducting metal (eg, aluminum); remove patch prior to MRI.

Pregnancy Risk Factor C

Lactation Enters breast milk/use caution (AAP rates "compatible")

Use

Scopolamine hydrobromide:

Injection: Preoperative medication to produce amnesia, sedation, and decrease salivary and respiratory secretions

Ophthalmic: Produce cycloplegia and mydriasis; treatment of iridocyclitis

Oral: Symptomatic treatment of postencephalitic parkinsonism and paralysis agitans; inhibits excessive motility and hypertonus of the genitourinary or gastrointestinal tract in such conditions as the irritable colon syndrome, mild dysentery, diverticulitis, pylorospasm, and cardiospasm

Transdermal: Prevention of nausea/vomiting associated with anesthesia or opiate analgesia; prevention of motion sickness

Scopolamine butylbromide:

Oral/Injection: Treatment of smooth muscle spasm of the genitourinary or gastrointestinal tract; injection may also be used to prior to radiological/diagnostic procedures to prevent spasm

Mechanism of Action/Effect Blocks the action of acetylcholine at parasympathetic sites in smooth muscle, secretory glands and the CNS; increases cardiac output, dries secretions, antagonizes histamine and serotonin

Contraindications Hypersensitivity to scopolamine or any component of the formulation; narrow-angle glaucoma; acute hemorrhage; paralytic ileus, GI or GU obstruction; thyrotoxicosis; tachycardia secondary to cardiac insufficiency; myasthenia gravis

Warnings/Precautions Use with caution with hepatic or renal impairment since adverse CNS effects occur more often in these patients; use with caution in infants and children since they may be more susceptible to adverse effects of scopolamine; use with caution in patients with GI obstruction, prostatic hyperplasia (nonobstructive), or urinary retention. Discontinue if patient reports unusual visual disturbances or pain within the eye. Use caution in hiatal hernia, reflux esophagitis, and ulcerative colitis. Scopolamine (hyoscine) hydrobromide should not be interchanged with scopolamine butylbromide formulations; dosages are not equivalent. Transdermal patch may contain conducting metal (eg, aluminum); remove patch prior to MRI.

Drug Interactions

Decreased Effect: Decreased effect of acetaminophen, levodopa, ketoconazole, digoxin, riboflavin, and potassium chloride in wax matrix preparations.

Increased Effect/Toxicity: Adverse anticholinergic effects may be additive with other anticholinergic agents (includes tricyclic antidepressants, antihistamines, and phenothiazines). Sedative effects of other CNS depressants may be additive with scopolamine.

Nutritional/Ethanol Interactions Ethanol: Avoid ethanol (may increase CNS depression).

Adverse Reactions Frequency not defined.

Ophthalmic: Note: Systemic adverse effects have been reported following ophthalmic administration.
Cardiovascular: Vascular congestion, edema
Central nervous system: Drowsiness
Dermatologic: Eczematoid dermatitis
Ocular: Blurred vision, photophobia, local irritation, increased intraocular pressure, follicular conjunctivitis, exudate
Respiratory: Congestion

Systemic:
Cardiovascular: Orthostatic hypotension, ventricular fibrillation, tachycardia, palpitation
Central nervous system: Confusion, drowsiness, headache, loss of memory, ataxia, fatigue
Dermatologic: Dry skin, increased sensitivity to light, rash
Endocrine & metabolic: Decreased flow of breast milk
Gastrointestinal: Constipation, xerostomia, dry throat, dysphagia, bloated feeling, nausea, vomiting
Genitourinary: Dysuria
Local: Irritation at injection site
Neuromuscular & skeletal: Weakness
Ocular: Increased intraocular pain, blurred vision
Respiratory: Dry nose
Miscellaneous: Diaphoresis (decreased)

Overdosage/Toxicology Symptoms of overdose include dilated pupils, flushed skin, tachycardia, hypertension, and ECG abnormalities. CNS manifestations resemble acute psychosis. CNS depression, circulatory collapse, respiratory failure, and death can occur. For a scopolamine overdose with severe life-threatening symptoms, physostigmine 1-2 mg SubQ or I.V. slowly should be given to reverse toxic effects.

Pharmacodynamics/Kinetics

Onset of Action: Oral, I.M.: 0.5-1 hour; I.V.: 10 minutes
Peak effect: 20-60 minutes; may take 3-7 days for full recovery; transdermal: 24 hours

Duration of Action: Oral, I.M.: 4-6 hours; I.V.: 2 hours

Half-Life Elimination: 4.8 hours

Metabolism: Hepatic

Excretion: Urine (as metabolites)

Available Dosage Forms [CAN] = Canadian brand name
Injection, solution, as hydrobromide: 0.4 mg/mL (1 mL)
Injection, solution, as hyoscine-N-butylbromide (Buscopan® [CAN]): 20 mg/mL [not available in U.S.]
Solution, ophthalmic, as hydrobromide (Isopto® Hyoscine): 0.25% (5 mL, 15 mL) [contains benzalkonium chloride]
Tablet, as hyoscine-N-butylbromide (Buscopan® [CAN]): 10 mg [not available in U.S.]
Tablet, soluble, as hydrobromide (Scopace™): 0.4 mg

Transdermal system (Transderm Scōp®): 1.5 mg (4s, 10s, 24s) [releases ~1 mg over 72 hours]

Dosing

Adults & Elderly: Note: Scopolamine (hyoscine) hydrobromide should not be interchanged with scopolamine butylbromide formulations. Dosages are not equivalent.

Scopolamine hydrobromide:
Preoperative:
I.M., I.V., SubQ: 0.3-0.65 mg; may be repeated every 4-6 hours
Transdermal patch: Apply 2.5 cm^2 patch to hairless area behind ear the night before surgery or 1 hour prior to cesarean section (the patch should be applied no sooner than 1 hour before surgery for best results and removed 24 hours after surgery)
Motion sickness: Transdermal: Apply 1 disc behind the ear at least 4 hours prior to exposure and every 3 days as needed; effective if applied as soon as 2-3 hours before anticipated need, best if 12 hours before
Refraction: Ophthalmic: Instill 1-2 drops of 0.25% to eye(s) 1 hour before procedure
Iridocyclitis: Ophthalmic: Instill 1-2 drops of 0.25% to eye(s) up to 4 times/day
Parkinsonism, spasticity, motion sickness: Oral: 0.4-0.8 mg as a range; the dosage may be cautiously increased in parkinsonism and spastic states.

Scopolamine butylbromide:
Gastrointestinal/genitourinary spasm (Buscopan® [CAN]; not available in the U.S.):
Oral: 10-20 mg daily (1-2 tablets); maximum: 6 tablets/day
I.M., I.V., SubQ: 10-20 mg; maximum: 100 mg/day. Intramuscular injections should be administered 10-15 minutes prior to radiological/diagnostic procedures

Pediatrics:
Scopolamine hydrobromide:
Preoperative: I.M., SubQ: 6 mcg/kg/dose (maximum: 0.3 mg/dose) every 6-8 hours
Refraction: Ophthalmic: Instill 1 drop of 0.25% to eye(s) twice daily for 2 days before procedure
Iridocyclitis: Ophthalmic: Instill 1 drop of 0.25% to eye(s) up to 3 times/day

Administration

I.V.:
Hydrobromide: Inject over 2-3 minutes
Butylbromide: Inject at a rate of 1 mL/minute

I.V. Detail:
Hydrobromide: Dilute with an equal volume of sterile water and administer by direct I.V.
pH: 3.5-6.5
Butylbromide: No dilution is necessary prior to injection
Topical: Topical disc is programmed to deliver *in vivo* 1 mg over 3 days. Once applied, do not remove the patch for 3 full days. Apply to hairless area of skin behind the ear. Wash hands before and after applying the disc to avoid drug contact with eyes.

Stability

Storage: Store tablets and/or injection at room temperature of 15°C to 30°C. Protect injection from light.
Hydrobromide injection: Avoid acid solutions, hydrolysis occurs at pH <3
Butylbromide injection: Stable in D_5W, NS, $D_{10}W$, and LR for up to 8 hours

Nursing Actions

Physical Assessment: Assess potential for interactions with other prescriptions, OTC medications, or herbal products patient may be taking (eg, ergot-containing drugs). When used preoperatively, safety precautions should be observed and patient should be advised about blurred vision. For all uses, (Continued)

Scopolamine Derivatives (Continued)

monitor therapeutic effectiveness and adverse reactions. Teach patient appropriate use (according to formulation and purpose), interventions to reduce side effects, and adverse symptoms to report. Systemic effects have been reported following ophthalmic administration.

Patient Education: Use as directed. May cause drowsiness, confusion, impaired judgment, or vision changes (use caution when driving or engaging in tasks requiring alertness until response to drug is known); dry mouth, nausea, or vomiting (small frequent meals, frequent mouth care, chewing gum, or sucking lozenges may help); orthostatic hypotension (use caution when climbing stairs and when rising from lying or sitting position); constipation (increased exercise, fluids, fruit, or fiber may help; if not effective consult prescriber); increased sensitivity to heat and decreased perspiration (avoid extremes of heat, reduce exercise in hot weather); or decreased milk if breast-feeding. Report hot, dry, flushed skin; blurred vision or vision changes; difficulty swallowing; chest pain, palpitations, or rapid heartbeat; painful or difficult urination; increased confusion, depression, or loss of memory; rapid or difficult respirations; muscle weakness or tremors; or eye pain. **Pregnancy precaution:** Inform prescriber if you are or intend to become pregnant.

Transdermal: Apply patch behind ear the day before traveling. Wash hands before and after applying, and avoid contact with the eyes. Do not remove for 3 days.

Ophthalmic: Instill as often as recommended. Wash hands before using. Do not let tip of applicator touch eye; do not contaminate tip of applicator (may cause eye infection, eye damage, or vision loss). Sit or lie down, open eye, look at ceiling, and instill prescribed amount of solution. Do not blink for 30 seconds, close eye and roll eye in all directions, and apply gentle pressure to inner corner of eye for 1-2 minutes. Temporary stinging or blurred vision may occur.

Geriatric Considerations Because of its long duration of action as a mydriatic agent, it should be avoided in elderly patients. Anticholinergic agents are not well tolerated in the elderly and their use should be avoided when possible.

Secobarbital (see koe BAR bi tal)

U.S. Brand Names Seconal®

Synonyms Quinalbarbitone Sodium; Secobarbital Sodium

Restrictions C-II

Pharmacologic Category Barbiturate

Medication Safety Issues
Sound-alike/look-alike issues:
Seconal® may be confused with Sectral®

Pregnancy Risk Factor D

Lactation Enters breast milk/use caution (AAP rates "compatible")

Use Preanesthetic agent; short-term treatment of insomnia

Mechanism of Action/Effect Interferes with transmission of impulses from the thalamus to the cortex of the brain resulting in an imbalance in central inhibitory and facilitatory mechanisms

Contraindications Hypersensitivity to barbiturates or any component of the formulation; marked hepatic impairment; dyspnea or airway obstruction; porphyria; pregnancy

Warnings/Precautions Should be used only after evaluation of potential causes of sleep disturbance. Failure of sleep disturbance to resolve after 7-10 days may indicate psychiatric or medical illness. Do not administer to patients in acute pain. Use caution in elderly patients, debilitated patients, hepatic impairment, renally impairment, or pediatric patients. May cause paradoxical responses, including agitation and hyperactivity, particularly in acute pain and pediatric patients. Use with caution in patients with depression or suicidal tendencies, or in patients with a history of drug abuse. Tolerance, psychological and physical dependence may occur with prolonged use. May cause CNS depression, which may impair physical or mental abilities. Effects with other sedative drugs or ethanol may be potentiated. May cause respiratory depression or hypotension, Use with caution in hemodynamically unstable patients or patients with respiratory disease.

Drug Interactions
Cytochrome P450 Effect: Induces CYP2A6 (strong), 2C8/9 (strong)

Decreased Effect: Barbiturates, such as secobarbital, are hepatic enzyme inducers, and may increase the metabolism of antipsychotics, some beta-blockers (unlikely with atenolol and nadolol), calcium channel blockers, chloramphenicol, cimetidine, corticosteroids, cyclosporine, disopyramide, doxycycline, ethosuximide, felbamate, furosemide, griseofulvin, lamotrigine, phenytoin, propafenone, quinidine, tacrolimus, TCAs, and theophylline. Barbiturates may increase the metabolism of estrogens and reduce the efficacy of oral contraceptives; an alternative method of contraception should be considered. Barbiturates inhibit the hypoprothrombinemic effects of oral anticoagulants via increased metabolism. Barbiturates may enhance the metabolism of methadone resulting in methadone withdrawal.

Increased Effect/Toxicity: Increased toxicity when combined with other CNS depressants, antidepressants, benzodiazepines, chloramphenicol, or valproic acid; respiratory and CNS depression may be additive. MAO inhibitors may prolong the effect of secobarbital. Barbiturates may enhance the hepatotoxic potential of acetaminophen (due to an increased formation of toxic metabolites). Chloramphenicol may inhibit the metabolism of barbiturates.

Nutritional/Ethanol Interactions
Ethanol: Avoid ethanol (may increase CNS depression).

Herb/Nutraceutical: Avoid valerian, St John's wort, kava kava, gotu kola (may increase CNS depression).

Adverse Reactions Frequency not defined.

Cardiovascular: Hypotension

Central nervous system: Dizziness, lightheadedness, "hangover" effect, drowsiness, CNS depression, fever, confusion, mental depression, unusual excitement, nervousness, faint feeling, headache, insomnia, nightmares, hallucinations

Dermatologic: Exfoliative dermatitis, rash, Stevens-Johnson syndrome

Gastrointestinal: Nausea, vomiting, constipation

Hematologic: Agranulocytosis, megaloblastic anemia, thrombocytopenia, thrombophlebitis, urticaria apnea

Local: Pain at injection site

Respiratory: Respiratory depression, laryngospasm

Overdosage/Toxicology Symptoms of overdose include unsteady gait, slurred speech, confusion, jaundice, hypothermia, fever, hypotension, respiratory depression, and coma. Charcoal hemoperfusion or hemodialysis may be useful, especially in the presence of very high serum barbiturate levels when the patient is in shock, coma, or renal failure. Forced alkaline diuresis is of no value in the treatment of intoxications with short-acting barbiturates.

Pharmacodynamics/Kinetics
Onset of Action: Onset of hypnosis: 15-30 minutes

Duration of Action: 3-4 hours with 100 mg dose

Time to Peak: Serum: Within 2-4 hours

Protein Binding: 45% to 60%

Half-Life Elimination: 15-40 hours, mean: 28 hours

Metabolism: Hepatic, by microsomal enzyme system

Excretion: Urine (as inactive metabolites, small amounts as unchanged drug)

Available Dosage Forms Capsule, as sodium: 100 mg

Dosing
Adults: Insomnia (hypnotic): Oral: 100 mg/dose at bedtime; range: 100-200 mg/dose

Elderly: Not recommended for use in the elderly (see Geriatric Considerations).

Pediatrics:

Preoperative sedation: Oral: Children: 2-6 mg/kg (maximum dose: 100 mg/dose) 1-2 hours before procedure

Sedation: Oral: Children: 6 mg/kg/day divided every 8 hours

Renal Impairment: Slightly dialyzable (5% to 20%)

Nursing Actions
Physical Assessment: Assess effectiveness and interactions of other medications patient may be taking. Patient should be assessed for history of addiction; long-term use can result in dependence, abuse, or tolerance. Evaluate periodically for need for continued use. Assess for CNS depression. Monitor vital signs and respiratory status. After long-term use, dosage should be tapered slowly. **Oral:** For inpatient use, institute safety measures (side rails, night light, call bell, assistance with ambulation). For outpatient use, monitor effectiveness and adverse reactions at beginning of therapy and periodically with long-term use. Assess knowledge/teach patient appropriate use, interventions to reduce side effects, and adverse symptoms to report.

Patient Education: Use exactly as directed; do not increase dose or frequency or discontinue without consulting prescriber. Drug may cause physical and/or psychological dependence. While using this medication, do not use alcohol or other prescription or OTC medications (especially, pain medications, sedatives, antihistamines, or hypnotics) without consulting prescriber. Maintain adequate hydration (2-3 L/day of fluids) unless instructed to restrict fluid intake. You may experience drowsiness, dizziness, or blurred vision (use caution when driving or engaging in tasks requiring alertness until response to drug is known); nausea or vomiting (small frequent meals, frequent mouth care, chewing gum, or sucking lozenges may help); or constipation (increased exercise, fluids, fruit, or fiber may help). Report skin rash or irritation; CNS changes (confusion, depression, increased sedation, excitation, headache, insomnia, or nightmares); respiratory difficulty or shortness of breath; difficulty swallowing or feeling of tightness in throat; unusual weakness or unusual bleeding in mouth, urine, or stool; or other unanticipated adverse effects. **Pregnancy/breast-feeding precautions:** Do not get pregnant while taking this medication. Use appropriate contraceptive measures. Consult prescriber if breast-feeding.

Geriatric Considerations Use of this agent in the elderly is not recommended due to its long half-life and addiction potential.

Related Information
Anxiolytic / Hypnotic Use in Long-Term Care Facilities *on page 1418*

Compatibility of Drugs in Syringe *on page 1372*

Federal OBRA Regulations Recommended Maximum Doses *on page 1421*

Selegiline (se LE ji leen)

U.S. Brand Names Eldepryl®; Emsam®

Synonyms Deprenyl; L-Deprenyl; Selegiline Hydrochloride

Pharmacologic Category Anti-Parkinson's Agent, MAO Type B Inhibitor; Antidepressant, Monoamine Oxidase Inhibitor

Medication Safety Issues
Sound-alike/look-alike issues:
Selegiline may be confused with Salagen®, Serentil®, sertraline, Serzone®, Stelazine®
Eldepryl® may be confused with Elavil®, enalapril

Pregnancy Risk Factor C

Lactation Excretion in breast milk unknown/use caution

Use Adjunct in the management of parkinsonian patients in which levodopa/carbidopa therapy is deteriorating; treatment of major depressive disorder

Unlabeled/Investigational Use Early Parkinson's disease; attention-deficit/hyperactivity disorder (ADHD); negative symptoms of schizophrenia; extrapyramidal symptoms; Alzheimer's disease (studies have shown some improvement in behavioral and cognitive performance)

Mechanism of Action/Effect At lower oral doses (≤10 mg/day), selegiline is a selective monoamine oxidase (MAO) type B inhibitor, which increases dopaminergic synaptic activity thus reducing symptoms of Parkinsonism. At higher oral doses or administered transdermally, selegiline nonselectively inhibits both MAO-B and MAO-A which blocks catabolism of other centrally-active biogenic amine neurotransmitters leading to improved mood

Contraindications Hypersensitivity to selegiline or any component of the formulation
Oral: Additional contraindication: Concomitant use of meperidine
Transdermal: Additional contraindications: Pheochromocytoma; concomitant use of meperidine, bupropion, selective or dual serotonin reuptake inhibitors (including SSRIs and SNRIs), tricyclic antidepressants, buspirone, tramadol, propoxyphene, methadone, dextromethorphan, St. John's Wort, mirtazapine, cyclobenzaprine, oral selegiline and other MAO inhibitors; sympathomimetic amines (eg, pseudoephedrine), carbamazepine, and oxcarbazepine; elective surgery requiring general anesthesia, local anesthesia containing sympathomimetic vasoconstrictors

Warnings/Precautions
Oral: MAO-B selective inhibition should not pose a problem with tyramine-containing products as long as the typical oral doses are employed, however, rare reactions have been reported. Increased risk of nonselective MAO inhibition occurs with oral doses >10 mg/day. Use of oral selgiline with tricyclic antidepressants and SSRIs has also been associated with rare reactions and should generally be avoided. Addition to levodopa therapy may result in exacerbation of levodopa adverse effects, requiring a reduction in levodopa dosage.

Transdermal: Nonselective MAO inhibition occurs with transdermal delivery and is necessary for antidepressant efficacy; dietary restrictions are recommended with doses >6 mg/24hours. Monitor for worsening of depression, suicidality and/or associated behaviors such as anxiety, agitation, panic attacks, insomnia, irritability, hostility, impulsivity, hypomania, and mania; worsening depression and severe abrupt suicidality that are not part of the presenting symptoms may require discontinuation or modification of drug therapy. Use caution in high-risk patients during initiation of therapy; prescriptions should be written for the smallest quantity.

Transdermal selegiline may worsen psychosis in some patients or precipitate a shift to mania or hypomania in
(Continued)

Selegiline (Continued)

patients with bipolar disorder. Patients presenting with depressive symptoms should be screened for bipolar disorder. Selegiline is not FDA approved for the treatment of bipolar depression. Do not use in combination with other antidepressants. Do not use within 1 week of other antidepressant discontinuation. Wait 2 weeks after discontinuing transdermal selegiline before initiating therapy with any contraindicated drug. May cause orthostatic hypotension- effects may be additive with other agents which cause orthostasis. Discontinue at least 10 days prior to elective surgery. Should not be stopped abruptly; taper off as rapidly as possible. Safety and efficacy in pediatric patients have not been established.

Drug Interactions

Cytochrome P450 Effect: Substrate of CYP1A2 (minor), 2A6 (minor), 2B6 (major), 2C9 (major), 2D6 (minor), 3A4 (minor); **Inhibits** CYP1A2 (weak), 2A6 (weak), 2C9 (weak), 2C19 (weak), 2D6 (weak), 2E1 (weak), 3A4 (weak)

Decreased Effect: CYP2B6 inducers may decrease the levels/effects of selegiline; example inducers include carbamazepine, nevirapine, phenobarbital, phenytoin, and rifampin. CYP2C9 inducers may decrease the levels/effects of selegiline; example inducers include carbamazepine, phenobarbital, phenytoin, rifampin, rifapentine, and secobarbital.

Increased Effect/Toxicity: CYP2B6 inhibitors may increase the levels/effects of selegiline; example inhibitors include desipramine, paroxetine, and sertraline. CYP2C9 inhibitors may increase the levels/effects of selegiline; example inhibitors include delavirdine, fluconazole, gemfibrozil, ketoconazole, nicardipine, NSAIDs, and sulfonamides. Concurrent use of oral selegiline (high dose) in combination with amphetamines, methylphenidate, dextromethorphan, fenfluramine, meperidine, nefazodone, sibutramine, tramadol, trazodone, tricyclic antidepressants, and venlafaxine may result in serotonin syndrome; these combinations are best avoided. Concurrent use of selegiline with an SSRI or SNRI may result in mania or hypertension; it is generally best to avoid these combinations. Transdermal selegiline is contraindicated with amphetamines, sympathomimetics or other CNS stimulants, dextromethorphan, meperidine, methadone, mirtazapine, propoxyphene, SSRIs/SNRIs, tramadol, tricyclic antidepressants. Oral selegiline (>10 mg/day) or transdermal doses ≥9 mg/24 hours in combination with tyramine (cheese, ethanol) may increase the pressor response; avoid high tyramine-containing foods in patients receiving >10 mg/day of oral selegiline or transdermal doses >6 mg/24 hours. The toxicity of levodopa (hypertension), lithium (hyperpyrexia), and reserpine may be increased by MAO inhibitors.

Nutritional/Ethanol Interactions

Ethanol: Avoid ethanol. Avoid beverages containing tyramine (hearty red wine and beer).

Food: Selegiline (>10 mg/day) may cause sudden and severe high blood pressure when taken with food high in tyramine (cheeses, sour cream, yogurt, pickled herring, chicken liver, canned figs, raisins, bananas, avocados, soy sauce, broad bean pods, yeast extracts, meats prepared with tenderizers, and many foods aged to improve flavor). Diet restriction of tyramine-rich foods are not necessary for lowest (6 mg) transdermal dose. Small amounts of caffeine may produce irregular heartbeat or high blood pressure and can interact with this medication for up to 2 weeks after stopping its use.

Herb/Nutraceutical: Avoid valerian, St John's wort, SAMe, kava kava (may increase risk of serotonin syndrome and/or excessive sedation).

Adverse Reactions Unless otherwise noted, the percentage of adverse events is reported for the transdermal patch:

>10%:
Central nervous system: Headache (18%), insomnia (12%)
Local: Application site reaction (24%)
1% to 10%:
Cardiovascular: Hypotension (including postural 3% to 10%), chest pain (≥1%), hypertension (≥1%), peripheral edema (≥1%)
Central nervous system: Dizziness (7% oral), hallucinations (3% oral), confusion (3% oral), headache (2% oral), agitation (≥1%), amnesia (≥1%), thinking abnormal (≥1%)
Dermatologic: Rash (4%), bruising (≥1%), pruritus (≥1%), acne (≥1%)
Endocrine and metabolic: Sexual side effects (≤1%), weight loss (5%)
Gastrointestinal: Nausea (10% oral), diarrhea (9%), xerostomia (8%), abdominal pain (4% oral), dyspepsia (4%), constipation (≥1%), flatulence (≥1%), anorexia (≥1%), gastroenteritis (≥1%), taste perversion (≥1%), vomiting (≥1%)
Genitourinary: Dysmenorrhea (≥1%), metrorrhagia (≥1%), UTI (≥1%), urinary frequency (≥1%)
Neuromuscular & skeletal: Myalgia (≥1%), neck pain (≥1%), paresthesia (≥1%)
Otic: Tinnitus (≥1%)
Respiratory: Pharyngitis (3%), sinusitis (3%), cough (≥1%), bronchitis (≥1%)
Miscellaneous: Diaphoresis (≥1%)

Overdosage/Toxicology Symptoms of overdose include tachycardia, palpitations, muscle twitching, and seizures. Both hypertension or hypotension can occur with intoxication. While treating hypertension, care is warranted to avoid sudden drops in blood pressure, since this may worsen MAO inhibitor toxicity. Cardiac arrhythmias are best treated with phenytoin or procainamide. Treatment is generally symptom-directed and supportive.

Pharmacodynamics/Kinetics

Onset of Action: Therapeutic: Oral: Within 1 hour
Duration of Action: Oral: 24-72 hours
Protein Binding: Protein binding: ~90%
Half-Life Elimination: 18-25 hours
Metabolism: Hepatic via CYP2D6, 2C9, and 3A4/5 to N-desmethylselegiline, methamphetamine and amphetamine
Excretion:
Urine; feces

Available Dosage Forms

Capsule, as hydrochloride (Eldepryl®): 5 mg
Tablet, as hydrochloride: 5 mg
Transdermal system [once-daily patch] (Emsam®): 6 mg/24 hours (30s) [20 cm², total selegiline 20 mg]; 9 mg/24 hours (30s) [30 cm², total selegiline 30 mg]; 12 mg/24 hours (30s) [40 cm², total selegiline 40 mg]

Dosing

Adults: Parkinson's disease: Oral: 5 mg twice daily with breakfast and lunch or 10 mg in the morning
Depression: Transdermal (Emsam®): Initial: 6 mg/24 hours once daily; may titrate based on clinical response in increments of 3 mg/day every 2 weeks up to a maximum of 12 mg/24 hours

Elderly:
Parkinson's disease: Oral: Initial: 5 mg in the morning; may increase to a total of 10 mg/day.
Depression: Transdermal (Emsam®): 6 mg/24 hours

Pediatrics: Children and Adolescents: ADHD (unlabeled use): Oral: 5-15 mg/day

Renal Impairment: No adjustment necessary.

Hepatic Impairment: No adjustment necessary in mild-moderate hepatic impairment.

Administration

Topical: Transdermal (Emsam®): Apply to clean, dry, intact skin to the upper torso (below the neck and above the waist), upper thigh, or outer surface of the upper arm. Avoid exposure of application site to external heat source, which may increase the amount of drug absorbed. Apply at the same time each day and rotate application sites. Wash hands with soap and water after handling. Avoid touching the sticky side of the patch.

Stability
Storage:
Tablet, capsule: Store at controlled room temperature 15°C to 30°C (59°F to 86°F).
Transdermal: Store at 20°C to 25°C (68°F to 77°F).

Nursing Actions
Physical Assessment: Assess effectiveness and interactions of other medications patient may be taking. Monitor therapeutic response (eg, mental status, involuntary movements), and adverse reactions at beginning of therapy and periodically throughout therapy. Monitor blood pressure. Be alert to thoughts of suicide. Patient should be cautioned against eating foods high in tyramine (see Tyramine Contents of Foods *on page 1406* list). Assess knowledge/teach patient appropriate use, interventions to reduce side effects, and adverse symptoms to report.

Patient Education: Take exactly as directed (may be prescribed in conjunction with levodopa/carbidopa); do not change dosage or discontinue without consulting prescriber. Therapeutic effects may take several weeks or months to achieve and you may need frequent monitoring during first weeks of therapy. Take with meals if GI upset occurs, before meals if dry mouth occurs, or after eating if drooling or if nausea occurs. Take at the same time each day. Avoid tyramine-containing foods (low potential for reaction). Maintain adequate hydration (2-3 L/day of fluids) unless instructed to restrict fluid intake; void before taking medication. Do not use alcohol and prescription or OTC sedatives or CNS depressants without consulting prescriber. You may experience drowsiness, dizziness, confusion, or vision changes (use caution when driving, climbing stairs, or engaging in tasks requiring alertness until response to drug is known); orthostatic hypotension (use caution when changing position - rising to standing from sitting or lying); constipation (increased exercise, fluids, fruit, or fiber may help); runny nose or flu-like symptoms (consult prescriber for appropriate relief); or nausea, vomiting, loss of appetite, or stomach discomfort (small frequent meals, frequent mouth care, chewing gum, or sucking lozenges may help). Report unresolved constipation or vomiting; chest pain, palpitations, irregular heartbeat; CNS changes (hallucination, loss of memory, seizures, acute headache, nervousness, thoughts of suicide, etc); painful or difficult urination; increased muscle spasticity, rigidity, or involuntary movements; skin rash; or significant worsening of condition. **Pregnancy/ breast-feeding precautions:** Inform prescriber if you are or intend to become pregnant. Consult prescriber if breast-feeding.

Dietary Considerations Emsam® 9 mg/24 hours or 12 mg/24 hours: Avoid tyramine-rich foods or beverages beginning the first day of treatment or for 2 weeks after discontinuation or dose reduction to 6 mg/24 hours.

Geriatric Considerations Selegiline is also being studied in Alzheimer's disease, but further studies are needed to assess its usefulness. Do not use at daily doses exceeding 10 mg/day because of the risks associated with nonselective inhibition of MAO.

Pregnancy Issues There are no adequate and well-controlled studies in pregnant women.

Additional Information When adding selegiline to levodopa/carbidopa, the dose of the latter can usually be decreased. Studies are investigating the use of selegiline in early Parkinson's disease to slow the progression of the disease.

Related Information
Tyramine Content of Foods *on page 1406*

Senna (SEN na)

U.S. Brand Names Black Draught Tablets [OTC]; Evac-U-Gen [OTC]; ex-lax® [OTC]; ex-lax® Maximum Strength [OTC]; Fletcher's® Castoria® [OTC]; Perdiem® Overnight Relief [OTC]; Senexon [OTC]; Senna-Gen® [OTC]; Sennatural™ [OTC]; Senokot® [OTC]; Uni-Senna [OTC]; X-Prep® [OTC] [DSC]

Pharmacologic Category Laxative, Stimulant

Medication Safety Issues
Sound-alike/look-alike issues:
Senexon® may be confused with Cenestin®
Senokot® may be confused with Depakote®

Use Short-term treatment of constipation; evacuate the colon for bowel or rectal examinations

Contraindications Per Commission E: Intestinal obstruction, acute intestinal inflammation (eg, Crohn's disease), colitis ulcerosa, appendicitis, abdominal pain of unknown origin; pregnancy

Warnings/Precautions Not recommended for over-the-counter (OTC) use in patients experiencing stomach pain, nausea, vomiting, or a sudden change in bowel movements which lasts >2 weeks. Not recommended for OTC use in children <2 years of age.

Adverse Reactions Frequency not defined: Gastrointestinal: Nausea, vomiting, diarrhea, abdominal cramps

Available Dosage Forms [DSC] = Discontinued product
Granules (Senokot®): Sennosides 15 mg/teaspoon (60 g, 180 g, 360 g) [cocoa flavor] [DSC]
Liquid:
Senexon: Sennosides 8.8 mg/5 mL (240 mL)
X-Prep®: Sennosides 8.8 mg/5 mL (75 mL) [alcohol free; contains sugar 50 g/75 mL; available individually or in a kit] [DSC]
Liquid concentrate (Fletcher's® Castoria®): Senna concentrate 33.3 mg/mL (75 mL) [alcohol free; contains sodium benzoate; root beer flavor]
Syrup (Uni-Senna): Sennosides 8.8 mg/5 mL (240 mL) [contains alcohol; butterscotch flavor]
Tablet: Sennosides 8.6 mg, 15 mg, 25 mg
ex-lax®: Sennosides USP 15 mg
ex-lax® Maximum Strength: Sennosides USP 25 mg
Perdiem® Overnight Relief: Sennosides USP 15 mg
Sennatural™, Senokot®, Senexon®, Senna-Gen®, Uni-Senna: Sennosides 8.6 mg
Tablet, chewable:
ex-lax®: Sennosides USP 15 mg [chocolate flavor]
Evac-U-Gen: Sennosides 10 mg

Dosing
Adults & Elderly:
Bowel evacuation: Oral: OTC labeling: Usual dose: Sennosides 130 mg (X-Prep® 75 mL) between 2-4 PM the afternoon of the day prior to procedure
Constipation: Oral: OTC ranges: Sennosides 15 mg once daily (maximum: 70-100 mg/day, divided twice daily)
Pediatrics:
Bowel evacuation: OTC labeling: Children ≥12 years: Refer to adult dosing.
Constipation: OTC ranges: Children:
2-6 years:
Sennosides: Initial: 3.75 mg once daily (maximum: 15 mg/day, divided twice daily)
Senna concentrate: 33.3 mg/mL: 5-10 mL up to twice daily
6-12 years:
Sennosides: Initial: 8.6 mg once daily (maximum: 50 mg/day, divided twice daily)
Senna concentrate: 33.3 mg/mL: 10-30 mL up to twice daily
≥12 years: Refer to adult dosing.
(Continued)

Senna (Continued)

Administration
Oral: Once daily doses should be taken at bedtime. Granules may be eaten plain, sprinkled on food, or mixed in liquids

Nursing Actions
Physical Assessment: Determine cause of constipation before treating. Teach patient proper use, side effects/interventions, and symptoms to report.

Patient Education: Take exactly as directed. DO NOT exceed recommended dosage; may cause dependence with prolonged or excessive use. Your urine may be discolored (red-brown) this is normal. Stop use and contact prescriber if you develop nausea, vomiting, persistent diarrhea, or abdominal cramps. If constipation worsens or you experience no relief contact prescriber. **Note:** Increased fluids, fruits, fiber, and exercise may help relieve constipation. OTC labeling does not recommend for use longer than 1 week in children <2 years of age or in women who are pregnant or nursing.

Dietary Considerations Liquid may be administered with fruit juice or milk to mask taste. X-Prep® liquid contains sugar 50 g/75 mL.

Additional Information Some products that may have previously been labeled as standardized senna concentrate are now labeled as sennosides. For example, Senokot® tablets, previously labeled as standardized senna concentrate 187 mg, are now labeled as sennosides 8.6 mg. The actual content of senna in this product did not change. Individual product labeling should be consulted prior to dosing.

Sertaconazole (ser ta KOE na zole)

U.S. Brand Names Ertaczo™
Synonyms Sertaconazole Nitrate
Pharmacologic Category Antifungal Agent, Topical
Pregnancy Risk Factor C
Lactation Excretion in breast milk unknown/use caution
Use Topical treatment of tinea pedis (athlete's foot)
Mechanism of Action/Effect Alters fungal cell wall membrane permeability
Contraindications Hypersensitivity to sertaconazole, other imidazoles (manufacturer-based contraindication), or any component of the formulation
Warnings/Precautions Discontinue drug if sensitivity or chemical irritation occurs. For external use only; not for ophthalmic or intravaginal use. Hypersensitivity to one imidazole antifungal may result in cross-reactivity with another. Safety and efficacy have not been established in pediatric patients <12 years of age.
Adverse Reactions 1% to 10%: Dermatologic: Burning, contact dermatitis, dry skin, tenderness
Available Dosage Forms Cream, topical, as nitrate: 2% (30 g)
Dosing
Adults & Elderly: Tinea pedis: Topical: Apply between toes and to surrounding healthy skin twice daily for 4 weeks
Pediatrics: Tinea pedis: Topical: Children ≥12 years: Refer to adult dosing.
Administration
Topical: For external use only. Apply to affected area between toes and to surrounding healthy skin. Make sure skin is dry before applying. Avoid use of occlusive dressing. Avoid contact with eyes, nose, mouth, and other mucous membranes.
Stability
Storage: Store at 25°C (77°F).
Nursing Actions
Physical Assessment: For external use only; not for ophthalmic or intravaginal use. Teach patient proper

use, appropriate interventions to reduce side effects, and adverse symptoms to report.

Patient Education: This medication is for topical use only. Avoid contact with eyes, nose, mouth, and other mucous membranes. Use exactly as directed. Wash feet and dry thoroughly. Apply to affected area between toes and to surrounding healthy skin. Avoid use of occlusive dressing. Wash hands thoroughly after application; infection can be spread to other parts of your body or to other persons. Wear socks that keep your feet dry, and change them frequently if you perspire heavily. Do not share foot wear with others. May cause dry skin, mild tenderness, or slight discomfort (burning) after application. Stop using and contact prescriber if burning or tenderness persists or if other adverse skin reactions occur. **Pregnancy/breast-feeding precautions:** Inform prescriber if you are or intend to become pregnant or breast-feed.

Sertraline (SER tra leen)

U.S. Brand Names Zoloft®
Synonyms Sertraline Hydrochloride
Restrictions A medication guide concerning the use of antidepressants in children and teenagers can be found on the FDA website at http://www.fda.gov/cder/Offices/ODS/labeling.htm. It should be dispensed to parents or guardians of children and teenagers receiving this medication.
Pharmacologic Category Antidepressant, Selective Serotonin Reuptake Inhibitor
Medication Safety Issues
Sound-alike/look-alike issues:
Sertraline may be confused with selegiline, Serentil® Zoloft® may be confused with Zocor®
Pregnancy Risk Factor C
Lactation Enters breast milk/not recommended (AAP rates "of concern")
Use Treatment of major depression; obsessive-compulsive disorder (OCD); panic disorder; post-traumatic stress disorder (PTSD); premenstrual dysphoric disorder (PMDD); social anxiety disorder
Unlabeled/Investigational Use Eating disorders; generalized anxiety disorder (GAD); impulse control disorders
Mechanism of Action/Effect Antidepressant with selective inhibitory effects on presynaptic serotonin (5-HT) reuptake and only very weak effects on norepinephrine and dopamine neuronal uptake
Contraindications Hypersensitivity to sertraline or any component of the formulation; use of MAO inhibitors within 14 days; concurrent use of pimozide; concurrent use of sertraline oral concentrate with disulfiram
Warnings/Precautions Antidepressants increase the risk of suicidal thinking and behavior in children and adolescents with major depressive disorder (MDD) and other depressive disorders; consider risk prior to prescribing. All patients must be closely monitored for clinical worsening, suicidality, or unusual changes in behavior, especially during the initiation of therapy or following an increase or decrease in dosage. When used in children, the child's family or caregiver should be instructed to closely observe the patient and communicate condition with healthcare provider. A medication guide should be dispensed with each prescription. **Sertraline is not FDA approved for use in children with major depressive disorder (MDD). However, it is approved for the treatment of obsessive-compulsive disorder (OCD) in children ≥6 years of age.**

The possibility of a suicide attempt is inherent in major depression and may persist until remission occurs. Use caution in high-risk patients. Worsening depression and severe abrupt suicidality that are not part of the presenting symptoms may require discontinuation or modification of drug therapy. The patient's family or caregiver should be alerted to monitor patients for the emergence of suicidality and associated behaviors (such as agitation, irritability, hostility, impulsivity, and hypomania) and call healthcare provider.

May worsen psychosis in some patients or precipitate a shift to mania or hypomania in patients with bipolar disorder. Patients presenting with depressive symptoms should be screened for bipolar disorder. Monotherapy in patients with bipolar disorder should be avoided. **Sertraline is not FDA approved for the treatment of bipolar depression.**

The potential for severe reaction exists when used with MAO inhibitors - serotonin syndrome (hyperthermia, muscular rigidity, mental status changes/agitation, autonomic instability) may occur. Has a very low potential to impair cognitive or motor performance. However, caution patients regarding activities requiring alertness until response to sertraline is known. Does not appear to potentiate the effects of alcohol, however, ethanol use is not advised.

Use caution in patients with a previous seizure disorder or condition predisposing to seizures such as brain damage, alcoholism, or concurrent therapy with other drugs which lower the seizure threshold. May increase the risks associated with electroconvulsive therapy. Use with caution in patients with hepatic or renal dysfunction and in elderly patients. May cause hyponatremia/SIADH. Use with caution in patients with renal insufficiency or other concurrent illness (due to limited experience). Sertraline acts as a mild uricosuric; use with caution in patients at risk of uric acid nephropathy. Use with caution in patients at risk of bleeding or receiving anticoagulant therapy; may cause impairment in platelet aggregation. Use with caution in patients where weight loss is undesirable. May cause or exacerbate sexual dysfunction.

Use oral concentrate formulation with caution in patients with latex sensitivity; dropper dispenser contains dry natural rubber. Monitor growth in pediatric patients. Discontinuation symptoms (eg, dysphoric mood, irritability, agitation, confusion, anxiety, insomnia, hypomania) may occur upon abrupt discontinuation. Taper dose when discontinuing therapy.

Drug Interactions

Cytochrome P450 Effect: Substrate of CYP2B6 (minor), 2C8/9 (minor), 2C19 (major), 2D6 (major), 3A4 (minor); **Inhibits** CYP1A2 (weak), 2B6 (moderate), 2C8/9 (weak), 2C19 (moderate), 2D6 (moderate), 3A4 (moderate)

Decreased Effect: The levels/effects of sertraline may be decreased by aminoglutethimide, carbamazepine, phenytoin, rifampin, and other CYP2C19 inducers. Sertraline may decrease the metabolism of tolbutamide; monitor for changes in glucose control. Sertraline may decrease the levels/effects of CYP2D6 prodrug substrates (eg, codeine, hydrocodone, oxycodone, tramadol).

Increased Effect/Toxicity: Sertraline should not be used with nonselective MAO inhibitors (phenelzine, isocarboxazid) or other drugs with MAO inhibition (linezolid); fatal reactions have been reported. Wait 5 weeks after stopping sertraline before starting a nonselective MAO inhibitor and 2 weeks after stopping an MAO inhibitor before starting sertraline. Concurrent selegiline has been associated with mania, hypertension, or serotonin syndrome (risk may be reduced relative to nonselective MAO inhibitors). Sertraline may increase serum concentrations of pimozide; concurrent use is contraindicated. Avoid use of oral concentrate with disulfiram.

Sertraline may inhibit the metabolism of thioridazine or mesoridazine, resulting in increased plasma levels and increasing the risk of QT$_c$ interval prolongation.

This may lead to serious ventricular arrhythmias, such as torsade de pointes-type arrhythmias and sudden death. Do not use together. Wait at least 5 weeks after discontinuing sertraline prior to starting thioridazine.

Sertraline may increase the levels/effects of levels/effects of amphetamines, selected beta-blockers, bupropion, selected benzodiazepines, calcium channel blockers, cisapride, cyclosporine, dextromethorphan, ergot alkaloids, fluoxetine, selected HMG-CoA reductase inhibitors, lidocaine, mesoridazine, mirtazapine, nateglinide, nefazodone, paroxetine, promethazine, propofol, risperidone, ritonavir, selegiline, sildenafil (and other PDE-5 inhibitors), tacrolimus, thioridazine, tricyclic antidepressants, venlafaxine, and other substrates of CYP2B6, 2D6 or 3A4. Sertraline may increase the hypoprothrombinemic response to warfarin.

The levels/effects of sertraline may be increased by chlorpromazine, delavirdine, fluconazole, fluoxetine, fluvoxamine, gemfibrozil, isoniazid, miconazole, omeprazole, paroxetine, pergolide, quinidine, quinine, ritonavir, ropinirole, ticlopidine, and other CYP2C19 or 2D6 inhibitors.

Combined use of SSRIs and amphetamines, buspirone, meperidine, nefazodone, serotonin agonists (such as sumatriptan), sibutramine, other SSRIs, sympathomimetics, ritonavir, tramadol, and venlafaxine may increase the risk of serotonin syndrome. Combined use of sumatriptan (and other serotonin agonists) may result in toxicity; weakness, hyper-reflexia, and incoordination have been observed with sumatriptan and SSRIs. In addition, concurrent use may theoretically increase the risk of serotonin syndrome; includes sumatriptan, naratriptan, rizatriptan, and zolmitriptan.

Concurrent lithium may increase risk of nephrotoxicity. Risk of hyponatremia may increase with concurrent use of loop diuretics (bumetanide, furosemide, torsemide). Concomitant use of sertraline and NSAIDs, aspirin, or other drugs affecting coagulation has been associated with an increased risk of bleeding; monitor.

Nutritional/Ethanol Interactions
Ethanol: Avoid ethanol (may increase CNS depression).
Food: Sertraline average peak serum levels may be increased if taken with food.
Herb/Nutraceutical: Avoid valerian, St John's wort, kava kava, gotu kola (may increase CNS depression).

Lab Interactions Increased (minor) triglycerides (S), LFTs; decreased uric acid (S)

Adverse Reactions
>10%:
  Central nervous system: Insomnia, somnolence, dizziness, headache, fatigue
  Gastrointestinal: Xerostomia, diarrhea, nausea
  Genitourinary: Ejaculatory disturbances
1% to 10%:
  Cardiovascular: Palpitations
  Central nervous system: Agitation, anxiety, nervousness
  Dermatologic: Rash
  Endocrine & metabolic: Decreased libido
  Gastrointestinal: Constipation, anorexia, dyspepsia, flatulence, vomiting, weight gain
  Genitourinary: Micturition disorders
  Neuromuscular & skeletal: Tremors, paresthesia
  Ocular: Visual difficulty, abnormal vision
  Otic: Tinnitus
  Miscellaneous: Diaphoresis (increased)

Additional adverse reactions reported in pediatric patients (frequency >2%): Aggressiveness, epistaxis, hyperkinesia, purpura, sinusitis, urinary incontinence

Overdosage/Toxicology Among 634 patients who overdosed on sertraline alone, 8 resulted in a fatal (Continued)

Sertraline *(Continued)*

outcome. Symptoms of overdose include somnolence, vomiting, tachycardia, nausea, dizziness, agitation, and tremor. Treatment is symptomatic and supportive.

Pharmacodynamics/Kinetics

Time to Peak: Plasma: 4.5-8.4 hours

Protein Binding: 98%

Half-Life Elimination: Parent drug: 26 hours; Metabolite N-desmethylsertraline: 66 hours (range: 62-104 hours)

Metabolism: Hepatic; extensive first-pass metabolism

Excretion: Urine and feces

Available Dosage Forms Note: Available as sertraline hydrochloride; mg strength refers to sertraline

Solution, oral concentrate: 20 mg/mL (60 mL) [contains alcohol 12%]

Tablet: 25 mg, 50 mg, 100 mg

Dosing

Adults:

Depression/OCD: Oral: Initial: 50 mg/day

Note: May increase daily dose, at intervals of not less than 1 week, to a maximum of 200 mg/day. If somnolence is noted, give at bedtime.

Panic disorder, PTSD, social anxiety disorder: Oral: Initial: 25 mg once daily; increased after 1 week to 50 mg once daily (see "Note" above)

Premenstrual dysphoric disorder (PMDD): 50 mg/day either daily throughout menstrual cycle **or** limited to the luteal phase of menstrual cycle, depending on physician assessment. Patients not responding to 50 mg/day may benefit from dose increases (50 mg increments per menstrual cycle) up to 150 mg/day when dosing throughout menstrual cycle **or** up to 100 mg day when dosing during luteal phase only. If a 100 mg/day dose has been established with luteal phase dosing, a 50 mg/day titration step for 3 days should be utilized at the beginning of each luteal phase dosing period.

Elderly: Oral: Initial: 25 mg/day in the morning; increase by 25 mg/day increments every 2-3 days if tolerated to 50-100 mg/day; additional increases may be necessary; maximum: 200 mg/day.

Pediatrics:

OCD: Oral: Children:

6-12 years: Initial: 25 mg once daily

13-17 years: Initial: 50 mg once daily

May increase daily dose, at intervals of not less than 1 week, to a maximum: 200 mg/day. If somnolence is noted, give at bedtime.

Renal Impairment: Multiple-dose pharmacokinetics are unaffected by renal impairment.

Hemodialysis effect: Not removed by hemodialysis

Hepatic Impairment: Sertraline is extensively metabolized by the liver. Caution should be used in patients with hepatic impairment. A lower dose or less frequent dosing should be used.

Administration

Oral: Oral concentrate: Must be diluted before use. Immediately before administration, use the dropper provided to measure the required amount of concentrate; mix with 4 ounces (1/2 cup) of water, ginger ale, lemon/lime soda, lemonade, or orange juice **only**. Do not mix with any other liquids than these. The dose should be taken immediately after mixing; do not mix in advance. A slight haze may appear after mixing; this is normal. **Note:** Use with caution in patients with latex sensitivity; dropper dispenser contains dry natural rubber.

Stability

Storage: Tablets and oral solution should be stored at controlled room temperature of 15°C to 30°C (59°F to 86°F).

Nursing Actions

Physical Assessment: Assess other medications patient may be taking for effectiveness and interactions. Assess mental status for worsening of depression, suicidal ideation, anxiety, social functioning, mania, or panic attack (especially during initiation of therapy and when dosage is changed). Taper dosage slowly when discontinuing. Assess knowledge/teach patient appropriate use, interventions to reduce side effects, and adverse symptoms to report. Pediatric patients: Monitor growth pattern.

Patient Education: Take exactly as directed; do not increase dose or frequency; or discontinue use abruptly. It may take 2-3 weeks to achieve desired results. Take in the morning to reduce the incidence of insomnia. Avoid alcohol, caffeine, and other prescription or OTC medications not approved by prescriber. Maintain adequate hydration (2-3 L/day of fluids) unless instructed to restrict fluid intake. You may experience drowsiness, dizziness, or lightheadedness (use caution when driving or engaging in tasks requiring alertness until response to drug is known); nausea, vomiting, anorexia, or dry mouth (small frequent meals, frequent mouth care, chewing gum, or sucking lozenges may help); postural hypotension (use caution when climbing stairs or changing position from sitting or lying to standing); urinary pattern changes (void before taking medication); or male sexual dysfunction (reversible). Report persistent insomnia or daytime sedation, agitation, nervousness, fatigue; muscle cramping, tremors, weakness, or change in gait; chest pain, palpitations, or swelling of extremities; vision changes or eye pain; hearing changes (ringing in ears); respiratory difficulty or breathlessness; skin rash or irritation; suicidal ideation; or worsening of condition. **Pregnancy/breast-feeding precautions:** Inform prescriber if you are or intend to become pregnant. Breast-feeding is not recommended.

Geriatric Considerations Sertraline's favorable side effect profile makes it a useful alternative to the traditional tricyclic antidepressants. Its potential stimulation effect and anorexia may be bothersome.

Pregnancy Issues Nonteratogenic effects including respiratory distress, cyanosis, apnea, seizures, temperature instability, feeding difficulty, vomiting, hypoglycemia, hypo- or hypertonia, hyper-reflexia, jitteriness, irritability, constant crying, and tremor have been reported in the neonate immediately following delivery after exposure of other SSRIs late in the third trimester. Adverse effects may be due to toxic effects of SSRI or drug discontinuation. In some cases, may present clinically as serotonin syndrome. There are no adequate and well-controlled studies in pregnant women. Use during pregnancy only if the potential benefit to the mother outweighs the possible risk to the fetus. If treatment during pregnancy is required, consider tapering therapy during the third trimester.

Additional Information Buspirone (15-60 mg/day) may be useful in treatment of sexual dysfunction during treatment with a selective serotonin reuptake inhibitor. May exacerbate tics in Tourette's syndrome.

Related Information

Antidepressant Medication Guidelines *on page 1414*

Sevelamer (se VEL a mer)

U.S. Brand Names Renagel®
Synonyms Sevelamer Hydrochloride
Pharmacologic Category Phosphate Binder
Medication Safety Issues
Sound-alike/look-alike issues:
Renagel® may be confused with Reglan®, Regonol®
Pregnancy Risk Factor C
Lactation Excretion in breast milk unknown/use caution (not absorbed systemically but may alter maternal nutrition)
Use Reduction of serum phosphorous in patients with chronic kidney disease on hemodialysis
Mechanism of Action/Effect Sevelamer (a polymeric compound) binds phosphate within the intestinal lumen, limiting absorption and decreasing serum phosphate concentrations without altering calcium, aluminum, or bicarbonate concentrations.
Contraindications Hypersensitivity to sevelamer or any component of the formulation; hypophosphatemia; bowel obstruction
Warnings/Precautions Use with caution in patients with gastrointestinal disorders including dysphagia, swallowing disorders, severe gastrointestinal motility disorders, or major gastrointestinal surgery. May cause reductions in vitamin D, E, K, and folic acid absorption. Long-term studies of carcinogenic potential have not been completed. Tablets should not be taken apart or chewed; broken or crushed tablets will rapidly expand in water/saliva and may be a choking hazard.
Drug Interactions
Decreased Effect: Sevelamer may bind to some drugs in the gastrointestinal tract and decrease their absorption. When changes in absorption of oral medications may have significant clinical consequences (such as antiarrhythmic and antiseizure medications), these medications should be taken at least 1 hour before or 3 hours after a dose of sevelamer. Sevelamer may decrease the bioavailability of ciprofloxacin by 50%.
Adverse Reactions
>10%:
Dermatologic: Rash (13%)
Gastrointestinal: Vomiting (22%), nausea (7% to 20%), diarrhea (4% to 19%), dyspepsia (5% to 16%)
Neuromuscular & skeletal: Limb pain (13%), arthralgia (12%)
Respiratory: Nasopharyngitis (14%), bronchitis (11%)
1% to 10%:
Cardiovascular: Hypertension (10%)
Central nervous system: Headache (9%), pyrexia (5%)
Gastrointestinal: Constipation (2% to 8%), flatulence (4%)
Neuromuscular & skeletal: Back pain (4%)
Respiratory: Dyspnea (10%), cough (7%), upper respiratory tract infection (5%)
Postmarketing and/or case reports: Abdominal pain
Overdosage/Toxicology Sevelamer is not absorbed systemically. Doses up to 14 g/day for 8 days have been administered without adverse effects. There are no reports of overdosage in patients.
Pharmacodynamics/Kinetics
Excretion: Feces
Available Dosage Forms Tablet, as hydrochloride: 400 mg, 800 mg
Dosing
Adults & Elderly: Reduction of serum phosphorous: Oral:
Patients not taking a phosphate binder: 800-1600 mg 3 times/day with meals; the initial dose may be based on serum phosphorous levels:
>5.5 mg/dL to <7.5 mg/dL: 800 mg 3 times/day

≥7.5 mg/dL to <9.0 mg/dL: 1200-1600 mg 3 times/day
≥9.0 mg/dL: 1600 mg 3 times/day
Maintenance dose adjustment based on serum phosphorous concentration (goal of lowering to <5.5 mg/dL; maximum daily dose studied was equivalent to 13 g/day):
>5.5 mg/dL: Increase by 1 tablet per meal every 2 weeks
3.5-5.5 mg/dL: Maintain current dose
<3.5 mg/dL: Decrease by 1 tablet per meal
Dosage adjustment when switching between phosphate binder products: 667 mg of calcium acetate is equivalent to 800 mg sevelamer
Stability
Storage: Store at controlled room temperature of 15°C to 30°C (59°F to 86°F).
Laboratory Monitoring Serum phosphorus, calcium, bicarbonate, chloride
Nursing Actions
Physical Assessment: Assess knowledge/teach patient appropriate use, possible side effects/interventions, and adverse symptoms to report. Monitor blood pressure.
Patient Education: Take as directed, with meals. Do not break or chew tablets (contents will expand in water). You may experience headache or dizziness (use caution when driving or engaging in tasks requiring alertness until response to drug is known); nausea or vomiting (small frequent meals, frequent mouth care, or sucking hard candy may help); diarrhea (yogurt or buttermilk may help); or mild neuromuscular pain or stiffness (mild analgesic may help). Report persistent adverse reactions. **Pregnancy/breast-feeding precautions:** Inform prescriber if you are or intend to become pregnant. Consult prescriber if breast-feeding.
Dietary Considerations Take with meals.
Breast-Feeding Issues It is not known whether sevelamer is excreted in human milk. Because sevelamer may cause a reduction in the absorption of some vitamins, it should be used with caution in nursing women.
Pregnancy Issues Because sevelamer may cause a reduction in the absorption of some vitamins, it should be used with caution in pregnant women.

Sibutramine (si BYOO tra meen)

U.S. Brand Names Meridia®
Synonyms Sibutramine Hydrochloride Monohydrate
Restrictions C-IV; recommended only for obese patients with a body mass index ≥30 kg/m² or ≥27 kg/m² in the presence of other risk factors such as hypertension, diabetes, and/or dyslipidemia; rule out obesity due to untreated hypothyroidism
Pharmacologic Category Anorexiant
Pregnancy Risk Factor C
Lactation Excretion in breast milk unknown/not recommended
Use Management of obesity, including weight loss and maintenance of weight loss; should be used in conjunction with a reduced-calorie diet
Mechanism of Action/Effect Sibutramine blocks the neuronal uptake of norepinephrine, serotonin, and (to a lesser extent) dopamine
Contraindications Hypersensitivity to sibutramine or any component of the formulation; during or within 2 weeks of MAO inhibitors (eg, phenelzine, selegiline) or concomitant centrally-acting appetite suppressants; anorexia nervosa; bulimia nervosa
Warnings/Precautions Use with caution in mild-moderate renal impairment or hepatic dysfunction, seizure disorder, hypertension, gallstones, narrow-angle glaucoma, nursing mothers, and elderly
(Continued)

Sibutramine *(Continued)*

patients; not for use in patients with severe renal or hepatic impairment or history of cardiovascular disorders (eg, CHF, stroke, arrhythmia). Primary pulmonary hypertension (PPH), a rare and frequently fatal pulmonary disease, has been reported to occur in patients receiving other agents with serotonergic activity which have been used as anorexiants. Although not reported in clinical trials, it is possible that sibutramine may share this potential, and patients should be monitored closely. Avoid concurrent use with other serotonergic agents, due to the risk of developing serotonin syndrome. Rare cases of bleeding have been reported; use caution in patients with bleeding disorders. Stimulants may unmask tics in individuals with coexisting Tourette's syndrome. Rare reports of depression, suicide and suicidal ideation have been documented; use caution and monitor closely in patients with history of psychiatric symptoms. Safety and efficacy have not been established in children <16 years of age.

Drug Interactions

Cytochrome P450 Effect: Substrate of CYP3A4 (major)

Decreased Effect: Inducers of CYP3A4 (including phenytoin, phenobarbital, carbamazepine, and rifampin) theoretically may reduce sibutramine serum concentrations.

Increased Effect/Toxicity: Serotonergic agents such as buspirone, selective serotonin reuptake inhibitors (eg, citalopram, fluoxetine, fluvoxamine, paroxetine, sertraline), sumatriptan (and similar serotonin agonists), dihydroergotamine, lithium, tryptophan, some opioid/analgesics (eg, meperidine, tramadol), and venlafaxine, when combined with sibutramine may result in serotonin syndrome. Dextromethorphan, MAO inhibitors and other drugs that can raise the blood pressure (eg decongestants, centrally-acting weight loss products, amphetamines, and amphetamine-like compounds) can increase the possibility of sibutramine-associated cardiovascular complications. Sibutramine may increase serum levels of tricyclic antidepressants. CYP3A4 inhibitors may increase the levels/effects of sibutramine; example inhibitors include azole antifungals, clarithromycin, diclofenac, doxycycline, erythromycin, imatinib, isoniazid, nefazodone, nicardipine, propofol, protease inhibitors, quinidine, telithromycin, and verapamil.

Nutritional/Ethanol Interactions

Ethanol: Avoid excess ethanol ingestion.

Herb/Nutraceutical: St John's wort may decrease sibutramine levels.

Adverse Reactions

>10%:

Central nervous system: Headache (30%), insomnia (11%)

Gastrointestinal: Xerostomia (17%), anorexia (13%), constipation (12%)

1% to 10%:

Cardiovascular: Tachycardia (3%), vasodilation (2%), hypertension (2%), palpitation (2%), chest pain (2%), edema (1%)

Central nervous system: Dizziness (7%), nervousness (5%), anxiety (5%), depression (4%), migraine (2%), somnolence (2%), CNS stimulation (2%), emotional lability (1%)

Dermatologic: Rash (4%), acne (1%), herpes simplex (1%)

Endocrine & metabolic: Dysmenorrhea (4%), metrorrhagia (1%)

Gastrointestinal: Appetite increased (9%), nausea (6%), abdominal pain (5%), dyspepsia (5%), gastritis (2%), vomiting (2%), taste perversion (2%), rectal disorder (1%)

Genitourinary: Urinary tract infection (2%), vaginal *Monilia* (1%)

Hepatic: Abnormal LFTs (2%)

Neuromuscular & skeletal: Back pain (8%), weakness (6%), arthralgia (6%), neck pain (2%), myalgia (2%), paresthesia (2%), tenosynovitis (1%), joint disorder (1%)

Otic: Ear disorder (2%), ear pain (1%)

Respiratory: Pharyngitis (10%), rhinitis (10%), sinusitis (5%), cough (4%), laryngitis (1%)

Miscellaneous: Flu-like syndrome (8%), diaphoresis (3%), allergic reactions (2), thirst (2%)

Frequency not defined:

Cardiovascular: Peripheral edema

Central nervous system: Thinking abnormal, agitation, fever

Dermatologic: Pruritus

Endocrine & metabolic: Menstrual disorders/irregularities

Gastrointestinal: Diarrhea, flatulence, gastroenteritis, tooth disorder

Neuromuscular & skeletal: Arthritis, hypertonia, leg cramps

Ocular: Amblyopia

Respiratory: Bronchitis, dyspnea

Overdosage/Toxicology Symptoms of overdose include hypertension, tachycardia, headache, and palpitations. Treatment is supportive. Monitor vitals; beta-blockers may be beneficial to control elevated pressure and heart rate; dialysis not likely to be effective.

Pharmacodynamics/Kinetics

Time to Peak: Sibutramine: 1.2 hours; Metabolites (M_1 and M_2): 3-4 hours

Protein Binding: Plasma: Parent drug and metabolites: >94%

Half-Life Elimination: Sibutramine: 1 hour; Metabolites: M_1: 14 hours; M_2: 16 hours

Metabolism: Hepatic; undergoes first-pass metabolism via CYP3A4; forms metabolites (active)

Excretion: Primarily urine (77%); feces

Available Dosage Forms Capsule, as hydrochloride: 5 mg, 10 mg, 15 mg

Dosing

Adults: Obesity: Oral: Initial: 10 mg once daily; after 4 weeks may titrate up to 15 mg once daily as needed and tolerated (may be used for up to 2 years, per manufacturer labeling).

Elderly: Use with caution; adjust dose based on renal or hepatic function.

Renal Impairment: Should not be used in patients with severe renal impairment.

Hepatic Impairment: No adjustment necessary for mild-to-moderate liver failure. Sibutramine should not be used in patients with severe liver failure.

Administration

Oral: May take with or without food.

Stability

Storage: Store at room temperature of 15°C to 30°C (59°F to 86°F).

Nursing Actions

Physical Assessment: Assess effectiveness and interactions of other medications patient may be taking. Monitor therapeutic response and periodically evaluate the need for continued use. Monitor vital signs, weight, and adverse reactions at start of therapy, when changing dosage, and at regular intervals during therapy. Assess knowledge/teach patient appropriate use, possible side effects, and symptoms to report.

Patient Education: Take exactly as directed; do not increase dose or frequency without consulting prescriber. May be taken with meals (do not take at bedtime). Avoid alcohol, caffeine, or OTC medications that act as stimulants. You may experience restlessness, dizziness, sleepiness (use caution when driving or engaging in tasks requiring alertness until response to drug is known); insomnia (taking medication early in morning may help, warm milk, and quiet environment at bedtime may help); increased appetite, nausea or vomiting (small frequent meals, frequent mouth care may help); constipation (increased exercise, fluids, fruit, or fiber may help); diarrhea (buttermilk, boiled milk, or yogurt may help); or altered menstrual periods (reversible when drug is discontinued). Report chest pain, palpitations, or irregular heartbeat; excessive nervousness, excitation, or sleepiness; back pain, muscle weakness, or tremors; CNS changes (acute headache, aggressiveness, restlessness, excitation, sleep disturbances); menstrual pattern changes; rash; blurred vision; runny nose, sinusitis, cough, or respiratory difficulty. **Pregnancy/breast-feeding precautions:** Inform prescriber if you are or intend to become pregnant. Breast-feeding is not recommended.

Dietary Considerations Sibutramine, as an appetite suppressant, is the most effective when combined with a low calorie diet and behavior modification counseling.

Additional Information Physicians should carefully evaluate patients for history of drug abuse and follow such patients closely, observing them for signs of misuse or abuse (eg, development of tolerance, excessive increases of doses, drug seeking behavior).

Unlike dexfenfluramine and fenfluramine, the medication does not cause the release of serotonin from neurons. Tests done on humans show no evidence of valvular heart disease and experiments done on animals show no evidence of the neurotoxicity which was found in similar testing using animals treated with fenfluramine and dexfenfluramine; has minimal potential for abuse.

Sildenafil (sil DEN a fil)

U.S. Brand Names Revatio™; Viagra®

Synonyms UK92480

Pharmacologic Category Phosphodiesterase-5 Enzyme Inhibitor

Medication Safety Issues
Sound-alike/look-alike issues:
Viagra® may be confused with Allegra®, Vaniqa™

Pregnancy Risk Factor B

Lactation Excretion in breast milk unknown/use caution

Use Treatment of erectile dysfunction; treatment of pulmonary arterial hypertension

Unlabeled/Investigational Use Psychotropic-induced sexual dysfunction; pulmonary arterial hypertension in children

Mechanism of Action/Effect Sildenafil enhances the effect of nitric oxide by inhibiting phosphodiesterase type 5 (PDE-5), resulting in smooth muscle relaxation. In erectile dysfunction, smooth muscle relaxation results in the inflow of blood into the corpus cavernosum with sexual stimulation. In pulmonary hypertension, smooth muscle relaxation results in pulmonary vasculature; vasodilation reducing pulmonary pressure.

Contraindications Hypersensitivity to sildenafil or any component of the formulation; concurrent use of organic nitrates (nitroglycerin) in any form (potentiates the hypotensive effects)

Warnings/Precautions Decreases in blood pressure may occur due to vasodilator effects; use caution in patients with resting hypotension (BP <90/50), hypertension (BP >170/110), fluid depletion, severe left ventricular outflow obstruction, autonomic dysfunction, or taking alpha-blockers. Not recommended for use with pulmonary veno-occlusive disease.

Use caution in patients with cardiovascular disease, including cardiac failure, unstable angina, or a recent history (within the last 6 months) of myocardial infarction, stroke, or life-threatening arrhythmia. Use caution in patients receiving concurrent bosentan.

There is a degree of cardiac risk associated with sexual activity; therefore, physicians may wish to consider the cardiovascular status of their patients prior to initiating any treatment for erectile dysfunction. Sildenafil should be used with caution in patients with anatomical deformation of the penis (angulation, cavernosal fibrosis, or Peyronie's disease), or in patients who have conditions which may predispose them to priapism (sickle cell anemia, multiple myeloma, leukemia).

Rare cases of nonarteritic ischemic optic neuropathy (NAION) have been reported; risk may be increased with history of vision loss. Other risk factors for NAION include low cup-to-disc ratio ("crowded disc"), coronary artery disease, diabetes, hypertension, hyperlipidemia, smoking, and age >50 years.

The safety and efficacy of sildenafil with other treatments for erectile dysfunction have not been established; use is not recommended. May cause dose-related impairment of color discrimination. Use caution in patients with retinitis pigmentosa; a minority have generic disorders of retinal phosphodiesterases (no safety information available). Safety and efficacy in pediatric patients have not been established.

Drug Interactions
Cytochrome P450 Effect: Substrate of CYP2C8/9 (minor), 3A4 (major); **Inhibits** CYP1A2 (weak), 2C8/9 (weak), 2C19 (weak), 2D6 (weak), 2E1 (weak), 3A4 (weak)

Decreased Effect: Enzyme inducers (including phenytoin, carbamazepine, phenobarbital, rifampin) may decrease the serum concentration and efficacy of sildenafil. Bosentan may decrease serum concentration and effect of sildenafil.

Increased Effect/Toxicity: Sildenafil potentiates the hypotensive effects of nitrates (amyl nitrate, isosorbide dinitrate, isosorbide mononitrate, nitroglycerin); severe reactions have occurred and concurrent use is contraindicated. Concomitant use of alpha-blockers (doxazosin) may lead to symptomatic hypotension in some patients (sildenafil in doses >25 mg should not be given within 4 hours of administering an alpha-blocker). Macrolide antibiotics may increase the effects of sildenafil.

CYP3A4 inhibitors may increase the levels/effects of sildenafil; example inhibitors include azole antifungals, clarithromycin, diclofenac, doxycycline, erythromycin, imatinib, isoniazid, nefazodone, nicardipine, propofol, protease inhibitors, quinidine, telithromycin, and verapamil. Sildenafil may potentiate the effect of other antihypertensives. Sildenafil may potentiate bleeding in patients receiving heparin. Reduce sildenafil dose to 25 mg/24 hours in patients receiving azole antifungals or protease inhibitors (use of Revatio™ with concurrent protease inhibitors is not recommended).

Nutritional/Ethanol Interactions
Food: Amount and rate of absorption of sildenafil is reduced when taken with a high-fat meal. Serum concentrations/toxicity may be increased with grapefruit juice; avoid concurrent use.
Herb/Nutraceutical: St John's wort may decrease sildenafil levels.

Adverse Reactions Based upon normal doses. (Adverse effects such as flushing, diarrhea, myalgia, and visual disturbances may be increased with doses >100 mg/24 hours.)
>10%:
Central nervous system: Headache (16% to 46%)
Gastrointestinal: Dyspepsia (7% to 17%)
1% to 10%:
Cardiovascular: Flushing (10%)
Central nervous system: Dizziness, insomnia, pyrexia
(Continued)

Sildenafil (Continued)

Dermatologic: Erythema, rash

Gastrointestinal: Diarrhea (3% to 9%), gastritis

Genitourinary: Urinary tract infection

Hematologic: Anemia, leukopenia

Hepatic: LFTs increased

Neuromuscular & skeletal: Myalgia, paresthesia

Ocular: Abnormal vision (color changes, blurred or increased sensitivity to light 3%; up to 11% with doses >100 mg)

Respiratory: Dyspnea exacerbated, epistaxis, nasal congestion, rhinitis, sinusitis

Overdosage/Toxicology In studies with healthy volunteers of single doses up to 800 mg, adverse events were similar to those seen at lower doses but incidence rates were increased. Dialysis not likely to be beneficial due to protein binding.

Pharmacodynamics/Kinetics

Onset of Action: ~60 minutes

Duration of Action: 2-4 hours

Time to Peak: 30-120 minutes; delayed by 60 minutes with a high-fat meal

Protein Binding: Plasma: ~96%

Half-Life Elimination: 4 hours

Metabolism: Hepatic via CYP3A4 (major) and CYP2C9 (minor route)

Excretion: Feces (80%); urine (13%)

Available Dosage Forms Tablet:

Revatio™: 20 mg

Viagra®: 25 mg, 50 mg, 100 mg

Dosing

Adults:

Erectile dysfunction (Viagra®): Oral: For most patients, the recommended dose is 50 mg taken as needed, approximately 1 hour before sexual activity. However, sildenafil may be taken anywhere from 30 minutes to 4 hours before sexual activity. Based on effectiveness and tolerance, the dose may be increased to a maximum recommended dose of 100 mg or decreased to 25 mg. The maximum recommended dosing frequency is once daily.

Pulmonary arterial hypertension (Revatio™): Oral: 20 mg 3 times/day, taken 4-6 hours apart

Dosage adjustment for patients >65 years of age: Hepatic impairment (cirrhosis), severe renal impairment (creatinine clearance <30 mL/minute): Higher plasma levels have been associated which may result in increase in efficacy and adverse effects; Viagra®: Starting dose of 25 mg should be considered

Dosage considerations for patients taking alpha blockers: Viagra®: Doses of 50 or 100 mg, should not be taken within 4 hours of an alpha blocker; doses of 25 mg may be given at any time

Dosage adjustment for concomitant use of potent CYP34A inhibitors:

Revatio™:

Erythromycin, saquinavir: No dosage adjustment

Itraconazole, ketoconazole, ritonavir: Not recommended

Viagra®:

Erythromycin, itraconazole, ketoconazole, saquinavir: Starting dose of 25 mg should be considered

Ritonavir: Maximum: 25 mg every 48 hours

Elderly: Initial: 25 mg, 1 hour before sexual activity. Age >65 years was associated with increased serum sildenafil concentrations which may increase side effects and efficacy.

Renal Impairment: Cl$_{cr}$ <30 mL/minute: Initial: 25 mg, 1 hour before sexual activity.

Hepatic Impairment: Hepatic impairment; cirrhosis: Initial: 25 mg, 1 hour before sexual activity.

Administration

Oral:

Revatio™: Administer tablets at least 4-6 hours apart

Viagra®: Administer orally ~1 hour before sexual activity (may be used anytime from 4 hours to 30 minutes before).

Stability

Storage: Store tablets at controlled room temperature of 15°C to 30°C (59°F to 86°F).

Nursing Actions

Physical Assessment: Monitor other medications patient may be taking for effectiveness and interactions. Instruct patient on appropriate use and cautions, possible side effects, and symptoms to report.

Patient Education: Inform prescriber of all other medications you are taking; serious side effects can result when sildenafil is used with nitrates and some other medications. Do not combine sildenafil with other approaches to treating erectile dysfunction without consulting prescriber. **Note:** Sildenafil provides no protection against sexually-transmitted diseases, including HIV. You may experience headache, flushing, or abnormal vision (color changes, blurred or increased sensitivity to light); use caution when driving at night or in poorly lit environments. Report immediately acute allergic reactions; chest pain or palpitations; persistent dizziness; sign of urinary tract infection; skin rash; respiratory difficulty; change in vision; genital swelling; or other adverse reactions. If erection lasts longer than 4 hours, contact prescriber immediately; permanent damage to the penis can occur.

Pregnancy Issues There are no adequate and well-controlled studies in pregnant women.

Additional Information Sildenafil is ~10 times more selective for PDE-5 as compared to PDE6. This enzyme is found in the retina and is involved in phototransduction. At higher plasma levels, interference with PDE6 is believed to be the basis for changes in color vision noted in some patients.

Silver Sulfadiazine (SIL ver sul fa DYE a zeen)

U.S. Brand Names Silvadene®; SSD®; SSD® AF; Thermazene®

Pharmacologic Category Antibiotic, Topical

Pregnancy Risk Factor B

Lactation For external use

Use Prevention and treatment of infection in second and third degree burns

Mechanism of Action/Effect Acts upon the bacterial cell wall and cell membrane. Bactericidal for many gram-negative and gram-positive bacteria and is effective against yeast. Active against *Pseudomonas aeruginosa*, *Pseudomonas maltophilia*, *Enterobacter* species, *Klebsiella* species, *Serratia* species, *Escherichia coli*, *Proteus mirabilis*, *Morganella morganii*, *Providencia rettgeri*, *Proteus vulgaris*, *Providencia* species, *Citrobacter* species, *Acinetobacter calcoaceticus*, *Staphylococcus aureus*, *Staphylococcus epidermidis*, *Enterococcus* species, *Candida albicans*, *Corynebacterium diphtheriae*, and *Clostridium perfringens*

Contraindications Hypersensitivity to silver sulfadiazine or any component of the formulation; premature infants or neonates <2 months of age (sulfonamides may displace bilirubin and cause kernicterus); pregnancy (approaching or at term)

Warnings/Precautions Use with caution in patients with G6PD deficiency, renal impairment, or history of allergy to other sulfonamides. Sulfadiazine may accumulate in patients with impaired hepatic or renal function. Use of analgesic might be needed before application. Systemic absorption is significant and adverse reactions may be due to sulfa component.

Drug Interactions
Decreased Effect: Topical proteolytic enzymes are inactivated by silver sulfadiazine.

Adverse Reactions Frequency not defined.
Dermatologic: Itching, rash, erythema multiforme, discoloration of skin, photosensitivity
Hematologic: Hemolytic anemia, leukopenia, agranulocytosis, aplastic anemia
Hepatic: Hepatitis
Renal: Interstitial nephritis
Miscellaneous: Allergic reactions may be related to sulfa component

Pharmacodynamics/Kinetics
Time to Peak: Serum: 3-11 days of continuous therapy
Half-Life Elimination: 10 hours; prolonged with renal impairment
Excretion: Urine (~50% as unchanged drug)

Available Dosage Forms
Cream, topical: 1% (25 g, 50 mg, 85 g, 400 g)
Silvadene®, Thermazene®: 1% (20 g, 50 g, 85 g, 400 g, 1000 g)
SSD®: 1% (25 g, 50 g, 85 g, 400 g)
SSD® AF: 1% (50 g, 400 g)

Dosing
Adults & Elderly: Antiseptic, burns: Topical: Apply once or twice daily
Pediatrics: Refer to adult dosing.

Administration
Topical: Apply with a sterile-gloved hand. Apply to a thickness $^1/_{16}$". Burned area should be covered with cream at all times.

Stability
Storage: Discard if cream is darkened (reacts with heavy metals resulting in release of silver).

Laboratory Monitoring Serum electrolytes, urinalysis, renal function, CBC in patients with extensive burns on long-term treatment

Nursing Actions
Physical Assessment: Assess allergy history before treatment (sulfonamides). Assess results of laboratory tests, therapeutic effectiveness (development of granulation), adverse response (eg, rash, irritation, burning, itching of unburned areas). Monitor for hepatic, renal, or hematological response effects with long-term use or use over large areas.

Patient Education: Usually applied by professional in burn care setting. Patient instruction should be appropriate to extent of burn, patient understanding, etc.

Additional Information Contains methylparaben and propylene glycol

---

Simvastatin (SIM va stat in)

U.S. Brand Names Zocor®
Pharmacologic Category Antilipemic Agent, HMG-CoA Reductase Inhibitor
Medication Safety Issues
Sound-alike/look-alike issues:
Zocor® may be confused with Cozaar®, Yocon®, Zoloft®
Pregnancy Risk Factor X
Lactation Excretion in breast milk unknown/contraindicated
Use Used with dietary therapy for the following:
Secondary prevention of cardiovascular events in hypercholesterolemic patients with established coronary heart disease (CHD) or at high risk for CHD: To reduce cardiovascular morbidity (myocardial infarction, coronary revascularization procedures) and

mortality; to reduce the risk of stroke and transient ischemic attacks
Hyperlipidemias: To reduce elevations in total cholesterol, LDL-C, apolipoprotein B, and triglycerides in patients with primary hypercholesterolemia (elevations of 1 or more components are present in Fredrickson type IIa, IIb, III, and IV hyperlipidemias); treatment of homozygous familial hypercholesterolemia
Heterozygous familial hypercholesterolemia (HeFH): In adolescent patients (10-17 years of age, females >1 year postmenarche) with HeFH having LDL-C ≥190 mg/dL or LDL ≥160 mg/dL with positive family history of premature cardiovascular disease (CVD), or 2 or more CVD risk factors in the adolescent patient

Mechanism of Action/Effect Simvastatin is a derivative of lovastatin that acts by competitively inhibiting 3-hydroxy-3-methylglutaryl-coenzyme A (HMG-CoA) reductase, the enzyme that catalyzes the rate-limiting step in cholesterol biosynthesis; lowers total and LDL-cholesterol with increase in HDL

Contraindications Hypersensitivity to simvastatin or any component of the formulation; acute liver disease; unexplained persistent elevations of serum transaminases; pregnancy; breast-feeding

Warnings/Precautions Secondary causes of hyperlipidemia should be ruled out prior to therapy. Liver function must be monitored by laboratory assessment. Rhabdomyolysis with acute renal failure has occurred. Risk is dose-related and is increased with concurrent use of lipid-lowering agents which may cause rhabdomyolysis (gemfibrozil, fibric acid derivatives, or niacin at doses ≥1 g/day), during concurrent use with danazol or strong CYP3A4 inhibitors (including amiodarone, clarithromycin, cyclosporine, erythromycin, telithromycin, itraconazole, ketoconazole, nefazodone, grapefruit juice in large quantities, verapamil, or protease inhibitors such as indinavir, nelfinavir, or ritonavir). Weigh the risk versus benefit when combining any of these drugs with simvastatin. Do not initiate simvastatin-containing treatment in a patient with pre-existing therapy of cyclosporine or danazol, unless the patient has previously demonstrated tolerance to ≥5 mg/day simvastatin. Temporarily discontinue in any patient experiencing an acute or serious major medical or surgical condition which may increase the risk of rhabdomyolysis. Discontinue temporarily for elective surgical procedures. Use caution in patients with renal insufficiency. Use with caution in patients who consume large amounts of ethanol or have a history of liver disease. Safety and efficacy have not been established in patients <10 years or in premenarcheal girls.

Drug Interactions
Cytochrome P450 Effect: Substrate of CYP3A4 (major); **Inhibits** CYP2C8/9 (weak), 2D6 (weak)
Decreased Effect: When taken within 1 before or up to 2 hours after cholestyramine, a decrease in absorption of simvastatin can occur.

Increased Effect/Toxicity: Risk of myopathy/rhabdomyolysis may be increased by concurrent use of lipid-lowering agents which may cause rhabdomyolysis (gemfibrozil, fibric acid derivatives, or niacin at doses ≥1 g/day), or during concurrent use of strong CYP3A4 inhibitors.

CYP3A4 inhibitors may increase the levels/effects of simvastatin; example inhibitors include azole antifungals, clarithromycin, diclofenac, doxycycline, erythromycin, imatinib, isoniazid, nefazodone, nicardipine, propofol, protease inhibitors, quinidine, telithromycin, and verapamil. In large quantities (ie, >1 quart/day), grapefruit juice may also increase simvastatin serum concentrations, increasing the risk of rhabdomyolysis. In general, concurrent use with CYP3A4 inhibitors is not recommended; manufacturer recommends limiting simvastatin dose to 20 mg/day when used
(Continued)

Simvastatin (Continued)

with amiodarone or verapamil, and 10 mg/day when used with cyclosporine, gemfibrozil, or fibric acid derivatives.

The anticoagulant effect of warfarin may be increased by simvastatin. Cholesterol-lowering effects are additive with bile-acid sequestrants (colestipol and cholestyramine).

Nutritional/Ethanol Interactions

Ethanol: Avoid excessive ethanol consumption (due to potential hepatic effects).

Food: Simvastatin serum concentration may be increased when taken with grapefruit juice; avoid concurrent intake of large quantities (>1 quart/day). Red yeast rice contains an estimated 2.4 mg lovastatin per 600 mg rice.

Herb/Nutraceutical: St John's wort may decrease simvastatin levels.

Adverse Reactions 1% to 10%:

Gastrointestinal: Constipation (2%), dyspepsia (1%), flatulence (2%)

Neuromuscular & skeletal: CPK elevation (>3x normal on one or more occasions - 5%)

Respiratory: Upper respiratory infection (2%)

Additional class-related events or case reports (not necessarily reported with simvastatin therapy): Alopecia, alteration in taste, anaphylaxis, angioedema, anorexia, anxiety, arthritis, cataracts, chills, cholestatic jaundice, cirrhosis, decreased libido, depression, dermatomyositis, dryness of skin/mucous membranes, dyspnea, elevated transaminases, eosinophilia, erectile dysfunction/impotence, erythema multiforme, facial paresis, fatty liver, fever, flushing, fulminant hepatic necrosis, gynecomastia, hemolytic anemia, hepatitis, hepatoma, hyperbilirubinemia, hypersensitivity reaction, impaired extraocular muscle movement, increased alkaline phosphatase, increased CPK (>10x normal), increased ESR, increased GGT, leukopenia, malaise, memory loss, myopathy, nail changes, nodules, ophthalmoplegia, pancreatitis, paresthesia, peripheral nerve palsy, peripheral neuropathy, photosensitivity, polymyalgia rheumatica, positive ANA, pruritus, psychic disturbance, purpura, rash, renal failure (secondary to rhabdomyolysis), rhabdomyolysis, skin discoloration, Stevens-Johnson syndrome, systemic lupus erythematosus-like syndrome, thrombocytopenia, thyroid dysfunction, toxic epidermal necrolysis, tremor, urticaria, vasculitis, vertigo, vomiting

Overdosage/Toxicology Very few adverse events. Treatment is symptomatic.

Pharmacodynamics/Kinetics

Onset of Action: >3 days; Peak effect: 2 weeks

Time to Peak: 1.3-2.4 hours

Protein Binding: ~95%

Half-Life Elimination: Unknown

Metabolism: Hepatic via CYP3A4; extensive first-pass effect

Excretion: Feces (60%); urine (13%)

Available Dosage Forms Tablet: 5 mg, 10 mg, 20 mg, 40 mg, 80 mg

Dosing

Adults: Note: Doses should be individualized according to the baseline LDL-cholesterol levels, the recommended goal of therapy, and the patient's response; adjustments should be made at intervals of 4 weeks or more; doses may need adjusted based on concomitant medications

Homozygous familial hypercholesterolemia: Oral: 40 mg once daily in the evening **or** 80 mg/day (given as 20 mg, 20 mg, and 40 mg evening dose)

Prevention of cardiovascular events, hyperlipidemias: Oral: 20-40 mg once daily in the evening; range: 5-80 mg/day

Patients requiring only moderate reduction of LDL-cholesterol: May be started at 10 mg once daily

Patients requiring reduction of >45% in low-density lipoprotein (LDL) cholesterol: May be started at 40 mg once daily in the evening

Patients with CHD or at high risk for CHD: Dosing should be started at 40 mg once daily in the evening; simvastatin may be started simultaneously with diet

Dosage adjustment for simvastatin with concomitant medications:

Cyclosporine or danazol: Patient must first demonstrate tolerance to simvastatin ≥5 mg once daily: Initial: 5 mg, should **not** exceed 10 mg/day

Fibrates or niacin: Dose should **not** exceed 10 mg/day

Amiodarone or verapamil: Dose should **not** exceed 20 mg/day

Elderly: Oral: Initial: Maximum reductions in LDL-cholesterol may be achieved with daily dose ≤20 mg.

Pediatrics: HeFH: Oral: Children 10-17 years (females >1 year postmenarche): 10 mg once daily in the evening; range: 10-40 mg/day (maximum: 40 mg/day)

Dosage adjustment with concomitant medications: With concomitant cyclosporine, danazol, fibrates, niacin, amiodarone, or verapamil: Refer to adult dosing.

Note: Doses should be individualized according to the baseline LDL-cholesterol levels, the recommended goal of therapy, and the patient's response; adjustments should be made at intervals of 4 weeks or more; doses may need adjusted based on concomitant medications

Renal Impairment: Because simvastatin does not undergo significant renal excretion, modification of dose should not be necessary in patients with mild to moderate renal insufficiency.

Severe renal impairment: Cl_{cr} <10 mL/minute: Initial: 5 mg/day with close monitoring.

Administration

Oral: May be taken without regard to meals.

Stability

Storage: Tablets should be stored in tightly-closed containers at temperatures between 5°C to 30°C (41°F to 86°F).

Laboratory Monitoring Creatine phosphokinase levels due to possibility of myopathy; serum cholesterol (total and fractionated)

Obtain liver function tests prior to initiation, dose, and thereafter when clinically indicated. Patients titrated to the 80 mg dose should be tested prior to initiation and 3 months after initiating the 80 mg dose. Thereafter, periodic monitoring (ie, semiannually) is recommended for the first year of treatment. Patients with elevated transaminase levels should have a second (confirmatory) test and frequent monitoring until values normalize. Discontinue if increase in ALT/AST is persistently >3 times ULN.

Nursing Actions

Physical Assessment: Assess potential for interactions with other pharmacological agents or herbal products patient may be taking (eg, gemfibrozil, fibric acid derivatives, niacin may increase risk of myopathy or rhabdomyolysis). Monitor laboratory tests and patient response on a regular basis throughout therapy (eg. rash, myalgia, blurred vision, abdominal pain, cough). Teach patient proper use (as addition to diet and exercise regimen), possible side effects/appropriate interventions, and adverse symptoms to report. **Pregnancy risk factor X:** Determine that patient is not pregnant before starting therapy. Do not give to women of childbearing age unless they are capable of complying with effective contraceptive use.

Instruct patient in appropriate contraceptive measures.

Patient Education: Do not take any new medication during therapy without consulting prescriber. Take at same time each day with or without food. Follow cholesterol-lowering diet and exercise regimen as prescribed. Avoid grapefruit juice and excessive alcohol while taking this medication. You will have periodic blood tests to assess effectiveness. May cause mild GI upset (should diminish with use); constipation (increased exercise, fluids, fiber, and fruit may help); headache, dizziness, insomnia (use caution when driving or engaged in potentially hazardous tasks until response to drug in known). Report unusual chest pain, swelling of extremities, weight gain of >5 lb/week, persistent cough; CNS changes (dizziness, memory loss, depression, or vision changes). Contact prescriber immediately with persistent muscle or skeletal pain, joint pain, or numbness, or any sign of allergic reactions (skin rash, difficulty breathing, tightness in throat, choking sensation, swelling of mouth or face). **Pregnancy/breast-feeding precautions:** Inform prescriber if you are pregnant. Do not get pregnant during and for 1 month following therapy. Consult prescriber for appropriate contraceptive measures. This drug may cause severe fetal defects. Do not donate blood during or for 1 month following therapy. Do not breast feed.

Dietary Considerations Red yeast rice contains an estimated 2.4 mg lovastatin per 600 mg rice.

Geriatric Considerations Effective and well tolerated in the elderly. The definition of and, therefore, when to treat hyperlipidemia in the elderly is a controversial issue. The National Cholesterol Education Program recommends that all adults maintain a plasma cholesterol <160 mg/dL. In elderly patients with one additional risk factor, goal LDL would decrease to <130 mg/dL. Pharmacologic treatment should be reserved for those who are unable to obtain a desirable plasma cholesterol concentration by diet alone and for whom the benefits of treatment are believed to outweigh the potential adverse effects, drug interactions, and cost of treatment.

Breast-Feeding Issues Excretion in breast milk is unknown, but would be expected; other medications in this class are excreted in human milk. Breast-feeding is contraindicated.

Pregnancy Issues Cholesterol biosynthesis may be important in fetal development. Contraindicated in pregnancy. Administer to women of childbearing potential only when conception is highly unlikely and patients have been informed of potential hazards.

Sirolimus (sir OH li mus)

U.S. Brand Names Rapamune®
Pharmacologic Category Immunosuppressant Agent
Pregnancy Risk Factor C
Lactation Excretion in breast milk unknown/not recommended
Use Prophylaxis of organ rejection in patients receiving renal transplants, in combination with corticosteroids and cyclosporine (cyclosporine may be withdrawn in low-to-moderate immunological risk patients after 2-4 months, in conjunction with an increase in sirolimus dosage)

Unlabeled/Investigational Use Investigational: Immunosuppression in other forms of solid organ transplantation and peripheral stem cell/bone marrow transplantation

Mechanism of Action/Effect Sirolimus inhibits T-lymphocyte activation and proliferation in response to antigenic and cytokine stimulation. Its mechanism differs from other immunosuppressants. It inhibits acute rejection of allografts and prolongs graft survival.

Contraindications Hypersensitivity to sirolimus or any component of the formulation

Warnings/Precautions Immunosuppressive agents, including sirolimus, increase the risk of infection and may be associated with the development of lymphoma. May increase serum lipids (cholesterol and triglycerides). Use with caution in patients with hyperlipidemia. May increase serum creatinine and decrease GFR. Use caution in patients with renal impairment, or when used concurrently with medications which may alter renal function. Monitor renal function closely when combined with cyclosporine; consider dosage adjustment or discontinue in patients with increasing serum creatinine. Has been associated with an increased risk of lymphocele. Cases of interstitial lung disease (eg, pneumonitis, bronchiolitis obliterans organizing pneumonia, pulmonary fibrosis) have been observed; risk may be increased with higher trough levels. Avoid concurrent use of strong CYP3A4 inhibitors or strong inducers of either CYP3A4 or P-glycoprotein. Concurrent use with a calcineurin inhibitor (cyclosporine, tacrolimus) may increase the risk of calcineurin inhibitor-induced hemolytic uremic syndrome/thrombotic thrombocytopenic purpura/thrombotic microangiopathy (HUS/TTP/TMA). Anaphylactic reactions, angioedema and hypersensitivity vasculitis have been reported. May increase sensitivity to UV light; use appropriate sun protection.

Sirolimus is not recommended for use in liver transplant patients; studies indicate an association with an increase risk of hepatic artery thrombosis and graft failure in these patients. Cases of bronchial anastomotic dehiscence have been reported in lung transplant patients when sirolimus was used as part of an immunosuppressive regimen; most of these reactions were fatal. Use in patients with lung transplants is not recommended. Safety and efficacy of cyclosporine withdrawal in high-risk patients is not currently recommended. Safety and efficacy in children <13 years of age, or in adolescent patients <18 years of age considered at high immunological risk, have not been established.

Drug Interactions
Cytochrome P450 Effect: Substrate of CYP3A4 (major); Inhibits CYP3A4 (weak)
Decreased Effect: CYP3A4 inducers may decrease the levels/effects of sirolimus; example inducers include aminoglutethimide, carbamazepine, nafcillin, nevirapine, phenobarbital, phenytoin, and rifamycins.

Increased Effect/Toxicity: Cyclosporine increases sirolimus concentrations during concurrent therapy, and cyclosporine levels may be increased; sirolimus should be taken 4 hours after cyclosporine oral solution (modified) and/or cyclosporine capsules (modified). CYP3A4 inhibitors may increase the levels/effects of sirolimus; example inhibitors include azole antifungals, clarithromycin, diclofenac, diltiazem, doxycycline, erythromycin, imatinib, isoniazid, nefazodone, nicardipine, propofol, protease inhibitors, quinidine, telithromycin, and verapamil; avoid concurrent use. Vaccination may be less effective and use of live vaccines should be avoided during sirolimus therapy. Concurrent therapy with calcineurin inhibitors (cyclosporine, tacrolimus) may increase the risk of HUS/TTP/TMA.

Nutritional/Ethanol Interactions
Food: Do not administer with grapefruit juice; may decrease clearance of sirolimus. Ingestion with high-fat meals decreases peak concentrations but increases AUC by 35%. Sirolimus should be taken consistently either with or without food to minimize variability.

Herb/Nutraceutical: St John's wort may decrease sirolimus levels; avoid concurrent use. Avoid cat's claw, echinacea (have immunostimulant properties; consider therapy modifications).

Adverse Reactions Incidence of many adverse effects is dose related
(Continued)

Sirolimus *(Continued)*

>20%:

Cardiovascular: Hypertension (39% to 49%), peripheral edema (54% to 64%), edema (16% to 24%), chest pain (16% to 24%)

Central nervous system: Fever (23% to 34%), headache (23% to 34%), pain (24% to 33%), insomnia (13% to 22%)

Dermatologic: Acne (20% to 31%)

Endocrine & metabolic: Hypercholesterolemia (38% to 46%), hypophosphatemia (15% to 23%), hyperlipidemia (38% to 57%), hypokalemia (11% to 21%)

Gastrointestinal: Abdominal pain (28% to 36%), nausea (25% to 36%), vomiting (19% to 25%), diarrhea (25% to 42%), constipation (28% to 38%), dyspepsia (17% to 25%), weight gain (8% to 21%)

Genitourinary: Urinary tract infection (20% to 33%)

Hematologic: Anemia (23% to 37%), thrombocytopenia (13% to 40%)

Neuromuscular & skeletal: Arthralgia (25% to 31%), weakness (22% to 40%), back pain (16% to 26%), tremor (21% to 31%)

Renal: Increased serum creatinine (35% to 40%)

Respiratory: Dyspnea (22% to 30%), upper respiratory infection (20% to 26%), pharyngitis (16% to 21%)

3% to 20%:

Cardiovascular: Atrial fibrillation, CHF, hypervolemia, hypotension, palpitation, peripheral vascular disorder, postural hypotension, syncope, tachycardia, thrombosis, vasodilation, venous thromboembolism

Central nervous system: Chills, malaise, anxiety, confusion, depression, dizziness, emotional lability, hypoesthesia, hypotonia, insomnia, neuropathy, somnolence

Dermatologic: Dermatitis (fungal), hirsutism, pruritus, skin hypertrophy, dermal ulcer, ecchymosis, cellulitis, rash (10% to 20%)

Endocrine & metabolic: Cushing's syndrome, diabetes mellitus, glycosuria, acidosis, dehydration, hypercalcemia, hyperglycemia, hyperphosphatemia, hypocalcemia, hypoglycemia, hypomagnesemia, hyponatremia, hyperkalemia (12% to 17%)

Gastrointestinal: Enlarged abdomen, anorexia, dysphagia, eructation, esophagitis, flatulence, gastritis, gastroenteritis, gingivitis, gingival hyperplasia, ileus, mouth ulceration, oral moniliasis, stomatitis, weight loss

Genitourinary: Pelvic pain, scrotal edema, testis disorder, impotence

Hematologic: Leukocytosis, polycythemia, TTP, hemolytic-uremic syndrome, hemorrhage, leukopenia (9% to 15%)

Hepatic: Abnormal liver function tests, alkaline phosphatase increased, ascites, LDH increased, transaminases increased

Local: Thrombophlebitis

Neuromuscular & skeletal: Increased CPK, arthrosis, bone necrosis, leg cramps, myalgia, osteoporosis, tetany, hypertonia, paresthesia

Ocular: Abnormal vision, cataract, conjunctivitis

Otic: Ear pain, deafness, otitis media, tinnitus

Renal: Increased BUN, albuminuria, bladder pain, dysuria, hematuria, hydronephrosis, kidney pain, tubular necrosis, nocturia, oliguria, pyuria, nephropathy (toxic), urinary frequency, urinary incontinence, urinary retention

Respiratory: Asthma, atelectasis, bronchitis, cough, epistaxis, hypoxia, lung edema, pleural effusion, pneumonia, rhinitis, sinusitis

Miscellaneous: Abscess, diaphoresis, facial edema, flu-like syndrome, hernia, infection, lymphadenopathy, lymphocele, peritonitis, sepsis

Overdosage/Toxicology Experience with overdosage has been limited. Dose-limiting toxicities include immune suppression. Reported symptoms of overdose include atrial fibrillation. Treatment is supportive, dialysis is not likely to facilitate removal.

Pharmacodynamics/Kinetics

Time to Peak: 1-2 hours

Protein Binding: 92%, primarily to albumin

Half-Life Elimination: Mean: 62 hours

Metabolism: Extensively hepatic via CYP3A4; P-glycoprotein-mediated efflux into gut lumen

Excretion: Feces (91%); urine (2%)

Available Dosage Forms

Solution, oral [bottle]: 1 mg/mL (60 mL) [contains ethanol 1.5% to 2.5%; packaged with oral syringes and a carrying case]

Tablet: 1 mg, 2 mg

Dosing

Adults & Elderly:

Immunosuppression: Oral:

Combination therapy with cyclosporine: For *de novo* transplant recipients, a loading dose of 3 times the daily maintenance dose should be administered on day 1 of dosing. Doses should be taken 4 hours after cyclosporine, and should be taken consistently either with or without food.

Dosing by body weight:

<40 kg: Loading dose: Loading dose: 3 mg/m² on day 1, followed by a maintenance dosing of 1 mg/m²/day

≥40 kg: Loading dose: 6 mg on day 1; maintenance: 2 mg/day

Maintenance therapy after withdrawal of cyclosporine:

Following 2-4 months of combined therapy, withdrawal of cyclosporine may be considered in low-to-moderate risk patients. Cyclosporine withdrawal in not recommended in high immunological risk patients. Cyclosporine should be discontinued over 4-8 weeks, and a necessary increase in the dosage of sirolimus (up to fourfold) should be anticipated due to removal of metabolic inhibition by cyclosporine and to maintain adequate immunosuppressive effects.

Sirolimus dosages should be adjusted to maintain trough concentrations of 12-24 ng/mL. Dosage should be adjusted at intervals of 7-14 days to account for the long half-life of sirolimus. Considerable increases in dosage may require an additional loading dose, calculated as the difference between the target concentration and the current concentration, multiplied by a factor of 3. Loading doses >40 mg may be administered over two days. Serum concentrations should not be used as the sole basis for dosage adjustment (monitor clinical signs/symptoms, tissue biopsy, and laboratory parameters).

Pediatrics:

Immunosuppression: Children ≥13 years: Oral: Refer to adult dosing.

Renal Impairment: No adjustment is necessary.

Hepatic Impairment: Reduce maintenance dose by approximately 33% in hepatic impairment. Loading dose is unchanged.

Administration

Oral: The solution should be mixed with at least 2 ounces of water or orange juice. No other liquids should be used for dilution. Patient should drink diluted solution immediately. The cup should then be refilled with an additional 4 ounces of water or orange juice, stirred vigorously, and the patient should drink the contents at once.

Stability

Storage:

Oral solution: Protect from light and store under refrigeration, 2°C to 8°C (36°F to 46°F). A slight haze may develop in refrigerated solutions, but the quality of the product is not affected. After opening, solution should be used in 1 month. If necessary, may be stored at temperatures up to 25°C (77°F) for several days after opening (up to 24 hours for pouches and not >15 days for bottles). Product may be stored in amber syringe for a maximum of 24 hours (at room temperature or refrigerated). Solution should be used immediately following dilution.

Tablet: Store at room temperature of 20°C to 25°C (68°F to 77°F). Protect from light.

Laboratory Monitoring Monitor sirolimus levels in pediatric patients, patients ≥13 years of age weighing <40 kg, patients with hepatic impairment, or on concurrent potent inhibitors or inducers of CYP3A4, and/or if cyclosporine dosing is markedly reduced or discontinued. Also monitor serum cholesterol and triglycerides and serum creatinine. Serum drug concentrations should be determined 3-4 days after loading doses; however, these concentrations should not be used as the sole basis for dosage adjustment, especially during withdrawal of cyclosporine (monitor clinical signs/symptoms, tissue biopsy, and laboratory parameters).

Nursing Actions
Physical Assessment: Assess effectiveness and interactions of other medications. Monitor laboratory tests at beginning and periodically during therapy. Monitor therapeutic response and adverse reactions and toxicity. Monitor blood pressure and renal function. Assess for signs of fluid retention and infection. Assess knowledge/teach patient appropriate use, interventions to reduce side effects, and adverse reactions to report.

Patient Education: Do not alter dose or discontinue without consulting prescriber. Do not ever mix sirolimus solution with anything other than water or orange juice (avoid taking with grapefruit juice). May be taken with or without food, but should be taken consistently with regard to food (always on an empty stomach or always with food). Consult prescriber about timing of any other prescribed or OTC medications. Maintain adequate hydration (2-3 L/day of fluids) unless instructed to restrict fluid intake. You will be susceptible to infection (avoid crowds and exposure to infection). If you have diabetes, monitor glucose levels closely (drug may alter glucose levels). Limit exposure to sunlight by wearing protective clothing or sunscreen. You may experience nausea, vomiting, loss of appetite (small frequent meals, good mouth care, chewing gum, or sucking hard candy may help); constipation (increase exercise, fluids, fruit, or fiber may help); or diarrhea (yogurt or buttermilk); or muscle or back pain (mild analgesic). Inform prescriber of any adverse effects including, but not limited to, unresolved GI problems; respiratory difficulty, cough, infection; skin rash or irritation; headache, insomnia, anxiety, confusion, emotional lability; changes in voiding pattern, burning, itching, or pain on urination; persistent bone, joint, or muscle cramping, pain or weakness; chest pain, palpitations, swelling of extremities; weight gain of 3-5 pounds per week; vision changes or hearing; or any other adverse reactions. **Pregnancy/breast-feeding precautions:** Inform prescriber if you are or intend to become pregnant. Breast-feeding is not recommended.

Dietary Considerations Take consistently, with or without food, to minimize variability of absorption.

Pregnancy Issues Effective contraception must be initiated before therapy with sirolimus and continued for 12 weeks after discontinuation.

Additional Information Sirolimus tablets and oral solution are not bioequivalent, due to differences in absorption. Clinical equivalence was seen using 2 mg tablet and 2 mg solution. It is not known if higher doses are also clinically equivalent.

Sodium Bicarbonate
(SOW dee um bye KAR bun ate)

U.S. Brand Names Brioschi® [OTC]; Neut®
Synonyms Baking Soda; NaHCO$_3$; Sodium Acid Carbonate; Sodium Hydrogen Carbonate
Pharmacologic Category Alkalinizing Agent; Antacid; Electrolyte Supplement, Oral; Electrolyte Supplement, Parenteral
Pregnancy Risk Factor C
Lactation Enters breast milk/compatible
Use Management of metabolic acidosis; gastric hyperacidity; as an alkalinization agent for the urine; treatment of hyperkalemia; management of overdose of certain drugs, including tricyclic antidepressants and aspirin
Mechanism of Action/Effect Dissociates to provide bicarbonate ion which neutralizes hydrogen ion concentration and raises blood and urinary pH
Contraindications Alkalosis, hypernatremia, severe pulmonary edema, hypocalcemia, unknown abdominal pain
Warnings/Precautions Use of I.V. NaHCO$_3$ should be reserved for documented metabolic acidosis and for hyperkalemia-induced cardiac arrest. Routine use in cardiac arrest is not recommended. Avoid extravasation, tissue necrosis can occur due to the hypertonicity of NaHCO$_3$. May cause sodium retention especially if renal function is impaired; not to be used in treatment of peptic ulcer; use with caution in patients with CHF, edema, cirrhosis, or renal failure. Not the antacid of choice for the elderly because of sodium content and potential for systemic alkalosis.
Drug Interactions
Decreased Effect: Decreased effect/levels of lithium, chlorpropamide, and salicylates due to urinary alkalinization.
Increased Effect/Toxicity: Increased toxicity/levels of amphetamines, ephedrine, pseudoephedrine, flecainide, quinidine, and quinine due to urinary alkalinization.
Nutritional/Ethanol Interactions Herb/Nutraceutical: Concurrent doses with iron may decrease iron absorption.
Adverse Reactions Frequency not defined.
Cardiovascular: Cerebral hemorrhage, CHF (aggravated), edema
Central nervous system: Tetany
Gastrointestinal: Belching, flatulence (with oral), gastric distension
Endocrine & metabolic: Hypernatremia, hyperosmolality, hypocalcemia, hypokalemia, increased affinity of hemoglobin for oxygen-reduced pH in myocardial tissue necrosis when extravasated, intracranial acidosis, metabolic alkalosis, milk-alkali syndrome (especially with renal dysfunction)
Respiratory: Pulmonary edema
Overdosage/Toxicology Symptoms of overdose include hypocalcemia, hypokalemia, hypernatremia, and seizures. Treatment is symptom-directed and supportive.
Pharmacodynamics/Kinetics
Onset of Action: Oral: Rapid; I.V.: 15 minutes
Duration of Action: Oral: 8-10 minutes; I.V.: 1-2 hours
Excretion: Urine (<1%)
Available Dosage Forms
Granules, effervescent (Brioschi®): 2.69 g/packet (6 g) [unit-dose packets; contains sodium 770 mg/packet; lemon flavor]; 2.69 g/capful (120 g, 240 g) [contains sodium 770 mg/capful; lemon flavor]
Infusion [premixed in sterile water]: 5% (500 mL)
Injection, solution:
4.2% [42 mg/mL = 5 mEq/10 mL] (10 mL)
7.5% [75 mg/mL = 8.92 mEq/10 mL] (50 mL)
(Continued)

Sodium Bicarbonate *(Continued)*

8.4% [84 mg/mL = 10 mEq/10 mL] (10 mL, 50 mL)

Neut®: 4% [40 mg/mL = 2.4 mEq/5 mL] (5 mL)

Powder: Sodium bicarbonate USP (120 g, 480 g) [contains sodium 30 mEq per ½ teaspoon]

Tablet: 325 mg [3.8 mEq]; 650 mg [7.6 mEq]

Dosing

Adults & Elderly:

Cardiac arrest: I.V.: Initial: 1 mEq/kg/dose one time; maintenance: 0.5 mEq/kg/dose every 10 minutes or as indicated by arterial blood gases

Note: Routine use of NaHCO₃ is not recommended and should be given only after adequate alveolar ventilation has been established and effective cardiac compressions are provided

Metabolic acidosis: I.V.: Dosage should be based on the following formula if blood gases and pH measurements are available:

$HCO_3^-(mEq) = 0.2 \times weight (kg) \times base\ deficit (mEq/L)$

Administer ½ dose initially, then remaining ½ dose over the next 24 hours; monitor pH, serum HCO_3^-, and clinical status

Note: If acid-base status is not available: 2-5 mEq/kg I.V. infusion over 4-8 hours; subsequent doses should be based on patient's acid-base status

Hyperkalemia: I.V.: 1 mEq/kg over 5 minutes

Chronic renal failure: I.V.: Initiate when plasma HCO_3^- <15 mEq/L Start with 20-36 mEq/day in divided doses, titrate to bicarbonate level of 18-20 mEq/L

Renal tubular acidosis: Oral:

Distal: 0.5-2 mEq/kg/day in 4-5 divided doses

Proximal: Initial: 5-10 mEq/kg/day; maintenance: Increase as required to maintain serum bicarbonate in the normal range

Urine alkalinization: Oral: Initial: 48 mEq (4 g), then 12-24 mEq (1-2 g) every 4 hours; dose should be titrated to desired urinary pH; doses up to 16 g/day (200 mEq) in patients <60 years and 8 g (100 mEq) in patients >60 years

Antacid: Oral: 325 mg to 2 g 1-4 times/day

Pediatrics:

Cardiac arrest: I.V.: Infants and Children: 0.5-1 mEq/kg/dose repeated every 10 minutes or as indicated by arterial blood gases; rate of infusion should not exceed 10 mEq/minute; neonates and children <2 years of age should receive 4.2% (0.5 mEq/mL) solution.

Note: Routine use of NaHCO₃ is not recommended and should be given only after adequate alveolar ventilation has been established and effective cardiac compressions are provided

Metabolic acidosis: I.V.: Infants and Children: Dosage should be based on the following formula if blood gases and pH measurements are available:

$HCO_3^-\ (mEq) = 0.3 \times weight (kg) \times base\ deficit (mEq/L)$

Administer ½ dose initially, then remaining ½ dose over the next 24 hours; monitor pH, serum HCO_3^-, and clinical status

Note: If acid-base status is not available: Dose for older Children: 2-5 mEq/kg I.V. infusion over 4-8 hours; subsequent doses should be based on patient's acid-base status.

Chronic renal failure: Oral: Children: Initiate when plasma HCO_3^- <15 mEq/L: 1-3 mEq/kg/day

Renal tubular acidosis, distal: Oral: Children: 2-3 mEq/kg/day

Renal tubular acidosis, proximal: Children: Initial: 5-10 mEq/kg/day; maintenance: Increase as required to maintain serum bicarbonate in the normal range

Urine alkalinization: Oral: Children: 1-10 mEq (84-840 mg)/kg/day in divided doses every 4-6 hours; dose should be titrated to desired urinary pH.

Administration

I.V. Detail: Observe for extravasation when giving I.V.

pH: 7.0-8.5

Stability

Compatibility: Stable in dextran 6% in dextrose, dextran 6% in NS, D₅¼NS, D₅½NS, D₅NS, D₅W, D₁₀W, ½NS, NS; incompatible with acids, acidic salts, alkaloid salts, calcium salts, catecholamines, and atropine

Y-site administration: Incompatible with allopurinol, amiodarone, amphotericin B cholesteryl sulfate complex, calcium chloride, doxorubicin liposome, idarubicin, imipenem/cilastatin inamrinone, leucovorin, midazolam, nalbuphine, ondansetron, oxacillin, sargramostim, verapamil, vincristine, vindesine, vinorelbine

Compatibility in syringe: Incompatible with etidocaine, glycopyrrolate, mepivacaine, metoclopramide, thiopental

Compatibility when admixed: Incompatible with amiodarone, ascorbic acid injection, carboplatin, carmustine, cefotaxime, ciprofloxacin, cisplatin, dobutamine, dopamine, epinephrine, hydromorphone, imipenem/cilastatin, isoproterenol, labetalol, levorphanol, magnesium sulfate, meropenem, morphine, norepinephrine, pentazocine, procaine, streptomycin, succinylcholine, ticarcillin/clavulanate potassium, vitamin B complex with C

Storage: Store injection at room temperature. Protect from heat and from freezing. Use only clear solutions.

Nursing Actions

Physical Assessment: Assess other medications patient may be taking for effectiveness and interactions (especially calcium channel blockers or cardiac glycosides). **I.V.:** Monitor therapeutic response (cardiac status, arterial blood gases, and electrolytes), adverse reactions (eg, CHF, tetany, intracranial acidosis), and monitor infusion site for patency (if extravasation occurs, elevate extravasation site and apply warm compresses). Teach patient adverse symptoms to report. **Oral:** Monitor effectiveness of treatment and adverse response. Assess knowledge/teach patient appropriate use, interventions to reduce side effects, and adverse symptoms to report.

Patient Education: Do not use for chronic gastric acidity. Take as directed. Chew tablets thoroughly and follow with a full glass of water, preferably on an empty stomach (2 hours before or after food). Report CNS effects (eg, irritability, confusion); muscle rigidity or tremors; swelling of feet or ankles; respiratory difficulty; chest pain or palpitations; respiratory changes; or tarry stools. **Pregnancy precaution:** Inform prescriber if you are or intend to become pregnant.

Dietary Considerations Oral product should be administered 1-3 hours after meals.

Sodium content:

Injection: 50 mL, 8.4% = 1150 mg = 50 mEq; each mL of 8.4% NaHCO₃ contains 23 mg sodium; 1 mEq NaHCO₃ = 84 mg

Granules: 2.69 g packet or capful = 770 mg sodium

Powder: 30 mEq sodium per ½ teaspoon

Geriatric Considerations Not the antacid of choice for the elderly because of sodium content and potential for systemic alkalosis (see maximum daily dose under Dosage).

Related Information

Compatibility of Drugs *on page 1370*

Sodium Citrate and Citric Acid
(SOW dee um SIT rate & SI trik AS id)

U.S. Brand Names Bicitra®; Cytra-2; Oracit®

Synonyms Modified Shohl's Solution

Pharmacologic Category Alkalinizing Agent, Oral

Pregnancy Risk Factor Not established

Lactation Excretion in breast milk unknown/compatible

Use Treatment of metabolic acidosis; alkalinizing agent in conditions where long-term maintenance of an alkaline urine is desirable

Available Dosage Forms Note: Contains sodium 1 mEq/mL and the equivalent to bicarbonate 1 mEq/mL
Solution, oral: Sodium citrate 500 mg and citric acid 334 mg per 5 mL (480 mL)
Bicitra®: Sodium citrate 500 mg and citric acid 334 mg per 5 mL (480 mL) [sugar free; grape flavor]
Cytra-2: Sodium citrate 500 mg and citric acid 334 mg per 5 mL (480 mL) [alcohol free, dye free, sugar free; grape flavor]
Oracit®: Sodium citrate 490 mg and citric acid 640 mg per 5 mL (15 mL, 30 mL, 500 mL, 3840 mL)

Dosing
Adults & Elderly: Systemic alkalization: Oral: 10-30 mL with water after meals and at bedtime
Pediatrics: Systemic alkalization: Oral: Infants and Children: 2-3 mEq/kg/day in divided doses 3-4 times/day **or** 5-15 mL with water after meals and at bedtime

Nursing Actions
Physical Assessment: Assess kidney function prior to starting therapy. Monitor cardiac status and serum potassium at beginning of therapy and at regular intervals with long-term therapy. Assess knowledge/teach patient appropriate use, possible side effects, and adverse symptoms to report.
Patient Education: Take as often as directed, after meals, and at least 2 hours before or after any other medications. Dilute with 1-3 oz of water and follow with additional water; chilling solution prior to taking will help to improve taste. You may experience diarrhea or nausea and vomiting; if severe, contact prescriber. Report CNS changes status (eg, irritability, tremors, confusion); swelling of feet or ankles; respiratory difficulty or palpitations; abdominal pain or tarry stools.

Sodium Polystyrene Sulfonate
(SOW dee um pol ee STYE reen SUL fon ate)

U.S. Brand Names Kayexalate®; Kionex™; SPS®

Pharmacologic Category Antidote

Medication Safety Issues
Sound-alike/look-alike issues:
Kayexalate® may be confused with Kaopectate®

Always prescribe either one-time doses or as a specific number of doses (eg, 15 g q6h x 2 doses). Scheduled doses with no dosage limit could be given for days leading to dangerous hypokalemia.

Pregnancy Risk Factor C

Lactation Excretion in breast milk unknown/use caution

Use Treatment of hyperkalemia

Mechanism of Action/Effect Removes potassium by exchanging sodium ions for potassium ions in the intestine before the resin is passed from the body; exchange capacity is 1 mEq/g in vivo, and in vitro capacity is 3.1 mEq/g, therefore, a wide range of exchange capacity exists such that close monitoring of serum electrolytes is necessary

Contraindications Hypersensitivity to sodium polystyrene sulfonate or any component of the formulation; hypernatremia, hypokalemia, obstructive bowel disease

Warnings/Precautions Use with caution in patients with severe CHF, hypertension, edema, or renal failure. Large oral doses may cause fecal impaction (especially in the elderly). Enema will reduce the serum potassium faster than oral administration, but the oral route will result in a greater reduction over several hours.

Drug Interactions
Increased Effect/Toxicity: Systemic alkalosis and seizure has occurred after cation-exchange resins were administered with nonabsorbable cation-donating antacids and laxatives (eg, magnesium hydroxide, aluminum carbonate). Digitalis toxicity may occur with hypokalemia.

Adverse Reactions Frequency not defined.
Endocrine & metabolic: Hypernatremia, hypokalemia, hypocalcemia, hypomagnesemia
Gastrointestinal: Anorexia, colonic necrosis (rare), constipation, fecal impaction, intestinal obstruction (due to concretions in association with aluminum hydroxide), nausea, vomiting

Overdosage/Toxicology Symptoms of overdose include hypokalemia including cardiac dysrhythmias, confusion, irritability, ECG changes, muscle weakness, and GI effects. Treatment is supportive, limited to management of fluid and electrolytes.

Pharmacodynamics/Kinetics
Onset of Action: 2-24 hours
Excretion: Completely feces (primarily as potassium polystyrene sulfonate)

Available Dosage Forms
Powder for suspension, oral/rectal:
Kayexalate®: 15 g/4 level teaspoons (480 g) [contains sodium 100 mg (4.1 mEq)/g]
Kionex™: 15 g/4 level teaspoons (454 g) [contains sodium 100 mg (4.1 mEq)/g]
Suspension, oral/rectal: 15 g/60 mL (60 mL, 120 mL, 200 mL, 500 mL) [contains sodium 1500 mg (65 mEq)/60 mL, sorbitol, and alcohol 0.1%; cherry/caramel flavor]
SPS®: 15 g/60 mL (60 mL, 120 mL, 480 mL) [contains alcohol 0.3%, sodium 1500 mg (65 mEq)/60 mL , and sorbitol; cherry flavor]

Dosing
Adults & Elderly: Hyperkalemia:
Oral: 15 g (60 mL) 1-4 times/day
Rectal: 30-50 g every 6 hours
Pediatrics: Hyperkalemia:
Oral: Children: 1 g/kg/dose every 6 hours
Rectal: Children: 1 g/kg/dose every 2-6 hours (in small children and infants, employ lower doses by using the practical exchange ratio of 1 mEq K⁺/g of resin as the basis for calculation)

Administration
Oral: Administer oral (or NG) as ~25% sorbitol solution; never mix in orange juice. Chilling the oral mixture will increase palatability.
Other: Rectal: Enema route is less effective than oral administration. Administer cleansing enema first. Retain enema in colon for at least 30-60 minutes and for several hours, if possible. Enema should be followed by irrigation with normal saline to prevent necrosis.

Stability
Storage: Store prepared suspensions at 15°C to 30°C (59°F to 86°F); store repackaged product in refrigerator and use within 14 days; freshly prepared suspensions should be used within 24 hours; do not heat resin suspension

Laboratory Monitoring Serum electrolytes, calcium, magnesium

Nursing Actions
Physical Assessment: Monitor laboratory tests. Monitor ECG until potassium levels are normal. Monitor for adverse reactions (eg, fecal impaction) and teach patient interventions and importance of reporting adverse symptoms promptly.
(Continued)

Sodium Polystyrene Sulfonate
(Continued)

Patient Education: Emergency instructions depend on patient's condition. You will be monitored for effects of this medication and frequent blood tests may be necessary. Oral: Take as directed. Mix well with a full glass of liquid (not orange juice). You may experience nausea or vomiting (small frequent meals, frequent mouth care, chewing gum, or sucking lozenges may help); or constipation or fecal impaction (increased dietary fluids and exercise may help). Report persistent constipation or GI distress; chest pain or rapid heartbeat; or mental confusion or muscle weakness. **Pregnancy/breast-feeding precautions:** Inform prescriber if you are pregnant. Consult prescriber if breast-feeding.

Dietary Considerations Do not mix in orange juice. Sodium content of 1 g: 31 mg (1.3 mEq).

Geriatric Considerations Large doses in the elderly may cause fecal impaction and intestinal obstruction. Best to administer using sorbitol 70% as vehicle.

Additional Information 1 g of resin binds approximately 1 mEq of potassium

---

Solifenacin (sol i FEN a sin)

U.S. Brand Names VESIcare®

Synonyms Solifenacin Succinate

Pharmacologic Category Anticholinergic Agent

Pregnancy Risk Factor C

Lactation Excretion in breast milk unknown/not recommended

Use Treatment of overactive bladder with symptoms of urinary frequency, urgency, or urge incontinence

Mechanism of Action/Effect Inhibits muscarinic receptors resulting in decreased urinary bladder contraction, increased residual urine volume, and decreased detrusor muscle pressure.

Contraindications Hypersensitivity to solifenacin or any component of the formulation; urinary retention; gastric retention; uncontrolled narrow-angle glaucoma.

Warnings/Precautions Use with caution in patients with bladder outflow obstruction, gastrointestinal obstructive disorders, and decreased gastrointestinal motility. Use with caution in patients with controlled (treated) narrow-angle glaucoma. Dosage adjustment is required for patients with renal or hepatic impairment. Patients on potent CYP3A4 inhibitors require lower dose. Safety and efficacy in pediatric patients have not been established.

Drug Interactions
Cytochrome P450 Effect: Substrate of CYP3A4 (major)

Decreased Effect: CYP3A4 inducers may decrease the levels/effects of solifenacin; example inducers include aminoglutethimide, carbamazepine, nafcillin, nevirapine, phenobarbital, and phenytoin.

Increased Effect/Toxicity: CYP3A4 inhibitors may increase the levels/effects of solifenacin; example inhibitors include azole antifungals, clarithromycin, diclofenac, doxycycline, erythromycin, ketoconazole, imatinib, isoniazid, nefazodone, nicardipine, propofol, protease inhibitors, quinidine, telithromycin, and verapamil; solifenacin dose should not exceed 5 mg/day.

Nutritional/Ethanol Interactions
Food: Grapefruit juice may increase the serum level effects of solifenacin.

Herb/Nutraceutical: St John's wort (*Hypericum*) may decrease the levels/effects of solifenacin.

Adverse Reactions Adverse reactions are dose related.
>10%: Gastrointestinal: Xerostomia (11% to 28%), constipation (5% to 13%)

1% to 10%:
Cardiovascular: Edema (up to 1%), hypertension (up to 1%)

Central nervous system: Dizziness (2%), fatigue (1% to 2%), depression (up to 1%)

Gastrointestinal: Nausea (2% to 3%), dyspepsia (1% to 4%), upper abdominal pain (1% to 2%), vomiting (up to 1%)

Genitourinary: Urinary tract infection (3% to 5%), urinary retention (up to 1%)

Ocular: Blurred vision (4% to 5%), dry eyes (up to 2%)

Respiratory: Cough (up to 1%), pharyngitis (up to 1%)

Miscellaneous: Influenza (1% to 2%)

Overdosage/Toxicology Overdosage can potentially result in severe central anticholinergic effects. Treatment should include gastric lavage and supportive measures.

Pharmacodynamics/Kinetics
Time to Peak: Plasma: 3-8 hours

Protein Binding: 98% bound to alpha$_1$-acid glycoprotein

Half-Life Elimination: 45-68 hours following chronic dosing

Metabolism: Extensively hepatic; via N-oxidation and 4 R-hydroxylation, forms one active and three inactive metabolites; primary pathway for elimination is via CYP3A4 route

Excretion: Urine 69% (<15% as unchanged drug); feces 23%

Available Dosage Forms Tablet: 5 mg, 10 mg

Dosing
Adults: Overactive bladder: Oral: 5 mg/day; if tolerated, may increase to 10 mg/day.

Elderly: Base dosing on renal/hepatic function.

Renal Impairment: Use with caution in reduced renal function; Cl$_{cr}$ <30 mL/minute: 5 mg/day

Hepatic Impairment: Use with caution in reduced hepatic function: Moderate: 5 mg/day; Severe: Not recommended

Administration
Oral: Swallow tablet whole; may take with liquids, without regard to food.

Stability
Storage: Store at room temperature between 15°C to 30°C (59°F to 86°F).

Nursing Actions
Physical Assessment: Assess other prescriptions and OTC medications the patient may be taking to avoid duplications and interactions. Assess knowledge/teach patient appropriate use, side effects, and symptoms to report. Monitor therapeutic response to medication; urination pattern.

Patient Education: Maintain adequate hydration (2-3 L/day) unless instructed to restrict fluid intake by prescriber. This medication may cause dry mouth (sucking on lozenges or hard candy may help). You may be more susceptible to heat prostration due to decreased ability to sweat. Use caution in hot weather (maintain adequate fluids, reduce exercise activity, rest frequently). You may experience constipation (increased exercise, fluids, fruit/fiber may help), nausea, vomiting, blurred vision and dry eyes. Report difficulty, pain, or burning on urination. **Pregnancy/breast-feeding precautions:** Inform prescriber if you are or intend to become pregnant. Consult prescriber before breast-feeding.

Geriatric Considerations In patients with Cl$_{cr}$ <30 mL/minute, doses >5 mg/day are not recommended.

Somatropin (soe ma TROE pin)

U.S. Brand Names Genotropin®; Genotropin Miniquick®; Humatrope®; Norditropin®; Norditropin® NordiFlex®; Nutropin®; Nutropin AQ®; Saizen®; Serostim®; Tev-Tropin™; Zorbtive™

Synonyms Human Growth Hormone; Somatrem

Pharmacologic Category Growth Hormone

Medication Safety Issues

Sound-alike/look-alike issues:

Somatrem may be confused with somatropin

Somatropin may be confused with somatrem, sumatriptan

Pregnancy Risk Factor B/C (depending upon manufacturer)

Lactation Excretion in breast milk unknown/not recommended

Use

Children:

Long-term treatment of growth failure due to inadequate endogenous growth hormone secretion (Genotropin®, Humatrope®, Norditropin®, Nutropin®, Nutropin AQ®, Saizen®, Tev-Tropin™)

Long-term treatment of short stature associated with Turner syndrome (Humatrope®, Nutropin®, Nutropin AQ®)

Treatment of Prader-Willi syndrome (Genotropin®)

Treatment of growth failure associated with chronic renal insufficiency (CRI) up until the time of renal transplantation (Nutropin®, Nutropin AQ®)

Long-term treatment of growth failure in children born small for gestational age who fail to manifest catch-up growth by 2 years of age (Genotropin®)

Long-term treatment of idiopathic short stature (nongrowth hormone-deficient short stature) defined by height standard deviation score (SDS) less than or equal to -2.25 and growth rate not likely to attain normal adult height (Humatrope®, Nutropin®, Nutropin AQ®)

Adults:

AIDS-wasting or cachexia with concomitant antiviral therapy (Serostim®)

Replacement of endogenous growth hormone in patients with adult growth hormone deficiency who meet both of the following criteria (Genotropin®, Humatrope®, Norditropin®, Nutropin®, Nutropin AQ®, Saizen®):

Biochemical diagnosis of adult growth hormone deficiency by means of a subnormal response to a standard growth hormone stimulation test (peak growth hormone ≤5 mcg/L)

and

Adult-onset: Patients who have adult growth hormone deficiency whether alone or with multiple hormone deficiencies (hypopituitarism) as a result of pituitary disease, hypothalamic disease, surgery, radiation therapy, or trauma

or

Childhood-onset: Patients who were growth hormone deficient during childhood, confirmed as an adult before replacement therapy is initiated

Treatment of short-bowel syndrome (Zorbtive™)

Unlabeled/Investigational Use Investigational: Congestive heart failure; AIDS-wasting/cachexia in children (Serostim®)

Mechanism of Action/Effect Human growth hormone stimulates growth of linear bone, skeletal muscle, and organs; stimulates erythropoietin which increases red blood cell mass; exerts both insulin-like and diabetogenic effects; enhances transmucosal transport of water, electrolytes, and nutrients across the gut

Contraindications Hypersensitivity to growth hormone or any component of the formulation; growth promotion in pediatric patients with closed epiphyses; progression of any underlying intracranial lesion or actively growing intracranial tumor; acute critical illness due to complications following open heart or abdominal surgery; multiple accidental trauma or acute respiratory failure; evidence of active malignancy; use in patients with Prader-Willi syndrome **without** growth hormone deficiency (except Genotropin®) or in patients with Prader-Willi syndrome **with** growth hormone deficiency who are severely obese or have severe respiratory impairment. Saizen® and Norditropin® are contraindicated with proliferative or preproliferative retinopathy.

Warnings/Precautions Use with caution in patients with diabetes or with risk factors for glucose intolerance. Intracranial hypertension has been reported with growth hormone product, funduscopic examinations are recommended; progression of scoliosis may occur in children experiencing rapid growth; patients with growth hormone deficiency may develop slipped capital epiphyses more frequently, evaluate any child with new onset of a limp or with complaints of hip or knee pain; patients with Turner syndrome are at increased risk for otitis media and other ear/hearing disorders, cardiovascular disorders (including stroke, aortic aneurysm, hypertension), and thyroid disease, monitor carefully. Concurrent glucocorticoid therapy may inhibit growth promotion effects; may require dosage adjustment or replacement glucocorticoid therapy in patients with ACTH deficiency. Products may contain benzyl alcohol, m-Cresol or glycerin, some products may be manufactured by recombinant DNA technology using E. coli as a host, consult specific product labeling. When administering to newborns, reconstitute with sterile water or saline for injection. Not for I.V. injection.

Fatalities have been reported in pediatric patients with Prader-Willi syndrome following the use of growth hormone. The reported fatalities occurred in patients with one or more risk factors, including severe obesity, sleep apnea, respiratory impairment, or unidentified respiratory infection; male patients with one or more of these factors may be at greater risk. Treatment interruption is recommended in patients who show signs of upper airway obstruction, including the onset of, or increased, snoring. In addition, evaluation of and/or monitoring for sleep apnea and respiratory infections are recommended.

Drug Interactions

Decreased Effect: Glucocorticoid therapy may inhibit growth-promoting effects. Growth hormone may induce insulin resistance in patients with diabetes mellitus; monitor glucose and adjust insulin dose as necessary.

Adverse Reactions

Growth hormone deficiency: Antigrowth hormone antibodies, carpal tunnel syndrome (rare), fluid balance disturbances, glucosuria, gynecomastia (rare), headache, hematuria, hyperglycemia (mild), hypoglycemia, hypothyroidism, leukemia, lipoatrophy, muscle pain, increased growth of pre-existing nevi (rare), pain/ local reactions at the injection site, pancreatitis (rare), peripheral edema, exacerbation of psoriasis, rash, seizure, weakness

Idiopathic short stature: (From ISS NCGS Cohort; all frequencies <1%): Arthralgia, avascular necrosis, bone growth (abnormal), carpal tunnel syndrome, diabetes mellitus, edema, fracture, gynecomastia, injection site reaction, intracranial hypertension, neoplasm (new onset or recurring), scoliosis (new onset or progression), slipped capital femoral epiphysis, tumor (new onset or recurring). Additional adverse effects noted in product literature (Humatrope®; frequency not established in large cohort): Hip pain, hyperlipidemia, hypertension, hypothyroidism, mylagia, otitis media.

Prader-Willi syndrome: Genotropin®: Aggressiveness, arthralgia, edema, hair loss, headache, benign intracranial hypertension, myalgia; fatalities associated with use in this population have been reported

(Continued)

Somatropin *(Continued)*

Turner syndrome: Humatrope®: Surgical procedures (45%), otitis media (43%), ear disorders (18%), hypothyroidism (13%), increased nevi (11%), peripheral edema (7%)

Adult growth hormone replacement: Increased ALT, increased AST, arthralgia, back pain, carpal tunnel syndrome, diabetes mellitus, fatigue, flu-like syndrome, gastritis, gastroenteritis, generalized edema, glucose intolerance, gynecomastia (rare), headache, hypertension, hypoesthesia, hypothyroidism, infection (nonviral), insomnia, joint disorder, laryngitis, myalgia, nausea, increased growth of pre-existing nevi, pain, pancreatitis (rare), paresthesia, peripheral edema, pharyngitis, rhinitis, stiffness in extremities, weakness

AIDS wasting or cachexia (limited): Serostim®: Musculoskeletal discomfort (54%), increased tissue turgor (27%), diarrhea (26%), neuropathy (26%), nausea (26%), fatigue (17%), albuminuria (15%), increased diaphoresis (14%), anorexia (12%), anemia (12%), increased AST (12%), insomnia (11%), tachycardia (11%), hyperglycemia (10%), increased ALT (10%)

Short-bowel syndrome: Zorbtive™: Peripheral edema (69% to 81%), edema (facial: 44% to 50%; peripheral 13%), arthralgia (13% to 44%), injection site reaction (19% to 31%), flatulence (25%), abdominal pain (20% to 25%), vomiting (19%), malaise (13%), nausea (13%), diaphoresis increased (13%), rhinitis (7%), dizziness (6%)

Small for gestational age: Genotropin®: Mild, transient hyperglycemia; benign intracranial hypertension (rare); central precocious puberty; jaw prominence (rare); aggravation of pre-existing scoliosis (rare); injection site reactions; progression of pigmented nevi

Overdosage/Toxicology Symptoms of acute overdose may include initial hypoglycemia (with subsequent hyperglycemia), fluid retention, headache, nausea, and vomiting. Long-term overdose may result in signs and symptoms of acromegaly.

Pharmacodynamics/Kinetics

Duration of Action: Maintains supraphysiologic levels for 18-20 hours

Half-Life Elimination: Preparation and route of administration dependent

Metabolism: Hepatic and renal (~90%)

Excretion: Urine

Available Dosage Forms [DSC] = Discontinued product

Injection, powder for reconstitution [rDNA origin]:

Genotropin® [preservative free]: 1.5 mg [4 int. units/mL] [delivers 1.3 mg/mL] [DSC]

Genotropin® [with preservative]:

5.8 mg [15 int. units/mL] [delivers 5 mg/mL]
13.8 mg [36 int. units/mL] [delivers 12 mg/mL]

Genotropin Miniquick® [preservative free]: 0.2 mg, 0.4 mg, 0.6 mg, 0.8 mg, 1 mg, 1.2 mg, 1.4 mg, 1.6 mg, 1.8 mg, 2 mg [each strength delivers 0.25 mL]

Humatrope®: 5 mg [~15 int. units], 6 mg [18 int. units], 12 mg [36 int. units], 24 mg [72 int. units]

Nutropin® [diluent contains benzyl alcohol]: 5 mg [~15 int. units]; 10 mg [~30 int. units]

Tev-Tropin™: 5 mg [15 int. units/mL] [diluent contains benzyl alcohol]

Saizen® [diluent contains benzyl alcohol]: 5 mg [~15 int. units; contains sucrose 34.2 mg]; 8.8 mg [~26.4 int. units; contains sucrose 60.2 mg]

Serostim®: 4 mg [12 int. units; contains sucrose 27.3 mg]; 5 mg [15 int. units; contains sucrose 34.2 mg]; 6 mg [18 int. units; contains sucrose 41 mg]

Zorbtive™: 8.8 mg [~26.4 int. units; contains sucrose 60.19 mg]; packaged with diluent containing benzyl alcohol]

Injection, solution [rDNA origin]:

Norditropin®: 5 mg/1.5 mL (1.5 mL); 15 mg/1.5 mL (1.5 mL) [cartridge]

Norditropin® NordiFlex®: 5 mg/1.5 mL (1.5 mL); 15 mg/1.5 mL (1.5 mL) [prefilled pen]

Nutropin AQ®: 5 mg/mL [~15 int. units/mL] (2 mL) [vial or cartridge]

Dosing

Adults:

Growth hormone deficiency: To minimize adverse events in older or overweight patients, reduced dosages may be necessary. During therapy, dosage should be decreased if required by the occurrence of side effects or excessive IGF-I levels.

Norditropin®: SubQ: Initial dose ≤0.004 mg/kg/day; after 6 weeks of therapy, may increase dose to 0.016 mg/kg/day

Nutropin®, Nutropin® AQ: SubQ: ≤0.006 mg/kg/day; dose may be increased according to individual requirements, up to a maximum of 0.025 mg/kg/day in patients <35 years of age, or up to a maximum of 0.0125 mg/kg/day in patients ≥35 years of age

Humatrope®: SubQ: ≤0.006 mg/kg/day; dose may be increased according to individual requirements, up to a maximum of 0.0125 mg/kg/day

Genotropin®: SubQ: Weekly dosage: ≤0.04 mg/kg divided into 6-7 doses; dose may be increased at 4- to 8-week intervals according to individual requirements, to a maximum of 0.08 mg/kg/week

Saizen®: SubQ: ≤0.005 mg/kg/day; dose may be increased to not more than 0.01 mg/kg/day after 4 weeks, based on individual requirements.

AIDS-wasting or cachexia:

Serostim®: SubQ: Dose should be given once daily at bedtime; patients who continue to lose weight after 2 weeks should be re-evaluated for opportunistic infections or other clinical events; rotate injection sites to avoid lipodystrophy

Daily dose based on body weight:
<35 kg: 0.1 mg/kg
35-45 kg: 4 mg
45-55 kg: 5 mg
>55 kg: 6 mg

Short-bowel syndrome (Zorbtive™): SubQ: 0.1 mg/kg once daily for 4 weeks (maximum: 8 mg/day)

Fluid retention (moderate) or arthralgias: Treat symptomatically or reduce dose by 50%

Severe toxicity: Discontinue therapy for up to 5 days; when symptoms resolve, restart at 50% of dose. If severe toxicity recurs or does not disappear within 5 days after discontinuation, permanently discontinue treatment.

Elderly: Patients ≥65 years of age may be more sensitive to the action of growth hormone and more prone to adverse effects; in general, dosing should be cautious, beginning at low end of dosing range.

Pediatrics:

Growth hormone deficiency:

Genotropin®: SubQ: Weekly dosage: 0.16-0.24 mg/kg divided into 6-7 doses

Humatrope®: I.M., SubQ: Weekly dosage: 0.18 mg/kg; maximum replacement dose: 0.3 mg/kg/week; dosing should be divided into equal doses given 3 times/week on alternating days, 6 times/week, or daily

Norditropin®: SubQ: 0.024-0.034 mg/kg/day, 6-7 times/week

Nutropin®, Nutropin® AQ: SubQ: Weekly dosage: 0.3 mg/kg divided into daily doses; pubertal patients: ≤0.7 mg/kg/week divided daily

Tev-Tropin™: SubQ: Up to 0.1 mg/kg administered 3 times/week

Saizen®: I.M., SubQ: 0.06 mg/kg/dose administered 3 times/week

Note: Therapy should be discontinued when patient has reached satisfactory adult height, when epiphyses have fused, or when the patient ceases to respond. Growth of 5 cm/year or more is expected, if growth rate does not exceed 2.5 cm in a 6-month period, double the dose for the next 6 months; if there is still no satisfactory response, discontinue therapy

Chronic renal insufficiency (CRI): *Nutropin®, Nutropin® AQ:* SubQ: Weekly dosage: 0.35 mg/kg divided into daily injections; continue until the time of renal transplantation

Dosage recommendations in patients treated for CRI who require dialysis:

Hemodialysis: Administer dose at night prior to bedtime or at least 3-4 hours after hemodialysis to prevent hematoma formation from heparin

CCPD: Administer dose in the morning following dialysis

CAPD: Administer dose in the evening at the time of overnight exchange

Turner syndrome: *Humatrope®, Nutropin®, Nutropin® AQ:* SubQ: Weekly dosage: ≤0.375 mg/kg divided into equal doses 3-7 times per week

Prader-Willi syndrome: *Genotropin®:* SubQ: Weekly dosage: 0.24 mg/kg divided into 6-7 doses

Small for gestational age: *Genotropin®:* SubQ: Weekly dosage: 0.48 mg/kg divided into 6-7 doses

Idiopathic short stature:

Humatrope®: SubQ: Weekly dosage: 0.37 mg/kg divided into equal doses 6-7 times per week

Nutropin®, Nutropin AQ®: SubQ: Weekly dosage: Up to 0.3 mg/kg divided into daily doses

AIDS-wasting or cachexia (unlabeled use): *Serostim®:* SubQ: Limited data; doses of 0.04 mg/kg/day were reported in five children, 6-17 years of age; doses of 0.07 mg/kg/day were reported in six children, 8-14 years of age

Renal Impairment: Reports indicate patients with chronic renal failure tend to have decreased clearance; specific dosing suggestions not available

Hepatic Impairment: Clearance may be reduced in patients with severe hepatic dysfunction; specific dosing suggestions are not available.

Administration

I.M.: Do not shake; administer SubQ or I.M. (rotate administration sites to avoid tissue atrophy); refer to product labeling. When administering to newborns, reconstitute with sterile water for injection. Cartridge must be administered using the corresponding color-coded NordiPen® injection pen.

Stability

Reconstitution:

Genotropin®: Reconstitute with diluent provided.

Genotropin MiniQuick®: Reconstitute with diluent provided. Consult the instructions provided with the reconstitution device.

Humatrope®:

Cartridge: Consult HumatroPen™ User Guide for complete instructions for reconstitution. **Do not use diluent provided with vials.**

Vial: 5 mg: Reconstitute with 1.5-5 mL diluent provided.

Nutropin®: Vial:

5 mg: Reconstitute with 1-5 mL bacteriostatic water for injection.

10 mg: Reconstitute with 1-10 mL bacteriostatic water for injection.

Saizen®: Vial:

5 mg: Reconstitute with 1-3 mL bacteriostatic water for injection or sterile water for injection; gently swirl; do not shake.

8.8 mg: Reconstitute with 2-3 mL bacteriostatic water for injection or sterile water for injection; gently swirl; do not shake.

Serostim®: Vial: Reconstitute with 0.5-1 mL sterile water for injection.

Tev-Tropin™: Reconstitute with 1-5 mL of diluent provided. Gently swirl; do not shake. May use preservative-free NS for use in newborns.

Zorbtive™: 8.8 mg vial: Reconstitute with 1-2 mL bacteriostatic water for injection; use within 14 days

Storage:

Genotropin®: Store at 2°C to 8°C (36°F to 46°F), do not freeze, protect from light

1.5 mg cartridge: Following reconstitution, store under refrigeration and use within 24 hours; discard unused portion

5.8 mg and 13.8 mg cartridge: Following reconstitution, store under refrigeration and use within 21 days

Miniquick®: Store in refrigerator prior to dispensing, but may be stored ≤25°C (77°F) for up to 3 months after dispensing; once reconstituted, solution must be refrigerated and used within 24 hours; discard unused portion

Humatrope®:

Vial: Before and after reconstitution, store at 2°C to 8°C (36°F to 46°F), avoid freezing; when reconstituted with bacteriostatic water for injection, use within 14 days; when reconstituted with sterile water for injection, use within 24 hours and discard unused portion

Cartridge: Before and after reconstitution, store at 2°C to 8°C (36°F to 46°F), avoid freezing; following reconstitution, stable for 14 days under refrigeration. Dilute with solution provided with cartridges **ONLY**; do not use diluent provided with vials

Norditropin®: Store at 2°C to 8°C (36°F to 46°F), do not freeze; avoid direct light

Cartridge: Must be used within 4 weeks once inserted into pen

Prefilled pen: Must be used within 4 weeks after initial injection

Nutropin®: Before and after reconstitution, store at 2°C to 8°C (36°F to 46°F), avoid freezing

Vial: Reconstitute with bacteriostatic water for injection; use reconstituted vials within 14 days; when reconstituted with sterile water for injection, use immediately and discard unused portion

AQ formulation: Use within 28 days following initial use

Saizen®: Prior to reconstitution, store at room temperature 15°C to 30°C (59°F to 86°F); following reconstitution with bacteriostatic water for injection, reconstituted solution should be refrigerated and used within 14 days; when reconstituted with sterile water for injection, use immediately and discard unused portion

Serostim®: Prior to reconstitution, store at room temperature 15°C to 30°C (59°F to 86°F); reconstitute with sterile water for injection; store reconstituted solution under refrigeration and use within 24 hours, avoid freezing. Do not use if cloudy

Tev-Tropin™: Prior to reconstitution, store at 2°C to 8°C (36°F to 46°F). Following reconstitution with bacteriostatic NS, solution should be refrigerated and used within 14 days. Some cloudiness may occur; do not use if cloudiness persists after warming to room temperature.

Zorbtive™: Store unopened vials and diluent at room temperature of 15°C to 30°C (59°F to 86°F). Store reconstituted 8.8 mg vial under refrigeration at 2°C to 8°C (36°F to 46°F); avoid freezing.

Laboratory Monitoring Periodic thyroid function tests, periodical urine testing for glucose, somatomedin C (IGF-I) levels; serum phosphorus, alkaline phosphatase and parathyroid hormone. If growth deceleration is observed in children treated for growth hormone deficiency, and not due to other causes, evaluate for presence of antibody formation. Strict blood glucose monitoring in diabetic patients.

(Continued)

Somatropin *(Continued)*

Somatrem (Protropin®): Consider changing to somatropin if antibody binding capacity is >2 mg/L

Nursing Actions

Physical Assessment: Assess potential for interactions with other prescriptions, OTC medications, or herbal products patient may be taking. Monitor laboratory tests. Monitor patient response (according to purpose for use) and adverse reactions. Instruct patients with diabetes to monitor glucose levels closely (may induce insulin intolerance). Encourage funduscopic examinations at initiation of therapy and periodically during treatment; Instruct patient in proper use if self-administered (storage, reconstitution, injection techniques, and syringe/needle disposal), possible side effects/appropriate interventions, and adverse symptoms to report. Pediatrics: Monitor growth curve; annually determine bone age.

Patient Education: This drug can only be administered by injection. If self-administered, you will be instructed by prescriber on proper storage, reconstitution, injection technique, and syringe/needle disposal. Use exactly as prescribed; do not discontinue or alter dose without consulting prescriber. Report immediately any pain, redness, burning, drainage, or swelling at injection site. If you have diabetes, monitor glucose levels closely; this medication may cause an alteration in your insulin levels. May cause side effects which are particular to purpose for use and formulation prescribed; your prescriber will instruct you in particular side effects for your medication. Report immediately unusual or persistent bleeding, excessive fatigue or swelling (edema) of extremities, joint or muscle pain or headache, nausea or vomiting, personality changes, or other persistent adverse effects. **Pregnancy/breast-feeding precaution:** Inform prescriber if you are or intend to become pregnant. Breast-feeding is not recommended.

Dietary Considerations

Prader-Willi syndrome: All patients should have effective weight control (use is contraindicated in severely-obese patients).

Short-bowel syndrome: Intravenous parenteral nutrition requirements may need reassessment as gastrointestinal absorption improves.

Sorafenib *(sor AF e nib)*

U.S. Brand Names Nexavar®

Synonyms BAY 43-9006; Sorafenib Tosylate

Pharmacologic Category Antineoplastic Agent, Tyrosine Kinase Inhibitor; Vascular Endothelial Growth Factor (VEGF) Inhibitor

Pregnancy Risk Factor D

Lactation Excretion in breast milk unknown/not recommended

Use Treatment of advanced renal cell cancer

Unlabeled/Investigational Use Treatment of hepatocellular, breast, colon, colorectal, nonsmall cell lung, ovarian, pancreatic and thyroid cancers; melanoma, sarcoma

Mechanism of Action/Effect Prevents tumor growth by inhibiting both tumor cell proliferation and tumor angiogenesis

Contraindications Hypersensitivity to sorafenib or any component of the formulation; pregnancy

Warnings/Precautions May cause hypertension, especially in the first 6 weeks of treatment; use caution in patients with underlying or poorly-controlled hypertension. May cause cardiac ischemia or infarction; avoid use in patients with unstable coronary artery disease or recent myocardial infarction. Serious bleeding events may occur; monitor PT/INR in patients on warfarin therapy. May complicate wound healing; temporarily withhold treatment for patients undergoing major surgical procedures. Use caution when administering sorafenib with compounds that are metabolized predominantly via UGT1A1 (eg, irinotecan). Hand-foot skin reaction and rash are the most common adverse events.

Drug Interactions

Cytochrome P450 Effect: Substrate of CYP3A4 (minor); **Inhibits** CYP2B6 (weak) and 2C8/9 (weak)

Increased Effect/Toxicity: Sorafenib may increase the levels/effects of doxorubicin.

Nutritional/Ethanol Interactions Herb/Nutraceutical: Avoid St John's wort (may decrease the levels/effects of sorafenib).

Adverse Reactions Note: Dose-limiting toxicities (diarrhea, fatigue, and hand-foot syndrome) were reversible upon discontinuation; rash and hand-foot syndrome are dose related; percentages not always reported.

>10%:

Cardiovascular: Hypertension (17%)

Central nervous system: Fatigue (32% to 33%; grade 3/4: 5% to <6%), sensory neuropathy (13%)

Dermatologic: Rash (38% to 40%), hand-foot syndrome (30% to 35%; grade 3/4: 6%), alopecia (27%), pruritus (19%), dry skin (11%), erythema

Endocrine & metabolic: Hypophosphatemia (45%; grade 3: 13%)

Gastrointestinal: Diarrhea (37% to 43%; grade 3/4: 2%), lipase increased (41%), amylase increased (30%), nausea (23%), anorexia (16%), vomiting (16%), constipation (15%), abdominal pain (11%), mouth pain

Hematologic: Lymphopenia (23%), neutropenia (<10% to 18%), hemorrhage (15%), thrombocytopenia (<10% to 12%), leukopenia

Neuromuscular & skeletal: Bone pain, muscle pain, weakness

Respiratory: Dyspnea (14%), cough (13%)

1% to 10%:

Cardiovascular: Flushing

Central nervous system: Headache (10%), depression, fever

Dermatologic: Acne, exfoliative dermatitis

Gastrointestinal: Weight loss (10%), appetite decreased, dyspepsia, dysphagia, glossodynia, mucositis, stomatitis, xerostomia

Genitourinary: Erectile dysfunction

Hematologic: Anemia

Hepatic: Transaminases increased

Neuromuscular & skeletal: Joint pain (10%), arthralgia, myalgia

Respiratory: Hoarseness

Miscellaneous: Influenza-like symptoms

Overdosage/Toxicology In clinical trials, doses of 800 mg twice daily produced diarrhea and dermatologic reactions. In the event of an overdose, treatment is symptomatic and supportive.

Pharmacodynamics/Kinetics

Time to Peak: 3 hours

Protein Binding: 99.5%

Half-Life Elimination: 25-48 hours

Metabolism: Hepatic, via CYP3A4 (primarily oxidated to the pyridine N-oxide; active, minor) and UGT1A9 (glucuronidation)

Excretion: Feces (77%, 51% as unchanged drug); urine (19%, as metabolites)

Available Dosage Forms Tablet, as tosylate: 200 mg

Dosing

Adults & Elderly:

Advanced renal cell carcinoma: Oral: 400 mg twice daily

Nonsmall cell lung cancer (unlabeled use): Oral: 400 mg twice daily

Pancreatic cancer (unlabeled use): Oral: 400 mg twice daily in combination with gemcitabine

Renal Impairment: Not studied in severe renal impairment (Cl_{cr} <30 mL/minute)

Hepatic Impairment: No adjustment required for mild (Child-Pugh class A) to moderate (Child-Pugh class B) hepatic impairment; not studied in severe hepatic impairment (Child-Pugh class C)

Dosing Adjustment for Toxicity: Temporary interruption and/or dosage reduction may be necessary for management of adverse drug reactions. The dose may be reduced to 400 mg once daily and then further reduced to 400 mg every other day.

Dose modification for skin toxicity:

Grade 1 (numbness, dysesthesia, paresthesia, tingling, painless swelling, erythema or discomfort of the hands or feet which do not disrupt normal activities): Continue sorafenib and consider symptomatic treatment with topical therapy.

Grade 2 (painful erythema and swelling of the hands or feet and/or discomfort affecting normal activities):

1st occurrence: Continue sorafenib and consider symptomatic treatment with topical therapy. **Note:** If no improvement, see dosing for 2nd or 3rd occurrence.

2nd or 3rd occurrence: Hold treatment until resolves to grade 0-1; resume treatment with dose reduced by one dose level (400 mg daily or 400 mg every other day)

4th occurrence: Discontinue treatment

Grade 3 (moist desquamation, ulceration, blistering, or severe pain of the hands or feet or severe discomfort that prevents working or performing daily activities):

1st or 2nd occurrence: Hold treatment until resolves to grade 0-1; resume treatment with dose reduced by one dose level (400 mg daily or 400 mg every other day)

3rd occurrence: Discontinue treatment

Administration

Oral: Administer without food, 1 hour before or 2 hours after eating.

Stability

Storage: Store at room temperature between 15°C and 30°C (59°F and 86°F). Protect from moisture.

Laboratory Monitoring CBC with differential, electrolytes, phosphorus

Nursing Actions

Physical Assessment: Assess potential for interactions with other pharmacological agents or herbal products patient may be taking (eg, increased or decreased levels/effects of sorafenib). Monitor laboratory tests, therapeutic effectiveness, and adverse reactions (especially blood pressure) on a regular basis during therapy. Teach patient proper use, possible side effects/appropriate interventions, and adverse symptoms to report.

Patient Education: Do not take any new medication during therapy without consulting prescriber. Take exactly as directed, 1 hour before or 2 hours after eating. You may need periodic laboratory tests while taking this medication. Maintain adequate hydration (2-3 L/day of fluids) unless instructed to restrict fluid intake. You may experience loss of appetite, nausea and vomiting (small, frequent meals and frequent mouth care may help), or diarrhea (buttermilk, boiled milk, or yogurt may help); or hair loss (may grow back when treatment is discontinued). Report immediately persistent headache, dizziness, vision changes (monitor blood pressure if recommended by prescriber). Report unusual skin rash; persistent gastrointestinal upset (diarrhea, constipation, abdominal pain); unusual or persistent cough; bone, joint, or muscle weakness, pain, or loss of sensation; flu-like symptoms; or other persistent adverse effects. **Pregnancy/breast-feeding precautions:** Inform prescriber is you are pregnant. Do not get pregnant. Consult prescriber for appropriate contraceptive measures while on this medications. Breast-feeding is not recommended.

Dietary Considerations Take without food (1 hour before or 2 hours after eating).

Geriatric Considerations No difference in efficacy or safety was observed between older and younger patients, but only 4% of patients studied were >75 years of age.

Pregnancy Issues There are no adequate and well-controlled studies in pregnant women. Because sorafenib inhibits angiogenesis, a critical component of fetal development, adverse effects on pregnancy would be expected. Women of childbearing potential should be advised to avoid pregnancy. Men and women should use effective birth control during treatment and for at least 2 weeks after treatment is discontinued.

Sorbitol (SOR bi tole)

Pharmacologic Category Genitourinary Irrigant; Laxative, Osmotic

Pregnancy Risk Factor C

Lactation Excretion in breast milk unknown

Use Genitourinary irrigant in transurethral prostatic resection or other transurethral resection or other transurethral surgical procedures; diuretic; humectant; sweetening agent; hyperosmotic laxative; facilitate the passage of sodium polystyrene sulfonate through the intestinal tract

Mechanism of Action/Effect A polyalcoholic sugar with osmotic cathartic actions

Contraindications Anuria

Warnings/Precautions Use with caution in patients with severe cardiopulmonary or renal impairment and in patients unable to metabolize sorbitol; large volumes may result in fluid overload and/or electrolyte changes.

Adverse Reactions Frequency not defined.

Cardiovascular: Edema

Endocrine & metabolic: Fluid and electrolyte losses, hyperglycemia, lactic acidosis

Gastrointestinal: Diarrhea, nausea, vomiting, abdominal discomfort, xerostomia

Overdosage/Toxicology Symptoms of overdose include nausea, diarrhea, fluid and electrolyte loss. Treatment is supportive to ensure fluid and electrolyte balance.

Pharmacodynamics/Kinetics

Onset of Action: 0.25-1 hour

Metabolism: Primarily hepatic to fructose

Available Dosage Forms

Solution, genitourinary irrigation: 3% (3000 mL, 5000 mL); 3.3% (2000 mL, 4000 mL)

Solution, oral: 70% (30 mL, 480 mL, 3840 mL)

Dosing

Adults & Elderly:

Hyperosmotic laxative (as single dose, at infrequent intervals):

Oral: 30-150 mL (as 70% solution)

Rectal enema: 120 mL as 25% to 30% solution

Adjunct to sodium polystyrene sulfonate: 15 mL as 70% solution orally until diarrhea occurs (10-20 mL/2 hours) or 20-100 mL as an oral vehicle for the sodium polystyrene sulfonate resin

When administered with charcoal:

Oral: 4.3 mL/kg of 70% sorbitol with 1 g/kg of activated charcoal every 4 hours until first stool containing charcoal is passed

Transurethral surgical procedures: Irrigation: Topical: 3% to 3.3% as transurethral surgical procedure irrigation

(Continued)

Sorbitol *(Continued)*

Pediatrics:
Hyperosmotic laxative (as single dose, at infrequent intervals):
Children 2-11 years:
Oral: 2 mL/kg (as 70% solution)
Rectal enema: 30-60 mL as 25% to 30% solution
Children >12 years: Oral, Rectal enema: Refer to adult dosing.

When administered with charcoal: Oral: Children: 4.3 mL/kg of 35% sorbitol with 1 g/kg of activated charcoal

Stability
Storage: Protect from freezing. Avoid storage in temperatures >150°F.

Laboratory Monitoring Electrolytes

Nursing Actions
Physical Assessment: When used as cathartic, determine cause of constipation before use. Assess knowledge/teach patient about use of nonpharmacological interventions to prevent constipation.

Patient Education: Cathartic: Use of cathartics on a regular basis will have adverse effects. Increased exercise, increased fluid intake, or increased dietary fruit and fiber may be effective in preventing and resolving constipation. **Breast-feeding precaution:** Consult prescriber if breast-feeding.

Geriatric Considerations Causes for constipation must be evaluated prior to initiating treatment. Nonpharmacological dietary treatment should be initiated before laxative use. Sorbitol is as effective as lactulose but is much less expensive.

Sotalol *(SOE ta lole)*

U.S. Brand Names Betapace®; Betapace AF®; Sorine®

Synonyms Sotalol Hydrochloride

Pharmacologic Category Antiarrhythmic Agent, Class II; Antiarrhythmic Agent, Class III; Beta-Adrenergic Blocker, Nonselective

Medication Safety Issues
Sound-alike/look-alike issues:
Sotalol may be confused with Stadol®
Betapace® may be confused with Betapace AF®
Betapace AF® may be confused with Betapace®

Pregnancy Risk Factor B

Lactation Enters breast milk/use caution (AAP rates "compatible")

Use Treatment of documented ventricular arrhythmias (ie, sustained ventricular tachycardia), that in the judgment of the physician are life-threatening; maintenance of normal sinus rhythm in patients with symptomatic atrial fibrillation and atrial flutter who are currently in sinus rhythm. Manufacturer states substitutions should not be made for Betapace AF® since Betapace AF® is distributed with a patient package insert specific for atrial fibrillation/flutter.

Mechanism of Action/Effect
Beta-blocker which contains both beta-adrenoreceptor-blocking (Vaughan Williams Class II) and cardiac action potential duration prolongation (Vaughan Williams Class III) properties

Class II effects: Increased sinus cycle length, slowed heart rate, decreased AV nodal conduction, and increased AV nodal refractoriness

Class III effects: Prolongation of the atrial and ventricular monophasic action potentials, and effective refractory prolongation of atrial muscle, ventricular muscle, and atrioventricular accessory pathways in both the antegrade and retrograde directions

Sotalol is a racemic mixture of d- and l-sotalol; both isomers have similar Class III antiarrhythmic effects while the l-isomer is responsible for virtually all of the beta-blocking activity

Sotalol has both beta$_1$- and beta$_2$-receptor blocking activity

The beta-blocking effect of sotalol is a noncardioselective [half maximal at about 80 mg/day and maximal at doses of 320-640 mg/day]. Significant beta blockade occurs at oral doses as low as 25 mg/day.

Significant Class III effects are seen only at oral doses ≥160 mg/day.

Contraindications Hypersensitivity to sotalol or any component of the formulation; bronchial asthma; sinus bradycardia; second- and third-degree AV block (unless a functioning pacemaker is present); congenital or acquired long QT syndromes; cardiogenic shock; uncontrolled congestive heart failure. Betapace AF® is contraindicated in patients with significantly reduced renal filtration (Cl_{cr} <40 mL/minute).

Warnings/Precautions Manufacturer recommends initiation (or reinitiation) and doses increased in a hospital setting with continuous monitoring and staff familiar with the recognition and treatment of life-threatening arrhythmias. Dosage of sotalol should be adjusted gradually with 3 days between dosing increments to achieve steady-state concentrations, and to allow time to monitor QT intervals. Some experts will initiate therapy on an outpatient basis in a patient without heart disease or bradycardia, who has a baseline uncorrected QT interval <450 msec, and normal serum potassium and magnesium levels; close EKG monitoring during this time is necessary. ACC/AHA guidelines for management of atrial fibrillation also recommend that for outpatient initiation the patient not have risk factors predisposing to drug-induced ventricular proarrhythmia (Fuster, 2001). Creatinine clearance must be calculated prior to dosing. Use cautiously in the renally-impaired (dosage adjustment required).

Monitor and adjust dose to prevent QT_c prolongation. Concurrent use with other QT_c-prolonging drugs (including Class I and Class III antiarrhythmics) is generally not recommended; withhold for 3 half-lives. Watch for proarrhythmic effects. Correct electrolyte imbalances before initiating (especially hypokalemia and hyperkalemia). Consider pre-existing conditions such as sick sinus syndrome before initiating. Conduction abnormalities can occur particularly sinus bradycardia. Use cautiously within the first 2 weeks post-MI (experience limited), in compensated heart failure, diabetes, or in patients with PVD. Beta-blocker therapy should not be withdrawn abruptly (particularly in patients with CAD), but gradually tapered to avoid acute tachycardia, hypertension, and/or ischemia. Use caution with concurrent use of beta-blockers and either verapamil or diltiazem; bradycardia or heart block can occur. Can mask signs of thyrotoxicosis. Use care with anesthetic agents which decrease myocardial function.

Drug Interactions
Decreased Effect: Decreased effect of sotalol may occur with aluminum-magnesium antacids (if taken within 2 hours), aluminum salts, barbiturates, calcium salts, cholestyramine, colestipol, NSAIDs, penicillins (ampicillin), rifampin, salicylates, and sulfinpyrazone due to decreased bioavailability and plasma levels. Beta-blockers may decrease the effect of sulfonylureas. Beta-agonists such as albuterol, terbutaline may have less of a therapeutic effect when administered concomitantly.

Increased Effect/Toxicity: Increased effect/toxicity of beta-blockers with calcium blockers since there may be additive effects on AV conduction or ventricular function. Other agents which prolong QT interval, including Class I antiarrhythmic agents, bepridil, cisapride, erythromycin, haloperidol, pimozide, phenothiazines, tricyclic antidepressants, and specific quinolones (including sparfloxacin, gatifloxacin, moxifloxacin) may increase the effect of sotalol on the prolongation of QT interval. Amiodarone may cause additive effects on QT_c prolongation as well as decreased heart rate, and has been associated with cardiac arrest in patients receiving some beta-blockers. When used concurrently with clonidine, sotalol may increase the risk of rebound hypertension after or during withdrawal of either agent. Beta-blocker and catecholamine depleting agents (reserpine or guanethidine) may result in additive hypotension or bradycardia. Beta-blockers may increase the action or levels of ethanol, nondepolarizing muscle relaxants, and theophylline although the effects are difficult to predict.

Nutritional/Ethanol Interactions

Food: Sotalol peak serum concentrations may be decreased if taken with food.

Herb/Nutraceutical: Avoid ephedra (may worsen arrhythmia).

Adverse Reactions

>10%:
Cardiovascular: Bradycardia (16%), chest pain (16%), palpitation (14%)
Central nervous system: Fatigue (20%), dizziness (20%), lightheadedness (12%)
Neuromuscular & skeletal: Weakness (13%)
Respiratory: Dyspnea (21%)

1% to 10%:
Cardiovascular: CHF (5%), peripheral vascular disorders (3%), edema (8%), abnormal ECG (7%), hypotension (6%), proarrhythmia (5%), syncope (5%)
Central nervous system: Mental confusion (6%), anxiety (4%), headache (8%), sleep problems (8%), depression (4%)
Dermatologic: Itching/rash (5%)
Endocrine & metabolic: Sexual ability decreased (3%)
Gastrointestinal: Diarrhea (7%), nausea/vomiting (10%), stomach discomfort (3% to 6%), flatulence (2%)
Genitourinary: Impotence (2%)
Hematologic: Bleeding (2%)
Neuromuscular & skeletal: Paresthesia (4%), extremity pain (7%), back pain (3%)
Ocular: Visual problems (5%)
Respiratory: Upper respiratory problems (5% to 8%), asthma (2%)

Overdosage/Toxicology Symptoms of intoxication include cardiac disturbances, CNS toxicity, bronchospasm, hypoglycemia and hyperkalemia. The most common cardiac symptoms include hypotension and bradycardia; atrioventricular block, intraventricular conduction disturbances, cardiogenic shock, and asystole may occur with severe overdose, especially with membrane-depressant drugs (eg, propranolol); CNS effects include convulsions, coma, and respiratory arrest is commonly seen with propranolol and other membrane-depressant and lipid-soluble drugs.

Treatment includes symptomatic treatment of seizures, hypotension, hyperkalemia and hypoglycemia. Bradycardia and hypotension resistant to atropine, isoproterenol or pacing may respond to glucagon. Wide QRS defects caused by the membrane-depressant poisoning may respond to hypertonic sodium bicarbonate. Repeat-dose charcoal, hemoperfusion, or hemodialysis may be helpful in removal of only those beta-blockers with a small V_d, long half-life, or low intrinsic clearance (acebutolol, atenolol, nadolol, sotalol).

Pharmacodynamics/Kinetics

Onset of Action: Rapid, 1-2 hours; Peak effect: 2.5-4 hours

Duration of Action: 8-16 hours

Protein Binding: None

Half-Life Elimination: 12 hours; Children: 9.5 hours; terminal half-life decreases with age <2 years (may by ≥1 week in neonates)

Metabolism: None

Excretion: Urine (as unchanged drug)

Available Dosage Forms

Tablet, as hydrochloride: 80 mg, 80 mg [AF], 120 mg, 120 mg [AF], 160 mg, 160 mg [AF], 240 mg
Betapace® [light blue]: 80 mg, 120 mg, 160 mg, 240 mg
Betapace AF® [white]: 80 mg, 120 mg, 160 mg
Sorine® [white]: 80 mg, 120 mg, 160 mg, 240 mg

Dosing

Adults & Elderly: Sotalol should be initiated and doses increased in a hospital with facilities for cardiac rhythm monitoring and assessment. Proarrhythmic events can occur after initiation of therapy and with each upward dosage adjustment.

Ventricular arrhythmias (Betapace®, Sorine®):
Oral:
Initial: 80 mg twice daily; dose may be increased gradually to 240-320 mg/day; allow 3 days between dosing increments (to attain steady-state plasma concentrations and to allow monitoring of QT intervals).
Usual range: Most patients respond to 160-320 mg/day in 2-3 divided doses.
Maximum: Some patients, with life-threatening refractory ventricular arrhythmias, may require doses as high as 480-640 mg/day; prescribed ONLY when the potential benefit outweighs the increased of adverse events.

Atrial fibrillation or atrial flutter (Betapace AF®):
Oral: Initial: 80 mg twice daily
Note: If the initial dose does not reduce the frequency of relapses of atrial fibrillation/flutter and is tolerated without excessive QT prolongation (not >520 msec) after 3 days, the dose may be increased to 120 mg twice daily. This may be further increased to 160 mg twice daily if response is inadequate and QT prolongation is not excessive.

Pediatrics: Sotalol should be initiated and doses increased in a hospital with facilities for cardiac rhythm monitoring and assessment. Proarrhythmic events can occur after initiation of therapy and with each upward dosage adjustment.

Note: The safety and efficacy of sotalol in children have not been established

Supraventricular arrhythmias: Oral: **Note:** Dosing per manufacturer, based on pediatric pharmacokinetic data; wait at least 36 hours between dosage adjustments to allow monitoring of QT intervals
Children ≤2 years: Dosage should be adjusted (decreased) by plotting of the child's age on a logarithmic scale; see graph on next page or refer to manufacturer's package labeling.
Children >2 years: Initial: 90 mg/m²/day in 3 divided doses; may be incrementally increased to a maximum of 180 mg/m²/day

Renal Impairment: Adults: Impaired renal function can increase the terminal half-life, resulting in increased drug accumulation. Sotalol (Betapace AF®) is contraindicated per the manufacturer for treatment of atrial fibrillation/flutter in patients with a Cl_{cr} <40 mL/minute.
Ventricular arrhythmias (Betapace®, Sorine®):
Cl_{cr} >60 mL/minute: Administer every 12 hours.
Cl_{cr} 30-60 mL/minute: Administer every 24 hours.
Cl_{cr} 10-30 mL/minute: Administer every 36-48 hours.
Cl_{cr} <10 mL/minute: Individualize dose.
Atrial fibrillation/flutter (Betapace AF®):
Cl_{cr} >60 mL/minute: Administer every 12 hours.
Cl_{cr} 40-60 mL/minute: Administer every 24 hours.
Cl_{cr} <40 mL/minute: Use is contraindicated.

Dialysis: Hemodialysis would be expected to reduce sotalol plasma concentrations because sotalol is
(Continued)

Sotalol *(Continued)*

**Sotalol Age Factor Nomogram
for Patients ≤2 Years of Age**

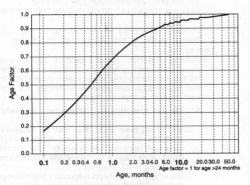

Age factor = 1 for age >24 months

Adapted from U.S. Food and Drug Administration.
http://www.fda.gov/cder/foi/label/2001/2115s3lbl.PDF

not bound to plasma proteins and does not undergo extensive metabolism. Administer dose postdialysis or administer supplemental 80 mg dose. Peritoneal dialysis does not remove sotalol; supplemental dose is not necessary.

Stability
Storage: Store at 25°C (77°F). Excursions permitted to 15°C to 30°C (59°F to 86°F).

Laboratory Monitoring Serum magnesium, potassium

Nursing Actions

Physical Assessment: Assess potential for interactions with other prescriptions, OTC medications, or herbal products patient may be taking. Monitor laboratory tests, blood pressure, and heart rate prior to and following first dose and with any change in dosage. Monitor for adverse effects (eg, cardiac and pulmonary status). Advise patients with diabetes to monitor glucose levels closely (beta-blockers may alter glucose tolerance). Should not be stopped abruptly; dose should be tapered gradually when discontinuing. Teach patient appropriate use, possible side effects/appropriate interventions (hypotension precautions), and adverse symptoms to report.

Patient Education: Do not take any new medications without consulting prescriber. Take exactly as directed; do not adjust dosage or discontinue without consulting prescriber. Take pulse daily (prior to medication) and follow prescriber's instruction about holding of medication. If you have diabetes, monitor serum sugar closely (drug may alter glucose tolerance or mask signs of hypoglycemia). May cause fatigue, dizziness, lightheadedness (use caution when driving or engaging in activities requiring alertness until response to drug is known), or postural hypotension (use caution when changing position from lying or sitting to standing, when driving, or climbing stairs until response to medication is known); alteration in sexual performance (reversible); nausea or vomiting (small frequent meals, frequent mouth care, sucking lozenges, or chewing gum may help); or diarrhea (boiled milk, buttermilk, or yogurt may help). Report immediately any chest pain, palpitations, irregular heartbeat; swelling of extremities, respiratory difficulty, new cough, or unusual fatigue; persistent

nausea, vomiting, or diarrhea; or unusual muscle weakness. **Breast-feeding precaution:** Consult prescriber if breast-feeding.

Dietary Considerations Administer on an empty stomach.

Geriatric Considerations Since elderly frequently have Cl_{cr} <60 mL/minute, attention to dose, creatinine clearance, and monitoring is important. Make dosage adjustments at 3-day intervals or after 5-6 doses at any dosage.

Breast-Feeding Issues Sotalol is considered compatible by the AAP. It is recommended that the infant be monitored for signs or symptoms of beta-blockade (hypotension, bradycardia, etc) with long-term use.

Pregnancy Issues There are no adequate and well-controlled studies in pregnant women. Beta-blockers have been associated with bradycardia, hypotension, and IUGR; IUGR is probably related to maternal hypertension. Sotalol has been shown to cross the placenta, and is found in amniotic fluid; therefore, sotalol should be used during pregnancy only if the potential benefit outweighs the potential risk. Cases of neonatal hypoglycemia have been reported following maternal use of beta-blockers at parturition or during breast-feeding. Monitor breast-fed infant for symptoms of beta-blockade.

Additional Information Pharmacokinetics in children are more relevant for BSA than age.

Sparfloxacin *(spar FLOKS a sin)*

U.S. Brand Names Zagam® [DSC]
Pharmacologic Category Antibiotic, Quinolone
Medication Safety Issues
Sound-alike/look-alike issues:
Zagam® may be confused with Zyban®

Pregnancy Risk Factor C
Lactation Enters breast milk/not recommended
Use Treatment of adults with community-acquired pneumonia caused by *C. pneumoniae, H. influenzae, H. parainfluenzae, M. catarrhalis, M. pneumoniae* or *S. pneumoniae*; treatment of acute bacterial exacerbations of chronic bronchitis caused by *C. pneumoniae, E. cloacae, H. influenzae, H. parainfluenzae, K. pneumoniae, M. catarrhalis, S. aureus* or *S. pneumoniae*
Mechanism of Action/Effect Inhibits DNA-gyrase in susceptible organisms; inhibits relaxation of supercoiled DNA and promotes breakage of double-stranded DNA
Contraindications Hypersensitivity to sparfloxacin, any component of the formulation, or other quinolones; a concurrent administration with drugs which increase the QT interval including amiodarone, bepridil, bretylium, cisapride, disopyramide, furosemide, procainamide, quinidine, sotalol, albuterol, chloroquine, halofantrine, phenothiazines, prednisone, and tricyclic antidepressants
Warnings/Precautions Not recommended in children <18 years of age; other quinolones have caused transient arthropathy in children; CNS stimulation may occur (tremor, restlessness, confusion, and very rarely hallucinations or seizures); use with caution in patients with known or suspected CNS disorder or renal dysfunction; prolonged use may result in superinfection. Moderate to severe photosensitivity reactions may occur in patients exposed to direct or indirect sunlight, or to artificial ultraviolet light. Patients should avoid unnecessary sunlight exposure during treatment and for 5 days following therapy. Pseudomembranous colitis may occur and should be considered in patients who present with diarrhea. Tendon inflammation and/or rupture have been reported with other quinolone antibiotics. Risk may be increased with concurrent corticosteroids, particularly in

the elderly. Discontinue at first sign of tendon inflammation or pain.

Severe hypersensitivity reactions, including anaphylaxis, have occurred with quinolone therapy. If an allergic reaction occurs (itching, urticaria, dyspnea, facial edema, loss of consciousness, tingling, cardiovascular collapse), discontinue drug immediately. Although quinolones may exacerbate myasthenia gravis, sparfloxacin appears to be an exception; caution is still warranted.

Drug Interactions
Decreased Effect: Concurrent administration of metal cations, including most antacids, oral electrolyte supplements, quinapril, sucralfate, some didanosine formulations (chewable/buffered tablets and pediatric powder for oral suspension), and other highly-buffered oral drugs, may decrease quinolone levels; separate doses.

Increased Effect/Toxicity: Sparfloxacin may increase the effects/toxicity of glyburide and warfarin. Concomitant use with corticosteroids may increase the risk of tendon rupture. Concomitant use with other QT_c-prolonging agents (eg, Class Ia and Class III antiarrhythmics, erythromycin, cisapride, antipsychotics, and cyclic antidepressants) may result in arrhythmias such as torsade de pointes. Probenecid may increase sparfloxacin levels.

Nutritional/Ethanol Interactions Herb/Nutraceutical: Avoid dong quai, St John's wort (may also cause photosensitization).

Adverse Reactions 1% to 10%:
Cardiovascular: QT_c interval prolongation (1%), vasodilation (1%)

Central nervous system: Insomnia (2%), dizziness (2%), headache (4%)

Dermatologic: Photosensitivity reaction (8%; severe <1%), pruritus (2%)

Gastrointestinal: Diarrhea (5%), dyspepsia (2%), nausea (4%), abdominal pain (2%), vomiting (1%), flatulence (1%), taste perversion (2%)

Hepatic: Increased LFTs

Overdosage/Toxicology Symptoms include acute renal failure and seizures. Treatment consists of GI decontamination and supportive care; it is not known if sparfloxacin is dialyzable.

Pharmacodynamics/Kinetics
Time to Peak: 3-5 hours

Protein Binding: 45%

Half-Life Elimination: Mean terminal: 20 hours (range: 16-30 hours)

Metabolism: Hepatic, primarily by phase II glucuronidation

Excretion: Excretion: Urine (50%; ~10% as unchanged drug); feces (50%)

Available Dosage Forms [DSC] = Discontinued product
Tablet: 200 mg [DSC]

Dosing
Adults & Elderly: Susceptible infections: Oral: Loading dose: 400 mg on day 1; maintenance dose: 200 mg/day for 10 days total therapy

Renal Impairment: Cl_{cr} <50 mL/minute: Administer 400 mg on day 1 as a loading dose, then 200 mg every 48 hours for a total of 8 additional days of therapy (total 6 tablets).

Administration
Oral: May be taken without regard to meals, however, should be administered at the same time each day. Antacids containing aluminum or magnesium; products containing iron, zinc, or calcium; and sucralfate and didanosine should all be given >4 hours after sparfloxacin.

Laboratory Monitoring Perform culture and sensitivity prior to beginning therapy. Monitor CBC, renal and hepatic function periodically if therapy is prolonged.

Nursing Actions
Physical Assessment: Culture and sensitivity tests should be assessed and patient's allergy history assessed before initiating therapy. Assess potential for interactions with other pharmacological agents and herbal products patient may be taking (eg, increased risk of arrhythmias). If severe allergic reaction occurs (itching, urticaria, dyspnea or facial edema, loss of consciousness, tingling, cardiovascular collapse) drug should be discontinued and prescriber notified immediately. Monitor laboratory tests, therapeutic effectiveness (resolution of infection), and adverse effects (photosensitivity, rash, gastrointestinal disturbance [diarrhea, nausea, vomiting, pain]).Teach patient proper use, possible side effects/appropriate interventions (eg, photosensitivity), and adverse symptoms to report (eg, opportunistic infection).

Patient Education: Do not take any new medication during therapy without consulting prescriber. Take as directed, at the same time each day. Antacids containing aluminum or magnesium and products containing iron, zinc, or calcium (vitamins) should be taken more than 4 hours after sparfloxacin. Take entire prescription even if feeling better. If dose is missed take as soon as possible, do not double doses. Maintain adequate hydration (2-3 L/day of fluids), unless instructed to restrict fluid intake. May cause photosensitivity (use sunscreen, wear protective clothing and eyewear, and avoid direct sunlight during and for several days following therapy); dizziness, lightheadedness, or anxiety (use caution when driving or engaging in tasks that require alertness until response to drug is known); nausea, vomiting, or dry mouth (small frequent meals, frequent mouth care, sucking lozenges, or chewing gum may help). If inflammation or tendon pain occurs, discontinue use immediately and report to prescriber. If allergic reaction occurs (itching urticaria, respiratory difficulty, facial edema or difficulty swallowing, loss of consciousness, tingling, chest pain, palpitations), discontinue immediately and report to prescriber. Report palpitations or chest pain; persistent diarrhea or constipation; or signs of superinfection (unusual fever or chills; vaginal itching or foul-smelling vaginal discharge; easy bruising or bleeding). **Pregnancy/breast-feeding precautions:** Inform prescriber if you are or intend to become pregnant. Do not breast-feed.

Dietary Considerations May be taken without regard to meals; should be taken at the same time each day.

Geriatric Considerations Elderly patients may be more susceptible to the cardiac adverse effects of sparfloxacin. Adjust dose based on renal function; evaluate patient's drug regimen prior to initiating therapy to avoid or make allowances for possible drug interactions since elderly frequently have diseases requiring medications that can interact with quinolones.

Breast-Feeding Issues The manufacturer recommends to discontinue nursing or to discontinue sparfloxacin.

Pregnancy Issues Reports of arthropathy (observed in immature animals and reported rarely in humans) have limited the use of fluoroquinolones in pregnancy. Teratogenic effects were not reported with sparfloxacin in animal studies. Based on limited data, quinolones are not expected to be a major human teratogen. Although quinolone antibiotics should not be used as first-line agents during pregnancy, when considering treatment for life-threatening infection and/or prolonged duration of therapy, the potential risk to the fetus must be balanced against the severity of the potential illness.

Spectinomycin (spek ti noe MYE sin)

U.S. Brand Names Trobicin® [DSC]

Synonyms Spectinomycin Hydrochloride

Pharmacologic Category Antibiotic, Miscellaneous

Medication Safety Issues
Sound-alike/look-alike issues:
Trobicin® may be confused with tobramycin

Pregnancy Risk Factor B

Lactation Enters breast milk/effect on infant unknown

Use Treatment of uncomplicated gonorrhea

Mechanism of Action/Effect A bacteriostatic antibiotic that selectively binds to the 30s subunits of ribosomes, and thereby inhibiting bacterial protein synthesis

Contraindications Hypersensitivity to spectinomycin or any component of the formulation

Warnings/Precautions Since spectinomycin is ineffective in the treatment of syphilis and may mask symptoms, all patients should be tested for syphilis at the time of diagnosis and 3 months later.

Overdosage/Toxicology Symptoms of overdose include paresthesia, dizziness, blurring of vision, ototoxicity, renal damage, nausea, sleeplessness, decrease in hemoglobin

Pharmacodynamics/Kinetics
Duration of Action: Up to 8 hours

Time to Peak: ~1 hour

Half-Life Elimination: 1.7 hours

Excretion: Urine (70% to 100% as unchanged drug)

Available Dosage Forms
Injection, powder for reconstitution, as hydrochloride:
Trobicin®: 2 g [diluent contains benzyl alcohol] [DSC]

Dosing
Adults & Elderly:
Uncomplicated gonorrhea (urethral, cervical, pharyngeal, or rectal): I.M.: 2 g deep I.M. or 4 g where antibiotic resistance is prevalent 1 time; 4 g (10 mL) dose should be given as two 5 mL injections, followed by adequate chlamydial treatment (doxycycline 100 mg twice daily for 7 days)

Disseminated gonococcal infection: I.M.: 2 g every 12 hours

Pediatrics: Gonorrhea: I.M.: Children:
<45 kg: 40 mg/kg/dose 1 time (ceftriaxone preferred)
≥45 kg: Refer to adult dosing.
Children >8 years who are allergic to PCNS/cephalosporins may be treated with oral tetracycline.

Renal Impairment: Hemodialysis effects: 50% removed by hemodialysis

Administration
I.M.: For I.M. use only.

Stability
Reconstitution: Use reconstituted solutions within 24 hours; reconstitute with supplied diluent only.

Laboratory Monitoring Test for syphilis before treatment and 3 months later (see Warnings/Precautions).

Nursing Actions
Physical Assessment: Assess knowledge/teach patient sexually transmitted diseases precautions. Monitor effectiveness and evaluate laboratory results.

Patient Education: This medication can only be administered I.M. You will need to return for follow-up blood tests. **Breast-feeding precaution:** Consult prescriber if breast-feeding.

Spironolactone (speer on oh LAK tone)

U.S. Brand Names Aldactone®

Pharmacologic Category Diuretic, Potassium-Sparing; Selective Aldosterone Blocker

Medication Safety Issues
Sound-alike/look-alike issues:
Aldactone® may be confused with Aldactazide®

Pregnancy Risk Factor C/D in pregnancy-induced hypertension (per expert analysis)

Lactation Enters breast milk/not recommended (AAP rates "compatible")

Use Management of edema associated with excessive aldosterone excretion; hypertension; congestive heart failure; primary hyperaldosteronism; hypokalemia; treatment of hirsutism; cirrhosis of liver accompanied by edema or ascites

Unlabeled/Investigational Use Female acne (adjunctive therapy); hirsutism; hypertension (pediatric); diuretic (pediatric)

Mechanism of Action/Effect Competes with aldosterone for receptor sites in the distal renal tubules, increasing sodium chloride and water excretion while conserving potassium and hydrogen ions; may block the effect of aldosterone on arteriolar smooth muscle as well

Contraindications Hypersensitivity to spironolactone or any component of the formulation; anuria; acute renal insufficiency; significant impairment of renal excretory function; hyperkalemia; pregnancy (pregnancy-induced hypertension - per expert analysis)

Warnings/Precautions Avoid potassium supplements, potassium-containing salt substitutes, a diet rich in potassium, or other drugs that can cause hyperkalemia. Monitor for fluid and electrolyte imbalances. Gynecomastia is related to dose and duration of therapy. Diuretic therapy should be carefully used in severe hepatic dysfunction; electrolyte and fluid shifts can cause or exacerbate encephalopathy. Discontinue use prior to adrenal vein catheterization. When evaluating a heart failure patient for spironolactone treatment, creatinine should be ≤2.5 mg/dL in men or ≤2 mg/dL in women and potassium <5 mEq/L.

Drug Interactions
Decreased Effect: The effects of digoxin (loss of positive inotropic effect) and mitotane may be reduced by spironolactone. Salicylates and NSAIDs (indomethacin) may decrease the natriuretic effect of spironolactone.

Increased Effect/Toxicity: Concurrent use of spironolactone with other potassium-sparing diuretics, potassium supplements, angiotensin receptor antagonists, co-trimoxazole (high dose), and ACE inhibitors can increase the risk of hyperkalemia, especially in patients with renal impairment. Cholestyramine can cause hyperchloremic acidosis in cirrhotic patients; avoid concurrent use.

Nutritional/Ethanol Interactions
Food: Food increases absorption.
Herb/Nutraceutical: Avoid natural licorice (due to mineralocorticoid activity)

Lab Interactions May cause false elevation in serum digoxin concentrations measured by RIA.

Adverse Reactions Incidence of adverse events is not always reported. (Mean daily dose: 26 mg)

Cardiovascular: Edema (2%, placebo 2%)
Central nervous system: Disorders (23%, placebo 21%) which may include drowsiness, lethargy, headache, mental confusion, drug fever, ataxia, fatigue
Dermatologic: Maculopapular, erythematous cutaneous eruptions, urticaria, hirsutism, eosinophilia
Endocrine & metabolic: Gynecomastia (men 9%; placebo 1%), breast pain (men 2%; placebo 0.1%),

serious hyperkalemia (2%, placebo 1%), hyponatremia, dehydration, hyperchloremic metabolic acidosis in decompensated hepatic cirrhosis, inability to achieve or maintain an erection, irregular menses, amenorrhea, postmenopausal bleeding

Gastrointestinal: Disorders (29%, placebo 29%) which may include anorexia, nausea, cramping, diarrhea, gastric bleeding, ulceration, gastritis, vomiting

Genitourinary: Disorders (12%, placebo 11%)

Hematologic: Agranulocytosis

Hepatic: Cholestatic/hepatocellular toxicity

Renal: Increased BUN concentration

Respiratory: Disorders (32%, placebo 34%)

Miscellaneous: Deepening of the voice, anaphylactic reaction, breast cancer

Overdosage/Toxicology Symptoms of overdose include drowsiness, confusion, clinical signs of dehydration and electrolyte imbalance, and hyperkalemia. Ingestion of large amounts of potassium-sparing diuretics may result in life-threatening hyperkalemia. This can be treated with I.V. glucose, with concurrent regular insulin. Sodium bicarbonate may also be used as a temporary measure. If needed, Kayexalate® oral or rectal solutions in sorbitol may also be used.

Pharmacodynamics/Kinetics

Duration of Action: 2-3 days

Time to Peak: Serum: 1-3 hours (primarily as the active metabolite)

Protein Binding: 91% to 98%

Half-Life Elimination: 78-84 minutes

Metabolism: Hepatic to multiple metabolites, including canrenone (active)

Excretion: Urine and feces

Available Dosage Forms Tablet: 25 mg, 50 mg, 100 mg

Dosing

Adults: To reduce delay in onset of effect, a loading dose of 2 or 3 times the daily dose may be administered on the first day of therapy. Oral:

Edema, hypokalemia: 25-200 mg/day in 1-2 divided doses

Hypertension (JNC 7): 25-50 mg/day in 1-2 divided doses

Diagnosis of primary aldosteronism: 100-400 mg/day in 1-2 divided doses

Acne in women (unlabeled use): 25-200 mg once daily

Hirsutism in women (unlabeled use): 50-200 mg/day in 1-2 divided doses

CHF, severe (with ACE inhibitor and a loop diuretic ± digoxin): 12.5-25 mg/day; maximum daily dose: 50 mg (higher doses may occasionallly be used). In the RALES trial, 25 mg every other day was the lowest maintenance dose possible.

Note: If potassium >5.4 mEq/L, consider dosage reduction.

Elderly: Oral: Initial: 25-50 mg/day in 1-2 divided doses; increase by 25-50 mg every 5 days as needed. Adjust for renal impairment.

Pediatrics: Administration with food increases absorption. To reduce delay in onset of effect, a loading dose of 2 or 3 times the daily dose may be administered on the first day of therapy.

Edema, hypertension (unlabeled use): Oral: Children 1-17 years: Initial: 1 mg/kg/day divided every 12-24 hours (maximum dose: 3.3 mg/kg/day, up to 100 mg/day)

Diagnosis of primary aldosteronism (unlabeled use): Oral: 125-375 mg/m²/day in divided doses

Renal Impairment:

Cl_{cr} 10-50 mL/minute: Administer every 12-24 hours.

Cl_{cr} <10 mL/minute: Avoid use.

Stability

Storage: Protect from light.

Laboratory Monitoring Serum electrolytes (potassium, sodium), renal function

Nursing Actions

Physical Assessment: Diuretic effect may be delayed 2-3 days and antihypertensive effect may be delayed 2-3 weeks (loading dose may be prescribed to reduce delay). Assess potential for interactions with other pharmacological agents patient may be taking (eg, anything that will increase risk of hyperkalemia). Monitor serum electrolytes and hepatic function on a regular basis during therapy. Monitor effectiveness (fluid status) and adverse reactions periodically (eg, CNS changes [drowsiness, headache, confusion], rash, gynecomastia, dehydration, hyperkalemia, jaundice). Teach patient appropriate use, possible side effects/appropriate interventions and symptoms to report.

Patient Education: Take as directed, with meals. Avoid any potassium supplements (vitamin/mineral products), potassium-containing salt substitutes, natural licorice, or extra dietary intake of potassium. Weigh yourself weekly at the same time, in the same clothes, and report weight loss >5 lb/week. May cause dizziness, drowsiness, confusion, or headache (use caution when driving or engaging in tasks requiring alertness until response to drug is known); nausea, vomiting, or dry mouth (small, frequent meals, frequent mouth care, sucking lozenges, or chewing gum may help); or decreased sexual ability, gynecomastia, impotence, menstrual irregularities (reversible with discontinuing of medication). Report mental confusion; clumsiness; persistent fatigue, chills, numbness, or muscle weakness in hands, feet, or face; acute persistent diarrhea; chest pain, rapid heartbeat, or palpitations; excessive thirst; or respiratory difficulty; breast tenderness or increased body hair in females; breast enlargement or inability to achieve erection in males. Pregnancy precaution: Do not get pregnant while taking this medication. Consult prescriber for appropriate contraceptive measures.

Dietary Considerations Should be taken with food to decrease gastrointestinal irritation and to increase absorption. Excessive potassium intake (eg, salt substitutes, low-salt foods, bananas, nuts) should be avoided.

Geriatric Considerations See Warnings/Precautions. When used in combination with ACE inhibitors, monitor patient for hyperkalemia.

Breast-Feeding Issues The active metabolite of spironolactone has been found in breast milk. Effects to humans are not known; however, this metabolite was found to be carcinogenic in rats. The manufacturer recommends discontinuing spironolactone or using an alternative method of feeding.

Pregnancy Issues Teratogenic effects were not observed in animal studies; however, doses used were less than or equal to equivalent doses in humans. The antiandrogen effects of spironolactone have been shown to cause feminization of the male fetus in animal studies. Two case reports did not demonstrate this effect in humans however, the authors caution that adequate data is lacking. Diuretics are generally avoided in pregnancy due to the theoretical risk that decreased plasma volume may cause placental insufficiency. Diuretics should not be used during pregnancy in the presence of reduced placental perfusion (eg, pre-eclampsia, intrauterine growth restriction).

Additional Information Maximum diuretic effect may be delayed 2-3 days and maximum hypertensive effects may be delayed 2-3 weeks.

Stavudine (STAV yoo deen)

U.S. Brand Names Zerit®

Synonyms d4T

Pharmacologic Category Antiretroviral Agent, Reverse Transcriptase Inhibitor (Nucleoside)

Medication Safety Issues
Sound-alike/look-alike issues:
Zerit® may be confused with Ziac®

Pregnancy Risk Factor C

Lactation Excretion in breast milk unknown/contraindicated

Use Treatment of HIV infection in combination with other antiretroviral agents

Mechanism of Action/Effect Inhibits reverse transcriptase of the human immunodeficiency virus (HIV)

Contraindications Hypersensitivity to stavudine or any component of the formulation

Warnings/Precautions Use with caution in patients who demonstrate previous hypersensitivity to zidovudine, didanosine, zalcitabine, pre-existing bone marrow suppression, renal insufficiency, or peripheral neuropathy. Peripheral neuropathy may be the dose-limiting side effect. Zidovudine should not be used in combination with stavudine. Lactic acidosis and severe hepatomegaly with steatosis have been reported with stavudine use, including fatal cases. Risk may be increased in obesity, prolonged nucleoside exposure, or in female patients. Suspend therapy in patients with suspected lactic acidosis; consider discontinuation of stavudine if lactic acidosis is confirmed. Pregnant women may be at increased risk of lactic acidosis and liver damage. Severe motor weakness (resembling Guillain-Barré syndrome) has also been reported (including fatal cases, usually in association with lactic acidosis); manufacturer recommends discontinuation if motor weakness develops (with or without lactic acidosis). Pancreatitis (including some fatal cases) has occurred during combination therapy (didanosine with or without hydroxyurea). Risk increased when used in combination regimen with didanosine and hydroxyurea. Suspend therapy with agents toxic to the pancreas (including stavudine, didanosine, or hydroxyurea) in patients with suspected pancreatitis.

Drug Interactions
Decreased Effect: Zidovudine inhibits intracellular phosphorylation of stavudine; concurrent use not recommended. Doxorubicin may inhibit intracellular phosphorylation of stavudine; use with caution. Ribavirin may inhibit intracellular phosphorylation of stavudine; use with caution.

Increased Effect/Toxicity: Risk of pancreatitis may be increased with concurrent didanosine use; cases of fatal lactic acidosis have been reported with this combination when used during pregnancy (use only if clearly needed). Risk of hepatotoxicity or pancreatitis may be increased with concurrent hydroxyurea use. Zalcitabine may increase risk of peripheral neuropathy; concurrent use not recommended.

Adverse Reactions All adverse reactions reported below were similar to comparative agent, zidovudine, except for peripheral neuropathy, which was greater for stavudine. Selected adverse events reported as monotherapy or in combination therapy include:

>10%:
Central nervous system: Headache
Dermatologic: Rash
Gastrointestinal: Nausea, vomiting, diarrhea
Hepatic: Hepatic transaminases increased
Neuromuscular & skeletal: Peripheral neuropathy
Miscellaneous: Amylase increased
1% to 10%: Hepatic: Bilirubin increased

Overdosage/Toxicology Acute toxicity was not reported following administration of 12-24 times the recommended dose in adults. Peripheral neuropathy and hepatic toxicity have been reported following chronic overdose. Stavudine may be removed by hemodialysis.

Pharmacodynamics/Kinetics
Time to Peak: Serum: 1 hour
Half-Life Elimination: 1-1.6 hours
Metabolism: Undergoes intracellular phosphorylation to an active metabolite
Excretion: Urine (40% as unchanged drug)

Available Dosage Forms
Capsule: 15 mg, 20 mg, 30 mg, 40 mg
Powder, for oral solution: 1 mg/mL (200 mL) [dye free; fruit flavor]

Dosing
Adults: HIV infection (in combination with other antiretrovirals): Oral:
≥60 kg: 40 mg every 12 hours
<60 kg: 30 mg every 12 hours

Elderly: Older patients should be closely monitored for signs and symptoms of peripheral neuropathy. Dosage should be carefully adjusted to renal function.

Pediatrics: HIV infection: Oral:
Newborns (Birth to 13 days): 0.5 mg/kg every 12 hours
Children:
>14 days and <30 kg: 1 mg/kg every 12 hours
≥30 kg: 30 mg every 12 hours

Renal Impairment:
Children: Specific recommendations not available. Reduction in dose or increase in dosing interval should be considered.
Adults:
Cl_{cr} >50 mL/minute:
≥60 kg: 40 mg every 12 hours
<60 kg: 30 mg every 12 hours
Cl_{cr} 26-50 mL/minute:
≥60 kg: 20 mg every 12 hours
<60 kg: 15 mg every 12 hours
Cl_{cr} 10-25 mL/minute, hemodialysis (administer dose after hemodialysis on day of dialysis):
≥60 kg: 20 mg every 24 hours
<60 kg: 15 mg every 24 hours

Dosing Adjustment for Toxicity: If symptoms of peripheral neuropathy occur, discontinue until symptoms resolve. Treatment may then be resumed at 50% the recommended dose. If symptoms recur at lower dose, permanent discontinuation should be considered.

Administration
Oral: May be administered without regard to meals. Oral solution should be shaken vigorously prior to use.

Stability
Storage: Capsules and powder for reconstitution may be stored at room temperature. Reconstituted oral solution should be refrigerated and is stable for 30 days.

Laboratory Monitoring Liver function, viral load

Nursing Actions
Physical Assessment: Allergy history should be assessed prior to beginning treatment. Assess other pharmacological or herbal products patient may be taking for potential interactions. **Note:** Monitor patient closely for any indication of adverse reactions (eg, peripheral neuropathy, lactic acidosis, hepatomegaly, motor weakness) that may require suspension of therapy. Monitor laboratory tests and effectiveness of therapy periodically during therapy. Teach patient proper use (eg, timing of multiple medications and drugs that should not be used concurrently), possible side effects/appropriate interventions, and adverse symptoms to report.

Patient Education: Do not take any new prescription, over-the-counter medications, or herbal products without consulting prescriber. This drug will not cure

HIV, nor has it been found to reduce transmission of HIV; use appropriate precautions to prevent spread to other persons. This drug is prescribed as one part of a multidrug combination; take exactly as directed, for full course of therapy. Maintain adequate hydration (2-3 L/day of fluids) unless advised by prescriber to restrict fluids. You may be susceptible to infection (avoid crowds and exposure to known infections and do not have any vaccinations without consulting prescriber). Frequent blood tests may be required with prolonged therapy. May cause dizziness or weakness (use caution when driving or engaging in tasks requiring alertness until response to drug is known); or nausea or vomiting (small frequent meals, frequent mouth care, chewing gum, or sucking lozenges may help). Report immediately any tingling, pain, or loss of sensation in toes, feet, muscles or joints; swollen glands; alterations in urinary pattern; swelling of extremities, weight gain, or other persistent adverse effects. If you are instructed to stop the medication, do not restart without specific instruction by your prescriber. **Pregnancy/breast-feeding precautions:** Inform prescriber if you are or intend to become pregnant. Do not breast-feed.

Dietary Considerations May be taken without regard to meals.

Breast-Feeding Issues HIV-infected mothers are discouraged from breast-feeding to decrease potential transmission of HIV.

Pregnancy Issues Cases of fatal and nonfatal lactic acidosis, with or without pancreatitis, have been reported in pregnant women. It is not known if pregnancy itself potentiates this known side effect; however, pregnant women may be at increased risk of lactic acidosis and liver damage. Hepatic enzymes and electrolytes should be monitored frequently during the 3rd trimester of pregnancy. Pharmacokinetics of stavudine are not significantly altered during pregnancy; dose adjustments are not needed. The Perinatal HIV Guidelines Working Group considers stavudine to be an alternative NRTI in dual nucleoside combination regimens; use with didanosine only if no alternatives are available, do not use with zidovudine. Health professionals are encouraged to contact the antiretroviral pregnancy registry to monitor outcomes of pregnant women exposed to antiretroviral medications (1-800-258-4263 or www.APRegistry.com).

Additional Information Potential compliance problems, frequency of administration and adverse effects should be discussed with patients before initiating therapy to help prevent the emergence of resistance.

Streptokinase (strep toe KYE nase)

U.S. Brand Names Streptase®
Synonyms SK
Pharmacologic Category Thrombolytic Agent
Pregnancy Risk Factor C
Lactation Excretion in breast milk unknown
Use Thrombolytic agent used in treatment of recent severe or massive deep vein thrombosis, pulmonary emboli, myocardial infarction, and occluded arteriovenous cannulas

Mechanism of Action/Effect Activates the conversion of plasminogen to plasmin by forming a complex, exposing plasminogen-activating site, and cleaving a peptide bond that converts plasminogen to plasmin; plasmin degrades fibrin, fibrinogen and other procoagulant proteins into soluble fragments; effective both outside and within the formed thrombus/embolus

Contraindications Hypersensitivity to anistreplase, streptokinase, or any component of the formulation; active internal bleeding; history of CVA; recent (within 2 months) intracranial or intraspinal surgery or trauma;

intracranial neoplasm, arteriovenous malformation, or aneurysm; known bleeding diathesis; severe uncontrolled hypertension

Warnings/Precautions Concurrent heparin anticoagulation can contribute to bleeding; careful attention to all potential bleeding sites. I.M. injections and nonessential handling of the patient should be avoided. Venipunctures should be performed carefully and only when necessary. If arterial puncture is necessary, use an upper extremity vessel that can be manually compressed. If serious bleeding occurs then the infusion of streptokinase and heparin should be stopped.

For the following conditions the risk of bleeding is higher with use of thrombolytics and should be weighed against the benefits of therapy: recent (within 10 days) major surgery (eg, CABG, obstetrical delivery, organ biopsy, previous puncture of noncompressible vessels), cerebrovascular disease, recent (within 10 days) gastrointestinal or genitourinary bleeding, recent trauma (within 10 days) including CPR, hypertension (systolic BP >180 mm Hg and/or diastolic BP >110 mm Hg), high likelihood of left heart thrombus (eg, mitral stenosis with atrial fibrillation), acute pericarditis, subacute bacterial endocarditis, hemostatic defects including ones caused by severe renal or hepatic dysfunction, significant hepatic dysfunction, pregnancy, diabetic hemorrhagic retinopathy or other hemorrhagic ophthalmic conditions, septic thrombophlebitis or occluded AV cannula at seriously infected site, advanced age (eg, >75 years), patients receiving oral anticoagulants, any other condition in which bleeding constitutes a significant hazard or would be particularly difficult to manage because of location.

Coronary thrombolysis may result in reperfusion arrhythmias. Hypotension, occasionally severe, can occur (not from bleeding or anaphylaxis). Follow standard MI management. Rare anaphylactic reactions can occur. Cautious repeat administration in patients who have received anistreplase or streptokinase within 1 year (streptokinase antibody may decrease effectiveness or risk of allergic reactions). Safety and efficacy in pediatric patients have not been established.

Streptokinase is not indicated for restoration of patency of intravenous catheters. Serious adverse events relating to the use of streptokinase in the restoration of patency of occluded intravenous catheters have involved the use of high doses of streptokinase in small volumes (250,000 international units in 2 mL). Uses of lower doses of streptokinase in infusions over several hours, generally into partially occluded catheters, or local instillation into the catheter lumen and subsequent aspiration, have been described in the medical literature. Healthcare providers should consider the risk for potentially life-threatening reactions (hypersensitivity, apnea, bleeding) associated with the use of streptokinase in the management of occluded intravenous catheters.

Drug Interactions
Decreased Effect: Antifibrinolytic agents (aminocaproic acid) may decrease effectiveness to thrombolytic agents.

Increased Effect/Toxicity: The risk of bleeding with streptokinase is increased by oral anticoagulants (warfarin), heparin, low molecular weight heparins, and drugs which affect platelet function (eg, NSAIDs, dipyridamole, ticlopidine, clopidogrel, IIb/IIIa antagonists). Although concurrent use with aspirin and heparin may increase the risk of bleeding. Aspirin and heparin were used concomitantly with streptokinase in the majority of patients in clinical studies of MI.

Nutritional/Ethanol Interactions Herb/Nutraceutical: Avoid cat's claw, dong quai, evening primrose, feverfew, red clover, horse chestnut, garlic, green tea, ginseng, ginkgo (all have additional antiplatelet activity). (Continued)

Streptokinase (Continued)

Adverse Reactions As with all drugs which may affect hemostasis, bleeding is the major adverse effect associated with streptokinase. Hemorrhage may occur at virtually any site. Risk is dependent on multiple variables, including the dosage administered, concurrent use of multiple agents which alter hemostasis, and patient predisposition (including hypertension). Rapid lysis of coronary artery thrombi by thrombolytic agents may be associated with reperfusion-related atrial and/or ventricular arrhythmia.

>10%:
    Cardiovascular: Hypotension
    Local: Injection site bleeding
1% to 10%:
    Central nervous system: Fever (1% to 4%)
    Dermatologic: Bruising, rash, pruritus
    Gastrointestinal: Gastrointestinal hemorrhage, nausea, vomiting
    Genitourinary: Genitourinary hemorrhage
    Hematologic: Anemia
    Neuromuscular & skeletal: Muscle pain
    Ocular: Eye hemorrhage, periorbital edema
    Respiratory: Bronchospasm, epistaxis
    Miscellaneous: Diaphoresis hemorrhage, gingival hemorrhage

Additional cardiovascular events associated with use in MI: Asystole, AV block, cardiac arrest, cardiac tamponade, cardiogenic shock, electromechanical dissociation, heart failure, mitral regurgitation, myocardial rupture, pericardial effusion, pericarditis, pulmonary edema, recurrent ischemia/infarction, thromboembolism, ventricular tachycardia

Overdosage/Toxicology Symptoms of overdose include epistaxis, bleeding gums, hematoma, spontaneous ecchymoses, and oozing at the catheter site. If uncontrollable bleeding occurs, discontinue infusion. Whole blood or blood products may be used to reverse bleeding.

Pharmacodynamics/Kinetics

Onset of Action: Activation of plasminogen occurs almost immediately

Duration of Action: Fibrinolytic effect: Several hours; Anticoagulant effect: 12-24 hours

Half-Life Elimination: 83 minutes

Excretion: By circulating antibodies and the reticuloendothelial system

Available Dosage Forms [DSC] = Discontinued product

Injection, powder for reconstitution: 250,000 int. units; 750,000 int. units; 1,500,000 int. units [DSC]

Dosing

Adults & Elderly: I.V.:
    Note: Antibodies to streptokinase remain for at least 3-6 months after initial dose: See Warnings/Precautions. An intradermal skin test of 100 units has been suggested to predict allergic response to streptokinase. If a positive reaction is not seen after 15-20 minutes, a therapeutic dose may be administered.
    Guidelines for acute myocardial infarction (AMI): I.V.: 1.5 million units over 60 minutes
    Administration:
        Dilute two 750,000 unit vials of streptokinase with 5 mL dextrose 5% in water (D₅W) each, gently swirl to dissolve.
        Add this dose of the 1.5 million units to 150 mL D₅W.
        This should be infused over 60 minutes; an in-line filter ≥0.45 micron should be used.
        Monitor for the first few hours for signs of anaphylaxis or allergic reaction. **Infusion should be slowed if lowering of 25 mm Hg in blood pressure or terminated if asthmatic symptoms appear.**

Note: If heparin is administered, start when aPTT is less than 2 times the upper limit of control; do not use a bolus, but initiate infusion adjusted to a target a PTT of 1.5-2 times the upper limit of control. If heparin is not administered by infusion, initiate 7500-12,500 units SubQ every 12 hours.

Guidelines for acute pulmonary embolism (APE): I.V.: 3 million unit dose over 24 hours
    Administration:
        Dilute four 750,000 unit vials of streptokinase with 5 mL dextrose 5% in water (D₅W) each, gently swirl to dissolve.
        Add this dose of 3 million units to 250 mL D₅W, an in-line filter ≥0.45 micron should be used.
        Administer 250,000 units (23 mL) over 30 minutes followed by 100,000 units/hour (9 mL/hour) for 24 hours.
        Monitor for the first few hours for signs of anaphylaxis or allergic reaction. **Infusion should be slowed if blood pressure is lowered by 25 mm Hg or if asthmatic symptoms appear.**
        Begin heparin 1000 units/hour about 3-4 hours after completion of streptokinase infusion or when PTT is <100 seconds.

Guidelines for thromboses: I.V.: Administer 250,000 units to start, then 100,000 units/hour for 24-72 hours depending on location.

Cannula occlusion: 250,000 units into cannula, clamp for 2 hours, then aspirate contents and flush with normal saline; **Not recommended; see Warnings/Precautions**

Pediatrics: Children: Safety and efficacy not established; limited studies have used the following doses.

Thromboses: I.V.: *Chest,* 1998 recommendations: Initial (loading dose): 2000 units/kg followed by 2000 units/kg/hour for 6-12 hours **or** initial (loading dose): 3500-4000 units/kg over 30 minutes followed by I.V. continuous infusion: 1000-1500 units/kg/hour; dose should be individualized based on response.

Clotted catheter: I.V.: **Note:** Not recommended due to possibility of allergic reactions with repeated doses: 10,000-25,000 units diluted in NS to a final volume equivalent to catheter volume; instill into catheter and leave in place for 1 hour, then aspirate contents out of catheter and flush catheter with normal saline.

Administration

I.M.: Do **not** administer by intramuscular injection.

I.V.: For I.V. or intracoronary use only. Infusion pump is required. Use in-line filter >0.8 micron.

I.V. Detail: pH: Dependent on diluent used

Stability

Reconstitution: Reconstituted solutions should be refrigerated and are stable for 24 hours.

Compatibility: Stable in D₅W, NS; **incompatible** with dextrans

Storage: Streptokinase, a white lyophilized powder, may have a slight yellow color in solution due to the presence of albumin. Intact vials should be stored at room temperature. Stability of parenteral admixture at room temperature (25°C) is 8 hours and at refrigeration (4°C) is 24 hours.

Laboratory Monitoring PT, aPTT, platelet count, hematocrit, fibrinogen concentration

Nursing Actions

Physical Assessment: **Note:** Streptokinase is not indicated for restoration of patency of intravenous catheters; life-threatening reactions are associated with this use. Assess potential for interactions with other pharmacological agents and herbal product patient may be taking (especially those medications that may affect coagulation [warfarin] or platelet function [NSAIDs, dipyridamole, ticlopidine, clopidogrel]) See Administration for infusion specifics (infusion pump is required). Monitor laboratory results. Monitor patient closely for bleeding during and following treatment; infusion site, neurological status (eg, intracranial hemorrhage), vital signs, ECG (reperfusion arrhythmias). Bedrest and bleeding precautions should be maintained; avoid I.M. injections, venipuncture (unless absolutely necessary) and nonessential handling of the patient. If arterial puncture is necessary, use an upper extremity vessel that can be manually compressed. Patient instructions determined by patient condition.

Patient Education: Inform prescriber of all medication or herbal products you are taking. This medication is only administered by infusion; you will be monitored closely during and after treatment. Immediately report burning, pain, redness, swelling, or oozing at infusion site, sudden acute headache, joint pain, chest pain, or altered vision. Following infusion you will have a tendency to bleed easily; use caution to prevent injury (use electric razor, soft toothbrush, and caution with knives, needles, or anything sharp) and follow instructions for strict bedrest to reduce the risk of injury. If bleeding does occur, report immediately and apply pressure to bleeding spot until bleeding stops completely. Report unusual pain (acute headache, joint pain, chest pain); unusual bruising or bleeding; blood in urine, stool, or vomitus; bleeding gums; vision changes; or respiratory difficulty. **Pregnancy/breast-feeding precautions:** Inform prescriber if you are or intend to become pregnant. Consult prescriber if breast-feeding.

Geriatric Considerations Investigators applied analysis to data for patients ≥75 years of age from two large trials studying the impact of streptokinase on patient outcome after acute myocardial infarction. Their conclusion was that age alone is not a contraindication to the use of streptokinase and that thrombolytic therapy is cost-effective and is beneficial toward the survival of elderly patients. Additional studies are needed to determine if a weight-adjusted dose will maintain efficacy but decrease adverse events such as stroke.

Streptomycin (strep toe MYE sin)

Synonyms Streptomycin Sulfate

Pharmacologic Category Antibiotic, Aminoglycoside; Antitubercular Agent

Medication Safety Issues

Sound-alike/look-alike issues:

Streptomycin may be confused with streptozocin

Pregnancy Risk Factor D

Lactation Enters breast milk/compatible

Use Part of combination therapy of active tuberculosis; used in combination with other agents for treatment of streptococcal or enterococcal endocarditis, mycobacterial infections, plague, tularemia, and brucellosis

Mechanism of Action/Effect Inhibits bacterial protein synthesis by binding directly to the 30S ribosomal subunits causing faulty peptide sequence to form in the protein chain

Contraindications Hypersensitivity to streptomycin or any component of the formulation; pregnancy

Warnings/Precautions Use with caution in patients with pre-existing vertigo, tinnitus, hearing loss, neuromuscular disorders, or renal impairment. Modify dosage in patients with renal impairment. Aminoglycosides are associated with nephrotoxicity or ototoxicity. The ototoxicity may be proportional to the amount of drug given and the duration of treatment. Tinnitus or vertigo are indications of vestibular injury and impending hearing damage. Renal damage is usually reversible.

Drug Interactions

Increased Effect/Toxicity: Increased/prolonged effect with depolarizing and nondepolarizing neuromuscular blocking agents. Concurrent use with amphotericin or loop diuretics may increase nephrotoxicity.

Lab Interactions False-positive urine glucose with Benedict's solution

Adverse Reactions Frequency not defined.

Cardiovascular: Hypotension

Central nervous system: Neurotoxicity, drowsiness, headache, drug fever, paresthesia

Dermatologic: Skin rash

Gastrointestinal: Nausea, vomiting

Hematologic: Eosinophilia, anemia

Neuromuscular & skeletal: Arthralgia, weakness, tremor

Otic: Ototoxicity (auditory), ototoxicity (vestibular)

Renal: Nephrotoxicity

Respiratory: Difficulty in breathing

Overdosage/Toxicology Symptoms of overdose include ototoxicity, nephrotoxicity, and neuromuscular toxicity. The treatment of choice following a single acute overdose appears to be maintenance of urine output of at least 3 mL/kg/hour during the acute treatment phase. Dialysis is of questionable value in enhancing aminoglycoside elimination. If required, hemodialysis is preferred over peritoneal dialysis in patients with normal renal function. Chelation with penicillins is experimental.

Pharmacodynamics/Kinetics

Time to Peak: I.M.: Within 1 hour

Protein Binding: 34%

Half-Life Elimination: Newborns: 4-10 hours; Adults: 2-4.7 hours, prolonged with renal impairment

Excretion: Urine (90% as unchanged drug); feces, saliva, sweat, and tears (<1%)

Available Dosage Forms Injection, powder for reconstitution: 1 g

Dosing

Adults:

Tuberculosis: I.M.:

Daily therapy: I.M.: 15 mg/kg/day (maximum: 1 g)

Directly observed therapy (DOT), twice weekly: I.M.: 25-30 mg/kg (maximum: 1.5 g)

Directly observed therapy (DOT), 3 times/week: I.M.: 25-30 mg/kg (maximum: 1 g)

Enterococcal endocarditis: I.M.: 1 g every 12 hours for 2 weeks, 500 mg every 12 hours for 4 weeks in combination with penicillin

Streptococcal endocarditis: I.M., I.V.: 1 g every 12 hours for 1 week, 500 mg every 12 hours for 1 week

Tularemia: I.M., I.V.: 1-2 g/day in divided doses for 7-10 days or until patient is afebrile for 5-7 days

Plague: I.M., I.V.: 2-4 g/day in divided doses until the patient is afebrile for at least 3 days

Elderly: Intramuscular: 10 mg/kg/day, not to exceed 750 mg/day; dosing interval should be adjusted for renal function. Some authors suggest not to give more than 5 days/week or give as 20-25 mg/kg/dose twice weekly.

Pediatrics:

Tuberculosis: I.M., I.V.: Children:

Daily therapy: 20-40 mg/kg/day (maximum: 1 g/day)

Directly observed therapy (DOT), twice weekly: 20-40 mg/kg (maximum: 1 g)

Directly observed therapy DOT, 3 times/week: 25-30 mg/kg (maximum: 1 g)

Renal Impairment:

Cl$_{cr}$ 10-50 mL/minute: Administer every 24-72 hours.

Cl$_{cr}$ <10 mL/minute: Administer every 72-96 hours.

Removed by hemo- and peritoneal dialysis: Administer dose postdialysis.

Administration

I.M.: Inject deep I.M. into large muscle mass.

I.V.: I.V. administration is not recommended. Has been administered intravenously over 30-60 minutes.

(Continued)

Streptomycin *(Continued)*

I.V. Detail: pH: 5-8 (injection)

Stability

Compatibility:

Compatibility in syringe: Incompatible with heparin

Compatibility when admixed: Incompatible with amobarbital, amphotericin B, chlorothiazide, heparin, methohexital, norepinephrine, pentobarbital, phenobarbital, phenytoin, sodium bicarbonate

Storage: Depending upon manufacturer, reconstituted solution remains stable for 2-4 weeks when refrigerated and 24 hours at room temperature. Exposure to light causes darkening of solution without apparent loss of potency.

Laboratory Monitoring Hearing (audiogram), BUN, creatinine; serum concentration of the drug should be monitored. Perform culture and sensitivity prior to initiating therapy.

Nursing Actions

Physical Assessment: Assess for allergy history prior to starting therapy. Assess potential for interactions with other pharmacological agents patient may be taking (eg, increased risk of toxicity with other nephrotoxic or ototoxic drugs). Monitor laboratory tests, effectiveness (resolution of infection), and adverse effects (eg, ototoxicity [auditory or vestibular], neurotoxicity [drowsiness, paresthesia], nephrotoxicity [I & O, hematuria, edema]) on a regular basis during therapy. Teach patient possible side effects/appropriate interventions and adverse symptoms to report.

Patient Education: Do not take any new medication during therapy without consulting prescriber. This medication can only be given by intramuscular injection. Therapy for TB may last several months. Do not discontinue even if you are feeling better. Maintain adequate hydration (2-3 L/day of fluids unless instructed to restrict fluid intake). May cause headache or dizziness (use caution when driving or engaging in tasks requiring alertness until response to drug is known); or nausea, vomiting, or loss of appetite (small, frequent meals, frequent mouth care, sucking lozenges, or chewing gum may help). Report immediately change in hearing or sense of fullness in ears; pain, weakness, tremors, or numbness in muscles; unusual clumsiness or change in strength or altered gait; change in urinary pattern or back pain; or respiratory difficulty or chest pain. **Pregnancy precaution:** Do not get pregnant while taking this medication. Consult prescriber for appropriate barrier contraceptive measures.

Geriatric Considerations Streptomycin is indicated for persons from endemic areas of drug-resistant *Mycobacterium tuberculosis* or who are HIV infected. Since most older patients acquired the *M. tuberculosis* infection prior to the availability of effective chemotherapy, isoniazid and rifampin are usually effective unless resistant organisms are suspected or the patient is HIV infected. Adjust dose interval for renal function.

Streptozocin *(strep toe ZOE sin)*

U.S. Brand Names Zanosar®

Synonyms NSC-85998

Pharmacologic Category Antineoplastic Agent, Alkylating Agent

Medication Safety Issues

Sound-alike/look-alike issues:

Streptozocin may be confused with streptomycin

Pregnancy Risk Factor D

Lactation Enters breast milk/contraindicated

Use Treatment of metastatic islet cell carcinoma of the pancreas, carcinoid tumor and syndrome, Hodgkin's disease, palliative treatment of colorectal cancer

Mechanism of Action/Effect Interferes with the normal function of DNA by alkylation and cross-linking the strands of DNA, and by possible protein modification

Contraindications Pregnancy

Warnings/Precautions Hazardous agent - use appropriate precautions for handling and disposal. Renal toxicity is dose-related and cumulative and may be severe or fatal.

Drug Interactions

Decreased Effect: Phenytoin results in negation of streptozocin cytotoxicity.

Increased Effect/Toxicity: Doxorubicin toxicity may be increased with concurrent use of streptozocin. Manufacturer recommends doxorubicin dosage adjustment be considered.

Adverse Reactions

>10%:

Gastrointestinal: Nausea and vomiting (100%)

Hepatic: Increased LFTs

Miscellaneous: Hypoalbuminemia

Renal: BUN increased, Cl_{cr} decreased, hypophosphatemia, nephrotoxicity (25% to 75%), proteinuria, renal dysfunction (65%), renal tubular acidosis

1% to 10%:

Endocrine & metabolic: Hypoglycemia (6%)

Gastrointestinal: Diarrhea (10%)

Local: Pain at injection site

Overdosage/Toxicology Symptoms of overdose include bone marrow suppression, nausea, and vomiting. Treatment of bone marrow suppression is supportive.

Pharmacodynamics/Kinetics

Duration of Action: Disappears from serum in 4 hours

Half-Life Elimination: 35-40 minutes

Metabolism: Rapidly hepatic

Excretion: Urine (60% to 70% as metabolites); exhaled gases (5%); feces (1%)

Available Dosage Forms Injection, powder for reconstitution: 1 g

Dosing

Adults & Elderly: Antineoplastic: Refer to individual protocols.

Single agent therapy: I.V.: 1-1.5 g/m^2 weekly for 6 weeks followed by a 4-week rest period

Combination therapy: I.V.: 0.5-1 g/m^2 for 5 consecutive days followed by a 4- to 6-week rest period

Pediatrics: Refer to adult dosing.

Renal Impairment:

Cl_{cr} 10-50 mL/minute: Administer 75% of dose.

Cl_{cr} <10 mL/minute: Administer 50% of dose.

Hepatic Impairment: Dose should be reduced in patients with severe liver disease.

Administration

I.V.: Administer as short (30-60 minutes) or 6-hour infusion; may be given by rapid I.V. push

I.V. Detail: pH: 3.5-4.5

Stability

Reconstitution: Dilute powder with 9.5 mL SWFI or NS to a concentration of 100 mg/mL.

Compatibility: Stable in D_5W, NS

Y-site administration: Incompatible with allopurinol, aztreonam, cefepime, piperacillin/tazobactam

Storage: Store intact vials under refrigeration; vials are stable for one year at room temperature. Solution reconstituted with 9.5 mL SWFI or NS to a concentration of 100 mg/mL is stable for 48 hours at room temperature and 96 hours under refrigeration. Further dilution in D_5W or NS is stable for 48 hours at room temperature and 96 hours under refrigeration when protected from light.

Laboratory Monitoring Liver function tests, CBC, renal function tests (BUN, serum creatinine) at baseline and weekly during therapy

Nursing Actions

Physical Assessment: Antiemetic should be administered prior to therapy (emetic potential 100%). Assess potential for interactions with other pharmacological agents. See Administration for infusion specifics. Infusion site should be monitored closely to prevent extravasation. Monitor laboratory tests, patient response, and adverse reactions (eg, nephrotoxicity [I & O, edema, hematuria, BUN], hepatotoxicity [jaundice, fatigue, LFTs], hypoglycemia, diarrhea [dehydration]) on a regular basis during therapy. Caution patients with diabetes to monitor glucose levels closely (may precipitate hypoglycemia). Teach patient (or caregiver) possible side effects/appropriate interventions, and adverse symptoms to report.

Patient Education: Do not take any new medication during therapy unless approved by prescriber. This drug can only be given I.V.; report immediately any redness, swelling, pain, or burning at infusion site. Maintain adequate hydration (2-3 L/day of fluids) unless instructed to restrict fluid intake. You will be more sensitive to infection (avoid crowds and exposure to infection and do not have any vaccinations without consulting prescriber). If you have diabetes, monitor glucose levels closely; may cause hypoglycemia. May cause nausea and vomiting (consult prescriber for antiemetic); nervousness, dizziness, confusion, or lethargy (use caution when driving or engaging in tasks requiring alertness until response to drug is known); or loss of body hair (reversible when treatment is finished). Report unusual back pain, change in urinary pattern; persistent fever, chills, or sore throat; unusual bleeding; blood in urine, vomitus, or stool; chest pain, palpitations, or respiratory difficulty; or swelling of feet or lower legs. **Pregnancy/breast-feeding precautions:** Inform prescriber if you are pregnant. Do not get pregnant during or for 1 month following therapy. Male: Do not cause a female to become pregnant. Male/female: Consult prescriber for instruction on appropriate barrier contraceptive measures. This drug may cause severe fetal damage. Do not breast-feed.

Succinylcholine (suks in il KOE leen)

U.S. Brand Names Quelicin®

Synonyms Succinylcholine Chloride; Suxamethonium Chloride

Pharmacologic Category Neuromuscular Blocker Agent, Depolarizing

Pregnancy Risk Factor C

Lactation Excretion in breast milk unknown/use caution

Use Adjunct to general anesthesia to facilitate both rapid sequence and routine endotracheal intubation and to relax skeletal muscles during surgery; to reduce the intensity of muscle contractions of pharmacologically- or electrically-induced convulsions; does not relieve pain or produce sedation

Mechanism of Action/Effect Acts similar to acetylcholine, produces depolarization of the motor endplate at the myoneural junction which causes sustained flaccid skeletal muscle paralysis produced by state of accommodation that developes in adjacent excitable muscle membranes

Contraindications Hypersensitivity to succinylcholine or any component of the formulation; personal or familial history of malignant hyperthermia; myopathies associated with elevated serum creatine phosphokinase (CPK) values; narrow-angle glaucoma, penetrating eye injuries; disorders of plasma pseudocholinesterase

Warnings/Precautions Use with caution in pediatrics and adolescents secondary to undiagnosed skeletal muscle myopathy and potential for ventricular dysrhythmias and cardiac arrest resulting from hyperkalemia; use with caution in patients with pre-existing hyperkalemia, paraplegia, extensive or severe burns, extensive denervation of skeletal muscle because of disease or injury to the CNS or with degenerative or dystrophic neuromuscular disease; may increase vagal tone

Drug Interactions

Increased Effect/Toxicity:

Increased toxicity: Anticholinesterase drugs (neostigmine, physostigmine, or pyridostigmine) in combination with succinylcholine can cause cardiorespiratory collapse; cyclophosphamide, oral contraceptives, lidocaine, thiotepa, pancuronium, lithium, magnesium salts, aprotinin, chloroquine, metoclopramide, terbutaline, and procaine enhance and prolong the effects of succinylcholine

Prolonged neuromuscular blockade: Inhaled anesthetics, local anesthetics, calcium channel blockers, antiarrhythmics (eg, quinidine or procainamide), antibiotics (eg, aminoglycosides, tetracyclines, vancomycin, clindamycin), immunosuppressants (eg, cyclosporine)

Lab Interactions Increased potassium (S)

Adverse Reactions

>10%:
Ocular: Increased intraocular pressure
Miscellaneous: Postoperative stiffness

1% to 10%:
Cardiovascular: Bradycardia, hypotension, cardiac arrhythmia, tachycardia
Gastrointestinal: Intragastric pressure, salivation

Causes of prolonged neuromuscular blockade: Excessive drug administration; cumulative drug effect, decreased metabolism/excretion (hepatic and/or renal impairment); accumulation of active metabolites; electrolyte imbalance (hypokalemia, hypocalcemia, hypermagnesemia, hypernatremia); hypothermia; drug interactions; increased sensitivity to muscle relaxants (eg, neuromuscular disorders such as myasthenia gravis or polymyositis)

Overdosage/Toxicology

Symptoms of overdose include respiratory paralysis and cardiac arrest.

Bradyarrhythmias can often be treated with atropine 0.1 mg (infants). Do not treat with anticholinesterase drugs (eg, neostigmine, physostigmine) since this may worsen its toxicity by interfering with its metabolism.

Pharmacodynamics/Kinetics

Onset of Action: I.M.: 2-3 minutes; I.V.: Complete muscular relaxation: 30-60 seconds

Duration of Action: I.M.: 10-30 minutes; I.V.: 4-6 minutes with single administration

Metabolism: Rapidly hydrolyzed by plasma pseudocholinesterase

Available Dosage Forms Injection, solution, as chloride: 20 mg/mL (5 mL, 10 mL); 50 mg/mL (10 mL); 100 mg/mL (10 mL)

Dosing

Adults & Elderly: Neuromuscular blockade: Dose to effect; doses will vary due to interpatient variability; use ideal body weight for obese patients

I.M.: 2.5-4 mg/kg, total dose should not exceed 150 mg

I.V.: 1-1.5 mg/kg, up to 150 mg total dose
Maintenance: 0.04-0.07 mg/kg every 5-10 minutes as needed
Continuous infusion: 10-100 mcg/kg/minute (or 0.5-10 mg/minute); dilute to concentration of 1-2 mg/mL in D_5W or NS

(Continued)

Succinylcholine *(Continued)*

Note: Initial dose of succinylcholine must be increased when nondepolarizing agent pretreatment used because of the antagonism between succinylcholine and nondepolarizing neuromuscular blocking agents

Pediatrics: Neuromuscular blockade: I.V.:

Note: Because of the risk of malignant hyperthermia, use of continuous infusions is not recommended in infants and children:

Small Children: Intermittent: Initial: 2 mg/kg/dose one time; maintenance: 0.3-0.6 mg/kg/dose at intervals of 5-10 minutes as necessary

Older Children and Adolescents: Intermittent: Initial: 1 mg/kg/dose one time; maintenance: 0.3-0.6 mg/kg every 5-10 minutes as needed

Hepatic Impairment: Dose should be reduced in patients with severe liver disease.

Administration

I.M.: I.M. injections should be made deeply, preferably high into deltoid muscle.

I.V.: May be given by rapid I.V. injection without further dilution.

I.V. Detail: pH: 3.0-4.5

Stability

Compatibility:

Stable in dextran 6% in dextrose, dextran 6% in NS, D_5LR, $D_5 1/4NS$, $D_5 1/2NS$, D_5NS, D_5W, $D_{10}W$, LR, $1/2NS$, NS

Y-site administration: Incompatible with thiopental

Compatibility when admixed: Incompatible with methohexital, nafcillin, sodium bicarbonate, thiopental

Storage: Refrigerate at 2°C to 8°C (36°F to 46°F); however, remains stable for ≤3 months unrefrigerated; powder form does not require refrigeration. Stability of parenteral admixture at refrigeration temperature (4°C) is 24 hours in D_5W or NS.

Laboratory Monitoring Serum potassium and calcium

Nursing Actions

Physical Assessment: Only clinicians experienced in the use of neuromuscular blocking drugs should administer and/or manage the use of succinylcholine. Ventilatory support must be instituted and maintained until adequate respiratory muscle function and/or airway protection are assured. Assess other medications for effectiveness and safety; other drugs that affect neuromuscular activity may increase/decrease neuromuscular block induced by succinylcholine. This drug does not cause anesthesia or analgesia; pain must be treated with appropriate analgesic agents. Continuous monitoring of vital signs, cardiac status, respiratory status, and degree of neuromuscular block (objective assessment with external nerve stimulator) is mandatory during infusion and until full muscle tone has returned. Muscle tone returns in a predictable pattern, starting with limbs, abdomen, chest diaphragm, intercostals, and finally muscles of the neck, face, and eyes. Safety precautions must be maintained until full muscle tone has returned. Provide appropriate patient teaching/support prior to and following administration.

Patient Education: Patient will usually be unconscious prior to administration. Education should be appropriate to individual situation. Reassurance of constant monitoring and emotional support to reduce fear and anxiety should precede and follow administration. Following return of muscle tone, do not attempt to change position or rise from bed without assistance. Report immediately any skin rash or hives, pounding heartbeat, respiratory difficulty, or muscle tremors. **Pregnancy/breast-feeding precautions:** Inform prescriber if you are pregnant. Consult prescriber if breast-feeding.

Related Information

Diagnostics and Surgical Aids *on page 1329*

Sucralfate (soo KRAL fate)

U.S. Brand Names Carafate®

Synonyms Aluminum Sucrose Sulfate, Basic

Pharmacologic Category Gastrointestinal Agent, Miscellaneous

Medication Safety Issues

Sound-alike/look-alike issues:

Sucralfate may be confused with salsalate

Carafate® may be confused with Cafergot®

Pregnancy Risk Factor B

Lactation Enters breast milk/compatible

Use Short-term management of duodenal ulcers; maintenance of duodenal ulcers

Unlabeled/Investigational Use Gastric ulcers; suspension may be used topically for treatment of stomatitis due to cancer chemotherapy and other causes of esophageal and gastric erosions; GERD, esophagitis; treatment of NSAID mucosal damage; prevention of stress ulcers; postsclerotherapy for esophageal variceal bleeding

Mechanism of Action/Effect Forms a complex by binding with positively charged proteins in exudates, forming a viscous paste-like, adhesive substance, when combined with gastric acid adheres to the damaged mucosal area. This selectively forms a protective coating that protects the lining against peptic acid, pepsin, and bile salts.

Contraindications Hypersensitivity to sucralfate or any component of the formulation

Warnings/Precautions Successful therapy with sucralfate should not be expected to alter the posthealing frequency of recurrence or the severity of duodenal ulceration. Use with caution in patients with chronic renal failure who have an impaired excretion of absorbed aluminum. Because of the potential for sucralfate to alter the absorption of some drugs, take other medications 2 hours before sucralfate when alterations in bioavailability are believed to be critical. Do not give antacids within 30 minutes of administration.

Drug Interactions

Decreased Effect: Sucralfate may alter the absorption of digoxin, phenytoin (hydantoins), warfarin, ketoconazole, quinidine, quinolones, tetracycline, theophylline. Because of the potential for sucralfate to alter the absorption of some drugs; separate administration (take other medications at least 2 hours before sucralfate). The potential for decreased absorption should be considered when alterations in bioavailability are believed to be critical.

Nutritional/Ethanol Interactions Food: Sucralfate may interfere with absorption of vitamin A, vitamin D, vitamin E, and vitamin K.

Adverse Reactions 1% to 10%: Gastrointestinal: Constipation

Overdosage/Toxicology Toxicity is minimal, may cause constipation

Pharmacodynamics/Kinetics

Onset of Action: Paste formation and ulcer adhesion: 1-2 hours

Duration of Action: Up to 6 hours

Metabolism: None

Excretion: Urine (small amounts as unchanged compounds)

Available Dosage Forms

Suspension, oral: 1 g/10 mL (10 mL) [DSC]

Carafate®: 1 g/10 mL (420 mL)

Tablet (Carafate®): 1 g

Dosing

Adults & Elderly:

Stress ulcer prophylaxis: Oral: 1 g 4 times/day

Stress ulcer treatment: Oral: 1 g every 4 hours

Treatment of duodenal ulcer: Oral:

Initial treatment: 1 g 4 times/day, 1 hour before meals or food and at bedtime for 4-8 weeks, or alternatively 2 g twice daily; treatment is recommended for 4-8 weeks in adults, the elderly will require 12 weeks.

Maintenance/prophylaxis of duodenal ulcer: 1 g twice daily

Stomatitis (unlabeled use): Oral: 1 g/10 mL suspension; swish and spit or swish and swallow 4 times/day.

Pediatrics: Dose not established, doses of 40-80 mg/kg/day divided every 6 hours have been used

Stomatitis (unlabeled use): Oral: Children: 2.5-5 mL (1 g/10 mL suspension), swish and spit or swish and swallow 4 times/day

Renal Impairment: Aluminum salt is minimally absorbed (<5%), however, may accumulate in renal failure.

Administration

Oral: Tablet may be broken or dissolved in water before ingestion. Administer with water on an empty stomach.

Stability

Storage: Suspension: Shake well. Refrigeration is **not** necessary; do **not** freeze.

Nursing Actions

Physical Assessment: Assess potential for interactions with other pharmacological agents patient may be taking (eg, will affect absorption of concurrently administered drugs). Monitor effectiveness (reduction in clinical symptoms) and adverse reactions. Teach patient proper use (eg, timing of other medications), possible side effects (eg, constipation) and interventions, and adverse symptoms to report.

Patient Education: Take recommended dose with water on an empty stomach, 1 hour before or 2 hours after meals. Take any other medications at least 2 hours before taking sucralfate. Do not take antacids (if prescribed) within 30 minutes of taking sucralfate. May cause constipation (increased exercise, fluids, fruit, or fiber may help). If constipation persists, consult prescriber for approved stool softener.

Dietary Considerations Administer with water on an empty stomach.

Geriatric Considerations Caution should be used in the elderly due to reduced renal function. Patients with Cl_{cr} <30 mL/minute may be at risk for aluminum intoxication. Due to low side effect profile, this may be an agent of choice in the elderly with PUD.

Sulfacetamide (sul fa SEE ta mide)

U.S. Brand Names Bleph®-10; Carmol® Scalp; Klaron®; Ovace™

Synonyms Sodium Sulfacetamide; Sulfacetamide Sodium

Pharmacologic Category Antibiotic, Ophthalmic; Antibiotic, Sulfonamide Derivative

Medication Safety Issues

Sound-alike/look-alike issues:

Bleph®-10 may be confused with Blephamide®

Klaron® may be confused with Klor-Con®

Pregnancy Risk Factor C

Lactation Excretion in breast milk unknown/use caution

Use

Ophthalmic: Treatment and prophylaxis of conjunctivitis due to susceptible organisms; corneal ulcers; adjunctive treatment with systemic sulfonamides for therapy of trachoma

Dermatologic: Scaling dermatosis (seborrheic); bacterial infections of the skin; acne vulgaris

Mechanism of Action/Effect Interferes with bacterial growth by inhibiting bacterial folic acid synthesis through competitive antagonism of PABA

Contraindications Hypersensitivity to sulfacetamide, sulfonamides, or any component of the formulation

Warnings/Precautions Severe reactions to sulfonamides have been reported, regardless of route of administration; reactions may include Stevens-Johnson syndrome, toxic epidermal necrolysis, fulminant hepatic necrosis, or blood dyscrasias. Chemical similarities are present among sulfonamides, sulfonylureas, carbonic anhydrase inhibitors, thiazides, and loop diuretics (except ethacrynic acid). Use in patients with sulfonamide allergy is specifically contraindicated in product labeling; however, a risk of cross-reaction exists in patients with allergy to any of these compounds; avoid use when previous reaction has been severe.

Ophthalmic: Inactivated by purulent exudates containing PABA; use with caution in severe dry eye; ointment may retard corneal epithelial healing. For topical application to the eye only; not for injection. Safety and efficacy have not been established in children <2 months of age.

Dermatologic: Use caution if applied to denuded or abraded skin. Some products contain sodium metabisulfite which may cause allergic reactions in certain individuals. For external use only; avoid contact with eyes. Safety and efficacy have not been established in children <12 years of age.

Drug Interactions

Decreased Effect: Silver containing products are incompatible with sulfacetamide solutions.

Adverse Reactions Frequency not defined.

Cardiovascular: Edema

Dermatologic: Burning, erythema, irritation, itching, stinging, Stevens-Johnson syndrome

Ocular (following ophthalmic application): Burning, conjunctivitis, conjunctival hyperemia, corneal ulcers, irritation, stinging

Miscellaneous: Allergic reactions, systemic lupus erythematosus

Pharmacodynamics/Kinetics

Half-Life Elimination: 7-13 hours

Excretion: When absorbed, primarily urine (as unchanged drug)

Available Dosage Forms [DSC] = Discontinued product

Cream, topical, as sodium (Ovace™): 10% (30 g, 60 g)

Foam, topical, as sodium (Ovace™): 10% (50 g, 100 g)

Gel, topical, as sodium (Ovace™): 10% (30 g, 60 g)

Lotion, as sodium:

Carmol® Scalp: 10% (85 g) [contains urea 10%]

Klaron®: 10% (120 mL) [contains sodium metabisulfite]

Ovace™: 10% (180 mL, 360 mL)

Ointment, ophthalmic, as sodium: 10% (3.5 g)

Solution, ophthalmic, as sodium: 10% (15 mL)

Bleph®-10: 10% (5 mL; 15 mL [DSC]) [contains benzalkonium chloride]

Dosing

Adults & Elderly:

Conjunctivitis: Ophthalmic:

Ointment: Apply to lower conjunctival sac 1-4 times/day and at bedtime

Solution: Instill 1-2 drops several times daily up to every 2-3 hours in lower conjunctival sac during waking hours and less frequently at night; increase dosing interval as condition responds. Usual duration of treatment: 7-10 days

Trachoma: Instill 2 drops into the conjunctival sac every 2 hours; must be used in conjunction with systemic therapy

Acne: Topical: Apply thin film to affected area twice daily

(Continued)

Sulfacetamide (Continued)

Seborrheic dermatitis: Topical: Apply at bedtime and allow to remain overnight; in severe cases, may apply twice daily. Duration of therapy is usually 8-10 applications; dosing interval may be increased as eruption subsides. Applications once or twice weekly, or every other week may be used to prevent eruptions.

Secondary cutaneous bacterial infections: Topical: Apply 2-4 times/day until infection clears

Pediatrics:

Conjunctivitis: Ophthalmic: Children >2 months: Refer to adult dosing.

Dermatologic: Topical: Children >12 years: Refer to adult dosing.

Administration

Topical:

Scalp lotion: Shampoo hair with a nonirritating shampoo prior to application. Part hair in sections and apply small quantities of lotion to scalp; rub in gently. Brush hair for 2-3 minutes. May discolor white fabric.

Acne lotion: Shake well before using.

Stability

Compatibility: Incompatible with silver and zinc sulfate. Sulfacetamide is inactivated by blood or purulent exudates.

Storage: Store at controlled room temperature.

Ophthalmic solution: Solution may be used if yellow; do not use if darkened.

Carmol® Scalp treatment: Do not freeze; may be used if slightly discolored.

Nursing Actions

Physical Assessment: Assess for previous sulfonamide allergy. Monitor effectiveness (resolutions of infection). Teach patient appropriate use (ophthalmic/topical), interventions to reduce side effects, and adverse symptoms to report.

Patient Education: Use as directed. Complete full course of therapy even if condition appears improved. **Pregnancy/breast-feeding precautions:** Inform prescriber if you are pregnant. Consult prescriber if breast-feeding.

Ophthalmic: Do not use other eye preparations at this time without consulting prescriber. Store at room temperature. Shake solution before using. Apply prescribed amount as often as directed. Wash hands before using. Do not let tip of applicator touch eye; do not contaminate tip of applicator (may cause eye infection, eye damage, or vision loss). When using solution, tilt head back and look upward. Gently pull down lower lid and put drop(s) in inner corner of eye. When using ointment, place medicine inside the lower lid, close eye, and roll eyeball in all directions. Do not blink for 1/2 minute. Apply gentle pressure to inner corner of eye for 30 seconds. Wipe away excess from skin around eye. Do not use any other eye preparation for at least 10 minutes. Do not share medication with anyone else. May cause sensitivity to bright light (dark glasses may help); temporary stinging or blurred vision may occur. Inform prescriber if you experience eye pain, redness, burning, watering, dryness, double vision, puffiness around eye, vision changes, or other adverse eye response; worsening of condition or lack of improvement within 3-4 days.

Topical: For external use only. Apply a thin film to affected area as often as directed. Do not cover with occlusive dressing; do not apply other lotions, creams, or medications to the area while using this medication. Report increased skin redness, irritation, or development of open sores; or if condition worsens or does not improve.

Geriatric Considerations Assess whether patient can adequately instill drops or ointment.

Breast-Feeding Issues The amount of systemic absorption following topical administration is not known. When used orally, small amounts of sulfonamides are excreted in breast milk.

Pregnancy Issues Use of systemic sulfonamides during pregnancy may cause kernicterus in the newborn; the amount of systemic absorption following topical administration is not known. Use during pregnancy only if clearly needed.

Sulfacetamide and Prednisolone
(sul fa SEE ta mide & pred NIS oh lone)

U.S. Brand Names Blephamide®
Synonyms Prednisolone and Sulfacetamide
Pharmacologic Category Antibiotic/Corticosteroid, Ophthalmic
Pregnancy Risk Factor C
Use Steroid-responsive inflammatory ocular conditions where infection is present or there is a risk of infection; ophthalmic suspension may be used as an otic preparation

Available Dosage Forms

Ointment, ophthalmic (Blephamide®): Sulfacetamide sodium 10% and prednisolone acetate 0.2% (3.5 g)

Solution, ophthalmic: Sulfacetamide sodium 10% and prednisolone sodium phosphate 0.25% (5 mL, 10 mL)

Suspension, ophthalmic (Blephamide®): Sulfacetamide sodium 10% and prednisolone acetate 0.2% (5 mL, 10 mL) [contains benzalkonium chloride]

Dosing

Adults & Elderly: Conjunctivitis: Ophthalmic:

Ointment: Apply to lower conjunctival sac 1-4 times/day

Solution, suspension: Instill 1-3 drops every 2-3 hours while awake

Pediatrics: Conjunctivitis: Ophthalmic: Children >2 months: Refer to adult dosing.

Nursing Actions

Physical Assessment: See individual agents.

Patient Education: Eye drops will burn upon instillation. Ointment will cause blurred vision. Do not touch container to eye. Wait at least 10 minutes before using another eye preparation. May cause sensitivity to sunlight. Notify physician if condition does not improve in 3-4 days. **Pregnancy precaution:** Notify prescriber if you are or intend to become pregnant.

Related Information

PrednisoLONE on page 1017
Sulfacetamide on page 1151

Sulfacetamide Sodium and Fluorometholone
(sul fa SEE ta mide SOW dee um & flure oh METH oh lone)

U.S. Brand Names FML-S®
Synonyms Fluorometholone and Sulfacetamide
Pharmacologic Category Antibiotic/Corticosteroid, Ophthalmic
Pregnancy Risk Factor C
Lactation

Enters breast milk/not recommended

Use Steroid-responsive inflammatory ocular conditions where infection is present or there is a risk of infection

Available Dosage Forms Suspension, ophthalmic: Sulfacetamide sodium 10% and fluorometholone 0.1% (5 mL, 10 mL) [contains benzalkonium chloride]

Dosing

Adults & Elderly: Conjunctivitis: Ophthalmic: Instill 1 drop into affected eye(s) 4 times/day

Note: Dose may be decreased but should not be discontinued prematurely; re-evaluation should occur if improvement is not seen within 2 days; in chronic conditions, dosing frequency should be gradually decreased prior to discontinuing treatment

Pediatrics: Conjunctivitis: Ophthalmic: Children >2 years: Refer to adult dosing.

Nursing Actions

Physical Assessment: See individual agents.

Patient Education: Pregnancy precaution: Notify prescriber if you are or intend to become pregnant.

Related Information

Fluorometholone *on page 529*

Sulfacetamide *on page 1151*

SulfaDIAZINE (sul fa DYE a zeen)

Pharmacologic Category Antibiotic, Sulfonamide Derivative

Medication Safety Issues

Sound-alike/look-alike issues:

SulfaDIAZINE may be confused with sulfasalazine, sulfiSOXAZOLE

Pregnancy Risk Factor B/D (at term)

Lactation Enters breast milk/contraindicated

Use Treatment of urinary tract infections and nocardiosis; adjunctive treatment in toxoplasmosis; uncomplicated attack of malaria

Unlabeled/Investigational Use Rheumatic fever prophylaxis

Mechanism of Action/Effect Interferes with bacterial growth by inhibiting bacterial folic acid synthesis through competitive antagonism of PABA

Contraindications Hypersensitivity to any sulfa drug or any component of the formulation; porphyria; children <2 months of age unless indicated for the treatment of congenital toxoplasmosis; sunscreens containing PABA; pregnancy (at term)

Warnings/Precautions Use with caution in patients with impaired hepatic function or impaired renal function, G6PD deficiency; dosage modification required in patients with renal impairment; fluid intake should be maintained ≥1500 mL/day, or administer sodium bicarbonate to keep urine alkaline; more likely to cause crystalluria because it is less soluble than other sulfonamides. Chemical similarities are present among sulfonamides, sulfonylureas, carbonic anhydrase inhibitors, thiazides, and loop diuretics (except ethacrynic acid). Use in patients with sulfonamide allergy is specifically contraindicated in product labeling, however, a risk of cross-reaction exists in patients with allergy to any of these compounds; avoid use when previous reaction has been severe.

Drug Interactions

Cytochrome P450 Effect: Substrate of CYP2C8/9 (major), 2E1 (minor), 3A4 (minor); **Inhibits** CYP2C8/9 (strong)

Decreased Effect: The levels/effects of sulfadiazine may be decreased by carbamazepine, phenobarbital, phenytoin, rifampin, rifapentine, secobarbital, and other CYP2C8/9 inducers. Decreased effect with PABA or PABA metabolites of drugs (eg, procaine, proparacaine, tetracaine, sunblock).

Increased Effect/Toxicity: Increased effect of oral anticoagulants and oral hypoglycemic agents. Sulfadiazine may increase the levels/effects of amiodarone, fluoxetine, glimepiride, glipizide, nateglinide, phenytoin, pioglitazone, rosiglitazone, sertraline, warfarin, and other CYP2C8/9 substrates.

Nutritional/Ethanol Interactions

Food: Avoid large quantities of vitamin C or acidifying agents (cranberry juice) to prevent crystalluria.

Herb/Nutraceutical: Avoid dong quai, St John's wort (may also cause photosensitization).

Adverse Reactions Frequency not defined.

Central nervous system: Fever, dizziness, headache

Dermatologic: Lyell's syndrome, Stevens-Johnson syndrome, itching, rash, photosensitivity

Endocrine & metabolic: Thyroid function disturbance

Gastrointestinal: Anorexia, nausea, vomiting, diarrhea

Genitourinary: Crystalluria

Hematologic: Granulocytopenia, leukopenia, thrombocytopenia, aplastic anemia, hemolytic anemia

Hepatic: Hepatitis, jaundice

Renal: Hematuria, acute nephropathy, interstitial nephritis

Miscellaneous: Serum sickness-like reactions

Overdosage/Toxicology Symptoms of overdose include drowsiness, dizziness, anorexia, abdominal pain, nausea, vomiting, hemolytic anemia, acidosis, jaundice, fever, and agranulocytosis. Doses as little as 2-5 g/day may produce toxicity. The aniline radical is responsible for hematologic toxicity. High volume diuresis may aid in elimination and prevention of renal failure. Leucovorin 5-15 mg/day has been used to speed recovery of bone marrow.

Pharmacodynamics/Kinetics

Time to Peak: Within 3-6 hours

Half-Life Elimination: 10 hours

Metabolism: Via N-acetylation

Excretion: Urine (43% to 60% as unchanged drug, 15% to 40% as metabolites)

Available Dosage Forms Tablet: 500 mg

Dosing

Adults & Elderly:

Toxoplasmosis: Oral: 2-6 g/day divided every 6 hours in conjunction with pyrimethamine 50-75 mg/day and with supplemental folinic acid

Asymptomatic meningococcal carriers: 1 g twice daily for 2 days

Nocardiosis: 4-8 g/day for a minimum of 6 weeks

Prevention of recurrent attacks of rheumatic fever (unlabeled use): 1 g/day

Pediatrics:

Asymptomatic meningococcal carriers: Oral:

Infants 1-12 months: 500 mg once daily for 2 days

Children 1-12 years: 500 mg twice daily for 2 days

Congenital toxoplasmosis: Oral:

Newborns and Children <2 months: 100 mg/kg/day divided every 6 hours in conjunction with pyrimethamine 1 mg/kg/day once daily and supplemental folinic acid 5 mg every 3 days for 6 months

Children >2 months: 25-50 mg/kg/dose 4 times/day

Toxoplasmosis: Oral:

Children >2 months: Loading dose: 75 mg/kg; maintenance dose: 120-150 mg/kg/day, maximum dose: 6 g/day; divided every 4-6 hours in conjunction with pyrimethamine 2 mg/kg/day divided every 12 hours for 3 days followed by 1 mg/kg/day once daily with supplemental folinic acid

Prevention of recurrent attacks of rheumatic fever (unlabeled use): Oral: >30 kg: 1 g/day; <30 kg: 0.5 g/day

Administration

Oral: Tablets may be crushed to prepare oral suspension of the drug in water or with a sucrose-containing solution. Aqueous suspension with concentrations of 100 mg/mL should be stored in the refrigerator and used within 7 days. Administer around-the-clock to promote less variation in peak and trough serum levels.

Laboratory Monitoring Perform culture and sensitivity prior to initiating therapy.

Nursing Actions

Physical Assessment: Allergy history should be assessed prior to starting therapy (sulfonamides). Assess potential for interactions with other pharmacological agents and herbal products patient may be taking (eg, increased or decreased levels/effects of

(Continued)

SulfaDIAZINE *(Continued)*

concurrently administered drugs). Monitor effectiveness (reduced clinical symptoms) and adverse reactions (eg, rash, photosensitivity, gastrointestinal disturbance [nausea, vomiting, anorexia], anemia, jaundice, hematuria). Teach patient proper use, possible side effects/appropriate interventions, and adverse symptoms to report.

Patient Education: Inform prescriber of any allergies you have. Do not take any new medication during therapy without consulting prescriber. Take as directed, at regular intervals around-the-clock. Take on an empty stomach, 1 hour before or 2 hours after meals with full glass of water. Complete full course of therapy even if you are feeling better. Take a missed dose as soon as possible. If almost time for next dose, skip the missed dose and return to your regular schedule. Do not take a double dose. Avoid large quantities of vitamin C. Maintain adequate hydration to prevent kidney damage (2-3 L/day of fluids unless instructed to restrict fluid intake). May cause dizziness or headache (use caution when driving or engaging in tasks requiring alertness until response to drug is known); photosensitivity (use sunblock, wear protective clothing and eyewear, and avoid direct sunlight); nausea, vomiting, or loss of appetite (small, frequent meals, frequent mouth care, sucking lozenges, or chewing gum may help). Report skin rash, persistent nausea, vomiting, or diarrhea; opportunistic infection (sore throat, fever, vaginal itching or discharge, unusual bruising or bleeding, fatigue); blood in urine or change in urinary pattern; persistent headache; abdominal pain; or respiratory difficulty. **Pregnancy/breast-feeding precautions:** Inform prescriber if you are or intend to become pregnant. Do not breast-feed.

Dietary Considerations Supplemental folinic acid should be administered to reverse symptoms or prevent problems due to folic acid deficiency.

Related Information

FDA Name Differentiation Project: The Use of Tall-Man Letters *on page 12*

Sulfamethoxazole and Trimethoprim
(sul fa meth OKS a zole & trye METH oh prim)

U.S. Brand Names Bactrim™; Bactrim™ DS; Septra®; Septra® DS

Synonyms Co-Trimoxazole; SMZ-TMP; Sulfatrim; TMP-SMZ; Trimethoprim and Sulfamethoxazole

Pharmacologic Category Antibiotic, Miscellaneous; Antibiotic, Sulfonamide Derivative

Medication Safety Issues

Sound-alike/look-alike issues:

Bactrim™ may be confused with bacitracin, Bactine®

Co-trimoxazole may be confused with clotrimazole

Septra® may be confused with Ceptaz®, Sectral®, Septa®

Pregnancy Risk Factor C/D (at term - expert analysis)

Lactation Enters breast milk/contraindicated (AAP rates "compatible with restrictions")

Use

Oral treatment of urinary tract infections due to *E. coli*, *Klebsiella* and *Enterobacter* sp, *M. morganii*, *P. mirabilis* and *P. vulgaris*; acute otitis media in children; acute exacerbations of chronic bronchitis in adults due to susceptible strains of *H. influenzae* or *S. pneumoniae*; treatment and prophylaxis of *Pneumocystis carinii* pneumonitis (PCP); traveler's diarrhea due to enterotoxigenic *E. coli*; treatment of enteritis caused by *Shigella flexneri* or *Shigella sonnei*

I.V. treatment or severe or complicated infections when oral therapy is not feasible, for documented PCP, empiric treatment of PCP in immune compromised patients; treatment of documented or suspected shigellosis, typhoid fever, *Nocardia asteroides* infection, or other infections caused by susceptible bacteria

Unlabeled/Investigational Use Cholera and *Salmonella*-type infections and nocardiosis; chronic prostatitis; as prophylaxis in neutropenic patients with *P. carinii* infections, in leukemics, and in patients following renal transplantation, to decrease incidence of PCP; treatment of *Cyclospora* infection, typhoid fever, *Nocardia asteroides* infection

Mechanism of Action/Effect Sulfamethoxazole interferes with bacterial folic acid synthesis; trimethoprim inhibits enzymes of the folic acid pathway

Contraindications Hypersensitivity to any sulfa drug, trimethoprim, or any component of the formulation; porphyria; megaloblastic anemia due to folate deficiency; infants <2 months of age; marked hepatic damage; severe renal disease; pregnancy (at term)

Warnings/Precautions Use with caution in patients with G6PD deficiency, impaired renal or hepatic function. Adjust dosage in patients with renal impairment. Injection vehicle contains benzyl alcohol and sodium metabisulfite. Fatalities associated with severe reactions including Stevens-Johnson syndrome, toxic epidermal necrolysis, hepatic necrosis, agranulocytosis, aplastic anemia, and other blood dyscrasias. Discontinue use at first sign of rash. Elderly patients and patients with HIV appear at greater risk for more severe adverse reactions. May cause hypoglycemia (particularly in malnourished, renal, or hepatic impairment). Use caution in patients with porphyria or thyroid dysfunction. May cause hyperkalemia. Slow acetylators may be more prone to adverse reactions.

Chemical similarities are present among sulfonamides, sulfonylureas, carbonic anhydrase inhibitors, thiazides, and loop diuretics (except ethacrynic acid). Use in patients with sulfonamide allergy is specifically contraindicated in product labeling, however, a risk of cross-reaction exists in patients with allergy to any of these compounds; avoid use when previous reaction has been severe.

Drug Interactions

Cytochrome P450 Effect:

Sulfamethoxazole: **Substrate** of CYP2C8/9 (major), 3A4 (minor); **Inhibits** CYP2C8/9 (moderate)

Trimethoprim: **Substrate** (major) of CYP2C8/9, 3A4; **Inhibits** CYP2C8/9 (moderate)

Decreased Effect: The levels/effects of sulfamethoxazole may be decreased by carbamazepine, phenobarbital, phenytoin, rifampin, rifapentine, secobarbital, and other CYP2C8/9 inducers. Although occasionally recommended to limit or reverse hematologic toxicity of high-dose sulfamethoxazole/trimethoprim, concurrent use has been associated with a decreased effectiveness in treating *Pneumocystis carinii*.

Increased Effect/Toxicity: Sulfamethoxazole/trimethoprim may increase toxicity of methotrexate. Sulfamethoxazole/trimethoprim may increase the serum levels of procainamide. Concurrent therapy with pyrimethamine (in doses >25 mg/week) may increase the risk of megaloblastic anemia. Sulfamethoxazole/trimethoprim may increase the levels/effects of amiodarone, fluoxetine, glimepiride, glipizide, nateglinide, phenytoin, pioglitazone, rosiglitazone, sertraline, warfarin, and other CYP2C8/9 substrates.

ACE Inhibitors, angiotensin receptor antagonists, or potassium-sparing diuretics may increase the risk of hyperkalemia. Concurrent use with cyclosporine may result in an increased risk of nephrotoxicity when used with sulfamethoxazole/trimethoprim. Trimethoprim may increase the serum concentration of dapsone.

Nutritional/Ethanol Interactions Herb/Nutraceutical: Avoid dong quai, St John's wort (may also cause photosensitization).

Lab Interactions Increased creatinine (Jaffé alkaline picrate reaction); increased serum methotrexate by dihydrofolate reductase method; does not interfere with RAI method

Adverse Reactions The most common adverse reactions include gastrointestinal upset (nausea, vomiting, anorexia) and dermatologic reactions (rash or urticaria). Rare, life-threatening reactions have been associated with co-trimoxazole, including severe dermatologic reactions and hepatotoxic reactions. Most other reactions listed are rare, however, frequency cannot be accurately estimated.

Cardiovascular: Allergic myocarditis

Central nervous system: Confusion, depression, hallucinations, seizure, aseptic meningitis, peripheral neuritis, fever, ataxia, kernicterus in neonates

Dermatologic: Rashes, pruritus, urticaria, photosensitivity; rare reactions include erythema multiforme, Stevens-Johnson syndrome, toxic epidermal necrolysis, exfoliative dermatitis, and Henoch-Schönlein purpura

Endocrine & metabolic: Hyperkalemia (generally at high dosages), hypoglycemia

Gastrointestinal: Nausea, vomiting, anorexia, stomatitis, diarrhea, pseudomembranous colitis, pancreatitis

Hematologic: Thrombocytopenia, megaloblastic anemia, granulocytopenia, eosinophilia, pancytopenia, aplastic anemia, methemoglobinemia, hemolysis (with G6PD deficiency), agranulocytosis

Hepatic: Hepatotoxicity (including hepatitis, cholestasis, and hepatic necrosis), hyperbilirubinemia, transaminases increased

Neuromuscular & skeletal: Arthralgia, myalgia, rhabdomyolysis

Renal: Interstitial nephritis, crystalluria, renal failure, nephrotoxicity (in association with cyclosporine), diuresis

Respiratory: Cough, dyspnea, pulmonary infiltrates

Miscellaneous: Serum sickness, angioedema, periarteritis nodosa (rare), systemic lupus erythematosus (rare)

Overdosage/Toxicology Symptoms of overdose include nausea, vomiting, GI distress, hematuria, and crystalluria. Bone marrow suppression may occur. Treatment is supportive. Adequate fluid intake is essential. Peritoneal dialysis is not effective and hemodialysis is only moderately effective in removing co-trimoxazole. Leucovorin 5-15 mg/day may accelerate hematologic recovery.

Pharmacodynamics/Kinetics

Time to Peak: Serum: Within 1-4 hours

Protein Binding: SMX: 68%, TMP: 45%

Half-Life Elimination: SMX: 9 hours, TMP: 6-17 hours; both are prolonged in renal failure

Metabolism: SMX: N-acetylated and glucuronidated; TMP: metabolized to oxide and hydroxylated metabolites

Excretion: Both are excreted in urine as metabolites and unchanged drug

Pharmacokinetic Note Effects of aging on the pharmacokinetics of both agents has been variable; increase in half-life and decreases in clearance have been associated with reduced creatinine clearance

Available Dosage Forms Note: The 5:1 ratio (SMX:TMP) remains constant in all dosage forms.

Injection, solution: Sulfamethoxazole 80 mg and trimethoprim 16 mg per mL (5 mL, 10 mL, 30 mL) [contains propylene glycol ~400 mg/mL, alcohol, benzyl alcohol, and sodium metabisulfite]

Suspension, oral: Sulfamethoxazole 200 mg and trimethoprim 40 mg per 5 mL (480 mL) [contains alcohol]

Septra®: Sulfamethoxazole 200 mg and trimethoprim 40 mg per 5 mL (480 mL) [contains alcohol 0.26% and sodium benzoate; cherry and grape flavors]

Tablet: Sulfamethoxazole 400 mg and trimethoprim 80 mg

Bactrim™: Sulfamethoxazole 400 mg and trimethoprim 80 mg [contains sodium benzoate]

Septra®: Sulfamethoxazole 400 mg and trimethoprim 80 mg

Tablet, double strength: Sulfamethoxazole 800 mg and trimethoprim 160 mg

Bactrim™ DS: Sulfamethoxazole 800 mg and trimethoprim 160 mg [contains sodium benzoate]

Septra® DS: Sulfamethoxazole 800 mg and trimethoprim 160 mg

Dosing

Adults & Elderly: Dosage recommendations are based on the trimethoprim component. Double-strength tablets are equivalent to sulfamethoxazole 800 mg and trimethoprim 160 mg.

Urinary tract infection:

Oral: One double-strength tablet every 12 hours for 10-14 days

Duration of therapy: Uncomplicated: 3-5 days; Complicated: 7-10 days

Pyelonephritis: 14 days

Prostatitis: Acute: 2 weeks; Chronic: 2-3 months

I.V.: 8-10 mg TMP/kg/day in divided doses every 6, 8, or 12 hours for up to 14 days with severe infections

Chronic bronchitis: Oral: One double-strength tablet every 12 hours for 10-14 days

Meningitis (bacterial): I.V.: 10-20 mg TMP/kg/day in divided doses every 6-12 hours

Shigellosis:

Oral: One double strength tablet every 12 hours for 5 days

I.V.: 8-10 mg TMP/kg/day in divided doses every 6, 8, or 12 hours for up to 5 days

Travelers' diarrhea: Oral: One double strength tablet every 12 hours for 5 days

Sepsis: I.V.: 20 TMP/kg/day divided every 6 hours

Pneumocystis carinii:

Prophylaxis: Oral: 1 double strength tablet daily or 3 times/week

Treatment: Oral, I.V.: 15-20 mg TMP/kg/day in 3-4 divided doses

Cyclospora (unlabeled use): Oral, I.V.: 160 mg TMP twice daily for 7-10 days

Nocardia (unlabeled use): Oral, I.V.:

Cutaneous infections: 5 mg TMP/kg/day in 2 divided doses

Severe infections (pulmonary/cerebral): 10-15 mg TMP/kg/day in 2-3 divided doses. Treatment duration is controversial; an average of 7 months has been reported.

Note: Therapy for severe infection may be initiated I.V. and converted to oral therapy (frequently converted to approximate dosages of oral solid dosage forms: 2 DS tablets every 8-12 hours). Although not widely available, sulfonamide levels should be considered in patients with questionable absorption, at risk for dose-related toxicity, or those with poor therapeutic response.

Pediatrics: Recommendations are based on the trimethoprim component.

General dosing guidelines: Children >2 months:

Mild-to-moderate infections: Oral: 8-12 mg TMP/kg/day in divided doses every 12 hours

Serious infection:

Oral: 20 mg TMP/kg/day in divided doses every 6 hours

I.V.: 8-12 mg TMP/kg/day in divided doses every 6 hours

Acute otitis media: Oral: 8 mg TMP/kg/day in divided doses every 12 hours for 10 days

(Continued)

Sulfamethoxazole and Trimethoprim
(Continued)

Urinary tract infection:
Treatment:
Oral: 6-12 mg TMP/kg/day in divided doses every 12 hours
I.V.: 8-10 mg TMP/kg/day in divided doses every 6, 8, or 12 hours for up to 4 days with serious infections
Prophylaxis: Oral: 2 mg TMP/kg/dose daily or 5 mg TMP/kg/dose twice weekly

***Pneumocystis*:**
Treatment: Oral, I.V.: 15-20 mg TMP/kg/day in divided doses every 6-8 hours
Prophylaxis: Oral, 150 mg TMP/m^2/day in divided doses every 12 hours for 3 days/week; dose should not exceed trimethoprim 320 mg and sulfamethoxazole 1600 mg daily
Alternative prophylaxis dosing schedules include:
150 mg TMP/m^2/day as a single daily dose 3 times/week on consecutive days
or
150 mg TMP/m^2/day in divided doses every 12 hours administered 7 days/week
or
150 mg TMP/m^2/day in divided doses every 12 hours administered 3 times/week on alternate days

Shigellosis:
Oral: 8 mg TMP/kg/day in divided doses every 12 hours for 5 days
I.V.: 8-10 mg TMP/kg/day in divided doses every 6, 8, or 12 hours for up to 5 days

Cyclospora (unlabeled use): Oral, I.V.: 5 mg TMP/kg twice daily for 7-10 days

Renal Impairment:
Cl$_{cr}$ 15-30 mL/minute: Administer 50% of recommended dose.
Cl$_{cr}$ <15 mL/minute: Not recommended

Administration
Oral:
May be taken with food and water.
I.V.: Infuse over 60-90 minutes, must dilute well before giving.
I.V. Detail: May be given less diluted in a central line. Not for I.M. injection. Administer around-the-clock every 6-12 hours.

pH: 10
Stability
Compatibility: Stable in D$_5$½NS, LR, ½NS
Y-site administration: Incompatible with fluconazole, midazolam, vinorelbine
Compatibility when admixed: Incompatible with fluconazole, verapamil

Storage:
Injection: Store at room temperature; do not refrigerate. Less soluble in more alkaline pH. Protect from light. Solution must be diluted prior to administration. Following dilution, store at room temperature; do not refrigerate. Manufacturer recommended dilutions and stability of parenteral admixture at room temperature (25°C):
5 mL/125 mL D$_5$W; stable for 6 hours
5 mL/100 mL D$_5$W; stable for 4 hours
5 mL/75 mL D$_5$W; stable for 2 hours
Studies have also confirmed limited stability in NS; detailed references should be consulted.
Suspension, tablet: Store at room temperature; protect from light
Laboratory Monitoring Perform culture and sensitivity testing prior to initiating therapy; serum potassium, creatinine, BUN

Nursing Actions
Physical Assessment: Results of culture and sensitivity tests and patient's allergy history should be assessed prior to therapy. Assess potential for interactions with other pharmacological agents or herbal products patient may be taking (eg, increased risk of hyperkalemia or nephrotoxicity). Monitor therapeutic response (according to purpose for use) and adverse effects (reactions are usually rare, however, severe dermatologic and hepatotoxic reactions have been reported). Advise patients with diabetes to monitor glucose levels closely; may cause hypoglycemia. Teach patient possible side effects/appropriate interventions and adverse symptoms to report (eg, rash, persistent gastrointestinal upset).

Patient Education: Do not take any new medication during therapy unless approved by prescriber. Take oral medication with 8 oz of water on an empty stomach, 1 hour before or 2 hours after meals, for best absorption. Finish all medication; do not skip doses. If you have diabetes, you should monitor your glucose levels closely; may cause hypoglycemia. May cause increased sensitivity to sunlight (use sunblock, wear protective clothing and dark glasses, and avoid direct exposure to sunlight); or nausea or vomiting (small frequent meals, frequent mouth care, sucking lozenges, or chewing gum may help). Report immediately rash; palpitations or chest pain; CNS changes (eg, hallucinations, abnormal anxiety, seizures); sore throat, unusual coughing, or shortness of breath; blackened stool; unusual bruising or bleeding; edema; or blood in urine or changes in urinary pattern. **Pregnancy/breast-feeding precautions:** Inform prescriber if you are or intend to become pregnant or breast-feed.

Dietary Considerations Should be taken with 8 oz of water on empty stomach.

Geriatric Considerations Elderly patients appear at greater risk for more severe adverse reactions. Adjust dose based on renal function.

Breast-Feeding Issues Sulfonamides are excreted in low concentrations in breast milk. Use during breast feeding in infants <2 months of age is contraindicated according to the manufacturer. The AAP considers use during breast-feeding "compatible" in full term neonates; however, breast-feeding is not recommended if the infant is ill, stressed, or premature **or** if the infant has glucose-6-phosphate dehydrogenase deficiency or hyperbilirubinemia.

Pregnancy Issues Do not use at term to avoid kernicterus in the newborn and use during pregnancy only if risks outweigh the benefits since folic acid metabolism may be affected.

Related Information
Trimethoprim *on page 1256*

Sulfasalazine (sul fa SAL a zeen)

U.S. Brand Names Azulfidine®; Azulfidine® EN-tabs®; Sulfazine; Sulfazine EC

Synonyms Salicylazosulfapyridine

Pharmacologic Category 5-Aminosalicylic Acid Derivative

Medication Safety Issues
Sound-alike/look-alike issues:
Sulfasalazine may be confused with salsalate, sulfaDIAZINE, sulfiSOXAZOLE
Azulfidine® may be confused with Augmentin®, azathioprine

Pregnancy Risk Factor B/D (at term)

Lactation Enters breast milk/use caution (AAP recommends use "with caution")

Use Management of ulcerative colitis; enteric coated tablets are also used for rheumatoid arthritis (including juvenile rheumatoid arthritis) in patients who inadequately respond to analgesics and NSAIDs

Unlabeled/Investigational Use Ankylosing spondylitis, collagenous colitis, Crohn's disease, psoriasis, psoriatic arthritis, juvenile chronic arthritis

Mechanism of Action/Effect Acts locally in the colon to decrease the inflammatory response and systemically interferes with secretion by inhibiting prostaglandin synthesis

Contraindications Hypersensitivity to sulfasalazine, sulfa drugs, salicylates, or any component of the formulation; porphyria; GI or GU obstruction; pregnancy (at term)

Warnings/Precautions Use with caution in patients with renal impairment; impaired hepatic function or urinary obstruction, blood dyscrasias, severe allergies or asthma, or G6PD deficiency; may cause folate deficiency (consider providing 1 mg/day folate supplement). Chemical similarities are present among sulfonamides, sulfonylureas, carbonic anhydrase inhibitors, thiazides, and loop diuretics (except ethacrynic acid). Use in patients with sulfonamide allergy is specifically contraindicated in product labeling, however, a risk of cross-reaction exists in patients with allergy to any of these compounds; avoid use when previous reaction has been severe. Safety and efficacy have not been established in children <2 years of age.

Drug Interactions

Decreased Effect: Decreased effect with iron, digoxin and PABA or PABA metabolites of drugs (eg, procaine, proparacaine, tetracaine).

Increased Effect/Toxicity: Sulfasalazine may increase hydantoin levels. Effects of thiopental, oral hypoglycemics, and oral anticoagulants may be increased. Sulfasalazine may increase the risk of myelosuppression with azathioprine, mercaptopurine, or thioguanine (due to TPMT inhibition); may also increase the toxicity of methotrexate. Risk of thrombocytopenia may be increased with thiazide diuretics. Concurrent methenamine may increase risk of crystalluria.

Nutritional/Ethanol Interactions

Food: May impair folate absorption.

Herb/Nutraceutical: Avoid dong quai, St John's wort (may also cause photosensitization)

Adverse Reactions

>10%:

Central nervous system: Headache (33%)

Dermatologic: Photosensitivity

Gastrointestinal: Anorexia, nausea, vomiting, diarrhea (33%), gastric distress

Genitourinary: Reversible oligospermia (33%)

<3%:

Dermatologic: Urticaria/pruritus (<3%)

Hematologic: Hemolytic anemia (<3%), Heinz body anemia (<3%)

Additional events reported with sulfonamides and/or 5-ASA derivatives: Cholestatic jaundice, eosinophilia pneumonitis, erythema multiforme, fibrosing alveolitis, hepatic necrosis, Kawasaki-like syndrome, SLE-like syndrome, pericarditis, seizure, transverse myelitis

Overdosage/Toxicology Symptoms of overdose include drowsiness, dizziness, anorexia, abdominal pain, nausea, vomiting, hemolytic anemia, acidosis, jaundice, fever, and agranulocytosis. The aniline radical is responsible for hematologic toxicity. High volume diuresis may aid in elimination and prevention of renal failure. Leucovorin 5-15 mg/day has been used to speed recovery of bone marrow.

Pharmacodynamics/Kinetics

Half-Life Elimination: 5.7-10 hours

Metabolism: Via colonic intestinal flora to sulfapyridine and 5-aminosalicylic acid (5-ASA); following absorption, sulfapyridine undergoes N-acetylation and ring hydroxylation while 5-ASA undergoes N-acetylation

Excretion: Primarily urine (as unchanged drug, components, and acetylated metabolites)

Available Dosage Forms

Tablet (Azulfidine®, Sulfazine): 500 mg

Tablet, delayed release, enteric coated (Azulfidine® EN-tabs®, Sulfazine EC): 500 mg

Dosing

Adults & Elderly:

Ulcerative colitis: Oral: Initial: 1 g 3-4 times/day, 2 g/day maintenance in divided doses; may initiate therapy with 0.5-1 g/day

Rheumatoid arthritis: Oral (enteric coated tablet): Initial: 0.5-1 g/day; increase weekly to maintenance dose of 2 g/day in 2 divided doses; maximum: 3 g/day (if response to 2 g/day is inadequate after 12 weeks of treatment)

Pediatrics:

Ulcerative colitis: Oral: Children ≥2 years: Initial: 40-60 mg/kg/day in 3-6 divided doses; maintenance dose: 20-30 mg/kg/day in 4 divided doses

Juvenile rheumatoid arthritis: Oral (enteric coated tablet): Children ≥6 years: 30-50 mg/kg/day in 2 divided doses; Initial: Begin with $1/4$ to $1/3$ of expected maintenance dose; increase weekly; maximum: 2 g/day typically

Renal Impairment:

Cl_{cr} 10-30 mL/minute: Administer twice daily.

Cl_{cr} <10 mL/minute: Administer once daily.

Hepatic Impairment: Avoid use.

Administration

Oral: GI intolerance is common during the first few days of therapy (give with meals).

Stability

Storage: Protect from light.

Nursing Actions

Physical Assessment: Assess for allergy history prior to starting therapy. See Contraindications and Warnings/Precautions for use cautions. Assess potential for interactions with other prescriptions, OTC medications, or herbal products patient may be taking (see Drug Interactions). Monitor patient response (see Adverse Reactions and Overdose/Toxicology). Caution patients with diabetes to monitor glucose levels closely (decreased effect of oral hypoglycemic agents). Teach patient proper use, possible side effects/appropriate interventions, and adverse symptoms to report (see Patient Education) on a regular basis during therapy. **Pregnancy risk factor B/D** - see Pregnancy Risk Factor for use cautions. Note breast-feeding caution.

Patient Education: Inform prescriber of all prescriptions, OTC medications, or herbal products you are taking, and any allergies you have. Take as directed, at regular intervals around-the-clock with food. Do not crush, chew, or dissolve coated tablets. Complete full course of therapy even if you are feeling better. Take a missed dose as soon as possible. If almost time for next dose, skip the missed dose and return to your regular schedule. Do not take a double dose. Maintain adequate hydration (2-3 L/day of fluids) to prevent kidney damage unless instructed to restrict fluid intake. If you have diabetes, monitor glucose levels closely (may cause decreased effect of oral hypoglycemic agents). Orange-yellow color of urine is normal. May cause dizziness or headache (use caution when driving or engaging in tasks requiring alertness until response to drug is known); photosensitivity (use sunblock, wear protective clothing and eyewear, and avoid direct sunlight); or nausea, vomiting, or loss of appetite (small, frequent meals, frequent mouth care, sucking lozenges, or chewing gum may help). Report rash; persistent nausea, vomiting, or diarrhea; opportunistic infection (sore throat, fever, vaginal itching or discharge, unusual bruising or bleeding, fatigue); blood in urine or change in urinary pattern; swelling of face, lips, or tongue, tightness in chest, bad cough, blue skin color, or other persistent adverse effects.

Pregnancy/breast-feeding precautions: Inform (Continued)

Sulfasalazine *(Continued)*

prescriber if you are or intend to become pregnant. Consult prescriber if breast-feeding.

Dietary Considerations Since sulfasalazine impairs folate absorption, consider providing 1 mg/day folate supplement.

Geriatric Considerations Adjust dose for renal function (see Additional Information).

Breast-Feeding Issues Sulfonamides are excreted in human breast milk and may cause kernicterus in the newborn. Although sulfapyridine has poor bilirubin-displacing ability, use with caution in women who are breast-feeding. The AAP classifies this agent to be used with caution since adverse effects have been reported in nursing infants.

Sulfinpyrazone *(sul fin PEER a zone)*

Synonyms Anturane

Restrictions Not available in U.S.

Pharmacologic Category Uricosuric Agent

Pregnancy Risk Factor C/D (near term - expert analysis)

Lactation Excretion in breast milk unknown

Use Treatment of chronic gouty arthritis and intermittent gouty arthritis

Unlabeled/Investigational Use To decrease the incidence of sudden death postmyocardial infarction

Mechanism of Action/Effect Acts by increasing the urinary excretion of uric acid, thereby decreasing blood urate levels; this effect is therapeutically useful in treating patients with acute intermittent gout, chronic tophaceous gout, and acts to promote resorption of tophi; also has antithrombic and platelet inhibitory effects

Contraindications Hypersensitivity to sulfinpyrazone, phenylbutazone, other pyrazoles, or any component of the formulation; active peptic ulcer; GI inflammation; blood dyscrasias; pregnancy (near term)

Warnings/Precautions Safety and efficacy are not established in children <18 years of age. Use with caution in patients with impaired renal function and urolithiasis.

Drug Interactions

Cytochrome P450 Effect: Substrate of CYP2C8/9 (major), 3A4 (minor); **Inhibits** CYP2C8/9 (moderate); **Induces** CYP3A4 (weak)

Decreased Effect: CYP2C8/9 inducers may decrease the levels/effects of sulfinpyrazone; example inducers include carbamazepine, phenobarbital, phenytoin, rifampin, rifapentine, and secobarbital. Decreased effect/levels of theophylline, verapamil. Decreased uricosuric activity with salicylates, niacins.

Increased Effect/Toxicity: Risk of acetaminophen hepatotoxicity is increased, while therapeutic effects may be reduced. Sulfinpyrazone may increase the levels/effects of CYP2C8/9 substrates (eg, amiodarone, fluoxetine, glimepiride, glipizide, nateglinide, phenytoin, pioglitazone, rosiglitazone, sertraline, warfarin).

Nutritional/Ethanol Interactions Herb/Nutraceutical: Avoid dong quai, St John's wort (may also cause photosensitization).

Lab Interactions Decreased uric acid (S)

Adverse Reactions Frequency not defined.

Cardiovascular: Flushing

Central nervous system: Dizziness, headache

Dermatologic: Dermatitis, rash

Gastrointestinal (most frequent adverse effects): Nausea, vomiting, stomach pain

Genitourinary: Polyuria

Hematologic: Anemia, leukopenia, increased bleeding time (decreased platelet aggregation)

Hepatic: Hepatic necrosis

Renal: Nephrotic syndrome, uric acid stones

Overdosage/Toxicology Symptoms of overdose include drowsiness, dizziness, anorexia, abdominal pain, nausea, vomiting, hemolytic anemia, acidosis, jaundice, fever, and agranulocytosis. The aniline radical is responsible for hematologic toxicity. High volume diuresis may aid in elimination and prevention of renal failure. Leucovorin 5-15 mg/day has been used to speed recovery of bone marrow.

Pharmacodynamics/Kinetics

Time to Peak: Serum: 1.6 hours

Half-Life Elimination: 2.7-6 hours

Metabolism: Hepatic to two active metabolites

Excretion: Urine (22% to 50% as unchanged drug)

Available Dosage Forms Tablet: 100 mg

Dosing

Adults & Elderly: Gouty arthritis: Oral: 100-200 mg twice daily increasing to 400 mg twice daily, monitoring uric acid concentrations; decrease to 200 mg/day as a maintenance dose; maximum daily dose: 800 mg

Renal Impairment: Cl$_{cr}$ <50 mL/minute: Avoid use.

Laboratory Monitoring Serum and urinary uric acid, CBC

Nursing Actions

Physical Assessment: Assess effectiveness and interactions of other medications patient may be taking. Monitor therapeutic response (eg, frequency and severity of gouty attacks), laboratory values, and adverse reactions at beginning of therapy and periodically with long-term use. Assess knowledge/teach patient appropriate use, interventions to reduce side effects, and adverse symptoms to report

Patient Education: Take as directed, with meals and a full glass of water. Avoid aspirin, aspirin-containing medications, or acetaminophen products. It is very important to maintain adequate hydration (2-3 L/day of fluids) to prevent kidney damage unless instructed to restrict fluid intake. You may experience nausea or vomiting (small frequent meals, frequent mouth care, chewing gum, or sucking lozenges may help). Report skin rash, persistent stomach pain, painful urination or bloody urine, unusual bruising or bleeding, fatigue, or yellowing of eyes or skin. **Pregnancy/breast-feeding precautions:** Inform prescriber if you are or intend to become pregnant. Consult prescriber if breast-feeding.

Dietary Considerations Should be taken with food or milk.

Geriatric Considerations Since sulfinpyrazone loses its effectiveness when the Cl$_{cr}$ is <50 mL/minute, its usefulness in the elderly is limited.

SulfiSOXAZOLE *(sul fi SOKS a zole)*

U.S. Brand Names Gantrisin®

Synonyms Sulfisoxazole Acetyl; Sulphafurazole

Pharmacologic Category Antibiotic, Sulfonamide Derivative

Medication Safety Issues

Sound-alike/look-alike issues:

SulfiSOXAZOLE may be confused with sulfaDIAZINE, sulfamethoxazole, sulfasalazine

Gantrisin® may be confused with Gastrosed™

Pregnancy Risk Factor B/D (near term)

Lactation Enters breast milk/compatible

Use Treatment of urinary tract infections, otitis media, *Chlamydia*; nocardiosis

Mechanism of Action/Effect Interferes with bacterial growth by inhibiting bacterial folic acid synthesis through competitive antagonism of PABA

Contraindications Hypersensitivity to sulfisoxazole, any sulfa drug, or any component of the formulation; porphyria; infants <2 months of age (sulfas compete with bilirubin for protein binding sites); patients with urinary obstruction; sunscreens containing PABA; pregnancy (at term)

Warnings/Precautions Use with caution in patients with G6PD deficiency (hemolysis may occur), hepatic or renal impairment; dosage modification required in patients with renal impairment; risk of crystalluria should be considered in patients with impaired renal function. Chemical similarities are present among sulfonamides, sulfonylureas, carbonic anhydrase inhibitors, thiazides, and loop diuretics (except ethacrynic acid). Use in patients with sulfonamide allergy is specifically contraindicated in product labeling, however, a risk of cross-reaction exists in patients with allergy to any of these compounds; avoid use when previous reaction has been severe.

Drug Interactions

Cytochrome P450 Effect: Substrate of CYP2C8/9 (major); **Inhibits** CYP2C8/9 (strong)

Decreased Effect: Decreased effect with PABA or PABA metabolites of drugs (eg, procaine, proparacaine, tetracaine), thiopental. May decrease cyclosporine levels.

Increased Effect/Toxicity: Sulfisoxazole may increase the levels/effects of amiodarone, fluoxetine, glimepiride, glipizide, nateglinide, phenytoin, pioglitazone, rosiglitazone, sertraline, warfarin, and other CYP2C8/9 substrates. May increase the effect of methotrexate. Risk of adverse reactions (thrombocytopenia purpura) may be increased by thiazide diuretics.

Nutritional/Ethanol Interactions

Food: Interferes with folate absorption.

Herb/Nutraceutical: Avoid dong quai, St John's wort (may also cause photosensitization).

Lab Interactions False-positive protein in urine; false-positive urine glucose with Clinitest®

Adverse Reactions Frequency not defined.

Cardiovascular: Vasculitis

Central nervous system: Fever, dizziness, headache

Dermatologic: Itching, rash, photosensitivity, Lyell's syndrome, Stevens-Johnson syndrome

Endocrine & metabolic: Thyroid function disturbance

Gastrointestinal: Anorexia, nausea, vomiting, diarrhea

Genitourinary: Crystalluria, hematuria,

Hematologic: Granulocytopenia, leukopenia, thrombocytopenia, aplastic anemia, hemolytic anemia

Hepatic: Jaundice, hepatitis

Renal: Interstitial nephritis

Miscellaneous: Serum sickness-like reactions

Overdosage/Toxicology Symptoms of overdose include drowsiness, dizziness, anorexia, abdominal pain, nausea, vomiting, hemolytic anemia, acidosis, jaundice, fever, and agranulocytosis. Doses as little as 2-5 g/day may produce toxicity. The aniline radical is responsible for hematologic toxicity. High volume diuresis may aid in elimination and prevention of renal failure. Leucovorin 5-15 mg/day has been used to speed recovery of bone marrow.

Pharmacodynamics/Kinetics

Time to Peak: Serum: 2-3 hours

Protein Binding: 85% to 88%

Half-Life Elimination: 4-7 hours; prolonged with renal impairment

Metabolism: Hepatic via acetylation and glucuronide conjugation to inactive compounds

Excretion: Urine (95%, 40% to 60% as unchanged drug) within 24 hours

Available Dosage Forms

Suspension, oral, pediatric, as acetyl (Gantrisin®): 500 mg/5 mL (480 mL) [contains alcohol 0.3%; raspberry flavor]

Tablet: 500 mg

Dosing

Adults & Elderly: Susceptible infections: Oral: 2-4 g stat, 4-8 g/day in divided doses every 4-6 hours

Pediatrics: Not for use in patients <2 months of age:

Children >2 months: Oral: Initial: 75 mg/kg, followed by 120-150 mg/kg/day in divided doses every 4-6 hours; not to exceed 6 g/day

Renal Impairment:

Cl_{cr} 10-50 mL/minutes: Administer every 8-12 hours.

Cl_{cr} <10 mL/minute: Administer every 12-24 hours.

Hemodialysis effects: >50% is removed by hemodialysis.

Administration

Oral: Administer around-the-clock to promote less variation in peak and trough serum levels.

Stability

Storage: Protect from light.

Laboratory Monitoring CBC, urinalysis, renal function. Obtain specimen for culture prior to first dose.

Nursing Actions

Physical Assessment: Allergy history should be assessed prior to starting therapy (sulfa drugs). Assess potential for interactions with other pharmacological agents patient may be taking (eg, increased or decreased levels/effects of concurrently administered drugs). Monitor effectiveness (reduced clinical symptoms) and adverse reactions (eg, photosensitivity, gastrointestinal disturbance [nausea, vomiting, anorexia], anemia, jaundice, hematuria). Caution patients with diabetes to monitor glucose levels closely (may cause altered response to oral hypoglycemics and may cause false-positive urine glucose with Clinitest®). Teach patient proper use, possible side effects/appropriate interventions, and adverse symptoms to report.

Patient Education: Take as directed with a full glass of water, at regular intervals around-the-clock, on an empty stomach (1 hour before or 2 hours after a meal). Complete full course of therapy even if you are feeling better. Take a missed dose as soon as possible. If almost time for next dose, skip the missed dose and return to your regular schedule. Do not take a double dose. Maintain adequate hydration (2-3 L/day of fluids) to prevent kidney damage unless instructed to restrict fluid intake. If you have diabetes, this medication may cause increased effect of oral hypoglycemics - monitor glucose levels closely; may alter Clinitest® response; use of alternative method of glucose monitoring is preferable. May cause dizziness or headache (use caution when driving or engaging in tasks requiring alertness until response to drug is known); photosensitivity (use sunblock, wear protective clothing and eyewear, and avoid direct sunlight); or nausea, vomiting, or loss of appetite (small, frequent meals, frequent mouth care, sucking lozenges, or chewing gum may help). Report persistent nausea, vomiting, or diarrhea; opportunistic infection (sore throat, fever, vaginal itching or discharge, unusual bruising or bleeding, fatigue); blood in urine or change in urinary pattern; swelling of face, lips, or tongue; tightness in chest; bad cough; or other persistent adverse effects. **Pregnancy precaution:** Inform prescriber if you are or intend to become pregnant.

Dietary Considerations Should be taken with a glass of water on an empty stomach.

Geriatric Considerations Sulfisoxazole is an effective anti-infective agent. Most prescribers prefer the combination of sulfamethoxazole and trimethoprim for its dual mechanism of action. Trimethoprim penetrates the prostate. Adjust dose for renal function.

Related Information

FDA Name Differentiation Project: The Use of Tall-Man Letters *on page 12*

Sulindac (sul IN dak)

U.S. Brand Names Clinoril®

Restrictions A medication guide should be dispensed with each prescription. A template for the required MedGuide can be found on the FDA website at: http://www.fda.gov/medwatch/SAFETY/2005/safety05.htm#NSAID

Pharmacologic Category Nonsteroidal Anti-inflammatory Drug (NSAID), Oral

Medication Safety Issues
Sound-alike/look-alike issues:
Clinoril® may be confused with Cleocin®, Clozaril®, Oruvail®

Pregnancy Risk Factor C/D (3rd trimester)

Lactation Excretion in breast milk unknown/not recommended

Use Management of inflammatory disease, osteoarthritis, rheumatoid arthritis, acute gouty arthritis, ankylosing spondylitis, bursitis/tendonitis of shoulder

Mechanism of Action/Effect Inhibits prostaglandin synthesis by decreasing the activity of the enzyme, cyclooxygenase, which results in decreased formation of prostaglandin precursors

Contraindications Hypersensitivity to sulindac, aspirin, other NSAIDs, or any component of the formulation; perioperative pain in the setting of coronary artery bypass surgery (CABG); pregnancy (3rd trimester)

Warnings/Precautions NSAIDs are associated with an increased risk of adverse cardiovascular events, including MI, stroke, and new onset or worsening of pre-existing hypertension. Risk may be increased with duration of use or pre-existing cardiovascular risk-factors or disease. Carefully evaluate individual cardiovascular risk profiles prior to prescribing. Use caution with fluid retention, CHF or hypertension.

Use of NSAIDs can compromise existing renal function. Renal toxicity can occur in patient with impaired renal function, dehydration, heart failure, liver dysfunction, those taking diuretics and ACEI and the elderly. Rehydrate patient before starting therapy. Monitor renal function closely. Sulindac is not recommended for patients with advanced renal disease. Use caution in patients with renal lithiasis; sulindac metabolites have been reported as components of renal stones. Use hydration in patients with a history of renal stones.

NSAIDs may increase risk of gastrointestinal irritation, ulceration, bleeding, and perforation. These events may occur at any time during therapy and without warning. Use caution with a history of GI disease (bleeding or ulcers), concurrent therapy with aspirin, anticoagulants and/or corticosteroids, smoking, use of alcohol, the elderly or debilitated patients.

Use the lowest effective dose for the shortest duration of time, consistent with individual patient goals, to reduce risk of cardiovascular or GI adverse events. Alternate therapies should be considered for patients at high risk.

NSAIDs may cause serious skin adverse events including exfoliative dermatitis, Stevens-Johnson syndrome (SJS) and toxic epidermal necrolysis (TEN). Anaphylactoid reactions may occur, even without prior exposure; patients with "aspirin triad" (bronchial asthma, aspirin intolerance, rhinitis) may be at increased risk. Do not use in patients who experience bronchospasm, asthma, rhinitis, or urticaria with NSAID or aspirin therapy.

Use with caution in patients with decreased hepatic function. Closely monitor patients with any abnormal LFT. Severe hepatic reactions (eg, fulminant hepatitis, liver failure) have occurred with NSAID use, rarely; discontinue if signs or symptoms of liver disease develop, or if systemic manifestations occur. May require dosage adjustment in hepatic dysfunction; sulfide and sulfone metabolites may accumulate.

Withhold for at least 4-6 half-lives prior to surgical or dental procedures.

Safety and efficacy in pediatric patients have not been established.

Drug Interactions
Decreased Effect: May reduce effect of some diuretics and antihypertensive effect of B-blockers, ACE inhibitors, angiotensin II inhibitors, hydralazine, verapamil. Cholestyramine and colestipol may reduce absorption of sulindac. Dimethyl sulfoxide may decrease active metabolite of sulindac; combination may cause peripheral neuropathy.

Increased Effect/Toxicity: Sulindac may increase effect/toxicity of anticoagulants (bleeding), antiplatelet agents (bleeding), aminoglycosides, bisphosphonates (GI irritation), corticosteroids (GI irritation), cyclosporine (nephrotoxicity), lithium, methotrexate, pemetrexed, treprostinil (bleeding), vancomycin.

Nutritional/Ethanol Interactions
Ethanol: Avoid ethanol (may enhance gastric mucosal irritation).
Food: Food may decrease the rate but not the extent of oral absorption. The therapeutic effect of sulindac may be decreased if taken with food.
Herb/Nutraceutical: Avoid alfalfa, anise, bilberry, bladderwrack, bromelain, cat's claw, celery, coleus, cordyceps, dong quai, evening primrose, feverfew, fenugreek, garlic, ginger, ginkgo biloba, red clover, horse chestnut, grapeseed, green tea, ginseng, guggul, horse chestnut seed, horseradish, licorice, prickly ash, red clover, reishi, SAMe, sweet clover, turmeric, white willow (all have additional antiplatelet activity).

Lab Interactions Increased chloride (S), sodium (S), bleeding time

Adverse Reactions
1% to 10%:
Cardiovascular: Edema (1% to 3%)
Central nervous system: Dizziness (3% to 9%), headache(3% to 9%), nervousness (1% to 3%)
Dermatologic: Rash (3% to 9%), pruritus (1% to 3%)
Gastrointestinal: Gastrointestinal: GI pain (10%), constipation (3% to 9%), diarrhea (3% to 9%), dyspepsia (3% to 9%), nausea (3% to 9%), abdominal cramps (1% to 3%), anorexia (1% to 3%), flatulence (1% to 3%), vomiting (1% to 3%)
Otic: Tinnitus (1% to 3%)

Overdosage/Toxicology Symptoms of overdose include dizziness, vomiting, nausea, abdominal pain, hypotension, coma, stupor, metabolic acidosis, leukocytosis, and renal failure. Management of NSAID intoxication is supportive and symptomatic. Seizures tend to be short-lived and often do not require drug treatment.

Pharmacodynamics/Kinetics
Onset of Action: Analgesic: ~1 hour
Duration of Action: 12-24 hours
Half-Life Elimination: Parent drug: ~8 hours; Active metabolite: ~16 hours
Metabolism: Hepatic; prodrug rmetabolized to sulfide metabolite (active) for therapeutic effects and to sulfone metabolites (inactive)
Excretion: Urine (50%, primarily as inactive metabolites); feces (25%, primarily as metabolites)

Available Dosage Forms
Tablet: 150 mg, 200 mg
Clinoril®: 200 mg

Dosing
Adults & Elderly: Note: Maximum daily dose: 400 mg
Osteoarthritis, rheumatoid arthritis, ankylosing spondylitis: 150 mg twice/daily
Bursitis/tendonitis: 200 mg twice daily; usual treatment: 7-14 days

Acute gouty arthritis: 200 mg twice daily; usual treatment: 7 days

Pediatrics: Dose not established

Renal Impairment: Not recommended with advanced renal impairment; if required, decrease dose and monitor closely.

Hepatic Impairment: Dose reduction is necessary; discontinue if abnormal liver function tests occur.

Administration

Oral: Should be administered with food or milk.

Laboratory Monitoring Liver enzymes, BUN, serum creatinine, CBC, platelets

Nursing Actions

Physical Assessment: Assess effectiveness and interactions of other medications patient may be taking. Monitor blood pressure at the beginning of therapy and periodically during use. Monitor laboratory tests, therapeutic response (eg, relief of pain and inflammation, increased activity tolerance), and adverse reactions (eg, GI and respiratory response, hepatotoxicity, ototoxicity) at beginning of therapy and periodically throughout therapy. Schedule ophthalmic evaluations for patients who develop eye complaints during long-term NSAID therapy. Assess knowledge/teach patient appropriate use, interventions to reduce side effects, and adverse symptoms to report.

Patient Education: Take this medication exactly as directed; do not increase dose without consulting prescriber. Take with food or milk to reduce GI distress. Maintain adequate hydration (2-3 L/day of fluids) unless instructed to restrict fluid intake. Do not use alcohol, aspirin or aspirin-containing medication, or any other anti-inflammatory medications without consulting prescriber. Regularly scheduled ophthalmic exams are advised with long-term use of NSAIDs. You may experience dizziness, nervousness, or headache (use caution when driving or engaging in tasks requiring alertness until response to drug is known); nausea, vomiting, or heartburn (small frequent meals, frequent mouth care, sucking lozenges, or chewing gum may help); or constipation (increased exercise, fluids, fruit, or fiber may help). GI bleeding, ulceration, or perforation can occur with or without pain; discontinue medication and contact prescriber if persistent abdominal pain, cramping, or blood in stool occurs. Report breathlessness or respiratory difficulty; chest pain; unusual bruising or bleeding; blood in urine, stool, mouth, or vomitus; unusual fatigue; skin rash or itching; change in urinary pattern; or change in hearing or ringing in ears. **Pregnancy/breast-feeding precautions:** Inform prescriber if you are or intend to become pregnant. This drug

Dietary Considerations Drug may cause GI upset, bleeding, ulceration, perforation; take with food or milk to minimize GI upset.

Geriatric Considerations Elderly are at high risk for adverse effects from NSAIDs. As much as 60% of elderly who develop GI complications can develop peptic ulceration and/or hemorrhage asymptomatically. The concomitant use of H₂ blockers, omeprazole, and sucralfate is not effective as prophylaxis with the exception of NSAID-induced duodenal ulcers which may be prevented by the use of ranitidine. Misoprostol is the only prophylactic agent proven effective. Also, concomitant disease and drug use contribute to the risk for GI adverse effects. Use lowest effective dose for shortest period possible. Consider renal function decline with age. Use of NSAIDs can compromise existing renal function especially when Cl$_{cr}$ is ≤30 mL/minute. Tinnitus may be a difficult and unreliable indication of toxicity due to age-related hearing loss or eighth cranial nerve damage. CNS adverse effects such as confusion, agitation, and hallucination are generally seen in overdose or high-dose situations, but elderly may demonstrate these adverse effects at lower doses than younger adults.

Sumatriptan (soo ma TRIP tan SUKS i nate)

U.S. Brand Names Imitrex®

Synonyms Sumatriptan Succinate

Pharmacologic Category Serotonin 5-HT$_{1D}$ Receptor Agonist

Medication Safety Issues

Sound-alike/look-alike issues:

Sumatriptan may be confused with somatropin, zolmitriptan

Pregnancy Risk Factor C

Lactation Enters breast milk/use caution (AAP rates "compatible")

Use

Oral, SubQ: Acute treatment of migraine with or without aura

SubQ: Acute treatment of cluster headache episodes

Mechanism of Action/Effect Selective agonist for serotonin (5-HT$_{1D}$ receptor) in cranial arteries to cause vasoconstriction and reduces sterile inflammation associated with antidromic neuronal transmission correlating with relief of migraine

Contraindications Hypersensitivity to sumatriptan or any component of the formulation; patients with ischemic heart disease or signs or symptoms of ischemic heart disease (including Prinzmetal's angina, angina pectoris, myocardial infarction, silent myocardial ischemia); cerebrovascular syndromes (including strokes, transient ischemic attacks); peripheral vascular syndromes (including ischemic bowel disease); uncontrolled hypertension; use within 24 hours of ergotamine derivatives; use within 24 hours of another 5-HT$_1$ agonist; concurrent administration or within 2 weeks of discontinuing an MAO inhibitor, specifically MAO type A inhibitors; management of hemiplegic or basilar migraine; prophylactic treatment of migraine; severe hepatic impairment; not for I.V. administration

Warnings/Precautions Sumatriptan is indicated only in patients ≥18 years of age with a clear diagnosis of migraine or cluster headache. Cardiac events, cerebral/subarachnoid hemorrhage, and stroke have been reported with 5-HT$_1$ agonist administration. Do not give to patients with risk factors for CAD until a cardiovascular evaluation has been performed. If the evaluation is satisfactory, the healthcare provider should administer the first dose and cardiovascular status should be periodically evaluated.

Significant elevation in blood pressure, including hypertensive crisis, has also been reported on rare occasions in patients with and without a history of hypertension. Vasospasm-related reactions have been reported other than coronary artery vasospasm. Peripheral vascular ischemia and colonic ischemia with abdominal pain and bloody diarrhea have occurred.

Use with caution in patients with history of seizure disorder or in patients with a lowered seizure threshold. Safety and efficacy in pediatric patients have not been established.

Drug Interactions

Increased Effect/Toxicity: Increased toxicity with ergot-containing drugs, avoid use, wait 24 hours from last ergot containing drug (dihydroergotamine, or methysergide) before administering sumatriptan. MAO inhibitors decrease clearance of sumatriptan increasing the risk of systemic sumatriptan toxic effects. Sumatriptan may enhance CNS toxic effects when taken with selective serotonin reuptake inhibitors (SSRIs) like fluoxetine, fluvoxamine, paroxetine, or sertraline. **Note:** Use cautiously in patients receiving concomitant medications that can lower the seizure threshold.

(Continued)

Sumatriptan (Continued)

Adverse Reactions

Injection:

>10%:

Central nervous system: Dizziness (12%), warm/hot sensation (11%)

Local: Pain at injection site (59%)

Neuromuscular & skeletal: Paresthesia (14%)

1% to 10%:

Cardiovascular: Chest pain/tightness/heaviness/pressure (2% to 3%), hyper-/hypotension (1%)

Central nervous system: Burning (7%), feeling of heaviness (7%), flushing (7%), pressure sensation (7%), feeling of tightness (5%), drowsiness (3%), malaise/fatigue (1%), feeling strange (2%), headache (2%), tight feeling in head (2%), cold sensation (1%), anxiety (1%)

Gastrointestinal: Abdominal discomfort (1%), dysphagia (1%)

Neuromuscular & skeletal: Neck, throat, and jaw pain/tightness/pressure (2% to 5%), mouth/tongue discomfort (5%), weakness (5%), myalgia (2%); muscle cramps (1%), numbness (5%)

Ocular: Vision alterations (1%)

Respiratory: Throat discomfort (3%), nasal disorder/discomfort (2%)

Miscellaneous: Diaphoresis (2%)

Nasal spray:

>10%: Gastrointestinal: Bad taste (13% to 24%), nausea (11% to 13%), vomiting (11% to 13%)

1% to 10%:

Central nervous system: Dizziness (1% to 2%)

Respiratory: Nasal disorder/discomfort (2% to 4%), throat discomfort (1% to 2%)

Tablet:

1% to 10%:

Cardiovascular: Chest pain/tightness/heaviness/pressure (1% to 2%), hyper-/hypotension (1%), palpitation (1%), syncope (1%)

Central nervous system: Burning (1%), dizziness (>1%), drowsiness (>1%), malaise/fatigue (2% to 3%), headache (>1%), nonspecified pain (1% to 2%, placebo 1%), vertigo (<1% to 2%), migraine (>1%), sleepiness (>1%)

Gastrointestinal: Diarrhea (1%), nausea (>1%), vomiting (>1%), hyposalivation (>1%)

Genitourinary: Hematuria (1%)

Hematologic: Hemolytic anemia (1%)

Neuromuscular & skeletal: Neck, throat, and jaw pain/tightness/pressure (2% to 3%), paresthesia (3% to 5%), myalgia (1%), numbness (1%)

Otic: Ear hemorrhage (1%), hearing loss (1%), sensitivity to noise (1%), tinnitus (1%)

Respiratory: Allergic rhinitis (1%), dyspnea (1%), nasal inflammation (1%), nose/throat hemorrhage (1%), sinusitis (1%), upper respiratory inflammation (1%)

Miscellaneous: Hypersensitivity reactions (1%), nonspecified pressure/tightness/heaviness (1% to 3%, placebo 2%); warm/cold sensation (2% to 3%, placebo 2%)

Overdosage/Toxicology Single oral doses ≤400 mg, injectable doses ≤16 mg, and nasal doses of 40 mg have been reported without adverse effects. Treatment of overdose should be supportive and symptomatic. Monitor for at least 12 hours or until signs and symptoms subside. It is not known if hemodialysis or peritoneal dialysis is effective.

Pharmacodynamics/Kinetics

Onset of Action: ~30 minutes

Time to Peak: Serum: 5-20 minutes

Protein Binding: 14% to 21%

Half-Life Elimination: Injection, tablet: 2.5 hours; Nasal spray: 2 hours

Metabolism: Hepatic, primarily via MAO-A isoenzyme

Excretion:

Injection: Urine (38% as indole acetic acid metabolite, 22% as unchanged drug)

Nasal spray: Urine (42% as indole acetic acid metabolite, 3% as unchanged drug)

Tablet: Urine (60% as indole acetic acid metabolite, 3% as unchanged drug); feces (40%)

Available Dosage Forms Note: Strength expressed as sumatriptan base

Injection, solution, as succinate: 8 mg/mL (0.5 mL) [disposable cartridge for use with STATdose System®]; 12 mg/mL (0.5 mL) [disposable cartridge for use with STATdose System® or vial]

Solution, intranasal spray: 5 mg (100 µL unit dose spray device); 20 mg (100 µL unit dose spray device)

Tablet, as succinate: 25 mg, 50 mg, 100 mg

Dosing

Adults:

Migraine:

Oral: A single dose of 25 mg, 50 mg, or 100 mg (taken with fluids). If a satisfactory response has not been obtained at 2 hours, a second dose may be administered. Results from clinical trials show that initial doses of 50 mg and 100 mg are more effective than doses of 25 mg, and that 100 mg doses do not provide a greater effect than 50 mg and may have increased incidence of side effects. Although doses of up to 300 mg/day have been studied, the total daily dose should not exceed 200 mg. The safety of treating an average of >4 headaches in a 30-day period have not been established.

Intranasal: Single dose of 5, 10, or 20 mg administered in one nostril; a 10 mg dose may be achieved by administration of a single 5 mg dose in each nostril; if headache returns, the dose may be repeated once after 2 hours, not to exceed a total daily dose of 40 mg. The safety of treating an average of >4 headaches in a 30-day period has not been established.

SubQ: Up to 6 mg; if side effects are dose-limiting, lower doses may be used. A second injection may be administered at least 1 hour after the initial dose, but not more than 2 injections in a 24-hour period.

Cluster headache: Refer to dosing under "Migraine, SubQ"

Renal Impairment: Dosage adjustment is not necessary.

Hepatic Impairment: Bioavailability of oral sumatriptan is increased with liver disease. If treatment is needed, do not exceed single doses of 50 mg. The nasal spray has not been studied in patients with hepatic impairment, however, because the spray does not undergo first-pass metabolism, levels would not be expected to alter. Use of all dosage forms is contraindicated with severe hepatic impairment.

Administration

Oral: Oral: Should be taken with fluids as soon as symptoms appear.

I.V.: Do **not** administer I.V.; may cause coronary vasospasm.

Other: Administer injection formulation subcutaneously. An autoinjection device (STATdose System®) is available for use with the 4 mg and 6 mg cartridges.

Stability

Storage: Store at 2°C to 20°C (36°F to 86°F). Protect from light.

Nursing Actions

Physical Assessment: For use only with a clear diagnosis of migraine or cluster headaches. Assess potential for interactions with other pharmacological agents patient may be taking (eg, ergot-containing drugs, MAO inhibitors, SSRIs). See Administration for specifics of SubQ, intranasal, oral formulation use. Monitor therapeutic effectiveness (relief of headaches) and adverse response (eg, dizziness, tingling, drowsiness, myalgia, vision alternation, nausea, vomiting; reactions differ according to formulation). Teach patient proper use according to formulation (eg, with SubQ, appropriate injection technique and syringe/needle disposal), possible side effects/appropriate interventions, and adverse symptoms to report.

Patient Education: Take at first sign of migraine attack. This drug is to be used to reduce your migraine, not to prevent or reduce the number of attacks. Follow exact instructions for use.

Nasal spray: Administer dose into one nostril. If headache returns or is not fully resolved after the first dose, the dose may be repeated after 2 hours. **Do not exceed 40 mg in 24 hours.**

Oral: If headache returns or is not fully resolved after first dose, the dose may be repeated after 2 hours. **Do not exceed 200 mg in 24 hours.** Take whole with fluids.

SubQ: If headache returns or is not fully resolved after first dose, the dose may be repeated after 1 hour. **Do not exceed two injections in 24 hours.**

All forms: Do not take any form of this drug within 24 hours of any other migraine medication without consulting prescriber. May cause dizziness, fatigue, or drowsiness (use caution when driving or engaging in tasks that require alertness until response to drug is known); or nausea or vomiting (small, frequent meals, frequent mouth care, chewing gum, or sucking on lozenges may help). Report chest tightness or pain; excessive drowsiness; acute abdominal pain; skin rash or burning sensation; muscle weakness, soreness, or numbness; respiratory difficulty; or any other persistent adverse reactions. **Pregnancy/ breast-feeding precautions:** Inform prescriber if you are or intend to become pregnant. Consult prescriber if breast-feeding.

Geriatric Considerations Use cautiously in the elderly, particularly since many elderly have cardiovascular disease which would put them at risk for cardiovascular adverse effects. Safety and efficacy in the elderly (>65 years) have not been established. Pharmacokinetic disposition is, however, similar to that in young adults.

Breast-Feeding Issues The amount of sumatriptan an infant would be exposed to following breast-feeding is considered to be small (although the mean milk-to-plasma ratio is ~4.9, weight adjusted doses estimates suggest breast-fed infants receive 3.5% of a maternal dose). Expressing and discarding the milk for 8-12 hours after a single dose is suggested to reduce the amount present even further. The half-life of sumatriptan in breast milk is 2.22 hours.

Tacrine (TAK reen)

U.S. Brand Names Cognex®

Synonyms Tacrine Hydrochloride; Tetrahydroaminoacrine; THA

Pharmacologic Category Acetylcholinesterase Inhibitor (Central)

Medication Safety Issues
Sound-alike/look-alike issues:
Cognex® may be confused with Corgard®

Pregnancy Risk Factor C

Lactation Excretion in breast milk unknown/not recommended

Use Treatment of mild to moderate dementia of the Alzheimer's type

Mechanism of Action/Effect Centrally-acting cholinesterase inhibitor. It elevates acetylcholine in cerebral cortex by slowing the degradation of acetylcholine.

Contraindications Hypersensitivity to tacrine, acridine derivatives, or any component of the formulation; patients previously treated with tacrine who developed jaundice

Warnings/Precautions The use of tacrine has been associated with elevations in serum transaminases; serum transaminases (specifically ALT) must be monitored throughout therapy; use extreme caution in patients with current evidence of a history of abnormal liver function tests; use caution in patients with urinary tract obstruction (bladder outlet obstruction or prostatic hyperplasia), asthma, and sick-sinus syndrome, bradycardia, or conduction abnormalities (tacrine may cause bradycardia and/or heart block). Also, patients with cardiovascular disease, asthma, or peptic ulcer should use cautiously. Adverse cardiovascular events may also occur in patients without known cardiac disease. Use with caution in patients with a history of seizures. May cause nausea, vomiting, or loose stools. Abrupt discontinuation or dosage decrease may worsen cognitive function. May be associated with neutropenia.

Drug Interactions

Cytochrome P450 Effect: Substrate of CYP1A2 (major); **Inhibits** CYP1A2 (weak)

Decreased Effect: CYP1A2 inducers may decrease the levels/effects of tacrine; example inducers include aminoglutethimide, carbamazepine, phenobarbital, rifampin, and cigarette smoking, Tacrine may worsen Parkinson's disease and inhibit the effects of levodopa. Tacrine may antagonize the therapeutic effect of anticholinergic agents (benztropine, trihexyphenidyl).

Increased Effect/Toxicity: CYP1A2 inhibitors may increase the levels/effects of tacrine; example inhibitors include amiodarone, ciprofloxacin, fluvoxamine, ketoconazole, norfloxacin, ofloxacin, and rofecoxib. Tacrine in combination with other cholinergic agents (eg, ambenonium, edrophonium, neostigmine, pyridostigmine, bethanechol), will likely produce additive cholinergic effects. Tacrine in combination with beta-blockers may produce additive bradycardia. Tacrine may increase the levels/effect of succinylcholine and theophylline. in elevated plasma levels. Fluvoxamine, enoxacin, and cimetidine increase tacrine concentrations via enzyme inhibition (CYP1A2). Acetylcholinesterase inhibitors (central) may increase the risk of antipsychotic-related extrapyramidal symptoms.

Nutritional/Ethanol Interactions Food: Food decreases bioavailability.

Adverse Reactions
>10%:
Central nervous system: Headache, dizziness
Gastrointestinal: Nausea, vomiting, diarrhea
Miscellaneous: Transaminases increased
1% to 10%:
Cardiovascular: Flushing
Central nervous system: Confusion, ataxia, insomnia, somnolence, depression, anxiety, fatigue
Dermatologic: Rash
Gastrointestinal: Dyspepsia, anorexia, abdominal pain, flatulence, constipation, weight loss
Neuromuscular & skeletal: Myalgia, tremor
Respiratory: Rhinitis

Overdosage/Toxicology Provide general supportive measures. Can cause cholinergic crisis characterized by severe nausea, vomiting, salivation, sweating, bradycardia, hypotension, collapse, and convulsions. Increased muscle weakness is a possibility and may result in death if respiratory muscles are involved.

Tertiary anticholinergics, such as atropine, may be used as an antidote for overdose. I.V. atropine sulfate titrated to effect is recommended at an initial dose of 1-2 mg I.V. with subsequent doses based upon clinical response. Atypical increases in blood pressure and heart rate have been reported with other cholinomimetics when (Continued)

Tacrine (Continued)

coadministered with quaternary anticholinergics such as glycopyrrolate.

Pharmacodynamics/Kinetics

Time to Peak: Plasma: 1-2 hours

Protein Binding: Plasma: 55%

Half-Life Elimination: Serum: 2-4 hours; Steady-state: 24-36 hours

Metabolism: Extensively by CYP450 to multiple metabolites; first pass effect

Available Dosage Forms Capsule, as hydrochloride: 10 mg, 20 mg, 30 mg, 40 mg

Dosing

Adults & Elderly:

Alzheimer's disease: Oral: Initial: 10 mg 4 times/day; may increase by 40 mg/day adjusted every 6 weeks; maximum: 160 mg/day; best administered separate from meal times.

Dose adjustment based upon transaminase elevations:

ALT ≤3 times ULN*: Continue titration

ALT >3 to ≤5 times ULN*: Decrease dose by 40 mg/day, resume when ALT returns to normal

ALT >5 times ULN*: Stop treatment, may rechallenge upon return of ALT to normal

*ULN = upper limit of normal

Note: Patients with clinical jaundice confirmed by elevated total bilirubin (>3 mg/dL) should not be rechallenged with tacrine

Hepatic Impairment: Patients with clinical jaundice confirmed by elevated total bilirubin (>3 mg/dL) should not be rechallenged with tacrine.

Laboratory Monitoring ALT (SGPT) levels and other liver enzymes at least every other week from weeks 4-16, then monitor once every 3 months

Nursing Actions

Physical Assessment: Assess bladder and sphincter adequacy prior to administering medication. Assess other medications patient may be taking for effectiveness and interactions. Monitor laboratory tests (ALT) throughout therapy, therapeutic effect, and adverse reactions (eg, cholinergic crisis [DUMBELS - diarrhea, urination, miosis, bronchospasm/bradycardia, excitability, lacrimation, and salivation/excessive sweating]). Assess knowledge/teach patient appropriate use, interventions to reduce side effects, and adverse symptoms to report.

Patient Education: This medication will not cure the disease, but may help reduce symptoms. Use as directed; do not increase dose or discontinue without consulting prescriber. Maintain adequate hydration (2-3 L/day of fluids) unless instructed to restrict fluid intake. May cause dizziness, sedation, or hypotension (rise slowly from sitting or lying position and use caution when driving or climbing stairs); vomiting or loss of appetite (small frequent meals, frequent mouth care, or chewing gum, or sucking lozenges may help); or diarrhea (boiled milk, yogurt, or buttermilk may help). Report persistent abdominal discomfort; significantly increased salivation, sweating, tearing, or urination; flushed skin; chest pain or palpitations; acute headache; unresolved diarrhea; excessive fatigue, insomnia, dizziness, or depression; increased muscle, joint, or body pain; vision changes or blurred vision; shortness of breath or wheezing; or signs of jaundice (yellowing of eyes or skin, dark colored urine or light colored stool, abdominal pain, or easy fatigue).

Pregnancy/breast-feeding precautions: Inform prescriber if you are or intend to become pregnant. Breast-feeding is not recommended.

Dietary Considerations Give with food if GI side effects are intolerable.

Geriatric Considerations Tacrine is currently FDA-approved for the treatment of Alzheimer's disease, it is clearly not a cure. At least 25% of patients may not tolerate the drug and only 50% of patients demonstrate some improvement in symptoms or a slowing of deterioration. While worth a trial in mild to moderate dementia of the Alzheimer's type, patients and their families must be counseled about the limitations of the drug and the importance of regular monitoring of liver function tests. No specific dosage adjustments are necessary due to age.

Tacrolimus (ta KROE li mus)

U.S. Brand Names Prograf®; Protopic®

Synonyms FK506

Restrictions An FDA-approved medication guide is available at http://www.fda.gov/cder/Offices/ODS/labeling.htm; distribute to each patient to whom the ointment is dispensed.

Pharmacologic Category Immunosuppressant Agent; Topical Skin Product

Medication Safety Issues

Sound-alike/look-alike issues:

Prograf® may be confused with Gengraf®

Pregnancy Risk Factor C

Lactation Enters breast milk/contraindicated

Use

Oral/injection: Potent immunosuppressive drug used in liver or kidney transplant recipients

Topical: Moderate to severe atopic dermatitis in patients not responsive to conventional therapy or when conventional therapy is not appropriate

Unlabeled/Investigational Use Potent immunosuppressive drug used in heart, lung, small bowel transplant recipients; immunosuppressive drug for peripheral stem cell/bone marrow transplantation

Mechanism of Action/Effect Suppresses cellular immunity (inhibits T-lymphocyte activation)

Contraindications Hypersensitivity to tacrolimus or any component of the formulation

Warnings/Precautions

Oral/injection: Insulin-dependent post-transplant diabetes mellitus (PTDM) has been reported (1% to 20%); risk increases in African-American and Hispanic kidney transplant patients. Increased susceptibility to infection and the possible development of lymphoma may occur after administration of tacrolimus. Nephrotoxicity and neurotoxicity have been reported, especially with higher doses; to avoid excess nephrotoxicity do not administer simultaneously with cyclosporine; monitoring of serum concentrations (trough for oral therapy) is essential to prevent organ rejection and reduce drug-related toxicity; tonic clonic seizures may have been triggered by tacrolimus. A period of 24 hours should elapse between discontinuation of cyclosporine and the initiation of tacrolimus. Use caution in renal or hepatic dysfunction, dosing adjustments may be required. Delay initiation if postoperative oliguria occurs. Use may be associated with the development of hypertension (common). Myocardial hypertrophy has been reported (rare). Each mL of injection contains polyoxyl 60 hydrogenated castor oil (HCO-60) (200 mg) and dehydrated alcohol USP 80% v/v. Anaphylaxis has been reported with the injection, use should be reserved for those patients not able to take oral medications.

Topical: Topical calcineurin inhibitors have been associated with rare cases of malignancy. Avoid use on malignant or premalignant skin conditions (eg cutaneous T-cell lymphoma). Topical calcineurin agents are considered second-line therapies in the treatment of atopic dermatitis/eczema, and should be limited to use in patients who have failed treatment with other therapies. They should be used for short-term and intermittent treatment using the minimum amount necessary for the control of symptoms should be used. Application should be limited to involved areas. Safety of intermittent use for >1 year has not been established.

Should not be used in immunocompromised patients. Do not apply to areas of active viral infection; infections at the treatment site should be cleared prior to therapy. Patients with atopic dermatitis are predisposed to skin infections, and tacrolimus therapy has been associated with risk of developing eczema herpeticum, varicella zoster, and herpes simplex. May be associated with development of lymphadenopathy; possible infectious causes should be investigated. Discontinue use in patients with unknown cause of lymphadenopathy or acute infectious mononucleosis. Not recommended for use in patients with skin disease which may increase systemic absorption (eg, Netherton's syndrome). Avoid artificial or natural sunlight exposure, even when Protopic® is not on the skin. Safety not established in patients with generalized erythroderma. The use of Protopic® in children <2 years of age is not recommended, particularly since the effect on immune system development is unknown.

Drug Interactions

Cytochrome P450 Effect: Substrate of CYP3A4 (major); **Inhibits** CYP3A4 (weak)

Decreased Effect: Antacids impair tacrolimus absorption (separate administration by at least 2 hours). St John's wort may reduce tacrolimus serum concentrations (avoid concurrent use). CYP3A4 inducers may decrease the levels/effects of tacrolimus; example inducers include aminoglutethimide, carbamazepine, nafcillin, nevirapine, phenobarbital, phenytoin, and rifamycins. Caspofungin and sirolimus may decrease the serum concentrations of tacrolimus.

Increased Effect/Toxicity: Amphotericin B and other nephrotoxic antibiotics have the potential to increase tacrolimus-associated nephrotoxicity. Cisapride and metoclopramide may increase tacrolimus levels. Synergistic immunosuppression results from concurrent use of cyclosporine. Voriconazole may increase tacrolimus serum concentrations; decrease tacrolimus dosage by 66% when initiating voriconazole. CYP3A4 inhibitors may increase the levels/effects of tacrolimus; example inhibitors include azole antifungals, clarithromycin, diclofenac, doxycycline, erythromycin, imatinib, isoniazid, nefazodone, nicardipine, propofol, protease inhibitors, quinidine, telithromycin, and verapamil. Azithromycin may increase tacrolimus concentration (limited documentation). Calcium channel blockers (dihydropyridine) may increase tacrolimus serum concentrations (monitor). Concurrent therapy with sirolimus may increase the risk of HUS/TTP/TMA.

Nutritional/Ethanol Interactions

Ethanol: Localized flushing (redness, warm sensation) may occur at application site of topical tacrolimus following ethanol consumption.

Food: Decreases rate and extent of absorption. High-fat meals have most pronounced effect (35% decrease in AUC, 77% decrease in C_{max}). Grapefruit juice, CYP3A4 inhibitor, may increase serum level and/or toxicity of tacrolimus; avoid concurrent use.

Herb/Nutraceutical: St John's wort: May reduce tacrolimus serum concentrations (avoid concurrent use).

Adverse Reactions

Oral, I.V.:

≥15%:

Cardiovascular: Chest pain, hypertension

Central nervous system: Dizziness, headache, insomnia, tremor (headache and tremor are associated with high whole blood concentrations and may respond to decreased dosage)

Dermatologic: Pruritus, rash

Endocrine & metabolic: Diabetes mellitus, hyperglycemia, hyper-/hypokalemia, hyperlipemia, hypomagnesemia, hypophosphatemia

Gastrointestinal: Abdominal pain, constipation, diarrhea, dyspepsia, nausea, vomiting

Genitourinary: Urinary tract infection

Hematologic: Anemia, leukocytosis, thrombocytopenia

Hepatic: Ascites

Neuromuscular & skeletal: Arthralgia, back pain, weakness, paresthesia

Renal: Abnormal kidney function, increased creatinine, oliguria, urinary tract infection, increased BUN

Respiratory: Atelectasis, dyspnea, increased cough, effusion

<15%:

Cardiovascular: Abnormal ECG (QRS or ST segment abnormal), angina pectoris, cardiopulmonary failure, deep thrombophlebitis, heart rate decreased, hemorrhage, hemorrhagic stroke, hypervolemia, hypotension, generalized edema, peripheral vascular disorder, phlebitis, postural hypotension, tachycardia, thrombosis, vasodilation

Central nervous system: Abnormal dreams, abnormal thinking, agitation, amnesia, anxiety, chills, confusion, depression, dizziness, elevated mood, emotional lability, encephalopathy, hallucinations, nervousness, paralysis, psychosis, quadriparesis, seizure, somnolence

Dermatologic: Acne, alopecia, cellulitis, exfoliative dermatitis, fungal dermatitis, hirsutism, increased diaphoresis, photosensitivity reaction, skin discoloration, skin disorder, skin ulcer

Endocrine & metabolic: Acidosis, alkalosis, Cushing's syndrome, decreased bicarbonate, decreased serum iron, diabetes mellitus, hypercalcemia, hypercholesterolemia, hyperphosphatemia, hypoproteinemia, increased alkaline phosphatase

Gastrointestinal: Anorexia, appetite increased, cramps, duodenitis, dysphagia, enlarged abdomen, esophagitis (including ulcerative), flatulence, gastritis, gastroesophagitis, GI perforation/hemorrhage, ileus, oral moniliasis, pancreatic pseudocyst, rectal disorder, stomatitis, weight gain

Genitourinary: Bladder spasm, cystitis, dysuria, nocturia, oliguria, urge incontinence, urinary frequency, urinary incontinence, urinary retention, vaginitis

Hematologic: Bruising, coagulation disorder, decreased prothrombin, hypochromic anemia, leukopenia, polycythemia

Hepatic: Abnormal liver function tests, ALT/AST increased, bilirubinemia, cholangitis, cholestatic jaundice, GGT increased, hepatitis (including granulomatous), jaundice, liver damage, increase LDH

Neuromuscular & skeletal: Hypertonia, incoordination, joint disorder, leg cramps, myalgia, myasthenia, myoclonus, nerve compression, neuropathy, osteoporosis

Ocular: Abnormal vision, amblyopia

Otic: Ear pain, otitis media, tinnitus

Renal: Albuminuria, renal tubular necrosis, toxic nephropathy

Respiratory: Asthma, bronchitis, lung disorder, pharyngitis, pneumonia, pneumothorax, pulmonary edema, respiratory disorder, rhinitis, sinusitis, voice alteration

Miscellaneous: Abscess, abnormal healing, allergic reaction, crying, flu-like syndrome, generalized spasm, hernia, herpes simplex, peritonitis, sepsis, writing impaired

Topical (as reported in children and adults, unless otherwise noted):

>10%:

Central nervous system: Headache (5% to 20%), fever (1% to 21%)

Dermatologic: Skin burning (43% to 58%; tends to improve as lesions resolve), pruritus (41% to 46%), erythema (12% to 28%)

(Continued)

Tacrolimus (Continued)

Respiratory: Increased cough (18% children)
Miscellaneous: Flu-like syndrome (23% to 28%), allergic reaction (4% to 12%)

1% to 10%:
Cardiovascular: Peripheral edema (3% to 4% adults)
Central nervous system: Hyperesthesia (3% to 7% adults), pain (1% to 2%)
Dermatologic: Skin tingling (2% to 8%), acne (4% to 7% adults), localized flushing (following ethanol consumption 3% to 7% adults), folliculitis (2% to 6%), urticaria (1% to 6%), rash (2% to 5%), pustular rash (2% to 4%), vesiculobullous rash (4% children), contact dermatitis (3% to 4%), cyst (1% to 3% adults), eczema herpeticum (1% to 2%), fungal dermatitis (1% to 2% adults), sunburn (1% to 2% adults), dry skin (1% children)
Endocrine & metabolic: Dysmenorrhea (4% women)
Gastrointestinal: Diarrhea (3% to 5%), dyspepsia (1% to 4% adults), abdominal pain (3% children), vomiting (1% adults), gastroenteritis (adults 2%), nausea (1% children)
Neuromuscular & skeletal: Myalgia (2% to 3% adults), weakness (2% to 3% adults), back pain (2% adults)
Ocular: Conjunctivitis (2% adults)
Otic: Otitis media (12% children)
Respiratory: Rhinitis (6% children), sinusitis (2% to 4% adults), bronchitis (2% adults), pneumonia (1% adults)
Miscellaneous: Varicella/herpes zoster (1% to 5%), lymphadenopathy (3% children)

Overdosage/Toxicology Symptoms are extensions of immunosuppressive activity and adverse effects. Symptomatic and supportive treatment is required. Hemodialysis is not effective.

Pharmacodynamics/Kinetics
Time to Peak: 0.5-4 hours
Protein Binding: 99%
Half-Life Elimination: Variable, 21-61 hours in healthy volunteers
Metabolism: Extensively hepatic via CYP3A4 to eight possible metabolites (major metabolite, 31-demethyl tacrolimus, shows same activity as tacrolimus *in vitro*)
Excretion: Feces (~92%); feces/urine (<1% as unchanged drug)

Available Dosage Forms
Capsule (Prograf®): 0.5 mg, 1 mg, 5 mg
Injection, solution (Prograf®): 5 mg/mL (1 mL) [contains dehydrated alcohol 80% and polyoxyl 60 hydrogenated castor oil]
Ointment, topical (Protopic®): 0.03% (30 g, 60 g, 100 g); 0.1% (30 g, 60 g, 100 g)

Dosing
Adults & Elderly:
Kidney transplant:
Oral: Initial dose: 0.2 mg/kg/day in 2 divided doses, given every 12 hours; initial dose may be given within 24 hours of transplant, but should be delayed until renal function has recovered; African-American patients may require larger doses to maintain trough concentration
Typical whole blood trough concentrations: Months 1-3: 7-20 ng/mL; months 4-12: 5-15 ng/mL
I.V.: Note: I.V. route should only be used in patients not able to take oral medications, anaphylaxis has been reported. Initial dose: 0.03-0.05 mg/kg/day as a continuous infusion; begin no sooner than 6 hours post-transplant, starting at lower end of the dosage range; adjunctive therapy with corticosteroids is recommended; continue only until oral medication can be tolerated

Liver transplant:
Oral: Initial dose: 0.1-0.15 mg/kg/day in 2 divided doses, given every 12 hours; begin oral dose no sooner than 6 hours post-transplant; adjunctive

therapy with corticosteroids is recommended; if switching from I.V. to oral, the oral dose should be started 8-12 hours after stopping the infusion
Typical whole blood trough concentrations: Months 1-12: 5-20 ng/mL
I.V.: Note: I.V. route should only be used in patients not able to take oral medications, anaphylaxis has been reported. Initial dose: 0.03-0.05 mg/kg/day as a continuous infusion; begin no sooner than 6 hours post-transplant starting at lower end of the dosage range; adjunctive therapy with corticosteroids is recommended; continue only until oral medication can be tolerated

Prevention of graft-vs-host disease: I.V.: 0.03 mg/kg/day as continuous infusion

Atopic dermatitis (moderate to severe): Topical: Apply minimum amount of 0.03% or 0.1% ointment to affected area twice daily; rub in gently and completely. Discontinue use when symptoms have cleared. If no improvement within 6 weeks, patients should be re-examined to confirm diagnosis.

Pediatrics:
Liver transplant:
Note: Patients without pre-existing renal or hepatic dysfunction have required and tolerated higher doses than adults to achieve similar blood concentrations. It is recommended that therapy be initiated at high end of the recommended adult I.V. and oral dosing ranges; dosage adjustments may be required.
Oral: Initial dose: 0.15-0.20 mg/kg/day in 2 divided doses, given every 12 hours; begin oral dose no sooner than 6 hours post-transplant; adjunctive therapy with corticosteroids is recommended; if switching from I.V. to oral, the oral dose should be started 8-12 hours after stopping the infusion
Typical whole blood trough concentrations: Months 1-12: 5-20 ng/mL
I.V.: Note: I.V. route should only be used in patients not able to take oral medications, anaphylaxis has been reported. Initial dose: 0.03-0.05 mg/kg/day as a continuous infusion; begin no sooner than 6 hours post-transplant; adjunctive therapy with corticosteroids is recommended; continue only until oral medication can be tolerated

Moderate-to-severe atopic dermatitis: Topical: Children ≥2 years: Apply 0.03% ointment to affected area twice daily; rub in gently and completely; discontinue applications when signs and symptoms of eczema have cleared

Renal Impairment: Evidence suggests that lower doses should be used. Patients should receive doses at the lowest value of the recommended I.V. and oral dosing ranges. Further reductions in dose below these ranges may be required. Tacrolimus therapy should usually be delayed up to 48 hours or longer in patients with postoperative oliguria.

Hemodialysis: Not removed by hemodialysis; supplemental dose is not necessary.

Peritoneal dialysis: Significant drug removal is unlikely based on physiochemical characteristics.

Hepatic Impairment: Use of tacrolimus in liver transplant recipients experiencing post-transplant hepatic impairment may be associated with increased risk of developing renal insufficiency related to high whole blood levels of tacrolimus. The presence of moderate-to-severe hepatic dysfunction (serum bilirubin >2 mg/dL) appears to affect the metabolism of FK506. The half-life of the drug was prolonged and the clearance reduced after I.V. administration. The bioavailability of FK506 was also increased after oral administration. The higher plasma concentrations as determined by ELISA, in patients with severe hepatic dysfunction are probably due to the accumulation of FK506 metabolites of lower activity. These patients should be monitored closely and dosage adjustments should be considered. Some evidence indicates that lower doses could be used in these patients.

Administration

Oral: If dosed once daily, administer in the morning. If dosed twice daily (not common), doses should be 12 hours apart. If the morning and evening doses differ, the larger dose (differences are never >0.5-1 mg) should be given in the morning. If dosed 3 times/day, separate doses by 8 hours.

I.V.: Administer by I.V. continuous infusion only. Do not use PVC tubing when administering dilute solutions. Tacrolimus is dispensed in a 50 mL glass container with no overfill. It is usually intended to be administered as a continuous infusion over 24 hours.

I.V. Detail: Do not mix with acyclovir or ganciclovir due to chemical degradation of tacrolimus (use different ports in multilumen lines). Do not alter dose with concurrent T-tube clamping. Adsorption of the drug to PVC tubing may become clinically significant with low concentrations.

Topical: Do not use with occlusive dressings. Burning at the application site is most common in first few days; improves as atopic dermatitis improves. Limit application to involved areas. Continue as long as signs and symptoms persist; discontinue if resolution occurs; re-evaluate if symptoms persist >6 weeks.

Stability

Reconstitution:

Dilute with 5% dextrose injection or 0.9% sodium chloride injection to a final concentration between 0.004 mg/mL and 0.02 mg/mL.

Storage:

Injection: Prior to dilution, store at 5°C to 25°C (41°F to 77°F). Stable for 24 hours in D_5W or NS in glass or polyolefin containers.

Capsules and ointment: Store at room temperature of 15°C to 30°C (59°F to 86°F).

Laboratory Monitoring Renal function, hepatic function, serum electrolytes, glucose. Since pharmacokinetics show great inter- and intrapatient variability over time, monitoring of serum concentrations (trough for oral therapy) has proven helpful to prevent organ rejection and reduce drug-related toxicity. Measure 3 times/week for first few weeks, then gradually decrease frequency as patient stabilizes.

Nursing Actions

Physical Assessment: Assess other medications patient may be taking for effectiveness and interactions. Monitor blood pressure frequently; can cause hypertension. Monitor laboratory tests prior to, during, and following therapy. Monitor response to therapy and adverse reactions. Patients with diabetes should monitor glucose levels closely (this medication may alter glucose levels). Monitor/instruct patient on appropriate use, interventions to reduce side effects, to monitor for signs of opportunistic infection (eg, persistent fever, malaise, sore throat, unusual bleeding or bruising), and adverse symptoms to report.

Patient Education: Take as directed, on an empty stomach. Be consistent with timing and consistency of meals if GI intolerance occurs (per manufacturer). Do not take within 2 hours before or after antacids. Do not alter dose and do not discontinue without consulting prescriber. Maintain adequate hydration (2-3 L/day of fluids) during entire course of therapy unless instructed to restrict fluid intake. You will be susceptible to infection (avoid crowds and exposure to infection). If you have diabetes, monitor glucose levels closely (drug may alter glucose levels). You may experience nausea, vomiting, loss of appetite (small frequent meals, frequent mouth care may help); diarrhea (boiled milk, yogurt, or buttermilk may help); constipation (increased exercise, fluids, fruit, fluid, or fiber may help; if unresolved, consult prescriber); or

muscle or back pain (mild analgesics may be recommended). Report chest pain; acute headache or dizziness; symptoms of respiratory infection, cough, or respiratory difficulty; unresolved GI effects; fatigue, chills, fever, unhealed sores, white plaques in mouth, irritation in genital area; unusual bruising or bleeding; pain or irritation on urination or change in urinary patterns; rash or skin irritation; or other unusual effects.

Topical: Before applying, wash area gently and thoroughly. Apply in thin film to affected area. Do not cover skin with bandages. Wash hands only if not treating skin on the hands. Protect skin from sunlight or exposure to UV light. Consult prescriber if breast-feeding

Pregnancy/breast-feeding precautions: Inform prescriber if you are or intend to become pregnant. Do not breast-feed.

Dietary Considerations Capsule: Take on an empty stomach; be consistent with timing and composition of meals if GI intolerance occurs (per manufacturer).

Breast-Feeding Issues Concentrations in breast milk are equivalent to plasma concentrations; breast-feeding is not advised.

Pregnancy Issues Tacrolimus crosses the placenta and reaches concentrations four times greater than maternal plasma concentrations. Neonatal hyperkalemia and renal dysfunction have been reported.

Additional Information Additional dosing considerations:

Switch from I.V. to oral therapy: Threefold increase in dose

Pediatric patients: About 2 times higher dose compared to adults

Liver dysfunction: Decrease I.V. dose; decrease oral dose

Renal dysfunction: Does not affect kinetics; decrease dose to decrease levels if renal dysfunction is related to the drug

---

Tadalafil (tah DA la fil)

U.S. Brand Names Cialis®

Synonyms GF196960

Pharmacologic Category Phosphodiesterase-5 Enzyme Inhibitor

Pregnancy Risk Factor B

Use Treatment of erectile dysfunction

Mechanism of Action/Effect Tadalafil enhances the effect of nitric oxide (NO) by inhibiting phosphodiesterase type 5 (PDE-5), which is responsible for degradation of cGMP in the corpus cavernosum; when sexual stimulation causes local release of NO, inhibition of PDE-5 by tadalafil causes increased levels of cGMP in the corpus cavernosum, resulting in smooth muscle relaxation and inflow of blood to the corpus cavernosum. At recommended doses, it has no effect in the absence of sexual stimulation.

Contraindications Hypersensitivity to tadalafil or any component of the formulation; concurrent use of organic nitrates (nitroglycerin) in any form

Warnings/Precautions There is a degree of cardiac risk associated with sexual activity; therefore, physicians may wish to consider the cardiovascular status of their patients prior to initiating any treatment for erectile dysfunction. Use caution in patients with left ventricular outflow obstruction (aortic stenosis or IHSS); may be more sensitive to hypotensive actions. Concurrent use with alpha-adrenergic antagonist therapy may cause symptomatic hypotension; patients should be hemodynamically stable prior to initiating tadalafil therapy at the lowest possible dose. Use caution in patients receiving strong CYP3A4 inhibitors, the elderly, (Continued)

Tadalafil (Continued)

or those with hepatic impairment or renal impairment; dosage adjustment/limitation is needed. Use caution in patients with peptic ulcer disease.

Agents for the treatment of erectile dysfunction should be used with caution in patients with anatomical deformation of the penis (angulation, cavernosal fibrosis, or Peyronie's disease), or in patients who have conditions which may predispose them to priapism (sickle cell anemia, multiple myeloma, leukemia). All patients should be instructed to seek medical attention if erection persists >4 hours. The safety and efficacy of tadalafil with other treatments for erectile dysfunction have not been studied and are, therefore, not recommended as combination therapy.

Rare cases of nonarteritic ischemic optic neuropathy (NAION) have been reported; risk may be increased with history of vision loss. Other risk factors for NAION include heart disease, diabetes, hypertension, smoking, age >50 years, or history of certain eye problems.

Safety and efficacy have not been studied in patients with the following conditions, therefore, use in these patients is not recommended: Arrhythmias, hypotension, uncontrolled hypertension, unstable angina or angina during intercourse, cardiac failure (NYHA Class II or greater), myocardial infarction within the last 3 months, or stroke within the last 6 months. A minority of patients with retinitis pigmentosa have genetic disorders of retinal phosphodiesterases; use is not recommended. Safety and efficacy in children have not been established.

Drug Interactions
Cytochrome P450 Effect: Substrate of CYP3A4 (major)

Increased Effect/Toxicity:

Tadalafil increases the hypotensive effects of alpha1-blockers. Concurrent use with organic nitrates may cause severe hypotension. Antifungals agents (imidazole), macrolide antibiotics (clarithromycin, erythromycin, telithromycin, troleandomycin), protease inhibitors (amprenavir, atazanavir, fosamprenavir, indinavir, lopinavir, nelfinavir, ritonavir, saquinavir), and other CYP3A4 inhibitors may increase tadalafil levels.

Nutritional/Ethanol Interactions

Ethanol: Substantial consumption of ethanol may increase the risk of hypotension and orthostasis. Lower ethanol consumption has not been associated with significant changes in blood pressure or increase in orthostatic symptoms.

Food: Rate and extent of absorption are not affected by food. Grapefruit juice may increase serum levels/toxicity of tadalafil. Do not give more than a single 10 mg dose of tadalafil more frequently than every 72 hours in patients who regularly consume grapefruit juice.

Adverse Reactions

>10%: Central nervous system: Headache (11% to 15%)

2% to 10%:

Cardiovascular: Flushing (2% to 3%)

Gastrointestinal: Dyspepsia (4% to 10%)

Neuromuscular & skeletal: CPK increased (2%), back pain (3% to 6%), myalgia (1% to 4%), limb pain (1% to 3%)

Respiratory: Nasal congestion (2% to 3%)

Overdosage/Toxicology Symptoms similar to those seen at lower doses (headache, back pain, myalgias). Treatment is symptomatic and supportive.

Pharmacodynamics/Kinetics
Onset of Action: Within 1 hour
Duration of Action: Up to 36 hours
Time to Peak: Plasma: 2 hours
Protein Binding: 94%
Half-Life Elimination: 17.5 hours
Metabolism: Hepatic, via CYP3A4 to metabolites (inactive)
Excretion: Feces (61%, as metabolites); urine (36%, as metabolites)
Available Dosage Forms Tablet: 5 mg, 10 mg, 20 mg
Dosing
Adults:
Erectile dysfunction: Oral: 10 mg prior to anticipated sexual activity (dosing range: 5-20 mg); to be given as one single dose and not given more than once daily. **Note:** Erectile function may be improved for up to 36 hours following a single dose; adjust dose.
Dosing adjustment with concomitant medications:
Alpha$_1$-blockers: If stabilized on either alpha blockers or tadalafil therapy, initiate new therapy with the other agent at the lowest possible dose.
CYP3A4 inhibitors: Dose reduction of tadalafil is recommended with strong CYP3A4 inhibitors. The dose of tadalafil should not exceed 10 mg, and tadalafil should not be taken more frequently than once every 72 hours. Examples of such inhibitors include amprenavir, atazanavir, clarithromycin, conivaptan, delavirdine, diclofenac, fosamprenavir, imatinib, indinavir, isoniazid, itraconazole, ketoconazole, miconazole, nefazodone, nelfinavir, nicardipine, propofol, quinidine, ritonavir, and telithromycin.

Elderly: Dosage is based on renal function; refer to dosing in renal impairment.
Renal Impairment:
Cl$_{cr}$ 31-50 mL/minute: Initial dose 5 mg once daily; maximum dose 10 mg not to be given more frequently than every 48 hours.
Cl$_{cr}$ <30 mL/minute or hemodialysis: Maximum dose 5 mg.
Hepatic Impairment:
Mild-to-moderate hepatic impairment (Child-Pugh class A or B): Dose should not exceed 10 mg once daily.
Severe hepatic impairment: Use is not recommended.
Administration
Oral: May be administered with or without food, prior to anticipated sexual activity.
Stability
Storage: Store at controlled room temperature of 15°C to 30°C (59°F to 86°F).
Nursing Actions
Physical Assessment: Assess potential for interactions with other prescription, OTC medications, or herbal products patient may be using. Instruct patient on appropriate use and cautions, possible side effects, and symptoms to report.
Patient Education: Inform prescriber of all other prescriptions, OTC medications, or herbal products you are taking and any allergies you have; serious side effects can result when tadalafil is used with some other medications. Avoid substantial consumption of alcohol. Do not combine tadalafil with other approaches to treating erectile dysfunction without consulting prescriber. **Note:** This drug provides no protection against sexually-transmitted diseases, including HIV. Take exactly as directed; do not take more often than prescribed. You may experience headache, fatigue, dizziness, or blurred vision (use caution when driving or engaging in hazardous tasks until response to drug is known); back or limb pain (consult prescriber for appropriate analgesic). Report immediately chest pain; palpitations; respiratory difficulty; unusual dizziness; change in vision; sign of

urinary tract infection; skin rash; genital swelling or priapism, erection lasting >4 hours, or other persistent adverse reactions.

Dietary Considerations May be taken with or without food.

Geriatric Considerations No significant differences in pharmacokinetics were seen in elderly men versus younger men. Dosing should be adjusted for renal function. Since older adults often have concomitant diseases, many of which may be contraindicated with the use of tadalafil, prescriber should complete a thorough review of diseases and medications prior to prescribing tadalafil.

Tamoxifen (ta MOKS i fen)

U.S. Brand Names Nolvadex® [DSC]; Soltamox™

Synonyms ICI-46474; NSC-180973; TAM; Tamoxifen Citrate

Restrictions An FDA-approved medication guide is available at www.AstraZeneca-us.com/pi/Nolvadex.pdf. Distribute to each female patient who is using tamoxifen to decrease risk of developing breast cancer or who has ductal carcinoma *in situ*.

Pharmacologic Category Antineoplastic Agent, Estrogen Receptor Antagonist

Medication Safety Issues
Sound-alike/look-alike issues:
Tamoxifen may be confused with pentoxifylline, Tambocor™

Pregnancy Risk Factor D

Lactation Excretion in breast milk unknown/contraindicated

Use Palliative or adjunctive treatment of advanced breast cancer; reduce the incidence of breast cancer in women at high risk; reduce risk of invasive breast cancer in women with ductal carcinoma *in situ* (DCIS); metastatic female and male breast cancer

Unlabeled/Investigational Use Treatment of mastalgia, gynecomastia, pancreatic carcinoma, melanoma and desmoid tumors; induction of ovulation; treatment of precocious puberty in females, secondary to McCune-Albright syndrome

Mechanism of Action/Effect Competitively binds to estrogen receptors on tumors and other tissue targets, producing a nuclear complex that decreases DNA synthesis and inhibits estrogen effects; nonsteroidal agent with potent antiestrogenic properties which compete with estrogen for binding sites in breast and other tissues; cells accumulate in the G_0 and G_1 phases; therefore, tamoxifen is cytostatic rather than cytocidal.

Contraindications Hypersensitivity to tamoxifen or any component of the formulation; concurrent warfarin therapy or history of deep vein thrombosis or pulmonary embolism (when tamoxifen is used for cancer risk reduction); pregnancy

Warnings/Precautions Hazardous agent - use appropriate precautions for handling and disposal. Serious and life-threatening events (including stroke, pulmonary emboli, and uterine malignancy) have occurred at an incidence greater than placebo during use for cancer risk reduction; these events are rare, but require consideration in risk:benefit evaluation. An increased incidence of thromboembolic events has been associated with use for breast cancer; risk may increase with chemotherapy addition; use caution in individuals with a history of thromboembolic events. Use with caution in patients with leukopenia, thrombocytopenia, or hyperlipidemias. Decreased visual acuity, retinopathy, corneal changes, and increased incidence of cataracts have been reported. Hypercalcemia has occurred in patients with bone metastasis. Significant bone loss of the

lumbar spine and hip was associated with use in premenopausal women. Liver abnormalities such as cholestasis, fatty liver, hepatitis, and hepatic necrosis have occurred. Hepatocellular carcinomas have been reported in some studies; relationship to treatment is unclear. Endometrial hyperplasia, polyps, endometriosis, uterine fibroids, and ovarian cysts have occurred. Increased risk of uterine or endometrial cancer; monitor. Safety and efficacy in children <2 years of age, or for treatment durations >1 year in children 2-10 years, have not been established.

Drug Interactions

Cytochrome P450 Effect: Substrate of CYP2A6 (minor), 2B6 (minor), 2C9 (major), 2D6 (major), 2E1 (minor), 3A4 (major); **Inhibits** CYP2B6 (weak), 2C8 (moderate), 2C9 (weak), 3A4 (weak)

Decreased Effect: CYP2C9 inducers may decrease the levels/effects of tamoxifen; example inducers include carbamazepine, phenobarbital, phenytoin, rifampin, rifapentine, and secobarbital. CYP3A4 inducers may decrease the levels/effects of tamoxifen; example inducers include aminoglutethimide, carbamazepine, nafcillin, nevirapine, phenobarbital, phenytoin, and rifamycins.

Increased Effect/Toxicity: Concomitant use of warfarin is contraindicated when used for risk reduction; results in significant enhancement of the anticoagulant effects of warfarin. Tamoxifen may increase the levels/effects of CYP2C8 substrates; example substrates include amiodarone, paclitaxel, pioglitazone, repaglinide, and rosiglitazone. CYP2C9 inhibitors may increase the levels/effects of tamoxifen; example inhibitors include delavirdine, fluconazole, gemfibrozil, ketoconazole, nicardipine, NSAIDs, sulfonamides, and tolbutamide. CYP2D6 inhibitors may increase the levels/effects of tamoxifen; example inhibitors include chlorpromazine, delavirdine, fluoxetine, miconazole, paroxetine, pergolide, quinidine, quinine, ritonavir, and ropinirole. CYP3A4 inhibitors may increase the levels/effects of tamoxifen; example inhibitors include azole antifungals, clarithromycin, diclofenac, doxycycline, erythromycin, imatinib, isoniazid, nefazodone, nicardipine, propofol, protease inhibitors, quinidine, telithromycin, and verapamil. Rifamycin derivatives may increase the metabolism (via CYP isoenzymes) of tamoxifen.

Nutritional/Ethanol Interactions Herb/Nutraceutical: Avoid black cohosh, dong quai in estrogen-dependent tumors. Avoid St John's wort (may decrease levels/effects of tamoxifen).

Lab Interactions T_4 elevations (which may be explained by increases in thyroid-binding globulin) have been reported; not accompanied by clinical hyperthyroidism

Adverse Reactions Note: Differences in the frequency of some adverse events may be related to use for a specific indication.

>10%:
Cardiovascular: Flushing (33% to 41%), hypertension (11%), peripheral edema (11%)
Central nervous system: Pain (3% to 16%), mood changes (12% to 18%), depression (2% to 12%)
Dermatologic: Skin changes (6% to 19%), rash (13%)
Endocrine & metabolic: Hot flashes (3% to 80%), fluid retention (32%), altered menses (13% to 25%), amenorrhea (16%)
Gastrointestinal: Nausea (5% to 26%), weight loss (23%)
Genitourinary: Vaginal bleeding (2% to 23%), vaginal discharge (13% to 55%)
Neuromuscular & skeletal: Weakness (19%), arthritis (14%), arthralgia (11%)
Respiratory: Pharyngitis (14%)
1% to 10%:
Cardiovascular: Chest pain (5%), venous thrombotic events (5%), edema (4%), cardiovascular ischemia
(Continued)

Tamoxifen (Continued)

(3%), cerebrovascular ischemia (3%), angina (2%), deep venous thrombus (2%), MI (1%)

Central nervous system: Insomnia (9%), dizziness (8%), headache (8%), anxiety (6%), fatigue (4%)

Dermatologic: Alopecia (<1% to 5%)

Endocrine & metabolic: Oligomenorrhea (9%), breast pain (6%), menstrual disorder (6%), breast neoplasm (5%), hypercholesterolemia (4%)

Gastrointestinal: Abdominal pain (9%), weight gain (9%), throat irritation (oral solution 5%), constipation (4% to 8%), diarrhea (7%), dyspepsia (6%), abdominal cramps (1%), anorexia (1%)

Genitourinary: Urinary tract infection (10%), leukorrhea (9%), vaginal hemorrhage (6%), vaginitis (5%), ovarian cyst (3%)

Hematologic: Thrombocytopenia (<1% to 10%), anemia (5%)

Hepatic: SGOT increased (5%), serum bilirubin increased (2%)

Neuromuscular & skeletal: Bone pain (6% to 10%), osteoporosis (7%), fracture (7%), arthrosis (5%), myalgia (5%), paresthesia (5%), musculoskeletal pain (3%)

Ocular: Cataract (7%)

Renal: Serum creatinine increased (up to 2%)

Respiratory: Cough (4% to 9%), dyspnea (8%), bronchitis (5%), sinusitis (5%)

Miscellaneous: Infection/sepsis (up to 9%), diaphoresis (6%), flu-like syndrome (6%), allergic reaction (3%)

Overdosage/Toxicology Overdose produced respiratory difficulties and seizure in animal studies. In humans, loading doses of 400 mg/m² followed by 150 mg/m² twice daily produced reversible neurotoxicity (tremor, hyperreflexia, unsteady gait, and dizziness). Loading doses of >250 mg/m² followed by 80 mg/m² twice daily produced QT prolongation in some patients. In the case of an overdose, treatment is symptom-directed and supportive.

Pharmacodynamics/Kinetics

Time to Peak: Serum: 5 hours

Protein Binding: 99%

Half-Life Elimination: Distribution: 7-14 hours; Elimination: 5-7 days; Metabolites: 14 days

Metabolism: Hepatic (via CYP3A4) to major metabolites, N-desmethyl tamoxifen (major) and 4-hydroxytamoxifen (minor), and a tamoxifen derivative (minor); undergoes enterohepatic recirculation

Excretion: Feces (26% to 51%); urine (9% to 13%)

Available Dosage Forms

Solution, oral:

Soltamox™: 10 mg/5 mL (150 mL) [licorice flavor]

Tablet: 10 mg, 20 mg

Nolvadex®: 10 mg, 20 mg [DSC]

Dosing

Adults & Elderly: Refer to individual protocols.

Breast cancer treatment:

Metastatic (males and females) or adjuvant therapy (females): Oral: 20-40 mg/day; daily doses >20 mg should be given in 2 divided doses (morning and evening)

DCIS (females): Oral: 20 mg once daily for 5 years

Breast cancer prevention (high-risk females): Oral: 20 mg/day for 5 years

Note: Higher dosages (up to 700 mg/day) have been investigated for use in modulation of multidrug resistance (MDR), but are not routinely used in clinical practice.

Induction of ovulation (unlabeled use): Oral: 5-40 mg twice daily for 4 days

Pediatrics: Female: Precocious puberty and McCune-Albright syndrome (unlabeled use): Oral: A dose of 20 mg/day has been reported in patients 2-10 years of age; safety and efficacy have not been established for treatment of longer than 1 year duration

Stability

Storage:

Solution: Store at room temperature at or below 25°C (77°F); do not refrigerate or freeze; protect from light. Use within 3 months of opening.

Tablet: Store at room temperature of 20°C to 25°C (68°F to 77°F).

Laboratory Monitoring CBC with platelets, serum calcium, LFTs

Nursing Actions

Physical Assessment: Assess potential for interactions with other pharmacological agents and herbal products patient may be taking (increased or decreased levels/effects of tamoxifen or other drugs administered concurrently). Monitor laboratory tests, therapeutic effectiveness (eg, complaints of bone pain is usually an indication of a good therapeutic effectiveness and will usually subside as treatment continues), and adverse reactions (eg, flushing, fluid retention, hot flashes, vaginal bleeding or discharge, constipation, rash, mood changes). Teach patient proper use, possible side effects/appropriate interventions (eg, periodic ophthalmic evaluations and annual gynecological exams and mammogram with long-term use), and adverse symptoms to report.

Patient Education: Do not take any new medication during therapy without consulting prescriber. Take exactly as directed. It is important to maintain adequate hydration (2-3 L/day of fluids) unless instructed to restrict fluid intake and adequate nutrition (small frequent meals may help). You should schedule an annual ophthalmic examination, gynecological exam, and mammogram if this medication is used long-term. You may experience hot flashes, hair loss, loss of libido (these will subside when treatment is completed). Bone pain may indicate a good therapeutic responses (consult prescriber for mild analgesics). May cause nausea, vomiting, loss of appetite (small frequent meals, frequent mouth care, sucking lozenges, or chewing gum may help); photosensitivity (use sunscreen, wear protective clothing and eyewear, and avoid direct sunlight); hot flashes (a cool room or cool compresses may help). Notify prescriber if menstrual irregularities, vaginal bleeding, or intolerable hot flashes occur. Report unusual bleeding or bruising; severe weakness or unusual fatigue; CNS changes (depression, mood changes); swelling or pain in calves; respiratory difficulty; vision changes; or other adverse effects. **Pregnancy/breast-feeding precautions:** Do not get pregnant while taking this medication and for 2 months after treatment is discontinued; consult prescriber for appropriate barrier or nonhormonal contraceptive measures. Do not breast-feed.

Geriatric Considerations Studies have shown tamoxifen to be effective in the treatment of primary breast cancer in elderly women. Comparative studies with other antineoplastic agents in elderly women with breast cancer had more favorable survival rates with tamoxifen. Initiation of hormone therapy rather than chemotherapy is justified for elderly patients with metastatic breast cancer who are responsive.

Breast-Feeding Issues Tamoxifen has been shown to inhibit lactation.

Pregnancy Issues Animal studies have demonstrated fetal adverse effects and fetal loss. There are no adequate and well-controlled studies in pregnant women. There have been reports of vaginal bleeding, birth defects and fetal loss in pregnant women. Tamoxifen use during pregnancy may have a potential long term risk to the fetus of a DES-like syndrome. For sexually-active women of childbearing age, initiate during menstruation (negative β-hCG immediately prior to initiation in women with irregular cycles). Tamoxifen may induce ovulation. Barrier or nonhormonal contraceptives are recommended. Pregnancy should be avoided during treatment and for 2 months after treatment has been discontinued.

Additional Information Oral clonidine is being studied for the treatment of tamoxifen-induced "hot flashes." The tumor flare reaction may indicate a good therapeutic response, and is often considered a good prognostic factor.

Tamsulosin (tam SOO loe sin)

U.S. Brand Names Flomax®
Synonyms Tamsulosin Hydrochloride
Pharmacologic Category Alpha₁ Blocker
Medication Safety Issues
Sound-alike/look-alike issues:
Flomax® may be confused with Fosamax®, Volmax®
Pregnancy Risk Factor B
Lactation Not indicated for use in women
Use Treatment of signs and symptoms of benign prostatic hyperplasia (BPH)
Mechanism of Action/Effect Antagonizes alpha₁ₐ adrenoreceptors in the prostate which mediate the dynamic component of urine flow obstruction by regulating smooth muscle tone of the bladder neck and prostate. When given to patients with BPH, blockade of alpha receptors leads to relaxation of these muscles, resulting in an improvement in urine flow rate and symptoms. Alpha blockade does not influence the static component of urinary obstruction, which is related to tissue proliferation.
Contraindications Hypersensitivity to tamsulosin or any component of the formulation; concurrent use with phosphodiesterase-5 (PDE-5) inhibitors including sildenafil (>25 mg), tadalafil (if tamsulosin dose >0.4 mg/day), or vardenafil
Warnings/Precautions Not intended for use as an antihypertensive drug. May cause orthostasis, syncope or dizziness. Patients should avoid situations where injury may occur as a result of syncope. Rule out prostatic carcinoma before beginning therapy with tamsulosin. Intraoperative Floppy Iris Syndrome occurred most often in patients taking their alpha-1 blocker at the time of cataract surgery, but some cases occurred when the alpha-1 blocker blocker was stopped 2-14 days prior to surgery and as long as 5 weeks to 9 months prior to surgery. The benefit of stopping an alpha-1blocker prior to cataract surgery has not been established. Rarely, patients with a sulfa allergy have also developed an allergic reaction to tamsulosin; avoid use when previous reaction has been severe.
Drug Interactions
Cytochrome P450 Effect: Substrate (major) of CYP2D6, 3A4
Decreased Effect: CYP3A4 inducers may decrease the levels/effects of tamsulosin; example inducers include aminoglutethimide, carbamazepine, nafcillin, nevirapine, phenobarbital, phenytoin, and rifamycins.
Increased Effect/Toxicity: Alpha-adrenergic blockers and calcium channel blockers may increase risk of hypotension. Risk of first-dose orthostatic hypotension may increase with beta-blockers. Cimetidine may decrease tamsulosin clearance. Blood pressure-lowering effects are additive with sildenafil (use with extreme caution), tadalafil (may be used when tamsulosin dose is ≤0.4 mg/day), and vardenafil (use is contraindicated by the manufacturer).

CYP2D6 inhibitors may increase the levels/effects of tamsulosin; example inhibitors include chlorpromazine, delavirdine, fluoxetine, miconazole, paroxetine, pergolide, quinidine, quinine, ritonavir, and ropinirole. CYP3A4 inhibitors may increase the levels/effects of

tamsulosin; example inhibitors include azole antifungals, clarithromycin, diclofenac, doxycycline, erythromycin, imatinib, isoniazid, nefazodone, nicardipine, propofol, protease inhibitors, quinidine, telithromycin, and verapamil.
Nutritional/Ethanol Interactions
Food: Fasting increases bioavailability by 30% and peak concentration 40% to 70%.
Herb/Nutraceutical: Avoid saw palmetto (due to limited experience with this combination).
Adverse Reactions
>10%:
Cardiovascular: Studies specific for orthostatic hypotension: Overall, at least one positive test was observed in 16% of patients receiving 0.4 mg and 19% of patients receiving the 0.8 mg dose. "First-dose" orthostatic hypotension following a 0.4 mg dose was reported as 7% at 4 hours postdose and 6% at 8 hours postdose.
Central nervous system: Headache (19% to 21%), dizziness (15% to 17%)
Genitourinary: Abnormal ejaculation (8% to 18%)
Respiratory: Rhinitis (13% to 18%)
1% to 10%:
Cardiovascular: Chest pain (~4%)
Central nervous system: Somnolence (3% to 4%), insomnia (1% to 2%), vertigo (0.6% to 1%)
Endocrine & metabolic: Libido decreased (1% to 2%)
Gastrointestinal: Diarrhea (4% to 6%), nausea (3% to 4%), stomach discomfort (2% to 3%), bitter taste (2% to 3%)
Neuromuscular & skeletal: Weakness (8% to 9%), back pain (7% to 8%)
Ocular: Amblyopia (0.2% to 2%)
Respiratory: Pharyngitis (5% to 6%), cough (3% to 5%), sinusitis (2% to 4%)
Miscellaneous: Infection (9% to 11%), tooth disorder (1% to 2%)
Overdosage/Toxicology Symptoms of overdose include headache and hypotension. Treatment is supportive.
Pharmacodynamics/Kinetics
Time to Peak: Fasting: 4-5 hours; With food: 6-7 hours Steady-state: By the fifth day of once daily dosing
Protein Binding: 94% to 99%, primarily to alpha₁ acid glycoprotein (AAG)
Half-Life Elimination: Healthy volunteers: 9-13 hours; Target population: 14-15 hours
Metabolism: Hepatic via CYP; metabolites undergo extensive conjugation to glucuronide or sulfate
Excretion: Urine (76%, <10% as unchanged drug); feces (21%)
Available Dosage Forms Capsule, as hydrochloride: 0.4 mg
Dosing
Adults & Elderly: Benign prostatic hyperplasia (BPH): Oral: 0.4 mg once daily ~30 minutes after the same meal each day; dose may be increased after 2-4 weeks to 0.8 mg once daily in patients who fail to respond. If therapy is interrupted for several days, restart with 0.4 mg once daily.
Renal Impairment:
Cl_cr ≥10 mL/minute: No adjustment needed.
Cl_cr <10 mL/minute: Not studied.
Administration
Oral: Capsules should be swallowed whole; do not crush, chew, or open.
Laboratory Monitoring Periodic lipid panels
Nursing Actions
Physical Assessment: Not for use as an antihypertensive. Assess potential for interactions with other pharmacological agents patient may be taking (eg, increased risk of hypotension). Monitor results of periodic lipid panels, therapeutic effectiveness (improved urine flow), and adverse reactions (eg, "first dose" orthostatic hypotension, headache, gastrointestinal (Continued)

Tamsulosin *(Continued)*

disturbance [nausea, vomiting], cough) at beginning of therapy and on a regular basis with long-term therapy. When discontinuing, dose should be tapered and blood pressure monitored closely. Teach patient proper use, possible side effects/appropriate interventions, and adverse symptoms to report.

Patient Education: Do not take any new medication during therapy without consulting prescriber. Take as directed; do not skip dose or discontinue without consulting prescriber. May cause drowsiness, dizziness, or impaired judgment with first doses (use caution when driving or engaging in tasks that require alertness until response to drug is known); postural hypotension (use caution when rising from sitting or lying position or when climbing stairs); nausea (frequent mouth care or sucking lozenges may help); urinary incontinence (void before taking medication); ejaculatory disturbance (reversible, may resolve with continued use of drug); diarrhea (buttermilk, boiled milk, or yogurt may help); palpitations or rapid heartbeat; respiratory difficulty, unusual cough, or sore throat; or other persistent side effects. Report palpitations or rapid heartbeat; respiratory difficulty; muscle weakness, fatigue, or pain; vision changes or hearing; rash; changes in urinary pattern; or other persistent side effects.

Dietary Considerations Take once daily, 30 minutes after the same meal each day.

Geriatric Considerations Metabolism of tamsulosin may be slower, and older patients may be more sensitive to the orthostatic hypotension caused by this medication. A 40% higher exposure (AUC) is anticipated in patients between 55 and 75 years of age as compared to younger subjects (20-32 years).

Tazarotene *(taz AR oh teen)*

U.S. Brand Names Avage™; Tazorac®
Pharmacologic Category Keratolytic Agent
Pregnancy Risk Factor X
Lactation Excretion in breast milk unknown/use caution
Use Topical treatment of facial acne vulgaris; topical treatment of stable plaque psoriasis of up to 20% body surface area involvement; mitigation (palliation) of facial skin wrinkling, facial mottled hyper/hypopigmentation, and benign facial lentigines

Contraindications Hypersensitivity to tazarotene, other retinoids or vitamin A derivatives (isotretinoin, tretinoin, etretinate), or any component of the formulation; use in women of childbearing potential who are unable to comply with birth control requirements; pregnancy (negative pregnancy test required)

Warnings/Precautions Women of childbearing potential must use adequate contraceptive measures because of potential teratogenicity. May cause photosensitivity; exposure to sunlight should be avoided unless deemed medically necessary, and in such cases, exposure should be minimized (including use of sunscreens/protective clothing) during use of tazarotene. Risk may be increased by concurrent therapy with known photosensitizers (thiazides, tetracyclines, fluoroquinolones, phenothiazines, sulfonamides). For external use only; avoid contact with eyes, eyelids, and mouth. Not for use on eczematous, broken, or sunburned skin; not for treatment of lentigo maligna. Avoid application over extensive areas; specifically, safety and efficacy of gel applied over >20% of BSA have not been established. Safety and efficacy in children <12 years of age have not been established.

Drug Interactions
Increased Effect/Toxicity: Increased toxicity may occur with sulfur, benzoyl peroxide, salicylic acid, resorcinol, or any product with strong drying effects (including alcohol-containing compounds) due to increased drying actions. May augment phototoxicity of sensitizing medications (thiazides, tetracyclines, fluoroquinolones, phenothiazines, sulfonamides).

Adverse Reactions Percentage of incidence varies with formulation and/or strength:

>10%: Dermatologic: Burning/stinging, desquamation, dry skin, erythema, pruritus, skin pain, worsening of psoriasis

1% to 10%: Dermatologic: Contact dermatitis, discoloration, fissuring, hypertriglyceridemia, inflammation, irritation, localized bleeding, rash

Frequency not defined:
Dermatologic: Photosensitization
Neuromuscular & skeletal: Peripheral neuropathy

Overdosage/Toxicology
Excessive topical use may lead to marked redness, peeling, or discomfort. Oral ingestion may lead to the same adverse effects as those associated with excessive oral intake of Vitamin A (hypervitaminosis A) or other retinoids.
Treatment: If oral ingestion occurs, monitor the patient and administer appropriate supportive measures as necessary

Pharmacodynamics/Kinetics
Duration of Action: Therapeutic: Psoriasis: Effects have been observed for up to 3 months after a 3-month course of topical treatment
Protein Binding: >99%
Half-Life Elimination: 18 hours
Metabolism: Prodrug, rapidly metabolized via esterases to an active metabolite (tazarotenic acid) following topical application and systemic absorption; tazarotenic acid undergoes further hepatic metabolism
Excretion: Urine and feces (as metabolites)

Available Dosage Forms
Cream:
Avage™: 0.1% (30 g) [contains benzyl alcohol]
Tazorac®: 0.05% (30 g, 60 g); 0.1% (30 g, 60 g) [contains benzyl alcohol]
Gel (Tazorac®): 0.05% (30 g, 100 g); 0.1% (30 g, 100 g) [contains benzyl alcohol]

Dosing
Adults & Elderly: Note: In patients experiencing excessive pruritus, burning, skin redness, or peeling, discontinue until integrity of the skin is restored, or reduce dosing to an interval the patient is able to tolerate.

Acne: Topical: Tazorac® cream/gel 0.1%: Cleanse the face gently. After the skin is dry, apply a thin film of tazarotene (2 mg/cm²) once daily, in the evening, to the skin where the acne lesions appear; use enough to cover the entire affected area

Palliation of fine facial wrinkles, facial mottled hyper/hypopigmentation, benign facial lentigines: Topical: Avage™: Apply a pea-sized amount once daily to clean dry face at bedtime; lightly cover entire face including eyelids if desired. Emollients or moisturizers may be applied before or after; if applied before tazarotene, ensure cream or lotion has absorbed into the skin and has dried completely.

Psoriasis: Topical:
Tazorac® cream/gel 0.05% or 0.1%: Apply once daily, in the evening, to psoriatic lesions using enough (2 mg/cm²) to cover only the lesion with a thin film to no more than 20% of body surface area. If a bath or shower is taken prior to application, dry the skin before applying. Unaffected skin may be more susceptible to irritation, avoid application to these areas. **Note:** In patients experiencing excessive pruritus, burning, skin redness, or peeling, discontinue until integrity of the skin is

restored, or reduce dosing to an interval the patient is able to tolerate.

Pediatrics: Note: In patients experiencing excessive pruritus, burning, skin redness, or peeling, discontinue until integrity of the skin is restored, or reduce dosing to an interval the patient is able to tolerate.

Acne: Children ≥12 years: Topical: Tazorac® cream/gel 0.1%: Cleanse the face gently. After the skin is dry, apply a thin film of tazarotene (2 mg/cm²) once daily, in the evening, to the skin where the acne lesions appear; use enough to cover the entire affected area

Psoriasis: Children ≥12 years: Topical: Tazorac® gel 0.05% or 0.1%: Apply once daily, in the evening, to psoriatic lesions using enough (2 mg/cm²) to cover only the lesion with a thin film to no more than 20% of body surface area. If a bath or shower is taken prior to application, dry the skin before applying. Unaffected skin may be more susceptible to irritation, avoid application to these areas.

Palliation of fine facial wrinkles, facial mottled hyper/hypopigmentation, benign facial lentigines: Children ≥17 years: Topical: Avage™: Refer to adult dosing.

Administration
Topical: Do not apply to eczematous or sunburned skin; apply thin film to affected areas; avoid eyes and mouth

Stability
Storage: Store at room temperature of 25°C (77°F), away from heat and direct light; do not freeze.

Nursing Actions
Physical Assessment: Assess potential for interactions with other prescriptions, OTC medications, or herbal products patient may be taking (eg, accumulated photosensitivity). Monitor patient response. Teach patient proper use, side effects/appropriate interventions, and adverse reactions to report. **Pregnancy risk factor X:** Determine that patient is not pregnant before beginning treatment. Do not give to women of childbearing age unless they are capable of complying with contraceptive use. Instruct patients of childbearing age about appropriate contraceptive measures..

Patient Education: This medication is for external use only; avoid using near eyes or mouth. Use exactly as directed; do not use more than recommended (severe skin reactions may occur). Avoid any other skin products (including cosmetics or personal products that may contain medications, spices, alcohols, or irritants) that are not approved by your prescriber. May cause photosensitivity, which will cause severe rash or burning (use sunblock SPF 15 or higher, wear protective clothing and eyewear, and avoid direct sunlight, sunlamps, or tanning beds). Report redness or discoloration, irritation, open sores, bleeding, burning, stinging, excessive dryness, or swelling of skin; or worsening of condition. **Pregnancy/breast-feeding precautions:** Inform prescriber if you are pregnant. Do not get pregnant during treatment. Consult prescriber for instruction on appropriate contraceptive measures. This drug may cause severe fetal defects. Do not allow anyone who may be or become pregnant to touch this medication. Consult prescriber if breast-feeding.

Application: Wash affected area gently and completely dry before applying medication. Apply a thin layer to cover affected area. Wash off any medication that gets on unaffected skin areas and wash hands thoroughly after application.

Geriatric Considerations No differences in safety or efficacy were seen when the cream formulation was administered to patients >65 years of age; may experience increased sensitivity. Increased incidence of

adverse effects and lower treatment success rates were observed with the gel formulation in the treatment of psoriasis.

Pregnancy Issues May cause fetal harm if administered to a pregnant woman. A negative pregnancy test should be obtained 2 weeks prior to treatment; treatment should begin during a normal menstrual period.

Tegaserod (teg a SER od)

U.S. Brand Names Zelnorm®

Synonyms HTF919; Tegaserod Maleate

Pharmacologic Category Serotonin 5-HT₄ Receptor Agonist

Pregnancy Risk Factor B

Lactation Excretion in breast milk unknown/not recommended

Use Short-term treatment of constipation-predominate irritable bowel syndrome (IBS) in women; treatment of chronic idiopathic constipation

Mechanism of Action/Effect Normalizes impaired motility by stimulating peristalsis and decreasing transit time in the gastrointestinal tract.

Contraindications Hypersensitivity to tegaserod or any component of the formulation; severe renal impairment; moderate or severe hepatic impairment; history of bowel obstruction, symptomatic gallbladder disease, suspected sphincter of Oddi dysfunction, or abdominal adhesions. Treatment should **not** be started in patients with diarrhea or in those who experience diarrhea frequently.

Warnings/Precautions Has been associated with rare intestinal ischemic events. Discontinue immediately with new or sudden worsening abdominal pain or rectal bleeding. Diarrhea may occur after the start of treatment, most cases reported as a single episode within the first week of therapy, and may resolve with continued dosing. However, serious consequences of diarrhea (hypovolemia, syncope) have been reported. Patients should be warned to contact healthcare provider immediately if they develop severe diarrhea, or diarrhea with severe cramping, abdominal pain, or dizziness. Use caution with mild hepatic impairment. Safety and efficacy have not been established in males with IBS or patients <18 years of age.

Nutritional/Ethanol Interactions Food: Bioavailability is decreased by 40% to 65% and C_{max} is decreased by 20% to 40% when taken with food. T_{max} is prolonged from 1 hour up to 2 hours when taken following a meal, but decreased to 0.7 hours when taken 30 minutes before a meal.

Adverse Reactions

>10%:
  Central nervous system: Headache (15%)
  Gastrointestinal: Abdominal pain (12%)

1% to 10%:
  Central nervous system: Dizziness (4%), migraine (2%)
  Gastrointestinal: Diarrhea (9%; severe <1%), nausea (8%), flatulence (6%)
  Neuromuscular & skeletal: Back pain (5%), arthropathy (2%), leg pain (1%)

Overdosage/Toxicology Treatment should be symptom-directed and supportive. Diarrhea, headache, abdominal pain, orthostatic hypotension, flatulence, nausea, and vomiting were reported in healthy volunteers with doses of 90-180 mg. Unlikely to be removed by dialysis.

Pharmacodynamics/Kinetics

Time to Peak: 1 hour

Protein Binding: 98% primarily to α₁-acid glycoprotein
(Continued)

Tegaserod *(Continued)*

Half-Life Elimination: I.V.: 11 ± 5 hours

Metabolism: GI: Hydrolysis in the stomach; Hepatic: oxidation, conjugation, and glucuronidation; metabolite (negligible activity); significant first-pass effect

Excretion: Feces (~66% as unchanged drug); urine (~33% as metabolites)

Available Dosage Forms Tablet: 2 mg, 6 mg

Dosing

Adults & Elderly:

IBS with constipation: Female: Oral: 6 mg twice daily, before meals, for 4-6 weeks; may consider continuing treatment for an additional 4-6 weeks in patients who respond initially.

Chronic idiopathic constipation: Oral: 6 mg twice daily, before meals; the need for continued therapy should be reassessed periodically

Renal Impairment: C_{max} and AUC of the inactive metabolite are increased with renal impairment.

Mild to moderate impairment: No dosage adjustment recommended

Severe impairment: Use is contraindicated

Hepatic Impairment: C_{max} and AUC of tegaserod are increased with hepatic impairment.

Mild impairment: No dosage adjustment recommended; however, user caution

Moderate to severe impairment: Use is contraindicated

Administration

Oral: Administer 30 minutes before meals.

Stability

Storage: Store at controlled room temperature of 15°C to 30°C (59°F to 86°F). Protect from moisture.

Nursing Actions

Physical Assessment: Monitor therapeutic effectiveness (improved bowel function) and adverse response (eg, clinically-significant diarrhea [hypovolemia, hypotension, syncope] or ischemic colitis [including rectal bleeding, bloody diarrhea, abdominal pain]) when beginning therapy and at regular intervals during treatment. Teach patient appropriate use, side effects/appropriate interventions, and adverse symptoms to report.

Patient Education: Do not take any new medication during therapy without consulting prescriber. Take exactly as directed, on an empty stomach, at least 30 minutes before meals. If you miss a dose, skip that dose and continue with regular schedule; do not double doses. May cause headache or dizziness (use caution when driving or engaging in tasks requiring alertness until response to drug is known); nausea or vomiting (small, frequent meals, frequent mouth care, chewing gum, or sucking lozenges may help); or diarrhea (should resolve within a week). Report immediately if you experience severe diarrhea, bloody diarrhea, rectal bleeding, abdominal cramping or pain, or dizziness. **Breast-feeding precaution:** Breast-feeding is not recommended.

Dietary Considerations Take on an empty stomach, 30 minutes before meals.

Additional Information In clinical trials, constipation was defined as <3 bowel movements per week, hard or lumpy stools, or straining with a bowel movement.

Telithromycin *(tel ith roe MYE sin)*

U.S. Brand Names Ketek®

Synonyms HMR 3647

Pharmacologic Category Antibiotic, Ketolide

Pregnancy Risk Factor C

Lactation Excretion in breast milk unknown/use caution

Use Treatment of community-acquired pneumonia (mild-to-moderate) caused by susceptible strains of *Streptococcus pneumoniae* (including multidrug-resistant isolates), *Haemophilus influenzae*, *Chlamydia pneumoniae*, *Moraxella catarrhalis*, and *Mycoplasma pneumoniae*; treatment of bacterial exacerbation of chronic bronchitis caused by susceptible strains of *S. pneumoniae*, *H. influenzae* and *Moraxella catarrhalis*; treatment of acute bacterial sinusitis caused by *Streptococcus pneumoniae*, *Haemophilus influenzae*, *Moraxella catarrhalis*, and *Staphylococcus aureus*

Unlabeled/Investigational Use Approved in Canada for use in the treatment of tonsillitis/pharyngitis due to *S. pyogenes* (as an alternative to beta-lactam antibiotics when necessary/appropriate)

Mechanism of Action/Effect Inhibits bacterial protein synthesis by binding to two sites on the 50S ribosomal subunit.

Contraindications Hypersensitivity to telithromycin, macrolide antibiotics, or any component of the formulation; concurrent use of cisapride or pimozide

Warnings/Precautions May prolong QT_c interval, leading to a risk of ventricular arrhythmias; closely-related antibiotics have been associated with malignant ventricular arrhythmias and torsade de pointes. Avoid in patients with prolongation of QT_c interval due to congenital causes, history of long QT syndrome, uncorrected electrolyte disturbances (hypokalemia or hypomagnesemia), significant bradycardia (<50 bpm), or concurrent therapy with QT_c-prolonging drugs (eg, class Ia and class III antiarrhythmics). Avoid use in patients with a prior history of confirmed cardiogenic syncope or ventricular arrhythmias while receiving macrolide antibiotics or other QT_c-prolonging drugs. Limited case reports have documented the occurrence of jaundice and serious liver damage; use caution with hepatic impairment or previous history of jaundice, and discontinue with signs/symptoms of liver damage. Use caution in renal impairment. Use caution in patients with myasthenia gravis (use only if suitable alternatives are not available). Inform patients of potential for blurred vision, which may interfere with ability to operate machinery or drive; use caution until effects are known. Safety and efficacy not established in pediatric patients <13 years of age per Canadian approved labeling and <18 years of age per U.S. approved labeling. Pseudomembranous colitis has been reported.

Drug Interactions

Cytochrome P450 Effect: Substrate of CYP1A2 (minor), 3A4 (major); **Inhibits** CYP2D6 (weak), 3A4 (strong)

Decreased Effect: The levels/effects of telithromycin may be decreased by aminoglutethimide, carbamazepine, nafcillin, nevirapine, phenobarbital, phenytoin, rifamycins, and other CYP3A4 inducers; avoid concurrent use.

Increased Effect/Toxicity: Concurrent use of cisapride or pimozide is contraindicated. Concurrent use with antiarrhythmics (eg, class Ia and class III) or other drugs which prolong QT_c (eg, gatifloxacin, mesoridazine, moxifloxacin, pimozide, sparfloxacin, thioridazine) may be additive; serious arrhythmias may occur. Neuromuscular-blocking agents may be potentiated by telithromycin.

Telithromycin may increase the levels/effects of selected benzodiazepines, calcium channel blockers, cyclosporine, ergot alkaloids, selected HMG-CoA reductase inhibitors, mirtazapine, nateglinide, nefazodone, pimozide, quinidine, sildenafil (and other PDE-5 inhibitors), tacrolimus, venlafaxine, warfarin (monitor), and other CYP3A4 substrates. Selected benzodiazepines (midazolam, triazolam), and selected HMG-CoA reductase inhibitors (atorvastatin, lovastatin and simvastatin) are generally contraindicated with strong CYP3A4 inhibitors. When used with strong CYP3A4 inhibitors, dosage adjustment/limits are recommended for sildenafil and other PDE-5 inhibitors; refer to individual monographs.

The levels/effects of telithromycin may be increased by azole antifungals, clarithromycin, diclofenac, doxycycline, erythromycin, imatinib, isoniazid, nefazodone, nicardipine, propofol, protease inhibitors, quinidine, verapamil, and other CYP3A4 inhibitors.

Adverse Reactions

2% to 10%:
Central nervous system: Headache (2% to 6%), dizziness (3% to 4%)
Gastrointestinal: Diarrhea (10%), nausea (7% to 8%), vomiting (2% to 3%), loose stools (2%), dysgeusia (2%)

≥0.2% to <2%:
Central nervous system: Vertigo, fatigue, somnolence, insomnia
Dermatologic: Rash
Gastrointestinal: Abdominal distension, abdominal pain, anorexia, constipation, dyspepsia, flatulence, gastritis, gastroenteritis, GI upset, glossitis, stomatitis, watery stools, xerostomia
Genitourinary: Vaginal candidiasis
Hematologic: Platelets increased
Hepatic: Transaminases increased, hepatitis
Ocular: Blurred vision, accommodation delayed, diplopia
Miscellaneous: Candidiasis, diaphoresis increased, exacerbation of myasthenia gravis (rare)

Additional effects also reported with telithromycin: Abnormal dreams, anemia, appetite decreased, bundle branch block, cholestasis, coagulation disorder, esophagitis, hyperkalemia, hypersensitivity, hypokalemia, leukopenia, lymphopenia, nervousness, neutropenia, palpitation, pharyngolaryngeal pain, polyuria, pseudomembranous colitis, QT_c prolongation, reflux esophagitis, serum creatinine increased, thrombocytopenia, tooth discoloration, tremor, urine discoloration, vaginal irritation, vasculitis, weakness

Overdosage/Toxicology Treatment should be symptomatic and supportive. ECG and electrolytes should be monitored.

Pharmacodynamics/Kinetics

Time to Peak: Plasma: 1 hour
Protein Binding: 60% to 70%
Half-Life Elimination: 10 hours
Metabolism: Hepatic, via CYP3A4 (50%) and non-CYP-mediated pathways
Excretion: Urine (13% unchanged drug, remainder as metabolites); feces (7%)

Available Dosage Forms

Tablet: 300 mg [not available in Canada], 400 mg
Ketek Pak™ [blister pack]: 400 mg (10s) [packaged as 10 tablets/card; 2 tablets/blister]

Dosing

Adults & Elderly:
Tonsillitis/pharyngitis (unlabeled U.S. indication): Oral: 800 mg once daily for 5 days
Acute exacerbation of chronic bronchitis, acute bacterial sinusitis: Oral: 800 mg once daily for 5 days
Community-acquired pneumonia: Oral: 800 mg once daily for 7-10 days

Pediatrics: Tonsillitis/pharyngitis (unlabeled U.S. indication): Children ≥13 years: Oral: Refer to adult dosing.

Renal Impairment:
Cl_{cr} <30 mL/minute:
U.S. product labeling: 600 mg once daily; when renal impairment is accompanied by hepatic impairment, reduce dosage to 400 mg once daily
Canadian product labeling: Reduce dose to 400 mg once daily
Hemodialysis: Administer following dialysis

Hepatic Impairment: No adjustment recommended, unless concurrent severe renal impairment is present.

Administration

Oral: May be administered with or without food.

Stability

Storage: Store at room temperature between 15°C and 30°C.

Laboratory Monitoring Culture and sensitivity; liver function tests

Nursing Actions

Physical Assessment: Culture and sensitivity report and previous allergy history should be assessed prior to therapy. Assess for potential interactions with other pharmacological agents patient may be using (eg, potential for increased risk of arrhythmias, decreased levels/effects of telithromycin). Monitor laboratory tests (LFTs), therapeutic effectiveness (resolution of infection) and adverse reactions (eg, jaundice, gastrointestinal disturbance [nausea, vomiting, diarrhea], CNS [vertigo, insomnia], rash, opportunistic infection, QT prolongation). Teach patient proper use, possible side effects/appropriate interventions, and adverse symptoms to report (especially any signs of jaundice or hepatic impairment).

Patient Education: Take as directed, with or without food. Do not chew or crush tablets. Take complete prescription even if you are feeling better. May cause headache, dizziness, or fatigue (use caution when driving or engaging in tasks that require alertness until response to drug is known); nausea or vomiting (small frequent meals and frequent mouth care may help), constipation (increased dietary fluid and fibers may help), diarrhea (consult prescribed if persistent). Report immediately dark urine, pale stool, yellowing of skin of eyes, or blurry vision. Report chest pain, palpitations, irregular heart beat, flushing or facial swelling; CNS disturbance (dizziness, headache, anxiety, abnormal dreams, tremor); unusual muscle weakness; skin rash; changes in vision; vaginal itching, burning, or discharge, or other adverse effects. **Pregnancy/breast-feeding precautions:** Inform prescriber if you are or intend to become pregnant or breast-feed.

Dietary Considerations May be taken with or without food.

Geriatric Considerations Bioavailability (57%) equivalent in persons ≥65 years compared to younger adults; although a 1.4- to 2-fold increase in AUC found in older adults. No dosage adjustment required. See dosing information.

Telmisartan (tel mi SAR tan)

U.S. Brand Names Micardis®
Pharmacologic Category Angiotensin II Receptor Blocker
Pregnancy Risk Factor C (1st trimester); D (2nd and 3rd trimesters)
Lactation Enters breast milk/not recommended
Use Treatment of hypertension; may be used alone or in combination with other antihypertensive agents
Mechanism of Action/Effect Telmisartan is a nonpeptide angiotensin receptor antagonist. Angiotensin II acts
(Continued)

Telmisartan *(Continued)*

as a vasoconstrictor. In addition to causing direct vaso-constriction, angiotensin II also stimulates the release of aldosterone. Once aldosterone is released, sodium as well as water are reabsorbed. The end result is an elevation in blood pressure. Telmisartan binds to the AT1 angiotensin II receptor. This binding prevents angiotensin II from binding to the receptor thereby blocking the vasoconstriction and the aldosterone secreting effects of angiotensin II.

Contraindications Hypersensitivity to telmisartan or any component of the formulation; hypersensitivity to other A-II receptor antagonists; bilateral renal artery stenosis; pregnancy (2nd and 3rd trimesters)

Warnings/Precautions Avoid use or use a smaller dose in patients who are volume depleted; correct depletion first. Deterioration in renal function can occur with initiation. Use with caution in unilateral renal artery stenosis and pre-existing renal insufficiency; significant aortic/mitral stenosis. Use with caution in patients who have biliary obstructive disorders or hepatic dysfunction.

Drug Interactions

Cytochrome P450 Effect: Inhibits CYP2C19 (weak)

Decreased Effect: Telmisartan decreased the trough concentrations of warfarin during concurrent therapy, however, INR was not changed.

Increased Effect/Toxicity: Telmisartan may increase serum digoxin concentrations. Potassium salts/supplements, co-trimoxazole (high dose), ACE inhibitors, and potassium-sparing diuretics (amiloride, spironolactone, triamterene) may increase the risk of hyperkalemia with telmisartan.

Nutritional/Ethanol Interactions Herb/Nutraceutical: Avoid dong quai if using for hypertension (has estrogenic activity). Avoid ephedra, yohimbe, ginseng (may worsen hypertension). Avoid garlic (may have increased antihypertensive effect).

Adverse Reactions May be associated with worsening of renal function in patients dependent on renin-angiotensin-aldosterone system.

1% to 10%:
Cardiovascular: Hypertension (1%), chest pain (1%), peripheral edema (1%)
Central nervous system: Headache (1%), dizziness (1%), pain (1%), fatigue (1%)
Gastrointestinal: Diarrhea (3%), dyspepsia (1%), nausea (1%), abdominal pain (1%)
Genitourinary: Urinary tract infection (1%)
Neuromuscular & skeletal: Back pain (3%), myalgia (1%)
Respiratory: Upper respiratory infection (7%), sinusitis (3%), pharyngitis (1%), cough (2%)
Miscellaneous: Flu-like syndrome (1%)

Overdosage/Toxicology Symptoms of overdose may include hypotension, dizziness, and tachycardia. Vagal stimulation may result in bradycardia. Treatment is supportive.

Pharmacodynamics/Kinetics

Onset of Action: 1-2 hours; Peak effect: 0.5-1 hours

Duration of Action: Up to 24 hours

Protein Binding: >99.5%

Half-Life Elimination: Terminal: 24 hours

Metabolism: Hepatic via conjugation to inactive metabolites; not metabolized via CYP

Excretion: Feces (97%)
Clearance: Total body: 800 mL/minute

Pharmacokinetic Note Orally active, not a prodrug.

Available Dosage Forms Tablet: 20 mg, 40 mg, 80 mg

Dosing

Adults: Hypertension: Oral: Initial: 40 mg once daily; usual maintenance dose range: 20-80 mg/day. Patients with volume depletion should be initiated on the lower dosage with close supervision.

Elderly: Initial: 20 mg/day; usual maintenance dose range: 20-80 mg/day

Hepatic Impairment: Supervise patients closely.

Laboratory Monitoring Monitor electrolytes, serum creatinine, BUN, urinalysis, symptomatic hypotension, and tachycardia

Nursing Actions

Physical Assessment: Assess potential for interactions with other pharmacological agents and herbal products patient may be taking (eg, increased risk of hypercalcemia or increased hypotensive effects). Monitor laboratory tests, therapeutic effectiveness (reduced hypertension), and adverse response (eg, hypotension, diarrhea, URI, cough) on a regular basis during therapy. Teach patient proper use, need for regular blood pressure monitoring, possible side effects/appropriate interventions, and adverse symptoms to report.

Patient Education: Do not take any new medication during therapy unless approved by prescriber. Take exactly as directed and do not alter dose or discontinue without consulting prescriber. Monitor blood pressure on a regular basis at same time of day, as advised by prescriber. This drug does not eliminate need for diet or exercise regimen as recommended by prescriber. May cause dizziness, fainting, or lightheadedness (use caution when driving or engaging in tasks that require alertness until response to drug is known); or postural hypotension (use caution when rising from lying or sitting position or climbing stairs). Report unusual weight gain and swelling of ankles, hands, face, lips, throat, or tongue; persistent fatigue; dry cough or respiratory difficulty; palpitations or chest pain; CNS changes; GI disturbances; muscle or bone pain, cramping, or tremors; change in urinary pattern; changes in hearing or vision; or other adverse response. **Pregnancy/breast-feeding precautions:** Inform prescriber if you are or intend to become pregnant. This drug should not be used in the 2nd or 3rd trimester of pregnancy. Consult prescriber for appropriate contraceptive measures if necessary. Breast-feeding is not recommended.

Dietary Considerations May be taken without regard to food.

Pregnancy Issues The drug should be discontinued as soon as possible when pregnancy is detected. Drugs which act directly on renin-angiotensin can cause fetal and neonatal morbidity and death.

Telmisartan and Hydrochlorothiazide
(tel mi SAR tan & hye droe klor oh THYE a zide)

U.S. Brand Names Micardis® HCT

Synonyms Hydrochlorothiazide and Telmisartan

Pharmacologic Category Angiotensin II Receptor Blocker Combination; Antihypertensive Agent, Combination; Diuretic, Thiazide

Pregnancy Risk Factor C (1st trimester); D (2nd and 3rd trimesters)

Lactation Enters breast milk/not recommended

Use Treatment of hypertension; combination product should not be used for initial therapy

Available Dosage Forms [CAN]: Canadian brand name
Tablet:
Micardis® HCT [available in U.S.]:
40/12.5: Telmisartan 40 mg and hydrochlorothiazide 12.5 mg
80/12.5: Telmisartan 80 mg and hydrochlorothiazide 12.5 mg
80/25: Telmisartan 80 mg and hydrochlorothiazide 25 mg
Micardis® Plus [CAN]: 80/25: Telmisartan 80 mg and hydrochlorothiazide 25 mg [Not available in U.S.]

Dosing

Adults: Hypertension: Oral: Replacement therapy: Combination product can be substituted for individual titrated agents. Initiation of combination therapy when monotherapy has failed to achieve desired effects:

Patients currently on telmisartan: Initial dose if blood pressure is not currently controlled on monotherapy of 80 mg telmisartan: Telmisartan 80 mg/hydrochlorothiazide 12.5 mg once daily; may titrate up to telmisartan 160 mg/hydrochlorothiazide 25 mg if needed.

Patients currently on HCTZ: Initial dose if blood pressure is not currently controlled on monotherapy of 25 mg once daily: Telmisartan 80 mg/hydrochlorothiazide 12.5 mg once daily or telmisartan 80 mg/hydrochlorothiazide 25 mg once daily; may titrate up to telmisartan 160 mg/hydrochlorothiazide 25 mg if blood pressure remains uncontrolled after 2-4 weeks of therapy. Patients who develop hypokalemia may be switched to telmisartan 80 mg/hydrochlorothiazide 12.5 mg.

Elderly: Refer to adult dosing. Monitor renal function.

Renal Impairment:
Cl_{cr} >30 mL/minute: Usual recommended dose
Cl_{cr} ≤30 mL/minute: Not recommended

Hepatic Impairment: Dosing should be started at telmisartan 40 mg/hydrochlorothiazide 12.5 mg. Do **not** use in patients with severe hepatic impairment.

Nursing Actions

Physical Assessment: See individual agents.

Patient Education: See individual agents. **Pregnancy/breast-feeding precautions:** Use appropriate contraceptive measures; do not get pregnant while taking this drug. Inform prescriber if you are or intend to become pregnant. Breast-feeding is not recommended.

Related Information

Hydrochlorothiazide *on page 610*
Telmisartan *on page 1175*

Temazepam (te MAZ e pam)

U.S. Brand Names Restoril®
Restrictions C-IV
Pharmacologic Category Hypnotic, Benzodiazepine
Medication Safety Issues
Sound-alike/look-alike issues:
Temazepam may be confused with flurazepam, lorazepam
Restoril® may be confused with Vistaril®, Zestril®
Pregnancy Risk Factor X
Lactation Enters breast milk/not recommended (AAP rates "of concern")
Use Short-term treatment of insomnia
Unlabeled/Investigational Use Treatment of anxiety; adjunct in the treatment of depression; management of panic attacks
Mechanism of Action/Effect Binds to stereospecific benzodiazepine receptors on the postsynaptic GABA neuron at several sites within the central nervous system, including the limbic system, reticular formation. Enhancement of the inhibitory effect of GABA on neuronal excitability results by increased neuronal membrane permeability to chloride ions. This shift in chloride ions results in hyperpolarization (a less excitable state) and stabilization.
Contraindications Hypersensitivity to temazepam or any component of the formulation (cross-sensitivity with other benzodiazepines may exist); narrow-angle glaucoma (not in product labeling, however, benzodiazepines are contraindicated); pregnancy
Warnings/Precautions As a hypnotic, should be used only after evaluation of potential causes of sleep disturbance. Failure of sleep disturbance to resolve after 7-10

days may indicate psychiatric or medical illness. Use is not recommended in patients with depressive disorders or psychoses. Avoid use in patients with sleep apnea. Use with caution in patients receiving concurrent CYP3A4 inhibitors, particularly when these agents are added to therapy. Use with caution in elderly or debilitated patients, patients with hepatic disease (including alcoholics), renal impairment, respiratory disease, impaired gag reflex, or obese patients.

Causes CNS depression (dose-related) which may impair physical and mental capabilities. Use with caution in patients receiving other CNS depressants or psychoactive agents. Benzodiazepines have been associated with falls and traumatic injury and should be used with extreme caution in patients who are at risk of these events (especially the elderly). May cause physical or psychological dependence - use with caution in patients with a history of drug dependence.

Benzodiazepines have been associated with anterograde amnesia. Paradoxical reactions, including hyperactive or aggressive behavior, have been reported with benzodiazepines, particularly in adolescent/pediatric or psychiatric patients. Does not have analgesic, antidepressant, or antipsychotic properties.

Drug Interactions

Cytochrome P450 Effect: Substrate (minor) of CYP2B6, 2C8/9, 2C19, 3A4

Decreased Effect: Oral contraceptives may increase the clearance of temazepam. Temazepam may decrease the antiparkinsonian efficacy of levodopa. Theophylline and other CNS stimulants may antagonize the sedative effects of temazepam. Carbamazepine, rifampin, rifabutin may enhance the metabolism of temazepam and decrease its therapeutic effect.

Increased Effect/Toxicity: Temazepam potentiates the CNS depressant effects of narcotic analgesics, barbiturates, phenothiazines, ethanol, antihistamines, MAO inhibitors, sedative-hypnotics, and cyclic antidepressants. Serum levels of temazepam may be increased by inhibitors of CYP3A4, including cimetidine, ciprofloxacin, clarithromycin, clozapine, diltiazem, disulfiram, digoxin, erythromycin, ethanol, fluconazole, fluoxetine, fluvoxamine, grapefruit juice, isoniazid, itraconazole, ketoconazole, labetalol, levodopa, loxapine, metoprolol, metronidazole, miconazole, nefazodone, omeprazole, phenytoin, rifabutin, rifampin, troleandomycin, valproic acid, and verapamil.

Nutritional/Ethanol Interactions

Ethanol: Avoid ethanol (may increase CNS depression).

Food: Serum levels may be increased by grapefruit juice.

Herb/Nutraceutical: St John's wort may decrease temazepam levels. Avoid valerian, St John's wort, kava kava, gotu kola (may increase CNS depression).

Adverse Reactions

1% to 10%:
Central nervous system: Confusion, dizziness, drowsiness, fatigue, anxiety, headache, lethargy, hangover, euphoria, vertigo
Dermatologic: Rash
Endocrine & metabolic: Decreased libido
Gastrointestinal: Diarrhea
Neuromuscular & skeletal: Dysarthria, weakness
Ocular: Blurred vision
Miscellaneous: Diaphoresis

Overdosage/Toxicology Symptoms of overdose include somnolence, confusion, coma, hypoactive reflexes, dyspnea, hypotension, slurred speech, and impaired coordination. Treatment for benzodiazepine overdose is supportive. Flumazenil has been shown to selectively block the binding of benzodiazepines to CNS receptors, resulting in a reversal of benzodiazepine-induced CNS depression but not always respiratory depression due to toxicity.
(Continued)

Temazepam *(Continued)*

Pharmacodynamics/Kinetics
Time to Peak: Serum: 2-3 hours
Protein Binding: 96%
Half-Life Elimination: 9.5-12.4 hours
Metabolism: Hepatic
Excretion: Urine (80% to 90% as inactive metabolites)

Available Dosage Forms
Capsule: 15 mg, 30 mg
Restoril®: 7.5 mg, 15 mg, 30 mg

Dosing
Adults: Insomnia: Oral: 15-30 mg at bedtime
Elderly: 15 mg in elderly or debilitated patients

Nursing Actions
Physical Assessment: For short-term use. Assess effectiveness and interactions of other medications patient may be taking. Assess for history of addiction; long-term use can result in dependence, abuse, or tolerance. For inpatient use, institute safety measures (side rails, night light, call bell, assistance with ambulation) and monitor effectiveness and adverse reactions. For outpatients, monitor for effectiveness of therapy and adverse reactions (eg, CNS depression) at beginning of therapy and periodically with long-term use. Assess knowledge/teach patient appropriate use, interventions to reduce side effects, and adverse symptoms to report. **Pregnancy risk factor X:** Determine that patient is not pregnant before starting therapy. Do not give to sexually-active female patients unless capable of complying with contraceptive use.

Patient Education: Use exactly as directed; do not increase dose or frequency or discontinue without consulting prescriber. Drug may cause physical and/or psychological dependence. May take with food to decrease GI upset. While using this medication, do not use alcohol or other prescription or OTC medications (especially, pain medications, sedatives, antihistamines, or hypnotics) without consulting prescriber. Maintain adequate hydration (2-3 L/day of fluids) unless instructed to restrict fluid intake. You may experience drowsiness, dizziness, lightheadedness, or blurred vision (use caution when driving or engaging in tasks requiring alertness until response to drug is known); or dry mouth or GI discomfort (small frequent meals, frequent mouth care, chewing gum, or sucking lozenges may help). Report CNS changes (confusion, depression, increased sedation, excitation, headache, abnormal thinking, insomnia, or nightmares, memory impairment, impaired coordination); muscle pain or weakness; respiratory difficulty; persistent dizziness, chest pain, or palpitations; alterations in normal gait; vision changes; or ineffectiveness of medication. **Pregnancy/breast-feeding precautions:** Inform prescriber if you are pregnant. Do not get pregnant during or for 1 month following therapy. Consult prescriber for instruction on appropriate contraceptive measures. This drug may cause severe fetal defects. Breast-feeding is not recommended.

Geriatric Considerations Because of its lack of active metabolites, temazepam is recommended in the elderly when a benzodiazepine hypnotic is indicated. Hypnotic use should be limited to 10-14 days. If insomnia persists, the patient should be evaluated for etiology.

Pregnancy Issues Benzodiazepines cross the placenta. The association between benzodiazepine exposure and malformations remains controversial. A number of types of malformation have been reported (oral cleft, inguinal hernia, cardiac defects, spina bifida, dysmorphic facial features, skeletal defects); however, confounding factors make a clear association difficult. Overall, the risk to the fetus may be low. Nonteratogenic effects (including neonatal flaccidity, respiratory and feeding problems, and withdrawal symptoms) during the postnatal period have also been reported with benzodiazepine use.

Other Issues Taper dosage gradually after long-term therapy. Abrupt withdrawal may cause tremors, nausea, vomiting, abdominal and/or muscle cramps.

Additional Information Abrupt discontinuation after sustained use (generally >10 days) may cause withdrawal symptoms.

Related Information
Anxiolytic / Hypnotic Use in Long-Term Care Facilities *on page 1418*
Federal OBRA Regulations Recommended Maximum Doses *on page 1421*

Temozolomide *(te moe ZOE loe mide)*

U.S. Brand Names Temodar®
Synonyms NSC-362856; TMZ
Pharmacologic Category Antineoplastic Agent, Alkylating Agent
Pregnancy Risk Factor D
Lactation Excretion in breast milk unknown/not recommended
Use Treatment of adult patients with refractory (first relapse) anaplastic astrocytoma who have experienced disease progression on nitrosourea and procarbazine; newly-diagnosed glioblastoma multiforme
Unlabeled/Investigational Use Glioma, melanoma
Mechanism of Action/Effect Prodrug, hydrolyzed to MTIC [(methyl-triazene-1-yl)-imidazole-4-carboxamide] (active form). The cytotoxic effects of MTIC are manifested through alkylation of DNA (O^6, N^7 of guanine).
Contraindications Hypersensitivity to temozolomide or any component of the formulation; hypersensitivity to dacarbazine (since both drugs are metabolized to MTIC); pregnancy
Warnings/Precautions The U.S. Food and Drug Administration (FDA) currently recommends that procedures for proper handling and disposal of antineoplastic agents be considered. *Pneumocystis carinii* pneumonia (PCP) may occur; risk is increased in those receiving steroids or longer dosing regimens; PCP prophylaxis is required with radiotherapy for the 42-day regimen. Myelosuppression may occur; an increased incidence has been reported in geriatric and female patients; prior to dosing, absolute neutrophil count (ANC) should be ≥1.5 X 10^9/L and platelet count ≥100 X 10^9/L. Use caution in patients with severe hepatic or renal impairment. Safety and efficacy in pediatric patients have not been established.
Nutritional/Ethanol Interactions Food: Food reduces rate and extent of absorption.
Adverse Reactions Adverse reactions are listed as the combined incidence in studies for treatment of newly-diagnosed glioblastoma multiforme during the maintenance phase (after radiotherapy) and refractory anaplastic astrocytoma in adults.
>10%:
Cardiovascular: Peripheral edema (up to 11%)
Central nervous system: Fatigue (34% to 61%), headache (23% to 41%), fatigue (34% to 61%), convulsions (6% to 23%), hemiparesis (18%), dizziness (5% to 12%), fever (up to 13%), coordination abnormality (up to 11%). In the case of CNS malignancies, it is difficult to distinguish the relative contributions of temozolomide and progressive disease to CNS symptoms.
Dermatologic: Alopecia (55% - maintenance phase after radiotherapy), rash (8% to 13%)
Gastrointestinal: Nausea (49% to 53%), vomiting (29% to 42%), constipation (22% to 33%), anorexia (9% to 27%), diarrhea (10% to 16%)
Hematologic: Lymphopenia (grade 3/4 in 55%), thrombocytopenia (grade 3/4 in 4% to 19%), neutropenia (grade 3/4 in 8% to 14%), leukopenia (grade 3/4 in 11%)

Neuromuscular & skeletal: Weakness (7% to 13%)

Miscellaneous: Viral infection (up to 11%)

1% to 10%:

Central nervous system: Ataxia (8%), memory impairment (up to 7%), confusion (5%), anxiety (7%), depression (up to 6%), amnesia (up to 10%), paresis (up to 8%), somnolence (up to 9%), insomnia (4% to 10%)

Dermatologic: Rash (8% to 13%), pruritus (5% to 8%), dry skin (up to 5%), radiation injury (2% - maintenance phase after radiotherapy), erythema (1%)

Endocrine & metabolic: Hypercorticism (8%), breast pain (up to 6%)

Gastrointestinal: Dysphagia (up to 7%), abdominal pain (5% to 9%), stomatitis (up to 9%), weight gain (up to 5%)

Genitourinary: Micturition frequency increased (up to 6%), incontinence (up to 8%), urinary tract infection (up to 8%)

Hematologic: Anemia (8%; grade 3/4 in up to 4%)

Neuromuscular & skeletal: Paresthesia (up to 9%), back pain (up to 8%), arthralgia (up to 6%), abnormal gait (up to 6%), myalgia (up to 5%),

Ocular: Diplopia (5%); vision abnormality (blurred vision, visual deficit, vision changes) (5% to 8%)

Respiratory: Pharyngitis (up to 8%), sinusitis (up to 6%), cough (5% to 8%), upper respiratory tract infection (up to 8%), dyspnea (5%)

Miscellaneous: Taste perversion (up to 5%), allergic reaction (up to 3%)

Overdosage/Toxicology Dose-limiting toxicity is hematological. In the event of an overdose, hematological evaluation is necessary. Treatment is supportive.

Pharmacodynamics/Kinetics

Time to Peak: Empty stomach: 1 hour

Protein Binding: 15%

Half-Life Elimination: Mean: Parent drug: 1.8 hours

Metabolism: Prodrug, hydrolyzed to the active form, MTIC; MTIC is eventually eliminated as CO_2 and 5-aminoimidazole-4-carboxamide (AIC), a natural constituent in urine

Excretion: Urine (~38%; parent drug 6%); feces 0.8%

Available Dosage Forms Capsule: 5 mg, 20 mg, 100 mg, 250 mg

Dosing

Adults: Oral (refer to individual protocols):

Anaplastic astrocytoma (refractory): Initial dose: 150 mg/m^2/day for 5 days; repeat every 28 days. Subsequent doses of 100-200 mg/m^2/day for 5 days per treatment cycle; based upon hematologic tolerance. This monthly-cycle regimen may be preceded by a 6- to 7-week regimen of 75 mg/m^2/day.

ANC <1000/mm^3 or platelets <50,000/mm^3 on day 22 or day 29 (day 1 of next cycle): Postpone therapy until ANC >1500/mm^3 and platelets >100,000/mm^3; reduce dose by 50 mg/m^2/day for subsequent cycle

ANC 1000-1500/mm^3 or platelets 50,000-100,000/mm^3 on day 22 or day 29 (day 1 of next cycle): Postpone therapy until ANC >1500/mm^3 and platelets >100,000/mm^3; maintain initial dose

ANC >1500/mm^3 and platelets >100,000/mm^3 on day 22 or day 29 (day 1 of next cycle): Increase dose to or maintain dose at 200 mg/m^2/day for 5 days for subsequent cycle

Glioblastoma multiforme (high-grade glioma):

Concomitant phase: 75 mg/m^2/day for 42 days with radiotherapy (60Gy administered in 30 fractions). **Note:** PCP prophylaxis is required during concomitant phase and should continue in patients who develop lymphocytopenia until recovery (common toxicity criteria [CTC] ≤1). Obtain weekly CBC.

ANC ≥1500/mm^3, platelet count ≥100,000/mm^3, and nonhematologic CTC ≤grade 1 (excludes alopecia, nausea/vomiting): Temodar® 75 mg/m^2/day may be continued throughout the 42-day concomitant period up to 49 days

Dosage modification:

ANC ≥500/mm^3 but <1500/mm^3 **or** platelet count ≥10,000/mm^3 but <100,000/mm^3 **or** nonhematologic CTC grade 2 (excludes alopecia, nausea/vomiting): Interrupt therapy

ANC <500/mm^3 **or** platelet count <10,000/mm^3 **or** nonhematologic CTC grade 3/4 (excludes alopecia, nausea/vomiting): Discontinue therapy

Maintenance phase (consists of 6 treatment cycles): Begin 4 weeks after concomitant phase completion. **Note:** Each subsequent cycle is 28 days (consisting of 5 days of drug treatment followed by 23 days without treatment). Draw CBC within 48 hours of day 22; hold next cycle and do weekly CBC until ANC >1500/mm^3 and platelet count >100,000/mm^3; dosing modification should be based on lowest blood counts and worst nonhematologic toxicity during the previous cycle.

Cycle 1: 150 mg/m^2/day for 5 days

Dosage modification for next cycle:

ANC <1000/mm^3, platelet count <50,000/mm^3, or nonhematologic CTC grade 3 (excludes for alopecia, nausea/vomiting) during previous cycle: Decrease dose by 50 mg/m^2/day for 5 days, unless dose has already been lowered to 100 mg/m^2/day, then discontinue therapy.

If dose reduction <100 mg/m^2/day is required or nonhematologic CTC grade 4 (excludes for alopecia, nausea/vomiting), or if the same grade 3 nonhematologic toxicity occurs after dose reduction: Discontinue therapy

Cycle 2: 200 mg/m^2/day for 5 days unless prior toxicity, then refer to Dosage Modifications under "Cycle 1" and give adjusted dose for 5 days

Cycles 3-6: Continue with previous cycle's dose for 5 days unless toxicity has occurred then, refer to Dosage Modifications under "Cycle 1" and give adjusted dose for 5 days

Elderly: Patients ≥70 years of age had a higher incidence of grade 4 neutropenia and thrombocytopenia in the first cycle of therapy than patients <70 years of age.

Renal Impairment: Caution should be used when administered to patients with severe renal impairment (Cl$_{cr}$ <39 mL/minute).

Hepatic Impairment: Caution should be used when administering to patients with severe hepatic impairment.

Administration

Oral: Capsules should not be opened or chewed but swallowed whole with a glass of water. May be administered on an empty stomach to reduce nausea and vomiting. Bedtime administration may be advised.

Stability

Storage: Store at controlled room temperature (15°C to 10°C/59°F to 86°F).

Laboratory Monitoring CBC

Nursing Actions

Physical Assessment: Use caution in presence of severe hepatic or renal. Monitor results of CBC, effectiveness (reduction in symptoms), and adverse effects (eg, CNS [convulsions, fatigue, impaired coordination, ataxia], gastrointestinal disturbance [nausea, vomiting, constipation], myelosuppression, rash, opportunistic infection, vision disturbance, cough). Teach patient proper use, possible side effects, and appropriate interventions.

Patient Education: Take exactly as directed. Take on an empty stomach (1 hour before or 2 hours after meals or at bedtime) to reduce GI upset. Do not open, crush, or chew capsules; swallow whole with full 8 oz of water. May cause headache, dizziness, confusion, fatigue, anxiety, insomnia, or impaired coordination (Continued)

Temozolomide *(Continued)*

(use caution when driving or engaging in tasks requiring alertness until response to medication is known); nausea, vomiting, or loss of appetite (small, frequent meals, good mouth care, chewing gum, or sucking hard candy may help); or hot flashes (cool dark room or cold compresses may help). Report chest pain, palpitations, acute headache, visual disturbances; unresolved GI problems; itching or burning on urination or vaginal discharge; acute joint, back, bone, or muscle pain; respiratory difficulty, unusual cough, or respiratory infection; or other adverse reactions. **Pregnancy/breast-feeding precautions:** Inform prescriber if you pregnant. Do not get pregnant while taking this medication. Consult prescriber for appropriate contraceptive measures. Breast-feeding is not recommended.

Dietary Considerations The incidence of nausea/ vomiting is decreased when the drug is taken on an empty stomach.

Pregnancy Issues May cause fetal harm when administered to pregnant women. Male and female patients should avoid pregnancy while receiving drug.

Tenecteplase *(ten EK te plase)*

U.S. Brand Names TNKase™

Pharmacologic Category Thrombolytic Agent

Medication Safety Issues
Sound-alike/look-alike issues:
TNKase™ may be confused with t-PA
TNK (occasional abbreviation for TNKase™) is an error-prone abbreviation (mistaken as TPA)

Pregnancy Risk Factor C

Lactation Use caution

Use Thrombolytic agent used in the management of acute myocardial infarction for the lysis of thrombi in the coronary vasculature to restore perfusion and reduce mortality.

Unlabeled/Investigational Use Acute MI — combination regimen of tenecteplase (unlabeled dose), abciximab, and heparin (unlabeled dose)

Mechanism of Action/Effect Initiates fibrinolysis by binding to fibrin and converting plasminogen to plasmin.

Contraindications Hypersensitivity to tenecteplase or any component of the formulation; active internal bleeding; history of stroke; intracranial/intraspinal surgery or trauma within 2 months; intracranial neoplasm; arteriovenous malformation or aneurysm; bleeding diathesis; severe uncontrolled hypertension

Warnings/Precautions Stop antiplatelet agents and heparin if serious bleeding occurs. Avoid I.M. injections and nonessential handling of the patient for a few hours after administration. Monitor for bleeding complications. Venipunctures should be performed carefully and only when necessary. If arterial puncture is necessary then use an upper extremity that can be compressed manually. For the following conditions the risk of bleeding is higher with use of tenecteplase and should be weighed against the benefits: recent major surgery, cerebrovascular disease, recent GI or GU bleed, recent trauma, uncontrolled HTN (systolic BP ≥180 mm Hg and/or diastolic BP ≥110 mm Hg), suspected left heart thrombus, acute pericarditis, subacute bacterial endocarditis, hemostatic defects, severe hepatic dysfunction, pregnancy, hemorrhagic diabetic retinopathy or other hemorrhagic ophthalmic conditions, septic thrombophlebitis or occluded AV cannula at seriously infected site, advanced age (>75 years of age), anticoagulants, recent administration of GP IIb/IIIa inhibitors. Coronary thrombolysis may result in reperfusion arrhythmias. Caution should be used with readministration of

tenecteplase. Safety and efficacy has not been established in pediatric patients. Cholesterol embolism has rarely been reported.

Drug Interactions
Decreased Effect: Aminocaproic acid (antifibrinolytic agent) may decrease effectiveness.
Increased Effect/Toxicity: Drugs which affect platelet function (eg, NSAIDs, dipyridamole, ticlopidine, clopidogrel, IIb/IIIa antagonists) may potentiate the risk of hemorrhage; use with caution.
Heparin and aspirin: Use with aspirin and heparin may increase bleeding. However, aspirin and heparin were used concomitantly with tenecteplase in the majority of patients in clinical studies.
Warfarin or oral anticoagulants: Risk of bleeding may be increased during concurrent therapy.

Adverse Reactions As with all drugs which may affect hemostasis, bleeding is the major adverse effect associated with tenecteplase. Hemorrhage may occur at virtually any site. Risk is dependent on multiple variables, including the dosage administered, concurrent use of multiple agents which alter hemostasis, and patient predisposition. Rapid lysis of coronary artery thrombi by thrombolytic agents may be associated with reperfusion-related arterial and/or ventricular arrhythmia. The incidence of stroke and bleeding increase in patients >65 years.

>10%:
Hematologic: Bleeding (22% minor: ASSENT-2 trial)
Local: Hematoma (12% minor)
1% to 10%:
Central nervous system: Stroke (2%)
Gastrointestinal: GI hemorrhage (1% major, 2% minor), epistaxis (2% minor)
Genitourinary: GU bleeding (4% minor)
Hematologic: Bleeding (5% major: ASSENT-2 trial)
Local: Bleeding at catheter puncture site (4% minor), hematoma (2% major)
Respiratory: Pharyngeal bleeding (3% minor)
Additional cardiovascular events associated with use in MI: Cardiogenic shock, arrhythmia, AV block, pulmonary edema, heart failure, cardiac arrest, recurrent myocardial ischemia, myocardial reinfarction, myocardial rupture, cardiac tamponade, pericarditis, pericardial effusion, mitral regurgitation, thrombosis, embolism, electromechanical dissociation, hypotension, fever, nausea, vomiting

Overdosage/Toxicology Increased incidence of bleeding

Pharmacodynamics/Kinetics
Half-Life Elimination: 90-130 minutes
Metabolism: Primarily hepatic
Excretion: Clearance: Plasma: 99-119 mL/minute

Available Dosage Forms Injection, powder for reconstitution, recombinant: 50 mg [packaged with diluent and syringe]

Dosing
Adults:
Coronary thrombosis/AMI: I.V.: The recommended total dose should not exceed 50 mg and is based on weight. Administer as a bolus over 5 seconds:
<60 kg: 30 mg dose
≥60 to <70 kg: 35 mg
≥70 to <80 kg: 40 mg
≥80 to <90 kg: 45 mg
≥90 kg: 50 mg
Note: All patients received 150-325 mg of aspirin as soon as possible and then daily. Intravenous heparin was initiated as soon as possible and PTT was maintained between 50-70 seconds.

Combination regimen (unlabeled): Half-dose tenecteplase (15-25 mg based on weight) and abciximab 0.25 mg/kg bolus then 0.125 mcg/kg/ minute (maximum 10 mcg/minute) for 12 hours with heparin dosing as follows: Concurrent bolus of 40 units/kg (maximum 3000 units), then 7 units/kg/hour (maximum 800 units/hour) as continuous infusion. Adjust to aPTT target of 50-70 seconds.

Elderly: Refer to adult dosing. Although dosage adjustments are not recommended, the elderly have a higher incidence of morbidity and mortality with the use of tenecteplase. The 30-day mortality in the ASSENT-2 trial was 2.5% for patients younger than 65 years, 8.5% for patients between 65 and 74 years, and 16.2% for patients 75 years and older. The intracranial hemorrhage rate was 0.4% for patient younger than 65 years, 1.6% for patients between 65 and 74 years, and 1.7% for patients 75 years and older. The risks and benefits of use should be weighted carefully in the elderly.

Renal Impairment: No adjustment is necessary.

Hepatic Impairment: Severe hepatic failure is a relative contraindication. Recommendations were not made for mild to moderate hepatic impairment.

Administration

I.V.: Tenecteplase should be reconstituted using the supplied 10 mL syringe with TwinPak™ Dual Cannula Device and 10 mL SWFI. Do not shake when reconstituting. Slight foaming is normal; will dissipate if left standing for several minutes. Any unused solution should be discarded. The reconstituted solution is 5 mg/mL. Dextrose-containing lines must be flushed with a saline solution before and after administration. Check frequently for signs of bleeding. Avoid I.M. injections and nonessential handling of patient.

Stability

Reconstitution: Tenecteplase should be reconstituted using the supplied 10 mL syringe with TwinPak™ Dual Cannula Device and 10 mL sterile water for injection. Tenecteplase is incompatible with dextrose solutions. Dextrose-containing lines must be flushed with a saline solution before and after administration. Administer as a single I.V. bolus over 5 seconds. If reconstituted and not used immediately, store in refrigerator and use within 8 hours.

Storage: Store at room temperature not to exceed 30°C (86°F) or under refrigeration 2°C to 8°C (36°F to 46°F).

Laboratory Monitoring CBC, PTT, signs and symptoms of bleeding, ECG monitoring

Nursing Actions

Physical Assessment: Assess potential for interactions with other pharmacological agents and herbal products patient may be taking (especially those medications that may affect coagulation [warfarin] or platelet function [NSAIDs, dipyridamole, ticlopidine, clopidogrel]). See Administration for infusion specifics. Monitor patient closely for bleeding during and following treatment. Monitor infusion site, neurological status (eg, intracranial hemorrhage), vital signs, and ECG (reperfusion arrhythmias). Arrhythmias may occur; antiarrhythmic drugs should be immediately available. Maintain bedrest and bleeding precautions. Avoid I.M. injections, venipuncture (unless absolutely necessary), and nonessential handling of the patient. If arterial puncture is necessary, an upper extremity vessel that can be manually compressed should be used. Patient instructions determined by patient condition.

Patient Education: This medication is only administered by infusion; you will be monitored closely during and after treatment. Immediately report burning, pain, redness, swelling, or oozing at infusion site. Following infusion you will have a tendency to bleed easily; use caution to prevent injury (use electric razor, soft toothbrush, and caution with knives, needles, or anything sharp) and follow instructions for strict bedrest to reduce the risk of injury. If bleeding does occur, report immediately and apply pressure to bleeding spot until bleeding stops completely. Report unusual pain (acute headache, joint pain, chest pain); unusual

bruising or bleeding; blood in urine, stool, or vomitus; bleeding gums; vision changes; or respiratory difficulty. **Pregnancy/breast-feeding precautions:** Inform prescriber if you are or intend to become pregnant or breast-feed.

Teniposide (ten i POE side)

U.S. Brand Names Vumon®
Synonyms EPT; VM-26
Pharmacologic Category Antineoplastic Agent, Miscellaneous
Medication Safety Issues
Sound-alike/look-alike issues:
  Teniposide may be confused with etoposide
Pregnancy Risk Factor D
Lactation Not recommended
Use Treatment of acute lymphocytic leukemia, small cell lung cancer
Mechanism of Action/Effect Inhibits mitotic activity; inhibits cells from entering mitosis
Contraindications Hypersensitivity to teniposide, Cremophor® EL (polyoxyethylated castor oil), or any component of the formulation; pregnancy
Warnings/Precautions Hazardous agent - use appropriate precautions for handling and disposal. Teniposide injection contains benzyl alcohol and should be avoided in neonates. The injection contains about 43% alcohol; the possible CNS depressant effect, especially with higher doses of teniposide, should be considered.

Drug Interactions

Cytochrome P450 Effect: Substrate of CYP3A4 (major); Inhibits CYP2C8/9 (weak), 3A4 (weak)

Decreased Effect: CYP3A4 inducers may decrease the levels/effects of teniposide; example inducers include aminoglutethimide, carbamazepine, nafcillin, nevirapine, phenobarbital, phenytoin, and rifamycins.

Increased Effect/Toxicity: May increase toxicity of methotrexate. Sodium salicylate, sulfamethizole, and tolbutamide displace teniposide from protein-binding sites which could cause substantial increases in free drug levels, resulting in potentiation of toxicity. Concurrent use of vincristine may increase the incidence of peripheral neuropathy. CYP3A4 inhibitors may increase the levels/effects of teniposide; example inhibitors include azole antifungals, clarithromycin, diclofenac, doxycycline, erythromycin, imatinib, isoniazid, nefazodone, nicardipine, propofol, protease inhibitors, quinidine, telithromycin, and verapamil.

Nutritional/Ethanol Interactions Herb/Nutraceutical: St John's wort may decrease teniposide levels.

Adverse Reactions

>10%:
  Gastrointestinal: Mucositis (75%); diarrhea, nausea, vomiting (20% to 30%); anorexia
  Hematologic: Myelosuppression, leukopenia, neutropenia (95%), thrombocytopenia (65% to 80%), anemia
    Onset: 5-7 days
    Nadir: 7-10 days
    Recovery: 21-28 days
1% to 10%:
  Cardiovascular: Hypotension (2%), associated with rapid (<30 minutes) infusions
  Dermatologic: Alopecia (9%), rash (3%)
  Miscellaneous: Anaphylactoid reactions (5%) (fever, rash, hyper-/hypotension, dyspnea, bronchospasm), usually seen with rapid (<30 minutes) infusions

Overdosage/Toxicology Symptoms of overdose include bone marrow suppression, leukopenia, thrombocytopenia, nausea, and vomiting. Treatment is supportive.
(Continued)

Teniposide *(Continued)*

Pharmacodynamics/Kinetics
Protein Binding: 99.4%
Half-Life Elimination: 5 hours
Metabolism: Extensively hepatic
Excretion: Urine (44%, 21% as unchanged drug); feces (≤10%)

Available Dosage Forms Injection, solution: 10 mg/mL (5 mL) [contains benzyl alcohol, dehydrated alcohol, and polyoxyethylated castor oil]

Dosing
Adults & Elderly:
Antineoplastic: I.V. (refer to individual protocols): 50-180 mg/m² once or twice weekly for 4-6 weeks or 20-60 mg/m²/day for 5 days
Small cell lung cancer: I.V.: 80-90 mg/m²/day for 5 days every 4-6 weeks
Dosage adjustment in Down syndrome patient: Reduce initial dosing give the first course at half the usual dose. Patients with both Down syndrome and leukemia may be especially sensitive to myelosuppressive chemotherapy.

Pediatrics:
Antineoplastic: I.V. (refer to individual protocols): 130 mg/m²/week, increasing to 150 mg/m² after 3 weeks and up to 180 mg/m² after 6 weeks
Acute lymphoblastic leukemia (ALL): I.V.: 165 mg/m² twice weekly for 8-9 doses **or** 250 mg/m² weekly for 4-8 weeks

Renal Impairment: Data is insufficient, but dose adjustments may be necessary in patient with significant renal impairment.

Hepatic Impairment: Data is insufficient, but dose adjustments may be necessary in patient with significant hepatic impairment.

Administration
I.V.: Irritant. Slow I.V. infusion over ≥30 minutes.
I.V. Detail: Hypotension or increased nausea and vomiting can occur if infused rapidly. Flush thoroughly before and after administration. Incompatible with heparin. Do not use in-line filter during I.V. infusion.

Teniposide must be diluted with either D₅W or 0.9% sodium chloride solutions to a final concentration of 0.1, 0.2, 0.4, or 1 mg/mL. In order to prevent extraction of the plasticizer DEHP, solutions should be prepared in non-DEHP-containing containers such as glass or polyolefin containers. **The use of polyvinyl chloride (PVC) containers is not recommended.**

pH: 5

Stability
Reconstitution: Teniposide must be diluted with either D₅W or 0.9% sodium chloride solutions to a final concentration of 0.1, 0.2, 0.4, or 1 mg/mL. **Solutions should be prepared in non-DEHP-containing containers such as glass or polyolefin containers.**
Compatibility: Stable in D₅W, LR, NS
Y-site administration: Incompatible with Idarubicin, heparin
Storage: Store ampuls in refrigerator at 2°C to 8°C (36°F to 46°F). Reconstituted solutions are stable at room temperature for up to 24 hours after preparation.

Laboratory Monitoring CBC, platelet count

Nursing Actions
Physical Assessment: Assess potential for interactions with other pharmacological agents or herbal products patient may be taking (eg, potential for increased or decreased levels/effects and risk of toxicity). Premedication with antiemetic may be beneficial. See Administration for infusion specifics. Infusion site should be closely monitored to prevent extravasation. Patient should be monitored closely during infusion for possible hypotension (may require discontinuing infusion and administering supportive

therapy) or hypersensitivity reactions (chills, fever, tachycardia, dyspnea, hypotension). Assess results of laboratory tests, therapeutic effectiveness, and adverse reactions (eg, mucositis, diarrhea, myelosuppression, leukopenia) prior to each infusion and throughout therapy. Teach patient possible side effects/appropriate interventions and adverse symptoms to report.

Patient Education: Do not take any new medication during therapy unless approved by prescriber. This medication can only be administered by infusion. Report immediately any swelling, pain, burning, or redness at infusion site. It is important to maintain adequate hydration (2-3 L/day of fluids) unless instructed to restrict fluid intake, and adequate nutrition (small, frequent meals may help). You will be more susceptible to infection (avoid crowds and exposure to infection and do not have any vaccinations without consulting prescriber). May cause nausea or vomiting (small, frequent meals, frequent mouth care, sucking lozenges, or chewing gum may help); diarrhea (buttermilk, boiled milk, or yogurt may help); or loss of hair (reversible). Report unusual bleeding or bruising, persistent fever or chills, sore throat, sores in mouth or vagina, or respiratory difficulty. **Pregnancy/breast-feeding precautions:** Do not get pregnant while taking this medication. Consult prescriber for appropriate barrier contraceptive measures. Breast-feeding is not recommended.

Tenofovir *(te NOE fo veer)*

U.S. Brand Names Viread®
Synonyms PMPA; TDF; Tenofovir Disoproxil Fumarate
Pharmacologic Category Antiretroviral Agent, Reverse Transcriptase Inhibitor (Nucleotide)
Pregnancy Risk Factor B
Lactation Excretion in breast milk unknown/contraindicated
Use Management of HIV infections in combination with at least two other antiretroviral agents
Mechanism of Action/Effect Tenofovir blocks replication of HIV virus by inhibiting the reverse transcriptase enzyme. It is chemically similar to adenosine 5'-monophosphate (a nucleotide), which is required to form DNA.
Contraindications Hypersensitivity to tenofovir or any component of the formulation
Warnings/Precautions Lactic acidosis and severe hepatomegaly with steatosis have been reported with nucleoside analogues, including fatal cases; use with caution in patients with risk factors for liver disease (risk may be increased in obese patients or prolonged exposure) and suspend treatment in any patient who develops clinical or laboratory findings suggestive of lactic acidosis (transaminase elevation may/may not accompany hepatomegaly and steatosis). Immune reconstitution syndrome may develop resulting in the occurrence of an inflammatory response to an indolent or residual opportunistic infection; further evaluation and treatment may be required.

May cause osteomalacia; increased biochemical markers of bone metabolism, serum parathyroid hormone levels, and 1,25 vitamin D levels have been noted with tenofovir use. A 5% to 7% loss of bone mineral density (BMD) has been reported in some patients. BMD monitoring should be considered in patients with a history of bone fracture or risk factors for osteopenia.

Use caution in renal impairment (Cl$_{cr}$ <50 mL/minute); dosage adjustment required. May cause acute renal failure or Fanconi syndrome; use caution with other nephrotoxic agents (especially those which compete for active tubular secretion), patients with low body weight, or concurrent medications which increase tenofovir levels. Use caution in hepatic impairment. All patients with HIV should be tested for HBV prior to initiation of treatment. Safety and efficacy of tenofovir during coinfection of HIV and HBV have not been established; acute, severe exacerbations of HBV have been reported following tenofovir discontinuation. In HBV coinfected patients, monitor hepatic function closely for several months following discontinuation. Safety and efficacy have not been established in pediatric patients.

Drug Interactions
Cytochrome P450 Effect: Inhibits CYP1A2 (weak)
Decreased Effect: Tenofovir may decrease serum concentrations of atazanavir and other protease inhibitors, resulting in a loss of virologic response (specific atazanavir dosing recommendations provided by manufacturer).
Increased Effect/Toxicity: Concurrent use has been noted to increase serum concentrations/exposure to didanosine and its metabolites, potentially increasing the risk of didanosine toxicity (hyperglycemia, pancreatitis, peripheral neuropathy, or lactic acidosis); decreased CD4 cell counts and decreased virologic response have been reported. Use caution and monitor closely; suspend therapy if signs/symptoms of toxicity are present. Drugs which may compete for renal tubule secretion (including acyclovir, cidofovir, ganciclovir, valacyclovir, valganciclovir) may increase the serum concentrations of tenofovir. Drugs causing nephrotoxicity may reduce elimination of tenofovir. Protease inhibitors (especially ritonavir and combinations with ritonavir) may increase serum concentrations of tenofovir.

Nutritional/Ethanol Interactions Food: Fatty meals may increase the bioavailability of tenofovir. Tenofovir may be taken with or without food.

Adverse Reactions
>10%:
    Central nervous system: Pain (7% to 12%)
    Gastrointestinal: Diarrhea (11% to 16%), nausea (8% to 11%),
    Neuromuscular & skeletal: Weakness (7% to 11%)
1% to 10%:
    Central nervous system: Headache (5% to 8%), depression (4% to 8%; treatment naïve 11%), insomnia (3% to 4%), fever (2% to 4%; treatment naïve 8%), dizziness (1% to 3%)
    Dermatologic: Rash event (maculopapular, pustular, or vesiculobullous rash, pruritus or urticaria 5% to 7%; treatment naïve 18%)
    Endocrine & metabolic: Amylase increased (9%, treatment naïve)
    Gastrointestinal: Vomiting (4% to 7%), abdominal pain (4% to 7%), dyspepsia (3% to 4%), flatulence (3% to 4%), anorexia (3% to 4%), weight loss (2% to 4%)
    Hematologic: Neutropenia (1% to 2%)
    Hepatic: Transaminases increased (2% to 4%)
    Neuromuscular & skeletal: Back pain (3% to 4%; treatment naïve 9%), myalgia (3% to 4%), neuropathy (peripheral 1% to 3%)
    Respiratory: Pneumonia (2% to 3%)
    Miscellaneous: Diaphoresis (3%)

Overdosage/Toxicology Limited experience with overdose. Treatment is supportive. Hemodialysis may be beneficial; reportedly 10% of an administered single dose of 300 mg was removed during a 4-hour session.

Pharmacodynamics/Kinetics
Time to Peak: Serum: Fasting: 36-84 minutes; With food: 96-144 minutes
Protein Binding: 7% to serum proteins
Half-Life Elimination:
    17 hours
Metabolism: Tenofovir disoproxil fumarate (TDF) is converted intracellularly by hydrolysis (by non-CYP

enzymes) to tenofovir, then phosphorylated to the active tenofovir diphosphate
Excretion: Urine (70% to 80%) via filtration and active secretion, primarily as unchanged tenofovir
Available Dosage Forms Tablet, as disoproxil fumarate: 300 mg [equivalent to 245 mg tenofovir disoproxil]
Dosing
Adults: HIV infection: Oral: 300 mg once daily
Renal Impairment:
    Cl_{cr} 30-49 mL/minute: 300 mg every 48 hours
    Cl_{cr} 10-29 mL/minute: 300 mg twice weekly
    Cl_{cr} <10 mL/minute without hemodialysis: No recommendation available.
    Hemodialysis: 300 mg every 7 days or after a total of 12 hours of dialysis (usually once weekly assuming 3 dialysis sessions lasting about 4 hours each)
Hepatic Impairment:
    No dosage adjustment required.

Administration
Oral: May be administered with or without food.
Stability
Storage: Store at 25°C (77°F); excursions permitted to 15°C to 30°C (59°F to 86°F).
Laboratory Monitoring CBC with differential, reticulocyte count, serum creatine kinase, CD4 cell count, HIV RNA plasma levels, renal and hepatic function tests, bone density (long-term), serum phosphorus; testing for HBV is recommended prior to the initiation of antiretroviral therapy
Patients with HIV and HBV coinfection should be monitored for several months following tenofovir discontinuation.

Nursing Actions
Physical Assessment: Allergy history should be assessed prior to beginning treatment. Assess other pharmacological or herbal products patient may be taking (concurrent use with other antiretroviral nephrotoxic or hepatotoxic drugs may increase potential for severe toxicities). Monitor laboratory tests, therapeutic response, and adverse reactions (eg, lactic acidosis [elevated transaminases]; osteomalacia, gastrointestinal disturbance [nausea, vomiting, diarrhea]; neutropenia, myalgia, peripheral neuropathy) on a regular basis throughout therapy. Teach patient proper use (eg, timing of multiple medications and drugs that should not be used concurrently), possible side effects/appropriate interventions, and adverse symptoms to report.
Patient Education: Do not take any new prescriptions, over-the-counter medications, or herbal products without consulting prescriber. This drug will not cure HIV, nor has it been found to reduce transmission of HIV; use appropriate precautions to prevent spread to other persons. This drug is prescribed as one part of a multidrug combination; take exactly as directed for full course of therapy. Maintain adequate hydration (2-3 L/day of fluids) unless advised by prescriber to restrict fluids. You may be susceptible to infection (avoid crowds and exposure to known infections and do not have any vaccinations without consulting prescriber). Frequent blood tests may be required with prolonged therapy. May cause dizziness or headache (use caution when driving or engaging in tasks requiring alertness until response to drug is known); or nausea or vomiting (small frequent meals, frequent mouth care, chewing gum, or sucking lozenges may help). Report immediately any tingling, pain, or loss of sensation in toes, feet, muscles or joints; swollen glands; alterations in urinary pattern; swelling of extremities; weight gain or loss; unusual weakness; signs of opportunistic infection (burning on urination, perineal itching, white plaques in mouth, unhealed sores, persistent sore throat or cough); or other persistent adverse effects. If you are instructed to stop the medication, do not restart without specific instruction by your prescriber.
(Continued)

Tenofovir (Continued)

Pregnancy/breast-feeding precautions: Inform prescriber if you are or intend to become pregnant. Do not breast-feed.

Dietary Considerations May be taken with or without food. Consider calcium and vitamin D supplementation in patients with history of bone fracture or osteopenia.

Breast-Feeding Issues HIV-infected mothers are discouraged from breast-feeding to decrease potential transmission of HIV.

Pregnancy Issues There are no adequate and well-controlled studies in pregnant women. Animal studies have shown decreased fetal growth and reduced fetal bone porosity. Clinical studies in children have shown bone demineralization with chronic use. Use in pregnancy only if clearly needed. Cases of lactic acidosis/hepatic steatosis syndrome have been reported in pregnant women receiving nucleoside analogues. It is not known if pregnancy itself potentiates this known side effect; however, pregnant women may be at increased risk of lactic acidosis and liver damage. Hepatic enzymes and electrolytes should be monitored frequently during the 3rd trimester of pregnancy in women receiving nucleoside analogues. Health professionals are encouraged to contact the Antiretroviral Pregnancy Registry to monitor outcomes of pregnant women exposed to antiretroviral medications (1-800-258-4263 or www.APRegistry.com).

Additional Information Approval was based on two clinical trials involving patients who were previously treated with antiretrovirals with continued evidence of HIV replication despite therapy. The risk:benefit ratio for untreated patients has not been established (studies currently ongoing), however, patients who received tenofovir showed significant decreases in HIV replication as compared to continuation of standard therapy.

A high rate of early virologic nonresponse was observed when abacavir, lamivudine, and tenofovir were used as the initial regimen in treatment-naïve patients. A high rate of early virologic nonresponse was also observed when didanosine, lamivudine, and tenofovir were used as the initial regimen in treatment-naïve patients. Use of either of these combinations is not recommended; patients currently on either of these regimens should be closely monitored for modification of therapy. Early virologic failure was also observed with tenofovir and didanosine delayed release capsules, plus either efavirenz or nevirapine; use caution in treatment-naïve patients with high baseline viral loads.

Terazosin (ter AY zoe sin)

U.S. Brand Names Hytrin®
Pharmacologic Category Alpha₁ Blocker
Pregnancy Risk Factor C
Lactation Excretion in breast milk unknown
Use Management of mild to moderate hypertension; alone or in combination with other agents such as diuretics or beta-blockers; benign prostate hyperplasia (BPH)

Mechanism of Action/Effect Alpha₁-specific blocking agent with minimal alpha₂ effects; this allows peripheral postsynaptic blockade, with the resultant decrease in arterial tone, while preserving the negative feedback loop which is mediated by the peripheral presynaptic alpha₂-receptors; terazosin relaxes the smooth muscle of the bladder neck, thus reducing bladder outlet obstruction

Contraindications Hypersensitivity to quinazolines (doxazosin, prazosin, terazosin) or any component of the formulation; concurrent use with phosphodiesterase-5 (PDE-5) inhibitors including sildenafil (>25 mg), tadalafil, or vardenafil

Warnings/Precautions Can cause significant orthostatic hypotension and syncope, especially with first dose. Prostate cancer should be ruled out before starting for BPH. Anticipate a similar effect if therapy is interrupted for a few days, if dosage is rapidly increased, or if another antihypertensive drug is introduced.

Drug Interactions
Decreased Effect: Decreased antihypertensive response with NSAIDs. Alpha-blockers reduce the response to pressor agents (norepinephrine).

Increased Effect/Toxicity: Terazosin's hypotensive effect is increased with beta-blockers, diuretics, ACE inhibitors, calcium channel blockers, other antihypertensive medications, sildenafil (use with extreme caution at a dose ≤25 mg), tadalafil (use is contraindicated by the manufacturer), and vardenafil (use is contraindicated by the manufacturer).

Nutritional/Ethanol Interactions Herb/Nutraceutical: Avoid dong quai if using for hypertension (has estrogenic activity). Avoid ephedra, yohimbe, ginseng (may worsen hypertension). Avoid saw palmetto. Avoid garlic (may have increased antihypertensive effect).

Adverse Reactions Asthenia, postural hypotension, dizziness, somnolence, nasal congestion/rhinitis, and impotence were the only events noted in clinical trials to occur at a frequency significantly greater than placebo (p <0.05).

>10%:
Central nervous system: Dizziness, headache
Neuromuscular & skeletal: Muscle weakness

1% to 10%:
Cardiovascular: Edema, palpitation, chest pain, peripheral edema (3%), orthostatic hypotension (3% to 4%), tachycardia
Central nervous system: Fatigue, nervousness, drowsiness
Gastrointestinal: Dry mouth
Genitourinary: Urinary incontinence
Ocular: Blurred vision
Respiratory: Dyspnea, nasal congestion

Overdosage/Toxicology Symptoms of overdose include hypotension, drowsiness, and shock. Treatment is supportive and symptomatic.

Pharmacodynamics/Kinetics
Onset of Action: 1-2 hours
Time to Peak: Serum: ~1 hour
Protein Binding: 90% to 95%
Half-Life Elimination: 9.2-12 hours
Metabolism: Extensively hepatic
Excretion: Feces (60%); urine (40%)

Available Dosage Forms Capsule: 1 mg, 2 mg, 5 mg, 10 mg

Dosing
Adults & Elderly:
Hypertension: Oral: Initial: 1 mg at bedtime; slowly increase dose to achieve desired blood pressure, up to 20 mg/day; usual dose range (JNC 7): 1-20 mg once daily
Benign prostatic hyperplasia: Oral: Initial: 1 mg at bedtime, increasing as needed; most patients require 10 mg day. If no response after 4-6 weeks of 10 mg/day, may increase to 20 mg/day.

Nursing Actions
Physical Assessment: Assess potential for interactions with other pharmacological agents and herbal products patient may be taking (especially anything that may decrease antihypertensive response [NSAIDS, ephedra, yohimbe, ginseng] or increase hypotensive effect [beta-blockers, diuretics, ACE inhibitors]. Monitor therapeutic effectiveness (blood pressure) and adverse reactions (eg, hypotension, dizziness, somnolence, and impotence) at beginning of therapy and on a regular basis with long-term therapy. When discontinuing, dose should be tapered and blood pressure monitored closely. Teach patient

proper use, possible side effects/appropriate interventions, and adverse symptoms to report.

Patient Education: Do not take any new medication during therapy unless approved by prescriber. Take as directed; at bedtime. Do not skip dose or discontinue without consulting prescriber. Follow recommended diet and exercise program. May cause drowsiness, dizziness, or impaired judgment (use caution when driving or engaging in tasks that require alertness until response to drug is known); postural hypotension (use caution when rising from sitting or lying position or when climbing stairs); dry mouth or nausea (frequent mouth care or sucking lozenges may help); urinary incontinence (void before taking medication); or sexual dysfunction (reversible, may resolve with continued use). Report altered CNS status (eg, fatigue, lethargy, confusion, nervousness); sudden weight gain (weigh yourself in the same clothes at the same time of day once a week); unusual or persistent swelling of ankles, feet, or extremities; palpitations or rapid heartbeat; respiratory difficulty; muscle weakness; or other persistent side effects. **Pregnancy/breast-feeding precautions:** Inform prescriber if you are or intend to become pregnant. Consult prescriber if breast-feeding.

Dietary Considerations May be taken without regard to meals at the same time each day.

Geriatric Considerations Adverse reactions such as dry mouth and urinary problems can be particularly bothersome in the elderly.

Terbinafine (TER bin a feen)

U.S. Brand Names Lamisil®; Lamisil® AT™ [OTC]
Synonyms Terbinafine Hydrochloride
Pharmacologic Category Antifungal Agent, Oral; Antifungal Agent, Topical
Medication Safety Issues
Sound-alike/look-alike issues:
Terbinafine may be confused with terbutaline
Lamisil® may be confused with Lamictal®, Lomotil®

Pregnancy Risk Factor B
Lactation Enters breast milk/not recommended
Use Active against most strains of *Trichophyton mentagrophytes*, *Trichophyton rubrum*; may be effective for infections of *Microsporum gypseum* and *M. nanum*, *Trichophyton verrucosum*, *Epidermophyton floccosum*, *Candida albicans*, and *Scopulariopsis brevicaulis*
Oral: Onychomycosis of the toenail or fingernail due to susceptible dermatophytes
Topical: Antifungal for the treatment of tinea pedis (athlete's foot), tinea cruris (jock itch), and tinea corporis (ringworm) [OTC/prescription formulations]; tinea versicolor [prescription formulations]

Contraindications Hypersensitivity to terbinafine, naftifine, or any component of the formulation

Warnings/Precautions While rare, the following complications have been reported and may require discontinuation of therapy: Changes in the ocular lens and retina, pancytopenia, neutropenia, Stevens-Johnson syndrome, toxic epidermal necrolysis. Rare cases of hepatic failure, including fatal cases, have been reported following oral treatment of onychomycosis. Not recommended for use in patients with active or chronic liver disease. Discontinue if symptoms or signs of hepatobiliary dysfunction or cholestatic hepatitis develop. If irritation/sensitivity develop with topical use, discontinue therapy. Oral products are not recommended for use with pre-existing liver or renal disease (≤50 mL/minute GFR). **Use caution in writing and/or filling prescription/orders. Confusion between Lamictal® (lamotrigine) and Lamisil® (terbinafine) has occurred.**

Drug Interactions
Cytochrome P450 Effect: Substrate (minor) of 1A2, 2C8/9, 2C19, 3A4; **Inhibits** CYP2D6 (strong); **Induces** CYP3A4 (weak)
Decreased Effect: Terbinafine may decrease the levels/effects of CYP2D6 prodrug substrates (eg, codeine, hydrocodone, oxycodone, tramadol).
Increased Effect/Toxicity: Terbinafine may increase the levels/effects of amphetamines, beta-blockers, dextromethorphan, fluoxetine, lidocaine, mirtazapine, nefazodone, paroxetine, risperidone, ritonavir, thioridazine, tricyclic antidepressants, venlafaxine, and other CYP2D6 substrates. The effects of warfarin may be increased.

Adverse Reactions
Oral: 1% to 10%:
Central nervous system: Headache, dizziness, vertigo
Dermatologic: Rash, pruritus, urticaria
Gastrointestinal: Diarrhea, dyspepsia, abdominal pain, appetite decrease, taste disturbance
Hematologic: Lymphocytopenia
Hepatic: Liver enzymes increased
Ocular: Visual disturbance

Topical: 1% to 10%:
Dermatologic: Pruritus, contact dermatitis, irritation, burning, dryness
Local: Irritation, stinging

Pharmacodynamics/Kinetics
Time to Peak: Plasma: 1-2 hours
Protein Binding: Plasma: >99%
Half-Life Elimination: Topical: 22-26 hours; Oral: Terminal half-life: 200-400 hours; very slow release of drug from skin and adipose tissues occurs; effective half-life: ~36 hours
Metabolism: Hepatic; no active metabolites; first-pass effect (40%); little effect on CYP
Excretion: Urine (70% to 75%)

Available Dosage Forms
Cream, as hydrochloride (Lamisil® AT™): 1% (12 g) [contains benzyl alcohol]
Solution, as hydrochloride [topical spray] (Lamisil®, Lamisil® AT™): 1% (30 mL)
Tablet (Lamisil®): 250 mg

Dosing
Adults & Elderly:
Superficial mycoses (onychomycosis): Oral:
Fingernail: 250 mg/day for up to 6 weeks; may be given in two divided doses
Toenail: 250 mg/day for 12 weeks; may be given in two divided doses
Systemic mycosis: Oral: 250-500 mg/day for up to 16 months
Athlete's foot (tinea pedis): Topical:
Cream: Apply to affected area twice daily for at least 1 week, not to exceed 4 weeks [OTC/prescription formulations]
Solution: Apply to affected area twice daily for 7 days [OTC/prescription formulations]
Ringworm and jock itch (tinea corporis, tinea cruris): Topical:
Cream: Apply to affected area once or twice daily for at least 1 week, not to exceed 4 weeks [OTC formulations]
Solution: Apply to affected area once daily for 7 days in tinea corporis and tinea cruris [OTC formulations]; apply to affected area twice daily for 7 days in tinea versicolor [prescription formulation]

Pediatrics:
Athlete's foot (tinea pedis), ringworm (tinea corporis), jock itch (tinea cruris): Children ≥12 years: Topical cream, solution: Refer to adult dosing.
Oral (unlabeled use in children):
10-20 kg: 62.5 mg/day
20-40 kg: 125 mg/day
>40 kg: 250 mg/day
(Continued)

Terbinafine *(Continued)*

Treatment duration:
Tinea pedis: 2 weeks
Tinea capitis: 2-4 weeks
Onychomycosis: Fingernails: 6 weeks; Toenails: 12 weeks

Renal Impairment: GFR <50 mL/minute: Oral administration is not recommended.

Hepatic Impairment: Clearance is decreased by ~50% with hepatic cirrhosis; use is not recommended.

Stability
Storage:
Cream: Store at 5°C to 30°C (41°F to 86°F).
Solution: Store at 5°C to 25°C (41°F to 77°F). Do not refrigerate.
Tablet: Store below 25°C (77°F). Protect from light.

Nursing Actions
Physical Assessment: Due to potential toxicity, the manufacturer recommends confirmation of diagnosis testing of nail specimens prior to treatment of onychomycosis. Assess potential for interactions with other pharmacological agents patient may be taking (may increase levels/effect of amphetamines, beta-blockers, ritonavir, risperidone, TCAs and other CYP2D6 substrates). Monitor laboratory tests, therapeutic effectiveness (according to purpose for use), and adverse reactions at beginning of therapy and on a regular basis with long-term therapy (will differ according to formulation and purpose for use). If irritation develops with topical use, discontinue therapy. If signs of hepatic dysfunction occur with oral formulation, discontinue use. Teach patient proper use, possible side effects/appropriate interventions, and adverse symptoms to report.

Patient Education: Do not take any new medication during therapy without consulting prescriber. Use exactly as directed. Take tablets at same time of day, with or without regard to meals. Take full prescription even if symptoms appear resolved, may take several months for full treatment (inadequate treatment may result in reinfection). May cause altered taste (normal). Report unusual fatigue; persistent loss of appetite, nausea or vomiting; dark urine/pale stool; or other persistent adverse response. **Breast-feeding precaution:** Breast-feeding is not recommended.
Topical (cream or spray): For topical use only. Wash and dry nails thoroughly before applying. Avoid contact with eyes, nose, or mouth. Do not use occlusive dressings. Report irritation, itching, burning or skin around nail. Full clinical effect may require several months due to the time required for a new nail to grow.

Breast-Feeding Issues Although minimal concentrations of terbinafine cross into breast milk after topical use, oral or topical treatment during lactation should be avoided.

Pregnancy Issues Avoid use in pregnancy since treatment of onychomycosis is postponable.

Additional Information Due to potential toxicity, the manufacturer recommends confirmation of diagnosis testing of nail specimens prior to treatment of onychomycosis. Patients should not be considered therapeutic failures until they have been symptom-free for 2-4 weeks off following a course of treatment; GI complaints usually subside with continued administration.

A meta-analysis of efficacy studies for toenail infections revealed that weighted average mycological cure rates for continuous therapy were 36.7% (griseofulvin), 54.7% (itraconazole), and 77% (terbinafine). Cure rate for 4-month pulse therapy for itraconazole and terbinafine were 73.3% and 80%. Additionally, the final outcome measure of final costs per cured infections for continuous therapy was significantly lower for terbinafine.

Terbutaline *(ter BYOO ta leen)*

U.S. Brand Names Brethine®
Synonyms Brethaire [DSC]; Bricanyl [DSC]
Pharmacologic Category Beta$_2$-Adrenergic Agonist
Medication Safety Issues
Sound-alike/look-alike issues:
Terbutaline may be confused with terbinafine, TOLBUTamide
Pregnancy Risk Factor B
Lactation Enters breast milk/compatible
Use Bronchodilator in reversible airway obstruction and bronchial asthma
Unlabeled/Investigational Use Tocolytic agent (management of preterm labor)
Mechanism of Action/Effect Relaxes bronchial smooth muscle by action on beta$_2$-receptors with less effect on heart rate
Contraindications Hypersensitivity to terbutaline or any component of the formulation; cardiac arrhythmias associated with tachycardia; tachycardia caused by digitalis intoxication
Warnings/Precautions When used for tocolysis, there is some risk of maternal pulmonary edema, which has been associated with the following risk factors, excessive hydration, multiple gestation, occult sepsis and underlying cardiac disease. To reduce risk, limit fluid intake to 2.5-3 L/day, limit sodium intake, maintain maternal pulse to <130 beats/minute.

Use caution in patients with cardiovascular disease (arrhythmia or hypertension or CHF), convulsive disorders, diabetes, glaucoma, hyperthyroidism, or hypokalemia. Beta agonists may cause elevation in blood pressure, heart rate, and result in CNS stimulation/excitation. Beta$_2$ agonists may increase risk of arrhythmia, increase serum glucose, or decrease serum potassium.

When used as a bronchodilator, optimize anti-inflammatory treatment before initiating maintenance treatment with terbutaline. Do not use as a component of chronic therapy without an anti-inflammatory agent. Only the mildest form of asthma (Step 1 and/or exercise-induced) would not require concurrent use based upon asthma guidelines. Patient must be instructed to seek medical attention in cases where acute symptoms are not relieved or a previous level of response is diminished. The need to increase frequency of use may indicate deterioration of asthma, and treatment must not be delayed.

Do not exceed recommended dose; serious adverse events including fatalities, have been associated with excessive use of inhaled sympathomimetics. Rarely, paradoxical bronchospasm may occur with use of inhaled bronchodilating agents; this should be distinguished from inadequate response.

Drug Interactions
Decreased Effect: Decreased effect with beta-blockers.
Increased Effect/Toxicity: Increased toxicity with MAO inhibitors, tricyclic antidepressants.
Nutritional/Ethanol Interactions Herb/Nutraceutical: Avoid ephedra, yohimbe (may cause CNS stimulation).
Adverse Reactions
>10%:
Central nervous system: Nervousness, restlessness
Endocrine & metabolic: Serum glucose increased, serum potassium decreased
Neuromuscular & skeletal: Trembling
1% to 10%:
Cardiovascular: Tachycardia, hypertension
Central nervous system: Dizziness, drowsiness, headache, insomnia
Gastrointestinal: Xerostomia, nausea, vomiting, bad taste in mouth

Neuromuscular & skeletal: Muscle cramps, weakness

Miscellaneous: Diaphoresis

Overdosage/Toxicology Symptoms of overdose include tachycardia, tremor, hypertension, angina, and seizures. Hypokalemia also may occur. Cardiac arrest and death may be associated with abuse of beta-agonist bronchodilators. Treatment includes immediate discontinuation and symptomatic and supportive therapies. Cautious use of beta-adrenergic blocking agents may be considered in severe cases.

Pharmacodynamics/Kinetics

Onset of Action: Oral: 30-45 minutes; SubQ: 6-15 minutes

Protein Binding: 25%

Half-Life Elimination: 11-16 hours

Metabolism: Hepatic to inactive sulfate conjugates

Excretion: Urine

Available Dosage Forms

Injection, solution, as sulfate: 1 mg/mL (1 mL)

Tablet, as sulfate: 2.5 mg, 5 mg

Additional dosage forms available in Canada: Powder for oral inhalation (Bricanyl® Turbuhaler): 500 mcg/actuation [50 or 200 metered doses]

Dosing

Adults & Elderly:

Asthma or bronchoconstriction:

Oral: 5 mg/dose every 6 hours 3 times/day; if side effects occur, reduce dose to 2.5 mg every 6 hours; not to exceed 15 mg in 24 hours.

SubQ: 0.25 mg/dose; may repeat in 15-30 minutes (maximum: 0.5 mg/4-hour period)

Bronchospasm (acute): *Inhalation* (Bricanyl® [CAN] MDI: 500 mcg/puff, *not labeled for use in the U.S.*): One puff as needed; may repeat with 1 inhalation (after 5 minutes); more than 6 inhalations should not be necessary in any 24 hour period. **Note:** If a previously effective dosage regimen fails to provide the usual relief, or the effects of a dose last for >3 hours, medical advice should be sought immediately; this is a sign of seriously worsening asthma that requires reassessment of therapy.

Premature labor (tocolysis; unlabeled use):

Acute: I.V. 2.5-10 mcg/minute; increased gradually every 10-20 minutes. Effective maximum dosages from 17.5-30 mcg/minute have been use with caution. Duration of infusion is at least 12 hours.

Maintenance: Oral: 2.5-10 mg every 4-6 hours for as long as necessary to prolong pregnancy depending on patient tolerance

Pediatrics:

Asthma or bronchoconstriction:

Oral: Children:

<12 years: Initial: 0.05 mg/kg/dose 3 times/day, increased gradually as required; maximum: 0.15 mg/kg/dose 3-4 times/day or a total of 5 mg/24 hours

12-15 years: 2.5 mg every 6 hours 3 times/day; not to exceed 7.5 mg in 24 hours

>15 years: 5 mg/dose every 6 hours 3 times/day; if side effects occur, reduce dose to 2.5 mg every 6 hours; not to exceed 15 mg in 24 hours

SubQ: Children:

<12 years: 0.005-0.01 mg/kg/dose to a maximum of 0.3 mg/dose; may repeat in 15-20 minutes

≥12 years: Refer to adult dosing.

Bronchospasm (acute): *Inhalation:* Bricanyl® [CAN] MDI: 500 mcg/puff, *not labeled for use in the U.S.*): Children ≥6 years: Refer to adult dosing.

Renal Impairment:

Cl$_{cr}$ 10-50 mL/minute: Administer 50% of normal dose.

Cl$_{cr}$ <10 mL/minute: Avoid use.

Administration

Oral: Administer around-the-clock to promote less variation in peak and trough serum levels.

I.V.: Use infusion pump.

I.V. Detail: pH: 3-5 (adjusted)

Stability

Compatibility: Stable in D$_5$W, ½NS, NS

Compatibility when admixed: Incompatible with bleomycin

Storage: Store injection at room temperature. Protect from heat, light, and from freezing. Use only clear solutions. Store powder for inhalation (Bricanyl® Turbuhaler [CAN]) at room temperature between 15°C and 30°C (58°F and 86°F).

Laboratory Monitoring FEV$_1$, peak flow, and/or other pulmonary function tests; serum potassium, serum glucose (in selected patients)

Tocolysis: If patient receives therapy for more than 1 week, monitor serum glucose.

Nursing Actions

Physical Assessment: Respiratory use: Assess effectiveness and interactions of other medications patient may be taking. Monitor effectiveness of therapy (relief of airway obstruction) and adverse reactions (eg, cardiac and CNS changes) at beginning of therapy and periodically with long-term use. If diabetic, monitor blood glucose (may cause elevation in serum glucose). For inpatient care, monitor vital signs and lung sounds prior to and periodically during therapy. Assess knowledge/teach patient appropriate use, interventions to reduce side effects, and adverse symptoms to report. **Preterm labor use: Inpatient:** Monitor maternal vital signs; respiratory, fluid status, cardiac, and electrolyte status; frequency, duration, and intensity of contractions; and fetal heart rate. **Outpatient:** Assess knowledge/teach patient appropriate use, interventions to reduce side effects, and adverse symptoms to report.

Patient Education: Use exactly as directed. Do not use more often than recommended (excessive use may result in tolerance, overdose may result in serious adverse effects) and do not discontinue without consulting prescriber. Maintain adequate hydration (2-3 L/day of fluids) unless instructed to restrict fluid intake. If you have diabetes, monitor blood sugar closely. Serum glucose may be elevated. You may experience nervousness, dizziness, or fatigue (use caution when driving or engaging in tasks requiring alertness until response to drug is known); or dry mouth, stomach upset (small frequent meals, frequent mouth care, chewing gum, or sucking hard candy may help). Report unresolved GI upset; dizziness or fatigue; vision changes; sudden weight gain; swelling of extremities; chest pain, rapid heartbeat, or palpitations; insomnia, nervousness, or hyperactivity; muscle cramping, tremors, or pain; unusual cough; or rash (hypersensitivity).

Preterm labor: Notify prescriber immediately if labor resumes or adverse side effects are noted

---

Terconazole (ter KONE a zole)

U.S. Brand Names Terazol® 3; Terazol® 7

Synonyms Triaconazole

Pharmacologic Category Antifungal Agent, Vaginal

Medication Safety Issues

Sound-alike/look-alike issues:

Terconazole may be confused with tioconazole

Pregnancy Risk Factor C

Lactation Excretion in breast milk unknown/not recommended

Use Local treatment of vulvovaginal candidiasis

Mechanism of Action/Effect Triazole ketal antifungal agent; involves inhibition of fungal cytochrome P450

Contraindications Hypersensitivity to terconazole or any component of the formulation

(Continued)

Terconazole (Continued)

Warnings/Precautions Should be discontinued if sensitization or irritation occurs. Microbiological studies (KOH smear and/or cultures) should be repeated in patients not responding to terconazole in order to confirm the diagnosis and rule out other pathogens.

Adverse Reactions 1% to 10%:
Central nervous system; Fever, chills
Gastrointestinal: Abdominal pain
Genitourinary: Vulvar/vaginal burning, dysmenorrhea

Available Dosage Forms
Cream, vaginal:
Terazol® 7: 0.4% (45 g) [packaged with measured-dose applicator]
Terazol® 3: 0.8% (20 g) [packaged with measured-dose applicator]
Suppository, vaginal (Terazol® 3): 80 mg (3s) [may contain coconut and/or palm kernel oil]

Dosing
Adults & Elderly: Vulvovaginal candidiasis: Intravaginal:
Terazol® 3 vaginal cream: Insert 1 applicatorful intravaginally at bedtime for 3 consecutive days.
Terazol® 7 vaginal cream: Insert 1 applicatorful intravaginally at bedtime for 7 consecutive days.
Terazol® 3 vaginal suppository: Insert 1 suppository intravaginally at bedtime for 3 consecutive days.

Stability
Storage: Store at room temperature of 13°C to 30°C (59°F to 86°F).

Nursing Actions
Physical Assessment: Assess knowledge/teach patient appropriate administration, possible side effects/interventions, and adverse symptoms to report.

Patient Education: Complete full course of therapy as directed. Insert vaginally as directed by prescriber or see package insert. Sexual partner may experience irritation of penis; best to refrain from intercourse during period of treatment. Suppositories may cause breakdown of rubber/latex products such as diaphragms; avoid concurrent use. Report persistent vaginal burning, itching, irritation, or discharge. **Pregnancy/breast-feeding precautions:** Inform prescriber if you are or intend to become pregnant. Consult prescriber if breast-feeding.

Geriatric Considerations Assess patient's ability to self-administer; may be difficult in patients with arthritis or limited range of motion.

Additional Information Watch for local irritation; assist patient in administration, if necessary; assess patient's ability to self-administer, may be difficult in patients with arthritis or limited range of motion

Teriparatide (ter i PAR a tide)

U.S. Brand Names Forteo™

Synonyms Parathyroid Hormone (1-34); Recombinant Human Parathyroid Hormone (1-34); rhPTH(1-34)

Restrictions An FDA-approved medication guide is available at http://www.fda.gov/cder/Offices/ODS/labeling.htm; distribute to each patient to whom this medication is dispensed.

Pharmacologic Category Parathyroid Hormone Analog

Pregnancy Risk Factor C

Lactation Excretion in breast milk unknown/not recommended

Use Treatment of osteoporosis in postmenopausal women at high risk of fracture; treatment of primary or hypogonadal osteoporosis in men at high risk of fracture

Mechanism of Action/Effect An analog of parathyroid hormone, teriparatide stimulates osteoblast function, increases gastrointestinal calcium absorption, and increases renal tubular reabsorption of calcium. Treatment with teriparatide increases bone mineral density, bone mass, and strength. In postmenopausal women, it has been shown to decrease osteoporosis-related fractures.

Contraindications Hypersensitivity to teriparatide or any component of the formulation

Warnings/Precautions In animal studies, teriparatide has been associated with an increase in osteosarcoma; risk was dependent on both dose and duration. Use of teriparatide for longer than 2 years is not recommended. Avoid use in patients with an increased risk of osteosarcoma (including Paget's disease, prior radiation, unexplained elevation of alkaline phosphatase, or in patients with open epiphyses). Do not use in patients with a history of skeletal metastases, hyperparathyroidism, or pre-existing hypercalcemia. Exclude metabolic bone disease other than osteoporosis prior to initiating therapy. Use caution in patients with active or recent urolithiasis. Use caution in patients at risk of orthostasis (including concurrent antihypertensive therapy), or in patients who may not tolerate transient hypotension (cardiovascular or cerebrovascular disease). Use caution in patients with renal or hepatic impairment (limited data available concerning safety and efficacy). Not approved for use in pediatric patients.

Drug Interactions
Increased Effect/Toxicity: Digitalis serum concentrations are not affected, however, transient hypercalcemia may increase risk of digitalis toxicity (case reports).

Nutritional/Ethanol Interactions
Ethanol: Excessive intake may increase risk of osteoporosis.
Herb/Nutraceutical: Ensure adequate calcium and vitamin D intake.

Adverse Reactions 1% to 10%:
Cardiovascular: Chest pain (3%), syncope (3%)
Central nervous system: Dizziness (8%), depression (4%), vertigo (4%)
Dermatologic: Rash (5%)
Endocrine & metabolic: Hypercalcemia (transient increases noted 4-6 hours postdose in 11% of women and 6% of men)
Gastrointestinal: Nausea (9%), dyspepsia (5%), vomiting (3%), tooth disorder (2%)
Genitourinary: Hyperuricemia (3%)
Neuromuscular & skeletal: Arthralgia (10%), weakness (9%), leg cramps (3%)
Respiratory: Rhinitis (10%), pharyngitis (6%), dyspnea (4%), pneumonia (4%)
Miscellaneous: Antibodies to teriparatide (3% of women in long-term treatment; hypersensitivity reactions or decreased efficacy were not associated in preclinical trials)

Overdosage/Toxicology No specific experience in overdose. Symptoms may include hypercalcemia, hypotension, headache, nausea, vomiting, and hypotension. Treatment is supportive (monitor serum calcium and phosphorus).

Pharmacodynamics/Kinetics
Half-Life Elimination: Serum: I.V.: 5 minutes; SubQ: 1 hour
Metabolism: Hepatic (nonspecific proteolysis)
Excretion: Urine (as metabolites)

Available Dosage Forms Injection, solution: 250 mcg/mL (3 mL) [prefilled syringe, delivers teriparatide 20 mcg/dose]

Dosing
Adults: Osteoporosis: SubQ: 20 mcg once daily; **Note:** Initial administration should occur under circumstances in which the patient may sit or lie down, in the event of orthostasis.

Renal Impairment: No dosage adjustment required. Bioavailability and half-life increase with Cl_{cr} <30 mL/minute.

Administration

Other: Administer by subcutaneous injection into the thigh or abdominal wall. Initial administration should occur under circumstances in which the patient may sit or lie down, in the event of orthostasis.

Stability

Storage: Store at 2°C to 8°C (36°F to 46°F). Protect from light. Do not freeze. Discard pen 28 days after first injection.

Laboratory Monitoring Serum calcium, serum phosphorus

Nursing Actions

Physical Assessment: Initial administration should occur where patient may sit or lie down, in the event of orthostasis. Monitor laboratory tests prior to and periodically during therapy. Monitor therapeutic effectiveness and adverse response at beginning of and regular intervals during therapy (eg, chest pain, hypotension, nausea, vomiting, arthralgia, leg cramps, dyspnea). Teach patient proper use (administration with injector "pen" and disposal), possible side effects/appropriate interventions (diet with adequate calcium and vitamin D), and adverse symptoms to report.

Patient Education: Do not take any new medication during therapy without consulting prescriber. Use injector pen and dispose of pen exactly as instructed (refer to Forteo™ user manual dispensed with the medication); rotate injection sites in thigh or abdominal wall. Sit when administering to reduce possibility of falling or injury. Avoid excess alcohol (may increase risk of osteoporosis) and follow dietary instructions of prescriber. May cause dizziness (use caution when driving or engaged in potentially hazardous tasks until response to drug is known); nausea, vomiting, or upset stomach (small frequent meals or frequent mouth care may help); muscle or skeletal pain, weakness, or cramping (consult prescriber for approved analgesic). Report chest pain or palpitations; respiratory difficulty; or other persistent adverse effects. **Pregnancy/breast-feeding precautions:** Inform prescriber if you are or intend to become pregnant. Breast-feeding is not recommended.

Geriatric Considerations No age-related differences in pharmacokinetics have been seen. In studies, no significant difference was seen in either efficacy or adverse effects between older patients and younger patients. Teriparatide should be considered as a last resort in patents who cannot tolerate or have not responded to other treatments for osteoporosis.

Breast-Feeding Issues Indicated for use in postmenopausal women. No studies have been conducted to determine excretion in breast milk. Not recommended for use in breast-feeding women.

Additional Information Teriparatide was formerly marketed as a diagnostic agent (Perithar™); that agent was withdrawn from the market in 1997. Teriparatide (Forteo™) is manufactured through recombinant DNA technology using a strain of *E. coli*.

Testolactone (tes toe LAK tone)

U.S. Brand Names Teslac®
Restrictions C-III
Pharmacologic Category Androgen
Medication Safety Issues
Sound-alike/look-alike issues:
Testolactone may be confused with testosterone
Pregnancy Risk Factor C
Lactation Excretion in breast milk unknown/not recommended

Use Palliative treatment of advanced or disseminated breast carcinoma

Mechanism of Action/Effect Testolactone is a synthetic testosterone derivative without significant androgen activity. The drug inhibits steroid aromatase activity, thereby blocking the production of estradiol and estrone from androgen precursors such as testosterone and androstenedione. Unfortunately, the enzymatic block provided by testolactone is transient and is usually limited to a period of 3 months.

Contraindications Hypersensitivity to testolactone or any component of the formulation; treatment of breast cancer in men

Warnings/Precautions Use with caution in hepatic, renal, or cardiac disease; prolonged use may cause drug-induced hepatic disease; history of porphyria. For use in postmenopausal women or in premenopausal women without ovarian function only. Safety and efficacy in pediatric patients have not been established.

Drug Interactions

Increased Effect/Toxicity: Increased effects of oral anticoagulants.

Lab Interactions Plasma estradiol concentrations by RIA

Adverse Reactions Frequency not defined.

Cardiovascular: Edema, blood pressure increased

Central nervous system: Malaise

Dermatologic: Maculopapular rash, alopecia (rare)

Endocrine & metabolic: Hypercalcemia

Gastrointestinal: Anorexia, diarrhea, nausea, edema of the tongue

Neuromuscular & skeletal: Paresthesias, peripheral neuropathies

Miscellaneous: Nail growth disturbance (rare)

Pharmacodynamics/Kinetics

Metabolism: Hepatic (forms metabolites)

Excretion: Urine

Available Dosage Forms Tablet: 50 mg

Dosing

Adults & Elderly: Breast carcinoma (palliative): Female: Oral: 250 mg 4 times/day for at least 3 months; desired response may take as long as 3 months.

Laboratory Monitoring Plasma calcium levels

Nursing Actions

Physical Assessment: For use in postmenopausal women or in premenopausal women without ovarian function only. May increase effects of oral anticoagulants. Monitor effectiveness of therapy, laboratory tests (calcium levels), and adverse reactions. Assess knowledge/teach patient appropriate use, possible side effects/appropriate interventions, and adverse symptoms to report.

Patient Education: Take as directed; do not discontinue without consulting prescriber. Effectiveness of therapy may take several months. Maintain adequate hydration (2-3 L/day of fluids) unless instructed to restrict fluid intake, and diet and exercise program recommended by prescriber. You may experience nausea or vomiting (small, frequent meals, frequent mouth care, sucking lozenges, or chewing gum may help). Report fluid retention (swelling of ankles, feet, or hands; respiratory difficulty or sudden weight gain); numbness, tingling, or swelling of fingers, toes, or face; skin rash, redness, or irritation; or other adverse reactions. **Pregnancy precaution:** Breast-feeding is not recommended.

Testosterone (tes TOS ter one)

U.S. Brand Names Androderm®; AndroGel®; Delatestryl®; Depo®-Testosterone; First® Testosterone; First® Testosterone MC; Striant®; Testim®; Testopel®

Synonyms Testosterone Cypionate; Testosterone Enanthate

Restrictions C-III

Pharmacologic Category Androgen

Medication Safety Issues
Sound-alike/look-alike issues:
Testosterone may be confused with testolactone
Testoderm® may be confused with Estraderm®

Transdermal patch may contain conducting metal (eg, aluminum); remove patch prior to MRI.

Pregnancy Risk Factor X

Lactation Enters breast milk/contraindicated

Use
Injection: Androgen replacement therapy in the treatment of delayed male puberty; male hypogonadism (primary or hypogonadotropic); inoperable female breast cancer (enanthate only)

Pellet: Androgen replacement therapy in the treatment of delayed male puberty; male hypogonadism (primary or hypogonadotropic)

Buccal, topical: Male hypogonadism (primary or hypogonadotropic)

Capsule (not available in U.S.): Management of congenital or acquired primary hypogonadism and hypogonadotropic hypogonadism; development and maintainenance of secondary sexual characteristics in males with testosterone deficiency; stimulation of puberty in carefully selected males with clearly delayed puberty not secondary to a pathological disorder; replacement therapy in syndromes with symptoms of deficiency or absence of endogenous testosterone; replacement therapy in impotence or for male climacteric symptoms when the conditions are due to a measured or documented androgen deficiency

Mechanism of Action/Effect Principal endogenous androgen responsible for promoting the growth and development of the male sex organs and maintaining secondary sex characteristics in androgen-deficient males

Contraindications Hypersensitivity to testosterone, soy, or any component of the formulation; males with carcinoma of the breast or prostate; pregnancy or women who may become pregnant

Systemic use is contraindicated in hepatic, renal, or cardiac disease; benign prostatic hyperplasia with obstruction; undiagnosed genital bleeding; hypercalcemia

Warnings/Precautions When used to treat delayed male puberty, perform radiographic examination of the hand and wrist every 6 months to determine the rate of bone maturation. May cause hypercalcemia in patients with prolonged immobilization. May accelerate bone maturation without producing compensating gain in linear growth. Has both androgenic and anabolic activity, the anabolic action may enhance hypoglycemia. Use caution in elderly patients or patients with other demographic factors which may increase the risk of prostatic carcinoma; careful monitoring is required. May cause fluid retention; use caution in patients with cardiovascular disease or other edematous conditions. Prolonged use of orally-active androgens has been associated with serious hepatic effects (hepatitis, hepatic neoplasms, cholestatic hepatitis, jaundice). May potentiate sleep apnea in some male patients (obesity or chronic lung disease). Transdermal patch may contain conducting metal (eg, aluminum); remove patch prior to MRI. Gels and buccal system have not been evaluated in males <18 years of age; safety and efficacy

of injection have not been established in males <12 years of age.

Drug Interactions
Cytochrome P450 Effect: Substrate (minor) of CYP2B6, 2C8/9, 2C19, 3A4; **Inhibits** CYP3A4 (weak)
Increased Effect/Toxicity: Testosterone may increase the effects warfarin.

Nutritional/Ethanol Interactions Herb/Nutraceutical: St John's wort may decrease testosterone levels.

Lab Interactions May cause a decrease in creatinine and creatine excretion and an increase in the excretion of 17-ketosteroids, thyroid function tests.

Adverse Reactions Frequency not defined.
Cardiovascular: Flushing, edema
Central nervous system: Excitation, aggressive behavior, sleeplessness, anxiety, mental depression, headache
Dermatologic: Hirsutism (increase in pubic hair growth), acne
Endocrine & metabolic: Menstrual problems (amenorrhea), virilism, breast soreness, gynecomastia, hypercalcemia, hypoglycemia
Gastrointestinal: Nausea, vomiting, GI irritation
Following buccal administration: Bitter taste, gum edema, gum or mouth irritation, gum tenderness, taste perversion
Genitourinary: Bladder irritability, epididymitis, impotence, priapism, prostatic carcinoma, prostatic hyperplasia, PSA increased (up to 18%), testicular atrophy, urination impaired
Hepatic: Hepatic dysfunction, cholestatic hepatitis, hepatic necrosis
Hematologic: Leukopenia, polycythemia, suppression of clotting factors
Miscellaneous: Hypersensitivity reactions

Pharmacodynamics/Kinetics
Duration of Action: Route and ester dependent; I.M.: Cypionate and enanthate esters have longest duration, ≤2-4 weeks
Protein Binding: 98% bound to sex hormone-binding globulin (40%) and albumin
Half-Life Elimination: 10-100 minutes
Metabolism: Hepatic; forms metabolites, including dihydrotestosterone (DHT) and estradiol (both active)
Excretion: Urine (90%); feces (6%)

Available Dosage Forms [CAN] = Canadian brand name
Capsule, gelatin, as deconate (Andriol™ [CAN]): 40 mg (10s) [not available in U.S.]
Gel, topical:
AndroGel®:
1.25 g/actuation (75 g) [1% metered-dose pump; delivers 5 g/4 actuations; provides 60 1.25 g actuations; contains ethanol]
2.5 g (30s) [1% unit dose packets; contains ethanol]
5 g (30s) [1% unit dose packets; contains ethanol]
Testim®: 5 g (30s) [1% unit-dose tube; contains ethanol]
Injection, in oil, as cypionate: 200 mg/mL (10 mL)
Depo®-Testosterone: 100 mg/mL (10 mL); 200 mg/mL (1 mL, 10 mL) [contains benzyl alcohol, benzyl benzoate, and cottonseed oil]
Injection, in oil, as enanthate: 200 mg/mL (5 mL)
Delatestryl®: 200 mg/mL (1 mL) [prefilled syringe; contains sesame oil]; (5 mL) [multidose vial; contains sesame oil]
Kit [for prescription compounding testosterone 2%; kits also contain mixing jar and stirrer]:
First® Testosterone:
Injection, in oil: Testosterone propionate 100 mg/mL (12 mL) [contains sesame oil and benzyl alcohol]
Ointment: White petroleum (48 g)
First® Testosterone MC:
Injection, in oil: Testosterone propionate 100 mg/mL (12 mL) [contains sesame oil and benzyl alcohol]
Cream: Moisturizing cream (48 g)

Mucoadhesive, for buccal application [buccal system] (Striant®): 30 mg (10s)

Pellet, for subcutaneous implantation (Testopel®): 75 mg (1 pellet/vial)

Transdermal system (Androderm®): 2.5 mg/day (60s); 5 mg/day (30s) [contains ethanol]

Dosing

Adults & Elderly:

Inoperable breast cancer (females): I.M.: Testosterone enanthate: 200-400 mg every 2-4 weeks

Male hypogonadism or hypogonadotropic hypogonadism:

Oral (buccal): 30 mg twice daily (every 12 hours) applied to the gum region above the incisor tooth

Capsule (Andriol®; not available in U.S.): Initial: 120-160 mg/day in 2 divided doses for 2-3 weeks; adjust according to individual response; usual maintenance dose: 40-120 mg/day (in divided doses)

I.M. (cypionate or enanthate ester): 50-400 mg every 2-4 weeks

Pellet (for subcutaneous implantation): 150-450 mg every 3-6 months

Transdermal:

Androderm®: Initial: Apply 5 mg/day once nightly to clean, dry area on the back, abdomen, upper arms, or thighs (do **not** apply to scrotum); dosing range: 2.5-7.5 mg/day; in nonvirilized patients, dose may be initiated at 2.5 mg/day

AndroGel®, Testim®: 5 g (to deliver 50 mg of testosterone with 5 mg systemically absorbed) applied once daily (preferably in the morning) to clean, dry, intact skin of the shoulder and upper arms. AndroGel® may also be applied to the abdomen. Dosage may be increased to a maximum of 10 g (100 mg). **(Do not apply testosterone gel to the genitals.)**

Delayed puberty in males:

I.M. (cypionate or enanthate ester): 50-200 mg every 2-4 weeks for a limited duration

Pellet (for subcutaneous implantation): 150-450 mg every 3-6 months

Pediatrics: Adolescents:

Male hypogonadism:

I.M.:

Initiation of pubertal growth: 40-50 mg/m²/dose (cypionate or enanthate ester) monthly until the growth rate falls to prepubertal levels

Terminal growth phase: 100 mg/m²/dose (cypionate or enanthate ester) monthly until growth ceases

Maintenance virilizing dose: 100 mg/m²/dose (cypionate or enanthate ester) twice monthly

SubQ: Pellet (for subcutaneous implantation): Refer to adult dosing.

Delayed puberty in males:

I.M.: 40-50 mg/m²/dose monthly (cypionate or enanthate ester) for 6 months

SubQ: Pellet (for subcutaneous implantation): Refer to adult dosing.

Oral capsule (Andriol®; not available in U.S.): Refer to adult dosing;

Hepatic Impairment: Reduce dose.

Administration

Oral:

Oral, buccal application (Striant®): One mucoadhesive for buccal application (buccal system) should be applied to a comfortable area above the incisor tooth. Apply flat side of system to gum. Rotate to alternate sides of mouth with each application. Hold buccal system firmly in place for 30 seconds to ensure adhesion. The buccal system should adhere to gum for 12 hours. If the buccal system falls out, replace with a new system. If the system falls out within 4 hours of next dose, the new buccal system should remain in place until the time of the following

scheduled dose. System will soften and mold to shape of gum as it absorbs moisture from mouth. Do not chew or swallow the buccal system. The buccal system will not dissolve; gently remove by sliding downwards from gum; avoid scratching gum.

Oral, capsule (Andriol®; not available in the U.S.): Should be administered with meals. Should be swallowed whole; do not crush or chew.

I.M.: Warm injection to room temperature and shaking vial will help redissolve crystals that have formed after storage. Administer by deep I.M. injection into the upper outer quadrant of the gluteus maximus.

Topical:

Transdermal patch: Androderm®: Apply patch to clean, dry area of skin on the arm, back, or upper buttocks. Following patch removal, mild skin irritation may be treated with OTC hydrocortisone cream. A small amount of triamcinolone acetonide 0.1% cream may be applied under the system to decrease irritation; do not use ointment. Patch should be applied nightly. Rotate administration sites, allowing 7 days between applying to the same site.

Gel: AndroGel®, Testim®: Apply gel (preferably in the morning) to clean, dry, intact skin of the shoulder and upper arms (AndroGel® may also be applied to the abdomen). Upon opening the packet(s), the entire contents should be squeezed into the palm of the hand and immediately applied to the application site(s). Alternatively, a portion may be squeezed onto palm of hand and applied, repeating the process until entire packet has been applied. Application sites should be allowed to dry for a few minutes prior to dressing. Hands should be washed with soap and water after application. **Do not apply testosterone gel to the genitals.** For optimal absorption, after application wait at least 5-6 hours prior to showering or swimming; however waiting at least 1 hour should have minimal affect on absorption if done infrequently. Alcohol-based gels are flammable; avoid fire or smoking until gel has dried.

Stability

Storage:

Androderm®: Store at room temperature. Do not store outside of pouch. Excessive heat may cause system to burst.

AndroGel®, Delatestryl®, Striant®, Testim®: Store at room temperature.

Depo® Testosterone: Store at room temperature. Protect from light.

Testopel®: Store in a cool location.

Laboratory Monitoring Periodic liver function tests, PSA, cholesterol, hemoglobin and hematocrit; radiologic examination of wrist and hand every 6 months (when using in prepubertal children)

Androderm®: Morning serum testosterone levels following application the previous evening

Gel: Morning serum testosterone levels 14 days after start of therapy

Nursing Actions

Physical Assessment: (For use in children see pediatric reference). See Contraindications and Warnings/Precautions for use cautions. Assess potential for interactions with other prescriptions, OTC medications, or herbal products patient may be taking (see Drug Interactions). Monitor laboratory tests, therapeutic effectiveness (according to purpose for use), and adverse reactions (see Adverse Reactions and Overdose/Toxicology) regularly during therapy. Caution patients with diabetes - may cause hypoglycemic reaction. Teach patient proper use (according to formulation), possible side effects/appropriate interventions, and adverse symptoms to report (see Patient Education). **Pregnancy risk factor X** - determine that patient is not pregnant before beginning treatment. Instruct patients of childbearing age or (Continued)

Testosterone *(Continued)*

males who may have intercourse with women of child-bearing age on appropriate barrier contraceptive measures. Breast-feeding is contraindicated.

Patient Education: If you have diabetes, monitor serum glucose closely and notify prescriber of changes; this medication may alter hypoglycemic requirements. You may experience acne, growth of body hair, loss of libido, impotence, or menstrual irregularity (usually reversible); nausea or vomiting (small frequent meals, frequent mouth care, sucking lozenges, or chewing gum may help). Report changes in menstrual pattern; enlarged or painful breasts; deepening of voice or unusual growth of body hair; persistent penile erection; fluid retention (swelling of ankles, feet, or hands, respiratory difficulty or sudden weight gain); unresolved changes in CNS (nervousness, chills, insomnia, depression, aggressiveness); altered urinary patterns; change in color of urine or stool; yellowing of eyes or skin; unusual bruising or bleeding; or other persistent adverse reactions.

Transdermal: Androderm®: Apply patch to clean, dry area of skin on the arm, back, or upper buttocks.

Topical gel: AndroGel®, Testim®: Apply gel (preferably in the morning) to clean, dry, intact skin of the shoulder and upper arms (AndroGel® may also be applied to the abdomen). Upon opening the packet(s), the entire contents should be squeezed into the palm of the hand and immediately applied to the application site(s). Alternatively, a portion may be squeezed onto palm of hand and applied, repeating the process until entire packet has been applied. Gel is flammable. Application sites should be allowed to dry for a few minutes prior to dressing. Hands should be washed with soap and water after application. **Do not apply testosterone gel to the genitals.**

Pregnancy/breast-feeding precautions: Inform prescriber if you are pregnant. Do not get pregnant during or for 1 month following therapy. Male: Do not cause a female to become pregnant. Male/female: Consult prescriber for instruction on appropriate contraceptive measures. This drug may cause severe fetal defects. Do not breast-feed.

Dietary Considerations Testosterone USP may be synthesized from soy. Food and beverages have not been found to interfere with buccal system; ensure system is in place following eating, drinking, or brushing teeth.

Geriatric Considerations Geriatric patients may have an increased risk of prostatic hyperplasia or prostatic carcinoma.

Pregnancy Issues Testosterone may cause adverse effects, including masculinization of the female fetus, if used during pregnancy. Females who are or may become pregnant should also avoid skin-to-skin contact to areas where testosterone has been applied topically on another person.

Tetracycline *(tet ra SYE kleen)*

U.S. Brand Names Sumycin®

Synonyms Achromycin; TCN; Tetracycline Hydrochloride

Pharmacologic Category Antibiotic, Tetracycline Derivative

Medication Safety Issues
Sound-alike/look-alike issues:
Tetracycline may be confused with tetradecyl sulfate
Achromycin may be confused with actinomycin, Adriamycin PFS®

Pregnancy Risk Factor D

Lactation Enters breast milk/not recommended (AAP rates "compatible")

Use Treatment of susceptible bacterial infections of both gram-positive and gram-negative organisms; also infections due to *Mycoplasma*, *Chlamydia*, and *Rickettsia*; indicated for acne, exacerbations of chronic bronchitis, and treatment of gonorrhea and syphilis in patients that are allergic to penicillin; as part of a multidrug regimen for *H. pylori* eradication to reduce the risk of duodenal ulcer recurrence

Mechanism of Action/Effect Inhibits protein synthesis of susceptible bacteria; bacteriostatic - causes call death.

Contraindications Hypersensitivity to tetracycline or any component of the formulation; do not administer to children ≤8 years of age; pregnancy

Warnings/Precautions Use of tetracyclines during tooth development may cause permanent discoloration of the teeth and enamel, hypoplasia and retardation of skeletal development and bone growth with risk being the greatest for children <4 years and those receiving high doses; use with caution in patients with renal or hepatic impairment (eg, elderly); dosage modification required in patients with renal impairment since it may increase BUN as an antianabolic agent; pseudotumor cerebri has been reported with tetracycline use (usually resolves with discontinuation); outdated drug can cause nephropathy; superinfection possible; use protective measure to avoid photosensitivity

Drug Interactions

Cytochrome P450 Effect: Substrate of CYP3A4 (major); **Inhibits** CYP3A4 (moderate)

Decreased Effect: Calcium, magnesium- or aluminum-containing antacids, iron, zinc, sodium bicarbonate, sucralfate, didanosine, or quinapril may decrease tetracycline absorption. Therapeutic effect of penicillins may be reduced with coadministration of tetracycline. Although anecdotal reports suggest oral contraceptive efficacy could be reduced by tetracyclines, this has been refuted by more rigorous scientific and clinical data. The levels/effects of tetracycline may be decreased by aminoglutethimide, carbamazepine, nafcillin, nevirapine, phenobarbital, phenytoin, rifamycins, and other CYP3A4 inducers.

Increased Effect/Toxicity: Methoxyflurane anesthesia when concurrent with tetracycline may cause fatal nephrotoxicity. Warfarin with tetracyclines may cause increased anticoagulation. Tetracycline may increase the levels/effects of selected benzodiazepines, calcium channel blockers, cisapride, cyclosporine, ergot alkaloids, selected HMG-CoA reductase inhibitors, mirtazapine, nateglinide, nefazodone, pimozide, quinidine, sildenafil (and other PDE-5 inhibitors), tacrolimus, venlafaxine, and other CYP3A4 substrates.

Nutritional/Ethanol Interactions

Food: Tetracycline serum concentrations may be decreased if taken with dairy products.

Herb/Nutraceutical: Avoid dong quai, St John's wort (may also cause photosensitization)

Lab Interactions False-negative urine glucose with Clinistix®

Adverse Reactions Frequency not defined.

Cardiovascular: Pericarditis

Central nervous system: Intracranial pressure increased, bulging fontanels in infants, pseudotumor cerebri, paresthesia

Dermatologic: Photosensitivity, pruritus, pigmentation of nails, exfoliative dermatitis

Endocrine & metabolic: Diabetes insipidus syndrome

Gastrointestinal: Discoloration of teeth and enamel hypoplasia (young children), nausea, diarrhea, vomiting, esophagitis, anorexia, abdominal cramps, antibiotic-associated pseudomembranous colitis, staphylococcal enterocolitis, pancreatitis

Hematologic: Thrombophlebitis

Hepatic: Hepatotoxicity

Renal: Acute renal failure, azotemia, renal damage

Miscellaneous: Superinfection, anaphylaxis, hypersensitivity reactions, candidal superinfection

Overdosage/Toxicology Symptoms of overdose include nausea, anorexia, and diarrhea. Treatment is supportive.

Pharmacodynamics/Kinetics

Time to Peak: Serum: Oral: 2-4 hours

Protein Binding: ~65%

Half-Life Elimination: Normal renal function: 8-11 hours; End-stage renal disease: 57-108 hours

Excretion: Urine (60% as unchanged drug); feces (as active form)

Available Dosage Forms

Capsule, as hydrochloride: 250 mg, 500 mg

Suspension, oral, as hydrochloride (Sumycin®): 125 mg/5 mL (480 mL) [contains sodium benzoate and sodium metabisulfite; fruit flavor]

Tablet, as hydrochloride (Sumycin®): 250 mg, 500 mg

Dosing

Adults & Elderly: Antibacterial: Oral:

Systemic infection: Oral: 250-500 mg/dose every 6 hours

Peptic ulcer disease: Eradication of *Helicobacter pylori*: 500 mg 2-4 times/day depending on regimen; requires combination therapy with at least one other antibiotic and an acid-suppressing agent (proton pump inhibitor or H_2 blocker)

Periodontitis: 250 mg every 6 hours until improvement (usually 10 days)

Pediatrics: Antibacterial, systemic: Children >8 years: Oral: 25-50 mg/kg/day in divided doses every 6 hours

Renal Impairment:

Cl_{cr} 50-80 mL/minute: Administer every 8-12 hours.

Cl_{cr} 10-50 mL/minute: Administer every 12-24 hours.

Cl_{cr} <10 mL/minute: Administer every 24 hours.

Slightly dialyzable (5% to 20%) via hemo- and peritoneal dialysis or via continuous arteriovenous or venovenous hemofiltration; supplemental dose is not necessary.

Hepatic Impairment: Avoid use or maximum dose is 1 g/day.

Administration

Oral: Oral should be given on an empty stomach (ie, 1 hour prior to, or 2 hours after meals) to increase total absorption. Administer at least 1-2 hours prior to, or 4 hours after antacid because aluminum and magnesium cations may chelate with tetracycline and reduce its total absorption. Administer around-the-clock to promote less variation in peak and trough serum levels.

Stability

Storage: Outdated tetracyclines have caused a Fanconi-like syndrome (nausea, vomiting, acidosis, proteinuria, glycosuria, aminoaciduria, polydipsia, polyuria, hypokalemia). Protect oral dosage forms from light.

Laboratory Monitoring Renal, hepatic, and hematologic function; WBC. Perform culture and sensitivity studies prior to initiating therapy to determine the causative organism and its susceptibility to tetracycline.

Nursing Actions

Physical Assessment: Assess effectiveness and interactions of other medications patient may be taking (see Drug Interactions). Monitor laboratory tests, therapeutic response, and adverse reactions (see Adverse Reactions) at beginning of therapy and periodically throughout therapy. Assess knowledge/teach patient appropriate use, interventions to reduce side effects, and adverse symptoms to report (see Patient Education). **Pregnancy risk factor B/D** - see Pregnancy Risk Factor for use cautions - assess knowledge/instruct patient on need to use appropriate barrier contraceptive measures and the need to avoid pregnancy. See Lactation for breast-feeding considerations.

Patient Education: Take this medication exactly as directed. Take all of the prescription even if you see an improvement in your condition. Do not use more or more often than recommended. Preferable to take on an empty stomach, 1 hour before or 2 hours after meals. Take at regularly scheduled times, around-the-clock. Avoid antacids, iron, or dairy products within 2 hours of taking tetracycline. You may experience photosensitivity (use sunscreen, wear protective clothing and eyewear, and avoid direct sunlight); dizziness or lightheadedness (use caution when driving or engaging in tasks requiring alertness until response to drug is known); or nausea/vomiting (small, frequent meals, frequent mouth care, chewing gum, or sucking lozenges may help). Report rash or intense itching, yellowing of skin or eyes, fever or chills, blackened stool, vaginal itching or discharge, foul-smelling stools, excessive thirst or urination, acute headache, unresolved diarrhea, respiratory difficulty, condition does not improve, or worsening of condition. **Pregnancy/breast-feeding precautions:** Do not get pregnant while taking this medication. Use appropriate barrier contraceptive measures. Breast-feeding is not recommended.

Geriatric Considerations The role of tetracycline has decreased because of the emergence of resistant organisms. Doxycycline is the tetracycline of choice when one is indicated because of its better GI absorption, less interactions with divalent cations, longer half-life, and the fact that the majority is cleared by nonrenal mechanisms.

Breast-Feeding Issues Negligible absorption by infant; potential to stain infants' unerupted teeth

Pregnancy Issues Tetracyclines cross the placenta and enter fetal circulation; may cause permanent discoloration of teeth if used during the last half of pregnancy.

Related Information

Compatibility of Drugs *on page 1370*

Thalidomide (tha LI doe mide)

U.S. Brand Names Thalomid®

Synonyms NSC-66847

Restrictions Thalidomide is approved for marketing only under a special distribution program. This program, called the "System for Thalidomide Education and Prescribing Safety" (STEPS® 1-888-423-5436), has been approved by the FDA. Prescribers and pharmacists must be registered with the program. No more than a 4-week supply should be dispensed. Blister packs should be dispensed intact (do not repackage capsules). Prescriptions must be filled within 7 days. Subsequent prescriptions may be filled only if fewer than 7 days of therapy remain on the previous prescription. A new prescription is required for further dispensing (a telephone prescription may not be accepted).

Pharmacologic Category Angiogenesis Inhibitor; Immunosuppressant Agent; Tumor Necrosis Factor (TNF) Blocking Agent

Medication Safety Issues

Sound-alike/look-alike issues:

Thalidomide may be confused with flutamide

Pregnancy Risk Factor X

Lactation Excretion in breast milk unknown/not recommended

Use Treatment and maintenance of cutaneous manifestations of erythema nodosum leprosum (ENL)

Unlabeled/Investigational Use Treatment of multiple myeloma; Crohn's disease; graft-versus-host reactions after bone marrow transplantation; AIDS-related aphthous stomatitis; Behçet's syndrome; Waldenström's

(Continued)

Thalidomide (Continued)

macroglobulinemia; Langerhans cell histiocytosis; may be effective in rheumatoid arthritis, discoid lupus erythematosus, and erythema multiforme

Mechanism of Action/Effect A derivative of glutethimide; mode of action for immunosuppression is unclear; inhibition of neutrophil chemotaxis and decreased monocyte phagocytosis may occur; may cause 50% to 80% reduction of tumor necrosis factor - alpha.

Contraindications Hypersensitivity to thalidomide or any component of the formulation; neuropathy (peripheral); patient unable to comply with STEPS® program; women of childbearing potential unless alternative therapies are inappropriate and adequate precautions are taken to avoid pregnancy; pregnancy

Warnings/Precautions Hazardous agent — use appropriate precautions for handling and disposal. Thalidomide is a known teratogen; effective contraception must be used for at least 4 weeks before initiating therapy, during therapy, and for 4 weeks following discontinuation of thalidomide for women of childbearing potential. Use caution with drugs which may decrease the efficacy of hormonal contraceptives. May cause sedation; patients must be warned to use caution when performing tasks which require alertness. Use caution in patients with renal or hepatic impairment, neurological disorders, or constipation.

Thalidomide has been associated with the development of peripheral neuropathy, which may be irreversible; use caution with other medications which may cause peripheral neuropathy. Consider immediate discontinuation (if clinically appropriate) in patients who develop neuropathy. May cause seizures; use caution in patients with a history of seizures, concurrent therapy with drugs which alter seizure threshold, or conditions which predispose to seizures. May cause neutropenia; discontinue therapy if absolute neutrophil count decreases to <750/mm³. Use caution in patients with HIV infection; has been associated with increased viral loads.

May cause orthostasis and/or bradycardia; use with caution in patients with cardiovascular disease or in patients who would not tolerate transient hypotensive episodes. Thrombotic events have been reported (generally in patients with other risk factors for thrombosis [neoplastic disease, inflammatory disease, or concurrent therapy with other drugs which may cause thrombosis]). Hypersensitivity, Stevens-Johnson syndrome (SJS) and toxic epidermal necrolyis (TEN) have been reported; withhold therapy and evaluate with skin rashes; permanently discontinued if rash is exfoliative, purpuric, bullous or if SJS or TEN is suspected. Safety and efficacy have not been established in children <12 years of age.

Drug Interactions

Decreased Effect: Thalidomide may decrease the effect of vaccines (dead organisms).

Increased Effect/Toxicity: Thalidomide may enhance the sedative activity of other drugs such as ethanol, barbiturates, reserpine, and chlorpromazine. Thalidomide may be associated with increased risk of serious infection when used in combination with abatacept or anakinra. Thalidomide may increase the risk of vaccinal infection with vaccine (live organism).

Nutritional/Ethanol Interactions

Ethanol: Avoid ethanol (may increase sedation).

Herb/Nutraceutical: Avoid cat's claw and echinacea (have immunostimulant properties; consider therapy modifications).

Adverse Reactions

Controlled clinical trials: ENL:
>10%:
Central nervous system: Somnolence (38%), headache (13%)
Dermatologic: Rash (21%)

1% to 10%:
Cardiovascular: Facial edema (4%), peripheral edema (4%)
Central nervous system: Malaise (8%), pain (8%), vertigo (8%), dizziness (4%)
Dermatologic: Pruritus (8%), dermatitis (fungal) (4%), maculopapular rash (4%), nail disorder (4%)
Gastrointestinal: Constipation (4%), diarrhea, (4%) nausea (4%), oral moniliasis (4%), tooth pain (4%)
Genitourinary: Impotence (8%)
Neuromuscular & skeletal: Weakness (8%), back pain (4%), neck pain (4%), neck rigidity (4%), tremor (4%)
Respiratory: Pharyngitis (4%), rhinitis (4%), sinusitis (4%)

HIV-seropositive:
General: An increased viral load has been noted in patients treated with thalidomide. This is of uncertain clinical significance - see Monitoring Parameters
>10%:
Central nervous system: Somnolence (36% to 38%), dizziness (19%), fever (19% to 22%), headache (17% to 19%)
Dermatologic: Rash (25%), maculopapular rash (17% to 19%), acne (3% to 11%)
Gastrointestinal: Diarrhea (11% to 19%), nausea (13%), oral moniliasis (6% to 11%)
Hematologic: Leukopenia (17% to 25%), anemia (6% to 13%), lymphadenopathy (6% to 13%)
Hepatic: AST increased (3% to 13%)
Neuromuscular & skeletal: Paresthesia (may be severe and/or irreversible) (6% to 16%), weakness (6% to 22%)
Renal: Hematuria (11%)
Miscellaneous: Diaphoresis (13%), lymphadenopathy (6% to 13%)
1% to 10%:
Cardiovascular: Peripheral edema (3% to 8%)
Central nervous system: Nervousness (3% to 9%), insomnia (9%), agitation (9%), pain (3%)
Dermatologic: Dermatitis (fungal) (6% to 9%), nail disorder (3%), pruritus (3% to 6%)
Endocrine & metabolic: Hyperlipemia (6% to 9%)
Gastrointestinal: Anorexia (3% to 9%), constipation (3% to 9%), xerostomia (8% to 9%), flatulence (8%)
Genitourinary: Impotence (3%)
Hepatic: LFTs abnormal (9%)
Neuromuscular & skeletal: Neuropathy (8%), back pain (6%)
Renal: Albuminuria (3% to 8%)
Respiratory: Pharyngitis (6% to 8%), sinusitis (3% to 8%)
Miscellaneous: Accidental injury (6%), infection (6% to 8%)

Overdosage/Toxicology Doses of up to 14.4 g have been reported (in suicide attempts) without fatalities. Treatment is symptom-directed and supportive.

Pharmacodynamics/Kinetics

Time to Peak: Plasma: 3-6 hours

Protein Binding: 55% to 66%

Half-Life Elimination: 5-7 hours

Metabolism: Nonenzymatic hydrolysis in plasma; forms multiple metabolites

Excretion: Urine (<1% as unchanged drug)

Available Dosage Forms Capsule: 50 mg, 100 mg, 200 mg

Dosing

Adults & Elderly:

Cutaneous ENL: Oral:

Initial: 100-300 mg/day taken once daily at bedtime with water (at least 1 hour after evening meal)

Adjustments to initial dose:
Patients weighing <50 kg: Initiate at lower end of the dosing range
Severe cutaneous reaction or patients previously requiring high dose: May be initiated at 400 mg/day; doses may be divided, but taken 1 hour after meals
Duration and tapering/maintenance:
Dosing should continue until active reaction subsides (usually at least 2 weeks), then tapered in 50 mg decrements every 2-4 weeks
Note: Patients who flare during tapering or with a history or requiring prolonged maintenance should be maintained on the minimum dosage necessary to control the reaction. Efforts to taper should be repeated every 3-6 months, in increments of 50 mg every 2-4 weeks.

Behçet's syndrome (unlabeled use): Oral: 100-400 mg/day

Graft-vs-host reactions (unlabeled use): Oral: 100-1600 mg/day; usual initial dose: 200 mg 4 times/day for use up to 700 days

AIDS-related aphthous stomatitis (unlabeled use): Oral: 200 mg twice daily for 5 days, then 200 mg/day for up to 8 weeks

Discoid lupus erythematosus (unlabeled use): Oral: 100-400 mg/day; maintenance dose: 25-50 mg

Pediatrics: Graft-vs-host reactions (unlabeled use): Oral: Children: 3 mg/kg 4 times/day

Administration

Oral: Avoid extensive handling of capsules; capsules should remain in blister pack until ingestion. If exposed to the powder content from broken capsules or body fluids from patients receiving thalidomide, the exposed area should be washed with soap and water.

Stability
Storage: Store at 15°C to 30°C (50°F to 86°F). Protect from light. Keep in original package.

Laboratory Monitoring Pregnancy testing (sensitivity of at least 50 mIU/mL) is required within 24 hours prior to initiation of therapy, weekly during the first 4 weeks, then every 4 weeks in women with regular menstrual cycles or every 2 weeks in women with irregular menstrual cycles. In HIV-seropositive patients; monitor viral load after 1 and 3 months, then every 3 months. CBC initially and periodically during therapy. Consider monitoring of sensory nerve application potential amplitudes at baseline and every 6 months to detect asymptomatic neuropathy.

Nursing Actions

Physical Assessment: Patient must be capable of complying with STEPS® program (see Use). Instruct patient on risks of pregnancy, appropriate contraceptive measures (see Patient Education), and necessity for frequent pregnancy testing (schedule pregnancy testing at time of dispensing and give patient schedule in writing). Assess other medications patient may be taking for possible interactions (see Drug Interactions). Monitor closely for signs of neuropathy (ie, numbness, tingling, and pain in extremities), CNS depression, and altered blood counts. Instruct patient on signs and symptoms to report (see Patient Education) and and appropriate interventions for adverse reactions.

Pregnancy risk factor X: Pregnancy test is required within 24 hours prior to beginning therapy, weekly during first month of therapy, and monthly thereafter for all women of childbearing age. Effective contraception with at least two reliable forms of contraception must be used for 1 month prior to beginning therapy, during therapy, and for 1 month following discontinuance of therapy. Women who have undergone a hysterectomy or have been postmenopausal for at least 24 consecutive months are the only exception. Do not prescribe, administer, or dispense to women of childbearing age or males who may have intercourse with women of childbearing age unless both female and male are capable of complying with contraceptive measures. Even males who have undergone vasectomy must acknowledge these risks in writing. Oral and written warnings concerning contraception and the hazards of thalidomide must be conveyed to females and males and they must acknowledge their understanding in writing. Parents or guardians must consent and sign acknowledgment for patients between 12 and 18 years of age following therapy. Breast-feeding is contraindicated.

Patient Education: You will be given oral and written instructions about the necessity of using two methods of contraception and the necessity of keeping return visits for pregnancy testing. Do not donate blood while taking this medicine. Male patients should not donate sperm. Avoid extensive handling of capsules; capsules should remain in blister pack until ingestion. If exposed to the powder content from broken capsules or body fluids from patients receiving thalidomide, the exposed area should be washed with soap and water. You may experience postural hypotension (use caution when rising from lying or sitting position); sleepiness; dizziness; headaches; lack of concentration (use caution when driving, climbing stairs, or engaging in tasks requiring alertness until response to drug is known); nausea or vomiting or loss of appetite (small frequent meals, frequent mouth care, chewing gum, or sucking lozenges may help); constipation or diarrhea; oral thrush (frequent mouth care is necessary); or sexual dysfunction (reversible). Report any of the above if persistent or severe. Report chest pain or palpitations or swelling of extremities; back, neck, or muscle pain or stiffness; numbness or pain in extremities; skin rash or eruptions; increased nervousness, anxiety, or insomnia; or any other symptom of adverse reactions. **Pregnancy/breast-feeding precautions:** Do not get pregnant (females) or cause pregnancy (males) during treatment. The use of two forms of contraception are required for 1 month prior to therapy, during therapy, and for 1 month following discontinuation of therapy. Pregnancy tests are routinely conducted during therapy. Do not breast-feed while taking this medication or for 1 month following discontinuation.

Dietary Considerations Should be taken at least 1 hour after the evening meal.

Breast-Feeding Issues Due to the potential for serious adverse reactions in the infant, a decision should be made to discontinue nursing or discontinue treatment with thalidomide.

Pregnancy Issues Embryotoxic with limb defects noted from the 27th to 40th gestational day of exposure; all cases of phocomelia occur from the 27th to 42nd gestational day; fetal cardiac, gastrointestinal, and genitourinary tract abnormalities have also been described. Either abstinence or two forms of effective contraception must be used for at least 4 weeks before initiating therapy, during therapy, and for 4 weeks following discontinuation of thalidomide. A negative pregnancy test (sensitivity of at least 50 mIU/mL) within 24 hours prior to beginning therapy, weekly during the first 4 weeks, and every 4 weeks (every 2 weeks for women with irregular menstrual cycles) thereafter is required for women of childbearing potential. Males (even those vasectomized) must use a latex condom during any sexual contact with women of childbearing age. Risk to the fetus from semen of male patients is unknown. Thalidomide must be immediately discontinued and the patient referred to a reproductive toxicity specialist if pregnancy occurs during treatment. Any suspected fetal exposure to thalidomide must be reported to the FDA via the MedWatch program (1-800-FDA-1088) and to Celgene Corporation (1-888-423-5436).

Theophylline (thee OFF i lin)

U.S. Brand Names Elixophyllin®; Quibron®-T; Quibron®-T/SR; Theo-24®; Theochron®; Theolair™; Theolair-SR® [DSC]; T-Phyl®; Uniphyl®

Synonyms Theophylline Anhydrous

Pharmacologic Category Theophylline Derivative

Medication Safety Issues
Sound-alike/look-alike issues:
Theolair™ may be confused with Thiola®, Thyrolar®

Pregnancy Risk Factor C

Lactation Enters breast milk/compatible (AAP rates "compatible")

Use Treatment of symptoms and reversible airway obstruction due to chronic asthma, chronic bronchitis, or COPD

Mechanism of Action/Effect Causes bronchodilatation, diuresis, CNS and cardiac stimulation, and gastric acid secretion by blocking phosphodiesterase which increases tissue concentrations of cyclic adenine monophosphate (cAMP) which in turn promotes catecholamine stimulation of lipolysis, glycogenolysis, and gluconeogenesis and induces release of epinephrine from adrenal medulla cells.

Contraindications Hypersensitivity to theophylline or any component of the formulation; premixed injection may contain corn-derived dextrose and its use is contraindicated in patients with allergy to corn-related products

Warnings/Precautions If a patient develops signs and symptoms of theophylline toxicity (eg, persistent, repetitive vomiting), a serum theophylline level should be measured and subsequent doses held. Due to potential saturation of theophylline clearance at serum levels in or (in some patients) less than the therapeutic range, dosage adjustment should be made in small increments (maximum: 25%). Due to wider interpatient variability, theophylline serum level measurements must be used to optimize therapy and prevent serious toxicity. Use with caution in patients with peptic ulcer, hyperthyroidism, seizure disorders, hypertension, and patients with cardiac arrhythmias (excluding bradyarrhythmias).

Drug Interactions
Cytochrome P450 Effect: Substrate of CYP1A2 (major), 2C8/9 (minor), 2D6 (minor), 2E1 (major), 3A4 (major); **Inhibits** CYP1A2 (weak)

Decreased Effect: CYP1A2 inducers may decrease the levels/effects of theophylline; example inducers include aminoglutethimide, carbamazepine, phenobarbital, and rifampin. CYP3A4 inducers may decrease the levels/effects of theophylline; example inducers include aminoglutethimide, carbamazepine, nafcillin, nevirapine, phenobarbital, phenytoin, and rifamycins.

Increased Effect/Toxicity: CYP1A2 inhibitors may increase the levels/effects of theophylline; example inhibitors include amiodarone, ciprofloxacin, fluvoxamine, ketoconazole, norfloxacin, ofloxacin, and rofecoxib. CYP2E1 inhibitors may increase the levels/effects of theophylline; example inhibitors include disulfiram, isoniazid, and miconazole. Changes in diet may affect the elimination of theophylline. CYP3A4 inhibitors may increase the levels/effects of theophylline; example inhibitors include azole antifungals, clarithromycin, diclofenac, doxycycline, erythromycin, imatinib, isoniazid, nefazodone, nicardipine, propofol, protease inhibitors, quinidine, telithromycin, and verapamil.

Nutritional/Ethanol Interactions Food: Food does not appreciably affect the absorption of liquid, fast-release products, and most sustained release products; however, food may induce a sudden release (dose-dumping) of once-daily sustained release products resulting in an increase in serum drug levels and potential toxicity. Avoid excessive amounts of caffeine. Avoid extremes of dietary protein and carbohydrate intake. Changes in diet may affect the elimination of theophylline; charbroiled foods may increase elimination, reducing half-life by 50%.

Adverse Reactions
Adverse reactions/theophylline serum level: (Adverse effects do not necessarily occur according to serum levels. Arrhythmia and seizure can occur without seeing the other adverse effects).
15-25 mcg/mL: GI upset, diarrhea, nausea/vomiting, abdominal pain, nervousness, headache, insomnia, agitation, dizziness, muscle cramp, tremor
25-35 mcg/mL: Tachycardia, occasional PVC
>35 mcg/mL: Ventricular tachycardia, frequent PVC, seizure

Uncommon at serum theophylline concentrations ≤20 mcg/mL:
1% to 10%:
Cardiovascular: Tachycardia
Central nervous system: Nervousness, restlessness
Gastrointestinal: Nausea, vomiting

Overdosage/Toxicology Symptoms of overdose include nausea, vomiting, insomnia, irritability, tachycardia, seizures, tonic-clonic seizures, insomnia, and circulatory failure. If seizures have not occurred, induce vomiting; ipecac syrup is preferred. Do not induce emesis in the presence of impaired consciousness. Repeated doses of charcoal have been shown to be effective in enhancing the total body clearance of theophylline. Do not repeat charcoal doses if an ileus is present. Charcoal hemoperfusion may be considered if serum theophylline levels exceed 40 mcg/mL, the patient is unable to tolerate repeat oral charcoal administrations, or if severe toxic symptoms are present. Clearance with hemoperfusion is better than clearance from hemodialysis. Administer a cathartic, especially if sustained release agents were used. Phenobarbital administered prophylactically may prevent seizures.

Pharmacodynamics/Kinetics
Onset of Action: I.V.: <30 minutes
Protein Binding: 40%, primarily to albumin
Half-Life Elimination: Highly variable and age, liver and cardiac function, lung disease, and smoking history dependent
Metabolism: Children >1 year and Adults: Hepatic; involves CYP1A2, 2E1 and 3A4; forms active metabolites (caffeine and 3-methylxanthine)
Excretion: Urine: Neonates: 50% unchanged; Children >3 months and Adults: 10% unchanged

Available Dosage Forms [DSC] = Discontinued product
Capsule, extended release (Theo-24®): 100 mg, 200 mg, 300 mg, 400 mg [24 hours]
Elixir (Elixophyllin®): 80 mg/15 mL (480 mL) [contains alcohol 20%; fruit flavor]
Infusion [premixed in D₅W]: 0.8 mg/mL (500 mL, 1000 mL); 1.6 mg/mL (250 mL, 500 mL); 2 mg/mL (100 mL); 3.2 mg/mL (250 mL); 4 mg/mL (50 mL, 100 mL)
Solution, oral: 80 mg/15 mL (15 mL, 18.75 mL, 500 mL) [dye free, sugar free; contains alcohol 0.4% and benzoic acid; orange flavor]
Tablet, controlled release:
T-Phyl®: 200 mg [12 hours; contains cetostearyl alcohol]
Uniphyl®: 400 mg, 600 mg [24 hours; contains cetostearyl alcohol]
Tablet, extended release: 100 mg, 200 mg, 300 mg, 450 mg
Theochron®: 100 mg, 200 mg, 300 mg [12-24 hours]
Tablet, immediate release:
Quibron®-T: 300 mg
Theolair™: 125 mg, 250 mg
Tablet, sustained release (Quibron®-T/SR): 300 mg [8-12 hours]
Tablet, timed release (Theolair™-SR [DSC]): 300 mg, 500 mg

Dosing

Adults: Bronchodilation/respiratory stimulant:

Initial dosage recommendation: Loading dose (to achieve a serum concentration of about 10 mcg/mL; loading doses should be given using a rapidly absorbed oral product **not** a sustained release product):

If no theophylline has been administered in the previous 24 hours: 4-6 mg/kg theophylline

If theophylline has been administered in the previous 24 hours: Administer ½ loading dose; 2-3 mg/kg theophylline can be given in emergencies when serum concentrations are not available

On the average, for every 1 mg/kg theophylline given, blood concentrations will rise 2 mcg/mL

Maintenance dose: See table.

Maintenance Dose for Acute Symptoms

Population Group	Oral Theophylline (mg/kg/day)	I.V. Aminophylline
Otherwise healthy nonsmoking adults (including elderly patients)	10 (not to exceed 900 mg/day)	0.5 mg/kg/h
Cardiac decompensation, cor pulmonale, and/ or liver dysfunction	5 (not to exceed 400 mg/day)	0.25 mg/kg/h

Note: For continuous I.V. infusion, divide total daily dose by 24 = mg/kg/h.

Bronchodilation: Oral:

Nonsustained release: 16-20 mg/kg/day divided into 4 doses/day

Sustained release: 9-13 mg/kg/day divided into 2-3 doses/day

Note: These recommendations, based on mean clearance rates for age or risk factors, were calculated to achieve a serum concentration of 10 mcg/mL. In healthy adults, a slow-release product can be used (9-13 mg/kg in divided dose). The total daily dose can be divided every 8-12 hours.

Dosage in obese patients: Use ideal body weight for obese patients. Dose should be adjusted further based on serum concentrations. Guidelines for obtaining theophylline serum concentrations are shown in the table under Monitoring Laboratory Tests.

Elderly: Elderly patients should be started with a 25% reduction in the adult dose.

Pediatrics:

Loading dose:

Apnea of prematurity: Neonates: Oral: 4 mg/kg/dose

Treatment of acute bronchospasm: Infants and Children: Oral (to achieve a serum level of about 10 mcg/mL; loading doses should be given using a rapidly absorbed oral product **not** a sustained release product):

If no theophylline has been administered in the previous 24 hours: 5 mg/kg theophylline

If theophylline has been administered in the previous 24 hours: 2.5 mg/kg theophylline may be given in emergencies when serum levels are not available

Note: A modified loading dose (mg/kg) may be calculated (when the serum level is known) by: [Blood level desired - blood level measured] divided by 2 (for every 1 mg/kg theophylline given, the blood level will rise by approximately 2 mcg/mL)

Maintenance dose: See table.

Note: These recommendations, based on mean clearance rates for age or risk factors, were calculated to achieve a serum level of 10 mcg/mL (5 mcg/mL for newborns with apnea/bradycardia).

Maintenance Dose for Acute Symptoms

Population Group	Oral Theophylline (mg/kg/day)
Premature infant or newborn to 6 wk (for apnea/bradycardia)[1]	4
6 wk to 6 mo[1]	10
Infants 6 mo to 1 y[1]	12-18
Children 1-9 y	20-24
Children 9-12 y, adolescent daily smokers of cigarettes or marijuana, and otherwise healthy adult smokers <50 y	16
Adolescents 12-16 y (nonsmokers)	13
Otherwise healthy nonsmoking adults (including elderly patients)	10 (not to exceed 900 mg/day)
Cardiac decompensation, cor pulmonale, and/or liver dysfunction	5 (not to exceed 400 mg/day)

[1]**Alternative dosing regimen for full-term infants <1 year of age:**

Total daily dose (mg) = [(0.2 x age in weeks) + 5] x weight (kg)

Postnatal age <26 weeks: Total daily dose divided every 8 hours

Postnatal age >26 weeks: Total daily dose divided every 6 hours

In newborns and infants, a fast-release oral product can be used. The total daily dose can be divided every 12 hours in newborns and every 6-8 hours in infants. In children and healthy adults, a slow-release product can be used. The total daily dose can be divided every 8-12 hours.

Note: Use ideal body weight for obese patients

Adjustment of dose: Dose should be further adjusted based on serum levels. Guidelines for drawing theophylline serum levels are shown in the table.

Administration

Oral: Long-acting preparations should be taken with a full glass of water, swallowed whole, or cut in half if scored. Do **not** crush. Extended release capsule forms can be opened and the contents sprinkled on soft foods; do **not** chew beads.

I.V. Detail: pH: 4.3

Stability

Compatibility: Stable in D₅W

Y-site administration: Incompatible with hetastarch, phenytoin

Compatibility when admixed: Incompatible with ascorbic acid injection, ceftriaxone, cimetidine

Laboratory Monitoring Therapeutic levels:

Asthma: 10-15 mg/mL (peak level)

Toxic concentration: >20 mg/mL

Nursing Actions

Physical Assessment: Assess effectiveness and interactions of other medications patient may be taking. Monitor effectiveness of therapy (respiratory rate, lung sounds, characteristics of cough and sputum) and adverse reactions (eg, cardiac and CNS changes) at beginning of therapy and periodically with long-term use. For inpatient care, monitor vital signs and lung sounds prior to and periodically during therapy. Assess knowledge/teach patient appropriate use, interventions to reduce side effects, and adverse symptoms to report.

Patient Education: Take exactly as directed; do not exceed recommended dosage. Avoid smoking (smoking may interfere with drug absorption as well as exacerbate condition for which medication is prescribed). If you are smoking when dosage is prescribed; inform prescriber if you stop smoking (dosage may need to be adjusted to prevent toxicity). (Continued)

Theophylline *(Continued)*

Preferable to take on empty stomach, 1 hour before or 2 hours after meals, with a full glass of water. Do not chew of crush sustained release forms; capsules may be opened and contents sprinkled on soft food (do not chew beads). Avoid dietary stimulants (eg, caffeine, tea, colas, or chocolate; may increase adverse side effects). Maintain adequate hydration (2-3 L/day of fluids) unless instructed to restrict fluid intake. You may experience nausea, vomiting, or lose of appetite (small frequent meals, frequent mouth care, chewing gum, or sucking lozenges may help). Report acute insomnia or restlessness, chest pain or rapid heartbeat, emotional lability or agitation, muscle tremors or cramping, acute headache, abdominal pain and cramping, blackened stool, or worsening of respiratory condition. **Pregnancy precaution:** Inform prescriber if you are or intend to become pregnant.

Dietary Considerations Should be taken with water 1 hour before or 2 hours after meals. Premixed injection may contain corn-derived dextrose and its use is contraindicated in patients with allergy to corn-related products.

Geriatric Considerations Although there is a great intersubject variability for half-lives of methylxanthines (2-10 hours), elderly as a group have slower hepatic clearance. Therefore, use lower initial doses and monitor closely for response and adverse reactions. Additionally, elderly are at greater risk for toxicity due to concomitant disease (eg, CHF, arrhythmias), and drug use (eg, cimetidine, ciprofloxacin); see Warnings/Precautions and Drug Interactions.

Breast-Feeding Issues Irritability may be observed in the nursing infant.

Pregnancy Issues Theophylline crosses the placenta; adverse effects may be seen in the newborn. Theophylline metabolism may change during pregnancy; monitor serum levels.

Additional Information Theophylline salt / theophylline content (percent)

Theophylline anhydrous (eg, most oral solids): 100% theophylline

Theophylline monohydrate (eg, oral solutions): 91% theophylline

Aminophylline (theophylline) (eg, injection): 80% (79% to 86%) theophylline

Oxtriphylline (choline theophylline) (eg, Choledyl®): 64% theophylline

Related Information

Peak and Trough Guidelines *on page 1387*

Thiabendazole *(thye a BEN da zole)*

U.S. Brand Names Mintezol®

Synonyms Tiabendazole

Pharmacologic Category Anthelmintic

Pregnancy Risk Factor C

Lactation Excretion in breast milk unknown/not recommended

Use Treatment of strongyloidiasis, cutaneous larva migrans, visceral larva migrans, dracunculiasis, trichinosis, and mixed helminthic infections

Unlabeled/Investigational Use Cutaneous larva migrans (topical application)

Mechanism of Action/Effect Inhibits helminth-specific mitochondrial fumarate reductase

Contraindications Hypersensitivity to thiabendazole or any component of the formulation; not for use as prophylactic treatment of enterobiasis (pinworm) infestation

Warnings/Precautions Use with caution in patients with renal or hepatic impairment, malnutrition or anemia, or dehydration. Causes sedation; caution must be used in performing tasks which require alertness. Not suitable treatment for mixed infections with *Ascaris*. Ophthalmic changes may occur and persist >1 year. Safety and efficacy are limited in children <14 kg (30 lb).

Drug Interactions

Cytochrome P450 Effect: Substrate of CYP1A2 (minor); **Inhibits** CYP1A2 (strong)

Increased Effect/Toxicity: Thiabendazole may increase the levels/effects of aminophylline, fluvoxamine, mexiletine, mirtazapine, ropinirole, theophylline, trifluoperazine, and other CYP1A2 substrates.

Lab Interactions Increased glucose

Adverse Reactions Frequency not defined.

Central nervous system: Seizures, hallucinations, delirium, dizziness, drowsiness, headache, chills

Dermatologic: Rash, Stevens-Johnson syndrome, pruritus, angioedema

Endocrine & metabolic: Hyperglycemia

Gastrointestinal: Anorexia, diarrhea, nausea, vomiting, drying of mucous membranes, abdominal pain

Genitourinary: Malodor of urine, hematuria, crystalluria, enuresis

Hematologic: Leukopenia

Hepatic: Jaundice, cholestasis, hepatic failure, hepatotoxicity

Neuromuscular & skeletal: Numbness, incoordination

Ocular: Abnormal sensation in eyes, blurred vision, dry eyes, Sicca syndrome, vision decreased, xanthopsia

Otic: Tinnitus

Renal: Nephrotoxicity

Miscellaneous: Anaphylaxis, hypersensitivity reactions, lymphadenopathy

Overdosage/Toxicology Symptoms of overdose include altered mental status and visual problems. Treatment is supportive.

Pharmacodynamics/Kinetics

Time to Peak: Oral suspension: Within 1-2 hours

Half-Life Elimination: 1.2 hours

Metabolism: Rapidly hepatic; metabolized to 5-hydroxy form

Excretion: Urine (90%) and feces (5%) primarily as conjugated metabolites

Available Dosage Forms [DSC] = Discontinued product

Suspension, oral: 500 mg/5 mL (120 mL) [DSC]

Tablet, chewable: 500 mg [orange flavor]

Dosing

Adults & Elderly: Note: Purgation is not required prior to use; drinking of fruit juice aids in expulsion of worms by removing the mucous to which the intestinal tapeworms attach themselves.

Parasitic infections: Oral: 50 mg/kg/day divided every 12 hours; maximum: 3 g/day

Treatment duration:

Strongyloidiasis: For 2 consecutive days

Cutaneous larva migrans: For 2 consecutive days; if active lesions are still present 2 days after completion, a second course of treatment is recommended.

Visceral larva migrans: For 7 consecutive days

Trichinosis: For 2-4 consecutive days; optimal dosage not established.

Dracunculosis: 50-75 mg/kg/day divided every 12 hours for 3 days

Cutaneous larva migrans: Topical (unlabeled): Apply directly to larval tracks 2-3 times/day for up to 2 weeks; application frequencies may range from 2-6 times/day. **Note:** Not available as a topical formulation; oral suspension (10% to 15%) has been used topically, as well as a number of extemporaneous formulations.

Pediatrics: Parasitic infections: Children: Refer to adult dosing.

Renal Impairment: Use with caution.
Hepatic Impairment: Use with caution.
Nursing Actions
Physical Assessment: Worm infestations are easily transmitted, all close family members should be treated. Instruct patient/caregiver on appropriate use, transmission prevention, possible side effects/appropriate interventions, and adverse symptoms to report.
Patient Education: Take exactly as directed for full course of medication. Tablets may be chewed, swallowed whole, or crushed and mixed with food. Increase dietary intake of fruit juices. All family members and close friends should also be treated. To reduce possibility of reinfection, wash hands and scrub nails carefully with soap and hot water before handling food, before eating, and before and after toileting. Keep hands out of mouth. Disinfect toilet daily and launder bed linens, undergarments, and nightclothes daily with hot water and soap. Do not go barefoot and do not sit directly on grass or ground. May cause dizziness, fainting, or lightheadedness (use caution when driving or engaging in tasks requiring alertness until response to drug is known); or abdominal pain, nausea, dry mouth, or vomiting (small, frequent meals, frequent mouth care, sucking lozenges, or chewing gum may help). Report skin rash or itching, unresolved diarrhea or vomiting, CNS changes (hallucinations, delirium, acute headache), change in color of urine or stool, or easy bruising or unusual bleeding. **Pregnancy/breast-feeding precautions:** Inform prescriber if you are pregnant. Breast-feeding is not recommended.

Thiamine (THYE a min)

Synonyms Aneurine Hydrochloride; Thiamine Hydrochloride; Thiaminium Chloride Hydrochloride; Vitamin B₁
Pharmacologic Category Vitamin, Water Soluble
Medication Safety Issues
Sound-alike/look-alike issues:
Thiamine may be confused with Tenormin®, Thorazine®
Pregnancy Risk Factor A/C (dose exceeding RDA recommendation)
Lactation Enters breast milk/compatible
Use Treatment of thiamine deficiency including beriberi, Wernicke's encephalopathy syndrome, and peripheral neuritis associated with pellagra, alcoholic patients with altered sensorium; various genetic metabolic disorders
Mechanism of Action/Effect An essential coenzyme in carbohydrate metabolism by combining with adenosine triphosphate to form thiamine pyrophosphate
Contraindications Hypersensitivity to thiamine or any component of the formulation
Warnings/Precautions Use with caution with parenteral route (especially I.V.) of administration.
Nutritional/Ethanol Interactions Food: High carbohydrate diets may increase thiamine requirement.
Lab Interactions False-positive for uric acid using the phosphotungstate method and for urobilinogen using the Ehrlich's reagent; large doses may interfere with the spectrophotometric determination of serum theophylline concentration

Pharmacodynamics/Kinetics
Excretion: Urine (as unchanged drug and as pyrimidine after body storage sites become saturated)
Available Dosage Forms
Injection, solution, as hydrochloride: 100 mg/mL (2 mL)
Tablet, as hydrochloride: 50 mg, 100 mg, 250 mg, 500 mg
Dosing
Adults & Elderly:
Recommended daily allowance: >14 years: 1-1.5 mg

Thiamine deficiency (beriberi): I.M. or I.V. 5-30 mg/dose 3 times/day (if critically ill); then orally 5-30 mg/day in single or divided doses 3 times/day for 1 month
Wernicke's encephalopathy: I.V., I.M.: Initial: 100 mg I.V., then 50-100 mg/day I.M. or I.V. until consuming a regular, balanced diet
Dietary supplement (depends on caloric or carbohydrate content of the diet): Oral: 1-2 mg/day
Note: The above doses can be found in multivitamin preparations.
Metabolic disorders: Oral: 10-20 mg/day (dosages up to 4 g/day in divided doses have been used)
Pediatrics:
Recommended daily allowance:
<6 months: 0.3 mg
6 months to 1 year: 0.4 mg
1-3 years: 0.7 mg
4-6 years: 0.9 mg
7-10 years: 1 mg
11-14 years: 1.1-1.3 mg
>14 years: 1-1.5 mg
Thiamine deficiency (beriberi):
Children: I.M., I.V.: 10-25 mg/dose daily (if critically ill), or 10-50 mg/dose orally every day for 2 weeks, then 5-10 mg/dose orally daily for 1 month
Dietary supplement (depends on caloric or carbohydrate content of the diet): Oral:
Infants: 0.3-0.5 mg/day
Children: 0.5-1 mg/day
Note: The above doses can be found in multivitamin preparations
Administration
I.M.: Parenteral form may be administered by I.M. or slow I.V. injection.
I.V.: Doses are usually administered over 1-2 minutes.
I.V. Detail: pH: 2.5-4.5
Stability
Compatibility: Stable in dextran 6% in dextrose, dextran 6% in NS, D₅LR, D₅¹/₄NS, D₅¹/₂NS, D₅NS, D₅W, D₁₀W, fat emulsion 10%, LR, ¹/₂NS, NS
Storage: Protect oral dosage forms from light.
Nursing Actions
Physical Assessment: Assess knowledge/teach patient appropriate administration (injection technique and needle disposal if I.M. self-administered) and dietary instruction.
Patient Education: Take exactly as directed; do not discontinue without consulting prescriber (deficiency state can occur in as little as 3 weeks). Follow dietary instructions (dietary sources include legumes, pork, beef, whole grains, yeast, fresh vegetables). **Pregnancy precaution:** Inform prescriber if you are or intend to become pregnant.
Dietary Considerations Dietary sources include legumes, pork, beef, whole grains, yeast, and fresh vegetables. A deficiency state can occur in as little as 3 weeks following total dietary absence.
Additional Information Single vitamin deficiency is rare; evaluate for other deficiencies

Thioguanine (thye oh GWAH neen)

U.S. Brand Names Tabloid®
Synonyms 2-Amino-6-Mercaptopurine; NSC-752; TG; 6-TG (error-prone abbreviation); 6-Thioguanine (error-prone abbreviation); Tioguanine
Restrictions The I.V. formulation is not available in U.S./Investigational
Pharmacologic Category Antineoplastic Agent, Antimetabolite (Purine Antagonist)
Medication Safety Issues
6-thioguanine and 6-TG are error-prone abbreviations (associated with six-fold overdoses of thioguanine)
(Continued)

Thioguanine (Continued)

Pregnancy Risk Factor D

Lactation Excretion in breast milk unknown

Use Treatment of acute myelogenous (nonlymphocytic) leukemia; treatment of chronic myelogenous leukemia and granulocytic leukemia

Mechanism of Action/Effect Purine analog that is incorporated into DNA and RNA resulting in the blockage of synthesis and metabolism of purine nucleotides

Contraindications Hypersensitivity to thioguanine or any component of the formulation; pregnancy

Warnings/Precautions Hazardous agent - use appropriate precautions for handling and disposal. Use with caution and reduce dose in patients with renal or hepatic impairment. Not recommended for long-term continuous therapy due to potential for hepatotoxicity (hepatic veno-occlusive disease). Discontinue in patients with evidence of hepatotoxicity. Caution with history of previous therapy resistance with either thioguanine or mercaptopurine (there is usually complete cross resistance between these two). Thioguanine is potentially carcinogenic and teratogenic. Patients with genetic deficiency of thiopurine methyltransferase (TPMT) or who are receiving drugs which inhibit this enzyme (mesalazine, olsalazine, sulfasalazine) may be highly sensitive to myelosuppressive effects.

Drug Interactions

Increased Effect/Toxicity: Allopurinol can be used in full doses with thioguanine unlike mercaptopurine. Use with busulfan may cause hepatotoxicity and esophageal varices. Aminosalicylates (olsalazine, mesalamine, sulfasalazine) may inhibit TPMT, increasing toxicity/myelosuppression of thioguanine.

Nutritional/Ethanol Interactions Food: Enhanced absorption if administered between meals.

Adverse Reactions

>10%: Hematologic: Myelosuppressive:

WBC: Moderate

Platelets: Moderate

Onset (days): 7-10

Nadir (days): 14

Recovery (days): 21

1% to 10%:

Dermatologic: Skin rash

Endocrine & metabolic: Hyperuricemia

Gastrointestinal: Mild nausea or vomiting, anorexia, stomatitis, diarrhea

Neuromuscular & skeletal: Unsteady gait

Overdosage/Toxicology Symptoms of overdose include bone marrow suppression, nausea, vomiting, malaise, hypertension, and sweating. Treatment is supportive. Dialysis is not useful.

Pharmacodynamics/Kinetics

Time to Peak: Serum: Within 8 hours

Half-Life Elimination: Terminal: 11 hours

Metabolism: Hepatic; rapidly and extensively via TPMT to 2-amino-6-methylthioguanine (active) and inactive compounds

Excretion: Urine

Available Dosage Forms

Injection, powder for reconstitution: 75 mg [investigational in U.S.]

Tablet [scored]: 40 mg

Dosing

Adults & Elderly: Total daily dose can be given at one time.

Antineoplastic: Oral: Refer to individual protocols: 2-3 mg/kg/day calculated to nearest 20 mg or 75-200 mg/m²/day in 1-2 divided doses for 5-7 days or until remission is attained

Pediatrics: Total daily dose can be given at one time.

Antineoplastic: Oral (refer to individual protocols):

Infants and Children <3 years: Combination drug therapy for acute nonlymphocytic leukemia: 3.3 mg/kg/day in divided doses twice daily for 4 days

Children >3 years: Refer to adult dosing.

Renal Impairment: Reduce dose.

Hepatic Impairment: Reduce dose.

Stability

Reconstitution: Reconstitute parenteral preparation with 5 mL SWFI, NS, or D₅W to yield a 15 mg/mL solution. Dilute in 50-500 mL D₅W or NS for infusion.

Storage:

Tablet: Store at room temperature.

Injection (investigational in U.S.): Store intact vials under refrigeration (2°C to 8°C). The reconstituted solution is stable for at least 24 hours under refrigeration. Further dilutions for infusion are stable for 24 hours at room temperature or under refrigeration.

Laboratory Monitoring CBC with differential and platelet count; liver function tests (weekly when beginning therapy then monthly, more frequently in patients with liver disease or concurrent hepatotoxic drugs); serum uric acid, renal function; some laboratories offer testing for TPMT deficiency

Nursing Actions

Physical Assessment: Assess potential for interactions with other pharmacological agents patient may be taking. Monitor laboratory tests, patient response, and adverse reactions (eg, myelosuppression, nausea, vomiting, malaise, rash, diarrhea) weekly when beginning therapy, then monthly. Teach patient appropriate use, possible side effects/appropriate interventions (eg, importance of adequate hydration), and adverse symptoms to report.

Patient Education: Do not take any new medication during therapy unless approved by prescriber. Take exactly as directed. Maintain adequate hydration (2-3 L/day of fluids) unless instructed to restrict fluid intake. May cause nausea and vomiting, diarrhea, or loss of appetite (small, frequent meals may help/request medication); weakness or lethargy (use caution when driving or engaging in tasks requiring alertness until response to drug is known); mouth sores (use good oral care); or headache (request medication). You will be susceptible to infection (avoid crowds and exposure to infection). Report signs or symptoms of infection (eg, fever, chills, sore throat, burning urination, fatigue); bleeding (eg, tarry stools, easy bruising); vision changes; unresolved mouth sores, nausea, or vomiting; CNS changes (hallucinations); or respiratory difficulty. **Pregnancy/breast-feeding precautions:** Do not get pregnant. Consult prescriber for appropriate contraceptive measures. The drug may cause permanent sterility and may cause birth defects. Consult prescriber if breast-feeding.

Thioridazine *(thye oh RID a zeen)*

Synonyms Thioridazine Hydrochloride

Pharmacologic Category Antipsychotic Agent, Typical, Phenothiazine

Medication Safety Issues

Sound-alike/look-alike issues:

Thioridazine may be confused with thiothixene, Thorazine®

Mellaril® may be confused with Elavil®, Mebaral®

Pregnancy Risk Factor C

Lactation Excretion in breast milk unknown/not recommended

Use Management of schizophrenic patients who fail to respond adequately to treatment with other antipsychotic drugs, either because of insufficient effectiveness or the inability to achieve an effective dose due to intolerable adverse effects from those medications

Unlabeled/Investigational Use Psychosis

Mechanism of Action/Effect Thioridazine is a piperidine phenothiazine which blocks postsynaptic mesolimbic dopaminergic receptors in the brain; exhibits a strong alpha-adrenergic blocking effect and depresses the release of hypothalamic and hypophyseal hormones

Contraindications Hypersensitivity to thioridazine or any component of the formulation (cross-reactivity between phenothiazines may occur); severe CNS depression; circulatory collapse; severe hypotension; bone marrow suppression; blood dyscrasias; coma; in combination with other drugs that are known to prolong the QT_c interval; in patients with congenital long QT syndrome or a history of cardiac arrhythmias; concurrent use with medications that inhibit the metabolism of thioridazine (fluoxetine, paroxetine, fluvoxamine, propranolol, pindolol); patients known to have genetic defect leading to reduced levels of activity of CYP2D6

Warnings/Precautions Thioridazine has dose-related effects on ventricular repolarization leading to QT_c prolongation, a potentially life-threatening effect. Therefore, it should be reserved for patients with schizophrenia who have failed to respond to adequate levels of other antipsychotic drugs. May cause orthostatic hypotension - use with caution in patients at risk of this effect or those who would tolerate transient hypotensive episodes (cerebrovascular disease, cardiovascular disease, or other medications which may predispose).

Highly sedating, use with caution in disorders where CNS depression is a feature. Use with caution in Parkinson's disease. Caution in patients with hemodynamic instability; bone marrow suppression; predisposition to seizures; subcortical brain damage; severe cardiac, hepatic, renal, or respiratory disease. Esophageal dysmotility and aspiration have been associated with antipsychotic use - use with caution in patients at risk of pneumonia (ie, Alzheimer's disease). Caution in breast cancer or other prolactin-dependent tumors (may elevate prolactin levels). May alter temperature regulation or mask toxicity of other drugs due to antiemetic effects.

Due to anticholinergic effects, use caution in patients with decreased gastrointestinal motility, urinary retention, BPH, xerostomia, visual problems, narrow-angle glaucoma (screening is recommended) and myasthenia gravis. Relative to other neuroleptics, thioridazine has a high potency of cholinergic blockade.

May cause extrapyramidal symptoms, including pseudoparkinsonism, acute dystonic reactions, akathisia, and tardive dyskinesia (risk of these reactions is low relative to other neuroleptics). May be associated with neuroleptic malignant syndrome (NMS). Doses exceeding recommended doses may cause pigmentary retinopathy.

Drug Interactions

Cytochrome P450 Effect: Substrate of CYP2C19 (minor), 2D6 (major); **Inhibits** CYP1A2 (weak), 2C8/9 (weak), 2D6 (moderate), 2E1 (weak)

Decreased Effect: Aluminum salts may decrease the absorption of phenothiazines. The efficacy of amphetamines may be diminished by antipsychotics; in addition, amphetamines may increase psychotic symptoms; avoid concurrent use. Anticholinergics may inhibit the therapeutic response to phenothiazines and excess anticholinergic effects may occur (includes benztropine, trihexyphenidyl, biperiden, and drugs with significant anticholinergic activity). Chlorpromazine (and possibly other low potency antipsychotics) may diminish the pressor effects of epinephrine. The antihypertensive effects of guanethidine or guanadrel may be inhibited by phenothiazines. Phenothiazines may inhibit the antiparkinsonian effect of levodopa. Enzyme inducers may enhance the hepatic metabolism of phenothiazines; larger doses may be required; includes rifampin, rifabutin, barbiturates, phenytoin, and cigarette smoking. Thioridazine may decrease the levels/effects of CYP2D6 prodrug substrates (eg, codeine, hydrocodone, oxycodone, tramadol).

Increased Effect/Toxicity: Concurrent use fluvoxamine, propranolol, and pindolol. The levels/effects of thioridazine may be increased by chlorpromazine, delavirdine, fluoxetine, miconazole, paroxetine, pergolide, quinidine, quinine, ritonavir, ropinirole, and other CYP2D6 inhibitors. **Thioridazine is contraindicated with strong inhibitors of this enzyme.**

Drugs which alter the QT_c interval may be additive with thioridazine, increasing the risk of malignant arrhythmias; includes type Ia antiarrhythmics, TCAs, and some quinolone antibiotics (sparfloxacin, moxifloxacin and gatifloxacin). **These agents are contraindicated with thioridazine.** Potassium depleting agents may increase the risk of serious arrhythmias with thioridazine (includes many diuretics, aminoglycosides, and amphotericin).

Phenothiazines inhibit the ability of bromocriptine to lower serum prolactin concentrations. The sedative effects of CNS depressants or ethanol may be additive with phenothiazines. Phenothiazines and trazodone may produce additive hypotensive effects. Metoclopramide may increase risk of extrapyramidal symptoms (EPS). Acetylcholinesterase inhibitors (central) may increase the risk of antipsychotic-related EPS. Concurrent use of antihypertensives may result in additive hypotensive effects (particularly orthostasis).

Thioridazine may increase the levels/effects of amphetamines, beta-blockers, dextromethorphan, fluoxetine, lidocaine, mirtazapine, nefazodone, paroxetine, risperidone, ritonavir, tricyclic antidepressants, venlafaxine, and other CYP2D6 substrates. **Concurrent use with fluvoxamine is contraindicated.**

Phenothiazines may produce neurotoxicity with lithium; this is a rare effect. Rare cases of respiratory paralysis have been reported with concurrent use of phenothiazines and polypeptide antibiotics. Naltrexone in combination with thioridazine has been reported to cause lethargy and somnolence. Phenylpropanolamine has been reported to result in cardiac arrhythmias when combined with thioridazine.

Nutritional/Ethanol Interactions

Ethanol: Avoid ethanol (may increase CNS depression).
Herb/Nutraceutical: Avoid kava kava, valerian, St John's wort, gotu kola (may increase CNS depression). Avoid dong quai, St John's wort (may also cause photosensitization).

Lab Interactions False-positives for phenylketonuria, urinary amylase, uroporphyrins, urobilinogen

Adverse Reactions Frequency not defined.
Cardiovascular: Hypotension, orthostatic hypotension, peripheral edema, ECG changes
Central nervous system: EPS (pseudoparkinsonism, akathisia, dystonias, tardive dyskinesia), dizziness, drowsiness, neuroleptic malignant syndrome (NMS), impairment of temperature regulation, lowering of seizure threshold, seizure
Dermatologic: Increased sensitivity to sun, rash, discoloration of skin (blue-gray)
Endocrine & metabolic: Changes in menstrual cycle, libido (changes in), breast pain, galactorrhea, amenorrhea
Gastrointestinal: Constipation, weight gain, nausea, vomiting, stomach pain, xerostomia, nausea, vomiting, diarrhea
Genitourinary: Difficulty in urination, ejaculatory disturbances, urinary retention, priapism
Hematologic: Agranulocytosis, leukopenia
Hepatic: Cholestatic jaundice, hepatotoxicity
(Continued)

Thioridazine *(Continued)*

Neuromuscular & skeletal: Tremor

Ocular: Pigmentary retinopathy, blurred vision, cornea and lens changes

Respiratory: Nasal congestion

Overdosage/Toxicology Symptoms of overdose include deep sleep, coma, extrapyramidal symptoms, abnormal involuntary muscle movements, hypotension, and arrhythmias.

Immediate cardiac monitoring, including continuous electrocardiographic monitoring, to detect arrhythmias. Avoid use of medications that also prolong the QT_c interval, such as disopyramide, procainamide, and quinidine. Following initiation of essential overdose management, toxic symptom treatment and supportive treatment should be initiated. Hypotension usually responds to I.V. fluids or Trendelenburg positioning. If unresponsive to these measures, the use of a parenteral inotrope may be required (eg, norepinephrine 0.1-0.2 mcg/kg/minute titrated to response); do not use epinephrine or dopamine. Seizures commonly respond to diazepam (I.V. 5-10 mg bolus in adults every 15 minutes if needed up to a total of 30 mg; I.V. 0.25-0.4 mg/kg/dose up to a total of 10 mg in children) or to phenytoin. Avoid barbiturates (may potentiate respiratory depression). Neuroleptics often cause extrapyramidal symptoms (eg, dystonic reactions) requiring management with diphenhydramine 1-2 mg/kg (adults) up to a maximum of 50 mg I.M. or I.V. slow push followed by a maintenance dose for 48-72 hours. When these reactions are unresponsive to diphenhydramine, benztropine mesylate I.V. 1-2 mg (adults) may be effective. These agents are generally effective within 2-5 minutes.

Pharmacodynamics/Kinetics

Duration of Action: 4-5 days

Time to Peak: Serum: ~1 hour

Half-Life Elimination: 21-25 hours

Available Dosage Forms Tablet, as hydrochloride: 10 mg, 15 mg, 25 mg, 50 mg, 100 mg, 150 mg, 200 mg

Dosing

Adults:

Schizophrenia/psychosis: Oral: Initial: 50-100 mg 3 times/day with gradual increments as needed and tolerated; maximum: 800 mg/day in 2-4 divided doses

Depressive disorders, dementia: Oral: Initial: 25 mg 3 times/day; maintenance dose: 20-200 mg/day

Elderly: Behavioral symptoms associated with dementia: Oral: Initial: 10-25 mg 1-2 times/day; increase at 4- to 7-day intervals by 10-25 mg/day; increase dose intervals (once daily, twice daily, etc) as necessary to control response or side effects. Maximum daily dose: 400 mg; gradual increases (titration) may prevent some side effects or decrease their severity.

Pediatrics:

Schizophrenia/psychosis: Oral:

Children >2-12 years: Range: 0.5-3 mg/kg/day in 2-3 divided doses; usual: 1 mg/kg/day; maximum: 3 mg/kg/day

Children >12 years: Refer to adult dosing.

Behavior problems: Oral:

Children >2-12 years: Initial: 10 mg 2-3 times/day, increase gradually.

Children >12 years: Refer to adult dosing.

Severe psychoses: Oral:

Children >2-12 years: Initial: 25 mg 2-3 times/day, increase gradually.

Children >12 years: Refer to adult dosing.

Renal Impairment: Not dialyzable (0% to 5%)

Administration

Oral: Do not take antacid within 2 hours of taking drug.

Stability

Storage: Protect from light.

Laboratory Monitoring Baseline ECG; serum potassium, lipid profile, fasting blood glucose and Hgb A_{1c}; BMI; do not initiate if QT_c >450 msec

Nursing Actions

Physical Assessment: Assess other medications patient is taking for effectiveness and interactions. Review ophthalmic exam and monitor laboratory results, therapeutic response (mental status, mood, affect, gait), and adverse reactions at beginning of therapy and periodically with long-term use (eg, excess sedation, extrapyramidal symptoms, tardive dyskinesia, CNS changes). Monitor for CNS depression/level of sedation. Avoid skin contact with liquid medication; may cause contact dermatitis (wash immediately with warm, soapy water). Assess knowledge/teach patient appropriate use, interventions to reduce side effects, and adverse symptoms to report.

Patient Education: Use exactly as directed; do not increase dose or frequency. Do not discontinue without consulting prescriber. Tablet may be taken with food. Mix oral solution with 2-4 oz of liquid (eg, juice, milk, water, pudding). Do not take within 2 hours of any antacid. Store away from light. Avoid alcohol or caffeine and other prescription or OTC medications not approved by prescriber. Maintain adequate hydration (2-3 L/day of fluids) unless instructed to restrict fluid intake. Avoid skin contact with liquid medication; may cause contact dermatitis (wash immediately with warm, soapy water). May turn urine red-brown (normal). You may experience excess drowsiness, lightheadedness, dizziness, or blurred vision (use caution driving or when engaging in tasks requiring alertness until response to drug is known); nausea, vomiting, or dry mouth (small frequent meals, frequent mouth care, chewing gum, or sucking lozenges may help); constipation (increased exercise, fluids, fruit, or fiber may help); postural hypotension (use caution climbing stairs or when changing position from lying or sitting to standing); urinary retention (void before taking medication); ejaculatory dysfunction (reversible); decreased perspiration (avoid strenuous exercise in hot environments); or photosensitivity (use sunscreen, wear protective clothing and eyewear, and avoid direct sunlight). Report persistent CNS effects (eg, trembling fingers, altered gait or balance, excessive sedation, seizures, unusual movements, anxiety, abnormal thoughts, confusion, personality changes); chest pain, palpitations, rapid heartbeat, severe dizziness; unresolved urinary retention or changes in urinary pattern; altered menstrual pattern, change in libido, swelling or pain in breasts (male or female); vision changes; skin rash, irritation, or changes in color of skin (gray-blue); or worsening of condition. **Pregnancy/breast-feeding precautions:** Inform prescriber if you are or intend to become pregnant. Breast-feeding is not recommended.

Geriatric Considerations (See Warnings/Precautions, Adverse Reactions, and Overdose/Toxicology.) Elderly patients have an increased risk of adverse response to side effects or adverse reactions to antipsychotics.

Related Information

Antipsychotic Medication Guidelines *on page 1415*

Federal OBRA Regulations Recommended Maximum Doses *on page 1421*

Thiotepa (thye oh TEP a)

Synonyms TESPA; Thiophosphoramide; Triethylenethiophosphoramide; TSPA

Pharmacologic Category Antineoplastic Agent, Alkylating Agent

Pregnancy Risk Factor D

Lactation Enters breast milk/not recommended

Use Treatment of superficial tumors of the bladder; palliative treatment of adenocarcinoma of breast or ovary; lymphomas and sarcomas; controlling intracavitary effusions caused by metastatic tumors; I.T. use: CNS leukemia/lymphoma, CNS metastases

Mechanism of Action/Effect Alkylating agent that reacts with DNA phosphate groups to produce cross-linking of DNA strands leading to inhibition of DNA, RNA, and protein synthesis; mechanism of action has not been explored as thoroughly as the other alkylating agents, it is presumed that the aziridine rings open and react as nitrogen mustard; reactivity is enhanced at a lower pH

Contraindications Hypersensitivity to thiotepa or any component of the formulation; pregnancy

Warnings/Precautions Hazardous agent — use appropriate precautions for handling and disposal. Potentially mutagenic, carcinogenic, and teratogenic. Reduce dosage and use caution in patients with hepatic, renal, or bone marrow damage. Use should be limited to cases where benefit outweighs risk.

Drug Interactions

Cytochrome P450 Effect: Inhibits CYP2B6 (weak)

Increased Effect/Toxicity: Other alkylating agents or irradiation used concomitantly with thiotepa intensifies toxicity rather than enhancing therapeutic response. Prolonged muscular paralysis and respiratory depression may occur when neuromuscular blocking agents are administered. Succinylcholine and other neuromuscular blocking agents' action can be prolonged due to thiotepa inhibiting plasma pseudocholinesterase.

Nutritional/Ethanol Interactions

Ethanol: Avoid ethanol (due to GI irritation).

Herb/Nutraceutical: Avoid black cohosh, dong quai in estrogen-dependent tumors.

Adverse Reactions

>10%:

Hematopoietic: Dose-limiting toxicity which is dose related and cumulative; moderate to severe leukopenia and severe thrombocytopenia have occurred. Anemia and pancytopenia may become fatal, so careful hematologic monitoring is required; intravesical administration may cause bone marrow suppression as well.

Hematologic: Myelosuppressive:

WBC: Moderate

Platelets: Severe

Onset: 7-10 days

Nadir: 14 days

Recovery: 28 days

Local: Pain at injection site

1% to 10%:

Central nervous system: Dizziness, fever, headache

Dermatologic: Alopecia, rash, pruritus, hyperpigmentation with high-dose therapy

Endocrine & metabolic: Hyperuricemia

Gastrointestinal: Anorexia, nausea and vomiting rarely occur

Emetic potential: Low (<10%)

Genitourinary: Hemorrhagic cystitis

Renal: Hematuria

Miscellaneous: Tightness of the throat, allergic reactions

Overdosage/Toxicology Symptoms of overdose include nausea, vomiting, precipitation of uric acid in kidney tubules, bone marrow suppression, and bleeding. Therapy is supportive only. Thiotepa is dialyzable. Transfusions of whole blood or platelets have been proven beneficial.

Pharmacodynamics/Kinetics

Half-Life Elimination: Terminal: Dose-dependent clearance: 109 minutes

Metabolism: Extensively hepatic

Excretion: Urine (as metabolites and unchanged drug)

Available Dosage Forms Injection, powder for reconstitution: 15 mg, 30 mg

Dosing

Adults & Elderly: Refer to individual protocols.

Usual dose (range):

I.M., I.V., SubQ: 30-60 mg/m^2 once weekly

I.V.: 0.3-0.4 mg/kg by rapid I.V. administration every 1-4 weeks, **or** 0.2 mg/kg or 6-8 mg/m^2/day for 4-5 days every 2-4 weeks

I.M.: 15-30 mg in various schedules have been given

Intracavitary: 0.6-0.8 mg/kg or 30-60 mg weekly

Intrapericardial: 15-30 mg

Intrathecal: 10-15 mg or 5-11.5 mg/m^2

Pediatrics: Refer to individual protocols. Children: Sarcomas: I.V.: 25-65 mg/m^2 as a single dose every 21 days.

Renal Impairment: Use with extreme caution, reduced dose may be warranted.

Administration

I.V.: Administer either as a short (10-60 minute) infusion or 1-2 minute push; a 1 mg/mL solution is considered isotonic; not a vesicant

I.V. Detail: A 1 mg/mL solution is considered isotonic; not a vesicant.

pH: 5.5-7.5

Other: Intravesical lavage: Instill directly into the bladder and retain for at least 2 hours; patient should be repositioned every 15-30 minutes for maximal exposure

Stability

Reconstitution: Reconstitute each vial to 10 mg/mL. Solutions for infusion should be diluted to a concentration ≥5 mg/mL in 5% dextrose or 1, 3, or 5 mg/mL in 0.9% sodium chloride injection. Solutions for intravesical administration should be diluted in 30-60 mL SWFI or NS. Solutions for intrathecal administration should be diluted in 1-5 mL NS or Elliott's B Solution.

Compatibility:

Y-site administration: Incompatible with cisplatin, filgrastim, minocycline, vinorelbine

Compatibility when admixed: Incompatible with cisplatin

Storage: Store intact vials under refrigeration (2°C to 8°C) and protect from light. Reconstituted solutions (10 mg/mL) are stable for up to 28 days under refrigeration (4°C to 8°C) or 7 days at room temperature (25°C).

Solutions for infusion in D$_5$W (≥5 mg/mL) are stable for 14 days under refrigeration (4°C) or 3 days at room temperature (23°C).

Solutions for infusion in NS (1, 3, or 5 mg/mL) are stable for 48 hours under refrigeration (4°C to 8°C) or 24 hours at room temperature (25°C). Solutions in NS at a concentration of ≤0.5 mg/mL are stable for <1 hour.

Laboratory Monitoring CBC with differential, platelet count, uric acid, urinalysis

Nursing Actions

Physical Assessment: Assess potential for interactions with other pharmacological agents patient may be taking (eg, other alkylating agents or irradiation used concomitantly with thiotepa intensifies toxicity; prolonged muscular paralysis and respiratory depression may occur when neuromuscular-blocking agents are administered). See Administration for infusion specifics. Monitor results of laboratory tests closely (Continued)

Thiotepa *(Continued)*

(eg, anemia and pancytopenia can become fatal). Monitor therapeutic effects and adverse response on a regular basis (eg, myelosuppression, leukopenia, hematuria), Teach patient possible side effects/appropriate interventions (eg, importance of adequate hydration) and adverse symptoms to report.

Patient Education: Do not take any new medication during therapy unless approved by prescriber (especially aspirin or aspirin-containing products). If administered by infusion, report immediately any redness, pain, swelling, or burning at infusion site. You will require regular blood tests to assess response to therapy. Maintain adequate hydration to prevent kidney damage (2-3 L/day of fluids unless instructed to restrict fluid intake). You may have increased sensitivity to infection (avoid crowds and exposure to infection and do not have any vaccinations unless approved by prescriber). May cause nausea, vomiting, or loss of appetite (small frequent meals, chewing gum, or sucking lozenges may help); rash; or hair loss. Report unusual bleeding or bruising; persistent fever or chills; sore throat; sores in mouth or vagina; blackened stool; or respiratory difficulty. **Pregnancy/breast-feeding precautions:** Inform prescriber if you are pregnant. Do not get pregnant (females) or cause a pregnancy (males) during therapy and for 1 month following completion of therapy. Consult prescriber for instruction on appropriate contraceptive measures. This drug may cause severe fetal defects. Breast-feeding is not recommended.

Additional Information A 1 mg/mL solution is considered isotonic.

Thiothixene *(thye oh THIKS een)*

U.S. Brand Names Navane®

Synonyms Tiotixene

Pharmacologic Category Antipsychotic Agent, Typical

Medication Safety Issues
Sound-alike/look-alike issues:
Thiothixene may be confused with thioridazine
Navane® may be confused with Norvasc®, Nubain®

Pregnancy Risk Factor C

Lactation Excretion in breast milk unknown/not recommended

Use Management of schizophrenia

Unlabeled/Investigational Use Psychotic disorders

Mechanism of Action/Effect Thiothixene is a thioxanthene antipsychotic which elicits antipsychotic activity by postsynaptic blockade of CNS dopamine receptors resulting in inhibition of dopamine-mediated effects; also has alpha-adrenergic blocking activity

Contraindications Hypersensitivity to thiothixene or any component of the formulation; severe CNS depression; circulatory collapse; blood dyscrasias; coma

Warnings/Precautions May be sedating, use with caution in disorders where CNS depression is a feature. Use with caution in Parkinson's disease. Caution in patients with hemodynamic instability; predisposition to seizures; subcortical brain damage; bone marrow suppression; severe cardiac, hepatic, renal, or respiratory disease. Esophageal dysmotility and aspiration have been associated with antipsychotic use - use with caution in patients at risk of pneumonia (ie, Alzheimer's disease). Caution in breast cancer or other prolactin-dependent tumors (may elevate prolactin levels). May alter temperature regulation or mask toxicity of other drugs due to antiemetic effects. May alter cardiac conduction - life-threatening arrhythmias have occurred with therapeutic doses of neuroleptics. May cause orthostatic hypotension - use with caution in

patients at risk of this effect or those who would tolerate transient hypotensive episodes (cerebrovascular disease, cardiovascular disease, or other medications which may predispose). Safety and efficacy in children <12 years of age have not been established.

May cause anticholinergic effects, use caution in patients with decreased gastrointestinal motility, urinary retention, BPH, xerostomia, visual problems, narrow-angle glaucoma (screening is recommended), and myasthenia gravis. Relative to other neuroleptics, thiothixene has a low potency of cholinergic blockade.

May cause extrapyramidal symptoms, including pseudoparkinsonism, acute dystonic reactions, akathisia, and tardive dyskinesia (risk of these reactions is high relative to other neuroleptics). May be associated with neuroleptic malignant syndrome (NMS) or pigmentary retinopathy.

Drug Interactions

Cytochrome P450 Effect: Substrate of CYP1A2 (major); **Inhibits** CYP2D6 (weak)

Decreased Effect: CYP1A2 inducers may decrease the levels/effects of thiothixene; example inducers include aminoglutethimide, carbamazepine, phenobarbital, and rifampin. Thiothixene inhibits the activity of guanadrel, guanethidine, levodopa, and bromocriptine. Benztropine (and other anticholinergics) may inhibit the therapeutic response to thiothixene. Thiothixene and low potency antipsychotics may reverse the pressor effects of epinephrine.

Increased Effect/Toxicity: CYP1A2 inhibitors may increase the levels/effects of thiothixene; example inhibitors include amiodarone, ciprofloxacin, fluvoxamine, ketoconazole, norfloxacin, ofloxacin, and rofecoxib. Thiothixene and CNS depressants (ethanol, narcotics) may produce additive CNS depressant effects. Thiothixene may increase the effect/toxicity of antihypertensives, benztropine (and other anticholinergic agents), lithium, trazodone, and TCAs. Thiothixene's concentrations may be increased by chloroquine, sulfadoxine-pyrimethamine, and propranolol. Metoclopramide may increase risk of extrapyramidal symptoms (EPS). Acetylcholinesterase inhibitors (central) may increase the risk of antipsychotic-related EPS.

Nutritional/Ethanol Interactions
Ethanol: Avoid ethanol (may increase CNS depression).
Herb/Nutraceutical: Avoid kava kava, valerian, St John's wort, gotu kola (may increase CNS depression).

Lab Interactions Increased cholesterol (S), glucose; decreased uric acid (S); may cause false-positive pregnancy test

Adverse Reactions Frequency not defined.
Cardiovascular: Hypotension, tachycardia, syncope, nonspecific ECG changes
Central nervous system: Extrapyramidal signs (pseudoparkinsonism, akathisia, dystonias, lightheadedness, tardive dyskinesia), dizziness, drowsiness, restlessness, agitation, insomnia
Dermatologic: Discoloration of skin (blue-gray), rash, pruritus, urticaria, photosensitivity
Endocrine & metabolic: Changes in menstrual cycle, libido (changes in), breast pain, galactorrhea, lactation, amenorrhea, gynecomastia, hyperglycemia, hypoglycemia
Gastrointestinal: Weight gain, nausea, vomiting, stomach pain, constipation, xerostomia, increased salivation
Genitourinary: Difficulty in urination, ejaculatory disturbances, impotence
Hematologic: Leukopenia, leukocytes
Neuromuscular & skeletal: Tremors
Ocular: Pigmentary retinopathy, blurred vision
Respiratory: Nasal congestion
Miscellaneous: Diaphoresis

Overdosage/Toxicology Symptoms of overdose include muscle twitching, drowsiness, dizziness, rigidity, tremor, hypotension, and cardiac arrhythmias. Treatment is symptom-directed and supportive.

Pharmacodynamics/Kinetics
Half-Life Elimination: >24 hours with chronic use
Metabolism: Extensively hepatic
Available Dosage Forms [DSC] = Discontinued product
Capsule: 1 mg, 2 mg, 5 mg, 10 mg
Navane®: 1 mg [DSC], 2 mg, 5 mg, 10 mg, 20 mg
Dosing
Adults:
Mild to moderate psychosis: Oral: 2 mg 3 times/day, up to 20-30 mg/day; more severe psychosis: Initial: 5 mg 2 times/day, may increase gradually, if necessary; maximum: 60 mg/day
Rapid tranquilization of the agitated patient (administered every 30-60 minutes): Oral: 5-10 mg; average total dose for tranquilization: 15-30 mg
Elderly: Nonpsychotic patients, dementia behavior: Initial: 1-2 mg 1-2 times/day; increase dose at 4- to 7-day intervals by 1-2 mg/day. Increase dosing intervals (bid, tid, etc) as necessary to control response or side effects; maximum daily dose: 30 mg. Gradual increases in dose may prevent some side effects or decrease their severity.
Pediatrics:
Children <12 years (unlabeled use): Oral: 0.25 mg/kg/24 hours in divided doses (dose not well established; use not recommended)
Children >12 years: Mild to moderate psychosis: Refer to adult dosing.
Renal Impairment: Not dialyzable (0% to 5%)
Laboratory Monitoring Lipid profile, fasting blood glucose/Hgb A_{1c}; BMI
Nursing Actions
Physical Assessment: Assess other medications patient is taking for effectiveness and interactions. Review ophthalmic exam and monitor laboratory results, therapeutic response (mental status, mood, affect, gait), and adverse reactions at beginning of therapy and periodically with long-term use (eg, excess sedation, extrapyramidal symptoms, tardive dyskinesia, CNS changes). Avoid skin contact with liquid medication; may cause contact dermatitis (wash immediately with warm, soapy water). Assess knowledge/teach patient appropriate use, interventions to reduce side effects, and adverse symptoms to report.
Patient Education: Use exactly as directed; do not increase dose or frequency. Do not discontinue without consulting prescriber. Capsules may be taken with food. Do not take within 2 hours of any antacid. Avoid alcohol or caffeine and other prescription or OTC medications not approved by prescriber. Maintain adequate hydration (2-3 L/day of fluids) unless instructed to restrict fluid intake. May turn urine red-brown (normal). You may experience excess drowsiness, lightheadedness, dizziness, or blurred vision (use caution driving or when engaging in tasks requiring alertness until response to drug is known); nausea or vomiting (small frequent meals, frequent mouth care, chewing gum, or sucking lozenges may help); constipation (increased exercise, fluids, fruit, or fiber may help); postural hypotension (use caution climbing stairs or when changing position from lying or sitting to standing); urinary retention (void before taking medication); ejaculatory dysfunction (reversible); decreased perspiration (avoid strenuous exercise in hot environments); or photosensitivity (use sunscreen, wear protective clothing and eyewear, and avoid direct sunlight). Report persistent CNS effects (eg, trembling fingers, altered gait or balance, excessive sedation, seizures, unusual movements, anxiety, abnormal thoughts, confusion, personality changes); chest pain, palpitations, rapid heartbeat, severe dizziness; unresolved urinary retention or changes in urinary pattern; altered menstrual pattern, change in

libido, swelling or pain in breasts (male or female); vision changes; skin rash, irritation, or changes in color of skin (gray-blue); or worsening of condition.
Pregnancy/breast-feeding precautions: Inform prescriber if you are or intend to become pregnant. Breast-feeding is not recommended.
Geriatric Considerations (See Warnings/Precautions, Adverse Reactions, and Overdose/Toxicology.) Elderly patients have an increased risk of adverse response to side effects or adverse reactions to antipsychotics.
Related Information
Federal OBRA Regulations Recommended Maximum Doses *on page 1421*

Thyroid (THYE roid)

U.S. Brand Names Armour® Thyroid; Nature-Throid® NT; Westhroid®
Synonyms Desiccated Thyroid; Thyroid Extract; Thyroid USP
Pharmacologic Category Thyroid Product
Pregnancy Risk Factor A
Lactation Enters breast milk/compatible
Use Replacement or supplemental therapy in hypothyroidism; pituitary TSH suppressants (thyroid nodules, thyroiditis, multinodular goiter, thyroid cancer), thyrotoxicosis, diagnostic suppression tests
Mechanism of Action/Effect The primary active compound is T_3 (triiodothyronine), which may be converted from T_4 (thyroxine) and then circulates throughout the body to influence growth and maturation of various tissues
Contraindications Hypersensitivity to beef or pork or any component of the formulation; recent myocardial infarction; thyrotoxicosis uncomplicated by hypothyroidism; uncorrected adrenal insufficiency
Warnings/Precautions Ineffective for weight reduction. High doses may produce serious or even life-threatening toxic effects particularly when used with some anorectic drugs. Use cautiously in patients with pre-existing cardiovascular disease (angina, CHD), elderly since they may be more likely to have compromised cardiovascular function. Chronic hypothyroidism predisposes patients to coronary artery disease. Desiccated thyroid contains variable amounts of T_3, T_4, and other triiodothyronine compounds which are more likely to cause cardiac signs or symptoms due to fluctuating levels. Should avoid use in the elderly for this reason. Many clinicians consider levothyroxine to be the drug of choice for thyroid replacement.
Drug Interactions
Decreased Effect: Thyroid hormones increase the therapeutic need for oral hypoglycemics or insulin. Cholestyramine can bind thyroid and reduce its absorption. Phenytoin may decrease thyroxine serum levels. Thyroid hormone may decrease effect of oral sulfonylureas.
Increased Effect/Toxicity: Thyroid may potentiate the hypoprothrombinemic effect of oral anticoagulants. Tricyclic antidepressants (TAD) coadministered with thyroid hormone may increase potential for toxicity of both drugs.
Lab Interactions Many drugs may have effects on thyroid function tests: para-aminosalicylic acid, aminoglutethimide, amiodarone, barbiturates, carbamazepine, chloral hydrate, clofibrate, colestipol, corticosteroids, danazol, diazepam, estrogens, ethionamide, fluorouracil, I.V. heparin, insulin, lithium, methadone, methimazole, mitotane, nitroprusside, oxyphenbutazone, phenylbutazone, PTU, perphenazine, phenytoin, propranolol, salicylates, sulfonylureas, and thiazides.
Overdosage/Toxicology Chronic excessive use results in signs and symptoms of hyperthyroidism, weight loss, nervousness, sweating, tachycardia, insomnia, heat
(Continued)

Thyroid (Continued)

intolerance, palpitations, vomiting, psychosis, fever, seizures, angina, arrhythmias, and CHF in those predisposed.

Reduce dose or temporarily discontinue therapy. Hypothalamic-pituitary-thyroid axis will return to normal in 6-8 weeks. Serum T_4 levels do not correlate well with toxicity. In massive acute ingestion, reduce GI absorption and give general supportive care.

Pharmacodynamics/Kinetics
Half-Life Elimination: Serum: Liothyronine: 1-2 days; Thyroxine: 6-7 days

Metabolism: Thyroxine: Largely converted to liothyronine

Available Dosage Forms
Tablet: 30 mg, 32.5 mg, 60 mg, 65 mg, 90 mg, 120 mg, 130 mg, 180 mg, 240 mg, 300 mg
Armour® Thyroid: 15 mg, 30 mg, 60 mg, 90 mg, 120 mg, 180 mg, 240 mg, 300 mg
Nature-Throid® NT, Westhroid®: 32.5 mg, 65 mg, 130 mg, 195 mg

Dosing
Adults: Hypothyroidism: Oral: Initial: 15-30 mg; increase with 15 mg increments every 2-4 weeks; use 15 mg in patients with cardiovascular disease or myxedema. Maintenance dose: Usually 60-120 mg/day; monitor TSH and clinical symptoms.

Note: Thyroid cancer requires larger amounts than replacement therapy.

Elderly: Not recommended for use in the elderly (see Geriatric Considerations).

Pediatrics: Hypothyroidism: Oral: See table.

Recommended Pediatric Dosage for Congenital Hypothyroidism

Age	Daily Dose (mg)	Daily Dose/ kg (mg)
0-6 mo	15-30	4.8-6
6-12 mo	30-45	3.6-4.8
1-5 y	45-60	3-3.6
6-12 y	60-90	2.4-3
>12 y	>90	1.2-1.8

Laboratory Monitoring Monitor T_4 and TSH. TSH is the most reliable guide for evaluating adequacy of thyroid replacement dosage. TSH may be elevated during the first few months of thyroid replacement despite patients being clinically euthyroid. In cases where T_4 remains low and TSH is within normal limits, an evaluation of "free" (unbound) T_4 is needed to evaluate further increase in dosage.

Nursing Actions
Physical Assessment: Ineffective for weight reduction. Assess potential for interactions with other pharmacological agents and herbal products patient may be taking (eg, may decrease level/effect of oral hypoglycemics, increase risk of toxicity with TCAs and some anorexics). Monitor laboratory tests at baseline and regularly during therapy. **Note:** Many drugs may effects thyroid function tests; when assessing results of thyroid function tests (see Lab Interactions). Monitor for hyperthyroidism (weight loss, nervousness, sweating, tachycardia, insomnia, heat intolerance, palpitations, vomiting, psychosis, fever, seizures, angina, arrhythmias). Caution patients with diabetes to monitor glucose levels closely (may increase need for oral hypoglycemics or insulin). Teach patient appropriate use, possible side effects/appropriate interventions, and adverse symptoms to report.

Patient Education: Do not take any new medication during therapy unless approved by prescriber. Thyroid replacement therapy is generally for life. Take as directed, in the morning before breakfast. Do not take antacids or iron preparations within 8 hours of thyroid medication. Do not change brands and do not discontinue without consulting prescriber. Consult prescriber if drastically increasing or decreasing intake of goitrogenic food (eg, asparagus, cabbage, peas, turnip greens, broccoli, spinach, Brussels sprouts, lettuce, soybeans). If you have diabetes, monitor glucose levels closely (may increase need for oral hypoglycemics or insulin). Report chest pain, rapid heart rate, palpitations, heat intolerance, excessive sweating, increased nervousness, agitation, or lethargy.

Dietary Considerations Should be taken on an empty stomach.

Geriatric Considerations Desiccated thyroid contains variable amounts of T_3, T_4, and other triiodothyronine compounds which are more likely to cause cardiac signs or symptoms due to fluctuating levels. Should avoid use in the elderly for this reason. Many clinicians consider levothyroxine to be the drug of choice.

Additional Information Equivalent doses: The following statement on relative potency of thyroid products is included in a joint statement by American Thyroid Association (ATA), American Association of Clinical Endocrinologists (AACE) and The Endocrine Society (TES): For purposes of conversion, levothyroxine sodium (T_4) 100 mcg is usually considered equivalent to desiccated thyroid 60 mg, thyroglobulin 60 mg, or liothyronine sodium (T_3) 25 mcg. However, these are rough guidelines only and do not obviate the careful re-evaluation of a patient when switching thyroid hormone preparations, including a change from one brand of levothyroxine to another. Joint position statement is available at http://www.thyroid.org/professionals/advocacy/04_12_08_thyroxine.html.

Tiagabine (tye AG a been)

U.S. Brand Names Gabitril®

Synonyms Tiagabine Hydrochloride

Pharmacologic Category Anticonvulsant, Miscellaneous

Medication Safety Issues
Sound-alike/look-alike issues:
Tiagabine may be confused with tizanidine

Pregnancy Risk Factor C

Lactation Enters breast milk/not recommended

Use Adjunctive therapy in adults and children ≥12 years of age in the treatment of partial seizures

Mechanism of Action/Effect The exact mechanism by which tiagabine exerts antiseizure activity is not definitively known; however, in vitro experiments demonstrate that it enhances the activity of gamma aminobutyric acid (GABA), the major neuroinhibitory transmitter in the nervous system; it is thought that binding to the GABA uptake carrier inhibits the uptake of GABA into presynaptic neurons, allowing an increased amount of GABA to be available to postsynaptic neurons; based on in vitro studies, tiagabine does not inhibit the uptake of dopamine, norepinephrine, serotonin, glutamate, or choline

Contraindications Hypersensitivity to tiagabine or any component of the formulation

Warnings/Precautions New-onset seizures and status epilepticus have been associated with tiagabine use when taken for unlabeled indications. Often these seizures have occurred shortly after the initiation of treatment or shortly after a dosage increase. Seizures have also occurred with very low doses or after several months of therapy. In most cases, patients were using concomitant medications (eg, antidepressants, antipsychotics, stimulants, narcotics). In these instances, the discontinuation of tiagabine, followed by an evaluation for an underlying seizure disorder, is suggested. Use for unapproved indications, however, has not been proven to be safe or effective and is not recommended. When tiagabine is used as an adjunct in partial seizures (an FDA-approved indication), it should not be abruptly discontinued because of the possibility of increasing seizure frequency, unless safety concerns require a more rapid withdrawal. Rarely, nonconvulsive status epilepticus has been reported following abrupt discontinuation or dosage reduction.

Use with caution in patients with hepatic impairment. Experience in patients not receiving enzyme-inducing drugs has been limited; caution should be used in treating any patient who is not receiving one of these medications (decreased dose and slower titration may be required). Weakness, sedation, and confusion may occur with tiagabine use. Patients must be cautioned about performing tasks which require mental alertness (eg, operating machinery or driving). Effects with other sedative drugs or ethanol may be potentiated. Animal studies suggest that tiagabine may bind to retina and uvea; however, no treatment-related ophthalmoscopic changes were seen long-term; periodic monitoring may be considered. May cause serious rash, including Stevens-Johnson syndrome. Safety and efficacy have not been established in children <12 years of age.

Drug Interactions

Cytochrome P450 Effect: Substrate of 3A4 (major)

Decreased Effect: CYP3A4 inducers may decrease the levels/effects of tiagabine; example inducers include aminoglutethimide, carbamazepine, nafcillin, nevirapine, phenobarbital, phenytoin, and rifamycins.

Increased Effect/Toxicity: CYP3A4 inhibitors may increase the levels/effects of tiagabine; example inhibitors include azole antifungals, clarithromycin, diclofenac, doxycycline, erythromycin, imatinib, isoniazid, nefazodone, nicardipine, propofol, protease inhibitors, quinidine, telithromycin, and verapamil. Valproate increased free tiagabine concentrations (*in vitro*) by 40%.

Nutritional/Ethanol Interactions

Ethanol: Avoid ethanol (may increase CNS depression).

Food: Food reduces the rate but not the extent of absorption.

Herb/Nutraceutical: St John's wort may decrease tiagabine levels. Avoid valerian, St John's wort, kava kava, gotu kola (may increase CNS depression).

Adverse Reactions

>10%:

Central nervous system: Concentration decreased, dizziness, nervousness, somnolence

Gastrointestinal: Nausea

Neuromuscular & skeletal: Weakness, tremor

1% to 10%:

Cardiovascular: Chest pain, edema, hypertension, palpitation, peripheral edema, syncope, tachycardia, vasodilation

Central nervous system: Agitation, ataxia, chills, confusion, difficulty with memory, confusion, depersonalization, depression, euphoria, hallucination, hostility, insomnia, malaise, migraine, paranoid reaction, personality disorder, speech disorder

Dermatologic: Alopecia, bruising, dry skin, pruritus, rash

Gastrointestinal: Abdominal pain, diarrhea, gingivitis, increased appetite, mouth ulceration, stomatitis, vomiting, weight gain/loss

Neuromuscular & skeletal: Abnormal gait, arthralgia, dysarthria, hyper-/hypokinesia, hyper-/hypotonia, myasthenia, myalgia, myoclonus, neck pain, paresthesia, reflexes decreased, stupor, twitching, vertigo

Ocular: Abnormal vision, amblyopia, nystagmus

Otic: Ear pain, hearing impairment, otitis media, tinnitus

Respiratory: Bronchitis, cough, dyspnea, epistaxis, pneumonia

Miscellaneous: Allergic reaction, cyst, diaphoresis, flu-like syndrome, lymphadenopathy

Overdosage/Toxicology Somnolence, impaired consciousness, agitation, confusion, speech difficulty, hostility, depression, weakness, myoclonus, and seizures may occur. Treatment is supportive.

Pharmacodynamics/Kinetics

Time to Peak: Plasma: 45 minutes

Protein Binding: 96%, primarily to albumin and α_1-acid glycoprotein

Half-Life Elimination: 2-5 hours when administered with enzyme inducers; 7-9 hours when administered without enzyme inducers

Metabolism: Hepatic via CYP (primarily 3A4)

Excretion: Feces (63%); urine (25%); 2% as unchanged drug; primarily as metabolites

Available Dosage Forms Tablet, as hydrochloride: 2 mg, 4 mg, 6 mg, 8 mg, 10 mg, 12 mg, 16 mg

Dosing

Adults & Elderly: Partial seizures (adjunct): Oral:

Patients receiving enzyme-inducing AED regimens: 4 mg once daily for 1 week; may increase by 4-8 mg weekly to response or up to 56 mg daily in 2-4 divided doses; usual maintenance: 32-56 mg/day

Patients **not** receiving enzyme-inducing AED regimens: The estimated plasma concentrations of tiagabine in patients not taking enzyme-inducing medications is twice that of patients receiving enzyme-inducing AEDs. Lower doses are required; slower titration may be necessary.

Pediatrics: Partial seizures: Oral:

Patients receiving enzyme-inducing AED regimens: Children 12-18 years: 4 mg once daily for 1 week; may increase to 8 mg daily in 2 divided doses for 1 week; then may increase by 4-8 mg weekly to response or up to 32 mg daily in 2-4 divided doses

Patients **not** receiving enzyme-inducing AED regimens: Refer to adult dosing.

Laboratory Monitoring A therapeutic range for tiagabine has not been established. Monitor complete blood counts, renal function tests, liver function tests, and routine blood chemistry.

Nursing Actions

Physical Assessment: Assess effectiveness and interactions of other medications patient may be taking. Monitor therapeutic response (seizure activity, force, type, duration), laboratory values, and adverse reactions at beginning of therapy and periodically with long-term use. Use and teach seizure/safety precaution. Assess knowledge/teach patient appropriate use, interventions to reduce side effects, and adverse symptoms to report.

Patient Education: Take exactly as directed; do not increase dose or frequency or discontinue without consulting prescriber. While using this medication, do not use alcohol and other prescription or OTC medications (especially pain medications, sedatives, antihistamines, or hypnotics) without consulting prescriber. Maintain adequate hydration (2-3 L/day of fluids) unless instructed to restrict fluid intake. You may experience drowsiness, dizziness, disturbed concentration, or blurred vision (use caution when driving or engaging in tasks requiring alertness until response to drug is known); or nausea, vomiting, or loss of appetite (small frequent meals, frequent mouth care, chewing gum, or sucking lozenges may help). Wear identification of epileptic status and medications. Report behavioral or CNS changes; skin rash; muscle cramping, weakness, tremors, changes in gait; vision difficulties; persistent GI distress (cramping, pain, vomiting); chest pain, irregular heartbeat, or palpitations; cough or respiratory difficulty; or worsening of seizure activity or loss of seizure control.

Pregnancy/breast-feeding precautions: Inform (Continued)

Tiagabine (Continued)

prescriber if you are or intend to become pregnant. Breast-feeding is not recommended.

Dietary Considerations Take with food.

Geriatric Considerations There has been limited clinical experience with geriatric patients during clinical evaluation - use with caution.

Ticarcillin (tye kar SIL in)

U.S. Brand Names Ticar®

Synonyms Ticarcillin Disodium

Pharmacologic Category Antibiotic, Penicillin

Medication Safety Issues

Sound-alike/look-alike issues:

Ticar® may be confused with Tigan®

Pregnancy Risk Factor B

Lactation Enters breast milk/compatible

Use Treatment of susceptible infections such as septicemia, acute and chronic respiratory tract infections, skin and soft tissue infections, and urinary tract infections due to susceptible strains of *Pseudomonas*, and other gram-negative bacteria

Mechanism of Action/Effect Interferes with bacterial cell wall synthesis during active multiplication, causing cell wall death and resultant bactericidal activity against susceptible bacteria

Contraindications Hypersensitivity to ticarcillin, any component of the formulation, or penicillins

Warnings/Precautions Due to sodium load and adverse effects (anemia, neuropsychological changes), use with caution and modify dosage in patients with renal impairment. Serious and occasionally severe or fatal hypersensitivity (anaphylactoid) reactions have been reported in patients on penicillin therapy (especially with a history of beta-lactam hypersensitivity and/or a history of sensitivity to multiple allergens). Use with caution in patients with seizures.

Drug Interactions

Decreased Effect: Tetracyclines may decrease penicillin effectiveness. Aminoglycosides may cause physical inactivation of aminoglycosides in the presence of high concentrations of ticarcillin and potential toxicity in patients with mild-moderate renal dysfunction. Although anecdotal reports suggest oral contraceptive efficacy could be reduced by penicillins, this has been refuted by more rigorous scientific and clinical data.

Increased Effect/Toxicity: Probenecid may increase penicillin levels. Neuromuscular blockers may have an increased duration of action (neuromuscular blockade). Penicillins may increase the exposure to methotrexate during concurrent therapy; monitor.

Lab Interactions May interfere with urinary glucose tests using cupric sulfate (Benedict's solution, Clinitest®); false-positive urinary or serum protein, positive Coombs' test

Some penicillin derivatives may accelerate the degradation of aminoglycosides *in vitro*, leading to a potential underestimation of aminoglycoside serum concentration.

Adverse Reactions Frequency not defined.

Central nervous system: Confusion, convulsions, drowsiness, fever, Jarisch-Herxheimer reaction

Dermatologic: Rash

Endocrine & metabolic: Electrolyte imbalance

Gastrointestinal: *Clostridium difficile* colitis

Hematologic: Bleeding, eosinophilia, hemolytic anemia, leukopenia, neutropenia, positive Coombs' reaction, thrombocytopenia

Hepatic: Hepatotoxicity, jaundice

Local: Thrombophlebitis

Neuromuscular & skeletal: Myoclonus

Renal: Interstitial nephritis (acute)

Miscellaneous: Anaphylaxis, hypersensitivity reactions

Overdosage/Toxicology Symptoms of penicillin overdose include neuromuscular hypersensitivity (eg, agitation, hallucinations, asterixis, encephalopathy, confusion, and seizures). Electrolyte imbalance may occur if the preparation contains potassium or sodium salts, especially in renal failure. Hemodialysis may be helpful to aid in removal of the drug from blood; otherwise, treatment is supportive or symptom-directed.

Pharmacodynamics/Kinetics

Time to Peak: Serum: I.M.: 30-75 minutes

Protein Binding: 45% to 65%

Half-Life Elimination:

Neonates: <1 week old: 3.5-5.6 hours; 1-8 weeks old: 1.3-2.2 hours

Children 5-13 years: 0.9 hour

Adults: 66-72 minutes; prolonged with renal and/or hepatic impairment

Excretion: Almost entirely urine (as unchanged drug and metabolites); feces (3.5%)

Available Dosage Forms Injection, powder for reconstitution, as disodium: 3 g

Dosing

Adults: *Note:* Ticarcillin is generally given I.V., I.M. injection is only for the treatment of uncomplicated urinary tract infections and dose should not exceed 2 g/injection when administered I.M.

Usual dosage range: I.M., I.V.: 1-4 g every 4-6 hours, usual dose: 3 g I.V. every 4-6 hours

Otitis externa (malignant): I.V.: 3 g every 4 hours with tobramycin

***Pseudomonas* infections:** I.V.: 3 g every 4 hours

Elderly: I.V.: 3 g every 4-6 hours; adjust dosing interval for renal impairment

Pediatrics: *Note:* Ticarcillin is generally given I.V., I.M. injection is only for the treatment of uncomplicated urinary tract infections and dose should not exceed 2 g/injection when administered I.M.

Susceptible infections: I.M., I.V.: Infants and Children:

Systemic infections: I.V.: 200-300 mg/kg/day in divided doses every 4-6 hours

Urinary tract infections: I.M., I.V.: 50-100 mg/kg/day in divided doses every 6-8 hours

Maximum dose: 24 g/day

Cystic fibrosis (acute pulmonary exacerbations): Infants and Children: I.V.: 100 mg/kg every 6 hours

Urinary tract infections: Infants and Children: I.M., I.V.: 50-100 mg/kg/day in divided doses every 6-8 hours

Renal Impairment:

Cl_{cr} 30-60 mL/minute: 2 g every 4 hours or 3 g every 8 hours

Cl_{cr} 10-30 mL/minute: 2 g every 8 hours or 3 g every 12 hours

Cl_{cr} <10 mL/minute: 2 g every 12 hours

Moderately dialyzable (20% to 50%)

Continuous arteriovenous or venovenous hemodiafiltration effects: Dose as for Cl_{cr} 10-50 mL/minute

Administration

I.M.: Do not give more than 2 g per injection.

I.V.: Intermittent infusion, over 30 minutes to 2 hours. Some penicillins (eg, carbenicillin, ticarcillin and piperacillin) have been shown to inactivate aminoglycosides *in vitro*. This has been observed to a greater extent with tobramycin and gentamicin, while amikacin has shown greater stability against inactivation. Concurrent use of these agents may pose a risk of reduced antibacterial efficacy *in vivo*, particularly in the setting of profound renal impairment. However, definitive clinical evidence is lacking. If combination penicillin/aminoglycoside therapy is desired in a patient with renal dysfunction, separation of doses (if feasible), and routine monitoring of aminoglycoside levels, CBC, and clinical response should be considered.

I.V. Detail: Too rapid of infusion may cause seizures.

pH: 6-8

Stability

Compatibility: Stable in D₅W, LR, NS, SWFI

Y-site administration: Incompatible with amphotericin B cholesteryl sulfate complex, fluconazole

Compatibility in syringe: Incompatible with doxapram

Compatibility when admixed: Incompatible with gentamicin, aminoglycosides

Storage: Reconstituted solution is stable for 72 hours at room temperature and 14 days when refrigerated or 30 days when frozen. For I.V. infusion in NS or D₅W.

Laboratory Monitoring Serum electrolytes, bleeding time, and periodic tests of renal, hepatic, and hematologic function; perform culture and sensitivity before administering first dose.

Nursing Actions

Physical Assessment: Patient's allergy history should be assessed prior to starting therapy. Assess potential for interactions with other pharmacological agents patient may be taking. See Administration for infusion/injection specifics. Monitor laboratory tests, therapeutic effectiveness, and adverse reactions (eg, hypersensitivity reactions, opportunistic infection). Advise patients with diabetes about use of Clinitest®; may cause false-positive. Teach patient possible side effects/appropriate interventions and adverse symptoms to report.

Patient Education: Do not take any new medication during therapy unless approved by prescriber. This drug can only be given by injection or infusion. Report immediately any redness, swelling, burning, or pain at infusion site or any signs of allergic reaction (eg, respiratory difficulty or swallowing, chest tightness, rash, hives, swelling of lips or mouth). Maintain adequate hydration (2-3 L/day of fluids) unless instructed to restrict fluid intake. If you have diabetes, drug may cause false test results with Clinitest®, consult prescriber for alternative method of glucose monitoring. May cause confusion or drowsiness (use caution when driving or engaging in tasks that require alertness until response to drug is known). Report persistent diarrhea or abdominal pain (do not use antidiarrheal medication without consulting prescriber); bloody urine or stool; muscle pain; mouth sores; respiratory difficulty; skin rash; or signs of opportunistic infection (eg, fever, chills, unhealed sores, white plaques in mouth or vagina, purulent vaginal discharge, fatigue).

Dietary Considerations Sodium content of 1 g: 119.6-149.5 mg (5.2-6.5 mEq)

Geriatric Considerations When used as empiric therapy or for documented pseudomonal pneumonia, it is best to combine with an aminoglycoside such as gentamicin or tobramycin. High sodium may limit use in patients with congestive heart failure. Adjust dose for renal function.

Ticarcillin and Clavulanate Potassium
(tye kar SIL in & klav yoo LAN ate poe TASS ee um)

U.S. Brand Names Timentin®

Synonyms Ticarcillin and Clavulanic Acid

Pharmacologic Category Antibiotic, Penicillin

Pregnancy Risk Factor B

Lactation Enters breast milk (other penicillins are compatible with breast-feeding)

Use Treatment of infections of lower respiratory tract, urinary tract, skin and skin structures, bone and joint, and septicemia caused by susceptible organisms. Clavulanate expands activity of ticarcillin to include beta-lactamase producing strains of *S. aureus, H. influenzae, Bacteroides* species, and some other gram-negative bacilli

Mechanism of Action/Effect Ticarcillin interferes with bacterial cell wall synthesis during active multiplication, causing cell wall death and resultant bactericidal activity against susceptible bacteria; clavulanic acid prevents degradation of ticarcillin by binding to the active site on beta-lactamase

Contraindications Hypersensitivity to ticarcillin, clavulanate, any penicillin, or any component of the formulation

Warnings/Precautions Use with caution and modify dosage in patients with renal impairment. Serious and occasionally fatal hypersensitivity (anaphylactoid) reactions have been reported in patients on penicillin therapy. These reactions are more likely to occur in individuals with a history of cephalosporin hypersensitivity and/or a history of sensitivity to multiple allergens.

Drug Interactions

Decreased Effect: Tetracyclines may decrease penicillin effectiveness. Aminoglycosides may cause physical inactivation of aminoglycosides in the presence of high concentrations of ticarcillin and potential toxicity in patients with mild-moderate renal dysfunction. Although anecdotal reports suggest oral contraceptive efficacy could be reduced by penicillins, this has been refuted by more rigorous scientific and clinical data.

Increased Effect/Toxicity: Probenecid may increase penicillin levels. Neuromuscular blockers may have an increased duration of action (neuromuscular blockade). Penicillins may increase the exposure to methotrexate during concurrent therapy; monitor.

Lab Interactions Positive Coombs' test, false-positive urinary proteins

Some penicillin derivatives may accelerate the degradation of aminoglycosides *in vitro*, leading to a potential underestimation of aminoglycoside serum concentration.

Adverse Reactions Frequency not defined.

Central nervous system: Confusion, convulsions, drowsiness, fever, Jarisch-Herxheimer reaction

Dermatologic: Rash, erythema multiforme, toxic epidermal necrolysis, Stevens-Johnson syndrome

Endocrine & metabolic: Electrolyte imbalance

Gastrointestinal: *Clostridium difficile* colitis

Hematologic: Bleeding, hemolytic anemia, leukopenia, neutropenia, positive Coombs' reaction, thrombocytopenia

Hepatic: Hepatotoxicity, jaundice

Local: Thrombophlebitis

Neuromuscular & skeletal: Myoclonus

Renal: Interstitial nephritis (acute)

Miscellaneous: Anaphylaxis, hypersensitivity reactions

Overdosage/Toxicology Symptoms of overdose include neuromuscular hypersensitivity and seizures. Hemodialysis may be helpful to aid in removal of the drug from blood; otherwise, treatment is supportive or symptom-directed.

Pharmacodynamics/Kinetics

Protein Binding:

Clavulanic acid: 9% to 30%

Half-Life Elimination:

Clavulanic acid: 66-90 minutes

Metabolism:

Clavulanic acid: Hepatic

Excretion:

Clavulanic acid: Urine (45% as unchanged drug)

Clearance: Does not affect clearance of ticarcillin

Pharmacokinetic Note See Ticarcillin monograph.

Available Dosage Forms

Infusion [premixed, frozen]: Ticarcillin 3 g and clavulanic acid 0.1 g (100 mL) [contains sodium 4.51 mEq and potassium 0.15 mEq per g]

(Continued)

Ticarcillin and Clavulanate Potassium
(Continued)

Injection, powder for reconstitution: Ticarcillin 3 g and clavulanic acid 0.1 g (3.1 g, 31 g) [contains sodium 4.51 mEq and potassium 0.15 mEq per g]

Dosing
Adults:
Systemic infections: I.V.: 3.1 g (ticarcillin 3 g plus clavulanic acid 0.1 g) every 4-6 hours (maximum: 18-24 g/day)

Amnionitis, cholangitis, diverticulitis, endometritis, epididymo-orchitis, mastoiditis, orbital cellulitis, peritonitis, pneumonia (aspiration): I.V.: 3.1 g every 6 hours

Liver abscess, parafascial space infections, septic thrombophlebitis: I.V.: 3.1 g every 4 hours

Pseudomonas **infections:** I.V.: 3.1 g every 4 hours

Urinary tract infections: I.V.: 3.1 g every 6-8 hours

Elderly: I.V.: 3.1 g every 4-6 hours; adjust for renal function.

Pediatrics:
Systemic infections:
Children <60 kg: 200-300 mg of ticarcillin component/kg/day in divided doses every 4-6 hours
Children ≥60 kg: 3.1 g (ticarcillin 3 g plus clavulanic acid 0.1 g) every 4-6 hours; maximum: 24 g/day

Bite wounds (animal): 200 mg/kg/day in divided doses

Neutropenic fever: 75 mg/kg every 6 hours (maximum 3.1 g)

Pneumonia (nosocomial): 300 mg/kg/day in 4 divided doses (maximum: 18-24 g/day)

Renal Impairment:
Cl_{cr} 30-60 mL/minute: Administer 2 g every 4 hours or 3.1 g every 8 hours.

Cl_{cr} 10-30 mL/minute: Administer 2 g every 8 hours or 3.1 g every 12 hours.

Cl_{cr} <10 mL/minute: Administer 2 g every 12 hours.

Cl_{cr} <10 mL/minute with hepatic dysfunction: 2 g every 24 hours.

Moderately dialyzable (20% to 50%)

Continuous arteriovenous or venovenous hemodiafiltration effects: Dose as for Cl_{cr} 10-50 mL/minute.

Peritoneal dialysis: Administer 3.1 g every 12 hours.

Hemodialysis: Administer 2 g every 12 hours; supplemented with 3.1 g after each dialysis.

Hepatic Impairment: Cl_{cr} <10 mL/minute with hepatic dysfunction: Administer 2 g every 24 hours.

Administration
I.V.: Infuse over 30 minutes.

Some penicillins (eg, carbenicillin, ticarcillin and piperacillin) have been shown to inactivate aminglycosides *in vitro*. This has been observed to a greater extent with tobramycin and gentamicin, while amikacin has shown greater stability against inactivation. Concurrent use of these agents may pose a risk of reduced antibacterial efficacy *in vivo*, particularly in the setting of profound renal impairment. However, definitive clinical evidence is lacking. If combination penicillin/aminoglycoside therapy is desired in a patient with renal dysfunction, separation of doses (if feasible), and routine monitoring of aminoglycoside levels, CBC, and clinical response should be considered.

I.V. Detail: pH: 5.5-7.5

Stability
Compatibility: Stable in D_5W, LR, NS, SWFI
Y-site administration: Incompatible with alatrofloxacin, amphotericin B cholesteryl sulfate complex
Compatibility when admixed: Incompatible with sodium bicarbonate, aminoglycosides

Storage: Reconstituted solution is stable for 6 hours at room temperature and 72 hours when refrigerated. I.V. infusion in NS is stable for 24 hours at room temperature, 7 days when refrigerated, or 30 days when frozen. Darkening of solution indicates loss of potency of clavulanate potassium.

Laboratory Monitoring Serum electrolytes, bleeding time, and periodic tests of renal, hepatic, and hematologic function; perform culture and sensitivity before administering first dose.

Nursing Actions
Physical Assessment: Assess for allergy history prior to starting therapy. Assess potential for interactions with other prescriptions, OTC medications, or herbal products patient may be taking. Advise patients with diabetes about use of Clinitest®. Monitor laboratory tests, therapeutic effectiveness, and adverse reactions (eg, hypersensitivity reactions, opportunistic infection). Teach patient possible side effects/appropriate interventions and adverse symptoms to report.

Patient Education: Do not take any new medication during therapy unless approved by prescriber. This drug can only be given by injection or infusion. Report immediately any redness, swelling, burning, or pain at infusion site or any signs of allergic reaction (eg, respiratory difficulty or swallowing, chest tightness, rash, hives, swelling of lips or mouth). Maintain adequate hydration (2-3 L/day of fluids) unless instructed to restrict fluid intake. If you have diabetes, drug may cause false test results with Clinitest®, consult prescriber for alternative method of glucose monitoring. May cause confusion or drowsiness (use caution when driving or engaging in tasks that require alertness until response to drug is known). Report persistent diarrhea or abdominal pain (do not use antidiarrheal medication without consulting prescriber), bloody urine or stool, muscle pain, mouth sores, respiratory difficulty, or skin rash; or signs of opportunistic infection (eg, fever, chills, unhealed sores, white plaques in mouth or vagina, purulent vaginal discharge, fatigue).

Dietary Considerations Sodium content of 1 g: 4.51 mEq; potassium content of 1 g: 0.15 mEq

Geriatric Considerations When used as empiric therapy or for a documented pseudomonal pneumonia, it is best to combine with an aminoglycoside such as gentamicin or tobramycin. High sodium content may limit use in patients with congestive heart failure. Adjust dose for renal function.

Related Information
Ticarcillin *on page 1208*

Ticlopidine *(tye KLOE pi deen)*

U.S. Brand Names Ticlid®
Synonyms Ticlopidine Hydrochloride
Pharmacologic Category Antiplatelet Agent
Pregnancy Risk Factor B
Lactation Excretion in breast milk unknown

Use Platelet aggregation inhibitor that reduces the risk of thrombotic stroke in patients who have had a stroke or stroke precursors. **Note:** Due to its association with life-threatening hematologic disorders, ticlopidine should be reserved for patients who are intolerant to aspirin, or who have failed aspirin therapy. Adjunctive therapy (with aspirin) following successful coronary stent implantation to reduce the incidence of subacute stent thrombosis.

Unlabeled/Investigational Use Protection of aortocoronary bypass grafts, diabetic microangiopathy, ischemic heart disease, prevention of postoperative DVT, reduction of graft loss following renal transplant

Mechanism of Action/Effect Ticlopidine is an inhibitor of platelet function with a mechanism which is different from other antiplatelet drugs. The drug significantly increases bleeding time. This effect may not be solely related to ticlopidine's effect on platelets. The prolongation of the bleeding time caused by ticlopidine is further increased by the addition of aspirin in *ex vivo* experiments. Although many metabolites of ticlopidine have been found, none have been shown to account for *in vivo* activity.

Contraindications Hypersensitivity to ticlopidine or any component of the formulation; active pathological bleeding such as PUD or intracranial hemorrhage; severe liver dysfunction; hematopoietic disorders (neutropenia, thrombocytopenia, a past history of TTP)

Warnings/Precautions Use with caution in patients who may have an increased risk of bleeding (such as, ulcers). Consider discontinuing 10-14 days before elective surgery. Use caution in mixing with other antiplatelet drugs. Use with caution in patients with severe liver disease or severe renal impairment (experience is limited). May cause life-threatening hematologic reactions, including neutropenia, agranulocytosis, thrombotic thrombocytopenia purpura (TTP), and aplastic anemia. Routine monitoring is required. Monitor for signs and symptoms of neutropenia including WBC count. Discontinue if the absolute neutrophil count falls to <1200/mm^3 or if the platelet count falls to <80,000/mm^3.

Drug Interactions

Cytochrome P450 Effect: Substrate of CYP3A4 (major); **Inhibits** CYP1A2 (weak), 2C8/9 (weak), 2C19 (strong), 2D6 (moderate), 2E1 (weak), 3A4 (weak)

Decreased Effect: Decreased effect of ticlopidine with antacids (decreased absorption). Ticlopidine may decrease the effect of digoxin or cyclosporine. The levels/effects of ticlopidine may be decreased by aminoglutethimide, carbamazepine, nafcillin, nevirapine, phenobarbital, phenytoin, rifamycins, and other CYP3A4 inducers. Ticlopidine may decrease the levels/effects of CYP2D6 prodrug substrates (eg, codeine, hydrocodone, oxycodone, tramadol).

Increased Effect/Toxicity: Ticlopidine may increase effect/toxicity of aspirin, anticoagulants, theophylline, and NSAIDs. Cimetidine may increase ticlopidine blood levels. Ticlopidine may increase the levels/effects of amphetamines, selected beta-blockers, citalopram, dextromethorphan, diazepam, fluoxetine, lidocaine, methsuximide, mirtazapine, nefazodone, paroxetine, phenytoin, sertraline, risperidone, ritonavir, thioridazine, tricyclic antidepressants, venlafaxine, and other CYP2C19 or 2D6 substrates.

Nutritional/Ethanol Interactions

Food: Ticlopidine bioavailability may be increased (20%) if taken with food. High-fat meals increase absorption, antacids decrease absorption.

Herb/Nutraceutical: Avoid cat's claw, dong quai, evening primrose, feverfew, garlic, ginkgo, ginger, red clover, horse chestnut, green tea, ginseng (all have additional antiplatelet activity).

Lab Interactions Increased cholesterol (S), alkaline phosphatase, transaminases (S)

Adverse Reactions As with all drugs which may affect hemostasis, bleeding is associated with ticlopidine. Hemorrhage may occur at virtually any site. Risk is dependent on multiple variables, including the use of multiple agents which alter hemostasis and patient susceptibility.

>10%:

Endocrine & metabolic: Increased total cholesterol (increases of ~8% to 10% within 1 month of therapy)

Gastrointestinal: Diarrhea (13%)

1% to 10%:

Central nervous system: Dizziness (1%)

Dermatologic: Rash (5%), purpura (2%), pruritus (1%)

Gastrointestinal: Nausea (7%), dyspepsia (7%), gastrointestinal pain (4%), vomiting (2%), flatulence (2%), anorexia (1%)

Hematologic: Neutropenia (2%)

Hepatic: Abnormal liver function test (1%)

Overdosage/Toxicology Symptoms of overdose include ataxia, seizures, vomiting, abdominal pain, and hematologic abnormalities. Specific treatments are lacking. Treatment is symptomatic and supportive.

Pharmacodynamics/Kinetics

Onset of Action: ~6 hours; Peak effect: 3-5 days; serum levels do not correlate with clinical antiplatelet activity

Half-Life Elimination: 24 hours

Metabolism: Extensively hepatic; has at least one active metabolite

Available Dosage Forms Tablet, as hydrochloride: 250 mg

Dosing
Adults:

Stroke prevention: Oral: 250 mg twice daily with food

Coronary artery stenting (initiate after successful implantation): Oral: 250 mg twice daily with food (in combination with antiplatelet doses of aspirin) for up to 30 days

Elderly: 250 mg twice daily with food; dosage in older patients has not been determined; however, in two large clinical trials, the average age of subjects was 63 and 66 years. A dosage decrease may be necessary if bleeding develops.

Administration
Oral: Administer with food.

Laboratory Monitoring CBC with differential and platelet counts every 2 weeks starting the second week through the third month of treatment; more frequent monitoring is recommended for patients whose absolute neutrophil counts have been consistently declining or are 30% less than baseline values. Liver function tests (alkaline phosphatase and transaminases) should be performed in the first 4 months of therapy if liver dysfunction is suspected.

Nursing Actions

Physical Assessment: Monitor effectiveness of therapy (laboratory results) frequently at beginning of treatment and regularly thereafter. Monitor and teach patient bleeding precautions, possible side effects, and adverse symptoms to report.

Patient Education: Take exact dosage prescribed, with food. Do not use aspirin or aspirin-containing medications and OTC medications without consulting prescriber. You may experience easy bleeding or bruising (use soft toothbrush or cotton swabs and frequent mouth care, use electric razor, avoid sharp knives or scissors). Report unusual bleeding or bruising, persistent fever, sore throat, weakness, paleness, changes in neurological status; blood in urine, stool, or vomitus; delayed healing of any wounds; skin rash; yellowing of skin or eyes; changes in color of urine or stool; pain or burning on urination; respiratory difficulty; or skin rash. **Breast-feeding precaution:** Consult prescriber if breast-feeding.

Dietary Considerations Should be taken with food to reduce stomach upset.

Geriatric Considerations Because of the risk of neutropenia and its relative expense as compared with aspirin, ticlopidine should only be used in patients with a documented intolerance to aspirin.

Tigecycline (tye ge SYE kleen)

U.S. Brand Names Tygacil™
Synonyms GAR-936
Pharmacologic Category Antibiotic, Glycylcycline
Pregnancy Risk Factor D
Lactation
Excretion in breast milk unknown/use caution
Use Treatment of complicated skin and skin structure infections caused by susceptible organisms, including methicillin-resistant *Staphylococcus aureus* and vancomycin-sensitive *Enterococcus faecalis*; treatment of complicated intra-abdominal infections
Mechanism of Action/Effect
A glycylcycline antibiotic, binds to the 30S ribosomal subunit of susceptible bacteria, inhibiting protein synthesis. Generally considered bacteriostatic. Tigecycline is a derivative of minocycline (9-t-butylglycylamido minocycline) but is not classified as a tetracycline. It has demonstrated activity against a variety of Gram-positive and -negative bacterial pathogens including methicillin-resistant staphylococci.
Contraindications Hypersensitivity to tigecycline or any component of the formulation
Warnings/Precautions Due to structural similarity with tetracyclines, use caution in patients with prior hypersensitivity and/or severe adverse reactions associated with tetracycline use. Due to structural similarities with tetracyclines, may be associated with photosensitivity, pseudotumor cerebri, pancreatitis, and antianabolic effects observed with this class. May cause fetal harm if used during pregnancy; patients should be advised of potential risks associated with use. Permanent discoloration of the teeth may occur if used during tooth development (fetal stage through children up to 8 years of age). Use caution in hepatic impairment; dosage adjustment may be required.

Tigecycline may be associated with the development of *C. difficile* colitis. Use caution in intestinal perforation (in the small sample of available cases, septic shock occurred more frequently than patients treated with imipenem/cilastatin comparator). Safety and efficacy in children <18 years of age have not been established.
Drug Interactions
Decreased Effect: Anecdotal reports of oral contraceptives suggesting decreased contraceptive efficacy with tetracyclines have been refuted by more rigorous scientific and clinical data.
Increased Effect/Toxicity: Retinoic acid derivatives may increase risk of pseudotumor cerebri (reported with tetracyclines). Hypoprothrombinemic response of warfarin may be increased with tigecycline; monitor INR closely during initiation or discontinuation.
Adverse Reactions Note: Frequencies relative to placebo are not available; some frequencies are lower than those experienced with comparator drugs.
>10%: Gastrointestinal: Nausea (25% to 30%; severe in 1%), vomiting (20%; severe in 1%), diarrhea (13%)
2% to 10%:
Cardiovascular: Hypertension (5%), peripheral edema (3%), hypotension (2%), phlebitis (2%)
Central nervous system: Fever (7%), headache (6%), dizziness (4%), pain (4%), insomnia (2%)
Dermatologic: Pruritus (3%), rash (2%)
Endocrine & metabolic: Hypoproteinemia (5%), hyperglycemia (2%), hypokalemia (2%)
Gastrointestinal: Abdominal pain (7%), constipation (3%), dyspepsia (3%)
Hematologic: Thrombocythemia (6%), anemia (4%), leukocytosis (4%)
Hepatic: SGPT increased (6%), SGOT increased (4%), alkaline phosphatase increased (4%), amylase increased (3%), bilirubin increased (2%), LDH increased (4%)
Local: Reaction to procedure (9%)

Neuromuscular & skeletal: Weakness (3%)
Renal: BUN increased (2%)
Respiratory: Cough increased (4%), dyspnea (3%), pulmonary physical finding (2%)
Miscellaneous: Abnormal healing (4%), infection (8%), abscess (3%), diaphoresis increased (2%)
Overdosage/Toxicology No specific experience in overdose. May experience increased nausea/vomiting. Not significantly removed by hemodialysis.
Pharmacodynamics/Kinetics
Protein Binding: 71% to 89%
Half-Life Elimination: Half-life elimination: Single dose: 27 hours; following multiple doses: 42 hours
Metabolism: Hepatic, via glucuronidation, N-acetylation, and epimerization to several metabolites, each <10% of the dose
Excretion: Urine (33%; with 22% as unchanged drug); feces (59%; primarily as unchanged drug)
Pharmacokinetic Note Systemic clearance is reduced by 55% and half-life increased by 43% in moderate hepatic impairment.
Available Dosage Forms Injection, powder for reconstitution: 50 mg
Dosing
Adults & Elderly: Complicated skin/skin structure or intra-abdominal infections: I.V.:
Initial: 100 mg as a single dose
Maintenance dose: 50 mg every 12 hours
Recommended duration of therapy: Intra-abdominal infections or complicated skin/skin structure infections: 5-14 days.
Renal Impairment:
No dosage adjustment required
Hepatic Impairment:
Mild-to-moderate hepatic disease: No dosage adjustment required
Severe hepatic impairment (Child-Pugh class C): Initial dose of 100 mg should be followed with 25 mg every 12 hours
Administration
I.V.: Infuse over 30-60 minutes through dedicated line or via Y-site
Stability
Reconstitution: Add 5.3 mL NS or D5W to each 50 mg vial. Swirl gently to dissolve. Resulting solution is 10 mg/mL. Transfer immediately to 100 mL I.V. bag for infusion (final concentration should not exceed 1 mg/mL). Reconstituted solution is red-orange.
Compatibility:
Stable in NS or D₅W; final concentration should not exceed 1 mg/mL
Y-site administration: Incompatible: Amphotericin B, chlorpromazine, methylprednisolone, voriconazole
Storage: Store at 20°C to 25°C prior to reconstitution, excursions permitted to 15°C to 30°C. Reconstituted solution must be immediately transferred (and further diluted) to allow I.V. administration. Following dilution, may be stored at room temperature for up to 6 hours, or up to 24 hours under refrigeration.
Nursing Actions
Physical Assessment: Results of culture and sensitivity tests and patient's allergy history should be assessed prior to beginning therapy. INR should be monitored when used concomitantly with warfarin. Assess results of therapeutic effectiveness (resolution of infection), and adverse reactions at beginning of and periodically throughout therapy (eg. nausea, vomiting, diarrhea, hypotention, peripheral edema, headache, rash, anemia, dyspnea, opportunistic infection [*C. difficile*], hypersensitivity). Teach patient purpose for use and adverse symptoms to report (refer to Patient Education).
Patient Education: This medication is only administered intravenously. Report immediately any burning,

pain, swelling at infusion site; difficulty breathing or swallowing, chest pain, or chills. Report an gastrointestinal upset (nausea, vomiting, diarrhea or constipation, stomach pain); headache, dizziness, difficulty breathing; increasing sweating, or other adverse reactions. **Pregnancy/breast-feeding precautions:** Inform prescriber in you are pregnant; this drug may cause fetal abnormalities.

Geriatric Considerations The manufacturer reports no significant differences in tigecycline's pharmacokinetics in small numbers of healthy older adults 65-75 years of age and >75 years compared to younger adults following a single 100 mg dose. No dosage adjustment is recommended.

Breast-Feeding Issues Glycylcyclines such as tigecycline are structurally related to tetracyclines, and are expected to share many of their properties. Although tetracyclines are excreted in limited amounts, the potential for staining of unerupted teeth has led some experts to recommend against breast-feeding. The AAP identified tetracyclines as "compatible" with breast-feeding.

Additional Information Generally considered bacteriostatic. Tigecycline is a derivative of minocycline (9-t-butylglycylamido minocycline), but is not classified as a tetracycline. It has demonstrated activity against a variety of Gram-positive and -negative bacterial pathogens.

Tiludronate (tye LOO droe nate)

U.S. Brand Names Skelid®

Synonyms Tiludronate Disodium

Pharmacologic Category Bisphosphonate Derivative

Pregnancy Risk Factor C

Lactation Excretion in breast milk unknown/use caution

Use Treatment of Paget's disease of the bone in patients who have a level of serum alkaline phosphatase (SAP) at least twice the upper limit of normal, or who are symptomatic, or who are at risk for future complications of their disease

Mechanism of Action/Effect A bisphosphonate which inhibits osteoclast activity, reducing enzymatic and transport processes that lead to resorption of bone. At least two possible mechanisms may be involved: detachment of osteoclasts from the bone surface (due to inhibition of protein-tyrosine-phosphatase) and inhibition of the osteoclastic proton pump, required to alter local pH to solubilize ions and bone matrix during resorption.

Contraindications Hypersensitivity to bisphosphonates or any component of the formulation

Warnings/Precautions Not recommended in severe renal impairment (Cl_{cr} <30 mL/minute). May cause upper gastrointestinal problems (eg, dysphagia, esophageal diseases, gastritis, duodenitis, ulcers). Bisphosphonate therapy has been associated with osteonecrosis, primarily of the jaw; this has been observed mostly in cancer patients, but also in patients with postmenopausal osteoporosis and other diagnoses. Dental exams and preventative dentistry should be performed prior to placing patients with risk factors on chronic bisphosphonate therapy. Invasive dental procedures should be avoided during treatment.

Drug Interactions

Decreased Effect: The following agents may decrease the absorption of oral bisphosphonate derivatives: Antacids (aluminum, calcium, magnesium), oral calcium salts, oral iron salts, and oral magnesium salts.

Increased Effect/Toxicity: Aminoglycosides may lower serum calcium levels with prolonged administration; concomitant use may have an additive hypocalcemic effect. NSAIDs may enhance the gastrointestinal adverse/toxic effects (increased incidence of GI ulcers) of bisphosphonate derivatives. Bisphosphonate derivatives may enhance the hypocalcemic effect of phosphate supplements.

Nutritional/Ethanol Interactions Food: In single-dose studies, the bioavailability of tiludronate was reduced by 90% when an oral dose was administered with, or 2 hours after, a standard breakfast compared to the same dose administered after an overnight fast and 4 hours before a standard breakfast.

Lab Interactions Bisphosphonates may interfere with diagnostic imaging agents such as technetium-99m-diphosphonate in bone scans.

Adverse Reactions The following events occurred >2% and at a frequency greater than placebo:

1% to 10%:

Cardiovascular: Chest pain (3%), edema (3%)

Central nervous system: Dizziness (4%), paresthesia (4%)

Dermatologic: Rash (3%), skin disorder (3%)

Gastrointestinal: Nausea (9%), diarrhea (9%), heartburn (5%), vomiting (4%), flatulence (3%)

Neuromuscular & skeletal: Arthrosis (3%)

Ocular: cataract (3%), conjunctivitis (3%), glaucoma (3%)

Respiratory: Rhinitis (5%), sinusitis (5%), cough (3%), pharyngitis (3%)

Overdosage/Toxicology Hypocalcemia is a potential consequence of overdose. Treatment is supportive.

Pharmacodynamics/Kinetics

Onset of Action: Delayed, may require several weeks

Time to Peak: Plasma: ~2 hours

Protein Binding: 90%, primarily to albumin

Half-Life Elimination: Healthy volunteers: 50 hours; Pagetic patients: 150 hours

Metabolism: Little, if any

Excretion: Urine (60% as unchanged drug) within 13 days

Available Dosage Forms Tablet, tiludronic acid: 200 mg [equivalent to 240 mg tiludronate disodium]

Dosing

Adults & Elderly: Paget's disease: Oral: 400 mg (2 tablets of tiludronic acid) daily for a period of 3 months

Renal Impairment: Tiludronate is excreted renally. It is not recommended for use in patients with severe renal impairment (Cl_{cr} <30 mL/minute) and is not removed by dialysis.

Administration

Oral: Take with 6-8 oz of plain water. Do not take within 2 hours of food, aspirin, indomethacin, or calcium-, magnesium-, or aluminum-containing medications.

Stability

Storage: Do not remove tablet from foil strips until they are to be used.

Laboratory Monitoring Serum calcium, alkaline phosphatase

Nursing Actions

Physical Assessment: Ascertain that patient is capable of complying with administration directions before starting treatment (eg, able to remain in standing or sitting position for 30 minutes). Monitor laboratory tests, therapeutic effectiveness, and adverse reactions (eg, rash, diarrhea, arthralgia, peripheral edema, gastrointestinal disturbance [nausea, vomiting, diarrhea], visual changes, hypocalcemia, hypophosphatemia). Teach patient appropriate use and administration of medication, lifestyle and dietary changes that will have a beneficial impact on Paget's disease, possible side effects, interventions to reduce side effects, and adverse reactions to report.

Patient Education: Do not take any new medication during therapy unless approved by prescriber. In order to be effective, this medication must be taken exactly as directed, with a full glass of water first thing (Continued)

Tiludronate *(Continued)*

in the morning, at least 30 minutes before the first food or beverage of the day. Remain standing or sitting for at least 30 minutes after taking this medication before eating. Do not remove medication from foil strip until ready to be used. Do not take aspirin, antacids or vitamin supplements containing calcium, magnesium, or aluminum within 2 hours. Consult prescriber to determine recommended lifestyle changes (eg, decreased smoking, decreased alcohol intake, dietary supplements of calcium, or increased dietary vitamin D). Notify prescriber at once if experiencing difficulty swallowing, pain when swallowing, or severe or persistent heartburn. May cause mild/temporary skin rash; or abdominal pain, diarrhea, or constipation (report if persistent). Report persistent muscle or bone pain or leg cramps; chest pain, palpitations, or swollen extremities; disturbed vision; ringing in the ears; unusual weakness or significantly increased perspiration. **Pregnancy/breast-feeding precautions:** Inform prescriber if you are or intend to become pregnant. Consult prescriber if breast-feeding.

Dietary Considerations Do not take within 2 hours of food.

Pregnancy Issues Teratogenic and nonteratogenic embryo/fetal effects have been reported in animal studies. There are no adequate and well-controlled studies in pregnant women. Bisphosphonates are incorporated into the bone matrix and gradually released over time. Theoretically, there may be a risk of fetal harm when pregnancy follows the completion of therapy. Based on limited case reports with pamidronate, serum calcium levels in the newborn may be altered if administered during pregnancy.

Timolol (TYE moe lole)

U.S. Brand Names Betimol®; Blocadren®; Istalol™; Timoptic®; Timoptic® OcuDose®; Timoptic-XE®

Synonyms Timolol Hemihydrate; Timolol Maleate

Pharmacologic Category Beta-Adrenergic Blocker, Nonselective; Ophthalmic Agent, Antiglaucoma

Medication Safety Issues

Sound-alike/look-alike issues:

Timolol may be confused with atenolol, Tylenol®

Timoptic® may be confused with Talacen®, Viroptic®

Bottle cap color change:

Timoptic®: Both the 0.25% and 0.5% strengths are now packaged in bottles with yellow caps; previously, the color of the cap on the product corresponded to different strengths.

Pregnancy Risk Factor C (manufacturer); D (2nd and 3rd trimesters - expert analysis)

Lactation Enters breast milk/use caution (AAP rates "compatible")

Use Ophthalmic dosage form used in treatment of elevated intraocular pressure such as glaucoma or ocular hypertension; oral dosage form used for treatment of hypertension and angina, to reduce mortality following myocardial infarction, and for prophylaxis of migraine

Mechanism of Action/Effect Blocks both beta$_1$- and beta$_2$-adrenergic receptors, reduces intraocular pressure by reducing aqueous humor production or possibly outflow; reduces blood pressure by blocking adrenergic receptors and decreasing sympathetic outflow, produces a negative chronotropic and inotropic activity through an unknown mechanism

Contraindications Hypersensitivity to timolol or any component of the formulation; sinus bradycardia; sinus node dysfunction; heart block greater than first degree

(except in patients with a functioning artificial pacemaker); cardiogenic shock; uncompensated cardiac failure; bronchospastic disease; pregnancy (2nd and 3rd trimesters)

Warnings/Precautions Administer cautiously in compensated heart failure and monitor for a worsening of the condition. Beta-blocker therapy should not be withdrawn abruptly (particularly in patients with CAD), but gradually tapered to avoid acute tachycardia, hypertension, and/or ischemia. Use caution with concurrent use of beta-blockers and either verapamil or diltiazem; bradycardia or heart block can occur. Beta-blockers can aggravate symptoms in patients with peripheral vascular disease. Patients with bronchospastic disease should generally not receive beta-blockers - monitor closely if used in patients at risk of bronchospasm. Use cautiously in patients with diabetes; may mask prominent hypoglycemic symptoms. May mask signs of thyrotoxicosis. Use cautiously in severe renal impairment: marked hypotension can occur in patients maintained on hemodialysis. Use care with anesthetic agents which decrease myocardial function. Can worsen myasthenia gravis. Similar reactions found with systemic administration may occur with topical (ophthalmic) administration.

Drug Interactions

Cytochrome P450 Effect: Substrate of CYP2D6 (major); **Inhibits** CYP2D6 (weak)

Decreased Effect: Decreased effect of timolol with aluminum salts, barbiturates, calcium salts, cholestyramine, colestipol, NSAIDs, penicillins (ampicillin), rifampin, salicylates, and sulfinpyrazone due to decreased bioavailability and plasma levels. Beta-blockers may decrease the effect of sulfonylureas. Beta-blockers may affect the action or levels of ethanol, disopyramide, nondepolarizing muscle relaxants, and theophylline, although the effects are difficult to predict.

Increased Effect/Toxicity: CYP2D6 inhibitors may increase the levels/effects of timolol; example inhibitors include chlorpromazine, delavirdine, fluoxetine, miconazole, paroxetine, pergolide, quinidine, quinine, ritonavir, and ropinirole. The heart rate-lowering effects of timolol are additive with other drugs which slow AV conduction (digoxin, verapamil, diltiazem). Reserpine increases the effects of timolol. Concurrent use of timolol may increase the effects of alpha-blockers (prazosin, terazosin), alpha-adrenergic stimulants (epinephrine, phenylephrine), and the vasoconstrictive effects of ergot alkaloids. Timolol may mask the tachycardia from hypoglycemia caused by insulin and oral hypoglycemics. In patients receiving concurrent therapy, the risk of hypertensive crisis is increased when either clonidine or the beta-blocker is withdrawn. Beta-blockers may increase the action or levels of ethanol, disopyramide, nondepolarizing muscle relaxants, and theophylline although the effects are difficult to predict.

Adverse Reactions

Ophthalmic:

>10%: Ocular: Burning, stinging

1% to 10%:

Cardiovascular: Hypertension

Central nervous system: Headache

Ocular: Blurred vision, cataract, conjunctival injection, itching, visual acuity decreased

Miscellaneous: Infection

Systemic:

1% to 10%:

Cardiovascular: Bradycardia

Central nervous system: Fatigue, dizziness

Respiratory: Dyspnea

Frequency not defined (reported with any dosage form):

Cardiovascular: Angina pectoris, arrhythmia, bradycardia, cardiac failure, cardiac arrest, cerebral vascular accident, cerebral ischemia, edema, hypotension, heart block, palpitation, Raynaud's phenomenon

Central nervous system: Anxiety, confusion, depression, disorientation, dizziness, hallucinations, insomnia, memory loss, nervousness, nightmares, somnolence

Dermatologic: Alopecia, angioedema, pseudopemphigoid, psoriasiform rash, psoriasis exacerbation, rash, urticaria

Endocrine & metabolic: Hypoglycemia masked, libido decreased

Gastrointestinal: Anorexia, diarrhea, dyspepsia, nausea, xerostomia

Genitourinary: Impotence, retoperitoneal fibrosis

Hematologic: Claudication

Neuromuscular & skeletal: Myasthenia gravis exacerbation, paresthesia

Ocular: Blepharitis, conjunctivitis, corneal sensitivity decreased, cystoid macular edema, diplopia, dry eyes, foreign body sensation, keratitis, ocular discharge, ocular pain, ptosis, refractive changes, tearing, visual disturbances

Otic: Tinnitus

Respiratory: Bronchospasm, cough, dyspnea, nasal congestion, pulmonary edema, respiratory failure

Miscellaneous: Allergic reactions, cold hands/feet, Peyronie's disease, systemic lupus erythematosus

Overdosage/Toxicology Symptoms of intoxication include cardiac disturbances, CNS toxicity, bronchospasm, hypoglycemia and hyperkalemia. The most common cardiac symptoms include hypotension and bradycardia. Atrioventricular block, intraventricular conduction disturbances, cardiogenic shock, and asystole may occur with severe overdose, especially with membrane-depressant drugs (eg, propranolol). CNS effects including convulsions, coma, and respiratory arrest are commonly seen with propranolol and other membrane-depressant and lipid-soluble drugs. Treatment is symptom-directed and supportive. Timolol is not readily dialyzable.

Pharmacodynamics/Kinetics
Onset of Action:
Hypotensive: Oral: 15-45 minutes; Peak effect: 0.5-2.5 hours
Intraocular pressure reduction: Ophthalmic: 30 minutes; Peak effect: 1-2 hours
Duration of Action: ~4 hours; Ophthalmic: Intraocular: 24 hours
Protein Binding: 60%
Half-Life Elimination: 2-2.7 hours; prolonged with renal impairment
Metabolism: Extensively hepatic; extensive first-pass effect
Excretion: Urine (15% to 20% as unchanged drug)
Available Dosage Forms Note: Unless otherwise specified, strength expressed as base.
Gel-forming solution, ophthalmic, as maleate: 0.25% (5 mL); 0.5% (2.5 mL, 5 mL)
Timoptic-XE®: 0.25% (5 mL); 0.5% (5 mL)
Solution, ophthalmic, as hemihydrate:
Betimol®: 0.25% (5 mL, 10 mL, 15 mL); 0.5% (5 mL, 10 mL, 15 mL) [contains benzalkonium chloride]
Solution, ophthalmic, as maleate: 0.25% (5 mL, 10 mL, 15 mL); 0.5% (5 mL, 10 mL, 15 mL) [contains benzalkonium chloride]
Istalol™: 0.5% (10 mL) [contains benzalkonium chloride and potassium sorbate]
Timoptic®: 0.25% (5 mL, 10 mL); 0.5% (5 mL, 10 mL) [contains benzalkonium chloride]
Solution, ophthalmic, as maleate [preservative free]:
Timoptic® OcuDose®: 0.25% (0.2 mL); 0.5% (0.2 mL) [single use]
Tablet, as maleate: 5 mg, 10 mg, 20 mg [strength expressed as salt]
Blocadren®: 20 mg [strength expressed as salt]

Dosing
Adults & Elderly:
Glaucoma: Ophthalmic:
Solution: Initial: 0.25% solution, instill 1 drop twice daily; increase to 0.5% solution if response not adequate; decrease to 1 drop/day if controlled; do not exceed 1 drop twice daily of 0.5% solution.
Istalol™: Instill 1 drop (0.5% solution) once daily in the morning.
Gel-forming solution (Timoptic-XE®): Instill 1 drop (either 0.25% or 0.5%) once daily
Hypertension: Oral: Initial: 10 mg twice daily, increase gradually every 7 days, usual dosage: 20-40 mg/day in 2 divided doses; maximum: 60 mg/day.
Prevention of myocardial infarction: Oral: 10 mg twice daily initiated within 1-4 weeks after infarction.
Migraine prophylaxis: Oral: Initial: 10 mg twice daily, increase to maximum of 30 mg/day.
Pediatrics: Children: Ophthalmic: Refer to adult dosing.
Administration
Other: Administer other topically-applied ophthalmic medications at least 10 minutes before Timoptic-XE®; wash hands before use; invert closed bottle and shake once before use; remove cap carefully so that tip does not touch anything; hold bottle between thumb and index finger; use index finger of other hand to pull down the lower eyelid to form a pocket for the eye drop and tilt head back; place the dispenser tip close to the eye and gently squeeze the bottle to administer 1 drop; remove pressure after a single drop has been released; **do not allow the dispenser tip to touch the eye**; replace cap and store bottle in an upright position in a clean area; do **not** enlarge hole of dispenser; do **not** wash tip with water, soap, or any other cleaner. Some ophthalmic solutions contain benzalkonium chloride; wait at least 10 minutes after instilling solution before inserting soft contact lenses.
Stability
Storage: Ophthalmic drops: Store at room temperature. Protect from light and freezing.
Timoptic Occudose®: Store in the protective foil wrap and use within 1 month after opening foil package.
Nursing Actions
Physical Assessment: Assess other medications patient may be taking for effectiveness and interactions. Monitor therapeutic effectiveness (appropriate for purpose of therapy [eg, migraine, ophthalmic, cardiac]) and adverse reactions (eg, adrenergic blocking effects) at beginning of therapy and regularly with long-term therapy. Monitor blood pressure periodically. Assess knowledge/teach patient appropriate use, interventions to reduce side effects, and adverse symptoms to report.
Patient Education: Oral: Take exact dose prescribed; do not increase, decrease, or discontinue dosage without consulting prescriber. Take at the same time each day. If you have diabetes, monitor serum glucose closely. May cause postural hypotension (use caution when rising from sitting or lying position or climbing stairs); dizziness, drowsiness, or blurred vision (use caution when driving or engaging in tasks requiring alertness until response to drug is known); decreased sexual ability (reversible); or nausea or vomiting (small frequent meals or frequent mouth care may help). Report swelling of extremities, respiratory difficulty, or new cough; weight gain (>3 lb/week); unresolved diarrhea or vomiting; or cold blue extremities. **Pregnancy/breast-feeding precautions:** Inform prescriber if you are or intend to become pregnant. Consult prescriber if breast-feeding.

Ophthalmic: For ophthalmic use only. Apply prescribed amount as often as directed. Wash hands before using. Do not let tip of applicator touch eye; do (Continued)

Timolol *(Continued)*

not contaminate tip of applicator (may cause eye infection, eye damage, or vision loss). Tilt head back and look upward. Gently pull down lower lid and put drop(s) inside lower eyelid at inner corner. Close eye and roll eyeball in all directions. Do not blink for ½ minute. Apply gentle pressure to inner corner of eye for 30 seconds. Wipe away excess from skin around eye. Do not use any other eye preparation for at least 10 minutes. Do not share medication with anyone else. Temporary stinging or blurred vision may occur. If using Istalol™, remove contact lenses prior to administration. Lenses may be reinserted 15 minutes following administration. Immediately report any adverse cardiac or CNS effects (usually signifies overdose). Report persistent eye pain, redness, burning, watering, dryness, double vision, puffiness around eye, vision changes, other adverse eye response, worsening of condition or lack of improvement.

Dietary Considerations Oral product should be administered with food at the same time each day.

Geriatric Considerations Due to alterations in the beta-adrenergic autonomic nervous system, beta-adrenergic blockade may result in less hemodynamic response than seen in younger adults.

Breast-Feeding Issues Timolol is excreted in breast milk following oral and ophthalmic administration, and is considered compatible by the AAP. It is recommended that the infant be monitored for signs or symptoms of beta-blockade (hypotension, bradycardia, etc) with long-term use.

Pregnancy Issues Timolol was shown to cross the placenta in an *in vitro* perfusion study. Beta-blockers have been associated with bradycardia, hypotension, hypoglycemia, and intrauterine growth rate (IUGR); IUGR is probably related to maternal hypertension. Available evidence suggests beta-blockers are generally safe during pregnancy (JNC 7). Cases of neonatal hypoglycemia have been reported following maternal use of beta-blockers at parturition or during breast-feeding. Bradycardia and arrhythmia have been reported in an infant following ophthalmic administration of timolol during pregnancy.

Tinidazole *(tye NI da zole)*

U.S. Brand Names Tindamax™

Pharmacologic Category Amebicide; Antibiotic, Miscellaneous; Antiprotozoal, Nitroimidazole

Pregnancy Risk Factor C

Lactation Enters breast milk/not recommended

Use Treatment of trichomoniasis caused by *T. vaginalis*; treatment of giardiasis caused by *G. duodenalis* (*G. lamblia*); treatment of intestinal amebiasis and amebic liver abscess caused by *E. histolytica*

Mechanism of Action/Effect After diffusing into the organism, it is proposed that tinidazole causes cytotoxicity by damaging DNA and preventing further DNA synthesis.

Contraindications Hypersensitivity to tinidazole, nitroimidazole derivatives (including metronidazole), or any component of the formulation; pregnancy (1st trimester); breast-feeding

Warnings/Precautions Use caution with CNS diseases; seizures and peripheral neuropathy have been reported with tinidazole and other nitroimidazole derivatives. Use caution with current or history of blood dyscrasias or hepatic impairment. When used for amebiasis, not indicated for the treatment of asymptomatic cyst passage. Safety and efficacy have not been established in children ≤3 years of age.

Drug Interactions
Cytochrome P450 Effect: Substrate of CYP3A4 (minor)
Decreased Effect: Specific interaction studies have not been conducted. Refer to Metronidazole monograph *on page 815*.
Increased Effect/Toxicity: Specific interaction studies have not been conducted. Refer to Metronidazole monograph *on page 815*.

Nutritional/Ethanol Interactions
Ethanol: The manufacturer recommends to avoid all ethanol or any ethanol-containing drugs (may cause disulfiram-like reaction characterized by flushing, headache, nausea, vomiting, sweating or tachycardia).
Food: Peak antibiotic serum concentration lowered and delayed, but total drug absorbed not affected.

Lab Interactions May interfere with AST, ALT, triglycerides, glucose, and LDH testing

Adverse Reactions
1% to 10%:
Central nervous system: Fatigue/malaise (1% to 2%), dizziness (≤1%), headache (≤1%)
Gastrointestinal: Metallic/bitter taste (4% to 6%), nausea (3% to 5%), anorexia (2% to 3%), dyspepsia/cramps/epigastric discomfort (1% to 2%), vomiting (1% to 2%), constipation (≤1%)
Neuromuscular & skeletal: Weakness (1% to 2%)
Frequency not defined.
Cardiovascular: Flushing, palpitation
Central nervous system: Ataxia, coma, confusion, convulsions, depression, drowsiness, fever, giddiness, insomnia, vertigo
Dermatologic: Angioedema, pruritus, rash, urticaria
Gastrointestinal: Diarrhea, furry tongue, oral candidiasis, salivation, stomatitis, thirst, tongue discoloration, xerostomia
Genitourinary: Urine darkened, vaginal discharge increased
Hematologic: Leukopenia (transient), neutropenia (transient), thrombocytopenia (reversible)
Hepatic: Transaminases increased
Neuromuscular & skeletal: Arthralgia, arthritis, myalgia, peripheral neuropathy (transient, includes numbness and paresthesia)
Respiratory: Bronchospasm, dyspnea, pharyngitis
Miscellaneous: Burning sensation, *Candida* overgrowth, diaphoresis

Overdosage/Toxicology Treatment should be symptomatic and supportive. Hemodialysis may be considered (43% removed during a 6-hour session).

Pharmacodynamics/Kinetics
Protein Binding: 12%
Half-Life Elimination: 13 hours
Metabolism: Hepatic via CYP3A4 (primarily); undergoes oxidation, hydroxylation and conjugation; forms a metabolite
Excretion: Urine (20% to 25%); feces (12%)
Available Dosage Forms Tablet [scored]: 250 mg, 500 mg

Dosing
Adults:
Amebiasis, intestinal: Oral: 2 g/day for 3 days
Amebiasis, liver abscess: Oral: 2 g/day for 3-5 days
Giardiasis: Oral: 2 g as a single dose
Trichomoniasis: Oral: 2 g as a single dose; sexual partners should be treated at the same time
Pediatrics:
Amebiasis, intestinal: Oral: Children >3 years: 50 mg/kg/day for 3 days (maximum dose: 2 g/day)
Amebiasis, liver abscess: Oral: Children >3 years: 50 mg/kg/day for 3-5 days (maximum dose: 2 g/day)
Giardiasis: Oral: Children >3 years: 50 mg/kg as a single dose (maximum dose: 2 g)

Renal Impairment: Adjustment not necessary. An additional dose equal to ¹/₂ the usual dose, should be administered at the end of hemodialysis if tinidazole is administered on a day hemodialysis occurs.

Hepatic Impairment: Specific recommendations are not available; use with caution.

Administration
Oral: Administer with food.

Stability
Storage: Store at controlled room temperature of 20°C to 25°C (68°F to 77°F). Protect from light.

Nursing Actions
Physical Assessment: Monitor therapeutic effectiveness (symptoms and laboratory tests) and adverse response. Teach patient appropriate use, interventions to reduce side effects, and adverse symptoms to report

Patient Education: Do not take any new medications during therapy without consulting prescriber. Take exactly as directed. Avoid all alcohol while taking this medication; may cause unpleasant reaction (flushing, nausea, vomiting, sweating, headache, rapid heart beat). Refrain from sexual intercourse or use contraceptive if being treated for trichomoniasis. May cause headache, drowsiness or dizziness (use caution when climbing stairs, driving, or engaged in potentially hazardous tasks until response to drug is known); mild gastrointestinal disturbance (nausea, vomiting, constipation, diarrhea, metallic/bitter taste, abdominal discomfort) small frequent meals, frequent mouth care, chewing gum or sucking lozenges may help. Report severe fatigue or weakness; chest pain or palpitations; swelling of lips or mouth, other persistent adverse reactions, lack of improvement or worsening of condition. **Pregnancy/breast-feeding precautions:** Inform prescriber if you are or intend to become pregnant. Breast-feeding is contraindicated.

Dietary Considerations Take with food. The manufacturer recommends that ethanol be avoided during treatment and for 3 days after therapy is complete.

Breast-Feeding Issues Breast-feeding should be discontinued during therapy and for 3 days after the last dose.

Pregnancy Issues Tinidazole crosses the placenta and enters the fetal circulation. Use during the first trimester is contraindicated.

Tinzaparin (tin ZA pa rin)

U.S. Brand Names Innohep®
Synonyms Tinzaparin Sodium
Pharmacologic Category Low Molecular Weight Heparin
Pregnancy Risk Factor B
Lactation Excretion in breast milk unknown/use caution
Use Treatment of acute symptomatic deep vein thrombosis, with or without pulmonary embolism, in conjunction with warfarin sodium

Mechanism of Action/Effect Standard heparin consists of components with molecular weights ranging from 4000-30,000 daltons with a mean of 16,000 daltons. Heparin acts as an anticoagulant by enhancing the inhibition rate of clotting proteases by antithrombin III, impairing normal hemostasis and inhibition of factor Xa. Low molecular weight heparins have a small effect on the activated partial thromboplastin time and strongly inhibit factor Xa. The primary inhibitory activity of tinzaparin is through antithrombin. Tinzaparin is derived from porcine heparin that undergoes controlled enzymatic depolymerization. The average molecular weight of tinzaparin ranges between 5500 and 7500 daltons which is distributed as (<10%) 2000 daltons (60% to 72%) 2000-8000 daltons, and (22% to 36%) >8000

daltons. The antifactor Xa activity is approximately 100 int. units/mg.

Contraindications Hypersensitivity to tinzaparin sodium, heparin, sulfites, benzyl alcohol, pork products, or any component of the formulation; active major bleeding; heparin-induced thrombocytopenia (current or history of)

Warnings/Precautions Patients with recent or anticipated neuraxial anesthesia (epidural or spinal anesthesia) are at risk of spinal or epidural hematoma and subsequent paralysis. Consider risk versus benefit prior to neuraxial anesthesia; risk is increased by concomitant agents which may alter hemostasis, as well as traumatic or repeated epidural or spinal puncture, and indwelling epidural catheters. Patient should be observed closely for signs and symptoms of neurological impairment. Not to be used interchangeably (unit for unit) with heparin or any other low molecular weight heparins.

Monitor patient closely for signs or symptoms of bleeding. Certain patients are at increased risk of bleeding. Risk factors include bacterial endocarditis; congenital or acquired bleeding disorders; active ulcerative or angiodysplastic GI diseases; severe uncontrolled hypertension; hemorrhagic stroke; use shortly after brain, spinal, or ophthalmologic surgery; patients treated concomitantly with platelet inhibitors; recent GI bleeding; thrombocytopenia or platelet defects; severe liver disease; hypertensive or diabetic retinopathy; or in patients undergoing invasive procedures. Monitor platelet count closely. Rare cases of thrombocytopenia have occurred. Manufacturer recommends discontinuation of therapy if platelets are <100,000/mm³.

Safety and efficacy in pediatric patients has not been established. Use with caution in the elderly (delayed elimination may occur). Heparin can cause hyperkalemia by affecting aldosterone; similar reactions could occur with LMWHs. Monitor for hyperkalemia. For subcutaneous injection only, do not mix with other injections or infusions. Clinical experience is limited in patients with BMI >40 kg.

Drug Interactions
Increased Effect/Toxicity: Drugs which affect platelet function (eg, aspirin, NSAIDs, dipyridamole, ticlopidine, clopidogrel, sulfinpyrazone, dextran) may potentiate the risk of hemorrhage. Thrombolytic agents increase the risk of hemorrhage.

Warfarin: Risk of bleeding may be increased during concurrent therapy. Tinzaparin is commonly continued during the initiation of warfarin therapy to assure anticoagulation and to protect against possible transient hypercoagulability

Lab Interactions Asymptomatic increases in AST (SGOT) (8.8%) and ALT (SGPT) (13%) have been reported. Elevations were >3 times the upper limit of normal and were reversible and rarely associated with increases in bilirubin.

Adverse Reactions As with all anticoagulants, bleeding is the major adverse effect of tinzaparin. Hemorrhage may occur at virtually any site. Risk is dependent on multiple variables.
>10%:
  Hepatic: Increased ALT (13%)
  Local: Injection site hematoma (16%)
1% to 10%:
  Cardiovascular: Angina pectoris, chest pain (2%), hyper-/hypotension, tachycardia
  Central nervous system: Confusion, dizziness, fever (2%), headache (2%), insomnia, pain (2%)
  Dermatologic: Bullous eruption, pruritus, rash (1%), skin disorder
  Gastrointestinal: Constipation (1%), dyspepsia, flatulence, nausea (2%), nonspecified gastrointestinal disorder, vomiting (1%)
  Genitourinary: Dysuria, urinary retention, urinary tract infection (4%)
(Continued)

Tinzaparin (Continued)

Hematologic: Anemia, hematoma, hemorrhage (2%), thrombocytopenia (1%)

Hepatic: Increased AST (9%)

Local: Deep vein thrombosis, injection site hematoma

Neuromuscular & skeletal: Back pain (2%)

Renal: Hematuria (1%)

Respiratory: Dyspnea (1%), epistaxis (2%), pneumonia, pulmonary embolism (2%), respiratory disorder

Miscellaneous: Impaired healing, infection, unclassified reactions

Overdosage/Toxicology Overdose may lead to bleeding; bleeding may occur at any site. In case of overdose, discontinue medication, apply pressure to bleeding site if possible, and replace volume and hemostatic blood elements as required. If these measures are ineffective, or if bleeding is severe, protamine sulfate may be administered at 1 mg per every 100 anti-Xa int. units of tinzaparin.

Pharmacodynamics/Kinetics

Onset of Action: 2-3 hours

Time to Peak: 4-5 hours

Half-Life Elimination: 3-4 hours

Metabolism: Partially metabolized by desulphation and depolymerization

Excretion: Urine

Available Dosage Forms Injection, solution, as sodium: 20,000 anti-Xa int. units/mL (2 mL) [contains benzyl alcohol and sodium metabisulfite]

Dosing

Adults & Elderly: Treatment of DVT: SubQ: 175 anti-Xa int. units/kg of body weight once daily. Warfarin sodium should be started when appropriate. Administer tinzaparin for at least 6 days and until patient is adequately anticoagulated with warfarin.

Note: To calculate the volume of solution to administer per dose: Volume to be administered (mL) = patient weight (kg) x 0.00875 mL/kg (may be rounded off to the nearest 0.05 mL)

Renal Impairment: Patients with severe renal impairment had a 24% decrease in clearance, use with caution.

Hepatic Impairment: No adjustment necessary.

Administration

I.V.: Patient should be lying down or sitting. Administer by deep SubQ injection, alternating between the left and right anterolateral and left and right posterolateral abdominal wall. Vary site daily. The entire needle should be introduced into the skin fold formed by the thumb and forefinger. Hold the skin fold until injection is complete. To minimize bruising, do not rub the injection site.

Stability

Storage: Store at 25°C (77°F). Excursions permitted to 15°C to 30°C (59°F to 86°F).

Laboratory Monitoring CBC including platelet count and hematocrit or hemoglobin, and stool for occult blood; the monitoring of PT and/or PTT is not necessary. Patients receiving both warfarin and tinzaparin should have their INR drawn just prior to the next scheduled dose of tinzaparin.

Nursing Actions

Physical Assessment: Assess potential for interactions with other pharmacological agents and herbal products patient may be taking (especially anything that will impact coagulation or platelet aggregation). Monitor laboratory tests on a regular basis. Monitor therapeutic effectiveness, and adverse response (eg, bleeding at any source, rash, angina, confusion, urinary retention, dyspnea. Observe and teach bleeding precautions. Teach patient use if self-administered (appropriate injection technique and syringe/needle disposal), possible side effects/appropriate interventions (eg, bleeding precautions), and adverse symptoms to report.

Patient Education: Do not take any new medication during therapy unless approved by prescriber. This drug can only be administered by injection. If self-administered, use exactly as directed and follow instructions for syringe disposal. Do not alter dosage or discontinue without consulting prescriber. You may have a tendency to bleed easily while taking this drug (brush teeth with soft brush, use waxed dental floss, use electric razor, avoid scissors or sharp knives, and avoid potentially harmful activities). Report immediately any unusual bleeding or bruising (eg, mouth, nose, blood in urine or stool); chest pain or palpitations; confusion, dizziness, or headache; skin rash or itching; persistent GI upset (eg, nausea, vomiting, abdominal pain, acute constipation); warmth, swelling, pain, or redness in calves or other areas; back or muscle pain; respiratory difficulties; or other persistent adverse reactions. **Pregnancy/breast-feeding precautions:** Inform prescriber if you are pregnant or intend to become pregnant or breast-feed.

Pregnancy Issues There are no adequate and well-controlled studies in pregnant women. Cases of teratogenic effects and/or fetal death have been reported (relationship to tinzaparin not established). Use during pregnancy only if clearly needed. Pregnant women, or those who become pregnant while receiving tinzaparin, should be informed of the potential risks to the fetus.

Additional Information Contains sodium metabisulfite and benzyl alcohol, 10 mg/mL

Tioconazole (tye oh KONE a zole)

U.S. Brand Names 1-Day™ [OTC]; Vagistat®-1 [OTC]

Pharmacologic Category Antifungal Agent, Vaginal

Medication Safety Issues

Sound-alike/look-alike issues:

Tioconazole may be confused with terconazole

Pregnancy Risk Factor C

Lactation Excretion in breast milk unknown/not recommended

Use Local treatment of vulvovaginal candidiasis

Mechanism of Action/Effect A 1-substituted imidazole derivative with a broad antifungal spectrum against a wide variety of dermatophytes and yeasts

Contraindications Hypersensitivity to tioconazole or any component of the formulation

Warnings/Precautions For vaginal use only. Petrolatum-based vaginal products may damage rubber or latex condoms or diaphragms. Separate use by 3 days.

Drug Interactions

Cytochrome P450 Effect: Inhibits CYP1A2 (weak), 2A6 (weak), 2C8/9 (weak), 2C19 (weak), 2D6 (weak), 2E1 (weak)

Adverse Reactions Frequency not defined.

Central nervous system: Headache

Gastrointestinal: Abdominal pain

Dermatologic: Burning, desquamation

Genitourinary: Discharge, dyspareunia, dysuria, irritation, itching, nocturia, vaginal pain, vaginitis, vulvar swelling

Pharmacodynamics/Kinetics

Onset of Action: Some improvement: Within 24 hours; Complete relief: Within 7 days

Excretion: Urine and feces

Available Dosage Forms Ointment, vaginal: 6.5% (4.6 g) [with applicator]

Dosing

Adults & Elderly: Vulvovaginal candidiasis: Vaginal: Insert 1 applicatorful in vagina, just prior to bedtime, as a single dose

Stability
Storage: Store at room temperature.

Nursing Actions
Physical Assessment: Assess knowledge/teach patient appropriate administration, possible side effects/interventions, and adverse symptoms to report

Patient Education: Consult with prescriber if treating a vaginal yeast infection for the first time. Insert high into the vagina. Refrain from intercourse during treatment. May interact with condoms and vaginal contraceptive diaphragms (ie, weaken latex); do not rely on these products for 3 days following treatment. Do not use tampons, douches, spermicides, or other vaginal products during treatment. Although product is used for a single day, relief from symptoms usually takes longer than 1 day. Report persistent (>3 days) vaginal burning, irritation, or discharge. **Breast-feeding precaution:** Breast-feeding is not recommended.

Tiotropium (ty oh TRO pee um)

U.S. Brand Names Spiriva®
Synonyms Tiotropium Bromide Monohydrate
Pharmacologic Category Anticholinergic Agent
Medication Safety Issues
Sound-alike/look-alike issues:
Spiriva® may be confused with Inspra™
Spiriva® capsules for inhalation are for administration via HandiHaler® device and are not for oral use
Pregnancy Risk Factor C
Lactation Excretion in breast milk unknown/use caution
Use Maintenance treatment of bronchospasm associated with COPD (bronchitis and emphysema)
Mechanism of Action/Effect Blocks the action of acetylcholine at parasympathetic sites in bronchial smooth muscle causing bronchodilation
Contraindications Hypersensitivity to tiotropium, its derivatives, or any component of the formulation (contains lactose); not for use as an acute ("rescue") bronchodilator
Warnings/Precautions Not indicated for the initial treatment of acute episodes of bronchospasm; use with caution in patients with myasthenia gravis, narrow-angle glaucoma, prostatic hyperplasia, or bladder neck obstruction; avoid inadvertent instillation of powder into the eyes. Immediate hypersensitivity reactions may occur. Use caution in renal impairment. Safety and efficacy have not been established in pediatric patients.
Drug Interactions
Cytochrome P450 Effect: Substrate (minor) of CYP2D6, 3A4
Increased Effect/Toxicity: Increased toxicity with anticholinergics or drugs with anticholinergic properties.
Adverse Reactions
>10%:
Gastrointestinal: Xerostomia (16%)
Respiratory: Upper respiratory tract infection (41% vs 37% with placebo), sinusitis (11% vs 9% with placebo), pharyngeal irritation (frequency not specified)
1% to 10%:
Cardiovascular: Angina, edema (dependent, 5%)
Central nervous system: Paresthesia, depression
Dermatologic: Rash (4%)
Endocrine & metabolic: Hypercholesterolemia, hyperglycemia
Gastrointestinal: Dyspepsia (6%), abdominal pain (5%), constipation (4%), vomiting (4%), reflux, ulcerative stomatitis
Genitourinary: Urinary tract infection (7%)
Neuromuscular & skeletal: Myalgia (4%), leg pain, skeletal pain
Ocular: Cataract

Respiratory: Pharyngitis (9%), rhinitis (6%), epistaxis (4%), dysphonia, laryngitis
Miscellaneous: Infection (4%), moniliasis (4%), allergic reaction, herpes zoster
Overdosage/Toxicology Conjunctivitis and xerostomia have been observed with doses up to 141 micrograms. Other symptoms of overdose include drying of respiratory secretions, cough, nausea, GI distress, blurred vision or impaired visual accommodation, headache, and nervousness. Acute overdose with tiotropium by inhalation is unlikely since it is so poorly absorbed. However, if poisoning occurs, it can be treated like any other anticholinergic toxicity. An anticholinergic overdose with severe life-threatening symptoms may be treated with physostigmine 1-2 mg SubQ or I.V. slowly.
Pharmacodynamics/Kinetics
Time to Peak: Plasma: 5 minutes (following inhalation)
Protein Binding: 72%
Half-Life Elimination: 5-6 days
Metabolism: Hepatic (minimal), via CYP2D6 and CYP3A4
Excretion: Urine (74% as unchanged drug)
Available Dosage Forms Powder for oral inhalation [capsule]: 18 mcg/capsule [contains lactose; packaged in 6s or 30s with HandiHaler® device]
Dosing
Adults & Elderly: COPD: Oral inhalation: Contents of 1 capsule (18 mcg) inhaled once daily using HandiHaler® device
Renal Impairment: Plasma concentrations increase in renal impairment. Use caution; no specific dosage adjustment recommended.
Administration
Oral: For inhalation, not to be swallowed
Inhalation: Administer once daily at the same time each day. Remove capsule from foil blister immediately before use. Place capsule in the capsule-chamber in the base of the HandiHaler® Inhaler. Must only use the HandiHaler® Inhaler. Close mouthpiece until a click is heard, leaving dustcap open. Exhale fully. Do not exhale into inhaler. Tilt head slightly back and inhale (rapidly, steadily and deeply); the capsule vibration may be heard within the device. Hold breath as long as possible. If any powder remains in capsule, exhale and inhale again. Repeat until capsule is empty. Throw away empty capsule; do not leave in inhaler. Do not use a spacer with the HandiHaler® Inhaler. Always keep capsules and inhaler dry.

Delivery of dose: Instruct patient to place mouthpiece gently between teeth, closing lips around inhaler. Instruct patient to inhale deeply and hold breath held for 5-10 seconds. The amount of drug delivered is small, and the individual will not sense the medication as it is inhaled. Remove mouthpiece prior to exhalation. Patient should not breathe out through the mouthpiece.
Stability
Storage: Store between 15°C and 25°C. Do not store capsules in HandiHaler® device. Capsules should be stored in the blister pack and only removed immediately before use. After first capsule in the strip is used, the 2 remaining capsules should be used over the next 2 days.
Laboratory Monitoring FEV$_1$, peak flow (or other pulmonary function studies)
Nursing Actions
Physical Assessment: Assess potential for interactions with other prescription or OTC medications or herbal products patient may be taking. Monitor pulmonary tests prior to and periodically during therapy. Monitor therapeutic effectiveness and adverse response at beginning of therapy and at regular intervals during therapy. Teach patient proper
(Continued)

Tiotropium *(Continued)*

use, appropriate interventions to reduce side effects, and adverse symptoms to report.

Patient Education: Use inhaler and medication as instructed - once daily, at same time each day. Do not use more often than prescribed. Do not use as an acute "rescue" bronchodilator. May cause nausea or vomiting (small frequent meals and frequent mouth care may help); hyperglycemia (if diabetic, monitor serum glucose closely); muscle or skeletal pain (consult prescriber for appropriate analgesic). Report swelling of face, mouth, or tongue; skin rash; chest pain or palpitations; persistent gastrointestinal effects; muscle or skeletal pain or weakness; change in vision; respiratory changes, sore throat, or flu-like symptoms. **Pregnancy/breast-feeding precautions:** Inform prescriber if you are or intent to be pregnant. Breast-feeding is not recommended.

Administration of HandiHaler® Inhaler: Remove capsule from blister pack immediately before using. Place capsule in capsule-chamber in the base of inhaler. Close mouthpiece until a click is heard, leaving dustcap open. Exhale fully (do not exhale into inhaler). Place mouthpiece gently between teeth, closing lips around inhaled, tilt head back slightly, and inhale once rapidly, steadily and deeply (the capsule vibration may be heard within the inhaler, but you will not sense the medication as it is inhaled.) Hold breath as long as possible. Remove inhaler from mouth before exhaling. If any powder remains in capsule, repeat inhalation again. Throw away empty capsule. Do not store capsule in inhaler and always keep inhaler and capsules dry.

Geriatric Considerations Assess patient's ability to use the HandiHaler®. In elderly patients, renal clearance of tiotropium was decreased and plasma concentrations were increased, due to decreased renal function. No significant difference in adverse effects were seen in young vs older patients. No dosage adjustments are recommended due to age or renal function. However, the manufacturer recommends monitoring patients with moderate-to-severe renal impairment.

Tipranavir *(tip RA na veer)*

U.S. Brand Names Aptivus®

Synonyms PNU-140690E; TPV

Pharmacologic Category Antiretroviral Agent, Protease Inhibitor

Pregnancy Risk Factor C

Lactation Excretion in breast milk unknown/contraindicated

Use Treatment of HIV-1 infections in combination with ritonavir and other antiretroviral agents; limited to highly treatment experienced or multi-protease inhibitor resistant patients.

Mechanism of Action/Effect Tipranavir is a nonpeptide inhibitor of HIV-1 protease. Inhibition of the viral protease prevents cleavage of the gag-pol polyprotein resulting in the production of immature, noninfectious virus

Contraindications Hypersensitivity to tipranavir or any component of the formulation or any contraindication to ritonavir therapy; concurrent therapy of tipranavir/ritonavir with alfuzosin, amiodarone, bepridil, cisapride, dihydroergotamine, ergonovine, ergotamine, flecainide, lovastatin, methylergonovine, midazolam, pimozide, propafenone, quinidine, simvastatin, St John's wort, triazolam, and voriconazole; patients with hepatic insufficiency (Child-Pugh Class B and C)

Warnings/Precautions Coadministration with ritonavir is required. May cause hepatitis or exacerbate pre-existing hepatic dysfunction; use with caution in patients with hepatitis B or C and in hepatic disease. May be associated with fat redistribution (buffalo hump, increased abdominal girth, breast engorgement, facial atrophy). Use caution in hemophilia. May increase cholesterol and/or triglycerides; hypertriglyceridemia may increase risk of pancreatitis. May cause hyperglycemia. Use with caution in patients with sulfonamide allergy or hemophilia. Tipranavir has been associated with dermatological adverse effects, including rash (sometimes accompanied by joint pain, throat tightness, or generalized pruritus) and photosensitivity. Immune reconstitution syndrome, including inflammatory responses to indolent infections, has been associated with antiretroviral therapy; additional evaluation and treatment may be required.

Tipranavir should be used with caution in combination with other agents metabolized by CYP3A4. Avoid concurrent use of lovastatin or simvastatin (risk of rhabdomyolysis may be increased). Avoid concurrent use of hormonal contraceptives, rifampin, and/or St John's wort (may lead to loss of virologic response and/or resistance). Use with caution with metronidazole or disulfiram (due to ethanol content of formulation). Safety and efficacy have not been established in children.

Drug Interactions

Cytochrome P450 Effect:

Substrate of CYP3A4 (major; minimal metabolism when coadministered with ritonavir)

Ritonavir: **Inhibits** CYP3A4 (strong) and 2D6

Decreased Effect: CYP3A4 inducers may decrease the levels/effects of tipranavir. Example inducers include aminoglutethimide, carbamazepine, nafcillin, nevirapine, phenobarbital, phenytoin, and rifamycins. When coadministered with ritonavir, reduction of tipranavir serum concentrations is unlikely. Rifampin may decrease serum concentrations of tipranavir. Concurrent use of rifampin is not recommended. The effect of methadone may be reduced by tipranavir (dosage increase may be required).

Serum concentrations of protease inhibitors may be decreased by tipranavir. Concurrent therapy with amprenavir, lopinavir, or saquinavir is not recommended. Tipranavir/ritonavir may decrease serum concentrations of nucleoside reverse transcriptase inhibitors (NRTIs, including abacavir, didanosine, and zidovudine); administer tipranavir/ritonavir 2 hours before or after didanosine.

Increased Effect/Toxicity: Note: Listed interactions include interactions resulting from coadministration with ritonavir. Refer to Ritonavir monograph *on page 1091* for additional interaction concerns. The serum concentrations of tipranavir may be increased by ritonavir. This combination is recommended to enhance the effect ("boost") tipranavir.

Tipranavir/ritonavir may increase the levels/effects of CYP3A4 substrates. Tipranavir/ritonavir may increase the toxicity of benzodiazepines; concurrent use of midazolam and triazolam is specifically contraindicated. Tipranavir may increase serum concentrations of cisapride, increasing the risk of malignant arrhythmias; use is contraindicated. Toxicity of pimozide is significantly increased by tipranavir/ritonavir; concurrent use is contraindicated. Tipranavir/ritonavir may increase serum concentrations/toxicity of several antiarrhythmic agents; contraindicated with amiodarone, bepridil, flecainide, propafenone, and quinidine (use extreme caution with lidocaine). Tipranavir/ritonavir may also increase serum concentrations/effects of calcium channel blockers and immunosuppressants (cyclosporine, sirolimus, tacrolimus).

Serum concentrations of HMG-CoA reductase inhibitors (atorvastatin, cerivastatin, lovastatin, simvastatin) may be increased by tipranavir/ritonavir, increasing the risk of myopathy/rhabdomyolysis. Lovastatin and simvastatin are not recommended. Use lowest possible dose of atorvastatin. Fluvastatin and prava-statin may be safer alternatives. Serum concentrations of rifabutin may be increased by tipranavir/ritonavir; dosage adjustment of rifabutin is required.

The toxicity of ergot alkaloids (dihydroergotamine, ergotamine, ergonovine, methylergonovine) is increased by tipranavir; concurrent use is contraindicated. Effects of hypoglycemic agents may be altered by tipranavir/ritonavir. Concurrent therapy with tipranavir may increase serum concentrations of normeperidine, and decrease serum concentrations of meperidine. The serum concentrations of sildenafil, tadalafil, and vardenafil may be increased by tipranavir/ritonavir; dose adjustment and limitations related to ritonavir coadministration must be recognized.

Concurrent use of disulfiram with tipranavir oral solution is contraindicated due to risk of adverse reaction (due to alcohol content of formulation). Clarithromycin may increase serum concentrations of tipranavir. Tipranavir/ritonavir may increase serum concentrations of clarithromycin. Use with caution and adjust dose of clarithromycin during concurrent therapy in renally impaired patients.

Nutritional/Ethanol Interactions
Ethanol: Capsules contain dehydrated alcohol 7% w/w (0.1g per capsule)
Food: Bioavailability is increased with a high-fat meal.

Adverse Reactions Protease inhibitors cause dyslipidemia which includes elevated cholesterol and triglycerides and a redistribution of body fat centrally to cause increased abdominal girth, buffalo hump, facial atrophy, and breast enlargement. These agents also cause hyperglycemia.

>10%:
Endocrine & metabolic: Hypercholesterolemia (>300 mg/dL: 11%), hypertriglyceridemia (>400 mg/dL: 26%)
Gastrointestinal: Diarrhea (11%)
Hepatic: Transaminase increased (ALT or AST: 24%)
2% to 10%:
Central nervous system: Fever (5%), fatigue (4%), headache (3%), depression (2%)
Dermatologic: Rash (2%)
Endocrine & metabolic: Amylase increased (3%)
Gastrointestinal: Nausea (7%), vomiting (3%), abdominal pain (3%), amylase increased (3%)
Hematologic: WBC decreased (grade 3-4: 4%)
Neuromuscular & skeletal: Weakness (2%)
Respiratory: Bronchitis (3%)

Pharmacodynamics/Kinetics
Protein Binding: 99%
Half-Life Elimination: 6 hours
Metabolism: Hepatic, via CYP3A4 (minimal when coadministered with ritonavir)
Excretion: Feces (82%); urine (4%); primarily as unchanged drug (when coadministered with ritonavir)
Available Dosage Forms Capsule, gelatin: 250 mg [contains dehydrated ethanol 7% per capsule]

Dosing
Adults & Elderly: HIV infection: Oral: 500 mg twice daily with a high-fat meal. Note: Coadministration with ritonavir (200 mg twice daily) is required.
Renal Impairment: No adjustment required.

Administration
Oral:
Should be administered with food (bioavailability is increased). Coadministration with ritonavir is standard.

Stability
Storage: Prior to opening bottle, store under refrigeration at 2°C to 8°C (36°F to 46°F). After bottle is opened, may be stored at 25°C (77°F), with excursions permitted to 15°C to 30°C (59°F to 86°F) for up to 60 days.

Laboratory Monitoring Viral load, CD4, serum glucose, liver function tests, bilirubin

Nursing Actions
Physical Assessment: Assess closely for potential interactions with other pharmacological agents or herbal products patient is taking (eg, ergot alkaloids, antiarrhythmics, HMG-CoA reductase inhibitors, hormonal contraceptives). Assess therapeutic response and adverse reactions (eg, gastrointestinal upset, diarrhea leading to dehydration and weight loss, hypercholesterolemia, hypertriglyceridemia, rash, bronchitis, myalgia, peripheral neuropathy) at regular intervals during therapy. Caution patients to monitor glucose levels closely; protease inhibitors may cause hyperglycemia or new-onset diabetes. Teach patient proper use, possible side effects/appropriate interventions, and adverse symptoms to report.(refer to Patient Education).

Patient Education:
Do not take any new medication during therapy unless approved by prescriber. This drug is not a cure for HIV, nor has it been found to reduce transmission. Take as directed, with a meal. This drug will usually be prescribed in combination with another medications; time medications as directed by prescriber. Maintain adequate hydration (2-3 L/day of fluids) unless instructed to restrict fluid intake. You may be advised to check your glucose levels (this drug can cause exacerbation or new-onset diabetes). You may be more susceptible to infection (avoid crowds and exposure to infection and do not have any vaccinations unless approved by prescriber). May cause body changes due to redistribution of body fat, facial atrophy, or breast enlargement (normal effects of drug); nausea, vomiting, or flatulence (small frequent meals, frequent mouth care, chewing gum, or sucking lozenges may help); muscle weakness or flank pain (consult prescriber for approved analgesic); headache or insomnia (consult prescriber for medication); or diarrhea (boiled milk, buttermilk, or yogurt may help). Inform prescriber if you experience muscle numbness or tingling; unresolved persistent vomiting, diarrhea, or abdominal pain; respiratory difficulty or chest pain; unusual skin rash; change in color of stool or urine or other persistent adverse effects. **Pregnancy/breast-feeding precautions:** Inform prescriber if you are or intent to be pregnant. This drug decreases the effect of oral contraceptives; consult prescriber for use of appropriate barrier contraceptives. Do not breast-feed.

Dietary Considerations Contains dehydrated alcohol 7% w/w (0.1 g per capsule)

Breast-Feeding Issues HIV-infected mothers are discouraged from breast-feeding to decrease potential transmission of HIV.

Tirofiban (tye roe FYE ban)

U.S. Brand Names Aggrastat®
Synonyms MK383; Tirofiban Hydrochloride
Pharmacologic Category Antiplatelet Agent, Glycoprotein IIb/IIIa Inhibitor
Medication Safety Issues
Sound-alike/look-alike issues:
Aggrastat® may be confused with Aggrenox®, argatroban
Pregnancy Risk Factor B
Lactation Excretion in breast milk unknown/contraindicated
Use In combination with heparin, is indicated for the treatment of acute coronary syndrome, including patients who are to be managed medically and those undergoing PTCA or atherectomy. In this setting, it has been shown to decrease the rate of a combined endpoint of death, (Continued)

Tirofiban (Continued)

new myocardial infarction or refractory ischemia/repeat cardiac procedure.

Mechanism of Action/Effect A reversible antagonist of fibrinogen binding to the GP IIb/IIIa receptor, the major platelet surface receptor involved in platelet aggregation. Platelet aggregation inhibition is reversible following cessation of the infusion.

Contraindications Hypersensitivity to tirofiban or any component of the formulation; active internal bleeding or a history of bleeding diathesis within the previous 30 days; history of intracranial hemorrhage, intracranial neoplasm, arteriovenous malformation, or aneurysm; history of thrombocytopenia following prior exposure; history of CVA within 30 days or any history of hemorrhagic stroke; major surgical procedure or severe physical trauma within the previous month; history, symptoms, or findings suggestive of aortic dissection; severe hypertension (systolic BP >180 mm Hg and/or diastolic BP >110 mm Hg); concomitant use of another parenteral GP IIb/IIIa inhibitor; acute pericarditis

Warnings/Precautions Bleeding is the most common complication. Watch closely for bleeding, especially the arterial access site for the cardiac catheterization. Prior to pulling the sheath, heparin should be discontinued for 3-4 hours and ACT <180 seconds or aPTT <45 seconds. Use standard compression techniques after sheath removal. Watch the site closely afterwards for further bleeding. Use with extreme caution in patients with platelet counts <150,000/mm^3, patients with hemorrhagic retinopathy, and chronic dialysis patients. Use caution with administration of other drugs affecting hemostasis. Adjust the dose with severe renal dysfunction (Cl$_{cr}$ <30 mL/minute). The use of tirofiban, aspirin and heparin together causes more bleeding than aspirin and heparin alone.

Drug Interactions

Decreased Effect: Levothyroxine and omeprazole decrease tirofiban levels; however, the clinical significance of this interaction remains to be demonstrated.

Increased Effect/Toxicity: Use of tirofiban with aspirin and heparin is associated with an increase in bleeding over aspirin and heparin alone; however, efficacy of tirofiban is improved. Risk of bleeding is increased when used with thrombolytics, oral anticoagulants, NSAIDs, dipyridamole, ticlopidine, and clopidogrel. Avoid concomitant use of other IIb/IIIa antagonists. Cephalosporins which contain the MTT side chain may theoretically increase the risk of hemorrhage.

Adverse Reactions Bleeding is the major drug-related adverse effect. Patients received background treatment with aspirin and heparin. Major bleeding was reported in 1.4% to 2.2%; minor bleeding in 10.5% to 12%; transfusion was required in 4% to 4.3%.

>1% (nonbleeding adverse events):

Cardiovascular: Bradycardia (4%), coronary artery dissection (5%), edema (2%)

Central nervous system: Dizziness (3%), fever (>1%), headache (>1%), vasovagal reaction (2%)

Gastrointestinal: Nausea (>1%)

Genitourinary: Pelvic pain (6%)

Hematologic: Thrombocytopenia: <90,000/mm^3 (1.5%), <50,000/mm^3 (0.3%)

Neuromuscular & skeletal: Leg pain (3%)

Miscellaneous: Diaphoresis (2%)

Overdosage/Toxicology The most frequent manifestation of overdose is bleeding. Treatment is cessation of therapy and assessment of transfusion. Tirofiban is dialyzable.

Pharmacodynamics/Kinetics

Half-Life Elimination: 2 hours

Metabolism: Minimally hepatic

Excretion: Urine (65%) and feces (25%) primarily as unchanged drug

Clearance: Elderly: Reduced by 19% to 26%

Available Dosage Forms

Infusion [premixed in sodium chloride]: 50 mcg/mL (100 mL, 250 mL)

Injection, solution: 250 mcg/mL (50 mL)

Dosing

Adults & Elderly: Acute coronary syndromes: I.V.: Initial rate of 0.4 mcg/kg/minute for 30 minutes and then continued at 0.1 mcg/kg/minute. Dosing should be continued through angiography and for 12-24 hours after angioplasty or atherectomy.

Renal Impairment: Cl$_{cr}$ <30 mL/minute: Reduce dose to 50% of normal rate.

Administration

I.V.: Infuse over 30 minutes. Tirofiban injection must be diluted to a concentration of 50 mcg/mL (premixed solution does not require dilution). Unused solution should be discarded. Do not administer via the same IV line as diazepam.

I.V. Detail: Intended for intravenous delivery using sterile equipment and technique. Do not add other drugs or remove solution directly from the bag with a syringe. Do not use plastic containers in series connections. Such use can result in air embolism by drawing air from the first container if it is empty of solution. Discard any unused solution. May be administered through the same catheter as heparin, lidocaine, dopamine, potassium chloride, and famotidine.

Stability

Compatibility: Stable in D$_5$¹/₂NS, D$_5$W, NS

Y-site administration: Incompatible with diazepam

Storage: Store at 25°C (77°F); do not freeze. Protect from light during storage.

Laboratory Monitoring Platelet count, persistent reductions <90,000/mm^3 may require interruption or discontinuation of infusion. Hemoglobin and hematocrit should be monitored prior to treatment, within 6 hours following loading infusion, and at least daily thereafter during therapy. Platelet count may need to be monitored earlier in patients who received prior glycoprotein IIb/IIIa antagonists. Because tirofiban requires concurrent heparin therapy, aPTT levels should also be followed.

Nursing Actions

Physical Assessment: Monitor vital signs and laboratory results prior to, during, and after therapy. Assess infusion insertion site during and after therapy (every 15 minutes or as institutional policy). Monitor closely for bleeding (eg, CNS changes; blood in urine, stool, or vomitus; unusual bruising or bleeding) and teach patient bleeding precautions (avoid invasive procedures and activities that could result in injury). Monitor closely for signs of unusual or excessive bleeding.

Patient Education: Emergency use may dictate depth of patient education. This medication can only be administered I.V. You will have a tendency to bleed easily following this medication. Use caution to prevent injury (use electric razor, use soft toothbrush, use caution with sharps). If bleeding occurs, apply pressure to bleeding spot until bleeding stops completely. Report unusual bruising or bleeding (eg, blood in urine, stool, or vomitus; bleeding gums, vaginal bleeding, nosebleeds); unusual and persistent fever; dizziness or vision changes; back, leg, or pelvic pain; or persistent nausea or vomiting. **Breast-feeding precaution:** Do not breast-feed.

Tizanidine (tye ZAN i deen)

U.S. Brand Names Zanaflex®
Synonyms Sirdalud®
Pharmacologic Category Alpha$_2$-Adrenergic Agonist
Medication Safety Issues
Sound-alike/look-alike issues:
Tizanidine may be confused with tiagabine
Pregnancy Risk Factor C
Lactation Excretion in breast milk unknown/not recommended
Use Skeletal muscle relaxant used for treatment of muscle spasticity
Unlabeled/Investigational Use Tension headaches, low back pain, and trigeminal neuralgia
Mechanism of Action/Effect
Acts within CNS at the level of the spinal cord to reduce excitation of motor neurons, resulting in muscle relaxation
Contraindications Hypersensitivity to tizanidine or any component of the formulation; concomitant therapy with ciprofloxacin or fluvoxamine
Warnings/Precautions
Reduce dose in patients with liver or renal disease. May cause significant orthostatic hypotension or bradycardia; use with caution in patients with hypotension or cardiac disease. Tizanidine clearance is reduced by more than 50% in elderly patients with renal insufficiency (Cl$_{cr}$ <25 mL/minute) compared to healthy elderly subjects; this may lead to a longer duration of effects and, therefore, should be used with caution in renally impaired patients.
Drug Interactions
Increased Effect/Toxicity:
Additive hypotensive effects may be seen with diuretics, other alpha adrenergic agonists, ciprofloxacin, or antihypertensives; CNS depression with baclofen or other CNS depressants. CYP1A2 Inhibitors may increase the levels/effects of tizanidine; example inhibitors include amiodarone, ciprofloxacin (contraindicated), fluvoxamine (contraindicated), ketoconazole, norfloxacin, ofloxacin, and rofecoxib. Oral contraceptives may decrease the clearance of tizanidine.
Nutritional/Ethanol Interactions
Ethanol: Avoid ethanol (may increase CNS depression).
Food: The tablet and capsule dosage forms are not bioequivalent when administered with food. Food increases both the time to peak concentration and the extent of absorption for both the tablet and capsule. However, maximal concentrations of tizanidine achieved when administered with food were increased by 30% for the tablet, but decreased by 20% for the capsule. Under fed conditions, the capsule is approximately 80% bioavailable relative to the tablet.
Herb/Nutraceutical: Avoid valerian, St John's wort, kava kava, gotu kola (may increase CNS depression). Avoid black cohosh, California poppy, coleus, golden seal, hawthorn, mistletoe, periwinkle, quinine, shepherd's purse (may increase hypotensive effects).
Adverse Reactions
>10%:
Cardiovascular: Hypotension (16% to 33%)
Central nervous system: Somnolence (48%), dizziness (16%)
Gastrointestinal: Xerostomia (49%)
Neuromuscular & skeletal: Weakness (41%)
1% to 10%:
Cardiovascular: Bradycardia (2% to 10%)
Central nervous system: Nervousness (3%), speech disorder (3%)
Gastrointestinal: Constipation (4%), vomiting (3%), pharyngitis (3%)
Genitourinary: UTI (10%), urinary frequency (3%)
Hepatic: Liver enzymes increased (3%)
Neuromuscular & skeletal: Dyskinesia (3%)
Ocular: Blurred vision (3%)
Respiratory: Rhinitis (3%)
Miscellaneous: Infection (6%), flu-like syndrome (3%)
Overdosage/Toxicology
Symptoms of overdose include dry mouth, bradycardia, hypotension
Treatment: Lavage (within 2 hours of ingestion) with activated charcoal; benzodiazepines for seizure control; atropine can be given for treatment of bradycardia; flumazenil has been used to reverse coma successfully; forced diuresis is not helpful; multiple dosing of activated charcoal may be helpful. Following attempts to enhance drug elimination, hypotension should be treated with I.V. fluids and/or Trendelenburg positioning.
Pharmacodynamics/Kinetics
Duration of Action: 3-6 hours
Time to Peak:
Fasting state: Capsule, tablet: 1 hour
Fed state: Capsule: 3-4 hours, Tablet: 1.5 hours
Half-Life Elimination: 2 hours
Metabolism:
Extensively hepatic
Excretion:
Urine (60%); feces (20%)
Available Dosage Forms
Capsule: 2 mg, 4 mg, 6 mg
Tablet: 2 mg, 4 mg
Dosing
Adults & Elderly:
Spasticity: Usual initial dose: 4 mg, may increase by 2-4 mg as needed for satisfactory reduction of muscle tone every 6-8 hours to a maximum of three doses in any 24 hour period
Range: 2-4 mg 3 times/day
Maximum dose: 36 mg/day
Renal Impairment: May require dose reductions or less frequent dosing
Hepatic Impairment: May require dose reductions or less frequent dosing.
Administration
Oral: Capsules may be opened and contents sprinkled on food; however, extent of absorption is increased up to 20% relative to administration of the capsule under fasted conditions.
Nursing Actions
Physical Assessment: Assess potential for interactions with other prescriptions, OTC medications, or herbal products patient may be taking. Assess results of laboratory tests, therapeutic response, and adverse reactions on a regular basis throughout therapy. Teach patient proper use, possible side effects/appropriate interventions, and adverse symptoms to report.
Patient Education: Take exactly as directed; do not change dosage or discontinue without consulting prescriber. If you miss a dose, take the missed dose as soon as possible if it is within an hour or so of the regular time. If not within an hour or so, skip the missed dose and go back to your regular dosing schedule. Do not double doses. Avoid alcohol. May cause dizziness, nervousness, insomnia, or daytime drowsiness (use caution when driving or engaging in tasks that require alertness until response to drug is known); postural hypotension (use caution and avoid quick moves when rising from sitting or lying position, climbing stairs, or engaging in activities that require quick movements); or nausea, vomiting, dry mouth, mouth sores, or upset stomach (small frequent meals, frequent mouth care, chewing gum, or sucking lozenges may help). Report persistent dizziness or GI symptoms; chest pain or palpitations; CNS disturbances (delusions, confusion); muscle weakness or tremors; rash; respiratory difficulty; or other persistent (Continued)

Tizanidine (Continued)

adverse effects. **Pregnancy/breast-feeding precautions:** Inform prescriber if you are or intend to become pregnant. Breast-feeding is not recommended.

Tobramycin (toe bra MYE sin)

U.S. Brand Names AKTob®; TOBI®; Tobrex®
Synonyms Tobramycin Sulfate
Pharmacologic Category Antibiotic, Aminoglycoside; Antibiotic, Ophthalmic
Medication Safety Issues
Sound-alike/look-alike issues:
Tobramycin may be confused with Trobicin®
AKTob® may be confused with AK-Trol®
Nebcin® may be confused with Inapsine®, Naprosyn®, Nubain®
Tobrex® may be confused with TobraDex®
Pregnancy Risk Factor D (injection, inhalation); B (ophthalmic)
Lactation Enters breast milk/not recommended
Use Treatment of documented or suspected infections caused by susceptible gram-negative bacilli including *Pseudomonas aeruginosa*; topically used to treat superficial ophthalmic infections caused by susceptible bacteria. Tobramycin solution for inhalation is indicated for the management of cystic fibrosis patients (>6 years of age) with *Pseudomonas aeruginosa*.
Mechanism of Action/Effect Interferes with bacterial protein synthesis by binding to 30S and 50S ribosomal subunits resulting in a defective bacterial cell membrane
Contraindications Hypersensitivity to tobramycin, other aminoglycosides, or any component of the formulation; pregnancy (injection/inhalation)
Warnings/Precautions Use with caution in patients with renal impairment, pre-existing auditory or vestibular impairment, and in patients with neuromuscular disorders. Dosage modification required in patients with impaired renal function (I.M. & I.V.). Aminoglycosides are associated with significant nephrotoxicity and ototoxicity; the ototoxicity is directly proportional to the amount of drug given and the duration of treatment. Tinnitus or vertigo are indications of vestibular injury. Ototoxicity is often irreversible, while renal damage is usually reversible.

Drug Interactions
Increased Effect/Toxicity: Increased antimicrobial effect of tobramycin with extended spectrum penicillins (synergistic). Neuromuscular blockers may have an increased duration of action (neuromuscular blockade). Amphotericin B, cephalosporins, and loop diuretics may increase the risk of nephrotoxicity.
Lab Interactions Some penicillin derivatives may accelerate the degradation of aminoglycosides *in vitro*, leading to a potential underestimation of aminoglycoside serum concentration.

Adverse Reactions
Injection: Frequency not defined:
Central nervous system: Confusion, disorientation, dizziness, fever, headache, lethargy, vertigo
Dermatologic: Exfoliative dermatitis, itching, rash, urticaria
Endocrine & metabolic: Serum calcium, magnesium, potassium, and/or sodium decreased
Gastrointestinal: Diarrhea, nausea, vomiting
Hematologic: Anemia, eosinophilia, granulocytopenia, leukocytosis, leukopenia, thrombocytopenia
Hepatic: ALT, AST, bilirubin, and/or LDH increased
Local: Pain at the injection site
Otic: Hearing loss, tinnitus, ototoxicity (auditory), ototoxicity (vestibular), roaring in the ears
Renal: BUN increased, cylindruria, serum creatinine increased, oliguria, proteinuria

Inhalation:
>10%:
Gastrointestinal: Sputum discoloration (21%)
Respiratory: Voice alteration (13%)
1% to 10%:
Central nervous system: Malaise (6%)
Otic: Tinnitus (3%)
Overdosage/Toxicology Symptoms of overdose include ototoxicity, nephrotoxicity, and neuromuscular toxicity. Treatment of choice following a single acute overdose appears to be maintenance of urine output of at least 3 mL/kg/hour during the acute treatment phase. Dialysis is of questionable value in enhancing aminoglycoside elimination. If required, hemodialysis is preferred over peritoneal dialysis in patients with normal renal function. Chelation with penicillins is investigational.

Pharmacodynamics/Kinetics
Time to Peak: Serum: I.M.: 30-60 minutes; I.V.: ~30 minutes
Protein Binding: <30%
Half-Life Elimination:
Neonates: ≤1200 g: 11 hours; >1200 g: 2-9 hours
Adults: 2-3 hours; directly dependent upon glomerular filtration rate
Adults with impaired renal function: 5-70 hours
Excretion: Normal renal function: Urine (~90% to 95%) within 24 hours

Available Dosage Forms
Infusion [premixed in NS]: 60 mg (50 mL); 80 mg (100 mL)
Injection, powder for reconstitution: 1.2 g
Injection, solution: 10 mg/mL (2 mL, 8 mL); 40 mg/mL (2 mL, 30 mL, 50 mL) [may contain sodium metabisulfite]
Ointment, ophthalmic (Tobrex®): 0.3% (3.5 g)
Solution for nebulization [preservative free] (TOBI®): 60 mg/mL (5 mL)
Solution, ophthalmic (AKTob®, Tobrex®): 0.3% (5 mL) [contains benzalkonium chloride]

Dosing
Adults: Individualization is **critical** because of the low therapeutic index.
Use of ideal body weight (IBW) for determining the mg/kg/dose appears to be more accurate than dosing on the basis of total body weight (TBW). In morbid obesity, dosage requirement may best be estimated using a dosing weight of IBW + 0.4 (TBW - IBW).
Initial and periodic plasma drug levels (eg, peak and trough with conventional dosing) should be determined, particularly in critically-ill patients with serious infections or in disease states known to significantly alter aminoglycoside pharmacokinetics (eg, cystic fibrosis, burns, or major surgery).
Severe life-threatening infections: I.M., I.V.:
Conventional dosing: 2-2.5 mg/kg/dose every 8-12 hours; to ensure adequate peak concentrations early in therapy, higher initial dosages may be considered in selected patients (eg, edema, septic shock, postsurgery, and/or trauma).
Once-daily dosing: Some clinicians suggest a daily dose of 4-7 mg/kg for all patients with normal renal function; this dose is at least as efficacious with similar, if not less, toxicity than conventional dosing.
Urinary tract infection: I.M., I.V.: 1.5 mg/kg/dose
Synergy (for gram-positive infections): I.M., I.V.: 1 mg/kg/dose
Hospital-acquired pneumonia (HAP): I.V.: 7 mg/kg/day once daily with antipseudomonal beta-lactam or carbapenem (American Thoracic Society/ATS guidelines)
Meningitis (*Pseudomonas aeruginosa*): I.V.: 5 mg/kg/day in divided doses every 8 hours (administered with another bacteriocidal drug)

Ocular infections: Ophthalmic:

Ointment: Apply 2-3 times/day; for severe infections, apply every 3-4 hours

Solution: Instill 1-2 drops every 4 hours; for severe infections, instill 2 drops every 30-60 minutes initially, then reduce to less frequent intervals

Pulmonary Infections: Inhalation:

Standard aerosolized tobramycin: 60-80 mg 3 times/day

High-dose regimen: 300 mg every 12 hours (do not administer doses <6 hours apart); administer in repeated cycles of 28 days on drug followed by 28 days off drug

Elderly: Dosage should be based on an estimate of ideal body weight.

I.M., I.V.: 1.5-5 mg/kg/day in 1-2 divided doses

I.V.: Once daily or extended interval: 5-7 mg/kg/dose given every 24, 36, or 48 hours based on Cl_{cr} (see Renal Impairment and Geriatric Considerations).

Pediatrics: Individualization is **critical** because of the low therapeutic index

Use of ideal body weight (IBW) for determining the mg/kg/dose appears to be more accurate than dosing on the basis of total body weight (TBW). In morbid obesity, dosage requirement may best be estimated using a dosing weight of IBW + 0.4 (TBW - IBW).

Susceptible systemic infections: I.M., I.V.:

Infants and Children <5 years: 2.5 mg/kg/dose every 8 hours

Children >5 years: 2-2.5 mg/kg/dose every 8 hours

Ocular infection: Ophthalmic: Children ≥2 months: See adult dosing.

Cystic fibrosis:

I.M., I.V.: 2.5-3.3 mg/kg every 6-8 hours

Inhalation:

Standard aerosolized tobramycin: 40-80 mg 2-3 times/day

High-dose regimen (TOBI®): Children ≥6 years: See adult dosing.

Note: Some patients may require larger or more frequent doses if serum levels document the need (eg, cystic fibrosis or febrile granulocytopenic patients). Also see drug level monitoring information in adult dosing.

Renal Impairment: I.M., I.V.:

Conventional dosing:

Cl_{cr} ≥60 mL/minute: Administer every 8 hours.

Cl_{cr} 40-60 mL/minute: Administer every 12 hours.

Cl_{cr} 20-40 mL/minute: Administer every 24 hours.

Cl_{cr} 10-20 mL/minute: Administer every 48 hours.

Cl_{cr} <10 mL/minute: Administer every 72 hours.

High-dose therapy: Interval may be extended (eg, every 48 hours) in patients with moderate renal impairment (Cl_{cr} 30-59 mL/minute) and/or adjusted based on serum level determinations.

Dialyzable; 30% removal of aminoglycosides occurs during 4 hours of HD - administer dose after dialysis and follow levels.

Continuous arteriovenous or venovenous hemofiltration: Dose as for Cl_{cr} of 10-40 mL/minute and follow levels.

Administration via CAPD fluid:

Gram-negative infection: 4-8 mg/L (4-8 mcg/mL) of CAPD fluid

Gram-positive infection (ie, synergy): 3-4 mg/L (3-4 mcg/mL) of CAPD fluid

Administration IVPB/I.M.: Dose as for Cl_{cr} <10 mL/ minute and follow levels.

Hepatic Impairment: Monitor plasma concentrations.

Administration

I.V.: Infuse over 30-60 minutes.

Some penicillins (eg, carbenicillin, ticarcillin and piperacillin) have been shown to inactivate aminglycosides *in vitro*. This has been observed to a greater extent with tobramycin and gentamicin, while

amikacin has shown greater stability against inactivation. Concurrent use of these agents may pose a risk of reduced antibacterial efficacy *in vivo*, particularly in the setting of profound renal impairment. However, definitive clinical evidence is lacking. If combination penicillin/aminoglycoside therapy is desired in a patient with renal dysfunction, separation of doses (if feasible), and routine monitoring of aminoglycoside levels, CBC, and clinical response should be considered.

I.V. Detail: Flush with saline before and after administration. **Incompatible** with heparin.

pH: 3.0-6.5 (injection, adjusted); 6-8 (reconstituted solution from powder)

Inhalation: TOBI®: To be inhaled over ~15 minutes using a handheld nebulizer.

Topical: Ophthalmic solution: Allow 5 minutes between application of "multiple-drop" therapy.

Other: Ophthalmic: Contact lenses should not be worn during treatment of ophthalmic infections.

Ointment: Do not touch tip of tube to eye. Instill ointment into pocket between eyeball and lower lid; patient should look downward before closing eye.

Solution: contact lenses should not be worn during treatment of ophthalmic infections. Allow 5 minutes between application of "multiple-drop" therapy.

Suspension: Shake well before using; Tilt head back, instill suspension in conjunctival sac and close eye(s). Do not touch dropper to eye. Apply light finger pressure on lacrimal sac for 1 minute following instillation.

Stability

Reconstitution: Dilute in 50-100 mL NS, D_5W for I.V. infusion

Compatibility: Stable in dextran 40 10% in dextrose, D_5NS, D_5W, $D_{10}W$, mannitol 20%, LR, NS

Y-site administration: Incompatible with allopurinol, amphotericin B cholesteryl sulfate complex, cefoperazone, heparin, hetastarch, indomethacin, propofol, sargramostim

Compatibility in syringe: Incompatible with cefamandole, clindamycin, heparin

Compatibility when admixed: Incompatible with cefamandole, cefepime, cefotaxime, cefotetan, floxacillin, heparin, penicillins

Storage:

Injection: Stable at room temperature both as the clear, colorless solution and as the dry powder. Reconstituted solutions remain stable for 24 hours at room temperature and 96 hours when refrigerated.

Ophthalmic solution: Store at 8°C to 27°C (46°F to 80°F).

Solution, for inhalation (TOBI®): Store under refrigeration at 2°C to 8°C (36°F to 46°F); may be stored in foil pouch at room temperature of 25°C (77°F) for up to 28 days. Avoid intense light. Solution may darken over time; however, do not use if cloudy or contains particles.

Laboratory Monitoring Urinalysis, BUN, serum creatinine, plasma tobramycin levels (as appropriate to dosing method). Peak levels are drawn 30 minutes after the end of a 30-minute infusion or 1 hour after initiation of infusion or I.M. injection. The trough is drawn just before the next dose. Levels are typically obtained after the third dose in conventional dosing. Perform culture and sensitivity studies prior to initiating therapy to determine the causative organism and its susceptibility to tobramycin. Some penicillin derivatives may accelerate the degradation of aminoglycosides.

Nursing Actions

Physical Assessment: Assess effectiveness and interactions of other medications patient may be taking. Assess patient's hearing level before, during, and following therapy; report changes to prescriber immediately. Monitor therapeutic response, laboratory (Continued)

Tobramycin *(Continued)*

values, and adverse reactions (neurotoxicity [vertigo, ataxia], opportunistic infection [fever, mouth and vaginal sores or plaques, unhealed wounds, etc]) at beginning of therapy and periodically throughout therapy. Assess knowledge/teach patient appropriate use, interventions to reduce side effects, and adverse symptoms to report.

Patient Education: Systemic: Maintain adequate hydration (2-3 L/day of fluids) unless instructed to restrict fluid intake. Report decreased urine output, swelling of extremities, respiratory difficulty, vaginal itching or discharge, rash, diarrhea, oral thrush, unhealed wounds, dizziness, change in hearing acuity or ringing in ears, or worsening of condition. **Pregnancy/breast-feeding precautions:** Inform prescriber if you are pregnant. Breast-feeding is not recommended.

Ophthalmic: Use as frequently as recommended; do not overuse. Do not let tip of applicator touch eye; do not contaminate tip of applicator (may cause eye infection, eye damage, or vision loss). Sit down, tilt head back, instill solution or drops inside lower eyelid, and roll eyeball in all directions. Close eye and apply gentle pressure to inner corner of eye for 30 seconds. May experience temporary stinging or blurred vision. Do not use any other eye preparation for 10 minutes. Inform prescriber if condition worsens or does not improve in 3-4 days.

Dietary Considerations May require supplementation of calcium, magnesium, potassium.

Geriatric Considerations Aminoglycosides are important therapeutic interventions for susceptible organisms and as empiric therapy in seriously ill patients. Their use is not without risk of toxicity; however, these risks can be minimized if initial dosing is adjusted for estimated renal function and appropriate monitoring is performed. High-dose, once-daily aminoglycosides have been advocated as an alternative to traditional dosing regimens. To date, there is little information on the safety and efficacy of these regimens in persons with a creatinine clearance <60 mL/minute/70 kg. A dosing nomogram based upon creatinine clearance has been proposed. Additional studies comparing high-dose, once-daily aminoglycosides to traditional dosing regimens in the elderly are needed before once-daily aminoglycoside dosing can be routinely adopted to this patient population.

Breast-Feeding Issues Tobramycin is excreted into breast milk. The actual amount following inhalation or topical therapy is not known. The AAP considers a related antibiotic, gentamicin, usually compatible with breast-feeding.

Pregnancy Issues Aminoglycosides, including tobramycin, cross the placenta. The manufacturers of Nebcin® and TOBI® have a labeled pregnancy category of D based on reports of bilateral congenital deafness in children whose mothers used streptomycin during pregnancy. The risk of teratogenic effects and deafness following *in utero* exposure to tobramycin is considered to be small and some resources consider the pregnancy risk factor to be C. The manufacturer of Tobrex® states that animal studies have not shown harm to the fetus; however, no adequate and well-controlled studies have been conducted in pregnant women.

Additional Information Once-daily dosing: Higher peak serum drug concentration to MIC ratios, demonstrated aminoglycoside postantibiotic effect, decreased renal cortex drug uptake, and improved cost-time efficiency are supportive reasons for the use of once daily dosing regimens for aminoglycosides. Current research indicates these regimens to be as effective for nonlife-threatening infections, with no higher incidence of nephrotoxicity, than those requiring multiple daily doses. Doses are determined by calculating the entire day's dose via usual multiple dose calculation techniques and administering this quantity as a single dose. Doses are then adjusted to maintain mean serum concentrations above the MIC(s) of the causative organism(s). (Example: 2.5-5 mg/kg as a single dose; expected Cp_{max}: 10-20 mcg/mL and Cp_{min}: <1 mcg/mL). Further research is needed for universal recommendation in all patient populations and gram-negative disease; exceptions may include those with known high clearance (eg, children, patients with cystic fibrosis, or burns who may require shorter dosage intervals) and patients with renal function impairment for whom longer than conventional dosage intervals are usually required.

Related Information
Peak and Trough Guidelines *on page 1387*

Tobramycin and Dexamethasone
(toe bra MYE sin & deks a METH a sone)

U.S. Brand Names TobraDex®
Synonyms Dexamethasone and Tobramycin
Pharmacologic Category Antibiotic/Corticosteroid, Ophthalmic
Pregnancy Risk Factor C
Lactation Excretion in breast milk unknown/use caution
Use Treatment of external ocular infection caused by susceptible gram-negative bacteria and steroid responsive inflammatory conditions of the palpebral and bulbar conjunctiva, lid, cornea, and anterior segment of the globe

Available Dosage Forms
Ointment, ophthalmic: Tobramycin 0.3% and dexamethasone 0.1% (3.5 g)
Suspension, ophthalmic: Tobramycin 0.3% and dexamethasone 0.1% (2.5 mL, 5 mL, 10 mL) [contains benzalkonium chloride]

Dosing
Adults & Elderly: Ocular infection/inflammation: Ophthalmic: Instill 1-2 drops of solution every 4 hours; apply ointment 2-3 times/day; for severe infections apply ointment every 3-4 hours, or solution 2 drops every 30-60 minutes initially, then reduce to less frequent intervals
Pediatrics: Ocular infection/inflammation: Children: Refer to adult dosing.

Nursing Actions
Physical Assessment: See individual agents.
Patient Education: Shake suspension well before using. Do not touch dropper to eye. Apply light finger pressure on lacrimal sac for one minute following instillation. Notify physician if condition fails to improve or worsens.

Related Information
Dexamethasone *on page 343*
Tobramycin *on page 1224*

Tolcapone *(TOLE ka pone)*

U.S. Brand Names Tasmar®
Restrictions A patient signed consent form acknowledging the risks of hepatic injury should be obtained by the treating physician.
Pharmacologic Category Anti-Parkinson's Agent, COMT Inhibitor
Pregnancy Risk Factor C
Lactation Excretion in breast milk unknown/contraindicated
Use Adjunct to levodopa and carbidopa for the treatment of signs and symptoms of idiopathic Parkinson's disease
Mechanism of Action/Effect Tolcapone is a selective and reversible inhibitor of catechol-o-methyltransferase

(COMT) which leads to more sustained blood levels of levodopa.

Contraindications Hypersensitivity to tolcapone or any component of the formulation; history of liver disease or tolcapone-induced hepatocellular injury; nontraumatic rhabdomyolysis or hyperpyrexia and confusion

Warnings/Precautions Due to reports of fatal liver injury, reserve for patients who are experiencing inadequate symptom control or who are not appropriate candidates for other available treatments. Patients must provide written consent acknowledging the risks of hepatic injury. Use with caution in patients with pre-existing dyskinesias, hepatic impairment, or severe renal impairment. Exacerbation of pre-existing dyskinesia and severe rhabdomyolysis has been reported. Has been associated with a syndrome resembling neuroleptic malignant syndrome (hyperpyrexia and confusion — some fatal) on abrupt withdrawal or dosage reduction.

Patients receiving tolcapone are predisposed to orthostatic hypotension, diarrhea (usually within the first 6-12 weeks of therapy), transient hallucinations (most commonly within the first 2 weeks of therapy), and new onset or worsened dyskinesia. Concomitant use of tolcapone and nonselective MAO inhibitors should be avoided. Selegiline is a selective MAO type B inhibitor (when given orally at ≤10 mg/day) and can be taken with tolcapone. Has also been associated with fibrotic complications, such as retroperitoneal fibrosis, pulmonary infiltrates or effusion and pleural thickening. Safety and efficacy in pediatric patients have not been established.

Drug Interactions
Cytochrome P450 Effect: Inhibits CYP2C9 (weak)
Increased Effect/Toxicity: Tolcapone may decrease the metabolism and increase the side effects of COMT substrates (eg, apomorphine, bitolterol, dobutamine, dopamine, epinephrine, norepinephrine, isoproterenol, isoetharine, and methyldopa). Effects on mental status may be additive with other CNS depressants; includes barbiturates, benzodiazepines, TCAs, antipsychotics, ethanol, narcotic analgesics, and other sedative-hypnotics. Concurrent use of nonselective MAO inhibitors with tolcapone may increase the risk of cardiovascular side effects; selective MAO inhibitors (eg, selegiline ≤10 mg/day) appear to pose limited risk.

Nutritional/Ethanol Interactions
Ethanol: Avoid ethanol (may increase CNS depression).
Food: Tolcapone, taken with food within 1 hour before or 2 hours after the dose, decreases bioavailability by 10% to 20%.
Avoid valerian, St John's wort, kava kava, gotu kola (may increase CNS depression).

Adverse Reactions
>10%:
Cardiovascular: Orthostatic hypotension (17%)
Central nervous system: Sleep disorder (24% to 25%), excessive dreaming (16% to 21%), somnolence (14% to 18%), dizziness (6% to 13%), headache (10% to 11%), confusion (10% to 11%)
Gastrointestinal: Nausea (30% to 35%), anorexia (19% to 23%), diarrhea (16% to 19%)
Neuromuscular & skeletal: Dyskinesia (42% to 51%), dystonia (19% to 22%), muscle cramps (17% to 18%)
1% to 10%:
Cardiovascular: Syncope (4% to 5%), chest pain (1% to 3%), hypotension (2%), palpitation
Central nervous system: Hallucinations (8% to 10%), fatigue (3% to 7%), loss of balance (2% to 3%), agitation (1%), euphoria (1%), hyperactivity (1%), malaise (1%), panic reaction (1%), irritability (1%), mental deficiency (1%), fever (1%), depression, hypoesthesia, tremor, speech disorder, vertigo, emotional lability, hyperkinesia

Dermatologic: Alopecia (1%), bleeding (1%), tumor (1%), rash
Gastrointestinal: Vomiting (8% to 10%), constipation (6% to 8%), xerostomia (5% to 6%), abdominal pain (5% to 6%), dyspepsia (3% to 4%), flatulence (2% to 4%) tooth disorder
Genitourinary: UTI (5%), hematuria (4% to 5%), urine discoloration (2% to 3%), urination disorder (1% to 2%), uterine tumor (1%), incontinence, impotence
Hepatic: Transaminases increased (1% to 3%; 3 times ULN, usually with first 6 months of therapy)
Neuromuscular & skeletal: Paresthesia (1% to 3%), hyper-/hypokinesia (1% to 3%), arthritis (1% to 2%), neck pain (2%), stiffness (2%), myalgia, rhabdomyolysis
Ocular: Cataract (1%), eye inflammation (1%)
Otic: Tinnitus
Respiratory: Upper respiratory infection (5% to 7%), dyspnea (3%), sinus congestion (1% to 2%), bronchitis, pharyngitis
Miscellaneous: Diaphoresis (4% to 7%), influenza (3% to 4%), burning (1% to 2%), flank pain, injury, infection

Overdosage/Toxicology No information is available regarding intentional overdose with tolcapone. The highest dose evaluated clinically was 800 mg 3 times/day, with side effects consisting primarily of nausea/vomiting, and dizziness. Treatment should be supportive and symptom-directed. Dialysis not likely to benefit.

Pharmacodynamics/Kinetics
Time to Peak: ~2 hours
Protein Binding: >99.0%
Half-Life Elimination: 2-3 hours
Metabolism: Glucuronidation to inactive metabolite
Excretion: Urine (60% as metabolites); feces (40%)
Available Dosage Forms Tablet: 100 mg, 200 mg
Dosing
Adults & Elderly: Parkinson's disease: Oral: Initial: 100 mg 3 times/day; may increase as tolerated to 200 mg 3 times/day, levodopa dose may need to be decreased upon initiation of tolcapone (average reduction in clinical trials was 30%)
Note: If clinical improvement is not observed after 3 weeks of therapy (regardless of dose), tolcapone treatment should be discontinued.
Renal Impairment: No adjustment necessary for mild-moderate impairment. Use caution with severe impairment; no safety information available in patients with Cl_cr<25 mL/minute.
Hepatic Impairment: Do not use.
Administration
Oral: May be administered with or without food.
Stability
Storage: Store at 20°C to 25°C (68°F to 77°F).
Laboratory Monitoring
Liver enzymes at baseline and then every 2-4 weeks for the first 6 months of therapy; thereafter, periodic monitoring should be conducted as deemed clinically relevant. If the dose is increased to 200 mg 3 times/day, reinitiate LFT monitoring every 2-4 weeks for 6 months, and then resume periodic monitoring. Discontinue therapy if the ALT or AST exceeds 2 times the upper limit of normal or if the clinical signs and symptoms suggest the onset of liver failure.
Nursing Actions
Physical Assessment: Assess effectiveness and interactions of other medications patient may be taking. Monitor therapeutic response (eg, mental status, involuntary movements) and adverse reactions (may exacerbate the adverse effects of levodopa including levodopa toxicity) at beginning of therapy and periodically throughout therapy. Monitor for CNS depression. Monitor blood pressure. Assess knowledge/teach patient appropriate use, interventions to reduce side effects, and adverse symptoms to report.
(Continued)

Tolcapone (Continued)

Patient Education: Take exactly as directed (may be prescribed in conjunction with levodopa/carbidopa); do not change dosage or discontinue without consulting prescriber. Therapeutic effects may take several weeks or months to achieve and you may need frequent monitoring during first weeks of therapy. Best to take 2 hours before or after a meal; however, may be taken with meals if GI upset occurs. Take at the same time each day. Maintain adequate hydration (2-3 L/day of fluids) unless instructed to restrict fluid intake. Do not use alcohol and prescription or OTC sedatives or CNS depressants without consulting prescriber. Urine or perspiration may appear darker. You may experience drowsiness, dizziness, confusion, or vision changes (use caution when driving, climbing stairs, or engaging in tasks requiring alertness until response to drug is known); orthostatic hypotension (use caution when changing position - rising to standing from sitting or lying); increased susceptibility to heat stroke, decreased perspiration (use caution in hot weather; maintain adequate fluids and reduce exercise activity); constipation (increased exercise, fluids, or fruit, or fiber may help); dry skin or nasal passages (consult prescriber for appropriate relief); or nausea, vomiting, loss of appetite, or stomach discomfort (small frequent meals, frequent mouth care, chewing gum, or sucking lozenges may help). Report unresolved constipation or vomiting; chest pain or irregular heartbeat; respiratory difficulty; acute headache or dizziness; CNS changes (hallucination, loss of memory, nervousness, etc); painful or difficult urination; abdominal pain or blood in stool; increased muscle spasticity, rigidity, or involuntary movements; skin rash; or significant worsening of condition. **Pregnancy/breast-feeding precautions:** Inform prescriber if you are or intend to become pregnant. Do not breast-feed.

Dietary Considerations May be taken without regard to food.

Tolterodine (tole TER oh deen)

U.S. Brand Names Detrol®; Detrol® LA

Synonyms Tolterodine Tartrate

Pharmacologic Category Anticholinergic Agent

Medication Safety Issues

Sound-alike/look-alike issues:

Detrol® may be confused with Ditropan®

Pregnancy Risk Factor C

Lactation Excretion in breast milk unknown/not recommended

Use Treatment of patients with an overactive bladder with symptoms of urinary frequency, urgency, or urge incontinence

Mechanism of Action/Effect Tolterodine is a competitive antagonist of muscarinic receptors. In animal models, tolterodine demonstrates selectivity for urinary bladder receptors over salivary receptors. Urinary bladder contraction is mediated by muscarinic receptors. Tolterodine increases residual urine volume and decreases detrusor muscle pressure.

Contraindications Hypersensitivity to tolterodine or any component of the formulation; urinary retention; gastric retention; uncontrolled narrow-angle glaucoma; myasthenia gravis

Warnings/Precautions Use with caution in patients with bladder flow obstruction, may increase the risk of urinary retention. Use with caution in patients with gastrointestinal obstructive disorders (ie, pyloric stenosis), may increase the risk of gastric retention. Use with caution in patients with controlled (treated) narrow-angle glaucoma; metabolized in the liver and

excreted in the urine and feces, dosage adjustment is required for patients with renal or hepatic impairment. Tolterodine has been associated with QT_c prolongation at high (supratherapeutic) doses. The manufacturer recommends caution in patients with congenital prolonged QT or in patients receiving concurrent therapy with QT_c-prolonging drugs (class Ia or III antiarrhythmics). However, the mean change in of QT_c even at supratherapeutic dosages was less than 15 msec. Individuals who are poor metabolizers via CYP2D6 or in the presence of inhibitors of CYP2D6 and CYP3A4 may be more likely to exhibit prolongation. Dosage adjustment is recommended in patients receiving CYP3A4 inhibitors (a lower dose of tolterodine is recommended). Safety and efficacy in pediatric patients have not been established.

Drug Interactions

Cytochrome P450 Effect: Substrate of CYP2C8/9 (minor), 2C19 (minor), 2D6 (major), 3A4 (major)

Decreased Effect: CYP3A4 inducers may decrease the levels/effects of tolterodine; example inducers include aminoglutethimide, carbamazepine, nafcillin, nevirapine, phenobarbital, phenytoin, and rifamycins. Use with acetylcholinesterase inhibitors may result in reduced therapeutic efficacy.

Increased Effect/Toxicity: CYP2D6 inhibitors may increase the levels/effects of tolterodine, which may include QT_c prolongation; example inhibitors include chlorpromazine, delavirdine, fluoxetine, miconazole, paroxetine, pergolide, quinidine, quinine, ritonavir, and ropinirole. No dosage adjustment was needed in patients coadministered tolterodine and fluoxetine. CYP3A4 inhibitors may increase the levels/effects of tolterodine, which may include QT_c prolongation; example inhibitors include azole antifungals, clarithromycin, diclofenac, doxycycline, erythromycin, imatinib, isoniazid, nefazodone, nicardipine, propofol, protease inhibitors, quinidine, telithromycin, and verapamil. Concomitant use with systemic anticholinergic agents may increase the risk of anticholinergic side effects. Use with pramlintide may result in increased slowing of gut motility. Additive effects on QT_c prolongation may occur with concurrent therapy with QT_c prolonging agents.

Nutritional/Ethanol Interactions

Food: Increases bioavailability (~53% increase) of tolterodine tablets, but does not affect the pharmacokinetics of tolterodine extended release capsules; adjustment of dose is not needed. As a CYP3A4 inhibitor, grapefruit juice may increase the serum level and/or toxicity of tolterodine, but unlikely secondary to high oral bioavailability.

Herb/Nutraceutical: St John's wort (*Hypericum*) appears to induce CYP3A enzymes.

Adverse Reactions As reported with immediate release tablet, unless otherwise specified

>10%: Gastrointestinal: Dry mouth (35%; extended release capsules 23%)

1% to 10%:

Cardiovascular: Chest pain (2%)

Central nervous system: Headache (7%; extended release capsules 6%), somnolence (3%; extended release capsules 3%), fatigue (4%; extended release capsules 2%), dizziness (5%; extended release capsules 2%), anxiety (extended release capsules 1%)

Dermatologic: Dry skin (1%)

Gastrointestinal: Abdominal pain (5%; extended release capsules 4%), constipation (7%; extended release capsules 6%), dyspepsia (4%; extended release capsules 3%), diarrhea (4%), weight gain (1%)

Genitourinary: Dysuria (2%; extended release capsules 1%)

Neuromuscular & skeletal: Arthralgia (2%)

Ocular: Abnormal vision (2%; extended release capsules 1%), dry eyes (3%; extended release capsules 3%)

Respiratory: Bronchitis (2%), sinusitis (extended release capsules 2%)

Miscellaneous: Flu-like syndrome (3%), infection (1%)

Overdosage/Toxicology Overdosage with tolterodine can potentially result in severe central anticholinergic effects and should be treated accordingly. ECG monitoring is recommended in the event of overdosage. QT_c prolongation has been observed at supratherapeutic doses; particularly in CYP2D6 poor metabolizers.

Pharmacodynamics/Kinetics

Time to Peak: Immediate release tablet: 1-2 hours; Extended release tablet: 2-6 hours

Protein Binding: >96% (primarily to alpha$_1$-acid glycoprotein)

Half-Life Elimination:

Immediate release tablet: Extensive metabolizers: ~2 hours; Poor metabolizers: ~10 hours

Extended release capsule: Extensive metabolizers: ~7 hours; Poor metabolizers: ~18 hours

Metabolism: Extensively hepatic, primarily via CYP2D6 (some metabolites share activity) and 3A4 usually (minor pathway). In patients with a genetic deficiency of CYP2D6, metabolism via 3A4 predominates. Forms three active metabolites.

Excretion: Urine (77%); feces (17%); excreted primarily as metabolites (<1% unchanged drug) of which the active 5-hydroxymethyl metabolite accounts for 5% to 14% (<1% in poor metabolizers)

Available Dosage Forms

Capsule, extended release, as tartrate (Detrol® LA): 2 mg, 4 mg

Tablet, as tartrate (Detrol®): 1 mg, 2 mg

Dosing

Adults & Elderly: Treatment of overactive bladder: Oral:

Immediate release tablet: 2 mg twice daily; the dose may be lowered to 1 mg twice daily based on individual response and tolerability

Dosing adjustment in patients concurrently taking CYP3A4 inhibitors: 1 mg twice daily

Extended release capsule: 4 mg once a day; dose may be lowered to 2 mg daily based on individual response and tolerability

Dosing adjustment in patients concurrently taking CYP3A4 inhibitors: 2 mg daily

Renal Impairment: Use with caution (studies conducted in patients with Cl_{cr} 10-30 mL/minute):

Immediate release tablet: 1 mg twice daily

Extended release capsule: 2 mg daily

Hepatic Impairment:

Immediate release tablet: 1 mg twice daily

Extended release capsule: 2 mg daily

Stability

Storage: Store at 15°C to 30°C (59°F to 86°F). Protect from light.

Nursing Actions

Physical Assessment: Assess potential for interactions with other prescriptions, OTC medications, or herbal products patient may be taking (eg, ergot-containing drugs). Monitor therapeutic effectiveness and adverse reactions. Teach patient appropriate use (according to formulation and purpose), interventions to reduce side effects, and adverse symptoms to report.

Patient Education: Take as directed, preferably with food. Do not break, crush, or chew extended release medication. May cause headache (consult prescriber for a mild analgesic); dizziness, nervousness, or sleepiness (use caution when driving, climbing stairs, or engaging in tasks requiring alertness until response to drug is known); or abdominal discomfort, diarrhea, constipation, nausea, or vomiting (small frequent meals, increased exercise, adequate hydration may

help). Report back pain, muscle spasms, alteration in gait, or numbness of extremities; unresolved or persistent constipation, diarrhea, or vomiting; or symptoms of upper respiratory infection or flu. Report immediately any chest pain or palpitations, difficulty urinating, or pain on urination. **Pregnancy/breast-feeding precautions:** Inform prescriber if you are or intend to become pregnant. Breast-feeding is not recommended.

Pregnancy Issues There are no adequate and well-controlled studies in pregnant women. Use during pregnancy only if the potential benefit to the mother outweighs the possible risk to the fetus.

Topiramate (toe PYRE a mate)

U.S. Brand Names Topamax®

Pharmacologic Category Anticonvulsant, Miscellaneous

Medication Safety Issues

Sound-alike/look-alike issues:

Topamax® may be confused with Tegretol®, Tegretol®-XR, Toprol-XL®

Pregnancy Risk Factor C

Lactation Enters breast milk/not recommended

Use Monotherapy or adjunctive therapy for partial onset seizures and primary generalized tonic-clonic seizures; adjunctive treatment of seizures associated with Lennox-Gastaut syndrome; prophylaxis of migraine headache

Unlabeled/Investigational Use Infantile spasms, neuropathic pain, cluster headache

Mechanism of Action/Effect Anticonvulsant activity may be due to a combination of potential mechanisms: Blocks neuronal voltage-dependent sodium channels, enhances GABA(A) activity, antagonizes AMPA/kainate glutamate receptors, and weakly inhibits carbonic anhydrase.

Contraindications Hypersensitivity to topiramate or any component of the formulation

Warnings/Precautions Use with caution in patients with hepatic, respiratory, or renal impairment. Topiramate may decrease serum bicarbonate concentrations (up to 67% of patients); treatment-emergent metabolic acidosis is less common. Risk may be increased in patients with a predisposing condition (organ dysfunction, ketogenic diet, or concurrent treatment with other drugs which may cause acidosis). Metabolic acidosis may occur at dosages as low as 50 mg/day. Monitor serum bicarbonate as well as potential complications of chronic acidosis (nephrolithiasis, osteomalacia, and reduced growth rates in children). The risk of kidney stones is about 2-4 times that of the untreated population, the risk of this event may be reduced by increasing fluid intake.

Cognitive dysfunction, psychiatric disturbances (mood disorders), and sedation (somnolence or fatigue) may occur with topiramate use; incidence may be related to rapid titration and higher doses. Topiramate may also cause paresthesia and ataxia. Topiramate has been associated with secondary angle-closure glaucoma in adults and children, typically within 1 month of initiation; discontinue in patients with acute onset of decreased visual acuity or ocular pain. Hyperammonemia with or without encephalopathy may occur with concomitant valproate administration; use with caution in patients with inborn errors of metabolism or decreased hepatic mitochondrial activity. Topiramate may be associated (rarely) with severe oligohydrosis and hyperthermia, most frequently in children; use caution and monitor closely during strenuous exercise, during exposure to high environmental temperature, or in patients receiving drugs with anticholinergic activity.

(Continued)

Topiramate *(Continued)*

Avoid abrupt withdrawal of topiramate therapy, it should be withdrawn/tapered slowly to minimize the potential of increased seizure frequency. Safety and efficacy have not been established in children <2 years of age for adjunctive treatment and <10 years of age for monotherapy. No adequate and well-controlled studies have been conducted in pregnant women; use only if benefit clearly outweighs risk.

Drug Interactions

Cytochrome P450 Effect: Inhibits CYP2C19 (weak); **Induces** CYP3A4 (weak)

Decreased Effect: Phenytoin can decrease topiramate levels by as much as 48%, carbamazepine reduces it by 40%. Digoxin levels and ethinyl estradiol blood levels are decreased when coadministered with topiramate. Hyperammonemia (with or without encephalopathy) has been reported in patients who tolerated valproic acid or topiramate alone; these drugs may modestly decrease the serum concentrations of the other drug.

Increased Effect/Toxicity: Concomitant administration with other CNS depressants will increase its sedative effects. Coadministration with acetazolamide: may increase the chance of nephrolithiasis and/ or hyperthermia. Topiramate may increase phenytoin concentration by 25%. Concurrent administration with anticholinergic drugs may increase the risk of oligohydrosis and/or hyperthermia (includes drugs with high anticholinergic activity such as antihistamines, cyclic antidepressants, and antipsychotics); use caution.

Nutritional/Ethanol Interactions

Ethanol: Avoid ethanol (may increase CNS depression).

Food: Ketogenic diet may increase the possibility of acidosis.

Herb/Nutraceutical: Avoid evening primrose (seizure threshold decreased).

Adverse Reactions Adverse events are reported for placebo-controlled trials of adjunctive therapy in adult and pediatric patients. Unless otherwise noted, the percentages refer to incidence in epilepsy trials. Note: A wide range of dosages were studied; incidence of adverse events was frequently lower in the pediatric population studied.

>10%:

Central nervous system: Dizziness (4% to 32%), ataxia (6% to 16%), somnolence (15% to 29%), psychomotor slowing (3% to 21%), nervousness (9% to 19%), memory difficulties (2% to 14%), speech problems (2% to 13%), fatigue (9% to 30%), difficulty concentrating (5% to 14%), depression (9% to 13%), confusion (4% to 14%)

Endocrine & metabolic: Serum bicarbonate decreased (dose-related: 7% to 67%; marked reductions [to <17 mEq/L] 1% to 11%)

Gastrointestinal: Nausea (6% to 12%; migraine trial: 14%), weight loss (8% to 13%), anorexia (4% to 24%)

Neuromuscular & skeletal: Paresthesia (1% to 19%; migraine trial: 35% to 51%)

Ocular: Nystagmus (10% to 11%), abnormal vision (<1% to 13%)

Respiratory: Upper respiratory infection (migraine trial: 12% to 13%)

Miscellaneous: Injury (6% to 14%)

1% to 10%:

Cardiovascular: Chest pain (2% to 4%), edema (1% to 2%), bradycardia (1%), pallor (up to 1%), hypertension (1% to 2%)

Central nervous system: Abnormal coordination (4%), hypoesthesia (1% to 2%; migraine trial: 8%), convulsions (1%), depersonalization (1% to 2%), apathy (1% to 3%), cognitive problems (3%), emotional lability (3%), agitation (3%), aggressive reactions (2% to 9%), tremor (3% to 9%), stupor (1% to 2%), mood problems (4% to 9%), anxiety (2% to 10%), insomnia (4% to 8%), appetite increased (1%), neurosis (1%), vertigo (1% to 2%)

Dermatologic: Pruritus (migraine trial: 2% to 4%), skin disorder (1% to 3%), alopecia (2%), dermatitis (up to 2%), hypertrichosis (up to 2%), rash erythematous (up to 2%), eczema (up to 1%), seborrhea (up to 1%), skin discoloration (up to 1%)

Endocrine & metabolic: Hot flashes (1% to 2%); metabolic acidosis (hyperchloremia, nonanion gap), dehydration, breast pain (up to 4%), menstrual irregularities (1% to 2%), hypoglycemia (1%), libido decreased (<1% to 2%)

Gastrointestinal: Dyspepsia (2% to 7%), abdominal pain (5% to 7%), constipation (3% to 5%), xerostomia (2% to 4%), fecal incontinence (1%), gingivitis (1%), diarrhea (2%; migraine trial: 11%), vomiting (1% to 3%), gastroenteritis (1% to 3%), GI disorder (1%), dysgeusia (2% to 4%; migraine trial: 12% to 15%), dysphagia (1%), flatulence (1%), GERD (1%), glossitis (1%), gum hyperplasia (1%), weight increase (1%)

Genitourinary: Impotence, dysuria/incontinence (<1% to 4%), prostatic disorder (2%), UTI (2% to 3%), premature ejaculation (migraine trial: 3%), cystitis (2%)

Hematologic: Leukopenia (1% to 2%), purpura (8%), hematoma (1%), prothrombin time increased (1%), thrombocytopenia (1%)

Neuromuscular & skeletal: Myalgia (2%), weakness (3% to 6%), back pain (1% to 5%), leg pain (2% to 4%), rigors (1%), hypertonia, arthralgia (1% to 7%), gait abnormal (2% to 8%), involuntary muscle contractions (2%; migraine trial: 4%), skeletal pain (1%), hyperkinesia (up to 5%), hyporeflexia (up to 2%)

Ocular: Conjunctivitis (1%), diplopia (2% to 10%), myopia (up to 1%)

Otic: Hearing decreased (1% to 2%), tinnitus (1% to 2%), otitis media (migraine trial: 1% to 2%)

Renal: Nephrolithiasis, renal calculus (migraine trial: 2%), hematuria (<1% to 2%)

Respiratory: Pharyngitis (3% to 6%), sinusitis (4% to 6%; migraine trial: 8% to 10%), epistaxis (1% to 4%) , rhinitis (4% to 7%), dyspnea (1% to 2%), pneumonia (5%), coughing (migraine trial: 2% to 3%), bronchitis (migraine trial: 3%)

Miscellaneous: Flu-like symptoms (3% to 7%), allergy (2% to 3%), body odor (up to 1%), fever (migraine trial: 1% to 2%), viral infection (migraine trial: 3% to 4%), infection (<1% to 2%), diaphoresis (≤1%), thirst (2%)

Overdosage/Toxicology Signs and symptoms of overdose include convulsions, drowsiness, speech disturbance, blurred vision, diplopia, impaired mentation, lethargy, and metabolic acidosis. Activated charcoal has not been shown to adsorb topiramate and is, therefore, not recommended; gastric contents should be emptied via lavage or emesis. Hemodialysis can remove approximately ~30% of the drug; however, most cases do not require removal and instead are best treated with supportive measures.

Pharmacodynamics/Kinetics

Time to Peak: Serum: ~2-4 hours

Protein Binding: 15% to 41% (inversely related to plasma concentrations)

Half-Life Elimination: Mean: Adults: Normal renal function: 21 hours; shorter in pediatric patients; clearance is 50% higher in pediatric patients

Metabolism: Hepatic via P450

Excretion: Urine (~70% to 80% as unchanged drug) Dialyzable: ~30%

Available Dosage Forms

Capsule, sprinkle: 15 mg, 25 mg

Tablet: 25 mg, 50 mg, 100 mg, 200 mg

Dosing

Adults:

Monotherapy: **Partial onset seizure and primary generalized tonic-clonic seizure:** Initial: 25 mg twice daily; may increase weekly by 50 mg/day up to 100 mg twice daily (week 4 dose); thereafter, may further increase weekly by 100 mg/day up to the recommended maximum of 200 mg twice daily.

Adjunctive therapy:

Migraine prophylaxis: Oral: Initial: 25 mg/day (in the evening), titrated at weekly intervals in 25 mg increments, up to the recommended total daily dose of 100 mg/day given in 2 divided doses

Partial onset seizures: Oral: Initial: 25-50 mg/day (given in 2 divided doses) for 1 week; increase at weekly intervals by 25-50 mg/day until response; usual maintenance dose: 100-200 mg twice daily. Doses >1600 mg/day have not been studied.

Primary generalized tonic-clonic seizures: Oral: Use initial dose as listed above for partial onset seizures, but use slower initial titration rate; titrate upwards to recommended dose by the end of 8 weeks; usual maintenance dose: 200 mg twice daily. Doses >1600 mg/day have not been studied.

Cluster headache (unlabeled use): Oral: Initial: 25 mg/day, titrated at weekly intervals in 25 mg increments, up to 200 mg/day

Neuropathic pain (unlabeled use): Oral: Initial: 25 mg/day, titrated at weekly intervals in 25-50 mg increments to target dose of 400 mg daily in 2 divided doses. Reported dosage range studied: 25-800 mg/day

Elderly: Most older adults have creatinine clearances <70 mL/min; obtain a serum creatinine and calculate creatinine clearance prior to initiation of therapy. An initial dose of 25 mg/day may be recommended, followed by incremental increases of 25 mg at weekly intervals until an effective dose is reached; refer to adult dosing for titration schedule.

Pediatrics:

Monotherapy: **Partial onset seizure and primary generalized tonic-clonic seizure:** Children ≥10 years: Oral: Refer to adult dosing.

Adjunctive therapy:

Partial onset seizure or seizure associated with Lennox-Gastaut syndrome: Children 2-16 years: Oral: Initial dose titration should begin at 25 mg (or less, based on a range of 1-3 mg/kg/day) nightly for the first week; dosage may be increased in increments of 1-3 mg/kg/day (administered in 2 divided doses) at 1- or 2-week intervals to a total daily dose of 5-9 mg/kg/day

Adolescents ≥17 years: Refer to adult dosing.

Primary generalized tonic-clonic seizure: Children 2-16 years: Oral: Use initial dose listed above, but use slower initial titration rate; titrate to recommended maintenance dose by the end of 8 weeks

Adolescents ≥17 years: Refer to adult dosing.

Renal Impairment: Cl$_{cr}$ <70 mL/minute: Administer 50% dose and titrate more slowly.

Hemodialysis: Supplemental dose may be needed during hemodialysis

Dialyzable: ~30%

Hepatic Impairment: Clearance may be reduced.

Administration

Oral: May be administered without regard to meals

Capsule sprinkles: May be swallowed whole or opened to sprinkle the contents on soft food (drug/food mixture should not be chewed).

Tablet: Because of bitter taste, tablets should not be broken.

Stability

Storage: Store at room temperature of 15°C to 30°C (59°F to 86°F). Protect from moisture

Laboratory Monitoring Recommended monitoring includes serum bicarbonate at baseline and periodically during treatment. Ammonia level in patients with unexplained lethargy, vomiting, or mental status changes.

Nursing Actions

Physical Assessment: Assess effectiveness and interactions of other medications patient may be taking. Monitor therapeutic response (seizure activity, force, type, duration), laboratory values, and adverse reactions at beginning of therapy and periodically with long-term use. Use and teach seizure/safety precautions. May cause weight loss; monitor weight periodically. Assess knowledge/teach patient appropriate use, interventions to reduce side effects, and adverse symptoms to report.

Patient Education: Take exactly as directed; do not increase dose or frequency or discontinue without consulting prescriber. While using this medication, do not use alcohol and other prescription or OTC medications (especially pain medications, sedatives, antihistamines, or hypnotics) without consulting prescriber. Maintain adequate hydration (2-3 L/day of fluids) unless instructed to restrict fluid intake; possibly to prevent the inflammation of kidney stones and dehydration. You may be at risk for decreased sweating and increased body temperature, especially in hot weather. You may experience drowsiness, dizziness, disturbed concentration, memory changes, or blurred vision (use caution when driving or engaging in tasks requiring alertness until response to drug is known); or mouth sores, nausea, vomiting, or loss of appetite (small frequent meals, frequent mouth care, chewing gum, or sucking lozenges may help). Wear identification of epileptic status and medications. Report behavioral or CNS changes; skin rash; muscle cramping, numbness in extremities, weakness, tremors, changes in gait; chest pain, irregular heartbeat, or palpitations; hearing loss; cough or respiratory difficulty; or worsening of seizure activity or loss of seizure control. Seek immediate medical evaluation if you experience sudden vision changes and/or periorbital pain. **Pregnancy/breast-feeding precautions:** Inform prescriber if you are pregnant or intend to become pregnant. Breast-feeding is not recommended.

Geriatric Considerations Since drug is renally excreted and most elderly will have creatinine clearance <70 mL/minute, doses must be reduced 50% and titrated more slowly. Obtain a serum creatinine and calculate creatinine clearance prior to starting therapy. Follow the recommended titration schedule and adjust time intervals to meet patient's needs.

Breast-Feeding Issues Based on limited data, topiramate was found in breast milk; low concentrations were detected in nursing infants.

Pregnancy Issues There are no adequate and well-controlled studies in pregnant women; use only if benefit to the mother outweighs the risk to the fetus. Postmarketing experience includes reports of hypospadias following *in vitro* exposure to topiramate.

Additional Information May be associated with weight loss in some patients

---

Topotecan (toe poe TEE kan)

U.S. Brand Names Hycamtin®

Synonyms Hycamptamine; NSC-609699; SK and F 104864; SKF 104864; SKF 104864-A; TOPO; Topotecan Hydrochloride; TPT

Pharmacologic Category Antineoplastic Agent, Natural Source (Plant) Derivative

Medication Safety Issues

Sound-alike/look-alike issues:

Hycamtin® may be confused with Hycomine®

(Continued)

Topotecan *(Continued)*

Pregnancy Risk Factor D

Lactation Excretion in breast milk unknown/contraindicated

Use Treatment of ovarian cancer, small cell lung cancer

Unlabeled/Investigational Use Investigational: Treatment of nonsmall cell lung cancer, sarcoma (pediatrics)

Mechanism of Action/Effect Binds to topoisomerase I and stabilizes the cleavable complex so that religation of the cleaved DNA strand cannot occur. This results in the accumulation of cleavable complexes and single-strand DNA breaks. Topotecan acts in S phase.

Contraindications Hypersensitivity to topotecan or any component of the formulation; severe bone marrow depression; pregnancy; breast-feeding

Warnings/Precautions Hazardous agent - use appropriate precautions for handling and disposal. Monitor bone marrow function. Should only administer to patients with adequate bone marrow reserves, baseline neutrophils at least 1500 cells/mm^3 and platelet counts at least 100,000/mm^3. Use caution in renal impairment.

Drug Interactions

Increased Effect/Toxicity: Concurrent administration of TPT and G-CSF in clinical trials results in severe myelosuppression. If G-CSF is to be used, manufacturer recommends that it should not be initiated until 24 hours after the completion of treatment with topotecan. Concurrent *in vitro* exposure to TPT and the topoisomerase II inhibitor etoposide results in no altered effect; sequential exposure results in potentiation. Concurrent exposure to TPT and 5-azacytidine results in potentiation both *in vitro* and *in vivo*. Myelosuppression was more severe when given in combination with cisplatin.

Nutritional/Ethanol Interactions Ethanol: Avoid ethanol (due to GI irritation).

Lab Interactions None known

Adverse Reactions

>10%:

Central nervous system: Headache, fatigue, fever, pain

Dermatologic: Alopecia (reversible), rash

Gastrointestinal: Nausea, vomiting, diarrhea, constipation, abdominal pain, stomatitis, anorexia

Hematologic: Myelosuppressive: Principle dose-limiting toxicity; white blood cell count nadir is 8-11 days and is more frequent than thrombocytopenia (at lower doses); recover is usually within 21 days and cumulative toxicity has not been noted.

Neuromuscular & skeletal: Weakness

Respiratory: Dyspnea (22%), cough

1% to 10%:

Hepatic: Transient increases in liver enzymes

Neuromuscular & skeletal: Paresthesia

Pharmacodynamics/Kinetics

Protein Binding: 35%

Half-Life Elimination: 2-3 hours

Metabolism: Undergoes a rapid, pH-dependent opening of the lactone ring to yield a relatively inactive hydroxy acid in plasma

Excretion: Urine (30%) within 24 hours

Available Dosage Forms Injection, powder for reconstitution, as hydrochloride: 4 mg [base]

Dosing

Adults & Elderly: Refer to individual protocols.

Metastatic ovarian cancer and small cell lung cancer:

IVPB: 1.5 mg/m^2/day for 5 days; repeated every 21 days (neutrophil count should be >1500/mm^3 and platelet count should be >100,000/mm^3)

I.V. continuous infusion: 0.2-0.7 mg/m^2/day for 7-21 days

Dosage adjustment for hematological effects: If neutrophil count <1500/mm^3, reduce dose by 0.25 mg/m^2/day for 5 days for next cycle

Renal Impairment:

Cl$_{cr}$ 20-39 mL/minute: Administer 50% of normal dose.

Cl$_{cr}$ <20 mL/minute: Do not use, insufficient data available.

Hemodialysis: Supplemental dose is not necessary.

CAPD effects: Unknown

CAVH effects: Unknown

Hepatic Impairment: Bilirubin 1.5-10 mg/dL: No adjustment necessary.

Administration

I.V.: Administer IVPB over 30 minutes or by 24-hour continuous infusion.

Stability

Reconstitution: Reconstitute vials with 4 mL SWFI, D$_5$, or NS; may be further diluted in 50-100 mL D$_5$W or NS for infusion.

Compatibility: Stable in D$_5$W, NS

Y-site administration: Incompatible with dexamethasone sodium phosphate, fluorouracil, mitomycin

Storage: Store intact vials of lyophilized powder for injection at room temperature and protected from light. Reconstituted solution is stable for 24 hours at room temperature or up to 7 days under refrigeration. Diluted in 50-100 mL D$_5$W or NS is stable for 24 hours at room temperature or up to 7 days under refrigeration.

Laboratory Monitoring CBC with differential and platelet count, renal function tests

Nursing Actions

Physical Assessment: See Contraindications, Warnings/Precautions, and Drug Interactions for use cautions. Monitor infusion site closely to prevent extravasation. Monitor laboratory tests (see above) and patient response prior to each infusion and throughout therapy (eg, signs of myelosuppression - see Adverse Reactions and Overdose/Toxicology). Teach patient possible side effects/appropriate interventions and adverse symptoms to report (see Patient Education). Pregnancy risk factor D - determine that patient is not pregnant before beginning treatment. Instruct patients of childbearing age on appropriate barrier contraceptive measures. Breast-feeding is contraindicated.

Patient Education: Inform prescriber of all prescriptions, OTC medications, or herbal products you are taking, and any allergies you have. Do not take any new medication during therapy unless approved by prescriber. This medication can only be administered I.V. Report immediately any redness, pain, swelling, or burning at infusion site. Maintain adequate hydration (2-3 L/day of fluids) unless instructed to restrict fluid intake. Maintain good oral hygiene (use soft toothbrush or cotton applicators several times a day and rinse mouth frequently). You will be susceptible to infection (avoid crowds and exposure to infection do not have any vaccinations unless approved by prescriber). May cause nausea, vomiting, or loss of appetite (small, frequent meals, frequent mouth care, sucking lozenges, or chewing gum may help, or consult prescriber); or hair loss (reversible). Report signs of opportunistic infection (eg, persistent fever or chills, unhealed sores, oral or vaginal sores, foul-smelling urine, painful urination, easy bruising or bleeding); unusual or persistent weakness or lethargy; numbness or tingling in extremities; or respiratory difficulty. **Pregnancy/breast-feeding precautions:** Inform prescriber if you are pregnant. Do not get pregnant while taking this medication. Consult prescriber for appropriate contraceptive measures. This medication may cause severe fetal harm. Do not breast-feed.

Pregnancy Issues May cause fetal harm in pregnant women.

Toremifene (TORE em i feen)

U.S. Brand Names Fareston®

Synonyms FC1157a; Toremifene Citrate

Pharmacologic Category Antineoplastic Agent, Estrogen Receptor Antagonist

Pregnancy Risk Factor D

Lactation Excretion in breast milk unknown/contraindicated

Use Treatment of advanced breast cancer; management of desmoid tumors and endometrial carcinoma

Mechanism of Action/Effect Nonsteroidal agent that competitively binds to estrogen receptors on tumors and other tissue targets (including breast and other tissues), producing a nuclear complex that decreases DNA synthesis and inhibits estrogen effects. Cells accumulate in the G_0 and G_1 phases; therefore, toremifene is cytostatic rather than cytocidal.

Contraindications Hypersensitivity to toremifene or any component of the formulation; pregnancy

Warnings/Precautions Hazardous agent — use appropriate precautions for handling and disposal. Hypercalcemia and tumor flare have been reported in some breast cancer patients with bone metastases during the first weeks of treatment. Tumor flare is a syndrome of diffuse musculoskeletal pain and erythema with increased size of tumor lesions that later regress. It is often accompanied by hypercalcemia. Tumor flare does not imply treatment failure or represent tumor progression. Institute appropriate measures if hypercalcemia occurs, and if severe, discontinue treatment. Drugs that decrease renal calcium excretion (eg, thiazide diuretics) may increase the risk of hypercalcemia in patients receiving toremifene. Leukopenia and thrombocytopenia have been reported rarely. Use cautiously in patients with anemia, hepatic failure, or thromboembolic disease.

Drug Interactions

Cytochrome P450 Effect: Substrate of CYP1A2 (minor), 3A4 (major)

Decreased Effect: CYP3A4 inducers may decrease the levels/effects of toremifene; example inducers include aminoglutethimide, carbamazepine, nafcillin, nevirapine, phenobarbital, phenytoin, and rifamycins.

Increased Effect/Toxicity: Concurrent therapy with warfarin results in significant enhancement of anticoagulant effects; has been speculated that a decrease in antitumor effect of tamoxifen may also occur due to alterations in the percentage of active tamoxifen metabolites.

Adverse Reactions

>10%:

Endocrine & metabolic: Vaginal discharge, hot flashes

Gastrointestinal: Nausea, vomiting

Miscellaneous: Diaphoresis

1% to 10%:

Cardiovascular: Thromboembolism: Toremifene has been associated with the occurrence of venous thrombosis and pulmonary embolism; arterial thrombosis has also been described in a few case reports; cardiac failure, MI, edema

Central nervous system: Dizziness

Endocrine & metabolic: Hypercalcemia may occur in patients with bone metastases; galactorrhea and vitamin deficiency, menstrual irregularities

Genitourinary: Vaginal bleeding or discharge, endometriosis, priapism, possible endometrial cancer

Ocular: Ophthalmologic effects (visual acuity changes, cataracts, or retinopathy), corneal opacities, dry eyes

Overdosage/Toxicology Theoretically, overdose may manifest as an increase of antiestrogenic effects such as hot flashes; estrogenic effects such as vaginal bleeding; or nervous system disorders such as vertigo, dizziness, ataxia, and nausea. No specific antidote exists and treatment is symptomatic.

Pharmacodynamics/Kinetics

Time to Peak: Serum: ~3 hours

Protein Binding: Plasma: >99.5%, primarily to albumin

Half-Life Elimination: ~5 days

Metabolism: Extensively hepatic, principally by CYP3A4 to N-demethyltoremifene, which is also antiestrogenic but with weak *in vivo* antitumor potency

Excretion: Primarily feces; urine (10%) during a 1-week period

Available Dosage Forms Tablet: 60 mg

Dosing

Adults & Elderly: Refer to individual protocols.

Metastatic breast carcinoma: Oral: 60 mg once daily, generally continued until disease progression is observed

Renal Impairment: No adjustment is necessary.

Hepatic Impairment: Toremifene is extensively metabolized in the liver and dosage adjustments may be indicated in patients with liver disease; however, no specific guidelines have been developed.

Stability

Storage: Store at 25°C (77°F); excursions permitted to 15°C to 30°C (59°F to 86°F). Protect from heat and light.

Laboratory Monitoring Obtain periodic complete blood counts, calcium levels, and liver function tests. Closely monitor patients with bone metastases for hypercalcemia during the first few weeks of treatment. Leukopenia and thrombocytopenia have been reported rarely; monitor leukocyte and platelet counts during treatment.

Nursing Actions

Physical Assessment: Assess potential for interactions with other pharmacological agents patient may be taking (drugs that decrease renal calcium excretion [eg, thiazide diuretics] may increase the risk of hypercalcemia, use with warfarin increases anticoagulant effect). Monitor laboratory tests on a regular basis throughout therapy. Monitor therapeutic effectiveness and adverse reactions regularly (eg, thromboembolism, MI, edema, hypercalcemia, endometriosis, nausea, vomiting, vision changes). Teach patient proper use, possible side effects/appropriate interventions and adverse symptoms to report.

Patient Education: Do not take any new medication during therapy unless approved by prescriber. Take as directed, without regard to food. You may experience an initial "flare" of this disease (eg, increased bone pain and hot flashes), which will subside with continued use. May cause nausea, vomiting, or loss of appetite (frequent mouth care, small, frequent meals, chewing gum, or sucking lozenges may help); dizziness (use caution when driving, climbing stairs, or engaging in tasks requiring alertness until response to drug is known); or loss of hair (reversible). Report vomiting that occurs immediately after taking medication; chest pain, palpitations, or swollen extremities; vaginal bleeding, hot flashes, or excessive perspiration; chest pain, unusual coughing, or respiratory difficulty; or any vision changes or dry eyes. **Pregnancy/breast-feeding precautions:** Do not get pregnant while taking this medication. Consult prescriber for appropriate contraceptive measures. Do not breast-feed.

Additional Information Increase of bone pain usually indicates a good therapeutic response

Torsemide (TORE se mide)

U.S. Brand Names Demadex®

Pharmacologic Category Diuretic, Loop

Medication Safety Issues

Sound-alike/look-alike issues:

Torsemide may be confused with furosemide

Demadex® may be confused with Denorex®

Pregnancy Risk Factor B

Lactation Excretion in breast milk unknown/use caution

Use Management of edema associated with congestive heart failure and hepatic or renal disease; used alone or in combination with antihypertensives in treatment of hypertension; I.V. form is indicated when rapid onset is desired

Mechanism of Action/Effect Inhibits reabsorption of sodium and chloride in the ascending loop of Henle and distal renal tubule, interfering with the chloride-binding cotransport system, thus causing increased excretion of water, sodium, chloride, magnesium, and calcium; does not alter GFR, renal plasma flow, or acid-base balance

Contraindications Hypersensitivity to torsemide, any component of the formulation, or any sulfonylureas; anuria

Warnings/Precautions Ototoxicity has been associated with loop diuretics and has been seen with oral torsemide. Do not administer intravenously in less than 2 minutes; single doses should not exceed 200 mg. Avoid electrolyte imbalances in cirrhosis that might lead to hepatic encephalopathy. Monitor fluid status and renal function in an attempt to prevent dehydration, oliguria, azotemia, and reversible increases in BUN and creatinine. Monitor closely for electrolyte imbalances particularly hypokalemia and correct when necessary. Coadministration with antihypertensives may increase the risk of hypotension.

Chemical similarities are present among sulfonamides, sulfonylureas, carbonic anhydrase inhibitors, thiazides, and loop diuretics (except ethacrynic acid). Use in patients with sulfonylurea allergy is specifically contraindicated in product labeling, however, a risk of cross-reaction exists in patients with allergy to any of these compounds; avoid use when previous reaction has been severe.

Drug Interactions

Cytochrome P450 Effect: Substrate of CYP2C8/9 (major); **Inhibits** CYP2C19 (weak)

Decreased Effect: Torsemide action may be reduced with probenecid. Diuretic action may be impaired in patients with cirrhosis and ascites if used with salicylates. Glucose tolerance may be decreased when used with sulfonylureas. CYP2C8/9 inducers may decrease the levels/effects of torsemide; example inducers include carbamazepine, phenobarbital, phenytoin, rifampin, rifapentine, and secobarbital. Torsemide efficacy may be decreased with NSAIDs.

Increased Effect/Toxicity: Torsemide-induced hypokalemia may predispose to digoxin toxicity and may increase the risk of arrhythmia with drugs which may prolong QT interval, including type Ia and type III antiarrhythmic agents, cisapride, and some quinolones (sparfloxacin, gatifloxacin, and moxifloxacin). The risk of toxicity from lithium and salicylates (high dose) may be increased by loop diuretics. Hypotensive effects and/or adverse renal effects of ACE inhibitors and NSAIDs are potentiated by bumetanide-induced hypovolemia. The effects of peripheral adrenergic-blocking drugs or ganglionic blockers may be increased by bumetanide.

Torsemide may increase the risk of ototoxicity with other ototoxic agents (aminoglycosides, cis-platinum), especially in patients with renal dysfunction. Synergistic diuretic effects occur with thiazide-type diuretics. Diuretics tend to be synergistic with other antihypertensive agents, and hypotension may occur.

Nutritional/Ethanol Interactions Herb/Nutraceutical: Avoid dong quai if using for hypertension (has estrogenic activity). Avoid ephedra, yohimbe, ginseng (may worsen hypertension). Avoid garlic (may have increased antihypertensive effect).

Adverse Reactions 1% to 10%:

Cardiovascular: Edema (1.1%), ECG abnormality (2%), chest pain (1.2%)

Central nervous system: Headache (7.3%), dizziness (3.2%), insomnia (1.2%), nervousness (1%)

Endocrine & metabolic: Hyperglycemia, hyperuricemia, hypokalemia

Gastrointestinal: Diarrhea (2%), constipation (1.8%), nausea (1.8%), dyspepsia (1.6%), sore throat (1.6%)

Genitourinary: Excessive urination (6.7%)

Neuromuscular & skeletal: Weakness (2%), arthralgia (1.8%), myalgia (1.6%)

Respiratory: Rhinitis (2.8%), cough increase (2%)

Overdosage/Toxicology Symptoms include electrolyte depletion, volume depletion, hypotension, dehydration, and circulatory collapse. Electrolyte depletion may manifest as weakness, dizziness, mental confusion, anorexia, lethargy, vomiting, and cramps. Treatment is supportive.

Pharmacodynamics/Kinetics

Onset of Action: Diuresis: 30-60 minutes; Peak effect: 1-4 hours

Duration of Action: ~6 hours

Protein Binding: Plasma: ~97% to 99%

Half-Life Elimination: 2-4; Cirrhosis: 7-8 hours

Metabolism: Hepatic (80%) via CYP

Excretion: Urine (20% as unchanged drug)

Available Dosage Forms

Injection, solution: 10 mg/mL (2 mL, 5 mL)

Tablet: 5 mg, 10 mg, 20 mg, 100 mg

Dosing

Adults:

Note: The oral form may be given regardless of meal times. Patients may be switched from the I.V. form to the oral and vice-versa with no change in dose.

Congestive heart failure: Oral, I.V.: 10-20 mg once daily; may increase gradually for chronic treatment by doubling dose until the diuretic response is apparent (for acute treatment. I.V. dose may be repeated every 2 hours with double the dose as needed). **Note:** ACC/AHA 2005 guidelines for chronic heart failure recommend a maximum daily oral dose of 200 mg; maximum single I.V. dose 100-200 mg

Continuous I.V. infusion: 20 mg I.V. load then 5-20 mg/hour

Chronic renal failure: Oral, I.V.: 20 mg once daily; increase as above.

Hepatic cirrhosis: Oral, I.V.: 5-10 mg once daily with an aldosterone antagonist or a potassium-sparing diuretic; increase as above.

Hypertension: Oral, I.V.: 2.5-5 mg once daily; increase to 10 mg after 4-6 weeks if an adequate hypotensive response is not apparent. If still not effective, an additional antihypertensive agent may be added.

Elderly: Usual starting dose should be 5 mg; refer to adult dosing.

Administration

I.V.: I.V. injections should be given over ≥2 minutes.

I.V. Detail: Ototoxicity has occurred with too rapid of injection.

pH: >8.3

Stability

Compatibility: Stable in D_5W, NS, ½NS

Laboratory Monitoring Renal function, electrolytes

Nursing Actions

Physical Assessment: Assess for allergy to sulfonylurea before beginning therapy. See Warnings/Precautions for use cautions. Assess potential for interactions with other pharmacological agents or herbal products the patient may be taking (especially anything that may impact fluid balance or increase potential for ototoxicity or hypotension). See Administration for infusion specifics. Monitor laboratory tests (electrolytes), therapeutic effectiveness, and adverse response (eg, dehydration, electrolyte imbalance, postural hypotension) on a regular basis during therapy. Caution patients with diabetes about closely monitoring glucose levels (glucose tolerance may be decreased). Teach patient appropriate use, possible side effects/appropriate interventions, and adverse symptoms to report.

Patient Education: Do not take any new medication during therapy unless approved by prescriber. Take as directed, with food or milk (to reduce GI distress), early in the day, or if twice daily, take last dose in late afternoon in order to avoid sleep disturbance and achieve maximum therapeutic effect. Include orange juice or bananas (or other potassium-rich foods) in daily diet. Do not take potassium supplements without consulting prescriber. Weigh yourself each day, at the same time, in the same clothes when beginning therapy, and weekly on long-term therapy; report unusual or unanticipated weight gain or loss. May cause postural hypotension (change position slowly when rising from sitting or lying); transient drowsiness, blurred vision, or dizziness (avoid driving or engaging in tasks that require alertness until response to drug is known); reduced tolerance to heat (avoid strenuous activity in hot weather or excessively hot showers); or constipation (increased exercise and increased dietary fiber, fruit, or fluids may help). Report unusual weight gain or loss (>5 lb/week), swelling of ankles and hands; persistent fatigue; unresolved constipation or diarrhea; weakness, fatigue, or dizziness; vomiting; cramps; change in hearing; or chest pain or palpitations. **Breast-feeding precaution:** Consult prescriber if breast-feeding.

Pregnancy Issues A decrease in fetal weight, an increase in fetal resorption, and delayed fetal ossification has occurred in animal studies.

Additional Information 10-20 mg torsemide is approximately equivalent to furosemide 40 mg or bumetanide 1 mg.

Tositumomab and Iodine I 131 Tositumomab

(toe si TYOO mo mab & EYE oh dyne eye one THUR tee one toe si TYOO mo mab)

U.S. Brand Names Bexxar®

Synonyms Anti-CD20-Murine Monoclonal Antibody I-131; B1; B1 Antibody; 131 I Anti-B1 Antibody; 131 I-Anti-B1 Monoclonal Antibody; Iodine I 131 Tositumomab and Tositumomab; Tositumomab I-131

Pharmacologic Category Antineoplastic Agent, Monoclonal Antibody; Radiopharmaceutical

Pregnancy Risk Factor X

Lactation Enters breast milk/contraindicated

Use Treatment of relapsed or refractory CD20 positive, low-grade, follicular, or transformed non-Hodgkin's lymphoma

Mechanism of Action/Effect Tositumomab is a murine IgG2a lambda monoclonal antibody which binds to the CD20 antigen, expressed on B-lymphocytes and on >90% of B-cell non-Hodgkin's lymphomas. Iodine I 131 tositumomab is a radio-iodinated derivative of tositumomab covalently linked to iodine 131. The possible actions of the regimen include apoptosis, complement-dependent cytotoxicity, antibody-dependent cellular cytotoxicity, and cell death. Administration results in depletion of CD20 positive cells.

Contraindications Hypersensitivity to murine proteins or any component of the formulation; pregnancy; breast-feeding

Warnings/Precautions Hypersensitivity reactions (including anaphylaxis) have been reported. Patients should be screened for human antimouse antibodies (HAMA); may be at increased risk of allergic or serious hypersensitivity reactions. Hematologic toxicity was reported to be the most common adverse effect with 27% patients requiring supportive care. Severe or life-threatening cytopenias (NCI CTC grade 3 or 4) have been reported in a large number of patients; may be prolonged and severe. Secondary malignancies have been reported following use.

Treatment involves radioactive isotopes; appropriate precautions in handling and administration must be followed. Patients must be instructed in measures to minimize exposure of others. Women of childbearing potential should be advised of potential fetal risk; effective contraceptive measures should be used for 12 months following treatment (males and females). Treatment may lead to hypothyroidism; patients should receive thyroid-blocking medications prior to the start of therapy. Patients should be premedicated to prevent infusion related reactions. For a single course of therapy only; multiple courses or use in combination with other chemotherapy or irradiation have not been studied.

Safety has not been established in patients with >25% lymphoma marrow involvement, platelet count <100,000 cells/mm^3 or neutrophil count <1500 cells/mm^3. Use caution with cardiovascular disease, renal, or hepatic impairment. Safety and efficacy have not been established with impaired renal function or in pediatric patients.

Drug Interactions

Decreased Effect: No formal drug interaction studies have been conducted. The ability of patients receiving tositumomab to generate humoral response (primary or anamnestic) to vaccination is unknown; safety of live vaccines has not been established.

Increased Effect/Toxicity: No formal drug interaction studies have been conducted.

Lab Interactions May interfere with tests using murine antibody technology.

Adverse Reactions

>10%:

Central nervous system: Fever (37%), pain (19%), chills (18%), headache (16%)

Dermatologic: Rash (17%)

Endocrine & metabolic: Hypothyroidism (7% to 19%)

Gastrointestinal: Nausea (36%), abdominal pain (15%), vomiting (15%), anorexia (14%), diarrhea (12%)

Hematologic:

Neutropenia (grade 3 or 4, 63%); thrombocytopenia (grade 3 or 4, 53%)

Time to nadir: 4-7 weeks

Duration: 30 days (>90 days in 5% to 7% of patients)

Neuromuscular & skeletal: Weakness (46%), myalgia (13%)

Respiratory: Cough (21%), pharyngitis (12%), dyspnea (11%)

Miscellaneous: Infusion-related reactions (26%, occurred within 14 days of infusion, included bronchospasm, chills, dyspnea, fever, hypotension, nausea, rigors, diaphoresis), infection (21%), HAMA-positive seroconversion (11%; up to 21% at 1 year)

1% to 10%:

Cardiovascular: Hypotension (7% to 10%), peripheral edema (9%), chest pain (7%), vasodilation (5%)

(Continued)

Tositumomab and Iodine I 131
Tositumomab (Continued)

Central nervous system: Dizziness (5%), somnolence (5%)

Dermatologic: Pruritus (10%)

Gastrointestinal: Constipation (6%), dyspepsia (6%), weight loss (6%)

Local: Injection site hypersensitivity

Neuromuscular & skeletal: Arthralgia (10%), back pain (8%), neck pain (6%)

Respiratory: Rhinitis (10%), pneumonia (6%), laryngismus

Miscellaneous: Diaphoresis (8%), hypersensitivity reaction (6%), secondary leukemia/myelodysplastic syndrome (3%; up to 6% at 5 years), anaphylactoid reaction, secondary malignancies, serum sickness

Overdosage/Toxicology Grade 4 hematologic toxicity lasting 18 days was reported in one patient accidentally receiving a total body dose of 88 cGy. Monitor for cytopenias and radiation-related toxicity.

Pharmacodynamics/Kinetics

Half-Life Elimination: Tositumomab:

Elimination: 36-48 hours

Terminal half-life decreased with high tumor burden, splenomegaly, or bone marrow involvement

Clearance: Blood: 68.2 mg/hour

Excretion: Iodine-131: Urine (98%) and decay

Available Dosage Forms Note: Not all components are shipped from the same facility. When ordering, ensure that all will arrive on the same day.

Kit [dosimetric package]: Tositumomab 225 mg/16.1 mL [2 vials], tositumomab 35 mg/2.5 mL [1 vial], and iodine I 131 tositumomab 0.1 mg/mL and 0.61mCi/mL (20 mL) [1 vial]

Kit [therapeutic package]: Tositumomab 225 mg/16.1 mL [2 vials], tositumomab 35 mg/2.5 mL [1 vial], and iodine I 131 tositumomab 1.1 mg/mL and 5.6 mCi/mL (20 mL) [1 or 2 vials]

Dosing

Adults: I.V.: Dosing consists of four components administered in 2 steps. Thyroid protective agents (SSKI, Lugol's solution or potassium iodide), acetaminophen and diphenhydramine should be given prior to or with treatment. Refer to Additional Information.

Step 1: Dosimetric step (Day 0):

Tositumomab 450 mg in NS 50 mL administered over 60 minutes

Iodine I 131 tositumomab (containing I-131 5.0 mCi and tositumomab 35mg) in NS 30 mL administered over 20 minutes

Note: Whole body dosimetry and biodistribution should be determined on Day 0; days 2, 3, or 4; and day 6 or 7 prior to administration of Step 2. If biodistribution is not acceptable, do not administer the therapeutic step. On day 6 or 7, calculate the patient specific activity of iodine I 131 tositumomab to deliver 75 cGy TBD or 65 cGy TBD (in mCi).

Step 2: Therapeutic step (Day 7):

Tositumomab 450 mg in NS 50 mL administered over 60 minutes

Iodine I 131 tositumomab:

Platelets ≥150,000/mm³: Iodine I 131 calculated to deliver 75 cGy total body irradiation and tositumomab 35 mg over 20 minutes

Platelets ≥100,000/mm³ and <150,000/mm³: Iodine I 131 calculated to deliver 65 cGy total body irradiation and tositumomab 35 mg over 20 minutes

Administration

I.V.:

Tositumomab: Infuse over 60 minutes

Iodine I 131 tositumomab: Infuse over 20 minutes

Reduce the rate of tositumomab or iodine 131 tositumomab infusion by 50% for mild-to-moderate infusion-related toxicities; interrupt for severe toxicity. Once severe toxicity has resolved, infusion may be restarted at half the previous rate. Prior to infusion, patients should be premedicated and a thyroid-protective agent should be started.

Stability
Reconstitution:

Tositumomab: Withdraw and discard 32 mL of saline from a 50 mL bag of NS. Add contents of both 225 mg vials of tositumomab (total 32 mL) to remaining NS to make a final volume of 50 mL. Gently mix by inverting bag, do not shake.

Iodine I 131 tositumomab: Calculate volume required for an iodine I 131 tositumomab activity of 5 mCi (specification sheet provided with product). If the amount of tositumomab contained in the iodine I 131 tositumomab solution contains <35 mg of tositumomab, use the 35 mg vial of tositumomab to prepare a final concentration of tositumomab 35 mg. Using NS, the final volume should equal 30 mL.

Storage:

Tositumomab: Store under refrigeration at 2°C to 8°C (36°F to 46°F); protect from strong light; do not freeze. Following dilution, tositumomab is stable for 24 hour when refrigerated or 8 hours at room temperature.

Iodine I 131 tositumomab: Store frozen at less than or equal to -20°C in the original lead pots. Allow 60 minutes for thawing at ambient temperature. Solutions for infusion are stable for up to 8 hours at 2°C to 8°C (36°F to 46°F) or room temperature.

Laboratory Monitoring CBC with differential (prior to therapy and at least weekly); TSH (prior to therapy and yearly); serum creatinine (immediately prior to administration)

Following infusion of the iodine I 131 tositumomab dosimetric dose, the total body gamma camera counts and whole body images should be taken within 1 hour of the infusion and prior to urination, and 2-4 days after the infusion and following urination, and 6-7 days after the infusion and following urination.

Nursing Actions

Physical Assessment: Premedication should be administered prior to infusion to reduce potential for infusion reactions. Monitor laboratory tests prior to therapy and immediately after therapy and regularly thereafter, as recommended. Monitor for any signs of any adverse response and notify prescriber immediately (eg, infusion related reactions have occurred up to 14 days of infusion. Teach patient possible side effects/appropriate interventions and adverse symptoms to report.

Patient Education: Do not take any new medications during therapy without consulting prescriber. This medication can only be administered by intravenous infusion. You will be closely monitored prior to, during, and following infusion. Report immediately any chills, nausea, diaphoresis; difficulty swallowing or breathing; tightness in chest or chest pain. You will have frequent laboratory tests following therapy to assess effectiveness and response. Other medication will be prescribed related to this therapy. Take as directed; do not stop or alter dosage without consulting prescriber. You may experience nausea, vomiting, abdominal pain (if persistent, contact prescriber for medication); loss of appetite (small, frequent meals and frequent mouth care may help). Report immediately any chills, persistent or acute headache, fever, rash, swelling of extremities, chest pain, muscle or back pain, upper respiratory symptoms (sore throat, runny nose, persistent cough, pneumonia), signs of infection, or other adverse reactions. **Pregnancy/breast-feeding precautions:** Inform prescriber if you are pregnant. Do not get pregnant (females) or cause a pregnancy (males) during therapy or for 12 months following therapy. Consult prescriber for appropriate contraceptives. This medication will cause severe fetal defects. Do not give blood during therapy of for 12 months following therapy. Do not breast-feed.

Breast-Feeding Issues Radioiodine and immunoglobulins are excreted in breast milk. Quantity of radioiodine may be greater than maternal serum concentrations. Women should be advised to discontinue nursing prior to therapy. The AAP considers radioactive iodine a compound which requires temporary cessation of breast-feeding.

Additional Information Thyroid protective agent: One of the following agents should be used starting at least 24 hours prior to the dosimetric dose and continued for 2 weeks after the therapeutic dose. Therapy should not begin without using one of the following agents:

SSKI: 4 drops 3 times/day

Lugol's solution: 20 drops 3 times/day

Potassium iodide: 130 mg once daily

Tramadol (TRA ma dole)

U.S. Brand Names Ultram®; Ultram® ER

Synonyms Tramadol Hydrochloride

Pharmacologic Category Analgesic, Non-narcotic

Medication Safety Issues

Sound-alike/look-alike issues:

Tramadol may be confused with Toradol®, Trandate®, Voltaren®

Ultram® may be confused with Ultane®, Voltaren®

Pregnancy Risk Factor C

Lactation Enters breast milk/contraindicated

Use Relief of moderate to moderately-severe pain

Mechanism of Action/Effect Binds to μ-opiate receptors in the CNS causing inhibition of ascending pain pathways, altering the perception of and response to pain; also inhibits the reuptake of norepinephrine and serotonin, which also modifies the ascending pain pathway

Contraindications Hypersensitivity to tramadol, opioids, or any component of the formulation; opioid-dependent patients; acute intoxication with alcohol, hypnotics, centrally-acting analgesics, opioids, or psychotropic drugs

Ultram® ER (extended release formulation): Additional contraindications: Severe (Cl$_{cr}$ <30 mL/minute) renal dysfunction, severe (Child-Pugh Class C) hepatic dysfunction

Warnings/Precautions Should be used only with extreme caution in patients receiving MAO inhibitors. May cause CNS depression and/or respiratory depression, particularly when combined with other CNS depressants. Use with caution and reduce dosage when administered to patients receiving other CNS depressants. An increased risk of seizures may occur in patients receiving serotonin reuptake inhibitors (SSRIs or anorectics), tricyclic antidepressants, other cyclic compounds (including cyclobenzaprine, promethazine), neuroleptics, MAO inhibitors, or drugs which may lower seizure threshold. Patients with a history of seizures, or with a risk of seizures (head trauma, metabolic disorders, CNS infection, or malignancy, or during ethanol/drug withdrawal) are also at increased risk.

Elderly patients and patients with chronic respiratory disorders may be at greater risk of adverse events. Use with caution in patients with increased intracranial pressure or head injury. Avoid use in patients who are suicidal or addiction prone. Use caution in heavy alcohol users. Use caution in treatment of acute abdominal conditions; may mask pain. Use tramadol with caution and reduce dosage in patients with liver disease or renal dysfunction. Not recommended during pregnancy or in nursing mothers. Tolerance or drug dependence may result from extended use (withdrawal symptoms have been reported); abrupt discontinuation should be avoided. Tapering of dose at the time of discontinuation limits the risk of withdrawal symptoms. Safety and efficacy in pediatric patients <18 years of age have not been established; use in this population is not recommended.

Drug Interactions

Cytochrome P450 Effect: Substrate of CYP2D6 (major), 3A4 (minor)

Decreased Effect: Carbamazepine may decrease analgesic efficacy of tramadol (increased metabolism) and tramadol may increase the risk of in patients on carbamazepine. CYP2D6 inhibitors may decrease the effects of tramadol; examples include chlorpromazine, delavirdine, fluoxetine, miconazole, paroxetine, pergolide, quinidine, quinine, ritonavir, and ropinirole. Quinidine may decrease M1 (active metabolite) serum concentrations.

Increased Effect/Toxicity: Tramadol may enhance the CNS depressant effect of ethanol and other CNS depressants. Cyclobenzaprine, MAO inhibitors, SSRIs, and tricyclic antidepressants may enhance the neuroexcitatory and/or seizure-potentiating effects of tramadol. Naloxone may increase the risk of seizures in tramadol overdose. Quinidine may increase tramadol serum concentrations. Naloxone may increase risk of seizures if administered in tramadol overdose. Serotonin modulators and sibutramine may enhance the serotonergic effects of tramadol.

Nutritional/Ethanol Interactions

Ethanol: Avoid ethanol (may increase CNS depression).

Food:

Immediate release: Does not affect the rate or extent of absorption.

Extended release: Reduced C$_{max}$ and AUC and T$_{max}$ occurred 3 hours earlier when taken with a high-fat meal.

Herb/Nutraceutical: Avoid valerian, St John's wort, kava kava, gotu kola (may increase CNS depression).

Adverse Reactions

>10%:

Cardiovascular: Flushing (8% to 16%)

Central nervous system: Dizziness (16% to 33%), headache (8% to 32%), insomnia (7% to 11%), somnolence (7% to 25%)

Dermatologic: Pruritus (6% to 12%)

Gastrointestinal: Constipation (12% to 46%), nausea (15% to 40%)

Neuromuscular & skeletal: Weakness (4% to 12%)

1% to 10%:

Cardiovascular: Chest pain (1% to <5%), postural hypotension (2% to 5%), vasodilation (1% to <5%)

Central nervous system: Agitation, anxiety (1% to <5%), confusion (1% to <5%), coordination impaired (1% to <5%), depression (1% to <5%), emotional lability, euphoria, hallucinations, hypoesthesia, lethargy, malaise, nervousness (1% to <5%), pain, pyrexia, restlessness

Dermatologic: Dermatitis, rash

Endocrine & metabolic: Hot flashes (2% to 9%), menopausal symptoms (1% to <5%)

Gastrointestinal: Abdominal pain, anorexia (<6%), diarrhea (5% to 10%), dry mouth (5% to 10%), dyspepsia, flatulence, vomiting (5% to 9%), weight loss

Genitourinary: Urinary frequency (1% to <5%), urinary retention (1% to <5%), urinary tract infection (1% to <5%)

Neuromuscular & skeletal: Arthralgia (1% to <5%), hypertonia (1% to <5%), rigors (<4%), paresthesia (1% to <5%), spasticity (1% to <5%), tremor (1% to <5%), creatinine phosphokinase increased

Ocular: Blurred vision (1% to <5%), miosis (1% to <5%)

Respiratory: Bronchitis (1% to <5%), cough (1% to <5%), dyspnea (1% to <5%), pharyngitis (1% to <5%),

(Continued)

Tramadol *(Continued)*

rhinorrhea (1% to <5%), sinusitis (1% to <5%)
Miscellaneous: Diaphoresis (2% to 6%), flu-like
syndrome (<2%)

A withdrawal syndrome may occur with abrupt discontinuation; includes anxiety, diarrhea, hallucinations
(rare), nausea, pain, piloerection, rigors, sweating,
and tremor. Uncommon discontinuation symptoms
may include severe anxiety, panic attacks, or paresthesia.

Overdosage/Toxicology Symptoms of overdose
include CNS and respiratory depression, lethargy,
coma, miosis, seizure, cardiac arrest, and death. Treatment may be symptom-directed and supportive.
Naloxone may reverse some overdose symptoms, but
may increase the risk of seizures. Hemodialysis is not
helpful in removal of tramadol.

Pharmacodynamics/Kinetics

Onset of Action: ~1 hour

Duration of Action: 9 hours

Time to Peak: Immediate release: 2 hours; Extended
release: 12 hours

Protein Binding: Plasma: 20%

Half-Life Elimination: Tramadol: ~6-8 hours; Active
metabolite: 7-9 hours; prolonged in elderly, hepatic or
renal impairment

Metabolism: Extensively hepatic via demethylation,
glucuronidation, and sulfation; has pharmacologically
active metabolite formed by CYP2D6 (M1;
O-desmethyl tramadol)

Excretion: Urine (30% as unchanged drug; 60% as
metabolites)

Available Dosage Forms

Tablet, as hydrochloride: 50 mg
Ultram®: 50 mg
Tablet, extended release, as hydrochloride:
Ultram® ER: 100 mg, 200 mg, 300 mg

Dosing

Adults: Moderate-to-severe chronic pain: Oral:
Immediate release formulation: 50-100 mg every 4-6
hours (not to exceed 400 mg/day)

For patients not requiring rapid onset of effect, tolerability may be improved by starting dose at 25
mg/day and titrating dose by 25 mg every 3 days,
until reaching 25 mg 4 times/day. Dose may then
be increased by 50 mg every 3 days as tolerated,
to reach dose of 50 mg 4 times/day.

Extended release formulation: 100 mg once daily;
titrate every 5 days (maximum: 300 mg/day)

Elderly: Oral: >75 years:
Immediate release: 50 mg every 6 hours (not to
exceed 300 mg/day); see dosing adjustments for
renal and hepatic impairment.
Extended release formulation: Refer to adult dosing.

Renal Impairment:
Immediate release: Cl_{cr} <30 mL/minute: Administer
50-100 mg dose every 12 hours (maximum: 200
mg/day).
Extended release: Should not be used in patients with
Cl_{cr} < 30 mL/minute.

Hepatic Impairment:
Immediate release: Cirrhosis: Recommended dose:
50 mg every 12 hours.
Extended release: Should not be used in patients with
severe (Child-Pugh Class C) hepatic dysfunction.

Administration

Oral: Do not crush or chew extended release tablet.

Stability

Storage: Store at 15°C to 30°C (59°F to 86°F).

Nursing Actions

Physical Assessment: Assess other medications
patient may be taking for additive or adverse interactions. Monitor therapeutic effectiveness and adverse
reactions or overdose at beginning of therapy and

periodically during therapy. May cause physical and/
or psychological dependence. Assess knowledge/
teach patient appropriate use. Teach patient to
monitor for adverse reactions, adverse reactions to
report, and appropriate interventions to reduce side
effects.

Patient Education: If self-administered, use exactly
as directed; do not increase dose or frequency. Drug
may cause physical and/or psychological dependence. While using this medication, do not use
alcohol and other prescription or OTC medications
(especially pain medications, sedatives, antihistamines, or cough preparations) without consulting
prescriber. Maintain adequate hydration (2-3 L/day of
fluids) unless instructed to restrict fluid intake. You
may experience drowsiness, dizziness, or blurred
vision (use caution when driving or engaging in tasks
requiring alertness until response to drug is known);
nausea, vomiting, or loss of appetite (small frequent
meals, frequent mouth care, chewing gum, or sucking
lozenges may help); or constipation (increased exercise, fluids, fruit, or fiber may help). Report severe
unresolved constipation, respiratory difficulty or shortness of breath, excessive sedation or increased
insomnia and restlessness, changes in urinary pattern
or menstrual pattern, seizures, muscle weakness or
tremors, or chest pain or palpitations. **Pregnancy/
breast-feeding precautions:** Inform prescriber if you
are or intend to become pregnant. Do not breast-feed.

Dietary Considerations May be taken with or without
food. Extended release formulation: Be consistent;
always give with food or always give on an empty
stomach.

Geriatric Considerations One study in the elderly
found that tramadol 50 mg was similar in efficacy as
acetaminophen 300 mg with codeine 30 mg.

Breast-Feeding Issues Not recommended for postde-
livery analgesia in nursing mothers.

Pregnancy Issues Tramadol has been shown to cross
the placenta. Postmarketing reports following tramadol
use during pregnancy include neonatal seizures, withdrawal syndrome, fetal death and stillbirth. Not recommended for use during labor and delivery.

Trandolapril *(tran DOE la pril)*

U.S. Brand Names Mavik®

Pharmacologic Category Angiotensin-Converting
Enzyme (ACE) Inhibitor

Pregnancy Risk Factor C (1st trimester)/D (2nd and
3rd trimesters)

Lactation Excretion in breast milk unknown/not recommended

Use Management of hypertension alone or in combination
with other antihypertensive agents; treatment of left
ventricular dysfunction after myocardial infarction

Unlabeled/Investigational Use As a class, ACE inhibitors are recommended in the treatment of systolic
congestive heart failure

Mechanism of Action/Effect Competitive inhibitor of
angiotensin-converting enzyme (ACE); prevents conversion of angiotensin I to angiotensin II, a potent vasoconstrictor; results in lower levels of angiotensin II which
causes an increase in plasma renin activity and a reduction in aldosterone secretion

Contraindications Hypersensitivity to trandolapril or
any component of the formulation; history of angioe-
dema-related to previous treatment with an ACE inhibitor; bilateral renal artery stenosis; pregnancy (2nd and
3rd trimesters)

Warnings/Precautions Angioedema can occur at any
time during treatment (especially following first dose). It
may involve head and neck (potentially affecting the
airway) or the intestine (presenting with abdominal

pain). Prolonged monitoring may be required especially if tongue, glottis, or larynx are involved as they are associated with airway obstruction. Those with a history of airway surgery in this situation have a higher risk. Careful blood pressure monitoring with first dose (hypotension can occur especially in volume-depleted patients). Dosage adjustment needed in severe renal dysfunction (Cl$_{cr}$ <30 mL/minute) or in hepatic cirrhosis. Use with caution in hypovolemia; collagen vascular diseases; valvular stenosis (particularly aortic stenosis); hyperkalemia; or before, during, or immediately after anesthesia. Avoid rapid dosage escalation, which may lead to renal insufficiency. Rare toxicities associated with ACE inhibitors include cholestatic jaundice (which may progress to hepatic necrosis) and neutropenia/agranulocytosis with myeloid hyperplasia. Use with caution in unilateral renal artery stenosis and pre-existing renal insufficiency.

Drug Interactions
Decreased Effect: Aspirin (high dose) may reduce the therapeutic effects of ACE inhibitors; at low dosages this does not appear to be significant. Rifampin may decrease the effect of ACE inhibitors. Antacids may decrease the bioavailability of ACE inhibitors (may be more likely to occur with captopril); separate administration times by 1-2 hours. NSAIDs, specifically indomethacin, may reduce the hypotensive effects of ACE inhibitors. More likely to occur in low renin or volume dependent hypertensive patients.

Increased Effect/Toxicity: Potassium supplements, co-trimoxazole (high dose), angiotensin II receptor antagonists (eg, candesartan, losartan, irbesartan), or potassium-sparing diuretics (amiloride, spironolactone, triamterene) may result in elevated serum potassium levels when combined with trandolapril. ACE inhibitor effects may be increased by phenothiazines or probenecid (increases levels of captopril). ACE inhibitors may increase serum concentrations/effects of lithium.

Diuretics have additive hypotensive effects with ACE inhibitors, and hypovolemia increases the potential for adverse renal effects of ACE inhibitors. In patients with compromised renal function, coadministration with NSAIDs may result in further deterioration of renal function. Allopurinol and ACE inhibitors may cause a higher risk of hypersensitivity reaction when taken concurrently.

Nutritional/Ethanol Interactions Herb/Nutraceutical: Avoid dong quai if using for hypertension (has estrogenic activity). Avoid ephedra, yohimbe, ginseng (may worsen hypertension). Avoid garlic (may have increased antihypertensive effect).

Adverse Reactions Note: Frequency ranges include data from hypertension and heart failure trials. Higher rates of adverse reactions have generally been noted in patients with CHF. However, the frequency of adverse effects associated with placebo is also increased in this population.

>1%:
Cardiovascular: Hypotension (<1% to 11%), bradycardia (<1% to 4.7%), intermittent claudication (3.8%), stroke (3.3%)
Central nervous system: Dizziness (1.3% to 23%), syncope (5.9%), asthenia (3.3%)
Endocrine & metabolic: Elevated uric acid (15%), hyperkalemia (5.3%), hypocalcemia (4.7%)
Gastrointestinal: Dyspepsia (6.4%), gastritis (4.2%)
Neuromuscular & skeletal: Myalgia (4.7%)
Renal: Elevated BUN (9%), elevated serum creatinine (1.1% to 4.7%), Cough (1.9% to 35%)

Overdosage/Toxicology Mild hypotension has been the primary toxic effect seen with acute overdose. Bradycardia may also occur. Hyperkalemia occurs even with therapeutic doses, especially in patients with renal insufficiency and those taking NSAIDs. Treatment is symptom-directed and supportive.

Pharmacodynamics/Kinetics
Onset of Action: 1-2 hours; Peak effect: Reduction in blood pressure: 6 hours
Duration of Action: Prolonged; 72 hours after single dose
Time to Peak: Parent: 1 hour; Active metabolite trandolaprilat: 4-10 hours
Protein Binding: 80%
Half-Life Elimination:
Trandolapril: 6 hours; Trandolaprilat: Effective: 10 hours, Terminal: 24 hours
Metabolism: Hepatically hydrolyzed to active metabolite, trandolaprilat
Excretion: Urine (as metabolites)
Clearance: Reduce dose in renal failure; creatinine clearances ≤30 mL/minute result in accumulation of active metabolite

Available Dosage Forms Tablet: 1 mg, 2 mg, 4 mg
Dosing
Adults & Elderly:
Hypertension: Oral; Initial dose in patients not receiving a diuretic: 1 mg/day (2 mg/day in black patients). Adjust dosage according to the blood pressure response. Make dosage adjustments at intervals of ≥1 week. Most patients have required dosages of 2-4 mg/day. There is a little experience with doses >8 mg/day. Patients inadequately treated with once daily dosing at 4 mg may be treated with twice daily dosing. If blood pressure is not adequately controlled with trandolapril monotherapy, a diuretic may be added.
Usual dose range (JNC 7): 1-4 mg once daily
Heart failure postmyocardial infarction or left ventricular dysfunction postmyocardial infarction: Oral: Initial: 1 mg/day; titrate patients (as tolerated) towards the target dose of 4 mg/day. If a 4 mg dose is not tolerated, patients can continue therapy with the greatest tolerated dose.
Renal Impairment: Cl$_{cr}$ ≤30 mL/minute: Administer lowest doses, starting at 0.5 mg/day.
Hepatic Impairment: Patients with hepatic cirrhosis: Start dose at 0.5 mg.
Laboratory Monitoring CBC, electrolytes, renal function; if patient has renal impairment, a baseline WBC with differential and serum creatinine should be evaluated and monitored closely during the first 3 months of therapy.

Nursing Actions
Physical Assessment: Assess potential for interactions with other pharmacological agents or herbal products patient may be taking (especially anything that may impact fluid balance or cardiac status). Monitor laboratory tests, therapeutic effectiveness, and adverse response (eg, hypovolemia, angioedema, postural hypotension) with first doses and on a regular basis during therapy. Teach patient proper use, possible side effects/appropriate interventions, and adverse symptoms to report.

Patient Education: Do not take any new medication during therapy unless approved by prescriber. Take exactly as directed; do not discontinue without consulting prescriber. Do not take antacids within 2 hours of this medication. Take first dose at bedtime. This drug does not eliminate need for diet or exercise regimen as recommended by prescriber. May cause dizziness, fainting, or lightheadedness (use caution when driving or engaging in tasks that require alertness until response to drug is known); postural hypotension (use caution when rising from lying or sitting position or climbing stairs); or diarrhea (buttermilk, boiled milk, yogurt may help). Report immediately any swelling of face, mouth, lips, tongue or throat. Report chest pain or palpitations; swelling of extremities, mouth, or tongue; skin rash; respiratory difficulty or unusual cough; or other persistent adverse reactions.
Pregnancy/breast-feeding precautions: Inform

(Continued)

Trandolapril (Continued)

prescriber if you are or intend to become pregnant. This drug should not be used in the 2nd or 3rd trimester of pregnancy. Consult prescriber for appropriate contraceptive measures if necessary. Do not breast-feed.

Geriatric Considerations Due to frequent decreases in glomerular filtration (also creatinine clearance) with aging, elderly patients may have exaggerated responses to ACE inhibitors. Differences in clinical response due to hepatic changes are not observed.

Pregnancy Issues ACE inhibitors can cause fetal injury or death if taken during the 2nd or 3rd trimester. Discontinue ACE inhibitors as soon as pregnancy is detected.

Trandolapril and Verapamil

(tran DOE la pril & ver AP a mil)

U.S. Brand Names Tarka®

Synonyms Verapamil and Trandolapril

Pharmacologic Category Antihypertensive Agent, Combination

Pregnancy Risk Factor C/D (2nd and 3rd trimesters)

Lactation Enters breast milk/contraindicated

Use Combination drug for the treatment of hypertension, however, not indicated for initial treatment of hypertension; replacement therapy in patients receiving separate dosage forms (for patient convenience); when monotherapy with one component fails to achieve desired antihypertensive effect, or when dose-limiting adverse effects limit upward titration of monotherapy

Available Dosage Forms Tablet, variable release:

1/240: Trandolapril 1 mg [immediate release] and verapamil hydrochloride 240 mg [sustained release]

2/180: Trandolapril 2 mg [immediate release] and verapamil hydrochloride 180 mg [sustained release]

2/240: Trandolapril 2 mg [immediate release] and verapamil hydrochloride 240 mg [sustained release]

4/240: Trandolapril 4 mg [immediate release] and verapamil hydrochloride 240 mg [sustained release]

Dosing

Adults: Hypertension: Oral: Individualize dose. Patients receiving trandolapril (up to 8 mg) and verapamil (up to 240 mg) in separate tablets may wish to receive Tarka® at equivalent dosages once daily.

Elderly: Refer to dosing in individual monographs.

Renal Impairment: Usual regimen need not be adjusted unless patient's creatinine clearance is <30 mL/minute. Titration of individual components must be done prior to switching to combination product

Hepatic Impairment: Has not been evaluated in hepatic impairment. Verapamil is hepatically metabolized, adjustment of dosage in hepatic impairment is recommended.

Nursing Actions

Physical Assessment: See individual agents.

Patient Education: See individual agents. **Pregnancy/breast-feeding precautions:** Inform prescriber if you are or intend to become pregnant. Do not breast-feed.

Related Information

Trandolapril *on page 1238*

Verapamil *on page 1281*

Tranylcypromine (tran il SIP roe meen)

U.S. Brand Names Parnate®

Synonyms Transamine Sulphate; Tranylcypromine Sulfate

Restrictions A medication guide concerning the use of antidepressants in children and teenagers can be found on the FDA website at http://www.fda.gov/cder/Offices/ODS/labeling.htm. It should be dispensed to parents or guardians of children and teenagers receiving this medication.

Pharmacologic Category Antidepressant, Monoamine Oxidase Inhibitor

Pregnancy Risk Factor C

Lactation Enters breast milk/not recommended

Use Treatment of major depressive episode without melancholia

Unlabeled/Investigational Use Post-traumatic stress disorder

Mechanism of Action/Effect Tranylcypromine is a nonhydrazine MAO inhibitor. It increases endogenous concentrations of epinephrine, norepinephrine, dopamine, and serotonin through inhibition of the enzyme (monoamine oxidase) responsible for the breakdown of these neurotransmitters.

Contraindications Hypersensitivity to tranylcypromine, other MAO inhibitors, dibenzazepine derivatives, or any component of the formulation; antiparkinson drugs, cardiovascular disease; cerebrovascular defect; headache history; hepatic disease; hypertension; pheochromocytoma; renal disease; concurrent use of antihistamines, antihypertensives, bupropion, buspirone, CNS depressants, dexfenfluramine, dextromethorphan, diuretics, ethanol, meperidine, SSRIs, and sympathomimetics; general anesthesia (discontinue 10 days prior to elective surgery); local vasoconstrictors; spinal anesthesia (hypotension may be exaggerated); foods which are high in tyramine, tryptophan, or dopamine, chocolate, or caffeine

Warnings/Precautions Risk of suicide: Antidepressants increase the risk of suicidal thinking and behavior in children and adolescents with major depressive disorder (MDD) and other depressive disorders; consider risk prior to prescribing. Closely monitor for clinical worsening, suicidality, or unusual changes in behavior. The child's family or caregiver should be instructed to closely observe the patient and communicate condition with healthcare provider. Such observation would generally include at least weekly face-to-face contact with patients or their family members or caregivers during the first 4 weeks of treatment, then every other week visits for the next 4 weeks, then at 12 weeks, and as clinically indicated beyond 12 weeks. Additional contact by telephone may be appropriate between face-to-face visits. A medication guide should be dispensed with each prescription. **Tranylcypromine is not FDA approved for treatment of children and adolescents.**

Adults treated with antidepressants should be observed similarly for clinical worsening and suicidality, especially during the initial few months of a course of drug therapy, or at times of dose changes (increases or decreases). The possibility of a suicide attempt is inherent in major depression and may persist until remission occurs. Use caution in high-risk patients. Prescriptions should be written for the smallest quantity.

Disease state precautions: Use with caution in patients who are hyperactive, hyperexcitable, or who have glaucoma, hyperthyroidism, diabetes or hypotension. May cause orthostatic hypotension (especially at dosages >30 mg/day). Use with caution in patients at risk of seizures, or in patients receiving other drugs which may lower seizure threshold. Discontinue at least 48 hours prior to myelography. May increase the risks associated with electroconvulsive therapy. Consider discontinuing, when possible, prior to elective surgery. Use with caution in patients with renal impairment. May worsen psychosis in some patients or precipitate a shift to mania or hypomania in patients with bipolar disorder. **Tranylcypromine is not FDA approved for the treatment of bipolar depression.**

Drug interactions: Hypertensive crisis may occur with tyramine, tryptophan, or dopamine-containing foods. Should not be used in combination with other antidepressants. Do not use within 5 weeks of fluoxetine discontinuation or 2 weeks of other antidepressant discontinuation. Hypotensive effects of antihypertensives may be exaggerated. Orthostasis may be additive when used with other agents also known to cause it. Use with caution in patients receiving disulfiram.

Elderly patients: Interactions with tyramine or tryptophan-containing foods and orthostasis have limited tranylcypromine's use.

Drug Interactions

Cytochrome P450 Effect: Inhibits CYP1A2 (moderate), 2A6 (strong), 2C8/9 (weak), 2C19 (moderate), 2D6 (moderate), 2E1 (weak), 3A4 (weak)

Decreased Effect: Acetylcholinesterase inhibitors decrease tranylcypromine's anticholinergic side effects. Tranylcypromine may decrease the effects of CYP2D6 prodrug substrates, and false neurotransmitters (guanadrel, methyldopa).

Increased Effect/Toxicity: Tranylcypromine may enhance the adverse effects of ethanol (CNS depression), amphetamines (hypertension), general anesthetics (hypotension), atomoxetine (CNS toxicity), buspirone (hypertension), CYP1A2 substrates, CYP2A6 substrates, CYP2C19 substrates, CYP2D6 substrates, dexmethylphenidate (hypertension), disulfiram (delirium), levodopa (hypertension), lithium (CNS toxicity), methylphenidate (hypertension), mirtazapine (CNS toxicity), rauwolfia alkaloids, and thioridazine. Tranylcypromine may enhance the vasopressor effects of alpha-/beta-agonists and enhance the hypertensive effects of alpha$_1$-agonists. Altretamine may enhance the orthostatic effects of tranylcypromine. Anticholinergics may enhance the side effects of tranylcypromine. Concurrent use of anorexiants, cyclobenzaprine, dextromethorphan, meperidine, SSRIs/SNRIs, serotonin 5-HT$_{1D}$ receptor agonist, sibutramine, and tricyclic antidepressants may result in a serotonin syndrome. Concurrent use of bupropion may lead to hypertension crisis. COMT inhibitors may cause adverse/toxic effects. Pramlintide may increase anticholinergic effects of tranylcypromine. Serotonin modulators may enhance the adverse/toxic effects of tranylcypromine. Tramadol may increase the neuroexcitatory and seizure-potentiating effects of tranylcypromine.

Nutritional/Ethanol Interactions

Ethanol: Avoid ethanol (many contain tyramine).

Food: Clinically-severe elevated blood pressure may occur if tranylcypromine is taken with tyramine-containing food. Avoid foods containing tryptophan or dopamine, chocolate or caffeine.

Herb/Nutraceutical: Avoid valerian, St John's wort, SAMe, ginseng. Avoid ginkgo (may lead to MAO inhibitor toxicity). Avoid ephedra, yohimbe (can cause hypertension).

Lab Interactions Decreased glucose

Adverse Reactions Frequency not defined.

Cardiovascular: Edema, orthostatic hypotension, palpitations, tachycardia

Central nervous system: Agitation, akinesia, anxiety, ataxia, chills, confusion, disorientation, dizziness, drowsiness, fatigue, headache, hyper-reflexia, insomnia, mania, memory loss, restlessness, sleep disturbances, twitching

Dermatologic: Alopecia, cystic acne (flare), pruritus, rash, urticaria, scleroderma (localized)

Endocrine & metabolic: Hypernatremia, hypermetabolic syndrome; sexual dysfunction (anorgasmia, ejaculatory disturbances, impotence); SIADH

Gastrointestinal: Abdominal pain, anorexia, constipation, diarrhea, nausea, vomiting, weight gain, xerostomia

Genitourinary: Incontinence, urinary retention

Hematologic: Agranulocytosis, anemia, leukopenia, thrombocytopenia

Hepatic: Hepatitis

Neuromuscular & skeletal: Akinesis, muscle spasm, myoclonus, numbness, paresthesia, tremor, weakness

Ocular: Blurred vision, glaucoma

Otic: Tinnitus

Miscellaneous: Diaphoresis

Overdosage/Toxicology Symptoms of overdose include headache, tachycardia or bradycardia, neck stiffness, nausea, vomiting, chest pain, sweating, photophobia, palpitations, muscle twitching, seizures, insomnia, orthostatic hypotension, hypertension, hypertensive crisis, hyperpyrexia, and coma. Treatment is symptom-directed and supportive. The manufacturer suggests phentolamine (5 mg given slowly I.V.) for treatment of hypertensive crisis. Other useful agents may be labetalol or nitroprusside.

Pharmacodynamics/Kinetics

Onset of Action: Therapeutic: 2 days to 3 weeks continued dosing

Time to Peak: Serum: ~2 hours

Half-Life Elimination: 90-190 minutes

Excretion: Urine

Available Dosage Forms Tablet: 10 mg

Dosing

Adults & Elderly: Depression: Oral: 10 mg twice daily, increase by 10 mg increments at 1- to 3-week intervals; maximum: 60 mg/day; usual effective dose: 30 mg/day

Laboratory Monitoring Blood glucose

Nursing Actions

Physical Assessment: Assess other medications patient may be taking for effectiveness and interactions. Monitor laboratory tests, therapeutic response (ie, mental status, mood, affect, suicidal ideation), and adverse reactions at beginning of therapy and periodically with long-term use. Monitor blood pressure. Observe for clinical worsening, suicidality, or unusual behavior changes, especially during the initial few months of therapy or during dosage changes. Assess knowledge/teach patient appropriate use, interventions to reduce side effects, and adverse symptoms to report.

Patient Education: Take exactly as directed; do not increase dose or frequency. It may take 2-3 weeks to achieve desired results. Take in the morning to reduce the incidence of insomnia. Avoid alcohol, caffeine, and other prescription or OTC medications not approved by prescriber. Avoid tyramine-containing foods (eg, pickles, aged cheese, wine); see prescriber for complete list of foods to be avoided. Maintain adequate hydration (2-3 L/day of fluids) unless instructed to restrict fluid intake. You may experience drowsiness, dizziness, or blurred vision (use caution when driving or engaging in tasks requiring alertness until response to drug is known); anorexia or dry mouth (small frequent meals, frequent mouth care, chewing gum, or sucking lozenges may help); constipation (increased exercise, fluids, fruit, or fiber may help); diarrhea (buttermilk, yogurt, or boiled milk may help); or orthostatic hypotension (use caution when climbing stairs or changing position from lying or sitting to standing); or altered sexual ability (reversible). Report persistent excessive sedation; muscle cramping, tremors, weakness, or change in gait; chest pain, palpitations, rapid heartbeat, or swelling of (Continued)

Tranylcypromine (Continued)

extremities; vision changes; suicidal ideation; or worsening of condition. **Pregnancy/breast-feeding precautions:** Inform prescriber if you are or intend to become pregnant. Breast-feeding is not recommended.

Dietary Considerations Avoid food which contains high amounts of tyramine. Avoid foods containing tryptophan or dopamine, including chocolate and caffeine.

Geriatric Considerations MAO inhibitors are effective and generally well tolerated by older patients. Potential interactions with tyramine- or tryptophan-containing foods (see Warnings/Precautions), other drugs, and adverse effects on blood pressure have limited use of MAO inhibitors. They are usually reserved for patients who do not tolerate or respond to traditional "cyclic" or "second generation" antidepressants. Tranylcypromine is the preferred MAO inhibitor because its enzymatic-blocking effects are more rapidly reversed. The brain activity of monoamine oxidase increases with age and even more so in patients with Alzheimer's disease. Therefore, MAO inhibitors may have an increased role in treating depressed patients with Alzheimer's disease.

Additional Information Tranylcypromine has a more rapid onset of therapeutic effect than other MAO inhibitors, but causes more severe hypertensive reactions.

Related Information
Antidepressant Medication Guidelines *on page 1414*
Tyramine Content of Foods *on page 1406*

Trastuzumab (tras TU zoo mab)

U.S. Brand Names Herceptin®
Pharmacologic Category Antineoplastic Agent, Monoclonal Antibody; Monoclonal Antibody
Pregnancy Risk Factor B
Lactation Excretion in breast milk unknown/not recommended
Use Treatment of metastatic breast cancer whose tumors overexpress the HER-2/*neu* protein
Unlabeled/Investigational Use Treatment of ovarian, gastric, colorectal, endometrial, lung, bladder, prostate, and salivary gland tumors
Mechanism of Action/Effect Trastuzumab is a monoclonal antibody which binds to the extracellular domain of the human epidermal growth factor receptor 2 protein (HER-2). It mediates antibody-dependent cellular cytotoxicity against cells which overproduce HER-2.
Contraindications Hypersensitivity to trastuzumab, Chinese hamster ovary cell proteins, or any component of the formulation
Warnings/Precautions Hazardous agent — use appropriate precautions for handling and disposal. Congestive heart failure associated with trastuzumab may be severe and has been associated with disabling cardiac failure, death, mural thrombus, and stroke. Left ventricular function should be evaluated in all patients prior to and during treatment with trastuzumab. Discontinuation should be strongly considered in patients who develop a clinically significant decrease in ejection fraction during therapy. Combination therapy with anthracyclines and cyclophosphamide increases the risk of cardiac dysfunction. Extreme caution should be used when treating patients with pre-existing cardiac disease or dysfunction, and in patients with previous exposure to anthracyclines or radiation therapy. Advanced age may also predispose to cardiac toxicity.

Serious adverse events, including hypersensitivity reaction (anaphylaxis), infusion reactions (including fatalities), and pulmonary events (including adult respiratory distress syndrome) have been associated with trastuzumab. Most of these events occur with the first infusion; pulmonary events may occur during or within 24 hours of administration; delayed reactions have occurred. Use with caution in pre-existing pulmonary disease. Discontinuation of trastuzumab should be strongly considered in any patient who develops anaphylaxis, angioedema, or acute respiratory distress syndrome. Retreatment of patients who experienced severe hypersensitivity reactions has been attempted (with premedication). Some patients tolerated retreatment, while others experienced a second severe reaction. When used in combination with myelosuppressive chemotherapy, trastuzumab may increase the incidence of neutropenia (moderate-to-severe) and febrile neutropenia. Safety and efficacy in children have not been established.

Drug Interactions
Increased Effect/Toxicity: Paclitaxel may result in a decrease in clearance of trastuzumab, increasing serum concentrations. Combined use with anthracyclines may increase the incidence/severity of cardiac dysfunction. Monoclonal antibodies may increase the risk for allergic reactions to trastuzumab due to the presence of HACA antibodies. Trastuzumab may increase the incidence of neutropenia and/or febrile neutropenia when used in combination with myelosuppressive chemotherapy.

Adverse Reactions Note: The most common adverse effects are infusion-related, occurring in up to 40% of patients, consisting of fever and chills (mild to moderate, often with other systemic symptoms). Treatment with acetaminophen, diphenhydramine, and/or meperidine is usually effective.

>10%:
Central nervous system: Pain (47%), fever (36%), chills (32%), headache (26%), insomnia (14%), dizziness (13%)
Dermatologic: Rash (18%)
Gastrointestinal: Nausea (33%), diarrhea (25%), vomiting (23%), abdominal pain (22%), anorexia (14%)
Neuromuscular & skeletal: Weakness (42%), back pain (22%)
Respiratory: Cough (26%), dyspnea (22%), rhinitis (14%), pharyngitis (12%)
Miscellaneous: Infection (20%); infusion reaction (40%, chills and fever most common)
1% to 10%:
Cardiovascular: Peripheral edema (10%), edema (8%), CHF (7%), tachycardia (5%)
Central nervous system: Paresthesia (9%), depression (6%), peripheral neuritis (2%), neuropathy (1%)
Dermatologic: Herpes simplex (2%), acne (2%)
Genitourinary: Urinary tract infection (5%)
Hematologic: Anemia (4%), leukopenia (3%)
Neuromuscular & skeletal: Bone pain (7%), arthralgia (6%)
Respiratory: Sinusitis (9%)
Miscellaneous: Flu syndrome (10%), accidental injury (6%), allergic reaction (3%)

Overdosage/Toxicology There is no experience with overdose in human clinical trials. Treatment is symptom-directed and supportive.

Pharmacodynamics/Kinetics
Half-Life Elimination: Mean: 5.8 days (range: 1-32 days)
Available Dosage Forms Injection, powder for reconstitution: 440 mg [packaged with bacteriostatic water for injection; diluent contains benzyl alcohol]
Dosing
Adults & Elderly:
Metastatic breast carcinoma: I.V.:
Loading dose: 4 mg/kg over 90 minutes; do not administer as an I.V. bolus or I.V. push.
Maintenance dose: 2 mg/kg once weekly (may be infused over 30 minutes if prior infusions are well tolerated).

or (unlabeled schedule)

Initial loading dose: 8 mg/kg intravenous infusion over 90 minutes

Maintenance dose: 6 mg/kg intravenous infusion over 90 minutes every 3 weeks

Renal Impairment: No adjustment is necessary.

Hepatic Impairment: No adjustment necessary.

Administration

I.V.: Administered by I.V. infusion; loading doses are infused over 90 minutes; maintenance doses may be infused over 30 minutes if tolerated.

I.V. Detail: Observe patients closely during the infusion for fever, chills, or other infusion-related symptoms.

Stability

Reconstitution: Reconstitute each vial with 20 mL of bacteriostatic sterile water for injection to a concentration of 21 mg/mL. Swirl gently, do not shake; allow vial to rest for ~5 minutes; avoid rapid expulsion from syringe. If patient has a known hypersensitivity to benzyl alcohol, it may be reconstituted with sterile water for injection. Further dilute in NS prior to administration. **Dextrose 5% solution CANNOT BE used.**

Compatibility: Stable in NS

Incompatible with D_5W

Storage: Store intact vials under refrigeration 2°C to 8°C (36°F to 46°F) prior to reconstitution. Stable for 28 days after reconstitution if refrigerated; do not freeze. If sterile water for injection without preservative is used for reconstitution, it must be used immediately. After dilution in 0.9% sodium chloride for injection in polyethylene bags, solution is stable for 24 hours at room temperature or refrigerated.

Nursing Actions

Physical Assessment: Monitor vital signs during infusion. Monitor response to therapy and adverse reactions (eg, infusion related symptoms such as fever, chills, headache, CHF, CNS changes, or opportunistic infection). Assess knowledge/teach patient interventions to reduce side effects, and adverse symptoms to report.

Patient Education: This medication can only be administered by infusion. Report immediately any adverse reactions during infusion (eg, respiratory difficulty, chills, fever, headache, backache, or nausea/vomiting) so appropriate medication can be administered. You will be susceptible to infection (avoid crowds and exposure to infection). You may experience dizziness or weakness (use caution when driving or engaging in tasks requiring alertness until response to drug is known); nausea or vomiting (small frequent meals, frequent mouth care, chewing gum, or sucking lozenges may help); diarrhea (boiled milk, yogurt, or buttermilk may help); or headache, back or joint pain (mild analgesics may offer relief). Report persistent GI effects; sore throat, runny nose, or respiratory difficulty; chest pain, irregular heartbeat, palpitations, swelling of extremities, or unusual weight gain; muscle or joint weakness, numbness, or pain; skin rash or irritation; itching or pain on urination; unhealed sores, white plaques in mouth or genital area, unusual bruising or bleeding; or other unusual adverse effects. **Breast-feeding precaution:** Breast-feeding is not recommended.

Breast-Feeding Issues It is not known whether trastuzumab is secreted in human milk. Because many immunoglobulins are secreted in milk, and the potential for serious adverse reactions exists, patients should discontinue nursing during treatment and for 6 months after the last dose.

Travoprost (TRA voe prost)

U.S. Brand Names Travatan®

Pharmacologic Category Ophthalmic Agent, Antiglaucoma; Prostaglandin, Ophthalmic

Medication Safety Issues
Sound-alike/look-alike issues:
Travatan® may be confused with Xalatan®

Pregnancy Risk Factor C

Lactation Excretion in breast milk unknown/use caution

Use Reduction of elevated intraocular pressure in patients with open-angle glaucoma or ocular hypertension who are intolerant of the other IOP-lowering medications or insufficiently responsive (failed to achieve target IOP determined after multiple measurements over time) to another IOP-lowering medication

Contraindications Hypersensitivity to travoprost or any component of the formulation; pregnancy

Warnings/Precautions May permanently change/increase brown pigmentation of the iris, the eyelid skin, and eyelashes. In addition, may increase the length and/or number of eyelashes (may vary between eyes); changes occur slowly and may not be noticeable for months or years. Bacterial keratitis may be caused by inadvertent contamination of multiple-dose ophthalmic solutions. Use caution in patients with intraocular inflammation, aphakic patients, pseudophakic patients with a torn posterior lens capsule, or patients with risk factors for macular edema. Contains benzalkonium chloride; remove contacts prior to administration and wait 15 minutes before reinserting. Contact with contents of vial should be avoided in women who are pregnant or attempting to become pregnant; in case of accidental exposure to the skin, wash the exposed area with soap and water immediately. Safety and efficacy have not been determined for use in patients with renal or hepatic impairment, angle-closure-, inflammatory-, or neovascular glaucoma. Safety and efficacy in pediatric patients have not been established.

Adverse Reactions
>10%: Ocular: Hyperemia (35% to 50%)
5% to 10%: Ocular: Decreased visual acuity, eye discomfort, foreign body sensation, pain, pruritus
1% to 5%:
Cardiovascular: Angina pectoris, bradycardia, hyper-/hypotension
Central nervous system: Depression, pain, anxiety, headache
Endocrine & metabolic: Hypercholesterolemia
Gastrointestinal: Dyspepsia
Genitourinary: Prostate disorder, urinary incontinence
Neuromuscular & skeletal: Arthritis, back pain, chest pain
Ocular (1% to 4%): Abnormal vision, blepharitis, blurred vision, conjunctivitis, dry eye, iris discoloration, keratitis, lid margin crusting, photophobia, subconjunctival hemorrhage, cataract, tearing, periorbital skin discoloration (darkening), eyelash darkening, eyelash growth increased
Respiratory: Bronchitis, sinusitis

Pharmacodynamics/Kinetics
Onset of Action: ~2 hours; Peak effect: 12 hours
Duration of Action: Plasma levels decrease to <10 pg/mL within 1 hour
Metabolism: Hydrolyzed by esterases in the cornea to active free acid; systemically; the free acid is metabolized to inactive metabolites

Available Dosage Forms Solution, ophthalmic: 0.004% (2.5 mL, 5 mL) [contains benzalkonium chloride]

Dosing
Adults & Elderly: Glaucoma (open angle) or ocular hypertension: Ophthalmic: Instill 1 drop into affected eye(s) once daily in the evening; do not exceed once-daily dosing (may decrease IOP-lowering (Continued)

Travoprost *(Continued)*

effect). If used with other topical ophthalmic agents, separate administration by at least 5 minutes.

Administration

Other: May be used with other eye drops to lower intraocular pressure. If using more than one ophthalmic product, wait at least 5 minutes in between application of each medication. Remove contact lenses prior to administration and wait 15 minutes before reinserting.

Stability

Storage: Store between 2°C to 25°C (36°F to 77°F); discard within 6 weeks of removing from sealed pouch

Nursing Actions

Physical Assessment: Assess potential for interactions with other prescriptions, OTC medications, or herbal products patient may be taking. Monitor patient response and adverse effects. Teach patient proper use, side effects/appropriate interventions, and symptoms to report.

Patient Education: For use in eyes only. Wash hands before instilling. Sit or lie down to instill. Open eye, look at ceiling, and instill prescribed amount of solution. Apply gentle pressure to inner corner of eye. Do not let tip of applicator touch eye; do not contaminate tip of applicator (may cause eye infection, eye damage, or vision loss). Contact prescriber concerning continued use of drops if eye infection develops, trauma occurs to the eye, and prior to eye surgery. This product contains benzalkonium chloride which may be adsorbed by contact lenses; remove contacts prior to administration and wait 15 minutes before reinserting. May cause permanent changes in eye color (increases the amount of brown pigment in the iris), eyelid, and eyelashes. May also increase the length and/or number of eyelashes. Changes may occur slowly (months to years). May be used with other eye drops to lower intraocular pressure. If using more than one eye drop medicine, wait at least 5 minutes in between application of each medication. Notify prescriber if conjunctivitis or eyelid reactions occur with use of this product. **Pregnancy precautions:** Do not use if you are pregnant or attempting to become pregnant. In case of accidental contact with the solution, wash skin with soap and water immediately. Consult prescriber if breast-feeding.

Pregnancy Issues May interfere with the maintenance of pregnancy. Do not use during pregnancy or in women attempting to become pregnant. Teratogenic effects in humans are not known.

Additional Information The IOP-lowering effect was shown to be 7-8 mm Hg in clinical studies. The mean IOP reduction in African-American patients was up to 1.8 mm Hg greater than in non-African-American patients. The reason for this effect is unknown.

Trazodone *(TRAZ oh done)*

U.S. Brand Names Desyrel®

Synonyms Trazodone Hydrochloride

Restrictions A medication guide concerning the use of antidepressants in children and teenagers can be found on the FDA website at http://www.fda.gov/cder/Offices/ODS/labeling.htm. It should be dispensed to parents or guardians of children and teenagers receiving this medication.

Pharmacologic Category Antidepressant, Serotonin Reuptake Inhibitor/Antagonist

Medication Safety Issues

Sound-alike/look-alike issues:

Desyrel® may be confused with Demerol®, Delsym®, Zestril®

Pregnancy Risk Factor C

Lactation Enters breast milk/use caution (AAP rates "of concern")

Use Treatment of depression

Unlabeled/Investigational Use Potential augmenting agent for antidepressants, hypnotic

Mechanism of Action/Effect Inhibits reuptake of serotonin, causes adrenoreceptor subsensitivity, and induces significant changes in 5HT presynaptic receptor adrenoreceptors. Trazodone also significantly blocks histamine (H1) and alpha$_1$ adrenergic receptors.

Contraindications Hypersensitivity to trazodone or any component of the formulation

Warnings/Precautions Antidepressants increase the risk of suicidal thinking and behavior in children and adolescents with major depressive disorder (MDD) and other depressive disorders; consider risk prior to prescribing. All patients must be closely monitored for clinical worsening, suicidality, or unusual changes in behavior, especially during the initiation of therapy or following an increase or decrease in dosage. When used in children, the child's family or caregiver should be instructed to closely observe the patient and communicate condition with healthcare provider. A medication guide should be dispensed with each prescription. **Trazodone is not FDA approved for use in children.**

The possibility of a suicide attempt is inherent in major depression and may persist until remission occurs. Use caution in high-risk patients. Worsening depression and severe abrupt suicidality that are not part of the presenting symptoms may require discontinuation or modification of drug therapy. The patient's family or caregiver should be alerted to monitor patients for the emergence of suicidality and associated behaviors (such as agitation, irritability, hostility, impulsivity, and hypomania) and call healthcare provider.

May worsen psychosis in some patients or precipitate a shift to mania or hypomania in patients with bipolar disorder. Patients presenting with depressive symptoms should be screened for bipolar disorder. Monotherapy in patients with bipolar disorder should be avoided. **Trazodone is not FDA approved for the treatment of bipolar depression.**

Priapism, including cases resulting in permanent dysfunction, has occurred with the use of trazodone. Not recommended for use in a patient during the acute recovery phase of MI. Trazodone should be initiated with caution in patients who are receiving concurrent or recent therapy with a MAO inhibitor.

The risks of sedation and/or postural hypotension are high relative to other antidepressants. Trazodone frequently causes sedation, which may result in impaired performance of tasks requiring alertness (eg, operating machinery or driving). Sedative effects may be additive with other CNS depressants and ethanol. Use with caution in patients with a history of cardiovascular disease (including previous MI, stroke, tachycardia, or conduction abnormalities). The risk of conduction abnormalities with this agent is low relative to other antidepressants.

Consider discontinuing, when possible, prior to elective surgery. Therapy should not be abruptly discontinued in patients receiving high doses for prolonged periods. Use caution in patients with a previous seizure disorder or condition predisposing to seizures such as brain damage, alcoholism, or concurrent therapy with other drugs which lower the seizure threshold. Use with caution in patients with hepatic or renal dysfunction and in elderly patients.

Drug Interactions

Cytochrome P450 Effect: Substrate of CYP2D6 (minor), 3A4 (major); **Inhibits** CYP2D6 (moderate), 3A4 (weak)

Decreased Effect: Trazodone inhibits the hypotensive response to clonidine. The levels/effects of trazodone may be decreased by aminoglutethimide, carbamazepine, nafcillin, nevirapine, phenobarbital, phenytoin, rifamycins, and other CYP3A4 inducers. Trazodone may decrease the levels/effects of CYP2D6 prodrug substrates (eg, codeine, hydrocodone, oxycodone, tramadol).

Increased Effect/Toxicity: Trazodone, in combination with other serotonergic agents (buspirone, MAO inhibitors), may produce additive serotonergic effects, including serotonin syndrome. Trazodone, in combination with other psychotropics (low potency antipsychotics), may result in additional hypotension. Fluoxetine may inhibit the metabolism of trazodone resulting in elevated plasma levels.

Trazodone may increase the levels/effects of amphetamines, beta-blockers, dextromethorphan, fluoxetine, lidocaine, mirtazapine, nefazodone, paroxetine, risperidone, ritonavir, thioridazine, tricyclic antidepressants, venlafaxine, and other CYP2D6 substrates. The levels/effects of trazodone may be increased by azole antifungals, clarithromycin, diclofenac, doxycycline, erythromycin, imatinib, isoniazid, nefazodone, nicardipine, propofol, protease inhibitors, quinidine, telithromycin, verapamil, and other CYP3A4 inhibitors.

Nutritional/Ethanol Interactions
Ethanol: Avoid ethanol (may increase CNS depression).
Food: Time to peak serum levels may be increased if trazodone is taken with food.
Herb/Nutraceutical: Avoid valerian, St John's wort, SAMe, kava kava (may increase risk of serotonin syndrome and/or excessive sedation).

Adverse Reactions
>10%:
Central nervous system: Dizziness, headache, sedation
Gastrointestinal: Nausea, xerostomia
Ocular: Blurred vision
1% to 10%:
Cardiovascular: Syncope, hyper-/hypotension, edema
Central nervous system: Confusion, decreased concentration, fatigue, incoordination
Gastrointestinal: Diarrhea, constipation, weight gain/loss
Neuromuscular & skeletal: Tremor, myalgia
Respiratory: Nasal congestion

Overdosage/Toxicology Symptoms of overdose include drowsiness, vomiting, hypotension, tachycardia, incontinence, coma, and priapism. Treatment is symptom-directed and supportive.

Pharmacodynamics/Kinetics
Onset of Action: Therapeutic (antidepressant): 1-3 weeks; sleep aid: 1-3 hours
Time to Peak: Serum: 30-100 minutes; delayed with food (up to 2.5 hours)
Protein Binding: 85% to 95%
Half-Life Elimination: 7-8 hours, two compartment kinetics
Metabolism: Hepatic via CYP3A4 to an active metabolite (mCPP)
Excretion: Primarily urine; secondarily feces
Available Dosage Forms Tablet, as hydrochloride: 50 mg, 100 mg, 150 mg, 300 mg
Dosing
Adults:
Depression: Oral: Initial: 150 mg/day in 3 divided doses (may increase by 50 mg/day every 3-7 days); maximum: 600 mg/day
Note: Therapeutic effects may take up to 6 weeks. Therapy is normally maintained for 6-12 months after optimum response is reached to prevent recurrence of depression.
Sedation/hypnotic (unlabeled use): Oral: 25-50 mg at bedtime (often in combination with daytime SSRIs). May increase up to 200 mg at bedtime.

Elderly: Oral: 25-50 mg at bedtime with 25-50 mg/day dose increase every 3 days for inpatients and weekly for outpatients, if tolerated; usual dose: 75-150 mg/day
Pediatrics:
Depression (unlabeled use):
Children 6-12 years: Initial: 1.5-2 mg/kg/day in divided doses; increase gradually every 3-4 days as needed; maximum: 6 mg/kg/day in 3 divided doses
Adolescents: Initial: 25-50 mg/day; increase to 100-150 mg/day in divided doses
Administration
Oral: Dosing after meals may decrease lightheadedness and postural hypotension.
Laboratory Monitoring Baseline liver function prior to and periodically during therapy
Nursing Actions
Physical Assessment: Assess other medications patient may be taking for effectiveness and interactions. Monitor laboratory tests, therapeutic response (ie, mental status, mood, affect, suicidal ideation), and adverse reactions at beginning of therapy and periodically with long-term use. Assess knowledge/teach patient appropriate use, interventions to reduce side effects, and adverse symptoms to report.
Patient Education: Do not take any new medication during therapy unless approved by prescriber. Take exactly as directed; do not increase dose or frequency. It may take 2-4 weeks to achieve desired results. Take after meals. Avoid excessive alcohol and caffeine. Maintain adequate hydration (2-3 L/day of fluids) unless instructed to restrict fluid intake. You may experience drowsiness, lightheadedness, dizziness (use caution when driving or engaging in tasks requiring alertness until response to drug is known); postural hypotension (use caution when climbing stairs or changing position from lying or sitting to standing); nausea, dry mouth (small frequent meals, frequent mouth care, chewing gum, or sucking lozenges may help); constipation (increased exercise, fluids, fruit, or fiber may help); or diarrhea (buttermilk, yogurt, or boiled milk may help). Report persistent dizziness or headache; muscle cramping, tremors, or altered gait; blurred vision or eye pain; chest pain or irregular heartbeat; suicidal ideation; or worsening of condition. Report prolonged or inappropriate erections. **Pregnancy/breast-feeding precautions:** Inform prescriber if you are or intend to become pregnant. Do not breast-feed.
Geriatric Considerations Very sedating, but little anticholinergic effects.
Related Information
Antidepressant Medication Guidelines *on page 1414*
Federal OBRA Regulations Recommended Maximum Doses *on page 1421*

Tretinoin (Oral) (TRET i noyn, oral)

U.S. Brand Names Vesanoid®
Synonyms All-*trans*-Retinoic Acid; ATRA; NSC-122758; Ro 5488; tRA; *trans*-Retinoic Acid
Pharmacologic Category Antineoplastic Agent, Miscellaneous
Medication Safety Issues
Sound-alike/look-alike issues:
Tretinoin may be confused with trientine
Pregnancy Risk Factor D
Lactation Enters breast milk/not recommended
Use Induction of remission in patients with acute promyelocytic leukemia (APL), French American British (FAB) classification M3 (including the M3 variant)
(Continued)

Tretinoin (Oral) *(Continued)*

Mechanism of Action/Effect Tretinoin appears to bind one or more nuclear receptors and inhibits clonal proliferation and/or granulocyte differentiation

Contraindications Sensitivity to parabens, vitamin A, other retinoids, or any component of the formulation; pregnancy

Warnings/Precautions Hazardous agent - use appropriate precautions for handling and disposal. Patients with acute promyelocytic leukemia (APL) are at high risk and can have severe adverse reactions to tretinoin.

May cause retinoic acid-APL (RA-APL) syndrome (fever, dyspnea, pulmonary infiltrates, pleural/pericardial effusions, cardiac dysfunction). May be treated with high-dose steroids. The majority of patients do not require termination of tretinoin therapy. During treatment, rapidly evolving leukocytosis is associated with a higher risk of life-threatening complications.

Not to be used in women of childbearing potential unless the woman is capable of complying with effective contraceptive measures. Repeat pregnancy testing and contraception counseling monthly throughout the period of treatment.

Retinoids have been associated with pseudotumor cerebri (benign intracranial hypertension), especially in children. Concurrent use of other drugs associated with this effect (eg, tetracyclines) may increase risk. Up to 60% of patients experienced reversible hypercholesterolemia or hypertriglyceridemia. Monitor liver function during treatment.

Drug Interactions

Cytochrome P450 Effect: Substrate (minor) of CYP2A6, 2B6, 2C8/9; **Inhibits** CYP2C8/9 (weak); **Induces** CYP2E1 (weak)

Increased Effect/Toxicity: Ketoconazole increases the mean plasma AUC of tretinoin. Concurrent use with antifibrinolytic agents (eg, aminocaproic acid, aprotinin, tranexamic acid) may increase risk of thrombosis. Concurrent use with tetracyclines may increase risk of pseudotumor cerebri.

Nutritional/Ethanol Interactions

Ethanol: Avoid ethanol (may increase CNS depression).

Food: Absorption of retinoids has been shown to be enhanced when taken with food.

Herb/Nutraceutical: St John's wort may decrease tretinoin levels. Avoid dong quai, St John's wort (may also cause photosensitization). Avoid additional vitamin A supplementation. May lead to vitamin A toxicity.

Adverse Reactions Virtually all patients experience some drug-related toxicity, especially headache, fever, weakness and fatigue. These adverse effects are seldom permanent or irreversible nor do they usually require therapy interruption.

>10%:

Cardiovascular: Peripheral edema (52%), chest discomfort (32%), edema (29%), arrhythmias (23%), flushing (23%), hypotension (14%), hypertension (11%)

Central nervous system: Headache (86%), fever (83%), malaise (66%), pain (37%), dizziness (20%), anxiety (17%), insomnia (14%), depression (14%), confusion (11%)

Dermatologic: Skin/mucous membrane dryness (77%), pruritus (20%), rash (54%), alopecia (14%)

Endocrine & metabolic: Hypercholesterolemia and/or hypertriglyceridemia (60%)

Gastrointestinal: Nausea/vomiting (57%), liver function tests increased (50% to 60%), GI hemorrhage (34%), abdominal pain (31%), mucositis (26%), diarrhea (23%), constipation (17%), dyspepsia (14%), abdominal distention (11%), weight gain (23%), weight loss (17%), xerostomia, anorexia (17%)

Hematologic: Hemorrhage (60%), leukocytosis (40%), disseminated intravascular coagulation (26%)

Local: Phlebitis (11%), injection site reactions (17%)

Neuromuscular & skeletal: Bone pain (77%), myalgia (14%), paresthesia (17%)

Ocular: Visual disturbances (17%)

Otic: Earache/ear fullness (23%)

Renal: Renal insufficiency (11%)

Respiratory: Upper respiratory tract disorders (63%), dyspnea (60%), respiratory insufficiency (26%), pleural effusion (20%), pneumonia (14%), rales (14%), expiratory wheezing (14%), dry nose

Miscellaneous: Infection (58%), shivering (63%), retinoic acid-acute promyelocytic leukemia syndrome (25%), diaphoresis increased (20%)

1% to 10%:

Cardiovascular: Cerebral hemorrhage (9%), pallor (6%), cardiac failure (6%), cardiac arrest (3%), MI (3%), enlarged heart (3%), heart murmur (3%), ischemia, stroke (3%), myocarditis (3%), pericarditis (3%), pulmonary hypertension (3%), secondary cardiomyopathy (3%)

Central nervous system: Intracranial hypertension (9%), agitation (9%), hallucination (6%), agnosia (3%), aphasia (3%), cerebellar edema (3%), cerebral hemorrhage (9%), seizures (3%), coma (3%), CNS depression (3%), dysarthria (3%), encephalopathy (3%), hypotaxia (3%), light reflex absent (3%), spinal cord disorder (3%), unconsciousness (3%), dementia (3%), forgetfulness (3%), somnolence (3%), slow speech (3%), hypothermia (3%)

Dermatologic: Cellulitis (8%), photosensitivity

Endocrine & metabolic: Acidosis (3%)

Gastrointestinal: Hepatosplenomegaly (9%), hepatitis (3%), ulcer (3%)

Genitourinary: Dysuria (9%), acute renal failure (3%), micturition frequency (3%), renal tubular necrosis (3%), enlarged prostate (3%)

Hepatic: Ascites (3%), hepatitis

Neuromuscular & skeletal: Tremor (3%), leg weakness (3%), hyporeflexia, dysarthria, facial paralysis, hemiplegia, flank pain, asterixis, abnormal gait (3%), bone inflammation (3%)

Ocular: Dry eyes, visual acuity change (6%), visual field deficit (3%)

Otic: Hearing loss

Renal: Acute renal failure, renal tubular necrosis

Respiratory: Lower respiratory tract disorders (9%), pulmonary infiltration (6%), bronchial asthma (3%), pulmonary/larynx edema

Miscellaneous: Face edema

Overdosage/Toxicology Symptoms of overdose include transient headache, facial flushing, cheilosis, abdominal pain, dizziness, and ataxia. All signs or symptoms have been transient and have resolved without apparent residual effects.

Pharmacodynamics/Kinetics

Time to Peak: Serum: 1-2 hours

Protein Binding: >95%

Half-Life Elimination: Terminal: Parent drug: 0.5-2 hours

Metabolism: Hepatic via CYP; primary metabolite: 4-oxo-all-*trans*-retinoic acid

Excretion: Urine (63%); feces (30%)

Available Dosage Forms Capsule: 10 mg [contains soybean oil and parabens]

Dosing

Adults & Elderly:

Acute promyelocytic leukemia (APL): Oral:

Remission induction: 45 mg/m^2/day in 2-3 divided doses for up to 30 days after complete remission (maximum duration of treatment: 90 days)

Remission maintenance: 45-200 mg/m^2/day in 2-3 divided doses for up to 12 months.

Pediatrics: APL induction of remission, remission maintenance: Oral: Refer to adult dosing.

Administration

Oral: Administer with meals; do not crush capsules

Stability

Storage: Store capsule at 15°C to 30°C (59°F to 86°F). Protect from light.

Laboratory Monitoring Monitor the patient's hematologic profile, coagulation profile, liver function results and triglyceride and cholesterol levels frequently. Consider temporary discontinuation if LFTs are >5 times the upper limit of normal.

Nursing Actions

Physical Assessment: To be administered under the supervision of a physician who is experienced in the management of patients with acute leukemia. Assess potential for interactions with other pharmacological agents and herbal products patient may be taking. Monitor laboratory tests and patient response (eg, cardiac, CNS, and respiratory status) on a frequent basis during therapy. Teach patient appropriate use, possible side effects/interventions, and adverse symptoms to report.

Patient Education: Do not take any new medication during therapy unless approved by prescriber. Take with food. Do not crush, chew, or dissolve capsules. Maintain adequate hydration (2-3 L/day of fluids) unless instructed to restrict fluid intake. Avoid alcohol and foods containing vitamin A, and foods with high fat content. May cause lethargy, dizziness, visual changes, confusion, anxiety (avoid driving or engaging in tasks requiring alertness until response to drug is known); nausea, vomiting, loss of appetite, or dry mouth (small, frequent meals, chewing gum, or sucking lozenges may help); photosensitivity (use sunscreen, wear protective clothing and eyewear, and avoid direct sunlight); dry, itchy skin; or dry or irritated eyes (avoid contact lenses). Report persistent vomiting or diarrhea, respiratory difficulty, unusual bleeding or bruising, acute GI pain, bone pain, swelling of extremities, unusual weight gain, or vision changes immediately. **Pregnancy/breast-feeding precautions:** Do not get pregnant (females) or cause a pregnancy (males) while taking this medication and for 1 month following completion of therapy. Consult prescriber for appropriate barrier contraceptive measures. Breast-feeding is not recommended.

Dietary Considerations To enhance absorption, some clinicians recommend giving with a fatty meal. Capsule contains soybean oil.

Pregnancy Issues Oral tretinoin is teratogenic and fetotoxic in rats at doses 1000 and 500 times the topical human dose, respectively.

Tretinoin (Topical) (TRET i noyn, TOP i kal)

U.S. Brand Names Avita®; Renova®; Retin-A®; Retin-A® Micro

Synonyms Retinoic Acid; *trans*-Retinoic Acid; Vitamin A Acid

Pharmacologic Category Retinoic Acid Derivative

Medication Safety Issues
Sound-alike/look-alike issues:
Tretinoin may be confused with trientine

Pregnancy Risk Factor C

Lactation Enters breast milk/compatible

Use Treatment of acne vulgaris; photodamaged skin; palliation of fine wrinkles, mottled hyperpigmentation, and tactile roughness of facial skin as part of a comprehensive skin care and sun avoidance program

Unlabeled/Investigational Use Some skin cancers

Mechanism of Action/Effect Keratinocytes in the sebaceous follicle become less adherent which allows for easy removal; decreases microcomedone formation

Contraindications Hypersensitivity to tretinoin or any component of the formulation; sunburn

Warnings/Precautions Use with caution in patients with eczema; avoid excessive exposure to sunlight and sunlamps; avoid contact with abraded skin, mucous membranes, eyes, mouth, angles of the nose. Palliation of fine wrinkles, mottled hyperpigmentation, and tactile roughness of facial skin: Do not use the 0.05% cream for longer than 48 weeks or the 0.02% cream for longer than 52 weeks. Not for use on moderate- to heavily-pigmented skin. Gel is flammable; do not expose to high temperatures or flame.

Drug Interactions

Cytochrome P450 Effect: Substrate (minor) of CYP2A6, 2B6, 2C8/9; **Inhibits** CYP2C8/9 (weak); **Induces** CYP2E1 (weak)

Increased Effect/Toxicity: Topical application of sulfur, benzoyl peroxide, salicylic acid, resorcinol, or any product with strong drying effects potentiates adverse reactions with tretinoin.

Photosensitizing medications (thiazides, tetracyclines, fluoroquinolones, phenothiazines, sulfonamides) augment phototoxicity and should not be used when treating palliation of fine wrinkles, mottled hyperpigmentation, and tactile roughness of facial skin.

Nutritional/Ethanol Interactions

Food: Avoid excessive intake of vitamin A (cod liver oil, halibut fish oil).

Herb/Nutraceutical: Avoid dong quai, St John's wort (may also cause photosensitization). Avoid excessive amounts of vitamin A supplements.

Adverse Reactions

>10%: Dermatologic: Excessive dryness, erythema, scaling of the skin, pruritus

1% to 10%:
Dermatologic: Hyperpigmentation or hypopigmentation, photosensitivity, initial acne flare-up
Local: Edema, blistering, stinging

Overdosage/Toxicology Excessive application may lead to marked redness, peeling or discomfort. Oral ingestion of the topical product may lead to the same adverse reactions seen with excessive vitamin A intake (increased intracranial pressure, jaundice, ascites, cutaneous desquamation; symptoms of acute overdose [12,000 units/kg] include nausea, vomiting, and diarrhea); toxic signs of an overdose commonly respond to drug discontinuation, and generally return to normal spontaneously within a few days to weeks. Toxic signs of a topical overdose commonly respond to drug discontinuation, and generally resolve spontaneously within a few days to weeks.

When confronted with signs of increased intracranial pressure, treatment with mannitol (0.25 g/kg I.V. up to 1 g/kg/dose repeated every 5 minutes as needed), dexamethasone (1.5 mg/kg I.V. load followed with 0.375 mg/kg every 6 hours for 5 days), and/or hyperventilation should be employed.

Pharmacodynamics/Kinetics

Metabolism: Hepatic for the small amount absorbed

Excretion: Urine and feces

Available Dosage Forms [DSC] = Discontinued product

Cream, topical: 0.025% (20 g, 45 g); 0.05% (20 g, 45 g); 0.1% (20 g, 45 g)
Avita®: 0.025% (20 g, 45 g)
Renova®: 0.02% (40 g); 0.05% (40 g, 60 g)
Retin-A®: 0.025% (20 g, 45 g); 0.05% (20 g, 45 g); 0.1% (20 g, 45 g)

Gel, topical: 0.025% (15 g, 45 g)
Avita®: 0.025% (20 g, 45 g) [contains ethanol 83%]
Retin-A®: 0.01% (15 g, 45 g); 0.025% (15 g, 45 g) [contains alcohol 90%]
Retin-A® Micro [microsphere gel]: 0.04% (20 g, 45 g); 0.1% (20 g, 45 g) [contains benzyl alcohol]

Liquid, topical (Retin-A®): 0.05% (28 mL) [contains alcohol 55%] [DSC]

(Continued)

Tretinoin (Topical) *(Continued)*

Dosing

Adults:

Acne vulgaris: Topical: Begin therapy with a weaker formulation of tretinoin (0.025% cream, 0.04% microsphere gel, or 0.01% gel) and increase the concentration as tolerated; apply once daily to acne lesions before retiring or on alternate days; if stinging or irritation develop, decrease frequency of application

Palliation of fine wrinkles, mottled hyperpigmentation, and tactile roughness of facial skin: Topical: Pea-sized amount of the 0.02% or 0.05% cream applied to entire face once daily in the evening

Elderly: Use of the 0.02% cream in patients 65-71 years of age showed similar improvement in fine wrinkles as seen in patients <65 years. Safety and efficacy of the 0.02% cream have not been established in patients >71 years of age. Safety and efficacy of the 0.05% cream have not been established in patients >50 years of age.

Pediatrics: Children >12 years: Acne vulgaris: Topical: Refer to adult dosing.

Administration

Topical: Palliation of fine wrinkles, mottled hyperpigmentation, and tactile roughness of facial skin: Cream: Prior to application, gently wash face with a mild soap. Pat dry. Wait 20-30 minutes to apply cream. Avoid eyes, ears, nostrils, and mouth.

Stability

Storage: Store at 25°C (77°F); gel is flammable, keep away from heat and flame

Nursing Actions

Physical Assessment: Assess knowledge/instruct patient on appropriate application, possible adverse effects, and symptoms to report.

Patient Education: For once-daily use, do not overuse. Avoid increased intake of vitamin A. Thoroughly wash hands before applying. Wash area to be treated at least 30 minutes before applying. Do not wash face more frequently than 2-3 times a day. Do not apply to areas near your mouth, eyes, corners of your nose, or open sores. Avoid using topical preparations that contain alcohol or harsh chemicals during treatment. It may take several weeks before the full benefit of the medication is seen. You may experience increased sensitivity to sunlight; protect skin with sunblock (minimum SPF 15), wear protective clothing, and avoid direct sunlight. Stop treatment and inform prescriber if rash, skin irritation, redness, scaling, or excessive dryness occurs. When used for hyperpigmentation and tactile redness of facial skin, wrinkles will not be eliminated. Must be used in combination with a comprehensive skin care program. **Pregnancy precaution:** Inform prescriber if you are pregnant.

Gel: Flammable; do not expose to flame and do not smoke during use.

Pregnancy Issues High doses may be teratogenic and fetotoxic. Tretinoin does not appear to be teratogenic when used topically since it is rapidly metabolized by the skin; however, there are rare reports of fetal defects. Use for acne only if benefit to mother outweighs potential risk to fetus. During pregnancy, do not use for palliation of fine wrinkles, mottled hyperpigmentation, and tactile roughness of facial skin.

Triamcinolone *(trye am SIN oh lone)*

U.S. Brand Names Aristocort®; Aristocort® A; Aristospan®; Azmacort®; Kenalog®; Kenalog-10®; Kenalog-40®; Nasacort® AQ; Triderm®; Tri-Nasal®

Synonyms Triamcinolone Acetonide, Aerosol; Triamcinolone Acetonide, Parenteral; Triamcinolone Diacetate, Oral; Triamcinolone Diacetate, Parenteral; Triamcinolone Hexacetonide; Triamcinolone, Oral

Pharmacologic Category Corticosteroid, Adrenal; Corticosteroid, Inhalant (Oral); Corticosteroid, Nasal; Corticosteroid, Systemic; Corticosteroid, Topical

Medication Safety Issues

Sound-alike/look-alike issues:

Kenalog® may be confused with Ketalar®

Nasacort® may be confused with NasalCrom®

TAC (occasional abbreviation for triamcinolone) is an error-prone abbreviation (mistaken as tetracaine-adrenaline-cocaine)

Pregnancy Risk Factor C

Lactation Excretion in breast milk unknown/use caution

Use

Nasal inhalation: Management of seasonal and perennial allergic rhinitis in patients ≥6 years of age

Oral inhalation: Control of bronchial asthma and related bronchospastic conditions

Oral topical: Adjunctive treatment and temporary relief of symptoms associated with oral inflammatory lesions and ulcerative lesions resulting from trauma

Systemic: Adrenocortical insufficiency, rheumatic disorders, allergic states, respiratory diseases, systemic lupus erythematosus (SLE), and other diseases requiring anti-inflammatory or immunosuppressive effects

Topical: Inflammatory dermatoses responsive to steroids

Mechanism of Action/Effect Decreases inflammation by suppression of migration of polymorphonuclear leukocytes and reversal of increased capillary permeability; suppresses the immune system by reducing activity and volume of the lymphatic system; suppresses adrenal function at high doses

Contraindications Hypersensitivity to triamcinolone or any component of the formulation; systemic fungal infections; serious infections (except septic shock or tuberculous meningitis); primary treatment of status asthmaticus; fungal, viral, or bacterial infections of the mouth or throat (oral topical formulation)

Warnings/Precautions Not to be used in status asthmaticus or for the relief of acute bronchospasm. May cause suppression of hypothalamic-pituitary-adrenal (HPA) axis, particularly in younger children or in patients receiving high doses for prolonged periods. Fatalities have occurred due to adrenal insufficiency in asthmatic patients during and after transfer from systemic corticosteroids to aerosol steroids; aerosol steroids do **not** provide the systemic steroid needed to treat patients having trauma, surgery, or infections. Withdrawal and discontinuation of the corticosteroid should be done slowly and carefully

Orally-inhaled and intranasal corticosteroids may cause a reduction in growth velocity in pediatric patients, which appears to be related to dose and duration of exposure.

May suppress the immune system, patients may be more susceptible to infection. Use with caution in patients with systemic infections or ocular herpes simplex. Avoid exposure to chickenpox and measles. Corticosteroids should be used with caution in patients with diabetes, hypertension, osteoporosis, peptic ulcer, glaucoma, cataracts, or tuberculosis. Use caution in hepatic impairment. Injection suspension contains benzyl alcohol; benzyl alcohol has been associated with the "gasping syndrome" in neonates and low-birth-weight infants.

Oral topical: Discontinue if local irritation or sensitization should develop. If significant regeneration or repair of oral tissues has not occurred in seven days, re-evaluation of the etiology of the oral lesion is advised.

Drug Interactions

Decreased Effect: Decreased effect with barbiturates and phenytoin. Rifampin increased metabolism of triamcinolone. Vaccine and toxoid effects may be reduced.

Increased Effect/Toxicity: Salicylates or NSAIDs coadministered oral corticosteroids may increase risk of GI ulceration.

Nutritional/Ethanol Interactions

Ethanol: Avoid ethanol (may enhance gastric mucosal irritation).

Food: Triamcinolone interferes with calcium absorption.

Herb/Nutraceutical: Avoid cat's claw, echinacea (have immunostimulant properties).

Adverse Reactions

Systemic: Frequency not defined:

Cardiovascular: Angioedema, bradycardia, CHF, hypertension, myocardial rupture (following recent MI), thrombophlebitis, vasculitis

Central nervous system: Convulsions, depression, emotional instability, fever, headache, intracranial pressure increased, neuropathy, paresthesia, personality changes, vertigo

Dermatologic: Acne, allergic dermatitis, bruising, cutaneous atrophy, dry/scaly skin, ecchymoses, facial erythema, petechiae, photosensitivity, rash, striae, thin/fragile skin, wound healing impaired

Endocrine & metabolic: Adrenocortical/pituitary unresponsiveness (particularly during stress), carbohydrate tolerance decreased, cushingoid state, diabetes mellitus (manifestations of latent disease), fluid retention, growth suppression (children), hirsutism, hypokalemic alkalosis, menstrual irregularities, negative nitrogen balance, potassium loss, sodium retention

Gastrointestinal: Abdominal distention, bowel perforation, diarrhea, dyspepsia, nausea, oral *Monilia* (oral inhaler), pancreatitis, peptic ulcer, ulcerative esophagitis, weight gain

Hepatic: Hepatomegaly

Local: Skin atrophy (at the injection site)

Neuromuscular & skeletal: Charcot-like arthropathy, femoral/humeral head aseptic necrosis, muscle mass decreased, muscle weakness, osteoporosis, pathologic fracture of long bones, steroid myopathy, tendon rupture, vertebral compression fractures

Ocular: Blindness (periocular injections), cataracts, intraocular pressure increased, exophthalmos, glaucoma, subcapsular cataract

Respiratory: Cough increased (nasal spray), epistaxis (nasal inhaler/spray), pharyngitis (nasal spray/oral inhaler), sinusitis (oral inhaler), voice alteration (oral inhaler)

Miscellaneous: Abnormal fat deposition (moon face), anaphylactoid reaction, anaphylaxis, diaphoresis increased, suppression to skin tests

Topical: Frequency not defined:

Dermatologic: Itching, allergic contact dermatitis, dryness, folliculitis, skin infection (secondary), itching, hypertrichosis, acneiform eruptions, hypopigmentation, skin maceration, skin atrophy, striae, miliaria, perioral dermatitis, atrophy of oral mucosa

Local: Burning, irritation

Overdosage/Toxicology
When consumed in high doses for prolonged periods, systemic hypercorticism and adrenal suppression may occur. In those cases, discontinuation of the corticosteroid should be done judiciously.

Pharmacodynamics/Kinetics

Duration of Action: Oral: 8-12 hours

Time to Peak: I.M.: 8-10 hours

Half-Life Elimination: Biologic: 18-36 hours

Available Dosage Forms

Aerosol for oral inhalation, as acetonide (Azmacort®): 100 mcg per actuation (20 g) [240 actuations]

Aerosol, topical, as acetonide (Kenalog®): 0.2 mg/2-second spray (63 g)

Cream, as acetonide: 0.025% (15 g, 80 g, 454 g); 0.1% (15 g, 80 g, 454 g, 2270 g); 0.5% (15 g)
Aristocort® A: 0.025% (15 g, 60 g); 0.1% (15 g, 60 g); 0.5% (15 g) [contains benzyl alcohol]
Triderm®: 0.1% (30 g, 85 g)

Injection, suspension, as acetonide:
Kenalog-10®: 10 mg/mL (5 mL) [contains benzyl alcohol; not for I.V. or I.M. use]
Kenalog-40®: 40 mg/mL (1 mL, 5 mL, 10 mL) [contains benzyl alcohol; not for I.V. or intradermal use]

Injection, suspension, as hexacetonide (Aristospan®): 5 mg/mL (5 mL); 20 mg/mL (1 mL, 5 mL) [contains benzyl alcohol; not for I.V. use]

Lotion, as acetonide: 0.025% (60 mL); 0.1% (60 mL)

Ointment, topical, as acetonide: 0.025% (15 g, 80 g, 454 g); 0.1% (15 g, 80 g, 454 g); 0.5% (15 g)
Aristocort® A: 0.1% (15 g, 60 g)

Paste, oral, topical, as acetonide: 0.1% (5 g)

Solution, intranasal, as acetonide [spray] (Tri-Nasal®): 50 mcg/inhalation (15 mL) [120 doses]

Suspension, intranasal, as acetonide [spray] (Nasacort® AQ): 55 mcg/inhalation (16.5 g) [120 doses]

Tablet (Aristocort®): 4 mg [contains lactose and sodium benzoate]

Dosing

Adults & Elderly: The lowest possible dose should be used to control the condition; when dose reduction is possible, the dose should be reduced gradually. Parenteral dose is usually $1/3$ to $1/2$ the oral dose given every 12 hours. In life-threatening situations, parenteral doses larger than the oral dose may be needed.

Adrenocortical insufficiency: Oral: Range: 4-12 mg/day

Allergic rhinitis (perennial or seasonal):
Nasal spray: 220 mcg/day as 2 sprays in each nostril once daily
Nasal inhaler: Initial: 220 mcg/day as 2 sprays in each nostril once daily; may increase dose to 440 mcg/day (given once daily or divided and given 2 or 4 times/day)
Oral (acute treatment only): Range: 8-12 mg/day

Asthma:
Oral: 8-16 mg/day
Oral inhalation: 200 mcg 3-4 times/day **or** 400 mcg twice daily; maximum dose: 1600 mcg/day

Carditis (acute rheumatic): Oral: Initial: 20-60 mg/day; reduce dose during maintenance therapy

Dermatoses (steroid-responsive, including contact/atopic dermatitis):
Oral: Initial: 8-16 mg/day
Injection:
Acetonide: Intradermal: Initial: 1 mg
Hexacetonide: Intralesional, sublesional: up to 0.5 mg/square inch of affected skin
Topical:
Cream, ointment: Apply thin film to affected areas 2-4 times/day
Spray: Apply to affected area 3-4 times/day

Ophthalmic disorders: Oral: 12-40 mg/day

Oral inflammatory lesions/ulcers: Oral topical: Press a small dab (about $1/4$ inch) to the lesion until a thin film develops; a larger quantity may be required for coverage of some lesions. For optimal results, use only enough to coat the lesion with a thin film; do not rub in.

(Continued)

Triamcinolone (Continued)

Rheumatic or arthritic disorders:
Oral: Range: 8-16 mg/day
> Lupus (SLE): Initial: 20-32 mg/day, some patients may need initial doses ≥48 mg; reduce dose during maintenance therapy

Intra-articular (or similar injection as designated):
> Acetonide: Intra-articular, intrabursal, tendon sheaths: Initial: Smaller joints: 2.5-5 mg, larger joints: 5-15 mg
>
> Hexacetonide: Intra-articular: Initial range: 2-20 mg/day

I.M.:
> Acetonide: Range: 2.5-60 mg/day; Initial: 60 mg

See table.

Triamcinolone Dosing

	Acetonide	Hexacetonide
Intrasynovial	5-40 mg	
Intralesional	1-30 mg (usually 1 mg per injection site); 10 mg/mL suspension usually used	Up to 0.5 mg/sq inch affected area
Sublesional	1-30 mg	
Systemic I.M.	2.5-60 mg/dose (usual adult dose: 60 mg; may repeat with 20-100 mg dose when symptoms recur)	
Intra-articular	2.5-40 mg	2-20 mg average
large joints	5-15 mg	10-20 mg
small joints	2.5-5 mg	2-6 mg
Tendon sheaths	2.5-10 mg	
Intradermal	1 mg/site	

Pediatrics:
Allergic rhinitis (perennial or seasonal):
Nasal spray:
> Children 6-11 years: 110 mcg/day as 1 spray in each nostril once daily.
> Children ≥12 years: Refer to adult dosing.

Nasal inhaler:
> Children 6-11 years: Initial: 220 mcg/day as 2 sprays in each nostril once daily
> Children ≥12 years: Refer to adult dosing.

Asthma:
Oral: 8-16 mg/day
Oral inhalation:
> Children 6-12 years: 100-200 mcg 3-4 times/day or 200-400 mcg twice daily; maximum dose: 1200 mcg/day
> Children >12 years: Refer to adult dosing.

Rheumatic conditions: I.M. (acetonide): Range: 2.5-60 mg/day
> Children 6-12 years: Initial: 40 mg
> Children ≥12 years: Refer to adult dosing.

Administration
Oral: Tablet: Once-daily doses should be given in the morning.
I.M.: Inject I.M. dose deep in large muscle mass, avoid deltoid.

Inhalation:
Intranasal: Spray/inhaler: Shake well prior to use. Gently blow nose to clear nostrils.

Oral: Shake well prior to use. Rinse mouth and throat after using inhaler to prevent candidiasis. Use spacer device provided with Azmacort®.

Topical:
Oral topical: Apply small dab to lesion until a thin film develops; do not rub in. Apply at bedtime or after meals if applications are needed throughout the day.

Topical: Apply a thin film sparingly and avoid topical application on the face. Do not use on open skin or wounds. Do not occlude area unless directed.

Other: Avoid subcutaneous administration.

Stability
Reconstitution: Injection, suspension: Hexacetonide: Avoid diluents containing parabens or preservatives (may cause flocculation). Diluted suspension stable ~1 week. Suspension for intralesional use, may be diluted with D_5NS, $D_{10}NS$ or SWFI to a 1:1, 1:2, or 1:4 concentration. Solutions for intra-articular use, may be diluted with lidocaine 1% or 2%.

Storage: Store at room temperature. Avoid freezing.

Injection, suspension: Shake well prior to use.

Topical spray: Avoid excessive heat.

Nursing Actions
Physical Assessment: Assess other medications patient may be taking for effectiveness and interactions. With systemic administration, patients with diabetes should monitor glucose levels closely (corticosteroids may alter glucose levels). Assess knowledge/teach patient appropriate use, interventions to reduce side effects, and adverse symptoms to report. When used for long-term therapy (>10-14 days), do not discontinue abruptly; decrease dosage incrementally.

Patient Education: Take exactly as directed; do not increase dose or discontinue abruptly without consulting prescriber. Take oral medication with or after meals. Avoid alcohol. Limit intake of caffeine or stimulants. Prescriber may recommend increased dietary vitamins, minerals, or iron. If you have diabetes, monitor glucose levels closely (antidiabetic medication may need to be adjusted). Inform prescriber if you are experiencing greater than normal levels of stress (medication may need adjustment). Some forms of this medication may cause GI upset (oral medication may be taken with meals to reduce GI upset; or small frequent meals and frequent mouth care may reduce GI upset). You may be more susceptible to infection (avoid crowds and exposure to infection). Report promptly excessive nervousness or sleep disturbances; any signs of infection (sore throat, unhealed injuries); excessive growth of body hair or loss of skin color; vision changes; excessive or sudden weight gain (>3 lb/week); swelling of face or extremities; respiratory difficulty; muscle weakness; change in color of stools (black or tarry) or persistent abdominal pain; or worsening of condition or failure to improve. **Pregnancy/breast-feeding precautions:** Inform prescriber if you are or intend to become pregnant. Consult prescriber if breast-feeding.

Aerosol: Shake gently before use. Use at regular intervals, no more frequently than directed. Not for use during acute asthmatic attack. Follow directions that accompany product. Rinse mouth and throat after use to prevent candidiasis. Do not use intranasal product if you have a nasal infection, nasal injury, or recent nasal surgery. If using two products, consult prescriber in which order to use the two products. Report unusual cough or spasm; persistent nasal bleeding, burning, or irritation; or worsening of condition.

Inhalation: Sit when using. Take deep breaths for 3-5 minutes, and clear nasal passages before administration (use decongestant as needed). Hold breath for 5-10 seconds after use, and wait 1-3 minutes between inhalations. Follow package insert instructions for use. Do not exceed maximum dosage. If also using inhaled bronchodilator, use before triamcinolone. Rinse mouth and throat after use to reduce aftertaste and prevent candidiasis.

Topical: For external use only. Not for eyes or mucous membranes or open wounds. Apply in very thin layer to occlusive dressing. Apply dressing to area being treated. Avoid prolonged or excessive use around sensitive tissues, genital, or rectal areas. Inform prescriber if condition worsens (swelling, redness, irritation, pain, open sores) or fails to improve.

Dietary Considerations May be taken with food to decrease GI distress.

Geriatric Considerations Because of the risk of adverse effects, systemic corticosteroids should be used cautiously in the elderly, in the smallest possible dose, and for the shortest possible time. Azmacort® (metered dose inhaler) comes with its own spacer device attached and may be easier to use in older patients.

Breast-Feeding Issues It is not known if triamcinolone is excreted in breast milk, however, other corticosteroids are excreted. Prednisone and prednisolone are excreted in breast milk; the AAP considers them to be "usually compatible" with breast-feeding. Hypertension was reported in a nursing infant when a topical corticosteroid was applied to the nipples of the mother.

Pregnancy Issues There are no adequate and well-controlled studies in pregnant women, however, triamcinolone is teratogenic in animals; use during pregnancy with caution. Increased incidence of cleft palate, neonatal adrenal suppression, low birth weight, and cataracts in the infant has been reported following corticosteroid use during pregnancy. In general, the use of large amounts, or prolonged use, of topical corticosteroids during pregnancy should be avoided. In the mother, corticosteroids may increase calcium and potassium excretion, elevate blood pressure, and cause salt and water retention.

Additional Information 16 mg triamcinolone is equivalent to 100 mg cortisone (no mineralocorticoid activity).

Effects of inhaled/intranasal steroids on growth have been observed in the absence of laboratory evidence of HPA axis suppression, suggesting that growth velocity is a more sensitive indicator of systemic corticosteroid exposure in pediatric patients than some commonly used tests of HPA axis function. The long-term effects of this reduction in growth velocity associated with orally-inhaled and intranasal corticosteroids, including the impact on final adult height, are unknown. The potential for "catch up" growth following discontinuation of treatment with inhaled corticosteroids has not been adequately studied.

Triazolam (trye AY zoe lam)

U.S. Brand Names Halcion®
Restrictions C-IV
Pharmacologic Category Hypnotic, Benzodiazepine
Medication Safety Issues
Sound-alike/look-alike issues:
Triazolam may be confused with alprazolam
Halcion® may be confused with halcinonide, Haldol®
Pregnancy Risk Factor X
Lactation Excretion in breast milk unknown/not recommended
Use Short-term treatment of insomnia

Mechanism of Action/Effect Binds to stereospecific benzodiazepine receptors on the postsynaptic GABA neuron at several sites within the central nervous system, including the limbic system, reticular formation. Enhancement of the inhibitory effect of GABA on neuronal excitability results by increased neuronal membrane permeability to chloride ions. This shift in chloride ions results in hyperpolarization (a less excitable state) and stabilization.

Contraindications Hypersensitivity to triazolam or any component of the formulation (cross-sensitivity with other benzodiazepines may exist); concurrent therapy with atazanavir, ketoconazole, itraconazole, nefazodone, and ritonavir; pregnancy

Warnings/Precautions As a hypnotic, should be used only after evaluation of potential causes of sleep disturbance. Failure of sleep disturbance to resolve after 7-10 days may indicate psychiatric or medical illness. Prescription should be written for a maximum of 7-10 days and should not be prescribed in quantities exceeding a 1-month supply. Abrupt discontinuation after sustained use (generally >10 days) may cause withdrawal symptoms. Use is not recommended in patients with depressive disorders or psychoses. Avoid use in patients with sleep apnea. Use with caution in elderly or debilitated patients, patients with hepatic disease (including alcoholics), renal impairment, respiratory disease, impaired gag reflex, or obese patients. Use caution with potent CYP3A4 inhibitors, as they may significantly decreased the clearance of triazolam.

Causes CNS depression (dose-related) which may impair physical and mental capabilities. Use with caution in patients receiving other CNS depressants or psychoactive agents. Benzodiazepines have been associated with falls and traumatic injury and should be used with extreme caution in patients who are at risk of these events (especially the elderly). May cause physical or psychological dependence - use with caution in patients with a history of drug dependence.

Benzodiazepines have been associated with anterograde amnesia. Paradoxical reactions, including hyperactive or aggressive behavior, have been reported with benzodiazepines, particularly in adolescent/pediatric or psychiatric patients. Does not have analgesic, antidepressant, or antipsychotic properties.

Drug Interactions
Cytochrome P450 Effect: Substrate of CYP3A4 (major); **Inhibits** CYP2C8/9 (weak)
Decreased Effect: CYP3A4 inducers may decrease the levels/effects of triazolam; example inducers include aminoglutethimide, carbamazepine, nafcillin, nevirapine, phenobarbital, phenytoin, and rifamycins.
Increased Effect/Toxicity: Sedative and/or respiratory depressive effects may be additive with other CNS depressants. CYP3A4 inhibitors may increase the levels/effects of triazolam; example inhibitors include azole antifungals, clarithromycin, diclofenac, doxycycline, erythromycin, imatinib, isoniazid, nefazodone, nicardipine, propofol, protease inhibitors, quinidine, telithromycin, and verapamil. Concurrent use of some strong CYP3A4 inhibitors (including azole antifungals, nefazodone, and protease inhibitors) has been contraindicated by the manufacturers. Oral contraceptives may decrease the clearance and increase the half-life of triazolam (monitor for increased triazolam effect).

Nutritional/Ethanol Interactions
Ethanol: Avoid ethanol (may increase CNS depression).
Food: Food may decrease the rate of absorption. Triazolam serum concentration may be increased by grapefruit juice; avoid concurrent use.
Herb/Nutraceutical: St John's wort may decrease levels. Avoid valerian, St John's wort, kava kava, gotu kola (may increase CNS depression).
(Continued)

Triazolam (Continued)

Adverse Reactions
>10%: Central nervous system: Drowsiness, anteriograde amnesia

1% to 10%:
Central nervous system: Headache, dizziness, nervousness, lightheadedness, ataxia

Gastrointestinal: Nausea, vomiting

Overdosage/Toxicology
Symptoms of overdose include somnolence, confusion, coma, diminished reflexes, dyspnea, and hypotension. Treatment for benzodiazepine overdose is supportive. Flumazenil has been shown to selectively block the binding of benzodiazepines to CNS receptors, resulting in reversal of benzodiazepine-induced CNS depression but not always respiratory depression.

Pharmacodynamics/Kinetics
Onset of Action: Hypnotic: 15-30 minutes

Duration of Action: 6-7 hours

Protein Binding: 89%

Half-Life Elimination: 1.7-5 hours

Metabolism: Extensively hepatic

Excretion: Urine (as unchanged drug and metabolites)

Available Dosage Forms Tablet: 0.125 mg, 0.25 mg [contains sodium benzoate]

Dosing
Adults: Note: Onset of action is rapid, patient should be in bed when taking medication.

Insomnia (short-term): Oral: 0.125-0.25 mg at bedtime (maximum dose: 0.5 mg/day)

Dental (preprocedure): Oral: 0.25 mg taken the evening before oral surgery; or 0.25 mg 1 hour before procedure

Elderly: Oral: Insomnia (short-term use): 0.0625-0.125 mg at bedtime; maximum dose: 0.25 mg/day (see Geriatric Considerations)

Hepatic Impairment: Reduce dose or avoid use in cirrhosis.

Administration
Oral: May take with food. Tablet may be crushed or swallowed whole. Onset of action is rapid, patient should be in bed when taking medication.

Nursing Actions
Physical Assessment: Assess other medications patient may be taking for effectiveness and interactions. Assess for history of addiction; long-term use can result in dependence, abuse, or tolerance. For inpatient use, institute safety measures and monitor effectiveness and adverse reactions. For outpatients, monitor therapeutic effectiveness and adverse reactions at beginning of therapy and periodically with long-term use. Assess knowledge/teach patient appropriate use, interventions to reduce side effects, and adverse symptoms to report. **Pregnancy risk factor X:** Determine that patient is not pregnant before starting therapy. Do not give to sexually-active female patients unless capable of complying with contraceptive use.

Patient Education: Take exactly as directed; do not increase dose or frequency. Drug may cause physical and/or psychological dependence. Do not use alcohol or other prescription or OTC medications (especially pain medications, sedatives, antihistamines, or hypnotics) without consulting prescriber. Maintain adequate hydration (2-3 L/day of fluids) unless instructed to restrict fluid intake. You may experience drowsiness, lightheadedness, impaired coordination, dizziness, or blurred vision (use caution when driving or engaging in tasks requiring alertness until response to drug is known); nausea, vomiting, or dry mouth (small frequent meals, frequent mouth care, chewing gum, or sucking lozenges may help); constipation (increased exercise, fluids, fruit, or fiber may help); altered sexual drive or ability (reversible); or photosensitivity (use sunscreen, wear protective clothing and eyewear, and avoid direct sunlight). Report persistent CNS effects (eg, memory impairment, confusion, depression, increased sedation, excitation, headache, agitation, insomnia or nightmares, dizziness, fatigue, impaired coordination, changes in personality, or changes in cognition); changes in urinary pattern; muscle cramping, weakness, tremors, or rigidity; ringing in ears or visual disturbances; chest pain, palpitations, or rapid heartbeat; excessive perspiration; excessive GI symptoms (cramping, constipation, vomiting, anorexia); or worsening of condition.

Pregnancy/breast-feeding precautions: Inform prescriber if you are pregnant. Do not get pregnant during or for 1 month following therapy. Consult prescriber for instruction on appropriate contraceptive measures. This drug may cause severe fetal defects. Breast-feeding is not recommended.

Geriatric Considerations
Due to the higher incidence of CNS adverse reactions and its short half-life, this benzodiazepine is not a drug of first choice. For short-term only.

Breast-Feeding Issues
It is not known if triazolam is excreted in breast milk; however, other benzodiazepines are known to be excreted in breast milk. The AAP rates use of related agents as "of concern" and breast-feeding is not recommended.

Pregnancy Issues
Benzodiazepines cross the placenta. The association between benzodiazepine exposure and malformations remains controversial. A number of types of malformation have been reported (oral cleft, inguinal hernia, cardiac defects, spina bifida, dysmorphic facial features, skeletal defects); however, confounding factors make a clear association difficult. Overall, the risk to the fetus may be low. Nonteratogenic effects (including neonatal flaccidity, respiratory and feeding problems, and withdrawal symptoms) during the postnatal period have also been reported with benzodiazepine use.

Related Information
Anxiolytic / Hypnotic Use in Long-Term Care Facilities on page 1418

Federal OBRA Regulations Recommended Maximum Doses on page 1421

Trifluoperazine (trye floo oh PER a zeen)

Synonyms Trifluoperazine Hydrochloride

Pharmacologic Category Antipsychotic Agent, Typical, Phenothiazine

Medication Safety Issues
Sound-alike/look-alike issues:
Trifluoperazine may be confused with triflupromazine, trihexyphenidyl

Stelazine® may be confused with selegiline

Pregnancy Risk Factor C

Lactation Enters breast milk/not recommended (AAP rates "of concern")

Use Treatment of schizophrenia

Unlabeled/Investigational Use Management of psychotic disorders

Mechanism of Action/Effect Trifluoperazine is a piperazine phenothiazine antipsychotic which blocks post-synaptic mesolimbic dopaminergic receptors in the brain; exhibits alpha-adrenergic blocking effect and depresses the release of hypothalamic and hypophyseal hormones

Contraindications Hypersensitivity to trifluoperazine or any component of the formulation (cross-reactivity between phenothiazines may occur); severe CNS depression; bone marrow suppression; blood dyscrasias; severe hepatic disease; coma

Warnings/Precautions May be sedating, use with caution in disorders where CNS depression is a feature. Use with caution in Parkinson's disease. Caution in patients with hemodynamic instability; predisposition to seizures; subcortical brain damage; hepatic impairment; severe cardiac, renal, or respiratory disease. Esophageal dysmotility and aspiration have been associated with antipsychotic use - use with caution in patients at risk of pneumonia (ie, Alzheimer's disease). Caution in breast cancer or other prolactin-dependent tumors (may elevate prolactin levels). May alter temperature regulation or mask toxicity of other drugs due to antiemetic effects. May alter cardiac conduction - life-threatening arrhythmias have occurred with therapeutic doses of phenothiazines. May cause orthostatic hypotension - use with caution in patients at risk of this effect or those who would tolerate transient hypotensive episodes (cerebrovascular disease, cardiovascular disease or other medications which may predispose). Safety in children <6 months of age has not been established.

Due to anticholinergic effects, should be used with caution in patients with decreased gastrointestinal motility, urinary retention, BPH, xerostomia, visual problems, narrow-angle glaucoma (screening is recommended) and myasthenia gravis. Relative to other antipsychotics, trifluoperazine has a low potency of cholinergic blockade.

May cause extrapyramidal symptoms, including pseudoparkinsonism, acute dystonic reactions, akathisia, and tardive dyskinesia (risk of these reactions is high relative to other neuroleptics). May be associated with neuroleptic malignant syndrome (NMS) or pigmentary retinopathy.

Drug Interactions
Cytochrome P450 Effect: Substrate of CYP1A2 (major)
Decreased Effect: CYP1A2 inducers may decrease the levels/effects of trifluoperazine; example inducers include aminoglutethimide, carbamazepine, phenobarbital, and rifampin. Phenothiazines inhibit the effects of levodopa, guanadrel, guanethidine, and bromocriptine. Benztropine (and other anticholinergics) may inhibit the therapeutic response to trifluoperazine and excess anticholinergic effects may occur. Cigarette smoking may enhance the hepatic metabolism of trifluoperazine. Trifluoperazine and possibly other low potency antipsychotics may reverse the pressor effects of epinephrine.
Increased Effect/Toxicity: CYP1A2 inhibitors may increase the levels/effects of trifluoperazine; example inhibitors include amiodarone, ciprofloxacin, fluvoxamine, ketoconazole, norfloxacin, ofloxacin, and rofecoxib. Trifluoperazine's effects on CNS depression may be additive when trifluoperazine is combined with CNS depressants (narcotic analgesics, ethanol, barbiturates, cyclic antidepressants, antihistamines, or sedative-hypnotics). Trifluoperazine may increase the effects/toxicity of anticholinergics, antihypertensives, lithium (rare neurotoxicity), trazodone, or valproic acid. Concurrent use with TCA may produce increased toxicity or altered therapeutic response. Chloroquine and propranolol may increase trifluoperazine concentrations. Hypotension may occur when trifluoperazine is combined with epinephrine. May increase the risk of arrhythmia when combined with antiarrhythmics, cisapride, pimozide, sparfloxacin, or other drugs which prolong QT interval. Metoclopramide may increase risk of extrapyramidal symptoms (EPS). Acetylcholinesterase inhibitors (central) may increase the risk of antipsychotic-related EPS.

Nutritional/Ethanol Interactions
Ethanol: Avoid ethanol (may increase CNS depression).
Herb/Nutraceutical: Avoid kava kava, gotu kola, valerian, St John's wort (may increase CNS depression). Avoid dong quai, St John's wort (may also cause photosensitization).

Lab Interactions False-positive for phenylketonuria; increased cholesterol (S), glucose; decreased uric acid (S)

Adverse Reactions Frequency not defined.
Cardiovascular: Hypotension, orthostatic hypotension, cardiac arrest
Central nervous system: Extrapyramidal signs (pseudoparkinsonism, akathisia, dystonias, tardive dyskinesia), dizziness, headache, neuroleptic malignant syndrome (NMS), impairment of temperature regulation, lowering of seizure threshold
Dermatologic: Increased sensitivity to sun, rash, discoloration of skin (blue-gray), photosensitivity
Endocrine & metabolic: Changes in menstrual cycle, libido (changes in), breast pain, hyperglycemia, hypoglycemia, gynecomastia, lactation, galactorrhea
Gastrointestinal: Constipation, weight gain, nausea, vomiting, stomach pain, xerostomia
Genitourinary: Difficulty in urination, ejaculatory disturbances, urinary retention, priapism
Hematologic: Agranulocytosis, leukopenia, pancytopenia, thrombocytopenic purpura, eosinophilia, hemolytic anemia, aplastic anemia
Hepatic: Cholestatic jaundice, hepatotoxicity
Neuromuscular & skeletal: Tremor
Ocular: Pigmentary retinopathy, cornea and lens changes
Respiratory: Nasal congestion
Overdosage/Toxicology Symptoms of overdose include deep sleep, coma, extrapyramidal symptoms, abnormal involuntary muscle movements, hypo- or hypertension, and cardiac arrhythmias. Treatment is symptom-directed and supportive.

Pharmacodynamics/Kinetics
Half-Life Elimination: >24 hours with chronic use
Metabolism: Extensively hepatic

Available Dosage Forms Tablet: 1 mg, 2 mg, 5 mg, 10 mg

Dosing
Adults:
Schizophrenia/psychoses: Oral:
Outpatients: 1-2 mg twice daily
Hospitalized or well supervised patient: Initial: 2-5 mg twice daily with optimum response in the 15-20 mg/day range; do not exceed 40 mg/day.
Nonpsychotic anxiety: Oral: 1-2 mg twice daily; maximum: 6 mg/day; therapy for anxiety should not exceed 12 weeks; do not exceed 6 mg/day for longer than 12 weeks when treating anxiety; agitation, jitteriness, or insomnia may be confused with original neurotic or psychotic symptoms.
Elderly:
Schizophrenia/psychoses: Oral: Refer to adult dosing. Dose selection should start at the low end of the dosage range and titration must be gradual.
Behavioral symptoms associated with dementia behavior: Oral: Initial: 0.5-1 mg 1-2 times/day; increase dose at 4- to 7-day intervals by 0.5-1 mg/day; increase dosing intervals (bid, tid, etc) as necessary to control response or side effects. Maximum daily dose: 40 mg. Gradual increases (titration) may prevent some side effects or decrease their severity.
Pediatrics: Schizophrenia/psychoses: Children 6-12 years: Oral: Hospitalized or well supervised patients: Initial: 1 mg 1-2 times/day, gradually increase until symptoms are controlled or adverse effects become troublesome; maximum: 15 mg/day.
Renal Impairment: Not dialyzable (0% to 5%)
Laboratory Monitoring Lipid profile, fasting blood glucose, Hgb A$_{1c}$; BMI

Nursing Actions
Physical Assessment: Assess other medications patient is taking for effectiveness and interactions. Review ophthalmic exam and monitor laboratory results, therapeutic response (mental status, mood, affect, gait), and adverse reactions at beginning of therapy and periodically with long-term use (eg, excess sedation, extrapyramidal symptoms, tardive (Continued)

Trifluoperazine *(Continued)*

dyskinesia, CNS changes). Initiate at lower doses (see Dosing) and taper dosage slowly when discontinuing. Assess knowledge/teach patient appropriate use, interventions to reduce side effects, and adverse symptoms to report.

Patient Education: Use exactly as directed; do not increase dose or frequency. Do not discontinue without consulting prescriber. Tablets may be taken with food. Do not take within 2 hours of any antacid. Avoid alcohol or caffeine and other prescription or OTC medications not approved by prescriber. Maintain adequate hydration (2-3 L/day of fluids) unless instructed to restrict fluid intake. You may experience excess drowsiness, lightheadedness, dizziness, or blurred vision (use caution driving or when engaging in tasks requiring alertness until response to drug is known); nausea or vomiting (small frequent meals, frequent mouth care, chewing gum, or sucking lozenges may help); constipation (increased exercise, fluids, fruit, or fiber may help); postural hypotension (use caution climbing stairs or when changing position from lying or sitting to standing); urinary retention (void before taking medication); ejaculatory dysfunction (reversible); decreased perspiration (avoid strenuous exercise in hot environments); or photosensitivity (use sunscreen, wear protective clothing and eyewear, and avoid direct sunlight). Report persistent CNS effects (eg, trembling fingers, altered gait or balance, excessive sedation, seizures, unusual movements, anxiety, abnormal thoughts, confusion, personality changes); chest pain, palpitations, rapid heartbeat, severe dizziness; unresolved urinary retention or changes in urinary pattern; altered menstrual pattern, changes in libido, swelling or pain in breasts (male or female); vision changes; skin rash, irritation, or changes in color of skin (gray-blue); or worsening of condition. **Pregnancy/breast-feeding precautions:** Inform prescriber if you are or intend to become pregnant. Breast-feeding is not recommended.

Dietary Considerations May be taken with food to decrease GI distress.

Geriatric Considerations (See Warnings/Precautions, Adverse Reactions, and Overdose/Toxicology.) Elderly patients have an increased risk of adverse response to side effects or adverse reactions to antipsychotics.

Additional Information Do not exceed 6 mg/day for longer than 12 weeks when treating anxiety. Agitation, jitteriness, or insomnia may be confused with original neurotic or psychotic symptoms.

Related Information
Antipsychotic Medication Guidelines *on page 1415*

Trifluridine *(trye FLURE i deen)*

U.S. Brand Names Viroptic®
Synonyms F_3T; Trifluorothymidine
Pharmacologic Category Antiviral Agent, Ophthalmic
Medication Safety Issues
Sound-alike/look-alike issues:
Viroptic® may be confused with Timoptic®
Pregnancy Risk Factor C
Lactation Excretion in breast milk unknown
Use Treatment of primary keratoconjunctivitis and recurrent epithelial keratitis caused by herpes simplex virus types I and II
Mechanism of Action/Effect Interferes with viral replication by incorporating into viral DNA in place of thymidine, inhibiting thymidylate synthetase resulting in the formation of defective proteins
Contraindications Hypersensitivity to trifluridine or any component of the formulation

Warnings/Precautions Mild local irritation of conjunctiva and cornea may occur when instilled but usually is a transient effect.
Adverse Reactions 1% to 10%: Local: Burning, stinging
Available Dosage Forms Solution, ophthalmic: 1% (7.5 mL)
Dosing
Adults & Elderly: Herpes keratoconjunctivitis, keratitis: Ophthalmic: Instill 1 drop into affected eye every 2 hours while awake, to a maximum of 9 drops/day, until re-epithelialization of corneal ulcer occurs. Then use 1 drop every 4 hours for another 7 days. Do **not** exceed 21 days of treatment. If improvement has not taken place in 7-14 days, consider another form of therapy.
Stability
Storage: Refrigerate at 2°C to 8°C (36°F to 46°F). Storage at room temperature may result in a solution altered pH which could result in ocular discomfort upon administration and/or decreased potency.

Nursing Actions
Physical Assessment: Monitor effectiveness of therapy, not for long-term use. Assess knowledge/teach patient appropriate use, interventions to reduce side effects, and adverse symptoms to report.
Patient Education: For ophthalmic use only. Store in refrigerator; do not use discolored solution. Apply prescribed amount as often as directed. Wash hands before using. Do not let tip of applicator touch eye; do not contaminate tip of applicator (may cause eye infection, eye damage, or vision loss). Tilt head back and look upward. Gently pull down lower lid and put drop(s) in inner corner of eye. Close eye and roll eyeball in all directions. Do not blink for 1/2 minute. Apply gentle pressure to inner corner of eye for 30 seconds. Wipe away excess from skin around eye. Do not use any other eye preparation for at least 10 minutes. Do not share medication with anyone else. May cause sensitivity to bright light (dark glasses may help); or temporary stinging or blurred vision may occur. Inform prescriber if you experience eye pain, redness, burning, watering, dryness, double vision, puffiness around eye, vision changes, or other adverse eye response; or worsening of condition or lack of improvement within 7-14 days. **Pregnancy/breast-feeding precautions:** Inform prescriber if you are pregnant. Consult prescriber if breast-feeding.
Geriatric Considerations Assess ability to self-administer.

Trihexyphenidyl *(trye heks ee FEN i dil)*

Synonyms Artane; Benzhexol Hydrochloride; Trihexyphenidyl Hydrochloride
Pharmacologic Category Anti-Parkinson's Agent, Anticholinergic; Anticholinergic Agent
Medication Safety Issues
Sound-alike/look-alike issues:
Trihexyphenidyl may be confused with trifluoperazine
Artane may be confused with Altace®, Anturane®, Aramine®
Pregnancy Risk Factor C
Lactation Excretion in breast milk unknown/use caution
Use Adjunctive treatment of Parkinson's disease; treatment of drug-induced extrapyramidal symptoms
Mechanism of Action/Effect Exerts a direct inhibitory effect on the parasympathetic nervous system. It also has a relaxing effect on smooth musculature; exerted both directly on the muscle itself and indirectly through parasympathetic nervous system (inhibitory effect)
Contraindications Hypersensitivity to trihexyphenidyl or any component of the formulation; narrow-angle glaucoma; pyloric or duodenal obstruction; stenosing peptic

ulcers; bladder neck obstructions; achalasia; myasthenia gravis

Warnings/Precautions Use with caution in hot weather or during exercise, especially when administered concomitantly with other atropine-like drugs to chronically-ill patients, alcoholics, patients with CNS disease, or persons doing manual labor in a hot environment. Elderly patients require strict dosage regulation. Use with caution in patients with tachycardia, cardiac arrhythmias, hypertension, hypotension, prostatic hyperplasia or any tendency toward urinary retention, liver or kidney disorders, and obstructive disease of the GI or GU tract. May exacerbate mental symptoms when used to treat extrapyramidal symptoms. When given in large doses or to susceptible patients, may cause weakness. Does not improve symptoms of tardive dyskinesias.

Drug Interactions

Decreased Effect: May increase gastric degradation of levodopa and decrease the amount of levodopa absorbed by delaying gastric emptying; the opposite may be true for digoxin. Therapeutic effects of cholinergic agents (tacrine, donepezil, rivastigmine, galantamine) and neuroleptics may be antagonized.

Increased Effect/Toxicity: Central and/or peripheral anticholinergic syndrome can occur when administered with amantadine, rimantadine, narcotic analgesics, phenothiazines and other antipsychotics (especially with high anticholinergic activity), tricyclic antidepressants, MAO inhibitors, quinidine and some other antiarrhythmics, and antihistamines. CNS depressants (cannabinoids, ethanol, barbiturates, and narcotic analgesics) may have additive effects with trihexyphenidyl; an abuse potential exits.

Nutritional/Ethanol Interactions Ethanol: Avoid ethanol (may increase CNS depression).

Adverse Reactions Frequency not defined.

Cardiovascular: Tachycardia

Central nervous system: Confusion, agitation, euphoria, drowsiness, headache, dizziness, nervousness, delusions, hallucinations, paranoia

Dermatologic: Dry skin, increased sensitivity to light, rash

Gastrointestinal: Constipation, xerostomia, dry throat, ileus, nausea, vomiting, parotitis

Genitourinary: Urinary retention

Neuromuscular & skeletal: Weakness

Ocular: Blurred vision, mydriasis, increase in intraocular pressure, glaucoma, blindness (long-term use in narrow-angle glaucoma)

Respiratory: Dry nose

Miscellaneous: Diaphoresis (decreased)

Overdosage/Toxicology Symptoms of overdose include blurred vision, urinary retention, and tachycardia. For anticholinergic overdose with severe life-threatening symptoms, physostigmine 1-2 mg SubQ or I.V. slowly, may be given to reverse these effects.

Pharmacodynamics/Kinetics

Onset of Action: Peak effect: Within 1 hour

Time to Peak: Serum: 1-1.5 hours

Half-Life Elimination: 3.3-4.1 hours

Excretion: Primarily urine

Available Dosage Forms

Elixir, as hydrochloride: 2 mg/5 mL (480 mL)

Tablet, as hydrochloride: 2 mg, 5 mg

Dosing

Adults: Parkinson's disease or drug-induced EPS: Oral: Initial: 1-2 mg/day, increase by 2 mg increments at intervals of 3-5 days; usual dose: 5-15 mg/day in 3-4 divided doses

Elderly: Parkinsonism: Oral: 1 mg on first day, increase by 2 mg every 3-5 days as needed until a total of 6-10 mg/day (in 3-4 divided doses) is reached. If the patient is on concomitant levodopa therapy, the daily dose is reduced to 1-2 mg 3 times/day. Avoid use if possible (see Geriatric Considerations).

Oral: Tolerated best if given in 3 daily doses and with food. High doses may be divided into 4 doses, at meal times and at bedtime. Patients may be switched to sustained-action capsules when stabilized on conventional dosage forms.

Physical Assessment: Assess effectiveness and interactions of other medications patient may be taking. Monitor renal function, therapeutic response (eg, parkinsonian symptoms), and adverse reactions such as anticholinergic syndrome (dry mouth and mucous membranes, constipation, epigastric distress, CNS disturbances, paralytic ileus) at beginning of therapy and periodically throughout therapy. Assess knowledge/teach patient appropriate use, interventions to reduce side effects, and adverse symptoms to report.

Patient Education: Take exactly as directed; with meals if GI upset occurs, before meals if dry mouth occurs, after eating if drooling or if nausea occurs. Take at the same time each day. Maintain adequate hydration (2-3 L/day of fluids) unless instructed to restrict fluid intake; void before taking medication. Do not use alcohol and all prescription or OTC sedatives or CNS depressants without consulting prescriber. You may experience drowsiness, confusion, or vision changes (use caution when driving, climbing stairs, or engaging in tasks requiring alertness until response to drug is known); increased susceptibility to heat stroke, decreased perspiration (use caution in hot weather; maintain adequate fluids and reduce exercise activity); constipation (increased exercise, fluids, fruit, or fiber may help); or dry skin or nasal passages (consult prescriber for appropriate relief). Report unresolved constipation; chest pain or palpitations; respiratory difficulty; CNS changes (hallucination, loss of memory, nervousness, etc); painful or difficult urination; increased muscle spasticity or rigidity; skin rash; or significant worsening of condition. **Pregnancy/breast-feeding precautions:** Inform prescriber if you are or intend to become pregnant. Consult prescriber if breast-feeding.

Geriatric Considerations Anticholinergic agents are generally not well tolerated in the elderly and their use should be avoided when possible. Elderly patients require strict dosage regulation. In the elderly, anticholinergic agents should not be used as prophylaxis against extrapyramidal symptoms.

Breast-Feeding Issues Anticholinergic agents may suppress lactation.

Additional Information Incidence and severity of side effects are dose related. Patients may be switched to sustained-action capsules when stabilized on conventional dosage forms.

Trimethobenzamide
(trye meth oh BEN za mide)

U.S. Brand Names Tebamide™; Tigan®; Trimazide [DSC]

Synonyms Trimethobenzamide Hydrochloride

Pharmacologic Category Anticholinergic Agent; Antiemetic

Medication Safety Issues

Sound-alike/look-alike issues:

Tigan® may be confused with Tiazac®, Ticar®

Pregnancy Risk Factor C

Lactation Excretion in breast milk unknown

Use Treatment of nausea and vomiting

Mechanism of Action/Effect Acts centrally to inhibit the medullary chemoreceptor trigger zone

Contraindications Hypersensitivity to trimethobenzamide, benzocaine (or similar local anesthetics), or any
(Continued)

Trimethobenzamide (Continued)

component of the formulation; injection contraindicated in children; suppositories contraindicated in premature infants or neonates

Warnings/Precautions May mask emesis due to Reye's syndrome or mimic CNS effects of Reye's syndrome in patients with emesis of other etiologies. Use in patients with acute vomiting should be avoided. May cause drowsiness; patient should avoid tasks requiring alertness (eg, driving, operating machinery). May cause extrapyramidal symptoms (EPS) which may be confused with CNS symptoms of primary disease responsible for emesis. Risk of adverse effects (eg, EPS, seizure) may be increased in patients with acute febrile illness, dehydration, or electrolyte imbalance; use caution.

Nutritional/Ethanol Interactions Ethanol: Concomitant use should be avoided (sedative effects may be additive).

Adverse Reactions Frequency not defined.

Cardiovascular: Hypotension

Central nervous system: Coma, depression, disorientation, dizziness, drowsiness, EPS, headache, opisthotonos, Parkinson-like syndrome, seizure

Gastrointestinal: Diarrhea

Hematologic: Blood dyscrasias

Hepatic: Jaundice

Neuromuscular & skeletal: Muscle cramps

Ocular: Blurred vision

Miscellaneous: Hypersensitivity reactions

Overdosage/Toxicology Symptoms of overdose include hypotension, seizures, CNS depression, cardiac arrhythmias, disorientation, and confusion. Treatment is symptom-directed and supportive.

Pharmacodynamics/Kinetics

Onset of Action: Antiemetic: Oral: 10-40 minutes; I.M.: 15-35 minutes

Duration of Action: 3-4 hours

Time to Peak: Oral: 45 minutes; I.M.: 30 minutes

Half-Life Elimination: 7-9 hours

Excretion: Urine (30% to 50%)

Available Dosage Forms

Capsule, as hydrochloride (Tigan®): 300 mg

Injection, solution, as hydrochloride: 100 mg/mL (2 mL)

Tigan®: 100 mg/mL (2 mL [preservative free], 20 mL)

Suppository, rectal, as hydrochloride: 100 mg, 200 mg

Tebamide™: 100 mg, 200 mg [contains benzocaine]

Tigan®, Trimazide [DSC]: 200 mg [contains benzocaine]

Dosing

Adults & Elderly:

Nausea, vomiting:

Oral: 300 mg 3-4 times/day

I.M., rectal: 200 mg 3-4 times/day

Postoperative nausea and vomiting (PONV): I.M.: 200 mg, followed 1 hour later by a second 200 mg dose

Pediatrics: Note: Rectal use is contraindicated in neonates and premature infants.

Nausea, vomiting: Children:

<14 kg: Rectal: 100 mg 3-4 times/day

14-40 kg: Rectal: 100-200 mg 3-4 times/day

>40 kg: Refer to adult dosing.

Administration

I.M.: Administer I.M. only. Inject deep into upper outer quadrant of gluteal muscle.

I.V.: Not for I.V. administration.

I.V. Detail: pH: 5

Stability

Storage: Store capsules, injection solution, and suppositories at room temperature.

Nursing Actions

Physical Assessment: Monitor therapeutic effectiveness, and adverse reactions with first dose and on a regular basis during therapy (eg, hypovolemia, angioedema, postural hypotension). Teach patient appropriate use (if self-administered injection, teach injection technique and syringe disposal), possible side effects/interventions, and adverse symptoms to report.

Patient Education: Do not take any new medication during therapy unless approved by prescriber. Take capsule as directed before meals; do not increase dose and do not discontinue without consulting prescriber. If using injection formulation, follow directions for injection and disposal of syringe. Follow directions for insertion of rectal suppositories. May cause drowsiness or blurred vision (use caution when driving or engaging in tasks that require alertness until response to drug is known) or diarrhea (buttermilk or yogurt may help). Report chest pain or palpitations, persistent dizziness or blurred vision, or CNS changes (disorientation, depression, confusion). **Pregnancy/breast-feeding precautions:** Inform prescriber if you are or intend to become pregnant. Consult prescriber if breast-feeding.

Trimethoprim (trye METH oh prim)

U.S. Brand Names Primsol®; Proloprim®

Synonyms TMP

Pharmacologic Category Antibiotic, Miscellaneous

Medication Safety Issues

Sound-alike/look-alike issues:

Trimethoprim may be confused with trimethaphan

Proloprim® may be confused with Prolixin®, Protropin®

Pregnancy Risk Factor C

Lactation Enters breast milk/use caution (AAP rates "compatible")

Use Treatment of urinary tract infections due to susceptible strains of *E. coli, P. mirabilis, K. pneumoniae, Enterobacter* sp and coagulase-negative *Staphylococcus* including *S. saprophyticus*; acute otitis media in children; acute exacerbations of chronic bronchitis in adults; in combination with other agents for treatment of toxoplasmosis, *Pneumocystis carinii*; treatment of superficial ocular infections involving the conjunctiva and cornea

Mechanism of Action/Effect Inhibits folic acid reduction to tetrahydrofolate, and thereby inhibits microbial growth

Contraindications Hypersensitivity to trimethoprim or any component of the formulation; megaloblastic anemia due to folate deficiency

Warnings/Precautions Use with caution in patients with impaired renal or hepatic function or with possible folate deficiency.

Drug Interactions

Cytochrome P450 Effect: Substrate (major) of CYP2C8/9, 3A4; **Inhibits** CYP2C8/9 (moderate)

Decreased Effect: The levels/effects of trimethoprim may be decreased by aminoglutethimide, carbamazepine, nafcillin, nevirapine, phenobarbital, phenytoin, rifampin, rifapentine, secobarbital, and other CYP2C8/9 or 3A4 inducers.

Increased Effect/Toxicity: Increased effect/toxicity/levels of phenytoin. Concurrent use with ACE inhibitors increases risk of hyperkalemia. Increased myelosuppression with methotrexate. May increase levels of digoxin. Concurrent use with dapsone may increase levels of dapsone and trimethoprim. Concurrent use with procainamide may increase levels of procainamide and trimethoprim. Trimethoprim may increase the levels/effects of amiodarone, fluoxetine, glimepiride, glipizide, nateglinide, phenytoin, pioglitazone, rosiglitazone, sertraline, warfarin, and other CYP2C8/9 substrates.

Adverse Reactions Frequency not defined.

Central nervous system: Aseptic meningitis (rare), fever

Dermatologic: Maculopapular rash (3% to 7% at 200 mg/day; incidence higher with larger daily doses), erythema multiforme (rare), exfoliative dermatitis (rare), pruritus (common), phototoxic skin eruptions, Stevens-Johnson syndrome (rare), toxic epidermal necrolysis (rare)

Endocrine & metabolic: Hyperkalemia, hyponatremia

Gastrointestinal: Epigastric distress, glossitis, nausea, vomiting

Hematologic: Leukopenia, megaloblastic anemia, methemoglobinemia, neutropenia, thrombocytopenia

Hepatic: Liver enzyme elevation, cholestatic jaundice (rare)

Renal: BUN and creatinine increased

Miscellaneous: Anaphylaxis, hypersensitivity reactions

Overdosage/Toxicology Symptoms of acute toxicity include nausea, vomiting, confusion, and dizziness. Chronic overdose results in bone marrow suppression. Treatment of acute overdose is supportive following GI decontamination. Use oral leucovorin 5-15 mg/day for treatment of chronic overdose. Hemodialysis is only moderately effective in eliminating drug.

Pharmacodynamics/Kinetics
Time to Peak: Serum: 1-4 hours
Protein Binding: 42% to 46%
Half-Life Elimination: 8-14 hours; prolonged with renal impairment
Metabolism: Partially hepatic
Excretion: Urine (60% to 80%) as unchanged drug
Available Dosage Forms [DSC] = Discontinued product
Solution, oral (Primsol®): 50 mg (base)/5 mL (480 mL) [contains sodium benzoate; bubble gum flavor]
Tablet: 100 mg
Proloprim®: 100 mg, 200 mg [DSC]

Dosing
Adults & Elderly: Susceptible infections: Oral: 100 mg every 12 hours or 200 mg every 24 hours for 10 days; longer treatment periods may be necessary for prostatitis (ie, 4-16 weeks)
Pediatrics: Oral: Children (>2 months or age): 4 mg/kg/day in divided doses every 12 hours
Renal Impairment:
Cl_{cr} 15-30 mL/minute: Administer 100 mg every 18 hours or 50 mg every 12 hours.
Cl_{cr} <15 mL/minute: Administer 100 mg every 24 hours or avoid use.
Moderately dialyzable (20% to 50%)

Administration
Oral: Administer with milk or food.

Stability
Storage: Protect the 200 mg tablet from light.
Laboratory Monitoring Periodic CBC and serum potassium during long-term therapy. Perform culture and sensitivity prior to initiating therapy.

Nursing Actions
Physical Assessment: Culture and sensitivity should be assessed prior to initiating therapy. Assess potential for interactions with other pharmacological agents patient may be taking (eg, risk of increased or decreased levels/effects with other medications). Monitor laboratory tests with long-term therapy. Monitor effectiveness (resolution of infection) and adverse reactions (eg, rash, electrolyte imbalance [K, NA], anemia, neutropenia, elevated LFTs, nausea, vomiting, confusion).Teach patient possible side effects/appropriate interventions and adverse symptoms to report.
Patient Education: Do not take any new medication during therapy unless approved by prescriber. Take per recommended schedule. Complete full course of therapy even if feeling better; do not skip doses. Maintain adequate hydration (2-3 L/day of fluids) unless instructed to restrict fluid intake. May cause nausea, vomiting, or GI upset (small, frequent meals, frequent

mouth care, sucking lozenges, or chewing gum may help). Report skin rash, redness, or irritation; feelings of acute fatigue or weakness; unusual bleeding or bruising; or other persistent adverse effects. **Pregnancy precaution:** Inform prescriber if you are or intend to become pregnant. Consult prescriber if breast-feeding.
Dietary Considerations May cause folic acid deficiency, supplements may be needed. Should be taken with milk or food.
Geriatric Considerations Trimethoprim is often used in combination with sulfamethoxazole; it can be used alone in patients who are allergic to sulfonamides; adjust dose for renal function (see Pharmacodynamics/Kinetics and Dosing).
Pregnancy Issues Because trimethoprim may interfere with folic acid metabolism, consider using only if the potential benefit to the mother outweighs the possible risk to the fetus.

Trimetrexate Glucuronate (tri me TREKS ate)

U.S. Brand Names NeuTrexin®
Synonyms NSC-352122; Trimetrexate Glucuronate
Pharmacologic Category Antineoplastic Agent, Miscellaneous
Pregnancy Risk Factor D
Lactation Excretion in breast milk unknown/not recommended
Use Alternative therapy for the treatment of moderate-to-severe *Pneumocystis jiroveci* pneumonia (PCP) in immunocompromised patients, including patients with acquired immunodeficiency syndrome (AIDS), who are intolerant of, or are refractory to, sulfamethoxazole/trimethoprim therapy or for whom sulfamethoxazole/trimethoprim and pentamidine are contraindicated
Unlabeled/Investigational Use Treatment of nonsmall cell lung cancer, metastatic colorectal cancer, metastatic head and neck cancer, pancreatic adenocarcinoma, cutaneous T-cell lymphoma
Mechanism of Action/Effect Exerts effects through potent inhibition of the enzyme dihydrofolate reductase (DHFR)
Contraindications Hypersensitivity to trimetrexate, methotrexate, leucovorin, or any component of the formulation; severe existing myelosuppression; pregnancy
Warnings/Precautions Hazardous agent - use appropriate precautions for handling and disposal. **Must be administered with concurrent leucovorin to avoid potentially serious or life-threatening toxicities.** Leucovorin therapy must extend for 72 hours past the last dose of trimetrexate. Hypersensitivity/allergic-type reactions have been reported, primarily when given as a bolus infusion, at higher than recommended doses for PCP, or in combination with fluorouracil or leucovorin. May cause anaphylactoid reactions (rarely) including acute hypotension and loss of consciousness. Epinephrine should be available for treatment of acute allergic symptoms. Use with caution in patients with mild myelosuppression, severe hepatic or renal dysfunction, hypoproteinemia, hypoalbuminemia, or previous extensive myelosuppressive therapies. Withhold zidovudine during trimetrexate treatment.
Drug Interactions
Increased Effect/Toxicity: Zidovudine may increase the myelotoxicity of trimetrexate; discontinue zidovudine during trimetrexate treatment. Trimetrexate may increase toxicity (infections) of live virus vaccines.
Adverse Reactions
>10%:
Hematologic: Neutropenia (30%)
Hepatic: AST increased (14%), ALT increased (11%)
(Continued)

Trimetrexate Glucuronate *(Continued)*

1% to 10%:
Central nervous system: Fever (8%), confusion (3%), fatigue (2%)
Dermatologic: Rash/pruritus (6%)
Endocrine & metabolic: Hyponatremia (5%), hypocalcemia (2%)
Gastrointestinal: Nausea/vomiting (5%), stomatitis
Hematologic: Thrombocytopenia (10%), anemia (7%)
Hepatic: Alkaline phosphatase increased (5%), bilirubin increased (2%)
Neuromuscular & skeletal: Peripheral neuropathy
Miscellaneous: Flu-like illness; hypersensitivity/allergic reactions (chills, rigors); anaphylactoid reactions (acute hypotension, loss of consciousness)

Overdosage/Toxicology Administration of trimetrexate without leucovorin may cause lethal complications. Toxicities observed at I.V. doses of 90 mg/m²/day with concurrent leucovorin were primarily hematologic. In the event of an overdose, trimetrexate should be discontinued and leucovorin should be administered at a dose of 40 mg/m² I.V. every 6 hours for 3 days.

Pharmacodynamics/Kinetics
Protein Binding: 80% to 90% (concentration dependent)
Half-Life Elimination: 9-18 hours (11 hours with leucovorin)
Metabolism: Extensively hepatic: O-demethylation followed by conjugation to glucuronide or sulfate (major); N-demethylation and oxidation (minor)
Excretion: Urine (10% to 40% as unchanged drug); feces (<1% to 8%)

Available Dosage Forms Injection, powder for reconstitution [preservative free]: 25 mg, 200 mg

Dosing
Adults & Elderly: Note: Concurrent leucovorin 20 mg/m² every 6 hours must be administered daily (oral or I.V.) during treatment and for 72 hours past the last dose of trimetrexate.

Pneumonia caused by *Pneumocystis jiroveci* (PCP): I.V.: 45 mg/m² once daily for 21 days; **alternative dosing based on weight:**
<50 kg: Trimetrexate 1.5 mg/kg/day; leucovorin 0.6 mg/kg 4 times/day

50-80 kg: Trimetrexate 1.2 mg/kg/day; leucovorin 0.5 mg/kg/4 times/day
>80 kg: Trimetrexate 1 mg/kg/day; leucovorin 0.5 mg/kg/4 times/day
Note: Oral doses of leucovorin should be rounded up to the next higher 25 mg increment.

Antineoplastic (unlabeled use): I.V.: 6-16 mg/m² once daily for 5 days every 21-28 days **or** 150-200 mg/m² every 2 weeks

Hepatic Impairment: Although it may be necessary to reduce the dose in patients with liver dysfunction, no specific recommendations exist.

Dosing Adjustment for Toxicity: Leucovorin therapy must be extended for 72 hours past the last dose of trimetrexate glucuronate.
Hematologic toxicity: See table.
Hepatic toxicity: Treatment should be interrupted if transaminase levels or alkaline phosphatase levels increase to >5 times the upper limit of normal.
Renal toxicity: Treatment should be interrupted if serum creatinine levels increase to >2.5 mg/dL and elevation is considered secondary to trimetrexate.
Other toxicities: Treatment should be interrupted in patients experiencing severe mucosal toxicity that interferes with oral intake. Treatment should be discontinued for fever that cannot be controlled with antipyretics (oral temperature ≥40.5°C/105°F).
In addition: If trimetrexate treatment is interrupted for toxicity, leucovorin therapy must continue for 72 hours past the last administered dose of trimetrexate.

Administration
I.V.: Infuse over 60-90 minutes.
I.V. Detail: Must be used with concurrent leucovorin; trimetrexate and leucovorin solutions **must** be administered separately. Intravenous lines should be flushed with at least 10 mL of D_5W before and after trimetrexate and between trimetrexate and leucovorin.

pH: 3.5-5.5
Stability
Reconstitution: Reconstitute with D_5W or SWFI to a concentration of 12.5 mg/mL. Do not use if cloudy or if precipitate forms. Prior to administration, solution should be further diluted with D_5W to a concentration of 0.25 mg/mL to 2 mg/mL.
Compatibility: Stable in D_5W, SWFI
Precipitate occurs with leucovorin or any solution containing chloride ion.
Y-site administration: Incompatible with foscarnet, indomethacin
Compatibility when admixed: Incompatible with chloride-containing solutions, leucovorin
Storage: Prior to reconstitution, vials should be stored at controlled room temperature of 20°C to 25°C (68°F to 77°F). Protect from light. Reconstituted solution is stable for 6 hours at room temperature and 24 hours under refrigeration. Diluted solutions for infusion are stable under refrigeration or at room temperature for 24 hours. Do not freeze.
Laboratory Monitoring Absolute neutrophil counts (ANC), platelet count, renal function tests (serum creatinine, BUN), and hepatic function (ALT, AST, alkaline phosphatase) twice weekly

Nursing Actions
Physical Assessment: Trimetrexate must be administered with concurrent leucovorin to avoid potentially serious or life-threatening toxicities. Leucovorin therapy must extend for 72 hours past the last dose of trimetrexate to reduce potential for life-threatening toxicities. Assess potential for interactions with other pharmacological agents patient may be taking. Patient must be monitored closely for anaphylactoid reactions; epinephrine should be available. Monitor laboratory tests at baseline and periodically during therapy. Assess therapeutic effectiveness and adverse reactions (eg, rash, gastrointestinal upset,

Dosage Adjustment in Hematologic Toxicity

Toxicity Grade	Neutrophils (Polys/Bands)	Platelets	Dosage Recommendations Trimetrexate	Leucovorin
1	>1000/mm³	>75,000/mm³	45 mg/m² once daily	20 mg/m² every 6 h
2	750-1000/mm³	50,000-75,000/mm³	45 mg/m² once daily	40 mg/m² every 6 h
3	500-749/mm³	25,000-49,999/mm³	22 mg/m² once daily	40 mg/m² every 6 h
4	<500/mm³	<25,000/mm³	Day 1-9: Discontinue Day 10-21: Interrupt up to 96 hours (see Note)	40 mg/m² every 6 h

Note:
If Grade 4 hematologic toxicity occurs prior to day 10: Trimetrexate should be discontinued and leucovorin administered for an additional 72 hours.

If Grade 4 hematologic toxicity occurs at day 10 or later: Trimetrexate may be held up to 96 hours to allow counts to recover.

If counts recover to Grade 3 within 96 hours, trimetrexate should be administered at a dose of 22 mg/m² and leucovorin 40 mg/m² every 6 hours.

When counts recover to Grade 2 toxicity, trimetrexate may be increased to 45 mg/m². Continue leucovorin at 40 mg/m² for duration of treatment.

Discontinue trimetrexate if counts do not improve to less than or equal to Grade 3 toxicity within 96 hours. Continue leucovorin at 40 mg/m² every 6 hours for 72 hours following last dose.

anemia, peripheral neuropathy, increased LFTs). Teach patient importance of maintaining prescribed schedule of leucovorin, possible side effects/appropriate interventions, and adverse symptoms to report.

Patient Education: Do not take any new medication during therapy unless approved by prescriber (especially aspirin or aspirin-containing products). This medication is only administered by intravenous infusion. Report immediately any redness, swelling, or pain at infusion site. This medication is administered concurrently with an oral medication (leucovorin); maintain exact schedule as prescribed for oral medication in order to reduce potential for serious reaction. Maintain adequate hydration (2-3 L/day of fluids unless instructed to restrict fluid intake). You may be more susceptible to infection (avoid crowds and exposure to infection and do not have any vaccinations unless approved by prescriber). Report unusual or persistent fever, chills, or joint pain; persistent gastrointestinal upset; changes in sensorium (eg, confusion, unusual or excessive fatigue); or other persistent adverse effects. **Pregnancy/breast-feeding precautions:** Inform prescriber if you are pregnant. Do not get pregnant while taking this medication or for 1 month after completing therapy. Consult prescriber for appropriate contraceptive measures. Do not breast-feed.

Geriatric Considerations No specific recommendations are available for the elderly. Use with caution in patients with liver dysfunction (see Dosing).

Breast-Feeding Issues It is recommended to discontinue breast-feeding during trimetrexate therapy.

Pregnancy Issues May cause fetal harm when administered to pregnant women. Women of childbearing potential should avoid becoming pregnant while receiving treatment. If used in pregnancy, or if patient becomes pregnant during treatment, the patient should be apprised of potential hazard to the fetus.

Additional Information Not a vesicant; methotrexate derivative

---

Trimipramine (trye MI pra meen)

U.S. Brand Names Surmontil®

Synonyms Trimipramine Maleate

Restrictions A medication guide concerning the use of antidepressants in children and teenagers can be found on the FDA website at http://www.fda.gov/cder/Offices/ODS/labeling.htm. It should be dispensed to parents or guardians of children and teenagers receiving this medication.

Pharmacologic Category Antidepressant, Tricyclic (Tertiary Amine)

Medication Safety Issues
Sound-alike/look-alike issues:
Trimipramine may be confused with triamterene, trimeprazine

Pregnancy Risk Factor C

Lactation Enters breast milk/contraindicated

Use Treatment of depression

Mechanism of Action/Effect Increases the synaptic concentration of serotonin and/or norepinephrine in the central nervous system by inhibition of their reuptake by the presynaptic neuronal membrane

Contraindications Hypersensitivity to trimipramine, any component of the formulation, or other dibenzodiazepines; use of MAO inhibitors within 14 days; use in a patient during the acute recovery phase of MI

Warnings/Precautions Antidepressants increase the risk of suicidal thinking and behavior in children and adolescents with major depressive disorder (MDD) and other depressive disorders; consider risk prior to prescribing. All patients must be closely monitored for clinical worsening, suicidality, or unusual changes in behavior, especially during the initiation of therapy or following an increase or decrease in dosage. When used in children, the child's family or caregiver should be instructed to closely observe the patient and communicate condition with healthcare provider. A medication guide should be dispensed with each prescription. **Trimipramine is not FDA approved for use in children.**

The possibility of a suicide attempt is inherent in major depression and may persist until remission occurs. Use caution in high-risk patients. Worsening depression and severe abrupt suicidality that are not part of the presenting symptoms may require discontinuation or modification of drug therapy. The patient's family or caregiver should be alerted to monitor patients for the emergence of suicidality and associated behaviors (such as agitation, irritability, hostility, impulsivity, and hypomania) and call healthcare provider.

May worsen psychosis in some patients or precipitate a shift to mania or hypomania in patients with bipolar disorder. Patients presenting with depressive symptoms should be screened for bipolar disorder. Monotherapy in patients with bipolar disorder should be avoided. **Trimipramine is not FDA approved for the treatment of bipolar depression.**

The degree of sedation, anticholinergic effects, orthostasis, and conduction abnormalities are high relative to other antidepressants. Trimipramine often causes drowsiness/sedation, resulting in impaired performance of tasks requiring alertness (eg, operating machinery or driving). Sedative effects may be additive with other CNS depressants and/or ethanol. Use with caution in patients with a history of cardiovascular disease (including previous MI, stroke, tachycardia, or conduction abnormalities). Use with caution in patients with urinary retention, benign prostatic hyperplasia, narrow-angle glaucoma, xerostomia, visual problems, constipation, or a history of bowel obstruction.

May alter glucose control - use with caution in patients with diabetes. Consider discontinuing, when possible, prior to elective surgery. Therapy should not be abruptly discontinued in patients receiving high doses for prolonged periods. May lower seizure threshold - use caution in patients with a previous seizure disorder or condition predisposing to seizures such as brain damage, alcoholism, or concurrent therapy with other drugs which lower the seizure threshold. May increase the risks associated with electroconvulsive therapy. Use with caution in hyperthyroid patients or those receiving thyroid supplementation. Use with caution in patients with hepatic or renal dysfunction and in elderly patients.

Drug Interactions

Cytochrome P450 Effect: Substrate (major) of CYP2C19, 2D6, 3A4

Decreased Effect: CYP2C19 inducers may decrease the levels/effects of trimipramine; example inducers include aminoglutethimide, carbamazepine, phenytoin, and rifampin. Trimipramine inhibits the antihypertensive response to bethanidine, clonidine, debrisoquin, guanadrel, guanethidine, guanabenz, and guanfacine. Cholestyramine and colestipol may bind TCAs and reduce their absorption; monitor for altered response. CYP3A4 inducers may decrease the levels/effects of trimipramine; example inducers include aminoglutethimide, carbamazepine, nafcillin, nevirapine, phenobarbital, phenytoin, and rifamycins.

Increased Effect/Toxicity: Pressor response to I.V. epinephrine, norepinephrine, and phenylephrine may be enhanced in patients receiving TCAs (**Note:** Effect is unlikely with epinephrine or levonordefrin dosages typically administered as infiltration in combination with local anesthetics). Trimipramine increases the effects of amphetamines, anticholinergics, other CNS (Continued)

Trimipramine (Continued)

depressants (sedatives, hypnotics, or ethanol), chlorpropamide, tolazamide, and warfarin. When used with MAO inhibitors, hyperpyrexia, hypertension, tachycardia, confusion, seizures, and **deaths have been reported** (serotonin syndrome). Serotonin syndrome has also been reported with ritonavir (rare).

CYP2C19 inhibitors may increase the levels/effects of trimipramine; example inhibitors include delavirdine, fluconazole, fluvoxamine, gemfibrozil, isoniazid, omeprazole, and ticlopidine. CYP2D6 inhibitors may increase the levels/effects of trimipramine; example inhibitors include chlorpromazine, delavirdine, fluoxetine, miconazole, paroxetine, pergolide, quinidine, quinine, ritonavir, and ropinirole. CYP3A4 inhibitors may increase the levels/effects of trimipramine; example inhibitors include azole antifungals, clarithromycin, diclofenac, doxycycline, erythromycin, imatinib, isoniazid, nefazodone, nicardipine, propofol, protease inhibitors, quinidine, telithromycin, and verapamil. Use of lithium with a TCA may increase the risk for neurotoxicity. Phenothiazines may increase concentration of some TCAs and TCAs may increase concentration of phenothiazines. Combined use of beta-agonists or drugs which prolong QT$_c$ (including quinidine, procainamide, disopyramide, cisapride, sparfloxacin, gatifloxacin, moxifloxacin) with TCAs may predispose patients to cardiac arrhythmias.

Nutritional/Ethanol Interactions

Ethanol: Avoid ethanol (may increase CNS depression).
Food: Grapefruit juice may inhibit the metabolism of some TCAs and clinical toxicity may result.
Herb/Nutraceutical: Avoid valerian, St John's wort, SAMe, kava kava (may increase risk of serotonin syndrome and/or excessive sedation).

Lab Interactions Increased glucose

Adverse Reactions Frequency not defined.
Cardiovascular: Arrhythmias, hyper-/hypotension, tachycardia, palpitation, heart block, stroke, MI
Central nervous system: Headache, exacerbation of psychosis, confusion, delirium, hallucinations, nervousness, restlessness, delusions, agitation, insomnia, nightmares, anxiety, seizure, drowsiness
Dermatologic: Photosensitivity, rash, petechiae, itching
Endocrine & metabolic: Sexual dysfunction, breast enlargement, galactorrhea, SIADH
Gastrointestinal: Xerostomia, constipation, increased appetite, nausea, unpleasant taste, weight gain, diarrhea, heartburn, vomiting, anorexia, trouble with gums, decreased lower esophageal sphincter tone may cause GE reflux
Genitourinary: Difficult urination, urinary retention, testicular edema
Hematologic: Agranulocytosis, eosinophilia, purpura, thrombocytopenia
Hepatic: Cholestatic jaundice, increased liver enzymes
Neuromuscular & skeletal: Tremors, numbness, tingling, paresthesia, incoordination, ataxia, peripheral neuropathy, extrapyramidal symptoms
Ocular: Blurred vision, eye pain, disturbances in accommodation, mydriasis, increased intraocular pressure
Otic: Tinnitus
Miscellaneous: Allergic reactions

Overdosage/Toxicology Symptoms of overdose include agitation, confusion, hallucinations, urinary retention, hypothermia, hypotension, tachycardia, and cardiac arrhythmias. Following initiation of essential overdose management, toxic symptoms should be treated.

Ventricular arrhythmias and ECG changes (QRS widening) often respond to systemic alkalinization (sodium bicarbonate 0.5-2 mEq/kg I.V.). Physostigmine (1-2 mg I.V. slowly for adults) may be indicated for reversing life-threatening cardiac arrhythmias. Treatment is symptomatic and supportive.

Pharmacodynamics/Kinetics

Protein Binding: 95%; free drug: 3% to 7%

Half-Life Elimination: 16-40 hours

Metabolism: Hepatic; significant first-pass effect

Excretion: Urine

Available Dosage Forms Capsule: 25 mg, 50 mg, 100 mg

Dosing

Adults: Depression: Oral: 50-150 mg/day as a single bedtime dose up to a maximum of 200 mg/day for outpatients and 300 mg/day for inpatients

Elderly: Oral: Initial: 25 mg at bedtime; increase by 25 mg/day every 3 days for inpatients and weekly for outpatients, as tolerated, to a maximum of 100 mg/day (see Geriatric Considerations).

Stability

Storage: Solutions stable at a pH of 4-5; turns yellowish or reddish on exposure to light. Slight discoloration does not affect potency; marked discoloration is associated with loss of potency. Capsules stable for 3 years following date of manufacture.

Nursing Actions

Physical Assessment: Assess other medications patient may be taking for effectiveness and interactions. Monitor therapeutic response (eg, mental status, mood, affect, suicidal ideation), and adverse reactions at beginning of therapy and periodically with long-term use. Assess knowledge/teach patient appropriate use, interventions to reduce side effects, and adverse symptoms to report.

Patient Education: Take exactly as directed; do not increase dose or frequency. It may take 2-3 weeks to achieve desired results. Take at bedtime. Avoid alcohol, caffeine, and other prescription or OTC medications not approved by prescriber. Maintain adequate hydration (2-3 L/day of fluids) unless instructed to restrict fluid intake. You may experience drowsiness, lightheadedness, dizziness, or blurred vision (use caution when driving or engaging in tasks requiring alertness until response to drug is known); nausea, altered taste, dry mouth (small frequent meals, frequent mouth care, chewing gum, or sucking lozenges may help); constipation (increased exercise, fluids, fruit, or fiber may help); diarrhea (buttermilk, yogurt, or boiled milk may help); increased appetite (monitor dietary intake to avoid excess weight gain); postural hypotension (use caution when climbing stairs or changing position from lying or sitting to standing); urinary retention (void before taking medication); or sexual dysfunction (reversible). Report persistent CNS effects (eg, insomnia, restlessness, fatigue, anxiety, impaired cognitive function, seizures, suicide ideation); muscle cramping or tremors; chest pain, palpitations, rapid heartbeat, swelling of extremities, or severe dizziness; unresolved urinary retention; vision changes or eye pain; yellowing of eyes or skin; pale stools/dark urine; suicidal ideation; or worsening of condition. **Pregnancy/breast-feeding precautions:** Inform prescriber if you are or intend to become pregnant. Do not breast-feed.

Geriatric Considerations Similar to doxepin in its side effect profile. Has not been well studied in the elderly. Very anticholinergic and, therefore, not considered a drug of first choice in the elderly when selecting an antidepressant.

Additional Information May cause alterations in bleeding time.

Related Information

Antidepressant Medication Guidelines on page 1414
Federal OBRA Regulations Recommended Maximum Doses on page 1421

Triptorelin (trip toe REL in)

U.S. Brand Names Trelstar™ Depot; Trelstar™ LA

Synonyms AY-25650; CL-118,532; D-Trp(6)-LHRH; Triptoraline; Triptorelin Pamoate; Tryptoreline

Pharmacologic Category Gonadotropin Releasing Hormone Agonist

Pregnancy Risk Factor X

Lactation Excretion in breast milk unknown/contraindicated

Use Palliative treatment of advanced prostate cancer as an alternative to orchiectomy or estrogen administration

Unlabeled/Investigational Use Treatment of endometriosis, growth hormone deficiency, hyperandrogenism, in vitro fertilization, ovarian carcinoma, pancreatic carcinoma, precocious puberty, uterine leiomyomata

Mechanism of Action/Effect Causes suppression of ovarian and testicular steroidogenesis due to decreased levels of LH and FSH with subsequent decrease in testosterone (male) and estrogen (female) levels. After chronic and continuous administration, usually 2-4 weeks after initiation, a sustained decrease in LH and FSH secretion occurs.

Contraindications Hypersensitivity to triptorelin or any component of the formulation, other LHRH agonists or LHRH; pregnancy

Warnings/Precautions Transient increases in testosterone can lead to worsening symptoms (bone pain, hematuria, bladder outlet obstruction) of prostate cancer during the first few weeks of therapy. Cases of spinal cord compression have been reported with LHRH agonists. Hypersensitivity reactions including angioedema and anaphylaxis have occurred. Rare cases of pituitary apoplexy (frequently secondary to pituitary adenoma) have been observed with leuprolide administration (onset from 1 hour to usually <2 weeks); may present as sudden headache, vomiting, visual or mental status changes, and infrequently cardiovascular collapse; immediate medical attention required. Safety and efficacy has not established in pediatric population.

Drug Interactions

Decreased Effect: Not studied. Hyperprolactinemic drugs (dopamine antagonists such as antipsychotics, and metoclopramide) are contraindicated.

Increased Effect/Toxicity: Not studied. Hyperprolactinemic drugs (dopamine antagonists such as antipsychotics, and metoclopramide) are contraindicated.

Lab Interactions Pituitary-gonadal function may be suppressed with chronic administration and for up to 8 weeks after triptorelin therapy has been discontinued.

Adverse Reactions As reported with Trelstar™ Depot and Trelstar™ LA; frequency of effect may vary by product:

>10%:

Central nervous system: Headache (30% to 60%)

Endocrine & metabolic: Hot flashes (95% to 100%), glucose increased, hemoglobin decreased, RBC count decreased

Hepatic: Alkaline phosphatase increased, ALT increased, AST increased

Neuromuscular & skeletal: Skeletal pain (12% to 13%)

Renal: BUN increased

1% to 10%:

Cardiovascular: Leg edema (6%), hypertension (4%), chest pain (2%), peripheral edema (1%)

Central nervous system: Dizziness (1% to 3%), pain (2% to 3%), emotional lability (1%), fatigue (2%), insomnia (2%)

Dermatologic: Rash (2%), pruritus (1%)

Endocrine & metabolic: Alkaline phosphatase increased (2%), breast pain (2%), gynecomastia (2%), libido decreased (2%), tumor flare (8%)

Gastrointestinal: Nausea (3%), anorexia (2%), constipation (2%), dyspepsia (2%), vomiting (2%), abdominal pain (1%), diarrhea (1%)

Genitourinary: Dysuria (5%), impotence (2% to 7%), urinary retention (1%), urinary tract infection (1%)

Hematologic: Anemia (1%)

Local: Injection site pain (4%)

Neuromuscular & skeletal: Leg pain (2% to 5%), back pain (3%), arthralgia (2%), leg cramps (2%), myalgia (1%), weakness (1%)

Ocular: Conjunctivitis (1%), eye pain (1%)

Respiratory: Cough (2%), dyspnea (1%), pharyngitis (1%)

Postmarketing and/or case reports: Anaphylaxis, angioedema, hypersensitivity reactions, spinal cord compression, renal dysfunction

Overdosage/Toxicology Accidental or intentional overdose unlikely. If it were to occur, supportive and symptomatic treatment would be indicated.

Pharmacodynamics/Kinetics

Time to Peak: 1-3 hours

Protein Binding: None

Half-Life Elimination: 2.8 ± 1.2 hours

Moderate to severe renal impairment: 6.5-7.7 hours

Hepatic impairment: 7.6 hours

Metabolism: Unknown; unlikely to involve CYP; no known metabolites

Excretion: Urine (42% as intact peptide); hepatic

Available Dosage Forms Injection, powder for reconstitution, as pamoate [also available packaged with Debioclip™ (prefilled syringe containing sterile water)]:

Trelstar™ Depot: 3.75 mg

Trelstar™ LA: 11.25 mg

Dosing

Adults & Elderly: Advanced prostate carcinoma:

Trelstar™ Depot: 3.75 mg once every 28 days

Trelstar™ LA: 11.25 mg once every 84 days

Renal Impairment: Specific guidelines are not available.

Hepatic Impairment: Specific guidelines are not available.

Administration

I.M.: Must be administered under the supervision of a physician. Administer by I.M. injection into the buttock; alternate injection sites.

Debioclip™: Follow manufacturer's instructions for mixing prior to use.

Stability

Reconstitution: Reconstitute with 2 mL sterile water for injection. Shake well to obtain a uniform suspension. Withdraw the entire contents into the syringe and inject immediately.

Storage:

Trelstar™ Depot: Store at 15°C to 30°C (59°F to 86°F)

Trelstar™ LA: Store at 20°C to 25°C (68°F to 77°F)

Laboratory Monitoring Serum testosterone levels, prostate-specific antigen

Nursing Actions

Physical Assessment: Monitor laboratory tests, therapeutic effectiveness, and adverse response. Teach patient possible side effects/appropriate interventions and adverse symptoms to report. **Pregnancy risk factor X.**

Patient Education: This medication can only be administered by injection. If diabetic, may alter blood glucose levels; monitor blood sugar closely. Report swelling, pain, or burning at injection site. May cause disease flare (increased bone pain), blood in urine, or urinary retention during early treatment (usually resolves within 1 week); impotence; or hot flashes (cool cloth on forehead, cool environment, and light, layered clothing may help; contact prescriber if these become intolerable). Report any persistent adverse GI upset; chest pain, rapid heartbeat, or palpations; numbness in extremities; acute headache; alterations in urinary pattern; or other persistent adverse effects. Report immediately sudden headache, severe (Continued)

Triptorelin (Continued)

vomiting, visual or mental status change, and cardio-vascular collapse. **Pregnancy/breast-feeding precautions:** This drug will cause severe fetal defects. Do not breast-feed.

Pregnancy Issues Contraindicated in women who are or may become pregnant.

Urokinase (yoor oh KIN ase)

U.S. Brand Names Abbokinase® [DSC]
Synonyms UK
Pharmacologic Category Thrombolytic Agent
Pregnancy Risk Factor B
Lactation Excretion in breast milk unknown/use caution
Use Thrombolytic agent for the lysis of acute massive pulmonary emboli or pulmonary emboli with unstable hemodynamics

Unlabeled/Investigational Use Thrombolytic agent used in treatment of recent severe or massive deep vein thrombosis, myocardial infarction, and occluded I.V. or dialysis cannulas

Mechanism of Action/Effect Promotes thrombolysis by directly activating plasminogen to plasmin, which degrades fibrin, fibrinogen, and other procoagulant plasma proteins

Contraindications Hypersensitivity to urokinase or any component of the formulation; active internal bleeding; history of CVA; recent (within 2 months) intracranial or intraspinal surgery or trauma; intracranial neoplasm, arteriovenous malformation, or aneurysm; known bleeding diathesis; severe uncontrolled hypertension

Warnings/Precautions Concurrent heparin anticoagulation can contribute to bleeding; careful attention to all potential bleeding sites. I.M. injections and nonessential handling of the patient should be avoided. Venipunctures should be performed carefully and only when necessary. If arterial puncture is necessary, use an upper extremity vessel that can be manually compressed. If serious bleeding occurs, then the infusion of urokinase and heparin should be stopped.

For the following conditions the risk of bleeding is higher with use of anistreplase and should be weighed against the benefits of therapy: recent (within 10 days) major surgery (eg, CABG, obstetrical delivery, organ biopsy, previous puncture of noncompressible vessels), cerebrovascular disease, recent (within 10 days) gastrointestinal or genitourinary bleeding, recent trauma (within 10 days) including CPR, hypertension (systolic BP >180 mm Hg and/or diastolic BP >110 mm Hg), high likelihood of left heart thrombus (eg, mitral stenosis with atrial fibrillation), acute pericarditis, subacute bacterial endocarditis, hemostatic defects including ones caused by severe renal or hepatic dysfunction, significant hepatic dysfunction, pregnancy, diabetic hemorrhagic retinopathy or other hemorrhagic ophthalmic conditions, septic thrombophlebitis or occluded AV cannula at seriously infected site, advanced age (eg, >75 years), patients receiving oral anticoagulants, any other condition in which bleeding constitutes a significant hazard or would be particularly difficult to manage because of location.

Coronary thrombolysis may result in reperfusion arrhythmias. Follow standard MI management. Rare anaphylactoid reactions can occur. Safety and efficacy in pediatric patients have not been established.

Drug Interactions
Decreased Effect: Aminocaproic acid (an antifibrinolytic agent) may decrease the effectiveness of thrombolytic therapy.

Increased Effect/Toxicity: Oral anticoagulants (warfarin), heparin, low molecular weight heparins, and drugs which affect platelet function (eg, NSAIDs,

dipyridamole, ticlopidine, clopidogrel, IIb/IIIa antagonists) may potentiate the risk of hemorrhage.

Adverse Reactions As with all drugs which may affect hemostasis, bleeding is the major adverse effect associated with urokinase. Hemorrhage may occur at virtually any site. Risk is dependent on multiple variables, including the dosage administered, concurrent use of multiple agents which alter hemostasis, and patient predisposition.

>10%: Local: Injection site: Bleeding (5% decrease in hematocrit reported in 37% patients; most bleeding occurring at external incisions or injection sites, but also reported in other areas)

Overdosage/Toxicology Symptoms of overdose include epistaxis, bleeding gums, hematoma, spontaneous ecchymoses, and oozing at the catheter site. In the event of overdose, stop the infusion and reverse bleeding with blood products that contain clotting factors.

Pharmacodynamics/Kinetics
Onset of Action: I.V.: Fibrinolysis occurs rapidly
Duration of Action: ≥4 hours
Half-Life Elimination: 6.4-18.8 minutes
Excretion: Urine and feces (small amounts)

Available Dosage Forms [DSC] = Discontinued product

Injection, powder for reconstitution: 250,000 int. units [contains human albumin 250 mg and mannitol 25 mg] [DSC]

Dosing
Adults & Elderly:

Acute pulmonary embolism: I.V.: Loading: 4400 int. units/kg over 10 minutes; maintenance: 4400 int. units/kg/hour for 12 hours. Following infusion, anticoagulation treatment is recommended to prevent recurrent thrombosis. Do not start anticoagulation until aPTT has decreased to less than twice the normal control value. If heparin is used, do not administer loading dose. Treatment should be followed with oral anticoagulants.

Deep vein thrombosis (unlabeled use): I.V.: Loading: 4400 units/kg over 10 minutes, then 4400 units/kg/hour for 12 hours

Myocardial infarction (unlabeled use): Intracoronary: 750,000 units over 2 hours (6000 units/minute over up to 2 hours)

Occluded I.V. catheters (unlabeled use):
5000 units in each lumen over 1-2 minutes, leave in lumen for 1-4 hours, then aspirate. May repeat with 10,000 units in each lumen if 5000 units fails to clear the catheter. **Do not infuse into the patient.** Volume to instill into catheter is equal to the volume of the catheter. Will not dissolve drug precipitate or anything other than blood products.

I.V. infusion: 200 units/kg/hour in each lumen for 12-48 hours at a rate of at least 20 mL/hour

Dialysis patient: 5000 units is administered in each lumen over 1-2 minutes; leave urokinase in lumen for 1-2 days, then aspirate.

Pediatrics: Children: Deep vein thrombosis, pulmonary embolus, or occluded catheter: I.V.: Refer to adult dosing.

Administration
I.V.: Solution may be filtered using a 0.22 or 0.45 micron filter during I.V. therapy. Administer using a pump which can deliver a total volume of 195 mL. The loading dose should be administered at 90 mL/hour over 10 minutes. The maintenance dose should be administered at 15 mL/hour over 12 hours. I.V. tubing should be flushed with NS or D₅W to ensure total dose is administered.

I.V. Detail: pH: 6.0-7.5

Stability
Reconstitution: Reconstitute vial with 5 mL sterile water for injection (preservative free) by gently rolling and tilting; do not shake. Contains no preservatives;

should not be reconstituted until immediately before using; discard unused portion. Solution will look pale and straw colored. May filter through ≤0.45 micron filter.

Compatibility: Stable in NS

Storage: Prior to reconstitution, store in refrigerator at 2°C to 8°C (36°F to 46°F). Prior to infusion, solution should be further diluted in D_5W or NS.

Laboratory Monitoring CBC, platelet count, aPTT, urinalysis

Nursing Actions

Physical Assessment: Assess potential for interactions with other pharmacological agents and herbal product patient may be taking (especially those medications that may affect coagulation [warfarin] or platelet function [NSAIDs, dipyridamole, ticlopidine, clopidogrel]). See Administration for infusion specifics (infusion pump is required). Monitor laboratory tests. Monitor patient closely for bleeding during and following treatment (infusion site, neurological status [eg, intracranial hemorrhage], vital signs, ECG [reperfusion arrhythmias]). Bedrest and bleeding precautions should be maintained; avoid I.M. injections, venipuncture (unless absolutely necessary), and nonessential handling of the patient. If arterial puncture is necessary, use an upper extremity vessel that can be manually compressed. Patient instructions determined by patient condition.

Patient Education: Inform prescriber of all medications or herbal products you are taking. This medication is only administered by infusion; you will be monitored closely during and after treatment. Immediately report burning, pain, redness, swelling, or oozing at infusion site; sudden acute headache; joint pain; chest pain; or altered vision. Following infusion, you will have a tendency to bleed easily; use caution to prevent injury (use electric razor, soft toothbrush, and caution with knives, needles, or anything sharp). Follow instructions for strict bedrest to reduce the risk of injury. If bleeding occurs, report immediately and apply pressure to bleeding spot until bleeding stops completely. Report unusual bruising or bleeding; blood in urine, stool, or vomitus; bleeding gums; or respiratory difficulty. **Pregnancy/breast-feeding precautions:** Inform prescriber if you are or intend to become pregnant. Consult prescriber if breast-feeding.

Ursodiol (ER soe dye ole)

U.S. Brand Names Actigall®; Urso 250™; Urso Forte™
Synonyms Ursodeoxycholic Acid
Pharmacologic Category Gallstone Dissolution Agent
Pregnancy Risk Factor B
Lactation Excretion in breast milk unknown
Use Actigall®: Gallbladder stone dissolution; prevention of gallstones in obese patients experiencing rapid weight loss; Urso®: Primary biliary cirrhosis
Unlabeled/Investigational Use Liver transplantation
Mechanism of Action/Effect Decreases the cholesterol content of bile and bile stones by reducing the secretion of cholesterol from the liver and the fractional reabsorption of cholesterol by the intestines. Mechanism of action in primary biliary cirrhosis is not clearly defined.
Contraindications Hypersensitivity to ursodiol, bile acids, or any component of the formulation; not to be used with cholesterol, radiopaque, bile pigment stones, or stones >20 mm in diameter; allergy to bile acids
Warnings/Precautions Gallbladder stone dissolution may take several months of therapy. Complete dissolution may not occur and recurrence of stones within 5 years has been observed in 50% of patients. Use with caution in patients with a nonvisualizing gallbladder and those with chronic liver disease.

Drug Interactions
Decreased Effect: Decreased effect with aluminum-containing antacids, cholestyramine, colestipol, clofibrate, and oral contraceptives (estrogens).

Adverse Reactions
>10%:
Central nervous system: Headache (up to 25%), dizziness (up to 17%)
Gastrointestinal: In treatment of primary biliary cirrhosis: Constipation (up to 26%)
1% to 10%:
Dermatologic: Rash (<1% to 3%), alopecia (<1% to 5%)
Gastrointestinal:
In gallstone dissolution: Most GI events (diarrhea, nausea, vomiting) are similar to placebo and attributable to gallstone disease.
In treatment of primary biliary cirrhosis: Diarrhea (1%)
Hematologic: Leukopenia (3%)
Miscellaneous: Allergy (5%)

Overdosage/Toxicology Symptoms of overdose include diarrhea. No specific therapy for diarrhea or overdose.

Pharmacodynamics/Kinetics
Half-Life Elimination: 100 hours
Metabolism: Undergoes extensive enterohepatic recycling; following hepatic conjugation and biliary secretion, the drug is hydrolyzed to active ursodiol, where it is recycled or transformed to lithocholic acid by colonic microbial flora
Excretion: Feces

Available Dosage Forms
Capsule (Actigall®): 300 mg
Tablet:
Urso 250™: 250 mg
Urso Forte™: 500 mg

Dosing
Adults & Elderly:
Gallstone dissolution: Oral: 8-10 mg/kg/day in 2-3 divided doses; use beyond 24 months is not established; obtain ultrasound images at 6-month intervals for the first year of therapy; 30% of patients have stone recurrence after dissolution
Gallstone prevention: Oral: 300 mg twice daily
Primary biliary cirrhosis: Oral: 13-15 mg/kg/day in 2-4 divided doses (with food)

Administration
Oral: Do not administer with aluminum-based antacids. If aluminum based antacids are needed, administer 2 hours after ursodiol. Urso® should be taken with food.

Stability
Storage: Do not store above 30°C (86°F)

Laboratory Monitoring
Gallstone disease: ALT, AST, ALP; sonogram may be required
Hepatic disease: Monitor hepatic function tests frequently

Nursing Actions
Physical Assessment: Assess results of laboratory tests, therapeutic effectiveness, and adverse reactions. Teach patient proper use, possible side effects signs to report.

Patient Education: Take medication as directed with food. Drug will need to be taken for 1-3 months after stone is dissolved and stones may recur. Report any persistent nausea, vomiting, abdominal pain, or yellowing of skin or eyes. **Breast-feeding precaution:** Consult prescriber if breast-feeding.

Dietary Considerations Urso® should be taken with food.

(Continued)

Ursodiol *(Continued)*

Geriatric Considerations No specific clinical studies in the elderly. Would recommend starting at lowest recommended dose with scheduled monitoring.

Valacyclovir *(val ay SYE kloe veer)*

U.S. Brand Names Valtrex®

Synonyms Valacyclovir Hydrochloride

Pharmacologic Category Antiviral Agent, Oral

Medication Safety Issues
Sound-alike/look-alike issues:
Valtrex® may be confused with Valcyte™
Valacyclovir may be confused with valganciclovir

Pregnancy Risk Factor B

Lactation Enters breast milk/use caution

Use Treatment of herpes zoster (shingles) in immunocompetent patients; treatment of first-episode genital herpes; episodic treatment of recurrent genital herpes; suppression of recurrent genital herpes and reduction of heterosexual transmission of genital herpes in immunocompetent patients; suppression of genital herpes in HIV-infected individuals; treatment of herpes labialis (cold sores)

Mechanism of Action/Effect Valacyclovir is rapidly converted to acyclovir before it exerts its antiviral activity against HSV-1, HSV-2, or VZV. Inhibits viral DNA synthesis and replication.

Contraindications Hypersensitivity to valacyclovir, acyclovir, or any component of the formulation

Warnings/Precautions Hazardous agent - use appropriate precautions for handling and disposal. Thrombotic thrombocytopenic purpura/hemolytic uremic syndrome has occurred in immunocompromised patients (at doses of 8 g/day); use caution and adjust the dose in elderly patients or those with renal insufficiency and in patients receiving concurrent nephrotoxic agents. For genital herpes, treatment should begin as soon as possible after the first signs and symptoms (within 72 hours of onset of first diagnosis or within 24 hours of onset of recurrent episodes). For herpes zoster, treatment should begin within 72 hours of onset of rash. For cold sores, treatment should begin at with earliest symptom (tingling, itching, burning). Safety and efficacy in prepubertal patients have not been established.

Drug Interactions

Decreased Effect: Cimetidine and/or probenecid has decreased the rate but not the extent of valacyclovir conversion to acyclovir leading to decreased effectiveness of valacyclovir.

Increased Effect/Toxicity: Valacyclovir and acyclovir have increased CNS side effects with zidovudine and probenecid.

Adverse Reactions
>10%: Central nervous system: Headache (14% to 35%)
1% to 10%:
Central nervous system: Dizziness (2% to 4%), depression (0% to 7%)
Endocrine: Dysmenorrhea (≤1% to 8%)
Gastrointestinal: Abdominal pain (2% to 11%), vomiting (<1% to 6%), nausea (6% to 15%)
Hematologic: Leukopenia (≤1%), thrombocytopenia (≤1%)
Hepatic: AST increased (1% to 4%)
Neuromuscular & skeletal: Arthralgia (≤1 to 6%)

Overdosage/Toxicology Precipitation in renal tubules may occur. Treatment is symptomatic and includes hemodialysis, especially if compromised renal function develops.

Pharmacodynamics/Kinetics

Protein Binding: 13.5% to 17.9%

Half-Life Elimination: Normal renal function: Adults: 2.5-3.3 hours (acyclovir), ~30 minutes (valacyclovir); End-stage renal disease: 14-20 hours (acyclovir)

Metabolism: Hepatic; valacyclovir is rapidly and nearly completely converted to acyclovir and L-valine by first-pass effect; acyclovir is hepatically metabolized to a very small extent by aldehyde oxidase and by alcohol and aldehyde dehydrogenase (inactive metabolites)

Excretion: Urine, primarily as acyclovir (88%); **Note:** Following oral administration of radiolabeled valacyclovir, 46% of the label is eliminated in the feces (corresponding to nonabsorbed drug), while 47% of the radiolabel is eliminated in the urine.

Available Dosage Forms Caplet: 500 mg, 1000 mg

Dosing

Adults & Elderly:

Herpes labialis (cold sores): Oral: 2 g twice daily for 1 day (separate doses by ~12 hours)

Herpes zoster (shingles): Oral: 1 g 3 times/day for 7 days

Genital herpes: Oral:
Initial episode: 1 g twice daily for 10 days
Recurrent episode: 500 mg twice daily for 3 days
Reduction of transmission: 500 mg once daily (source partner)
Suppressive therapy:
Immunocompetent patients: 1000 mg once daily (500 mg once daily in patients with <9 recurrences per year)
HIV-infected patients (CD4 ≥100 cells/mm³): 500 mg twice daily

Pediatrics: Herpes labialis (cold sores): Adolescents: Refer to adult dosing.

Renal Impairment:
Herpes zoster: Adults:
Cl_{cr} 30-49 mL/minute: 1 g every 12 hours
Cl_{cr} 10-29 mL/minute: 1 g every 24 hours
Cl_{cr} <10 mL/minute: 500 mg every 24 hours
Genital herpes: Adults:
Initial episode:
Cl_{cr} 10-29 mL/minute: 1 g every 24 hours
Cl_{cr} <10 mL/minute: 500 mg every 24 hours
Recurrent episode: Cl_{cr} <10-29 mL/minute: 500 mg every 24 hours
Suppressive therapy: Cl_{cr} <10-29 mL/minute:
For usual dose of 1 g every 24 hours, decrease dose to 500 mg every 24 hours
For usual dose of 500 mg every 24 hours, decrease dose to 500 mg every 48 hours
HIV-infected patients: 500 mg every 24 hours
Herpes labialis: Adolescents and Adults:
Cl_{cr} 30-49 mL/minute: 1 g every 12 hours for 2 doses
Cl_{cr} 10-29 mL/minute: 500 mg every 12 hours for 2 doses
Cl_{cr} <10 mL/minute: 500 mg as a single dose
Hemodialysis: Dialyzable (~33% removed during 4-hour session); administer dose postdialysis
Chronic ambulatory peritoneal dialysis/continuous arteriovenous hemofiltration dialysis: Pharmacokinetic parameters are similar to those in patients with ESRD; supplemental dose not needed following dialysis

Administration

Oral: If GI upset occurs, administer with meals.

Stability

Storage: Store at 15°C to 25°C (59°F to 77°F).

Laboratory Monitoring Urinalysis, BUN, serum creatinine, liver enzymes, and CBC

Nursing Actions

Physical Assessment: Monitor therapeutic effectiveness (resolution of clinical symptoms) and adverse responses (eg, CNS changes [dizziness, depression], nausea, vomiting, dysmenorrhea, arthralgia). Teach patient appropriate use, possible side effects/appropriate interventions, and adverse symptoms to report.

Patient Education: This medication is not a cure for genital herpes; it is not known if it will prevent transmission to others. Take as directed, with or without food. Begin use at first sign of herpes. Maintain adequate hydration (2-3 L/day of fluids) unless instructed to restrict fluid intake. May cause headache, dizziness (use caution when driving or engaging in potentially hazardous tasks until response to drug is known); or nausea, vomiting, abdominal pain (small, frequent meals, frequent mouth care, chewing gum, or sucking lozenges may help). Immediately report difficulty swallowing or breathing; rash or hives; or changes in menses. **Breast-feeding precaution:** Consult prescriber if breast-feeding.

Dietary Considerations May be taken with or without food.

Geriatric Considerations More convenient dosing and increased bioavailability, without increasing side effects, make valacyclovir a favorable choice compared to acyclovir. Has been shown to accelerate resolution of postherpetic pain. Adjust dose for renal impairment.

Breast-Feeding Issues Peak concentrations in breast milk range from 0.5-2.3 times the corresponding maternal acyclovir serum concentration. This is expected to provide a nursing infant with a dose of acyclovir equivalent to ~0.6 mg/kg/day following ingestion of valacyclovir 500 mg twice daily by the mother. Use with caution while breast-feeding.

Pregnancy Issues Teratogenicity registry has shown no increased rate of birth defects than that of the general population; however, the registry is small and use during pregnancy is only warranted if the potential benefit to the mother justifies the risk of the fetus.

Valdecoxib (val de KOKS ib)

U.S. Brand Names Bextra® *[Withdrawn from Market]*

Pharmacologic Category Nonsteroidal Anti-inflammatory Drug (NSAID), COX-2 Selective

Pregnancy Risk Factor C/D (3rd trimester)

Lactation Excretion in breast milk unknown/not recommended

Use Relief of signs and symptoms of osteoarthritis and adult rheumatoid arthritis; treatment of primary dysmenorrhea

Mechanism of Action/Effect Inhibits cyclooxygenase-2 (COX-2) and as a result, prostaglandin synthesis resulting in decreased pain.

Contraindications Hypersensitivity to valdecoxib, sulfonamides, or any component of the formulation; patients who have experienced asthma, urticaria, or allergic-type reactions to aspirin or NSAIDs; acute pain following CABG; pregnancy (3rd trimester)

Warnings/Precautions Gastrointestinal irritation, ulceration, bleeding, and perforation may occur with NSAIDs. Use with caution in patients with a history of GI bleeding, ulcers, or risk factor for GI bleeding. Anaphylactic/anaphylactoid reactions may occur, even with no prior exposure to valdecoxib. Serious dermatologic reactions (including life-threatening Stevens-Johnson syndrome and erythema multiforme) have been reported; discontinue in any patients who develop rash or any signs of hypersensitivity. Use with caution in patients with decreased renal function, hepatic disease, CHF, hypertension, fluid retention, dehydration, or asthma. Carefully evaluate individual cardiovascular risk profiles prior to prescribing COX-2 inhibitors. COX-2 inhibitors may not be appropriate in patients with cardiovascular disease or in patients with significant risk factors for cardiovascular disease. Use caution in

patients with known or suspected deficiency of cytochrome P450 isoenzyme 2C9. Use in patients with severe hepatic impairment (Child-Pugh Class C) is not recommended. Use in patients following CABG has been associated with an increase in thromboembolic events, including MI, stroke, DVT, and PE. Safety and efficacy have not been established for patients <18 years of age.

Drug Interactions

Cytochrome P450 Effect: Substrate (minor) of CYP2C8/9, 3A4; Inhibits CYP2C8/9 (weak), 2C19 (weak)

Decreased Effect: ACE inhibitors, angiotensin II antagonists, hydralazine, loop and thiazide diuretics effects reduced.

Increased Effect/Toxicity: Anticoagulants and antiplatelet drugs may increase risk of bleeding. Warfarin efficacy may increase. Corticosteroids may increase risk of GI ulceration. Cyclosporine, dextromethorphan, lithium levels increased. Serum concentrations/toxicity of methotrexate may be increased. Azole antifungals may increase valdecoxib concentrations.

Nutritional/Ethanol Interactions

Ethanol: Avoid ethanol (may enhance gastric mucosal irritation).

Food: Time to peak level is delayed by 1-2 hours when taken with high-fat meal, but other parameters are unaffected.

Herb/Nutraceutical: Avoid cat's claw, dong quai, evening primrose, feverfew, garlic, ginger, ginkgo, red clover, horse chestnut, green tea, ginseng (may cause increased risk of bleeding).

Adverse Reactions 2% to 10%:

Cardiovascular: Peripheral edema (2% to 3%), hypertension (2%)

Central nervous system: Headache (5% to 9%), dizziness (3%)

Dermatologic: Rash (1% to 2%)

Gastrointestinal: Dyspepsia (8% to 9%), abdominal pain (7% to 8%), nausea (6% to 7%), diarrhea (5% to 6%), flatulence (3% to 4%), abdominal fullness (2%)

Neuromuscular & skeletal: Back pain (2% to 3%), myalgia (2%)

Otic: Earache, tinnitus

Respiratory: Upper respiratory tract infection (6% to 7%), sinusitis (2% to 3%)

Miscellaneous: Influenza-like symptoms (2%)

Overdosage/Toxicology Symptoms of overdose may include epigastric pain, drowsiness, lethargy, nausea, and vomiting; gastrointestinal bleeding may occur. Rare manifestations include hypertension, respiratory depression, coma, and acute renal failure. Treatment is symptomatic and supportive. Forced diuresis, hemodialysis, hemoperfusion, and/or urinary alkalinization may not be useful.

Pharmacodynamics/Kinetics

Onset of Action: Dysmenorrhea: 60 minutes

Time to Peak: 2.25-3 hours

Protein Binding: 98%

Half-Life Elimination: 8-11 hours

Metabolism: Extensively hepatic via CYP3A4 and 2C9; glucuronidation; forms metabolite (active)

Excretion: Primarily urine (as metabolites)

Available Dosage Forms Tablet: 10 mg, 20 mg

Dosing

Adults & Elderly:

Osteoarthritis and rheumatoid arthritis: Oral: 10 mg once daily; **Note:** No additional benefits seen with 20 mg/day

Primary dysmenorrhea: Oral: 20 mg twice daily as needed

Pediatrics: Not indicated for pediatric patients.

Renal Impairment: Not recommended for use in advanced disease.

Hepatic Impairment: Not recommended for use in advanced liver dysfunction (Child-Pugh Class C). (Continued)

Valdecoxib *(Continued)*

Administration
Oral: Avoid dehydration. Encourage patient to drink plenty of fluids.

Stability
Storage: Store at 15°C to 30°C (59°F to 86°F).

Nursing Actions
Physical Assessment: Assess effectiveness and interactions of other prescription, OTC, or herbal medication patient may be taking. Assess allergy history (salicylates, NSAIDs). Monitor blood pressure at the beginning of therapy and periodically during use. Monitor for effectiveness of therapy and adverse reactions. Assess knowledge/teach patient appropriate use, interventions to reduce side effects, and adverse symptoms to report.

Patient Education: Use exactly as directed. May be taken with food to reduce GI upset. Do not take with antacids. Avoid alcohol, aspirin, or other medication unless approved by prescriber. Maintain adequate hydration (2-3 L/day of fluids) unless instructed to restrict fluid intake. GI bleeding, ulceration, or perforation can occur with or without pain. Stop taking medication and report immediately abdominal tenderness, stomach pain or cramping; unusual bleeding or bruising; or blood in vomitus, stool, or urine. You may experience dizziness, confusion, or blurred vision (avoid driving or engaging in tasks requiring alertness until response to drug is known); or anorexia, nausea, vomiting (small frequent meals, frequent mouth care, chewing gum or sucking lozenges may help). Report any skin rash, muscle aches, unusual fatigue, lethargy, yellowing of skin or eyes, flu-like symptoms, easy bruising or bleeding, sudden weight gain, changes in urinary pattern, respiratory difficulty, shortness of breath, chest pain, or signs of upper respiratory infection. **Pregnancy/breast-feeding precautions:** Inform prescriber if you are or intend to become pregnant. This drug should not be used in the 3rd trimester of pregnancy. Breast-feeding is not recommended.

Dietary Considerations May be taken with or without food.

Geriatric Considerations The elderly are at increased risk for adverse effects from NSAIDs. As many as 60% of elderly can develop peptic ulceration and/or hemorrhage asymptomatically. CNS adverse effects such as confusion, agitation, and hallucination are generally seen in overdose or high-dose situations; however, elderly patients may demonstrate these adverse effects at lower doses than younger adults. The elderly are also at increased risk of renal toxicity.

Pregnancy Issues Use should be avoided in late pregnancy because it may cause premature closure of the ductus arteriosus.

Valganciclovir *(val gan SYE kloh veer)*

U.S. Brand Names Valcyte™

Synonyms Valganciclovir Hydrochloride

Pharmacologic Category Antiviral Agent

Medication Safety Issues
Sound-alike/look-alike issues:
Valcyte™ may be confused with Valium®, Valtrex®
Valganciclovir may be confused with valacyclovir

Pregnancy Risk Factor C

Lactation Excretion in breast milk unknown/contraindicated

Use Treatment of cytomegalovirus (CMV) retinitis in patients with acquired immunodeficiency syndrome (AIDS); prevention of CMV disease in high-risk patients (donor CMV positive/recipient CMV negative) undergoing kidney, heart, or kidney/pancreas transplantation

Mechanism of Action/Effect Valganciclovir is a prodrug of ganciclovir, and is rapidly metabolized in the body to form ganciclovir. Ganciclovir inhibits the formation of viral DNA within infected cells, blocking reproduction of the virus.

Contraindications Hypersensitivity to valganciclovir, ganciclovir, acyclovir, or any component of the formulation; absolute neutrophil count <500/mm³; platelet count <25,000/mm³; hemoglobin <8 g/dL

Warnings/Precautions Dosage adjustment or interruption of valganciclovir therapy may be necessary in patients with neutropenia and/or thrombocytopenia and patients with impaired renal function. Not approved for use in children. Due to differences in bioavailability, valganciclovir tablets cannot be substituted for ganciclovir capsules on a one-to-one basis. Not indicated for use in liver transplant patients (higher incidence of tissue-invasive CMV relative to oral ganciclovir was observed in trials). Safety and efficacy not established in pediatric patients.

Drug Interactions
Decreased Effect: Reported for ganciclovir: A decrease in blood levels of ganciclovir AUC may occur when used with didanosine.

Increased Effect/Toxicity: Reported for ganciclovir: Immunosuppressive agents may increase hematologic toxicity of ganciclovir. Imipenem/cilastatin may increase seizure potential. Oral ganciclovir increases blood levels of zidovudine, although zidovudine decreases steady-state levels of ganciclovir. Since both drugs have the potential to cause neutropenia and anemia, some patients may not tolerate concomitant therapy with these drugs at full dosage. Didanosine levels are increased with concurrent ganciclovir. Other nephrotoxic drugs (eg, amphotericin and cyclosporine) may have additive nephrotoxicity with ganciclovir.

Nutritional/Ethanol Interactions Food: Coadministration with a high-fat meal increased AUC by 30%.

Adverse Reactions
>10%:
Central nervous system: Fever (31%), headache (9% to 22%), insomnia (16%)
Gastrointestinal: Diarrhea (16% to 41%), nausea (8% to 30%), vomiting (21%), abdominal pain (15%)
Hematologic: Granulocytopenia (11% to 27%), anemia (8% to 26%)
Ocular: Retinal detachment (15%)
1% to 10%:
Central nervous system: Peripheral neuropathy (9%), paresthesia (8%), seizure (<5%), psychosis, hallucinations (<5%), confusion (<5%), agitation (<5%)
Hematologic: Thrombocytopenia (8%), pancytopenia (<5%), bone marrow depression (<5%), aplastic anemia (<5%), bleeding (potentially life-threatening due to thrombocytopenia <5%)
Renal: Decreased renal function (<5%)
Miscellaneous: Local and systemic infection, including sepsis (<5%); allergic reaction (<5%)

Overdosage/Toxicology Symptoms of overdose with ganciclovir include neutropenia, vomiting, hypersalivation, bloody diarrhea, cytopenia, and testicular atrophy. Treatment is supportive. Hemodialysis removes 50% of the drug. Hydration may be of some benefit.

Pharmacodynamics/Kinetics
Protein Binding: 1% to 2%
Half-Life Elimination: Ganciclovir: 4.08 hours, prolonged with renal impairment; Severe renal impairment: Up to 68 hours
Metabolism: Converted to ganciclovir by intestinal mucosal cells and hepatocytes
Excretion: Urine (primarily as ganciclovir)

Available Dosage Forms Tablet, as hydrochloride: 450 mg [valganciclovir hydrochloride 496.3 mg equivalent to valganciclovir 450 mg]

Dosing

Adults & Elderly:

CMV retinitis: Oral:

Induction (active retinitis): 900 mg twice daily for 21 days (with food)

Maintenance: Following induction treatment, or for patients with inactive CMV retinitis who require maintenance therapy: Recommended dose: 900 mg once daily (with food)

Prevention of CMV disease following transplantation: Oral: 900 mg once daily (with food) beginning within 10 days of transplantation; continue therapy until 100 days post-transplantation.

Renal Impairment:

Induction dose:

Cl_{cr} 40-59 mL/minute: 450 mg twice daily

Cl_{cr} 25-39 mL/minute: 450 mg once daily

Cl_{cr} 10-24 mL/minute: 450 mg every 2 days

Maintenance dose:

Cl_{cr} 40-59 mL/minute: 450 mg once daily

Cl_{cr} 25-39 mL/minute: 450 mg every 2 days

Cl_{cr} 10-24 mL/minute: 450 mg twice weekly

Note: Valganciclovir is not recommended in patients receiving hemodialysis. For patients on hemodialysis (Cl_{cr} <10 mL/minute), it is recommended that ganciclovir be used (dose adjusted as specified for ganciclovir).

Administration

Oral: Avoid direct contact with broken or crushed tablets. Consideration should be given to handling and disposal according to guidelines issued for antineoplastic drugs. However, there is no consensus on the need for these precautions.

Stability

Storage: Store at 25°C (77°F), excursions permitted to 15°C to 30°C (59°F to 86°F).

Laboratory Monitoring Retinal exam (at least every 4-6 weeks), CBC, platelet counts, serum creatinine

Nursing Actions

Physical Assessment: Assess potential for interactions with other pharmacological agents patient may be taking (eg, increased risk of nephrotoxicity and hematologic toxicity). Monitor laboratory tests, therapeutic effectiveness (reduction in clinical symptoms), and adverse response (eg, peripheral neuropathy, neutropenia, anemia, nephrotoxicity, retinal detachment, vomiting, bloody diarrhea) on a regular basis during therapy. Teach proper use, possible side effects/appropriate interventions, and adverse symptoms to report.

Patient Education: Do not take any new medication during therapy unless approved by prescriber. This medication is not a cure for CMV retinitis. Take exactly as directed; do not alter dosage or discontinue without consulting prescriber. You will need frequent and regular laboratory tests and ophthalmic exams while taking this medication. Maintain adequate hydration (2-3 L/day of fluids) unless instructed to restrict fluid intake. You may be more susceptible to infection (avoid crowds or exposure to infection and do not have any vaccinations unless approved by prescriber). May cause headache or insomnia (use caution when driving or engaging in hazardous tasks until response to drug is known); nausea or vomiting (small, frequent meals, good mouth care, sucking lozenges, or chewing gum may help); diarrhea (boiled milk, yogurt, or buttermilk may help); or photosensitivity (use sunscreen, wear protective clothing and eyewear, and avoid direct sunlight). Report fever; chills; unusual bleeding or bruising; infection or unhealed sores; white plaques in mouth or vaginal discharge; CNS disturbances (eg, hallucinations, confusion, nightmares); or weakness or loss of feeling in nerves or muscles. **Pregnancy/breast-feeding precautions:** Inform prescriber if you are pregnant. Males and females should use appropriate barrier contraceptive measures during and for 90 days following end of therapy. Do not breast-feed.

Dietary Considerations Should be taken with meals.

Breast-Feeding Issues HIV-infected mothers are discouraged from breast-feeding to decrease the potential transmission of HIV.

Pregnancy Issues Valganciclovir is converted to ganciclovir and shares its reproductive toxicity. Ganciclovir may adversely affect spermatogenesis and fertility; due to its mutagenic potential, contraceptive precautions for female and male patients need to be followed during and for at least 90 days after therapy with this drug.

Valproic Acid and Derivatives

(val PROE ik AS id & dah RIV ah tives)

U.S. Brand Names Depacon®; Depakene®; Depakote® Delayed Release; Depakote® ER; Depakote® Sprinkle®

Synonyms Dipropylacetic Acid; Divalproex Sodium; DPA; 2-Propylpentanoic Acid; 2-Propylvaleric Acid; Valproate Semisodium; Valproate Sodium; Valproic Acid

Pharmacologic Category Anticonvulsant, Miscellaneous

Medication Safety Issues

Sound-alike/look-alike issues:

Depakene® may be confused with Depakote®

Depakote® may be confused with Depakene®, Depakote® ER, Senokot®

Pregnancy Risk Factor D

Lactation Enters breast milk/use caution (AAP considers "compatible")

Use Monotherapy and adjunctive therapy in the treatment of patients with complex partial seizures; monotherapy and adjunctive therapy of simple and complex absence seizures; adjunctive therapy patients with multiple seizure types that include absence seizures; treatment of acute or mixed manic episodes associated with bipolar disorder; migraine prophylaxis

Mania associated with bipolar disorder (Depakote®)

Migraine prophylaxis (Depakote®, Depakote® ER)

Unlabeled/Investigational Use Behavior disorders (eg, agitation, aggression) in patients with dementia (based on the results of several randomized, controlled trials, there is little evidence to support this use); status epilepticus

Mechanism of Action/Effect Causes increased availability of gamma-aminobutyric acid (GABA), an inhibitory neurotransmitter, to brain neurons or may enhance the action of GABA or mimic its action at postsynaptic receptor sites

Contraindications Hypersensitivity to valproic acid, derivatives, or any component of the formulation; hepatic dysfunction; urea cycle disorders

Warnings/Precautions Hepatic failure resulting in fatalities has occurred in patients; children <2 years of age are at considerable risk; other risk factors include organic brain disease, mental retardation with severe seizure disorders, congenital metabolic disorders, and patients on multiple anticonvulsants. Hepatotoxicity has been reported after 3 days to 6 months of therapy. Monitor patients closely for appearance of malaise, weakness, facial edema, anorexia, jaundice, and vomiting; may cause severe thrombocytopenia, inhibition of platelet aggregation and bleeding; tremors may indicate overdosage; use with caution in patients receiving other anticonvulsants.

Cases of life-threatening pancreatitis, occurring at the start of therapy or following years of use, have been reported in adults and children. Some cases have been hemorrhagic with rapid progression of initial symptoms to death.

(Continued)

Valproic Acid and Derivatives
(Continued)

May cause teratogenic effects such as neural tube defects (eg, spina bifida). Use in women of childbearing potential requires that benefits of use in mother be weighed against the potential risk to fetus, especially when used for conditions not associated with permanent injury or risk of death (eg, migraine).

Hyperammonemic encephalopathy, sometimes fatal, has been reported following the initiation of valproate therapy in patients with known or suspected urea cycle disorders (UCD), particularly those with ornithine trans-carbamylase deficiency. Although a rare genetic disorder, UCD evaluation should be considered for the following patients, prior to the start of therapy: History of unexplained encephalopathy or coma; encephalopathy associated with protein load; pregnancy or postpartum encephalopathy; unexplained mental retardation; history of elevated plasma ammonia or glutamine; history of cyclical vomiting and lethargy; episodic extreme irrita-bility, ataxia; low BUN or protein avoidance; family history of UCD or unexplained infant deaths (particularly male); signs or symptoms of UCD (hyperammonemia, encephalopathy, respiratory alkalosis). Patients who develop symptoms of hyperammonemic encephalop-athy during therapy with valproate should receive prompt evaluation for UCD and valproate should be discontinued.

Hyperammonemia may occur with therapy and may be present with normal liver function tests. Ammonia levels should be measured in patients who develop unex-plained lethargy and vomiting, or changes in mental status. Discontinue therapy if ammonia levels are increased and evaluate for possible UCD.

In vitro studies have suggested valproate stimulates the replication of HIV and CMV viruses under experimental conditions. The clinical consequence of this is unknown, but should be considered when monitoring affected patients.

Anticonvulsants should not be discontinued abruptly because of the possibility of increasing seizure frequency; valproate should be withdrawn gradually to minimize the potential of increased seizure frequency, unless safety concerns require a more rapid withdrawal. Concomitant use with clonazepam may induce absence status.

CNS depression may occur with valproate use. Patients must be cautioned about performing tasks which require mental alertness (operating machinery or driving). Effects with other sedative drugs or ethanol may be potentiated.

Drug Interactions

Cytochrome P450 Effect: For valproic acid: **Substrate** (minor) of CYP2A6, 2B6, 2C8/9, 2C19, 2E1; **Inhibits** CYP2C8/9 (weak), 2C19 (weak), 2D6 (weak), 3A4 (weak); **Induces** CYP2A6 (weak)

Decreased Effect: Carbapenem antibiotics (ertapenem, imipenem, meropenem) may decrease valproic acid concentrations to subtherapeutic levels; monitor.

Increased Effect/Toxicity: Absence seizures have been reported in patients receiving VPA and clona-zepam. Valproic acid may increase, decrease, or have no effect on carbamazepine and phenytoin levels. Valproic acid may increase serum concentra-tions of carbamazepine - epoxide (active metabolite). Valproic acid may increase serum concentrations of lamotrigine, phenobarbital, tricyclic antidepressants, and zidovudine. Macrolide antibiotics (clarithromycin, erythromycin, troleandomycin), felbamate, and isoni-azid may inhibit the metabolism of valproic acid. Aspirin or other salicylates may displace valproic acid from protein-binding sites, leading to acute toxicity.

Nutritional/Ethanol Interactions
Ethanol: Avoid ethanol (may increase CNS depression).
Food: Food may delay but does not affect the extent of absorption. Valproic acid serum concentrations may be decreased if taken with food. Milk has no effect on absorption.
Herb/Nutraceutical: Avoid evening primrose (seizure threshold decreased)

Lab Interactions Valproic acid may cause abnormalities in liver function tests; false-positive result for urine ketones; accuracy of thyroid function tests

Adverse Reactions

Adverse reactions reported when used as monotherapy for complex partial seizure:
>10%:
Central nervous system: Headache (up to 31%), somnolence (7% to 30%), dizziness (12% to 25%), insomnia (1% to 15%), nervousness (1% to 11%), pain (up to 11%)
Dermatologic: Alopecia (6% to 24%)
Gastrointestinal: Nausea (15% to 48%), vomiting (7% to 27%), diarrhea (7% to 23%), abdominal pain (7% to 23%), dyspepsia (7% to 23%), anorexia (11% to 12%)
Hematologic: Thrombocytopenia (1% to 24%)
Neuromuscular & skeletal: Tremor (1% to 57%), weakness (6% to 27%)
Ocular: Diplopia (up to 16%), amblyopia/blurred vision (8% to 12%)
Miscellaneous: Infection (1% to 20%), flu-like symp-toms (1% to 12%)
1% to 10%:
Cardiovascular: Arrhythmia, chest pain, edema, hyper-/hypotension, palpitation, peripheral edema (1% to 8%), postural hypotension, tachycardia, vasodilatation
Central nervous system: Abnormal dreams, agitation, amnesia (5% to 7%), anxiety, catatonic reaction, chills, confusion, depression, emotional lability, hallucinations, hypokinesia, malaise, personality disorder, psychosis, reflexes increased, sleep disorder, speech disorder, tardive dyskinesia, thinking abnormal (up to 6%), vertigo
Dermatologic: Bruising, discoid lupus erythematosus, dry skin, erythema nodosum, furunculosis, macropapular rash, petechia, pruritus, rash, sebor-rhea, vesiculobullous rash
Endocrine & metabolic: Amenorrhea, dysmenorrhea, hypoproteinemia, metrorrhagia
Gastrointestinal: Dysphagia, eructation, fecal inconti-nence, flatulence, gastroenteritis, glossitis, gum hemorrhage, hematemesis, appetite increased, mouth ulceration, pancreatitis, periodontal abscess, taste perversion, weight gain (1% to 9%), stomatitis, constipation, dry mouth, tooth disorder, weight loss (up to 6%)
Genitourinary: Cystitis, urinary frequency, urinary incontinence, UTI, vaginitis
Hematologic: Anemia, bleeding time increased, leuko-penia
Hepatic: AST/ALT increased
Neuromuscular & skeletal: Abnormal gait, arthralgia, arthrosis, ataxia (up to 8%), back pain (1% to 8%), hypertonia, leg cramps, myalgia, myasthenia, neck rigidity, paresthesia, twitching
Ocular: Abnormal vision, conjunctivitis, dry eye, eye pain, nystagmus (7% to 8%), photophobia
Otic: Deafness, otitis media, tinnitus (1% to 7%)
Respiratory: Bronchitis, epistaxis, hiccup, increased cough, pneumonia, rhinitis, sinusitis

Additional adverse effects: Frequency not defined:
Cardiovascular: Bradycardia
Central nervous system: Aggression, behavioral dete-rioration, cerebral atrophy (reversible), dementia, encephalopathy (rare), hostility, hyperactivity, hypo-esthesia, parkinsonism

Dermatologic: Cutaneous vasculitis, erythema multiforme, photosensitivity, Stevens-Johnson syndrome, toxic epidermal necrolysis (rare)

Endocrine & metabolic: Breast enlargement, galactorrhea, hyperammonemia, hyponatremia, inappropriate ADH secretion, parotid gland swelling, polycystic ovary disease (rare), abnormal thyroid function tests

Genitourinary: Enuresis

Hematologic: Anemia, aplastic anemia, bone marrow suppression, eosinophilia, hematoma formation, hemorrhage, hypofibrinogenemia, intermittent porphyria, lymphocytosis, macrocytosis, pancytopenia

Hepatic: Bilirubin increased, hyperammonemic encephalopathy (in patients with UCD)

Neuromuscular & skeletal: Asterixis, bone pain, dysarthria

Ocular: Seeing "spots before the eyes"

Renal: Fanconi-like syndrome (rare, in children)

Miscellaneous: Anaphylaxis, carnitine decreased, hyperglycinemia, lupus

Postmarketing and/or case reports: Life-threatening pancreatitis (2 cases out of 2416 patients), occurring at the start of therapy or following years of use, has been reported in adults and children. Some cases have been hemorrhagic with rapid progression of initial symptoms to death. Cases have also been reported upon rechallenge.

Overdosage/Toxicology Symptoms of overdose include coma, deep sleep, motor restlessness, and visual hallucinations. Supportive treatment is indicated. Naloxone has been used to reverse CNS depressant effects, but may block the action of other anticonvulsants.

Pharmacodynamics/Kinetics

Time to Peak: Serum: 1-4 hours; Divalproex (enteric coated): 3-5 hours

Protein Binding: Dose dependent: 80% to 90%

Half-Life Elimination: Increased in neonates and with liver disease; Children: 4-14 hours; Adults: 9-16 hours

Metabolism: Extensively hepatic via glucuronide conjugation and mitochondrial beta-oxidation. The relationship between dose and total valproate concentration is nonlinear; concentration does not increase proportionally with the dose, but increases to a lesser extent due to saturable plasma protein binding. The kinetics of unbound drug are linear.

Excretion: Urine (30% to 50% as glucuronide conjugate, 3% as unchanged drug)

Available Dosage Forms Note: Strength expressed as valproic acid

Capsule, as valproic acid (Depakene®): 250 mg

Capsule, sprinkles, as divalproex sodium (Depakote® Sprinkle®): 125 mg

Injection, solution, as valproate sodium (Depacon®): 100 mg/mL (5 mL) [contains edetate disodium]

Syrup, as valproic acid: 250 mg/5 mL (480 mL)
Depakene®: 250 mg/5 mL (480 mL)

Tablet, delayed release, as divalproex sodium (Depakote®): 125 mg, 250 mg, 500 mg

Tablet, extended release, as divalproex sodium (Depakote® ER): 250 mg, 500 mg

Dosing

Adults & Elderly:

Seizures:

Oral: Initial: 10-15 mg/kg/day in 1-3 divided doses; increase by 5-10 mg/kg/day at weekly intervals until therapeutic levels are achieved; maintenance: 30-60 mg/kg/day. Adult usual dose: 1000-2500 mg/day. **Note:** Regular release and delayed release formulations are usually given in 2-4 divided doses/day, extended release formulation (Depakote® ER) is usually given once daily. Conversion to Depakote® ER from a stable dose of Depakote® may require an increase in the total

daily dose between 8% and 20% to maintain similar serum concentrations.

I.V.: Administer as a 60-minute infusion (≤20 mg/minute) with the same frequency as oral products; switch patient to oral products as soon as possible. Alternatively, rapid infusions have been given: ≤15 mg/kg over 5-10 minutes (1.5-3 mg/kg/minute).

Rectal (unlabeled): Dilute syrup 1:1 with water for use as a retention enema; loading dose: 17-20 mg/kg one time; maintenance: 10-15 mg/kg/dose every 8 hours

Status epilepticus (unlabeled use):

Loading dose: I.V.: 15-25 mg/kg administered at 3 mg/kg/minute

Maintenance dose: I.V. infusion: 1-4 mg/kg/hour; titrate dose as needed based upon patient response and evaluation of drug-drug interactions

Mania:

Oral: 750-1500 mg/day in divided doses; dose should be adjusted as rapidly as possible to desired clinical effect; a loading dose of 20 mg/kg may be used; maximum recommended dosage: 60 mg/kg/day

Extended release tablets: Initial: 25 mg/kg/day given once daily; dose should be adjusted as rapidly as possible to desired clinical effect; maximum recommended dose: 60 mg/kg/day.

Migraine prophylaxis: Oral:

Extended release tablets: 500 mg once daily for 7 days, then increase to 1000 mg once daily; adjust dose based on patient response; usual dosage range 500-1000 mg/day

Delayed release tablets: 250 mg twice daily; adjust dose based on patient response, up to 1000 mg/day

Pediatrics: Seizures: Oral, I.V., Rectal: Children ≥10 years: Refer to adult dosing.

Renal Impairment: A 27% reduction in clearance of unbound valproate is seen in patients with Cl_{cr} <10 mL/minute. Hemodialysis reduces valproate concentrations by 20%, therefore no dose adjustment is needed in patients with renal failure. Protein binding is reduced, monitoring only total valproate concentrations may be misleading.

Hepatic Impairment: Dosage reduction is required. Clearance is decreased with liver impairment. Hepatic disease is also associated with decreased albumin concentrations and 2- to 2.6-fold increase in the unbound fraction. Free concentrations of valproate may be elevated while total concentrations appear normal.

Administration

Oral: Do not crush delayed release or extended release drug product or capsules.

I.V.: Depacon®: Following dilution to final concentration, administer over 60 minutes at a rate of ≤20 mg/minute. Alternatively, single doses up to 15 mg/kg have been administered as a rapid infusion over 5-10 minutes (1.5-3 mg/kg/minute).

Stability

Reconstitution: Injection should be diluted in 50 mL of a compatible diluent; is physically compatible and chemically stable in D_5W, NS, and LR for at least 24 hours when stored in glass or PVC.

Storage: Store vials at room temperature 15°C to 30°C (59°F to 86°F).

Laboratory Monitoring Liver enzymes, CBC with platelets, PT/PTT, serum ammonia (with symptoms of lethargy, mental status change)

Nursing Actions

Physical Assessment: Assess effectiveness and interactions of other medications patient may be taking. **I.V.:** Keep patient under observation (vital signs; neurological, cardiac, and respiratory status), (Continued)

Valproic Acid and Derivatives
(Continued)

observe safety/seizure precautions, and monitor therapeutic response (seizure activity, force, type, duration). For outpatients, monitor therapeutic effect (seizure activity, frequency, force, type, duration), laboratory values, and adverse reactions at beginning of therapy and periodically with long-term use. Assess knowledge/teach patient seizure safety precautions, appropriate use, interventions to reduce side effects, and adverse symptoms to report. **Note:** Valproic acid will alter results of urine ketones (use serum glucose testing) and reduce effectiveness of oral contraceptives (use alternative form of contraception to prevent pregnancy). Some adverse reactions including hepatic failure and thrombocytopenia can occur 3 days to 6 months after beginning therapy.

Patient Education: When used to treat generalized seizures, patient instructions are determined by patient's condition and ability to understand. **Oral:** Take as directed; do not alter dose or timing of medication. Do not increase dose or take more than recommended. Do not crush or chew capsule or enteric-coated pill. While using this medication, do not use alcohol and other prescription or OTC medications (especially pain medications, sedatives, antihistamines, or hypnotics) without consulting prescriber. Maintain adequate hydration (2-3 L/day of fluids) unless instructed to restrict fluid intake. If you have diabetes, monitor serum glucose closely (valproic acid will alter results of urine ketones). You may experience headache; sleepiness or dizziness (use caution when driving or engaging in tasks requiring alertness until response to drug is known); visual changes; and hair loss. Report alterations in menstrual cycle; abdominal cramps, unresolved diarrhea, vomiting, or constipation; skin rash; unusual bruising or bleeding; blood in urine, stool, or vomitus; malaise; weakness; facial swelling; yellowing of skin or eyes; persistent abdominal pain; excessive sedation; or restlessness. **Pregnancy/breast-feeding precautions:** Do not get pregnant while taking this medication; use appropriate contraceptive measures. Consult prescriber if breast-feeding.

Dietary Considerations Valproic acid may cause GI upset; take with large amount of water or food to decrease GI upset. May need to split doses to avoid GI upset.

Coated particles of divalproex sodium may be mixed with semisolid food (eg, applesauce or pudding) in patients having difficulty swallowing; particles should be swallowed and not chewed

Valproate sodium oral solution will generate valproic acid in carbonated beverages and may cause mouth and throat irritation; do not mix valproate sodium oral solution with carbonated beverages; sodium content of valproate sodium syrup (5 mL): 23 mg (1 mEq)

Breast-Feeding Issues Crosses into breast milk. AAP considers **compatible** with breast-feeding.

Pregnancy Issues Crosses the placenta. Neural tube, cardiac, facial (characteristic pattern of dysmorphic facial features), skeletal, multiple other defects reported. Epilepsy itself, number of medications, genetic factors, or a combination of these probably influence the teratogenicity of anticonvulsant therapy. Risk of neural tube defects with use during first 30 days of pregnancy warrants discontinuation prior to pregnancy and through this period of possible. Use in women of childbearing potential requires that benefits of use in mother be weighed against the potential risk to fetus, especially when used for conditions not associated with permanent injury or risk of death (eg, migraine).

Additional Information Extended release tablets have 10% to 20% less fluctuation in serum concentration than delayed release tablets. Extended release tablets are not bioequivalent to delayed release tablets.

Related Information
Peak and Trough Guidelines *on page 1387*

Valrubicin (val ROO bi sin)

U.S. Brand Names Valstar® [DSC]

Synonyms AD3L; N-trifluoroacetyladriamycin-14-valerate

Pharmacologic Category Antineoplastic Agent, Anthracycline

Medication Safety Issues
Sound-alike/look-alike issues:
Valstar® may be confused with valsartan

Pregnancy Risk Factor C

Lactation Excretion in breast milk unknown/not recommended

Use Intravesical therapy of BCG-refractory carcinoma *in situ* of the urinary bladder

Mechanism of Action/Effect Blocks function of DNA topoisomerase II; inhibits DNA synthesis, causes extensive chromosomal damage, and arrests cell development; unlike other anthracyclines, does not appear to intercalate DNA

Contraindications Hypersensitivity to anthracyclines, Cremophor® EL, or any component of the formulation; concurrent urinary tract infection or small bladder capacity (unable to tolerate a 75 mL instillation)

Warnings/Precautions Hazardous agent - use appropriate precautions for handling and disposal. Do not administer if mucosal integrity of bladder has been compromised or bladder perforation is present. Irritable bladder symptoms may occur during instillation and retention. Caution in patients with severe irritable bladder symptoms. Valrubicin should be used cautiously (if at all) in patients having a history of hypersensitivity reactions to other medications prepared with Cremophor® EL.

Drug Interactions
Decreased Effect: No specific drug interactions studies have been performed. Systemic exposure to valrubicin is negligible, and interactions are unlikely.

Increased Effect/Toxicity: No specific drug interactions studies have been performed. Systemic exposure to valrubicin is negligible, and interactions are unlikely.

Adverse Reactions
>10%: Genitourinary: Frequency (61%), dysuria (56%), urgency (57%), bladder spasm (31%), hematuria (29%), bladder pain (28%), urinary incontinence (22%), cystitis (15%), urinary tract infection (15%)
1% to 10%:
Cardiovascular: Chest pain (2%), vasodilation (2%), peripheral edema (1%)
Central nervous system: Headache (4%), malaise (4%), dizziness (3%), fever (2%)
Dermatologic: Rash (3%)
Endocrine & metabolic: Hyperglycemia (1%)
Gastrointestinal: Abdominal pain (5%), nausea (5%), diarrhea (3%), vomiting (2%), flatulence (1%)
Genitourinary: Nocturia (7%), burning symptoms (5%), urinary retention (4%), urethral pain (3%), pelvic pain (1%), hematuria (microscopic) (3%)
Hematologic: Anemia (2%)
Neuromuscular & skeletal: Weakness (4%), back pain (3%), myalgia (1%)
Respiratory: Pneumonia (1%)

Overdosage/Toxicology Inadvertent paravenous extravasation has not been associated with skin ulceration or necrosis. Myelosuppression is possible following inadvertent systemic administration, or following significant systemic absorption from intravesical instillation.

Pharmacodynamics/Kinetics

Metabolism: Negligible after intravesical instillation and 2 hour retention

Excretion: Urine when expelled from urinary bladder (98.6% as intact drug; 0.4% as N-trifluoroacetyladriamycin)

Available Dosage Forms [DSC] = Discontinued product

Injection, solution [DSC]: 40 mg/mL (5 mL) [contains Cremophor® EL 50% (polyoxyethyleneglycol trini-noleate) and dehydrated alcohol 50%]

Dosing

Adults & Elderly: Urinary carcinoma *in situ*: Intravesical: 800 mg once weekly for 6 weeks

Renal Impairment: No adjustment is necessary.

Hepatic Impairment: No adjustment necessary.

Administration

I.V.: Valrubicin is administered as an intravesicular bladder lavage, usually in 75 mL of 0.9% sodium chloride injection. The drug is retained in the bladder for 2 hours, then voided. Due to the Cremophor® EL diluent, valrubicin should be administered through non-PVC tubing.

Stability

Reconstitution: Allow vial to warm to room temperature without heating. Dilute 800 mg (20 mL) with 55 mL NS.

Storage: Store unopened vials under refrigeration at 2°C to 8°C (36°F to 48°F). Stable for 12 hours when diluted in 0.9% sodium chloride.

Laboratory Monitoring Cystoscopy, biopsy, and urine cytology every 3 months for recurrence or progression

Nursing Actions

Physical Assessment: This medication is administered by a physician through a urinary bladder catheter, using aseptic technique. **Note:** Caution must be used to prevent exposure to this mediation. Monitor patient response during and following instillation (genitourinary [frequency, urgency, incontinence or dysuria, bladder spasm or pain, hematuria, urinary tract infection], rash, nausea, vomiting, myalgia, hyperglycemia). Instruct patient on appropriate interventions to reduce side effects and adverse symptoms to report.

Patient Education: This medication will be instilled into your bladder through a catheter to be retained for as long as possible. Your urine will be red tinged for the next 24 hours; report promptly if this continues for a longer period. May cause altered urination patterns (frequency, dysuria, or incontinence), some bladder pain, pain on urination, or pelvic pain; report if these persist. If you have diabetes, monitor glucose levels closely (may cause hyperglycemia). It is important that you maintain adequate hydration (2-3 L/day of fluids) unless instructed to restrict fluid intake. May cause dizziness or fatigue (use caution when driving or engaging in tasks requiring alertness until response to drug is known); or nausea, vomiting, or taste disturbance (small, frequent meals, frequent mouth care, chewing gum, or sucking lozenges may help). Report chest pain or palpitations; persistent dizziness; swelling of extremities; persistent nausea, vomiting, diarrhea, or abdominal pain; muscle weakness, pain, or tremors; unusual cough or respiratory difficulty; or other adverse effects. **Pregnancy/breast-feeding precautions:** Inform prescriber if you are pregnant. Do not get pregnant while taking this medication and for 1 month following therapy; consult prescriber for appropriate barrier contraceptives. Breast-feeding is not recommended.

Breast-Feeding Issues It is not known whether valrubicin is secreted in human milk. Because many immunoglobulins are secreted in milk, and the potential for serious adverse reactions exists, a decision should be made whether to discontinue nursing or discontinue the drug, taking into account the importance of the drug to the mother.

Valsartan (val SAR tan)

U.S. Brand Names Diovan®

Pharmacologic Category Angiotensin II Receptor Blocker

Medication Safety Issues

Sound-alike/look-alike issues:

Valsartan may be confused with losartan, Valstar™

Diovan® may be confused with Darvon®, Dioval®, Zyban®

Pregnancy Risk Factor C/D (2nd and 3rd trimesters)

Lactation Excretion in breast milk unknown/contraindicated

Use Alone or in combination with other antihypertensive agents in the treatment of essential hypertension; treatment of heart failure (NYHA Class II-IV); reduction of cardiovascular mortality in patients with left ventricular dysfunction postmyocardial infarction

Mechanism of Action/Effect Valsartan produces direct antagonism of the angiotensin II (AT2) receptors. Valsartan blocks the vasoconstrictor and aldosterone-secreting effects of angiotensin II. It displaces angiotensin II from the AT1 receptor and produces its blood pressure lowering effects by antagonizing AT1-induced vasoconstriction, aldosterone release, catecholamine release, arginine vasopressin release, water intake, and hypertrophic responses. This action results in more efficient blockade of the cardiovascular effects of angiotensin II and fewer side effects than the ACE inhibitors.

Contraindications Hypersensitivity to valsartan or any component of the formulation; hypersensitivity to other A-II receptor antagonists; bilateral renal artery stenosis; pregnancy (2nd and 3rd trimesters)

Warnings/Precautions During the initiation of therapy, hypotension may occur, particularly in patients with heart failure or post-MI patients. Avoid use or use a smaller dose in patients who are volume depleted; correct depletion first.

Deterioration in renal function can occur with initiation. Use with caution in unilateral renal artery stenosis and pre-existing renal insufficiency; significant aortic/mitral stenosis. Use caution in patients with severe renal impairment or significant hepatic dysfunction. Monitor renal function closely in patients with severe heart failure; changes in renal function should be anticipated and dosage adjustments of valsartan or concomitant medications may be needed.

Drug Interactions

Cytochrome P450 Effect: Inhibits CYP2C8/9 (weak)

Decreased Effect: Phenobarbital, ketoconazole, troleandomycin, sulfaphenazole

Increased Effect/Toxicity: Valsartan blood levels may be increased by cimetidine and monoxidine; clinical effect is unknown. Concurrent use of potassium salts/supplements, co-trimoxazole (high dose), ACE inhibitors, and potassium-sparing diuretics (amiloride, spironolactone, triamterene) may increase the risk of hyperkalemia.

Nutritional/Ethanol Interactions

Food: Decreases rate and extent of absorption by 50% and 40%, respectively.

Herb/Nutraceutical: Avoid dong quai if using for hypertension (has estrogenic activity). Avoid ephedra, yohimbe, ginseng (may worsen hypertension). Avoid garlic (may have increased antihypertensive effect).

Adverse Reactions

>10%: Central nervous system: Dizziness (2% to 17%)

1% to 10%:

Cardiovascular: Hypotension (6% to 7%), postural hypotension (2%)

(Continued)

Valsartan *(Continued)*

Central nervous system: Fatigue (2% to 3%)
Endocrine & metabolic: Serum potassium increased (4% to 10%), hyperkalemia (<1% to 2%)
Gastrointestinal: Diarrhea (5%), abdominal pain (2%)
Hematologic: Neutropenia (2%)
Neuromuscular & skeletal: Arthralgia (3%), back pain (3%)
Renal: Creatinine increased >50% (4%)
Respiratory: Cough (3%)
Miscellaneous: Viral infection (3%)

Overdosage/Toxicology Only mild toxicity (hypotension, bradycardia, hyperkalemia) has been reported with large overdoses (up to 5 g of captopril and 300 mg of enalapril). No fatalities have been reported. Treatment is symptomatic. Not removed by hemodialysis.

Pharmacodynamics/Kinetics
Onset of Action: Antihypertensive effect: 2 weeks (maximal: 4 weeks)
Time to Peak: 2-4 hours
Protein Binding: 95%, primarily albumin
Half-Life Elimination: 6 hours
Metabolism: To inactive metabolite
Excretion: Feces (83%) and urine (13%) as unchanged drug
Available Dosage Forms Tablet: 40 mg, 80 mg, 160 mg, 320 mg

Dosing
Adults & Elderly:
Hypertension: Initial: 80 mg or 160 mg once daily (in patients who are not volume depleted); dose may be increased to achieve desired effect; maximum recommended dose: 320 mg/day
Heart failure: Initial: 40 mg twice daily; titrate dose to 80-160 mg twice daily, as tolerated; maximum daily dose: 320 mg
Left ventricular dysfunction after MI: Initial: 20 mg twice daily; titrate dose to target of 160 mg twice daily as tolerated; may initiate ≥12 hours following MI
Renal Impairment:
Cl$_{cr}$ >10 mL/minute: No dosage adjustment necessary.
Dialysis: Not significantly removed.
Hepatic Impairment: Mild to moderate liver disease: ≤80 mg/day

Administration
Oral: Administer with or without food.
Stability
Storage: Store at controlled room temperature of 15°C to 30°C (59°F to 86°F). Protect from moisture.
Laboratory Monitoring Baseline and periodic electrolyte panels, renal and liver function, urinalysis

Nursing Actions
Physical Assessment: Assess effectiveness and interactions with other pharmacological agents and herbal products patients may be taking (eg, concurrent use of potassium supplements, ACE inhibitors, potassium-sparing diuretics may increase risk of hyperkalemia). Monitor laboratory tests at baseline and periodically during therapy. Monitor therapeutic effectiveness (reduced hypertension) and adverse response on a regular basis during therapy (eg, changes in renal function, dizziness, bradycardia, cough, headache, nausea, hypotension, hyperkalemia). Teach patient appropriate use according to drug form and purpose of therapy, possible side effects/appropriate interventions, and adverse symptoms to report.
Patient Education: Do not take any new medication during therapy unless approved by prescriber (especially sleep remedies or antisleep products, cough or cold remedies, or weight-loss products). Take exactly as directed and do not discontinue without consulting prescriber. This drug does not eliminate need for diet or exercise regimen as recommended by prescriber. May cause dizziness or lightheadedness (use caution when driving or engaging in tasks that require alertness until response to drug is known); postural hypotension (use caution when rising from lying or sitting position or climbing stairs); diarrhea (boiled milk, buttermilk, or yogurt may help). Report changes in urinary pattern; swelling of extremities; unusual back ache; chest pain or palpitations; unrelenting headache; muscle weakness or pain; unusual cough; or other persistent adverse reactions. **Pregnancy/breast-feeding precautions:** Inform prescriber if you are or intend to become pregnant. This drug should not be used in the 2nd or 3rd trimester of pregnancy. Consult prescriber for appropriate contraceptive measures if necessary. Do not breast-feed.

Dietary Considerations Avoid salt substitutes which contain potassium. May be taken with or without food.

Pregnancy Issues Medications which act on the renin-angiotensin system are reported to have the following fetal/neonatal effects: Hypotension, neonatal skull hypoplasia, anuria, renal failure, and death; oligohydramnios is also reported. These effects are reported to occur with exposure during the 2nd and 3rd trimesters. Valsartan should be discontinued as soon as possible after pregnancy is detected.

Additional Information Valsartan may have an advantage over losartan due to minimal metabolism requirements and consequent use in mild to moderate hepatic impairment.

Valsartan and Hydrochlorothiazide
(val SAR tan & hye droe klor oh THYE a zide)

U.S. Brand Names Diovan HCT®
Synonyms Hydrochlorothiazide and Valsartan
Pharmacologic Category Angiotensin II Receptor Blocker Combination; Antihypertensive Agent, Combination; Diuretic, Thiazide
Pregnancy Risk Factor C/D (2nd and 3rd trimester)
Lactation Excretion in breast milk unknown/not recommended
Use Treatment of hypertension (not indicated for initial therapy)
Available Dosage Forms Tablet:
80 mg/12.5 mg: Valsartan 80 mg and hydrochlorothiazide 12.5 mg
160 mg/12.5 mg: Valsartan 160 mg and hydrochlorothiazide 12.5 mg
160 mg/25 mg: Valsartan 160 mg and hydrochlorothiazide 25 mg

Dosing
Adults & Elderly: Hypertension: Oral: Dose is individualized (combination substituted for individual components); dose may be titrated after 3-4 weeks of therapy.
Usual recommended starting dose of valsartan: 80 mg or 160 mg once daily when used as monotherapy in patients who are not volume depleted
Renal Impairment: Cl$_{cr}$ ≤30 mL/minute: Use of combination not recommended. Contraindicated in patients with anuria.
Hepatic Impairment: Use with caution.
Nursing Actions
Physical Assessment: See individual agents.
Patient Education: See individual agents. **Pregnancy/breast-feeding precautions:** Inform prescriber if you are or intend to become pregnant. Breast-feeding is not recommended.
Related Information
Hydrochlorothiazide *on page 610*
Valsartan *on page 1271*

Vancomycin (van koe MYE sin)

U.S. Brand Names Vancocin®

Synonyms Vancomycin Hydrochloride

Pharmacologic Category Antibiotic, Miscellaneous

Medication Safety Issues
Sound-alike/look-alike issues:
I.V. vancomycin may be confused with Invanz®
Vancomycin may be confused with vecuronium

Pregnancy Risk Factor C

Lactation Enters breast milk/use caution

Use Treatment of patients with infections caused by staphylococcal species and streptococcal species; used orally for staphylococcal enterocolitis or for antibiotic-associated pseudomembranous colitis produced by *C. difficile*

Mechanism of Action/Effect Inhibits bacterial cell wall synthesis

Contraindications Hypersensitivity to vancomycin or any component of the formulation; avoid in patients with previous severe hearing loss

Warnings/Precautions Use with caution in patients with renal impairment or those receiving other nephrotoxic or ototoxic drugs. Dosage modification is required in patients with impaired renal function (especially elderly).

Drug Interactions
Increased Effect/Toxicity: Increased toxicity with other ototoxic or nephrotoxic drugs. Increased neuromuscular blockade with most neuromuscular blocking agents.

Adverse Reactions
Oral:
>10%: Gastrointestinal: Bitter taste, nausea, vomiting
1% to 10%:
Central nervous system: Chills, drug fever
Hematologic: Eosinophilia
Parenteral:
>10%:
Cardiovascular: Hypotension accompanied by flushing
Dermatologic: Erythematous rash on face and upper body (red neck or red man syndrome - infusion rate related)
1% to 10%:
Central nervous system: Chills, drug fever
Dermatologic: Rash
Hematologic: Eosinophilia, reversible neutropenia

Overdosage/Toxicology Symptoms of overdose include ototoxicity and nephrotoxicity. There is no specific therapy for overdose with vancomycin. Care is symptomatic and supportive. Peritoneal filtration and hemofiltration (not dialysis) have been shown to reduce the serum concentration of vancomycin. High flux dialysis may remove up to 25% of the drug.

Pharmacodynamics/Kinetics
Time to Peak: Serum: I.V.: 45-65 minutes
Protein Binding: 10% to 50%
Half-Life Elimination: Biphasic: Terminal:
Newborns: 6-10 hours
Infants and Children 3 months to 4 years: 4 hours
Children >3 years: 2.2-3 hours
Adults: 5-11 hours; significantly prolonged with renal impairment
End-stage renal disease: 200-250 hours
Excretion: I.V.: Urine (80% to 90% as unchanged drug); Oral: Primarily feces

Available Dosage Forms
Capsule (Vancocin®): 125 mg, 250 mg
Infusion [premixed in iso-osmotic dextrose] (Vancocin®): 500 mg (100 mL); 1 g (200 mL)
Injection, powder for reconstitution: 500 mg, 1 g, 5 g, 10 g

Dosing
Adults:
Systemic infections: I.V.: Initial dosage recommendation: Normal renal function: 1 g every 12 hours **or** select individualized dosage based on weight (10-15 mg/kg)
Note: Select interval based on estimated Cl$_{cr}$ >60 mL/minute every 12 hours, 40-60 mL/minute every 24 hours, <40 mL/minute >24 hours; monitor levels.
Hospital"acquired pneumonia (HAP): 15 mg/kg/dose every 12 hours (American Thoracic Society/ATS guidelines)
Meningitis *(Pneumococcus or Staphylococcus)*: I.V.: 30-45 mg/kg/day in divided doses every 8-12 hours **or** 500-750 mg every 6 hours (with third-generation cephalosporin for PCN-resistant *Streptococcus pneumoniae*); maximum dose: 2-3 g/day
Prophylaxis for bacterial endocarditis: I.V.:
Dental, oral, or upper respiratory tract surgery: 1 g 1 hour before surgery
GI/GU procedure: 1 g plus 1.5 mg/kg gentamicin 1 hour prior to surgery
CNS infections:
Intrathecal: Dose: Up to 20 mg/day
Antibiotic lock technique (for catheter infections): 2 mg/mL in SWI/NS or D$_5$W; instill 3-5 mL into catheter port as a flush solution instead of heparin lock. **(Note:** Do not mix with any other solutions.)
Pseudomembranous colitis produced by *C. difficile*: Oral: 125 mg 4 times/day for 10 days. **Note:** Due to the emergence of resistant enterococci, the use of vancomycin is limited in most settings
Elderly: Elderly patients may require greater dosage reduction than expected. Best to individualize therapy; dose (mg/kg/24 hours) = (0.227 x Cl$_{cr}$) + 5.67. Refer to adult dosing.
Pediatrics:
Systemic infections: Initial dosage recommendation: I.V.:
Neonates:
Postnatal age ≤7 days:
<1200 g: 15 mg/kg/dose every 24 hours
≥1200 g: 10 mg/kg/dose divided every 8 hours
>2000 g: 15 mg/kg/dose every 12 hours
Postnatal age >7 days:
<1200 g: 15 mg/kg/dose every 24 hours
≥1200 g: 10 mg/kg/dose divided every 8 hours
Infants >1 month and Children: 40 mg/kg/day in divided doses every 6 hours
Prophylaxis for bacterial endocarditis: I.V.:
Dental, oral, or upper respiratory tract surgery: 20 mg/kg 1 hour prior to the procedure
GI/GU procedure: 20 mg/kg plus gentamicin 2 mg/kg 1 hour prior to surgery
CNS infections:
Intrathecal: **Note:** Vancomycin is available as a powder for injection and may be diluted to 1-5 mg/mL concentration in preservative-free 0.9% sodium chloride for administration into the CSF
Neonates: 5-10 mg/day
Children: 5-20 mg/day
I.V.: Infants >1 month and Children with staphylococcal central nervous system infection: 60 mg/kg/day in divided doses every 6 hours
Antibiotic lock technique (for catheter infections): 2 mg/mL in SWI/NS or D$_5$W; instill 3-5 mL into catheter port as a flush solution instead of heparin lock **(Note:** Do not mix with any other solutions)
Pseudomembranous colitis produced by *C. difficile*: Oral:
Neonates: 10 mg/kg/day in divided doses
Children: 40 mg/kg/day in divided doses, added to fluids
Note: Use is restricted in most settings
(Continued)

Vancomycin (Continued)

Renal Impairment: Vancomycin levels should be monitored in patients with any renal impairment.

Cl_{cr} >60 mL/minute: Start with 1 g or 10-15 mg/kg/dose every 12 hours.

Cl_{cr} 40-60 mL/minute: Start with 1 g or 10-15 mg/kg/dose every 24 hours.

Cl_{cr} <40 mL/minute: Will need longer intervals; determine by serum concentration monitoring.

Hemodialysis: Not dialyzable (0% to 5%); generally not removed; exception minimal-moderate removal by some of the newer high-flux filters. Dose may need to be administered more frequently. Monitor serum concentrations.

Continuous ambulatory peritoneal dialysis (CAPD): Not significantly removed; administration via CAPD fluid: 15-30 mg/L (15-30 mcg/mL) of CAPD fluid.

Continuous arteriovenous hemofiltration: Dose as for Cl_{cr} 10-40 mL/minute.

Antibiotic lock technique (for catheter infections): 2 mg/mL in SWI/NS or D_5W; instill 3-5 mL into catheter port as a flush solution instead of heparin lock (**Note:** Do not mix with any other solutions).

Hepatic Impairment: Reduce dose by 60%.

Administration

Oral: May be administered with food.

I.M.: Do not administer I.M.

I.V.: Administer vancomycin by I.V. intermittent infusion over at least 60 minutes at a final concentration not to exceed 5 mg/mL.

If a maculopapular rash appears on the face, neck, trunk, and/or upper extremities (Red man syndrome), slow the infusion rate to over 1½ to 2 hours and increase the dilution volume. Hypotension, shock, and cardiac arrest (rare) have also been reported with too rapid of infusion. Reactions are often treated with antihistamines and steroids.

Extravasation treatment: Monitor I.V. site closely; extravasation will cause serious injury with possible necrosis and tissue sloughing. Rotate infusion site frequently.

I.V. Detail:
pH: 3.9 (in distilled water or sodium chloride 0.9%); 2.5-4.5 (5% solution in water)

Stability

Reconstitution: Reconstitute vials with 20 mL of SWFI for each 1 g of vancomycin (10 mL/500 mg vial; 20 mL/1 g vial; 100 mL/5 g vial; 200 mL/10 g vial). The reconstituted solution must be further diluted with at least 100 mL of a compatible diluent per 500 mg of vancomycin prior to parenteral administration.

Compatibility: Stable in dextran 6% in NS, D_5LR, D_5NS, D_5W, $D_{10}W$, LR, NS

Y-site administration: Incompatible with albumin, amphotericin B cholesteryl sulfate complex, cefepime, gatifloxacin, heparin, idarubicin, omeprazole

Compatibility in syringe: Incompatible with heparin

Compatibility when admixed: Incompatible with amobarbital, chloramphenicol, chlorothiazide, dexamethasone sodium phosphate, penicillin G potassium, pentobarbital, phenobarbital, phenytoin

Storage: Reconstituted 500 mg and 1 g vials are stable for at either room temperature or under refrigeration for 14 days. **Note:** Vials contain no bacteriostatic agent. Solutions diluted for administration in either D_5W or NS are stable under refrigeration for 14 days or at room temperature for 7 days.

Laboratory Monitoring Perform culture and sensitivity studies prior to first dose. Periodic renal function, urinalysis, serum vancomycin concentrations, WBC, audiogram with prolonged use. Obtain drug levels after the third dose unless otherwise directed. Peaks are drawn 1 hour after the completion of a 1- to 2-hour infusion. Troughs are obtained just before the next dose.

Nursing Actions

Physical Assessment: Assess results of culture and sensitivity tests and patient's allergy history prior to first dose. Use caution with renal impairment. Assess potential for interactions with other pharmacological agents patient may be taking (eg, concurrent use with anything that is ototoxic or nephrotoxic increases risk of toxicity). See Administration for infusion specifics (premedication with antihistamines may prevent or minimize "red man" reaction). Monitor infusion site closely to prevent extravasation. Assess results of laboratory tests, therapeutic effectiveness (resolution of infection), and adverse response (eg, hypotension, rash, neutropenia, nausea, vomiting, auditory changes) on a regular basis during therapy. Teach patient appropriate use (oral), possible side effects/appropriate interventions, and adverse symptoms to report.

Patient Education: Do not take any new medication during therapy unless approved by prescriber. With I.V. use, report immediately any chills; pain, swelling, or redness at infusion site; or respiratory difficulty. Take as directed with food, for as long as prescribed. Maintain adequate hydration (2-3 L/day of fluids) unless instructed to restrict fluid intake.

Oral/I.V.: May cause nausea, vomiting, or GI upset (small, frequent meals, frequent mouth care, sucking lozenges, or chewing gum may help). Report rash or hives; chills or fever; persistent GI disturbances; opportunistic infection (sore throat, chills, fever, burning, itching on urination, vaginal discharge, white plaques in mouth); respiratory difficulty; decreased urine output; chest pain or palpitations; changes in hearing or fullness in ears; or worsening of condition.

Pregnancy/breast-feeding precautions: Inform prescriber if you are or intend to become pregnant. Consult prescriber if breast-feeding.

Dietary Considerations May be taken with food.

Geriatric Considerations As a result of age-related changes in renal function and volume of distribution, accumulation and toxicity are a risk in the elderly. Careful monitoring and dosing adjustment is necessary.

Breast-Feeding Issues Vancomycin is excreted in breast milk but is poorly absorbed from the gastrointestinal tract. Therefore, systemic absorption would not be expected. Theoretically, vancomycin in the GI tract may affect the normal bowel flora in the infant, resulting in diarrhea.

Additional Information Because of its long half-life, vancomycin should be dosed on an every 12 hour basis; monitoring of peak and trough serum levels is advisable. The "red man syndrome" characterized by skin rash and hypotension is not an allergic reaction but rather is associated with too rapid infusion of the drug. To alleviate or prevent the reaction, infuse vancomycin at a rate of ≥30 minutes for each 500 mg of drug being administered (eg, 1 g over ≥60 minutes); 1.5 g over ≥90 minutes.

Related Information
Compatibility of Drugs on page 1370
Peak and Trough Guidelines on page 1387

Vardenafil (var DEN a fil)

U.S. Brand Names Levitra®

Synonyms Vardenafil Hydrochloride

Pharmacologic Category Phosphodiesterase-5 Enzyme Inhibitor

Medication Safety Issues
Sound-alike/look-alike issues:
Levitra® may be confused with Lexiva™

Pregnancy Risk Factor B

Lactation Excretion in breast milk unknown/not indicated for use in women.

Use Treatment of erectile dysfunction

Mechanism of Action/Effect Vardenafil enhances the effect of nitric oxide by inhibiting phosphodiesterase type 5 (PDE-5), resulting in smooth muscle relaxation and inflow of blood into the corpus cavernosum with sexual stimulation.

Contraindications Hypersensitivity to vardenafil or any component of the formulation; concurrent use of organic nitrates (nitroglycerin; scheduled dosing or as needed)

Warnings/Precautions There is a degree of cardiac risk associated with sexual activity; therefore, physicians may wish to consider the patient's cardiovascular status prior to initiating any treatment for erectile dysfunction. Use caution in patients with anatomical deformation of the penis (angulation, cavernosal fibrosis, or Peyronie's disease) and in patients who have conditions which may predispose them to priapism (sickle cell anemia, multiple myeloma, leukemia). Patients should be instructed to seek medical attention if erection persists >4 hours.

Not recommended for use in patients with congenital QT prolongation or those taking Class Ia or III antiarrhythmics. Concomitant use with alpha blockers may cause hypotension; safety of this combination may be affected by other antihypertensives and intravascular volume depletion. Patients should be hemodynamically stable prior to initiating therapy. Use caution with effective CYP3A4 inhibitors, the elderly, or those with hepatic impairment (Child-Pugh class B); dosage adjustment is needed.

Rare cases of nonarteritic ischemic optic neuropathy (NAION) have been reported; risk may be increased with history of vision loss. Other risk factors for NAION include heart disease, diabetes, hypertension, smoking, age >50 years, or history of certain eye problems.

Safety and efficacy have not been studied in patients with the following conditions, therefore, use in these patients is not recommended at this time: Hypotension, uncontrolled hypertension, unstable angina, severe cardiac failure; a life-threatening arrhythmia, myocardial infarction, or stroke within the last 6 months; severe hepatic impairment (Child-Pugh class C); end-stage renal disease requiring dialysis; retinitis pigmentosa or other degenerative retinal disorders. The safety and efficacy of vardenafil with other treatments for erectile dysfunction have not been studied and are not recommended as combination therapy.

Drug Interactions

Cytochrome P450 Effect: Substrate of CYP2C (minor), 3A5 (minor), 3A4 (major)

Increased Effect/Toxicity: CYP3A4 inhibitors may increase the levels/effects of vardenafil; example inhibitors include azole antifungals, clarithromycin, diclofenac, doxycycline, erythromycin, imatinib, isoniazid, nefazodone, nicardipine, propofol, protease inhibitors, quinidine, telithromycin, and verapamil. Nitroglycerin may lead to excessive hypotension; concomitant use is contraindicated. Alpha-blockers may also lead to excessive hypotension; initiate vardenafil at lowest possible dose if patient is stabilized on alpha blocker; initiate alpha-blocker at lowest possible dose and titrate cautiously in patients on a stable dose of vardenafil.

Nutritional/Ethanol Interactions

Food: High-fat meals decrease maximum serum concentration 18% to 50%. Serum concentrations/toxicity may be increased with grapefruit juice; avoid concurrent use.

Adverse Reactions

>10%:

Cardiovascular: Flushing (11%)

Central nervous system: Headache (15%)

2% to 10%:

Central nervous system: Dizziness (2%)

Gastrointestinal: Dyspepsia (4%), nausea (2%)

Neuromuscular & skeletal: CPK increased (2%)

Respiratory: Rhinitis (9%), sinusitis (3%)

Miscellaneous: Flu-like syndrome (3%)

Overdosage/Toxicology Doses of up to 120 mg caused back pain, myalgia, and/or abnormal vision in healthy volunteers. Treatment should be symptomatic and supportive.

Pharmacodynamics/Kinetics

Time to Peak: Plasma: 0.5-2 hours

Half-Life Elimination: Terminal: Vardenafil and metabolite: 4-5 hours

Metabolism: Hepatic via CYP3A4 (major), CYP2C and 3A5 (minor); forms metabolite (active)

Excretion: Feces (91% to 95% as metabolites); urine (2% to 6%)

Clearance: 56 L/hour

Available Dosage Forms Tablet: 2.5 mg, 5 mg, 10 mg, 20 mg

Dosing

Adults:

Erectile dysfunction: Oral: 10 mg 60 minutes prior to sexual activity; dosing range: 5-20 mg; to be given as one single dose and not given more than once daily

Dosing adjustment with concomitant medications:

Alpha blocker (dose should be stable at time of vardenafil initiation): Initial vardenafil dose: 5 mg/24 hours; if an alpha blocker is added to vardenafil therapy, it should be initiated at the smallest possible dose, and titrated carefully.

Erythromycin: Maximum vardenafil dose: 5 mg/24 hours

Indinavir: Maximum vardenafil dose: 2.5 mg/24 hours

Itraconazole:

200 mg/day: Maximum vardenafil dose: 5 mg/24 hours

400 mg/day: Maximum vardenafil dose: 2.5 mg/24 hours

Ketoconazole:

200 mg/day: Maximum vardenafil dose: 5 mg/24 hours

400 mg/day: Maximum vardenafil dose: 2.5 mg/24 hours

Ritonavir: Maximum vardenafil dose: 2.5 mg/72 hours

Elderly: Erectile dysfunction: Elderly ≥65 years: Oral: Initial: 5 mg 60 minutes prior to sexual activity; to be given as one single dose and not given more than once daily.

Renal Impairment: Dose adjustment not needed for mild, moderate, or severe impairment; use has not been studied in patients on renal dialysis.

Hepatic Impairment: Child-Pugh class B: Initial: 5 mg 60 minutes prior to sexual activity (maximum dose: 10 mg); to be given as one single dose and not given more than once daily.

Oral: May be administered with or without food, 60 minutes prior to sexual activity.

Stability

Storage: Store at controlled room temperature of 15°C to 30°C (59°F to 86°F).

Nursing Actions

Physical Assessment: Assess potential for interactions with other prescriptions, OTC medications, and herbal products patient may be taking. Teach patient proper use, possible side effects/appropriate interventions, and adverse symptoms to report.

Patient Education: Do not take any new medication during therapy without consulting prescriber. Use (Continued)

Vardenafil *(Continued)*

exactly as directed 60 minutes prior to sexual activity without regard to meals; avoid taking with high-fat meals or grapefruit juice. Do not combine with other approaches to treating erectile dysfunction without consulting prescriber. **Note:** This medication does not provide protection against sexually-transmitted diseases, including HIV. You may experience headache, flushing, or blurred vision (use caution when driving at night or in poorly lit environments until response is known). Report immediately chest pain; acute head pain; respiratory difficulty; change in vision (seeing a blue tinge to objects or having difficulty telling the difference between the colors blue and green); allergic response (chills, fever, respiratory difficulty, rash); genital swelling; erection lasting >4 hours; or other adverse reactions.

Dietary Considerations May take with or without food

Geriatric Considerations In adults ≥65 years of age, vardenafil plasma concentrations were higher than younger males (mean C_{max} was 34% higher), therefore, initial dose should be lower than the usual adult dose. See Pharmacodynamics/Kinetics and Dosing. Since older adults often have concomitant diseases, many of which may be contraindicated with the use of vardenafil, the prescriber should complete a thorough review of diseases and medications prior to prescribing vardenafil.

Vasopressin *(vay soe PRES in)*

U.S. Brand Names Pitressin®

Synonyms ADH; Antidiuretic Hormone; 8-Arginine Vasopressin

Pharmacologic Category Antidiuretic Hormone Analog; Hormone, Posterior Pituitary

Medication Safety Issues
Sound-alike/look-alike issues:
Pitressin® may be confused with Pitocin®

Pregnancy Risk Factor C

Lactation Enters breast milk/use caution

Use Treatment of diabetes insipidus; prevention and treatment of postoperative abdominal distention; differential diagnosis of diabetes insipidus

Unlabeled/Investigational Use Adjunct in the treatment of GI hemorrhage and esophageal varices; pulseless arrest (ventricular tachycardia [VT]/ventricular fibrillation [VF], asystole/pulseless electrical activity [PEA]); vasodilatory shock (septic shock)

Mechanism of Action/Effect Increases cyclic adenosine monophosphate (cAMP) which increases water permeability at the renal tubule resulting in decreased urine volume and increased osmolality; causes peristalsis by directly stimulating the smooth muscle in the GI tract; direct vasoconstrictor without inotropic or chronotropic effects

Contraindications Hypersensitivity to vasopressin or any component of the formulation

Warnings/Precautions Use with caution in patients with seizure disorders, migraine, asthma, vascular disease, renal disease, cardiac disease, chronic nephritis with nitrogen retention, goiter with cardiac complications, arteriosclerosis. I.V. infiltration may lead to severe vasoconstriction and localized tissue necrosis, gangrene of extremities or tongue, and ischemic colitis.

Drug Interactions
Decreased Effect: Lithium, epinephrine, demeclocycline, heparin, and ethanol block antidiuretic activity to varying degrees.
Increased Effect/Toxicity: Chlorpropamide, urea, clofibrate, carbamazepine, and fludrocortisone potentiate antidiuretic response.

Nutritional/Ethanol Interactions Ethanol: Avoid ethanol (due to effects on ADH).

Adverse Reactions Frequency not defined.
Cardiovascular: Arrhythmia, asystole (>0.4 units/minute), blood pressure increased, cardiac output decreased (>0.4 units/minute), chest pain, MI, vasoconstriction (with higher doses), venous thrombosis
Central nervous system: Pounding in the head, fever, vertigo
Dermatologic: Ischemic skin lesions, circumoral pallor, urticaria
Gastrointestinal: Abdominal cramps, flatulence, mesenteric ischemia, nausea, vomiting
Genitourinary: Uterine contraction
Neuromuscular & skeletal: Tremor
Respiratory: Bronchial constriction
Miscellaneous: Diaphoresis

Overdosage/Toxicology Symptoms of overdose include drowsiness, weight gain, confusion, listlessness, and water intoxication. Water intoxication requires withdrawal of the drug. Severe intoxication may require osmotic diuresis and loop diuretics.

Pharmacodynamics/Kinetics
Onset of Action: Nasal: 1 hour
Duration of Action: Nasal: 3-8 hours; I.M., SubQ: 2-8 hours
Half-Life Elimination: Nasal: 15 minutes; Parenteral: 10-20 minutes
Metabolism: Nasal/Parenteral: Hepatic, renal
Excretion: Nasal: Urine; Parenteral: SubQ: Urine (5% as unchanged drug) after 4 hours

Available Dosage Forms
Injection, solution: 20 units/mL (0.5 mL, 1 mL, 10 mL)
Pitressin®: 20 units/mL (1 mL)

Dosing
Adults & Elderly:
Diabetes insipidus:
Note: Dosage is highly variable; titrated based on serum and urine sodium and osmolality in addition to fluid balance and urine output
I.M., SubQ: 5-10 units 2-4 times/day as needed (dosage range 5-60 units/day)
Continuous I.V. infusion: 0.5 milliunit/kg/hour (0.0005 unit/kg/hour); double dosage as needed every 30 minutes to a maximum of 0.01 unit/kg/hour
Intranasal: Administer on cotton pledget, as nasal spray, or by dropper
Abdominal distention: I.M.: 5 units stat, 10 units every 3-4 hours
GI hemorrhage (unlabeled use):
Continuous I.V. infusion: 0.5 milliunits/kg/hour (0.0005 unit/kg/hour); double dosage as needed every 30 minutes to a maximum of 10 milliunits/kg/hour
I.V.: Initial: 0.2-0.4 unit/minute, then titrate dose as needed; if bleeding stops, continue at same dose for 12 hours, taper off over 24-48 hours.
Pulseless arrest (unlabeled use) [ACLS protocol]:
I.V; I.O.: 40 units; may give one dose to replace first or second dose of epinephrine. I.V./I.O. drug administration is preferred, but if no access, may give endotracheally at 2 to 2 ½ times the I.V. dose. Mix with 5-10 mL of water or normal saline, and administer down the endotracheal tube.
Vasodilatory shock/septic shock (unlabeled use):
I.V.: Vasopressin has been used in doses of 0.01-0.1 units/minute for the treatment of septic shock. Doses >0.05 units/minute may have more cardiovascular side effects. Most case reports have used 0.04 units/minute continuous infusion as a fixed dose.

Pediatrics:

Diabetes insipidus:

Note: Dosage is highly variable; titrated based on serum and urine sodium and osmolality in addition to fluid balance and urine output

I.M., SubQ:

Children: 2.5-10 units 2-4 times/day as needed

Continuous I.V. infusion: Children: 0.5 milliunit/kg/hour (0.0005 unit/kg/hour); double dosage as needed every 30 minutes to a maximum of 0.01 unit/kg/hour

Intranasal: Administer on cotton pledget, as nasal spray, or by dropper

GI hemorrhage (unlabeled use): I.V. infusion: Dilute in NS or D₅W to 0.1-1 unit/mL

Children: Initial: 0.002-0.005 units/kg/minute; titrate dose as needed; maximum: 0.01 unit/kg/minute; continue at same dosage (if bleeding stops) for 12 hours, then taper off over 24-48 hours

Hepatic Impairment: Some patients respond to much lower doses with cirrhosis.

Administration

I.V.:

GI hemorrhage: Administration requires the use of an infusion pump and should be administered in a peripheral line.

Vasodilatory shock: Administration through a central catheter is recommended.

Infusion rates:

100 units in 500 mL D₅W rate

0.1 unit/minute: 30 mL/hour

0.2 units/minute: 60 mL/hour

0.3 units/minute: 90 mL/hour

0.4 units/minute: 120 mL/hour

0.5 units/minute: 150 mL/hour

0.6 units/minute: 180 mL/hour

I.V. Detail: Use extreme caution to avoid extravasation because of risk of necrosis and gangrene. In treatment of varices, infusions are often supplemented with nitroglycerin infusions to minimize cardiac effects.

Topical: Topical administration on nasal mucosa: Administer injectable vasopressin on cotton plugs, as nasal spray, or by dropper. Should not be inhaled.

Other: If no I.V. /I.O. access may give endotracheally at 2 to 2½ times the I.V. dose. Mix with 5-10 mL of water or normal saline, and administer down the endotracheal tube.

Stability

Compatibility: Stable in D₅W, NS

Storage: Store injection at room temperature. Protect from heat and from freezing. Use only clear solutions.

Laboratory Monitoring Serum and urine sodium, urine specific gravity, urine and serum osmolality

Nursing Actions

Physical Assessment: Assess potential for interactions with other pharmacological agents patient may be taking (eg, concurrent use that will block or enhance antidiuretic response). Note Administration for intravenous or intranasal use. I.V. requires use of infusion pump and close monitoring to prevent extravasation (may cause severe necrosis and gangrene). Monitor laboratory tests and adverse response (eg, cardiac status, blood pressure, CNS status, fluid balance, signs or symptoms of water intoxication, intranasal irritation) on a regular basis during therapy. Teach patient possible side effects/appropriate interventions and adverse symptoms to report.

Patient Education: Do not take any new medication during therapy unless approved by prescriber. Avoid alcohol. This drug will usually be administered by infusion or injection. Report immediately any redness, swelling, pain, or burning at infusion/injection site. When self-administered follow directions exactly. May cause dizziness, drowsiness (use caution when driving or engaging in potentially hazardous tasks

until response to drug is known); nausea, vomiting, cramping (small, frequent meals, frequent mouth care, chewing gum, or sucking lozenges may help), Report persistent nausea, vomiting, abdominal cramps; tremor, acute headache, or dizziness; chest pain or irregular heartbeat; respiratory difficulty or excess perspiration; CNS changes (confusion, drowsiness); or runny nose or painful nasal membranes (intranasal).

Geriatric Considerations Elderly patients should be cautioned not to increase their fluid intake beyond that sufficient to satisfy their thirst in order to avoid water intoxication and hyponatremia. Under experimental conditions, the elderly have shown to have a decreased responsiveness to vasopressin with respect to its effects on water homeostasis.

Breast-Feeding Issues Based on case reports, vasopressin and desmopressin have been used safely during nursing.

Pregnancy Issues Animal reproduction studies have not been conducted. Vasopressin and desmopressin have been used safely during pregnancy based on case reports.

Additional Information Vasopressin increases factor VIII levels and may be useful in hemophiliacs.

Vecuronium (ve KYOO roe ni um)

U.S. Brand Names Norcuron® [DSC]

Synonyms ORG NC 45

Pharmacologic Category Neuromuscular Blocker Agent, Nondepolarizing

Medication Safety Issues

Sound-alike/look-alike issues:

Vecuronium may be confused with vancomycin

Norcuron® may be confused with Narcan®

Pregnancy Risk Factor C

Lactation Excretion in breast milk unknown/use caution

Use Adjunct to general anesthesia to facilitate endotracheal intubation and to relax skeletal muscles during surgery; to facilitate mechanical ventilation in ICU patients; does not relieve pain or produce sedation

Mechanism of Action/Effect Blocks acetylcholine from binding to receptors on motor endplate inhibiting depolarization

Contraindications Hypersensitivity to vecuronium or any component of the formulation

Warnings/Precautions Ventilation must be supported during neuromuscular blockade; certain clinical conditions may result in potentiation or antagonism of neuromuscular blockade:

Potentiation: Electrolyte abnormalities, severe hyponatremia, severe hypocalcemia, severe hypokalemia, hypermagnesemia, neuromuscular diseases, acidosis, acute intermittent porphyria, renal failure, hepatic failure

Antagonism: Alkalosis, hypercalcemia, demyelinating lesions, peripheral neuropathies, diabetes mellitus

Increased sensitivity in patients with myasthenia gravis, Eaton-Lambert syndrome; resistance in burn patients (>30% of body) for period of 5-70 days postinjury; resistance in patients with muscle trauma, denervation, immobilization, infection; use with caution in patients with hepatic or renal impairment; does not counteract bradycardia produced by anesthetics/vagal stimulation. Cross-sensitivity with other neuromuscular-blocking agents may occur; use extreme caution in patients with previous anaphylactic reactions.

Drug Interactions

Increased Effect/Toxicity: Increased effects are possible with aminoglycosides, beta-blockers, clindamycin, calcium channel blockers, halogenated anesthetics, imipenem, ketamine, lidocaine, loop diuretics (Continued)

Vecuronium (Continued)

(furosemide), macrolides (case reports), magnesium sulfate, procainamide, quinidine, quinolones, tetracyclines, and vancomycin. May increase risk of myopathy when used with high- dose corticosteroids for extended periods.

Overdosage/Toxicology

Symptoms of overdose include prolonged skeletal muscle weakness and apnea cardiovascular collapse. Use neostigmine, edrophonium, or pyridostigmine with atropine to antagonize skeletal muscle relaxation; support of ventilation and the cardiovascular system through mechanical means, fluids, and pressors may be necessary.

Pharmacodynamics/Kinetics

Onset of Action: Good intubation conditions: Within 2.5-3 minutes; Maximum neuromuscular blockade: Within 3-5 minutes

Duration of Action: 20-40 minutes

Half-Life Elimination: 51-80 minutes

Metabolism: Active metabolite: 3-desacetyl vecuronium ($\frac{1}{2}$ the activity of parent drug)

Excretion: Primarily feces (40% to 75%); urine (30% as unchanged drug and metabolites)

Available Dosage Forms Injection, powder for reconstitution, as bromide: 10 mg, 20 mg [may be supplied with diluent containing benzyl alcohol]

Dosing

Adults & Elderly:

Neuromuscular blockade: I.V. (do not administer I.M.):

Initial: 0.08-0.1 mg/kg or 0.04-0.06 mg/kg after initial dose of succinylcholine for intubation

Maintenance: 0.01-0.015 mg/kg 25-40 minutes after initial dose, then 0.01-0.015 mg/kg every 12-15 minutes (higher doses will allow less frequent maintenance doses); may be administered as a continuous infusion at 0.8-2 mcg/kg/minute

Pretreatment/priming: Adults: 10% of intubating dose given 3-5 minutes before initial dose

Neuromuscular blockade in ICU patients: Adults: 0.05-0.1 mg/kg bolus followed by 0.8-1.7 mcg/kg/minute once initial recovery from bolus observed or 0.1-0.2 mg/kg/dose every 1 hour

Pediatrics:

Neuromuscular blockade: I.V. (do not administer I.M.):

Infants >7 weeks to 1 year: Initial: 0.08-0.1 mg/kg/dose; maintenance: 0.05-0.1 mg/kg/every 60 minutes as needed

Children >1 year: Refer to adult dosing.

Hepatic Impairment: Dose reductions are necessary in patients with liver disease.

Administration

I.V.: Concentration of 1 mg/mL may be administered by rapid I.V. injection. May further dilute reconstituted vial to 0.1-0.2 mg/mL in a compatible solution for I.V. infusion. Concentration of 1 mg/mL may be used for I.V. infusion in fluid-restricted patients.

I.V. Detail: pH: 4

Stability

Reconstitution: Reconstitute with compatible solution for injection to final concentration of 1 mg/mL.

Compatibility:

Incompatible with alkaline solutions/medications.

Y-Site administration: Incompatible with thiopental

Compatibility in syringe: Incompatible with thiopental

Storage: Store intact vials of powder for injection at room temperature 15°C to 30°C (59°F to 86°F). Vials reconstituted with bacteriostatic water for injection (BWFI) may be stored for 5 days under refrigeration or at room temperature. Vials reconstituted with other compatible diluents (nonbacteriostatic) should be stored under refrigeration and used within 24 hours.

Nursing Actions

Physical Assessment: Only clinicians experienced in the use of neuromuscular-blocking drugs should administer and/or manage the use of vecuronium. Ventilatory support must be instituted and maintained until adequate respiratory muscle function and/or airway protection are assured. Assess other medications for effectiveness and safety. Other drugs that affect neuromuscular activity may increase/decrease neuromuscular block induced by vecuronium. This drug does not cause anesthesia or analgesia; pain must be treated with appropriate analgesic agents. Continuous monitoring of vital signs, cardiac status, respiratory status, and degree of neuromuscular block (objective assessment with peripheral external nerve stimulator) is mandatory during infusion and until full muscle tone has returned. Muscle tone returns in predictable a pattern, starting with diaphragm, abdomen, chest, limbs, and finally muscles of the neck, face, and eyes. Safety precautions must be maintained until full muscle tone has returned. **Note:** It may take longer for return of muscle tone in obese or elderly patients or patients with renal or hepatic disease, dehydration, electrolyte imbalance, or severe acid/base imbalance. Provide appropriate patient teaching/support prior to and following administration.

Long-term use: Monitor fluid levels (intake and output) during and following infusion. Reposition patient and provide appropriate skin care, mouth care, and care of patient's eyes every 2-3 hours while sedated. Provide appropriate emotional and sensory support (auditory and environmental).

Patient Education: Patient will usually be unconscious prior to administration. Patient education should be appropriate to individual situation. Reassurance of constant monitoring and emotional support to reduce fear and anxiety should precede and follow administration. Following return of muscle tone, do not attempt to change position or rise from bed without assistance. Report immediately any skin rash or hives, pounding heartbeat, respiratory difficulty, or muscle tremors. **Pregnancy/breast-feeding precautions:** Inform prescriber if you are or intend to become pregnant. Consult prescriber if breast-feeding.

Pregnancy Issues Use in cesarean section has been reported. Umbilical venous concentrations were 11% of maternal.

Additional Information Vecuronium is classified as an intermediate-duration neuromuscular-blocking agent. It produces minimal, if any, histamine release; does not relieve pain or produce sedation. It may produce cumulative effect on duration of blockade.

Venlafaxine (VEN la faks een)

U.S. Brand Names Effexor®; Effexor® XR

Restrictions A medication guide concerning the use of antidepressants in children and teenagers can be found on the FDA website at http://www.fda.gov/cder/Offices/ODS/labeling.htm. It should be dispensed to parents or guardians of children and teenagers receiving this medication.

Pharmacologic Category Antidepressant, Serotonin/Norepinephrine Reuptake Inhibitor

Pregnancy Risk Factor C

Lactation Enters breast milk/not recommended

Use Treatment of major depressive disorder; generalized anxiety disorder (GAD), social anxiety disorder (social phobia); panic disorder

Unlabeled/Investigational Use Obsessive-compulsive disorder (OCD); hot flashes; neuropathic pain; attention-deficit/hyperactivity disorder (ADHD)

Mechanism of Action/Effect Venlafaxine and its active metabolite o-desmethylvenlafaxine (ODV) are potent inhibitors of neuronal serotonin and norepinephrine reuptake and weak inhibitors of dopamine reuptake. Venlafaxine and ODV have no significant activity for muscarinic cholinergic, H_1-histaminergic, or alpha$_2$-adrenergic receptors. Venlafaxine and ODV do not possess MAO-inhibitory activity.

Contraindications Hypersensitivity to venlafaxine or any component of the formulation; use of MAO inhibitors within 14 days; should not initiate MAO inhibitor within 7 days of discontinuing venlafaxine

Warnings/Precautions Antidepressants increase the risk of suicidal thinking and behavior in children and adolescents with major depressive disorder (MDD) and other depressive disorders; consider risk prior to prescribing. All patients must be closely monitored for clinical worsening, suicidality, or unusual changes in behavior, especially during the initiation of therapy or following an increase or decrease in dosage. When used in children, the child's family or caregiver should be instructed to closely observe the patient and communicate condition with healthcare provider. Reduced growth rate has been observed with venlafaxine therapy in children. A medication guide should be dispensed with each prescription. **Venlafaxine is not FDA approved for use in children.**

The possibility of a suicide attempt is inherent in major depression and may persist until remission occurs. Use caution in high-risk patients. Worsening depression and severe abrupt suicidality that are not part of the presenting symptoms may require discontinuation or modification of drug therapy. The patient's family or caregiver should be alerted to monitor patients for the emergence of suicidality and associated behaviors (such as agitation, irritability, hostility, impulsivity, and hypomania) and call healthcare provider.

May worsen psychosis in some patients or precipitate a shift to mania or hypomania in patients with bipolar disorder. Patients presenting with depressive symptoms should be screened for bipolar disorder. Monotherapy in patients with bipolar disorder should be avoided. **Venlafaxine is not FDA approved for the treatment of bipolar depression.**

The potential for severe reactions exists when used with MAO inhibitors (myoclonus, diaphoresis, hyperthermia, NMS features, seizures, and death). May cause sustained increase in blood pressure or tachycardia; dose related and increases are generally modest (12-15 mmHg diastolic). Use caution in patients with recent history of MI, unstable heart disease, or hyperthyroidism; may cause increase in anxiety, nervousness, insomnia; may cause weight loss (use with caution in patients where weight loss is undesirable); may cause increases in serum cholesterol. Use caution with hepatic or renal impairment. Venlafaxine has been associated with the development of SIADH and hyponatremia.

May increase the risks associated with electroconvulsive therapy. Use cautiously in patients with a history of seizures. The risks of cognitive or motor impairment, as well as the potential for anticholinergic effects are very low. May cause or exacerbate sexual dysfunction. May impair platelet aggregation, resulting in bleeding.

Abrupt discontinuation or dosage reduction after extended (≥6 weeks) therapy may lead to agitation, dysphoria, nervousness, anxiety, and other symptoms. When discontinuing therapy, dosage should be tapered gradually over at least a 2-week period. If intolerable symptoms occur following a decrease in dosage or upon discontinuation of therapy, then resuming the previous dose with a more gradual taper should be considered. Use caution in patients with increased intraocular pressure or at risk of acute narrow-angle glaucoma.

Drug Interactions

Cytochrome P450 Effect: Substrate of CYP2C8/9 (minor), 2C19 (minor), 2D6 (major), 3A4 (major); **Inhibits** CYP2B6 (weak), 2D6 (weak), 3A4 (weak)

Decreased Effect: Serum levels of indinavir may be reduced be venlafaxine (AUC reduced by 28%); clinical significance not determined. CYP3A4 inducers may decrease the levels/effects of venlafaxine; example inducers include aminoglutethimide, carbamazepine, nafcillin, nevirapine, phenobarbital, phenytoin, and rifamycins.

Increased Effect/Toxicity: Concurrent use of MAO inhibitors (phenelzine, isocarboxazid), or drugs with MAO inhibitor activity (linezolid) may result in serotonin syndrome; should not be used within 2 weeks of each other. Selegiline may have a lower risk of this effect, particularly at low dosages, due to selectivity for MAO type B. In addition, concurrent use of buspirone, lithium, meperidine, nefazodone, selegiline, serotonin agonists (sumatriptan, naratriptan), sibutramine, SSRIs, trazodone, or tricyclic antidepressants may increase the risk of serotonin syndrome. Serum levels of haloperidol may be increased by venlafaxine. CYP2D6 inhibitors may increase the levels/effects of venlafaxine; example inhibitors include chlorpromazine, delavirdine, fluoxetine, miconazole, paroxetine, pergolide, quinidine, quinine, ritonavir, and ropinirole. CYP3A4 inhibitors may increase the levels/effects of venlafaxine; example inhibitors include azole antifungals, clarithromycin, diclofenac, doxycycline, erythromycin, imatinib, isoniazid, nefazodone, nicardipine, propofol, protease inhibitors, quinidine, telithromycin, and verapamil.

Nutritional/Ethanol Interactions
Ethanol: Avoid ethanol (may increase CNS effects).
Herb/Nutraceutical: Avoid valerian, St John's wort, SAMe, kava kava, tryptophan (may increase risk of serotonin syndrome and/or excessive sedation).

Lab Interactions Increased thyroid, uric acid, glucose, potassium, AST, cholesterol (S)

Adverse Reactions
>10%:
Central nervous system: Headache (25% to 34%), insomnia (15% to 23%), somnolence (12% to 23%), dizziness (11% to 20%), nervousness (6% to 13%)
Gastrointestinal: Nausea (21% to 37%), xerostomia (12% to 22%), anorexia (8% to 20%), constipation (8% to 15%)
Genitourinary: Abnormal ejaculation/orgasm (2% to 16%)
Neuromuscular & skeletal: Weakness (8% to 17%)
Miscellaneous: Diaphoresis (10% to 14%)
1% to 10%:
Cardiovascular: Vasodilation (3% to 4%); hypertension (dose related; 3% in patients receiving <100 mg/day, up to 13% in patients receiving >300 mg/day); palpitation (3%), tachycardia (2%), chest pain (2%), postural hypotension (1%), edema
Central nervous system: Abnormal dreams (3% to 7%), anxiety (5% to 6%), yawning (3% to 5%), agitation (2% to 4%), chills (3%), confusion (2%), abnormal thinking (2%), depersonalization (1%), depression (1% to 3%), chills, fever, migraine, amnesia, hypoethesia, trismus, vertigo
Dermatologic: Rash (3%), pruritus (1%), bruising
Endocrine & metabolic: Libido decreased (3% to 9%)
Gastrointestinal: Diarrhea (6% to 8%), vomiting (3% to 6%), dyspepsia (5%), abdominal pain (4%), flatulence (3% to 4%), taste perversion (2%), weight loss (1% to 4%), appetite increased, weight gain
Genitourinary: Impotence (4% to 10%), urinary frequency (3%), impaired urination (2%), urinary retention (1%), prostatic disorder
Neuromuscular & skeletal: Tremor (4% to 5%), hypertonia (3%), paresthesia (2% to 3%), twitching (1% to 2%), neck pain, arthralgia
Ocular: Abnormal or blurred vision (4% to 6%), mydriasis (2%
Otic: Tinnitus (2%)
Respiratory: Pharyngitis (7%), sinusitis (2%), cough increased, dyspnea
(Continued)

Venlafaxine *(Continued)*

Miscellaneous: Infection (6%), flu-like syndrome (6%), trauma (2%)

Overdosage/Toxicology Symptoms of overdose include somnolence and occasionally tachycardia. Predominantly occurs in combination with ethanol and/or other drug use. Most overdoses resolve with only supportive treatment, though ECG monitoring would be prudent considering the risk of arrythmia. Use of activated charcoal, inductions of emesis, or gastric lavage should be considered for acute ingestion. Forced diuresis, dialysis, and hemoperfusion not effective due to large volume of distribution.

Pharmacodynamics/Kinetics

Time to Peak:

Immediate release: Venlafaxine: 2 hours, ODV: 3 hours

Extended release: Venlafaxine: 5.5 hours, ODV: 9 hours

Protein Binding: Bound to human plasma protein: Venlafaxine 27%, ODV 30%

Half-Life Elimination: Venlafaxine: 3-7 hours; ODV: 9-13 hours; Steady-state plasma: Venlafaxine/ODV: Within 3 days of multiple dose therapy

Prolonged with cirrhosis and dialysis:

Adults: Cirrhosis: Venlafaxine: ~30%, ODV: ~60%

Adults: Dialysis: Venlafaxine: ~180%, ODV: ~142%

Metabolism: Hepatic via CYP2D6 to active metabolite, O-desmethylvenlafaxine (ODV); other metabolites include N-desmethylvenlafaxine and N,O-didesmethylvenlafaxine

Excretion: Urine (~87%, 5% as unchanged drug, 29% as unconjugated ODV, 26% as conjugated ODV, 27% as minor inactive metabolites) within 48 hours

Clearance at steady state: Venlafaxine: 1.3 ± 0.6 L/hour/kg, ODV: 0.4 ± 0.2 L/hour/kg

Clearance decreased with:

Cirrhosis: Adults: Venlafaxine: ~50%, ODV: ~30%

Severe cirrhosis: Adults: Venlafaxine: ~90%

Renal impairment (Cl_{cr} 10-70 mL/minute): Adults: Venlafaxine: ~24%

Dialysis: Adults: Venlafaxine: ~57%, ODV: ~56%; due to large volume of distribution, a significant amount of drug is not likely to be removed.

Available Dosage Forms

Capsule, extended release (Effexor® XR): 37.5 mg, 75 mg, 150 mg

Tablet (Effexor®): 25 mg, 37.5 mg, 50 mg, 75 mg, 100 mg

Dosing

Adults:

Depression:

Immediate-release tablets: 75 mg/day, administered in 2 or 3 divided doses, taken with food; dose may be increased in 75 mg/day increments at intervals of at least 4 days, up to 225-375 mg/day

Extended-release capsules: 75 mg once daily taken with food; for some new patients, it may be desirable to start at 37.5 mg/day for 4-7 days before increasing to 75 mg once daily; dose may be increased by up to 75 mg/day increments every 4 days as tolerated, up to a maximum of 225 mg/day

GAD, social anxiety disorder: *Extended-release capsules:* 75 mg once daily taken with food; for some new patients, it may be desirable to start at 37.5 mg/day for 4-7 days before increasing to 75 mg once daily; dose may be increased by up to 75 mg/day increments every 4 days as tolerated, up to a maximum of 225 mg/day

Panic disorder: *Extended-release capsules:* 37.5 mg once daily for 1 week; may increase to 75 mg daily, with subsequent weekly increases of 75 mg/day up to a maximum of 225 mg/day.

Obsessive-compulsive disorder (unlabeled use): Titrate to usual dosage range of 150-300 mg/day; however, doses up to 375 mg daily have been used; response may be seen in 4 weeks

Neuropathic pain (unlabeled use): Dosages evaluated varied considerably based on etiology of chronic pain, but efficacy has been shown for many conditions in the range of 75-225 mg/day; onset of relief may occur in 1-2 weeks, or take up to 6 weeks for full benefit.

Hot flashes (unlabeled use): Doses of 37.5-75 mg/day have demonstrated significant improvement of vasomotor symptoms after 4-8 weeks of treatment; in one study, doses >75 mg/day offered no additional benefit; however, higher doses (225 mg/day) may be beneficial in patients with perimenopausal depression.

Attention-deficit disorder (unlabeled use): Initial: Doses vary between 18.75 to 75 mg/day; may increase after 4 weeks to 150 mg/day; if tolerated, doses up to 225 mg/day have been used

Note: When discontinuing this medication after more than 1 week of treatment, it is generally recommended that the dose be tapered. If venlafaxine is used for 6 weeks or longer, the dose should be tapered over 2 weeks when discontinuing its use.

Elderly: No specific recommendations for elderly, but may be best to start lower at 25-50 mg twice daily and increase as tolerated by 25 mg/dose. Extended-release formulation: 37.5 mg once daily, increase by 37.5 mg every 4-7 days as tolerated

Pediatrics: ADHD (unlabeled use): Children and Adolescents: Oral: Initial: 12.5 mg/day

Children <40 kg: Increase by 12.5 mg/week to maximum of 50 mg/day in 2 divided doses

Children ≥40 kg: Increase by 25 mg/week to maximum of 75 mg/day in 3 divided doses

Mean dose: 60 mg or 1.4 mg/kg administered in 2-3 divided doses

Renal Impairment:

Cl_{cr} 10-70 mL/minute: Decrease dose by 25%.

Hemodialysis: Decrease total daily dose by 50% given after completion of dialysis.

Hepatic Impairment: Reduce total dosage by 50%.

Administration

Oral: Administer with food.

Extended release capsule: Swallow capsule whole; do not crush or chew. Alternatively, contents may be sprinkled on a spoonful of applesauce and swallowed immediately without chewing; followed with a glass of water to ensure complete swallowing of the pellets.

Laboratory Monitoring Cholesterol

Nursing Actions

Physical Assessment: Assess other medications patient may be taking for effectiveness and interactions. Monitor therapeutic response (ie, mental status, mood, affect, clinical worsening, suicidal ideation), and adverse reactions at beginning of therapy and periodically with long-term use. Observe for clinical worsening, suicidality, or unusual behavior changes; especially during the initial few months of therapy or during dosage changes. Assess knowledge/teach patient appropriate use, interventions to reduce side effects, and adverse symptoms to report.

Patient Education: Take exactly as directed; do not increase dose or frequency. It may take 2-3 weeks to achieve desired results. Take with food. Extended release capsules should be swallowed whole; do not crush or chew. Alternatively, contents may be emptied onto a spoonful of applesauce and swallowed without chewing. Avoid alcohol, caffeine, and other prescription or OTC medications not approved by prescriber. Maintain adequate hydration (2-3 L/day of fluids) unless instructed to restrict fluid intake. You may experience excess drowsiness or insomnia, lightheadedness, dizziness, or blurred vision (use caution when driving or engaging in tasks requiring alertness until response to drug is known); headache, nausea, vomiting, anorexia, altered taste, dry mouth (small frequent meals, frequent mouth care, chewing gum, or sucking lozenges may help); constipation (increased exercise, fluids, fruit, or fiber may help); diarrhea (buttermilk, yogurt, or boiled milk may help); postural hypotension (use caution when climbing stairs or changing position from lying or sitting to standing); urinary retention (void before taking medication); or sexual dysfunction (reversible). Report persistent CNS effects (eg, insomnia, restlessness, fatigue, anxiety, abnormal thoughts, suicidal ideation, confusion, personality changes, impaired cognitive function); muscle cramping or tremors; chest pain, palpitations, rapid heartbeat, swelling of extremities, or severe dizziness; unresolved urinary retention; vision changes or eye pain; hearing changes or ringing in ears; skin rash or irritation; or worsening of condition. **Pregnancy/breast-feeding precautions:** Inform prescriber if you are or intend to become pregnant. Do not breast-feed.

Dietary Considerations Should be taken with food.

Geriatric Considerations Has not been studied exclusively in the elderly, however, its low anticholinergic activity, minimal sedative and hypotensive effects make this a potentially valuable antidepressant in treating elderly with depression. No dose adjustment is necessary for age alone, additional studies are necessary; adjust dose for renal function in the elderly.

Breast-Feeding Issues The manufacturer recommends discontinuing nursing or discontinuing venlafaxine, depending upon the importance of the drug to the mother.

Pregnancy Issues Teratogenic effects were not observed in animal studies. Nonteratogenic effects including respiratory distress, cyanosis, apnea, seizures, temperature instability, feeding difficulty, vomiting, hypoglycemia, hypo- or hypertonia, hyper-reflexia, jitteriness, irritability, constant crying, and tremor have been reported in the neonate immediately following delivery after exposure late in the third trimester. Adverse effects may be due to toxic effects of SNRI or drug discontinuation. There are no adequate and well-controlled studies in pregnant women. Use during pregnancy only if the potential benefit to the mother outweighs the possible risk to the fetus. If treatment during pregnancy is required, consider tapering therapy during the third trimester.

Related Information
Antidepressant Medication Guidelines *on page 1414*

Verapamil *(ver AP a mil)*

U.S. Brand Names Calan®; Calan® SR; Covera-HS®; Isoptin® SR; Verelan®; Verelan® PM

Synonyms Iproveratril Hydrochloride; Verapamil Hydrochloride

Pharmacologic Category Antiarrhythmic Agent, Class IV; Calcium Channel Blocker

Medication Safety Issues
Sound-alike/look-alike issues:
Verapamil may be confused with Verelan®
Calan® may be confused with Colace®
Covera-HS® may be confused with Provera®
Isoptin® may be confused with Isopto® Tears
Verelan® may be confused with verapamil, Virilon®, Voltaren®

Pregnancy Risk Factor C

Lactation Enters breast milk (small amounts)/not recommended

Use Orally for treatment of angina pectoris (vasospastic, chronic stable, unstable) and hypertension; I.V. for supraventricular tachyarrhythmias (PSVT, atrial fibrillation, atrial flutter)

Unlabeled/Investigational Use Migraine; hypertrophic cardiomyopathy; bipolar disorder (manic manifestations)

Mechanism of Action/Effect Inhibits calcium ion from entering the "slow channels" or select voltage-sensitive areas of vascular smooth muscle and myocardium during depolarization. Produces a relaxation of coronary vascular smooth muscle and coronary vasodilation. Increases myocardial oxygen delivery in patients with vasospastic (Prinzmetal's) angina. Slows automaticity and conduction of AV node.

Contraindications Hypersensitivity to verapamil or any component of the formulation; severe left ventricular dysfunction; hypotension (systolic pressure <90 mm Hg) or cardiogenic shock; sick sinus syndrome (except in patients with a functioning artificial pacemaker); second- or third-degree AV block (except in patients with a functioning artificial pacemaker); atrial flutter or fibrillation and an accessory bypass tract (WPW, Lown-Ganong-Levine syndrome)

Warnings/Precautions Avoid use in heart failure; can exacerbate condition. Can cause hypotension. Rare increases in liver function tests can be observed. Can cause first-degree AV block or sinus bradycardia. Other conduction abnormalities are rare. Use caution when using verapamil together with a beta-blocker. Avoid use of I.V. verapamil with an I.V. beta-blocker; can result in asystole. Use caution in patients with hypertrophic cardiomyopathy (IHSS). Use with caution in patients with attenuated neuromuscular transmission (Duchenne's muscular dystrophy, myasthenia gravis). Adjust the dose in severe renal dysfunction and hepatic dysfunction. Verapamil significantly increases digoxin serum concentrations (adjust digoxin's dose). May prolong recovery from nondepolarizing neuromuscular-blocking agents.

Drug Interactions
Cytochrome P450 Effect: Substrate of CYP1A2 (minor), 2B6 (minor), 2C8/9 (minor), 2C18 (minor), 2E1 (minor), 3A4 (major); **Inhibits** CYP1A2 (weak), 2C8/9 (weak), 2D6 (weak), 3A4 (moderate)

Decreased Effect: The levels/effects of verapamil may be decreased by aminoglutethimide, carbamazepine, nafcillin, nevirapine, phenobarbital, phenytoin, rifamycins, and other CYP3A4 inducers. Lithium levels may be decreased by verapamil. Nafcillin decreases plasma concentration of verapamil.

Increased Effect/Toxicity: Use of verapamil with amiodarone, beta-blockers, or flecainide may lead to bradycardia and decreased cardiac output. Aspirin and concurrent verapamil use may increase bleeding times. Lithium neurotoxicity may result when verapamil is added. Effect of nondepolarizing neuromuscular blocker is prolonged by verapamil. Grapefruit juice may increase verapamil serum concentrations. Blood pressure-lowering effects may be additive with sildenafil, tadalafil, and vardenafil (use caution).

Cisapride levels may be increased by verapamil, potentially resulting in life-threatening arrhythmias; avoid concurrent use. Verapamil may increase the levels/effects of selected benzodiazepines, other calcium channel blockers, cyclosporine, ergot alkaloids, selected HMG-CoA reductase inhibitors, mirtazapine, nateglinide, nefazodone, pimozide, quinidine, risperidone, sildenafil (and other PDE-5 inhibitors), tacrolimus, telithromycin, venlafaxine, and other CYP3A4 substrates. In addition, serum concentrations of the following drugs may be increased by verapamil: Alfentanil, digoxin, doxorubicin, ethanol, (Continued)

Verapamil *(Continued)*

prazosin, and theophylline. Verapamil may increase colchicine toxicity (especially nephrotoxicity).

The levels/effects of verapamil may be increased by azole antifungals, clarithromycin, diclofenac, doxycycline, erythromycin, imatinib, isoniazid, nefazodone, nicardipine, propofol, protease inhibitors, quinidine, telithromycin, and other CYP3A4 inhibitors.

Nutritional/Ethanol Interactions

Ethanol: Avoid or limit ethanol (may increase ethanol levels).

Food: Grapefruit juice may increase the serum concentration of verapamil; avoid concurrent use.

Herb/Nutraceutical: St John's wort may decrease levels. Avoid dong quai if using for hypertension (has estrogenic activity). Avoid ephedra, yohimbe, ginseng (may worsen arrhythmia or hypertension). Avoid garlic (may have increased antihypertensive effect).

Lab Interactions Increased alkaline phosphatase, CPK, LDH, aminotransferase [AST (SGOT)/ALT (SGPT)] (S)

Adverse Reactions

>10%: Gastrointestinal: Gingival hyperplasia (19%)

1% to 10%:

Cardiovascular: Bradycardia (1.4% oral, 1.2% I.V.); first-, second-, or third-degree AV block (1.2% oral, unknown I.V.); CHF (1.8% oral); hypotension (2.5% oral, 3% I.V.); peripheral edema (1.9% oral), symptomatic hypotension (1.5% I.V.); severe tachycardia (1% I.V.)

Central nervous system: Dizziness (3.3% oral, 1.2% I.V.), fatigue (1.7% oral), headache (2.2% oral, 1.2% I.V.)

Dermatologic: Rash (1.2% oral)

Gastrointestinal: Constipation (12% up to 42% in clinical trials), nausea (2.7% oral, 0.9% I.V.)

Respiratory: Dyspnea (1.4% oral)

Overdosage/Toxicology Primary cardiac symptoms of calcium blocker overdose include hypotension and bradycardia (second- or third-degree atrioventricular block, or sinus arrest with junctional rhythm). Intraventricular conduction is usually not affected so QRS duration is normal (verapamil does prolong the PR interval).

Noncardiac symptoms include confusion, stupor, nausea, vomiting, metabolic acidosis and hyperglycemia. Following initial gastric decontamination, if possible, repeated calcium administration may promptly reverse depressed cardiac contractility (but not sinus node depression or peripheral vasodilation). Large doses of calcium chloride (up to 1 g/hour for 24 hours) have been used in refractory cases. Glucagon, epinephrine, and amrinone may treat refractory hypotension. Glucagon and epinephrine also increase heart rate (outside the U.S., 4-aminopyridine may be available as an antidote). Dialysis and hemoperfusion are not effective in enhancing elimination although repeat-dose activated charcoal may serve as an adjunct with sustained-release preparations.

Pharmacodynamics/Kinetics

Onset of Action: Oral (immediate release tablets): Peak effect: 1-2 hours; I.V.: Peak effect: 1-5 minutes

Duration of Action: Oral: Immediate release tablets: 6-8 hours; I.V.: 10-20 minutes

Protein Binding: 90%

Half-Life Elimination: Infants: 4.4-6.9 hours; Adults: Single dose: 2-8 hours, Multiple doses: 4.5-12 hours; prolonged with hepatic cirrhosis

Metabolism: Hepatic via multiple CYP isoenzymes; extensive first-pass effect

Excretion: Urine (70%, 3% to 4% as unchanged drug); feces (16%)

Available Dosage Forms

Caplet, sustained release: 120 mg, 180 mg, 240 mg

Calan® SR: 120 mg, 180 mg, 240 mg

Capsule, extended release, controlled onset, as hydrochloride:

Verelan® PM: 100 mg, 200 mg, 300 mg

Capsule, sustained release, as hydrochloride: 120 mg, 180 mg, 240 mg, 360 mg

Verelan®: 120 mg, 180 mg, 240 mg, 360 mg

Injection, solution, as hydrochloride: 2.5 mg/mL (2 mL, 4 mL)

Tablet, as hydrochloride: 80 mg, 120 mg

Calan®: 40 mg, 80 mg, 120 mg

Tablet, extended release: 120 mg, 180 mg, 240 mg

Tablet, extended release, controlled onset, as hydrochloride:

Covera-HS®: 180 mg, 240 mg

Tablet, sustained release, as hydrochloride: 120 mg, 180 mg, 240 mg

Isoptin® SR: 120 mg, 180 mg, 240 mg

Dosing

Adults:

Angina: Oral: Initial: 80-120 mg twice daily (elderly or small stature: 40 mg twice daily); range: 240-480 mg/day in 3-4 divided doses

Hypertension: Oral:

Immediate release: 80 mg 3 times/day; usual dose range (JNC 7): 80-320 mg/day in 2 divided doses

Sustained release: 240 mg/day; usual dose range (JNC 7): 120-360 mg/day in 1-2 divided doses; 120 mg/day in the elderly or small patients (no evidence of additional benefit in doses >360 mg/day).

Extended release:

Covera-HS®: Usual dose range (JNC 7): 120-360 mg once daily (once-daily dosing is recommended at bedtime)

Verelan® PM: Usual dose range: 200-400 mg once daily at bedtime

Arrhythmia (SVT): I.V.: 2.5-5 mg (over 2 minutes); second dose of 5-10 mg (~0.15 mg/kg) may be given 15-30 minutes after the initial dose if patient tolerates, but does not respond to initial dose; maximum total dose: 20 mg

Elderly:

Oral: 120-480 mg/24 hours divided 3-4 times/day

Sustained release: 120 mg/day; adjust dose after 24 hours by increases of 120 mg/day. When switching from immediate release forms, total daily dose may remain the same. Controlled onset: initiate therapy with 180 mg in the evening; titrate upward as needed to obtain desired response and avoiding adverse effects.

Pediatrics: Children: SVT:

I.V.:

<1 year: 0.1-0.2 mg/kg over 2 minutes; repeat every 30 minutes as needed

1-15 years: 0.1-0.3 mg/kg over 2 minutes; maximum: 5 mg/dose, may repeat dose in 15 minutes if adequate response not achieved; maximum for second dose: 10 mg/dose

Oral (dose not well established):

1-5 years: 4-8 mg/kg/day in 3 divided doses **or** 40-80 mg every 8 hours

>5 years: 80 mg every 6-8 hours

Renal Impairment: Cl$_{cr}$ <10 mL/minute: Administer 50% to 75% of normal dose.

Hepatic Impairment: In cirrhosis, reduce dose to 20% to 50% of normal and monitor ECG.

Administration

Oral: Do not crush or chew sustained or extended release products.

Calan® SR, Isoptin® SR: Administer with food.

Verelan®, Verelan® PM: Capsules may be opened and the contents sprinkled on 1 tablespoonful of applesauce, then swallowed without chewing.

I.V.: Rate of infusion: Over 2 minutes

I.V. Detail: pH: 4.1-6.0

Stability

Compatibility: Stable in dextran 40 10% in NS, dextran 75 6% in NS, D₅LR, D₅½NS, D₅NS, D₅W, LR, ½NS, NS

Y-site administration: Incompatible with albumin, amphotericin B cholesteryl sulfate complex, ampicillin, nafcillin, oxacillin, propofol, sodium bicarbonate

Compatibility when admixed: Incompatible with albumin, amphotericin B, floxacillin, hydralazine, trimethoprim/sulfamethoxazole

Storage: Store injection at room temperature. Protect from heat and from freezing. Use only clear solutions. Protect I.V. solution from light.

Nursing Actions

Physical Assessment: Assess other medications patient may be taking for effectiveness and interactions. I.V. requires use of infusion pump and continuous cardiac and hemodynamic monitoring. Monitor laboratory tests, therapeutic response (cardiac status), and adverse reactions when beginning therapy, when titrating dosage, and periodically during long-term oral therapy. Assess knowledge/teach patient appropriate use (oral), interventions to reduce side effects, and adverse symptoms to report.

Patient Education: Oral: Take as directed. Do not alter dosage or discontinue therapy without consulting prescriber. Do not crush or chew sustained or extended release forms. Avoid grapefruit juice; avoid (or limit) alcohol and caffeine. You may experience dizziness or lightheadedness (use caution when driving or engaging in tasks requiring alertness until response to drug is known); nausea or vomiting (small frequent meals, frequent mouth care, chewing gum, or sucking lozenges may help); constipation (increased exercise, fluids, fruit, or fiber may help); or diarrhea (buttermilk, boiled milk, or yogurt may help). Report chest pain, palpitations, or irregular heartbeat; unusual cough, respiratory difficulty, or swelling of extremities (feet/ankles); muscle tremors or weakness; confusion or acute lethargy; or skin irritation or rash. **Pregnancy precaution:** Inform prescriber if you are or intend to become pregnant.

Dietary Considerations Calan® SR and Isoptin® SR products may be taken with food or milk, other formulations may be administered without regard to meals; sprinkling contents of Verelan® or Verelan® PM capsule onto applesauce does not affect oral absorption.

Geriatric Considerations Elderly may experience a greater hypotensive response. Theoretically, constipation may be more of a problem in the elderly. Calcium channel blockers are no more effective in the elderly than other therapies, however, they do not cause significant CNS effects, which is an advantage over some antihypertensive agents. Generic verapamil products which are bioequivalent in young adults may not be bioequivalent in the elderly. Use generics cautiously.

Breast-Feeding Issues Crosses into breast milk; manufacturer recommends to discontinue breast-feeding while taking verapamil. AAP considers **compatible** with breast-feeding.

Pregnancy Issues Crosses the placenta. One report of suspected heart block when used to control fetal supraventricular tachycardia. May exhibit tocolytic effects.

Related Information

Compatibility of Drugs *on page 1370*

VinBLAStine (vin BLAS teen)

Synonyms NSC-49842; Vinblastine Sulfate; VLB

Pharmacologic Category Antineoplastic Agent, Natural Source (Plant) Derivative; Antineoplastic Agent, Vinca Alkaloid

Medication Safety Issues

Sound-alike/look-alike issues:

VinBLAStine may be confused with vinCRIStine, vinorelbine

Note: Must be dispensed in overwrap which bears the statement **"Do not remove covering until the moment of injection. Fatal if given intrathecally. For I.V. use only."** Syringes should be labeled: **"Fatal if given intrathecally. For I.V. use only."**

Pregnancy Risk Factor D

Lactation Enters breast milk/not recommended

Use Treatment of Hodgkin's and non-Hodgkin's lymphoma, testicular, lung, head and neck, breast, and renal carcinomas, Mycosis fungoides, Kaposi's sarcoma, histiocytosis, choriocarcinoma, and idiopathic thrombocytopenic purpura

Mechanism of Action/Effect Vinblastine arrests cell cycle growth in metaphase. Also inhibits RNA synthesis and amino acid metabolism resulting in inhibition of metabolic pathways and cell growth.

Contraindications For I.V. use only; **I.T. use may result in death**; hypersensitivity to vinblastine or any component of the formulation; pregnancy

Warnings/Precautions Hazardous agent - use appropriate precautions for handling and disposal. Vinblastine is a moderate vesicant; avoid extravasation. Dosage modification required in patients with impaired liver function and neurotoxicity. Using small amounts of drug daily for long periods may cause neurotoxicity and is therefore not advised. For I.V. use only. **Intrathecal administration results in death.** Use with caution in patients with cachexia or ulcerated skin. Monitor closely for shortness of breath or bronchospasm in patients receiving mitomycin C.

Drug Interactions

Cytochrome P450 Effect: Substrate of CYP2D6 (minor), 3A4 (major); **Inhibits** CYP2D6 (weak), 3A4 (weak)

Decreased Effect: CYP3A4 inducers may decrease the levels/effects of vinblastine; example inducers include aminoglutethimide, carbamazepine, nafcillin, nevirapine, phenobarbital, phenytoin (may reduce vinblastine serum concentrations), and rifamycins.

Increased Effect/Toxicity: CYP3A4 inhibitors may increase the levels/effects of vinblastine; example inhibitors include azole antifungals, clarithromycin, diclofenac, doxycycline, erythromycin, imatinib, isoniazid, nefazodone, nicardipine, propofol, protease inhibitors, quinidine, telithromycin, and verapamil.

Previous or simultaneous use with mitomycin-C has resulted in acute shortness of breath and severe bronchospasm within minutes or several hours after vinca alkaloid injection and may occur up to 2 weeks after the dose of mitomycin. Mitomycin-C in combination with administration of VLB may cause acute shortness of breath and severe bronchospasm, onset may be within minutes or several hours after VLB injection.

Nutritional/Ethanol Interactions Herb/Nutraceutical: St John's wort may decrease vinblastine levels. Avoid black cohosh, dong quai in estrogen-dependent tumors.

Adverse Reactions

>10%:

Dermatologic: Alopecia

Endocrine & metabolic: SIADH

Gastrointestinal: Diarrhea (less common), stomatitis, anorexia, metallic taste

Hematologic: May cause severe bone marrow suppression and is the dose-limiting toxicity of VLB

(Continued)

VinBLAStine *(Continued)*

(unlike vincristine); severe granulocytopenia and thrombocytopenia may occur following the administration of VLB and nadir 5-10 days after treatment

Myelosuppression (primarily leukopenia, may be dose limiting)

Onset: 4-7 days

Nadir: 5-10 days

Recovery: 4-21 days

1% to 10%:

Cardiovascular: Hypertension, Raynaud's phenomenon

Central nervous system: Depression, malaise, headache, seizure

Dermatologic: Rash, photosensitivity, dermatitis

Endocrine & metabolic: Hyperuricemia

Gastrointestinal: Constipation, abdominal pain, nausea (mild), vomiting (mild), paralytic ileus, stomatitis

Genitourinary: Urinary retention

Neuromuscular & skeletal: Jaw pain, myalgia, paresthesia

Respiratory: Bronchospasm

Overdosage/Toxicology Symptoms of overdose include bone marrow suppression, mental depression, paresthesia, loss of deep tendon reflexes, and neurotoxicity. There are no antidotes for vinblastine. Treatment is supportive and symptomatic, including fluid restriction or hypertonic saline (3% sodium chloride) for drug-induced secretion of inappropriate antidiuretic hormone (SIADH).

Pharmacodynamics/Kinetics

Protein Binding: 99%

Half-Life Elimination: Biphasic: Initial: 0.164 hours; Terminal: 25 hours

Metabolism: Hepatic to active metabolite

Excretion: Feces (95%); urine (<1% as unchanged drug)

Available Dosage Forms

Injection, powder for reconstitution, as sulfate: 10 mg

Injection, solution, as sulfate: 1 mg/mL (10 mL) [contains benzyl alcohol]

Dosing

Adults & Elderly: Refer to individual protocols.

Antineoplastic (typical dosages): I.V.: 4-20 mg/m^2 (0.1-0.5 mg/kg) every 7-10 days **or** 5-day continuous infusion of 1.5-2 mg/m^2/day **or** 0.1-0.5 mg/kg/week

Pediatrics: Refer to adult dosing.

Renal Impairment: Not removed by hemodialysis

Hepatic Impairment:

Serum bilirubin 1.5-3.0 mg/dL or AST 60-180 units: Administer 50% of normal dose.

Serum bilirubin 3.0-5.0 mg/dL: Administer 25% of dose.

Serum bilirubin >5.0 mg/dL or AST >180 units: Omit dose.

Administration

I.V.: Vesicant. **Fatal if given intrathecally.** For I.V. administration only, usually as a slow (2-3 minutes) push, or a bolus (5- to 15-minute) infusion. It is occasionally given as a 24-hour continuous infusion.

I.V. Detail: Follow guidelines for handling cytotoxic agents.

Extravasation management: Mix 250 units hyaluronidase with 6 mL of NS. Inject the hyaluronidase solution subcutaneously through 6 clockwise injections into the infiltrated area using a 25-gauge needle; change the needle with each new injection. Apply heat immediately for 1 hour. Repeat 4 times/day for 3-5 days. Elevate extremity. Application of cold or hydrocortisone is contraindicated.

pH: 3.5-5.0

Stability

Reconstitution: Reconstitute to a concentration of 1 mg/mL with bacteriostatic water, bacteriostatic NS, SWFI, NS, or D$_5$W; for infusion, may be diluted with 50-1000 mL Ns or D$_5$W.

Compatibility: Stable in D$_5$W, LR, NS, bacteriostatic water

Y-site administration: Incompatible with cefepime, furosemide

Compatibility in syringe: Incompatible with furosemide

Storage: Store intact vials under refrigeration (2°C to 8°C) and protect from light. Solutions reconstituted in bacteriostatic water or bacteriostatic NS are stable for 21 days at room temperature or under refrigeration.

Note: Must be dispensed in overwrap which bears the statement "Do not remove covering until the moment of injection. Fatal if given intrathecally. For I.V. use only." Syringes should be labeled: "Fatal if given intrathecally. For I.V. use only."

Laboratory Monitoring CBC with differential and platelet count, serum uric acid, hepatic function

Nursing Actions

Physical Assessment: Assess potential for interactions with other pharmacological agents and herbal products patient may be taking (eg, previous or concurrent use mitomycin"C can cause severe reaction). Premedication with antiemetic is advisable. Monitor infusion site closely to prevent extravasation (vesicant will cause tissues damage and necrosis). Monitor laboratory tests, renal function, and adverse reactions (eg, SIADH, bone marrow suppression, leukopenia, hypertension, gastrointestinal disturbance, myalgia, depression, paresthesia) prior to each infusion and throughout therapy. Teach patient possible side effects/appropriate interventions and adverse symptoms to report.

Patient Education: Do not take any new medication during therapy unless approved by prescriber. This medication can only be administered by infusion; report immediately any redness, swelling, burning, or pain at infusion site; sudden difficulty breathing; swelling; chest pain; or chills. Maintain adequate hydration (2-3 L/day of fluids) unless instructed to restrict fluid intake, and nutrition (small, frequent meals will help). You will be more susceptible to infection (avoid crowds and exposure to infection and do not have any vaccinations unless approved by prescriber). May cause hair loss (will grow back after therapy); nausea or vomiting (request antiemetic); photosensitivity (use sunscreen, wear protective clothing and eyewear, and avoid direct sunlight); feelings of extreme weakness or lethargy (use caution when driving or engaging in tasks requiring alertness until response to drug is known); or mouth sores (use soft toothbrush, waxed dental floss, and frequent oral care). Report persistent constipation or abdominal pain; numbness or tingling in fingers or toes (use care to prevent injury); weakness or pain in muscles or jaw; signs of infection (eg, fever, chills, sore throat, burning urination, fatigue); unusual bleeding (eg, tarry stools, easy bruising, blood in stool, urine, or mouth); unresolved mouth sores; skin rash or itching; or respiratory difficulty. **Pregnancy/breast-feeding precautions:** Do not get pregnant (females) or cause a pregnancy (males) during this therapy. Consult prescriber for appropriate contraceptive measures. Breast-feeding is not recommended.

Related Information

FDA Name Differentiation Project: The Use of Tall-Man Letters *on page 12*

VinCRIStine (vin KRIS teen)

U.S. Brand Names Vincasar PFS®
Synonyms LCR; Leurocristine Sulfate; NSC-67574; VCR; Vincristine Sulfate
Pharmacologic Category Antineoplastic Agent, Natural Source (Plant) Derivative; Antineoplastic Agent, Vinca Alkaloid
Medication Safety Issues
Sound-alike/look-alike issues:
VinCRIStine may be confused with vinBLAStine
Oncovin® may be confused with Ancobon®

To prevent fatal inadvertent intrathecal injection, it is recommended that all doses be dispensed in a small minibag. When dispensing vincristine in a syringe, vincristine must be packaged in the manufacturer-provided overwrap which bears the statement **"Do not remove covering until the moment of injection. For intravenous use only. Fatal if given intrathecally."**

Pregnancy Risk Factor D
Lactation Enters breast milk/not recommended
Use Treatment of leukemias, Hodgkin's disease, non-Hodgkin's lymphomas, Wilms' tumor, neuroblastoma, rhabdomyosarcoma
Mechanism of Action/Effect Binds to microtubular protein of the mitotic spindle causing metaphase arrest; cell-cycle phase specific in the M and S phases
Contraindications Hypersensitivity to vincristine or any component of the formulation; **for I.V. use only, fatal if given intrathecally**; patients with demyelinating form of Charcot-Marie-Tooth syndrome; pregnancy
Warnings/Precautions Hazardous agent — use appropriate precautions for handling and disposal. Vincristine is a moderate vesicant; avoid extravasation.
Dosage modification required in patients with impaired hepatic function or who have pre-existing neuromuscular disease. Vincristine is a vesicant; avoid extravasation. Use with caution in the elderly; avoid eye contamination; observe closely for shortness of breath, bronchospasm, especially in patients treated with mitomycin C. Alterations in mental status such as depression, confusion, or insomnia; constipation, paralytic ileus, and urinary tract disturbances may occur. All patients should be on a prophylactic bowel management regimen.
Intrathecal administration of vincristine has uniformly caused death; vincristine should never be administered by this route. Neurologic effects of vincristine may be additive with those of other neurotoxic agents and spinal cord irradiation.

Drug Interactions
Cytochrome P450 Effect: Substrate of CYP3A4 (major); **Inhibits** CYP3A4 (weak)
Decreased Effect: Digoxin levels may decrease with combination chemotherapy. CYP3A4 inducers may decrease the levels/effects of vincristine; example inducers include aminoglutethimide, carbamazepine, nafcillin, nevirapine, phenobarbital, phenytoin, and rifamycins.
Increased Effect/Toxicity: Vincristine should be given 12-24 hours before asparaginase to minimize toxicity (may decrease the hepatic clearance of vincristine). Acute pulmonary reactions may occur with mitomycin-C. Previous or simultaneous use with mitomycin-C has resulted in acute shortness of breath and severe bronchospasm within minutes or several hours after vinca alkaloid injection and may occur up to 2 weeks after the dose of mitomycin.

CYP3A4 inhibitors may increase the levels/effects of vincristine. Example inhibitors include azole antifungals, clarithromycin, diclofenac, doxycycline, erythromycin, imatinib, isoniazid, nefazodone, nicardipine, propofol, protease inhibitors, quinidine, telithromycin,

and verapamil. Digoxin plasma levels and renal excretion may decrease with combination chemotherapy including vincristine. Nifedipine may increase the levels/effects of vincristine.
Nutritional/Ethanol Interactions Herb/Nutraceutical: St John's wort may decrease vincristine levels.
Adverse Reactions
>10%: Dermatologic: Alopecia (20% to 70%)
1% to 10%:
Cardiovascular: Orthostatic hypotension or hypertension, hyper-/hypotension
Central nervous system: CNS depression, confusion, cranial nerve paralysis, fever, headache, insomnia, motor difficulties, seizure
Intrathecal administration of vincristine has uniformly caused death; vincristine should never be administered by this route. Neurologic effects of vincristine may be additive with those of other neurotoxic agents and spinal cord irradiation.
Dermatologic: Rash
Endocrine & metabolic: Hyperuricemia
Gastrointestinal: Abdominal cramps, anorexia, bloating, constipation (and possible paralytic ileus secondary to neurologic toxicity), diarrhea, metallic taste, nausea (mild), oral ulceration, vomiting, weight loss
Genitourinary: Bladder atony (related to neurotoxicity), dysuria, polyuria, urinary retention
Hematologic: Leukopenia (mild), thrombocytopenia, myelosuppression (onset: 7 days; nadir: 10 days; recovery: 21 days)
Local: Phlebitis, tissue irritation and necrosis if infiltrated
Neuromuscular & skeletal: Cramping, jaw pain, leg pain, myalgia, numbness, weakness
Peripheral neuropathy: Frequently the dose-limiting toxicity of vincristine. Most frequent in patients >40 years of age; occurs usually after an average of 3 weekly doses, but may occur after just one dose. Manifested as loss of the deep tendon reflexes in the lower extremities, numbness, tingling, pain, paresthesia of the fingers and toes (stocking glove sensation), and "foot drop" or "wrist drop."
Ocular: Optic atrophy, photophobia
Overdosage/Toxicology Symptoms of overdose include bone marrow suppression, mental depression, paresthesia, loss of deep tendon reflexes, alopecia, and nausea. Severe symptoms may occur with 3-4 mg/m^2.

There are no antidotes for vincristine. Treatment is supportive and symptomatic, including fluid restriction or hypertonic saline (3% sodium chloride) for drug-induced secretion of inappropriate antidiuretic hormone (SIADH). Case reports suggest that folinic acid may be helpful in treating vincristine overdose. It is suggested that 100 mg folinic acid be given I.V. every 3 hours for 24 hours, then every 6 hours for 48 hours. This is in addition to supportive care. The use of pyridoxine, leucovorin factor, cyanocobalamin, or thiamine has been used with little success for drug-induced peripheral neuropathy.
Pharmacodynamics/Kinetics
Protein Binding: 75%
Half-Life Elimination: Terminal: 24 hours
Metabolism: Extensively hepatic
Excretion: Feces (~80%); urine (<1% as unchanged drug)
Available Dosage Forms Injection, solution, as sulfate: 1 mg/mL (1 mL, 2 mL)
Dosing
Adults & Elderly: Note: Doses are often capped at 2 mg; however, this may reduce the efficacy of the therapy and may not be advisable. Refer to individual protocols; orders for single doses >2.5 mg or >5 mg/ treatment cycle should be verified with the specific treatment regimen and/or an experienced oncologist prior to dispensing.
(Continued)

VinCRIStine *(Continued)*

Antineoplastic (typical dosages): I.V.: 0.4-1.4 mg/m^2, may repeat every week **or**

0.4-0.5 mg/day continuous infusion for 4 days every 4 weeks **or**

0.25-0.5 mg/m^2/day continuous infusion for 5 days every 4 weeks

Pediatrics: Refer to individual protocols. **Note:** Doses are often capped at 2 mg; however, this may reduce the efficacy of the therapy and may not be advisable. Orders for single doses >2.5 mg or >5 mg/treatment cycle should be verified with the specific treatment regimen and/or an experienced oncologist prior to dispensing.

Antineoplastic (typical dosages): I.V.:

Children ≤10 kg or BSA <1 m^2: Initial therapy: 0.05 mg/kg once weekly then titrate dose

Children >10 kg or BSA ≥1 m^2: 1-2 mg/m^2, may repeat once weekly for 3-6 weeks; maximum single dose: 2 mg

Neuroblastoma: I.V. continuous infusion with doxorubicin: 1 mg/m^2/day for 72 hours

Hepatic Impairment:

Serum bilirubin 1.5-3.0 mg/dL or AST 60-180 units: Administer 50% of normal dose.

Serum bilirubin 3.0-5.0 mg/dL: Administer 25% of dose.

Serum bilirubin >5.0 mg/dL or AST >180 units: Omit dose.

Administration

I.V.: Vesicant. For I.V. use only. **Fatal if given intrathecally.** Usually administered as slow (1-2 minutes) push or short (10-15 minutes) infusion; 24-hour continuous infusions are occasionally used

I.V. Detail: Follow guidelines for handling cytotoxic agents. Drug should be administered by qualified personnel. Do not allow to come in contact with skin. If contact occurs, wash thoroughly with soap and water. Avoid extravasation; agent is a vesicant and will cause sloughing.

Extravasation management: Mix 250 units hyaluronidase with 6 mL of NS. Inject the hyaluronidase solution subcutaneously through 6 clockwise injections into the infiltrated area using a 25-gauge needle. Change the needle with each new injection. Elevate extremity. Apply heat immediately for 1 hour. Repeat 4 times/day for 3-5 days. Application of cold or hydrocortisone is contraindicated.

pH: 3.5-5.5

Other: Intralesional injection has been reported for Kaposi's sarcoma

Stability

Reconstitution: Solutions for I.V. infusion may be mixed in NS or D$_5$W.

Compatibility: Stable in D$_5$W, LR, NS

Y-site administration: Incompatible with cefepime, furosemide, idarubicin, sodium bicarbonate

Compatibility in syringe: Incompatible with furosemide

Storage:

Undiluted vials: Store under refrigeration; may be stable for up to 30 days at room temperature

I.V. solution: Diluted in 20-50 mL NS or D$_5$W, stable for 7 days under refrigeration, or 2 days at room temperature. In ambulatory pumps, solution is stable for 7-10 days at room temperature.

Laboratory Monitoring Serum electrolytes (sodium), hepatic function, CBC, serum uric acid

Nursing Actions

Physical Assessment: Assess potential for interactions with other pharmacological agents and herbal products patient may be taking (eg, CYP3A4 inducers; previous or concurrent use with mitomycin-C can cause severe reaction). Premedication

with antiemetic is advisable. May cause severe constipation, paralytic ileus, intestinal obstruction, necrosis, and/or perforation; prophylactic bowel management regimen may be advisable. Monitor infusion site closely to prevent extravasation (vesicant will cause tissue damage and necrosis). Monitor laboratory tests, hepatic function, and adverse reactions prior to each infusion and throughout therapy (eg, CNS [motor difficulties, seizure, depression], neuromuscular [myalgia, cramping], peripheral neuropathy, photophobia). Teach patient possible side effects/appropriate interventions and adverse symptoms to report.

Patient Education: Do not take any new medication during therapy unless approved by prescriber. This medication can only be administered by infusion; report immediately any redness, swelling, burning, or pain at infusion site. Maintain adequate hydration (2-3 L/day of fluids) unless instructed to restrict fluid intake and nutrition (small frequent meals will help). You will be more susceptible to infection (avoid crowds and exposure to infection and do not have any vaccinations unless approved by prescriber). May cause postural hypotension (use caution when rising from sitting or lying position or when climbing steps); hair loss (will grow back after therapy); nausea or vomiting (request antiemetic if persistent); photosensitivity (use sunscreen, wear protective clothing and eyewear, and avoid direct sunlight); feelings of extreme weakness or lethargy (use caution when driving or engaging in tasks requiring alertness until response to drug is known); mouth sores (use soft toothbrush, waxed dental floss, and frequent oral care). Report persistent gastrointestinal changes (eg, constipation, abdominal cramps, bloating); numbness, tingling, or pain in legs, fingers, or toes (use care to prevent injury); signs of infection (eg, fever, chills, sore throat, burning urination, fatigue); unusual bleeding (eg, tarry stools, easy bruising, blood in stool, urine, or mouth); unresolved mouth sores; skin rash or itching; respiratory difficulty; or other persistent adverse effects. **Pregnancy/breast-feeding precautions:** Do not get pregnant (females) or cause a pregnancy (males) during this therapy. Consult prescriber for appropriate contraceptive measures. Breast-feeding is not recommended.

Related Information

FDA Name Differentiation Project: The Use of Tall-Man Letters *on page 12*

Vinorelbine *(vi NOR el been)*

U.S. Brand Names Navelbine®

Synonyms Dihydroxydeoxynorvinkaleukoblastine; NVB; Vinorelbine Tartrate

Pharmacologic Category Antineoplastic Agent, Natural Source (Plant) Derivative; Antineoplastic Agent, Vinca Alkaloid

Medication Safety Issues

Sound-alike/look-alike issues:

Vinorelbine may be confused with vinBLAStine

Pregnancy Risk Factor D

Lactation Excretion in breast milk unknown/contraindicated

Use Treatment of nonsmall cell lung cancer

Unlabeled/Investigational Use Treatment of breast cancer, ovarian carcinoma, Hodgkin's disease, non-Hodgkin's lymphoma

Mechanism of Action/Effect Mitotic inhibition that causes metaphase arrest in neoplastic cells

Contraindications For I.V. use only; **I.T. use may result in death;** hypersensitivity to vinorelbine or any component of the formulation; pregnancy

Warnings/Precautions Hazardous agent - use appropriate precautions for handling and disposal. Avoid extravasation; dosage modification required in patients with impaired liver function and neurotoxicity. Frequently monitor patients for myelosuppression both during and after therapy. Granulocytopenia is dose-limiting. **Intrathecal administration may result in death**. Use with caution in patients with cachexia or ulcerated skin.

Acute shortness of breath and severe bronchospasm have been reported, most commonly when administered with mitomycin. Fatal cases of interstitial pulmonary changes and ARDS have also been reported. May cause severe constipation (grade 3-4), paralytic ileus, intestinal obstruction, necrosis, and/or perforation.

Drug Interactions

Cytochrome P450 Effect: Substrate of CYP2D6 (minor), 3A4 (major); **Inhibits** CYP2D6 (weak), 3A4 (weak)

Decreased Effect: CYP3A4 inducers may decrease the levels/effects of vinorelbine; example inducers include aminoglutethimide, carbamazepine, nafcillin, nevirapine, phenobarbital, phenytoin, and rifamycins.

Increased Effect/Toxicity: Previous or simultaneous use with mitomycin-C has resulted in acute shortness of breath and severe bronchospasm within minutes or several hours after vinca alkaloid injection and may occur up to 2 weeks after the dose of mitomycin. CYP3A4 inhibitors may increase the levels/effects of vinorelbine; example inhibitors include azole antifungals, clarithromycin, diclofenac, doxycycline, erythromycin, imatinib, isoniazid, nefazodone, nicardipine, propofol, protease inhibitors, quinidine, telithromycin, and verapamil. Incidence of granulocytopenia is significantly higher in cisplatin/vinorelbine combination therapy than with single-agent vinorelbine.

Nutritional/Ethanol Interactions Herb/Nutraceutical: St John's wort may decrease vinorelbine levels.

Adverse Reactions

>10%:
Central nervous system: Fatigue (27%)
Dermatologic: Alopecia (12%)
Gastrointestinal: Nausea (44%, severe <2%) and vomiting (20%) are most common and are easily controlled with standard antiemetics; constipation (35%), diarrhea (17%)
Emetic potential: Moderate (30% to 60%)
Hematologic: May cause severe bone marrow suppression and is the dose-limiting toxicity of vinorelbine; severe granulocytopenia (90%) may occur following the administration of vinorelbine; leukopenia (92%), anemia (83%)
Myelosuppressive:
WBC: Moderate - severe
Onset: 4-7 days
Nadir: 7-10 days
Recovery: 14-21 days
Hepatic: Elevated SGOT (67%), elevated total bilirubin (13%)
Local: Injection site reaction (28%), injection site pain (16%)
Neuromuscular & skeletal: Weakness (36%), peripheral neuropathy (20% to 25%)
1% to 10%:
Cardiovascular: Chest pain (5%)
Gastrointestinal: Paralytic ileus (1%)
Hematologic: Thrombocytopenia (5%)
Local: Phlebitis (7%)
Neuromuscular & skeletal: Mild to moderate peripheral neuropathy manifested by paresthesia and hyperesthesia, loss of deep tendon reflexes (<5%); myalgia (<5%), arthralgia (<5%), jaw pain (<5%)
Respiratory: Dyspnea (3% to 7%)

Overdosage/Toxicology Symptoms of overdose include bone marrow suppression, mental depression, paresthesia, loss of deep tendon reflexes, and neurotoxicity. There are no antidotes for vinorelbine. Treatment is supportive and symptomatic, including fluid restriction or hypertonic saline (3% sodium chloride) for

drug-induced secretion of inappropriate antidiuretic hormone (SIADH).

Pharmacodynamics/Kinetics

Protein Binding: 80% to 90%
Half-Life Elimination: Triphasic: Terminal: 27.7-43.6 hours
Metabolism: Extensively hepatic to two metabolites, deacetylvinorelbine (active) and vinorelbine N-oxide
Excretion: Feces (46%); urine (18%, 10% to 12% as unchanged drug)
Clearance: Plasma: Mean: 0.97-1.26 L/hour/kg

Available Dosage Forms Injection, solution [preservative free]: 10 mg/mL (1 mL, 5 mL)

Dosing

Adults & Elderly: Refer to individual protocols.
Nonsmall cell lung cancer: I.V.:
Single-agent therapy: 30 mg/m^2 every 7 days
Combination therapy with cisplatin: 25 mg/m^2 every 7 days (with cisplatin 100 mg/m^2 every 4 weeks); **Alternatively:** 30 mg/m^2 in combination with cisplatin 120 mg/m^2 on days 1 and 29, then every 6 weeks.

Dosage adjustment in hematological toxicity (based on granulocyte counts):
Granulocytes ≥1500 cells/mm^3 on day of treatment: Administer 100% of starting dose.
Granulocytes 1000-1499 cells/mm^3 on day of treatment: Administer 50% of starting dose.
Granulocytes <1000 cells/mm^3 on day of treatment: Do not administer. Repeat granulocyte count in 1 week. If 3 consecutive doses are held because granulocyte count is <1000 cells/mm^3, discontinue vinorelbine.

Adjustment: For patients who, during treatment, have experienced fever or sepsis while granulocytopenic or had 2 consecutive weekly doses held due to granulocytopenia, subsequent doses of vinorelbine should be:
75% of starting dose for granulocytes ≥1500 cells/mm^3
37.5% of starting dose for granulocytes 1000-1499 cells/mm^3

Renal Impairment: No dose adjustments are required for renal insufficiency.

Hepatic Impairment:
Serum bilirubin ≤2 mg/dL: Administer 100% of starting dose.
Serum bilirubin 2.1-3 mg/dL: Administer 50% of starting dose.
Serum bilirubin >3 mg/dL: Administer 25% of starting dose.
In patients with concurrent hematologic toxicity and hepatic impairment, administer the lower doses determined from the above recommendations under Adult Dosing.

Administration

I.V.: FATAL IF GIVEN INTRATHECALLY. Administer as a direct intravenous push or rapid bolus, over 6-10 minutes (up to 30 minutes). Longer infusions may increase the risk of pain and phlebitis. Intravenous doses should be followed by 150-250 mL of saline or dextrose to reduce the incidence of phlebitis and inflammation.

I.V. Detail: Do not administer in an extremity with poor circulation or repeatedly into the same vein.

Extravasation management: Mix 250 units hyaluronidase with 6 mL of NS. Inject the hyaluronidase solution subcutaneously through 6 clockwise injections into the infiltrated area using a 25-gauge needle. Change the needle with each new injection. Elevate extremities. Apply heat immediately for 1 hour. Repeat 4 times/day for 3-5 days. Application of cold or hydrocortisone is contraindicated.

pH: 3.5 (injection)
(Continued)

Vinorelbine (Continued)

Stability

Reconstitution: Dilute in 10-50 mL D_5W or NS.

Compatibility: Stable in $D_5\frac{1}{2}NS$, D_5W, LR, NS, $\frac{1}{2}NS$

Y-site administration: Incompatible with acyclovir, allopurinol, aminophylline, amphotericin B, amphotericin B cholesteryl sulfate complex, ampicillin, cefazolin, cefoperazone, cefotetan, ceftriaxone, cefuroxime, co-trimoxazole, fluorouracil, furosemide, ganciclovir, methylprednisolone sodium succinate, mitomycin, piperacillin, sodium bicarbonate, thiotepa

Storage: Store intact vials under refrigeration (2°C to 8°C) and protect from light; vials are stable at room temperature for up to 72 hours. Dilutions in D_5W or NS are stable for 24 hours at room temperature.

Laboratory Monitoring CBC with differential and platelet count, hepatic function

Nursing Actions

Physical Assessment: Assess potential for interactions with other pharmacological agents and herbal products patient may be taking. Premedication with antiemetic is advisable. May cause severe constipation, paralytic ileus, intestinal obstruction, necrosis, and/or perforation; prophylactic bowel management regimen may be advisable. See Administration for infusion specifics. Monitor infusion site closely to prevent extravasation (may cause tissue damage and necrosis). Monitor laboratory tests, therapeutic effectiveness, and adverse reactions prior to each infusion and throughout therapy. Teach patient possible side effects/appropriate interventions and adverse symptoms to report..

Patient Education: Do not take any new medication during therapy unless approved by prescriber. This medication can only be administered by infusion; report immediately any redness, swelling, burning, or pain at infusion site. Maintain adequate hydration (2-3 L/day of fluids) unless instructed to restrict fluid intake, and nutrition (small, frequent meals will help). You will be more susceptible to infection (avoid crowds and exposure to infection and do not have any vaccinations unless approved by prescriber). May cause hair loss (will grow back after therapy); nausea or vomiting (request antiemetic); photosensitivity (use sunscreen, wear protective clothing and eyewear, and avoid direct sunlight); feelings of weakness or lethargy (use caution when driving or engaging in tasks requiring alertness until response to drug is known); or mouth sores (use soft toothbrush, waxed dental floss and frequent oral care). Report persistent constipation or abdominal pain; numbness or tingling in fingers or toes (use care to prevent injury); weakness, numbness, or pain in muscles or extremities; signs of infection (eg, fever, chills, sore throat, burning urination, fatigue); unusual bleeding (eg, tarry stools, easy bruising, blood in stool, urine, or mouth); unresolved mouth sores; skin rash or itching; or respiratory difficulty. **Pregnancy/breast-feeding precautions:** Do not get pregnant (females) or cause a pregnancy (males) during this therapy. Consult prescriber for appropriate contraceptive measures. Do not breast-feed.

Vitamin E (VYE ta min ee)

U.S. Brand Names Alph-E [OTC]; Alph-E-Mixed [OTC]; Aquasol E® [OTC]; Aquavit-E [OTC]; d-Alpha-Gems™ [OTC]; E-Gems® [OTC]; E-Gems Elite® [OTC]; E-Gems Plus® [OTC]; Ester-E™ [OTC]; Gamma E-Gems® [OTC]; Gamma-E Plus [OTC]; High Gamma Vitamin E Complete™ [OTC]; Key-E® [OTC]; Key-E® Kaps [OTC]

Synonyms d-Alpha Tocopherol; dl-Alpha Tocopherol

Pharmacologic Category Vitamin, Fat Soluble

Medication Safety Issues
Sound-alike/look-alike issues:
Aquasol E® may be confused with Anusol®

Pregnancy Risk Factor A/C (dose exceeding RDA recommendation)

Lactation Enters breast milk/compatible

Use Dietary supplement

Unlabeled/Investigational Use To reduce the risk of bronchopulmonary dysplasia or retrolental fibroplasia in infants exposed to high concentrations of oxygen; prevention and treatment of tardive dyskinesia and Alzheimer's disease; prevention and treatment of hemolytic anemia secondary to vitamin E deficiency

Mechanism of Action/Effect Prevents oxidation of vitamin A and C; protects polyunsaturated fatty acids in membranes from attack by free radicals and protects red blood cells against hemolysis

Contraindications Hypersensitivity to vitamin E or any component of the formulation

Warnings/Precautions May induce vitamin K deficiency. Necrotizing enterocolitis has been associated with oral administration of large dosages (eg, >200 units/day) of a hyperosmolar vitamin E preparation in low birth weight infants.

Drug Interactions
Decreased Effect: Vitamin E may impair the hematologic response to iron in children with iron-deficiency anemia; monitor.

Increased Effect/Toxicity: Vitamin E may alter the effect of vitamin K actions on clotting factors resulting in an increase hypoprothrombinemic response to warfarin; monitor.

Adverse Reactions Frequency not defined.
Central nervous system: Fatigue, headache, weakness
Dermatologic: Contact dermatitis with topical preparation
Endocrine & metabolic: Gonadal dysfunction
Gastrointestinal: Diarrhea, intestinal cramps, nausea
Neuromuscular & skeletal: Weakness
Ocular: Blurred vision

Pharmacodynamics/Kinetics
Metabolism: Hepatic to glucuronides
Excretion: Feces

Available Dosage Forms
Capsule: 400 int. units, 1000 int. units
Key-E® Kaps: 200 int. units, 400 int. units
Capsule, softgel: 200 int. units, 400 int. units, 600 int. units, 1000 int. units
Alph-E: 200 int. units, 400 int. units
Alph-E-Mixed: 200 int. units [contains mixed tocopherols]; 400 int. units [contains mixed tocopherols], 1000 int. units [sugar free; contains mixed tocopherols]
Aqua Gem E®: 200 units, 400 units
d-Alpha-Gems™: 400 int. units [derived from soybean oil]
E-Gems®: 30 int. units, 100 int. units, 200 int. units, 400 int. units, 600 int. units, 800 int. units, 1000 int. units, 1200 int. units [derived from soybean oil]
E-Gems Plus®: 200 int. units, 400 int. units, 800 int. units [contains mixed tocopherols]
E-Gems Elite®: 400 int. units [contains mixed tocopherols]
Ester-E™: 400 int. units

Gamma E-Gems®: 90 int. units [also contains mixed tocopherols]

Gamma-E Plus: 200 int. units [contains soybean oil]

High Gamma Vitamin E Complete™: 200 int. units [contains soybean oil, mixed tocopherols]

Cream: 50 int. units/g (60 g), 100 int. units/g (60 g), 1000 int. units/120 g (120 g), 30,000 int. units/57 g (57 g)

Key-E®: 30 int. units/g (60 g, 120 g, 600 g)

Lip balm (E-Gem® Lip Care): 1000 int. units/tube [contains vitamin A and aloe]

Oil, oral/topical: 100 int. units/0.25 mL (60 mL, 75 mL); 1150 units/0.25 mL (30 mL, 60 mL, 120 mL); 28,000 int. units/30 mL (30 mL)

Alph-E: 28,000 int. units/30 mL (30 mL) [topical]

E-Gems®: 100 units/10 drops (15 mL, 60 mL)

Ointment, topical (Key-E®): 30 units/g (60 g, 120 g, 480 g)

Powder (Key-E®): 700 int. units per 1/4 teaspoon (15 g, 75 g, 1000 g) [derived from soybean oil]

Solution, oral drops: 15 int. units/0.3 mL (30 mL)

Aquasol E®: 15 int. units/0.3 mL (12 mL, 30 mL) [latex free]

Aquavit-E: 15 int. units/0.3 mL (30 mL) [butterscotch flavor]

Suppository, rectal/vaginal (Key-E®): 30 int. units (12s, 24s) [contains coconut oil]

Tablet: 100 int. units, 200 int. units, 400 int. units, 500 int. units

Key-E®: 200 int. units, 400 int. units

Dosing

Adults & Elderly: Vitamin E may be expressed as alpha-tocopherol equivalents (ATE), which refer to the biologically active (R) stereoisomer content. Oral:

Recommended daily allowance (RDA): 15 mg; upper limit of intake should not exceed 1000 mg/day

Pregnant female:

≤18 years: 15 mg; upper level of intake should not exceed 800 mg/day

19-50 years: 15 mg; upper level of intake should not exceed 1000 mg/day

Lactating female:

≤18 years: 19 mg; upper level of intake should not exceed 800 mg/day

19-50 years: 19 mg; upper level of intake should not exceed 1000 mg/day

Vitamin E deficiency: 60-75 units/day

Prevention of vitamin E deficiency: Oral: 30 units/day

Cystic fibrosis: Oral: 100-400 units/day

Beta-thalassemia: Oral: 750 units/day

Sickle cell disease: Oral: 450 units/day

Alzheimer's disease: Oral: 1000 units twice daily

Tardive dyskinesia: Oral: 1600 units/day

Superficial dermatologic irritation: Topical: Apply a thin layer over affected area.

Pediatrics: Vitamin E may be expressed as alpha-tocopherol equivalents (ATE), which refer to the biologically active (R) stereoisomer content. Oral:

Recommended daily allowance (RDA):

Premature infants ≤3 months: 17 mg

Infants (adequate intake; RDA not establshed):

≤6 months: 4 mg

7-12 months: 6 mg

Children:

1-3 years: 6 mg; upper limit of intake should not exceed 200 mg/day

4-8 years: 7 mg; upper limit of intake should not exceed 300 mg/day

9-13 years: 11 mg; upper limit of intake should not exceed 600 mg/day

14-18 years: 15 mg; upper limit of intake should not exceed 800 mg/day

Vitamin E deficiency:

Children (with malabsorption syndrome): 1 unit/kg/day of water miscible vitamin E (to raise plasma tocopherol concentrations to the normal range within 2 months and to maintain normal plasma concentrations)

Cystic fibrosis, beta-thalassemia may require higher daily maintenance doses:

Cystic fibrosis: Oral: 100-400 units/day

Beta-thalassemia: Oral: 750 units/day

Administration

Oral: Swallow capsules whole, do not crush or chew.

Stability

Storage: Protect from light.

Laboratory Monitoring

Monitor plasma tocopherol concentrations (normal range: 6-14 mcg/mL).

Nursing Actions

Physical Assessment: Assess effectiveness and interactions of other medications patient may be taking. Assess knowledge/teach patient appropriate use (according to formulation prescribed) and adverse symptoms to report.

Patient Education: Take exactly as directed; do not take more than the recommended dose. Do not use mineral oil or other vitamin E supplements without consulting prescriber. Report persistent nausea, vomiting, or cramping; or gonadal dysfunction. **Pregnancy precaution:** Inform prescriber if you are pregnant.

Additional Information The 2R-stereoisomeric forms of α-tocopherol are used to define vitamine E intake and RDA. While international units are no longer recognized, many fortified foods and supplements continue to use this term although USP units are now used by the pharmaceutical industry when labeling vitamin E supplements. Both IUs and USP units are based on the same equivalency. The following can be used to convert international units (IU) of vitamin E (and esters) to milligrams α-tocopherol in order to meet recommended daily intake:

Synthetic (eg, all-racemic α-tocopherol):

dl-α-tocopherol:

USP: 1.10 IU / mg; 0.91 mg / IU

Molar: 2.12 μmol / IU

α-tocopherol: 0.45 mg / IU

dl-α-tocopherol acetate:

USP: 1 IU / mg; 1 mg / IU

Molar: 2.12 μmol / IU

α-tocopherol: 0.45 mg / IU

dl-α-tocopherol succinate:

USP: 0.89 IU / mg; 1.12 mg / IU

Molar: 2.12 μmol / IU

α-tocopherol: 0.45 mg / IU

Natural (eg, RRR-α-tocopherol):

d-α-tocopherol:

USP: 1.49 IU / mg; 0.67 mg / IU

Molar: 1.56 μmol / IU

α-tocopherol: 0.67 mg / IU

d-α-tocopherol acetate:

USP: 1.36 IU / mg; 0.74mg / IU

Molar: 1.56 μmol / IU

α-tocopherol: 0.67 mg / IU

d-α-tocopherol succinate:

USP: 1.21 IU / mg; 0.83 mg / IU

Molar: 1.56 μmol / IU

α-tocopherol: 0.67 mg / IU

Historically, vitamin E supplements have been labeled (incorrectly) as *d-* or *dl-*α-tocopherol. Synthetic vitamin E compounds are racemic mixtures, and may be designated as all-racemic (all rac-α-tocopherol). The natural form contains the only RRR-α-tocopherol. All of these compounds may be present in fortified foods and multivitamins. Not all stereoisomers are capable of performing physiological (Continued)

Vitamin E (Continued)

functions in humans; therefore, cannot be considered to meet vitamin E requirements.

Voriconazole (vor i KOE na zole)

U.S. Brand Names VFEND®

Synonyms UK109496

Pharmacologic Category Antifungal Agent, Oral; Antifungal Agent, Parenteral

Pregnancy Risk Factor D

Lactation Excretion in breast milk unknown/not recommended

Use Treatment of invasive aspergillosis; treatment of esophageal candidiasis; treatment of candidemia (in non-neutropenic patients); treatment of *Candida* deep tissue infections; treatment of serious fungal infections caused by *Scedosporium apiospermum* and *Fusarium* spp (including *Fusarium solani*) in patients intolerant of, or refractory to, other therapy

Mechanism of Action/Effect Interferes with fungal cytochrome P450 activity, decreasing ergosterol synthesis (principal sterol in fungal cell membrane) and inhibiting fungal cell membrane formation.

Contraindications Hypersensitivity to voriconazole or any component of the formulation (cross-reaction with other azole antifungal agents may occur but has not been established, use caution); coadministration of CYP3A4 substrates which may lead to QT_c prolongation (cisapride, pimozide, or quinidine); coadministration with barbiturates (long acting), carbamazepine, efavirenz, ergot alkaloids, rifampin, rifabutin, ritonavir (≥800 mg/day), and sirolimus; pregnancy (unless risk:benefit justifies use)

Warnings/Precautions Visual changes are commonly associated with treatment. Patients should be warned to avoid tasks which depend on vision, including operating machinery or driving. Changes are reversible on discontinuation following brief exposure/treatment regimens (≤28 days).

Serious hepatic reactions (including hepatitis, cholestasis, and fulminant hepatic failure) have occurred during treatment, primarily in patients with serious concomitant medical conditions. However, hepatotoxicity has occurred in patients with no identifiable risk factors. Use caution in patients with pre-existing hepatic impairment (dose adjustment required).

Voriconazole tablets contain lactose; avoid administration in hereditary galactose intolerance, Lapp lactase deficiency, or glucose-galactose malabsorption. Suspension contains sucrose; use caution with fructose intolerance, sucrose-isomaltase deficiency, or glucose-galactose malabsorption. Avoid/limit use of intravenous formulation in patients with renal impairment; intravenous formulation contains excipient sulfobutyl ether beta-cyclodextrin (SBECD), which may accumulate in renal insufficiency. Infusion-related reactions may occur with intravenous dosing. Consider discontinuation of infusion if reaction is severe.

Use caution in patients with an increased risk of arrhythmia (concurrent QT_c-prolonging drugs, hypokalemia, cardiomyopathy, or prior cardiotoxic therapy). Correct electrolyte abnormalities (low levels of calcium, magnesium, and potassium) before initiating therapy. Use caution in patients receiving concurrent non-nucleoside reverse transcriptase inhibitors (efavirenz is contraindicated).

Avoid use in pregnancy, unless an evaluation of the potential benefit justifies possible risk to the fetus. Safety and efficacy have not been established in children <12 years of age.

Drug Interactions

Cytochrome P450 Effect: Substrate of CYP2C9 (major), 2C19 (major), 3A4 (minor); **Inhibits** CYP2C9 (weak), 2C19 (weak), 3A4 (moderate)

Decreased Effect: Barbiturates (phenobarbital, secobarbital), carbamazepine, efavirenz, rifampin, and ritonavir (≥800 mg/day) decrease serum levels/effects of voriconazole; concurrent use is contraindicated. CYP2C9 inducers, CYP2C19 inducers, and phenytoin decrease serum levels/effects of voriconazole.

Increased Effect/Toxicity: Voriconazole increases serum levels/effects of efavirenz, ergot alkaloids, pimozide, quinidine, rifabutin, and sirolimus; concurrent use contraindicated. Voriconazole increases serum levels/effects of benzodiazepines (metabolized by oxidation; eg, alprazolam, diazepam, triazolam, midazolam), buspirone, busulfan, calcium channel blockers (eg, felodipine, nifedipine, verapamil), cisapride, CYP2C9 substrates, CYP3A4 substrates, cyclosporine, HMG-CoA reductase inhibitors (except pravastatin and fluvastatin), methadone, omeprazole, phenytoin, sulfonylureas, tacrolimus, trimetrexate, warfarin, and vinca alkaloids. Use with QT_c-prolonging agents may increase risk of malignant arrhythmia

Nutritional/Ethanol Interactions

Food: May decrease voriconazole absorption. Voriconazole should be taken 1 hour before or 1 hour after a meal.

Herb/Nutraceutical: St John's wort may decrease voriconazole levels.

Adverse Reactions

>10%: Ocular: Visual changes (photophobia, color changes, increased or decreased visual acuity, or blurred vision occur in ~21%)

1% to 10%:

Cardiovascular: Tachycardia (2% to 3%), hyper-/hypotension (2%), vasodilation (2%), peripheral edema (1%)

Central nervous system: Fever (6%), chills (4%), headache (3%), hallucinations (3%), dizziness (1%)

Dermatologic: Rash (6%), pruritus (1%)

Endocrine & metabolic: Hypokalemia (2%), hypomagnesemia (1%)

Gastrointestinal: Nausea (5% to 6%), vomiting (4% to 5%), abdominal pain (2%), diarrhea (1%), xerostomia (1%)

Hematologic: Thrombocytopenia (1%)

Hepatic: Alkaline phosphatase increased (4%), transaminases increased (2% to 3%), AST increased (2%), ALT increased (2%), cholestatic jaundice (1%)

Ocular: Chromatopsia (1%), photophobia (2% to 3%)

Overdosage/Toxicology Visual changes may occur; one patient had photophobia for 10 minutes. Treatment is symptom-directed and supportive. Following intravenous overdose, toxicity from the vehicle, SBECD, may also occur. Both voriconazole and the intravenous vehicle can be eliminated via hemodialysis.

Pharmacodynamics/Kinetics

Time to Peak: 1-2 hours

Protein Binding: 58%

Half-Life Elimination: Variable, dose dependent

Metabolism: Hepatic, nonlinear (via CYP isoenzymes)

Excretion: Urine (as inactive metabolites)

Available Dosage Forms

Injection, powder for reconstitution: 200 mg [contains SBECD 3200 mg]

Powder for oral suspension: 200 mg/5 mL (70 mL) [contains sodium benzoate and sucrose; orange flavor]

Tablet: 50 mg, 200 mg [contains lactose]

Dosing

Adults & Elderly:

Invasive aspergillosis and other serious fungal infections: I.V.: Initial: Loading dose: 6 mg/kg every 12 hours for 2 doses; followed by maintenance dose of 4 mg/kg every 12 hours

Candidemia and other deep tissue *Candida* infections: I.V.: Initial: Loading dose 6 mg/kg every 12 hours for 2 doses; followed by maintenance dose of 3-4 mg/kg every 12 hours

Note: *Conversion to oral dosing:*

Patients <40 kg: 100 mg every 12 hours; increase to 150 mg every 12 hours in patients who fail to respond adequately

Patients ≥40 kg: 200 mg every 12 hours; increase to 300 mg every 12 hours in patients who fail to respond adequately

Endophthalmitis, fungal: I.V.: 6 mg/kg every 12 hours for 2 doses, then 200 mg orally twice daily

Esophageal candidiasis: Oral:

Patients <40 kg: 100 mg every 12 hours

Patients ≥40 kg: 200 mg every 12 hours

Note: Treatment should continue for a minimum of 14 days, and for at least 7 days following resolution of symptoms.

Dosage adjustment in patients unable to tolerate treatment:

I.V.: Dose may be reduced to 3 mg/kg every 12 hours

Oral: Dose may be reduced in 50 mg increments to a minimum dosage of 200 mg every 12 hours in patients weighing ≥40 kg (100 mg every 12 hours in patients <40 kg)

Dosage adjustment in patients receiving concomitant phenytoin:

I.V.: Increase maintenance dosage to 5 mg/kg every 12 hours

Oral: Increase dose from 200 mg to 400 mg every 12 hours in patients ≥40 kg (100 mg to 200 mg every 12 hours in patients <40 kg)

Dosage adjustment in patients receiving concomitant cyclosporine: Reduce cyclosporine dose by ½ and monitor closely.

Pediatrics:

Children <12 years: No data available

Children ≥12 years: Refer to adult dosing.

Renal Impairment: In patients with Cl$_{cr}$ <50 mL/minute, accumulation of the intravenous vehicle (SBECD) occurs. After initial loading dose, oral voriconazole should be administered to these patients, unless an assessment of the benefit:risk to the patient justifies the use of I.V. voriconazole. Monitor serum creatinine and change to oral voriconazole therapy when possible.

Hemodialysis: Oral dosage adjustment not required.

Hepatic Impairment:

Mild to moderate hepatic dysfunction (Child-Pugh class A and B): Following standard loading dose, reduce maintenance dosage by 50%

Severe hepatic impairment: Should only be used if benefit outweighs risk; monitor closely for toxicity

Administration

Oral: Administer 1 hour before or 1 hour after a meal.

I.V.: Infuse over 1-2 hours (rate not to exceed 3 mg/kg/hour). Do not infuse concomitantly into same line or cannula with other drug infusions, including TPN.

Stability

Reconstitution:

Powder for injection: Reconstitute 200 mg vial with 19 mL of sterile water for injection (use of automated syringe is not recommended). Resultant solution (20 mL) has a concentration of 10 mg/mL. Prior to infusion, must dilute to 0.5-5 mg/mL with NS, LR, D$_5$WLR, D$_5$½NS, D$_5$W, D$_5$W with KCl 20 mEq, ½NS, or D$_5$WNS. Do not dilute with 4.2% sodium bicarbonate infusion.

Powder for oral suspension: Add 46 mL of water to the bottle to make 40 mg/mL suspension. Discard unused portion after 14 days.

Compatibility:

Stable in NS, LR, D$_5$WLR, D$_5$½NS, D$_5$W, D$_5$W with KCl 20 mEq, ½NS, or D$_5$WNS½NS

Incompatible: Do not infuse simultaneously with blood products.

Incompatible with alkaline solutions, bicarbonate, aminofusin 10%, electrolyte solutions; do not infuse **concomitantly** into same line or cannula with other drug infusions, including TPN.

Storage:

Powder for injection: Store at 15°C to 30°C (59°F to 86°F). Reconstituted solutions are stable for up to 24 hours under refrigeration at 2°C to 8°C (36°F to 46°F).

Powder for oral suspension: Store at 2°C to 8°C (36°F to 46°F). Reconstituted oral suspension may be stored at 15°C to 30°C (59°F to 86°F).

Tablets: Store at 15°C to 30°C (59°F to 86°F).

Laboratory Monitoring Hepatic function at initiation and during course of treatment; renal function

Nursing Actions

Physical Assessment: Allergy history should be assessed prior to beginning therapy. Assess potential for interactions with other pharmacological agents and herbal products patient may be taking (eg, risk for increased or decreased levels/effects of voriconazole). Assess results of laboratory tests, therapeutic effectiveness (resolution of fungal infection), and adverse response (eg, vision changes [photophobia, changed visual acuity, blurred vision], hepatic toxicity [increased liver enzymes, jaundice], tachycardia) on a regular basis. Teach patient use, possible side effects (eg, vision changes) and interventions, and adverse symptoms to report.

Patient Education: Do not take any new medication during therapy unless approved by prescriber. Take full course of medication as ordered. Preferable to take on empty stomach (1 hour before or 2 hours after a meal). Avoid grapefruit juice while taking this medication. Maintain adequate hydration (2-3 L/day of fluids) unless instructed to restrict fluid intake. You may experience headache, dizziness, blurred vision, photophobia, or changes in visual acuity (use caution when driving or engaging in tasks that require alertness until response to drug is known - vision changes are reversible on discontinuation following brief treatment); or nausea or vomiting (small, frequent meals, frequent mouth care, sucking lozenges, or chewing gum may help). Report immediately any change in vision. Report skin rash; chest pain, palpitations, or rapid heartbeat; fever, chills, or hallucinations; persistent GI upset; urinary pattern changes; yellowing of skin or eyes; changes in color of stool or urine; or any other persistent side effects. **Pregnancy/breast-feeding precautions:** Inform prescriber if you are pregnant. Do not get pregnant while taking this drug. Fetal harm can occur. Consult prescriber for appropriate contraceptive measures. Breast-feeding is not recommended.

Dietary Considerations Oral: Should be taken 1 hour before or 1 hour after a meal. Voriconazole tablets contain lactose; avoid administration in hereditary galactose intolerance, Lapp lactase deficiency, or glucose-galactose malabsorption. Suspension contains sucrose; use caution with fructose intolerance, sucrose-isomaltase deficiency, or glucose-galactose malabsorption.

Breast-Feeding Issues Excretion in breast milk has not been investigated; avoid breast-feeding until additional data are available.

Pregnancy Issues Voriconazole can cause fetal harm when administered to a pregnant woman. Should be used in pregnant woman only if benefit to mother justifies potential risk to the fetus.

Warfarin (WAR far in)

U.S. Brand Names Coumadin®; Jantoven™

Synonyms Warfarin Sodium

Pharmacologic Category Anticoagulant, Coumarin Derivative

Medication Safety Issues

Sound-alike/look-alike issues:

Coumadin® may be confused with Avandia®, Cardura®, Compazine®, Kemadrin®

High alert medication: The Institute for Safe Medication Practices (ISMP) includes this medication among its list of drugs which have a heightened risk of causing significant patient harm when used in error.

Pregnancy Risk Factor X

Lactation Does not enter breast milk, only metabolites are excreted (AAP rates "compatible")

Use Prophylaxis and treatment of venous thrombosis, pulmonary embolism and thromboembolic disorders; atrial fibrillation with risk of embolism and as an adjunct in the prophylaxis of systemic embolism after myocardial infarction

Unlabeled/Investigational Use Prevention of recurrent transient ischemic attacks and to reduce risk of recurrent myocardial infarction

Mechanism of Action/Effect Interferes with hepatic synthesis of vitamin K-dependent coagulation factors (II, VII, IX, X)

Contraindications Hypersensitivity to warfarin or any component of the formulation; hemorrhagic tendencies; hemophilia; thrombocytopenia purpura; leukemia; recent or potential surgery of the eye or CNS; major regional lumbar block anesthesia or surgery resulting in large, open surfaces; patients bleeding from the GI, respiratory, or GU tract; threatened abortion; aneurysm; ascorbic acid deficiency; history of bleeding diathesis; prostatectomy; continuous tube drainage of the small intestine; polyarthritis; diverticulitis; emaciation; malnutrition; cerebrovascular hemorrhage; eclampsia/pre-eclampsia; blood dyscrasias; severe uncontrolled or malignant hypertension; severe hepatic disease; pericarditis or pericardial effusion; subacute bacterial endocarditis; visceral carcinoma; following spinal puncture and other diagnostic or therapeutic procedures with potential for significant bleeding; history of warfarin-induced necrosis; an unreliable, noncompliant patient; alcoholism; patient who has a history of falls or is a significant fall risk; pregnancy

Warnings/Precautions Use care in the selection of patients appropriate for this treatment. Ensure patient cooperation especially from the alcoholic, illicit drug user, demented, or psychotic patient. Use with caution in trauma, acute infection (antibiotics and fever may alter affects), renal insufficiency, prolonged dietary insufficiencies (vitamin K deficiency), moderate-severe hypertension, polycythemia vera, vasculitis, open wound, active TB, history of PUD, anaphylactic disorders, indwelling catheters, severe diabetes, thyroid disease, severe renal disease, and menstruating and postpartum women. Use with caution in protein C deficiency.

Hemorrhage is the most serious risk of therapy. Patient must be instructed to report bleeding, accidents, or falls. Patient must also report any new or discontinued medications, herbal or alternative products used, significant changes in smoking or dietary habits. Necrosis or gangrene of the skin and other tissues can occur (rarely) due to early hypercoagulability. "Purple toes syndrome," due to cholesterol microembolization, may rarely occur (often after several weeks of therapy). Women may be at risk of developing ovarian hemorrhage at the time of ovulation. The elderly may be more sensitive to anticoagulant therapy.

Drug Interactions

Cytochrome P450 Effect: Substrate of CYP1A2 (minor), 2C8/9 (major), 2C19 (minor), 3A4 (minor); **Inhibits** CYP2C8/9 (moderate), 2C19 (weak)

Decreased Effect: Serum levels/effects of warfarin may be decreased by: aminoglutethimide, antithyroid agents, aprepitant, azathioprine, barbiturates, bile acid sequestrants, bosentan, carbamazepine, CYP2C8/9 inducers (strong), dicloxacillin, glutethimide, griseofulvin, hormonal contraceptives (estrogens and progestins), mercaptopurine, nafcillin, phytonadione, rifamycin derivatives, and sulfasalazine.

Increased Effect/Toxicity: Serum levels/effects of warfarin may be increased by: acetaminophen (>1.3 g for > 1 week), allopurinol, amiodarone, androgens, antifungal agents (imidazole), capecitabine, cephalosporins, cimetidine, COX-2 inhibitors, CYP2C8/9 inhibitors (moderate/strong), disulfiram, drotrecogin alfa, etoposide, fibric acid derivatives, fluconazole, fluorouracil, glucagon, HMG-CoA reductase inhibitors, ifosfamide, leflunomide, macrolide antibiotics, metronidazole, NSAIDs (nonselective), orlistat, phenytoin, propafenone, propoxyphene, proton pump inhibitors (omeprazole), quinidine, quinolone antibiotics, ropinirole, salicylates, SSRIs, sulfinpyrazone, sulfonamide derivatives, tetracycline derivatives, thyroid products, tigecycline, treprostinil, tricyclic antidepressants, vitamin A, vitamin E, voriconazole, zafirlukast, and zileuton.

Nutritional/Ethanol Interactions

Ethanol: Avoid ethanol. Acute ethanol ingestion (binge drinking) decreases the metabolism of warfarin and increases PT/INR. Chronic daily ethanol use increases the metabolism of warfarin and decreases PT/INR.

Food: The anticoagulant effects of warfarin may be decreased if taken with foods rich in vitamin K. Vitamin E may increase warfarin effect. Cranberry juice may increase warfarin effect.

Herb/Nutraceutical: Cranberry, fenugreek, ginkgo biloba, glucosamine, may enhance bleeding or increase warfarin's effect. Ginseng (American), coenzyme Q_{10}, and St John's wort may decrease warfarin levels and effects. Avoid alfalfa, anise, bilberry, bladderwrack, bromelain, cat's claw, celery, coleus, cordyceps, dong quai, evening primrose oil, fenugreek, feverfew, garlic, ginger, ginkgo biloba, ginseng (American), ginseng (Panax), ginseng (Siberian), grape seed, green tea, guggul, horse chestnut seed, horseradish, licorice, prickly ash, red clover, reishi, same (s-adenosylmethionine), sweet clover, turmeric,and white willow (all have additional antiplatelet activity).

Adverse Reactions As with all anticoagulants, bleeding is the major adverse effect of warfarin. Hemorrhage may occur at virtually any site. Risk is dependent on multiple variables, including the intensity of anticoagulation and patient susceptibility.

Additional adverse effects are often related to idiosyncratic reactions, and the frequency cannot be accurately estimated.

Cardiovascular: Vasculitis, edema, hemorrhagic shock

Central nervous system: Fever, lethargy, malaise, asthenia, pain, headache, dizziness, stroke

Dermatologic: Rash, dermatitis, bullous eruptions, urticaria, pruritus, alopecia

Gastrointestinal: Anorexia, nausea, vomiting, stomach cramps, abdominal pain, diarrhea, flatulence, gastrointestinal bleeding, taste disturbance, mouth ulcers

Genitourinary: Priapism, hematuria

Hematologic: Hemorrhage, leukopenia, unrecognized bleeding sites (eg, colon cancer) may be uncovered by anticoagulation, retroperitoneal hematoma, agranulocytosis

Hepatic: Hepatic injury, jaundice, transaminases increased

Neuromuscular & skeletal: Paresthesia, osteoporosis

Respiratory: Hemoptysis, epistaxis, pulmonary hemorrhage, tracheobronchial calcification

Miscellaneous: Hypersensitivity/allergic reactions

Skin necrosis/gangrene, due to paradoxical local thrombosis, is a known but rare risk of warfarin therapy. Its onset is usually within the first few days of therapy and is frequently localized to the limbs, breast or penis. The risk of this effect is increased in patients with protein C or S deficiency.

"Purple toes syndrome," caused by cholesterol microembolization, also occurs rarely. Typically, this occurs after several weeks of therapy, and may present as a dark, purplish, mottled discoloration of the plantar and lateral surfaces. Other manifestations of cholesterol microembolization may include rash; livedo reticularis; gangrene; abrupt and intense pain in lower extremities; abdominal, flank, or back pain; hematuria, renal insufficiency; hypertension; cerebral ischemia; spinal cord infarction; or other symptom of vascular compromise.

Overdosage/Toxicology Symptoms of overdose include internal or external hemorrhage and hematuria. Avoid emesis and lavage to avoid possible trauma and incidental bleeding. When an overdose occurs, the drug should be immediately discontinued and vitamin K_1 (phytonadione) may be administered, up to 25 mg I.V. for adults. When hemorrhage occurs, fresh frozen plasma transfusions can help control bleeding by replacing clotting factors. In urgent bleeding, prothrombin complex concentrates may be needed.

Management of elevated INR: See table.

Pharmacodynamics/Kinetics
Onset of Action: Anticoagulation: Oral: 36-72 hours; Peak effect: Full therapeutic effect: 5-7 days; INR may increase in 36-72 hours

Duration of Action: 2-5 days

Half-Life Elimination: 20-60 hours; Mean: 40 hours; highly variable among individuals

Metabolism: Hepatic

Available Dosage Forms

Injection, powder for reconstitution, as sodium (Coumadin®): 5 mg

Tablet, as sodium (Coumadin®, Jantoven™): 1 mg, 2 mg, 2.5 mg, 3 mg, 4 mg, 5 mg, 6 mg, 7.5 mg, 10 mg

Dosing
Adults:
Prevention/treatment of thrombosis/embolism:
I.V. (administer as a slow bolus injection): 2-5 mg/day

Oral: Initial dosing must be individualized. Consider the patient (hepatic function, cardiac function, age, nutritional status, concurrent therapy, risk of bleeding) in addition to prior dose response (if available) and the clinical situation. Start 5-10 mg daily for 2 days. Adjust dose according to INR results; usual maintenance dose ranges from 2-10 mg daily (individual patients may require loading and maintenance doses outside these general guidelines).

Note: Lower starting doses may be required for patients with hepatic impairment, poor nutrition, CHF, elderly, high risk of bleeding, or patients that are debilitated. Higher initial doses may be reasonable in selected patients (ie, receiving enzyme-inducing agents and with low risk of bleeding).

Elderly: Oral: Initial dose ≤5 mg. Usual maintenance dose: 2-5 mg/day. The elderly tend to require lower dosages to produce a therapeutic level of anticoagulation (due to changes in the pattern of warfarin metabolism).

Management of Elevated INR

INR	Symptom	Action
Above therapeutic range to <5	No significant bleeding	Lower or hold the next dose and monitor frequently; when INR approaches desired range, may resume dosing with a lower dose if INR was significantly above therapeutic range.
≥5 and <9	No significant bleeding	Omit the next 1 or 2 doses; monitor INR and resume with a lower dose when the INR approaches the desired range.
		Alternatively, if there are other risk factors for bleeding, omit the next dose and give vitamin K_1 orally ≤5 mg; resume with a lower dose when the INR approaches the desired range.
		If rapid reversal is required for surgery, then given vitamin K_1 orally 2-4 mg and hold warfarin. Expect a response within 24 hours; another 1-2 mg may be given orally if needed.
≥9	No significant bleeding	Hold warfarin, give vitamin K_1 orally 5-10 mg, expect the INR to be reduced within 24-48 hours; monitor INR and administer additional vitamin K if necessary. Resume warfarin at lower doses when INR is in the desired range.
Any INR elevation	Serious bleeding	Hold warfarin, give vitamin K_1 (10 mg by slow I.V. infusion), and supplement with fresh plasma transfusion or prothrombin complex concentrate (Factor X complex); recombinant factor VIIa is an alternative to prothrombin complex concentrate. Vitamin K_1 injection can be repeated every 12 hours.
Any INR elevation	Life-threatening bleeding	Hold warfarin, give prothrombin complex concentrate, supplemented with vitamin K_1 (10 mg by slow I.V. infusion); repeat if necessary. Recombinant factor VIIa is an alternative to prothrombin complex concentrate.

Note: Use of high doses of vitamin K_1 (10.0-15.0) may cause resistance to warfarin for up to a week. Heparin or low molecular weight heparin can be given until the patient becomes responsive to warfarin.

Reference: Ansell J, Hirsh J, Poller L et al. "The Pharmacology and Management of the Vitamin K Antagonists," *Chest*, 2004, 126 (3 Suppl):204-33.

(Continued)

Warfarin (Continued)

Pediatrics:

Prevention/treatment of thrombosis: Oral: Infants and Children: 0.05-0.34 mg/kg/day; infants <12 months of age may require doses at or near the high end of this range; consistent anticoagulation may be difficult to maintain in children <5 years of age.

Hepatic Impairment: Monitor effect at usual doses. The response to oral anticoagulants may be markedly enhanced in obstructive jaundice, hepatitis, and cirrhosis. Prothrombin index should be closely monitored.

Administration

Oral: Do not take with food. Take at the same time each day.

I.V.: Administer as a slow bolus injection over 1-2 minutes. Avoid all I.M. injections.

I.V. Detail: pH: 8.1-8.3

Stability

Reconstitution: Injection is stable for 4 hours at room temperature after reconstitution with 2.7 mL of sterile water (yields 2 mg/mL solution).

Compatibility: Stable in D_5LR, $D_5^{1}/_2NS$, D_5NS, D_5W, $D_{10}W$

Y-site administration: Incompatible with aminophylline, bretylium, ceftazidime, cimetidine, ciprofloxacin, dobutamine, esmolol, gentamicin, labetalol, metronidazole, promazine, lactated Ringer's

Compatibility in syringe: Incompatible with heparin

Storage: Protect from light.

Laboratory Monitoring Prothrombin time (desirable range usually 1.5-2 times the control), hematocrit, INR (desirable range usually 2.0-3.0 with standard therapy, 2.5-3.5 with high-dose therapy)

Nursing Actions

Physical Assessment: Use caution with any condition that increases risk of bleeding (eg, renal impairment, dietary vitamin K or C deficiency, hypertension, open wounds, TB, PUD, diabetes, thyroid or renal disease, recent surgery). Assess potential for interactions with other pharmacological agents and herbal products patient may be taking (especially those medications that may affect coagulation or platelet). Monitor laboratory tests closely. Monitor patient frequently for adverse reactions (eg, bleeding from any site, rash, urticaria, gastrointestinal upset, abdominal pain, diarrhea, hypersensitivity reaction). Teach patient possible side effects/appropriate interventions (eg, safety precautions) and adverse symptoms to report. **Pregnancy risk factor X:** Determine that patient is not pregnant before beginning treatment. Teach patients of childbearing age appropriate use of contraceptives.

Patient Education: It is imperative that you inform prescriber of all prescriptions, OTC medications, or herbal products you are taking. Do not take any new medication during therapy unless approved by prescriber. Take exactly as directed; if dose is missed, take as soon as possible. Do not double dose. Follow diet and activity as recommended by prescriber; check with prescriber before changing diet. Avoid alcohol. Do not make major changes in your dietary intake of vitamin K (green vegetables). You will have a tendency to bleed easily while taking this drug (use soft toothbrush, waxed dental floss, electric razor, and avoid scissors or sharp knives and potentially harmful activities). May cause nausea, vomiting, disturbed taste (small frequent meals, frequent mouth care, sucking lozenges, or chewing gum may help). Report any unusual bleeding or bruising (eg, bleeding gums, nosebleed, blood in urine, dark stool, bloody emesis, heavier than usual menses, or menstrual irregularities); skin rash or irritation; unusual fever; persistent nausea or GI upset; pain in joints or back; swelling or

pain at injection site; or unhealed wounds. **Pregnancy precautions:** Do not get pregnant while taking this medication. Consult prescriber for appropriate barrier contraceptive measures.

Dietary Considerations Foods high in vitamin K (eg, beef liver, pork liver, green tea and leafy green vegetables) inhibit anticoagulant effect. Do not change dietary habits once stabilized on warfarin therapy; a balanced diet with a consistent intake of vitamin K is essential; avoid large amounts of alfalfa, asparagus, broccoli, Brussels sprouts, cabbage, cauliflower, green teas, kale, lettuce, spinach, turnip greens, watercress decrease efficacy of warfarin. It is recommended that the diet contain a CONSISTENT vitamin K content of 70-140 mcg/day. Check with healthcare provider before changing diet.

Geriatric Considerations Before committing an elderly patient to long-term anticoagulation therapy, their risk for bleeding complications secondary to falls, drug interactions, living situation, and cognitive status should be considered. A risk of bleeding complications has been associated with increased age.

Breast-Feeding Issues Warfarin does not pass into breast milk and can be given to nursing mothers (AAP rates "compatible"). However, limited data suggests prolonged PT may occur in some infants. Women who are breast-feeding should be carefully monitored to avoid excessive anticoagulation. Evaluation of coagulation tests and vitamin K status of breast-feeding infant is considered prudent.

Pregnancy Issues Oral anticoagulants cross the placenta and produce fetal abnormalities. Warfarin should not be used during pregnancy because of significant risks. Adjusted-dose heparin can be given safely throughout pregnancy in patients with venous thromboembolism.

Related Information

Overdose and Toxicology *on page 1423*
Peak and Trough Guidelines *on page 1387*

Zafirlukast (za FIR loo kast)

U.S. Brand Names Accolate®

Synonyms ICI-204,219

Pharmacologic Category Leukotriene-Receptor Antagonist

Medication Safety Issues

Sound-alike/look-alike issues:

Accolate® may be confused with Accupril®, Accutane®, Aclovate®

Pregnancy Risk Factor B

Lactation Enters breast milk/contraindicated

Use Prophylaxis and chronic treatment of asthma in adults and children ≥5 years of age

Mechanism of Action/Effect Leukotrienes are inflammatory mediators of asthma. Zafirlukast blocks leukotriene receptors and is able to reduce bronchoconstriction and inflammatory cell infiltration.

Contraindications Hypersensitivity to zafirlukast or any component of the formulation

Warnings/Precautions Zafirlukast is not indicated for use in the reversal of bronchospasm in acute asthma attacks, including status asthmaticus. Therapy with zafirlukast can be continued during acute exacerbations of asthma.

Hepatic adverse events (including hepatitis, hyperbilirubinemia, and hepatic failure) have been reported; female patients may be at greater risk. Discontinue immediately if liver dysfunction is suspected. Periodic testing of liver function may be considered (early detection is generally believed to improve the likelihood of recovery). If hepatic dysfunction is suspected (due to clinical signs/symptoms), liver function tests should be measured immediately. Do not resume or restart if hepatic function studies are consistent with dysfunction. Use caution in patients with alcoholic cirrhosis; clearance is reduced.

Rare cases of eosinophilic vasculitis (Churg-Strauss) have been reported in patients receiving zafirlukast (usually, but not always, associated with reduction in concurrent steroid dosage). No causal relationship established. Monitor for eosinophilic vasculitis, rash, pulmonary symptoms, cardiac symptoms, or neuropathy.

An increased proportion of zafirlukast patients >55 years of age reported infections as compared to placebo-treated patients. These infections were mostly mild or moderate in intensity and predominantly affected the respiratory tract. Infections occurred equally in both sexes, were dose-proportional to total milligrams of zafirlukast exposure, and were associated with coadministration of inhaled corticosteroids.

Drug Interactions
Cytochrome P450 Effect: Substrate of CYP2C8/9 (major); **Inhibits** CYP1A2 (weak), 2C8/9 (moderate), 2C19 (weak), 2D6 (weak), 3A4 (weak)
Decreased Effect: The levels/effects of zafirlukast may be decreased by carbamazepine, phenobarbital, phenytoin, rifampin, rifapentine, secobarbital, and other CYP2C8/9 inducers. Zafirlukast concentrations may be reduced by erythromycin.
Increased Effect/Toxicity: Zafirlukast concentrations are increased by aspirin. Zafirlukast may increase theophylline levels. Zafirlukast may increase the levels/effects of amiodarone, fluoxetine, glimepiride, glipizide, nateglinide, phenytoin, pioglitazone, rosiglitazone, sertraline, warfarin, and other CYP2C8/9 substrates.

Nutritional/Ethanol Interactions Food: Decreases bioavailability of zafirlukast by 40%.

Adverse Reactions
>10%: Central nervous system: Headache (13%)
1% to 10%:
    Central nervous system: Dizziness (2%), pain (2%), fever (2%)
    Gastrointestinal: Nausea (3%), diarrhea (3%), abdominal pain (2%), vomiting (2%), dyspepsia (1%)
    Hepatic: SGPT increased (2%)
    Neuromuscular & skeletal: Back pain (2%), myalgia (2%), weakness (2%)
    Miscellaneous: Infection (4%)

Overdose/Toxicology There is no experience with overdose in humans to date. Treatment is supportive.

Pharmacodynamics/Kinetics
Time to Peak: Serum: 3 hours
Protein Binding: >99%, primarily to albumin
Half-Life Elimination: 10 hours
Metabolism: Extensively hepatic via CYP2C9
Excretion: Urine (10%); feces

Available Dosage Forms Tablet: 10 mg, 20 mg

Dosing
Adults & Elderly: Asthma: Oral: 20 mg twice daily
Pediatrics: Asthma: Oral:
    Children 5-11 years: 10 mg twice daily. Safety and effectiveness have not been established in children <5 years of age.
    Children ≥12 years: Refer to adult dosing.
Renal Impairment:
    Dosage adjustment not required.
Hepatic Impairment: Clearance of zafirlukast is reduced with a greater C_{max} and AUC of 50% to 60% in patients with alcoholic cirrhosis.

Administration
Oral: Administer 1 hour before or 2 hours after meals.

Stability
Storage: Store tablets at controlled room temperature (20°C to 25°C; 68°F to 77°F); protect from light and moisture; dispense in original airtight container

Laboratory Monitoring Monitor for improvements in air flow; periodic monitoring of LFTs may be considered (not proved to prevent serious injury, but early detection may enhance recovery)

Nursing Actions
Physical Assessment: Not for use in acute asthma attack. Assess effectiveness and interactions of other medications patient may be taking. Monitor effectiveness of therapy and adverse reactions at beginning of therapy and periodically with long-term use. Monitor for liver dysfunction. Assess knowledge/teach patient appropriate use, interventions to reduce side effects, and adverse symptoms to report.

Patient Education: Do not use during acute bronchospasm. Take regularly as prescribed, even during symptom-free periods. This medication should be taken on an empty stomach, 1 hour before or 2 hours after meals. Do not take more than recommended or discontinue use without consulting prescriber. Do not stop taking other antiasthmatic medications unless instructed by prescriber. Avoid aspirin or aspirin-containing medications unless approved by prescriber. You may experience headache, drowsiness, dizziness, or blurred vision (use caution when driving or engaging in tasks requiring alertness until response to drug is known); or gastric upset, nausea, or vomiting (small frequent meals, frequent mouth care, chewing gum, or sucking lozenges may help). Report persistent CNS or GI symptoms; muscle or back pain; weakness, fever, chills; yellowing of skin or eyes; dark urine or pale stool; or skin rash. Contact prescriber immediately if experiencing right upper abdominal pain, nausea, fatigue, itching, flu-like symptoms; swelling of the eyes, face, neck, or throat; anorexia; or worsening of condition. **Breast-feeding precaution:** Do not breast-feed.

Dietary Considerations Should be taken on an empty stomach (1 hour before or 2 hours after meals).

Geriatric Considerations The mean dose (mg/kg) normalized AUC and C_{max} increase and plasma clearance decreases with increasing age. In patients >65 years of age, there is a two- to threefold greater C_{max} and AUC compared to younger adults. Some studies have demonstrated slightly higher adverse effect reports in elderly compared to younger adults: Headache (4.7%), diarrhea and nausea (1.8%), and pharyngitis (1.3%). No changes in dose recommended for elderly.

Breast-Feeding Issues The manufacturer does not recommend breast-feeding due to tumorigenicity observed in animal studies.

Zalcitabine (zal SITE a been)

U.S. Brand Names Hivid®
Synonyms ddC; Dideoxycytidine
Pharmacologic Category Antiretroviral Agent, Reverse Transcriptase Inhibitor (Nucleoside)
Pregnancy Risk Factor C
Lactation Excretion in breast milk unknown/contraindicated
Use In combination with at least two other antiretrovirals in the treatment of patients with HIV infection; it is not recommended that zalcitabine be given in combination with didanosine, stavudine, or lamivudine due to overlapping toxicities, virologic interactions, or lack of clinical data
Mechanism of Action/Effect Inhibits cell protein synthesis leading to cell death with viral replication.
Contraindications Hypersensitivity to zalcitabine or any component of the formulation
Warnings/Precautions Careful monitoring of pancreatic enzymes and liver function tests in patients with a history of pancreatitis, increased amylase, those on parenteral nutrition or with a history of ethanol abuse; (Continued)

Zalcitabine *(Continued)*

discontinue use immediately if pancreatitis is suspected; lactic acidosis and severe hepatomegaly and failure have rarely occurred with zalcitabine resulting in fatality (stop treatment if lactic acidosis or hepatotoxicity occur); some cases may possibly be related to underlying hepatitis B; use with caution in patients on digitalis, or with CHF, renal failure, or hyperphosphatemia; zalcitabine can cause severe peripheral neuropathy; avoid use, if possible, in patients with pre-existing neuropathy or at risk of developing neuropathy. Risk factors include CD4 counts <50 cells/mm^3, diabetes mellitus, weight loss, other drugs known to cause peripheral neuropathy.

Drug Interactions

Decreased Effect: It is not recommended that zalcitabine be given in combination with didanosine, stavudine, or lamivudine due to overlapping toxicities, virologic interactions, or lack of clinical data. Doxorubicin and lamivudine have been shown *in vitro* to decrease zalcitabine phosphorylation. Magnesium/aluminum-containing antacids and metoclopramide may decrease the absorption of zalcitabine.

Increased Effect/Toxicity: Amphotericin, foscarnet, and aminoglycosides may potentiate the risk of developing peripheral neuropathy or other toxicities associated with zalcitabine by interfering with the renal elimination of zalcitabine. Other drugs associated with peripheral neuropathy include chloramphenicol, cisplatin, dapsone, disulfiram, ethionamide, glutethimide, gold, hydralazine, iodoquinol, isoniazid, metronidazole, nitrofurantoin, phenytoin, ribavirin, and vincristine. Concomitant use with zalcitabine may increase risk of peripheral neuropathy. Concomitant use of zalcitabine with didanosine is not recommended. Concomitant use of ribavirin and nucleoside analogues may increase the risk of developing lactic acidosis (includes adefovir, didanosine, lamivudine, stavudine, zalcitabine, zidovudine).

Nutritional/Ethanol Interactions Food: Food decreases peak plasma concentrations by 39%. Extent and rate of absorption may be decreased with food.

Lab Interactions May cause abnormalities in CBC, WBC, hemoglobin, platelet count, AST, ALT, or alkaline phosphatase.

Adverse Reactions

>10%:

Central nervous system: Fever (5% to 17%), malaise (2% to 13%)

Neuromuscular & skeletal: Peripheral neuropathy (28%)

1% to 10%:

Central nervous system: Headache (2%), dizziness (1%), fatigue (4%), seizure (1.3%)

Dermatologic: Rash (2% to 11%), pruritus (3% to 5%)

Endocrine & metabolic: Hypoglycemia (2% to 6%), hyponatremia (4%), hyperglycemia (1% to 6%)

Gastrointestinal: Nausea (3%), dysphagia (1% to 4%), anorexia (4%), abdominal pain (3% to 8%), vomiting (1% to 3%), diarrhea (<1% to 10%), weight loss, oral ulcers (3% to 7%), increased amylase (3% to 8%)

Hematologic: Anemia (occurs as early as 2-4 weeks), granulocytopenia (usually after 6-8 weeks)

Hepatic: Abnormal hepatic function (9%), hyperbilirubinemia (2% to 5%)

Neuromuscular & skeletal: Myalgia (1% to 6%), foot pain

Respiratory: Pharyngitis (2%), cough (6%), nasal discharge (4%)

Overdosage/Toxicology Symptoms of overdose include delayed peripheral neurotoxicity. Treatment is supportive.

Pharmacodynamics/Kinetics

Protein Binding: <4%

Half-Life Elimination: 2.9 hours; Renal impairment: ≤8.5 hours

Metabolism: Intracellularly to active triphosphorylated agent

Excretion: Urine (>70% as unchanged drug)

Available Dosage Forms Tablet: 0.375 mg, 0.75 mg

Dosing

Adults & Elderly: HIV infection (component of combination therapy): Oral: Daily dose: 0.75 mg every 8 hours

Pediatrics: HIV infection: Oral:

Children <13 years: Safety and efficacy have not been established; investigational dose: 0.01 mg/kg every 8 hours

Adolescents: Refer to adult dosing.

Renal Impairment:

Cl$_{cr}$ 10-40 mL/minute: Administer 0.75 mg every 12 hours.

Cl$_{cr}$ <10 mL/minute: Administer 0.75 mg every 24 hours.

Moderately dialyzable (20% to 50%)

Administration

Oral: Food decreases absorption; take on an empty stomach. Administer around-the-clock. Do not take at the same time with dapsone.

Stability

Storage: Tablets should be stored in tightly closed bottles at room temperature (59°F to 86°F)

Laboratory Monitoring CBC and serum chemistry (prior to initiation and appropriate intervals), renal function, CD4 counts, serum amylase, triglyceride, calcium, viral load

Nursing Actions

Physical Assessment: Allergy history should be assessed prior to beginning treatment. Assess other pharmacological or herbal products patient may be taking (especially those that increase risk of peripheral neuropathy). Monitor laboratory tests, therapeutic response, and adverse reactions (lactic acidosis [elevated transaminases]; gastrointestinal disturbance [nausea, vomiting, diarrhea]; myalgia; peripheral neuropathy) on a regular basis throughout therapy. Teach patient proper use (eg, timing of multiple medications and drugs that should not be used concurrently), possible side effects/appropriate interventions, and adverse symptoms to report.

Patient Education: Do not take any new prescriptions, over-the-counter medications, or herbal products without consulting prescriber. This drug will not cure HIV, nor has it been found to reduce transmission of HIV; use appropriate precautions to prevent spread to other persons. This drug is prescribed as one part of a multidrug combination; take exactly as directed; preferably on an empty stomach, 1 hour before or 2 hours after meals. Do not take antacids or other medication within 1 hour of taking this medication. Maintain adequate hydration (2-3 L/day of fluids) unless advised by prescriber to restrict fluids. You may be susceptible to infection (avoid crowds and exposure to known infections and do not have any vaccinations without consulting prescriber). Frequent blood tests may be required with prolonged therapy. May cause dizziness, fatigue, or headache (use caution when driving or engaging in tasks requiring alertness until response to drug is known); nausea, vomiting, lack of appetite (small frequent meals, frequent mouth care, chewing gum, or sucking lozenges may help). Report muscle weakness or pain; tingling, numbness, or pain in toes or fingers; weakness of extremities; chest pain, palpitations, or rapid heartbeat; swelling of extremities; weight gain or loss >5 lb/week; signs of infection (eg, fever, chills, sore throat, burning urination, fatigue); unusual bleeding (eg, tarry stools, easy bruising, or blood in stool, urine, or mouth); skin rash, irritation; or any other persistent adverse effects. **Pregnancy/breast-feeding precautions:** Inform prescriber if you are or intend to become pregnant. Do not breast-feed.

Breast-Feeding Issues HIV-infected mothers are discouraged from breast-feeding to decrease potential transmission of HIV.

Pregnancy Issues It is not known if zalcitabine crosses the human placenta. Animal studies have shown zalcitabine to be teratogenic; developmental toxicities were also observed. Cases of lactic acidosis/hepatic steatosis syndrome have been reported in pregnant women receiving nucleoside analogue drugs. It is not known if pregnancy itself potentiates this known side effect; however, pregnant women may be at increased risk of lactic acidosis and liver damage. Hepatic enzymes and electrolytes should be monitored frequently during the 3rd trimester of pregnancy in women receiving nucleoside analogues. Health professionals are encouraged to contact the antiretroviral pregnancy registry to monitor outcomes of pregnant women exposed to antiretroviral medications (1-800-258-4263 or www.APRegistry.com).

Additional Information Potential compliance problems, frequency of administration and adverse effects should be discussed with patients before initiating therapy to help prevent the emergence of resistance.

Zaleplon (ZAL e plon)

U.S. Brand Names Sonata®
Restrictions C-IV

Pharmacologic Category Hypnotic, Nonbenzodiazepine

Pregnancy Risk Factor C

Lactation Enters breast milk/not recommended

Use Short-term (7-10 days) treatment of insomnia (has been demonstrated to be effective for up to 5 weeks in controlled trial)

Mechanism of Action/Effect Zaleplon is unrelated to benzodiazepines, barbiturates, or other hypnotics. However, it interacts with the benzodiazepine GABA receptor complex. Nonclinical studies have shown that it binds selectively to the brain omega-1 receptor situated on the alpha subunit of the GABA-A receptor complex.

Contraindications Hypersensitivity to zaleplon or any component of the formulation

Warnings/Precautions Failure of sleep disturbance to resolve after 7-10 days may indicate psychiatric and/or medical illness. Use with caution in patients with depression, particularly if suicidal risk may be present. Use with caution in patients with a history of drug dependence. Abrupt discontinuance may lead to withdrawal symptoms. May impair physical and mental capabilities; caution in patients receiving other CNS depressants or psychoactive medications. Effects with other sedative drugs or ethanol may be potentiated. Use with caution in the elderly, those with compromised respiratory function, or renal and hepatic impairment. Because of the rapid onset of action, zaleplon should be administered immediately prior to bedtime or after the patient has gone to bed and is having difficulty falling asleep. Capsules contain tartrazine (FDC yellow #5); avoid in patients with sensitivity (caution in patients with asthma).

Drug Interactions
Cytochrome P450 Effect: Substrate of CYP3A4 (minor)

Increased Effect/Toxicity: Zaleplon potentiates the CNS effects of CNS depressants, including ethanol, anticonvulsants, antipsychotics, barbiturates, benzodiazepines, narcotic agonists, and other sedative agents. Cimetidine increases concentrations of zaleplon. Avoid concurrent use or use 5 mg zaleplon as starting dose in patient receiving cimetidine.

Nutritional/Ethanol Interactions
Ethanol: Avoid ethanol (may increase CNS depression).

Food: High fat meal prolonged absorption; delayed t_{max} by 2 hours, and reduced C_{max} by 35%.

Herb/Nutraceutical: St John's wort may decrease zaleplon levels. Avoid valerian, St John's wort, kava kava, gotu kola (may increase CNS depression).

Adverse Reactions
1% to 10%:
Cardiovascular: Peripheral edema, chest pain
Central nervous system: Amnesia, anxiety, depersonalization, dizziness, hallucinations, hypoesthesia, somnolence, vertigo, malaise, depression, lightheadedness, impaired coordination, fever, migraine
Dermatologic: Photosensitivity reaction, rash, pruritus
Gastrointestinal: Abdominal pain, anorexia, colitis, dyspepsia, nausea, constipation, xerostomia
Genitourinary: Dysmenorrhea
Neuromuscular & skeletal: Paresthesia, tremor, myalgia, weakness, back pain, arthralgia
Ocular: Abnormal vision, eye pain
Otic: Hyperacusis
Miscellaneous: Parosmia

Overdosage/Toxicology Symptoms include CNS depression, ranging from drowsiness to coma. Mild overdose is associated with drowsiness, confusion, and lethargy. Serious case may result in ataxia, respiratory depression, hypotension, hypotonia, coma, and rarely death. Treatment is supportive.

Pharmacodynamics/Kinetics
Onset of Action: Rapid; Peak effect: ~1 hour
Duration of Action: 6-8 hours
Time to Peak: Serum: 1 hour
Protein Binding: 60% ± 15%
Half-Life Elimination: 1 hour
Metabolism: Extensive, primarily via aldehyde oxidase to form 5-oxo-zaleplon and to a lesser extent by CYP3A4 to desethylzaleplon; all metabolites are pharmacologically inactive
Excretion: Urine (primarily metabolites, <1% as unchanged drug)
Clearance: Plasma: Oral: 3 L/hour/kg

Available Dosage Forms Capsule: 5 mg, 10 mg [contains tartrazine]

Dosing
Adults: Insomnia (short-term use): Oral: 10 mg at bedtime (range: 5-20 mg)
Elderly: Reduce dose to 5 mg at bedtime
Renal Impairment: No adjustment for mild to moderate renal impairment; use in severe renal impairment has not been adequately studied.
Hepatic Impairment: Mild to moderate impairment: 5 mg; not recommended for use in patients with severe hepatic impairment.

Administration
Oral: Administer immediately before bedtime or when the patient is in bed and cannot fall asleep.

Stability
Storage: Store at controlled room temperature of 20°C to 25°C (68°F to 77°F); protect from light

Nursing Actions
Physical Assessment: Assess effectiveness and interactions of other medications. Assess for history of addiction (long-term use may result in dependence, abuse, or tolerance). For inpatient use, institute safety measures and monitor effectiveness and adverse reactions. For outpatients, monitor therapeutic effectiveness and adverse reactions at beginning of therapy and periodically with long-term use. Assess knowledge/teach patient appropriate use, interventions to reduce side effects, and adverse reactions to report.

Patient Education: Take exactly as directed; immediately before bedtime, or when you cannot fall asleep. Do not alter dosage or frequency; may be habit forming. Avoid alcohol and other prescription or OTC medications (especially medications to relieve pain, (Continued)

Zaleplon *(Continued)*

induce sleep, reduce anxiety, treat or prevent cold, coughs, or allergies) unless approved by prescriber. You may experience drowsiness, dizziness, somnolence, vertigo, lightheadedness, blurred vision (avoid driving or engaging in activities that require alertness until response to drug is known); photosensitivity (avoid exposure to direct sunlight, wear protective clothing, and sunscreen); nausea or GI discomfort (small frequent meals, good mouth care, chewing gum, or sucking hard candy may help); constipation (increase exercise, fluids, fruit, or fiber may help); or menstrual disturbances (reversible when drug is discontinued). Discontinue drug and report any severe CNS disturbances (hallucinations, acute nervousness or anxiety, persistent sleepiness or lethargy, impaired coordination, amnesia, or impaired thought processes); skin rash or irritation; eye pain or major vision changes; respiratory difficulty; chest pain; ear pain; or muscle weakness or pain. **Pregnancy/ breast-feeding precautions:** Inform prescriber if you are or intend to become pregnant. Breast-feeding is not recommended.

Pregnancy Issues Benzodiazepines cross the placenta. The association between benzodiazepine exposure and malformations remains controversial. A number of types of malformation have been reported (oral cleft, inguinal hernia, cardiac defects, spina bifida, dysmorphic facial features, skeletal defects); however, confounding factors make a clear association difficult. Overall, the risk to the fetus may be low. Nonteratogenic effects (including neonatal flaccidity, respiratory and feeding problems, and withdrawal symptoms) during the postnatal period have also been reported with benzodiazepine use.

Additional Information Prescription quantities should not exceed a 1-month supply.

Related Information

Anxiolytic / Hypnotic Use in Long-Term Care Facilities *on page 1418*

Zanamivir *(za NA mi veer)*

U.S. Brand Names Relenza®

Pharmacologic Category Antiviral Agent; Neuraminidase Inhibitor

Pregnancy Risk Factor C

Lactation Excretion in breast milk unknown/use caution

Use Treatment of uncomplicated acute illness due to influenza virus A and B; treatment should only be initiated in patients who have been symptomatic for no more than 2 days. Prophylaxis against influenza virus A and B

Mechanism of Action/Effect Zanamivir inhibits influenza virus neuraminidase enzymes, potentially altering virus particle aggregation and release.

Contraindications Hypersensitivity to zanamivir or any component of the formulation

Warnings/Precautions Patients must be instructed in the use of the delivery system. No data are available to support the use of this drug in patients who begin use for treatment after 48 hours of symptoms. Effectiveness has not been established in patients with significant underlying medical conditions or for prophylaxis of influenza in nursing home patients. Not recommended for use in patients with underlying respiratory disease, such as asthma or COPD, due to lack of efficacy and risk of serious adverse effects. Bronchospasm, decreased lung function, and other serious adverse reactions, including those with fatal outcomes, have been reported in patients with and without airway disease; discontinue with bronchospasm or signs of decreased lung function. For a patient with an underlying airway disease where a medical decision has been made to use zanamivir, a

fast-acting bronchodilator should be made available, and used prior to each dose. Not a substitute for the flu vaccine. Consider primary or concomitant bacterial infections. Powder for oral inhalation contains lactose. Safety and efficacy of repeated courses or use with severe renal impairment have not been established; efficacy in children <5 years of age have not been established.

Drug Interactions

Decreased Effect: Zanamivir may diminish the therapeutic effect of live, attenuated influenza virus vaccine (FluMist™). The manufacturer of FluMist™ recommends that the administration of anti-influenza virus medications be avoided during the period beginning 48 hours prior to vaccine administration and ending 2 weeks after vaccine.

Adverse Reactions Most adverse reactions occurred at a frequency which was less than or equal to the control (lactose vehicle).

>10%:

Central nervous system: Headache (prophylaxis 13% to 24%; treatment 2%)

Gastrointestinal: Throat/tonsil discomfort/pain (prophylaxis 8% to 19%)

Respiratory: Cough (prophylaxis 7% to 17%; treatment ≤2%), nasal signs and symptoms (prophylaxis 12%; treatment 2%)

Miscellaneous: Viral infection (prophylaxis 3% to 13%)

1% to 10%:

Central nervous system: Fever/chills (prophylaxis 5% to 9%; treatment <1.5%), fatigue (prophylaxis 5% to 8%; treatment <1.5%), malaise (prophylaxis 5% to 8%; treatment <1.5%), dizziness (treatment 1% to 2%)

Dermatologic: Urticaria (treatment <1.5%)

Gastrointestinal: Anorexia/appetite decreased (prophylaxis 2% to 4%), nausea (prophylaxis 1% to 2%; treatment ≤3%), diarrhea (prophylaxis 2%; treatment 2% to 3%), vomiting (prophylaxis 1% to 2%; treatment 1% to 2%) abdominal pain (treatment <1.5%)

Neuromuscular & skeletal: Muscle pain (prophylaxis 3% to 8%), musculoskeletal pain (prophylaxis 6%), arthralgia/articular rheumatism (prophylaxis 2%), arthralgia (treatment <1.5%), myalgia (treatment <1.5%)

Respiratory: Infection (ear/nose/throat; prophylaxis 2%; treatment 2% to 5%), sinusitis (treatment 3%), bronchitis (treatment 2%), nasal inflammation (prophylaxis 1%)

Overdosage/Toxicology Information is limited, and symptoms appear similar to reported adverse events from clinical studies. Treatment should be symptom-directed and supportive

Pharmacodynamics/Kinetics

Protein Binding: Plasma: <10%

Half-Life Elimination: Serum: 2.5-5.1 hours

Metabolism: None

Excretion: Urine (as unchanged drug); feces (unabsorbed drug)

Available Dosage Forms Powder for oral inhalation: 5 mg/blister (20s) [4 blisters per Rotadisk® foil pack, 5 Rotadisk® per package; packaged with Diskhaler® inhalation device; contains lactose]

Dosing

Adults & Elderly: Influenza virus A and B:

Prophylaxis: Oral inhalation:

Household setting: Two inhalations (10 mg) once daily for 10 days. Begin within 1½ days following onset of signs or symptoms of index case.

Community outbreak: Two inhalations (10 mg) once daily for 28 days. Begin within 5 days of outbreak.

Treatment: Oral inhalation: Two inhalations (10 mg total) twice daily for 5 days. Doses on first day should be separated by at least 2 hours; on subsequent days, doses should be spaced by ~12 hours. Begin within 2 days of signs or symptoms.

Pediatrics: Influenza virus A and B:

Prophylaxis: Oral inhalation:

Household setting: Children ≥5 years: Refer to adult dosing.

Community outbreak: Adolescents: Refer to adult dosing.

Treatment: Oral inhalation: Children ≥7 years: Refer to adult dosing.

Administration

Inhalation: Must be used with Diskhaler® delivery device. Patients who are scheduled to use an inhaled bronchodilator should use their bronchodilator prior to zanamivir. With the exception of the initial dose when used for treatment, administer at the same time each day.

Stability

Storage: Store at room temperature (25°C) 77°F. Do not puncture blister until taking a dose using the Diskhaler®.

Nursing Actions

Physical Assessment: Therapy for treatment must be started within 48 hours of first influenza symptoms. Teach patient appropriate use (inhalation device), interventions to reduce side effects, and adverse reactions to report.

Patient Education: This is **not** a substitute for the influenza vaccine. Use delivery device exactly as directed; complete full regimen, even if symptoms improve sooner. If you have asthma or COPD you may be at risk for bronchospasm; see prescriber for appropriate bronchodilator before using zanamivir. Stop using this medication and contact your physician if you experience shortness of breath, increased wheezing, or other signs of bronchospasm. You may experience dizziness or headache (use caution when driving or engaging in hazardous tasks until response to drug is known). Report unresolved diarrhea, vomiting, or nausea; acute fever or muscle pain; or other acute and persistent adverse effects. **Pregnancy/breast-feeding precautions:** Inform prescriber if you are or intend to become pregnant. Consult prescriber if breast-feeding.

Breast-Feeding Issues Zanamivir has been shown to be excreted in the milk of animals, but its excretion in human milk is unknown. Caution should be used when zanamivir is administered to a nursing mother.

Additional Information Majority of patients included in clinical trials were infected with influenza A, however, a number of patients with influenza B infections were also enrolled. Patients with lower temperature or less severe symptoms appeared to derive less benefit from therapy. No consistent treatment benefit was demonstrated in patients with chronic underlying medical conditions.

Ziconotide (zi KOE no tide)

U.S. Brand Names Prialt®

Pharmacologic Category Analgesic, Non-narcotic; Calcium Channel Blocker, N-Type

Pregnancy Risk Factor C

Lactation Excretion in breast milk unknown/not recommended

Use Management of severe chronic pain in patients requiring intrathecal (I.T.) therapy and are intolerant or refractory to other therapies

Mechanism of Action/Effect Ziconotide selectively binds to N-type voltage sensitive calcium channels located on the afferent nerves of the dorsal horn in the spinal cord. This binding is thought to block N-type calcium channels, leading to a blockade of excitatory neurotransmitter release and reducing sensitivity to painful stimuli.

Contraindications Hypersensitivity to ziconotide or any component of the formulation; history of psychosis; I.V. administration

I.T. administration is contraindicated in patients with infection at the injection site, uncontrolled bleeding, or spinal canal obstruction that impairs CSF circulation

Warnings/Precautions Severe psychiatric symptoms and neurological impairment have been reported; interrupt or discontinue therapy if cognitive impairment, hallucinations, mood changes, or changes in consciousness occur. Cognitive impairment may appear gradually during treatment and is generally reversible after discontinuation. Use caution in the elderly; may experience confusion. Patients should be instructed to use caution in performing tasks which require alertness (eg, operating machinery or driving). May have additive effects with opiates or other CNS-depressant medications. Does not potentiate opiate-induced respiratory depression. Will not prevent or relieve symptoms associated with opiate withdrawal and opiates should not be abruptly discontinued. Unlike opioids, ziconotide therapy can be interrupted abruptly or discontinued without evidence of withdrawal. Meningitis may occur with use of I.T. pumps and treatment may require removal of system and discontinuation of therapy. Safety and efficacy have not been established with renal or hepatic dysfunction, or in pediatric patients.

Drug Interactions

Increased Effect/Toxicity: May enhance the adverse/toxic effects of other CNS depressants

Adverse Reactions Percentages reported when using the slow (21-day) titration schedule; frequencies may be higher with faster titration.

>10%:

Central nervous system: Dizziness (47%), somnolence (22%), confusion (18%), ataxia (16%), headache (15%), memory impairment (12%), pain (11%)

Gastrointestinal: Nausea (41%), diarrhea (19%), vomiting (15%)

Neuromuscular & skeletal: Weakness (22%), gait disturbances (15%), hypertonia (11%)

2% to 10%:

Cardiovascular: Chest pain, edema, hyper-/hypotension, postural hypotension, tachycardia, vasodilation

Central nervous system: Anxiety (9%), speech disorder (9%), aphasia (8%), dysesthesia (7%), fever (7%), hallucinations (7%), nervousness (7%), vertigo (7%), agitation, chills, depression, dreams abnormal, emotional lability, hostility, hyperesthesia, insomnia, malaise, meningitis, paranoid reaction, stupor

Dermatologic: Bruising, cellulitis, dry skin, pruritus, rash

Endocrine & metabolic: Hypokalemia

Gastrointestinal: Anorexia (10%), abdominal pain, constipation, dehydration, dyspepsia, taste perversion, weight loss, xerostomia

Genitourinary: Urinary retention (9%), dysuria, urinary incontinence, urinary tract infection, urination impaired

Hematologic: Anemia

Local: Catheter complication, catheter site pain, pump site complication, pump site mass, pump site pain

Neuromuscular & skeletal: Paresthesia (7%), arthralgia, arthritis, back pain, CPK increased (<2%), incoordination, leg cramps, myalgia, myasthenia, neck pain, neck rigidity, neuralgia, reflexes decreased, tremor

Ocular: Vision abnormal (10%), nystagmus (8%), diplopia, photophobia,

Otic: Tinnitus

Respiratory: Bronchitis, cough, dyspnea, pharyngitis, pneumonia, rhinitis, sinusitis

Miscellaneous: CSF abnormalities, diaphoresis, flu-like syndrome, infection

(Continued)

Ziconotide *(Continued)*

Overdosage/Toxicology Exaggerated pharmacological effects, including ataxia, confusion, dizziness, garbled speech, hypotension, nausea, nystagmus, sedation, spinal myoclonus, stupor, unresponsiveness, vomiting and word-finding difficulty, are reported at doses >19.2 mcg/day. Respiratory depression was not observed. In case of overdose, ziconotide can be discontinued temporarily or withdrawn; additional treatment should be symptom directed and supportive. Opioid antagonists are not effective. Most patients recover within 24 hours of discontinuing ziconotide therapy.

Pharmacodynamics/Kinetics

Protein Binding: 50%

Half-Life Elimination: I.V.: 1-1.6 hours (plasma); I.T.: 2.9-6.5 hours (CSF)

Metabolism: Metabolized via endopeptidases and exopeptidases present on multiple organs including kidney, liver, lung; degraded to peptide fragments and free amino acids

Excretion: I.V.: Urine (<1%)

Available Dosage Forms Injection, solution, as acetate [preservative free]: 25 mcg/mL (20 mL); 100 mcg/mL (1 mL, 2 mL, 5 mL)

Dosing

Adults: Chronic pain: I.T.: Initial dose: 2.4 mcg/day (0.1 mcg/hour)

Dose may be titrated by ≤2.4 mcg/day (0.1 mcg/hour) at intervals ≥2-3 times/week to a maximum dose of 19.2 mcg/day (0.8 mcg/hour) by day 21; average dose at day 21: 6.9 mcg/day (0.29 mcg/hour). A faster titration should be used only if the urgent need for analgesia outweighs the possible risk to patient safety.

Dosage adjustment for toxicity: Cognitive impairment: Reduce dose or discontinue. Effects are generally reversible within 2 weeks of discontinuation.

Elderly: Refer to adult dosing. Use with caution.

Dosing Adjustment for Toxicity: Cognitive impairment: Reduce dose or discontinue. Effects are generally reversible within 2 weeks of discontinuation.

Administration

I.V.: Not for I.V. administration

I.V. Detail: pH: 4-5

Other: Not for I.V. administration. **For I.T. administration only** using Medtronic SynchroMed® EL, SynchroMed® II Infusion System, or CADD-Micro® ambulatory infusion pump.

Medtronic SynchroMed® EL or SynchroMed® II Infusion Systems:

Naive pump priming (first time use with ziconotide): Use 2 mL of undiluted ziconotide 25 mcg/mL solution to rinse the internal surfaces of the pump; repeat twice for a total of 3 rinses

Initial pump fill: Use only undiluted 25 mcg/mL solution and fill pump after priming. Following the initial fill only, adsorption on internal device surfaces will occur, requiring the use of the undiluted solution and refill within 14 days.

Pump refills: Contents should be emptied prior to refill. Subsequent pump refills should occur at least every 40 days if using diluted solution or every 60 days if using undiluted solution

CADD-Micro® ambulatory infusion pump: Refer to manufacturers' manual for initial fill and refill instructions

Stability

Reconstitution: Preservative free NS should be used when dilution is needed.

CADD-Micro® ambulatory infusion pump: Initial fill: Dilute to final concentration of 5 mcg/mL

Storage: Prior to use, store vials at 2°C to 8°C (36°F to 46°F); once diluted, may be stored at 2°C to 8°C (36°F to 46°F) for 24 hours. Do not freeze. Protect from light.

When using the Medtronic SynchroMed® EL or SynchroMed® II Infusion System, solutions expire as follows:

25 mcg/mL: Undiluted:
Initial fill: Use within 14 days
Refill: use within 60 days
100 mcg/mL
Undiluted: Refill: Use within 60 days
Diluted: Refill: Use within 40 days

Nursing Actions

Physical Assessment:

Assess other medications patient may be taking for effectiveness and interactions. This medication is given intrathecally via an implanted pump. Monitor for therapeutic response. Monitor for changes in behavior, cognitive impairment, hallucinations, or changes in mood or consciousness. Assess knowledge/teach patient appropriate use, interventions to reduce side effects, and adverse symptoms to report.

Patient Education:

Avoid alcohol, other prescriptions, or OTC medications (especially sedatives, tranquilizers, antihistamines, and other pain medications) without consulting prescriber. You may experience dizziness, sleepiness, or lightheadedness (use caution when driving or engaging in tasks requiring alertness until response to drug is known); nausea or vomiting (small frequent meals, frequent mouth care, chewing gum, or sucking lozenges may help); constipation (increased exercise, fluids, fruit, or fiber may help); or diarrhea (buttermilk, boiled milk, or yogurt may help), loss of appetite. Report chest pain, swelling of extremities (feet/ankles); muscle weakness and poor coordination; hallucinations, confusion, or extreme weakness. **Pregnancy/breast-feeding precaution:** Inform prescriber if you are or intend to become pregnant. Breast-feeding not recommended.

Geriatric Considerations See Warnings/Precautions, Adverse Reactions, and Dosing. Manufacturer reports that in all trials there was a higher incidence of confusion in the elderly compared to younger adults.

Breast-Feeding Issues The manufacturer recommends discontinuing breast-feeding or discontinuing ziconotide.

Zidovudine *(zye DOE vyoo deen)*

U.S. Brand Names Retrovir®

Synonyms Azidothymidine; AZT (error-prone abbreviation); Compound S; ZDV

Pharmacologic Category Antiretroviral Agent, Reverse Transcriptase Inhibitor (Nucleoside)

Medication Safety Issues

Sound-alike/look-alike issues:

Azidothymidine may be confused with azathioprine, aztreonam

Retrovir® may be confused with ritonavir

AZT is an error-prone abbreviation (mistaken as azathioprine, aztreonam)

Pregnancy Risk Factor C

Lactation Enters breast milk/not recommended

Use Management of patients with HIV infections in combination with at least two other antiretroviral agents; for prevention of maternal/fetal HIV transmission as monotherapy

Unlabeled/Investigational Use Postexposure prophylaxis for HIV exposure as part of a multidrug regimen

Mechanism of Action/Effect Zidovudine is a thymidine analog which interferes with the HIV virus that results in inhibition of viral replication.

Contraindications Life-threatening hypersensitivity to zidovudine or any component of the formulation

Warnings/Precautions Often associated with hematologic toxicity including granulocytopenia, severe anemia requiring transfusions, or (rarely) pancytopenia. Use with caution in patients with bone marrow compromise (granulocytes <1000 cells/mm^3 or hemoglobin <9.5 mg/dL); dosage adjustment may be required in patients who develop anemia or neutropenia. Lactic acidosis and severe hepatomegaly with steatosis have been reported, including fatal cases; use with caution in patients with risk factors for liver disease (risk may be increased in obese patients or prolonged exposure) and suspend treatment with zidovudine in any patient who develops clinical or laboratory findings suggestive of lactic acidosis (transaminase elevation may/may not accompany hepatomegaly and steatosis). Prolonged use has been associated with symptomatic myopathy. Reduce dose in patients with renal impairment.

Drug Interactions
Cytochrome P450 Effect: Substrate (minor) of CYP2A6, 2C8/9, 2C19, 3A4

Decreased Effect: *In vitro* evidence suggests zidovudine's antiretroviral activity may be antagonized by doxorubicin and ribavirin; avoid concurrent use. Zidovudine may decrease the antiviral activity of stavudine (based on *in vitro* data); avoid concurrent use.

Increased Effect/Toxicity: Coadministration of zidovudine with drugs that are nephrotoxic (amphotericin B), cytotoxic (flucytosine, vincristine, vinblastine, doxorubicin, interferon), inhibit glucuronidation or excretion (acetaminophen, cimetidine, indomethacin, lorazepam, probenecid, aspirin), or interfere with RBC/WBC number or function (acyclovir, ganciclovir, pentamidine, dapsone). Clarithromycin may increase blood levels of zidovudine (although total body exposure was unaffected, peak plasma concentrations were increased). Valproic acid significantly increases zidovudine's blood levels (believed due to inhibition first pass metabolism). Concomitant use of ribavirin and nucleoside analogues may increase the risk of developing lactic acidosis (includes adefovir, didanosine, lamivudine, stavudine, zalcitabine, zidovudine).

Adverse Reactions
>10%:
Central nervous system: Severe headache (42%), fever (16%)
Dermatologic: Rash (17%)
Gastrointestinal: Nausea (46% to 61%), anorexia (11%), diarrhea (17%), pain (20%), vomiting (6% to 25%)
Hematologic: Anemia (23% in children), leukopenia, granulocytopenia (39% in children)
Neuromuscular & skeletal: Weakness (19%)
1% to 10%:
Central nervous system: Malaise (8%), dizziness (6%), insomnia (5%), somnolence (8%)
Dermatologic: Hyperpigmentation of nails (bluish-brown)
Gastrointestinal: Dyspepsia (5%)
Hematologic: Changes in platelet count
Neuromuscular & skeletal: Paresthesia (6%)

Overdosage/Toxicology Symptoms of overdose include nausea, vomiting, ataxia, and granulocytopenia. Erythropoietin, thymidine, and cyanocobalamin have been used experimentally to treat zidovudine-induced hematopoietic toxicity, yet none are presently specified as the agent of choice. Treatment is supportive.

Pharmacodynamics/Kinetics
Time to Peak: Serum: 30-90 minutes
Protein Binding: 25% to 38%
Half-Life Elimination: Terminal: 60 minutes
Metabolism: Hepatic via glucuronidation to inactive metabolites; extensive first-pass effect
Excretion:
Oral: Urine (72% to 74% as metabolites, 14% to 18% as unchanged drug)
I.V.: Urine (45% to 60% as metabolites, 18% to 29% as unchanged drug)

Available Dosage Forms
Capsule (Retrovir®): 100 mg
Injection, solution [preservative free] (Retrovir®): 10 mg/mL (20 mL)
Syrup (Retrovir®): 50 mg/5 mL (240 mL) [contains sodium benzoate; strawberry flavor]
Tablet (Retrovir®): 300 mg

Dosing
Adults & Elderly:
Prevention of maternal-fetal HIV transmission:
Maternal (per AIDSinfo guidelines): 100 mg 5 times/day **or** 200 mg 3 times/day **or** 300 mg twice daily. Begin at 14-34 weeks gestation and continue until start of labor.
During labor and delivery, administer zidovudine I.V. at 2 mg/kg over 1 hour followed by a continuous I.V. infusion of 1 mg/kg/hour until the umbilical cord is clamped
HIV infection:
Oral: 300 mg twice daily or 200 mg 3 times/day
I.V.: 1-2 mg/kg/dose (infused over 1 hour) administered every 4 hours around-the-clock (6 doses/day)
Prevention of HIV following needlesticks (unlabeled use): Oral: 200 mg 3 times/day plus lamivudine 150 mg twice daily; a protease inhibitor (eg, indinavir) may be added for high risk exposures; begin therapy within 2 hours of exposure if possible
Note: Patients should receive I.V. therapy only until oral therapy can be administered

Pediatrics:
Prevention of maternal-fetal HIV transmission (in neonates):
Note: Dosing should begin 8-12 hours after birth and continue for the first 6 weeks of life.
Oral:
Full-term infants: 2 mg/kg/dose every 6 hours
Infants ≥30 weeks and <35 weeks gestation at birth: 2 mg/kg/dose every 12 hours; at 2 weeks of age, advance to 2 mg/kg/dose every 8 hours
Infants <30 weeks gestation at birth: 2 mg/kg/dose every 12 hours; at 4 weeks of age, advance to 2 mg/kg/dose every 8 hours
I.V. (infants unable to receive oral dosing):
Full term: 1.5 mg/kg/dose every 6 hours
Infants ≥30 weeks and <35 weeks gestation at birth: 1.5 mg/kg/dose every 12 hours; at 2 weeks of age, advance to 1.5 mg/kg/dose every 8 hours
Infants <30 weeks gestation at birth: 1.5 mg/kg/dose every 12 hours; at 4 weeks of age, advance to 1.5 mg/kg/dose every 8 hours
During labor and delivery, administer zidovudine I.V. at 2 mg/kg over 1 hour followed by a continuous I.V. infusion of 1 mg/kg/hour until the umbilical cord is clamped
Treatment of HIV infection:
Oral: Children 3 months to 12 years:
160 mg/m^2/dose every 8 hours; dosage range: 90 mg/m^2/dose to 180 mg/m^2/dose every 6-8 hours; some Working Group members use a dose of 180 mg/m^2 to 240 mg/m^2 every 12 hours when using in drug combinations with other antiretroviral compounds, but data on this dosing in children is limited
I.V. continuous infusion: 20 mg/m^2/hour
I.V. intermittent infusion: 120 mg/m^2/dose every 6 hours

Renal Impairment: Cl$_{cr}$ <10 mL/minute: May require minor dose adjustment.
Hemodialysis: At least partially removed by hemo- and peritoneal dialysis. Administer dose after hemodialysis or administer 100 mg supplemental dose. During CAPD, dose as for Cl$_{cr}$ <10 mL/minute.
Continuous arteriovenous or venovenous hemodiafiltration effects: Administer 100 mg every 8 hours.
(Continued)

Zidovudine *(Continued)*

Hepatic Impairment: Reduce dose by 50% or double dosing interval in patients with cirrhosis.

Administration

Oral: Administer around-the-clock to promote less variation in peak and trough serum levels. Oral zidovudine may be administered without regard to food.

I.M.: Do not give I.M.

I.V.: Avoid rapid infusion or bolus injection
Neonates: Infuse over 30 minutes
Adults: Infuse over 1 hour

I.V. Detail: pH: 5.5

Stability

Reconstitution: Solution for injection should be diluted with D_5W to a concentration of ≤4 mg/mL; the solution is physically and chemically stable for 24 hours at room temperature and 48 hours if refrigerated. Attempt to administer diluted solution within 8 hours, if stored at room temperature or 24 hours if refrigerated to minimize potential for microbially contaminated solutions.

Compatibility: Stable in D_5W, NS; incompatible with blood products and protein solutions

Storage: Store undiluted vials at room temperature and protect from light.

Laboratory Monitoring Monitor CBC and platelet count at least every 2 weeks, MCV, serum creatinine kinase, CD4 cell count, viral load

Nursing Actions

Physical Assessment: Allergy history should be assessed prior to beginning treatment. Assess other pharmacological or herbal products patient may be taking (eg, increased risk of nephrotoxicity, hepatotoxicity, lactic acidosis). Monitor laboratory tests, therapeutic response, and adverse reactions (eg, lactic acidosis [elevated transaminases]; gastrointestinal disturbance [nausea, vomiting, diarrhea]; myalgia, peripheral neuropathy) on a regular basis throughout therapy. Teach patient proper use (eg, timing of multiple medications and drugs that should not be used concurrently), possible side effects/appropriate interventions, and adverse symptoms to report.

Patient Education: Do not take any new prescriptions, over-the-counter medications, or herbal products without consulting prescriber. This drug will not cure HIV, nor has it been found to reduce transmission of HIV; use appropriate precautions to prevent spread to other persons. This drug is prescribed as one part of a multidrug combination; take oral preparation exactly as directed. Maintain adequate hydration (2-3 L/day of fluids) unless advised by prescriber to restrict fluids. You may be susceptible to infection (avoid crowds and exposure to known infections and do not have any vaccinations without consulting prescriber). Frequent blood tests may be required with prolonged therapy. May cause dizziness, fatigue, or headache (use caution when driving or engaging in tasks requiring alertness until response to drug is known); nausea, vomiting, lack of appetite (small frequent meals, frequent mouth care, chewing gum, or sucking lozenges may help). Report unresolved nausea or vomiting; signs of infection (eg, fever, chills, sore throat, burning urination, flu-like symptoms, fatigue); unusual bleeding (eg, tarry stools, easy bruising, blood in stool, urine, or mouth); skin rash or irritation; muscle weakness or tremors; or any other persistent adverse effects. **Pregnancy/breast-feeding precautions:** Inform prescriber if you are or intend to become pregnant. Do not breast-feed.

Dietary Considerations May be taken without regard to food.

Breast-Feeding Issues HIV-infected mothers are discouraged from breast-feeding to decrease potential transmission of HIV.

Pregnancy Issues Zidovudine crosses the placenta. The use of zidovudine reduces the maternal-fetal transmission of HIV by ~70% and should be considered for antenatal and intrapartum therapy whenever possible. The Perinatal HIV Guidelines Working Group considers zidovudine the preferred NRTI for use in combination regimens during pregnancy. In HIV infected mothers not previously on antiretroviral therapy, treatment may be delayed until after 10-12 weeks gestation. Cases of lactic acidosis/hepatic steatosis syndrome have been reported in pregnant women receiving nucleoside analogues. It is not known if pregnancy itself potentiates this known side effect; however, pregnant women may be at increased risk of lactic acidosis and liver damage. Hepatic enzymes and electrolytes should be monitored frequently during the 3rd trimester of pregnancy in women receiving nucleoside analogues. Health professionals are encouraged to contact the antiretroviral pregnancy registry to monitor outcomes of pregnant women exposed to antiretroviral medications (1-800-258-4263 or www.APRegistry.com).

Other Issues Anemia occurs usually after 4-6 weeks of therapy. Dose adjustments and/or transfusions may be required.

Additional Information Potential compliance problems, frequency of administration and adverse effects should be discussed with patients before initiating therapy to help prevent the emergence of resistance.

Zidovudine and Lamivudine

(zye DOE vyoo deen & la MI vyoo deen)

U.S. Brand Names Combivir®

Synonyms AZT + 3TC (error-prone abbreviation); Lamivudine and Zidovudine

Pharmacologic Category Antiretroviral Agent, Reverse Transcriptase Inhibitor (Nucleoside)

Pregnancy Risk Factor C

Lactation See individual agents.

Use Treatment of HIV infection when therapy is warranted based on clinical and/or immunological evidence of disease progression. Combivir® given twice daily, provides an alternative regimen to lamivudine 150 mg twice daily plus zidovudine 600 mg/day in divided doses; this drug form reduces capsule/tablet intake for these two drugs to 2 per day instead of up to 8.

Available Dosage Forms Tablet: Zidovudine 300 mg and lamivudine 150 mg

Dosing

Adults: Treatment of HIV infection: Oral: 1 tablet twice daily. Because this is a fixed-dose combination product, avoid use in patients requiring dosage reduction including children <12 years of age, renally impaired patients with a creatinine clearance ≤50 mL/minute, patients with low body weight (<50 kg or 110 pounds), or those experiencing dose-limiting adverse effects.

Pediatrics: Children >12 years: Refer to adult dosing.

Nursing Actions

Physical Assessment: See individual agents.

Patient Education: Do not take any new prescriptions, over-the-counter medications, or herbal products without consulting prescriber. This drug will not cure HIV, nor has it been found to reduce transmission of HIV; use appropriate precautions to prevent spread to other persons. Maintain adequate hydration (2-3 L/day of fluids) unless advised by prescriber to restrict fluids. You may be susceptible to infection (avoid crowds and exposure to known infections and do not have any vaccinations without consulting prescriber). Frequent blood tests may be required with prolonged therapy. May cause dizziness, fatigue, or headache (use caution when driving or engaging in tasks requiring alertness until response to drug is known); nausea, vomiting, lack of appetite (small frequent meals, frequent mouth care, chewing gum, or sucking lozenges may help). Report unresolved nausea or vomiting; signs of infection (eg, fever, chills, sore throat, burning urination, flu-like symptoms, fatigue); unusual bleeding (eg, tarry stools, easy bruising, or blood in stool, urine, or mouth); skin rash or irritation; muscle weakness or tremors; or any other persistent adverse effects. **Pregnancy/breast-feeding precautions:** Inform prescriber if you are or intend to become pregnant. Do not breast-feed.

Related Information
Lamivudine *on page 704*
Zidovudine *on page 1300*

Zileuton (zye LOO ton)

U.S. Brand Names Zyflo®
Pharmacologic Category 5-Lipoxygenase Inhibitor
Pregnancy Risk Factor C
Lactation Excretion in breast milk unknown/not recommended
Use Prophylaxis and chronic treatment of asthma in children ≥12 years of age and adults
Mechanism of Action/Effect Inhibits leukotriene formation which contributes to inflammation, edema, mucous secretion, and bronchoconstriction in the airway of the asthmatic.
Contraindications Hypersensitivity to zileuton or any component of the formulation; active liver disease or transaminase elevations greater than or equal to three times the upper limit of normal (≥3 times ULN)
Warnings/Precautions Not indicated for the reversal of bronchospasm in acute asthma attacks; therapy may be continued during acute asthma exacerbations. Hepatic adverse effects have been reported (elevated transaminase levels); females >65 years and patients with pre-existing elevated transaminases may be at greater risk. Serum ALT should be monitored. Discontinue zileuton and follow transaminases until normal if patients develop clinical signs/symptoms of liver dysfunction or with transaminase levels >5 times ULN (use caution with history of liver disease and/or in those patients who consume substantial quantities of ethanol.)
Drug Interactions
Cytochrome P450 Effect: Substrate (minor) of CYP1A2, 2C8/9, 3A4; **Inhibits** CYP1A2 (weak)
Increased Effect/Toxicity: Zileuton may increase the serum concentration/effects of theophylline, propranolol, and warfarin; monitor and reduce doses accordingly.
Nutritional/Ethanol Interactions
Ethanol: Avoid ethanol (may increase CNS depression; may increase risk of hepatic toxicity).
Herb/Nutraceutical: St John's wort may decrease zileuton levels.
Adverse Reactions
>10%: Central nervous system: Headache (25%)
1% to 10%:
Central nervous system: Pain (8%)
Gastrointestinal: Dyspepsia (8%), nausea (6%), abdominal pain (5%)
Hematologic: Leukopenia (1%)
Hepatic: ALT increased (2%)
Neuromuscular & skeletal: Asthenia (4%), myalgia (3%)
Frequency not defined:
Cardiovascular: Chest pain
Central nervous system: Dizziness, fever, insomnia, malaise, nervousness, somnolence
Dermatologic: Pruritus
Gastrointestinal: Constipation, flatulence, vomiting

Genitourinary: Urinary tract infection, vaginitis
Neuromuscular & skeletal: Arthralgia, hypertonia, neck pain/rigidity
Ocular: Conjunctivitis
Miscellaneous: Lymphadenopathy
Overdosage/Toxicology Symptoms of overdose: Human experience is limited. Oral minimum lethal doses in mice and rats were 500-1000 mg/kg and 300-1000 mg/kg, respectively (providing >3 and 9 times the systemic exposure achieved at the maximum recommended human daily oral dose, respectively). No deaths occurred, but nephritis was reported in dogs at an oral dose of 1000 mg/kg. Treat symptomatically; institute supportive measures as required.
Pharmacodynamics/Kinetics
Time to Peak: Serum: 1.7 hours
Protein Binding: 93%
Half-Life Elimination: 2.5 hours
Metabolism: Several metabolites in plasma and urine; metabolized via CYP1A2, 2C9, and 3A4
Excretion: Urine (~95% primarily as metabolites); feces (~2%)
Available Dosage Forms Tablet: 600 mg
Dosing
Adults & Elderly:
Asthma: Oral: 600 mg 4 times/day
Pediatrics: Asthma: Oral:
Children <12 years: Safety and effectiveness have not been established.
Children ≥12 years: Refer to adult dosing.
Renal Impairment: Adjustment not necessary.
Hepatic Impairment: Contraindicated with hepatic dysfunction.
Administration
Oral: May be administered without regard to meals (eg, with or without food).
Stability
Storage: Store tablets at controlled room temperature of 20°C to 25°C (68°F to 77°F). Protect from light.
Laboratory Monitoring Liver function tests
Nursing Actions
Physical Assessment: Not for use to relieve acute asthmatic attacks. Assess effectiveness and interactions of other medications patient may be taking. Monitor results of laboratory tests, effectiveness of therapy (relief of airway obstruction), and adverse reactions at beginning of therapy and periodically with long-term use. For inpatient care, monitor vital signs and lung sounds prior to and periodically during therapy. Assess knowledge/teach patient appropriate use, interventions to reduce side effects, and adverse symptoms to report.
Patient Education: This medication is not for an acute asthmatic attack; in acute attack, follow instructions of prescriber. Do not stop other asthma medication unless advised by prescriber. Take with meals and at bedtime on a continuous bases; do not discontinue even if feeling better (this medication may help reduce incidence of acute attacks). Avoid alcohol and other medications unless approved by your prescriber. You may experience mild headache (mild analgesic may help); fatigue or dizziness (use caution when driving); or nausea or heartburn (small frequent meals, frequent mouth care, sucking lozenges, or chewing gum may help). Report persistent headache, chest pain, rapid heartbeat, or palpitations; skin rash or itching; unusual bleeding (eg, tarry stools, easy bruising, or blood in stool, urine, or mouth); skin rash or irritation; muscle weakness or tremors; redness, irritation, or infections of the eye; flu-like symptoms; itching; jaundice or dark urine; or worsening of asthmatic condition. **Pregnancy/breast-feeding precautions:** Inform prescriber if you are or intend to become pregnant. Breast-feeding is not recommended.
(Continued)

Zileuton *(Continued)*

Dietary Considerations May be taken with or without food.

Geriatric Considerations No differences in the pharmacokinetics found between younger adults and elderly; no dosage adjustments necessary. However, monitor liver effects closely as with any patient regardless of age.

Breast-Feeding Issues Due to the potential tumorigenicity of zileuton in animal studies, the manufacturer does not recommend breast-feeding.

Ziprasidone *(zi PRAY si done)*

U.S. Brand Names Geodon®

Synonyms Zeldox; Ziprasidone Hydrochloride; Ziprasidone Mesylate

Pharmacologic Category Antipsychotic Agent, Atypical

Pregnancy Risk Factor C

Lactation Excretion in breast milk unknown/not recommended

Use Treatment of schizophrenia; treatment of acute manic or mixed episodes associated with bipolar disorder with or without psychosis; acute agitation in patients with schizophrenia

Unlabeled/Investigational Use Tourette's syndrome

Mechanism of Action/Effect Ziprasidone is a benzylisothiazolylpiperazine antipsychotic which blocks a number of CNS receptors, including dopamine, serotonin, alpha$_1$ adrenergic, and histamine receptors. Also inhibits reuptake of serotonin and epinephrine. Results in improvement in positive and negative symptoms of schizophrenia.

Contraindications Hypersensitivity to ziprasidone or any component of the formulation; history (or current) prolonged QT; congenital long QT syndrome; recent myocardial infarction; history of arrhythmias; uncompensated heart failure; concurrent use of other QT$_c$-prolonging agents including amiodarone, arsenic trioxide, bretylium, chlorpromazine, cisapride, class Ia antiarrhythmics (quinidine, procainamide), dofetilide, dolasetron, droperidol, halofantrine, ibutilide, levomethadyl, mefloquine, mesoridazine, pentamidine, pimozide, probucol, some quinolone antibiotics (moxifloxacin, sparfloxacin, gatifloxacin), sotalol, tacrolimus, and thioridazine

Warnings/Precautions Patients with dementia-related behavioral disorders treated with atypical antipsychotics are at an increased risk of death compared to placebo. Ziprasidone is not approved for this indication.

May result in QT$_c$ prolongation (dose-related), which has been associated with the development of malignant ventricular arrhythmias (torsade de pointes) and sudden death. Observed prolongation was greater than with other atypical antipsychotic agents (risperidone, olanzapine, quetiapine), but less than with thioridazine. Avoid hypokalemia, hypomagnesemia. Use caution in patients with bradycardia. Discontinue in patients found to have persistent QT$_c$ intervals >500 msec. Patients with symptoms of dizziness, palpitations, or syncope should receive further cardiac evaluation.

May cause extrapyramidal symptoms. Antipsychotic use may also be associated with neuroleptic malignant syndrome (NMS). Use with caution in patients at risk of seizures.

May cause orthostatic hypotension. Atypical antipsychotics have been associated with development of hyperglycemia. There is limited documentation with ziprasidone and specific risk associated with this agent is not known. Use caution in patients with diabetes or other disorders of glucose regulation; monitor for worsening of glucose control.

Cognitive and/or motor impairment (sedation) is common with ziprasidone. Use with caution in disorders where CNS depression is a feature. Use with caution in Parkinson's disease. Use with caution in patients at risk of aspiration pneumonia (ie, Alzheimer's disease). Caution in breast cancer or other prolactin-dependent tumors. Use caution in renal or hepatic impairment. Ziprasidone has been associated with a fairly high incidence of rash (5%). Safety and efficacy have not been established in pediatric patients.

The possibility of a suicide attempt is inherent in psychotic illness or bipolar disorder; use caution in high-risk patients during initiation of therapy. Prescriptions should be written for the smallest quantity consistent with good patient care.

Drug Interactions

Cytochrome P450 Effect: Substrate (minor) of CYP1A2, 3A4; **Inhibits** CYP2D6 (weak), 3A4 (weak)

Decreased Effect: Carbamazepine may decrease serum concentrations of ziprasidone. Other enzyme-inducing agents may share this potential. Amphetamines may decrease the efficacy of ziprasidone. Ziprasidone may inhibit the efficacy of levodopa.

Increased Effect/Toxicity:

Ketoconazole may increase serum concentrations of ziprasidone. Other CYP3A4 inhibitors may share this potential.

Concurrent use with QT$_c$-prolonging agents may result in additive effects on cardiac conduction, potentially resulting in malignant or lethal arrhythmias. Concurrent use is contraindicated; includes amiodarone, arsenic trioxide, bretylium, chlorpromazine, cisapride; class Ia antiarrhythmics (quinidine, procainamide); dofetilide, dolasetron, droperidol, halofantrine, ibutilide, levomethadyl, mefloquine, mesoridazine, pentamidine, pimozide, probucol; some quinolone antibiotics (moxifloxacin, sparfloxacin, gatifloxacin); sotalol, tacrolimus, and thioridazine. Potassium- or magnesium-depleting agents (diuretics, aminoglycosides, cyclosporine, and amphotericin B) may increase the risk of QT$_c$ prolongation. Antihypertensive agents may increase the risk of orthostatic hypotension. CNS depressants may increase the degree of sedation caused by ziprasidone. Metoclopramide may increase risk of extrapyramidal symptoms (EPS). Acetylcholinesterase inhibitors (central) may increase the risk of antipsychotic-related EPS.

Nutritional/Ethanol Interactions

Ethanol: Avoid ethanol (may increase CNS depression).

Food: Administration with food increases serum levels twofold. Grapefruit juice may increase serum concentration of ziprasidone.

Herb/Nutraceutical: St John's wort may decrease serum levels of ziprasidone, due to a potential effect on CYP3A4. This has not been specifically studied. Avoid kava kava, chamomile (may increase CNS depression).

Lab Interactions Increased cholesterol, triglycerides, eosinophils

Adverse Reactions Note: Although minor QT$_c$ prolongation (mean 10 msec at 160 mg/day) may occur more frequently (incidence not specified), clinically-relevant prolongation (>500 msec) was rare (0.06%) and less than placebo (0.23%).

>10%:

Central nervous system: Extrapyramidal symptoms (2% to 31%), somnolence (8% to 31%), headache (3% to 18%), dizziness (3% to 16%)

Gastrointestinal: Nausea (4% to 12%)

1% to 10%:

Cardiovascular: Chest pain (5%), postural hypotension (5%), hypertension (2% to 3%), bradycardia (2%), tachycardia (2%), vasodilation (1%), facial edema, orthostatic hypotension

Central nervous system: Akathisia (2% to 10%), anxiety (2% to 5%) insomnia (3%), agitation (2%), speech disorder (2%), personality disorder (2%), psychosis (1%), akinesia, amnesia, ataxia, chills, confusion, coordination abnormal, delirium, dystonia, fever, hostility, hypothermia, oculogyric crisis, vertigo

Dermatologic: Rash (4%), fungal dermatitis (2%)

Endocrine & metabolic: Dysmenorrhea (2%)

Gastrointestinal: Weight gain (10%), constipation (2% to 9%), dyspepsia (1% to 8%), diarrhea (3% to 5%), vomiting (3% to 5%), salivation increased (4%), xerostomia (1% to 5%), tongue edema (3%), abdominal pain (2%), anorexia (2%), dysphagia (2%), rectal hemorrhage (2%), tooth disorder (1%), buccoglossal syndrome

Genitourinary: Priapism (1%)

Local: Injection site pain (7% to 9%)

Neuromuscular & skeletal: Weakness (2% to 6%), hypoesthesia (2%), myalgia (2%), paresthesia (2%), back pain (1%), cogwheel rigidity (1%), hypertonia (1%), abnormal gait, choreoathetosis, dysarthria, dyskinesia, hyper-/hypokinesia, hypotonia, neuropathy, tremor, twitching

Ocular: Vision abnormal (3% to 6%), diplopia

Respiratory: Infection (8%), rhinitis (1% to 4%), cough (3%), pharyngitis (3%), dyspnea (2%)

Miscellaneous: Diaphoresis (2%), furunculosis (2%), flu-like syndrome (1%), photosensitivity reaction, withdrawal syndrome

Overdosage/Toxicology Reported symptoms include somnolence, slurring of speech, tremor, and anxiety. Acute extrapyramidal symptoms may also occur. Cardiac monitoring should be initiated immediately. Treatment is symptom-directed and supportive. Not removed by dialysis.

Pharmacodynamics/Kinetics

Time to Peak: Oral: 6-8 hours; I.M.: ≤60 minutes

Protein Binding: 99%, primarily to albumin and alpha$_1$-acid glycoprotein

Half-Life Elimination: Oral: 7 hours; I.M.: 2-5 hours

Metabolism: Extensively hepatic, primarily via aldehyde oxidase; less than 1/3 of total metabolism via CYP3A4 and CYP1A2 (minor)

Excretion: Feces (66%) and urine (20%) as metabolites; little as unchanged drug (1% urine, 4% feces) Clearance: 7.5 mL/minute/kg

Available Dosage Forms

Capsule, as hydrochloride: 20 mg, 40 mg, 60 mg, 80 mg

Injection, powder for reconstitution, as mesylate: 20 mg

Dosing

Adults:

Bipolar mania: Oral: Initial: 40 mg twice daily (with food)

Adjustment: May increase to 60 or 80 mg twice daily on second day of treatment; average dose 40-80 mg twice daily.

Schizophrenia: Oral: Initial: 20 mg twice daily (with food)

Adjustment: Increases (if indicated) should be made no more frequently than every 2 days; ordinarily patients should be observed for improvement over several weeks before adjusting the dose.

Maintenance: Range 20-100 mg twice daily; however, dosages >80 mg twice daily are generally not recommended.

Acute agitation (schizophrenia): I.M.: 10 mg every 2 hours **or** 20 mg every 4 hours (maximum: 40 mg/day). Oral therapy should replace I.M. administration as soon as possible.

Elderly: No dosage adjustment is recommended; consider initiating at a low end of the dosage range, with slower titration.

Pediatrics:

Tourette's syndrome (unlabeled use): Children and adolescents: Oral: 5-40 mg/day

Renal Impairment:

Oral: No dosage adjustment is recommended

I.M.: Cyclodextrin, an excipient in the I.M. formulation, is cleared by renal filtration; use with caution.

Ziprasidone is not removed by hemodialysis.

Hepatic Impairment: No adjustment necessary.

Administration

Oral: Administer with food.

I.M.: Injection: For I.M. administration only.

Stability

Reconstitution: Each vial should be reconstituted with 1.2 mL SWI; shake vigorously; will form a pale, pink solution containing 20 mg/mL ziprasidone.

Storage:

Capsule: Store at controlled room temperature of 15°C to 30°C (59°F to 86°F).

Vials for injection: Prior to reconstitution, store at controlled room temperature of 15°C to 30°C (59°F to 86°F); protect from light. Following reconstitution, injection may be stored at room temperature up to 24 hours, or up to 7 days if refrigerated; protect from light.

Laboratory Monitoring Serum potassium and magnesium; fasting lipid profile and fasting blood glucose, Hgb A$_{1c}$ (prior to treatment, at 3 months, then annually).

Nursing Actions

Physical Assessment: Assess other medications patient may be taking for effectiveness and interactions. Monitor therapeutic response and adverse reactions at beginning and at regular periods throughout therapy. Monitor weight prior to initiating therapy and at least monthly. Assess knowledge/teach appropriate use of this medication, interventions to reduce side effects, and adverse symptoms to report.

Patient Education: Use this mediation exactly as directed; do not alter dosage or discontinue without consulting prescriber; may take 2-3 weeks to achieve desired results. Do not share this medication with anyone else. Avoid alcohol, caffeine, other prescription or OTC medication unless approved by prescriber. Maintain adequate hydration (2-3 L/day of fluids) unless instructed to restrict fluid intake. If diabetic, you may experience increased blood sugars. Monitor blood sugars closely. You may experience drowsiness, lightheadedness, impaired coordination, dizziness, or blurred vision (use caution when driving or engaging in tasks hazardous until response to drug is known); dry mouth, nausea, or GI upset (small frequent meals, good mouth care, sucking lozenges or chewing gum may help); postural hypotension (rise slowly when changing position from lying or sitting to standing or when climbing stairs); urinary retention (void before taking medication); or constipation (increased exercise, fluids, fruit, or fiber may help). Report immediately persistent CNS effects (eg, trembling, altered gait or balance, excessive sedation, seizures, unusual muscle or skeletal movements, excessive anxiety, hallucinations, nightmares, suicidal thoughts, or confusion); swelling or pain in breasts (male or female); altered menstrual pattern; sexual dysfunction; alteration in urinary pattern; vision changes; rash; respiratory difficulty; or chest pain or palpitations. **Pregnancy/breast-feeding precautions:** Inform prescriber if you are or intend to become pregnant. Breast-feeding is not recommended.

Pregnancy Issues Developmental toxicity demonstrated in animals. There are no adequate and well-controlled studies in pregnant women. Use only if potential benefit justifies risk to the fetus.

Additional Information The increased potential to prolong QT$_c$, as compared to other available antipsychotic agents, should be considered in the evaluation of available alternatives.

Zoledronic Acid (ZOE le dron ik AS id)

U.S. Brand Names Zometa®

Synonyms CGP-42446; Zoledronate

Pharmacologic Category Antidote; Bisphosphonate Derivative

Pregnancy Risk Factor D

Lactation Excretion in breast milk unknown/not recommended

Use Treatment of hypercalcemia of malignancy, multiple myeloma, bone metastases of solid tumors

Unlabeled/Investigational Use Investigational: Prevention of bone metastases from breast or prostate cancer; treatment of metabolic bone diseases

Mechanism of Action/Effect A bisphosphonate which inhibits bone resorption via actions on osteoclasts or on osteoclast precursors; inhibits osteoclastic activity and skeletal calcium release induced by tumors. Decreases serum calcium and phosphorus, and increases their elimination.

Contraindications Hypersensitivity to zoledronic acid, other bisphosphonates, or any component of the formulation; pregnancy

Warnings/Precautions Bisphosphonate therapy has been associated with osteonecrosis, primarily of the jaw; this has been observed mostly in cancer patients, but also in patients with postmenopausal osteoporosis and other diagnoses. Dental exams and preventative dentistry should be performed prior to placing patients with risk factors on chronic bisphosphonate therapy. Invasive dental procedures should be avoided during treatment.

Use caution in renal dysfunction; dosage adjustment required. In cancer patients, renal toxicity has been reported with doses >4 mg or infusions administered over 15 minutes. Risk factors for renal deterioration include pre-existing renal insufficiency and repeated doses of zoledronic acid and other bisphosphonates. Dehydration and the use of other nephrotoxic drugs which may contribute to renal deterioration should be identified and managed. Use is not recommended in patients with severe renal impairment (serum creatinine >3 mg/dL) and bone metastases (limited data); use in patients with hypercalcemia of malignancy and severe renal impairment should only be done if the benefits outweigh the risks. Renal function should be assessed prior to treatment; if decreased after treatment, additional treatments should be withheld until renal function returns to within 10% of baseline. Adequate hydration is required during treatment (urine output ~2 L/day); avoid overhydration, especially in patients with heart failure; diuretics should not be used before correcting hypovolemia. Renal deterioration, resulting in renal failure and dialysis has occurred in patients treated with zoledronic acid after single and multiple infusions at recommended doses of 4 mg over 15 minutes. **Note:** When used in the treatment of Paget's disease (Aclasta® — not available in the U.S.), significant renal deterioration has not been observed with the usual 5 mg unit-dose.

Infrequent reports of severe (and occasionally debilitating) bone, joint, and/or muscle pain during bisphosphonate treatment; onset of pain ranged from a single day to several months, with relief in most cases upon discontinuation of the drug. Some patients experienced recurrence when rechallenged with same drug or another bisphosphonate.

Use caution in patients with aspirin-sensitive asthma (may cause bronchoconstriction), hepatic dysfunction, and the elderly. Women of childbearing age should be advised against becoming pregnant. Safety and efficacy in pediatric patients have not been established.

Drug Interactions

Decreased Effect: The following agents may decrease the absorption of oral bisphosphonate derivatives: Antacids (aluminum, calcium, magnesium), oral calcium salts, oral iron salts, and oral magnesium salts.

Increased Effect/Toxicity: Aminoglycosides may lower serum calcium levels with prolonged administration; concomitant use may have an additive hypocalcemic effect. NSAIDs may enhance the gastrointestinal adverse/toxic effects (increased incidence of GI ulcers) of bisphosphonate derivatives. Bisphosphonate derivatives may enhance the hypocalcemic effect of phosphate supplements.

Lab Interactions Bisphosphonates may interfere with diagnostic imaging agents such as technetium-99m-diphosphonate in bone scans.

Adverse Reactions

>10%:

Cardiovascular: Leg edema (5% to 21%), hypotension (11%)

Central nervous system: Fatigue (39%), fever (32% to 44%), headache (5% to 19%), dizziness (18%), insomnia (15% to 16%), anxiety (11% to 14%), depression (14%), agitation (13%), confusion (7% to 13%), hypoesthesia (12%)

Dermatologic: Alopecia (12%), dermatitis (11%)

Endocrine & metabolic: Dehydration (14%), hypophosphatemia (12% to 13%), hypokalemia (12%), hypomagnesemia (11%)

Gastrointestinal: Nausea (29% to 46%), constipation (27% to 31%), vomiting (14% to 32%), diarrhea (17% to 24%), anorexia (9% to 22%), abdominal pain (14% to 16%), weight loss (16%), appetite decreased (13%)

Genitourinary: Urinary tract infection (12% to 14%)

Hematologic: Anemia (22% to 33%), neutropenia (12%)

Neuromuscular & skeletal: Bone pain (55%), weakness (24%), myalgia (23%), arthralgia (5% to 21%), back pain (15%), paresthesia (15%), limb pain (14%), skeletal pain (12%), rigors (11%)

Renal: Renal deterioration (8% to 40%)

Respiratory: Dyspnea (22% to 27%), cough (12% to 22%)

Miscellaneous: Cancer progression (16%), moniliasis (12%)

1% to 10%:

Cardiovascular: Chest pain

Central nervous system: Somnolence

Endocrine & metabolic: Hypocalcemia (1%), hypermagnesemia (2%)

Gastrointestinal: Dysphagia (5% to 10%), dyspepsia (10%), mucositis, stomatitis (8%), sore throat (8%)

Hematologic: Thrombocytopenia (10%), pancytopenia, granulocytopenia

Neuromuscular & skeletal: Asthenia

Renal: Serum creatinine increased (2%)

Respiratory: Pleural effusion, upper respiratory tract infection (10%)

Miscellaneous: Metastases, nonspecifc infection

Symptoms of hypercalcemia include polyuria, nephrolithiasis, anorexia, nausea, vomiting, constipation, weakness, fatigue, confusion, stupor, and coma. These may not be drug-related adverse events, but related to the underlying metabolic condition.

Overdosage/Toxicology Clinically significant hypocalcemia, hypophosphatemia, and hypomagnesemia may occur.

Pharmacodynamics/Kinetics

Onset of Action: Maximum effect may not been seen for 7 days.

Protein Binding: ~22%

Half-Life Elimination: Triphasic; Terminal: 146 hours

Excretion: Urine (39% ± 16% as unchanged drug) within 24 hours; feces (<3%)

Available Dosage Forms [CAN] = Canadian brand name

Infusion, solution [premixed] (Aclasta® [CAN]): 5 mg (100 mL) [not available in U.S.]

Injection, solution: 4 mg/5 mL (5 mL) [as monohydrate 4.264 mg]

Dosing

Adults & Elderly:

Hypercalcemia of malignancy (albumin-corrected serum calcium ≥12 mg/dL): I.V.: 4 mg (maximum) given as a single dose. Wait at least 7 days before considering retreatment. Dosage adjustment may be needed in patients with decreased renal function following treatment.

Multiple myeloma or metastatic bone lesions from solid tumors: I.V.: 4 mg every 3-4 weeks

Note: Patients should receive a daily calcium supplement and multivitamin containing vitamin D

Paget's disease (Aclasta®, not available in U.S.): 5 mg infused over at least 15 minutes. **Note:** Data concerning retreatment is not available.

Renal Impairment:

Zometa®: Mild-to-moderate renal impairment:

Cl_{cr} >60 mL/minute: 4 mg

Cl_{cr} 50-60 mL/minute: 3.5 mg

Cl_{cr} 40-49 mL/minute: 3.3 mg

Cl_{cr} 30-39 mL/minute: 3 mg

Cl_{cr} <30 mL/minute: Not recommended

Aclasta® [not available in U.S.]: Cl_{cr} >30 mL/minute: No adjustment recommended.

Renal toxicity:

Hypercalcemia of malignancy: Evidence of renal deterioration: Evaluate risk versus benefit.

Bone metastases: Evidence of renal deterioration: Discontinue further dosing until renal function returns to within 10% of baseline: renal deterioration defined as follows:

Normal baseline creatinine: Increase of 0.5 mg/dL

Abnormal baseline creatinine: Increase of 1 mg/dL

Reinitiate dose at the same dose administered prior to treatment interruption.

Hepatic Impairment: Specific guidelines are not available.

Administration

I.V.: Infuse over 15-30 minutes.

I.V. Detail: Infuse in a line separate from other medications. Patients should be appropriately hydrated prior to treatment.

Stability

Reconstitution: Dilute solution for injection in 100 mL NS or D_5W prior to administration. Infusion of solution must be completed within 24 hours

Compatibility: Incompatible with calcium-containing solutions (eg, LR)

Storage: Store intact vials at 25°C (77°F).

Laboratory Monitoring Monitor serum creatinine prior to each dose. Serum electrolytes, phosphate, magnesium, and hemoglobin/hematocrit should be evaluated regularly. Monitor serum calcium to assess response and avoid overtreatment.

Nursing Actions

Physical Assessment: Patients at risk for osteonecrosis (eg, chemotherapy, corticosteroids, poor oral hygiene) should have dental exams and necessary preventive dentistry should be done before beginning bisphosphonate therapy. Assess potential for interactions with other pharmacological agents and herbal products patient may be taking. Calcium and vitamin D supplements may be recommended. Monitor laboratory tests and patient response on a regular basis during therapy. Teach patient possible side effects/appropriate interventions (eg, need for adequate hydration) and adverse symptoms to report.

Patient Education: This medication is only administered intravenously. Avoid vitamins during infusion or for 2-3 hours after completion. Maintain adequate hydration (2-3 L/day of fluids unless instructed to restrict fluid intake). You may experience nausea, vomiting, or loss of appetite (small, frequent meals, good mouth care, sucking lozenges, or chewing gum may help); headache, dizziness, insomnia, confusion ((use caution when driving or engaging in tasks that require alertness until response to drug is known) or recurrent bone pain (consult prescriber for analgesic). Report unusual muscle twitching or spasms, severe diarrhea/constipation, acute bone, joint or muscle pain; changes in urinary pattern, burning or itching on urination; skin rash; difficulty breathing; chest pain; or other persistent adverse effects. **Pregnancy/breast-feeding precautions:** Inform prescriber if you are or intend to become pregnant. Do not get pregnant during therapy. Consult prescriber for instructions on appropriate contraceptive measures. This drug may cause fetal defects. Breast-feeding is not recommended.

Dietary Considerations Multiple myeloma or metastatic bone lesions from solid tumors: Take daily calcium supplement (500 mg) and daily multivitamin (with 400 int. units vitamin D).

Geriatric Considerations

This drug requires adequate hydration and adjustments for creatine clearance for its use. Older adults are often volume depleted secondary to drugs and a blunted thirst reflex. See Special Alerts and Warnings/Precautions.

Pregnancy Issues Animal studies resulted in embryotoxicity and losses. May cause fetal harm when administered to a pregnant woman. Use only if the benefit to the mother outweighs the potential risk to the fetus.

Zolmitriptan (zohl mi TRIP tan)

U.S. Brand Names Zomig®; Zomig-ZMT™

Synonyms 311C90

Pharmacologic Category Serotonin 5-HT$_{1D}$ Receptor Agonist

Medication Safety Issues

Sound-alike/look-alike issues:

Zolmitriptan may be confused with sumatriptan

Pregnancy Risk Factor C

Lactation Excretion in breast milk unknown/use caution

Use Acute treatment of migraine with or without aura

Mechanism of Action/Effect Zolmitriptan is a selective 5-HT$_{1B/1D}$ agonist

Contraindications Hypersensitivity to zolmitriptan or any component of the formulation; ischemic heart disease or Prinzmetal's angina; signs or symptoms of ischemic heart disease; uncontrolled hypertension; symptomatic Wolff-Parkinson-White syndrome or arrhythmias associated with other cardiac accessory conduction pathway disorders; use with ergotamine derivatives (within 24 hours of); use within 24 hours of another 5-HT$_1$ agonist; concurrent administration or within 2 weeks of discontinuing an MAO inhibitor; management of hemiplegic or basilar migraine

Warnings/Precautions Zolmitriptan is indicated only in patient populations with a clear diagnosis of migraine. Not for prophylactic treatment of migraine headaches. Cardiac events (including myocardial infarction, ventricular arrhythmia, cardiac arrest, and death) have been reported with 5-HT$_1$ agonist administration. Should not be given to patients who have risk factors for CAD without adequate cardiac evaluation. Patients with suspected CAD should have cardiovascular evaluation to rule out CAD before considering zolmitriptan's use; if cardiovascular evaluation negative, first dose would be safest if given in the healthcare provider's office. Periodic evaluation of those without cardiovascular disease, (Continued)

Zolmitriptan *(Continued)*

but with continued risk factors should be done. Significant elevation in blood pressure, including hypertensive crisis, has also been reported. Vasospasm-related reactions have been reported other than coronary artery vasospasm. Peripheral vascular ischemia and colonic ischemia with abdominal pain and bloody diarrhea have occurred. Use with caution in patients with hepatic impairment. Zomig-ZMT™ tablets contain phenylalanine. Safety and efficacy not established in patients <18 years of age.

Drug Interactions

Cytochrome P450 Effect: Substrate of CYP1A2 (minor)

Increased Effect/Toxicity: Ergot-containing drugs may lead to vasospasm; cimetidine, MAO inhibitors, oral contraceptives, propranolol increase levels of zolmitriptan; concurrent use with SSRIs and sibutramine may lead to serotonin syndrome.

Nutritional/Ethanol Interactions Ethanol: Limit use (may have additive CNS toxicity)

Lab Interactions No interferences have been identified

Adverse Reactions Percentages noted from oral preparations.

1% to 10%:

Cardiovascular: Chest pain (2% to 4%), palpitation (up to 2%)

Central nervous system: Dizziness (6% to 10%), somnolence (5% to 8%), pain (2% to 3%), vertigo (≤2%)

Gastrointestinal: Nausea (4% to 9%), xerostomia (3% to 5%), dyspepsia (1% to 3%), dysphagia (≤2%)

Neuromuscular & skeletal: Paresthesia (5% to 9%), weakness (3% to 9%), warm/cold sensation (5% to 7%), hypoesthesia (1% to 2%), myalgia (1% to 2%), myasthenia (up to 2%)

Miscellaneous: Neck/throat/jaw pain (4% to 10%), diaphoresis (up to 3%), allergic reaction (up to 1%)

Overdosage/Toxicology Treatment is symptom-directed and supportive. It is not known if hemodialysis or peritoneal dialysis is effective.

Pharmacodynamics/Kinetics

Onset of Action: 0.5-1 hour

Time to Peak: Serum: Tablet: 1.5 hours; Orally-disintegrating tablet and nasal spray: 3 hours

Protein Binding: 25%

Half-Life Elimination: 2.8-3.7 hours

Metabolism: Converted to an active N-desmethyl metabolite (2-6 times more potent than zolmitriptan)

Excretion: Urine (~60% to 65% total dose); feces (30% to 40%)

Available Dosage Forms

Solution, nasal spray [single dose] (Zomig®): 5 mg/0.1 mL (0.1 mL)

Tablet (Zomig®): 2.5 mg, 5 mg

Tablet, orally disintegrating (Zomig-ZMT™): 2.5 mg [contains phenylalanine 2.81 mg/tablet; orange flavor]; 5 mg [contains phenylalanine 5.62 mg/tablet; orange flavor]

Dosing

Adults:

Migraine headache:

Oral:

Tablet: Initial: ≤2.5 mg at the onset of migraine headache; may break 2.5 mg tablet in half

Orally-disintegrating tablet: Initial: 2.5 mg at the onset of migraine headache

Nasal spray: Initial: 1 spray (5 mg) at the onset of migraine headache

Note: Use the lowest possible dose to minimize adverse events. If the headache returns, the dose may be repeated after 2 hours; do not exceed 10 mg within a 24-hour period. Controlled trials have not established the effectiveness of a second dose if the initial one was ineffective

Elderly: No dosage adjustment needed, but elderly patients are more likely to have underlying cardiovascular disease and should have careful evaluation of cardiovascular system before prescribing.

Renal Impairment: No dosage adjustment recommended. There is a 25% reduction in zolmitriptan's clearance in patients with severe renal impairment (Cl$_{cr}$ 5-25 mL/minute)

Hepatic Impairment: Administer with caution in patients with liver disease, generally using doses <2.5 mg. Patients with moderate-to-severe hepatic impairment may have decreased clearance of zolmitriptan, and significant elevation in blood pressure was observed in some patients.

Administration

Oral: Administer as soon as migraine headache starts. Tablets may be broken. Orally-disintegrating tablets: Must be taken whole; do not break, crush or chew; place on tongue and allow to dissolve; administration with liquid is not required

Other: Nasal spray: Administer as soon as migraine headache starts. Blow nose gently prior to use. After removing protective cap, instill device into nostril. Block opposite nostril; breathe in gently through nose while pressing plunger of spray device. One dose (5 mg) is equal to 1 spray in 1 nostril.

Stability

Storage: Store at 20°C to 25°C (68°F to 77°F); protect from light and moisture

Nursing Actions

Physical Assessment: For use only with a clear diagnosis of migraine headaches. Assess potential for interactions with other pharmacological agents and herbal products patient may be taking (eg, ergot-containing drugs). Monitor effectiveness and adverse response (eg, chest pain, nausea, dizziness, paresthesia, myalgia, pain). Teach patient proper use (according to formulation), possible side effects/appropriate interventions, and adverse symptoms to report..

Patient Education: This drug is to be used to reduce your migraine, not to prevent or reduce the number of attacks. Follow exact instructions for use. Remove orally-disintegrating tablet from blister package just before using, place on tongue, and allow to dissolve. Do not crush, break, or chew. Regular tablet may be broken in half for use. Do not remove protective cap from nasal spray until ready to use. Do not take within 24 hours of any other migraine medication without first consulting prescriber. If first dose brings relief, second dose may be taken anytime after 2 hours if migraine returns. If you have no relief with first dose, do not take a second dose without consulting prescriber. Do not exceed 10 mg in 24 hours. May cause dizziness or drowsiness (use caution when driving or engaging in tasks requiring alertness until response to drug is known); or dry mouth (frequent mouth care and sucking on lozenges may help). Report immediately any chest pain, heart throbbing, or tightness in throat; swelling of eyelids, face, or lips; skin rash or hives; easy bruising; blood in urine, stool, or vomitus; pain or itching with urination; or pain, warmth, or numbness in extremities. **Pregnancy/breast-feeding precautions:** Inform prescriber if you are or intend to become pregnant. Consult prescriber if breast-feeding.

Geriatric Considerations Zolmitriptan use in the elderly patient has not been studied.

Pregnancy Issues In pregnant animals, zolmitriptan caused embryolethality and fetal abnormalities at doses ≥11 times the equivalent human dose.

Additional Information Not recommended if the patient has risk factors for heart disease (high blood pressure, high cholesterol, obesity, diabetes, smoking, strong family history of heart disease, postmenopausal woman, or a male >40 years of age).

This agent is intended to relieve migraine, but not to prevent or reduce the number of attacks. Use only to treat an actual migraine attack.

Zolpidem (zole PI dem)

U.S. Brand Names Ambien®; Ambien CR™
Synonyms Zolpidem Tartrate
Restrictions C-IV; not available in Canada
Pharmacologic Category Hypnotic, Nonbenzodiazepine
Medication Safety Issues
Sound-alike/look-alike issues:
Ambien® may be confused with Ambi 10®
Pregnancy Risk Factor C
Lactation Enters breast milk/not recommended (AAP rates "compatible")
Use Short-term treatment of insomnia (sleep onset and/or sleep maintenance)
Mechanism of Action/Effect Structurally dissimilar to benzodiazepines. Selective hypnotic effects (with minor anxiolytic, myorelaxant and anticovulsant properties) mediated through selective affinity for the alpha-1 subunit of the omega-1 (benzodiazepine) receptor located on the GABA$_A$ receptor complex. Agonism at this site enhances GABA-ergic chloride conductance hyperpolarizing neuronal membranes thereby reducing the responsiveness to excitatory signals.
Contraindications Hypersensitivity to zolpidem or any component of the formulation
Warnings/Precautions Should be used only after evaluation of potential causes of sleep disturbance. Failure of sleep disturbance to resolve after 7-10 days may indicate psychiatric or medical illness. Use with caution in patients with depression. Abnormal thinking and behavioral changes have been associated with sedative-hypnotics. Sedative/hypnotics may produce withdrawal symptoms following abrupt discontinuation. Causes CNS depression, which may impair physical and mental capabilities. Effects with other sedative drugs or ethanol may be potentiated. Use caution in the elderly; dose adjustment recommended. Closely monitor elderly or debilitated patients for impaired cognitive or motor performance. Avoid use in patients with sleep apnea or a history of sedative-hypnotic abuse. Use caution with hepatic impairment; dose adjustment required. Prescriptions should be written for the smallest effective dose (especially in the elderly) and for the smallest quantity consistent with good patient care (especially with depression). Safety and efficacy have not been established in pediatric patients.

Drug Interactions
Cytochrome P450 Effect: Substrate of CYP1A2 (minor), 2C8/9 (minor), 2C19 (minor), 2D6 (minor), 3A4 (major)
Decreased Effect: CYP3A4 inducers may decrease the levels/effects of zolpidem; example inducers include aminoglutethimide, carbamazepine, nafcillin, nevirapine, phenobarbital, phenytoin, and rifamycins.
Increased Effect/Toxicity: Use of zolpidem in combination with other centrally-acting drugs may produce additive CNS depression. CYP3A4 inhibitors may increase the levels/effects of zolpidem; example inhibitors include azole antifungals, clarithromycin, diclofenac, doxycycline, erythromycin, imatinib, isoniazid, nefazodone, nicardipine, propofol, protease inhibitors, quinidine, telithromycin, troleandomycin, and verapamil.
Nutritional/Ethanol Interactions
Ethanol: Avoid ethanol (may increase CNS depression).
Food: Maximum plasma concentration and bioavailability are decreased with food; time to peak plasma concentration is increased; half-life remains unchanged.

Herb/Nutraceutical: St John's wort may decrease zolpidem levels. Avoid valerian, St John's wort, kava kava, gotu kola (may increase CNS depression).
Lab Interactions Increased aminotransferase [ALT (SGPT)/AST (SGOT)], bilirubin (S); decreased RAI uptake
Adverse Reactions Actual frequency may be dosage form, dose and/or age dependent
>10%: Central nervous system: Dizziness, headache, somnolence
1% to 10%:
Cardiovascular: Blood pressure increased, chest discomfort, palpitation
Central nervous system: Anxiety, apathy, amnesia, ataxia, attention disturbance, body temperature increased, confusion, depersonalization, depression, disinhibition, disorientation, drowsiness, drugged feeling, euphoria, fatigue, fever, hallucinations, hypoesthesia, insomnia, memory disorder, lethargy, lightheadedness, mood swings, stress
Dermatologic: Rash, urticaria, wrinkling
Endocrine & metabolic: Menorrhagia
Gastrointestinal: Abdominal discomfort, abdominal pain, abdominal tenderness, appetite disorder, constipation, diarrhea, dyspepsia, flatulence, gastroenteritis, gastroesophageal reflux, hiccup, nausea, vomiting, xerostomia
Genitourinary: Urinary tract infection
Neuromuscular & skeletal: Arthralgia, back pain, balance disorder, myalgia, neck pain, paresthesia, psychomotor retardation, tremor, weakness
Ocular: Asthenopia, blurred vision, depth perception altered, diplopia, visual disturbance, red eye
Otic: Labyrinthitis, tinnitus, vertigo
Renal: Dysuria
Respiratory: Pharyngitis, sinusitis, upper respiratory tract infection, throat irritation
Miscellaneous: Allergy, binge eating, flu-like symptoms
Overdosage/Toxicology Symptoms of overdose include coma and hypotension. Treatment for overdose is supportive. Rarely is mechanical ventilation required. Flumazenil has been shown to selectively block binding to CNS receptors, resulting in a reversal of CNS depression, but not always respiratory depression. Hemodialysis is not likely to be of benefit.
Pharmacodynamics/Kinetics
Onset of Action: 30 minutes
Duration of Action: 6-8 hours
Time to Peak:
2 hours; 4 hours with food
Protein Binding: 92%
Half-Life Elimination: 2.5-2.8 hours (range 1.4-4.5 hours); Cirrhosis: Up to 9.9 hours
Metabolism: Hepatic, primarily via CYP3A4 (~60%), to inactive metabolites
Excretion: As metabolites in urine, bile, feces
Available Dosage Forms [DSC] = Discontinued product
Tablet, as tartrate:
Ambien®: 5 mg, 10 mg
Ambien® PAK™ [dose pack]: 5 mg (30s); 10 mg (30s) [DSC]
Tablet, extended release, as tartrate (Ambien CR™): 6.25 mg, 12.5 mg
Dosing
Adults: Insomnia: Oral:
Ambien®: 10 mg immediately before bedtime; maximum dose: 10 mg
Ambien CR™: 12.5 mg immediately before bedtime
Elderly:
Ambien®: 5 mg immediately before bedtime
Ambien CR™: 6.25 mg immediately before bedtime
Renal Impairment: Dose adjustment not required; monitor closely.
Not dialyzable
(Continued)

Zolpidem (Continued)

Hepatic Impairment:
Ambien®: 5 mg
Ambien CR™: 6.25 mg

Administration
Oral: Ingest immediately before bedtime due to rapid onset of action. Ambien CR™ tablets should not be divided, crushed, or chewed.

Nursing Actions
Physical Assessment: For short-term use. Assess effectiveness and interactions of other medications patient may be taking Assess for history of addiction; long-term use can result in dependence, abuse, or tolerance. After long-term use, taper dosage slowly when discontinuing. Monitor for CNS depression. For inpatient use, institute safety measures and monitor effectiveness and adverse reactions. For outpatients, monitor therapeutic effectiveness and adverse reactions at beginning of therapy and periodically with long-term use. Assess knowledge/teach patient appropriate use, interventions to reduce side effects, and adverse symptoms to report.

Patient Education: Use exactly as directed; do not increase dose or frequency or discontinue without consulting prescriber. Drug may cause physical and/or psychological dependence. While using this medication, do not use alcohol or other prescription or OTC medications (especially, pain medications, sedatives, antihistamines, or hypnotics) without consulting prescriber. Maintain adequate hydration (2-3 L/day of fluids) unless instructed to restrict fluid intake. You may experience drowsiness, dizziness, or blurred vision (use caution when driving or engaging in tasks requiring alertness until response to drug is known); nausea (small frequent meals, frequent mouth care, chewing gum, or sucking lozenges may help); or diarrhea (buttermilk, boiled milk, yogurt may help). Report CNS changes (confusion, depression, increased sedation, excitation, headache, abnormal thinking, insomnia, or nightmares); muscle pain or weakness; respiratory difficulty; chest pain or palpitations; or ineffectiveness of medication. **Breast-feeding precaution:** Consult prescriber if breast-feeding

Dietary Considerations For faster sleep onset, do not administer with (or immediately after) a meal.

Geriatric Considerations In doses >5 mg, there was subjective evidence of impaired sleep on the first post-treatment night. There have been few reports of increased hypotension and/or falls in the elderly with this drug. Can be considered a drug of choice in the elderly when a hypnotic is indicated.

Pregnancy Issues Children born of mothers taking sedative/hypnotics may be at risk for withdrawal; neonatal flaccidity has been reported in infants following maternal use of sedative/hypnotics during pregnancy.

Additional Information Causes less disturbances in sleep stages as compared to benzodiazepines. Time spent in sleep stages 3 and 4 are maintained; decreases sleep latency. Should not be prescribed in quantities exceeding a 1-month supply.

Related Information
Anxiolytic / Hypnotic Use in Long-Term Care Facilities on page 1418

Zonisamide (zoe NIS a mide)

U.S. Brand Names Zonegran®
Pharmacologic Category Anticonvulsant, Miscellaneous

Pregnancy Risk Factor C
Lactation Excretion in breast milk unknown/contraindicated
Use Adjunct treatment of partial seizures in children >16 years of age and adults with epilepsy
Unlabeled/Investigational Use Bipolar disorder
Mechanism of Action/Effect The exact mechanism of action is not known. May stabilize neuronal membranes and suppress neuronal hypersynchronization through action at sodium and calcium channels. Does not affect GABA activity.
Contraindications Hypersensitivity to zonisamide, sulfonamides, or any component of the formulation
Warnings/Precautions Rare, but potentially fatal sulfonamide reactions have occurred following the use of zonisamide. These reactions include Stevens-Johnson syndrome and toxic epidermal necrolysis, usually appearing within 2-16 weeks of drug initiation. Discontinue zonisamide if rash develops. Chemical similarities are present among sulfonamides, sulfonylureas, carbonic anhydrase inhibitors, thiazides, and loop diuretics (except ethacrynic acid). Use in patients with sulfonamide allergy is specifically contraindicated in product labeling, however, a risk of cross-reaction exists in patients with allergy to any of these compounds; avoid use when previous reaction has been severe.

Decreased sweating (oligohydrosis) and hyperthermia requiring hospitalization have been reported in children. Discontinue zonisamide in patients who develop acute renal failure or a significant sustained increase in creatinine/BUN concentration. Kidney stones have been reported. Use cautiously in patients with renal or hepatic dysfunction. Significant CNS effects include psychiatric symptoms, psychomotor slowing, and fatigue or somnolence. Fatigue and somnolence occur within the first month of treatment, most commonly at doses of 300-500 mg/day. Abrupt withdrawal may precipitate seizures; discontinue or reduce doses gradually. Safety and efficacy in children <16 years of age has not been established.

Drug Interactions
Cytochrome P450 Effect: Substrate of CYP2C19 (minor), 3A4 (major)

Decreased Effect: CYP3A4 inducers may decrease the levels/effects of zonisamide; example inducers include aminoglutethimide, carbamazepine, nafcillin, nevirapine, phenobarbital, phenytoin, and rifamycins.

Increased Effect/Toxicity: Sedative effects may be additive with other CNS depressants; monitor for increased effect (includes barbiturates, benzodiazepines, narcotic analgesics, ethanol, and other sedative agents). CYP3A4 inhibitors may increase the levels/effects of zonisamide; example inhibitors include azole antifungals, clarithromycin, diclofenac, doxycycline, erythromycin, imatinib, isoniazid, nefazodone, nicardipine, propofol, protease inhibitors, quinidine, telithromycin, and verapamil.

Nutritional/Ethanol Interactions
Ethanol: Avoid ethanol (may increase CNS depression).
Food: Food delays time to maximum concentration, but does not affect bioavailability.

Adverse Reactions Adjunctive Therapy: Frequencies noted in patients receiving other anticonvulsants:

>10%:
Central nervous system: Somnolence (17%), dizziness (13%)

Gastrointestinal: Anorexia (13%)

1% to 10%:
Central nervous system: Headache (10%), agitation/irritability (9%), fatigue (8%), tiredness (7%), ataxia (6%), confusion (6%), decreased concentration (6%), memory impairment (6%), depression (6%), insomnia (6%), speech disorders (5%), mental slowing (4%), anxiety (3%), nervousness (2%), schizophrenic/schizophreniform behavior (2%), difficulty in verbal expression (2%), status epilepticus (1%), tremor (1%), convulsion (1%), hyperesthesia (1%), incoordination (1%)
Dermatologic: Rash (3%), bruising (2%), pruritus (1%)
Gastrointestinal: Nausea (9%), abdominal pain (6%), diarrhea (5%), dyspepsia (3%), weight loss (3%), constipation (2%), dry mouth (2%), taste perversion (2%), vomiting (1%)
Neuromuscular & skeletal: Paresthesia (4%), weakness (1%), abnormal gait (1%)
Ocular: Diplopia (6%), nystagmus (4%), amblyopia (1%)
Otic: Tinnitus (1%)
Respiratory: Rhinitis (2%), pharyngitis (1%), increased cough (1%)
Miscellaneous: Flu-like syndrome (4%) accidental injury (1%)

Overdosage/Toxicology No specific antidotes are available; experience with doses >800 mg/day is limited. Emesis or gastric lavage, with airway protection, should be done following a recent overdose. General supportive care and close observation are indicated. Renal dialysis may not be effective due to low protein binding (40%).

Pharmacodynamics/Kinetics
Time to Peak: 2-6 hours
Protein Binding: 40%
Half-Life Elimination: 63 hours
Metabolism: Hepatic via CYP3A4; forms N-acetyl zonisamide and 2-sulfamoylacetyl phenol (SMAP)
Excretion: Urine (62%, 35% as unchanged drug, 65% as metabolites); feces (3%)

Available Dosage Forms [DSC] = Discontinued product
Capsule: 25 mg, 50 mg, 100 mg
Zonegran®: 25 mg, 50 mg [DSC], 100 mg

Dosing
Adults:
Adjunctive treatment of partial seizures: Oral: Initial: 100 mg/day. Dose may be increased to 200 mg/day after 2 weeks. Further dosage increases to 300 mg and 400 mg/day can then be made with a minimum of 2 weeks between adjustments, in order to reach steady state at each dosage level. Doses of up to 600 mg/day have been studied, however, there is no evidence of increased response with doses >400 mg/day.
Mania (unlabeled use): Oral: Initial: 100-200 mg/day; maximum: 600 mg/day (Kanba, 1994)
Elderly: Data from clinical trials is insufficient for patients older than 65. Begin dosing at the low end of the dosing range.
Pediatrics: Children >16 years: Refer to adult dosing.
Renal Impairment: Slower titration and frequent monitoring are indicated in patients with renal or hepatic disease. There is insufficient experience regarding dosing/toxicity in patients with estimated GFR <50 mL/minute. Marked renal impairment (Cl$_{cr}$ <20 mL/minute) was associated with a 35% increase in AUC.
Hepatic Impairment: Slower titration and frequent monitoring are indicated.

Stability
Storage: Store at controlled room temperature 25°C (77°F). Protect from moisture and light.

Nursing Actions
Physical Assessment: Assess other medications patient may be taking for increased risk of drug/drug interactions. Monitor therapeutic response, laboratory results, and adverse reactions at beginning of therapy and periodically with long-term use. Observe and teach seizure precautions. Assess knowledge/teach patient appropriate use, interventions to reduce side effects, and adverse symptoms to report.
Patient Education: Take exactly as directed, as the same time each day, with or without food. Do not increase frequency, alter dose, or discontinue without consulting prescriber. If you miss a dose, take as soon as possible. If it is almost time for your next dose, skip the missed dose. Do not chew, crush, or open capsules; swallow whole. Maintain adequate hydration (2-3 L/day of fluids) unless instructed to restrict fluid intake. Avoid grapefruit juice while on this medication. While using this medication, avoid alcohol, herbal remedies, OTC or prescriptions drugs (especially pain medication, antihistamines, psychiatric medications, sedatives, or hypnotics) unless approved by your prescriber. Wear/carry identification of epileptic status and medications. You may experience drowsiness, dizziness, or blurred vision (use caution when driving or engaging in tasks requiring alertness until response to drug is known); or nausea, vomiting, constipation, dry mouth, or loss of appetite (small frequent meals, frequent mouth care, chewing gum, or sucking hard candy may help). Report CNS changes (changes in speech patterns, mentation changes, changes in cognition or memory, unusual thought patterns, coordination difficulties, or excessive drowsiness); respiratory difficulty or tightening of the throat; swelling of mouth, lips, or tongue; muscle cramping, weakness, or pain; rash or skin irritations; unusual bruising or bleeding (mouth, urine, stool); fever, sore throat, sores in your mouth; swelling of extremities; sudden back pain, pain on urination, or dark/bloody urine (signs of kidney stones); or other adverse response including change in seizure type or frequency. **Pregnancy/breast-feeding precautions:** Inform prescriber if you are or intend to become pregnant. Do not breast-feed.
Dietary Considerations May be taken with or without food.
Breast-Feeding Issues Based on limited case reports, it appears zonisamide is excreted in breast milk. Use during lactation only if the potential benefits outweigh the potential risks.
Pregnancy Issues Fetal abnormalities and death have been reported in animals, however, there are no studies in pregnant women.

APPENDIX
TABLE OF CONTENTS

APPENDIX *(Continued)*

COMMON SYMBOLS AND ABBREVIATIONS USED IN MEDICAL ORDERS[1]

Abbreviation	Meaning
āā, aa	of each
ac	before meals or food
ad	to, up to
a.d.	right ear
ADD	attention-deficit disorder
ADHD	attention-deficit/hyperactivity disorder
ADLs	activities of daily living
ad lib	at pleasure
a.l.	left ear
AM	morning
amp	ampul
amt	amount
aq	water
aq. dest.	distilled water
ARDS	adult respiratory distress syndrome
a.s.	left ear
ASAP	as soon as possible
a.u.	each ear
AUC	area under the curve
bid	twice daily
bm	bowel movement
bp	blood pressure
BPH	benign prostatic hyperplasia
BSA	body surface area
c	a gallon
c̄	with
cal	calorie
cap	capsule
CBT	cognitive behavioral therapy
cc	cubic centimeter
CHF	congestive heart failure
CIV	continuous I.V. infusion
cm	centimeter
comp	compound
cont	continue
CRF	chronic renal failure
CT	computed tomography
d	day
d/c	discontinue
dil	dilute
disp	dispense
div	divide
DTs	delirium tremens
dtd	give of such a dose
ECT	electroconvulsive therapy
EEG	electroencephalogram
EKG	electrocardiogram
elix, el	elixir
emp	as directed
EPS	extrapyramidal side effects
ESRD	end stage renal disease
et	and
EtOH	alcohol
ex aq	in water
f, ft	make, let be made

COMMON SYMBOLS AND ABBREVIATIONS USED IN MEDICAL ORDERS[1] *(Continued)*

Abbreviation	Meaning
FMS	fibromyalgia syndrome
g	gram
GAD	generalized anxiety disorder
GABA	gamma-aminobutyric acid
GERD	gastroesophageal reflux disease
GITS	gastrointestinal therapeutic system
GFR	glomerular filtration rate
gr	grain
gtt	a drop
GVHD	graft versus host disease
h	hour
hs	at bedtime
HSV	herpes simplex virus
HTN	hypertension
IBD	inflammatory bowel disease
IBS	irritable bowel syndrome
ICH	intracranial hemorrhage
IHSS	idiopathic hypertrophic subaortic stenosis
I.M.	intramuscular
IOP	intraocular pressure
IU	international unit
I.V.	intravenous
kcal	kilocalorie
kg	kilogram
KIU	kallikrein inhibitor unit
L	liter
liq	a liquor, solution
M	mix; Molar
MAOIs	monamine oxidase inhibitors
mcg	microgram
m. dict	as directed
mEq	milliequivalent
mg	milligram
mixt	a mixture
mL	milliliter
mm	millimeter
mM	millimolar
MRI	magnetic resonance imaging
MS	multiple sclerosis
NKA	no known allergies
NMS	neuroleptic malignant syndrome
no.	number
noc	in the night
non rep	do not repeat, no refills
NPO	nothing by mouth
NSAID	nonsteroidal anti-inflammatory drug
NV	nausea and vomiting
O, Oct	a pint
OA	osteoarthritis
OCD	obsessive-compulsive disorder
o.d.	right eye
o.l.	left eye
o.s.	left eye
o.u.	each eye
PAT	paroxysmal artrial tachycardia
pc, post cib	after meals
PD	Parkinson's disease

Abbreviation	Meaning
per	through or by
PID	pelvic inflammatory disease
PM	afternoon or evening
P.O.	by mouth
P.R.	rectally
prn	as needed
PSVT	paroxysmal supraventricular tachycardia
PTA	prior to admission
PTSD	post-traumatic stress disorder
PUD	peptic ulcer disease
pulv	a powder
PVD	peripheral vascular disease
q	every
qad	every other day
qd	every day
qh	every hour
qid	four times a day
qod	every other day
qs	a sufficient quantity
qs ad	a sufficient quantity to make
qty	quantity
qv	as much as you wish
RA	rheumatoid arthritis
Rx	take, a recipe
rep	let it be repeated
s̄	without
sa	according to art
sat	saturated
S.C.	subcutaneous
sig	label, or let it be printed
sol	solution
solv	dissolve
s̄s̄	one-half
sos	if there is need
SSRIs	selective serotonin reuptake inhibitors
stat	at once, immediately
STD	sexually-transmitted disease
supp	suppository
syr	syrup
tab	tablet
tal	such
TCA	tricyclic antidepressant
TD	tardive dyskinesia
tid	three times a day
tr, tinct	tincture
trit	triturate
tsp	teaspoonful
ULN	upper limits of normal
ung	ointment
u.d., ut dict	as directed
v.o.	verbal order
VZV	varicella zoster virus
w.a.	while awake
x3	3 times
x4	4 times

[1]Other than drug synonyms

APOTHECARY / METRIC EQUIVALENTS

Approximate Liquid Measures

Basic equivalent: 1 fluid ounce = 30 mL

Examples:

1 gallon .... 3800 mL	1 gallon .... 128 fluid ounces
1 quart .... 960 mL	1 quart .... 32 fluid ounces
1 pint .... 480 mL	1 pint .... 16 fluid ounces
8 fluid oz .... 240 mL	15 minims .... 1 mL
4 fluid oz .... 120 mL	10 minims .... 0.6 mL

Approximate Household Equivalents

1 teaspoonful .... 5 mL	1 tablespoonful .... 15 mL

Weights

Basic equivalents:

1 oz .... 30 g	15 gr .... 1 g

Examples:

4 oz .... 120 g	1 gr .... 60 mg
2 oz .... 60 g	1/100 gr .... 600 mcg
10 gr .... 600 mg	1/150 gr .... 400 mcg
7½ gr .... 500 mg	1/200 gr .... 300 mcg
16 oz .... 1 lb	

Metric Conversions

Basic equivalents:

1 g .... 1000 mg	1 mg .... 1000 mcg

Examples:

5 g .... 5000 mg	5 mg .... 5000 mcg
0.5 g .... 500 mg	0.5 mg .... 500 mcg
0.05 g .... 50 mg	0.05 mg .... 50 mcg

Exact Equivalents

1 g	=	15.43 gr	0.1 mg	=	1/600 gr
1 mL	=	16.23 minims	0.12 mg	=	1/500 gr
1 minim	=	0.06 mL	0.15 mg	=	1/400 gr
1 gr	=	64.8 mg	0.2 mg	=	1/300 gr
1 pint (pt)	=	473.2 mL	0.3 mg	=	1/200 gr
1 oz	=	28.35 g	0.4 mg	=	1/150 gr
1 lb	=	453.6 g	0.5 mg	=	1/120 gr
1 kg	=	2.2 lb	0.6 mg	=	1/100 gr
1 qt	=	946.4 mL	0.8 mg	=	1/80 gr
			1 mg	=	1/65 gr

Solids[1]

¼ grain	=	15 mg
½ grain	=	30 mg
1 grain	=	60 mg
1½ grains	=	90 mg
5 grains	=	300 mg
10 grains	=	600 mg

[1]Use exact equivalents for compounding and calculations requiring a high degree of accuracy.

AVERAGE WEIGHTS AND SURFACE AREAS

**Average Weight and Surface Area of Preterm Infants,
Term Infants, and Children**

Age	Average Weight (kg)[1]	Approximate Surface Area (m²)
Weeks Gestation		
26	0.9-1	0.1
30	1.3-1.5	0.12
32	1.6-2	0.15
38	2.9-3	0.2
40 (term infant at birth)	3.1-4	0.25
Months		
3	5	0.29
6	7	0.38
9	8	0.42
Years		
1	10	0.49
2	12	0.55
3	15	0.64
4	17	0.74
5	18	0.76
6	20	0.82
7	23	0.90
8	25	0.95
9	28	1.06
10	33	1.18
11	35	1.23
12	40	1.34
Adults	70	1.73

[1]Weights from age 3 months and older are rounded off to the nearest kilogram.

BODY MASS INDEX (BMI)

$$BMI = \frac{weight\ (kg)}{[height\ (m)]^2}$$

BODY SURFACE AREA OF ADULTS AND CHILDREN

Calculating Body Surface Area in Children

In a child of average size, find weight and corresponding surface area on the boxed scale to the left; or, use the nomogram to the right. Lay a straightedge on the correct height and weight points for the child, then read the intersecting point on the surface area scale. (**Note:** 2.2 lb = 1 kg)

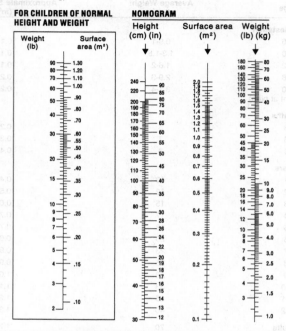

BODY SURFACE AREA FORMULA
(Adult and Pediatric)

$$BSA\ (m^2) = \sqrt{\frac{Ht\ (in) \times Wt\ (lb)}{3131}} \quad \text{or, in metric: } BSA\ (m^2) = \sqrt{\frac{Ht\ (cm) \times Wt\ (kg)}{3600}}$$

References

Lam TK and Leung DT, "More on Simplified Calculation of Body Surface Area," *N Engl J Med*, 1988, 318(17):1130 (Letter).
Mosteller RD, "Simplified Calculation of Body Surface Area", *N Engl J Med*, 1987, 317(17):1098 (Letter).

PEDIATRIC DOSAGE ESTIMATIONS

Dosage Estimations Based on Weight:

Augsberger's rule:

$$\frac{(1.5 \times \text{weight in kg} + 10)}{\% \text{ of adult dose}} = \text{child's approximate dose}$$

Clark's rule:

$$\frac{\text{weight (in pounds)}}{150} \times \text{adult dose} = \text{child's approximate dose}$$

Dosage Estimations Based on Age:

Augsberger's rule:

$$\frac{(4 \times \text{age in years} + 20)}{\% \text{ of adult dose}} = \text{child's approximate dose}$$

Bastedo's rule:

$$\frac{\text{age in years} + 3}{30} \times \text{adult dose} = \text{child's approximate dose}$$

Cowling's rule:

$$\frac{\text{age at next birthday (in years)}}{24} \times \text{adult dose} = \text{child's approximate dose}$$

Dilling's rule:

$$\frac{\text{age (in years)}}{20} \times \text{adult dose} = \text{child's approximate dose}$$

Fried's rule for infants (younger than 1 year):

$$\frac{\text{age (in months)}}{150} \times \text{adult dose} = \text{infant's approximate dose}$$

Young's rule:

$$\frac{\text{age (in years)}}{\text{age} + 12} \times \text{adult dose} = \text{child's approximate dose}$$

POUNDS / KILOGRAMS CONVERSION

1 pound = 0.45359 kilograms
1 kilogram = 2.2 pounds

lb	=	kg		lb	=	kg		lb	=	kg
1	=	0.45		70	=	31.75		140	=	63.50
5		2.27		75		34.02		145		65.77
10		4.54		80		36.29		150		68.04
15		6.80		85		38.56		155		70.31
20		9.07		90		40.82		160		72.58
25		11.34		95		43.09		165		74.84
30		13.61		100		45.36		170		77.11
35		15.88		105		47.63		175		79.38
40		18.14		110		49.90		180		81.65
45		20.41		115		52.16		185		83.92
50		22.68		120		54.43		190		86.18
55		24.95		125		56.70		195		88.45
60		27.22		130		58.91		200		90.72
65		29.48		135		61.24				

TEMPERATURE CONVERSION

Celsius to Fahrenheit = (°C x 9/5) + 32 = °F
Fahrenheit to Celsius = (°F − 32) x 5/9 = °C

°C	=	°F		°C	=	°F		°C	=	°F
100.0	=	212.0		39.0	=	102.2		36.8	=	98.2
50.0		122.0		38.8		101.8		36.6		97.9
41.0		105.8		38.6		101.5		36.4		97.5
40.8		105.4		38.4		101.1		36.2		97.2
40.6		105.1		38.2		100.8		36.0		96.8
40.4		104.7		38.0		100.4		35.8		96.4
40.2		104.4		37.8		100.1		35.6		96.1
40.0		104.0		37.6		99.7		35.4		95.7
39.8		103.6		37.4		99.3		35.2		95.4
39.6		103.3		37.2		99.0		35.0		95.0
39.4		102.9		37.0		98.6		0		32.0
39.2		102.6								

REFERENCE VALUES FOR ADULTS

Automated Chemistry (CHEMISTRY A)

Test	Values	Remarks
SERUM / PLASMA		
Acetone	Negative	
Albumin	3.2-5 g/dL	
Alcohol, ethyl	Negative	
Aldolase	1.2-7.6 IU/L	
Ammonia	20-70 mcg/dL	Specimen to be placed on ice as soon as collected.
Amylase	30-110 units/L	
Bilirubin, direct	0-0.3 mg/dL	
Bilirubin, total	0.1-1.2 mg/dL	
Calcium	8.6-10.3 mg/dL	
Calcium, ionized	2.24-2.46 mEq/L	
Chloride	95-108 mEq/L	
Cholesterol, total	≤200 mg/dL	Fasted blood required – normal value affected by dietary habits. This reference range is for a general adult population.
HDL cholesterol	40-60 mg/dL	Fasted blood required – normal value affected by dietary habits.
LDL cholesterol	<160 mg/dL	If triglyceride is >400 mg/dL, LDL cannot be calculated accurately (Friedewald equation). Target LDL-C depends on patient's risk factors.
CO_2	23-30 mEq/L	
Creatine kinase (CK) isoenzymes		
CK-BB	0%	
CK-MB (cardiac)	0%-3.9%	
CK-MM (muscle)	96%-100%	
CK-MB levels must be both ≥4% and 10 IU/L to meet diagnostic criteria for CK-MB positive result consistent with myocardial injury.		
Creatine phosphokinase (CPK)	8-150 IU/L	
Creatinine	0.5-1.4 mg/dL	
Ferritin	13-300 ng/mL	
Folate	3.6-20 ng/dL	
GGT (gamma-glutamyltranspeptidase)		
male	11-63 IU/L	
female	8-35 IU/L	
GLDH	To be determined	
Glucose (preprandial)	<115 mg/dL	Goals different for diabetics.
Glucose, fasting	60-110 mg/dL	Goals different for diabetics.
Glucose, nonfasting (2-h postprandial)	<120 mg/dL	Goals different for diabetics.
Hemoglobin A_{1c}	<8	
Hemoglobin, plasma free	<2.5 mg/100 mL	
Hemoglobin, total glycosolated (Hb A_1)	4%-8%	
Iron	65-150 mcg/dL	
Iron binding capacity, total (TIBC)	250-420 mcg/dL	
Lactic acid	0.7-2.1 mEq/L	Specimen to be kept on ice and sent to lab as soon as possible.
Lactate dehydrogenase (LDH)	56-194 IU/L	
Lactate dehydrogenase (LDH) isoenzymes		
LD_1	20%-34%	
LD_2	29%-41%	
LD_3	15%-25%	
LD_4	1%-12%	
LD_5	1%-15%	
Flipped LD_1/LD_2 ratios (>1 may be consistent with myocardial injury) particularly when considered in combination with a recent CK-MB positive result.		
Lipase	23-208 units/L	
Magnesium	1.6-2.5 mg/dL	Increased by slight hemolysis.
Osmolality	289-308 mOsm/kg	
Phosphatase, alkaline		
adults 25-60 y	33-131 IU/L	
adults 61 y or older	51-153 IU/L	
infancy-adolescence	Values range up to 3-5 times higher than adults	
Phosphate, inorganic	2.8-4.2 mg/dL	
Potassium	3.5-5.2 mEq/L	Increased by slight hemolysis.
Prealbumin	>15 mg/dL	

REFERENCE VALUES FOR ADULTS *(Continued)*

Automated Chemistry (CHEMISTRY A) *(continued)*

Test	Values	Remarks
Protein, total	6.5-7.9 g/dL	
SGOT (AST)	<35 IU/L (20-48)	
SGPT (ALT) (10-35)	<35 IU/L	
Sodium	134-149 mEq/L	
Transferrin	>200 mg/dL	
Triglycerides	45-155 mg/dL	Fasted blood required.
Troponin I	<1.5 ng/mL	
Urea nitrogen (BUN)	7-20 mg/dL	
Uric acid		
male	2-8 mg/dL	
female	2-7.5 mg/dL	
CEREBROSPINAL FLUID		
Glucose	50-70 mg/dL	
Protein		
adults and children	15-45 mg/dL	CSF obtained by lumbar puncture.
newborn infants	60-90 mg/dL	

On CSF obtained by cisternal puncture: About 25 mg/dL
On CSF obtained by ventricular puncture: About 10 mg/dL
Note: Bloody specimen gives erroneously high value due to contamination with blood proteins

URINE		
(24-hour specimen is required for all these tests unless specified)		
Amylase	32-641 units/L	The value is in units/L and **not** calculated for total volume.
Amylase, fluid (random samples)		Interpretation of value left for physician, depends on the nature of fluid.
Calcium	Depends upon dietary intake	
Creatine		
male	150 mg/24 h	Higher value on children and during pregnancy.
female	250 mg/24 h	
Creatinine	1000-2000 mg/24 h	
Creatinine clearance (endogenous)		
male	85-125 mL/min	A blood sample must accompany urine specimen.
female	75-115 mL/min	
Glucose	1 g/24 h	
5-hydroxyindoleacetic acid	2-8 mg/24 h	
Iron	0.15 mg/24 h	Acid washed container required.
Magnesium	146-209 mg/24 h	
Osmolality	500-800 mOsm/kg	With normal fluid intake.
Oxalate	10-40 mg/24 h	
Phosphate	400-1300 mg/24 h	
Potassium	25-120 mEq/24 h	Varies with diet; the interpretation of urine electrolytes and osmolality should be left for the physician.
Sodium	40-220 mEq/24 h	
Porphobilinogen, qualitative ·	Negative	
Porphyrins, qualitative	Negative	
Proteins	0.05-0.1 g/24 h	
Salicylate	Negative	
Urea clearance	60-95 mL/min	A blood sample must accompany specimen.
Urea N	10-40 g/24 h	Dependent on protein intake.
Uric acid	250-750 mg/24 h	Dependent on diet and therapy.
Urobilinogen	0.5-3.5 mg/24 h	For qualitative determination on random urine, send sample to urinalysis section in Hematology Lab.
Xylose absorption test		
children	16%-33% of ingested xylose	
FECES		
Fat, 3-day collection	<5 g/d	Value depends on fat intake of 100 g/d for 3 days preceding and during collection.
GASTRIC ACIDITY		
Acidity, total, 12 h	10-60 mEq/L	Titrated at pH 7.

Blood Gases

	Arterial	Capillary	Venous
pH	7.35-7.45	7.35-7.45	7.32-7.42
pCO$_2$ (mm Hg)	35-45	35-45	38-52
pO$_2$ (mm Hg)	70-100	60-80	24-48
HCO$_3$ (mEq/L)	19-25	19-25	19-25
TCO$_2$ (mEq/L)	19-29	19-29	23-33
O$_2$ saturation (%)	90-95	90-95	40-70
Base excess (mEq/L)	-5 to +5	-5 to +5	-5 to +5

HEMATOLOGY

Complete Blood Count

Age	Hgb (g/dL)	Hct (%)	RBC (mill/mm^3)	RDW
0-3 d	15.0-20.0	45-61	4.0-5.9	<18
1-2 wk	12.5-18.5	39-57	3.6-5.5	<17
1-6 mo	10.0-13.0	29-42	3.1-4.3	<16.5
7 mo to 2 y	10.5-13.0	33-38	3.7-4.9	<16
2-5 y	11.5-13.0	34-39	3.9-5.0	<15
5-8 y	11.5-14.5	35-42	4.0-4.9	<15
13-18 y	12.0-15.2	36-47	4.5-5.1	<14.5
Adult male	13.5-16.5	41-50	4.5-5.5	<14.5
Adult female	12.0-15.0	36-44	4.0-4.9	<14.5

Age	MCV (fL)	MCH (pg)	MCHC (%)	Plts (x 10^3/mm^3)
0-3 d	95-115	31-37	29-37	250-450
1-2 wk	86-110	28-36	28-38	250-450
1-6 mo	74-96	25-35	30-36	300-700
7 mo to 2 y	70-84	23-30	31-37	250-600
2-5 y	75-87	24-30	31-37	250-550
5-8 y	77-95	25-33	31-37	250-550
13-18 y	78-96	25-35	31-37	150-450
Adult male	80-100	26-34	31-37	150-450
Adult female	80-100	26-34	31-37	150-450

REFERENCE VALUES FOR ADULTS *(Continued)*

WBC and Differential

Age	WBC (x 10³/mm³)	Segs	Bands	Lymphs	Monos
0-3 d	9.0-35.0	32-62	10-18	19-29	5-7
1-2 wk	5.0-20.0	14-34	6-14	36-45	6-10
1-6 mo	6.0-17.5	13-33	4-12	41-71	4-7
7 mo to 2 y	6.0-17.0	15-35	5-11	45-76	3-6
2-5 y	5.5-15.5	23-45	5-11	35-65	3-6
5-8 y	5.0-14.5	32-54	5-11	28-48	3-6
13-18 y	4.5-13.0	34-64	5-11	25-45	3-6
Adults	4.5-11.0	35-66	5-11	24-44	3-6

Age	Eosinophils	Basophils	Atypical Lymphs	No. of NRBCs
0-3 d	0-2	0-1	0-8	0-2
1-2 wk	0-2	0-1	0-8	0
1-6 mo	0-3	0-1	0-8	0
7 mo to 2 y	0-3	0-1	0-8	0
2-5 y	0-3	0-1	0-8	0
5-8 y	0-3	0-1	0-8	0
13-18 y	0-3	0-1	0-8	0
Adults	0-3	0-1	0-8	0

Segs = segmented neutrophils.
Bands = band neutrophils.
Lymphs = lymphocytes.
Monos = monocytes.

Erythrocyte Sedimentation Rates and Reticulocyte Counts

Sedimentation rate, Westergren	Children	0-20 mm/hour
	Adult male	0-15 mm/hour
	Adult female	0-20 mm/hour
Sedimentation rate, Wintrobe	Children	0-13 mm/hour
	Adult male	0-10 mm/hour
	Adult female	0-15 mm/hour
Reticulocyte count	Newborns	2%-6%
	1-6 mo	0%-2.8%
	Adults	0.5%-1.5%

REFERENCE VALUES FOR CHILDREN

		Normal Values
CHEMISTRY		
Albumin	0-1 y	2-4 g/dL
	1 y to adult	3.5-5.5 g/dL
Ammonia	Newborns	90-150 mcg/dL
	Children	40-120 mcg/dL
	Adults	18-54 mcg/dL
Amylase	Newborns	0-60 units/L
	Adults	30-110 units/L
Bilirubin, conjugated, direct	Newborns	<1.5 mg/dL
	1 mo to adult	0-0.5 mg/dL
Bilirubin, total	0-3 d	2-10 mg/dL
	1 mo to adult	0-1.5 mg/dL
Bilirubin, unconjugated, indirect		0.6-10.5 mg/dL
Calcium	Newborns	7-12 mg/dL
	0-2 y	8.8-11.2 mg/dL
	2 y to adult	9-11 mg/dL
Calcium, ionized, whole blood		4.4-5.4 mg/dL
Carbon dioxide, total		23-33 mEq/L
Chloride		95-105 mEq/L
Cholesterol	Newborns	45-170 mg/dL
	0-1 y	65-175 mg/dL
	1-20 y	120-230 mg/dL
Creatinine	0-1 y	≤0.6 mg/dL
	1 y to adult	0.5-1.5 mg/dL
Glucose	Newborns	30-90 mg/dL
	0-2 y	60-105 mg/dL
	Children to adults	70-110 mg/dL
Iron		
	Newborns	110-270 mcg/dL
	Infants	30-70 mcg/dL
	Children	55-120 mcg/dL
	Adults	70-180 mcg/dL
Iron binding	Newborns	59-175 mcg/dL
	Infants	100-400 mcg/dL
	Adults	250-400 mcg/dL
Lactic acid, lactate		2-20 mg/dL
Lead, whole blood		<10 mcg/dL
Lipase		
	Children	20-140 units/L
	Adults	0-190 units/L
Magnesium		1.5-2.5 mEq/L
Osmolality, serum		275-296 mOsm/kg
Osmolality, urine		50-1400 mOsm/kg
Phosphorus	Newborns	4.2-9 mg/dL
	6 wk to 19 mo	3.8-6.7 mg/dL
	19 mo to 3 y	2.9-5.9 mg/dL
	3-15 y	3.6-5.6 mg/dL
	>15 y	2.5-5 mg/dL
Potassium, plasma	Newborns	4.5-7.2 mEq/L
	2 d to 3 mo	4-6.2 mEq/L
	3 mo to 1 y	3.7-5.6 mEq/L
	1-16 y	3.5-5 mEq/L
Protein, total	0-2 y	4.2-7.4 g/dL
	>2 y	6-8 g/dL
Sodium		136-145 mEq/L
Triglycerides	Infants	0-171 mg/dL
	Children	20-130 mg/dL
	Adults	30-200 mg/dL
Urea nitrogen, blood	0-2 y	4-15 mg/dL
	2 y to adult	5-20 mg/dL

REFERENCE VALUES FOR CHILDREN (Continued)

		Normal Values
Uric acid	Male	3-7 mg/dL
	Female	2-6 mg/dL
ENZYMES		
Alanine aminotransferase (ALT) (SGPT)	0-2 mo	8-78 units/L
	>2 mo	8-36 units/L
Alkaline phosphatase (ALKP)	Newborns	60-130 units/L
	0-16 y	85-400 units/L
	>16 y	30-115 units/L
Aspartate aminotransferase (AST)	Infants	18-74 units/L
(SGOT)	Children	15-46 units/L
	Adults	5-35 units/L
Creatine kinase (CK)	Infants	20-200 units/L
	Children	10-90 units/L
	Adult male	0-206 units/L
	Adult female	0-175 units/L
Lactate dehydrogenase (LDH)	Newborns	290-501 units/L
	1 mo to 2 y	110-144 units/L
	>16 y	60-170 units/L

Blood Gases

	Arterial	Capillary	Venous
pH	7.35-7.45	7.35-7.45	7.32-7.42
pCO$_2$ (mm Hg)	35-45	35-45	38-52
pO$_2$ (mm Hg)	70-100	60-80	24-48
HCO$_3$ (mEq/L)	19-25	19-25	19-25
TCO$_2$ (mEq/L)	19-29	19-29	23-33
O$_2$ saturation (%)	90-95	90-95	40-70
Base excess (mEq/L)	-5 to +5	-5 to +5	-5 to +5

Thyroid Function Tests

T$_4$ (thyroxine)	1-7 d	10.1-20.9 mcg/dL
	8-14 d	9.8-16.6 mcg/dL
	1 mo to 1 y	5.5-16 mcg/dL
	>1 y	4-12 mcg/dL
FTI	1-3 d	9.3-26.6
	1-4 wk	7.6-20.8
	1-4 mo	7.4-17.9
	4-12 mo	5.1-14.5
	1-6 y	5.7-13.3
	>6 y	4.8-14
T$_3$ by RIA	Newborns	100-470 ng/dL
	1-5 y	100-260 ng/dL
	5-10 y	90-240 ng/dL
	10 y to adult	70-210 ng/dL
T$_3$ uptake		35%-45%
TSH	Cord	3-22 µIU/mL
	1-3 d	<40 µIU/mL
	3-7 d	<25 µIU/mL
	>7 d	0-10 µIU/mL

DIAGNOSTICS AND SURGICAL AIDS

Agent	Use
Apraclonidine (Iopidine®)	Prevention and treatment of postsurgical intraocular pressure elevation
Benzylpenicilloyl-polylysine (Pre-Pen® [DSC])	Adjunct in assessing the risk of administering penicillin (penicillin or benzylpenicillin) in adults with a history of clinical penicillin hypersensitivity
Candida albicans (Monilia) (Candin®)	Screen for the detection of nonresponsiveness to antigens in immunocompromised individuals
Cellulose (oxidized regenerated) (Surgicel®)	Temporary packing for the control of capillary, venous, or small arterial hemorrhage
Chondroitin sulfate – sodium hyaluronate (Viscoat®)	Surgical aid in anterior segment procedures, protects corneal endothelium and coats intraocular lens thus protecting it
Collagen hemostat (Avitene®; Helistat®)	Adjunct to hemostasis when control of bleeding by ligature is ineffective or impractical
Corticotropin (H.P. Acthar® Gel)	Diagnostic aid in adrenocortical insufficiency; repository dosage form is used for acute exacerbations of multiple sclerosis or severe muscle weakness in myasthenia gravis; cosyntropin is preferred
Cosyntropin (Cortrosyn® Injection)	Diagnostic test to differentiate primary adrenal from secondary (pituitary) adrenocortical insufficiency
Cyclopentolate (AK-Pentolate® [DSC]; Cyclogyl®)	Diagnostic procedures requiring mydriasis and cycloplegia
Cyclopentolate and phenylephrine (Cyclomydril® Ophthalmic)	Induce mydriasis greater than that produced with cyclopentolate alone
Dapiprazole (Rev-Eyes™)	Reverse dilation due to drugs (adrenergic or parasympathomimetic) after eye exams
Dimercaprol (BAL in Oil®)	Antidote to gold, arsenic (except arsine), and mercury poisoning (except nonalkyl mercury); adjunct to edetate calcium disodium in lead poisoning; possibly effective for antimony, bismuth, chromium, copper, nickel, tungsten, or zinc
Dinoprost	Abort 2nd trimester pregnancy
Fluorescein sodium (AK-Fluor® Injection; Fluorescite® Injection; Fluorets® Ophthalmic Strips; Fluor-I-Strip®; Fluor-I-Strip-AT®; Ful-Glo® Ophthalmic Strips)	Demonstrates defects of corneal epithelium; diagnostic aid in ophthalmic angiography
Gelatin, absorbable (Gelfilm® Ophthalmic; Gelfoam® Topical)	Adjunct to provide hemostasis in surgery; used in open prostatic surgery
Histoplasmin (Histolyn-CYL® Injection)	Diagnose histoplasmosis; assess cell-mediated immunity
Hydroxyamphetamine and tropicamide (Paremyd® Ophthalmic)	Diagnostic mydriasis with cycloplegia
Hydroxypropyl methylcellulose (Gonak™; Goniosol®)	Ophthalmic surgical aid in cataract extraction and intraocular implantation; gonioscopic examination
Indocyanine green (IC-Green®)	Determine hepatic function, cardiac output, and liver blood flow and for ophthalmic angiography
Methacholine (Provocholine®)	Diagnosis of bronchial airway hyperactivity
Methylene blue (Urolene Blue®)	Antidote for cyanide poisoning and drug-induced methemoglobinemia, indicator dye, chronic urolithiasis. **Unlabeled use:** Has been used topically (0.1% solutions) in conjunction with polychromatic light to photoinactivate viruses such as herpes simplex; has been used alone or in combination with vitamin C for the management of chronic urolithiasis.
Mumps skin test antigen	Assess the status of cell-mediated immunity
Proparacaine (Alcaine®; Ophthetic®)	Anesthesia for tonometry, gonioscopy; suture removal from cornea; removal of corneal foreign body; cataract extraction, glaucoma surgery; short operative procedure involving the cornea and conjunctiva
Proparacaine and fluorescein (Flucaine®; Fluoracaine® Ophthalmic)	Anesthesia for tonometry, gonioscopy; suture removal from cornea; removal of corneal foreign body; cataract extraction, glaucoma surgery
Protirelin (Thyrel® TRH [DSC])	Adjunct in the diagnostic assessment of thyroid function, and an adjunct to other diagnostic procedures in assessment of patients with pituitary or hypothalamic dysfunction; causes release of prolactin from the pituitary and is used to detect defective control of prolactin secretion
Secretin (SecreFlo™)	Diagnose Zollinger-Ellison syndrome, chronic pancreatic dysfunction, and some hepatobiliary diseases such as obstructive jaundice resulting from cancer or stones in the biliary tract
Sermorelin acetate (Geref® Diagnostic)	Geref® Diagnostic: For the evaluation of short children whose height is at least 2 standard deviations below the mean height for their chronological age and sex, presenting with low basal serum levels of IGF-1 and IGF-1-BP3. A single intravenous injection of sermorelin is indicated for evaluating the ability of the somatotroph of the pituitary gland to secrete growth hormone (GH). A normal plasma GH response demonstrates that the somatotroph is intact. Geref® injection: Treatment of idiopathic growth hormone deficiency
Sincalide (Kinevac®)	Postevacuation cholecystography; gallbladder bile sampling; stimulate pancreatic secretion for analysis
Skin test antigens, multiple (Multitest CMI®)	Detection of nonresponsiveness to antigens by means of delayed hypersensitivity skin testing
Sodium hyaluronate (Healon®; Healon® GV)	Surgical aid in cataract extraction, intraocular implantation, corneal transplant, glaucoma filtration, and retinal attachment surgery
Succinylcholine (Quelicin® Injection)	Produces skeletal muscle relaxation in procedures of short duration such as endotracheal intubation or endoscopic exams
Thrombin, topical (Thrombin-JMI®)	Hemostasis whenever minor bleeding from capillaries and small venules is accessible
Thyrotropin Alpha (Thyrogen®)	As an adjunctive diagnostic tool for serum thyroglobulin (Tg) testing with or without radioiodine imaging in the follow-up of patients with well-differentiated thyroid cancer
Trichophyton skin test	Assess cell-mediated immunity
Tropicamide (Mydral™; Mydriacyl®; Tropicacyl®)	Short-acting mydriatic used in diagnostic procedures, as well as preoperatively and postoperatively; treatment of some cases of acute ititis, iridocyclitis, and keratitis

HERBAL AND NUTRITIONAL PRODUCTS

TOP HERBAL PRODUCTS

This section contains general information on commonly encountered herbal or nutritional products. A more complete listing of products follows.

Alpha-Lipoic Acid
Synonyms: Alpha-Lipoate; Lipoic Acid; Thioctic acid
Use: Treatment of glaucoma and neuropathies
Mechanism of Action/Effect: Sulfur-containing cofactor normally synthesized in humans; potent antioxidant
Warnings: Use with caution in individuals who may be predisposed to hypoglycemia (including individuals receiving antidiabetic agents).
Drug Interactions: Oral hypoglycemics or insulin
Adverse Reactions: Rash
Dosing: Oral: 20-600 mg/day (common dose: 25-50 mg twice daily)

Androstenedione
Use: Increase strength and muscle mass
Mechanism of Action/Effect: Weak androgenic steroid hormone believed to facilitate faster recovery from exercise and to promote muscle development in response to training
Contraindication: Hypertension
Warnings: Use with caution in individuals with CHF, prostate conditions, and hormone-sensitive tumors. The FDA requires specific labeling on this supplement, noting that these supplements "contain steroid hormones that may cause breast enlargement, testicular shrinkage, and infertility in males, and increased facial and body hair, voice deepening and clitoral enlargement in females."
Drug Interactions: Estrogens and androgenic drugs
Dosing: Oral: 50-100 mg/day (usually about 1 hour before exercising)

Arginine
Synonyms: L-Arginine
Use: Treatment of high cholesterol, poor circulation, inflammatory bowel disease, immunity enhancement, male infertility; promotes lean body mass, surgery and wound healing, sexual vitality and enhancement
Mechanism of Action/Effect: Precursor to nitric oxide; plays a key role in the urea cycle, which is the biochemical pathway that metabolized protein and other nitrogen-containing compounds
Warnings: Use caution in individuals with herpes simplex; may stimulate growth of virus.
Drug Interactions: Nitroglycerin and sildenafil
Dosing: Oral: 3-6 g/day

Bifidobacterium bifidum / Lactobacillus acidophilus
Use:
  B. bifidum: Treatment of Crohn's disease, diarrhea, ulcerative colitis; maintenance of anaerobic microflora in the colon
  L. acidophilus: Treatment of constipation, infant diarrhea, lactose intolerance; recolonization of the GI tract with beneficial bacteria during and after antibiotic use
Mechanism of Action/Effect: Natural components of colonic flora, used to facilitate recolonization with benign symbiotic organisms; promote vitamin K synthesis and absorption
Drug Interactions: Antibiotics eliminate *B. bifidum* and *L. acidophilus*
Adverse Reactions: No known toxicity or serious side effect
Dosing: Oral: 5-10 billion colony forming units (CFU) per day (dairy free); refrigerate to maintain optimum potency

Bilberry
Synonym: *Vaccinium myrtillus*
Use: Treatment of ophthalmologic disorders (eg, macular degeneration, diabetic retinopathy, cataracts) and vascular disorders (eg, varicose veins, phlebitis)
Mechanism of Action/Effect: Reportedly inhibits a variety of inflammatory mediators, including histamine, proteases, leukotrienes, and prostaglandins; may decrease capillary permeability and inhibit platelet aggregation
Contraindication: Active bleeding (eg, peptic ulcer, intracranial bleeding)
Warnings: Use with caution in individuals with a history of bleeding, hemostatic disorders, or drug-related hemostatic problems. Use with caution in individuals taking anticoagulants (eg, warfarin, aspirin, aspirin-containing products, NSAIDs) or antiplatelet agents (eg, ticlopidine, clopidogrel, dipyridamole). Discontinue use prior to dental or surgical procedures (generally at least 14 days before).
Drug Interactions: Oral hypoglycemics, anticoagulants, NSAIDs, aspirin, or insulin (effects may be altered)
Dosing: Oral: 80 mg 2-3 times/day

Black Cohosh
Synonym: *Cimicifuga racemosa*
Use: Treatment of vasomotor symptoms of menopause, premenstrual syndrome (PMS), mild depression, arthritis
Mechanism of Action/Effect: Contains multiple phytoestrogens and salicylic acid (small amounts)
Contraindications: Pregnancy (may stimulate uterine contractions) and lactation; history of estrogen-dependent tumors or endometrial cancer
Warnings: Use with caution in individuals allergic to salicylates (unknown whether the amount of salicylic acid is likely to affect platelet aggregation or have other effects associated with salicylates); those receiving hormone replacement therapy, taking oral contraceptives, or with a history of thromboembolic disease or stroke
Drug Interactions: Oral contraceptives, hormonal replacement therapy
Adverse Reactions: High doses: Nausea, vomiting, headache, hypotension
Dosing: Oral: 20-40 mg twice daily

Chamomile

Synonyms: *Matricaria chamomilla*; *Matricaria recutita*
Use: Topical anti-inflammatory with hypnotic properties; treatment of hemorrhoids, irritable bowel, eczema, mastitis and leg ulcers; cigarette tobacco flavoring
Mechanism of Action/Effect: Antispasmodic; anti-inflammatory; antiulcer; antibacterial and sedative effects also documented
Contraindications: Hypersensitivity to *Asteraceae/Compositae* family or ragweed pollens
Warnings: Use with caution in asthmatics; cross sensitivity may occur in individuals allergic to ragweed pollens, asters, or chrysanthemums.
Drug Interactions: May increase effect of coumarin-type anticoagulants at high doses; may potentiate sedatives (benzodiazepines, barbiturates)
Adverse Reactions: Contact dermatitis, emesis (from dried flowering heads), anaphylaxis, hypersensitivity reactions (especially in atopic individuals)
Dosing:
Tea: ±150 mL H_2O poured over heaping tablespoon (±3 g) of chamomile, covered and steeped 5-10 minutes; tea is used 3-4 times/day for GI upset
Liquid extract: 1-4 mL 3 times/day
Pregnancy Implications: Excessive use should be avoided due to potential teratogenicity.

Chasteberry

Synonyms: Chastetree; *Vitex agnus-castus*
Use: Treatment of acne vulgaris, corpus luteum insufficiency, hyperprolactinemia, insufficient lactation, menopause, menstrual disorders (eg, amenorrhea, endometriosis, premenstrual syndrome)
Mechanism of Action/Effect: Noted to possess significant effect on pituitary function; demonstrated to have progesterone-like effects (may stimulate luteinizing hormone [LH] and inhibit follicle-stimulating hormone [FSH]
Contraindications: Pregnancy and lactation (based on case reports of uterine stimulation and emmenagogue effects)
Warnings: Use with caution in individuals receiving hormonal therapy.
Drug Interactions: Hormonal replacement therapy, oral contraceptives, dopamine antagonists (eg, metoclopramide and antipsychotics)
Dosing: Oral: 400 mg/day in the morning (preferably on an empty stomach)

Chondroitin Sulfate

Use: Treatment of osteoarthritis
Mechanism of Action/Effect: Reported to act synergistically with glucosamine to support the maintenance of strong, healthy cartilage and maintain joint function; inhibits synovial enzymes (elastase, hyaluronidase) which may contribute to cartilage destruction and loss of joint function (studies inconclusive)
Adverse Reactions: No known toxicity or serious side effects.
Dosing: Oral: 300-1500 mg/day

Chromium

Use: Improves glycemic control; increases lean body mass; reduces obesity; improves lipid profile by decreasing total cholesterol and triglycerides, increasing HDL (dosages in excess of >300 mg/day reported to benefit breast cancer, diabetes, and cardiovascular diseases)
Mechanism of Action/Effect: Chromium picolinate is the only active form of chromium. It appears that chromium, in its trivalent form, increases insulin sensitivity and improves glucose transport into cells. The mechanism by which this happens could include one or more of the following: Increase the number of insulin receptors, enhance insulin binding to target tissues, promote activation of insulin-receptor tyrosine dinase activity, enhance beta-cell sensitivity in the pancreas.
Drug Interactions: Any medications that may also affect blood sugars (eg, beta-blockers, thiazides, oral hypoglycemics, and insulin); discuss chromium use prior to initiating
Adverse Reactions: Nausea, loose stools, flatulence, changes in appetite; isolated reports of anemia, cognitive impairment, renal failure
Dosing: 50-600 mcg/day

Coenzyme Q10

Synonym: Ubiquinone
Use: Treatment of angina, chronic fatigue syndrome, CHF, hypertension, muscular dystrophy, obesity, Parkinson's disease, periodontal disease
Mechanism of Action/Effect: Functions as a lipid-soluble antioxidant, providing protection against free radical damage; involved in ATP generation, the primary source of energy in human physiology
Drug Interactions: Drugs which can cause depletion of CoQ_{10}: Hydralazine, thiazide diuretics, HMG-CoA reductase inhibitors, sulfonylureas, beta-blockers, tricyclic antidepressants, chlorpromazine, clonidine, methyldopa, diazoxide, biguanides, haloperidol; CoQ_{10} may decrease response to warfarin
Contraindications: Doxorubicin
Warnings: Controlled trials have not demonstrated benefit in heart failure.
Dosing: Oral: 30-200 mg/day

Cranberry

Synonym: *Vaccinium macrocarpon*
Use: Prevention of nephrolithiasis, prevention and treatment of urinary tract infection
Mechanism of Action/Effect: Although early research indicated that cranberry worked through urinary acidification, current research indicates that a cranberry-derived glycoprotein inhibits *E. coli* adherence to the epithelial cells of the urinary tract.
Dosing: Oral: 300-400 mg twice daily or 8-16 oz/day of 100% cranberry juice

HERBAL AND NUTRITIONAL PRODUCTS *(Continued)*

Dehydroepiandosterone

Synonym: DHEA

Use: Treatment of depression, diabetes, fatigue, aging, lupus

Mechanism of Action/Effect: Precursor for the synthesis of over 50 hormones (including estrogen and testosterone); secreted by the adrenal glands, DHEA has been shown to stimulate production of insulin growth factor-1 (IGF-1) and change the response to insulin, decreasing the insulin requirement in individuals with diabetes. Supplementation may also increase circulating testosterone levels.

Contraindications: History of prostate or breast cancer

Warnings: Use with caution in individuals with hepatic dysfunction, diabetes, or those predisposed to hypoglycemia. Blood glucose should be closely monitored in diabetics and the dosage of antidiabetic agents should be closely monitored among health care providers.

Drug Interactions: May interact with androgens, estrogens, corticosteroids, insulin, oral hypoglycemic agents

Adverse Reactions: No known toxicity or serious side effects; long-term human studies have not been conducted

Dosing: Oral: 5-50 mg/day; 100 mg/day has been used in elderly individuals

Dong Quai

Synonyms: *Angelica sinensis*; Chinese angelica

Use: Treatment of anemia, hypertension, menopause, dysmenorrhea, PMS, amenorrhea; improves energy (particularly in females)

Mechanism of Action/Effect: Reported to cause vasodilation and may have hematopoietic properties; rich in phytoestrogens which may demonstrate similar pharmacological effects, but are less potent than pure estrogenic compounds

Contraindications: Active bleeding (eg, peptic ulcer, intracranial bleeding); may alter hemostasis, based on potential interference with platelet aggregation (observed with related species)

Warnings: Use with caution in individuals at risk of hypotension and those who would tolerate hypotension poorly (eg, cerebrovascular or cardiovascular disease); individuals taking antihypertensive medications, hormone replacement therapy, oral contraceptives, or with a history of estrogen-dependent tumors, endometrial cancer, thromboembolic disease, or stroke; individuals with a history of bleeding, hemostatic disorders, or drug-related hemostatic problems; those taking anticoagulants (may potentiate effects of warfarin) or antiplatelet agents (eg, ticlopidine, clopidogrel, dipyridamole); and in pregnant and lactating women. May cause photosensitization; avoid prolonged exposure to sunlight or other sources of ultraviolet radiation (ie, tanning booths). Discontinue use prior to dental or surgical procedures (generally at least 14 days before).

Drug Interactions: Antihypertensives, anticoagulants, antiplatelet drugs, hormonal replacement therapy, oral contraceptives, photosensitizing medications

Dosing: Oral: 200 mg twice daily

Echinacea

Synonyms: American Coneflower; Black Susans; Comb Flower; *Echinacea angustifolia*; Indian Head; Purple Coneflower; Scury Root; Snakeroot

Use: Treatment of cold and flu, upper respiratory tract infections, urinary tract infections

Mechanism of Action/Effect: Has antihyaluronidase and anti-inflammatory activity; caffeic acid glycosides and isolutylamides associated with the plant can cause immune stimulation (leukocyte phagocytosis and T-cell activation)

Contraindications: Allergy to sunflowers, daisies, ragweed; autoimmune diseases (eg, collagen vascular disease [lupus, RA], HIV/AIDS), multiple sclerosis, tuberculosis, pregnancy; per Commission E: Parenteral administration is contraindicated, but oral use is not contraindicated during pregnancy

Warnings: May alter immunosuppression; long-term use may cause immunosuppression. Persons allergic to sunflowers may display cross-allergy potential. Use as a preventative treatment should be discouraged.

Drug Interactions: May alter response to immunosuppressive therapy

Adverse Reactions: Tingling sensation of tongue, allergic reactions (rare); may become immunosuppressive with continuous use over 6-8 weeks

Per Commission E: None known for oral and external use

Dosing: Continuous use should not exceed 8 weeks

    Capsule: 500 mg 3 times/day on day 1, then 250 mg 4 times/day, standardized to contain 4% echinacosides *(E. angustifolia)* or 4% sesquiterpene esters *(E. purpurea)* per dose

    Plant juice: Freshly expressed *(E. purpurea)*: 60 drops 3 times/day with food for 1 day, then 40 drops 3 times/day with food for up to 10 days, standardized to contain not less than 2.4% soluble beta-1,2 D-5 fructofuranosides per dose

    Topical: Apply to affected area as needed

Evening Primrose

Synonyms: Evening Primrose Oil; *Oenothera biennis*

Use: Treatment of diabetic neuropathy, endometriosis, hyperglycemia, irritable bowel syndrome, multiple sclerosis, omega-6-fatty acid supplementation, PMS, menopause, rheumatoid arthritis

Mechanism of Action/Effect: Contains high amounts of gamma-linolenic acid, or GLA, an essential omega-6 fatty acid which reportedly reduces generation of arachidonic acid metabolites in short-term use, improving symptoms of various inflammatory and immune conditions; reported to stimulate hormone synthesis

Contraindications: Seizure disorders (may lower seizure threshold, based on animal studies), schizophrenia, active bleeding (may inhibit platelet aggregation), individuals receiving anticonvulsant or antipsychotic medications

Warnings: Use with caution in individuals with a history of bleeding, hemostatic disorders, or drug-related hemostatic problems; individuals taking anticoagulants (eg, warfarin, aspirin, aspirin-containing products, NSAIDs) or antiplatelet agents (eg, ticlopidine, clopidogrel, dipyridamole). Discontinue use prior to dental or surgical procedures (generally at least 14 days before).

Drug Interactions: Anticonvulsants (seizure threshold decreased), anticoagulants, antiplatelet agents

Dosing: Oral: 500 mg to 8 g/day

Feverfew

Synonyms: Altamisa; Bachelor's Buttons; Featherfew; Featherfoil; Nosebleed; *Tanacetum parthenium*; Wild Quinine

Use: Prophylaxis and treatment of migraine headaches; treatment of menstrual complaints and fever

Mechanism of Action/Effect: Active ingredient is parthenolide (~0.2% concentration), which is a serotonin antagonist; also, the plant may be an inhibitor of prostaglandin synthesis and platelet aggregation; may have spasmolytic activity

Contraindications: Pregnancy and lactation; children <2 years of age; allergies to feverfew and other members of Asteraceae, daisy, ragweed, chamomile

Warning: Use with caution in patients taking medications with serotonergic properties.

Drug Interactions: Anticoagulants (eg, aspirin, aspirin-containing products, NSAIDs)

Adverse Reactions: Mouth ulcerations, contact dermatitis, abdominal pain, nausea, vomiting, loss of taste; postfeverfew syndrome on discontinuation (nervousness, insomnia, still joints, headache)

Dosing: 125 mg 1-2 times/day

Garlic

Synonyms: *Allium savitum*; Comphor of the Poor; Nectar of the Gods; Poor Mans Treacle; Rustic Treacle; Stinking Rose

Use: Treatment of hypertension; lowers LDL cholesterol and triglycerides and raises HDL cholesterol; may lower blood glucose and decrease thrombosis; potential anti-inflammatory and antitumor effects

Mechanism of Action/Effect: Allinin garlic is converted to allicin (after the bulb is ground), which is odoriferous and may have some antioxidant activity; ajoene (a byproduct of allicin) has potent platelet inhibition effects; garlic can also decrease LDL cholesterol levels and increase fibrinolytic activity. The LDL benefit of garlic is modest.

Contraindication: Pregnancy

Warnings: Onset of cholesterol-lowering and hypotensive effects may require months. Use with caution in patients receiving treatment for hyperglycemia or hypertension.

Drug Interactions: Iodine uptake may be reduced with garlic ingestion; can exacerbate bleeding in patients taking aspirin or anticoagulant agents; may increase the risk of hypoglycemia; may increase response to antihypertensives

Adverse Reactions: Skin blistering, eczema, systemic contact dermatitis, immunologic contact urticaria, GI upset and changes in intestinal flora (rare) per Commission E, lacrimation, asthma (upon inhalation of garlic dust), allergic reactions (rare), change in odor of skin and breath (per Commission E)

Half-Life Elimination: N-acetyl-S-allyl-L-cysteine: 6 hours

Excretion: Pulmonary and renal

Dosing: Adults: 4-12 mg allicin/day

Average daily dose for cardiovascular benefit: 0.25-1 g/kg or 1-4 cloves daily in an 80 kg individual in divided doses

Toxic dose: >5 cloves or >25 mL of extract can cause GI symptoms

Additional Information: 1% as active as penicillin as an antibiotic; number one over-the-counter medication in Germany; enteric-coated products may demonstrate best results.

Ginger

Synonym: *Zingiber officinale*

Pregnancy Risk Factor: Per Commission E, not to be used for morning sickness during pregnancy (some contradictory recommendations exist); high doses may be abortifacient

Use: Antiemetic; digestive aid; treatment of nausea and motion sickness, headaches, colds and flu, osteoarthritis; flavoring agent in beverages and mouthwashes

Mechanism of Action/Effect: Unknown; appears to decrease prostaglandin synthesismay increase GI motility; may have cardiotonic activity and inhibit platelet aggregation (very high doses)

Contraindication: Gallstones (per Commission E)

Warnings: Use with caution in diabetics, patients on cardiac glycosides, and those receiving anticoagulants.

Drug Interactions: May alter response to cardiotonic, hypoglycemic, anticoagulant, and antiplatelet agents

Dosing:

Prevention of motion sickness or digestive aid: 1-4 g/day (250 mg of ginger root powder 3-4 times/day)

Per Commission E: 2-4 g/day or equivalent preparations

HERBAL AND NUTRITIONAL PRODUCTS *(Continued)*

Ginkgo Biloba

Synonyms: Kew Tree; Maidenhair Tree

Use: Treatment of tinnitus, visual disorders, traumatic brain injury, vertigo of vascular origin

Europe: Treatment of intermittent claudication, arterial insufficiency, and cerebral vascular disease (dementia)

Per Commission E: Demential syndromes including memory deficits, etc (tinnitus, headache); depressive emotional conditions, primary degenerative dementia, vascular dementia, or both

Mechanism of Action/Effect: Dilates blood vessels and inhibits platelet aggregation; leaf extract contain terpenoids and flavonoids which can allegedly inactivate oxygen-free radicals causing vasodilatation and antagonize effects of platelet activating factor (PAF); fruit pulp contains ginkolic acids which are allergens (seeds are not sensitizing)

Contraindications: Pregnancy, clotting disorders, hypersensitivity to ginkgo biloba preparations (per Commission E)

Warnings: Use with caution following recent surgery or trauma. Effects may require 1-2 months. Controlled studies have not demonstrated consistent efficacy in dementia.

Drug Interactions: Due to effects on PAF, use with caution in patients receiving anticoagulants or platelet inhibitors.

Adverse Reactions: Palpitations, bilateral subdural hematomas, dizziness, seizures (in children), restlessness, urticaria, cheilitis, nausea, diarrhea, vomiting, stomatitis, proctitis, stomach or intestinal upsets, hyphema

Rare (per Commission E): Headache, allergic skin reactions, stomach or GI upset

Onset of Effect: 1 hour

Peak Absorption: 2-3 hours

Duration of Action: 7 hours

Bioavailability: 70% to 100%

Half-life: Ginkgolide A: 4 hours; ginkgolide B: 10.6 hours; bilobalide: 3.2 hours

Dosing: ~40 mg 3 times/day with meals; 60-80 mg twice daily to 3 times/day (depending on indication); maximum dose: 360 mg/day

Cerebral ischemia: 120 mg/day in 2-3 divided doses (24% flavonoid-glycoside extract, 6% terpene glycosides); beneficial effects for cerebral ischemia in the elderly occur after 1 month of use

Ginseng, Panax

Synonyms: Asian Ginseng; *Panax ginseng*

Use: Adrenal tonic; immunosupportive; enhances physical/mental performance and energy levels; adjunct support for chemotherapy/radiation

Mechanism of Action/Effect: Ginsenosides are believed to act via hormone receptors in the hypothalamus, pituitary glands, and other tissues. Ginsenosides stimulate secretion of adrenocorticotropic hormone (ACTH), leading to production of increased release of adrenal hormones, including cortisol. Specific triterpenoid saponins (diols) are claimed to be mediate improvements in endurance and learning. These compounds are also believed to contribute to sedative and antihypertensive properties. A second group (triols) reportedly increase blood pressure and function as central nervous system stimulants. *Panax ginseng* is reported to have immunostimulating effects. *Panax ginseng* has been claimed to facilitate adaptation to stress caused by chemotherapy and radiation.

Contraindications: Renal failure, acute infection, active bleeding (may alter hemostasis), pregnancy and lactation

Adverse Reactions: Mastalgia, vaginal breakthrough bleeding **Note:** Prolonged use or high dosages may cause Ginseng Abuse Syndrome (diarrhea, hypertension, nervousness, dermatologic eruptions, insomnia) and/or palpitations and tachycardia in sensitive individuals

Warnings: Use with caution in individuals with hyper- or hypotension; those with a history of bleeding, hemostatic disorders, or drug-related hemostatic problems; those receiving MAO inhibitors or stimulants (eg, decongestants, caffeine). Discontinue use prior to dental or surgical procedures (generally at least 14 days before).

Drug Interactions: Antihypertensives, MAO inhibitors, central nervous stimulants (caffeine), sympathomimetics, and hormonal therapies; anticoagulant medications, including warfarin, aspirin, aspirin-containing products, NSAIDs, or antiplatelet agents (eg, ticlopidine, clopidogrel, dipyridamole).

Dosing: Oral: 100-600 mg/day in divided doses

Ginseng, Siberian

Synonyms: *Eleutherococcus senticosus;* Siberian Ginseng

Use: Believed to facilitate adaptation to stress and to act as an immune stimulant.; reported to enhance athletic performance and physical endurance, increase mental alertness and amount of quality work performed, and decrease sick days

Contraindication: Active bleeding; hemostasis may be affected

Warnings: Use with caution in individuals with hypertension or those receiving antihypertensive medications (may potentiate effects); individuals at risk of hypotension, elderly , or those who would not tolerate transient hyper- or hypotensive episodes (ie, cerebrovascular or cardiovascular disease); diabetics; those with a history of bleeding, hemostatic disorders, or drug-related hemostatic problems. Discontinue use prior to dental or surgical procedures (generally at least 14 days before). Extensive or prolonged use may heighten estrogenic activity (based on pharmacological activity).

Drug Interactions: Barbiturates, antihypertensives, insulin, oral hypoglycemics, digoxin, stimulants (including OTC); anticoagulants (eg, warfarin, aspirin, aspirin-containing products, NSAIDs) or antiplatelet agents (eg, ticlopidine, clopidogrel, dipyridamole)

Dosing: Oral: 100-200 mg twice daily

Glucosamine

Use: Treatment of osteoarthritis, rheumatoid arthritis, tendonitis, gout, bursitis

Mechanism of Action/Effect: An amino sugar, which is a key component in the synthesis of proteoglycans, a group of proteins found in cartilage which are negatively charged, and attract water so they can produce synovial fluid in the joints; the theory is that supplying the body with these precursors will replenish important synovial fluid, and lead to production of new cartilage. Glucosamine also appears to inhibit cartilage-destroying enzymes (eg, collagenase and phospholipase A2), thus stopping the degenerative processes of osteoarthritis. A third mechanism may be glucosamine's ability to prevent production of damaging superoxide radicals, which may lead to cartilage destruction.

Adverse Reactions: Flatulence, nausea

Warnings: Use caution in patients with diabetes; may cause insulin resistance

Drug Interactions: May increase effect of oral anticoagulants and alter response to insulin or oral hypoglycemics

Dosing: 500 mg 3-4 times/day (sulfate form)

Golden Seal

Synonyms: Eye Balm; Eye Root; *Hydrastis canadensis*; Indian Eye; Jaundice Root; Orange Root; Turmeric Root; Yellow Indian Paint; Yellow Root

Use: Treatment of hemorrhoids, postpartum hemorrhage, mucosal inflammation/gastritis (efficacy not established in clinical studies); produces GI and peripheral vascular activity; used in sterile eyewashes; used as a mouthwash and laxative

Mechanism of Action/Effect: Contains the alkaloids hydrastine (4%) and berberine (6%), which at higher doses can cause vasoconstriction, hypertension, and mucosal irritation. Berberine can produce hypotension.

Contraindications: Pregnancy and lactation

Warnings: Should not be used in patients with hypertension, glaucoma, diabetes, history of stroke, seizures, or heart disease.

Drug Interaction: May interfere with vitamin B absorption

Adverse Reactions: High doses: Stimulation/agitation, nausea, vomiting, diarrhea, mouth and throat irritation, extremity numbness, respiratory failure

Dosing:
Root: 0.5-1 g 3 times/day
Solid form: Usual dose: 5-10 grains

Green Tea

Synonym: *Camellia sinensis*

Use: Platelet-aggregation inhibitor; antioxidant with anticarcinogenic activity; supportive in cancer prevention and cardiovascular disease; may lower cholesterol

Mechanism of Action/Effect: Reportedly has antioxidant properties and protects against oxidative damage to cells and tissues. Demonstrated to increase HDL cholesterol, decrease LDL cholesterol, and decrease triglycerides. Green tea has also been reported to block the peroxidation of LDL, inhibit formation of thromboxane formation, and block platelet aggregation. Human studies have noted a correlation between consumption of green tea and improvement in prognosis in some forms of breast cancer.

Contraindications: Active bleeding (eg, peptic ulcer, intracerebral bleeding)

Warnings: Nondecaffeinated products should be used with caution in individuals with peptic ulcer disease or cardiovascular disease. Use with caution in individuals with a history of bleeding, hemostatic disorders, or drug-related hemostatic problems; those receiving anticoagulants (reported to antagonize the effects of warfarin) or antiplatelet agents (eg, ticlopidine, clopidogrel, dipyridamole). Discontinue use prior to dental or surgical procedures (generally at least 14 days before). Use with caution when taking other stimulants (caffeine, decongestants), unless a caffeine-free product is used. **Note:** Addition of milk to tea may significantly lower the antioxidant potential of this agent.

Drug Interactions: Anticoagulants (eg, warfarin, aspirin, aspirin-containing products, NSAIDs), antiplatelet agents (eg, ticlopidine, clopidogrel, dipyridamole), stimulants (including OTC decongestants)

Adverse Reactions: If product is not decaffeinated, caffeine may cause gastric irritation, decreased appetite, insomnia, tachycardia, palpitations, and nervousness in sensitive individuals.

Dosing: Oral: 250-500 mg/day

Hawthorn

Synonyms: *Crataegus laevigata; Crataegus monogyna; Crataegus oxyacantha; Crataegus pinnatifida*; English Hawthorn; Haw; Maybush; Whitethorn

Use: Sedative; treatment of cardiovascular abnormalities (eg, arrhythmia, angina), increased cardiac output, increased contractility of heart muscle

Mechanism of Action/Effect: Contains flavonoids, catechin, and epicatechin which may be cardioprotective and have vasodilatory properties; shown to dilate coronary vessels

Contraindications: Pregnancy and lactation

Drug Interactions: Antihypertensives (effect enhanced), ACE inhibitors, digoxin; effects with Viagra® are unknown

Adverse Reactions: Hypotension, bradycardia, hypertension, depression, fatigue, rash, nausea

Dosing: Daily dose of total flavonoids: 10 mg
Per Commission E: 160-900 mg native water-ethanol extract (ethanol 45% v/v or methanol 70% v/v, drug-extract ratio: 4-7:1, with defined flavonoid or procyanidin content), corresponding to 30-168.7 mg procyanidins, calculated as epicatechin, or 3.5-19.8 mg flavonoids, calculated as hyperoside in accordance with DAB 10 (German pharmacopoeia #10) in 2 or 3 individual doses; duration of administration: 6 weeks minimum

HERBAL AND NUTRITIONAL PRODUCTS *(Continued)*

Horse Chestnut

Synonym: *Aesculus hippocastanum*

Use: Treatment of varicose veins, hemorrhoids, other venous insufficiencies, deep venous thrombosis, lower extremity edema

Mechanism of Action/Effect: Reportedly functions as an anti-inflammatory, which may be related to quercetin's reported ability to inhibit cyclo-oxygenase and lipoxygenase, the enzymes which form inflammatory prostaglandins and leukotrienes; quercetin is also an inhibitor of phosphodiesterase, which has been correlated to cardiotonic, hypotensive, spasmolytic, antiplatelet, and sedative actions; inhibits platelet aggregation and supports collagen structures

Contraindications: Active bleeding (eg, peptic ulcer, intracranial bleeding)

Warnings: Use with caution in individuals with hepatic or renal impairment, a history of bleeding, hemostatic disorders, or drug-related hemostatic problems. Discontinue use prior to dental or surgical procedures (generally at least 14 days before).

Drug Interactions: Anticoagulants (eg, warfarin, aspirin, aspirin-containing products, NSAIDs) and antiplatelet agents (eg, ticlopidine, clopidogrel, dipyridamole)

Adverse Reaction: GI upset

Dosing:
Oral: 300 mg 1-2 times/day, standardized to 50 mg escin per dose
Topical: Apply 2% escin gel 1-2 times/day to affected area

Kava

Synonyms: Awa; Kew; *Piper methysticum*; Tonga; Kava kava

Use: Treatment of anxiety, stress, and restlessness (per Commission E); sleep inducement

Mechanism of Action/Effect: Contains alpha-pyrones in root extracts; may possess central dopaminergic antagonistic properties

Contraindications: Per Commission E: Pregnancy, endogenous depression

Warnings: Extended continuous intake can cause a temporary yellow discoloration of skin, hair, and nails. In this case, further application must be discontinued. In rare cases, allergic skin reactions occur. Also, accommodative disturbances (eg, enlargement of the pupils and disturbances of the oculomotor equilibrium) have been described.

Drug Interactions: Coma can occur from concomitant administration of alprazolam; may potentiate alcohol or CNS depressants, barbiturates, psychopharmacological agents

Adverse Reactions: Euphoria, depression, somnolence, skin discoloration (prolonged use), muscle weakness, eye disturbances, hepatotoxicity

Dosing: Per Commission E: Do not use for >3 months without medical advice. Herb and preparations equivalent to 60-120 mg kavalactones

Melaleuca Oil

Use: Dermal agent for burns; marketed as fungicidal, bactericidal

Mechanism of Action/Effect: Consists of plant terpenes, pinenes, and cineole, derived from the *Melaleuca alternifolia* tree, the colorless or pale yellow oil can cause CNS depression; may be bacteriostatic

Adverse Reactions: Allergic reactions or dermatitis (rare)

Dosing: Topical: Minimal toxic dose: Infant: <10 mL

Melatonin

Use: Treatment of sleep disorders (eg, jet lag, insomnia, neurologic problems, shift work), aging, cancer, immune system support

Mechanism of Action/Effect: Hormone responsible for regulating the body's circadian rhythm and sleep patterns; release is prompted by darkness and inhibited by light. Secretion appears to peak during childhood, and declines gradually through adolescence and adulthood. Melatonin receptors have been found in blood cells, the brain, gut, and ovaries; may also have a role in regulating cardiovascular and reproductive function through its antioxidant properties.

Contraindications: Immune disorders; pregnancy and lactation

Warnings: Avoid prolonged use. Persistent sleep difficulties may be a sign of medical illness.

Drug Interactions: Medications commonly used as sedatives or hypnotics, or those that induce sedation, drowsiness (eg, benzodiazepines, narcotics); CNS depressants (prescription, supplements such as 5-HTP); other herbs known to cause sedation include kava, valerian

Adverse Reactions: Reduced alertness, headache, irritability, increased fatigue, drowsiness, sedation

Dosing: Sleep disturbances: 0.3-5 mg/day

Red Yeast Rice

Synonym: *Monascus purpureus*

Use: Hypercholesterolemic agent; may lower triglycerides and LDL cholesterol and raise HDL cholesterol

Mechanism of Action/Effect: Eight compounds with HMG-CoA reductase inhibitory activity have been identified, including lovastatin and its active hydroxy acid metabolite.

Contraindications: Pregnancy, or if trying to become pregnant, and lactation (based on pharmacological activity); known hypersensitivity to rice or yeast; children and adults <20 years of age; hepatic disease, history of liver disease, or those who may be at risk of liver disease; serious infection, recent major surgery, other serious disease, or organ transplant individuals; any individual who consumes more than 1-2 alcohol-containing drinks per day

Warnings: Use with caution in individuals currently receiving other cholesterol-lowering medications. HMG-CoA reductase inhibitors have been associated with rare (less than 1% to 2% incidence) but serious adverse effects, including hepatic and skeletal muscle disorders (myopathy, rhabdomyolysis). The risk of these disorders may be increased by concomitant therapy with specific medications. Discontinue use at the first sign of hepatic dysfunction.

Drug Interactions: HMG-CoA reductase inhibitors, other cholesterol-lowering agents, anticoagulants, gemfibrozil, erythromycin, itraconazole, ketoconazole, cyclosporine, niacin, clofibrate, fenofibrate

Adverse Reaction: GI upset

Dosing: Oral: 1200 mg twice daily

SAMe

Synonym: S-Adenosylmethionine

Use: Treatment of depression

Mechanism of Action/Effect: Not defined; functions as a cofactor in many synthetic pathways

Contraindication: Active bleeding (eg, peptic ulcer, intracranial bleeding)

Warnings: Use caution when combining with other antidepressants, tryptophan, or 5-HTP. SAMe is not effective in the treatment of depressive symptoms associated with bipolar disorder.

Drug Interactions: May potentiate activity and/or toxicities of MAO inhibitors, tricyclic antidepressants, or SSRIs; may potentiate the antidepressant effects of 5-HTP, tryptophan, and St John's wort

Adverse Reactions: Dry mouth, nausea, restlessness

Dosing: Oral: 400-1600 mg/day

Sassafras Oil

Synonym: *Sassafras albidum*

Use: Mild counterirritant on the skin (ie, lice or insect bites)

Mechanism of Action/Effect: Contains safrole (up to 80%) which inhibits liver microsomal enzymes; its metabolite may cause hepatic tumors

Adverse Reactions: Primarily related to sassafras oil and safrole: Tachycardia, flushing, hypotension, sinus tachycardia, anxiety, hallucinations, vertigo, aphasia, contact dermatitis, vomiting, fatty changes of liver, hepatic necrosis, mydriasis, diaphoresis; little documentation of adverse effects due to ingestion of herbal tea

Absorption: Orally

Metabolism: Hepatic

Excretion: Renal primarily

Warnings: Considered unsafe by the FDA; should not be ingested (banned in food by FDA since 1960)

Dosing: Tea can contain as much as 200 mg (3 mg/kg) of safrole.
Toxic: 0.66 mg/kg (based on rodent studies); Lethal: ~5 mL

Saw Palmetto

Synonyms: Palmetto Scrub; *Sabal serrulata; Sabasilis serrulatae; Serenoa repens*

Use: Treatment of benign prostatic hyperplasia

Mechanism of Action/Effect: Liposterolic extract of the berries may inhibit the enzymes 5α-reductase, along with cyclo-oxygenase and 5-lipoxygenase, thus exhibiting antiandrogen and anti-inflammatory effects; does not reduce prostatic enlargement but may help increase urinary flow (not FDA approved)

Contraindications: Pregnancy and lactation

Adverse Reactions: Headache, gynecomastia, stomach problems (rare, per Commission E)

Absorption: Oral: Low

Dosing: Adults: Dried fruit: 0.5-1 g 3 times/day

Schisandra

Synonym: *Schizandra chinensis*

Use: Promoted as an adaptogen/health tonic; hepatic protection and detoxification; increased endurance, stamina, and work performance

Mechanism of Action/Effect: Stimulates hepatic glycogen synthesis, protein synthesis, and increases microsomal enzyme activity; functions as an antioxidant

Contraindication: Pregnancy (based on uterine stimulation in animal studies)

Drug Interactions: Cytochrome P450 enzyme induction may alter the metabolism of many drugs (calcium channel blockers noted to be decreased)

Dosing: Oral: 100 mg twice daily

Soy Isoflavones

Synonym: Isoflavones

Use: Treatment of decreased bone loss, hypercholesterolemia, menopausal symptoms

Mechanism of Action/Effect: Contains plant-derived estrogenic compounds, however, the estrogenic potency has been estimated to be only 1/1000 to 1/100,000 that of estradiol; reported to inhibit bone reabsorption in postmenopausal women and lower serum lipids, including LDL cholesterol and triglycerides, along with increases in HDL cholesterol

Contraindication: History of estrogenic tumors (endometrial or breast cancer)

Warnings: May alter response to hormonal therapy; use with caution in individuals with history of thromboembolism or stroke

Drug Interactions: Weak estrogenic effect; may interact with estrogen-containing medications (close monitoring is recommended)

Dosing: Oral: 500-1000 mg/day soy extract

HERBAL AND NUTRITIONAL PRODUCTS *(Continued)*

St John's Wort

Synonyms: Amber Touch-and-Feel; Goatweed; *Hypercium perforatum*; Klamath Weed; Rosin Rose

Use: Treatment of mild-moderate depression, stress, anxiety, insomnia, vitiligo (topical); popular drug for AIDS patients due to possible antiretroviral activity; topically for wound healing

Per Commission E: Psychovegetative disorders, depressive moods, anxiety and/or nervous unrest; oily preparations for dyspeptic complaints; oily preparations externally for treatment of post-therapy of acute and contused injuries, myalgia, first degree burns

Mechanism of Action/Effect: Active ingredients are xanthones, flavonoids (hypericin) which can act as monoamine oxidase inhibitors, although *in vitro* activity is minimal; majority of activity appears to be related to GABA modulation; may be related to dopamine, serotonin, norepinephrine modulation also

Contraindications: Endogenous depression, pregnancy, children <2 years of age; concurrent use of indinavir or therapeutic immunosuppressants (cyclosporine)

Warnings: May be photosensitizing; use caution with tyramine-containing foods; appears to induce hepatic cytochrome P450 3A3/4 enzymes, potentially reducing effect of many medications.

Drug Interactions: Avoid amphetamines or other stimulants and concurrent use with SSRI or other antidepressants. Use caution with MAO inhibitors, levodopa, 5-hydroxytryptophan, and drugs metabolized by CYP3A3/4. Treatment failure with HIV medications and immunosuppressants has been associated with use.

Adverse Reactions: Sinus tachycardia, photosensitization (especially in fair-skinned person, per Commission E), stomach pains, abdominal pain

Dosing: Based on hypericin extract content: Oral: 300 mg 3 times/day

Valerian

Synonyms: Radix; Red Valerian; *Valeriana edulis*; *Valeriana wallichi*

Use: Sleep-promoting agent and minor tranquilizer; treatment of anxiety, panic attacks, intestinal cramps, headache

Per Commission E: Restlessness, sleep disorders based on nervous conditions

Mechanism of Action/Effect: May affect neurotransmitter levels (serotonin, GABA, and norepinephrine); also has antispasmodic properties

Drug Interactions: Not synergistic with alcohol; potentiation of other CNS depressants is possible

Adverse Reactions: Cardiac disturbances (unspecified), lightheadedness, restlessness, fatigue, nausea, tremor, blurred vision

Dosing:

Sedative: 1-3 g (1-3 mL of tincture)

Sleep aid: 1-3 mL of tincture at bedtime

Dried root: 0.3-1 g

Vanadium

Use: Treatment of type 1 and type 2 diabetes

Mechanism of Action/Effect: Reported to be a cofactor in nicotinamide adenine dinucleotide phosphate (NADPH) oxidation reactions, lipoprotein lipase activity, amino acid transport, and hematopoiesis; may improve/augment glucose regulation

Warning: Use with caution in diabetics or in those predisposed to hypoglycemia; may alter glucose regulation. Effects of drugs with hypoglycemic activity may be potentiated (including insulin and oral hypoglycemics). Closely monitor blood sugar, dosage of these agents (including insulin) may require adjustment. This should be carefully coordinated among the individual's healthcare providers.

Drug Interactions: Oral hypoglycemics or insulin

Adverse Reactions: No dietary toxicity or serious side effects reported, however industrial exposure has resulted in toxicity.

Dosing: Oral: RDI: 250 mcg 1-3 times/day

HERBS AND COMMON NATURAL AGENTS

The authors have chosen to include this list of natural products and proposed medical claims. However, due to limited scientific investigation to support these claims, this list is not intended to imply that these claims have been scientifically proven.

Proposed Medicinal Claims

Herb	Medicinal Claim
Agrimony	Digestive disorders
Alfalfa	Source of carotene (vitamin A); contains natural fluoride
Allspice	General health
Aloe	Healing agent
Anise (seed)	Prevent gas
Astragalus	Enhance energy reserves; immune system modulation; adaptogen
Barberry (bark)	Treat halitosis
Bayberry (bark)	Relieve and prevent varicose veins
Bay (leaf)	Relieves cramps
Bee pollen	Renewal of enzymes, hormones, vitamins, amino acids, and others
Bergamot	Calming effect
Bilberry (leaf)	Increases night vision; reduces eye fatigue; antioxidant; circulation
Birch (bark)	Treat urinary problems; used for rheumatism
Blackberry (leaf)	Treat diarrhea
Black cohosh	Relieves menstrual cramps; phytoestrogen
Blueberry (leaf)	Diarrhea
Blue cohosh	Regulate menstrual flow
Blue flag	Treatment of skin diseases and constipation
Boldo (leaf)	Stimulates digestion; treatment of gallstones
Boneset	Treatment of colds and flu
Bromelain	Digestive enzyme
Buchu (leaf)	Diuretic
Buckthorn (bark)	Expels worms; laxative
Burdock (leaf and root)	Treatment of severe skin problems; cases of arthritis
Butternut (bark)	Works well for constipation
Calendula (flower)	Mending and healing of cuts or wounds topically
Capsicum (cayenne)	Normalizes blood pressure; circulation
Caraway (seed)	Aids digestion
Cascara sagrada (bark)	Remedies for chronic constipation
Catnip	Calming effect in children
Celery (leaf and seed)	Blood pressure; diuretic
Centaury	Stimulates the salivary gland
Chamomile (flower)	Excellent for a nervous stomach; relieves cramping associated with the menstrual cycle
Chickweed	Rich in vitamin C and minerals (calcium, magnesium, and potassium); diuretic; thyroid stimulant
Chicory (root)	Effective in disorders of the kidneys, liver, and urinary canal
Cinnamon (bark)	Prevents infection and indigestion; helps break down fats during digestion
Cleavers	Treatment of kidney and bladder disorders; useful in obstructions of the urinary organ
Cloves	General medicinal
Coriander (seed)	Stomach tonic
Cornsilk	Diuretic
Cranberry	Urinary tract health
Cubeb (berry)	Chronic bladder trouble; increases flow of urine
Damiana (leaf)	Sexual impotency
Dandelion (leaf)	Diuretic
Dandelion (root)	Detoxify poisons in the liver; beneficial in lowering blood pressure
Dill weed	Digestive health

HERBAL AND NUTRITIONAL PRODUCTS *(Continued)*

Proposed Medicinal Claims *(continued)*

Herb	Medicinal Claim
Dong quai (root)	Female troubles; menopause and PMS symptoms; anemia; blood pressure
Echinacea (root)	Treat strep throat, lymph glands; immune modulating
Eucalyptus (leaf)	Mucolytic
Elder	Antiviral
Elecampane (root)	Cough with mucus
Eyebright	Eyesight
Fennel (seed)	Remedies for gas and acid stomach
Fenugreek (seed)	Allergies, coughs, digestion, emphysema, headaches, migraines, intestinal inflammation, ulcers, lungs, mucous membranes, and sore throat
Feverfew	Migraines; helps reduce inflammation in arthritis joints
Garlic (bulb)	Lowers blood cholesterol; anti-infective
Gentian	Digestive health
Ginger (root)	Antiemetic
Ginkgo biloba	Improves blood circulation to the brain; asthma; vertigo; tinnitus; impotence
Ginseng, Siberian (root)	Resistance against stress; slows the aging process; adaptogen
Goldenseal	Treatment of bladder infections, cankers, mouth sores, mucous membranes, and ulcers
Gota kola	"Memory herb"; nerve tonic; wound healing
Gravelroot (queen of the meadow)	Remedy for stones in the kidney and bladder
Green barley	Antioxidant
Hawthorn	Antioxidant; cardiotonic
Henna	External use only
Hibiscus (flower)	Diuretic
Hops (flower)	Insomnia; used to decrease the desire for alcohol
Horehound	Acute or chronic sore throat and coughs
Horsetail (shavegrass)	Rich in minerals, especially silica; used to develop strong fingernails and hair, good for split ends; diuretic
Ho shou wu	Rejuvenator
Hydrangea (root)	Backaches
Juniper (berry)	Diuretic
Kava (root)	Calm nervousness; anxiety; pain
Kelp	High contents of natural plant iodine, for proper function of the thyroid; high levels of natural calcium, potassium, and magnesium
Lavender (oil)	Wound healing; decrease scarring (topical)
Lecithin	Break up cholesterol; prevent arteriosclerosis
Licorice (root)	Expectorant; used in peptic ulceration; adrenal exhaustion
Malva (flower)	Soothes inflammation in the mouth and throat; helpful for earaches
Marjoram	Beneficial for a sour stomach or loss of appetite
Marshmallow (leaf)	Demulcent
Milk thistle	Liver detoxifier; antioxidant
Motherwort	Nervousness
Mugwort	Used for rheumatism and gout
Mullein (leaf)	High in iron, magnesium, and potassium; sinuses; relieves swollen joints; soothing bronchial tissue
Mustard (seed)	General medicinal
Myrrh (gum)	Removes bad breath; sinus problems
Nettle (leaf)	Remedy for dandruff; antihistaminic qualities
Nettle (root)	Used in benign prostatic hyperplasia (BPH)
Nutmeg	Gas
Oregano (leaf)	Settles the stomach after meals; helps treat colds
Oregon grape (root)	Gallbladder problems
Papaya (leaf)	Digestive stimulant; contains the enzyme papain

Proposed Medicinal Claims *(continued)*

Herb	Medicinal Claim
Paprika (sweet)	Stimulates the appetite and gastric secretions
Passion (flower)	Mild sedative
Pau d'arco	Protects immune system; antifungal
Peppermint (leaf)	Excellent for headaches; digestive stimulation
Pleurisy (root)	Mucolytic
Poppy seed blue	Excellent in the making of breads and desserts
Prickly ash (bark)	Increases circulation
Psyllium (seed)	Lubricant to the intestinal tract
Red clover	Phytoestrogenic properties
Red raspberry (leaf)	Decreases menstrual bleeding
Rhubarb (root)	Powerful laxative
Rose hips	High content of vitamin C
Saw palmetto (berry)	Used in benign prostatic hyperplasia (BPH)
Scullcap	Nerve sedative
Seawrack (bladderwrack)	Combat obesity; contains iodine
Senna (leaf)	Laxative
Shepherd's purse	Female reproductive health
Sheep sorrel	Diuretic
Slippery elm (bark)	Normalize bowel movement; beneficial for hemorrhoids and constipation
Solomon's seal (root)	Poultice for bruises
Spikenard	Skin ailments such as acne, pimples, blackheads, rashes, and general skin problems
Star anise	Promotes appetite and relieves flatulence
St John's wort	Mild to moderate depression
Summer savory (leaf)	Treats diarrhea, upset stomach, and sore throat
Thyme (leaf)	Ulcers (peptic)
Uva-ursi (leaf)	Diuretic; used in urinary tract health
Valerian (root)	Promotes sleep
Vervain	Remedy for fevers
White oak (bark)	Strong astringent
White willow (bark)	Used for minor aches and pains in the body; aspirin content
Wild alum (root)	Powerful astringent; used as rinse for sores in mouth and bleeding gums
Wild cherry	Cough suppressant
Wild Oregon grape (root)	Chronic skin disease
Wild yam (root)	Used in female reproductive health
Wintergreen (leaf)	Valuable for colic and gas in the bowels
Witch hazel (bark and leaf)	Hemorrhoids
Wormwood	Antiparasitic
Yarrow (root)	Fevers
Yellow dock (root)	Good in all skin problems
Yerba santa	Bronchial congestion
Yohimbe	Natural aphrodisiac
Yucca (root)	Reduces inflammation of the joints

HERBAL AND NUTRITIONAL PRODUCTS *(Continued)*

HERB-DRUG INTERACTIONS / CAUTIONS

Herb	Drug Interaction / Caution
Acidophilus / bifidobacterium	Antibiotics (oral)
Activated charcoal	Vitamins or oral medications may be adsorbed
Alfalfa	Do not use with lupus due to amino acid L-canavanine; causes pancytopenia at high doses; warfarin (alfalfa contains a large amount of vitamin K)
Aloe vera	Caution in pregnancy, may cause uterine contractions; digoxin, diuretics (hypokalemia)
Ashwagandha	May cause sedation and other CNS effects
Asparagus root	Causes diuresis
Barberry	Normal metabolism of vitamin B may be altered with high doses
Birch	If taking a diuretic, drink plenty of fluids
Black cohosh	Estrogen-like component; pregnant and nursing women should probably avoid this herb; also women with estrogen-dependent cancer and women who are taking birth control pills or estrogen supplements after menopause; caution also in people taking sedatives or blood pressure medications
Black haw	Do not give to children <6 years of age (salicin content) with flu or chickenpox due to potential Reye's syndrome; do not take if allergic to aspirin
Black pepper (*Piper nigrum*)	Antiasthmatic drugs (decreases metabolism)
Black tea	May inhibit body's utilization of thiamine
Blessed thistle	Do not use with gastritis, ulcers, or hyperacidity since herb stimulates gastric juices
Blood root	Large doses can cause nausea, vomiting, CNS sedation, low BP, shock, coma, and death
Broom (*Cytisus scoparius*)	MAO inhibitors lead to sudden blood pressure changes
Bugleweed (*Lycopus virginicus*)	May interfere with nuclear imaging studies of the thyroid gland (thyroid uptake scan)
Cat's claw (*Uncaria tomentosa*)	Avoid in organ transplant patients or patients on ulcer medications, antiplatelet drugs, NSAIDs, anticoagulants, immunosuppressive therapy, intravenous immunoglobulin therapy
Chaste tree berry (*Vitex agnus-castus*)	Interferes with actions of oral contraceptives, HRT, and other endocrine therapies; may interfere with metabolism of dopamine-receptor antagonists
Chicory (*Cichorium intybus*)	Avoid with gallstones due to bile-stimulating properties
Chlorella (*Chlorella vulgaris*)	Contains significant amounts of vitamin K
Chromium picolinate	Picolinic acid causes notable changes in brain chemicals (serotonin, dopamine, norepinephrine); do not use if patient has behavioral disorders or diabetes
Cinnabar root (*Salviae miltiorrhizae*)	Warfarin (increases INR)
Deadly nightshade (*Atropa belladonna*)	Contains atropine
Dong quai	Warfarin (increases INR), estrogens, oral contraceptives, photosensitizing drugs, histamine replacement therapy, anticoagulants, antiplatelet drugs, antihypertensives
Echinacea	Caution with other immunosuppressive therapies; stimulates TNF and interferons
Evening primrose oil	May lower seizure threshold; do not combine with anticonvulsants or phenothiazines
Fennel	Do not use in women who have had breast cancer or who have been told not to take birth control pills
Fenugreek	Practice moderation in patients on diabetes drugs, MAO inhibitors, cardiovascular agents, hormonal medicines, or warfarin due to the many components of fenugreek
Feverfew	Antiplatelets, anticoagulants, NSAIDs
Forskolin, coleonol	This herb lowers blood pressure (vasodilator) and is a bronchodilator and increases the contractility of the heart, inhibits platelet aggregation, and increases gastric acid secretion
Foxglove	Digitalis-containing herb
Garlic	Blood sugar-lowering medications, warfarin, and aspirin at medicinal doses of garlic

Herb	Drug Interaction / Caution
Ginger	May inhibit platelet aggregation by inhibiting thromboxane synthetase at large doses; *in vitro* and animal studies indicate that ginger may interfere with diabetics; has anticoagulant effect, so avoid in medicinal amounts in patients on warfarin or heart medicines
Ginkgo biloba	Warfarin (ginkgo decreases blood clotting rate); NSAIDs, MAO inhibitors
Ginseng	Blood sugar-lowering medications (additive effects) and other stimulants
Ginseng (American, Korean)	Furosemide (decreases efficacy)
Ginseng (Siberian)	Digoxin (increases digoxin level)
Glucomannan	Diabetics (herb delays absorption of glucose from intestines, decreasing mean fasting sugar levels)
Goldenrod	Diuretics (additive properties)
Gymnema	Blood sugar-lowering medications (additive effects)
Hawthorn	Digoxin or other heart medications (herb dilates coronary vessels and other blood vessels, also inotropic)
Hibiscus	Chloroquine (reduced effectiveness of chloroquine)
Hops	Those with estrogen-dependent breast cancer should not take hops (contains estrogen-like chemicals); patients with depression (accentuate symptoms); alcohol or sedative (additive effects)
Horehound	May cause arrhythmias at high doses
Horseradish	In medicinal amounts with thyroid medications
Kava	CNS depressants (additive effects, eg, alcohol, barbiturates, etc); benzodiazepines
Kelp	Thyroid medications (additive effects or opposite effects by negative feedback); kelp contains a high amount of sodium
Labrador tea	Plant has narcotic properties, possible additive effects with other CNS depressants
Lemon balm	Do not use with Graves disease since it inhibits certain thyroid hormones
Licorice	Acts as a corticosteroid at high doses (about 1.5 lbs candy in 9 days) which can lead to hypertension, edema, hypernatremia, and hypokalemia (pseudoaldosteronism); do not use in persons with hypertension, glaucoma, diabetes, kidney or liver disease, or those on hormonal therapy; may interact with digitalis (due to hypokalemia)
Lobelia	Contains lobeline which has nicotinic activity; may mask withdrawal symptoms from nicotine; it can act as a polarizing neuromuscular blocker
Lovage	Is a diuretic
Ma huang	MAO inhibitors, digoxin, beta-blockers, methyldopa, caffeine, theophylline, decongestants (increases toxicity)
Marshmallow	May delay absorption of other drugs taken at the same time; may interfere with treatments of lowering blood sugar
Meadowsweet	Contains salicylates
Melatonin	Acts as contraceptive at high doses; antidepressants (decreases efficacy)
Mistletoe	May interfere with medications for blood pressure, depression, and heart disease
L-phenylalanine	MAO inhibitors
Pleurisy root	Digoxin (plant contains cardiac glycosides); also contains estrogen-like compounds; may alter amine concentrations in the brain and interact with antidepressants
Prickly ash (Northern)	Contains coumarin-like compounds
Prickly ash (Southern)	Contains neuromuscular blockers
Psyllium	Digoxin (decreases absorption)
Quassia	High doses may complicate heart or blood-thinning treatments (quassia may be inotropic)
Red clover	May have estrogen-like actions; avoid when taking birth control pills, HRT, people with heart disease or at risk for blood clots, patients who suffer from estrogen-dependent cancer; do not take with warfarin
Red pepper	May increase liver metabolism of other medications and may interfere with high blood pressure medications or MAO inhibitors
Rhubarb, Chinese	Do not use with digoxin (enhanced effects)

HERBAL AND NUTRITIONAL PRODUCTS *(Continued)*

Herb	Drug Interaction / Caution
St John's wort	Indinavir, cyclosporine, SSRIs or any antidepressants, tetracycline (increases sun sensitivity); digoxin (decreases digoxin concentration); may also interact with diltiazem, nicardipine, verapamil, etoposide, paclitaxel, vinblastine, vincristine, glucocorticoids, cyclosporine, dextromethorphan, ephedrine, lithium, meperidine, pseudoephedrine, selegiline, yohimbine, ACE inhibitors (serotonin syndrome, hypertension, possible exacerbation of allergic reaction)
Saw palmetto	Acts an antiandrogen; do not take with prostate medicines or HRT
Squill	Digoxin or persons with potassium deficiency; also not with quinidine, calcium, laxatives, saluretics, prednisone (long-term)
Tonka bean	Contains coumarin, interacts with warfarin
Vervain	Avoid large amounts of herb with blood pressure medications or HRT
Wild Oregon grape	High doses may alter metabolism of vitamin B
Wild yam	May interfere with hormone precursors
Wintergreen	Warfarin, increased bleeding
Sweet woodruff	Contains coumarin
Yarrow	Interferes with anticoagulants and blood pressure medications
Yohimbe	Do not consume tyramine-rich foods; do not take with nasal decongestants, PPA-containing diet aids, antidepressants, or mood-altering drugs

Herbs Contraindicated During Lactation
According to German Commission E

Aloe
(*Aloe vera*)

Basil
(*Ocimum basillicum*)

Buckthorn (bark and berry)
(*Rhamnus frangula, R. cathartica*)

Cascara sagrada
(*Rhamnus purshiana*)

Coltsfoot (leaf)
(*Tussilago farfara*)

Combination of senna, peppermint oil, and
caraway oil

Kava (root)
(*Piper methysticum*)

Petasite (root)
(*Petasites* spp)

Indian snakeroot (*Rauwolfia serpentina*)

Rhubarb (root)
(*Rheum palmatum*)

Senna
(*Cassia senna*)

Herbs Contraindicated During Pregnancy
According to German Commission E

Aloe
(*Aloe vera*)

Autumn crocus
(*Colchicum autumnale*)

Black cohosh (root)
(*Cimicifuga racemosa*)

Buckthorn (bark and berry)
(*Rhamnus frangula, R. cathartica*)

Cascara sagrada (bark)
(*Rhamnus purshiana*)

Chaste tree (fruit)
(*Vitex agnus-castus*)

Cinchona (bark)
(*Cinchona* spp)

Cinnamon (bark)
(*Cinnamomum zeylanicum*)

Coltsfoot (leaf)
(*Tussliago farfara*)

Echinacea purpurea
(*Echinacea purpurea*)

Fennel (oil)
(*Foeniculum vulgare*)

Combination of licorice, peppermint, and chamomile

Combination of licorice, primrose, marshmallow, and
anise

Combination of senna, peppermint oil, and
caraway oil

Ginger (root)[1]
(*Zingiber officinale*)

Indian snakeroot
(*Rauwolfia serpentina*)

Juniper (berry)
(*Juniperus comunis*)

Kava (root)
(*Piper methysticum*)

Licorice (root)
(*Glycyrrhiza glabra*)

Marsh tea
(*Ledum palustre*)

Mayapple (root)
(*Podophyllum peltatum*)

Petasite (root)
(*Petasites* spp)

Rhubarb (root)
(*Rheum palmatum*)

Sage (leaf)
(*Salvia officinalis*)

Senna
(*Cassia senna*)

[1]A subsequent review of the clinical literature could find no basis for the contraindication of ginger, a common spice, during pregnancy (Fulder and Tenne, 1996).

IMMUNIZATION RECOMMENDATIONS

Recommended Childhood and Adolescent Immunization Schedule, by Vaccine and Age – United States, 2006

Vaccine ▼ / Age ▶	Birth	1 mo	2 mo	4 mo	6 mo	12 mo	15 mo	18 mo	24 mo	4-6 y	11-12 y	13-14 y	15 y	16-18 y
Hepatitis B[1]	HepB	HepB		HepB[1]		HepB					HepB series			
Diphtheria, tetanus, pertussis[2]			DTaP	DTaP	DTaP		DTaP			DTaP	Tdap	Tdap		
Haemophilus influenzae type b[3]			Hib	Hib	Hib[3]	Hib								
Inactivated poliovirus[4]			IPV	IPV		IPV				IPV				
Measles, mumps, rubella[4]						MMR				MMR	MMR			
Varicella[5]						Varicella					Varicella			
Meningococcal[6]							Vaccines with broken line are for selected populations				MCV4	MCV4		
											MPSV4	MCV4		
Pneumococcal[7]			PCV	PCV	PCV	PCV				PCV	PCV	PPV		
Influenza[8]						Influenza (yearly)				Influenza (yearly)				
Hepatitis A[9]						HepA series				HepA series				

☐ Range of recommended ages   ▨ Catch-up immunization   ▦ Assessment at age 11-12 years

This schedule indicates the recommended ages for routine administration of currently licensed childhood vaccines, as of December 1, 2005, for children through age 18 years. Any dose not administered at the recommended age should be administered at any subsequent visit, when indicated and feasible. ▨ Indicates age groups that warrant special effort to administer those vaccines not previously administered. Additional vaccines might be licensed and recommended during the year. Licensed combination vaccines may be used whenever any components of the combination are indicated and other components of the vaccine are not contraindicated and if approved by the Food and Drug Administration for that dose of the series. Providers should consult respective Advisory Committee on Immunization Practices (ACIP) statements for detailed recommendations. Clinically significant adverse events that follow vaccination should be reported to the Vaccine Adverse Event Reporting System (VAERS). Guidance about how to obtain and complete a VAERS form is available at http://www.vaers.hhs.gov or by telephone, 800-822-7967.

1. **Hepatitis B vaccine (HepB).** *AT BIRTH:* All newborns should receive monovalent HepB soon after birth and before hospital discharge. Infants born to mothers who are hepatitis B surface antigen (HBsAg)-positive should receive HepB and 0.5 mL of hepatitis B immune globulin (HBIG) within 12 hours of birth. Infants born to mothers whose HBsAg status is unknown should receive HepB within 12 hours of birth. The mother should have blood drawn as soon as possible to determine her HBsAg status; if HBsAg-positive, the infant should receive HBIG as soon as possible (no later than age 1 week). For infants born to HBsAg-negative mothers, the birth dose can be delayed in rare circumstances but only if a physician's order to withhold the vaccine and a copy of the mother's original HBsAg-negative laboratory report are documented in the infant's medical record. *FOLLOWING THE BIRTH DOSE:* The HepB series should be completed with either monovalent HepB or a combination vaccine containing HepB. The second dose should be administered at age 1-2 months. The final dose should be administered at age ≥24 weeks. Administering four doses of HepB is permissible (eg, when combination vaccines are administered after the birth dose); however, if monovalent HepB is used, a dose at age 4 months is not needed. Infants born to HBsAg-positive mothers should be tested for HBsAg and antibody to HBsAg after completion of the HepB series at age 9-18 months (generally at the next well-child visit after completion of the vaccine series).

2. **Diphtheria, tetanus toxoids, and acellular pertussis vaccine (DTaP).** The fourth dose of DTaP may be administered as early as age 12 months, provided 6 months have elapsed since the third dose and the child is unlikely to return at age 15-18 months. The final dose in the series should be administered at age ≥4 years. Tetanus toxoid, reduced diphtheria toxoid, and acellular pertussis vaccine (Tdap adolescent preparation) is recommended at age 11-12 years for those who have completed the recommended childhood DTP/DTaP vaccination series and have not received a tetanus and diphtheria toxoids (Td) booster dose. Adolescents aged 13-18 years who missed the age 11-12 year Td/Tdap booster dose should also receive a single dose of Tdap if they have completed the recommended childhood DTP/DTaP vaccination series. Subsequent Td boosters are recommended every 10 years.

3. **Haemophilus influenzae type b conjugate vaccine (Hib).** Three Hib conjugate vaccines are licensed for infant use. If PRP-OMP (PedvaxHIB® or ComVax® [Merck]) is administered at ages 2 and 4 months, a dose at age 6 months is not required. DTaP/Hib combination products should not be used for primary immunization in infants at ages 2, 4, or 6 months, but may be used as boosters after any Hib vaccine. The final dose in the series should be administered at age ≥12 months.

4. **Measles, mumps, and rubella vaccine (MMR).** The second dose of MMR is recommended routinely at age 4-6 years but may be administered during any visit, provided at least 4 weeks have elapsed since the first dose and both doses are administered at or after age 12 months. Those who have not previously received the second dose should complete the schedule by age 11-12 years.

5. **Varicella vaccine.** Varicella vaccine is recommended at any visit at or after age 12 months for susceptible children (ie, those who lack a reliable history of varicella). Susceptible persons age ≥13 years should receive 2 doses, administered at least 4 weeks apart.

6. **Meningococcal vaccine (MCV4).** Meningococcal conjugate vaccine (MCV4) should be administered to all children at age 11-12 years as well as to unvaccinated adolescents at high school entry (age 15 years). Other adolescents who wish to decrease their risk for meningococcal disease may also be vaccinated. All college freshmen living in dormitories should also be vaccinated, preferably with MCV4, although meningococcal polysaccharide vaccine (MPSV4) is an acceptable alternative. Vaccination against invasive meningococcal disease is recommended for children and adolescents age ≥2 years with terminal complement deficiencies or anatomic or functional asplenia and for certain other high risk groups (see MMWR, 2005, 54(RR-7); use MPSV4 for children age 2-10 years and MCV4 for older children, although MPSV4 is an acceptable alternative.

7. **Pneumococcal vaccine.** The heptavalent pneumococcal conjugate vaccine (PCV) is recommended for all children age 2-23 months and for certain children age 24-59 months. The final dose in the series should be administered at age ≥12 months. Pneumococcal polysaccharide vaccine (PPV) is recommended in addition to PCV for certain high-risk groups. See MMWR, 2000, 49(RR-9):1-35.

8. **Influenza vaccine** is recommended annually for children age ≥6 months with certain risk factors (including, but not limited to, asthma, cardiac disease, sickle cell disease, HIV infection, diabetes, and conditions that can compromise respiratory function or handling of respiratory secretions or that can increase the risk for aspiration), healthcare workers, and other persons (including household members) in close contact with persons in groups at high risk (see MMWR, 2005, 54(RR-8). In addition, healthy children age 6-23 months and close contacts of healthy children age 0-5 months are recommended to receive influenza vaccine because children in this age group are at substantially increased risk for influenza-related hospitalizations. For healthy nonpregnant persons age 5-49 years, the intranasally administered, live, attenuated influenza vaccine (LAIV) is an acceptable alternative to the intramuscular trivalent inactivated influenza vaccine (TIV). See MMWR, 2005, 54(RR-8). Children receiving TIV should receive an age-appropriate dosage (0.25 mL for children age 6-35 months or 0.5 mL for children age ≥3 years). Children age ≤8 years who are receiving influenza vaccine for the first time should receive two doses (separated by at least 4 weeks for TIV and at least 6 weeks for LAIV).

9. **Hepatitis A vaccine (HepA).** Hepatitis A vaccine is recommended for all children at age 1 year (ie, 12-23 months). The two doses in the series should be administered at least 6 months apart. States, counties, and communities with existing HepA vaccination programs for children age 2-18 years are encouraged to maintain these programs. In these areas, new efforts focused on routine vaccination of children age 1 year should enhance, not replace, ongoing programs directed at a broader population of children. HepA is also recommended for certain high risk groups (see MMWR, 1999, 48(RR-12):1-37.

Approved by the Advisory Committee on Immunization Practices (http://www.cdc.gov/nip/acip), the American Academy of Pediatrics (http://www.aap.org), and the American Academy of Family Physicians (http://www.aafp.org). Additional information about vaccines, including precautions and contraindications for vaccination and vaccine shortages, is available in English and Spanish from the National Immunization Program at http://www.cdc.gov/nip or by telephone, 800-232-4646).

Reference:
"Recommended Childhood and Adolescent Immunization Schedule — United States, 2006," MMWR, 2005, 54(51 & 52):Q1-4.

CATCH-UP IMMUNIZATION SCHEDULE FOR CHILDREN AND ADOLESCENTS WHO START LATE OR WHO ARE ≥1 MONTH BEHIND, BY AGE GROUP, VACCINE, AND DOSAGE INTERVAL – UNITED STATES, 2006

Tables 1 and 2 provide catch-up schedules and minimum intervals between doses for children whose vaccinations have been delayed. A vaccine series does not need to be restarted, regardless of the time that has elapsed between doses. Use the chart appropriate for the child's age.

Table 1. Catch-up Schedule for Children Age 4 Months - 6 Years

Vaccine (Minimum Age for Dose 1)	Minimum Interval Between Doses			
	Dose 1 to Dose 2	Dose 2 to Dose 3	Dose 3 to Dose 4	Dose 4 to Dose 5
DTaP (6 wk)	4 weeks	4 weeks	6 months	6 months[1]
IPV (6 wk)	4 weeks	4 weeks	4 weeks[2]	
HepB[3] (birth)	4 weeks	8 weeks (and 16 weeks after 1st dose)		
MMR (12 mo)	4 weeks[4]			
Varicella (12 mo)				
Hib[5] (6 wk)	**4 weeks:** If 1st dose administered at age <12 months **8 weeks (as final dose):** If 1st dose administered at age 12-14 months **No further doses needed** if 1st dose administered at age ≥15 months	**4 weeks**[6]**:** If current age <12 months **8 weeks (as final dose)**[6]**:** If current age ≥12 months and 2nd dose administered at age <15 months **No further doses needed** if previous dose administered at age ≥15 months	**8 weeks (as final dose):** This dose only necessary for children age 12 months - 5 years who received 3 doses before age 12 months	
PCV[7] (6 wk)	**4 weeks:** If 1st dose administered at age <12 months and current age <24 months **8 weeks (as final dose):** If 1st dose administered at age ≥12 months or current age 24-59 months **No further doses needed** for healthy children if 1st dose administered at age ≥24 months	**4 weeks:** If current age <12 months **8 weeks (as final dose):** If current age ≥12 months **No further doses needed** for healthy children if previous dose administered at age ≥24 months	**8 weeks (as final dose):** This dose only necessary for children age 12 months - 5 years who received 3 doses before age 12 months	

Table 2. Catch-up Schedule for Children Age 7-18 Years

Vaccine	Minimum Interval Between Doses		
	Dose 1 to Dose 2	Dose 2 to Dose 3	Dose 3 to Booster Dose
Td[8]	4 weeks	6 months	**6 months:** If first dose administered at age <12 months and current age <11 years; otherwise **5 years**
IPV[9]	4 weeks	4 weeks	IPV[2,9]
HepB	4 weeks	8 weeks (and 16 weeks after first dose)	
MMR	4 weeks		
Varicella[10]	4 weeks		

IMMUNIZATION RECOMMENDATIONS *(Continued)*

Footnotes to Table 1 and Table 2

[1]DTaP (diphtheria, tetanus, pertussis): The fifth dose is not necessary if the fourth dose was administered after the fourth birthday.

[2]IPV (inactivated poliovirus): For children who received an all-IPV or all-oral poliovirus (OPV) series, a fourth dose is not necessary if third dose was administered at age ≥4 years. If both OPV and IPV were administered as part of a series, a total of four doses should be administered, regardless of the child's current age.

[3]HepB (hepatitis B): Administer the 3-dose series to all persons age <19 years if they were not previously vaccinated.

[4]MMR (measles, mumps, rubella): The second dose of MMR is recommended routinely at age 4-6 years, but may be administered earlier if desired.

[5]Hib *(Haemophilus influenzae* type b): Vaccine is not generally recommended for children age ≥5 years.

[6]Hib: If current age <12 months and the first two doses were PRP-OMP (PedvaxHIB® or ComVax® [Merck]), the third (and final) dose should be administered at age 12-15 months and at least 8 weeks after the second dose.

[7]PCV (pneumococcal conjugate vaccine): Vaccine is not generally recommended for children age ≥5 years.

[8]Td (tetanus, diphtheria): Tdap adolescent preparation may be substituted for any dose in a primary catch-up series or as a booster if age appropriate for Tdap. A 5-year interval from the last Td dose is encouraged when Tdap is used as a booster dose. See ACIP recommendations for additional information.

[9]IPV (inactivated poliovirus): Vaccine is not generally recommended for persons age ≥18 years.

[10]Varicella: Administer the 2-dose series to all susceptible adolescents age ≥13 years.

Reporting Adverse Reactions

Adverse reactions to vaccines should be reported through the Vaccine Adverse Event Reporting System (VAERS). Information on reporting reactions after vaccination is available at **http://www.vaers.hhs.gov** or by telephone, **800-822-7967**. Suspected cases of vaccine-preventable diseases should be reported to the state or local health department.

Additional information about vaccines, including precautions and contraindications for vaccination and vaccine shortages, is available in English and Spanish from the National Immunization Program at **http://www.cdc.gov/nip** or by telephone, **800-CDC-INFO (800-232-4636)**.

Recommended Adult Immunization Schedule, by Vaccine and Age Group
United States, October 2005 - September 2006

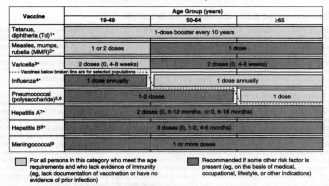

Vaccine	Age Group (years)		
	19-49	50-64	≥65
Tetanus, diphtheria (Td)[1]*	1-dose booster every 10 years		
Measles, mumps, rubella (MMR)[2]*	1 or 2 doses	1 dose	
Varicella[3]*	2 doses (0, 4-8 weeks)	2 doses (0, 4-8 weeks)	
	--- Vaccines below broken line are for selected populations ---		
Influenza[4]*	1 dose annually	1 dose annually	
Pneumococcal (polysaccharide)[5,6]	1-2 doses		1 dose
Hepatitis A[7]*	2 doses (0, 6-12 months, or 0, 6-18 months)		
Hepatitis B[8]*	3 doses (0, 1-2, 4-6 months)		
Meningococcal[9]	1 or more doses		

☐ For all persons in this category who meet the age requirements and who lack evidence of immunity (eg, lack documentation of vaccination or have no evidence of prior infection)

■ Recommended if some other risk factor is present (eg, on the basis of medical, occupational, lifestyle, or other indications)

*Covered by the Vaccine Injury Compensation Program.
Note: These recommendations must be read along with the footnotes, which can be found following this schedule.

Recommended Adult Immunization Schedule, by Vaccine and Medical and
Other Indications — United States, October 2005 - September 2006

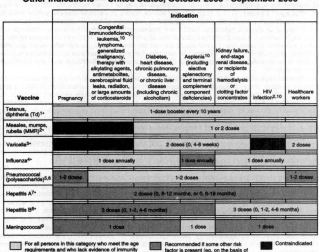

Vaccine	Pregnancy	Congenital immunodeficiency, leukemia,[10] lymphoma, generalized malignancy, therapy with alkylating agents, antimetabolites, cerebrospinal fluid leaks, radiation, or large amounts of corticosteroids	Diabetes, heart disease, chronic pulmonary disease, or chronic liver disease (including chronic alcoholism)	Asplenia[10] (including elective splenectomy and terminal complement component deficiencies)	Kidney failure, end-stage renal disease, or recipients of hemodialysis or clotting factor concentrates	HIV infection[2,10]	Healthcare workers
Tetanus, diphtheria (Td)[1]*	1-dose booster every 10 years						
Measles, mumps, rubella (MMR)[2]*			1 or 2 doses				
Varicella[3]*			2 doses (0, 4-8 weeks)				2 doses
Influenza[4]*	1 dose annually		1 dose annually		1 dose annually		
Pneumococcal (polysaccharide)[5,6]	1-2 doses		1-2 doses				1-2 doses
Hepatitis A[7]*	2 doses (0, 6-12 months, or 0, 6-18 months)						
Hepatitis B[8]*	3 doses (0, 1-2, 4-6 months)				3 doses (0, 1-2, 4-6 months)		
Meningococcal[9]	1 dose		1 dose		1 dose		

☐ For all persons in this category who meet the age requirements and who lack evidence of immunity (eg, lack documentation of vaccination or have no evidence of prior infection)

■ Recommended if some other risk factor is present (eg, on the basis of medical, occupational, lifestyle, or other indications)

■ Contraindicated

*Covered by the Vaccine Injury Compensation Program.
Note: These recommendations must be read along with the footnotes, which can be found following this schedule.

IMMUNIZATION RECOMMENDATIONS *(Continued)*

Footnotes to Recommended Adult Immunization Schedule

[1]**Tetanus and diphtheria (Td) vaccination.** Adults with uncertain histories of a complete primary vaccination series with diphtheria and tetanus toxoid-containing vaccines should receive a primary series using combined Td toxoid. A primary series for adults is 3 doses; administer the first 2 doses at least 4 weeks apart and the third dose 6-12 months after the second. Administer 1 dose if the person received the primary series and if the last vaccination was received ≥10 years previously. Consult the ACIP statement for recommendations for administering Td as prophylaxis in wound management (http://www.cdc.gov/mmwr/preview/mmwrhtml/00041645.htm). The American College of Physicians Task Force on Adult Immunization supports a second option for Td use in adults – a single Td booster at age 50 years for persons who have completed the full pediatric series, including the teenage/young adult booster. A newly licensed tetanus-diphtheria-acellular-pertussis vaccine is available for adults. ACIP recommendations for its use will be published.

[2]**Measles, mumps, rubella (MMR) vaccination.** *Measles component:* Adults born before 1957 can be considered immune to measles. Adults born during or after 1957 should receive ≥1 dose of MMR unless they have a medical contraindication, documentation of ≥1 dose, history of measles based on healthcare provider diagnosis, or laboratory evidence of immunity. A second dose of MMR is recommended for adults who 1) were recently exposed to measles or in an outbreak setting; 2) were previously vaccinated with killed measles vaccine; 3) were vaccinated with an unknown type of measles vaccine during 1963-1967; 4) are students in postsecondary educational institutions; 5) work in a healthcare facility; or 6) plan to travel internationally. Withhold MMR or other measles-containing vaccines from HIV-infected persons with severe immunosuppression. *Mumps component:* 1 dose of MMR vaccine should be adequate for protection for those born during or after 1957 who lack a history of mumps based on healthcare provider diagnosis or who lack laboratory evidence of immunity. *Rubella component:* Administer 1 dose of MMR vaccine to women whose rubella vaccination history is unreliable or who lack laboratory evidence of immunity. For women of childbearing age, regardless of birth year, routinely determine rubella immunity and counsel women regarding congenital rubella syndrome. Do not vaccinate women who are pregnant or who might become pregnant within 4 weeks of receiving vaccine. Women who do not have evidence of immunity should receive MMR vaccine upon completion or termination of pregnancy and before discharge from the healthcare facility.

[3]**Varicella vaccination.** Varicella vaccination is recommended for all adults without evidence of immunity to varicella. Special consideration should be given to those who 1) have close contact with persons at high risk for severe disease (healthcare workers and family contacts of immunocompromised persons) or 2) are at high risk for exposure or transmission (eg, teachers of young children; child care employees; residents and staff members of institutional settings, including correctional institutions; college students; military personnel; adolescents and adults living in households with children; nonpregnant women of childbearing age; and international travelers). Evidence of immunity to varicella in adults includes any of the following: 1) documented age-appropriate varicella vaccination (ie, receipt of 1 dose before age 13 years or receipt of 2 doses [administered at least 4 weeks apart] after age 13 years); 2) U.S.-born before 1966 or history of varicella disease before 1966 for non-U.S.-born persons; 3) history of varicella based on healthcare provider diagnosis or parental or self-report of typical varicella disease for persons born during 1966-1997 (for a patient reporting a history of an atypical, mild case, healthcare providers should seek either an epidemiologic link with a typical varicella case or evidence of laboratory confirmation, if it was performed at the time of acute disease); 4) history of herpes zoster based on healthcare provider diagnosis; or 5) laboratory evidence of immunity. Do not vaccinate women who are pregnant or who might become pregnant within 4 weeks of receiving the vaccine. Assess pregnant women for evidence of varicella immunity. Women who do not have evidence of immunity should receive dose 1 of varicella vaccine upon completion or termination of pregnancy and before discharge from the healthcare facility. Dose 2 should be administered 48 weeks after dose 1.

[4]**Influenza vaccination.** *Medical indications:* Chronic disorders of the cardiovascular or pulmonary systems, including asthma; chronic metabolic diseases, including diabetes mellitus, renal dysfunction, hemoglobinopathies, or immunosuppression (including immunosuppression caused by medications or HIV); any condition (eg, cognitive dysfunction, spinal cord injury, seizure disorder, or other neuromuscular disorder) that compromises respiratory function or the handling of respiratory secretions or that can increase the risk for aspiration; and pregnancy during the influenza season. No data exist on the risk for severe or complicated influenza disease among persons with asplenia; however, influenza is a risk factor for secondary bacterial infections that can cause severe disease among persons with asplenia. *Occupational indications:* Healthcare workers and employees of long-term-care and assisted living facilities. *Other indications:* Residents of nursing homes and other long-term-care and assisted living facilities; persons likely to transmit influenza to persons at high risk (ie, in-home household contacts and caregivers of children aged 0-23 months, or persons of all ages with high-risk conditions), and anyone who wishes to be vaccinated. For healthy, nonpregnant persons aged 5-49 years without high-risk conditions who are not contacts of severely immunocompromised persons in special care units, intranasally administered influenza vaccine (FluMist®) may be administered in lieu of inactivated vaccine.

[5]**Pneumococcal polysaccharide vaccination.** *Medical indications:* Chronic disorders of the pulmonary system (excluding asthma); cardiovascular diseases; diabetes mellitus; chronic liver diseases, including liver disease as a result of alcohol abuse (eg, cirrhosis); chronic renal failure or nephrotic syndrome; functional or anatomic asplenia (eg, sickle cell disease or splenectomy [if elective splenectomy is planned, vaccinate at least 2 weeks before surgery]); immunosuppressive conditions (eg, congenital immunodeficiency, HIV infection [vaccinate as close to diagnosis as possible when CD4 cell counts are highest], leukemia, lymphoma, multiple myeloma, Hodgkin disease, generalized malignancy, or organ or bone marrow transplantation); chemotherapy with alkylating agents, antimetabolites, or long-term systemic corticosteroids; and cochlear implants. *Other indications:* Alaska Natives and certain American Indian populations; residents of nursing homes and other long-term-care facilities.

[6]**Revaccination with pneumococcal polysaccharide vaccine.** One-time revaccination after 5 years for persons with chronic renal failure or nephritic syndrome; functional or anatomic asplenia (eg, sickle cell disease or splenectomy); immunosuppressive conditions (eg, congenital immunodeficiency, HIV infection, leukemia, lymphoma, multiple myeloma, Hodgkin disease, generalized malignancy, or organ or bone marrow transplantation); or chemotherapy with alkylating agents, antimetabolites, or long-term systemic corticosteroids. For persons aged ≥65 years, one-time revaccination if they were vaccinated ≥5 years previously and were aged <65 years at the time of primary vaccination.

[7]**Hepatitis A vaccination.** *Medical indications:* Persons with clotting-factor disorders or chronic liver disease. *Behavioral indications:* Men who have sex with men or users of illegal drugs. *Occupational indications:* Persons working with hepatitis A virus (HAV)-infected primates or with HAV in a research laboratory setting. *Other indications:* Persons traveling to or working in countries that have high or intermediate endemicity of hepatitis A (for list of countries, see http://www.cdc.gov/travel/diseases.htm#hepa) as well as any person wishing to obtain immunity. Current vaccines should be administered in a 2-dose series at either 0 and 6-12 months, or 0 and 6-18 months. If the combined hepatitis A and hepatitis B vaccine is used, administer 3 doses at 0, 1, and 6 months.

[8]**Hepatitis B vaccination.** *Medical indications:* Hemodialysis patients (use special formulation [40 µg/mL] or two 20 µg/mL doses) or patients who receive clotting-factor concentrates. *Occupational indications:* Healthcare workers and public-safety workers who have exposure to blood in the workplace and persons in training in schools of medicine, dentistry, nursing, laboratory technology, and other allied health professions. *Behavioral indications:* Injection-drug users; persons with more than one sex partner during the previous 6 months; persons with a recently acquired sexually transmitted disease (STD); and men who have sex with men. *Other indications:* Household contacts and sex partners of persons with chronic hepatitis B virus (HBV) infection; clients and staff members of institutions for developmentally disabled persons; all clients of STD clinics; inmates of correctional facilities; and international travelers who will be in countries with high or intermediate prevalence of chronic HBV infection for more than 6 months (for list of countries, see http://www.cdc.gov/travel/diseases.htm#hepa).

[9]**Meningococcal vaccination.** *Medical indications:* Adults with anatomic or functional asplenia or terminal complement component deficiencies. *Other indications:* First-year college students living in dormitories; microbiologists who are routinely exposed to isolates of *Neisseria meningitidis*; military recruits; and persons who travel to or reside in countries in which meningococcal disease is hyperendemic or epidemic (eg, the "meningitis belt" of sub-Saharan Africa during the dry season [December-June]), particularly if contact with local populations will be prolonged. Vaccination is required by the government of Saudi Arabia for all travelers to Mecca during the annual Hajj. Meningococcal conjugate vaccine is preferred for adults meeting any of the above indications who are aged ≤55 years, although meningococcal polysaccharide vaccine (MPSV4) is an acceptable alternative. Revaccination after 5 years might be indicated for adults previously vaccinated with MPSV4 who remain at high risk for infection (eg, persons residing in areas in which disease is epidemic).

[10]**Selected conditions for which *Haemophilus influenzae* type b (Hib) vaccine may be used.** Hib conjugate vaccines are licensed for children aged 6-71 months. No efficacy data are available on which to base a recommendation concerning use of Hib vaccine for older children and adults

with the chronic conditions associated with an increased risk for Hib disease. However, studies suggest good immunogenicity in patients who have sickle cell disease, leukemia, or HIV infection or who have had splenectomies; administering vaccine to these patients is not contraindicated.

Adapted from "Recommended Adult Immunization Schedule – United States, October 2005 - September 2006," *MMWR*, 2005, 54(40)Q1-4.

The Recommended Adult Immunization Schedule has been approved by the Advisory Committee on Immunization Practices (ACIP), the American College of Obstetricians and Gynecologists (ACOG), and the American Academy of Family Physicians (AAFP).

This schedule indicates the recommended age groups and medical indications for routine administration of currently licensed vaccines for persons ≥19 years of age. Licensed combination vaccines may be used whenever any components of the combination are indicated and when the vaccine's other components are not contraindicated. For detailed recommendations, consult manufacturers' package inserts and the complete statements from ACIP (http://www.cdc.gov/nip/publications/acip-list.htm).

Additional information about the vaccines listed above and contraindications for vaccination is also available at http://www.cdc.gov/nip or from the CDC-INFO Contact Center at 800-CDC-INFO (232-4636) in English or Spanish, 24 hours a day, 7 days a week.

IMMUNIZATION RECOMMENDATIONS *(Continued)*

RECOMMENDATIONS OF THE ADVISORY COMMITTEE ON IMMUNIZATION PRACTICES (ACIP)

Recommendations for Measles Immunization

Category	Recommendations
Unimmunized, no history of measles (12-15 mo)	A 2-dose schedule (with MMR) is recommended. The first dose is recommended at 12-15 mo; the second is recommended at 4-6 y.
Children 6-11 mo in epidemic situations	Immunize (with monovalent measles vaccine or, if not available, MMR); reimmunization (with MMR) at 12-15 mo is necessary, and a third dose is indicated at 4-6 y
Children 4-12 y who have received 1 dose of measles vaccine at ≥12 mo	Reimmunize (1 dose)
Students in college and other post-high school institutions who have received 1 dose of measles vaccine at ≥12 mo	Reimmunize (1 dose)
History of vaccination before the first birthday	Consider susceptible and immunize (2 doses)
History of receipt of inactivated measles vaccine or unknown type of vaccine, 1963-1967	Consider susceptible and immunize (2 doses)
Further attenuated or unknown vaccine given with IG	Consider susceptible and immunize (2 doses)
Allergy to eggs	Immunize; no reactions likely
Neomycin allergy, nonanaphylactic	Immunize; no reactions likely
Severe hypersensitivity (anaphylaxis) to neomycin or gelatin	Avoid immunization
Tuberculosis	Immunize; vaccine does not exacerbate infection
Measles exposure	Immunize and/or give IG, depending on circumstances
HIV-infected	Immunize (2 doses) unless severely immunocompromised
Personal or family history of seizures	Immunize; advise parents of slightly increased risk of seizures
Immunoglobulin or blood recipient	Immunize at the appropriate interval

MMR = measles-mumps-rubella vaccine; IG = immune globulin; HIV = human immunodeficiency virus.
Adapted from "Report of the Committee on Infectious Diseases," *2003 Red Book*®, 26th ed.

Immunization in HIV-Infected Persons

Vaccination of immunocompromised patients depends on the characteristics of the vaccine and the patient. Vaccines are typically divided into two broad categories: those which contain live virus/bacteria or those which are derived from a component of the organism (or an inactivated organism). Live virus or live bacterial vaccines have been associated with severe complications in immunocompromised patients, and should generally be avoided [(except in selected circumstances (noted below)]. Inactivated, recombinant, subunit, polysaccharide, and conjugate vaccines and toxoids can be administered to all immunocompromised patients. However, it should be recognized that the response to these vaccines may be suboptimal. If indicated, all inactivated vaccines are recommended in usual doses and according to prescribed schedules. Pneumococcal, meningococcal, and Hib vaccines are recommended only for specific subpopulations, including functional or anatomic asplenia.

Special consideration must be given to immunization with measles and/or varicella vaccines. Persons with HIV are at a higher risk for severe complications from measles infection. In patients without severe immunocompromise, measles vaccination in HIV-infected persons has not been reported to cause severe and/or unusual adverse events. MMR vaccination is recommended for all HIV-infected persons who do not have evidence of severe immunocompromise (defined as a low age-specific total CD4+ T-lymphocyte count or a low CD4+ T-lymphocyte count as a percentage of total lymphocytes).

Varicella and/or herpes zoster infections are also associated with an increased risk of severe complications in children with HIV infection. Asymptomatic or mildly symptomatic HIV-infected children receiving varicella vaccination have demonstrated adequate response to the vaccine without evidence of severe and/or unusual events. However, experience has been limited. Varicella vaccine should be considered for children who are classified as CDC class N1 or A1 with age-specific CD4+ T-lymphocyte percentages ≥25%.

HIV-infected persons who are receiving IVIG may not respond to MMR or varicella vaccines (or an individual component) due to the presence of a passively acquired antibody. Measles vaccine should be considered approximately 2 weeks before the next scheduled dose of IVIG (unless otherwise contraindicated). Unless serologic testing confirms the production of specific antibodies, the vaccination should be repeated at the recommended interval. In patients receiving maintenance IVIG therapy, an additional dose of IVIG should be considered if the exposure to measles occurs ≥3 weeks following a standard dose. Persons with cellular immunodeficiency should not receive varicella vaccine; however, persons with humoral immunodeficiency should be vaccinated (including persons with dysgammaglobulinemia or hypogammaglobulinemia).

Summarized/adapted from Atkinson WL, Pickering LK, Schwartz B, et al, "General Recommendations on Immunization. Recommendations of the Advisory Committee on Immunization Practices (ACIP) and the American Academy of Family Physicians (AAFP)," *MMWR Recomm Rep*, 2002, 51(RR-2):1-35.

Recommendations for Pneumococcal Conjugate Vaccine Use Among Healthy Children During Moderate and Severe Shortages

Age at First Vaccination (mo)	No Shortage[1]	Moderate Shortage	Severe Shortage
<6	2, 4, 6, and 12-15 months	2, 4, and 6 months (defer fourth dose)	2 doses at 2-month interval in first 6 months of life (defer third and fourth doses)
7-11	2 doses at 2-month interval; 12-15 month dose	2 doses at 2-month interval; 12-15-month dose	2 doses at 2-month interval (defer third dose)
12-23	2 doses at 2-month interval	2 doses at 2-month interval	1 dose (defer second dose)
>24	1 dose should be considered	No vaccination	No vaccination
Reduction in vaccine doses used[2]		21%	46%

[1]The vaccine schedule for no shortage is included as a reference. Providers should not use the no shortage schedule regardless of their vaccine supply until the national shortage is resolved.

[2]Assumes that approximately 85% of vaccine is administered to healthy infants beginning at age <7 months; approximately 5% is administered to high-risk infants beginning at age <7 months; and approximately 10% is administered to healthy children beginning at age 7-24 months. Actual vaccine savings will depend on a provider's vaccine use.

Adapted from the Advisory Committee on Immunization Practices, "Updated Recommendations on Use of Pneumococcal Conjugate Vaccine in a Setting of Vaccine Shortage," *MMWR Morb Mortal Wkly Rep*, 2001, 50(50):1140-2.

Recommended Regimens for Pneumococcal Conjugate Vaccine Among Children With a Late Start or Lapse in Vaccine Administration

Age at Examination (mo)	Previous Pneumococcal Conjugate Vaccination History	Recommended Regimen[1]
2-6	0 doses	3 doses 2 months apart, 4th dose at 12-15 months
	1 dose	2 doses 2 months apart, 4th dose at 12-15 months
	2 doses	1 dose, 4th dose at 12-15 months
7-11	0 doses	2 doses 2 months apart, 3rd dose at 12-15 months
	1 or 2 doses before age 7 months	1 dose at 7-11 months, with another dose at 12-15 months (≥2 months later)
12-23	0 doses	2 doses ≥2 months apart
	1 dose before age 12 months	2 doses ≥2 months apart
	1 dose at ≥12 months	1 dose ≥2 months after the most recent dose
	2 or 3 doses before age 12 months	1 dose ≥2 months after the most recent dose
24-59		
Healthy children[2]	Any incomplete schedule	Consider 1 dose ≥2 months after the most recent dose
High risk[3]	<3 doses	1 dose ≥2 months after the most recent dose and another dose ≥2 months later
	3 doses	1 dose ≥2 months after the most recent dose

[1]For children vaccinated at age <1 year, the minimum interval between doses is 4 weeks. Doses administered at ≥12 months should be at least 8 weeks apart.

[2]Providers should consider 1 dose for healthy children 24-59 months, with priority to children 24-35 months, American Indian/Alaska native and black children, and those who attend group child care centers.

[3]Children with sickle cell disease, asplenia, human immunodeficiency virus infection, chronic illness, cochlear implant, or immunocompromising condition.

Adapted from "CDC. Notice to Readers: Pneumococcal Conjugate Vaccine Shortage Resolved," *MMWR Morb Mortal Wkly Rep*, 2003, 52(19):446-7.

IMMUNIZATION RECOMMENDATIONS *(Continued)*

POSTEXPOSURE PROPHYLAXIS FOR HEPATITIS B[1]

Exposure	Hepatitis B Immune Globulin	Hepatitis B Vaccine
Perinatal	0.5 mL I.M. within 12 h of birth	0.5 mL[2] I.M. within 12 h of birth (no later than 7 d), and at 1 and 6 mo[3]; test for HB_sAg and anti-HB_s at 12-15 mo
Sexual	0.06 mL/kg I.M. within 14 d of sexual contact; a second dose should be given if the index patient remains HB_sAg-positive after 3 mo and hepatitis B vaccine was not given initially	1 mL I.M. at 0, 1, and 6 mo for homosexual and bisexual men and regular sexual contacts of persons with acute and chronic hepatitis B
Percutaneous; exposed person unvaccinated		
Source known HB_sAg-positive	0.06 mL/kg I.M. within 24 h	1 mL I.M. within 7 d, and at 1 and 6 mo[4]
Source known, HB_sAg status not known	Test source for HB_sAg; if source is positive, give exposed person 0.06 mL/kg I.M. once within 7 d	1 mL I.M. within 7 d, and at 1 and 6 mo[4]
Source not tested or unknown	Nothing required	1 mL I.M. within 7 d, and at 1 and 6 mo
Percutaneous; exposed person vaccinated		
Source known HB_sAg-positive	Test exposed person for anti-HB_s.[5] If titer is protective, nothing is required; if titer is not protective, give 0.06 mL/kg within 24 h.	Review vaccination status[6]
Source known, HB_sAg status not known	Test source for HB_sAg and exposed person for anti-HB_s. If source is HB_sAg-negative, or if source is HB_sAg-positive but anti-HB_s titer is protective, nothing is required. If source is HB_sAg-positive and anti-HB_s titer is not protective or if exposed person is a known nonresponder, give 0.06 mL/kg I.M. within 24 h. A second dose of hepatitis B immune globulin can be given 1 mo later if a booster dose of hepatitis B vaccine is not given.	Review vaccination status[6]
Source not tested or unknown	Test exposed person for anti-HB_s. If anti-HB_s titer is protective, nothing is required. If anti-HB_s titer is not protective, 0.06 mL/kg may be given along with a booster dose of hepatitis B vaccine.	Review vaccination status[6]

[1]HB_sAg = hepatitis B surface antigen; anti-HB_s = antibody to hepatitis B surface antigen; I.M. = intramuscularly; SRU = standard ratio units.
[2]Each 0.5 mL dose of plasma-derived hepatitis B vaccine contains 10 mcg of HB_sAg; each 0.5 mL dose of recombinant hepatitis B vaccine contains 5 mcg (Merck Sharp & Dohme) or 10 mcg (SmithKline Beecham) of HB_sAg.
[3]If hepatitis B immune globulin and hepatitis B vaccine are given simultaneously, they should be given at separate sites.
[4]If hepatitis B vaccine is not given, a second dose of hepatitis B immune globulin should be given 1 month later.
[5]Anti-HB_s titers <10 SRU by radioimmunoassay or negative by enzyme immunoassay indicate lack of protection. Testing the exposed person for anti-HB_s is not necessary if a protective level of antibody has been shown within the previous 24 months.
[6]If the exposed person has not completed a three-dose series of hepatitis B vaccine, the series should be completed. Test the exposed person for anti-HB_s. If the antibody level is protective, nothing is required. If an adequate antibody response in the past is shown on retesting to have declined to an inadequate level, a booster dose (1 mL) of hepatitis B vaccine should be given. If the exposed person has inadequate antibody or is a known nonresponder to vaccination, a booster dose can be given along with one dose of hepatitis B immune globulin.

PREVENTION OF HEPATITIS A THROUGH ACTIVE OR PASSIVE IMMUNIZATION: RECOMMENDATIONS OF THE ADVISORY COMMITTEE ON IMMUNIZATION PRACTICES (ACIP)

PROPHYLAXIS AGAINST HEPATITIS A VIRUS INFECTION

Recommended Doses of Immune Globulin (IG) for Hepatitis A Pre-exposure and Postexposure Prophylaxis[1]

Setting	Duration of Coverage	IG Dose[2]
Pre-exposure	Short-term (1-2 months)	0.02 mL/kg
	Long-term (3-5 months)	0.06 mL/kg[3]
Postexposure	—	0.02 mL/kg

[1]Infants and pregnant women should receive a preparation that does not include thimerosal.

[2]IG should be administered by intramuscular injection into either the deltoid or gluteal muscle. For children <24 months of age, IG can be administered in the anterolateral thigh muscle.

[3]Repeat every 5 months if continued exposure to HAV occurs.

Recommended Dosages of Havrix®[1]

Vaccinee's Age (y)	Dose (EL.U.)[2]	Volume (mL)	No. Doses	Schedule (mo)[3]
2-18	720	0.5	2	0, 6-12
>18	1440	1.0	2	0, 6-12

[1]Hepatitis A vaccine, inactivated, SmithKline Beecham Biologicals.

[2]Enzyme-linked immunosorbent assay (ELISA) units.

[3]0 months represents timing of the initial dose; subsequent numbers represent months after the initial dose.

Recommended Dosages of VAQTA®[1]

Vaccinee's Age (y)	Dose (units)	Volume (mL)	No. Doses	Schedule (mo)[2]
2-17	25	0.5	2	0, 6-18
>17	50	1.0	2	0, 6

[1]Hepatitis A vaccine, inactivated, Merck & Company, Inc.

[2]0 months represents timing of the initial dose; subsequent numbers represent months after the initial dose.

Adapted from "Prevention of Hepatitis A Through Active or Passive Immunization: Recommendations of the Advisory Committee on Immunization Practices (ACIP)," *MMWR Recomm Rep*, 1999, 48(RR-12):1-37.

IMMUNIZATION RECOMMENDATIONS *(Continued)*

RECOMMENDATIONS FOR TRAVELERS

Recommended Immunizations for Travelers to Developing Countries[1]

Immunizations	Length of Travel		
	Brief, <2 wk	Intermediate, 2 wk - 3 mo	Long-term Residential, >3 mo
Review and complete age-appropriate childhood schedule	+	+	+
• DTaP; poliovirus vaccine, and *H. influenzae* type b vaccine may be given at 4-wk intervals if necessary to complete the recommended schedule before departure			
• Measles: 2 additional doses given if younger than 12 mo of age at first dose			
• Varicella			
• Hepatitis B[2]			
Yellow fever[3]	+	+	+
Hepatitis A[4]	+	+	+
Typhoid fever[4]	±	+	+
Meningococcal disease[5]	±	±	+
Rabies[6]	±	+	+
Japanese encephalitis[3]	±	±	+

[1]+ = recommended; ± = consider.

[2]If insufficient time to complete 6-month primary series, accelerated series can be given.

[3]For endemic regions, see *Health Information for International Travel* in *Red Book*®. For high-risk activities in areas experiencing outbreaks, vaccine is recommended even for brief travel.

[4]Indicated for travelers who will consume food and liquids in areas of poor sanitation.

[5]For endemic regions of Africa, during local epidemics, and travel to Saudi Arabia for the Hajj.

[6]Indicated for person with high risk of animal exposure, and for travelers to endemic countries.

Adapted from "Report of the Committee on Infectious Diseases," *2003 Red Book*®, 26th ed, 94.

Recommendations for Pre-exposure Immunoprophylaxis of Hepatitis A Virus Infection for Travelers[1]

Age (y)	Likely Exposure (mo)	Recommended Prophylaxis
<2	<3	IG, 0.02 mL/kg[2]
	3-5	IG, 0.06 mL/kg[2]
	Long-term	IG, 0.06 mL/kg at departure and every 5 mo if exposure to HAV continues[2]
≥2	<3[3]	HAV vaccine[4,5] or IG, 0.02 mL/kg[2]
	3-5[3]	HAV vaccine[4,5] or IG, 0.06 mL/kg[2]
	Long-term	HAV vaccine[4,5]

[1]IG = immune globulin; HAV = hepatitis A virus.

[2]IG should be administered deep into a large muscle mass. Ordinarily, no more than 5 mL should be administered in one site in an adult or large child; lesser amounts (maximum 3 mL) should be given to small children and infants.

[3]Vaccine is preferable, but IG is an acceptable alternative.

[4]To ensure protection in travelers whose departure is imminent, IG also may be given.

[5]Dose and schedule of hepatitis A vaccine as recommended according to age.

Adapted from "Report of the Committee on Infectious Diseases," *2003 Red Book*®, 26th ed, 312.

Prevention of Malaria[1]

Drug	Adult Dosage	Pediatric Dosage
	Chloroquine-Sensitive Areas[2]	
Chloroquine phosphate[3,4]	500 mg (300 mg base), once/week[5]	5 mg/kg base once/week, up to adult dose of 300 mg base[5]
	Chloroquine-Resistant Areas[2]	
Mefloquine[4,6,7]	250 mg once/week[5]	<15 kg: 5 mg/kg[5]
		15-19 kg: ¼ tablet[5]
		20-30 kg: ½ tablet[5]
		31-45 kg: ¾ tablet[5]
		>45 kg: 1 tablet[5]
or		
Doxycycline[4,8]	100 mg/d[9]	2 mg/kg/d, up to 100 mg/d[9]
or		
Atovaquone/proguanil[4,10]	250 mg/100 mg (1 tablet) daily[11]	11-20 kg: 62.5 mg/25 mg[10,11]
		21-30 kg: 125 mg/50 mg[10,11]
		31-40 kg: 187.5 mg/75 mg[10,11]
		>40 kg: 250 mg/100 mg[10,11]
Alternative:		
Primaquine[8,12,13]	30 mg base daily	0.5 mg/kg base daily
Chloroquine phosphate[3]	500 mg (300 mg base) once/week[5]	5 mg/kg base once/week, up to adult dose of 300 mg base[5]
plus		
Proguanil[14]	200 mg once/day	<2 y: 50 mg once/day
		2-6 y: 100 mg once/day
		7-10 y: 150 mg once/day
		>10 y: 200 mg once/day

[1]No drug regimen guarantees protection against malaria. If fever develops within a year (particularly within the first 2 months) after travel to malarious areas, travelers should be advised to seek medical attention. Insect repellents, insecticide-impregnated bed nets, and proper clothing are important adjuncts for malaria prophylaxis.

[2]Chloroquine-resistant *P. falciparum* occurs in all malarious areas except Central America west of the Panama Canal Zone, Mexico, Haiti, the Dominican Republic, and most of the Middle East (chloroquine resistance has been reported in Yemen, Oman, Saudi Arabia, and Iran).

[3]In pregnancy, chloroquine prophylaxis has been used extensively and safely.

[4]For prevention of attack after departure from areas where *P. vivax* and *P. ovale* are endemic, which includes almost all areas where malaria is found (except Haiti), some experts prescribe in addition primaquine phosphate 26.3 mg (15 mg base)/day or, for children, 0.3 mg base/kg/day during the last 2 weeks of prophylaxis. Others prefer to avoid the toxicity of primaquine and rely on surveillance to detect cases when they occur; particularly when exposure was limited or doubtful.

[5]Beginning 1-2 weeks before travel and continuing weekly for the duration of stay and for 4 weeks after leaving.

[6]In the U.S., a 250 mg tablet of mefloquine contains 228 mg mefloquine base. Outside the U.S., each 275 mg tablet contains 250 mg base.

[7]The pediatric dosage has not been approved by the FDA, and the drug has not been approved for use during pregnancy. However, it has been reported to be safe for prophylactic use during the second or third trimester of pregnancy and possibly during early pregnancy as well (CDC Health Information for International Travel, 2001-2003, 113; BL Smoak, Writer JV, Keep LW, et al, "The Effects of Inadvertent Exposure of Mefloquine Chemoprophylaxis on Pregnancy Outcomes and Infants of US Army Servicewomen," *J Infect Dis*, 1997, 176(3):831-3). Mefloquine is not recommended for patients with cardiac conduction abnormalities. Patients with a history of seizures or psychiatric disorders should avoid mefloquine (*Medical Letter*, 1990, 32:13). Resistance to mefloquine has been reported in some areas, such as Thailand; in these areas, doxycycline should be used for prophylaxis. In children <8 years of age, proguanil plus sulfisoxazole has been used (KN Suh and JS Keystone, *Infect Dis Clin Pract*, 1996, 5:541).

[8]An approved drug, but considered investigational for this condition by the U.S. Food and Drug Administration.

[9]Beginning 1-2 days before travel and continuing for the duration of stay and for 4 weeks after leaving. Use of tetracyclines is contraindicated in pregnancy and in children <8 years of age. Doxycycline can cause gastrointestinal disturbances, vaginal moniliasis, and photosensitivity reactions.

[10]Atovaquone plus proguanil is available as a fixed-dose combination tablet: adult tablets (250 mg atovaquone/100 mg proguanil, *Malarone*) and pediatric tablets (62.5 mg atovaquone/25 mg proguanil, *Malarone Pediatric*). To enhance absorption, it should be taken within 45 minutes after eating (Looareesuwan S, Chulay JD, Canfield CJ, et al, "Malarone (Atovaquone and Proguanil Hydrochloride): A Review of Its Clinical Development for Treatment of Malaria. Malarone Clinical Trials Study Group," *Am J Trop Med Hyg*, 1999, 60(4):533-41). Although approved for once daily dosing, to decrease nausea and vomiting the dose for treatment is usually divided in two.

[11]Shanks GE et al, *Clin Infect Dis*, 1998, 27:494; Lell B, Luckner D, Ndjave M, et al, "Randomised Placebo-Controlled Study of Atovaquone Plus Proguanil for Malaria Prophylaxis in Children," *Lancet*, 1998, 351(9104):709-13. Beginning 1-2 days before travel and continuing for the duration of stay and for 1 week after leaving. In one study of malaria prophylaxis, atovaquone/proguanil was better tolerated than mefloquine in nonimmune travelers (Overbosch D, Schilthuis H, Bienzle U, et al, "Atovaquone-Proguanil Versus Mefloquine for Malaria Prophylaxis in Nonimmune Travelers: Results From a Randomized, Double-Blind Study," *Clin Infect Dis*, 2001, 33(7):1015-21).

[12]Primaquine phosphate can cause hemolytic anemia, especially in patients whose red cells are deficient in glucose-6-phosphate dehydrogenase. This deficiency is most common in African, Asian, and Mediterranean peoples. Patients should be screened for G6PD deficiency before treatment. Primaquine should not be used during pregnancy.

[13]Several studies have shown that daily primaquine, beginning 1 day before departure and continued until 7 days after leaving the malaria area, provides effective prophylaxis against chloroquine-resistant *P. falciparum* (Baird JK, Lacy MD, Basri H, et al, "Randomized, Parallel Placebo-Controlled Trial of Primaquine for Malaria Prophylaxis in Papua, Indonesia," *Clin Infect Dis*, 2001, 33(12):1990-7). Some studies have shown less efficacy against *P. vivax*. Nausea and abdominal pain can be diminished by taking with food.

[14]Proguanil (Paludrine – Wyeth Ayerst, Canada; AstraZeneca, United Kingdom), which is not available alone in the U.S.A. but is widely available in Canada and Europe, is recommended mainly for use in Africa south of the Sahara. Prophylaxis is recommended during exposure and for 4 weeks afterwards. Proguanil has been used in pregnancy without evidence of toxicity (Phillips-Howard PA and Wood D, "The Safety of Antimalarial Drugs in Pregnancy," *Drug Saf*, 1996, 14(3):131-45).

Adapted from "Report of the Committee on Infectious Diseases," *2003 Red Book®*, 26th ed, 760-1.

IMMUNIZATION RECOMMENDATIONS *(Continued)*

ADVERSE EVENTS AND VACCINATION

Reportable Events Following Vaccination[1]

Vaccine / Toxoid		Event	Onset Interval
Tetanus in any combination; DTaP, DTP, DTP-Hib, DT, Td, TT	A.	Anaphylaxis or anaphylactic shock	7 days
	B.	Brachial neuritis	28 days
	C.	Any sequela (including death) of above events	Not applicable
	D.	Events described in manufacturer's package insert as contraindications to additional doses of vaccine	See package insert
Pertussis in any combination; DTaP, DTP, DTP-Hib, P	A.	Anaphylaxis or anaphylactic shock	7 days
	B.	Encephalopathy (or encephalitis)	7 days
	C.	Any sequela (including death) of above events	Not applicable
	D.	Events described in manufacturer's package insert as contraindications to additional doses of vaccine	See package insert
Measles, mumps, and rubella in any combination; MMR, MR, M, R	A.	Anaphylaxis or anaphylactic shock	7 days
	B.	Encephalopathy (or encephalitis)	15 days
	C.	Any sequela (including death) of above events	Not applicable
	D.	Events described in manufacturer's package insert as contraindications to additional doses of vaccine	See package insert
Rubella in any combination; MMR, MR, R	A.	Chronic arthritis	42 days
	B.	Any sequela (including death) of above events	Not applicable
	C.	Events described in manufacturer's package insert as contraindications to additional doses of vaccine	See package insert
Measles in any combination; MMR, MR, M	A.	Thrombocytopenic purpura	7-30 days
	B.	Vaccine-strain measles viral infection in an immunodeficient recipient	6 months
	C.	Any sequela (including death) of above events	Not applicable
	D.	Events described in manufacturer's package insert as contraindications to additional doses of vaccine	See package insert
Inactivated polio (IPV)	A.	Anaphylaxis or anaphylactic shock	7 days
	B.	Any sequela (including death) of above events	Not applicable
	C.	Events described in manufacturer's package insert as contraindications to additional doses of vaccine	See package insert
Hepatitis B	A.	Anaphylaxis or anaphylactic shock	7 days
	B.	Any sequela (including death) of above events	Not applicable
	C.	Events described in manufacturer's package insert as contraindications to additional doses of vaccine	See package insert
Haemophilus influenzae type b (conjugate)	A.	Events described in manufacturer's package insert as contraindications to additional doses of vaccine	See package insert
Varicella	A.	Events described in manufacturer's package insert as contraindications to additional doses of vaccine	See package insert
Rotavirus	A.	Intussusception	30 days
	B.	Any sequela (including death) of above events	Not applicable
	C.	Events described in manufacturer's package insert as contraindications to additional doses of vaccine	See package insert
Pneumococcal conjugate	A.	Events described in manufacturer's package insert as contraindications to additional doses of vaccine	See package insert

[1]Effective date: August 26, 2002.

The Reportable Events Table (RET) reflects what is reportable by law (42 USC 300aa-25) to the Vaccine Adverse Event Reporting System (VAERS), including conditions found in the manufacturer's package insert. In addition, individuals are encouraged to report **any** clinically significant or unexpected events (even if you are not certain the vaccine caused the event) for **any** vaccine, whether or not it is listed on the RET. Manufacturers are also required by regulation (21CFR 600.80) to report to the VAERS program all adverse events made known to them for any vaccine.

Adapted from the website http://www.vaers.org/reportable.htm. For further information, contact VAERS at 1-800-822-7967.

IMMUNIZATIONS[1] (VACCINES[2])

Drug	Use	Stability	Dosage and Administration
Anthrax vaccine (adsorbed)[2,3] BioThrax™	Immunization against *Bacillus anthracis*, recommended for individuals who may come in contact with animal products which come from anthrax endemic areas and may be contaminated with *Bacillus anthracis* spores; postexposure prophylaxis in combination with antibiotics, recommended for high-risk persons such as veterinarians and others handling potentially infected animals; routine immunization for the general population is not recommended. The Department of Defense is implementing an anthrax vaccination program against the biological warfare agent anthrax, which will be administered to all active duty and reserve personnel. **Note:** Safety and efficacy not established for adults >65 years of age.	Store under refrigeration at 2°C to 8°C (36°F to 46°F). Do not freeze. Do not mix with other injections or use the same site. Shake well before use; do not use if discolored or contains particulate matter.	SubQ: Children ≥18 years and Adults: Three injections of 0.5 mL each given 2 weeks apart, followed by three additional injections given at 6-, 12-, and 18 months; booster at 1-year intervals Massage site to disperse the vaccine postinjection. It is not necessary to restart the series if a dose is not given on time; resume as soon as practical.
BCG vaccine[6] TheraCys®; TICE® BCG	Immunization against tuberculosis and immunotherapy for cancer; treatment of bladder cancer; strongly recommended for infants and children with negative tuberculin skin tests who are at high risk of intimate and prolonged exposure to persistently untreated or ineffectively treated patients with infectious pulmonary tuberculosis; cannot be removed from the source of exposure; cannot be placed on long-term preventive therapy; and are continuously exposed with tuberculosis who have bacilli resistant to isoniazid and rifampin; recommended for tuberculin-negative infants and children in groups in which the rate of new infections exceeds 1% per year and for whom the usual surveillance and treatment programs have been attempted but are not operationally feasible	Refrigerate; protect from light. Use TICE® BCG within 2 hours of mixing.	Children >1 month and Adults: **Immunization against tuberculosis** (TICE® BCG): 0.2-0.3 mL percutaneous; initial lesion usually appears after 10-14 days consisting of small red papule at injection site and reaches maximum diameter of 3 mm in 4-6 weeks. Conduct postvaccinal tuberculin test (ie, 5 TU of PPD) in 2-3 months; if test is negative, repeat vaccination. **Immunotherapy for bladder cancer:** *Intravesical treatment:* Instill into bladder for 2 hours *TheraCys®:* One dose instilled into bladder once weekly for 6 weeks followed by one treatment at 3, 6, 12, 18, and 24 months *TICE® BCG:* One dose instilled into the bladder once weekly for 6 weeks followed by once monthly for 6-12 months (should only be given intravesicularly or percutaneously)
Diphtheria and tetanus toxoid[5,6]	Active immunity against diphtheria and tetanus when pertussis vaccine is contraindicated; tetanus prophylaxis in wound management	Refrigerate.	I.M.: **Children: 6 weeks to 1 year of age:** DT: Three 0.5 mL doses at least 4 weeks apart; administer a reinforcing dose 6-12 months after third injection. **Children >1-6 years:** DT: Two 0.5 mL doses at least 4 weeks apart; reinforcing dose 6-12 months after second injection **Children 4-6 years:** Booster: DT: 0.5 mL; not necessary if all 4 doses were given after fourth birthday; administer doses at 10-year intervals with adult preparation. **Children ≥7 years and Adults:** Td: 2 primary doses of 0.5 mL each, given at an interval of 4-6 weeks; third (reinforcing) dose of 0.5 mL 6-12 months later; booster every 10 years
Diphtheria, tetanus toxoids, and acellular pertussis vaccine[5,6] Daptacel®; Infanrix®; Tripedia®	Active immunization of children from 6 weeks of age through seventh birthday for prevention of diphtheria, tetanus, and pertussis	Refrigerate at 2°C to 8°C (35°F to 46°F); do not freeze.	I.M. (anterolateral aspect of thigh or deltoid muscle of upper arm): **Children 6 weeks through 6 years of age** (use same product for all 3 doses): Three doses of 0.5 mL, usually given at 2-, 4-, and 6 months of age; may be repeated every 4-8 weeks; booster: fourth dose given at ~15-20 months of age, but at least 6 months after third dose. Fifth dose given at 5-6 years of age, prior to starting school or kindergarten (if the fourth dose is given at 4 years of age, the fifth dose may be omitted.) **Children ≥7 years and Adults:** Adult Td preparation is the preferred agent.
Diphtheria, tetanus toxoids, acellular pertussis vaccine and *Haemophilus influenzae* b conjugate vaccine (combined)[2,3] TriHIBit®	Active immunization of children 15-18 months of age for prevention of diphtheria, tetanus, pertussis, and invasive disease caused by *H. influenzae* type b	Should be used within 30 minutes of reconstitution.	I.M.: Children >15 months of age: 0.5 mL;TriHIBit® is Tripedia® vaccine used to reconstitute ActHIB® (*Haemophilus* b conjugate) vaccine. The combination can be used for the DTaP dose given at 15-18 months when Tripedia® was used for the initial doses and a primary series of HIB vaccine has been given.

IMMUNIZATIONS[1] (VACCINES[2]) *(Continued)*

Drug	Use	Stability	Dosage and Administration
Diphtheria, tetanus toxoids, acellular pertussis, hepatitis B (recombinant), and poliovirus (inactivated) vaccine[5,6] Pediarix™	Active immunization against diphtheria, tetanus, pertussis, hepatitis B virus (all known subtypes), and poliomyelitis (caused by poliovirus types 1, 2, and 3)	Store under refrigeration of 2°C to 8°C (36°F to 46°F). Do not freeze; discard if frozen. Do not administer additional vaccines or immunoglobulins at the same site, or use the same syringe. Shake well prior to use; do not use unless a homogeneous, turbid, white suspension forms.	I.M. (anterolateral aspects of the thigh or the deltoid muscle of the upper arm): Immunization: Vaccination usually begins at 2 months, but may be started as early as 6 weeks of age: 0.5 mL; repeat in 6-8 week intervals (preferably 8-week) for a total of 3 doses. Children previously vaccinated with one or more components and who are also scheduled to receive all vaccine components (safety and efficacy not established): Hepatitis B vaccine: Infants born of HBsAg-negative mothers who received 1 dose of hepatitis B vaccine at birth may be given Pediarix™. Infants who received 1 or more doses of hepatitis B vaccine (recombinant) may be given Pediarix™ to complete the hepatitis B series. Diphtheria and tetanus toxoids, and acellular pertussis vaccine (DTaP): Infants previously vaccinated with 1 or 2 doses of Infanrix® may use Pediarix™ to complete the first 3 doses of the series; use of Pediarix™ to complete DTaP vaccination started with products other than Infanrix® is not recommended. Inactivated polio vaccine (IPV): Infants previously vaccinated with 1 or 2 doses of IPV may use Pediarix™ to complete the first 3 doses of the series.
Haemophilus b conjugate vaccine[2,6] ActHIB®, HibTITER®, PedvaxHIB®	Routine immunization of children 2 months to 5 years of age against invasive disease caused by H. influenzae ; unimmunized children 5 years of age with a chronic illness known to be associated with increased risk of Haemophilus influenzae type b disease, specifically, persons with anatomic or functional asplenia or sickle cell anemia or those who have undergone splenectomy, should receive Hib vaccine. Haemophilus b conjugate vaccines are not indicated for prevention of bronchitis or other infections due to H. influenzae in adults; adults with specific dysfunction or certain complement deficiencies who are at especially high risk of H. influenzae type b infection (HIV-infected adults); patients with Hodgkin's disease (vaccinated at least 2 weeks before the initiation of chemotherapy or 3 months after the end of chemotherapy)	Keep in refrigerator; may be frozen (not diluent) without affecting potency. Reconstituted Hib-Imune® remains stable for only 8 hours, whereas HibVAX® remain stable for 30 days when refrigerated.	Note: The same brand drug should be used throughout the vaccination series. If vaccine previously used is unknown, infants (2-6 months of age) should be given a primary series of three doses. Have epinephrine 1:1000 available. I.M.: Children: 0.5 mL as a single dose administered according to one of the following "brand-specific" schedules (boosters to be given at least 2 months after previous dose): HibTITER®: Age at 1st dose: 2-6 months: 3 doses, 2 months apart; booster in 15 months 7-11 months: 2 doses, 2 months apart; booster in 15 months 12-14 months: 1 dose; booster in 15 months 15-60 months: 1 dose; no booster PedvaxHIB®: Age at 1st dose: 2-6 months: 2 doses, 2 months apart; booster in 12 months 7-11 months: 2 doses, 2 months apart; booster in 15 months 12-14 months: 1 dose; booster in 15 months 15-60 months: 1 dose; no booster ProHIBIT®: Age at 1st dose: 15-60 months: 1 dose; no booster
Hepatitis A vaccine[2,5,6] Havrix®, VAQTA®	Protection against hepatitis A or for populations at risk: travelers to developing countries, household and sexual contact with persons infected with hepatitis A, child day care employees, patients with chronic liver disease, illicit drug users, male homosexuals, institutional workers (eg, institutions for the mentally and physically handicapped persons, prisons, etc), and healthcare workers who may be exposed to hepatitis A virus (eg, laboratory employees); protection lasts for ~15 years		Note: Use caution in patients with serious active infection, cardiovascular disease, or pulmonary disorders; treatment for anaphylactic reactions should be immediately available. I.M. (deltoid muscle): Havrix®: Children 12 months -18 years: 720 ELISA units (0.5 mL) with a booster dose of 720 ELISA units 6-12 months following primary immunization Adults: 1440 ELISA units (1 mL) with a booster 6-12 months following primary immunization VAQTA®: Children 12 months - 18 years: 25 units (0.5 mL) with 25 units (0.5 mL); booster in 6-18 months Adults: 50 units (1 mL) with 50 units (1 mL); booster in 6-18 months

Drug	Use	Stability	Dosage and Administration
Hepatitis A (inactivated) and hepatitis B (recombinant) vaccine[2,5,6] Twinrix®	Active immunization against disease caused by hepatitis A virus and hepatitis B virus (all known subtypes) in populations desiring protection against or at high risk of exposure to these viruses; travelers to areas of intermediate/high endemicity for **both** HAV and HBV; those at increased risk of HBV infection due to behavioral or occupational factors; patients with chronic liver disease; laboratory workers who handle live HAV and HBV; healthcare workers, police, and other personnel who render first aid or medical assistance; workers who come in contact with sewage; employees of day care centers and correctional facilities; patients/staff of hemodialysis units; male homosexuals; patients frequently receiving blood products; military personnel; users of injectable illicit drugs; close household contacts of patients with hepatitis A and hepatitis B infection	Store in refrigerator at 2°C to 8°C (36°F to 46°F). Do not freeze (discard if frozen). Do not use the same syringe or site as additional vaccines or immunoglobulins. Shake well prior to use; do not dilute.	I.M. (deltoid muscle): Adults: Three doses (1 mL each) given on a 0-, 1-, and 6-month schedule
Hepatitis B immune globulin BayHep B®; HepaGam B™; Nabi-HB®	Provide prophylactic passive immunity to hepatitis B infection to those individuals exposed; newborns of mothers known to be hepatitis B surface antigen positive; not indicated for treatment of active hepatitis B infections; ineffective in the treatment of chronic active hepatitis B infection	Refrigerate at 2°C to 8°C (36°F to 46°F); do not freeze.	HBIG may be administered at the same time (but at a different site) or up to 1 month preceding hepatitis B vaccination without impairing the active immune response. I.M. (gluteal or deltoid region): Newborns: Hepatitis B: 0.5 mL as soon after birth as possible (within 12 hours); may repeat at 3 months in order for a higher rate of prevention of the carrier state to be achieved. At this time, an active vaccination program with the vaccine may begin. Infants <12 months: Household exposure prophylaxis: 0.5 mL (to be administered if mother or primary caregiver has acute HBV infection) Adults: Postexposure prophylaxis: 0.06 mL/kg as soon as possible after exposure (ie, within 24 hours of needlestick, ocular, or mucosal exposure or within 14 days of sexual exposure); usual dose: 3-5 mL; repeat at 28-30 days after exposure

IMMUNIZATIONS[1] (VACCINES[2]) *(Continued)*

Drug	Use	Stability	Dosage and Administration
Hepatitis B vaccine Engerix-B®; Recombivax HB®	Immunization against infection caused by all known subtypes of hepatitis B virus in individuals considered at high risk of potential exposure to hepatitis B virus or HB$_s$Ag-positive materials. Immunity will last~5-7 years.	Refrigerate at 2°C to 8°C (36°F to 46°F); do not freeze. Shake well prior to withdrawal and use.	It is possible to interchange the vaccines for completion of a series or for booster doses; the antibody produced in response to each type of vaccine is comparable, however, the quantity of the vaccine will vary. Administer with caution in patients receiving anticoagulant therapy. SubQ injection may be administered in patients at risk of hemorrhage which may result in an increased incidence of local reactions and a reduced therapeutic effect. Refer to specific product labeling for dosing. **I.M.** (deltoid muscle): Adults: Immunization regimen consists of 3 doses (0, 1, and 6 months); first dose given on the elected date; second dose given 1 month later; third dose given 6 months after the first dose *Alternative dosing schedule:* **Recombivax HB®:** *Children 11-15 years* (10 mcg/mL adult formulation): First dose of 1 mL, given on the elected date, second dose given 4-6 months later **Engerix-B®:** *Children ≥10 years:* (10 mcg/0.5 mL formulation): High-risk children: 0.5 mL at 0, 1, 2, and 12 months; lower-risk children ages 5-10 who are candidates for an extended administration schedule may receive an alternative regimen of 0.5 mL at 0, 12, and 24 months; if booster is needed, revaccinate with 0.5 mL *Adolescents 11-19 years* (20 mcg/mL formulation): 1 mL, at 0, 1, and 6 months. High-risk adolescents: 1 mL at 0, 1, 2, and 12 months; lower-risk adolescents 11-16 years who are candidates for an extended administration schedule may receive an alternative regimen of 0.5 mL (using the 10 mcg/0.5 mL) formulation at 0, 12, and 24 months; if booster is needed, revaccinate with 20 mcg *Adults ≥ 20 years:* High-risk adults (20 mcg/mL formulation): 1 mL at 0, 1, 2, and 12 months; if booster dose is needed, revaccinate with 1 mL
Immune globulin (intramuscular) BayGam®	Household and sexual contacts of persons with hepatitis A, measles, varicella, and possibly rubella; travelers to high-risk areas outside tourist routes; staff, attendees, and parents of diapered attendees in daycare center outbreaks For travelers, IG is not an alternative to careful selection of foods and water; frequent travelers should be tested for hepatitis A antibody, immune hemolytic anemia, and neutropenia (with TTP, I.V. route is usually used).	Refrigerate; do not freeze. Do not mix with other medications.	Skin testing should not be performed as local irritation can occur and be misinterpreted as a positive reaction. Immune globulin can interfere with the antibody response to parenterally administered live virus vaccines. I.M.: **Hepatitis A:** *Pre-exposure prophylaxis upon travel into endemic areas (hepatitis A vaccine preferred):* 0.02 mL/kg for anticipated risk 1-3 months; 0.06 mL/kg for anticipated risk >3 months; repeat approximate dose every 4-6 months if exposure continues. *Postexposure prophylaxis:* 0.02 mL/kg given within 2 weeks of exposure **Measles:** Prophylaxis: 0.25 mL/kg/dose (max: 15 mL) given within 6 days of exposure followed by live attenuated measles vaccine in 3 months or at 15 months of age (whichever is later) **Leukemia, lymphoma, immunodeficiency disorders, generalized malignancy, or those receiving immunosuppressive therapy:** 0.5 mL/kg (max: 15 mL). **Poliomyelitis:** Prophylaxis: 0.3 mL/kg/dose as a single dose **Rubella:** Prophylaxis: 0.55 mL/kg/dose within 72 hours of exposure **Varicella:** Prophylaxis: 0.6-1.2 mL/kg (varicella-zoster immune globulin preferred) within 72 hours of exposure **IgG deficiency:** 1.3 mL/kg, then 0.66 mL/kg in 3-4 weeks **Hepatitis B:** Prophylaxis: 0.06 mL/kg/dose (HBIG preferred)

Drug	Use	Stability	Dosage and Administration
Influenza virus vaccine Fluarix™; fluMist®; Fluvirin®; Fluzone®	Provide active immunity to influenza virus strains contained in the vaccine; for high-risk persons including those ≥65 years of age; residents of nursing homes and other chronic-care facilities that house persons of any age with chronic medical conditions; adults and children with chronic disorders of the pulmonary or cardiovascular systems (asthma); adults and children who have required regular medical follow-up or hospitalization during the preceding year because of chronic metabolic diseases (including diabetes mellitus), renal dysfunction, hemoglobinopathies, or immunosuppression (including immunosuppression caused by medications); children and adolescents (6 months to 18 years of age) who are receiving long-term aspirin therapy and therefore, may be at risk for developing Reye's syndrome after influenza; women who will be in the 2nd or 3rd trimester of pregnancy during the influenza season. Otherwise healthy children aged 6-23 months, healthy persons who may transmit influenza to those at risk, and others who are interested in immunization to influenza virus should receive the vaccine as long as supply is available.	Store between 2°C to 8°C (36°F to 46°F). Potency is destroyed by freezing; do not use if product has been frozen. Suspension should be shaken well prior to use; inspect for particulate matter and discoloration prior to administration. **Note:** Previous year vaccines should not be used to prevent present year influenza.	I.M.: (deltoid muscle in adults and older children; anterolateral aspect of the thigh in infants and young children): *Previously unvaccinated children <9 years:* 2 doses given >1 month apart **Fluarix™:** *Adults:* 0.5 mL/dose (1 dose) **Fluzone®:** *Children 6-35 months:* 0.25 mL/dose (1 or 2 doses) *Children 3-8 years:* 0.5 mL/dose (1 or 2 doses) *Children ≥9 years and Adults:* 0.5 mL/dose (1 dose) **Fluvirin®:** *Children 4-8 years:* 0.5 mL/dose (1 or 2 doses) *Children ≥9 years and Adults:* 0.5 mL/dose (1 dose) **Intranasal: fluMist®:** *Children 5-8 years, previously not vaccinated with influenza vaccine:* Initial season: Two 0.5 mL doses separated by 6-10 weeks *Children 5-8 years, previously vaccinated with influenza vaccine:* 0.5 mL/dose (1 dose) *Children ≥9 years and Adults ≤49 years:* 0.5 mL/dose (1 dose)
Japanese encephalitis virus vaccine (inactivated) JE-VAX®	Active immunization against Japanese encephalitis for children ≥ 1 year of age and adults who plan to spend 1 month or more in endemic areas in Asia (especially persons traveling during the transmission season or visiting rural area); older adults >55 years of age should be considered for vaccination (due to increased risk of developing symptomatic illness after infection) Those planning travel to or residence in endemic areas should consult the Travel Advisory Service (Central Campus) for specific advice; consider vaccination for shorter trips to epidemic areas or extensive outdoor activities in rural endemic areas. Because of the potential for severe adverse reactions, Japanese encephalitis vaccine is not recommended for **all** persons traveling to or residing in Asia.	Refrigerate at 2°C to 8°C. Do not freeze. Discard 8 hours after reconstitution.	Severe adverse reactions may occur within minutes following vaccination or up to 17 days later; most reactions occur within 10 days (majority within 48 hours). Observe vaccinees for 30 minutes after vaccination; warn them of the possibility of delayed generalized urticaria and to remain where medical care is readily available for 10 days following any dose of the vaccine. U.S. recommended primary immunization schedule: **SubQ:** **Children 1-3 years:** Three 0.5 mL doses given on days 0, 7, and 30 **Children >3 years and Adults:** Three 1 mL doses given on days 0, 7, and 30; give third dose on day 14 when time does not permit waiting **Booster:** After 2 years, or according to current recommendation **Note:** Abbreviated schedules should be used only when necessary due to time constraints. Two doses a week apart produce immunity in about 80% of recipients; the longest regimen yields highest titers after 6 months. Travel should not commence ≤10 days after the last dose of vaccine, to allow adequate antibody formation and recognition of any delayed adverse reaction. Advise concurrent use of other means to reduce the risk of mosquito exposure when possible, including bed nets, insect repellents, protective clothing, avoidance of travel in endemic areas, and avoidance of outdoor activity during twilight and evening periods.
Measles, mumps, and rubella vaccines (combined) M-M-R® II	Prophylaxis for measles, mumps, and rubella	Prior to reconstitution, store the powder at 2°C to 8°C (36°F to 46°F) or colder (freezing does not affect potency). Protect from light. Diluent may be stored with powder or at room temperature.	SubQ (outer aspect of the upper arm): Infants >12 months: Administer 0.5 mL, then repeat at 4-6 years of age. If the second dose was not received, the schedule should be completed by the 11- to 12-year-old visit. If there is risk of exposure to measles, single-antigen measles vaccine should be administered at 6-11 months of age with a second dose (of MMR) at >12 months of age. **Note:** MMR vaccine should not be given within 3 months of immune globulin or whole blood. Have epinephrine available during and after administration. Should not be administered to severely immunocompromised persons with the exception of asymptomatic children with HIV (ACIP and AAP recommendation); Severely immunocompromised patients and symptomatic HIV-infected patients who are exposed to measles should receive immune globulin, regardless of prior vaccination status. Defer immunization during any acute illness. Females should not become pregnant within 3 months of vaccination.

IMMUNIZATIONS[1] (VACCINES[2]) *(Continued)*

Drug	Use	Stability	Dosage and Administration
Measles virus vaccine (live) Attenuvax®	Immunization for adults born after 1957 without documentation of live vaccine on or after first birthday, physician-diagnosed measles, or laboratory evidence of immunity should be vaccinated, ideally with two doses of vaccine separated by no less than 1 month; for those previously vaccinated with one dose of measles vaccine, revaccination is recommended for students entering colleges and other institutions of higher education, for healthcare workers at the time of employment, and for international travelers who visit endemic areas.	Refrigerate at 2°C to 8°C. Discard if left at room temperature for over 8 hours. Protect from light.	SubQ (outer aspect of upper arm): Children ≥15 months and Adults: 0.5 mL; no routine booster.
Meningococcal polysaccharide vaccine (groups A, C, Y, and W-135) Menomune®- A/C/Y/W-135	Immunization of children≥2 years of age and adults in epidemic or endemic areas as might be determined in a population delineated by neighborhood, school, dormitory, or other reasonable boundary; the prevalent serogroup in such a situation should match a serogroup in the vaccine. Individuals at particular high-risk include persons with terminal component complement deficiencies and those with anatomic or function asplenia. For use with travelers visiting areas of a country that are recognized as having hyperendemic or epidemic meningococcal disease. Vaccinations should be considered for household or institutional contacts of persons with meningococcal disease as an adjunct to appropriate antibiotic chemoprophylaxis as well as medical and laboratory personnel at risk of exposure to meningococcal disease.	Store at 2°C to 8°C (35°F to 46°F).	SubQ: One dose (0.5 mL); individuals who are sensitive to thimerosal should receive single-dose pack (reconstituted with 0.78 mL vial without preservative); the need for booster is unknown; have epinephrine 1:1000 available
Mumps virus vaccine (live/attenuated) Mumpsvax®	Mumps prophylaxis by promoting active immunity **Note:** Trivalent measles-mumps-rubella (M-M-R®) vaccine is the preferred agent for most children and many adults. Persons born prior to 1957 are generally considered immune and need not be vaccinated.	Refrigerate; protect from light. Discard within 8 hours after reconstitution.	SubQ (outer aspect of upper arm): Children ≥15 months and Adults: 0.5 mL; no booster
Plague vaccine	Vaccinate selected travelers to countries where avoidance of rodents and fleas is impossible; laboratory and field personnel working with *Yersinia pestis* organisms possibly resistant to antimicrobials; those engaged in *Yersinia pestis* aerosol experiments or in field operations in areas with enzootic plague where regular exposure to potentially infected wild rodents, rabbits, or their fleas cannot be prevented; prophylactic antibiotics may be indicated following definite exposure, whether or not the exposed persons have been vaccinated.		I.M.: Three doses: First dose 1 mL, second dose (0.2 mL) 1 month later, third dose (0.2 mL) 5 months after the second dose; booster at 1- to 2-year intervals if exposure continues

Drug	Use	Stability	Dosage and Administration
Pneumococcal conjugate vaccine (7-valent) Prevnar®	Immunization of infants and toddlers against active disease caused by *Streptococcus pneumoniae* due to serotypes included in the vaccine	Store refrigerated at 2°C to 8°C (36°F to 46°F).	Use of the pneumococcal conjugate vaccine does not replace the use of the 23-valent vaccine in children >24 months of age with sickle cell disease, asplenia, HIV infection, chronic illness, or if immunocompromised. I.M. **Infants: 2-6 months:** 0.5 mL at approximately 2 month-interval for 3 consecutive doses, followed by a fourth dose of 0.5 mL at 12-15 months of age. The first dose may be given as young as 2 months of age, but is typically given at 6 weeks of age. In case of a moderate shortage of vaccine, defer the fourth dose until shortage is resolved; in case of a severe shortage of vaccine, defer third and fourth doses until shortage is resolved. **Infants and Children (previously unvaccinated):** *7-11 months:* 0.5 mL for a total of 3 doses; 2 doses at least 4 weeks apart, followed by a third dose after the 1-year birthday, separated from the second dose by at least 2 months *12-23 months:* 0.5 mL for a total of two doses, separated by at least 2 months *24-59 months:* Healthy Children: 0.5 mL as a single dose. Children with sickle cell disease, asplenia, HIV infection, chronic illness, or immunocompromising conditions (not including bone marrow transplants with results pending): Use PPV23 (pneumococcal polysaccharide vaccine, polyvalent) at 12- and 24-months until studies are complete): 0.5 mL for a total of 2 doses, separated by 2 months **Children (previously vaccinated with a lapse in vaccination administration):** *7-11 months:* Previously received 1 or 2 doses PCV7: 0.5 mL dose at 7-11 months of age, followed by a second dose ≥2 months later at 12-15 months of age. *12-23 months:* Previously received 1 dose before 12 months: 0.5 mL dose, followed by a second dose ≥2 months later. Previously received 2 doses before 12 months: 0.5 mL dose ≥2 months after the most recent dose. *24-59 months:* Any incomplete schedule: 0.5 mL as a single dose. **Note:** Patients with chronic diseases or immunosuppressing conditions should receive 2 doses ≥2 months apart.

IMMUNIZATIONS[1] (VACCINES[2]) *(Continued)*

Drug	Use	Stability	Dosage and Administration
Pneumococcal polysaccharide vaccine (polyvalent) Pneumovax® 23	For children >2 years of age and adults who are at increased risk of pneumococcal disease and its complications because of underlying health conditions; older adults, including those ≥65 years of age	Refrigerate.	SubQ, I.M. (deltoid muscle or lateral migthigh): **Children >2 years and Adults:** 0.5 mL; have epinephrine (1:1000) available. **Revaccination** should be considered if: ≥6 years have elapsed since initial vaccination; for patients who received 14-valent pneumococcal vaccine and are at highest risk (asplenic) for fatal infection; at ≥6 years in patients with nephrotic syndrome, renal failure, or transplant recipients; and 3-5 years in children with nephrotic syndrome, asplenia, or sickle cell disease. Use with caution in individuals who have had episodes of pneumococcal infection within the preceeding 3 years; may result in increased reactions to vaccine or cause relapse in patients with stable idiopathic thrombocytopenia purpura. **Previously vaccinated with PCV7 vaccine:** *With sickle cell disease, asplenia, immunocompromised or HIV infection:* 0.5 mL at 2 years of age and 2 months after last dose of PCV7; revaccination with PPV23 should be given 5 years for children >10 years of age and every 3-5 years for children 10 years of age; revaccination should not be administered <3 years after the previous PPV23 dose *With chronic illness:* 0.5 mL at 2 years of age and 2 months after last dose of PCV7; revaccination with PPV23 is not recommended *Following bone marrow transplant (use of PCV7 under study):* Administer one dose PPV23 at 12- and 24-months following BMT.
Poliovirus vaccine (inactivated) IPOL®	All children should receive four doses of IPV (at age 2 months, age 4 months, between ages 6-18 months, and between ages 4-6 years). OPV supplies are expected to be very limited in the United States after inventories are depleted. ACIP reaffirms its support for the global eradication initiative and use of OPV as the vaccine of choice to eradicate polio where it is endemic. Oral poliovirus vaccine (OPV), if available, may be used only for the following special circumstances: Mass vaccination campaigns to control outbreaks of paralytic polio; unvaccinated children who will be traveling within 4 weeks to areas where polio is endemic or epidemic; children of parents who do not accept the recommended number of vaccine injections (these children may receive OPV only for the third or fourth dose or both; healthcare providers should administer OPV only after discussing the risk for VAPP with parents or caregivers)		**Infants 6-12 weeks of age:** Oral: 0.5 mL; second dose 6-8 weeks after first dose (commonly at 4 months); third dose 8-12 months after second dose (commonly at 18 months) **Older Children and Adults** (adolescents through 18 years of age): SubQ: Two 0.5 mL doses 4-8 weeks apart and a third dose of 0.5 mL 6-12 months after second dose. Enhanced-potency inactivated poliovirus vaccine (E-IPV) is preferred for primary vaccination of adults, two doses 4-8 weeks apart, a third dose 6-12 months after the second. For adults with a completed primary series and/or for whom a booster is indicated, either OPV or E-IPV can be given (E-IPV preferred). If immediate protection is needed, either OPV or E-IPV is recommended. **Booster:** All children who have received primary immunization series, should receive a single follow-up dose and all children who have not should complete primary series.
Rabies immune globulin (human) BayRab®, Imogam® Rabies-HT	Part of postexposure prophylaxis of persons with rabies exposure who lack a history of pre-exposure or postexposure prophylaxis with rabies vaccine or a recently documented neutralizing antibody response to previous rabies vaccination; it is preferable to give RIG with the first dose of vaccine, but it can be given up to 8 days after vaccination. **Note:** RIG should always be administered in conjunction with rabies vaccine (HDCV) regimen (as soon as possible after the first dose of vaccine, up to 8 days). Persons with an adequate titer and those who have been completely immunized with rabies vaccine should not receive RIG, only booster doses of HDCV.	Refrigerate.	I.M. (gluteal muscle): 20 units/kg in a single dose Infiltrate half of the dose locally around the wound; administer the remainder I.M.

Drug	Use	Stability	Dosage and Administration
Rabies virus vaccine Imovax® Rabies; RabAvert®	**Pre-exposure immunization:** Vaccinate persons with greater than usual risk due to occupation or avocation including veterinarians, rangers, animal handlers, certain laboratory workers, and persons living in or visiting countries for >1 month where rabies is a constant threat. Complete pre-exposure prophylaxis does not eliminate the need for additional therapy with rabies vaccine after a rabies exposure. **Postexposure prophylaxis:** If a bite from a carrier animal is unprovoked and it is not captured and rabies is present in that species and area, administer rabies immune globulin (RIG) and the vaccine as indicated.	Refrigerate at 2°–8°C (36°–46°F); do not freeze. Protect from light. Use reconstituted vaccine immediately.	I.M. (deltoid muscle, in adults and older children; outer aspect of the thigh for younger children): **Pre-exposure prophylaxis:** 1 mL on days 0, 7, and 21-28; prolonging the interval between doses does not interfere with immunity achieved after concluding dose of the basic series. **Postexposure prophylaxis (Cleanse wound with soap and water first.):** *Persons not previously immunized:* 20 units/kg body weight, half infiltrated at bite site if possible, remainder I.M. and 5 doses of rabies vaccine, 1 mL on days 0, 3, 7, 14, and 28 *Persons who have previously received postexposure prophylaxis, pre-exposure series, or have a documented adequate rabies antibody titer:* 1 mL of either vaccine on days 0 and 3; do not administer RIG *Booster* (for occupational or other continuing risk): 1 mL every 2-5 years (or based on antibody titers)
Rubella virus vaccine (live) Meruvax® II	Selective active immunization against rubella; recommended for persons from 12 months of age to puberty; all adults lacking documentation of live vaccine on or after first birthday, or laboratory evidence of immunity should be vaccinated (particularly women of childbearing age; young adults who work in or congregate in hospitals, colleges, and on military bases; susceptible travelers) **Note:** Trivalent measles-mumps-rubella (M-M-R® II) vaccine is the preferred agent for most children and many adults. Persons born prior to 1957 are generally considered immune and need not be vaccinated.	Refrigerate; store at 2°C to 8°C (36°F to 46°F). Discard reconstituted vaccine after 8 hours. Ship vaccine at 10°C; may use dry ice. Protect from light.	Children ≥12 months and Adults: SubQ (outer aspect of upper arm): 0.5 mL; avoid injection into blood vessel.
Smallpox vaccine[4] Dryvax®	Active immunization against vaccinia virus, the causative agent of smallpox ACIP recommends vaccination of laboratory workers at risk of exposure from cultures or contaminated animals which may be a source of vaccinia or related Orthopoxviruses capable of causing infections in humans (monkeypox, cowpox, or variola). Revaccination is recommended every 10 years. In October 2002, the FDA approved the licensing of the current stockpile of smallpox vaccine. This approval allows the vaccine to be distributed and administered in the event of a smallpox attack.	Store at 2°C to 8°C (36°F to 46°F). Do not freeze.	Using a bifurcated needle, 1 drop of vaccine is introduced into the superficial layers of the skin using a multiple-puncture technique. The skin over the insertion of the deltoid muscle or the posterior aspect of the arm over the triceps are the preferred sites for vaccination. A single-use bifurcated needle should be dipped carefully into the reconstituted vaccine (following removal of rubber stopper). Visually confirm that the needle picks up a drop of vaccine solution. Deposit the drop of vaccine onto clean, dry skin at the vaccination site. Holding the bifurcated needle perpendicular to the skin, punctures are to be made rapidly into the superficial skin of the vaccination site. The puncture strokes should be vigorous enough to allow a trace of blood to appear after approximately 15-20 seconds. Wipe off any remaining vaccine with dry sterile gauze. To prevent transmission of the virus, cover vaccination site with gauze and cover gauze with a semipermeable barrier or clothing. Good handwashing prevents inadvertent inoculation. Dispose of all materials in a biohazard waste container. All materials must be burned, boiled, or autoclaved. If no evidence of vaccine take is apparent after 7 days, the individual may be vaccinated again.
Tetanus immune globulin (human) BayTet™	Passive immunization against tetanus (tetanus immune globulin is preferred over tetanus antitoxin for treatment of active tetanus); part of the management of an unclean wound in a person whose history of previous receipt of tetanus toxoid is unknown or who has received less than three doses of tetanus toxoid; elderly may require TIG more often than younger patients with tetanus infection due to declining antibody titers with age.	Refrigerate at 2°C to 8°C (36°F to 46°F). Never administer tetanus toxoid (Td) and TIG in the same syringe (toxoid will be neutralized).	Toxoid may be given at a separate site. Have epinephrine 1:1000 available. Boosters will be necessary. I.M.: **Prophylaxis:** Children: 4 units/kg (some recommend administering 250 units to small children) Adults: 250 units **Treatment:** Children: 500-3000 units (infiltrate some solution locally around the wound) Adults: 3000-6000 units

IMMUNIZATIONS[1] (VACCINES[2]) *(Continued)*

Drug	Use	Stability	Dosage and Administration
Tetanus toxoid (adsorbed)	Selective induction of active immunity against tetanus in selected patients. **Note:** Not equivalent to tetanus toxoid fluid. Tetanus and diphtheria toxoids for adult use (Td) is the preferred immunizing agent for most adults and for children after 7 years of age. Young children should receive trivalent DTwP or DTaP (diphtheria/tetanus/pertussis – whole cell or acellular), as part of their childhood immunization program, unless pertussis is contraindicated, then TD is warranted.	Refrigerate; do not freeze.	Have epinephrine 1:1000 available. Avoid injection into a blood vessel. I.M. (midthigh laterally or deltoid): Adults: 0.5 mL; repeat 0.5 mL at 4-8 weeks after the first dose and at 6-12 months after the second dose; booster every 5-10 years
Tetanus toxoid (fluid)	Detection of delayed hypersensitivity and assessment of cell-mediated immunity; active immunization against tetanus in the rare adult or child who is allergic to the aluminum adjuvant (a product containing adsorbed tetanus toxoid is preferred)	Refrigerate.	Have epinephrine 1:1000 available. Anergy testing: Adults: Intradermal: 0.1 mL (Td, TD, DTaP/DTwP recommended): Three doses of 0.5 mL I.M. or SubQ at 4- to 8-week intervals; give fourth dose 6-12 months after third dose; booster: 0.5 mL I.M., SubQ every 10 years
Typhoid vaccine Typhim Vi®; Vivotif Berna®	**Parenteral:** Promotes active immunity to typhoid fever for patients intimately exposed to a typhoid carrier or foreign travel to a typhoid fever endemic area. **Oral:** Immunization of children >6 years and adults who expect intimate exposure of or household contact with typhoid fever, travelers to areas of the world with a risk of exposure to typhoid fever, and workers in microbiology laboratories with expected frequent contact with *S. typhi.* **Typhoid vaccine:** Live, attenuated typhoid vaccine should not be administered to immunocompromised persons, including those known to be infected with HIV (parenteral inactivated vaccine is a theoretically safer alternative for this group)	Refrigerate, do not freeze; if mistakenly placed in a freezer, remove as soon as possible and place in refrigerator (potency unaffected). Can be used if exposed to temperature ≤80°F.	**I.M.** (deltoid muscle): Typhim Vi®: Children ≥2 years and Adults: 0.5 mL (25 mcg) injection in given at least 2 weeks prior to expected exposure; reimmunization: 0.5 mL single dose every 2 years is currently recommended for repeated or continued exposure **Oral:** Children ≥6 years and Adults: Swallow 1 capsule whole (do not chew) 1 hour before a meal with cold or lukewarm drink on alternate days (day 1, 3, 5, and 7) for a total of 4 doses; booster every 5 years (full course). **Note:** Not all recipients of typhoid vaccine will be fully protected against typhoid fever. Unless a complete immunization schedule is followed, an optimum immune response may not be achieved.
Varicella virus vaccine Varivax®	The American Association of Pediatrics recommends that the chickenpox vaccine should be given to all healthy children between 12 months of age to 18 years. Children 12 months of age to 13 years who have not been immunized or who have not had chickenpox should receive 1 vaccination while children 13-18 years of age require 2 vaccinations 4-8 weeks apart. The vaccine has been added to the childhood immunization schedule for infants 12-28 months of age and children 11-12 years of age who have not been vaccinated previously or who have not had the disease. It is recommended to be given with the measles, mumps, and rubella (MMR) vaccine.	Store powder in freezer at -15°C (5°F); may be stored under refrigeration for up to 72 continuous hours prior to reconstitution. Protect from light. Discard vaccine if not used within 72 hours. Store diluent separately at room temperature or in refrigerator.	SubQ: Children 12 months to 12 years: 0.5 mL Children ≥12 years to Adults: SubQ: 2 doses of 0.5 mL separated by 4-8 weeks.

Drug	Use	Stability	Dosage and Administration
Varicella-zoster immune globulin (human)	Passive immunization of susceptible immunodeficient patients after exposure to varicella. Most effective if begun within 96 hours of exposure. There is no evidence that VZIG modifies established varicella-zoster infections. **Restrict administration to:** Patients with neoplastic disease (leukemia, lymphoma); congenital or acquired immunodeficiency; immunosuppressive therapy with steroids, antimetabolites, or other immunosuppressive treatment regimens; newborns or mothers who had onset of chickenpox within 5 days before delivery or within 48 hours after delivery; premature infant (≥28 weeks gestation) whose mother has no history of chickenpox; premature infants (<28 weeks gestation or ≤1000 g VZIG) regardless of maternal history. **One of the following types of exposure to chickenpox or zoster patients may warrant administration:** Continuous household contact; playmate contact (>1 hour play indoors); hospital contact (in same 2-4 bedroom or adjacent beds in a large ward or prolonged face-to-face contact with an infectious staff member of patient); susceptible to varicella-zoster, age <15 years (administer to immunocompromised adolescents and adults and to other older patients on an individual basis). An acceptable alternative to VZIG prophylaxis is to treat varicella, if it occurs, with high-dose I.V. acyclovir.	Refrigerate at 2°C to 8°C.	I.M. (gluteal muscle or large muscle mass): 125 units/10 kg (22 lb); maximum dose: 625 units (5 vials); minimum dose: 125 units; do not administer fractional doses. High-risk susceptible patients who are exposed again more than 3 weeks after a prior dose of VZIG should receive another full dose; there is no evidence VZIG modifies established varicella-zoster infections.
Yellow fever vaccine YF-VAX®	Induction of active immunity against yellow fever virus, primarily among persons traveling or living in areas where yellow fever infection exists. (Some countries require a valid international Certification of Vaccination showing receipt of vaccine; if a pregnant woman is to be vaccinated only to satisfy an international requirement, efforts should be made to obtain a waiver letter.) The WHO requires revaccination every 10 years to maintain traveler's vaccination certificate.	Do not use vaccine unless shipping case contains some dry ice on arrival; must be shipped on dry ice. Maintain vaccine at continuous temperature of -30°C to 5°C (-22°F to 41°F). Use within 1 hour of reconstitution.	SubQ: 0.5 mL single dose 10 days to 10 years before travel; booster every 10 years

¹Contact Poison Control Center.

²Federal law requires that date of administration, name of vaccine manufacturer, lot number of vaccine, and administering person's name, title, and address be entered into the patient's permanent medical record.

³Not commercially available in the U.S.; presently, all anthrax vaccine lots are owned by the U.S. Department of Defense. The Centers for Disease Control (CDC) does not currently recommend routine vaccination of the general public.

⁴The bulk of current supplies have been designated for use by the U.S. military. Bioterrorism experts have proposed immunization of first responders (including police, fire, and emergency workers), but these plans may not be implemented until additional stocks of vaccine are licensed. Recommendations for use in response to bioterrorism are regularly updated by the CDC, and may be found at www.cdc.gov.

⁵For patients at risk of hemorrhage following intramuscular injection, the ACIP recommends "it should be administered intramuscularly if, in the opinion of the physician familiar with the patients bleeding risk, the vaccine can be administered with reasonable safety by this route. If the patient receives antihemophilia or other similar therapy, intramuscular vaccination can be scheduled shortly after such therapy is administered. A fine needle (23 gauge or smaller) can be used for the vaccination and firm pressure applied to the site (without rubbing) for at least 2 minutes. The patient should be instructed concerning the risk of hematoma from the injection."

⁶All serious adverse reactions must be reported to the U.S. Department of Health and Human Services (DHHS) Vaccine Adverse Event Reporting System (VAERS), 1-800-822-7967.

COMPATIBILITY OF DRUGS

Drug Compatibility Guide

KEY

Y = Compatible
N = Incompatible
Blank = Information about compatibility was not available

	aminophylline	amphotericin B	ampicillin	atropine	calcium gluconate	carbenicillin	cefazolin	cimetidine	clindamycin	diazepam	dopamine	epinephrine	erythromycin	fentanyl	furosemide	gentamicin
aminophylline	□		Y		Y	N	N		N	Y	Y	Y	N	N		
amphotericin B		□	N		N	N		N			N					N
ampicillin	Y	N	□	N	N	Y	Y		N		N		N			N
atropine			N	□				Y		N		N		Y		
calcium gluconate	Y	N	N		□		N		N		Y	N	Y			
carbenicillin	N	N	Y			□	Y	Y		Y	N	N				N
cefazolin	N		Y		N		□	N		Y			N			N
cimetidine		N		Y		Y	N	□	Y			Y	Y		Y	Y
clindamycin	N		N		N	Y		Y	□							Y
diazepam	Y		N			Y				□		N			N	
dopamine	Y	N	N		Y	Y					□					N
epinephrine	N		N	N	N		Y		N			□	N		N	
erythromycin	N		N		Y	N	N	Y				N	□			
fentanyl			Y											□		
furosemide							Y			N		N			□	N
gentamicin		N	N			N	N		Y		Y				N	□
glycopyrrolate			Y								N					
heparin sodium	Y	Y	Y	N	Y			Y	Y	Y	Y	Y	N		Y	N
hydrocortisone	Y	Y	N		Y	Y	Y		Y		Y		Y			
hydroxyzine	N		Y								N			Y		
levarterenol	N			N	Y	N	N	Y		N		N			N	
lidocaine	Y	N	Y		Y	Y	N	Y		N	Y	N	Y			
meperidine	N		Y							N		Y		Y		
morphine	N		Y							N		Y		Y		
nitroglycerin	Y											Y		Y		
pentobarbital	Y		N			N	N	N	N				N	N		
potassium chloride	Y	N	Y	Y	Y	Y	Y	Y	Y	Y	N	Y	N	Y	Y	
sodium bicarbonate	Y	Y		N	N				Y	N		N	Y			
tetracycline	N	N	N			N	N	N	Y			Y		N		N
vancomycin	N		Y					Y					Y			
verapamil	Y	N	Y	Y	Y	Y	Y	Y	Y	Y	Y	Y	Y	Y		Y	Y
vitamin B & C complex	N		Y	Y	Y	N	Y	Y	Y	N	Y	Y	N			Y	Y

NOTE: Because the compatibility of two or more drugs in solution depends on several variables such as the solution itself, drug concentration and the method of mixing (bottle, syringe, or Y-site), this table is intended to be used solely as a guide to general drug compatibilities. Before mixing any drugs, the healthcare professional should ascertain if a potential incompatibility exists by referring to an appropriate information source.

(continued)

KEY

Y = Compatible
N = Incompatible
Blank = Information about compatibility was not available

	glycopyrrolate	heparin sodium	hydrocortisone	hydroxyzine	levarterenol	lidocaine	meperidine	morphine	nitroglycerin	pentobarbital	potassium chloride	sodium bicarbonate	tetracycline	vancomycin	verapamil	vitamin B & C complex
aminophylline		Y	Y	N	N	Y	N	N	Y	Y	Y	Y	N	N	Y	N
amphotericin B		Y	Y			N					N	Y	N		N	
ampicillin		Y	N			Y					Y		N		Y	Y
atrophine	Y	N		Y	N		Y	Y		N	Y	N			Y	Y
calcium gluconate		Y	Y		Y	Y					Y	N	N	Y	Y	Y
carbenicillin		Y		N	Y						Y		N		Y	N
cefazolin		Y		N	N					N	Y		N		Y	Y
cimetidine		Y		Y	Y					N	Y		Y	Y	Y	Y
clindamycin		Y	Y							N	Y	Y			Y	Y
diazepam	N	N		N	N	N	N	N		N	N	N			Y	N
dopamine		Y	Y		Y				Y		Y		Y		Y	Y
epinephrine		Y		N	N	Y					N	N			Y	Y
erythromycin		N	Y		Y					N	Y	Y	N	Y	Y	N
fentanyl			Y				Y	Y		N						
furosemide		Y			N				Y		Y		N		Y	Y
gentamicin		N													Y	Y
glycopyrrolate	□		Y			Y	Y	Y		N		N				
heparin sodium		□	N	N	Y	Y	N	N			Y	Y	N	N	Y	Y
hydrocortisone		N	□	Y	Y					N	Y	Y	N	Y	Y	Y
hydroxyzine	Y	N		□		Y	Y	Y		N						N
levarterenol		Y	Y		□					N	Y		Y		Y	Y
lidocaine	Y	Y	Y	Y		□			Y	Y	Y	Y	Y		Y	Y
meperidine	Y	N	Y				□	N		N		N			Y	
morphine	Y	N	Y				N	□		N	Y	N			Y	Y
nitroglycerin						Y			□						Y	
pentobarbital	N		N	N	N	Y	N	N		□		N	N	N	Y	
potassium chloride		Y	Y		Y	Y		Y			□	Y	Y	Y	Y	
sodium bicarbonate	N	Y	Y			Y	N	N		N	Y	□	N	N	Y	N
tetracycline		N	N	Y	Y					N	Y	N	□			Y
vancomycin		N	Y							N	Y	N		□	Y	Y
verapamil		Y	Y	Y	Y	Y	Y	Y	Y	Y	Y	Y		Y	□	Y
vitamin B & C complex		Y	Y	N	Y	Y		Y			N	Y	Y	Y	Y	□

COMPATIBILITY OF DRUGS IN SYRINGE

Compatibility of Drugs in Syringe

	atropine	butorphanol	chlorpromazine	cimetidine	dimenhydrinate	diphenhydramine	fentanyl	glycopyrrolate	heparin	hydroxyzine	meperidine
atropine	□	Y	Y	Y	M	M	M	Y	M	Y	Y
butorphanol	Y	□	Y	Y	N	Y	Y			Y	M
chlorpromazine	Y	Y	□	N	N	M	M	Y	N	M	M
cimetidine	Y	Y	N	□		Y	Y	Y	Y	Y	Y
dimenhydrinate	M	N	N		□	M	M	N	M	N	M
diphenhydramine	M	Y		Y	M	□		Y		M	M
fentanyl	M	Y	M		M	M	□		M	Y	M
glycopyrrolate	Y		Y	Y	N	Y		□		Y	Y
heparin	M		N		M		M		□		N
hydroxyzine	Y	Y	M	Y	N	M	Y	Y		□	M
meperidine	Y	M	M	Y	M	M	M	Y	N	M	□
metoclopramide	M		M		M	Y	M			M	M
midazolam	Y	Y	Y	Y	N	Y	Y	Y		Y	Y
morphine	M	Y	M	Y	M	M	M	Y	N	Y	N
nalbuphine	Y			Y						Y	
pentazocine	M	Y	M	Y	M	M	M	N	N	Y	M
pentobarbital	M	N	N	N	N	N	N	N		N	N
prochlorperazine	M	Y	Y	Y	N	M	M	Y		M	M
promethazine	M	Y	M	Y	N	M	M	Y	N	M	Y
ranitidine	Y		Y		Y	Y	Y	Y		N	Y
secobarbital				N				N			
thiopental			N		N	N		N			N

KEY
Y = Compatible in a syringe
M = Moderately compatible, inject immediately after combining
N = Incompatible, do not mix in syringe
Blank = Information about compatibility is not currently available

(continued)

	metoclopramide	midazolam	morphine	nalbuphine	pentazocine	pentobarbital	prochlorperazine	promethazine	ranitidine	secobarbital	thiopental
atropine	M	Y	M	Y	M	M	M	M	Y		
butorphanol		Y	Y		Y	N	Y	Y			
chlorpromazine	M	Y	M		M	N	Y	M	Y		N
cimetidine		Y	Y	Y	Y	N	Y	Y		N	
dimenhydrinate	M	N	M		M	N	N	N	Y		N
diphenhydramine	Y	Y	M		M	N	M	M	Y		N
fentanyl	M	Y	M		M	N	M	M	Y		
glycopyrrolate		Y	Y		N	N	Y	Y	Y	N	
heparin	M		N		N			N			
hydroxyzine	M	Y	Y	Y	Y	N	M	M	N		
meperidine	M	Y	N		M	N	M	Y	Y		N
metoclopramide	□	Y	M		M		M	M	Y		
midazolam	Y	□	Y	Y		N	N	Y	N		
morphine	M	Y	□		M	N	M	M	Y		N
nalbuphine		Y		□		N	Y	Y	Y		
pentazocine	M		M		□	N	M	Y	Y		
pentobarbital	N	N	N	N	N	□	N	N			Y
prochlorperazine	M	N	M	Y	M	N	□	M	Y		N
promethazine	M	Y	M	Y	Y	N	M	□	Y		N
ranitidine	Y	N	Y	Y	Y		Y	Y	□		
secobarbital										□	
thiopental			N			Y	N	N			□

Reprinted from Malseed RT, Goldstein FJ, & Balkon N, *Pharmacology: Drug Therapy and Nursing Management* (4th ed), Philadelphia: JB Lippincott Co (1995). Used with permission.

MANAGEMENT OF DRUG EXTRAVASATIONS

Vesicant: Causes tissue destruction.

Irritant: Causes aching, tightness, and phlebitis with or without inflammation.

Extravasation: Leakage of fluid out of a blood vessel.

Vesicant extravasation: Leakage of a drug that causes pain, necrosis, or tissue sloughing.

Delayed extravasation: Symptoms occur 48 hours after drug administration.

Flare: Local, nonpainful, possibly allergic reaction often accompanied by reddening along the vein.

A potential, and potentially highly morbid, complication of drug therapy is soft tissue damage caused by leakage of the drug solution out of the vein. A variety of complications, including erythema, ulceration, pain, tissue sloughing, and necrosis are possible. This problem is not unique to antineoplastic therapy; a variety of drugs have been reported to cause tissue damage if extravasated.

Vesicant Agents

Hyperosmotic Agents (>280 mOsm/L)	Ischemia Inducers	Direct Cellular Toxins	
		Nonantineoplastic Agents	**Antineoplastic Agents**
Calcium chloride (>10%)	Dobutamine	Aminophylline	Amsacrine
Contrast media	Dopamine	Chlordiazepoxide	Dactinomycin
Crystalline amino acids (4.25%)	Epinephrine	Diazepam	Daunorubicin
Dextrose (>10%)		Digoxin	Doxorubicin
Mannitol (>5%)	Norepinephrine	Ethanol	Epirubicin
Potassium chloride (>2 mEq/mL)	Phenylephrine	Nafcillin	Idarubicin
Sodium bicarbonate (8.4%)	Vasopressin	Nitroglycerine	Mechlorethamine
Sodium chloride (>1%)		Phenytoin Propylene glycol Sodium thiopental Tetracycline	Mitomycin Streptozocin (?) Vinblastine Vincristine Vindesine Vinorelbine

In addition to the known vesicants, a number of other antineoplastic agents, not generally considered to be vesicants, have been associated with isolated reports of tissue damage following extravasation.

Agents Associated With Occasional Extravasation Reactions

Aclacinomycin

Bleomycin

Carmustine

Cisplatin

Dacarbazine

Esorubicin

Etoposide

Floxuridine

Fluorouracil

Menogaril

Mitoxantrone

Paclitaxel

Teniposide

The actual incidence of drug extravasations is unknown. Some of the uncertainty stems from varying definitions of incidence. Incidence rates have been reported based on total number of drug doses administered, number of vesicant doses administered, number of treatments, number of patients treated with vesicants, and total number of patients treated. Most estimates place the incidence of extravasations with cytotoxic agents in the range of 1% to 7%.

The optimal treatment of drug extravasations is uncertain. A variety of antidotes have been proposed; however, objective clinical evidence to support these recommendations frequently is not available. There are no well done randomized prospective trials of potential treatments. Controlled clinical trials are not feasible, limiting efforts to identify optimal management of these reactions. Extant reports are based on animal models, anecdotal cases, and/or small uncontrolled series of patients. Many of the existing reports, both animal and human, used more than one therapeutic intervention, adding to the difficulty of identifying the efficacy of any single approach.

The best "treatment" for extravasation reactions is prevention. Although it is not possible to prevent all accidents, a few simple precautions can minimize the risk to the patient. The vein used should be a large, intact vessel with good blood flow. To minimize the risk of dislodging the catheter, veins in the hands and in the vicinity of joints (eg, antecubital) should be avoided. Veins in the forearm (ie, the basilic, cephalic, and median antebrachial, basilic and cephalic) are usually good options for peripheral infusions. Prior to drug administration, the patency of the I.V. line should be verified. The line should be flushed with 5-10 mL of a saline or dextrose solution; and the drug(s) infused through the side of a free-flowing isotonic saline or dextrose infusion.

A frequently recommended precaution against drug extravasation is the use of a central venous catheter. Use of a central line has several advantages, including high patient satisfaction, reliable venous access, high flow rates, and rapid dilution of the drug. A wide variety of devices are readily available. Many institutions encourage or require use of a vascular access device for administration of vesicant agents.

Despite their benefit, central lines are not an absolute solution. Vascular access devices are subject to a number of complications. The catheter tip may not be properly positioned in the superior vena cava/right atrium, or may migrate out of position. Additionally, these catheters require routine care to maintain patency and avoid infections. Finally, extravasation of drugs from venous access devices is possible. Misplacement/migration of the catheter tip, improper placement of the needle in accessing injection ports, and cuts, punctures, or rupture of the catheter itself have all been reported. One report found a 6.4% extravasation rate from subcutaneous ports, quite similar to extravasation rates reported from peripheral lines.

When a drug extravasation does occur, a variety of immediate actions have been recommended. Although there is considerable uncertainty regarding the value of some potential treatments, a few initial steps seem to be generally accepted.

1. **Stop the infusion.** At the first suspicion of infiltration, the drug infusion should be stopped. If infiltration is not certain, the line can be tested by attempting to aspirate blood, and careful infusion of a few milliliters of saline or dextrose solution.

2. **Do NOT remove the catheter/needle.** The infiltrated catheter should not be removed immediately. It should be left in place to facilitate aspiration of fluid from the extravasation site, and, if appropriate, administration of an antidote.

3. **Aspirate fluid.** To the extent possible, the extravasated drug solution should be removed from the subcutaneous tissues.

4. **Do NOT flush the line.** Flooding the infiltration site with saline or dextrose in an attempt to dilute the drug solution generally is not recommended. Rather than minimizing damage, such a procedure may have the opposite effect by distributing the vesicant solution over a wider area.

5. **Remove the catheter/needle.** If an antidote is not going to be injected into the extravasation site, the infiltrated catheter should be removed. If an antidote is to be injected into the area, it should be injected through the catheter to ensure delivery of the antidote to the infiltration site. When this has been accomplished, the catheter should then be removed.

Two issues for which there is less consensus are the application of heat or cold, and the use of various antidotes. A variety of recommendations exist for each of these concerns; there is no consensus concerning the proper approach.

Cold. Intermittent cooling of the area of infiltration results in vasoconstriction, which tends to restrict the spread of the drug. It may also inhibit the local effects of some drugs (eg, anthracyclines). Application of cold is usually recommended as immediate treatment for most cytotoxic drug extravasations, except the vinca alkaloids. In one report of extravasation treatment, almost 90% of the extravasations treated only with ice required no further therapy.

The largest single published series of cytotoxic drug extravasations was 175 patients reported by Larson in 1985. This series includes some of the more commonly used vesicants, including the anthracyclines, mechlorethamine, mitomycin, and the vinca alkaloids. For 119 patients, local application of ice (15 minutes four times a day for 3 days) and close observation was the sole treatment. The remaining 56 patients received a variety of antidotes. In 89% of the patients treated with ice alone, the extravasation resolved without further treatment. Of the patients treated by other methods, only 53% resolved without further treatment.

Helpful as it may be, Larson's report does have some limitations. Agents such as the podophyllotoxins and taxanes which are occasionally associated with soft tissue damage were not included. The report included infiltrations of the vinca alkaloids, even though the literature recommends use of heat to treat these. Also, except for doxorubicin extravasations in the group treated with ice and observation, responses for the individual drugs were not indicated. In this group, 72% of the doxorubicin extravasations resolved completely.

Heat. Application of heat results in a localized vasodilation and increased blood flow. Increased circulation is believed to facilitate removal of the drug from the area of infiltration. The data supporting use of heat are less convincing than for cold. One report of the application of heat for nonantineoplastic drug extravasations suggested application of heat increased the risk of skin maceration and necrosis. Most data are from animal studies, with relatively few human case reports. Animal models indicate application of heat exacerbates the damage from anthracycline extravasations. No large series of extravasations managed with the application of heat has been published. Heat is generally recommended for treatment for vinca alkaloid extravasations; a few reports recommend it for podophyllotoxin and paclitaxel infiltrations. There are conflicting reports on the initial management of paclitaxel infiltrations. The Oncology Nursing Society recommends applying ice, a report from MD Anderson Institute recommends heat, other reports indicate neither approach is effective.

ANTIDOTES

A very wide variety of agents have been reported as possible antidotes for extravasated drugs, with no consensus on their proper use. For a number of reasons, evaluation of the various reports is difficult.

1. **Mechanism of action.** For many drugs, the underlying mechanism responsible for the tissue damage is not certain. For some of the antidotes, the purported mechanism of action of the antidote is also unclear.

2. **Controlled trials.** Prospective, randomized controlled trials are not practical. Information concerning treatment of extravasations is based almost exclusively on animal models, anecdotal reports, and small, uncontrolled studies.

MANAGEMENT OF DRUG EXTRAVASATIONS *(Continued)*

3. **Outcomes definitions.** Published reports use a number of different end-points and outcomes to define efficacy of a given treatment.

4. **Confounding factors.** A number of confounding factors exist which make assessment of various antidotes difficult. Among these are:

   a. Response to nonpharmacologic therapy. Application of heat or cold alone, especially the latter, appears to have a significant protective effect.

   b. Multiple therapies. A number of reports used more than one therapeutic modality to treat drug extravasations. In many cases, cold or heat is applied along with the antidote. In some cases, more than one antidote is used, sometimes in conjunction with heat or cold. Use of multiple approaches further complicates the determination of the possible effect of a particular antidote, or the additive effect of various combinations.

   c. Variable applications. For some proposed antidotes, different doses, concentrations, methods of application, and duration of therapy have been reported.

Agents Used as Antidotes

Albumin	Fluorescein
Antihistamines	Iron dextran
Antioxidants	Isoproterenol
Beta-adrenergics	Radical dimer
Carnitine	Saline
Corticosteroids[1]	Sodium bicarbonate
Dextranomer	Sodium hypochlorite
Dimethylsulfoxide	Sodium thiosulfate[1]
Dopamine	Vitamin E

[1]Listed in the package insert of at least one agent.

Sodium bicarbonate. An 8.4% solution of sodium bicarbonate was briefly recommended for treatment of anthracycline extravasations. The recommendation was based on a case report of its use in a single patient. The proposed mechanism of action was that the high pH of the bicarbonate solution would break the glycosidic bond of the anthracycline; thereby, inactivating it. Follow-up studies in a variety of animal models failed to confirm the original report. Also, the concentrated sodium bicarbonate may itself be a vesicant. See the Vesicant Agents table. At present, most reviews discourage its use and the Oncology Nursing Society (ONS) guidelines for treating extravasations do not include sodium bicarbonate to treat anthracycline infiltrations.

Corticosteroids. Steroids are most commonly used to treat anthracycline extravasations. Hydrocortisone is the steroid most frequently recommended, although dexamethasone has also been used. It is suggested that steroids reduce local inflammation from the extravasated drug. Such activity has not been confirmed; nor has it been demonstrated that the tissue damage from drug infiltrations is the result of an inflammatory process. Interpretation of steroid efficacy is complicated by the multiple doses, routes of administration, duration of therapy, and outcome measurements used. Reports of animal trials offer little additional information, being plagued by many of the limitations of the clinical case reports. The official labeling of only one of the three suppliers of doxorubicin includes a steroid as part of the treatment for drug extravasations. The product labeling from two doxorubicin suppliers, as well as the suppliers of daunorubicin, idarubicin, and liposome-encapsulated anthracyclines do not mention corticosteroids to treat drug infiltrations. The ONS extravasation guidelines also do not include a steroid as part of the treatment of anthracycline extravasations.

Dimethyl sulfoxide (DMSO). A number of reports have suggested application of DMSO is an effective treatment for infiltrations of a number of different drugs. It is believed DMSO's protective effect is due to its ability to act as a free radical scavenger (one theory suggests tissue damage from vesicants, particularly anthracyclines, is due to formation of hydroxyl free radicals). Results in animal models have been equivocal, with some reports indicating DMSO is beneficial, and some showing little or no effect. Clinical reports of its use are extremely difficult to interpret due to variations in DMSO concentration, number of applications/day, duration of therapy, and concomitant treatments. A number of different treatments, including cold, steroids, vitamin E, and sodium bicarbonate have been used in conjunction with DMSO. Also, most studies used DMSO concentrations >90% which is not available for clinical use in the United States.

A further complication to interpretation of DMSO's efficacy is that some series included infiltrations of agents not generally considered to be vesicants. The largest clinical series included infiltrations in 75 patients; but only 31 of the extravasations involved vesicants (doxorubicin, epirubicin, or mitomycin). The remaining incidents involved drugs not usually associated with tissue damage (cisplatin, ifosfamide, and mitoxantrone). Application of 99% DMSO for 7 days and ice for 3 days resulted in a 93.5% success rate in the patients with vesicant extravasations. Only two patients (6.5%) had complications requiring further therapy. Whether the addition of DMSO represented a real improvement over ice alone is difficult to assess.

Sodium thiosulfate. A freshly prepared 1/6 M (~4%) solution of sodium thiosulfate has been recommended for treatment of mechlorethamine and cisplatin infiltrations. This recommendation is based on *in vitro* data demonstrating an interaction between sodium thiosulfate and cisplatin, dacarbazine, and mechlorethamine; and very limited animal data on thiosulfate's ability to inactivate dacarbazine and mechlorethamine. At present, no clinical reports of its efficacy for treating cisplatin or dacarbazine extravasations have been published. Since cisplatin and dacarbazine are generally not considered to be vesicants, the use of thiosulfate to treat infiltrations of these drugs may not be required.

The use of sodium thiosulfate to treat mechlorethamine infiltrations is based almost exclusively on the *in vitro* and animal data. A single case report of successful thiosulfate treatment of an accidental intramuscular mechlorethamine injection has been published. Thus far, no reports of thiosulfate treatment of mechlorethamine infiltrations have been published.

One study of thiosulfate therapy of antineoplastic drug extravasations has been published. In a series of 63 patients with extravasation of doxorubicin, epirubicin, mitomycin, or vinblastine, 31 were treated with subcutaneous hydrocortisone and topical dexamethasone. The remaining 32 patients received subcutaneous injection of a 2% thiosulfate solution in addition to the subcutaneous and topical steroids. No patient in either group developed skin ulceration or required surgery; but the patients who received the thiosulfate healed in about half the time as the patients who received only the steroid therapy.

Selected Readings

Barlock AL, Howser DM, and Hubbard SM, "Nursing Management of Adriamycin Extravasation," *Am J Nurs*, 1979, 137:94-6.

Bertelli G, "Prevention and Management of Extravasation of Cytotoxic Drugs," *Drug Safety*, 1995, 12(4):245-55.

Boyle DM and Engelking C, "Vesicant Extravasation: Myths and Realities," *Oncol Nurs Forum*, 1995, 22(1):57-67.

Brothers TE, Von Moll LK, Niederhuber JE, et al, "Experience With Subcutaneous Infusion Ports in Three Hundred Patients," *Surg Gynecol Obstet*, 1988, 166(4):295-301.

Dorr RT, "Antidotes to Vesicant Chemotherapy Extravasations," *Blood Rev*, 1990, 4(1):41-60.

Dorr RT, "Pharmacologic Management of Vesicant Chemotherapy Extravasations," *Cancer Chemotherapy Handbook*, 2nd ed, Dorr RT and Von Hoff, DD, Norwalk, CT: Appleton & Lange, 1994, 109-18.

Dorr RT and Alberts DS, "Vinca Alkaloid Skin Toxicity: Antidote and Drug Disposition Studies in the Mouse," *J Natl Cancer Inst*, 1985, 74(1):113-20.

Dorr RT, Alberts DS, and Stone A, "Cold Protection and Heat Enhancement of Doxorubicin Skin Toxicity in the Mouse," *Cancer Treat Rep*, 1985, 69(4):431-7.

Larson DL, "What Is the Appropriate Management of Tissue Extravasation by Antitumor Agents?" *J Plast Reconstr Surg*, 1985, 75:397-402.

Larson DL, "Treatment of Tissue Extravasation by Antitumor Agents," *Cancer*, 1982, 49:1796-9.

Larson DL, "Alterations in Wound Healing Secondary to Infusion Injury," *Clin Plast Surg*, 1990, 17(3):509-17.

Rudolph R and Larson DL, "Etiology and Treatment of Chemotherapeutic Agent Extravasation Injuries: A Review," *J Clin Oncol*, 1987, 5(7):1116-26.

"Vesicants and Irritants," *Cancer Chemotherapy Guidelines and Recommendations for Practice*, Oncology Nursing Society, 1996, 55-9.

MANAGEMENT OF DRUG EXTRAVASATIONS (Continued)

Reported Treatment Regimens for Cytotoxic Drug Extravasations

Treatment	Dose	Route	Duration	Concomitant Therapy	Used to Treat
Cold[1]	15 min qid	Topical	3-4 days	None	All agents[2]
Heat[1]	15 min on; 15 min off	Topical	1 day	None	Vinca alkaloids
Heat	NS	Topical	NS	None	Epipodophyllotoxins, taxanes[3]
Hydrocortisone	100 mg	I.V., SubQ, I.D.	One time	Ice	All agents except vinca alkaloids
Dimethylsulfoxide[4]	99% q8h	Topical	1 week	Ice for 3 days	Doxorubicin
Dimethylsulfoxide[4]	99% q2-4h	Topical	3 days	None	Doxorubicin
Dimethylsulfoxide[4]	99% q6-24h	Topical	14 days	None	Doxorubicin
Dimethylsulfoxide[4]	90% q12h	Topical	2 days	Vitamin E 10%	Doxorubicin, esorubicin, mitomycin
Dimethylsulfoxide[4]	99% q6-12h	Topical	1-5 weeks	None	Mitomycin
Sodium thiosulfate	2%	SubQ	One time	SubQ and topical steroids	Doxorubicin, epirubicin, vinblastine, mitomycin
Sodium thiosulfate[1]	1/6 M (~4%)	I.V., SubQ	One time	Ice or heat	Mechlorethamine, cisplatin

NS = not specified; I.V. = intravenous; SubQ = subcutaneous; I.D. = intradermal.

[1]Listed in the package insert of at least one product.

[2]Most guidelines discourage application of cold to treat infiltrations of vinca alkaloids. Some reports discourage its use to treat infiltrations of epipodophyllotoxins and/or taxanes.

[3]There are conflicting data on the efficacy or heat or cold for infiltrations of epipodophyllotoxins and taxanes. Each approach has been reported to be effective, harmful, and of no discernable effect.

[4]DMSO concentrations >50% are not available for human use in the U.S.

MANAGEMENT OF NAUSEA AND VOMITING

> **Nausea:** The feeling or sensation of an imminent desire to vomit.
>
> **Vomiting:** The forceful upward expulsion of gastric contents.
>
> **Retching:** Rhythmic, labored, spasmodic respiratory movements involving the diaphragm, chest wall, and abdominal muscles.

Nausea and vomiting are common side effects of many antineoplastic agents and are often the effects patients fear most. Uncontrolled nausea and vomiting can have a significant impact on a patient's overall therapy and response to treatment. In addition to the deleterious effect on the patient's attitude and quality of life, nausea and vomiting can cause significant, potentially fatal complications. Uncontrolled nausea and vomiting can result in dehydration, electrolyte imbalances, weight loss, and malnutrition. Prolonged vomiting and retching can cause esophageal and/or gastric ruptures (Mallory-Weiss tears, Boerhaave's syndrome) and bleeding. Patients with poorly-controlled nausea or vomiting often require interruptions or delays in therapy. This can also lead to development of anticipatory nausea and vomiting, the patient's loss of confidence in the overall therapy, noncompliance, and refusal of further therapy.

Table 1. Causes of Nausea or Vomiting

Abdominal Emergencies
- Appendicitis
- Cholecystitis
- Peritonitis
- GI obstruction

Acute Systemic Infections
- Bacterial
- Parasitic
- Viral

Cardiovascular Disorders
- Congestive heart failure
- Myocardial infarction

CNS Disorders
- Hypotension
- Increased intracranial pressure
- Mènière's disease
- Otitis interna
- Syncope

Drugs
- Antibiotics
- Antineoplastics
- Aspirin
- Cardiac glycosides
- Levodopa
- Nonsteroidal anti-inflammatory agents
- Opiates
- Quinidine
- Steroids
- Theophylline

Endocrine Disorders
- Adrenal insufficiency
- Diabetes mellitus

Gastrointestinal Disorders

Pregnancy

Psychogenic Stimuli

Uremia

Emesis is controlled by a complex system, centering on the vomiting (or emetic) center in the medulla, and the chemoreceptor trigger zone (CTZ) located in the area postrema in the fourth ventricle of the brain. A network of various neuroreceptors, located throughout the gastrointestinal tract and CNS, processes signals to and from the emetic center and CTZ. When stimulated by impulses from visceral afferents, vestibular or limbic systems, cerebral cortex, or chemoreceptor trigger zone, the emetic center transmits signals that initiate the vomiting cascade. These impulses from the emetic center stimulate the salivary, vasomotor, respiratory centers, and cranial nerves, and initiate the vomiting reflex. Activation of the vomiting center appears to be crucial to initiation of vomiting. Elimination of the vomiting center, or failure to stimulate it, completely eliminates vomiting.

Receptors for a large number of different neurotransmitters, including dopamine, serotonin, acetylcholine, histamine, opiates, and benzodiazepines, are involved in the vomiting reflex. Blockade of one or more of these receptors is the basic mechanism of action of most antiemetic agents. Most drug-induced nausea, including that provoked by the antineoplastic drugs, appears to be caused by activation of the emetic center by impulses from the peripheral afferents and/or the CTZ. Blockade of these impulses is a primary focus of antiemetic therapy.

Nausea and vomiting caused by cytotoxic therapy generally falls into one of three categories: immediate, acute, or delayed. While not drug-induced *per se*, a fourth syndrome, anticipatory nausea and vomiting, is also a relatively common complication of antineoplastic therapy. Immediate nausea/vomiting occurs within the first 30-120 minutes of drug administration. Acute nausea/vomiting is seen within the first 24 hours of drug administration. These two syndromes are often grouped together under the term acute nausea/vomiting. Delayed nausea/vomiting begins after the first 24 hours of drug administration; however, in some cases, onset may be delayed for as long as 3-5 days. Even in the absence of actual emesis, patients may experience varying degrees of nausea, often accompanied by anorexia.

Table 2 describes the emetogenic potential of many of the antineoplastic agents. Several factors affect the emetic potential of these agents. For some drugs, such as cyclophosphamide or methotrexate, the dose given has a significant effect on the drug's emetogenicity. Higher doses of these agents are much more emetogenic than low doses. The method of administration can also affect the incidence of nausea. Cytarabine, when given as a continuous infusion, is generally moderately emetogenic; higher doses given as short infusions usually produce a much higher incidence and severity of nausea and vomiting.

MANAGEMENT OF NAUSEA AND VOMITING *(Continued)*

Management of Nausea and Vomiting

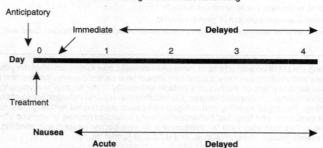

Patterns of drug-induced nausea/vomiting

Table 2. Emetogenic Potential of Antineoplastic Agents

Very High (>90%)

Cisplatin	Dacarbazine	JM-216	Melphalan (I.V.)
Cytarabine (>2 g)	Didemnin-B	Mechlorethamine	Streptozocin

High (60% to 90%)

Aldesleukin	Dactinomycin	Gemtuzumab ozogamicin	Mitotane
Amifostine	Denileukin diftitox	Hydroxyurea	Mitoxantorone
Arsenic trioxide	Elsamitrucin	Idarubicin	Oxaliplatin
Bortezomib	Epirubicin	Irinotecan	Pemetrexed
Carmustine	Estramustine	Lomustine	Toremifene
Cyclophosphamide (>1 g)	Etoposide	Mitomycin	Tretinoin
Cytarabine (<2 g)	Gemcitabine		

Moderate (30% to 60%)

Alemtuzumab	Daunorubicin	Ibritumomab	Raltitrexed
Altretamine	Daunorubicin (liposomal)	Ifosfamide	Temozolomide
Aminocamptothecin	Dexrazoxane	Imatinib	Teniposide
Amonafide	Diazequone	Interferons	Tomudex
Amsacrine	Docetaxel	Interleukin-6	Topotecan
Asparaginase	Doxorubicin	Mitoguazone	Tositumomab
Azacitidine	Epirubicin	PALA	Trastuzumab
Bevacizumab	Floxuridine	Pegaspargase	Trimetrexate
Carboplatin	Flutamide	Pentostatin	UFT
Cetuximab	Fulvestrant	Plicamycin	Vinblastine
Cladribine	Gefitinib	Procarbazine	Vinorelbine
Cyclophosphamide (<1 g)			

Low (10% to 30%)

Abarelix	Exemestane	Letrozole	Rituximab
BCG vaccine	Floxuridine	Levamisole	Steroids
Bexarotene	Fluorouracil	Melphalan (oral)	Suramin
Cetuximab	Flutamide	Methotrexate (high dose)	Tamoxifen
Cytarabine (liposomal)	Fulvestrant	Nilutamide	Thioguanine
Doxorubicin (liposomal)	Gefitinib	Porfimer	Vindesine
Etoposide phosphate	Gemcitabine		

Very Low (<10%)

Alitretinoin	Busulfan	Leucovorin	Paclitaxel
Androgens	Chlorambucil	Leuprolide	Thalidomide
Aminoglutethimide	Estrogens	Megestrol	Thiotepa
Anastrozole	Fludarabine	Mercaptopurine	Triptorelin
Bicalutamide	Goserelin	Mesna	Valrubicin
Bleomycin	Homoharringtonine	Methotrexate (low dose)	Vincristine

Drugs With a High Incidence But Low Severity of Nausea / Vomiting

Amonafide	Docetaxel	Mitoguazone
Carboplatin	Gemcitabine	Mitoxantrone
Cyclophosphamide (<1 g)	Hydroxyurea	Tretinoin
Dexrazoxane	Interferons	Vinblastine

Drugs With a Low Incidence But High Severity of Nausea / Vomiting

Lomustine	Methotrexate (high dose)	Semustine

DELAYED NAUSEA AND VOMITING

The problem of delayed nausea and vomiting has become more obvious within the last few years. As more effective drugs and combination regimens were developed to control acute nausea/vomiting, the delayed syndrome has emerged as a more significant problem. Although it is most commonly associated with cisplatin, delayed nausea may also be seen in patients receiving mitomycin, cyclophosphamide, or ifosfamide. The nausea or vomiting generally begins within 48-72 hours after chemotherapy administration, but may be seen as early as 16-18 hours after drug administration, or as late as 4 or 5 days. The nausea/vomiting usually resolves over 2 or 3 days. The exact cause of this effect is not clear; however, it is believed to have a separate mechanism from acute nausea or vomiting. Gastritis, tissue destruction, electrolyte fluctuations, or effects on the central or peripheral nervous system have all been postulated as possible mechanisms for delayed nausea.

Appropriate therapy for delayed nausea and vomiting remains problematic. Current information seems to support early prophylactic therapy with a steroid, steroid/serotonin antagonist, or steroid/dopamine antagonist combination as the most effective therapy for delayed nausea and vomiting. In patients refractory to a steroid/serotonin regimen, aprepitant, a neurokinin receptor antagonist, may be added. The current approach to delayed nausea and vomiting tends to favor a scheduled, prophylactic regimen of dexamethasone, or dexamethasone/serotonin or dopamine antagonist combination, beginning 16-24 hours after administration of the chemotherapy, and continuing for 2-5 days. This approach is more advantageous than intermittent intervention with a 5HT$_3$ antagonist.

BREAKTHROUGH NAUSEA AND VOMITING

Continuing the same regimen that failed to prevent vomiting usually is not desirable. There is little evidence that breakthrough vomiting may respond to an additional dose(s) of a serotonin blocker. A scheduled regimen of "conventional" antiemetics is probably more effective than intermittent administration of a 5HT$_3$ antagonist. Merely increasing the dose of the serotonin antagonist may not be an option either. The currently available serotonin antagonists have relatively flat dose/response curves. Dose response studies have demonstrated that granisetron's efficacy seems to reach a plateau at 10 mcg/kg. There appears to be no difference in efficacy between granisetron doses of 10 mcg/kg and 40 mcg/kg. A similar limitation exists for dolasetron, ondansetron, and palonosetron. A number of reports suggests that ondansetron doses between 20-32 mg have comparable efficacy in preventing nausea induced by a variety of antineoplastic drugs. Daily doses >32 mg seem to provide no increase in response. Data are also lacking on the value of using a different serotonin antagonist to treat nausea/vomiting resulting from the failure of the initial serotonin antagonist regimen.

Likewise, there is minimal information regarding the appropriate prophylactic antiemetic regimen for subsequent chemotherapy cycles, both in patients who responded well during the initial treatment cycle, and in patients who do not respond well to the initial serotonin antagonist/steroid regimen. Several reports suggest the efficacy of the initial antiemetic regimen diminishes over time. Patients often experience gradual increased incidences of nausea and vomiting during subsequent treatment cycles. A number of possible alternatives exist, including switching to another serotonin antagonist, switching to a nonserotonin modulating antiemetic, adding a nonserotonin blocking antiemetic to the original regimen, and altering the schedule of drug administration. The addition of a neurokinin receptor antagonist (eg, aprepitant) to the previous serotonin antagonist/steroid regimen is recommended. One study suggests that the addition of low-dose propofol to the steroid/serotonin antagonist may be useful.

MANAGEMENT OF NAUSEA AND VOMITING (Continued)

Table 3. Classification of Antiemetic Agents

Antihistamines	Diphenhydramine, hydroxyzine, promethazine
Anticholinergics	Scopolamine
Benzodiazepines	Diazepam, lorazepam
Butyrophenones	Droperidol, haloperidol
Cannabinoids	Dronabinol, nabilone
Corticosteroids	Dexamethasone, methylprednisolone
Neurokinin antagonists	Aprepitant, ezlopitant,[1] vofopitant,[1] L-758298,[1] CP-122721[1]
Phenothiazines	Chlorpromazine, perphenazine, prochlorperazine, thiethylperazine,[1] triflupromazine, (promethazine)
Serotonin antagonists	Dolasetron, granisetron, ondansetron, palonosetron, tropesitron[1]
Substituted benzamides	Metoclopramide, trimethobenzamide

[1]Not commercially available in the U.S.

Table 4. Site of Action of Antiemetic Agents

Emetic center	Antihistamines, anticholinergics, serotonin antagonists
Chemoreceptor trigger zone (CTZ)	Benzamides, butyrophenones, phenothiazines
Cerebral cortex	Antihistamines, benzodiazepines, cannabinoids, (corticosteroids), neurokinin antagonists(?)
Peripheral	Metoclopramide, neurokinin antagonists, serotonin antagonists
Unknown	Corticosteroids

Table 5. Equitherapeutic Serotonin Antagonist Doses

Drug	Oral	I.V.
Dolasetron	100-200 mg	1.8 mg/kg or 100 mg
Granisetron	2 mg	10 mcg/kg or 1 mg
Ondansetron	8-24 mg	8-10 mg
Palonosetron	–	0.25 mg

Anticholinergics. Alkaloids (eg, atropine and scopolamine) exhibit some antiemetic activity, primarily postoperative nausea and vomiting, and motion sickness. The apparent mechanism of action is blockage of central muscarinic receptors. Toxicities such as sedation, restlessness, blurred vision, and dry mouth limit the systemic use of these agents. Transdermal application of scopolamine is sometimes helpful as an adjunct in delayed nausea, or in treating prolonged mild nausea seen occasionally. The recent lack of availability of the transdermal scopolamine formulation effectively precludes use of this drug for chemotherapy-induced nausea.

Antihistamines. The antihistamines block H_1 receptors both centrally and in the middle ear. A number of drugs in this class are effective against motion sickness and labyrinth disorders; but only diphenhydramine, hydroxyzine, and promethazine seem to have any activity against chemotherapy-induced nausea or vomiting. The major toxicities seen with these drugs are drowsiness, sedation, and dry mouth. These agents are most commonly used to enhance the efficacy of combination antiemetic regimens, although hydroxyzine or promethazine are occasionally used to treat mild-to-moderate nausea in patients who cannot tolerate, or are refractory to, other antiemetics. Diphenhydramine is frequently used in combination with dopamine antagonists to prevent extrapyramidal reactions often seen with those agents.

Benzodiazepines. The exact antiemetic mechanism or location of action of the benzodiazepines is unclear. An inhibitory effect on the vomiting center, anxiolytic activity, and general CNS depression have all been postulated. Possible sites of action include the limbic system, vomiting center, cerebrum, and brain stem. The most common side effects include sedation, drowsiness, and amnesia. Lorazepam is the most commonly used benzodiazepine, but midazolam and diazepam have also been used. As single agents, the benzodiazepines have only mild antiemetic activity. Benzodiazepines are commonly used as adjuncts to conventional antiemetics in the prophylaxis and treatment of acute nausea and vomiting. In this setting, the anterograde amnesia induced by the benzodiazepine is usually considered a desired therapeutic effect rather than an adverse reaction. The benzodiazepines are also highly effective in the prevention of anticipatory nausea and vomiting, possibly due to their anxiolytic effect.

Butyrophenones. A group of dopamine antagonists that is occasionally useful in treating chemotherapy-induced nausea and vomiting is the butyrophenones. Both haloperidol and droperidol have been reported to have antiemetic activity against moderate-to-highly emetogenic chemotherapy. Domperidone, a related drug, is also reported to have antiemetic activity; however, significant cardiovascular toxicities have limited trials with this drug. As with most other antiemetics, the optimum response to the butyrophenones is seen in multidrug regimens. Like other dopamine blockers, extrapyramidal reactions, restlessness, sedation, and hypotension are relatively common side effects.

Cannabinoids. Proper evaluation of the antiemetic activity of cannabinoid derivatives has been hindered by social and political stigmas associated with marijuana use. Tetrahydrocannabinol, levonantradol, and nabilone are all reported to be effective in treating chemotherapy-induced nausea and vomiting. The specific site and mechanism of activity is unclear. Inhibition of endorphins in the emetic center, suppression of prostaglandin synthesis, and inhibition of medullary activity through an unspecified cortical action have all been postulated. Cannabinoids can inhibit buildup of cyclic adenosine monophosphate, and cannabinoid receptors have been identified in the hippocampus, hypothalamus, and cortex. What role, if any, these have in the control of nausea and vomiting is not known. Cannabinoids seem to be most effective against mild-to-moderately emetogenic chemotherapy. Blurred vision, hypotension, and tachycardia, and a number of CNS complications, including euphoria, dysphoria, hallucinations, and sedation are seen with cannabinoid therapy. Cannabinoids are not often used as initial antiemetic therapy, but do offer an alternative in patients unable to tolerate, or who are refractory to, other antiemetic agents.

Corticosteroids. The mechanism of antiemetic activity for the steroids is unknown, although alterations of cell permeability and inhibition of prostaglandin synthesis have been postulated. In spite of this uncertainty, corticosteroids, particularly dexamethasone, are frequent components of combination antiemetic regimens for high-to-moderately emetogenic chemotherapy. As a single agent, dexamethasone appears to be equal to, or more effective than, $5HT_3$ antagonists for delayed nausea and vomiting. For patients in whom a corticosteroid is not clearly contraindicated, these agents are an important component of antiemetic therapy.

Neurokinin-1 (NK$_1$) Receptor Antagonists. Neurokinin, or substance P, antagonists are the latest class of antiemetics. Substance P is a tachykinin (neurokinin) located in neurons of the central and peripheral nervous system. It is associated with a variety of functions, including emesis, depression, inflammatory pain and inflammatory/immune responses in asthma, and other diseases. Substance P's activity is mediated by the NK_1 receptor, a G-protein receptor coupled to the inositol phosphate signal pathway. Blocking this receptor is a mechanism to treat conditions mediated at least in part by substance P. Several neurokinin receptor antagonists, including aprepitant (MK-869, L-754030), its prodrug L-758298, ezlopitant (CJ-11974), vofopitant (GR-205171), and CP-122721 have been studied, but aprepitant is the only one that has been approved for marketing. NK$_1$ antagonists are effective in preventing cisplatin-induced nausea and vomiting, when used in conjunction with a serotonin antagonist and steroid. Addition of a neurokinin antagonist to a serotonin ($5HT_3$) antagonist and steroid combination increases control of acute nausea by 10% to 15%, and control of delayed nausea by 20% to 30%. Most studies indicate the neurokinin receptors are less effective then serotonin antagonists, particularly for prevention of acute nausea within the first 8-12 hours. However, the neurokinin antagonists appear to be more effective than serotonin antagonists in preventing delayed nausea (days 2-5). Although the National Cancer Coordinating Network (NCCN) and Multinational Association of Supportive Cancer Care (MASCC) guidelines include use of aprepitant as initial therapy for highly emetogenic regimens, other guidelines [American Society of Clinical Oncology (ASCO), American Society of Health-System Pharmacists (ASHP)], and most practitioners reserve these agents for patients who develop vomiting after receiving an appropriate serotonin antagonist and steroid antiemetic regimen.

Phenothiazines. Phenothiazines were the first class of drugs accepted as antiemetic therapy for antineoplastic chemotherapy. Blockade of dopamine (D_2) receptors in the area postrema (chemoreceptor trigger zone and vomiting center) appears to be their primary mechanism of action. A number of different drugs, including chlorpromazine, perphenazine, prochlorperazine, promethazine, and thiethylperazine (no longer marketed in the United States), have antiemetic activity. Common toxicities such as extrapyramidal reactions, restlessness, sedation, and hypotension limit the use of these drugs. In generally tolerated doses, the phenothiazines are most effective against mild-to-moderate nausea or vomiting, but have little impact on emesis from highly emetogenic agents such as dacarbazine or cisplatin. Higher doses of these agents may have increased activity, but the increased incidence and severity of side effects usually prohibits their use. Since the serotonin antagonists became available, use of the phenothiazines generally has been limited to prevention of nausea from mildly emetogenic chemotherapy, treatment of breakthrough nausea/vomiting in patients refractory to a serotonin blocker, or in association with dexamethasone to treat delayed nausea.

Serotonin ($5HT_3$) Antagonists. A major advance in antiemetic therapy was the introduction of the serotonin ($5HT_3$) antagonists. The high efficacy rate of these agents in preventing acute nausea and vomiting, coupled with low incidence of side effects, has made them the preferred choice in this setting. The major limitation to their use has been economic. The high cost of serotonin antagonists has resulted in many institutions placing severe limitations on their use. Most comparisons have shown that a serotonin antagonist/steroid combination is significantly better than either agent alone. For prevention of acute nausea and vomiting caused by highly emetogenic antineoplastic regimens, a serotonin antagonist/steroid combination usually represents the most effective antiemetic therapy. Since there seems to be little difference in efficacy or toxicity among the available serotonin antagonists, selection of a specific agent is a matter of institutional or prescriber preference.

In spite of their popularity, the serotonin antagonists are not the complete solution to treatment-induced emesis. Some trials have found no difference in efficacy between serotonin antagonist-based regimens and previously used combinations, leaving toxicity, convenience, and economic issues as the discriminating factors in drug selection. Two particular questions concerning serotonin antagonist use remain unanswered: appropriate second-line therapy for treatment failures, and use in noncisplatin regimens.

Like any medication, serotonin antagonists are not 100% effective. Approximately 40% to 60% of patients receiving serotonin antagonist monotherapy will experience some nausea, or have at least one episode of vomiting. Addition of a steroid to the regimen reduces the failure rate significantly, with some trials reporting only 10% to 15% of patients failing the initial therapy. Regardless of the initial antiemetic therapy, some patients will experience one or more episodes of vomiting following administration of the cytotoxic therapy. Choice of a salvage antiemetic regimen for these patients is problematic. Controlled trials of the serotonin antagonists have focused primarily on prevention of nausea/vomiting. Only a few small uncontrolled reports relate to their utility as salvage therapy to terminate vomiting once it begins.

Most studies in patients receiving chemotherapy over several consecutive days suggest the serotonin antagonists have their greatest protective effect in the initial 24 hours, and possibly the initial 16-18 hours, of a chemotherapy cycle. These factors further limit the usefulness of serotonin antagonists in patients who experience nausea/vomiting following prophylactic antiemetic therapy with one of these agents.

MANAGEMENT OF NAUSEA AND VOMITING *(Continued)*

Substituted Benzamides. Metoclopramide is the most commonly used antiemetic drug in this category. Prior to introduction of the 5HT$_3$ antagonists, high-dose (2-3 mg/kg) metoclopramide was the preferred drug for prevention of nausea/vomiting from highly emetogenic chemotherapy. Metoclopramide's ability to block central and peripheral dopamine receptors was believed to be the mechanism of it's antiemetic activity. Recognition that high doses also blocked serotonin receptors led to identification of the role serotonin inhibition has in preventing nausea/vomiting, and, ultimately, to development of the 5HT$_3$ antagonists. Like the phenothiazines, use of metoclopramide is complicated by extrapyramidal reactions, restlessness, sedation, and hypotension. Diarrhea is also a significant side effect, especially with the high doses used for antiemetic therapy. Also like the phenothiazines, the current use of metoclopramide is generally limited to prevention of nausea from mild-to-moderately emetogenic chemotherapy, treatment of breakthrough nausea/vomiting, or to treat delayed nausea.

REPRESENTATIVE ANTIEMETIC REGIMENS

HIGHLY EMETOGENIC CHEMOTHERAPY

Dexamethasone 10-20 mg P.O. or I.V. + a serotonin antagonist daily 15-30 minutes before treatment on each day of chemotherapy

> Recommended serotonin antagonist regimens:
> **Dolasetron 100-200 mg P.O.** once daily
> **Dolasetron 1.8 mg/kg I.V.** once daily
> **Dolasetron 100 mg I.V.** once daily
> **Granisetron 2 mg P.O.** once daily
> **Granisetron 1 mg P.O.** q12h
> **Granisetron 10 mcg/kg I.V.** once daily
> **Granisetron 1 mg I.V.** once daily
> **Ondansetron 0.45 mg/kg I.V.** once daily
> **Ondansetron 8-16 mg I.V.** once daily
> **Ondansetron 8-10 mg I.V.** q8h
> **Ondansetron 16-24 mg P.O.** q12-24h
> **Palonosetron 0.25 mg I.V.** day 1 of each cycle
> *(doses should not be given more than once weekly)*

For continuous infusion therapy, carboplatin and high-dose (>1 g/m^2) cyclophosphamide regimens, the following regimen may be preferred:

> **Dexamethasone 10 mg P.O. or I.V. + a serotonin antagonist** q12h

> Recommended serotonin antagonist regimens:
> **Granisetron 1 mg P.O.**
> **Granisetron 10 mcg/kg I.V.**
> **Ondansetron 8-16 mg I.V.**
> **Ondansetron 16-24 mg P.O.**
> **Palonosetron 0.25 mg I.V.** day 1 of each cycle
> *(doses should not be given more than once weekly)*

> **Refractory patients:** Add:
> **Aprepitant 125 mg** P.O. 30-60 minutes before treatment, then
> **Aprepitant 80 mg** P.O. days 2 and 3

MODERATELY EMETOGENIC CHEMOTHERAPY

Dexamethasone 10 mg P.O. or I.V. + a serotonin antagonist daily 15-30 minutes before treatment on each day of chemotherapy

> Recommended serotonin antagonist regimens:
> **Ondansetron 8-16 mg P.O.** once daily
> **Ondansetron 8 mg P.O.** q12h
> **Ondansetron 8-10 mg I.V.** once daily

For continuous infusion therapy, the following regimen may be preferred:

> **Dexamethasone 4 mg P.O. or I.V. + ondansetron 8 mg P.O. or I.V.** q12h on each day of chemotherapy

MILDLY EMETOGENIC CHEMOTHERAPY

All agents are given 15-30 minutes before treatment and may be repeated every 4-6 hours, if necessary. With the exceptions of dexamethasone (given over 5-15 minutes) and droperidol (given by I.V. push), intravenous doses should be given over 30 minutes.

> **Dexamethasone 4 mg P.O./I.V./I.M.**
> **Droperidol 1.25-5 mg I.M./I.V. push**
> **Haloperidol 2 mg P.O./I.V./I.M.**
> **Metoclopramide 20-40 mg P.O./I.V./I.M.**
> **Prochlorperazine 10-20 mg P.O./I.V./I.M.**

DELAYED NAUSEA AND VOMITING

Dexamethasone + a dopamine, neurokinen, or serotonin antagonist. Therapy should start within 12-24 hours of administration of the emetogenic chemotherapy.

Recommended regimens:

Dexamethasone

8 mg P.O. q12h for 2 days, then 4 mg P.O. q12h for 2 days

or

20 mg P.O. 1 hour before chemotherapy; 10 mg P.O. 12 hours after chemotherapy, then 8 mg P.O. q12h for 4 doses, then 4 mg P.O. q12h for 4 doses

Recommended dopamine/neurokinin/serotonin antagonist regimens:

Droperidol 1.25-2.5 mg I.V./I.M. q4h for 2-4 days

Metoclopramide 0.5 mg/kg P.O. q6h for 2-4 days

Ondansetron 8 mg P.O. q8h for 2-4 days

Prochlorperazine 10 mg P.O. q6h for 2-4 days

Aprepitant 125 mg P.O. day 1, 80 mg P.O. days 2 and 3

GENERAL PRINCIPLES FOR MANAGING NAUSEA AND VOMITING

1. **Prophylaxis is *MUCH* better than treatment of actual vomiting.** For agents with a moderate-to-high (30% to 100%) incidence of nausea, patients should be pretreated with an antiemetic. Depending on the antiemetic agent(s) and route(s) of administration, pretreatment may range from 1 hour to 5 minutes prior to administration of the antineoplastic agent(s).

2. **Doses and intervals of the antiemetic regimen need to be individualized for each patient.** "PRN" regimens should **not** be used. A fixed schedule of drug administration is preferable.

3. **If a patient has had no nausea for 24 hours** while on their scheduled antiemetic regimen, **it is usually possible to switch to a "PRN" regimen.** The patient should be advised to resume the fixed schedule *at the FIRST sign of recurrent nausea*, and continue it until they have had at least 24 hours without nausea.

4. **Titrate antiemetic dose to patient tolerance.**

5. In most cases, **combination regimens are required for optimum control of nausea.** Do not be afraid to use two or more agents, *from different pharmacologic categories*, to achieve optimal results.

6. To the extent possible, **avoid duplication of agents from the same pharmacologic category.**

7. **Anticipatory nausea and vomiting can often be minimized if the patient receives effective prophylaxis against nausea from the first cycle of therapy.**

8. **If anticipatory nausea does develop, an anxiolytic agent is usually the drug of choice.**

9. **"If it's not broken – DON'T fix it!"** Regardless of your own preferences, if the patient's current antiemetic regimen is working, don't change it.

10. **For moderately emetogenic regimens, a steroid and dopamine blocker** (eg, metoclopramide, prochlorperazine) **is usually the most cost-effective regimen.**

11. **For highly emetogenic regimens, a steroid and serotonin receptor blocker** (eg, dolasetron, granisetron, ondansetron) **combination is the preferred regimen.**

12. **A neurokinin blocker** (eg, aprepitant) **is a good first alternative if the serotonin blocker fails.** A dopamine antagonist (eg, metoclopramide, prochlorperazine) may also be effective.

13. Although most nausea or vomiting develops within the first 24 hours after treatment, **delayed reactions (1-7 days after chemotherapy) are not uncommon.**

14. **Other antiemetics, such as cannabinoids, antihistamines, or anticholinergics) have limited use as initial therapy.** They are best used in combination with more effective agents (steroids, dopamine, or serotonin blockers); or, as second- or third-line therapy.

15. **Serotonin and neurokinin blockers are most effective in scheduled prophylactic regimens**; rather than in "PRN" regimens to chase existing vomiting.

16. **Serotonin and neurokinin antagonists have limited efficacy in stopping nausea or vomiting once it has begun.** A dopamine blocker may be more effective.

17. **The serotonin blockers appear to have a "ceiling" dose,** above which there is little or no added antiemetic effect.

18. **Serotonin antagonists are most effective within the first 24-48 hours.** Most studies of multiple day dosing show a sharp decline in the efficacy of the serotonin antagonists after the second or third day.

19. **Neurokinin antagonists are not very effective as single agents,** and should only be used in combination with a serotonin antagonist and steroid.

MANAGEMENT OF NAUSEA AND VOMITING *(Continued)*

Selected References

"ASHP Therapeutic Guidelines on the Pharmacologic Management of Nausea and Vomiting in Adult and Pediatric Patients Receiving Chemotherapy or Radiation Therapy or Undergoing Surgery", *Am J Health Syst Pharm*, 1999, 56(8):729-64.

De Wit R, "Current Position of 5HT$_3$ Antagonists and the Additional Value of NK$_1$ Antagonists; A New Class of Antiemetics, *Br J Cancer*, 2003, 88(12):1823-7.

Gralla RJ, Osoba D, Kris MG, et al, "Recommendations for the Use of Antiemetics: Evidence-Based, Clinical Practice Guidelines," *J Clin Oncol*, 1999, 17(9):2971-94.

Graves T, "Emesis as a Complication of Cancer Chemotherapy: Pathophysiology, Importance, and Treatment," *Pharmacotherapy*, 1992, 12(4):337-45.

Grunberg SM and Hesketh PJ, —Control of Chemotherapy-Induced Emesis," *N Engl J Med*, 1993, 329(24):1790-6.

Hesketh PJ, Kris MG, Grunberg SM, et al, "Proposal for Classifying the Acute Emetogenicity of Cancer Chemotherapy," *J Clin Oncol*, 1997, 15(1):103-9.

Hesketh PJ, Van Belle S, Aapro M, et al, "Differential Involvement of Neurotransmitters Through the Time Course of Cisplatin-Induced Emesis as Revealed by Therapy With Specific Receptor Antagonists," *Eur J Cancer*, 2003, 39(8):1074-80.

Holdsworth MT, "Ethical Issues Regarding Study Designs Used in Serotonin-Antagonist Drug Development," *Ann Pharmacother*, 1996, 30(10):1182-4.

NCCN Antiemesis Practice Guidelines, The Complete Library of NCCN Oncology Practice Guidelines, Rockledge, PA: National Comprehensive Cancer Network, 2004; www.nccn.org.

"Prevention of Chemotherapy- and Radiotherapy-Induced Emesis: Results of Perugia Consensus Conference. Antiemetic Subcommittee of the Multinational Association of Supportive Care in Cancer (MASCO)," *Ann Oncol*, 1998, 9(8):811-9.

PEAK AND TROUGH GUIDELINES

Drug	When to Sample	Therapeutic Levels*	Usual Half-Life	Steady State (Ideal Sampling Time)	Potentially Toxic Levels*
Antibiotics					
Gentamicin Tobramycin	30 min after 30 min infusion Trough: <0.5 h before next dose	Peak: 4-10 mcg/mL Trough: <2.0 mcg/mL	2 h	15 h	Peak: >12 mcg/mL Trough: >2 mcg/mL
Amikacin		Peak: 20-35 mcg/mL Trough: <8 mcg/mL			Peak: >35 mcg/mL Trough: >8 mcg/mL
Vancomycin	Peak: 1 h after 1 h infusion Trough: <0.5 h before next dose	Peak: 30-40 mcg/mL Trough: 5-10 mcg/mL	6-8 h	24 h	Peak: >80 mcg/mL Trough: >13 mcg/mL
Anticonvulsants					
Carbamazepine	Trough: Just before next oral dose In combination with other anticonvulsants	4-12 mcg/mL 4-8 mcg/mL	15-20 h	7-12 d	>12 mcg/mL
Ethosuximide	Trough: Just before next oral dose	40-100 mcg/mL	30-60 h	10-13 d	>100 mcg/mL
Phenobarbital	Trough: Just before next dose	15-40 mcg/mL	40-120 h	20 d	>40 mcg/mL
Phenytoin Free phenytoin	Trough: Just before next dose Draw at same time as total level.	10-20 mcg/mL 1-2 mcg/mL	Concentration dependent	5-14 d	>20 mcg/mL
Primidone	Trough: Just before next dose (**Note:** Primidone is metabolized to phenobarb; order levels separately.)	5-12 mcg/mL	10-12 h	5 d	>12 mcg/mL
Valproic acid	Trough: Just before next dose	50-100 mcg/mL	5-20 h	4 d	>150 mcg/mL
Bronchodilators					
Aminophylline (I.V.)	18-24 h after starting or changing a maintenance dose; given as a constant infusion	10-20 mcg/mL	Nonsmoking adult: 8 h Children and smoking adults: 4 h	2 d	>20 mcg/mL
Theophylline (P.O.)	Peak levels: Not recommended Trough level: Just before next dose				
Cardiovascular Agents					
Digoxin	Trough: Just before next dose (levels drawn earlier than 6 h after a dose will be artificially elevated)	0.5-2 ng/mL	36 h	5 d	>2 ng/mL
Lidocaine	Steady-state levels are usually achieved after 6-12 h	1.2-5.0 mcg/mL	1.5 h	5-10 h	>6 mcg/mL
Procainamide	Trough: Just before next oral dose I.V.: 6-12 h after infusion started Combined procainamide plus NAPA	4-10 mcg/mL NAPA: 6-10 h 5-30 mcg/mL	Procain: 2.7-5 h >30 (NAPA + procain)	20 h	>10 mcg/mL
Quinidine	Trough: Just before next oral dose	2-5 mcg/mL	6 h	24 h	>10 mcg/mL
Warfarin	Same time of day each draw	See Warfarin monograph.	42 h	5-7 d	See Warfarin monograph.

PEAK AND TROUGH GUIDELINES *(Continued)*

Drug	When to Sample	Therapeutic Levels*	Usual Half-Life	Steady State (Ideal Sampling Time)	Potentially Toxic Levels*
Other Agents					
Amitriptyline plus nortriptyline	Trough: Just before next dose	120-250 ng/mL		4-80 d	
Cyclosporine		Months post-transplant: Plasma: 50-150 ng/mL Whole blood: 150-450 ng/mL		Variable	
Desipramine		50-300 ng/mL	12-54 h	3-11 d	
Imipramine plus desipramine		150-300 ng/mL	9-24 h	2-5 d	
Lithium		0.6-1.2 mEq/mL (acute)	18-20 h	2-7 d	>3 mEq/mL
Nortriptyline		50-140 ng/mL		4-19 d	

*Due to methodology differences, reference ranges may vary from laboratory to laboratory; check with the laboratory service used for their appropriate levels.

ORAL MEDICATIONS THAT SHOULD NOT BE CRUSHED

There are a variety of reasons for crushing tablets or capsule contents prior to administering to the patient. Patients may have nasogastric tubes which do not permit the administration of tablets or capsules; an oral solution for a particular medication may not be available from the manufacturer or readily prepared by pharmacy; patients may have difficulty swallowing capsules or tablets; or mixing of powdered medication with food or drink may make the drug more palatable.

Generally, medications which should not be crushed fall into one of the following categories.

- **Extended-Release Products**. The formulation of some tablets is specialized as to allow the medication within it to be slowly released into the body. This is sometimes accomplished by centering the drug within the core of the tablet, with a subsequent shedding of multiple layers around the core. Wax melts in the GI tract. Slow-K® is an example of this. Capsules may contain beads which have multiple layers which are slowly dissolved with time.

Common Abbreviations for Extended-Release Products

CD	Controlled dose
CR	Controlled release
CRT	Controlled-release tablet
LA	Long-acting
SR	Sustained release
TR	Timed release
TD	Time delay
SA	Sustained action
XL	Extended release
XR	Extended release

- **Medications Which Are Irritating to the Stomach**. Tablets which are irritating to the stomach may be enteric-coated which delays release of the drug until the time when it reaches the small intestine. Enteric-coated aspirin is an example of this.

- **Foul-Tasting Medication**. Some drugs are quite unpleasant to taste so the manufacturer coats the tablet in a sugar coating to increase its palatability. By crushing the tablet, this sugar coating is lost and the patient tastes the unpleasant tasting medication.

- **Sublingual Medication**. Medication intended for use under the tongue should not be crushed. While it appears to be obvious, it is not always easy to determine if a medication is to be used sublingually. Sublingual medications should indicate on the package that they are intended for sublingual use.

- **Effervescent Tablets**. These are tablets which, when dropped into a liquid, quickly dissolve to yield a solution. Many effervescent tablets, when crushed, lose their ability to quickly dissolve.

Recommendations

1. It is not advisable to crush certain medications.

2. Consult individual monographs prior to crushing capsule or tablet.

3. If crushing a tablet or capsule is contraindicated, consult with your pharmacist to determine whether an oral solution exists or can be compounded.

ORAL MEDICATIONS THAT SHOULD NOT BE CRUSHED *(Continued)*

Drug Product	Dosage Form	Dosage Reasons / Comments
Accuhist®	Tablet	Slow release⁸
Accutane®	Capsule	Mucous membrane irritant
Aciphex™	Tablet	Slow release
Adalat® CC	Tablet	Slow release
Adderall XR™	Capsule	Slow release¹
Advicor®	Tablet	Slow release
Afeditab™ CR	Tablet	Slow release
Aggrenox®	Capsule	Slow release **Note:** Capsule may be opened; contents include an aspirin tablet that may be chewed and dipyridamole pellets that may be sprinkled on applesauce
Alavert™ Allergy Sinus 12 Hour	Tablet	Slow release
Allegra-D®	Tablet	Slow release
Altocor™	Tablet	Slow release
Arthritis Bayer® Time Release	Capsule	Slow release
Arthrotec®	Tablet	Enteric-coated
A.S.A.® Enseals®	Tablet	Enteric-coated
Asacol®	Tablet	Slow release
Ascriptin® A/D	Tablet	Enteric-coated
Ascriptin® Extra Strength	Tablet	Enteric-coated
Augmentin XR™	Tablet	Slow release², ⁸
Avinza™	Capsule	Slow release¹ (not pudding)
Avodart™	Capsule	Teratogenic potential⁹
Azulfidine® EN-tabs®	Tablet	Enteric-coated
Bayer® Aspirin EC	Caplet	Enteric-coated
Bayer® Aspirin, Low Adult 81 mg	Tablet	Enteric-coated
Bayer® Aspirin, Regular Strength 325 mg	Caplet	Enteric-coated
Biaxin® XL	Tablet	Slow release
Biltricide®	Tablet	Taste⁸
Bisacodyl	Tablet	Enteric-coated³
Bontril® Slow-Release	Capsule	Slow release
Calan® SR	Tablet	Slow release⁸
Carbatrol®	Capsule	Slow release¹
Cardene® SR	Capsule	Slow release
Cardizem®	Tablet	Slow release
Cardizem® CD	Capsule	Slow release¹
Cardizem® LA	Tablet	Slow release
Cardizem® SR	Capsule	Slow release¹
Carter's Little Pills®	Tablet	Enteric-coated
Cartia® XT	Capsule	Slow release
Ceclor® CD	Tablet	Slow release
Ceftin®	Tablet	Taste² **Note:** Use suspension for children
CellCept®	Capsule, tablet	Teratogenic potential⁹
Charcoal Plus®	Tablet	Enteric-coated
Chloral Hydrate	Capsule	**Note:** Product is in liquid form within a special capsule²
Chlor-Trimeton® 12-Hour	Tablet	Slow release²
Cipro™	Tablet	Taste⁵
Cipro® XR	Tablet	Slow release
Claritin-D® 12-Hour	Tablet	Slow release
Claritin-D® 24-Hour	Tablet	Slow release
Colace®	Capsule	Taste⁵
Colestid®	Tablet	Slow release
Comhist® LA	Capsule	Slow release¹
Commit™	Lozenge	**Note:** Integrity compromised by chewing or crushing
Compazine® Spansule®	Capsule	Slow release²
Concerta®	Tablet	Slow release
Contac® 12-Hour	Tablet	Slow release
Cotazym-S®	Capsule	Enteric-coated¹

(continued)

Drug Product	Dosage Form	Dosage Reasons / Comments
Covera-HS™	Tablet	Slow release
Creon® 5, 10, 20	Capsule	Slow release[1]
Crixivan®	Capsule	Taste **Note:** Capsule may be opened and mixed with fruit puree (eg, banana)
Cymbalta®	Capsule	Enteric-coated
Cytovene®	Capsule	Skin irritant
Cytoxan®	Tablet	**Note:** Drug may be crushed, but maker recommends using injection
Dallergy®	Capsule	Slow release
Dallergy-JR®	Capsule	Slow release
Deconamine® SR	Capsule	Slow release[2]
Defen L.A.®	Tablet	Slow release[8]
Depakene®	Capsule	Slow release mucous membrane irritant[2]
Depakote®	Tablet	Slow release
Depakote® ER	Tablet	Slow release
Desoxyn®	Tablet	Slow release
Desyrel®	Tablet	Taste[5]
Detrol® LA	Capsule	Slow release
Dexedrine® Spansule®	Capsule	Slow release
Diamox® Sequels®	Capsule	Slow release
Dilacor® XR	Capsule	Slow release
Dilatrate-SR®	Capsule	Slow release
Diltia XT®	Capsule	Slow release
Ditropan® XL	Tablet	Slow release
Dolobid®	Tablet	Irritant
Donnatal® Extentab®	Tablet	Slow release[2]
Drisdol®	Capsule	Liquid filled[4]
Drixoral®	Tablet	Slow release[2]
Drixoral® Plus	Tablet	Slow release
Drixoral® Sinus	Tablet	Slow release
Dulcolax®	Capsule	Liquid-filled
Dulcolax®	Tablet	Enteric-coated[3]
Duratuss® G	Tablet	Slow release[9]
Duratuss® GP	Tablet	Slow release[8]
Dynabac®	Tablet	Enteric-coated
DynaCirc® CR	Tablet	Slow release
Easprin®	Tablet	Enteric-coated
EC-Naprosyn®	Tablet	Enteric-coated
Ecotrin® Adult Low Strength	Tablet	Enteric-coated
Ecotrin® Maximum Strength	Tablet	Enteric-coated
Ecotrin® Regular Strength	Tablet	Enteric-coated
E.E.S.® 400	Tablet	Enteric-coated[2]
Effexor® XR	Capsule	Slow release
Efidac/24® Pseudoephedrine	Tablet	Slow release
Efidac® 24	Tablet	Slow release
E-Mycin®	Tablet	Enteric-coated
Entex® LA	Capsule	Slow release[2]
Entex® PSE	Capsule	Slow release
Entocort™ EC	Capsule	Enteric-coated[1]
Ergomar®	Tablet	Sublingual form[7]
Eryc®	Capsule	Enteric-coated[1]
Ery-Tab®	Tablet	Enteric-coated
Erythrocin Stearate	Tablet	Enteric-coated
Erythromycin Base	Tablet	Enteric-coated
Eskalith CR®	Tablet	Slow release
Evista®	Tablet	Taste; teratogenic potential[9]
Extendryl JR	Capsule	Slow release
Extendryl SR	Capsule	Slow release[2]
Feldene®	Capsule	Mucous membrane irritant
Feosol®	Tablet	Enteric-coated[2]
Feratab®	Tablet	Enteric-coated[2]

ORAL MEDICATIONS THAT SHOULD NOT BE CRUSHED *(Continued)*

Drug Product	Dosage Form	Dosage Reasons / Comments
Fergon®	Tablet	Enteric-coated
Fero-Grad 500®	Tablet	Slow release
Ferro-Sequels®	Tablet	Slow release
Flagyl ER®	Tablet	Slow release
Flomax®	Capsule	Enteric-coated[1]
Fosamax®	Tablet	Mucous membrane irritant
Fumatinic®	Capsule	Slow release
Geocillin®	Tablet	Taste
Gleevec®	Tablet	Taste[8] **Note:** May be dissolved in mineral oil or apple juice
Glucophage® XR	Tablet	Slow release
Glucotrol® XL	Tablet	Slow release
Gris-PEG®	Tablet	**Note:** Crushing may result in precipitation of larger particles.
Guaifed®	Capsule	Slow release
Guaifed®-PD	Capsule	Slow release
Guaifenex® DM	Tablet	Slow release[8]
Guaifenex® LA	Tablet	Slow release[8]
Guaifenex® PSE	Tablet	Slow release[8]
Guaimax-D®	Tablet	Slow release
Hista-Vent® DA	Tablet	Slow release[8]
Humibid® DM	Tablet	Slow release
Humibid® LA	Tablet	Slow release
Iberet® Filmtab	Tablet	Slow release[2]
Iberet®-500	Tablet	Slow release[2]
Iberet-Folic-500®	Tablet	Slow release
ICAPS® Time Release	Tablet	Slow release
Imdur™	Tablet	Slow release[8]
Inderal® LA	Capsule	Slow release
Inderide® LA	Capsule	Slow release
Indocin® SR	Capsule	Slow release[1,2]
InnoPran XL™	Capsule	Slow release
Ionamin®	Capsule	Slow release
Isoptin® SR	Tablet	Slow release
Isordil® Sublingual	Tablet	Sublingual form[7]
Isosorbide Dinitrate Sublingual	Tablet	Sublingual form[7]
Isosorbide SR	Tablet	Slow release
K+ 8®	Tablet	Slow release[2]
K+ 10®	Tablet	Slow release[2]
Kadian®	Capsule	Slow release[1] **Note:** Do not give via N/G tubes
Kaon-Cl®	Tablet	Slow release[2]
K-Dur®	Tablet	Slow release
Klor-Con®	Tablet	Slow release[2]
Klor-Con® M	Tablet	Slow release[2]
Klotrix®	Tablet	Slow release[2]
K-Lyte®	Tablet	Effervescent tablet[6]
K-Lyte/Cl®	Tablet	Effervescent tablet[6]
K-Lyte DS®	Tablet	Effervescent tablet[6]
K-Tab®	Tablet	Slow release[2]
Lescol® XL	Tablet	Slow release
Levbid®	Tablet	Slow release[8]
Levsinex® Timecaps®	Capsule	Slow release
Lexxel®	Tablet	Slow release
Lipram 4500	Capsule	Enteric-coated[1]
Lipram-CR	Capsule	Enteric-coated[1]
Lipram-PN	Capsule	Enteric-coated[1]
Lipram-UL	Capsule	Enteric-coated[1]
Lipram (all products)	Capsule	Slow release[1]

(continued)

Drug Product	Dosage Form	Dosage Reasons / Comments
Liquibid-PD	Tablet	Slow release[8]
Lithobid®	Tablet	Slow release
Lodine® XL	Tablet	Slow release
Lodrane® LD	Capsule	Slow release[1]
Mag-Tab® SR	Tablet	Slow release
Maxifed®	Tablet	Slow release
Maxifed® DM	Tablet	Slow release
Maxifed-G®	Tablet	Slow release
Mestinon® Timespan®	Tablet	Slow release[2]
Metadate® CD	Capsule	Slow release[1]
Metadate™ ER	Tablet	Slow release
Methylin™ ER	Tablet	Slow release
Micro-K®	Capsule	Slow release
Motrin®	Tablet	Taste[5]
MS Contin®	Tablet	Slow release[2]
Mucinex®	Tablet	Slow release
Myfortic®	Tablet	Slow release
Naprelan®	Tablet	Slow release
Nasatab® LA	Tablet	Slow release[8]
Nexium®	Capsule	Slow release[1]
Niaspan®	Tablet	Slow release
Nicotinic Acid	Capsule, tablet	Slow release
Nifediac™ CC	Tablet	Slow release
Nitrostat®	Tablet	Sublingual route[7]
Norflex™	Tablet	Slow release
Norpace® CR	Capsule	Slow release form within a special capsule
Oramorph SR®	Tablet	Slow release[2]
Oruvail®	Capsule	Slow release
OxyContin®	Tablet	Slow release
Palgic®-D	Tablet	Slow release[8]
Pancrease®	Capsule	Enteric-coated[1]
Pancrease® MT	Capsule	Enteric-coated[1]
Pancrecarb MS®	Capsule	Enteric-coated[1]
PanMist®-DM	Tablet	Slow release[8]
PanMist®-Jr	Tablet	Slow release[8]
PanMist®-LA	Tablet	Slow release[8]
Pannaz®	Tablet	Slow release[8]
Papaverine Sustained Action	Capsule	Slow release
Paxil CR™	Tablet	Slow release
Pentasa®	Capsule	Slow release
Perdiem® Fiber Therapy	Granules	Wax coated
PhenaVent™ D	Tablet	Slow release
Plendil®	Tablet	Slow release
Prelu-2®	Capsule	Slow release
Prevacid®	Capsule	Slow release
Prevacid®	Suspension	Slow release Note: Contains enteric-coated granules
Prilosec®	Capsule	Slow release
Procainamide HCl SR	Tablet	Slow release
Procanbid®	Tablet	Slow release
Procardia®	Capsule	Delays absorption[2, 5]
Procardia XL®	Tablet	Slow release Note: AUC is unaffected.
Profen II®	Tablet	Slow release[8]
Profen II DM®	Tablet	Slow release[8]
Profen Forte™ DM	Tablet	Slow release[8]
Pronestyl®-SR	Tablet	Slow release
Propecia®	Tablet	Note: Women who are, or may become, pregnant, should not handle crushed or broken tablets
Proscar®	Tablet	Note: Women who are, or may become, pregnant, should not handle crushed or broken tablets

ORAL MEDICATIONS THAT SHOULD NOT BE CRUSHED (Continued)

Drug Product	Dosage Form	Dosage Reasons / Comments
Protonix®	Tablet	Slow release
Quibron-T/SR®	Tablet	Slow release[2]
Rescon-Jr	Tablet	Slow release
Respa-DM®	Tablet	Slow release[8]
Respaire®-120 SR	Capsule	Slow release
Ritalin-SR®	Tablet	Slow release
Rondec-TR®	Tablet	Slow release[2]
Rythmol® SR	Capsule	Slow release
Sinemet® CR	Tablet	Slow release
SINUvent® PE	Tablet	Slow release[8]
Slo-Niacin®	Tablet	Slow release[8]
Slow-Mag®	Tablet	Slow release
Somnote™	Capsule	Liquid filled
Sudafed® 12-Hour	Capsule	Slow release[2]
Sular®	Tablet	Slow release
Symax SR	Tablet	Slow release
Taztia XT™	Capsule	Slow release
Tegretol®-XR	Tablet	Slow release
Temodar®	Capsule	**Note:** If capsules are accidentally opened or damaged, rigorous precautions should be taken to avoid inhalation or contact of contents with the skin or mucous membranes[9]
Tessalon®	Capsule	Slow release
Theo-24®	Tablet	Slow release[2]
Theochron®	Tablet	Slow release
Tiazac®	Capsule	Slow release
Topamax®	Capsule	Taste[1]
Topamax®	Tablet	Taste
Touro™ CC	Tablet	Slow release
Touro EX®	Tablet	Slow release
Touro LA®	Tablet	Slow release
Trental®	Tablet	Slow release
TripTone®	Tablet	Slow release
Tylenol® Arthritis Pain	Tablet	Slow release
Tylenol® 8 Hour	Tablet	Slow release
Ultrase®	Capsule	Enteric-coated[1]
Ultrase® MT	Capsule	Enteric-coated[1]
Uniphyl®	Tablet	Slow release
Urocit®-K	Tablet	Wax-coated
Verelan®	Capsule	Slow release[1]
Videx® EC	Capsule	Slow release
Voltaren®-XR	Tablet	Slow release
VoSpire ER™	Tablet	Slow release
Wellbutrin SR®	Tablet	Slow release
Wellbutrin XL™	Tablet	Slow release
Xanax XR®	Tablet	Slow release
Z-Cof LA	Tablet	Slow release[8]
Zephrex LA®	Tablet	Slow release
ZORprin®	Tablet	Slow release
Zyban®	Tablet	Slow release

See footnotes on next page.

[1]Capsule may be opened and the contents taken without crushing or chewing; soft food such as applesauce or pudding may facilitate administration; contents may generally be administered via nasogastric tube using an appropriate fluid, provided entire contents are washed down the tube.

[2]Liquid dosage forms of the product are available; however, dose, frequency of administration, and manufacturers may differ from that of the solid dosage form.

[3]Antacids and/or milk may prematurely dissolve the coating of the tablet.

[4]Capsule may be opened and the liquid contents removed for administration.

[5]The taste of this product in a liquid form would likely be unacceptable to the patient; administration via nasogastric tube should be acceptable.

[6]Effervescent tablets must be dissolved in the amount of diluent recommended by the manufacturer.

[7]Tablets are made to disintegrate under the tongue.

[8]Tablet is scored and may be broken in half without affecting release characteristics.

[9]Skin contact may enhance tumor production; avoid direct contact.

Adapted from Mitchell JF, "Oral Dosage Forms That Should Not Be Crushed-2004," available at www.hospitalpharmacyjournal.com.

SELECTED ADVERSE EFFECTS

Adverse drug reactions can range from inconvenient to life-threatening. The type of effects, the severity, and frequency of occurrence is dependent on the medication and dosage of the medication being used, as well as the individual's response to the therapy. Early recognition by healthcare providers or patients of these adverse side effects is a major factor if appropriate intervention is to implemented. The following are definitions of selected adverse effects, and examples of some (by no means all) medications associated with these adverse effects.

Name	Description
Acute tubular necrosis	Acute renal failure characterized by direct toxicity to tubular cells. Cellular debris (casts) are a prominent feature of urinary sediment. Usually requires several days of treatment. **Examples of associated drugs:** Aminoglycosides
Ageusia	Loss of sense of taste. **Examples of associated drugs:** Bleomycin, cisplatin, diltiazem
Akathisia	Evidenced by an uncontrollable constant need for motion, pacing, and squirming or restlessness; usually develops within first 2 months of antipsychotic treatment. **Examples of associated drugs:** Promethazine, haloperidol
Alopecia	Loss of body hair. **Examples of associated drugs:** Chemotherapeutic agents, beta-blockers
Anemia	A condition in which the number of red blood cells, the amount of hemoglobin, and the volume of packed red blood cells of blood is less than normal; manifested by pallor of the skin and mucus membranes, shortness of breath, palpitation of the heart, soft systolic murmurs, lethargy, fatigability, nosebleeds, bleeding gums, easy bruising, hematuria or blood in stool. **Examples of associated drugs:** Amoxicillin, warfarin
Angioedema	Localized swelling of the subcutaneous tissue of face, hands, feet, and genitalia. **Examples of associated drugs:** ACE inhibitors
Anhidrosis	Deficiency of or absence of sweat; since sweating is necessary for cooling, persons with anhidrosis are at increased risk for hyperthermia
Anorexia	Loss of desire for food. **Examples of associated drugs:** CNS stimulants
Anticholinergic effects	Usually used to describe blockade of muscarinic receptors. Symptoms include blurred vision, mydriasis, increased intraocular pressure, headache, flushing, tachycardia, nervousness, constipation, dizziness, insomnia, mental confusion or excitement, dry mouth, altered taste perception, dysphagia, constipation, palpitations, bradycardia, urinary hesitancy or retention, impotence, decreased sweating, susceptibility to heat prostration, thickening or drying of bronchial secretions. **Examples of associated drugs:** Tricyclic antidepressants, antihistamines
Anticoagulant skin necrosis	Occurs early in therapy (3-5) days with oral anticoagulants (eg, warfarin). A paradoxical effect of oral anticoagulant therapy which involves microembolization and necrosis of skin often localized to the abdomen, breast, buttock, and thigh regions. Genetic deficiency of protein C appears to be a risk factor. **Examples of associated drugs:** Oral anticoagulants (eg, warfarin)
Cushing's syndrome	Usually a response to excess levels of circulating glucocorticoids; resembles Cushing's disease (pituitary tumor); characterized by obesity, hyperglycemia, glycosuria, muscle weakness, menstrual irregularities, fluid and electrolyte disturbances, hirsutism, myopathy, and decreased resistance to infection. **Examples of associated drugs:** Prednisone
Disulfiram reaction	Many drugs will produce a disulfiram-type reaction when the patient ingests alcohol. Symptoms includes nausea and/or vomiting, pounding or throbbing headache, systemic flushing, respiratory difficulties (dyspnea, hyperventilation), sweating, excessive thirst, cardiac disturbances (chest pain, palpitations), vertigo, visual disturbances (blurred or double vision), and CNS disturbances (confusion, convulsions). **Examples of associated drugs:** Metronidazole, cephalosporins with MTT side chains
Drug fever	Persistent fever which may be associated with low-grade allergic reaction to a drug entity. Often develops several days after initial defervescence from antibiotics. Other causes of fever related to drugs may be due to dopamine inhibition (see neuroleptic malignant syndrome). **Examples of associated drugs:** Beta-lactams, macrolides
Dysgeusia	Impairment of or perversion of sense of taste **Examples of associated drugs:** Captopril, telithromycin
Dystonia	Develops early in therapy – sometimes within hours of first dose. Typically, appears as severe spasms of the muscles of face, neck, tongue, and back. Oculogyric crisis (upward deviation of the eyes) and opisthotonus (tetanic spasm of back muscles cause trunk to arch forward, with head and lower extremities thrown backward. Acute cramping can cause dislocation of joints and laryngeal dystonia can impair respiration (can be fatal, requires emergency treatment). **Examples of associated drugs:** Haloperidol, phenothiazines
Eosinophilic pneumonitis	Development of interstitial pneumonitis due to eosinophilic infiltrates. Shortness of breath and inflammation are prominent features. **Examples of associated drugs:** Mesalamine
Erythema multiforme	Cutaneous eruption of macules, papules, and/or subdermal vesicles (multiform appearance), including characteristic "target" or "iris" lesions over the dorsal aspect of the hands and forearms. Self-limiting eruptions are termed "minor", while major eruptions may be referred to as Stevens-Johnson syndrome. **Examples of associated drugs:** Phenytoin, sulfonamides
Extrapyramidal movement disorders	Movement disorders associated with antipsychotic effects: Dystonia, pseudoparkinsonism, akathisia, tardive dyskinesia. **Examples of associated drugs:** Metoclopramide, haloperidol, phenothiazines
Hallucinations	**Examples of associated drugs:** Opiates

Name	Description
Hepatotoxicity	Hepatocellular damage or multilobular hepatic necrosis can result in liver dysfunction manifested as jaundice or hepatitis; yellowing of skin or eyes is usually a later manifestation; anorexia, fatigue or malaise, nausea, darkening in color of urine or light colored stool may occur first. **Examples of associated drugs:** Acetaminophen (overdose), carbamazepine
Interstitial nephritis	Acute renal failure characterized by localized inflammatory/allergic reaction, pronounced eosinophilic collection in interstitial cells of kidney. Eosinophils may appear in urine. Usually develops after several days of therapy. **Examples of associated drugs:** Beta-lactams, NSAIDs
Methemoglobinemia	Rare reaction in which the hemoglobin molecule is altered, rendering it unable to effectively carry oxygen after exposure to a chemical initiator. Cyanosis, respiratory distress, lactic acidosis, and shock may progress rapidly after exposure. May occur with any route of administration, including topical. **Examples of associated drugs:** Nitrates, local anesthetics
Myositis / rhabdomyolysis	Inflammation/toxicity to muscle cells characterized by muscle pain/stiffness. Pronounced lysis of muscle cells leads to dramatic increase in serum CPK and possible precipitation of myoglobin in urine. **Examples of associated drugs:** HMG CoA reductase inhibitors (particularly when combined with drugs like erythromycin or cyclosporine)
Neuroleptic malignant syndrome	Rare, but may cause 30% to 50% fatality, response to antipsychotic therapy – usually with high-potency drugs. Manifests as extremely rigid musculoskeletal posturing, extremely high fevers, sweating, dysrhythmias, and acute fluctuations of blood pressure and consciousness, respiratory failure and/or cardiac collapse (requires immediate supportive care and withdrawal of antipsychotic medication). **Examples of associated drugs:** Haloperidol, phenothiazines
Neuromuscular blockade	Weakness, respiratory failure as neuromuscular transmission may be interrupted. Patients with decreased neuromuscular transmission (eg, myasthenia gravis) are at particular risk. **Examples of associated drugs:** Aminoglycosides, macrolides
Neutropenia	A decrease in circulating neutrophils, usually defined as an absolute neutrophil count (ANC) less than 1.5×10^9/L. The ANC can be calculated using the following formula: Total WBC x % neutrophils. Mild neutropenia confers little risk for infection in an otherwise healthy individual but as the neutrophil count drops below 1.0×10^9 cells/L, the risk of infection increases. **Examples of associated drugs:** Beta-lactams, procainamide, carbamazepine
Opportunistic infection	Many medications reduce the natural resistance to infection and/or mask the more obvious indications of an infection when persons are receiving antineoplastics, antivirals, antibiotics, and glucocorticoids. Symptoms include sore throat, fever, chills, unhealed sores, purulent vaginal discharge, white plaques in mouth, fatigue, and joint pain. **Examples of associated drugs:** Chemotherapeutic agents, broad-spectrum antibiotics, immunosuppressants
Optic neuritis	Blurred vision, altered color discrimination, and constriction of visual fields. **Examples of associated drugs:** Quinidine, cisplatin
Orthostatic hypotension	Reduced muscle tone in the venous wall which causes blood to pool in lower extremity veins when the person assumes an erect position from lying or sitting; blood return to the heart is decreased because of this pooling, resulting in decreased cardiac output, and abrupt fall in blood pressure. **Examples of associated drugs:** Tricyclic antidepressants, beta-blockers
Paradoxical response	A response to a medication that is opposite of the anticipated response or side effects (eg, a paradoxical response to CNS depressants may be CNS excitation such as hyperactivity, aggression, decreased ability to concentrate). **Examples of associated drugs:** Benzodiazepines, phenobarbital
Photophobia	Blocking muscarinic receptors on the sphincter of the iris decreases ability to adapt to bright light with intolerance for any bright light; both artificial lighting and outside sunlight. **Examples of associated drugs:** Anticholinergics
Photosensitization / phototoxicity	Phototoxic and photoallergic reactions result from a combination of a sensitizing agent and ultraviolet light. The sensitizing agent in phototoxic reactions may be systemically ingested or locally applied. The reaction occurs within hours of exposure. Photoallergy results from chemical change to the structure of a sensitizing agent, and may require several days before symptoms appear. **Examples of associated drugs:** Fluoroquinolones, tetracyclines
Postural hypotension	See orthostatic hypotension.
Pseudoparkinsonism	Blocking of dopamine receptors produces symptoms that resemble Parkinson's disease: Bradycardia, facies, drooling, tremors, rigidity, gait disturbance, and stooped posture (usually develops within first month of therapy). **Examples of associated drugs:** Antipsychotic medications, haloperidol
Pulmonary fibrosis	Restrictive airway disease due to fibrous changes in the lungs, often manifest only after long-term drug administration. **Examples of associated drugs:** Nitrofurantoin, melphalan, amiodarone
Purple toes syndrome	Peripheral ischemia and cyanosis generally localized to the plantar surfaces and sides of the toes which may occasionally progress to necrosis or gangrene. The effect is believed to be caused by cholesterol microemboli. Effects are noted after weeks to months of therapy. **Examples of associated drugs:** Oral anticoagulants
QTc prolongation	Lengthening of the corrected Q-T interval (on ECG) which may predispose to the development of polymorphic ventricular tachycardia (torsade de pointes). **Examples of associated drugs:** Type Ia and III antiarrhythmics, selected fluoroquinolones, erythromycin, thioridazine, mesoridazine
Seizures (drug-induced)	An infrequent, nonspecific effect of a variety of medications, particularly at high concentrations. Drug-induced seizures may occur due to lowering of seizure threshold, blockade of inhibitory neurotransmitters (GABA) or direct neuroexcitatory effects. **Examples of associated drugs:** Tricyclic antidepressants (lower seizure threshold), high-dose beta-lactam or fluoroquinolone antibiotics (GABA blockade); theophylline or accumulation of normeperidine (neuroexcitation)

SELECTED ADVERSE EFFECTS *(Continued)*

Name	Description
Serotonin syndrome	Presence of three or more of the following: Altered mental status (40% - primarily confusion or hypomania), agitation, tremor (50%), shivering, diarrhea, hyperreflexia (pronounced) in lower extremities, myoclonus (50%), ataxia or incoordination, fever (50% incidence; temperature >105°F associated with grave prognosis), diaphoresis. **Examples of associated drugs:** Serotonin reuptake inhibitors, MOMA (ecstasy), clomipramine, combinations of many drugs
Stevens-Johnson syndrome (SJS)	Rare reaction; symptoms include widespread lesions of the skin and mucous membranes, fever, malaise, and toxemia; reducing or discontinuing the sulfonamide at the first sign of skin rash may reduce the incidence of SJS. **Examples of associated drugs:** Associated primarily with sulfonamides and associated compounds such as sulfonylureas, thiazide diuretics, and loop diuretics; anticonvulsants
Stomatitis	Mucositis is a general term for erythema, edema, desquamation, and ulceration of the gastrointestinal tract. Stomatitis refers to the finding of mucositis in the mouth or oropharynx. **Examples of associated drugs:** Chemotherapeutic agents
Sulfite hypersensitivity	Reactions occur within 2-15 minutes after ingestion of inhalation and include nasal pruritus, rhinorrhea, conjunctivitis, generalized urticaria, dyspnea, wheezing, angioedema, flushing, weakness, and anaphylaxis; patients frequently have underlying allergies or asthmatic disease. **Examples of associated drugs:** Sulfite derivatives are common antioxidant preservatives used in foods and medications. Sulfite derivatives include sodium bisulfite, potassium bisulfite, sodium metabisulfite, sodium sulfites, potassium metabisulfite, and sulfur dioxide. Most common food sources are fresh fruits and vegetables, shellfish, soft drinks, beer, wine, dried foods, and fruit drinks. Sympathomimetic medications are very susceptible to oxidation and frequently contain bisulfites in concentrations of 0.3% to 0.75%.
Tardive dyskinesia	Usually develops with long-term therapy - symptoms may be irreversible. Characterized by wormlike, writhing movements of tongue and facial muscles, lip-smacking, or flicking tongue movements; can progress to involuntary movements of digits or limbs. **Examples of associated drugs:** Haldol®, phenothiazines
Tendonitis / Achilles' tendon rupture	Pain associated with tendon area, most commonly in the Achilles' region, which may progress to tendon rupture, particularly if the effect is not recognized and therapy is continued. **Examples of associated drugs:** Fluoroquinolones
Teratogenic effects	Neonatal abnormalities (physical and mental) that result from impaired development at some stage in the fetal development; specificity of defects depends on several factors, including the period of fetal development when the medication was used (eg, some drugs are teratogenic during the early period of fetal development, some are teratogenic during later periods of development, and some have negative impact on fetal development during any period of the pregnancy). **Examples of associated drugs:** Phenytoin, metronidazole
Thrombocytopenia	A decrease in the circulating platelet count to levels which may impair coagulation. Generally a count <100,000 cells/microliter is considered thrombocytopenia. Counts <20,000 cells/microliter are considered severe thrombocytopenia, and may result in spontaneous bleeding. **Examples of associated drugs:** H_2 antagonists, beta-lactams
Tyramine reaction	Specific foods in the presence of MAO inhibitors. Normally, dietary tyramine is inactivated by MAO (monamine oxidase) in the intestinal wall and by hepatic MAO. In the presence of MAO inhibitors, dietary tyramine is not inactivated, passes without metabolism into the circulation to promote the release of accumulated norepinephrine stores in the sympathetic nerve terminals, thereby causing massive vasoconstriction and acute stimulation of the heart. Reactions can be severe and usually require emergency treatment. **Examples of associated drugs:** MAO inhibitors
Vestibulotoxicity	Form of ototoxicity which affects vestibular function, as opposed to hearing. Primary symptom is ataxia or difficulty maintaining balance. **Examples of associated drugs:** Aminoglycosides
Virilization	Acne, deepening of voice, increased body and facial hair, baldness, clitoral enlargement, increased libido, menstrual irregularities (hair loss, voice changes, and enlargement of clitoris may be irreversible). **Examples of associated drugs:** Minoxidil, phenytoin
Xerostomia	Dry mouth results from blockade of muscarinic receptors on salivary glands. Decreased salivation and excessively dry mouth are extremely uncomfortable but also interfere with mastication and swallowing, resulting in poor nutrition. **Examples of associated drugs:** Clonidine, anticholinergics

DISCOLORATION OF FECES DUE TO DRUGS

Black
Acetazolamide
Alcohols
Alkalies
Aluminum hydroxide
Aminophylline
Aminosalicylic acid
Amphetamine
Amphotericin
Antacids
Anticoagulants
Aspirin
Betamethasone
Bismuth
Charcoal
Chloramphenicol
Chlorpropamide
Clindamycin
Corticosteroids
Cortisone
Cyclophosphamide
Cytarabine
Digitalis
Ethacrynic acid
Ferrous salts
Floxuridine
Fluorides
Fluorouracil
Halothane
Heparin
Hydralazine
Hydrocortisone
Ibuprofen
Indomethacin
Iodine drugs
Iron salts
Levarterenol
Levodopa
Manganese
Melphalan
Methylprednisolone
Methotrexate

Methylene blue
Oxyphenbutazone
Phenacetin
Phenolphthalein
Phenylbutazone
Phenylephrine
Phosphorous
Potassium salts
Prednisolone
Procarbazine
Pyrvinium
Reserpine
Salicylates
Sulfonamides
Tetracycline
Theophylline
Thiotepa
Triamcinolone
Warfarin

Blue
Chloramphenicol
Methylene blue

Dark Brown
Dexamethasone

Gray
Colchicine

Green
Indomethacin
Iron
Medroxyprogesterone

Greenish Gray
Oral antibiotics
Oxyphenbutazone
Phenylbutazone

Light Brown
Anticoagulants

Orange-Red
Phenazopyridine
Rifampin

Pink
Anticoagulants
Aspirin
Heparin
Oxyphenbutazone
Phenylbutazone
Salicylates

Red
Anticoagulants
Aspirin
Heparin
Oxyphenbutazone
Phenolphthalein
Phenylbutazone
Pyrvinium
Salicylates
Tetracycline syrup

Red-Brown
Oxyphenbutazone
Phenylbutazone
Rifampin

Tarry
Ergot preparations
Ibuprofen
Salicylates
Warfarin

White / Speckling
Aluminum hydroxide
Antibiotics (oral)
Indocyanine green

Yellow
Senna

Yellow-Green
Senna

Adapted from Drugdex® — Drug Consults, Micromedex, Vol 62, Denver, CO: Rocky Mountain Drug Consultation Center, 1998.

DISCOLORATION OF URINE DUE TO DRUGS

Black
Cascara
Cotrimoxazole
Ferrous salts
Iron dextran
Levodopa
Methocarbamol
Methyldopa
Naphthalene
Pamaquine
Phenacetin
Phenols
Quinine
Sulfonamides

Blue
Anthraquinone
DeWitt's pills
Indigo blue
Indigo carmine
Methocarbamol
Methylene blue
Mitoxantrone
Nitrofurans
Resorcinol
Triamterene

Blue-Green
Amitriptyline
Anthraquinone
DeWitt's pills
Doan's® pills
Indigo blue
Indigo carmine
Magnesium salicylate
Methylene blue
Resorcinol

Brown
Anthraquinone dyes
Cascara
Chloroquine
Hydroquinone
Levodopa
Methocarbamol
Methyldopa
Metronidazole
Nitrofurans
Nitrofurantoin
Pamaquine
Phenacetin
Phenols
Primaquine
Quinine
Rifabutin
Rifampin
Senna
Sodium diatrizoate
Sulfonamides

Brown-Black
Isosorbide mono- or dinitrate
Methyldopa
Metronidazole
Nitrates
Nitrofurans
Phenacetin
Povidone iodine
Quinine
Senna

Dark
p-Aminosalicylic acid
Cascara
Levodopa
Metronidazole
Nitrites
Phenacetin
Phenol
Primaquine
Quinine
Resorcinol
Riboflavin
Senna

Green
Amitriptyline
Anthraquinone
DeWitt's pills
Indigo blue
Indigo carmine
Indomethacin
Methocarbamol
Methylene blue
Nitrofurans
Phenols
Propofol
Resorcinol
Suprofen

Green-Yellow
DeWitt's pills
Methylene blue

Milky
Phosphates

Orange
Chlorzoxazone
Dihydroergotamine mesylate
Heparin sodium
Phenazopyridine
Phenindione
Rifabutin
Rifampin
Sulfasalazine
Warfarin

Orange-Red-Brown
Chlorzoxazone
Doxidan
Phenazopyridine
Rifampin
Warfarin

Orange-Yellow
Fluorescein sodium
Rifampin
Sulfasalazine

Pink
Aminopyrine
Anthraquinone dyes
Aspirin
Cascara
Danthron
Deferoxamine
Methyldopa
Phenazopyridone
Phenolphthalein
Phenothiazines
Phenytoin
Salicylates
Senna

Purple
Phenolphthalein

Red
Anthraquinone
Cascara
Chlorpromazine
Daunorubicin
Deferoxamine
Dihydroergotamine mesylate
Dimethyl sulfoxide
DMSO
Doxorubicin
Heparin
Ibuprofen
Methyldopa
Oxyphenbutazone
Phenacetin
Phenazopyridine
Phenolphthalein
Phenothiazines
Phensuximide
Phenylbutazone
Phenytoin
Rifampin
Senna

Red-Brown
Cascara
Deferoxamine
Methyldopa
Oxyphenbutazone
Pamaquine
Phenacetin
Phenazopyridine
Phenolphthalein
Phenothiazines
Phenylbutazone
Phenytoin
Quinine
Senna

Red-Purple
Chlorzoxazone
Ibuprofen
Phenacetin
Senna

Rust
Cascara
Chloroquine
Metronidazole
Nitrofurantoin
Pamaquine
Phenacetin
Quinacrine
Riboflavin
Senna
Sulfonamides

Yellow
Nitrofurantoin
Phenacetin
Quinacrine
Riboflavin
Sulfasalazine

Yellow-Brown
Aminosalicylate acid
Bismuth
Cascara
Chloroquine
DeWitt's pills
Methylene blue
Metronidazole
Nitrofurantoin
Pamaquine
Primaquine
Quinacrine
Senna
Sulfonamides

Yellow-Pink
Cascara
Senna

Adapted from Drugdex® — Drug Consults, Micromedex, Vol 62, Denver, CO: Rocky Mountain Drug Consultation Center, 1998.

FEVER DUE TO DRUGS

Most Common

Atropine	Cephalosporins	Procainamide
Amphotericin B	Interferon	Quinidine
Asparaginase	Methyldopa	Salicylates (high doses)
Barbiturates	Penicillins	Streptomycin
Bleomycin	Phenytoin	Sulfonamides

Less Common

Allopurinol	Hydralazine	Nitrofurantoin
Antihistamines	Hydroxyurea	Pentazocine
Azathioprine	Imipenem	Procarbazine
Carbamazepine	Iodides	Propylthiouracil
Cimetidine	Isoniazid	Rifampin
Cisplatin	Mercaptopurine	Streptokinase
Colistimethate	Metoclopramide	Triamterene
Diazoxide	Nifedipine	Vancomycin
Folic acid	NSAIDs	

References

Cunha BA, "Antibiotic Side Effects," *Med Clin North Am*, 2001, 85(1):149-85.
Mackowiak PA and LeMaistre CF, "Drug Fever: A Critical Appraisal of Conventional Concepts. An Analysis of 51 Episodes in Two Dallas Hospitals and 97 Episodes Reported in the English Literature," *Ann Intern Med*, 1987, 106(5):728-33.
Tabor PA, "Drug-Induced Fever," Table 2, "Drugs Implicated in Causing a Fever," *Drug Intell Clin Pharm*, 1986, 20(6):416.

SEROTONIN SYNDROME

Diagnostic Criteria for Serotonin Syndrome

- Recent addition or dosage increase of any agent increasing serotonin activity or availability (usually within 1 day)
- Absence of abused substances, metabolic infectious etiology, or withdrawal
- No recent addition or dosage increase of a neuroleptic agent prior to onset of signs and symptoms
- Presence of three or more of the following: (% incidence)

Agitation (34%)
Abdominal pain (4%)
Ataxia/incoordination (40%)
Diaphoresis (45%)
Diarrhea (8%)
Hyperpyrexia (45%)
Hypertension/hypotension (35%)
Hyperthermia
Hyperreflexia (52%)
Mental status change – cognitive behavioral changes:
   Anxiety (15%)
   Euphoria/hypomania (21%)
   Confusion (51%)
   Agitation (34%)
   Disorientation
   Coma/unresponsiveness (29%)
Muscle rigidity (51%)

Mydriasis
Myoclonus (58%)
Nausea (23%)
Nystagmus (15%)
Restlessness/hyperactivity (48%)
Salivation (2%)
Seizures (12%)
Shivering (26%)
Sinus tachycardia (36%)
Tachypnea (26%)
Tremor (43%)
Unreactive pupils (20%)

Drugs (as Single Causative Agent)
Which Can Induce Serotonin Syndrome

Specific serotonin reuptake inhibitors (SSRI)
MDMA (Ecstasy)
Clomipramine

Drug Combinations Which Can Induce Serotonin Syndrome[1]

Alprazolam – Clomipramine
Amphetamines – MAO inhibitors
Amphetamines – SSRIs (Citalopram, Fluoxetine, Fluvoxamine, Paroxetine, Sertraline)
Amphetamines – Tricyclic antidepressants
Amitriptyline – Dihydroergotamine
Amitriptyline – Lithium – Trazodone
Amitriptyline – Sertraline
Anorexiants – MAO inhibitors
Bromocriptine – Levodopa/Carbidopa
Buspirone – Nefazodone
Buspirone – SSRIs (Citalopram, Fluoxetine, Fluvoxamine, Paroxetine, Sertraline)
Buspirone – Trazodone
Buspirone – Tricyclic antidepressants
Carbamazepine – Fluoxetine
Citalopram – Moclobemide
Clomipramine – Alprazolam
Clomipramine – Clorgiline
Clomipramine – Lithium
Clomipramine – MAO inhibitors
Clomipramine – Moclobemide
Clomipramine – S-adenosylmethionine
Clomipramine – Tranylcypromine
Clorgiline – Clomipramine
Dextromethorphan – MAO inhibitors
Dextromethorphan – SSRIs (Citalopram, Fluoxetine, Fluvoxamine, Paroxetine, Sertraline)
Dextropropoxyphene – Phenelzine – Trazodone
Dihydroergotamine – Amitriptyline
Dihydroergotamine – Paroxetine
Dihydroergotamine – SSRIs (Citalopram, Fluoxetine, Fluvoxamine, Paroxetine, Sertraline)
Dihydroergotamine – Tricyclic antidepressants
Fentanyl – SSRIs (Citalopram, Fluoxetine, Fluvoxamine, Paroxetine, Sertraline)
Fluoxetine – Carbamazepine

Fluoxetine – Remoxipride
Fluoxetine – Tryptophan
Levodopa/Carbidopa – Bromocriptine
Linezolid - SSRIs (Citalopram, Fluoxetine, Fluvoxamine, Paroxetine, Sertraline)
Linezolid – Tramadol
Linezolid – Tricyclic antidepressants
Lithium – Amitriptyline – Trazodone
Lithium – Clomipramine
Lithium – SSRIs (Citalopram, Fluoxetine, Fluvoxamine, Paroxetine, Sertraline)
Lithium – Tricyclic antidepressants
Lithium – Venlafaxine
Lysergic acid diethylamide (LSD) – SSRIs (Citalopram, Fluoxetine, Fluvoxamine, Paroxetine, Sertraline)
Metoclopramide – Sertraline
Metoclopramide – Venlafaxine
MAO inhibitors – Amphetamines
MAO inhibitors – Anorexiants
MAO inhibitors – Clomipramine
MAO inhibitors – Dextromethorphan
MAO inhibitors – Meperidine
MAO inhibitors – Nefazodone
MAO inhibitors – Serotonin agonists
MAO inhibitors – S-adenosylmethionine
MAO inhibitors – SSRIs (Citalopram, Fluoxetine, Fluvoxamine, Paroxetine, Sertraline)
MAO inhibitors – St John's Wort
MAO inhibitors – Tramadol
MAO inhibitors – Trazodone
MAO inhibitors – Tricyclic antidepressants
MAO inhibitors – Tryptophan
MAO inhibitors – Venlafaxine
Meperidine – MAO inhibitors
Meperidine – Moclobemide
Meperidine – Nefazodone

SEROTONIN SYNDROME *(Continued)*

Meperidine – SSRIs (Citalopram, Fluoxetine, Fluvoxamine, Paroxetine, Sertraline)

Moclobemide – Citalopram

Moclobemide – Clomipramine

Moclobemide – Meperidine

Moclobemide – Pethidine

Moclobemide – SSRIs (Citalopram, Fluoxetine, Fluvoxamine, Paroxetine, Sertraline)

Moclobemide – Tricyclic antidepressants

Nefazodone – Buspirone

Nefazodone – MAO inhibitors

Nefazodone – Meperidine

Nefazodone – Serotonin agonists

Nefazodone – SSRIs (Citalopram, Fluoxetine, Fluvoxamine, Paroxetine, Sertraline)

Nefazodone – Trazodone

Nefazodone – Tramadol

Nefazodone – Valproic Acid

Nortriptyline – Trazodone

Paroxetine – Dihydroergotamine

Paroxetine – Trazodone

Pethidine – Moclobemide

Phenelzine – Trazodone – Dextropropoxyphene

Remoxipride – Fluoxetine

S-adenosylmethionine – Clomipramine

S-adenosylmethionine – MAO inhibitors

S-adenosylmethionine – SSRIs (Citalopram, Fluoxetine, Fluvoxamine, Paroxetine, Sertraline)

S-adenosylmethionine – Tricyclic antidepressants

Selegiline (high-dose) – SSRIs (Citalopram, Fluoxetine, Fluvoxamine, Paroxetine, Sertraline)

Selegiline (high-dose) – Tricyclic antidepressants

Selegiline (high-dose) – Venlafaxine

Serotonin agonists (Sumatriptan, others) – MAO inhibitors

Serotonin agonists (Sumatriptan, others) – Nefazodone

Serotonin agonists (Sumatriptan, others) – SSRIs (Citalopram, Fluoxetine, Fluvoxamine, Paroxetine, Sertraline)

Serotonin agonists (Sumatriptan, others) – TCAs

Serotonin agonists (Sumatriptan, others) – Tramadol

Sertraline – Amitriptyline

Sibutramine – SSRIs (Citalopram, Fluoxetine, Fluvoxamine, Paroxetine, Sertraline)

SSRIs – Amphetamines

SSRIs – Buspirone

SSRIs – Dextromethorphan

SSRIs – Dihydroergotamine

SSRIs – Fentanyl

SSRIs – Linezolid

SSRIs – Lithium

SSRIs – Lysergic acid diethylamide (LSD)

SSRIs – MAO inhibitors

SSRIs – Meperidine

SSRIs – Moclobemide

SSRIs – Nefazodone

SSRIs – S-adenosylmethionine

SSRIs – Selegiline (high-dose)

SSRIs – Serotonin agonists

SSRIs – Sibutramine

SSRIs – St John's Wort

SSRIs – Tramadol

SSRIs – Trazodone

SSRIs – Tricyclic antidepressants

SSRIs – Tryptophan

St John's Wort – MAO inhibitors

St John's Wort – SSRIs (Citalopram, Fluoxetine, Fluvoxamine, Paroxetine, Sertraline)

St John's Wort – Tricyclic antidepressants

Sympathomimetics – Tricyclic antidepressants

Tramadol – Linezolid

Tramadol – MAO inhibitors

Tramadol – Nefazodone

Tramadol – Serotonin agonists

Tramadol – SSRIs (Citalopram, Fluoxetine, Fluvoxamine, Paroxetine, Sertraline)

Tramadol – TCAs

Tranylcypromine – Clomipramine

Trazodone – Buspirone

Trazodone – Lithium – Amitriptyline

Trazodone – MAO inhibitors

Trazodone – Nefazodone

Trazodone – Nortriptyline

Trazodone – Paroxetine

Trazodone – SSRIs (Citalopram, Fluoxetine, Fluvoxamine, Paroxetine, Sertraline) (theoretical)

Tricyclic antidepressants – Amphetamines

Tricyclic antidepressants – Buspirone

Tricyclic antidepressants – Dihydroergotamine

Tricyclic antidepressants – Linezolid

Tricyclic antidepressants – Lithium

Tricyclic antidepressants – MAO inhibitors

Tricyclic antidepressants – Moclobemide

Tricyclic antidepressants – S-adenosylmethionine

Tricyclic antidepressants – Serotonin agonists

Tricyclic antidepressants – SSRIs (Citalopram, Fluoxetine, Fluvoxamine, Paroxetine, Sertraline)

Tricyclic antidepressants – St John's Wort

Tricyclic antidepressants – Sympathomimetics

Tricyclic antidepressants – Tramadol

Tryptophan – Fluoxetine

Tryptophan – MAO inhibitors

Tryptophan – SSRIs (Citalopram, Fluoxetine, Fluvoxamine, Paroxetine, Sertraline)

Valproic acid – Nefazodone

Venlafaxine – Lithium

Venlafaxine – MAO inhibitors

Venlafaxine – Selegiline (high-dose)

[1]When administered within 2 weeks of each other.

Guidelines for Treatment of Serotonin Syndrome

Therapy is primarily supportive with intravenous crystalloid solutions utilized for hypotension and cooling blankets for mild hyperthermia. Norepinephrine is the preferred vasopressor. Chlorpromazine (25 mg I.M.) or dantrolene sodium (1 mg/kg I.V. – maximum dose 10 mg/kg) may have a role in controlling fevers, although there is no proven benefit. Benzodiazepines are the first-line treatment in controlling rigors and thus, limiting fever and rhabdomyolysis, while clonazepam may be specifically useful in treating myoclonus. Endotracheal intubation and paralysis may be required to treat refractory muscular contractions. Tachycardia or tremor can be treated with beta-blocking agents; although due to its blockade of 5-HTIA receptors, the syndrome may worsen. Serotonin blockers such as diphenhydramine (50 mg I.M.), cyproheptadine (adults: 4-8 mg every 2-4 hours up to 0.5 mg/kg/day; children: up to 0.25 mg/kg/day), or chlorpromazine (25 mg I.M.) have been used with variable efficacy. Nitroglycerin (I.V. infusion of 2 mg/kg/minute with lorazepam) also has been utilized with variable efficacy in case reports. It appears that cyproheptadine is most consistently beneficial.

Recovery seen within 1 day in 70% of cases; mortality rate is about 11%.

Pharmacokinetics of Selective Serotonin-Reuptake Inhibitors (SSRIs)

SSRI	Half-life (h)	Metabolite Half-life	Peak Plasma Level (h)	% Protein Bound	Bioavailability (%)
Citalopram	35	N/A	4	80	80
Fluoxetine	Initial: 24-72 Chronic: 96-144	Norfluoxetine 4-16 days	6-8	95	72
Fluvoxamine	16	N/A	3	80	53
Paroxetine	21	N/A	5	95	>90
Sertraline	26	N-desmethyl-sertraline 2-4 days	5-8	98	—

References

Gardner DM and Lynd LD, "Sumatriptan Contraindications and the Serotonin Syndrome," *Ann Pharmacother*, 1998, 32(1):33-8
Gitlin MJ, "Venlafaxine, Monoamine Oxidase Inhibitors, and the Serotonin Syndrome," *J Clin Psychopharmacol*, 1997, 17:66-7.
Heisler MA, Guidery JR, and Arnecke B, "Serotonin Syndrome Induced by Administration of Venlafaxine and Phenelzine," *Ann Pharmacother*, 1996, 30:84.
Hodgman MJ, Martin TG, and Krenzelok EP, "Serotonin Syndrome Due to Venlafaxine and Maintenance Tranylcypromine Therapy," *Hum Exp Toxicol*, 1997, 16:14-7.
John L, Perreault MM, Tao T, et al, "Serotonin Syndrome Associated With Nefazodone and Paroxetine," *Ann Emerg Med*, 1997, 29:287-9.
LoCurto MJ, "The Serotonin Syndrome," *Emerg Clin North Am*, 1997, 15(3):665-75.
Martin TG, "Serotonin Syndrome," *Ann Emerg Med*, 1996, 28:520-6.
Mills K, "Serotonin Toxicity: A Comprehensive Review for Emergency Medicine," *Top Emerg Med*, 1993, 15:54-73.
Mills KC, "Serotonin Syndrome: A Clinical Update," *Crit Care Clin*, 1997, 13(4):763-83.
Nisijima K, Shimizu M, Abe T, et al, "A Case of Serotonin Syndrome Induced by Concomitant Treatment With Low-Dose Trazodone, and Amitriptyline and Lithium," *Int Clin Psychopharmacol*, 1996, 11:289-90.
Sobanski T, Bagli M, Laux G, et al, "Serotonin Syndrome After Lithium Add-On Medication to Paroxetine," *Pharmacopsychiatry*, 1997, 30:106-7.
Sporer, "The Serotonin Syndrome: Implicated Drugs, Pathophysiology and Management," *Drug Safety*, 1995, 13(2):94-104.
Sternbach H, "The Serotonin Syndrome," *Am J Psychiatry*, 1991, 146:705-7.
Van Berkum MM, Thiel J, Leikin JB, et al, "A Fatality Due to Serotonin Syndrome," *Medical Update for Psychiatrists*, 1997, 2:55-7.

TYRAMINE CONTENT OF FOODS

Food	Allowed	Minimize Intake	Not Allowed
Beverages	Milk, decaffeinated coffee, tea, soda	Chocolate beverage, caffeine-containing drinks, clear spirits	Acidophilus milk, beer, ale, wine, malted beverages
Breads/cereals	All except those containing cheese	None	Cheese bread and crackers
Dairy products	Cottage cheese, farmers or pot cheese, cream cheese, ricotta cheese, all milk, eggs, ice cream, pudding (except chocolate)	Yogurt (limit to 4 oz per day)	All other cheeses (aged cheese, American, Camembert, cheddar, Gouda, gruyere, mozzarella, parmesan, provolone, romano, Roquefort, stilton)
Meat, fish, and poultry	All fresh or frozen	Aged meats, hot dogs, canned fish and meat	Chicken and beef liver, dried and pickled fish, summer or dry sausage, pepperoni, dried meats, meat extracts, bologna, liverwurst
Starches – potatoes/rice	All	None	Soybean (including paste)
Vegetables	All fresh, frozen, canned, or dried vegetable juices except those not allowed	Chili peppers, Chinese pea pods	Fava beans, sauerkraut, pickles, olives, Italian broad beans
Fruit	Fresh, frozen, or canned fruits and fruit juices	Avocado, banana, raspberries, figs	Banana peel extract
Soups	All soups not listed to limit or avoid	Commercially canned soups	Soups which contain broad beans, fava beans, cheese, beer, wine, any made with flavor cubes or meat extract, miso soup
Fats	All except fermented	Sour cream	Packaged gravy
Sweets	Sugar, hard candy, honey, molasses, syrups	Chocolate candies	None
Desserts	Cakes, cookies, gelatin, pastries, sherbets, sorbets	Chocolate desserts	Cheese-filled desserts
Miscellaneous	Salt, nuts, spices, herbs, flavorings, Worcestershire sauce	Soy sauce, peanuts	Brewer's yeast, yeast concentrates, all aged and fermented products, monosodium glutamate, vitamins with Brewer's yeast

VITAMIN K CONTENT IN SELECTED FOODS

The following lists describe the relative amounts of vitamin K in selected foods. The abbreviations for vitamin K are "H" for high amounts, "M" for medium amounts, and "L" for low amounts.

Foods[1]	Portion Size[2]	Vitamin K Content
Coffee brewed	10 cups	L
Cola, regular and diet	3½ fl oz	L
Fruit juices, assorted types	3½ fl oz	L
Milk	3½ fl oz	L
Tea, black, brewed	3½ fl oz	L
Bread, assorted types	4 slices	L
Cereal, assorted types	3½ oz	L
Flour, assorted types	1 cup	L
Oatmeal, instant, dry	1 cup	L
Rice, white	½ cup	L
Spaghetti, dry	3½ oz	L
Butter	6 Tbsp	L
Cheddar cheese	3½ oz	L
Eggs	2 large	L
Margarine	7 Tbsp	M
Mayonnaise	7 Tbsp	H
Oils		
Canola, salad, soybean	7 Tbsp	H
Olive	7 Tbsp	M
Corn, peanut, safflower, sesame, sunflower	7 Tbsp	L
Sour cream	8 Tbsp	L
Yogurt	3½ oz	L
Apple	1 medium	L
Banana	1 medium	L
Blueberries	⅔ cup	L
Cantaloupe pieces	⅔ cup	L
Grapes	1 cup	L
Grapefruit	½ medium	L
Lemon	2 medium	L
Orange	1 medium	L
Peach	1 medium	L
Abalone	3½ oz	L
Beef, ground	3½ oz	L
Chicken	3½ oz	L
Mackerel	3½ oz	L
Meatloaf	3½ oz	L
Pork, meat	3½ oz	L
Tuna	3½ oz	L
Turkey, meat	3½ oz	L
Asparagus, raw	7 spears	M
Avocado, peeled	1 small	M
Beans, pod, raw	1 cup	M
Broccoli, raw and cooked	½ cup	H
Brussel sprout, sprout and top leaf	5 sprouts	H
Cabbage, raw	1½ cups shredded	H
Cabbage, red, raw	1½ cups shredded	M
Carrot	⅔ cup	L
Cauliflower	1 cup	L
Celery	2½ stalks	L
Coleslaw	¾ cup	M
Collard greens	½ cup chopped	H
Cucumber peel, raw	1 cup	H
Cucumber, peel removed	1 cup	L

VITAMIN K CONTENT IN SELECTED FOODS *(Continued)*

Foods[1]	Portion Size[2]	Vitamin K Content
Eggplant	1¼ cups pieces	L
Endive, raw	2 cups chopped	H
Green scallion, raw	⅔ cup chopped	H
Kale, raw leaf	¾ cup	H
Lettuce, raw, heading, bib, red leaf	1¾ cups shredded	H
Mushroom	1½ cups	L
Mustard greens, raw	1½ cups	H
Onion, white	⅔ cup chopped	L
Parsley, raw and cooked	1½ cups chopped	H
Peas, green, cooked	⅔ cup	M
Pepper, green, raw	1 cup chopped	L
Potato	1 medium	L
Pumpkin	½ cup	L
Spinach, raw leaf	1½ cups	H
Tomato	1 medium	L
Turnip greens, raw	1½ cups chopped	H
Watercress, raw	3 cups chopped	H
Honey	5 Tbsp	L
Jell-O® Gelatin	⅓ cup	L
Peanut butter	6 Tbsp	L
Pickle, dill	1 medium	M
Sauerkraut	1 cup	M
Soybean, dry	½ cup	M

[1]This list is a partial listing of foods. For more complete information, refer to references 1-2.
[2]Portions in chart are calculated from estimated portions provided in reference 4.

References

Booth SL, Sadowski JA, Weihrauch JL, et al, "Vitamin K₁ (Phylloquinone) Content of Foods a Provisional Table," *J Food Comp Anal*, 1993, 6:109-20.
Ferland G, MacDonald DL, and Sadowski JA, "Development of a Diet Low in Vitamin K₁ (Phylloquinone)," *J Am Diet Assoc*, 1992, 92, 593-7.
Hogan RP, "Hemorrhagic Diathesis Caused by Drinking an Herbal Tea," *JAMA*, 1983, 249:2679-80.
Pennington JA, *Bowes and Church's Food Values of Portions Commonly Used*, 15th ed, JP Lippincott Co, 1985.

DRUGS IN PREGNANCY

Medications Known to Be Teratogens

Alcohol	Isotretinoin
Androgens	Lithium
Anticonvulsants	Live vaccines
Antineoplastics	Methimazole
Cocaine	Penicillamine
Diethylstilbestrol	Tetracyclines
Etretinate	Warfarin
Iodides (including radioactive iodine)	

Medications Suspected to Be Teratogens

ACE inhibitors	Oral hypoglycemic drugs
Benzodiazepines	Progestogens
Estrogens	Quinolones

Medications With No Known Teratogenic Effects[1]

Acetaminophen	Narcotic analgesics
Cephalosporins	Penicillins
Corticosteroids	Phenothiazines
Docusate sodium	Thyroid hormones
Erythromycin	Tricyclic antidepressants
Multiple vitamins	

[1]No drug is absolutely without risk during pregnancy. These drugs appear to have a minimal risk when used judiciously in usual doses under the supervision of a medical professional.

Medications With Nonteratogenic Adverse Effects in Pregnancy

Antithyroid drugs	Diuretics
Aminoglycosides	Isoniazid
Aspirin	Narcotic analgesics (chronic use)
Barbiturates (chronic use)	Nicotine
Benzodiazepines	Nonsteroidal anti-inflammatory agents
Beta-blockers	Oral hypoglycemic agents
Caffeine	Propylthiouracil
Chloramphenicol	Sulfonamides
Cocaine	

Adapted from DiPiro JT, Talbert RL, Hayes PE, et al, "Therapeutic Considerations During Pregnancy and Lactation," *Pharmacotherapy: A Pathophysiologic Approach*, 4th ed, Stamford, CT: Appleton & Lange, 1999.

DRUGS IN PREGNANCY *(Continued)*

MATERNAL / FETAL MEDICATIONS

Adapted from Briggs GG, "Medication Use During the Perinatal Period,"
J Am Pharm Assoc, 1998, 38:717-27.

Antibiotics in Pregnancy

Antibiotic	Comments
Antibiotics to Be Avoided	
Aminoglycosides (prolonged use)	Eighth cranial nerve damage (hearing loss, vestibulotoxicity)
Erythromycin estolate	Hepatotoxic in mother
Fluoroquinolones	Potentially mutagenic, cartilage damage, arthropathy, and teratogenicity
Ribavirin	Possibly fetotoxic
Tetracyclines	Staining of deciduous teeth (4th month through term)
Antibiotics Which Are Generally Regarded as Safe	
Aminoglycosides (limited use)	
Cephalosporins	
Clindamycin	
Erythromycin	
Penicillins	

Treatment and Prevention of Infection in Pregnancy

Prophylaxis	
Preterm premature rupture of membranes	Ampicillin, amoxicillin, cefazolin, amoxicillin/clavulanate, ampicillin/sulbactam, erythromycin
Prevention of bacterial endocarditis	Ampicillin 2 g and gentamicin 1.5 mg/kg (max: 120 mg) within 30 min of delivery, followed by 1 g ampicillin (I.V.) or amoxicillin (oral) 6 hours later
Cesarean section	Cefazolin (I.V. or uterine irrigation) or clindamycin/gentamicin
Treatment	
Bacterial vaginosis	Clindamycin (oral or gel) in first trimester (gel has been associated with higher rate of preterm deliveries) Metronidazole (oral) for 7 days or gel for 5 days (after first trimester)
Chorioamnionitis	Ampicillin plus gentamicin (clindamycin, erythromycin, or vancomycin if PCN allergic)
Genital herpes	First episode: Oral acyclovir Near term treatment may reduce Cesarian sections I.V. therapy for disseminated infection
Group B streptococci	Penicillin G 5 million units once, then 2.5 million units q4h Ampicillin 2 g once, then 1 g q4h Clindamycin or erythromycin if PCN allergic
HIV*	*Note: Always consult HIV guidelines (www.aidsinfo.nih.gov) Zidovudine (limits maternal-fetal transmission) Oral dosing during pregnancy/I.V. prior to delivery Other antiretroviral agents - effects unknown Lamivudine during labor used in combination with zidovudine in women who have not received prior antiretroviral therapy
Postpartum endometritis	Ampicillin (vancomycin if PCN allergic) plus clindamycin (or metronidazole) plus gentamicin until afebrile
Pyelonephritis	Ampicillin-gentamicin Cefazolin Co-trimoxazole
Urinary tract infection	Amoxicillin/ampicillin (resistance has increased) Co-trimoxazole Nitrofurantoin Cephalexin
Vaginal candidiasis	Buconizole for 7 days Clotrimazole for 7 days Miconazole for 7 days Terconazole for 7 days

Preterm Labor: Tocolytic Agents

Drug Class	Route	Fetal/Neonatal Toxicities	Maternal Toxicities
Beta-adrenergic agonists Ritodrine, terbutaline	Oral, I.V., SubQ	Fetal tachycardia, intraventricular septal hypertrophy, neonatal hyperinsulinemia/hypoglycemia	Pulmonary, edema, myocardial infarction, hypokalemia, hypotension, hyperglycemia, tachycardia
Magnesium	I.V.	Neurologic depression in newborn (loss of reflexes, hypotonia, respiratory depression); fetal hypocalcemia and hypercalcuria; abnormal fetal bone mineralization and enamel hypoplasia	Hypotension, respiratory depression, ileus/constipation, hypocalcemia, pulmonary edema, hypotension, headache/dizziness
NSAIDs Indomethacin	Oral, P.R.	Ductus arteriosis: premature closure, tricuspid regurgitation, primary pulmonary hypertension of the newborn, PDA; intraventricular hemorrhage, necrotizing enterocolitis, renal failure	GI bleeding, oligohydramnios, pulmonary edema, acute renal failure
Calcium channel blockers Nifedipine	Oral	Hypoxia secondary to maternal hypotension	Hypotension, flushing, tachycardia, headache
Nitrates Nitroglycerin	I.V./S.L.	Hypoxia secondary to maternal hypotension	Hypotension, headache, dizziness

Pregnancy-Induced Hypertension[1]

Drug Class	Maternal / Fetal Effects
Antihypertensives Contraindicated in PIH	
Diuretics	Reduction of maternal plasma volume exacerbates disease; use in chronic hypertension acceptable (if no superimposed pregnancy-induced hypertension)
ACE inhibitors	Teratogenic in second and third trimester; fetal/newborn anuria and hypotension, fetal oligohydramnios; neonatal death (congenital abnormalities of skull and renal failure)
Hypertension Treatment[2]	
Central-acting Methyldopa	Relatively safe in second/third trimester
Beta-blockers Acebutolol, atenolol, metoprolol, pindolol, propranolol	Increased risk of IUGR
Alpha-/beta-blocking Labetolol	See beta-blockers
Vasodilators Hydralazine	Relatively safe in second/third trimester
Nitrates Nitroglycerin	Relatively safe in second/third trimester
Calcium channel blockers Nifedipine	Relatively safe in second/third trimester

[1]Includes management of pre-eclampsia/eclampsia and HELLP syndrome. **Note:** Prevention may include low-dose aspirin (81 mg/day) or calcium supplementation (2 g/day).

[2]All agents must be carefully titrated to avoid fetal hypoxia.

BREAST-FEEDING AND DRUGS

Prior to recommending or prescribing medications to a lactating woman, the following should be considered:

- Is drug therapy necessary?
- Can drug exposure to the infant be minimized? (Using a different route of administration, timing of the dose in relation to breast-feeding, length of therapy, using breast milk stored prior to treatment, etc)
- The infants age and health status (their own ability to metabolize the medication)
- The pharmacokinetics of the drug
- Will the drug interact with a medication the infant is prescribed?
- If medications must be used, pick the safest drug possible.
- In situations where the only drug available may have adverse effects in the nursing infant, consider measuring the infants blood levels.

The tables presented below have been adapted from the American Academy of Pediatrics Committee on Drugs report "Transfer of Drugs and Other Chemicals Into Human Milk," September 2001. It should not be inferred that if a medication is not in the tables it is considered safe for administration to a lactating woman; only that published reports concerning their use were not available at the time the report was published.

Table 1. Cytotoxic Drugs

Cyclophosphamide	Doxorubicin
Cyclosporine	Methotrexate

These are medications thought to interfere with cellular metabolism in the nursing infant. Immune suppression may be possible; effects on growth or carcinogenesis are not known. In addition, doxorubicin is concentrated in human milk; methotrexate is associated with neutropenia in the nursing infant.

Table 2. Drugs of Abuse

Amphetamine	Marijuana
Cocaine	Phencyclidine
Heroin	

Drugs of abuse are not only dangerous to the nursing infant, but also to the mother. Women should be encouraged to avoid their use completely. Effects to the infant reported with amphetamine use in the mother include irritability and poor sleeping; it is also a substance that is concentrated in human milk. Cocaine may cause irritability, vomiting, diarrhea, tremors, or seizures in the infant. Heroin may also cause tremors as well as restlessness, vomiting, and poor feeding.

Nicotine, which was previously on this list, is associated with decreased milk production, decreased weight gain in the infant, and possible increased respiratory illness in the infant. Although there are still questions outstanding regarding smoking and breast-feeding, women should be counseled on the possible effects to their infants and offered aid to smoking cessation if appropriate.

Table 3. Radioactive Compounds That Require Temporary Cessation of Breast-Feeding

Drug	Recommended Time for Cessation of Breast-Feeding
Copper 64 (^{64}Cu)	Radioactivity in milk present at 50 h
Gallium 67 (^{67}Ga)	Radioactivity in milk present for 2 wk
Indium 111 (^{111}In)	Very small amount present at 20 h
Iodine 123 (^{123}I)	Radioactivity in milk present up to 36 h
Iodine 125 (^{125}I)	Radioactivity in milk present for 12 d
Iodine 131 (^{131}I)	Radioactivity in milk present 2-14 d, depending on study
Iodine^{131}	If used for thyroid cancer, high radioactivity may prolong exposure to infant
Radioactive sodium	Radioactivity in milk present 96 h
Technetium-99m (^{99m}Tc), ^{99m}Tc macroaggregates, ^{99m}Tc O4	Radioactivity in milk present 15 h to 3 d

Consider pumping and storing milk prior to study for use during the radioactive period. Pumping should continue after the study to maintain milk production; however, this milk should be discarded until radioactivity is gone. Notify nuclear medicine physician prior to study that the mother is breast-feeding; a short-acting radionuclide may be appropriate. Contact Radiology Department after testing is complete to screen milk samples before resuming feeding.

Table 4a. Psychotropic Drugs Whose Effect on Nursing Infants Is Unknown But May Be of Concern

Antianxiety	Antidepressant	Antipsychotic
Alprazolam	Amitriptyline	Chlorpromazine
Diazepam	Amoxapine	Clozapine[1]
Lorazepam	Bupropion	Haloperidol
Midazolam	Clomipramine	Mesoridazine
Perphenazine	Desipramine	Trifluoperazine
Prazepam[1]	Doxepin	
Quazepam	Fluoxetine	
Temazepam	Fluvoxamine	
	Imipramine	
	Nortriptyline	
	Paroxetine	
	Sertraline[1]	
	Trazodone	

[1]Drug is concentrated in human milk.

Psychotropic medications usually appear in the breast milk in low concentrations. Although adverse effects in the infant may be limited to a few case reports, the long half-life of these medications and their metabolites should be considered. In addition, measurable amounts may be found in the infants plasma and also brain tissue. Long-term effects are not known. Colic, irritability, feeding and sleep disorders, and slow weight gain are effects reported with fluoxetine. Chlorpromazine may cause galactorrhea in the mother, while drowsiness and lethargy have been reported in the nursing infant. A decline in developmental scores has been reported with chlorpromazine and haloperidol.

Table 4b. Additional Drugs Whose Effect on Nursing Infants Is Unknown But May Be of Concern

Drug	Reported Effect in Nursing Infant
Amiodarone	Hypothyroidism
Chloramphenicol	Idiosyncratic bone marrow suppression
Clofazimine	Increase in skin pigmentation; high transfer of mothers dose to infant is possible
Lamotrigine	Therapeutic serum concentrations in infant
Metoclopramide[1]	
Metronidazole	
Tinidazole	

[1]Drug is concentrated in human milk.

No adverse effects to the infant have been reported for metoclopramide; however, it should be recognized that it is a dopaminergic agent. Metronidazole and tinidazole are *in vitro* mutagenic agents. In cases where single dose therapy is appropriate for the mother, breast-feeding may be discontinued for 12-24 hours to allow excretion of the medication.

Table 5. Drugs That Have Been Associated With Significant Effects on Some Nursing Infants and Should Be Given to Nursing Mothers With Caution[1]

Drug	Reported Effect
Acebutolol	Hypotension, bradycardia, tachypnea
5-Aminosalicylic acid	Diarrhea (one case)
Atenolol	Cyanosis, bradycardia
Bromocriptine	Suppresses lactation; may be hazardous to the mother
Aspirin (salicylates)	Metabolic acidosis (one case)
Clemastine	Drowsiness, irritability, refusal to feed, high-pitched cry, neck stiffness (one case)
Ergotamine	Vomiting, diarrhea, convulsions (doses used in migraine medications
Lithium	One-third to one-half therapeutic blood concentration in infants
Phenindione	Anticoagulant: increased prothrombin and partial thromboplastin time in one infant; not used in the United States
Phenobarbital	Sedation; infantile spasms after weaning from milk-containing phenobarbital, methemoglobinemia (one case)
Primidone	Sedation, feeding problems
Sulfasalazine (salicylazosulfapyridine)	Bloody diarrhea (one case)

[1]Blood concentration in the infant may be of clinical importance; measure when possible.

References

American Academy of Pediatrics Committee on Drugs, "Transfer of Drugs and Other Chemicals Into Human Milk," *Pediatrics*, 2001, 108(3): 776-89.
2000 Red Book: Report of the Committee on Infectious Diseases, 25th ed, Elk Grove Village, IL: American Academy of Pediatrics, 2000, 98-104.

ANTIDEPRESSANT MEDICATION GUIDELINES

The under-diagnosis and under-treatment of depression in nursing homes has been documented in a *Journal of the American Medical Association* paper entitled, "Depression and Mortality in the Nursing Home" [*JAMA*, February 27, 1991, 265(8)]. The Centers for Medicare and Medicaid Services (CMS), formerly known as the Health Care Financing Administration (HCFA), continues to support the accurate identification and treatment of depression in nursing homes.

The surveyor should not urge a facility to use behavioral monitoring charts (documenting quantitatively [eg, number of episodes] and objectively [eg, withdrawn behavior such as, staying in their room, refusal to speak, etc]) when antidepressant drugs are used in nursing homes. Such charts are promoted in the interpretative guidelines for antipsychotic and benzodiazepine and other anxiolytic/sedative drugs, but **not** for antidepressant drugs. These charts may be helpful for monitoring the effects of antidepressant drugs in nursing homes, but they may place additional paperwork burden on the facility, and thus act as a deterrent to the appropriate diagnosis and treatment of this condition.

The following is a list of commonly used antidepressant drugs:

Generic Name	Brand Name
Amitriptyline[1]	Elavil®
Amoxapine	Asendin®
Bupropion	Wellbutrin®
Citalopram[1]	Celexa®
Clomipramine[1]	Anafranil®
Desipramine	Norpramin®
Doxepin[1]	Sinequan®
Fluoxetine	Prozac®
Fluvoxamine	Luvox®
Imipramine[1]	Tofranil
Maprotiline	Ludiomil®
Mirtazapine	Remeron®
Nefazodone	Serzone®
Nortriptyline	Aventyl®, Pamelor®
Paroxetine	Paxil®
Phenelzine[1]	Nardil®
Protriptyline	Vivactil®
Sertraline	Zoloft®
Tranylcypromine[1]	Parnate®
Trazodone	Desyrel®
Trimipramine[1]	Surmontil®
Venlafaxine	Effexor®

[1]These are not necessarily drugs of choice for depression in the elderly. They are listed here only in the event of their potential use.

ANTIPSYCHOTIC MEDICATION GUIDELINES

Appropriate indications for use of antipsychotic medications are outlined in the Health Care Finance Administration's Omnibus Reconciliation Act (OBRA) of 1987. These regulations require that antipsychotics be used to treat specific conditions (listed below) and not solely for behavior control.

Approved indications include:

- acute psychotic episode
- atypical psychosis
- brief reactive psychosis
- delusional disorder
- Huntington's disease
- psychotic mood disorder (including manic depression and depression with psychotic features)
- schizo-affective disorder
- schizophrenia
- schizophrenic form disorder
- Tourette's disease
- short-term (7 days) for hiccups, nausea, vomiting, or pruritus
- organic mental syndrome with psychotic or agitated features:

    – behaviors are quantitatively and objectively documented
    – behaviors must be **persistent**
    – behaviors are not caused by preventable reasons
    – patient presents a danger to self or others
    – continuous crying or screaming if this impairs functional status
    – psychotic symptoms (hallucinations, paranoia, delusions) which cause resident distress or impaired functional capacity

"Clinically contraindicated" means that a resident with a "specific condition" who has had a history of recurrence of psychotic symptoms (eg, delusions, hallucinations) which have been stabilized with a maintenance dose of an antipsychotic drug without incurring significant side effects (eg, tardive dyskinesia) **should not receive gradual dose reductions.** In residents with organic mental syndromes (eg, dementia, delirium), "clinically contraindicated" means that a gradual dose reduction has been attempted **twice** in 1 year and that attempt resulted in the return of symptoms for which the drug was prescribed to a degree that a cessation in the gradual dose reduction, or a return to previous dose levels was necessary.

If the medication is being used outside the guidelines, the physician must provide justification why the continued use of the drug and the dose of the drug is clinically appropriate.

Antipsychotics should not be used if one or more of the following is/are the **only** indication:

- wandering
- poor self care
- restlessness
- impaired memory
- anxiety
- depression (without psychotic features)
- insomnia
- unsociability
- indifference to surroundings
- fidgeting
- nervousness
- uncooperativeness
- agitated behaviors which do **not** represent danger to the resident or others

Selection of an antipsychotic agent should be based on the side effect profile since all antipsychotic agents are equally effective at equivalent doses. Coadministration of two or more antipsychotics does not have any pharmacological basis or clinical advantage and increases the potential for side effects.

ANTIPSYCHOTIC MEDICATION GUIDELINES *(Continued)*

DOSING GUIDELINES

1. Daily dosages should be equal to or less than those listed below, unless documentation exists to support the need for higher doses to maintain or improve functional status.

Generic	Brand	Daily Dose for Patients With Organic Mental Syndrome
Chlorpromazine	Thorazine®	75 mg
Clozapine	Clozaril®	50 mg
Fluphenazine	Prolixin®	4 mg
Haloperidol	Haldol®	4 mg
Loxapine	Loxitane®	10 mg
Mesoridazine	Serentil®	25 mg
Molindone	Moban®	10 mg
Olanzapine	Zyprexa®	5 mg
Perphenazine	Trilafon®	8 mg
Pimozide	Orap™	4 mg
Prochlorperazine	Compazine®	10 mg
Quetiapine	Seroquel®	100 mg
Risperidone	Risperdal®	2 mg
Thioridazine	Mellaril®	75 mg
Thiothixene	Navane®	7 mg
Trifluoperazine	Stelazine® [DSC]	8 mg

2. The dose of prochlorperazine may be exceeded for short-term (up to 7 days) for treatment of nausea and vomiting. Residents with nausea and vomiting secondary to cancer or cancer chemotherapy can also be treated with higher doses for longer periods of time.

3. The residents must receive adequate monitoring for significant side effects such as tardive dyskinesia, postural hypotension, cognitive-behavioral impairment, akathisia, and parkinsonism.

4. Gradual dosage reductions are to be attempted twice in 1 year if prescribed for OMS. If symptoms for which the drug has been prescribed return and both reduction attempts have proven unsuccessful, the physician may indicate further reductions are clinically contraindicated.

5. "Clinically contraindicated" means that a resident **need not undergo** a "gradual dose reduction" or "behavioral interventions" if:

   - The resident has a "specific condition" and has a history of recurrence of psychotic symptoms (eg, delusions, hallucinations), which have been stabilized with a maintenance dose of an antipsychotic drug without incurring significant side effects.

   - The resident has organic mental syndrome (now called "delirium, dementia, and amnestic and other cognitive disorders" by DSM IV) and has had a gradual dose reduction attempted **twice** in 1 year and that attempt resulted in the return of symptoms for which the drug was prescribed to a degree that a cessation in the gradual dose reduction, or a return to previous dose reduction was necessary.

   - The resident's physician provides a justification why the continued use of the drug and the dose of the drug is clinically appropriate. This justification should include: a) a diagnosis, but not simply a diagnostic label or code, but the description of symptoms, b) a discussion of the differential psychiatric and medical diagnosis (eg, why the resident's behavioral symptom is thought to be a result of a dementia with associated psychosis and/or agitated behaviors, and not the result of an unrecognized painful medical condition or a psychosocial or environmental stressor), c) a description of the justification for the choice of a particular treatment, or treatments, and d) a discussion of why the present dose is necessary to manage the symptoms of the resident. This information need not necessarily be in the physician's progress notes, but must be a part of the resident's clinical record.

Examples of evidence that would support a justification of why a drug is being used outside these guidelines but in the best interests of the resident may include, but are not limited to the following.

- A physician's note indicating for example, that the dosage, duration, indication, and monitoring are clinically appropriate, **and the reasons why they are clinically appropriate**; this note should demonstrate that the physician has carefully considered the risk/benefit to the resident in using drugs outside the guidelines.

- A medical or psychiatric consultation or evaluation (eg, Geriatric Depression Scale) that confirms the physician's judgment that use of a drug outside the guidelines is in the best interest of the resident.

- Physician, nursing, or other health professional documentation indicating that the resident is being monitored for adverse consequences or complications of the drug therapy.

- Documentation confirming that previous attempts at dosage reduction have been unsuccessful.

- Documentation (including MDS documentation) showing resident's subjective or objective improvement, or maintenance of function while taking the medication.

- Documentation showing that a resident's decline or deterioration is evaluated by the interdisciplinary team to determine whether a particular drug, or a particular dose, or duration of therapy, may be the cause.

- Documentation showing why the resident's age, weight, or other factors would require a unique drug dose or drug duration, indication, or monitoring.

- Other evidence you may deem appropriate.

ANXIOLYTIC / HYPNOTIC USE IN LONG-TERM CARE FACILITIES

One of the regulations regarding medication use in long-term care facilities concerns "unnecessary drugs." The regulation states, "Each resident's drug regimen must be free from unnecessary drugs." The Health Care Financing Administration (HCFA), now known as Centers for Medicaid and Medicare Services (CMS), issued the final interpretive guidelines on this regulation (*State Operations Manual: Provider Certification, Transmittal 232,* Washington, DC: HCFA, Department of Health and Human Services, September 1989). The following is a summary of these guidelines as they pertain to anxiolytic/hypnotic agents.

A. **Long-Acting Benzodiazepines**

Long-acting benzodiazepine drugs should not be used in residents unless an attempt with a shorter-acting drug has failed. If they are used, the doses must be no higher than the listed dose, unless higher doses are necessary for maintenance or improvement in the resident's functional status. Daily use should be less than 4 continuous months unless an attempt at a gradual dose reduction is unsuccessful. Residents on diazepam for seizure disorders or for the treatment of tardive dyskinesia are exempt from this restriction. Residents on clonazepam for bipolar disorder, tardive dyskinesia, nocturnal myoclonus, or seizure disorder are also exempt. Residents on long-acting benzodiazepines should have a gradual dose reduction at least twice within 1 year before it can be concluded that the gradual dose reduction is "clinically contraindicated."

Generic	Brand	Maximum Daily Geriatric Dose (mg)
Chlordiazepoxide	Librium®	20
Clonazepam	Klonopin™	1.5
Clorazepate	Tranxene®	15
Diazepam	Valium®	5
Flurazepam	Dalmane®	15
Halazepam	Paxipam®	40
Quazepam	Doral®	7.5

B. **Benzodiazepine or Other Anxiolytic / Sedative Drugs**

Anxiolytic/sedative drugs should be used for purposes other than sleep induction only when other possible causes of the resident's distress have been ruled out and the use results in maintenance or improvement in the resident's functional status. Daily use should not exceed 4 continuous months unless an attempt at gradual dose reduction has failed. Anxiolytics should only be used for generalized anxiety disorder, dementia with agitated states that either endangers the resident or others, or is a source of distress or dysfunction; panic disorder or symptomatic anxiety associated with other psychiatric disorders. The dose should not exceed those listed below unless a higher dose is needed as evidenced by the resident's response. Gradual dosage reductions should be attempted at least twice within 1 year before it can be concluded that a gradual dose reduction is "clinically contraindicated."

Short-Acting Benzodiazepines

Generic	Brand	Maximum Daily Geriatric Dose (mg)
Alprazolam	Xanax®	0.75
Estazolam[1]	ProSom®	0.5
Lorazepam	Ativan®	2
Oxazepam	Serax®	30

[1]Primarily used as a hypnotic agent.

Other Anxiolytic and Sedative Drugs

Generic	Brand	Maximum Daily Geriatric Dose (mg)
Chloral hydrate	Noctec®, etc	750
Diphenhydramine	Benadryl®	50
Hydroxyzine	Atarax®, Vistaril®	50

Note: Chloral hydrate, diphenhydramine, and hydroxyzine are not necessarily drugs of choice for treatment of anxiety disorders. CMS lists them only in the event of their possible use.

C. **Drugs Used for Sleep Induction**

Drugs for sleep induction should only be used when all possible reasons for insomnia have been ruled out (ie, pain, noise, caffeine). The use of the drug must result in the maintenance or improvement of the resident's functional status. Daily use of a hypnotic should not exceed 10 consecutive days unless an attempt at a gradual dose reduction is unsuccessful. The dose should not exceed those listed below unless a higher dose has been deemed necessary. Gradual dose reductions should be attempted at least three times within 6 months before it can be concluded that a gradual dose reduction is "clinically contraindicated."

Hypnotic Drugs

Generic	Brand	Daily Geriatric Dose (mg)
Alprazolam[1]	Xanax®	0.25
Chloral hydrate	Noctec®	500
Diphenhydramine	Benadryl®	25
Estazolam	ProSom®	0.5
Hydroxyzine	Atarax®, Vistaril®	50
Lorazepam[1]	Ativan®	1
Oxazepam[1]	Serax®	15
Temazepam	Restoril®	7.5
Triazolam	Halcion®	0.125
Zaleplon	Sonata®	5
Zolpidem	Ambien®	5

[1]Not officially indicated as a hypnotic agent.

Note: Chloral hydrate, diphenhydramine, and hydroxyzine are not necessarily drugs of choice for sleep disorders. CMS lists them only in the event of their possible use.

D. **Miscellaneous Hypnotic / Sedative / Anxiolytic Drugs**

The initiation of the following medications should not occur in any dose in any resident. Residents currently using these drugs or residents admitted to the facility while using these drugs should receive gradual dose reductions. Newly admitted residents should have a period of adjustment before attempting reduction. Dose reductions should be attempted at least twice within 1 year before it can be concluded that it is "clinically contraindicated."

Examples of Barbiturates

Generic	Brand
Amobarbital	Amytal®
Amobarbital/secobarbital	Tuinal®
Butabarbital	Butisol Sodium®
Combinations	Fiorinal®, etc
Pentobarbital	Nembutal®
Secobarbital	Seconal®

Miscellaneous Hypnotic / Sedative / Anxiolytic Agents

Generic	Brand
Ethchlorvynol	Placidyl®
Glutethimide	Doriden®
Meprobamate	Equanil®, Miltown®
Methyprylon	Noludar®

CMS[1] GUIDELINES FOR UNNECESSARY DRUGS IN LONG-TERM CARE FACILITIES

Procedures: Section 483.25(1)(1)

Omnibus Budget Reconciliation Act of 1987. PL100-203, December 22, 1987.

Consider drug therapy "unnecessary" only after determining that the facility's use of the drug is:

- in excessive dose (including duplicate drug therapy)
- for excessive duration
- without adequate monitoring
- without adequate indications of use
- in the presence of adverse consequences which indicate the dose should be reduced or discontinued, or
- any combination of the reasons above

Allow the facility the opportunity to provide a rationale for the use of drugs prescribed outside the preceding guidelines. The facility may not justify the use of a drug prescribed outside the proceeding guidelines solely on the basis of "the doctor ordered it." This justification would render the regulation meaningless. The rationale must be based on sound risk-benefit analysis of the resident's symptoms and potential adverse effects of the drug. Examples of evidence that would support a justification of why a drug is being used outside these guidelines but in the best interests of the resident may include, but are not limited to:

- a physician's note indicating for example, that the dosage, duration, indication, and monitoring are clinically appropriate, **and the reasons why they are clinically appropriate**; this note should demonstrate that the physician has carefully considered the risk/benefit to the resident in using drugs outside the guidelines

- a medical or psychiatric consultation or evaluation (eg, geriatric depression scale) that confirms the physician's judgment that use of a drug outside the guidelines is in the best interest of the resident

- physician, nursing, or other health professional documentation indicating that the resident is being monitored for adverse consequences or complications of the drug therapy

- documentation confirming that previous attempts at dosage reduction have been unsuccessful

- documentation (including MDS documentation) showing resident's subjective or objective improvement, or maintenance of function while taking the medication

- documentation showing that a resident's decline or deterioration is evaluated by the interdisciplinary team to determine whether a particular drug, or a particular dose, or duration of therapy, may be the cause

- documentation showing why the resident's age, weight, or other factors would require a unique drug dose or drug duration, indication, monitoring, and

- other evidence the survey team may deem appropriate

If the survey team determines that there is a deficiency in the use of antipsychotics, cite the facility under either the "unnecessary drug" regulation or the "antipsychotic drug" regulation, but not both.

Note: The unnecessary drug criterion of "adequate indications for use" does not simply mean that the **physician's order** must include a reason for using the drug (although such order-writing is encouraged). It means that the **resident** lacks a valid clinical reason for use of the drug, as evidenced by the survey team's evaluation of some, but not necessarily all, of the following:

- observation, assessment, and interview of the resident
- plan of care
- progress notes/reports of significant change
- laboratory reports
- professional consults
- drug orders

[1]The Health Care Financing Administration (HCFA) has been renamed **Centers for Medicare and Medicaid Services (CMS).**

FEDERAL OBRA REGULATIONS RECOMMENDED MAXIMUM DOSES

Antidepressants

Drug	Brand Name	Usual Max Daily Dose for Age ≥65	Usual Max Daily Dose
Amitriptyline	Elavil®	150 mg	300 mg
Amoxapine	Asendin®	200 mg	400 mg
Desipramine	Norpramin®	150 mg	300 mg
Doxepin	Adapin®, Sinequan®	150 mg	300 mg
Imipramine	Tofranil®	150 mg	300 mg
Maprotiline	Ludiomil®	150 mg	300 mg
Nortriptyline	Aventyl®, Pamelor®	75 mg	150 mg
Protriptyline	Vivactil®	30 mg	60 mg
Trazodone	Desyrel®	300 mg	600 mg
Trimipramine	Surmontil®	150 mg	300 mg

Antipsychotics

Drug	Brand Name	Usual Max Daily Dose for Age ≥65	Usual Max Daily Dose	Daily Oral Dose for Residents With Organic Mental Syndromes
Chlorpromazine	Thorazine®	800 mg	1600 mg	75 mg
Chlorprothixene	Taractan®	800 mg	1600 mg	75 mg
Clozapine	Clozaril®	25 mg	450 mg	50 mg
Fluphenazine	Prolixin®	20 mg	40 mg	4 mg
Haloperidol	Haldol®	50 mg	100 mg	4 mg
Loxapine	Loxitane®	125 mg	250 mg	10 mg
Mesoridazine	Serentil®	250 mg	500 mg	25 mg
Molindone	Moban®	112 mg	225 mg	10 mg
Perphenazine	Trilafon®	32 mg	64 mg	8 mg
Promazine	Sparine®	50 mg	500 mg	150 mg
Risperidone	Risperdal®	1 mg	16 mg	2 mg
Thioridazine	Mellaril®	400 mg	800 mg	75 mg
Thiothixene	Navane®	30 mg	60 mg	7 mg
Trifluoperazine	Stelazine®	40 mg	80 mg	8 mg
Trifluopromazine	Vesprin®	100 mg	20 mg	–
Quetiapine	Seroquel®		800 mg	200 mg

FEDERAL OBRA REGULATIONS RECOMMENDED MAXIMUM DOSES *(Continued)*

Anxiolytics[1]

Drug	Brand Name	Usual Daily Dose for Age ≥65	Usual Daily Dose for Age ≤65
Alprazolam	Xanax®	2 mg	4 mg
Chlordiazepoxide	Librium®	40 mg	100 mg
Clorazepate	Tranxene®	30 mg	60 mg
Diazepam	Valium®	20 mg	60 mg
Halazepam	Paxipam®	80 mg	160 mg
Lorazepam	Ativan®	3 mg	6 mg
Meprobamate	Miltown®	600 mg	1600 mg
Oxazepam	Serax®	60 mg	90 mg

[1]**Note:** CMS-OBRA (formerly HCFA-OBRA) guidelines strongly urge clinicians not to use barbiturates, glutethimide, and ethchlorvynol due to their side effects, pharmacokinetics, and addiction potential in the elderly. Also, CMS (formerly HCFA) discourages use of long-acting benzodiazepines in the elderly.

Hypnotics[1]
(Should not be used for more than 10 continuous days)

Drug	Brand Name	Usual Max Single Dose for Age ≥65	Usual Max Single Dose
Alprazolam	Xanax®	0.25 mg	1.5 mg
Amobarbital	Amytal®	105 mg	300 mg
Butabarbital	Butisol®	100 mg	200 mg
Chloral hydrate	Noctec®	750 mg	1500 mg
Chloral hydrate	Various	500 mg	1000 mg
Diphenhydramine	Benadryl®	25 mg	50 mg
Ethchlorvynol	Placidyl®	500 mg	1000 mg
Flurazepam	Dalmane®	15 mg	30 mg
Glutethimide	Doriden®	500 mg	1000 mg
Halazepam	Paxipam®	20 mg	40 mg
Hydroxyzine	Atarax®	50 mg	100 mg
Lorazepam	Ativan®	1 mg	2 mg
Oxazepam	Serax®	15 mg	30 mg
Pentobarbital	Nembutal®	100 mg	200 mg
Secobarbital	Seconal®	100 mg	200 mg
Temazepam	Restoril®	15 mg	30 mg
Triazolam	Halcion®	0.125 mg	0.5 mg

[1]**Note:** CMS-OBRA (formerly known as HCFA-OBRA) guidelines strongly urge clinicians not to use barbiturates, glutethimide, and ethchlorvynol due to their side effects, pharmacokinetics, and addiction potential in the elderly. Also, CMS (formerly known as HCFA) discourages use of long-acting benzodiazepines in the elderly and also discourages the use of diphenhydramine and hydroxyzine.

OVERDOSE AND TOXICOLOGY

GENERAL STABILIZATION OF THE PATIENT

The recommended treatment plan for the poisoned patient is not unlike general treatment plans taught in advanced cardiac life support (ACLS) or advanced trauma life support (ATLS) courses. In this manner, the initial approach to the poisoned patient should be essentially similar in every case, irrespective of the toxin ingested, just as the initial approach to the trauma patient is the same, irrespective of the mechanism of injury. This approach, which can be termed as routine poison management, essentially includes the following aspects.

- Stabilization: ABCs (airway, breathing, circulation; administration of glucose, thiamine, oxygen, and naloxone)
- History, physical examination leading toward the identification of class of toxin (toxidrome recognition)
- Prevention of absorption (decontamination)
- Specific antidote, if available
- Removal of absorbed toxin (enhancing excretion)
- Support and monitoring for adverse effects

Drug	Effect	Comment
25-50 g **dextrose** (D_{50}W) intravenously to reverse the effects of drug-induced hypoglycemia (adult); 1 mL/kg D_{50}W diluted 1:1 (child)	This can be especially effective in patients with limited glycogen stores (ie, neonates and patients with cirrhosis)	Extravasation into the extremity of this hyperosmolar solution can cause Volkmann's contractures
50-100 mg intravenous **thiamine**	Prevent Wernicke's encephalopathy	A water-soluble vitamin with low toxicity; rare anaphylactoid reactions have been reported
Initial dosage of **naloxone** should be 2 mg in adult patients preferably by the intravenous route, although intramuscular, subcutaneous, intralingual, and endotracheal routes may also be utilized. Pediatric dose is 0.1 mg/kg from birth until 5 years of age.	Specific opioid antagonist without any agent properties	It should be noted that some semisynthetic opiates (such as meperidine or propoxyphene) may require higher initial doses for reversal, so that a total dose of 6-10 mg is not unusual for the adults. If the patient responds to a bolus dose and then relapses to a lethargic or comatose state, a naloxone drip can be considered. This can be accomplished by administering two-thirds of the bolus dose that revives the patient per hour or injecting 4 mg naloxone in 1 L crystalloid solution and administering at a rate of 100 mL/ hour 0.4 mg/hour)
Oxygen, utilized in 100% concentration	Useful for carbon monoxide, hydrogen, sulfide, and asphyxiants	While oxygen is antidotal for carbon monoxide intoxication, the only relative toxic contraindication is in paraquat intoxication (in that it can promote pulmonary fibrosis)
Flumazenil	Benzodiazepine antagonist	Not routinely recommended due to increased risk of seizures

OVERDOSE AND TOXICOLOGY (Continued)

LABORATORY EVALUATION OF OVERDOSE

Unknown Ingestion: Electrolytes, anion gap, serum osmolality, arterial blood gases, serum drug concentration

Known Ingestion: Labs tailored to agent

ANION GAP

Definition: The difference in concentration between unmeasured cation and anion equivalents in serum

Anion gap = $Na^+ - Cl^- + HCO_3^-$
(The normal anion gap is 10-14 mEq/L)

DIFFERENTIAL DIAGNOSIS

Increased Anion Gap Acidosis

Organic anions:
 Lactate (sepsis, hypovolemia, seizures, large tumor burden)
 Pyruvate
 Uremia
 Ketoacidosis (β-hydroxybutyrate and acetoacetate)
 Amino acids and their metabolites
 Other organic acids

Inorganic anions:
 Hyperphosphatemia
 Sulfates
 Nitrates

Decreased Anion Gap

Organic cations:
 Hypergammaglobulinemia

Inorganic cations:
 Hyperkalemia
 Hypercalcemia
 Hypermagnesemia

Medications and toxins:
 Lithium

Hypoalbuminemia

TOXINS AFFECTING THE ANION GAP

Drugs Causing Increased Anion Gap (>12 mEq/L)

Nonacidotic
 Carbenicillin

Metabolic Acidosis
 Acetaminophen
 (ingestion >75-100 g)
 Acetazolamide
 Amiloride
 Ascorbic acid
 Benzalkonium chloride
 Benzyl alcohol
 Beta-adrenergic drugs
 Bialaphos
 2-Butanone
 Carbon monoxide
 Centrimonium bromide
 Chloramphenicol
 Colchicine
 Cyanide
 Dapsone
 Dimethyl sulfate
 Dinitrophenol
 Endosulfan
 Epinephrine (I.V. overdose)
 Ethanol
 Ethylene dibromide
 Ethylene glycol

Sodium salts

Fenoprofen
Fluoroacetate
Formaldehyde
Fructose (I.V.)
Glycol ethers
Hydrogen sulfide
Ibuprofen (ingestion >300 mg/kg)
Inorganic acid
Iodine
Iron
Isoniazid
Ketamine
Ketoprofen
Metaldehyde
Metformin
Methanol
Methenamine mandelate
Monochloracetic acid
Nalidixic acid
Naproxen
Niacin
Papaverine
Pennyroyal oil

Pentachlorophenol
Phenelzine
Phenformin (off the market)
Phenol
Phenylbutazone
Phosphoric acid
Potassium chloroplatinite
Propylene glycol
Salicylates
Sorbitol (I.V.)

Strychnine
Surfactant herbicide
Tetracycline (outdated)
Theophylline
Tienilic acid
Toluene
Tranylcypromine
Vacor
Verapamil

Drugs Causing Decreased Anion Gap (<6 mEq/L)

Acidosis

Ammonium chloride
Bromide
Iodide

Lithium
Polymyxin B
Tromethamine

OSMOLALITY

Definition: The summed concentrations of all osmotically active solute particles

Predicted serum osmolality =

$2 Na^+ + glucose (mg/dL) / 18 + BUN (mg/dL) / 2.8$

The normal range of serum osmolality is 285-295 mOsm/L.

Differential diagnosis of increased serum osmolal gap (>10 mOsm/L)

Medications and toxins
Alcohols (ethanol, methanol, isopropanol, glycerol, ethylene glycol)
Mannitol

Calculated Osm

Osmolal gap = measured Osm − calculated Osm

0 to +10: Normal
>10: Abnormal
<0: Probable lab or calculation error

Drugs Causing Increased Osmolar Gap

(by freezing-point depression, gap is >10 mOsm)

Ethanol[1]
Ethylene glycol[1]
Glycerol
Hypermagnesemia (>9.5 mEq/L)
Isopropanol[1] (acetone)
Iodine (questionable)

Mannitol
Methanol[1]
Propylene glycol
Severe alcoholic ketoacidosis or lactic acidosis
Sorbitol[1]

[1]Toxins increasing both anion and osmolar gap.

Toxins Associated With Oxygen Saturation Gap

(>5% difference between measured and calculated value)

Carbon monoxide
Cyanide (questionable)

Hydrogen sulfide (possible)
Methemoglobin

OVERDOSE AND TOXICOLOGY *(Continued)*

Toxins Eliminated by Multiple Dosing of Activated Charcoal

Acetaminophen	Meprobamate
Amitriptyline	Methotrexate
Atrazine (?)	Methyprylon
Baclofen (?)	Nadolol
Bupropion (?)	Nortriptyline
Carbamazepine	Phencyclidine (?)
Chlordecone	Phenobarbital
Cyclosporine	Phenylbutazone
Dapsone	Phenytoin (?)
Dextropropoxyphene	Piroxicam
Diazepam (desmethyldiazepam)	Propoxyphene
Digitoxin	Propranolol (?)
Digoxin (with renal impairment)	Salicylates (?)
Disopyramide	Theophylline
Glutethimide	Valproic acid
Maprotiline	Vancomycin (?)

The following agents have been studied and have not been demonstrated to result in enhanced elimination:

Amiodarone	Imipramine
Chlopropamide	Tobramycin

Toxins Eliminated by Forced Saline Diuresis

Barium	Isoniazid (?)
Bromides	Meprobamate
Chromium	Methyl iodide
Cimetidine (?)	Mushrooms (Group I)
Cis-platinum	Nickel
Cyclophosphamide	Potassium chloroplatinite
Hydrazine	Thallium
Iodide	Valproic acid (?)
Iodine	

Toxins Eliminated by Alkaline Diuresis

2,4-D-chlorophenoxyacetic acid	2-Methyl-4-chlorophenoxyacetic acid (MCPA)
Barbital (serum levels >10 mg/dL)	Orellanine (?)
Chlorpropamide	Phenobarbital
Fluoride	Primidone
Iopanoic Acid (?)	Quinolones antibiotic
Isoniazid (?)	Salicylates
Mephobarbital	Sulfisoxazole
Methotrexate	Uranium

A urine flow of 3-5 mL/kg/hour should be achieved with a combination of isotonic fluids or diuretics. Alkalinization can be achieved by administration of 44-88 mEq of sodium bicarbonate per liter to titrate a urine pH of 7.5; 20-40 mEq/L of potassium chloride may also be required (potassium should not be administered in patients with renal insufficiency). It should be noted that the efficacy of forced diuresis has only been studied for salicylates and phenobarbital. Although several drugs can exhibit enhanced elimination through an acidic urine (tranylcypromine, quinine, chlorpheniramine, fenfluramine, strychnine, cathinone or khat, amphetamines, phencyclidine, nicotine, bismuth, diethylcarbamazine citrate, ephedrine, flecainide, local anesthetics), the practice of acidifying the urine should be discouraged in that it can produce metabolic acidosis and promote renal failure in the presence of rhabdomyolysis.

Drugs and Toxins Removed by Hemoperfusion (Charcoal)

Amanita phalloides (?)

Atenolol (?)

Bromisoval

Bromoethylbutyramide

Caffeine

Carbamazepine

Carbon tetrachloride (?)

Carbromal

Chloral hydrate (trichloroethanol)

Chloramphenicol

Chlorfenvinfos (?)

Chlorpropamide

Clonidine

Colchicine (?)

Creosote (?)

Dapsone

Demeton-S-methyl sulfoxide

Diltiazem (?)

Dimethoate

Disopyramide

Ethylene oxide

Glutethimide

Levothyroxine (?)

Lindane

Liotrix

Meprobamate

Methaqualone

Methotrexate

Methsuximide

Methyprylon (?)

Metoprolol (?)

Nadolol (?)

Orellanine (?)

Oxalic acid (?)

Paraquat

Parathion (?)

Pentamidine

Phenelzine (?)

Phenobarbital

Phenol

Phenytoin

Podophyllin (?)

Procainamide (?)

Quinidine (?)

Rifabutin (?)

Sotalol (?)

Thallium

Thyroglobulin/thyroid hormone

Theophylline

Valproic acid

Verapamil (?)

Continuous arteriovenous hemofiltration has been used to treat lithium, paraquat, N-acetyl-procainamide, and vancomycin ingestions with varying results. It is capable of filtering molecules with a molecular weight up to 50,000 but some substances such as thallium and formaldehyde cannot be removed by this method despite their low molecular weight.

Exchange transfusion is a useful modality to enhance drug elimination in neonatal or infant drug toxicity. Usually double or triple volume exchanges are performed. It has been utilized to treat barbiturate, acetaminophen, iron, caffeine, methyl salicylate, propafenone, ganciclovir, sodium nitrite, lead, phenazopyridine hydrochloride, pine oil, theophylline overdose, and nitrate exposure in pediatric patients. Exchange transfusions (500-2000 mL) volume replacement have also been used to treat adults with 80-150 g ingestions of parathion.

OVERDOSE AND TOXICOLOGY *(Continued)*

TREATMENTS[1]

Drug or Drug Class	Signs / Symptoms	Treatment / Comments
Acetaminophen	Nausea, vomiting, diaphoresis, delirium, fever, coma, vascular collapse, hepatic necrosis, transient azotemia, renal tubular necrosis	Assess severity of ingestion; adult doses ≥140 mg/kg are thought to be toxic. Obtain serum concentration ≥4 hours postingestion and use acetaminophen nomogram to evaluate need for acetylcysteine. Gastric decontamination within 2-4 hours after ingestion. May administer activated charcoal for one dose; this may decrease absorption of acetylcysteine if given within 1 hour of acetylcysteine. For unknown ingested quantities and for significant ingestion, give acetylcysteine orally (diluted 1:4 with juice or carbonated beverage); initial: 140 mg/kg then give 70 mg/kg every 4 hours for 17 doses. I.V. protocols are used in some institutions.
Alpha-adrenergic blocking agents	Hypotension, drowsiness	Give activated charcoal, additional treatment if symptomatic; use I.V. fluids, dopamine, or norepinephrine to treat hypotension. Epinephrine may worsen hypotension due to beta effects.
Aminoglycosides	Ototoxicity, nephrotoxicity, neuromuscular toxicity	Hemodialysis or peritoneal dialysis may be useful in patients with decreased renal function; calcium may reverse the neuromuscular toxicity.
Anticholinergics, antihistamines	Coma, hallucinations, delirium, tachycardia, dry skin, urinary retention, dilated pupils	For life-threatening arrhythmias or seizures. Adults: 2 mg/dose physostigmine, may repeat 1-2 mg in 20 minutes and give 1-4 mg slow I.V. over 5-10 minutes if signs and symptoms recur (relatively contraindicated if QRS >0.1 msec).
Barbiturates	Respiratory depression, circulatory collapse, bradycardia, hypotension, hypothermia, slurred speech, confusion, coma	Repeated oral doses of activated charcoal given every 3-6 hours will increase clearance. Adults: 30-60 g. Assure GI motility, adequate hydration, and renal function. Urinary alkalinization with I.V. sodium bicarbonate will increase renal elimination of longer-acting barbiturates (eg, phenobarbital). Charcoal hemoperfusion may be required in severe overdose.
Benzodiazepines	Respiratory depression, apnea (after rapid I.V.), hypoactive reflexes, hypotension, slurred speech, unsteady gait, coma	Dialysis is of limited value; support blood pressure and respiration until symptoms subside. Flumazenil: Initial dose: 0.2 mg given I.V. over 30 seconds. If further response is desired after 30 seconds, give 0.3 mg over another 30 seconds. Further doses of 0.5 mg can be given over 30 seconds at 1-minute intervals up to a total of 3 mg. Continuous infusions may be used in rare instances since duration of benzodiazepines is longer than flumazenil.
Beta-adrenergic blockers	Hypotension, bronchospasm, bradycardia, hypoglycemia, seizures	Activated charcoal; treat symptomatically; glucagon, atropine, isoproterenol, dobutamine, or cardiac pacing may be needed to treat bradycardia, conduction defects, or hypotension.
Carbamazepine	Dizziness, drowsiness, ataxia, involuntary movements, opisthotonos, seizures, nausea, vomiting, agitation, nystagmus, coma, urinary retention, respiratory depression, tachycardia, arrhythmias	Use supportive therapy, general poisoning management as needed. Use repeated oral doses of activated charcoal given every 3-6 hours to decrease serum concentrations. Charcoal hemoperfusion may be needed. Treat hypotension with I.V. fluids, dopamine, or norepinephrine. Monitor EKG. Diazepam may control convulsions but may exacerbate respiratory depression.

TREATMENTS[1] *(continued)*

Drug or Drug Class	Signs / Symptoms	Treatment / Comments
Cardiac glycosides	Hyperkalemia may develop rapidly and result in life-threatening cardiac arrhythmias, progressive bradyarrhythmias, second or third degree heart block unresponsive to atropine, ventricular fibrillation, asystole	Obtain serum drug level, induce emesis, or perform gastric lavage. Give activated charcoal to reduce further absorption. Atropine may reverse heart block. Digoxin immune Fab (digoxin-specific antibody fragments) is used in serious cases. Each 40 mg of digoxin immune Fab binds with 0.6 mg of digoxin.
Cholinergic	Nausea, vomiting, diarrhea, miosis, CNS depression, excessive salivation, excessive sweating, muscle weakness	Suction oral secretions, decontaminate skin, atropinize patient. Atropine dose must be individualized. Adults: Initial atropine dose: 1 mg; titrate dose upward. Pralidoxime (2-PAM) may need to be added for moderate to severe intoxications.
Cyanide	Myocardial depression, lactic acidosis, hypotension, respiratory depression, shock, and cyanosis despite high oxygen saturation	Cyanide antidote kit: 1) Inhale vapor from 0.3 mL amyl nitrate ampul until I.V. sodium nitrite available; 2) sodium nitrite 300 mg I.V. then 3) sodium thiosulfate 12.5 g I.V. over 10 minutes
Heparin	Severe hemorrhage	1 mg of protamine sulfate will neutralize approximately 90 units of heparin sodium (bovine) or 115 units of heparin sodium (porcine) or 100 units of heparin calcium (porcine).
Hydantoin derivatives	Nausea, vomiting, nystagmus, slurred speech, ataxia, coma	Gastric lavage or emesis; repeated oral doses of activated charcoal may increase clearance of phenytoin. Use 0.5-1 g/kg (30-60 g/dose) activated charcoal every 3-6 hours until nontoxic serum concentration is obtained. Assure adequate GI motility, supportive therapy.
Iron	Lethargy, nausea, vomiting, green or tarry stools, hypotension, weak rapid pulse, metabolic acidosis, shock, coma, hepatic necrosis, renal failure, local GI erosions	If immediately after ingestion and not already vomiting, give ipecac or lavage with saline solution. Give deferoxamine mesylate I.V. at 15 mg/kg/hour in cases of severe poisoning (serum iron >350 μg/mL) until the urine color is normal, the patient is asymptomatic, or a maximum daily dose of 8 g is reached. Urine output should be maintained >2 mL/kg/hour to avoid hypovolemic shock.
Isoniazid	Nausea, vomiting, blurred vision, CNS depression, intractable seizures, coma, metabolic acidosis	Control seizures with diazepam. Give pyridoxine I.V. equal dose to the suspected overdose of isoniazid or up to 5 g empirically. Give activated charcoal.
Nonsteroidal anti-inflammatory drugs	Dizziness, abdominal pain, sweating, apnea, nystagmus, cyanosis, hypotension, coma, seizures (rarely)	Induce emesis. Give activated charcoal via NG tube. Fluid therapy is commonly effective in managing the hypotension that may occur following an acute NSAIDs overdose, except when this is due to an acute blood loss. Seizures tend to be very short-lived and often do not require drug treatment, although, recurrent seizures should be treated with I.V. diazepam. Since many of the NSAIDs undergo enterohepatic cycling, multiple doses of charcoal may be needed to reduce the potential for delayed toxicities. Provide symptomatic and supportive care.
Opioids and morphine analogs	Respiratory depression, miosis, hypothermia, bradycardia, circulatory collapse, pulmonary edema, apnea	Establish airway and adequate ventilation. Give naloxone 0.4 mg and titrate to a maximum of 10 mg. Additional doses may be needed every 20-60 minutes. May need to institute continuous infusion, as duration of action of opiates can be longer than duration of action of naloxone.
Organophosphates (insecticides, pyridostigmine, neostigmine)	Bronchospasm, diarrhea, diaphoresis, ventricular dysrhythmia, fasiculations, flacid paralysis, lethargy, coma	Atropine 2-5 mg every 15 minutes until symptoms abate (0.05 mg/kg children). If severe, may add pralidoxime 1-2 g over 15-30 minutes (20-50 mg/kg children); may repeat every 8-12 hours or continuous infusion 0.5 g/hour (10-20 mg/kg/hour children).

OVERDOSE AND TOXICOLOGY *(Continued)*

TREATMENTS[1] *(continued)*

Drug or Drug Class	Signs / Symptoms	Treatment / Comments
Phenothiazines	Deep, unarousable sleep, anticholinergic symptoms, extrapyramidal signs, diaphoresis, rigidity, tachycardia, cardiac dysrhythmias, hypotension	Activated charcoal; do **not** dialyze. Use I.V. benztropine mesylate 1-2 mg/dose slowly over 3-6 minutes for extrapyramidal signs. Use I.V. fluids and norepinephrine to treat hypotension. Avoid epinephrine which may cause hypotension due to phenothiazine-induced alpha-adrenergic blockade and unopposed epinephrine B_2 action. Use benzodiazepines for seizure management and to decrease rigidity.
Salicylates	Nausea, vomiting, respiratory alkalosis, hyperthermia, dehydration, hyperapnea, tinnitus, headache, dizziness, metabolic acidosis, coma, hypoglycemia, seizures	Induce emesis or gastric lavage immediately. Give several doses of activated charcoal, rehydrate, and use sodium bicarbonate to correct metabolic acidosis and enhance renal elimination by alkalinizing the urine. Control hyperthermia by cooling blankets or sponge baths. Correct coagulopathy with vitamin K I.V. and platelet transfusions as necessary. Hypoglycemia may be treated with I.V. dextrose. Seizures should be treated with I.V. benzodiazepines (diazepam 5-10 mg I.V.). Give supplemental potassium after renal function has been determined to be adequate. Monitor electrolytes; obtain stat serum salicylate level and follow.
Tricyclic antidepressants	Agitation, confusion, hallucinations, urinary retention, hypothermia, hypotension, tachycardia, arrhythmias, seizures	Give activated charcoal ± lavage. Use sodium bicarbonate for QRS >0.1 msec; alkalinization by hyperventilation has been used in patients on mechanical ventilation; I.V. fluids and norepinephrine may be used for hypotension; benzodiazepines may be used for seizure management.
Warfarin	Internal or external hemorrhage, hematuria	For moderate overdoses, give oral, SubQ, or I.D., or slow I.V. (I.V. associated with anaphylactoid reactions) phytonadione; usual dose: 2.5-10 mg, adjust per prothrombin time. For severe hemorrhage, give fresh frozen plasma or whole blood. See Warfarin monograph.
Xanthine derivatives	Vomiting, abdominal pain, bloody diarrhea, tachycardia, extrasystoles, tachypnea, tonic/clonic seizures	Give activated charcoal orally. Repeated oral doses of activated charcoal increase clearance. Use 0.5-1 g/kg (30-60 g/dose) of activated charcoal every 1-4 hours (depending on the severity of ingestion) until nontoxic serum concentrations are obtained. Assure adequate GI motility, supportive therapy. Charcoal hemoperfusion or hemodialysis can also be effective in decreasing serum concentrations and should be used if the serum concentration approaches 90-100 mcg/mL in acute overdoses.

[1]Consult more specific toxicology references (eg, Leikin JB and Paloucek FP, *Poisoning & Toxicology Handbook*, Hudson, OH: Lexi-Comp Inc, 1998, and Poisondex®) for further information.

CONTROLLED SUBSTANCE INDEX

ALPHABETICAL INDEX

NOTES

NOTES

NOTES

NOTES

NOTES

NOTES

NOTES

NOTES

Other Products Offered by Lexi-Comp®

Drug Information Handbook

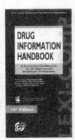

This easy-to-use reference is compiled especially for the pharmacist, physician, or other healthcare professional needing quick access to drug information. The book is organized in four sections for easy retrieval of critical information. Includes drug monographs, listed alphabetically, with extensive cross-referencing.

Includes: Over 1300 drug monographs; Drug Interaction information; Labeled and Investigational indications; Up to 33 key fields per monograph including Medication Safety Issues; Pharmacodynamics/Kinetics; Dosing for renal/hepatic impairment; and a Pharmacologic Category Index

The valuable Appendix information includes hundreds of charts and reviews of special topics such as guidelines for treatment and therapy recommendations.

Published in cooperation with APhA.

Drug Interactions Handbook

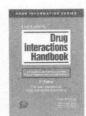

The new standard for evaluating drug and herbal interactions, this comprehensive handbook was designed to allow convenient access to interaction data. More than 150,000 interactions are documented in a user-friendly structure that is extensively indexed and fully cross referenced by page number. Includes: The most comprehensive and clinically-relevant table of Cytochrome P450 enzyme substrates, inducers, and inhibitors in the industry;the greatest number of potential interactions compared to any other interactions references; Drug, food, herbal, and alcohol interactions; Reliability Rating - Indicating the quality and nature of documentation for an interaction; Risk Rating - A: No Known Interaction, B: No Action Needed, C: Monitor Therapy, D: Consider Therapy Modification, X: Avoid; and Severity Rating - Indicating the reported or possible magnitude of an interaction

Pediatric Dosage Handbook

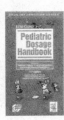

Designed for any healthcare professional requiring quick access to comprehensive, pediatric drug information. Includes: Over 745 drug monographs, including vaccines; Extemporaneous preparation formulas; Up to 35 key fields of information per monograph including Medication Safety Issues, Neonatal and Pediatric Dosing

Geriatric Dosage Handbook

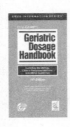

Designed for any healthcare professional managing geriatric patients.
Includes: Complete adult and geriatric dosing; Special geriatric considerations; Up to 36 key fields of information in each monograph including Medication Safety Issues; and Extensive information on drug interactions as well as dosing for patients with renal/hepatic impairment

Other Products Offered by Lexi-Comp®

Pharmacology Companion Guide

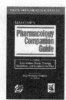

This guide supplies the best of Lexi-Comp's comparative charts, therapy guidelines, and supplemental data. Ideal for healthcare providers who require a quick reference to all the key appendix information found in our popular *Drug Information Handbook* or as a companion to our PDA software.

Includes: Abbreviations and measurements; ACLS Algorithms; Cytochrome P450 and Drug Interactions; and Laboratory Values

Pediatric Pharmacology Companion Guide

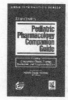

This guide supplies the best of Lexi-Comp's comparative charts, therapy guidelines, and supplemental data. Ideal as a quick reference to all the key appendix information found in our popular *Pediatric Dosage Handbook* or as a companion to our PDA software.

Includes: Apgar Scoring System; CPR Pediatric Drug Dosages; Immunization Guidelines; and Pediatric ALS Algorithms

Drug-Induced Nutrient Depletion Handbook

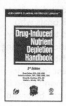

Provides a complete listing of drugs known to deplete the body of nutritional compounds.

Includes: Alphabetical listing of drugs most commonly prescribed (by Brand and Generic name) cross-referenced by page number to nutrients depleted; Key points of information include Abstract & Studies section; and Nutrient monographs with concise descriptions of the effects of depletion, biological function and effect, sources of repletion, RDA, dosage range, and dietary sources for nutrients

Pharmacogenomics Handbook

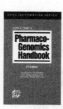

Ideal for any healthcare professional or student wishing to gain insight into the emerging field of pharmacogenomics.

Includes: Information concerning key genetic variations that may influence drug disposition and/or sensitivity; brief introductions to fundamental concepts in genetics and genomics. A foundation for all clinicians who will be called on to integrate rapidly-expanding genomic knowledge into the management of drug therapy,

Other Products Offered by Lexi-Comp®

Drug Information Handbook for Perioperative Nursing

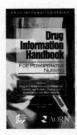

Designed especially for perioperative nurses, Registered Nurses practicing in operative and interventional procedure settings, and upper-division nursing students seeking a distinctive reference for dosing, administration, monitoring, and patient education criteria for perioperative patient care environments

Includes: Up to 40 fields per monograph including Medication Safety data; Adult, Pediatric, and Geriatric Dosing guidelines; and information on each phase of the perioperative encounter and how it is addressed, with emphasis on special situations central to perioperative patient care

Drug Information Handbook for the Allied Health Professional

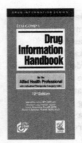

Designed for medical secretaries, transcriptionists, pharmacy technicians, and other allied health professionals requiring quick access to basic information regarding medications.

Includes: Over 1600 monographs offering up to 13 key fields of information and 125 pages of updated, valuable charts and tables

Anesthesiology & Critical Care Drug Handbook

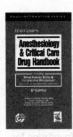

Designed for anesthesiologists, critical care practitioners, and all healthcare professionals involved in the care of surgical or ICU patients.

Includes: Comprehensive drug information to ensure the appropriate clinical management of patients; Intensivist and Anesthesiologist perspective; Over 2000 medications most commonly used in the preoperative and critical care setting; and Special Topics/Issues section with frequently encountered patient conditions

Drug Information Handbook for Dentistry

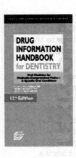

Specifically compiled and designed for all dental professionals who require quick access to concisely-stated drug information pertaining to commonly prescribed medications. Excellent for chairside use, each drug monograph is alphabetically organized by brand and generic names.

Contains over 7500 drugs and herbal products, including dental, medical, OTCs, Canadian, and Mexican drugs. Lists Local Anesthetic/Vasoconstrictor Precautions and Effects on Dental Treatment for each monograph. Includes Drug Interactions, Contraindications, Warnings/Precautions, Common Adverse Effects, Use, Dosage, and Pregnancy Risk Factor.

Other Products Offered by Lexi-Comp®

Clinician's Guide to Internal Medicine

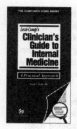

Quick access to essential information covering diagnosis, treatment, and management of commonly-encountered patient conditions in Internal Medicine.

Includes: Practical approaches ideal for point-of-care use; Algorithms to establish a diagnosis and select the appropriate therapy; and Tables to summarize diagnostic and therapeutic strategies

Clinician's Guide to Laboratory Medicine

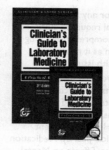

A resource providing a logical step-by-step process from an abnormal lab test to diagnosis. This two-book set provides you with a full size guide and a portable pocket version for convenient referencing.

Includes: 137 chapters; 700 charts, tables, and algorithms; and sections such as neurology, infectious diseases, and obstetrics/gynecology

Clinician's Guide to Diagnosis

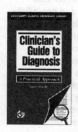

A reference with a practical approach to commonly-encountered symptoms, designed to follow the logical thought process of a seasoned clinician.

Includes: Evidence-based, easy-to-find answers to the questions that commonly arise in the symptom evaluation process; Over 35 algorithms that provide parallel references to the information in each chapter

Laboratory Test Handbook

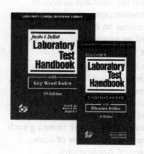

An invaluable source of information for anyone interested in diagnostic laboratory testing.

Includes: 960 tests; Up to 25 fields per test; Extensive cross-referencing; Over 12,000 references; and Key Word Index: test result, disease, organ system and syndrome

Clinicians, nurse practitioners, residents, nurses, and students will appreciate the Concise version of the *Laboratory Test Handbook* for its convenience as a quick reference. This abridged version includes 876 tests.

Other Products Offered by Lexi-Comp®

Drug Information Handbook for Psychiatry

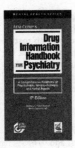

Designed for any healthcare professional requiring quick access to comprehensive drug information as it relates to mental health issues.

Includes: Detailed drug monographs for psychotropic, nonpsychotropic, and herbal medications; Special fields such as Mental Health Comment (useful clinical pearls), Medication Safety Issues, Effects on Mental Status, and Effects on Psychiatric Treatment

Psychotropic Drug Information Handbook

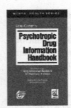

Designed for any healthcare professional requiring a small, portable, quick reference to psychotropic drug information. This is a pocket-sized companion to the *Drug Information Handbook for Psychiatry*.

Includes: All psychotropic agents; Adult and pediatric dosing; FDA-approved and unlabeled uses; Medication safety issues; and Useful clinical pearls

Rating Scales for Mental Health

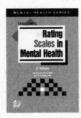

Ideal for clinicians as well as administrators, this book provides an overview of over 100 recommended rating scales for mental assessment.

Includes: Rating scales for conditions such as General Anxiety, Social/Family Functioning, Eating Disorders, and Sleep Disorders; and Monograph format covering such topics as Overview of Scale, General Applications, Psychometric Properties, and References

A Patient Guide to Mental Health

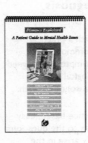

Fully laminated, durable construction, and beautifully illustrated, this flip chart was designed specifically for healthcare professionals dealing with mental health patients. This patient education tool will assist in explaining the 8 most common mental health issues to your patients on a level that they will understand.

❶ Alzheimer's Disease
❷ Anxiety
❸ Bipolar Disorder
❹ Depression
❺ Insomnia
❻ Obsessive-Compulsive Disorder
❼ Panic Attacks
❽ Schizophrenia

To order call Customer Service at 1-866-397-3433 or go to www.lexi.com.
Outside of the U.S. call: 330-650-6506 or www.lexi.com

Other Products Offered by Lexi-Comp®

Lexi-Comp ONLINE

Seven of the Top 10 hospitals ranked in the *U.S. News and World Report's* Best Hospitals of 2005 use Lexi-Comp's clinical databases and technology. These include Johns Hopkins, Cleveland Clinic, Massachusetts General, Stanford, UCLA and many others.

Lexi-Comp® ONLINE™ integrates industry-leading databases and enhanced searching technology to bring you time-sensitive clinical information at the point-of-care. Our interface eliminates the need to navigate through multiple pages or make unnecessary mouse clicks.

ONLINE includes 14 unique databases and six modules that include the following topic areas:

- Core drug information with specialty fields
- Pediatrics and Geriatrics
- Pharmacogenomics
- Infectious Diseases
- Laboratory Tests and Diagnostic Procedures
- Natural Products
- Interactions: Lexi-Interact analysis application for Rx, OTC, and natural products
- Patient Education leaflets: Lexi-PALS™ for adults and Pedi-PALS™ for pediatric patients, available in 18 languages
- Lexi-Drug ID™ drug identification system
- Lexi-CALC™ over 50 medical calculations for drug dosing and organ function assessment

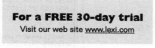

For a FREE 30-day trial
Visit our web site www.lexi.com

Academic and Institutional
licenses available.

**Integration with
CPOE/EMR/Pharmacy Information
Systems available**

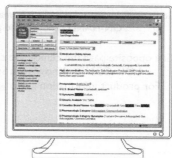

To order call Customer Service at 1-866-397-3433 or go to www.lexi.com.
Outside of the U.S. call: 330-650-6506 or www.lexi.com

Other Products Offered by Lexi-Comp®

Lexi-Comp ON-HAND
For Palm OS® and
Windows™ Powered Pocket PC Devices

Lexi-Comp prides itself on creating and delivering timely and quality information for use at the point-of-care. Our content is not subject to third party recommendations or suggestions, but is based upon the hard work contributed by our respected authors, internal clinical team, and the thousands of professionals within the healthcare industry who constantly review and validate our data.

With Lexi-Comp® ON-HAND™ you can synchronize your handheld device multiple times per week, giving you up-to-date information on the latest warnings and new drug information. All updates are included with your annual subscription.

Lexi-Comp ON-HAND databases include:

- Lexi-Drugs®
- Pediatric Lexi-Drugs®
- Lexi-Interact™
- Griffith's 5-Minute Clinical Consult™
- Lexi-Natural Products™
- Lexi-Poisoning & Toxicology™
- Lexi-Infectious Diseases™
- Lexi-Lab & Diagnostic Procedures™
- Nursing Lexi-Drugs®
- Perioperative Nursing Lexi-Drugs®

- Dental Lexi-Drugs®
- Lexi-Pharmacogenomics™
- Medical Abbreviations by Neil Davis
- Stedman's Medical Dictionary
- Lexi-NBCA™ (Nuclear, Biological, & Chemical Agent Exposures)
- Lexi-PALS™ (Patient Advisory Leaflets)
- Lexi-CALC™
- Lexi-I.V. Compatibility™
- Lexi-Companion Guides™
- Pharmacotherapy Handbook by Wells

Go to www.lexi.com for more information on Lexi-Comp's
ON-HAND products and packages.

See opposite page for clinical areas covered by the
LEXI-COMP® Knowledge Solution™.
For product information go to www.lexi.com.

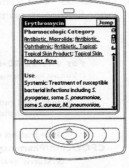

Palm OS®   Pocket PC

To order call Customer Service at 1-866-397-3433 or go to www.lexi.com.
Outside of the U.S. call: 330-650-6506 or www.lexi.com